Swaiman's Pediatric Neurology: Principles and Practice 6e

With pleasure and appreciation we dedicate this book to our spouses and children, who made it possible for us to bring this text to fruition and who taught us what was really important in development over the lifespan. It is impossible to adequately describe the value of their encouragement and support. We also would like to express our appreciation to the Elsevier editorial staff who are extremely talented and helpful in keeping track of all the details necessary to complete such a task as well as their judicious editorial skills. Furthermore, no dedication of a book embracing this field would be meaningful without a tribute to the courage and perseverance of neurologically impaired children and their caretakers.

Content Strategist: Lotta Kryhl/Sarah Barth
Content Development Specialist: Humayra Rahman Khan
Content Coordinator: Joshua Mearns
Project Manager: Andrew Riley
Design: Miles Hitchen
Marketing Manager: Michele Milano

Swaiman's Pediatric Neurology
Principles and Practice

SIXTH EDITION

KENNETH F. SWAIMAN, MD
Director Emeritus, Division of Pediatric Neurology;
Professor Emeritus of Neurology and Pediatrics
University of Minnesota Medical School
Minneapolis, MN, USA

STEPHEN ASHWAL, MD
Distinguished Professor of Pediatrics;
Chief, Division of Child Neurology
Department of Pediatrics
Loma Linda University School of Medicine
Loma Linda, CA, USA

DONNA M. FERRIERO, MD, MS
W.H. And Marie Wattis Distinguished
Professor and Chair
Department of Pediatrics;
Physician-in-Chief
UCSF Benioff Children's Hospital
San Francisco, CA, USA

NINA F. SCHOR, MD, PHD
William H. Eilinger Professor and Chair
Department of Pediatrics;
Professor, Departments of Neurology and Neuroscience;
Pediatrician-in-Chief, Golisano Children's Hospital
University of Rochester School of Medicine and Dentistry
Rochester, NY, USA

RICHARD S. FINKEL, MD
Chief, Division of Neurology
Nemours Children's Hospital;
Professor of Neurology
University of Central Florida College of Medicine
Orlando, FL, USA

ANDREA L. GROPMAN, MD
Chief, Neurogenetics and Neurodevelopmental Disabilities
Department of Neurology
Children's National Medical Center
George Washington University of the Health Sciences
Washington, DC, USA

PHILLIP L. PEARL, MD
Director of Epilepsy and Clinical Neurophysiology
Boston Children's Hospital;
William G. Lennox Chair and Professor of Neurology
Harvard Medical School
Boston, MA, USA

MICHAEL I. SHEVELL, MDCM, FRCP(C), FCAHS
Professor, Departments of Pediatrics, Neurology and
Neurosurgery;
Chair, McGill Department of Pediatrics;
Pediatrician-in-Chief, Montreal Children's Hospital-McGill
University Health Centre (MUHC)
Harvey Guyda Professor
Department of Pediatrics, Faculty of Medicine,
McGill University
Montreal, QC, Canada

Search full text online at ExpertConsult.com

ELSEVIER   Edinburgh   London   New York   Oxford   Philadelphia   St Louis   Sydney   Toronto   2018

ELSEVIER

© 2017, Elsevier Inc. All rights reserved.
First edition 1989
Second edition 1994
Third edition 1999
Fourth edition 2006
Fifth edition 2012
Sixth edition 2018

Notices

Knowledge and best practice in this field are constantly changing. As new research and experience broaden our understanding, changes in research methods, professional practices, or medical treatment may become necessary.

Practitioners and researchers must always rely on their own experience and knowledge in evaluating and using any information, methods, compounds, or experiments described herein. In using such information or methods they should be mindful of their own safety and the safety of others, including parties for whom they have a professional responsibility.

With respect to any drug or pharmaceutical products identified, readers are advised to check the most current information provided (i) on procedures featured or (ii) by the manufacturer of each product to be administered, to verify the recommended dose or formula, the method and duration of administration, and contraindications. It is the responsibility of practitioners, relying on their own experience and knowledge of their patients, to make diagnoses, to determine dosages and the best treatment for each individual patient, and to take all appropriate safety precautions.

To the fullest extent of the law, neither the Publisher nor the authors, contributors, or editors, assume any liability for any injury and/or damage to persons or property as a matter of products liability, negligence or otherwise, or from any use or operation of any methods, products, instructions, or ideas contained in the material herein.

ISBN: 978-0-323-37101-8
eISBN: 978-0-323-37481-1

Printed in China

Last digit is the print number: 9   8   7   6   5   4   3   2   1

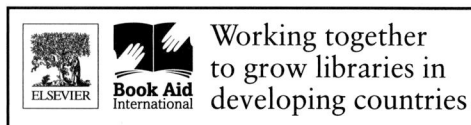

Contents

Preface to the First Edition

It is concurrently tiring, humiliating, and intellectually revitalizing to compile a book containing the essence of the information that embraces one's life work and professional preoccupation. For me, there is a certain moth-to-the-flame phenomenon that cannot be resisted; therefore this new book has been produced.

Pediatric neurology has come of age since my initial interest and subsequent immersion in the field. Concentrated attention to the details of brain development and function has brought much progress and understanding. Studies of disease processes by dedicated and intelligent individuals accompanied by a cascade of new technology (e.g., neuroimaging techniques, positron emission tomography, DNA probes, synthesis of gene products, sophisticated lipid chemistry) have propelled the field forward. The simultaneous increase of knowledge and capability of pediatric neurologists and others who diagnose and treat children with nervous system dysfunction has been extremely gratifying.

Although once within the realm of honest delusion of a seemingly sane (but unrealistic) devotee of the field, it is no longer possible to believe that a single individual can fathom, much less explore, the innumerable rivulets that coalesce to form the river of knowledge that currently is pediatric neurology. Streams of information in certain areas sometimes peacefully meander for years; suddenly, when knowledge of previously obscure areas is advanced and the newly gained information becomes central to understanding basic pathophysiologic entities, a once small stream gains momentum and abruptly flows with torrential force.

This text is an attempt to gather the most important aspects of current pediatric neurology and display them in a comprehensible manner. The task, although consuming great energies and concentration, cannot be accomplished completely because new conditions are described daily.

The advancement of the field necessitated that preparation of this text keep pace with current knowledge and present new and valuable techniques. My colleagues and I have made every effort to discharge this responsibility. Because of continuous scientific progress, controversies are extant in some areas for varying periods; wherever possible, these areas of conflict are indicated.

This book is divided into four unequal parts. Part I contains a discussion of the historic and clinical examination. Part II contains information concerning laboratory examination. Chapters relating to the symptom complexes that often reflect the chief complaints of neurologically impaired children compose Part III. Part IV provides detailed discussion of various neurologic diseases that afflict children.

Although every precaution has been taken to avoid error, bias, and prejudice, inevitably some of these demons have become embedded in the text. The editor assumes full responsibility for these indiscretions.

It is my fervent hope that the reader will find this book informative and stimulating and that the contents will provide an introduction to the understanding of many of the conditions that remain mysterious and poorly explained.

Kenneth F. Swaiman, MD
Autumn 1988

Preface to the Sixth Edition

In 1975, a little over 40 years ago, the first two-volume reference text concerning Pediatric Neurology was published. In 1971, Dr Swaiman was approached by an executive editor of C.V. Mosby to discuss publishing a book on pediatric neurology based on papers he had read from a University of Minnesota Continuing Medical Education Course. This was a year before the first Child Neurology Society meeting and thus before the formal organization of pediatric neurologists. Drs. Ken Swaiman and Frank Wright began this project, immediately facing the challenge of delineating the field. At that time, the importance of neurochemistry and genetics was being emphasized, there were questions as to whether learning disabilities or autism were legitimate components of child neurology, and recruiting authors for various chapters was difficult as sub-specialties of the discipline were in their infancy or under- or undeveloped.

The first edition preface of *The Practice of Pediatric Neurology* stated, "*We have aspired to create a well-illustrated book that stresses the mainstays of modern pediatric neurology—the staggering array of neuromuscular and metabolic diseases described in the past 30 years, the relationship of embryology to congenital malformations, the growing number of recognized but yet unexplained degenerative diseases of childhood, and higher cortical function as related to learning capabilities of the child.*" The book and the subsequent 1982 edition were internationally well received. *Pediatric Neurology* and subsequently *Swaiman's Pediatric Neurology* were first published in 1989 and then in 1994, 1999, 2005 and 2012. Elsevier succeeded C.V. Mosby as the publisher in 2012. The growth of the discipline is documented by the fact that the number of pages and chapters has grown greatly: from 40 chapters/1082 pages in 1975 to 108 chapters/2290 pages in 2012.

This sixth edition of *Swaiman's Pediatric Neurology: Principles & Practice* reflects the remarkable increase in knowledge and complexity of the field since the fifth edition. Keeping abreast of all new information required us to increase the size and scope of this book from 108 to 170 chapters. To avoid publishing an overwhelming and oversized tome, we meticulously curated the most immediately necessary information and guidance in the print book, while providing the full text, our most comprehensive edition ever, online. We are proud of our mobile-optimized, downloadable e-book, which is included with your print purchase, and which provides easy and complete searchable and annotatable access to the content. Between the portable print book and the expansive online text, this reference offers a remarkable collection of well written chapters on topics of importance to professionals around the world who care for children with neurological disorders.

To accomplish these goals, we have increased the number of editors from four in the last edition (Ken Swaiman, Stephen Ashwal, Donna Ferriero, Nina Schor) to eight by adding four new and accomplished individuals with expertise in specific areas: Andrea Gropman (neurogenetics and metabolic disorders); Richard Finkel (neuromuscular disorders); Phillip Pearl (pediatric epilepsy); and Michael Shevell (neurodevelopmental disabilities). We also had some unofficial expert guidance for specific sections of the book on neurodevelopmental malformations (Bill Dobyns); pediatric movement disorders (Jon Mink); and pediatric neurooncology (Roger Packer).

Major changes in the book that the reader will find of interest include:

- Completely new sections on pediatric immune mediated nervous system disorders (4 chapters), cerebrovacular diseases (6 chapters), neurooncology (13 chapters), neuromuscular disorders (18 chapters), and clinical care care of the child with neurologic disorders (11 chapters).
- Major expansions of the sections on perinatal acquired and congenital disorders (7 chapters), neurodevelopmental disabilities (11 chapters), pediatric epilepsy (23 chapters), and nonepiletiform paroxysmal disorders and disorders of sleep (7 chapters).
- Three new chapters for the section on emerging concepts in child neurology including topics related to the developmental connectome, stem cell transplantation, and cellular and animal models of neurological disease.
- Updates of all remaining chapters by an international group of authors who are experts in their respective fields.
- Other new chapters in different sections of the book include: neuropsychological assessement; development of a neonatal neurointensive care unit; neonatal traumatic brain, spine and peripheral nervous system injury; an overview of the conceptual framework of the developmental encephalopathies; an overview of how to evaluate patients with a suspected metabolic disorder; a review of conditions associated with vitamin metabolism; and a chapter on nutrition and malnutrition and the developing brain.

We hope that the reader will find this book a useful resource and that the information will benefit the many children who suffer from these conditions. It is our wish that the greater world community will increase support for the care of neurologically impaired children and the research necessary to provide further understanding of, and improved treatment and preventive measures for, neurologic diseases. This support will improve the survival and quality of life of these brave children and their families.

Kenneth F. Swaiman
Stephen Ashwal
Donna M. Ferriero
Nina F. Schor
Richard S. Finkel
Andrea L. Gropman
Phillip L. Pearl
Michael I. Shevell

Acknowledgments

We wish to thank all of the authors who graciously gave of their time to prepare and review their chapters, as well as the editorial and publishing staff at Elsevier, especially Charlotta Kryhl, Humayra Rahman Khan, Joshua Mearns, Andrew Riley and many others. Without their diligence and persistence, we would have never been able to complete this project.

Contributors

The editors would like to acknowledge and offer grateful thanks for the input of all previous editions' contributors, without whom this new edition would not have been possible.

Gregory S. Aaen, MD
Assistant Professor of Pediatrics and
  Neurology
Loma Linda University School of
  Medicine
Loma Linda, CA, USA

Nicholas Scott Abend, MD MSCE
Associate Professor of Neurology and
  Pediatrics
Departments of Neurology and
  Pediatrics
University of Pennsylvania and
  Children's Hospital of Philadelphia
Philadelphia, PA, USA

Amal Abou-Hamden, FRACS
Neurosurgeon
University of Adelaide, Wakefield
  Hospital
Royal Adelaide Hospital
Adelaide, SA, Australia

Jeffrey C. Allen, MD
Professor of Pediatrics and Neurology
NYU Langone Medical Center
New York, NY, USA

Anthony A. Amato, MD
Vice-chairman, Department of
  Neurology
Chief, Neuromuscular Division
Brigham and Women's Hospital
Professor of Neurology
Harvard Medical School
Boston, MA, USA

Catherine Amlie-Lefond, MD
Professor of Neurology
University of Washington;
Director
Pediatric Vascular Neurology Program
Seattle Children's Hospital
Seattle, WA, USA

Stephen Ashwal, MD
Distinguished Professor of Pediatrics
  and Neurology;
Chief, Division of Pediatric Neurology
Loma Linda University School of
  Medicine
Loma Linda, CA, USA

Russell C. Bailey, MD
Assistant Professor of Neurology and
  Pediatrics
Department of Neurology
University of Virginia
Charlottesville, VA, USA

James F. Bale, Jr., MD
Professor of Pediatrics and Neurology;
Vice Chair-Education, Department of
  Pediatrics
University of Utah Health Care
Salt Lake City, UT, USA

Brenda Banwell, MD
Chief of Neurology
The Children's Hospital of Philadelphia
Professor of Neurology and Pediatrics
Perelman School of Medicine
University of Pennsylvania
Philadelphia, PA, USA

Kristin W. Barañano, MD, PhD
Assistant Professor of Neurology;
Clinical Associate
Johns Hopkins University School of
  Medicine
Department of Neurology
Baltimore, MD, USA

A. James Barkovich, MD
Professor of Radiology and Biomedical
  Imaging, Neurology, Pediatrics and
  Neurosurgery
University of California
San Francisco, CA, USA

Richard J. Barohn, MD
Gertrude and Dewey Ziegler Professor
  of Neurology;
Chair, Department of Neurology
University of Kansas Medical Center
Kansas City, KS, USA

Ute K. Bartels, MD
Professor
The Paediatric Brain Tumour Program
The Hospital for Sick Children
University of Toronto
Toronto, ON, Canada

Brenda Bartnik-Olson, PhD
Associate Professor of Radiology
Radiology
Loma Linda University School of
  Medicine
Loma Linda, CA, USA

Ori Barzilai
Resident Neurosurgeon
Tel Aviv Medical Center
Tel Aviv, Israel

Alexander Bassuk, MD, PhD
Associate Professor
Pediatrics
University of Iowa Graduate College
Iowa City, IA, USA

David R. Bearden, MD
Assistant Professor of Neurology and
  Pediatrics
Department of Neurology,
Division of Child Neurology
University of Rochester School of
  Medicine
Rochester, NY, USA

Liat Ben-Sira, MD
Director
Imaging (Pediatrics)
Tel Aviv Sourasky Medical Center
Tel Aviv, Israel

Timothy J. Bernard, MD, MSCS
Associate Professor
Department of Pediatrics, Section of
  Child Neurology
University of Colorado School of
  Medicine
Aurora, CO, USA

Elizabeth Berry-Kravis, MD, PhD
Professor
Departments of Pediatrics, Neurological
  Sciences, and Biochemistry
Rush University Medical Center
Chicago, IL, USA

Lauren A. Beslow, MD, MSCE
Assistant Professor of Neurology and
  Pediatrics
The Perelman School of Medicine of
  The University of Pennsylvania
Division of Neurology
The Children's Hospital of Philadelphia
Philadelphia, PA, USA

Jaclyn A. Biegel, PhD
Chief, Division of Genomic Medicine;
Director, Center for Personalized
    Medicine
Department of Pathology and
    Laboratory Medicine
Children's Hospital Los Angeles;
Professor of Clinical Pathology
    (Clinical Scholar)
University of Southern California Keck
    School of Medicine
Los Angeles, CA, USA

Lori Billinghurst, MD, MSc, FRCPC
Attending Physician
Division of Neurology
The Children's Hospital of
    Philadelphia;
Clinical Assistant Professor of
    Neurology
Perelman School of Medicine
The University of Pennsylvania
Philadelphia, PA, USA

Angela K. Birnbaum, PhD
Professor
PHARM Experimental and Clinical
    Pharm
University of Minnesota
Twin Cities, MN, USA

Joanna S. Blackburn, MD
Assistant Professor
Department of Pediatrics
Ann, Robert H. Lurie Children's
    Hospital of Chicago
Northwestern Feinberg School of
    Medicine
Chicago, IL, USA

Nuala Bobowski, PhD
Postdoctoral Fellow
Monell Chemical Senses Center
Philadelphia, PA, USA

Adrienne Boire, MD, PhD
Neuro-Oncologist
Neurology
Memorial Sloan Kettering Cancer
    Center
New York, NY, USA

Carsten G. Bönnemann, MD
Senior Investigator
Division of Intramural Research
National Institute of Neurological
    Disorders and Stroke
Bethesda, MD, USA

Sonia L. Bonifacio, MD
Clinical Associate Professor of
    Pediatrics;
Associate Medical Director, NeuroNICU
Stanford University School of Medicine
Division of Neonatal, Developmental
    Medicine
Palo Alto, CA, USA

Daniel J. Bonthius, MD, PhD
Professor
Departments of Pediatrics and
    Neurology
University of Iowa
Iowa City, IA, USA

Breck Borcherding, MD
Assistant Professor
Department of Psychiatry
Weill Cornell Medicine
New York, NY, USA

Brian R. Branchford, MD
Assistant Professor
Center for Cancer and Blood Disorders
Children's Hospital Colorado
Hemophilia and Thrombosis Center
University of Colorado School of
    Medicine
Aurora, CO, USA

John Brandsema, MD
Assistant Professor of Clinical
    Neurology
Perelman School of Medicine at the
    University of Pennsylvania;
Attending Physician
The Children's Hospital of Philadelphia
Philadelphia, PA, USA

Kathryn M. Brennan, MBChB, PhD
Consultant Neurologist
Department of Neurology
Queen Elizabeth University Hospital
Glasgow, Scotland, UK

J. Nicholas Brenton, MD
Assistant Professor
Department of Neurology, Division of
    Pediatrics
University of Virginia
Charlottesville, VA, USA

Amy R. Brooks-Kayal, MD
Professor, Departments of Pediatrics
    and Neurology, University of
    Colorado, School of Medicine,
    Aurora;
Department of Pharmaceutical Sciences,
    Skaggs School of Pharmacy and
    Pharmaceutical Sciences, San Diego;
Chief and Ponzio Family Chair,
    Pediatric Neurology, Children's
    Hospital Colorado
Colorado Aurora, CO, USA

Lawrence W. Brown, MD
Associate Professor
Departments of Neurology and
    Pediatrics
The Children's Hospital of Philadelphia
Perelman School of Medicine University
    of Pennsylvania
Philadelphia, PA, USA

Jeffrey Buchalter, MD
Chairman
Pain Management
Gulf Coast Pain Institute
Pensacola, FL, USA

Carol S. Camfield, MD, FRCPC
Researcher
Department of Pediatrics, Dalhousie
    University
IWK Health Centre,
Halifax, NS, Canada

Peter R. Camfield, MD, FRCPC
Researcher
Department of Pediatrics, Dalhousie
    University
IWK Health Centre
Halifax, NS, Canada

Cristina Campoy, MD, PhD
Professor of Pediatrics
University of Granada
Granada, Spain

Jessica L. Carpenter, MD
Assistant Professor
Department of Neurology
Children's National Health System
    (CNHS)
George Washington University
Washington, DC, USA

Taeun Chang, MD
Associate Professor
Child Neurology
Children's National Health System
Washington, DC, USA

Vann Chau, MD, FRCPC
Assistant Professor of Pediatrics
Department of Pediatrics (Neurology)
The Hospital for Sick Children,
    University of Toronto
Toronto, ON, Canada

Susan N. Chi, MD
Assistant Professor of Pediatrics
Dana-Farber Cancer Institute
Boston Children's Hospital
Harvard Medical School
Boston, MA, USA

Claudia A. Chiriboga, MD, MPH
Professor of Neurology and Pediatrics
Division of Pediatric Neurology
Columbia University Medical Center
New York, NY, USA

Yoon-Jae Cho, MD
Assistant Professor
Neurology
Stanford University
Stanford, CA, USA

Cindy W. Christian, MD
Professor, Department of Pediatrics
The Perelman School of Medicine
University of Pennsylvania
Philadelphia, PA, USA

Nicolas Chrestian, MD, FRCPC
Department of Child Neurology
Centre Hospitalier Mère-Enfant-Soleil
  Université Laval (CHUL)
Quebec City
Quebec, Canada

Maria Roberta Cilio, MD, PhD
Professor, Neurology and Pediatrics;
Director of Pediatric Epilepsy Research
Division of Epilepsy and Clinical
  Neurophysiology
University of California
San Francisco, CA, USA

Robin D. Clark, MD
Professor
Department of Pediatrics, Medical
  Genetics
Loma Linda University School of
  Medicine
Loma Linda, CA, USA

Bruce H. Cohen, MD
Professor of Pediatrics, Northeast Ohio
  Medical University;
Director, NeuroDevelopmental Science
  Center and Neurology
Department of Pediatrics
Children's Hospital Medical Center of
  Akron
Akron, OH, USA

Ronald D. Cohn, MD, FACMG
Paediatrician in Chief, The Hospital for
  Sick Children
Professor and Chair
Department of Paediatrics
The University of Toronto
Toronto, ON, Canada

Anne M. Connolly, MD
Professor of Neurology and Pediatrics
Washington University School of
  Medicine
Saint Louis, MO, USA

Todd Constable, PhD
Professor of Radiology and Biomedical
  Imaging and of Neurosurgery;
Director MRI Research
Yale University
New Haven, CT, USA

Shlomi Constantini, MD
Department of Pediatric Neurosurgery
The Israeli Neurofibromatosis Center
Dana Children's Hospital
Tel Aviv Medical Center
Tel Aviv, Israel

Jeannine M. Conway, PharmD
Associate Professor
Department of Experimental and
  Clinical Pharmacology
College of Pharmacy, University of
  Minnesota
Minneapolis, MN, USA

David L. Coulter, MD
Senior Associate in Neurology;
Associate Professor of Neurology
Harvard Medical School
Boston, MA, USA

Tina M. Cowan, PhD
Associate Professor
Department of Pathology
Stanford University
Stanford, CA, USA

Russell C. Dale, MRCP, PhD
Professor of Paediatric Neurology
Child and Adolescent Health
University of Sydney
Sydney, NSW, Australia

Benjamin Darbro, MD, PhD
Director, Shivanand R. Patil
  Cytogenetics and Molecular
  Laboratory;
Assistant Professor of Pediatrics -
  Medical Genetics
University of Iowa
Iowa City, IA, USA

Basil T. Darras, MD
Joseph J. Volpe Professor of Neurology
Harvard Medical School;
Associate Neurologist-in-Chief;
Chief, Division of Clinical Neurology;
Director, Neuromuscular Program;
Boston Children's Hospital
Boston, MA, USA

Jahannaz Dastgir, DO
Department of Pediatric Neurology
Goryeb Children's Hospital/Atlantic
  Health System
Morristown, NJ, USA
Assistant Professor, Department of
  Pediatrics
Sidney Kimmel Medical College of
  Thomas Jefferson University,
  Philadelphia, PA, USA

Linda De Meirleir, MD, PhD
Professor
Neurology and Pediatric Neurology
Catholic University of Leuven
Leuven, Belgium

Darryl C. De Vivo, MD
Sidney Carter Professor of Neurology
  and Pediatrics
Department of Neurology
Columbia University Medical Center
New York, NY, USA

Linda S. de Vries, MD, PhD
Professor
Department of Neonatology
University Medical Centre Utrecht/
  Wilhelmina Children's Hospital
Utrecht, The Netherlands

Jeremy K. Deisch, MD
Assistant Professor of Pathology
Loma Linda University
Loma Linda, CA, USA

Paul Deltenre, MD, PhD
Professor, Department of Neurology
Laboratoire de Neurophysiologie
CHU Brugmann – Université Libre de
  Bruxelles
Bruxelles, Belgium

Jay Desai, MD
Assistant Professor of Clinical
  Neurology
Keck School of Medicine
University of Southern California
Los Angeles, CA, USA

Maria Descartes, MD
Professor
Department of Genetics
University of Alabama in Birmingham
Birmingham, AL, USA

Gabrielle deVeber, MD
Professor of Pediatrics
University of Toronto;
Director, Children's Stroke Program,
  Division of Neurology
Hospital for Sick Children;
Senior Scientist, Research Institute,
  Hospital for Sick Children
Toronto, ON, Canada

Sameer C. Dhamne
Biomedical Research Manager
Boston Children's Hospital
Harvard Medical School
Boston, MA, USA

Jullianne Diaz
Clinic Coordinator
Children's National Health System
Washington, DC, USA

Salvatore DiMauro, MD
Lucy G. Moses Professor of Neurology
Department of Neurology
Columbia University Medical Center
New York, NY, USA

William B. Dobyns, MD
Center for Integrative Brain Research
Seattle Children's Research Institute
Seattle, WA, USA

Dan Doherty, MD, PhD
Associate Professor
Department of Pediatrics
Divisions of Genetic and
  Developmental Medicine
Seattle Children's Hospital
University of Washington School of
  Medicine
Seattle, WA, USA

Elizabeth J. Donner, MD MSc FRCPC
Director, Comprehensive Epilepsy
  Program
Division of Neurology, The Hospital for
  Sick Children
Associate Professor, Department of
  Paediatrics
University of Toronto
Toronto, ON, Canada

Nico U.F. Dosenbach, MD, PhD
Assistant Professor
Department of Neurology
Washington University School of
  Medicine
St. Louis, MO, USA

James J. Dowling, MD, PhD
Senior Scientist, Program for Genetics
  and Genome Biology;
Staff Clinician, Division of Neurology
Hospital for Sick Children;
Associate Professor, Departments of
  Paediatrics and Molecular Genetics
University of Toronto
Toronto, ON, Canada

**James M. Drake, BSE, MB, BCh, MSc,
FRCSC**
Head
Neurosurgery
The Hospital for Sick Children
Toronto, ON, Canada

Cecile Ejerskov, MD
Department of Pediatrics
Aarhus University Hospital
Aarhus, Denmark

Andrew G. Engel, MD
McKnight-3M Professor of Neuroscience
Department of Neurology
Mayo Clinic College of Medicine
Rochester, MN, USA

Gregory M. Enns, MB, ChB
Professor
Department of Pediatrics
Stanford University
Stanford, CA, USA

María Victoria Escolano-Margarit, MD
Professor
Department of Pediatrics
University of Granada
Granada, Spain

Iris Etzion, MD
Senior visiting fellow
Department of Neurology
Division of Neurogenetics and
  Developmental Pediatrics
Children's National Medical Center and
  the George Washington University of
  the Health Sciences, Washington, DC,
  USA

S. Ali Fatemi, MD
Director
Neurogenics and Moser Centre for
  Leukodystrophies
Kennedy Krieger Institute
Baltimore, MD, USA

Darcy L. Fehlings, MD, FRCPC, MSc
Professor
Division of Developmental Paediatrics,
  Department of Paediatrics
Holland Bloorview Kids Rehabilitation
  Hospital
University of Toronto
Toronto, ON, Canada

Michelle Lauren Feinberg, MD
Resident
Department of Neurosurgery
George Washington University
Washington, DC, USA

Donna M. Ferriero, MD MS
W.H. And Marie Wattis Distinguished
  Professor;
Chair, Department of Pediatrics;
Physician-in-Chief UCSF Benioff
  Children's Hospital
San Francisco, CA, USA

Pauline A. Filipek, MD
Director, The Autism Center at CLI;
Professor of Pediatrics
Children's Learning Institute and the
  Division of Child, Adolescent
  Neurology
University of Texas Health Science
  Center
Houston, TX, USA

Richard S. Finkel, MD
Chief, Division of Neurology
Nemours Children's Hospital;
Professor of Neurology
University of Central Florida College of
  Medicine
Orlando, FL, USA

Paul G. Fisher, MD
Professor, Neurology and Pediatrics,
  and by courtesy Neurosurgery and
  Human Biology;
Beirne Family Professor of Pediatric
  Neuro-Oncology;
Bing Director of Human Biology
Stanford University
Stanford, CA, USA

Kevin Flanigan, MD
Robert F. and Edgar T. Wolfe
  Foundation Endowed Chair In
  Neuromuscular Research
Professor of Pediatrics and Neurology,
  The Ohio State University;
Director, Center for Gene Therapy
The Research Institute of Nationwide
  Children's Hospital
Columbus, OH, USA

Nicholas K. Foreman, MB.ChB. MRCP
Seebaum-Tschetter Chair of
  Neuro-Oncology
Professor, Department of Pediatrics;
University of Colorado
Denver, CO, USA

Israel Franco, MD, FACS, FAAP
Director Yale New Haven Children's
  Bladder and Continence Program
New Haven, CT, USA;
Professor of Urology
New York Medical College
Valhalla, NY, USA

Yitzchak Frank, MD
Clinical Professor
Pediatrics, Neurology, Psychiatry
Icahn School of Medicine at Mount
  Sinai
New York, NY, USA

Douglas R. Fredrick, MD
Clinical Professor
Department of Ophthalmology
Byers Eye Institute
Stanford University
Palo Alto, CA, USA

Hudson H. Freeze, PhD
Director
Human Genetics Program
Sanford Burnham Prebys Medical
  Discovery Institute
La Jolla, CA, USA

Cristina Fuente-Mora, PhD
Research Scientist
Department of Neurology
New York University School of
  Medicine
New York, NY, USA

Joseph M. Furman, MD, PhD
Professor
Departments of Otolaryngology and
  Neurology
University of Pittsburgh
Pittsburgh, PA, USA

Renata C. Gallagher, MD, PhD
Associate Professor of Clinical
  Pediatrics;
Director, Biochemical Genetics
Department of Pediatrics
UCSF Benioff Children's Hospital
San Francisco, CA, USA

Catherine Garel, MD
Hôpital d'enfants Armand-Trousseau
Department of Radiology
Paris, France

Emily Gertsch, MD
Referring Physician
Raleigh Neurology Associates
Raleigh, NC, USA

Donald L. Gilbert, MD MS FAAN FAAP
Professor of Pediatrics and Neurology;
Program Director;
Child Neurology Residency Director
Tourette Syndrome and Movement
  Disorders Clinics Director
Transcranial Magnetic Stimulation
  Laboratory
Cincinnati Children's Hospital Medical
  Center
Cincinnati, OH, USA

Elizabeth E. Gilles, MD
Pediatric Neurologist
Child Neurology Solutions, PLLC
Saint Paul, MN, USA

Christopher C. Giza, MD
Physician
Pediatrics, Pediatric Neurology
Ronald Reagan UCLA Medical Center
Los Angeles, CA, USA

Carol A. Glaser, MD
Chief, Encephalitis and Special
  Investigations Section
Division of Communicable Disease
  Control
Richmond, CA, USA

Hannah C. Glass, MDCM, MAS
Associate Professor
Departments of Neurology, Pediatrics
  and Epidemiology, Biostatistics
University of California, San Francisco
San Francisco, CA, USA

Tracy Glauser, MD
Associate Director, Cincinnati
  Children's Research Foundation;
Director, Comprehensive Epilepsy
  Center;
Co-Director, Genetic Pharmacology
  Service
Cincinnati Children's Hospital Medical
  Center
Cincinnati, OH, USA

Joseph Glykys, MD, PhD
Instructor in Neurology
Department of Neurology
Division of Child Neurology
Massachusetts General Hospital
Harvard Medical School
Boston, MA, USA

Amy Goldstein, MD
Director, Neurogenetics, Metabolism;
Assistant Professor of Pediatrics
University of Pittsburgh School of
  Medicine
Division of Child Neurology Children's
  Hospital of Pittsburgh
Pittsburgh, PA, USA

Hernan Dario Gonorazky, MD
Clinical and Research Neuromuscular
  Fellow
Division of Neurology
Genetics and Genome Biology Program
PGCRL, Hospital for Sick Children
University of Toronto
Toronto, ON, Canada

Rodolfo Gonzalez, PhD
Principal Scientist
International Stem Cell Corporation
Carlsbad, CA, USA

Howard P. Goodkin, MD, PhD
The Shure Professor of Neurology and
  Pediatrics
Department of Neurology
University of Virginia
Charlottesville, VA, USA

John M. Graham, Jr., MD, ScD
Professor Emeritus
Department of Pediatrics
Cedars-Sinai Medical Center and
  Harbor-UCLA Medical Center
David Geffen School of Medicine at
  UCLA
Los Angeles, CA, USA

Alexander L. Greninger, MD, PhD
Laboratory of Medicine
University of Washington
Seattle, WA, USA

Gary Gronseth, MD
Professor and Vice-Chairman
Department of Neurology
University of Kansas Medical Center
Kansas City, KS, USA

Andrea L. Gropman, MD
Chief, Neurogenetics and
  Neurodevelopmental Disabilities
Department of Neurology
Children's National Medical Center
George Washington University of the
  Health Sciences
Washington, DC, USA

Richard Grundy, MD
Professor of Paediatric Neuro-Oncology
  and Cancer Biology
Children's Brain Tumour Research
  Centre
University of Nottingham
Nottingham, UK

Renzo Guerrini, MD, FRCP
Professor and Head
Neuroscience Department
University of Florence and Children's
  Hospital Anna Meyer
Florence, Italy

Nalin Gupta, MD, PhD
UCSF Benioff Professor in Children's
  Health
Departments of Neurological Surgery
  and Pediatrics
University of California San Francisco
San Francisco, CA, USA

Jin S. Hahn, MD
Professor
Department of Neurology and
  Pediatrics
Stanford University, School of Medicine
Stanford, CA, USA

Milton H. Hamblin, PhD
Assistant Professor
Department of Pharmacology
Tulane University School of Medicine,
New Orleans, LA, USA

Abeer J. Hani, MD
Assistant Professor of Pediatrics and
  Neurology
Lebanese American University
Beirut, Lebanon

Sharyu Hanmantgad
Department of Radiology
Memorial Sloan-Kettering Cancer
  Center
New York, NY, USA

Mary J. Harbert, MD
Director of Neonatal Neurology
Sharp Mary Birch Hospital for Women
  and Newborns;
Assistant Professor of Neurosciences
University of California San Diego
San Diego, CA, USA

Chellamani Harini, MBBS, MD
Instructor
Department of Neurology
Boston Children's Hospital
Boston, MA, USA

Andrea M. Harriott, MD
Fellow
Department of Neurology
Brigham and Women's Hospital
  Massachusetts General Hospital
Boston, MA, USA

Chad Heatwole, MD, MS-CI
Associate Professor of Neurology
Department of Neurology
University of Rochester
Rochester, MN, USA

Andrew D. Hershey, MD, PhD, FAHS
Endowed Chair and Director of
  Neurology;
Director, Headache Center
Cincinnati Children's Hospital Medical
  Center;
Professor of Pediatrics and Neurology
University of Cincinnati, College of
  Medicine
Cincinnati, OH, USA

Deborah G. Hirtz, MD
Professor
Neurological Sciences and Pediatrics
University of Vermont School of
  Medicine
Burlington, VT, USA

Gregory L. Holmes, MD
Professor of Neurological Sciences and
 Pediatrics;
Chair, Department of Neurological
 Sciences
University of Vermont College of
 Medicine
Burlington, VT, USA

Barbara A. Holshouser, PhD
Professor
Department of Radiology
Loma Linda University School of
 Medicine
Loma Linda, CA, USA

Kathleen A. Hurwitz, MD
Physician
Hurwitz Pediatrics
Murrieta, CA, USA

Eugene Hwang, MD
Attending, Pediatric Neuro-oncology
Director, Clinical Neuro-oncology
 Immunotherapeutics Program
Center for Cancer and Blood Disorders
Children's National Medical Center
Washington, DC, USA

Rebecca N. Ichord, MD
Associate Professor, Neurology
University of Pennsylvania School of
 Medicine;
Director, Pediatric Stroke Program
Philadelphia, PA, USA

Paymaan Jafar-Nejad, MD
Assistant Director
Department of Neuro Drug Discovery
Ionis Pharmaceuticals, Inc.
Carlsbad, CA, USA

Sejal V. Jain, MD
Associate Director of the Sleep Center;
Director, Neurology-Sleep Program;
Assistant Professor of Pediatrics and
 Neurology
Cincinnati Children's Hospital Medical
 Center
Cincinnati, OH, USA

Lori Jordan, MD, PhD
Assistant Professor
Departments of Pediatrics and
 Neurology
Vanderbilt University Medical Center
Nashville, TN, USA

Marielle A. Kabbouche, MD, FAHS
Professor of Pediatrics and Neurology
University of Cincinnati, College of
 Medicine;
Director, Inpatient Headache Program
Department of Pediatrics and
 Neurology
Cincinnati Children's Hospital Medical
 Center
Cincinnati, OH, USA

Joanne Kacperski, MD
Assistant Professor of Neurology and
 Pediatrics
University of Cincinnati, College of
 Medicine
Department of Pediatrics and
 Neurology
Cincinnati Children's Hospital Medical
 Center
Cincinnati, OH, USA

Peter B. Kang, MD
Associate Professor of Pediatrics and
 Chief, Division of Pediatric
 Neurology
Department of Pediatrics
University of Florida College of
 Medicine
Gainesville, FL, USA

Matthias A. Kariannis, MD, MS
Associate Professor of Pediatrics and
 Otolaryngology
Division of Pediatric Hematology/
 Oncology
NYU Langone Medical Center and
 Perlmutter Cancer Center
New York, NY, USA

Horacio Kaufmann, MD
Felicia B. Axelrod Professor of
 Dysautonomia Research
Department of Neurology
NYU School of Medicine
New York, NY, USA

Harper L. Kaye, MD
Neurologist
Clinical Neuromodulation
Boston Children's Hospital
Boston, MA, USA

Robert Keating, MD
Chief
Neurosurgery
Children's National
Washington, DC, USA

Colin R. Kennedy, MBBS, MD
Professor in Neurology and Paediatrics
Faculty of Medicine
University of Southampton
Southampton, UK

Yasmin Khakoo, MD
Child Neurology Director;
Associate Attending Pediatric
 Neurologist/Neuro-oncologist
Memorial Sloan Kettering Cancer
 Center
New York, NY, USA

Adam Kirton, MD, MSc, FRCPC
Associate Professor
Pediatrics and Clinical Neurosciences
 Cumming School of Medicine
University of Calgary Alberta Children's
 Hospital Research Institute
Calgary, AB, Canada

John T. Kissel, MD
Professor of Neurology, Pediatrics,
 Neuroscience;
Chairman, Department of Neurology
The Gilbert and Kathryn Mitchell Chair
 in Neurology
The Ohio State University Wexner
 Medical Center
Department of Neurology
Columbus, OH, USA

Kelly G. Knupp, MD
Associate Professor of Neurology and
 Pediatrics
University of Colorado School of
 Medicine Children's Hospital
Colorado Aurora, CO, USA

Bruce R. Korf, MD, PhD
Wayne H. and Sara Crews Finley Chair
 in Medical Genetics;
Professor and Chair, Department of
 Genetics;
Director, Heflin Center for Genomic
 Sciences
University of Alabama at Birmingham
Birmingham, AL, USA

Eric H. Kossoff, MD
Professor
Departments of Neurology and
 Pediatrics
Johns Hopkins Hospital
Baltimore, MD, USA

Sanjeev V. Kothare, MD
Director, Pediatric Sleep Program
New York University Langone Medical
 Center;
Pediatric Neurologist and Epileptologist
NYU Comprehensive Epilepsy Center
Department of Neurology
New York, NY, USA

Oren Kupfer, MD
Assistant Professor of Pediatrics
Pediatric Pulmonary Medicine
University of Colorado School of
 Medicine
Children's Hospital Colorado
Aurora, CO, USA

**W. Curt LaFrance, Jr., MD, MPH,
FAAN, FANPA, DFAPA**
Director
Neuropsychiatry and Behavioral
 Neurology
Rhode Island Hospital
Providence, RI, USA

Beatrice Latal, MD, MPH
Professor
Child Development Center
University Children's Hospital Zurich
Zurich, Switzerland

Steven M. Leber, MD, PhD
Professor
Departments of Pediatrics and
    Neurology
University of Michigan
Ann Arbor, MI, USA

Jean-Pyo Lee, PhD
Assistant Professor
Department of Neurology
Tulane University School of Medicine
New Orleans, LA, USA

Ilo E. Leppik, MD
Professor of Neurology and Pharmacy
University of Minnsota
Minneapolis, MN, USA

Tally Lerman-Sagie, MD
Professor
Neurosurgery
Edith Wolfson Medical Center
Jerusalem, Israel

Jason T. Lerner, MD
Associate Professor
Division of Pediatric Neurology
David Geffen School of Medicine at
    UCLA
Los Angeles, CA, USA

Richard J. Leventer, MD
Professor
Division of Medicine
The Royal Children's Hospital
    Melbourne
Melbourne, Australia

Daniel J. Licht, MD
Associate Professor of Neurology;
Director of the Wolfson Family
    Laboratory for Clinical and
    Biomedical Optics
Department of Neurology
The Children's Hospital of Philadelphia
Philadelphia, PA, USA

Uta Lichter-Konecki, MD, PhD
Visiting Professor of Pediatrics
Director of the Metabolism Program
Division of Medical Genetics/PKU
    Program
Children's Hospital of Pittsburgh
Pittsburgh, PA, USA

Zvi Lidar, MD
Consultant Physician
Neurosurgery
Herzliya Medical Center
Tel Aviv-Yafo, Israel

Djin Gie Liem, PhD
Senior Lecturer
School of Exercise, Nutrition Sciences
Deakin University
Burwood, NSW, Australia

Tobias Loddenkemper, MD
Director of Clinical Epilepsy Research;
Associate Professor, Harvard Medical
    School
Division of Epilepsy and Clinical
    Neurophysiology
Boston Children's Hospital
Boston, MA, USA

Roger K. Long, MD
Associate Professor
Department of Pediatrics
University of California, San Francisco
San Francisco, CA, USA

Quyen N. Luc, MD
Clinical Assistant Professor of
    Neurology
Keck School of Medicine
University of Southern California
Los Angeles, CA, USA

Mark Mackay, MBBS, PhD, FRACP
Director, Children's Stroke Program
Department of Neurology, Royal
    Children's Hospital;
Honorary Research Fellow, Clinical
    Sciences Theme,
Murdoch Childrens Research Institute;
Honorary Professorial Research Fellow
Florey Institute of Neurosciences and
    Mental Health
University of Melbourne
Melbourne, VIC, Australia

Annette Majnemer, MD
Professor; Director and Associate Dean
School of Physical and Occupational
    Therapy
McGill University
Montreal, Canada

Naila Makhani, MD, MPH
Assistant Professor
Departments of Pediatrics and
    Neurology
Yale University School of Medicine
New Haven, CT, USA

Gustavo Malinger, MD
Associate Professor
Obstetrics and Gynecology
Tel-Aviv University
Tel-Aviv, Israel

David E. Mandelbaum, MD
Professor
Neurology, Pediatrics
Brown University
Providence, RI, USA

Stephen M. Maricich, PhD, MD
Mellon Foundation Scholar
Assistant Professor
Department of Pediatrics
Division of Neurology
Pittsburgh, PA, USA

Kiran P. Maski, MD
Instructor, Harvard Medical School
Department of Neurology
Boston Children's Hospital
Boston, MA, USA

Mudit Mathur, MD, MBA, FAAP, FCCM
Associate Professor
Department of Pediatrics, Division of
    Pediatric Critical Care
Loma Linda University School of
    Medicine
Loma Linda, CA, USA

Dennis J. Matthews, MD
Professor; Chairman
Physical Medicine and Rehabilitation
University of Colorado
Denver, CO, USA

Kelly McMahon, MD
Genetic Counselor
University of Rochester Medical Center
Rochester, NY, USA

Megan B. DeMara-Hoth
Clinical Research Associate (Volunteer)
Neurology
Medical College of Wisconsin
Milwaukee, WI, USA

Bryce Mendelsohn, MD, PhD
Assistant Clinical Professor
Department of Pediatrics, Division of
    Medical Genetics
University of California
San Francisco, CA, USA

Julie A. Mennella, PhD
Member
Monell Chemical Senses Center
Philadelphia, PA, USA

Laura R. Ment, MD
Professor, Departments of Pediatrics
    and Neurology;
Associate Dean
Yale School of Medicine
New Haven, CT, USA

Eugenio Mercuri, MD
Professor of Pediatric Neurology
Catholic University Sacred Heart
Rome, Italy

David J. Michelson, MD
Assistant Professor
Departments of Pediatrics and
    Neurology
Loma Linda University Health
Loma Linda, CA, USA

Mohamad A. Mikati, MD
Wilburt C. Davison Professor of
    Pediatrics;
Professor of Neurobiology;
Chief, Division of Pediatric Neurology
Duke University Medical Center
Durham, NC, USA

Fady M. Mikhail, MD
Co-Director
Department of Genetics
University of Birmingham
Birmingham, AL, USA

Steven Paul Miller, MDCM, MAS
Division Head and Professor of
    Pediatrics
Bloorview Children's Hospital Chair in
    Pediatric Neuroscience
Department of Pediatrics (Neurology)
The Hospital for Sick Children,
    University of Toronto
Toronto, ON, Canada

Jeff M. Milunsky, MD
Co-Director, Center for Human
    Genetics;
Director, Clinical Genetics;
Senior Director, Molecular Genetics
Center for Human Genetics
Cambridge, MA, USA

Jonathan W. Mink, MD, PhD
Frederick A. Horner, MD Endowed
    Professor in Pediatric Neurology
Departments of Neurology,
    Neuroscience, and Pediatrics
University of Rochester
Rochester, NY, USA

Ghayda M. Mirzaa, MD
Assistant Professor
Center for Integrative Brain Research
Children's Research Institute
Seattle, WA, USA

Wendy G. Mitchell, MD
Professor, Clinical Neurology
Keck School of Medicine
University of Southern California
Children's Hospital Los Angeles
Los Angeles, CA, USA

Michael A. Mohan, MD
Department of Sleep Medicine
Boston Children's Hospital
Beth Israel Deaconess Medical Center
Boston, MA, USA

Payam Mohassel, MD
Clinical Fellow
National Institutes of Health, National
    Institute of Neurological Disorders
    and Stroke
Bethesda, MD, USA

**Mahendranath Moharir, MD, MSc,
FRACP**
Pediatric Neurologist and Associate
    Professor
Division of Neurology, Department of
    Pediatrics
The Hospital for Sick Children and
    University of Toronto
Toronto, ON, Canada

Umrao R. Monani, PhD
Associate Professor
Pathology, Cell Biology
Columbia University Medical Center
New York, NY, USA

Michelle Monje Deisseroth, MD, PhD
Anne T. and Robert M. Bass Endowed
    Faculty Scholar in Pediatric Cancer
    and Blood Diseases
Assistant Professor of Neurology, and
    by courtesy, Neurosurgery, Pathology
    and Pediatrics
Stanford University
Palo Alto, CA, USA

Manikum Moodley, MD, FCP, FRCP
Staff Pediatric Neurologist
Center for Pediatric Neurology
Neurological Institute, Cleveland Clinic
Cleveland, OH, USA

Andrew Mower, MD
Neurology
Children's Hospital of Orange County
Orange County, CA, USA

Richard T. Moxley III, MD
Professor of Neurology and Pediatrics
University of Rochester Medical Center
School of Medicine and Dentistry
Rochester, NY, USA

Sabine Mueller, MD, PhD, MAS
Associate Professor
Department of Neurology,
    Neurosurgery and Pediatrics
University of California, San Francisco
San Francisco, CA, USA

Alysson R. Muotri, PhD
Associate Professor
Departments of Pediatrics and Cellular,
    Molecular Medicine
University of California San Diego
La Jolla, CA, USA

Sandesh C.S. Nagamani, MBBS, MD
Assistant Professor
Molecular and Human Genetics
Baylor College of Medicine
Houston, TX, US

Mohan J. Narayanan, MD
Barrow Neurological Institute
Phoenix, AZ, USA

Vinodh Narayanan, MD
Medical Director
Center for Rare Childhood Disorders
The Translational Genomics Research
    Institute (TGen)
Phoenix, AZ, USA

Ruth D. Nass, MD
Nancy Glickenhaus Pier Professor of
    Pediatric Neuropsychiatry;
Professor, Department of Child and
    Adolescent Psychiatry;
Professor, Department of Pediatrics
NYU Langone Medical Center
NYU Child Study Center
New York, NY, USA

Jeffrey L. Neul, MD, PhD
Chief of Child Neurology;
Professor and Vice Chair
Department of Neurosciences
University of California
San Diego, CA, USA

Yoram Nevo, MD
Professor and chair
Institute of Neurology
Schneider Children's Medical Center of
    Israel
Tel-Aviv University
Tel Aviv, Israel

Bobby G. Ng, BS
Scientist
Genetic Disease Program
Sanford - Burnham - Prebys Medical
    Discovery Institute
La Jolla, CA, USA

Katherine C. Nickels, MD
Assistant Professor
Department of Neurology
Mayo Clinic
Rochester, MN, USA

Graeme A.M. Nimmo, MBBS, MSc
Resident
Clinical and Metabolic Genetics
The Hospital for Sick Children
University of Toronto
Toronto, ON, Canada

Michael J. Noetzel, MD
Professor of Neurology and Pediatrics;
Vice Chair, Division of Pediatric and
    Developmental Neurology
Washington University School of
    Medicine;
Medical Director, Clinical and
    Diagnostic Neuroscience Services
St. Louis Children's Hospital
St. Louis, MO, USA

Lucy Norcliffe-Kaufmann, PhD
Assistant Professor, Physiology and
    Neuroscience
NYU Langone Medical Center
New York, NY, USA

Douglas R. Nordli, Jr., MD
Chief of the Division of Pediatric
    Neurology and co-director of the
    Neuroscience Institute
Children's Hospital Los Angeles
Los Angeles, CA, USA

Ulrike Nowak-Göttl, MD
Professor;
Deputy Director Campus Kiel
Institute of Clinical Chemistry
Universitätsklinikum
    Schleswig-Holstein
Kiel, Germany

Hope L. O'Brien, MD, FAHS
Associate Professor of Pediatrics and
  Neurology
University of Cincinnati, College of
  Medicine;
Director, Young Adult Headache Clinic;
Program Director, Headache Medicine
  Education
Department of Pediatrics and
  Neurology
Cincinnati Children's Hospital Medical
  Center
Cincinnati, OH, USA

Joyce Oleszek, MD
Associate Professor
Department of Rehabilitation
University of Colorado at Denver
Denver, CO, USA

Maryam Oskoui, MDCM, MSc, FRCPC
Assistant Professor
Departments of Pediatrics and
  Neurology/Neurosurgery
McGill University
Montreal, QC, Canada

Alex R. Paciorkowski, MD
Assistant Professor
Department of Neurology
University of Rochester Medical Center
Rochester, MN, USA

Roger J. Packer, MD
Senior Vice-President, Center for
  Neuroscience and Behavioral
  Medicine;
Gilbert Family Neurofibromatosis
  Family Distinguished Professor in
  Neurofibromatosis;
Director, Brain Tumor Institute;
Director, Neurofibromatosis Institute
Children's National Health System;
Professor, Neurology and Pediatrics
George Washington University
Washington, DC, USA

Seymour Packman, MD
Professor Emeritus
Department of Pediatrics, Division of
  Medical Genetics
University of California
San Francisco, CA, USA

Jose-Alberto Palma, MD
Assistant Professor, Department of
  Neurology;
Assistant Director, Dysautonomia
  Research Laboratory
NYU Langone Medical Center
New York, NY, USA

Andrea C. Pardo, MD, FAAP
Assistant Professor
Department of Pediatrics and
  Neurology
Ann and Robert H. Lurie Children's
  Hospital of Chicago
Northwestern Feinberg School of
  Medicine
Chicago, IL, USA

Julie A. Parsons, MD
Associate Professor of Pediatrics and
  Neurology
Child Neurology
University of Colorado School of
  Medicine
Aurora, CO, USA

John Colin Partridge, MD
Professor, Emeritus
Pediatrics (Neonatology)
University of California San Francisco
UCSF Benioff Children's Hospital
San Francisco, CA, USA

Gregory M. Pastores, MD
Clinical Professor, Medicine (Genetics)
University College Dublin
Dublin, Ireland

Marc C. Patterson, MD
Chair, Division of Child and Adolescent
  Neurology
Professor of Neurology, Pediatrics and
  Medical Genetics
Director, Child Neurology Training
  Program
Mayo Clinic
Rochester, MMN, USA

William J. Pearce, PhD
Professor of Physiology
Center for Perinatal Biology
Loma Linda University School of
  Medicine
Loma Linda, CA, USA

Phillip L. Pearl, MD
Director of Epilepsy and Clinical
  Neurophysiology
Boston Children's Hospital;
William G. Lennox Professor of
  Neurology
Harvard Medical School
Boston, MA, USA

Melanie Penner, MD, FRCP(C)
Clinician Investigator and
  Developmental Pediatrician
Holland Bloorview Kids Rehabilitation
  Hospital
Toronto, ON, Canada

Leila Percival, RN
Clinical Research Nurse
NYU Langone Medical Center
New York, NY, USA

Marcia Pereira, PhD
Instructor
Department of Neurology
Tulane University School of Medicine
New Orleans, LA, USA

Stefan M. Pfister, MD
Professor of Pediatrics
Division of Pediatric Neurooncology
German Cancer Research Center
  (DKFZ)
Heidelberg, Germany

John Phillips, MD
Professor and Director of Child
  Neurology
Department of Neurology
University of New Mexico Health
  Science Center
Albuquerque, NM, USA

Barbara Plecko, MD
Professor
Department of Child Neurology
University Children's Hospital Zurich
Zurich, Switzerland

Sigita Plioplys, MD
Head, Pediatric Neuropsychiatry
  Program
Child and Adolescent Psychiatry;
Associate Professor of Psychiatry and
  Behavioral Sciences
Northwestern University Feinberg
  School of Medicine
Ann & Robert H. Lurie Children's
  Hospital of Chicago
Chicago, IL, USA

Annapurna Poduri, MD, MPH
Associate Professor
Department of Neurology
Boston Children's Hospital, Harvard
  Medical School
Boston, MA, USA

Sharon Poisson, MD
Assistant Professor
Neurology Clinic
University of Colorado Hospital
Aurora, CO, USA

Scott L. Pomeroy, MD, PhD
Bronson Crothers Professor and
  Chairman
Department of Neurology
Harvard Medical School
Boston, MA, USA

Andrea Poretti, MD
Assistant Professor
Division of Pediatric Radiology
Russell H. Morgan Department of
  Radiology and Radiological Science
The John Hopkins University School of
  Medicine
Baltimore, MD, USA

Scott W. Powers, PhD, ABPP, FAHS
Professor of Pediatrics and CCRF
  Endowed Chair
University of Cincinnati College of
  Medicine;
Director of Clinical and Translational
  Research
Cincinnati Children's Research
  Foundation;
Co-Director, Headache Center;
Director, Center for Child Behavior and
  Nutrition Research and Training
Division of Behavioral Medicine and
  Clinical Psychology
Cincinnati Children's Hospital Medical
  Center
Cincinnati, OH, USA

Michael R. Pranzatelli, MD
Courtesy Professor of Neurology
  University of Central Florida College
  of Medicine
Orlando, FL, USA;
Adjoint Professor of Neurology
  University of Colorado School of
  Medicine
Founder and President
National Pediatric Neuroinflammation
  Organization, Inc.
Orlando, FL, USA

Allison Przekop, DO
Associate Professor
Pediatrics, Division of Pediatric
  Neurology
Loma Linda University Children's
  Hospital
Loma Linda, CA, USA

**Malcolm Rabie, MB BCh, FCP (SA)
(Neurol.)**
Staff Physician
Institute of Neurology, Schneider
  Children's Medical Center of Israel
Tel Aviv University
Tel Aviv, Israel

Sampathkumar Rangasamy, PhD
Research Assistant Professor
Neurogenomics Division and The
  Dorrance Center for Rare Childhood
  Disorders,
The Translational Genomics Research
  Institute (TGen)
Phoenix, AZ, USA

Gerald V. Raymond, MD
Professor, Department of Neurology
The University of Minnesota
Minneapolis, MN, USA

Alyssa T. Reddy, MD
Professor of Pediatrics;
Director, Neuro-Oncology Program
UAB Cancer Prevention and Control
  Training Program
University of Alabama
Birmingham, AL, USA

Rebecca L. Rendleman, MD, CM
Assistant Professor of Clinical
  Psychiatry
Weill Cornell Medical College;
Assistant Attending Psychiatry
NewYork-Presbyterian Hospital
New York, NY, USA

Jong M. Rho, MD
Professor, Departments of Paediatrics,
  Clinical Neurology;
Division Head, Paediatric Neurology
Alberta Children's Hospital;
Dr. Robert Haslam Chair in Child
  Neurology;
Alberta Children's Hospital
Calgary, AB, USA

Lance H. Rodan, MD
Instructor in Pediatrics, Harvard
  Medical School
Department of Neurology, Boston
  Children's Hospital, Boston MA
Department of Medicine, Division of
  Genetics and Genomics, Boston
  Children's Hospital
Boston, MA, USA

Sarah M. Roddy, MD
Associate Professor of Pediatrics and
  Neurology;
Associate Dean of Admissions
Loma Linda University School of
  Medicine
Loma Linda, CA, USA

Elizabeth E. Rogers
Associate Professor of Pediatrics
Director, Intensive Care Nursery Follow
  Up Program
Associate Clinical Director, Intensive
  Care Nursery
UCSF – Benioff Children's Hospital San
  Francisco
San Francisco, CA, USA

Stephen M. Rosenthal, MD
Professor of Pediatrics
Division of Pediatric Endocrinology
Medical Director, Child and Adolescent
  Gender Center
University of California, San Francisco
San Francisco, CA, USA

N. Paul Rosman, MD
Professor of Pediatrics and Neurology
Pediatrics, Neurology; Division of
  Pediatric Neurology
Boston Medical Center
Boston University School of Medicine
Boston, MA, USA

M. Elizabeth Ross, MD, PhD
Nathan Cummings Professor of
  Neurology and Neuroscience;
Director, Center for Neurogenetics
Brain and Mind Research Institute
Weill Cornell Medical College
New York, NY, USA

Alexander Rotenberg, MD, PhD
Associate in Neurology;
Research Associate in Neurology;
Director, Neuromodulation Program
F.M. Kirby Neurobiology Center
Boston Children's Hospital
Boston, MA, USA

Robert S. Rust, MA, MD
Professor
Neurology
University of Virginia Medical Center
Charlottesville, VA, USA

Cheryl P. Sanchez, MD
Associate Professor
Department of Pediatrics
Loma Linda University Children's
  Hospital
Loma Linda, CA, USA

**Pedro Sanchez, MD, FAAP, MSCE,
FACMG**
Director of Craniofacial Genetics
  Children's Hospital Los Angeles;
Assistant Professor of Clinical Pediatrics
University of Southern California;
Assistant Professor of Clinical
  Pathology
University of Southern California
Los Angeles, CA, USA

Iván Sánchez Fernández, MD
Epilepsy Fellow
Division of Epilepsy and Clinical
  Neurophysiology
Boston Children's Hospital
Boston, MA, USA

Tristan T. Sands, MD, PhD
Assistant Professor of Neurology
Columbia University Medical Center
New York City, NY, USA

Terence D. Sanger, MD PhD
Associate Professor
University of Southern California
Department Biomedical Engineering,
  Biokinesiology, Child Neurology
Los Angeles, CA, USA

**Kumar Sannagowdara, MD DCH,
MRCPCH (UK)**
Assistant Professor of Pediatric
  Neurology and Epilepsy
Medical College of Wisconsin
Milwaukee, WI, USA

Dustin Scheinost, MD
Associate Research Scientist
Department of Radiology, Biomedical
  Imaging
Yale School of Medicine
New Haven, CT, USA

Mark S. Scher, MD
Tenured Professor of Pediatrics and
  Neurology;
Chief, Division of Pediatric Neurology;
Director, Fetal and Neonatal Neurology
  Program
Pediatrics, Rainbow Babies and
  Children's Hospital
Case Western Reserve University, School
  of Medicine
Cleveland, OH, USA

Nina F. Schor, MD, PhD
William H. Eilinger Professor and Chair
Department of Pediatrics;
Professor, Department of Neurology
  and Neuroscience;
Pediatrician-in-Chief, Golisano
  Children's Hospital
University of Rochester School of
  Medicine and Dentistry
Rochester, NY, USA

Isabelle Schrauwen, PhD
Research Assistant Professor
Neurogenomics Division
The Translational Genomics Research
    Institute (TGen)
Phoenix, AZ, USA

Michael M. Segal, MD, PhD
Founder and Chief Scientist
SimulConsult, Inc.
Chestnut Hill, MA, USA

Syndi Seinfeld, DO, MS
Assistant Professor
Child Neurology
Virginia Commonwealth University
Richmond, VA, USA

Duygu Selcen, MD
Associate Professor of Neurology and
    Pediatrics
Department of Neurology
Mayo Clinic College of Medicine
Rochester, MN, USA

Laurie E. Seltzer, DO
Senior Instructor of Child Neurology;
Epilepsy Fellow
University of Rochester Medical Center
Rochester, NY, USA

**Margaret Semrud-Clikeman, PhD, LP
ABPdN**
Professor of Pediatrics
University of Minnesota Medical School
Minneapolis, MN, USA

Dennis W. Shaw, MD
Professor of Radiology
Department of Radiology
University of Washington
Seattle Children's Hospital
Seattle, WA, USA

Bennett A. Shaywitz, MD
Charles and Helen Schwab Professor of
    Pediatrics (Neurology);
Co-Director, Yale Center for Dyslexia
    and Creativity
Yale School of Medicine
New Haven, CT, USA

Sally E. Shaywitz, MD
Audrey G. Ratner Professor of Learning
    Development;
Co-Director, Yale Center for Dyslexia
    and Creativity
Yale School of Medicine
New Haven, CT, USA

Renée A. Shellhaas, MD, MS
Clinical associate professor
Department of pediatrics and
    communicable diseases (division of
    pediatric neurology)
University of Michigan
Ann Arbor, MI, USA

Elliott H. Sherr, MD, PhD
Professor
UCSF School of Medicine
San Francisco, CA, USA

Rita D. Sheth, MD MPH
Assistant Professor of Pediatrics
Pediatric Nephrology
Department of Pediatrics
Loma Linda University School of
    Medicine
Loma Linda, CA, USA

**Michael I. Shevell, MDCM, FRCP(C),
FCAHS**
Professor, Departments of Pediatrics,
    Neurology and Neurosurgery;
Chair, McGill Department of Pediatrics;
Pediatrician-in-Chief, Montreal
    Children's Hospital-McGill University
    Health Centre (MUHC);
Harvey Guyda Professor
Department of Pediatrics, Faculty of
    Medicine, McGill University
Montreal, QC, Canada

Shlomo Shinnar, MD, PhD
Professor Neurology, Pediatrics and
    Epidemiology and Population
    Health;
Hyman Climenko Professor of
    Neuroscience Research;
Director, Comprehensive Epilepsy
    Management Center
Montefiore Medical Center, Albert
    Einstein College of Medicine
Bronx, NY, USA

Ben Shofty, MD
Resident
Division of Neurosurgery
Tel Aviv Medical Center
Tel Aviv, Israel

Stanford K. Shu, MD
Assistant Professor of Pediatrics
Division of Child Neurology
Department of Pediatrics
Loma Linda University School of
    Medicine;
Pediatric Neurologist
Loma Linda University Children's
    Hospital
Loma Linda, CA, USA

Michael E. Shy, MD
Professor of Neurology, Pediatrics and
    Physiology
Carver College of Medicine
University of Iowa
Iowa City, IA, USA

Laura Silveira Moriyama, MD
Professor, Department Posgraduate
    Program in Medicine
Institute Ciências da Saúde
Universidade Nove de Julho (Uninove)
São Paulo, SP, Brazil

Nicholas J. Silvestri, MD
Assistant Professor
Department of Neurology
University at Buffalo Jacobs School of
    Medicine and Biomedical Sciences
Buffalo, New York, NY, USA

Katherine B. Sims, MD
Professor of Neurology
Department of Neurology, Division of
    Child Neurology
Massachusetts General Hospital and
    Harvard Medical School
Boston, MA, USA

Harvey S. Singer, MD
Professor
Departments of Neurology and
    Pediatrics
Johns Hopkins University School of
    Medicine
Johns Hopkins Hospital
Baltimore, MD, USA

Nilika Shah Singhal, MD
Assistant Professor
Department of Neurology, Pediatrics
University of California San Francisco
San Francisco, CA, USA

Craig M. Smith, MD
Attending Physician, Critical Care;
Instructor in Pediatrics
Northwestern University
Feinberg School of Medicine
Ann & Robert H. Lurie Children's
    Hospital of Chicago
Chicago, IL, USA

Edward Smith, MD
Director of Cerebrovascular Surgery;
    Associate Professor,
Department of Neurosurgery
Boston Children's Hospital, Harvard
    Medical School
Boston, MA, USA

Stephen A. Smith, MD
Medical Director, Neuromuscular
    Program
Gillette Children's Specialty Healthcare
Saint Paul, MN, USA

Evan Y. Snyder, MD, PhD
Professor
Department of Stem Cells and
    Regenerative Medicine
Sanford-Burnham-Prebys Medical
    Discovery Institute
La Jolla, CA, USA

Janet Soul, MDCM, FRCPC
Associate Professor of Neurology
Department of Neurology
Harvard Medical School
Boston, MA, USA

**Christy L. Spalink, RN, MSN,
ACNP-BC**
Complex Medical Care Coordinator
Department of Neurology
New York University School of
    Medicine
New York, NY, USA

Karen A. Spencer, MD, MS, MPH
Instructor
Department of Neurology
Boston Children's Hospital
Boston, MA, USA

Carl E. Stafstrom, MD, PhD
Professor of Neurology and Pediatrics
Lederer Chair in Pediatric Epilpesy
Division of Pediatric Neurology
Johns Hopkins University Cchool of
    Medicine
Baltimore, MD, USA

Robert Steinfeld, MD, PhD
Professor
Department of Pediatrics
University Medical Center Goettingen
Goettingen, Germany

Jonathan B. Strober, MD
Professor
Departments of Neurology, Pediatrics
UCSF Benioff Children's Hospital San
    Francisco
San Francisco, CA, USA

Joseph Sullivan, MD
Associate Professor of Neurology,
    Pediatrics;
Director, UCSF Pediatric Epilepsy
    Center
University of California San Francisco
San Francisco, CA, USA

Kenneth F. Swaiman, MD
Director Emeritus, Division of Pediatric
    Neurology;
Professor Emeritus of Neurology and
    Pediatrics
University of Minnesota Medical School
Minneapolis, MN, USA

Kathryn J. Swoboda, MD
Director
Neurogenetics Unit
Center for Genomic Medicine
Department of Neurology
Massachusetts General Hospital
Boston, MA, USA

Elizabeth D. Tate, MN, ARNP, BC-FNP
Nurse Practitioner
National Pediatric Neuroinflammation
    Organization, Inc.
Orlando, FL, USA

William O. Tatum IV, DO
Professor
Department of Neurology
Mayo Clinic College of Medicine
Jacksonville, FL, USA

Ingrid Tein, MD, FRCP (C)
Director, Neurometabolic Clinic and
    Research Laboratory, Division of
    Neurology;
Associate Professor, Department of
    Pediatrics, Laboratory Medicine and
    Pathobiology;
Senior Associate Scientist, Genetics and
    Genome Biology Program
The Hospital for Sick Children
The University of Toronto
Toronto, ON, Canada

Kristyn Tekulve, MD
Assistant Professor of Child Neurology
Department of Neurology, Division of
    Child Neurology
Riley Hospital for Children at Indiana
    University School of Medicine
Indianapolis, IN, USA

Jeffrey R. Tenney, MD, PhD
Pediatric Epileptologist
Division of Neurology;
Assistant Professor
UC Department of Pediatrics
Cincinnati Children's Hospital Medical
    Center
Cincinnati, OH, USA

Elizabeth A. Thiele, MD, PhD
Director, Pediatric Epilepsy Program;
Director, Carol and James Herscot
    Center for Tuberous Sclerosis
    Complex;
Professor of Neurology, Harvard
    Medical School
Massachusetts General Hospital
Boston, MA, USA

Robert Thompson-Stone, MD
Assistant Professor
Department of Neurology
University of Rochester
Rochester, NY, USA

Laura Tochen, MD
Assistant Professor
Department of Neurology
Children's National Medical Center
Washington, DC, USA

Laura M. Tormoehlen, MD
Associate Professor of Clinical
    Neurology and Emergency Medicine
Indiana University School of Medicine
Indianapolis, IN, USA

Lily Tran, MD
Assistant Clinical Professor, Department
    of Pediatrics
University of California- Irvine;
CHOC Children's Specialist, Pediatric
    Neurology
Orange, CA, USA

Doris A. Trauner, MD
Distinguished Professor
Departments of Neurosciences and
    Pediatrics
UCSD School of Medicine
La Jolla, CA, USA

Sinan O. Turnacioglu, MD
Assistant Professor
Neurogenetics and Neurodevelopmental
    Pediatrics
Children's National Health System
George Washington University
Washington, DC, USA

Nicole J. Ullrich, MD, PhD
Associate Professor of Neurology
Department of Neurology
Boston Children's Hospital
Harvard Medical School
Boston, MA, USA

David K. Urion, MD, FAAN
Director, Behavioral Neurology Clinics
    and Programs;
Director of Education and Residency
    Training Programs in Child
    Neurology and Neurodevelopmental
    Disabilities;
Charles F. Barlow Chair
Boston Children's Hospital;
Associate Professor of Neurology
Harvard Medical School
Boston, MA, USA

Guy Van Camp, PhD
Senior research scientist
Centre of Medical Genetics
University of Antwerp
Antwerp, Belgium

Michèle Van Hirtum-Das, MD
Neurologist
Children's Hospital Los Angeles;
University of California Los Angeles
    Medical Center
Los Angeles, CA, USA

Clara D.M. van Karnebeek, MD, PhD
Associate Professor
Department of Paediatrics
Academic Medical Center
Amsterdam, The Netherlands;
Department of Pediatrics
Centre for Molecular Medicine and
    Therapeutics
University of British Columbia
Vancouver, BC, Canada

Lionel Van Maldergem, MD, PhD
Professor
Centre for Human Genetics
University of Franche-Comté
Besançon, France

Adeline Vanderver, MD
Associate Professor
Division of Neurology
Program Director of the
    Leukodystrophy Center of Excellence
Jacob A. Kamens Endowed Chair in
    Neurological Disorders and
    Translational NeuroTherapeutics
Children's Hospital of Philadelphia
Philadelphia, PA, USA

Nicholas A. Vitanza, MD
Acting Assistant Professor of Pediatrics
University of Washington School of
    Medicine
Seattle Children's Hospital
Seattle, WA, USA

Michael von Rhein, MD
Head, Division of Developmental
    Pediatrics
Department of Pediatrics Kantonal
    Hospital Winterthur;
Child Development Center
University Childrens Hospital
Zurich, Switzerland

Emily von Scheven, MD, MAS
Professor of Clinical Pediatrics
Chief, Division of Pediatric
    Rheumatology
University of California, San Francisco
San Francisco, CA, USA

Ann Wagner, PhD
Chief, Neurobehavioral Mechanisms of
    Mental Disorders Branch
Division of Translational Research
National Institute of Mental Health
National Institutes of Health
Bethesda, MD, USA

Mark S. Wainwright, MD, PhD
Founders' Board Chair in Neurocritical
    Care;
Professor of Pediatrics and Neurology
Ann, Robert H Lurie Children's
    Hospital of Chicago
Northwestern University Feinberg
    School of Medicine
Chicago, IL, USA

Melissa A. Walker, MD, PhD
Assistant in Neurology
Massachusetts General Hospital
Boston, MA, USA

John T. Walkup, MD
Professor
Department of Psychiatry
Weill Cornell Medical College
New York-Presbyterian Hospital
New York, NY, USA

Laurence Walsh, MD
Associate Professor of Clinical
    Neurology, Genetics and Pediatrics
Departments of Neurology, Medical
    and Molecular Genetics and
    Pediatrics
Indiana University School of Medicine
Riley Hospital for Children at Indiana
    University Health
Indianapolis, IN, USA

Lauren C. Walters-Sen, MD
Geneticist
Center for Human Genetics, Inc.
Cambridge, MA, USA

Raymond Y. Wang, MD
Director, Multidisciplinary Lysosomal
    Disorder Program
Division of Metabolic Disorders
CHOC Children's Hospital;
Assistant Clinical Professor
Department of Pediatrics
University of California-Irvine
Orange, CA, USA

**Thomas T. Warner, BA, BM, BCh,
PhD, FRCP**
Professor and Director Reta Lila Weston
    Institute of Neurological Studies
UCL Institute of Neurology
National Hospital for Neurology and
    Neurosurgery
London, UK

Harry T. Whelan, MD
Bleser Professor, Neurology, Pediatrics
    and Hyperbaric Medicine;
Director of Hyperbaric Medicine
Medical College of Wisconsin
Milwaukee, WI, USA

Geoffrey A. Weinberg, MD
Professor of Pediatrics
Director, Pediatric HIV Program
Division of Pediatric Infectious Diseases
Department of Pediatrics
University of Rochester School of
    Medicine, Dentistry
Rochester, NY, USA

Elizabeth M. Wells, MD
Assistant Professor
George Washington University;
Medical Director
Inpatient Neurology
Center for Neuroscience and the Brain
    Tumor Institute
Children's National Health System
Washington, DC, USA

James W. Wheless, MD, FAAP, FAAN
Professor and Chief of Pediatric
    Neurology;
Le Bonheur Chair in Pediatric
    Neurology
University of Tennessee Health Science
    Center;
Director, Le Bonheur Comprehensive
    Epilepsy Program, Neuroscience
    Institute
Le Bonheur Children's Hospital
Memphis, TN, USA

Elaine C. Wirrell, MD
Professor and Director of Pediatric
    Epilepsy
Department of Neurology
Mayo Clinic
Rochester, MN, USA

Jeffrey H. Wisoff, MD
Professor of Neurosurgery and
    Pediatrics
Director, Division of Pediatric
    Neurosurgery
Department of Neurosurgery
NYU Langone Medical Center
New York, NY, USA

Nicole I. Wolf, MD, PhD
Assistant Professor
Child Neurology
VU University Medical Center
Amsterdam, The Netherlands

Gil I. Wolfe, MD
Irvin and Rosemary Smith Professor
    and Chairman
Department of Neurology
University at Buffalo, State University of
    New York
Jacobs School of Medicine and
    Biomedical Sciences
Buffalo, NY, USA

F. Virginia Wright, PT, PhD
Senior Scientist
Bloorview Research Institute Holland
    Bloorview Kids Rehabilitation
    Hospital Bloorview Children's
    Hospital Foundation Chair in
    Pediatric Rehabilitation.
Toronto, ON, Canada

Nathaniel D. Wycliffe, MD
Associate Professor of Radiology
Loma Linda University School of
    Medicine
Loma Linda, CA, USA

Michele L. Yang, MD
Assistant Professor
Department of Pediatrics; Section of
    Child Neurology
Children's Hospital Colorado
Aurora, CO, USA

Christopher J. Yuskaitis, MD, PhD
Department of Neurology, Boston
    Children's Hospital
Instructor in Neurology
Harvard Medical School
Boston, MA, USA

Huda Y. Zoghbi, MD
Ralph D. Feigin Professor;
Director, Jan and Dan Duncan
    Neurological Research Institute at
    Texas Children's Hospital;
Investigator, Howard Hughes Medical
    Institute
Pediatrics and Molecular and Human
    Genetics
Baylor College of Medicine
Houston, TX, USA

Mary L. Zupanc, MD
Professor and Division Chief
Department of Pediatrics and
    Neurology
Children's Hospital of Orange County
University of California–Irvine
Orange, CA, USA

1 General Aspects of the Patient's Neurologic History

Kenneth F. Swaiman and John Phillips

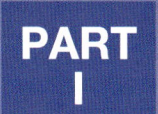 An expanded version of this chapter is available on www.expertconsult.com. See inside cover for registration details.

When presented with a challenging patient in 1885, with students Josef Babinski, Sigmund Freud, and others looking on, Dr. Charcot used the most important tools he had at his disposal: a careful history and a detailed examination. If he were alive today, Dr. Charcot would use those same tools.

There is no substitute for an accurate and thorough history. The patient or parent begins with an explanation of his or her concern. In most medical settings this opening statement lasts less than 60 seconds if not interrupted, as it unfortunately generally is, by the physician (Beckman and Frankel, 1984). More focused questions follow as a differential diagnosis is developed. In some cases language can be a barrier, particularly with the growing multiculturalism in the United States and other countries, and it is important that the interview be conducted in the native language of the patient. This may require the use of interpreters. Using a nonprofessional or poorly trained medical interpreter should be avoided because this has a much higher risk of causing clinically significant errors than using an experienced professional interpreter (Flores et al., 2012). In addition, an effective medical interview requires eye contact to help establish patient rapport (Cole and Bird, 2014), and the near-ubiquitous presence of computers in examination rooms, with an electronic medical record at the physician's fingertips, can be a problem. Compared with using paper medical records, there is now significantly more time spent looking at the medical record (now on a computer screen) and less time looking at the patient (Asan et al., 2014). However, although there is no turning back on the electronic medical record, and the pressure to see more patients may be increasing, the balance of new technology is certainly favorable. Once adopted, the electronic medical record improves physician's productivity and portable telemedicine equipment allows access to virtually any language needed in a medical setting (Cheriff et al., 2010).

Arriving at an appropriate differential diagnosis is an active process. As information is obtained suggesting specific disease categories, further questioning helps narrow the possible diagnostic possibilities. This process is assisted by considering general groups of neurologic diseases. Memory aides are often used to recall differential diagnostic categories—VINDICATE and VITAMIN C are two common examples (Table 1-1). Overlap exists between categories, and within each disease category are multiple subcategories and then specific diseases that become more or less likely as the patient interview proceeds. For example, recurrent strokes from MELAS (a disorder of energy metabolism) could be considered both a vascular and a metabolic process. The important issue is that, if focal weakness is the presenting concern, then the patient interview continues in an effort to discern whether the weakness is recurrent or triggered by fever or dehydration (which might make a metabolic disorder more likely). Further questioning may disclose a history of lactic acidosis that narrows the differential diagnosis further to a possible mitochondrial disorder such as MELAS, which can then be confirmed with genetic testing. The point is to begin broadly. Cast a wide net. Consider all disease categories until a more focused differential diagnosis is possible based on the detailed history.

Part of clarifying the history of the current illness is to answer four basic questions:

1. Is the process acute or insidious?
2. Is it focal or generalized?
3. Is it progressive or static?
4. At what age did the problem begin?

The order in which disease findings develop and the precise **age of onset** of symptoms and signs may be critical factors in the process of accurate diagnosis. Many degenerative disorders have specific ages of onset that can help narrow the differential diagnosis; cognitive regression in an 8-year-old may raise the question of adrenoleukodystrophy, whereas in a 2-year-old one might consider neuronal ceroid lipofuscinosis. The presence of repeated episodes or associated phenomena should also be determined. For example, although the clinical manifestations of cerebrovascular events such as an acute stroke normally develop over minutes to hours, the underlying process may be long-standing; therefore, acute onset of vascular symptoms may be the result of a subacute or chronic process. On the other hand, infections, electrolyte imbalances, and toxic processes (such as exposure to over-the-counter drugs, prescription medications, insecticides, and other toxins found around the home) usually progress over a day to several days before maximum symptoms occur. More chronic are degenerative diseases, inborn metabolic disorders, and neoplastic conditions that usually progress insidiously over weeks to months.

Evaluation of whether a condition is **focal or generalized** is central to the diagnostic process. A focal neurologic lesion is not necessarily one that causes focal manifestations but is one that can be related to dysfunction in a circumscribed neuroanatomic location. For example, a focal lesion in the brainstem may cause ipsilateral cranial nerve and contralateral corticospinal tract involvement. If the problem is not focal, it usually results from a generalized process or from several lesions (i.e., multifocal). Neoplastic and vascular diseases frequently result in focal processes; occasionally, trauma results in such abnormalities. Generalized or multifocal conditions are usually associated with degenerative, congenital, metabolic, or toxic abnormalities.

In child neurology, it is particularly important that the clinician always attempt to determine whether the condition

TABLE 1-1 Disease Category Acronyms

Vindicate	
V	Vascular
I	Inflammatory
N	Neoplastic
D	Degenerative
I	Infectious
C	Congenital
A	Allergy or autoimmune
T	Trauma or toxin
E	Endocrine
Vitamin C	
V	Vascular
I	Infectious
T	Trauma
A	Autoimmune
M	Metabolic
I	Idiopathic
N	Neoplastic
C	Congenital

is **progressive or static**. This is best accomplished by taking a detailed developmental history. Documenting the age of acquisition of major motor, language, and social milestones allows characterization of a child's developmental progress compared with age-based norms. To address the critical issue of developmental regression, questions are posed that determine whether the child is no longer capable of motor or intellectual activities that were previously performed. This information is essential to the diagnosis of progressive disease, which is usually preceded by a period of normal development. Occasionally, prior formal neurologic and psychometric evaluations may be available that help enormously in providing objective documentation of prior developmental status. Reviewing family photographs, videos, baby books, or old Facebook postings can be helpful. In progressive conditions, such as those caused by metabolic or neoplastic disorders, documentation of increasing loss of normal function or an increase in any symptoms is essential. Static conditions can be the result of traumatic or anoxic injury, a congenital abnormality, or perhaps a resolving acute toxic ingestion.

Reviewing the **medical history** is an essential part of any interview and often provides information that is critical in arriving at an appropriate diagnosis, extending information gleaned from the history of current illness. In child neurology, medical history begins with the moment of conception. Was conception achieved with reproductive technology, the long-term consequences of which are not clear? Was the mother older than 35 years at the time of conception, a possible risk factor for adverse outcome? During gestation, were there exposures to toxins such as alcohol, nicotine, or prescription or illicit drugs? Was the pregnancy planned and was the mother healthy throughout gestation? At what point was fetal movement first noted (i.e., quickening), which should be at approximately 4 to 5 months' gestation, and did it continue throughout the entire pregnancy? Were there problems with poverty, nutrition, or exposure to violence and stress? Obtaining some of this important information could be difficult because of privacy concerns, and may require a confidential interview with mother.

Details of the delivery are critical and may not be entirely recalled by parents; therefore, reviewing birth records if available is important. Information such as duration of labor, medications or assistive devices (forceps and vacuum extraction) used, presence of meconium at delivery, and gestational age may have direct relevance to later brain development. The general status of the newborn immediately after delivery should also be understood. Objective information is important such as birth weight, Apgar scores, head circumference, and any neonatal complications encountered. Obtaining accurate information may require interviewing all caregivers, particularly with children whose mothers had pregnancy-related health problems and may have been sick. An enormously important piece of information that needs to be confirmed and not just assumed is the status of neonatal screening. Depending on the state or country of birth, most children are screened as a public health measure for certain treatable metabolic conditions. In the United States (http://www.babysfirsttest.org/newborn-screening/states) and Canada (http://raredisorders.ca/documents/CanadaNBSstatus updatedNov.112010.pdf), it varies by state and province, but all screen for at least some disorders of amino acid metabolism, fatty acid oxidation diseases, organic acid conditions, and hemoglobin and endocrine disorders.

Family history is particularly important as many disorders encountered by the clinician may have a genetic basis. Begin by asking if any family members suffer from the same problems that affect the patient. Autosomal-dominant traits may be present in successive generations, although the degree of expressivity may vary. Autosomal-recessive traits often do not manifest in successive generations but may be present in siblings. Consanguinity must be considered when autosomal-recessive disease is part of the differential diagnosis, even if it is not forthcoming from interviewing parents (the incidence of false paternity has been reported to be from 1% to 30% depending on the population studied).

Cognitive and behavioral development is influenced by the child's home environment. A social history helps identify whether risk factors such as exposure to poverty, violence, parental depression, or bullying are present. Some clinics find the SEEK parent screening questionnaire helpful to identify potential challenges in the home environment (Fig. 1-2).

Caregivers should be questioned carefully about the nature and results of previously performed tests, including electrodiagnostic tests, brain-imaging studies, biochemical studies (e.g., quantitative assays of amino acids, organic acids, lactic acid, and lysosomal enzymes), biopsies, and chromosomal or gene studies. It is particularly important to review the full report of prior comprehensive genetic tests such as microarray analysis, exome sequencing, or genome-wide association studies (GWAS). Even when these tests fail to establish a clear diagnosis, they usually identify abnormalities of unknown clinical significance, and what was once unclear may have over time been found to have clear clinical implications. Therefore it may be helpful to perform an updated review of abnormalities identified on prior genetic testing. Use of prior medication should also be documented, including those medications that may have been prescribed but not taken, with note made of results of such therapies. If prior imaging has been performed, reviewing the study and not simply relying on the report is helpful to confirm findings (this is particularly important if the radiology interpretation is by someone without pediatric experience, or whose experience is not known as may occur with an on-call teleradiology service).

Thus, history taking is an active process. Beginning with a presenting complaint, the clinician broadly considers multiple diagnostic categories, which are narrowed as open-ended questions and followed by more specific queries. An exhaustive, all-encompassing neurologic history is impossible to obtain, particularly under the time constraints most clinicians face in today's environment. Therefore a skilled clinician is able to focus the interview on relevant information, often following up details that are more important than the patient or caregiver is aware of, and likewise, gently steering the conversation

SEEK Parent Questionnaire   No. ____
A Safe Environment for Every Kid

Dear Parent or Caregiver: **Being a parent is not easy.** *We want to help families have a safe environment for kids. We are asking everyone these questions. Please answer the questions about your* **child being seen today** *for a check-up. They are about issues that affect many families. If there's a problem, we'll try to help.*

Today's Date: ____/____/200_
Child's Date of Birth: ____/____/____
Sex of Child: ☐ Male   ☐ Female

PLEASE CHECK

☐ Yes	☐ No	Do you need the telephone number for **Poison Control**?
☐ Yes	☐ No	Do you need a **smoke alarm** for your home?
☐ Yes	☐ No	Does **anyone** smoke **tobacco** at home?
☐ Yes	☐ No	Is there a **gun** in your home?
☐ Yes	☐ No	In the last year, did **you** worry that your food would **run out** before you got money, or food stamps to buy more?
☐ Yes	☐ No	Do you worry that your **child** may have been **physically** abused?
☐ Yes	☐ No	Do you worry that your **child** may have been **sexually** abused?
☐ Yes	☐ No	Lately, do **you** often feel **down, depressed,** or **hopeless**?
☐ Yes	☐ No	Do **you** often feel **lonely**?
☐ Yes	☐ No	During the past month, have **you** felt **little interest** or **pleasure** in the things you used to enjoy?
☐ Yes	☐ No	Do you often feel your **child** is **difficult** to take care of?
☐ Yes	☐ No	Do you wish you had more **help** with your **child**?
☐ Yes	☐ No	Do **you** feel so **stressed** you can't take another day?
☐ Yes	☐ No	Do **you** sometimes find you need to **hit/spank** your child?
☐ Yes	☐ No	In the past year, have **you** or **your partner** had a problem with **drugs** or **alcohol?**
☐ Yes	☐ No	In the past year, have **you** or **your partner** felt the need to cut back on **drinking** or **drug use**?
☐ Yes	☐ No	Have **you ever** been in a relationship in which you were physically **hurt** or **threatened** by a partner?
☐ Yes	☐ No	In the past year, have **you** been **afraid** of a partner?
☐ Yes	☐ No	In the past year have **you** thought of getting a **court order** for protection?
☐ Yes	☐ No	**Are there any problems you'd like help with today?**

Please give this form to the doctor or nurse you're seeing today. Thank you

_____ _____
Provider's name, PRINTED   Provider's Signature   Date

Figure 1-2. SEEK questionnaire. *[With permission from Dubowitz et al. (2007).]*

away from trivial discussion. Carefully listening to what is stated and how it is stated is important. Directly questioning the child when possible provides unique information, particularly if done at the onset of the interview before the adults start talking. Documenting exact quotes, using the vocabulary of the child or caregiver, improves accuracy of the medical record and avoids relying on an observer's interpretation of events when first-hand information is available. Bringing this information together is then the job of the clinician, who assembles all relevant facts into a cogent story that characterizes the neurologic process.

A child's developmental status is critically important in any neurologic assessment, and using a valid developmental screening test is helpful. Several assessment tools are available. These can be divided into provider-administered tools, such as the **Denver developmental screening test-II** (DDST-II) (see Fig. A-1ab in Appendix A), and parent questionnaires (Tervo, 2005), such as the **ages and stages questionnaire** and the **parents' evaluation of developmental status**.

Using the DDST-II, development is plotted over four broad domains of gross motor, fine motor, personal-social, and language skills from birth through 6 years of age. The age distribution for passing at the 25th, 50th, and 90th percentile is noted for each of 125 items. The DDST-II can be performed in a busy office setting; however, it is only a screening test, and any concerns should be followed up with more extensive developmental assessments. Also, adaptations must be made based on the cultural context. For example, the DDST-II items "using a spoon and fork" and "playing board games" are not relevant in cultures in which no one does these activities, and may need to be substituted by more appropriate developmental items. Concerns have been raised about the lack of validity of the DDST-II, and in the United States some states do not recommend using the DDST-II as a result of poor sensitivity and specificity (Minnesota Department of Health, http://www.health.state.mn.us/divs/fh/mch/devscrn/).

The **ages and stages questionnaire** is a preferred screening tool of many pediatric clinics and public health departments for children from 4 months to 5 years old, utilizing the insight that parents and caregivers offer regarding their child's development (Thompson et al., 2010). It requires responses from parents and caregivers to answer questions regarding whether specific developmental skills are demonstrated (yes, sometimes, and not yet). Five broad developmental domains are covered: communication, gross motor, fine motor, problem solving, and personal-social. Similarly, the **parents' evaluation of developmental status** is used for children from birth to 8 years old and relies on parent report through a 10-item standardized questionnaire covering expressive and receptive language, fine motor, gross motor, behavior, socialization, self-care, and learning, which identifies risk based on parental assessment. Both the ages and stages questionnaire and the parents' evaluation of developmental status are appropriate screening tools for child development and can be completed in a busy office setting.

Often it is not development but behavior that is of concern to parents. Clarifying as much as possible the nature of the behavioral concern helps. More helpful than hearing "He's acting out" is knowing if there is a problem with attention, impulsivity, aggression, or mood swings. Is there social withdrawal? Are there compulsions? Is the maladaptive behavior triggered by something or does it occur without warning?

Assessment tools are available that can help clarify problem behavior. For young children, one of the few available standardized measures is the **infant toddler social emotional assessment** or its abbreviated version, the **brief infant toddler social emotional assessment**, both of which are designed for children from 1 to 3 years old. The Brief Infant Toddler Social Emotional Assessment includes separate forms for parents and

for childcare providers, each of which can be completed in less than 10 minutes. Two general types of behavior are assessed: 1) social emotional problems, including aggression, anxiety, dysregulation, and atypical behavior, and 2) social emotional competence such as attention, motivation, empathy, and positive peer relationships. For older children, the **child symptom inventory** provides parent and teacher checklists to help screen for a broad number of behavioral concerns in children from 5 to 18 years of age such as anxiety, attention deficit hyperactivity disorder, depression, oppositional defiant disorder, and conduct disorder. Likewise, the **Swanson, Nolan and Pelham qestionnaire** (SNAP) for children from 6 to 18 years old has forms available for teachers or parents that help distinguish between attention deficit hyperactivity disorder and other childhood behavioral disorders. Other general behavior assessment tools commonly used are the **Achenbach system of empirically based assessment** for children from 6 to 18 years old (this includes the **child behavior checklist**, which is a parent-report questionnaire, and the **youth self-report** to be completed by the child), and the **behavioral assessment system for children, second edition**, for age 2 to 25 years (this also includes questionnaires for parents and teachers, as well as a self-report questionnaire). In all instances in which behavior is a concern, it is helpful to use assessment tools that characterize behavior across environments (i.e., home, school, and daycare).

A common behavioral question is whether there is attention deficit hyperactivity disorder, in which case the **revised Conners parent rating scale** (age 3 to 17 years) or the **Vanderbilt** (age 6 to 12 years) is commonly used. Another common question that arises is whether a child has autistic spectrum disorder, which can be screened for using the **modified checklist for autism in toddlers** (Fig. 1-5) completed by a caregiver or via physician interview. Screening all children for autism is now recommended by the American Academy of Pediatrics at age 18 and 24 months.

Developmental screening is an enormously important part of the neurologic evaluation, but it must be interpreted carefully. For example, language delay may be caused by a congenital brain malformation or could be entirely the result of an impoverished environment (Fernald et al., 2013). Also, a single developmental screening is not as accurate as repeated assessments over time, and any abnormal screening results should prompt an immediate referral for more complete developmental testing by an appropriate professional.

Thus, a careful and informed history is at the core of the neurologic assessment of a child. The presenting complaint is explored in detail, followed by relevant aspects of the medical history, family history, and review of prior investigations or treatments. Assessment of the developmental status of the child is an essential component of this process, which eventually guides the examination to follow.

Child neurology is a unique and inherently complex endeavor, and at times the initial history uncovers information requiring clarification through a follow-up literature search. Commonly used general medical search engines include PubMed (http://www.ncbi.nlm.nih.gov/pubmed) or Google Scholar (http://scholar.google.com/). Specific websites might be considered such as Treatable Intellectual Disorder (http://www.treatable-id.org/) for metabolic conditions, or the Online Mendelian Inheritance in Man (http://www.omim.org/) for genetic disorders. As always, a tincture of humility is helpful for even the experienced clinician, knowing that a diagnosis can be frustratingly elusive at first. But what is initially confusing may be clarified as a child is followed over time and new information obtained, and through a partnership with the family and careful attention to neurologic detail, the correct diagnosis can be identified.

M-CHAT

Please fill out the following about how your child usually is. Please try to answer every question. If the behavior is rare (e.g., you've seen it once or twice), please answer as if the child does not do it.

1.	Does your child enjoy being swung, bounced on your knee, etc.?	Yes No
2.	Does your child take an interest in other children?	Yes No
3.	Does your child like climbing on things, such as up stairs?	Yes No
4.	Does your child enjoy playing peek-a-boo/hide-and-seek?	Yes No
5.	Does your child ever pretend, for example, to talk on the phone or take care of a doll or pretend other things?	Yes No
6.	Does your child ever use his/her index finger to point, to ask for something?	Yes No
7.	Does your child ever use his/her index finger to point, to indicate interest in something?	Yes No
8.	Can your child play properly with small toys (e.g. cars or blocks) without just mouthing, fiddling, or dropping them?	Yes No
9.	Does your child ever bring objects over to you (parent) to show you something?	Yes No
10.	Does your child look you in the eye for more than a second or two?	Yes No
11.	Does your child ever seem oversensitive to noise? (e.g., plugging ears)	Yes No
12.	Does your child smile in response to your face or your smile?	Yes No
13.	Does your child imitate you? (e.g., you make a face-will your child imitate it?)	Yes No
14.	Does your child respond to his/her name when you call?	Yes No
15.	If you point at a toy across the room, does your child look at it?	Yes No
16.	Does your child walk?	Yes No
17.	Does your child look at things you are looking at?	Yes No
18.	Does your child make unusual finger movements near his/her face?	Yes No
19.	Does your child try to attract your attention to his/her own activity?	Yes No
20.	Have you ever wondered if your child is deaf?	Yes No
21.	Does your child understand what people say?	Yes No
22.	Does your child sometimes stare at nothing or wander with no purpose?	Yes No
23.	Does your child look at your face to check your reaction when faced with something unfamiliar?	Yes No

© 1999 Diana Robins, Deborah Fein, & Marianne Barton

Figure 1-5. Modified checklist for autism in toddlers. *[With permission from Robins et al. (1999).]*

REFERENCES

The complete list of references for this chapter is available in the e-book at www.expertconsult.com.
  See inside cover for registration details.

SELECTED REFERENCES

Asan, O., Smith, P., Montague, E., 2014. More screen time, less face time—implications for EHR design. J. Eval. Clin. Pract. 20, 896–901.

Beckman, H.B., Frankel, R.M., 1984. The effect of physician behavior on the collection of data. Ann. Intern. Med. 101, 692–696.

Cheriff, A.D., Kapur, A.G., Qui, M., et al., 2010. Physician productivity and the ambulatory EHR in a large academic multi-specialty physician group. Int. J. Med. Inform. 79, 492–500.

Cole, S.A., Bird, J., 2014. The Medical Interview, third ed. Saunders, Philadelphia.

Dubowitz, H., Felgelman, S., Lane, W., et al., 2007. Screening for depression in an urban pediatric primary care clinic. Pediatrics 119, 435–443.

Fernald, A., Marchman, V.A., Weisleder, A., 2013. SES differences in language processing skill and vocabulary are evident at 18 months. Dev. Sci. 16, 234–248.

Flores, G., Abreu, M., Barone, C.P., et al., 2012. Errors of medical interpretation and their potential clinical consequences: a comparison of professional versus ad hoc versus no interpreters. Ann. Intern. Med. 60, 545–553.

Robins, D.L., Fein, D., Barton, M.L., 1999. Modified checklist for autism in toddlers (M-CHAT) follow-up interview. Self-published. Available at <http://www.mchatscreen.com/Official_M-CHAT_Website.html>.

Tervo, R.C., 2005. Parent's reports predict their child's developmental problems. Clin. Pediatr. 44, 601–611.

Thompson, L.A., Tuli, S.Y., Saliba, H., et al., 2010. Improving developmental screening in pediatric resident education. Clin. Pediatr. 49, 737–742.

E-BOOK FIGURES AND TABLES

2 Neurologic Examination of the Older Child

Kenneth F. Swaiman and John Phillips

An expanded version of this chapter is available on www.expertconsult.com. See inside cover for registration details.

The neurologic examination provides critical and unique information that cannot be acquired otherwise (Campbell, 2013). Regardless of patient age, the essence of this information is the same: mental status, cranial nerves, motor, reflexes, sensory, and coordination/cerebellar testing. *How* this information is obtained is very age-dependent, however (Egan, 1990).

OBSERVATION/MENTAL STATUS

Observation during history-taking is helpful, even when a child isn't being directly questioned (Menkes et al., 2005). Abnormal movements might suggest epilepsy, motor tic disorder, or a behavioral diagnosis such as attention deficit hyperactivity disorder (Pina-Garza, 2013). Caregiver–child interactions during the interview may offer clues into what the home environment is like. During this period the examiner surreptitiously assesses mental status, making note of language, attention, affect, and general developmental status (see Table 2-1).

SCREENING GROSS MOTOR FUNCTION

Consider beginning with a rapid screening examination in case the child later becomes uncooperative. Start with the child standing. Ask the child to hop in place on each foot, tandem-walk forward and backward, toe-walk, and heel-walk. Then, checking for Gowers' maneuver, the child is asked to rise quickly from a squatting position, followed by asking the child to stand with the feet close together, eyes closed, and arms and hands outstretched. This maneuver allows simultaneous assessment of Romberg's sign and adventitious movements. Finally, finger-nose-finger movements help assess cerebellar function.

PHYSICAL EXAMINATION
Cranial Nerve Examination

Examination of the cranial nerves in infants and younger children usually requires some modification of the sequence and may need some ingenious improvisation of the procedure, according to the degree of cooperation of the child (Volpe, 2008). As is the case with all examinations of infants and young children, the less threatening portions of the examination should be performed first.

Olfactory Nerve: Cranial Nerve I

Cranial nerve I can be evaluated by having the child smell pleasant aromas (e.g., chocolate, vanilla, peppermint) through each nostril while the other is manually occluded. Anosmia may occur after head trauma, with a severe upper respiratory tract infection, or in the rare instance of a frontal lobe mass involving the cribriform plate region.

Optic Nerve: Cranial Nerve II

Begin with formal visual acuity testing using a Snellen chart or a "near card" in older children. Younger children are more difficult and many times only gross vision can be evaluated. Beyond 4 years of age, the E test is useful. The child is taught to recognize the E, and to discern the direction in which the three "arms" are pointing and point a finger accordingly.

Peripheral visual field testing is accomplished using a small (3-mm) white or red test object, a toy, or in a pinch, the examiner's fingers can be used. The test object is moved from the temporal to the nasal fields and then from the superior and inferior portions of the temporal and nasal fields while the child looks directly at the examiner's nose. Finger counting can be used if acuity is grossly distorted. In cases of extreme impairment, perception of a rapidly moving finger can be used.

The optic disc (i.e., optic nerve head) of the older child is sharply defined and often salmon-colored, which differs from the pale gray color of the disc in an infant. In the presence of a deep cup in the optic disc, the color may appear pale, but the pallor is localized to the center of the disc. The pallor of optic atrophy occurs centrally and peripherally, and is accompanied by a decreased number of arterioles in the disc margins. Most commonly, papilledema is associated with elevation of the optic disc, distended veins, and lack of venous pulsations. Hemorrhages may surround the disc. Before papilledema is obvious, there may be blurring of the nasal disc margins and hyperemia of the nerve head.

The presence or absence of the pupillary light reflex differentiates between peripheral and cortical blindness. Lesions of the anterior visual pathway (i.e., retina to lateral geniculate body) result in the interruption of the afferent limb of the pupillary light reflex, producing an absent or decreased reflex. Anterior visual pathway interruption can cause amblyopia in one eye. In this situation, the pupil fails to constrict when stimulated with direct light; however, the consensual pupillary response (i.e., response when the other eye is illuminated) is intact. The deficient pupillary reflex is revealed by alternately aiming a light source toward one eye and then the other. In the eye with decreased vision, consensual pupillary constriction is greater than the response to direct light stimulation (Marcus Gunn pupil); the pupil of the affected eye may dilate slightly during direct stimulation (Haymaker, 1969).

Oculomotor, Trochlear, and Abducens Nerves: Cranial Nerves III, IV, and VI

The oculomotor, trochlear, and abducens cranial nerves control extraocular motor movements; these nerves must operate synchronously or diplopia ensues. Cranial nerve III innervates the superior, inferior, and medial recti; the inferior oblique; and the eyelid elevator (levator palpebrae superioris). Cranial nerves IV and VI innervate the superior oblique muscle and the lateral rectus muscle, respectively. Unfortunately for

TABLE 2-1 Emerging Patterns of Behavior from 1 to 5 Years of Age

15 Months

Motor:	Walks alone; crawls up stairs
Adaptive:	Makes tower of two cubes; makes line with crayon; inserts pellet into bottle
Language:	Jargon; follows simple commands; may name familiar object (ball)
Social:	Indicates some desires or needs by pointing; hugs parents

18 Months

Motor:	Runs stiffly; sits on small chair; walks up stairs with one hand held; explores drawers and waste baskets
Adaptive:	Piles three cubes; initiates scribbling; imitates vertical stroke; dumps pellet from bottle
Language:	Ten words (average); names pictures; identifies one or more parts of body
Social:	Feeds self; seeks help when in trouble; may complain when wet or soiled; kisses parents with pucker

24 Months

Motor:	Runs well; walks up and down stairs one step at a time; opens doors; climbs on furniture
Adaptive:	Makes tower of six cubes; circular scribbling; imitates horizontal strokes; folds paper once imitatively
Language:	Puts three words together (subject, verb, object)
Social:	Handles spoon well; tells immediate experiences; helps to undress; listens to stories with pictures

30 Months

Motor:	Jumps
Adaptive:	Makes tower of eight cubes; makes vertical and horizontal strokes but generally will not join them to make a cross; imitates circular stroke, forming closed figure
Language:	Refers to self by pronoun "I"; knows full name
Social:	Helps put things away; pretends in play

36 Months

Motor:	Goes up stairs alternating feet; rides tricycle; stands momentarily on one foot
Adaptive:	Makes tower of nine cubes; imitates construction of "bridge" of three cubes; copies circle; imitates cross
Language:	Knows age and gender; counts three objects correctly; repeats three numbers or sentence of six syllables
Social:	Plays simple games (in "parallel" with other children); helps in dressing (unbuttons clothing and puts on shoes); washes hands

48 Months

Motor:	Hops on one foot; throws ball overhand; uses scissors to cut out pictures; climbs well
Adaptive:	Copies bridge from model; imitates construction of "gate" of five cubes; copies cross and square; draws man with 2–4 parts besides head; names longer of two lines
Language:	Counts four pennies accurately; tells a story
Social:	Plays with several children with beginning of social interaction and role playing; goes to toilet alone

60 Months

Motor:	Skips
Adaptive:	Draws triangle from copy; names heavier of two weights
Language:	Names four colors; repeats sentences of ten syllables; counts ten pennies correctly
Social:	Dresses and undresses; asks questions about meanings of words; domestic role playing

(Adapted with permission from Behrman RE, et al. Nelson Textbook of Pediatrics, 14th edn. Philadelphia: WB Saunders, 1992.)

purposes of understanding, the function of extraocular muscles depends somewhat on the direction of gaze. The lateral and medial recti are abductors and adductors of the globe, respectively. The superior rectus and inferior oblique are elevators, and the inferior rectus and superior oblique are depressors. The oblique muscles act in the vertical plane while an eye is adducted. The recti muscles serve this function when an eye is abducted (Figure 2-2). When directed forward (i.e., primary position), the oblique muscles effect torsion around the anteroposterior axis (rotation) of the globes.

In heterophorias, also called phorias, both globes are directed normally on near or far objects during fixation; however, one or both deviate when one eye is occluded while the other eye fixes. Forcing fixation of the uncovered eye by alternately covering each eye confirms the diagnosis of heterophorias. Exophoria is a predisposition to divergence, whereas esophoria is a predisposition to convergence.

Eye deviations detectable during binocular vision are heterotropias, also called tropias. Adduction tropias are esotropias; abduction tropias are exotropias. Tropias are most often caused by compromised extraocular muscle innervation. Extraocular palsies can frequently be detected by observation of eye movements. A red glass is placed in front of an eye, and a focused, relatively intense white light is aimed at the eyes from various visual fields while the child fixes on the light. A merged, solitary, red–white image is perceived when extraocular movements are normal; however, when muscle paresis is present, the child reports a separation of the red and white images when looking in the direction of action of the affected

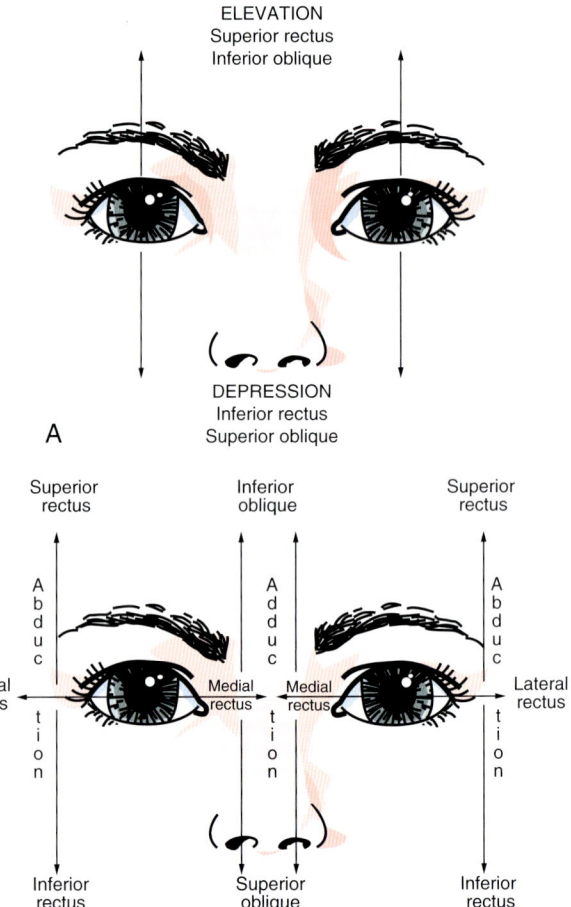

Figure 2-2. Extraocular muscle movement. A, In primary position. **B,** In abduction and adduction. *(Courtesy of the Division of Pediatric Neurology, University of Minnesota Medical School.)*

muscle. The farthest peripheral image is the one perceived by the abnormal eye; this eye can be identified by the color of the image. Volitional turning of the head accompanies paresis of the lateral rectus muscle to forestall diplopia; the head is deviated toward the paretic muscle, and the eyes are directed ahead. In superior oblique or superior rectus muscle palsies, tilting of the head toward the shoulder opposite the side of the paretic eye muscle occurs.

Extraocular muscle dysfunction is associated with many conditions that affect the brainstem, cranial nerves, neuromuscular junction, or muscles. Cranial nerve VI function may be impaired by increased intracranial pressure, irrespective of cause. Squint, usually esotropia, often accompanies decreased visual acuity in infants and young children.

Ptosis and extraocular muscle paralysis accompany dysfunction of cranial nerve III. Ptosis resulting from oculomotor nerve compromise is usually more pronounced than is the malposition of the lid associated with Horner syndrome. Complete oculomotor nerve paralysis, although uncommon, causes the eye to position downward and outward. Poor adduction and elevation are also evident.

Eye deviation is often the harbinger of a serious neurologic problem. Destructive lesions of the brainstem nuclei cause conjugate eye deviation toward the opposite side. Destructive cerebral hemispheral lesions cause eye deviation toward the side of the lesion; conversely, an irritative cerebral hemispheral lesion (such as a seizure focus) causes the eyes to turn away from the side of the lesion. Hence for a cortical lesion, "the patient looks at their stroke but away from their seizure." Vertical gaze paresis results from dysfunction of the tectal area of the midbrain. Patients with a pineal tumor or hydrocephalus may be unable to elevate the eyes for upward gaze.

Brainstem lesions, especially those in the midbrain or pons, may disrupt the medial longitudinal fasciculus. The resultant impairment of conjugate eye movement is referred to as an internuclear ophthalmoplegia. There is weakness of medial rectus muscle contraction of the adducting eye, which is accompanied by a monocular nystagmus in the abducting eye. Occasionally, paresis of lateral rectus muscle movement in the abducting eye may occur. Medial longitudinal fasciculus involvement may be unilateral or bilateral.

Internal ophthalmoplegia consists of a fully dilated pupil that is unreactive to light or accommodation. Extraocular muscle function is normal when each muscle is tested separately. The oculomotor nerve, nucleus, or the parasympathetic ciliary ganglion may be a site of involvement.

External ophthalmoplegia results in ptosis and paralysis of all extraocular muscles. Pupillary reactivity is normal.

Opticokinetic nystagmus is a useful test in evaluating the eye movements of children. A drum or tape with stripes or figures is slowly rotated or drawn before the child's eyes in horizontal and vertical directions. With fixation, the child should visually track the object in the direction the tape is being drawn, with a rapid, rhythmic movement (refixation) of the eyes in the reverse direction to enable fixation on the next figure or stripe. Absence of such a response may result from failure of fixation, amaurosis, or disturbed saccadic eye movements.

The child who appears clinically blind because of a conversion reaction usually exhibits a normal opticokinetic nystagmus response. Children who manifest congenital nystagmus and have an opticokinetic nystagmus response in the vertical plane likely have adequate functional sight.

Spontaneous nystagmus (i.e., involuntary oscillatory movements of the eye) may be horizontal, vertical, or rotary; a patient can exhibit all three types. The movements may consist of a slow and a fast phase, giving rise to the term jerk nystag- mus. However, the phases may be of equal duration and amplitude, appearing pendular. In general, vertical nystagmus is associated with either medication or brainstem dysfunction. While a few beats of horizontal nystagmus with extreme lateral gaze are normal, persistent horizontal nystagmus indicates dysfunction of the cerebellum or brainstem vestibular system components; the nystagmus is coarser (i.e., the amplitude of movements are greater) when the direction of gaze is toward the side of the lesion. Seesaw nystagmus is characterized by disconjugate (alternating) movement of the eyes, which move upward and downward in a seesaw motion. This type of nystagmus may accompany lesions in the region of the optic chiasm (see Chapter 6).

Trigeminal Nerve: Cranial Nerve V

Cranial nerve V, the trigeminal nerve, has motor and sensory functions. The motor division of the trigeminal nerve innervates the masticatory muscles: masseter, pterygoid, and temporalis. Temporalis muscle atrophy manifests as scalloping of the temporal fossa. The masseter muscle bulk may be assessed by palpation while the patient firmly closes the jaw. Pterygoid muscle strength is evaluated by having the patient open the mouth and "slide" the jaw from one side to the other while the examiner resists movements with the hand to assess muscle strength. The jaw reflex is elicited when the examiner places a finger on the patient's chin while the mouth is slightly open and taps the finger to stretch the masticatory muscles. A rapid muscle contraction with closure of the mouth is the reflex response. This stretch reflex receives its afferent and efferent nerve control from cranial nerve V; the segmental level is located in the midpons. The expected reflex reaction is absent with motor nucleus and peripheral trigeminal nerve compromise. Conversely, this reflex is overactive in the presence of supranuclear lesions; rarely, jaw clonus may be evident. Because of weakness of the ipsilateral pterygoid muscles, unilateral impairment of the trigeminal nerve causes deviation of the jaw toward the side of the lesion. Cranial nerve V is also responsible for sensation involving the face, including eye and the anterior half of the scalp.

Facial Nerve: Cranial Nerve VII

Taste sensation over the anterior two-thirds of the tongue, secretory fibers (parasympathetic) innervating the lacrimal and salivary glands, and innervation of all facial muscles are accomplished by cranial nerve VII. Complete motor dysfunction on one side of the face ensues when the cranial nerve VII pathway is disrupted in the nucleus, pons, or peripheral nerve. The patient is unable to move the forehead upward, close the eye forcefully, or elevate the corner of the mouth on the side of the affected nerve.

Central (supranuclear) facial nerve impairment produces only paresis of the muscles involving the lower face, with resultant drooping of the angle of the mouth, disappearance or diminution of the nasal labial fold, and widened palpebral fissure. The muscles of the forehead, which are innervated bilaterally, are unaffected.

Taste sensation in the anterior two-thirds of the tongue is in part provided by the chorda tympani nerve, which traverses the path of the facial nerve for a short distance. Testing of taste sensation is difficult. Evaluation of taste requires that the patient extend the tongue and that the examiner hold the tip of the tongue with a piece of gauze and place salty, sweet, acidic, and sour and bitter materials, usually represented by salt, sugar, vinegar, and quinine, on the anterior portion of the tongue. The patient's tongue must remain outside of the mouth until the test is completed. An older patient should be able to identify each substance.

Auditory Nerve: Cranial Nerve VIII

Function and evaluation of cranial nerve VIII are discussed in detail in Chapters 7 and 8. Although cranial nerve VIII is known as the auditory nerve, it has auditory and vestibular functions.

Patients who fail to develop speech or who have slow speech development, as well as those who have difficulty with fluency and articulation, may have hearing impairment. Older children can cooperate with formal audiometric testing. Such testing may not be possible in younger infants, but brainstem auditory-evoked potentials may provide the necessary information concerning hearing impairment and the level of dysfunction within the nervous system.

Clinical evaluation and caloric testing can be used for gross assessment of vestibular function. To perform caloric testing, the patient is in the supine position, with head flexed at 30 degrees. Ice water (10 mL) is injected over 30 seconds into one external auditory canal at a time. The conscious patient develops coarse nystagmus toward the ipsilateral ear; no eye deviation occurs. If the patient has some degree of obtundation, there is a modification of the response. The eyes become tonically deviated ipsilaterally, with accompanying nystagmus occurring contralaterally. If the patient is comatose, cold water stimulation usually causes tonic deviation ipsilaterally and no nystagmus; if the coma is profound or the patient is brain-dead, no eye changes occur.

Glossopharyngeal and Vagus Nerves: Cranial Nerves IX and X

Examination of the larynx, pharynx, and palate provides most of the desired information concerning the function of cranial nerves IX and X. Unilateral paresis of the soft palate causes an ipsilateral droop, even when the patient is expelling air through the open mouth or gagging in response to a tongue blade. Bilateral involvement causes a flaccid soft palate bilaterally.

The gag reflex is mediated through cranial nerve IX and is elicited by touching the posterior pharyngeal mucosa with a tongue blade. Normal individuals may have absence or a seemingly disproportionately violent response; assessing the importance of changes in the gag reflex is difficult in the absence of other findings. The integrity of cranial nerves IX and X is necessary for a gag response; sensation of the soft palate and uvula travels via cranial nerve IX, and motor function is carried by cranial nerve X. Thus unilateral weakness causes deviation of the uvula *away* from the weak side (unlike unilateral weakness of cranial nerve XII, discussed later, which causes deviation of the tongue *toward* the weak side).

Spinal Accessory Nerve: Cranial Nerve XI

Cranial nerve XI provides innervation for the trapezius and sternocleidomastoid muscles. Cranial nerve XI comprises some fibers from C1 and C2, and some from the motor nucleus in the brainstem, and is unique in combining brainstem and cervical cord origins. The trapezius muscles are assessed when the patient is asked to shrug the shoulders against resistance while the sternocleidomastoid muscle is tested by asking the child to rotate their head to one side against resistance. Weakness of the sternocleidomastoid muscle results in an inability to rotate the head to the contralateral side.

Hypoglossal Nerve: Cranial Nerve XII

The tongue muscle is the primary responsibility of cranial nerve XII. Atrophy and fasciculation of the tongue occur when the ipsilateral hypoglossal nucleus or hypoglossal nerve is involved. The protruded tongue deviates toward the involved side because contraction of the normally innervated tongue muscle causes protrusion and is unopposed.

Skeletal Muscles

Tone, bulk, and strength of the skeletal muscles should be determined during this portion of the examination. Motor functions of the spinal nerves are described in Table 2-3.

The strength of limb muscles is assessed, when possible, by testing the child's ability to counteract resistance imposed by the examiner on proximal and distal muscle groups or individual muscles.

Muscle Testing

The following scoring system is useful for recording muscle power:

5: normal power
4: inability to maintain position against moderate resistance
3: inability to maintain position against slight resistance or gravity
2: active movement with gravity eliminated
1: trace of contraction
0: no contraction.

Arm and shoulder strength can also be assessed by asking the child to lean against a wall with legs placed a foot or two from the wall edge and arms outstretched with the palms against the wall. Testing lower extremity strength can be assessed by asking the child to sit on the floor then rapidly stand; the normal child will spring erect. With weakness of the hip extensors, however, Gowers' maneuver will be engaged, and the patient climbs up their own legs, pushing themselves into the erect position.

Muscle bulk is evaluated by gentle palpation and observation. Muscle tenderness, nerve tenderness, and nerve hypertrophy can also be assessed by palpation. Myotonia can be elicited by tapping over the thenar eminence and deltoid muscles.

Muscle tone is evaluated when the child is relaxed so that resistance to passive movement can be monitored. Aside from passive movement of limbs at joints, the examiner also assesses the extensibility of muscles by shaking the limbs and determining the range of motion.

Tone may be decreased in the presence of cerebellar disease and anterior horn cell disease. Tone may be increased because of the rigidity associated with basal ganglia disease and spasticity associated with corticospinal tract dysfunction.

Deep Tendon Reflexes

Standard deep tendon reflexes (i.e., muscle stretch reflexes) are elicited: biceps, triceps, brachioradialis, patellar, and Achilles reflexes.

The response to elicitation of deep tendon reflexes can be characterized as follows:

0: absent
1: hyporeflexic (trace, or only seen with reinforcement)
2: normal
3: hyperreflexic
4: unsustained clonus
5: sustained clonus.

Enhancement of tendon reflex responses when reflexes are seemingly absent can be promoted by having the child squeeze an object such as a block or ball or perform the more

TABLE 2-3 Extraocular Muscle Paralysis

Nerves	Muscles*	Function
Cervical Plexus (C1–C4)		
Cervical	Deep cervical	Flexion, extension, and rotation of neck
Phrenic	Scalene	Elevation of ribs (inspiration)
	Diaphragm	Inspiration
Brachial Plexus (C5–T1)		
Anterior	Pectorales major and minor	Adduction and depression of arm downward and medially
Long thoracic	Serratus anterior	Fixation of scapula on raising arm
Dorsal scapular	Levator scapulae	Elevation of scapula
	Rhomboid	Drawing scapula upward and inward
Suprascapular	Supraspinatus	Outward rotation of arm
	Infraspinatus	Elevation and outward rotation of arm
Subscapular	Latissimus dorsi	
	Teres major	Inward rotation and abduction of arm toward the back
	Subscapularis	Inward rotation of arm
Axillary	Deltoid	Raising of arm to horizontal
	Teres minor	Outward rotation of arm
Musculocutaneous	Biceps brachii	Flexion and supination of forearm
	Coracobrachialis	Elevation and adduction of arm
	Brachialis	Flexion of forearm
Median	Flexor carpi radialis	Flexion and radial deviation of hand
	Palmaris longus	Flexion of hand
	Flexor digitorum sublimis	Flexion of middle phalanges of second through fifth fingers
	Flexor pollicis longus	Flexion of distal phalanx of thumb
	Flexor digitorum profundus (radial half)	Flexion of distal phalanges of second and third fingers
	Pronator quadratus	Pronation
	Pronator teres	Pronation
	Abductor pollicis brevis	Abduction of metacarpus I at right angles to palm
	Flexor pollicis brevis	Flexion of proximal phalanx of thumb
	Lumbricals I, II, III	Flexion of proximal phalanges and extension of other phalanges of first, second, and third fingers
	Opponens pollicis brevis	Opposition of metacarpus I
Ulnar	Flexor carpi ulnaris	Flexion and ulnar deviation of hand
	Flexor digitorum profundus (ulnar half)	Flexion of distal phalanges of fourth and fifth fingers
	Adductor pollicis	Adduction of metacarpus I
	Hypothenar	Abduction, opposition, and flexion of little finger
	Lumbricals III, IV	Flexion of first phalanx and extension of other phalanges of fourth and fifth fingers
	Interossei	Same action as preceding. Also spreading apart and bringing together of fingers
Radial	Triceps brachii	Extension of forearm
	Brachioradialis	Flexion of forearm
	Extensor carpi radialis	Extension and radial flexion of hand
	Extensor digitorum communis	Extension of proximal phalanges of second through fifth fingers
	Extensor digiti quinti proprius	Extension of proximal phalanx of little finger
	Extensor carpi ulnaris	Extension and ulnar deviation of hand
	Supinator	Supination of forearm
	Abductor pollicis longus	Abduction of metacarpus I
	Extensor pollicis brevis	Extension of proximal phalanx of thumb
	Extensor pollicis longus	Abduction of metacarpus I and extension of distal phalanges of thumb
	Extensor indicis proprius	Extension of proximal phalanx of index finger
Thoracic Nerves		
Thoracic	Thoracic and abdominal	Elevation of ribs, expiration, abdominal compression, etc.
Lumbar Plexus (T12–L4)		
Femoral	Iliopsoas	Flexion of leg at hip
	Sartorius	Inward rotation of leg together with flexion of upper and lower leg
	Quadriceps femoris	Extension of lower leg
Obturator	Pectineus	
	Adductor longus	
	Adductor brevis	Adduction of leg
	Adductor magnus	
	Gracilis	
	Obturator externis	Adduction and outward rotation of leg

Continued on following page

TABLE 2-3 Extraocular Muscle Paralysis *(Continued)*

Sacral Plexus (L5–S5)		
Superior gluteal	Gluteus medius Gluteus minimus }	Abduction and inward rotation of leg; also, under certain circumstances, outward rotation
	Tensor fasciae latae	Flexion of leg at hip
	Piriformis	Outward rotation of leg
	Gluteus maximus	Extension of leg at hip
Inferior gluteal		
Sciatic	Obturator internus Gemelli Quadratus femoris }	Outward rotation of leg
	Biceps femoris	Flexion of leg at hip
	Semitendinosus	
	Semimembranosus	
Peroneal	Tibialis anterior	Dorsiflexion and supination of foot
Deep	Extensor digitorum longus	Extension of toes
	Extensor hallucis brevis	Extension of great toe
Superficial	Peroneus	Pronation of foot
Tibialis	Gastrocnemius Soleus }	Plantar flexion of foot
	Tibialis posterior	Adduction of foot
	Flexor digitorum longus	Flexion of distal phalanges II–V
	Flexor hallucis longus	Flexion of distal phalanx I
	Flexor digitorum brevis	Flexion of middle phalanges II–V
	Flexor hallucis brevis	Flexion of middle phalanx I
	Plantar	Spreading, bringing together, and flexion of proximal phalanges of toes
Pudendal	Perineal anal sphincters	Closure of sphincters of pelvic organs; participation in sexual act; contraction of pelvic floor

*Various muscles may receive still other nerve supplies than those mentioned. The following are the principal accessory nerve supplies: the brachial muscle receives fibers from the radial nerve; the flexor digitorum sublimis, from the ulnar; the adductor pollicis, from the median; the pectineus, from the femoral; the adductor magnus, from the tibial.
(With permission from Haymaker W. Bing's Local Diagnosis in Neurological Diseases, 15th edn. St. Louis: Mosby, 1969.)

traditional Jendrassik maneuver (i.e., hooking the fingers together while flexed and then attempting to pull them apart). Hyperreflexia may be indicated by an abnormal "spread" of responses, which includes contraction of muscle groups that usually do not contract when a specific reflex is being elicited (i.e., crossed thigh adductor or finger flexor reflexes).

Other Reflexes

A flexor (plantar) toe sign response is normal in children. The Babinski reflex is elicited by firm, steady, slow stroking from posterior to anterior of the lateral margin of the sole with an object such as a key or a tongue blade. The stimulus should not be painful. A positive response is a slow, tonic hyperextension of the great toe. A similar response is elicited using maneuvers such as the Chaddock (firmly stroking the lateral aspect of the foot) or Oppenheim (downward pressure on the medial aspect of the tibia).

Flicking the patient's nail (second or third finger) downward with the examiner's nail (i.e., the Hoffmann reflex) results in flexion of the distal phalanx of the thumb. No response or a muted response occurs in normal children; a brisk or asymmetric response occurs in the presence of corticospinal tract involvement.

Abdominal reflexes are obtained by stroking the abdomen from lateral to medial with strokes beginning just above the umbilicus, lateral to the umbilicus, and just below the umbilicus directed toward the umbilicus. Unilateral absence of the reflex can be associated with acquired corticospinal tract dysfunction.

The cremasteric reflex is elicited in males by stroking the inner aspects of the thigh in a caudal–rostral direction and observing the contraction of the scrotum. The reflex is normally present and symmetric. Absence or asymmetry may indicate corticospinal tract involvement.

Sensory System

Cooperation is necessary for a successful sensory examination. Vibration and proprioception can be assessed in all four limbs. Touch may be assessed by a single stimulus or by double simultaneous stimulation of two skin areas, which involves touching two parts of the body simultaneously (i.e., double simultaneous stimulation test). Extinction is the term used to denote failure of the child to perceive both stimuli. The contralateral parietal lobe to the side on which the unidentified stimulus was applied is the site of dysfunction. Pain, as tested with a pinprick, must be assessed gently, rapidly, and in a nonthreatening and playful manner. Segmental sensory innervations of the arm and leg should be noted. For example, the nipples are at approximately the T5 level and the umbilicus at the T10 level.

Cortical sensory function can be tested in the older child. Stereognosis is the recognition of familiar objects by touch. After the patient closes the eyes, objects are placed by the examiner in one of the child's hands and then the other. The patient should recognize the objects by size, texture, and form. Objects may include a button, coins, safety pin, or key. Absence of stereognosis is astereognosis. Astereognosis usually results from lesions of the parietal lobe.

Graphesthesia is the ability to recognize numbers, letters, or other readily identifiable symbols traced on the skin. This ability can be determined best by tracing the symbols in a preliminary trial while the child's eyes are open. When the patient's eyes are closed, the figures are traced over the palm or forearm. Failure to identify the symbols is dysgraphesthesia. By 8 years of age, most children are able to identify all single digits correctly.

The ability to distinguish between closely approximated stimulation at two points is two-point discrimination. Normal findings have been reported for children 2 to 12 years old.

Testing of this modality is frequently performed over the fingertips. Absence or impairment of two-point discrimination results from parietal lobe dysfunction.

Cerebellar Function

Cerebellar function is assessed in a number of ways. Hand patting (i.e., alternating pronation and supination of the hand on the thigh while the other hand remains stationary on the other thigh) is a good method for assessing dysdiadochokinesis. The maneuver is repeated with each hand separately to assess the presence of mirror movements (i.e., synkinesis). Other cerebellar tests include repetitive finger tapping (thumb to forefinger), foot tapping, and finger-to-nose, finger-to-finger (examiner's)-to-nose, and heel-to-knee-to-shin stroking. Several signs of cerebellar disease include head tilt, tremor when approaching a target (intention tremor), overshooting or undershooting a target (dysmetria), speech with an unusual cadence or prosody (cerebellar speech), or gait ataxia.

GAIT EVALUATION

The evaluation of gait is discussed in detail in Chapter 5.

REFERENCES

The complete list of references for this chapter is available in the e-book at www.expertconsult.com.

See inside cover for registration details.

SELECTED REFERENCES

Campbell, W.W., 2013. DeJong's The Neurologic Examination, seventh ed. Lippincott, Philadelphia.

Egan, D.F., 1990. Developmental examination of infants and pre-school children. Clinics in developmental medicine, vol. 112. MacKeith Press, Oxford.

Haymaker, W., 1969. Bing's local diagnosis in neurological diseases, fifteenth ed. CV Mosby, St. Louis.

Menkes, J.H., Sarnat, H.B., Maria, B., 2005. Textbook of Child Neurology, seventh ed. Williams & Wilkins, Baltimore.

Pina-Garza, J.E., 2013. Fenichel's Clinical Pediatric Neurology: a Signs and Symptoms Approach, seventh ed. WB Saunders, Philadelphia.

Volpe, J.J., 2008. The neurological examination: normal and abnormal features. In: Volpe, J.J. (Ed.), Neurology of the Newborn, fifth ed. WB Saunders, Philadelphia.

E-BOOK FIGURES AND TABLES

The following figures and tables are available in the e-book at www.expertconsult.com. See inside cover for registration details.

Fig 2-1 Bilateral oculomotor nerve paralysis.

Fig 2-3 Facial sensation supplied by the trigeminal nerve.

Fig 2-4 Right facial paralysis of the peripheral type.

Fig 2-5 Möbius' syndrome is manifested by bilateral palsy of cranial nerves VI and VII.

Fig 2-6 Fasciculation of the tongue, especially of the right lateral border, in a patient with group 2 Werdnig–Hoffmann disease.

Fig 2-7 Position of the limbs for muscle strength (see Table 2-6).

Fig 2-8 Gowers' maneuver indicates weakness of truncal and proximal lower extremity muscles.

Fig 2-9 Radicular cutaneous fields.

Fig 2-10 Segmental sensory innervation of the leg.

Fig 2-11 Segmental sensory innervation of the arm.

Table 2-2 Extraocular Muscle Paralysis

Table 2-4 Segmental Innervation of Muscles of Extremities

Table 2-5 Segmental Innervation of Trunk Muscles

Table 2-6 Muscle Testing

Table 2-7 Muscle Stretch (Tendon) Reflexes

3 Neurologic Examination after the Newborn Period Until 2 Years of Age

Kenneth F. Swaiman and John Phillips

There is no one way to organize the examination of an infant. Experienced examiners develop individual techniques and sequences that are flexible depending on the child's level of cooperation (Jan, 2007). The technique presented here, which has worked for many clinicians, is a four-stage examination sequence, beginning with the least intrusive maneuvers. Developmental assessment is an integral part of this examination; norms are well established (Box 3-1), and when development lags, referral for more detailed testing may be considered.

The **first stage** of the examination is observation. In the **second stage**, the head, muscle tone, superficial and deep sensation, gross response to sound, and visual fields can be evaluated while the child remains on the caregiver's lap. The **third stage** becomes more invasive, and may require help from a caregiver or assistant. At this point, a general examination is performed, including measurement of the occipitofrontal circumference and optic fundi. In the **fourth stage** of the examination, the child is placed on the floor and encouraged to crawl, walk, and run, if possible.

EVALUATION OF THE PATIENT
Stage 1

Because many children at this age need a few minutes to feel comfortable with a stranger, it is preferable not to rush into the examination. It is often helpful to have the child sit on the caregiver's lap facing the examiner during this history-taking session to encourage familiarity. The point is to try to help the child become comfortable with the examination room and the examiner.

The sequence of examination should be flexible and determined by the child's comfort level and temperament, although eventually a complete examination must be conducted (Campbell, 2013). Most importantly, it is imperative that the clinician comprehensively conduct that aspect of the examination related to the chief complaint.

Observations done at this stage include an assessment of the child's level of alertness, awareness of surroundings, and affect. Communication skills can be noted and compared with age-appropriate expectations (Egan, 1990). Movement should be evident as well, particularly of the face, eyes, and extremities, and the examiner should look specifically for any asymmetry or abnormalities of control or posture.

Head

Examination of the head is done systematically, looking for asymmetry, indentations, and protuberances. Evaluation of the fontanels and cranial sutures should be performed with gentle palpation. Hair color, distribution, texture, and pattern, including unusual whorl patterns, also should be assessed.

The occipitofrontal circumference should always be measured. If the child becomes agitated, this can be deferred until later in the examination (stage 3), but it must be taken at some point. Change over time, rather than a single measurement, provides the most useful information. In addition, the size of the anterior fontanel, which is typically closed by 12 months of age, should be recorded, along with any tenseness when the child is sitting comfortably in an upright position. Other fontanels are usually difficult to palpate, except in pathologic states. Finally, the head should be auscultated for the presence of unusual intracranial bruits.

Cranial Nerves

Most of the examination of cranial nerve function of the infant and toddler can be completed by observation with minimal invasive procedures. Details concerning examination of each cranial nerve can be found in Chapter 2. Toys or colorful objects can facilitate the assessment of extraocular movements in young children. If the child appears uninterested in bright objects, the possibility of a visual defect or an underlying intellectual defect must be considered. Double simultaneous stimulation (i.e., simultaneously bringing two bright objects into both temporal fields) normally causes the child to look from one object to the other; failure to take notice of one object may indicate homonymous hemianopsia. An optokinetic tape (with repetitive bars or objects) should be drawn horizontally and then vertically across the child's field of vision. An absent response may result from lack of visual fixation or from gross impairment of vision.

A beam from a small flashlight directed at each eye allows evaluation of pupil size, pupillary responses, and the red retinal reflex. Eye features to be noted include symmetry of the palpebral fissures, relative size of the two globes, angulation of the eyes compared with other facial components (i.e., mongoloid or antimongoloid slant) and with the ears, cataracts, conjunctival telangiectases, colobomas of the iris, ptosis, proptosis, and malformed or eccentrically placed pupils.

Observing the child's facial movements throughout the entire examination is helpful (Nelson and Eng, 1972). Widening of the ipsilateral palpebral fissure or inability to bury the limbus when crying is indicative of facial nerve weakness. In the younger infant, sucking and rooting reflexes should be obtained. Sometimes, the child can be induced to protrude the tongue if the examiner urges the child to imitate the examiner's tongue movements. Deformity, atrophy, or abnormal positioning of the tongue can be observed. Tongue fasciculations should be evaluated with the tongue in the resting position, and by gently elevating the tongue with a depressor and examining the undersurface.

Basic responses to the sound made by a tuning fork, rubbing fingers together, ringing a bell, or using a toy noise-maker that generates noise at a modest volume may provide much information. The examiner must be careful not to confuse response to a visual cue (e.g., the movement needed to elicit noise from a toy) with response to the sound.

BOX 3-1 Child Development from 2 Months through 2 Years

2 MONTHS
- Keeps hands predominantly fisted
- Lifts head up for several seconds while prone
- Startles in response to loud noise
- Follows with eyes and head over 90-degree arc
- Smiles responsively
- Begins to vocalize single sounds

3 MONTHS
- Occasionally holds hands fisted
- Lifts head up above body plane and holds position
- Holds an object briefly when placed in hand
- Turns head toward object, fixes and follows fully in all directions with eyes
- Smiles and vocalizes when talked to
- Watches own hands, stares at faces
- Laughs

4 MONTHS
- Holds head steady while in sitting position
- Reaches for an object, grasps it, brings it to mouth
- Turns head in direction of sound
- Smiles spontaneously

5–6 MONTHS
- Lifts head while supine
- Rolls from prone to supine
- Lifts head and chest up in prone position
- Exhibits no head lag
- Transfers object from hand to hand
- Babbles
- Sits with support
- Localizes direction of sound

7–8 MONTHS
- Sits in tripod fashion without support
- Stands briefly with support
- Bangs object on table
- Reaches out for people

- Mouths all objects
- Says "da-da," "ba-ba"

9–10 MONTHS
- Sits well without support, pulls self to sit
- Stands holding on
- Waves "bye-bye"
- Drinks from cup with assistance
- Uses pincer grasp

11–12 MONTHS
- Walks with assistance
- Uses two to four words with meaning
- Creeps well
- Assists in dressing
- Understands a few simple commands

13–15 MONTHS
- Walks by self, falls easily
- Says several words, uses jargon
- Scribbles with crayon
- Points to things wanted

18 MONTHS
- Climbs stairs with assistance, climbs up on chair
- Throws ball
- Builds two to four-block tower
- Feeds self
- Takes off clothes
- Points to two or three body parts
- Uses many intelligible words

24 MONTHS
- Runs, walks up and down stairs alone (both feet per step)
- Speaks in two- to three-word sentences
- Turns single pages of book
- Builds four- to six-block tower
- Kicks ball
- Uses pronouns "you," "me," and "I"

(Data from Frankenburg WK, Dodds J, Archer P, et al. Pediatrics. 1992;89:91; Illingsworth RS. The development of the infant and young child. 9th ed. Baltimore: Williams & Wilkins; 1987; and Knobloch H, Stevens F, Malone A. The revised developmental screening inventory. Houston, Texas: Gesell Developmental Test Materials; 1980.)

Motor Evaluation

As with all other parts of the evaluation, the motor examination begins with observation. Even before touching the child, general posture and the symmetry of movements of the arms and legs are observed, with note made of any gross discrepancies in muscle bulk or limb length. Definite hand preference (such as reaching across the midline to avoid using the contralateral hand) before 24 months is abnormal.

Decreased muscle bulk may not be appreciated because of the large amount of subcutaneous fat at this age, and muscle atrophy may be undetected. Careful palpation helps distinguish between fat and muscle.

The next step is evaluation of muscle tone, which is defined as resistance of muscle to passive stretch. This also requires palpation. Muscle tone and range of motion of the arms and legs are best assessed when the child is in the relaxed state by gently shaking and moving the hands and feet in flexion and extension. Pronation and supination of the hands and forearms provide further information about range of motion and the presence of spasticity or rigidity. Greater-than-normal resistance to passive movement indicates hypertonia, whereas less-than-normal resistance indicates hypotonia. It is important to distinguish increased *tone* from limitation of movement due to joint *contracture*. It is also important to note when the child is actively resisting the examiner, which is a reflection of *strength*. Spontaneous muscle movements, particularly those against gravity, provide the most information concerning muscle strength. Further assessment of strength is provided by judging the degree of resistance that occurs when active movement is attempted against the examiner. Experience helps in this part of the examination, particularly in cases of mild abnormalities, but even a novice should be able to make a reasonable judgment about both tone and strength in most instances.

Upper motor neuron unit involvement may cause decreased movement of an entire extremity or more focal abnormalities, such as limited flexion of the arm at the elbow, persistent fisting, or adduction of the thumb against the palm. Erb's brachial plexus injury is a lower motor neuron disorder commonly causing internal rotation and adduction at the shoulder, often with the "waiter's tip" posture (Pina-Garza, 2013). Interacting with the infant using toys and other interesting objects may facilitate the evaluation of limb strength, range of motion, and coordination. In the older cooperative child, individual muscle testing should be carried out when appropriate.

There is a normal developmental sequence of fine motor control as the child becomes more adept at reaching for objects. Grasping things with both hands and holding the object before the face or immediately placing it in the mouth is later superseded by transferring the object from hand to hand and manipulating the toy. The infant's grasping skills are best demonstrated in response to small objects. The 4- to 5-month-old infant is able to grasp an object with the entire hand, at 7 months the thumb and the neighboring two fingers are used, and the pincer grasp (using only the thumb and forefinger) should be present by 9 to 11 months. The palmar grasp reflex (i.e., obligate grasp reflex) should gradually diminish from 3 to 6 months of age. The persistence of the obligate grasp reflex beyond 6 months of age may signal corticospinal tract dysfunction. Observation of the child's ability to raise the arms while reaching for an object helps assess proximal muscle strength. Congenital malformations of the fingers and hands from webbing to clinodactyly can be readily determined during this portion of the examination.

Direct examination of the hips should include assessment of the range of motion; decreased excursion may signify spasticity or subluxation of the hip joints. Galeazzi's sign is performed in a supine child by flexing the hips 90 degrees with feet on the examination table, noting any asymmetry of femur length. Hip disease such as subluxation often results in a shorter leg and may exist separately or as a result of spasticity. Conversely, increased excursion may represent hypotonia or ligamental laxity.

Initial examination of the legs consists of assessment of muscle symmetry and mass. Spontaneous motor movements are also evaluated, making note of the quality and symmetry of any movement. Assessment of tone is similar to that done with the arms and hands; one should gently shake the feet and passively move the joints of the lower extremities from hip to knee to ankle.

Deep tendon reflexes that are excessively brisk may indicate upper motor neuron unit disease, especially when associated with clonus. Asymmetry is particularly worrisome because of the association with pathologic conditions. Absent deep tendon reflexes are seen with anterior horn cell disease or peripheral neuropathy. The crossed adductor reflex is elicited when the patellar reflex is stimulated and resultant contraction of the adductor muscles occurs in the opposite leg. This response can be normal until approximately 1 year of age. However, persistence of the response, particularly unilaterally, suggests the presence of corticospinal tract involvement.

The plantar response can be as important in infants as in adults. There is no consensus about when an extensor response is a normal finding, although an asymmetric extensor toe sign is always abnormal, as is an extensor toe sign that persists beyond 12 months of age (Hogan and Milligan, 1971). A pathologic extensor plantar sign is indicative of upper motor neuron unit disease. Several beats of ankle clonus are often present in the neonatal period and should disappear by 2 months of age. The persistence of ankle clonus and extensor plantar responses in an older child suggests upper motor neuron unit disease even in the absence of hyperreflexia.

Cerebellar function is difficult to assess in infants; it is easiest when a cooperative child can be observed sitting, standing, walking, or reaching for objects. The examiner can also observe the child during play to see resting or intention tremor, dysmetria, titubation or truncal sway while sitting, and fine motor coordination. Decreased tone may accompany other signs of cerebellar dysfunction.

Sensory Testing and Cutaneous Examination

Light touch can be tested by gently stroking the extremities; this should lead to a reaction, with signs of recognition ranging from eye deviation and facial response to anxious withdrawal of the limbs (Figure 3-4). Application of a tuning fork often causes arrest of motion and a wide-eyed look of wonder in the child who cannot otherwise describe the feeling.

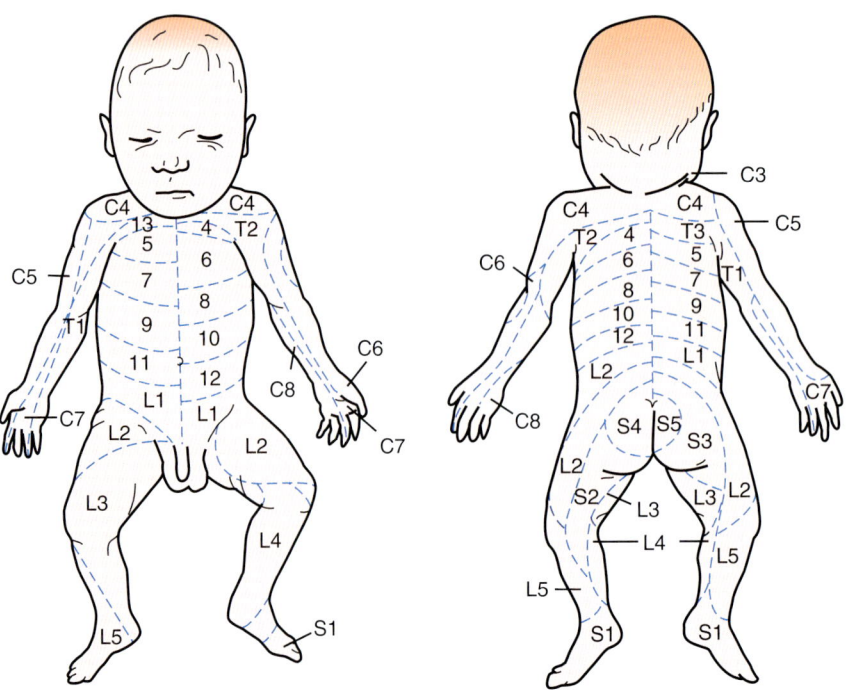

Figure 3-4. Segmental distribution of the cutaneous nerves of an infant. *(Modified from Fanaroff AA, Martin RJ. Neonatal-perinatal medicine: diseases of the fetus and infant, 5th ed. St. Louis: Mosby, 1992.)*

Proprioception cannot be directly evaluated at this age, but observations of sitting positions, gait, and posture may provide some clues. Pain response from light application of a pin or gentle pinching should be reserved until late in the examination, lest causing pain confirms a child's suspicions about the examiner, and upsets an already worried parent.

During the sensory examination, careful observation of the child's skin is important to rule out a neurocutaneous disorder. Are there hypopigmented macules of tuberous sclerosis present, café au lait spots as seen in neurofibromatosis, or a port wine stain in the area of the first division of the trigeminal nerve that might suggest Sturge-Weber syndrome? Particular examination of the spine is necessary to check for scoliosis, sinus tracts, scars, dimples, and hemangiomas. Unusual skin lesions or hair growth over the spine suggest the presence of an underlying mesodermal defect, such as diastematomyelia or spina bifida occulta. The spine should be palpated along its entire course for defects.

Abdominal and cremasteric reflexes are present at birth. The abdominal reflex is elicited by stroking the skin of the upper, middle, and lower portions of the abdomen laterally from the midline. Each stroke elicits a muscle contraction mediated by a different group of thoracic nerves from T8 to T12. The response results in the retraction of the umbilicus toward the stimulated side. The cremasteric reflex is elicited by upwardly stroking the inner thigh, beginning 3 to 5 cm below the inguinal crease. The cremasteric reflex results in an elevation of the testicles due to contraction of the overlying smooth muscles. Cremasteric reflexes are mediated by spinal nerves L1 to L2.

Stage 2

For stage 2 of the evaluation the child should be placed on an examination table with the caregiver close by to provide reassurance to the child and assistance to the examiner, if necessary. Motor evaluation of the older child can also be carried out on a larger, carpeted surface. By 3 months of age, an infant in the prone position should be able to hold the head and chest off the table. Good head control when held in the sitting position should be evident by 4 months of age. The child should be able to sit unsupported and maintain adequate balance by 8 to 9 months of age. Independent achievement of the sitting position should occur by 10 months of age. The child should crawl by 10 months, pull to a standing position by 10 months, and creep by 11 months. The child should walk with support by 12 months and without support by 13 to 14 months.

Trunk, shoulder, and pelvic girdle tone and strength are directly evaluated. The child is observed while held in vertical and horizontal suspension. A hypotonic infant often droops over the examiner's arm when held in horizontal suspension. In vertical suspension, the hypotonic child may slide through the examiner's hands (Volpe, 2008). The child may be unable to maintain a standing posture when the feet are placed on the table surface; this must be distinguished from active withdrawal of the legs that may also prevent successful standing. If spasticity is present, there may be arching of the extended head, neck, and back while in horizontal suspension. Spasticity may also cause extension of the lower extremities with "scissoring" (excessive abduction) and toe walking.

Motor Performance Instruments

Through the years, several instruments have been devised that are useful for evaluating motor performance in relation to chronologic age. These instruments have provided norms for evaluating the expected rate of motor development for a number of different assessments and maneuvers.

Developmental Reflexes

Developmental reflexes represent maturational stages of the developing nervous system (Prechtl, 1997). Occasionally, developmental reflexes can have localizing value, but usually they are nonspecific. Abnormal findings include the absence or poor manifestation of the expected response, persistence of a reflex that should have disappeared, or an asymmetric response (Table 3-1).

Correctly eliciting the **Moro reflex** requires holding the infant in the supine position, lifting the head, and then allowing the head to fall approximately 30 degrees while cradling the head in the examiner's hands. The expected response is initial extension and abduction of the arms with extension of the fingers, followed by adduction of the arms at the shoulder. Asymmetry at any age, or persistence beyond 5 to 6 months, is always abnormal.

The **asymmetric tonic neck reflex** (ATNR) may be detected in the neonatal period but reaches its peak at 2 months and is absent by 6 months of age. To elicit the reflex, the head is turned to one side while the infant is lying in the supine position. There is extension of the arm and leg on the side toward which the face is turned, while the contralateral extremities flex ("fencer's posture"). A normal infant should not maintain the position beyond a few seconds (i.e., obligate ATNR).

The **palmar grasp reflex** is elicited by placing an object or the examiner's finger in the palm of the infant's hand; this leads to an involuntary flexion response. This reflex subsides by 3 to 6 months of age and is replaced by voluntary grasping, which is necessary to allow transfer of objects from hand to hand.

In slightly older infants, the **Landau reflex** can first be elicited between 5 and 10 months of age, and can usually be seen up to 2 years of age. With one hand supporting the abdomen in the prone position, the examiner flexes the infant's head with his or her other hand. The normal response is flexion of the legs and trunk.

The **placing reflex** response can be demonstrated by holding the upright infant in a manner that causes the dorsal surface of the infant's feet to touch the underside of a tabletop. The infant flexes the legs at the hips and knees so that contact with the underside of the surface ceases.

One of the most useful maneuvers is the **traction response** (Zafeiriou, 2004). This is elicited with the infant in the supine position; the examiner grasps both hands and pulls the infant gently and slowly upward, to a sitting position. Marked head lag with little resistance to the examiner's pulling efforts characterizes the newborn response. By 1 month, the infant's head shows transient neck flexion followed by extension as the infant is pulled forward. Usually, by 3 to 5 months of age at the latest, the infant is able to participate actively with arm flexion at the elbow, and by holding the head and trunk in a straight line as the examiner pulls the child to the upright position. At this point there should be no head lag, and little or no forward motion of the head as the child reaches the upright position.

A valuable measure of vestibular function in the newborn can be obtained by holding the infant in a supine position with the feet closest to the examiner. As the examiner rotates the infant laterally in each direction, the eyes of the infant deviate in the direction of rotation, accompanied by intermittent nystagmus to the opposite side. This maneuver also allows extraocular movements to be assessed.

TABLE 3-1 Eliciting Primitive Reflexes

Reflex	Position	Method	Response	Age at Disappearance
Palmar grip	Supine	Placing the index finger in the palm of the infant	Flexion of fingers, fist making	6 months
Plantar grip	Supine	Pressing a thumb against the sole just behind the toes	Flexion of toes	15 months
Galant	Prone	Scratching the skin of the infant's back from the shoulder downward, 2–3 cm lateral to the spinous processes	Incurvation of the trunk, with the concavity on the stimulated side	4 months
Asymmetric tonic neck	Supine	Rotation of the infant's head to one side for 15 seconds	Extension of the extremities on the chin side and flexion of those on the occipital side	3 months
Suprapubic extensor	Supine	Pressing the skin over the pubic bone with the fingers	Reflex extension of both lower extremities, with adduction and internal rotation into talipes equinus	4 weeks
Crossed extensor	Supine	Passive total flexion of one lower extremity	Extension of the other lower limb, with adduction and internal rotation into talipes equinus	6 weeks
Rossolimo	Supine	Light tapping of toes 2–4 at their plantar surfaces	Tonic flexion of the toes at the first metacarpophalangeal joint	4 weeks
Heel	Supine	Tapping on the heel with a hammer, with the infant's hip and knee joints flexed and the ankle joint in neutral position	Rapid reflex extension of the lower extremity in question	3 weeks
Moro	Supine	Sudden head extension produced by a light drop of the head	Abduction followed by adduction and flexion of upper extremities	6 months
Babinski	Supine	Striking along the lateral aspect of the sole, extending from the heel to the head of the fifth metatarsal	Combined extensor response: simultaneous dorsiflexion of the great toe and fanning of the remaining toes	Presence always abnormal

(Data from multiple sources: Futagi Y, Tagawa T, Otani K. Brain Dev. 1992;14:294; Vojta V. Die cerebralen Bewegungstoerungen im Kindesalter, 4te Auflage. Stuttgart: Ferdinand Enke Verlag; 1988; Zafeiriou DI, Tsikoulas IG, Kremenopoulos GM. Pediatr Neurol. 1995;13:148; Zafeiriou DI, Tsikoulas I, Kremenopoulos G, et al. Brain Dev. 1999a;21:216; Zafeiriou DI, Tsikoulas I, Kremenopoulos G, et al. J Child Neurol. 1999b;14:514; Zafeiriou DI, Tsikoulas I, Kremenopoulos G, et al. Brain and Development. 1998;20:307; and Zafeiriou DI. Pediatr Neurol. 2000;22:75.)

There are other developmental reflexes, but those discussed here appear to be the most often evaluated and the most useful.

Stage 3

Examination of the optic fundi should be performed with the infant supine, possibly lying in the caregiver's lap or held over the caregiver's shoulder with the infant's head held tightly against the caregiver's head. Abnormalities of the fundi, including vascular changes, elevation of the optic disc, and retinal changes, along with abnormalities of the lens and media, should be assessed. Mydriatic agents and sedation are rarely employed in the office evaluation, although they are both occasionally necessary. During the first few months of life, the optic discs may be somewhat gray. This normal finding should not be confused with optic atrophy.

The general portion of the examination follows. A heart murmur may signify congenital structural anomalies more widespread than just in the heart. Stridor heard on auscultation may accompany weakness of the upper respiratory musculature. The presence of hepatosplenomegaly should be determined because many storage diseases, which also affect the brain, may be the cause of organ enlargement. When spinal lesions are suspected, the anal sphincter should be examined for tone and the presence of an anal cutaneous reflex (the so-called "anal wink"). Congenital anomalies of the genitalia should be noted. The remainder of the general examination, particularly the intrusive aspects, such as evaluation of the auditory meati, tympanic membranes, mouth, and teeth, can be done at this time.

Stage 4

Spontaneous motor abilities are assessed in this stage of the examination. The crawling child can be put on a carpeted floor or a suitable pad; if the child stands, or walks, he or she should be placed on the floor. The child should be allowed to ambulate or encouraged by rolling a ball across the room or having the child follow a parent across the room. Spastic diparesis, hemiplegia, waddling, footdrop, limp, or ataxia may be evident. The manner in which the child stoops and bends to retrieve a ball or block may show premature hand dominance, athetosis, tremor, or weakness of the legs. Whenever there is a question of proximal weakness, the child should be observed when arising from the floor to a standing position to determine the presence of Gowers' maneuver.

Unlike in the examination of older children, the testing of individual muscle groups in infants is usually impracticable. Nevertheless, evaluation of spontaneous movements and use of some specific maneuvers (e.g., traction response, wheelbarrow maneuver, standing from the floor or a seated position) can provide information about spasticity, weakness, and incoordination. As always, a comparison of the examination findings must be made with expected age-related norms.

Further examination of muscle strength can be accomplished by using the parachute response; the examiner holds the child in the prone position over an examination table and gently thrusts the patient toward the table surface. A fully developed response (expected at 8 months) consists of arm and wrist extension, allowing the outstretched palms to make contact with the table as the infant supports his or her body weight with the arms and shoulders. Formal individual muscle testing can be used in the older child whenever necessary.

The sensory examination can be difficult. Begin with examination of touch, position sense, and vibration sense. A tuning fork placed on the appropriate bony prominence may elicit a look of surprise or bemusement. Evaluation of pain should be done last and only after the examiner demonstrates to the child the method that will be used.

During this phase of the examination, the Romberg maneuver can be performed. The older child is asked to stand in one place with the feet together and close the eyes; a positive Romberg's sign occurs when the child sways or falls with the eyes closed. The examiner should also observe the child for titubation, nystagmus, and dysmetria while reaching for objects. Cooperative children older than 3 years should be able to perform finger-to-nose testing with the eyes closed. The heel-shin test is frequently not possible in children younger than 4 years.

Assessment of the deep tendon reflexes is best carried out with the infant or toddler in the caregiver's lap. The biceps response in most infants can be difficult to elicit, but the triceps and brachioradialis reflexes are usually readily detected. The patellar and Achilles responses are typically present and easy to elicit. Toe signs can be evaluated as in older children.

GENERAL CONSIDERATIONS

Throughout the examination, the clinician should evaluate the child's alertness, interest in the surroundings, and ability to learn during the examination. The child's speech pattern should also be assessed. By 15 months of age, the child should have a consistent vocabulary of 2 to 6 words, and by 18 months, up to 20 words. Short phrases consisting of two or three words are usually part of the child's repertoire by 21 to 24 months. By 2 years of age, most children have a vocabulary of up to 50 words. Using specific scales to evaluate intelligence and development levels is of some help, but a single office assessment may not be reliable. It is therefore important that the examiner become proficient in informal means of evaluating these characteristics (Maria and English, 1993).

Young children are not always easy to examine. However, taking a staged approach as suggested here, and being sensitive to the child's temperament, often results in a successful examination.

REFERENCES

The complete list of references for this chapter is available in the e-book at www.expertconsult.com.
   See inside cover for registration details.

SELECTED REFERENCES

Campbell, W.W., 2013. DeJong's The Neurologic Examination, seventh ed. Lippincott, Philadelphia.

Egan, D.F., 1990. Developmental examination of infants and preschool children. Clinical Developmental Medicine, vol. 112. MacKeith Press, Oxford.

Hogan, G.R., Milligan, J.E., 1971. The plantar reflex of the newborn. N. Engl. J. Med. 285, 502.

Jan, M.M., 2007. Neurological examination of difficult and poorly cooperative children. J. Child Neurol. 22, 1209.

Maria, B.L., English, W., 1993. Do pediatricians independently manage common neurological problems? J. Child Neurol. 8, 73.

Nelson, K.B., Eng, G.D., 1972. Congenital hypoplasia of depressor anguli oris muscle: differentiation from congenital facial palsy. J. Pediatr. 81, 16.

Pina-Garza, J.E., 2013. Fenichel's Clinical Pediatric Neurology: A Signs and Symptoms Approach, seventh ed. WB Saunders, Philadelphia.

Prechtl, H.F., 1997. State of the art of a new functional assessment of the young nervous system. An early predictor of cerebral palsy. Early Hum. Dev. 24, 1.

Volpe, J.J., 2008. The neurological examination: normal and abnormal features. In: Volpe, J.J. (Ed.), Neurology of the Newborn, fifth ed. WB Saunders, Philadelphia.

Zafeiriou, D.I., 2004. Primitive reflexes and postural reactions in the neurodevelopmental examination. Pediatr. Neurol. 31, 1.

E-BOOK FIGURES AND TABLES

The following figures and tables are available in the e-book at www.expertconsult.com. See inside cover for registration details.

Fig. 3-1 Entire hand grasp of a 4-month-old infant.

Fig. 3-2 Use of two fingers and thumb in the grasp of a 7-month-old infant.

Fig. 3-3 Pincer grasp with the thumb and forefinger of an 11-month-old infant.

Fig. 3-5 Extended legs, scissoring, toe stance, and fisting in an infant with spastic quadriplegia.

Fig. 3-6 The Moro response to rapid extension of the neck in a 2-day-old infant. The abduction phase of arm movement is illustrated. A cry usually accompanies the response, and the leg position varies.

Fig. 3-7 The traction maneuver causes little response in a 2-day-old infant. There is little or no perceptible flexion of the neck or the arms at the elbows.

Fig. 3-8 Abnormal parachute response.

Box 3-2 Most Commonly Used Motor Performance Tools

Box 3-3 Tips for Examining Noncooperative Children

Table 3-2 Eliciting Postural Reactions

4 Neurologic Examination of the Term and Preterm Infant

Kenneth F. Swaiman and John Phillips

THE TERM INFANT

The essence of the newborn neurologic examination, whether for a premature or a term-born child, remains exactly the same as with older children. It begins with observation, followed by an examination that may need to be done "out of order" depending on circumstances. Several examinations done over time may be required to most accurately characterize an infant's neurologic status.

Observation

Careful observation begins the examination, noting any congenital abnormalities that are present and the general level of alertness. Cranial nerve assessment can be largely obtained via observation, making note of spontaneous eye movement, facial symmetry, and response to sounds and light. Observation also provides much information regarding the motor system. For example, term infants have predominantly flexor tone with frequent flexion at the knees and elbows. Intermittent fisting of the hands, including adduction and infolding of the thumbs (i.e., cortical thumbs), is often present. Limb position and posturing should be roughly symmetric. While supine, a healthy infant may have spontaneous limb movements that are asymmetric with a jerking quality—this is normal. Excessive jitteriness or tremulousness, however, particularly of the hands or jaw may suggest hyperexcitability of the central nervous system (CNS).

Cranial Vault Evaluation

The occipitofrontal circumference should be plotted on a graph standardized for gender, race, and gestational age to determine whether the measurement falls within the normal range (i.e., two standard deviations above or below the mean). Variances within two standard deviations may be due in part to head shape; for example, the same volume will require a larger circumference in an oblong head compared with a round head. Significant deviation from normal always requires further evaluation.

Some deformities of the cranium are related to the birthing process. Vaginal deliveries may be associated with scalp and subcutaneous edema causing *caput succedaneum*, particularly if vacuum extraction is used. *Cephalohematomas* are hemorrhages within the periosteum of individual cranial bones and therefore do not cross suture lines. *Subgaleal hematomas* result from bleeding under the scalp aponeurosis and are often preceded by forceps or vacuum-assisted delivery space. The scalp may be edematous and boggy because of underlying blood. Although most subgaleal hematomas are benign, if large enough they can cause hypovolemic shock. Infants delivered by cesarean section usually have relatively round heads.

The anterior fontanel, readily palpable at birth and often pulsating with the infants heart rate, is concave or flat in relation to the surrounding cranium. The fontanel should be assessed with the child held in the sitting position if there is any question of increased pressure. A bulging fontanel without the child crying raises a concern regarding increased intracranial pressure. The anterior fontanel varies in size but usually ranges from 1 to 3 cm in its longest dimension (Popich and Smith, 1972). The posterior fontanel in the neonate usually is open but admits only a fingertip.

Cranial sutures (e.g., sagittal, metopic, lambdoidal, and squamosal) are readily palpable in the newborn. Overriding sutures, often the sagittal and lambdoidal, are sometimes seen in the first week of life. Gentle palpation should demonstrate that sutures readily separate from one another unless premature closure has occurred, which may cause asymmetric skull growth.

Auscultation over the infant skull, particularly the anterior fontanel and neck vessels, usually reveals a venous hum in a number of locations. Rarely, systolic-diastolic bruits, particularly those that are focal and asymmetric, indicate the presence of an arteriovenous malformation; however, at times these bruits may be heard in normal infants.

Developmental Reflexes

Developmental reflexes are primitive reflexes with complex responses, and largely reflect the integrity of the brainstem and spinal cord; the role of higher centers, although of importance, is not fully known. This includes the Moro, rooting, grasping, tonic neck, stepping, and placing reflexes. Many of these reflexes are present at birth and undergo modification during the first 6 months of life. Detailed discussion of these reflexes is presented in Chapter 3.

Motor Function

Gentle manipulation of the infant's limbs allows for assessment of muscle tone and strength. *Tone* is resistance to passive movement and should be evaluated while the infant is awake but at rest. *Strength* is resistance to active movement, which can be assessed in an infant by noting resistance to spontaneous movements. The optimal position to assess tone and strength is supine with the head in the midposition so that the tonic neck reflex does not augment tone unilaterally.

Horizontal and vertical suspensions are helpful maneuvers when assessing infant motor function. When held in the vertical position, the hypotonic and weak infant tends to slide through the examiner's hands. In the horizontal position, the hypotonic infant droops over the examiner's arms without raising head or legs. Conversely, increased tone may cause opisthotonus, with persistent extension in both vertical and horizontal positions. Scissoring (i.e., crossing of the legs because of excessive, involuntary adductor magnus contraction) may also be evident with increased tone, but usually does not occur until after the neonatal period. The most common cause of generalized decreased tone is depression of CNS function, congenital malformations, or neuromuscular disorders. Increased muscle tone may be seen in a variety of conditions that cause neonatal encephalopathy. Indeed, there are myriad causes of abnormalities of tone and strength, and careful serial examinations over time are often required to arrive at the correct diagnosis.

While the infant is being handled, stimulation may cause jittery or tremulous movements of the jaw or limbs. The movements usually terminate when stimulation ends, although noises or abrupt changes in light may trigger them. Brief and mild tremulousness can be normal; however, when increased, these movements may indicate metabolic abnormalities (e.g., electrolyte imbalance), bleeding, congenital CNS defects (structural or functional), infections, or drug withdrawal syndromes.

Deep tendon reflexes are assessed just as with older children. Although they may be brisk or absent in the newborn (Critchley, 1968), asymmetry is always abnormal.

Typically, the plantar response is extensor for at least the first month of life and usually through the first year of life. Persistence of extensor toe-sign responses beyond infancy or any asymmetry suggests corticospinal tract impairment and may be associated with alterations in tone and other deep tendon reflex abnormalities.

Several beats of ankle clonus are frequently elicited in the newborn, often enhanced by crying. Increased clonus, however, often with other examination abnormalities, may be the harbinger of serious CNS disease.

Cranial Nerve Examination

A more detailed discussion of the cranial nerve examination is found in Chapter 2. Cranial nerve I, the olfactory nerve, is infrequently tested but may be evaluated by the use of pleasant but definitive aromatic substances; virtually, all neonates born after 32 weeks' gestation respond.

Evaluation of cranial nerves II, III, IV, and VI involves assessment of the eyes. Pupils should be symmetric, with equal response to light. A bright light causes the infant to blink or hold the lids closed. The presence of ptosis or increased height of the palpebral fissure should be evaluated.

Examination of the optic fundi may be difficult but is necessary. Numerous changes, including chorioretinitis (i.e., salt-and-pepper pigmentary changes), may be observed. Hemorrhages are commonly detected after vaginal delivery, even in the absence of traumatic delivery. The optic nerve may be hypoplastic, as manifested by a small, pearl-colored optic disc. The color of the optic disc in the newborn infant is grayish white. Retinal hemorrhages may be found in a large percentage of otherwise normal infants who have no history of abnormal delivery and who later prove to be neurologically normal.

The newborn infant turns toward a light of moderate intensity and fixes on a bright object or the examiner's face. Most often, the newborn's eyes are symmetrically open or closed. If one eye is open and the other closed, there should be a shifting from one side to the other. Width of palpebral fissures should be equal; if not, the presence of ptosis may suggest an abnormality of cranial nerve III function, sympathetic innervation dysfunction, neuromuscular junction difficulty, weakness of the levator muscle of the lid, or abnormality of the lid connective tissue. Occasionally, central or peripheral seventh nerve paresis may result in asymmetry of the palpebral fissure.

Extraocular movements are monitored while a child is lying quietly. Slight lapses of conjugate gaze are common in the newborn period. Newborn visual acuity is difficult to assess, but black and white–patterned objects can be used. The examiner's face is often the best "target." The intended object of focus is moved slowly in the infant's field of vision, less than a foot from the infant's eyes. The infant slowly follows

with eye movement, particularly in lateral directions. Prolonged gaze may occur in the newborn period (Brazelton et al., 1976). Opticokinetic nystagmus may be elicited by using a striped, rotating drum or striped cloth strip, which is slowly pulled across the infant's visual field in the vertical and horizontal directions. The response is the same as in older children (Chapter 2).

Although small-excursion, lateral-gaze nystagmus may be present in the newborn, the coarser to-and-fro pattern of congenital nystagmus, which is oscillatory in nature, is usually unmistakable. Although unusual, nystagmus associated with mild esotropia or exotropia may be evident in the newborn. Wild, jerky nystagmus of congenital opsoclonus is a startling and readily discernible finding suggesting midbrain involvement.

Doll's-eye movement is elicited by the examiner by gently rotating the infant's head from one side to the other. The eyes move conjugately in the direction opposite to the rotation of the head. Movement of the head in the vertical position (upward and downward) causes similar movements in the vertical plane. Failure of the eyes to move in the expected manner may suggest abnormalities of cranial nerves or brainstem nuclei.

To gain further information, the infant may be held supine on the examiner's arm as the examiner rotates and watches the infant's eyes. This oculovestibular maneuver causes movement so that there is lateral conjugate deviation in the direction of the rotation. When the rotational movement is terminated abruptly, the eye movements reverse. It is possible to assess the integrity of cranial nerves III and VI with this maneuver.

Facial movements are readily observed during crying. Asymmetry should be carefully assessed to determine whether it is related to an upper motor neuron lesion (such as the so-called central seventh nerve palsy causing contralateral lower face weakness), a peripheral nerve lesion (causing unilateral weakness of both the upper and lower face), or a muscle problem such as hypoplasia of the depressor anguli oris that causes weakness of a lower lip and is also referred to as asymmetric crying facies (Nelson and Eng, 1972). This syndrome is a congenital abnormality that does not involve cranial nerve VII, but may be associated with somatic atrophy, vertebral and rib abnormalities, renal dysgenesis, or cardiac defects. Thus, careful observation makes an enormous difference in helping localize abnormalities of facial movement.

Meaningful hearing evaluation during routine neurologic examination is difficult because of simultaneous visual cues and variable responses.

Crying should not be intentionally elicited by the examiner; however, when it does occur, as it often the case, there is an opportunity to assess cranial nerves IX, X, and XII. During the lusty segments of crying, the infant's tongue and palate may be readily inspected. Asymmetry or loss of tongue bulk may indicate abnormalities of cranial nerve XII or its nucleus. Tongue fasciculations are best identified when the child is quiet and not crying and often occur along the lateral margins and underside of the tongue.

Furthermore, the quality of crying may reflect general neurologic status. An infant with generally depressed CNS function often cries infrequently, and the cry is weak and may be high-pitched. An irritable child with a hyperexcitable nervous system may have a high-pitched shriek.

Cranial nerves V, VII, IX, X, and XII are involved in sucking and swallowing. Swallowing dysfunction requires close scrutiny to determine which cranial nerve or nerves are involved. The gag reflex is present in term newborns and requires normal function of cranial nerves IX and X.

Tests for pain and sensation are imprecise at this age, and the gross response of infants to stroking and pinprick with withdrawal, crying, and change in sucking rates may be the only information possible. More sophisticated testing can be devised during which heart and respiratory rates are monitored.

If necessary, in the presence of olfactory, gustatory, visual, tactile, or auditory stimuli, sophisticated monitoring and scoring of body activity may be performed. All such sensory stimuli produce habituation in the newborn.

THE PRETERM INFANT

The designation of an infant as preterm is related primarily to length of gestation. Term gestation is 38 to 42 weeks from conception. Late prematurity is used to describe infants born between 34 and 37 weeks' gestation. Gestational age must be estimated to appropriately interpret the neurologic examination (Mercuri et al., 2003). Normally, birth weight reflects gestational age; infants born before 28 weeks' gestation usually weigh less than 1000 g (so-called *extremely low birth weight*), and infants born after 31 to 32 weeks' gestation often weigh between 1000 and 1500 g (*low birth weight*).

General Examination

It is sometimes difficult (as well as inaccurate) to estimate gestational age from the date of the first day of the mother's last menstrual period. Examination findings can be helpful when determining gestational age such as skin texture and color, quantity of breast tissue and ear cartilage, and the stage of development of the external genitalia (Table 4-3) (Dubowitz et al., 1970).

Neurologic Examination

Although estimation of gestational age should be made as soon after birth as possible, the neurologic examination may be postponed for 1 to 2 days, depending on the condition of the infant and the need for physiologic support. The examination should be performed while the infant is awake and approximately 1 hour before the next scheduled feeding. Otherwise the child may seem fussy if examined when hungry, or hypotonic and lethargic if examined shortly after a feeding.

Environmental Interaction

Responsiveness increases with CNS maturation. Periods of apparent wakefulness are rare before 28 weeks' gestation. By 31 weeks' gestation, a readily recognizable level of alertness during wakeful stages occurs and by 32 weeks, external stimulation is usually unnecessary to provoke wakefulness. In those born after 37 weeks' gestation, crying is commonly present during wakefulness. By 40 weeks' gestational age, the preterm infant continues to be alert for reasonable periods and responds to visual, auditory, and tactile stimulation. Sleep and wakeful periods are easily identified.

Formal Scale of Gestational Assessment

Using a systematic evaluation of body and neurologic characteristics, Dubowitz et al. (1970) were able to achieve a high correlation with gestational age (Fig. 4-3).

Deep Tendon Reflex Assessment

Deep tendon reflexes vary with maturity (Kuban et al., 1986). In a study of preterm infants of more than 27 weeks' postconceptional age, the pectoralis major reflex was elicited in all, and by 33 weeks' gestation, essentially all demonstrated the Achilles, patellar, biceps, thigh adductor, and brachioradialis reflexes. Infants of less than 33 weeks' gestation had decreased elicitation rates for patellar and biceps reflexes and had overall decreases in reflex intensity compared with their older counterparts. Contrary to conventional wisdom, head position had no effect on the reflexes.

Body Attitude

During maturation, preterm infants adopt typical postures that correspond to gestational age. These postures have been charted and are useful for evaluation of gestational age (Dubowitz et al., 1970).

Muscle Tone

At 26 to 28 weeks' gestation, the infant is extremely hypotonic. When held by the examiner in vertical suspension, the infant does not extend the head, limbs, or trunk. The change from the hypotonia of the preterm infant to the flexion posture of the term infant manifests first in the legs and then in the arms and head. At 34 weeks' gestation, the infant lies in the frogleg position while supine; the legs are flexed at the hip and knee, but the arms remain extended and relatively hypotonic.

Measurement of various limb angles offers some objective evidence for the degree of tone. The popliteal angle, measured by maximum extension of the leg at the knee with the hip fully flexed, decreases from 180 degrees at 28 weeks' gestation to less than 90 degrees at term, and further decreases through the first year of life.

During the traction maneuver, the head lags considerably, with little resistance until after 30 weeks' gestation. The head

TABLE 4-3 External Characteristics Useful for Estimation of Gestational Age

External Characteristics	Gestational Age			
	28 Weeks	**32 Weeks**	**36 Weeks**	**40 Weeks**
Ear cartilage	Pinna soft, remains folded	Pinna slightly harder but remains folded	Pinna harder, springs back	Pinna firm, stands erect from head
Breast tissue	None	None	1- to 2-mm nodule	6- to 7-mm nodule
Male external genitalia	Testes undescended; smooth scrotum	Testes in inguinal canal; few scrotal rugae	Testes high in scrotum; more scrotal rugae	Testes descended; pendulous scrotum covered with rugae
Female external genitalia	Prominent clitoris; small, widely separated labia	Prominent clitoris; larger separated labia	Clitoris less prominent; labia majora cover labia minora	Clitoris covered by labia majora
Plantar surface	Smooth	1–2 anterior creases	2–3 anterior creases	Creases cover sole

(With permission from Volpe JJ. Neurology of the newborn, 4th edn. Philadelphia: WB Saunders, 2001.)

extensors develop gradually, followed by the flexors. By 38 weeks, the head follows the trunk, is maintained briefly, and then falls forward when the infant is pulled from a supine to a sitting position during the traction maneuver.

In small preterm infants, the scarf sign, which is elicited by folding the arm across the chest toward the opposite shoulder, is present if the elbow reaches the opposite shoulder. In term infants, the elbow cannot be brought beyond the midline.

The extreme hypotonia of preterm infants permits the legs to be flexed at the hip so that the heel can be passively brought to the side of the face (i.e., heel-to-ear maneuver). Understandably, this positioning is restricted in the older infant because of increasing tone.

Tone may also be monitored while postural and righting reflexes are assessed. During the stepping maneuver, the 28-week preterm infant will not support weight. However, over the next few weeks, there is gradual support of weight, and by 34 weeks, a good supporting response is present. Tremors and even clonic movements may occur in the small preterm infant but are not normally present after 32 weeks' gestation. Stretching movements of the limbs are common in small preterm infants while they are awake but somewhat less common during sleep. These movements may spread to include the trunk and head.

Cranial Nerves

Some features of the preterm infant examination are different from features of the older infant's examination. Head position is unpredictable in the small preterm infant, but by 35 weeks' gestation, there is a preference for the head to be held to the right, which is normal.

Neuromuscular Maturity

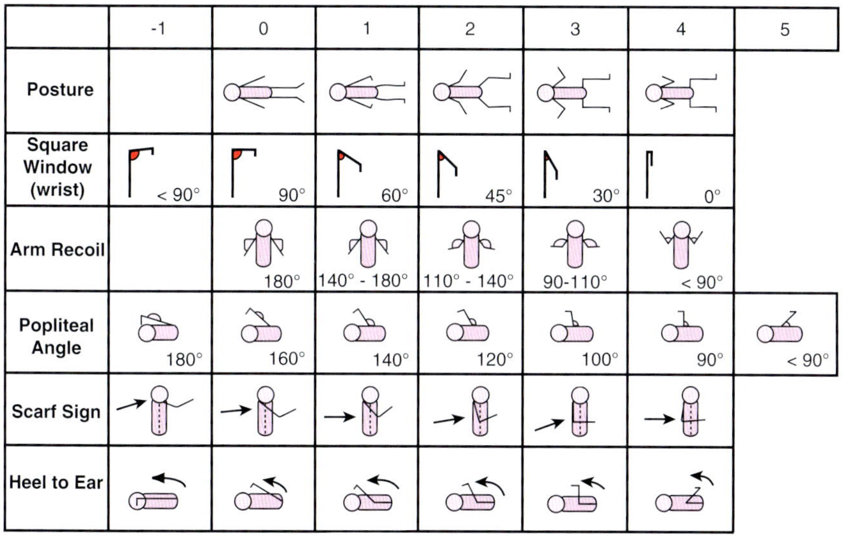

Physical Maturity

Skin	sticky friable transparent	gelatinous red, translucent	smooth pink, visible veins	superficial peeling &/or rash, few veins	cracking pale areas rare veins	parchment deep cracking no vessels	leathery cracked wrinkled
Lanugo	none	sparse	abundant	thinning	bald areas	mostly bald	
Plantar Surface	heel-toe 40–50 mm: -1 <40 mm:-2	>50 mm no crease	faint red marks	anterior transverse crease only	creases ant. 2/3	creases over entire sole	
Breast	imperceptible	barely perceptible	flat areola no bud	stippled areola 1–2 mm bud	raised areola 3–4 mm bud	full areola 5–10 mm bud	
Eye/Ear	lids fused loosely:-1 lightly:-2	lids open pinna flat stays folded	sl. curved pinna; soft: slow recoil	well-curved pinna; soft but ready recoil	formed & firm instant recoil	thick cartilage ear stiff	
Genitals Male	scrotum flat, smooth	scrotum empty faint rugae	testes in upper canal rare rugae	testes descending few rugae	testes down good rugae	testes pendulous deep rugae	
Genitals Female	clitoris prominent labia flat	prominent clitoris small labia minora	prominent clitoris enlarging minora	majora & minora equally prominent	majora large minora small	majora cover clitoris & minora	

Maturity Rating

score	weeks
-10	20
-5	22
0	24
5	26
10	28
15	30
20	32
25	34
30	36
35	38
40	40
45	42
50	44

A

Figure 4-3. A, Scoring system for neurologic criteria.

Continued

SOME NOTES ON TECHNIQUES OF ASSESSMENT OF NEUROLOGIC CRITERIA

POSTURE: Observed with infant quiet and in supine position. Score 0: Arms and legs extended; 1: Beginning of flexion of hips and knees, arms extended; 2: Stronger flexion of legs, arms extended; 3: Arms slightly flexed, legs flexed and abducted; 4: Full flexion of arms and legs.

SQUARE WINDOW: The hand is flexed on the forearm between the thumb and index finger of the examiner. Enough pressure is applied to get as full a flexion as possible, and the angle between the hypothenar eminence and the ventral aspect of the forearm is measured and graded according to diagram. (Care is taken not to rotate the infant's wrist while doing this maneuver.)

ARM RECOIL: With the infant in the supine position the forearms are first flexed for 5 seconds, then fully extended by pulling on the hands, and then released. The sign is fully positive if the arms return briskly to full flexion (Score 2). If the arms return to incomplete flexion or the response is sluggish it is graded as Score 1. If they remain extended or are only followed by random movements the score is 0.

LEG RECOIL: With the infant supine, the hips and knees are fully flexed for 5 seconds, then extended by traction on the feet, and released. A maximal response is one of full flexion of the hips and knees (Score 2). A partial flexion scores 1, and minimal or no movement scores 0.

POPLITEAL ANGLE: With the infant supine and the pelvis flat on the examining couch, the thigh is held in the knee–chest position by the examiner's left index finger and thumb supporting the knee. The leg is then extended by gentle pressure from the examiner's right index finger behind the ankle and the popliteal angle is measured.

SCARF SIGN: With the infant supine, take the infant's hand and try to put it around the neck and as far posteriorly as possible around the opposite shoulder. Assist this maneuver by lifting the elbow across the body. See how far the elbow will go across and grade according to illustrations. Score 0: Elbow reaches opposite axillary line; 1: Elbow between midline and opposite axillary line; 2: Elbow reaches midline; 3: Elbow will not reach midline.

HEEL TO EAR MANEUVER: With the infant supine, draw the infant's foot as near to the head as it will go without forcing it. Observe the distance between the foot and the head as well as the degree of extension at the knee. Grade according to diagram. Note that the knee is left free and may draw down alongside the abdomen.

B

Figure 4-3, cont'd B, Description of techniques used to assess neurologic signs.

The small preterm infant may cry in response to provocation (Fenichel, 1978), but crying often occurs when the infant is unprovoked. By 36 to 37 weeks' gestation, the cry is more vigorous, frequent, and persistent, and it is easily elicited by noxious stimuli.

The pupillary light reflex is not fully mature before 29 to 30 weeks' gestation, and in the resting state, the infant's pupils are usually miotic. The reflex becomes progressively evident and is mature by 32 weeks.

Although they may forcefully close their eyes when a bright light is directed toward them, infants of 28 weeks' gestation or less do not turn in the direction of the light. By using a large target (e.g., large, red ball; hoop; and handful of yarn), visual fixation and even rudimentary scanning and tracking may be evident in infants of 31 to 32 weeks' gestation (Hack et al., 1976). Associated with this response, there may be widening of the palpebral fissure. By 36 to 38 weeks' gestation, the infant rotates the head toward a light and closes the eyes forcefully when a strong light stimulus is presented.

The doll's-eye reflex is elicited in the 28- to 32-week preterm infant who has no compromise of consciousness. The ease of eliciting a response is enhanced because infants do not visually fixate. By 36 weeks' gestation, this response is not elicited in the normal infant.

Developmental Reflexes

Observation and description of the major reflex changes peculiar to the preterm infant have been undertaken by many investigators (Table 4-7).

The *rooting and sucking reflexes* in small preterm infants are perfunctory but become vigorous in infants of 34 weeks' gestation. The Moro reflex, first present in fragmentary form at 24 weeks, is well developed by 28 weeks, although it fatigues easily and lacks a complete adduction phase. Not until 38 weeks' gestation is the entire response characteristic of the term infant observed.

At 28 weeks' gestation, the *grasp reflex* is evident just in the fingers, and by 32 weeks, the palm and fingers participate. Slightly later, contraction of the muscles of the shoulder girdle and elbows occurs during the traction maneuver when the infant is pulled from a supine to a sitting position.

The *tonic reflex* is elicited by turning of the head to one side. The arm on the side to which the head is turned extends, and the other arm flexes. The legs may follow suit, but the response is often absent or subtle. This "fencing" position often can be elicited in the 35-week preterm infant.

The *crossed-extensor reflex* is obtained by stroking the sole of one foot while holding the leg firmly in extension. The response occurs in the opposite leg and comprises rapid flexion at the hips and knees with attendant withdrawal, followed by extension, adduction, and fanning of the toes. The complete response, elicited in infants of about 36 weeks' gestation, is informative when asymmetric. Otherwise, it only establishes that some degree of primitive function is present.

The *stepping response* (i.e., automatic walking) is usually present by 37 weeks' gestation and can be induced by resting the infant's soles on a mattress and rocking the infant gently from one foot to the other. This procedure usually initiates

TABLE 4-7 Neurologic Maturation

Function	26 Weeks	30 Weeks	34 Weeks	38 Weeks
Resting posture	Flexion of arms Flexion or extension of legs	Flexion of arms Flexion or extension of legs	Flexion of all limbs	Flexion of all limbs
Arousal	Unable to maintain	Maintain briefly	Remain awake	Remain awake
Rooting	Absent	Long latency	Present	Present
Sucking	Absent	Long latency	Weak	Vigorous
Pupillary reflex	Absent	Variable	Present	Present
Traction	No response	No response	Head lag	Mild head lag
Moro	No response	Extension; no adduction	Adduction variable	Complete
Withdrawal	Absent	Withdrawal only	Crossed extension	Crossed extension

(With permission from Fenichel GM. The neurological consultation. In: Fenichel GM, ed. Neonatal neurology, 4th edn. New York: WB Saunders, 2001.)

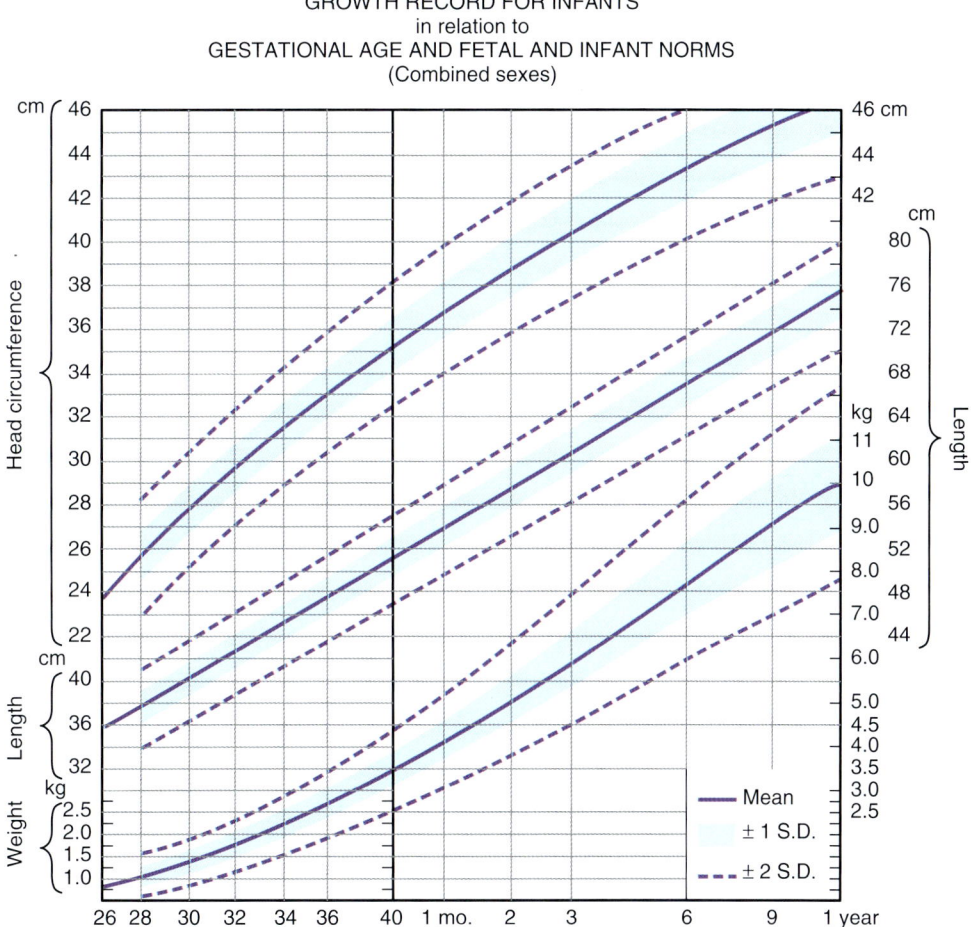

GROWTH RECORD FOR INFANTS
in relation to
GESTATIONAL AGE AND FETAL AND INFANT NORMS
(Combined sexes)

Figure 4-15. A fetal-infant growth graph for infants of various gestational ages. This can be used for plotting growth from birth until 1 year of age after term status has been reached. *(With permission from Babson SG, Benda GI. Growth graphs for the clinical assessment of infants of varying gestational age. J Pediatr 1976;89:814.)*

a walking sequence, which is facilitated by the examiner supporting the infant's weight and tilting the infant forward and begins at approximately 32 to 34 weeks' gestation. The preterm infant usually walks on the toes, whereas a term infant typically uses a heel-to-toe gait pattern.

Ongoing neurologic examinations of the preterm infant are most important for the assessment of development and neurologic status. When the preterm infant reaches the equivalent of 40 weeks' gestation, the neurologic examination results are not the same as those of a term newborn. After reaching 40 weeks' gestation the preterm infant lies with relatively less elevation of the pelvis, and so the prone body profile is flatter than that of the term newborn. The preterm infant continues toe-walking and, even at 40 weeks, often has hypotonia, incomplete dorsiflexion of the foot, and a greater popliteal angle compared with the term newborn.

Assessment of Head Growth Patterns

There are expected changes in head growth. Naturally, size should increase with age, but the shape also changes, becoming more elongated during the first few months of life. Abnormalities of head growth such as microcephaly or hydrocephalus often develop over time, and therefore serial measurements are required to make such diagnoses. A standard plotting curve is necessary to monitor head growth in the preterm infant such as depicted in Fig. 4-15 (Babson and Benda, 1976).

Thus with flexibility and persistence, a newborn neurologic examination is accomplished. As always, it is helpful to be aware of the range of normal variation among children, and any abnormal findings need to be carefully replicated. Involving the family when possible during the examination provides an opportunity to build trust and establish rapport. This is essential to the job of the child neurologist, who not only characterizes the neurologic status and helps guide a diagnostic and therapeutic plan, but must also engage in that most human of endeavors, providing support and empathy to a family facing an unexpected and often frightening future.

REFERENCES

The complete list of references for this chapter is available in the e-book at www.expertconsult.com.
See inside cover for registration details.

SELECTED REFERENCES

Babson, S.G., Benda, G.I., 1976. Growth graphs for the clinical assessment of infants of varying gestational age. J. Pediatr. 89, 814.

Brazelton, T.B., Parker, W.B., Zuckerman, B., 1976. Importance of behavioral assessment of the neonate. Curr. Probl. Pediatr. 2, 49.

Critchley, E.M., 1968. The neurological examination of neonates. J. Neurol. Sci. 7, 427.

Dubowitz, L., Dubowitz, V., Goldberg, C., 1970. Clinical assessment of gestational age in the newborn infant. J. Pediatr. 77, 1.

Fenichel, G.M., 1978. Neurological assessment of the 25 to 30 week premature infant. Ann. Neurol. 4, 92.

Hack, M., Mostow, A., Miranda, S.B., 1976. Development of attention in preterm infants. Pediatrics 58, 669.

Kuban, K.C.K., Skouteli, H.N., Urion, D.K., et al., 1986. Deep tendon reflexes in premature infants. Pediatr. Neurol. 2, 266.

Mercuri, E., Guzzetta, A., Laroche, S., et al., 2003. Neurologic examination of preterm infants at term age: comparison with term infants. Pediatrics 142, 647.

Nelson, K.B., Eng, G.D., 1972. Congenital hypoplasia of depressor anguli oris muscle: differentiation from congenital facial palsy. J. Pediatr. 81, 16.

Popich, G.A., Smith, D.W., 1972. Fontanels: range of normal size. J. Pediatr. 80, 749.

E-BOOK FIGURES AND TABLES

Muscular Tone and Gait Disturbances

Kenneth F. Swaiman and John Phillips

An expanded version of this chapter is available on www.expertconsult.com. See inside cover for registration details.

TONE

Muscle tone is defined as resistance to passive stretch (Sanger et al., 2003). It is conventionally separated into postural and phasic types. **Postural tone** is the result of a steady, restrained stretch on tendons and attached muscles, resulting in protracted muscle contraction. Gravity is the most common stimulus for this response. The axial muscles are primarily involved with postural tone. **Phasic tone** is the result of rapid stretching of a tendon, attached muscle, and most importantly, the muscle spindle. Muscles of the extremities are primarily involved in phasic tone. The response is rapid and short-lived. Phasic tone is the topic primarily discussed in this chapter, and it is referred to simply as tone.

Abnormalities of tone can be broadly defined as hypertonia (increased tone) or hypotonia (decreased tone). Common forms of hypertonia are spasticity, dystonia, and rigidity. **Spasticity** is velocity-dependent resistance to passive stretch. **Dystonia** includes velocity-independent resistance to passive stretch, often with simultaneous contraction of agonist and antagonistic muscles and fluctuating involuntary extremity movement or postures. With dystonia, tone may increase if another body part is moved or touched. **Rigidity** is also velocity-independent resistance to passive stretch in all directions of joint movement, but unlike dystonia there is no involuntary movement or extremity postures (Sanger et al., 2003).

PATHOLOGY

The final common pathway of upper or lower motor unit modification of tone is through the gamma loop (fusimotor) system. Intimately involved with monitoring and effecting tone are the two stretch-sensitive muscle receptors—the muscle spindles and the Golgi tendon organs (Figure 5-1). Spinal cord reflex responses depend on ongoing activity in interneurons.

Stationed in all areas of the skeletal muscle is the muscle spindle, a fusiform-shaped receptor structure. Sensory endings wrap around the central sections of the intrafusal fibers and monitor the stretch of these fibers. Through efferent axons, gamma neurons within the anterior horn of the spinal cord innervate the contractile muscle portions on each end of the intrafusal fiber and enhance the sensitivity of the sensory endings to stretch.

The intrafusal muscle fibers are divided into three types: nuclear chain fibers, dynamic nuclear bag fibers, and static nuclear bag fibers. A solitary Ia afferent fiber provides primary sensory innervation for all three types of intrafusal fibers. A group II afferent fiber innervates chain and static bag fibers, providing secondary sensory endings. The various sensory endings on the different types of intrafusal fibers have different sensitivities to the rate of the change of length. This intricate system of muscle spindle innervation allows the muscle stretch receptors to monitor muscle tension, length, and velocity of stretch, and provide input for maintenance of tone.

It is through their effect on the gamma motor neuron that portions of the central nervous system (CNS) (i.e., motor cortex, thalamus, basal ganglia, vestibular nuclei, reticular formation, and cerebellum) modify tone, with ensuing hypotonia or hypertonia (i.e., spasticity).

The Golgi tendon organs, unlike the muscle spindles, are found in series with the skeletal muscle fibers and are attached at one end to the muscle and at the other to the tendon. Tendon organs are much more sensitive to muscle contraction than muscle spindles. Conversely, tendon organs are much less sensitive to stretch than muscle spindles. Each of these relative sensitivities plays a specific role during the performance of various motor tasks.

EVALUATION OF THE PATIENT
History

It is critical to establish when an abnormality first became evident, and what changes, if any, have occurred over time.

Examination

Preterm infants, even when healthy, are normally hypotonic relative to a term newborn; therefore, corrected ages must be considered when assessing preterm infants during the first months of life.

The infant's tendency to assume unusual postures may indicate the presence of hypotonia—especially the "frogleg" position, in which the supine infant lies with the lower limbs externally rotated and abducted. Hypotonia is often associated with generalized weakness, with resultant poor suck, cry, and respiratory effort in addition to a paucity of spontaneous limb movements. Observation of the chest may disclose pectus excavatum and a bell-shaped chest, indicating relative weakness of intercostal muscles compared with the better-preserved strength of the diaphragm during respiratory efforts.

Tone should be assessed both when the neonate is active and also when at rest. Passive pronation, supination, flexion, and extension of the limbs and gently shaking the hands and feet is required. The scarf sign (wrapping the infant's arm across the chest) and the traction can be helpful as well.

The hypotonic infant will slip through the hands of the examiner when held under the axillae (i.e., vertical suspension maneuver). If the hypotonic infant is supported by the trunk in an outstretched prone position (i.e., horizontal suspension maneuver), gravity causes flexion, or droop of the head and extremities ("inverted comma"). The infant with *hyper*tonia responds differently to these maneuvers. In vertical suspension the infant with spasticity may demonstrate extension and scissoring of the legs with fisting, and in horizontal suspension there can be persistent hyperextension of the legs and neck.

Weakness is often readily diagnosed in the infant and younger child by observation; in the older child, more formal

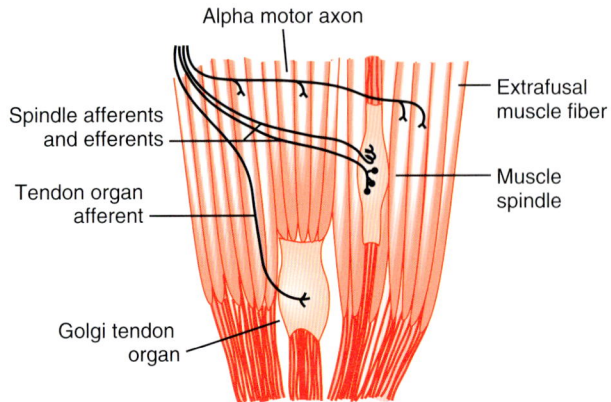

Figure 5-1. Muscle spindles and Golgi tendon organs are encapsulated structures found in skeletal muscle. The main skeletal muscle fibers, or extrafusal fibers, are innervated by large-diameter alpha motor axons. The muscle spindle has a fusiform shape and is arranged in parallel with extrafusal fibers. It is innervated by afferent and efferent fibers. The Golgi tendon organ is found at the junction between a group of extrafusal fibers and the tendon; it is therefore in series with extrafusal fibers. Each tendon organ is innervated by a single afferent axon. *(Adapted from Granit R., 1975. The functional role of the muscle spindles–facts and hypotheses. Brain 98, 531.)*

and discrete muscle testing is possible, as described in Chapter 2.

Deep tendon reflexes should always be elicited. When the lower motor unit is involved, the deep tendon reflexes range from hypoactive to absent.

Whereas hypotonia may occur due to pathology in either the peripheral or CNS, increased tone always involves the CNS. In general terms, dystonia and rigidity are usually related to involvement of the basal ganglia or their output tracts and are associated with normal or decreased deep tendon reflexes. Spasticity can be conceptualized as involving the pyramidal tract system and is associated with hyperreflexia, the sometimes abnormal spread of the reflex (crossed adductor response or Hoffman sign) and extensor plantar responses. An exception is in the acute phase of traumatic injury when transient hypotonia and decreased reflexes can occur (for example, as seen in the so-called "spinal shock").

Specific laboratory studies may be essential in establishing the diagnosis. There is increasing reliance for specific diagnosis on genetic analysis, which has been replacing the need for biopsy in most cases. When upper motor unit diseases are involved, a careful history, electroencephalography, evoked potentials, brain imaging, specific endocrine evaluations, and specific enzyme determinations may be required.

DIAGNOSIS

For didactic purposes and simplification, the motor pathway from the motor neuron in the motor strip to the skeletal muscle fiber can be divided into upper and lower motor neuron units. The upper motor neuron (unit) includes the pyramidal neuron in the motor cortex and the myelinated nerve fiber, which traverses the corticospinal tract and eventually terminates in the internuncial pool in the spinal cord adjacent to the anterior horn cell. The lower motor neuron (unit) consists of the anterior horn cell, peripheral nerve, neuromuscular junction, and muscle. Upper motor unit disease may result in increased or diminished muscle tone in infants and young children, whereas lower motor unit disease generally results in decreased tone.

When assessing a child with hypotonia, it is important to distinguish whether there is a central or peripheral etiology. Impairment of the lower motor unit causes hypotonia and weakness. Hyporeflexia, fasciculations, and muscle atrophy also result.

Inadequate brain control of the motor pathways, or central hypotonia, is the most common cause of decreased tone. The presence of normoactive or brisk deep tendon reflexes suggests that the child is probably not suffering from lower motor unit impairment. The examiner should be alert for other signs of brain dysfunction, such as lethargy, unresponsiveness to the environment (i.e., visual and auditory stimuli), lack of development of social skills in the early months of life, and delayed development of language and reasoning skills in older children.

Diseases of the upper motor unit may be classified according to pathophysiologic causes (i.e., metabolic, degenerative, traumatic, congenital–structural, infectious, or toxic). A similar classification may be used for lower motor unit diseases; such diseases also may be categorized by the anatomic site of involvement.

Increased muscle tone needs to be characterized as spasticity, dystonia, or rigidity. The Hypertonia Assessment Tool provides a convenient approach to patient evaluation, particularly when mixed tone exists (Figure 5-4) (Jethwa et al., 2010). More detailed evaluation of spasticity is possible using the Modified Ashworth Scale (Bohannon and Smith, 1987) and the Tardieu assessment (Patrick and Ada, 2006).

CLINICAL LABORATORY STUDIES

Conventional laboratory studies are rarely helpful, although creatine kinase and thyroid studies should be performed in the presence of hypotonia. Abnormalities of increased or decreased tone may require specific enzyme testing or genetic analysis.

Magnetic resonance imaging (MRI) is the standard imaging modality for the diagnosis of structural CNS abnormalities. Cerebrospinal fluid studies may demonstrate pleocytosis, increased levels of protein, or abnormal proteins, and specific patterns may point to demyelinating conditions or peripheral neuropathy. Spinal fluid neurotransmitter metabolite assessment may be helpful in the evaluation of dystonia. Assessment for leukocyte enzyme activities associated with certain lipid storage diseases may provide definitive diagnoses for conditions that affect the brain alone, the brain and anterior horn cells, or the brain and peripheral nerves.

Some neuromuscular and mitochondrial diseases are associated with cardiomyopathies, and electrocardiography or echocardiography may be of assistance in establishing a diagnosis. Electromyography differentiates neurogenic from myopathic conditions.

The diagnosis of peripheral neuropathy, particularly in conditions that involve the central and peripheral nervous systems, may be readily overlooked without the determination of nerve conduction velocities. Normative data are available for all age groups.

GAIT IMPAIRMENT
Physiologic Considerations

Conventionally, the period from one heel–ground contact to the next heel–ground contact of one foot is one gait cycle; walking can be divided into stance and swing phases. The instant from which heel–ground contact occurs until the instant when contact terminates is the stance phase. The period beginning immediately after the toe leaves the ground

Holland Bloorview
Kids Rehabilitation Hospital

Bloorview
RESEARCH INSTITUTE

HYPERTONIA ASSESSMENT TOOL (HAT) - SCORING CHART

Name:_____   Chart/File #:_____

Clinical Diagnosis:_____   Date of Birth: _____

Limb Assessed: Gender: ☐ Male   ☐ Female

☐ Arm   ☐ Left   ☐ Right   HAT Assessor:_____

☐ Leg   ☐ Left   ☐ Right   Date of Assessment: _____

HYPERTONIA ASSESSMENT TOOL (HAT)

HAT ITEM	SCORING GUIDELINES (0=negative or 1=positive)	SCORE 0=negative 1=positive (circle score)	TYPE OF HYPERTONIA
1. Increased involuntary movements/postures of the designated limb with tactile stimulus of another body part	0= No involuntary movements or postures observed	0	DYSTONIA
	1= Involuntary movements or postures observed	1	
2. Increased involuntary movements/postures with purposeful movements of another body part	0= No involuntary movements or postures observed	0	DYSTONIA
	1= Involuntary movements or postures observed	1	
3. Velocity-dependent resistance to stretch	0= No increased resistance noticed during fast stretch compared to slow stretch	0	
	1= Increased resistance noticed during fast stretch compared to slow stretch	1	
4. Presence of a spastic catch	0= No spastic catch noted	0	SPASTICITY
	1= Spastic catch noted	1	
5. Equal resistance to passive stretch during bidirectional movement of a joint	0= Equal resistance not noted with bi-directional movement	0	RIGIDITY
	1= Equal resistance noted with bi-directional movement	1	
6. Increased tone with movement of another body part	0= No increased tone noted with purposeful movement	0	DYSTONIA
	1= Greater tone noted with purposeful movement	1	
7. Maintenance of limb position after passive movement	0= Limb returns (partially or fully) to original position	0	RIGIDITY
	1= Limb remains in final position of stretch	1	

SUMMARY SCORE – HAT DIAGNOSIS

		Check box:
DYSTONIA →	Positive score (1) on at least one of the Items #1, 2, or 6	☐ Yes ☐ No
SPASTICITY →	Positive score (1) on either one or both of the Items #3 or 4	☐ Yes ☐ No
RIGIDITY →	Positive score (1) on either one or both of the Items #5 or 7	☐ Yes ☐ No
MIXED TONE →	Presence of 1 or more subgroups (e.g. dystonia, spasticity, rigidity)	☐ Yes ☐ No

HAT
DIAGNOSIS:
(Fill in all that apply) _____

HAT Manual can be accessed at http://www.hollandbloorview.ca/research/scientistprofiles/fehlings.php

Figure 5-4. Hypertonia Assessment Scale. *(From: Jethwa, A., Mink, J., Macarthur, C., Knights, S., Fehlings, T., Fehlings, D., 2010. Development of the Hypertonia Assessment Tool (HAT): a discriminative tool for hypertonia in children. Dev. Med. Child Neurol. 52, e83–e87.)*

until the heel contacts the ground is the swing phase. Normally, the stance phase occupies 60% of the duration of the cycle, and the swing phase occupies 40%.

Evaluation of the Patient

Specific aspects of the neurologic examination are particularly relevant to gait. It is important to determine whether abnormalities are focal or diffuse and to note whether there is abnormal muscle tone, weakness, extrapyramidal movements, extensor toe signs, or abnormalities of deep tendon reflexes.

To evaluate gait fully, it is important that the examiner be able to see the entire picture, so the patient should be unencumbered by clothing and is best tested wearing only underwear (or, for more modest older children, short pants and an undershirt). The child's back should be carefully examined with special attention to the lower spine, looking for cutaneous lesions or scoliosis.

The hip, knee, and ankle joints should be moved through their entire range of motion, and the presence of contractures determined. Any pain associated with joint movement should be evaluated. In infants, congenital dislocation or subluxation of the hip is often associated with skin fold asymmetry along the medial thigh. Before the patient's walk is observed, the Romberg test should be performed. Walking should be assessed while the patient is barefoot and also while the patient is wearing shoes. Patients who wear braces should be examined both with and without braces. Among the important characteristics are symmetry of gait from leg to leg; whether walking occurs on the balls of the feet, flat-footed, or on the heels; and the relative stability of the pelvis.

Fluctuating upper extremity postures triggered by walking may suggest a dystonic component. Reduced arm swing is often seen in hemiparesis. The arms should move so that the contralateral arm swings forward synchronously with the swing phase of each leg (see Figure 5-5). When the child runs, abnormal arm and hand postures and movements are frequently accentuated.

An older child should be asked to tandem-walk forward and backward (heel-to-toe); the examiner can facilitate compliance by demonstration. The child should be asked to pivot quickly when changing direction. The backward heel-to-toe walk should also be executed. The child should walk on the toes and reverse direction, remaining on the toes. This process needs to be repeated on the heels.

The clinician should ask the child to circle the examiner, first in one direction and then in the other. If the child has hemispheric cerebellar disease, the child will tend to depart from the circular path toward the examiner or away from the examiner, depending on the side of the lesion.

It is advantageous to have the child climb steps to observe pelvic strength and stamina. Hip girdle strength can be assessed when the child is asked to squat and then stand rapidly. Evidence of hip girdle weakness may also be gained by asking the child to lie down in the supine position and sit up by flexing at the hip. Gowers' maneuver can help identify proximal leg weakness.

While the child walks and runs with shoes on, the examiner should listen and observe for evidence of scraping, scuffing, and slapping sounds. Formal gait analysis may be obtained, which assesses various facets of gait in children.

DIFFERENTIAL DIAGNOSIS
Spastic Hemiplegic Gait

Hemiplegia typically results from disruption of the corticospinal tract above the medulla. Tone is often increased, and posture is characterized by leg extension or slight knee flexion. Hemiplegic gait includes impaired natural swing at the hip and knee with leg circumduction. The pelvis is often tilted upward on the involved side to permit adequate circumduction. With ambulation, the leg moves forward and then swings back toward the midline in a circular movement. The heel-walking exercise is impaired as the patient scuffs the lateral sole and the toe of the shoe while dragging the foot.

The affected leg bears weight for less time than the normal leg during ambulation. The expected rhythmic reciprocal swing of the arm with the stance phase of the opposite leg is absent. Dystonia rather than spasticity should be considered if the arm is held behind the plane of the body on a routine basis.

The etiology of hemiplegic gait cannot always be determined, but one should look for focal brain lesions such as porencephalic cysts, subdural hematomas, cerebral masses, and cerebrovascular accidents.

Spastic Diplegic Gait

Spastic diplegia implies bilateral corticospinal tract dysfunction involving both legs out of proportion to arms. Sutherland and Davids (1993) provided the classic description of four types of pathologic gait patterns seen with spastic diplegia.

Jump gait is characterized by excessive flexion throughout the gait cycle of the hip and knee with plantar flexion of the ankle, resulting in a jumping quality to each step. **Crouch gait** has excessive hip and knee flexion with the ankle in excessive dorsiflexion through the gait cycle and is often seen in patients with severe spastic diplegia or quadriplegia. In the **stiff knee gait** pattern, the knee is stiff with insufficient flexion in the swing phase, causing difficulty with foot clearance, resulting in compensatory hip circumduction and external rotation of the affected leg and a vaulting quality to the contralateral leg during stance. **Recurvatum gait** is less common and occurs

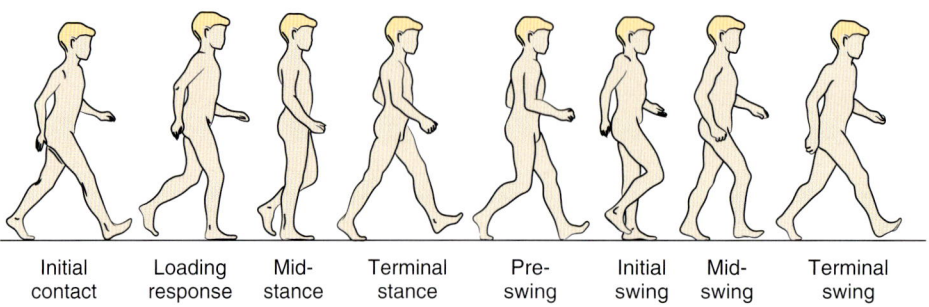

| Initial contact | Loading response | Mid-stance | Terminal stance | Pre-swing | Initial swing | Mid-swing | Terminal swing |

Figure 5-5. Schematic representation of various phases of a child walking. *(Adapted from Õunpuu, S., Gage, J.R., Davis, R.B, 1991. Three-dimensional lower extremity joint kinetics in normal pediatric gait. J Pediatr Orthop. 11, 341.)*

with excessive knee extension in the stance phase of the gait cycle with or without an equinus ankle contracture.

Cerebellar Gait

An unsteady, wide-based, often lurching gait signifies cerebellar pathway dysfunction. Cerebellar hemispheric lesions result in veering to the ipsilateral side. For example, if a child with a right cerebellar lesion is asked to circle the examiner in a clockwise direction, he or she will collide with the examiner within a few circles.

In order for cerebellar impairment to be better observed, the child should be asked to rise from a chair, walk a straight line, and suddenly reverse direction while walking in a tight circle. The child should be asked to tandem-walk along a straight line to facilitate observation of ataxia. The child should be asked to stand with feet close together, first with eyes open and then with eyes closed. This is the Romberg test, and the child with cerebellar difficulties will maintain a stable or mildly unsteady stance with eyes open, but sway or fall toward the involved cerebellar hemisphere with eyes closed.

Compromise of the cerebellar hemisphere is associated with abnormal movement of the ipsilateral limbs. If the anterior lobe of the cerebellum or midline cerebellar structures are compromised, only gait may be involved, without abnormalities of the upper extremities.

The clinical presentation of **sensory ataxia** can be similar to ataxia due to a midline cerebellar lesion. With sensory ataxia, the cerebellum lacks normal sensory input from various portions of the sensory system, including peripheral nerves, posterior roots, posterior columns, or connections leading from the posterior columns to the parietal lobes through the medial lemnisci. This results in marked instability during standing, and when walking there is a wide-based gait. Muscle power remains unaffected.

The patient with sensory ataxia lacks position sense and avoids obstacles by raising the legs inordinately and stepping sharply downward, the heel striking the ground first ("steppage gait"). A fraction of a second later the toe makes contact and produces the second part of a split sound. The child often compensates for loss of sensory awareness by looking at the ground during walking. The child usually has no complaint of sensory abnormality unless ataxia is caused by a global peripheral neuropathy (i.e., one severely affecting all sensory modalities). However, examination will reveal abnormal position and vibratory sense primarily in the lower extremities. The Romberg test is positive as well, just as it is with lesions of the cerebellum.

The **differential diagnosis** of a cerebellar gait depends on time course. Chronic or slowly progressive ataxia may be caused by congenital malformations, inherited cerebellar atrophies, aminoacidurias, mitochondrial diseases, lipid storage diseases, anoxic encephalopathy, demyelinating diseases, posterior fossa tumors, or hydrocephalus. Whole exome sequencing may provide a diagnosis in more than half of patients without a clear etiology for their ataxia (Pyle et al., 2015). Some causes of sensory ataxia include subacute combined degeneration, polyneuritis, demyelinating disease, and Friedreich's ataxia.

Acute onset of ataxia can be frightening for parents as well as clinicians. Although the process is most often benign and self-limited, the differential diagnosis is broad and includes a number of serious conditions. A careful, systematic, neurologic evaluation helps ensure dangerous processes are not missed.

Evaluation of acute ataxia requires neuroimaging to rule out a growing structural lesion such as a posterior fossa tumor. MRI is required for best visualization of the posterior fossa structures. Obtaining urine for catecholamine metabolites might be considered to rule out neuroblastoma, which can present with opsoclonus and myoclonus or "dancing eyes, dancing feet." Urine should also be obtained for toxicology screening (Onders et al., 2015; Monte et al., 2015).

Episodic ataxia might be see with inborn errors of metabolism such as Hartnup disease or maple syrup urine disease; therefore, serum amino acid testing might be considered in the appropriate setting. Epileptic seizures may also appear as episodic clumsiness or ataxia, therefore an electroencephalogram (EEG) might be considered as part of the workup. The extensive differential diagnosis of ataxia is found in Chapter 67.

Acute cerebellar ataxia of childhood is a diagnosis of exclusion, generally felt to be an autoimmune disorder involving the cerebellum. The patient is usually between 1 and 4 years old with a peak in the second year of life (Connolly et al., 1994). The attacks may be so severe that the patient is bedridden, but more often present with unsteadiness and truncal ataxia.

Lumbar puncture usually includes normal opening pressure, mild pleocytosis, and normal glucose and protein, although a slight increase in protein content may be evident after several weeks.

There is no standard therapy for acute cerebellar ataxia of childhood. Full recovery without treatment typically occurs within several weeks. Acyclovir does not appear beneficial; although, there are several case reports of using steroids and intravenous immunoglobulin. Long-term neurologic sequelae can occur.

Extrapyramidal Gait

Extrapyramidal gait disturbance is identified by decreased automatic movements, rigidity, and bradykinesia. The patient often leans forward, with a subsequent anterior shift of the center of gravity; this results in propulsion or festinating gait. The child may lose control and fall if the steps become more rapid and the center of gravity shifts unduly forward.

Characteristically, the affected child may have difficulty with the initial step and may take a few short steps or actually hop and shuffle forward before the walking sequence is established. In addition to the gait difficulties, children with extrapyramidal involvement may have reduced blinking, be devoid of normal facial expression ("mask facies"), and seldom fold their arms or cross their legs.

Other Dyskinetic Gaits

A number of other movement disorders cause unusual gait patterns. Athetosis, when profound, may be associated with overall stiffness and bizarre body postures. The walk may have an associated dance-like or prancing appearance and may be incorrectly diagnosed as a form of conversion reaction. Arms, hands, wrists, and fingers frequently move in deliberate, writhing movements about the long axis of the limb and then slowly reverse the rotational movement with irregular pace.

Other uncommon gait manifestations may accompany torsion dystonia. The foot may be held in plantar flexion or inversion. Manifestations may fluctuate in intensity; therefore, the clinician should be careful not to diagnose a conversion reaction. Children with this condition walk better backward than forward, including during the tandem-walk examination. This pattern of walking better backward than forward also may be found in patients who have quadriceps muscle weakness.

Chorea may also impair proximal hip muscle and trunk muscle action. The result is a rapidly shifting positioning of the trunk and body. The head may also move quickly along, with associated grimacing of the facial muscles, choreiform movements of the trunk and limbs, and irregular breathing patterns and sounds.

Steppage Gait

Weakness of dorsiflexion of the feet and toes and fixed contracture in plantar flexion result in a steppage gait. The contracture most often accompanies weakness of the peroneal and anterior tibial muscles. To avoid stumbling, the child lifts the foot disproportionately high at the start of each stride. Flexion at the hip and knee is exaggerated, followed by a forward flinging of the foot. The toe precedes the heel or ball of the foot in hitting the ground, emitting the first portion of a split sound.

Hip Weakness Gait

Severe weakness of the abductors and extensors of the hip leads to a pathologic "waddling" gait caused when the child walks with a marked lordosis of the thoracolumbar spine with a forward center of gravity to compensate for pelvic instability and a wide-based gait. The pelvis markedly pivots and rotates sharply from side to side as weight shifts. This unusual movement pattern allows balance to be maintained despite hip muscle weakness.

Gait Apraxia

Severe frontal lobe disease can result in gait disturbance despite absence of any direct motor or sensory impairment. Although the child may successfully complete certain simple and automatic movements with the legs, he or she is unable to implement more complex activities, such as tracing a circle with the feet, kicking an object, or attempting to walk in a prescribed pattern. The patient may have difficulty initiating the walking process when already standing and have further problems with execution of the serial acts of rising, standing, or walking. Other frontal lobe manifestations, such as dementia and reappearance of primitive grasp reflexes, rooting, and palmomental reflexes, may be present.

Antalgic Gait (Painful Gait)

Pain can arise from any leg and foot structure, including nails, skin, joints, bone, and muscles. The associated limp is caused by a decreased weight support on the painful leg and increased duration of weight support on the unaffected leg.

Conversion Disorder

Various terms have been used for nonneurologic gait abnormalities such as psychogenic gait disorder, functional gait disorder, hysterical paralysis, and conversion disorder. Presentations are diverse. Characteristic of the gait pattern with conversion disorder is that it may vary from one moment to the next, and there is often a distractible component to the movement disorder. Usually the clinician will find no associated abnormalities of coordination, tone, or strength when the patient is sitting or lying down.

Pediatric patients with conversion reaction gait difficulties are almost never malingerers. Rather, they have physical manifestations of underlying psychological disorders and require supportive and empathetic intervention. Confronting the patient and family with a diagnosis that appears to trivialize their pain and fear is never helpful. Accurate, prompt diagnosis leading to early treatment in a multidisciplinary setting offers the best chance of a successful outcome in pediatric conversion disorders (Schwingenschuh et al., 2008).

It is therefore with careful observation and a systematic approach that abnormalities of tone and gait are appropriately addressed. A thoughtful examination can often avoid the need for extensive diagnostic testing, or can identify patients in whom an expedient workup is required because of serious pathology. Addressing such problems requires an understanding of basic neuroanatomy and neurophysiology, as well as possessing the compassion required to calm a nervous child or listen carefully to a worried parent. This is indeed part of the challenge and satisfaction that comes from the practice of child neurology.

REFERENCES

The complete list of references for this chapter is available in the e-book at www.expertconsult.com.
See inside cover for registration details.

SELECTED REFERENCES

Bohannon, R.W., Smith, M.B., 1987. Interrater reliability of a modified Ashworth scale of muscle spasticity. Phys. Ther. 67 (2), 206–207.
Connolly, A.M., Dodson, W.E., Prensky, A.L., et al., 1994. Course and outcome of acute cerebellar ataxia. Ann. Neurol. 35 (6), 673–679.
Jethwa, A., Mink, J., Macarthur, C., et al., 2010. Development of the Hypertonia Assessment Tool (HAT): a discriminative tool for hypertonia in children. Dev. Med. Child Neurol. 52 (5), e83–e87.
Monte, A.A., Zane, R.D., Heard, K.J., 2015. The implications of marijuana legalization in Colorado. JAMA. 313 (3), 241–242.
Onders, B., Casavant, M.J., Spiller, H.A., et al., 2015. Marijuana exposure among children younger than six years in the United States. Clin. Pediatr. (Phila) 0009922815589912.
Patrick, E., Ada, L., 2006. The Tardieu Scale differentiates contracture from spasticity whereas the Ashworth Scale is confounded by it. Clin. Rehabil. 20 (2), 173–182.
Pyle, A., Smertenko, T., Bargiela, D., et al., 2015. Exome sequencing in undiagnosed inherited and sporadic ataxias. Brain. 138 (2), 276–283.
Sanger, T.D., Delgado, M.R., Gaebler-Spira, D., et al., 2003. Classification and definition of disorders causing hypertonia in childhood. Pediatrics. 111 (1), e89–e97.
Schwingenschuh, P., Pont-Sunyer, C., Surtees, R., et al., 2008. Psychogenic movement disorders in children: a report of 15 cases and a review of the literature. Mov. Disord. 23 (13), 1882–1888.
Sutherland, D.H., Davids, J.R., 1993. Common gait abnormalities of the knee in cerebral palsy. Clin. Orthop. Relat. Res. 288, 139–147.

E-BOOK FIGURES AND TABLES

The following figures and tables are available in the e-book at www.expertconsult.com. See inside cover for registration details.

6 Vision Loss

Douglas R. Fredrick

 An expanded version of this chapter is available on www.expertconsult.com. See inside cover for registration details.

In children, the complaint of blurred vision or vision loss is often nonspecific and may be difficult to elicit. Although most causes of vision loss in children result from ocular problems, neurologic disorders may have vision loss as a characteristic and early manifesting feature. The ability to determine the cause of vision loss frequently aids in the diagnosis of the underlying neurologic disorder, may help determine prognosis, and can be used to monitor treatment efficacy.

VISUAL DEVELOPMENT

Of all the sensory systems, the visual system is perhaps the most immature at birth. Postnatal developmental reorganization of the retina takes place during the first several months of life, with intercellular connections forming between the photoreceptors and inner retinal cells. Myelination of the optic radiations through the temporal, parietal, and occipital lobes occurs in the first year of life. The most dramatic structural reorganization occurs in the striate cortex, where cortical cells responsible for the first stages of visual processing require normal focused visual input to develop in the correct orientation and to achieve maximum visual acuity. As described by Hubel and Wiesel in 1962, visual deprivation occurring in an immature brain causes abnormal formation of the striate cortical cells and decreased synaptic connections and leads to amblyopia. For vision to develop normally, all of the anatomic components of the visual system must be properly formed during development. A structurally intact neurologic substrate must receive properly focused visual information consistently over the first several years of life if normal, maximal visual acuity is to be achieved.

ASSESSMENT AND QUANTIFICATION OF VISUAL ACUITY
Vision Assessment in Infancy

At term, healthy infants display a wide range of visual behaviors, with some infants lying awake and alert and tracking faces from the first day of life, whereas others are seemingly disinterested in their visual world for the first several weeks. Most infants can visually fix on a face and follow by 2 months of age. It is possible to assess vision before this time in the office with no special tools or techniques. The most important requisite for assessing visual acuity is that the infant is fully awake (Huo et al., 1999).

For infants, light is usually an aversive stimulus, and turning on the lights or shining a light in the eye causes the infant to wince. This response is an indication that the child is experiencing some light stimuli. The best stimulus to elicit visual behavior is the face of a parent or caretaker. Positional changes can also be used to the examiner's advantage, because an infant who keeps his or her eyes closed often opens the eyes when held in the supine position and rotated gently about the observer. Another method is to grasp the infant under the arms and lift her or him above the observer's head. The infant reflexively opens the eyes, allowing the observer to attract the infant's attention. As most infants fix and follow by 2 months of age, those who do not should be referred to an ophthalmologist.

Although fixation behavior allows the clinician to determine whether the infant can see, it does not quantify visual acuity. Two techniques have been devised for this purpose. The visual evoked potential is an electrophysiologic test in which visual stimuli are presented to an alert and focused infant, and the cortical response to the visual stimulus is measured in a repeatable and quantifiable fashion (see Chapter 12) (Fulton et al., 1981). The pattern may be an alternating checkerboard, or horizontally or vertically aligned black-and-white stripes. The size of the stripes or checkerboard is described as cycles per degree or cycles per centimeter, which can be correlated to standard methods of visual or decimal visual acuity. Large targets are initially used to confirm that a cortical signal is recorded by occipitally placed scalp electrodes. The stimulus pattern is then slowly decreased in size until a recordable response can no longer be elicited.

A second test used to quantify visual acuity is the forced-choice preferential looking test (PLT) (see Figure 6-1). Instead of using a cortically recorded electrical response, visual stimuli are presented and the child's ability to see is determined by the ability to move the eyes toward the visual stimulus. Vertically or horizontally aligned black-and-white stripes are presented to the child on a test card. When given a choice between a pattern background and a homogeneous background, infants instinctively are interested in the pattern background and make an eye movement or saccade toward the black and white stripes. An observer who is watching through a peephole in the middle of the card records in a masked fashion whether he or she sees the infant make the saccade. Limitations of this test include the need for an infant who is not irritable and a trained observer.

Both techniques have been validated in older children and are reliable and accurate methods to assess visual acuity. Using these techniques, it can be estimated that a neonate's visual acuity is approximately 20/2000. By 2 months of age, acuity has improved to 20/200, and by 1 year of age, it is approximately 20/60. By 4 years of age, infants should see 20/25. At this age, more reliable tests of visual acuity can be used.

Vision Assessment in Children

Once a child becomes verbal but is still preliterate, matching tests can be used to quantify visual acuity (Figure 6-2). In the past, the tumbling E has been used; the examiner asks the child to show the direction of the letter E as it is presented in numerous different positions. These tests have been replaced by matching games such as HOTV cards and child recognition symbols or Lea symbols that ask a child to match test optotypes that are presented in progressively smaller sizes (Figure 6-2). These tests have been validated and are consistent with Snellen visual acuity, which is the gold standard for measurement of visual acuity in children and adults. Snellen visual acuity can be recorded in numerous forms using notations such as 20/20, decimal notation, or *logmar* notation, a method of quantification that allows more useful statistical analysis when conducting studies of visual acuity in children and adults.

ASSESSMENT OF COLOR VISION

Assessment of color vision can be useful in determining the cause of vision loss. Optic nerve injury often causes decreased color vision as its first presenting sign, even before distance visual acuity or the size of the visual field has been affected. The most useful tests for this purpose are the Hardy-Rand-Rittler (HRR) test plates and the Ishihara color plates. The combination of these techniques can separate those children who simply have red–green color deficiency from those with impaired color vision caused by optic nerve injury.

ASSESSMENT OF VISUAL FIELDS

It is not possible to quantify small visual-field deficits in young children. It is possible to diagnose significant hemianopias in small infants using a two-person examination technique. With this technique, one examiner sits in front of the child, maintaining fixation through use of a toy or verbal stimulus. A second tester stands behind the child and introduces a toy or colored object silently in the periphery of the child's vision. When the child sees the toy, he or she generates a saccade or a head movement toward the toy. In this fashion, hemianopias can be detected, aiding in the diagnosis of underlying neurologic problems and determining rehabilitation strategies for children with vision impairment associated with neurologic disease. Older patients can be tested with kinetic perimetry using the Goldmann perimeter or automated visual fields. These tests are particularly useful for patients who are being monitored for visual-field changes associated with benign intracranial hypertension, low-grade gliomas, or midline tumors that, before treatment, may induce ocular or central nervous system (CNS) injury.

ASSESSMENT OF OCULAR MOTILITY

Assessment of ocular motility allows the examiner to assess function of cranial nerves III, IV, and VI (see Chapters 2–4). Ductions and versions can be tested using brightly colored toys and objects. It is important to check the child binocularly first before patching the infant's eye because patching may be distracting and preclude acquiring useful information. Alignment should be checked using the alternate cover test where fixation is maintained and the visual axis of each eye is occluded alternately. Refixation of the eyes during alternate occlusion may indicate the presence of strabismus such as esotropia, exotropia, or hypertropia (Figure 6-3).

Assessment of Optic Nerve and Retinal Nerve Fiber Layer Integrity

Assessment of the health of the optic nerve is an essential task when evaluating a child with vision loss. Either the direct ophthalmoscope or the indirect ophthalmoscope can be used, and when examining a cooperative child through a dilated pupil, this can be simple. However, when examining an unhappy infant with nystagmus and an undilated pupil, this can be a challenge even for experienced ophthalmologists, let alone the pediatric neurologist. The color, contour, and clarity of the peripapillary vessels should be evaluated. If the nerve is pale and flat, that may indicate optic atrophy; if the optic cup is enlarged, that may indicate glaucoma or transynaptic degeneration; if the nerve is elevated and disc margins are blurred, that may indicate papilledema or nerve head drusen. In the past, the description of the nerve was qualitative, or could be documented by photographs, which could be compared in a longitudinal serial fashion. In recent years, spectral domain ocular coherence tomography (sd-OCT) has been used to objectively quantify the contour of the optic nerve and the thickness of the retinal nerve fiber layer (Avery et al., 2015). This technology will be standard of care for following children with demyelinating disorders and children with compressive optic neuropathy and degenerative neurometabolic disorders.

CLINICAL FEATURES ASSOCIATED WITH VISION LOSS

The three features that must be characterized in assessing vision loss are laterality of vision impairment, temporal nature of vision loss, and associated ocular and neurologic abnormalities. Children with unilateral vision loss are frequently asymptomatic. When a child does realize that there is unilateral decreased visual acuity, it is usually because of the sudden discovery of this problem rather than its sudden onset. Mild degrees of vision loss are not usually recognized by the child but are detected by a teacher or healthcare provider at the time of a vision-screening examination. The rapidity of onset of the vision loss also depends on whether the loss is unilateral or bilateral; long-standing unilateral vision loss may not be noticed until the unaffected eye is covered. In contrast, bilateral sudden vision impairment, as can occur with compressive or rapidly demyelinating lesions, may be noticed by the child or caretaker immediately. Associated neurologic signs and symptoms often allow the clinician to localize the disease process before neuroimaging and help the neuroradiologist determine the best type of study to perform.

Because symptoms are inconsistently reported, clinicians must be familiar with the physical signs of unilateral vision loss. During the newborn's physical examination, pediatricians must look for the presence of a red pupillary reflex in each eye. The presence of a white pupil is called leukocoria, and it is associated with poorly developed vision in one or both affected eyes in the infant (Figure 6-4). The causes of leukocoria are variable, and at a minimum, the condition can cause loss of vision; in more serious situations, leukocoria can be associated with life-threatening conditions such as retinoblastoma. Poor vision in one eye from birth often leads to strabismus that is noticed by the caretaker. Nystagmus is common when there is decreased visual acuity in one or both eyes resulting from a structural anomaly or to a functional deficit preventing visual information from being transmitted from the eye to the cortex. In an infant, bilateral vision loss is manifested by strabismus or nystagmus and visual inattention with poor fixation after 2 months of age. Older children with mild vision loss are usually asymptomatic and their problems are not detected until vision is screened by their pediatrician or family practitioner. Children who have progressive loss of visual acuity exhibit behaviors such as sitting extremely close to the television, being disinterested in distant objects or activities, and having difficulty with tasks that require fine visual acuity.

Associated ocular features of vision loss are important to confirm. Infants with poor vision often develop nystagmus by 2 months of age. They are visually inattentive and do not fix and follow well by this age, and they frequently manifest strabismus or a "wandering eye." Older children usually do not complain of vision problems but have strabismus. They often close one eye or squint the eye in different lighting conditions, rub their eyes frequently, and occasionally complain of double vision when strabismus occurs suddenly. Children with significant vision loss have disrupted circadian rhythms and disturbed sleep–wake cycles. Other associated neurologic symptoms include headache, nausea, and vomiting.

EXAMINATION OF CHILDREN WITH VISION LOSS

It is the role of the neurologist or the primary care physician to document decreased visual acuity in children who are suspected of having vision loss or found to have vision loss during a screening examination. Infants should have their visual acuity assessed by their fixation behavior. Extraocular movements should be tested to evaluate cranial nerve function, and pupils should be tested to determine the response to light and presence or absence of an afferent pupillary defect. A direct ophthalmoscope should be used to check for a red reflex, because absence of the red reflex indicates a corneal or lenticular opacity or an intraocular tumor such as retinoblastoma. If the patient has any of these abnormalities, she or he should be seen by an ophthalmologist to assess for structural abnormalities and to recommend additional diagnostic tests. Older children can have their acuity assessed as described earlier. They should have a full motility examination, and an attempt should be made to examine the fundus. The neurologist should feel comfortable using dilating eye drops such as tropicamide. This procedure facilitates examination of the optic nerve head and macula. Any child with abnormal visual acuity, motility, pupillary reflexes, or retinal examination should be referred to an ophthalmologist for further examination.

VISION LOSS IN INFANTS
Clinical Manifestations

Whereas most adults and older children with neurologic disease involving the visual pathways have alterations in visual acuity or visual function, infants usually have problems resulting from failure of vision to develop normally after birth. Parents are concerned that their children fail to use their vision appropriately or never develop normal visual fixation behaviors. These children have no symptoms because they cannot articulate their complaints, but they manifest many signs that can be useful in diagnosing and localizing the cause of the decreased visual acuity. Signs of decreased visual acuity in an infant include failure to fix and follow an object by 2 months of age or visual inattention manifested by the complaint that the infant looks through the caretaker or indirectly at the caretaker's face.

Strabismus is another common complaint in children and infants who have poor visual acuity. Strabismus early in life is not rare. Up to 30% of infants manifest intermittent deviations in the first 2 months of life, with exotropia occurring more commonly than esotropia. The deviation is usually intermittent and decreases in frequency over the first few months of life. Any child who has a strabismus lasting longer than a few months should be assessed for an underlying ocular anomaly.

Nystagmus is commonly seen in children who have bilateral structural anomalies, leading to abnormal visual development. Nystagmus rarely exists at birth. At birth, there may be other movements such as ocular flutter, square wave jerks, or saccadic intrusions that are short-lived and become infrequent over time. In contrast, when a child has a structural anomaly such as bilateral optic nerve hypoplasia, lack of visual stimulation of the striate cortex leads to a sensory nystagmus. The

amplitude of the nystagmus can be quite large between the ages of 2 and 6 months, with the amplitude decreasing and the frequency increasing with time.

Infants with visual problems also often demonstrate behavioral mannerisms that help suggest the cause of the vision loss. Children with retinal dysfunction from congenital dysfunction of the photoreceptors or from retinopathy of prematurity often press their eyes to generate some sort of photic stimulation. Children with cortical visual impairment may demonstrate overlooking behavior, an eccentric fixation, to maximize visual function in the visual fields that are least damaged from the underlying cortical injury. Patients with achromatopsia or congenital glaucoma may be quite photosensitive and demonstrate behaviors to shield their eyes from the light to minimize the dysphoric sensation they receive from visual stimulation.

Differential Diagnosis of Vision Loss in Infants

As with every physical sign and symptom, the history and general physical examination often determine the diagnosis, even before ophthalmologic and neurologic examination. If vision loss is suspected by the pediatrician or family practitioner, the child should be seen by an ophthalmologist before being referred to a neurologist. Most infants with vision loss have underlying ocular anomalies that can be diagnosed and obviate the need for expensive neuroimaging or genetic and metabolic testing. The ophthalmologist can direct the neurologist and geneticist toward the most likely diagnosis to minimize the inconvenience, cost, and morbidity associated with diagnostic evaluation in children with vision loss resulting from neurologic disease.

Structural Anomalies

Retinopathy of Prematurity. Retinopathy of prematurity remains a common cause of vision impairment in infants, causing blindness in more than 500 infants each year in the United States. These patients develop cicatricial changes in the retina leading to vision impairment. Premature infants who do not develop retinopathy of prematurity are still at risk for cerebral vision impairment because of periventricular leukomalacia. Prematurity is the most common cause of pediatric vision impairment in developed countries and the vision loss can be caused by damage to the retina or injury to gray or white matter involving the visual pathways (Dutton and Jacobson, 2001). Children with periventricular leukomalacia can sometimes have enlargement of the optic cup, mimicking glaucoma, but representing loss of nerve fiber layer because of transsynaptic degeneration.

Congenital Cataracts. All infants should be screened for cataracts at birth by their pediatrician or family practitioner. The presence of a clear red reflex makes it unlikely that cataracts are present. An abnormal red reflex should prompt ophthalmologic evaluation to determine the location of the optical opacity.

Treatment involves prompt recognition, removal of visually significant cataracts, and visual rehabilitation with intraocular lens implantation, extended-wear soft contact lenses, or aphakic spectacles.

Corneal Opacity. Corneal opacities usually are easily detected by pediatricians or parents at birth when a white spot, or leukoma, is detected within the cornea (see Figure 6-5). These opacities are associated with other structural anomalies, such as microphthalmos, or small eye, and anterior segment dysgenesis, which may also be associated with glaucoma or birth trauma. These corneal opacities can cause significant vision impairment and are difficult to correct, because the success rate of corneal transplantation is poor in infants.

Ocular Coloboma. Coloboma, or absence of tissue, can affect vision profoundly. If the coloboma involves the iris but not deeper tissues, visual acuity can be normal (Figure 6-6). However, when the coloboma involves the central retina, macula, or the optic nerve, vision can be severely impaired. Children with bilateral colobomata are at high risk for underlying neurologic problems. Any child with bilateral colobomata should be evaluated for chromosomal trisomies and the CHARGE association (i.e., coloboma, heart defects, atresia choanae, retardation of growth and development, genitourinary problems, and ear anomalies). Aicardi syndrome should be considered in any female with a seizure disorder and ocular colobomata (Figure 6-7). Patients with Aicardi syndrome have ectopic gray matter and other CNS malformations; the disorder is X-linked and lethal for males. Coloboma of the optic nerve can also be associated with underlying renal disease, known as the papillorenal syndrome; this diagnosis is made by genetic testing for mutations in the *PAX6* gene.

Retinal Dysplasia. Structural anomalies of the retina not associated with retinopathy of prematurity can lead to significant vision impairment. These forms of retinal dysplasia are frequently associated with a variety of neurologic malformations. An example is Walker–Warburg syndrome, in which congenital retinal dysplasia is associated with cerebral structural abnormalities such as hydrocephalus, agyria, and occasionally encephalocele (see Chapters 25–30) (Liu, 2001). Muscle–eye–brain disease is another example of neurologic and retinal dysplasia resulting from abnormal glial development caused by defective glycosylation of α-dystroglycan. This results in profound CNS involvement and significant vision loss. Norrie disease is an X-linked condition in which retinal dysplasia is associated with mental retardation and deafness.

Optic Nerve Hypoplasia. Failure of the optic nerves to form properly leads to a small dysfunctional optic nerve. In optic nerve hypoplasia, the nerve is small and its morphology abnormal (Figure 6-8). Frequently, there is a double-ring sign; the scleral canal of the optic nerve is present, but the optic nerve tissues comprise only a small portion of the canal, leading to two distinct rings. Children with optic nerve hypoplasia frequently have nystagmus. Children with optic nerve hypoplasia may have de Morsier syndrome, or septo-optic dysplasia, characterized by midline structural defects of the CNS (e.g., absence of the septum pellucidum and agenesis of the corpus callosum) in addition to neuroendocrine dysfunction (see Chapter 97). All children with optic nerve hypoplasia should undergo neuroimaging, with particular attention to the septum pellucidum, corpus callosum, and pituitary body. The presence of an ectopic bright spot places the child at higher risk for neuroendocrine dysfunction. The absence of cerebral developmental anomalies does not mean that endocrine abnormalities will not occur, and children require continued endocrinologic follow-up. There have been numerous cases of sudden death associated with septo-optic dysplasia, in which affected children develop a febrile illness that leads to rapid decompensation and death as a result of adrenal insufficiency. Parents should be advised concerning these potential risks and treat all illnesses seriously.

Ocular or Oculocutaneous Albinism. Normal pigment formation is essential for normal ocular development and normal function of the retinal pigment epithelium. Albinism may involve the eye and skin (oculocutaneous albinism), or only the eye (ocular albinism); both forms are associated with decreased visual acuity. Patients with oculocutaneous albinism are more severely affected, with visual acuity in the

20/200 range, whereas those with ocular albinism have acuity in the range of 20/60 to 20/80. Both conditions manifest with nystagmus early in life. The diagnosis of ocular albinism is made by documenting transillumination defects in the iris during slit-lamp examination. This test can be performed in infants, and it obviates the need for further evaluation.

Leber Congenital Amaurosis. Leber congenital amaurosis is a disorder of the photoreceptors and the retinal pigment epithelium in which photoreceptor function is extinguished. Infants have large-amplitude, slow-frequency, roving nystagmus. They frequently begin to press on their eyes by 2 to 3 months of age, and they may have a completely normal ophthalmoscopic examination with normal-appearing optic nerve and retina. The diagnosis is established by electroretinography. In this test, the electrical amplitude of the retina is measured using a contact lens placed on the eye that is stimulated by bright lights to elicit a cone response and dim lights to stimulate a rod response (Figure 6-9). In congenital amaurosis, both rod and cone responses are extinguished.

Vision Loss Caused by Cortical Visual Impairment

In developed countries, decreased vision caused by cortical or cerebral visual impairment is the leading cause of vision impairment in infants. Damage to the visually immature brain impedes normal visual development and leads to lifelong subnormal vision. The most common causes of cortical visual impairment in developed countries are neonatal encephalopathies (see Chapter 17). The second most common cause of cortical visual impairment is periventricular leukomalacia (see Chapter 19). Injury and ischemia lead to damage in the periventricular white matter and frequently affect visual development.

Clinical features of cortical visual impairment are those of an infant who fails to develop visual fixation behavior after 2 to 3 months of age. These children are often neurologically impaired and have delayed motor milestones and abnormal findings for the neurologic examination. Magnetic resonance imaging (MRI) in affected children usually provides evidence of leukoencephalopathy. Infants with cortical visual impairment do not fix or follow, and appear to be visually disinterested in the environment. Infants commonly demonstrate off and on visual behavior, during which there are moments of what appears to be normal visual fixation interspersed with longer periods of visual inattention. Infants respond well to high-contrast targets such as black-and-white toys and large pattern images. Children with profound cortical visual impairment early in infancy can demonstrate a progressive increase in visual function over several years and may become quite visually proficient. It is important to refer children with cortical visual impairment for low-vision services that can provide sensory stimulation exercises, which improve the visual performance of infants and provide emotional, social, and educational support for parents.

Structural Cerebral Anomalies Causing Cortical Visual Impairment

Hydrocephalus. Ophthalmic signs of hydrocephalus and increased intracranial pressure include the setting sun sign, which describes the infant's gaze held in a downward fixed position, with the eyelids retracted and the infant unable to elevate the eyes willfully. Because the cranial sutures are not closed, papilledema usually does not occur early in infancy. After the cranial vault is closed, papilledema can occur as with any child with increased intracranial pressure (see Chapter 77). Children with hydrocephalus require surgical relief of their obstruction by ventriculostomy or ventriculoperitoneal shunt placement. An ophthalmologic examination should be obtained to document the presence of normal optic nerves or the absence of optic atrophy. Many older children with chronic hydrocephalus have optic atrophy that precludes future useful information about the presence of intracranial pressure because atrophic optic nerves do not swell and cannot reflect increased intracranial pressure. Other ocular signs of increased intracranial pressure include cranial nerve VI paresis, often manifesting as new-onset esotropia.

Structural Brain Anomalies. Children with schizencephaly frequently have decreased visual acuity as a result of damage to the optic radiations and pathways. Contralateral hemianopias and epilepsy are common clinical manifestations. Visual function in children with large schizencephalic clefts, as well as those with porencephaly or hydrocephalus, may improve despite a very abnormal appearance on neuroimaging once the patient is shunted and the cortex re-expands.

There are numerous congenital disorders associated with brain malformations, such as the Walker–Warburg syndrome, Dandy–Walker syndrome, and muscle–eye–brain disease, in which structural brain anomalies (see Chapters 22–27) are accompanied by decreased visual function because of striate cortex involvement or associated ocular anomalies such as retinal dysplasia.

Vision Loss Caused by Epilepsy. Children with epilepsy frequently have poor visual function. When the seizure disorder results from a structural abnormality, there is often concomitant strabismus, nystagmus, and developmental delay. Patients with seizures may develop visual auras before the seizure (see Chapter 54), and functional blindness during the postictal period. Children with frequent seizures throughout the day often have poor visual fixation development. The use of antiepileptic drugs may sedate the child to the point where general development is delayed, and this can affect development of visual acuity. Optimizing antiepileptic drug therapy should be encouraged, because visual acuity can markedly improve when seizures are well controlled. Certain antiepileptic drugs such as vigabatrin may be associated with specific retinal or ophthalmic abnormalities (see Chapter 59).

Delayed Visual Maturation. Occasionally, a healthy infant older than 2 months is referred because of failure of development of visual fixation behaviors. Results of ophthalmologic and neurologic examinations may be completely normal. Such infants may have the condition of delayed visual maturation, a diagnosis of exclusion in which visual development is delayed but eventually becomes normal. Often, the onset of visual fixation is dramatic and usually occurs by 6 months of age.

Diagnostic Evaluation of Infants with Poor Vision

An infant who fails to develop visual fixation should first be referred to an ophthalmologist. Examination by an ophthalmologist most often uncovers the causes of decreased vision, which may be caused by any of the congenital structural anomalies described previously. If examination findings are completely normal, the next considerations are a neurologic examination and possibly neuroimaging.. Neurometabolic testing should be performed to exclude reversible and potentially treatable inborn errors of metabolism involving carbohydrate or urea cycle metabolism or mitochondrial disorders. These conditions are described in detail in various chapters in this textbook.

In an infant with poor visual function but normal neurologic examination results and normal neuroimaging findings,

electroretinography may be used to determine the presence of photoreceptor dysfunction. Such patients usually demonstrate signs of retinal disease, including nystagmus and eye-pressing behavior. Depending on the response to different light stimuli, determination can be made whether there is rod-related (affecting night vision) or cone-related dysfunction that affects central vision or color, or both (Figure 6-9).

VISION LOSS IN CHILDREN

The disease processes leading to vision loss in children are quite different from those affecting infants. Children often demonstrate different signs of vision loss and are frequently able to complain of symptoms associated with vision loss, thus aiding in the evaluation and guiding diagnostic strategies.

Symptoms and Signs of Vision Loss

Children with vision loss frequently do not complain about vision loss unless it is bilateral. Children often do not use the term *blurred vision,* but may say, "I can't see," "things are fuzzy," or "things are double." Signs of vision loss are much more helpful. When the child squints and closes the eyelids, the pinhole effect helps focus out-of-focus light. This behavior is common in children with refractive errors. Those with acute bilateral loss of vision will sit close to the television or become disinterested in activities occurring at a distance. They may hold objects very close to their faces to see them clearly. Children with new-onset strabismus associated with vision loss frequently close one eye to avoid diplopia. They may be sensitive to sunlight and shield their eyes because bright light may markedly decrease their visual acuity, especially when there is associated retinal dysfunction. Children may also tilt their heads when vision is reduced in one eye.

Differential Diagnosis of Vision Loss in Children

Refractive errors are the most common cause of vision loss in children. This form of vision loss is usually detected by a pediatrician, who does a vision screening examination in the office, or by the school district that mandates vision checks in kindergarten or first grade. Vision loss may be unilateral or bilateral. When vision loss is caused by refractive error, correcting the refractive error yields 20/20 vision in each eye.

Amblyopia

Amblyopia is a functional and structural condition wherein an abnormal visual stimulus leads to abnormal development of cortical visual processing cells with smaller cell size and abnormal intercellular connections. Amblyopia results from early visual deprivation, strabismus, or unequal refractive errors. These structural changes are reversible if detected early in life and treated with occlusion therapy. By removing the visual impairment, straightening the eye, or focusing the vision through spectacles, and then patching the unaffected eye to stimulate the immature visual system, amblyopia can be reversed. Whether or not vision can be restored depends on the age of detection. As a rule, most children with amblyopia should be detected and treated by the age of 6 months for the best visual prognosis.

Ocular Anomalies Causing Vision Loss

In an infant with vision loss, it is helpful to approach the eye systematically from an external to an internal point to evaluate for causes of vision impairment.

Eyelid Abnormalities: Ptosis. Ptosis can be a cause of vision loss and a localizing sign of underlying impairment. It may be so profound that it occludes the visual axis, leading to deprivation amblyopia. The eyelid may rest over the cornea and be associated with significant astigmatism that can lead to anisometropic amblyopia. Other forms of congenital ptosis include congenital third nerve palsy and the congenital fibrosis syndrome, which are associated with abnormalities of all extraocular muscles with very abnormal eye movements. Neurologic causes of ptosis in children include infant botulism, congenital Horner syndrome (associated with congenital neuroblastoma), or Marcus Gunn jaw wink syndrome, a synkinesis with eyelid bobbing occurring during masseter muscle function and chewing as a result of synkinesis of cranial nerves V and III.

Corneal Anomalies. Although most corneal anomalies are structural anomalies seen in infants, such as Peters syndrome or scleralization of the cornea, acquired corneal dystrophies and degenerations can lead to vision loss. Some metabolic diseases manifest with corneal changes leading to vision loss. These include the mucopolysaccharidoses such as Hurler syndrome, which is associated with corneal clouding, and Fabry disease, which can lead to deposition of material in the cornea, decreasing visual acuity.

Anomalies of the Retina. Degenerative diseases of the retina can cause gradual loss of visual acuity and may be extremely difficult to diagnose in young children (Table 6-1).

Unlike congenital retinal dysfunction that leads to large-amplitude nystagmus, marked vision impairment, and clear-cut electroretinographic findings, retinal degeneration in older children may be insidious in onset, unaccompanied by significant visual symptoms and with equivocal findings on electroretinography.

One of the most common causes of visual dysfunction resulting from retinal dysfunction is Stargardt disease, also known as fundus flavimaculatus. This disease is a degenerative condition of the retinal pigment epithelium leading to photoreceptor dysfunction. Children have slowly decreasing visual acuity. There are characteristic changes on funduscopic examination, and diagnostic tests such as fluorescein angiography, visual-field testing, and electroretinography can help confirm the diagnosis (Figure 6-10).

Retinitis Pigmentosa. In retinitis pigmentosa, abnormalities of the retinal pigment epithelium can lead to photoreceptor dysfunction and death. Retinitis pigmentosa typically affects rods before affecting cones. This process leads to initial symptoms of night blindness and constriction of the peripheral visual field, eventually affecting cones and central visual acuity. A typical *bone spicule* pattern of the retinal pigment epithelium is diagnostic. Electrodiagnostic tests, such as electroretinography, may be helpful. Retinitis pigmentosa has been characterized as involving rods or cones, or both. All modes of inheritance patterns have been described, and there may be variations of phenotypic expression within families.

TABLE 6-1 Neurologic Disease Associated with Vision Loss and Retinal Abnormalities

Condition	Cherry-Red Spot	Macular Dystrophy	Pigmentary Changes
Neuronal ceroid lipofuscinosis		+	+
Abetalipoproteinemia			+
Refsum disease			+
Cockayne syndrome			+
Bardet–Biedl syndrome			+
Kearns–Sayre syndrome			+
Hallervorden–Spatz syndrome			+
Aicardi syndrome			+
Alström syndrome			+
Gangliosidoses			
Tay–Sachs disease	+		
Sandhoff disease	+		
Mucopolysaccharidoses			
Hunter syndrome			+
Hurler syndrome			+
Sanfilippo syndrome			+
Scheie syndrome			+
Zellweger syndrome			+
Friedreich ataxia		+	+
Niemann–Pick disease	+		
Sialidosis	+		
Farber syndrome	+		
Metachromatic leukodystrophy	+		
Spinocerebellar ataxia		+	+
Gaucher disease	+		
Adrenoleukodystrophy			+

+, Positive association.

Neurometabolic Retinal Dysfunction. Several neurometabolic disorders have been associated with retinal dysfunction and secondary vision loss. In neuronal ceroid lipofuscinosis, abnormal accumulation of neurotoxic products within the retina leads to cell dysfunction and death (see Chapter 41). There are multiple forms of neuronal ceroid lipofuscinosis occurring in different age groups. Characteristic of all forms of neuronal ceroid lipofuscinosis is the development of decreased visual acuity resulting from poor retinal function. Degeneration of the ganglion cell layer results in a typical funduscopic appearance, and ophthalmoscopic examination coupled with electrophysiologic testing can help diagnose these children who have seizures and progressive loss of milestones (Figure 6-10). Retinal dysfunction occurs in inherited mitochondrial cytopathies such as Kearns–Sayre syndrome, in which a pigmentary retinopathy is associated with decreased visual acuity, external ophthalmoplegia, and cardiac conduction defects.

Optic Nerve Disorders

Papilledema. The presence of increased intracranial pressure leads to edema of the optic nerve (i.e., papilledema). The borders of the optic nerve are indistinct and the vessels are swollen; the nerve itself is elevated, with surrounding hemorrhage or exudates (Figure 6-11). Papilledema in children can be caused by obstruction of the ventricular system, craniosynostosis, or communicating hydrocephalus. Whereas early papilledema in adults rarely causes visual symptoms, papilledema can be chronic in children, with slow onset and relatively late discovery of disease, and decreased visual acuity can be a presenting complaint. Usually, this does not occur unless the increase in intracranial pressure is rapid and significant in onset or has been of long duration, leading to chronic axonal compression and edema formation in the retina and causing decreased visual acuity or cell death and incipient optic atrophy. For papilledema in children, mandatory neuroimaging should be followed by lumbar puncture. Pseudotumor cerebri or benign intracranial hypertension is not an infrequent cause of papilledema in overweight children. The diagnosis is made after neuroimaging excludes an obstructive lesion and lumbar puncture reveals increased intracranial pressure and no abnormal cytology. Occasionally, pseudotumor cerebri may be associated with sinovenous thrombosis that can be detected with magnetic resonance venography (MRV). Because many drugs can cause benign intracranial hypertension, the treatment is withdrawal of inciting agents such as tetracycline and its derivatives, and vitamin A analogs. Visual dysfunction associated with possible secondary ischemic optic neuropathic changes should prompt consideration for optic nerve sheath fenestration or lumbar or ventriculoperitoneal shunting to relieve pressure to prevent permanent loss of visual acuity.

Pseudopapilledema. In pseudopapilledema, the optic nerve appears to be elevated, but there is a lack of edema surrounding the nerve, which is seen with true papilledema (Figure 6-12). Pseudopapilledema can be seen with optic nerve head drusen. Optic nerve drusen are extracellular deposits of material within the nerve fiber layer that cause a lumpy elevation of the optic nerve. Later in childhood, the material develops a glistening calcific appearance and can be easily detected by autofluorescence angiography or by ultrasonography. In earlier stages of the disease, the bright signal intensity and reflective characteristics are not as evident, making the diagnosis one of exclusion considered only after lumbar puncture and neuroimaging have eliminated more dangerous conditions. The absence of hemorrhages and of blurred disc margins suggests that pseudopapilledema is more likely to be present. Serial examinations and documentation by photography can help differentiate true papilledema from pseudopapilledema.

Optic Neuritis. Whereas adults with optic neuritis usually have unilateral disease, bilateral presentation is more common in children. Children rarely complain of decreased vision in one eye. Optic neuritis in children frequently follows viral illnesses; it is most commonly associated with inflammation and swelling of the optic nerve head, and may be accompanied by vasculitis (Figure 6-13). In children, there is usually edema of the optic nerve associated with loss of vision and an afferent pupillary defect, whereas in adults, most cases of optic neuropathy are retrobulbar with no visible changes on ophthalmoscopy. Any demyelinating episode may be the first sign of multiple sclerosis, and the risk of a pediatric patient eventually developing multiple sclerosis varies from 7% to 56% (Waldman et al., 2011). Children who have white matter changes on neuroimaging have a higher risk of developing multiple sclerosis and require close observation so that use of interferons may be considered. A particular form of optic neuritis that occurs more frequently in children than in adults is acute disseminated encephalomyelitis (ADEM), as described in Chapter 72. Neuromyelitis optica, or Devic disease, is a rare but debilitating form of optic neuritis that occurs in association with transverse myelitis; diagnosis is made by serologic detection of aquaporin-4 autoimmunity (NMO-IgG), a test that should be performed on all children with optic neuritis.

Optic Atrophy. In children, optic atrophy is often not diagnosed until both eyes are affected (Table 6-2). The most worrisome cause of optic atrophy is compressive disease of the optic nerve. Atrophy may occur from increased intracranial pressure caused by obstructive intracranial lesions, or from compression of the optic nerve from orbital processes or intrinsic tumors of the optic nerve (e.g., optic nerve gliomas). Children with optic atrophy should undergo neuroimaging to establish a specific diagnosis. Children with neurofibromatosis type 1 and optic gliomas require close ophthalmic monitoring, as these tumors may demonstrate spontaneous regression, and treatment should be considered only if there is documented progressive loss of visual acuity or peripheral visual field.

When neuroimaging fails to demonstrate compressive lesions, hereditary optic atrophy should be considered. Kjer optic atrophy is transmitted in an autosomal-dominant pattern; it presents with slow onset of visual acuity loss, first in a 20/80 to 20/100 range and then stabilizing in the 20/400 range. Wolfram syndrome includes optic atrophy as one of its clinical features (i.e., diabetes insipidus, diabetes mellitus, optic atrophy deafness [DIDMOAD]), and this autosomal-recessive condition maps to *WFS1* on chromosome 4p. Neurometabolic diseases may cause optic atrophy and are usually diagnosed by the constellation of neurologic and physical findings associated with the disease. Ischemic optic neuropathy has been described in children with underlying renal insufficiency in which the patient develops sudden changes in blood pressure because of illness or blood loss.

Other disorders that can lead to optic atrophy are the mitochondrial encephalopathies (see Chapter 37). Patients with maternally transmitted Leber hereditary optic neuropathy have loss of visual acuity in the second decade of life. This is associated with characteristic unilateral changes in the optic nerve head and telangiectatic changes in the optic nerve head vessels. There have been numerous genetic polymorphisms described in patients with Leber optic atrophy, and molecular DNA testing is available. Included in this group of

TABLE 6-2 Neurologic Disease Associated with Vision Loss and Optic Atrophy

Category	Disease or Syndrome	Category	Disease or Syndrome

Developmental anomalies	Optic nerve hypoplasia
	  Septo-optic dysplasia or de Morsier syndrome
	Prenatal or perinatal ischemia
	  Infarction
	  Periventricular leukomalacia
	  White matter disease of prematurity
	Cerebral structural anomalies
	  Hydrocephalus
	  Schizencephaly
	  Walker–Warburg syndrome
	  Encephalocele
	  Holoprosencephaly
		Inflammatory conditions	Sarcoidosis
			Systemic lupus erythematosus
			Sjögren syndrome
			Collagen–vascular disease
			Autoimmune disorders
			Postvaccination inflammatory reaction

		Ischemic conditions	Renal disease Sickle cell disease Moyamoya disease
		Trauma	Direct Indirect

Degenerative disease	Leukodystrophies
	  Adrenoleukodystrophy
	  Krabbe leukodystrophy
	  Pelizaeus–Merzbacher disease
	  Alexander disease
	  Canavan disease
	  Leigh disease
	Lysosomal disorders
	  Gangliosidoses GM_1 and GM_2
	  Mucopolysaccharidoses
	  Niemann–Pick disease
	Ataxias
	  Friedreich ataxia
	  Charcot–Marie–Tooth disease
	Miscellaneous conditions
	  Neuronal ceroid lipofuscinosis
	  Wolfram syndrome
	  Zellweger syndrome
		Demyelinating conditions	Optic neuritis
			Acute disseminated encephalomyelopathy
			Multiple sclerosis
			Leigh disease
			Aquaporin channelopathies

		Compressive conditions	Pituitary tumor Hypothalamic tumor Craniopharyngioma Optic nerve glioma Optic nerve meningioma Rhabdomyosarcoma Papilledema Idiopathic intracranial hypertension Craniosynostosis or craniofacial dysostosis Germinoma Primitive neuroectodermal tumor
		Hereditary conditions	Kjer optic atrophy Leber congenital amaurosis Mitochondrial cytopathies Congenital disorders of glycosolation Leber hereditary optic neuropathy
Infectious diseases	Lyme disease—*Borrelia burgdorferi* Cat-scratch disease—*Bartonella henselae* Syphilis Tuberculosis West Nile virus Epstein-Barr virus Cryptococcus Human immunodeficiency virus (HIV)	Toxicities	Lead Copper Streptomycin Hydroxyquinolones Methanol Ethambutol

disorders is Kearns–Sayre syndrome, mitochondrial encephalomyopathy with lactic acidosis and strokelike syndrome (MELAS), and myoclonic epilepsy with ragged red fiber disease (MERRF) (see Chapter 37).

Cerebral Vision Impairment

Whereas cerebral vision impairment in infants results from ischemic encephalopathy or white matter disease, impairment in older children usually is traumatic in nature. An ischemic episode such as a near-drowning, meningitis, or stroke can also cause cortical vision impairment. Toxic cortical blindness can be caused by vincristine, cyclosporine, and tacrolimus. Visual acuity can be profoundly affected and show slow, progressive improvement over 1 to 2 years. The diagnosis is made by a combination of history, neuroimaging, and normal ocular examination findings.

NYSTAGMUS IN INFANCY

Like the visual system, the ocular motor system is immature at birth. Abnormal eye movement such as ocular flutter, bobbing, saccadic intrusions, or saccadic paresis may be transient in the first few weeks of life, but they usually resolve completely. Nystagmus, or oscillation of the eyes in a stereotypic fashion, is rarely seen at birth but usually develops by 2 months of age. There are three primary causes of nystagmus in infancy—problem with the eyes, problem with the brain, or infantile nystagmus—each having different visual consequences and health considerations (Papageorgiou et al., 2014). The presence of nystagmus can make assessment of visual function difficult, as normal fixation responses will be abnormal. All infants and children with nystagmus without a previous neurologic diagnosis should be seen by an ophthalmologist to determine whether there is an ocular cause for the abnormal eye movements (Table 6-3).

TRANSIENT EPISODIC VISION LOSS IN CHILDREN

To hear a child complain about occasional abnormal vision is not a rare phenomenon. School-aged children frequently complain about blurred vision after prolonged distance or near-visual tasks such as reading, taking tests, or taking notes from the white board. These symptoms are usually brief and

TABLE 6-3 Causes of Bilateral Infantile Vision Impairment Manifesting with Nystagmus by Age 2 Months

Category	Cause of Impairment
Disorders of corneal clarity	Developmental anomalies Peters syndrome Rieger syndrome Sclerocornea Congenital glaucoma Forceps birth trauma
Crystalline lens opacity	Congenital cataract
Uveal anomalies	Aniridia Oculocutaneous or ocular albinism
Vitreous anomalies	Vitreous hemorrhage Persistent hyperplastic primary vitreous
Retinal anomalies	Leber congenital amaurosis Achromatopsia or monochromatopsia Retinopathy of prematurity Retinal dysplasia Chorioretinal scarring Congenital toxoplasmosis Chorioretinal coloboma
Optic nerve anomalies	Optic nerve hypoplasia Optic nerve atrophy Optic nerve coloboma Morning glory disc

resolve after a short period of rest. Complaints of more profound transient and episodic visual loss or blindness should make the clinician consider three causes: intracranial hypertension, migraine, and functional vision loss. Increased intracranial pressure can cause transient obscuration of vision, especially when children change position from supine to standing. They may also complain of positive scotoma and "black-out spells." Migraines in children do not usually manifest as classic migraines but frequently have an atypical presentation with vision loss, frequent episodes of abdominal pain, and absence of headache. A child may complain about decreased visual acuity but have normal vision without ocular pathology. This form of functional visual loss has a variety of causes and may be difficult to diagnose and detect. Children most often complain about bilateral vision loss and initially report visual acuity in the 20/400 range. Their symptoms may be exaggerated, but the children rarely bump into objects when entering a room despite reports of markedly diminished visual acuity. This is a diagnosis of exclusion, and children should be carefully examined, perhaps on repeated occasions, before the diagnosis is made (Table 6-4).

TABLE 6-4 Causes of Vision Loss, Associated Findings, and Diagnostic Recommendations

Cause of Vision Loss	Associated Findings/Syndrome	Diagnostic Evaluation
Leber congenital amaurosis	Large-amplitude, slow-frequency, roving nystagmus at 2 months of age; eye pressing (oculodigital sign)	Electroretinogram for photoreceptor function; renal consultation to rule out Senior syndrome
Ocular albinism/ oculocutaneous albinism	Moderate-amplitude nystagmus by 2 months, fair skin, X-linked inheritance; rule out Chediak–Higashi and Hermansky–Pudlak syndromes	Slit-lamp examination for iris transillumination defects; examine mother for signs of retinal hypopigmentation
Aniridia	Nystagmus at 2 months; consider WAGR syndrome	Slit-lamp examination shows lack of iris development; obtain genetic consult and urologic consultation to rule out and follow for Wilms tumor
Achromatopsia	High-frequency, low-amplitude nystagmus caused by lack of cone photoreceptor development; photophobia	Electroretinogram for photoreceptor function
Optic nerve coloboma	Nystagmus if severe and bilateral, strabismus if unilateral; CHARGE sequence, papillorenal syndrome	MRI of brain to rule out encephalocele and other structural anomalies; genetic and renal consultation to rule out other syndromes
Optic nerve hypoplasia	Nystagmus by 2 months if bilateral, strabismus if unilateral; septo-optic dysplasia/Aicardi syndrome; hypoglycemic at birth, signs of panhypopituitarism	MRI of brain—look for agenesis of corpus callosum, absence of septum pellucidum, absence or ectopy of pituitary bright spot, gray matter heterotopia in Aicardi syndrome
Retinopathy of prematurity	History of prematurity, oculodigital sign	Ophthalmic examination
Norrie disease	Nystagmus at 2 months, X-linked, bilateral retinal detachment with cataract	Ophthalmic examination; genetic consultation
Congenital cataract	Nystagmus at 2 months if complete cataract, strabismus if unilateral; stigmata of trisomies; metabolic signs if enzymatic or mitochondrial	Ophthalmic examination; if bilateral, consider galatosemia screen, urine amino acids (Lowe syndrome), urine for reducing substances, genetic consultation; examine parents to rule out autosomal-dominant cataract; TORCH evaluation

Continued on following page

TABLE 6-4 Causes of Vision Loss, Associated Findings, and Diagnostic Recommendations *(Continued)*

Cause of Vision Loss	Associated Findings/Syndrome	Diagnostic Evaluation
Optic neuritis	Vision loss, possible pain with eye movements, afferent pupil defect, focal neurologic findings; ADEM, neuromyelitis optica (Devic disease), multiple sclerosis, syphilis, Lyme disease, cat-scratch disease, toxin (nutritional, ethambutol, methanol), Leber hereditary optic neuropathy	Ophthalmic examination, MRI, lumbar puncture with opening pressure, serology and monoclonal bands, infectious disease consultation, genetic evaluation if positive family history; test for Leber hereditary optic neuropathy
Optic atrophy	Vision loss, strabismus, associated focal neurologic findings, endocrine signs/symptoms, deafness, loss of milestones in NCL/neurometabolic disorders/Leigh disease; family history	Attention to pre- and perinatal history, neuroimaging, genetic consultation, endocrinologic consultation, assess for mitochondrial dysfunction
Cerebral visual impairment	Vision loss, sterotypic features: off/on, saccadic paresis; history of pre-/perinatal ischemia, intraventricular hemorrhage/prematurity, meningitis, cerebral developmental anomaly, cerebral palsy, seizure disorder	Neuroimaging; genetics if no known etiology
Refractive errors/amblyopia	Often sudden discovery or during screening examination; family history common; nonfocal neurologic examination; refractive errors correct with pinhole	Ophthalmic examination
Papilledema	Vision loss only if chronic or rapid onset, scotoma on change in position, constricted fields, esotropia with abducens paresis, headache, nausea; risk factors for idiopathic intracranial hypertension—obese, female, estrogen use, tetracycline, vitamin A, steroids, growth hormone, cerebral venous thrombosis	Ophthalmic examination—loss of spontaneous venous pulsations and edema of optic nerve, MRI and MRV, lumbar puncture with opening pressure

ADEM, acute disseminated encephalomyelitis; CHARGE, coloboma, heart defects, atresia choanae, retardation of growth and development, genitourinary problems, and ear anomalies; MRI, magnetic resonance imaging; MRV, magnetic resonance venography; NCL, neuronal ceroid lipofuscinosis; TORCH, toxoplasmosis, rubella, cytomegalovirus, herpes simplex virus; WAGR, Wilms tumor, genitourinary abnormalities, and mental retardation.

REFERENCES

The complete list of references for this chapter is available in the e-book at www.expertconsult.com.
See inside cover for registration details.

SELECTED REFERENCES

Avery, R.A., Rajjoub, R.D., Trimboli-Heidler, C., et al., 2015. Applications of optical coherence tomography in pediatric clinical neuroscience. Neuropediatrics 46 (2), 88–97.

Dutton, G.N., Jacobson, L.K., 2001. Cerebral visual impairment in children. Semin. Neonatol. 6 (6), 477–485.

Fulton, A.B., Hansen, R.M., Manning, K.A., 1981. Measuring visual acuity in infants. Surv. Ophthalmol. 25 (5), 325–332.

Hubel, D.N., Wiesel, T.N., 1962. Receptive fields, binocular interactions and functional architecture in the cats visual cortex. J. Physiol. 160, 106.

Huo, R., Burden, S.K., Hoyt, C.S., et al., 1999. Chronic cortical visual impairment in children: aetiology, prognosis, and associated neurological deficits. Br. J. Ophthalmol. 83 (6), 670–675.

Liu, G.T., 2001. Visual loss in childhood. Surv. Ophthalmol. 46 (1), 35–42.

Papageorgiou, E., McLean, R.J., Gottlob, I., 2014. Nystagmus in childhood. Pediatr. Neonatol. 55 (5), 341–351.

Waldman, A.T., Stull, L.B., Galetta, S.L., et al., 2011. Pediatric optic neuritis and risk of multiple sclerosis: meta-analysis of observational studies. J. AAPOS 15 (5), 441–446.

E-BOOK FIGURES AND TABLES

The following figures and tables are available in the e-book at www.expertconsult.com. See inside cover for registration details.

Fig. 6-1 Vision assessment in infancy.
Fig. 6-2 Vision assessment in children.
Fig. 6-3 Assessment of ocular motility.
Fig. 6-4 Spectral domain optical coherence tomography.
Fig. 6-5 Corneal edema caused by a forceps injury at the time of delivery.
Fig. 6-6 Ocular coloboma.
Fig. 6-7 Optic nerve hypoplasia and chorioretinal lacunas seen in patients with Aicardi syndrome.
Fig. 6-8 Optic nerve hypoplasia.
Fig. 6-9 Electroretinogram for a normal child (left) and a child with Leber congenital amaurosis (right).
Fig. 6-10 Degenerative retinal disease.
Fig. 6-11 Severe papilledema in a patient with idiopathic intracranial hypertension.
Fig. 6-12 Optic disc drusen.
Fig. 6-13 Frosted angiitis in an immunosuppressed patient with cytomegalovirus retinitis and neuritis.

7 Hearing Impairment

Lionel Van Maldergem, Guy Van Camp, and Paul Deltenre

An expanded version of this chapter is available on www.expertconsult.com. See inside cover for registration details.

INTRODUCTION

The terms "hearing loss" (HL) and "hearing impairment" designate an abnormal auditory function whatever its type, localization, or the mechanism underlying it. In most circumstances the term "hearing loss" is used after a standard clinical audiogram has indicated elevated thresholds for detection of sound waves. But the hearing process cannot be reduced to this quantitative assessment. To fulfill its two main ecological functions, namely, keeping us aware of what is happening in our surroundings and sound-based communication, a normal auditory function must be able to influence behavior in a way appropriate to the meaning of the physical event having produced the detected sound. In real life, we do not perceive sound waves; we perceive mental images of their sources. Not only do we identify the sources around us, but also we are able to localize them in space. In case they are moving, we perceive whether they are approaching us or moving away. In most real-life situations there are several simultaneously active sound sources. The ears receive a mixture of sound waves, which our auditory system interprets to reconstruct the mental images of their respective sources. Our peripheral sensory organ named the cochlea provides the brain with a neural representation of sounds through the cochlear nerve. The cochlea does not perform source reconstruction: it has an analytic role based on filtering of complex multisource environmental sound waves, parsing them into an array of narrow frequency bands. The neural code conveyed by each afferent fiber of the cochlear nerve represents fluctuations in time of environmental sound intensities within a specific tonotopic frequency channel. As shown in Figure 7-1, the output of each cochlear filter comprises two components: the temporal fine structure that represents the instantaneous acoustic pressure variations and the envelope describing the overall amplitude variations over time.

The central auditory nervous system (CANS) is faced with the enormous neurocomputing challenge of reconstructing sound sources from these individual spectro-temporal profiles. Processes by which the brain reconstructs our auditory environment from cochlear output have been named auditory scene analysis (ASA). These processes allow us to selectively attend to one among several speakers, a situation described as the cocktail party problem (McDermott, 2009). Deterioration of ASA mechanisms can occur in the absence of measurable threshold elevation and lead to auditory complaints taking the general form of poor understanding in noise despite normal thresholds, a combination recognized as obscure auditory dysfunction, King–Kopetzky syndrome, or central auditory processing disorder (CAPD). Efficiency of ASA processes can also be reduced as a consequence of peripheral sensory defects that not only cause a threshold elevation but also distort the primary neural code conveying the details of suprathreshold sound components.

ANATOMY AND PHYSIOLOGY OF THE EAR AND AUDITORY SYSTEM

Interested readers will find information on the anatomy and physiology of the auditory system in the online version of this chapter as well as in recent books (e.g., Pickles, 2012) or on the Cochlea and Neuroreille websites (http://www.cochlea.eu/en; http://www.neuroreille.com/promenade/english/start_gb.htm).

HEARING LOSS
HL Classification

Multiple descriptive dimensions of HL are used to provide a comprehensive evaluation in a given patient:

Classification by Definition of Impairment Site

Current clinical and electrophysiological tools allow delineating four main categories:

1. Conductive HL. This type of impairment is caused by defective transmission of sound to the cochlea. It can occur because of an external ear or middle ear defect. By definition, the inner ear remains normal. Owing to bone conduction, conductive HL never exceeds 60 dB.

2. Sensorineural HL. This term points to a defect anywhere along the auditory pathway between the cochlea and the cerebral cortex. The vast majority are of endocochlear origin, a term referring to nonconductive HL secondary to cochlear defects, including the cochlear nerve in its intracochlear segment. Clinical and electrophysiological tools often do not allow precise identification of the defective structure involved in endocochlear deafness in contrast with major genetic advances made in recent years. Improved imaging and electrophysiological tools allow proper detection of many of the central defects.

3. Auditory Neuropathy Spectrum Disorder. Preserved outer hair cell (OHC) responses (cochlear microphonic and/or otoacoustic emissions [OAEs]) and absent or severely disrupted auditory brainstem responses (ABR) including wave I are mandatory to make a diagnosis of auditory neuropathy spectrum disorder (ANSD). Many mechanisms interfering with the normal synchrony of the primary neural code sent to the brain by the cochlear nerves can lead to an ANSD profile (Starr et al., 2008). These include inner hair cell defects, ribbon synapse defects, or a defect of the cochlear nerve itself. Clinical manifestations are dominated by speech misunderstanding, usually worse than that which could be anticipated from the audiogram. Whenever the cochlear nerve alone is involved, a diagnosis of true neuropathy can be made.

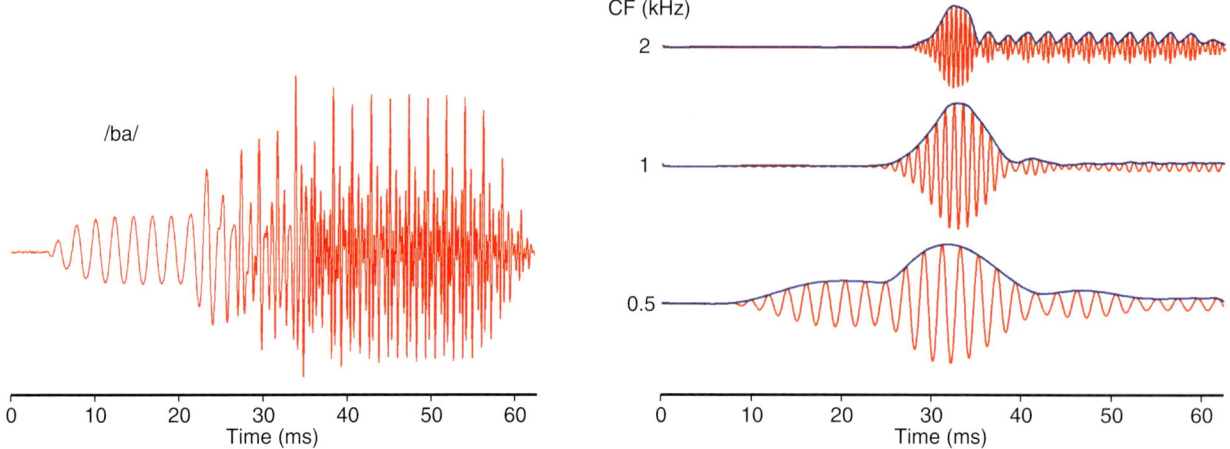

Figure 7-1. Original acoustic waveform of the French synthetic syllable /ba/ (*courtesy W. Serniclaes, ULB, Brussels*) (**A**) compared with simulation of the output of three normal cochlear filters, respectively, centered on 0.5, 1, and 2 kHz (**B**), fed with the /ba/ waveform. Each cochlear filter extracts a spectral portion of the syllable and yields a composite signal describing variations of the temporal fine structure *(red)* and envelope *(blue)* components over time. CF, central frequency; ENV, envelope; TFS, temporal fine structure.

TABLE 7-1 Hearing Loss Classification by Degree: ASHA and BIAP Schemes

Degree of HL	ASHA Average Loss (dB HL)	BIAP	Speech Perception
Normal to *normal-subnormal*	−10 to 15	*<20*	
Slight	16 to 25	*21 to 40*	Normally voiced speech perceived; whispered/distant speech missed
Mild	26 to 40	—	
Moderate to *moderate 1st degree*	41 to 55	*41 to 55*	Voice level must be raised above normal to be perceived. Lip reading
Moderately severe to *moderate 2nd degree*	56 to 70	*56 to 70*	may be used to compensate.
Severe	71 to 90	*70 to 90*	Voice level must be raised and delivered close to the ear.
Profound	>90	*>90*	No speech perception

ASHA, American Speech-Language-Hearing Association; BIAP, European Bureau International d'Audio-Phonologie; HL, hearing loss.

4. Central HL. Compression of brainstem auditory pathways by neighboring tumors is rare in children. Intrinsic tumors such as brainstem gliomas may interfere with auditory function. Hypomyelinating and demyelinating diseases may occasionally cause central HL (Pelizaeus–Merzbacher disease, adrenoleukodystrophy, multiple sclerosis, acute disseminated encephalomyelitis). Cortical deafness describes very rare instances of abnormal auditory reactivity caused by extensive bilateral auditory cortex destruction or deafferentation. Electrophysiological recordings exclude a cochlear origin, whereas behavioral testing is indicative of auditory agnosia. Most cases are attributable to cerebrovascular diseases and usually occur in adults. Landau–Kleffner syndrome produces similar central disturbances, affecting children who often appear to have HL of various severities related to auditory agnosia. Classical kernicterus and mild forms often called bilirubin-induced neurologic dysfunction spare the cochlea but affect the auditory nerve and central auditory pathways depending on the degree of hyperbilirubinemia. Resulting hearing deficits may range from normal thresholds with defective central processing to profound deafness.

Classification by Severity and Profile of Thresholds Elevation

Most severity scales categorize HL severity on the basis of average audiometric pure-tones thresholds obtained at three to four frequencies: 0.5, 1, 2, and 4 kHz. Thresholds are expressed in dB on the hearing level scale used in clinical audiometry, and so 0 dB represents the average threshold of normal subjects whatever the frequency. Most systems share four main descriptive categories: mild, moderate, severe, and profound, but may vary in their details. Table 7-1 illustrates a simplified version of the classifications recommended by the American Speech-Language-Hearing Association (ASHA; http://www.asha.org/public/hearing/Degree-of-Hearing-Loss/) and the European Bureau International d'Audio-Phonologie (BIAP; http://www.biap.org/index.php).

EVALUATION OF AUDITORY FUNCTION

Hearing tests are either behavioral (i.e., they seek a behavioral reaction to stimulus) or objective (i.e., independent from the subject's willingness and cognitive state), being based on stimulus-induced physiological responses.

The Cross-Check Principle

The cross-check principle, a cornerstone of pediatric audiology, states that a battery of independent tests is needed to provide an accurate description of hearing problems.

Behavioral Methods

Behavioral methods depend on the developmental age and neurologic status, and reliable thresholds are often impossible to obtain in pediatric patients with moderate to profound intellectual disability. Even in normally developing children, one must wait until 36 months of age before reliable thresholds can be obtained across the entire population.

Objective Methods

Tympanometry

Acoustic immittance measurements by tympanometry yield a series of objective parameters: tympanic admittance or compliance, related to tympanic membrane mobility, Eustachian tube function, and external auditory ear canal volume, which is increased in case of perforated eardrum or permeable transtympanic ventilating tubes.

Objective Audiometry

Otoacoustic emissions. OAEs are byproducts of sound processing by OHCs that lose control of a small fraction of incident energy and send it back to middle ear. OAEs are rapidly abolished with threshold elevation (≥35 dB) in sensorineural HL (SNHL) involving OHCs, which is the case of most endocochlear HLs, but not of retrocochlear HLs and ANSD.

Auditory evoked potentials. They are classified according to three main characteristics: their latency range, time course, and dependency on cognitive processing. Early auditory evoked potentials (AEPs) represent the cornerstone of pediatric objective audiometry. Click-evoked ABRs are the centerpiece of electrophysiological evaluation of children at risk for hearing and complex neurologic disorders. Figure 7-6 illustrates how ABR morphology, amplitude, and latency evolve according to click level in a normal subject.

IMAGING

Magnetic resonance imaging (MRI) is the main technique used for patients with SNHL for defining intralabyrinthine and intracranial anomalies. Computed tomography (CT) is more useful for middle ear and temporal bone assessment.

HEARING PROBLEMS IN THE PEDIATRIC POPULATION

Conductive HL and External Ear Malformations

Conductive HL is the most common cause of HL in children. Eighty percent of all children have had at least one episode of otitis media with effusion by age 10 years. Reversible conductive HL often coexists with cochlear HL, the combination being designated as mixed HL. An additional conductive loss may severely reduce auditory performances in the case of cochlear HL.

Congenital malformations of the external or middle ear are often unilateral. Congenital anomalies of the external ear have an incidence of about 1:6000. Inner ear malformations are present in 11% to 30% of individuals with outer and middle ear malformations. External and inner ear malformations frequently have a genetic basis and are rarely acquired. Syndromes associated with pinnae malformation include the branchio-oto-renal syndrome (OMIM 113650); auriculo-facio-vertebral syndrome or Goldenhar syndrome (OMIM 164210); coloboma, heart defect, atresia choanae, retarded growth, genital and ear anomalies (CHARGE) syndrome (OMIM 214800); Treacher–Collins syndrome (OMIM

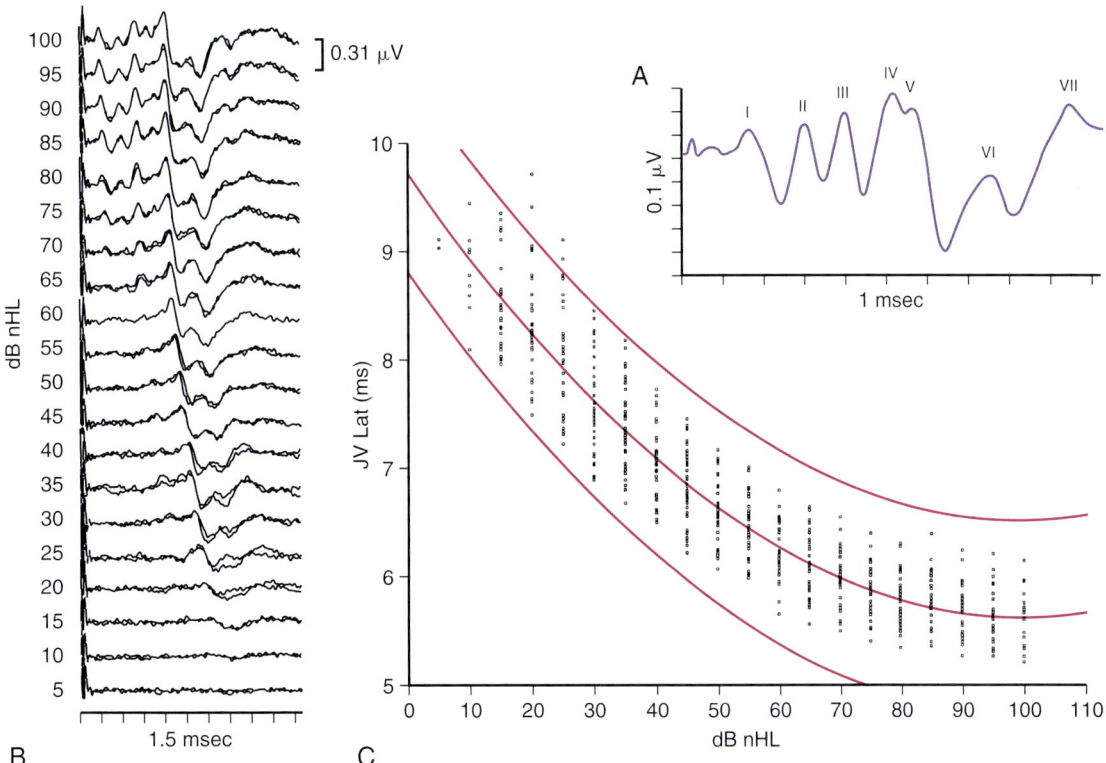

Figure 7-6. A, A normal click-evoked ABR waveform as it can be obtained from a normally hearing young subject. Stimulus level is 75 dB nHL. For brief stimuli such as clicks and tone-bursts, the nHL scale refers to the average threshold of a small group of normal subjects for a given stimulus. **B,** Effect of click intensity on ABR parameters: rise in latencies, drop in amplitudes, and progressive disappearance of early waves with reduction of intensity toward threshold. **C,** ABR wave V correlation between latency and intensity: individual data from 32 normal young subjects fitted by a quadratic function and 99% upper and lower confidence limits. Wave V is sometimes referred to as JV after D.L. Jewett, one of the ABR discoverers. ABR, auditory brainstem responses.

154500); and Townes–Brocks syndrome (OMIM 107480). The size and morphological alterations in these conditions are more frequently bilateral and rather symmetric. Chromosomal anomalies are also associated with external ear malformations as seen with autosomal aneuploidies, namely, Down syndrome, Patau syndrome (trisomy 13), and Edwards syndrome (trisomy 18), but also for more complex chromosomal rearrangements.

Sensorineural HL

Permanent SNHL is the most prevalent sensory impairment in childhood, affecting 1/700 infants. SNHL may result from genetic or environmental factors and can be syndromic or nonsyndromic.

An enlarged vestibular aqueduct (EVA) is the most common inner ear malformation found in children with cochlear HL. The associated HL is variable in severity, may be asymmetric or unilateral, may be pre- or postlingual, and can fluctuate over time or suddenly progress.

It is frequently observed in *SLC26A4*-related autosomal recessive nonsyndromic hearing loss (ARNSHL) and Pendred syndrome, and rarely in CHARGE syndrome, Waardenburg syndrome (WS), or Branchio-Oto-Renal syndrome.

Toxoplasmosis, other (viruses), rubella, cytomegalovirus, herpes simplex (infection) (TORCH) infections may cause HL, often not isolated but associated with CNS involvement, including intracranial calcifications and destructive lesions seen on MRI and CT. CMV infection remains a frequent cause of acquired SNHL in neonates worldwide. Its prevalence is 0.58% in developed countries. CMV explains up to 21% of acquired HL at birth and up to 25% at the age of 4 years. Congenital toxoplasmosis and bacterial meningitis remain a concern, as up to 5% to 35% of survivors experience bilateral SNHL when infection occurs before the age of 2 years.

Ototoxicity

Aminoglycosides antibiotics, mainly gentamycin, streptomycin, and vancomycin, are major ototoxic drugs, their deleterious role being modulated by the presence of m.1555A>G mutation. Macrolides may also be associated with some drug-induced deafness, as are antineoplastic cis- and carboplatin agents, rarely used in infancy and childhood. Nonsteroidal antiinflammatory drugs and antimalarial medications may also cause a reversible ototoxicity. High doses of ionizing radiation used in cranial radiotherapy have been reported to cause HL, as can excessive noise exposure.

Auditory Neuropathy Spectrum Disorder

ANSD is not a rare entity: it is associated with 8% of newly diagnosed pediatric cases of HL and 10% of children with permanent HL. Both genetic and nongenetic causes have been established.

GENETIC HEARING LOSS

Genetic HL can be divided into syndromic (SHL) and nonsyndromic forms (NSHL). Both have a monogenic cause in many cases, and all major types of inheritance patterns are observed. The most frequent type is autosomal recessive HL (ARNSHL) that accounts for almost 80% of cases. ARNSHL is typically congenital and severe to profound in nature, although at a later age at onset, milder forms or a progressive character is described in a minority of cases. Approximately 20% of cases are dominantly inherited, mostly of later onset and usually progressive (autosomal dominant nonsyndromic hearing loss;

ADNSHL). Infrequently, HL follows the rules of X-linked or mitochondrial inheritance. NSHL is a highly heterogeneous trait, with more than 80 genes identified. It is likely that many more gene abnormalities remain to be identified. A continuously updated overview of genes associated with hereditary HL is available online at the Hereditary Hearing Loss Homepage (HHLH; http://www.hereditaryhearingloss.org).

Nonsyndromic Hearing Loss

Genes that have been associated with NSHL fall into different categories. Most show an expression pattern largely restricted to the inner ear, as they encode proteins involved in cochlea development or function. Others have a broad expression pattern, encoding proteins present in other organs. The frequency of HL mutation carriage in unaffected individuals varies across populations and ethnicities. Data are only available for a small number of genes.

Autosomal Recessive Inheritance

ARNSHL is caused by mutations in a limited set of genes, including *GJB2*, *SLC26A4*, *MYO15A*, *OTOF*, *CDH23*, and *TMC1*. *GJB2* mutations represent the most frequently reported cause of ARNSHL. Over 100 different mutations have been reported in this gene (http://davinci.crg.es/deafness/index .php). It is frequent in European countries close to the Mediterranean (up to 50% of ARNSHL cases). One is particularly prevalent in European populations because of a founder effect: 35delG.

Another common mutation is *SLC26A4*, which also is involved in a syndromic form of ARNSHL, Pendred syndrome, in which HL is accompanied by a thyroid goiter. However, as goiter usually appears later in life, or in some cases never appears, it is also considered an NSHL gene. An ARNSHL gene in which mutations are associated with a recognizable audiological phenotype is that encoding otoferlin (*OTOF*). Mutations in this audiological gene often result in prelingual, profound ARNSHL associated with an ANSD electrophysiological profile.

Autosomal Dominant Inheritance

In contrast to ARNSHL where *GJB2*-related and *SLC26A4*-related HL are overrepresented, none of the ADNSHL genes is particularly frequent. Dominant mutations in *WFS1* encoding wolframin and those in *COCH* encoding cochlin are associated with a recognizable phenotype.

X-Linked and Mitochondrial Inheritance

Although X-linked and mitochondrial inherited HL are not frequent, representing together less than 3% of cases, a couple of mutations are often included in diagnostic panels because of their nature (point mutations) or their associated anomalies (see syndromic HL section). Mutations in *POU3F4* cause an X-linked form of HL characterized by a mixed or purely sensorineural HL and temporal bone malformation on MRI. Its diagnosis has therapeutic consequences because the presence of a *POU3F4* mutation can represent a contraindication for stapes surgery, hence the importance of temporal bone imaging in any basic workup of congenital HL. One mitochondrial gene is especially noteworthy. This is *MT-RNRI*, encoding the mitochondrial small subunit ribosomal RNA. The 1555A>G substitution causes HL induced by administration of clinically appropriate doses of aminoglycosides. In some individuals, HL can be present without exposure to aminoglycosides, suggesting involvement of modifier genes.

Genetic Diagnostics for Nonsyndromic Hearing Loss

For more than two decades, attempts at establishing the molecular basis of HL have been made by Sanger sequencing. Although genes routinely analyzed for NSHL may differ between countries and labs, some are more common (e.g., GJB2, GJB6, and SLC26A4), or those giving rise to a recognizable audiological or clinical phenotype when mutated (Table 7-2).

Traditional DNA diagnostic strategies usually deal with a small number of genes and a one-by-one sequential basis, meaning that the vast majority of HL genes remain unexplored outside a research setting. However, as next-generation sequencing (NGS) is becoming more available, it is now possible to sequence a large number of genes. Universities and private labs are able to offer testing for up to 125 HL genes, including both syndromic and nonsyndromic forms. In addition, multiple family members can be analyzed by NGS, allowing segregation studies, that is, characterization of those individuals from the family that inherited different genetic markers. This approach allows diagnosis of a specific HL type in a family, but also in up to 15% of families establishing a digenic inheritance by diagnosing a combination of two different types of deafness within the same family. However, although Sanger sequencing has a claimed sensitivity of 99%, the sensitivity of NGS-related techniques remains dependent on the number of reads, and a small percentage of mutations will be missed.

Syndromic Hearing Loss

Syndromes in which deafness is not isolated but associated with other anomalies or involving other systems represent a significant part (about one third) of the so-called genetic deafness. Two points deserve consideration (Toriello and Smith, 2013). The first is that of an enhanced interest in nonsyndromic deafness through availability of gene panels has rendered more frequent extensive audiological and imaging work-ups in previously unexplored children, thus dramatically increasing our knowledge of previously obscure rare conditions and drawing attention to new entities. This extended workup also led to reassignment of a number of nonsyndromic cases to the syndromic group by recognition of new entities and recognition of unsuspected known syndromes and subtle unreported clinical signs by reverse phenotyping. The other point pertains to the dramatic increase in the number of HL syndromes that has to be considered, and it is beyond the scope of this chapter to provide a detailed description of the clinical features of these syndromes (Hennekam et al., 2010).

Because of the large number of conditions causing HL, there is a need for differentiating the vast majority of conditions in which deafness is an occasional finding, entities remaining private by the small number of families described so far from *bona fide* regular and frequent HL syndromes. These, less than two dozen major deafness syndromes, most, if not all, following the rules of mendelian inheritance, will be the subject of this section (Table 7-3).

Waardenburg syndrome. WS is a clinically and genetically heterogeneous condition that manifests with HSNHL and abnormal pigmentation of the hair, skin, and iris. Four subtypes have been described. A neurologic variant (peripheral demyelinating neuropathy, central dysmyelinating leukodystrophy, Waardenburg syndrome, Hirschsprung disease, PCWH) has also been delineated. Its classical phenotype includes WS type 1 with telecanthus and *PAX3* mutations, WS type 2 without telecanthus and *MITF* or *SOX10* mutations, and

TABLE 7-2 Frequently Analyzed NSHL Genes in Routine Genetic Diagnostics

Gene	Inheritance Pattern	Phenotype
GJB2	AR	Most frequent gene associated with ARNSHL in many populations. Its mutations in GJB2 give rise to severe to profound HL in most cases, although rarely mild to moderate HL is observed. It may be combined with GJB6 deletion.
SLC26A4	AR	Both a frequent gene and a recognizable phenotype. Enlargement of vestibular aqueduct or Mondini dysplasia is seen on inner ear imaging. Mutations in this gene are also determining Pendred syndrome.
OTOF	AR	Congenital severe hearing loss caused by auditory synaptopathy, characterized by initially normal otoacoustic emission responses and preserved cochlear microphonic, whereas auditory brainstem responses are absent.
TECTA	AR/AD	By contrast to most cases of ARNSHL, which are severe to profound in nature, a milder phenotype is observed in TECTA-related ARNSHL (OMIM 603629). HL is typically moderate to severe, mainly affecting the midfrequencies. There is heterogeneity of mode of inheritance for TECTA-related HL, because some mutations give rise to an autosomal dominant transmission (ADNSHL; OMIM 601543).
WFS1	AD	Mild or moderate nonprogressive HL, only affecting the low frequencies. An autosomal recessive syndrome with multisystemic involvement is observed in case of homozygosity or compound heterozygosity (Wolfram Syndrome; OMIM 222300).
COCH	AD	Usually onset in the third decade with progressive hearing loss, accompanied by vestibular dysfunction, leading to absence of cochlear and vestibular function after during the fourth decade. The condition is particularly frequent in Belgium and the Netherlands because of a founder effect of P51S mutation (OMIM 603196).
POU3F4	XL	Sensorineural or mixed hearing loss associated with defects in bony labyrinth, including enlargement of the auditory canal, Mondini dysplasia, and/or stapes fixation (OMIM 300039).
MT-RNR1	Mitochondrial	m.1555A>G mutation in this gene is a relatively frequent cause of an aminoglycoside-induced HL, although in some cases it causes HL without aminoglycoside exposure.

This table contains a list of frequently analyzed NSHL genes in routine genetic diagnostics because of their high prevalence like GJB2 and SLC26A4 or as a result of the distinctive recognizable pattern of the HL they are associated with, differing from the severe to profound sensorineural HL caused by most genes. ADNSHL, autosomal dominant nonsyndromic hearing loss; ARNSHL, autosomal recessive nonsyndromic hearing loss; CM, cochlear microphonic; HL, hearing loss; NSHL, nonsyndromic hearing loss.

TABLE 7-3 Examples of Syndromes Involving Hearing Loss

Syndrome	Syndromic Features
Alport syndrome (OMIM 301050, 203780, 104200)	Kidney
Branchio-oto-renal syndrome (OMIM 113650)	Kidney, external ear
Treacher–Collins syndrome (OMIM 154500)	Craniofacial
Pendred syndrome (OMIM 274600)	Endocrine
Waardenburg syndrome (OMIM 193500, 193510, 148820, 277580)	Integuments, eye
Jervell–Lange–Nielsen syndrome (OMIM 220400)	Heart
Usher syndrome (OMIM 276900, 276901, 276902)	Eye

This table contains a list of syndromes associated with hearing loss and their syndromic feature. For additional information, please refer to the following section and/or to specific (http://www.ncbi.nlm.nih.gov/omim) and (http://www.ncbi.nlm.nih.gov/books/NBK1434/).

type 4, sometimes called WS, recessive phenotype, which is a severe, early-onset subtype often associated to Hirschsprung syndrome. There is genetic heterogeneity of this subtype, with mutations in genes encoding endothelin 3, its receptor, and mutations in *SOX10*, encoding a transcription factor being also at cause in recessive forms. In *SOX10*-related type 4 WS, temporal bone imaging studies frequently show an enlarged vestibular aqueduct that could point to the diagnosis. Interestingly, some *SOX10*-mutated patients have instead of WS, a Kallmann disease phenotype, and some others have a sporadic deafness-only phenotype, without any pigmentary, olfactive, or dysmorphic features, that can be diagnosed by appropriate interpretation of temporal bone MRI. Since 1998, approximately 100 heterozygous point mutations or deletions of *SOX10* have been reported, first in WS4 (WS with Hirschsprung disease), then in its neurologic variant, and recently in WS2. Although very rare, mutations in genes encoding endothelin 3 or receptor (*EDN3*-related, *EDNRB*-related) are also described. The common features of WS syndrome are SNHL and depigmentation of scalp, skin, and irides. A white forelock is the most remarkable sign, but premature, widespread graying of hair or depigmented skin macules are seen. Because of variable expressivity common to AD disorders, asking for the presence of this type of anomalies in relatives during the taking of a patient's history is of value in cases of apparently sporadic deafness: it is not uncommon to have a hearing relative with one or several of these signs. Type 3 WS is an exceedingly rare occurrence of homozygosity for *PAX3* mutations determining a more severe phenotype that includes short stature and bone deformity.

Usher syndrome. US is another instance in which the differential timing at onset of different components of the syndrome may critically delay diagnosis. US comprises three main phenotypes. US type I combines congenital profound HL with vestibular areflexia, followed by delayed progressive retinitis pigmentosa (RP). Vestibular function is preserved in types II and III. Because vision is doomed to extinction in US, it is particularly important to perform cochlear implantation at an early age in order to optimize speech development before the visual channel is lost. Visual impairment can be diagnosed by fundoscopy and by electroretinography (ERG), the latter allowing a more reliable and earlier detection of RP. In US type I, the earliest clinical signs are delayed walking and hypotonia because of the vestibular deficit, and so these

findings in a congenitally profoundly deaf child should prompt ERG investigations. US is the principal cause of deaf-blindness.

Treacher–Collins syndrome. Also known as Franceschetti–Klein syndrome, Treacher–Collins syndrome is the most frequent mandibulofacial dysostosis. It has a very characteristic facial dysmorphia that combines hypoplasia of zygomatic bones and mandible, external ear abnormalities, notching of lower eyelid, malar hypoplasia, downward slant of palpebral fissures, and microretrognathia. It is often associated with medial cleft palate. HL is present in nearly 50% affected individuals. It is of the conductive type, with fusion or undermodeling of the ossicles being at cause. Although dysmorphic features of variable severity are present at birth, conductive deafness may become obvious only later in life. Besides a prevalent autosomal dominant form caused by heterozygous mutations in *TCOF*, autosomal recessive forms have been demonstrated to be caused by mutations in genes encoding subunits of the polymerase complex *POLR1D* and *POLR1C*.

Refsum disease and infantile Refsum disease. Although very rare, Refsum disease deserves mention because early diagnosis, often based on detection of visual impairment associated with anosmia and neurologic features, can lead to specific treatment and prevent otherwise irreversible complications. This is a singular inborn error of metabolism linked to a single peroxisomal enzyme deficiency, either the one encoding phytanoyl-CoA hydroxylase or *PEX7*. It induces signs and symptoms that include peripheral neuropathy, ichthyosis, visual impairment due to retinitis pigmentosa and, lately, hearing loss. Dietary lowering plasma concentration of phytanic acid or iterative plasmapheresis allows a partial control of progression of ichthyosis, peripheral neuropathy, and/or RP.

There are other inborn errors of metabolism in which progressive HL has been linked to accumulation of toxic metabolites. Very-long-chain fatty acids, biliary acids, and phytanic acid are such metabolites thought to play such a role in much more severe conditions belonging to the group of generalized peroxisomal disorders or peroxisome biogenesis defects. For historical reasons, one of these severe diseases has been unfortunately given the name infantile Refsum disease, resembling too closely to the completely different adult Refsum disease and a source of confusion, as the neurodevelopmental outcome of the former is much more severe than that of the latter. More than 40 different enzyme deficiencies versus a single enzyme deficiency explain this discrepancy. Stabilization or even regression of HL has been achieved after orthotopic liver or hepatocyte transplantation in infantile Refsum disease.

SLC26A4-related deafness, Pendred syndrome. This mixed type of autosomal recessive deafness is usually nonsyndromal, accounting for *about* 12% of AR cases and is the second cause after connexin 26–related deafness. However, a small percentage of mutated patients have thyroid gland dysfunction and goiter, usually manifest during the second decade of life, defining one of the first deafness syndromes described by Pendred in 1896.

CHARGE syndrome. Elucidation of the molecular basis of what has been called CHARGE association (and not syndrome) for decades, an acronym for <u>c</u>oloboma, <u>h</u>eart defects, <u>a</u>tresia choanae, <u>r</u>etardation of growth and development, <u>g</u>enitourinary problems, and <u>e</u>ar malformation by a Dutch group in 2004, resulted in considerable expansion of its clinical phenotype, *CHD7* heterozygous mutation, now being observed not only in a number of incomplete phenotypes, but also in case of sporadic deafness observed in association with isolated or multiple cranial nerve palsies.

Also, it does not occur as a *de novo* mutation, but as a mutation inherited from an asymptomatic parent in up to 10% of the cases. In terms of genetic counseling, to differentiate between these distinct situations is of importance (<1% vs. 50% recurrence risk). Deafness in this syndrome can be caused by a cochlear malformation or auditory nerve absence. In contrast to other causes of deafness, moderate to severe intellectual disability is very common and makes prenatal diagnosis and early family counseling concerning quality of life issues an option.

Mitochondrial deafness. Maternal inheritance occurs commonly but not universally in mitochondrial disorders, partly due to the fact that genotype does not predict phenotype, by contrast to disorders resulting from mutations in nuclear-encoded genes. It is worth noting that an important part of mitochondrial disorders are due to mutations in these nuclearly-encioded genes. From a clinical point of view, mt.3243G>A mutation is important as it may induce deafness in association with a wide spectrum of other symptoms. In intermediate situations, deafness is found in association with insulin-dependent diabetes mellitus, or more complex phenotypes with either ataxia or stroke-like episodes, in the context of lactic acidosis.

Another interesting deafness/mitochondrial mutation is the m.1555A>G mutation, for its double-sided expression: on the one hand, it may give rise to a classical postlingual deafness in the absence of any triggering factor; on the other hand, it is associated with deafness related to aminoglycoside exposure. There are many other mitochondrial DNA mutations that are associated with deafness (OMIM). Co-occurrence of an associated movement disorder, cardiomyopathy, and elevated creatinine kinase level, presence of a tubulopathy, or lactic acidosis should prompt consideration of this possibility.

Alport syndrome. In this condition, postlingual HL is associated with kidney disease detected by hematuria prior to end-stage renal insufficiency. It is important to recognize because it is inherited in most cases as an X-linked recessive condition, with up to 15% of carrier females eventually becoming symptomatic. Its cardinal features are hematuria with subsequent renal insufficiency leading to dialysis and renal transplantation in a majority of patients. SNHL deafness generally occurs after the onset of renal disease. Carrier females are at risk of giving birth to affected male offspring, and in addition to determination of whether or not they have deafness, a urinalysis to screen for hematuria is indicated. Additional genetic studies of the family may be helpful as the mutation may not occur *de novo*. The alpha 5 chains of type 4 collagen are deficient, because of mutations in the corresponding gene *COL4A5*. Rarely, the disease is transmitted in an autosomal recessive manner, with an increased severity and mutations affecting *COL4A3 and COL4A4*.

Marshall–Stickler spectrum. This syndromic autosomal dominant condition, also because of a collagen deficiency, is remarkable by its distinctive dysmorphic features that include flattening of the face, nasal hypoplasia and upturned nares, eye involvement (high myopia, retinal detachment), high arched palate and/or cleft palate, micrognathia, and short stature. Mutations are usually identified in the gene encoding the alpha 1 chain of type 2 collagen *(COL2A1)*, but have also been described in association to involvement of type 9 collagens.

Jervell–Lange–Nielsen syndrome. Autosomal dominant and recessive forms of a similar condition coexist and are characterized by the long QT syndrome, which is inconstantly associated with HSNHL in the context of the presence of voltage-gated potassium channelopathies (KCNQ1 and KCNE1). Because profound to moderate deafness is the clinical presentation and prolonged QT interval can only be diagnosed after recording an electrocardiogram (ECG), it is of paramount importance to include this test in the evaluation of a congenitally deaf patient or even in children or older

patients with postlingual deafness. In patients with Jervell–Lange–Nielsen Syndrome, appropriate treatment (beta-blockers) and surveillance could be initiated, keeping in mind that sudden death because of ventricular fibrillation is the most severe complication. In some families, there is a history of intrauterine fetal death.

CONSEQUENCES OF HEARING IMPAIRMENT

Consequences of HL are to be understood in the context of speech development during critical maturational periods (Kral, 2013). Lack of auditory reference to real words, objects, and events leads to adverse cognitive effects. Uncorrected congenital or early acquired profound HL has far reaching consequences impinging on literacy development and cognitive abilities. There is accumulating evidence that this is also true for mild losses and even unilateral ones. Intervention programs recommend screening before 1 month, definite diagnosis no later than 3 months, and intervention by 6 months (Joint Committee on Infant Hearing). Any provider of pediatric healthcare involved with a child whose diagnosis or intervention program is not secured could play a major role in this respect. It cannot be overemphasized that in caring for a child with suspected HL or who has known risk factors (e.g., congenital CMV infection, positive family history), passed neonatal screening does not exclude significant HL as it may be delayed in onset or progressive in nature (Kral and O'Donoghue, 2010).

CLINICAL EVALUATION AND SPECIALIZED TESTING OF SUSPECTED HL
Patient and Family Histories

A detailed family history and pedigree are an integral part of the evaluation of every newly identified hearing-impaired child. Of importance is the pedigree reconstruction. Each parent should be questioned on his/her sibship with first name, maiden name, year of birth, number of offspring, and miscarriage(s). Special attention should be paid to grandparents, the place where they were born, and any history of hearing impairment, keeping in mind that presbyacusia is physiological after age 50. Of significance is any kind of relationship between the parents, pointing to autosomal recessive inheritance.

Clinical Evaluation and Specialized Testing

Once the pedigree and a detailed clinical history have been completed, a suspected mode of inheritance can usually be ascertained. If HL is thought to be of sporadic occurrence, one must still consider that autosomal recessive inheritance is possible as is autosomal dominant inheritance as a *de novo* mutation, or when a parent is mildly affected (variable expressivity). In addition, nonpenetrance, as well as mitochondrial inheritance or X-linked inheritance remains to be considered. Likewise, the absence of family history does not preclude a genetic basis and the possibility of an environmental etiology must also be looked for.

The clinical examination is of great importance and may yield diagnostic clues. In addition to growth parameters, attention should be paid to whether there are facial dysmorphic features, abnormal pinnae, branchial cleft pits, cysts or fistulae, preauricular pits or nodules, telecanthus, heterochromia iridis and pigmentary anomalies, high myopia, pigmentary retinopathy, increased or decreased occipitofrontal head circumference, nasolabial folds, submucous cleft palate, goiter, limb anomalies, organomegaly, disproportionate short or tall stature, muscle wasting, ataxia, and so on. Neurologic examination should determine the presence or absence of pyramidal signs, cranial nerve involvement, a movement disorder, and abnormal deep tendon reflexes. In autosomal dominant forms of syndromic HL that tend to have a variable expression, a key diagnostic feature may be found in a relative rather than in the proband. A complete blood count is important, including platelets size, as megathrombocytopenia is a good marker of *MYH9*-related deafness (OMIM 153650). The presence of hematuria on a urinalysis may suggest Alport syndrome (OMIM 301050, 203780, 104200) and Fanconi syndrome.

Screening for inborn errors of metabolism, especially mitochondrial when diabetes mellitus, ptosis, cardiomyopathy, failure to thrive, or seizures are present. Screening for disorders of amino acid and organic acid metabolism, obtaining plasma lactate and pyruvate levels, and chemistry profiles, including liver enzymes, are all helpful.

A muscle biopsy with biochemical and immunological study of the respiratory chain can be instrumental if additional clinical signs and symptoms are compatible with a mitochondrial cytopathy. Elevation of liver enzymes, associated with a visual deficiency or the presence of retinitis pigmentosa in an infant or toddler, should elicit a search for a peroxisomal biogenesis defect, including assessment of very-long-chain fatty acids, bile acids, and phytanic acid followed by a skin/liver biopsy in case of positive findings. A lysosomal storage disorder must be considered if the liver or spleen is enlarged, and if there are coarse facial features or stiff joints, distended abdomen, or a history of chronic otitis media assessment for a storage disorder should be considered. A search for vacuolized lymphocytes is a basic test, as is the search for an accumulation of urinary glycosaminoglycans. However, the first one requires expertise and the latter has a low specificity. Hence, asking for direct assessment of suspected enzyme deficiency in fresh leukocytes may accelerate the diagnostic process. For example, detection of iduronate-sulfatase is indicative of Hunter disease and alpha-iduronidase is indicative of Hurler syndrome. In a different set of conditions, skin lesions may provide diagnostic clues. Examples include the presence of angiokeratoma in patients with Fabry disease or an oligosaccharidosis like beta-mannosidosis and H syndrome, a recently described histiocytosis with cutaneous rash and frequently associated HL. It introduces a new class of genetic deafness where inflammatory cutaneous lesions can give suggest a different category of diagnostic entities. A second example includes the pigmentary anomalies seen in patients with WS.

Audiological Evaluation

Recommendations on techniques that should be applied and information that should be gathered have been issued for the audiological assessment of infants between birth and 6 months. Recommendations to fit the needs of older subjects with delayed development, multiple handicaps, or increased risk of auditory nervous system anomalies may be summarized and commented on as follows:

1. External and middle ears assessment by otoscopy and tympanometry, including acoustic reflexes and appropriate selection of probe frequency according to age
2. Evoked potentials recording to define type, degree, and configuration of HL and detect abnormal neural conduction along the cochlear nerve and/or brainstem pathways
3. Otoacoustic emissions
4. Behavioral audiometry
5. Speech detection and recognition

6. Follow up and monitoring of the infant's communication skills. Several forms of HL are delayed or progressive. It has been estimated that 1/56 children with permanent HL at 1 year had delayed-onset HL.

MANAGEMENT OF HEARING LOSS

A primary aim of rehabilitation efforts is promoting or restoring an infant's or child's communication skills and optimizing the level of language development on which cognitive and socioemotional behavior is contingent. A secondary aim is to provide environmental auditory object identification and localization. Efficient management often requires the combined expertise of otologists, audiologists, speech and language therapists, psychologists, special educators, and social workers. Currently available assistive devices (conventional hearing aids, cochlear implants, frequency modulation systems) allow many severe to profound HL children to be to a regular classroom setting.

Reconstructive Surgery for External and Middle Ears Malformation

Surgery is usually performed after the age of 8 years. Meanwhile, at least in children with HL, bone conduction hearing aids must be fitted early to avoid hearing deprivation during critical developmental periods.

Choice of Communication Mode for Severe to Profound HL

Among the two main communication strategies, namely, speech-based (oralism) and sign-based (sign language), the oral mode is usually preferred to sign communication to promote integration in the hearing population. In some individuals, parents will make the choice of acculturation of their child to the deaf signing world rather than to the hearing, speaking one, because, being profoundly deaf themselves, they use sign language in daily life or because they wish to respect and protect the communicative and social modes developed by their child. Choosing between these options is not a simple matter and has to be thoroughly discussed with the parents and the multidisciplinary rehabilitation team, before selecting what appears most appropriate for an individual child and his/her family.

Assistive Devices

Two main types of assistive devices are used to restore or improve auditory perception: conventional hearing aids (amplification devices) and cochlear implants. Frequency modulation systems are of great help: acquiring the teacher's speech by a collar-worn directional microphone, the system sends the target signal to the child's hearing aid by radio waves, and so ambient noise surrounding the subject is not amplified as it would have been with a child-worn microphone. Binaural amplification is recommended because it improves sound source localization and hearing in noise performances.

Cochlear Implants

Cochlear implants are now well established as the gold standard for restoring useful hearing in bilateral severe-to-profound HL for which amplification fails to allow satisfactory progress. The best results are obtained in two situations: cases of postlingually acquired deafness and early implantation of congenital cases. The optimal age for implanting congenital cases is between 6 months and 2 years.

Brainstem Implants

An auditory brainstem implant stimulating the surface of cochlear nucleus can be indicated when cochlear implantation is impossible. The main indication for auditory brainstem implantation is type 2 neurofibromatosis.

FUTURE DEVELOPMENTS

Advances in HL research over the next decade will focus on electrophysiological applications to better understand the mechanisms of speech development, use of newer imaging technologies, improvement of conventional hearing aid functionality, and in the implementation of hearing restoration therapies. Measurement of the quality of neural coding within the CANS using digital signal processing techniques and perceptual training will possibly improve central representation of speech items. Functional imaging and diffusion tensor imaging are likely to be useful in the study of functionally or structurally abnormal CANS pathways. Digital signal processing techniques that can now be implemented in conventional hearing aids should contribute to alleviate the consequences of at least some forms of neural code distortion. Gene, stem cells, and molecular therapies are beginning to show efficiency in animal models, and it is hoped that they will be applied to use in humans in the forthcoming decades.

REFERENCES

The complete list of references for this chapter is available in the e-book at www.expertconsult.com.
    See inside cover for registration details.

SELECTED REFERENCES

Hennekam, R., Allanson, J., Krantz, I., 2010. Gorlin's Syndromes of the Head and Neck, fifth ed. Oxford Monographs on Medical Genetics. Oxford University Press, New York.

Kral, A., O'Donoghue, G.M., 2010. Profound deafness in childhood. N. Engl. J. Med. 363, 1438–1450.

Kral, A., 2013. Auditory critical periods: a review from system's perspective. Neuroscience 247, 117–133.

McDermott, J.H., 2009. The cocktail party problem. Curr. Biol. 19, R1024–R1027.

Pickles, J.O., 2012. An Introduction to the Physiology of Hearing, fourth ed. Emerald, Bingley, UK.

Starr, A., Zeng, F.G., Michalewski, H.G., et al., 2008. Perspectives on auditory neuropathy: disorders of inner hair cell, auditory nerve and their synapse. In: Basbaum, A.I., Kaneko, A.Shepherd, G.M. (Eds.), The Senses: A Comprehensive Reference Audition. Academic Press, San Diego, pp. 347–412.

Toriello, H., Smith, S.D. (Eds.), 2013. Hereditary Hearing Loss and Its Syndromes. Oxford Monographs on Medical Genetics. Oxford University Press, New York.

E-BOOK FIGURES AND TABLES

The following figures and tables are available in the e-book at www.expertconsult.com. See inside cover for registration details.

Fig. 7-2 Acoustic pressure variation time course for a sinusoidally amplitude-modulated pure tone at 1 kHz.

Fig. 7-3 The intricate relationship of the semicircular canals, vestibule, and cochlea.

Fig. 7-4 Microphotograph of the inner hair cell ribbon synapse.

Fig. 7-5 Air conduction thresholds.

Fig. 7-7 Auditory brainstem response differential diagnosis between conductive and sensorineural hearing loss.

Fig. 7-8 Data from a 2-year-old girl with pontine tegmental cap dysplasia.

Fig. 7-9 Midsagittal T2-weighted MR imaging.

8 Vertigo

Joseph M. Furman and Amy Goldstein

INTRODUCTION

Vertigo in children may escape recognition because of the child's inability to describe the symptoms, the short duration of most vertiginous episodes, the presence of overwhelming autonomic symptoms, or the mistaken idea that an episode of vertigo may be a manifestation of a behavioral disorder.

Vertigo is defined in clinical practice as a subjective sensation of movement, such as spinning, turning, tilting, or whirling, of the patient or the surroundings. Dizziness is a nonspecific term used by patients to describe sensations of altered orientation to the environment that may or may not include vertigo, and often is used to describe lightheadedness or presyncopal symptoms.

Although vertigo may be a symptom of a vestibular disorder in the pediatric population, patients react to and describe dizziness in different ways in relation to their age. For instance, young children cannot accurately relate symptoms of dizziness. Preschool children rarely complain of vertigo or dizziness but may feel clumsy or be perceived as such by family or teachers. Older children and adolescents are usually able to explain their symptoms well, with their explanations differing little from the explanations of adults.

In any case, a vestibular abnormality should be suspected in a child who is observed to be clumsy or displays unprovoked fright, or who spontaneously clings to a parent. Sudden and recurrent bouts of unexplained nausea and vomiting also are suggestive of a vestibular abnormality.

In children, as well as in adults, a careful history, physical examination, and laboratory testing can establish the cause of dizziness in most patients.

PHYSIOLOGIC BASIS OF BALANCE

When a hair cell is stimulated by rotation, translation, or change in orientation with respect to gravity, the firing rate in the eighth nerve fiber innervating that particular hair cell either increases or decreases. Movements that cause the stereocilia to bend toward the kinocilium result in a depolarization of the hair cell and cause the eighth nerve fiber to increase its firing rate, whereas movements that bend the stereocilia away from the kinocilium decrease the neural firing in the eighth nerve. The eighth nerve synapses in the vestibular nuclei, which consist of superior, medial, lateral, and inferior divisions. In addition to the input from the labyrinth, the vestibular nuclei receive input from other sensory systems, such as vision, somatic sensation, and hearing. The sensory information is integrated and the output from the vestibular nuclei influences eye movements, truncal stability, and spatial orientation.

The oculovestibular reflex is a mechanism by which a head movement automatically results in an eye movement that is equal to and opposite of the head movement so that the visual axis of the eye stays on target: that is, a leftward head movement is associated with a rightward eye movement and vice versa. Another feature of the oculovestibular reflex is that the two vestibular nuclear complexes on either side of the brainstem cooperate with one another in such a way that, for the horizontal system, when one nucleus is excited, the other is inhibited. The central nervous system (CNS) responds to differences in neural activity between the two vestibular complexes. When there is no head movement, the neural activity, i.e., the resting discharge, is symmetrical in the two vestibular nuclei. The brain detects no differences in neural activity and concludes that the head is not moving (Fig. 8-1A). When the head moves, e.g., to the left, endolymph flow produces an excitatory response in the labyrinth on the side toward which the head moves, e.g., on the left, and an inhibitory response on the opposite side, e.g., on the right. Thus neural activity in the vestibular nerve and nuclei, e.g., on the left and right, increases and decreases respectively (Fig. 8-1B). The brain interprets this difference in neural activity between the two vestibular complexes as a head movement and generates appropriate oculovestibular and postural responses. This reciprocal push-pull balance between the two labyrinths is disrupted as a result of labyrinthine injury.

An acute loss of peripheral vestibular function unilaterally, e.g., on the right, causes a loss of resting neural discharge activity in that vestibular nerve and the ipsilateral nucleus (Fig. 8-1C). Because the brain responds to differences between the two labyrinths, this will be interpreted by the brain as a rapid head movement toward the healthy labyrinth, i.e. vertigo. "Corrective" eye movements are produced toward the opposite side, resulting in nystagmus, with the slow component moving toward the abnormal side, e.g., the right, and the quick components of nystagmus moving toward the healthy labyrinth, e.g., the left.

EVALUATION OF PATIENTS WITH DIZZINESS

At the initial visit, in addition to the chief complaint, a complete medical history that includes associated symptoms, medical history, family history, and medication use is mandatory.

After the interview, a complete physical examination should be performed, with particular emphasis on the cranial nerves, including an examination of eye movements.

In some patients, further testing may be medically necessary if the diagnosis is not clear, including the use of vestibular testing in a specialized laboratory.

History
Chief Complaint

It is important that the child explain the symptoms in his or her own vocabulary and describe associated sensations, such as headache, nausea, vomiting, or motion sickness. It might be helpful to relate the patient's symptoms to experiences, such as being on a merry-go-round or a boat. It is important to establish the onset, duration, and frequency of dizziness episodes and to associate the episodes with certain activities. Triggering factors include change in position, coughing or sneezing, sleep deprivation, and psychological stressors.

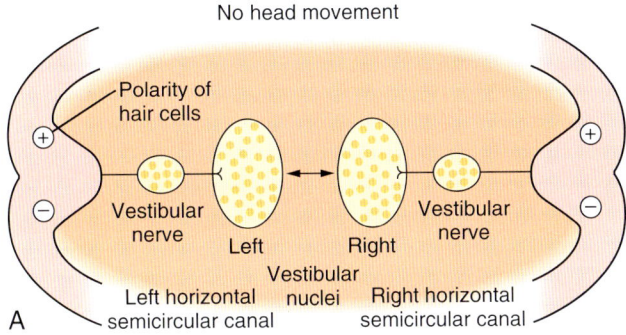

No head movement

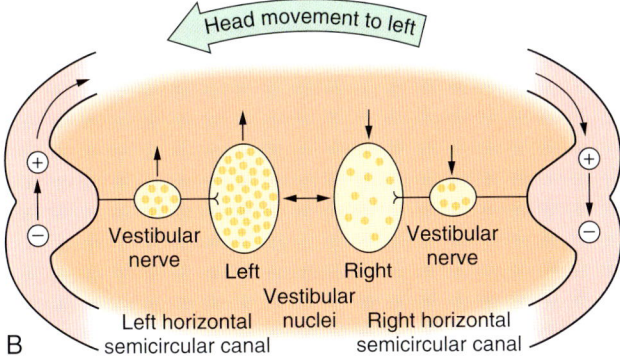

Head movement to left

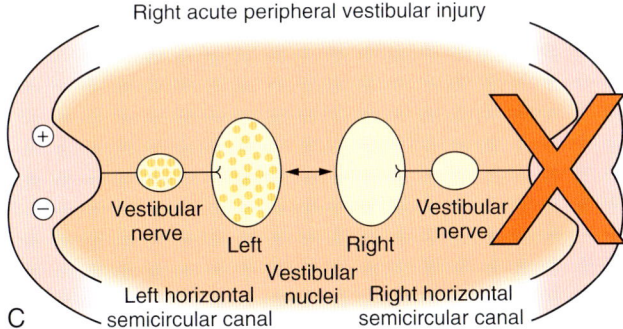

Right acute peripheral vestibular injury

Figure 8-1. Schematic illustrations of the "push-pull" effect of the oculovestibular reflex. **A,** No head movement in healthy subject. **B,** Head movement to the left in healthy subject. **C,** Right acute peripheral vestibular injury.

The clinician should inquire about the presence of hearing loss, its onset, evolution or progression, fluctuation and worsening, and improving or stable status. Does the patient have tinnitus or a feeling of fullness? Is the hearing loss bilateral or unilateral? To establish the presence of neurologic symptoms, the clinician should determine whether there have been instances of seizure activity, altered mental status, ataxia, weakness, numbness, disturbances of swallowing or taste, coughing, facial paralysis, or blurring and loss of vision.

Physical Examination

In addition to a complete neurologic examination, the child should also be observed when walking or running for incoordination of movements, i.e., ataxia. Also, an assessment of nystagmus is especially important. Spontaneous nystagmus is an involuntary, rhythmic movement of the eyes not induced by any external stimulation. Spontaneous nystagmus has two components: slow and fast. Nystagmus is named by the fast component, which is easily identified. Spontaneous nystag-

mus is tested by having the patient look straight ahead with and without fixation (i.e., in primary gaze). Gaze-evoked nystagmus is assessed by having the patient deviate the eyes laterally (no greater than 30 degrees) with fixation. End-gaze nystagmus with eyes fully deviated laterally is a normal finding. Positional testing is performed with the use of maneuvers that may produce nystagmus or vertigo. Static positional nystagmus is assessed by placing the patient in each of the these six positions: sitting, supine, supine with the head turned to the right, supine with the head turned to the left, and right and left lateral positions. Positional nystagmus presents as soon as the patient assumes the position and persists for as long as the patient remains in the provocative position. Assessment of vestibulospinal function with a foam pad should be performed with or without a visual conflict dome.

In addition to a history and physical examination, an assessment may include vestibular testing. Vestibular laboratory testing is recommended in any child with a history of vertigo in whom a thorough history and physical examination have not established a diagnosis, in order to differentiate between a peripheral or central vestibular lesion, and to identify the side of the lesion in a peripheral abnormality. In addition, vestibular laboratory testing provides permanent documentation, and changes can be followed by repeat testing. Vestibular laboratory testing includes oculovestibular and vestibulospinal tests. Both types of tests provide only an indirect measure of the function of the vestibular end organs, in that they rely on measures of motor response, e.g, eye movements or postural sway, resulting from vestibular sensory input.

Videonystagmography

Videonystagmography is currently the most widely used method of recording eye movements; it uses infrared light. Ocular motor testing, positional testing, and caloric testing constitute a common test battery that requires about 1 hour. Sedatives and vestibular suppressant medications should be discontinued for 2 days before testing. Ocular motor testing evaluates neural motor output independent of the vestibular system. Abnormalities in the ocular motor system may cause misleading conclusions from vestibular testing that relies on eye movements. Testing saccades uses a computer-controlled sequence of target jumps. Saccade abnormalities are defined as overshooting the target (hypermetric saccades) and undershooting the target (hypometric saccades). Disorders in the saccadic system suggest a CNS abnormality. Spontaneous nystagmus and gaze-evoked nystagmus are recorded with and without fixation (closing the eyes or darkness), and by asking the patient to look 30 degrees to the right and left. Spontaneous nystagmus present in darkness without fixation, which decreases or resolves with visual fixation, suggests a peripheral vestibular disorder. However, spontaneous nystagmus that is present with fixation and does not significantly decrease with loss of fixation is most likely a CNS abnormality. Ocular pursuit involves asking the patient to follow a moving target back and forth along a slow, pendular path. Normal subjects can follow a target smoothly without interruption. Abnormalities of pursuit tracking are caused by lesions in the CNS. Laboratory testing of optokinetic nystagmus uses black-and-white stripes moving left and right. Abnormalities include asymmetries or absence of responses, which suggest a CNS abnormality.

Positional testing includes both static and paroxysmal (dynamic) testing. As in the clinical assessment, during static positional testing, the patient is placed in the sitting, supine, head left, head right, left lateral, and right lateral positions in darkness. Static positional nystagmus, contrary to paroxysmal nystagmus, presents as soon as the patient assumes the provocative position and persists for as long as the patient stays in that position. Static positional nystagmus is a nonspecific, nonlocalizing vestibular sign. Paroxysmal positional testing employs the Dix–Hallpike maneuver, a maneuver that involves bringing the patient from sitting with the head straight to sitting with the head turned 45 degrees to one side to lying down with the head still turned and the neck extended 20 degrees below the horizontal. The patient is then seated upright again, and the maneuver is repeated with the head turning to the opposite side. Upon attainment and maintenance of each head-back stance, the eye movements are noted. Latency to onset of nystagmus, a rotational component to the nystagmus, and attenuation of the nystagmus with maintenance of the position all suggest the diagnosis of benign paroxysmal positional vertigo, especially if this maneuver reproduces the patient's symptoms. This condition is rare in children and, when present, is thought to be a childhood migraine variant.

Caloric Testing

Caloric testing aims to assess each labyrinth separately by producing nystagmus via thermal stimulation of the vestibular system. The patient is placed in a position in which the horizontal semicircular canals lie in the vertical plane (head elevated 30 degrees). Caloric stimulation causes a convection current in the horizontal semicircular canal that causes a deflection of the cupula (into which the hairs of the hair cells are embedded) and a change in activity of the vestibular nerve. Cold irrigation produces a fast nystagmus component away from the irrigated ear; warm irrigation produces a fast nystagmus component toward the irrigated ear. The common mnemonic *COWS* "cold opposite, warm same," refers to the direction of the fast-beating nystagmus. Binaural bithermal caloric testing uses stimuli of 30° C and 44° C, and each canal is irrigated for 30 seconds with 250 mL of water. There is a rest period of 5 minutes between irrigations. The most common method of measuring the caloric response is to compute the peak slow-component velocity of the nystagmus induced by the thermal stimulus, which reflects the intensity of the vestibular response. To compare the responsiveness of one ear to the other ear, it is established practice to use Jongkees' formula to compute a percentage of reduced vestibular response:

$$[[(R30° + R44°) - (L30° + L44°)]/$$
$$[R30° + R44° + L30° + L44°]] \times 100 \text{ percent}$$

For many laboratories, normal limits are considered to be a reduced vestibular response of more than 24%. A reduced vestibular response suggests a peripheral vestibular lesion.

Rotational Testing

Rotation is the natural stimulus to the semicircular canals. Rotational testing causes minimal discomfort and is precise and well tolerated, even by infants and young children (who can be placed on a parent's lap). Rotation stimulates both labyrinths at the same time and thus does not provide lateralizing information. Caloric response and rotational testing are complementary. The most common type of rotational testing uses sinusoidal harmonic acceleration. The eye velocity produced by the rotation is compared with stimulus velocity.

Three parameters are derived from rotational testing: gain, phase, and symmetry. Gain is a measure of the size of the response. Reduced gain indicates decreased vestibular sensitivity. Unilateral vestibular loss may or may not reduce gain. Thus reduced gain usually indicates bilateral vestibular loss. Phase describes the timing relationship between the rotational chair

velocity and the eye velocity. Ideal eye movements have zero phase lead, whereas large phase leads are usually abnormal. Phase is a highly sensitive but nonspecific measure of vestibular system abnormalities. The directional preponderance (i.e., deviation from symmetry) of the eye movements is derived by comparing the velocity of the eye movement to right and left. Directional preponderance is a nonspecific sign. Note that gain, phase, and degree of symmetry do not indicate the site or the side of the lesion. However, rotational testing measures change in response to vestibular disease and can be used to monitor a child's progress.

Computerized Dynamic Platform Posturography

Computerized dynamic posturography, known commercially as EquiTest® (NeuroCom International, Inc.), consists of a floor and a visual scene that can move (Fig. 8-6A). By combining visual and floor conditions, six different sensory conditions can be used to assess the patient's ability to use combinations of sensory inputs (Fig. 8-6B). Conditions 5 and 6 assess how patients use vestibular information when it is the only available sense providing reliable information; reduced or distorted sensory information from the visual system and somatosensory system forces patients to rely on their vestibular sensations to maintain upright balance.

Posturography and Vestibular Disorders—Results from the Medical Literature

Several studies have suggested that, after successful vestibular compensation, posturography test results normalize and patients lose their "5, 6 pattern" (i.e., their abnormal response to conditions 5 and 6 on posturography testing) and may, in fact, have normal postural sway (Furman, 1995). Thus posturography may provide valuable information regarding the status of compensation for a peripheral vestibular deficit.

Vestibular-Evoked Myogenic Potentials

Vestibular-evoked myogenic potentials (VEMPs) refer to electrical activity recorded from neck muscles in response to intense auditory clicks. VEMPs provide information about the status of the sacculus and inferior vestibular nerve. A limitation of VEMPs is that it requires normal middle ear function when performed using air-conducted stimuli. VEMPs have been performed successfully in children. Children as young as age 3 can tolerate testing.

DISORDERS PRODUCING VERTIGO

Vertigo in children can be divided into three broad categories:

1. Acute nonrecurring spontaneous vertigo
2. Recurrent vertigo
3. Nonvertiginous dizziness, disequilibrium, and ataxia (Table 8-1)

A recent study of 2000 children found that vertigo in children was caused by: a migrainous equivalent, 25%; benign paroxysmal vertigo of childhood, 20%; head trauma, 10%; ocular disorders, 10%; inner ear malformations, 10%; vestibular neuronitis, 5%; labyrinthitis, 5%; and posterior fossa tumors, less than 1% (Wiener-Vacher, 2008). A more recent study of 6965 10 year olds in the United Kingdom found a 5.7% prevalence of vertigo. Of these children, vertigo symptoms made them stop their activity, and 60% of them also had headache. A change in hearing while vertiginous was reported in 20% (Humphriss and Hall, 2011).

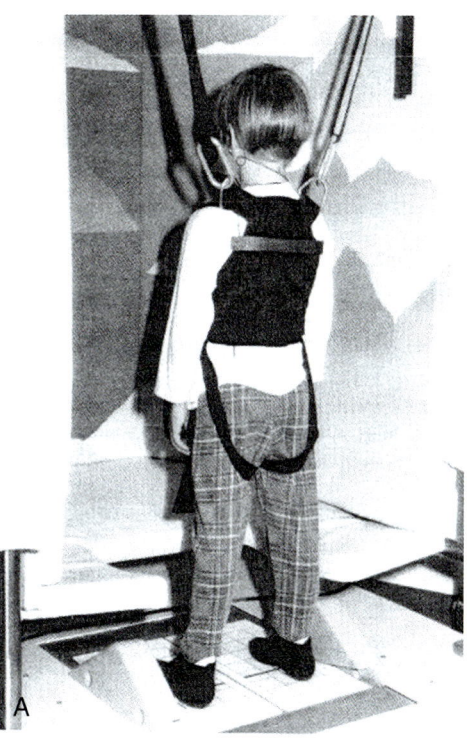

EquiTest® conditions

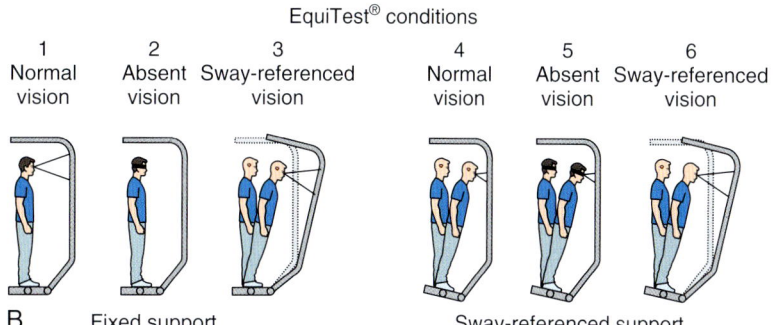

Figure 8-6. The EquiTest® system. A, EquiTest® system (NeuroCom International, Inc.) shows the child standing on the platform surrounded by a visual scene. A safety harness is attached to the child in case loss of balance should occur. The platform surface and visual surround are capable of moving independently or simultaneously. Pressure-sensing strain gauges beneath the platform surface detect the patient's sway by measuring vertical and horizontal forces applied to the surface. **B,** The six sensory testing conditions of the EquiTest® posturography platform. *(With permission from Neuro-Com International, Inc., Clackman, Ore.)*

TABLE 8-1 Comparison of Disorders Causing Childhood Dizziness

Disorders	Duration of Symptoms/Episodes	Hearing	Vestibular Laboratory Abnormalities
Nonrecurrent Vertigo			
Vestibular neuritis	Days	Normal	Unilateral caloric reduction
Trauma-labyrinthine concussion	Days	Often impaired SNHL*	Possible unilateral caloric reduction
Perilymphatic fistula	Variable	Often impaired SNHL	Possible unilateral caloric reduction
Recurrent Vertigo			
Ménière's disease	Minutes to hours	Low-frequency SNHL	Unilateral caloric reduction
Migraine	Variable	Normal	Directional preponderance
Anxiety	Minutes	Normal	Directional preponderance
Seizure disorder	Seconds to minutes	Normal	Normal
Periodic ataxia	Hours to days	Normal	Normal
Nonvertiginous Dizziness			
Bilateral vestibular loss	Constant	Usually normal but may be impaired	Bilateral caloric reduction/reduced gain on rotation
Otitis media	Constant	Conductive	Abnormal posturography
Cerebellar lesions	Constant	Normal	Abnormal ocular motor testing

*SNHL; sensorineural hearing loss.
(Modified with permission from Tusa RS et al. Dizziness in childhood. J Child Neurol. 1994;9:261.)

Acute Nonrecurring Spontaneous Vertigo

Acute nonrecurring spontaneous vertigo is unusual in children. In an acute vestibular syndrome, the vertigo that is experienced results in a reduction in the normal baseline activity in the ipsilateral vestibular nerve. Because the brain responds to differences in activity between the two vestibular nuclear complexes, the patient experiences vertigo. Additionally, the child may experience autonomic symptoms, including nausea and vomiting. Typically, children adapt to an acute loss of unilateral peripheral vestibular function within several days.

Head Trauma

Head trauma can cause an acute episode of vertigo via a labyrinthine concussion. The mechanism of injury in labyrinthine concussion is poorly understood but may relate to pressure waves transmitted to the labyrinth. Other mechanisms of vertigo after head trauma include injury of the CNS, specifically, a brainstem or cerebellar contusion, or a temporal bone fracture. Another diagnostic consideration for a patient with head trauma followed by vertigo or nonspecific dizziness is that of perilymphatic fistula, i.e., an anomalous connection between the inner ear and middle ear spaces that has been well documented in children.

Vertigo is a common complaint in patients with postconcussion syndrome, with 81% reporting dizziness.

Vestibular Neuritis

Vestibular neuritis is rarely seen in children younger than 10 years old. It should be considered when a viral syndrome is followed by symptoms suggestive of an acute unilateral peripheral vestibular loss. It presents with acute severe vertigo, nystagmus, nausea, and vomiting. The vertigo is worsened by head movements, and patients often prefer to lie down, usually with the affected ear up. There is no hearing loss or tinnitus. Management is supportive and symptomatic, with early ambulation. Vestibular suppressants such as meclizine may be given, but only for a short course, as they may delay long-term recovery.

Recurrent Vertigo

Recurrent vertigo in children can be a result of disease of the peripheral or central vestibular system. However, most recurrent vertigo in children is due to a CNS disorder rather than a peripheral vestibular disorder.

Migraine-Related Dizziness

Migraine is probably the most common cause of recurrent vertigo in children. Whereas migraine typically presents as headache in adults, other manifestations of migraine, including recurrent vertigo and disequilibrium, are more common in children. Benign paroxysmal vertigo of childhood, which is likely to be of migrainous origin, as well as paroxysmal torticollis of infancy, can present with recurrent vertigo in children. Nonvertiginous symptoms of vestibular dysfunction can also be related to migraine. The manifestations of migraine in childhood are quite varied (Balkany and Finkel, 1986).

Benign paroxysmal vertigo of childhood was first described by Basser (Basser, 1964). Vertigo occurs in isolation, without tinnitus and hearing loss. The age of onset is usually by 4 years, but can be as late as 12 years. Vertigo usually lasts less than 1 minute but may last only seconds. Vertigo may occur while sitting, standing, or lying. Pallor, nausea, sweating, and occasionally vomiting occur. Consciousness is not impaired, and the child can recall the episode. There may be no pain or headache associated with the attacks. Immediately after the

attack, the child resumes normal activities. The interval between the attacks varies from weekly to every 6 months. Vertigo attacks usually cease spontaneously after a few years. Physical examination, including a neurologic evaluation, is normal, as is imaging of the skull and temporal bones. Basser reported a moderate or complete canal paresis on caloric testing. However, the response to bithermal caloric testing has been found to be highly variable (Finkelhor and Harker, 1987; Mira et al., 1984). Other testing is normal. Children with benign paroxysmal vertigo of childhood often have a positive family history of migraine, and migraine headaches may develop in later years (Koehler, 1980; Lanzi et al., 1994) and may respond positively to antimigraine treatment. The initial treatment of migrainous vertigo in children is dietary restrictions of foods known to provoke migraine. If this is unsuccessful, the next step is symptomatic treatment with a vestibular suppressant, such as meclizine, during episodes. However, the episodes are usually very brief. If the spells are frequent and especially if they impair school performance, use of a prophylactic antimigraine agent, such as propranolol or topiramate, should strongly be considered (Cass et al., 1997). In younger children, cyproheptadine has also been used successfully.

Ménière's Disease

Ménière's disease, a syndrome presumably caused by endolymphatic hydrops, can occur spontaneously or as a delayed sequela of a previous insult from trauma or viral infection. The disorder rarely occurs in children. Ménière's disease is characterized by a combination of dizziness, unilateral hearing loss, and unilateral tinnitus, which are usually preceded by a feeling of fullness in the affected ear. Following episodes, children are more likely to recover auditory function than are adults. Ménière's disease can be bilateral. Also, with time, a reduction in the responsiveness of the involved peripheral vestibular system occurs. Management of endolymphatic hydrops in children includes reassurance and explanation of the condition to the parents, in addition to salt restriction and a diuretic (Cyr et al., 1985).

Seizure Disorders

Seizure disorders are often accompanied by some sense of dizziness and disequilibrium, although seizures are not frequently associated with true vertigo. However, the term *tornado epilepsy* has been used to describe seizures that are associated with a sense of spinning that can mimic the symptoms of a peripheral vestibular ailment. If a typical vertiginous spell is followed by a generalized tonic-clonic seizure, the diagnosis becomes clearer.

Familial Episodic Ataxia

Familial episodic ataxia is a rare syndrome with autosomal-dominant inheritance and is characterized by episodes of dizziness, disequilibrium, and gait instability that may last for several hours. At least eight types of the syndrome have been identified, and genetic testing is available. These syndromes differ in the duration of the paroxysms of ataxia and associated features. Treatment with acetazolamide can be very helpful for those responsive to it.

Nonvertiginous Disequilibrium

Patients with both peripheral and central vestibular disorders can have nonvertiginous disequilibrium, imbalance, and ataxia. Indeed, many disorders affecting the CNS are symptomatic in this way. Bilateral peripheral vestibular disorders typically occur without vertigo and thus may mimic a central disorder. Numerous CNS abnormalities can be associated with nonvertiginous dizziness. Many of these abnormalities involve the cerebellum and include cerebellar hypoplasia or atrophy, posterior fossa tumors, and Chiari malformations. Also, medication side effects should not be overlooked when evaluating a child with dizziness and disequilibrium.

Bilateral Peripheral Vestibular Loss

Bilateral peripheral vestibular loss can be either congenital and due to inner ear malformations or acquired from meningitis, ototoxicity, and autoimmune disease of the inner ear. Regardless of etiology, bilateral vestibular loss, if severe, is called Dandy's syndrome. Dandy's syndrome is characterized by two specific symptoms: oscillopsia (i.e., jumbling of the visual surround during head motion) and severe gait instability in darkness. Children with bilateral vestibular loss often learn to use alternative sensory inputs, such as vision and proprioception. Also, they modify strategies of eye movements. Environments and tasks that require vestibular function, such as ambulating in dimly lit spaces or trying to maintain stable vision during walking, are extremely challenging for individuals with bilateral vestibular loss.

Central Nervous System Disorders

Numerous CNS disorders cause dizziness, disequilibrium, imbalance, and ataxia. In childhood, cerebellar abnormalities, such as cerebellar vermian hypoplasia, posterior fossa tumors, and Chiari malformation, are the most common disorders encountered. Cerebellar atrophy and ataxia syndromes, such as those caused by familial spinocerebellar ataxia disorders, can also cause these symptoms and are typically progressive. The clinical presentation of such patients may be confusing because they are unlikely to have vertigo and may not display evidence of limb ataxia if their abnormalities affect solely midline cerebellar structures.

Drug-Induced Dizziness

Many drugs can cause nonvertiginous dizziness. For example, the aminoglycosides, especially gentamicin, can cause ototoxicity, which may result in bilateral peripheral vestibular loss. In the pediatric age group, phenytoin is used in the treatment of epilepsy and may produce dizziness and nystagmus as signs of intoxication. With this in mind, any child in whom dizziness develops while on a regular medication should be viewed as a possible case of iatrogenic dizziness.

Nonneurotologic Disorders

Another cause of dizziness in children is psychosomatic dizziness, which usually occurs in children of school age. It may be associated with depression, adjustment reaction of adolescence, and behavior problems. Such children usually have normal vestibular and auditory testing, normal electroencephalograms, and normal imaging studies. When evaluating a child with dizziness, it is essential to determine whether the patient has an associated anxiety disorder, either as the sole cause of their vertiginous complaints, as an accompaniment to an underlying balance system abnormality, or indirectly related to the dizziness, e.g., through a common brainstem ailment causing both disequilibrium and an anxiety disorder.

Treating anxiety disorders in children is challenging because of medication side effects. If the anxiety symptoms are severe, patients should be referred to a child psychiatrist.

Some children with sensory integration disorder, with or without developmental delay, may be overly responsive to vestibular stimulation. An early intervention therapeutic program that helps desensitize the child may help immensely.

Treatments

In addition to the medications that have been discussed, vestibular rehabilitation therapy (VRT) may also be helpful in the treatment of vertigo. Exercises designed to help compensate for an inner ear deficit are taught by specialized physical therapists. VRT can be helpful for benign paroxysmal positional vertigo (BPPV), Ménière's disease, labyrinthitis, vestibular neuritis, and postconcussion vertigo when the symptoms persist for more than a few weeks.

REFERENCES

The complete list of references for this chapter is available in the e-book at www.expertconsult.com.
    See inside cover for registration details.

SELECTED REFERENCES

Balkany, T.J., Finkel, R.S., 1986. The dizzy child. Ear Hear. 7 (3), 138–142.

Basser, L., 1964. Benign paroxysmal vertigo of childhood. Brain 87, 141–152.

Cass, S.P., et al., 1997. Migraine-related vestibulopathy. Ann. Otol. Rhinol. Laryngol. 106 (3), 182–189.

Cyr, D.G., et al., 1985. Vestibular evaluation of infants and preschool children. Otolaryngol. Head Neck Surg. 93 (4), 463–468.

Finkelhor, B.K., Harker, L.A., 1987. Benign paroxysmal vertigo of childhood. Laryngoscope 97 (10), 1161–1163.

Furman, J.M., 1995. Role of posturography in the management of vestibular patients. Otolaryngol. Head Neck Surg. 112 (1), 8–15.

Humphriss, R.L., Hall, A.J., 2011. Dizziness in 10 year old children: an epidemiological study. Int. J. Pediatr. Otorhinolaryngol. 75 (3), 395–400.

Koehler, B., 1980. Benign paroxysmal vertigo of childhood: a migraine equivalent. Eur. J. Pediatr. 134 (2), 149–151.

Lanzi, G., et al., 1994. Benign paroxysmal vertigo of childhood: a long-term follow-up. Cephalalgia 14 (6), 458–460.

Mira, E., et al., 1984. Benign paroxysmal vertigo in childhood. Diagnostic significance of vestibular examination and headache provocation tests. Acta Otolaryngol Suppl. 406, 271–274.

Wiener-Vacher, S.R., 2008. Vestibular disorders in children. Int. J. Audiol. 47 (9), 578–583.

E-BOOK TABLES AND FIGURES

The following figures and tables are available in the e-book at www.expertconsult.com. See inside cover for registration details.

9 Taste and Smell

Julie A. Mennella, Nuala Bobowski, and Djin Gie Liem

CHEMICAL SENSES

The chemical senses of taste, smell, and chemical irritation convey a range of information, warning us of environmental hazards and determining the flavor—good or bad—of ingested foods and liquids (Doty, 2015). The pleasure or displeasure experienced upon ingesting food results from a complex process mediated by the chemical senses in the periphery and then by multiple brain substrates, which are remarkably well conserved phylogenetically. The degree to which the chemicals that stimulate these flavor senses are liked or disliked is determined by interactions of innate factors and experience. Hardwired from birth, the basic biology of humans steers us to seek out sweet foods dense with energy, salty foods dense with minerals, and savory foods rich in proteins and to reject bitter-tasting toxins and unripe sour foods (Mennella, 2014). In essence, these senses function as gatekeepers throughout the life span: they control one of the most important decisions an animal is required to make—whether to reject a foreign substance or consume it.

Taste, Smell, and Flavor

The Taste System

Taste, or gustation, refers to the sensation that occurs when chemicals stimulate taste receptors located on a large portion of the tongue's dorsum and other parts of the oropharynx, such as the larynx, pharynx, and epiglottis. The taste system is attuned to a small number of perceptual classes of experience, the so-called basic tastes (i.e., sweet, salty, savory, bitter, and sour), each of which specifies crucial information about nutrients or dangerous substances. These basic tastes either stimulate intake (sweet, salty, and savory) or inhibit it (bitter and perhaps sour). From an evolutionary perspective, these taste qualities likely evolved to detect and reject that which is harmful (e.g., bitter) and to seek out and ingest that which is beneficial (e.g., sweet, salty). Unlike our modern, commercially produced diet, which has led to the widespread use of added sugars and salts in many parts of the world, the diet of our primitive past was drastically different: salt and sugar were rare and difficult to obtain. Thus the preference for salty and sweet tastes, which is heightened during childhood (Mennella, 2014), is thought to have evolved to attract us to minerals and energy-producing sugars (and their accompanying vitamins) during periods of maximal growth, whereas rejection of bitter-tasting and irritating substances evolved to protect us from poisons, and rejection of concentrated sours evolved to protect us from unripe fruits.

The hedonics of taste are intimately connected to the ingestion or rejection of foods and beverages and thus can pose a nutritional risk when foods and beverages containing highly preferred tastes (sweet, salty) are consumed in excess. Indeed, many chronic diseases (e.g., hypertension, obesity) that plague modern society derive in large part from poor food choices, dictated by our taste preferences. The senses can also pose a risk when healthful foods such as bitter-tasting vegetables are avoided and when children fail to comply with a medication regimen due to the bad taste of the drugs. Many active pharmaceutical ingredients taste bitter or irritate the mouth and throat. Although encapsulating the medicine in pill or tablet form to avoid unpleasant tastes is effective for adults, this is problematic for children, many of whom cannot or will not swallow pills and thus often consume their medication in a liquid formulation. Children cannot benefit from medicines they will not take, and their heightened sensitivity to some bitter tastes makes this especially challenging (Mennella et al., 2013).

The taste receptors in the oral cavity are localized in taste buds, which are innervated by branches of three cranial nerves: the facial (VII), glossopharyngeal (IX), and vagal (X) nerves (Fig. 9-1). Major progress has been made in identifying the initial events in taste recognition. It appears that two different strategies have evolved to detect taste molecules (Bachmanov et al., 2014). For salty and sour tastes, it is widely believed that ion channels serve as receptors. Here H+ (sour) and Na+ (salty) ions are thought to flow through the channels into the cell. However, for both of these taste qualities, the molecular identity of the receptors and their exact mechanisms are still under investigation.

For sweet, umami (savory), and bitter tastes, G-protein-coupled receptors (GPCRs) appear to play the most prominent roles. These GPCRs bind taste molecules in a sort of lock-and-key mechanism. For sweet and umami, a family of three GPCRs, named T1R1, T1R2, and T1R3, act in pairs (T1R1 + T1R3 for umami, and T1R2 + T1R3 for sweet) to detect molecules imparting these taste qualities. The bitter receptors, the T2Rs, comprise a substantially larger family of GPCRs, with about 25 members (Bachmanov et al., 2014). Not only are the chemicals that elicit these three taste qualities detected by specialized receptors on the tongue and other parts of the oral cavity, but many of these receptor proteins are expressed in a wide variety of other tissues, including the gastrointestinal tract, testes, respiratory epithelium, brain, and heart. Although their function in these tissues is still under investigation, this is an emerging area of research. For example, it was recently discovered that bitter receptors expressed in the ciliated cells of the sinonasal epithelium can trigger immune responses when stimulated with chemical signals from bacteria. Thus the expression of these bitter taste receptors in respiratory epithelium may also play a vigilant role in upper airway immunity.

The Olfactory System

Smell, or olfaction, occurs when chemicals stimulate olfactory receptors located on a relatively small patch of tissue high in the nasal cavity. Odor stimuli can reach the olfactory receptors in two ways: by entering the nostrils during inhalation (orthonasal route) or by traveling from the back of the oral cavity toward the roof of the nasal pharynx (retronasal route). Individual experiences largely determine how much a person

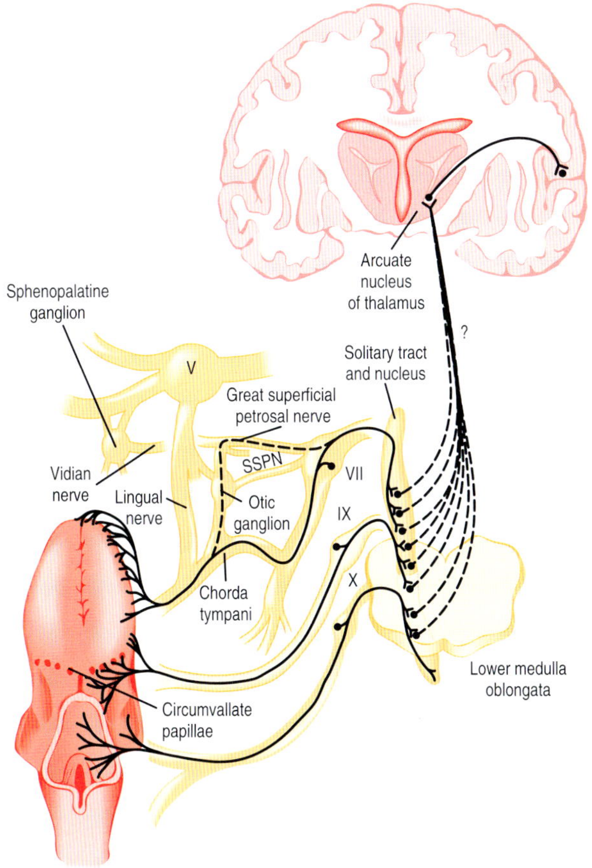

Figure 9-1. Taste innervation is supplied by cranial nerves VII, IX, and X. Filiform, fungiform, and circumvallate papillae are present, with most taste sensation originating from the fungiform and circumvallate papillae. The anterior two thirds of the tongue is innervated by the chorda tympani, a branch of cranial nerve VII; the posterior one third of the tongue and palate are innervated by cranial nerves IX and X. Central connections of the pathways of the cranial nerves in the nucleus solitarius ascend through the thalamus to the parietal operculum. SSPN, small superficial petrosal nerve.

likes or dislikes an odor, although there is some evidence that some odors may be innately biased in a positive or negative direction.

Flavor

Flavor, as an attribute of foods and beverages, is defined as the integration of multiple sensory inputs of the taste, retronasal olfaction, and irritation (e.g., sensations of burn, viscosity, and temperature, resulting from stimulation of nerve endings in the soft membranes of the buccal and nasal cavities of a substance in the oral and nasal cavities. However, the perceptions arising from the taste and smell senses are often confused and misappropriated—odors perceived through the mouth (retronasally) are referred to the oral cavity, whereas odors perceived through the nose (orthonasally) are referred to the external world. For example, the sensations of vanilla, fish, chocolate, and coffee are often erroneously attributed only to the taste system, but much of the sensory input results from retronasal olfaction. Holding the nose while eating interrupts retronasal olfaction and thereby eliminates many of the subtleties of food or medicines, leaving only the taste components.

Clinical Disorders of Taste and Smell

The common confusion between taste and retronasal olfaction is highlighted when patients, young and old, report they cannot taste when they suffer only from olfactory loss. Approximately two thirds of patients who present to specialized chemosensory clinics complain of taste loss, but most patients are diagnosed with a measurable smell dysfunction, rather than a gustatory one, as the basis of their "taste" complaint. A retrospective review of patients evaluated for chemosensory dysfunction complaints revealed that severe, generalized taste deficits (i.e., complete or nearly complete taste loss) do occur but are extremely rare, whereas profound olfactory deficits are more common.

Although complete taste loss is rare, clinical disorders that influence taste and smell perception are more common (Mott and Leopold, 1991; Cowart et al., 1997). As shown in Box 9-1 and Box 9-2, disorders of taste and smell can arise from a variety of sources (Mott and Leopold, 1991; Schecklmann et al., 2013; Doty, 2015); however, many of the conditions listed are based on adult patients' reports and not on standardized test assessments of chemosensory functioning or controlled clinical trials. This lack of systematic analysis, as well as patient confusion between taste and retronasal olfaction, underscores the need for careful sensory evaluation of these causes. Moreover, clinical disorders that influence taste and olfactory perception involve multiple organ systems and require a multidisciplinary approach for appropriate diagnosis and management.

Despite advances in our understanding of the mechanisms and functions of the chemical senses, there are no internationally accepted standards of impairment for the chemical senses, and the treatment options for taste and smell disorders remain limited. Olfactory dysfunctions resulting from impairment of odor access to the olfactory receptors may be treated. For example, patients may experience improvements in olfactory ability after adenoidectomy or surgical management of nasal polyps, which can reestablish nasal airflow. However, individuals whose deficit involves the olfactory neuroepithelium or central olfactory or cortical pathways typically have no treatment options other than time and possible spontaneous recovery. Similarly, the prognosis for severe taste loss is mixed, and gradual recovery was the most common pattern observed in such patients.

In addition to a careful medical history and otolaryngologic examination, assessment of a smell or taste complaint should involve standardized testing using a variety of psychophysical techniques (e.g., detection thresholds, magnitude estimates, quality identification) in a clinical setting. This is particularly important for evaluating olfactory and taste functioning in young children (younger than 5 years of age), who are more prone to attention lapses, tend to answer questions in the affirmative, have limited ability to read and identify labeled choices, and are likely to be unfamiliar with many stimuli used in adult tests. To address the need for brief, comprehensive assessment tools that can be used by clinicians and researchers in a variety of settings, the National Institutes of Health (NIH) Blueprint for Neuroscience Research established and then funded the Toolbox Initiative to assemble tools to assess the domains of cognition, emotion, motor function, and sensation. Included in the sensation tool set is a validated, specialized battery of tests to assess taste and smell for diverse populations from 3 to 85 years of age (Coldwell et al., 2013). Information on the NIH Toolbox tests to assess taste and olfaction can be obtained from the NIH website (www.nihtoolbox.org) and from a special issue of the journal, *Neurology* (vol. 80, no. 11, suppl. 3).

BOX 9-1 Conditions Associated with Disturbances of Taste

- Genetic conditions
  - Familial dysautonomia
  - Turner syndrome
- Endocrine, metabolic, and autoimmune conditions
  - Adrenal insufficiency
  - Cronkhite-Canada syndrome
  - Diabetes mellitus
  - Hypothyroidism, pseudohypoparathyroidism
  - Hyperthyroidism
  - Lupus erythematosus
  - Primary amyloidosis (affecting tongue)
  - Reiter syndrome
  - Scleroderma
  - Sjögren syndrome
- Gastrointestinal and liver diseases
  - Acute hepatitis
  - Chronic liver disease
  - Obstructive jaundice
- Hypertension
- Iatrogenic conditions
  - Acoustic tumor removal
  - Hypophysectomy
  - Laryngectomy
  - Tonsillectomy
  - Cerebellopontine angle meningioma removal
  - Chorda tympani injury or stretching
  - Radiation or chemotherapy
  - Temporal lobectomy
- Infectious conditions
  - Upper respiratory tract infection
  - Candidiasis

- Ulcerative lesions (e.g., gonorrhea, herpes simplex, mycoses, syphilis, varicella zoster)
- Local processes
  - Glossitis
  - Hansen disease
  - Oral mycosis
  - Otitis media
  - Parotid infection or tumor
  - Submandibular gland carcinoma
- Neurologic conditions
  - Bell palsy
  - Brain tumor
  - Guillain-Barré syndrome
  - Head trauma
  - High-altitude syndrome
  - Migraine
  - Multiple sclerosis
  - Seizure disorders
- Uremia or dialysis
- Miscellaneous conditions
  - Bulimia
  - Acquired immunodeficiency syndrome (AIDS)-related periodontitis
  - Cancer
  - Dental caries
  - Gastric reflux disease
  - Gingivitis (acute and chronic)
  - Occupational exposure

(Data taken with permission from Mott AE, Leopold DA. Disorders in taste and smell. Med Clin North Am 1991;75:1321; and from Bromley SM, Doty RL. Clinical disorders affecting taste: Evaluation and management. In: Doty RL, ed. Handbook of olfaction and gustation, 2nd ed. New York: Marcel Dekker, 2003:935.)

For further information about taste and smell disorders, see the National Institute on Deafness and Other Communication Disorders (NIDCD) Information Clearinghouse, a national resource center for information about hearing, balance, smell, taste, voice, speech, and language for health professionals, patients, industry, and the public (www.nidcd.nih.gov/health/misc/pages/clearinghouse.aspx), as well as the NIDCD website (www.nidcd.nih.gov) and the National Institute of Dental and Craniofacial Research website (www.nidcr.nih.gov). Specific clinical questions can be addressed to the NIDCD, the Monell Chemical Senses Center, or the University of Pennsylvania Health Taste and Smell Clinic.

THE ONTOGENY OF TASTE PERCEPTION AND PREFERENCES

The convergence of findings from the scientific literature suggests that human infants, as well as children, have functioning gustatory and olfactory systems that modulate their feeding and expressive behaviors. This responsiveness is not the same as that of adults; these chemosensory systems mature postnatally (Table 9-1) and are influenced by experiences in ways we are just beginning to understand (Mennella, 2014). Little is known about the infant's perception of chemical irritation (e.g., sensations of burn, viscosity, and temperature). Thus this section focuses on the senses of taste and smell, but we acknowledge that other chemical senses may play important roles in the behavior of infants.

The fetus and newborn infants have functioning chemosensory systems, and infants' feeding and expressive behaviors are modulated by taste and smell stimuli. Although these sensory systems are operable early in ontogeny, the fetus and newborns are not merely miniature adults because their sensory systems mature postnatally and are influenced by experience in ways not yet fully understood. Like other sensory systems, taste is experienced through a "sensory window" that changes with age and experience and is partially defined by genetics. Children have well-developed sensory systems for detecting tastes, as well as smells and chemical irritants, and their basic biological preferences for sweet and salty and rejection of bitter tastes are heightened during childhood until late adolescence, when they decline to levels observed in adults. These sensory and biological considerations shed light on why children are so vulnerable to the current food environment rich in added sugars and salt (Mennella, 2014) and why children often reject the bad taste of medicines (Mennella et al., 2013).

Clinical Significance of Taste in Infants and Children

Taste dysfunctions are described by several terms (Cowart et al., 1997). Ageusia refers to a complete loss of gustatory function, whereas hypogeusia refers to diminished sensitivity to detect a specific taste quality or class of compounds (e.g., phenylthiocarbamide). Dysgeusia and phantogeusia refer,

BOX 9-2 Conditions Associated with Disturbances of Olfaction

- Genetic conditions
  - Cleft palate (males)
  - Down syndrome
  - Familial dysautonomia
  - Kallmann syndrome
  - Turner syndrome
- Central nervous system malformations
  - Septo-optic dysplasia
  - Holoprosencephaly
- Endocrine or metabolic conditions
  - Adrenal insufficiency
  - Diabetes mellitus
  - Hypothyroidism
  - Pseudohypoparathyroidism
- Iatrogenic conditions
  - Laryngectomy
  - Ethmoidectomy
  - Hypertelorism procedures
  - Orbitofrontal lobectomy
  - Radiotherapy
  - Rhinoplasty
  - Submucous resection, nasal septum
  - Temporal lobectomy
- Infectious conditions
  - Herpes simplex meningoencephalitis
  - Human immunodeficiency virus (HIV) infection
  - Upper respiratory tract infection
- Liver disease
  - Acute viral hepatitis
  - Cirrhosis
- Local processes
  - Hansen disease
  - Nasal obstruction (adenoid hypertrophy, large inferior turbinates)
  - Polyposis
  - Sjögren syndrome
  - Tumors
- Neurologic conditions
  - Alzheimer disease
  - Head trauma
  - Huntington disease
  - Korsakoff syndrome
  - Multiple sclerosis
  - Meningiomas
  - Migraines
  - Parkinson disease
  - Seizure disorders
  - Temporal lobe tumors
  - Myasthenia gravis
- Psychiatric conditions
  - Hypochondriasis
  - Major depression
  - Posttraumatic stress disorder
  - Schizophrenia
- Uremia or dialysis
- Miscellaneous conditions
  - Cystic fibrosis
  - Giant cell arteritis
  - Occupational exposure
  - Sarcoidosis

(Adapted with permission from Mott AE, Leopold DA. Disorders in taste and smell. Med Clin North Am 1991;75:1321–53; psychiatric conditions updated from Schecklmann, et al. J Neural Transm 2013;120:121–30.)

TABLE 9-1 Developmental Changes in Response to Tastes

Primary Taste	Taste Example	Fetuses and Premature Infants	Newborns	Older Infants (1–24 months)	Children
Sweet	Sugars	Preference*†	Preference*†	Preference*†	Preference*†
Sour	Citric acid	Not known	Rejection*	Rejection*	Preference*†
Bitter	Quinine Urea	Not known Not known	Rejection* Indifference* Rejection‡	Not known Rejection	Rejection*
Salty	NaCl	Not known	Indifference* Rejection§	Indifference Preference*¶	Preference*†
Umami	MSG	Not known	Preference‖	Preference‖	Not known

*Responses to various taste solutions relative to water or diluent.
†Heightened preference compared with adults.
‡Facial expressions suggest rejection, whereas intake studies suggest indifference.
§Sucking measures suggest rejection, whereas intake and facial expression studies suggest indifference.
¶Preference emerges at approximately 4 months of age; before that, indifference or rejection occurs, depending on the methods used.
‖Preference seen only when monosodium glutamate (MSG) is mixed with soup; MSG solution alone is rejected relative to plain water.

respectively, to distortion in the perceived qualities of a taste stimulus and the experience of a taste sensation in the apparent absence of a gustatory stimulus. The study of clinical abnormalities in taste perception in pediatric populations has received little scientific attention, in part because, as discussed earlier, the clinical assessment of taste is not well developed. Some reports in these age groups, although limited, are highlighted here. Box 9-1 lists conditions that sometimes are associated with taste disorders in adults.

A few disorders with neurologic symptoms have been associated with taste disturbances in infants and children. Familial dysautonomia is a hereditary autonomic and sensory neuropathy that affects almost exclusively Jewish children of Ashkenazi extraction. Patients with this disorder could detect but failed to label correctly salty, bitter, sweet, and water stimuli, but sour taste and the sense of smell were preserved. Surgical procedures of the head or neck may sometimes result in taste distortion. For example, tonsillectomy has been associated with taste dysfunction, perhaps because of damage to the lingual branch of the glossopharyngeal nerve. Approximately one third of patients experience taste disturbance 2 weeks after undergoing a tonsillectomy; levels decrease to 8% at 6 months and 2% at 18 months after surgery.

Surgical procedures that involve the middle ear may damage the chorda tympani nerve (branch of cranial nerve VII), which mediates taste perception on the anterior tongue. Damage to or anesthesia of the chorda tympani nerve can increase taste sensations (particularly bitter) from the glossopharyngeal branch of cranial nerve IX and cranial nerve X and blunt retronasal olfactory sensations from cranial nerve I. Likewise, middle ear infections or oral infections that reach the middle ear through the eustachian tubes may affect the chorda tympani nerve as it passes between the malleus and incus and thus affect taste perception. Insults to the chorda tympani nerve may explain some taste disruptions. In particular, occurrence of otitis media during childhood was associated with losses of bitter taste on the tip of the tongue and, when severe, reduced perception of sweetness throughout the mouth, which was associated with a higher risk for obesity.

Endocrine, metabolic, and nutritional disorders causing loss of taste are rare in adults and presumably in pediatric populations. Children with chronic renal failure exhibited reduced preference for sweet-tasting foods, which was unrelated to plasma zinc levels, whereas infants and children diagnosed with second- and third-degree protein-energy malnutrition preferred soup to which savory tastes (e.g., casein hydrolysate) had been added over soup alone. Such findings provide information that may be useful for clinicians in planning palatable diets for these patients.

The most common etiologic factor contributing to taste disturbances in adults appears to be medication use (Schiffman, 1983), but there are few reports regarding similar effects in pediatric populations. Not all individuals taking a particular drug are affected, and the mechanisms by which these medications alter chemosensory function are not well understood. Nevertheless, a variety of medications have been reported sometimes to cause taste (and smell) dysfunction in adults (see Table 9-2).

TABLE 9-2 Drugs Associated with Taste and Smell Dysfunction*

Medication Class	Specific Drug	Chemosensory Dysfunction
Anesthetic	Benzocaine	Ageusia
	Lidocaine	Anosmia
	Cocaine	Anosmia
	Tetracaine	Ageusia
Antibacterial	Procaine penicillin	Metallic dysgeusia
	Metronidazole	Metallic dysgeusia
	Tetracycline	Metallic dysgeusia
	Doxycycline	Anosmia, parosmia
Antiepileptic	Carbamazepine	Hypogeusia
	Tegretol	Hypogeusia
Antidiabetic	Biguanide	Metallic dysgeusia
Antifungal	Amphotericin B	Hypogeusia
Antiinflammatory	Phenylbutazone	Ageusia
	Azelastine	Bitter, metallic dysgeusia
Immunosuppressive/antineoplastic	5-Fluorouracil	Sour, bitter dysgeusia
	Methotrexate	Sour, metallic dysgeusia; ageusia
	Cisplatin	Ageusia
Antirheumatic	Allopurinol	Metallic dysgeusia
	Penicillamine	Metallic dysgeusia
Antithyroid	Methylthiouracil	Ageusia and anosmia
Cardiovascular	Captopril	Increased taste thresholds
	Diltiazem	Hypogeusia, hyposmia
	Nifedipine	Dysgeusia and parosmia
Dental products	Chlorhexidine	Ageusia, loss of salty taste, persistent aftertaste
	Hexidine	Altered taste
	Sodium lauryl sulfate	Loss of sweet and salty taste; dysgeusia
Muscle relaxant	Baclofen	Ageusia, hypogeusia
Opiate	Codeine	Olfactory depression
	Morphine	Olfactory depression
Sympathomimetic	Amphetamines	Bitter dysgeusia; parosmia
Tranquilizers	Chlormezanone	Ageusia; metallic and bitter dysgeusia
Vasopressors	Midodrine	Metallic dysgeusia; antiseptic ("Dettol/Pine-Sol") parosmia

*This is a partial listing of the medications associated with taste and smell disturbances in adults. Not all individuals taking a particular drug are affected, and the mechanisms by which these medications alter chemosensory function are not well understood.

THE ONTOGENY OF OLFACTORY AND FLAVOR PERCEPTION

Infants are able to detect and discriminate a wide variety of odors shortly after birth. They hedonically respond to differences in odor quality, appear to be as sensitive to odors as adults (if not more so), and are capable of retaining complex olfactory and flavor memories.

The early state of maturity and plasticity of the olfactory system favor is related to its involvement in adaptive responses to development. First, experience-induced plasticity in response to odors is a means to tune the olfactory system to stimuli deemed relevant in an individual's environment. Second, salient memories formed during the first 10 years of life will likely be olfactory. Autobiographical memories triggered by olfactory information mainly occurred during the first decade of life, whereas those associated with verbal and visual cues more often occurred later in adolescence and early adulthood.

The normal fetus has open airway passages that are bathed in amniotic fluid and inhales more than twice the volume it swallows during the latter stages of gestation; thus the fetus may be exposed to a unique olfactory environment before birth. This experience represents the first exposure to flavors (tastes and retronasally perceived odors) that will subsequently be provided in mother's milk and then in table foods. Such retronasal perception of odors in amniotic fluid and then in mother's milk provides the infant with the potential for a rich source of various chemosensory experiences and facilitates transition from a diet consisting exclusively of human milk to a mixed diet by providing the infant with bridges of familiarity, such that the infant experiences common flavors in the two feeding situations (Mennella, 2014). Because the infant's first flavor experiences occur before birth in amniotic fluid, breast milk forms a bridge between the experiences of flavors in utero and those in solid foods. The types and intensity of flavors experienced in breast milk may be unique for each infant and serve to identify the culture to which the child is born and raised. When an infant is exposed to a flavor in the amniotic fluid or breast milk and is tested sometime later, the exposed infants accept the flavor more than infants without such experience. This pattern makes evolutionary sense because the foods that a woman eats when she is pregnant and nursing are likely the ones to which her infant will have the earliest exposure.

Breastfeeding conferred an advantage when infants first tasted a food, but only if their mothers regularly eat similar-tasting foods. If their mothers eat fruits and vegetables, breast-fed infants will learn about these dietary choices by experiencing the flavors in mother's milk, thus highlighting the importance of a varied diet for both pregnant and lactating women. These varied sensory experiences with food flavors may help explain why children who are breastfed are less picky and more willing to try new foods; this, in turn, contributes to greater fruit and vegetable consumption in childhood.

Learning about foods and flavors continues during and after weaning. Regardless of whether infants are breastfed or formula-fed, they can learn through repeated dietary experience and dietary variety. Both formula-fed and breastfed infants ingest significantly more of a particular pureed fruit or vegetable after repeated exposure (8 to 10 days) to that particular food. Merely looking at the food does not appear to be sufficient because children have to taste the food to learn to like it. Furthermore, the dietary experience does not have to include the specific food, because exposure to a variety of foods between and within a meal, not just repeated exposure to a single food, facilitates acceptance of novel fruits and vegetables within that particular food category.

The food habits established during infancy track into childhood and adolescence for both nutrient-dense and nutrient-poor foods. Such dietary patterns, which begin to be identified during childhood, are significant determinants of the quality of the adult diet. This raises important issues about high-risk neonates, whose early sensory experiences are often drastically different from those of a typical infant, lacking continuity with prenatal sensory experiences. For example, preterm infants are often unable to coordinate sucking, swallowing, and breathing, so nasogastric or orogastric tube feeding is used to provide adequate nutrition. When fed by a tube, infants likely have a relatively constrained olfactory and flavor experience in the context of feeding because their nutrition bypasses the oral and nasal cavities.

High-risk infants are also faced with a wide array of medical conditions that contribute to temporary or permanent alteration of taste and smell as adults. Many medications, including antibiotics and antiinflammatory agents (Schiffman, 1983), have been shown to alter taste and smell (see Table 9-2), and these medications are commonly given to high-risk neonates. Gastroesophageal reflux disease is another common problem in preterm infants and results in a sour or bitter taste in the mouth from reflux of stomach acid up the esophagus and into the throat. The long-term effects of these alterations on the development of flavor preferences in the child are not known.

Clinical Significance of Olfaction in Infants and Children

The terminology used to describe olfactory dysfunction parallels that used for taste disorders (Doty, 2015). Anosmia refers to the complete absence of olfactory functioning, whereas hyposmia refers to diminished olfactory functioning. In some patients, there may be a deficit in the perception of only a specific odorous compound (e.g., androsterone) or a class of compounds; this condition is commonly referred to as specific anosmia. Hyperosmia refers to an increased sensitivity to smell, dysosmia or parosmia refers to distortions in the perceived qualities of an odor stimulus, and phantosmia refers to the perception of an odor when the odor stimulus is not present.

Box 9-2 lists several conditions that are associated with olfactory disorders in adults. Paranasal sinus disease, prior upper respiratory tract infection, and head trauma account for more than two-thirds of adult cases of olfactory dysfunction. One of the more common forms of head trauma among athletes, concussion, is also associated with olfactory dysfunction, particularly difficulty in identifying odors. Of particular relevance to the neurologist is the fact that a cardinal feature of several neurodegenerative diseases (e.g., Alzheimer, Parkinson) is an olfactory deficit. The loss of smell (and hearing) is less common after head trauma in children than in adults. Common causes associated with impaired olfactory sensitivity in children include nasal obstruction; allergic, chronic, or hypertrophic rhinitis; and nasal polyps (frequently seen in children suffering from cystic fibrosis). Olfactory functioning improves after adenoidectomy in children with nasal obstruction caused by adenoid hypertrophy. Evaluating a child with partial or complete loss of smell may require referral to an otorhinolaryngologist to determine whether there are any local pathologic findings (e.g., foreign body, nasal polyp). Shearing of the olfactory nerves, hemorrhage into the olfactory bulb, fractures of the cribriform plate, and frontal lobe contusions have all been reported in children, but their effects on chemosensory functions remain unknown.

As for the sense of taste, little is known about genetic and congenital disorders of smell perception in infants and children. Although the majority of cases of anosmia are acquired, a small minority of individuals is born anosmic; however, the exact cause for this congenital condition remains unknown (Feldmesser et al., 2007). The principal genetic syndrome associated with permanent anosmia, Kallmann syndrome, is associated with mutations in a variety of genes, many of which are related to defects in neuronal migration. Like the sense of taste, a variety of medications can affect olfactory perception in adults (Schiffman, 1983) (Table 9-2). Moreover, certain metals (e.g., cadmium, zinc, mercury), tobacco products, and a variety of industrial substances cause olfactory loss or distortion.

Several psychiatric conditions are associated with olfactory dysfunction among adults (Box 9-2). Although many posit that relationships exist between olfactory dysfunction and neuropsychiatric disorders among children (Schecklmann et al., 2013), the lack of standardized methodologies and control measures, and potential confounds such as attention and medication use make definitive diagnoses or conclusions difficult. Nevertheless, many disorders are often associated with changes in feeding behaviors (e.g., "picky" eating), which may involve each of the chemical senses.

In assessing picky eating, a thorough medical history and physical examination are recommended to assess the child's growth and nutritional status and to determine the presence of underlying conditions that may result in feeding problems, such as premature birth, gastroesophageal reflux, swollen tonsils, viral infection, or food allergies. A focused feeding history should be completed, including the duration of the feeding problem, whether the child has shown signs of difficulty swallowing, whether the child was ever placed on nothing-by-mouth (nil per os [NPO]) for prolonged periods of time, and whether associated medical interventions centered on the mouth area. Parents should be asked to report on the child's behaviors associated with the feeding problem, including whether anything specific aggravates or alleviates the problem, whether the child indicates hunger or demonstrates an appetite, typical meal duration, and even parental temperament and expectations during feeding times. Because underlying causes of picky eating are oftentimes not due to a medical condition but may be due to lack of prior experience—for example, limited exposure to particular foods or a variety of foods and flavors—understanding all aspects of a child's feeding history is imperative to developing treatment strategies to help the child improve eating behavior.

SUMMARY

The chemical senses of taste, smell, and chemical irritation convey information that warns us of environmental hazards and determines the flavor of ingested foodstuffs. The complex process that generates pleasure or displeasure upon ingesting food is mediated both by the chemical senses in the periphery and by multiple brain substrates, which are remarkably well conserved phylogenetically. Hardwired from birth, the basic biology of humans steers us to seek out sweet (energy-dense), salty (mineral-dense), and savory (protein-rich) foods and to reject bitter-tasting toxins and unripe sour foods.

The fetus and newborn infants have functioning chemosensory systems, and infants' feeding and expressive behaviors are modulated by taste and smell stimuli. Although these sensory systems are operable early in ontogeny, the fetus and newborns are not merely miniature adults, because their sensory systems mature postnatally and are influenced by experience in ways not yet fully understood. Like other sensory systems, taste is experienced through a "sensory window" that changes with age and experience and is partially defined by genetics. Children's basic biological preferences for sweet and salty and rejection of bitter tastes are heightened during childhood. These sensory and biological considerations shed light on why it is difficult to make lifestyle changes in young children and why it is difficult for children to eat nutritious foods when these foods do not taste good to them or take medicines that taste extremely bitter. We cannot easily change the basic ingrained biology of liking sweets and avoiding bitterness.

What we can do is modulate children's flavor preferences by providing early exposure, starting in utero, to a wide variety of healthy flavors and moderating exposure to salt. The reward systems that encourage us to seek out pleasurable sensations and the emotional potency of food- and flavor-related memories initiated early in life together play a role in the strong emotional component of food habits throughout the life span. An appreciation of the complexity of early feeding and a greater understanding of the cultural and biological mechanisms underlying the development of food preferences will aid in our development of evidence-based strategies and programs to improve the diets of our children. Better understanding of the scientific basis for distaste and how to ameliorate it is a public health priority for advancing availability of formulations of drug products that will be accepted by children and getting children off to a good start in food choices and preferences. The study of smell and taste perception in clinical populations of infants and children and the influence of chemosensory dysfunction on nutritional status have received little scientific attention, and they remain important areas for future investigations.

REFERENCES

The complete list of references for this chapter is available in the e-book at www.expertconsult.com.
See inside cover for registration details.

SELECTED REFERENCES

Bachmanov, A.A., Bosak, N.P., Lin, C., et al., 2014. Genetics of taste receptors. Curr. Pharm. Des. 20 (16), 2669–2683.

Coldwell, S.E., Mennella, J.A., Duffy, V.B., et al., 2013. Gustation assessment using the NIH Toolbox. Neurology 80 (11 Suppl. 3), S20–S24.

Cowart, B.J., Young, I.M., Feldman, R.S., et al., 1997. Clinical disorders of smell and taste. Occup. Med. 12 (3), 465–483.

Doty, R.L. (Ed.), 2015. Handbook of Olfaction and Gustation, third ed. Wiley Blackwell, New York.

Feldmesser, E., Bercovich, D., Avidan, N., et al., 2007. Mutations in olfactory signal transduction genes are not a major cause of human congenital general anosmia. Chem. Senses 32 (1), 21–30.

Mennella, J.A., 2014. Ontogeny of taste preferences: Basic biology and implications for health. Am. J. Clin. Nutr. 99 (3), 704S–711S.

Mennella, J.A., Spector, A.C., Reed, D.R., et al., 2013. The bad taste of medicines: Overview of basic research on bitter taste. Clin. Ther. 35 (8), 1225–1246.

Mott, A.E., Leopold, D.A., 1991. Disorders in taste and smell. Med. Clin. North Am. 75 (6), 1321–1353.

Schecklmann, M., Schwenck, C., Taurines, R., et al., 2013. A systematic review on olfaction in child and adolescent psychiatric disorders. J. Neural Transm. 120 (1), 121–130.

Schiffman, S.S., 1983. Taste and smell in disease (second of two parts). N. Engl. J. Med. 308 (22), 1337–1343.

E-BOOK FIGURES AND TABLES

The following figures and tables are available in the e-book at www.expertconsult.com. See inside cover for registration details.

Fig. 9-2 Lateral depiction of the innervation of cranial nerves.
Fig. 9-3 Major structures involved in olfaction.

10 Neuropsychological Assessment

Margaret Semrud-Clikeman and Kenneth F. Swaiman

 An expanded version of this chapter is available on www.expertconsult.com. See inside cover for registration details.

INTRODUCTION

Pediatric neuropsychology differs from adult neuropsychology because development is incomplete and brain differences emerge through childhood and adolescence that interact with the environment changing brain structure and neural pathways (Giedd, 2004). A discussion of neuropsychological assessment can be found in several excellent texts (Lezak et al., 2004). The teaming of neurology and neuropsychology can provide state-of-the-art service to children, particularly those with complex and refractory disorders.

Because development is an important aspect at both ends of the life span, it is important to recognize the neuropsychological differences that may occur and the manner in which they may relate to interventions. Moreover, an important aspect for children is the ability to do well in school. Executive functioning is an important aspect of academic and social success. Executive functioning in the areas of planning, organization, emotional control, and inhibition are all important skills for success. Frequently physicians are consulted about difficulties in these areas. An important reference to assist physicians, teachers, and parents in working with children with difficulties in this area has been published by Lynn Meltzer (Meltzer, 2007). Finally, studies that link brain imaging differences in children with autism (Adolphs, 2002) and attention-deficit/hyperactivity disorder (ADHD) (Semrud-Clikeman et al., 2006) are providing new windows into our understanding of these disorders.

NEUROPSYCHOLOGICAL ASSESSMENT
What is a Neuropsychological Assessment?

Neuropsychological assessments are frequently completed to provide additional information about a variety of developmental disorders. The most common referral questions concern medical disorders including genetic disorders, concussion/traumatic brain injury, recovery from cancer/brain tumors, and other neurologic concerns such as epilepsy and movement disorders. In addition, children who have acquired disorders such as those resulting from exposure to lead or other teratogenic substances are also frequently referred for an evaluation. Disorders such as dyslexia, ADHD, autism spectrum disorder, and fetal alcohol spectrum disorder are common reasons for referral for assessment, particularly when typical interventions have not been successful. Psychiatric disorders such as obsessive-compulsive disorder, anxiety and depression, and behavioral dysregulation are referred for evaluation to more fully understand the child's difficulty and to provide recommendations for intervention in the home and at school.

Child clinical neuropsychology is best viewed within an integrative perspective for the study and treatment of child and adolescent disorders. By addressing brain functions and the environmental influences inherent in complex human behaviors, such as thinking, feeling, reasoning, planning, and executive functioning, clinicians can assist neurologists and pediatricians in providing the most appropriate service to children with severe learning, psychiatric, developmental, and acquired disorders (Chapters 50 and 58 and chapters in part XIX). Although clinical psychologists and neuropsychologists use similar measures, the interpretation differs. A neuropsychologist views test findings through the lens of neurodevelopment. With our burgeoning knowledge of neural development from studies of serial magnetic resonance imaging, we are able to more fully understand how the environment, genetics, age, gender, and experience can alter brain activity and brain development (Shaywitz et al., 2004). Attention to the scope and sequence of development of cortical structures and related behaviors that emerge during childhood allows further understanding of the effect of interventions, instructional opportunities, and enrichment on the neurodevelopmental process.

Due to the complexity of the brain, and in particular the developing brain, it is most appropriate to utilize a transactional approach to the study and treatment of childhood and adolescent disorders. A description of a transactional approach is that it takes into consideration how abnormalities or developmental complications interact with the environment, how development itself affects the nature and severity of impairment, how to most efficiently assess these difficulties, and how to determine the most appropriate interventions. In this model, neuropsychological assessment—correctly completed—is therapeutic. In this view, the child's performance on appropriate measures plus the feedback to the medical professional, parent, and school provide a basis for understanding the child's strengths and weaknesses and for participating in the development of appropriate interventions. A transactional approach stresses consultation and collaboration with the caregivers of the child (as well as assisting the child in adjusting to his/her areas of challenge) but also with medical practitioners. In summary, child clinical neuropsychology is best viewed within an integrated framework, incorporating behavioral, psychosocial, cognitive, and environmental factors into a comprehensive model for the assessment and treatment of brain-related disorders in children and adolescents.

Current theory posits that regions of the brain have a bidirectional influence on various neural functional systems, which in turn affect the intellectual and perceptual capacity of the child. The child's behavioral, psychological, and cognitive manifestation of a childhood disorder is likely influenced by the interaction of these functional systems. In addition, the child's neurologic functioning also interacts with his/her social, family, and school environments that facilitate compensatory or coping skills in the individual child, which are either helpful or problematic.

Theorists have hypothesized that developmental regulation underlies behavioral and biological functioning. In other words, biological vulnerabilities influence and are influenced by coping skills and stresses experienced in the child's life. Such adaptation may or may not be efficient or "healthy" but can be viewed as the child's attempt to achieve self-stabilization. In such a paradigm, the individual reacts to both internal and external environments as he or she attempts to make his or her way in the world. Children who experience severe neglect and/or abuse in utero have been found to exhibit significant dysregulation and disruption of the hypothalamic-pituitary-adrenal axis affecting emotional and neuropsychological development (Tarullo and Gunnar, 2006).

The transactional model incorporates these findings by assuming a dynamic interaction among the biogenetic, neuropsychological, environmental, cognitive, and psychosocial systems. Further, biogenetic forces shape the child's experiences and are most predominant during embryogenesis and early infancy. As the child develops, the social and cultural environment in which he or she lives begins to influence the child's neurologic development. Moreover, the child's temperament also interacts with all of these environments and causes changes in these environments.

The quality of fit between the caregiver's and the child's temperaments can result in adaptation to difficult behavior or exacerbation of this behavior. For example, a child who is fussy and difficult will not fare as well with an anxious or domineering parent as with a more even-tempered parent. Similarly, an "easy" child will generally work well with any parent. A "difficult" child-"easy" parent match may be advantageous in that the parent can help reduce the adverse effects of the child's inborn biological tendencies. So, although parental caretaking may not change the biological tendencies of the child, it may buffer biological vulnerabilities (Rothbart and Sheese, 2007). For those children who experience early deprivation and/or abuse, parental caretaking begun at later ages may not be able to fully buffer neurologic differences that are laid down early on. Rather, the child may always have these difficulties and will need additional support to develop appropriate coping mechanisms. The physician is well placed to understand neurologic development within the lens of transactional theory.

MULTICULTURAL FACTORS

It is important to note that most neuropsychological measures have not been standardized on ethnicities beyond middle-class whites. Cultural expectations and mores have just begun to be studied in neuropsychology. In the past, neuropsychology has suggested that the brain may not be culturally bound. Currently, culture and neurodevelopment has been implicated in handedness, specialization of the cerebral hemispheres for tasks, and self-reports of behavioral functioning (Carlson et al., 2000). Differences in language may also affect neuropsychological assessment even when an interpreter is utilized. Some words or concepts do not readily translate from English. Moreover, the standardized norms may not apply to the patient's ethnicity.

An example of these difficulties is exemplified in a study by Keith and Fine (2005) which focused on possible ethnic differences in learning. Quality and quantity of instruction, previous achievement, and motivation were statistically evaluated across Anglo-American, African American, Hispanic, Native American, and Asian American groups. Although higher quality of instruction was found to lead to better achievement across the groups, quality of instruction appeared to be less important for Native American groups than quantity of instruction. Quantity of instruction was also found to be important for the Asian American population. In contrast, academic motivation and prior achievement were the best predictors for learning for the Anglo-American students. There were also differences for African American and Hispanic students where motivation, previous achievement and coursework were the strongest influences on their resultant learning. These findings indicate that children of different ethnicities

may benefit from differing strategies and that cultural differences may play a major role in task performance.

NEUROPSYCHOLOGICAL TESTING

Neuropsychological testing can be very useful to the neurologist in assisting in developing appropriate interventions. Neuropsychological testing is generally an adjunct to the neurologic assessment and can be helpful in establishing areas of strengths and weaknesses that can then be translated into assistance in the school setting. Most neuropsychologists use a flexible battery that covers the main domains of functioning to assess children. Generally, the focus in neuropsychological assessment with children and adolescents revolves around the following tenets:

a. It is important to discriminate between behaviors present within a normal neurodevelopmental framework from those which are delayed or which are a result of alterations of the central nervous system given the child's social-environmental context.
b. Learning deficits/disorders and behavioral difficulties are examined within the context of brain function.
c. Recovery of function after brain injury, neurosurgery, and radiologic/chemotherapy treatment is monitored to assess the effect of these treatments on normal development and emotional/behavioral adjustment.
d. Focus is present on the different neuropsychological domains of functioning, particularly in the areas of cognition, executive functioning, memory, motor, behavior, and emotion during recovery or during a neurodevelopmental course.
e. Neuropsychology investigates the psychiatric disorders of children with severe neurologic disorders.
f. Neuropsychology assists in the design of remediation programs, particularly when used within an integrated clinical framework.

Scores on neuropsychological measures are generally one of four types. *Scaled scores* are generally found on the subtests of major measures including the Wechsler Intelligence Scales, executive functioning scales, as well as some of the achievement batteries. *Average scaled scores* are between 7 and 13 with a mean at 10. Scores between 5 and 7 are below average and those 4 and lower are considered significantly below average. Scaled scores between 13 and 15 are above average and those above 15 are significantly above average. Figure 10-1 illustrates these different types of scores. *Standard scores* are those with a mean of 100 and average performance between 85 and 115. Most overall IQ measures, adaptive functioning, and executive functioning measures are based on these standard scores. As seen in Figure 10-1, scores 116 to 130 are considered high average and those above 130 superior. Scores from 70 to 84 are considered low average and those below 70 are considered significantly below average. *T scores* are used with some ability measures (Kaufman Assessment Battery for Children and Differential Ability Scales) and with developmental measures (Mullen Scales of Early Learning) as well as with many behavioral rating scales. Average T scores range from 40 to 60 with scores above 60 classified as high or above average and those below 40 as below average or low average.

In some cases, scores will be presented with percentiles. Percentiles cannot be used as precisely as scaled, standard, or T scores and cannot be subtracted or added. Rather, they give an idea of how the child compares to other children his/her age. At times, age equivalents and grade equivalents may be reported, but these are only rough estimates and should be used with extreme caution. A child in third grade who scores at a first grade level is not performing as a first grader would

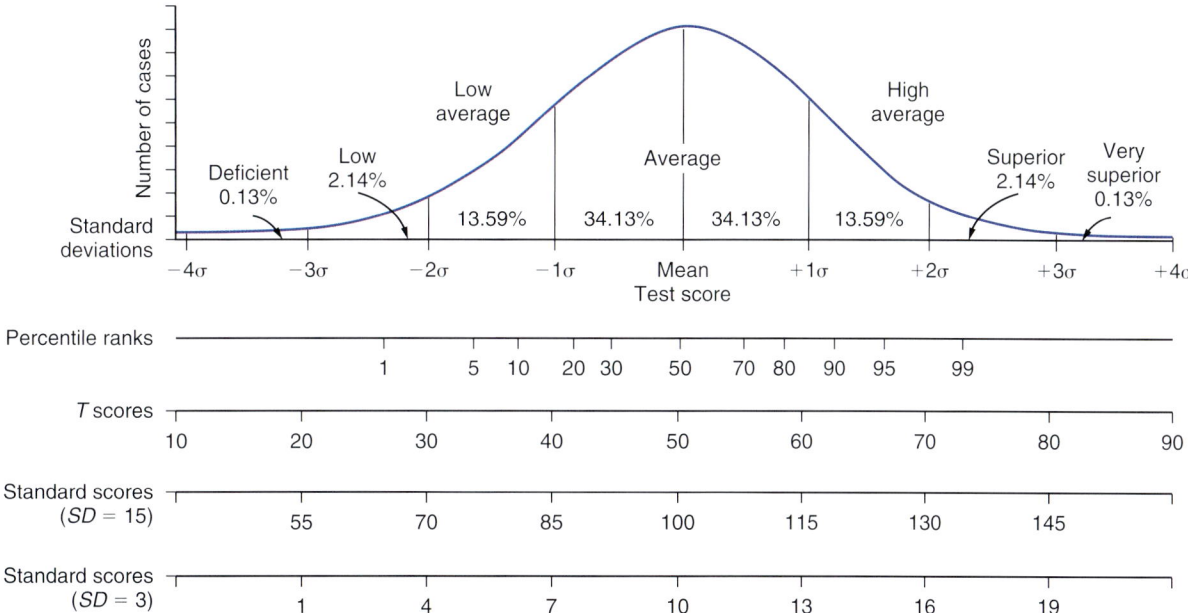

Figure 10-1. Normal curve showing standard scores, T Scores, Percentiles, and Z-Scores. *(Modified from* www.assessmentpsychology.com. *©2005–2014. William E. Benet, PhD, PsyD. All rights reserved.)*

on the material; rather, it means that the child shares with the average first grader the number of items correct on the test and should only be interpreted in reference to the child's current grade comparison group. Similarly, age equivalents are obtained by computing the average raw score obtained by children at different ages.

Table 10-1 describes the major measures used by most child neuropsychologists. It is not meant to be an exhaustive list of all available measures as that is beyond the scope of this chapter. Table 10-1 is intended to provide basic information about the measures frequently reported in neuropsychological assessments. Unless noted otherwise, higher scores are desirable.

WHEN TO REFER FOR NEUROPSYCHOLOGICAL EVALUATION

Neuropsychological evaluations are generally recommended under the following conditions:

1. Conditions affecting the central nervous system, such as head trauma, chemotherapy/radiation treatment, genetic disorder, neurodegenerative disorders, transplant (solid organ or bone marrow), and seizures. Serial evaluations are particularly important for these children in order to monitor recovery as well as to assess treatment efficacy.
2. Learning difficulties that have not responded to traditional educational intervention, particularly when there are soft neurologic signs present. Soft signs include toe-walking, concurrent movement in a body part not required for a motor task (synkinesia), problems with perception of finger location as well as tactile sensations (agnosia), problems with completing rapid alternating movement in a limb or body part (dysdiadochokinesis), and tactile localization as well as minor reflex asymmetries in the presence of normal cognitive development.
3. Severe mood and behavioral dysregulation that have been resistant to traditional psychopharmacological, psychological, or behavioral interventions.

4. Acute onset of memory, cognitive, academic, motor, speech/language, behavioral, and behavioral dysregulation disorders.
5. Regression of skills previously mastered.

THE NEUROPSYCHOLOGICAL REPORT

A good neuropsychological evaluation and report will include measures of cognition, executive functioning, learning/memory (visual and oral), fine motor, visual-motor, behavior, and emotion. Generally, neuropsychological reports begin with an explanation of the referral question and then move into background information concerning the child's gestation, delivery, early development, and medical history.

One of the most important aspects of the neuropsychological report is the section describing the behavioral observations. This section describes the child's reaction during the session as well as any unusual observed behaviors. Particular emphasis is given to the child's attention to task, frustration tolerance, and the ease with which rapport is established. These aspects of the child's behavior affect the results that are found and are very important for understanding the validity and reliability of the assessment. Good neuropsychological reports not only synthesize in an understandable manner the findings from tests, but they also incorporate the background information, medical history, and behavioral observations into a coherent story to assist with treatment. In addition, the report should provide tailored recommendations for home, school, and if appropriate, medical treatment. Table 10-2 provides the aspects of a good neuropsychological report. A Roman numeral will highlight these aspects in the following excerpts.

The sample report contained in this section is representative of a report that was found to be useful by the neurologist who referred the child:

I. ***Reason for Evaluation:*** *Sasha Small is a 9-year, 10-month old, right-handed male who was referred to the Pediatric*

TABLE 10-1 Most Commonly Used Neuropsychological Measures

Neuropsychological Measure	Age Range	Description	Comments
DEVELOPMENTAL SCALES			
Bayley Scales of Infant Development III (BSID III)	1–42 mos	Provides overall cognitive scores as well as scores in the areas of language, motor, and behavior.	Excellent overall measure. Reliability and validity are very good. Must be administered by a trained professional.
Mullen Scales of Early Learning	Birth to 68 mos	Provides scores and age equivalents for expressive language, receptive language, fine motor, gross motor, and visual reception (measure of problem solving).	Very child friendly—attractive tasks which are quite hands on. Can be administered by trained nurses as well as psychologists.
Denver Developmental Screening Test II	Birth to 6 yrs	Provides age equivalents in the areas of motor, language, and social.	Good screening measure and should be used to refer for further testing if needed. Nurses and nurse practitioners can administer.
COGNITIVE			
Wechsler Primary and Preschool Scale of Intelligence (WPPSI) IV	2–6:7–3	Provides overall score as well as scores on verbal comprehension, perceptual reasoning, working memory, and processing speed.	Excellent measure of cognitive ability for children without language difficulties.
Wechsler Intelligence Scale for Children V	6.0:16–11	Similar to WPPSI.	One of the best measures of overall ability, providing information about working memory and processing speed as well as general language and perception. Very strong psychometric properties. Requires advanced training for administration and interpretation.
Kaufman Assessment Battery for Children II	3–18	Provides a measure of cognitive functioning with less dependence on language. Results in scores for planning, knowledge, simultaneous, and sequential reasoning; also has a nonverbal score.	Good measure for children of different cultures or whose first language is not English. Is relatively easy to administer and score. Usually administered by psychologists/neuropsychologists.
Stanford-Binet Intelligence Scale 5	2–85+	Provides scores for verbal ability, perceptual reasoning, working memory, and overall ability.	Excellent measure for younger children with difficulty with attention and motor control. With older ages, the load on language is substantial.
Differential Abilities Scale II	2–6:17–11	Provides measures of verbal skills, memory, and nonverbal processing. Also has an achievement scale.	Excellent measure for children with reduced attentional skills, autism, and behavioral regulation difficulties.
Woodcock-Johnson Test of Cognitive Abilities Cognitive Battery IV	2–85+	Measures of fluid reasoning, auditory processing, memory, attention, visual-motor skills. More like an academic test.	Very long battery than can take over 90 min to administer. Not frequently used by neuropsychologists—more often used in education.
Universal Nonverbal Intelligence Test	5–0:17–11	Provides an overall measure of ability—does not use language.	Excellent measure for hard-of-hearing children as well as English-as-a-second-language learners.
Leiter International Intelligence Scale-3	3–75+	Nonverbal test.	Good for deaf, hard-of-hearing and English-as-a-second-language learners.
Comprehensive Test of Nonverbal Intelligence 4	6–0:89–11	Nonverbal measure.	Fairly good screen for ability but as defined there is no language component.
EXECUTIVE FUNCTIONING			
A Developmental NEuroPSYchological Assessment (NEPSY II)	3–16	Comprehensive test of measures of memory (verbal and visual), attention, inhibition, verbal fluency, sensorimotor skills.	Excellent measure for executive functioning as well as for memory and motor skills. Most clinicians do not use the full battery as it can take more than 2 hours to administer. Requires a psychologist/neuropsychologist to administer.
Delis-Kaplan Executive Function System	8–89	Comprehensive measure of executive functioning including measures of working memory, metacognition, perspective taking, attention, planning, and organization.	Excellent measure of executive functioning. Requires a skilled neuropsychologist for interpretation. Most clinicians use some subtests rather than full battery as it can take more than 2 hours to administer.
Behavior Rating Inventory of Executive Functioning	2–18	Parent, teacher, and self-rating of basic executive functioning skills.	Provides measure of emotional control, behavioral regulation, and metacognition. Computer scored. Can be administered by medical personnel as well as psychology.
Wisconsin Card Sorting Test	6–6:89	Measure of cognitive flexibility, attention, distractibility, and problem solving.	Complex administration and scoring require additional training—generally administered by neuropsychologists.

TABLE 10-1 Most Commonly Used Neuropsychological Measures *(Continued)*

Neuropsychological Measure	Age Range	Description	Comments
MEMORY			
California Verbal Learning Test—Children's version	5–16.11	Requires the child to learn a list of words and provides 4 additional practice trials. Also provides a delay as well as cues to remembering the list.	Good and relatively easy measure of short- and long-term memory as well as learning rate.
Wechsler Memory Scale-IV	16–0:90–11	Appropriate for patients 16 yrs and older. Provides a comprehensive evaluation of memory as well as individual scores of visual and auditory memory.	Good measure of memory, both long and short-term. Full test requires more than 1 hour to administer. Most clinicians use a part of the measure. Generally administered by psychologists.
Rey-Osterrieth Complex Figure Test	5–0 to adult	Requires the patient to copy a very complex figure and then 20 minutes later to draw from memory.	Easy to administer—requires some training for interpretation. Measures planning and organization as well as visual-motor skills.
Test of Memory and Learning-2	5–0:59–11	Measures of visual and auditory memory as well as the patient's ability to learn a novel task.	Good measure of overall memory.
MOTOR			
Purdue Pegboard Test	3–adult	Measure of fine motor dexterity.	Can compare dominant, nondominant, and both [hands] together scores. Easy to administer and score.
Grooved Pegboard Test	5–adult	Measure of fine motor dexterity.	Can compare dominant and nondominant hands. More complex than Purdue as it has pegs that fit only one way into the hole.
Tapping	5–adult	Measure of fine motor speed.	Provides scores for dominant and nondominant hands. Patient must tap quickly on a key. Easy to administer and score.
Grip Strength	6–adult	Measure of hand strength.	Provides measure of hand strength for dominant and nondominant hands. Easy to administer and score.
ACHIEVEMENT			
Gray Oral Reading Tests IV	6–0:23–11	Measure of reading accuracy, rate, and comprehension.	Good and fairly quick measure of overall reading ability.
Woodcock-Johnson Test of Achievement Battery V	2–85+	Provides a detailed measure of reading ability, mathematics, written language, and auditory comprehension.	Requires some training for administration. Must be computer scored.
Wechsler Individual Achievement Test III	4–0:50–11	Provides a detailed measure of reading, mathematics, and written language as well as oral comprehension.	Requires some training for administration, scoring, and interpretation.
BEHAVIOR RATING SCALES			
Behavior Assessment System for Children-2	2–adult	This is a comprehensive measure of behavior and emotional development. Provides T scores for externalizing, internalizing, and adaptive behaviors.	Has a parent, teacher, and self-report form. Easy to administer and relatively easy to interpret. Has computer scoring. Is unique as it also has adaptive behavior scales. Different forms for preschool, ages 8–11, ages 12–21, and adults.
Achenbach System of Empirically Based Assessment (Child Behavior Checklist)	18 mos–90+	This is a comprehensive measure of behavior and emotional skills. T scores are available for internalizing and externalizing behaviors.	Widely used. Has a teacher, parent, and self-report form. Easy to administer and relatively easy to interpret with computer scoring. Assessment has multicultural applications in Africa, Asia and South America.
ADAPTIVE BEHAVIOR SCALES			
Vineland Adaptive Behavior Scale	0–90	This measure provides parent, caregiver, and/or teacher input as to the child's performance in communication, daily living skills, socialization and for children ages 5 and under, fine and gross motor skills. There is also a measure of problematic behaviors.	Relatively easy to administer and score. The scale can be compared with ability scores as well as to language skills. There are two forms—the rating scale completed independently by the parent or the interview scale. The interview scale requires additional training.
Adaptive Behavior Assessment System, 3rd edition	0–89	Has 5 forms based on age. Is completed by parents and teachers. Provides 3 adaptive domains (communication, socialization, daily living skills).	Very easy for parents to complete. Has parent, teacher/day care provider forms as well as an adult form.

TABLE 10-2 Details of an Optimal Neuropsychological Report

Report Aspect	What is Included
I. Reason for Referral	Clear, concise, explanation for referral; name of referring professional; relevant medical information.
II. History	Provides relevant information about parental education, family composition and history, current stressors, medical and social history.
III. Behavioral Observation	This very important section provides information about how the child approached the tasks, attention, language, mood, and how easily rapport was established. It also includes a statement as to how valid and reliable the results are which were obtained.
IV. Tests Administered	This is a brief list of what measures were utilized.
V. Test Interpretation and Impressions	This is the body of the report and includes information as to how the child scored on measures of cognition, language, attention, memory, and motor skills. It concludes with a summary statement that not only provides information as to what these findings mean and what diagnoses are appropriate, it also links these findings to neurologic and psychological functioning.
VI. Recommendations	This section provides recommendations and is generally grouped into three sections: school, medical, and home.

Neuropsychology Clinic by the Neurofibromatosis Clinic. Sasha has a history of neurofibromatosis type 1 (NF1), a genetic syndrome that is associated with physical manifestations such as skin abnormalities, as well as increased risk for learning disabilities and behavioral problems. At present, Sasha attends fourth grade in a regular education classroom. He receives speech therapy to address concerns related to articulation. His parents reported several behavioral concerns, including immature behaviors, difficulty making friends, and frequent angry outbursts. The purpose of the current evaluation was to assess Sasha's neurocognitive functioning and to assist with educational and treatment planning.

The next part of the report should provide a short synopsis of the family and social history. This section should include information about the parents and their education, the family makeup, and any stressors currently being experienced. In addition, the developmental and medical history should provide information about the pregnancy and delivery as well as developmental milestones and any concerns that were present during infancy and toddlerhood. It should also provide information as to whether the child has had any head injuries, experienced any domestic violence or other trauma, and information about the child's vision, hearing, sleep, and appetite. After this section, information about the child's school history is very helpful, particularly outlining whether the child has any special accommodations, has been evaluated by his or her school or another clinician, and what reports the teachers have made as to the child's academic progress and social and behavioral functioning. It should also provide information about what psychological services (therapy) have been put into place for this child. Finally, within this section,

it is optimal to have a summary section that concisely discusses the child's current level of functioning. The following excerpt illustrates this summary:

> *II. **Current Functioning**: Sasha's parents reported primary concern regarding Sasha's difficulties with behavioral regulation and social development. His mother indicated that Sasha's behavior can be difficult to manage when he is angry or he does not get his way. He will have long "fits" if his parents tell him to do things he does not want to do (e.g., brush teeth, change clothes, take a shower, turn off electronics, or practice math/reading). Sasha frequently becomes angry or jealous of his sister, who does not tend to misbehave or get into trouble. He will frequently yell at her and sometimes he will become aggressive and hit her. His parents noted that despite these behaviors, Sasha can also be sweet, kind-hearted and gentle at times.*

As stated, the behavioral observations section is very important for understanding how the child was during the assessment, his/her level of engagement, how difficult/easy it was to establish rapport, and to describe areas of functioning such as language, attention, and mood. By reading the next excerpt one should be able to picture Sasha during the assessment and whether to have faith in the results.

> *III. **Behavioral Observations**: Sasha's mother accompanied him to the evaluation. Sasha presented as a casually dressed boy who appeared his chronological age. He was appropriately dressed, but frequently walked around with untied shoelaces. He willingly accompanied the examiner and his mother to the testing room. After being seated and beginning the testing, Sasha did not take off his heavy winter coat until the examiner had prompted him to do so. Sasha was able to transition into testing without difficulty. Rapport was easily established and maintained. Sasha's speech was fluent, but he had difficulties with articulation and made several sound substitutions particularly the "r" sound (e.g., "three" = "thwee," "break" = "bwake"). His speech was usually intelligible, although the examiner occasionally needed to prompt him to repeat himself to understand what he said. Sasha asked questions or commented on the tests frequently, and occasionally made requests (e.g., asking for a break or a snack). Sasha frequently made comments when he felt that a test item was difficult. Sasha's eye contact was appropriate. No problems were apparent with fine or gross motor skills, and no unusual motor movements were observed. He wrote and drew with his right hand. It was notable that during a pegboard task, Sasha dropped pegs several times when trying to place them in the board.*

> *Sasha was generally pleasant and cooperative throughout the evaluation. He had some difficulty regulating his body and would frequently stand up in his chair during the tasks. On some tasks he had difficulty waiting for directions to be completed before attempting to start the task, and the examiner often needed to prompt him to listen to all of the instructions. He was generally attentive to the tasks, although toward the end of the session he appeared more distracted and often looked elsewhere when the examiner talked with him. He was occasionally distracted by looking at some playground equipment outside the testing room window. His affect varied according to the topic but was appropriate to the situation. He appeared fatigued toward the end of testing and occasionally asked how much time was left. He took multiple long bathroom breaks during testing. Sasha showed a few behaviors that seemed more typical of a younger child. For example, when asked a question about whether he had ever purposefully hurt himself, he began hitting his head and joked that it was*

"fun." When the examiner followed up with additional questions, he denied a desire to hurt himself. Overall, Sasha seemed to put forth good effort on the testing and worked to the best of his abilities. Therefore the results of testing are thought to be a valid and accurate indicator of Sasha's functioning in the areas assessed.

The next section discusses the findings and should provide a concise and systematic review of the measures. Discussion of cognitive ability, memory, executive functioning, and behavioral/emotional functioning should be discussed. It is also important to tie these results to whatever medical, genetic, or brain difference is present. The following is very short excerpts of a much longer report to give a flavor of what should be included in a good neuropsychological report. Tests that were used are in italics and underlined allowing more efficient use of Table 10-1.

*IV. **Result and Impressions:** Sasha Small is a 9-year, 10-month old boy with a history of **neurofibromatosis type 1 (NF1)**. NF1 is an inherited neurologic disorder that can affect multiple systems of the body. It is associated with symptoms such as skin changes, neurofibromas (tumors that form on the nerves under the skin), skeletal abnormalities, and other complications. Additionally, problems with behavioral health can be one of the most significant features of the syndrome for many individuals. Research indicates that children with NF1 are at higher risk for cognitive and learning disabilities than unaffected children, as well as for social and behavioral difficulties. Due to this increased risk, it can be useful to obtain periodic developmental assessments to inform educational and treatment planning.*

This paragraph sets the stage for understanding the relationship between NF1 and the neuropsychological findings. The report then moves into the various domains that were assessed beginning with cognition:

Results of the current evaluation indicate that Sasha's overall intellectual abilities are broadly within the average range (Wechsler Intelligence Scale for Children-V). Sasha performed slightly weaker on verbal tests (i.e., those assessing his knowledge of verbal concepts and his ability to reason with words), scoring mildly below average. Finally, like many individuals with NF1, Sasha performed below average range on tests of working memory, suggesting a relative weakness in the ability to hold information in mind for short periods of time while solving a problem. Taken together, Sasha's profile suggests that he has intact intellectual functioning, but he does better on tasks that require him to process visual information than tasks that depend on verbal or working memory abilities. Consistent with his overall average cognitive abilities, Sasha performed within the average range on a measure assessing his verbal learning and memory (California Verbal Learning Test-Children's Version).

The next section begins to characterize attention and executive functioning, two areas that significantly impacted children with NF. These findings did not result in a diagnosis of ADHD but did result in a finding of frontal lobe executive dysfunction. Frontal lobe executive dysfunction is a disorder characterized by difficulties with organization, working memory, and planning. These difficulties often translate into problems in academic skills particularly in the areas of mathematics:

*Attention skills are an area of concern for many children with NF1, and many children with this diagnosis also qualify for a diagnosis of attention-deficit/hyperactivity disorder (ADHD). Results of the current assessment indicate that Sasha does demonstrate some weaknesses in attention, but at the current time these symptoms are not sufficiently impairing to warrant a diagnosis of ADHD (Test of Variables of Attention). Sasha does show evidence of difficulties with managing his impulses. On a questionnaire measure of executive functioning skills Behavior Rating Inventory of Executive Function (BRIEF), Sasha's mother indicated significant concerns related to initiating tasks, managing his emotions, and monitoring his behaviors. On a similar questionnaire (BRIEF), his teacher indicated significant concerns related to inhibiting behaviors and self-monitoring. Sasha performed within normal limits on clinic-based measures of executive functioning (e.g., his ability to quickly generate words according to letter and category cues and his ability to rapidly scan and sequences sets of numbers and letters) (Delis Kaplan Tests of Executive Function). Results of the current evaluation suggest that Sasha does well with tasks when provided guidance and prompting by the examiner, but struggles with impulse control and self-monitoring when working independently. These results are consistent with a **frontal lobe and executive function deficit**, which is commonly seen in children who exhibit ADHD symptoms and encompasses Sasha's difficulties with organizing an approach to schoolwork tasks.*

A good neuropsychological report also addresses the child's psychological/emotional/behavioral functioning. The following section is an example of how a diagnosis of NF1 can affect the child's adjustment.

Emotionally, parent and teacher ratings did not indicate problems severe enough to indicate a mood or anxiety disorder, although his NF1 diagnosis and family history indicates that Sasha is at risk for these problems in the future. Therefore his social-emotional well-being should be monitored over time. On a questionnaire measure, his mother reported significant aggressive behaviors (e.g., often argues with parents, loses temper too easily, annoys others on purpose) and has depressive symptoms (e.g., is easily upset, complains about not having friends, is negative about things), suggesting that Sasha may be developing frustration surrounding his difficulties managing his behaviors and directs this frustration toward others (Behavior Assessment System for Children-2). Indeed, Sasha's responses to a self-report measure indicated mild concerns related to negative thinking patterns and depression (e.g., feeling that he has too many problems, doesn't seem to do anything right, and is not understood by others).

Finally, a summary of the test results is very useful, and it is frequently the paragraph that most physicians turn to as the bottom line for the child:

In summary, we are pleased to note that Sasha is functioning at age-expected levels in a variety of areas including intellectual functioning, his ability to learn and retain new information, and his mental flexibility. Overall, Sasha does not show significant intellectual or learning problems seen in some children with NF1, consistent with his overall mild features. These strengths suggest that Sasha has the capability to continue to do well academically. Sasha's weaknesses with impulse control, social awareness, and mood regulation are commonly seen in children with NF1 and can be addressed in the classroom, at home or in recreational settings.

The final section of the report should include recommendations that are reasonable and which can be implemented (Part VI in Table 10-2). Generally, recommendations in three areas are provided: academic, behavioral, and psychological. The academic recommendations are written to assist schools in providing appropriate services for children and may recommend assessment for an Individual Educational Plan required under law for children suspected of a disability. In Sasha's case, he may qualify under the category of "Other Health Impaired" or, in some states, "Other Health Disability" due to his diagnosis of NF1. If he does not qualify for special education, he may qualify for assistance under the Americans with Disabilities Act that allows for support within the regular classroom for children with medical disorders.

The behavioral section often addresses the need for psychotherapy as well as for additional supports for emotional development. In this section, recommendations for parental support are also provided as well as directions for further evaluation if the child experiences more difficulty. For example we made the following recommendations:

V. We recommend that Sasha's family, school professionals, and therapist continue to monitor Sasha for symptoms of a mood disorder. In the future, if his caregivers observe an increase in behavioral outbursts, diminished interest or pleasure in activities, withdrawal from activities he previously enjoyed, increased irritability, or if Sasha is experiencing increased worries that become distressing or difficult to control, they may wish to have him re-evaluated by a psychologist or a neuropsychologist to determine whether further mental health supports are needed.

We recommend that Sasha's caregivers focus on praising/rewarding Sasha for his effort and for improvements in his ability to regulate his behavior (e.g., "Wow! I liked how you kept thinking about that problem until you figured out a solution; nice work, buddy!," or "Awesome job listening!") rather than praising him for specific achievements or successes. For children like Sasha, too much focus on outcomes (e.g., grades, test scores, athletic achievements such as points scored in a game) may serve to create high levels of competitiveness and self-doubt. Praise that is focused on accomplishments and achievements can actually serve to increase negative self-perceptions if the child finds himself struggling to meet a goal. Instead, reinforcement of things like Sasha's effort, persistence and good attitude can help to take his focus off of "winning" and "achieving" and will likely result in Sasha being able experience more fun and enjoyment in his daily activities.

As a follow-up to this case, the school used this report to develop a treatment plan to provide Sasha with appropriate interventions to assist with his development. Sasha had been participating in play therapy, which was not providing any success in changing his behaviors or mood. After our discussion, therapy was shifted from play therapy to a more directed therapy that provided Sasha with tools to manage his behaviors.

CONCLUSION

Pediatric neuropsychological assessments can serve as an important adjunct to clinical practice. A good neuropsychological report will not only provide a summary of the findings but will also provide appropriate interventions and support. The feedback to the parents of the results is an important therapeutic tool that can assist them in adjusting to some of the child's difficulties while also emphasizing the strengths that the child possesses. Neurology and neuropsychology are a natural alliance that can assist with appropriate support for children and their families.

REFERENCES

The complete list of references for this chapter is available in the e-book at www.expertconsult.com.
    See inside cover for registration details.

SELECTED REFERENCES

Adolphs, R., 2002. Neural systems for recognizing emotion. Curr. Opin. Neurobiol. 12 (2), 169–177.

Carlson, C.I., Uppal, S., Prosser, M., 2000. Ethnic differences in processes contributing to the self-esteem of early adolescent girls. J. Early Adolesc. 20 (1), 44–67.

Giedd, J.N., 2004. Structural magnetic resonance imaging of the adolescent brain. Ann. N. Y. Acad. Sci. 1021, 77–85.

Keith, T.Z., Fine, J.G., 2005. Multicultural influences on school learning: similarities and differences across groups. In: Frisby, C.L., Reynolds, C.R. (Eds.), Comprehensive Handbook of Multicultural School Psychology. John Wiley & Sons, Hoboken, NJ, pp. 457–482.

Lezak, M.D., Howieson, D.B., Loring, D.W., 2004. Neuropsychological Assessment, fourth ed. Oxford University Press, New York.

Meltzer, L., 2007. Executive Function in the Classroom. Guilford, New York.

Rothbart, M.K., Sheese, B.E., 2007. Temperament and emotion regulation. In: Gross, J.J. (Ed.), Handbook of Emotion Regulation. Guilford Press, New York, pp. 331–350.

Semrud-Clikeman, M., Pliszka, S.R., Lancaster, J., et al., 2006. Volumetric MRI differences in treatment—naïve vs chronically treated children with ADHD. Neurology 67, 1023–1027.

Shaywitz, B.A., Shaywitz, S.E., Blachman, B.A., et al., 2004. Development of left occipitotemporal systems for skilled reading in children after a phonologically-based intervention. Biol. Psychiatry 55, 926–933.

Tarullo, A.R., Gunnar, M.R., 2006. Child maltreatment and the developing HPA axis. Horm. Behav. 50, 632–639.

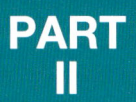
11 Spinal Fluid Examination

David J. Michelson

INTRODUCTION

For more than a century, physicians have employed lumbar puncture (LP) and examination of the cerebrospinal fluid (CSF) in the diagnosis and management of neurologic diseases. Major and lasting contributions to the study of CSF are represented by the textbooks written by Merritt and Fremont-Smith (1938) and Fishman (1992). CSF evaluation is contributing to our still-evolving understanding of the pathophysiology of central nervous system (CNS) disorders, while continuing to play an as yet indispensable role in the clinical management of many of those disorders.

CEREBROSPINAL FLUID FORMATION, FLOW, AND ABSORPTION

CSF is principally formed by secretion from the choroid plexus, villous invaginations of the walls of the lateral, third, and fourth ventricles that are richly vascularized and lined by a ciliated epithelium. The choroid plexus of the lateral ventricles is continuous through the foramina of Monro with the choroid plexus of the roof of the third ventricle. The arterial supply to this portion of the choroid plexus originates from the anterior choroidal arteries, which branch off from the internal carotid arteries, and from the posterior choroidal arteries, which are branches of the posterior cerebral arteries. The posterior inferior cerebellar arteries usually supply the choroid plexus of the fourth ventricle. Blood flow to choroidal vessels is almost 10 times greater than that to the cerebral cortex.

The capillaries of the choroid plexus, unlike those found in most other areas of the brain, have large fenestrations that offer little resistance to the passage of fluid, ions, and small macromolecules. Passage of blood past these capillaries creates an ultrafiltrate of plasma within the interstitial space at the basolateral surface of the epithelial cells.

CSF secretion depends on active transport proteins that are differentially localized on the apical and basolateral membranes of the choroid plexus epithelial cells. Water follows the flow of sodium (Na^+) and chloride (Cl^-) ions from the interstitial fluid (ISF) into the CSF. Carbonic anhydrase within the epithelial cells catalyzes the formation of carbonic acid (H_2CO_3) from water (H_2O) and carbon dioxide (CO_2). Carbon dioxide diffuses freely into the epithelial cells from the bloodstream, but the dissociation products of carbonic acid, bicarbonate (HCO_3^-), and hydrogen (H^+), are exported across the basolateral membrane by Na^+/H^+ and Cl^-/HCO_3^- exchangers. Sodium is then transported across the apical membrane, into the CSF, via Na^+/K^+ ATPases (Figure 11-2). Water flows passively along the osmotic gradient created by this net ion flux from the ISF to the ventricles through aquaporin-1 channels.

Other specific active transport proteins present along the basolateral membrane allow transport into the CSF of essential hydrophilic micronutrients, including glucose, amino acids, purines, nucleosides, and vitamins. Transport proteins along the apical membrane work to clear the CSF of potentially toxic metabolites, such as organic acids and bases.

Tight junctions link the choroid plexus epithelial cells, limiting the free diffusion of ionic molecules and creating the blood–CSF barrier. Although protein diffusion is largely restricted, most of the small amount of protein found in the CSF is nevertheless of plasma origin. Maintenance of a relatively stable CSF composition, despite wide variation in the composition of the plasma, reflects the integrity of the blood–CSF barrier and the work of active transporters against concentration gradients.

The choroid plexus produces from 70% to 90% of the CSF, with the remainder deriving from movement of brain parenchymal ISF across the ependyma into the ventricles and across the pial membrane into the subarachnoid space. The rate of CSF formation in healthy adults averages 0.35 mL per minute, or roughly 500 mL each day. Children produce proportionally less CSF, depending on their height and weight, with as little as 25 mL produced per day in newborns. Postmortem studies have provided estimates that total CSF volume ranges from 50 mL in term neonates to 150 mL in adults, with only a small percentage contained within normal-sized ventricles. The total volume of the CSF undergoes complete replacement three to four times each day.

CSF production can be greatly reduced in experimental animals given the sodium–potassium ATPase inhibitor ouabain. Carbonic anhydrase inhibitors, such as acetazolamide, can reduce CSF production by 50% to 100% in rats. Acetazolamide reduces CSF production in humans just 6% to 50%, which explains the limited clinical effectiveness of this medication in the treatment of increased intracranial pressure. Furosemide and other loop diuretics also weakly inhibit carbonic anhydrase activity but also reduce CSF production through inhibition of sodium, potassium, and chloride cotransporters.

CSF produced in the lateral ventricles passes through the foramina of Monro into the third ventricle and then flows through the aqueduct of Sylvius into the fourth ventricle. CSF exits the ventricular system through the lateral foramina of Luschka to enter the prepontine cistern and cerebellopontine angles. Alternatively, CSF can leave the fourth ventricle through the midline foramen of Magendie, entering the cisterna magna, from which it can flow upward over the cerebellar hemispheres or downward into the spinal subarachnoid space and around the brainstem into the basal cisterns, including the interpeduncular cistern. CSF flows predominantly

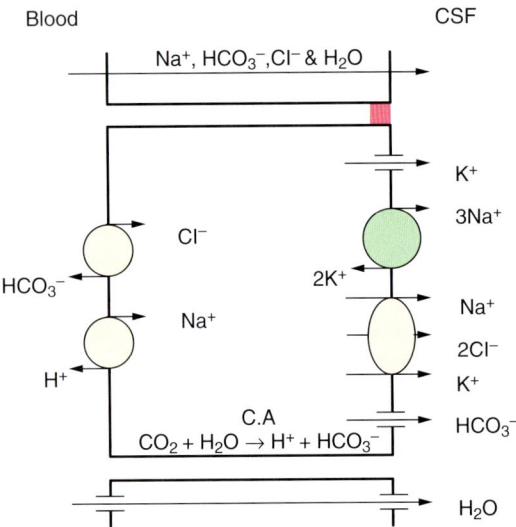

Blood   CSF

Na^+, HCO_3^-, Cl^- & H_2O

K^+

$3Na^+$

Cl^-

$2K^+$

Na^+

Na^+

$2Cl^-$

H^+

K^+

C.A

$CO_2 + H_2O \rightarrow H^+ + HCO_3^-$

HCO_3^-

H_2O

HCO_3^-

Figure 11-2. Major processes involved in cerebrospinal fluid secretion. 1, Carbonic anhydrase catalyzes the production of bicarbonate (HCO_3) ions and protons (H^+) from water (H_2O) and carbon dioxide (CO_2). **2,** Bicarbonate is exchanged for chloride (Cl^-) across the basolateral membrane. **3,** Bicarbonate and chloride flow into the CSF through anion channels, down an electrochemical gradient, and through sodium (Na^+)–potassium (K^+)–chloride cotransport. **4,** Sodium is exchanged for protons across the basolateral membrane and for potassium across the apical membrane. **5,** Water follows the osmotic gradient created by the combined secretion of sodium, chloride, and bicarbonate into the CSF. *(With permission from Damkier HH, Brown PD, Praetorius J. Physiology [Bethesda]. 2010;25[4]:239–49.)*

downward posterior to the spinal cord and upward anterior to the cord. The fluid eventually reaches the basal cisterns, from which flow is mainly upward over the brain convexity.

In the steady state, the rate of CSF absorption is equal to that of its production. Most CSF is absorbed into the venous sinuses across the arachnoid villi and granulations, arachnoid membrane invaginations through the dural lining of the sinuses that are concentrated near the sagittal sinus. Absorption across the arachnoid villi occurs by vesicular transport. This action demonstrates a dependence on the hydrostatic pressure gradient across the villous surface, such that the villi act as one-way pressure valves that open above a threshold pressure, usually 20 to 50 mm H_2O. Modern research utilizing radioactive tracers has shown that significant CSF absorption also occurs across the capillaries, veins, and lymphatics of the spinal cord and spinal roots, and, via the perineural subarachnoid space around olfactory nerve rootlets, through the cribriform plate and nasal lymphatics (Kapoor et al., 2008).

CEREBROSPINAL FLUID FUNCTION

The CSF provides buoyancy and physical protection to the brain, absorbing the stretching and compressive forces generated by normal head movement and lessening the impact of the deceleration and rotational forces created by head trauma. A second protective function derives from the ability of the CSF to redistribute in response to acute changes in other intracranial contents, helping to maintain normal intracranial pressure. The CSF is also thought to serve as a route for the transport of centrally acting hormones, such as for the diffusion of hypothalamic releasing factors across the third ventricle.

The CSF aids in the excretion of metabolites through bulk absorption of the ISF of the brain and spinal cord. This "sink

action," along with the various mechanisms by which the CSF composition is maintained, suggests that the CSF plays a significant role in normal physiology and in the compensatory response to pathologic situations.

DIAGNOSTIC SAMPLING OF CEREBROSPINAL FLUID
Indications

Changes in the composition of the CSF have been associated with a wide variety of neurologic conditions. Sampling of the CSF is considered helpful in the diagnosis and management of several such conditions in children, and may be most useful in cases of suspected meningitis, encephalitis, subarachnoid hemorrhage, intracranial hypertension (as in pseudotumor cerebri), leptomeningeal carcinomatosis, pediatric neurotransmitter diseases, and neurodegenerative diseases. In each case, the potential benefits of the information that can be obtained should be weighed against the risks of the procedures used for CSF sampling. Families should be involved as much as possible in the decision-making process to allow them to provide truly informed consent.

Contraindications and Cautions

LP through a soft tissue infection such as cellulitis is discouraged because of concern that this can introduce bacteria into deeper tissues and cause an epidural abscess, osteomyelitis, or meningitis. The risk of a bleeding complication, other than a bloody tap, from a diagnostic or therapeutic lumbar puncture in patients with even severe thrombocytopenia is very low. Many pediatric hospitals follow a protocol for holding anticoagulants prior to lumbar puncture (low-molecular-weight heparin [LMWH] for 24 hours and unfractionated heparin [UH] for 4 hours) and restarting several hours afterward (4-6 hours for UH and 6-9 hours for LMWH), with a low risk of complications reported (Avila et al., 2014).

There is considerable and understandable fear that LP in patients with a CSF obstruction can unbalance the pressure across the area of obstruction and contribute to cerebral herniation or spinal cord compression. Neuroimaging, usually with cranial computed tomography (CT), is often performed before LP, especially in patients with suspected meningitis. However, herniation has been reported after normal neuroimaging, and LP has been performed safely in patients with abnormal CT scans, leading many to continue to debate the appropriate use of neuroimaging before LP. Because it is considered essential that antibiotic administration not be delayed when meningitis is suspected, especially with meningococcal disease, current recommendations are to start antibiotics as soon as possible, regardless of when LP can be performed (Gaieski et al., 2012).

Procedure

The success of an LP is determined by the correct positioning of the needle and the patient, and depends almost as much on the relaxation of the patient and on the skill and experience of the assistants as it does on that of the needle-wielding physician. Local analgesia, with or without the use of additional anxiolytics, may be sufficient for cooperative older children, but moderate to deep sedation is often necessary for younger children. Although aggressive assistants can easily overpower neonates and young infants, obviating the need for sedation, they must take care not to cause airway compromise. Patients with abnormal lumbar spine anatomy, such as that resulting from a congenital defect such as spina bifida or an acquired deformity such as scoliosis, may require direct imaging of the spine with fluoroscopy or ultrasound.

The lower end of the spinal cord, the conus medullaris, is found by MRI to be at the L1-L2 vertebral interspace in most subjects and safely above the L3 vertebral body in all subjects without spinal deformity. To avoid damaging the conus, only the interspaces below L3 are used for LP. With a patient lying in the lateral recumbent position, the L3-L4 interspace can be found at the level of the superior iliac crests. This area should be carefully palpated and marked to ensure that it can be identified after the patient is cleaned and draped. Having the patient curl with the neck and hips flexed can maximize the size of the interspace. Whether the patient is placed in a lateral recumbent or seated position, care should be taken to maintain the alignment of the shoulders and hips, avoiding rotation of the spine. Having the patient's back near the edge of the bed and at a proper height can aid in the comfort and success of the physician.

The patient's skin should be prepared using a microbicidal agent, such as a 10% solution of povidone-iodine. The skin should be given time to dry and then wiped clean and draped with sterile towels. A local anesthetic, such as a 1% solution of lidocaine, can be injected into the area to minimize the pain of repeated needlesticks. Anesthesia provides little benefit when the LP can be accomplished with a single needlestick, because the pain of the anesthetic injection often equals or exceeds that of the spinal needle insertion. A reasonable alternative is the use of a topical analgesic cream, such as the 5% emulsion of lidocaine and prilocaine commonly referred to as eutectic mixture of local anesthetics (EMLA). EMLA requires 20 to 30 minutes of application but has been associated with a decreased pain response, even in neonates.

The most commonly used spinal needles are 2.5- or 5-cm-long, 20- or 22-gauge Quincke needles, which are beveled and fitted with a stylet. The sharply beveled tip of the Quincke needle should be turned to face the patient's side so that its cutting edge can push between, rather than cut, the longitudinal fibers of the dura. Atraumatic needles, such as the Whitacre and Sprotte needles, have duller tips that make dural injury less likely. These needles are also more flexible, encounter more tissue resistance, and require the use of an introducer, making them more difficult to position. Advancing the needle without its stylet in place may increase the chances of successful and nontraumatic CSF collection, but has been discouraged because of concern that this will introduce cells that might later form a spinal epidermoid tumor.

The needle is gradually advanced, the ligamentum flavum and dura are pierced, and a slight popping sensation is felt as the subarachnoid space is entered. The stylet is removed to allow CSF to drain to the needle hub. If no fluid appears, the needle should be rotated a quarter-turn in case a nerve rootlet or strand of arachnoid is obstructing the opening. If this does not initiate CSF flow, the needle can be introduced a few millimeters more, sometimes resulting in a second popping sensation. If there is still no CSF, the stylet should be replaced and the needle slowly withdrawn for redirection of the needle toward the same interspace or for selection of another interspace.

After CSF is flowing from the needle, a stopcock and manometer should be attached to the needle hub. The opening pressure should be measured with the child relaxed and in the lateral decubitus position. There should be no direct pressure on the abdomen during the measurement. Slow CSF flow may be caused by partial needle obstruction or by low CSF pressure. One way to ensure that a low manometry reading is a true reflection of the CSF pressure is to apply firm pressure to the patient's abdomen. In the absence of an outflow obstruction or disconnection between the needle and manometer,

there should be a rapid rise in the manometer reading, followed by a rapid fall as abdominal pressure is released. An accurate manometry reading should also be accompanied by small fluctuations in the height of the fluid column with the pulse and respirations.

Opening pressures in adults and older children have historically been considered normal between 120 and 200 mm H_2O, with pressures as high as 250 mm H_2O considered normal for obese adults. A prospective multicenter study of opening pressures in children without medical conditions found a mean of 196 mm H_2O, with the 90th percentile being 280 mm H_2O (Avery, 2014). Pathologic elevations of the CSF pressure are discussed in Chapter 105.

After the opening pressure has been recorded, CSF can be collected for analysis. Abdominal pressure or Valsalva maneuvers can be used to increase slow flow. In the case of very slow flow, gentle aspiration with a syringe may be attempted, although this may increase the risk of pulling a nerve rootlet or strand of arachnoid into the needle. At least 5 mL of CSF should be collected; the first three tubes of 1 to 2 mL are sufficient for routine studies: Gram stain, bacterial culture, cell count and differential, and glucose and protein concentrations. If the first tubes are grossly bloody, a fourth tube of at least 2 mL should be collected to aid in the differentiation of subarachnoid hemorrhage from a traumatic tap. This tube can also be held in reserve for additional studies, such as special microbiologic, immunologic, or metabolic tests.

Replacing the stylet before withdrawing the spinal needle is recommended to avoid pulling a strand of arachnoid through the dura, creating a channel for continued CSF leakage and increasing the risk of postprocedural headache.

In special situations, CSF can be obtained by ventricular shunt or by ventricular or cisternal puncture, usually with the assistance of a neurosurgeon.

Complications

Transient complications during the procedure include pain and paresthesias in the distribution of a lumbar nerve root resulting from contact with the needle. The discomfort should subside with repositioning of the needle toward the midline, and permanent nerve injury is highly unlikely.

More serious complications of LP do occur, although rarely. These mainly involve subarachnoid, subdural, and epidural hematomas resulting from a breach of the epidural venous plexus, radicular arteries, or radicular veins. Patients commonly have signs and symptoms of meningeal irritation or local pain. Severe symptoms, such as sensory, motor, or sphincter dysfunction, suggest the need for surgical hematoma evacuation.

Infectious complications, including meningitis, epidural abscess, and osteomyelitis, can result from the use of incompletely aseptic technique. LP in the setting of bacteremia or active hematologic malignancy is not strictly contraindicated.

The most common complications of LP are back pain and postprocedural headache. Postprocedural headache may occur within 72 hours of the puncture, may be worsened by an upright position and relieved by recumbency (orthostatic), and may be associated with neck stiffness, nausea, vomiting, and cranial nerve palsies. Pathologic reductions of the CSF pressure are discussed in Chapter 105.

Several technical aspects and patient factors appear to lessen the incidence and severity of postprocedural headache in adults, including the use of small-diameter needles or atraumatic needles, low body mass index, male gender, and lack of a history of headache. Bed rest after LP has not been found to prevent headache, but it is effective in reducing pain after it has developed. Similarly, prophylactic epidural blood patches do not prevent headaches but are very successful in the treatment of refractory postprocedural headaches. Studies have been contradictory or negative regarding the use of steroids, hydration, or caffeine for the prevention or treatment of postprocedural headaches.

CEREBROSPINAL FLUID ANALYSIS

Appearance

Normal CSF is clear and colorless, indistinguishable from water when held up to white light in identical tubes. A cell count greater than 50 cells/mm^3 can cause a snowy scattering of light, but the eye cannot easily distinguish between white blood cells (WBCs) and red blood cells (RBCs). With RBC counts between 500 and 6000 cells/mm^3, the CSF color becomes pink or xanthochromic.

Cells

Counting chambers can provide CSF WBC and RBC counts, with a pathologist reviewing a stained slide for confirmation. Normal values for infants have been difficult to obtain, in part because LP is rarely done without an indication such as fever, but also because many early studies had small samples and included children with conditions known to elevate CSF cell counts, such as viral meningitis (Chadwick et al., 2011). Older infants and children have normal values similar to those of adults (Table 11-2).

Centrifugation and staining of the CSF are suitable for most clinical cytology. The WBCs found in normal CSF are typically 70% lymphocytes and 30% monocytes. An elevated WBC count or more than a few polymorphonuclear cells may indicate inflammation or infection within the CNS, but counts are not specific enough to allow ready differentiation, for example, of bacterial from viral meningitis. Neoplastic cells, plasma cells, stem cells, and eosinophils within the CSF are always considered abnormal. However, because cytologic analysis has such a low sensitivity, CSF testing for leptomeningeal metastasis of a systemic malignancy should be repeated multiple times and should employ large collection volumes. These points are examined in detail in Chapters 114 to 116, which discuss CNS infections, and Chapters 122 to 133, which discuss CNS malignancies.

Excessive RBCs in CSF can be diagnostic of subarachnoid hemorrhage (SAH), but can also occur with a traumatic LP.

TABLE 11-2 Total White Blood Cell Counts in the Cerebrospinal Fluid of Children without Central Nervous System Disease

Age	N*	WBC Mean ± SD†	95th Percentile
Neonate			
Premature (28-37 wk GA)	38	5.1 ± 5.8	16.7
Term (38-42 wk GA)	25	4.5 ± 3.6	11.7
Infant			
<6 weeks	64	3.7 ± 3.4	10.5
6 weeks to 3 months	67	2.9 ± 2.9	8.7
3-6 months	84	1.9 ± 2.0	5.9
6-12 months	75	2.6 ± 2.5	7.6
Child	81	1.9 ± 2.7	7.3
Juvenile and adult‡		2.6 ± 1.7	6.0

*N, the number of samples studied; SD, standard deviation; WBC, white blood cell; wk GA, gestational age in weeks.
†White blood cell counts (cells/mm^3) are reported as means ± standard deviations.
‡The juvenile and adult level is provided for comparison.

Clot formation within the tube of CSF suggests a traumatic LP. RBC counts in serial tubes always decrease in cases of traumatic LP, but this should not be used to exclude the possibility of SAH unless the later tubes have a RBC count approaching zero.

A formula for the correction of the CSF WBC count in patients with suspected traumatic LP is widely used, in which 1 WBC is subtracted for every 500 to 700 RBCs found in the CSF. However, the use of corrections of this kind is unhelpful in the clinical diagnosis of meningitis.

Microorganisms

The first 1 to 2 mL of CSF, even if contaminated with blood from a traumatic puncture, should be stained and cultured for microorganisms. Gram staining allows for an early bacteriologic diagnosis, and results may influence the choice of antibiotic treatment. Outside of a strong clinical suspicion, there is probably no benefit to the routine use of acid-fast stains and mycobacterial cultures, India ink preparations and fungal cultures, or viral cultures.

Latex agglutination tests for common bacterial antigens have shown diagnostic value in patients who had been treated with antibiotics before LP for suspected meningitis. Other studies have strongly questioned the value of such tests, finding high false-positive rates, low sensitivity, or no added benefit over Gram staining and culture. Several biomarkers, such as serum procalcitonin, have been tested for their ability to distinguish bacterial meningitis from viral meningitis in patients with a negative CSF Gram stain (Viallon et al., 2011)

Immunologic tests for antigens and antibodies and polymerase chain reaction tests for DNA and RNA can greatly aid in the identification of organisms that are difficult to culture. These techniques can be applied to cases of bacterial meningitis but are particularly useful in the evaluation of immunocompromised hosts, encephalitis, and chronic meningitis, when viral, fungal, rickettsial, and other unusual organisms are more likely to be identified (Baron et al., 2013).

Glucose

Facilitated transporters on the membranes of capillary endothelial cells are responsible for the entry of glucose into the brain ISF. Normal CSF glucose concentrations range between 45 and 80 mg/dL, or about two thirds of the plasma glucose concentration. A CSF glucose concentration less than 40 mg/dL (i.e., hypoglycorrhachia) or a ratio of less than two thirds of the plasma glucose level is considered abnormal.

Very low CSF glucose values, sometimes below the limits of laboratory detection, are seen with diverse causes of severe meningeal inflammation, probably resulting from a combination of increased glucose use by the brain and spinal cord, glucose use by leukocytes within the CSF, and inhibition of glucose transport into the CSF.

Patients with defective transport of glucose across the blood–brain barrier resulting from mutations in the *SLCA1* gene encoding the GLUT-1 transporter typically present with low CSF glucose levels (<40 mg/dL), a low ratio of CSF glucose to plasma glucose (<0.6), and a medically refractory epileptic encephalopathy that shows response to treatment with the ketogenic diet. Patients may have fixed and/or paroxysmal movement disorders, sometimes as an isolated phenotype.

Protein

The protein content of CSF is very low relative to plasma concentrations, with most plasma proteins excluded from the CSF by the blood–CSF barrier. The total protein content of the

TABLE 11-3 Total Protein Content in the Cerebrospinal Fluid of Healthy Children

Age	N*	Mean ± SD†	95th Percentile
0-6 days	11	80.9 ± 20.8	122.5
7-13 days	7	70.4 ± 23.6	117.6
14-27 days	13	53.9 ± 17.8	89.5
28-41 days	10	46.5 ± 15.4	77.3
42-59 days	11	45.6 ± 14.2	74
2-4 months	9	34.8 ± 12	58.8
5-8 months	7	20.4 ± 2.4	25.2
9-11 months	5	16.6 ± 2.6	21.8
12-23 months	8	16.8 ± 2.7	22.2
2-7 years	21	17.7 ± 3.1	23.9
8-13 years	19	20.8 ± 4.1	29

*N, the number of samples studied; SD, standard deviation.
†Protein concentrations (mg/dL) are reported as means ± standard deviations.

CSF is higher in neonates than in older infants and children (Table 11-3).

Combination of established techniques of two-dimensional gel electrophoresis with advances in mass spectrometry is leading to the development of a new field of study, quantitative neuroproteomics (Craft et al., 2013). Detailed CSF analysis of a variety of small molecules is advancing our understanding of the pathophysiology of CNS disorders and holds great potential for future clinical use in diagnosis and prognosis.

Immunologic Analysis

CSF immunoglobulins, particularly immunoglobulin G (IgG), are increased with many inflammatory, infectious, and neoplastic conditions of the CNS. This increase is in large part a reflection of the impaired blood–CSF barrier, permitting increased entry into the CSF of all proteins, including albumin. Specific intrathecal production of IgG may also occur in these conditions, as can be demonstrated qualitatively with tests for oligoclonal banding and quantitatively with calculations such as the IgG index:

$$([IgG]_{CSF}/[IgG]_{plasma})/([Alb]_{CSF}/[Alb]_{plasma})$$

Among patients with clinically definite multiple sclerosis, for example, up to 95% have intrathecal oligoclonal bands, and more than 70% have an elevated IgG index. Positive intrathecal oligoclonal bands are demonstrated for patients with other inflammatory disorders, from which multiple sclerosis must sometimes be differentiated. The utility of CSF analysis in the diagnosis of acquired demyelinating diseases is discussed in Chapter 100.

Neurometabolic Studies

The usual laboratory evaluation of a child with unexplained encephalopathy consists of plasma, urine, and radiologic studies. When CSF is collected as a part of the evaluation, metabolic tests can be expanded to include lactate, pyruvate, 5-methyltetrahydrofolate, and quantitative amino acid measurement. The appropriate patient selection and testing is discussed in Chapter 36, which provides an overview regarding metabolic disorders, and Chapter 44, which reviews neurotransmitter-related disorders.

REFERENCES

The complete list of references for this chapter is available in the e-book at www.expertconsult.com.
See inside cover for registration details.

SELECTED REFERENCES

Avery, R.A., 2014. Reference range of cerebrospinal fluid opening pressure in children: historical overview and current data. Neuropediatrics 45 (4), 206–211.

Avila, M.L., Macartney, C.A., Hitzler, J.K., et al., 2014. Assessment of the outcomes associated with periprocedural anticoagulation management in children with acute lymphoblastic leukemia. J. Pediatr. 164 (5), 1201–1207.

Baron, E.J., Miller, J.M., Weinstein, M.P., et al., 2013. A guide to utilization of the microbiology laboratory for diagnosis of infectious diseases: 2013 recommendations by the Infectious Diseases Society of America (IDSA) and the American Society for Microbiology (ASM) (a). Clin. Infect. Dis. 57 (4), e22–e121.

Chadwick, S.L., Wilson, J.W., Levin, J.E., et al., 2011. Cerebrospinal fluid characteristics of infants who present to the emergency department with fever: establishing normal values by week of age. Pediatr. Infect. Dis. J. 30 (4), e63–e67.

Craft, G.E., Chen, A., Nairn, A.C., 2013. Recent advances in quantitative neuroproteomics. Methods 61 (3), 186–218.

Fishman, R.A., 1992. Cerebrospinal Fluid in Diseases of the Nervous System, second ed. W.B. Saunders, Philadelphia.

Gaieski, D.F., Nathan, B.R., Weingart, S.D., et al., 2012. Emergency neurologic life support: meningitis and encephalitis. Neurocrit. Care 17 (Suppl. 1), S66–S72.

Kapoor, K.G., Katz, S.E., Grzybowski, D.M., et al., 2008. Cerebrospinal fluid outflow: an evolving perspective. Brain Res. Bull. 77 (6), 327–334.

Merritt, H.H., Fremont-Smith, F., 1938. The Cerebrospinal Fluid. W.B. Saunders, Philadelphia.

Viallon, A., Desseigne, N., Marjollet, O., et al., 2011. Meningitis in adult patients with a negative direct cerebrospinal fluid examination: value of cytochemical markers for differential diagnosis. Crit. Care 15 (3), R136.

E-BOOK FIGURES AND TABLES

The following figures and tables are available in the e-book at www.expertconsult.com. See inside cover for registration details.

12 Pediatric Neuroimaging

Nathaniel D. Wycliffe, Barbara A. Holshouser, Brenda Bartnik-Olson, and Stephen Ashwal

A clear understanding of various clinical signs and symptoms of neurologic diseases in children and knowledge of normal neuroanatomy and its alterations in various disease processes are prerequisites for the correct performance and interpretation of the many powerful neuroimaging techniques available. In this chapter we provide an overview of the strengths and weaknesses of pediatric ultrasound, computed tomography (CT), and magnetic resonance imaging (MRI). A discussion of the neuroimaging changes associated with normal brain development is beyond the scope of this chapter, but several excellent monographs are available (Barkovich and Raybaud, 2001; Provenzale, 2009; Tortori-Donati Rossi, 2005). Figures for this chapter appear solely in the online chapter version.

CRANIAL ULTRASOUND

In the prenatal and perinatal period, real-time sonography is currently the most frequently used neuroimaging modality. The various methods of acquiring ultrasound images are discussed in the online chapter. Fetal sonography has had a marked effect on patient counseling and management but is limited by (*i*) nonspecific sonographic appearance of some anomalies, (*ii*) technical factors that make visualization of the side of the brain near the transducer and of the posterior fossa difficult to assess, and (*iii*) subtle parenchymal abnormalities that cannot be visualized sonographically. Figures 12-1 to 12-9 demonstrate some of the normal and abnormal features that can be detected. A wide array of central nervous system (CNS) pathology detected by prenatal sonography includes fetal seizures via abnormal movements, holoprosencephaly, encephalocele, schizencephaly, lissencephaly, hydrocephaly, Dandy–Walker malformation, spina bifida, and congenital astrocytoma.

In newborns, the open anterior fontanel provides an excellent window for the evaluation of the infant brain. Postnatally, sonography is helpful in the evaluation of hypoxic-ischemic encephalopathy, including complications of hemorrhage into the germinal matrix, ventricles, or surrounding parenchyma. For infants younger than 30 weeks' gestation, routine cranial ultrasonography screening should be performed once between 7 and 14 days of age, and should be repeated optimally between 36 and 40 weeks' postmenstrual age to detect lesions such as intraventricular hemorrhage, periventricular leukomalacia, ventriculomegaly, and intrauterine infections. Major migrational anomalies, such as agyria-pachygyria and lissencephaly, or tuberous sclerosis may be delineated; however, smaller heterotopias or other subcortical dysplasias may be overlooked. Sonography can be used to screen for myelodysplasia (see Chapter 19). It can also reveal the presence or absence of cord pulsations, a sign of tethering as well as other dysraphic lesions, such as meningocele, lipoma, hydromyelia, Arnold–Chiari II malformation, diastematomyelia, and lipomyelomeningocele.

Intraoperative sonography is an important modality for the safe and specific guidance of neurosurgical biopsy or lesion resection, for the accurate placement of ventricular shunts, drainage of intraparenchymal fluid collections, localization of brain or cord tumors, drainage of hydrosyringomyelias, delineation of posttraumatic intraspinal bone fragments, and for monitoring resection of arteriovenous malformations.

COMPUTED TOMOGRAPHY

CT has been available since the 1970s for clinical use in children. Ionizing radiation resulting from x-ray CT is effectively restricted to the immediate body part and several generations of scanners are available, including the helical CT introduced in the early 1990s and the multidetector or multislice scanner. This availability has resulted in an increased number of computed tomographic scans of children, increasing the potential for inappropriate use and excessive radiation dosing. The risk of cancer from low-level radiation such as from a single CT scan is unproven. The life-saving benefits of these examinations in the care for individuals of all ages are proven and widely known. The cancer risk from CT is cumulative and special consideration must be given to children, who have a longer lifetime in which to manifest radiation-related cancer. It is necessary to limit radiation from CT in children and follow the ALARA ("as low as reasonably achievable") principle as discussed in the online chapter. All new CT scanners sold in the United States now comply with the National Electrical Manufacturers Association XR 25 CT Dose-Check Standard. Compliant CT scanners can be configured to inform operators when scan settings would likely yield radiation doses that would exceed preassigned values, allowing users to confirm or correct settings that might otherwise lead to unnecessarily high exposures.

The digital tomographic image is composed of a matrix of voxels (i.e., pixels with volume resulting from the finite thickness of the tomogram). Each voxel is assigned a numeric value called a CT number, which is related to tissue density. CT has good soft-tissue resolution and is especially useful along high-contrast interfaces, such as air–water, fat–water, and bone–water in the orbits, sinuses, and temporal bones. CT is limited by streaking artifacts in areas adjacent to thick bone or metallic objects such as dental fillings and gunshot wound pellets. These artifacts are particularly troublesome in the posterior fossa because of the dense temporal petrous bones.

CT scanners are fast and widely available for emergencies and for medically unstable patients. Direct scanning is routinely performed in the axial plane and if needed in the coronal plane. Multiplanar reformatting of axial image data can be accomplished; however, reformatted images have less resolution. Direct coronal computed tomographic examinations can be obtained for the enhanced evaluation of the orbits, sinuses, temporal bones, and temporomandibular joints. Coronal plane images can be used to evaluate patients for intrasellar, skull-based, midline, or vertex intracranial lesions. Three-dimensional reconstructions have been useful for surgical planning of craniofacial reconstructions.

Abnormalities can be characterized with CT as having low density, isodensity, or high density in relation to the brain.

Lesions that appear lower in density include edema, necrosis, infarction (Figure 12-10), neoplasms, leukodystrophies, inflammation, and cysts. Loss of gray–white matter differentiation may be seen with diffuse brain edema after hypoxic-ischemic injury or a demyelinating process. Fat-containing lesions usually appear less dense than water or of mixed density, as in patients with a teratodermoid type of tumor. Air appears as the lowest density (posttraumatic or postsurgical pneumocephalus). Isodense lesions are difficult to recognize unless there are changes that demonstrate displacement or replacement of normal structures or intravenous contrast materials that separate the lesion from normal structures. High-density lesions usually indicate hemorrhage or the presence of calcium (Figure 12-11). Pathologic intracranial calcifications can be seen with congenital infections, neurocysticercosis, intracranial tumors, tuberous sclerosis, Sturge–Weber syndrome, neurofibromatosis, Cockayne syndrome, hypoparathyroidism, arteriovenous malformations, Galen's vein malformations, encephalomalacia, cerebral infarction, or the sequelae of perinatal asphyxia. Hypercellular neoplasms may also appear as high-density lesions on CT. Computed tomographic imaging can be used for precise localization during needle-biopsy procedures or volumetric resection of pediatric brain tumors. In neonates, non–contrast-enhanced CT after ultrasound is helpful in evaluating acute hemorrhage (Figures 12-12 and 12-13), developmental anomalies (Figures 12-14 and 12-15), acute trauma (Figures 12-16 and 12-17), suspected infarction (see Figure 12-10A), and hydrocephalus.

In childhood neurodegenerative diseases, CT may reveal decreased basal ganglia attenuation and cerebral white matter or focal or generalized cerebral atrophy. Noncontrast CT can evaluate patients with neurocutaneous syndromes to detect calcifications as in tuberous sclerosis (see Figure 12-15) and for the evaluation of patients with acute onset of seizures. After closed-head injury (accidental or nonaccidental), CT without contrast material is usually optimal for evaluation of the skull, intracranial hemorrhage, orbits, sinuses, facial or temporal bones, and osseous spine for fractures. Imaging patterns of intracranial hemorrhage in children younger than 3 years have been reported to predict whether the injury was intentional and include convexity or interhemispheric subdural hemorrhages, hygromas (i.e., nonhemic subdural fluid) with intracranial hemorrhage, and/or absence of a skull fracture with intracranial hemorrhage.

Iodinated contrast enhancement is normally seen as a high-density area within the brain and other normal tissues, including vascular and dural structures, pituitary gland, infundibulum, pineal gland, and choroid plexus, but normal parenchymal enhancement usually is too subtle to appreciate. Mechanisms of contrast enhancement include blood–brain barrier disruption, extravasation of intravascular contrast material, or accumulation of contrast material in hyperperfused regions.

Contrast-enhanced CT is helpful in the evaluation of suspected or known vascular malformations, neoplasms (Figure 12-18 and 12-11A), abscesses (Figure 12-19), and empyemas. In infants and children with chronic subdural hematomas, contrast enhancement may reveal an enhancing membrane and may differentiate infarction from neoplasm or abscess. In patients with suspected metastases or seeding of neoplasms, contrast-only CT scan may be sufficient. However, in all the clinical situations previously described, MRI is considered more definitive.

MAGNETIC RESONANCE IMAGING

MRI is the most powerful neuroimaging modality for adults and children. It involves no ionizing radiation as in CT and no acoustic window that restricts cranial ultrasound to the period of infancy before the fontanels close. MRI provides multiplanar imaging with excellent resolution without repositioning of the patient or the machine. Bone does not interfere with soft-tissue resolution; however, metallic objects often produce signal void or field distortion artifacts. Some ferromagnetic or electronic devices, such as non-MR safe aneurysm clips, pacemakers, and implanted defibrillators, contraindicate the use of MRI. MRI has less tolerance for patient movement and sedation is required for most young children. Sedated and intubated patients require MR-compatible monitoring of vital signs and ventilator support. MRI is generally more expensive than CT; however, it is less expensive than more invasive procedures such as angiography, CT myelography, and cisternography.

MRI uses magnetic fields and radiofrequency pulses to obtain high-resolution images. Hydrogen nuclei (protons) are used to generate detectable signals in MRI. MR images are created by sending radiofrequency pulses into a patient lying in an external magnetic field, thereby perturbing hydrogen nuclei into producing signals of various intensities from different body tissues. The resulting signals are mapped on to a grayscale digital image and the intensity MRI signals is determined by several intrinsic factors, such as the proton density, the mobility of the protons within the molecular lattice (T1 relaxation), the effect of local magnetic fields produced by magnetic nuclei within the tissue (T2 relaxation), and susceptibility effects (i.e., from paramagnetic biologic substances such as hemorrhage) on local magnetic fields within tissue (T2* relaxation). Programmed sequences, such as spin echo (SE), inversion recovery, and gradient-recalled echo (GRE), use a sequence of radiofrequency and gradient magnetic field pulses to acquire images weighted with one of the aforementioned factors. On T1-weighted (T1W) images, typically produced with SE or GRE sequences, tissues with short T1 relaxation times, such as fat and intracellular and extracellular methemoglobin, produce a high signal intensity (i.e., bright or hyperintense). Cerebrospinal fluid (CSF), muscle, deoxyhemoglobin, hemosiderin, tissues, and substances with long T1 relaxation times appear dark on T1W images.

On T2-weighted (T2W) images, tissues or structures with long T2 relaxation times, such as CSF, edema, many tumors, extracellular methemoglobin, infarcts, and multiple sclerosis plaques are bright, whereas tissues or substances such as muscle, cortical bone, deoxyhemoglobin, and hemosiderin are dark as a result of short T2 relaxation times (see Figures 12-22, 12-25, and 12-29). Inversion recovery sequences are used to nullify or eliminate signal from a particular tissue. Fluid-attenuated inversion recovery (FLAIR) sequences nullify signal from fluids, causing CSF to appear dark rather than bright as on T2W images. This sequence is used to increase conspicuity of lesions that are bright on T2 (multiple sclerosis plaques, infarcts) and located near the ventricles, and is particularly useful for identifying subacute subdural hemorrhage. Another sequence called short tau inversion recovery (STIR) nullifies signal from fat and can be used to identify lesions in fatty areas such as the orbits or neck. GRE sequences are used to provide T2W contrast to identify hemorrhage. Because of the increased use of higher-field-strength clinical imaging magnets at 3T, GRE is routinely used to provide T1W contrast. Routinely, T1W and T2W images in various planes are acquired and followed by T1W images with contrast, if needed. The most commonly used contrast agent for MRI contains gadolinium, which shortens the T1 relaxation time of tissues that take up gadolinium contrast agent and thus produce a bright or hyperintense signal on T1W images.

GRE sequences, also routinely used to perform magnetic resonance angiography (MRA), are programmed to show moving protons as bright and are often added to image the vasculature.

MRI is the only modality that provides accurate assessment of brain myelination. Contrast-enhanced MRI is also more sensitive than contrast-enhanced CT for detection of encephalitis, brain abscess (Figure 12-20), ventriculitis, or small foci of leptomeningeal involvement. MRI is often better than CT in demonstrating traumatic injuries, particularly diffuse axonal shearing injury, posttraumatic olfactory injury, brainstem contusion, subacute hemorrhage, encephalomalacia, gliosis, migrational anomalies such as gray matter heterotopias, closed-lip schizencephaly, lissencephaly (Figure 12-21), pachygyria, and hemimegalencephaly, and neurocutaneous disorders such as neurofibromatosis.

MRI is useful in the evaluation of patients with movement disorders, such as Wilson disease, because it demonstrates abnormal T2 signal in the basal ganglia, especially the outer rim of the putamen and in the substantia nigra; in juvenile Huntington disease, it reveals atrophy of the caudate nuclei and increased T2 signal in atrophic caudate nuclei. In pantothenate kinase deficiency (formerly designated as Hallervorden–Spatz syndrome), MRI demonstrates areas of symmetric low-signal intensity in T2W images with high signal intensity in the anteromedial aspect of the globus pallidus, the so-called eye of the tiger sign. MRI shows multifocal cortical infarctions and the presence of lactate peaks in proton magnetic resonance spectroscopy (MRS) in mitochondrial disorders, such as mitochondrial encephalomyopathy, lactic acidosis, and stroke-like episodes (MELAS) syndrome. In other mitochondrial disorders, such as myoclonic epilepsy with ragged red fibers (MERRF) syndrome, Kearns–Sayre syndrome, Leigh disease, Alpers disease, and Menkes disease, symmetric white matter T2 hyperintensities with involvement of deep cerebral nuclei are observed.

For focal (Figure 12-22) and diffuse white matter disease, T2W MRI is more sensitive than CT. MRI should preferentially be used to evaluate children with acute disseminated encephalomyelitis (Figure 12-23), human immunodeficiency virus (HIV) encephalitis, sickle cell disease, vasculitis such as systemic lupus erythematosus, Lyme disease, progressive multifocal leukoencephalopathy, and multiple sclerosis. Patterns of white matter involvement can be seen in certain inherited leukodystrophies. Early, diffuse involvement of the peripheral subcortical white matter is seen in Pelizaeus–Merzbacher disease, Canavan disease, and Alexander disease. In Canavan disease, patients have macrocephaly, and on proton MRS, a larger-than-normal *N*-acetyl-aspartate (NAA) peak is produced. In Alexander disease, there is predilection for T2 lengthening in frontal white matter and enhancement after contrast administration. A predilection for occipital white matter involvement is seen with adrenoleukodystrophy. In globoid cell leukodystrophy, T2 hyperintensity can be seen in the cerebellum and deep cerebral white matter, whereas the thalami and basal ganglia may be hypointense.

MRI can demonstrate mesial temporal sclerosis (Figure 12-24) in patients with epilepsy and can reveal small tumors in the aqueduct, sella turcica, or brainstem (Figure 12-25). MRI can also detect hippocampal dysplasia, hippocampal atrophy, and dual pathology with cortical dysplasia. These high-resolution scans help in the surgical evaluation and treatment for refractory epilepsy. MRI is also the preferred procedure when children have symptoms and signs that suggest a CNS tumor (Figures 12-11 and 12-25 to 12-27). Figure 12-28 shows an unusual presentation of subependymal giant cell astrocytoma in a newborn. In the evaluation of pediatric head and neck lesions, MRI is essential for assessment of possible intracranial extension of disease.

MRA has added a new dimension to the evaluation of pediatric cerebrovascular disease and can be used to evaluate vascular malformations, vasoocclusive disease (see Figures 12-13C and 12-22B), and vascular neoplasms. MRA may demonstrate occlusions or stenoses of the supraclinoid internal carotid arteries, the proximal anterior and middle cerebral arteries, collateral vessels, and parenchymal lesions in moyamoya disease, as well as proximal large-vessel stenotic lesions in children with sickle cell disease.

MRI may detect silent infarctions in children with Kawasaki or sickle cell disease as well as small white matter and basal ganglia infarctions in children with migraine or sickle cell disease (Figure 12-22). MRI is helpful in identifying and staging hemorrhage and clot formation as a function of the evolution of hemoglobin breakdown products (Figure 12-29) and can differentiate arterial from venous occlusive disease. It is also useful in identifying sinovenous thrombosis and associated venous infarction or dural sinus thrombosis. In evaluating intracranial hemorrhage caused by angiographically occult lesions such as cavernomas (see Figure 12-29), MRI is the procedure of choice. MRI can differentiate between various infantile extra-axial fluid collections and may distinguish effusions and hygromas from subdural hematomas. Special MRI sequences (FLAIR) can differentiate CSF–containing lesions (e.g., arachnoid cysts) from other lesions (e.g., epidermoid tumors). MRI is excellent in delineating midline abnormalities (Figure 12-30). Absence of T1 hyperintensity in the posterior pituitary on a sagittal MR image is diagnostic of central diabetes insipidus in children. For evaluation of hypopituitarism in children, MRI is critical. Hydrocephalus also may be evaluated with MRI (Figure 12-31). Likewise, in patients with CNS tumors and CSF seeding, MRI with gadolinium enhancement is very sensitive and is used for planning surgery, radiotherapy, and chemotherapy.

MAGNETIC RESONANCE SPECTROSCOPY

MRS is a clinically useful, noninvasive tool for identifying the biochemical state of the CNS (Bluml, S., Panigrahy, A., 2012). Certain atomic nuclei such as ^{1}H (protons) are magnetic, and when exposed to a strong magnetic field, they align in a particular orientation. If the nuclei are then excited by a radiofrequency pulse at their resonant frequency, they produce a detectable signal during relaxation back to equilibrium. Because of their local chemical environment, each proton produces a signal at a slightly different frequency, called a chemical shift. After a Fourier transform analysis, the plots of the resulting nuclear magnetic resonance spectra appear as peaks of signal intensity versus signal frequency or chemical shift and the area underneath the peak represents the relative concentration of the metabolite.

MRI uses the strong signals from ^{1}H nuclei of water and their spatial location to reconstruct anatomic images, whereas proton MRS is interested in the much weaker signals from nonwater protons to obtain quantitative information about biologic molecules within tissue. Small concentrations of brain metabolites can be detected using acquisition sequences, such as stimulated-echo acquisition mode and point-resolved spectroscopy. Initial studies in children used phosphorus (^{31}P) MRS to investigate spectral changes seen after neonatal asphyxia. Now the majority of studies focus on the use of proton MRS.

Spectral Metabolites Using Proton Magnetic Resonance Spectroscopy

Proton MRS (^{1}H-MRS) is used to investigate a wide range of neurologic disorders. Unlike ^{31}P MRS, ^{1}H-MRS can be obtained using the same coils as imaging. Metabolites measured with ^{1}H-MRS include NAA, a neuronal marker; creatine (Cre) composed of phosphocreatine and creatine, which are bioenergetic metabolites; choline-containing compounds (Cho), including free choline and phosphoryl and glycerophosphoryl choline that are released during membrane disruption; lactate (Lac), which accumulates in response to tissue damage or anaerobic glycolysis; and other metabolites only seen when acquired with short echo time sequences, such as the neurotransmitters glutamate and immediately formed glutamine (Glx) and myoinositol (mI or Ins), an osmolyte and astrocyte marker. During normal maturation of the brain, NAA, Cre, and Glx levels increase, and Cho and Ins levels decrease (Figure 12-32). It is not uncommon to detect small lactate peaks in spectra from normal newborn brain, but if lactate levels are high or appear after the neonatal period, it may indicate possible hypoxic-ischemic injury, a metabolic disorder, or infection.

Diseases Studied with Proton Magnetic Resonance Spectroscopy

Characteristic proton spectra in adults have been described in stroke, hepatic encephalopathy, dementia, diabetic ketoacidosis, tumor, multiple sclerosis, acquired immunodeficiency syndrome–related leukodystrophies, and trauma. In children, abnormalities have been observed in a variety of metabolic and mitochondrial encephalopathies, brain tumors, and certain neurodegenerative conditions (Bluml, S., Panigrahy, A., 2012).

Proton MRS has been used after acute traumatic and nontraumatic injuries. Typically, NAA is reduced as a result of neuronal loss or dysfunction and Cho is elevated because of diffuse axonal injury (DAI) shearing of myelin and cellular membranes and/or repair. Lac elevation is more common in children with nonaccidental trauma. Reduced NAA/Cho and elevated Cho/Cre ratios correlate with impaired neuropsychologic functioning after traumatic brain injury. Spectral sampling in areas of the brain that did not appear to be visibly injured has shown altered metabolite ratios that suggested definite injury. The time interval before MRS acquisition after injury and location of sample within the brain might affect findings. MRS also holds great promise for research of mild traumatic brain injury and sports-related concussion as it provides a sensitive, noninvasive assessment of neurochemical alterations. Several studies suggest the strong potential for using MRS to provide accurate estimates of long-term neurologic and neuropsychologic function after traumatic brain injury. More recently, a longitudinal study using more advanced MR imaging techniques such as susceptibility-weighted imaging (SWI) and diffusion tensor imaging (DTI) along with MRS has shown these techniques to be capable of detecting posttraumatic hemorrhagic lesions and the corresponding abnormalities on DTI, as well as metabolite abnormalities on MR spectroscopic imaging (MRSI) (Figure 12-33).

MRS with diffusion-weighted imaging (DWI) has been used to evaluate children with stroke and hypoxic-ischemic injury. Confirmation of the death of tissue is provided on proton MRS by a rise in Lac from anaerobic glycolysis and a loss of NAA from neuronal death. The combination of MRI and MRS can provide prognostic information in children after near-drowning. MRI and MRS have been found particularly useful in the evaluation of neonates with perinatal encephalopathy. Reduced NAA-derived metabolite ratios, elevated Cho or Ins, as well as abnormalities on DWI have been shown to reflect the severity of injury. Neonates with elevated Lac levels and decreased NAA/Cre ratios have been more likely to have a poor outcome compared with age-matched control subjects (Figure 12-34).

Proton MRS combined with MRI is useful in screening patients for metabolic and mitochondrial disorders based on the detection of increased cerebral lactate or the presence of other elevated metabolite peaks. Disorders include glutaric aciduria type 2, pyruvate dehydrogenase deficiency, Leigh disease, X-linked adrenoleukodystrophy, MELAS, and a variety of other conditions. In phenylketonuria, elevated phenylalanine levels can be seen with MRS, and in Canavan disease, MRS shows marked elevation of the NAA peaks. In Leigh disease, as in other mitochondrial or metabolic disorders, MRS reveals an abnormally high Lac peak and a decreased NAA peak in the basal ganglia and occipital gray matter (Figure 12-35). In some metabolic diseases, Lac is present during the acute illness, and with improvement, serial spectra can demonstrate its resolution. Elevated cerebral Lac has also been detected when blood Lac levels have been normal in symptomatic patients. In children with global developmental delay, proton MRS has also been useful in detecting creatine deficiency associated with disorders of creatine synthesis or transport.

Proton MRS also has been used in the evaluation of children with epilepsy showing decreased NAA, increased Cho, and increased Lac levels in epileptic foci compared with nonictal or contralateral regions. It is likely that studies will demonstrate a role for proton MRS in the selection of patients with intractable seizures for surgery.

The use of proton MRS has been examined in children and adults with CNS tumors. Malignant tumors are characterized by an increase in Cho caused by an increase in active cell proliferation and a decrease in NAA because of replacement of neurons with tumor cells. In one study, the pretreatment total Cho peak was the most reliable indicator of malignancy. In another study, Cho signal intensities were highest in astrocytomas and anaplastic astrocytomas, and creatine signal intensities were lowest in glioblastomas. However, tumoral metabolic characteristics exhibited large variations, precluding diagnostic accuracy of MRS in differentiating low- and high-grade lesions. In children, it has been suggested that proton MRS may be useful in differentiating various types of cerebellar tumors.

An acquisition technique commonly used to evaluate CNS tumors is MR spectroscopic imaging (MRSI) or chemical shift imaging (CSI); it allows simultaneous acquisition of multiple spectra within a single imaging plane (2D MRSI), or in multiple planes to cover the entire brain (3D MRSI). This allows evaluation of the entire tumor volume and surrounding brain to determine the extent of involvement outside an enhancing area or spectroscopic differences in a nonhomogeneous tumor.

MRS is useful in differentiating tumor recurrence from radiation necrosis. Patients with postirradiation necrosis are more likely to have reduced NAA, Cre, and Cho peaks with presence of lactate and lipids, compared with patients with tumor recurrence in which Cho is increased. MRS has prognostic significance in predicting outcome in children with certain brain tumors. Patients with a Cho/NAA ratio greater than 4.5 were found to have a higher mortality rate. In adults, MRS has been used to determine whether metastatic CNS tumors from distal primary sites are present. However, MRS data cannot be used alone because of significant overlap and nonspecificity of the results. It is difficult to distinguish nonneoplastic lesions such as hamartomas, histiocytic lesions, or dysplastic lesions from low-grade neoplasms by MRS. Part XVI of this book reviews imaging and spectroscopy data across the different tumor types that occur in children.

DIFFUSION-WEIGHTED IMAGING

Diffusion-weighted imaging (DWI) uses MRI to measure the diffusion of water through tissues. Random displacements of water molecules (i.e., diffusion) are modified by structural and physiologic factors in a medium. In a medium in which diffusion of water molecules is identical in all directions, the process is called isotropic diffusion. When the process depends on direction, it is called anisotropic diffusion. In brain white matter, diffusivity of water molecules is not the same in all directions. DWI has been used to investigate stroke and hypoxic-ischemic injury in children, to differentiate solid (e.g., epidermoid tumors) from cystic CNS lesions, and to evaluate patients with demyelinating disease. The most important factors regulating diffusion include tissue and fluid viscosity, membrane barriers to the free movement of water, chemical interaction of water with macromolecules, and local tissue temperature. MRI can be used to measure apparent diffusion by using an additional pair of strong gradient pulses to the standard pulse sequence. Such data are used to calculate apparent diffusion coefficient (ADC) maps. On an ADC map, the signal intensity corresponds to the ADC value; thus, low ADC values (representing restricted diffusion) correspond to a dark signal on an ADC map. The same area of restricted diffusion would show up bright on a corresponding diffusion-weighted image.

The ADC of water protons is greater in regions of unimpeded water molecular motion, such as that from CSF from the ventricular system or cystic brain lesions. In normal brain parenchyma, where diffusion of water molecules is relatively restricted, the ADC is lower. Regions of restricted or slower molecular motion appear hyperintense. For example, with ischemic injury, water accumulates intracellularly and is reflected as hyperintense regions on DWI with a corresponding hypointense signal on the ADC map. The hyperacute decrease in the ADC seen during ischemia is related to the development of cytotoxic edema associated with an increase in intracellular volume because of sodium and water influx. DWI is useful in differentiating cystic brain lesions (high ADC) from epidermoid tumors (lower ADC). In high-grade cerebral gliomas, DWI can differentiate components of the tumor and distinguish areas of nonenhancing tumor from areas of peritumoral edema.

DWI has been used to study aspects of myelination. In white matter, diffusion has been found to be anisotropic; there is greater water mobility along myelinated fiber tracts than perpendicular to them. By measuring these differences, DWI allows investigation of myelin orientation and development. This finding may be of particular interest in evaluating children with closed-head injuries. In one report, DWI was found to have increased utility in detection of brain injury in children with nonaccidental trauma. DWI may also identify evidence of corpus callosal and subcortical white matter injury, and restricted diffusion in white matter has been associated with poor neurologic and neuropsychological outcomes.

During early brain myelination, anisotropy in DWI precedes myelination changes and is helpful in evaluating the normal progression of myelination in infants. DWI obtained during the acute phase of periventricular leukomalacia is more sensitive than conventional MRI and ultrasound in detecting hyperintensities that evolve to damaging lesions at follow-up MRI. In neonates, DWI is useful in the evaluation of acute ischemic brain injury and seizures. In children younger than 2 years, DWI is useful for evaluating acute ischemic injuries, metabolic disorders, and leukodystrophies. In patients with sickle cell disease and an acute CNS event, DWI is an essential part of the investigation. DWI is helpful for earlier identification of the changes in acute carbon monoxide poisoning or dural sinus thrombosis. In patients with posterior reversible encephalopathy syndrome, DWI shows reversible vasogenic edema and, in severe cases, its conversion to cytotoxic edema, which is associated with a poorer outcome.

Children with new-onset prolonged seizures can develop unilateral hippocampal sclerosis. The presence of diffusion restriction in the affected hippocampal region can herald subsequent development of mesial temporal sclerosis. DWI can be helpful in the evaluation of CNS tumors, as it may show diffusion restriction. However, hyperintensity on DWI has been observed in solid portions of glioblastomas, and in combination with spectroscopy, may be helpful in determining an appropriate site for biopsy and in evaluating tumor recurrence. Hyperintensity also can be seen in lymphomas on DWI.

DWI is useful for evaluating children with intracranial infection. Cerebral abscesses, tuberculomas, subdural empyemas, and epidural abscesses demonstrate hyperintensity with DWI. Neurocysticercosis cysts and encephalitis appear hyperintense on DWI, whereas toxoplasmosis lesions produce variable signal intensity. In pyogenic ventriculitis, DWI shows signal intensity in dependent intraventricular fluid. DWI may be of some prognostic value in children with herpes simplex encephalitis. These lesions can exhibit low or high signal intensity indicating vasogenic or cytotoxic edema. Patients with cytotoxic edema have fulminating disease and are more likely to have a complicated clinical course and poorer outcome. Patients with vasogenic edema are less seriously ill.

DWI has assumed an important role in the early evaluation of patients with stroke. DWI reveals hyperintensity in an acute infarct soon after the onset of ischemia. Significant DWI lesions have been associated with little clinical recovery. Stroke in children is an unexpected event, and the causes are more diverse than in older populations. Imaging plays an important role in the evaluation and management of children with stroke (see Part XIII Cerebrovascular Disease in Children).

The combination of MRI, DWI, DTI, perfusion-weighted imaging (PWI), MRA, and MR venography, as clinically indicated, offers the best sensitivity for the detection of the lesion, determination of its extent, and evaluation of the degree of underlying vascular compromise. In neonates, DWI is helpful for the early diagnosis of stroke, and findings may be more pronounced than those seen on conventional MRI. It is not unusual in the evaluation of neonatal strokes to have positive findings on DWI and MRI but negative findings on MRA or MR venography. Venous infarcts are common in newborns. They are usually adjacent to the dural sinuses and show hemorrhagic components (Figure 12-38). Stroke in the newborn can also be hemorrhagic (Figures 12-39 and 12-40).

DIFFUSION TENSOR IMAGING

With diffusion tensor imaging (DTI) it is possible to have in vivo localization of neuronal fiber tracts. DTI uses the anisotrophy inherent within white matter axons of the brain. Alignment of fiber tracts determines the water diffusion anisotrophy or directionality. Diffusion of water is preferential along the longitudinal axis of the axon; at the same time, the diffusion of water along the perpendicular axis is restricted. In DTI, each voxel has one or more pairs of parameters—a rate of diffusion and a preferred direction of diffusion—described in terms of three-dimensional space. Three gradient directions are applied, sufficient to estimate the trace of the diffusion tensor or "average diffusivity," whereas DTI derives neural tract directional information from the data using three-dimensional or multidimensional vector algorithms based on a minimum of 6 and up to 256 diffusion-sensitized gradient directions, sufficient to compute the diffusion tensor. Mathematically, the preferred direction of diffusion is described as the diffusion ellipsoid or tensor. The tensor has three Eigen values: λ_1, λ_2, and λ_3. The λ_1 value points to the direction of the axon and is called the longitudinal, axial, or parallel diffusivity. The λ_2 and λ_3 values are the two small axes tensors, which are often averaged to produce a measure of the radial diffusivity, also called the perpendicular diffusivity. Longitudinal or radial diffusivity can reflect pathologic processes; for example, during evaluation of white matter infarct, radial diffusivity is considered to be related to membrane integrity.

The directional information can be exploited to select and follow neural tracts through the brain—a process called tractography. From the diffusion tensor, diffusion anisotropy measures, such as the fractional anisotropy (FA), can be computed. Fractional anisotropy is a scaler value between 0 and 1 that describes the degree of anisotropy of a diffusion process. A value of 0 means that diffusion is isotropic; that is, it is unrestricted in all directions. An FA value of 1 means that diffusion occurs along one axis only and is fully restricted along all other directions. FA is a measure often used in diffusion imaging, where it is thought to reflect fiber density, axonal diameter, and myelination in white matter.

DTI is increasingly used to evaluate normal brain development and changes associated with a wide variety of neonatal and pediatric neurologic disorders, as well as the brain's response to injury. DTI has been highly instrumental in advancing knowledge regarding early structural cerebral organization and maturation. DTI has been used in preterm and term infants to evaluate changes in cortical connectivity after white matter injury.

DTI has been found to be valuable in surgical planning for resection of brain tumors to map tracts associated with motor and language cortex (Figure 12-41) or temporal lobectomy for intractable epilepsy. Eloquent white matter tracts, such as the pyramidal tracts and optic radiations, can be assessed in relation to the tumor. When temporal lobectomy is contemplated for epilepsy surgery, DTI may be used to predict visual field deficits after temporal lobe resection. DTI has been found to be valuable in imaging of stroke to assess the relation between eloquent fiber tracts and infarcts, and in the prognosis of gross motor functions. It also has been found to be useful in the evaluation of various adult diseases, such as Alzheimer disease, multiple sclerosis, amyotrophic lateral sclerosis, spinocerebellar atrophy, and Parkinson disease.

DTI has been useful in evaluation of spinal cord lesions in differentiating traumatic from neoplastic and inflammatory causes. Patients with trauma may show reduced FA values (Figure 12-42). DTI has also been used to study axonal injury of the corticospinal tract in patients with Arnold–Chiari II malformations, suggesting developmental white matter damage in the corpus callosum beside that exerted by hydrocephalus. DTI also has been studied in children with global developmental delay. In one study, bilateral absence of the arcuate fasciculus was observed in some patients and FA was reduced in the right inferior longitudinal fasciculus.

Challenges for tractography remain. Validations of the tractography images are mostly based on known neuroanatomy. This remains a limitation of this technique. Intraoperative electrophysiological testing has been used to correlate preoperative tractography, which indicated that tractography might underestimate the fiber tracts. Ongoing development of tractography must be pursued to increase the signal-to-noise ratio while shortening the scan time, improving the in-plane image resolution, and reducing partial volume averaging because of slice thickness. Higher-field-strength scanners using multi-channel head coils and parallel imaging techniques are being used to provide some of these crucial improvements.

PERFUSION MAGNETIC RESONANCE IMAGING

Perfusion-weighted imaging (PWI) is an extension of MR technology that allows evaluation of blood volume, blood transit time, and blood flow as relative measures. PWI is used in the evaluation of patients early after symptoms of cerebral ischemia, although other clinical applications are being investigated. Two techniques have been developed based on the magnetic susceptibility effect of gadolinium-containing contrast agents and on the noninvasive magnetic labeling of arterial blood. The first, referred to as contrast-enhanced dynamic susceptibility-weighted perfusion imaging (DSC-PWI), can image relative differences in blood volume over time. Paramagnetic compounds (e.g., gadolinium-DTPA), which are used as MRI contrast agents, possess strong magnetic susceptibility, and susceptibility differences between the contrast agent and the surrounding tissue create local magnetic field gradients that can be used to acquire images after contrast injection. Images can be viewed dynamically to assess contrast entry and clearance through the tissue, with calculation of the transit time. The relative cerebral blood volume can be estimated by measuring the area under the tracer concentration–time curve, as can the relative cerebral blood flow from the ratio of the cerebral blood volume and mean brain transit time.

The second method involves blood flow imaging by magnetically labeled protons of the arterial inflow using a radiofrequency pulse and following the label through the brain's circulation. This method is known as arterial spin labeling (ASL). Deoxyhemoglobin contained within erythrocytes is paramagnetic, and on deoxygenation, the magnetic susceptibility of deoxyhemoglobin is increased and creates local field gradients, the so-called *BOLD* effect. The blood oxygen level–dependent (BOLD) technique takes advantage of this phenomenon to quantify cerebral blood flow. Although not widely used because of technical issues (low spatial resolution, difficulties with quantification, etc.), this technique has an advantage in the pediatric population as it does not involve the injection of intravenous contrast agents. Figure 12-43 shows cerebral blood flow (CBF) maps derived from a pulsed arterial spin labeling sequence in a pediatric patient being evaluated for a possible head injury.

Several studies have suggested that PWI can aid in the evaluation of acute ischemic injury, particularly by determining which patients have the potential for recovery and which may benefit from thrombolytic therapy. In patients with sickle cell disease, abnormalities on PWI are associated with neurologic symptoms although the areas of abnormality may not be seen in conventional MRI, MR angiography, or transcranial Doppler examination. PWI has also been used to differentiate tumor types. In one study, differences were observed in patients with glioblastomas, anaplastic gliomas, and low-grade gliomas. Combined with spectroscopy, PWI findings can help differentiate progression from stable tumors. Another area of interest for DWI and PWI is in children with acute disseminated encephalomyelitis. In children with cerebral arteriovenous malformation and other proliferative angiopathies, PWI may be helpful in determining areas of hyperperfusion, hypoperfusion, or venous congestion adjacent to the lesion.

SUSCEPTIBILITY-WEIGHTED IMAGING

A sequence using a high-spatial-resolution, three-dimensional, fast, low-angle MRI technique that is extremely sensitive to susceptibility has been described (Tong et al., 2008). This sequence, which can be performed on conventional scanners, was originally designed for MR venography using the paramagnetic property of intravascular deoxyhemoglobin.

This technique, known as SWI, has been very useful in detecting hemorrhagic lesions associated with diffuse axonal injury, and it has depicted significantly more small hemorrhagic lesions than conventional T2*-weighted, gradient-echo techniques. In children with traumatic brain injury and diffuse axonal injury, the number and volume of hemorrhagic lesions detected with SWI have correlated with the initial severity of injury as measured by the Glasgow Coma Scale scores, duration of coma, and long-term outcome. SWI can also be used to categorize tissue as normal-appearing or with nonhemorrhagic or hemorrhagic injury.

Neonatal strokes, which are sometimes related to dural sinus thrombosis, can be hemorrhagic (Chapter 20). SWI is more sensitive than CT or conventional MRI sequences (including GRE T2*) in detecting hemorrhage in patients with acute strokes. This blood-sensitive sequence has been found to be extremely valuable in detection of hemorrhage in children with accidental or nonaccidental trauma, infarctions, tumors, proliferative angiopathies, and vascular malformations, including Sturge–Weber syndrome and cavernous angioma (Figure 12-44), and in patients with hypertensive encephalopathy (Figure 12-45). In the examples of SWI (see Figures 12-44 and 12-45), both cases exhibit a markedly increased number and more intense abnormal signal on SWI than with other MRI sequences.

FUNCTIONAL MAGNETIC RESONANCE IMAGING

Functional MRI (fMRI) is a technique that measures changes in tissue perfusion based on changes in blood oxygenation. It is used to study regional brain activity in response to sensory, motor, and cognitive stimulation based on the assumption that neuronal activation induces an increase in glucose metabolism and blood flow. fMRI can be used to study the distribution of cerebral hemodynamic changes associated with various sensory stimuli, including vision, sensorimotor, olfactory, and auditory function, and to investigate complex cognitive functions, such as speech and language processing and reading (see Part VII: Neurodevelopmental Disorders).

Echoplanar fMRI combined with appreciation of the BOLD contrast mechanism is the most frequently used technique. The BOLD contrast mechanism relies on the fact that an increase in regional blood flow (and oxyhemoglobin) occurs in response to task performance or stimulation but is not accompanied by a concomitant increase in local tissue oxygen extraction. Because of this inflow of oxyhemoglobin, the amount of deoxyhemoglobin in the stimulated cortex does not significantly increase. This regional imbalance of oxyhemoglobin and deoxyhemoglobin reduces the net "susceptibility effect" of deoxyhemoglobin, which can be detected by magnetic susceptibility-sensitive imaging techniques using GRE methods. MRI scanners equipped with echoplanar imaging can obtain gradient images of the stimulated cortex within seconds of stimulation and display increased signal in the stimulated cortex. More-detailed technical descriptions and applications of this technique are beyond the scope of this chapter, but several sources provide excellent reviews of this technology (Viallon et al., 2015).

With the aid of fMRI, the development of brain function can be followed, and deviation from the normal pattern can be established. Early diagnosis of functional deficits has the potential to reduce residual deficits because of the earlier implementation of cognitive or other forms of rehabilitation. Acquisition of fMRI data from children is associated with a number of methodological challenges, primarily compliance and head motion; however, good data can be obtained.

fMRI is being used in patients with various neurologic diseases, including medically refractory epilepsy and brain tumors. Preoperative evaluation of such patients includes MRI and scalp, subdural, or depth electrode electroencephalography (EEG), and often includes endovascular amobarbital testing to determine which cerebral hemisphere is dominant (Wada test). Preoperative fMRI has been used to determine the feasibility of a proposed surgical resection and to select patients for invasive surgical functional mapping. fMRI appears to be as sensitive and specific as the Wada test for speech localization, preoperative memory lateralization, and intraoperative cortical mapping. fMRI performed immediately before surgery can help determine the location of neighboring eloquent functional area of concern. Some have used fMRI and DTI together with anatomic imaging to improve functional outcomes after tumor resection (see Figure 12-41).

MAGNETIC SOURCE IMAGING

Magnetic source imaging uses magnetoencephalography (MEG). When source localizations modeled from the magnetoencephalographic signal are registered with high-resolution MRI, the resulting images display functional information in an anatomic context. In functional mapping of the sensorimotor cortex, a combination of magnetic source imaging and fMRI allows improved sensitivity, fewer false-positive results, and high spatial and temporal resolution. One of the important clinical applications of functional brain imaging is pretreatment mapping to allow definition of eloquent cortex in relation to mass lesions that may be surgically resected or treated with focused irradiation (e.g., gamma knife and protons) or combinations of irradiation and chemotherapy. Magnetic source imaging may also have future applications in studying developmental plasticity after injury.

MEG is a powerful and accurate tool for the presurgical evaluation of children with refractory epilepsy and helpful in evaluating patients with dyslexia. Studies have demonstrated aberrant activation maps consisting of reduced activity in left temporoparietal areas (including the posterior part of the superotemporal, angular, and supratemporal gyri) and increased activity in homologous cortex from the right hemisphere. Studies using MEG in patients with normal MRI scans who had acquired aphasia and suspected Landau–Kleffner syndrome have demonstrated unilateral and bilateral perisylvian MEG spikes, as well as spikes from nonsylvian regions. MEG is also being used in association with three-dimensional MRI in neuronavigational systems and is a promising tool that can potentially be used in more extensive surgical procedures to lessen injury to eloquent brain areas.

Among the advantages of fMRI, magnetic source imaging, and MRS are noninvasiveness, absence of ionizing radiation, and superior spatial resolution. Functional MRI is also complementary to anatomic MRI because functional imaging takes into account normal individual variations in the functional topography of the brain. It can detect altered topography or functional plasticity, which may present because of functional reorganization in patients with various forms of cerebral injury.

SPINAL IMAGING

Initial assessment of spinal abnormalities in children includes plain films or, in the very young child, ultrasound. CT is usually indicated for acute spine injuries to determine whether a fracture, dislocation, or spondylolysis is present. CT is also helpful for the evaluation of benign tumors or vertebral body anomalies (Chapter 106). For most infants and children, MRI has replaced myelography and CT myelography as the definitive procedure for spinal neuroaxis imaging, including spinal dysraphism, other developmental anomalies of the spine (Figures 12-46 and 12-47), and acquired processes, such as neoplasms. CT myelography may have an advantage over MRI in patients with spinal dysraphism for demonstrating the location of cord tethering and for demonstrating nerve root avulsions after trauma. In the evaluation of the spinal bone marrow for metastatic disease, MRI is the procedure of choice (Figure 12-48). Detailed information on spine imaging of children is beyond the scope of this chapter, but several excellent reviews (Van Goethem et al., 2007) are available and Chapter 106 reviews spinal cord injuries.

ANGIOGRAPHY

The role of angiography has diminished since the emergence of CT, MRI, and MRA in pediatric neuroimaging. Contrast angiography in children requires sedation and anesthesia, and may have complications such as death, stroke, and thrombosis of the femoral artery. It is usually restricted to the evaluation of vascular malformations, vasculopathy, vasculitis, and vaso-occlusive disease (see Figure 12-10E) (Part XIII, Cerebrovascular Disease in Children), and occasionally to CNS tumors (Part XVI: Pediatric Neurooncology).

SINGLE-PHOTON EMISSION COMPUTED TOMOGRAPHY AND POSITRON EMISSION TOMOGRAPHY

Single-photon emission computed tomography (SPECT) uses one or more gamma cameras rotating around the patient and acquiring numerous transmission scans after injection of a labeled radiopharmaceutical. Technetium 99m ethylene cysteinate dimer, a radiopharmaceutical used for brain perfusion, and Tc 99m hexamethylpropyleneamine oxime are the main radiotracers used for clinical brain SPECT imaging. They have the advantage of a Tc 99m label with its optimal imaging characteristics. The indications for brain SPECT imaging in children include planning for epilepsy surgery, evaluation of brain death, acute neurologic loss (including stroke), language disorders, hypertension resulting from renal vascular disease, traumatic brain injury, and migraine. Pediatric psychological conditions in which regional cerebral blood flow studies are occasionally obtained include anorexia nervosa, autism, Gilles de la Tourette syndrome, and attention-deficit/hyperactivity disorder. Considerable research is taking place in neuroreceptor imaging using iodinated- and technetium-labeled neuroligands to measure certain critical components of neurotransmission. Ongoing research is using SPECT and positron emission tomography (PET) in the study of psychiatric disorders such as schizophrenia, anxiety disorders, depression, autism, and stress and mood disorders. Iodine-131-labeled metaiodobenzylguanidine (MIBG) localizes in adrenergic neurons and is helpful in evaluating patients with neural crest tumors or neuroblastoma.

Studies using PET scanning have made major contributions during the past decade to understanding the developmental neurobiology of the nervous system, particularly with reference to cerebral and cerebellar glucose, and oxidative metabolism and blood flow. However, because of its limited availability, a comprehensive review of the technology and its clinical applications is not included here; several good sources are available (Purz et al., 2014).

PET has been used to study patients with many different pediatric neurologic disorders, including various forms of epilepsy (Figure 12-24), Rasmussen encephalitis, autism, language disorders, attention-deficit disorders, movement disorders, neonatal hypoxic-ischemic encephalopathy, moyamoya disease, tuberous sclerosis, Langerhans cell histiocytosis, and CNS tumors.

The most common clinical application is for pediatric epilepsy, particularly those with drug-resistant epilepsy (Chapter 78). Such patients frequently have infantile spasms, focal ictal abnormalities in the frontal or temporal regions, or CNS malformations. PET is most useful for patients who have normal neuroimaging studies but clinically and electrographically have a focal seizure disorder or a generalized seizure disorder with significant asymmetries of activity. Interictal PET studies demonstrate areas of hypometabolic glucose metabolism using 2-deoxy-[^{18}F] fluoro-D-glucose in areas considered epileptogenic. Ictal PET scans demonstrate more variable metabolic changes. In patients with refractory localization–related seizures, temporal lobe abnormalities can frequently be detected with PET. Studies have indicated congruence between focal temporal EEG abnormalities, hippocampal atrophy on MRI, hypometabolism in corresponding interictal regions with PET, and reductions in the metabolite ratios using proton MRS.

Patients with infantile spasms may also have significant EEG and PET cortical or subcortical asymmetries that have been shown useful in the evaluation for epilepsy surgery. PET may reveal lateralized or localized regions of hypometabolic glucose use that corresponds to localized EEG abnormalities and cortical dysplasias or other structural abnormalities. Surgical resection of regions with one hypometabolic area usually results in improved seizure control; patients with multiple hypometabolic regions are unlikely to benefit from such treatment.

PET has also been of particular value in children with intractable seizures who have subtle or major CNS malformations. These cases include children with tuberous sclerosis, Sturge–Weber syndrome, hemimegalencephaly, and focal cortical dysplasias and other migrational disorders. PET imaging of children with CNS tumors is useful. Brain tumors can be histologically heterogeneous, and stereotactic biopsies may lead to inaccurate diagnosis or grading. Increased uptake with fluoro-D-glucose–PET may represent more malignant or aggressive tumors. By combining PET and MRI in the planning of a stereotactic brain biopsy, it may be possible to improve the diagnostic yield and reduce sampling from high-risk or functional areas.

Acknowledgments

Imaging figures in this chapter were provided by Dr. Nathaniel D. Wycliffe and spectra by Dr. Barbara Holshouser from the Division of Neuroradiology, Department of Radiology, Loma Linda University School of Medicine, Loma Linda, California.

REFERENCES

The complete list of references for this chapter is available in the e-book at www.expertconsult.com.
See inside cover for registration details.

SELECTED REFERENCES

Barkovich, A.J., Raybaud, C., 2001. Pediatric Neuroimaging, fifth ed. Lippincott Williams & Wilkins, New York.

Bluml, S., Panigrahy, A. (Eds.), 2012. MR Spectroscopy of Pediatric Brain Disorders. Springer Verlag, Berlin.

Provenzale, J.M., 2009. Advances in pediatric neuroradiology: highlights of the recent medical literature. AJR Am. J. Roentgenol. 192, 19–25.

Purz, S., Sabri, O., Viehweger, A., et al., 2014. Potential pediatric applications of PET/MR. J. Nucl. Med. 55, 32S–39S.

Tong, K.A., Ashwal, S., Obenaus, A., et al., 2008. Susceptibility-weighted MR imaging: a review of clinical applications in children. AJNR Am. J. Neuroradiol. 29, 9–17.

Tortori-Donati, P., Rossi, A., Bianchen, R. (Eds.), 2005. Pediatric Neuroradiology. Springer-Verlag, Berlin.

Van Goethem, J.W.M., van den Hauwe, L., Parizel, P.M., et al. (Eds.), 2007. Spinal Imaging: Diagnostic Imaging of the Spine and Spinal Cord. Springer-Verlag, Berlin.

Viallon, M., Cuvinciuc, V., Delattre, B., et al., 2015. State-of-the-art MRI techniques in neuroradiology: principles, pitfalls, and clinical applications. Neuroradiology 57, 441–467.

E-BOOK FIGURES AND TABLES

The following figures and tables are available in the e-book at www.expertconsult.com. See inside cover for registration details.

13 Pediatric Neurophysiologic Evaluation

Mark S. Scher

An expanded version of this chapter is available on www.expertconsult.com. See inside cover for registration details.

Pediatric neurophysiologic studies are an integral part of the diagnostic evaluation of the infant or child with suspected brain dysfunction; electroencephalography (EEG), polysomnography, evoked responses, and computerized neurophysiological analyses comprise four general diagnostic modalities. Genotype-phenotype comparisons are now being investigated that will redefine neurophysiological studies as endophenotypes to study gene–environment interactions (Scher and Loparo, 2009). Several excellent reviews supplement this discussion and can assist the physician with the evaluation of children who exhibit these phenomena (Kaminska et al., 2015).

UTILITY OF PEDIATRIC NEUROPHYSIOLOGICAL STUDIES

Guidelines for Interpretation

EEG analysis requires a systematic, orderly process in which a series of steps are followed to reach a proper interpretation. The rhythmicity of spontaneous EEG signals gives a continuous admixture of scalp-generated oscillatory potentials. EEG frequencies used for clinical studies are classified in four band ranges. Delta activity is less than 4 Hz; theta activity is 4 to less than 7 Hz; alpha activity is 8 to less than 14 Hz; and beta activity is greater than 14 to 30 Hz. Although DC (usually lower than 3 Hz) and gamma-frequencies (higher than 30 Hz) can be recorded with appropriate filter settings, these rhythms are currently applied only to research recordings. In general, the amplitude of EEG activity is inversely proportional to frequency.

For pediatric EEG studies, the amount of slow activity decreases with increasing age, and the persistence and frequency of slow activity vary in different brain regions. It is important to appreciate the presence and degree of expression of frequencies in various regions at different ages, and other parameters such as waveform, manner of occurrence (e.g., random, continuous), and amplitude are essential to visual analysis.

Newborn Electroencephalographic Patterns

There are expected changes in the scalp-generated EEG patterns for neonates of different gestational ages. The experienced encephalographer can approximate the electrical maturity within 2 weeks of the gestational age. Changing electrical patterns reflect the postconceptional age of the neonate independent of birth weight. Maturation of the neonate's sleep-wake behavior follows maturation of the CNS and is independent of the birth weight. Preterm neonates, when corrected to term postconceptional age, should have EEG patterns and sleep behavior similar to those of term, appropriate-for-gestational-age newborns.

Normal Electroencephalographic Patterns in Infancy Through Adolescence

Waking Patterns

Although sleep patterns predominate for the newborn, state development during infancy prepares the child for sustained periods of wakefulness. Waking EEG patterns are the first part of the discussion of normal EEG patterns in childhood.

One of the fundamental characteristics of the waking EEG pattern is the dominant background activity. Berger initially described how the dominant frequency increased as ages advanced during childhood. By 3 to 4 months of age, a discernible occipitoparietal rhythm of 3 to 4 Hz is observed (Fig. 13-11A). The activity approximates 5 Hz by 6 months and increases to 6 to 7 Hz by 9 to 18 months of age (Fig. 13-11B). The 6-Hz to 7-Hz frequency remains fairly stable until 2 years of age, when it varies between 7 and 8 Hz. By 3 years of age, the dominant waking rhythm of childhood is within the alpha range in 82% of children (Fig. 13-11C). The mean frequency is 9 Hz by 7 years of age and 10 Hz by 15 years of age (Fig. 13-11D). Quantitative analysis of the EEG posterior-dominant rhythms in healthy adolescents has documented that the maturation of the posterior dominant rhythm is nearly complete by age 16. Further, the frequency range of this rhythm is substantially narrower than the alpha range.

The amplitude, asymmetry, and locus of the dominant rhythm also change with increasing age. Higher amplitudes are seen at younger ages, with maximum amplitudes at 6 to 9 years that subsequently decline during adolescence. Asymmetries of this activity can be expected, with higher amplitude on the right in 20% of children, although differences of 50% or greater must be considered with suspicion. No correlation to hand dominance has been demonstrated. About 70% of adults and 95% of children have an occipital location to the dominant rhythm, but at least three independent alpha rhythms can be recorded over the scalp—occipital, temporal, and central regions—which may differ in frequency as much as 2 Hz. More anterior expression of the dominant rhythm becomes evident during adulthood.

Mu Rhythm

The mu, or central, rhythm commonly is 9 to 10 Hz and should not be confused with the central dominant rhythm of 7 to 9 Hz in infants. Although the mu rhythm is observed in less than 5% of children younger than 4 years, it can be observed in 18% of children between 8 and 16 years of age and occurs somewhat more frequently in females. It can be blocked by movement of the opposite limb rather than eye opening. Although the mu rhythm may frequently appear asymmetrically and alternately in either hemisphere, a persistent asymmetry suggests a structural lesion on the attenuated side or irritation on the predominant side (e.g., after head injury).

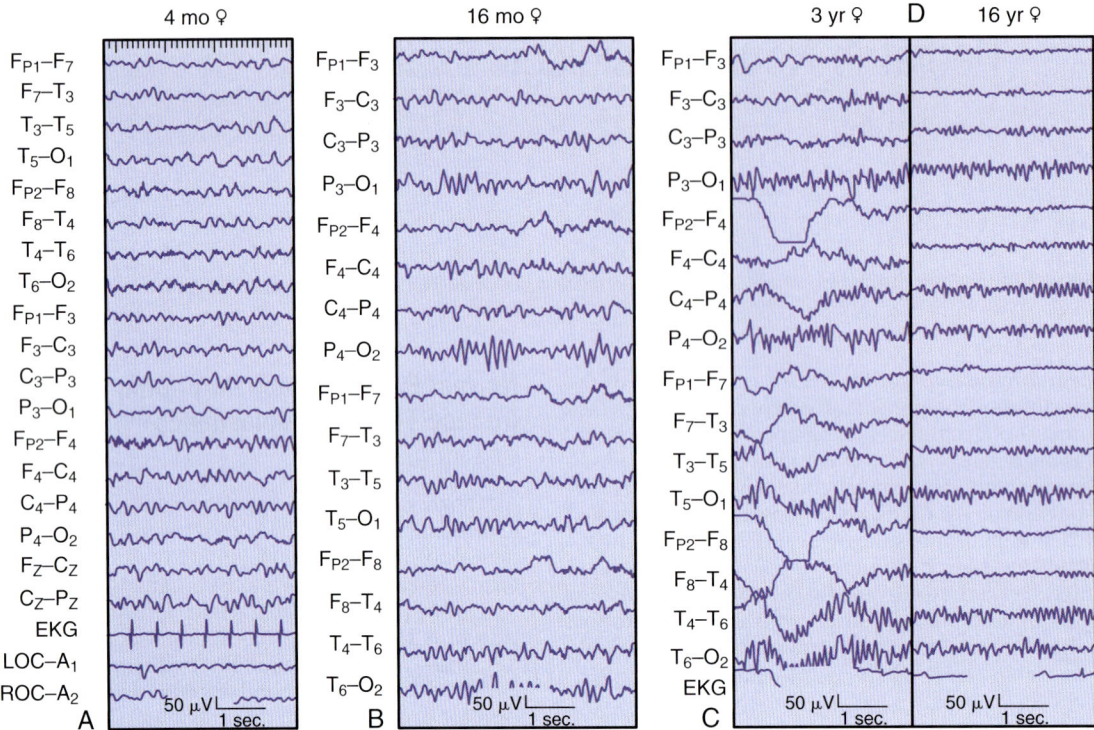

Figure 13-11. Posterior dominant rhythms (line markings) at four different ages during childhood while the patient was awake with eyes closed. **A,** A 4-Hz dominant rhythm at 4 months of age. **B,** Dominant rhythm of 6 to 7 Hz at 16 months of age. **C,** Dominant rhythm of 9 Hz at 3 years of age. **D,** Dominant rhythm of 10 to 12 Hz that is well regulated in a 16-year-old adolescent.

Beta Activity

Three distinctive band ranges are described for beta frequencies in waking EEG recordings of children. Limited diagnostic use can be applied to the overall description of fast activity. Beta activity in the range of 18 to 25 Hz is most commonly encountered, with ranges of 14 to 16 Hz and 35 to 40 Hz observed less frequently. Symmetric distribution over each anterior head region is usually observed. Asymmetries of as much as 30% to 40% can be encountered without the presence of a structural lesion. Important diagnostic conclusions can be assigned if beta activity is reduced by more than 50%, especially when associated with delta or theta slowing in the same head region. Prominent scalp edema can also attenuate the high-frequency EEG signals in the absence of cerebral pathologic conditions. Symmetric prominence of beta activity is commonly encountered with the administration of certain sedative medications, especially barbiturates or benzodiazepines. Skull defects can contribute to an asymmetric exaggeration of beta activity over the bony defect—that is, breach rhythm.

Theta and Delta Slowing

Theta rhythms are commonly encountered in the frontocentral regions and are usually related to drowsiness or heightened emotional states. In the past, theta rhythms were associated with a variety of clinical conditions, including epilepsy, but their common occurrence is now better appreciated as a normal variant.

Posterior slow waves located in the parieto-occipital regions, commonly referred to as posterior slow waves of youth, constitute the most frequently observed normal delta slow activity in the waking EEG record of children (Fig. 13-12). Commonly located in the occipitoparietal or occipitotemporal

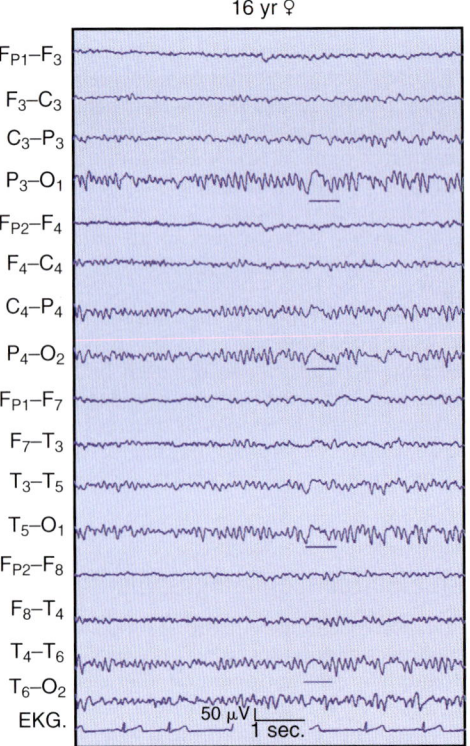

Figure 13-12. EEG of a 16-year-old female who is awake with her eyes closed demonstrates a biooccipital posterior slow wave of youth (line marking).

regions is a 2.5-Hz to 4.5-Hz monorhythmic or polymorphic delta wave with an amplitude of less than 100 μV. Superimposed alpha activities are also observed with these delta waves, which can have symmetric or asymmetric occurrences. The neurologist should view an asymmetry of greater than 50% between regions with suspicion. It will block with eye opening and disappear with the alpha rhythm during drowsiness. Rarely seen before 2 years of age, it has maximum expression between 8 and 14 years, especially in females. Approximately 25% of normal children have this pattern. The distinction between this pattern and other abnormal slow-wave activity should be based on complexity of the waveform, persistence, symmetry, and amplitude, all in the context of closed-head injury, hypoxia, or other encephalitides.

Lambda Waves

Lambda waves can be observed in normal patients when they are viewing a well-illuminated picture of complex design. Sharply contoured occipital transients with a prominent surface-positive phase lasting 75 to 150 msec are described, although an extremely sharp appearance may cause suspicion of an abnormality. Eye closure or darkening of the room eliminates lambda waves, whereas occipital spike discharges persist. These transients are observed in young infants and can be seen occasionally in neonates.

Hyperventilatory Response

In the past, a response to hyperventilation was considered evidence of a brain abnormality in children. However, it has become commonplace to observe prominent high-amplitude slowing in normal children, with maximum expression between 8 and 12 years that persists as a less significant electrographic change into adulthood. A greater degree of response has been associated with lower blood glucose or carbon dioxide concentrations. Standardization of hyperventilation is necessary for the clinician to best judge the EEG slowing relative to age differences reported for children. This activation maneuver, as well as photic stimulation, continues to be an important part of the EEG reviewing for children (Ahdab and Riachi, 2014).

Proper testing procedure usually requires 3 to 5 minutes of overbreathing by the child to elicit the response, although shorter time intervals have been suggested for specific purposes (Watemberg et al., 2015). Careful notation of artifact and an anticipation of spikelike, high-amplitude sharp waves are emphasized. Superimposed faster frequencies that may appear to be spike discharges are followed by slow waves during hyperventilation and are commonly overinterpreted as an abnormal finding (Fig. 13-13).

Photic Stimulation

Photic stimulation may produce a variety of electrographic phenomena that can be useful to the neurologist. It is suggested that a strobe light be used with 500,000-foot to 2 million-foot candles of intensity at a distance of 12 inches from the face and at multiple flash frequencies. Both occipital and parietal channels should be included, with one channel recording the output signal from the light source.

Two artifacts should be anticipated. The photoelectric effect usually appears in the frontopolar electrodes and is caused by high resistance or defective grounding of these electrodes. Simply shielding these electrodes from the light source may be sufficient to determine whether it is present. A second artifact results from the photomyoclonic effect. Muscle contractions, usually around the anterotemporal, frontal, and frontopolar electrodes, are recorded in response to the light flashes.

Taking these possible sources of artifact into consideration, the normal phenomenon is a sharp surface-positive waveform, maximal in the parietal and occipital electrodes, which matches the flash frequency (Fig. 13-14A). Photic stimulation might induce drowsiness, including a normal sharp-wave phenomenon known as posterior occipital sharp transients (Fig. 13-16C). Slower flash frequencies result in more prominent responses in younger children. However, the spike discharges in these posterior leads can be diffusely distinguished by their waveform, field, symmetry, and persistence relative to the start and end of the flash of light. The abnormal photoparoxysmal response (Fig. 13-14B and C) is discussed in a subsequent section, including its relationship to epilepsy and withdrawal states.

Drowsy Patterns

A drowsy state represents a transition from wakefulness associated with the disappearance of the occipital alpha rhythm and the emergence of central-parietal theta activities. Pendular eye movements may be detected in the anterior, temporal, or frontopolar channels. EEG changes may precede behavioral evidence of sleepiness, especially in the younger child. This period of successively greater amounts of rhythmic and paroxysmal slow activity has been called hypnagogic hypersynchrony and may be overinterpreted by the inexperienced clinician. Similar to the notched, sharp-wave activity during hyperventilation, superimposed activity may be seen during drowsiness and misinterpreted as abnormal spike or sharp-wave discharges.

The EEG recording should be obtained continuously from wakefulness through drowsiness into sleep so that the complete succession of changes in background activities can be

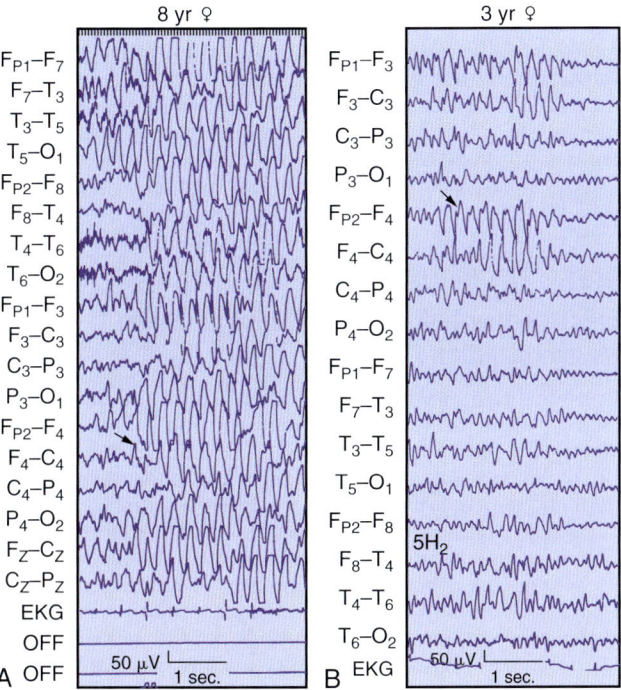

Figure 13-13. A, EEG of an 8-year-old female during hyperventilation. Arrow indicates notching of the high-amplitude slow activity in the absence of epileptiform discharges. **B,** EEG of a 3-year-old female during drowsy, light sleep. Notched, high-amplitude delta activity occurs (arrow) in the absence of epileptiform discharges.

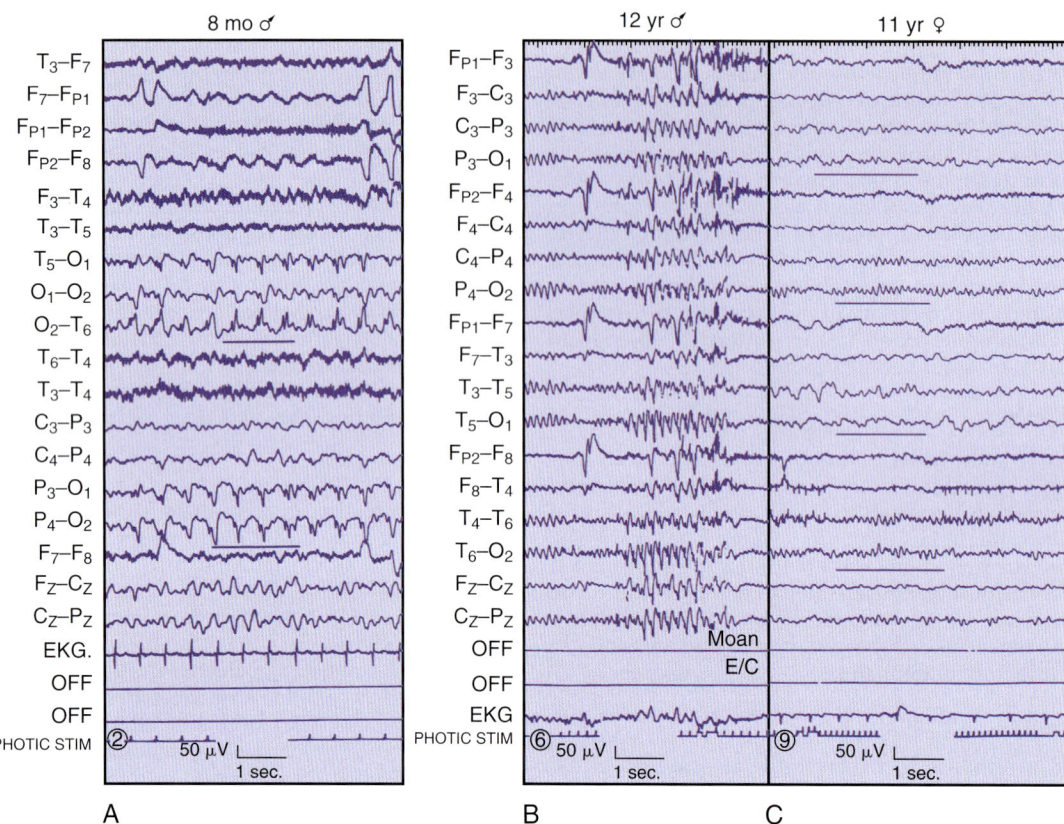

Figure 13-14. Types of EEG photic responses. **A,** EEG of an 8-month-old male with prominent driving in a slow-flash frequency in the occipital regions. **B,** EEG of a 12-year-old male with a photoparoxysmal response confined within the duration of the stimulus at six flashes per second. **C,** EEG of an 11-year-old female with suppression of driving in the left hemisphere and with intermixed slowing in the same head region. Encephalomalacia in the left posterior quadrant was demonstrated on imaging studies. (**A,** *Courtesy of Dr. P Crumrine, Children's Hospital, Pittsburgh.*)

observed. A slowing in the alpha rhythm with an increase in amplitude already described can be seen in a diffuse distribution or regionally over the anterior or posterior scalp areas in association with more prominent beta activity.

The first and more common pattern is rhythmic beta activities over the central or frontocentral region of approximately 200 μV. It is most pronounced between 3 months and 4 years of age, and is not encountered after 7 years of age. Typically, the frequency of this rhythmic pattern will increase to 6 Hz with age. A second pattern consists of prominent bisynchronous bursts of 2 to 5 Hz greater than 350 μV from 6 months to 5 years of age. This pattern is commonly misinterpreted as spike-and-wave discharges because of the superimposition of the faster frequencies.

Sleep Activation Procedures

Based on an extensive review of the subject of sleep and sleep deprivation, there is general agreement that sleep and sleep deprivation have a substantial activating effect on the occurrence of interictal epileptiform discharges. Recent updates addressed the activating effect of sleep deprivation over and beyond the effect of only sleep. Most published guidelines do not recommend sleep deprivation for the initial study because of the burden to the patient. However, sleep deprivation has been considered superior to sleep alone in one study, although other investigators suggest that sleep state can be better achieved during routine EEGs by simply ordering the sequence of activation procedures. By performing hyperventilation first with photic stimulation at the end of the study the

neurophysiologist can maximize the yield of attaining sleep during a routine recording. The inclusion of sleep as part of the child's study ensures a greater likelihood for the activation of specific epileptiform features associated with specific epileptic syndromes such as benign rolandic epilepsy of childhood, Landau-Kleffner syndrome, and electrical status during slow-wave sleep.

SLEEP PATTERNS

Electroencephalographic Neonatal Sleep as an Ultradian Rhythm

In normal term newborns, sleep alternates with waking states over a 3-hour to 4-hour cycle at night and during the day. Within the first month or two of life after birth for the term infant, sleep-wake state organization begins to adapt to the light and dark cycles, as well as regularly recurring social cues. Circadian rhythmicity of body temperature and heart rate occurs in approximately 50% of preterm infants at 29 to 35 weeks conceptional age. However, longer-run ultradian rhythms of 3 to 4 hours duration correspond to feeding and social interventions. Increases in body movement activity and heart rate and decreases in rectal skin temperature are present during interventions, reflecting changes in the infant's microenvironment and the infant-caretaker interactions. Even the ultradian EEG sleep cycle length of the preterm infant, as defined by changes in EEG discontinuity, shows a positive correlation of cycle length and increasing postconceptional age. By postconceptional term age, the ultradian EEG sleep cycle is longer for the preterm than for the term infant. Regardless of the cycle length, the architecture remains the same between preterm and term groups and is composed of active sleep segments interrupted by transitional or indeterminate sleep segments. Reactivity or arousal periods punctuate within and between sleep segments. Indeterminate sleep and arousal phenomena represent important expressions of sleep continuity.

The neonatal ultradian EEG sleep cycle is approximately 30 to 70 minutes. The sleep segments that constitute this cycle include two active and two quiet sleep segments, usually beginning as an active sleep portion on falling asleep. Transitional sleep segments within and between active sleep segments are commonly called indeterminate sleep segments. Reactivity or arousal periods also punctuate within and between sleep segments. Indeterminate sleep and arousal phenomena represent important expressions of sleep continuity.

Infant and Childhood Sleep

The infant's ultradian sleep cycle lengthens with maturation to 75 to 90 minutes. The idealized sleep architecture after sleep onset consists of one REM sleep segment that follows four non-REM (or quiet sleep) segments. Regional EEG patterns are identified during these sleep segments, which assists in the assessment of sleep organization.

Vertex Waves and Sleep Spindles

The transitional state of drowsiness is sometimes referred to as stage 1 of sleep and may include sharp-wave discharges that are maximal in amplitude over the vertex and central regions. Commonly, symmetric central diphasic waveforms become better expressed and more abundant during stage 2 sleep, which coincides with the appearance of sleep spindles. These waveforms usually have an initial surface-negative wave, followed by a surface-positive phase. The onset of vertex waves can be between 2 and 5 months of age and can appear asymmetric, particularly at younger ages. If this asymmetry exceeds 20%, the neurologist must consider the presence of a lesion on the attenuated side. Excessively asynchronous appearance of vertex waves has been associated with increased intracranial pressure or structural midline defects such as agenesis of the corpus callosum.

Sleep spindles primarily define stage 2 of sleep and are not clearly expressed until 3 to 4 months of age. Synchrony is gradually achieved with increasing age, and most spindles are bilaterally synchronous by 18 months. The waveform morphology of sleep spindles in infants differs from that of older patients. The duration of spindles is 1.5 to 1.8 seconds at 4 to 6 months. At this age, they frequently reach 4 to 6 seconds, which subsequently shortens to 0.5 second by 25 to 54 months.

Spindles lasting as long as 4 to 6 seconds are frequently observed in infants younger than 1 year, but "extreme" spindles have been described in neurologically abnormal children of older ages (Fig. 13-15B). The common frequency range is 13 to 14 Hz, but slower spindle frequencies of 10 to 12 Hz are also documented in about 5% of children older than 5 years. Spindle density is highest at 3 to 9 months and at a minimum at 27 to 54 months. Faster bursts of 18 to 22 Hz may resemble spindles but are usually associated with medications such as benzodiazepines and barbiturates. Sleep spindle evolution from infancy to adolescence has been described. Sleep spindle activity changes with maturation in terms of length and density. The establishment of age-related normative data of sleep spindle activity will improve the identification of non-REM 2 in infancy, childhood, and adolescence and will enable detection of delayed neuronal maturation and/or sleep stability.

Occipital Sharp Transients

Two types of sharp transients can occur in the occipital region during sleep. Posterior sharp transients of sleep are surface-positive, checkmark-like waveforms, which usually occur in runs of 4 to 5 Hz but may occur singly. Although appearing asymmetrically, these waveforms are bilaterally synchronous. Although posterior sharp transients of sleep can appear between 4 and 5 years of age, they are most commonly encountered during the early sleep of young adults 15 to 35 years of age. The other form of occipital transients in children also appears during drowsiness. It has a cone-shaped configuration or a diphasic sharp wave resembling a vertex transient.

Frequency Distribution During Sleep

More pronounced beta activity can accompany drowsiness. As stage 2 sleep emerges, a definite frequency and amplitude gradient can be appreciated between the anterior and posterior head regions. Higher-frequency, lower-amplitude activity predominates in anterior head regions, with the converse situation occurring in posterior head regions. With deeper sleep, this gradient is less well defined. Its absence or poor organization has been observed in children with developmental delays. The quantitative measure of slow-wave sleep provides a measurable biomarker of developmental neuroplasticity (Wilhelm et al., 2014).

Arousal Patterns

Infants younger than 2 months of age have only a diminution of background amplitude with arousal. By 2 to 3 months of age, diphasic slow waves accompany this desynchronization and may merge with delta waves by 5 months of age. With further arousal, 4-Hz to 8-Hz rhythmic waveforms appear diffusely or in the frontocentral regions, last for several seconds, and disappear by 4 years of age. More monorhythmic 4-Hz to 5-Hz activity may persist into young adulthood and can be seen in 40% of children 10 to 14 years old. Postarousal hypersynchrony of 2.5 to 3.5 Hz generally appears frontally but may also be expressed posteriorly with further arousals. Such electrographic changes cease at any time, with the recording reverting back to the previous sleep pattern.

Patterns of Uncertain Significance

The most commonly encountered pattern is the 14-positive and 6-positive spike discharge (Fig. 13-16A). Although initially assigned clinical significance, this pattern subsequently has been identified in several control populations. These surface-positive waveforms appear in the posterotemporal regions or adjacent areas during sleep, with a 60-μV to 70-μV, comb-shaped configuration that may last as long as 3 seconds. It is best demonstrated with a referential montage and has a peak incidence during adolescence.

The 6-Hz spike-wave complexes are less common waveforms, having maximal amplitude in the centroparietal regions. Historically considered clinically important in patients with headache and autonomic symptoms, they can be seen in normal control subjects, especially adolescents. These complexes can be induced by diphenhydramine in 30% of normal volunteers (Fig. 13-16B). Small, sharp spikes and psychomotor variants, benign epileptiform variants, are uncommonly observed in children. Small, sharp spikes occur more frequently in a normal rather than a patient population. Psychomotor variant patterns also are described in as many normal, asymptomatic individuals as in study patients.

ABNORMAL ELECTROENCEPHALOGRAPHIC PATTERNS

Abnormal Neonatal Electroencephalographic Patterns

Numerous medical complications can contribute to an encephalopathic state in the sick neonate, consisting of diffuse, multifocal, or focal brain dysfunction. Many times, focal and diffuse processes exist simultaneously, creating a more difficult interpretative situation. EEG findings can substantially add to clinical assessments, given the limited clinical repertoire of the immature infant and the practical limitations of a sick neonate who is confined by catheters, intubation, pharmacologic paralysis, and an isolette. Visual and computerized analyses of EEG patterns will assume greater significance as outcome measures are developed that will assess the efficacy of neuroprotective interventions. Comparison of the neonate's EEG background activity with that expected for a particular gestational or postconceptional age can rapidly estimate the severity of a neonatal encephalopathy.

Four general guidelines must be recognized before applying EEG analysis to the assessment of the newborn with suspected CNS dysfunction. First, neonatal EEG abnormalities are nonspecific with respect to etiology; a specific diagnosis is only infrequently associated with a particular EEG pattern. Second, it is difficult to determine by only a single EEG study if the observed EEG abnormalities are reflective of a transient or more permanent encephalopathy unless serial studies are obtained. Third, EEG abnormalities alone cannot be interpreted by the clinician with respect to the timing of the brain insult. Fourth, despite the degree of severity regarding EEG patterns, abnormalities usually disappear rapidly over time. This "normalization" of EEG disturbances can occur even in infants who will later suffer severe neurologic sequelae. Obtaining several EEG studies is recommended for all high-risk infants, beginning during the acute phase of the illness and repeated judiciously over the first days of life into the second week until normal studies are obtained, or alternatively, electrographic abnormalities are noted to persist.

Assessment of Prognosis

Serial EEG studies during the neonatal period offer more information than can be obtained from an isolated recording. None the less, some reports emphasize the prognostic significance of single recordings with severely abnormal features (Watanabe et al., 1980), whereas other reports suggest that serial studies provide the clinician with a sensitive prognostic indication of neurodevelopmental outcome. Monod and colleagues analyzed 691 neonatal EEG studies of 270 children whose clinical conditions were documented from 3 to 14 years. Certain EEG abnormalities were related to neurologic sequelae. Examples of suppression-burst (paroxysmal), isoelectric, multifocal sharp-wave patterns, and an invariant pattern are shown in Figures 13-17 to 13-20. Tharp and colleagues subsequently adapted these abnormalities to preterm neonates. From a retrospective analysis of 184 neonatal EEG studies of 81 infants born at or before 36 weeks gestation, and subsequent clinical assessment of 64 survivors, a severely abnormal pattern was of prognostic value. Table 13-1 summarizes the major EEG abnormalities discussed in these two studies. Severe EEG disturbances help establish a reference point for the neonatologist. Improving or worsening trends may have important prognostic implications in the context of the neonate's evolving clinical condition.

Focal Abnormalities

Neonatal EEG patterns assessments have been shown to be helpful in the evaluation of focal, regional, or hemispheric brain abnormalities. Parasagittal and lateralized EEG abnormalities (central or midline regions) have been correlated with a variety of brain lesions. In a population of 60 neonates with midline EEG abnormalities and cerebral lesions identified with neuroimaging or neuropathologic studies, intraventricular hemorrhage was the most common hemorrhagic lesion, whereas periventricular leukomalacia and cerebral infarction were the most common ischemic lesions associated with parasagittal abnormal patterns. Midline EEG abnormalities include amplitude attenuation, positive sharp waves, seizures, and discharges associated with myoclonus. Other studies have also demonstrated the association of positive vertex sharp waves with intraventricular hemorrhage (Fig. 13-21) or periventricular leukomalacia, and the association of midline electrographic seizures with infarction. Late chronologic changes in neonatal EEG findings with periventricular leukomalacia have also been described, after positive sharp waves and other midline or rolandic abnormalities have been noted in the acute time period. Chronic stage changes consist of persistent amplitude and frequency suppression of varying degrees of severity, emphasizing the greater efficacy of serial recordings.

Lateralized EEG abnormalities, including neonatal seizures, have been associated with congenital or acquired brain lesions (Fig. 13-22). After the seizure, the prominent abnormality is an attenuation of background frequencies or amplitude.

Transient asymmetries have also been described in asymptomatic neonates during the initial portion of quiet sleep. Judgment must be used before proceeding to imaging procedures to assess such patients for structural lesions.

Neonatal Seizures

Despite the need to diagnose neonatal seizures promptly, unique clinical and electrographic features may delay timely recognition and treatment. The varied and less organized clinical expression of neonatal seizures makes the diagnosis more difficult. Accepted clinical criteria may not always distinguish seizure movements from pathologic nonseizure movements. Classifications have been developed that have improved the clinical accuracy of the observer. Technologies using prolonged EEG or synchronized video EEG-monitoring sessions will likely prove more valuable in diagnosing clinical and electrographic seizures (Shellhaas, 2015). Computer-assisted and automated detection systems continue to be presented with varying degrees of specificity and sensitivity for seizure detection, as exemplified by several reports. Amplitude-integrated EEG in neonates has also been compared with conventional EEG for a variety of neonatal diagnostic and prognostic purposes. This simplified technology will need to be combined with more extensive neurophysiological monitoring paradigms; several proposed classification schemes have been discussed.

Neonates may have seizures that are not detected unless an EEG is performed. Some of these patients are pharmacologically paralyzed for ventilatory care, whereas others fail to demonstrate clinical seizures despite the appearance of electrographic seizures in the absence of a paralytic agent. Electroclinical uncoupling after antiseizure medication use can suppress clinical signs associated with seizures. EEG seizures are recognized by the electroencephalographer based on the evolution of discharges that can be clearly distinguished from the background and are not related to artifact. The frequency of these discharges is usually in the slow range with a variety of waveforms. The evolution of discharges implies a gradual change in the location, amplitude, waveform, or distribution. The arbitrary definition for the minimum duration of a seizure is 10 seconds, with the average duration being 1–5 minutes for term or preterm neonates, unless status epilepticus occurs. Clinical ictal activity may accompany the electrical seizure (Fig. 13-23A and B). Only a few patterns are associated with a particular clinical presentation. For example, alpha-range rhythms have been associated with respiratory disturbances such as apnea as the clinical correlate appearing with an electrographic seizure.

Five categories of clinical seizure types have been historically described and may be associated with any number of EEG seizure patterns. These five categories are subtle, focal clonic, multifocal clonic, tonic, and myoclonic. Focal or multifocal EEG seizures can be observed, and generalized discharges are seen rarely. The infrequent occurrence of a clinical seizure without a coincident EEG accompaniment has been described (Fig. 13-23C). Although one explanation is that this is a nonseizure movement disorder originating from a subcortical location, the possibility of a subcortical seizure focus may also exist.

Focal Periodic Patterns

Focal and multifocal periodic abnormalities have been described in neonatal recordings. These discharges do not have an acceptable evolution in EEG features to be identified as an electrographic seizure. Instead, stereotypic, repetitive discharges at slow frequencies are observed, and they are usually brief (Fig. 13-24). More prolonged and lateralized periodic discharges have also been described for many clinical situations, specifically for neonates with asphyxia and herpes encephalitis. Short runs of periodic discharges are more commonly observed. Parasagittal discharges occur in preterm and temporal patterns in term neonates, and they are associated with EEG seizures and brain lesions such as infarction. This association of periodic patterns with brain lesions is reminiscent of the association between periodic lateralized discharges and brain lesions in adults and children. Repetitive EEG patterns such as periodic discharges do not satisfy arbitrarily defined descriptions of electrographic seizures but may have important relationships to clinically observed seizures.

Spikes and Sharp Waves

In most situations, the electroencephalographer has difficulty assigning clinical significance to sporadic epileptiform features on neonatal recordings. These epileptiform characteristics may be seen in asymptomatic, apparently healthy infants. Several features, however, may help distinguish normal from abnormal spike or sharp waves. Epileptiform discharges that are frequent and multifocal and persistently occur throughout sleep may have pathologic significance. Several investigators have proposed that five-spike or sharp-wave discharges per hour suggest an abnormality. Other features such as positive sharp waves, periodic discharges, and midline discharges commonly are associated with CNS insults.

Spike and sharp-wave discharges have been described in specific neonatal populations based on serious medical disorders, principally seizures. Hughes and colleagues described spike and sharp-wave discharges in 236 neonates whose postconceptional age ranged from 24 to 48 weeks. Approxi-

mately 55% had recordings because of a clinical suspicion of neonatal seizures. Sporadic sharp waves, more frequent in the right hemisphere, were found primarily in the centrotemporal regions in 85% of the total population. An additional 15% had positive sharp waves or repetitive sharp waves. No control group in which epileptiform discharges were observed was included nor was follow-up reported. Rowe and associates documented sharp-wave discharges in 51% of 74 neonates. These infants were followed up to 33 months of age, and the presence of sharp waves on the neonatal EEG correlated with early developmental outcome. However, the investigators stress that EEG background abnormalities were more predictive than isolated epileptiform features. Spike discharges rarely occur in the neonate at any gestational age. Sharp-wave discharges are, however, common in frontopolar, right temporal, and left central regions in otherwise asymptomatic neonates. Sharp waves in occipital or midline locations are rarely seen in healthy neonates and may have greater clinical significance.

Epileptiform Abnormalities

EEG remains the principal investigation for children with epilepsy. However, the technique has been historically accepted, without strict reliability assessments. The clinician's classification of a child's seizure disorder, as well as possible diagnostic and therapeutic decisions, is based on interictal EEG results. The neurologist relies on interictal EEG recordings performed particularly close in time to the occurrence of the seizure event. However, demonstration of epileptiform abnormalities in the EEG patterns of patients with seizures does not occur in approximately 50% of the first routine interictal EEG recording. Repeated EEG recordings may increase the diagnostic yield. A retrospective study of adults with the diagnosis of epilepsy found the chance of detecting interictal epileptiform activities to be approximately 20% for the second EEG and less than 10% after the fourth negative repeat EEG recording. In a study of children between the ages of 1 month and 16 years with one or more idiopathic or symptomatic newly diagnosed seizures, a repeat EEG was obtained in children who expressed no epileptiform activity on their initial EEG recording. Of 552 children studied, 56% had epileptiform activity on the initial EEG; for the overall group who had a repeat EEG recording, 30% had epileptiform activity when the initial EEG pattern was normal. Epileptiform activities were more likely if the repeat EEG included sleep. These findings are in accord with earlier reports in the literature on repeat EEG recordings after sleep deprivation in children with suspected epilepsy; between 32% and 75% of children had epileptiform activity on repeat EEGs after sleep deprivation. Other reports warn against obtaining a repeat EEG that may yield different and sometimes conflicting information for the clinician in children with absence seizures or generalized motor seizures. These investigators describe repeat EEG recordings in 159 infants, with 40% to 70% discordance for the type of abnormality on the second EEG compared with the first.

Among a variety of abnormal EEG patterns, certain features have been associated in patients with seizure disorders and are commonly referred to as epileptiform. Epileptiform waveforms include spikes, sharp waves, spikes and waves, sharp and slow waves, and multiple spikes. The sharp wave has a waveform that is characteristically negative in polarity with a duration of 70 to 200 msec. This finding is contrasted with the spike morphology, which is of shorter duration (20 to 70 msec) and sharper morphology. The slow-wave complex that may accompany either waveform generally is between 1 and 5 Hz (i.e., 200 to 1000 msec).

Epileptiform features are not necessarily associated with clinical seizures. One study found that 2.7% of 743 normal children had epileptiform EEG activity. This percentage increased to 8.7% during sleep. Although a more recent study claimed a lower percentage of 0.70% (Bihege et al., 2014), digital EEG studies may detect a higher percentage than analog studies used historically (Borusiak et al., 2010).

In certain forms of genetic epilepsy, family members are asymptomatic but have abnormal EEG discharges. Conversely, patients with well-documented seizures may have normal EEG studies, particularly children younger than 2 years. Only 56% of patients with seizures in one study had epileptiform activity on the first EEG recording.

Epileptiform discharges not accompanied by obvious clinical events usually are regarded as subclinical or interictal. However, careful observation with psychometric testing can reveal brief episodes of impaired cognitive function during such discharges. This feature has been observed in 50% of patients who exhibit discharges during testing, and it may contribute to behavioral and cognitive deficits. Limited evidence-based analyses suggest that suppression of discharges is associated with improved psychosocial function. Specific pediatric epileptic syndromes may have a greater association with such deficits.

After a patient with recurrent epileptic seizures is treated with antiseizure medication and becomes seizure-free for some period, the clinician is eventually challenged with the decision about whether treatment should be continued. In making this decision, the neurologist must weigh the risk of side effects of drugs against the risk of seizure relapse. Certain indicators of prognosis continue to be of important clinical value. The EEG study has remained one predictor of outcome after withdrawal of treatment, but many children who become seizure-free during drug treatment continue to manifest epileptiform activity in their EEG recordings. Correlations between EEG findings and clinical outcome after discontinuation of treatment have been reported in many studies, as reviewed by Andersson and colleagues, but there is a lack of unanimity, given the fact that different EEG variables have been assigned prognostic importance. Children whose last EEG before discontinuation of treatment displays generalized irregular spike-and-wave activity relapse more often than other children; 67% of children with such activity in their final EEG studies relapsed, compared with a relapse rate of 33% for children without epileptiform activity or with other epileptiform abnormalities. Children who were treated for only 1 year and in whom irregular, generalized spike-and-wave activities were present in one or more recordings had a high relapse rate. Apart from treatment of children with irregular, generalized spike-and-wave activity, most physicians discontinue treatment after 6 months to 2 years of seizure control. The presence of epileptiform activity does not necessarily influence the prognosis for the recurrence of seizures, with the exception of certain types of abnormal epileptiform activity or patient groups. For example, in a cohort of children with cryptogenic localization-related epilepsy who were followed for more than 5 years after drug withdrawal, 8 of 82 (9.8%) experienced seizure recurrence. Two independent risk factors were 6 years of age or older at seizure onset and 5 years or more from the start of drug therapy. Another report of children with cryptogenic partial epilepsy recommended EEG studies during drug withdrawal, even with a previously normal EEG study, because the presence of EEG abnormalities was associated with a high probability of seizures.

Spike-and-Wave Patterns. The most frequently encountered spike-and-wave pattern is a bilaterally synchronous, single or polyspike discharge, followed in frequency by rhythmic slow waves. Both features are surface-negative, and these discharges can be 100 to 200 msec long. Discharges in certain regions (e.g., frontal) appear slightly before the generalized burst or are maximally expressed in one particular location. The examiner may see fragments of the spike-and-wave pattern, depending on the montage or sensitivity setting, because of cancellation effects of bipolar recordings or the low amplitude of the complexes. The fastest frequency of the discharges (3 to 6 Hz) is at the onset of seizures, with slowing to 2.5 to 4 Hz during the electrographic seizure. Augmentation of the discharges can be seen with hyperventilation or non-REM sleep, although the spike-and-wave pattern can become slower and more complex in morphology during sleep. Two nonspecific phenomena are often associated with a generalized spike-and-wave pattern and consist of bursts of 2-Hz to 4-Hz, rhythmic slow waves or a more monorhythmic, occipital delta activity.

Photic stimulation may elicit a spike-and-wave discharge (Fig. 13-14B) but can only support the evidence for seizures suggested by the clinical evaluation. This pattern also appears in 3.4% of normal control subjects and in 20% of siblings of patients with photoparoxysmal seizures who have never had clinical seizures. Only 10% of these siblings had clinical seizures. A prolonged response that outlasts the stimulus may be a stronger indication that a seizure disorder is present, but there is also an age-dependent expression of this abnormal pattern between 5 and 15 years. Even self-limited photoparoxysmal responses that do not outlast the stimulus can be highly correlated with epilepsy. This pattern is most easily elicited with a frequency of 10 to 16 flashes per second. Clinicians must anticipate that children with photosensitive epilepsy can still have an excellent prognosis that is independent of the persistence or disappearance of photosensitivity on the EEG study.

Patients on dialysis, with electrolyte disturbances, or exhibiting withdrawal from drugs such as barbiturates and alcohol are more susceptible to photoparoxysmal responses with or without clinical accompaniment. Even for the nonepileptic pediatric patient, photoparoxysmal responses may be present in the absence of acute encephalopathies, with persistence for as long as 6 years after the initial documentation. Suppression of photic driving responses may also occur in the presence of structural nervous system disorders (Fig. 13-14C).

Sharp-Wave and Slow-Wave Complexes. The sharp-wave and slow-wave complex pattern consists of a sharp wave of negative polarity lasting 100 to 200 msec and slow waves lasting 350 to 400 msec at a frequency of 1 to 2 Hz. Although diffusely distributed over the scalp in most patients, it may be asymmetric or confined to anterior or posterior quadrants. This waveform is augmented only during sleep and can be associated with sudden desynchronization of the record, which is associated with a burst of beta activity called an electrodecremental response. Although the highest incidence of sharp-wave and slow-wave complexes occurs between 1 and 5 years of age, they are also evident well into adulthood. Hypsarrhythmia can precede the sharp-wave and slow-wave complex during the first year of life.

Of clinical seizures with sharp-wave and slow-wave complexes, 90% are tonic, and these seizures are resistant to therapy, persisting at least 15 years after beginning treatment. Other types of clinical seizures can also occur, depending on the age of onset: tonic seizures at 16 months, absence seizures at 32 months, myoclonic seizures at 39 months, and tonic-clonic seizures after 43 months.

Mental subnormality is identified in 30% of patients at diagnosis. When seizures are present before 2 years of age and are caused by CNS disease, the child will more likely exhibit delayed development. The clinical and EEG syndrome that includes the three features of seizures—mental subnormality, and sharp-wave and slow-wave complexes—is called the Lennox-Gastaut syndrome.

Hypsarrhythmia. Hypsarrhythmia is the most common interictal EEG pattern associated with infantile spasms. The most common clinical description is a sudden, symmetric, tonic muscle contraction producing flexion/extension of the trunk and extremities, although a variety of movement patterns have been described. The EEG pattern is a chaotic mixture of high-amplitude slow waves, multifocal spikes, and intrahemispheric-interhemispheric asynchrony. This EEG pattern usually is observed in children 3 months to 5 years old, and it can be preceded by a burst-suppression or low-voltage invariant pattern in the newborn period. Hypsarrhythmia can also be preceded by a normal EEG pattern. During a spasm, an electrodecremental response interrupts the high-amplitude slowing by a sudden diminution of all activity with a duration of 1 second to 1 minute. The role of EEG is limited to diagnosis only, with no reliable correlation with cause, course, or prognosis, including mental development.

Generalized Periodic Discharges. Generalized periodic discharges are distinguished from bilateral synchronous spike-and-wave discharges by the broader waveforms in the context of a periodic quality. This pattern has been historically identified with two clinical situations: Creutzfeldt-Jakob disease in adults and subacute sclerosing panencephalitis in children.

The periodic complexes in subacute sclerosing panencephalitis appear at approximately 4-second to 14-second intervals but have no relation with the clinical progression of the disease. Similarly, there is no relation between the myoclonic movements and these discharges. The periodic discharges may first arise from a normal background and may initially be observed only during sleep.

Focal Epileptiform Patterns

The incidence of focal-spike discharges in the normal population (1.5% of 1000 children) has been previously estimated. More recently, an overall prevalence of 6.5% was detected in 383 healthy children 6 to 13 years of age; 4 showed generalized or bifrontal spikes, 12 showed constant focal localized discharges, and 9 showed multifocal discharges. Spike discharges in symptomatic patients should be correlated with the clinical context in which the discharges are observed. Focal spikes are identified in children with cerebral palsy in the absence of clinical seizures; however, the presence of focal spikes in children younger than 2 years of age implies severe neurologic impairment. Spike foci on a single EEG examination are not a reliable indicator of structural brain lesions because the location of the spike discharges on subsequent EEG studies may be shifted to different foci. However, the absence or rare occurrence of a spike discharge on a routine EEG usually predicts better outcome, compared with more frequent spikes in any head region associated with EEG background slowing.

Rolandic Spikes. Rolandic spikes are associated with the most common genetic epilepsy of childhood. High-amplitude spike and slow waves are prominently observed singly or in runs in the central and midtemporal regions Shifting laterality occurs in the same or subsequent EEG studies, and these focal discharges may be associated with generalized spike-and-wave discharges in 5% of children. The EEG background activity is otherwise normal, and certain patients have rolandic spikes that appear only during sleep, commonly during non-REM sleep. An unusual polarity relationship is associated with the discharges, consisting of a simultaneous negative and positive phase-reversal in two different locations of the spike discharge. This polarity may represent a horizontal rather than the more common vertical dipole, and is associated with abnormal EEG activity.

Occipital Spikes. Benign childhood epilepsy with occipital paroxysms (benign occipital epilepsy) typically presents between 4 and 12 years of age. One study by Panayiotopoulos suggests that this is a common form of epilepsy in children. Of 94 patients, 18 (20%) fulfilled the criteria for benign epilepsy of childhood with occipital paroxysms. The clinical presentation may be emesis and visual phenomena in older children with simple or complex visual hallucinations or distortions with preservation of consciousness. In younger children, seizures are less frequent and are often nocturnal but may be dramatic with periods of prolonged unresponsiveness. The EEG patterns for both clinical presentations are composed of repetitive occipital spike discharges on eye closure. It has been debated whether this syndrome is related to the reflex epilepsies in which generalized seizures and EEG abnormalities can be initiated by video games and other visual stimuli. However, the presence of occipital epileptiform EEG abnormalities may be associated with children with migraine headaches, with or without accompanying epilepsy. Specific electroclinical features help distinguish these two groups.

Besides the benign occipital epilepsy syndrome, a greater proportion of children with occipital discharges have symptomatic epilepsy, although neonates may also reflect occipital spike discharges after as a result of brain disorders and the EEG study can assist in predicting better outcome based on the presence of generalized spike-and-wave discharges or normal EEG background rhythms.

Temporal Spikes and Sharp Waves

Although not associated with a distinctive epileptic syndrome, temporal spike discharges must be distinguished from the spikes associated with rolandic epilepsy. The electroencephalographer can ascertain a difference by determining whether there is a more limited temporal location to the spike discharge without expression of a dipole, as described previously. According to a study by Eeg-Oloffsson, temporal spikes are rarely seen in normal children (2 of 743 patients) but are frequently seen in epileptic patients (92% of 666), including children with complex partial seizures.

Complex partial seizures commonly begin during childhood, and anatomic abnormalities have been detected in some of these patients. Static lesions, such as mesial temporal sclerosis, hippocampal herniation, or hamartoma, have all been described, and several of these patients also demonstrate homonymous hemianopsia or quadrantanopsia on visual field testing, presumably because of perinatal occlusion of the posterior cerebral artery.

Multiple Independent Spike Foci

Patients with spike discharges in at least three noncontiguous electrode positions are considered to have multiple independent spike foci. No patients in a normal population have this pattern, whereas 63 of 1500 patients with seizures and EEG recordings demonstrate this pattern. Of patients with multiple independent spike foci, 90% had clinical seizures, most of which were generalized motor seizures. Although 66% of patients had subnormal intelligence, normal cognitive abilities were more likely if there were few spike discharges and a normal EEG background. Sleep can augment spikes and activate new foci, but hyperventilation or photic stimulation cannot. Of these patients, 25% had previous EEG studies with hypsarrhythmia or sharp-wave and slow-wave complexes.

Periodic Discharges

Generalized periodic discharges and neonatal periodic patterns have already been discussed. The present description pertains to the EEG phenomenon that consists of repetitive stereotypic focal discharges that remain lateralized with a duration of at least 10 minutes, or 20% of the recording time. Waveform morphologies can be varied and are collectively referred to as periodic lateralized epileptiform discharges. This phenomenon represents an acute or a subacute process in adults or children. Usually, a brain lesion such as infarction, contusion, or cerebritis can be identified. Periodic discharges in the temporal region may suggest an encephalitic process caused by a herpetic infection.

Biphasic or polyphasic discharges of 100 to 200 msec and 100 to 200 μV have a frequency of 1 to 2 Hz .These discharges persist for a limited number of days or weeks in adults and are replaced by focal polymorphic delta slowing. Multifocal periodic patterns can also occur. In children, more subacute or chronic processes have been associated with focal or multifocal periodic lateralized epileptiform discharges. Similar to adults, periodic lateralized epileptiform discharges can also be seen in acutely encephalopathic children from infection or toxin exposure and are highly associated with seizures. Stimulus-induced rhythmic, periodic, or ictal discharges can be documented in older patients undergoing continuous EEG monitoring in the intensive care setting, which need to be distinguished from spontaneous seizures. Stimulus-evoked seizures have been described for neonates, but older pediatric populations have not been systematically identified. In adults, 90% exhibit a depressed level of consciousness, whereas 70% demonstrate focal neurologic defects. Periodic discharges are commonly observed after a seizure, particularly if it is focal in onset; about 80% of these patients have frequent seizures. An unusual seizure disorder in children has been described, consisting of agitation and confusion, in which periodic discharges in the frontal regions are observed when the patient is awake or asleep.

REFERENCES

 The complete list of references for this chapter is available in the e-book at www.expertconsult.com.

See inside cover for registration details.

SELECTED REFERENCES

Ahdab, R., Riachi, N., 2014. Reexamining the added value of intermittent photic stimulation and hyperventilation in routine EEG practice. Eur. Neurol. 71 (1–2), 93–98.

Bihege, C.J., Langer, T., Jenke, A.C., et al., 2014. Prevalence of epileptiform discharges in healthy infants. J. Child Neurol. 30 (11), 1409–1413.

Borusiak, P., Zilbauer, M., Jenke, A.C., 2010. Prevalence of epileptiform discharges in healthy children—new data from a prospective study using digital EEG. Epilepsia 51 (7), 1185–1188.

Kaminska, A., Cheliout-Heraut, F., Eisermann, M., et al., 2015. EEG in children, in the laboratory or at the patient's bedside. Neurophysiol. Clin. 45 (1), 65–74.

Scher, M.S., Loparo, K.A., 2009. Neonatal EEG/sleep state analyses: a complex phenotype of developmental neural plasticity. Dev. Neurosci. 31, 259–275.

Shellhaas, R.A., 2015. Continuous long-term electroencephalography: the gold standard for neonatal seizure diagnosis. Semin. Fetal Neonatal Med. 20 (3), 149–153.

Watanabe, K., Miyazaki, S., Hara, K., et al., 1980. Behavioral state cycles, background EEGs and prognosis of newborns with perinatal hypoxia. Electroencephalogr. Clin. Neurophysiol. 49 (5–6), 618–625.

Watemberg, N., Farkash, M., Har-Gil, M., et al., 2015. Hyperventilation during routine electroencephalography: are three minutes really necessary? Pediatr. Neurol. 52 (4), 410–413.

Wilhelm, I., Kurth, S., Ringli, M., et al., 2014. Sleep slow-wave activity reveals developmental changes in experience-dependent plasticity. J. Neurosci. 34 (37), 12568–12575.

E-BOOK FIGURES AND TABLES

The following figures and tables are available in the e-book at www.expertconsult.com. See inside cover for registration details.

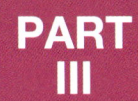

14 Microstructural and Functional Connectivity in the Developing Brain

Laura R. Ment, Dustin Scheinost, and Todd Constable

 An expanded version of this chapter is available on www.expertconsult.com. See inside cover for registration details.

ABBREVIATIONS

ADC	Apparent diffusion coefficient
ADHD	Attention-deficit/hyperactivity disorder
ASD	Autistic spectrum disorder
DMN	Default mode network
dMRI	Diffusion tensor MRI
FA	Fractional anisotropy
fMRI	Functional MRI
ICA	Independent component analysis
ICN	Intrinsic connectivity network
MD	Mean diffusivity
PMA	Postmenstrual age
PT	Preterm
ROI	Region of interest
rs-fMRI	Resting state functional MRI
TBSS	Tract-based spatial statistics
TEA	Term-equivalent age
t-fMRI	Task-based functional MRI
VBM	Voxel-by-voxel morphometry

INTRODUCTION

Neurobehavioral disorders are a major pediatric public health problem. Of the world's children, 10% suffer intellectual and developmental disabilities, 1 in 68 is diagnosed with autism spectrum disorder (ASD), as many as 9% are affected with attention-deficit/hyperactivity disorder (ADHD), and 2 to 2.5 per 1000 live births suffer cerebral palsy. The annual lifetime care costs for children and adolescents with these diagnoses in the United States alone exceeds $50 billion, reflecting both educational and medical costs in addition to loss of productivity. Organization of structural and functional brain networks is necessary for typical neurodevelopment, and converging data suggest that many neurodevelopmental disorders are attributable to alterations in connectivity (Dennis and Thompson, 2013; Di Martino et al., 2014).

The nervous system is a network of interconnected neurons, and the architecture of cerebral circuits is influenced by both the genetically determined program of cortical development and the environment. A major goal is to create a comprehensive map of these connections, or connectome. Noninvasive neuroimaging technologies provide important information about microstructural and functional neural connectivity, and when combined with powerful network modeling tools, these methods offer new opportunities to understand the developing connectome.

Cerebral network studies include both microstructural, functional, and effective connectivity. Diffusion tensor magnetic resonance imaging (dMRI) techniques combined with graph-theory analysis permits the mapping of anatomic regions and their interconnecting pathways with high spatial resolution, and the resulting networks provide large-scale maps of the brain's microstructural connectivity (Sporns et al., 2005). Similarly, maps of functional connectivity derived from MRI provide important information about neural regions that are functionally coupled, whether or not they are structurally connected (Friston, 2011). Finally, effective connectivity attempts to capture a network of "directed causal effects" between neural elements, and allows identification of models that best fit the data. Together, these strategies offer the opportunity to examine the influence of both genetic and epigenetic influences on the developing brain.

Assessment Strategies for Connectivity

Tools of network science include microstructural, functional, and effective connectivity as defined by noninvasive MRI strategies (Table 14-1). Although it is less commonly employed, anatomic covariance is also reviewed in this chapter.

Microstructural connectivity describes the anatomic connections linking a set of neural elements. Diffusion-weighted imaging assesses the diffusion of water along axons and thus permits visualization of axonal pathways (Sporns, 2013). By modeling the directional diffusion of water as an ellipsoidal shape, or *tensor*, at each voxel in the brain, dMRI permits the assessment of major white matter fiber bundles. Eigenvector maps can be color-coded to indicate the orientation of the major eigenvector and thus provide a visible indicator of the axis in which water diffusion is the highest. The first eigenvector, $\lambda 1$, describes the direction of maximal diffusion, and the second and third eigenvectors define diffusivity perpendicular to this principle axis. Radial diffusivity represents the average of $\lambda 2$ and $\lambda 3$, and is affected by changes in axon caliber and myelination. FA is the ratio of $\lambda 1$ to $\lambda 2$, and $\lambda 3$ is dependent on axonal integrity. Fractional anisotropy (FA), the degree to which water diffuses in one direction (along the axon), is the most common measure used to assess axonal integrity.

The apparent diffusion coefficient (ADC) is a measure of the magnitude of the diffusion of water in a tissue, independent of direction. In contrast, mean diffusivity (MD) is a measure of the degree of restriction to diffusion of water molecules, irrespective of direction. Low values for MD are consistent with greater organization, whereas high values of FA suggest more highly organized, strongly myelinated tracts. Studies comparing FA and ADC in subjects with a wide variety of diseases to healthy controls show lower FA and higher ADC in the affected group, but this is not universally applicable.

TABLE 14-1 Methods for Assessing Connectivity

Strategy	Variables	Definitions
dMRI	Fractional anisotropy (FA)	Degree to which water diffuses in one direction (along the axon)
	Apparent diffusion coefficient (ADC)	Measure of the magnitude of diffusion of water, independent of direction
	Mean diffusivity (MD)	Measure of the degree of restriction to diffusion of water molecules irrespective of direction
	Axial diffusivity	Magnitude of diffusion along the axon
	Radial diffusivity	Magnitude of diffusion perpendicular to the axon
	Fiber tracking	Matrix-based connectivity analysis—white-matter connections between gray-matter nodes
fMRI	Spatial-temporal patterns	Similarity of spontaneous brain signal fluctuations reflecting functional connections between distinct brain regions
	Measures of brain activity	Task-driven changes in local activity

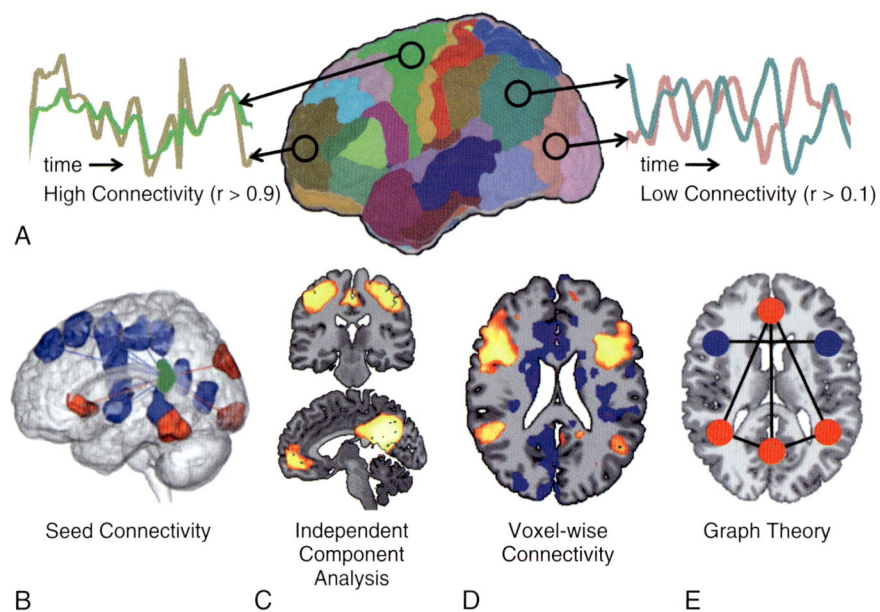

Figure 14-1. Overview of functional connectivity. A, Functional connectivity is defined as the correlation between blood-oxygen-level-dependent (BOLD) time course for any two regions or voxels in the brain. A higher correlation between time courses implies higher functional connectivity between the regions. Common methods for functional connectivity include seed, matrix, and voxel-wise connectivity. **B,** Seed connectivity involves identifying key regions or "seeds" and assessing connectivity between these seeds and all other voxels in the brain. This analysis is the most common. **C,** Independent component analysis (ICA) is a statistical approach in which resting-state data are decomposed into time courses and associated maps describing the temporal and spatial characteristics of the components comprising the data. **D,** Voxel-wise connectivity involves assessing connectivity for every voxel in the brain to every other voxel in the brain and summarizing these correlations with a summary statistic. This method is highly data driven because no a priori region needs to be specified (unlike in seed and matrix connectivity). However, any information about a specific connection is lost. **E,** Graph theory provides models for connectivity that best explain empirical data and is characterized by the set of definitions shown in Table 14-2. A network is composed of a set of nodes (or neural elements) and edges, their mutual connections.

Importantly, microstructural connectivity data do not provide information on the direction in which information travels along fiber pathways.

The three main approaches to analyzing dMRI data, region-of-interest (ROI) quantification, tract-based analysis, and tractography, are shown in Figure 14-1, but recent studies also demonstrate the importance of whole-brain voxel-by-voxel morphometry (VBM). ROI selection and quantification is the most frequently used, whereas VBM is an alternative method designed to quantify regional changes in volume measured with high-resolution three-dimensional anatomic MRI. Tract-based spatial statistics (TBSS) is based on the realignment of the FA maps of all subjects projected onto an FA map skeleton. Tractography permits the reconstruction of white-matter pathways from point to point and demonstrates the brain's global connectivity.

Functional connectivity is based on the blood-oxygen-level-dependent (BOLD) signal and is derived from time-series data. It assesses "temporal correlations between spatially remote neurophysiological events" (Friston, 2011). fMRI data can be collected either in the presence of a task (t-fMRI) or in the resting state (rs-fMRI). Temporal variations in fMRI signals appear to arise spontaneously, and the synchronicity in these temporal variations indicates functional connectivity, the strength of which may be modulated by tasks and/or sensory stimuli.

The four major methods to assess fMRI data are also shown in Figure14-1 and include seed-based, independent components analysis (ICA), voxel-wise connectivity, and graph theory. In the seed-based approach, the time course of a seed placed in an ROI is correlated with time courses for the rest of the voxels in the brain to search for synchronous temporal patterns. Brain regions with a high degree of positive correlation with the seed are thought to be "functionally coupled" (Friston, 2011). In contrast, ICA is a statistical approach in which resting-state data are decomposed into time courses and associated maps, describing the temporal and spatial characteristics of the components comprising the data. Voxel-wise connectivity is a model-free, whole-brain voxel-by-voxel analysis strategy.

Effective connectivity defines networks of directed causal effects between neural elements. This strategy provides a model that best accounts for the observed data, and recent advances in effective connectivity have been employed for network discovery. Although effective connectivity offers much promise, most studies investigating the connectome are accomplished using either microstructural or functional connectivity data, and these strategies are the focus of this chapter.

Anatomic Covariance

Morphologic features of different brain regions are not independent of those of other areas, and the brain shows a high level of coordination between different structures. This co-ordination, or covariance, of morphologic features is often referred to as *anatomic covariance* and is a key marker of typical development in early childhood. Using ROIs, patterns of anatomic covariance have been linked to developmental disorders. Similarly, network-level approaches investigate the covariance patterns of every pairwise combination of brain regions, forming a network to provide a more complete anatomic description of the candidate disorder.

Tools of Network Science

Similar to ROI strategies, graph-theory analyses are suitable for both microstructural and functional connectivity data. Graph theory provides models for connectivity that best explain empirical data and is characterized by the set of definitions shown Table 14-2. A network is composed of a set of nodes (or neural elements) and edges, their mutual connections. Nodes may be derived by parcellating cortical and subcortical gray matter according to anatomic borders or by defining a random parcellation scheme in which the brain is divided into evenly spaced and sized clusters. Following the definition of nodes, structural or functional couplings can be estimated, and the full set of couplings can be assembled into a connectivity matrix, as shown in Figure 14-2. Three important measures are *integration, segregation,* and *small-worldness.* Network *integration* refers to how densely connected all nodes are to one another. Networks with nodes that are all connected to one another exhibit high integration, whereas those with few connections show low integration. Network *segregation* refers to the extent

to which a network is organized into a collection of subnetworks. A fully connected network in which each node is connected to all others has low segregation; a network formed of disconnected parts has high segregation. Finally, a *small-world* network has evidence of both segregation and integration. A small-world network has nodes grouped into subnetworks, with efficient travel between these subnetworks.

Rich club (RC) organization is another graph-theory measure for summarizing connectivity; important (or "rich") nodes connect preferentially to other important nodes. Whereas microstructural RCs remain largely consistent over the lifespan, functional RCs evolve during development as hubs mature to accomplish the efficient long-range transfer of information.

TABLE 14-2 Graph-Theory Tools for Assessing Connectivity

Variables	Definitions
Nodes	Neural elements
Edges	Connections between nodes
Integration	Measure assessing how densely connected all nodes are to one another
Path	Unique sequence of edges that connects one node to another
Characteristic path length (CPL)	Global average of all distances across the entire network
Global efficiency (GE)	Average of the inverse of all distances
Segregation	Measure of the extent to which a network is organized into a collection of subnetworks
Modularity (ML)	Measure of the strength of division of a network into communities
Clustering coefficient (CC)	Density of connections among a node's topological neighbors
Small-worldness	Measure combining both segregation and integration to assess network efficiency
Influence	Statistical attempt to quantify the importance of a given node or edge for a network
Degree	Number of edges attached to a given node
Rich club (RC)	Nodes that connect preferentially to other important nodes

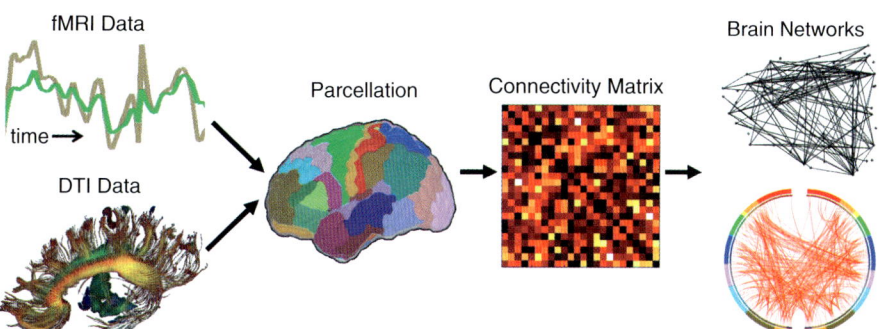

Figure 14-2. Schematic of connectivity analysis. To construct a brain network, dMRI or fMRI data are conventionally put into a parcellation scheme whereby the gray matter is subdivided into 100 to 400 regions of interest. The pairwise association between each gray-matter regions is then computed, forming a connectivity matrix. For dMRI data, this association is typically based on the number of white-matter fibers connecting the gray-matter regions. For fMRI data, this association is the correlation between BOLD time courses for the gray-matter regions. A brain network is then constructed from the nodes (gray-matter regions) and the edges (pairwise associations). These brain networks may be converted to sparser networks by removing edges with an association below a chosen threshold.

Intrinsic Connectivity Networks

Spontaneous intrinsic coherent low-frequency (<0.1 Hz) fluctuations between distant neuronal regions measured using fMRI suggest functional connections, and these identify intrinsic connectivity networks (ICNs). ICNs detected during rs-fMRI correspond to networks observed across functional tasks and are present during mild anesthesia and sleep, making them advantageous for studying infants and young children.

In adults, ICNs include the visual, default mode, cerebellar, sensorimotor, auditory, executive control, and salience networks. There are three visual networks; these correspond to the medial, occipital pole, and lateral visual areas. Visual behaviors correspond to specific networks, and cognition–language–orthography and cognition–space have been found to lateralize to the occipital pole and lateral visual maps, respectively. The default model network (DMN) is the most studied ICN and includes the posterior cingulate cortex/precuneus, medial prefrontal cortex, inferior parietal cortex, and medial temporal lobe. The DMN most commonly "deactivates" in t-fMRI experiments, subserves internally directed mentation, and is inversely correlated with networks supporting externally directed attention.

Resting-state networks emerge during the 21st to 38th weeks of gestation, and fragmentary networks resembling adult ICNs have been demonstrated in typically developing children shortly after birth. Maturation profiles of these networks are both genetic and environment dependent.

Categorization of Disorders of Connectivity

During development of the human brain from fetal life to adulthood, white-matter tracts undergo significant changes. Likewise, functional connections develop, mature, and respond to environmental perturbations. The source of alterations in connectivity may include genetic, epigenetic, or traumatic disorders. Conditions such as autism are widely believed to represent connectivity disorders of genetic origin. In contrast, the alterations in functional organization that characterize the preterm population are most likely attributable to environmental changes. Finally, injuries such as stroke and concussion are reported to result in acquired disturbances of connectivity.

Fetal Development
Microstructural Studies

Important anatomic and functional networks are established in the fetal brain during the second and third trimesters (Ouyang et al., 2015). Defining these networks during the different stages of human fetal brain development provides insight not only into typical development, but also into the neurobiological foundations of developmental disorders (Dennis and Thompson, 2013), and the emergence of fetal dMRI studies followed by rs-fMRI has permitted examination of human fetuses in real time.

dMRI studies in human fetuses between 18 and 37 weeks postmenstrual age (PMA) with no structural brain pathologies have visualized bilateral, cranio-caudally oriented, and callosal trajectories in addition to sensorimotor tracts and smaller fiber bundles such as thalamocortical fibers, corticopontine fibers, and corticospinal tracts. FA values are highest in the splenium of the corpus callosum, followed by the genu and the posterior limbs of the internal capsules. Limbic system tracts including the fornix and the cingulum bundle are present as early as 14 to 17 weeks PMA. Likewise, internal capsule fibers also appear as early as 14 weeks, and the general maturation pattern for the internal capsule is anterior-posterior from weeks 14 to 37.

The anterior commissure and the corpus callosum comprise the major *commissural tracts* and are also observed at 14 to 17 weeks, and an anterior-to-posterior maturation pattern for the corpus callosum from 17 to 37 weeks PMA has been described. Finally, the uncinate fasciculus and inferior longitudinal fasciculus represent the earliest association fiber tracts and can both be traced at 19 weeks. In contrast, the arcuate fasciculus is not detectable during fetal development.

Fetal Functional Imaging

Recent developments in magnetic resonance (MR) techniques permit the identification of processes that underlie the development of the fetal functional connectome. Cross-sectional examination of connectivity in healthy human fetuses of 24 to 38 weeks PMA has demonstrated increasing interhemispheric connectivity with advancing fetal age, and the strength of fetal functional connectivity has been significantly correlated with the spatial location of the ROI on the medial-lateral but not the anterior-posterior axis, in contrast to dMRI data. Long-range functional connections exhibit a linear increase with no periods of peaking development, whereas a region-specific increase of functional connectivity is reported to follow a sequence of occipital, temporal, frontal, and parietal expansion.

Likewise, graph-theory analyses demonstrate that the fetal brain is organized in a modular structure, wherein connections are much stronger within than among modules. With advancing PMA intermodule connection strength increases, sensorimotor modules become more connected to the cerebellum, prefrontal areas become more connected to the posterior parietal cortex, and a ventral-frontal-temporal cortex module becomes more left lateralized and functionally integrated with regions that develop into Broca's and Wernicke's areas, which are critical for language acquisition in the developing brain. Finally, motor, visual, default mode, thalamic, and temporal networks have been reported in the human fetal brain between 24 and 38 weeks PMA.

Environmental Perturbations

Environmental influences ranging from socioeconomic status to prenatal drug exposure may influence connectivity. Although it is difficult to parse the contributions of parental education, household food insecurity, and maternal stress, preliminary studies suggest that connectivity decreases in the frontotemporal regions subserving language and behavior in infants and toddlers from the most affected homes.

Connectivity in Typically Developing Children

The advent of sophisticated neuroimaging strategies is propelling the study of brain maturation in older children and adolescents. However, early brain growth and connectivity in typically developing infants and young children have not been extensively studied, leaving considerable gaps in knowledge about these important periods. The cerebrum increases in size through early adulthood, and white-matter volumes continue to expand throughout adolescence and into middle age. In addition, a recent longitudinal MRI analysis across the first 3 months of life suggested that brain development is most rapid in the days immediately following birth, when the whole-brain growth rate is approximately 1% per day, slowing to 0.4% per day by the end of the first 3 months, with overall growth of 64% in 90 days.

Maturation of Microstructural Networks: Increases in Anisotropy, Decreases in Diffusivity

White-matter myelination is intense throughout the first year of life, and increases in FA and decreases in ADC are rapid in the first postnatal year and continue throughout the second, reflecting increasing myelination and coherence of fiber tracts. These changes continue across development and have been most frequently reported in the corpus callosum, internal capsule, white matter of the frontal and prefrontal cortex, and subcortical regions. Different white-matter regions follow different developmental trajectories, and the age at peak FA for varying tracts ranges from 23 years for the fibers connecting the subcortical, temporal, and occipital regions to 39 years for the cingulum (Dennis and Thompson, 2013). The last tracts to reach maturity are those responsible for executive control of behavior and interhemispheric connectivity.

Although there are few developmental studies using structural graph theory in typically developing children, increases in both local and global efficiency have been reported with age in children across the first 18 years of life. Additionally, a single study reported the presence of a microstructural RC network similar to that in older subjects from adolescence through adulthood.

Finally, FA is highly heritable; genetic influences are reported to be greater in adolescence than in adulthood and greater in males than females, and heritability is higher in those with higher socioeconomic status. In contrast, environmental factors contributing to FA in typically developing children and adolescents have been less well defined.

Functional Maturation: Increases in Integration and Segregation

The developmental trajectories of functional networks studied in infants, children and adolescents employ both seed-based and ICN approaches (Power et al., 2010). Typically developing term neonates show networks in the visual, auditory, motor, somatosensory, and prefrontal cortices, and a recent investigation employing rs-fMRI in infants ranging in age from birth to 2 years suggested a maturation sequence from primary sensorimotor/auditory to visual, to attention/default mode, and finally to executive control networks. The sensorimotor and auditory networks are relatively mature at birth; likewise, the salience-thalamus connectivity network is also present in neonates. In contrast, the executive network shows limited maturation in network topology and is far from adultlike at the end of the first postnatal year, whereas the DMN is detected in neonates in the first weeks of life and matures across the first 2 years.

Children have sparser connections between DMN seeds and fewer long-range connections than do adults, mainly in areas responsible for conflict monitoring, emotion regulation, and processing of complex information. Similarly, graph-theory analyses show that children have both lower intranetwork integration and less internetwork segregation than do adults. With development, there is a shift from stronger short-range connections in children to stronger long-range connections in adolescents and young adults.

Influence of Genes and the Environment

The extent to which genes influence the functional brain network early in development is just beginning to be explored. Emerging heritability analyses suggest that global efficiency among brain regions is under strong genetic control (h2 lambda = 42%), irrespective of the total number of brain connections. Likewise, the molecular mechanisms supporting functional connectivity are just beginning to be defined. Recent data suggest, however, that many genes contributing to functional connectivity subserve ion channels and synaptogenesis (Richiardi et al., 2015). Likewise, environmental factors ranging from nutrition to maternal education to child neglect and maltreatment alter connectivity in typically developing children.

Preterm Birth Results in Long-Term Alterations in Connectivity

Preterm (PT) birth represents a global health problem, with PT infants at high risk of brain injury, altered brain development, and future neurobehavioral impairment. Language delays and problems with executive function are common in PT individuals; alterations in connectivity have been postulated as contributing to these developmental outcomes, suggesting that PT birth is a developmental disorder.

dMRI Studies Provide Evidence of Widespread Microstructural Abnormalities

FA values in the white matter of PT neonates are lower than those of PMA-matched term controls in several regions, including the centrum semiovale, frontal white matter, genu of the corpus callosum, and both external and internal capsules. Likewise, ADC values are significantly higher in both frontal and occipital white matter, suggesting widespread microstructural abnormalities, even in the absence of major focal lesions.

dMRI measures are related to gestational age at birth, PMA, comorbidities such as bronchopulmonary dysplasia, sepsis, and painful procedures. dMRI is also helpful for assessing ischemic white-matter lesions, characterized by restricted diffusion and low ADC values during the acute phase of injury detectable on diffusion-weighed imaging and dMRI before they are noted on conventional MRI. In infants with cystic periventricular leukomalacia, dMRI changes are seen in areas distant from the focal lesions at term-equivalent age (TEA); in more diffuse injury, ADC values are elevated in periventricular and subcortical white matter, suggesting widespread dysmaturation of white matter in the prematurely born.

dMRI measures correlate with neurodevelopmental performance in the prematurely born. FA in the optic radiations correlates with visual performance at TEA, and increased ADC values in white matter at TEA are associated with adverse neurodevelopmental outcome at 2 years corrected age. Likewise, FA values in the posterior limb of the internal capsule are associated with cognitive outcomes in the first postnatal year.

Finally, PT birth is associated with long-lasting and widespread alterations in white matter, and these alterations correlate with a variety of behavioral sequelae, ranging from language to executive function and, in young adulthood, psychiatric symptomatology.

Functional Studies: Alterations in Neural Networks in the Prematurely Born

Resting-state ICNs have been identified in PT infants at TEA; these are fragmentary at PMA 25 through 27 weeks and form at significantly different rates across the putative third trimester of gestation. Additionally, although these ICNs mirror those of term control infants, network analyses suggest less complexity in the neural systems of PT neonates.

These differences persist into childhood in the prematurely born. ROI studies demonstrate auxiliary right hemisphere connections for language and increased connectivity between both frontal cortices and the salience, default mode, and executive networks, suggesting alterations in neural networks for language, attention, and behavior in the prematurely born. Similarly, ICA analyses suggest global increases in connectivity in PT subjects compared with term controls, consistent with the ROI data. Finally, both years of maternal education and language testing scores are predictors of connectivity in PT subjects at young adulthood, suggesting that the alterations in functional connectivity unique to the PT population have significant functional implications.

Graph-Theory Analyses Support These Data

The topology of ICNs in PT neonates is positively correlated with structural networks, and this coupling increases with PMA. In contrast, PT subjects show reduced covariance in both language and frontoparietal functional networks compared with controls at TEA, suggesting that functional connections in PT subjects are less complex than those in term neonates. Similarly, RC analyses of microstructural networks confirm altered network architecture and reduced network capacity in PT subjects at TEA.

Graph-theory evidence for altered network function persists in adolescents and young adults born preterm. Increased functional connectivity within the posterior DMN and increased anticorrelation within the executive network have been reported in adolescents who were born PT. In contrast, Granger causality analysis reveals widespread reduction in between-network connectivity in preterm infants, particularly in connections between the salience network and the DMN.

Environmental Factors Alter Connectivity in the Prematurely Born

Pain and neonatal stress influence microstructural connectivity, as does housing in single rooms and daily exposure to the mother's voice during the critical putative third trimester of gestation. PT infants with white-matter injury show reduced connectivity between homologues compared with those without injury, and the severity of injury correlates with the loss of connectivity.

Autism Spectrum Disorder

Autism spectrum disorder (ASD) affects nearly 1 in 88 children and is widely thought to represent a disorder of connectivity, in which the environment may interact with the genome. dMRI studies report widespread disruptions in microstructural connectivity, particularly in those tracts subserving social cognition, in children, adolescents, and young adults with ASD. (Ameis and Catani, 2015).

dMRI studies across the past decade demonstrate both increases and reductions in FA across frontal, parietal, and temporal regions in subjects with ASD compared with age-matched typically developing controls, and little consistency had been noted across patient populations until the advent of two longitudinal analyses. Both supported altered early development and age-related changes that may underlie impaired brain functioning, particularly in social behavior and communication in children, with ASD. A first study of infants at risk for autism showed that those subsequently diagnosed with autism exhibited increased FA for a majority of sampled white-matter tracts at age 6 months, no FA differences compared with no-autism subjects at 12 months, and decreased FA at 24 months, demonstrating altered brain growth in ASD across corticocortical, projection, and interhemispheric white-matter tracts over the first 2 years of life. A second, larger investigation confirmed that the frontal tracts in toddlers with ASD showed greater FA values and volume than normal at younger ages, but an overall impaired rate of development subsequent to that time. As shown in Table 14-3, dMRI studies of ASD suggest far-ranging alterations in FA. Both long-range and short-range connections are reported to be involved, and fibers that mediate both frontal and temporal connectivity are most frequently affected. Microstructural changes differ in younger subjects with ASD compared with those found in affected adolescents and young adults, suggesting that ASD alters the developmental trajectory of interregional connections.

TBSS studies confirm these findings. Older individuals are most likely to demonstrate widespread decreases in FA, whereas young children with ASD show increases in this parameter. Studies using an ROI approach in younger children

---

TABLE 14-3 Disorders of Development

Developmental Disorder	Microstructural and Functional Alterations	Network Perturbations

Autistic spectrum disorder (ASD)	Age-related changes in both
	    Younger subjects—hyperconnectivity
	    Older subjects—hypoconnectivity
	    Preferential involvement of frontal and temporal regions
		Hyperconnectivity within the default mode network (DMN)

Attention-deficit/ hyperactivity disorder (ADHD)	Decreased fractional anisotropy (FA) in fronto-striato-cerebellar tracts Decreased FA in fronto-temporal tracts Decreased functional connectivity in frontal, striatal, temporo-parietal, and cerebellar regions	Reduced default mode network (DMN) segregation Alterations in intranetwork connectivity in DMN, dorsal attention network, and visual network
Tourette syndrome (TS)	Decreased FA in the corpus callosum and frontal-caudate connections Decreased functional connectivity in frontal-parietal and cingulo-opercular regions	Hypoconnectivity within networks subserving adaptive online control and set maintenance
Preterm (PT) birth	Decreased FA in centrum semiovale, frontal white matter, genu corpus callosum, internal, and external capsules; increased apparent diffusion coefficient (ADC) in frontal and occipital white matter Resting-state intrinsic connectivity networks (ICNs) present at term-equivalent age (TEA), but less complex than in term controls In older subjects, increased functional connectivity in language centers; also between frontal cortex and salience network, executive network, and DMN	Reduced covariance in language and fronto-parietal networks at TEA; rich club demonstrates reduced network capacity In older PT children, increased intranetwork connectivity for both executive network and DMN

demonstrated increased FA in the anterior cingulate and superior temporal gyrus, changes that correlate with behavioral measures, whereas ROI studies of older subjects revealed decreases in FA in the corpus callosum, left uncinate, and longitudinal fasciculus. Alterations within the left uncinate forecast autism symptoms, and recent data suggest left-hemisphere impairment, particularly in the thalamic and fronto-parietal networks, in high-functioning children with ASD.

Recent work has investigated functional networks in children, adolescents, and young adults with ASD. Early studies suggested reduced network integration in autism, especially in areas important for social behavior, but other studies report hyperconnectivity. Further, although functional connectivity studies of older subjects support the hypoconnectivity theory, several recent studies of school-aged subjects with ASD compared with control children demonstrated hyperconnectivity in ASD subjects at the whole-brain and subsystems levels. Regions of greatest significance included the primary sensory, paralimbic, and association areas, and greater frontal connectivity was positively associated with severity of social deficits. Similarly, graph-theory analyses suggest preferential involvement of the DMN in adolescent subjects with ASD, and hyperconnectivity within the DMN has been related to Autism Diagnostic Observation Schedule scores in adolescents with ASD.

Together, the reported age-related changes in microstructural and functional data in children with ASD suggest the need for longitudinal, standardized imaging investigations with genetic analyses to optimize diagnosis and intervention strategies.

Tourette Syndrome

Tourette syndrome (TS) is a neurodevelopmental disorder characterized by the presence of multiple unwanted and irresistible motor and phonic tics, and imaging studies across the past decade suggest that it is in part attributable to abnormal processing in major cortical control networks. Volumetric MRI studies of children and adolescents with TS report reductions in the corpus callosum and the putamen, globus pallidus, and lenticular nuclei bilaterally. Volumetric abnormalities have also been reported in the frontal and parietal cortices, suggesting involvement of both corticocortical and corticosubcortical circuitry.

Because the corpus callosum is the major commissure connecting homologous cortical regions and cortical networks are thought to be altered in TS, researchers have investigated microstructural connectivity in the corpus callosum in children with TS. dMRI studies have demonstrated decreased FA throughout all subregions of the corpus callosum in TS subjects compared with controls, although FA values do not correlate with the severity of tic symptoms. Similarly, tractography studies have shown decreased connectivity between the caudate nucleus and the left anterior-dorsolateral frontal cortex.

Likewise, fMRI analyses suggest impaired functional connectivity throughout the brain in adolescents with TS. Significant alterations have been reported in the frontoparietal network subserving rapid, adaptive online control and a cingulo-opercular network important for set maintenance in TS subjects compared with controls, suggesting that TS is a developmental movement disorder that alters adaptive, rapid control signaling. Together, published data suggest widespread alterations in microstructural and functional networks subserving cerebral control systems in children and adolescents with TS, but the clinical implications of these findings remain largely unexplored (Table 14-3).

Attention-Deficit/Hyperactivity Disorder

Attention deficit hyperactivity disorder (ADHD) is characterized by age-inappropriate inattention, hyperactivity, and impulsivity. Although ADHD is disproportionately diagnosed in males and is a heterogeneous disorder, ADHD patients exhibit deficits in executive functions long attributed to alterations in fronto-striato-parietal and fronto-cerebellar networks, and—similar to other developmental disorders—ADHD is thought to be a disorder of connectivity.

Whole-brain cross-sectional analyses have demonstrated reduced subcortical gray matter in subjects with ADHD, and microstructural studies of children and adults with ADHD report reduced white-matter microstructure integrity in ADHD patients relative to healthy controls in several fronto-striato-cerebellar white-matter tracts, including the right anterior corona radiata, left cerebellar white matter, internal capsule, forceps minor close to the genu of the corpus callosum, and cingulum. Similarly, graph-theory analyses have shown that males (but not females) with ADHD have decreased FA in prefrontal circuits, but increased FA in the orbito-fronto-cerebellar-striatal circuitries; these FA levels reportedly correlate with inattention and hyperactivity/impulsivity symptoms.

fMRI studies demonstrate that ADHD subjects exhibit deficits in function of specific frontal, striatal, temporoparietal, and cerebellar regions, and that ADHD patients also have abnormalities in functional interregional connectivity between these regions during both rest and task conditions. rs-fMRI studies of 757 participants in the ADHD-200 study showed altered connectivity between the DMN and ventral attention network, including significantly increased connectivity between the posterior cingulate cortex in the DMN and right anterior insula and supplementary motor area in the ventral attention network.

Recent studies have addressed the functional organization of subjects with ADHD, as shown in Table 14-3. ICA analyses of participants in the ADHD-200 sample demonstrated reduced DMN segregation co-occurring with structural abnormalities in the dorsolateral prefrontal cortex and anterior cingulate cortex, two important cognitive control regions. ADHD subjects also showed altered intranetwork connectivity in the DMN, dorsal attention network, and visual network, with co-occurring distributed structural deficits. In these analyses, gray-matter changes predicted alterations in fMRI. Likewise, ADHD subjects exhibited lower FA and functional connectivity inside RC networks, but a higher number of axonal fibers outside the RC compared with typically developing controls.

Sports-Related Concussion

The incidence of reported concussion in the pediatric population has been steadily increasing, and approximately one-fifth of pediatric patients with sports-related concussions will have persistent cognitive symptoms at 4 weeks following injury. These symptoms include slowed processing speed, poor concentration, and difficulties with memory, and emerging MRI studies suggest that these symptoms are attributable not only to changes in neuronal metabolism and perfusion but also alterations in neural connectivity. (Ashwal et al., 2014).

Recent data suggest both regional and network vulnerability in the pediatric population. Microstructural analyses of adolescents 1 month following concussion demonstrated higher FA values in multiple regions in the concussed group compared with age-matched control subjects; these include primarily frontal white-matter regions bilaterally. In contrast, when pediatric subjects 8 to 17 years of age with persistent neurocognitive deficits 3 to 12 months following a sports-related concussion were compared with control subjects, they showed decreased FA in the right anterior and posterior internal capsules. Furthermore, differences in dMRI metrics differentiated patients with persistent cognitive symptoms; FA values were lower and diffusivity values higher in subjects with cognitive symptoms.

Similarly, fMRI studies of adults have demonstrated frontal vulnerability to mild traumatic brain injury. Connectivity is decreased within the DMN during the acute, subacute, and chronic phases of injury, with additional findings of increased connectivity between the rostral anterior cingulate gyrus and ventrolateral prefrontal cortex. Interhemispheric connectivity is disrupted in the visual cortex, hippocampus, and dorsolateral prefrontal cortex, and longitudinal studies have demonstrated long-lasting decreases in frontal connectivity.

Likewise, an fMRI study in adolescents 1 month following sports-related concussion demonstrated alterations in the DMN, increased connectivity in the right frontal executive function network, and increased connectivity in the left frontal operculum cortex associated with the ventral attention network. Microstructural studies of this cohort demonstrate abnormalities within the anterior corona radiata bilaterally, the anatomic connection for the primary nodes of the DMN.

Epilepsy

Children with epilepsy are at high risk for developmental delay, ADHD, and behavioral problems such as depression and anxiety. In adult subjects epilepsy disrupts microstructural and functional connectivity, and these measures correlate with cognition and behavior. Although there are fewer studies of neural connectivity in children with epilepsy, emerging data suggest that epilepsy syndromes are associated with focal and widespread influences on the developing brain. Reported findings differ for different epilepsy syndromes, and published genetic correlations are not yet available.

Childhood absence epilepsy is a nonconvulsive, idiopathic epilepsy characterized by sudden and brief changes in consciousness. Clinical findings are accompanied by bilateral, synchronous, 2.5- to 4-Hz generalized spike wave discharges, and children with this disorder are at high risk for impairment in attention and executive function. Preliminary microstructural studies of children with absence epilepsy have demonstrated decreases in network strength and global and local efficiency, particularly in the orbitofrontal region, subcortical structures, and limbic cortex. fMRI investigations have shown significant alterations in functional connectivity within the salience network in patients compared with controls, with decreased connectivity in the right anterior insula, anterior temporoparietal junction, and bilateral dorsolateral frontal cortex, and increased connectivity in the anterior and middle cingulate gyri and caudate nucleus. The salience network subserves attention, and, together, data from both microstructural and functional connectivity studies support alterations in this important network as a possible cause of attentional dysfunction in children with absence epilepsy.

Rolandic epilepsy is a focal childhood epilepsy, presumably genetic, characterized by language impairment, inattention, and impulsivity. Although these seizures largely resolve during adolescence, interictal electroencephalogram (EEG) rolandic discharges may interfere with local brain maturation, resulting in alterations in cognition and behavior. Microstructural studies of children with rolandic epilepsy have shown reduced FA and decreased connectivity compared with controls, predominantly over the left pre- and postcentral gyri ipsilateral to the electroencephalographic focus; significant negative correlations between FA in these regions and measures of attention and anxiety have also been reported. fMRI investigations have demonstrated reduced connectivity in the left inferior frontal gyrus, or Broca's area, compared with controls, suggesting alterations in systems for both attention and language.

Children with *frontal-lobe epilepsy* have lower FA values in both the posterior white matter and in the second component of the superior longitudinal fasciculus. The latter tract connects parietal association areas with the prefrontal lobe and is frequently associated with spatial attention and perception of visual space. In contrast, a single study examining dMRI and fMRI in children with frontal-lobe epilepsy suggested more global changes. Microstructural network alterations included increased clustering, increased path length, stronger within-module connectivity, and weaker between-module connectivity compared with healthy controls. Functional connectivity within networks was related to cognitive performance, and structural modularity increased with decreased cognitive performance, suggesting decreased coupling between large-scale functional network modules in childhood frontal-lobe epilepsy.

Perinatal Stroke

Perinatal arterial ischemic infarcts preferentially involve the anterior circulation, and most occur within the left hemisphere, although there is considerable variability in terms of lesion etiology, onset, size, and location. Many children with early injury demonstrate remarkable recovery of language function, but there are considerable differences in the degree of recovery. There are few studies available, but t-fMRI and rs-fMRI assessments suggest refinement of the prevailing notion that language recovery following left-hemisphere perinatal stroke relies on the contribution of the contralateral hemisphere. Preliminary reports demonstrate no difference in functional imaging during language tasks. Similarly, the few published t-fMRI studies argue against the "right-hemisphere takeover" theory of recovery and suggest that increasing interhemispheric connectivity between posterior-superior-temporal language regions may be of benefit for testing scores, although these data require rigorous replication.

Imaging Genetics

The emergence of sophisticated imaging strategies has permitted not only the more accurate phenotyping of developmental disorders, but also the large-scale investigation of the role of genetic variants in neural connectivity. Emerging data across the past decade suggest the strong influence of the genome on the underlying architecture of functional brain communication during development, and both the Human Connectome Project and the Enhancing Neuroimaging Genetics through Meta-Analysis (ENIGMA) Consortium provide large data sets valuable for assessing the degree of genetic influence contributing to neural connectivity. The former will soon enroll neonates, children, and adolescents, and the ENIGMA Consortium is an effort coordinated by 125 institutions in 12 countries.

Likewise, pediatric populations with imaging and genetic data are now becoming available. One excellent example is the Pediatric Imaging, Neurocognition and Genetics (PING) study, which already has been employed to demonstrate that genetic variation in the neuregulin-1 gene alters brain developmental trajectories as assessed by dMRI in typically developing children. The PING study is a cross-sectional database of 1400 typically developing children ages 3 to 18 years collected at 10 academic institutions in the United States.

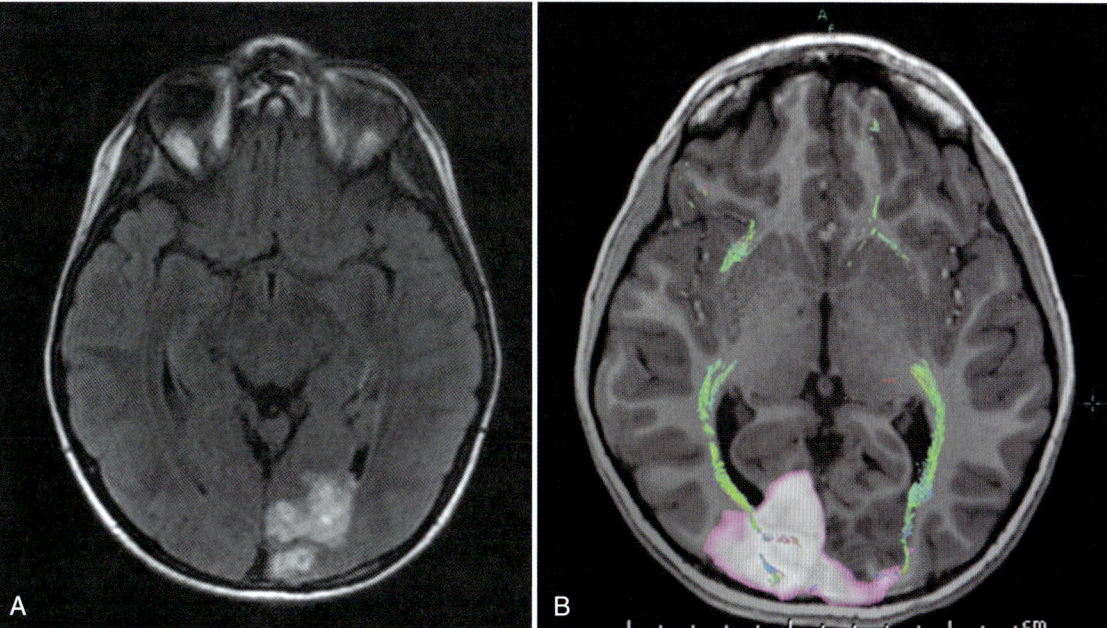

Figure 14-7. Microstructural connectivity in a 10-year-old male with occipital glioma. A 10-year-old male presented with seizures and headache. Brain MRI *(left panel)* demonstrated a left occipital mass, later diagnosed as a glioma. The photic-stimulation task fMRI and dMRI *(right panel)* shows a typical activation pattern *(white region with pink borders)* in the left hemisphere, but not the right. Similarly, dMRI microstructural imaging demonstrates occipital fiber tracts in green in the left hemisphere, but displacement of these visual fibers around the tumor in the left occiput. *(Figure courtesy of CC Duncan, MD, Yale School of Medicine.)*

Undiagnosed Developmental Disorders: The Role of Connectivity

Global developmental delay, intellectual disability, and neurobehavioral disorders are relatively common conditions, ut state-of-the-art strategies, including genetic, imaging, and metabolic assessments, provide diagnoses for less than 3 to 4 in 10 children. These data suggest that other strategies must be employed, and MRI-based connectomics has the potential to develop biomarkers for adverse neurodevelopmental outcomes in children with prenatal or perinatal disorders. Additionally, the monitoring of brain plasticity changes could provide a basis for the development and testing of therapies to improve outcomes in children with disorders of connectivity.

Current Clinical Applications

Functional and microstructural MR imaging have become part of routine brain mapping in pediatric patients with epilepsy or supratentorial tumors requiring surgery, as shown in Figure 14-7. fMRI protocols can localize most relevant language, visual, and/or motor regions in individual children and appear to be a valuable complementary tool for surgical planning of epileptogenic foci and brain tumors. In contrast, the role of fMRI and dMRI strategies in cerebral plasticity and intervention/treatment studies is just beginning to be evaluated. Recent data from an ongoing intervention trial of children with cerebral palsy suggest that microstructural connectivity increases concurrently with functional improvement, pilot data from a cognitive-behavioral therapy trial suggest that rs-fMRI data forecast symptom severity in obsessive-compulsive disorder up to 1 year after treatment, and fMRI has recently been employed to demonstrate widespread changes in functional connectivity of the brain's reading network as a result of

intervention in children with ASD, suggesting the clinical potential of this strategy.

CONCLUSIONS

The role of neuroimaging studies in developmental disorders of childhood is transitioning from a basic science tool to an integral part of the translational research cycle, with promise not only for early identification of disorders of connectivity, but also for the monitoring of therapeutic interventions.

Acknowledgments

The authors thank Ms. Cheryl Lacadie and Ms. Marie Campbell for technical and administrative assistance. The authors are supported by NIH NS27116, NS53865, T32 DA022975, and the Gates Foundation OPP1119263.

REFERENCES

The complete list of references for this chapter is available in the e-book at www.expertconsult.com.
    See inside cover for registration details.

SELECTED REFERENCES

Ameis, S.H., Catani, M., 2015. Altered white matter connectivity as a neural substrate for social impairment in Autism Spectrum Disorder. Cortex 62, 158–181.

Ashwal, S., Tong, K.A., Ghosh, N., et al., 2014. Application of advanced neuroimaging modalities in pediatric traumatic brain injury. J. Child Neurol. 29 (12), 1704–1717.

Dennis, E.L., Thompson, P.M., 2013. Typical and atypical brain development: a review of neuroimaging studies. Dialogues Clin. Neurosci. 15 (3), 359–384.

Di Martino, A., Fair, D.A., Kelly, C., et al., 2014. Unraveling the miswired connectome: A developmental perspective. Neuron. 83 (6), 1335–1553.

Friston, K.J., 2011. Functional and effective connectivity: a review. Brain Connect. 1 (1), 13–36.

Ouyang, A., Jeon, T., Sunkin, S.M., et al., 2015. Spatial mapping of structural and connectional imaging data for the developing human brain with diffusion tensor imaging. Methods 73, 27–37.

Power, J.D., Fair, D.A., Schlaggar, B.L., et al., 2010. The development of human functional brain networks. Neuron 67 (5), 735–748.

Richiardi, J., Altmann, A., Milazzo, A.C., et al., 2015. BRAIN NETWORKS. Correlated gene expression supports synchronous activity in brain networks. Science 348 (6240), 1241–1244.

Sporns, O., 2013. Structure and function of complex brain networks. Dialogues Clin. Neurosci. 15 (3), 247–262.

Sporns, O., Tononi, G., Kotter, R., 2005. The human connectome: A structural descriiption of the human brain. PLoS Comput. Biol. 1, 245–251.

E-BOOK FIGURES

The following figures and tables are available in the e-book at www.expertconsult.com. See inside cover for registration details.

15 Stem Cell Transplantation for Childhood Neurologic Disorders

Jean-Pyo Lee, Marcia Pereira, Rodolfo Gonzalez, Milton H. Hamblin, and Evan Y. Snyder

 An expanded version of this chapter is available on www.expertconsult.com. See inside cover for registration details.

Research into neural stem cells (NSCs) and their potential therapeutic applications for the central nervous system (CNS) has grown dramatically in the past decade. In pediatric neurologic disorders, NSCs show promise as therapy against lysosomal storage disorders (LSDs) and inborn errors of metabolism, including Tay–Sachs disease (TSD) and Sandhoff disease (SD). Moreover, NSCs may have potential benefit as a treatment against cerebral hypoxia and stroke.

The goal of stem cell transplantation for childhood neurologic disorders is to protect host cells and/or replace damaged cells with healthy cells and, in doing so, restore the functioning of original tissues and organs. NSCs may be derived from human embryonic stem cells (hESCs) or induced pluripotent stem cells (iPSCs). Whatever the benefits of each of these derived cell types, there are trade-offs between safety, effectiveness, and cost.

In this chapter, we review the methods used in studying NSCs and outcomes discovered from NSCs transplanted into the mammalian brain of animal models (mainly mouse and rat) of pediatric disorders. This information will provide insight into using NSCs in clinical trials for pediatric diseases.

NEURAL STEM CELL BIOLOGY
Definition of Neural Stem Cells

NSCs are the most primordial and least committed cells of the nervous system. Because immunocytochemically detectable markers that are sufficiently specific have not yet been fully defined, an NSC is still best defined operationally. NSCs must have the following properties: (1) *self-renewal* (produces unaltered daughter cells in response to mitogens) and (2) *multipotency* (generates all three fundamental neuroectodermal lineages—neurons, astrocytes, and oligodendrocytes—in a regional and developmental stage-appropriate manner). There is no consensus yet about how many intermediary steps exist between the stem cell stage and the emergence of a mature functional cell. If a cell type appears to show a more limited self-renewal capacity and a narrower range of fate, it is by convention called a *progenitor* or *precursor* rather than a stem cell.

Stem Cell Niche and Function of Neural Stem Cells in the Developing Central Nervous System

The population of NSCs in the adult brain is harbored in special locations called *niches*. To sustain homeostasis of NSC populations, NSCs proliferate and differentiate following an innate genetic program and respond to signals from this specialized microenvironment.

In the early stages of mammalian cerebrogenesis, NSCs are located in a primary germinal zone known as the ventricular zone (VZ). It is estimated that stem cells account for 5%

to 20% of the cells in the VZ of the telencephalon of an embryonic day 10 (E10) mouse. The earliest NSCs divide symmetrically to amplify identical daughter cells. A stem cell retains continuous mitotic potential while remaining multipotent. In response to specific developmental signals, somewhat later in cerebrogenesis, NSCs divide asymmetrically to generate partially differentiated neural progenitor cells. Neural precursor cells then begin to express differentiation markers while remaining mitotically active. They differentiate once they exit from the cell cycle, with the final fate of a given progenitor cell depending on extrinsic morphogenic signals, specific patterns of transcriptional activation, and growth factors. Neurons are generated before the generation of glia during development.

The secondary germinal zone, believed to develop from the VZ, includes the subventricular zone (SVZ) of the forebrain, external germinal layer of the cerebellum, and the subgranule layer of the hippocampus. NSCs are believed to populate these areas as well and maintain homeostasis in the brain. The SVZ is known to serve as an endogenous source of multipotent neural precursors that give rise to neurons and glia to replace dead cells and support cell turnover. In rodent SVZ, newly generated neural precursors reach their final destination in the olfactory bulb after long-distance migration through a well-defined path called the rostral migratory stream. However, it is debatable whether the human SVZ can give rise to neurons.

Although endogenous NSCs are present in the mammalian brain, where major neurologic damage occurs, endogenous NSCs are shown to be inadequate or ineffective for repair. One reason the brain does a poor job regenerating function may be that endogenous NSCs are surrounded by a microenvironment that does not promote the differentiation or survival of NSCs. The news is not all bad. Results of several NSC transplantation experiments suggest that neurogenic cues are temporarily transmitted during degenerative processes and that exogenous NSCs are able to sense, home in, and respond appropriately to those cues. Although these mechanisms are not fully understood, it seems that some neurodegenerative processes broadcast neurogenic signals, and these send out developmental and migration cues to which NSCs can respond. For effective stem cell therapy, NSCs must widely distribute throughout the brain. To this end, various methods have been developed to extract and induce NSCs to their optimal proficiency.

Isolation and Propagation of Neural Stem Cells in Vitro

Several in vitro methods exist to isolate and expand human or mouse NSC populations in a manner that maintains their stem-like qualities. For example, NSCs can be isolated directly from the neuroectoderm, the primary germinal zone (VZ) of fetuses, or from residual secondary germinal zones such as the subventricular or subgerminal zone in adults. However,

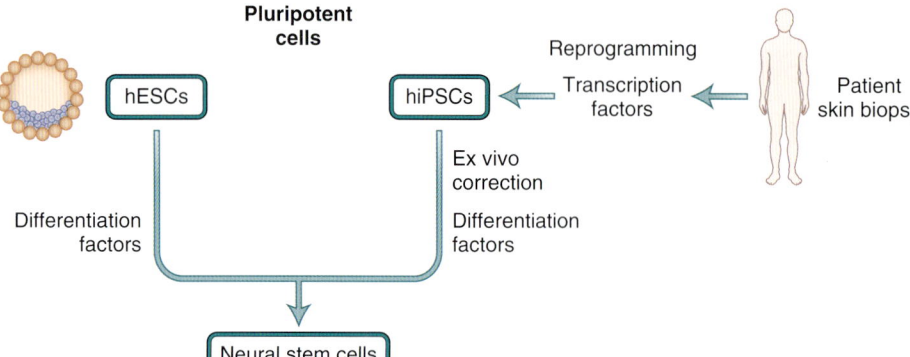

Figure 15-1. Diagram of generating human iPSC-derived NSCs from patients. hiPSCs can be generated by reprogramming of patient skin fibroblasts through transduction of four pluripotency genes, *OCT4*, *SOX2*, *KLF4*, and *C-MYC*. hiPSCs can then be genetically engineered using ex vivo gene correction and differentiated into hiPSC-NSCs. hESCs, human embryonic stem cells; hiPSCs, human-induced pluripotent stem cells; NSCs, neural stem cells.

it remains unclear whether adult-derived NSCs can make projection neurons and necessary connections as precisely as that of naturally generated neurons during development.

NSCs can be isolated and propagated in growth medium containing basic fibroblast growth factor (bFGF) and epidermal growth factor (EGF). In vitro, these cells express markers characteristic of undifferentiated NSCs such as nestin, and musashi, which can then differentiate when appropriate induction factors are added. In vivo, these cells have been tested in a variety of neurodegenerative disease models and have proven to be therapeutically beneficial in some cases (Taylor et al., 2006). To achieve optimal migration and engraftment, it is preferable to transplant undifferentiated NSCs than cells that have undergone varying degrees of differentiation ex vivo. NSCs can also be derived secondarily in vitro from human pluripotent stem cells, such as ESCs and iPSCs.

Generation of Human and Murine Neural Stem Cells from Embryonic Stem Cells

For hESC differentiation in vitro, neural differentiation appears to be a primary default lineage for hESC differentiation under conditions that do not maintain pluripotency. Therefore the earliest methods for generating NSCs from hESCs, although with very low efficiency, were by spontaneous differentiation in the absence of conditions that promote self-renewal (Reubinoff et al., 2001). In subsequent studies, specific stimuli can be added to mimic embryonic neurogenesis as a way of improving the yield of NSCs derived from hESCs (Chambers et al., 2009).

For murine ESCs, retinoic acid signaling promotes generation of NSC. ESCs, which are derived from the inner cell mass of a blastocyst, are capable of giving rise to differentiated progeny from all three embryonic germ layers. Although ESCs, by definition, never senesce, they require a great deal of instruction to direct them toward the NSC lineage fate.

Efficient neural induction of hESCs involves growing them under monolayer feeder-free defined culture conditions and dual SMA and MAD related protein (SMAD) inhibition of the TGFβ/BMP signaling pathways. After neural induction, NSCs can be derived and expanded under defined culture medium conditions with bFGF and EGF and be used for transplantation studies. The tumorigenic risk can be removed by extending the in vitro culture time of ESC-NSCs for several passages before transplantation.

Generation of Neural Stem Cells from Induced Pluriporent Stem Cells

NSCs derived from iPSCs are particularly interesting. Direct reprogramming of somatic cells into pluripotent-state cells is an alternative to traditional nuclear transfer and somatic cell

fusion using ESCs. In this way, it has circumvented the ethics controversies of hESCs and therapeutic cloning. Unlike hESCs, iPSCs show no immunologic incompatibility, making them a desirable NSC line for use in therapy. It is anticipated that iPSCs could replace many applications in regenerative medicine suggested for hESCs.

To generate iPSCs, somatic cells are subjected to epigenetic reprogramming by forcing exogenous expression of specific transcription factors. Many different somatic cell types have been reprogrammed to create iPSCs (Takahashi and Yamanaka, 2006). These include foreskin fibroblasts, wherein iPSCs are generated by ectopic expression of chromatin-remodeling transcription factors (e.g., OCT4, SOX2, KLF4, and C-MYC) (Figure 15-1).

Fibroblasts, which can be easily obtained from human biopsies, are readily expanded in number and reprogrammed. However, clinical use of these first-generation iPSCs is limited because of risks imposed by insertional mutagenesis by these transcription factors, some of which are oncogenes. Efforts to eliminate these concerns have led to experimentation using transient expression of reprogramming factors with plasmids, adenoviruses, transposon vectors, and even purified recombinant proteins. Although these methods have proven experimentally successful for iPSC generation, their reprogramming efficiency is prohibitively low for practical applications.

Studies show low efficiency of generating iPSCs; resources are thus sufficient but less efficient because of variability in the differentiated state and the age of somatic cells. Residual DNA methylation states inherited from original differentiated cells remain in iPSCs, therefore, the plasticity of iPSC fate can be limited. Additionally, a caveat associated with iPSC generation is overexpression of c-myc and viral transduction. Using nonviral techniques and adding chemicals to increase production efficiency would be expected to provide a better approach.

An in-depth analysis using genome-wide transcriptional profiling of iPSCs and ESCs demonstrated that both cell types share a common pluripotency and self-renewal network. iPSCs can differentiate into derivatives representing all three embryonic germ layers and produce nearly identical progeny from neural, hepatic, and mesenchymal lineages.

The differentiation process of iPSCs can be divided into stages. First, embryoid bodies are formed. These are cell aggregates that appear when they are detached from the feeder layer and put into serum containing medium. To enrich for particular cell types, certain exogenous factors influencing the differentiation program need to be supplemented. Next, molecular markers can be selected for detection of expressed cell markers to identify specific cell types and subsequent generation of progenitor cells. As with ESCs, iPSCs can be used to derive NSCs using a monolayer culture and dual inhibition of

SMAD signaling. Alternately and potentially most promising is the ability to generate self-renewable and multipotent NSCs directly from fibroblasts bypassing iPSCs by expression of a single transcription factor, SOX2 or OCT4.

In vitro microarray analysis indicates that iPSC-NSCs (NSCs derived from iPSCs) and ESC-NSCs show similar but not identical gene expression and epigenetic patterns. It would be ideal to be able to use iPSCs derived from a given patient (and corrected ex vivo) because this strategy offers a way to potentially eliminate some degree of inflammation (because of immuno-incompatibility). Therefore, with future improvements in the derivation, quality, and validation, we can be optimistic that an improved version of iPSCs will become available for cell therapy–based regenerative medicine in the times ahead. In the last stage, certain progenitor cells such as NSCs can generate specific cell types. NSCs can further differentiate into neurons, astrocytes, and oligodendrocytes by modifying culture conditions.

Transplantation of Neural Stem Cells

Whether NSCs are sourced from embryonic or neonatal cells, or the adult CNS of either humans or rodents, once they are transplanted into mouse brains, they can integrate throughout the CNS (Lee et al., 2009; Huang et al., 2014). Unfortunately, differentiated or postmitotic neurons derived from NSCs neither engraft robustly nor migrate extensively. Successful engraftment and integration requires adhering to the following principles: stem cells enter the CNS in an undifferentiated state during the active log growth phase and then they exit the cell cycle in the brain, where they are receptive to environmental cues. For example, NSCs derived from various sources have been transplanted to pediatric or adult neurologic disease mouse brains, demonstrating their ability to migrate and improve the pathophysiology of the brain, oxidative stress, and the damage of blood–brain barrier (BBB).

Regarding optimal transplantation time in many pediatric neurologic disorders, administrating NSCs presymptomatically may decrease the demand on host NSCs to replace neurons and reconstruct circuitry. Although neuronal replacement receives more attention, its effects can be complemented, and even surpassed by the range of homeostatic factors and actions that NSCs intrinsically express. It has been demonstrated that NSCs are able to direct their fate in response to an abnormal environment and interact reciprocally with the host CNS (Yandava et al., 1999). The main caveat to this interaction is through exogenous NSCs "reprogramming" host circuitry to correct dysfunction and deficiencies. It may be more efficacious to focus on preserving established circuitry than to attempt to build new connections. Thus transplanting NSCs into cerebral ventricles of newborn mice is proven to be a good strategy in terms of timing (presymptomatic) and achieving extensive stem cell migration in a mouse model of pediatric disease. There has also been evidence that multiple NSC transplantations into different regions of the brain may prove to be more beneficial than a single transplantation. For example, NSCs were transplanted into the cerebral ventricles and the cerebellum of neonate mouse models of SD. The results showed that there was an added benefit to the increased pool of available NSCs and also to the introduction of NSCs to new regions of the brain. Further investigation is of interest because NSC transplantations into multiple regions, or multiple transplantations into the same region, may be necessary for certain diseases that have a global pathology. However, it is uncertain whether increasing the number of transplanted NSCs is safe or if appropriate connections will be made. A more practical application of NSC transplantation therefore lies in the potential to protect and maintain existing neuronal connections, rather than neuronal replacement.

To evaluate the impact of stem cells on mouse models of pediatric diseases with global brain pathology, NSCs can be transplanted into the cerebral ventricles of newborn mice. Newborn mice are easy to inject, with their soft skulls facilitating penetration. Transplanted NSCs gain access to most regions of the ventricular and SVZ. Cells then migrate to distant CNS regions and participate in normal development of different brain regions at multiple stages of brain development. When NSC transplantation is performed in utero, disease progression may be more effectively arrested. Prenatally or neonatally transplanted NSCs can survive for a long time in the recipient mouse brain without requiring immunosuppressant treatment. The impact of NSCs in engrafted mice can be determined in terms of survival and motor function and varies according to disease models. Electrophysiology on acute slices from engrafted brains can be performed to assess functional integration of donor NSC-derived cells (Figure 15-2).

Detection of Donor Neural Stem Cells in the Host Mouse Brain

There are many ways to track and identify transplanted donor cells in a recipient brain. One of the most commonly used in vitro stem cell labeling techniques is bromodeoxyuridine (BrdU), which incorporates into DNA during the S phase and can prelabel mitotically active donor cells. Labeled cells can be identified by the anti-BrdU antibody and can be instrumental to determine the number of cell divisions that engrafted cells have undergone in vivo posttransplantation. Donor cells can also be marked by constitutive viral markers such as LacZ or GFP, or other markers using tissue-specific and inducible promoters. Sex mismatch between donor and recipient can be instrumental to detect the cells. For example, donor cells can also be identified by the presence of the Y chromosome if male cells are transplanted into a female host. This detection technique is very useful when donor cells and recipients are the same species. In addition, species mismatch can be instrumental to identify donor cells. For example, human donor cells in the mouse brain can be identified by a human-specific antibody.

In vivo, several molecular imaging techniques are used for noninvasive stem cell tracking. For example, donor cells transduced with vectors encoding Luciferase make it possible to track living donor cells, after injection of animals with D-luciferin, in the recipient brain. Alternatively, in vivo tracking of cells can be done with in vitro labeling with ferromagnetic beads and magnetic resonance imaging (MRI). This MRI setup is expensive and can be technically challenging when nanoparticles leak out of dead cells. These imaging techniques can be efficiently utilized in preclinical studies track the migration of NSCs.

Homing of Neural Stem Cells

In mammalian brains of all ages, NSCs may be attracted even at a great distance to injury sites and regions of neurodegeneration. Both human and mouse NSCs express many chemokines and chemokine receptors (including CXCR4 and adhesion molecules and immunoglobulins) that mediate homing to sources of proinflammatory chemokines such as chemokine stromal cell derived factor-1α (SDF-1α, also known as CXCL12). SDF-1α signaling through CXCR4 has previously been identified as a key step in the homing of stem cells. Expression of SDF-1α is often up-regulated within

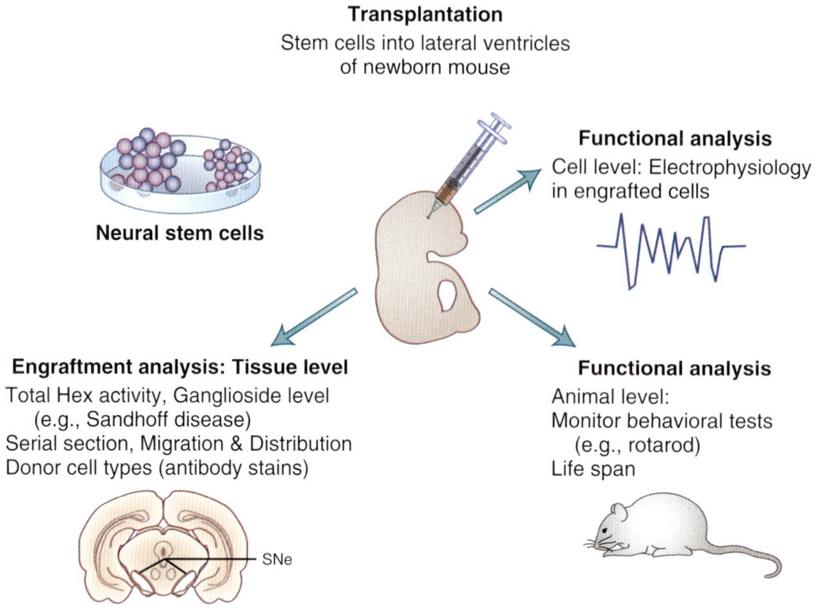

Transplantation
Stem cells into lateral ventricles
of newborn mouse

Neural stem cells

Functional analysis
Cell level: Electrophysiology
in engrafted cells

Engraftment analysis: Tissue level
Total Hex activity, Ganglioside level
    (e.g., Sandhoff disease)
Serial section, Migration & Distribution
Donor cell types (antibody stains)

SNe

Functional analysis
Animal level:
Monitor behavioral tests
    (e.g., rotarod)
Life span

Figure 15-2. Flow scheme of neural stem cell transplantation. Engrafted NSCs into the cerebral ventricles of a newborn mouse model of CNS disease (e.g., Sandhoff mice) migrate extensively to distant CNS regions. Engrafted cells survive for a long time, as determined by *lac*Z (encodes β-galactosidase) staining, which traces donor cells histochemically (X-gal reaction, blue). Effects of engrafted NSCs can then be analyzed at animal, tissue, and cellular levels. Functional integration of engrafted NSC-derived cells can be assessed by electrophysiological recording in acute brain slices. CNS, central nervous system; NSCs, neural stem cells.

injuries in areas such as the brain, heart, and kidney. SDF-1α is shown to be involved in the pathophysiological process of neurologic disorders and in promoting the directed migration of stem cells and regeneration of injured tissues (Imitola et al., 2004).

The migration of NSCs activated by the chemotactic effect of SDF-1α is also reported in vitro, showing that SDF-1α significantly induced the migration of NSCs in a dose-dependent manner. The relevance of SDF-1α in the migration of endogenous NSCs after brain injury and the contribution of the SDF-1α–CXCR4 system to NSC homing in traumatic brain injury is also implicated. Thus exploitation of the SDF-1α–CXCR4 system can be instrumental to improve brain repair.

Bystander Effects of Engrafted Neural Stem Cells

NSCs do much more than neuronal replacement. NSCs actually possess an array of actions that are potentially therapeutic. In addition to replacing the neural elements of the brain, NSCs have been shown to reduce inflammation in the CNS, secrete trophic factors, provide inherently derived gene products to host cells, and reduce toxic damage. Initially, the goal of NSC transplantation therapy was to replace or replenish dead or dying host cells, but the "chaperone" actions of NSCs prove to be more impactful than neuronal replacement itself and contribute to the many improvements seen in experimental models. Paracrine effects of these neurotrophic factors include alteration of the brain microenvironment by improving host regenerative processes, such as angiogenesis and migration, or by reducing destructive processes, such as apoptosis. CNS inflammation is characterized by both microglial activation and macrophage infiltration. Thus present recognition of inflammation as a key common factor in the pathology of neurologic disorders has further characterized the innate anti-inflammatory capabilities of NSCs (Lee et al., 2007).

THERAPEUTIC POTENTIAL OF NSCS
Lysosomal Storage Disorders

Lysosomal storage disorders (LSDs) (Chapter 41), a group of more than 50 autosomal recessive metabolic neurodegenerative diseases, are caused by deficiencies of specific acid hydrolases. Currently, no effective treatments are available for infantile onset forms of these diseases.

There is a growing appreciation of the multifaceted actions of NSCs in CNS repair. Although functional neuronal replacement has received the most attention, this action can be complemented by a range of other stem cell actions that exert various homeostatic forces. These aspects of therapeutic potential of NSCs are particularly relevant for treating LSDs. LSDs serve as an "easy" target for NSC treatment because of the following factors: (1) most LSDs with CNS pathologies quickly progress to eventual morbidity; (2) the etiology and pathophysiology of most LSDs, which are typically monogenic, are better understood than the more publicized diseases that are typically polygenic or manifest spontaneously in adults; (3) LSDs can be detected early (prenatal/neonatal) presymptomatically when intervention may have a more effective long-term impact; (4) the mutation typically results in a single deficient enzyme that can be cross-corrected to sufficient levels to sustain normal metabolism; (5) the ability of NSCs to diffuse through the BBB and naturally integrate into existing CNS circuitry while producing intrinsic gene products fills in major gaps in effective LSD therapy; (6) the biology of NSCs coincides well with the biology of the pediatric brain; that is, exogenous NSCs transplanted prenatally/neonatally would diffuse and differentiate with host (mutant) cells in response to microenvironmental cues.

Bystander Effects of Neural Stem Cells in Lysosomal Storage Disorders

In mouse models of LSDs, transplantation of genetically modified NSCs encoding missing enzyme genes is shown to be beneficial. (1) MPS VII mouse models, caused by a frameshift mutation in the *B-glucuronidase* (GUSB) gene, demonstrated the potential for treatment of LSDs using enzyme replacement therapies. (2) A mouse model has been used for TSD, a gangliosidosis, which results in the mutation of the α-subunit of the β-hexosaminidase enzyme (consisting of HexA and HexB isozymes). The pathology of TSD results in progressive and fatal neurodegeneration that is caused by buildup of the ganglioside GM2 in the CNS. It was first demonstrated that cross-corrective enzymes (HexA) produced from exogenous NSCs could function to reduce pathologic accumulation of GM2 in vitro. The same principal has been applied to the TSD mouse model by overexpressing HexA production, where NSC engraftment in vivo has shown reduction in neuropathology. It has also been observed that overexpression of lysosomal enzymes does not seem to have deleterious effects, although overexpression of other factors may or may not be problematic.

Reduction of neuropathology through NSC transplantation depends on (1) whether the corrective enzyme is required in small amounts to maintain normal function, (2) whether it is secreted, and (3) whether it can be taken up by mannose-6-phosphate (M6P) receptors. These traits have been demonstrated in the mouse model of SD, a gangliosidosis caused by a mutation of the β-subunit of Hex. SD is characterized by the deficiency of both HexA and HexB, resulting in the accumulation of the gangliosides GM2 and GA2 in the CNS. The pathologic accumulation of GM2 and GA2 causes rapid and progressive neurodegeneration that is fatal typically in infancy. Evidence in SD mouse models has shown that both human and mouse NSCs transplanted into the brains of neonates have migrated extensively throughout the brain while providing cross-correcting Hex enzyme, resulting in reduced ganglioside storage (both GM2 and GA2) in lysosomes. Engraftment was measured using LacZ-labeled NSCs traced by X-gal, and functionality was measured using electrophysiological methods to detect electrophysiologically active neurons in the CNS after NSC transplantation (see Figure 15-2). These exogenous NSCs incorporated into the host circuitry through cytoarchitectural interactions and distributed intrinsic homeostatic gene products and, also to a lesser extent, provided neuronal replacement. Transplanted mice showed an increase in lifespan and an improvement in motor function.

Of particular note, in combination with substrate reduction therapy (SRT), the potential for synergistic effects with NSC transplantation was examined in the SD mouse model. SRT is a pharmacologic treatment strategy that targets the amount of substrate to be metabolized. Iminosugars such as *N*-butyldeoxynojirimycin (NB-DNJ) and *N*-butyldeoxygalactonojirimycin (NB-DGJ) are used in SRT to inhibit glycosphingolipid synthesis, thus reducing the amount of substrate available and decreasing storage in lysosomes. This is of particular interest because the addition of an oral pharmacologic agent in combination with NSC transplantation in SD mice improved the enzymatic action of NSCs without the need for genetic manipulation (Figure 15-3). These results suggest that combination therapies that utilize the inherent capabilities of NSCs can provide improved outcomes compared with each method administered separately. Only a small percentage (less than 5%) of donor-derived cells that were neurons probably had the smallest impact. These results show a bystander effect of NSCs and also encourage combination therapy along with NSC transplantation.

Cell Replacement of NSCs in LSDs

In addition to widespread molecular therapy, there is cell replacement therapy. Neonatal brain injury is accompanied by a broad range of factors, including activation of oxidative stress, inflammation, and excitotoxicity pathways that can lead to damage. In addition to neuronal damage, injury to nonneuronal cell types such as astrocytes and oligodendrocytes might also impair neurodevelopment.

The prospect of replacing oligodendrocytes may be a bit more achievable than neurons, yet, even then, a number of considerations may make this goal less than straightforward.

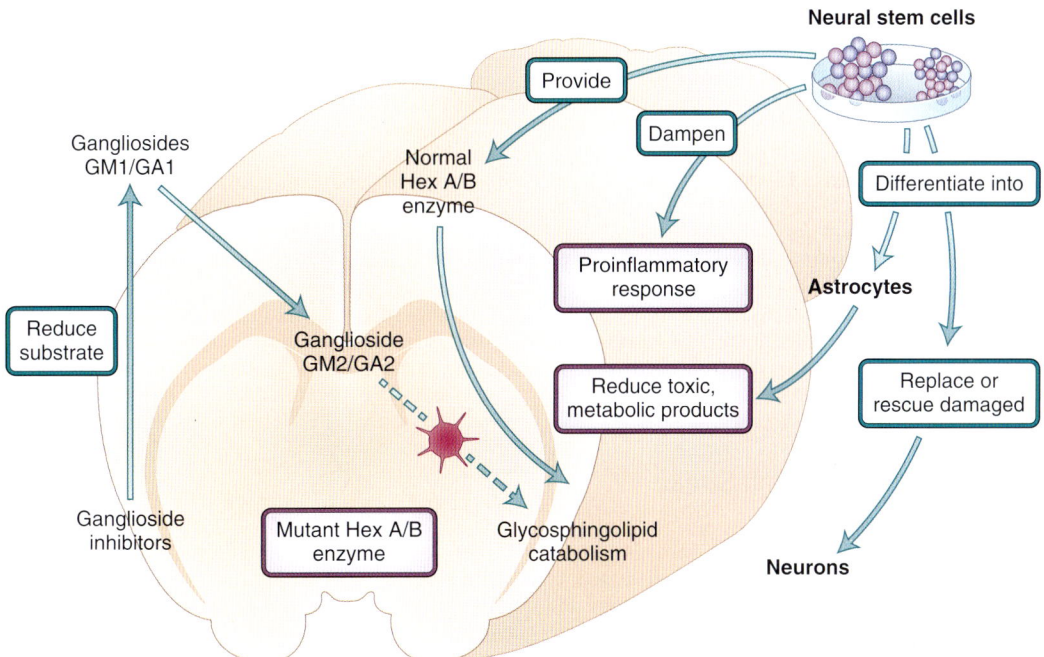

Figure 15-3. Diagram of multimodal therapeutic potential of NSCs in pediatric neurodegenerative diseases. The beneficial effects of transplanted NSCs are mediated by multiple actions, including their ability to produce trophic factors, preserve neuronal function, and reduce astrogliosis and inflammation. NSCs, neural stem cells.

There have been demonstrations of NSC transplantation to replace oligodendrocytes in disorders of CNS dysmyelination. Dysmyelination plays an important role in many genetic (i.e., inborn metabolic errors and leukodystrophies) and acquired (i.e., traumatic, ischemic, and inflammatory) neurodegenerative processes.

The first application of using NSCs to replenish myelin in the CNS occurred with the *shiverer* (*shi*) mouse model. *Shi* mice have dysfunctional oligodendrocytes and dysmyelination of the CNS because of a deletion mutation in the myelin basic protein (MBP), which is required for myelin function. Both human and mouse NSCs were transplanted into the cerebral ventricles of neonatal *shi* mice. Widespread engraftment throughout the CNS was observed as was an increase in levels of MBP, resulting in decreased tremors in the mice (Snyder and Flax, 1995). The fact that human NSCs were effective is critical because dysmyelination is central to many genetic and acquired neurodegenerative processes in humans. While there is no human version of "shiverer" disease, oligodendrocyte dysfunction and the consequent dysmyelination are prominent features of some important LSDs.

An example of CNS dysmyelination in humans is *Krabbe leukodystrophy,* also known as *globoid cell leukodystrophy* (GCL). GCL is caused by deficient galactosylceramidase (GalC) activity, whose primary substrate is a component of the myelin sheath. GCL presents with CNS dysmyelination, oligodendrocyte degeneration, and macrophage infiltration.

The pathophysiology of GCL has been debated. Whether it is caused by a cell autonomous defect or by a toxic environment that would kill all cells (including host and transplanted cells) is in question. It has been hypothesized that the toxic environment might be caused by the buildup of the glycolipid psychosine because of the deficiency of GalC. Loss of GalC causes the buildup of the toxic glycolipid psychosine. The toxicity of psychosine to neural cells has been shown in in vitro experiments, where oligodendrocytes were especially susceptible. An animal model using *twitcher* (*twi*) mice has been used to examine whether transplantation of NSCs could be therapeutic in this toxic environment. Results of NSC transplantation into neonatal *twi* mice showed that NSCs were capable of surviving and differentiating into oligodendrocytes in the CNS. This showed that the toxic environment created by psychosine did not rule out cell transplantation therapies for GCL. The innate resistance that NSCs possess to the toxic environment is also more pronounced in the undifferentiated state. However, although the exogenous NSCs are able to engraft and differentiate into existing circuitry, little to no appreciable relief of symptoms is observed in *twi* mice. Of particular interest though is that a larger proportion (than normal) of NSCs differentiated into oligodendrocytes, suggesting that NSCs may be able to detect what cell type or niche is deficient and act to restore homeostasis by directing its fate. These studies indicated that NSCs may be able to detect what cell type or niche is deficient, and then act to alter its fate. It has become clear that ongoing reciprocal interactions occur between NSCs and damaged host cells.

Hypoxic Ischemic Brain Injury and Stroke

Hypoxic ischemic injury (HII) during the perinatal period may lead long-term neurologic deficits. HII damages brain parenchymal cells and their connections, causes vascular and BBB dysfunction, and produces an extensive inflammatory response, but it also initiates endogenous protective processes.

NSC transplantation in rodent models of neonatal HII shows that NSCs are successfully engrafted, extensively migrate to injury sites, and replace lost tissue by differentiating into neurons that integrate with host neuronal networks. Engrafted NSCs migrate toward damaged regions in the neonatal brain in response to endogenous chemokines and can move at a rate of approximately 100 μm/day where they can survive for up to 52 weeks after transplantation NSC-engrafted brains showed reduced activation of resident microglia, and increased expression of growth factors for FGF2, GDNF, IGF-1, and the neuroblast marker doublecortin, and oligodendrocyte markers Olig2 and MBP. The driving force of the functional improvements seen after NSC engraftment could be widespread changes in gene expression.

In stroke animal models, it has been shown that NSCs, when injected intravenously 3 days after reperfusion, survived in the brain for at least 1 month, and engrafted mice showed improvement of neurologic deficits. However, most of the cells remained in an undifferentiated state, suggesting that cell replacement was not the main mechanism responsible for the improvement. Undifferentiated NSCs had an anti-inflammatory effect, reduced glial scar formation, and protected striatal neurons. Similar beneficial effects of hNSCs are reported in the early stage of the adult cerebral ischemic-reperfusion mouse model. Engrafted hNSCs 1 day poststroke migrated rapidly and extensively to damaged regions after transplantation into a neurogenic site where migration cues are already underway during stroke onset. The hNSCs then counteracted a number of pathologic processes of stroke and repaired BBB damage. Although long-term effects of transplanted hNSCs on the amelioration of ischemic stroke–induced behavioral dysfunction in a rodent model have been reported, this study is the first to show rapid beneficial impacts on behavioral function (within 24 hours) upon early delivery of hNSCs into the hippocampus. Transplantation of hiPSC-NSCs in the same experimental stroke model showed a similar beneficial effect in the early stage of stroke injury. Transplantation of hESC-derived NSCs into the infarct boundary zone in a rat model of ischemic stroke improved impaired forelimb function. These studies show that the therapeutic effect of hNSCs demonstrated in pediatric disorders can be extended to adult neurologic and neurovascular disorders.

SUMMARY

The regenerative and homeostatic capabilities that NSCs possess make them prime candidates for use in treating childhood neurologic disorders, including LSDs. Although cell replacement receives more attention, its effects can be complemented by bystander actions of factors secreted by NSCs. The intrinsic qualities of NSCs include anti-inflammatory, anti-apoptotic, proregenerative, proangiogenic, and neurotrophic growth factors. NSC transplantation may work synergistically with other therapies such as substrate reduction, enzyme replacement, gene therapy, and other pharmacologic interventions. For example, the synergistic potential of NSCs in combination with SRT was shown in a mouse model of SD. In such multimodal strategies, NSCs seem to serve as the "glue" that synchronizes different therapeutic actions for childhood neurologic disorders.

FUTURE APPLICATIONS

The future of NSC therapy in pediatric neurologic disorders is sufficiently encouraging and has the potential to circumvent the onset and/or progression of neurodegenerative processes. Although we may be far away from being able to fully reverse established disease processes that will require cell replacement and reconstruction of damaged CNS, there is great potential for NSCs to circumvent the progression of disease before it manifests. Ideally, early intervention presymptomatically and/or in utero would provide optimal results. Such an intervention brings up the premise that an early diagnosis, either prenatal or neonatal, has been confirmed. Early detection may be difficult because it would require a high level of suspicion and an extensive knowledge of family history on the part of the clinician and/or a good prenatal/neonatal screening program. However, the ability to translate these findings from animal models to successful human therapies is still ongoing. The successful translation of NSC therapy from animal models to use in human clinical trials will require further characterization of NSC biology and the pathophysiology of diseases in question. Important aspects of NSC biology to be explored further include the following: (1) characterization of the hNSCs to be used, with detailed protocols for their propagation and phenotype determination; (2) Comprehensive examination of the fate of transplanted hNSCs in vivo (i.e., Do they become electrophysiologically active neurons that make proper connections without making improper connections? Do they survive as differentiated glial cells or as undifferentiated progenitors? Do they survive at all in the environment, and if so how long?); (3) determination of whether the amount of enzyme expressed intrinsically by the hNSC enough to establish normal metabolic function, or whether genetic manipulation will be required to increase the production and secretion of the target enzyme; (4) determination of whether there is a measurable improvement in behavioral function after NSC engraftment and whether this is long-term; and (5) determination of how NSCs should be administered in order to reach all areas of the nervous system requiring treatment. Although administration of NSCs directly into cerebral ventricles has shown widespread diffusion throughout the cortex and cerebrum, diffusion to other parts of the CNS, including the cerebellum and spinal cord, and also to the peripheral nervous system may be required in order to fully prevent pathologies. This is of particular interest for some forms of LSDs with infantile onset. However, methods for NSC administration into areas other than the cerebrum and cortex require further examination in animal models.

Extensive characterization of human-derived NSCs, particularly hiPSCs, is needed to pave the way for clinical applications. Some of the key questions are as follows: Should NSCs be obtained from areas of neuroectodermal origin? If so, should they be from a fetal or adult source? Will an adult source be equally as effective? Will nonneural sources be as effective? Should a stable pool of NSCs be used for all patients, or should patient-derived NSCs be used as an autologous source for each patient. Finding the most effective way to obtain NSCs for transplantation therapy will be required to derive an efficacious treatment in humans.

There are many pathologic manifestations that make up individual diseases. In all, if we are to achieve success in treating pediatric CNS diseases, we need to embrace a wide variety of approaches that include genetics; molecular science; pharmacology; tissue engineering; cell replacement therapy; and antiapoptotic, angiogenic, and anti-inflammatory methods. Although upregulated proinflammatory cytokines can be deleterious in some disease stages, they also serve as a signal for homing of exogenous stem cells into CNS injury sites. What role does inflammation play in different stages of disease progression? Answering this question will be critical for determining how inflammation contributes to brain injury and regenerating damaged tissue. Determining how these methods and factors can be coupled with NSC transplantation in a safe and efficacious manner is essential in the translation to clinical practice.

REFERENCES

The complete list of references for this chapter is available in the e-book at www.expertconsult.com.
 See inside cover for registration details.

SUGGESTED REFERENCES

Chambers, S.M., Fasano, C.A., Papapetrou, E.P., et al., 2009. Highly efficient neural conversion of human ES and iPS cells by dual inhibition of SMAD signaling. Nat. Biotechnol. 27 (3), 275–280.

Huang, L., Wong, S., Snyder, E.Y., et al., 2014. Human neural stem cells rapidly ameliorate symptomatic inflammation in early-stage ischemic-reperfusion cerebral injury. Stem Cell Res. Ther. 5 (6), 129.

Imitola, J., Raddassi, K., Park, K.I., et al., 2004. Directed migration of neural stem cells to sites of CNS injury by the stromal cell-derived factor 1alpha/CXC chemokine receptor 4 pathway. Proc. Natl. Acad. Sci. U.S.A. 101 (52), 18117–18122.

Lee, J.P., Jeyakumar, M., Gonzalez, R., et al., 2007. Stem cells act through multiple mechanisms to benefit mice with neurodegenerative metabolic disease. Nat. Med. 13, 439–447.

Lee, J.P., Tsai, D.J., In Park, K., et al., 2009. The dynamics of long-term transgene expression in engrafted neural stem cells. J. Comp. Neurol. 515 (1), 83–92.

Reubinoff, B.E., Itsykson, P., Turetsky, T., et al., 2001. Neural progenitors from human embryonic stem cells. Nat. Biotechnol. 19, 1134–1140.

Snyder, E.Y., Flax, J.D., 1995. Transplantation of neural progenitor and stem-like cells as a strategy for gene therapy and repair of neurodegenerative diseases. Ment. Retard. Dev. Disabil. Res. Rev. 1, 27–38.

Takahashi, K., Yamanaka, S., 2006. Induction of pluripotent stem cells from mouse embryonic and adult fibroblast cultures by defined factors. Cell 126, 663–676.

Taylor, R.M., Lee, J.P., Palacino, J.J., et al., 2006. Intrinsic resistance of neural stem cells to toxic metabolites may make them well suited for cell non-autonomous disorders: evidence from a mouse model of Krabbe leukodystrophy. J. Neurochem. 97 (6), 1585–1599.

Yandava, B.D., Billinghurst, L.L., Snyder, E.Y., 1999. "Global" cell replacement is feasible via neural stem cell transplantation: evidence from the dysmyelinated shiverer mouse brain. Proc. Natl. Acad. Sci. U.S.A. 96 (12), 7029–7034.

16 Cellular and Animal Models of Neurologic Disease

Sampathkumar Rangasamy, Mohan J. Narayanan, Isabelle Schrauwen,
Alysson R. Muotri, and Vinodh Narayanan

INTRODUCTION

Animal models of neurologic disease have played a crucial role in improving our understanding of disease pathology and biological mechanisms, and in the development of treatment approaches. This is true for acquired disorders (such as traumatic injury to the brain or spinal cord, infection or immune-mediated attacks on the nervous system, and vascular lesions) as well as genetic disorders. In this chapter, we review selected topics that pertain to the use of animal and cellular models specifically of *genetic* neurologic disease. We start with a discussion of spontaneously occurring mutations (e.g., mouse models of leukodystrophies) and then move to genetically engineered mouse models. We provide an overview of transgenic mouse technology used to overexpress genes of interest, to "knock out" specific target genes, to "knock in" specific mutations, and to introduce mutations in a tissue-specific and developmental age–specific manner (conditional alleles). We then discuss the latest methods for gene editing (CRISPR-Cas9 RNA-editing technology) for introducing mutations at specifically targeted locations. Finally, we turn to the use of cellular model systems derived from mutant animals and the use of patient-derived stem cells, again for improved understanding of biology and as tools in large-scale compound screens in searches for novel therapeutic agents.

SPONTANEOUSLY OCCURRING MUTANT ANIMALS

Although mice are probably the most frequently used animals when it comes to modeling human disease, there are other species that have played a key role in the understanding of specific neurologic disorders. Examples include American Quarter Horses with hyperkalemic periodic paralysis, and Irish wolfhounds with hyperekplexia or startle disease. In these cases, parallel studies in humans and in mutant animals have resulted in an improved understanding of the role of sodium channels or glycinergic synaptic transmission, respectively, in these disorders.

The organisms most often used for the study of early development are the fruit fly, *Drosophila melanogaster,* and the roundworm, *Caenorhabditis elegans.* Short generation time; the ease with which large numbers of organisms can be generated, maintained, and studied; and methods for selection of mutations based on specific morphologic or behavioral phenotypes made these ideal organisms for genetic studies. Phenotype-driven screens for mutations allowed for the discovery of many genes that were involved in the determination of the body plan (e.g., segmentation genes and homeobox genes), specific aspects of neural development (e.g., structure of the eye, axon pathfinding, dendrite growth, muscle and nerve development, and learning and memory), regulation of growth and size, and genes encoding families of ion channels. In fact, the unusual and interesting names for many genes important in neural development, including "dunce," "shaker," "numb," "big brain," "roundabout," "commissureless," and "inebriated," come from studies in mutant *Drosophila.*

An example of studies in *Drosophila* that were critical to the advancement of our understanding of human disease pathogenesis relates to tuberous sclerosis complex (TSC). Linkage studies in families with TSC led to the identification of the *TSC1* and *TSC2* genes, but the function of the encoded proteins was not clear. Deletion of these genes in mice by gene targeting recapitulated the tumor suppressor function of the *TSC* genes. The breakthrough came with the study of *Drosophila* mutants with altered insulin signaling and a disordered cellular growth phenotype (Pan et al., 2004). In a genetic screen for mutants affecting the structure of the *Drosophila* compound eye, several lines were isolated with enlarged ommatidia, of normal structure, but with enlarged cells. These were shown to be allelic to a previously identified mutant, *gigas.* Cloning of the *gigas* gene showed that it was homologous to the human *TSC2* gene. A series of studies of *Drosophila Tsc1* and *Tsc2* mutants were critical in placing the TSC1-TSC2 complex downstream of AKT/PKB and upstream of mTOR in a critical cell growth pathway.

Christiane Nusslein-Volhard, who shared the 1995 Nobel Prize in Physiology and Medicine with Edward B. Lewis and Eric F. Wieschaus for their "discoveries concerning genetic control of early embryonic development," transitioned from studies in *Drosophila* to zebrafish *(Danio rerio)* to see if her ideas applied to vertebrate development (Nobel lecture, December 8, 1995). With the advances in methods of genetic engineering (described later in section "Genome Engineering Using CRISPR-Cas9 Technology"), zebrafish have become a very useful system in which to model human disorders affecting many organ systems, including the nervous system, and a variety of disorders (Kabashi et al., 2010).

A large number of naturally occurring mouse mutants have been described over the years.

The shiverer *(shi)* mouse was first reported as a naturally occurring mutant in 1973, and its shivering phenotype was shown to be an autosomal recessive trait. Shiverer mice develop a generalized tremor (shiver) during activity by 14 days of age. Tonic seizures develop by 30 days and death usually occurs by 50 to 100 days. There is a severe abnormality of central myelin, with abnormal structure (fewer layers of myelin lamellae and absent major dense line) ascribed to a lack of the myelin basic protein (MBP). In one of the earliest successes of gene therapy in mice, introduction of a wild-type *Mbp* transgene into the shiverer resulted in an almost complete rescue of the phenotype.

Although there are no known human diseases caused by mutation of the *Mbp* gene, the shiverer remains a useful model system for studying novel therapies (transplantation of oligodendrocytes, oligodendrocyte precursors, or stem cells) for dysmyelinating disorders.

Twitcher *(twi)* is a model for human autosomal recessive Krabbe disease or globoid cell leukodystrophy, caused by deficiency of galactosylceramidase (GALC). Twitcher mice are

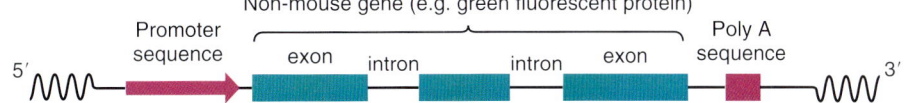

Figure 16-1. Diagram of a DNA construct for transgenic mice. The template for a simple transgenic construct includes (1) a promoter sequence (5′ regulatory sequences) that drives the expression of transgene, (2) a coding sequence (e.g., green fluorescent protein) with introns and exons, and (3) a polyadenylation signal sequence (3′ regulatory sequences) for the stability of mRNA. Transgenic DNA constructs are prepared and cloned into a vector for propagation. The transgene is cut out by appropriate restriction enzymes in linear form before injecting into mouse eggs.

normal at birth, but become hypoactive by 15 to 20 days; by 3 weeks there is rapid deterioration of motor function, with weight loss, progressive weakness, paralysis of hind limbs, and death by 3 months. Pathologic studies show a severe lack of myelin, astrocytic gliosis, and infiltration with macrophages containing periodic acid-Schiff–positive material (globoid cells). Surprisingly, the major substrate of GALC, galactosylceramide, does not accumulate within the brain. There is a significant accumulation of galactosylsphingosine (psychosine), also a substrate for GALC, in brain and other tissues. It is thought that psychosine is cytotoxic and leads to degeneration of oligodendrocytes, leading to myelin degradation. The twitcher mouse has been useful for testing a variety of therapeutic approaches for the leukodystrophies such as bone marrow transplantation or transgenic rescue.

GENETICALLY ENGINEERED MOUSE MODELS

Models generated by expressing selected genes integrated into the mouse genome (transgenic mice), or by replacing endogenous loci with altered genes (gene targeting) have been useful for studies in neural development and neurologic disease (Joyner, 2000; Arbeit, 2001).

Transgenic Mice

Animals that carry a foreign gene, such as the one encoding the jellyfish green fluorescent protein (GFP), in their genome are called transgenic animals. The expression of the transgene is usually controlled by promoters or enhancers included as part of the transgene, or by regulatory elements that are located within the integration site. Transgenes such as GFP are useful for tagging and tracing cells expressing the transgene. The transgenic approach is also useful to model a gain-of-function phenotype by overexpression of the gene (e.g., expression of a mutant Huntington disease allele), to examine the effect of gene copy number, to study the function and specificity of gene regulatory elements (promoters and enhancers), or even to detect and clone regulatory elements (enhancer trap methods). A particularly useful application of this technology is the generation of transgenic mice expressing Cre recombinase under the control of a promoter that directs expression of Cre in specific tissues at specific developmental ages. Such animals are used in the production of conditional knock-out animals by breeding with "floxed" animals (as described in the next section).

Key steps in the generation of transgenic mice are as follows: (1) construction and purification of the transgene vector DNA, which includes certain important elements; (2) collection of fertilized mouse eggs (zygote) within 12 hours of fertilization, before fusion of the male and female pronuclei; (3) microinjection of transgene DNA into the male pronucleus of the fertilized egg; (4) implantation of microinjected zygotes into a pseudopregnant host female mouse; (5) genotyping and analysis to detect transgene expression in the newborn pups; (6) comparison and selection of different transgenic lines for study (which may differ by copy number of transgenes and integration site).

The transgene DNA construct is similar to expression vectors used for protein expression in mammalian cells. It typically contains a 5′ region including a promoter or enhancer; the coding sequence for the gene of interest, which may include short introns; and a 3′ region that includes a polyadenylation signal for the encoded mRNA (Figure 16-1).

The 5′ region including the promoter is a crucial part of the transgene, as it regulates the spatial and temporal pattern of transgene expression. Promoter–enhancer combinations from ubiquitously expressed genes drive transgene expression in all the cells. These include the metallothionein, myosin heavy chain (MHC) class I, RNA polymerase II, or beta-actin promoters. Cell type or tissue-specific transgene expression can be driven by using promoter–enhancer elements derived from genes expressed in select tissues and cell types. Examples include the myosin light chain (MLC), or MHC promoter to direct expression in the heart, nestin promoter to drive expression in the brain, and glial fibrillary acidic protein (GFAP) promoter to direct expression in astrocytes.

The coding region may be a complementary DNA (cDNA) corresponding to a specific RNA isoform of a gene of interest, or include an entire gene with exons and introns. In cases where the intent of the experiment is to characterize the 5′ region (promoter and enhancer sequences), the coding region might consist only of a reporter gene. In other cases, a reporter gene may be included in addition to a distinct transgene of interest, to track cells in which the transgene is expressed. Commonly used reporters include the bacterial *lacZ* gene encoding β-galactosidase, and GFP and its variants red fluorescent protein (RFP), cyan fluorescent protein (CFP), and yellow fluorescent protein (YFP). The fluorescent reporters having different spectral properties are used in transgenic mice models for identification of cell types, colocalization experiments, electrophysiological studies on specific cell populations in the brain, and high-resolution studies for detailed measures of dendritic spine density, dendrite width, and axonal length. The 3′ region typically includes transcription termination signals and polyadenylation signals, which confer mRNA stability.

In spite of the optimal design of a transgenic expression vector, there are often unexpected effects related to sequences at the integration site—these may counter the selected promoter and enhancer elements. Integration might in fact disrupt some other critical genes resulting in a novel phenotype. In addition, transgene expression during early development may cause untoward defects and may not allow the planned studies in older animals. Inducible transgenes were devised to circumvent some of these problems. In such a system, transgene expression is regulated by an exogenous compound administered to the animal.

The tet-operon–repressor bitransgenic system, the ecdysone receptor, the estrogen receptor (ER) ligand–binding domain, the progesterone receptor, and the lac and GAL4 systems have been used to control gene expression in transgenic mice. One transgene expresses a tetracycline operon transactivator or hormone receptor (ER, mutated ER, ecdysone receptor, and progesterone receptor) under control of a selected promoter. A second transgene is engineered that contains a promoter that is regulated by the appropriate transactivator or hormone receptor (which binds to DNA). In such animals, drug treatment (with tetracycline, estrogen, tamoxifen, and ecdysone) results in suppression or activation of the other transgene of interest.

Once a transgenic expression construct is created and validated, it is purified and a known concentration of DNA is injected as a linear piece of DNA into the male pronucleus (larger of the two pronuclei) of newly fertilized eggs (zygotes) (Figure 16-3). Injection before fusion of the male and female pronuclei greatly increases the rate of transgene integration. Random insertion of the transgenic DNA will occur into the genome of the embryo at the one-cell stage. The integrated transgene will generally be present in all cell types of the developing embryo and be transmitted through the germline. Microinjected zygotes are then implanted into the oviduct of pseudopregnant females, resulting in birth of both wild-type and transgenic founder mice, each of which represents the first generation of a new line of mice. Each transgenic line has to be genotyped, and expression of the transgene at the protein level has to be confirmed.

Knock-out and Knock-in Mice

The ability to generate "designer mice" in which specific genes are altered was a result of several key discoveries: (1) isolation of pluripotent mouse embryonic stem cells (ES cells), (2) the generation of transgenic chimeric by mice introducing ES cells into host blastocysts, (3) the ability to alter the genome of ES cells by homologous recombination, and (4) the ability to introduce genetically altered ES cells into blastocysts and transmit such genetic modifications through the germline (Capecchi, 2005).

ES cells are derived from the inner cell mass of a blastocyst-stage mouse embryo. Cells are maintained in appropriate culture conditions to propagate them in an undifferentiated, diploid state. Male (40, XY) ES cells are now available from a number of different mouse strains. As depicted in Figure 16-4, ES cells of a specific genotype (A, depicted by dark color) are injected into host embryos (blastocysts) of a different strain (typically a different coat color). These modified embryos are implanted into pseudopregnant surrogate females. Chimeric offspring (composite coat color) often have different compositions (host genotype or modified ES cell genotype) in their germ cells. Chimeras are crossed with wild-type animals and offspring genotyped for transmission of the ES cell genotype. These founder animals can then be bred to homozygosity for phenotypic studies.

Homologous recombination was shown to occur in mammalian cells, and used to introduce mutations into a specifically targeted location of a gene in ES cells. These genetically modified ES cells then could be used to produce chimeric mice, as described earlier. If the intention was to create a null mutant (one in which the encoded protein is not expressed), then we would "knock out" the corresponding gene. If the intention is to reproduce a missense mutation, then one would "knock in" that particular mutation.

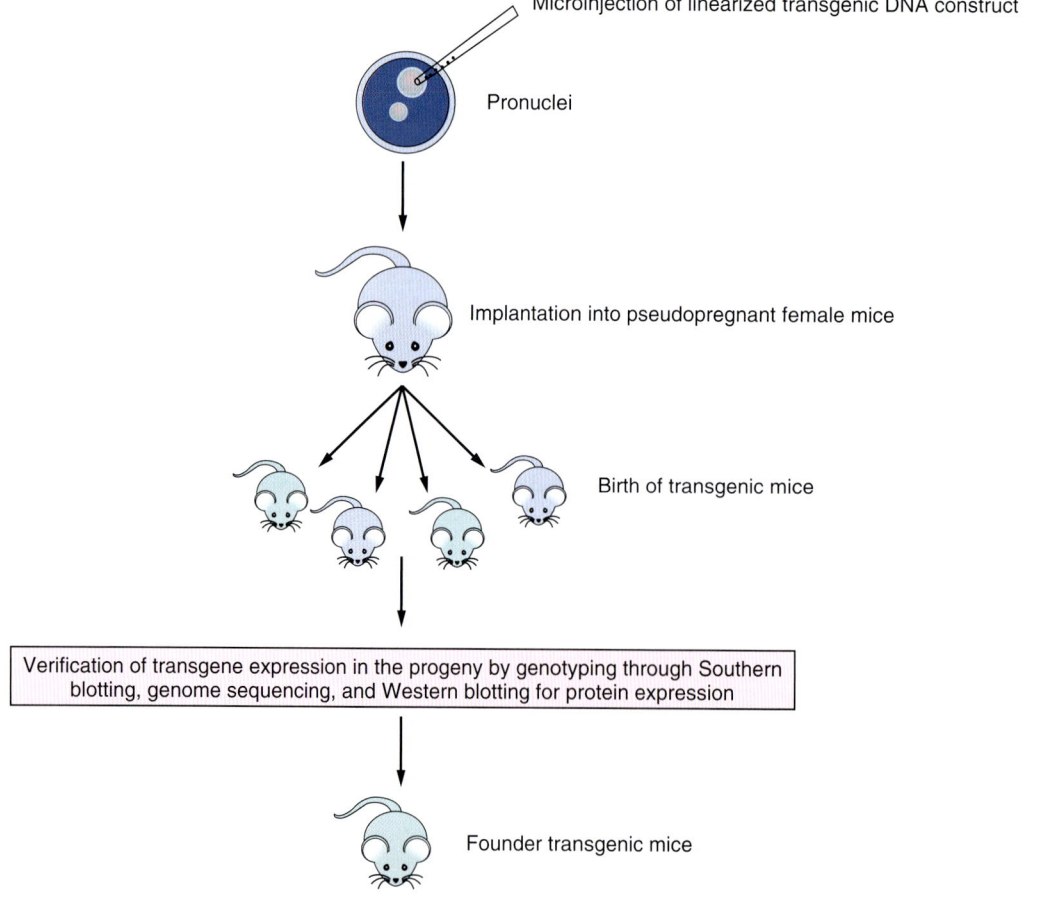

Figure 16-3. Outline of transgenic mice production through transgene microinjection. A transgenic linear DNA construct is physically microinjected into a male pronucleus of newly fertilized egg. Microinjected eggs are transplanted into the oviduct of a pseudopregnant female host. Random insertion of the transgenic DNA will result in birth of transgenic founder mice.

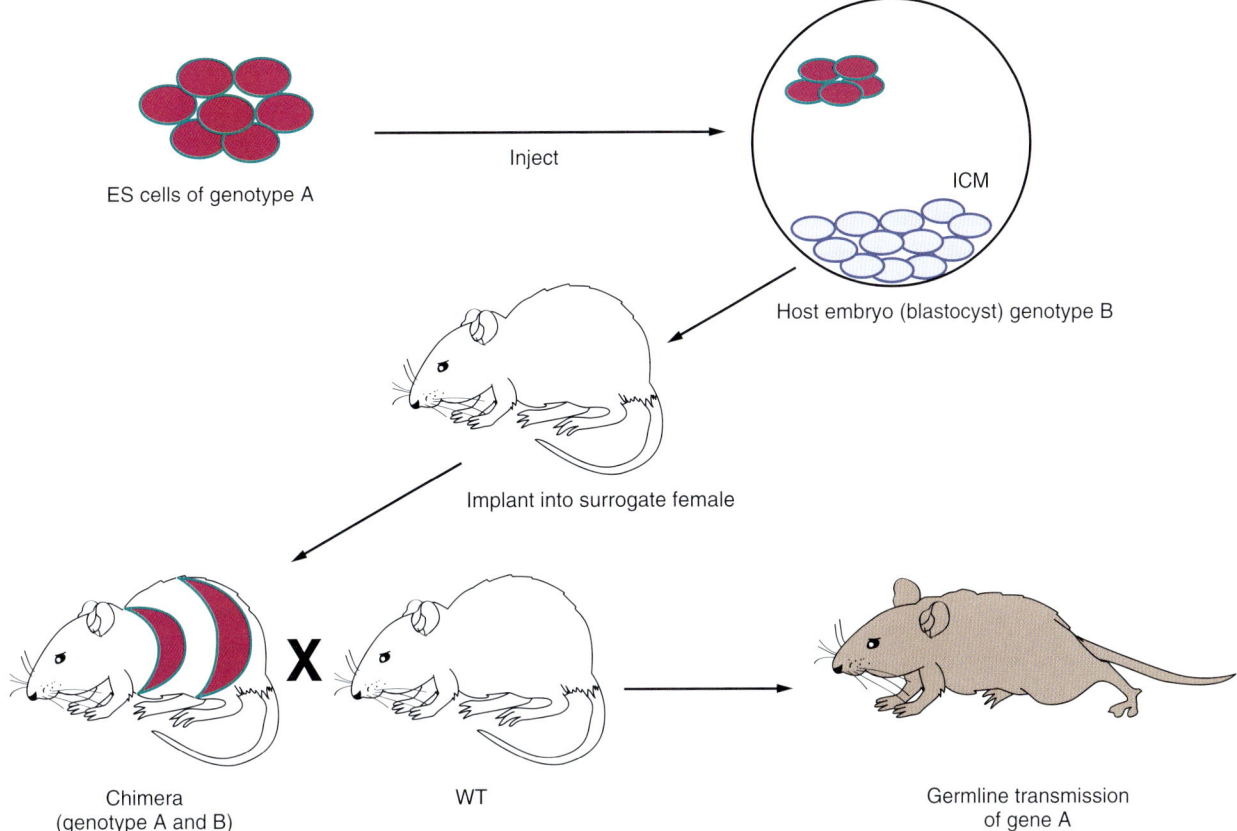

Figure 16-4. **Generation of embryonic stem (ES) cell–derived chimeras.** Cartoon depicting the injection of ES cells of a specific genotype (A) into host blastocyst followed by implantation into a pseudopregnant host. Chimeric offspring are often detected based on coat color. Chimeras are crossed with wild-type animals and offspring are tested for germline transmission of the desired genotype (A). Founder mice are then maintained in the desired genetic background by breeding.

Null mutations are frequently created by eliminating one or more critical exons of a gene. An important element of experimental design is to consider the multiple RNA molecules that may be generated from the gene of interest by alternative splicing, and making sure that eliminating the targeted exon(s) will in fact produce the desired result, and not simply result in a different transcript encoding a different protein isoform.

The first step in creating a gene-targeting vector is the cloning of a segment of mouse genomic DNA containing the targeted exon. This exon is then replaced by a positive selection marker; a commonly used marker is an expression cassette that confers neomycin resistance. As shown in Figure 16-5A, the targeting vector contains long segments (typically longer than 1 kbp) of homologous DNA flanking the targeted site, with the positive selection marker cassette in place of the targeted exon. The targeting vector (linearized DNA) is then electroporated into ES cells. The positive selection marker can be used to select for events in which the targeting vector has integrated into the ES cell genome, but this does not differentiate between random integration and homologous recombination events. Random integration of the targeting vector DNA is a much more frequent event than homologous recombination. A negative selection marker can be included in the vector, outside of the regions of homology, for selection against random integration events. ES cell clones that survive the selection pressure (cultured in the presence of a neomycin analog, for instance) can be expanded, and split for genotyping and storage. DNA is extracted from individual ES cell clones and tested to determine whether only the desired targeting event has occurred, or whether random integration of the transgene has occurred. This is frequently done by PCR-based assays that detect unique DNA fragments that result from proper recombination on the 5'- side and the 3'- side of the targeted exon.

The cartoon in Figure 16-5 shows several possible targeting vectors. When the targeted exon is either replaced or disrupted by a positive selection cassette (see Figure 16-5A), the result of homologous recombination is usually a null allele ("knockout") from which no corresponding protein is made. When the targeting vector is synthesized to include a specific point mutation inserted into the targeted exon, with the positive selection marker in close proximity, flanked by regions of sequence homology, the result is a "knock-in" of that specific point mutation (Figure 16-5B).

In some cases, a complete knock-out of the gene of interest (null allele) may be lethal during embryogenesis, making it impossible to study the effect of this mutation in adult animals. A system, called conditional gene targeting, that has adapted site-specific recombinases from bacteria gets around this problem. Two commonly used recombinase systems are the Cre-Lox system and the Flp-Frt system. The Cre recombinase, a protein encoded by a bacteriophage, recognizes a specific 34-bp *lox* sequence and catalyzes recombination between two *lox* sites. Cre-mediated recombination between two directly repeated *lox* sites (oriented in the same direction) results in excision of the intervening DNA (deletion), whereas recombination between two inverted lox sites causes inversion of the intervening DNA segment. If the targeting vector is designed to introduce *lox* sites flanking a specific exon, the

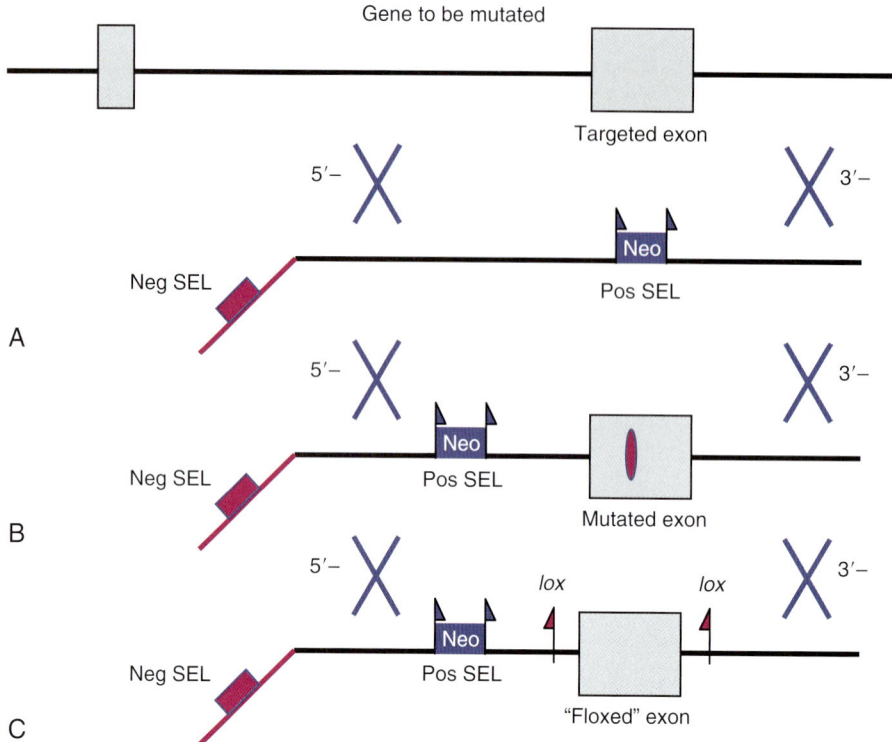

Figure 16-5. Homologous recombination strategies. The gene to be targeted for mutation is diagrammed at the top. **A,** Targeting vector designed to replace the targeted exon with a selection marker (Neo = neomycin resistance expression cassette with flanking Frt sites, denoted by blue "flags"). 5′ and 3′ stretches of homologous DNA favoring recombination are indicated. A negative selection marker is shown located outside of the segments of homologous DNA. **B,** Targeting vector designed to "knock in" a point mutation into the targeted exon. **C,** Targeting vector designed to generate a "floxed" allele. Lox sites flanking the targeted exon are indicated as red "flags." SEL, selection.

result of homologous recombination is a "floxed" allele (Figure 16-5C). Transgenic mice generated in which these "floxed" alleles are transmitted through the germline are called "floxed" mice, and usually have no abnormal phenotype. A number of transgenic mice are readily available in which Cre recombinase is expressed in restricted cell populations at specific ages, dictated by the promoter driving Cre expression. These include Cre expressed ubiquitously all during development, in specific tissues (liver, immune cells, and nerve tissue), in specific regions of the brain (cerebellum, hypothalamus, and cortex), and during specific developmental stages. There are also transgenic mice in which Cre expression is inducible. When "floxed" mice are crossed with a Cre-expressing mouse, offspring containing both alleles will have the targeted allele excised in a spatially and temporally restricted manner. The availability of a large number of mice bearing "floxed" alleles, and a variety of Cre-expressing transgenic mice has greatly facilitated the study of gene function in specific cell populations within the brain.

Genome Engineering Using CRISPR-Cas9 Technology

Clustered regularly interspaced palindromic repeats (CRISPR)–associated Cas9 is a recently developed genome-editing technology, and shows promise to be a highly efficient system for manipulating the genome sequence of living cells and organisms (Hsu et al., 2014). Advancement of CRISPR technology allows researchers to "edit" the gene (DNA) sequence on a chromosome in cells and tissues more quickly and precisely. The basic idea is to introduce double-strand breaks in a targeted fashion in the genome of a cell, which is then repaired using endogenous cellular machinery to produce a mutation.

This technology allows a wide range of biological and disease modeling applications, including the modeling or rescue of monogenic disorders and more complex neurologic disorders such as autism. The CRISPR-Cas9 system was first observed in unicellular organisms (archaea and bacteria) as a group of DNA short sequence repeats of 20 bp, which played an important role in bacterial acquired immunity against viral/phage infections. Bacteria, upon a viral infection, can precisely incorporate the viral DNA as short sequence repeats, separated by a short palindromic repeat into a region of its genome, designated as CRISPR. In subsequent infections, these sequences will be transcribed as small RNAs called CRISPR targeting RNA (crRNA), which hybridizes to the target DNA of virus. This in turn activates and guides a multifunctional endonuclease (Cas9) to cleave the hybridized viral DNA.

Because of its conceptual simplicity, a modified version of CRSIPR-Cas9 is swiftly becoming the method of choice for genome engineering in living systems. Compared with previous methods of genome editing, such as zinc-finger nucleases (ZFNs) and transcription activator–like effector nucleases (TALENs), which depend on protein–DNA interactions instead of DNA–RNA interactions, this system offers several advantages, including target design simplicity, target efficiency, and the possibility of high-throughput screening and multiplexing. CRISPR-Cas9 consists of a Cas endonuclease that is directed to cleave a target sequence by a single-guide RNA (sgRNA) when followed by a 5′- protospacer-adjacent motif (PAM) in a eukaryotic cell. The sgRNA is a 100-nucleotide molecule formed by fusion of a CRISPR RNA (crRNA) with a transactivating CRISPR RNA (tracrRNA). After Cas9 cuts the double-stranded target DNA, three to four nucleotides upstream of the PAM sequence, two different repairing pathways can be activated, which can be selected based on the desired genome editing: nonhomologous end-joining (NHEJ) and homology-directed repair (HDR). NHEJ can lead to a "loss of function" by introducing insertion/deletion mutations (indels) of various lengths, which in turn can disrupt the reading frame of target genes or the binding sites of *trans*-acting factors in promoters or enhancers. HDR-mediated repair can be used to modify the gene of interest by introducing specific point mutations or other desired sequences through recombination of the target locus with exogenously supplied DNA donor templates (Figure 16-7A).

The CRISPR-Cas9 system has a wide variety of applications and has been used for the introduction of single point mutations, deletions, or insertions in a particular target gene or transcriptional regulator sequences, either as a knock-in or knock-out models. Other applications of CRISPR-Cas9 include the simultaneous activation of multiple endogenous genes by transcriptional activation (CRISPR-on), the imaging of genomic loci, and epigenetic modification.

Cas9-mediated genome editing has enabled an accelerated generation of transgenic and cellular models. CRISPR-Cas9 can be used to genome-edit primary, immortalized, human induced pluripotent stem cells (iPSCs) and other cells by the transfection of plasmids carrying Cas9 and the appropriately designed sgRNA. There are several advantages to this technology, including the multiplexing ability that allows the study of polygenic disease models and the ability to correct existing mutations in patient-derived cell lines. A major advantage of CRISPR-Cas9 is that it is not limited to mutagenesis in ES cells for the generation of knock-out or knock-in animal models. The Cas9 protein and transcribed sgRNA can be directly injected into fertilized zygotes, bypassing the typical ES cell targeting stage, allowing the fast generation of mutant animals.

Although CRISPR-Cas9 is an easy and efficient strategy for the generation of genetically modified cells, there are some limitations. There are specific sequence limitations on the targeting range of sgRNAs and a careful design is required that is both target specific and shows limited off-target effects. Off-target cleavage is a major concern in CRISPR-Cas9, as several studies show that RNA-guided Cas9 nuclease cleaves genomic DNA sequences containing several mismatches to the guide strand. Several methods have been developed to minimize these off-target effects. A promising study showed that a double-nicking strategy using the Cas9 nickase mutant with paired guide RNAs (Figure 16-7B) has shown efficient genome modification with minimal off-target effects. CRISPR-Cas9 is thus a versatile genome-editing technology that can be used to study and model both monogenic and polygenic disorders and shows potential for the development of therapeutic genome-editing techniques.

CELLULAR MODEL SYSTEMS: CELL LINES AND PRIMARY NEURONAL CULTURES

Once a specifically targeted transgenic mouse model has been created, the first step is to validate its gene structure and ensure that the mutant allele is indeed expressed as designed. Once this is done, the next step is to phenotype the animals at several levels. This includes measurement of animal growth and survival, appearance of neurologic symptoms (such as seizures or ataxia), studies of strength and coordination, detailed behavioral analysis, tests of learning and memory, tests of social behavior, histopathological studies of various tissues and brain regions, fine structure analysis of neurons from different brain regions, electrophysiological studies in tissue sections or dissociated cells, and studies of gene and

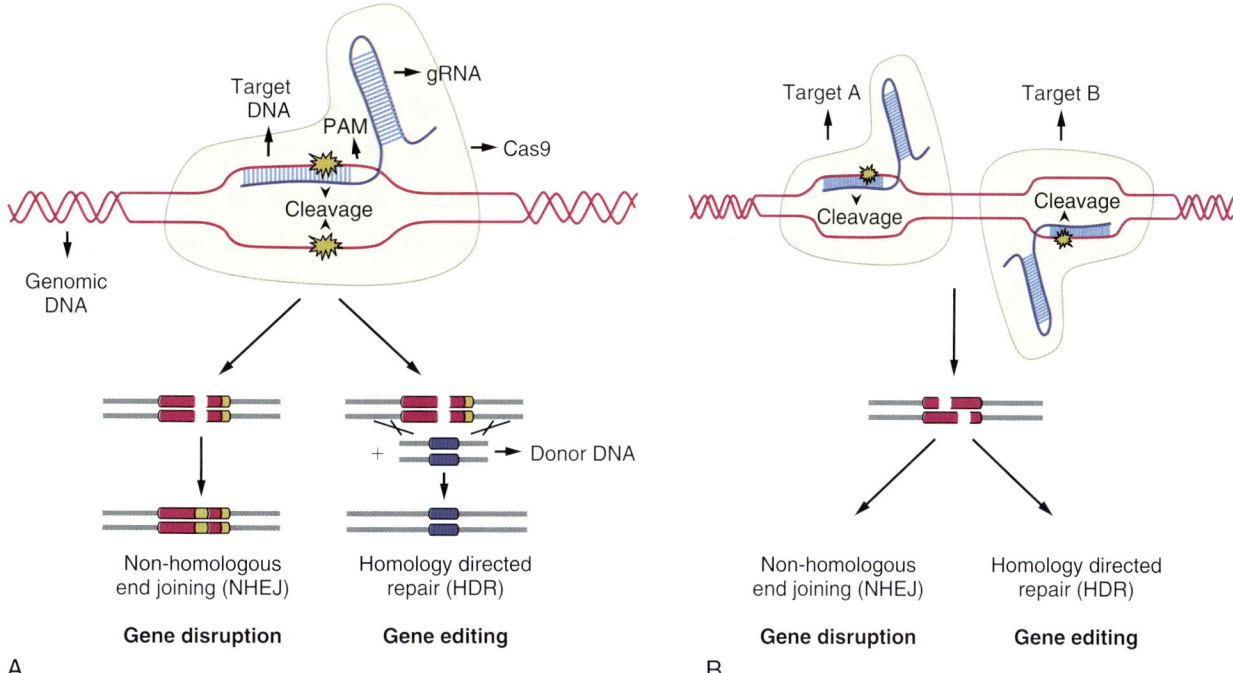

Figure 16-7. CRISPR-Cas9–mediated targeted DNA mutation. **A,** Wild-type Cas9 cleaves double-stranded DNA 3 to 4 bp upstream of the 5′-protospacer-adjacent motif (PAM) sequence, activating double-strand break (DSB) repair machinery. In the absence of a homologous repair donor, single DSBs generated by CRISPR-Cas9 are repaired through the error-prone nonhomologous end-joining (NHEJ), which results in insertion or deletion (indel) mutations, disrupting the target sequence. Alternatively, precise mutations and knock-ins can be made by providing a homologous repair template (single or double stranded) through the homology-directed repair (HDR) pathway. **B,** Double nicking mediates genome editing with improved specificity: a D10A mutant nickase version of Cas9 makes a site-specific single-strand nick. Two different guide RNA (gRNA) can be used to introduce breaks, which can be repaired through HDR or NHEJ.

protein expression. Preclinical trials of a small number of candidate compounds are possible in such animals, but it is not practical to do large-scale therapeutic screens of hundreds or thousands of compounds using in vivo systems.

One attractive option for large-scale compound screens involves use of cultured cells isolated from genetically engineered mice. Cell lines from most tissues can be established and used for biological studies and therapeutic screens. These include ES cells, which in turn can be differentiated into any desired cell type. For the study of neurologic disease, one could use neuronal cultures prepared from specific mouse brain regions such as the cortex, hippocampus, or cerebellum following established protocols.

An example of the successful use of a genetically engineered mouse model is in the identification of compounds that may potentially be used to treat Angelman syndrome, caused by mutation of the *Ube3A* gene. A transgenic Ube3a-YFP (yellow fluorescent protein) knock-in mouse model has been developed as a reporter of *Ube3a* gene imprinting. In cultured embryonic cortical neurons prepared from these mice, Ube3a-YFP expression was suppressed when Ube3a-YFP was *paternally* inherited (Ube3a$^{m+/pYFP}$), but was expressed when Ube3a-YFP was *maternally* inherited (Ube3a$^{mYFP/p+}$). Neurons from Ube3a$^{m+/pYFP}$ animals were used to screen for drugs that upregulated YFP fluorescence, as a marker of activation of the imprinted allele. Topoisomerase inhibitors (such as topotecan) were found to unsilence the paternal *Ube3a* allele. Topotecan was then tested in an AS mouse (maternally derived Ube3a-null allele) both in primary neuronal cultures and in vivo. Topotecan unsilenced and upregulated expression of the paternal *Ube3a* allele in several regions of the nervous system, suggesting that these were potential therapeutic agents for treatment of AS (Huang et al., 2011).

Using well-characterized mutant and wild-type cultures allows for neuronal phenotypic and molecular comparisons. Features such as neuronal size, axon growth, dendrite branching, spine structure, and even development of functional synapses can be studied in vitro. These in vitro phenotypes may replicate what is seen in vivo, but are now amenable to manipulation by gene transfection or siRNA-mediated knockdown. For instance, using cultures prepared from a "floxed" animal, one can study the cellular phenotype of eliminating the targeted gene in vitro by transfection with a Cre expression vector.

As with any system, the use of primary cultures of neurons from genetically engineered mice has certain limitations. Neurons have a limited lifespan in vitro. If the focus is on neurons from a small brain region (hypothalamus or brainstem), then the number of cells that can be isolated from a single animal may be small, and this may limit the type of experiments that can be done. In some cases where cultures are relatively homogeneous (cerebellar granule neurons, for instance), one could pool together cell preparations from several genotypically identical animals for large-scale high-throughput screens (HTS).

When using primary neuronal cultures in an HTS compound screen, it is important to have a phenotypic biomarker that can be adapted to an HTS system (An and Tolliday, 2010). With a focus on searching for novel small-molecule therapies for Rett syndrome (RTT), such an approach has been used in the development of an HTS assay using cultured hippocampal and cerebellar granule neurons from MeCP2 mutant animals. In the MeCP2 A140V knock-in mutant model for X-linked mental retardation, we demonstrated increased cell packing density in various brain regions, a reduction in neuronal size, and reduction in dendrite branching. Quantification and comparison of soma size in cultured hippocampal neurons from MeCP2 A140V and wild-type mice revealed that soma size was significantly reduced in mutant hippocampal neurons compared with wild type. The definition of neuronal size as a quantifiable cellular phenotype supports its uses as a biomarker in the development of a high throughput in vitro assay to screen for compounds that rescue the small neuronal phenotype ("phenotypic assay"). This offers a novel approach to identification of potential small-molecule drugs for treating RTT and other neurodevelopmental disorders.

HTS rely on the development of an assay that uses a simple and quantifiable phenotypic or biochemical marker. Assays are standardized in traditional laboratory bench-top experiments, and then miniaturized and automated for 96-, 384-, or 1536-well microplate formats. New technologies such as high-throughput, high-content image analysis enable research labs to develop miniaturized cell-based assays to screen tens of thousands of compounds per day. Well-designed secondary and tertiary screens are used to validate the hits detected in the primary screen. For instance, for studies in MeCP2 mutant animals, cerebellar granule neurons prepared from male mutant and wild-type animals were initially used. As the vast majority of patients with RTT are female, however, any potential therapeutic agent has to be tested in females. Female transgenic mice are engineered to carry the mutant *MeCP2* gene on the maternal X-chromosome and a transgene for GFP on the paternal X-chromosome (wild-type MeCP2 sequence). Because of X-inactivation, neurons expressing the wild-type *MeCP2* allele from the paternal X-chromosome are GFP(+) and fluorescent, whereas neurons expressing the mutant *MeCP2* allele are GFP(−). Such a system permits the identification of compounds that rescue the size phenotype in mutant neurons, without adversely affecting wild-type neurons. Tertiary screens in culture might include a different phenotype (dendrite growth and branching), leading to tests in patient-derived iPSCs (as described in the next section). Eventually, a small number of selected compounds from such in vitro screens can be tested in genetically engineered animal models in vivo, with appropriate biological or behavioral phenotypic markers.

Recent advances in HTS have enabled automation in every step of the assay. Integration of robotic systems for plate handling, cell loading in microwell plates, live cell fluorescence image capture, microelectrode arrays for electrophysiological phenotypes, and high-content data analysis has significantly increased the efficiency and shortened time for HTS. HTS approaches in primary cortical neuronal cultures have been utilized to identify small-molecule modulators of synaptic proteins that alter neurotransmission, potentially useful as a novel therapeutic strategy for psychiatric and neurologic disorders. HTS methods are already being used in primary neuronal cultures and cell lines to develop therapies for Huntington and Alzheimer disease. Availability of large compound libraries, sophisticated data acquisition and image analysis tools, and efficient HTS assays will result in rapid identification of potential therapies that can then be tested in secondary screens and preclinical animal models.

INDUCED PLURIPOTENT STEM CELLS: A NOVEL HUMAN CELL MODEL FOR NEUROLOGIC DISEASES

Pluripotent human embryonic stem cells (hESCs) have been isolated from early stage human embryos (blastocysts), can self-renew, and differentiate into various cell types, offering an unlimited source of cell types for research. By taking advantage of preimplantation genetic diagnosis, hESCs carrying mutations in specific genes known to cause human diseases, including cystic fibrosis, Huntington disease, Marfan syndrome, fragile X syndrome, and other monogenetic diseases, have been created. Reverse genetics can be used to generate hESC disease models by homologous recombination. Unfortunately, apart from the ethics and political concerns related to hESC line derivation, this strategy is also limited by the availability of human blastocysts and by the number of genes one can manipulate in hESCs. Moreover, complex disorders in which multiple genes are affected, or "sporadic" diseases such as autism spectrum disorders, schizophrenia, or amyotrophic lateral sclerosis, in which the genetic alteration is not known, cannot be modeled using reverse genetics in hESCs.

Reprogramming technology provides a possible solution to this problem as it allows the genomes of human individuals afflicted with neurologic disorders to be captured in a pluripotent stem cell line. Reprogramming of somatic cells to a pluripotent state by overexpression of specific genes was first accomplished using mouse embryonic fibroblasts. Four retroviral-mediated transcription factors, the octamer binding protein 4 (OCT4, also known as POU5F1), SOX2, Krüppel-like factor 4 (KLF4), and MYC, were sufficient to induce the expression of endogenous pluripotency genes in somatic cells. These reprogrammed cells were able to form embryoid bodies in vitro and teratomas in vivo, and contributed to several tissues in chimeric embryos when injected into mouse blastocysts. The report of human reprogrammed cells using the same set of transcriptional factors happened soon after. These cells, named iPSCs, can be derived from cells isolated from peripheral tissues of normal individuals or people affected from several conditions (Marchetto et al., 2010). Differentiation of human iPSCs allows for the recapitulation of brain development in-a-dish, providing a platform with greater accessibility to experimental manipulation and high-throughput assays for drug screening. Ideally, such an in vitro platform should maximize translational potential by recapitulating in vivo brain development and function as much as possible.

As with other models, the iPSC system also has important limitations. Although the iPSC models show great promise, their use in many cases is implicitly based on the assumption that they recapitulate neurodevelopmental milestones of a specified developmental maturity and neuroanatomical region in vitro. Current limitations include nonoptimized culture conditions and differentiation protocols, the intrinsic cellular variability (likely related to the nonoptimal conditions), and the choice of proper controls. Genome-editing technology is becoming a popular method to alleviate concerns about confounding clonal variation from reprogramming and differentiation techniques. Obviously, genome editing will work only where the genetic alterations are previously known. Finally, another big challenge for iPSC models is the validation of phenotypes observed in human neurons. Unquestionably, the iPSC technology still requires a series of optimization steps. Future work will help to answer how well human iPSCs match in vivo development, what level of developmental maturity is achieved after differentiation, and what specific neurodevelopmental processes and molecular mechanisms are preserved, providing a guide for future disease modeling in-a-dish systems. Nonetheless, even with all these caveats, the iPSC is already generating novel insights that should be seen with an open mind for novel perspectives.

INSIGHTS FROM INDUCED PLURIPOTENT STEM CELLS TO MODEL NEURODEVELOPMENTAL DISORDERS

The utility of iPSCs in the investigation of the functional consequences of mutations in the gene encoding the methyl-CpG-binding protein-2 (MeCP2) in neurons from patients with RTT has been demonstrated. Neurons derived from RTT-iPSCs

carrying different MeCP2 mutations showed several alterations compared with five healthy nonaffected individuals, such as decreased soma size, altered dendritic spine density, and reduced excitatory synapses (Kim et al., 2011). Defects in the number of glutamatergic synapses could be reversed using two candidate drugs, insulin growth factor 1 (IGF1) and gentamicin. IGF1 is considered to be a candidate for pharmacologic treatment of RTT and potentially other central nervous sytem (CNS) disorders in ongoing clinical trials. These observations bring valued information for RTT because they suggest that presymptomatic defects may represent novel biomarkers to be exploited as diagnostic tools and therapeutic targets.

Recently progress has been made toward analogous modeling of nonsyndromic autism in studies from a patient with a TRPC6 gene mutation. The biological impact of the gene mutation and its functional relationship to autism etiology were evaluated through several analyses using cortical neurons derived from iPSCs. Taken together, these findings suggest that TRPC6 is a novel predisposing gene for autism that may act in a multiple-hit model. This was the first study to use iPSC-derived human neurons to model nonsyndromic autism spectrum disorders and illustrate the potential of modeling genetically complex sporadic diseases using iPSCs.

Drug-screening platforms using iPSC-derived cell types require robust phenotypes and large numbers of target cells. Whereas most research has focused on neurons, the transition to an HTS platform has intrinsic challenges, mainly because iPSC neurons are particularly difficult to produce in a homogenous population and challenged to behave in the high-throughput format. Glial cells may also represent exciting novel therapeutic targets. Previous studies have established that astrocytes secrete signaling molecules that stimulate the formation and function of synapses. Thus it is likely that astrocytes also contribute to disease and could be an alternative cell type for some neurologic disorders. Independent of the cell type used, read outs such as cellular morphology can be measured using high-content imaging software, whereas biochemical and gene expression read outs could be valuable alternatives because of the simplicity of these assays.

IPSCs are now a valuable tool for the understanding of the fundamental molecular and cellular mechanisms underlying neurologic disorders. Moreover, they can nicely complement studies using other models, such as animals or postmortem brain tissues. The iPSC system has also the potential to speed and improve drug development, facilitating the identification of ineffective or unsafe drugs earlier in the development process. Human patient–derived iPSCs offer the opportunity for genetics-based personalized medicine, for both understanding disease specifics in a given patient and developing relevant individualized therapeutic strategies.

REFERENCES

The complete list of references for this chapter is available in the e-book at www.expertconsult.com.
See inside cover for registration details.

SELECTED REFERENCES

An, W.F., Tolliday, N., 2010. Cell-based assays for high-throughput screening. Mol. Biotechnol. 45 (2), 180–186.

Arbeit, J.M., 2001. Strategies, principles, and techniques using transgenic and knockout mouse models. In: Souba, W.W., Wilmore, D.W. (Eds.), Guide to Research Techniques in Neuroscience. Academic Press, New York, p. 175–191.

Capecchi, M.R., 2005. Gene targeting in mice: functional analysis of the mammalian genome for the twenty-first century. Nat. Rev. Genet. 6 (6), 507–512.

Hsu, P.D., Lander, E.S., Zhang, F., 2014. Development and applications of CRISPR-Cas9 for genome engineering. Cell 157 (6), 1262–1278.

Huang, H.S., Allen, J.A., Mabb, A.M., et al., 2011. Topoisomerase inhibitors unsilence the dormant allele of Ube3a in neurons. Nature 481 (7380), 185–189.

Joyner, A.L. (Ed.), 2000. In: Hames, B.D. (Ed.), Gene Targeting: A Practical Approach, second ed. Practical Approach Series, series. Oxford University Press, Oxford.

Kabashi, E., Champagne, N., Brustein, E., et al., 2010. In the swim of things: recent insights to neurogenetic disorders from zebrafish. Trends Genet. 26 (8), 373–381.

Kim, K.Y., Hysolli, E., Park, I.H., 2011. Neuronal maturation defect in induced pluripotent stem cells from patients with Rett syndrome. Proc. Natl. Acad. Sci. U.S.A. 108 (34), 14169–14174.

Marchetto, M.C., Winner, B., Gage, F.H., 2010. Pluripotent stem cells in neurodegenerative and neurodevelopmental diseases. Hum. Mol. Genet. 19 (R1), R71–R76.

Pan, D., Dong, J., Zhang, Y., et al., 2004. Tuberous sclerosis complex: from *Drosophila* to human disease. Trends Cell Biol. 14 (2), 78–85.

E-BOOK FIGURES AND TABLES

The following figures and tables are available in the e-book at www.expertconsult.com. See inside cover for registration details.

Fig. 16-2 Tet system for inducible transgene expression.

Fig. 16-6 Cre-Lox and Flp-Frt site-specific recombinase systems.

Fig. 16-8 High-throughput compound screens.

Table 16-1 Selected Naturally Occurring Mouse Mutant Models

17 Neonatal Neurointensive Care

Hannah C. Glass and Sonia L. Bonifacio

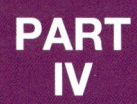 An expanded version of this chapter is available on www.expertconsult.com. See inside cover for registration details.

INTRODUCTION

The 20th century has brought significant advances in neonatal cardiopulmonary resuscitation and critical care. There are now very high rates of survival among neonates with previously life-threatening conditions, for example, perinatal asphyxia, extreme prematurity, and congenital malformations of the heart and lungs. Despite advances in cardiopulmonary care, neonates continue to suffer neurologic complications of critical illness. Up to 25% of children at high-level intensive care nurseries may be diagnosed with encephalopathy, brain injury, seizures, and other neurologic conditions (Glass et al., 2010). These children are at high risk for long-term disabilities, including cerebral palsy and epilepsy, as well as intellectual and behavioral disabilities.

Neonatal neurocritical care (also called neurointensive or brain-focused care) is a subspecialty that has developed in response to recent advances in brain care and improved understanding of the impact of critical illness on the developing brain. It is now well known that brain injury is exacerbated by alterations in temperature (especially hyperthermia), and glucose (especially hypoglycemia), and that infection is a risk factor for injury and altered brain development in preterm neonates. In addition, technological advances—for example, digital electroencephalography (EEG) with bedside trending (such as amplitude-integrated EEG [aEEG]) and remote access availability—allow the bedside team to assess brain function in real time. Furthermore, safe, high-resolution brain imaging techniques using magnetic resonance (MR) are available to assess the impact of critical illness on brain structure and development.

This important focus on the brain during the period of critical illness allows for medical (including possible neuroprotective) interventions, developmentally supportive care, communication with parents, and decision making while the patient is in the nursery. In principle, neurocritical care can lead to improved outcomes through the following mechanisms: (1) earlier recognition and treatment of neurologic conditions, (2) prevention of secondary brain injury through attention to basic physiology (temperature regulation, glucose homeostasis, oxygenation, and blood pressure support), (3) consistent management using guidelines and protocols, and (4) use of experienced specialized teams at dedicated referral centers.

As the field of neonatal neurocritical care has developed, it has become apparent that certain diseases warrant consideration for having newborns more intensively monitored. Infants who suffer from acute or chronic neurologic conditions may benefit from the teamwork, guidelines, and brain-focused approach of a neurocritical care service. The most common conditions include encephalopathy (and hypoxic-ischemic encephalopathy [HIE]), seizures (both acute symptomatic seizures and neonatal onset epilepsies), stroke (both arterial and venous), intracranial hemorrhage, and intracranial infection (Glass et al., 2010). Patients who are at high risk for brain injury, such as those who are of extremely low gestational age (<28 weeks' gestation at birth), or have hydrocephalus, congenital heart malformations, need for extracorporeal membrane oxygenation (ECMO), vascular malformations of the central nervous system, or symptomatic hypoglycemia will also benefit from monitoring, imaging, and a team approach as they are at high risk for seizures, and optimal brain care may minimize injury. Finally, children with developmental anomalies, such as brain malformations, multiple congenital anomalies, or dysmorphisms can also benefit from the multidisciplinary neurocritical care approach.

ESTABLISHING A MULTIDISCIPLINARY NEUROINTENSIVE CARE NURSERY

Establishing a neurointensive care nursery involves a culture change for the entire intensive care nursery toward brain-focused care, such that all patient care providers are continually aware of the neurologic implications of critical illnesses and the impact of management strategies on the developing brain. This can be accomplished by (1) developing a strong leadership team with representatives from neonatology, neurology, and nursing; (2) providing training and education to all providers, including physicians, nurses, nurse practitioners, and respiratory therapists, among others; (3) developing local guidelines for common neurologic conditions; and (4) ensuring adequate technology for brain monitoring, imaging, and application of hypothermia. With these changes, bedside providers learn to consider the brain to be as important as the heart and lungs in day-to-day management.

Leaders from neonatology, neurology, and nursing must work together to develop guidelines and protocols, as well as training and educational programs for their respective specialties. Guidelines and protocols can help to standardize the approach to the neurologic evaluation and treatment and reduce practice variation that can occur in large units with high turnover of medical and nursing staff (Figure 17-1). Buy-in from all team members, especially nurses, who are present at all hours, is critical for promoting the mission of minimizing brain injury and providing brain-focused care and, ultimately, will lead to culture change.

Most neurointensive care nurseries are closed units with the neonatologist acting as the MD of record and the neurologist acting to comanage patients, taking an equal role in decision making and communication with the family. The neonatologist identifies patients at risk of brain injury and provides optimized resuscitation and supportive care to prevent secondary injuries. The neurologist takes an early active role from the time of the initial presentation of neurologic signs or symptoms. The neurologist can help to guide the initial investigation and management decisions, including rapid implementation of medical treatment, as well as coordinating with the neurophysiology service for application and interpretation of EEG, and with the neuroradiologist for appropriate imaging protocols. The neurologist perspective is important when discussing prognosis and follow-up with the family, especially if the child is expected to have a long-term disabling neurologic condition.

The bedside nurse plays a critical role in the management of neonates with neurologic conditions. Specialized education will help the nurse to become expert in neurologic care. The nurse will learn to recognize signs and symptoms of injury, quickly triage patients and equipment (e.g., EEG machines and the cooling blanket) for faster care, adhere to management guidelines and anticipate next steps in care, safely transport critically ill neonates to the MR scanner, and communicate effectively with families. Other key members of the multidisciplinary team include neurophysiologists or epileptologists, neuroradiologists, developmental care practitioners, physical and occupational therapists, pharmacists, and social workers. The unit itself may be a virtual space or a specific area within the neonatal intensive care unit.

RESUSCITATION AND SUPPORTIVE CARE TO PREVENT BRAIN INJURY

The concept of the golden hour originated in the adult trauma literature and referred to the hour between identification of the patient and admission to the emergency room. In neonates, the concept of the golden hour can be applied to guide the complex care required for all premature very low-birth-weight (<1500 g) neonates, as well as for preterm and term neonates who are born after signs of perinatal distress and in whom the initial examination demonstrates encephalopathy. During the golden hour, multiple measures are simultaneously performed to resuscitate the neonate. For preterm neonates, birth represents a period of transition that is complicated by physiologic immaturity, which results in a high-risk period for acquired brain injury. In encephalopathic neonates, end organ failure may put the neonate at risk for secondary injury as a result of inadequate brain perfusion or hypoglycemia.

After performing resuscitation guided by Neonatal Resuscitation Program (NRP) practices, care providers should apply brain protective strategies by maintaining physiologic homeostasis to help prevent secondary brain injury. Ventilation must be carefully controlled as both hypo- and hypercarbia can affect cerebral blood flow. Blood pressure should be maintained in the appropriate range for the gestational age to support cerebral blood flow as there may be poor cerebral autoregulation in critically ill and preterm neonates (Kasdorf and Perlman, 2013). Temperature stability is important: hyperthermia is associated with worse outcomes in term neonates with brain injury and hypothermia is associated with worse outcomes in preterm neonates. Finally, glucose levels need to be monitored closely to avoid hypoglycemia, as this is associated with both de novo brain injury and worse outcome in the setting of existing brain injury.

CURRENT TREATMENT OPTIONS FOR NEONATES WITH HYPOXIC-ISCHEMIC ENCEPHALOPATHY

Neonatal encephalopathy caused by suspected or confirmed HIE is among the common diagnoses encountered in the neurointensive care nursery (Glass et al., 2010). Therapeutic hypothermia treatment is the only clinically available neuroprotective therapy for neonatal encephalopathy secondary to perinatal asphyxia. Multiple randomized controlled trials (RCTs) have demonstrated benefit with reduction in death or disability at 18 to 24 months of age (RR 0.75, 95% CI 0.68–0.83), and sustained benefits now being observed at school age (Jacobs et al., 2013). For any one child to benefit from treatment, on average 7 (5–10) need to be treated. Therapeutic hypothermia is now accepted as the standard of care for neonates who meet criteria established by the RCTs.

Because neonates who meet criteria must be initiated on treatment within 6 hours after birth, decision making regarding whom to treat must be implemented rapidly and through coordinated efforts between the referring center and the cooling center if the child is born at a smaller center. Outreach to referring centers by a neurocritical care program will include education regarding eligibility criteria, as well as how to perform a neurologic examination to determine eligibility as soon as possible after the resuscitation. Cord gas should be obtained in any neonate with a high-risk event before delivery (e.g., uterine rupture and cord accident) or low Apgar scores. Formal neurologic examination for signs of moderate to severe encephalopathy must be performed after the resuscitation period. Abnormal aEEG background pattern or aEEG seizures can be used as additional criteria, but hypothermia should not be delayed for neonates who qualify by standard criteria. If physiologic criteria are met (i.e., Apgars, gas, and need for resuscitation) but the neonate is not encephalopathic, serial neurologic examinations over the first 6 hours after birth should be clearly documented in the medical record, and neonates who demonstrate signs of encephalopathy initiated on hypothermia as soon as possible.

Once a patient meets criteria, if not already in a center with an established hypothermia treatment program, the treating physician should consult with a hypothermia center and initiate passive cooling by removing or reducing external heat sources as soon as possible. Both animal and human studies show that earlier initiation of therapeutic hypothermia is associated with better outcomes (Gunn and Thoresen, 2006). Before implementation of a servocontrolled device for temperature control, frequent monitoring of core temperature is essential to prevent the temperature from falling rapidly below 33.0°C (which is more common in severely encephalopathic neonates), as this carries an increased risk of cardiovascular compromise. Passive cooling can be safely initiated or maintained on transport, although devices to provide servoregulated treatment during medical transport are now available and appear to effectively reduce the time to achieving therapeutic hypothermia, as well as prevent large temperature fluctuations and severe hypothermia.

In animal models, therapeutic hypothermia has limited efficacy unless the animal receives sedation. One approach is to use a morphine infusion throughout hypothermia starting at a dose of 20 mcg/kg/hr and titrating down each day by 5 to 10 mcg/kg/hr and off once cooling is complete. Shivering can be treated with magnesium boluses (to achieve high normal levels), acral warming, or additional doses of morphine or benzodiazepine.

During hypothermia, neonates should be monitored with continuous, prolonged monitoring, preferably using continuous video EEG. The risk of seizures in neonates undergoing hypothermia is approximately 50%. Clinical indicators such as resuscitation parameters and degree of encephalopathy are not associated with the risk of seizures in neonates undergoing hypothermia. However, the initial EEG background can help to stratify risk of seizures: neonates whose EEG background is abnormal at the onset of recording have the highest risk (70%

for neonates with EEG background that is excessively discontinuous, and >60% if the EEG background is severely abnormal), whereas those with normal EEG background have a lower risk (~10%). In addition to providing information regarding risk of seizures, the early EEG recording provides important prognostic information that can be used to start counseling parents regarding goals of care. Early normal or mildly abnormal EEG is associated with a good prognosis, and parents can be informed even on the first day after birth that there are no signs of severe brain injury. An early severely abnormal EEG (e.g., burst suppression, depressed and undifferentiated, extremely low voltage, or status epilepticus at the onset of recording) is associated with a poor prognosis and brain injury if it persists beyond 24 to 36 hours after birth. This information is useful for counseling families early in the course of hypothermia so that they may process the information and begin to make decisions regarding goals of care before onset of rewarming. Not all neonates who have electrographic seizures will have brain injury, and so if seizures are few, brief, focal, and easily treated with first-line medications and occur in the setting of a normal or mildly abnormal EEG, the prognosis may be good.

Neonates undergoing hypothermia should be imaged with magnetic resonance imaging (MRI) at least once before discharge because MRI is associated with developmental outcome with an accuracy of ~80% for moderate to severe abnormalities indicating death or disability (Rutherford et al., 2010). The optimal timing of imaging may depend on the experience and resources of the center; each center should aim to standardize the timing so as to become experienced with the appearance of images at a given time point. One approach is to image neonates just after cooling has ended (days 4–6). This approach has several advantages: (1) the neonate may need less or no sedation to achieve good-quality images as many remain encephalopathic because of brain injury and or delayed metabolism of morphine or other sedatives; (2) the MRI can serve as a good turning point between the acute phase of the admission and recovery and planning for home, and counseling regarding prognosis and follow-up care can be completed using results of the clinical examination, monitoring, and MRI results; and (3) MRI can be performed before discharge home; many neonates treated with hypothermia are ready for discharge home between 8 and 10 days after birth. Some centers prefer to complete MRI in the second week after birth (days 10–14) as there are reports of evolution of brain injury that is apparent only on a later scan and the patient may be more clinically stable at this time point, although this may require bringing the patient back for imaging after discharge. Another approach is to perform an early (days 4–6) scan and repeat imaging in the second week after birth if the results are discordant (i.e., very abnormal neurologic examination finding or difficulty establishing feeding and EEG results with a normal MRI).

Treatment of HIE in the setting of a specialized neurointensive care nursery may offer the following benefits: (1) quicker onset of cooling by an experienced team; (2) rapid, around-the-clock detection and treatment of seizures; and (3) counseling for parents by experienced physicians and nurses.

Unfortunately, hypothermia does not prevent all patients with HIE from death or developmental disabilities; the rate of such adverse outcomes was approximately 50% in the RCTs. There are multiple ongoing preclinical and clinical investigations of adjunctive treatments to hypothermia. These adjunctive agents target additional mechanistic pathways that are involved in the evolution of hypoxic-ischemic injury. Agents under investigation include erythropoietin, xenon, and melatonin (Johnston et al., 2011).

BRAIN MONITORING AND SEIZURE MANAGEMENT

Continuous, real-time brain monitoring is increasingly used to assess background brain function and for accurate diagnosis of seizures, and is recommended for a large number of high-risk populations (Shellhaas et al., 2011). Increased use of monitoring has shown that paroxysmal events at the bedside may or may not have an electrographic correlate, and seizures without obvious clinical correlate (subclinical seizures) are common among critically ill neonates. There are three main indications for monitoring: (1) to assess the differential diagnosis of paroxysmal events (i.e., patients with one or more events that are concerning for seizure), (2) to detect seizures in selected high-risk populations (e.g., neonates with encephalopathy, neonates receiving therapeutic hypothermia, known intracranial hemorrhage or infection, and need for ECMO), and/or (3) to assess for background abnormalities in neonates who are encephalopathic.

Whereas conventional video electroencephalogram (EEG) is the gold standard for seizure diagnosis, bedside monitoring using trending algorithms such as aEEG allow the bedside providers to observe longitudinal trends in brain health, including the impact of medications and procedures, and are useful for detecting some seizures. Both conventional EEG and aEEG are useful and complementary tools, and, used concurrently (and optimally recorded on the same machine), can inform management for both bedside team and the neurologist or neurophysiologist (Glass et al., 2013).

Neurologists working in the neonatal intensive care unit (NICU) should become familiar with the advantages and limitations of aEEG, and be prepared to interpret bedside recordings (Figures 17-2 and 17-3) (Glass et al., 2013). Most pediatric neurologists will find the aEEG relatively easy to interpret, even without formal training in neonatal neurophysiology. aEEG can be very helpful for quickly visualizing changes in encephalopathy (reflected as a change in the background pattern) over time, and can also be useful for quickly identifying seizures. There is fair to good agreement between aEEG and EEG background classification in term newborns with encephalopathy. Reported seizure detection by aEEG ranges from about 25% to 85% and depends largely on the study design, population, and technique. Seizure detection is improved with training and experience, high seizure amplitude and burden, central or parietal positioning of the electrodes, multichannel recording, and use of the raw EEG trace. Like EEG, aEEG is subject to electrical and mechanical artifacts, and so the neurologist should become familiar with the appearance of common artifacts on aEEG. The primary advantage of using aEEG for seizure detection is the enhanced ability for real-time detection and treatment: at most centers, there is only one neurophysiologist available to review the EEG intermittently, whereas the aEEG displayed at the bedside can be continuously reviewed by the bedside nurse, as well as the attending neonatologists and house staff.

EEG and aEEG background patterns provide prognostic information for neonates with encephalopathy. Among neonates with encephalopathy caused by presumed hypoxic-ischemic injury who are not cooled, an abnormal aEEG background within 3 to 6 hours after birth is highly predictive of adverse neurodevelopmental outcome. Among cooled neonates, an abnormal early aEEG/EEG background has a lower specificity for adverse outcome, whereas a normal early aEEG/EEG is reassuring as it is associated with a good outcome. A persistently abnormal aEEG/EEG background at 24 to 48 hours is highly predictive of adverse neurodevelopmental outcome (Bonifacio et al., 2015).

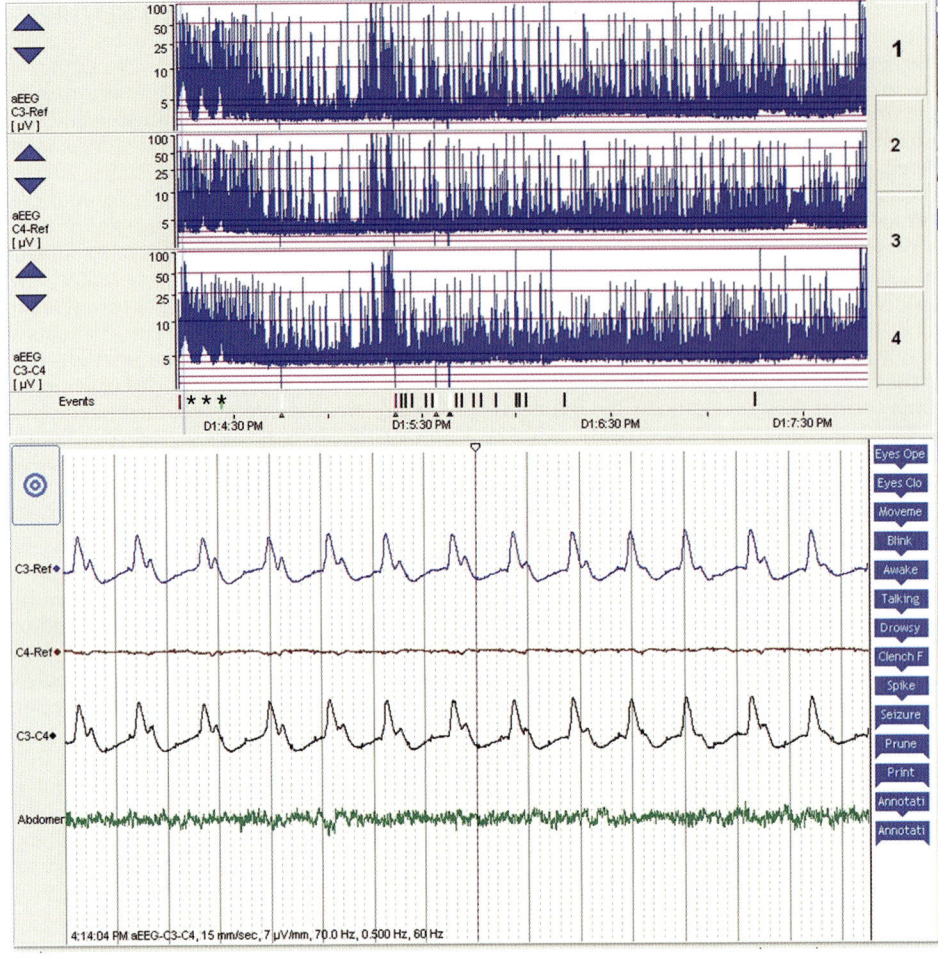

Figure 17-2. Seizures in a neonate with a burst suppression background. The repetitive sudden rise in the lower margin at the beginning of the compressed aEEG trace (marked with an *) corresponds to seizures on the raw EEG trace in the lower panel of the image. EEG, electroencephalography; aEEG, amplitude-integrated EEG.

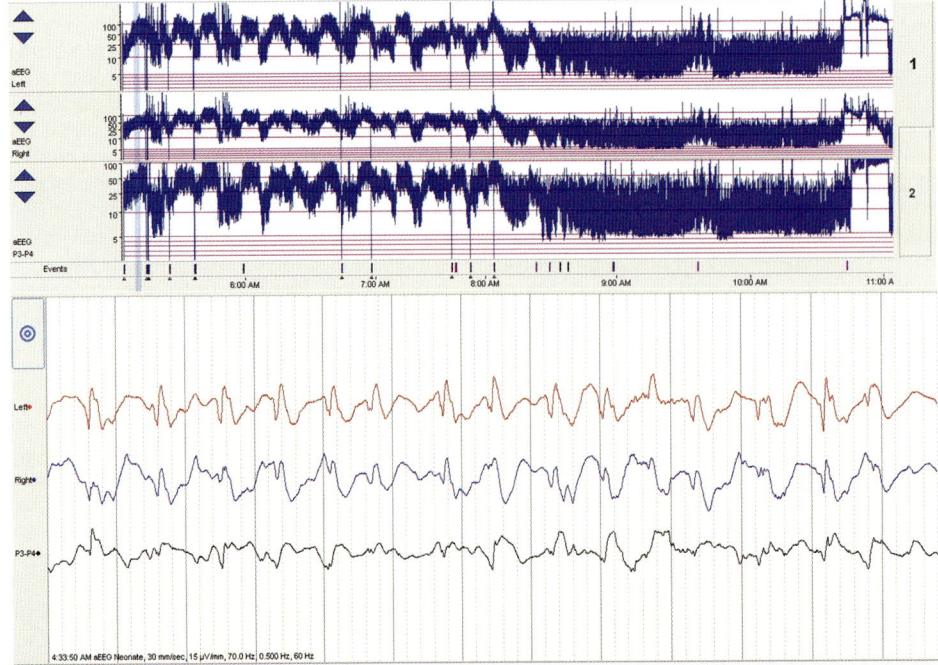

Figure 17-3. Status epilepticus (or saw-tooth pattern) followed by a discontinuous background pattern after treatment with phenobarbital. A high-voltage tracing in an encephalopathic neonate should be carefully examined for repetitive seizures indicating status epilepticus.

Seizures are often the first sign of a serious neurologic condition in a neonate, and are among the most common causes for neurologic consultation by a neonatal neurocritical care service (Glass et al., 2010). Phenobarbital and phenytoin are the only drugs that have been tested in randomized neonatal trials, and both have approximately equal efficacy (~50%) as first-line treatment. Some neurologists favor levetiracetam for its low-side-effect profile; however, there are no good efficacy data to support its use. The traditional approach to seizure treatment, that is, to treat clinical events with or without confirmation of electrographic seizures and to perform brief EEGs every few days or weeks, fails to adequately treat acute symptomatic seizures in neonates. When this paradigm is used, neonates may be exposed to harmful medication by overtreatment of paroxysmal events that are not seizures, or undertreatment of seizures without clear clinical correlate, which may be missed without continuous monitoring. Recurrent seizures and status epilepticus are harder to control than isolated seizures, and so the bedside team should aim for rapid treatment. Seizure medications should be available on the unit for rapid administration that bypasses the hospital pharmacy. Having seizure guidelines for medications for treatment of acute symptomatic seizures can improve the speed of administration by limiting the need for discussion about medication choice. Drug levels are rarely helpful in the setting of acute symptomatic seizures, which should be treated before the results of a level are available. Acute symptomatic seizures in neonates follow a clear tempo, with rapid onset in the first day after birth, fluctuation in frequency, and then seizure termination by 72 to 96 hours after birth. For this reason, prolonged treatment is rarely warranted. Discontinuation of medications within 24 to 72 hours of the last electrographic seizure is safe and can reduce exposure to potentially harmful medications such as phenobarbital.

BRAIN IMAGING

Brain imaging modalities for neonates include head ultrasonography (HUS), MRI, and computed tomography (CT). HUS is commonly utilized for first-line evaluation of neonates with suspected neurologic conditions or critical illness as it can be easily and safely performed at the bedside in most centers. In preterm neonates HUS is used to evaluate for intraventricular hemorrhages, posthemorrhagic ventricular dilatation, and hydrocephalus, and in the assessment of cystic periventricular leukomalacia. In critically ill term neonates, HUS is useful to evaluate for hemorrhage and hydrocephalus, and can be used to detect some ischemic injuries (mature ischemic stroke and global hypoxic-ischemic injuries), but its sensitivity and specificity are dependent on the timing of imaging, as well as the experience of the examiner and interpreter. In the highest risk preterm neonates (<30 weeks' gestation at birth), HUS is typically performed routinely within the first week after birth, at 3 to 7 days of age, and then serially until term-equivalent age to evaluate for changes in the white matter. Cerebellar hemorrhages are increasingly identified in preterm neonates, and are associated with adverse motor and cognitive outcomes. Large cerebellar hemorrhages can be identified with HUS using a mastoid view, but smaller hemorrhages are not apparent on HUS and, unless the neonate undergoes MRI (and especially blood-sensitive sequences with thin cuts), cerebellar hemorrhages may go undiagnosed. CT scan can be used to evaluate for neurosurgical conditions if HUS is not available, but its use is discouraged because of the poor resolution of gray and white matter pathologies and it exposes the neonate to unnecessary ionizing radiation.

MRI is the best tool to image the neonatal brain as it does not employ ionizing radiation and has high resolution for congenital and acquired abnormalities in the gray and white matter (Counsell et al., 2010). MRI can be performed safely without sedation in many children. In addition, conventional T1- and T2-weighted MRI, diffusion-weighted imaging, susceptibility-weighted imaging, and MR spectroscopy are important to identify areas of acute injury, and characteristic patterns can facilitate the diagnosis of metabolic or infectious processes. Fluid-attenuated inversion recovery (FLAIR) sequences are less useful given the high water content of the neonatal brain. All MR sequences must be optimized for newborn imaging; utilizing a stroke or seizure imaging protocol that has been defined by the MR manufacturer or by the neuroradiologist for adults or older children is inadequate. MRI is prognostic for developmental disabilities in both preterm and term neonates, and is increasingly performed before discharge from intensive care.

PALLIATIVE CARE

Neurologic conditions that are encountered in the NICU carry high mortality (~20% compared with 7% of overall NICU admissions in one tertiary care center) (Glass et al., 2010). When a child has a neurologic condition that is not compatible with life, or is expected to develop severe and permanent developmental disabilities, in many centers, providers will offer the parents a palliative approach to care. Early predictors of adverse outcome include neurologic examination (persistent severe encephalopathy), EEG (burst suppression pattern or worse persisting 48 hours), severe seizures (status epilepticus, multifocal seizures, and seizures not responding to first- or second-line medications), and MRI (extensive injury) (Bonifacio et al., 2015). Although neonates with severe brain injury may initially be severely encephalopathic, the brainstem usually recovers and the child has eye opening and/or semipurposeful movements that do not necessarily indicate meaningful recovery. Counseling families to anticipate these changes can help build trust. Careful use of clear language can help with communication to families, including avoiding terms that are easily confused, such as "vegetative state" and especially "near brain death." Describing clinical features and ancillary testing that indicate likely adverse prognosis, as well as a range of possible outcomes, can help the family to understand what the future may hold for the child and family if the child survives.

Palliative care requires a team approach with the neonatologist, neurologist, and bedside nurse and house staff providing a consistent message to the family. Involvement of the hospital pediatric palliative care team can be helpful, especially if the infant is expected to survive for longer than a day or two. Team members who are not comfortable with palliative care can be excused from caring for the child. Burnout and compassion fatigue are common among nurses who care for a high percentage of children with adverse outcomes, and so provisions should be made to increase the pool of nurses to ensure adequate breaks for those caring for critically ill children, to provide education about common neurologic conditions such as HIE and updates on children with good outcomes, and to ensure communication between the bedside nurse and the team members so that the nurse is aware of the daily plan and plans for communication with the parents.

REFERENCES

The complete list of references for this chapter is available in the e-book at www.expertconsult.com.

See inside cover for registration details.

SELECTED REFERENCES

Bonifacio, S.L., deVries, L.S., Groenendaal, F., 2015. Impact of hypothermia on predictors of poor outcome: how do we decide to redirect care? Semin. Fetal Neonatal Med. 20 (2), 122–127.

Counsell, S.J., Tranter, S.L., Rutherford, M.A., 2010. Magnetic resonance imaging of brain injury in the high-risk term infant. Semin. Perinatol. 34 (1), 67–78.

Glass, H.C., Bonifacio, S.L., Peloquin, S., et al., 2010. Neurocritical care for neonates. Neurocrit. Care 12 (3), 421–429.

Glass, H.C., Wusthoff, C.J., Shellhaas, R.A., 2013. Amplitude-integrated electro-encephalography: the child neurologist's perspective. J. Child Neurol. 28 (10), 1342–1350.

Gunn, A.J., Thoresen, M., 2006. Hypothermic neuroprotection. NeuroRx. 3 (2), 154–169.

Jacobs, S.E., Berg, M., Hunt, R., et al., 2013. Cooling for newborns with hypoxic ischaemic encephalopathy. Cochrane Database Syst. Rev. (1), CD003311.

Johnston, M.V., Fatemi, A., Wilson, M.A., et al., 2011. Treatment advances in neonatal neuroprotection and neurointensive care. Lancet Neurol. 10 (4), 372–382.

Kasdorf, E., Perlman, J.M., 2013. Strategies to prevent reperfusion injury to the brain following intrapartum hypoxia-ischemia. Semin. Fetal Neonatal Med. 18 (6), 379–384.

Rutherford, M., Ramenghi, L.A., Edwards, A.D., et al., 2010. Assessment of brain tissue injury after moderate hypothermia in neonates with hypoxic-ischaemic encephalopathy: a nested substudy of a randomised controlled trial. Lancet Neurol. 9 (1), 39–45.

Shellhaas, R.A., Chang, T., Tsuchida, T., et al., 2011. The American Clinical Neurophysiology Society's guideline on continuous electroencephalography monitoring in neonates. J. Clin. Neurophysiol. 28 (6), 611–617.

E-BOOK FIGURES AND TABLES

The following figures and tables are available in the e-book at www.expertconsult.com. See inside cover for registration details.

Fig. 17-1 Examples of local guidelines for hypothermia and stroke management.

Table 17-1 Acuity-Based Guidelines for Neonatal Neurocritical Care Comanagement

18 Neonatal Seizures

Renée A. Shellhaas, Hannah C. Glass, and Taeun Chang

An expanded version of this chapter is available on www.expertconsult.com. See inside cover for registration details.

INTRODUCTION

Children are at highest risk for seizures during the first month of life. Seizures in newborns are usually symptomatic of an underlying acute injury (such as hypoxic-ischemic injury or stroke) and are only rarely manifestations of epilepsy syndromes. Similar to other critically ill patient populations, most neonatal seizures are subclinical—they have no outward manifestation and are most accurately diagnosed by electro-encephalography (EEG). Herein, we review the pathophysiology, epidemiology, diagnosis, treatment, and long-term implications of seizures in neonates.

PATHOPHYSIOLOGY

The neonatal period presents the highest lifetime risk for seizures. Acute symptomatic seizures caused by birth trauma and hemorrhage, hypoxic-ischemic injury, perinatal infections, and metabolic disturbances account for more than 80% of seizures. Less commonly, congenital brain malformations, inborn errors of metabolism, and epileptic encephalopathies can present in the neonatal period with seizures as the first sign of neonatal onset epilepsy.

The immature brain is highly susceptible to acute symptomatic seizures because of age-dependent mechanisms that lead to excess excitation and reduced inhibition. Results from animal models suggest that acute symptomatic seizures are deleterious to the developing brain. In humans, seizures in the newborn period are associated with brain injury and adverse neurodevelopment. In addition, among neonates with hypoxic-ischemic encephalopathy (HIE), seizures are associated with higher lactate on magnetic resonance (MR) spectroscopy (indicating injury) and higher rates of adverse neurodevelopmental outcome that are independent of the severity of brain injury. These data suggest that seizures may also be harmful to human newborns with underlying brain injury.

Mechanisms of Excitability in the Developing Brain

The developing brain's propensity to generate seizures is multifactorial. The primary mechanisms of inhibition (through gamma-amino-butyric acid [GABA]) and excitation (through glutamatergic system) favor excitability during the neonatal period.

GABA is the primary inhibitory mechanism of the adult brain. In mature neurons, $GABA_A$ receptor activation leads to chloride *influx* to produce membrane hyperpolarization and inhibits the neuron's ability to fire action potentials. In immature neurons, however, there is a net chloride *efflux* with $GABA_A$ receptor activation, which leads to membrane depolarization and increases the likelihood of the neuron to fire an action potential. The developmental changes in neuronal chloride gradients are mediated largely by membrane ion transporters, NKCC1 and KCC2.

In early life, a relatively higher expression of NKCC1 leads to a high intracellular chloride concentration, and subsequent depolarization upon activation of the $GABA_A$ receptor. With increasing age, the expression of the KCC2 chloride co-transporter becomes dominant, which leads neurons to display the mature pattern of low intracellular chloride and hyperpolarization with activation of the $GABA_A$ receptor. Thus GABAergic medications (such as benzodiazapines and barbiturates), which are commonly used to treat seizures in neonates, could, in theory, cause a paradoxical excitatory response. Nonetheless, the response to phenobarbital as a first-line agent is approximately 50%, which is similar to the effect of first-line agents in the pediatric intensive care unit and suggests that GABA agents are inhibitory in some populations of neurons in the neonatal period. Bumetanide, a potent diuretic that acts to alter the intracellular chloride concentration in favor of hyperpolarization, has been proposed as an adjunct to improve the efficacy of phenobarbital, but safety and efficacy data are not yet available.

Glutamate is the primary excitatory neurotransmitter. The glutamate receptors are developmentally regulated, and lead to enhanced excitability of the immature brain. N-methyl-d-aspartate (NMDA) receptors are relatively abundant in newborns, and their subunits are configured with a high level of the NR2B subunit, which leads to greater excitability through prolonged current delay and excitatory postsynaptic potentials, as well as a relative insensitivity to magnesium ions.

Finally, excitability is enhanced during the neonatal period as a result of physiologic, use-dependent synaptogenesis, when both synapse and dendritic spine density are at their peak.

The Effect of Seizures on Early Brain Development

Seizures during early development can lead to developmental changes that alter neuronal circuitry and may impair learning and memory in animal models. Developmental alterations that have been observed in neonatal animal models after induced seizures include (1) reduced density of dendritic spines in hippocampal pyramidal neurons, (2) decreased neurogenesis, (3) delayed neuronal loss, and (4) changes in hippocampal plasticity (e.g., decreased capacity for long-term potentiation, reduced susceptibility to kindling and enhanced paired-pulse inhibition). Furthermore, in the setting of brain injury and hyperthermia, seizures can lead to hippocampal necrosis in animal models. In addition, neonatal seizures increase the susceptibility to unprovoked recurrent seizures (epilepsy) later in the animal's life (Holmes, 2009).

EPIDEMIOLOGY
Incidence of Neonatal Seizures

Current estimates of the incidence of seizures in newborns range from 1 to 3.5 per 1000 live births, or approximately 14,000 newborns annually in the United States (Table 18-1).

Estimates as high as 1 per 20 have been reported for preterm or very low-birth-weight newborns, with incidence inversely related to birth weight and gestational age. Males are more often affected than females, and infants of African American origin have a higher incidence of seizures than those of other races and ethnicities. Seizures in the newborn usually occur in the first week of life (approximately 70% to 85%), particularly in the first 2 days of life.

Although seizure incidence reported in more recent studies is lower than that reported in older studies, differences in case ascertainment or study site(s) may be responsible for this variation. The true incidence of seizures in the newborn is difficult to ascertain as population studies have been based on clinically observed or reported seizure-like activity, without EEG confirmation. Newer data suggest that such case ascertainment may include infants whose events were not, in fact, seizures, while excluding those with exclusively subclinical seizures. Most studies use a case definition of seizures in infants up to 44 weeks' postmenstrual age.

Seizure duration in newborns has not commonly been examined in the published population-based studies as seizures were defined clinically and often retrospectively. Limited data suggest that, similar to EEG-based case cohort studies of newborns with seizures, 85% of seizures lasted less than 5 minutes. Though rare, 5% of affected newborns were clinically observed to have seizures lasting more than 30 minutes. Emergence of continuous prolonged video-EEG recordings with the conversion from pen-and-paper to digital EEG technology has improved our ability to capture and characterize neonatal seizures. Seizures and status epilepticus may be more common than previously realized, but most neonatal seizures remain brief with 60% lasting less than 90 seconds.

Risk Factors for Neonatal Seizures

Risk factors for neonatal seizures are related to their long list of underlying etiologies (Table 18-2). In addition to low birth weight and gestational age, risks for seizures in a newborn include preexisting maternal diabetes, maternal fever or infection, perinatal or postnatal infection, major morbidities or surgical interventions in the infant, evidence of fetal distress, and postterm delivery. Possible risk factors also include advanced maternal age, maternal nulliparity, and male gender.

ETIOLOGY

The causes of seizures in newborns are numerous and diverse (see Table 18-2); a single newborn can have more than one cause of seizures. Most neonatal seizure etiologies reflect underlying acute brain injury rather than epilepsy. Our ability to determine etiology has improved with enhanced access to EEG monitoring and brain magnetic resonance imaging (MRI), as well as advances in genetic testing. Determination of seizure etiology is critical, as treatment of the underlying cause may be life-saving (e.g., antibiotics for a newborn with bacterial meningitis), and combining seizure burden with etiology can assist in assessing prognosis.

Etiologies of neonatal seizures can be divided into three broad categories: (1) acute symptomatic seizures (by far the most common), (2) developmental brain abnormalities, and (3) genetic or neonatal epilepsy syndromes.

Acute Symptomatic Seizures

Hypoxic ischemic encephalopathy (HIE) is the most frequent cause and accounts for up to 40% to 45% of neonatal seizures. Therapeutic hypothermia is now standard care for HIE in newborns 36 weeks' or greater gestation and EEG monitoring is recommended for cooled newborns. Prolonged continuous video EEG throughout cooling and rewarming is preferred. If continuous EEG is not available, then continuous amplitude-integrated EEG (aEEG), or daily serial routine EEGs for the first 4 days of life are suggested. Even though cooling may decrease seizure burden, about half of treated newborns still have seizures during therapeutic hypothermia. Seizure onset continues to be within the first 24 hours of life (Boylan et al., 2015).

Cerebrovascular events, including *arterial and venous infarctions and intracranial hemorrhages,* are the second most common cause of neonatal seizures (7% to 18%). Arterial ischemic perinatal strokes (AIS) occur in 1 in 2300 to 5000 live births and are typically the result of embolism from the placenta or umbilical cord, carotid artery or heart. Seizures are their most frequent presenting symptom of androgen insensitivity syndrome (AIS). Almost two thirds involve the left middle cerebral artery territory. Maternal risk factors for perinatal arterial ischemic strokes include oligohydramnios, clinical or histologic chorioamnionitis, premature rupture of membranes, preeclampsia, diabetes, and smoking. Neonatal risk factors include congenital cardiac abnormalities, systemic infections,

TABLE 18-2 Distribution of Neonatal Seizure Etiologies

	Loman et al. [2014] (2002–2009), N = 221	Pisani et al. [2008] (1999–2004), N = 106	Tekgul et al. [2006] (1997–2000), N = 89	Mastrangelo et al. [2005] (1990–1998), N = 94	Ronen et al. [1999] (1990–1994), N = 89
Hypoxic-ischemic encephalopathy, %	57.5	43.4	40	44.7	40
Metabolic or electrolyte disturbances, %	10.9	6.6	3	3.2	19
Intracranial hemorrhage, %	9.0	23.6	17	4.3	11
Cerebrovascular disorders, %	7.7	—	18	7.4	7
Infections, %	6.3	7.5	3	10.6	20
Congenital central nervous system abnormalities, %	3.2	5.7	5	9.6	10
Inborn errors of metabolism, %	2.3	6.6	1	7.4	—
Epilepsy syndromes, %	2.3	—	—	5.3	6
Intoxications, %	0.5	—	—	—	—
Unknown, %	0.5	6.6	12	1.1	14

coagulation disorders in the infant, placental abnormalities, and male gender.

Cerebral sinovenous thrombosis (CSVT) usually involves the superior sagittal sinus and/or transverse sinus in term infants and medullary vein thrombosis in preterm infants. The incidence is 1 to 2.69 per 100,000 newborns. Venous infarction occurs in approximately 60% of reported cases. Two thirds of affected neonates present with seizures during the first week of life. Maternal, fetal, and neonatal risk factors are similar to arterial strokes. Many infants have a combination of predisposing factors, including neonatal sepsis and dehydration.

Intracranial hemorrhages can result in neonatal seizures. Diagnosis typically requires neuroimaging, and head ultrasonography and brain MRI are the preferred modalities. Computed tomography is not preferred for newborns, given the risk of radiation and lack of benefit relative to ultrasonography for identification of conditions for which neurosurgical interventions are required. Hemorrhages in term neonates may be caused by trauma, coagulopathy, or vascular malformations. Intraventricular hemorrhages (IVH) are common in preterm infants less than 30 weeks' gestation but on occasion can present in term infants with sinovenous thrombosis. IVH is the primary seizure etiology in preterm infants. Seizures are associated with IVH grade 3 or periventricular hemorrhagic infarct (IVH grade 4) and typically occur in the first 3 days of life.

Systemic or central nervous system (CNS) infections are the third most common cause of seizure in newborns (3–10%). This category includes in utero or postnatal infections, meningitis, and meningoencephalitis. Viral etiologies include herpes simplex virus (HSV), cytomegalovirus (CMV), parechovirus, lymphocytic choriomeningitis virus (LCMV), disseminated enterovirus, and parvovirus. Bacterial sources include group B streptococcus (early and late), *Escherichia coli*, and toxoplasmosis. *Lumbar puncture is recommended in all neonates with suspected infection.* Infants too unstable to undergo lumbar puncture should be treated empirically for CNS infection.

Seizures caused by primary *metabolic disturbances*, or metabolic abnormalities associated with acute medical illness, account for 3% to 7% of EEG-confirmed seizures. Such disturbances most often include abnormal glucose, calcium, or sodium levels. Typically, reversal of the abnormal level results in resolution of the neonatal seizures.

Hypoglycemia occurs in 1 to 3 out of 1000 live births. In general, hypoglycemia is defined as less than 45 mg/dL in term infants and less than 30 mg/dL in preterm infants. Risk factors include maternal diabetes, small for gestational age, in conjunction with illness, feeding issues, and/or pancreatic insulinoma. Initial treatment is to provide supplemental glucose. Antiseizure drug administration is necessary only if seizures persist despite glucose boluses. Severe hypoglycemia may result in brain parenchymal injury, which is most often localized to the posterior brain quadrants.

Hypocalcemia is the cause of 1% of all neonatal seizures. It is defined based on free ionized calcium levels rather than total serum calcium. Hypocalcemia within the first 3 days of life is associated with low-birth-weight infants, maternal diabetes, HIE, and endocrinopathies. Late-onset hypocalcemia, after 1 week of life, is now rare but is associated with maternal hyperparathyroidism or maternal vitamin D deficiency, or may be a manifestation of DiGeorge syndrome. Hypocalcemia caused by high-phosphorus–containing formulas or use of cow's milk is uncommon in the United States.

Hyponatremia or hypernatremia is seen most commonly in extremely premature infants. Among term infants, sodium imbalance can be caused by incorrect mixing, because of incorrect mixing of formula or severe dehydration, or can be a complication of intracranial injury. Severe dehydration with hypernatremia and seizures may be associated with CSVT.

Inborn errors of metabolism cause 1% to 7% of neonatal seizures. Prompt diagnosis is necessary to correct the underlying metabolic disorder and minimize irreversible brain injury (Chapter 23). The presence of seizure is related to the degree of metabolic derangement and resultant injury to the brain. Seizures can be associated with urea cycle defects (hyperammonemia), organic acidurias, and aminoacidopathies (metabolic acidosis).

Metabolic epileptic encephalopathies are uncommon, but sometimes treatable, causes of seizures in newborns. These disorders can be divided into three broad categories: (1) disorders of neurotransmitter metabolism, (2) disorders of energy metabolism, and (3) biosynthetic defects causing brain malformation, dysfunction, and degeneration.

Disorders of neurotransmitter metabolism include nonketotic hyperglycinemia, pyridoxal-5'-phosphate–responsive encephalopathy, pyridoxine-dependent epilepsy (PDE), folinic acid–responsive seizures, mitochondrial glutamate transporter, aromatic amino acid decarboxylase deficiency, D-2-hydroxyglutaric aciduria, and GABA disorders.

Nonketotic hyperglycinemia is a defect in the glycine cleavage system. Newborns often present with apnea, hypotonia, encephalopathy, and refractory seizures. Seizures are believed to be the result of overactivation of NMDA excitatory amino acid receptors. Diagnosis is by elevated cerebrospinal fluid (CSF)–to–serum glycine ratio.

PDE is caused by a rare autosomal recessive antiquitin deficiency (*ALDH7A1* gene). The seizures rapidly respond to intravenous (IV) pyridoxine, and so a pyridoxine administration trial is warranted for newborns with unexplained treatment-resistant seizures (see Treatment section later). Folinic acid–dependent seizures are an allelic phenotype. Diagnosis is by examining alpha-aminoadipic semialdehyde levels in urine, and by observation of seizure remittance with pyridoxine treatment. Pyridoxine-5'-phosphate deficiency is related to PDE, but often presents with severe epileptic encephalopathy and is responsive to oral pyridoxal phosphate and not to pyridoxine.

Disorders of energy metabolism include glucose transporter deficiency, pyruvate dehydrogenase deficiency, pyruvate carboxylase deficiency, biotinidase deficiency, respiratory chain disorders (Leigh disease and Alpers disease), Menkes disease, fumarase deficiency, sulfite oxidase deficiency, purine disorders, and creatine synthesis and transporter defects. *Molybdenum cofactor deficiency* and *isolated sulfite oxidase deficiency* are rare but can mimic HIE in clinical presentation.

Biosynthetic defects causing brain malformation and cerebral dysfunction include peroxisomal disorders, congenital disorders of glycosylation, glycolipid synthesis (GM3 synthase deficiency), cholesterol synthesis (Smith–Lemli–Opitz syndrome), serine and glutamine deficiency syndromes (rare), methylation disorders (homocysteine and folate disorders), neuronal ceroid lipofuscinosis, and lysosomal disorders. *Peroxisomal biogenesis disorders* include Zellweger syndrome, neonatal adrenoleukodystrophy, and infantile Refsum disease. Presentation includes severe encephalopathy, refractory neonatal seizures, and subtle dysmorphic features. The diagnosis is made by measurement of very long-chain fatty acids and phytanic acid.

Developmental Brain Abnormalities

Congenital CNS abnormalities are relatively common causes of neonatal seizures (5–10%). Diagnosis requires neuroimaging, with MRI the preferred imaging modality. Recognition and precise classification have increased with brain MR imaging. Affected newborns may have comorbid HIE as they may not tolerate labor and delivery. Common developmental brain abnormalities include focal cortical dysplasia, hemimegalencephaly, lissencephaly, heterotopias, schizencephaly, and polymicrogyria. Neonatal brain abnormalities can also be seen in patients with tuberous sclerosis. Neonatal seizures in the context of developmental brain abnormalities are associated with intractable seizures, chronic epilepsy, and poor neurodevelopmental outcome.

Epilepsy Syndromes

Neonatal epilepsy syndromes can range from benign (seizures expected to resolve quickly and long-term neurodevelopment likely to be normal) to severe early onset epileptic encephalopathies (seizures expected to be treatment-resistant and long-term neurodevelopment likely to be abnormal).

Severe epilepsy syndromes should be suspected for neonates with no obvious acute symptomatic cause of seizures, especially if the EEG background shows burst suppression. Initial diagnostic testing should include brain MRI, often with MR spectroscopy. MRI findings may help narrow the differential diagnosis and tailor the subsequent workup. An IV pyridoxine challenge (as outlined below in the Treatment section) should be performed while serum, urine, CSF, and genetic studies are collected and processed.

Familial epilepsies include benign familial neonatal epilepsy (BFNE) and benign idiopathic neonatal seizures (BINS). BFNE is an autosomal dominant epilepsy syndrome with 85% penetrance that is related to KCNQ2 or KCNQ3 voltage-gated potassium channel mutations. Seizure onset is usually in the first week of life and the semiology is commonly focal tonic seizures. Seizures resolve spontaneously in early infancy. Infants have a normal neurologic examination, normal interictal EEG, and a family history of neonatal seizures. BINS usually occur between 4 and 6 days of life and resolve within 2 weeks, and the infant has no family history of neonatal seizures. Some affected individuals have been reported to have KCNQ2 mutations.

A more severe phenotype is also associated with KCNQ2 mutations. KCNQ2 encephalopathy presents with frequent pharmacoresistant seizures in the first week of life. Seizures often have a tonic semiology. The interictal EEG is markedly abnormal and often meets criteria for burst suppression. Brain MRI reveals subtle T1 and T2 hyperintensities in the basal ganglia and thalami—findings that may resolve after the neonatal period. Affected children typically have severe global neurodevelopmental disabilities.

There are two classic neonatal epileptic encephalopathy syndromes (Beal et al., 2012). *Early myoclonic encephalopathy (EME)* has neonatal onset with erratic focal myoclonic jerks, often accompanied by focal seizures and occasionally by tonic seizures. The typical interictal EEG shows a burst–suppression pattern during sleep. Later, the EEG evolves into atypical hypsarrhythmia or multifocal sharp waves or spikes. EME is typically caused by metabolic disorders, such as nonketotic hyperglycinemia, pyridoxine dependency, and propionic aciduria; molybdenum cofactor deficiency; sulfite oxidase deficiency; Menkes disease; and Zellweger syndrome. *Ohtahara syndrome* presents with frequent tonic spasms in newborns or young infants. It is associated with a burst–suppression EEG pattern during *both* the awake and sleep states, along with severe encephalopathy and treatment-resistant epilepsy. Causes typically include structural brain abnormalities (cerebral dysgenesis, porencephaly, hemimegalencephaly, and Aicardi syndrome) and monogenic mutations (e.g., ARX, SLC25A22, PLCβ1, and PNKP).

DIAGNOSIS

Traditionally, neonatal seizures were diagnosed by clinical observation, with their semiology categorized according to the motor manifestations—focal clonic, multifocal clonic, generalized tonic, myoclonic, and subtle. The "subtle" semiology refers to seizures with signs such as abnormal eye movements, lip smacking, swimming or pedaling movements, or apnea.

Although classic research relied on recognition of clinical signs for the diagnosis of neonatal seizures, modern EEG data have demonstrated that not all clinically suspicious events are epileptic seizures—indeed, most are not. In one study, bedside clinicians (nurses and physicians) were trained to record any events that were suspicious for seizures for a sample of high-risk neonates who were undergoing conventional EEG recording. Only 9% (48 of 526) of all EEG-confirmed seizures had clinical signs that were noted in the bedside logs, whereas 78% (129 of 177) of the abnormal paroxysmal events documented by NICU staff had no EEG correlate (i.e., the events were not seizures) (Murray et al., 2008).

Imprecise seizure diagnosis has significant consequences: newborns with primarily subclinical seizures may be undertreated, whereas many infants whose paroxysmal events are, in fact, not caused by seizures, may be exposed unnecessarily to potentially detrimental anticonvulsant medications.

Although some neonatal seizures have associated clinical signs, multiple studies of critically ill newborns have highlighted the fact that most neonatal seizures are subclinical. Subclinical seizures have no outward manifestation, and are therefore only detectable with EEG. That most neonatal seizures are subclinical should not be surprising. Preverbal children cannot communicate their experiences of sensory phenomena caused by seizures (e.g., visual changes associated with occipital seizures, or déjà vu because of temporal lobe seizures), and unless the seizure originates from, or propagates to, the motor cortex, there will be no abnormal movements. Isolated paroxysmal changes in blood pressure or heart rate, without other associated clinical signs, often raise concern for seizures in high-risk newborns, but these events are rarely because of seizures. Even neonates who present with clinically apparent seizure semiologies often experience electroclinical dissociation when medication is administered (e.g., EEG seizures persist even after resolution of the clinical signs).

Because clinical signs of neonatal seizures are uncommon and difficult to identify, EEG monitoring is required for precise diagnosis of paroxysmal events and for quantification of seizure burden. Neonatal seizures are most properly defined by their EEG patterns and they need not have a clinical semiology. A seizure is an abnormal EEG pattern that evolves, is of greater than 2-μV amplitude, and has a duration of 10 seconds or greater (Figure 18-1). Distinct seizures are separated by a 10-second or greater seizure-free interval. It is very uncommon for individual neonatal seizures to be more than a few minutes in duration, but the seizures are often very frequent. Therefore neonatal status epilepticus is defined as seizures that occupy more than 50% of any 1-hour EEG epoch (e.g., a newborn with 30 1-minute seizures in an hour would meet criteria for status epilepticus, as would an infant with a single seizure that lasts 30 minutes or greater) (Tsuchida et al., 2013).

Neonatal Electroencephalogram Monitoring
Conventional Video Electroencephalogram

Video EEG monitoring remains the gold standard for neonatal seizure detection and is indispensible for research studies that

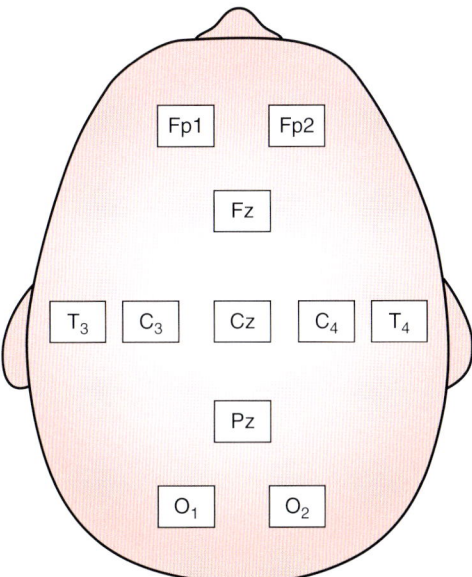

Figure 18-2. The international 10–20 system for electroencephalography electrode placement, modified for neonates, includes the electrode positions indicated by the boxes. By convention, the odd and even numbers designate the left and right sides of the head, respectively, and "z" labels the midline positions. Additional extracerebral channels, including respiratory and electrocardiogram tracings, are also necessary to exclude artifact and determine behavioral state. Extraocular and surface electromyography leads are often useful, but not always required.

attempt to quantify seizure burden and/or treatment responses. Standard electrode positions, using the international 10–20 system, modified for neonates are recommended (Figure 18-2). In addition to the scalp electrodes, extracerebral leads for respiratory and electrocardiogram recording are required for accurate evaluation of behavioral state and exclusion of extracerebral artifacts. Time-locked video monitoring is highly recommended during the EEG recording to assist in the differential diagnosis of abnormal paroxysmal events. Video is critical to distinguish sources of artifact, such as handling or patting the infant, or electronic interference from intensive care unit (ICU) equipment. Surface electromyography and extraoculography leads are often utilized, but these are not mandatory. A bedside observer (typically the bedside nurse) is also important, as this person can press a patient event marker, or enter information directly onto the digital file through a bedside computer, to alert the neurophysiologist to clinically important events, such as the occurrence of target paroxysmal events or administration of neuroactive medications. Minimum standards for neonatal EEG recording have been defined by the American Clinical Neurophysiology Society.

Indications for Electroencephalogram Monitoring

Not every sick newborn requires EEG monitoring. Rather, this resource-intensive monitoring should be targeted at those at highest risk for seizures. In general, consideration for EEG monitoring is recommended for neonates with paroxysmal clinical events that are suspicious for seizures, as well as those with proven or suspected acute brain injury *and* clinical encephalopathy. The American Clinical Neurophysiology Society also provides guidelines on selection of newborns for EEG monitoring (Shellhaas et al., 2011).

Duration of EEG Recording

A routine-length, 60-minute, neonatal EEG is inadequate to screen for neonatal seizures. High-risk newborns should ideally be monitored with at least 24 hours of conventional EEG if seizures are suspected, because nearly all neonates with seizures will be identified within 24 hours of monitoring. If seizures are identified, experts suggest that they be monitored with EEG until the infant is seizure-free for at least 24 hours. In some circumstances this duration of monitoring is not feasible, or is not in the infant's best interests (e.g., an infant with a severe neonatal epilepsy syndrome might not be expected to remain seizure-free, or monitoring might be appropriately suspended to allow for neuroimaging).

A 60-minute routine-length neonatal EEG *is* typically sufficient to assess the EEG background, which might be of interest as a marker of prognosis or as an adjunctive tool for estimating gestational age. The suggested 60-minute duration is longer than routine-length EEGs for older infants or children, because it is imperative that all behavioral states be recorded. It is not unusual for a newborn to have a relatively normal awake EEG background but have clinically significant abnormalities detected during quiet sleep.

If EEG monitoring is initiated in order to clarify whether a newborn's paroxysmal clinical events are caused by seizures, then the EEG should be recorded until several typical episodes are captured. If the EEG background is stable and the target events are not seizures, then monitoring for this purpose can be terminated.

As discussed under the Acute Symptomatic Seizures subheading, HIE is the most common etiology of neonatal seizures. These newborns are now treated with therapeutic hypothermia for neuroprotection. Since at least half of neonates treated with therapeutic hypothermia for HIE have EEG-confirmed seizures, many neonatal neurointensive care programs recommend that EEG monitoring continue throughout cooling and rewarming. EEG background patterns and their prognostic significance are altered by therapeutic hypothermia. Sleep–wake cycling, for example, emerges later in infants who are cooled than those who do not receive therapeutic hypothermia, and not all neonates with a suppressed EEG background in the first day of life will have a poor prognosis. Despite therapeutic hypothermia, severe interictal EEG abnormalities, especially burst suppression, remain ominous if they persist beyond 24 to 30 hours of life.

Because conventional EEG monitoring is resource-intensive and requires specialized equipment, available technologists, and trained electroencephalographers, a reduced-montage EEG has gained popularity in many Neonatal Intensive Care Units (NICUs). aEEG is a simplified trend monitor that displays one or two channels of time-compressed, processed EEG signal on a semilogarithmic scale. Interpretation of the aEEG signal is enhanced by concurrent display of the raw single or multichannel EEG. aEEG background patterns have predictive value for neonates with HIE and other causes of encephalopathy. The use of aEEG for seizure detection is controversial, as this tool is specific but not sensitive in this capacity. There is substantial variability in the reported sensitivity of aEEG for seizure detection (usually 25–35%, but occasionally reported 85% sensitivity for individual seizure detection).

Diagnostic Considerations for Neonates with Seizures

If the diagnosis of neonatal seizures is being entertained, a complete evaluation for the etiology is warranted (Figures 18-3 and 18-4). The great majority of neonatal seizures are acute symptomatic manifestations of brain injury and many

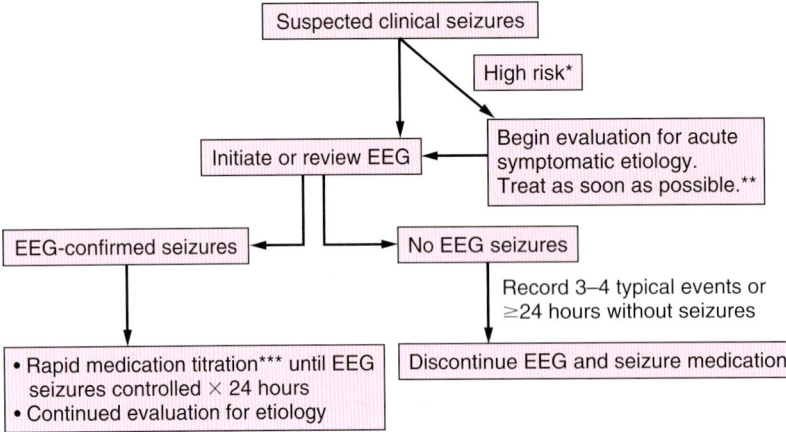

* High-risk scenarios: known or suspected acute brain injury, encephalopathy, previous EEG seizures, first 72 hours of life
** Reverse glucose or electrolyte abnormalities, and/or administer lorazepam 0.1 mg/kg IV, and/or administer
phenobarbital loading dose.
*** Refer to Figure 18.5

Figure 18-3. Assessment algorithm for newborns with suspected seizures.

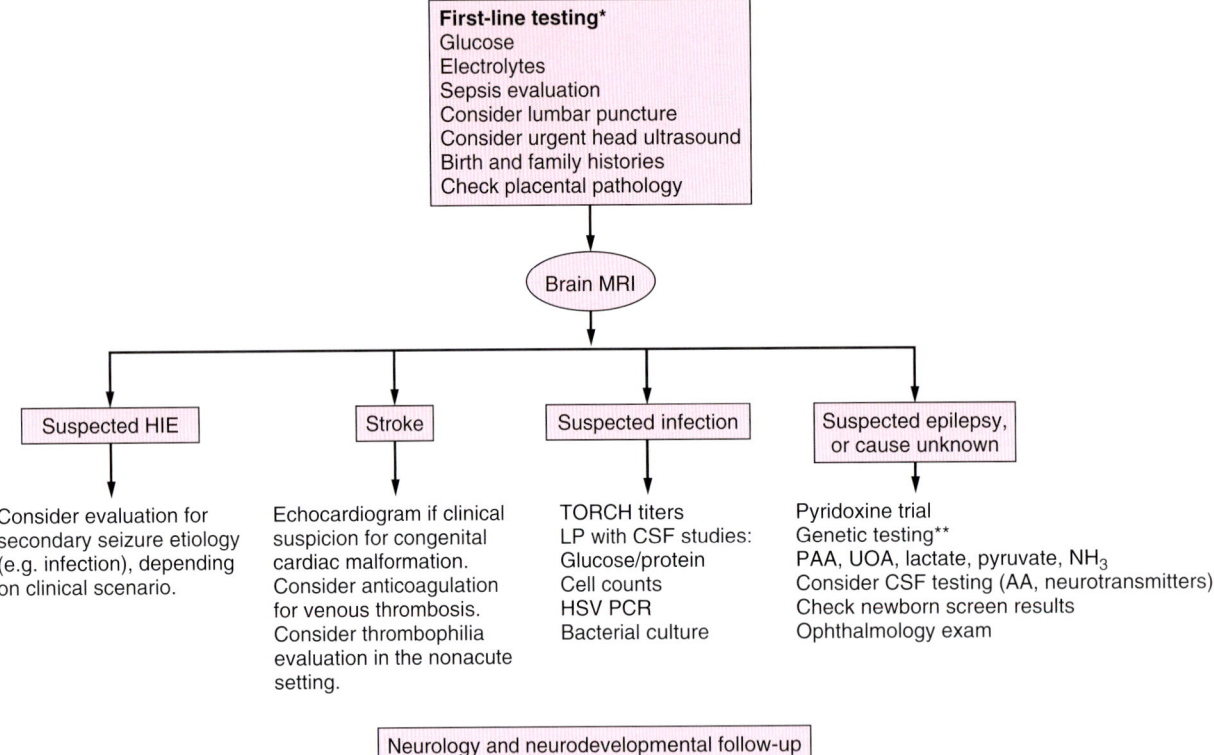

**Genetic testing can include: karyotype, chromosomal microarray, epilepsy gene panel, or single gene testing.

Figure 18-4. Assessment algorithm for newborns with seizures. First-line testing should occur simultaneously with initiation of electroencephalography (and empiric seizure treatment in high-risk clinical scenarios). Most infants should receive neuroimaging, and brain magnetic resonance imaging (MRI) is the preferred neuroimaging modality. Second-line testing depends on the clinical scenario and MRI findings. Newborns with seizures are at high risk for long-term neurodevelopmental disability and epilepsy, and so they require careful follow-up by appropriate clinicians.

require urgent, specific treatment. This diagnostic evaluation should occur in tandem with treatment of seizures. Glucose and electrolyte levels should be measured and any abnormality corrected emergently. A full sepsis evaluation, including cultures of blood, urine, and CSF, is strongly recommended (unless the infant is too unstable to undergo a lumbar puncture or a definite alternative diagnosis is made). Empiric

antibiotics should usually be administered until the cultures are negative.

In most hospitals and emergency departments, it is straightforward to obtain a head ultrasound. Despite its low resolution, cranial ultrasonography can be used to screen for obvious hydrocephalus or intracranial hemorrhage. Computed tomography is usually avoided in neonates, because of the concern about radiation exposure. Rather, MRI is the standard neuroimaging modality for neonates with seizures. If arterial ischemic stroke or vascular malformations are suspected, MR angiogram is recommended. If a venous sinus thrombosis is suspected (e.g., in a term neonate with intraventricular or thalamic hemorrhage), MR venogram may be diagnostic and concurrent MRI may reveal venous strokes.

The maternal and family history must be reviewed. The use of maternal selective serotonin reuptake inhibitors (SSRI) in the third trimester is a common cause of abnormal movements during the first 12 hours of life, but these are usually not seizures. Serotonin–norepinephrine reuptake inhibitors (SNRI) withdrawal may be associated with electroclinical seizures starting in the first 3 days of life. Even if withdrawal from SSRIs, SNRIs, or drugs of abuse is suspected, other serious causes of seizure should be ruled out. Although seizures can occur in the setting of withdrawal from prescribed or illicit drugs used during pregnancy, and neonatal abstinence syndrome incidence is rising, most affected newborns do not have seizures. Convulsions or other abnormal movements *without electrographic correlate* need not be treated with seizure medications. Family history may reveal BFNE as the likely cause in an otherwise well-appearing infant.

Further diagnostic testing depends on the clinical scenario. If the evaluation for infection is negative and there is no other immediately obvious cause of seizures after MRI and basic metabolic workup, then testing for inborn errors of metabolism is reasonable for newborns with abnormal neurologic examinations and pharmacoresistant seizures. This testing may include measurement of lactate, pyruvate, ammonia, plasma amino acids, urine organic acids, and sometime advanced testing of the CSF. If the infant has congenital anomalies and/or dysmorphic features, or if a neonatal epilepsy syndrome is suspected, genetic testing and consultation should be considered. Single-gene testing is occasionally helpful, but clinical availability of early onset epilepsy gene panels is improving and may be more cost-effective. Chromosomal microarray may also reveal clinically significant abnormalities.

TREATMENT
Acute Treatment

Because new-onset seizures in a neonate often reflect a serious underlying neurologic condition, they should be treated as a medical emergency. Once the bedside clinician has established that the vital signs are stable and taken note of the clinical manifestations of a suspected seizure, glucose must be checked immediately and electrolytes (including calcium and magnesium) drawn to rule out rapidly treatable causes of seizures. Video EEG should be initiated as soon as possible to confirm that clinical events have an electrographic correlate. If infection is suspected, appropriate cultures should be drawn and treatment initiated, including acyclovir for herpes simplex virus and broad spectrum antibiotics for a suspected bacterial infection.

Treatment of Acute Symptomatic Seizures

Treatment with antiseizure medications should be initiated as soon as possible once electrographic seizures are confirmed (or immediately in a patient with a high-risk condition such as HIE, acute intracranial hemorrhage, or clonic motor hemiconvulsions indicating a likely stroke; see Figure 18-3). Medication should be administered in adequate bolus doses titrated to abolish electrographic seizures (including electrographic seizures without clinical correlate) as quickly as possible (Figure 18-5) (Hellström-Westas et al., 2015).

Few data from clinical trials are available to guide anticonvulsant management decisions. A suggested treatment algorithm is presented in Figure 18-5. According to international surveys, phenobarbital remains the most commonly used agent for first-line treatment of seizures in newborn infants. Seizures are controlled in roughly half of patients after a single phenobarbital loading dose of 20 mg/kg (Painter et al., 1999). Phenytoin (or, preferably, IV fosphenytoin in the acute setting) has similar efficacy to phenobarbital when used at a loading dose of 20 mg/kg, but maintenance dosing—particularly with oral administration—is challenging in neonates because of less predictable absorption and pharmacokinetics than phenobarbital. Levetiracetam is increasingly used in spite of limited safety and efficacy data. Initial pharmacokinetic data suggest use of a levetiracetam loading dose (40 mg/kg) followed by maintenance dosing (10 mg/kg/dose or greater administered every 8 hours) may be considered.

If seizures are not controlled after repeated loading doses of standard medications, infusions are sometimes indicated. Midazolam infusion is an alternative or add-on agent in refractory cases in the setting of acute brain injury and status epilepticus. Lidocaine infusions can be used for refractory acute symptomatic neonatal seizures. Note that lidocaine is contraindicated for neonates with congenital heart disease and for those who have previously been treated with phenytoin/fosphenytoin, because of the risk of arrhythmia. Additionally, lidocaine dosing must be adjusted for neonates treated with therapeutic hypothermia (phenobarbital dosing does not need to be adjusted).

Maintenance anticonvulsant medication dosing should be initiated for neonates who have confirmed electrographic seizures. For newborns with clinical events without proven electrographic seizures, maintenance dosing may be discontinued and the EEG reviewed frequently to ensure that the neonate does not subsequently develop electrographic seizures.

Discontinuation of Medication for Acute Symptomatic Seizures

Acute symptomatic seizures typically arise within the first 24 to 48 hours of life, after which there is a short period of high seizure burden, followed by a longer period of lower seizure burden. Overall duration of acute symptomatic seizures is typically 48 to 96 hours. Knowing the seizure tempo and careful use of video-EEG monitoring to determine when seizures arise and resolve can help guide duration of seizure medications. Because the recurrence risk in the neonatal period is low, many neonates can be safely discontinued from medications after resolution of acute symptomatic seizures. There is no need to wean medications that have been used for only a short duration (less than 1 week). If the child is to be maintained on medications, the regimen should be simplified and a plan put in place to reassess the infant after discharge from hospital so that anticonvulsants may be discontinued during the first few months of life.

Treatment of Early Onset Epilepsy Syndromes

If the diagnostic evaluation rules out an acute symptomatic cause for neonatal seizures, early onset epilepsy should be suspected. The treatment of epilepsy in the neonatal period is different from the approach for acute symptomatic seizures. First, rapid treatment of seizures probably does not affect seizure burden or long-term outcome, and so medications should be carefully titrated to maximally tolerated doses to ensure efficacy or failure. Second, neonates with epilepsy must

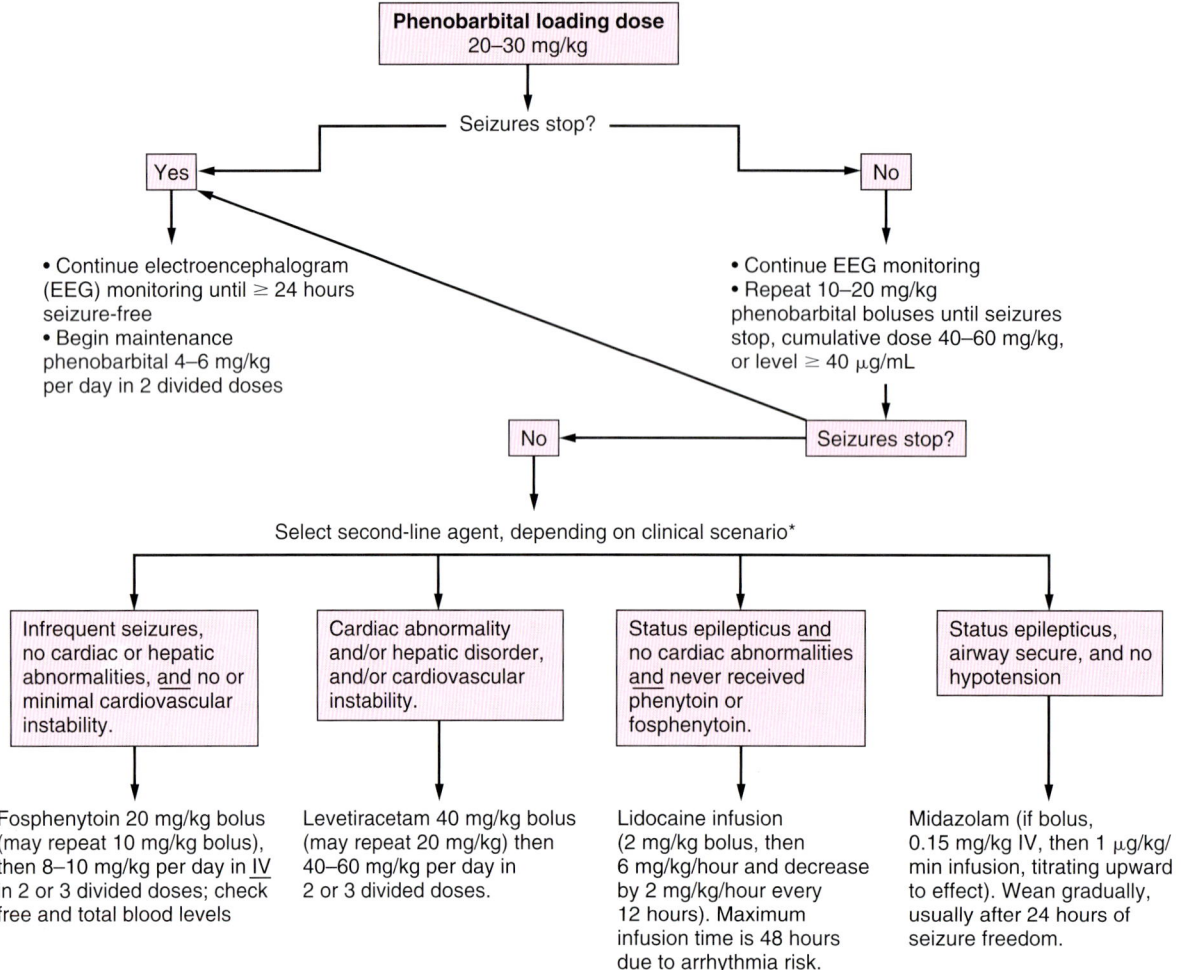

Figure 18-5. Suggested treatment algorithm for neonatal seizures. The rapidity of medication administration will depend on local guidelines and resources. Frequent assessment of treatment response is recommended.

continue medications after discharge home, even if seizures have been controlled with medical management.

Vitamin-responsive inborn errors of metabolism may present with neonatal encephalopathy and refractory seizures, and so pharmacologic doses of pyridoxine, folinic acid, and pyridoxal 5′-phosphate are indicated in this setting. Neonates with suspected PDE should be administered a trial of IV pyridoxine (100 mg IV while EEG is recording). The infant must be monitored during this trial, as apnea and bradycardia can be provoked. If there is a clear response, test urine alpha-AASA and/or plasma pipecolic acid levels and consider confirmation with ALDH7A1 mutation analysis. If there is no response to pyridoxine, a trial of pyridoxal 5′-phostphate (60 mg/kg/day divided 3 times/day for 2–3 days) and then folinic acid (2.5 mg IV) may be attempted.

Carbamazepine and oxcarbazepine are effective and well tolerated for neonates with seizures caused by KCNQ2/3 mutations (either BFNE or KCNQ2 encephalopathy). If carbamazepine or oxcarbazepine is not effective, a trial of retigabine, which selectively affects the K+ channel, may be worthwhile.

OUTCOMES AFTER NEONATAL SEIZURES

Neonatal seizures are associated with an array of adverse outcomes, including intellectual disability, cerebral palsy, postneonatal epilepsy, and death (Uria-Avellanal et al., 2013). Most often in the literature, cognitive and behavioral outcomes are not reported separately from cerebral palsy. Instead, outcomes are grouped into "favorable" (survival without impairment) or "unfavorable" (death, or intellectual disability, and/or cerebral palsy, and/or epilepsy). The risk for unfavorable outcomes related to neonatal seizures is difficult to isolate from the underlying cause of the seizures. Additionally, because many infants with neonatal seizures are critically ill, they often have multiple comorbidities that affect long-term outcomes. As an example, a newborn whose seizures are caused by HIE is at risk for impaired neurodevelopment because of the acute brain injury, as well as the seizures, but might also have neonatal sepsis or feeding problems that lead to suboptimal nutrition, all of which may elevate the risk for adverse outcomes.

Mortality After Neonatal Seizures

Despite modern neonatal intensive care, 10% to 30% of newborns with seizures die during the neonatal period. Risk of death is higher in certain subgroups (e.g., preterm infants). Geographic variation in reported mortality may reflect cultural differences regarding decisions to withdraw intensive care for neonates with extremely poor prognosis. Among survivors of neonatal seizures, those with abnormal neurodevelopment remain at elevated risk of death throughout childhood.

Cognitive Outcomes After Neonatal Seizures

The longest-term follow-up studies included infants with clinically diagnosed neonatal seizures. Among survivors, 40% to 50% have global developmental delays, and preterm infants are at higher risk than full-term neonates. Among neonates with HIE, a diagnosis of neonatal seizures increases the risk for developmental delays and intellectual disability, after controlling for the degree of encephalopathy. Severe seizure burden increases this risk.

Cerebral Palsy After Neonatal Seizures

About 25% to 35% of long-term neonatal seizure survivors develop cerebral palsy. Most of those with severe cerebral palsy have comorbid global developmental delays, including intellectual disability. Among survivors of neonatal seizures, having cerebral palsy is also a significant risk factor for postneonatal epilepsy.

Postneonatal Epilepsy

Postneonatal epilepsy—in which the acute symptomatic seizures subside, but recurrent unprovoked seizures develop later in life—affects 20% to 30% of survivors of neonatal seizures. Most often, epilepsy develops in the first few years of life. Children can have a range of epilepsy syndromes, depending on the etiology of the neonatal seizures. Most studies have not been powered to describe details of the epilepsy syndromes, but several groups have reported a 10% to 16% incidence of West syndrome after clinical neonatal seizures.

Clinical risk factors for postneonatal epilepsy include requirement of more than one medication to control the acute neonatal seizures, moderate or severe neonatal encephalopathy, abnormal neuroimaging, and low birth weight. EEG risk factors include status epilepticus, persistently abnormal interictal EEG background, multifocal (vs. focal) seizures, and ictal spread to the contralateral hemisphere.

Among people with chronic epilepsy, a history of clinical neonatal seizures is a definite risk factor for long-term non-remission of the epilepsy. By extension, because treatment-resistant epilepsy is associated with cognitive and behavioral challenges, early life seizures may predispose to long-term intellectual and behavioral difficulties.

CONCLUSIONS

The immature brain is predisposed to seizures. Neonatal seizures usually reflect acute underlying brain injury, rather than epilepsy. Thus evaluations to confirm the diagnosis of seizures (with EEG) and to determine and treat their etiology must occur simultaneously. There are very few data from clinical trials to guide treatment decisions. Phenobarbital is the most commonly prescribed first-line agent. Controversy remains regarding the ideal duration of treatment. However, it is clear that neonatal seizures are associated with substantial risk of mortality and of long-term neurodevelopmental disability and epilepsy. High-quality research is urgently needed in order to determine the best treatment algorithms and, ultimately, to improve long-term outcomes.

REFERENCES

The complete list of references for this chapter is available in the e-book at www.expertconsult.com.

 See inside cover for registration details.

SELECTED REFERENCES

Beal, J.C., Cherian, K., Moshé, S.L., 2012. Early-onset epileptic encephalopathies: Ohtahara syndrome and early myoclonic encephalopathy. Pediatr. Neurol. 47, 317–323.

Boylan, G.B., Kharoshankaya, L., Wusthoff, C.J., 2015. Seizures and hypothermia: Importance of electroencephalographic monitoring and considerations for treatment. Semin. Fetal Neonatal Med. 20, 103–109.

Hellström-Westas, L., Boylan, G., Ågren, J., 2015. Systematic review of neonatal seizure management strategies provides guidance on antiepileptic treatment. Acta Paediatr. 104, 123–129.

Holmes, G.L., 2009. The long-term effects of neonatal seizures. Clin. Perinatol. 36, 901–914.

Loman, A.M., ter Horst, H.J., Lambrechtsen, F.A., et al., 2014. Neonatal seizures: Aetiology by means of a standardized work-up. Eur. J. Paediatr. Neurol. 8, 360–367.

Mastrangelo, M., van Lierde, A., Bray, M., et al., 2005. Epileptic seizures, epilepsy, and epileptic syndromes in newborns: A nosological approach to 94 new cases by the 2001 proposed diagnostic scheme for people with epileptic seizures and with epilepsy. Seizure 14, 304–311.

Murray, D.M., Boylan, G.B., Ali, I., et al., 2008. Defining the gap between electrographic seizure burden, clinical expression and staff recognition of neonatal seizures. Arch. Dis. Child. Fetal Neonatal Ed. 93, F187–F191.

Painter, M.J., et al., 1999. Phenobarbital compared with phenytoin for the treatment of neonatal seizures. N. Engl. J. Med. 341, 485–489.

Pisani, F., Copioli, C., Di Gioia, C., et al., 2008. Neonatal seizures: Relation of ictal video-electroencephalography (EEG) findings with neurodevelopmental outcome. J. Child Neurol. 23, 394–398.

Ronen, G.M., Penney, S., Andrews, W., 1999. The epidemiology of clinical neonatal seizures in Newfoundland: A population-based study. J. Pediatr. 134, 71–75.

Shellhaas, R.A., Chang, T., Tsuchida, T., et al., 2011. The American Clinical Neurophysiology Society's guideline on continuous electroencephalography monitoring in neonates. J. Clin. Neurophysiol. 28, 611–617.

Tekgul, H., Gauvreau, K., Soul, J., et al., 2006. The current etiologic profile and neurodevelopmental outcome of seizures in term newborn infants. Pediatrics 117, 1270–1280.

Tsuchida, T.N., Wusthoff, C.J., Shellhaas, R.A., et al., 2013. American clinical neurophysiology society standardized EEG terminology and categorization for the description of continuous EEG monitoring in neonates: Report of the American Clinical Neurophysiology Society critical care monitoring committee. J. Clin. Neurophysiol. 30, 161–173.

Uria-Avellanal, C., Marlow, N., Rennie, J.M., 2013. Outcome following neonatal seizures. Semin. Fetal Neonatal Med. 18, 224–232.

E-BOOK FIGURES AND TABLES

The following figures and tables are available in the e-book at www.expertconsult.com. See inside cover for registration details.

Fig. 18-1 Electroencephalography recorded from a 3-day-old male, born at 38 weeks' gestation, who presented with apnea associated with focal tonic stiffening.
Box 18-1 Neonatal Seizure Pearls.
Table 18-1 Estimates of Neonatal Seizure Incidence

19 Hypoxic-Ischemic Brain Injury in the Term Newborn

Vann Chau, Donna M. Ferriero, and Steven P. Miller

An expanded version of this chapter is available on www.expertconsult.com. See inside cover for registration details.

SCOPE OF THE PROBLEM

Neonatal encephalopathy (NE) is a clinical syndrome characterized by "a subnormal level of consciousness or seizures, and often accompanied by difficulty with initiating and maintaining respiration and depression of tone and reflexes," in the earliest days of life of a term newborn (Douglas-Escobar and Weiss, 2015). Hospital-based estimates note that it affects up to 6 to 8 per 1000 live births. With the increasing recognition that hypoxia-ischemia is a critical contributor to NE, therapeutic hypothermia has emerged as standard practice in the care of the term neonate with hypoxic-ischemic encephalopathy (HIE). Equally relevant is the emergence of *neonatal neurocritical care units*, which combine the synergistic expertise of neonatologists, neurologists, neuroradiologists, nursing staff, and others involved in the care of the sick neonate (Bonifacio et al., 2011).

ETIOLOGY OF BRAIN INJURY IN THE TERM NEWBORN

There is increasing recognition that neonatal brain injury is related to antenatal, perinatal, and postnatal factors, and is not always the result of "birth asphyxia." Many risk factors for neonatal encephalopathy are clearly prenatal. However, recent cohorts evaluated with magnetic resonance imaging (MRI) studies demonstrate that *brain injury actually happens at or near the time of birth.* The revised 2014 American College of Obstetricians and Gynecologists (ACOG) guidelines clearly articulate several pathways to NE, including proximate and distal risk factors that may occur during the prepartum, intrapartum, and postpartum periods (ACOG, 2014). More specifically, postnatal causes may account for up to 10% of neonatal encephalopathy in the *term* infant.

CLINICAL SYNDROME AND NATURAL HISTORY
Clinical Syndrome

Neonatal encephalopathy is usually evidenced by alterations in alertness, tone, respiratory status, reflexes, and feeding, and seizures (Table 19-1). The severity of brain injury, reflecting the duration and magnitude of the hypoxic-ischemic insult, determines the nature of the evolution of this clinical encephalopathy. In newborns with moderate to severe encephalopathy, symptoms usually evolve over days, making *serial* detailed examinations important. As with any neurologically ill newborn, the baby's gestational age must be considered in the interpretation of physical findings. There is a characteristic progression of signs in newborns with a severe hypoxic-ischemic insult (Table 19-2). The affected neonate exhibits a depressed level of consciousness from the very first hours of life. Periodic breathing with apnea and bradycardia often heralds this initial presentation. Hypotonia is almost universally found. In the first day of life, the pupillary response is often preserved, and abnormalities of eye movements are not detected. In severely injured newborns, seizures may be seen within 6 to 12 hours of birth. Seizures at this stage are often subtle, manifesting as ocular movements, lip smacking, apneas, or bicycling movements of the extremities. Focal clonic seizures may also occur and often indicate focal cerebral infarction. Seizures in the term neonate with HIE can be difficult to diagnose based on clinical features alone, particularly in those with an abnormal electroencephalogram (EEG) background. Seizures continue to be common in neonates with HIE treated with hypothermia and are seen in almost one third of affected babies.

As described by Volpe, in latter hours of the first day of life, there may be a transient increase in the level of alertness that is not accompanied by other signs of neurologic improvement. This can be falsely reassuring because this apparent increase in alertness is frequently accompanied by more seizures and apnea, shrill cry, and jitteriness. With careful bedside examination, weakness in the proximal limbs and increased muscle stretch reflexes may be observed, but in the very severely injured newborn, diffuse weakness with absent movements and reflexes is common (Volpe, 2008).

By the third day of life in newborns with severe brain injury, the level of consciousness deteriorates, with manifestation of respiratory arrest and other signs of brainstem dysfunction. During this period, cerebral edema resulting from hypoxia-ischemia is maximal and can further impair cerebral blood flow secondary to increased vascular pressure. Those newborns surviving beyond the third day of life begin to show an improved alertness. Yet hypotonia and weakness in the proximal limbs, face, and bulbar musculature persist.

Documenting this clinical evolution is a critical component of the evaluation of an encephalopathic newborn. The use of a simple encephalopathy score as a bedside tool can help the clinician standardize the assessment and monitoring of encephalopathic newborns. In infants with moderate encephalopathy on the fourth day of life, those treated with hypothermia were shown to have a more favorable outcome than those receiving standard care (Azzopardi et al., 2014).

Management of Neonatal Encephalopathy

Because many etiologies of neonatal encephalopathy have specific therapies, the clinician's initial task is to determine the underlying etiology through careful history taking, neurologic examination, laboratory testing, and brain imaging studies. The history should elicit indicators of intrauterine distress that may have contributed to decreased placental or fetal blood flow: fetal heart tracing abnormalities, passage of meconium, or a history of a difficulty in labor or delivery. The details of the delivery-room resuscitation, medications, and ventilatory support should be noted. Laboratory tests are critical to exclude reversible causes of neonatal encephalopathy. The management of moderate or severe encephalopathy should occur in a neonatal intensive care unit, with close collaboration between the neurologist and neonatologist. Prompt consideration of the initiation of therapeutic hypothermia is critical because earlier cooling is most effective.

Immediate management requires securing an appropriate airway and maintaining adequate circulation. Ventilatory support with mechanical ventilation or continuous positive airway pressure (CPAP) is often required. Metabolic complications such as hypoglycemia, hypocalcemia, hyponatremia, and acidosis frequently accompany hypoxic-ischemic encephalopathy and should be identified and treated. Liver enzymes and serum creatinine are performed to detect injury in other end organs, and serum ammonia and lactate levels can expedite the investigation of an inborn error of metabolism. Lumbar puncture to evaluate for intracranial infections should be performed if the history is not typical for HIE or if a clinical suspicion of infection exists. If infection is suspected, ampicillin and gentamicin are started, and acyclovir is added if herpes simplex virus is a consideration. The clinician should also be vigilant to diagnose and treat postnatal sepsis given the negative association with outcomes in this population. If the history, examination, or initial laboratory investigations point to an inborn error of metabolism, early treatment is crucial, and a biochemical geneticist should be consulted. The diagnosis of a severe intracranial hemorrhage requires monitoring of platelet levels and coagulation function and should prompt consultation with a neurosurgeon. Because the clinical syndrome evolves considerably over the first 72 hours of life, management of specific complications, such as respiratory compromise or seizures, can often be anticipated.

The investigation of term newborns with encephalopathy addresses three primary concerns: (1) identifying the underlying etiology, (2) determining the timing of the brain injury, and (3) predicting the neurodevelopmental outcome of the affected newborn. Addressing these concerns is critical for the application of "neuroprotection" strategies, such as hypothermia (Papile et al., 2014). Although the severity of brain injury in term asphyxiated newborns is not reliably predicted by clinical indicators, the severity of clinical encephalopathy is a strong predictor of neurodevelopmental outcome. The risk of motor and cognitive deficits appears to be minimal in mild encephalopathy and pronounced in the severe end of the spectrum, but inconsistent in moderate encephalopathy. Newborns with moderate encephalopathy are thus the most likely to benefit from neuroimaging.

Brain Imaging of Newborns With Encephalopathy

Brain imaging has revealed patterns of brain injury following a hypoxic-ischemic insult that are unique to the immature brain and that depend on the age at which it occurs and the severity and duration of the insult (Fig. 19-1). Neonatal brain injury evolves over days or weeks. This time course "opens the door" for therapeutic interventions, with different interventions needed in the evolution of the injury.

To confirm the diagnosis of hypoxic-ischemic brain injury and determine the extent of injury, MRI and diffusion-weighted imaging (DWI) are optimally obtained between 3 and 5 days of life in term newborns with encephalopathy. In newborns treated with hypothermia, further studies are needed to determine the *optimal* timing of MRI. Cranial ultrasound can be used for the detection of antenatal injury and severe

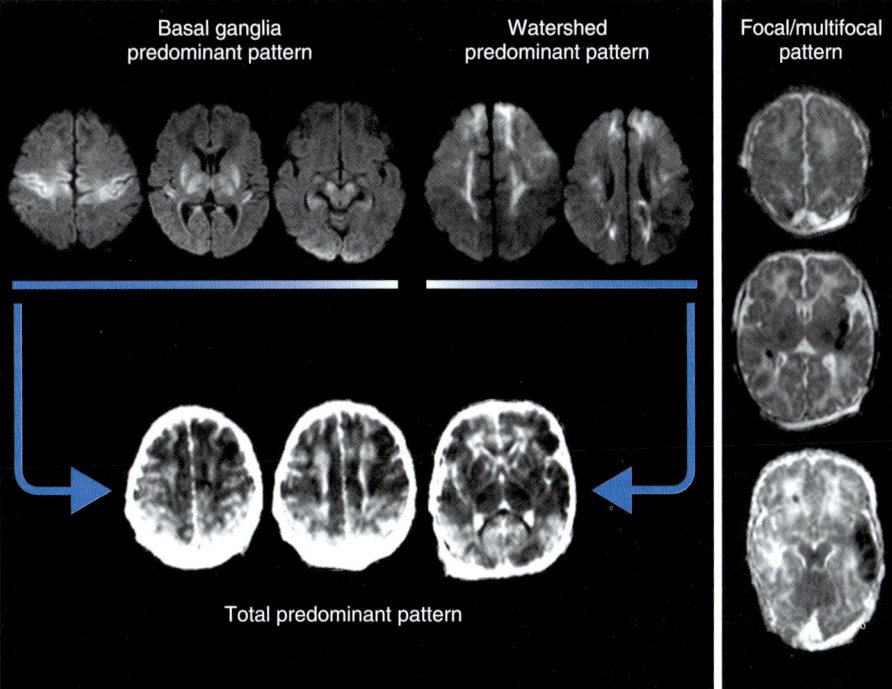

Figure 19-1. Predominant patterns of brain injury in term hypoxic-ischemic encephalopathy. **A,** Basal-ganglia-predominant pattern of injury in a newborn with perinatal asphyxia imaged on the third day of life. Brain injury is demonstrated on diffusion-weighted imaging (DWI) as areas of restricted diffusion (hyperintense, bright areas) in the motor cortex around the central sulcus, thalami, basal ganglia, optic radiations, hippocampi, and midbrain. **B,** Watershed-predominant pattern of injury in a newborn with perinatal asphyxia imaged on the third day of life. Cortical and subcortical brain injury is demonstrated on DWI in the watershed regions, affecting both the cortex and the white matter. Both the basal-nuclei-predominant and watershed-predominant patterns can lead to the total predominant pattern (**C**) if severe enough, as shown on these apparent diffusion coefficient (ADC) maps as areas of restricted diffusion (hypointense, dark areas). **D,** Multifocal white-matter injury in the periventricular and subcortical white matter in a newborn, seen as areas of restricted diffusion identified by arrows (hypointense, dark areas) on the ADC maps. **E,** Stroke: Focal infarct in the left middle cerebral artery territory in the same newborn with perinatal asphyxia, demonstrated on the ADC as an area of restricted diffusion marked by the star (hypointense, dark areas).

intracranial hemorrhage, followed by MRI for comprehensive diagnostic and prognostic evaluation.

Advanced Magnetic Resonance Techniques. Advanced magnetic resonance (MR) techniques, such as diffusion and spectroscopic imaging, allow for the observation of the progression of brain injury in the newborn (Counsell et al., 2014).

Magnetic Resonance Spectroscopy. MR spectroscopy (MRS) can be used to measure changes in certain brain metabolites from a given region of the brain. N-acetylaspartate (NAA) and lactate are the most useful in assessing brain injury. NAA is found in high concentrations in neurons, and levels increase with advancing cerebral maturity. NAA levels decrease with cerebral injury or impaired cerebral metabolism. Lactate is normally produced by astrocytes and used as fuel by neurons to replenish energy stores via oxidative phosphorylation. Lactate levels are elevated with the disturbed oxidative metabolism seen with hypoxia-ischemia. Elevated lactate and reduced NAA levels are highly predictive of neurodevelopmental outcome. Given this, lactate/NAA ratios are especially discriminatory of newborns with adverse outcomes. Myo-inositol is elevated with neonatal hypoxic-ischemic brain injury.

Diffusion Imaging. Diffusion-weighted MR imaging (DWI) detects alterations in free-water diffusion. Diffusion-tensor imaging (DTI) measures the amount (apparent diffusion coefficient [ADC] or average diffusivity) and the directionality of water motion (fractional anisotropy [FA]). With acute injury, intracellular water increases, and water movement is "restricted" by the cell membrane. The ADC or average diffusivity map (D_{av}) is a quantitative water diffusion map that shows restricted diffusion as areas of diminished signal intensity. Reduced ADC values in the posterior limb of the internal capsule are associated with a greater risk of adverse neurodevelopmental outcome. FA values in the white matter and basal ganglia are decreased with significant injury during the first week of life in term newborns with encephalopathy. Therapeutic hypothermia is associated with preserved brain microstructure, particularly in the basal ganglia and thalamus. Therapeutic hypothermia modifies the significance of restricted diffusion, such that greater restriction is needed for an adverse outcome.

Brain Perfusion. Brain perfusion in the neonate with HIE can be quantified with MR arterial spin labeling techniques. Recent data suggest that higher perfusion values in neonates with HIE predict worse neurodevelopmental outcomes, and that therapeutic hypothermia may be less effective when hyperperfusion is found early after neonatal HIE. These MR assessments can also be complemented by bedside measures using frequency domain near-infrared spectroscopy (FDNIRS) and diffuse correlation spectroscopy (DCS) to measure cerebral hemodynamics.

Patterns of Brain Injury

In a primate model, the distribution of injury was shown to be associated with the duration and severity of ischemia. Acute-profound asphyxia produces injury in the basal ganglia and thalamus, and partial asphyxia causes white-matter injury. Similar patterns of injury are found in term newborns following hypoxia-ischemia (Fig. 19-1). The basal-ganglia-predominant pattern involves the basal ganglia, thalamus, and perirolandic cortex. The *watershed* pattern predominantly involves the vascular watershed, from the white matter and extending to the cerebral cortex. Maximal injury in both the watershed region and basal ganglia results in the total pattern of brain injury. The predominant pattern of injury appears to be more strongly associated with neurodevelopmental

outcome than the severity of injury in any given region. The focal or multifocal pattern of injury is increasingly recognized in cohorts studied with MRI, especially with stroke or white-matter injury. Recent data suggest that strokes (arterial or venous) are also associated with neonatal encephalopathy in the term newborn. White-matter injury (WMI) is recognized in up to 23% of term newborns with encephalopathy (Fig. 19-1) and tends to be seen in infants with lower gestational age at birth, within the range of term birth. In sequential studies of term newborns with encephalopathy, delayed white-matter degeneration extending past the first week of life is also seen. This delayed white-matter injury might follow injury to the basal ganglia, just as Wallerian degeneration of the corticospinal tract degeneration is found following some middle cerebral artery strokes in the term newborn.

Progression of Neonatal Brain Injury

Timing the onset and determining the progression of brain injury has been greatly facilitated with the use of diffusion MR techniques and MRS. Recent studies have shown that the reduction in ADC resulting from brain injury seen on diffusion imaging evolves over the initial days of life, reaching its nadir by 2 to 4 days after injury. Thus MR diffusion images obtained before the nadir may not show the full extent of injury. Importantly, diffusion abnormalities persist for 7 to 8 days in the newborn before returning toward normal values (pseudonormalization) and ultimately reflect increased diffusion with tissue degeneration. In the first 24 hours following brain injury in the term newborn, lactate increases, followed by a decrease in NAA in the 3 days following injury. In a proportion of patients, brain injury will progressively worsen over the first 2 weeks of life to involve new brain areas, particularly the white-matter tracts. The prolonged progression of neonatal brain injury is consistent with the mechanisms of cell injury that persist for days following hypoxic-ischemic brain injury in the newborn.

OUTCOMES

The neurodevelopmental outcome following neonatal encephalopathy depends on the etiology of the encephalopathy and the pattern and severity of the brain injury. Neurodevelopmental deficits resulting from HIE typically involve motor, visual, and/or cognitive functions (Table 19-3). Both genetic and postnatal factors, such as socioeconomic factors (e.g., environmental exposures and parental education), likely modify of an individual's neurodevelopmental outcome following neonatal brain injury. Postneonatal epilepsy is identified in up to half of the survivors of moderate to severe neonatal encephalopathy, and is particularly common in those with cerebral palsy and developmental delay.

Cognitive deficits may feature prominently following hypoxic-ischemic brain injury (Pappas et al., 2015), even in the absence of cerebral palsy, particularly with the watershed pattern of injury. The ACOG task force on neonatal encephalopathy now concludes that the outcomes following an acute intrapartum event may include cerebral palsy of the spastic quadriplegic or dyskinetic type, and other subtypes of cerebral palsy are less likely. Developmental coordination disorder, autism spectrum disorder, or specific language impairments should also be considered as possibilities in follow up of encephalopathic newborns.

Motor Function

In term survivors of hypoxic-ischemic brain injury, the risk of cerebral palsy or severe disability may involve more than one

TABLE 19-3 Summary of Published Trials of Hypothermia for Neuroprotection in the Newborn*

Outcomes	CoolCap 112/118 18 months[†]	ICE 107/101 2 years	NICHD 97/93 6–7 years	TOBY 163/162 6–7 years
Death	29% vs. 39%[‡]		28% vs. 44%[§]	29% vs. 30%
Death or major disability	48% vs. 66%[§]	55% vs. 67%[§]	41% vs. 60%[§]	
Cerebral palsy		21% vs. 17%	17% vs. 29%	21% vs. 36%[§]
GMFCS disability 2-5		16% vs. 12%	59% vs. 58%	22% vs. 41%[§]
Motor score on Bayley scales ≤ 2 SD	24% vs. 39%	19% vs. 14%		
Visual impairment	7% vs. 14%	1% vs. 0%	1% vs. 4%	1% vs. 1%
Hearing impairment	6% vs. 2%	2% vs. 2%	5% vs. 2%	4% vs. 10%
Epilepsy	13% vs. 15%		10% vs. 16%	
Survival free of disability		42% vs. 22%[§]	41% vs. 42%	45% vs. 28%[§]

*aEEG, amplitude-integrated electroencephalogram; GMFCS, Gross Motor Function Classification System; ICE, Infant Cooling Evaluation; NICHD, National Institute of Child Health and Human Development; SD, standard deviation; TOBY, Total Body Hypothermia for Neonatal Encephalopathy.
[†]First and second percentages are from hypothermic and control groups, respectively.
[‡]Comparisons in the entire cohort did not show statistical significance. However, analysis in the subgroup of newborns with less severe aEEG changes. Numbers shown are for subgroup analysis.
[§]Statistically significant.

third of affected newborns and is most common in those with a severe encephalopathy. Spastic quadriparesis is the most common type of cerebral palsy, although athetoid or spastic hemiparesis also occur. Minor motor impairments that do not meet diagnostic criteria for cerebral palsy are diagnosed in more than one third of children with moderate encephalopathy and in more than one fourth of those with mild encephalopathy.

Vision and Hearing

Severe visual impairment or blindness occurs in up to one fourth of children after moderate or severe encephalopathy, especially in the setting of hypoglycemia. Visual dysfunction may result from injury to the posterior visual pathway, including the primary visual cortex, resulting in cortical visual impairment. The pattern of brain injury involving the basal ganglia and thalamus is associated with deficits of visual acuity, visual field deficits, and stereopsis. Sensorineural hearing loss, likely secondary to brainstem injury, is also seen following neonatal encephalopathy, even affecting up to 18% of survivors of moderate encephalopathy without cerebral palsy.

Cognition

Overall, cognitive deficits are seen in 30% to 50% of childhood survivors of moderate HIE. Intellectual performance in children with severe encephalopathy *without* cerebral palsy is also affected. School-age survivors of moderate neonatal encephalopathy are more likely to have difficulties with reading, spelling, and arithmetic or require additional school resources. Cognitive deficits such as those in language and memory may be seen even when IQ scores are "normal." Behavioral difficulties such as hyperactivity and emotional problems should also be considered even in those children without motor disability.

Outcome and Therapeutic Hypothermia

Therapeutic hypothermia, using selective head cooling or whole-body cooling, is now considered the standard of care for infants of at least 35 weeks of gestation with moderate to severe HIE who meet inclusion criteria used in clinical trials. Therapeutic hypothermia should be continued for 72 hours, with a target rectal (or esophageal) temperature of 33°C to 34°C for whole-body cooling or 34°C to 35°C for selective head cooling. Rewarming should occur over 6 to 12 hours (0.5°C every 1-2 hours).

An initial meta-analysis clearly demonstrated that hypothermia is neuroprotective. Both mortality and disability were reduced at 18 months of age, and survival without disability was increased. Because of concerns that hypothermia may be less beneficial for infants with severe encephalopathy, further analysis showed benefits of hypothermia (death or moderate to severe disability) for both infants with moderate encephalopathy (risk ratio [RR] 0.67; 95% confidence interval [CI], 0.56-0.81) and those with severe encephalopathy (RR 0.83; 95% CI, 0.74-0.92). Survival without neurodevelopmental delay was increased (RR 1.63; 95% CI, 1.36–1.95).

Longer-term outcomes were described in two main multicenter randomized trials. The first trial found that hypothermia resulted in lower death rates and did not increase rates of severe disability among survivors. Moderate or severe disability occurred in 24 of 69 hypothermia children (35%) and 19 of 50 control children (38%) ($P = 0.87$). Attentional or executive dysfunction occurred in 4% children receiving hypothermia and 13% of those receiving usual care ($P = 0.19$), and visuospatial dysfunction occurred in 4% of the hypothermia group and 3% of controls ($P = 0.80$). Hypothermia resulted in lower death rates and did not increase rates of severe disability among survivors. The second trial found that more children in the hypothermia group than in the control group survived without neurologic abnormalities (65 of 145 [45%] vs. 37 of 132 [28%]; relative risk, 1.60; 95% confidence interval, 1.15-2.22). Among the survivors, children in the hypothermia group had significant reductions in the risk of cerebral palsy (21% vs. 36%, $P = 0.03$) and the risk of moderate or severe disability (22% vs. 37%, $P = 0.03$).

OUTCOME PREDICTION

Several authors reported the utility of evoked potentials, mainly visual evoked potentials (VEPs) and somatosensory evoked potentials (SSEPs), in outcome prediction. Delayed latencies and absent cortical responses seem to be associated with adverse outcomes. The background of EEG and amplitude-integrated EEG (aEEG) was also found to be associated with long-term outcomes. Abnormal backgrounds (flat trace, continuous low-voltage and burst-suppression patterns) that persist beyond the first 24 hours of life seem to correlate best with outcomes.

The pattern of brain injury on neuroimaging conveys important prognostic information regarding the pattern of neurodevelopmental abnormalities. The basal ganglia pattern of injury and abnormal signal intensity in the posterior limb of the internal capsule are both predictive of severely impaired

motor and cognitive outcomes. The cognitive deficits associated with this pattern are not surprising given the common involvement of the cerebral cortex and cerebellum. In contrast, the watershed pattern is associated with cognitive impairments that are not necessarily accompanied by major motor deficits. In asphyxiated survivors without functional motor deficits, the severity of watershed-distribution injury was most strongly associated with impaired language skills. Neurologic deficits may also be found with normal brain imaging. In these patients, subtle brain injuries may only be detectable with quantitative brain imaging techniques.

The predictive values of these different tests were summarized in a recent meta-analysis (Fig. 19-2) (van Laerhoven

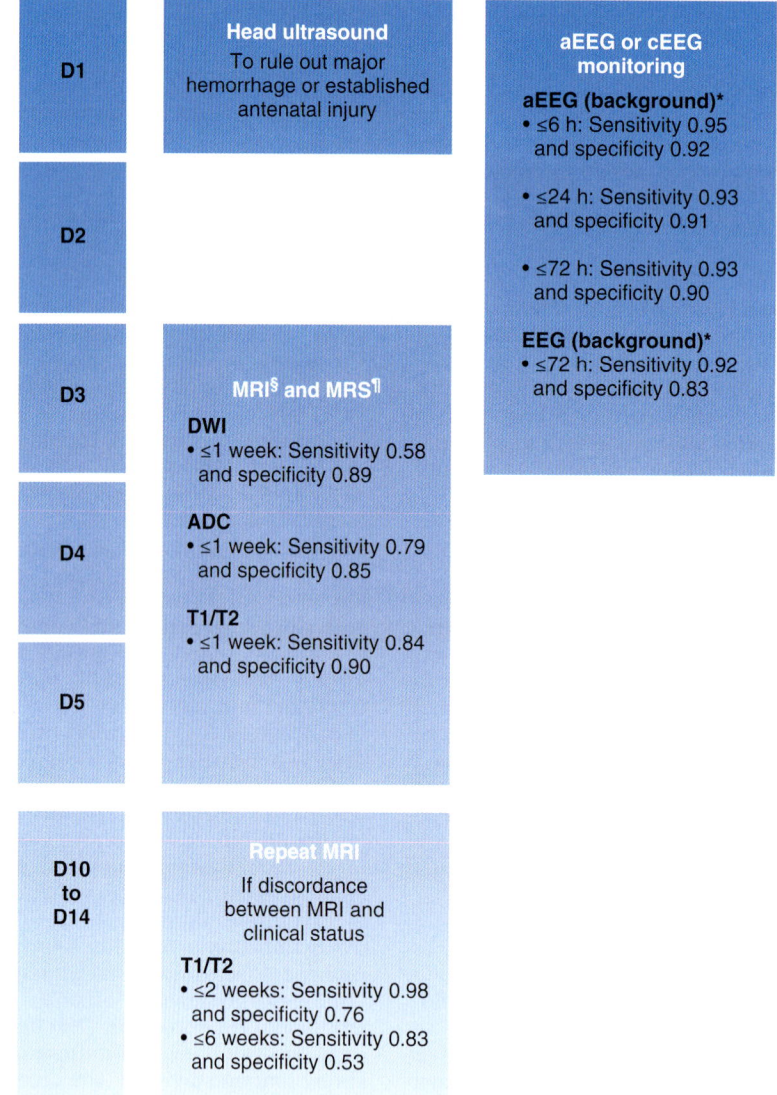

Figure 19-2. Suggested diagnostic tests for newborns with suspected hypoxic-ischemic encephalopathy. Pooled sensitivities and specificities are for adverse outcome tested at less than 18 months of age. Adverse outcome is defined by one or more of the following: (1) cerebral palsy; (2) score greater than or equal to 2 standard deviations below the mean on the Bayley Mental and Developmental Scales or Griffiths Mental Developmental Index; (3) death during the specified follow-up period. ADC, apparent diffusion coefficient; aEEG, amplitude-integrated electroencephalogram; DWI, diffusion-weighted imaging; EEG, electroencephalogram; MRI, magnetic resonance imaging; MRS, magnetic resonance spectroscopy; NAA, N-acetylaspartate; PLIC, posterior limb of the internal capsule. *Abnormal aEEG and EEG background includes flat trace, continuous low-voltage or burst-suppression pattern, and seizures. §Abnormal MRI findings include low ADC values in basal ganglia (≤1031 or 1018.5 × 10^{-6} mm^2/s, depending on studies); abnormal T1/T2/DWI in basal ganglia, watershed, cortex, PLIC, diffuse, brainstem, or cerebellum; or atypical patterns. ¶Abnormal MRS ratios include basal ganglia lactate/NAA > 0.08, ratio lactate/creatine > 0.3, ratio NAA/creatine < 0.5, and elevated lactate/NAA in basal ganglia. *(Pooled sensitivities and specificities data from van Laerhoven H, de Haan TR, Offringa M, et al, Prognostic tests in term neonates with hypoxic-ischemic encephalopathy: a systematic review. Pediatrics. 2013 Jan;131(1):88–98.)*

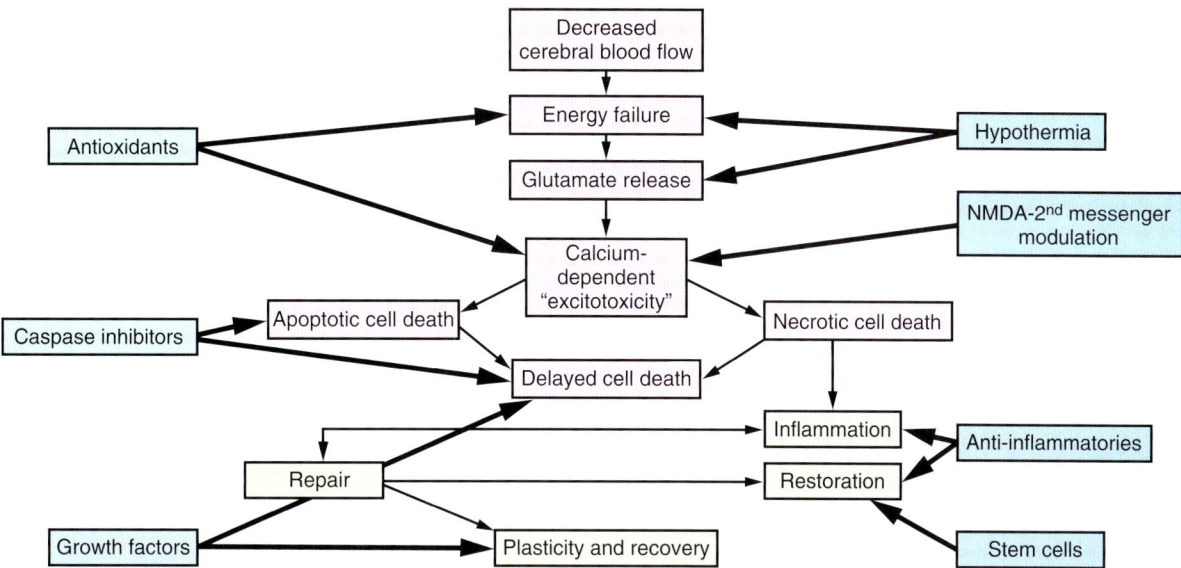

Figure 19-3. Key molecular mechanisms that contribute to hypoxic-ischemic neurodegeneration. NMDA, N-methyl-d-aspartate.

et al., 2013). In the era of therapeutic hypothermia, the optimal timing of these tests warrants further investigations.

PATHOPHYSIOLOGY OF NEONATAL HYPOXIC-ISCHEMIC BRAIN INJURY AND NEUROPROTECTION

The adverse consequences of cerebral ischemia include deprivation of energy substrates and oxygen and an inability to clear potentially toxic accumulated metabolites. Although linear flow charts cannot accurately convey the complex cascade of interrelated molecular pathways that lead to hypoxic-ischemic neurodegeneration, Figure 19-3 highlights some of the critical mechanisms.

Over the past 25 years, considerable information has emerged about the cellular and molecular consequences of cerebral hypoxia-ischemia and the molecular events that lead to neuronal cell death. Despite the traditional view of greater resistance to central nervous system (CNS) injury in the neonate because of lower metabolic demands and the greater plasticity of the developing CNS, susceptibility to hypoxia-ischemia may be amplified. Specific brain structures and neural cells in the developing brain may be selectively vulnerable to hypoxic-ischemic injury. The following reviews information about the pathophysiology of hypoxic-ischemic brain injury. Several reviews can provide complementary perspectives.

Cerebral Blood Flow and Energy Metabolism

It is widely accepted that preterm infants have a "pressure-passive" cerebral circulation; however, term infants may remain at risk for impairment of cerebrovascular autoregulation. Several basic physiologic mechanisms may contribute to impairment. Increased expression of inducible and neuronal isoforms of nitric oxide synthase (iNOS and nNOS) may narrow the autoregulatory window, and downregulation of prostaglandin receptors in response to high circulating prostaglandin levels may blunt the prostaglandin-mediated vasoconstrictive response to hypertension and thereby contribute to inappropriately increased cerebral blood flow. A recent

study found an upregulation of proangiogenic proteins in term neonates exposed to hypoxia-ischemia who do not acquire injury relative to those who develop brain injury. After an ischemic insult has occurred, the neonate remains at high risk for further damage in the acute recovery phase, because severe brain injury is often associated with major blood pressure fluctuations postnatally. However, aggressive management of blood pressure may not necessarily affect outcome because these fluctuations may also result from the brain insult and reflect the underlying severity of the brain injury.

An inadequate supply of glucose or alternate substrates plays a pivotal role in hypoxic-ischemic neuronal cell death. Although overall metabolic demands are lower in the neonatal brain than in the adult brain, metabolic needs rise during periods of rapid brain growth. The brain regions most susceptible to hypoxic-ischemic injury in the term infant (e.g., basal ganglia, thalamus) are the same regions that are most vulnerable to mitochondrial toxins. Brain development is associated with a transition from the ability to use glucose and ketones as energy substrates in the neonate to an absolute requirement for glucose in the adult. The deleterious effects of lactate accumulation after hypoxia-ischemia therefore may be attenuated in the neonate compared with the adult.

Excitotoxicity

Glutamate can activate a variety of excitatory amino acid receptors that are broadly classified based on their selective responses to specific agonists (e.g., NMDA, AMPA, kainate) or their signaling mechanisms (i.e., ionotropic [ligand-gated ion channel] or metabotropic [G-protein coupled]). Excitatory amino acid neurotransmission plays a pivotal role in brain development and in learning and memory. A substantial body of data has emerged documenting that overactivation of excitatory amino acid receptors (i.e., excitotoxicity) contributes to neurodegeneration. Hypoxic-ischemic brain injury disrupts brain glutamate metabolism. Elevated levels of cerebrospinal fluid glutamate have been documented in infants with severe hypoxic-ischemic injury.

Two closely linked mechanisms contribute to ischemia-induced increases in synaptic glutamate: increased efflux from presynaptic nerve terminals and impaired reuptake by glia and neurons. Any pathophysiologic process that depletes energy supply (e.g., hypoxia-ischemia, hypoglycemia, prolonged seizures) will disrupt these mechanisms and result in increased synaptic glutamate accumulation.

The structure and function of the NMDA receptor channel complex is developmentally regulated. There is compelling evidence that susceptibility to NMDA- and AMPA-mediated excitotoxicity peaks in the immature rodent and that treatment with NMDA and AMPA receptor antagonists confers robust protection against neonatal hypoxic-ischemic brain injury. However, concerns have been raised that NMDA receptor antagonists might have specific risks in the immature brain; blockade of NMDA synaptic activity could disrupt critical neurodevelopmental processes. AMPA antagonists seemingly have fewer potential risks in the immature brain than do NMDA antagonists, but negative data with the AMPA receptor antagonist, such as topiramate, showed no efficacy in a near-term sheep model of cerebral ischemia with delayed administration.

There has been considerable interest in evaluating the neuroprotective efficacy of magnesium sulfate. This interest stems from the intrinsic potentially neuroprotective properties of Mg^{2+}, including blockade of NMDA receptor activation. In experimental studies, pretreatment with magnesium sulfate was shown to limit subsequent neonatal hypoxic-ischemic injury, but treatment after hypoxia-ischemia was shown to be of limited benefit. Magnesium sulfate has been found to protect in some animal models of white-matter damage, but did not affect CSF levels of excitatory neurotransmitters in asphyxiated human neonates. However, a recent trial showed that exposure to magnesium sulfate before anticipated early preterm delivery did not reduce the combined risk of moderate or severe cerebral palsy or death, although the rate of cerebral palsy was reduced among survivors.

Oxidative Stress

Oxidative stress describes the alterations in cellular milieu that result from an increase in free-radical production as a result of oxidative metabolism under pathologic conditions. In the brain injured by hypoxia-ischemia, excitotoxicity and oxidative stress are inextricably linked. In cells with normally functioning mitochondria, more than 80% of available oxygen is reduced to energy equivalents (ATP) by cytochrome oxidase. The rest is converted to superoxide anions that under physiologic conditions are reduced to water by enzymatic and nonenzymatic antioxidant mechanisms. An inevitable consequence of mitochondrial dysfunction is an accumulation of superoxide, and any process that depletes antioxidant defenses will result in the default conversion of superoxide to even more reactive species, such as the hydroxyl radical.

With reoxygenation, mitochondrial oxidative phosphorylation is overwhelmed, and reactive oxygen species accumulate. The immature brain is particularly susceptible to free-radical attack and lipid peroxidation. Free-radical scavengers (e.g., alpha-phenyl-n-tert-butyl-nitrone [PBN], a spin-trap agent that converts free radicals to stable adducts) and metal chelators (e.g., deferoxamine) can protect neurons from injury mediated by hydrogen peroxide in vitro and in vivo. These agents also protect neurons from NMDA-induced toxicity.

Nitric oxide (produced constitutively in endothelium, astrocytes, and neurons) metabolism provides another critical link between excitotoxicity and oxidative injury in the brain with hypoxia-ischemia injury. Hypoxic-ischemic increases in nitric oxide (NO) production have multiple potential beneficial and detrimental effects. Nitric oxide regulates vascular tone, influences inflammatory responses to injury, and directly modulates NMDA receptor function. Early endothelial NO is protective by maintaining blood flow, but early neuronal NO and late inducible NO are neurotoxic by promoting cell death.

Neuroprotection by selective inhibition of nNOS or iNOS has been demonstrated. Regions expressing nNOS correspond to those that express NMDA receptors and correlate with regions of neurotoxicity both in vivo and in vitro. Few studies have been performed in asphyxiated human newborns in relation to cerebral NO production. Initial results in premature infants treated with inhaled NO for prevention of bronchopulmonary dysplasia showed reductions in ultrasound-diagnosed brain injury and improvements in neurodevelopmental outcomes at 2 years of age; however, in a large European trial, low-dose (5 ppm) iNO started early (<24 hours after birth) for a median of 20 days did not affect neurodevelopmental or other health outcomes at 2 years of age.

Several other antioxidant strategies that either block free-radical production or increase antioxidant defenses have been studied. The most promising of the antioxidant agents appears to be melatonin, which has many targets along the injury cascade, including oxidative stress, inflammation, apoptosis, mitochondrial failure, and nuclear effect. It is a direct scavenger of reactive oxygen species (ROS) and NO. Human neonates treated with melatonin were found to have decreased proinflammatory cytokines. Allopurinol has mixed effects. Early allopurinol in asphyxiated infants improved short-term neurodevelopmental outcomes and decreased serum NO levels after administration; however, no improvement in long-term outcomes was seen for later treatment after birth asphyxia.

Independent of brain injury, oxidative stress is also linked to procedural pain. In asphyxiated term newborns, tissue-damaging procedures without treatment may be more detrimental than treatment with opioids. Compared with opioid-treated neonates, untreated infants showed more impaired brain metabolites in the basal ganglia, thalami, and occipital gray matter, suggesting a certain degree of brain protection.

Inflammation

Perinatal brain injury activates the immune system and triggers responses that involve mediators such as cytokines and chemokines that act in concert with free radicals and NO in contributing to the excitotoxic cascade (Fig. 19-3) (Hagberg et al., 2015). Cytokines that have been strongly implicated as mediators of brain inflammation in neonates include interleukin-1b, tumor necrosis factor-a, interleukin-6, and membrane cofactor protein-1. Measurements of cerebrospinal fluid and plasma levels of several cytokines in asphyxiated term infants suggest that the injured brain can be the source of acutely elevated cytokine levels. A more recent study linked Il-6 with cerebral palsy, giving credence to the fact that there is an underlying genetic susceptibility in at-risk newborns.

The observed relationship between maternal infection and neonatal brain injury has been documented, but controversy still exists. In a case-control study from the Kaiser Permanente Medical Care Program, it was found that chorioamnionitis or placental infection conferred a fourfold overall risk for cerebral palsy in term infants. Neonates exposed to chorioamnionitis had a lower risk of brain injury and adverse outcomes than did newborns with sepsis. In an independent cohort of term neonates with HIE, decreased placental maturation predicted an increased risk of white-matter watershed injury, whereas chronic villitis was associated with injury to the basal ganglia and thalamus irrespective of white-matter injury.

Several compounds that block microglial activation or cytokine release, such as corticosteroids, melatonin, erythropoietin, Cox inhibitors, cromolyn, histamine receptor blockers, N-acetyl-cysteine, etanercept, IL-1ra, and simvastatin, have shown promising neuroprotective properties.

Cell Death

Apoptosis is critical for normal brain development, but it is also an important component of injury following neonatal HI and stroke. Activation of intrinsic or extrinsic apoptotic pathways leads to cleavage and activation of caspase 3, which is maximally produced in the neonatal period. Proapoptotic Bax is present in high concentrations during the first two postnatal weeks. Although necrosis plays a major role in early neuronal death in both the immature and mature brain, there appears to be some aspect of apoptosis within the first 24 hours following neonatal HI. It is likely that apoptosis is not the cause of most acute cell death, but rather of delayed phases of injury and neurodegeneration. This delayed apoptotic cell death likely relates to target deprivation and loss of neurotrophic support. Specific and nonspecific inhibition of caspases or cysteine proteases, which are highly activated after HI, has also been attempted, with some success. Another form of cell death recently implicated in neonatal brain injury is necroptosis, or programmed necrosis.

OTHER NEUROPROTECTION STRATEGIES

Although neuroprotective interventions consisting of pharmacologic antagonism of glutamate, free radicals, inflammatory mediators, and apoptosis have been successful to some degree in experimental animal models of hypoxic-ischemic brain injury, none of these other strategies has been successfully translated into clinical practice (Juul and Ferriero, 2014). Even if short-term studies of newborns treated with hypothermia showed benefit, improvements in the rate of death or the occurrence of an IQ score of less than 70 at 6 to 7 years of age were not significant. Therefore combinatorial therapy may provide more long-lasting neuroprotection, salvaging the brain from severe injury and deficits while also enhancing repair and regeneration, hopefully providing additive, if not synergistic, protection.

Xenon is approved for use as a general anesthetic in Europe and has shown promise as a protective agent. It is an NMDA antagonist, preventing progression of excitotoxic damage. It appears to be superior to other NMDA antagonists, possibly through inhibition of AMPA and kainite receptors, reduction of neurotransmitter release, or effects on other ion channels, and because of its action as a preconditioning agent. Combination xenon and hypothermia initiated 4 hours after neonatal HI was shown to provide synergistic histologic and functional protection when evaluated at 30 days after injury. More recently, a study delaying both hypothermia and xenon for 5 hours after neonatal HI also showed long-term improvement into adulthood.

N-acetylcysteine (NAC) is a medication approved for neonates that is a scavenger of oxygen radicals and restores intracellular glutathione levels, attenuating reperfusion injury and decreasing inflammation and NO production. Adding NAC therapy to systemic hypothermia was shown to reduce brain volume loss at both 2 and 4 weeks after neonatal rodent HI, with increased myelin expression and improved reflexes.

Neurotrophic Factors

Erythropoietin (EPO) is a glycoprotein that was originally identified for its role in erythropoiesis. Its functions include modulation of the inflammatory and immune responses, vasogenic and proangiogenic effects through its interaction with vascular endothelial growth factor (VEGF), and effects on CNS development and repair. EPO plays a vital role in neural differentiation and neurogenesis early in development. Recent evidence suggests that exogenously administered EPO has a protective effect in a variety of different models of immature brain injury. Single- and multiple-dose treatment regimens of EPO following neonatal focal ischemic stroke in rats also were shown to reduce infarct volume and to improve short-term sensorimotor outcomes, but there may be more long-term behavioral benefits in female rats. EPO treatment that was delayed 24 hours after neonatal HI also was shown to attenuate brain injury. A recent trial of EPO for neonatal asphyxia showed that repeated low-dose therapy (300-500 U/kg every other day for 2 weeks) reduced the risk of disability for infants with moderate HIE, and no negative hematopoietic side effects were observed.

VEGF is a regulator of angiogenesis that also promotes neuronal cell proliferation and migration. VEGF-A expression occurs in cortical neurons during early development. Following exposure to hypoxia, there is increased neuronal and glial expression, directing vascularization and stimulating proliferation of astrocytes, microglia, and neuronal cell types. VEGF also has chemotactic effects on neurogenic zones in the brain. VEGF appears to play an essential role in the beneficial and protective effects of hypoxic preconditioning in neonatal mice.

Stem Cells

Neural stem cells (NSCs) are multipotent precursors that self-renew and retain the ability to differentiate into a variety of neuronal and nonneuronal cell types in the CNS. They reside in neurogenic zones throughout life. In neonatal models, intraventricular implantation of NSCs after HI results in their migration to areas of injury. In both rodent and primate models, these cells were shown to promote regeneration, and nonneuronal phenotypes were shown to inhibit inflammation and scar formation while promoting angiogenesis and neuronal cell survival. Intranasal administration of BDNF-overexpressing mesenchymal cells 3 days after stroke in neonatal rats resulted in reduced gray- and white-matter loss and improved motor function at 14 days after stroke. Although no adverse effects have been noted, efficacy is dependent on time of implantation, and the therapeutic window is not known.

HYPOXIC-ISCHEMIC BRAIN INJURY IN THE PRETERM INFANT

In preterm infants, the clinical presentation of neonatal encephalopathy is less stereotyped than in full-term newborns, making the identification of eligible candidates for therapeutic hypothermia more challenging.

Among preterm infants born at 33 to 35 weeks of gestation, 2.5% met physiologic criteria for perinatal acidosis (defined as pH < 7.0), and only 27% had neurologic signs of moderate to severe HIE on the first day of life, a proportion similar to that seen in term newborns.

In a retrospective cohort, 55 encephalopathic preterm infants were described. Placental abruption was the commonest identifiable etiology. On MRI, the main sites of injury included the basal ganglia (75%), white matter (89%), brainstem (44%), and cortex (58%). Injury in the basal ganglia was mostly severe, whereas white-matter injury was mild and diffuse. Brainstem lesions were more commonly seen with severe cases. In this series, 2-year outcomes were worse than would have been expected in term newborns. The mortality rate of 32% suggests this was a severely affected cohort. Of the survivors, 26% had cerebral palsy, with severe spastic quadriplegia most common. Mild impairment was seen in 10%. Only 32% of the surviving children were normal. Clinical seizures preceded quadriplegic cerebral palsy and death in 65%; clinical seizures were more strongly predictive of poor outcome than was infection.

Currently, hypothermia is not recommended in the preterm population. It is thought that immature thermoregulation may predispose preterm newborns to higher risk of cold-related complications. However, studies in preterm animals demonstrated hypothermia to be safe. In a study of asphyxiated preterm sheep fetuses, exposure to prolonged head cooling was associated with significantly less loss of neurons and immature oligodendroglia. Recent studies of mild hypothermia in newborns of very low birth weight with necrotizing enterocolitis demonstrated no increase in mortality, bleeding, infection, and need of inotropes, and no alteration in clot formation. New trials are under way to study the effectiveness of therapeutic hypothermia in late-preterm infants.

FUTURE DIRECTIONS

Sources of genetic variation that contribute to differential susceptibility to a broad range of illnesses are a subject of intense investigation. Brain imaging, and particularly advanced MRI techniques, may provide important insight into how therapeutic hypothermia operates so that its use can be optimized and synergistic therapies added. Studies are needed to determine whether applying a specific method of cooling to a defined pattern of injury will enable individualized treatment.

REFERENCES

The complete list of references for this chapter is available in the e-book at www.expertconsult.com.

   See inside cover for registration details.

SELECTED REFERENCES

ACOG, 2014. Executive summary: Neonatal encephalopathy and neurologic outcome, second edition. Report of the American College of Obstetricians and Gynecologists' Task Force on Neonatal Encephalopathy. Obstet. Gynecol. 123, 896–901.

Azzopardi, D., Strohm, B., Marlow, N., et al., 2014. Effects of hypothermia for perinatal asphyxia on childhood outcomes. N. Engl. J. Med. 371, 140–149.

Bonifacio, S.L., Glass, H.C., Peloquin, S., et al., 2011. A new neurological focus in neonatal intensive care. Nat. Rev. Neurol. 7, 485–494.

Counsell, S.J., Ball, G., Edwards, A.D., 2014. New imaging approaches to evaluate newborn brain injury and their role in predicting developmental disorders. Curr. Opin. Neurol. 27, 168–175.

Douglas-Escobar, M., Weiss, M.D., 2015. Hypoxic-ischemic encephalopathy: a review for the clinician. JAMA Pediatr 169, 397–403.

Hagberg, H., Mallard, C., Ferriero, D.M., et al., 2015. The role of inflammation in perinatal brain injury. Nat. Rev. Neurol. 11, 192–208.

Juul, S.E., Ferriero, D.M., 2014. Pharmacologic neuroprotective strategies in neonatal brain injury. Clin. Perinatol. 41, 119–131.

Papile, L.A., Baley, J.E., Bentiz, W., et al., 2014. Hypothermia and neonatal encephalopathy. Pediatrics 133, 1146–1150.

Pappas, A., Shankaran, S., McDonald, S.A., et al., 2015. Cognitive outcomes after neonatal encephalopathy. Pediatrics 135, e624–e634.

van Laerhoven, H., de Haan, T.R., Offringa, M., et al., 2013. Prognostic tests in term neonates with hypoxic-ischemic encephalopathy: a systematic review. Pediatrics 131, 88–98.

Volpe, J.J., 2008. In: Ferriero, D., (Ed.), Neurology of the Newborn, fifth ed. W. B. Saunders Company, Philadelphia.

E-BOOK FIGURES AND TABLES

The following figures and tables are available in the e-book at www.expertconsult.com. See inside cover for registration details.

Table 19-1 Encephalopathy Score

Table 19-2 Distinguishing Features of the Three Clinical Stages of Postanoxic Encephalopathy in the Full-Term Infant

20 Cerebrovascular Disorders in the Newborn

Adam Kirton, Lori Jordan, and Linda S. de Vries

 An expanded version of this chapter is available on www.expertconsult.com. See inside cover for registration details.

INTRODUCTION

Stroke is brain injury secondary to focal disease of the cerebral vasculature. The perinatal period may be the most focused lifetime period of risk for stroke. Perinatal stroke accounts for most hemiparetic cerebral palsy, and survivors often suffer additional lifelong morbidities. Due to neuroimaging, specific perinatal stroke diseases are now definable by considering mechanism (ischemia or hemorrhage), vessels affected (arteries or veins), and timing (fetal versus neonatal). Pathophysiology remains poorly understood, but outcomes and management are increasingly defined. This chapter reviews the clinical epidemiology of each perinatal stroke disease.

Definitions

A National Institute of Neurologic Disorders and Stroke workshop on perinatal stroke provided consensus recommendations on the definition of ischemic perinatal stroke (Raju et al., 2007). The working definition for perinatal stroke was "a group of heterogeneous conditions in which there is a focal disruption of cerebral blood flow secondary to arterial or cerebral venous thrombosis or embolization, occurring between 20 weeks of fetal life through the 28th postnatal day and confirmed by neuroimaging or neuropathology studies." This covers ischemic stroke, but here we will also include perinatal intracerebral hemorrhage (ICH).

Timing of injury cannot always accurately be determined but accepted terminologies include "perinatal" (28 weeks gestation to 7 days after birth), "neonatal" (0 to 28 days after birth), and "presumed perinatal" (presenting beyond day 28 of life). Adding consideration of mechanism (ischemia or hemorrhage) and vessels affected (arteries or veins) to these time windows defines five specific perinatal stroke diseases. Acute symptomatic perinatal arterial ischemic stroke (PAIS), the most common and well-studied, provides the template for the remaining disorders of presumed perinatal ischemic stroke (PPS), including fetal periventricular venous infarction (PVI), neonatal cerebral sinovenous thrombosis (CSVT), and perinatal intracerebral hemorrhage (ICH).

ACUTE SYMPTOMATIC PERINATAL ARTERIAL ISCHEMIC STROKE (PAIS)

Epidemiology

Brain infarction due to arterial occlusion occurs in 1 per 1600 to 4000 live births. The first week may carry the most focused lifetime risk for stroke. Perinatal stroke may have a male predominance. Most PAIS are large artery occlusions occurring in the middle cerebral artery (Fig. 20-1). Left-sided lesions are more common and may relate to asymmetries in hemodynamics. Lesions may occur in any arterial territory and populations of posterior cerebral artery and perforating artery PAIS are described.

Pathophysiology and Potential Risk Factors

Many maternal, fetal, and neonatal risk factors have been associated with PAIS, but evidence for true causation is lacking in most cases (Kirton et al., 2011). Discovery of one potential factor should not lead to definitive conclusions. The best evidence comes from four published case-control studies. There is no evidence that PAIS can be anticipated or prevented. There are no modifiable factors a mother can control to prevent perinatal stroke though maternal blame and guilt appear to be common. Most studies have examined similar groups of clinical associations including maternal, antepartum, peripartum, placental, prothrombotic, cardiac, infectious, and genetic factors.

Placental disorders are a suspicious but unproven cause of PAIS. Multiple factors support placental involvement including lack of recurrence and multifocal lesions in 20% to 30% suggesting proximal embolization. Placentas are often discarded before diagnosis but pathological studies support and association with multiple placental disorders including chorioamnionitis, fetal thrombotic vasculopathy, and villitis of unknown etiology. Thrombosis is common in placental disease and strokes are common in fetal thrombotic vasculopathy. Placental disease should be highly considered with tissue pathology acquired when possible.

Maternal and antepartum factors include primiparity and maternal history of infertility. Maternal smoking during pregnancy has been identified as an independent risk factor in one study. The role of other modifiable maternal factors such as nutrition, medications, and substance abuse, remains undetermined. Preeclampsia has been independently associated with PAIS, but evidence for other common disorders such as oligohydramnios and gestational diabetes has been limited. Complicated labor and delivery are more common in PAIS but do not imply causation. Neonatal encephalopathy and global hypoxic-ischemic encephalopathy may occur with PAIS and may reflect common pathogenesis. Many peripartum factors have been inconsistently associated with PAIS including prolonged second stage, prolonged rupture of membranes, maternal fever, meconium-stained amniotic fluid, 5 minute APGAR scores less than 7, cord abnormalities, and the need for intervention during delivery. A relationship with both large and small birth weight has been suggested.

Prothrombotic factors have been associated with PAIS though estimates vary widely. Studies have been limited by variable disease classification, laboratory methods, and age at testing. A meta-analysis including perinatal stroke populations described consistent associations with protein C deficiency, elevated lipoprotein a, factor V Leiden, and prothrombin 20210 mutation (Kenet et al., 2010). Other large studies specific to PAIS have found little or minimal evidence of thrombophilia. Other factors are increasingly disproven such as antiphospholipid antibodies and MTHFR mutations.

Maternal thrombophilia is poorly studied but may also play a role. Evaluation for thrombophilia is complicated in

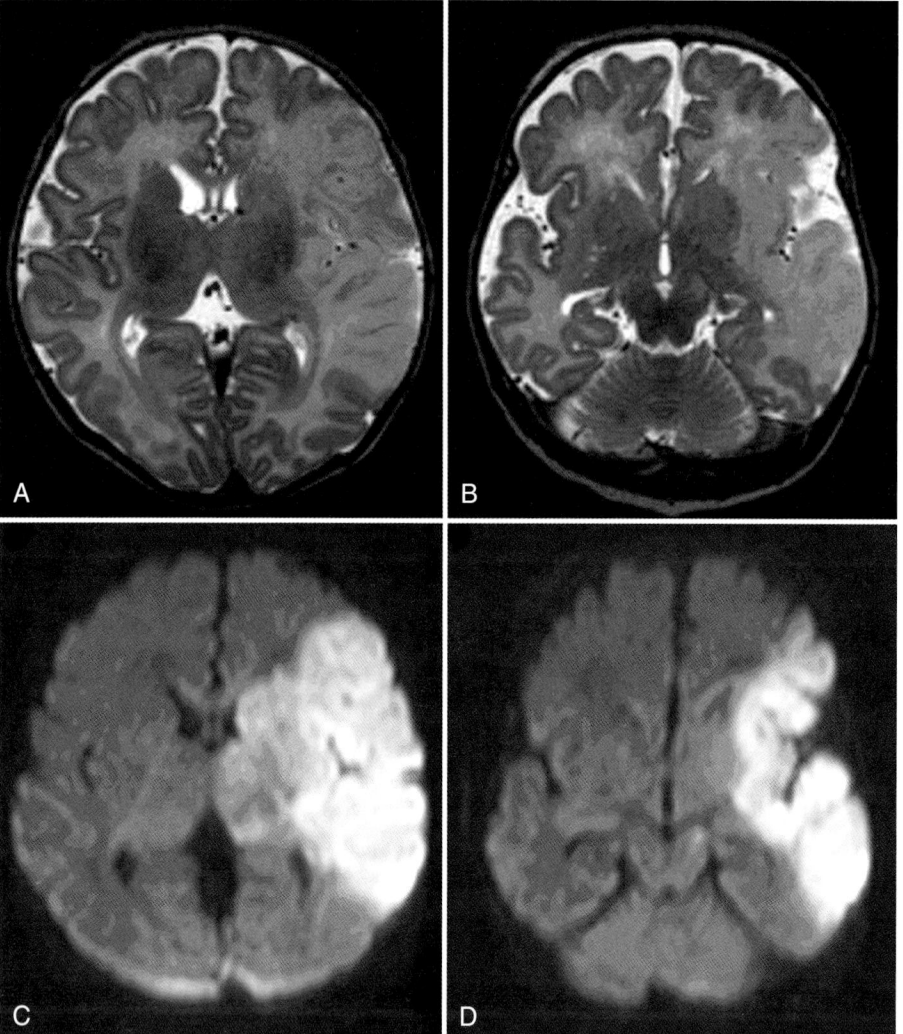

Figure 20-1. Acute Symptomatic Perinatal Arterial Ischemic Stroke (PAIS). Main branch left middle cerebral artery infarct in a term infant with hemiconvulsions. **A, B,** T2 weighted spin eccho sequence (T2SE) (TR/TE = 7650/150). **C, D,** Diffusion-weighted images (b = 800). Involvement of basal ganglia and cerebral peduncle is best appreciated with DWI.

the newborn, and whether such testing should be deferred to a later age or done at all remains controversial. Complex congenital heart disease is associated with 15% to 20% of PAIS cases with specific treatment implications. Arterial stroke was found in nearly 40% of infants preceding congenital heart disease repair. Certain procedures further increase the risk. Evaluation including echocardiography is indicated in acute PAIS though yield may be low when examination is normal.

Perinatal infection has been well associated with both arterial and venous perinatal stroke.

Neonatal sepsis and bacterial meningitis carry high risk with specific patterns of injury. Maternal fever alone has been independently associated with PAIS. Placental infection is a highly suspicious PAIS mechanism. With readily available treatments, most acute PAIS will be investigated and treated empirically for bacterial infection. Familial recurrence of PAIS is uncommon, but genetic mechanisms may contribute. Single gene mutations such as *COL4A1* are increasingly linked to perinatal stroke (see Fig. 20-7). A case–control study of candidate polymorphisms, involving thrombosis, cytokine, vascular, and cell adhesion function, was negative. Unique risk factors may be present in preterm infants with PAIS, including twin-to-twin transfusion syndrome and hypoglycemia.

Clinical Presentation

Recognition and diagnosis of acute symptomatic PAIS is usually not complicated. Most neonates present with seizures during the first 72 hours of life. Infants are often initially well, staying with their mother on the ward. Seizures that are focal and present at later than 12 hours of age are clinical predictors of PAIS. Focal neurologic signs such as hemiparesis are rarely seen. Other clinical signs include poor feeding, decreased level of consciousness, hypotonia, and apnea. Preterm PAIS presents with similar signs. Perforator artery PAIS may be less likely to have a typical presentation.

Diagnosis: Neuroimaging

PAIS is a clinical and neuroradiographic diagnosis. Cranial ultrasound is often the first investigation but is relatively insensitive and nonspecific. Ultrasound can reveal a wedge-shaped area of increased echogenicity within the middle cerebral artery territory diagnostic of PAIS. A CT scan of the head can exclude hemorrhage and accurately diagnose PAIS with hypodensity within an arterial territory but has limited sensitivity and includes radiation.

Modern neuroimaging with MRI has enhanced the detection and classification of perinatal stroke. MRI with diffusion-weighted imaging (DWI) is sensitive and specific and should be performed in any newborn with focal seizures. DWI quickly confirms recent (within days), acute, focal brain infarction with restricted diffusion in an arterial territory (see Fig. 20-1). Most PAIS are large, middle cerebral artery occlusions with combined cortical and subcortical injuries. Multifocal or bilateral lesions are present in up to 30% of cases, suggesting a proximal embolic source. Acute DWI changes may extend to other brain structures connected to a stroke. Restricted diffusion down the corticospinal tract is associated with poor motor outcome (hemiparetic cerebral palsy) (see Fig. 20-1). Hemorrhagic transformation of PAIS may be detected with blood-sensitive MRI. Neuroimaging in PAIS should include assessment of the cerebral vasculature. MR angiography (MRA) of the head and neck may demonstrate focal arterial occlusions. Simple division of lesions by level of middle cerebral artery occlusion may help predict neurologic outcome. For example, proximal M1 middle cerebral artery PAIS includes the lateral lenticulostriate arteries, resulting in infarction of the basal ganglia as well as distal major territories of the frontal, parietal, and temporal lobes. Such main branch involvement is less common in preterm infants. Advanced MRI techniques such as diffusion tensor imaging may also help predict early pathway injury and functional outcomes. Chronic versions of these and other advanced neuroimaging methods such as volumetrics, voxel-based lesion symptom mapping, functional MRI, resting-state functional MRI, and noninvasive brain stimulation are advancing the understanding of developmental plasticity after perinatal stroke with implications for rehabilitation (see later in this chapter).

Acute Management

Evidence-based management strategies for PAIS are limited within published consensus-based guidelines. Neuroprotective approaches are based on first principles and extrapolation of animal models, adult stroke studies, and neonatal hypoxic-ischemic encephalopathy.

Examples include maintenance of normal blood sugar, ventilation/oxygenation, blood pressure, and temperature. Hyperthermia worsens neonatal ischemic brain injury in animal models and although hypothermia has not been studied in human perinatal stroke, sources of fever should be sought and treated. Consensus guidelines only recommend administration of unfractionated or low molecular weight heparin in neonates with ongoing cardioembolic risk. Thrombolytic agents are not recommended. Evidence from perinatal stroke animal models has advanced the first neuroprotective trials of erythropoietin in PAIS in which early trials are establishing safety data to advance further studies. Continuous or amplitude-integrated EEG may be helpful for recognizing and treating neonatal seizures as they are often subclinical. Prompt recognition and treatment of seizures may prevent secondary brain injury although the ideal agents and duration of treatment have not been established. Acute seizures typically cease within days, suggesting that long-term anticonvulsants are usually not required. Additional investigational considerations relate to possible risk factors and include exclusion of infection, cardiac evaluations, including echocardiography, and placental pathology when possible.

Outcomes and Rehabilitation

Most survivors of perinatal stroke suffer lifelong neurologic disability (Kirton et al., 2013). Deficits span all areas of development and function, affecting both child and family. Motor deficits and cerebral palsy predominate, but disorders of sensation, language, cognition, epilepsy, behavior, and mental health are common. Evidence-based rehabilitation strategies are limited but increasing. With most knowledge of outcomes and their management arising from the PAIS literature, the major morbidities and relevant rehabilitation strategies are reviewed here in detail. Outcomes and management are similar in the remaining perinatal stroke diseases that follow in which specific differences are highlighted.

Recovery from early injury to the immature brain is a complex process that occurs continually across development. Outcomes from perinatal stroke and the factors that determine them differ from those of older children or adults with stroke. It is erroneous to assume that the potentially increased plasticity of the very young brain portends better outcomes from perinatal stroke.

Motor: Cerebral Palsy

Perinatal stroke accounts for most hemiparetic cerebral palsy. Motor deficits affect 25% to 50% of children with PAIS. Most PAIS involve the middle cerebral artery, injuring key components of the motor network and resulting in hemiparesis affecting the upper more than lower extremity. Motor deficits emerge around 4 to 6 months with asymmetry and early hand preference. Unless infarcts are bilateral, most achieve independent walking on time. Motor dysfunction is a complex interaction of brain injury location, developmental plastic adaptation, and multiple physical factors over time such as weakness, dexterity, tone, musculoskeletal issues, and factors inherent to the individual child. A focal injury of defined timing in a healthy brain makes perinatal stroke an ideal human model of developmental plasticity. Combining animal and human neurophysiology and imaging studies has generated new models of developmental motor plasticity after perinatal stroke. The degree of control of affected extremities by the ipsilateral (contralesional) hemisphere is a major determinant of motor function. These models also identify potential targets for neuromodulation.

Validated measures and evidence-based management for perinatal stroke hemiparesis are poorly defined. Early initiation of rehabilitation therapy is considered beneficial. Multidisciplinary teams typically include physical, occupational, and speech therapists, orthopedic surgeons, and pediatric physiatrists. Emerging evidence-based interventions for children with cerebral palsy are applicable and have recently undergone systematic review (Sakzewski et al., 2009). Recommendations for improving motor function include constraint-induced movement therapy (CIMT), bimanual training, goal-directed training, occupational therapy after botulinum toxin, and home programs. Additional recommendations can be found for outcomes, including spasticity, contractures, muscle strengthening, and various psychosocial outcomes. The same guidelines provide evidence on clearly disproven and potentially harmful interventions.

Multiple randomized controlled trials support the efficacy of CIMT in congenital hemiparesis without studies specific to perinatal stroke. The primary tenets include induced constraint of the unaffected upper limb with a removable cast or splint combined with intensive, goal-directed therapy, usually over a period of 1 to 3 weeks. Intensive bimanual approaches to motor rehabilitation in hemiplegic children have also been developed with evidence of similar efficacy. All such interventions should adhere to the principles of the WHO International Classification of Functioning, Disability, and Health, use objective and validated outcome measures, and monitor achievement of child-specific functional goals.

Noninvasive brain stimulation such as transcranial magnetic stimulation (TMS) represents an opportunity for neuromodulation to enhance function. Safety and tolerability of TMS is well established in children. In adults, many randomized, controlled trials of brain stimulation have demonstrated efficacy for stroke-induced hemiparesis. A trial of repetitive TMS (rTMS) in 19 children with hemiparetic cerebral palsy over 2 weeks demonstrated favorable safety and tolerability with early evidence of efficacy. A recently completed factorial trial of 45 school-aged children with perinatal stroke hemiparesis randomized to inhibitory rTMS or sham and CIMT or not. After an intensive, 2-week, peer-supported, goal-directed motor learning day camp, all children perceived significant functional gains. The chances of achieving significant change doubled with rTMS or CIMT with additive effects.

Nonmotor Disabilities

Dysfunctional sensation is an understudied but important contributor to disability in perinatal stroke. The sensation of position, motion, and force or proprioception provides afferent input that is essential for integrated limb control. Studies of children with cerebral palsy have suggested proprioceptive dysfunction is common. In adults with stroke, proprioception is a major determinant of upper extremity hemiparesis recovery. New evidence studying robotic position matching suggests marked deficits in position sense in children with perinatal stroke (Kuczynski et al., 2016).

Visuospatial deficits can occur after perinatal stroke. Deficits may parallel patterns in older children and adults such as contralateral quadrantanopsia with visual pathway injuries though robust plasticity in visual cortex often seems to minimize such problems. Right hemisphere lesions may be more likely to impair spatial integration (organizing elements into a unified whole) whereas left-sided injuries may impair processing detail. Using a block-design test, children with perinatal stroke in the right hemisphere made more global errors (overall design shape) whereas children with left-sided lesions tended to make local errors (precise internal pattern). Visuospatial neglect may also occur but without the predilection for right hemisphere lesions seen in adults.

Deficits in higher brain functions occur in more than half of children with PAIS. The study of neuropsychological outcomes faces numerous challenges, including delayed timing of appearance of deficits to later in childhood. Standardized IQ testing studies suggest mean intelligence is usually within the low-normal range but prospective longitudinal studies have demonstrated specific disorders of cognitive function. Age at testing is critical and deficits emerge over time. Verbal abilities may be relatively preserved compared with performance abilities. Children with epilepsy may be particularly at risk (see later in this chapter). Carefully developmental follow up is required with neuropsychological and educational testing over time to define learning needs and optimal educational environments.

Behavioral and emotional self-regulation included in executive functions (e.g., attention, inhibition, mental flexibility, working memory, and metacognitive skills) may be altered after perinatal stroke. Routine cognitive testing may suggest relative sparing of some executive functions. Studies of children with congenital hemiplegia as well as perinatal stroke describe higher rates of attention disorders. Attention deficit hyperactivity disorder (ADHD) is also increased after early childhood stroke. With implications for academic success and readily available treatments, attention disorders should be screened for.

Disorders of language represent a stark contrast from adult stroke. Developmental language disorders may occur in 20% to 25%, but lesion laterality makes little or no difference. Subtle lateralization effects may include left-sided lesions in school-aged children, leading to increased morphologic errors, less use of complex syntax, and reduced detailed story settings when relaying a personal narrative. Functional MRI (fMRI) studies suggest most children have bilateral language representation for both expressive and receptive functions. This balance may dictate function as preservation of ipsilesional frontal areas, but bilateral representation of temporal-parietal language areas has been associated with better function. Language is a prominent component of preschool developmental assessments in which early speech therapy may be indicated.

Children with PAIS risk later epilepsy though estimates vary from 15% to 54%. Although lesions are unilateral, diffuse epileptic encephalopathies such as infantile spasms can occur. Many children may "outgrow" their epilepsy, only incurring seizures during a window of development.

Anticonvulsant or other treatments specific to perinatal stroke have not been determined though lesion focality makes such children excellent epilepsy surgery candidates. Possible associations between early acute seizures and later epilepsy may emphasize the importance of early management.

Accumulating evidence suggests that epilepsy may adversely influence neuropsychological outcomes. Emerging data from a population-based perinatal stroke study suggests a strong association between continuous discharges in slow-wave sleep and poor neuropsychological outcomes. Such pathological EEG activity may be both a biomarker and potentially modifiable modulator of neuropsychological outcomes. Screening for such abnormalities may be indicated, particularly in children with poor developmental trajectories or regression. Beyond this, treatment is based on best practices for childhood epilepsy.

Outcome Prediction

Estimating long-term outcomes in the acute setting is important to counsel families and select patients for trials. The ability of early clinical, laboratory, and EEG markers to predict outcomes has been disappointing. Neuroimaging variables, including lesion size and location, have been associated primarily with outcomes. Injury to major components of the motor system (rolandic cortex, posterior limb of internal capsule, basal ganglia) can estimate risk of cerebral palsy. Restricted diffusion in the corticospinal tract or "pre-Wallerian degeneration" also helps predict long-term hemiparesis. Most remaining brain functions are more difficult to estimate. When counseling families, it should be remembered that even for motor outcomes, only approximations can be made. This is particularly true for more complex developmental outcomes in which only years of observation will determine the outcome in most cases.

Recurrence

The most predictable outcome from perinatal stroke is the lack of recurrence. Lifetime occurrence of ischemic stroke is exceedingly rare, estimated at less than 1% for both the child and future pregnancies. An exception is neonates with congenital heart disease in which recurrence rates approach 14%. In the remaining neonates, secondary stroke prevention is not usually required. With no established maternal risk factors, primary prevention strategies do not exist. This message of extremely low risk of recurrence for child and mother must be repeatedly stated to families to alleviate worry and inform family planning.

Psychology and Mental Health

Family-centered education, support, and counseling are essential. Quality of life may be underestimated by parents, and

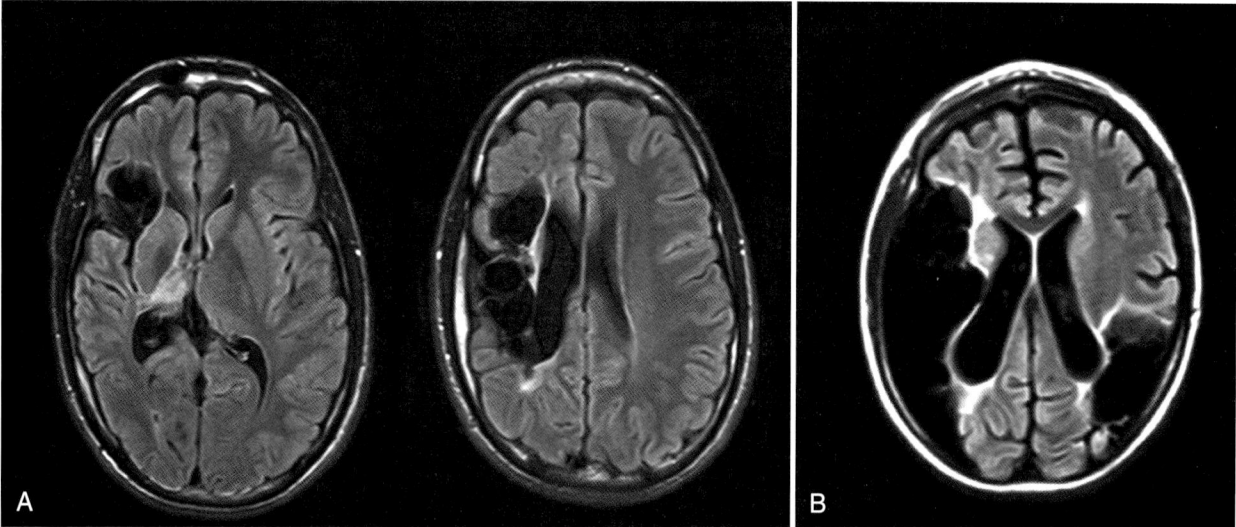

Figure 20-2. Arterial Presumed Perinatal Stroke. A, Parents noted their 6-month-old was not using the left upper extremity. FLAIR MRI at 9 months demonstrates a large cystic area with surrounding gliosis in the distribution of the right middle cerebral artery (MCA). Sparing of the putamen suggests the site of occlusion was the distal M1 segment. **B,** A 2-month-old with failure to thrive and microcephaly underwent MRI. Well demarcated, cystic areas with surrounding gliosis are shown in the distributions of the entire right MCA and posterior trunk of the left MCA.

inversely related to degree of cognitive dysfunction. Recent interventional clinical trials suggest meaningful psychological and quality-of-life benefits may be realized. Parental psychological morbidity can easily be missed but disabling to the entire family. The Alberta Perinatal Stroke Parental Outcome Measure (POM) was recently developed and validated to screen for parental psychological morbidity. As a definitive cause can usually not be identified, mothers may harbor unjustified feelings of guilt and/or blame with implications for maternal mental health and family life. Simple educational counseling, connecting parents with information, and establishing support resources with the help of best-practice documents now available can have a major influence. Families also require help interpreting the abundance of misinformation currently available to make informed decisions.

PRESUMED PERINATAL ISCHEMIC STROKE (PPS)

Many perinatal strokes will not manifest clinical signs during newborn period (Kirton et al., 2008). Diagnosis instead occurs retrospectively when congenital hemiparesis, new-onset seizures, or other deficits appear later in infancy. The most common presentation is motor asymmetry or early hand preference at 4 to 6 months. There is often a diagnostic delay up to 2 years as parental concerns may be minimized. Neuroimaging with MRI is the definitive diagnostic test. This scenario is referred to as presumed perinatal ischemic stroke (PPS), defined as a term (longer than 36 weeks) infant older than 28 days with a normal neonatal neurologic history presenting with a neurologic deficit or seizure referable to focal, chronic infarction on neuroimaging. As some lesions involve both ischemic and hemorrhagic mechanisms (see later in this chapter), the more general term of presumed perinatal stroke (PPS) is used here. Precise timing is not possible but is presumed to be either fetal or immediately proximate to delivery with acute signs being absent or missed. The clinical syndrome of PPS has long been recognized, but imaging can now define specific PPS diseases. Late-presenting versions of the arterial PAIS described previously can be differentiated from fetal venous lesions.

ARTERIAL PRESUMED PERINATAL STROKE

Many PPS are well demarcated, wedge-shaped areas of encephalomalacia within an arterial territory, typically the middle cerebral artery (Fig. 20-2). Lesions are indistinguishable from chronic PAIS imaging. Infants with arterial PPS are more likely to show isolated deep lesions. Pathophysiology of arterial PPS is poorly understood. Categories of risk factors similar to PAIS are suggested, including acute perinatal factors and prothrombotic conditions. These similarities support the suggestion that symptomatic PAIS and arterial PPS are often the same disease, differing only in the timing of clinical presentation. Only limited associations have been suggested between cardiac disease, arterial PPS, and the yield of cardiac evaluations when examination is normal is probably very low. As only those children with deficits will typically be diagnosed, there is a strong selection bias whereby most arterial PPS cases have long-term morbidity. This creates an effect whereby arterial PPS outcomes appear relatively severe compared with the other perinatal stroke syndromes. As hemiparetic cerebral palsy is the most common presenting sign, it is not surprising that more than 70% to 80% have motor deficits. Compared with subcortical venous PPS (see later in this chapter), arterial PPS is associated with risk of seizures and nonmotor developmental delays. Cortical involvement appears to predict nonmotor outcomes, including language and cognitive morbidities, as well as epilepsy.

PERIVENTRICULAR VENOUS INFARCTION (PVI)

Modern neuroimaging of PPS has defined a specific fetal perinatal stroke. PVI defines term-born children with preterm, in utero germinal matrix hemorrhage, and secondary venous infarction. Germinal matrix hemorrhage obstructs medullary venous drainage of the periventricular white matter with resulting venous infarction damaging the corticospinal tracts. Children are normal at birth but present with hemiparetic cerebral palsy at 4 to 6 months. The same mechanism of injury is well established in delivered preterm infants (see Chapter 22). Modern MRI can confirm such remote germinal matrix hemorrhage using blood-sensitive sequences (Fig. 20-3).

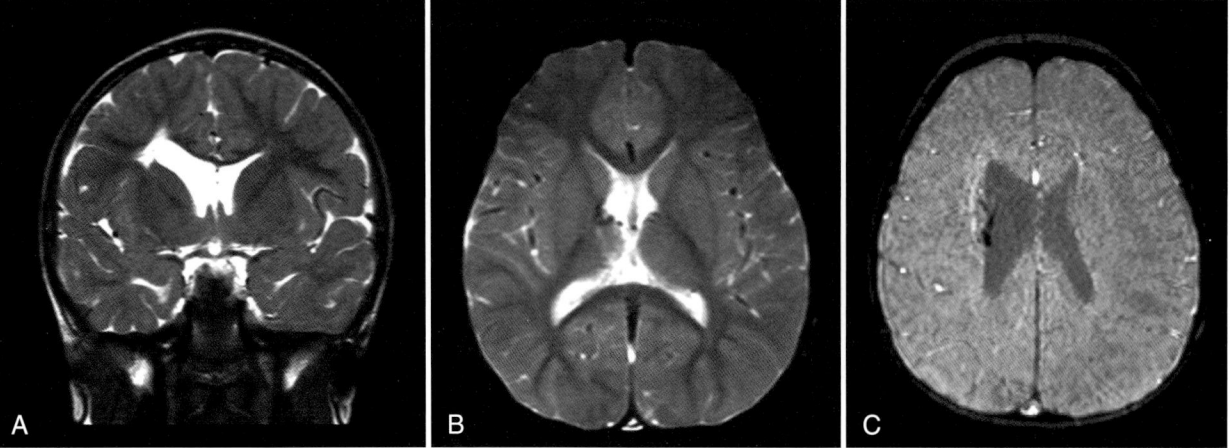

Figure 20-3. Fetal Periventricular Venous Infarction (PVI). Parents noted a right hand preference at 4 months and left-sided weakness of arm and leg by 12 months. **A,** T2-weighted MRI at 24 months demonstrates a focal area of encephalomalacia and gliosis in the periventricular white matter with sparing of the basal ganglia. Blood-sensitive imaging shows hemosiderin in the region of the germinal matrix (**B,** Gradient ECHO) and white matter lesion (**C,** Susceptibility-weighted imaging) consistent with PVI.

Validated diagnostic imaging criteria for PVI include isolated, cystic porencephaly of the periventricular white matter with gliosis and ex vacuo ventricular dilatation, sparing of the basal ganglia and subcortical white matter, and increased T2/FLAIR down the posterior limb of the internal capsule. Compared with arterial PPS, the lower extremity is more often affected in PVI. In a PPS series, PVI accounted for 75% of subcortical injuries. Case-control risk factors studies for PVI are limited. With timing removed from the immediate perinatal period, no associations with recognizable clinical factors have been identified. A contribution of thrombophilia has been suggested. Genetic alterations influencing vascular stability such as *COL4A1* and *COL4A2* mutations are increasingly recognized. Risk factors for germinal matrix hemorrhage in preterm infants described elsewhere (see Chapter 22) that often relate to neonatal intensive care are avoided in term-born PVI.

Consistent with the small, subcortical location of PVI, most incur only a "pure," isolated motor impairment. The lower extremity is more often affected in PVI. Risk of cognitive and behavioral disorders as well as epilepsy is very low. For both arterial PPS and PVI, the general principles of neurorehabilitation outlined previously are applicable.

NEONATAL CEREBRAL SINOVENOUS THROMBOSIS (CSVT)
Epidemiology

Cerebral venous drainage occurs through superficial and deep systems of cerebral veins that converge to form dural venous sinuses. CSVT is the pathological formation of thrombus within this venous system which may or may not lead to venous congestion and infarction. The incidence of neonatal CSVT is approximately 0.4 per 100,000 (deVeber et al., 2001).

Pathophysiology and Risk Factors

With limited prospective or case-control data, evidence for neonatal CSVT pathophysiology is lacking. Reduced flow results in venous congestion progressing to venous infarction, often with prominent hemorrhagic transformation. This process can mimic intracerebral hemorrhage, particularly in term neonates with intraventricular hemorrhage, many of whom have deep CSVT with thalamic injury.

A consistent list of associations includes thrombophilia in which relative risk is highest for antithrombin III, protein C, and protein S deficiencies. Nonspecific perinatal complications and systemic diseases associated with neonatal CSVT include hypoxic-ischemic encephalopathy, sepsis and other infections (including meningitis), disseminated intravascular coagulation, meconium aspiration, and dehydration. Extracorporeal membrane oxygenation—but not cardiac disease alone—may be a risk. Slower flow and stasis within the cerebral veins and dural venous sinuses may contribute to thrombosis. The proximity of the dural sinuses to suture lines may create vulnerability to trauma at the time of birth. Occipital bone compression of the superior sagittal sinus related to supine positioning is associated with neonatal CSVT and may be amendable to simple positioning.

Clinical Presentation and Diagnosis

Seizures are the most common presentation of neonatal CSVT (Berfelo et al., 2010). Focal signs are uncommon, but diffuse neurologic dysfunction is often evident, including lethargy, hypotonia, feeding difficulties, and apnea. The majority of cases present in the first week of life. Extensive CSVT may result in impaired venous drainage and/or hydrocephalus secondary to arachnoid granulation dysfunction and impaired cerebrospinal fluid resorption. Resulting increased intracranial pressure may manifest with bulging fontanel, splayed sutures, impaired upgaze, and prominent scalp veins.

Neuroimaging is required to confirm CSVT and parenchymal involvement. Cranial ultrasound may detect midline thrombus or unilateral thalamic hemorrhage whereas power Doppler can image sinus flow. Additional imaging is required to exclude CSVT in peripheral locations and confirm the extent of thrombosis and brain tissue involvement. Unenhanced CT is insensitive, but contrast-enhanced CT venography can effectively diagnose CSVT by demonstrating filling defects. CT alone lacks accuracy with the added risk of radiation.

An MRI is the investigation of choice with superior ability to define venous edema, infarction, and hemorrhage (Figs 20-4, 20-5, 20-6). Blood-sensitive sequences may be particularly useful, including specific biomarkers such as the "iris" sign in the frontal white matter of neonates with deep CSVT (Fig. 20-6). MR venography (MRV) can confirm the location,

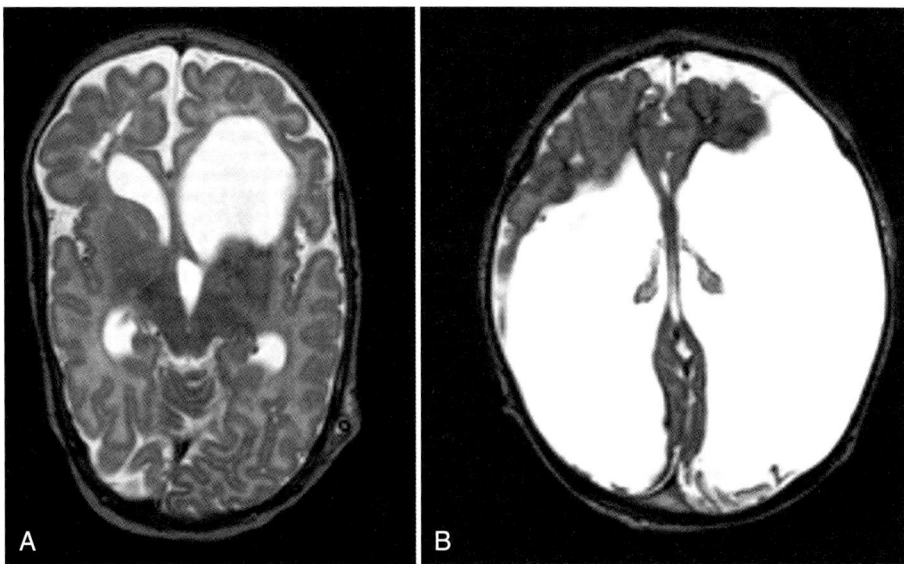

Figure 20-4. Neonatal Cerebral Sinovenous Thrombosis (CSVT). Sagittal T1 MRI shows extensive T1 hyperintense thrombus within the superior sagittal sinus, straight sinus, and the vein of Galen in a 2-week-old neonate who presented with seizure.

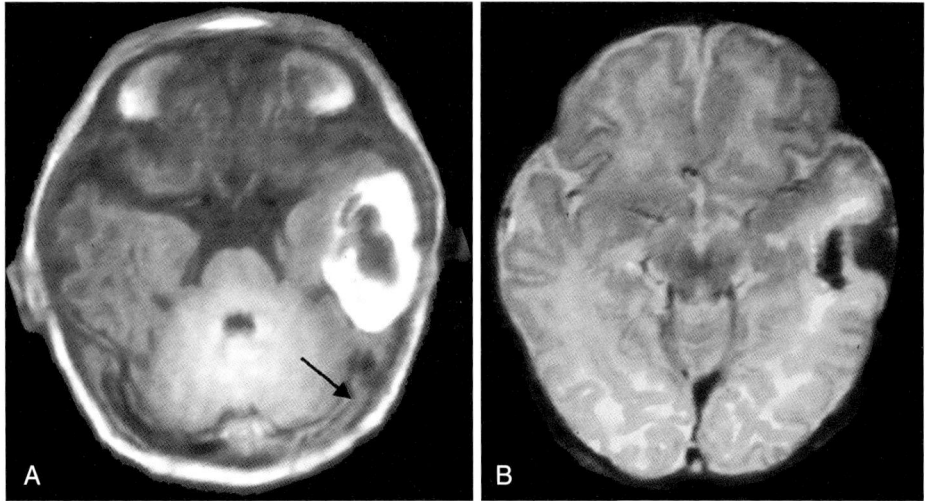

Figure 20-6. Deep system neonatal CSVT with hemorrhage. A term neonate presented with seizures on day 6. The MRV (not shown) confirmed CSVT involving the straight sinus. **A,** T2 MRI demonstrates hemorrhage in the left thalamus with intraventricular extension and punctate white matter lesions in the frontal white matter. **B,** SWI confirms hemorrhage in the same territory (iris sign).

extent, and degree of occlusion. Gadolinium-based or three-dimensional (3D) MRV may have significant advantages over time-of-flight studies. Imaging signs of deep CSVT can be difficult to interpret but must not be missed for risk of bilateral deep injury and poor outcome.

Management

Evidence supports the consideration of anticoagulation for neonatal CSVT (Moharir et al., 2010). However, consensus-based guidelines and treatment practices among pediatric stroke experts are inconsistent. The American College of Chest Physicians guidelines suggest anticoagulation for infants without significant intracranial hemorrhage. For those with hemorrhage, they suggest either (1) anticoagulation or (2) supportive care with radiological monitoring at 5 to 7 days with anticoagulation if thrombus extension occurs. The American Heart Association (AHA) guidelines recommend antico-

agulation only with evidence of thrombus propagation. Significant experience supports the safety of anticoagulation in neonates with CSVT.

Without controlled trials, the best evidence for efficacy comes from a large study of 83 neonates with CSVT. All were diagnosed, serially imaged, and treated according to protocol with 35% receiving anticoagulation. Follow-up imaging at 5 to 7 days demonstrated propagation in 28% of untreated newborns compared with 4% of those anticoagulated. Propagation was associated with new infarcts in 10% whereas hemorrhage in 3 of 21 was not associated with outcome. Anticoagulation treatment should therefore be considered, and if not initiated, early repeat imaging to exclude propagation is indicated. Duration of therapy is typically 6 to 12 weeks with 90% demonstrating full recanalization. Additional early management should adhere to the neuroprotective strategies described previously, including correction of dehydration and the treatment of infection and seizures.

Outcomes

Neonatal CSVT outcomes are abnormal in most survivors. In a systematically evaluated cohort of 90 neonates followed for a median of 2.5 years, most (more than 60%) incurred neurologic morbidity with language and sensorimotor deficits being most common. Predictors of poor outcome include parenchymal injury and bilateral lesions. Hemiparesis and cerebral palsy estimates range from 25% to 67%. Most children will walk unless they have bilateral injuries. Cognitive and neuropsychological deficits are consistently described though long-term outcome studies are limited. The risk of epilepsy after neonatal CSVT is 15% to 40%, and those with thalamic injury may be at high risk of sleep-related epileptic encephalopathy. Rehabilitation strategies are comparable to those outlined previously. Recurrence risk is very low with long-term prevention typically only required for children with chronic high-risk conditions such as severe thrombophilia.

PERINATAL INTRACEREBRAL HEMORRHAGE
Definitions and Epidemiology

Inconsistent terms for neonatal brain bleeding include neonatal hemorrhagic stroke, perinatal hemorrhagic stroke, and perinatal intracerebral hemorrhage (ICH). According to the NIH Common Data Elements, perinatal ICH is "a condition in a term (longer than 36 weeks) neonate with encephalopathy, manifest as seizures, altered mental status, and/or neurologic deficit occurring before the 29th postnatal day confirmed by neuroimaging or autopsy showing a focal collection of blood within the brain parenchyma." This term is distinct from intraventricular hemorrhage in a preterm infant (see Chapter 22), but term-born intraventricular hemorrhage is included here. Pathological bleeding can extend across multiple intracranial compartments, but pure extraaxial hemorrhage is not considered here (see Chapter 19). It should be noted however that modern neuroimaging has shown that mild extraaxial bleeding occurs in up to 50% of term neonates.

Research of perinatal ICH has been limited and complicated by terminology issues with the four largest series reporting different proportions of ICH types. Precise incidence estimates for term ICH are unknown, but one population-based, administrative data set suggested a prevalence of 6.2 per 100,000 (1 in 16,000) live births for intraparenchymal and subarachnoid hemorrhage (Bruno et al., 2014).

Pathophysiology and Risk Factors

The mechanisms of perinatal ICH are idiopathic in more than 50% of cases. The primary differential diagnoses include vascular malformations (e.g., arteriovenous malformations) and hematological disorders (e.g., thrombocytopenia, hemophilia). Trauma should be considered but not assumed simply due to the presence of blood combined with normal neonatal bruising or assisted delivery as this disassociation has long been established. Clinical variables, including maternal, antenatal, and neonatal factors, have not been consistently associated. Vitamin K-dependent bleeding may be increasing due to refusal of vitamin K at birth but is easily treatable. Hemorrhagic transformation of ischemic injuries can mimic perinatal ICH and is common. Genetic disorders such as *COL4A1* mutations can cause perinatal hemorrhage. Cutaneous vascular lesions or family history may suggest a genetic vascular malformation syndrome such as hereditary hemorrhagic telangiectasia (HHT).

Clinical Presentation and Diagnosis

The most common presentation for perinatal ICH is seizures within 48 hours of birth. Compared with the ischemic perinatal stroke syndromes discussed previously, prevalence of neonatal encephalopathy, decreased level of consciousness, poor feeding, apnea, and signs of increased intracranial pressure are more common. Electrographic-only seizures often occur, suggesting a role for continuous video EEG monitoring. Accurate diagnosis and assignment of mechanism depend on neuroimaging (Figs. 20-8 and 20-9). MRI is the investigation of choice though an unstable neonate may require urgent cranial ultrasound or CT. An MRI includes sequences with exquisite sensitivity to blood such as susceptibility-weighted imaging. Most perinatal ICH lesions are single and unilateral, and the presence of diffuse bilateral lesions should alter the differential diagnosis (e.g., bleeding diathesis). Routine MRI sequences can help age blood although the rules for doing so are based on adult studies. An MRI avoids radiation and can usually be completed without sedation. Vascular imaging with angiography (MRA) to screen for malformations and venography (MRV) to exclude CSVT are usually indicated. Conventional angiography may eventually be required in some children to exclude or characterize vascular malformations. Additional investigations include blood work to screen for bleeding disorders.

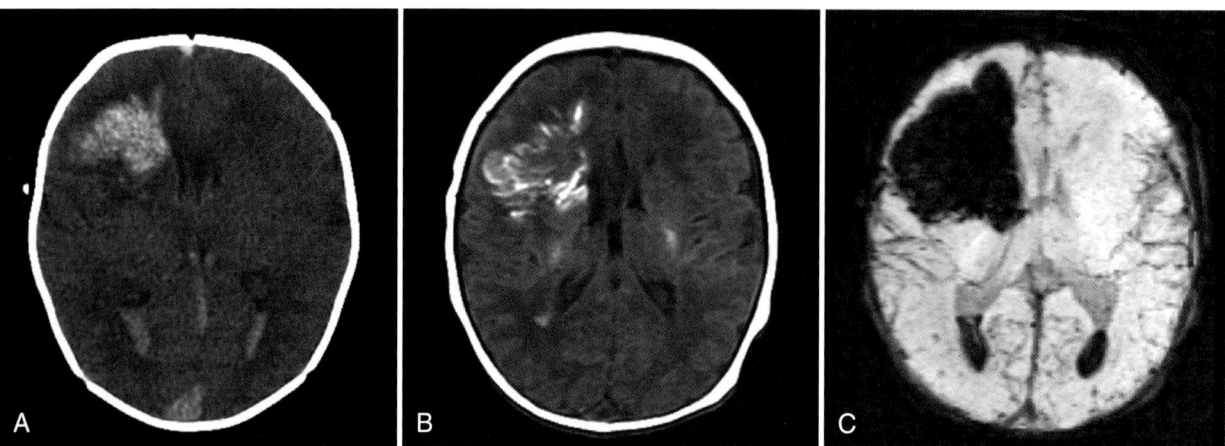

Figure 20-8. Perinatal intracerebral hemorrhage (ICH). A term baby presented with seizures and encephalopathy on day 1. **A,** CT demonstrates a large intracerebral hemorrhage in the right frontal lobe with spillage into the ventricles. **B,** T1-weighted MRI confirms the same whereas blooming on SWI MRI (**C**) exaggerates the appearance of hemorrhage.

Management

The American Heart Association guidelines offer several recommendations for the treatment of perinatal ICH. These include immediate correction of hematological abnormalities, giving Vitamin K to those at risk, replacement of coagulation factors in neonates with known deficiency, and consideration of ventricular drainage for posthemorrhagic hydrocephalus. Larger bleeds require immediate neurosurgical consultation. The general principles of neuroprotection outlined previously apply.

Outcomes

Studies on outcomes from perinatal ICH are limited with short follow-up durations. They suggest an increased mortality but lower long-term morbidity compared with other perinatal stroke types. The larger series suggest mortality rates of 13% to 25% but no neurologic deficits for most survivors (60% to 80%). Epilepsy occurs, but prevalence and risk factors have not been well described. Recurrence risk for perinatal ICH is very low unless there are persisting risk factors such as a bleeding disorder or vascular malformation. With a low recurrence and such a high proportion of "idiopathic" cases, it has been suggested that many perinatal ICH may be "one-time" events secondary to small vascular malformations that rupture and obliterate during transition to extrauterine life.

REFERENCES

 The complete list of references for this chapter is available in the e-book at www.expertconsult.com.
See inside cover for registration details.

SELECTED REFERENCES

Berfelo, F.J., Kersbergen, K.J., van Ommen, C.H., et al., 2010. Neonatal cerebral sinovenous thrombosis from symptom to outcome. Stroke 41, 1382–1388.

Bruno, C.J., Beslow, L.A., Witmer, C.M., et al., 2014. Haemorrhagic stroke in term and late preterm neonates. Arch. Dis. Child. Fetal Neonatal Ed. 99, F48–F53.

deVeber, G., Andrew, M., Adams, C., et al., 2001. Cerebral sinovenous thrombosis in children. N. Engl. J. Med. 345 (6), 417–423.

Kenet, G., Lutkhoff, L.K., Albisetti, M., et al., 2010. Impact of thrombophilia on risk of arterial ischemic stroke or cerebral sinovenous thrombosis in neonates and children: a systematic review and meta-analysis of observational studies. Circulation 121, 1838–1847.

Kirton, A., Armstrong-Wells, J., Chang, T., et al., 2011. Symptomatic neonatal arterial ischemic stroke: the International Pediatric Stroke Study. Pediatrics 128, e1402–e1410.

Kirton, A., deVeber, G., 2013. Life after perinatal stroke. Stroke 44 (11), 3265–3271.

Kirton, A., deVeber, G., Pontigon, A.M., et al., 2008. Presumed perinatal ischemic stroke: vascular classification predicts outcomes. Ann. Neurol. 63 (4), 436–443.

Kuczynski, A.M., Dukelow, S.P., Semrau, J.A., et al., 2016. Robotic quantification of position sense in children with perinatal stroke. Neurorehabil Neural Repair. pii: 1545968315624781. [Epub ahead of print] PMID: 26747126.

Moharir, M.D., Shroff, M., Stephens, D., et al., 2010. Anticoagulants in pediatric cerebral sinovenous thrombosis: a safety and outcome study. Ann. Neurol. 67, 590–599.

Raju, T.N., Nelson, K.B., Ferriero, D., et al., 2007. Ischemic perinatal stroke: summary of a workshop sponsored by the National Institute of Child Health and Human Development and the National Institute of Neurological Disorders and Stroke. Pediatrics 120, 609–616.

Sakzewski, L., Ziviani, J., Boyd, R., 2009. Systematic review and meta-analysis of therapeutic management of upper-limb dysfunction in children with congenital hemiplegia. Pediatrics 123 (6), e1111–e1122.

E-BOOK FIGURES AND TABLES

The following figures and tables are available in the e-book at www.expertconsult.com. See inside cover for registration details.

Fig. 20-5 Neonatal Cerebral Sinovenous Thrombosis (CSVT).

Fig. 20-7 Deep system neonatal CSVT with hemorrhage.

Fig. 20-9 Parenchymal involvement in extraaxial hemorrhage.

Table 20-1 Levels of Evidence-based Knowledge in Perinatal Stroke.

Table 20-2 Evaluation of Perinatal Stroke.

21 Neonatal Nervous System Trauma

Mary J. Harbert and Andrea C. Pardo

An expanded version of this chapter is available on www.expertconsult.com. See inside cover for registration details.

INTRODUCTION

Obstetric and perinatal trauma resulting in neonatal death or severe disability was a very common problem until the late 20th century; these were described at length in classic textbooks and journal articles. Methods to assess the fetus and improved obstetric techniques have significantly decreased birth-related trauma today. Accidental and abusive traumas have now gained more prominence. The neurologist has an important role in the assessment and evaluation of neonates that have suffered central or peripheral nervous system injury caused by trauma.

The neurologist is expected to provide guidance for prognosis as well as to determine the etiology of the suspected injury. As cases of perinatal trauma often become litigious, particularly ones involving labor and delivery management, the neurologist should take care when discussing the causality of an injury. A detailed history and physical examination are critical. The neurologist must note the events of pregnancy, labor, and delivery as this time window is one of high potential for nervous system injury. Gestational age is critical as preterm newborns are more vulnerable to injury than a term newborn and their manifestations of brain injury are often different. Consideration of nontraumatic disorders that clinically manifest similarly to traumatic injury is crucial, particularly if the cause of the injury is unclear. Knowledge of incidental nervous system findings that can be associated with labor and delivery is also vital; not all intracranial hemorrhage seen after delivery is traumatic (Rutherford, 2015; Volpe, 2008).

INTRAUTERINE TRAUMA

Pregnancies are complicated by trauma in about 5% to 7% of the cases. The most common causes of trauma in pregnant women are motor vehicle accidents (MVAs), accidental falls, and violence.

Blunt trauma to the abdomen during pregnancy is a known trigger of preterm labor and placental abruption, and begets a higher incidence of cesarean delivery. Catastrophic labor events such as maternal trauma, placental abruption, and uterine rupture are considered "sentinel events" for intrapartum asphyxia and these newborns may require evaluation for therapeutic hypothermia.

The incidence of MVAs during pregnancy is high; in a multiyear retrospective study of over 320,000 singleton live births, 2.8% of pregnant mothers had been in a car accident. MVAs during pregnancy significantly increase risk for preterm labor and placental abruption regardless of maternal injury, and women who sustain injury are at higher risk for cesarean delivery and fetal demise. Fetal neurologic trauma as a result of MVAs includes intracranial hemorrhages, skull fractures, and even fetal transection. There are case reports of fetal injury and fatality even when the mother has not sustained significant trauma (ACOG, 2014).

Domestic violence is a frequent cause of blunt trauma sustained during pregnancy and is also associated with repeated trauma during pregnancy, heightening the risk of injury to both mother and newborn. There is association between physical abuse during gestation and adverse neonatal outcomes such as prematurity, low birth weight, and, possibly, the need for cesarean delivery. There are no large-scale studies that have evaluated neonatal outcomes specifically involving the nervous system in the context of physical abuse during pregnancy. If trauma caused by physical abuse is suspected, the mother should be asked confidentially, as women who are asked about battering are more likely to answer in the affirmative without others present. Engagement of the social work team is paramount.

Penetrating trauma accounts for 10% of all traumas in pregnancy. Up to 6% of all fetal deaths are related to gunshot wounds. The incidence of fetal injury is about 70%, with fetal demise in 65% of the cases of gunshot wound to a pregnant mother. Death results from direct injury, uteroplacental damage, or shock. In cases of uterine injury with a viable fetus, delivery is recommended. Fetal intracranial gunshot wounds are extremely rare and often fatal; with survival, there is risk of encephalopathy, seizures, and long-term developmental impairment.

PERINATAL TRAUMA BY LOCATION
Extracranial Injury

Caput succedaneum is a self-limited collection of serosanguineous fluid infiltrating the connective tissue beneath the skin. The position of the caput depends on the presentation of the fetus and is most commonly seen in the occipital midline. The reported prevalence is between 1.8% and 33.6% of all vaginal births, with the most common risk factors being maternal nulliparity and the use of vacuum delivery. Caput succedaneum may be an indicator of prolonged labor. It is rarely associated with intracranial injury. No treatment is required because it normally resolves spontaneously within a few days of birth.

Cephalohematoma is a relatively common extraaxial injury in the neonate, occurring in up to 2.5% of all births. Instrumented vaginal delivery (with forceps or vacuum) increases the incidence to about 10%, and both nulliparity and prolonged labor are additional risk factors. Cephalohematomas, however, do not usually represent a problem to the neonate. Bleeding occurs because of the rupture of the diploid veins beneath the periosteum. Most cephalohematomas are recognized within 24 hours after birth and are firm, well-demarcated and are bounded by the suture lines given the dense attachment of the periosteum to the bone. Cephalohematomas may calcify and very rarely may become a source of infection if punctured. They may require excision if they are cosmetically deforming or invading. Cephalohematomas may be associated to skull fractures in up to 25% of the cases and a skull radiograph may help determine the presence of a fracture. Further imaging or testing is usually not needed unless other injuries are considered based on the neurologic examination.

Cephalohematomas tend to disappear spontaneously by the first month of age.

Subgaleal (or subaponeurotic) hemorrhage is a potentially lethal complication of vacuum delivery. It develops when emissary veins connecting the dural sinuses and scalp veins rupture and bleed into the potential space between the scalp aponeurosis and the periosteum. This space in term newborns may hold up to 260 mL of blood and there are several reports of subgaleal hemorrhage causing exsanguination and hypovolemic shock. This space is not limited by cranial suture lines and can extend from the nape of the neck to the orbits, which differentiates it from cephalohematomas. Subgaleal hematomas may progress over the first 24 hours and usually resolve after 2 to 3 weeks. Problematic subgaleal hematomas may not manifest until significant blood volume has been lost and altered mental status, pallor, hypotonia, apnea, and other symptoms related to hemorrhagic shock develop. Cranial ultrasonography may identify the hematoma as a hypoechoic or hyperechoic collection in the subgaleal space and a skull radiograph may be needed to rule out fractures. Mortality is high and reported in up to 25% of neonates mostly because of hemorrhagic shock, coagulopathy, and multiorgan failure. Management consists of adequate fluid resuscitation, control of the coagulopathy, and supportive care. It is not clear if neurosurgical intervention may be helpful in subgaleal hemorrhage, although there is a case report of a newborn with massive subgaleal hemorrhage and shock who made a good recovery after evacuation of the hematoma through a scalp incision.

Skull fractures have a wide-ranging incidence in the neonatal period, being reported in 0.5% to 10% of births. Skull fractures may be caused by compression during instrumented vaginal delivery or by compression from the maternal pelvis, and they are extremely rare when the fetus is delivered by cesarean section. Some skull fractures in the neonatal period present without an inciting event and may be a result of intrauterine mechanical stresses such as fibroids or other pelvic abnormalities. Risk factors for skull fractures include nulliparity, elderly multiparity, and dislodgement of the vacuum cup, and they should be suspected in cases of cephalohematoma and subarachnoid hemorrhage. Skull fractures may be linear or depressed (also known as "ping-pong" fractures). Linear fractures may radiographically present as linear lucencies. Depressed skull fractures may present as linear hyperdensities at the rim of the skull. A "growing skull fracture" is a pathologic splitting along a suture line and can be a result of vacuum- or forceps-aided delivery. The meninges can herniate through this defect, creating a fluid-filled collection known as a leptomeningeal cyst, or "growing fontanelle" when in proximity to a fontanelle. These typically need surgical repair. Nongrowing linear fractures do not require any treatment. Treatment of depressed skull fractures is controversial and may include surgical elevation when deeper than 5 mm. Surgical reduction is recommended when there is radiologic evidence of bone fragments within the parenchyma, neurologic deficits related to the fracture, increased intracranial pressure, or signs of cerebrospinal fluid (CSF) leakage under the galea.

Spinal cord injuries associated with birth are uncommon. Although more cord injuries are reported with instrumented delivery, particularly with forceps and rotation of the forceps, spinal cord injury has also been reported in newborns after uneventful deliveries, implicating in utero injury. There are several case reports of intrauterine injury to the spinal cord presumably because of neck hyperextension and breech positioning. Injury to the cervical cord has been documented with breech delivery, mostly when the fetal head is hyperextended (Reichard, 2008).

Intracranial Hemorrhage

The incidence of intracranial hemorrhage secondary to birth trauma is declining, likely because of improved obstetric care (Werner et al., 2011). Etiologies other than traumatic injury related to birth should be kept in mind when evaluating an infant with intracranial hemorrhage (see section Trauma mimics). Abusive head trauma should always be considered in the differential diagnosis if the newborn has returned to the hospital (Pollina et al., 2001).

Epidural hemorrhage (bleeding between the dura and the skull) is rare in neonates. It is unclear whether the hemorrhage comes from branches of the meningeal arteries or the venous sinuses and this remains a topic of controversy. Epidural hemorrhage can present with seizures and hypotonia, usually within the first 24 hours of life. The most common risk factors are maternal nulliparity and the use of forceps. Skull fractures may be present. Head ultrasonography may not show evidence of epidural hemorrhage unless the bleeding is significant or causes significant midline shift. Computed tomography (CT) and magnetic resonance imaging (MRI) are more accurate in detecting epidural hemorrhage. Treatment is supportive. The need for decompressive surgery is rare, but indicated when there is neurologic deterioration or evidence of significant mass effect or midline shift of brain structures.

Subdural hemorrhage (SDH) is present in roughly a quarter of asymptomatic term newborns. The proposed mechanism of the bleeding is tearing of the falx and tentorium or the bridging cortical veins. Associated risk factors include difficult delivery, prolonged labor, and vacuum extraction. The presentation is variable depending on location and extent of the hemorrhage, and symptoms include pallor, lethargy, irritability, tense fontanelle, irregular respiration, apnea, hypotonia, and seizures. Most SDH found in asymptomatic infants secondary to birth trauma are less than 3 mm in diameter and resolve by 4 weeks of age. Asymptomatic SDH has an excellent prognosis. Symptomatic posterior fossa SDH in the term neonate is rare, but is clinically important as it can cause brainstem compression or hydrocephalus, which may require surgery. MRI is superior to CT in identification of posterior fossa SDH in neonates (Figure 21-2); ultrasonography usually fails to identify a posterior fossa hemorrhage but is able to identify hydrocephalus.

Subarachnoid hemorrhages are more common in preterm newborns. Suspicion for subarachnoid bleed arises when lumbar puncture reveals blood that fails to remit with drainage and elevated CSF protein. Symptomatic subarachnoid hemorrhage can also present with neonatal seizures, irritability, feeding difficulties, and occasionally hyperthermia because of cortical irritation.

Intraparenchymal hemorrhages in the term neonate are rare and usually asymptomatic, unless they are extensive. Intraparenchymal bleeding can arise from small cortical contusions, shear injury, or diffuse axonal injury. When symptomatic, features include seizures, hypotonia, apnea, and altered mental status. Intracranial ultrasonography reveals focal areas of hyperechogenicity that may have mass effect. The presentation of intraparenchymal hemorrhage in term neonates may be associated with coagulopathy, as well as sepsis and hypoxic ischemic injury. Most newborns with intraparenchymal hemorrhage do not require acute neurosurgical intervention (Figure 21-3).

Peripheral Nerve Injuries

Facial nerve injury from perinatal trauma occurs in 0.5 to 7.5 per 1000 live births. Risk factors include fetal macrosomia, nulliparity, and use of forceps. Forceps can directly compress

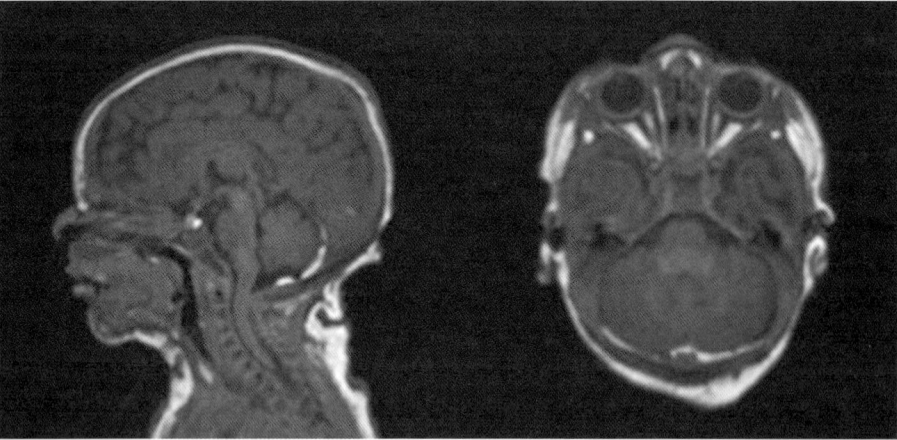

Figure 21-2. Term infant presented with seizures and somnolence. Magnetic resonance imaging T1-weighted image showing hyperintense hemorrhage layering posterior to the cerebellum, along the tentorium bilaterally and the cisterna magna. *(Courtesy of Dr. Andrea C. Pardo, MD, Loma Linda University School of Medicine.)*

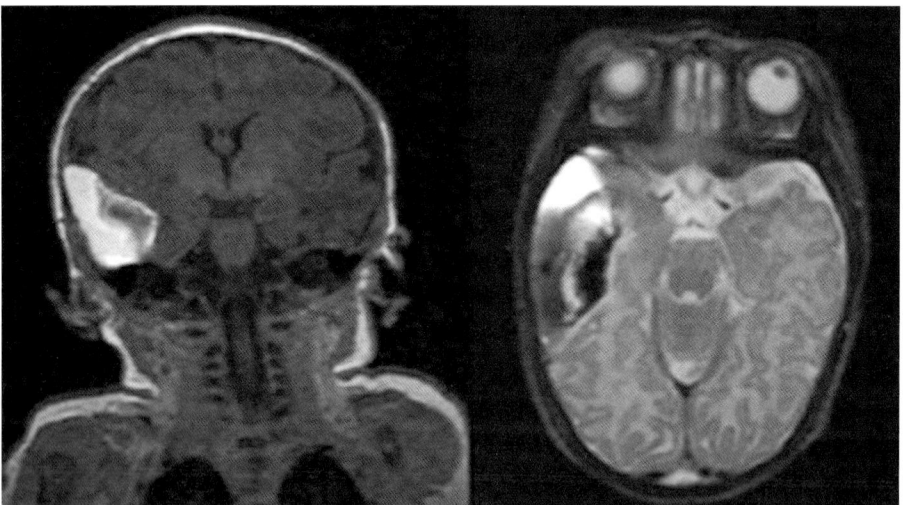

Figure 21-3. Coronal T2-weighted and axial T1-weighted magnetic resonance images of a 2-week-old newborn with right temporal intraparenchymal and extra-axial hemorrhage. *(Courtesy of Dr. Paggie Kim, MD, Loma Linda University School of Medicine.)*

the facial nerve at the stylomastoid foramen, or the nerve can be compressed against the maternal sacral promontory or ischial spines. The typical presentation is hemifacial weakness with inability to close the eye and flattening of the nasolabial fold at rest. Mimics of facial nerve injury include Möbius syndrome, hypoplasia of the anguli oris muscle, and hemifacial microsomia. MRI or high-resolution CT imaging can assist in evaluating neonates in whom the etiology is uncertain. Birth-related facial nerve palsy spontaneously resolves in 90% of infants by 1 month of age, and treatment is usually conservative before 4 weeks of age. Surgery is indicated if there is complete absence of voluntary and evoked motor unit responses in all muscles innervated by the facial nerve, if there is no functional or electrophysiologic recovery present after 5 weeks of age, or if there is hemotympanum with a displaced petrous bone fracture (Bergman et al., 1986).

Brachial plexus injury is a common perinatal injury, occurring in 1 to 3 neonates per 1000 live births. The most important risk factor is shoulder dystocia, but other risk factors include malposition, labor induction, prolonged second stage, instrumented vaginal delivery, and fetal macrosomia. Erb's palsy is an injury to the upper plexus and accounts for 80%

of brachial plexus injuries. The newborn displays lack of movement of the affected arm and the classic "waiter's tip" posture because of the loss of wrist extension. During examination, the lack of movement of the upper extremity is confirmed with tactile stimulation, Moro reflex, asymmetric tonic neck reflex, and palmar grasp. Fracture of the clavicle or humerus, subluxation of the shoulder, or cervical spine may be present. Klumpke's paralysis is defined by injury isolated to the C8 and T1 roots and accounts for 1% of brachial plexus injuries. Klumpke's paralysis is recognized by a flaccid hand in an otherwise active arm. Usually, there is evidence of injury to the entire plexus rather than just upper or lower plexus involvement (Abzug and Kozin, 2014).

There are several clinical classifications in the literature, but the Narakas classification may be the most useful for prognosis (Table 21-2).

A common mechanism of perinatal brachial plexus injury is lateral traction of the head at delivery with the anterior shoulder caught behind the maternal symphysis pubis. This may result in bleeding, edema, tearing of the branches of the brachial plexus, or even root avulsion. Avulsion injury is the most severe and should be suspected with complete

TABLE 21-2 Narakas Classification for Brachial Plexopathy

Group	Nerve Roots	Examination	Recovery
I	C5, C6	Paresis of deltoid and biceps without involvement of the wrist or hand	>90%
II	C5, C6, C7	Paresis of deltoid, biceps, triceps, and wrist extensors. Long flexors and intrinsic hand muscles unaffected	~65%
III	C5, C6, C7, C8, T1	Flail arm (total arm weakness)	<50%
IV	C5, C6, C7, C8, T1 with Horner syndrome	Flail arm in association to Horner syndrome ipsilateral to the affected arm	0%

plexopathy, Horner syndrome, or hemidiaphragm paralysis. Nontraumatic causes of brachial plexus injury, such as cervical ribs, amniotic bands, and congenital aplasia of the brachial plexus, should be considered in the differential diagnosis.

A chest radiograph should be obtained for newborns with plexopathy to rule out fractures, cervical ribs, and investigate concomitant hemidiaphragm paralysis, although hemidiaphragm elevation may not be seen if the baby is receiving positive-pressure ventilation. Visualization of the brachial plexus for perioperative planning can be performed with a CT myelogram, although recent data have shown that high-resolution MRI is equally sensitive and specific, and can spare the infant the radiation exposure and the injection of intrathecal contrast. Electrodiagnostic testing can describe the location and extent of injury, but the clinical utility remains controversial as it may overestimate recovery.

Treatment of neonates with brachial plexus injures in the absence of a fracture may commence immediately with passive range of motion of the upper extremity in order to avoid contractures. If there is a fracture present, the passive range of motion treatment may commence after 3 weeks, when the fracture has healed. Nonsurgical management is indicated when there is antigravity biceps strength at 3 months of age and a greater likelihood of recovery. Surgical management is indicated when there is absence of biceps function at 3 months of age. Nerve grafting transfer is the most commonly used microsurgical technique for the repair brachial plexus injuries, with good functional outcomes in 60% to 80% of infants.

Phrenic nerve injury is rare in the perinatal period, occurring in 1 per 15,000 live births, and it is usually concomitant with brachial plexus palsy in 75% of patients. The mechanism of injury is overextension of the cervical cord during birth. Most commonly, the right phrenic nerve and subsequently the right hemidiaphragm are affected. The diagnosis is usually suspected because of paradoxical chest rise during respiration. Chest x-ray identifies an elevated hemidiaphragm. There may be spontaneous recovery from 1 to 6 months of age, but failure to wean ventilator support and persistent respiratory distress are indications for diaphragmatic plication.

TRAUMA ASSOCIATED WITH SPECIFIC OBSTETRIC MANEUVERS

Delivery via vacuum extraction has been linked to many types of nervous system trauma. Documentation of delivery via cesarean section does not preclude the use of vacuum extraction. Debate about the safety of vacuum extraction exists in the obstetric literature dating back to the 1960s. In 1998 the U.S. Food and Drug Administration issued a health advisory reporting newborn deaths and injuries in the wake of vacuum delivery. After the advisory was released, reports of adverse events attributed to vacuum delivery increased 22-fold. Overall, rates of instrumented delivery in the United States have recently declined (ACOG, 1994).

Most guidelines recommend against the use of vacuum extraction in neonates of less than 34 weeks' gestation. There are few studies documenting the outcomes of preterm infants delivered via vacuum extraction, and so this recommendation is based upon the reasonable assertion that vacuum extraction is not a good choice for delivering preterm neonates with a tendency toward spontaneous intracranial hemorrhage. A Swedish study compared preterm infants delivered via vacuum against those delivered via cesarean section and noninstrumented vaginal delivery, and found that preterm neonates delivered via vacuum extraction suffered significantly higher rates of intracranial and extracranial bleeding, as well as higher rates of brachial plexus injuries.

Extracranial complications of vacuum extraction include caput succedaneum, cephalohematoma, subgaleal hematoma, and skull fractures. Higher rates of retinal hemorrhages are seen in newborns delivered via vacuum extraction, with one study finding retinal hemorrhages in 75% of vacuum-delivered newborns. Other less common extracranial injuries attributed to vacuum extraction include scalp subcutaneous emphysema, skull lacerations, and corneal injuries. Newborns delivered via vacuum extraction have a higher rate of shoulder dystocia and brachial plexus palsy. Although this could reflect confounding by increased birth weight, this association also has been seen in preterm newborns delivered by vacuum extraction (Doumouchtsis and Arulkumaran, 2008).

Vacuum extraction has been associated with every type of intracranial hemorrhage, although the most commonly observed types of bleeds are extracranial hemorrhages. Subdural hematomas of the posterior fossa are of particular concern because expansion of the hemorrhage can cause brainstem compression and may require surgical evacuation. Dural tears, tentorial laceration, and venous sinus rupture have been reported as a consequence of vacuum extraction as have focal ischemic strokes. Although cerebral herniation is uncommon in newborns that underwent vacuum extraction because of the mobility of the cranial sutures, it can occur; medial herniation of the parietal lobes has been reported in association with vacuum extraction.

Usage of forceps in operative vaginal delivery has been declining in recent years for a number of reasons: the availability of blood products and a wider variety of antibiotics increasing the safety of cesarean delivery; possible increased fetal morbidity with forceps delivery; increased consumer emphasis on natural childbirth; and fear of litigation. Injury to the facial nerve is a well-known complication of forceps utilization. Spinal cord injury, as well as in some cases even transection, has been attributed to forceps delivery, particularly when the forceps are used to rotate the fetal head into the desired occiput anterior position. There are many reports of ocular trauma with forceps; contact between the blade of the forceps and the eye can result in direct trauma to the eye or compression of the globe between the orbit and the forceps blade.

Fetal scalp electrodes have been associated with increased rates of infection and maternofetal transfer of infections such as herpes. Fetal scalp electrodes have been associated with puncture of the meninges and CSF leaks.

PERINATAL COUNSELING FOR AVOIDANCE OF BIRTH-ASSOCIATED TRAUMA

Neurologists are increasingly involved in perinatal consultation for fetal neurologic problems, especially as the use of fetal MRI becomes more common. The particular ethics challenges of fetal neurologic diagnosis are beyond the scope of this chapter, and they are important and are discussed in Chapter 33.

Birth-related injuries are not easily predicted based solely on the presence of a fetal brain malformation, although there are some congenital disorders that predispose to birth trauma. The American College of Obstetrics and Gynecology has noted that fetal congenital anomalies are a relative contraindication for vaginal delivery, such as hydrocephalus with increased biparietal diameter and some skeletal dysplasias. Fetal conditions must be considered on an individual basis, as not all fetal anomalies confer the same risk of birth trauma.

IATROGENIC NEUROTRAUMA DURING THE NEWBORN PERIOD

Infants admitted to the neonatal intensive care unit may be hospitalized for a prolonged time period and undergo multiple interventions, making them susceptible to iatrogenic trauma. Intravascular catheters in the setting of an immature clotting system place infants at risk for venous and arterial clots, which may result in stroke or paraplegia. Intravascular catheters can puncture the ascending lumbar veins, creating a pathway for infusion of nonblood substances into the dural space. Central venous lines can puncture the subarachnoid space. Scalp venous catheters have been associated with venous dural air emboli, which may be prevented by using the supine or Trendelenburg position to avoid the pressure gradients that increase the risk of air embolism. Epidural catheters for regional anesthesia have been implicated in causing epidural bleeding and paraplegia.

Peripheral nerves may also be subject to iatrogenic damage. Internal jugular lines damaging the phrenic nerve can result in respiratory failure and prolonged need for ventilation. Brachial artery puncture has been associated with median nerve injury resulting in pincer grasp impairment in later infancy. Carpal tunnel syndrome secondary to radial artery catheterization has also been reported. Umbilical arterial catheters can migrate into the inferior gluteal artery and cause ischemic necrosis of the gluteal region with subsequent sciatic and peroneal neuropathy.

TRAUMA MIMICS

Rare disorders that predispose to bone fractures such as osteogenesis imperfecta and Menkes disease can present as fractures and/or intracranial hemorrhages that can be erroneously attributed to perinatal trauma. Bleeding disorders may also be mistaken with trauma in the neonatal population, and 3% to 5% of newborns with hemophilia present around birth with intracranial bleeding, including intraparenchymal hemorrhage, cephalohematoma, and SDHs. Vacuum-assisted delivery and rotational and mid cavity forceps are associated with a higher risk of intracranial hemorrhage in patients with neonatal hemophilia and should be avoided. Other primary bleeding disorders that can present in newborns

with intracranial hemorrhage mimicking birth trauma include congenital afibrinogenemia, von Willebrand disease, and neonatal autoimmune thrombocytopenia. Parental refusal of vitamin K administration for prophylaxis against late vitamin K deficiency bleeding can also result in spontaneous intracranial hemorrhage. Intracranial hemorrhage in the neonate can (rarely) be caused by rupture of an aneurysm or arteriovenous malformation. Normal routine prenatal imaging does not rule out intracranial vascular malformation, as these malformations have been reported to develop relatively late in gestation. There are also reports of arteriovenous malformations of the spinal cord in which the presenting symptom is paralysis caudal to the lesion.

Neonates with nervous system trauma should be followed closely by a child neurologist. Neurologists may become the medical home for providing interventions, referring to physical or occupational therapies, and establishing long-term relationships with the caretakers as they may face challenges during the school years.

REFERENCES

The complete list of references for this chapter is available in the e-book at www.expertconsult.com.
See inside cover for registration details.

SELECTED REFERENCES

Abzug, J.M., Kozin, S.H., 2014. Evaluation and management of brachial plexus birth palsy. Orthop. Clin. North Am. 45, 225–232.

ACOG. 1994. Practice bulletin: operative vaginal delivery: American College of Obstetrics and Gynecology cited 2015 Jan 5. Available at: <http://www.acog.org/Womens-Health/Labor-and-Delivery>.

ACOG. 2014. Car safety for pregnant women, babies and children cited 2014 December 15. Available at: <http://www.acog.org/Patients/FAQs/Car-Safety-for-Pregnant-Women-Babies-and-Children>.

Bergman, I., May, M., Wessel, H.B., et al., 1986. Management of facial palsy caused by birth trauma. Laryngoscope 96, 381–384.

Doumouchtsis, S.K., Arulkumaran, S., 2008. Head trauma after instrumental births. Clin. Perinatol. 35, 69–83, viii.

Pollina, J., Dias, M.S., Li, V., et al., 2001. Cranial birth injuries in term newborn infants. Pediatr. Neurosurg. 35, 113–119.

Reichard, R., 2008. Birth injury of the cranium and central nervous system. Brain Pathol. 18, 565–570.

Rutherford, M.A., 2015. MRI of the neonatal brain. London, UK. 2005–2015. Available at: <http://www.mrineonatalbrain.com>.

Volpe, J.J., 2008. Neurology of the Newborn, fifth ed. Saunders/Elsevier, Philadelphia, PA, p. xiv, 1094.

Werner, E.F., Janevic, T.M., Illuzzi, J., et al., 2011. Mode of delivery in nulliparous women and neonatal intracranial injury. Obstet. Gynecol. 118, 1239–1246.

E-BOOK FIGURES AND TABLES

The following figures and tables are available in the e-book at www.expertconsult.com. See inside cover for registration details.

22 Injury to the Developing Preterm Brain: Intraventricular Hemorrhage and White Matter Injury

Janet S. Soul and Laura R. Ment

 An expanded version of this chapter is available on www.expertconsult.com. See inside cover for registration details.

INTRODUCTION

Preterm birth represents one of the most important public health problems in the world today. There were an estimated 140 million live births worldwide in 2012, and 11.5% of them were premature, or born at less than 37 completed weeks of gestation (Blencowe et al., 2013). Worldwide, over half of neonates born at younger than 28 weeks' gestation and 24% of those born at 28 to 31 weeks are estimated to have neurodevelopmental impairment. Survival is increasing for neonates of all gestational ages, and thus the prevalence of prematurely born children with cognitive impairments, behavioral disorders, and motor handicaps at school age continues to rise.

Brain injury is common in preterm neonates, and the two most common neuropathologic processes include intraventricular hemorrhage (IVH) and white matter injury (WMI). IVH, or hemorrhage into the germinal matrix tissues of the developing brain, is detected in 10% to 25% of very low birth weight preterm neonates, whereas WMI and the global neuronal and axonal deficits that may accompany it are found in 50% or more of this vulnerable population. Because both processes are unique to preterm neonates and represent a significant burden of disease, the pathophysiology, outcome, and prevention of these injuries will be reviewed separately.

INTRAVENTRICULAR HEMORRHAGE

IVH is a problem for infants at the lowest limits of viability. Both the incidence and severity of hemorrhage are inversely related to gestational age (GA); the highest grades of hemorrhage occur in 37% of neonates of 22 to 23 weeks' gestation but only 9% of those born at 26 to 28 weeks of gestation. High-grade IVH is more common in males than females, and, although the risk period for IVH is in the first 4 to 5 postnatal days, the timing of IVH is bimodal. Half occur within the first 6 postnatal hours, whereas one third occur after the first postnatal day, suggesting differing etiologies.

Cranial ultrasounds are routinely used to screen preterm neonates for IVH, and the most commonly employed grading systems for hemorrhage are shown in Table 22-1. When associated with grades 1 to 3 IVH, unilateral grade 4 hemorrhages most likely represent periventricular hemorrhagic infarctions (PVHI).

During the first three postnatal days, 75% of infants with IVH suffer seizures detected by amplitude-integrated EEG monitoring. Approximately one third develop posthemorrhagic ventricular dilation (PHVD), defined as ventricular enlargement higher than the 97th percentile for gestational age, and 15% of infants with grades 3 to 4 IVH require permanent CSF diversion. Finally, although preterm neonates with parenchymal involvement of hemorrhage are at high risk for neurodevelopmental handicap, even those with low-grade hemorrhage (i.e., grades 1 to 2 IVH) perform less well at school age than their nonhemorrhage preterm peers.

PATHOPHYSIOLOGY

Intraventricular Hemorrhage Is a Complex Disorder

IVH is a complex developmental disorder, with contributions from both the environment and the genome of the child. IVH occurs in that critical period of time before week 32 to 33 postconception and has been attributed to changes in cerebral blood flow to the immature germinal matrix microvasculature. Genetic vulnerability and healthcare disparities may also play a role.

Multiple lines of data support the hypothesis that the etiology of IVH is multifactorial. Maternal transport, antenatal steroid administration, and improved resuscitation techniques have become the standard of care worldwide, but the incidence of grade 3 to 4 hemorrhage has remained 14% to 17% for almost 20 years. In addition, the risk period for hemorrhage is independent of GA, suggesting that either the transition to extrauterine life and/or the triggers to which the neonates are exposed contribute to hemorrhage. Twin studies show that 41.3% of the variance in IVH risk is attributable to familial and environmental factors. Finally, candidate gene studies implicate the inflammatory, coagulation, and vascular pathways.

Clinical Risk Factors

Clinical studies suggest numerous environmental and medical risk factors for IVH, as shown in Box 22-1. In addition, maternal race and healthcare disparities influence the risk for IVH in preterm neonates. Women of African ancestry are at greater risk for preterm delivery compared with white women, and more women of African ancestry who deliver prematurely receive inadequate prenatal care. Further, their neonates are less likely to receive surfactant or assisted ventilation. The rate of IVH-related mortality in neonates of African ancestry is twice that in white neonates, and, relative to white infants, those of African ancestry are at significantly increased risk for hemorrhage.

Anatomic Factors Are Permissive for Hemorrhage

The germinal matrix remains relatively robust through 32 to 33 weeks' gestation, and its microvessels are the source of hemorrhage in the brain of the prematurely born. Proliferation of glial and neuronal precursors occur in both the germinal matrix and the subventricular zone, and the metabolically active germinal matrix requires a rich blood supply, yet its vessels are neuropathologically immature and thus at risk for hemorrhage. (For review, see Ballabh, 2010).

The blood-brain barrier is composed of basement membrane proteins, endothelial tight junctions, capillary pericytes, and astrocytic endfeet. In comparison to microvessels within

TABLE 22-1 Grading Systems for Germinal Matrix Intraventricular Hemorrhages

Papile*		Volpe†	
Grade	Description	Grade	Description
Grade 1	Germinal matrix hemorrhage	Grade I	Germinal matrix hemorrhage with no or minimal hemorrhage
Grade 2	Blood within but not distending ventricular system	Grade II	IVH (10–50% of ventricular area)
Grade 3	Blood filling and distending ventricular system	Grade III	IVH (>50% of ventricular area; usually distends ventricle)
Grade 4	Parenchymal involvement of hemorrhage	Severe + periventricular hemorrhagic infarction	Grade III IVH with periventricular hemorrhagic infarction

*(Data from: Papile LS, Burstein J, Burstein R. Incidence and evolution of the subependymal intraventricular hemorrhage: a study of infants with weights less than 1500 grams. J Pediatr 1978;92:529–34.)
†(Data from: Volpe JJ. Neurology of the newborn, 3rd edition. Philadelphia: WB Saunders, 1995; p. 424–428.)

BOX 22-1 Clinical Risk Factors for Intraventricular Hemorrhage

EARLY ONSET HEMORRHAGE
- Low birth weight, low gestational age
- Maternal fertility treatment
- No prenatal care
- No antenatal steroid exposure
- Maternal antenatal hemorrhage
- No maternal preeclampsia
- Maternal chorioamnionitis and/or infection
- No tertiary care delivery
- Early clamping of the umbilical cord
- Vigorous resuscitation
- No CPAP ventilation
- Neonatal transport after delivery

ONSET AFTER 6 TO 8 POSTNATAL HOURS
- Hypotension requiring medical therapy
- Respiratory distress syndrome
- Acidosis
- Hypoxemia
- Extremes of P_{CO_2} levels (both high and low)
- Sodium bicarbonate exposure
- Pneumothoraces
- Seizures

---

the gray and white matter, germinal matrix microvessels demonstrate a paucity of fibronectin, fewer pericytes, and decreased perivascular coverage by glial endfeet, consistent with regional vulnerability of the blood-brain barrier. The germinal matrix also has a greater vascular density than other brain regions, suggesting rapid angiogenesis to support its greater metabolic rate requirement. This angiogenesis is induced by high levels of vascular endothelial growth factor (VEGF) and angiopoietin (ANGPT)-2 found selectively in the germinal matrix compared with both cortical and white matter regions. Together, these factors promote sprouting of immature vessels lacking both basement membrane proteins and pericyte investiture, providing further evidence for microvascular vulnerability.

The venous circulation may also contribute to the susceptibility to intraparenchymal hemorrhage. Venous blood from the periventricular white matter flows through a fan-shaped array of medullary veins into the veins of the germinal matrix, and subsequently into the terminal veins. This tortuous anatomy results in venous stasis, permitting periventricular hemorrhagic infarction (PVHI).

Alterations in Cerebral Blood Flow Contribute to IVH

Alterations in cerebral blood flow (CBF) may also play a role. CBF was reported to be pressure-passive in the asphyxiated preterm infant over four decades ago, yet the physiologic factors that contribute to cerebral autoregulatory systems in the prematurely born are just beginning to be understood. Further, the definition of the cerebral pressure-flow autoregulatory plateau, or that range of cerebral perfusion pressures over which CBF is normally maintained, is poorly defined for the extremely low GA neonate. Nonetheless, preclinical data suggest that at perfusion pressures both higher than and lower than this reportedly relatively narrow plateau, cerebral blood flow becomes pressure-passive.

Changes in perfusion pressure, alterations in circulating oxygen and carbon dioxide levels, and in the magnitude of these fluctuations are important regulators of CBF in the preterm neonate, and CBF remains stable in preterm neonates who do not develop IVH. In contrast, lower systemic perfusion pressure followed by cerebral hyperperfusion, a fluctuating perfusion pattern, and lack of autoregulation are all associated with IVH. In response to these alterations, hemorrhage begins within the germinal matrix, and blood may rupture into the ventricular system. After ventricular distension by an acute hemorrhage event, cerebral blood flow falls. Venous stasis within the periventricular white matter ensues, and periventricular hemorrhagic infarction may soon develop.

Prostaglandins, and particularly the cyclo-oxygenase 2 (COX-2) system, are important modulators of CBF. Hypoxia, hypotension, growth factors, and inflammatory modulators may all induce COX-2. An increase in prostanoids results in release of VEGF, the potent angiogenic factor associated with hemorrhage.

Clinical events associated with increases in cerebral blood flow include vigorous resuscitation, rapid volume reexpansion, endotracheal tube repositioning, recurrent suctioning, complex nursing care procedures, and the administration of sodium bicarbonate, as well as respiratory distress syndrome, hypoxemia, extremes of P_{CO_2} levels (i.e., both hypocapnia and hypercapnia), and acidosis. Similarly, IVH has been reported after seizures and pneumothoraces in infants with no previous hemorrhage. In contrast, a delay of at least 30 seconds (and to 180 seconds) to clamp the umbilical cord after birth stabilizes blood pressure and decreases the incidence of IVH.

Candidate Genes for IVH

IVH has been attributed to the interaction of the environment and the genome. Preclinical candidate gene studies implicate microvascular proteins, whereas clinical data suggest variants in inflammatory, coagulation, and vascular pathways.

Preclinical studies suggest that variants in one or more microvascular proteins confer vulnerability to environmental triggers. Mice with mutations in COL4A1 experience IVH after the stress accompanying vaginal delivery. These are preventable by surgical delivery, suggesting an interaction between an environmental trigger and the genome. Similarly, mice with mutations in activin receptor-like kinase 5, alpha v integrins, annexin 7, CREB binding protein, death receptor, Id proteins 1 and 3, or Tgfbr2 also develop hemorrhage mimicking grade 4 IVH. All are implicated in angiogenesis and vascular maturation. (For review, see Ment et al., 2014). In addition, autoregulation relies on smooth muscle cells, pericytes, and proteins ranging from Ca++ and K+ channels, phospholipase A1, arachidonic acid, and adenosine to nitric oxide and cytokines among others. Mice with mutations in annexin 7, a gene encoding a Ca++-activated GTPase supporting Ca++ channel activity, experience IVH, suggesting that variants in genes controlling CBF may also contribute to hemorrhage.

Coagulation factors have long been considered clinical candidate genes for IVH, both because of the pathophysiology of hemorrhage and their putative role in perinatal stroke. The most widely studied include the factor V Leiden (F5) variant, polymorphisms of methylene-tetrahydrofolate reductase (MTHFR) and the prothrombin 20210G>A variant (F2).

The contribution of the F5 polymorphism to IVH has been interrogated in different populations with varying results. A point mutation results in replacement of amino acid 506 arginine to glutamine in an activated protein C cleavage site. Activated protein C cleaves the peptide bonds in activated F5, resulting in inhibition of the coagulation pathway, and the variant presents with hypercoagulability. In four different studies, the F5 variant was reported to be associated with IVH, protect against hemorrhage or show no effect.

MTHFR, a second candidate, catalyzes the reduction of 5,10-methylenetrahydrofolate to 5-methyltetrahydrofolate and is necessary for conversion of homocysteine to methionine. Hyperhomocysteinemia is associated with polymorphisms at -677 and -1298 and results in endothelial cell injury and alterations in coagulation including stroke, thrombosis and vascular disorders. A recent investigation of these polymorphisms in preterms with atypical PVHI suggested a high incidence of deleterious variants.

Cytokines are also postulated to play a role in IVH. Hypoxia results in the loss of blood-brain barrier function, permitting cytokines from the peripheral circulation direct access to the preterm brain. Cytokines secreted may also be synthesized by CNS glia. Interleukin-1β (Il-1β) is the major cytokine involved in activation of the hypothalamic-pituitary-adrenal axis. In response to hypoxic ischemic injury, Il-1β increases across the brain, and both the Il-1β -511 T and the Il-1β-31 C allele have been associated with an increased risk for hemorrhage.

Similarly, in a single study the CC genotype of IL-6-174 significantly increased risk for IVH. Finally, TNF-α plays a pivotal role in the acute phase proinflammatory cytokine cascade and the −308 A allele in the TNF-α promoter region has been associated with IVH in preterm neonates.

Proteins contributing to the integrity of the developing CNS vasculature and those mediating cerebral blood flow are also excellent targets. COL4A1 encodes type IV collagen alpha chain 1A, a principal component of basement membranes expressed during development. Mutations in COL4A1 have been reported in infants with congenital porencephaly, fetal IVH, and preterm neonates with hemorrhage. Likewise, nitric oxide (NO) promotes cerebral vasodilation, and variants in the promoter of endothelial NO synthase have also been associated with hemorrhage.

NEUROPATHOLOGY

Over 90% of all IVH in preterm infants originate in germinal matrix tissues between the caudate nucleus and the thalamus at the level of, or slightly posterior to, the foramen of Monro. A small percentage may also originate from the choroid plexus, a common site of IVH in term infants.

Periventricular hemorrhagic infarction (PVHI), germinal matrix destruction, porencephaly, and posthemorrhagic hydrocephalus (PHH) are the direct neuropathologic consequences of hemorrhage. In contrast, WMI with associated atrophic ventriculomegaly is frequently detected in infants with IVH but is multifactorial in etiology.

Ten percent to 20% of infants with GMH develop intraparenchymal abnormalities, or PVHI. These venous infarctions arise not only from the acute increase in intracranial pressure attributable to the GMH itself, but also from the tortuous anatomy of the periventricular venous system. In addition, some investigators believe that the parenchymal involvement of IVH represents a direct pressure-mediated extension of hemorrhage from either a massive GMH or blood within the ventricular system. These lesions are difficult to distinguish and have been variously named PVHI, parenchymal involvement of hemorrhage, or grade 4 IVH.

Further, whereas germinal matrix hemorrhage may result in the destruction of the germinal matrix and loss of neuronal and glial cells residing there, extension of hemorrhage into the subventricular zone and periventricular white matter is associated with not only the loss of additional precursor cells but also axonal necrosis. After grade 4 IVH, a cavitary lesion, or porencephaly, may result. Porencephalies have hemosiderin in the walls lining them and are freely communicating with the ventricular system.

Finally, PHH represents a not uncommon sequela of IVH. The meninges are thickened and show an infiltration by hemosiderin-laden macrophages, resulting in occlusion of the arachnoid villi, obstruction to flow of CSF through the foramina of Luschka and Magendie, and impairment of flow through the tentorial notch. Occasionally, aqueductal obstruction is caused by an acute blood clot, ependymal disruption, or reactive gliosis.

NEUROIMAGING

Cranial ultrasonography is the current method of choice for the diagnosis and monitoring of IVH in preterm infants. Many nurseries use the standard grading system found in Table 22-1. Although grades 3 to 4 IVH are easily imaged by ultrasonography, grades 1 to 2 hemorrhage may be more difficult to both diagnose and differentiate, and interobserver agreement is reportedly poor with these lesions. Use of the posterior fontanelle or the appreciation of posthemorrhagic ventricular dilation may facilitate diagnosis of grade 2 IVH, but this distinction may also be made by the use of newer MRI sequences including susceptibility-weighted imaging.

Rarely found without IVH, intraparenchymal echodensities (IPE) are believed to represent PVHI and generally occur in infants of the youngest GAs during the first postnatal week. The ultrasound appearance is an echogenic juxtaventricular white matter lesion, superior and lateral to the lateral ventricle and extending toward the cortex in a flare pattern without evidence for mass effect on the surrounding brain. IPE eventually cavitate or atrophy to form either a porencephaly or adjacent *ex vacuo* ventriculomegaly, and MR studies demonstrate a single hemorrhagic lesion adjacent to or communicating with the lateral ventricle in addition to IVH.

CLINICAL FINDINGS

The clinical manifestations of IVH are variable, and in one large series, over 75% of hemorrhages were clinically unrecognized. Nonetheless, infants with large hemorrhages may suffer a significant decrease in hematocrit and experience coma, seizures, changes in tone and reflexes, and unremitting metabolic acidosis. Apneic and bradycardic spells may be attributable to either increased intracranial pressure or changes in CBF to brainstem respiratory control centers. In addition, infants with even low-grade IVH may have significantly elevated serum glucose values and evidence for inappropriate secretion of antidiuretic hormone.

Examination of the CSF in preterms undergoing unremarkable sepsis evaluations reveals 0 to 20 WBC, absence of RBC, and protein values of 100 to 200 mg/dL. In patients with new-onset IVH, findings include large numbers of RBC, WBC in direct proportion to the peripheral RBC/WBC ratio, elevations of protein, and low glucose values. Although infants with grade 1 IVH have no CSF abnormalities, for neonates with grade 2 to 4 hemorrhage CSF protein levels and red blood cell counts correlate with grade of IVH. Profound hypoglycorrhachia, with CSF glucose values lower than 10 mg/dL, may be found in infants with all grades of hemorrhage, although this is also more common with high-grade hemorrhage.

Days to weeks after hemorrhage, the CSF demonstrates decreasing red blood cell numbers but elevated white blood cell counts in excess of 500 to 1000/mm^3 and persistent hypoglycorrhachia. The latter two findings may lead to a suspicion of bacterial meningitis, a diagnosis only determined by CSF cultures.

NEONATAL OUTCOME

In the neonatal period, infants with IVH are at risk for the development of seizures and posthemorrhagic ventricular dilation (PHVD). The incidence of seizures in infants with IVH ranges from 5% to 75%, and diagnosis is facilitated by continuous amplitude-integrated EEG.

Approximately one third of infants with IVH develop PHVD, defined as ventricular enlargement greater than the 97% for GA. In addition, as many as 25% to 50% of infants with grades 3 to 4 IVH experience PHH, or the presence of intraventricular blood, increasing ventriculomegaly, and increased intracranial pressure; 15% of neonates with grades 3 to 4 IVH and PHH require permanent CSF diversion (Mazzola et al., 2014). Infants with IVH may also develop acute obstruction at either the foramen of Monro or the aqueduct; they present with signs of acutely increased intracranial pressure and require immediate neurosurgical attention, as shown in Video 20-1. Randomized controlled trials for PHH include intraventricular streptokinase or tissue plasminogen activator, repeated lumbar punctures, and DRIFT (drainage, irrigation and fibrinolytic therapy), but none of these strategies has proven effective.

Infants with IVH and/or PVHI should undergo regular ultrasonographic determinations of ventricular size. If ventricular size and ICP increase, neurosurgical consultation is recommended. Temporizing measures, including subgaleal shunts, ventricular reservoir placement, or third ventriculostomy (Video 20-2) aim to avoid permanent ventriculoperitoneal shunt placement, but future multicenter randomized trials are required to explore these treatment options.

LONG-TERM OUTCOME

Cerebral palsy has long been recognized as a sequela of IVH, and significant cognitive and neuropsychiatric abnormalities are also being recognized at school age and beyond.

For preterm children, the incidence of CP is reported to increase with the grade of hemorrhage. CP is diagnosed in 30% of children with grade 3 to 4 IVH, 10.4% with grades 1 to 2 IVH, and 6.5% with no hemorrhage. Recent data indicate that CP among preterm infants is almost equally divided among spastic diplegia, hemiplegia, and quadriplegia.

IVH is also a significant cause of disability in the prematurely born. Preterm subjects with grades 3 to 4 IVH have significantly worse cognitive abilities and educational performance compared with those without hemorrhage. They are also at high risk for executive function, memory and behavioral disorders. In a recent large study, over three fourths of subjects with grade 3 to 4 IVH had full scale IQ scores more than 2 SD lower than the mean, compared with 12% of subjects with no hemorrhage. However, even survivors with low-grade IVH experience alterations in cognition and behavior, and recent reports note significantly more deficits in cognitive abilities and executive function in preterm subjects with grade 2 IVH compared with those without hemorrhage at childhood and adolescence.

Finally, gray and white matter volumes are decreased during childhood and adolescence in preterms with IVH. Similarly, diffusion tensor imaging shows impaired cerebral myelination in those with high-grade hemorrhage, suggesting that IVH irreversibly alters corticogenesis in the prematurely born.

PREVENTION OF INTRAVENTRICULAR HEMORRHAGE

Although the most efficacious means for preventing IVH would be the prevention of preterm birth, environmental and pharmacologic interventions must be considered (Table 22-5).

When preterm birth is certain, transport of the mother and fetus to a tertiary perinatal center specializing in high-risk obstetric care is advisable; infants who are "outborn" and require transport have consistently higher rates of hemorrhage than "inborn" neonates. Blood pressure and transcutaneous oxygen pressure should be continuously monitored to prevent hypoxemia, hypotension, and acidosis. Abrupt changes in

TABLE 22-5 Prevention of IVH in Preterm Neonates

Etiology	Strategies
Environmental	Universal prenatal care
	Maternal transport
	Tertiary care center delivery
	Delayed cord clamping (when feasible for 30–60 seconds after birth)*
	Bag and mask ventilation, early CPAP
	Monitoring of blood gases to prevent hypoxemia, hypocarbia, hypercarbia, and/or acidosis
	Continuous blood pressure monitoring— prevention of arterial hypotension
	No routine tracheal suctioning or chest physical therapy
	No early neonatal transport
Pharmacologic	Complete course of antenatal steroid exposure
	Early administration of surfactant (within first 30 postnatal minutes)
	Postnatal indomethacin
	Avoid sodium bicarbonate exposure

CPAP, continuous positive airways pressure.
*American College of Obstetricians and Gynecologists (Obstet Gynecol 2012;120:1522–1526)

blood pressure, hypocarbia with PCO_2 levels lower than 30 mm Hg, and sodium bicarbonate administration should be avoided. Finally, delayed cord clamping significantly decreases the incidence of IVH, and the WHO recommends delayed cord clamping, when feasible, for at least 30 to 60 seconds after birth in preterm neonates.

In addition, corticosteroids administered before preterm birth lower the incidence of IVH and decrease mortality. Fetal exposure to antenatal steroids decreases the relative risk of any IVH by half, and the relative risk for severe IVH is approximately 25% compared with preterms without exposure. These benefits extend to a broad range of gestational ages, are not limited by gender or race, and are not associated with adverse side effects.

Likewise, postnatal indomethacin treatment significantly decreases the overall risk for IVH, and particularly that for grade 3 to 4 hemorrhage. Meta-analyses show no increase in necrotizing enterocolitis, excessive bleeding, or renal complications in treated infants compared with controls, and follow-up studies demonstrate no adverse outcomes. Current recommendations suggest that infants of 32 weeks and younger GA who are at high risk for IVH and lack contraindications for therapy be treated with prophylactic indomethacin 0.1 mg/kg/dose beginning at 6 to 12 postnatal hours, with two additional doses 24 and 48 hours thereafter.

Finally, protocols, including both pharmacologic and environment interventions (antenatal steroids), resuscitation by an attending neonatologist to include bag and mask ventilation with air only, early CPAP, administration of surfactant without intubation and avoidance of routine tracheal suctioning, and arterial hypotension significantly decrease hemorrhage.

CEREBELLAR HEMORRHAGE

Cerebellar hemorrhage (CBH) occurs in 20% or more of preterm neonates, and as many as three-fourths of infants with cerebellar hemorrhages experience IVH. The timing of injury may differ, however, suggesting differences in pathophysiology; the mean age for diagnosis of CBH is 5.2 days, compared with 1.7 days for IVH. Risk factors for CBH include lack of antenatal steroid exposure, emergent cesarean section, hypotension requiring therapy, sepsis, PDA, and acidosis. Finally, infants who experience CBH are at high risk for neurodevelopmental disability.

WHITE MATTER INJURY OF THE PREMATURE NEWBORN

White matter injury (WMI) is the predominant lesion of the premature newborn brain, resulting in much of the cognitive, behavioral, and motor impairments seen in children born prematurely. The true incidence of this injury is not known, largely because detection of the diffuse, noncystic form of this lesion is difficult using conventional neuroimaging and because a threshold for defining clinically important signal abnormality in the cerebral white matter has not been rigorously defined either by US or MRI. White matter injury is used increasingly in place of the traditional term periventricular leukomalacia (PVL) as it describes better the more common diffuse lesion of the cerebral white matter that extends beyond the periventricular regions. A more encompassing term, "encephalopathy of prematurity," has been proposed by Volpe to include the findings of cortical and subcortical gray matter abnormalities associated with WMI (Volpe, 2009). This term is not yet in widespread use in the literature, but it reflects increasing evidence that premature newborns suffer a diffuse brain injury that affects many gray matter structures as well as cerebral white matter.

Neuropathology

The neuropathology of WMI consists of two components: focal necrosis (leading to cyst formation) in the deep periventricular white matter and a diffuse gliosis of the cerebral white matter, often extending well beyond the periventricular region. The acute lesions of WMI are characterized by axonal swellings, microglial activation, and reactive astrocytosis. Older lesions of remote WMI consist of astrogliosis, microgliosis, hypomyelination, and sometimes cysts which may be quite small (less than 1 mm), hence not detectable by conventional imaging studies. Failure of oligodendrocyte maturation results in hypomyelination, which together with axonal loss/injury, causes the decrease in cerebral white matter volume with accompanying increase in ventricular volume (atrophic ventriculomegaly).

Gray matter (neuronal) loss and injury in association with WMI has been demonstrated by quantitative neuroimaging studies showing marked reductions in cortical and subcortical gray matter volume and neuropathologic studies showing significant neuronal loss and gliosis in the thalamus, basal ganglia, and cerebral cortex. In addition, gliosis and neuronal loss were found in the cerebellar white matter, cortex, and nuclei, and selected brainstem nuclei of some infants with WMI. It remains unclear whether the neuronal loss and gliosis are predominantly a consequence of primary injury to axons of the cerebral white matter, or whether there is a separate direct injury to neurons of the cortical, subcortical, and cerebellar gray matter, or both. Volpe elegantly synthesized the neuropathologic findings together with concurrent events in human brain development to present a comprehensive thesis of how the interaction of both destructive and altered developmental processes produces the "encephalopathy of prematurity." He proposed that WMI in the preterm brain involves primary destructive effects as well as widespread disturbances of brain maturation and development, producing a diffuse brain "lesion" (Volpe, 2009). This review is a must read for understanding injury to the developing brain, as he describes how injury and loss of cerebral axons, subplate neurons and migrating cortical GABAergic neurons, and impaired cerebellar growth and injury all may contribute to the diffuse encephalopathy of prematurity that extends beyond the well-recognized white matter pathology.

Pathogenesis

The distinctive lesion found in the immature white matter of preterm newborns likely results from the interaction of multiple pathogenetic factors whose relative contributions likely differ among individuals and populations of newborns (Volpe, 2008). Numerous risk factors for the development of WMI have been identified, but in most cases three major categories of factors contribute to the pathogenesis of WMI in premature newborns (Box 22-3):

1. Hypoxia-ischemia
2. Inflammation/infection
3. Vulnerability of immature white matter

These three categories, as well as additional risk factors for WMI, are discussed in detail.

Hypoxia-Ischemia

Neuropathologic studies employing postmortem injections of the vessels demonstrated vascular border and end zones in the periventricular white matter in which WMI is typically found, suggesting a major role for hypoxia-ischemia. In addition, cerebral blood flow is quite low in the white matter of preterm newborns, and data show that critically ill premature newborns frequently have pressure-passive circulation at least intermittently, putting them at risk for cerebral ischemia. Notably, the fluctuations in pressure-passivity do not necessarily correlate with periods of hypotension, suggesting that a normal blood pressure does not necessarily indicate adequate cerebral perfusion. In addition to the intrinsic immaturity of the cerebral circulation in preterm newborns, a patent ductus arteriosus, as well as serious perinatal or postnatal infections such as necrotizing enterocolitis (NEC), sepsis, and/or meningitis, can all adversely affect cerebral hemodynamics. Hypoxia and hypocarbia, ventilation strategies, suctioning, medications such as indomethacin or caffeine, infusions, transfusions, and other interventions have all been shown to exert a deleterious effect on cerebral hemodynamics and may contribute to the pathogenesis of WMI.

Inflammation/Infection

Both epidemiologic and experimental studies support a role for inflammation and/or infection in the pathogenesis of WMI. Studies show an association between maternal infection, prolonged rupture of membranes, cord blood IL-6 levels, placental inflammation/infection, and WMI, suggesting that maternal infection is an etiologic factor in the pathogenesis of WMI. Similarly, significant postnatal infections such as sepsis or NEC have been associated with WMI. Neuropathologic data show an abundance of activated microglia in the white matter of the preterm brain, suggesting that infection/inflammation is a potential mechanism in the pathogenesis of WMI. Rodent data show involvement of activated microglia and a role of cytokines such as interferon-γ, suggesting mechanisms by which inflammation/infection may play a role in the pathogenesis of WMI (Back and Rosenberg, 2014). Additionally, an interaction or synergism between hypoxia-ischemia and infection/inflammation is likely, as hypoxia-ischemia may result in activation of microglia, and conversely, systemic infection may result in hypoxia-ischemia.

Vulnerability of Immature White Matter

WMI occurs much more commonly in the preterm newborn than in the term newborn, and its diffuse gliotic lesion affects the immature (premyelinating) oligodendrocyte predominantly. These findings point to a maturational vulnerability of the immature cerebral white matter in which this cell type is most vulnerable to injury at this age. Immature oligodendrocytes are susceptible to injury and apoptotic cell death by free radical attack, cytokines, and excitotoxicity.

Additional Risk Factors

Numerous risk factors for WMI and/or long-term neurologic impairments have been identified in epidemiologic and prospective studies of preterm newborns, although the specific mechanism by which each risk factor exerts its effect is not always clear. Many known risk factors—for example, lower gestational age at birth and chronic ventilation for chronic lung disease in preterm newborns—may mediate their effect through one or more of the three major pathogenetic mechanisms described previously. Additional risk factors deserve mention.

Intraventricular Hemorrhage. As described in the previous section on IVH, IVH and WMI are often both present in many neuropathology, imaging, and clinical studies of preterm newborns and are difficult to separate. IVH likely increases the risk of WMI, not only because these two entities share some of the same pathogenetic risk factors (e.g., hypoxia-ischemia) but also because IVH may exacerbate WMI. Given their frequent cooccurrence, it is difficult to differentiate the etiologic factors and separate effects of IVH and PVL on long-term neurologic outcome.

Postnatal Corticosteroid Use. Clinical studies of postnatal steroids (particularly dexamethasone) given to treat lung disease have shown an association with worse neurodevelopmental outcome in treated compared with untreated preterm newborns, although the mechanism is unclear. Data showing an adverse effect of dexamethasone on brain development and neurodevelopmental outcome led to a change from frequent use of postnatal steroids to treat lung disease, to a careful weighing of the risks of steroid use against the risk of severe lung disease, and to consideration of using hydrocortisone rather than dexamethasone.

Nutrition. Nutritional factors such as total caloric intake, as well as specific vitamins and nutrients, are likely extremely important for optimal brain development and neurologic outcome. Data suggest that undernutrition during a vulnerable period of brain development can result in hypomyelination (rodent) or smaller brain volumes (human). Further work is needed in this critically important field of early life nutrition and its influence on brain development.

Clinical Presentation

WMI is typically a clinically silent lesion, evolving over days to weeks with few or no outward neurologic signs, until spasticity is first detected weeks to months later or when children present at an even later age with cognitive difficulties at preschool or school age, sometimes without preceding motor abnormalities. With moderate to severe WMI, some degree of spasticity in the lower extremities may be detected by careful examination by term age or earlier, and there may be axial flexor and proximal appendicular weakness or feeding difficulties when WMI is severe. Because detection of WMI is not possible by routine clinical examination during the newborn period in most cases, imaging studies are needed to detect WMI (and IVH), as recommended in standard published imaging guidelines (Ment et al., 2002).

EEG

EEG is useful in the identification of brain injury by demonstrating background abnormalities in the first days after birth or by demonstrating focal abnormalities such as transient positive rolandic sharp waves (a highly specific but not highly sensitive marker of WMI). Serial EEG studies are more useful than a single EEG for the identification of abnormalities that correlate with WMI and long-term neurologic deficits. Interestingly, WMI is associated with early acute EEG changes followed by later chronic abnormalities (coinciding with cyst formation, when that occurs), supporting the idea that the insult resulting in WMI occurs around or very soon after birth.

Neuroimaging

Ultrasound

The evolution of echogenic (or hyperechoic) lesions in the periventricular white matter over the first few weeks after birth, with or without cyst formation, is the classic description of WMI detected by serial cranial ultrasound (US) studies (Fig. 22-15). The diagnosis of noncystic WMI is difficult with US, partly because the interobserver variability is high even in rigorous, prospective US studies and partly because there is no general agreement regarding the number, size, location, and persistence of hyperechoic lesions defining WMI by US. Cerebral atrophy (i.e., volume loss) associated with WMI results in eventual atrophic ventriculomegaly and enlarged extraaxial

CSF spaces, which are usually present within weeks after birth (see Fig. 22-15).

Magnetic Resonance Imaging

MRI is used to detect WMI in newborns and children born prematurely, particularly for research studies but increasingly for clinical purposes. Conventional T1- or T2-weighted (T1w, T2w) MRI sequences easily demonstrate cystic lesions, but noncystic WMI is also detected by MRI, evident as high T2w signal intensity and low T1w signal intensity in the cerebral white matter in newborns (Kwon et al., 2014). Punctate lesions have been reported particularly in the corona radiata and posterior periventricular white matter (and occasionally the gray matter) (Fig. 22-15). Notably, cystic lesions may collapse over time and may appear as punctate lesions or other patterns of signal abnormality in the white matter, highlighting the utility of serial imaging studies. Although MRI is more difficult to obtain than US in the early acute period, it is more sensitive than cranial ultrasound for the detection of WMI in preterm newborns, especially for the noncystic form of WMI and small cerebellar hemorrhage. As for US studies, no universally accepted measure of the severity, pattern, or location of signal abnormality by MRI defines WMI for clinical purposes. Although clearly a greater severity of WMI correlates with a higher incidence of later neurodevelopmental deficits in general, a broad range of neurologic outcome exists for mild, moderate, and severe WMI.

Research MRI studies have been particularly helpful in elucidating the timing, distribution, and clinical correlates of WMI in children born prematurely. For example, volumetric MRI data analysis demonstrated the marked reduction in cortical and subcortical gray matter volumes accompanying WMI that had been underappreciated before the availability of these quantitative measurement techniques. Volumetric, DTI, and functional MRI studies of older children born preterm have been particularly useful in determining the clinical correlates

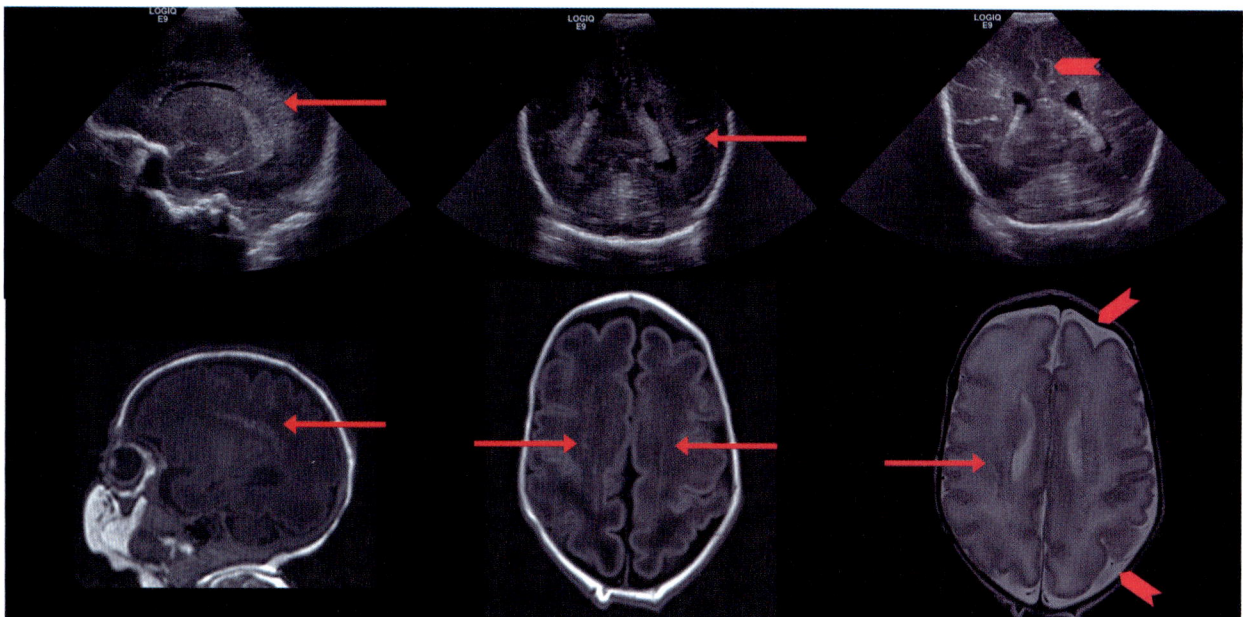

Figure 22-15. Ultrasound and MRI correlation of white matter injury. Sagittal and coronal US at 2 days (**A, B**) and 1 month (**C**), and MRI at 2 months (**D**, Sag T1; **E,** Ax T1 FLAIR; **F,** Ax T2) of baby born at 28 weeks, showing PVL with echogenicity in periventricular white matter bilaterally by US *(arrows)* that evolves to bilateral linear punctate lesions by MRI and enlargement of extraaxial CSF spaces *(notched arrowheads).*

of MRI findings because the larger, mostly myelinated brain of the older child allows many brain structures to be analyzed in greater detail and more precisely than in the newborn, and cognitive, social, and behavioral outcome measures are also more definitive and specific than at the young ages often used in neonatal outcome studies.

Recommendations for Imaging the Preterm Neonate and Child Born Preterm

Current recommendations for imaging the preterm neonate state that screening cranial ultrasound should be performed on all infants with gestational ages younger than 30 weeks at 7 to 14 days of age and should be repeated at 36 to 40 weeks' postmenstrual age (Ment et al., 2002). This recommendation by the Quality Standards Subcommittee of the American Academy of Neurology and the Practice Committee of the Child Neurology Society is designed to detect both clinically silent IVH, which may require additional clinical and/or radiologic monitoring and changes in management, and

evidence of PVL +/- ventriculomegaly. Emerging data suggest that cerebral MRI with DTI at term equivalent age may provide important prognostic information about injury not detected by US and may help predict motor outcome and, to a lesser degree, risk of cognitive, social, or sensory impairments. The largest study to date of 480 newborns born at younger than 28 weeks confirmed that severity of WMI and cerebellar injury predicted neurologic outcome at 18 to 22 months of age, and that late US or MRI (35 to 42 weeks) were more predictive than early US (4 to 14 days). Brain MRI may also be performed in an older infant or child born prematurely to confirm clinically suspected WMI when there are cognitive, motor, and/or sensory impairments of unclear etiology (see Fig. 22-16), for example, when neonatal cranial US studies were reportedly normal. MRI studies beyond the newborn period rarely show cysts but may show increased signal intensity on T2w as well as fluid-attenuated inversion-recovery images in areas of gliotic white matter with delayed or decreased myelination, thinning of the corpus callosum, and enlarged ventricles, indicating a decrease in cerebral white (and likely gray) matter

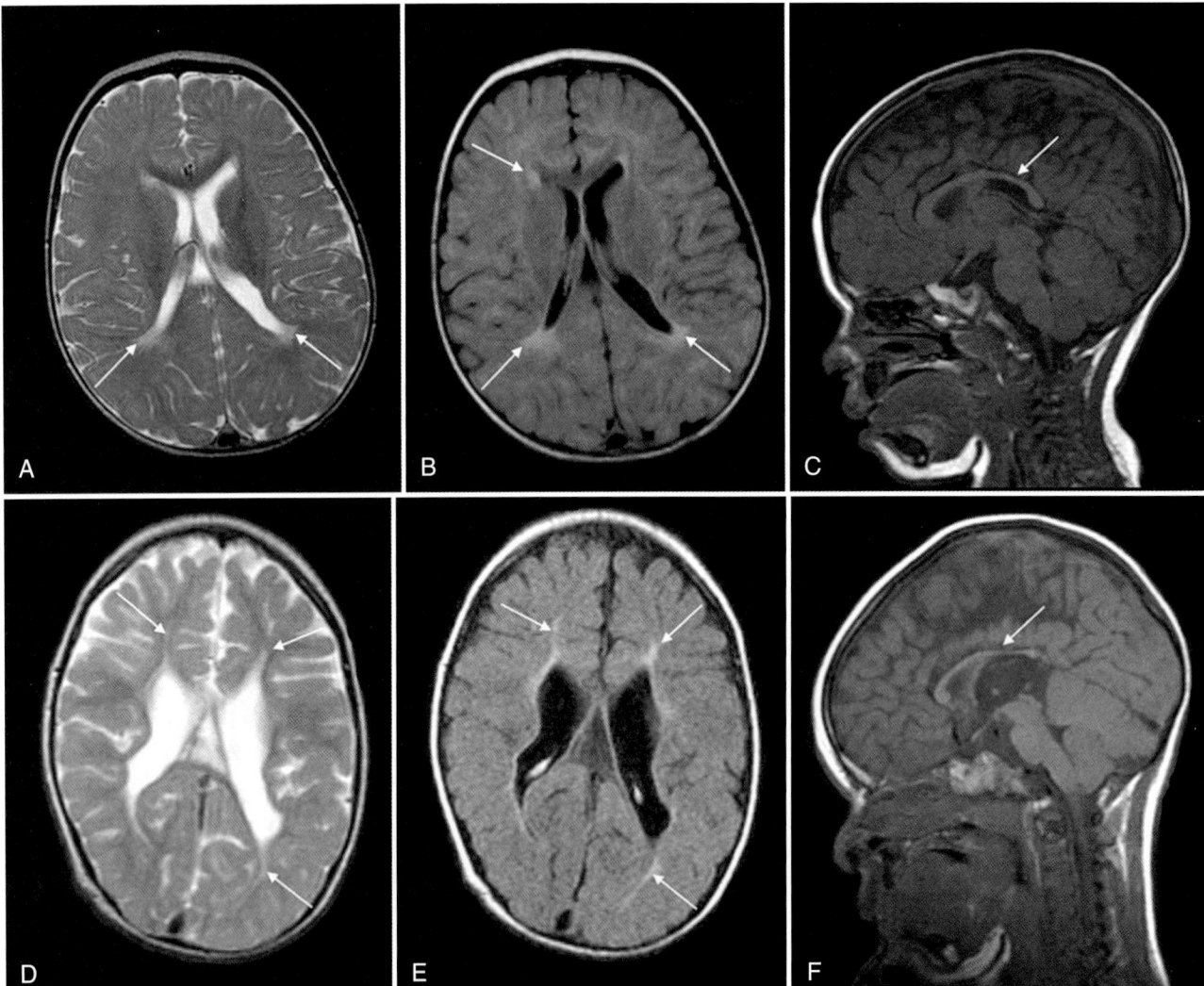

Figure 22-16. MRI of mild and severe white matter injury in young children. A–C, Axial T2-weighted. **(A)** T2 fluid-attenuated inversion-recovery (FLAIR) **(B)** and sagittal T1-weighted **(C)** images demonstrating mild WMI in an 12-month-old born at 30 weeks' gestational age; at age 3 years this patient had mild spastic diparesis with accompanying gross and fine motor impairments/delays. **D–F,** Axial T2-weighted. **(D),** T2 FLAIR **(E)** and sagittal T1-weighted **(F)** images demonstrating severe WMI in a 2-year-old boy born at 29 weeks' gestational age; this patient had severe diplegia (quadriplegia), infantile spasms, severe cognitive impairment with IQ lower than 70, and cerebral visual impairment. *Arrows* demonstrate areas of signal abnormality in the white matter on axial sequences and thinning of the corpus callosum on the sagittal sequence.

volume (Fig. 22-16). Abnormal signal intensity may be detected in gray matter structures, but volume loss in cortical and subcortical gray matter structures is difficult to detect without quantitative measurement.

Outcome

WMI is the principal cause of the cognitive, behavioral, motor, and sensory impairments found in children born at younger than 32 weeks' gestational age. Most outcome studies of children born prematurely include children with all types of brain lesions, so it is difficult to determine the specific outcome attributable to WMI alone. That being said, it is likely that WMI and hemorrhagic venous infarction (grade 4 IVH) are the major lesions contributing to neurologic disabilities in children born prematurely. The incidence and severity of neurologic impairments increases with lower gestational age at birth, but many other antenatal, neonatal, and postneonatal risk factors relate to later neurodevelopmental impairments, such as chronic medical illness, socioeconomic status, and parental education.

Cognitive

Lower overall IQ and specific types of cognitive impairments have been found in children born prematurely compared with term-born children. Lower gestational age and birth weight are major risk factors for cognitive impairments, in addition to identified brain injury. Deficits of attention and organization, math skills, and reading comprehension are much more common in children born extremely preterm than in term-born controls. Most large prospective studies of the cognitive outcome of older children born prematurely do not associate cognitive measures with specific brain lesions (such as WMI), but quantitative imaging data suggest that it is indeed WMI and associated gray matter correlates that underlie most of these cognitive impairments.

Social/Behavioral

Children born prematurely have higher rates of social and behavioral difficulties than do term-born children, including attention deficit/hyperactivity, emotional, anxiety, autism spectrum, and behavioral disorders. Of these, attention problems are commonly recognized, although anxiety and other social and emotional disorders are increasingly identified. Children born preterm appear to be at higher risk of autism than term-born children, but the reported incidence of autism is highly variable, depending on the population studied, age at assessment and the tool used to identify autistic traits.

Motor

WMI and lower gestational age at birth are major risk factors for motor disability. The incidence of CP is much higher in children born extremely prematurely, occurring in approximately 20% of children born at 26 weeks or younger gestational age, but in only 4% of children born at 32 weeks' gestational age. Spastic diparesis is the most common form of CP in preterm infants with WMI, which may present as quadriparesis when severe. Some dystonia is frequently part of spastic diparesis caused by PVL, and occasionally hypotonia, ataxia, or some other motor abnormality may be observed. Hemiparesis is found less frequently than spastic diparesis and usually results from periventricular hemorrhagic infarction but may occasionally result from markedly asymmetric WMI. Even in the absence of overt CP, coordination difficulties, and other more subtle abnormalities of motor function or development are often found in children born prematurely.

Visual

Whereas some children born prematurely have retinopathy of prematurity affecting their vision, WMI and other cerebral lesions can result in strabismus, nystagmus, and other disorders of ocular motility, low acuity, visual field deficits (largely inferior fields), and perceptual difficulties, some of which may not be recognized until school age or later. Children with WMI may have visual perceptual defects or other higher order visual impairments that worsen their cognitive and school function, so these are particularly important to detect and address with therapy.

Epilepsy

Children with severe WMI occasionally develop epilepsy (e.g., Fig. 22-16), although epilepsy is more commonly related to gray matter lesions, and most long-term studies reporting epilepsy rates do not specify associated brain lesions. Reported rates of epilepsy vary from 2% to 6%, and are associated with lower gestational age at birth.

Prevention and Management

Preventive efforts should begin antenatally whenever possible, with administration of medications known to reduce morbidity in preterm newborns. Antenatal steroid administration has been associated with approximately 50% decrease in cerebral white matter lesions and a decrease in neonatal death (odds ratio 0.69), with no change or decreased rate of adverse neurodevelopmental outcome, and thus is recommended for women with preterm labor. Meta-analyses of five trials of antenatal magnesium showed a 32% reduction in the risk of CP and improved motor outcome.

NICU Management

After birth, maintenance of normal cerebral perfusion and oxygenation should be attempted by careful management of systemic hemodynamics and oxygenation, including blood pressure, intravascular volume, oxygenation, and ventilation, and avoidance of treatments or procedures that result in sudden or deleterious changes in hemodynamics or oxygenation. Avoidance and prompt treatment of infection may minimize WMI, although no prospective studies have demonstrated the effect of such interventions on reducing WMI. Adequate nutrition is also important for normal brain development, but the specific type and amount of nutrients also remain an active area of research.

At the time of writing, no specific neuroprotective therapies or medications prevent or minimize WMI during the newborn period, but promising neuroprotective agents shown to prevent or minimize WMI in animal models are currently being tested in clinical trials (Juul SE and Ferriero, 2014). Erythropoietin is being tested in two ongoing trials to determine whether it can improve neurologic outcome in preterm newborns, and melatonin is being tested to determine whether it has neuroprotective effects in IUGR fetuses and preterm newborns. Results of these trials will likely be available after publication of this textbook with further trials of neuroprotective agents in the coming years.

Management After NICU Discharge

Management of infants with WMI after discharge from the neonatal intensive care unit should include careful monitoring to identify any cognitive, behavioral, sensory, or motor delays or impairments, with implementation of appropriate therapies. Follow up by pediatric neurologists or other pediatric physicians trained in infant and child development should be provided for children born prematurely, particularly those born at younger than 32 weeks' gestational age. Early intervention services, including physical, occupational, speech and language, behavioral/social, and visual therapies, should be provided as needed to address specific developmental delays or impairments. Auditory and visual evaluations should be performed at older ages to ensure normal specialized sensory function because subtle sensory and perceptual difficulties may not be apparent without specific testing. Similarly, assessment of cognitive and social function of school-age children may be needed even in the absence of early developmental delay or other sensorimotor impairments.

Acknowledgments

This work was supported by NS 27116 (LRM), NS 53865 (LRM), NINDS 1P01-NS38475, the Charles H Dana Foundation (JSS), the March of Dimes (JSS), and P30 HD18655, the Boston Children's Hospital Intellectual and Developmental Disabilities Research Center (BCH IDDRC) (JSS). The authors thank Walter C Allan, M.D., Praveen Ballabh, M.D., Charles C Duncan, M.D., Gordon Sze, M.D., and Joseph J Volpe, M.D., for scientific advice.

REFERENCES

The complete list of references for this chapter is available online at www.expertconsult.com.

See inside cover for registration details.

SELECTED REFERENCES

Back, S.A., Rosenberg, P.A., 2014. Pathophysiology of glia in perinatal white matter injury. Glia 62 (11), 1790–1815.

Ballabh, P., 2010. Intraventricular hemorrhage in premature infants: mechanism of disease. Pediatr. Res. 67 (1), 1–8.

Blencowe, H., Lee, A.C., Cousens, S., et al., 2013. Preterm birth-associated neurodevelopmental impairment estimates at regional and global levels for 2010. Pediatr. Res. 74 (Suppl. 1), 17–34.

Juul, S.E., Ferriero, D.M., 2014. Pharmacologic neuroprotective strategies in neonatal brain injury. Clin. Perinatol. 41 (1), 119–131.

Kwon, S.H., Vasung, L., Ment, L.R., et al., 2014. The role of neuroimaging in predicting neurodevelopmental outcomes of preterm neonates. Clin. Perinatol. 41 (1), 257–283.

Mazzola, C.A., Choudhri, A.F., Auguste, K.I., et al., 2014. Pediatric hydrocephalus: systematic literature review and evidence-based guidelines. Part 2: Management of posthemorrhagic hydrocephalus in premature infants. J. Neurosurg. Pediatr. 14 (Suppl. 1), 8–23.

Ment, L.R., Aden, U., Lin, A., et al., 2014. Gene-environment interactions in severe intraventricular hemorrhage of preterm neonates. Pediatr. Res. 75 (1–2), 241–250.

Ment, L.R., Bada, H.S., Barnes, P., et al., 2002. Practice parameter: neuroimaging of the neonate: report of the Quality Standards Subcommittee of the American Academy of Neurology and the Practice Committee of the Child Neurology Society. Neurology 58 (12), 1726–1738.

Volpe, J.J., 2009. Brain injury in premature infants: a complex amalgam of destructive and developmental disturbances. Lancet Neurol. 8, 110–124.

Volpe, J.J., 2008. Neurology of the Newborn. WB Saunders Co., Philadelphia. Chapter 6, Hypoxic-Ischemic Encephalopathy: Biochemical and Physiological Aspects, 247–324. Chapter 7, Hypoxic-Ischemic Encephalopathy: Intrauterine Assessment, 325–346. Chapter 8, Hypoxic-Ischemic Encephalopathy: Neuropathology and Pathogenesis, 347–399. Chapter 9, Hypoxic-Ischemic Encephalopathy: Clinical Aspects, 400–480. Chapter 11, Intracranial Hemorrhage: Germinal Matrix-Intraventricular Hemorrhage of the Premature Infant, 517–588.

E-BOOK FIGURES AND TABLES

23 Perinatal Metabolic Encephalopathies

Rebecca N. Ichord and David R. Bearden

An expanded version of this chapter is available on www.expertconsult.com. See inside cover for registration details.

INTRODUCTION

This chapter reviews perinatal metabolic encephalopathies under two categories: (1) correctable disturbances in glucose and ion balance, and (2) genetically determined inborn errors of metabolism (IEMs), grouped according to clinical symptomatology into the following four types (Box 23-1):

- Fulminant metabolic crisis
- Epileptic encephalopathies
- Chronic encephalopathies with multiorgan involvement
- Chronic encephalopathies without multiorgan involvement

A brief synopsis of each condition is provided, emphasizing distinctive clinical features, diagnosis, and management (Hoffman, Zschocke, and Nyhan, 2010; Ficicioglu and Bearden, 2011).

GENERAL APPROACH

Metabolic disease should be considered in any newborn with encephalopathy. Acute reversible metabolic perturbations are monophasic and resolve after metabolic correction, whereas presentation in IEMs is delayed or progressive, often with diffuse nonspecific symptoms evolving to malignant symptoms (seizures, movement disorder). Neonatal-onset chronic static encephalopathies are increasingly linked to genetic metabolic disease, and may have few features distinguishing them as metabolic. Suspicion of IEM should increase with any of the following factors:

- Multiple components of the nervous system affected (brain, peripheral nerves, skeletal muscle)
- Multiple organ systems affected
- Systemic symptoms (vomiting, autonomic instability)

The most common nongenetic acute neonatal metabolic encephalopathies can be identified from history and results of first-stage studies. Encephalopathic newborns often are assumed incorrectly to have suffered asphyxia when, in fact, they have a static disease of prenatal origin or a metabolic disease that decompensated at birth. Perinatal hypoxic-ischemic encephalopathy should be diagnosed only with unequivocal evidence of ischemic or hypoxemic exposure. Without this, the differential diagnosis should remain broad until a comprehensive evaluation is complete. Evaluation involves staged diagnostic testing while simultaneously treating potentially life-threatening conditions (Table 23-2, Fig. 23-1).

CORRECTABLE DISTURBANCES OF GLUCOSE AND SALT BALANCE

Hypoglycemia

Neonatal hypoglycemia falls into five categories: (1) extrauterine maladaptation, (2) hyperinsulinism, (3) increased glucose consumption, (4) congenital endocrinopathies, and (5) IEMs. Clinical presentation is variable and nonspecific, featuring tachycardia, irritability, and altered consciousness; with blood glucose levels less than 1.0 μM, symptoms may progress to coma and circulatory collapse. Mild symptoms rapidly reverse with glucose administration, whereas severe encephalopathy does not. In severely symptomatic cases, imaging may show acute injury preferentially affecting the parietal-occipital cortex and periventricular white matter. Symptomatic infants should be treated while evaluation proceeds. Poor outcome is associated with severe acute encephalopathy or when the cause is a fatty acid oxidation defect or hyperinsulinism.

Disturbances of Sodium Balance

Sodium plays a critical role in regulating cell volume, water flux, membrane excitability, and synaptic transmission. Causes of hyponatremia or hypernatremia are numerous.

Hyponatremia

Hyponatremia is common in sick neonates, often as a result of excess arginine vasopressin secretion with other organ disease (lung disease, intracranial hemorrhage, surgery), and rarely congenital adrenal insufficiency. Mild symptoms appear at 120 to 130 mEq/L and severe symptoms at less than 120 mEq/L, with somnolence and hypotonia progressing to seizures and coma. Mild subacute chronic hyponatremia is treated by correcting the underlying cause. Treatment of acute severe hyponatremic encephalopathy is challenging. Seizures are resistant to anticonvulsants, and the encephalopathy frequently depresses respiratory function and warrants rapid correction, which can be accomplished with 3% saline, generally without neurologic complications.

Hypernatremia

Hypernatremic encephalopathy arises from hypertonic dehydration of neurons and glia, sometimes compounded by hyperviscosity, cerebral venous thrombosis, or intracranial hemorrhage. Hypernatremia is caused by excess sodium intake, excess water losses, or both. Management requires repleting volume deficits with isotonic solutions or plasma expanders, correcting hypernatremia over 48 to 72 hours, and lowering serum sodium approximately 10 to 15 mEq/L/24 hours.

INBORN ERRORS OF METABOLISM

Perinatal genetic metabolic encephalopathies are divided into the following four groups (Box 23-2):

1. Acute fulminant illnesses with metabolic crisis
2. Subacute epileptic encephalopathies
3. Chronic encephalopathies with multiorgan involvement
4. Chronic encephalopathies without multiorgan involvement

Clinical features, magnetic resonance imaging (MRI) findings, and results of first-stage tests may suggest specific disorders, verified by definitive second- or third-stage tests, including

---

BOX 23-1 Predominant Presenting Clinical Features in Neonatal Genetic Metabolic Disorders

ACUTE FULMINANT METABOLIC CRISIS

- Urea cycle defects
- Maple syrup urine disease (MSUD)
- Organic acidopathies: isovaleric, propionic, methylmalonic
- Oxidative phosphorylation disorders (OxPhos defects): pyruvate dehydrogenase (PDH) deficiency, pyruvate carboxylase (PC) deficiency, electron transport defects
- Fructose-1,6-biphosphatase deficiency
- Glutamine synthetase deficiency
- Fatty acid oxidation defects: carnitine palmitoyltransferase deficiency type II (CPT II), mitochondrial trifunctional protein deficiency (MTP defects), malonyl-CoA decarboxylase (MCD)

SUBACUTE PROGRESSIVE EPILEPTIC ENCEPHALOPATHY

- Glycine cleavage defects
- Pyridoxine and pyridoxal 5'-phosphate (PLP) dependency
- Sulfite oxidase and molybdenum cofactor deficiency (Sulf Ox, Moco)
- Menkes' disease
- Cytochrome oxidase (COX) deficiency
- L-amino acid decarboxylase (L-AAD) deficiency
- Methyl-CpG-binding protein-2 (MECP2)
- Glucose transporter type 1 deficiency syndrome (GLUT1 DS)
- 5-amino-4-imidazolecarboxamide ribosiduria/succinyl-5-amino-4-imidazolecarboxamide ribosiduria (AICAR/SAICAR)
- Serine biosynthesis defects

CHRONIC ENCEPHALOPATHY WITH MULTIORGAN INVOLVEMENT

- Mitochondrial disorders
- Congenital defects of glycosylation (CDGs)
- Peroxisomal disorders
- Cholesterol biosynthesis defects

CHRONIC ENCEPHALOPATHY WITHOUT MULTIORGAN INVOLVEMENT

- L-amino acid decarboxylase (L-AAD) deficiency
- Glutaric aciduria
- GTP cyclohydrolase deficiency
- Phenylketonuria (PKU)
- Succinic semialdehyde dehydrogenase (SSADH) deficiency

BOX 23-2 Causes of Hyponatremia and Hypernatremia in Neonates

CAUSES OF HYPONATREMIA

Disorders Causing Positive Water Balance

- Excessive AVP secretion
  - Systemic hypoxia, ischemia
  - Mechanical ventilation
  - Pneumothorax
  - Intracranial hemorrhage
  - Septic shock
  - Neonatal drug withdrawal
  - Hypothyroidism
- Water intoxication
  - Inappropriately dilute intravenous fluids
  - Inappropriately dilute formula feedings

Disorders Causing Negative Sodium Balance

- Abnormal renal salt handling
  - Chronic renal insufficiency
  - Adrenal insufficiency
  - Acute pyelonephritis
  - Acute obstructive uropathy
  - Urinary ascites
- Insufficient salt intake relative to losses
  - High insensible fluid/electrolyte losses
  - Vomiting, diarrhea
  - Low-salt-containing infant formulas

CAUSES OF HYPERNATREMIA

Disorders Causing Negative Water Balance

- Deficient AVP secretion (central diabetes insipidus)
  - Meningitis, encephalitis
  - Hypoxic-ischemic encephalopathy
  - Midline CNS malformations with pituitary insufficiency
- Renal unresponsiveness to AVP
  - Obstructive uropathy
  - Renal dysplasia
  - Drugs
- Excess water losses
  - Extensive skin disease
  - Osmotic diuresis

DISORDERS CAUSING POSITIVE SODIUM BALANCE

- Administration of hypertonic salt solutions
- Ingestion of hypertonic feedings

AVP, arginine vasopressin; CNS, central nervous system.

---

genetic and molecular studies (Xue, Ankala, Wilcox, and Hegde, 2014). See Table 23-2 and Figure 23-1.

Acute Fulminant Metabolic Diseases

Maple Syrup Urine Disease

Maple syrup urine disease (MSUD) is an autosomal-recessive defect of branched-chain keto acid dehydrogenase (BCKAD) causing elevated plasma leucine, isoleucine, and valine, and their corresponding keto acids. The severe neonatal form is most common, presenting 4 to 7 days after birth with progressive lethargy, dystonia, and seizures, evolving to coma and decerebrate posturing. MRI features include T2 hyperintensity and restricted diffusion of brainstem, dentate nuclei, deep gray nuclei, and periventricular white matter. Biochemical abnormalities include ketoacidosis, ketonuria, hypoglycemia, and hyponatremia. Elevated plasma leucine, isoleucine, and valine, and elevated urinary 3-hydroxyvaleric acid, should suggest the diagnosis. BCKAD enzyme activity in skin fibroblasts is low. Treatment for severe decompensation requires peritoneal dialysis or hemodialysis, along with supportive and nutritional measures to induce an anabolic state. Long-term management requires dietary restriction of leucine, good nutritional support, and avoidance of catabolic stresses. Long-term outcome is related to the number and severity of metabolic decompensations.

Other Organic Acidopathies

Organic acidopathies involve defects in amino acid catabolism resulting in elevated urinary organic acids (Knerr et al., 2012). MSUD is a prominent example, as described in the preceding section. Defective degradation of leucine, valine, and isoleucine causes accumulation of branched-chain organic acid intermediates, most commonly isovaleric (IVA), propionic (PA), and methylmalonic aciduria (MMA). Newborn screening detects many cases. Symptoms in neonates include vomiting and lethargy, progressing to seizures and coma. These disorders should be suspected when first-stage screening reveals ketosis, lactic acidosis, hypoglycemia, and hyperammonemia. Diagnosis rests on urinary organic acid profiles and

TABLE 23-2 Laboratory Evaluation of the Infant With Suspected Metabolic Encephalopathy

First Stage: Survey and Screening	Second Stage: Identify Category of Metabolic Defect	Third Stage: Verify Enzyme or Gene Defect
Blood Glucose Electrolytes Mg^{++}, Ca^{++}, PO_4 BUN, creatinine Liver enzymes CBC, platelets, PT, PTT Arterial blood gas Ammonia Lactate, pyruvate	Blood Quantitative plasma amino acids Very-long-chain fatty acids Acyl carnitine profile Carbohydrate-deficient transferrin level Copper, ceruloplasmin levels Cholesterol Uric acid Lysosomal enzyme analysis	Tissue biopsy (muscle, liver) for enzyme assay Skin fibroblast culture for enzyme assay Specific gene mutation and/or panel testing Genome-wide array Whole-exome sequencing
Urine Ketone bodies, reducing substances Protein, blood Cells	Urine Quantitative amino acids Organic acids Galactose Sulfites Xanthine, hypoxanthine Uric acid Ribosides	
CSF Glucose, protein Cell count Microbiology	CSF Quantitative amino acids Neurotransmitters and pterin metabolites Folic acid Lactate, pyruvate	

BUN, blood urea nitrogen; CBC, complete blood count; CSF, cerebrospinal fluid; PT, prothrombin time; PTT, partial thromboplastin time.

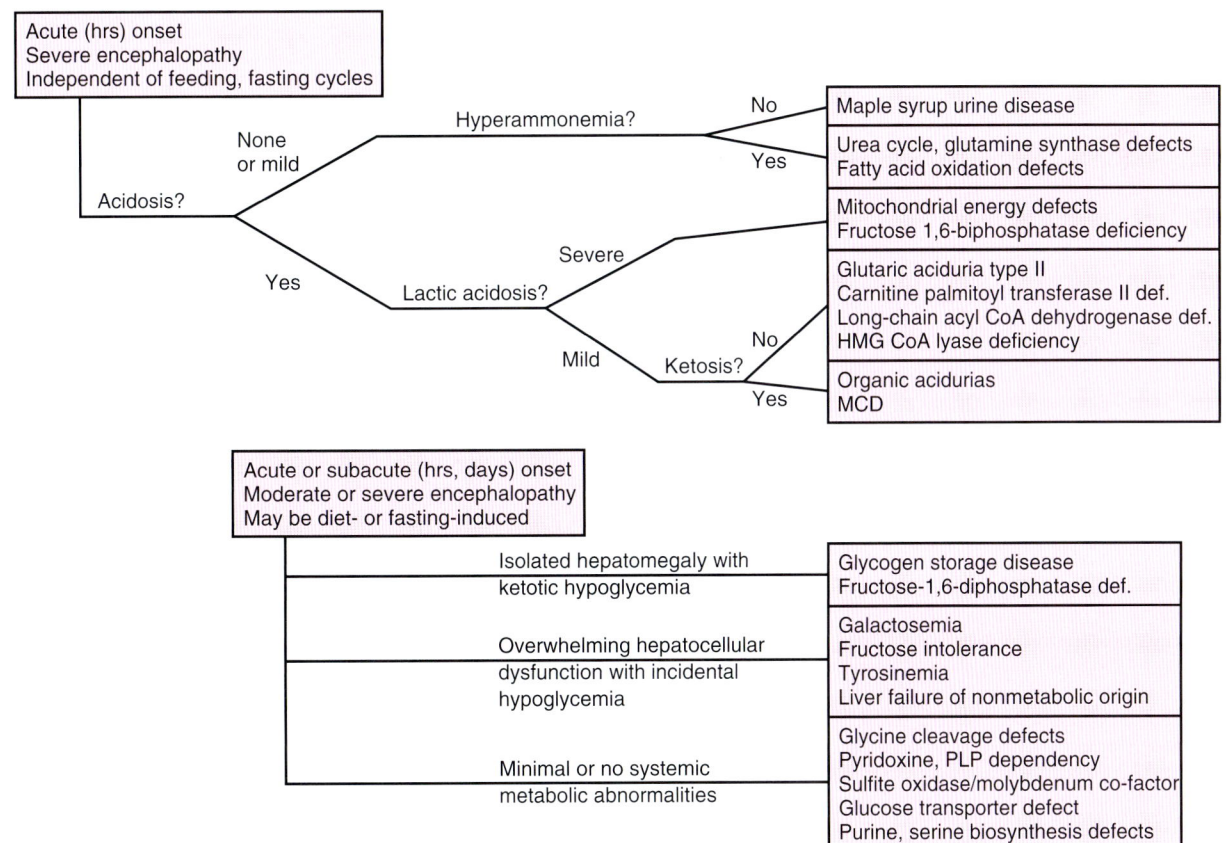

Figure 23-1. Algorithm for evaluation of suspected metabolic encephalopathy in neonates. MCD, malonyl-CoA decarboxylase deficiency; PLP, pyridoxine and pyridoxal 5′-phosphate dependency.

measurement of serum amino acids and acylcarnitines, confirmed by enzyme assay and/or genetic testing. Management involves glucose administration and protein restriction. Peritoneal dialysis may be necessary. Cofactor supplementation may be helpful using L-carnitine and N-carbamylglutamate and biotin for PA, glycine for IVA, and cobalamin for MMA. Creatine and ornithine alpha-ketoglutarate replacement has been suggested. Long-term management involves protein-restricted, high-carbohydrate diets and avoidance of catabolic stresses. Long-term outcome can be normal if decompensations are minimized in frequency and treated aggressively.

Primary Lactic Acidosis Resulting From Defects in Oxidative Phosphorylation

Primary lactic acidosis causes severe encephalopathy in neonates, with defects in pyruvate oxidation involving the pyruvate dehydrogenase (PDH) enzyme complex, pyruvate carboxylase (PC), and the respiratory chain. Secondary lactic acidosis is common in hypoxia or ischemia and in other IEMs secondarily affecting energy metabolism.

Pyruvate oxidation disorders related to PDH deficiency include multiple subtypes. The most common E_1 component defects are X-linked dominants, presenting in newborns with permanent lactic acidosis and fulminant encephalopathy progressing to death. Intrauterine growth retardation, facial and limb anomalies, and minor brain dysgenesis are common. Neuroimaging findings include necrosis and cavitation in cortical white matter, basal ganglia, and brainstem nuclei. Treatment is limited. Some success has been reported with the ketogenic diet and thiamine and carnitine supplements.

Several subtypes of PC deficiency exist, with a spectrum of clinical manifestations. Type B is the severe neonatal form, presenting as fulminant neonatal encephalopathy with permanent lactic acidosis, hypoglycemia, citrullinemia, and hyperammonemia, and is usually fatal in early infancy. Symptoms include depressed mental status, hypotonia, tremors and dystonic movements, and paroxysmal eye-movement abnormalities. Imaging shows cystic periventricular leukomalacia. Diagnosis is challenging because of similarities to other IEMs and hypoxic-ischemic encephalopathy. Treatment involves use of high-carbohydrate diets.

Respiratory chain defects comprise a large spectrum of biochemical and genetic disorders with variable phenotypes. These disorders should be considered in infants with severe intractable lactic acidosis or encephalopathy combined with a cardinal clinical feature (external ophthalmoplegia, myopathy, or cardiomyopathy). Growth failure and other organ dysfunction are common. When lactic acidosis is present, the lactate:pyruvate ratio is increased (>25) in disorders of oxidative phosphorylation as compared with PDH complex disorders, in which the lactate:pyruvate ratio is usually normal. Clinical course may be benign in cases with only skeletal muscle involvement (benign infantile mitochondrial myopathy) or fatal in cases with intractable acidosis. Treatment options are limited and rely on supportive strategies to minimize catabolic stresses, and administration of cofactors (carnitine, nicotinamide, riboflavin).

Diagnosis of primary genetic defects of mitochondrial function involving pyruvate metabolism and respiratory chain is difficult because of the extreme phenotypic and genotypic variability and because histologic and histochemical diagnostic techniques are difficult and not widely available. These conditions should be suspected in infants with persistent severe lactic acidosis combined with other organ disease, especially myopathy and/or cardiomyopathy. Confirmation and further biochemical definition of the diagnosis are complex and may require detailed biochemical studies to isolate the functional defect, followed by identification of specific pathogenic gene mutations (Honzik et al., 2012).

Glutamine Synthetase Deficiency

Glutamine synthetase (GS) plays a critical role in the brain to detoxify ammonia and regulate concentration and compartmentalization of neurotransmitter pools of glutamate and gamma-aminobutyric acid (GABA). GS deficiency is a rare autosomal-recessive condition manifest as profound neonatal encephalopathy with coma, quadriparesis, severe bulbar dysfunction, lissencephaly, and death shortly after birth as a result of multiorgan failure. Diagnosis in this clinical setting is suggested by moderate hyperammonemia with very low or absent glutamine concentration in blood, cerebrospinal fluid (CSF), and urine, and is confirmed by deficient enzyme activity in cultured fibroblasts. There are no effective treatments.

Fructose-1,6-Biphosphatase Deficiency

Fructose-1,6-biphosphatase (FDPase) deficiency is an autosomal-recessive defect in gluconeogenesis. It presents as early infantile-onset severe acute encephalopathy, with fasting-induced lactic acidosis, ketoacidosis, and hypoglycemia, usually without other organ involvement, except hepatomegaly. The clinical and biochemical features should suggest the diagnosis, confirmed by enzyme assay on a liver biopsy specimen. Treatment is similar to that for type I glycogenosis, in addition to restriction of fructose and sucrose intake.

Fatty Acid Oxidation Defects

Fatty acid oxidation disorders involve several enzymes in the degradation of lipids to fatty acids to acetyl-CoA or ketone-body production. These include carnitine palmitoyl transferase II (CPT II) deficiency, mitochondrial trifunctional protein deficiency (MTP), malonyl-CoA decarboxylase deficiency (MCD), multiple acyl-CoA dehydrogenase deficiency (MADD), and classic acyl-CoA dehydrogenase deficiencies (long-chain, or LCAD; medium-chain, or MCAD; short-chain, or SCAD). Although most of these present beyond the neonatal period, several have distinctive presentations in neonates, involving rapid onset of a fulminant metabolic encephalopathy with hypoglycemia, hyperammonemia, low or moderate ketonuria, and metabolic acidosis. Associated features include hepatomegaly, cardiomyopathy, and myopathy. Patients with MCD and MADD have cortical dysgenesis with pachygyria, white-matter atrophy, and gray-matter heterotopias. Characteristic clinical features should suggest the diagnosis, supported by decreased total plasma carnitine and elevated plasma acylcarnitine intermediates. Definitive diagnosis rests on measuring enzyme activity and genomic sequence analysis. Treatment involves supportive measures, glucose administration, carnitine supplementation, and modification of feeding schedules to minimize fasting states. Long-term outcome depends on the frequency and severity of decompensation.

MTP deficiency predominantly presents in neonates, with rapid onset of depressed consciousness, heart failure, diffuse hypotonia and weakness with absent tendon reflexes, severe lactic acidosis, and death in a majority of patients as a result of heart failure. Multisystem involvement may include retinopathy, peripheral neuropathy, myopathy, cardiomyopathy, and liver disease.

CPT II deficiency has several phenotypes presenting at different ages. The neonatal-onset form is the least common and most severe form and is almost always fatal. Affected infants have prenatally detected cerebral lesions and malformations. Neurologic symptoms appear shortly after birth, including seizures, depressed consciousness, hypotonia with myopathic features, and cardiomyopathy leading to circulatory failure. Metabolic features are typical of fatty acid oxidation defects. Management is supportive and symptomatic, but ineffective in most cases. Definitive biochemical diagnosis is a prelude to confirmatory genetic testing.

Urea Cycle Disorders

Neonates with urea cycle defects (UCDs) develop severe hyperammonemia, rapidly progressive lethargy, and vomiting, progressing to coma (Häberle et al., 2012). First-stage testing reveals no other major biochemical abnormalities. Diagnosis rests on plasma amino acid and urine organic acid and urinary orotate excretion profiles. Definitive diagnosis is confirmed by genetic testing. Elevated plasma glutamine levels are common to all of the UCDs. Transient hyperammonemia of the newborn resembles UCDs, featuring severe transient hyperammonemia associated with respiratory distress syndromes or herpes simplex infection. It differs from UCDs in its earlier onset (first 24 hours of life) and association with prematurity and pulmonary disease. Treatment includes discontinuing protein intake and administering intravenous dextrose and ammonia-scavenging drugs—sodium benzoate, phenylacetate, and arginine. Infants unresponsive to these measures or those presenting with coma may require hemodialysis. Long-term outcome is variable, with motor and cognitive deficits dependent on the severity and frequency of hyperammonemic decompensations.

Subacute Epileptic Encephalopathies

Glycine Cleavage Defects

Glycine cleavage defects are autosomal-recessive disorders causing glycine accumulation. The most common form is a neonatal-onset progressive encephalopathy with depressed consciousness, apnea, and seizures, usually myoclonic, and burst suppression on electroencephalogram (EEG). Lifelong severe cognitive and motor disabilities and intractable epilepsy are the rule among survivors. Factors predicting poorer outcome include early age of symptom onset, presence of cerebral dysgenesis, and degree of glycine elevation. Neuroimaging abnormalities include cerebral dysgenesis of prenatal origin, compounded by acute new foci of injury in acutely symptomatic neonates appearing as restricted diffusion in the posterior limbs of the internal capsule, lateral thalami, and dorsal midbrain and pontine nuclei, evolving to a progressive vacuolating myelinopathy in the postnatal period. Biochemical abnormalities are limited to elevated glycine levels in plasma and CSF, with CSF:plasma ratio less than 0.06. Definitive diagnosis rests on finding absent or very low activity of the glycine cleavage system enzyme in liver biopsy or autopsy, confirmed by genetic studies. Glycine cleavage defects differ from the hyperglycinemia that accompanies organic acidopathies in the presence of ketosis in the latter, and in characteristic organic acid excretion profiles. There are no proven therapies. Seizures are resistant to standard anticonvulsants. Treatment with dextromethorphan, ketamine, benzoate, and the ketogenic diet has been reported, with limited success.

Pyridoxine-Dependent and Pyridoxal Phosphate-Dependent Epileptic Encephalopathies

Pyridoxine is the precursor for pyridoxal-5-phosphate (PLP), an essential cofactor for multiple enzymes in brain metabolism. Two enzyme defects with distinct gene mutations cause deficient PLP production: pyridoxine-dependent epilepsy (PDE) and pyridoxal phosphate-dependency disorder (Plecko, 2013). Pyridoxal phosphate-dependency disorder involves mutations in the gene for pyridox(am)ine-5′-phosphate oxidase (PNPO), which converts pyridoxine to PLP. The spectrum of PDE includes gene mutations leading to partial loss of PNPO activity, presenting as pyridoxine-responsive neonatal-onset epilepsy with normal levels of PDE biomarkers.

Affected infants present with prenatal- or neonatal-onset drug-resistant epilepsy and chronic encephalopathy, with no other metabolic abnormalities. EEG is severely abnormal, with several types of epileptiform patterns (hypsarrhythmia, burst suppression, generalized spike-wave). Diagnosis in PDE rests on finding elevated levels of α-aminoadipic semialdehyde and pipecolic acid in urine, blood, and CSF, confirmed by mutation analysis of the *antiquitin* gene. Diagnosis of PNPO deficiency should be considered in infants with the clinical features of PDE, but who are not fully responsive to pyridoxine, lack the confirmatory biochemical markers (elevated urinary alpha-aminoadipic semialdehyde dehydrogenase [AASA]), and respond to PLP. Genetic testing of the PNPO gene confirms the diagnosis.

Folinic acid–responsive neonatal epileptic encephalopathy (FARNE) resembles PDE clinically and electrographically. Although FARNE is identical biochemically and genetically to PDE, these patients have a better response to either a combination of pyridoxine and folinic acid or folinic acid alone.

Treatment in pyridoxine-dependency disorders includes supplementation with both pyridoxine and folinic acid because there is variable response to either agent alone. Dietary restriction of lysine has been suggested. Infants with clinical features PDE who are unresponsive to pyridoxine and folinic acid may be given pyridoxal supplementation while awaiting genetic testing for PNPO deficiency.

Sulfite Oxidase and Molybdenum Cofactor Deficiency

Molybdenum cofactor (Moco) deficiency and isolated sulfite oxidase deficiency are related autosomal-recessive diseases affecting xanthine and sulfite metabolism. These defects share a similar clinical presentation that involves severe neonatal-onset epileptic encephalopathy with diffuse severe cavitary leukomalacia (Schwarz, Mendel, and Ribbe, 2009). Infants are born at term uneventfully and develop seizures in the first week, followed by arrested development, acquired microcephaly, and early appearance of generalized hypertonicity. Clinical and radiographic features in the early stages mimic hypoxic-ischemic encephalopathy. Distinctive neuroimaging features include symmetric acute lesions affecting the globus pallidi and subthalamic regions coexisting with chronic-appearing cerebral infarction, pontocerebellar hypoplasia, and severe cavitary leukomalacia. There are no associated malformative anomalies, systemic metabolic perturbations, or abnormalities affecting other organ systems.

Diagnosis is suggested by increased urinary excretion of sulfites, thiosulfate, S-sulfocysteine, and taurine. Patients with Moco deficiency have low serum and urinary uric acid levels and increased urinary xanthine and hypoxanthine levels. Patients with isolated sulfite oxidase deficiency have normal uric acid metabolite levels. Diagnosis may be confirmed by enzyme assay of biopsied liver or cultured skin fibroblasts. Treatment is supportive, with an emphasis on optimizing anticonvulsant therapy.

Serine Biosynthesis Defects

Serine biosynthesis defects may present as neonatal-onset chronic encephalopathies with prominent refractory epilepsy, and most commonly result from 3-phosphoglycerate dehydrogenase deficiency. Affected infants are neurologically abnormal at birth, with intrauterine growth retardation, congenital microcephaly, cataracts, seizures, and neurodevelopmental impairment. They have a distinctive leukoencephalopathy with hypomyelination, vacuolar changes, and gliosis, which may improve after treatment with serine and glycine supplementation. Diagnosis rests on finding low CSF concentrations of serine, glycine, and 5-methyltetrahydrofolate. This disorder is treatable with high-dose dietary supplementation of serine (500-700 mg/kg/day) and glycine (200 mg/kg/day).

Purine Biosynthesis Defects

Purine biosynthesis disorders manifesting in the neonatal period involve adenylosuccinate lyase or riboside transformylase enzyme deficiencies (Jurecka, 2009). Affected infants are born uneventfully at term and develop severe neonatal encephalopathy with hypotonia and seizures. Neuroimaging may be normal initially, followed later by diffuse atrophy. These infants develop severe static encephalopathy with profound mental retardation, blindness as a result of optic atrophy, refractory epilepsy, and growth failure. The cardinal biochemical feature is elevated riboside metabolites 5-amino-4-imidazolecarboxamide ribosiduria (AICA) and succinyl-5-amino-4-imidazolecarboxamide ribosiduria (SAICA) in urine and CSF. Affected infants may have disturbed glucose and lipid metabolism as a result of impaired hepatic gluconeogenesis and fatty acid and cholesterol synthesis. Treatment with D-ribose and uridine supplementation has been shown to be of limited benefit. Management is symptomatic and supportive because there is no definitive or curative treatment.

L-Amino Acid Decarboxylase Deficiency

L-amino acid decarboxylase deficiency (L-ADD) is a defect of biogenic amine neurotransmitter metabolism that results in deficient brain dopamine, serotonin, norepinephrine, and epinephrine. Patients present in the first weeks of life with lethargy, hypotonia, dysphagia, and seizures, and sometimes with hypoglycemia and acidosis. Autonomic dysfunction leads to ptosis, hypotension, gastric and intestinal dysmotility, and impaired thermoregulation. Movement disorders are common, with dystonia, athetosis, oculogyric crises, and nonepileptic myoclonus. Diagnosis rests on finding increased L-DOPA and 5-hydroxytryptophan and decreased homovanillic acid (HVA) and 5-hydroxy-indole-acetic acid (5-HIAA) levels in CSF. Vanillactic acid (VLA) levels are elevated on urine organic acid profile. Management is symptomatic and supportive. Outcome is poor in most patients, who develop mixed severe motor and cognitive disability and chronic movement disorders that are refractory to symptomatic treatment.

Asparagine Synthetase Deficiency

Asparagine modulates the cell cycle, cell proliferation, and neuronal hyperexcitability. Asparagine synthetase (AS) deficiency causes a progressive neonatal-onset encephalopathy featuring quadriplegia, profound intellectual disability, refractory epilepsy, and progressive diffuse cerebral atrophy. CSF levels of asparagine in affected patients are low compared with normal patients. Diagnosis is confirmed with molecular genetic analysis. Treatment rests on supportive and anticonvulsant therapies. Nutritional supplementation with asparagine has been suggested, with uncertain benefit.

Chronic Encephalopathies Without Multiorgan Involvement
Hyperphenylalaninemia

Hyperphenylalaninemia causes a neonatal-onset chronic encephalopathy as a result of defects in phenylalanine metabolism, including phenylalanine hydroxylase (PAH) deficiency, tetrahydrobiopterin (BH$_4$) synthesis deficiency, and GTP cyclohydrolase (GTPC) deficiency. In classical phenylketonuria (PKU) caused by PAH deficiency, plasma phenylalanine levels exceed 1000 μM, and PAH activity in liver biopsy is severely deficient. Non-PKU hyperphenylalaninemia is a milder form, with plasma phenylalanine less than 1000 μM and less severely deficient PAH activity. Clinical symptoms in untreated classical PKU include irritability, hyperkinesis, acquired microcephaly, and severe cognitive deficiency. Infants with GTPC deficiency have a neonatal-onset chronic encephalopathy with severe hypotonia, bulbar dysfunction, and seizures. Treatment with L-DOPA has been beneficial in some patients. Diagnosis is made through newborn metabolic screening followed by quantitation of plasma phenylalanine and tyrosine and urinary and CSF biopterin metabolites. Treatment involves dietary restriction of phenylalanine, and folate and BH$_4$ replacement in patients with BH$_4$ disorders.

Succinic Semialdehyde Dehydrogenase Deficiency

Succinic semialdehyde dehydrogenase deficiency is a defect of GABA degradation causing elevated brain GABA. Some patients present as neonates with a chronic encephalopathy and later develop diffuse hypotonia, neurodevelopmental impairment, and epilepsy. MRI finding of T2 hyperintensity in the globus pallidus may suggest the diagnosis, which rests on finding high levels of GABA in CSF and urine and elevated urinary 4-hydroxybutyric acid. Treatment with vigabatrin has been suggested, with variable results.

Glutaric Aciduria

Glutaric aciduria (GA) is an autosomal-recessive defect in degradation of 2-keto-adipic acid, a metabolite in lysine and tryptophan degradation pathways. Neonatal and early infantile presentation occurs in type I GA, caused by glutaryl-CoA dehydrogenase deficiency. Affected infants have chronic progressive encephalopathy of neonatal or early infantile onset with macrocephaly, hypotonia evolving to rigidity and dystonia, developmental regression, and epilepsy. There may be episodic decompensations triggered by intercurrent illness, with vomiting, ketotic hypoglycemia, acidosis, hyperammonemia, hepatomegaly, and depressed consciousness. MRI shows frontotemporal atrophy with prominent extraaxial CSF collections and, in some cases, subdural hemorrhage. Metabolic crises are associated with acute bilaterally symmetric striatal necrosis, leading to permanent neuromotor disability. Diagnosis rests on finding elevated urinary glutaric acid and 3-OH-glutaric acid, confirmed by enzyme assay. Treatment involves dietary protein restriction, in particular L-lysine and tryptophan, and supplementation with L-carnitine and riboflavin. Type II GA involves multiple acyl-CoA dehydrogenase deficiencies, causing elevations of multiple organic acids. The clinical picture in neonatal-onset type II GA is severe, with nonketotic hypoglycemia, metabolic acidosis, vomiting, depressed consciousness, and multiorgan dysfunction.

Chronic Encephalopathies With Multiorgan Involvement
Congenital Disorders of Glycosylation

Congenital disorders of glycosylation (CDGs) involve defective protein glycosylation, affecting cotranslational modification of numerous secretory and membrane-bound proteins (Funke et al., 2013). Type I involves oligosaccharide precursor assembly; type II involves oligosaccharide processing. A new classification system based on genetic and molecular features uses the gene symbol followed by the extension "CGD." CDG type Ia is the most common and has two presentation types: a neurologic and a multisystem pattern. The neurologic presentation involves chronic severe neurologic disability with prominent hypotonia and cerebellar dysfunction, punctuated by episodic acute deterioration resembling stroke. MRI shows cerebellar atrophy. Usually normal at birth, some patients present with hypotonia and oculomotor abnormalities, with later ataxic hypotonic motor impairment and severe cognitive deficiency, retinopathy, epilepsy, acquired microcephaly, thromboembolic strokes, and weakness resulting from polyneuropathy. Associated nonneurologic findings include growth failure, protein-losing enteropathy, obstructive cardiomyopathy, and nephrotic syndrome. Diagnosis rests on the measurement of transferrin isoelectric focusing (TIEF) and molecular genetic testing. Associated biochemical findings include elevated liver transaminases, low serum proteins, anemia, leukopenia, and low serum cholesterol. Treatment includes supplementation of mannose for MPI-CDG, fucose for SLC35C1-CDG, and butyrate for PIBM-CDG, with variable benefit.

Peroxisomal Disorders

Peroxisomal disorders are progressive neurologic diseases with variable age of onset and severity. Neonatal forms with prominent neurologic involvement are autosomal-recessive disorders, including Zellweger syndrome (ZS) and neonatal adrenoleukodystrophy (NALD). ZS involves multiorgan dysfunction, with typical facial dysmorphism, ocular anomalies (cataracts, glaucoma, pigmentary retinopathy), hepatic fibrosis, cystic kidney disease, subclinical adrenocortical insufficiency, and cardiac anomalies. Neurologic features include seizures, cranial nerve dysfunction, optic atrophy, and diffuse myopathic weakness. Survivors are profoundly handicapped. Neuroimaging and pathological studies reveal cortical and cerebellar migrational abnormalities and central white-matter demyelination. Biochemical studies reveal elevated very-long-chain fatty acids (VLCFAs), phytanic acid, and pipecolic acids, and deficient synthesis of plasmalogens. Diagnosis can be confirmed by gene sequencing. NALD resembles ZS in many respects but is less severe. There are no proven treatments.

Cholesterol Biosynthesis Defects (Smith–Lemli–Opitz Syndrome)

Smith–Lemli–Opitz syndrome is a disorder of cholesterol biosynthesis and presents in the neonatal period with multiple congenital anomalies and a chronic static encephalopathy, with hypotonia, sensorineural deafness, dysphagia, severe cognitive deficiency, microcephaly. Nonneurologic problems include abnormal facies with ptosis and micrognathia, genital anomalies, growth retardation, cataracts, congenital heart defects, digital anomalies, and cleft palate. Cerebral malformations (holoprosencephaly, agenesis of the corpus callosum, frontal hypoplasia, cerebellar hypoplasia) are common. Diagnosis is suggested by low serum cholesterol, confirmed by finding elevated serum 7-and 8-dehydrocholesterol. Treatment is supportive and symptomatic.

REFERENCES

 The complete list of references for this chapter is available in the e-book at www.expertconsult.com.
See inside cover for registration details.

SELECTED REFERENCES

Ficicioglu, C., Bearden, D., 2011. Isolated neonatal seizures: when to suspect inborn errors of metabolism. Pediatr. Neurol. 45 (5), 283–291.

Funke, S., Gardeitchik, T., Kouwenberg, D., et al., 2013. Perinatal and early infantile symptoms in congenital disorders of glycosylation. Am. J. Med. Genet. A 161A (3), 578–584.

Häberle, J., Boddaert, N., Burlina, A., et al., 2012. Suggested guidelines for the diagnosis and management of urea cycle disorders. Orphanet J. Rare Dis. 7, 32.

Hoffman, G.F., Zschocke, J., Nyhan, W.L., 2010. Inherited Metabolic Diseases: A Clinical Approach. Springer, Heidelberg.

Honzik, T., Tesarova, M., Magner, M., et al., 2012. Neonatal onset of mitochondrial disorders in 129 patients: clinical and laboratory characteristics and a new approach to diagnosis. J. Inherit. Metab. Dis. 35 (5), 749–759.

Jurecka, A., 2009. Inborn errors of purine and pyrimidine metabolism. J. Inherit. Metab. Dis. 32 (2), 247–263.

Knerr, I., Weinhold, N., Vockley, J., et al., 2012. Advances and challenges in the treatment of branched-chain amino/keto acid metabolic defects. J. Inherit. Metab. Dis. 35 (1), 29–40.

Plecko, B., 2013. Pyridoxine and pyridoxalphosphate-dependent epilepsies. Handb Clin Neurol 113, 1811–1817.

Schwarz, G., Mendel, R.R., Ribbe, M.W., 2009. Molybdenum cofactors, enzymes and pathways. Nature 460 (7257), 839–847.

Xue, Y., Ankala, A., Wilcox, W.R., et al., 2014. Solving the molecular diagnostic testing conundrum for Mendelian disorders in the era of next-generation sequencing: single-gene, gene panel, or exome/genome sequencing. Genet. Med.

E-BOOK FIGURES AND TABLES

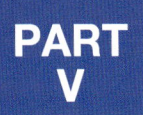
24 Overview of Human Brain Malformations

William B. Dobyns, Renzo Guerrini, and A. James Barkovich

 An expanded version of this chapter is available on www.expertconsult.com. See inside cover for registration details.

INTRODUCTION

This section (Part V) on congenital structural defects reviews a large and growing number of complex developmental disorders of the brain, spinal cord, and skull. They represent the tip of the iceberg of developmental brain disorders more broadly, as they present with many of the same clinical features and involve many of the same molecular pathways—and sometimes the same genes—as more common and less specific disorders such as intellectual disability, early life epilepsy and autism. They collectively encompass a field of knowledge that has expanded dramatically over the past several decades. But the field has not expanded in isolation. Brain malformations:

- Largely represent defects during the earliest stages of brain development, and thus reflect the underlying embryology and developmental genetics of the nervous system;
- Provide an important window into normal brain development and into the genetic regulation of brain development and function;
- Frequently co-occur with other diverse developmental brain disorders both with and without recognized structural defects; and
- Are associated with a wide spectrum of functional deficits including intellectual disability (mental retardation), developmental language disorders, epilepsy, social and behavioral disabilities, numerous other specific learning disabilities, attention deficits, motor deficits associated with abnormal motor tone and posture or dyskinesias, and a host of problems associated with sleep, feeding, mood, hormonal and autonomic dysregulation.

Thus an understanding of brain malformations is important in assessing almost all types of neurologic disorders in children. They are separated into disorders involving defects in development of primary brain stages and regions including neural tube (Chapter 25); forebrain (Chapter 26) and mid-hindbrain (Chapter 27) defects; malformations of cortical development involving brain size (Chapter 28) and other malformations of cortical development (Chapter 29); diverse disorders resulting in hydrocephalus (Chapter 30) or skull development (Chapter 31); and an important new chapter on clinically and genetically overlapping disorders without consistent brain malformations that we designate "developmental encephalopathies" (Chapter 32) with Angelman and Rett syndromes as paradigms. This section ends with a detailed look at prenatal diagnosis for this group of disorders (Chapter 33). In the sections that follow, brain malformations are reviewed including epidemiology, classification, clinical recog-

nition, relationship to other neurologic disorders and selected environmental factors, and genetic counseling.

EPIDEMIOLOGY

The incidence of brain malformations has been estimated to be approximately 3.32 per 1000 and the prevalence approximately 2.21 per 1000 at age 14 years from studies of a 1-year birth cohort from northern Finland (Von Wendt and Rantakallio, 1986). These are much higher rates than were recognized in the era before MRI and recent increases in surgical treatment of hydrocephalus and epilepsy. Not surprisingly, the incidence is much higher in studies of children with cerebral palsy. This is an important point. To emphasize this, boy with apparent cerebral palsy attributed to prematurity at approximately 29 weeks gestation had a brain MRI that revealed mild callosal and cerebellar vermis hypoplasia, and chromosome microarray revealed a deletion 22q11.2, which implies either a genetic cause or possibly combined genetic and acquired pathogenesis.

CLASSIFICATION

Although the chapters that follow review many different malformations, they are not complete as the number of recognized malformations continues to expand. Presenting these data is also complicated by the tendency for malformations to co-occur in some patients. For example, Figure 24-1 shows a striking example of a boy with malformations of the forebrain (agenesis of the corpus callosum), mid-hindbrain (severe cerebellar hypoplasia and mega-cisterna magna), brain size (megalencephaly), neuronal migration (periventricular nodular heterotopia), and cortical organization (polymicrogyria overlying the heterotopia).

We have from time to time constructed flexible classification schemes for many of these malformations that primarily rely on traditional concepts such as embryology and anatomy with a contribution from genetic discoveries. Whereas recent discoveries lead to genes and gene pathways more than to embryology and anatomy, a more traditional classification scheme is listed in this and the following chapters. Outlines for brainstem and cerebellar (mid-hindbrain) malformations and for cortical malformations are shown in Boxes 24-1 and 24-2. Further details regarding most subgroups of malformations and the basis for the classification are given in the primary references (Barkovich et al., 2005; Barkovich et al., 2009). These schemes rely on—in decreasing order of priority—the underlying genetic basis when known, the

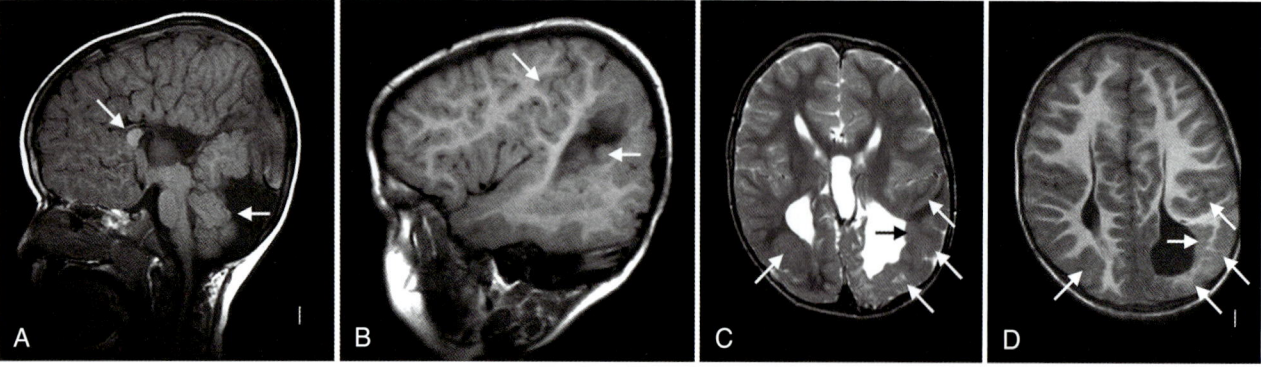

Figure 24-1. Brain images from a single patient showing multiple malformations. T1–weighted sagittal images demonstrate severe callosal hypogenesis with a small anterior remnant (angled arrow in **A**), very small cerebellar vermis (horizontal arrow in **A**) in an enlarged posterior fossa, extended Sylvian fissure with cortex connecting the perisylvian and superior parietal regions (angled arrow in **B**), and periventricular nodular heterotopia in the trigone (horizontal arrow in **B**). T2– and T1–weighted axial images show periventricular nodular heterotopia adjacent to the posterior portion of the lateral ventricles (horizontal arrows in **C** and **D**), and infolded gyri with mildly thick cortex overlying the heterotopia (angled arrows in **C** and **D**). *(Courtesy of W.B. Dobyns, research subject LR00-086.)*

BOX 24-1 Classification for Mid-Hindbrain Malformations

I. Malformations secondary to early anteroposterior and dorsoventral patterning defects, or to misspecification of mid-hindbrain germinal zones
  A. Anteroposterior patterning defects
    1. Gain, loss, or transformation of the diencephalon and midbrain
    2. Gain, loss, or transformation of the midbrain and rhombomere 1
    3. Gain, loss, or transformation of lower hindbrain structures
  B. Dorsoventral patterning defects
    1. Defects of alar and basal ventricular zones
    2. Defects of alar ventricular zones only
    3. Defects of basal ventricular zones only
II. Malformations associated with later generalized developmental disorders that significantly affect the brainstem and cerebellum (and have pathogenesis at least partly understood)
  A. Developmental encephalopathies associated with MHM
  B. Mesenchymal-neuroepithelial signaling defects associated with MHM
  C. Malformations of neuronal and glial proliferation that prominently affect the brainstem and cerebellum
  D. Malformation of neuronal migration that prominently affect the brainstem and cerebellum
    1. Lissencephaly with cerebellar hypoplasia
    2. Neuronal heterotopia with prominent brainstem and cerebellar hypoplasia
    3. Polymicrogyria with cerebellar hypoplasia

    4. Malformations with basement membrane and neuronal migration deficits
  E. Diffuse molar tooth type dysplasias associated with defects in ciliary proteins
    1. Syndromes affecting the brain with low frequency involvement of the retina and kidney
    2. Syndromes affecting the brain, eyes, kidneys, liver and variable other systems
III. Localized brain malformations that significantly affect the brainstem and cerebellum (pathogenesis partly or largely understood, includes local proliferation, cell specification, migration and axonal guidance)
  A. Multiple levels of mid-hindbrain
  B. Midbrain malformations
  C. Malformations of rhombomere 1 including cerebellar malformations
  D. Pons malformations
  E. Medulla malformations
IV. Combined hypoplasia and atrophy in putative prenatal onset degenerative disorders
  A. Pontocerebellar hypoplasia
  B. Mid-hindbrain malformations with congenital disorders of glycosylation
  C. Other metabolic disorders with cerebellar or brainstem hypoplasia or disruption
  D. Cerebellar hemisphere hypoplasia (rare, more commonly acquired than genetic, often associated with clefts or cortical malformation)

---

relevant embryology, brain imaging features, and miscellaneous other clinical features. Future revisions of these systems will rely more and more on the molecular pathways and genes.

Brain Imaging Recognition

The improved quality of brain imaging studies, especially advances in MRI technology, has led directly to increased recognition and more accurate classification of brain malformations. Still, several recurrent types of classification errors continue to occur based on studies sent to the authors for review. First, pachgyria appears to be the best known of the severe cortical

malformations, and accordingly, all types of severe cortical malformations are often interpreted as "pachgyria." The prime examples of malformations mistaken for pachgyria include severe congenital microcephaly (but here the cortex is usually thin rather than thick), tubulinopathies, polymicrogyria, and cobblestone malformations (for these, the cortex is moderately thick, but the surface and cortical-white matter interface are irregular rather than smooth). This unfortunately often leads to testing of the "lissencephaly" genes in patients with other cortical malformations, with negative results. Second, a thin corpus callosum may result from reduced volume of white matter due to abnormal development of white matter,

BOX 24-2 Classification for Malformations of
Cortical Development

MALFORMATIONS OF CORTICAL DEVELOPMENT

I. Malformations due to abnormal neuronal and glial proliferation or apoptosis
   A. Decreased proliferation or increased apoptosis, or increased proliferation or decreased apoptosis
      1. Microcephaly with normal to thin cortex
      2. Microlissencephaly (extreme microcephaly with thick cortex)
      3. Microcephaly with polymicrogyria
      4. Megalencephaly
   B. Abnormal proliferation (abnormal cell types)
      1. Nonneoplastic
         a. Cortical hamartomas of tuberous sclerosis
         b. Cortical dysplasia with balloon cells
         c. Hemimegalencephaly
      2. Neoplastic (with disordered cortex)
         a. Dysembryoplastic neuroepithelial tumor
         b. Ganglioglioma
         c. Gangliocytoma

II. Malformations due to abnormal neuronal migration
   A. Lissencephaly and subcortical band heterotopia spectrum
   B. Cobblestone malformation syndromes
   C. Heterotopia
      1. Subependymal (periventricular)
      2. Subcortical (other than band heterotopia)
      3. Marginal glioneuronal

III. Malformations due to abnormal cortical organization (including late neuronal migration)
   A. Polymicrogyria and schizencephaly
      1. Bilateral polymicrogyria syndromes
      2. Schizencephaly (polymicrogyria with clefts)
      3. Polymicrogyria as part of multiple congenital anomaly/mental retardation syndromes
   B. Cortical dysplasia without balloon cells
   C. Microdysgenesis

IV. Malformations of cortical development, not otherwise classified
   A. Malformations secondary to inborn errors of metabolism
      1. Mitochondrial and pyruvate metabolic disorders
      2. Peroxisomal disorders
   B. Other unclassified malformations
      1. Sublobar dysplasia
      2. Others

progressive white matter dysgenesis, or white matter injury. However, this appearance is sometimes interpreted as agenesis of the corpus callosum. Next, diverse causes of cerebellar hypoplasia are often interpreted as Dandy-Walker malformation (when associated with a large posterior fossa and an enlarged fourth ventricle) or the so-called "Dandy-Walker variant" (equated with isolated cerebellar vermis hypoplasia). The latter is so overused and misapplied that the term should be abandoned. Finally, enlarged fluid collections below and especially behind the cerebellum are interpreted as arachnoid cysts or as "mega-cisterna magna" considering the latter a non-pathogenic variant. In our experience, mega-cisterna magna with fluid both below and behind the cerebellum sometimes represents a developmental disorder that belongs in the Dandy-Walker spectrum, and may be incorrectly interpreted as an arachnoid cyst.

Relationships to Other Neurologic Disorders

The close connection between brain malformations and other classes of developmental disorders is conceptually important. A few examples include agenesis of the corpus callosum associated with nonketotic hyperglycinemia; cerebellar vermis hypoplasia or heterotopia with multiple acyl-CoA dehydrogenase deficiency known as glutaric aciduria type 2; cobblestone malformations and cerebellar hypoplasia with congenital disorders of glycosylation; pachygyria variants with severe peroxisomal disorders such as Zellweger syndrome; and cerebellar hypoplasia or agenesis of the corpus callosum with either autism or infantile spasms. Further, most malformations of cortical development are associated with epilepsy, which may be severe. Observations in these and many other disorders suggest that brain malformations represent the most severe expression or "tip of the iceberg" of a host of developmental brain disorders. One of the best examples involves disorders associated with mutations of the ARX gene, which can cause lissencephaly, agenesis of the corpus callosum, hydrocephalus, developmental encephalopathy with epilepsy (i.e., epileptic encephalopathy), or mental retardation with dyskinesia.

Relationship to Environmental Factors

The genetic basis for many brain malformations has been known for years, and new genes are constantly being discovered. The question arises: are all brain malformations genetic? Although easy to overlook, substantial data exists to support environmental (extrinsic) causes for several brain malformations. Both microcephaly and hydrocephalus can result from numerous prenatal and early life diseases such as intraventricular hemorrhage in premature infants, other causes of intracranial bleeding, hypoxic-ischemic injury, central nervous system infections, and a host of other disorders reviewed throughout this text. Holoprosencephaly has been associated with pregestational diabetes and with structural analogs of cholesterol that interfere with cholesterol metabolism in humans and animals. Periventricular nodular heterotopia have been seen in mice and rats after prenatal exposure to high-dose ionizing radiation and possibly in humans as well. Schizencephaly and polymicrogyria, usually with microcephaly as well, have been associated with second trimester (13 to 21 weeks gestation) prenatal vascular disruption and with intrauterine cytomegalovirus infections. Numerous reports in the lay press from mid-2015 on, as well as one report of prenatal diagnosis have recently implicated the Zika virus as a cause of microcephaly, sometimes with additional evidence of prenatal brain injury. It has been blamed for a dramatic increase in the frequency of congenital microcephaly in Brazil and is rapidly spreading to other countries and regions.

GENETIC COUNSELING

Although the genetic basis for more and more brain malformations and related syndromes are being uncovered, few studies examining the overall contribution of genetic disorders to brain malformations have been reported. Accordingly, only partial and selective information about the genetic recurrence risk for different brain malformations is available. However, some general guidelines are listed in Table 24-1.

For example, the recurrence risk for holoprosencephaly reported in the literature is approximately 6%, but we have become aware of frequent mild expression or "formes fruste" of this malformation and, accordingly, suggest using a higher recurrence risk of 13% for isolated holoprosencephaly without

TABLE 24-1 Probable Genetic Recurrence Risks for Major Classes of Brain Malformations

Malformation Groups	Sp	Ch	AD	AR	XL	Recurrence Risk Comments
	Pattern of Inheritance					
FOREBRAIN MALFORMATIONS						
Holoprosencephaly	++	++	++	±	±	Risk is variable, may be high
Agenesis of corpus callosum	++	++	±	±	++	Risk is generally low
Septo-optic dysplasia	++	–	–	±	–	Risk is very low, has occurred
MID-HINDBRAIN MALFORMATIONS						
Pontocerebellar hypoplasia	–	–	–	++	–	Risk is 25%, all forms are AR
Cerebellar hypoplasia (diffuse)	++	++	±	++	+	Risk is variable, need diagnosis
Cerebellar hypoplasia (vermis)	++	++	±	+	+	Risk is variable, need diagnosis
Dandy-Walker malformation	++	+	±	±	±	Risk is very low, has occurred
Molar tooth malformation	–	–	–	++	–	Risk is 25%, all forms are AR
Rhombencephalosynapsis	++	–	–	–	–	No recurrences reported
CORTICAL MALFORMATIONS						
Microcephaly, congenital	–	–	–	++	–	Risk is 25%, most forms are AR
Microcephaly, postnatal	++	++	+	+	+	Risk is variable, includes XL
Megalencephaly	++	–	–	–	–	Risk is low (except for PTEN)
Lissencephaly and SBH	++	++	–	+	++	Risk is variable, includes XL
Cobblestone malformation	–	–	–	++	–	Risk is 25%, all forms are AR
Heterotopia, periventricular	++	++	+	±	++	Risk is variable, may be high
Heterotopia, subcortical	++	–	–	–	–	No recurrences reported
Polymicrogyria, perisylvian	++	++	±	±	+	Risk is low, XL may be important
Polymicrogyria, other forms						Risk is generally low
Schizencephaly	++	–	–	±	–	Risk is very low, has occurred
Focal cortical dysplasias	++	–	–	–	–	No recurrences reported
Hemimegalencephaly	++	–	–	–	–	No recurrences reported

Abbreviations: AD, autosomal dominant; AR, autosomal recessive; Ch, chromosome imbalance; Risk, recurrence risk for siblings or other relatives; Sp, sporadic occurrence; XL, X–linked; ++, commonly observed; +, occasionally observed; ±, rarely observed and often poorly documented; –, never observed

known chromosome imbalances. For several malformations such as agenesis of the corpus callosum and polymicrogyria, single gene inheritance has been reported but only rarely and no formal studies are available. This implies a "generally low" risk and counseling with some uncertainty given that the experience is limited and exceptions occur. For some other malformations such as rhombencephalosynapsis and hemimegalencephaly, no examples of familial recurrence have ever been reported despite clinical recognition for decades. The first reports of familial focal cortical dysplasia have appeared, but this must be very rare, suggesting that the recurrence risk is very low. The most difficult malformations are those with significantly different recurrence risks for different subtypes and syndromes such as diffuse and vermis predominant cerebellar hypoplasia. These estimates are largely anecdotal in origin, so treating physicians and genetic counselors are encouraged to review information on the specific disorder at hand when counseling families.

REFERENCES

The complete list of references for this chapter is available in the e-book at www.expertconsult.com.
See inside cover for registration details.

SELECTED REFERENCES

Barkovich, A.J., Kuzniecky, R.I., Jackson, G.D., et al., 2005. A developmental and genetic classification for malformations of cortical development. Neurology 65 (12), 1873–1887.

Barkovich, A.J., Millen, K.J., Dobyns, W.B., 2009. A developmental and genetic classification for midbrain-hindbrain malformations. Brain 132 (Pt 12), 3199–3230.

von Wendt, L., Rantakallio, P., 1986. Congenital malformations of the central nervous system in a 1-year birth cohort followed to the age of 14 years. Childs Nerv. Syst. 2 (2), 80–82.

25 Disorders of Neural Tube Development

Nalin Gupta and M. Elizabeth Ross

An expanded version of this chapter is available on www.expertconsult.com. See inside cover for registration details.

INTRODUCTION

Neural tube defects (NTDs) are second only to congenital heart defects as the most common serious birth defect, affecting between 0.3 and 10 per 1000 live births, depending on geographic region. NTDs result from complex interactions of genes and environmental conditions. A significant proportion of NTDs may be preventable with measures such as prenatal maternal folic acid (FA) supplementation or by avoiding prenatal exposure to known teratogenic drugs or toxins. Here we discuss the NTD pathogenesis, risk factors, complications, and management.

ANATOMY AND EMBRYOLOGY
Formation of the Neural Tube

Among the earliest morphologic specializations in the embryo is the neural placode, followed by neural plate and then neural tube. In the late second gestational week, the human embryo is a bilaminar disc of epiblast cells overlying hypoblast cells. By the third week, the disc develops a midline groove, the primitive streak, in the caudal third (Fig. 25-1A), which marks the initiation of gastrulation and the formation of three germ layers—ectoderm (giving rise to skin and the nervous system), mesoderm (providing inductive signals to ectoderm and contributing to morphogenesis), and endoderm (giving rise to viscera). The primitive node at the cranial end of the streak contains cells that act to organize the embryonic axes (Fig. 25-1). At the same stage, thickening of the rostral ectoderm by the apical-basal elongation of cells into a pseudostratified columnar shape produces the neural placode that marks the initiation of neurulation (see Fig. 25-1B). Cells migrating through the primitive streak and node displace the hypoblast cells to form endoderm and subsequently middle layer mesoderm. Cells that migrate through the node in the midline form the prechordal plate and notochord, which are important for induction of the ventral CNS structures, starting with the neural plate.

Neural plate formation is actually a default state of the ectoderm, and formation of epidermis involves the inhibition of bone morphogenetic protein (BMP) and the wingless (Wnt) signaling pathway. As the plate begins to emerge, morphogenesis, or shape changes, involving groups of cells in the neuroepithelium and surround, is essential to formation of brain and spinal cord. By 20 days of gestation, the neural plate appears indented in the midline, forming a groove or medial hinge region flanked by ridges–the neural folds. These folds elevate from the plane of the neural plate through the combined influences of proliferation of neural cells and underlying mesenchymal cells. Bending inward of the neural folds at the dorsolateral hinge points occurs through morphologic shape changes of the neural cells, which become radially elongated while their apical (luminal) poles constrict, through a combination of cell-cycle regulation that moves nuclei to the basal end of cells in the hinge region and actin-myosin contraction at the apical poles of cells in the hinge region, to bring the tips of the neural folds to touch. In the head region, the proliferation and movement of epidermis and mesenchyme cells also help to push the neural folds into apposition because at spinal levels, neighboring mesenchyme may be less critical to neural tube closure. In addition to cell elongation and proliferation, the shape changes in the neural plate are affected by cell motility in the form of convergent extension, in which laterally placed cells move to the midline and migrate rostro-caudally in a process that is mediated by noncanonical Wnt signaling (Fig. 25-4). Thus once elevation and bending of the neural folds occur, the lateral margins or tips of the folds join and then fuse in the midline to become the neural tube.

In order to achieve this rising and bending inward of the neural folds, the cells of the neural plate must proliferate in an ordered manner, called interkinetic nuclear migration of progenitors, forming a pseudostratified epithelium in which S-phase occurs at the basal (outer) surface of the neural folds, mitosis (M-phase) occurs at the apical (central or luminal) surface, and G1 and G2 phase nuclei are positioned at intermediate locations. In addition, in the process of convergent extension, cells move medially and through the medial hinge region to migrate rostrocaudally and elongate the neuraxis, narrowing the ventral floor plate. If the floor plate is too wide or the neural folds fail to elevate and bend, the folds will not appose and NTDs will ensue (see Fig. 25-4). When apposition is successful, midline fusion of the neural folds, a process known as neurulation, occurs first at primary closure points and progresses by adding multiple closure points such as the teeth of a zipper to extend rostrally and caudally from each node to complete neural tube closure (Copp et al., 2003).

In humans, the anterior neuropore, the region that will eventually give rise to the brain, closes approximately by day 26 of human gestation. The posterior neuropore, the region that will give rise to the caudal spinal column, closes approximately by day 29 of human embryogenesis. After the neural tube closes, it separates from the overlying ectoderm in a process termed dysjunction. Cells of the somitic mesoderm invade the space between the ectoderm and neural tube to form somites that eventually give rise to the posterior elements of the vertebral bodies and the paraspinal muscles. Specific neural cells at the tips of the folds are excluded from the neural tube; these cells form the neural crest, which is the anlage of the peripheral sensory and autonomic nervous systems and which also contributes the meninges and portions of the skull and face.

Molecular Patterning of the Neural Tube

Work in animal models has identified a host of factors required for proper neurulation and neural tube closure. A key observation was that a small fragment of nonneural tissue (mesoderm), when transplanted, could duplicate the neural tube, indicating that secreted factors from mesoderm are sufficient to induce neurulation. These factors include chordin, noggin, sonic hedgehog (SHH), and several others, which are both necessary and sufficient for proper neurulation and control of the amount and fate of the neuroectoderm. In mammals, two distinct groups of nonneural cells appear to provide these early patterning signals: axial mesodermal cells of the

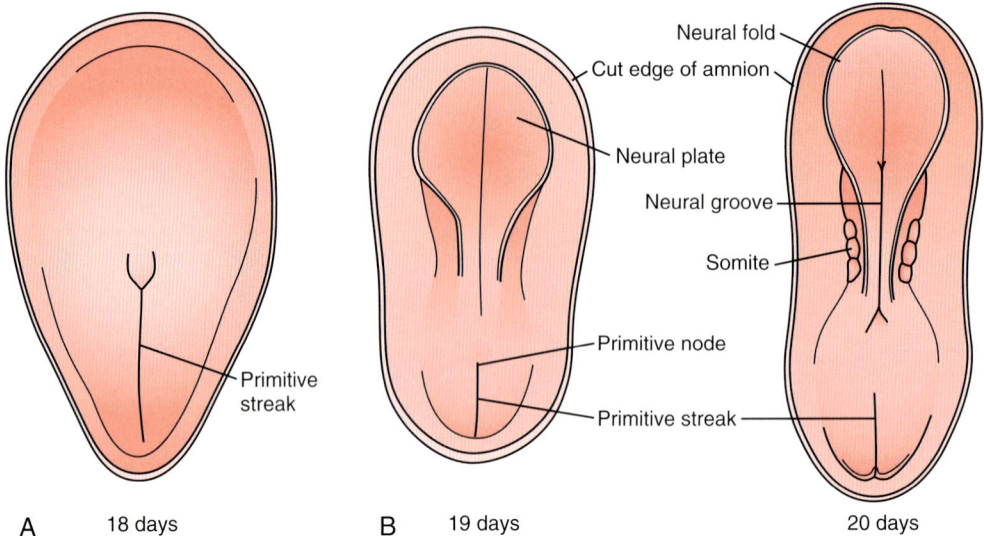

Figure 25-1. Early stages of gastrulation and neurulation in human embryogenesis: views of the dorsal surface. **A,** The primitive streak emerges as a groove at the caudal pole of the embryo, with the primitive node at the cranial pole. Epiblast cells moving through the primitive streak and node form the three germ layers—ectoderm, mesoderm, and endoderm. **B,** A thickening of the ectoderm forms the neural plate, initiated at the cranial pole, whereas the primitive streak at the caudal end initiates gastrulation. By 20 days' gestation, the neural folds have elevated from the neural plate, and tips of the folds are closing. Somites, comprised of mesoderm cells, support the elevation of the neural folds and are the precursors of vertebrae. *(Adapted from Sadler, T.W., 2005. Embryology of neural tube development. Am J Med Genet C Semin Med Genet 135C, 2–8.)*

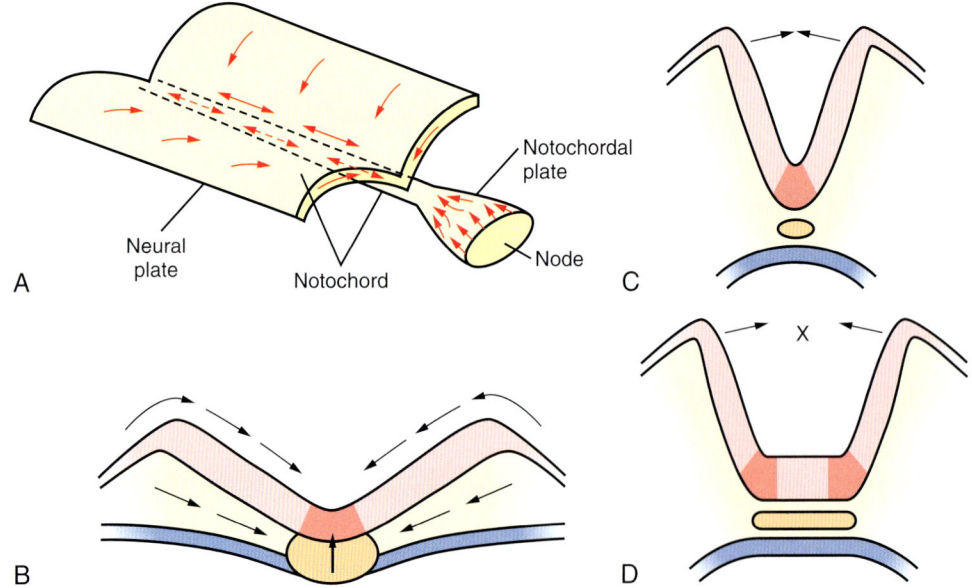

Figure 25-4. Cell movements affecting planar cell polarity (PCP) signaling in the early developing nervous system. **A** and **B,** Schematics showing cell movement toward the midline into the neural groove and longitudinally to narrow and elongate the embryo. **C,** This movement serves to narrow the ventral floor plate (red), facilitating median hinge-point bending and apposition of the neural folds. **D,** When PCP signaling is impaired, as in the looptail mouse-bearing mutation in *Vangl2*, the floor plate is wider (intervening cells remain in the floor plate region), which prevents the folds from meeting in the midline. *(**A,** With permission from Ybot-Gonzalez, P., et al., 2007. Convergent extension, planar-cell-polarity signaling and initiation of mouse neural tube closure. Development 134, 789–799. **B–D,** With permission from Copp, A.J., et al., 2003. Dishevelled: linking convergent extension with neural tube closure. Trends Neurosci 26, 453–455.)*

notochord, which underlie the midline of the neural plate; and the cells of the epidermal ectoderm, which flank its lateral edges. The notochord is the source of ventralizing inductive factor, and the epidermal ectoderm is the source of dorsalizing factors. Opposing actions of these two signals establish the identity and pattern of cell types generated along the dorsal-ventral axis of the neural tube.

The nervous system is organized in response to intrinsic patterning genes and critical embryonic signaling pathways involving secreted factors and cell-cell interactions. The homeotic, Hox, transcription factor genes provide a positional "address" or identity of spinal cord and hindbrain neurons. Fate determination along the dorsal-ventral axis also requires the action of three opposing signaling pathways:

1. Sonic hedgehog (SHH), produced ventrally by the notochord
2. Wnt, in which pathway different Wnts define dorsoventral regions of neural tube
3. Bone morphogenetic protein (BMP), in which pathway different BMPs are secreted by dorsally placed cells from the boundary of the neural and nonneural ectoderm

In this model, SHH released by the notochord diffuses toward the ventral neural tube and induces the differentiation of the floor plate. The floor plate then produces additional SHH, which diffuses and establishes a gradient along the dorsal-ventral axis of the neural tube. Differentiation of cells in the dorsal half of the neural tube depends on signals such as BMPs provided by the lateral epidermal ectoderm. BMP4 and BMP7, released by the epidermal ectoderm, diffuse toward the dorsal neural tube and induce the differentiation of the roof plate. Regions of the spinal cord that are exposed to the highest concentrations of SHH and lowest concentrations of BMPs give rise to ventral motor neurons, whereas cells exposed to lowest SHH and highest BMP concentrations give rise to dorsal cells, such as commissural projection neurons. Rostro-caudally, the neural tube is regionalized into four major divisions: forebrain, midbrain, hindbrain, and spinal cord. Actions of FGF, Wnt, and retinoic acid (RA) pathways confer a caudal identity and also influence telencephalic patterning.

EPIDEMIOLOGY AND PATHOGENESIS
Incidence

Among live births, females are more affected by NTDs than males by 2 to 1. Additionally, the prevalence of NTDs varies across time, by region, and by ethnicity and approximates 0.5 cases per 1000 in the United States but 10 per 1000 in parts of China and India. FA fortification of the United States food supply and/or the availability of prenatal diagnosis and the elective termination has reduced NTD prevalence in the United States to 0.37 cases per 1000 reported. The twin concordance rate among same-sex twins (presumed monozygotic) is significantly increased (to 6.8%), supporting a genetic contribution. Furthermore, compared with an incidence in the general population of 1 per 1000, the risk of NTD recurrence in a family with one affected child increases to 1.8 per 100 but does not approach the 1 in 4 recurrence risk of an autosomal-recessive mutation with complete penetrance.

Complex Genetic Contributions

The complexity of the genetic underpinnings of neurulation is reflected in the NTD-prone mouse lines, for which over 250 mutations have been associated with failure of neural tube closure (Harris and Juriloff, 2010). Despite this wealth of information, there is no single-gene polymorphism in the human homologs of these mouse genes that confers a robust, broadly reproducible enhanced risk of developing an NTD. This has led to the supposition that the genesis of NTDs requires the compounding of multiple gene polymorphisms.

The several hundred genes that have been associated with NTDs in mouse models are beginning to provide insights into molecular networks that are critically important for neurulation and may become clinically useful (Ross, 2010). For example, just as mutation in *Vangl2* renders the looptail mouse prone to NTD, polymorphisms in human *Vangl1* and *Vangl2* have been implicated in NTD patients. The complexity of the genetic underpinnings of NTD indicates that meeting the challenge for determining individual risk—and the optimal preventative therapy—will require evaluation of multiple genes (in signaling, metabolic, and transcriptional pathways)

in a single person to detect compounding effects of gene polymorphisms that alone might not be significant. Advanced technologies for high-throughput genomic DNA sequencing and analysis and detection of the epigenome and perhaps the microbiome, as well as untargeted metabolomic screening, will all play a role in the clinical evaluation of individual patient assessments of NTD risk and prevention.

Gene-Environment Interactions in Neural Tube Defects

The environmental variables that have been implicated as risk factors for nonsyndromic forms of spina bifida are listed in Table 25-1. Risk factors include maternal diabetes, maternal obesity, and prepregnancy weight gain. Moreover, maternal periconceptional elevations in simple sugars that raise the glycemic index have been associated with increased NTD risk, even among nondiabetic women. In animal models, exposing rat embryos to a hyperglycemic environment induces dysmorphisms, accompanied by increases in biomarkers of oxidative stress and inositol depletion.

Studies in the United Kingdom, later corroborated in Eastern Europe and elsewhere, indicated that the prevalence of NTDs could be reduced by 70% or more by prenatal supplementation with FA, even in the absence of maternal folate deficiency. However, some populations demonstrated only a small or no significant reduction in NTD rates with prenatal FA supplementation, suggesting that differences in genetic background, diet, or other environmental exposures could influence the efficacy of folate supplementation. Inadequate intake of natural folate before and during early pregnancy is associated with a 2- to 8-fold increased risk of MMC and anencephaly, as indicated by several series of case-controlled, randomized clinical trials and community-based interventions.

Teratogens

RA is a well-known teratogen when administered to nonhuman embryos, in which one of its many effects is to induce

TABLE 25-1 Risk Factors for Spina Bifida

Risk Factor	Relative Risk (-Fold Increase)
ESTABLISHED RISK FACTORS	
History of previous affected pregnancy with same partner	30
Inadequate maternal intake of folic acid	2–8
Pregestational maternal diabetes	2–10
Valproic acid and carbamazepine	10–20
SUSPECTED RISK FACTORS	
Maternal vitamin B_{12} status	3
Maternal obesity	1.5–3.5
Maternal hyperthermia	2
Maternal diarrhea	3–4
Gestational diabetes	NE
Fumonisins	NE
Paternal exposure to Agent Orange	NE
Chlorination disinfection byproducts in drinking water	NE
Electromagnetic fields	NE
Hazardous waste sites	NE
Pesticides	NE

NE, not established.
(With permission from Mitchell, L.E. et al., 2004. Spina bifida. Lancet 364, 1885–1895.)

NTDs, including spina bifida, exencephaly, and anencephaly in several different species. Most, if not all, antiepileptic drugs (AEDs) are known teratogens. Different AEDs, however, are associated with different constellations of malformations. An increased risk of MMC is associated with in utero exposure to valproic acid or carbamazepine alone, or in combination with other AEDs. In infants exposed to valproic acid or carbamazepine, the risk of MMC can be as high as 1% to 2% (Wlodarczyk et al., 2012). The mechanisms by which valproic acid and carbamazepine increase the risk of NTD have not been established, but there is general consensus that genetic predisposition to its teratogenic effect is required for valproate to promote NTDs. Folate administration does not appear to protect against the effects of valproic acid or carbamazepine on neural tube closure.

CLASSIFICATION OF NEURAL TUBE DEFECTS
Nomenclature

Broadly speaking, it is useful to separate those anomalies that arise from an early failure of neural tube formation and those that arise from defects in subsequent developmental steps. MMC refers to the commonest form of spina bifida, which comprises a flat neural placode, the unfolded derivative of the neural plate, elevated above a sac containing cerebrospinal fluid and continuous with the skin.

Neural tube closure is required for subsequent steps, including formation of mesodermal structures (e.g., dura, posterior spinal elements, and muscle). Milder NTDs often result in near-normal formation of mesodermal structures and closure of the overlying skin. This basic difference, the presence or absence of skin, has led to the designation of spina bifida into open forms, spina bifida aperta, or closed forms, spina bifida occulta. Spina bifida occulta is a confusing term because it can refer to either a broader group of anomalies that have normal skin overlying the spinal defect or a specific anomaly that indicates a lack of fusion of the spinous processes in the lumbar area and has limited clinical significance

(see later in this chapter). Fortunately, both of these terms are not common in current use.

Embryologic Classification of Neural Tube Defects

Neurulation is first visible as ectodermal thickening into the neural plate and proceeds in steps outlined previously. The commonly encountered NDs may be classified on the basis of the embryologic anomalies due to:

- Defects of neural folding and formation—myelomeningocele and anencephaly
- Disordered postneurulation development—encephaloceles
- Incomplete dysjunction—dermal sinus and associated dermoid and epidermoid tumors
- Premature dysjunction—spinal cord lipomas
- Disorders of gastrulation—split cord malformation, neurenteric cysts
- Disordered secondary neurulation—thickened filum terminale, myelocystocele
- Failure of caudal neuraxial development—sacral agenesis

MYELOMENINGOCELE

Myelomeningocele (MMC), the most complex of congenital spinal deformities, involves all tissue layers dorsal to and including the neural tube (i.e., spinal cord, nerve roots, meninges, vertebral bodies, skin). The dysplastic neural tube observed in newborns with MMC is a flat, disorganized segment of tissue located at the middle and most superficial portion of a cerebrospinal fluid-containing sac (Fig. 25-14).

Antenatal Diagnosis

Maternal serum α-fetoprotein (AFP) determination and ultrasound examination are used to identify fetuses that have or are likely to have spina bifida or anencephaly. Elevated amniotic AFP concentrations correlate with open NTDs, whereas

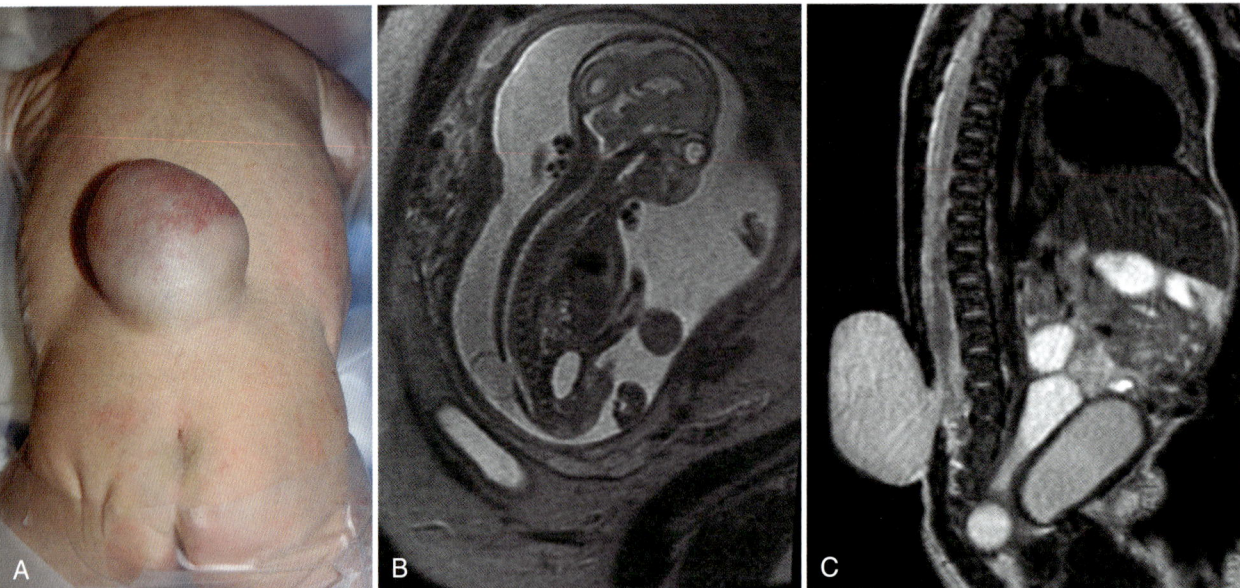

Figure 25-14. Lumbar meningocele in a newborn. A, External appearance of the skin. **B,** Midline sagittal view from a fetal T2-weighted MRI study depicts a fluid-filled cystic lesion. Note homogeneous water signal within the lesion, suggesting the diagnosis of meningocele, rather than meningomyelocele. **C,** Midline sagittal T2-weighted image from the postnatal MRI showing the fluid-filled sac and the spinal cord within the spinal canal.

closed lesions usually do not lead to increased AFP concentration. Detection of NTDs correlates with the magnitude of increase in the amniotic fluid AFP level; NTDs are associated in a minority of pregnancies with mildly elevated AFP levels, in a majority of those with moderately elevated levels, and overwhelmingly in those with very elevated AFP levels.

Sonography can differentiate between ventral wall defects and NTDs and can identify additional structural malformations that are characteristic of fetuses with chromosomal abnormalities. It is 60% accurate in low-risk pregnancies, which is equivalent to the accuracy of serum AFP screening (64%), 89% accurate in high-risk pregnancies, and 100% accurate for women referred for confirmation of a suspected spina bifida by another ultrasonographer. The data indicate that neither sonography nor AFP screening alone provides sufficient sensitivity or specificity but that, when these studies are used together, the predictive value is much higher.

Clinical Features

The mortality rate for MMC is approximately 50% in the absence of therapy. The primary goal of surgery for closure of the lumbosacral defect is to prevent meningitis. The location and extent of the defect determine the nature and degree of neurologic impairment; rating scales attempt to standardize the evaluation of affected children. Lumbosacral involvement is most common. Thoracic defects are the most complex and frequently are associated with serious complications. Cervical cord involvement is different from MMC of the lower spine and can be differentiated into two types:

1. Myelocystocele herniating posteriorly into a meningocele
2. Meningocele with or without an underlying split cord malformation

Varying degrees of leg paresis, usually profound, and sphincter dysfunction are the major clinical manifestations. Congenital dislocation of the hips or deformities of the feet such as clubbing may also occur. Severe sensory loss and accompanying trophic ulcers may complicate the condition. Occasionally, only sphincter disturbances are present.

Hydrocephalus is present in about 70% to 85% of patients with MMC and occurs most frequently with thoracolumbar lesions, which accounts for 90% of patients. Most persons with spina bifida have normal intelligence, but specific cognitive disabilities and language difficulties are common and can adversely affect educational and occupational achievements and the ability to live independently.

Secondary Abnormalities
Central Nervous System Complications

Seizures have been reported in up to 17% of patients with MMC and almost always occur in those with shunted hydrocephalus. Additional CNS abnormalities seen in these patients may underlie seizures and include encephalomalacia, previous stroke, malformations, and intracranial calcifications. Seizures may be difficult to control, and frequently, seizure exacerbation is associated with shunt malfunction or ventriculitis.

Bladder and Bowel Dysfunction

Bladder dysfunction and urinary incontinence pose major management problems and may be present at birth in the form of hydronephrosis. Interruption of sacral nerve roots and fiber connections between the brainstem and sacral cord causes the dysfunction. Loss of sphincter tone, overflow incontinence, sacral and rectal loss of sensation, and loss of detrusor activity on cystometry are seen. Normal bladder control occurs in 10% of children with MMC. Prevention of bladder infection requires intermittent catheterization to maintain low residual urine volumes and prophylactic antibacterial drugs. Vesicoureteral reflux often develops during the second and third years of life, and assessment for this problem must be ongoing.

Orthopedic Problems

Orthopedic defects associated with this paralysis, muscle imbalance, and accompanying regional spasticity may be severe and necessitate early intervention. Severe foot deformities afflict 80% of children and are treated with splinting or casting. Sensory deficits of the casted skin areas increase risk of skin ulcers. Physical therapy may help to preserve and extend the range of motion of the joints.

Progressive leg or foot deformity, weakness, pain, or deterioration of gait or bladder function implies restricted growth or tethering of the spinal cord. Cord tethering affects many older children with spina bifida who are neurologically stable. Surgical repair of a worsening tethered spinal cord and shunting or fenestration of syringomyelia can prevent decline of function.

Chiari II Malformation

Classification. Multiple hindbrain malformations are associated with congenital hydrocephalus. Four types of Chiari malformation have been characterized. Chiari I malformation is a downward displacement of the cerebellum and cerebellar tonsils. Chiari II malformation is a complex malformation that includes downward displacement of the cerebellar vermis and tonsils and is encountered almost exclusively in patients with MMC. Chiari III is an encephalocervical meningocele, and Chiari IV refers to hypoplasia of the cerebellum.

The major features of the Chiari II malformation include:

1. Inferior displacement of the medulla and the fourth ventricle into the upper cervical canal
2. Elongation and thinning of the upper medulla and lower pons, persistence of the embryonic flexure of these structures, and the appearance of a "beaking" of the tectum
3. Inferior displacement of the lower cerebellum through the foramen magnum into the upper cervical regions
4. A variety of bone defects of the foramen magnum, occiput, and upper cervical vertebrae

Hydromyelia and syringomyelia of the cervical spinal cord occur in 20% to 50% of patients.

Clinical Features. The symptoms associated with Chiari II malformations include apnea, swallowing difficulties, and stridor in the newborn and headache, quadriparesis, scoliosis, and balance and coordination difficulties in the older child; they are present in up to one-third of persons with the disorder (Box 25-1). It is often difficult to differentiate between symptoms related to the hydrocephalus versus cerebellar malformation, but many symptoms are directly referable to cerebellar, brainstem, and cranial nerve dysfunction. More than one-third of affected infants display feeding disturbances with reflux and aspiration. Vocal cord paralysis with stridor and abnormalities of ventilation, including both obstructive and central apnea may occur.

The causes of the clinical abnormalities of brainstem function are threefold. First, they relate in part to the brainstem malformation, which involves cranial nerves and other nuclei, present in most cases. Second, compression and traction of the anomalous caudal brainstem by hydrocephalus and

BOX 25-1 Clinical Manifestations of Chiari II Malformation

- Apnea
- Tongue fasciculations
- Stridor
- Facial palsy
- Gastroesophageal reflux
- Swallowing difficulties
- Poor feeding
- Ataxia
- Hypotonia
- Upper extremity weakness
- Hydrocephalus
- Syringomyelia
- Attention deficit
- Seizures
- Extraocular movement abnormalities
- Nystagmus
- Increased mortality

(With permission from McLone, D.G., Dias, M.S., 2003. The Chiari II malformation: cause and impact. Childs Nerv Syst 19, 540–550.)

increased intracranial pressure also may play a role, especially in the vagal nerve disturbance that results in vocal cord paralysis and stridor. Third, ischemic and hemorrhagic necrosis of the brainstem often is present also and may be secondary to the disturbed arterial architecture of the caudally displaced vertebrobasilar circulation.

Management

Management of MMC requires multidisciplinary efforts involving many specialists. Treatment includes surgical reduction and other associated defects such as syringomyelia, prevention of infection, covering of the MMC, control of hydrocephalus, management of urinary dysfunction, and treatment of the paralysis and abnormalities of the hips and feet.

Fetal Repair of Myelomeningocele

Compared with historical controls, infants given treatment in utero have a lower incidence of moderate to severe hindbrain herniation and hydrocephalus requiring shunting. A randomized, prospective clinical trial examined the efficacy of fetal repair of MMC between 22 and 26 weeks gestational age compared with standard postnatal repair. After inclusion of 183 subjects and analysis of 158 children at 12 months of age, the study was closed because of demonstrated benefit in the fetal treatment arm (Adzick et al, 2011; Gupta et al, 2012). In particular, there was a reduced rate of hydrocephalus requiring shunting, an improvement in motor function, and an improvement in hindbrain herniation in the group who underwent fetal repair. These benefits were balanced by the increased risk of preterm delivery and a number of maternal risks. The long-term outcomes are still undefined, but the patients recruited for the study described previously are being evaluated.

Management in the Newborn Period

Standard treatment includes closure of skin lesions overlying MMCs and treatment of hydrocephalus. The value of immediate correction of the defect within 48 hours of birth is widely accepted. Even when cerebrospinal fluid leakage occurs, however, a delay in closure for up to 48 hours does not increase the risk of infection or worsen the neurologic deficit. In such cases, the patient is given antibiotics, and the exposed placode is kept clean and moist. Ultrasonography and urodynamic studies should be carried out to assess the status of the urinary tract and provide a baseline for continuing assessment. At this age, bowel function is usually not difficult because affected infants have the gastrocolic reflex and pass stools with most feedings. The decision to give vigorous therapy for the most severely affected infants with MMC is beset by moral and medical considerations; restricted therapy often is associated with survival but poor outcome.

Treatment of Chiari II Malformation

Evaluation with MRI is the procedure of choice to evaluate a Chiari II malformation. Before considering surgical decompression of the posterior fossa, it is important to treat hydrocephalus if present. A properly functioning ventricular shunt often can obviate the need for decompression of hindbrain herniation. Many patients will resolve brainstem symptomatology with shunting. Significant improvement in the size of an accompanying spinal syrinx may occur after ventriculoperitoneal shunting or shunt revision. Suboccipital craniectomy may be warranted to decompress neural and vascular structures.

Outcome

Short-term and long-term survival of patients with spina bifida has increased with improvements in medical and surgical management. Patients with MMC are at substantial risk for leg weakness and paralysis, sensory, bowel and bladder dysfunction, and orthopedic abnormalities (e.g., clubfoot, contractures, hip dislocation, scoliosis, kyphosis). In general, the functional level corresponds to the anatomic level of the bony spinal defect. Patients with MMC also develop symptoms from associated malformations of the CNS, including hydrocephalus, syringomyelia, and Chiari II malformations.

ANENCEPHALY

Anencephaly is a congenital malformation in which both cerebral hemispheres are absent. Most anencephalic infants are stillborn, and those infants born alive die shortly after birth. Epidemiologic studies demonstrate a striking variation in prevalence rates. The highest incidence is in Great Britain and Ireland, and the lowest incidence is in Asia, Africa, and South America.

In the past two decades, prenatal screening with ultrasound examination during the first trimester, which is nearly 100% accurate, and maternal AFP determinations have resulted in earlier detection of anencephaly. Earlier detection has resulted in a dramatic decrease in the average gestational age at birth, from 35.6 weeks in the 1970s to 19.6 weeks in 1988 to 1990, with virtually no term liveborn anencephalic infants born after 1990 in those pregnancies in which a prenatal diagnosis of anencephaly had been made (Drugan, 2001).

Pathogenesis

The causes of anencephaly remain unknown; however, of importance, they mirror the causes of spina bifida, and similarly, folate has reduced the incidence of disease significantly. Indeed, both spina bifida and anencephaly can occur in the same family, reflecting the stochastic nature of where and when neural tube closure may fail. Risk factors discussed previously apply to both spina bifida and anencephaly.

Differential Diagnosis

In anencephaly, the absence of the brain and calvaria can be total or partial. Acrania is defined as congenital partial or total absence of the skull. Craniorachischisis is characterized by anencephaly, accompanied by a contiguous bony defect of the spine and exposure of neural tissue. In iniencephaly, dysraphism in the occipital region is accompanied by severe retroflexion of the neck and trunk, with three cardinal features: deficiency of the occipital bone; cervicothoracic spinal retroflexion; and rachischisis. Iniencephaly differs from anencephaly in that the cranial cavity is present and skin covers the head and retroflexed region. A majority of the patients also have visceral and other severe CNS malformations. In encephalocele, the brain and meninges herniate through a defect in the calvaria.

Pathology

The cranial vault is defective over the vertex, exposing a soft, angiomatous mass of neural tissue covered by a thin membrane continuous with the skin. The cranial abnormality may extend inferiorly to the cervical region, with formation of a complete spina bifida. The extremely thin and flattened spinal cord is readily observed. The optic globes usually are protuberant because of inadequate bony orbits.

ENCEPHALOCELE

An encephalocele is a herniation of intracranial contents through a midline skull defect. Also known as cephaloceles, these lesions are classified by their contents and location. Cranial meningoceles contain only leptomeninges and cerebrospinal fluid, whereas encephaloceles also contain brain parenchyma. The incidence of cephaloceles is approximately 0.8 to 5 per 10,000 live births, with encephaloceles being the most common form.

Encephaloceles occur in the occipital (75%) or frontal areas (25%). Basal and transsphenoidal encephaloceles are rare; they may appear between the ethmoid and sphenoid bones and extend into the upper pharynx. Encephaloceles extending from the orbit, nose, or forehead are termed sincipital encephaloceles; those in the occipital region are termed notencephaloceles.

Etiology

The etiology of encephaloceles is likely is multifactorial. Studies have indicated that consumption of FA during the periconceptional period can reduce the risk of anencephaly, as well as spina bifida. A similar protective effect, however, has not been noted for encephalocele.

Clinical Characteristics

A fluctuant, round, balloon-like mass that protrudes from the cranium, usually posteriorly, is the most typical manifestation of encephaloceles. The mass may pulsate and be covered by an erythematous, translucent, or opaque membrane, or by normal skin. The amount of compromised and deformed neural tissue and the degree of resultant microcephaly determine the extent of cerebral dysfunction. Brain tissue not extending into the encephalocele (i.e., retained within the intracranial cavity) may be deformed and functionally impaired.

Severe intellectual and motor delays typically occur in association with microcephaly; motor delay is accompanied by weakness and spasticity. Intellectual impairment is more prevalent in patients with posterior encephaloceles than in those with anterior encephaloceles. Some patients, however, may have fairly normal development. When the deformity extends into the ventricle, hydrocephalus is almost inevitable.

Management

Prenatal diagnosis of encephaloceles may be established with determination of increased amniotic AFP content and ultrasound studies. Surgical correction of all but the smallest encephaloceles is necessary. Accompanying hydrocephalus may require ventriculoperitoneal shunting. Associated systemic abnormalities are present in approximately half of the patients, depending on the syndromic nature of the condition. A full battery of endocrinologic screens should be performed to evaluate basal encephaloceles.

OCCULT FORMS OF SPINAL DYSRAPHISM

The spectrum of occult spinal dysraphism includes anomalies in which the overlying skin is mostly normal and covers the underlying NTD. These anomalies include distortion of the spinal cord or roots by fibrous bands and adhesions, intraspinal lipomas, dermoid or epidermoid cysts, fibrolipomas, spinal cord lipomas, lipomyelomeningocele, and split cord malformations.

Symptoms of occult spinal dysraphism may be absent, minimal, or severe, depending on the degree of neural involvement. The patient may exhibit static or slowly progressive weakness, spasticity, or sensory loss in the legs or feet, gait difficulty, and foot deformity. Bowel and bladder dysfunction such as incontinence, repeated bladder infection, and enuresis also may occur. Common findings include diminished Achilles tendon reflexes, contracted heel cords, high arches, equinovarus deformity of the feet, decreased rectal sphincter tone, unequal leg or foot length, scattered sensory loss, Babinski signs, and trophic ulcers. Ultrasonography and MRI have greatly facilitated the diagnosis and management of these occult lesions. A tethered spinal cord, lipoma, or fatty filum terminale can be detected without invasive myelography. Ultrasonography can demonstrate a poorly pulsatile, low-lying, or thickened conus medullaris in infants. The decision to proceed to surgery is based on progressive symptomatology.

Spinal Cord Lipoma

Spinal cord lipomas are developmental anomalies that range from a small fatty mass attached to the distal spinal cord to very complex anomalies that involve all spinal structures. In some cases, the lipoma is entirely intraspinal and extends through a limited defect in the posterior elements of the spine into the subcutaneous tissues. When involving subcutaneous tissues along with a cerebrospinal fluid-containing space, this is usually referred to as a lipomyelomeningocele.

Spinal cord lipomas are considered more complex forms of spinal dysraphism. Despite this, they can present with either no symptoms or symptoms over long periods of time. If untethering of the spinal cord can be accomplished with low morbidity, then a surgical procedure should be considered early in life. For large and complex lesions, particularly in patients with normal function, serious consideration should be given to observation, as deficits can evolve slowly.

Dermal Sinus Tract

Recurrent meningitis from external contamination of cerebrospinal fluid may result from occult congenital malformations along the spinal canal and neuraxis such as dermal sinus tracts. From an embryologic perspective, sinus tracts consist of epithelial-lined canals that probably represent persistence of an ectodermal-derived pathway from the skin to the CNS. In most cases, the spinal cord appears largely normal, implying that neural tube formation is complete but a persistent communication is still present. Dermal sinus tracts are seen in approximately 1 in 2500 live births. An MRI scan should be obtained, followed by surgical treatment to eliminate this connection and remove the risk of meningitis.

Spina Bifida Occulta

Spina bifida occulta, a confusing term, is defined as a defect in the posterior bony components of the vertebral column without involvement of the cord or meninges. It occurs in at least 5% of the population but most often is asymptomatic. The presence of a cutaneous lesion, tuft of hair, or a cutaneous angioma or lipoma in the midline of the back, is associated with spina bifida occulta in only approximately 10% of cases, although the percentage increases to approximately 50% when two or more skin lesions are present.

Meningocele

Meningocele, a protrusion of meninges without accompanying nervous tissue, is not associated with neurologic deficit. The mass usually is evident as a fluid-filled protrusion covered by skin or membrane in the midline. An MRI is essential to determine the contents of a mass along the spine and in differentiating meningocele from MMC (Fig. 22-14). Very small subcutaneous lesions may remain undetected for prolonged periods and typically require no specific treatment.

When careful examination of patients with suspected meningocele reveals significant neurologic abnormality (e.g., equinovarus deformity, gait disturbance, abnormal bladder function), the diagnosis of MMC is appropriate. These patients likely have entrapped nerve roots within the defect that can be identified during surgery.

Split Cord Malformations

Embryology

In split cord malformations, previously known as diastematomyelia, a midline septum divides the spinal cord longitudinally into two, usually unequal portions extending up to 10 thoracolumbar segments. The septum may span the entire width of the spinal canal and is anchored to the ventral dura mater on the posterior aspect of the vertebral bodies. Split cord malformations can be divided into two different types. In type I, present in 50% of cases, a split spinal cord is surrounded by a normal undivided arachnoid-dural sleeve without a septum. In type II, present in the other 50%, each hemicord is invested by a separate dural sleeve, divided by a fibrous, cartilaginous, or bony septum.

Clinical Characteristics

Patients with split cord malformations present with a congenital scoliosis, hydrocephalus, or cutaneous lesion such as hairy patch, dimple, hemangioma, subcutaneous mass, or teratoma. A progressive myelopathy with deformities of the feet, scoliosis, kyphosis, or discrepancy in leg length may develop. The intervening mesenchymal elements appear to contribute to progressive neurologic, urologic, and orthopedic deterioration from spinal cord tethering. Resection of the spur should be performed in patients who have progressive neurologic manifestations; those without worsening symptoms should be observed until progression occurs and then resection performed.

DISORDERS OF SECONDARY NEURULATION
Fibrofatty Filum Terminale

The filum terminale is the nonfunctional continuation of the end of the spinal cord. It usually consists of fibrous tissue without functional nervous tissue. Although its embryologic origin is unclear, it probably represents the termination of the neural tube and its most caudal link to the rest of the embryonic tissues. The filum can be enlarged either with fibrous tissue only or with fat. A thickened or fatty filum terminale may be associated with a low conus and a spectrum of clinical findings, including bladder dysfunction, leg numbness and weakness, and scoliosis. In the presence of neurologic findings and a fatty filum, an untethering procedure may be considered.

Sacral Agenesis

Sacral agenesis is a congenital absence of all or part of the sacrum. In its classic form, often described as the caudal regression syndrome, malformations of most or all structures derived from the caudal region of the embryo, including the urogenital system, the hindgut, caudal spine, spinal cord, and the lower limbs, may be seen. Approximately 15% to 25% of mothers of these children have insulin-dependent diabetes mellitus.

REFERENCES

The complete list of references for this chapter is available online at www.expertconsult.com.
See inside cover for registration details.

SELECTED REFERENCES

Adzick, N.S., Thom, E.A., Spong, C.Y., et al., 2011. A randomized trial of prenatal versus postnatal repair of myelomeningocele. N. Engl. J. Med. 364, 993–1004. doi:10.1056/NEJMoa1014379.

Copp, A.J., Greene, N.D., Murdoch, J.N., 2003. The genetic basis of mammalian neurulation. Nat. Rev. Genet. 4, 784–793.

Drugan A, Weissman A, Evans MI. Screening for neural tube defects. Clin Perinatol 2001;28:279–87, vii.

Gupta, N., Rand, L., Farrell, J., et al., 2012. Open fetal repair for myelomeningocele. J. Neurosurg. Pediatr. 9, 265–273.

Harris, M.J., Juriloff, D.M., 2010. An update to the list of mouse mutants with neural tube closure defects and advances toward a complete genetic perspective of neural tube closure. Birth Defects Res. A. Clin Mol. Teratol. 88, 653–669.

Ross, M.E., 2010. Gene-environment interactions: folate metabolism and the embryonic nervous system. Wiley Interdiscip. Rev. Syst. Biol. Med. 2 (4), 471–480.

Wlodarczyk, B.J., Palacios, A.M., George, T.M., et al., 2012. Antiepileptic drugs and pregnancy outcomes. Am. J. Med. Genet. A 158A, 2071–2090.

⊛ E-BOOK FIGURES AND TABLES

26 Disorders of Forebrain Development

Elliott H. Sherr and Jin S. Hahn

An expanded version of this chapter is available on www.expertconsult.com. See inside cover for registration details.

INTRODUCTION

The prosencephalon forms at the end of primary neurulation as one of three principal vesicles: the hindbrain, the midbrain, and the forebrain (prosencephalon). The major disorders of prosencephalic formation, holoprosencephaly, agenesis of the corpus callosum, and septooptic dysplasia, are discussed in the next sections, after a brief introduction to prosencephalic development.

Prosencephalon Patterning

Prosencephalic development occurs by inductive interactions from the prechordal mesoderm. The peak time period of development is the second and third months of gestation. Prosencephalon development occurs as three sequential events: prosencephalic formation, prosencephalic cleavage, and midline prosencephalic development (Fig. 26-1). Prosencephalic formation segments this structure into three prosomeres (P1–P3). P1 becomes the pretectum, P2 the thalamus, and P3 the prethalamus. More rostral brain regions, including the telencephalon, are also divided into prosomeric boundaries. The neocortex itself exhibits regionally restricted gene expression; however, data argue against anatomically and regionally restricted boundaries because cell lineage experiments demonstrate that sibling cells can occupy multiple nuclei throughout the anteroposterior axis.

Prosencephalic Cleavage

Prosencephalic cleavage occurs in the fifth and sixth weeks of gestation and includes three basic cleavages:

1. Horizontal, to form the paired optic vesicles, and olfactory bulbs and tracts
2. Transverse, to separate the telencephalon from the diencephalons
3. Sagittal, to form the paired cerebral hemispheres, lateral ventricles, and the basal ganglia from the telencephalon

Three crucial thickenings or plates of tissue become apparent around the end of the second month; these are the commissural, the chiasmatic, and the hypothalamic plates. These structures are important in the formation, respectively, of the corpus callosum, anterior commissure and septum pellucidum, the optic nerve chiasm, and the hypothalamic structures. Disorders associated with abnormal development of the prosencephalon are outlined in Table 26-1.

HOLOPROSENCEPHALY

Holoprosencephaly (HPE) is a complex brain malformation characterized by a failure of the forebrain (prosencephalon) to separate completely into two distinct cerebral hemispheres, a process normally complete by the fifth week of gestation. HPE is typically associated with midline facial anomalies.

Epidemiology

HPE is the most common developmental defect of the forebrain and midface in humans and occurs in 1 in 250 pregnancies, but because only 3% of the fetuses with HPE survive to delivery, the incidence in live births is only approximately 1 in 10,000. There also appears to be a slight female preponderance in some case series. A few studies of limited size suggest a higher than average prevalence of HPE in Far East Asians and Filipinos.

Definition and Subtypes of Holoprosencephaly

The sine qua non of HPE is incomplete cleavage of midline structures involving the telencephalon and diencephalon. HPE typically is divided into three main subtypes and distinguished by the degree of separation of the cerebral hemispheres (Fig. 26-2).

In the most severe type, *alobar HPE*, nearly complete lack of separation of the cerebral hemispheres is characteristic, with a single midline ventricle very often communicating with a dorsal cyst. The interhemispheric fissure and corpus callosum are completely absent. In the intermediate form, *semilobar HPE*, the anterior hemispheres are not separated, but some degree of separation of the posterior hemispheres is seen. Similarly, the genu and body of the corpus callosum are absent, but the splenium is present. The frontal horns of the lateral ventricles are not developed, but the posterior horns are present. The mildest form, *lobar HPE*, is characterized by lack of separation of the most rostral and ventral aspects of the cerebral hemispheres. The splenium and body of the corpus callosum are present, but the genu is absent. Rudimentary frontal horns may be present.

In addition to these types, another subtype is identifiable: the *middle interhemispheric variant*. In this variant, the midportion of the cerebral hemispheres is continuous across the midline, with absence of the corpus callosum seen only in this region. There is separation of the anterior frontal lobes, basal forebrain, and occipital lobes. Evidence for this malformation being a subtype of HPE is bolstered by mutation of the ZIC2 gene, which has been implicated in causing the classic forms of HPE.

Failure of separation also is common in the hypothalamic, caudate, lentiform, and thalamic nuclei. About one fourth of patients have some degree of midbrain nonseparation. Occasionally, isolated neuronal heterotopias are seen, particularly in the middle interhemispheric variant. The gyri often are normally developed, although in alobar and semilobar HPE, the gyri may be excessively smooth or broad. Although for discussion HPE is divided into subtypes, the degree of

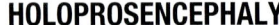

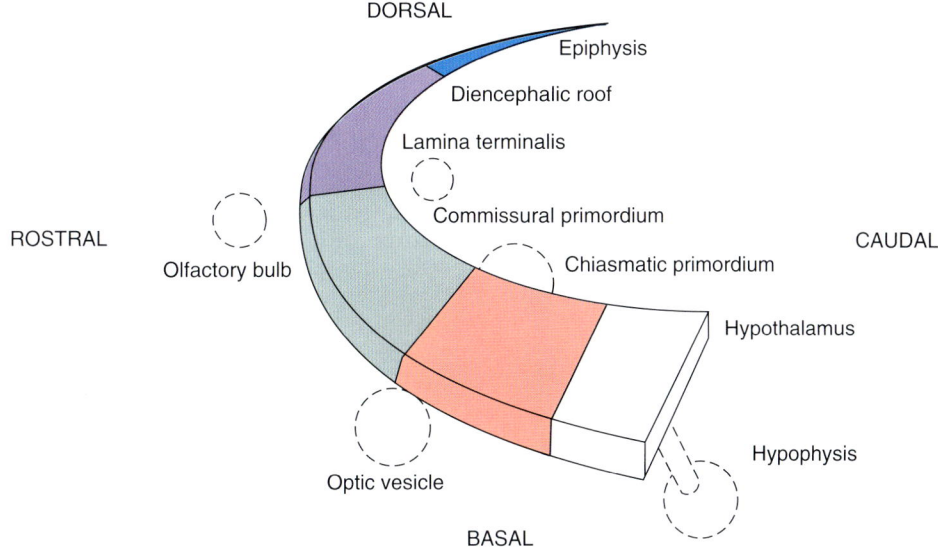

Figure 26-1. Prosencephalic midline development. The prosencephalic midline is presented by a series of independent but closely related segments. Note particularly the commissural, chiasmatic, and hypothalamic primordia or plates. The proximity of these structures in the developing brain and their derivation from a common primordium explain the spectrum of midline defects associated with septooptic dysplasia, which include optic nerve hypoplasia and hypothalamic and corpus callosum defects. *(With permission from Leech RW, Shuman RM. Holoprosencephaly and related midline cerebral anomalies: A review. J Child Neurol 1986;1:3.)*

malformation occurs along a spectrum, and individual patients do not fall neatly into categories.

Etiology

Multiple environmental and genetic factors have been implicated in causing HPE. Prenatal exposures to a variety of toxins, medications, and infections also have been reported. The strongest teratogenic evidence exists for maternal diabetes and exposure to alcohol and retinoic acid. A diabetic mother's risk of having a child with HPE is approximately 1%, a greater than 100-fold increase over the general population. A recent population study confirmed the risks of preexisting maternal diabetes and salicylates (aspirin) but also noted an increased risk with artificial reproductive therapy. Some teratogens are thought to produce HPE via interference with the sonic hedgehog gene signaling pathways, or cholesterol biosynthesis.

Approximately 30% to 50% of live births with HPE have chromosomal abnormalities, but this is likely an overestimation based on underreporting of milder cases. HPE can be seen in association with trisomy 13, trisomy 18, or triploidy. Various deletions or duplications of chromosomal regions have also been associated with HPE. HPE is also seen in single gene syndromes, such as Pallister-Hall syndrome, Rubinstein-Taybi syndrome, Smith-Lemli-Opitz, and Goldenhar syndromes. An updated list of genetic disorders associated with HPE can be found on the online Mendelian Inheritance in Man (OMIM) website (http://www.ncbi.nlm.nih.gov/omim).

In nonsyndromic and nonchromosomal HPE, autosomal-dominant and autosomal-recessive pedigrees have been reported. At least nine genes have been associated with HPE, including: SHH (7q36); ZIC2 (13q32); SIX3 (2p21); TGIF (18p11.3); PATCHED-1 (9q22); GLI2 (2q14); DISP1 (1q24); NODAL (10q); and FOXH1 (8q24.3). Of these genes, the four most commonly affected (SHH, ZIC2, SIX3, and TGIF) account for only 25% of the cases of HPE with normal chromosomes and approximately 5% to 10% of all HPE patients (Roessler and Muenke, 2010).

SHH (sonic hedgehog) was the first identified HPE-associated mutated gene, and the SHH protein is a secreted intercellular signaling molecule involved in establishing cell fates at several points during development. SHH is expressed early in development in the ventral forebrain and is critical for ventral patterning of the developing neural tube. Disruption of SHH signaling in animal models mimics the brain and facial malformations in HPE.

The SHH signaling network is the common pathway through which multiple environmental and genetic influences interact to cause HPE. For example, PTCH is a receptor for SHH, and GLI2 is a mediator of SHH target gene transcription. Environmental influences link the SHH signaling network with hypocholesterolemia. For example, maternal hypocholesterolemia has been implicated in HPE. Also, HPE is seen in Smith-Lemli-Opitz syndrome, which is due to a defect in 7-dehydrocholesterol reductase, the final enzyme in cholesterol synthesis.

Clinical Manifestations and Outcomes

Along with the midline brain malformation seen in HPE, a corresponding midline facial malformation may be present. In its most severe and usually lethal form, cyclopia with the presence of a single midline eye and a proboscis (rudimentary single-nostril nose) above the eye can be present. Survivors may have hypotelorism, a flattened nasal bridge, median cleft lip and palate, or a single median maxillary central incisor. The oft-quoted statement "the face predicts the brain" refers to the observation that the degree of facial malformation frequently reflects the degree of brain malformation. This was amended later to "the face predicts the brain approximately 80% of the time," in recognition of individuals with alobar HPE with a normal facial appearance, as well as cases of milder brain malformation associated with abnormal facies.

Previous studies indicated that children with HPE do not survive beyond early infancy. This may have been due to the identification of only the most severe cases. Early death is typical for most cytogenetically abnormal children and those individuals with the most severe facial features (cyclopia or ethmocephaly). In children without these risk factors, more recent studies have indicated that long-term survival is not uncommon. In one series of 104 HPE patients, the mean age at the time of study was 4 years, and 15% were between 10 and 19 years of age. When death did occur, causes included brainstem dysfunction, pneumonia, dehydration from diabetes insipidus, and rarely, intractable seizures.

Children with HPE may experience a variety of medical and neurologic problems. A significant proportion develops hydrocephalus, with 60% of alobar and 8% of semilobar requiring a VP shunt. As in children with other midline brain defects, endocrinologic problems are very common. Diabetes insipidus is particularly frequent, growth hormone deficiency, hypocortisolism, and hypothyroidism also may occur. The endocrinopathies may be due to midline defects involving the hypothalamus and are rarely due to a dysgenetic (e.g., hypoplastic or ectopic) pituitary gland.

Approximately half of the children with HPE have epilepsy, and the likelihood of developing seizures does not correlate with the severity of the brain malformation. The most common seizure type is complex partial seizures, with or without secondary generalization, but seizures can include generalized tonic-clonic, tonic, atonic, myoclonic, or infantile spasms. In 50% of affected children, the seizures are relatively easy to control with antiepileptic medication but with increased risk associated with cortical dysplasia.

Feeding problems and swallowing dysfunction are common in children with HPE and are correlated with the severity of the brain malformation. Two thirds of patients with alobar and semilobar HPE require gastrostomy tubes.

Developmental disability affects nearly all patients with HPE. The severity of the brain malformation determines the degree of delay and neurologic impairments (including hypotonia and spasticity). Severe developmental delay is present in alobar HPE. There is no reported case of a child with alobar HPE who is able to sit independently. In lobar HPE, approximately 50% of children ambulate (with or without assistance), use their hands functionally, and have some verbal communication. Neuropsychologic evaluation in HPE demonstrates relative strengths in receptive language and socialization and weaknesses in visual reasoning and nonverbal problem skills.

In the middle interhemispheric variant, the incidence of endocrinopathies is much lower than has been attributed to the more normally separated hypothalamus seen on MRI. The degree of motor complications (hypotonia evolving into spasticity and dystonia) and developmental dysfunction is similar to that seen in lobar HPE.

Management

Children with alobar HPE, a dorsal cyst, or normocephaly or macrocephaly should be closely observed for the development of hydrocephalus and perhaps shunting early given the high risk, as hydrocephalus can lead to progressive head enlargement and greater difficulty in caring for the child. Electrolyte screening should be performed for diabetes insipidus surveillance. Screening for other endocrine abnormalities should be considered, including assays of cortisol, thyroid-stimulating hormone, free thyroxine, and insulin-like growth factor-1 (IGF-1). If seizures develop, the possibility of acute reactive seizures should be evaluated for and a serum sodium level checked. MRI also should be considered to evaluate for focal heterotopia. Gastrostomy tubes often are necessary to address the complex management issues of ensuring adequate calories related to feeding dysfunction and delivery of adequate free water necessary for management of diabetes insipidus. Motor difficulties and dystonia may be partially responsive to trihexyphenidyl. This agent may improve upper extremity and oromotor function. Motor dysfunction, including hypertonia and dystonia, is common and may require physical, pharmacologic, or surgical therapies.

Prenatal Diagnosis and Imaging

The first-trimester ultrasound can detect alobar HPE but may be much less sensitive in detecting milder cases. The presence of large dorsal cysts, hydrocephalus, or midline craniofacial defects may provide clues that eventually lead to the recognition of the associated HPE. Fetal MRI has been used to diagnosis a range of HPE. Other midline anomalies, such as agenesis of the corpus callosum, absence of the septum pellucidum, and hydrocephalus with communication of the lateral ventricles, are sometimes misdiagnosed prenatally as HPE (Fig. 26-3).

Genetic Counseling and Testing

The recurrence risk of isolated HPE is estimated to be 6%. Special attention should be given to the family history to identify "microforms" such as anosmia or a single central incisor. Such a finding indicates higher recurrence risk. Genetic sequence analysis is commercially available and should be considered. Prenatal testing for HPE risk genes is possible by means of amniocentesis or chorionic villus sampling. The gene tests, in conjunction with fetal MRI, have been found to be helpful in prenatal diagnosis and counseling in a series of pregnancies. High-resolution cytogenetic analysis can detect abnormalities in 24% to 45% of all individuals with HPE. Chromosomal microarray has a higher yield in detecting chromosomal deletions, duplications, and unbalanced rearrangements and is the preferred chromosomal test in fetuses and newborns suspected of having HPE.

AGENESIS OF THE CORPUS CALLOSUM

The corpus callosum forms between the 8th and 14th weeks of fetal development. Nearly 200 million axons course through this structure and innervate opposing hemispheres in a homotopic manner; that is, each axon innervates structures in the mirror location in the opposing hemisphere. Absence or diminution of this structure is found in 1 in 3000 live births and is the most common birth defect of the central nervous system after spina bifida. Callosal abnormalities are frequently seen with other malformations of brain development but can present in an isolated manner (Fig. 26-4). Many cases are also associated with birth defects in other organ systems and can be caused by chromosomal disorders. There is also recognition that subtle chromosomal copy number variants (CNVs) play a critical role in the etiology of ACC (Sajan et al., 2013). Single-gene mutations and metabolic disorders can also disrupt callosal development. Fetal alcohol syndrome, the best-known and most studied environmental cause of ACC, can also result in a significant reduction in white-matter volume. There is a great diversity of clinical outcomes for patients with ACC. Many individuals with ACC have deficits in social cognition, even with a normal IQ. Many of these individuals carry clinical diagnoses that place their phenotype on the autism spectrum. In children with ACC and associated brain anomalies, many have seizures and more significant developmental impairment, including intellectual disability and cerebral palsy. In some individuals with ACC due to chromosomal, metabolic, or single-gene disorders, the outcome can be quite severe, including a significantly shortened life expectancy.

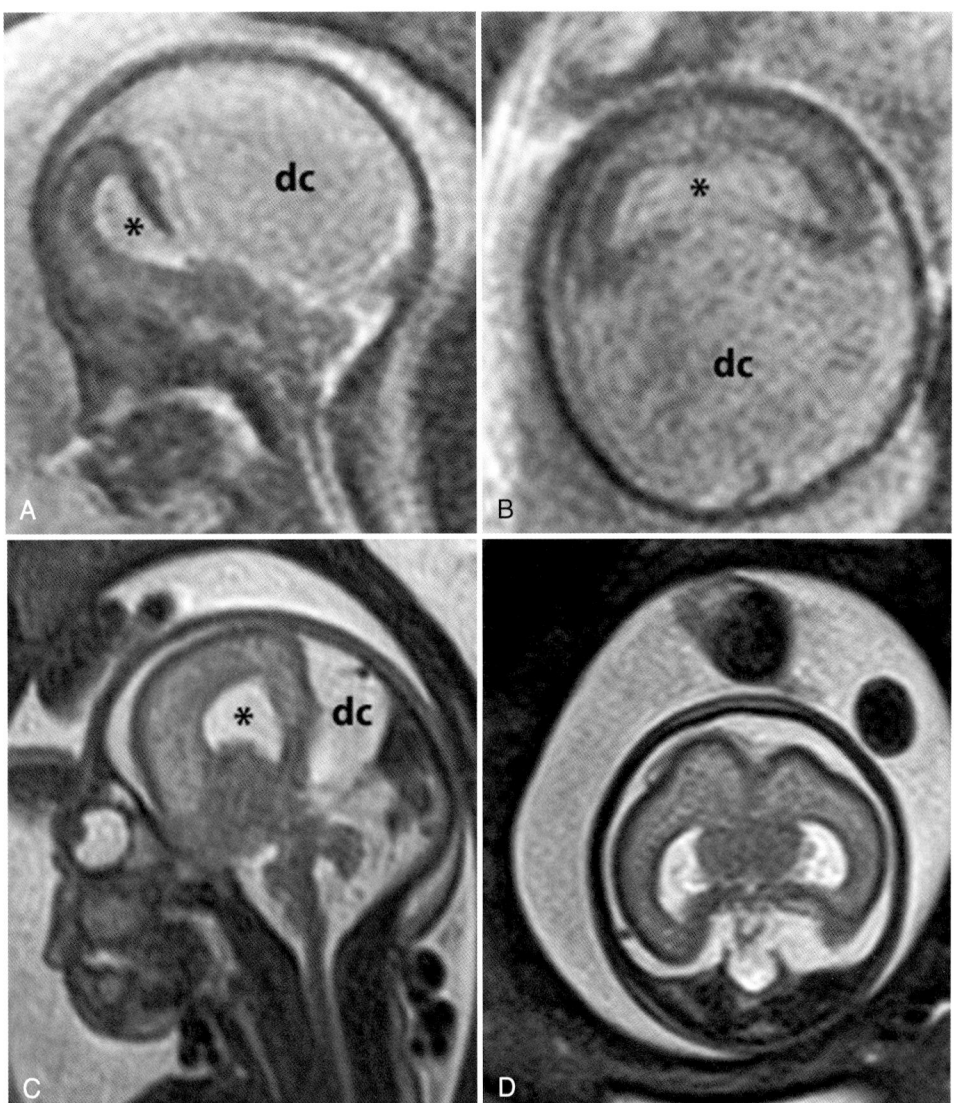

Figure 26-3. Fetal magnetic resonance imaging in holoprosencephaly. **A** and **B,** Fetal MRI (single-shot fast spin echo) of a 21-week- and 5-day-old fetus with alobar HPE. The thalami, basal ganglia, and midbrain structures are incompletely delineated on the midline sagittal image **(A)**. A large dorsal cyst (dc) communicates with the monoventricle (*asterisk*). The hemispheres are not separated, resulting in a holosphere **(B)**. **C** and **D,** Fetal MRI of a 26-week gestational age fetus with trisomy 13 and semilobar HPE. The HASTE fetal sequence in the midsagittal plane **(C)** shows a monoventricle (*asterisk*), a moderate size dorsal cyst (dc), and inferior cerebellar vermis hypoplasia (Dandy-Walker complex). On the axial image **(D)**, the thalami and basal ganglia appear fused, whereas the posterior hemispheres are separated. *(With permission from Hahn JS, Barnes PD. Neuroimaging advances in holoprosencephaly: refining the spectrum of the midline malformation. Am J Med Genet Part C 2010;154C:120–132.)*

Epidemiology

Population studies suggest a birth incidence for ACC of 1 in 3000 (Glass et al., 2008). Like many birth defects, the incidence rate of ACC is higher in births from mothers over age 40, with a nearly three-fold increased risk compared with women in their 20s. There is also a slightly higher prevalence in children born to older fathers, as has also been reported recently for autism. Babies with ACC are nearly four times more likely to be born prematurely than the general population. It should be noted that detection of ACC occurs more commonly with better ultrasound surveillance, and its detection in utero may alert physicians to the increased probability of premature birth (Glass et al., 2008). In addition, identifying ACC should also alert the clinician to screen for other organ malformations, including musculoskeletal, renal, and gastrointestinal.

Prenatal Diagnosis and Prediction of Outcomes

The majority of information on the epidemiology of callosal agenesis comes from studies of postnatally diagnosed cases. However, in the studies that investigated all types of ACC in large fetal cohorts, approximately 70% of individuals had other associated anomalies in the central nervous system, including white matter deficits, cortical malformations, cysts, and posterior fossa abnormalities (Hetts et al., 2006). Isolated ACC only accounted for approximately 30% of the total number of cases. In these cases of prenatally detected, isolated ACC, approximately 50% show neurologic impairment in the first few years of life, and many of the remainder show cognitive and behavioral deficits during school years. Current standard ultrasonography can reliably detect callosal agenesis at 22 weeks' gestation; however, many pregnant women receive a single ultrasound at 18 weeks to evaluate fetal anatomy as part of standard prenatal care. There are recommendations within the obstetric community to perform two ultrasounds, one transvaginally at 14 weeks to assess nuchal translucency and other early visible anatomic changes and a second study at 20 to 22 weeks to better visualize later-developing structures, such as the corpus callosum.

Development of the Corpus Callosum

The corpus callosum is the largest white-matter tract in the brain, with over 190 million axons crossing the midline to innervate principally homotopic structures. The disproportionate increase in white-matter volume in mammalian and, specifically, in primate evolution points to the importance of long-range connectivity (particularly of the frontal lobes) in brain evolution and function. The first callosal fibers can be seen crossing the midline around the 14th week of gestation. The midline is composed of a number of structures that likely assist in guiding these callosal fibers, including the glial wedge, midline zipper glia, glial sling, and indusium griseum glia (Fig. 26-5). The full complexity of molecular and cellular events necessary for callosal development is not yet known, but these events can be seen within a general framework of developmental steps that include: birth and specification of commissural neurons; guidance of these neurons to the midline; midline fusion and development of key midline structures (as outlined in Fig. 26-5); and axonal crossing of the midline with guidance of crossed neurons to the final site of connectivity. In patients with ACC, it can be difficult to determine which one of these steps is altered. However, in one group, patients with microcephaly and absent Probst bundles, there are likely defects in the initial birth and specification of commissural neurons. In contrast, it is more likely that patients who have Probst bundles (and normal or near-normal cerebral white-matter volume) have deficits in axonal guidance or midline fusion.

Imaging and the Corpus Callosum

Imaging of children and adults with ACC has shown that the missing corpus callosum is frequently only one component of the spectrum of brain malformations found in an individual patient. In a retrospective study of 142 cases of callosal agenesis, only five had truly "isolated" ACC, whereas over half had malformations of cortical development, one third had cerebellar malformations, and one fourth had brainstem anomalies. Advanced techniques such as diffusion tensor imaging (DTI) have demonstrated that the ventral cingulum bundle (CB) is smaller and has lower fractional anisotropy in ACC patients, which may explain the behavioral deficits observed in ACC.

Etiology

Genetic

Many molecular and cellular processes are necessary for normal callosal formation. As such, many single-gene recessive disorders can be associated with callosal agenesis (Table 26-2). Whole exome sequencing has accelerated this discovery and new genes such EPG5 for Vici syndrome, C12orf57 for Temtamy syndrome, and GPSM2 for Chudley-McCullough syndrome were recently discovered. Autosomal dominant disorders associated with callosal agenesis and dysgenesis,

such as mutations in the DEAD-box gene DDX3X were also recently identified (Snijders Blok et al., 2015). In many disorders, the degree of callosal dysgenesis can be quite variable as in Sotos syndrome, in which complete ACC is present in a minority of cases, but other versions of callosal dysgenesis are prevalent in these patients (Schaefer et al., 1997).

There is also evidence that de novo chromosomal disorders play a significant role in callosal dysgenesis. A recent publication cataloged de novo deletions and duplications at recurrent genetic loci from nearly 400 ACC patients. These include regions in 1p36, 1q4, 6p25, 6q2, 8p, 13q, and 14q. A subsequent publication suggested that over 15% of ACC patients have a large de novo CNV that may be causative. Although the initial presumption has been that most cases of ACC have a genetic etiology, it is possible that nongenetic causes may play an important etiologic role.

Nongenetic

The best example of environmental causes of ACC is fetal alcohol syndrome (FAS). Despite this linkage, there is clearly variability in the expression of callosal deficits in fetal alcohol syndrome. The cell surface molecule L1, which is involved in both axon guidance and fasciculation, is a proposed target for alcohol toxicity and signaling through this pathway may explain the variable expressivity of fetal EtOH exposure. There are a few reports of heavy metal toxicity and ACC, but without many reports, it is difficult to attribute a significant percentage of ACC cases to these causes.

Clinical Manifestations

Association of Agenesis of the Corpus Callosum With Autism and Related Neurodevelopmental Disorders

A wide range of clinical deficits can be seen in individuals with callosal agenesis including autism, intellectual disability, epilepsy, and cerebral palsy. However, it is difficult to know the precise prevalence of these associated features because most individuals with ACC are evaluated specifically because of their clinical difficulties, introducing ascertainment bias. With that limitation in mind, many studies have reported that patients with ACC have significant cognitive and neuromotor impairment. Epilepsy is common and is more prevalent in patients who have other associated brain malformations. Autistic features are present in approximately 40% of patients with ACC who have normal IQs, and a more detailed analysis shows that high-functioning ACC individuals also have problems with social cognition, paralinguistic communication, and executive function skills. Thus they have difficulties holding down jobs, finding partners, and living independently, even though they may have normal intelligence.

Management

Currently, the mainstay of management for patients with ACC includes symptomatic measures that may include use of antiepileptic drugs for epilepsy, physical and occupational therapy for hypotonia and cerebral palsy, and speech therapy. Patients with ACC, including apparently high-functioning individuals, often have difficulty with more complex cognitive and behavioral tasks and need explicit behavioral training and education, which is often lacking in school settings. Anecdotal reports suggest that these individuals do better with therapy targeted at simplifying these tasks, providing repetition, and supporting a slower learning pace. Although many individuals with ACC have social deficits, they generally desire social

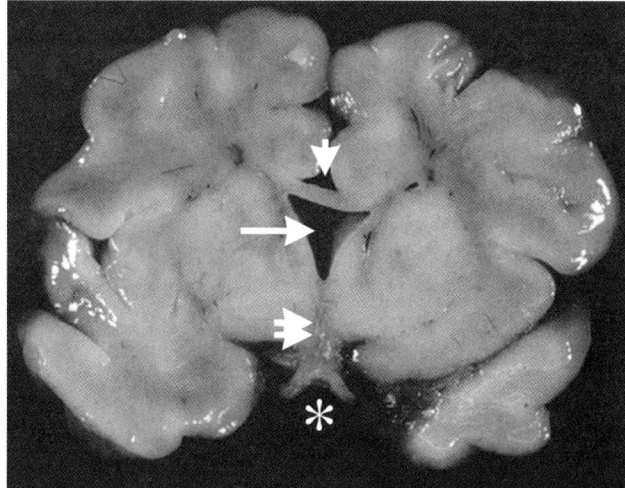

Figure 26-8. Septooptic dysplasia. In this brain of a newborn, note corpus callosum thinning (*short arrow*), absent septum pellucidum (*long arrow*), hypothalamic hypoplasia (*double arrows*), and optic nerve hypoplasia (*asterisk*).

interactions. With recent reports of the potential benefits of intranasal oxytocin treatment for autistic individuals with social deficits, some have hypothesized that similar approaches may have long-lasting benefits in ACC patients. This approach remains to be formally tested.

SEPTOOPTIC DYSPLASIA

The constellation of symptoms that comprise septooptic dysplasia (SOD) is presumed to result from failure of formation of the optic nerves, septum pellucidum, pituitary gland, and all midline structures within the prosencephalon (Fig. 26-8). Patients typically present with pituitary hormone abnormalities that can result in hypoglycemia or microphallus at birth or growth failure and other endocrine manifestations throughout childhood. It is a rare condition, with an estimated incidence of 1 to 10 in 100,000; known genetic etiologies contribute to only a small percentage of cases. Also, data suggest that young maternal age contributes to the risk of developing SOD. SOD is better viewed as a complex (SOD complex), with variable etiology and clinical presentation.

Definition and Subtypes

There are three cardinal features of SOD: optic nerve hypoplasia, pituitary abnormalities, and midline brain defects (involving primarily the septum pellucidum and, at times, the corpus callosum). The diagnosis of SOD is typically made when two of the three features are present; however, given the heterogeneity intrinsic to this constellation of symptoms, most investigators have initiated their analysis by ascertaining patients with optic nerve hypoplasia (ONH) and then grouping those that had both pituitary dysfunction and absence of the septum pellucidum. From a clinical perspective, those that had ONH and pituitary anomalies but a normal septum pellucidum will have similar management issues. In contrast, those that have ONH and an absent septum pellucidum without pituitary abnormalities often have other brain malformations and likely represent a separate group.

Etiology

SOD and ONH have been associated with primiparous birth and young maternal age. Additional risk factors that have been consistently reported include maternal smoking and low socioeconomic status. Two genes were initially found in association with SOD, the homeobox gene, HESX1, and the transcription factor gene, SOX2. Chromosomal changes also have rarely been reported in SOD cases. More recently, data suggested an overlap between Kallmann syndrome and SOD. Thus most patients with SOD are hypothesized to result from a combination of genetic and environmental factors, recognizing that other mechanisms are yet to be discovered.

Clinical Manifestations

SOD can present at birth with manifestations of pituitary insufficiency, including hypoglycemia, hypogonadotropic hypogonadism, and midline birth defects, including cleft lip and palate, as well as other brain malformations such as a thin corpus callosum. SOD patients are also at risk for adrenocorticotropic hormone, thyroid-stimulating hormone, and growth hormone deficiency. As with HPE and ACC, many patients with SOD have developmental delay and cerebral palsy.

Management

Symptom management is essential in individuals with SOD, and careful attention should be paid to the heterogeneity of this complex disorder. Any child presenting with nystagmus should be evaluated for optic nerve involvement, and if ONH is detected, the patient should be assessed for anterior pituitary hormone deficiency. Additionally, many children with SOD can have developmental delay and seizures and should be evaluated for these possible concerns. Because children are at risk for adrenocorticotropic hormone, thyroid-stimulating hormone, and growth hormone deficiency (as well as hypothalamic dysfunction and poor production of the posterior pituitary hormones, antidiuretic hormone and oxytocin), they can present with hypoglycemia, diabetes insipidus, and poor thermoregulation. Multiple case reports of sudden death in SOD patients have described these complications (Kauvar and Muenke, 2010).

REFERENCES

The complete list of references for this chapter is available in the e-book at www.expertconsult.com.
 See inside cover for registration details.

SELECTED REFERENCES

Glass, H.C., Shaw, G.M., Ma, C., et al., 2008. Agenesis of the corpus callosum in California 1983–2003: a population-based study. Am. J. Med. Genet. A 146A (19), 2495–2500.

Hetts, S.W., Sherr, E.H., Chao, S., et al., 2006. Anomalies of the corpus callosum: an MR analysis of the phenotypic spectrum of associated malformations. AJR Am. J. Roentgenol. 187 (5), 1343–1348.

Kauvar, E.F., Muenke, M., 2010. Holoprosencephaly: recommendations for diagnosis and management. Curr. Opin. Pediatr. 22 (6), 687–695.

Roessler, E., Muenke, M., 2010. The molecular genetics of holoprosencephaly. Am. J. Med. Genet. C Semin. Med. Genet. 154C (1), 52–61.

Sajan, S.A., Fernandez, L., Nieh, S.E., et al., 2013. Both rare and de novo copy number variants are prevalent in agenesis of the corpus callosum but not in cerebellar hypoplasia or polymicrogyria. PLoS Genet. 9 (10), e1003823.

Schaefer, G.B., Bodensteiner, J.B., Buehler, B.A., et al., 1997. The neuroimaging findings in Sotos syndrome. Am. J. Med. Genet. 68 (4), 462–465.

Snijders Blok, L., Madsen, E., Juusola, J., et al., 2015. Mutations in DDX3X Are a Common Cause of Unexplained Intellectual Disability with Gender-Specific Effects on Wnt Signaling. Am. J. Hum. Genet. 97 (2), 343–352.

✪ E-BOOK FIGURES AND TABLES

27 Disorders of Cerebellar and Brainstem Development

Dan Doherty and Andrea Poretti

An expanded version of this chapter is available on www.expertconsult.com. See inside cover for registration details.

INTRODUCTION

Advances in brain imaging, neuropathology, clinical phenotyping, genetics, and developmental biology have markedly improved the diagnosis of patients with structural disorders of the cerebellum and brainstem (SDCB) (Barkovich et al., 2009; Doherty et al., 2013; Robinson et al., 2014). It is now possible to recognize dozens of specific conditions by their clinical and imaging features, facilitating the identification of genetic and environmental (nongenetic) causes (Table 27-1).

SDCB include malformations (genetic) and disruptions (acquired due to prenatal infection, hemorrhage, or ischemia). The differentiation between a malformation (genetic) and a disruption (acquired) implies a huge difference in the recurrence risk with implications for genetic counseling and family planning (Poretti et al., 2009). The majority of disruptions are acquired lesions without recurrence risk; however, a genetic predisposition to disruptive lesions may be present in some cases, such as dominant mutations in *COL4A1*.

In addition to specifying recurrence risk, precise diagnosis is essential for providing accurate prognostic information and guiding surveillance for associated medical issues, supportive therapies, genetic testing, and emerging gene-specific therapies. Furthermore, a specific diagnosis can relieve parental guilt and allow families affected by rare disorders to connect with each other for support.

CLINICAL FEATURES

The clinical features of SDCB are usually nonspecific and include hypotonia, motor delay, ataxia, and abnormal eye movements (Table 27-2). Cognitive impairment is common, but the range is broad (Bolduc et al., 2011). Although characteristic clinical features help identify patients with posterior fossa abnormalities, clinical features point to a specific diagnosis only in a minority (e.g., "figure-of-eight" head-shaking pattern for rhombencephalosynapsis). In the majority of patients, identifying the final diagnosis requires integration of history, clinical examination, neuroimaging, and laboratory testing.

APPROACH TO NEUROIMAGING

Magnetic resonance imaging (MRI) is the neuroimaging tool of choice (Jissendi-Tchofo et al., 2015). Evaluation in multiple imaging planes and familiarity with the normal age-dependent anatomy of the pediatric mid-hindbrain is essential (Table 27-3).

Advanced neuroimaging techniques may be useful in selected cases. Susceptibility-weighted imaging (SWI) is highly sensitive for blood products and calcifications and is helpful in disruptive lesions. ^{1}H-MR spectroscopy can be useful in the diagnosis of mitochondrial and other metabolic disorders. Diffusion tensor imaging (DTI) provides information about the microarchitecture of cerebellar structures, the course of cerebellar white matter tracts, and their connections with other brain structures. In addition, DTI may reveal new diseases due to axon guidance defects that are not detectable by conventional structural MRI. Functional MRI (task-based and resting state) remains largely a research tool but shows promise for improving diagnostic specificity, guiding treatment, and monitoring treatment response.

APPROACH TO GENETIC TESTING

Given the incredible advances in sequencing technologies and other methods for identifying mutations across the entire genome, clinical genetic testing is very much a moving target. The different SDCB can be caused by large chromosome abnormalities, as well as recessive and dominant simple nucleotide variants. The importance of *de novo* and mosaic dominant mutations has only recently been appreciated. Repeat expansion has only been described in the spinocerebellar ataxias (rare in children), and imprinting defects have not been shown to cause SDCB.

DISORDERS PRIMARILY AFFECTING CEREBELLUM

Cerebellar Hypoplasias Primarily Affecting Vermis

Dandy-Walker Malformation

Clinical characteristics: Dandy-Walker malformation (DWM, OMIM 220200) is the most prevalent human cerebellar malformation (about 1 in 30,000 live births). The majority of children present prenatally or during the first year. Macrocephaly affects 90% to 100% of children during infancy. The outcome is variable and at least one third of patients have normal cognitive function, but the risk of abnormal neurodevelopmental outcome is increased in patients with extra-CNS abnormalities.

Differential diagnosis and evaluation: The diagnosis of DWM is based on the neuroimaging findings: 1) hypoplasia and anticlockwise rotation of the cerebellar vermis on sagittal view; and 2) cystic dilation of the fourth ventricle, filling nearly the entire posterior fossa. In most patients, the tentorium is elevated, the posterior fossa is enlarged, and the cerebellar hemispheres are hypoplastic and splayed. Frequently, hydrocephalus is also present, whereas brainstem hypoplasia and other malformations (e.g., callosal dysgenesis and migrational abnormalities) are less common. Abnormal vermian lobulation and additional brain malformations may be associated with poorer cognitive outcome.

Additional terms such as "Dandy-Walker variant," "Dandy-Walker complex," or "Dandy-Walker spectrum" have been variably used to refer to related constellations of imaging findings. If full criteria for DWM are not met, a detailed anatomic description (e.g., inferior cerebellar vermis hypoplasia or global CH) should be used, and nonspecific terms such as Dandy-Walker variant should be abandoned.

DWM can be distinguished from other posterior fossa cystic malformations through detailed neuroimaging assessment. Blake's pouch cyst (BPC) is characterized by an infraretrocerebellar cyst that communicates with an enlarged fourth

TABLE 27-1 Typical Clinical, Imaging, and Genetic Characteristics of Midbrain and Hindbrain Malformations Involving the Cerebellum

Disease	Clinical Features	Neuroimaging Features	Causes (genes)	Inheritance
DISORDERS PRIMARILY AFFECTING THE CEREBELLUM				
Dandy-Walker malformation	Macrocephaly common, variable intellectual disability, systemic involvement possible	Hypoplastic upwardly rotated vermis, fourth ventricle dilatation, large posterior fossa, hydrocephalus	ZIC1, ZIC4, FOXC1, FGF17, LAMC1, NID1 (rare), most unknown	Sporadic (recurrence risk <5%)
Joubert syndrome	Hypotonia, ataxia, alternating apnea and tachypnea (improves with age), intellectual disability, retinal dystrophy, coloboma, nephronophthisis, liver fibrosis, polydactyly	Molar tooth sign, vermis hypoplasia, encephalocele (rare), foramen magnum cephalocele (occasional), anterior midbrain and dorsal medulla heterotopia (occasional), polymicrogyria, agenesis of the corpus callosum (rare)	More than 30 genes including AHI1, ARL13B, C2CD3, C5ORF42, CC2D2A, CEP41, CEP290, HYLS1, INPP5E, KIAA0586, KIF7, MKS1, NPHP1, NPHP4, OFD1, RPGRIP1L, TCTN1, TCTN2, TCTN3, TMEM67, TMEM138, TMEM216, TMEM237	AR, X-linked (OFD1 only)
Rhombencephalosynapsis	Alopecia, trigeminal anesthesia (GLH), head shaking (figure-of-eight pattern), hyperactivity and impulsivity, VACTERL features (<50%), variable ataxia, variable cognitive function	Continuity of cerebellar hemispheres, absence of the cerebellar vermis, absent septum pellucidum, aqueductal stenosis, fused colliculi, holoprosencephaly (rare), absent olfactory bulbs (<50%)	Unknown	Sporadic
X-linked intellectual disability with cerebellar hypoplasia	Moderate intellectual disability	Mild vermis hypoplasia, mild cerebellar hemisphere hypoplasia, variable ventriculomegaly	OPHN1	X-linked
Oculocerebrocutaneous syndrome	Orbital cysts, microphthalmia or anophthalmia, focal skin defects and appendages	Severely hypoplastic vermis, normal or hypoplastic cerebellar hemispheres, enlarged dysplastic tectum, thick, vertical superior cerebellar peduncles, agenesis of the corpus callosum, frontal polymicrogyria	Unknown	Sporadic
Unilateral cerebellar hypoplasia	Developmental and speech delay, hypotonia, ataxia, abnormal ocular movements, variable cognitive outcome, segmental head and neck hemangioma in PHACE syndrome	Hypoplasia of one cerebellar hemisphere, vermis may be involved, affected hemisphere may be dysplastic, variable volume of the posterior fossa, brainstem asymmetry, supratentorial disruptive lesions possible	Prenatal hemorrhage	Sporadic
Cerebellar hyperplasia	Highly variable features of Alexander disease, fucosidosis, Sotos syndrome, Williams syndrome, Costello syndrome, MCAP syndrome, MPPH syndrome	Large cerebellum, cerebellum wrapped around brainstem	Genes for associated disorders	Various depending on specific disorder
GPR56-related bilateral frontoparietal polymicrogyria	Seizures, moderate-severe intellectual disability, ataxia	Frontoparietal or generalized polymicrogyria, patchy or diffuse white matter signal changes, cerebellar dysplasia with cerebellar cysts	GPR56	AR
Chudley-McCullough syndrome	Hearing loss, mild or no ataxia, mild neurodevelopmental impairment	Cerebellar hemisphere dysplasia, inferior cerebellar vermis hypoplasia, partial agenesis of the corpus callosum, frontal subcortical heterotopia, frontal polymicrogyria, arachnoid cysts	GPSM2	AR
Poretti-Boltshauser syndrome	Ataxia, ocular motor apraxia, strabismus, speech delay, intellectual disability, high myopia, non-progressive retinal dystrophy	Cerebellar dysplasia with cysts (may be absent), vermis hypoplasia, abnormal configuration of the fourth ventricle	LAMA1	AR

TABLE 27-1 Typical Clinical, Imaging, and Genetic Characteristics of Midbrain and Hindbrain Malformations Involving the Cerebellum *(Continued)*

Disease	Clinical Features	Neuroimaging Features	Causes (genes)	Inheritance
PHACE syndrome	Segmental hemangioma (usually head and neck), intracranial and great vessel abnormalities, variable intellectual disability in <50% of patients (usually mild)	Unilateral cerebellar hypoplasia with or without vermis involvement, Dandy-Walker malformation, dysmorphic or absent major vessels, occasional heterotopia, polymicrogyria	Unknown	Sporadic
Lissencephaly-related midbrain and hindbrain malformations	Spasticity, seizures, severe cognitive impairment in patients with *RELN* mutations, broad range of cognitive outcomes in patients with tubulinopathies and *ARX* mutations	Heterogeneous: pachygyria with mildly thickened cortex (*RELN*); variable spectrum, lissencephaly with moderately thick cortex (more severe posteriorly), small or absent basal ganglia, agenesis of the corpus callosum, small pons with normal cerebellum (*ARX*); highly variable range of polymicrogyria to lissencephaly, enlarged tectum, dysmorphic basal ganglia, thin or absent corpus callosum (tubulinopathies)	*RELN, ARX, TUBA1A, TUBB2B, TUBB3*	AR (*RELN*), X-linked (*ARX*), de novo AD (*TUBA1A, TUBB2B, TUBB3*)
DISORDERS AFFECTING CEREBELLUM AND BRAINSTEM				
VLDLR-related cerebellar hypoplasia	Ataxia, moderate-severe intellectual disability, quadripedal locomotion in some patients	Cerebellar hypoplasia with decreased foliation (vermis more severe than hemispheres), pontine hypoplasia, simplified cortical gyral pattern	*VLDLR*	AR
Pontocerebellar hypoplasia type 1	Spinal muscular atrophy	Hypoplastic pons, proportional hypoplasia of vermis and hemispheres	*EXOSC3, VRK1, RARS2*	AR
TSEN-related pontocerebellar hypoplasia (types 2, 4, and 5)	Neonatal encephalopathy, severe progressive microcephaly, increased tone, dyskinesia, seizures, cortical visual impairment, usually severe intellectual disability	Postmigrational microcephaly, small pons and cerebellum, seemingly atrophic cortex, thin corpus callosum, vermis less hypoplastic than hemispheres (dragonfly appearance)	*TSEN54, TSEN2, TSEN34*	AR
Pontocerebellar hypoplasia type 6	Increased lactate concentration in CSF	Small pons and cerebellum, vermis more severely hypoplastic than hemispheres	*RARS2*	AR
CASK-related pontocerebellar hypoplasia	Typically female (rarely male), progressive microcephaly, variable hearing loss, intellectual disability	Small pons and cerebellum (can be mild), proportionate cerebellar vermis and hemisphere hypoplasia	*CASK*	X-linked
CHMP1A-related pontocerebellar hypoplasia	Acquired microcephaly, increased extremity tone and contractures, moderate-severe intellectual disability	Small pons and cerebellum, proportionate vermis and hemisphere hypoplasia	*CHMP1A*	AR
Congenital disorders of glycosylation type 1a	Abnormal fat distribution, retinitis pigmentosa, failure to thrive, increased transaminase, coagulopathy, hypothyroidism, hypogonadism, seizures, stroke-like episodes, ataxia, mild-severe intellectual disability	Pontocerebellar hypoplasia with progressive atrophy, T2-hyperintense cerebellar cortex and cortical atrophy in some patients	*PMM2*	AR
Dystroglycanopathies (Walker-Warburg syndrome, muscle-eye-brain disease, Fukuyama muscular dystrophy)	Seizures, severe intellectual disability, eye involvement (cataracts, coloboma, high myopia), muscle involvement (weakness, contractures, variably increased creatine kinase)	Kinked brainstem, large tectum, cerebellar hypoplasia, subcortical cerebellar cysts, cobblestone cortex, abnormal myelination, ventriculomegaly	15 genes including *POMT, POMGnT1, FKRP, POMT1, POMT2, FKTN, LARGE, ISPD, GTDC2*	AR

Continued on following page

TABLE 27-1 Typical Clinical, Imaging, and Genetic Characteristics of Midbrain and Hindbrain Malformations Involving the Cerebellum *(Continued)*

Disease	Clinical Features	Neuroimaging Features	Causes (genes)	Inheritance
Pontine tegmental cap dysplasia	Hearing loss, trigeminal anesthesia, corneal scarring, dysphagia, variable cardiac, vertebral, and rib defects, substantial ataxia, moderate-severe intellectual disability	Hypoplastic pons, mildly hypoplastic cerebellum, cap of white matter on dorsum of pons, hypoplastic middle and inferior cerebellar peduncles	Unknown	Sporadic
Cerebellar agenesis	Ataxia, dysarthria, hypotonia, variable degree of intellectual disability, neonatal diabetes mellitus (*PTF1A* mutation)	Small to absent cerebellum, small pons	Variable, including malformations (*PTF1A* mutation) and prenatal disruptions	Variable, AR (*PTF1A* mutation) or sporadic
DISORDERS PRIMARILY AFFECTING THE BRAINSTEM				
Brainstem disconnection	Absent or weak suck and swallowing, central respiratory insufficiency, increased or decreased muscle tone, poor visual fixation, seizures, unstable body temperature	Nearly complete absence of a brainstem segment with intact rostral and caudal portions connected only by a thin cord of tissue, cerebellar hypoplasia, basilar artery may be absent	Unknown	Sporadic

AD, autosomal dominant; AR, autosomal recessive; CSF, cerebrospinal fluid; GLH, Gómez-López-Hernández syndrome; MCAP, megalencephaly capillary malformation-polymicrogyria; MPPH, megalencephaly polydactyly polymicrogyria-hydrocephalus; PHACE, posterior fossa brain malformations, hemangioma, arterial lesions, cardiac defects, and eye abnormalities; VACTERL, vertebral defects, anal atresia, cardiac defects, tracheo-oesophageal fistula, renal defects, and limb defects.

(Modified with permission from Doherty. D., Millen, K.J., Barkovich, A.J., 2013. Midbrain and hindbrain malformations: advances in clinical diagnosis, imaging, and genetics. Lancet Neurology 12(4), 381–93. PMID: 23518331; PMCID: PMC4158743.)

TABLE 27-3 Role of the MRI Planes for the Evaluation of Cerebellar Hypoplasia

MRI Planes	Key Points
Coronal	1. Excellent overview of vermis and hemispheres (severity of vermis vs. hemispheric involvement, hemispheric asymmetry). 2. Normally, cerebellar fissures radiate from the cerebellar nuclei to the surface. 3. The orientation and curvature of the cerebellar fissures is abnormal in cerebellar dysplasia.
Sagittal	1. Assess vermis, brainstem and fourth ventricle morphology, posterior fossa size, and supratentorial midline structures. 2. The dorsal margin of the brainstem should be almost straight. 3. The fastigium of the fourth ventricle should be just below the midpoint of the ventral pons. 4. The rostrocaudal height of the vermis should be almost equal to the distance from the caudal tectum to the obex. 5. In cerebellar hypoplasia, the fastigium is upwardly displaced and the rostrocaudal height of the vermis is reduced. 6. Major vermis fissures are less prominent or absent in rhombencephalosynapsis.
Axial	1. Assess the morphology of vermis and hemispheres. 2. Essential to assess the supratentorial structures. 3. Normally, the cerebellar fissures have an "onion-like" orientation parallel to the calvarium.

(Modified with permission from Poretti, A., Boltshauser, E., Doherty, D., 2014. Cerebellar hypoplasia: differential diagnosis and diagnostic approach. Am J Med Genet C Semin Med Genet 166C(2), 211–26. PMID: 24839100.)

ventricle. A normal cerebellar vermis differentiates BPC from DWM, whereas an enlarged fourth ventricle differentiates BPC from arachnoid cysts and mega cisterna magna (MCM). Arachnoid cysts do not communicate with the fourth ventricle and may cause obstructive hydrocephalus. MCM is an enlarged cisterna magna with otherwise normal vermis, fourth ventricle, and posterior fossa.

Pathophysiology: In most patients, the cause of DWM remains unknown; however, DWM may occur as part of a Mendelian syndrome (e.g., Ritscher-Schinzel or Ellis-van Creveld syndromes), aneuploidies (e.g., trisomy 9, 13, 18), or other chromosome abnormalities. In small subsets of patients, mutations in *ZIC1*, *ZIC4*, *FOXC1*, *FGF17*, *LAMC1*, and *NID1* have been identified. The function of these genes suggests that DWM may result from defects in the interaction between the developing cerebellum and the surrounding mesenchyme. DWM occurs mostly sporadically and overall the recurrence risk is low (1% to 5%); however, in a given family with a specific genetic disorder, the recurrence risk may be substantially higher.

Management: Correction of hydrocephalus is the main treatment in DWM. Considerable debate still exists regarding the best CSF diversion strategy. Options include shunt placement and endoscopic third ventriculostomy with or without choroid plexus cauterization.

Joubert Syndrome

Joubert syndrome (JS) was first described in 1969, and the pathognomonic "molar tooth sign" was identified in 1997 (Romani et al., 2013). We favor using the terms JS or Molar Tooth Malformation disorder for all patients who have the molar tooth malformation (MTM) and describing any additional features present in each patient.

Clinical characteristics: Patients with JS are often identified prenatally with vermis hypoplasia and diagnosed with DWM or DWV. After birth, hypotonia is uniformly present, whereas the characteristic abnormal breathing pattern (episodes of tachypnea followed by apnea) and abnormal eye movements (ocular motor apraxia) are common. Ataxia develops later, and intellectual disability of varying degrees is present in the majority of the patients. Polydactyly, cystic or echogenic kidneys, chorioretinal coloboma, encephalocele, and other features are less common but can be helpful clues to the diagnosis.

Differential diagnosis and evaluation: The MTM on brain MRI is pathognomonic, comprising vermis hypoplasia, long, thick and horizontally oriented superior cerebellar peduncles (SCP), and a deep interpeduncular fossa; however, the components of the MTM can be present without an obvious molar tooth appearance on MRI due to the plane of section (Fig. 27-1). In addition, superior cerebellar dysplasia is often present and can be very helpful for diagnosis. Patients may also have other brain abnormalities, including polymicrogyria, agenesis of the corpus callosum, as well as cortical and brainstem heterotopia (Fig. 27-1D).

Other disorders associated with neonatal hypotonia (Prader Willi syndrome, spinal muscular atrophy, myopathies) or cerebellar ataxia can be distinguished from JS by the features listed previously when they are present. Polydactyly, retinal dystrophy, cystic kidney disease, and liver fibrosis result in clinical overlap with other ciliopathies. Infrequently, mildly affected patients can also present with "isolated" ocular motor apraxia or retinal dystrophy.

Pathophysiology: The distinctive MTM imaging phenotype has facilitated the identification of mutations in more than 30 genes, all of which encode proteins that function in and around a subcellular organelle called the primary cilium. Primary cilia are membrane-enclosed microtubule-based "antennae" that project from most cells. They are decorated with receptor proteins that detect light, mechanical, and chemical inputs, including ligands for sonic hedgehog, G-protein coupled receptor, and other signaling pathways. Based on these diverse functions in many cell types, the wide variety of phenotypes observed in JS patients is not surprising.

Management: Diagnosing JS is essential because of the progressive retinal, kidney, and liver involvement. Identifying the genetic cause facilitates prognostic and reproductive counseling, and guides the frequency of medical monitoring. Early diagnosis of extra-CNS involvement ensures early treatment to avoid secondary complications such as anemia, malnutrition, osteoporosis, and catastrophic gastrointestinal bleeding. Many patients have sleep disordered breathing, requiring careful monitoring and in some cases tonsillectomy and adenoidectomy or positive airway pressure support during sleep.

Global CH with Involvement of Both Vermis and Hemispheres

Global CH refers to involvement of both vermis and cerebellar hemispheres (Poretti et al., 2014). The clinical and neuroimaging findings associated with CH may suggest a specific disease (such as prenatal infection or neurometabolic disease) or help to plan further investigations and interpret their results (Table 27-4). Chromosome array and whole-exome sequencing are indicated if dysmorphic signs or other features suggest a genetic disorder.

Global CH may be the neuroimaging feature of nonprogressive cerebellar ataxia (NPCA). Patients present with hypotonia and motor and language delays that often evolve into ataxia and intellectual disability. The brain MRI may be normal or reveal widened interfolial spaces, giving the impression of cerebellar atrophy. An increasing number of genes (e.g., *CA8*, *ZNF592*, *WDR81*, *ATP8A2*, and *WWOX*) have been associated with NPCA.

Unilateral Cerebellar Hypoplasia

Unilateral cerebellar hypoplasia (UCH) ranges from complete aplasia to mild asymmetry in cerebellar hemisphere size. UCH may be an incidental finding or occur in patients with developmental delay and cerebellar signs. Generally, UCH represents a residual change after a disruptive prenatal cerebellar insult, most likely a hemorrhage, so recurrence is rare. The role for thrombophilia workup in these patients is controversial but should be considered. UCH is the most common posterior fossa feature of PHACE(S) (OMIM 606519), usually associated with an abnormal ipsilateral internal carotid artery.

Cerebellar Atrophy

Cerebellar atrophy (CA) is defined as enlarged fissures (interfolial spaces) in comparison to the folia (Poretti et al., 2008). This pattern implies loss of cerebellar parenchyma caused by a progressive disease or a single severe insult (infection or toxic exposure). Distinguishing CA from CH can be problematic or impossible based on a single imaging study. In addition, atrophy can be superimposed on hypoplasia, as documented in pontocerebellar hypoplasia and congenital disorders of glycosylation type 1a.

Typically, CA is more pronounced in the vermis, but the cerebellar hemispheres can be more affected in some pontocerebellar hypoplasias and extremely premature infants. In contrast to prenatal-onset conditions, the pons is preserved in CA.

A pattern-recognition approach based on neuroimaging findings (Table 27-5) may allow the diagnosis in some patients, whereas CA can be isolated or associated with other infratentorial or supratentorial findings such as hypomyelination, progressive white matter abnormalities (e.g., diffuse, multifocal, with cerebellar, brainstem, or periventricular predominance), involvement of the basal ganglia (e.g., calcifications, atrophy, and signal changes), signal changes of the dentate nuclei, and hyperintense T2-signal in the cerebellar cortex (Fig. 27-2).

Cerebellar Dysplasias

Cerebellar dysplasia is defined by abnormal cerebellar foliation, white matter arborization, and gray-white matter junction. For specific diagnosis, it is important to determine the pattern of dysplasia, whether cysts are present, and whether the patient has other clinical features (Table 27-6). Diagnosing cerebellar dysplasia is important because most of the genetic causes are autosomal recessive with 25% recurrence risk.

Clinical Characteristics: The clinical presentation of cerebellar dysplasia is similar to other SDCB, although frequently more subtle.

Differential diagnosis and evaluation: Cerebellar dysplasia disorders have distinguishing features such as frequent seizures, polymicrogyria, and white matter signal changes (Fig. 27-3A) with *GPR56* mutations (OMIM 606854), high myopia, retinal abnormalities, and cerebellar cysts (Fig. 27-3B), without cortical involvement or elevated creatine kinase in Poretti-Boltshauser syndrome (OMIM 615960), and sensorineural hearing loss, partial or complete callosal agenesis, frontal subcortical heterotopia, and frontal polymicrogyria (Fig. 27-3C) in Chudley-McCullough syndrome (OMIM 604213).

Pathophysiology: Multiple mechanisms underlie cerebellar dysplasia including abnormal precursor cell division and neuronal migration. In particular, the α-dystroglycanopathies, Poretti-Boltshauser syndrome (*LAMA1* mutations), and

GPR56-associated cerebellar dysplasia are thought to be due to basement membrane defects that result in abnormal neuronal migration. Chudley-McCullough syndrome is caused by recessive mutations in *GPSM2*, which encodes a GTPase regulator needed for correct orientation of stem cell division.

Management: As with other diagnostic categories, patients with cerebellar dysplasia disorders should be monitored for associated medical issues. This is most pertinent to patients with JS as described previously, Poretti-Boltshauser syndrome (high myopia and abnormal retinal development), and Chudley-McCullough syndrome (sensorineural hearing loss).

Cerebellar Hyperplasia and Chiari Type I Malformation

Cerebellar Hyperplasia

Cerebellar hyperplasia (macrocerebellum) is rare and characterized by excessive cerebellar volume with preserved shape. The cerebellar hemispheres are usually more affected than the vermis and may expand into adjacent anatomic regions by wrapping around the brainstem.

Clinical characteristics: Ataxia, hypotonia, intellectual disability, and ocular movement disorders are common, but other clinical features depend on the underlying disease.

Differential diagnosis and evaluation: Macrocerebellum may be isolated or part of well-defined syndromes (e.g., Costello, Sotos, Proteus, megalencephaly syndromes) or neurometabolic diseases (e.g., fucosidosis, Alexander disease, and mucopolysaccharidoses).

Pathophysiology: Macrocerebellum is not a nosologic entity but represents the shared structural manifestation resulting from a variety of biological disturbances. The recurrence risk depends on the underlying disorder but is low in children with isolated macrocerebellum.

Management: Treatment depends on the underlying disease. In isolated, idiopathic macrocerebellum, treatment is symptomatic.

Chiari I Malformation

Clinical characteristics: Chiari I malformation (CIM) is defined by ectopia/herniation of at least one cerebellar tonsil 5 mm or more below the foramen magnum, although this can be seen in a substantial number of asymptomatic individuals. Children may present with a variety of symptoms ranging from headache to severe myelopathy and brainstem dysfunction. Headache affects approximately 80% of patients and is usually occipital in location and induced or exacerbated by Valsalva maneuvers. Other common symptoms include neck pain, weakness, numbness, and loss of temperature sensation. Ocular (e.g., downbeat nystagmus) and otological signs and symptoms are reported in approximately 70% of patients. Lower cranial nerve dysfunction (e.g., dysphagia and stridor) is typical in children younger than 3 years of age. Progressive scoliosis associated with syringohydromyelia is relatively common.

Differential diagnosis and evaluation: CIM is diagnosed by measuring the position of the cerebellar tonsils relative to the line from the basion to the opisthion on midsagittal images. Tonsillar herniation has been shown to be larger than 5mm in more than 90% of symptomatic children (Fig. 27-4). Tonsillar compression, increased movement of the brainstem and tonsils due to abnormal CSF pulsation, effaced cerebrospinal fluid (CSF) spaces, and decreased flow at the foramen magnum may help identify symptomatic patients. Syringohydromyelia occurs in 30% to 70% of patients and should be assessed by spine MRI. CIM is also seen in a subset of patients

with rhombencephalosynapsis, requiring specific evaluation of imaging for this malformation.

Pathophysiology: Pediatric CIM is due to a mismatch between the size of the cerebellum and posterior fossa, that may result from abnormal skull base (e.g. short clivus) or premature closure of cranial sutures such as in Crouzon syndrome.

Management: Surgical decompression is the only effective therapeutic approach for CIM and is usually offered if syringohydromyelia, severe characteristic headache, or bulbar symptoms are present. Hydrocephalus should be resolved before decompression is considered. Minimal tonsillar herniation, lack of objective neurologic findings, and mild headache support a conservative approach.

Rhombencephalosynapsis

Rhombencephalosynapsis (RES) is defined by continuity of the cerebellar hemispheres across the midline with partial or complete absence of the cerebellar vermis (Fig. 27-5).

Clinical characteristics: Patients with RES most often present with ventriculomegaly, hydrocephalus, motor delays, and/or ataxia during childhood. Side-to-side or figure-of-eight headshaking, typical facial features (flat midface, prominent forehead, hypertelorism, low set, posteriorly rotated ears), congenital scalp alopecia, towering skull shape, trigeminal anesthesia, and short stature can be clues to the diagnosis. RES can be also associated with features of VACTERL association (vertebral anomalies, anal atresia, cardiac malformations, tracheoesophageal fistula, renal anomalies, and limb defects) or an unusual form of posterior holoprosencephaly. The triad of RES, trigeminal anesthesia, and congenital scalp alopecia, often with abnormal towering head shape, has been named Gómez-López-Hernández syndrome.

Differential diagnosis and evaluation: When not immediately recognized, RES should be suspected in patients with ventriculomegaly and a small cerebellum, aqueductal stenosis, or CIM.

Pathophysiology: RES is sporadic, and no genetic causes have been identified; therefore, the recurrence risk is considered to be very low. Disruption of dorsal-ventral patterning is a proposed mechanism underlying RES; however, no animal model has been identified, limiting the understanding of underlying mechanisms.

Management: Once diagnosed, patients should be evaluated for the features described above, particularly hydrocephalus and trigeminal anesthesia, which can result in blindness from corneal scarring. Evaluation for cardiac and renal abnormalities is also indicated. ADHD symptoms and behavioral issues can be challenging and may respond atypically to medications.

DISORDERS AFFECTING CEREBELLUM AND BRAINSTEM
Pontocerebellar Hypoplasias

The term pontocerebellar hypoplasia (PCH) can be used descriptively for reduced volume of both cerebellum and pons; however, PCH has also been used as a diagnostic category, encompassing numbered subtypes with clinical and genetic overlap (Fig. 27-6 and Table 27-1).

Clinical characteristics: Patients with PCH can present prenatally with polyhydramnios, microcephaly, ventriculomegaly, or posterior fossa fluid collection, or in the newborn period with abnormal tone, poor feeding, respiratory difficulties, or seizures. Many patients have severe neurodevelopmental disability, with a few notable exceptions. Congenital or postnatal microcephaly is common. Anterior horn cell

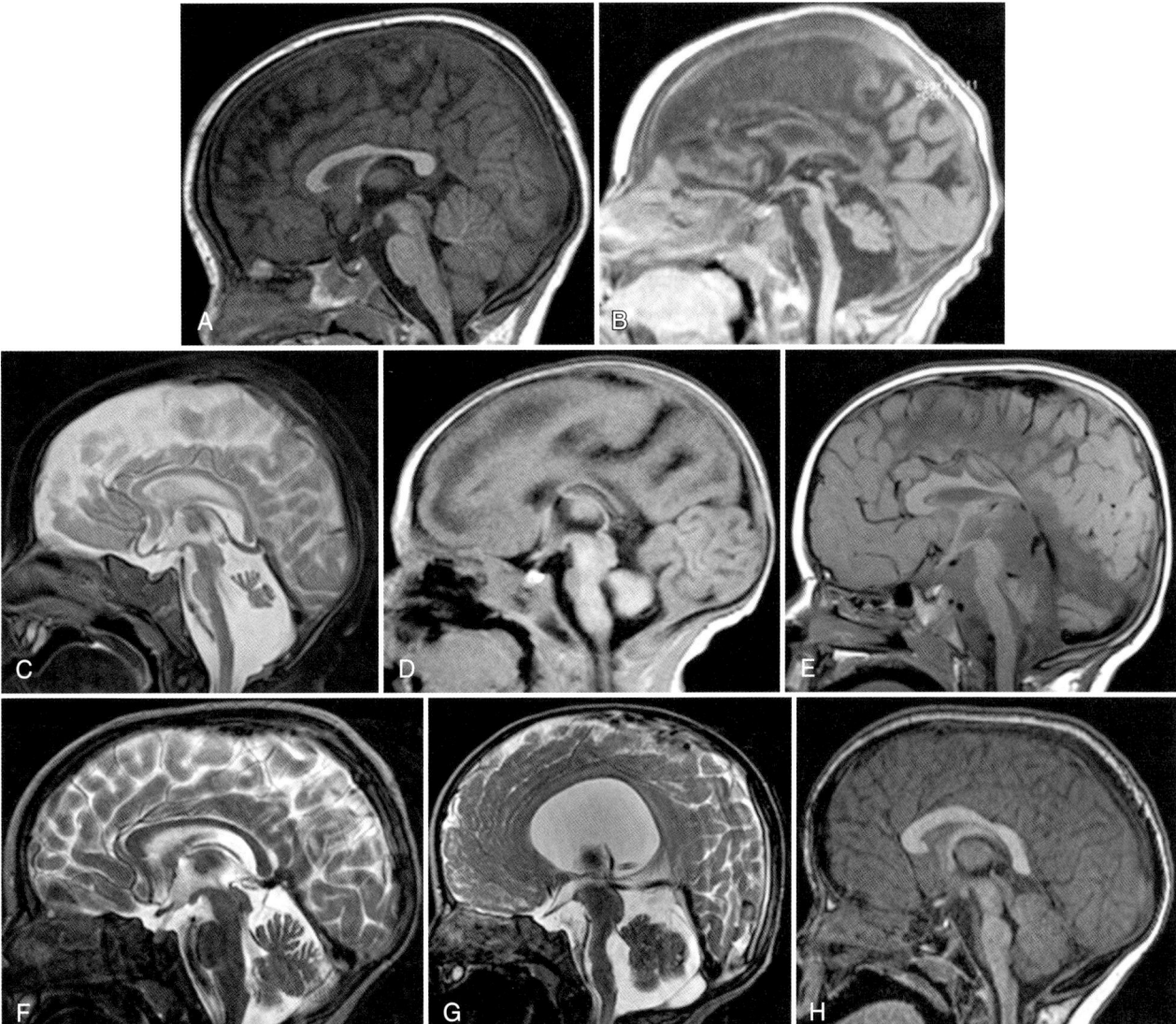

Figure 27-6. Pontocerebellar hypoplasias. A, Midsagittal T1-weighted image of a 6-year-old girl with headache shows normal morphology of the brainstem and cerebellum. **B,** Midsagittal T1-weighted image of a 1-year-old child with postnatal progressive microcephaly, dyskinetic movement disorders, and mutations in *TSEN54* reveals hypoplasia of the pons and cerebellar vermis, as well as a thin corpus callosum and cortical atrophy. **C,** Midsagittal T2-weighted image of a 2.5-year-old girl with developmental delay, seizures, and *CASK* mutation reveals hypoplasia of the pons and cerebellar vermis. **D,** Midsagittal T1-weighted image of an infant with hypotonia and severe developmental delay due to *RELN* mutations reveals hypoplasia of the pons and cerebellar vermis, unfoliated vermis, thickened and simplified gyral pattern in the frontal and parietal lobes, and more normal gyral pattern of the occipital lobe. **E,** Midsagittal T1-weighted image of a 3-year-old boy born at 25 weeks of gestation reveals a small posterior fossa, small cerebellar vermis, small pons, and thin corpus callosum. **F,** Midsagittal T2-weighted image of a 9-month-old girl with congenital disorder of glycosylation type 1a, developmental delay, microcephaly, strabismus, nystagmus, increased liver enzymes, and *PMM2* mutations reveals cerebellar atrophy that is more prominent in the anterior part of the vermis. **G,** Midsagittal T2-weighted image of a 5-month-old child with muscle-eye-brain disease and *POMGnT1* mutations, who presented with developmental delay, seizures, and proximal weakness. Cerebellar hypoplasia, flattening of ventral pons, dysmorphic tectum and midbrain, abnormally concave dorsal brainstem, enlarged fourth ventricle, and supratentorial ventriculomegaly are apparent. **H,** Midsagittal T1-weighted image of a 3-year-old girl with pontine tegmental cap dysplasia, sensorineural hearing loss, and global developmental delay, reveals a flat ventral pons, a cap protruding from the dorsal pons into the fourth ventricle, and mild vermis hypoplasia. *(**A** and **B,** With permission from Lee, R.W., et al. A diagnostic approach for cerebral palsy in the genomic era. Neuromolecular Med 2014;16(4):821–44. **C,** Courtesy of Prof. Dr. Eugen Boltshauser, University Children's Hospital of Zurich, Switzerland. **D,** Courtesy of Prof. Dr. William B. Dobyns, Seattle Children's Research Institute, Seattle, WA. **E,** With permission from Poretti, A., et al, Cerebellar hypoplasia: differential diagnosis and diagnostic approach. Am J Med Genet C Semin Med Genet 2014;166(2):211–26. **F,** Courtesy of Prof. Dr. Eugen Boltshauser, University Children's Hospital of Zurich, Switzerland. **G,** With permission from Poretti A et al, Cerebellar hypoplasia: differential diagnosis and diagnostic approach. Am J Med Genet C Semin Med Genet 2014;166(2):211–26). **H,** With permission from Poretti A et al, Cerebellar hypoplasia: differential diagnosis and diagnostic approach. Am J Med Genet C Semin Med Genet 2014;166(2):211–26.)*

involvement with weakness and areflexia favors *EXOSC3* and *VRK164* mutations. Increased CSF lactate suggests *RARS2* mutations, whereas sensorineural hearing loss in girls suggests X-linked *CASK* mutations.

Differential diagnosis and evaluation: PCHs are difficult to distinguish by neuroimaging features alone, and mutations in the same gene have been reported in different numbered PCH types; therefore, we favor referring to the PCHs by the associated gene rather than by number. A relatively preserved vermis compared with hemispheres ("dragonfly pattern" on coronal view) is typically associated with mutations in *TSEN54*. Simplified cortical gyral pattern and vermis without folia are characteristic features of *RELN-* and *VLDLR*-related PCHs.

PCH may be also seen in patients with tubulinopathies, α-dystroglycanopathies, congenital disorders of glycosylation type 1, and pontine tegmental cap dysplasia, as well as with severe prematurity.

Pathophysiology: Multiple mechanisms lead to the appearance of PCH on imaging. The *TSEN* and *RARS2* genes are involved in tRNA production, and the rapidly developing hindbrain may be particularly sensitive to the resulting impaired protein synthesis. *CASK*, *RELN*, and *VLDLR* (a coreceptor for the RELN pathway) may function with *TBR1* to regulate cerebellar neuronal migration and lamination.

Management: Patients with PCH are particularly prone to feeding problems, seizures, and tone abnormalities. As yet, PCH-specific treatments have not been developed.

Congenital Muscular Dystrophies Due to Defective α-Dystroglycan Glycosylation

The "α-dystroglycanopathies" are a group of congenital muscular dystrophies.

Clinical characteristics: The phenotype is characterized by muscle (weakness, hypotonia, and increased CK), brain (intellectual disability, seizures, and tetraspasticity), and eye (microphthalmia, chorioretinal coloboma, cataract, glaucoma, or high myopia) involvement. Based on the severity of the findings, overlapping phenotypes have been described including Fukuyama disease, muscle-eye-brain disease, and Walker-Warburg syndrome.

Differential diagnosis and evaluation: Neuroimaging findings may include PCH, cerebellar dysplasia with cysts, dysplastic tectum, pontomesencephalic kinking, ventriculomegaly, white matter signal changes, and cobblestone cortex. The diagnosis can be confirmed by muscle biopsy and genetic testing.

Pathophysiology: Mutations in 15 genes responsible for the O- and rarely N-glycosylation of α-dystroglycan, an extracellular protein required for basement membrane integrity without which neurons overmigrate, have been associated with α-dystroglycanopathies.

Management: Treatment is symptomatic.

Tubulinopathies

Tubulinopathies are a recently reported group of brain malformations caused by mutations in tubulin genes (Bahi-Buisson et al., 2014).

Clinical characteristics: The clinical phenotype is wide and includes variable intellectual disability, spastic cerebral palsy, postnatal microcephaly, and early onset of therapy resistant seizures. Dysmorphic features are rare, and other organs are not affected.

Differential diagnosis and evaluation: Neuroimaging findings include malformations of cortical development (lissencephaly and polymicrogyria), dysmorphic basal ganglia with abnormal anterior limb of the internal capsule, ventriculomegaly, agenesis/dysgenesis of the corpus callosum and anterior commissure, PCH, and dysplasia of the cerebellum, tectum, and brainstem.

Pathophysiology: Tubulinopathies are caused by mutations in neuron-expressed tubulin genes (*TUBA1A, TUBA8, TUBB2B, TUBB3,* and *TUBB5*). The majority of mutations are *de novo*, but germline mosaicism and autosomal recessive inheritance have been observed.

Management: Treatment is symptomatic.

Pontine Tegmental Cap Dysplasia

Clinical characteristics: Pontine tegmental cap dysplasia (PTCD, OMIM 614688) is sporadic and characterized by bilateral sensorineural deafness, trigeminal anesthesia, facial paralysis, and difficulty swallowing. Ataxia, nystagmus, developmental delay, and intellectual disability are ubiquitous. Trigeminal anesthesia can result in corneal scarring with severe visual impairment. Vertebral segmentation anomalies, rib malformations, congenital heart defects, and cyclic vomiting have been reported.

Differential diagnosis and evaluation: Diagnosis is based on a flattened ventral pons, abnormal transverse white matter ("cap") on the pontine tegmentum, very thin middle cerebellar peduncles (MCP), and absent inferior cerebellar peduncles. Hypoplastic or absent facial and cochlear nerves and duplicated internal auditory canals may be present.

Pathophysiology: The (presumed genetic) cause of PTCD is unknown, and the lack of familial recurrence supports *de novo* dominant or complex causes. The absent transverse pontine fibers and SCP decussation, ectopic transverse fibers on the dorsal pons, and ectopic prepontine arcuate fibers are highly suggestive of an underlying axon guidance defect.

Management: Treatment is symptomatic. Based on limited experience, the prognosis for cochlear implantation is poor. Keratoplasty may be considered for corneal opacities, but due to the lack of sensation, corneal transplantation should be approached with caution.

Cerebellar Agenesis

Cerebellar agenesis implies near complete absence of cerebellar structures; pontine hypoplasia is consistently present. The diagnosis is made by neuroimaging showing only a tiny remnant of cerebellar tissue that likely corresponds to the MCPs, anterior vermian lobules, or flocculi. Cerebellar agenesis may be due to a primary malformation (mostly *PTF1A* mutation) or a disruption. Symptoms include ataxia, dysarthria, hypotonia, and variable cognitive impairment. A small subset of patients with myelomeningocele has cerebellar agenesis thought to be due to vascular insufficiency associated with Chiari II malformation.

DISORDERS PRIMARILY AFFECTING BRAINSTEM
Horizontal Gaze Palsy and Progressive Scoliosis

Clinical characteristics: Horizontal gaze palsy and progressive scoliosis (HGPPS, OMIM 607313) is an autosomal recessive disorder characterized by congenital absence of horizontal eye movements, preservation of vertical gaze, and progressive scoliosis.

Differential diagnosis and evaluation: The diagnosis is based on characteristic neuroimaging findings including a "butterfly"-shaped medulla and a dorsal midline pontine cleft. DTI typically shows absence decussation of the corticospinal tracts, pontine sensory tracts, and SCP.

Pathophysiology: HGPPS is caused by mutations in *ROBO3*, which encodes a receptor required for axonal guidance.

Management: Scoliosis progresses when children begin to walk and almost all patients require early surgical correction.

Brainstem Disconnection

Brainstem disconnection (BD) is defined by nearly complete absence of a brainstem segment with intact rostral and caudal portions connected only by a thin cord of tissue.

Clinical characteristics: All children are symptomatic at birth, with absent or weak suck and swallowing, central respiratory insufficiency, increased or decreased muscle tone, and reduced visual fixation. Seizures and unstable body temperature may also occur. The majority of children die before 2 months of age and do not achieve any developmental milestones. Extracerebral involvement (congenital cardiac abnormalities, hydronephrosis, and vertebral body anomalies) may occur.

Differential diagnosis and evaluation: The diagnosis is based on the characteristic neuroimaging findings, and the basilar artery is absent in most patients. Supratentorial abnormalities are unusual.

Pathophysiology: The pathogenesis is unknown. Both malformative and disruptive pathomechanisms have been proposed.

Management: Parents should be counseled about the grave prognosis in clear lay terms and given a range of treatment options including comfort care. Invasive treatments should be carefully considered and offered with caution because they will not improve brain function and may not improve quality of life.

Other Disorders with Predominantly Brainstem Involvement

Athabascan brainstem dysgenesis syndrome (ABDS, OMIM 601536) and Bosley-Salih-Alorainy syndrome (BSAS, OMIM 601536) are brainstem patterning disorders with normal brain MRI caused by loss of *HOXA1* function. In mouse models, *HOXA1* is needed for correct specification of hindbrain rhombomeres 4 and 5, as well as inner ear and heart development. ABDS and BSAS share the same phenotype including cranial nerve palsies, sensorineural hearing loss, abnormal intracranial blood vessels, and cardiac outflow tract defects.

CHN1-related Duane retraction syndrome (OMIM 604356), *SALL4*-related Duane radial ray syndrome (OMIM 607323), and congenital fibrosis of the extraocular muscles types 1 to 3 (OMIM 135700, 602078, 600638, 609384) caused by mutations in *KIF21A*, *PHOX2A*, *TUBB3*, and *TUBB2B* are other cranial dysinnervation disorders characterized by abnormal eye movements.

Moebius syndrome (OMIM 157900) is mostly sporadic and defined by the combination of congenital nonprogressive abducens and facial nerve palsies. It is a heterogeneous disorder presumably caused by malformative and disruptive etiologies and has been associated with prenatal exposure to misoprostol.

REFERENCES

The complete list of references for this chapter is available in the e-book at www.expertconsult.com.
See inside cover for registration details.

SELECTED REFERENCES

Bahi-Buisson, N., Poirier, K., Fourniol, F., et al., 2014. The wide spectrum of tubulinopathies: what are the key features for the diagnosis? Brain 137 (Pt 6), 1676–1700.

Barkovich, A.J., Millen, K.J., Dobyns, W.B., 2009. A developmental and genetic classification for midbrain-hindbrain malformations. Brain 132 (Pt 12), 3199–3230.

Bolduc, M.E., Du Plessis, A.J., Sullivan, N., et al., 2011. Spectrum of neurodevelopmental disabilities in children with cerebellar malformations. Dev. Med. Child Neurol. 53 (5), 409–416.

Doherty, D., Millen, K.J., Barkovich, A.J., 2013. Midbrain and hindbrain malformations: advances in clinical diagnosis, imaging, and genetics. Lancet Neurol. 12 (4), 381–393.

Jissendi-Tchofo, P., Severino, M., Nguema-Edzang, B., et al., 2015. Update on neuroimaging phenotypes of mid-hindbrain malformations. Neuroradiology 57 (2), 113–138.

Poretti, A., Wolf, N.I., Boltshauser, E., 2008. Differential diagnosis of cerebellar atrophy in childhood. Eur. J. Paediatr. Neurol. 12 (3), 155–167.

Poretti, A., Prayer, D., Boltshauser, E., 2009. Morphological spectrum of prenatal cerebellar disruptions. Eur. J. Paediatr. Neurol. 13 (5), 397–407.

Poretti, A., Boltshauser, E., Doherty, D., 2014. Cerebellar hypoplasia: Differential diagnosis and diagnostic approach. Am. J. Med. Genet. C Semin. Med. Genet. 166 (2), 211–226.

Robinson, A.J., 2014. Inferior vermian hypoplasia—preconception, misconception. Ultrasound Obstet. Gynecol. 43 (2), 123–136.

Romani, M., Micalizzi, A., Valente, E.M., 2013. Joubert syndrome: congenital cerebellar ataxia with the molar tooth. Lancet Neurol. 12 (9), 894–905.

E-BOOK FIGURES AND TABLES

28 Disorders of Brain Size

Ghayda M. Mirzaa and William B. Dobyns

INTRODUCTION

Disorders of abnormal brain size—microcephaly (too small) and macrocephaly (too large)—are very common or relatively common disorders. Microcephaly and macrocephaly are traditionally defined as head circumference—or more formally "occipitofrontal circumference" (OFC)—two or more standard deviations (SD) lower than or higher than the mean for age and gender, respectively. However, this criterion includes many developmentally normal individuals and a host of underlying causes. Researchers studying both usually define severe microcephaly or macrocephaly as OFC 3 SD or 4 SD (or more) lower than or higher than the mean, respectively. In this chapter, microcephaly, and megalencephaly will be discussed separately.

MICROCEPHALY

Microcephaly (MIC) refers to a cranium significantly smaller than the standard for the individual's age and sex. It is considered a neurologic sign rather than a disorder per se, as it may result from many different causes that affect several stages of brain development, and occurs in isolation as well as in association with other features in numerous genetic syndromes (Ashwal et al., 2009). Approximately 1% of referrals to child neurologists are specifically for evaluation of microcephaly, and approximately 15% of children referred to child neurologists for evaluation of developmental disabilities have MIC.

Historically, a confusing plethora of terms have been used to describe and classify various types of microcephaly. When severe congenital microcephaly is seen without other major brain or somatic malformations, the term *primary microcephaly* has been used in the literature. However, primary microcephaly is not a distinct etiologic category in and of itself, but rather a term that describes an increasingly broad group of disorders, many with etiologies not yet well understood. The most clinically useful classification of microcephaly from the clinical and molecular diagnostic perspectives is by age of onset into *congenital* and *postnatal onset* microcephaly. Table 28-1 summarizes the common disorders associated with these two groups of microcephaly.

Advances in neuroimaging and molecular genetic technologies, particularly the increasing use of next generation sequencing (NGS), have resulted in dramatically better understanding of the types and causes of microcephaly, suggesting that a reappraisal of schemes for classification and diagnostic testing is warranted. NGS methods in particular, including whole exome sequencing, have uncovered a large number of novel genes associated with microcephaly (Alcantara and O'Driscoll, 2014).

Pathology

Microcephaly broadly results from decreased neuronal proliferation or increased programmed cell death (apoptosis). However, the pathologic changes described in various types of microcephaly are diverse, which is not surprising given the genetic heterogeneity of microcephaly and large number of associated conditions. This section is confined to the description to severe congenital microcephaly. The macroscopic changes described in most pathologic reports include a very small cerebral volume, normal or minimally altered pattern of convolutions, and normal size of the third and lateral ventricles. However, our brain imaging experience shows that this is not consistently true as in many forms the frontal lobes are disproportionately small, and the number and complexity of the gyral pattern and the depth of sulci are generally reduced. The microscopic changes, especially involving the cerebral cortex, are also heterogeneous.

In one group, the cortex has normal thickness and lamination, but the number of neurons is dramatically reduced. In several other types of microcephaly, the cortex appears abnormally thin, presumably resulting from premature exhaustion of the germinal zone (Barkovich et al., 1992). In the latter, abnormalities of cellular architecture predominate in the first two layers of the cortex, referred to as "type I familial microcephaly." Layer 2 is almost devoid of granule neurons and may be fragmented into small nests (sometimes called "glomeruli") or small columns that protrude into the molecular layer. In a few individuals, the vertical bands of neurons arising in layer 2 cross the molecular layer to protrude into the meninges. Neurons may be seen in the molecular layer, either as scattered large pyramidal or stellate neurons, or as persistence of a fetal monolayer of granule neurons found just beneath the pia. The lower cortical layers are less affected but have abnormal distribution of cells in some areas. In some brains, persistence of fetal wavy or "combed" monocellular bands in the middle of the cortex has been seen. In these types of microcephaly, the cerebellum is typically small but proportionate to the reduced size of the cerebrum or relatively larger.

Severe congenital microcephaly has been observed with several other types of brain malformations including holoprosencephaly, disproportionate brainstem and cerebellar hypoplasia, abnormalities of neuronal migration including true lissencephaly, periventricular nodular heterotopia, and polymicrogyria (Table 28-2). Agenesis of the corpus callosum is commonly seen in different types of microcephaly. We therefore suspect that it is a nonspecific feature of decreased brain growth in most individuals, as the growing cerebral hemispheres must be apposed closely enough for the precallosal sling to cross the gap, which requires growth. We have therefore not included microcephaly and agenesis of the corpus callosum as a category in its own right, although this may need to be added in the future as our delineation and classification of microcephaly syndromes evolve.

Neuroimaging

In most patients with isolated congenital microcephaly, brain magnetic resonance imaging (MRI) reveals characteristic abnormalities that are collectively designated "microcephaly with simplified gyral pattern" (Basel-Vanagaite and Dobyns,

2010). This pattern consists of a reduced number of gyri separated by abnormally shallow sulci. Commonly associated abnormalities include foreshortened frontal lobes, mildly enlarged lateral ventricles, and a thin corpus callosum or even partial agenesis of the corpus callosum in some individuals. Although interpretation of brain imaging studies in microcephaly would seem straightforward, this has proved challenging in clinical practice, primarily for severe congenital microcephaly, due to a number of factors. First, brain MRI scans of children with microcephaly are often interpreted as normal other than for the small size. However, close inspection of MRI scans will invariably show some of the features noted previously. Although these changes can be subtle, they are not normal and can be of diagnostic importance. Further, brain imaging in individuals with more severe forms of microcephaly may show fewer convolutions, some broader than 2 cm, leading to the misinterpretation of "pachygyria." But imaging in the large majority of these patients shows a normal or thin cortex, whereas true lissencephaly (agyria and pachygyria) is always associated with an abnormally thick cortex. In these situations, misdiagnoses may result as clinicians often respond to such reports by ordering tests for lissencephaly disorders (such as LIS1 gene analysis, for example), which are almost always negative. There are few disorders that are associated with true microlissencephaly, including the tubulinopathies (such as the TUBA1A-related disorders, for example) and NDE1-related microcephaly.

Whereas most of the genes associated with severe congenital microcephaly are associated with nonspecific brain imaging patterns that can be collectively grouped under the category of microcephaly with simplified gyral pattern, there are numerous microcephaly syndromes associated with recognizable patterns of abnormalities. These additional abnormalities can be broadly divided into the following groups: (1) microcephaly with simplified gyri and pontocerebellar hypoplasia; (2) microcephaly with simplified gyri and enlarged extraaxial space; (3) microcephaly with simplified gyri and both pontocerebellar hypoplasia and enlarged extraaxial space; and (4) microcephaly with additional cortical malformations. Table 28-3, lists the most common genetic causes of various forms of microcephaly.

Clinical Features

The clinical manifestations associated with microcephaly are heterogeneous, partly depending on the underlying cause. Most individuals with severe congenital microcephaly have an obviously small head, often with a low, sloping forehead and a flat occiput. The face and ears are normal but may appear disproportionately large due to small head size. Intellectual disability is moderate in some types but severe to profound in others. In moderately affected patients, hyperactivity may dominate the patient's behavior even though tone is typically normal. In severely affected children, spasticity, and epilepsy predominate. In children with milder forms of syndromic microcephaly, a variety of dysmorphic features may be present and may be helpful in identifying a specific underlying syndrome.

Cognitive impairment and intellectual disability. A correlation between microcephaly and intellectual disability (ID) has been recognized since studies in the late 1800s and subsequent research has explored the strength of this correlation in a number of ways, although rarely in a prospective manner among a broad cohort of subjects. The incidence of microcephaly has varied in studies depending on the population studied. Prevalence estimates of microcephaly in institutionalized patients reported a rate of microcephaly from 6.5% to 53%. In contrast, the prevalence of microcephaly

in children seen in neurodevelopmental clinics averaged 24.7% (range 6%-40.4%). Other studies have looked at the incidence and significance of microcephaly in children who were functioning normally or had normal intelligence. One report of 1006 students in mainstream classrooms found that 1.9% had mild (2 to 3 SD lower than the mean) and none had severe microcephaly (greater than 3 SD lower than the mean). The microcephalic subjects had similar mean IQ (99.5) to the normocephalic group (105) but lower mean academic achievement scores (49 versus 70). Another report looking at the records of 1775 normally intelligent patients aged 11 to 21 years followed in adolescent medicine clinics found 11 (0.6%) with severe microcephaly (greater than 3 SD lower than the mean).

Numerous studies underscore the fact that microcephaly is common in developmentally delayed children with the incidence greater in those with more severe ID. Even in low risk populations (e.g., children with normal school placement), 1.9% has microcephaly and in many of these children, subtle cognitive deficits are detected. In addition, there is a 50% increased risk for being developmentally delayed in children with microcephaly compared with children without microcephaly (e.g., 15.3% versus 7%) and a strong correlation between the severity of microcephaly and developmental outcome (i.e., ID occurs in 10.5% of children with mild microcephaly (less than 2 SD) and in 51.2% of children with severe microcephaly (greater than 3 SD lower than the mean). Given these observations, serial developmental screening should be performed in children with microcephaly.

Epilepsy. The relation between microcephaly and epilepsy is of great clinical importance: (a) the incidence of epilepsy is much higher in microcephalic children; (b) a greater number of children with epilepsy are likely to be microcephalic; (c) microcephaly is a significant risk factor for medically refractory epilepsy; and (d) the presence of microcephaly (whether congenital or postnatal) may help determine the underlying etiology of a child's epilepsy.

One study involving 66 microcephalic children (greater than 2 SD lower than the mean) found an overall prevalence of epilepsy of 40.9%. It has also been suggested that epilepsy is more common in postnatal onset than in congenital microcephaly. In one study, epilepsy occurred in 50% of children with postnatal compared with only 35.7% with congenital microcephaly. Microcephaly also is a significant risk factor for medically refractory epilepsy.

In one study of 30 children, microcephaly was found in 58% of those with medically refractory epilepsy compared with 2% in whom seizures were well controlled.

Although children with microcephaly are generally at greater risk for epilepsy, many do not have epilepsy. There are, however, certain microcephaly syndromes in which epilepsy is a prominent feature (Table 28-4). Knowledge of these disorders and their genetic basis can help establish a diagnosis and determine prognosis.

Overall, it is important to be aware that epilepsy is more common in children with microcephaly and when it occurs, it is more difficult to treat. Certain microcephaly syndromes are associated with a much higher incidence of epilepsy. Increasingly, genetic etiologies defining the relation between microcephaly and epilepsy are being identified. In addition, there are no systematic studies regarding EEG findings in children with microcephaly who have or do not have epilepsy.

Ophthalmologic abnormalities. Limited studies have surveyed the incidence of vision loss or specific ophthalmologic disorders in children with microcephaly. One study found an incidence of 145 cases of congenital eye malformations (microphthalmia, anophthalmia, cataracts, coloboma, etc.) in 212,479 consecutive births. Microcephaly was among the malformations in 56% of these children. Another study of 360 children with severe microcephaly (greater than 3 SD lower than the mean) found eye abnormalities in 6.4% but in only 0.2% of 3600 age-matched normocephalic controls. Other reported eye abnormalities in microcephalic children include anophthalmia-microphthalmia, blindness or visual loss, cataracts, colobomas, nystagmus, optic atrophy, ptosis, and retinal disorders. Table 28-5 lists some of the more common microcephaly syndromes associated with ophthalmologic involvement.

Audiological abnormalities. No studies have surveyed the incidence of hearing loss or audiological disorders in children with microcephaly broadly. One study of 100 children with complex ear anomalies reported that 85 had neurologic involvement and 13 children were microcephalic. Hearing loss is likely the most common audiological disorder associated with microcephaly. Table 28-6 summarizes the most common microcephaly syndromes listed in OMIM in which prominent audiological involvement is reported.

Etiology

Mild MIC, which we define as OFC 2 to 3 SD lower than the mean, is associated with a variety of maternal and other prenatal disorders, prenatal and postnatal brain injuries, familial forms, chromosomal disorders, and numerous genetic syndromes. Among the chromosomal disorders, the most commonly associated with microcephaly are trisomies (trisomies 13, 18, and 21) and structural rearrangements such as Cri du Chat syndrome (deletion 5p15). For most individuals, this presents as mild congenital microcephaly that is often followed by more severe postnatal microcephaly. An OMIM search for "microcephaly" lists more than 400 syndromic associations, making this a nonspecific search term. Among the rapidly growing list of disorders, some of the best known include Angelman syndrome, MECP2-related disorders, and Cornelia de Lange syndrome. Here we will review only a small selection of the more common causes of microcephaly.

Extrinsic causes. Extrinsic (acquired) injuries before birth or early in life can lead to microcephaly. The developing nervous system is highly vulnerable to infections, including cytomegalovirus, toxoplasmosis, rubella, herpes simplex, and group B coxsackievirus. Intrauterine infections of any of these can result in microcephaly (Norman et al., 1995). Most recently, infections of the Zika virus have been reported in association with severe congenital microcephaly in Brazil and other countries in South America.

Maternal metabolic disorders during pregnancy such as diabetes mellitus, uremia, and undiagnosed or inadequately treated phenylketonuria may result in neonatal microcephaly. These complications are now generally seen less frequently due to improved early detection and treatment of these disorders. Malnutrition, hypertension, and placental insufficiency may also result in intrauterine growth retardation and microcephaly.

Maternal alcoholism during pregnancy has also been linked with microcephaly as part of fetal alcohol syndrome (FAS). The clinical features of FAS include growth and mental retardation, midface hypoplasia, short palpebral fissures, epicanthal folds, and behavioral problems. Neuropathologic findings include microcephaly, heterotopia, widespread cortical and white matter dysplasias, and defects of neuronal and glial migration. MIC has also been reported with maternal exposure to cocaine.

Isolated congenital (previously termed "primary") microcephaly. When congenital MIC is the only abnormality on evaluation, the disorder has been designated "primary microcephaly." As discussed previously, this designation becomes much more useful when restricted to children with birth OFC lower than 3 SD. Most patients with primary microcephaly also have mild growth deficiency with statures typically 2 to 3 SD lower than the mean, which may be part of the syndrome or due to nutritional factors. The body growth profile is much less striking than head size, the latter of which is typically 4 to 8 SD lower than the mean after early childhood. Most affected individuals fall into one of two somewhat heterogeneous, clinical subgroups (Dobyns, 2002).

The first group is composed of children with extreme microcephaly but only moderate neurologic problems, usually with only moderate ID and no spasticity or epilepsy. Neonatal examinations are usually normal except for microcephaly, but many children initially have poor feeding and weight gain. They may have normal tone or mild distal spasticity but typically do not have moderate or severe spasticity. Seizures are uncommon and are easily controlled, if present. Febrile seizures occur and should be managed as in any other child. Early development is only mildly delayed and many infants progress to walking between 1 and 2 years of age and develop limited language skills. This group is genetically very heterogenous (Table 28-3).

The second group consists of congenital microcephaly with a severe neurologic phenotype that includes severe spasticity and epilepsy. Neonatal examination demonstrates abnormal neonatal reflexes and generalized spasticity, and these children subsequently develop impaired feeding and recurrent vomiting leading to poor weight gain, profound ID, and severe spastic quadriparesis. Most of these infants have early-onset intractable epilepsy. In addition to a simplified gyral pattern, brain MRI may demonstrate other abnormalities as summarized previously (Fig. 28-1). Children with Amish lethal microcephaly, for example, fall within this group, except that hypotonia predominates rather than spasticity, and seizures are generally not prominent.

The wide clinical spectrum suggests pathogenetically heterogeneous conditions, and several syndromes and genes have been identified (Table 28-3).

Severe microcephaly with cortical brain malformations. Severe microcephaly has been reported in association with several other types of brain malformation. Severe microcephaly and true lissencephaly (with an abnormally thick cortex) have been reported with at least three different patterns The most common of these very rare syndromes is probably the Barth microlissencephaly syndrome, which consists of severe microcephaly, diffuse complete agyria, and severe brainstem and cerebellar hypoplasia. Severe microcephaly with diffuse periventricular nodular heterotopia has been described and clearly differs from other forms of heterotopia. Other subsets of patients with severe microcephaly also have diffuse polymicrogyria.

With the advent of next generation sequencing, a rapidly growing number of syndromes with microcephaly and additional, often severe, brain malformations, are now known such as the tubulin-related disorders and microcephaly with cortical malformations due to mutations of RTTN, WDR62, KATNB1, to name a few.

Severe microcephaly with proportionate growth deficiency. Several syndromes with severe intrauterine and postnatal growth deficiency and proportionate microcephaly have been described, although the head size does not keep up with slow body growth, leading to disproportionate microcephaly in childhood and later on in most affected children. The best known of these disorders are Seckel syndrome, Majewski syndrome, microcephalic osteodysplastic primordial dwarfism type 1 (MOPD1), also known as Taybi-Linder syndrome, and microcephalic osteodysplastic primordial dwarfism type

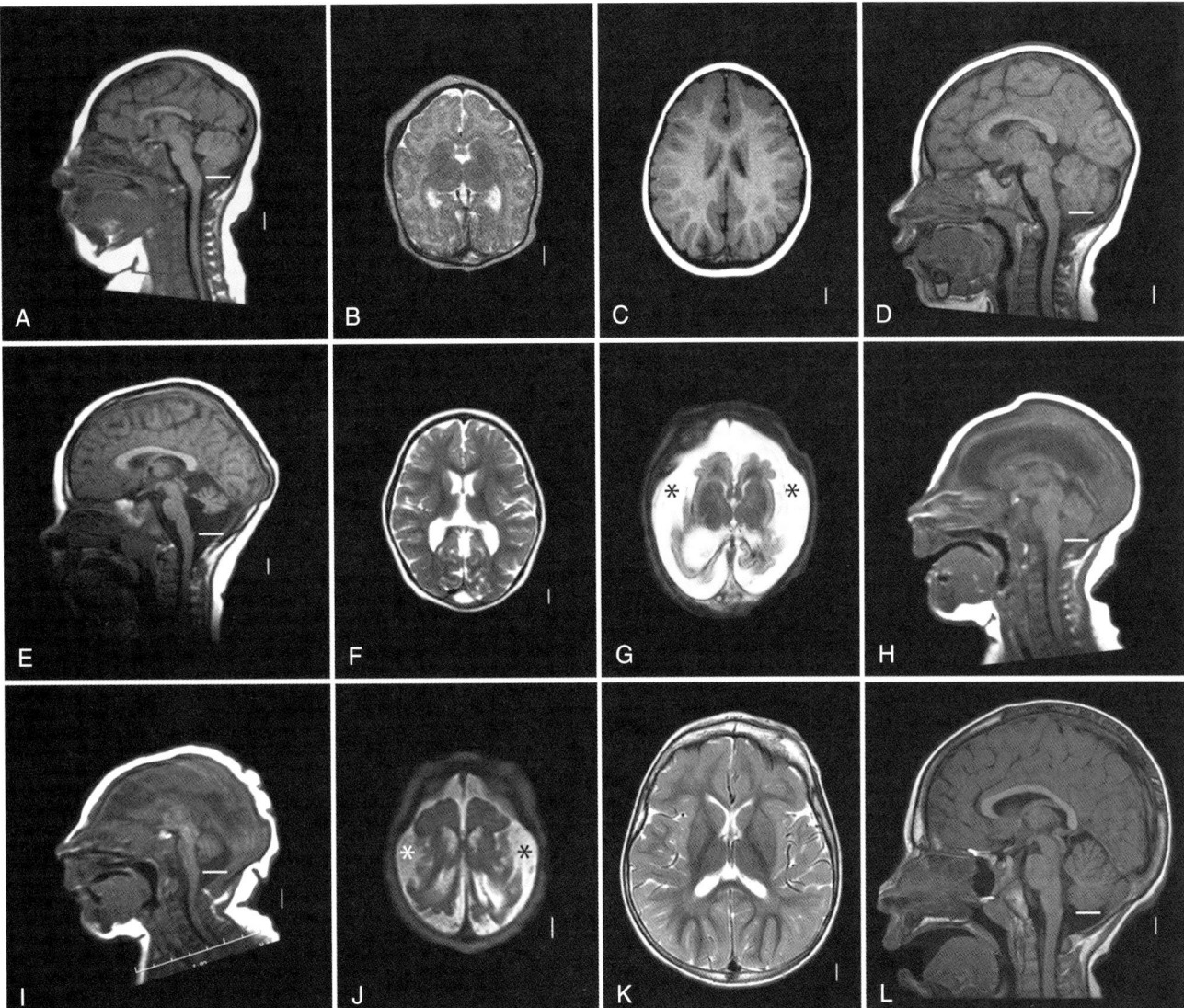

Figure 28-1. Representative magnetic resonance imaging from each microcephaly subgroup. **A–D** Microcephaly with simplified gyral pattern only. **E–F** Microcephaly with simplified gyri and pontocerebellar hypoplasia. **G–H** Microcephaly with simplified gyri and enlarged extraaxial space and proportionate cerebellum. **I–J** Microcephaly with simplifed gyri, enlarged extraaxial space, and marked pontocerebellar hypoplasia. **K–L** Normal brain magnetic resonance images for comparison purposes. *Asterisks* indicate enlarged extraaxial space. *(Adapted from: Basel-Vanagaite, L., Dobyns, W.B., 2010. Clinical and brain imaging heterogeneity of severe microcephaly. Pediatr Neurol 43, 7–16.)*

2 (MOPD2). Several other syndromes with severe growth deficiency and microcephaly have been described in a few patients. In some children, the skeletal changes may be absent or less prominent than in Seckel syndrome or the MOPD syndromes.

Seckel syndrome consists of severe intrauterine and postnatal growth deficiency and abnormal facial features, including large eyes, beaklike protrusion of the nose, narrow face, and receding lower jaw. All affected individuals have severe ID, although severity varies considerably. Abnormalities of the brain seen on postmortem examination or brain imaging demonstrate pure microcephaly with deficient production of neurons and other cell types in some patients, whereas other patients have severe brain malformations including lissencephaly. Some patients have various hematological abnormalities such as pancytopenia or acute myeloid leukemia.

MOPD1, or Taybi-Linder syndrome, consists of similar severe intrauterine and postnatal growth deficiency, combined with abnormal body proportions and short limbs. Typical skeletal changes consist of low and broad pelvis with poor formation of the acetabulum, short and bowed humerus and femur, dislocated hips and elbows, retarded epiphyseal maturation, cleft vertebral arches, platyspondyly, horizontal acetabular roofs, and short long bones with enlarged metaphyses. Patients with MOPD1 may also have skin abnormalities, including hyperkeratosis and sparsity of hair and eyebrows. Brain malformations are common and include lissencephaly, heterotopia, callosal agenesis, and cerebellar vermis hypoplasia.

MOPD2 consists of similar severe intrauterine and postnatal growth deficiency, proportionate microcephaly at birth that progresses to disproportionate microcephaly, shortening of the middle and distal segments of the limbs, progressive bony dysplasia, abnormal facial appearance—including prominent nose and malformed ears—and a high-pitched voice. Patients may have dilated arteries in the brain that resemble aneurysms or moyamoya disease.

Microlissencephaly (MLIS) MOPD1-type. MLIS occurs in some patients with microcephalic osteodysplastic primordial dwarfism type 1 (MOPD1), a syndrome that is difficult to distinguish from severe forms of Seckel syndrome. The phenotype consists of severe prenatal growth deficiency, microcephaly, sparse hair, dry scaling skin, skeletal anomalies such as platyspondyly, slender ribs, short and bowed proximal humeri and femurs, small iliac wings, dysplastic acetabulum and small hands and feet, and profound ID. A few have aplastic anemia, another overlap with Seckel syndrome. The neuropathology consists of a variant form of LIS-3L with frontal predominance.

Genetics

Microcephaly is genetically very heterogeneous, and the rate of identification of novel microcephaly genes has increased dramatically with the advent of clinical next generation sequencing (NGS). The majority of microcephaly genes are key regulators of critical cellular processes, including mitotic spindle assembly and structure, centrosome formation and function, cilia function, and DNA repair and damage response (DDR) pathways. The most common genes are listed in Table 28-3.

Antenatal Diagnosis

Microcephaly can often be diagnosed by second trimester fetal ultrasonography. This is likely due to variable onset of deceleration of head growth. When this occurs early, as it often does in severe microcephaly, ultrasound examination should be able to detect the abnormality but not when it begins in the late second or third trimester. The diagnosis of more complex microcephaly syndromes associated with malformations of cortical development is difficult prenatally, as the resolution of fetal MRI scans is often inadequate to fully delineate the nature and extent of cerebral malformations.

Genetic Counseling

Most forms of severe congenital microcephaly (with or without intrauterine growth retardation [IUGR]) are genetic, and the majority of these disorders are inherited in an autosomal recessive manner, with a 25% recurrence risk. Disorders associated with postnatal microcephaly are much more genetically heterogeneous, with some inherited in de novo/autosomal dominant (familial or sporadic), autosomal recessive, and X-linked inheritance (Table 28-3).

Summary

With potentially hundreds of causes of microcephaly, including prenatal and postnatal onset disorders, as well as genetic and acquired etiologies, diagnostic evaluations of affected children are often complex. Investigations of patients with microcephaly include evaluation for prenatal exposure to teratogens, especially alcohol, drugs, and isotretinoin (a vitamin A analog), assessment of the family history, birth history, and associated malformations. Laboratory studies should include: titers for toxoplasmosis, syphilis, rubella virus, cytomegalovirus, and herpes simplex virus; neuroimaging; evaluation for maternal and childhood metabolic disorders; and genetic testing, including chromosome analysis and testing for small deletions or duplications, followed by single gene disorders. Algorithms for the evaluation of the infant and child with congenital (Fig. 28-2) and postnatal (Fig. 28-3) microcephaly are available to serve as a generalized approach to the diagnostic evaluation.

MEGALENCEPHALY (AND MACROCEPHALY)
Definition and Classification

Macrocephaly is defined as an occipitofrontal circumference (OFC) 2 SD or more higher than the mean for age, gender, and ethnicity measured over the greatest frontal circumference.

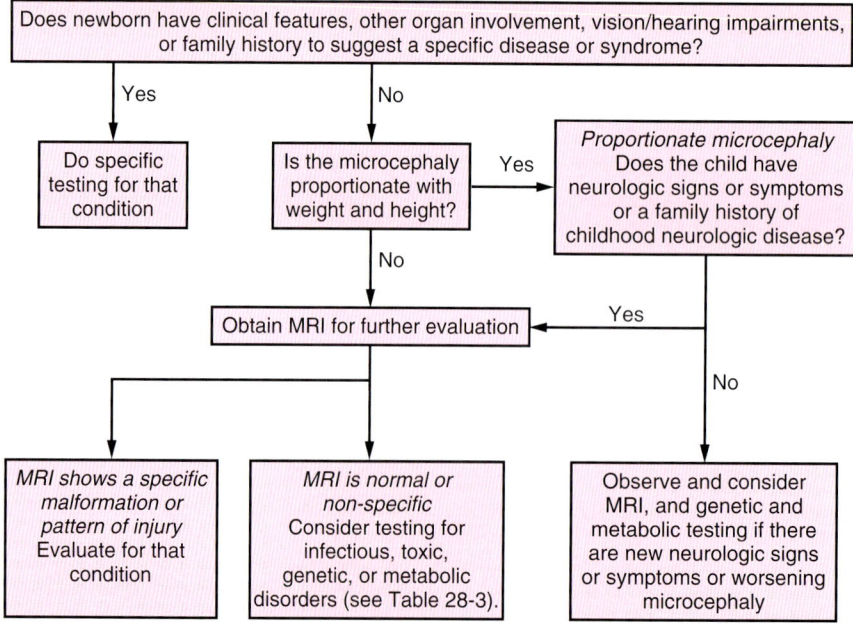

Figure 28-2. Algorithm for the diagnostic evaluation of the infant or child with congenital microcephaly. *(Adapted from: Ashwal, S., Michelson, D., Plawner, L., Dobyns, W.B., 2009. Practice parameter: evaluation of the child with microcephaly (an evidence-based review): report of the Quality Standards Subcommittee of the American Academy of Neurology and the Practice Committee of the Child Neurology Society. Neurology 73, 887–897.)*

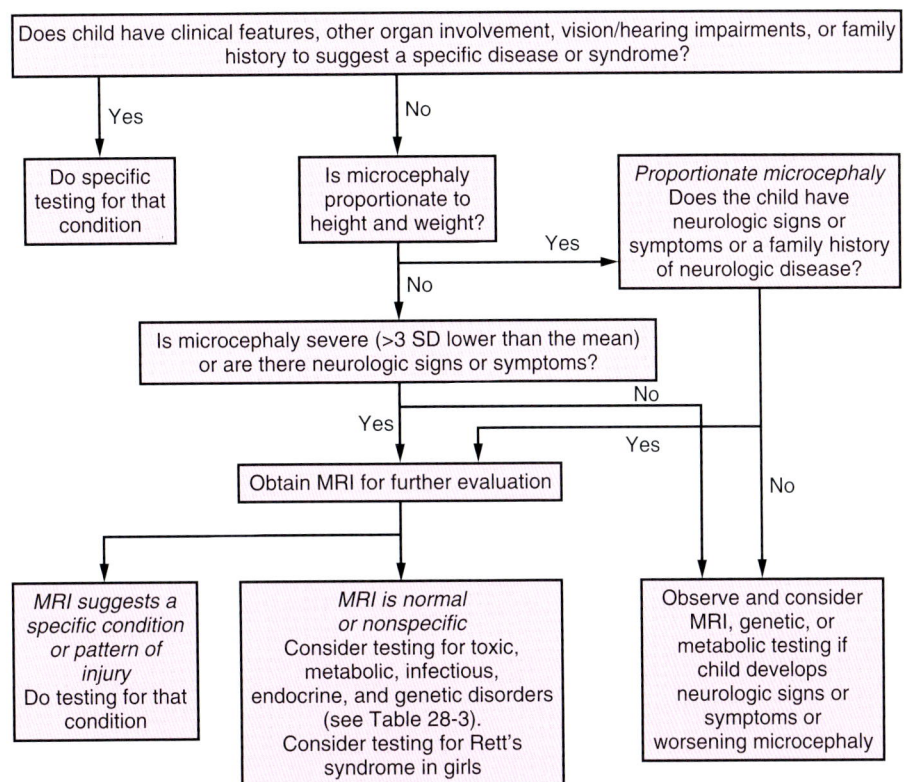

Figure 28-3. Algorithm for the diagnostic evaluation of the infant or child with postnatal onset microcephaly. *(Adapted from: Ashwal, S., Michelson, D., Plawner, L., Dobyns, W.B., 2009. Practice parameter: evaluation of the child with microcephaly (an evidence-based review): report of the Quality Standards Subcommittee of the American Academy of Neurology and the Practice Committee of the Child Neurology Society. Neurology 73, 887–897.)*

Macrocephaly is caused by a myriad of conditions, including hydrocephalus, cerebral edema, space-occupying lesions, subdural fluid collection, thickening or enlargement of the skull (or hyperostosis), and a truly enlarged brain or megalencephaly (Box 28-1). The classic definition of *megalencephaly* first proposed by DeMyer in 1986 stands as an oversized and overweight brain (or an increased brain mass) that exceeds the mean by 2 SD or more for age, gender, and ethnicity.

Megalencephaly is associated with diverse syndromes and etiologies. DeMyer first divided it in 1972 into anatomic and metabolic subtypes. *Metabolic megalencephalies* result from cellular edema or abnormal accumulation of metabolic substrates within the neurons and glia secondary to an underlying biochemical defect (most commonly an enzyme deficiency), without an increase in cell number. The most common causes of metabolic megalencephalies are listed in Table 28-7 and include cerebral organic acid disorders such as Canavan disease, glutaric aciduria type I, lysosomal storage disorders, such generalized gangliosidosis, Tay-Sachs disease, Krabbe disease, some mucopolysaccharidoses, among others. Canavan, Krabbe, Alexander diseases, and megalencephalic leukoencephalopathy with subcortical cysts are leukoencephalopathies—that is, demyelinating disorders whereby the underlying biochemical or genetic defect alters myelin formation and function. The metabolic megalencephalies are not true cortical malformations per se and will therefore not be discussed further in this chapter but are discussed in Chapter 99.

Anatomic megalencephalies, on the other hand, are secondary to an increase in the size or number of cells, or both, and are disorders of neuronal development resulting from either increased neuronal proliferation or failure of programmed cell death, or apoptosis. These disorders are quite numerous and will be the focus of the remainder of this chapter. Anatomic megalencephaly varies by distribution or degree of involvement from diffuse to focal megalencephaly. This latter group includes classic unilateral megalencephaly or hemimegalencephaly (Table 28-8). The presence of true megalencephaly (versus absolute or relative macrocephaly) is indicated in the table. Focal forms of brain overgrowth, including classic hemimegalencephaly, are characterized by segmental brain overgrowth with unique clinical and neuroimaging characteristics and syndromic associations. The recent molecular discoveries of megalencephaly, hemimegalencephaly, and other segmental forms of cortical dysplasia, including focal cortical dysplasia, highlight that these disorders constitute a continuum or spectrum with shared etiologies, as will be discussed later in this chapter.

Pathology and Pathogenesis

Numerous animal models of syndromic and nonsyndromic megalencephaly display neuronal and glial hypertrophy, increased neuronal proliferation, and decreased apoptosis. Most of the animal models and studies of human tissues studying megalencephaly have involved important growth signaling pathways, most prominently the phosphatidylinositol-4,5-bisphosphate-3-kinase (PI3K)-protein kinase B (AKT)-mammalian target of rapamycin (mTOR) pathway (PI3K-AKT-MTOR), and Ras/mitogen-activated protein kinase (MAPK) pathways.

Pten (phosphatase and tensin homolog on chromosome ten) mutant mice were found to develop macrocephaly and behavioral abnormalities reminiscent of human autism spectrum disorders such as reduced social activity, increased anxiety and sporadic seizures. These closely resemble the human phenotype of Pten-related disorders described in this chapter. At the cellular level, in vivo effects of loss of Pten include loss of neuronal polarity, neuronal hypertrophy, and, in one study, increased astrocyte proliferation and hypertrophy.

The mammalian target of rapamycin (mTOR) is a serine/threonine kinase that has well-known functions in regulation of cellular proliferation and growth and crucial roles in neuronal development and synaptic plasticity. It also contributes to Pten-mediated growth regulation in the mammalian nervous system. In studies, mTOR inhibition reversed neuronal hypertrophy in Pten-deficient mice and also resulted in amelioration of a subset of Pten-associated abnormal behaviors, thereby substantiating evidence that the mTOR pathway downstream of Pten is critical for its complex phenotype.

Loss of Tsc1 and Tsc2, two downstream negative regulators of the mTOR pathway, has been shown to cause neuronal hypertrophy in vitro and in vivo, supporting a role of TSC1 and TSC2 in neuronal growth regulation and synaptic function. Interruptions of TSC1 and TSC2 cause tuberous sclerosis complex, known to be associated with megalencephaly, hemimegalencephaly, and focal megalencephaly.

Most recently, studies of other components of the PI3K-AKT-MTOR pathway have been identified in association with megalencephaly, including PIK3CA, PIK3R2, AKT3, and CCND2. CCND2 is one of the D-group of cyclins responsible for regulation the G1-S transition of the cell cycle. In utero electroporation of mutant CCND2 in mouse demonstrated increased proliferation of neuroprogenitor cells, as well as decreased cell cycle exit. A mouse model of an Akt3 gain of function mutation has electrographic seizures and showed abnormal hemispheric architecture. Another recent mouse model of a Pik3ca gain of function mutation demonstrates megalencephaly, hydrocephalus, and increased predisposition to epilepsy. In these animal models, treatment with PI3K-AKT-MTOR pathway inhibitors partially rescued several aspects of the phenotypes, including acutely treating epilepsy in the latter model. Further, the Nf1 knockout mouse was found to have increased neuroglial progenitor/stem cells (NSC) proliferation and gliogenesis in the brainstem, also driven by mTOR-mediated activation. All of these studies and many others clearly implicate aberrations of the PI3K-AKT-MTOR signaling pathway as the most critical mediators of brain growth dysregulation.

Other animal models of megalencephaly include mouse mutants with loss-of-function mutations in genes regulating programmed cell death, or apoptosis, such as Caspase-3, Caspase-9, and Apaf-1, which were found to have gross brain malformations and neuronal hyperplasia. These mutations are embryonically lethal when germline. Transgenic mice overexpressing insulin-like growth factor (IGF-1) exhibit brain overgrowth characterized by increased numbers of neurons and oligodendrocytes, as well as excessive myelin formation. IGF-1 stimulates: (1) proliferation of neural progenitors and possibly pluripotent neural stem cells (NSCs); (2) survival of neurons and oligodendrocytes; and (3) differentiation of neurons, including neuritic outgrowth and synaptogenesis, and of oligodendrocytes, including expression of myelin gene proteins and myelination. As a result of these events, brain growth is increased with IGF-1 overexpression and reduced with decreased IGF-1 signaling. Although much less information is available in man, individuals with IGF1 gene deletions or mutations that result in severe deficits in IGF-1 expression are microcephalic and intellectually disabled.

Etiology

The most common megalencephaly/macrocephaly syndromes are listed in Table 28-8 with a brief overview of their clinical features, MRI findings, and genetic causes. These include classic overgrowth syndromes such as Sotos, Weaver, and Simpson-Golabi-Behmel syndromes, *PTEN*-related disorders, the macrocephaly capillary malformation (MCAP) syndrome, skeletal dysplasias, as well as chromosomal disorders. The majority of these disorders are inherited in a de novo/autosomal dominant fashion. Their clinical features and neurodevelopmental outcome are quite variable and dependent on the ensuing neuronal dysfunction caused by the specific underlying disorder. The most notable megalencephaly/macrocephaly disorders are discussed briefly here.

Overgrowth Syndromes. Macrocephaly frequently occurs in conjunction with body overgrowth (height and weight more than 2 SD higher than the mean for age) as in Sotos, Weaver, and Simpson-Golabi-Behmel syndromes. Many of these overgrowth disorders are characterized by excessive growth in fetal life and infancy with subsequent decline in growth rate and normalization of growth in adulthood. Partial (or focal) and unilateral overgrowth (or hemihypertrophy) is occasionally seen in other megalencephaly syndromes such as MCAP, *PTEN*-related disorders, among others. Children who are macrocephalic at birth may become normocephalic or relatively microcephalic when older if body overgrowth supersedes brain growth, as typically occurs in Beckwith-Wiedemann syndrome.

Sotos syndrome is an autosomal dominant disorder caused by heterozygous mutations or deletions of *NSD1*. Macrocephaly is usually present at all ages in more than 90% of children and is considered to be a cardinal feature. In some series, macrocephaly was present at birth in 50% of children, with birth OFCs as high as 4 SD higher than the mean and later OFCs ranging between 2 and 7 SD. Most patients have a nonprogressive neurologic dysfunction characterized by clumsiness and poor coordination. Delays in expressive language and motor development during infancy are particularly common, and in some instances, may be followed by attainment of normal or near-normal intelligence. Several patients with Sotos and autistic features have been reported. Seizures and tone abnormalities are occasionally present. Brain MRI abnormalities present in patients with Sotos and NSD1 mutations include enlarged extraaxial fluid and lateral ventricles in 70% and 60% of patients, respectively. It has been suggested that these increased CSF spaces are primarily responsible for macrocephaly in Sotos syndrome rather than true brain overgrowth. Eighty percent to 90% of patients have a demonstrable NSD1 abnormality. NSD1 (nuclear receptor-binding SET domain protein-1) is involved in an intricate regulatory network of genes that appear to have a concerted role in various processes including cell growth and tumorigenesis.

Weaver syndrome (WS) is a rare overgrowth disorder characterized by macrocephaly, dysmorphic facial features (especially prominent hypertelorism), metaphyseal flaring of the femurs, camptodactyly, deep-set nails, and hoarse low-pitched cry. Heterozygous mutations of EZH2 have been identified in WS. EZH2 catalyzes the methylation of lysine residue 27 of histone 3 (H3K27) as part of the polycomb repressive complex 2 (PCR2), resulting in chromatin compaction and repression of transcription. EZH2 activity is inhibited by AKT (v-akt murine thymoma viral oncogene homolog 1), a key component of the PI3K-AKT-MTOR pathway, which blocks binding of EZH2 to histone 3.

Simpson-Golabi-Behmel syndrome (SGBS) is an X-linked disorder characterized by congenital overgrowth, macroglossia, renal and skeletal abnormalities, and an increased risk of

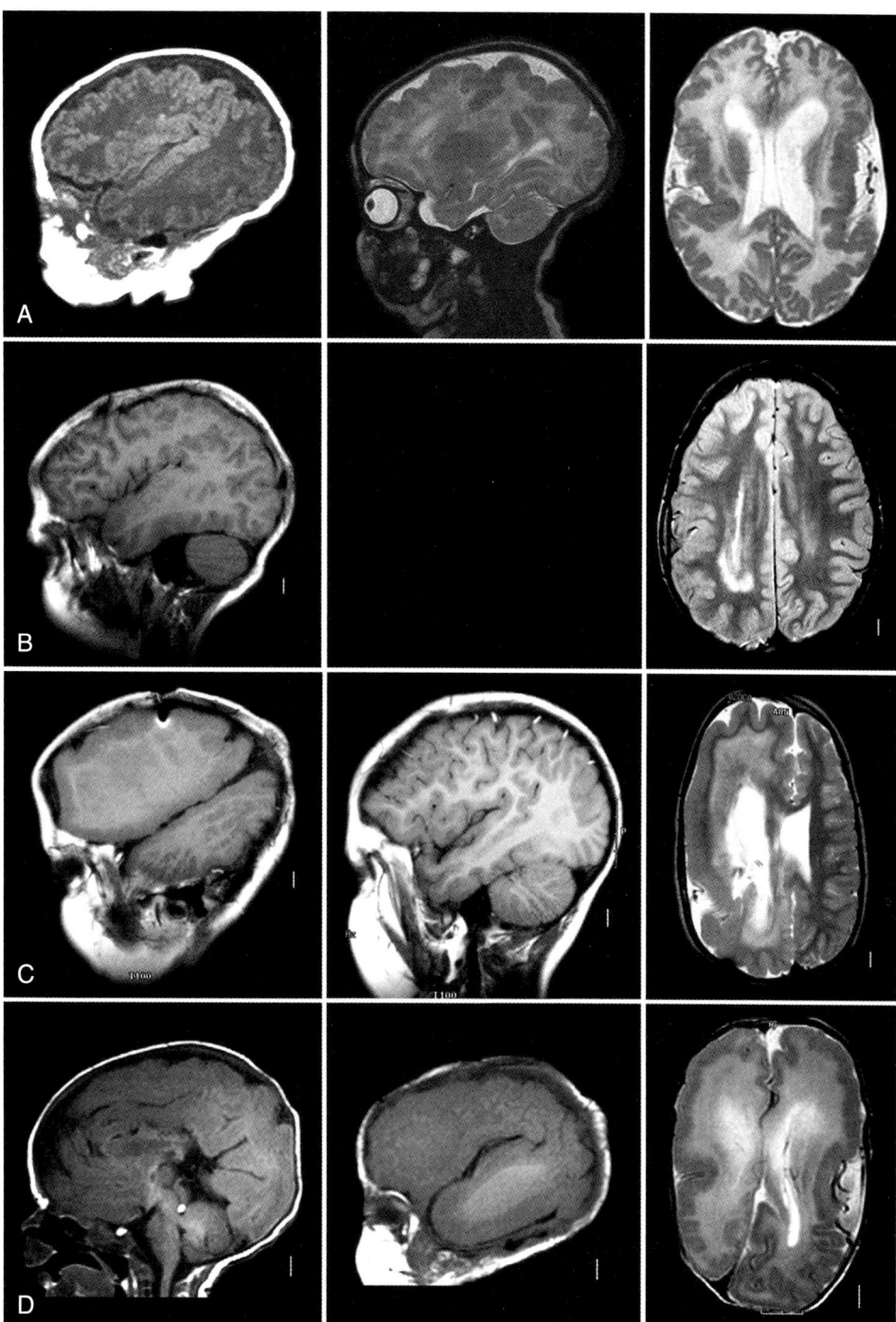

Figure 28-4. Subtypes of megalencephaly and hemimegalencephaly. Right parasagittal (left column except midsagittal in **D**), left parasagittal (middle column), and axial (right column) magnetic resonance images from four patients with megalencephaly (MEG) or hemimegalencephaly (HMEG) variants. **A** The top row images depict symmetric MEG and perisylvian polymicrogyria with normal white matter. The patient was a female with the originally described "megalencephaly polymicrogyria-polydactyly hydrocephalus" (MPPH) syndrome (Mirzaa et al., 2004). The symmetry and normal white matter distinguish this malformation from HMEG. **B** The second row images show partial HMEG, with enlargement of the posterior frontal, temporal, and parietal lobes on the right. The abnormal white matter typical of HMEG is seen circling the back of the right lateral ventricle. **C** The third row images demonstrate severe HMEG involving the entire right hemisphere, but sparing the left. The central and deep white matter has diffusely bright signal, sparing only the superficial U fibers. **D** The bottom row images show a very rare malformation consisting of bilateral HMEG that is more severe on the left side. *(Courtesy of Dr. Ghayda Mirzaa, William B. Dobyns, Center for Integrative Brain Research, Seattle Children's Research Institute, Seattle, WA.)*

embryonal tumors. Macrocephaly is often congenital. Patients may have hypotonia and mild developmental delay, although most have normal intelligence. Most cases of SGBS are due to mutations or deletions of the glypican-3 (GPC3) gene at Xq26, a member of a multigene family encoding at least six distinct glycosylphosphatidylinositol-linked cell surface heparan sulfate proteoglycans (HSPGs) that act as coreceptors for multiple families of growth factors that have been shown to regulate cell proliferation, differentiation, and patterning, including that of the brain. In support of the glypicans' role in development, mice with null mutations in glypican-1 (Gpc1) have a severely reduced brain size and an abnormally small-sized cerebellum. Therefore Gpc1 may have a role in early neurogenesis, possibly through regulation of fibroblast growth factor (FGF) signaling.

The megalencephaly capillary malformation syndrome (MCAP). MCAP is a distinct syndrome characterized by megalencephaly, vascular malformations (most often cutis marmorata), hemihypertrophy, digit anomalies, and skin and connective tissue laxity. Its neuroimaging findings have been thoroughly reviewed in the literature and include cortical malformations (polymicrogyria), ventriculomegaly leading to hydrocephalus, and cerebellar tonsillar ectopia. Vascular anomalies are characteristic features, and most commonly consist of cutis marmorata, the cutaneous marbled appearance frequently seen in Caucasian newborns that tends to fade with time but often persists. Other vascular anomalies include a midline nevus flammeus, vascular rings, and telangiectasias. Digital anomalies include the common 2 to 3 toe syndactyly (greater than 25% syndactyly), 2 to 3 to 4 finger syndactyly, and postaxial polydactyly. MCAP is predominantly caused by mosaic (or postzygotic) mutations of the catalytic subunit of the PI3K enzymatic complex, PIK3CA. Mosaic mutations of the same gene are now known to be associated with segmental cortical malformations, including focal cortical dysplasia and hemimegalencephaly, as well as a spectrum of somatic overgrowth disorders, including CLOVES syndrome, isolated macrodactyly, and isolated lymphatic malformations.

The megalencephaly perisylvian polymicrogyria-postaxial polydactyly hydrocephalus syndrome (MPPH). MPPH is a megalencephaly disorder that resembles MCAP. Megalencephaly is most often congenital, with OFCs ranging from 2 to 4 SD higher than the mean at birth, reaching up to 8 SD later in life. Variable degrees of ID, hypotonia, and seizures occur. MRI abnormalities common to both MCAP and MPPH include diffuse megalencephaly that is symmetric or mildly asymmetric, a high rate of hydrocephalus that is often shunted, or ventriculomegaly, progressive posterior fossa crowding with cerebellar tonsillar herniation that may require decompression, polymicrogyria that is by far bilateral perisylvian in distribution, and white matter abnormalities (Fig. 28-4A). A distinct subset of patients has a very thick (or mega-) corpus callosum. All reported cases to date appear sporadic. MPPH is caused by mutations in three core components of the PI3K-AKT-MTOR pathway including PIK3R2, AKT3, and CCND2.

PTEN-related disorders. PTEN is a tumor suppressor gene, somatic mutations of which have been reported to varying degrees in multiple sporadic malignancies (such as glioblastoma multiforme). De novo or inherited constitutional mutations of *PTEN* have been found in a set of disorders of macrocephaly and hamartomatous overgrowth, namely Cowden (CS) and Bannayan-Riley-Ruvalcaba (BRRS). Cowden and Bannayan-Riley-Ruvalcaba syndromes have a high degree of clinical overlap and are believed to constitute a single clinical spectrum called the *PTEN*-hamartoma tumor syndrome (PHTS). Macrocephaly is a prominent and progressive feature with OFCs typically 4.5 SD or more higher than the mean and reaching up to 8 SD. Hypotonia and delayed gross motor

skills are common findings. Sixty percent of patients have a mild proximal myopathy, and 25% have seizures. Additional features include hamartomas, lipomas, intestinal polyps, and various types of cutaneous vascular malformations. *PTEN* mutation carriers are at an increased risk of various tumors (most notably of the breast, thyroid, and endometrium). *PTEN* mediates cell cycle arrest and/or apoptosis by negatively regulating the phosophinositide-3-kinase-Akt serine/threonine protein kinase (PI3K/Akt) pathway. Accumulating evidence suggests that *PTEN* also regulates cell survival pathways such as the MAPK pathway. *PTEN* mutations have recently been identified in patients with isolated macrocephaly and autism spectrum disorders (ASD) and/or ID, with an overall estimated *PTEN* mutation frequency in macrocephaly autism of 20%.

RASopathies. The Ras/mitogen-activated protein kinase (MAPK) pathway is essential in the regulation of the cell cycle, cell differentiation, growth, and cell senescence, each of which are critical to normal development. The "RASopathies" are a class of developmental disorders caused by germline mutations in genes that encode protein components of the Ras/MAPK pathway, which result in dysregulation of the pathway and profound deleterious effects on development. These disorders include neurofibromatosis type 1 (NF1), Costello syndrome (HRAS), cardio-facio-cutaneous (CFC) syndrome (KRAS, BRAF, and MEK1), Noonan syndrome (PTPN11, KRAS, SOS1, RAF1, NRAS, BRAF, SHOC2), and others. Costello syndrome is a unique combination of failure to thrive, cardiac abnormalities, and a predisposition to papillomata and malignant tumors. In a systematic review of 28 patients, absolute or relative macrocephaly was found in 100% of patients and, more specifically, an evolving megalencephaly and cerebellar enlargement, overlapping with MCAP syndrome. Neurologic abnormalities include developmental delay/ID, nystagmus and hypotonia.

Neurofibromatosis type 1 (NF1) shares features of other overgrowth syndromes such as the presence of macrocephaly, various types of tumors, and, occasionally, hemihyperplasia of a limb or digit, despite an increased incidence of short stature. Macrocephaly in the absence of hydrocephalus occurs in 50% of individuals with NF1. Quantitative MRI studies have demonstrated the presence of true megalencephaly, largely secondary to increased white matter volume. Learning disabilities have been reported in up to 70% of individuals, and 3% have severe developmental delay. Their neurocognitive profile may also include easy distractibility, impulsiveness, and deficient visual-motor coordination. Seizures occur in approximately 6% to 7% of patients. Frank hydrocephalus with aqueductal stenosis, as well as asymptomatic ventricular dilation, has been observed in approximately 4% of patients. *NF1* is a tumor suppressor gene expressed in neurons and glial cells and encodes neurofibromin, one of the earliest identified regulators of the RAS-MAPK pathway, and thus it has important roles in cellular proliferation and differentiation.

Other syndromes, including skeletal dysplasia, as well as chromosomal abnormalities, associated with megalencephaly are listed in Table 28-8.

REFERENCES

The complete list of references for this chapter is available in the e-book at www.expertconsult.com.
See inside cover for registration details.

SELECTED REFERENCES

Alcantara, D., O'Driscoll, M., 2014. Congenital microcephaly. Am. J. Med. Genet. C Semin. Med. Genet. 166C (2), 124–139.

Ashwal, S., Michelson, D., Plawner, L., et al., 2009. Practice parameter: evaluation of the child with microcephaly (an evidence-based review): report of the Quality Standards Subcommittee of the American Academy of Neurology and the Practice Committee of the Child Neurology Society. Neurology 73, 887–897.

Barkovich, A.J., Gressens, P., Evrard, P., 1992. Formation, maturation, and disorders of brain neocortex. AJNR 13, 423–446.

Basel-Vanagaite, L., Dobyns, W.B., 2010. Clinical and brain imaging heterogeneity of severe microcephaly. Pediatr. Neurol. 43, 7–16.

Dobyns, W.B., 2002. Primary microcephaly: new approaches for an old disorder. Am. J. Med. Genet. 112, 315–317.

Mirzaa, G., et al., 2004. Megalencephaly and perisylvian polymicrogyria with postaxial polydactyly and hydrocephalus: a rare brain malformation syndrome associated with mental retardation and seizures. Neuropediatrics 35(6):353–359.

Norman, M.G., McGillivray, B.C., Kalousek, D.K., et al., 1995. Congenital Malformations of the Brain: Pathological, Embryological, Clinical, Radiological, and Genetic Aspects. Oxford University Press, New York.

E-BOOK FIGURES AND TABLES

The following figures and tables are available in the e-book at www.expertconsult.com. See inside cover for registration details.

29 Malformations of Cortical Development

William B. Dobyns, Richard J. Leventer, and Renzo Guerrini

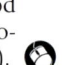 An expanded version of this chapter is available on www.expertconsult.com. See inside cover for registration details.

INTRODUCTION

Development of the human cerebral cortex is a complex and tightly regulated process that can be divided into three broad and overlapping steps, including (I) neural stem cell proliferation and cell type differentiation, (II) neuronal migration, and (III) final neuronal positioning, further cortical organization, and connectivity. Disruption of any one of these processes may result in a wide range of developmental disorders in humans. Many of these are recognized as malformations on brain imaging studies or visual inspection at autopsy and, collectively, comprise a class of disorders that we designate as malformations of cortical development (MCD).

Barkovich and associates developed a classification scheme for MCD based on the developmental steps at which the process was first disturbed, the underlying genes and biological pathways disrupted, and–when more objective data was not available–on brain imaging features (Barkovich et al., 2012). This system classifies MCD into three major groups as noted previously. Disorders presenting with abnormal brain size—microcephaly and megalencephaly—were reviewed in the previous chapter (see Chapter 28). Here we consider the subset of developmental disorders of the cortex in which alterations in brain size are not the dominant or only feature. These include several well-known cortical malformations—lissencephaly (LIS) and related tubulinopathies (with features intermediatge between LIS and polymicrogyria), cobblestone cortical malformations (COB), classic four-layer (or unlayered) polymicrogyria (PMG) as described in schizencephaly and other conditions, as well as periventricular nodular heterotopia (PNH) and a growing number of predominately subcortical malformations. Although this classification system has proven helpful for recognizing specific MCD and sending appropriate diagnostic testing in affected individuals, it has not consistently fit with new gene discoveries. This has led us to take the first steps in developing a parallel system based on the underlying biological pathways.

EMBRYOLOGY

The online summary touches on several; of the advances made over the past decade; here we include a summary of the key pathways of migration and their primary neurotransmitters in Figure 29-1. Many reviews are available, including a recent recent collection of papers in a symposium on "Patterning and Evolving the Vertebrate Forebrain" (Retaux, 2009).

BIOLOGIC PATHWAYS

By last count, at least 20 different biological pathways have been associated with MCD. Several are obvious candidates. For example, several MCD-associated genes function in early forebrain patterning, regulation of the cell cycle (neurogenesis and likely gliogenesis as well), intracellular structural changes necessary for cell movement (i.e., neuronal migration), and central pathways that regulate these processes. But for others the connection with MCD was initially less obvious, such as defects in messenger RNA splicing, intracellular trafficking, and protein glycosylation. Even as the underlying mechanisms are defined, it often remains unclear why some of these pathways have a disproportionate effect on the brain and why they result in a particular type of MCD. As a first step in developing a parallel classification system for MCD based on biologic pathways, we have organized many of the best understood mechanisms into groups based loosely on head size, a surrogate for control of the cell cycle, and apoptosis (Table 29-1).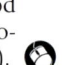

LISSENCEPHALY AND SUBCORTICAL BAND HETEROTOPIA

Lissencephaly (LIS) or "smooth brain" and the related malformation known as subcortical band heterotopia (SBH) are the classic malformations associated with deficient neuronal migration. LIS is recognized based on an abnormal gyral pattern consisting of absent or abnormally wide gyri and an abnormally thick cortex. SBH is less obvious, consisting of a normal or mildly "simplified" gyral pattern associated with a variably thick layer of gray matter replacing the central and upper portions of white matter.

Brain Imaging

Most of the distinguishing features seen on the macroscopic pathologic examination can be seen by brain imaging as well (Fig. 29-2). The different types of LIS and SBH may be distinguished by both the pattern and severity of the malformation. Recognition of these patterns has become essential for syndrome and molecular diagnosis and for assessing prognosis and genetic risk.

For all forms of true LIS, the brain surface appears smooth, with areas of absent (agyria) and abnormally wide gyri (pachygyria) and abnormally thick cerebral cortex. In normal brains, most gyri are approximately 1 to 1.5 cm wide and the normal cortex 3 to 4 mm thick, but thicker in the primary motor cortex and thinner in the primary visual cortex. In most types of LIS, gyri are typically 3 cm wide or more, and the cortex 8 to 20 mm thick. The exceptions are some tubulinopathies, three-layered LIS, and uncommon variants with an unusual undulating gyral pattern and mildly thick cortex (5 to 10 mm). This pattern can occur with severe cerebellar hypoplasia in the reelinopathies or with normal cerebellar size. Several distinct types of LIS are associated with agenesis of the corpus callosum, moderate to severe cerebellar hypoplasia (designated lissencephaly with cerebellar hypoplasia, LCH), or both.

In SBH, the brain surface appears superficially normal, except that the sulci or crevices between gyri tend to be very shallow, and the cortex is normal and not thick. But just beneath the cortex, often separated from it by just a few millimeters of white matter, lies a smooth band of neurons that never reached the true cortex. The inner margin of the band is usually smooth, whereas the outer margin may appear smooth (with thick bands) or follow interdigitations of the overlying cortex (with thin bands). Both LIS and SBH may be seen with anterior or posterior predominant distribution. Thus the gradient of LIS and SBH can be anterior equal to posterior (a = p), anterior more severe than posterior (a > p), or posterior more severe than anterior (p > a). In four-layered LIS, the cortex is usually 12 to 20 mm thick, whereas in other variants it may be only 8 to 12 mm thick. Common associated malformations include thick, under rotated and rounded hippocampi, enlarged posterior portions of the lateral ventricles, and flat anterior portion of the corpus callosum. Several other types of LCH may be differentiated based on brain imaging.

Clinical Features

The clinical features in children with common and severe forms of LIS are similar and can be helpful in differentiating LIS from other cortical malformations (Guerrini and Dobyns, 2014). Children with the most common types of LIS (or SBH) typically appear normal as newborns, although a few have a history of polyhydramnios, apnea, hypotonia, poor feeding, and mildly elevated newborn bilirubin levels that may reflect poor swallowing. With most types of LIS, seizures are uncommon during the first days of life. Most affected children come to medical attention during the first year of life due to (1) neurologic deficits in the first weeks or months consisting of poor feeding, mild hypotonia, and abnormal arching behavior or opisthotonus, (2) delayed motor milestones later in the first year of life, or (3) onset of seizures during the first year of life, which is by far the most common. In all affected children, the major medical problems encountered are feeding problems and gastroesophageal reflux, epilepsy of many different types, and recurrent aspiration and pneumonia due to the feeding problems.

A few children feed poorly from the first weeks of life, but this often improves unless they have one of the severe LIS variants. Most feed reasonably well for the first several years, except that many have difficulty during intercurrent illnesses. Feeding often worsens later, especially after about 3 years, with increased aspiration, decreased feeding tolerance, and recurrent pneumonia. These problems are frequently related to worsening epilepsy, use of some antiepileptic drugs (especially benzodiazepines), and gastroesophageal reflux, whether obviously symptomatic or not. They lead to placement of gastrostomy tubes and operations to reduce reflux (fundal plications) in many affected children, although the age varies widely within the first decade. Other clinical features seen with LIS include minimal pyramidal signs and dysarthria.

Epilepsy

Most and probably all children with LIS have seizures (Christian et al., 2015). The onset is usually between three and 12 months but may be later. Between 35% and 85% of children with classic LIS develop infantile spasms in the first year of life, although hypsarrhythmia is usually absent. After 1 year, they typically have continued mixed seizure types including epileptic spasms, typically presenting on awakening, myoclonic, tonic, and tonic-clonic seizures. Many meet criteria for Lennox-Gastaut syndrome, which can be associated with a decline in skills with poor seizure control. In general, the same treatment strategies used for Lennox-Gastaut syndrome generally may be used in patients with LIS or SBH. In children with XLAG, epilepsy is nearly continuous. In both classic LIS and XLAG, studies in mouse mutants have shown deficiencies in cortical interneurons that use gamma-aminobutyric acid (GABA) as their primary neurotransmitter. Thus GABAergic medications have some theoretical basis for use in these children. Early diagnosis of seizure disorders and aggressive attempts to control seizures and abate severe

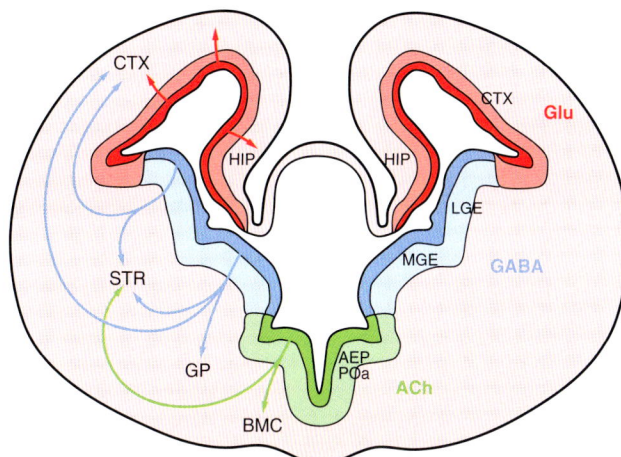

Figure 29-1. Representation of a coronal section of the brain from an embryonic day 14 mouse (equivalent to a week 15 human embryo). **Right half,** The major subdivisions of the telencephalic proliferative zones, with the probable regions of origin of neurons expresssing specific neurotransmitters, including glutamate, GABA, and acetylcholine. **Left half,** The migration pathways followed by neurons from the various proliferative zones, with straight arrows representing radial migration in all three major zones and curved arrows representing nonradial migration. Most projection neurons follow radial migration, whereas most interneurons follow nonradial pathways. Ach, acetylcholine; aep, anterior entopeduncular area; bmc, basal magnocellular complex; ctx, cortex; gaba, γ-aminobutyric acid; glu, glutamate; gp, globus pallidus; hip, hippocampus; lge, lateral ganglionic eminence; mge, medial ganglionic eminence; poa, anterior preoptic area; str, striatum. See also color plate. *(Modified from Wilson, S.W., Rubenstein, J.L.R., 2000. Induction and dorsoventral patterning of the telencephalon. Neuron 28, 641–651. Reprinted with permission from Elsevier.)*

EEG abnormalies usually prove helpful in maintaining function.

Survival

For children with the most common forms of classic LIS, the mortality rate is 50% or higher by 10 years, and few live past 20 years. Children with the most severe LIS syndromes, especially MDS, severe forms of LCH, XLAG, MOPD1, or Barth microlissencephaly syndrome, have an even more severe course and higher mortality rate. However, these rates do not apply to children with less severe forms including partial (partial frontal or partial posterior) LIS or pachygyria, SBH, Baraitser-Winter syndrome, or variants with only mildly thick cortex (reelinopathies and the new "thin" LIS variants), as these subtypes all have better cognitive function and much longer survival.

These last several groups, including SBH, have mild to moderate cognitive impairment, although both normal intelligence and severe cognitive impairment have been seen in some individuals. Cognitive development may slow after onset of seizures. The frequency and severity vary greatly. EEG investigations usually demonstrate generalized spike-and-wave discharges or multifocal abnormalities. Neurologic outcome usually correlates with the thickness of the subcortical band heterotopia and severity of the gyral pattern as seen on MRI.

TUBULINOPATHIES

Mutations of tubulin genes were first reported as causing LIS (for TUBA1A) or PMG with several other genes. Mutations of TUBA1A were subsequently associated with both classic four-layered LIS and LCH, and mutations of TUBB2B rarely with LCH. With further experience however, the cortical malformations seen in most individuals with mutations of tubulin or tubulin motor genes comprise a recognizable spectrum of malformations that can be distinguished from both LIS and PMG by brain imaging and neuropathology. Thus we have begun to classify them as a group that overlaps with LIS but is distinct from PMG.

Brain Imaging

The most severe tubulinopathies present with severe LCH that corresponds to two-layered LIS, and some mutations of tubulin or tubulin motor genes cause classic LIS that likely corresponds to four-layered (posterior predominant) LIS. The most common pattern was first described as a form of polymicrogyria, but with further experience, tubulinopathies have features intermediate between LIS and PMG and can be distinguished from both. The gyral pattern is abnormal with patchy and mildly asymmetric abnormalities in gyral size and orientation and varying sulcal depth. A pattern involving a cluster of multiple shallow sulci was frequently observed, especially in the frontal lobes. We will define this as "tubulinopathy-associated dysgyria" until a clearer terminology emerges. This pattern differs from simplified gyral pattern, in which the gyri are too few in number. Cortical thickness varies and can be mildly thin, normal, or mildly thick. The basal ganglia and thalami are dysplastic and mildly asymmetric with a bulbous appearance and diffuse, branched, or absent anterior limb of the internal capsule. The lateral ventricles have an irregular contour and abnormal rounding of the frontal horns, likely related to the basal ganglia dysplasia. The corpus callosum is variably affected from almost complete agenesis to normal. Most have brainstem dysplasia although the severity varies. The most typical features are a mildly enlarged midbrain tectum, flat pons, and globular medulla with indistinct demarcation between the pyramids and olives. Most patients have a striking dysplasia of the anterior (superior) cerebellum that consists of "diagonal" folia on axial views. The vermis, especially the anterior vermis, is usually small with normal or mildly small cerebellar hemispheres.

Clinical Features

The clinical features of tubulinopathies are generally comparable to LIS. Children with severe LCH with two-layered LIS have profound handicaps and short survival. Children with obvious cortical malformations (the typical appearance described previously that resembles PMG) have severe handicaps. Children with subtle gyral malformations usually have better development, but still with moderate handicaps. Further details are lacking as this group is just now being separated from LIS and PMG.

COBBLESTONE MALFORMATIONS

Cobblestone malformation or lissencephaly is a severe brain malformation associated with abnormal migration from the brain into the leptomeninges, and frequently with eye anomalies and congenital muscular dystrophy (CMD). The older term "type 2" lissencephaly should be abandoned. These malformations comprise the severe end of a graded series of disorders associated with defective glycosylation of alpha-dystroglycan, that include—from most to least severe—Walker-Warburg syndrome (WWS), muscle-eye-brain disease (MEB), Fukuyama congenital muscular dystrophy (FCMD), CMD with mental retardation and isolated cerebellar hypoplasia and dysplasia, CMD with mental retardation but no recognized cortical malformation, and limb girdle muscular dystrophy. These are referred to as dystroglycanopathies. Although neuropathological confirmation is sparse, cobblestone or cobblestone-like malformations also occur in a growing group of other disorders, including isolated bilateral frontoparietal cobblestone malformation (previously called bilateral fronto-parietal polymicrogyria) associated with mutations of the GPR56 gene, at least two congenital disorders of glycosylation—Debré type autosomal recessive cutis laxa and CHIME-like syndrome—and a small group of disorders associated with mutations of laminin-coding genes.

Brain Imaging

The brain imaging changes of CMD-associated cobblestone malformation present a continuous series of malformations that begins with the severe changes of WWS and ends with normal brain imaging. But most patients cluster into one of the defined syndromes, which consist of WWS, an intermediate group classified as MEB, and progressively less severe forms ending with normal brain imaging. The key imaging features are most easily recognized for WWS and are collectively pathognomonic for this spectrum of disorders.

The imaging abnormalities seen in WWS, shown in an online figure, begin with macrocephaly and prominent forehead, resulting from existing or prior hydrocephalus, and reduced size and partial obliteration of extraaxial spaces, which is especially prominent between the cerebral hemispheres. The cerebral surface is undersulcated, usually with diffuse apparent agyria. The cerebral cortex is moderately thick, usually about 7 to 10 mm unless thinned by hydrocephalus. The cortical-white matter border is jagged with frequent vertical (perpendicular to the cortical-white matter border) striations, which differs from lissencephaly and from the chaotic striations seen in classic polymicrogyria. Just beneath the cortex, streaks of laminar subcortical heterotopia are seen that differ from typical subcortical band heterotopia based on their beaded and discontinuous appearance. The white matter has very abnormal signal (bright on T2 and dark on T1 MRI sequences; dark on CT scan) and may have small cysts. The white matter volume may be normal or thinned by hydrocephalus. The third and lateral ventricles are enlarged and may be very large and rounded reflecting active hydrocephalus. Very rarely, the ventricles may be small. The corpus callosum is present, although frequently thin.

The brainstem and cerebellum in WWS are remarkably dysplastic with a kink at the midbrain-pons junction in which the midbrain is angled dorsally with respect to the pons. The lower brainstem appears small with moderate to severe hypoplasia of the medulla and pons, near absence of the basis points, and ventral midline clefts of the ventral pons. But the midbrain and especially the tectum are abnormally large. The cerebellum is small with the vermis more severely involved than the hemispheres, a dysplastic foliar pattern, and often small cysts within or near the cerebellar cortex. The posterior fossa may be enlarged and a few patients have small occipital meningoceles.

The imaging abnormalities in MEB are similar but consistently less severe than in WWS. The macrocephaly and hydrocephalus are common in MEB as well, although partial obliteration of extraaxial spaces is less extensive. The cerebral surface is again undersulcated but with frontal predominant cobblestone-type dysgyria that resembles pachygyria but with the intracortical striations noted for WWS. Some areas resembling classic polymicrogyria may be seen. The jagged cortical-white matter border and vertical striations are similar to WWS, although fewer streaks of subcortical heterotopia are seen. The white matter has a very abnormal signal similar to WWS in infants, but over time, this evolves from diffuse to patchy to minimal signal changes. The frequency of hydrocephalus and thinning of the white matter and corpus callosum is probably similar.

The brainstem and cerebellum in MEB are also dysplastic but less severe than WWS. The brainstem lacks the kink, but the lower brainstem, especially the pons, appears small, whereas the midbrain and tectum are enlarged. The cerebellar changes are similar but on average less severe than in WWS, except that cerebellar cortical cysts may be more common. This may be due to a high frequency of cerebellar cysts in MEB patients with mutations of the *POMGnT1* gene.

The imaging abnormalities in FCMD are similar to MEB but overall less severe. Hydrocephalus is uncommon. The dysgryia is less severe but still frontal predominant, although some patients have severe temporal lobe near agyria. The brainstem and cerebellum most often appear normal. Next on the spectrum, patients with mental retardation and cerebellar cysts have relatively normal forebrain structures and cerebral cortex; however, review of some published images shows that the cortex is mildly abnormal. The cerebellum mimics the appearance seen in MEB.

The brain imaging abnormalities in other cobblestone disorders, especially GPR56-associated brain malformation, are similar to MEB, including moderate frontal-predominant cobblestone-type dysgyria, moderately thick cortex with vertical striations, patchy white matter abnormalities, hydrocephalus, and brainstem and vermis predominant cerebellar hypoplasia and dysplasia. The brainstem is usually not as thin as seen in MEB. Similar imaging features with a posterior predominant (parietooccipital) distribution, including the beaded subcortical heterotopia, have been described with mutations of several laminin genes defining a new "lamininopathy" group of MCD.

Clinical Features

Cobblestone malformations occur in a graded series of congenital muscular dystrophies with brain involvement associated with reduced glycosylation of alpha-dystroglycan that include—from least to most severe—CMD with mental retardation without obvious cortical malformation, CMD with mental retardation and isolated cerebellar hypoplasia and dysplasia, Fukuyama congenital muscular dystrophy (FCMD), muscle-eye-brain disease (MEB), and Walker-Warburg syndrome (WWS). In all of the cobblestone malformation syndromes associated with CMD, the phenotype consists of moderate to profound mental retardation, severe hypotonia, mild distal spasticity, and poor vision.

Prognosis and Management

Children with most of these syndromes have both cobblestone brain malformation and progressive muscle disease, which lead to combined hypotonia (from the brain and muscle disease) and spasticity (from the brain malformation). The combination makes orthopedic and rehabilitation management difficult. Although the causative genes may be the same, it is important to distinguish between the various clinical syndromes, as the prognosis and management differ. WWS is a severe disorder associated with profound mental retardation and congenital hypotonia. Few children with WWS survive past 3 years. MEB and FCMD are less severe with variable survival from later in the first decade into the teens and beyond; some patients have survived into the fifth decade. Some children with WWS reported to live longer than 3 years may be better classified as having MEB.

Optimal management begins with early recognition and accurate counseling regarding the prognosis, as some parents of children with WWS choose to limit life-sustaining interventions. Most children with WWS and some with MEB have congenital hydrocephalus that can only be managed with a shunt. Children with WWS who have occipital cephaloceles may not have hydrocephalus at birth, but excision of the cephaloceles may be followed by hydrocephalus. Thus placement of a shunt should be considered at the time of cephalocele removal. Seizures occur but are rarely as severe as those seen in patients with lissencephaly or subcortical band heterotopia. In WWS and MEB, congenital glaucoma and buphthalmos require care by an ophthalmologist. Treatment of other eye anomalies that can interfere with vision, such as retinal nonattachment or detachment, cataracts and corneal opacities, should be assessed on an individual basis in view of the poor prognosis. Children with FCMD and other cobblestone syndromes have no or only minor eye anomalies.

The muscle disease progresses slowly, so that frequent evaluations to assess orthopedic and other rehabilitation needs are important. Careful seating is essential owing to severe hypotonia, and contractures need to be managed with physical therapy and splinting as needed. In WWS, the CMD probably progresses slowly over time, but this is not apparent clinically owing to the severe hypotonia and short survival period. Children with FCMD who learn to walk typically lose this skill several years later.

Individuals with GPR56-associated "frontoparietal" cobblestone malformation have global developmental delay, later moderate to severe intellectual disability, dysconjugate gaze, and bilateral pyramidal and cerebellar signs. Seizures have been reported in more than 90% of patients, most often generalized epilepsy.

NEURONAL HETEROTOPIA

Neuronal heterotopia consists of groups of neurons in an abnormal location. The most common subtype is periventricular nodular heterotopia (PNH) lining the lateral ventricles. Other less frequent forms include many types of subcortical heterotopia, in which the major portion of the malformation is located in the subcortical white matter, and glioneuronal heterotopia found over the surface of the brain, often described as leptomeningeal. These are also known as brain warts. Examples of several types are shown in the online version.

Periventricular Nodular Heterotopia. PNH consist of nodular masses of gray matter that line the ventricular walls and protrude into the lumen, resulting in an irregular outline. They are recognized as a relatively common malformation that may occur as a single nodule or heterotopion or as multiple contiguous or noncontiguous nodules or heterotopia. When the nodules are single or few in number, they may be associated with seizures or learning problems but are unlikely to help with diagnosis. When the lesions are bilateral and numerous, a genetic basis is likely. When the nodules are diffuse and contiguous, they may be associated with other brain malformations, especially hypogenesis of the corpus callosum, cerebellar hypoplasia or polymicrogyria.

Brain Imaging

Brain imaging using MRI demonstrates typical nodules along the ventricular walls, with different patterns of involvement that can be used to help to distinguish different syndromes. Patients with the classic X-linked form typically have bilateral contiguous or nearly contiguous periventricular nodular heterotopia that spare the temporal horns, associated with mildly thin corpus callosum, cerebellar vermis hypoplasia, and megacisterna magna. Patients with autosomal recessive severe congenital microcephaly and periventricular nodular heterotopia have symmetric nodular heterotopia lining the ventricles, thin overlying cortex with abnormal gyri, mildly enlarged lateral ventricles and delayed myelination. In the frontal predominant form, heterotopias are limited to the frontal horns and bodies of the lateral ventricles. They may occur alone or with overlying polymicrogyria. In the more common and usually syndromic posterior predominant forms, heterotopias are limited to the trigones, temporal, and occipital horns. Posterior heterotopia may be associated with overlying polymicrogyria and cerebellar hypoplasia, hippocampal and cerebellar hypoplasia, or hydrocephalus.

Clinical Features

The clinical presentation and course found in patients with PNH varies among the recognized syndromes. In individuals with PNH but no other brain malformations, seizures and learning problems are common, whereas more severe developmental problems are not, although exceptions certainly occur. When microcephaly or any other brain malformations is found, the likelihood of mental retardation increases greatly. Patients with BPNH and severe cerebellar hypoplasia often are brought to medical attention due to developmental ataxia.

Among all forms of PNH, the most common and often the presenting symptom is epilepsy, which has been reported in 80% to 90% of patients, although an ascertainment bias appears likely. The age at seizure onset is variable but at times delayed until early adulthood. Most patients have one or more types of partial seizures, which may be easily controlled or refractory. There is no clear relationship between the epilepsy severity and extent of nodular heterotopia. The associated EEG abnormalities are not specific, consisting of infrequent interictal discharges that may be generalized, multifocal, or focal. Pseudotemporal lobe localization has also been reported. Studies using depth electrodes in patients with periventricular nodular heterotopia and epilepsy have found the nodules to be intrinsically epileptogenic. However, seizure onset most often begins within a complex epileptogenic zone that includes both the heterotopia and overlying cortex. Intractable seizures associated with heterotpia should be treated aggressively. Temporal lobe surgery for patients with periventricular nodular heterotopia and associated hippocampal sclerosis has not generally been successful.

POLYMICROGYRIA AND SCHIZENCEPHALY

The term "polymicrogyria (PMG)" was first used to describe a cerebral or cerebellar cortex with multiple excessive small convolutions, which may or may not be appreciated macroscopically. Synonymous terms in the literature include status verrucosus deformis, micropolygyria, and microgyria. As most often used in practice, the definition of PMG does not encompass a specific histologic cortical abnormality, but it is generally accepted that PMG is both an abnormality of excessive gyration and a microscopic abnormality of cortical structure. The most recognized and specific pattern of PMG occurs in schizencephaly (SCH), a term first used by Yakovlev and Wadsworth to describe full thickness clefts in the brain that are lined by PMG. The presence of gray matter lining the cleft and usually surrounding the opening on the cortical surface is one of the main distinguishing features between SCH and porencephalic cysts, the latter being lined by white matter or gliosis. SCH often occurs in the same central and perisylvian regions

as other forms of PMG, and many reports in the imaging and pathology literature have described unilateral SCH and contralateral PMG. SCH should be considered a subtype of PMG, and therefore it is presented in this section.

Brain Imaging

Using CT and low field strength MRI, PMG is difficult to discern and may only appear as mildly thickened cortex. For this reason, PMG is frequently misdiagnosed as pachygyria or lissencephaly. The only current role for CT in the evaluation of PMG is to assess for evidence of intracerebral calcifications, which are seen in PMG resulting from congenital cytomegalovirus infection and a few rare disorders. Using high-quality MRI at 1.5T or greater with appropriate age-specific protocols, it is now possible to reliably differentiate PMG from other malformations of cortical development (MCDs), provided that the individual interpreting the MRI has knowledge of the imaging features of MCDs. Sagittal imaging extending laterally to involve the Sylvian fissures is of great value, as PMG often affects the opercular regions. Examples of several types are shown in the online version.

Polymicrogyric cortex often appears mildly thickened (usually 6 to 10 mm) on imaging due to cortical overfolding rather than true cortical thickening. This compares with lissencephaly in which the cortex is usually 10 to 20 mm thick. With thick slices, the cortex may appear mildly thickened with an irregular or "stippled" gray-white junction and with better imaging (such as inversion recovery) using thin contiguous slices microgyri and microsulci may be appreciated. In younger children with PMG, the cortex may not appear particularly thickened. This is thought due to the immature state of myelination in subcortical and intracortical fibers. T2 signal within the cortex is usually normal, although delayed myelination or high T2 signal in the underlying white matter may be seen. Diffusely abnormal white matter signal should raise the question of an in utero infection such as cytomegalovirus, or a peroxisomal disorder. The subarachnoid space may be enlarged over PMG and may contain excessive or anomalous venous drainage, especially in the Sylvian regions. Other developmental anomalies may include gray matter heterotopia, ventricular enlargement or dysmorphism, and abnormalities of the corpus callosum and cerebellum.

CT or MRI scanning is usually sufficient to diagnose SCH and determine whether the SCH is associated with an open-lip or closed-lip, although MRI is the modality of choice. The gray matter lining the cleft has the imaging appearance of PMG with apparent mild cortical thickening, an irregular surface and stippling of the gray-white interface. Subtle SCH may recognizable by a "puckering" or "dimple" outwards of the lateral ventricle at the point at which the cleft reaches the ventricular margin. By definition, SCH clefts are always lined by gray matter. SCH is frequently asymmetric, and the contralateral hemisphere should be closely evaluated for the presence of a milder SCH or PMG without a cleft. Agenesis of the septum pellucidum and hypoplasia of the optic nerves are common and are present in as many as 30% of patients with SCH.

Several types of white matter abnormalities can be seen with PMG or PMG-like malformations. In typical PMG and SCH, prominent perivascular spaces are common. Extensive white matter signal changes characteristic of gliosis lining a cleft suggest that the lesion is porencephaly rather than SCH. More extensive white matter signal changes are seen in cobblestone cortical malformations. Abnormal vascular drainage is an extremely common finding, which is detected using MRI imaging sequences for depiction of cerebral veins such as susceptibility-weighted angiography.

PMG has been described in a number of topographic patterns. Most of these are bilateral and symmetric, the most common of which is bilateral perisylvian PMG, although the perisylvian form may be asymmetric or unilateral. Other bilateral symmetric forms are generalized, bilateral frontal, and parasagittal parietooccipital PMG, although little or no neuropathologic data is available to support the classification. PMG has also been described in association with periventricular nodular heterotopia.

Clinical Features

The clinical sequelae of PMG are highly variable, and depend on several factors. The most consistent predictors of a poor developmental outcome include: microcephaly, especially severe microcephaly of −3 standard deviations or smaller; abnormal neurologic examination, especially spasticity; widespread distribution of PMG, especially when bilateral and frontal; and additional brain malformations such as heterotopia or cerebellar hypoplasia.

PMG is reported as an occasional component in many different conditions, including metabolic disorders, chromosome deletion syndromes, and multiple congenital anomaly syndromes. These patients may have a variety of clinical problems other than those attributable to the PMG. Some patients with PMG or SCH have fewer clinical problems than would be expected for the location and extent of cortex involved (for example, perisylvian PMG with deletion 22q11.2), whereas others have more severe problems (for example, perisylvian PMG with deletion 1p36.3). PMG may involve eloquent cortical areas representing language or primary motor functions, yet these functions may occasionally be retained with minimal or no disability. This is especially true with lesions such as unilateral perisylvian PMG.

Perisylvian Polymicrogyria. The most common form of PMG involves the perisylvian regions in a bilateral and relatively symmetric pattern. The combination of bilateral perisylvian PMG, oromotor dysfunction, and seizure disorder has been called the "congenital bilateral perisylvian syndrome" and is the best described syndrome of PMG. Patients with perisylvian PMG typically have oromotor dysfunction, including difficulties with tongue (tongue protrusion and side to side movement), facial and pharyngeal motor function resulting in problems with speech production, sucking and swallowing, excessive drooling, and facial diplegia. They may also have dysarthria and an expressive dysphasia. More severely affected patients have minimal or no expressive speech, necessitating the use of alternate methods of communication such as signing or langage assistive devices such as picture boards or computer-assisted devices. Examination demonstrates facial diplegia, limited tongue movements, brisk jaw jerk, and frequent absence of the gag reflex. Patients presenting in childhood may have other abnormalities including arthrogryposis, hemiplegia, and hearing loss, although the data available on children is limited. Up to 75% of affected individuals have mild to moderate intellectual disability. Motor dysfunction may include limb spasticity, although this is rarely severe if present. A smaller group of patients have unilateral perisylvian PMG and present with hemiparesis or seizures. Their developmental and neurologic deficits are typically less severe.

Other Patterns. Several other patterns of PMG have been described, including bilateral frontal, bilateral parasagittal parietooccipital, bilateral parietooccipital, multilobar, and bilateral generalized PMG, as well as PMG associated with periventricular gray matter heterotopia. The clinical features of these less common forms of PMG vary from BPP, although

epilepsy, developmental delay, and spasticity are common accompaniments. Unsurprisingly, spasticity appears to be more frequent when the frontal lobes are involved. Note that the subtype described as "bilateral frontoparietal PMG" is in our view better classified as bilateral frontoparietal cobblestone malformation, and was discussed in a previous section.

Epilepsy. The data regarding epilepsy in PMG is largely based on the study of patients with perisylvian PMG. The frequency of epilepsy in these patients is 60% to 85%, although seizure onset may not occur until the second decade, usually between 4 and 12 years of age. Seizure types include atypical absence, atonic and tonic drop attacks, generalized tonic-clonic, and partial. It is rare for partial seizures to secondarily generalize. Occasionally patients may develop bilateral facial motor seizures with retained awareness. The occurrence of infantile spasms is uncommon in PMG, in contrast to patients with lissencephaly, tubulinopathies, tuberous sclerosis, or focal cortical dysplasia in which the frequency of spasms is much higher. Seizures may be daily and intractable in at least 50% of patients, and EEG typically shows generalized spike and wave or multifocal discharges with a centroparietal emphasis. Polymicrogyria is a frequent cause of epilepsy with continuous spikes and waves during sleep, a form of age related epileptic encephalopathy.

Schizencephaly. Patients with closed-lip SCH typically present with hemiparesis or motor delay, whereas patients with open-lip SCH typically present with hydrocephalus, seizures, and intellectual disability, which can be severe. Seizure types include complex partial seizures, as well as infantile spasms, tonic, atonic, and tonic-clonic seizures, although these are less common. The severity and type of seizures do not appear to correlate with topography of the SCH. The outcome is worst for those with bilateral open-lipped SCH and best for those with unilateral closed-lip SC. Many patients have associated brain abnormalities such as agenesis of the septum pellucidum that probably contribute to the disability in some patients.

FOCAL CORTICAL DYSPLASIA AND HEMIMEGALENCEPHALY

Hemimegalencephaly (HMEG) and focal cortical dysplasia (FCD) constitute a spectrum of malformations of cortical development with shared neuropathology features. The former is primarily defined by macroscopic enlargement of (more or less) one hemisphere, whereas FCD is primarily defined by histopathology. FCD was first described as a histologic abnormality seen in surgical specimens from 10 patients with epilepsy that is now referred to as FCD type 2b, but use of the term has gradually expanded. As currently classified (Blumcke et al., 2011), FCD encompasses a wide spectrum of cortical malformations with variable features including microscopic neuronal heterotopia, dyslamination, and abnormal cell types. It has been divided into three major types and nine subtypes based on histopathological features. Type 1 consists of abnormal cortical lamination without large or dysmorphic neurons or any other primary pathologic process. Type 2 consists of abnormal cortical lamination with large, dysmorphic neurons and several other features. Type 3 consists of abnormal cortical lamination without large or dysmorphic neurons that occurs immediately adjacent to another principal pathologic process such as hippocampal sclerosis, glial or neuroglial tumor, or vascular malformations. The histopathology in HMEG is essentially the same as FCD type 2, both discussed with megalencephaly in a previous chapter.

Brain Imaging

FCD is rarely visible by CT and may not be visible even with high quality MRI, especially FCD type 1. Subtle abnormalities in the gyral pattern, cortical thickness, and gray-white junction are best seen using thin slice T1-weighted images. Some forms of FCD may show increased signal on FLAIR and T2-weighted images. White matter signal may be abnormal in the region of FCD, producing intractable seizures, but it is not clear whether this represents dysplastic white matter, or a consequence of abnormal or advanced myelination secondary to frequent seizure activity.

In FCD type 1, typical features consist of subtle cortical thickening and irregular sulcation or gyration. Other features may include lobar hypoplasia or atrophy and hippocampal sclerosis. The most striking imaging features of FCD are seen in FCD type 2. The lesions in these patients typically show increased cortical thickness, blurring of the gray-white junction, abnormal sulcal and gyral patterns, and high signal at the base of the lesion and in the underlying white matter on T2 and FLAIR sequences.

Several specific named patterns of FCD have been described based primarily on brain imaging features. FCD has also been shown to occur at the base of a sulcus with cortical thickening and poor gray-white differentiation, often with a linear band of high signal from the base of the lesion to the lateral ventricle, known as the "transmantle sign," shown for FCD types Ib and IIb. In focal transmantle dysplasia, a wedge of dysplastic tissue extends from the lateral ventricle up to the cortical surface. Histology shows features of FCD with balloon cells plus white matter astrogliosis, and MRI shows a wedge of disorganized tissue with increased T2 signal. These lesions have collectively been called "bottom of the sulcus" dysplasias. Sublobar dysplasia is characterised by a deep infolding of the cortex with a thickened cortex and possible poor gray-white differentiation in the malformed region. Associated brain abnormalities include ventricular dysmorphism and callosal and cerebellar dysgenesis. Another form of FCD affecting one posterior quadrant of the brain has been designated posterior quadrantic dysplasia.

Presurgical localization of these lesions often requires advanced MRI imaging techniques and analysis such as the use of surface coils, volume averaging, curvilinear reformatting, or 3T imaging. Functional studies, including SPECT and FDG-PET scanning, are also often required to maximise the likelihood of identifying and defining the boundaries of FCD. New MRI methods for lesion detection are being evaluated including multichannel coils, high field strength (greater than 3T), arterial spin labeling, susceptibility-weighted imaging, and diffusion tensor/spectrum imaging.

Clinical Features

Apart from tuberous sclerosis, the cortical malformation typically occurs as an isolated feature with no particular dysmorphic, neurocutaneous, or congenital anomalies. However, HMEG and FCD can occur with several well-known syndromes. These include the linear nevus sebaceous (Schimmelpenning) syndrome, Sturge-Weber syndrome, the PTEN hamartoma tumor (Cowden) syndrome, and pigmentary mosaicism sometimes designated as "hypomelanosis of Ito."

The most common clinical sequelae of FCD are seizures. Developmental delay, cognitive disability, and focal neurologic deficits are only observed with extensive dysplasias. Seizures from FCD may arise at any age from *in utero* seizures until adulthood, although most patients present in childhood. Some studies have shown consistent clinical differences between patients with FCD types 1 and 2. FCD type 2 usually has extratemporal location and is manifested with a younger age of seizure onset and higher seizure frequencies. Seizure semiology varies, depending on the location of the FCD and age of the patient. Younger children often present with asymmetric infantile spasms. The seizure disorder may be intractable and life threatening so that surgical resection may be appropriate. Much of the developmental delay and cognitive disabilities associated with FCD may be due to the effects of repeated seizure activity. As complete as possible surgical resection of the FCD is consistently the most important variable for long-term seizure control in epilepsy secondary to FCD that is unresponsive to anticonvulsants; accordingly, surgery is being performed at increasingly younger ages in an attempt to protect the child against the deleterious effect of uncontrolled epilepsy and multiple medications.

Etiology, Genetic, and Molecular Basis

Since the last edition of this text, substantial progress has been made in understanding the pathogenesis for FCD. In FCD type 1, not much is known. In one large study, prenatal and perinatal brain injuries, especially prematurity, intraventricular hemorrhage with hydrocephalus, and perinatal asphyxia, were found in 25 of 200 (12.5%) of children with FCD, mostly FCD1a and FCD1b. Much more progress has been made for FCD type 2. The PI3K-AKT-MTOR pathway is involved in the control of cell proliferation and growth, protein synthesis, synaptic plasticity, and other key cellular functions. Several studies have shown upregulation of this pathway (especially of MTOR and AKT) in resected brain tissue from patients with FCD type 2, as well as in tuberous sclerosis, hemimegalencephaly, and some low-grade, epilepsy-associated tumors (Jansen et al., 2015). Subsequent genetic analysis has demonstrated germline or mosaic mutations in several genes in the PI3K-AKT-MTOR pathway in both FCD2a and FCD2b, as well as in hemimegalencephaly with FCD type 2 histopathology. The genes implicated to date include PIK3CA, PTEN, MTOR, DEPDC5, and BRAF, as well as AKT3 in hemimegalencephaly (Jansen et al., 2015; D'Gama et al., 2015).

Treatment

Most patients with epilepsy due to FCD do not respond to conventional antiepileptic drugs, and many remain either surgically inaccessible or surgical failures. A subset of patients are treated surgically with rates of success that can reach up to around 80%, depending on the extent and location of the lesion, its histologic subtype, presurgical assessment, and completeness of resection. The most successfull operations are conducted in children with infantile spasms and FCD in whom remission of spasms is often accompanied by overall clinical improvement or in children with FCD of the anterior temporal pole in whom rates of postoperative seizure freedom are very high. High resolution imaging, multimodal fusion imaging, and novel neurophysiological approaches, such as the study of high frequency oscillations, as well as a more precise characterization of eloquent cortical regions, have provided in recent years considerable improvements for less invasive and more precise surgical planning (Guerrini et al., 2015). Although many patients with refractory epilepsy caused by FCD cannot be adequately treated, novel therapeutic avenues based on mTOR inhibitors are opening new perspectives.

SUMMARY

Researchers in the field of human MCD have made assumptions as to the likely timing of the etiologies of different malformations based on their appearance using both pathologic and neuroimaging techniques. For example, heterotopic gray matter is assumed to result from disordered neuronal migration, as the heterotopic neurons appear to have arrested their migration to the cortex prematurely. Assumptions such as these were proposed well before a basic understanding of the genetic and molecular mechanisms of normal cortical development were established. In many instances, these assumptions have proved correct, yet it is now appreciated that many cortical malformations are likely secondary to abnormalities occurring at stages other than that of neuroblast migration. Our understanding of the genetic and molecular basis of cortical development is advancing rapidly, with new genes or new roles for known genes being discovered. A more complete understanding of the key genes involved in human cortical development will be required in order to understand the possible timing and molecular basis of many malformations of cortical development.

REFERENCES

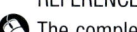 The complete list of references for this chapter is available in the e-book at www.expertconsult.com.
See inside cover for registration details.

SELECTED REFERENCES

Barkovich, A.J., Guerrini, R., Kuzniecky, R.I., et al., 2012. A developmental and genetic classification for malformations of cortical development: update 2012. Brain 135, 1348–1369.

Blumcke, I., Thom, M., Aronica, E., et al., 2011. The clinicopathologic spectrum of focal cortical dysplasias: a consensus classification proposed by an ad hoc Task Force of the ILAE Diagnostic Methods Commission. Epilepsia 52, 158–174.

Christian, S.L., Collins, S., Adams, C., et al., 2015. PI3K/AKT pathway mutations cause a spectrum of brain malformations from megalencephaly to focal cortical dysplasia. Brain 138, 1613–1628.

D'Gama, A.M., Geng, Y., Couto, J.A., et al., 2015. mTOR pathway mutations cause hemimegalencephaly and focal cortical dysplasia. Ann. Neurol.

Guerrini, R., Dobyns, W.B., 2014. Malformations of cortical development: clinical features and genetic causes. Lancet Neurol. 13, 710–726.

Guerrini, R., Duchowny, M., Jayakar, P., et al., 2015. Diagnostic methods and treatment options for focal cortical dysplasia. Epilepsia 56, 1669–1686.

Jansen, L.A., Mirzaa, G.M., Ishak, G.E., et al., 2015. PI3K/AKT pathway mutations cause a spectrum of brain malformations from megalencephaly to focal cortical dysplasia. Brain 138, 1613–1628.

Retaux, S., 2009. Editorial: the vertebrate forebrain. Semin. Cell Dev. Biol. 20, 697.

E-BOOK FIGURES AND TABLES

The following figures and tables are available in the e-book at www.expertconsult.com. See inside cover for registration details.

Fig. 29-2. Subtypes of lissencephaly.
Fig. 29-3. Subtypes of cobblestone cortical malformations.
Fig. 29-4. Subtypes of heterotopia.
Fig. 29-5. Microscopic features of polymicrogyria.
Fig. 29-6. Subtypes of polymicrogyria.
Fig. 29-7. Microscopic features and subtypes of focal cortical dysplasia.
Table 29-1. Biological pathways implicated in malformations of cortical development
Table 29-2. Lissencephaly patterns, syndromes, inheritance, and genes
Table 29-3. Mutation frequencies for lissencephaly syndromes with known causal genes
Table 29-4. Cobblestone patterns, syndromes, inheritance, and genes
Table 29-5. Heterotopia patterns, syndromes, inheritance, and genes
Table 29-6. Clinical and imaging features of the polymicrogyria syndromes
Table 29-7. Polymicrogyria and polymicrogyria-like cortical malformations: patterns syndromes, inheritance, and genes
Table 29-8. Current classification system for focal cortical dysplasia

Hydrocephalus and Arachnoid Cysts

Amal Abou-Hamden and James M. Drake

HYDROCEPHALUS

Definition

Hydrocephalus is most simply defined as an increase in the fluid containing spaces of the brain at increased pressure, resulting from an imbalance between cerebrospinal fluid (CSF) production and absorption or flow (Rekate, 2009). This definition excludes other abnormalities of CSF dynamics such as benign intracranial hypertension in which the ventricles are not enlarged, or "hydrocephalus ex-vacuo," where cerebral atrophy and focal destructive lesions also lead to an abnormal increase of CSF passively.

Classification

There is no universally accepted classification system, and a number of classification systems for hydrocephalus have been suggested (Boaz and Edwards-Brown, 1999). These include

- Communicating versus noncommunicating
- Obstructive versus absorptive
- Acquired versus congenital
- Genetic or central nervous system (CNS) malformation-associated versus isolated
- Intraventricular-obstructive versus extraventricular
- Simple versus complicated

The terms *compensated hydrocephalus* and *uncompensated hydrocephalus* generally refer to whether an increase in ventricular size is associated with evidence of raised intracranial pressure. In some cases a gradual increase in ventricular size stabilizes by reaching a new equilibrium and the patient has no symptoms or signs of raised intracranial pressure. However, patients with apparently arrested hydrocephalus may still develop symptoms and signs at a later date, and so the process is not entirely static.

In communicating hydrocephalus, the flow is not obstructed but CSF is inadequately reabsorbed in the subarachnoid space, whereas in noncommunicating or obstructive hydrocephalus, the flow of CSF from the ventricles to the subarachnoid space is obstructed.

Congenital hydrocephalus is present at birth and often associated with developmental defects, whereas acquired hydrocephalus occurs after the development of the brain and ventricles. Hydrocephalus also has been classified based on the stage of development at the time that the ventricles became dilated. The various subtypes of fetal hydrocephalus are classified according to the mechanism of obstruction to the flow of CSF. These include: primary or simple hydrocephalus with a single point of obstruction to flow; dysgenetic hydrocephalus with complex abnormalities of the CNS, such as the Arnold–Chiari malformation; and secondary hydrocephalus from tumor or bleeding. This classification is cross-referenced to the stage of fetal development (e.g., neuronal maturation, cell migration) and may prove useful in deciding when treatment may be futile if beyond the legal period for terminating a pregnancy, and in identifying potential candidates for early delivery or fetal surgery.

Extraventricular obstructive hydrocephalus is now recognized to represent, almost universally, benign pericerebral collections of infancy that are usually familial, resolve with time, and almost never require treatment (Drake, 2008). Exceptions include genetic conditions, such as certain mucopolysaccharidoses, achondroplasia, Sotos syndrome, and glutaric aciduria type I, often associated with developmental delay. In these cases, identification is important as therapeutic options exist for many forms of mucopolysaccharidoses and for glutaric aciduria type I.

Epidemiology

In newborns, cited incidence of hydrocephalus ranges from 0.3 to 4 per 1000 live births. Occurring as a single congenital disorder, the incidence of hydrocephalus has been reported as 0.9 to 1.5 per 1000 births. The incidence of pediatric hydrocephalus has declined in many developed countries as antenatal screening, genetic testing, and pregnancy termination have reduced the incidence of congenital malformations of the brain that cause hydrocephalus. The incidence of open neural tube defects also has decreased precipitously as a result of maternal folate supplementation, antenatal screening, and termination of pregnancy based on superior antenatal imaging with ultrasound and magnetic resonance imaging (MRI) (Chakraborty et al., 2008). The incidence of intraventricular hemorrhage (IVH) also has decreased as a result of better perinatal management of prematurity.

Cerebrospinal Fluid Production, Circulation, and Absorption

CSF is produced by two mechanisms: Most of the CSF is thought to be secreted by the choroid plexus within the cerebral ventricles. Extrachoroidal CSF production in subarachnoid sites and by way of a transependymal route also has been documented. About 20% or more of CSF is derived from brain extracellular fluid created as a byproduct of cerebral metabolism. Normally, rates of production (0.35 mL/min or approximately 400 to 500 mL/day) and absorption of CSF are equal. Total CSF volume is 65 to 140 mL in children, and 90 to 150 mL in adults.

CSF production has been reported to remain constant across the normal intracranial pressure range and to decrease when intracranial pressure approaches mean arterial pressure. There have been reports, however, of downregulation of CSF production in patients with chronic hydrocephalus.

Information gained from MRI analysis of CSF movement demonstrates pulsatile to-and-fro motion of CSF within the lateral ventricles, produced from a brain-pumping motion that ejects the CSF and causes a net downward flow.

Historically, it has been held that CSF is absorbed into the vascular system mainly through the arachnoid villi within the arachnoid granulations covering the brain and spinal cord leptomeninges. There is normally 5- to 7-mm Hg difference in pressure between the dural venous sinuses and the subarachnoid space, which is presumed to be the hydrostatic force behind the absorption of CSF. Newborn infants do not have visible arachnoid granulations, suggesting that the maximum capacity for reabsorption is less than that in the adult, or that CSF is absorbed by different mechanisms in the neonate.

More recently, olfactory nerves, the cribriform plate, and nasal lymphatics have been identified as important sites for CSF absorption. Absorption of CSF across brain tissue into capillaries also has been proposed (Greitz, 2004).

Etiology and Pathophysiology

Hydrocephalus can be a symptom of a large number of disorders (Greitz, 2004), and a list of conditions in which it has been reported is summarized in Box 30-1. It is associated with tumors and infections, and may be a complication of prematurity and trauma (Renier et al., 1988). It is also seen in apparent isolation. High-resolution MRI of postnatal life has provided clues to the etiology of hydrocephalus, which in the past would have been labeled as idiopathic; some of these include IVH, aqueductal stenosis (Figure 30-3), and migrational abnormalities.

Hydrocephalus is caused by either abnormal CSF reabsorption, or flow, or, rarely, overproduction. Its etiology depends on the age of the child. During the neonatal to late infancy period (0 to 2 years), hydrocephalus is usually caused by a perinatal hemorrhage, meningitis, and developmental abnormalities, the most common being aqueductal stenosis. The hydrocephalus seen in babies with spina bifida usually results from an associated Chiari malformation. In early to late childhood (2 to 10 years), the most common causes of hydrocephalus are posterior fossa tumors and aqueductal stenosis.

Congenital Causes in Infants and Children

Approximately 55% of all cases of hydrocephalus are congenital. Primary aqueductal stenosis accounts for approximately 5% of congenital hydrocephalus, whereas aqueductal stenosis secondary to neoplasm, infection, or hemorrhage accounts for another 5%. Primary aqueductal stenosis usually presents in infancy. Its morphology may be that of "forking" of the aqueduct, an aqueductal septum, "true" narrowing of the aqueduct, or X-linked aqueductal stenosis. Secondary aqueductal stenosis is caused by gliosis secondary to intrauterine infection or germinal matrix hemorrhage.

Anatomic malformations frequently observed with idiopathic congenital hydrocephalus are associated with abnormalities of hindbrain development, and include Chiari malformations, Dandy–Walker malformation (DWM), and others. DWM is associated with atresia of the foramen of Luschka and Magendie, and affects 2% to 4% of newborns with hydrocephalus. About 50% of all patients with DWM develop hydrocephalus. The dilated fourth ventricle does not communicate effectively with the subarachnoid space. In patients with Chiari malformations, hydrocephalus may occur, with fourth ventricle outlet obstruction in Chiari type 1 malformation; it is commonly associated with myelomeningocele in the Chiari type 2 malformation. Hydrocephalus occurs in approximately 80% to 90% of patients with myelomeningocele; of these cases, 50% are obvious at birth (Tuli et al., 2003).

Neonatal hydrocephalus can also be part of a major cerebral malformation, such as an encephalocele or holoprosencephaly, or can be associated with inherited metabolic diseases, such as achondroplasia and Hurler disease. Other causes of congenital hydrocephalus include agenesis of the foramen of Monro, congenital tumors, arachnoid cysts, vascular malformations (vein of Galen), and intrauterine toxoplasmosis.

Acquired Causes in Infants and Children

Infective causes of hydrocephalus include meningitis, especially bacterial, which can lead to hydrocephalus by either inflammatory aqueductal stenosis or leptomeningeal fibrosis. In some geographic areas, parasitic disease, such as intraventricular cysticercosis, can cause hydrocephalus by mechanical obstruction.

Posthemorrhagic hydrocephalus (PHH) occurs after IVH and can be related to prematurity, head injury, or rupture of a vascular malformation. Approximately one third of extremely low-birth-weight infants with an IVH develop PHH.

Mass lesions account for 20% of all cases of hydrocephalus in children. These are usually tumors, such as medulloblastoma, astrocytoma, and ependymoma, but cysts, abscesses, vascular malformations, or hematomas also can be the cause. Approximately 20% of children develop hydrocephalus requiring shunting after posterior fossa tumor removal.

Increased venous sinus pressure can also lead to hydrocephalus. This can be related to achondroplasia, some craniosynostosis, or venous sinus thrombosis.

Iatrogenic causes of hydrocephalus include hypervitaminosis A, which can lead to hydrocephalus by increasing secretion of CSF or by increasing permeability of the blood–brain barrier. Hyper-vitaminosis A is a more common cause of idiopathic intracranial hypertension.

Clinical Characteristics

The clinical features of hydrocephalus depend on the age of the child at presentation and the time of onset in relation to closure of the cranial sutures. With the current advances in antenatal monitoring, the majority of congenital cases of hydrocephalus are diagnosed early (Figure 30-4), allowing for planned cesarean delivery in the moderate to severe cases in which cephalopelvic disproportion is expected.

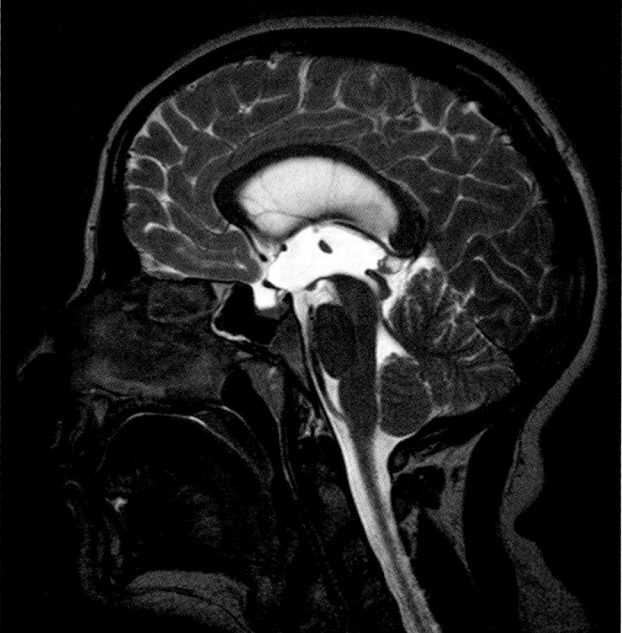

Figure 30-3. Aqueductal stenosis. Occlusion of the aqueduct of Sylvius results in enlargement of the lateral and third ventricles (proximal to the aqueduct), with relative normalcy of the fourth ventricle (distal to the aqueduct).

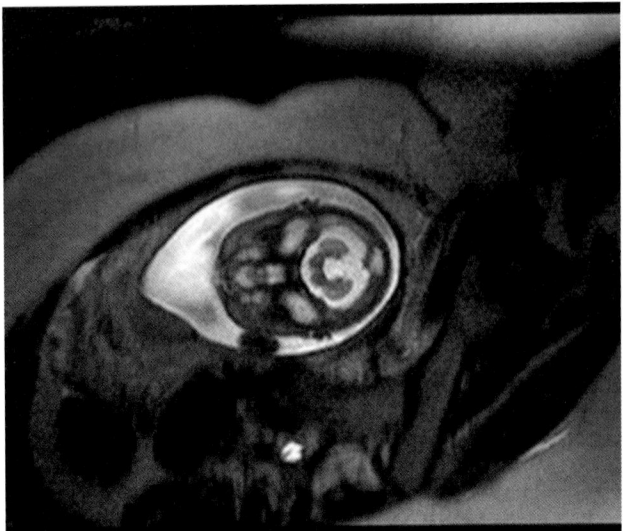

Figure 30-4. Antenatal magnetic resonance imaging showing fetal hydrocephalus. Asymmetric enlargement of the ventricular system is readily seen in the brain of this fetus.

Symptoms and Signs in Infants

Hydrocephalus can present as acute raised intracranial pressure but, because of the relative distensibility of the infant skull, the presentation may be more subtle, with symptoms of failure to thrive or delayed development. Infants with hydrocephalus may be drowsy and irritable. Poor feeding and vomiting are common. These infants may have apneic spells, episodes of bradycardia, and a bulging, tense anterior fontanel. Head circumference increases abnormally across centiles, and the head circumference is at or above the 98th percentile for age. Scalp veins may be distended, scalp skin thin and shiny, and cranial sutures splayed. In most children, the hydrocephalus only gradually becomes obvious. In advanced cases, clinical examination reveals a significant craniofacial disproportion, with expansion of the dome and low-set ears and eyes. In very severe cases, where the cerebral cortex is thinned, transillumination of the cranial cavity may be possible. Epileptic seizures are rarely seen as a result of hydrocephalus alone.

Papilledema is rare in this age group, although funduscopy may reveal retinal venous engorgement. Oculomotor abnormalities may include abducens nerve palsy. Upgaze palsy, from third ventricular pressure on the midbrain tectum producing a "setting-sun" sign, can be observed, although this is usually absent in premature infants. Some infants with definite hydrocephalus exhibit no such signs, as hydrocephalus may have developed slowly and the splaying of the sutures may have prevented the intracranial pressure from rising considerably.

Symptoms and Signs in Older Children

In children older than 2 years, the head circumference is usually within normal limits if hydrocephalus develops after closure of the cranial sutures, or may be increased in children with preexisting (infantile) but unrecognized progressive hydrocephalus.

Learning problems and reduced intellectual function are common, and neurologic development may be delayed. School-aged children may have deteriorating school performance as a result of headaches, failing mental function, memory loss, or behavioral disturbances. More acutely, these children present with symptoms and signs of increased intracranial pressure, such as headache, nausea, vomiting, drowsiness, gait changes, papilledema, or impaired upward or lateral gaze. Failure of upward gaze is caused by pressure on the tectal plate through the suprapineal recess. When intracranial pressure is significantly increased, other elements of the dorsal midbrain syndrome (Parinaud syndrome) may be observed.

Abnormal hypothalamic functions (e.g., short stature, gigantism, obesity, delayed puberty, primary amenorrhea, menstrual irregularity, and diabetes insipidus) may occur secondary to increased intracranial pressure or dilatation of the third ventricle. Difficulty in walking may develop secondary to truncal and limb ataxia or limb spasticity. This affects the lower limbs preferentially because the periventricular pyramidal tracts are stretched by the enlarged ventricles. Neck pain may indicate associated tonsillar herniation; blurred vision may be present as a consequence of papilledema, which, if left untreated, leads to optic atrophy.

Genetics

Although commonly considered a single disorder, hydrocephalus is a collection of heterogeneous complex and multifactorial disorders. A growing body of evidence suggests that genetic factors play a major role in its pathogenesis.

Congenital hydrocephalus may occur alone (nonsyndromic) or as part of a syndrome with other anomalies (syndromic). It is estimated that about 40% of individuals with hydrocephalus have a genetic etiology. The isolated (nonsyndromic) form of congenital hydrocephalus is a primary and major phenotype caused by a specific faulty gene. In syndromic forms, it is difficult to define the defective gene because of the association with other anomalies.

Autosomal-recessive, autosomal-dominant, X-linked recessive, and X-linked dominant forms of hydrocephalus are recognized.

At least 43 gene mutations linked to hereditary hydrocephalus have been identified in animal models and humans. To date, nine genes associated with hydrocephalus have been identified in animal models, whereas only one such gene has been identified in humans: the hydrocephalus (X-linked) gene. X-linked hydrocephalus (HSAS1, OMIM) occurs in approximately 5% to 15% of congenital cases in which a genetic etiology is determined. The gene responsible for X-linked human congenital hydrocephalus is at Xq28, encoding for L1CAM (L1 cell adhesion molecule). Congenital aqueductal stenosis can also be inherited as an autosomal-recessive disorder (OMIM 236635).

In general, the recurrence risk for congenital hydrocephalus excluding X-linked hydrocephalus is low. Empiric risk rates range from less than 1% to 4%, indicating the rarity of autosomal-recessive congenital hydrocephalus.

Neuroimaging
Cranial Ultrasound

Ultrasound is by far the quickest, cheapest, and most convenient method to demonstrate ventricular enlargement in infants with an open fontanel, particularly for posthemorrhagic hydrocephalus in premature infants and as serial imaging in follow-up. Ventricular width measured from the midline to the lateral border of the lateral ventricle in the midcoronal view is the measurement with the least interobserver variability, and centiles for gestational age have been compiled. Sedation is not required for acquiring ultrasound images, and the procedure can be repeated frequently without any adverse effects. It may not visualize the posterior fossa well, and may not always establish an etiologic diagnosis.

Computed Tomography

Computed tomography (CT) demonstrates ventricular size and morphology and periventricular lucency, and can reveal underlying pathologies, such as hemorrhage or posterior fossa tumors. Imaging of asymptomatic patients (especially after shunt revision) may serve as a reliable baseline study for comparison with subsequent imaging studies when patients become symptomatic. CT is widely available and often does not require sedation of the child. The limitations of CT are exposure to radiation, particularly with serial CT imaging so that alternative imaging such as ultrasound or rapid sequence MRI is frequently preferred.

Magnetic Resonance Imaging

MRI provides better morphologic definition and etiologic diagnosis, such as the presence of low-grade gliomas or colloid cysts, which may not be demonstrated on CT. It is better for evaluating Chiari malformations or cerebellar or periaqueductal tumors. Cine MRI is an MRI technique to measure CSF stroke volume in the cerebral aqueduct and can be used for demonstrating patency of third ventriculostomy fenestration. Limitations of MRI are that children often require general anesthesia and programmable shunt valves require reprogramming after MRI.

In patients with acute hydrocephalus characterized by ventricular enlargement and transependymal edema, with loss of sulci, the diagnosis is usually very obvious. Serial imaging demonstrating an increase in ventricular size may be required in equivocal cases. Conversely, an apparently normal ventricular size cannot exclude active hydrocephalus in a patient with a preexisting shunt, for example. Hydrostatic hydrocephalus is suggested when either the size of both temporal horns is 2 mm or greater in width, and the sylvian and interhemispheric fissures are not visible, or when both temporal horns are 2 mm or greater, and the ratio of the largest width of the frontal horns to the internal diameter from inner table to inner table at this level is greater than 0.5 mm.

The Evans ratio is the ratio of largest width of the frontal horns to the maximal biparietal diameter. A ratio greater than 30% is suggestive of hydrostatic hydrocephalus. A modification of Evans ratio, the frontal occipital horn ratio, may be more accurate and has been used in a number of prospective studies to quantify the degree of hydrocephalus and the response to treatment.

In communicating hydrocephalus, all ventricles are dilated. If the lateral and third ventricles are dilated and the fourth ventricle is small, it is likely that the obstruction is at the level of the aqueduct of Sylvius.

Diagnosis

Modern ultrasonography and, since the late 1980s, fetal MRI have significantly improved the ability to detect ventricular enlargement as a result of hydrocephalus in utero. Antenatal ultrasound and MRI provide reasonably detailed fetal brain anatomy, and can detect malformations and fetal ventriculomegaly as early as 17 to 21 weeks and 8 to 21 weeks, respectively. Anatomic ventriculomegaly is not sufficient to diagnose hydrocephalus. When diagnosing hydrocephalus in neonates or infants, it is essential to establish that there is a truly abnormal rate of skull growth. Records of head circumference measurements and its comparison with body weight and length centile charts are an integral part of postnatal follow-up of any child. Head circumference must be recorded and plotted on an accepted growth curve chart, with the patient's exact age. In the presence of hydrocephalus, any of the following may be observed: head circumference more than 2 standard deviations above normal or disproportionate to body length or weight, accelerated growth crossing centile curves, or continued head growth of more than 1.25 cm/week.

Evaluation of the patient with an enlarged head entails consideration of the many causes of macrocephaly, including hydrocephalus. Evaluation should include a history of trauma or CNS infection. The family history may demonstrate X-linked hydrocephalus caused by stenosis of the aqueduct of Sylvius or may reveal familial macrocephaly.

After a full review of the pregnancy, delivery, and neonatal history, as well as the clinical examination and ultrasound examination, it is usually possible to classify hydrocephalus into an etiologic group. If no obvious explanation can be determined, then the possibility of an intrauterine infection should be investigated. Coagulation factor deficiencies, as well as thrombocytopenia, should be excluded, as isoimmune thrombocytopenia and coagulation factor V deficiency can present as congenital hydrocephalus resulting from congenital IVH.

Differential Diagnosis

Besides hydrocephalus, causes of increasing head size include chronic subdural effusions or hematomas, pseudotumor cerebri, neurofibromatosis, metabolic abnormalities of bone or brain, cerebral gigantism (Sotos syndrome), and benign familial forms.

Benign extracranial hydrocephalus is a condition in infants and children with enlarged subarachnoid spaces accompanied by increasing head circumference with normal or mildly dilated ventricles. This condition is also known as "benign subdural collections of infancy," "pericerebral CSF collections," or "benign macrocrania." This has been postulated by some to be a variant of communicating hydrocephalus, but tends to run a benign course and stabilize by 12 to 18 months of age. Close serial monitoring of head circumference and serial imaging with CT or MRI are recommended to monitor for ventriculomegaly. Shunting is rarely, if ever, required.

A rare but striking condition that can mimic hydrocephalus is hydranencephaly or anencephaly, a postneurulation defect that results in total or near-total absence of the cerebral tissue, with the intracranial cavity being filled with CSF. This is usually caused by fetal bilateral internal carotid artery infarction or infection.

Hydrocephalus ex-vacuo is caused by atrophy rather than altered CSF dynamics. Certain metabolic and degenerative disorders, such as glycogen storage and Alexander disease, can cause macrocephaly. Finally, there may be a family history of large heads.

Pathology

The precise pathologic features of hydrocephalus vary, depending on the age of onset, the rate of ventricular enlargement, and the degree of ventriculomegaly. Typically, elevated CSF pressure initially enlarges the frontal horns of the lateral ventricles, followed by enlargement of the entire ventricular system above the site of obstruction. Hydrocephalus is associated with flattening and destruction of the ventricular ependymal lining, as well as edema and necrosis of the periventricular white matter. Periventricular glial cells proliferate, resulting in a layer of reactive gliosis. The pathologic findings may be a result of reduced blood flow to the white matter, causing hypoxic injury or toxicity to the white matter as a result of build-up of waste products not removed appropriately because of changes in the extracellular matrix.

Separation of the ependymal lining of the ventricles enhances permeability, which increases edema formation in adjacent white matter (transependymal fluid absorption). The expanding ventricles flatten the cerebral gyri and obliterate the sulci over the cortical surface. Unless the acute obstruction is relieved, increasing pressure may hinder cerebral blood flow, cause cerebral herniation, and compromise brainstem function.

Increasing pressure and ventricular enlargement are associated with necrosis of brain parenchyma. White matter is more vulnerable to destruction than gray matter in the presence of progressive hydrocephalus.

Management

The management of hydrocephalus is the most common problem in pediatric neurosurgery. In infants and children with symptomatic or progressive ventriculomegaly, the decision to treat with a CSF diversion procedure poses no therapeutic dilemma. However, not all patients with enlarged ventricles require treatment.

In patients with obstructive hydrocephalus secondary to a mass that is surgically accessible, resection of the mass may lead to resolution of the hydrocephalus and a shunt might not be necessary. This situation occurs infrequently in comparison with communicating hydrocephalus. If no documented obstruction or operable lesion is present and the hydrocephalus is mild and slowly progressive, a trial period of observation or medical management may be indicated, especially in preterm infants.

Another situation in which observation is reasonable is arrested hydrocephalus, which is an uncommon state of chronic hydrocephalus in which the CSF pressure has returned to normal and there is no pressure gradient between the cerebral ventricles and the brain parenchyma. Patients should be followed carefully, with neurologic examinations, neuropsychological assessments, and careful assessment of their development. A shunt will be necessary if there is any deterioration of those parameters (Figure 30-5).

Rapid-onset hydrocephalus with increased intracranial pressure is an emergency. Depending on the specific patient, any of the following procedures can be performed: Ventricular tap in infants, external ventricular drainage, lumbar puncture in posthemorrhagic and postmeningitic hydrocephalus, endoscopic third ventriculostomy, or placement of a ventriculoperitoneal shunt.

Prognosis

Before the 1950s, the outlook of untreated hydrocephalus was extremely poor. The development of satisfactory shunting substantially improved the outlook of children with hydrocephalus but brought its own set of problems and complications. Most children with hydrocephalus will require multiple shunt revisions. Shunt dependence carries a 1% per year mortality. Another series of 907 patients reported a mortality rate of 12% at 10 years from the time of initial shunt insertion, with the main risk factor for death being a history of shunt infection. Shunt-related complications, including death, have been reported to be greater in patients with myelomeningocele than in those who required shunt placement for the treatment of other conditions.

The neurologic and intellectual disabilities among patients with hydrocephalus depend on many factors, including etiology and degree of hydrocephalus, thickness of the cortical mantle and corpus callosum, requirement for a shunt, and

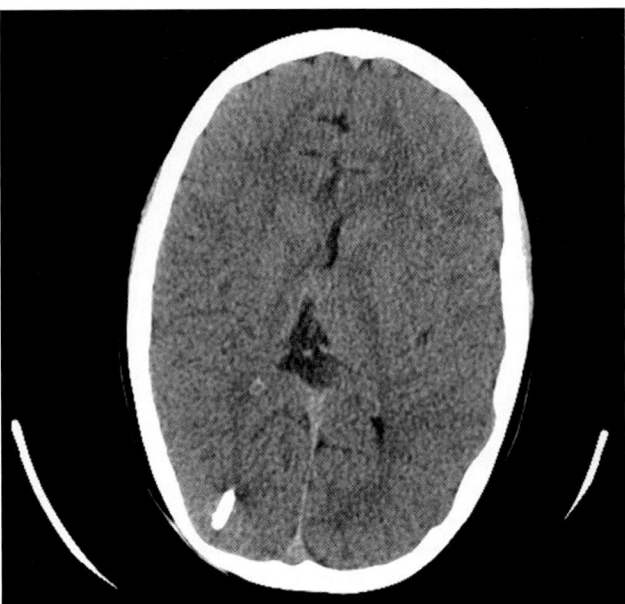

Figure 30-5. Slit ventricle syndrome. Patients who have undergone ventricular shunting for hydrocephalus and develop severe headache may have normal or small (as seen in this figure) ventricles on imaging studies. The etiology of this syndrome is best determined in the individual patient by intracranial pressure measurement and can include severe intracranial hypotension analogous to spinal headaches, intermittent obstruction of the ventricular catheter, intracranial hypertension with small ventricles and a failed shunt (normal-volume hydrocephalus), intracranial hypertension with a working shunt (cephalocranial hypertension), or shunt-related migraine.

presence of other brain anomalies. Associated conditions, such as IVH, CNS infection, and hypoxia, may dictate the ultimate prognosis more than the hydrocephalus.

A series of 233 patients with congenital hydrocephalus evaluated for longer than 20 years reported a mortality rate of 13.7%. In this series, 115 patients underwent psychological evaluation; approximately 63% showed normal performance, whereas 30% had mild retardation, and 7% had severe retardation. Another study found that children with congenital hydrocephalus were less likely to require special education placement (29%) than those in whom hydrocephalus was caused by meningitis (52%) or IVH (60 %) (Kestle et al., 2000).

Intellectual sequelae include significant scatter among Wechsler Intelligence Scale for Children—Revised (WISC-R) subtest scores, often with greater impairment of performance and motor tasks, as well as of nonverbal compared with verbal skills. Normal intellectual function is present in 40% to 65% of patients who received appropriate treatment. The probability of normal intelligence is enhanced if shunts are placed early and proper function is maintained.

INTRACRANIAL ARACHNOID CYSTS
Definition

Intracranial arachnoid cysts are benign, nongenetic developmental cysts that contain spinal fluid and occur within the arachnoid membrane (Gosalakkal, 2002). The mechanism of formation during embryogenesis is uncertain. Several mechanisms could account for the enlargement of these cysts, including secretion by the cells forming the cyst walls, a unidirectional valve, or liquid movements secondary to pulsations

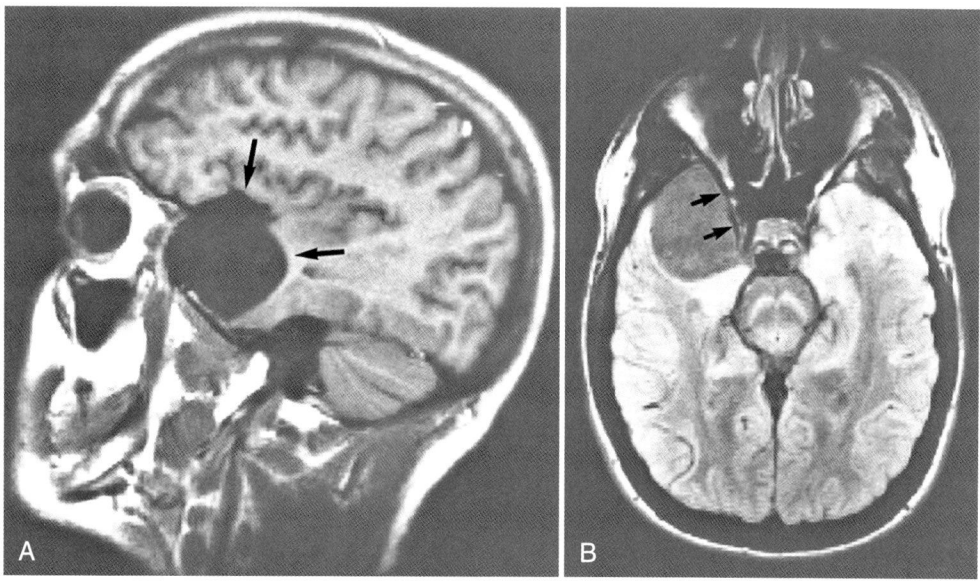

Figure 30-6. Arachnoid cyst. A, A cystic mass with signal intensity suggestive of cerebrospinal fluid is seen to deform the right temporal lobe *(arrows)* on this parasagittal image from a T1-weighted magnetic resonance imaging (MRI) study. **B,** Note the eroded appearance of the greater sphenoid wing *(arrows)* from the arachnoid cyst on this axial image from a spin density-weighted MRI study. *(Courtesy of Joseph R. Thompson, Department of Radiation Sciences, Loma Linda University School of Medicine, Loma Linda, California.)*

of the veins. The cysts occur in proximity to arachnoid cisterns, most often in the sylvian fissure. Common neurologic features are headache, seizures, hydrocephalus, focal enlargement of the skull, and signs and symptoms of elevated intracranial pressure and developmental delay, as well as specific signs or symptoms resulting from neural compression. Some arachnoid cysts remain asymptomatic. Progressive enlargement and intracystic or subdural hemorrhage are potential complications. Suprasellar arachnoid cysts may produce neuroendocrine dysfunction, hydrocephalus, and optic nerve compression. Posterior fossa cysts are now more frequently recognized with the use of MRI and CT, and frequently require surgical treatment.

In a series of 61 children with arachnoid cysts, 42% were supratentorial and 46% infratentorial. Macrocephaly was the presenting symptom in 72%, and associated features included cranial asymmetry in 39%, aqueductal stenosis in 16%, and agenesis of the corpus callosum in 13%. Developmental delay was a common finding. Skull radiographs may suggest the diagnosis; CT or MRI is the definitive diagnostic procedure (Figure 30-6).

Clinical Characteristics

Symptoms vary, depending on the size of the cyst and its location. Several common locations have been well described in the literature.

Sylvian Fissure/Middle Cranial Fossa

Nearly two thirds of pediatric arachnoid cysts are located in the sylvian fissure/middle cranial fossa. They may increase in volume, opening the fissure and exposing the middle cerebral artery. This exposure may result in compression and underdevelopment of the anterior superior surface of the temporal lobe. Controversy remains concerning whether they originate directly from the meninges adjacent to the temporal pole, or whether partial agenesis of the temporal lobe favors secondary formation of the cyst. Headaches are the most common presenting symptom; proptosis, contralateral motor weakness,

and seizures also may occur. In 10% of children, developmental delay may be present. Treatment depends on clinical symptoms. Recent studies have suggested some cognitive improvement after surgical treatment. Children with bitemporal arachnoid cysts also should be evaluated for the possibility of glutaricaciduria type 1 or neurofibromatosis.

Sellar Region

Both suprasellar and intrasellar cysts can occur in children. Suprasellar cysts can cause third ventricular obstructive hydrocephalus at the level of the foramen of Monro, and may be associated with visual impairment and endocrine dysfunction. Progressive head enlargement, growth retardation, developmental delay, and bitemporal hemianopsia have all been described. A bobble-head doll syndrome, with involuntary head movements secondary to increased pressure on the third ventricle and dorsomedial thalamic nuclei, is responsible. Endoscopic surgical approaches are now preferred.

Posterior Fossa

Arachnoid cysts of the posterior fossa are uncommon and must be differentiated from other cystic malformations of the posterior fossa, such as the DWM. Macrocrania and raised intracranial pressure are frequently observed. Cerebellar cysts demonstrate nystagmus and other cerebellar signs. Other rare manifestations reported include cervical spinal cord compression, which may improve after posterior fossa cystoperitoneal shunting or endoscopic surgery. In such patients, gait disturbances and headache are commonly seen.

Complications

Several clinical complications are believed to be associated with arachnoid cysts, although the relation between cyst presence and development of symptoms remains controversial; thus, the decision to operate is difficult and must be made on a patient-by-patient basis. Surgery is indicated when the cyst is causing obstructive hydrocephalus or if neuroimaging demonstrates mass effect, with compression of normal brain or brainstem structures. The relation between symptoms such as attention-deficit disorder, aphasia, or migraine-like headaches is uncertain, and correlation between cyst location and specific symptoms or congruent electroencephalogram (EEG) abnormalities is necessary before symptoms can be attributed to the cyst.

Epilepsy

Anecdotal studies suggest a relation between seizure reduction and removal of arachnoid cysts. The relation between the presence of arachnoid cysts and occurrence of seizures when the intracranial pressure is normal is uncertain, however, and outcomes, whether patients are managed medically or surgically, are similar. In addition, interictal and ictal EEG may not correspond to the site of the arachnoid cyst, raising the question whether the presence of an EEG abnormality is incidental.

Subdural Hematoma and Hygroma

Subdural hematomas and hygromas are infrequently encountered complications of arachnoid cysts of the middle cranial fossa and are particularly rare with cysts in other regions. Minor head trauma has been suggested to be a precipitating factor. Arachnoid cysts of the middle cranial fossa were found in 2.4% of patients with chronic subdural hematomas or hygromas in one report.

Neuropsychiatric Disorders

Attention-deficit/hyperactivity disorder, speech delay, and developmental delay have been found in association with arachnoid cysts, particularly in the temporal lobe, but a causal relation remains uncertain. Mental impairment and developmental delay have been associated with large arachnoid cysts, and the presence of cysts and developmental delay may be part of a common developmental process. Recent studies have suggested improvements in cognition after surgical treatment. The increased incidence of arachnoid cysts in conditions such as Down syndrome, mucopolysaccharidoses, schizencephaly, and neurofibromatosis suggests a higher incidence in children with underlying abnormalities of the brain. Aphasia, including that of Landau–Kleffner syndrome, also has been associated with the presence of left sylvian arachnoid cysts. Even in patients in whom CT and MRI failed to reveal mass effect, positron emission tomography (PET) has demonstrated hypometabolism in speech areas. Postoperative improvement in PET studies corresponded to improvement in vocabulary.

Management

When symptoms warrant, surgical intervention to decompress the cyst, including endoscopic management or shunting procedures, is required. Arachnoid cysts may occur with or without hydrocephalus. The success rate of fenestration is higher in those patients without hydrocephalus (i.e., 73% required no additional treatment) than in hydrocephalus patients (32%). About 12% of patients with hydrocephalus treated with fenestration alone may require a cystoperitoneal shunt. In general, cyst fenestration should be the primary procedure in patients without hydrocephalus. If hydrocephalus is present, cyst fenestration is still recommended, but a ventriculoperitoneal (VP) shunt should be placed if hydrocephalus is marked or after fenestration if the hydrocephalus is progressive.

CONCLUSIONS

Pediatric hydrocephalus, arachnoid cysts, and benign extra-axial collections are common, complex, and, in many ways, poorly understood disorders. Whereas persistent efforts over the last century to improve understanding and, where required, treatment of these disorders have had modest success, recent advances in imaging, neurophysiology, and molecular biology have led to important discoveries, suggesting that significant advances are imminent.

REFERENCES

The complete list of references for this chapter is available in the e-book at www.expertconsult.com.
    See inside cover for registration details.

SELECTED REFERENCES

Boaz, J.C., Edwards-Brown, M.K., 1999. Hydrocephalus in children: neurosurgical and neuroimaging concerns. Neuroimaging Clin. N. Am. 9, 73–91.

Chakraborty, A., Crimmins, D., et al., 2008. Toward reducing shunt placement rates in patients with myelomeningocele. J. Neurosurg. Pediatr. 1, 361–365.

Drake, J.M., 2008. The surgical management of pediatric hydrocephalus. Neurosurgery 62, 633–640, discussion 640–642.

Gosalakkal, J.A., 2002. Intracranial arachnoid cysts in children: a review of pathogenesis, clinical features, and management. Pediatr. Neurol. 26, 93.

Greitz, D., 2004. Radiological assessment of hydrocephalus: new theories and implications for therapy. Neurosurg. Rev. 27, 145–165, discussion 166–167.

Kestle, J., Drake, J., et al., 2000. Long-term follow-up data from the Shunt Design Trial. Pediatr. Neurosurg. 33, 230–236.

Rekate, H.L., 2009. A contemporary definition and classification of hydrocephalus. Semin. Pediatr. Neurol. 16, 9–15.

Renier, D., Sainte-Rose, C., et al., 1988. Prenatal hydrocephalus: outcome and prognosis. Childs Nerv. Syst. 4, 213–222.

Tuli, S., Drake, J., et al., 2003. Long-term outcome of hydrocephalus management in myelomeningoceles. Childs Nerv. Syst. 19, 286–291.

E-BOOK FIGURES AND TABLES

The following figures and tables are available in the e-book at www.expertconsult.com. See inside cover for registration details.

31 Congenital Anomalies of the Skull

Pedro Sanchez and John M. Graham, Jr.

An expanded version of this chapter is available on www.expertconsult.com. See inside cover for registration details.

INTRODUCTION

Congenital anomalies of the skull can arise any time during gestation. During the first 4 to 6 weeks of development from conception, neural crest cells in the fetal head region migrate and differentiate into mesenchymal cells that form the bones of the face, whereas the cranial base and base of the skull are derived from the occipital somitomeres. The viscerocranium is derived from neural crest and it forms the cartilaginous bones of the face (Sadler and Langman, 2009). The neurocranium develops directly from mesenchyme derived from the occipital somitomeres through membranous ossification and is divided into the membranous part, forming the flat bones of the cranial vault, and the chondrocranium, forming the cartilaginous bones of the base of the skull.

There are six fibrous areas where two or more cranial bones meet (fontanels). The five major sutures are the metopic, sagittal, coronal, squamosal, and lambdoid sutures; the six fontanels are the anterior (one), anterolateral (sphenoidal) (two), posterolateral (two), and posterior (one) fontanels (Figure 31-1). The presence of the sutures and fontanels allows the bones of the skull to overlap each other (termed *molding*) during the birth process. Different sutures become ossified at different times, with the metopic suture being the first to ossify at 4 to 7 months and the remaining sutures not completely ossifying until adulthood.

CRANIOSYNOSTOSIS VERSUS DEFORMATIONAL PLAGIOCEPHALY

Craniosynostosis is the process of premature sutural fusion that results in craniostenosis (literally "cranial narrowing"). *Plagiocephaly* is a nonspecific term used to describe an asymmetric head shape, which can result from either craniosynostosis or positional cranial deformation, and differentiation between these two causes is critical to determining the proper mode of treatment (i.e., surgery vs. physical or molding techniques). Craniosynostosis is usually treated with a neurosurgical procedure involving partial calvariectomy, whereas deformational plagiocephaly usually responds to early physical therapy, repositioning, and/or cranial orthotic therapy if those measures are unsuccessful.

In an otherwise structurally normal fetus, prenatal relaxation of normal growth-stretch tensile forces in the underlying dura across a suture for a significant period during late fetal life can result in craniosynostosis. This may also occur when the lack of growth stretch is caused by a deficit in brain growth, as in severe primary microcephaly. The most common cause of craniosynostosis in otherwise normal infants is constraint of the fetal head in utero. Factors that influence fetal constraint may include multiple birth gestation, macrosomia, oligohydramnios, and maternal uterine malformations (e.g., uterine fibroids, bicornuate uterus). When external fetal head constraint limits growth stretch parallel to a cranial suture, it may lead to craniosynostosis of an intervening suture between the constraining points. Sagittal craniosynostosis (the most common type of craniosynostosis) usually is isolated and occurs in an otherwise normal child. The constrained suture tends to develop a bony ridge, especially at the point of maximal constraint between the biparietal eminences. Such ridging can easily be palpated or visualized on skull radiographs, and three-dimensional cranial computed tomography (3D-CT) allows the ridge to be seen even more clearly (Figure 31-2).

Craniosynostosis is usually recognized shortly after birth from the abnormal shape of the head and lack of molding resolving to normal. Early closure of a fontanel, head asymmetry, and/or palpable ridging along a closed suture can be presenting features. If there is uncertainty whether sutures are truly synostotic, 3D-CT can provide a more accurate appraisal (see Figure 31-2).

Synostosis prevents future expansion at that site, and the rapidly growing brain then distorts the calvarium into an aberrant shape, depending on which sutures have become synostotic (Figure 31-2). The earlier the synostosis takes place, the greater the effect on skull shape. Craniosynostosis may be caused by many different mechanisms, such as mutant genes, chromosome disorders, storage disorders, hyperthyroidism, or failure of normal brain growth (Table 31-1). The entire topic of craniosynostosis has been comprehensively reviewed Cohen and MacLean (2000).

Sutural Anatomy and Head Shape

Different terms have been used to describe the varying head shape alterations caused by craniosynostosis, with the resultant head shape dependent on the suture involved. An elongated keel-shaped skull with prominent forehead and occiput is termed *dolichocephaly* or *scaphocephaly*. This head shape is usually associated with premature sagittal suture closure and a palpable ridge toward the posterior end of the suture (see Figure 31-2).

Premature fusion of both coronal sutures produces a high, wide forehead with a short skull, resulting in brachycephaly, whereas fusion of one coronal suture produces an asymmetric head shape. When coronal craniosynostosis occurs, it is important to examine the patient carefully for associated anomalies that might suggest a recognizable genetic syndrome such as thumb anomalies in Pfeiffer syndrome, ambiguous genitalia in Antley-Bixler syndrome, or polysyndactyly in Apert syndrome. Synostosis of multiple cranial sutures is more likely to result in elevated intracranial pressure and to require shunting for hydrocephalus. In extreme cases, a cloverleaf head shape can result from multiple suture synostosis, usually with signs of increased intracranial pressure and a "beaten copper" radiographic appearance of the inner table of the skull.

A triangle-shaped skull (trigonocephaly) is caused by premature fusion of the metopic suture (see Figure 31-2). Syndromic metopic synostosis can also occur, and trigonocephaly is seen in a variety of syndromes, some of which are associated with mental retardation or chromosome anomalies.

Unilateral lambdoid synostosis results in trapezoidal plagiocephaly, which differs from deformational posterior

233

plagiocephaly because of supine positioning and torticollis, and from synostotic anterior plagiocephaly because of unicoronal synostosis (see Figure 31-2). Radiographic signs include trapezoidal cranial asymmetry, small posterior fossa, and sutural sclerosis with ridging; however, sole reliance on skull radiographs and clinical signs can lead to misdiagnosis, so it is best to confirm the diagnosis of suspected lambdoid synostosis with a 3D-CT scan.

Plagiocephaly (which translates literally from the Greek term *plagio kephale* as "oblique head") is a term used to describe asymmetry of the head shape, when viewed from the top (Graham and Sanchez-Lara, 2016). The term *deformational plagiocephaly* should suffice to distinguish this type of defect and its proper type of management. The side of the plagiocephaly is usually indicated by the bone that has been most flattened by the deforming forces (usually the occiput for infants who sleep on their backs). Deformational plagio-

cephaly is usually not associated with premature closure of a cranial suture, but because craniosynostosis can also be caused by fetal head constraint, when both deformational plagiocephaly and craniosynostosis occur together, the diagnosis can be difficult, requiring complex management.

Infants with limited mobility because of hypotonia, hydrocephalus, macrocephaly, or limb anomalies are also more likely to develop deformational plagiocephaly, which can complicate syndromes with these features. Predisposing factors resulting in excessive or asymmetric head deformation include restrictive intrauterine environments, poor muscle tone, torticollis, clavicular fracture, cervical-vertebral abnormalities, sleeping position, multiple gestation, and incomplete bone mineralization. The development of excessive positional brachycephaly, with or without plagiocephaly, can be an early indication of hypotonia or that parents are not providing their infants with adequate "tummy time."

Epidemiology of Craniosynostosis

The incidence of craniosynostosis is 3.4 per 10,000 births, and it is usually an isolated, sporadic anomaly in an otherwise normal child. A specific genetic etiology can be identified in approximately 21% of cases. About 8% of all craniosynostosis cases are familial. Familial types of craniosynostosis are seen frequently in coronal synostosis, accounting for 14.4% of coronal synostosis, 6% of sagittal synostosis, and 5.6% of metopic synostosis, whereas lambdoidal synostosis is almost never familial. The frequency of associated twinning is increased, and most twin pairs are discordant, especially with sagittal and metopic synostosis, which would tend to support fetal crowding as a cause for these types of synostosis; concordance for coronal synostosis is much higher for monozygotic twins than for dizygotic twins, suggesting that many cases of coronal synostosis have a genetic basis.

Sagittal synostosis is the most common type of craniosynostosis, accounting for 50% to 60% of cases and occurring in 1.9 per 10,000 births, with a 3.5 : 1 male-to-female sex ratio.

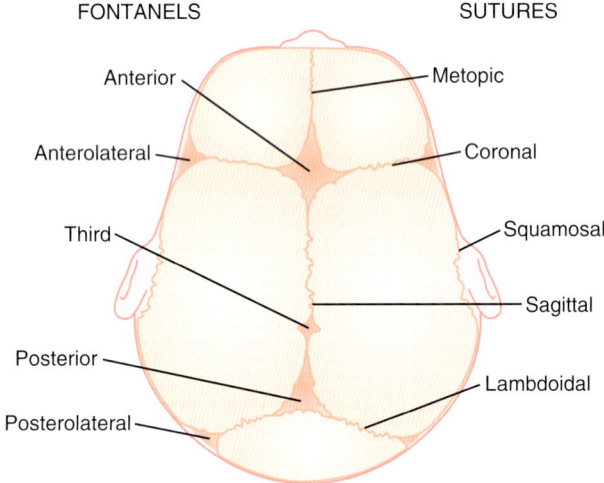

Figure 31-1. Schematic showing name and location of cranial sutures and fontanels.

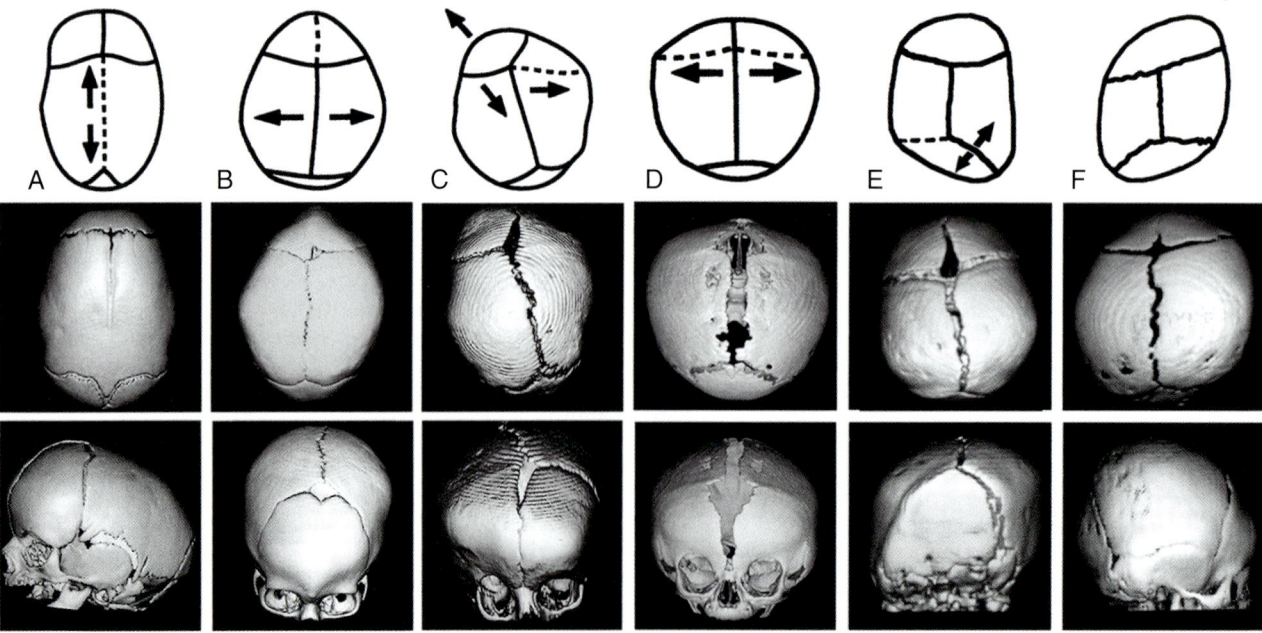

Figure 31-2. Schematic drawing and three-dimensional computed tomography reconstructions of synostosis and plagiocephaly. **A,** Sagittal synostosis with dolichocephaly. **B,** Metopic synostosis. **C,** Right coronal synostosis. **D,** Bilateral coronal synostosis. **E,** Left lambdoid synostosis. **F,** Right occipital deformational plagiocephaly.

TABLE 31-1 Syndromes Associated With Craniosynostosis

Metopic	**Multiple**
Trigonocephaly (*FGFR1*)	Trigonocephaly (*FGFR1*)
Metopic craniosynostosis (*FREM1*)	Metopic craniosynostosis (*FREM1*)
Opitz C trigonocephaly (*CD96*)	Opitz C trigonocephaly (*CD96*)
Say-Meyer	Say-Meyer 3MC (*COLEC11, MASP1*)
Sagittal	Antley-Bixler (*POR*)
Berant	Baller-Gerold (*RECQL4*)
Chitayat hypophosphatemia	Barber-Say
Cranioectodermal dysplasia (*ITF43, WDR35, WDR19, IFT122*)	Beare-Stevenson cutis gyrata (*FGFR2*)
Craniosynostosis, Philadelphia type (Dup 2q34)	Boston type (*MSX2*)
Hydrocephalus, autosomal dominant	Carpenter (*RAB23, MEGF8*)
Loeys-Dietz (*TGFB2, TGFBR1, TGFBR2, SMAD3*)	Cole-Carpenter
Pfeiffer cardiocranial syndrome	Craniofacial dyssynostosis
Richieri-Costa overgrowth	Craniosynostosis and dental anomalies (*IL11RA*)
Sensenbrenner (*IFT122*)	Craniosynostosis type 4 (*ERF*)
Shprintzen-Goldberg (*SKI*)	Craniosynostosis type 5 (*ALX4*)
Tricho-dento-osseous type I (*DLX3*)	Craniotelencephalic dysplasia
Coronal	Crouzon (*FGFR2*)
Acrocraniofacial dysostosis	Crouzon with acanthosis nigricans (crouzonodermoskeletal) (*FGFR3*)
Alagille (*JAG1, NOTCH2*)	Curry-Jones
Apert (*FGFR2*)	Elejalde: acrocephalopolydactylous
Auralcephalosyndactyly	dysplasia (*MYO5A*)
Brachydactyly, type C (*GDF5*)	Fontaine-Farriaux
Coronal craniosynostosis (*TCF12*)	Fryns type
Cranio-fronto-nasal dysplasia (*EFNB1*)	Gomez-Lopez-Hernandez
Craniomicromelic dysplasia	Grieg (*GLI3*)
Craniorhiny	Holoprosencephaly with craniosynostosis
Craniosynostosis-mental retardation-clefting syndrome	Hunter-McAlpine (del 17q23)
Gorlin-Chaudhry-Moss	Jackson-Weiss (*FGFR2*)
Hersh	Lin-Gettig
Hypomandibular faciocranial dysostosis	Lowry-Craniosynostosis with fibular aplasia
Muenke (*FGFR3*)	Lowry-MacLean
Nonsyndromal coronal cranioosynostosis (*FGFR3, EFN4*)	Microcephaly Micromelia
Spondyloepiphyseal dysplasia with craniosynostosis	Osteoglophonic dysplasia (*FGFR1*)
	Pfeiffer (*FGFR1, FGFR2*)
	Saethre-Chotzen (*TWIST*)
	Sakati-Nyhan
	San Francisco
	Say-Poznanski
	SCARF
	Seckel (*ATR*)
	Thanatophoric dysplasia (*FGFR3*)

Only 6% of cases are familial, with 72% of cases sporadic and no paternal or maternal age effects noted. Twinning occurred in 4.8% of 366 cases, with only one monozygotic twin pair being concordant.

Coronal craniosynostosis is the second most frequent type of craniosynostosis (accounting for 20% to 30% of cases). Unilateral coronal craniosynostosis can be either genetic or caused by fetal head constraint from an aberrant fetal lie, multiple gestation, or small uterine cavity. Approximately 71% of unilateral coronal craniosynostosis is right-sided, and 67% of vertex presentations are in the left occiput transverse position, possibly explaining the prevalence of right-sided, unilateral, coronal craniostenosis. Nonsyndromic coronal craniosynostosis occurs 0.94 per 10,000 births, with 61% of cases sporadic, and 14.4% of 180 pedigrees familial. Bilateral cases occur much more frequently than unilateral cases, and coronal synostosis is more frequent in females (male-to-female ratio 1:2). The paternal age is statistically older than average (32.7 years), and these data have been interpreted as being consistent with fresh dominant mutation and autosomal-dominant inheritance with 60% penetrance, when the synostosis has a genetic basis.

Metopic synostosis occurs in about 0.67 per 10,000 births, making it the third most frequent type of craniosynostosis (accounting for 10% to 20% of patients). Like sagittal synostosis, metopic synostosis is more frequent in males (3.3:1

male-to-female ratio) and seldom familial (5.6% of cases). There is no maternal or paternal age effect, and the frequency of associated twinning was 7.8% of 179 pedigrees studied, with only 2 twin monozygotic pairs concordant.

Familial craniosynostosis is usually transmitted as an autosomal-dominant trait with incomplete penetrance and variable expressivity. A wide variety of chromosomal anomalies have also been associated with craniosynostosis with microdeletions and duplications detected by karyotype or chromosome microarray analysis. Deletions of 9p and 11q, microdeletions, and translocations disrupting TWIST1 on chromosome 7p have all been described. In addition, craniosynostosis can also occur as a feature of several genetic syndromes, many of which manifest phenotypic overlap and genetic heterogeneity. Single-gene disorders associated with craniosynostosis include Apert syndrome, Crouzon syndrome, Pfeiffer syndrome, Saethre-Chotzen syndrome, Jackson-Weiss syndrome, Boston craniosynostosis, Beare-Stevenson cutis gyrata syndrome, and Muenke syndrome.

Secondary craniosynostosis can occur with certain primary metabolic disorders (e.g., hyperthyroidism, rickets), storage disorders (e.g., mucopolysaccharidosis), hematological disorders (thalassemia, sickle cell anemia, polycythemia vera), brain malformations, and selected teratogenic exposures (e.g., diphenylhydantoin, retinoic acid, valproic acid, aminopterin, fluconazole, cyclophosphamide) (Cohen and MacLean, 2000).

Bilateral coronal synostosis often lacks sutural ridging and usually has a genetic pathogenesis. Some have suggested that all patients should be screened for mutations in one or more of the following genes: *CD96*, *EFNB1*, *ERF*, *FGFR1*, *FGFR2*, *FGFR3*, *GLI3*, *IFT122*, *MEGF8*, *MSX2*, *POR*, *RAB23*, *RECQL4*, *RUNX2*, *SKI*, *TCF12*, and *TWIST1*. In 2010 Wilkie et al. established a genetic diagnosis in 21% of cases (86% monogenic disorders, and 14% chromosomal disorders), with the most frequently involved genes *FGFR2* (32%), *FGFR3* (25%), *TWIST1* (19%), and *EFNB1* (7%) (Wilkie et al., 2010). Inability to demonstrate a mutation does not rule out a genetic basis for the craniosynostosis, and not every person with a pathogenic mutation manifests craniosynostosis.

Kleeblattschädel (Cloverleaf Skull)

Kleeblattschädel is a term used to describe a cloverleaf skull configuration consisting of protrusion of each of the cranial bones, with broadening of the temporal region and face. These cranial protrusions are separated into focal bulges by furrows along the suture lines. The eyes often protrude, leading to corneal ulceration, scarring, and subsequent blindness, if the corneal surface remains unprotected. Occipital encephaloceles can occur, and associated hydrocephalus is common. The presence of kleeblattschädel indicates that multiple sutural fusions occurred during early prenatal life. Increased thickening of the base of the occipital bone prevents lengthening of the skull, thus yielding the typical shape.

Multiple sutural synostosis is much more likely to result from genetic mutations in *FGFR* genes, *TWIST*, or *MSX2*, all of which result in syndromes that can present with cloverleaf skull (Cohen and MacLean, 2000).

Patients with kleeblattschädel need to be followed carefully for hydrocephalus, which may be part of the syndrome, rather than attributable to the multiple suture synostosis. The purpose of surgery should be to decompress the brain, expand the bony orbits to accommodate the globes, and open airway passages.

Treatment and Outcomes of Craniosynostosis

Mild degrees of craniosynostosis may not always require surgery. The usual indication for surgery is to restore normal craniofacial shape and growth. When both the coronal and sagittal sutures are synostotic, impairing brain growth early in infancy, surgery is indicated to prevent neurologic and ophthalmologic complications associated with increased intracranial pressure and inadequate orbital volume. Several neurosurgical techniques have been developed for the treatment of craniosynostosis. Most of these techniques involve removing the aberrant portion of the bony calvarium from its underlying dura, including the area surrounding the synostotic suture(s). Newer endoscopic repair techniques have been developed, followed by postoperative orthotic molding. Such procedures are most effective if performed relatively early in infancy. These techniques are most effective in normal infants without a syndromic type of craniosynostosis.

One comorbidity of synostosis is hydrocephalus, which may occur secondarily, or be a part of a genetic craniosynostosis syndrome. This occurs in 4% to 10% of patients with craniosynostosis and is more frequent with syndromic and multiple sutural craniosynostosis. In nonsyndromic patients, the rate of cerebral ventricular dilatation is the same as that observed in the general population. Such dilatation usually stabilizes spontaneously and rarely requires shunting. Some cases of progressive hydrocephalus in syndromic craniosynostosis cases were related to multiple sutural involvement, thereby constricting cranial volume, constricting the skull base, crowding the posterior fossa, and causing jugular foraminal stenosis. These findings were most frequent among patients with Crouzon, Pfeiffer, or Apert syndrome, especially in association with cloverleaf skull abnormalities. A diffuse beaten copper pattern on skull radiographs, along with obliteration of anterior sulci or narrowing of basal cisterns in children under the age of 18 months, is predictive of increased intracranial pressure in over 95% of cases.

Nonsyndromic Craniosynostosis
Neurocognitive Development

There is a growing body of evidence that single-suture craniosynostosis is associated with neurobehavioral problems. Syndromes with multiple-suture fusions have more commonly been associated with elevated rates for intellectual disability and learning disabilities. Most studies have found adverse neurocognitive outcomes in about 35% to 40% of assessed cases, with an occasional study finding this number to be as high as 50%. A few studies have reported a 3- to 5-times higher-than-average risk of poor neurobehavioral outcome. In studies that directly measured the IQs of children with sagittal synostosis, a discrepancy of greater than 20 standard score points between language and nonverbal IQ scores was found.

Sagittal synostosis has not been found to affect the neurologic function of the infant or toddler significantly (Kapp-Simon et al., 1993). However, some studies conducted in older children have found moderate to severe speech and language difficulties in up to 37% of cases, and the tendency toward such problems is associated with a positive family history for such difficulties and later age of surgical correction.

In a long-term neurodevelopmental outcome study of nonsyndromic cases, correlation was found between outcomes and timing of surgery, with 22.6% of those operated on before 12 months showing impaired mental development versus 52.2% impaired mental development in those who underwent surgery after age 12 months. Overall, 31% of cases of trigonocephaly were observed to have delayed development, and this appeared to be related to the severity of the malformation and the presence of associated malformations. There is preliminary evidence that surgical management with whole-vault cranioplasty performed before 6 months of age provides the most favorable long-term intellectual outcomes in patients with isolated sagittal synostosis.

WIDE CRANIAL SUTURES

Cranial sutures are considered to be widened when the sutural separation is more than 2 SD above the mean sutural width for age. Wide cranial sutures in themselves cause no impairment, but they can be an indication of increased intracranial pressure or caused by craniosynostosis in another part of the skull. The younger an infant begins to have increased intracranial pressure, the earlier sutural diastasis will appear. If the wide cranial sutures are caused by defective or delayed ossification, no treatment is generally indicated as the ossification will improve and sutural width will decrease with age.

ANOMALIES OF FONTANELS

A fontanel measuring either 2 SD above or 2 SD below the mean for age is termed large or small, respectively. Closure of the anterior fontanel before 6 months is considered early, whereas closure after 18 months is considered late. The other fontanels are normally closed at term gestation.

The anterior fontanel is the largest of the fontanels and normally closes by 18 months. A small or absent anterior fontanel usually indicates some type of underlying pathology, with the most common etiologies including any cause of congenital microcephaly, craniosynostosis (particularly involving the metopic suture), or accelerated bone maturation such as that occurs in hyperthyroidism.

Large fontanels may be noted at birth by palpation and confirmed by measurement. Causes of both large fontanels and delayed closure include increased intracranial pressure or delayed ossification of the cranium caused by an underlying genetic, nutritional, or metabolic etiology. Cleidocranial dysplasia typically results in delayed closure of the anterior fontanel with widened cranial sutures and hypoplastic clavicles. Although early or late closure of the fontanel is reasonably common, care must be taken to rule out underlying pathology.

CRANIAL DERMAL SINUS

A cranial dermal sinus is a midline depression or tract lined by stratified squamous epithelium that extends from the skin toward the central nervous system or its coverings. Cranial dermal sinuses are most common in the occipital region, but can be found anywhere. Clinical presentation is often as a cutaneous localized swelling that presents an infection or cystic expansion of the sinus tract beneath the skin surface, occasionally with drainage. Occasionally, cystic expansion occurs within the cranial cavity, which obstructs cerebrospinal fluid flow, compresses the adjacent neural structures, and/or ruptures to cause sterile meningitis, which can be recurrent.

In the facial region, the most frequent congenital midline mass is a nasal dermoid sinus cyst, which can have intracranial extension and be associated with other anomalies. Nasal dermoid sinus cysts usually arise sporadically, although reports of familial occurrence have been documented. Nasal pits are present in 50% of patients with nasal dermoids and intracranial extension noted in 36% to 45% of cases. Associated anomalies were present in 41% of one series examined by a multidisciplinary team, and they were associated with many different syndromes and chromosome anomalies. Complications can result from enlargement of the cyst, skeletal distortion, and recurrent infection. The recommended treatment of the tract and any associated dermoid tumor or cyst is surgery.

PARIETAL FORAMINA (INCLUDING CRANIUM BIFIDUM)

Parietal foramina are small defects in the superoposterior angles of the parietal bones through which emissary veins may pass through the calvarium (Figure 31-5). Usually, parietal foramina present as symmetric oval defects situated on each side of the sagittal suture, and their size diminishes with age. They are covered with normal scalp and hair, and are detected through palpation and radiography. Occasionally, brain covered by dura and intact scalp can bulge through extensive lesions, suggesting the possibility of an encephalocele, but the location of these lesions off the midline differentiates them from neural tube closure defects (Epstein and Epstein, 1967).

Parietal foramina are usually small and only detectable radiographically; however, 10% are 5 mm or more and can be as large as 50 mm in diameter. Small parietal foramina are found in 60% to 70% of all adults, whereas large parietal foramina are present in less than 1% of adults. Small unilateral defects are more common than bilateral defects. When the defect is unilateral, it more often involves the right side, and males are more commonly affected than females, with a ratio of 5:3. Parietal foramina themselves cause no impairment, usually manifest autosomal-dominant inheritance with

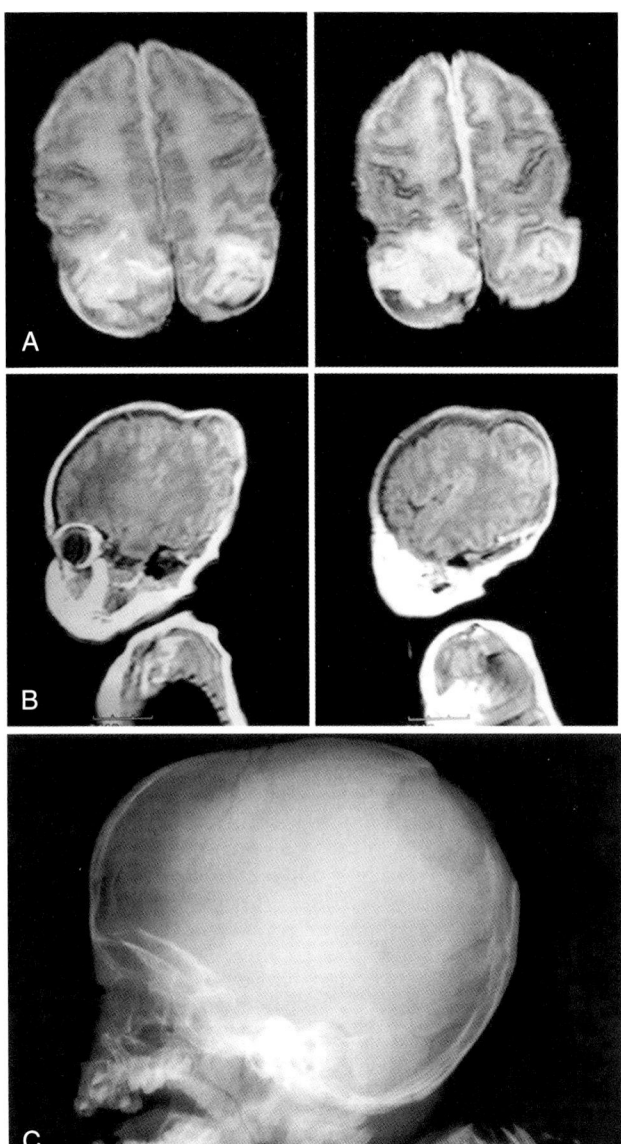

Figure 31-5. Parietal foramina. A and **B,** Large parietal defects at birth detected by MRI. **C,** Partial closure by age 16 months on skull radiograph.

variable expression, and can occur as part of the phenotype in a few syndromes.

WORMIAN BONES

Wormian bones were named after Dr. Worm, who initially described them as accessory bones that occur within cranial suture lines or fontanels. They can occur singly, or in large numbers, and are diagnosed radiographically. Wormian bones could be mistaken for a skull fracture, but experienced radiographic interpretation should resolve this error. They can occur within any suture but are rare in coronal or sagittal sutures. Although they do not cause any impairment themselves, their significance is variable.

The pathogenesis of Wormian bones is thought to be related to intracranial strain along with open sutures causing ossification defects. Although the prevalence of Wormian bones in the general population is as high as 17%, the prevalence varies with age. Males are more often affected than females, and differences between ethnic groups have been noted. Wormian bones are commonly seen in osteogenesis imperfecta and other disorders resulting in defective cranial bone mineralization. The more severe the defective mineralization, the more numerous the Wormian bones, and such infants can also become quite brachycephalic as a consequence of postnatal supine positioning with soft cranial bones.

SCALP VERTEX APLASIA

Scalp vertex aplasia, or aplasia cutis congenita (ACC), is a relatively common congenital defect resulting in localized absence of skin, usually occurring on the scalp as an isolated finding not associated with other abnormalities. Scalp vertex aplasia begins as multiple or solitary, sharply marginated, raw areas with absence of skin. These lesions mature into atrophic scars devoid of adnexal structures, usually in the vertex area or midline superior occipital region. The cause of these lesions is heterogeneous and includes vascular disruption, trauma, teratogens, and genetic factors. The frequency is 1 per 3000 live births, and a classification system of subtypes for ACC has been suggested by Frieden. With prompt closure and a healthy underlying dura, cranial bone growth will occur after prompt early wound closure, and the risk of fatal hemorrhage or meningitis is greatly lessened.

THIN CRANIAL BONES

Thin cranial bones have little or no diploë, which is the spongy intervening bone separating the outer and inner layers. The diagnosis of thin cranial bones is made radiographically and is usually subjective. Thin calvarial bones can be secondary to craniosynostosis (particularly adjacent to the ridging in sagittal synostosis) and hydrocephalus, or can occur as part of several syndromes in which undermineralization is a feature. Areas of radiolucency are called craniolacunae (luckenschadel) and are often secondary to spinal dysraphism. These generally disappear by age 1 year. Regionally thinned areas can also occur in association with porencephaly, subdural hygroma, arachnoid cyst, and some tumors. Craniolacunae probably do not occur as isolated traits. Prognosis depends on the underlying etiology, and lacunar skull defects themselves have no direct effects on the infant.

UNDERMINERALIZATION OF THE SKULL

Undermineralization of the skull results in increased radiolucency of the cranial bones and is attributable to decreased calcium deposition. Congenital under mineralization occurs in several syndromes, particularly osteogenesis imperfecta and hypophosphatasia. Hypophosphatasia occurs in at least three forms, including infantile, childhood, and adult forms. Undermineralization is most pronounced in the infantile form and is least evident in the adult form. The infantile form can usually be diagnosed by fetal ultrasonography, whereas the other forms are often diagnosed after birth by radiographs and measurement of serum alkaline phosphatase levels (Goodman and Gorlin, 1983). Fluorosis and vitamin D–dependent rickets can also produce postnatal undermineralization of the skull, but areas of sclerosis are also present in fluorosis. The incidence of undermineralization is low, and prognosis is dependent on cause, varying widely from stillbirth or death during infancy to little effect at all.

CRANIOTABES

Prolonged forceful pressure on the fetal vertex may result in diminished cranial mineralization affecting the superior portions of the parietal bones. Such craniotabes is more likely to occur in first-born infants, especially with early fetal head descent into a vertex presentation for a prolonged period. Mild degrees of craniotabes occur in about 2% of newborn babies, and more extensive degrees of craniotabes are less common. Craniotabes was first described in congenital syphilis, and it can also be seen with subclinical rickets because of vitamin D deficiency. Rickets should be considered in any infant with a nonvertex presentation, whose mother might be at risk for nutritional deficiency, and such infants usually manifest generalized craniotabes with osteomalacia.

With compression-related craniotabes, the prognosis is excellent, and the calvarium usually mineralizes in a normal fashion within 2 to 3 months after birth. If the mother has vitamin D–deficient rickets and there is more generalized craniotabes and osteomalacia, this condition usually manifests a prompt response to vitamin D therapy over the next few months. As in other defects of skeletal mineralization, such as osteogenesis imperfecta and hypophosphatasia, initial care must be taken to avoid fractures. Infants with osteogenesis imperfecta or hypophosphatasia usually show generalized osteomalacia, brittle bones, and Wormian bones.

THICK CRANIAL BONES

Increased thickness of cranial bones is detected on radiographic examination, and there may be normal or increased cranial density. The diagnosis of a thickened cranium is made radiographically, although no formal criteria have been established for determining whether cranial bones are thick. Although there is wide variability among different individuals, the thickest part of a normal cranium is not, in general, any greater than 1 cm. There are both ethnic- and sex-related variations in skull thickness. Women have thicker skulls than men, and blacks have thicker skulls than whites.

Several syndromes with thick calvarial bones have been described, including Pyle disease, Robinow syndrome, Fountain syndrome, autosomal-dominant osteopetrosis, and pseudohypoparathyoidism. It is unknown whether thick cranial bones can occur as an isolated trait, and the prognosis depends on the underlying condition. In hemolytic diseases, such as thalassemia, vertical striations ("hair-on-end" appearance) occur, whereas in bone diseases such as osteopetrosis, sclerosis occurs. Overgrowth of the middle table can also occur in microcephaly. In situations in which a shunt has been placed to relieve hydrocephalus, thickening of both inner and middle tables can occur.

SCLEROSIS AND HYPEROSTOSIS OF THE SKULL

Increased density or overmineralization of the cranial bones can be generalized or localized, and this is termed *sclerosis* or *hyperostosis of the skull*. Sclerosis generally refers to an increase in bone density without an alteration in width, whereas hyperostosis is caused by bone overgrowth that leads to an increase in density and width, though not all cases fit cleanly into one category or the other (Kozlowski and Beighton, 1995). Hyperostosis is distinct from thick cranial bones, although hyperostosis and occasionally sclerosis can also cause thick cranial bones. Most of the sclerosing bone dysplasias manifest generalized changes, which are classified on the basis of the distribution and configuration of these abnormalities (Kozlowski and Beighton, 1995).

The presence of sclerosis or hyperostosis can be diagnosed radiographically or by CT, and scintigraphy may provide information on disease progression (Figure 31-8). Radiologic changes are age related, and definitive diagnosis may be difficult in early childhood (Kozlowski and Beighton, 1995). All

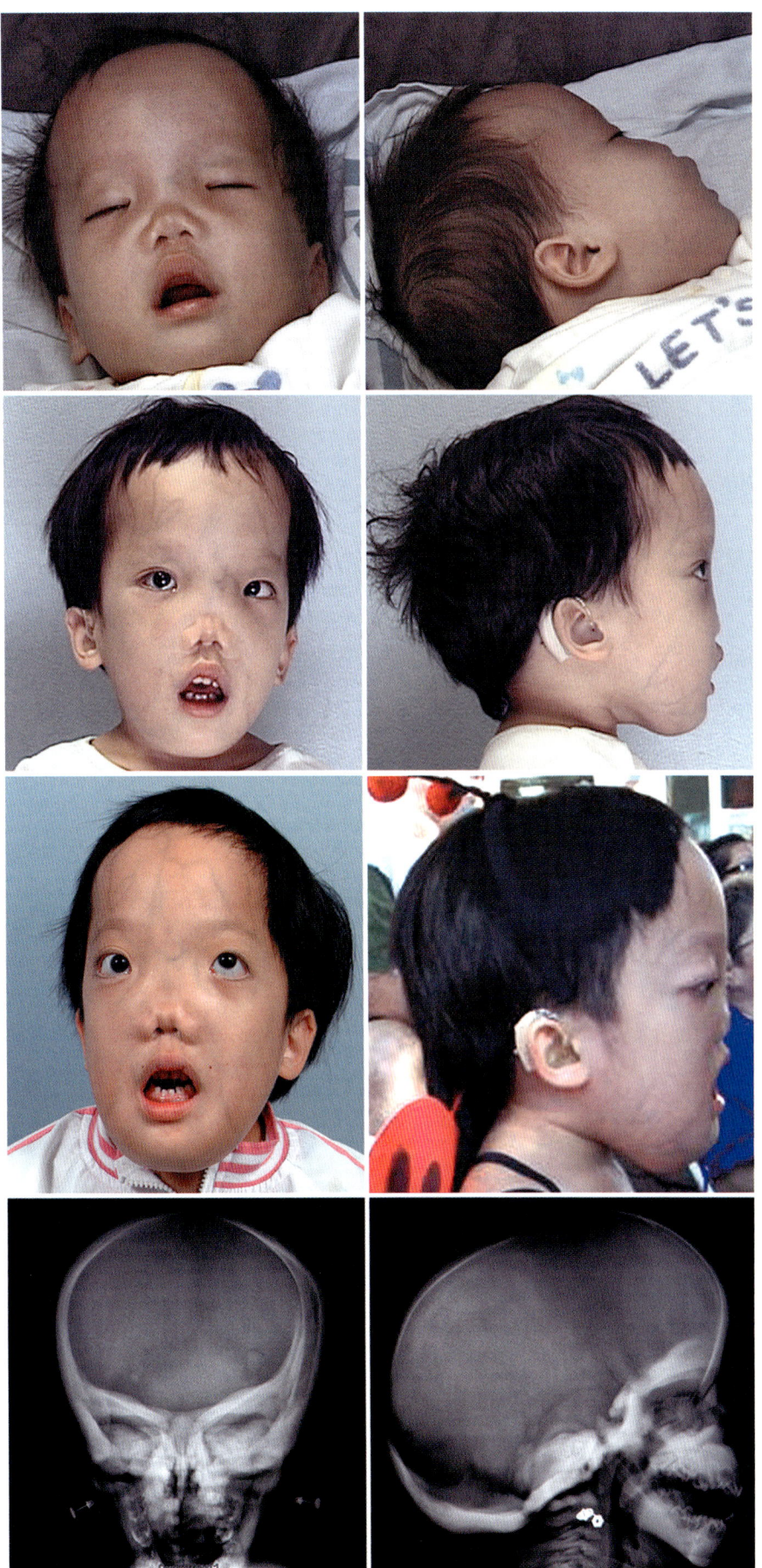

Figure 31-8. Craniometaphyseal dysplasia presenting with progressive craniofacial changes and hearing loss.

conditions that cause generalized osteosclerosis affect the skull (Kozlowski and Beighton, 1995). Localized sclerosis of the base of the skull can occur in polyostotic fibrous dysplasia, Jansen-type metaphyseal dysplasia, severe anemia, hypercalciuria, and Paget's disease. It may also be seen with a meningioma or inflammation (Kozlowski and Beighton, 1995). Symptoms include narrowing of cranial nerve foramina, which in turn can cause nerve palsy, deafness, or vision defects. Increased intracranial pressure is not uncommon, and papilledema can also occur as a complication. Two primary pathologic processes can lead to sclerosis: overproduction of bone and failure of osteoclastic absorption of bone. The prognosis depends on the underlying cause and varies from individuals being asymptomatic to sudden death from medullary compression. In addition, facial palsy, as well as hearing and vision loss, may occur because of cranial nerve compression within stenotic foramina, which may require surgical decompression. Craniotomy to relieve increased intracranial pressure may also be indicated.

ANOMALIES OF THE SELLA TURCICA

Anomalies include abnormal size and/or shape of the sella turcica, which is the central depression within the sphenoid bone that contains the pituitary gland. Assessment of the sella turcica can be best established radiographically using a lateral skull x-ray or by CT scan using the "bone window" setting. It is a critical landmark for orthodontics and craniofacial morphology, and variants in shape should be noted in orthodontic planning. A small or absent sella has been described in patients with hypopituitarism and myotonic dystrophy, whereas a large sella occurs in patients with storage disorders, pituitary tumors, empty sella syndrome, craniopharyngioma, intrasellar aneurysm, untreated hypogonadism, and hypothyroidism.

A J-shaped sella describes the lateral profile of the sella turcica, in which the sella resembles a "J" lying on its side. A J-shaped sella can occur as a normal variant, but may also occur in individuals with calvarial enlargement or optic nerve gliomas (Swischuk, 1972). Bridged sella is caused by bony bridging between anterior and posterior clinoids and can be a normal variant. It can also be seen in nevoid basal cell carcinoma syndrome (Gorlin syndrome), craiofaciofrontodigital syndrome, geleophysic dysplasia, and lysosomal storage disorders.

ANOMALIES OF TEMPORAL BONE

Congenital anomalies of the temporal bone (including external, middle, and inner ear abnormalities) can cause significant morbidity in children such as hearing loss and balance problems. A complete discussion of the myriad of congenital temporal bone anomalies is beyond the scope of this chapter. Jackler et al. proposed the most commonly used classification of inner ear abnormalities. Inner ear malformations consist of complete labyrinthine aplasia, cochlear aplasia, common cavity, incomplete partition type I & II, cochlea hypoplasia, semicircular canal abnormalities, and enlarged vestibular aqueduct (Yiin et al., 2011).

ANOMALIES OF FORAMEN MAGNUM

The foramen magnum is an oval-shaped opening in the occipital bone bound by the basiocciput anteriorly, the occipital condyles laterally, and the supraocciput posteriorly. If premature suture fusion occurs and/or endochondral ossification is abnormal, a small foramen magnum is the result. Anomalies of the foramen magnum include either small or large size, or a keyhole shape. In a retrospective review of

3D-CT on 101 patients, Göçmez ranked their frequency. MRI best achieves diagnostic assessment of foramen magnum size or shape, although x-ray or CT may also be used. Reference tables have been published indicating normal foramen magnum size. The clinical effects of a small foramen magnum vary from asymptomatic individuals to those with weakness, apneic spells, hyperreflexia, hydrocephalus, and abnormal somatosensory-evoked potentials and/or polysomnograms. Achondroplasia is the most common syndrome with a small foramen magnum, but other skeletal dysplasias and disorders associated with sclerosis of the skull can also lead to a small foramen magnum. A large foramen magnum usually results from chronic increased intracranial pressure or from direct effects of an expanding process within the foramen magnum (syringomyelia, Arnold-Chiari malformation). Asymmetry of the foramen magnum occurs with craniovertebral anomalies or premature synostosis of one or more of the occipital synchondroses. Children with the latter may tend to hold their heads obliquely. A keyhole-shaped foramen magnum has been described in the hydrolethalus syndrome.

Prognosis for a small foramen magnum is variable, but the most serious outcome of brainstem compression may be sudden death. Recommended treatment is suboccipital craniectomy. The prognosis for a large or abnormally shaped foramen magnum is dependent on the underlying cause.

ANOMALIES OF THE OTHER BASAL FORAMINA AND CANALS

There are at least 11 foramina and canals in the base of the cranium through which blood vessels and nerves enter or leave the intracranial space. Congenital anomalies include asymmetry of paired foramina, communication with other foramina, and absence if the transmitted structure is absent. Anomalies of any of these foramina can include abnormal opening size or configuration and are typically incidental findings discovered on scans obtained for other purposes.

BASILAR IMPRESSION

Basilar impression is a malformation or deformation of the cranial base consisting of indentation of the base of the skull at the craniospinal junction. Basilar impression may be suspected when there is limited movement and shortening of the neck, but definitive diagnosis requires radiography, CT scan, or MRI scan. In basilar impression, the odontoid moves cephalad and can protrude into the foramen magnum, thus compromising function of the spinal cord, brainstem, and cerebellum, as well as impeding the flow of cerebrospinal fluid. Symptoms include pain, limitation of movement, increased intracranial pressure, hydrocephalus, and cranial nerve symptoms. Symptoms may appear suddenly or develop over several months.

Primary basilar impression is caused by a congenital defect of osseous structures in the cervico-occipital region, and can occur as an autosomal-dominant trait. Secondary basilar impression is related to disease of the skull and has been reported in association with osteogenesis imperfecta, Hajdu-Cheney syndrome, and several endocrine disorders.

Affected individuals may be asymptomatic, develop sudden or progressive symptoms, or die suddenly. Treatment consists of immobilization or, in severe cases, decompression of the foramen magnum, laminectomy of the first and second cervical vertebrae, and cervico-occipital fusion. Shunting for hydrocephalus may also be indicated. Cranial base pathology is a serious complication of osteogenesis imperfecta, and early bisphosphonate treatment may delay development of craniocervical junction pathology.

Bathrocephaly

Bathrocephaly is a skull deformation that appears as a step-like deformity at the back of the skull, and it is also termed *an occipital shelf*. It is not associated with craniosynostosis, but can occur secondary to breech position in utero and has been associated with a persistent mendosal suture. In general, this anomaly is of no significance, and spontaneous improvement usually occurs. Prognosis is poor only if breech position is secondary to malformation or neurologic dysfunction.

Occipital Horns

Occipital horns are bony protuberances situated on both sides of the foramen magnum and pointing caudad. They have been described only in individuals with an X-linked syndrome, Ehlers-Danlos type IX, or a mild form of Menkes disease caused by mutation in the gene encoding Cu(2+)-transporting ATPase, alpha polypeptide (*ATP7A*).

REFERENCES

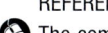 The complete list of references for this chapter is available online at www.expertconsult.com.
 See inside cover for registration details.

SELECTED REFERENCES

Cohen, M.M., MacLean, R.E., 2000. Craniosynostosis: Diagnosis, Evaluation, and Management, second ed. Oxford University Press, New York.
Epstein, J.A., Epstein, B.S., 1967. Deformities of the skull surfaces in infancy and childhood. J. Pediatr. 70, 636–647.
Goodman, R.M., Gorlin, R.J., 1983. The Malformed Infant and Child: An Illustrated Guide. Oxford University Press, New York.
Graham, J.M. Jr., Sanchez-Lara, P.A., 2016. Smith's Recognizable Patterns of Human Deformation. Saunders/Elsevier, Philadelphia.
Kapp-Simon, K.A., Figueroa, A., Jocher, C.A., et al., 1993. Longitudinal assessment of mental development in infants with nonsyndromic craniosynostosis with and without cranial release and reconstruction. Plast. Reconstr. Surg. 92, 831–839, discussion 40–41.
Kozlowski, K., Beighton, P., 1995. Gamut Index of Skeletal Dysplasias: An Aid to Radiodiagnosis, second ed. Springer, New York.
Sadler, T.W., Langman, J., 2009. Langman's Medical Embryology, eleventh ed. Lippincott William & Wilkins, Baltimore, MD.
Swischuk, L.E., 1972. The normal pediatric skull. Variations and artefacts. Radiol. Clin. North Am. 10, 277–290.
Wilkie, A.O., Byren, J.C., Hurst, J.A., et al., 2010. Prevalence and complications of single-gene and chromosomal disorders in craniosynostosis. Pediatrics 126, e391.
Yiin, R.S., Tang, P.H., Tan, T.Y., 2011. Review of congenital inner ear abnormalities on CT temporal bone. Br. J. Radiol. 84, 859–863.

E-BOOK FIGURES AND TABLES

The following figures and tables are available in the e-book at www.expertconsult.com. See inside cover for registration details.

Fig. 31-3 A, Multiple suture synostosis resulting in a cloverleaf skull. **B,** Three-dimensional CT scans show multiple sutural synostosis with multiple areas of cranial thinning, which would yield a "beaten copper" appearance on skull radiographs.

Fig. 31-4 Three-dimensional CT scan demonstrating excessive Wormian bones and wide cranial sutures in a child with cleidocranial dysplasia.

Fig. 31-6 Osteogenesis type IV with marked osteopenia of the skull and spine, and multiple Wormian bones. The patient also had a history of multiple fractures with minimal trauma.

Fig. 31-7 Aplasia cutis congenita in association with trisomy 13.

Fig. 31-9 Three-dimensional CT images and frontal MRI of a 6-year-old with polyostotic fibrous dysplasia or McCune-Albright syndrome.

32 Developmental Encephalopathies

Alex R. Paciorkowski, Laurie E. Seltzer, and Jeffrey L. Neul

An expanded version of this chapter is available on www.expertconsult.com. See inside cover for registration details.

DEFINITION OF DEVELOPMENTAL ENCEPHALOPATHIES

This chapter addresses a group of disorders that share a common constellation of features. These are disorders that have not fit neatly into the traditional classifications of autism spectrum disorder, perhaps because of concomitant severe intellectual disability, or have not quite been captured by the category of "intellectual disability" because of the obvious and profound abnormalities of social interaction, language development, and repetitive behaviors more consistent with a diagnosis of autism. Many of these disorders also may present with a severe early-life epileptic encephalopathy—yet on follow-up at a later age, the epilepsy is not a prominent part of the phenotype. A common feature is also that, aside from hypotonia, many of these disorders are not overly apparent at birth. Head size at birth is frequently normal, but in many of these disorders, microcephaly emerges over time. Brain magnetic resonance imaging (MRI) usually does not show classic malformations, but subtle features typically involving the corpus callosum and cerebellum can be seen. During infancy, these disorders may resemble one another, making clinical diagnosis difficult. Sentinel features then emerge over time. All of these disorders commonly include the development of multiple elements of dysfunction in the neurologic axis, and they can include breathing dysfunction, gastrointestinal motility disorders, mood disorders, and other severe impairments that are in excess of those usually seen in individuals with intellectual disability alone or autism alone. These affected domains are illustrated in Figure 32-1. We therefore introduce the term *developmental encephalopathy* to more effectively describe the severe patterns of disabilities seen in these individuals (Table 32-1).

RELATIONSHIP TO EPILEPTIC ENCEPHALOPATHIES

Epileptic encephalopathies were originally defined as disorders with prominent seizures, in which neurologic function deteriorates as a consequence of epileptic activity, usually combined with a severe signature interictal pattern (Dulac, 2001). Canonical examples of epileptic encephalopathies include early myoclonic encephalopathy, Ohtahara syndrome, malignant migrating partial seizures of infancy, infantile spasms, and Lennox-Gastaut syndrome. More recently, epileptic encephalopathies have been defined as electroclinical syndromes associated with a high probability of encephalopathic features that present or worsen after the onset of epilepsy (Berg et al., 2010). The implication in these disorders is that the epileptic activity itself may contribute to severe impairment beyond what might be expected, and this impairment may worsen over time. However, the discovery of mutations in numerous genes for epileptic encephalopathies has led to the hypothesis that the overall disorder may be the product of the underlying genetic cause or a combination of the genetic cause and the epileptic process itself. An example of this phenomenon is individuals with duplications of 14q12 that include the gene *FOXG1*, who typically present with infantile spasms, respond to adrenocorticotropic hormone with cessation of spasms and resolution of hypsarrhythmia, do not develop subsequent epilepsy, yet on follow-up have severe intellectual disability, impaired language, socialization, and repetitive movements. The case of duplications of *FOXG1* suggests the epilepsy course is not the primary determinant of the natural history of the disorder, and what may begin as an epileptic encephalopathy can emerge in later childhood as a developmental encephalopathy. Therefore most epileptic encephalopathies are best understood to be a subset of developmental encephalopathies that present with prominent seizure symptoms.

RELATIONSHIP TO DISORDERS WITH PROMINENT BRAIN MALFORMATIONS

Polyalanine expansion mutations in *ARX* were the first genetic cause of epileptic encephalopathy to be described, and these mutations are one of the best-understood causes of a spectrum of developmental brain disorders that includes intellectual disability, dystonia, infantile spasms, and agenesis of the corpus callosum, with individuals with null mutations having the brain malformation–multiple congenital anomaly syndrome X-linked lissencephaly with abnormal genitalia. The milder mutations found in individuals with polyalanine expansions in *ARX* fit the diagnostic criteria for a developmental encephalopathy (with an emphasis on the subgroup of epileptic encephalopathy), illustrating how different mutations within the same gene can result in different classes of developmental brain disorders. However, individuals with developmental encephalopathies do not typically have major brain malformations but much more commonly have disorders of head size, such as postnatal microcephaly, agenesis of the corpus callosum, and cerebellar vermis hypoplasia.

RELATIONSHIP TO AUTISM SPECTRUM DISORDERS

Angelman syndrome and Rett syndrome, two classical examples of developmental encephalopathies, were previously termed "genetic forms of autism." However, as our knowledge of the natural history of both Angelman and Rett syndromes has advanced we are now aware of additional features, such as characteristic breathing rhythm abnormalities and cardiac complications seen in girls and women with *MECP2* mutations and characteristic electroencephalogram and epilepsy findings in individuals with Angelman syndrome that are not seen in individuals with more typical autism spectrum disorders. Furthermore, aspects of the standardized autism diagnostic tools, such as the Autism Diagnostic Observation Schedule (ADOS) and the Autism Diagnostic Interview (ADI-R), are difficult to test in children with Angelman or Rett syndrome as a result of the concomitant cognitive impairment. The fifth edition of the *Diagnostic and Statistical Manual of Mental Disorders* (DSM-V) removed genetic causes from the diagnostic definition of autism spectrum disorders in an attempt to less

TABLE 32-1 Neurofunctional Domains That Are Commonly Disordered in Individuals With Developmental Encephalopathies

Many of the Domains That Are More Severely Impaired in Developmental Encephalopathies, When Milder, Are Core Features of Autism Spectrum Disorders

Neurofunctional Domain	Severe Examples	More Common Examples
Ambulation	Inability to attain walking in several disorders	Abnormal gait in Angelman syndrome
Autonomic nervous system	Cardiac rhythm disturbances in Rett syndrome; severe constipation in Mowat-Wilson syndrome	Difficulties with temperature regulation in many disorders
Awareness of self and environment	Inability to respond when name is called or to orient toward a caregiver in several disorders	May also be a common feature of autism
Breathing	Hyperventilation in Pitt-Hopkins syndrome; breathing dysrhythmia in Rett syndrome	
Epilepsy	Epileptic encephalopathy in *CDKL5* disorder; infantile spasms in *FOXG1* duplications	Nonspecific epilepsy in many disorders
Fine motor	Absence of functional hand use in *FOXG1*-related disorder	Fine motor development impeded by frequent hand stereotypies
Food behavior	Hyperphagia in Prader-Willi syndrome	Anorexic symptoms in many disorders
Language (expressive)	Absence of verbal language in many disorders	Core feature of autism spectrum disorders
Language (receptive)	Delays in receptive language in many disorders, although many caregivers report receptive language skills are stronger than expressive language skills	Impairment also seen in autism spectrum disorders
Mood	Persistent irritability may be a feature of many disorders and can affect activities of daily living	Inappropriate laughter in Angelman syndrome
Movement disorder	Chorea/dystonia in *FOXG1* disorder; parkinsonism in Rett syndrome	Hyperkinesis in *MEF2C*-disorder
Reciprocity	Impairment of social "give-and-take" in many disorders	Core feature of autism spectrum disorders
Sensory	Increased pain threshold in many disorders may lead to injuries	
Sleep	Abnormal sleep-wake cycles in Angelman syndrome	

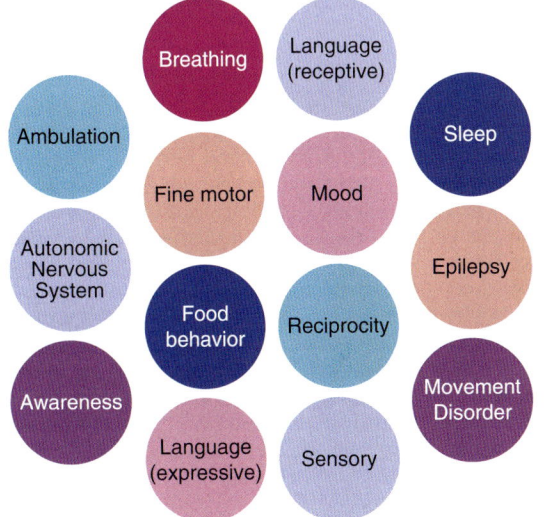

Figure 32-1. Fourteen neurobehavioral and neurofunctional domains that may be affected with disability in individuals with developmental encephalopathies.

TABLE 32-2 Genes and Biological Pathways Associated With Developmental Encephalopathies

Gene	Protein Function	Syndrome(s)
TRANSCRIPTIONAL REGULATORS		
ARX	Transcription factor	X-linked infantile spasms syndrome; X-linked lissencephaly with abnormal genitalia; Partington syndrome
FOXG1	Transcription factor	*FOXG1* disorders
MEF2C	Transcription factor	*MEF2C* disorder
MECP2	Methyl-CpG-binding domain protein	Rett syndrome
PURA	Transcription factor	*PURA* disorder
TCF4	Transcription factor	Pitt-Hopkins syndrome
ZEB2	Transcription factor	Mowat-Wilson syndrome
SYNAPTIC STRUCTURAL SUPPORT		
CDKL5	Serine-threonine protein kinase	*CDKL5* disorder
CNTNAP2	Cell adhesion, ion channel localization	*CNTNAP2* disorder
NRXN1	Cell adhesion	*NRXN1* disorder
UNKNOWN BIOLOGICAL PATHWAY		
UBE3A	Ubiquitin-protein ligase	Angelman syndrome

the confusion about overlap among these developmental conditions. We now see a hypothesis emerging that genetic mutation class can influence where on the spectrum a patient falls between autism spectrum disorder and developmental encephalopathy; for example, such a spectrum of disability has been observed in individuals with mutations in *CNTNAP2* ranging from classic autistic features to a more severe Pitt-Hopkins syndrome phenotype.

BIOLOGICAL PATHWAYS INVOLVED

Mutations in numerous novel genes have been discovered recently in individuals with all forms of developmental brain disorders, including developmental encephalopathies, providing an emerging landscape of the biological pathways involved in the pathogenesis of these disorders. Table 32-2 summarizes some of the key genes, biological pathways, and the syndromes with which they are associated. This is an area of active research and new genes are being added to this list with high frequency. One observation is the prominence of transcription factors (genes that encode proteins that bind DNA and regulate the expression of other genes) or regulators of transcription factors among these pathways. Several of these transcription factors have known critical roles in forebrain development, suggesting that mutations in these genes lead to abnormal patterning, and specific impairments of neuronal development such as migration, neurite outgrowth, and synapse development and function. Other biological pathways clearly involved in the pathogenesis of this class of disorders include synapse structural support (i.e., *CDKL5*) and synaptic function (i.e., *SCN1A*, *SCN2A*, *STXBP1*), and it is not surprising that these pathways also overlap with disorders that often present as epileptic encephalopathies.

SPECIFIC DEVELOPMENTAL ENCEPHALOPATHIES
Rett Syndrome

Rett syndrome, initially described by Andreas Rett in 1966 but not widely recognized until several decades later, is in many respects the prototypical developmental encephalopathy. Caused by loss-of-function mutations in *MECP2* (Amir et al., 1999), Rett syndrome manifests as a combination of intellectual disability, autistic features, abnormal movements, and a spectrum of additional neurofunctional deficits. Affected individuals often have a period of normal development, although hypotonia can be present early on. Deceleration in head growth, loss of verbal language, and stereotypic hand movements usually start in toddlerhood, but may be present as early as 6 months of age. Other distinguishing features include breathing abnormalities, bruxism, abnormal sleep patterns, abnormal muscle tone (including spasticity), and scoliosis. The associated movement disorder appears to be complex, and has a natural history of hyperkinesis in younger individuals, with bradykinesis with parkinsonian features emerging in older patients. The breathing abnormalities are also distinctive, and include both hyperventilation and breath holding. Cardiac rhythm abnormalities, dysautonomia, and biventricular myocardial dysfunction can also occur in patients with Rett syndrome, and affected individuals have a 300-fold increased risk of sudden cardiac death.

Multiple forms of epilepsy have been reported in individuals with Rett syndrome, and up to 60% can be affected with seizures. Complex partial, generalized tonic-clonic, atypical absence, atonic, tonic, and myoclonic seizures have all been described. Epilepsy usually develops at a mean age of 4.7 years. Four characteristic stages of electroencephalogram (EEG) abnormalities that reflect the progression of epilepsy and encephalopathy have been described. One challenge in the care of individuals with Rett syndrome and seizures is the common prevalence of nonepileptic behavioral spells.

CDKL5 Disorder

During the characterization of Rett syndrome, a group of girls were identified with epileptic encephalopathy, usually infantile spasms, who went on to have some symptoms reminiscent of Rett syndrome. Mutations in *CDKL5* were subsequently discovered in these patients (Weaving et al., 2004). Since then, much has been learned about the natural history that departs from the clinical course of Rett syndrome, and it is no longer appropriate to refer to *CDKL5* disorder as a "Rett variant" or "congenital Rett syndrome."

Unlike in Rett syndrome, infantile spasms and early infantile myoclonic seizures are common in individuals with mutations in *CDKL5*. Infants show developmental delays early that are associated with their epileptic encephalopathy and do not have a period of normal development followed by regression as can be seen in Rett syndrome. Deceleration of head growth is common, with 55% of individuals in one study manifesting postnatal microcephaly. Similar to Rett syndrome, those with mutations in *CDKL5* also have severely delayed motor development and poor functional hand use, and most are nonambulatory. Many have disordered breathing and sleep disturbance. Mutations of *CDKL5* do occur in surviving males, and in one cohort of boys presenting with epileptic encephalopathy 3% had mutations in *CDKL5*.

FOXG1 Disorders

FOXG1 found on chromosome 14q12 is a transcription factor that regulates dorsal-ventral brain patterning. It is necessary for the development of Cajal-Retzius cells and inhibits gliogenesis and promotes neurogenesis. Disorders involving *FOXG1* were first described in 2005 in a female patient with agenesis of the corpus callosum, severe cognitive impairment, and microcephaly. Children with mutations of *FOXG1* are often thought to have a variant of Rett syndrome; however, it has become increasingly clear that individuals with mutations of *FOXG1* have a clearly distinct phenotype.

There are two clinical syndromes recognized in *FOXG1*, deletions/intragenic loss-of-function mutations and duplications. Each of these has distinct developmental and behavioral characteristics. Individuals with deletions or intragenic mutations of *FOXG1* have global developmental delay and cognitive impairment starting early in infancy. These individuals are typically nonverbal with little expressive or receptive language, have severely impaired motor development, and do not attain ambulation. Oftentimes a chorea-dystonia movement disorder is evident. Sleep dysfunction is common as a result of frequent awakenings and GI disturbances such as gastroesophageal reflux can be severe, even requiring surgical treatment with a fundoplication and feeding tube placement. Individuals with deletions/intragenic mutations of *FOXG1* have low to borderline normal head circumferences at birth and often develop postnatal microcephaly by 2 years old. Epilepsy is very common in these children, with seizures developing early in childhood, and they have a variety of seizure types, including complex partial seizures, myoclonic seizures, and generalized tonic-clonic seizures. The patterns of seizures and epileptiform activity do not fit a typical epilepsy syndrome, and the seizures are often refractory to treatment. On MRI, individuals with deletions or intragenic mutations of *FOXG1* often have abnormalities of the corpus callosum, ranging from hypoplasia of the genu to agenesis of the corpus callosum, which are associated with larger deletions. Also evident are foreshortened frontal lobes and reduced white-matter volumes.

Duplications of *FOXG1* have different clinical features. These children also have developmental delay but are not always as impaired as seen in the deletions/intragenic mutations. Individuals with duplications of *FOXG1* frequently have language delay, but they are more likely to attain ambulation compared with the deletions/intragenic mutations. Fine motor skills are not as severely affected in the duplications *FOXG1* group. These individuals do not have the same choreiform movement disorder and are normocephalic. MRI scans are typically normal. Children with duplications of *FOXG1* have epilepsy but it is distinctive from the mutations/intragenic mutations. Duplications of *FOXG1* are associated with a younger age of onset of epilepsy and more specifically with infantile spasms. What is perhaps most interesting about this subgroup with infantile spasms and duplications of *FOXG1* is that the spasms typically respond to adrenocorticotropic hormone (ACTH), and the children do not go on to develop other types of epilepsy.

MEF2C Disorder

Deletions and loss-of-function mutations in *MEF2C* on chromosome 5q14.3 are associated with intellectual disability and epilepsy with additional autistic features such as absent speech and impaired social interactions. Several observers have commented on the abnormal tone and movement patterns that emerge during infancy in individuals with *MEF2C* disorder, with profound hypotonia being common, coupled with the emergence of a hyperkinetic ("always in motion") pattern prevalent with frequent hand stereotypies that can be accompanied by dystonia and/or chorea. Available data on the natural history of the *MEF2C* movement disorder are sparse, but one 46 year-old individual was described with hypokinesis, spasticity, and intermittent hand-wringing stereotypies.

Just over half of individuals with *MEF2C* disorder are diagnosed with epilepsy during infancy, with myoclonic seizures and infantile spasms being the most common semiology. The remainder of individuals will usually develop epilepsy later in childhood, although several individuals have been described without seizures, and these tend to be those with partial deletions of *MEF2C*. *MEF2C* disorder is therefore another developmental encephalopathy where many (but not all) patients present with an epileptic encephalopathy, but the epilepsy is ultimately variable and not a distinctive feature of the phenotype.

Children with *MEF2C* disorder have a range of other neurofunctional and behavioral impairments that describe the class of developmental encephalopathies. Individuals are usually nonverbal with severe impairment of language and reciprocal communication. Visual tracking is usually poor, and some individuals have avoidance of eye contact. Most manifest inappropriate laughter. Gastrointestinal motility is often abnormal, with clinically significant reflux disease, dysphagia, and constipation. Many parents report their children had high pain tolerance, for example not crying during immunizations or after injuries. Two subjects have been reported with persistent episodes of breathing dysrhythmia, but this behavior does not appear to be a widespread phenomenon.

Brain MRI findings are usually nonspecific in *MEF2C* disorder, with patients generally having normal head size and no cortical malformations. One report documented periventricular nodular heterotopia in three patients with chromosome 5q14.3q15 deletions, but *MEF2C* was considered outside the heterotopia critical region, and this association has not been reported in other patients. Other nonspecific findings on MRI, such as corpus callosum dysmorphology, increased extraaxial spaces, enlarged lateral ventricles, white-matter hyperintensities, and mild cerebellar vermis hypoplasia, have also been described.

Pitt-Hopkins Syndrome

Pitt-Hopkins syndrome is characterized by intellectual disability, postnatal microcephaly, and a characteristic respiratory dysrhythmia (Pitt and Hopkins, 1978). The breathing pattern is usually a combination of hyperventilation mixed with breath-holding behavior that can worsen with excitement, usually appears during early childhood but may not emerge until after the second half of the first decade.

Pitt-Hopkins syndrome is caused by *de novo* loss-of-function mutations in the transcription factor *TCF4*. TCF4 protein forms heterodimers with HASH1, another helix-loop-helix transcription factor important in the development of noradrenergic neurons that control respiratory drive in the brainstem, possibly explaining the prominent breathing dysrhythmia associated with this syndrome.

Most individuals with Pitt-Hopkins syndrome develop epilepsy after 2 years of age, although seizures during infancy are not uncommon. Seizure types described are nonspecific, but can be intractable. Brain MRI findings are nonspecific and can include hypoplasia of the corpus callosum, mild-moderate dilation of the lateral ventricles, and cerebellar hypoplasia with the only really characteristic observation in some patients being an unusual "bulging" of the caudate nuclei into the lateral ventricles.

Mowat-Wilson Syndrome

Mowat-Wilson syndrome is a multiple congenital anomaly syndrome with prominent intellectual disability, agenesis of the corpus callosum, microcephaly, and seizures (Mowat et al., 1998). Affected individuals have characteristic facial dysmorphology including hypertelorism, medially flared and broad eyebrows, prominent columella, (i.e., tissue linking nasal tip to nasal base) pointed chin and uplifted, cupped earlobes. Congenital heart defects and Hirschsprung disease are also core features of the phenotype. *De novo* mutations in *ZEB2* (previously known as *ZFHX1B* and *SIP1*) and deletions of chromosome 2q22 cause Mowat-Wilson syndrome.

Between 70% and 75% of individuals with Mowat-Wilson syndrome have epilepsy, with onset of seizures occurring at a median age of 14.5 months. Atypical absence seizures were common, as were focal seizures, and status epilepticus also reported. Frequent additional neurofunctional deficits included oral and repetitive behaviors, pain insensitivity, and emotional disturbances.

ZEB2 is a transcriptional inhibitor that mediates axonal growth and plays a role in ipsilateral intracortical brain formation. Mice deficient in Sip1 lack a corpus callosum, anterior commissure, and corticospinal tracts. The protein is highly expressed in pyramidal neurons in the hippocampus and dentate gyrus and in postmitotic neurons in the cerebral cortex, and it also controls a feedback signaling mechanism promoting fate switch in cortical progenitors from neurogenesis to gliogenesis. Finally, Zeb2 appears to be positioned downstream of Dlx1/2 in a pathway required to generate cortical GABAergic interneurons, which may play a role in the frequent epilepsy seen in Mowat-Wilson syndrome.

Chromosome 15q Disorders

Three distinct disorders are mediated by mutations or structural rearrangements occurring on chromosome 15q11q13, providing a fascinating window into the pathogenesis and differential symptomatology of developmental encephalopathies. The proximal chromosome 15q is subject to unequal crossover, resulting in rearrangements, and there are several well-described breakpoint regions. The scope of abnormalities seen in the chromosome 15q disorders is illustrated in Figure 32-3.

Angelman Syndrome

Angelman syndrome was first described in 1965 and the associated phenotypes of inappropriate laughter, developmental disability, and ataxic gait are well recognized (Angelman, 2008). Although four mechanisms can lead to Angelman syndrome (Table 32-3), the common genetic etiology is the loss of expression of the maternally inherited copy of the

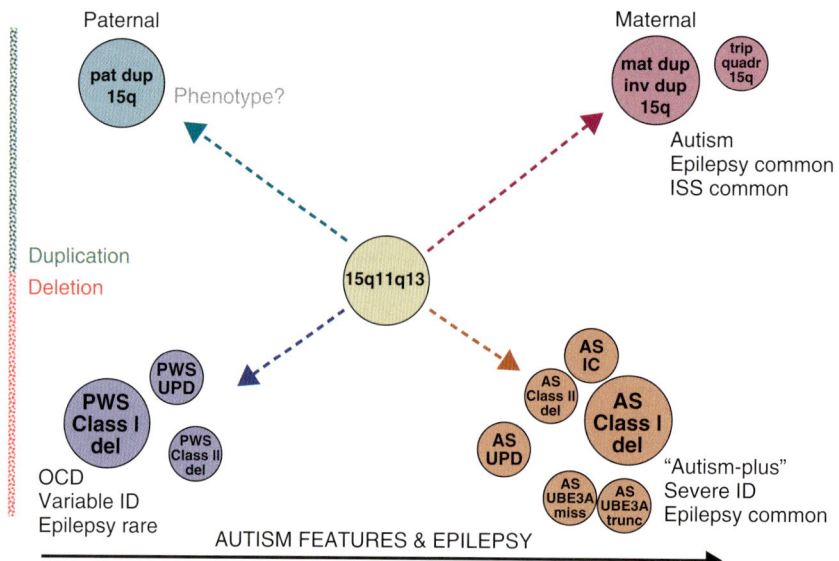

Figure 32-3. Interrelationships among the disorders associated with chromosome 15q11q13. Duplications of chromosome 15q from paternal origin (top left) are not described, and it is not known if they manifest a phenotype. Duplications of 15q from maternal origin (top right) are associated with autism and epilepsy, including frequent infantile spasms (ISS). Deletions of 15q from paternal origin (lower left) are associated with Prader-Willi syndrome (PWS), with frequent obsessive-compulsive disorder (OCD) symptoms, variable intellectual disability (ID), and, rarely, epilepsy. Deletions of 15q from maternal origin (lower right) and mutations in *UBE3A* cause Angelman syndrome (AS), which is associated with autism features, severe ID, and, commonly, epilepsy. There is overall a trend toward more severe autism features and epilepsy in maternal duplication of 15q11q13 and Angelman syndrome and less of these phenotypic features in Prader-Willi syndrome. Mat dup, maternal duplication; inv dup, inverted duplication; trip, triplication; quad, quadruplication.

TABLE 32-3 Genetic Mechanisms Leading to Angelman Syndrome

Class	Genetic Event	Angelman Syndrome Cases, %
I	De novo deletion in maternally inherited chromosome 15q11q13	70–75
II	Uniparental disomy chromosome 15	2–3
III	Imprinting center defects	3–5
IV	*UBE3A* mutations	5–10

imprinted gene *UBE3A* on chromosome 15q11q13. This may occur through de novo deletion in the maternally inherited chromosome 15q11q13 (70%–75% of individuals with Angelman syndrome), uniparental disomy of chromosome 15 with a failure to inherit the maternal copy of *UBE3A* (2%–3% of individuals with Angelman syndrome), abnormal 15q11q13 methylation resulting from mutations in the imprinting center (3%–5% of individuals with Angelman syndrome), and mutations in *UBE3A* itself (5%–10% of individuals with Angelman syndrome).

Physical and behavioral features that include intellectual disability and absent language characterize Angelman Syndrome. Individuals with Angelman syndrome typically have a happy demeanor with inappropriate laughter, but hyperactivity and aggression are frequent behavioral complications. Several abnormal movement patterns have been described in Angelman syndrome, including ataxic gait and jerk-like limb movements. Tremor has been commonly reported, and may represent semirhythmic cortical myoclonus. One individual has been reported with paroxysmal tonic upward gaze. Sleep disturbance is also a significant clinical finding in 72% of

individuals with Angelman syndrome, with abnormal sleep-wake cycle impairment. There are data suggesting that behavioral therapy may be helpful in addressing disordered sleep. Intractable epilepsy is common in Angelman syndrome, with 80% to 90% of individuals affected. The average age of seizure onset was 1 year old, with a range of 4 months to 2 years 11 months. Multiple seizure types have been observed, including atypical absence, myoclonic, partial, complex partial, generalized tonic-clonic, and status epilepticus. Angelman syndrome therefore is an example of a developmental encephalopathy in which seizures can be prominent, although no single electroclinical epilepsy syndrome is dominant in the phenotype. The natural history of epilepsy in Angelman syndrome has been studied, and seizures usually persist into adulthood.

Prader-Willi Syndrome

The inclusion of Prader-Willi syndrome within the category of developmental encephalopathy may appear at first glance to be surprising. Yet when one contemplates the phenotype of this disorder mediated by abnormal imprinting of the paternal copy of 15q11q13, it is evident that the criteria for developmental encephalopathy are met. Individuals with Prader-Willi syndrome can present in infancy with marked hypotonia and failure to thrive. Characteristic dysmorphologic findings of eye shape, small hands, and small feet are usually seen. However, many affected children are not diagnosed at this stage although the importance of recognizing this disorder early is paramount for the option of growth hormone therapy to be offered to the family. Growth hormone therapy has resulted in a dramatic change in the outcome of Prader-Will syndrome, and in many cases, the morbid obesity is a consequence of unchecked hyperphagia that can be avoided. Older individuals have a characteristic neurobehavioral phenotype that includes frequent ritualistic obsessive-compulsive behaviors. Affective psychiatric disorders are common, and individuals with the maternal uniparental disomy genetic subtype appeared to be especially vulnerable to these behavioral complications.

Epilepsy is a rare complication of Prader-Willi syndrome, which is remarkable given the high density of GABAergic genes (*GABRA5*, *GABRB3*, and *GABRG3*) on chromosome 15q11q13 and the high prevalence of epilepsy in Angelman and duplication of maternal 15q11q13 syndromes. It appears likely that the effect of loss of paternal imprinting on these genes is not epileptogenic.

Duplication of Maternal 15q11q13

Duplications of the maternally inherited copy of chromosome 15q11q13 region are the most frequently reported chromosomal aberration in individuals with autism spectrum disorders (0.5%-3%) (Bolton et al., 2001; Depienne et al., 2009). Epilepsy is common, with infantile spasms having a high incidence, and Lennox-Gastaut syndrome reported as well. Some individuals have been described with tetrasomy and pentasomy 15q11q13, severe intellectual disability with autism, and mild dysmorphism.

CNTNAP2 and *NRXN1* Disorders

Autosomal recessive mutations in *CNTNAP2* and *NRXN1* have been described in individuals with intellectual disability, severely limited verbal language, and respiratory dysrhythmia similar to Pitt-Hopkins syndrome. Both of these genes have emerged as candidates for autism spectrum disorders, although the evidence supporting pathogenicity of variants in autism is not very strong. *CNTNAP2* variants have also segregated with learning disability and dyslexia in some families. Others have identified heterozygous variants in both *CNTNAP2* and *NRNX1*; however, in most cases, the variant was inherited from a normal parent and no second mutation in the gene was identified. Therefore the full spectrum of *CNTNAP2* and *NRXN1* disorders and their relationship to Pitt-Hopkins syndrome, autism spectrum disorders, or other learning disabilities remain unclear.

DYRK1A Disorder

DYRK1A is a tyrosine-(Y)-phosphorylation regulated kinase encoded on chromosome 21 that has been implicated as responsible for the cognitive abnormalities common in Down syndrome. Recently de novo loss-of-function mutations in *DYRK1A* and chromosome 21q22.13 microdeletions have been identified in individuals with congenital microcephaly, intellectual disability, and autistic features. Additional clinical findings include ataxia, intrauterine growth restriction, and characteristic facial features. Impaired speech and stereotyped behaviors were common findings. Mutations in *DYRK1A* were found recurrently in a series of individuals with intellectual disability, suggesting the disorder may be more frequent than currently recognized.

PURA Disorder

PURA disorder is one of the most recent diagnoses discovered that fits within the definition of developmental encephalopathy. De novo loss-of-function mutations in this transcriptional regulator have been found in individuals presenting with neonatal hypotonia, poor feeding, and epilepsy. Affected individuals with deletions of chromosome 5q31.3 including *PURA* were previously described. Initial genotype–phenotype correlations suggest that mutations disrupting the Pur repeat III result in a more severe phenotype. Brain MRI findings appear to include nonspecific white matter dysmaturation and increased extraaxial spaces.

Conclusions

We use the term *developmental encephalopathy* to capture the full spectrum of phenotypes in conditions where intellectual disability coexists with autistic features and other abnormalities of the autonomic nervous system, changes in gastrointestinal motility and breathing rhythm, specific types of epilepsy, and movement disorders. This new conceptual framework is necessary to differentiate these conditions from neurodevelopmental disorders that primarily present with global developmental delay, isolated intellectual disability, and epilepsy syndromes. When initially described, the clinical features of affected individuals may be complex and overlap with intellectual disability, autism spectrum disorders, and other neurobehavioral characteristics such that one disorder is superficially difficult to distinguish from another. For this reason, close attention to differentiating signs and symptoms is important. Some of these disorders have specific abnormalities seen on brain imaging. In some cases, specific epilepsy types or movement disorder patterns are common.

As more genetic causes of developmental encephalopathies are discovered, we can begin to understand the associated underlying biological mechanisms. An emerging common theme is that of abnormal transcriptional regulation at the critical early stages of brain development; many of the causative genes are transcription factors that bind specific DNA sequences and regulate the expression of other genes. Synapse structural support is another biological grouping that appears to be important in the causation of developmental encephalopathies. Ultimately, the molecular circuitry underlying these disorders may create common features among various disorders, offering the potential that common novel therapeutic strategies may be applied to multiple disorders. It is interesting that both of these pathways overlap with the emerging biological mechanisms for epilepsy and autism spectrum disorders, which certainly share similar phenotypic features. A better understanding of the specific pathophysiological mechanisms by which the mutations cause the developmental encephalopathies outlined in this chapter will likely provide insight into the pathologic mechanisms underlying these common disorders.

As advanced genetic technologies are increasingly being used to make diagnoses in the child neurology clinic, it is not surprising that these approaches are helpful in making a molecular diagnosis in children with developmental encephalopathies as well. Identification of a genetic cause for an individual's disorder may allow recommendations to be made for surveillance for known medical complications and affect decisions about choice of medications. Identification of a genetic diagnosis may also open the door for affected individuals to participate in clinical trials and/or natural history studies available for that disorder.

Appropriate genetic evaluation of a patient with a developmental encephalopathy will include specific genetic studies for clinically identifiable disorders. For example, for girls with developmental regression with loss of hand skills and language, Rett Syndrome should be considered and mutation analysis of *MECP2* performed. Rett Syndrome-like features with early seizures suggest mutation testing in *CDKL5* and DNA methylation studies of chromosome 15q to evaluate for Angelman and Prader-Willi syndromes if clinical features suggest these disorders. Chromosomal microarray (CMA) tests for pathogenic microdeletions or microduplications, such as duplication 15q11q13 syndrome. Also, CMA may detect microdeletions involving any of the single-gene disorders discussed in this chapter. Should methylation studies and

CMA be negative, a clinician can either proceed to an appropriate next-generation sequencing gene panel, if it includes the likely genes of interest, or whole-exome sequencing. The use and interpretation of these technologies are discussed in Chapter 30.

REFERENCES

The complete list of references for this chapter is available in the e-book at www.expertconsult.com.

See inside cover for registration details.

REFERENCES

Amir, R.E., Van den Veyver, I.B., Wan, M., et al., 1999. Rett syndrome is caused by mutations in X-linked MECP2, encoding methyl-CpG-binding protein 2. Nat. Genet. 23, 185–188.

Angelman, H., 2008. "Puppet" Children A Report on Three Cases. Dev. Med. Child Neurol. 7, 681–688.

Berg, A.T., Berkovic, S.F., Brodie, M.J., et al., 2010. Revised terminology and concepts for organization of seizures and epilepsies: report of the ILAE Commission on Classification and Terminology, 2005-2009. Epilepsia 51, 676–685.

Bolton, P.F., Dennis, N.R., Browne, C.E., et al., 2001. The phenotypic manifestations of interstitial duplications of proximal 15q with special reference to the autistic spectrum disorders. Am. J. Med. Genet. 105, 675–685.

Depienne, C., Moreno-De-Luca, D., Heron, D., et al., 2009. Screening for genomic rearrangements and methylation abnormalities of the 15q11-q13 region in autism spectrum disorders. Biol. Psychiatry 66, 349–359.

Dulac, O., 2001. Epileptic encephalopathy. Epilepsia 42 (Suppl. 3), 23–26.

Mowat, D.R., Croaker, G.D., Cass, D.T., et al., 1998. Hirschsprung disease, microcephaly, mental retardation, and characteristic facial features: delineation of a new syndrome and identification of a locus at chromosome 2q22-q23. J. Med. Genet. 35, 617–623.

Pitt, D., Hopkins, I., 1978. A syndrome of mental retardation, wide mouth and intermittent overbreathing. Aust. Paediatr. J. 14, 182–184.

Weaving, L.S., Christodoulou, J., Williamson, S.L., et al., 2004. Mutations of CDKL5 cause a severe neurodevelopmental disorder with infantile spasms and mental retardation. Am. J. Hum. Genet. 75, 1079–1093.

E-BOOK FIGURES AND TABLES

The following figures and tables are available in the e-book at www.expertconsult.com. See inside cover for registration details.

Fig. 32-2 Hypogenesis of the anterior (genu) of the corpus callosum in an individual with an intragenic loss-of-function mutation in *FOXG1*.

Fig. 32-4 When mutated, genes acting in the nucleus (*ARX, FOXG1, MECP2, PURA, TCF4, ZEB2*) and at the synapse (*CDKL5, CNTNAP2, NRXN1*) are known causes of developmental encephalopathies.

33 Prenatal Diagnosis of Structural Brain Anomalies

Tally Lerman-Sagie, Liat Ben-Sira, Catherine Garel, and Gustavo Malinger

An expanded version of this chapter is available on www.expertconsult.com. See inside cover for registration details.

INTRODUCTION

The fetal brain develops during the course of pregnancy, from its primitive three-vesicle stage into a complex structure with an array of sulci and gyri resembling the adult brain by the end of gestation. Fetal brain development can be studied by ultrasound (US), starting from gestational weeks 6 to 7 until delivery. Fetal magnetic resonance imaging (MRI) further enables demonstration of anatomy, particularly of cortical development and diverse anomalies, starting at around 18 to 20 weeks of pregnancy.

Sonography is the most important imaging method for prenatal malformation screening. The use of a comprehensive, multiplanar approach, in which coronal and sagittal planes are added to the classical axial planes, and addition of a transvaginal approach enable depiction of the cortex, midline brain structures, and the posterior fossa.

Fetal MRI is complementary to US and is used primarily to confirm and characterize brain abnormalities detected by prenatal sonography. The higher contrast resolution allows better differentiation of normal from abnormal tissue.

An understanding of embryologic development and the correlation between US and MRI is critical in order to be able to diagnose structural brain defects prenatally.

PRENATAL ASSESSMENT OF NORMAL BRAIN DEVELOPMENT IN THE FIRST TRIMESTER

Brain development in the embryonic phase is assessed only by US. Cortical development starts at about 7 weeks of gestation and other brain structures develop synchronously with the cortex, including the commissures and the cerebellum.

By the end of the first trimester (weeks 10 to 12), the cortex is about 1 to 2 mm thick and the crescent hemispheres fill the anterior part of the head. The insula appears as a slight depression on the lateral surface of the hemispheres. The corpus callosum is not yet visible. The cerebellar hemispheres seem to meet in the midline (Blaas and Eik-Nes, 2009).

Major structural defects, particularly malformations of dorsal induction and prosencephalic development, can be identified in first-trimester studies.

PRENATAL ASSESSMENT OF NORMAL DEVELOPMENT OF THE CORTEX

Gyration can be observed by the second month of intrauterine life and continues to develop even after delivery. The primary sulci appear as shallow grooves on the surface of the brain that become progressively more deeply infolded and then develop side branches. The major fissures and sulci develop in predictable patterns, starting at about 16 weeks, and therefore the timing of their appearance is a reliable estimate of gestational age.

At 18 to 20 weeks, the brain surface is almost completely smooth, with only the major fissures present. The most active period of cortical development, as demonstrated by US, is between 27 and 30 weeks. During this time, most sulci become detectable (Cohen-Sacher et al., 2006) (Table 33-1 and Figure 33-6).

MRI after about 20 weeks of gestation provides excellent information unimpeded by calvarial calcification. Brain MRI can depict the walls of the ventricles, which are lined by the ventricular zone (germinal matrix), which is very thick earlier in gestation, and appears as a smooth band of dark T2 signal and bright T1 signal lining the lateral ventricles. The cerebral mantle is seen on fetal MRI until about 28 weeks of gestation in a multilayered pattern (see Figure 33-6).

The development of the cortex can be visualized from mid-pregnancy. On MRI, gyration starts with the appearance of a shallow indentation of the fetal brain in the temporal regions at the 18th gestational week. The central sulcus begins to be visible at 24 weeks of gestation. Fissures then become deeper and tighter, and gyri bulge into the subarachnoid space. Until the 35th gestational week, all primary and most of the secondary sulci are present (Garel et al., 2001) (see Figure 33-6 and Table 33-1).

The development of the sylvian fissure is one of the major brain maturational processes occurring in fetal life, and abnormalities in this process are frequent in children with developmental delay. It is observed in all fetuses at 22 to 23 weeks of gestation as a shallow depression at the surface of the brain, and the insula is wide open at this time. There is progressive closure that begins posteriorly and extends anteriorly. By 33 weeks of gestation, insular sulci are recognizable and the surface of the sylvian fissure becomes more and more indented (Figures 33-1 and 33-2).

PRENATAL ASSESSMENT OF NORMAL DEVELOPMENT OF THE CORPUS CALLOSUM

The corpus callosum develops between gestational weeks 8 and 20. A complete demonstration by US necessitates obtaining sagittal planes through the fontanels with the transvaginal approach. Coronal planes are useful for studying the relationship between the corpus callosum and neighboring structures. The completely formed corpus callosum may be depicted using high-resolution transducers by 21 to 22 weeks of gestation, as an arched hypoechogenic structure delimited by the more echogenic callosal sulcus cranially and the anechogenic cavum septi pelucidi caudally. At this age, its shape is already very similar to that of the mature corpus callosum, and the genu, body, and splenium can be well demonstrated.

The corpus callosum can be depicted by MRI on midline sagittal T2 images by gestational week 20 as a band of low signal intensity superior to the fornix.

PRENATAL ASSESSMENT OF NORMAL DEVELOPMENT OF THE POSTERIOR FOSSA

The ultrasonographic evaluation should include multiplanar images of the cerebellum. The cerebellar vermis can be detected by US in the midsagittal plane as early as 18 weeks of gestation. The midsagittal anterior–posterior diameters increase in a linear fashion.

TABLE 33-1 Chronology of Sulcation According to Neuropathological, Sonographic, and Magnetic Resonance Imaging Studies

	Anatomic Appearance	Detectable in 25–75% of Brains by MRI	Detectable in 25–75% of Brains by Ultrasound	Present in > 75% of Brains by MRI	Present in > 75% of Brains by Ultrasound
Interhemispheric fissure	10			22–23	18
Sylvian fissure	14	24–25		29	18
Parieto-occipital fissure	16		18	22–23	20
Hippocampal fissure				22–23	18
Callosal sulcus	14			22–23	18
Calcarine fissure	16	22–23	20	24–25	22
Cingular sulcus	18	22–23	20	24–25	24
Central sulcus	20	24–25	26	27	28
Postcentral sulcus	25	27	28	28	30
Precentral sulcus	24	26	28	27	30
Superior temporal sulcus	23	26	28	27	30
Inferior temporal sulcus	30	30	28	33	30
Superior frontal sulcus	25	24–25	28	29	30
Inferior frontal sulcus	28	26	28	29	30
Secondary cingular sulcus	32	31	30	33	32
Insular sulcus	34–35	33	30	34	32
Secondary occipital sulcus	34	32	26	34	30
Olfactory sulcus	16		24		30
Marginal sulcus		22–23	26	27	30

The primary fissure is observed between 27 and 30 weeks of pregnancy. Some degree of differentiation between lobules is possible, starting from 30 to 32 weeks of gestation.

The fourth ventricle is uniformly observed as a triangular structure anterocaudal to the vermis. The cerebellar vermis is best assessed by MRI on direct midline sagittal images and on coronal images. The cerebellar hemispheres are best assessed on axial and coronal views.

Fetal MRI shows gestational age-specific changes in signal intensity in the normal development and maturation of the cerebellar hemispheres and brainstem. The cerebellar cortex, dentate nucleus, tectum, dorsal pons, and medulla are T1-hyperintense and T2-hypointense. By 26–27 weeks of gestation, a three-layered pattern is noted in the cerebellar hemispheres. Fetal brain MRI can show the fissures of the cerebellum, depending on the gestational age. The primary fissure is identified on sagittal images at 22 weeks but the cerebellar surface is smooth. From 24 to 29 weeks, foliation of the vermis and posterior lobes of the cerebellum is seen on sagittal images. The convoluted pattern of the cerebellum is well identified from 30 weeks on and is always seen beyond 33 weeks (Fogliarini et al., 2005a).

PRENATAL DIAGNOSIS OF VENTRICULOMEGALY

Assessment of the width of the atria of the lateral cerebral ventricles is recommended as part of the routine anomaly scan.

The lateral ventricle should be measured by US in the axial plane, at the level of the frontal horns and cavum septi pellucidi, with the calipers positioned at the level of the internal margin of the medial and lateral wall of the atria.

Ventriculomegaly is defined as a lateral ventricular width ≥10 mm. Fetal ventriculomegaly may be classified as mild when the lateral ventricular width is between 10 and 15 mm, and severe when larger than 15 mm; it may be unilateral or bilateral.

Ventriculomegaly is defined as isolated if there is no additional evidence of associated malformations or markers of aneuploidy. Mild ventriculomegaly represents a diagnostic and counseling difficulty, as it can be an apparently benign finding, but can also be associated with chromosomal abnormalities, congenital infection, cerebral vascular accidents, and other fetal cerebral and extracerebral abnormalities; it may also have implications regarding long-term neurodevelopmental outcome (Melchiorre et al., 2009). Therefore, upon confirmation of ventriculomegaly, a complete search for associated central nervous system (CNS) and non-CNS anomalies should be attempted, including a study of the brain in a multiplanar approach. The investigation should also include screening for in utero infection, amniocentesis, and fetal echocardiography. MRI can add important information to that obtained by US imaging. Information relevant enough to modify obstetric management can be obtained in 10% of cases.

Follow-up examinations at 3- to 4-week intervals are indicated to assess progressive enlargement of ventricles or to diagnose associated pathologies not previously detected.

When mild ventriculomegaly is isolated, the outcome is usually good. The risk for abnormal outcome increases when there are associated anomalies, the atrial width is greater than 12 mm, or there is a progressive increase of the lateral ventricular width.

The outcome of severe ventriculomegaly depends mainly on the presence of associated pathologies. When associated pathologies are diagnosed, the prognosis is usually poor unless the cause is intraventricular hemorrhage. Even when isolated, the risk of perinatal death or severe neurologic sequelae is in the range of 50% of survivors.

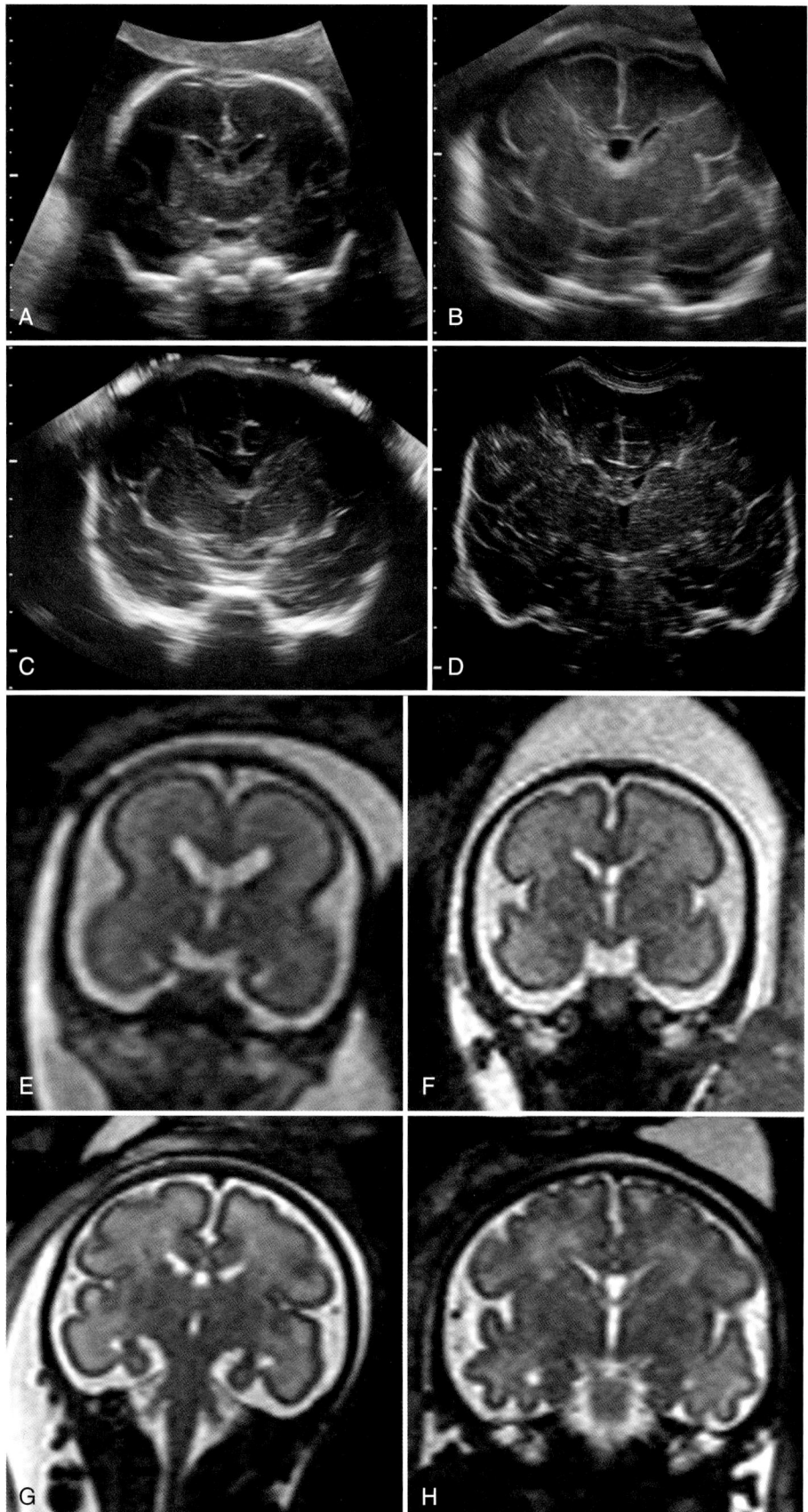

Figure 33-6. A–D, Maturation of the normal fetal cortex by ultrasound. Coronal slices at 23 **(A)**, 27.5 **(B)**, 31.5 **(C)**, and 35 **(D)** weeks. **E–H,** Maturation of the normal fetal cortex by magnetic resonance imaging (MRI) (note opercularization). Coronal T2-weighted slices at 23 **(E)**, 27 **(F)**, 31 **(G)**, and 35 **(H)** weeks. *(A–D: Courtesy of Dr. Zvi Leibovitz.)*

PRENATAL DIAGNOSIS OF ABNORMALITIES OF THE CORPUS CALLOSUM

Developmental abnormalities of the corpus callosum include agenesis, hypogenesis (or partial agenesis), dysgenesis, hypoplasia, and secondary destruction. Agenesis of the corpus callosum (ACC) can be detected prenatally by routine sonography, for which the important signs include absence of the cavum septum pellucidum, colpocephaly, high-riding third ventricle, widening of the interhemispheric fissure, and radiating medial hemispheric sulci. US can also depict an abnormally thick corpus callosum, which may signify a poor prognosis.

Fetal MRI is clinically helpful in suspected cases of ACC because it can confirm the absence of the corpus callosum and diagnose associated anomalies. ACC is rarely isolated. Additional abnormalities occur frequently (46%). The most common findings are sulcation and posterior fossa abnormalities. Abnormal sulcal morphology can be detected as early as 19 gestational weeks. The gyral abnormalities include polymicrogyria, lissencephaly, pachygyria, and schizencephaly.

Interestingly, in 10% of fetuses with ACC, there may be evidence of destructive changes in the brain parenchyma, suggesting either an acquired etiology or a genetic/metabolic abnormality (Prasad et al., 2009).

PRENATAL DIAGNOSIS OF MALFORMATIONS OF CORTICAL DEVELOPMENT

Although the migration process terminates around the end of the first half of pregnancy, malformations of cortical development are seldom diagnosed in utero, possibly because the time of appearance of significant morphologic changes is beyond the recommended time of the anatomic scan (19 to 23 weeks), and because US evaluation of the brain is often limited to visualization of the lateral ventricles and cerebellum.

Abnormal sulcation landmarks have been observed as early as the 22nd week of gestation in fetuses suffering from lissencephaly. In fetuses with migration disorders, US usually demonstrates one of the following patterns: delayed or premature appearance of sulcation, a thin and irregular cortical mantle, wide abnormal overdeveloped or underdeveloped gyri, wide opening of isolated sulci, nodular bulging into the lateral ventricles, cortical clefts, and intraparenchymal echogenic nodules (Malinger et al., 2007).

A definitive diagnosis is hard to reach prenatally; US can identify abnormal migration but cannot definitively differentiate between different pathologies.

MRI can identify cortical malformations more accurately, particularly late in pregnancy. The imaging signs suggestive of abnormal sulcation are: mild ventriculomegaly associated with delayed cortical development; dysgenesis of the sylvian fissure; delayed or abnormal sulcal appearance; callosal abnormality; cortical thickening; heterotopias; absence or abnormal appearance of fissures; irregular, abnormal, asymmetric gyri; and noncontinuous cortex in schizencephaly (Fogliarini et al., 2005b).

When the operculum is abnormally formed, the prognosis is usually poor and an underlying malformation of cortical development can be detected. An underdeveloped operculum for gestational age is usually associated with an abnormal head circumference or other brain anomalies. When it is an isolated finding, it may represent a metabolic disease, chromosomal anomaly, or benign delayed maturation of the operculum, usually associated with macrocephaly and enlargement of the subarachnoid spaces (Prasad et al., 2009).

Prenatal Diagnosis of Lissencephaly Type I

Fetuses with lissencephaly type 1 can be diagnosed after 27 to 30 weeks of gestation when most of the primary sulci are already present, either by detailed neurosonography or by MRI, by demonstration of dysgenesis of the sylvian fissure, delayed sulcal appearance, callosal abnormality, and cortical thickening. Sometimes, zones of normal cortex and zones of pachygyric or agyric cortex alternate. The bilateral opercular dysplasia is responsible for a figure-eight-shaped brain.

Fetuses with Miller–Dieker syndrome have abnormal parieto-occipital and sylvian fissures by the time of the second-trimester US examination.

Prenatal Diagnosis of Cobblestone Complex

Findings suggestive of cobblestone complex are early enlargement of the lateral ventricles, abnormal sulcation, abnormal vermis, a Z-shaped brainstem, retinal detachment, and cataract.

MRI can better visualize the posterior fossa, brainstem, and gyration pattern (Fogliarini et al., 2005b).

Prenatal Diagnosis of Complex Cortical Malformations

Mutations in tubulin genes cause complex cortical malformations. Three subtypes of cortical malformations have been described in fetuses: microlissencephaly with corpus callosum agenesis, severely hypoplastic brainstem and cerebellum; lissencephaly, either classical or associated with cerebellar hypoplasia, with corpus callosum agenesis; and polymicrogyria-like cortical dysplasia with inconstant corpus callosum agenesis and hypoplastic brainstem and cerebellum.

Prenatal Diagnosis of Periventricular Nodular Heterotopia

Periventricular nodular heterotopia should be considered when US depicts an irregular lateral ventricular wall with indentations of periventricular tissue and a signal similar to that of the cortex. The sonographic diagnosis is difficult, particularly when the lateral ventricle width is normal. MRI demonstrates multiple small nodular subependymal foci of low signal intensity, isointense to the germinal matrix, located in the margins of the lateral ventricles. They cannot be distinguished reliably from the subependymal nodules seen in tuberous sclerosis; therefore, it is important to search for other manifestations of tuberous sclerosis. A posterior fossa cyst, which can be seen in females with filamin A mutations, may be the initial abnormality and, in association with periventricular nodules, may suggest the prenatal diagnosis.

Heterotopia may go unrecognized when the nodules are small or subcortical.

Prenatal Diagnosis of Polymicrogyria

The cortical changes of polymicrogyria take place late in pregnancy and appear as localized and/or generalized absence of normal sulcation with multiple abnormal infoldings of the affected cortex. It is more apparent on MRI than on US. In young fetuses (24 weeks), the identification of the cortical malformation is quite difficult, and the manifestations in both US and MRI are subtle (Adamsbaum et al., 2005). They include presence of sulci that are not as expected, according to the gestational age; an irregular surface of the brain; and absence of the normal signal of the cortical ribbon. Late in pregnancy, the MRI features are similar to what is known in the postnatal period: packed and serrated microgyri, irregular cortex–white-matter junction, and an aberrant and asymmetric sulcal pattern (Fogliarini et al., 2005b). Because the MRI pattern of polymicrogyria changes with increasing gestational age, it is important to follow young fetuses and repeat the US and MRI examinations in order to confirm the diagnosis.

Prenatal Diagnosis of Schizencephaly

Prenatal US enables diagnosis of schizencephaly, although prenatal MRI is more specific in detection of the gray matter lining the defect, communication with the ventricle, and other associated structural abnormalities. The prenatal diagnosis of schizencephaly depends on the extent of cleft separation; closed-lip and open-lip variants with a very small gap remain undiagnosed. The prenatal diagnosis of schizencephaly has been described as early as 21 weeks. Neurosonography demonstrates bilateral or unilateral open-lip wedge-shaped defects, usually in the parietotemporal regions, frequently accompanied by absence of the cavum septum pellucidum. Fetal MRI shows schizencephalic clefts extending from the pial surface to the ventricle lined with gray matter, which is seen as a low-signal-intensity line covering the edge of the remaining brain parenchyma. This finding allows differentiation of the defect from porencephaly (Fogliarini et al., 2005b).

PRENATAL DIAGNOSIS OF POSTERIOR FOSSA ANOMALIES

Infratentorial anomalies are usually diagnosed in utero when associated with enlarged posterior fossa fluid spaces, with or without an abnormal fourth ventricle. The suspicion of abnormal cerebellar development is usually raised after the visualization of a small cerebellum or a large communication between the fourth ventricle and the cisterna magna, using the transcerebellar axial plane. Severe anomalies, such as Arnold–Chiari malformation type 2, Dandy–Walker malformation, and cerebellar hypoplasia, are usually detected during routine second-trimester US examinations.

Particular care should be taken in order to differentiate between the vermis and the cerebellar hemisphere in cases of suspected vermian agenesis or hypoplasia. Visualization of the normal triangular shape of the fourth ventricle, and of the primary vermian fissure, facilitates exclusion of vermian pathologies.

The in utero diagnosis of the pontocerebellar hypoplasias necessitates measurements of the pons diameter in addition to the cerebellar dimensions. It is important to note the relationship of the size of the midbrain to pons and medulla. In cases of diagnostic uncertainties, a follow-up examination is pertinent, because a false-positive diagnosis of partial vermian agenesis may be made before 24 weeks of pregnancy, because of delayed closure of the fourth ventricle owing to a persistent Blake pouch cyst, and cerebellar hypoplasia may be missed early in pregnancy because the arrest of growth occurs later.

A dysplastic cerebellum, which refers to disorganized development, such as an abnormal folial pattern or the presence of heterotopic nodules of gray matter, is rarely diagnosed in utero, even with MRI, because it does not produce signal abnormalities.

Prenatal Diagnosis of Chiari Type II Malformation

The posterior fossa is relatively small in Chiari II malformation, and spinal neural tube defects are present with variable hindbrain herniation. The Chiari II malformation may be associated with callosal anomalies, fenestration of the falx, and cortical malformations. The cisterna magna is obliterated by a low-lying torcula, vermian herniation through the foramen magnum, and a small slitlike fourth ventricle. The herniated cerebellum often degenerates. The cerebellum is banana shaped because of the herniation and small posterior fossa. The fetus may demonstrate a lemon-shaped skull.

Prenatal Diagnosis of Dandy–Walker Malformation

Prenatal diagnosis of Dandy–Walker malformation is usually possible during the second trimester; midsagittal planes enable visualization of the abnormal vermis, the communication between the fourth ventricle and the enlarged cisterna magna, and the elevated torcula and tentorium. It should not be confused with partial vermian agenesis. Dandy–Walker malformation may be associated with other CNS anomalies, such as callosal dysgenesis, occipital encephalocele, polymicrogyria, or heterotopias. Hydrocephalus may develop only late in pregnancy or postnatally.

The prognosis after a prenatal diagnosis of Dandy–Walker malformation is variable; however, the prognosis is worse when there are associated brain anomalies (Bolduc and Limperopoulos, 2009).

Prenatal Diagnosis of Mega Cisterna Magna, Posterior Fossa Arachnoid Cyst, and Blake's Pouch Cyst

Isolated enlargement of the posterior fossa is frequently diagnosed by fetal US or MRI. It may be seen in three situations: mega cisterna magna, posterior fossa arachnoid cyst, and Blake's pouch cyst. The prognosis in all three entities is usually good.

In mega cisterna magna, the posterior fossa depth is greater than 10 mm, but the vermis and torcula location are normal. The term has been loosely applied to a large-appearing retrocerebellar cerebrospinal fluid space with a normal vermis and cerebellar hemispheres. It is usually an incidental finding, but it can be associated with other anomalies. Mega cisterna magna can be difficult to distinguish from an arachnoid cyst, as both are anechoic fluid spaces. Congenital arachnoid cysts are extraaxial, and 10% to 45% occur in the posterior fossa. They present on US as anechoic avascular cysts with mass effect on the cerebellum or internal table of the skull. Associated congenital anomalies are rare.

Blake's pouches have the same radiographic appearance as do arachnoid cysts, with the exception that, in some cases, the choroid plexus can be identified, as it extends through the median aperture along the superior cyst wall, carrying the anterior lip of the median aperture far up the vallecula. Blake's pouches communicate with the fourth ventricle and may or may not produce mass effect on the cerebellum. Occasionally, there is the appearance of compression or absence of the inferior vermis. It may be hard to differentiate between inferior vermis hypoplasia and a Blake's pouch cyst.

Prenatal Diagnosis of Vermis Hypoplasia/Agenesis

The term *Dandy–Walker variant* has been used to describe a heterogeneous group of disorders with different degrees of cerebellar vermis agenesis, slight or absent upward rotation of the vermis, and variably sized posterior fossa fluid collections, but without enlargement of the posterior fossa. However, in recent years, it has been strongly advocated that the term be abandoned altogether, given its multiple and variable definitions. The terms *hypoplasia* and *agenesis* are used interchangeably in the literature on fetal vermian abnormalities, but the definitions of these entities are completely different. Vermian agenesis means either complete or partial absence of the vermis. In partial vermian agenesis, part of the vermis is absent and the remaining part is anatomically of normal volume. Because of the craniocaudal development of the vermis, partial agenesis involves its inferior part. Vermian hypoplasia means a small but complete vermis with congenital volume diminution.

Vermis agenesis is associated with CNS and non-CNS anomalies in up to 71% of children, with the most common being ventriculomegaly and agenesis of corpus callosum. Extra-CNS anomalies have also been reported in up to 65%, with cardiac, renal, extremity, and facial anomalies occurring most frequently (Bolduc and Limperopoulos, 2009).

Vermian development is assessed in the midline sagittal view from the caudal extent of the inferior vermis over the fourth ventricle. The diagnosis of inferior vermis agenesis is made when there is partial absence of the inferior portion of the cerebellar vermis with normal- or near-normal-shaped cerebellar hemispheres, a normal-sized posterior fossa without obvious cystic lesions, and normal supratentorial structures. The normal proportion of anterior vermis to posterior vermis (1 : 2) is lost. A correct diagnosis of inferior vermian agenesis is difficult and, even with MRI, there is a false-positive rate of 32%.

Inferior vermian agenesis should be differentiated from failure of "closure" of the vermis with normal morphology and biometry; this probably represents isolated elevation or rotation of the vermis because of a persistent Blake's pouch. Failure of "closure" seems to result from two potential processes: arrest of vermian development so that it does not cover the fourth ventricle at its inferior extent, or failure of adequate fenestration of the fourth ventricular outflow foramina, leading to a secondary elevation of an otherwise normal vermis. The prognosis in these situations is completely different.

Prenatal Diagnosis of Cerebellar Hypoplasia

Cerebellar hypoplasia implies abnormal development rather than atrophy. Diagnosis is made by measurement of the transverse cerebellar diameter.

Severe cerebellar hypoplasia is easily identified in utero after 22 weeks as a very small cerebellum associated with a shallow brainstem and absence of the anterior bulging of the pons, resulting in pontocerebellar atrophy/hypoplasia of extremely poor prognosis. Isolated cerebellar hypoplasia is more challenging, and difficulty in distinguishing malformation from necrosis can occur, especially in unilateral hypoplasia. An intact cerebellar cortex is most likely seen in cerebellar hypoplasia, as opposed to cerebellar necrosis, in which the cortical ribbon is usually absent (Fogliarini et al., 2005b).

Prenatal Diagnosis of Rhombencephalosynapsis

The diagnosis of rhombencephalosynapsis is raised, after demonstration of a small transcerebellar diameter. US and MRI both demonstrate a hypoplastic, single-lobed cerebellum with fused cerebellar hemispheres, no vermis, and transverse folia. Associated cerebral abnormalities are usually found. Coronal and axial planes are superior for diagnosis of rhombencephalosynapsis, because a midline sagittal cut through the cerebellum can be mistaken for a vermis.

Prenatal Diagnosis of Molar Tooth-Related Syndromes

The diagnosis of the molar tooth (deep interpeduncular fossa, thick and elongated superior cerebellar peduncles, vermian agenesis) is difficult to visualize in utero. However, the prenatal diagnosis of Joubert syndrome or related disorders usually follows a positive family history and the finding of abnormal posterior fossa anatomy on fetal ultrasonography or the presence of associated suggestive features, such as kidney anomalies, polydactyly. The molar tooth features can be visualized in the axial plane, including the interpeduncular fossa, cerebellar peduncles, and brainstem.

Prenatal Diagnosis of Brainstem Anomalies

Brainstem malformations are usually described in utero when they are associated with cerebellar and cerebral anomalies. Fetuses with cobblestone malformations show a prominent elongation of the tectum, a thin pons, a small dysplastic vermis, and a kinked brainstem. Fetuses with pontocerebellar hypoplasia demonstrate a reduction of all midbrain and hindbrain measurements in addition to a short transcerebellar diameter.

REFERENCES

The complete list of references for this chapter is available in the e-book at www.expertconsult.com.
    See inside cover for registration details.

SELECTED REFERENCES

Adamsbaum, C., Moutard, M.L., Andre, C., et al., 2005. MRI of the fetal posterior fossa. Pediatr. Radiol. 35, 124–140.

Blaas, H.G., Eik-Nes, S.H., 2009. Sonoembryology and early prenatal diagnosis of neural anomalies. Prenat. Diagn. 29, 312–325.

Bolduc, M.E., Limperopoulos, C., 2009. Neurodevelopmental outcomes in children with cerebellar malformations: a systematic review. Dev. Med. Child Neurol. 51, 256–267.

Cohen-Sacher, B., Lerman-Sagie, T., Lev, D., et al., 2006. Sonographic developmental milestones of the fetal cerebral cortex: a longitudinal study. Ultrasound Obstet. Gynecol. 27, 494–502.

Fogliarini, C., Chaumoitre, K., Chapon, F., et al., 2005a. Assessment of cortical maturation with prenatal MRI. Part I: normal cortical maturation. Eur. Radiol. 15, 1671–1685.

Fogliarini, C., Chaumoitre, K., Chapon, F., et al., 2005b. Assessment of cortical maturation with prenatal MRI. Part II: abnormalities of cortical maturation. Eur. Radiol. 15, 1781–1789.

Garel, C., Chantrel, E., Brisse, H., et al., 2001. Fetal cerebral cortex: normal gestational landmarks identified using prenatal MR imaging. Am. J. Neuroradiol. 22, 184–189.

Malinger, G., Kidron, D., Schreiber, L., et al., 2007. Prenatal diagnosis of malformations of cortical development by dedicated neurosonography. Ultrasound Obstet. Gynecol. 29, 178–191.

Melchiorre, K., Bhide, A., Gika, A.D., et al., 2009. Counseling in isolated mild fetal ventriculomegaly. Ultrasound Obstet. Gynecol. 34, 212–224.

Prasad, A.N., Malinger, G., Lerman-Sagie, T., 2009. Primary disorders of metabolism and disturbed fetal brain development. Clin. Perinatol. 36, 621–638.

⊗ E-BOOK FIGURES AND TABLES

The following figures and tables are available in the e-book at www.expertconsult.com. See inside cover for registration details.

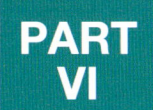

34 Neurogenetics in the Genome Era

Kelly McMahon, Alex R. Paciorkowski, Lauren C. Walters-Sen, Jeff M. Milunsky, Alexander Bassuk, Benjamin Darbro, Jullianne Diaz, William B. Dobyns, and Andrea Gropman

 An expanded version of this chapter is available on www.expertconsult.com. See inside cover for registration details.

INTRODUCTION TO THE HUMAN GENOME

The human genome consists of approximately 3.08 billion base pairs of deoxyribonucleic acid (DNA) divided into 22 numbered chromosomes and two sex chromosomes (X, Y). Nearly 3% of the genome is protein coding, or exonic, and has come to be termed the exome. This coding region is responsible for some 20,000 genes, the primary units of heredity. The remainder of the genome (approximately 97%) is comprised of regions of repeats and segmental duplications (50%), and some highly conserved regulatory regions. Compared with many other organisms, the genome of Homo sapiens is modest in size, and the diversity of protein products in humans is greatly increased through the process of alternative splicing.

Chromosomes reside in the cell nucleus in a three-dimensional structure called a fractal globule with important consequences for short-range and long-range regulation of gene expression. The nucleotide sequence of the genome is the principle determinant of gene activity, but chromosomes are comprised of DNA upon a protein scaffold, the combination of which is termed chromatin. The proteins within chromatin include histones, which are strongly evolutionarily conserved DNA-associated proteins. Chromatin that is less condensed is termed euchromatin and contains coding DNA. The more condensed heterochromatin contains noncoding DNA. Epigenetic factors, defined as factors independent of the nucleotide sequence that affect gene expression, include methylation of DNA and histone acetylation. Taken together, the journey from primary DNA sequence to biological effect is a complex one with numerous opportunities for the introduction of pathology.

The numbered chromosomes are referred to as autosomes and exist in pairs in every cell, each member of the pair being derived from a parent. Chromosome X and Y have pseudoautosomal regions with distinct recombinatory properties. Through the process of X-inactivation, women selectively inactivate one X chromosome in every cell, leading to the observation that in this sense all females are mosaic.

In addition to the nuclear genome, cells have an additional mitochondrial genome that resides in those organelles and whose division and replication are regulated semiautonomously. The mitochondrial genome comprises 14 genes, and several well-characterized human disorders are associated with mutations in those genes. Many of the genes encoded in the mitochondrial genome produce proteins essential for function of the electron transport chain. Due to the lack of mitochondria in paternal sperm, an individual's mitochondrial genome is generally derived maternally. Mutations within the mitochondrial genome can occur somatically with the result that any one cell may host several copies of that genome, some with mutations and some without, a phenomenon called heteroplasmy.

Genomic Variation

The terminology used to describe genomic variation can be complex, and a glossary of terms is included in Table 34-1.

Chromosomal Structural Rearrangements

A variety of chromosomal structural rearrangements has been known to geneticists for many decades and includes translocations of part of one chromosomal arm onto another. Translocations are often visible on karyotype and are classified as balanced or unbalanced, depending on whether or not they result in net loss or gain of genomic material. On the whole balanced translocations are generally regarded as nonpathogenic, unless the translocation disrupts a critical locus. Balanced translocations can, however, result in chromosomal breakage and can mediate a chromosomal deletion or duplication in an offspring—for example Robertsonian translocations as a cause of Trisomy 21. These examples change recurrence risk inform the need to perform karyotypes in parents of children with chromosomal abnormalities.

History of Cytogenetics

The origins of human cytogenetics can be attributed to Walther Flemming, who first described human chromosomes in the early 1880s. Improvements in technology in the early 20th century led to research into the number of human chromosomes and the configuration of sex chromosomes between males and females. However, it was not until the accidental "discovery" of hypotonic treatment in the early 1950s that the diploid complement of chromosomes was set at 46. This key step, which caused the cells to swell and allowed chromosomes to separate, was necessary to fully visualize each homolog pair. At the same time, the use of colchicine to destroy the mitotic spindle permitted scientists to view the chromosomes at the stage of maximal contraction. This combined hypotonic/colchicine technique led to the modern field of cytogenetic analysis that we know today (Gerson and Keagle, 2013).

With accurate visualization of chromosomes, various defects in chromosome number and structure were discovered. The first such discovery was made by Lejeune and colleagues in 1959 with the observation of an additional chromosome in the fibroblasts of patients with Down

TABLE 34-1 Glossary of Terms Used to Describe Genomic Variation

Term	Definition
Aneuploidy	A chromosomal numerical abnormality, such as a trisomy or monosomy
Balanced translocation	A type of chromosomal structural rearrangement where there is no apparent loss or gain of genetic material
Heteroplasmy	Presence of more than one mitochondrial genome within a cell
Indel	An insertion or deletion of DNA.
Missense mutation	A coding single nucleotide variant that results in a change in amino acid sequence; a type of nonsynonymous variant
Mosaic	Presence of more than one populations of cells with different genotypes within an organism.
Mutation	A genetic variant that causes abnormal biologic function and is pathogenic, disease-causing; this can include any pathogenic genetic variant but is most commonly used to refer to pathogenic single nucleotide variants
Nonsense mutation	A coding variant that results in the premature introduction of a stop codon
Nonsynonymous variant	A coding variant that results in a change in amino acid sequenc.
Regions of homozygosity	Chromosomal regions where the pattern of DNA polymorphisms indicates decreased genetic diversity
Segmental duplication	Genomic sequences sharing >90% similarity over >1 kb with another genomic location
Short tandem repeats	Tracks of tandemly repeated short (1–6 bp) DNA sequence motifs; also called microsatellites
Single nucleotide polymorphism	Single nucleotide variant that is found in the general population and is considered benign; a type of single nucleotide variant
Single nucleotide variant	A single change in the nucleotide sequence that may be benign (polymorphism) or pathogenic (mutation)
Somatic mosaic	A form of mosaicism that occurs due to mitotic errors after fertilization
Structural rearrangements	Deletion, duplication, or translocation of chromosomal material
Synonymous variant	A coding variant that does not result in a change in amino acid sequence. Can affect exon splicing
Unbalanced translocation	A type of chromosomal structural rearrangement where there is loss or gain of genetic material
Uniparental disomy	The inheritance of both copies of a chromosome, or a chromosomal region, from one parent only
Variant of unknown significance	A variant whose pathogenicity is unknown

syndrome, later identified as chromosome 21. The sex chromosome abnormalities of Turner syndrome, Klinefelter syndrome, and Triple X syndrome were also defined in 1959, by Ford and colleagues, Jacobs and Strong, and Jacobs and associates, respectively. The next year brought the description of Patau syndrome and Edwards syndrome, later defined as trisomy 13 and trisomy 18, respectively. No additional advances in the field could be made until improvement in staining techniques.

When methods for examining chromosomes under the microscope were first developed, individual chromosomes could not be identified because of solid staining. Instead, they were separated into seven groups (A to G), based on their length and centromere position. Although not ideal, this was suitable for the analysis of simple monosomies and trisomies. However, the discovery of quinacrine mustard staining by Caspersson and colleagues in 1971 allowed the identification of individual chromosomes, the foundation of the numbering system in use today. The ability to positively identify a chromosome, along with the possibility of visualizing "bands" within each homolog, led to an explosion of defined chromosomal syndromes, including deletions, duplications, inversions, translocations, and other rearrangements.

The field has expanded, with development of new technologies that allow even finer resolution of the chromosomal complement. Several of these techniques use molecular genetics methodologies as discussed further in this chapter. Thus the distinction between cytogenetics and molecular genetics has become blurred. In general, traditional cytogenetic analyses examine large regions of the genome such as chromosomes or regions of chromosomes, whereas standard molecular genetics

methods focus on smaller regions of the genome, from single nucleotides to genes and gene regions. However, even in this era of nucleotide-level resolution, traditional cytogenetics remains critical for the study of rearrangements not routinely detected by new technologies, most importantly balanced rearrangements that disrupt crucial genes in development.

A uniform system of human chromosome classification and nomenclature is used to describe abnormalities. This system was developed at a series of international conferences and was most recently revised in 2013. In this system, the chromosomes are separated into bands, which are placed into regions defined by landmarks. As resolution increases, bands can be subdivided into subbands, which are designated with a decimal point. All bands are described in relation to the centromere, with higher region and subband numbers corresponding with more telomeric positions. The four required components of a band description are: (1) chromosome number; (2) arm symbol (p for short arm or q for long arm); (3) region number; and (4) band number within the region. Thus the designation 17p13.3 (read as "17-p-one-three-point-three") corresponds to chromosome 17, short arm, region 1, band 3, subband 3. The use of this standardized system allows consistent description of chromosomal abnormalities regardless of the laboratory performing the analysis.

As with any technique, there are limitations to traditional cytogenetic analysis. Even with high-resolution banding techniques genomic imbalances smaller than three megabases cannot be visualized. In addition, cryptic rearrangements involving bands of similar size and staining density may not be recognized. On the other hand, polymorphic variations in banding, aside from common sites, can be confused for pathogenic changes if not further explored through family studies. Mosaicism for multiple cell lines may not be recognized if the level of the secondary cell line is low (typically lower than 20%). Finally, the genetic composition of chromosomal material of unknown origin, either in the form of markers or material added on to existing chromosomes often cannot be confirmed through standard analysis. Additional techniques, such as fluorescent in situ hybridization (discussed later in this chapter) or microarray analysis, are often necessary to fully elucidate the genomic origin of such material (Haines et al., 2012).

Fluorescence in Situ Hybridization

Fluorescence in situ hybridization (FISH) is a technique used to detect specific chromosomes or chromosomal regions through hybridization (attachment) of fluorescently labeled DNA probes to denatured chromosomal DNA. Examination under fluorescent lighting detects the presence or absence of the hybridized fluorescent signal (and hence presence or absence of the chromosome material). Described as a "molecular cytogenetic" technique, FISH has been accepted as the standard-of-care for a variety of chromosomal aberrations. These abnormalities are too small to be visualized using standard cytogenetic techniques and too large to be analyzed with standard DNA sequencing.

FISH studies can be performed on metaphase chromosomes or interphase cells, depending on the type of abnormality being considered and the probe type being used. Probes can be divided into three major categories: repetitive sequence, whole chromosome, or unique sequence. Repetitive sequence probes include those covering the alpha satellite regions at the centromeres of chromosomes. These probes can be used to detect aneuploidy in both metaphase and interphase cells. Whole chromosome probes, or chromosome painting probes, are comprised of both unique and mildly repetitive sequences covering the entire length of a particular chromosome. These are most often used in metaphase cells for the study of structural abnormalities.

The most widely used probe type, unique sequence, is used to study a particular genomic region, ranging in size from 1 kb to larger than 1 Mb. These probes can be used in interphase or metaphase cells to detect deletions, duplications, or other abnormalities. However, in contrast with metaphase FISH, interphase FISH does not permit visualization of the actual chromosomes; therefore most types of structural rearrangements cannot be reliably detected. An additional type of unique sequence probe that is commonly used is telomere-specific probes. These probes correspond to the telomeres of all of the chromosomes and are used to detect abnormalities at the ends of chromosomes that are not visible by routine chromosome analysis. The previous utility of these probes has now generally been replaced by microarray analysis or MPLA analysis (see later section). Most FISH analyses examine one to two chromosomal regions at once, although it is possible to multiplex probes with special fluorescent markers to increase the number of regions that can be assayed.

FISH analyses are also used in conjunction with microarray studies that have identified copy number variations. Although microarrays can provide the highest resolution of genomic gains and losses, FISH analysis is still necessary to identify the underlying mechanism of the genomic alteration. For example, FISH studies can discriminate between tandem duplication and duplication due to an unbalanced rearrangement. Even though the outcome of the two abnormalities is the same (gain of a particular region), the mechanism of the abnormality could have a substantial influence on family planning. In addition, FISH analysis is often less expensive and faster than additional microarray studies when determining the inheritance pattern of a microarray abnormality. This can lead to a more rapid clinical assessment of the patient, given the possible pathogenicity of a de novo variant versus a likely benign familial copy number change.

Copy Number Variations

The completion of the draft human genome sequence in 2000 inaugurated a new era of appreciation for the patterns of genomic variation. It was soon discovered that the human genome contains numerous areas of segmental duplication, which are nucleotide sequences sharing greater than 90% similarity over larger than1 kb in size with another genomic location. There are over 1400 copy number variable regions in the human genome (about 12% of the entire genome), and 25% of these copy number variable regions are associated with segmental duplications. Segmental duplications are therefore an important mechanism mediating copy number variation. Copy number variants range in size from small insertions or deletions of single nucleotides, through duplication or deletion of chromosomal regions hundreds of kilobases (kb) in size or larger, all the way to include trisomies (duplications of entire chromosomes) or monosomies (loss of entire chromosomes). However, most copy number variants are benign and number in the hundreds of kb in size (Cooper et al., 2011; Kearney et al., 2011).

Indels

Among genomic variants, insertions/deletions (indels) are the second most common type and the most common type of structural variant. Collectively, between 1.6 and 2.5 million indel polymorphisms are present in the human population, with approximately 0.4 million short indels (1 to 16 bp) present per individual. The presence of an indel may be associated with disease, particularly if the inserted or deleted nucleotides result in a frameshift in a coding region. In contrast, the biological function of indels located within noncoding regions, intragenic regions, introns, and untranslated regions are more likely to be benign variants.

Short Tandem Repeats

Short tandem repeats (STRs), or "microsatellites," are tracks of tandemly repeated short (1 to 6 bp) DNA sequence motifs. STRs may occur in both intergenic and intragenic regions, including within genes, and account for approximately 3% of the human genome. Some microsatellites are highly mutable and show both sequence and length polymorphism whereas others are more conserved and can be informative markers in population genetics, mapping, and linkage studies. A specific subclass of trinucleotide repeats are combinations of nucleotides arranged repetitively (i.e., CAG or CGG repeats).

Mutations, Single Nucleotide Variants, and Single Nucleotide Polymorphisms

A word regarding nomenclature is important at the outset here. For geneticists, there are important distinctions between mutations, single nucleotide variants, and single nucleotide polymorphisms. All refer to alterations in a single nucleotide. The term mutation is best reserved for nucleotide changes that are clearly associated with a deleterious biological effect or a disease. Single nucleotide variants (or SNVs) are those nucleotide changes not clearly associated with abnormal biology or disease but not clearly benign population variants either. SNVs therefore may be understood to include variants of unknown significance. Finally, single nucleotide polymorphisms (or SNPs) are a special group of common nucleotide variants present in a significant (generally greater than 0.05%) percentage of the human population and are widely understood not to be associated with abnormal biology or disease. SNPs that have been documented in the general population will have catalog numbers (beginning with "rs") and will be present in the Database of Single Nucleotide Polymorphisms (dbSNP; http://www.ncbi.nlm.nih.gov/SNP/), often with an associated mean allele frequency.

Single nucleotide variants are the most common form of genomic variation, with 3 million SNVs typically present per individual. Of these, nearly 20,000 are located within coding regions. When SNVs located within coding regions do not result in a change in the amino acid sequence encoded, they are termed synonymous variants. There have usually no identifiable biological effects of synonymous SNVs except when they are located in splice regions at the exon-intron boundaries. When an SNV results in a change in the amino acid encoded, it is referred to as a nonsynonymous variant. These variants that alter the amino acid sequence may prove to be pathogenic if the change significantly affects the conformation or biological activity of the protein.

Methods of General Mutation Detection

DNA Sequence Analysis

Sanger Sequencing. DNA sequence analysis is the most sensitive and direct method to detect mutations at the level of individual nucleotides. The most widely used method of DNA sequencing is the Sanger method, also known as dideoxy sequencing or chain termination. It is based on the use of synthetic nucleotide analogs—2, 3-dideoxynucleoside triphosphates (ddNTPs). Dideoxy NTPs differ from nucleotides found in natural DNA in that they lack the 3′-hydroxyl group. When integrated into a sequence, they prevent the addition of further nucleotides as phosphodiester bonds cannot form between a dideoxynucleotide and the next incoming nucleotide. Thus the DNA chain is terminated.

DNA sequencing most commonly is performed by the method of cycle sequencing, in which the DNA region to be sequenced (which is first generated by PCR) is denatured, and a short oligonucleotide is annealed to one of the template strands. DNA synthesis occurs in the presence of DNA polymerase, ddNTPs, and normal (deoxy) nucleotides and starts from the 3′ end of the annealed oligonucleotide. As the DNA is synthesized, nucleotides are added on to the growing chain by the DNA polymerase; however, on occasion, a ddNTP is incorporated into the chain in place of a normal nucleotide, resulting in a chain-terminating event. At the end of the sequencing reaction, multiple DNA molecules are present such that, at each nucleotide position, a proportion of molecules are terminated because of the incorporation of a ddNTP. These products are separated by size on capillary or polyacrylamide gel electrophoresis systems, and the fluorescently labeled ddNTPs are detected. Each ddNTP is labeled with a different fluorophore. Shorter DNA molecules migrate faster than longer molecules on electrophoresis, and by analyzing the different fluorescent signal of all of the different-sized molecules, the DNA sequence can be determined. For example, ddCTP is labeled with a blue fluorophore. Everywhere a G residue exists in the template DNA, either a dCTP or a ddCTP will be incorporated into the synthesized strand. For every G residue in the template DNA, a proportion of molecules with a ddCTP at that site will be present. Each of these molecules will be of a different size, depending on where a G residue resides in the sequence and will be distinguished by electrophoresis. The same applies for the other ddNTPs. Specialized DNA sequencing software exists that can convert the different fluorescent signals to different-color peaks that constitute a DNA sequence chromatogram.

After performing the necessary laboratory techniques, the sequence is analyzed by a trained molecular technician. Computer programs are used to facilitate the comparison of generated sequence with the reference sequence for the region of interest. If differences are discovered, they should ideally be confirmed. Such differences are then described using both nucleotide and amino acid designations in the standardized fashion. The nucleotide change is defined as the position in the coding sequence, with the adenine nucleotide of the initiator ATG designated as the first base, followed by the nucleotide change, all beginning with a "c" identifier. For example, a guanine to cytosine change at the fiftieth nucleotide in the coding sequence would be defined as "c.50G>C." The amino acid change is then defined as the original amino acid (either three letter or single letter code), the numerical identifier of the amino acid in question, and the new amino acid, all beginning with a "p" identifier. For example, using the previous nucleotide change, the seventeenth codon changes from CCA to CGA, which results in a change from proline to arginine; this would be defined as "p.Pro17Arg" (alternatively "p.P17R").

The next stage of analysis involves bioinformatics techniques. The variant identified through sequencing may be a known population polymorphism, a known pathogenic mutation, a completely novel variant, or a reported variant without clear phenotypic consequences. In order to determine which class contains the identified variant, a molecular geneticist queries public databases such as dbSNP, ClinVar, or HGMD. If the pathogenicity of the variant is unknown, this aspect can be explored using web-based prediction programs, such as PolyPhen, SIFT, MutPred, Condel, or FATHMM. However, it should be remembered that these are predictions only and are not definitive evidence of the functional effect of a given variant. A sequence variant is typically reported as pathogenic, of uncertain significance, or benign, and the final report should include all pertinent information regarding this designation.

The use of the Sanger technique to study the sequence of a genomic region of interest is limited only by the ability of the user to design appropriate oligonucleotides, or primers, to be used in PCR amplification and subsequent sequencing. However, several limitations exist for this technique and must be taken into account. First, as the Sanger technique relies on an initial PCR amplification, it is subject to PCR errors. These events are rare, but they can cause significant problems in final analysis if they occur early in the PCR cycling process. Second, Sanger sequencing is not well-adapted to analyzing mosaicism, again due to the initial PCR step. This is not a quantitative method, and a target sequence in a smaller proportion can be overwhelmed by another sequence present in the template. Third, care must be taken in the design of primers to ensure that the proper target is amplified, which is especially vital when considering genes with closely related pseudogenes. Finally, Sanger sequencing can only detect changes in sequence, not changes in copy number. If one allele carries a deletion or duplication, it will not be detected; the final chromatogram will be consistent with two homozygous alleles. These caveats must be considered when using Sanger sequencing.

Deletion/Duplication Analysis. The most common method of deletion/duplication analysis is Multiplex Ligation-dependent Probe Amplification, or MPLA. MLPA is used to detect copy number changes of small DNA fragments. This technique is most often used to assay individual exons of genes but can also be used to study the subtelomeric regions of chromosomes or multiple regions of specific chromosomes to detect aneuploidy. In this technique, special MLPA probes are hybridized to the ends of sequences under study; if both ends are present, the probes are ligated together. Only then can PCR be used to amplify the complete sequences. The unique MLPA probes are comprised of a sequence compatible to the target sequence, a stuffer sequence for size variation, and a common PCR primer sequence. The combination of variable size products and a single set of PCR amplification primers allow this technique to assay up to fifty separate targets in a single reaction. MLPA utilizes the same laboratory equipment as PCR-based Sanger sequencing, specifically a thermocycler and a fluorescent capillary electrophoresis system.

MLPA is often the first-tier test in disorders primarily caused by exon or gene deletions/duplications, such as Duchenne muscular dystrophy (DMD), spinal muscular atrophy (SMN1), and Charcot-Marie-Tooth neuropathy (PMP22). In addition, the use of MLPA in conjunction with traditional gene sequencing can increase the rate of detection of pathogenic variants, typically up to an additional 10%.

MLPA is advantageous in that it can detect very small imbalances, to the level of 50 to 75 nucleotides, which is much smaller than the resolution of oligonucleotide microarrays or FISH analysis. In addition, the exact location of the imbalance does not need to be known a priori, as is required with standard PCR-based methods of deletion/duplication analysis. However, kits are only available commercially for defined genomic locations, without the ability to study less commonly affected regions. In addition, care must be taken when interpreting results that are indicative of deletions. Sequence variation within the probe target site can either abolish or reduce probe binding, which would generate an electrophoretic profile consistent with a deletion. As such, results must be considered in conjunction with clinical information, and ideally all results should be confirmed with a separate methodology.

Methylation Studies. Methylation of cytosine is a DNA modification associated with several biological processes, including imprinting, X chromosome inactivation, and silencing of repetitive DNA sequences. The most recent studies suggested approximately 151 genes in the mouse genome were subject to imprinting, and a similar number estimated for the human genome, despite some recent methodological controversy. Of these, the 15q11q13 region, associated with the Angelman, Prader-Willi, and Duplication of Maternal 15q11q13 syndromes is most notable. These are imprinting disorders, in which the phenotype is determined by the pattern of parental methylation of 15q11q13. Individuals with loss of the paternal methylation pattern present with Prader-Willi syndrome, whereas those with loss of the maternal methylation pattern present with Angelman syndrome.

This may occur through a number of molecular mechanisms, and for Angelman syndrome includes de novo deletion of 15q11q13 (70% to 75% of individuals) uniparental disomy for chromosome 15 (2% to 3% of individuals), imprinting center mutations (3–5% of individuals), or mutations in UBE3A (5% to 10% of individuals) a gene on 15q11q13 whose expression is directed by parent-of-origin allele-specific methylation. Therefore the best first test for diagnosis of Angelman syndrome is bisulfide methylation sensitive polymerase chain reaction (PCR), which will detect any of the methylation defects, whether caused by chromosomal deletion, uniparental disomy, or imprinting center mutation. Chromosomal microarray will only detect 15q11q13 deletions, will miss approximately 25% of Angelman patients and should not be used as the first diagnostic test. In individuals with normal 15q11q13 methylation studies, but who have a phenotype consistent with Angelman syndrome, UBE3A sequencing should be the second test sent.

Chromosomal Microarray. Copy number variants (CNVs) are identified by array-based methods that use comparative genome hybridization (CGH). CGH determines copy number of genomic DNA sequencing using varying intensity patterns between hybridized patient and control DNA. Control DNA used in microarray either represents the whole genome or contains cloned fragments (targeted microarray) from the genome. Bacterial artificial chromosomes (BAC) probes are approximately 75,000 to 150,000 base pairs in length whereas oligonucleotide probes, used for oligonucleotide and single-nucleotide polymorphism (SNP) arrays, are approximately 50 to 60 base pairs in length, allowing for increased breakpoint specificity and improved accuracy of copy number variants. The resolution of the array depends on the number and types of probes used and whether the probes are targeted or cover the whole genome (Manning and Hudgins, 2010). SNP arrays can detect copy number neutral regions of homozygosity that can be associated with uniparental disomy or consanguinity by comparing reference DNA to hybridized patient DNA. Identifying a copy neutral region of homozygosity may suggest an autosomal recessive disease in the patient. Typically, clinical chromosomal microarrays can detect chromosomal imbalances of 20 to 50 kb in targeted regions.

Copy number variants (CNVs) are classified as either pathogenic/abnormal, variant of unknown significance (VUS), or likely benign. It should be kept in mind when interpreting results that the estimated mean number of benign CNVs per individual is 800 or more. When a copy number variant is identified by chromosomal microarray, fluorescence in-situ hybridization (FISH) studies to confirm the finding in the patient, parental FISH studies, clinical genetic evaluation, and genetic counseling are recommended. In general, when a CNV is found to be inherited from a healthy parent, is gene poor, or is a duplication with no known dosage-sensitive genes involved, this indicates that the variant is likely benign. Likely pathogenic CNVs include those which are inherited from an affected parent, are gene rich, or overlap a genomic coordinates for a known genomic-imbalance syndrome.

Several studies have validated chromosomal microarray as a first tier test, over G-banded karyotype, in the evaluation of developmental delay, intellectual disability, autism spectrum disorders, and multiple congenital abnormalities. In a study of 21,698 patients with developmental delay, intellectual disability, autism spectrum disorders, or multiple congenital abnormalities, chromosomal microarray was found to have a diagnostic yield of 12.2%.

Pathogenic CNVs have been shown to play a role in the etiology of epilepsy, providing evidence to support that chromosomal microarray be a part of the diagnostic evaluation for patients with unexplained epilepsy. It is estimated that up to 40% of epilepsies have a genetic component. Chromosomal microarray can identify recurrent CNVs for epilepsy "hotspots," deletions, or duplications in known epilepsy genes, or nonrecurrent CNVs involving epilepsy genes. Chromosomal microarray has an even higher diagnostic yield in individuals with epilepsy and additional findings such as intellectual disabilities, dysmorphic features, malformations, developmental delay, and autism spectrum disorders. In a study of 102 patients with different types of epilepsy, either isolated or with intellectual disability/developmental delay, dysmorphic features, autism or other neurologic signs, 10 of 102 (9.8%) were found to have pathogenic CNVs associated with epilepsy. Limitations of chromosomal microarray include poor detection of low-level mosaicism, balanced rearrangement, and, in some arrays, polyploidy. Chromosomal microarray should not be used when a rapid turnaround time is needed, when a chromosomal trisomy such as Trisomy 21 is suspected, or when a well-described syndrome is suspected as a diagnosis.

Southern Blot. The Southern blot is a technique that uses gel electrophoresis combined with labeled probes for a DNA sequence of interest that allows for the detection of repeat expansions within specific genes. The technique is used to detect the triplet repeat expansions seen in neurologic diseases such as myotonic dystrophy, fragile X syndrome, and many spinocerebellar ataxias. Despite advances in sequencing technologies, this technique remains the standard for direct molecular diagnosis of these disorders.

Next-Generation Sequencing. The term "next-generation sequencing," or "high-throughput sequencing," has become synonymous with the most recent appearance on the clinical and research scene of massively parallel sequencing of regions of interest. In 2009 the first use of next-generation sequencing, specifically whole-exome sequencing, as a proof-of-principle to confirm mutations in MYH3 as the causative gene for Freeman-Sheldon syndrome. Soon after, a similar technique was employed to identify DHODH as the causative gene for Miller syndrome, followed by the identification of MLL2 as the first causative gene for Kabuki syndrome. Of note, the identification of MLL2 highlighted the challenging bioinformatics aspects of next-generation sequencing analysis, as several iterations of analysis were required before mutations were found. In the years since those findings, an evolution of the technological platforms for next-generation sequencing has occurred, with the Illumina platform producing 100 bp paired-end reads, currently the most prevalent in research and clinical diagnostic settings, although alternatives exist.

Next-generation sequencing involves the targeted capture of defined genomic regions of interest. At the most narrow— for example, those available in disease gene panels such as epilepsy or intellectual disability panels—the region of interest may be the coding exons of several dozen genes. Larger regions of interest such as the exome include the coding regions of all genes. Variability in the percentage coverage of each gene is a factor in the capture of regions of interest and should be taken into account during the selection of a sequencing method. The bioinformatics analysis of next-generation sequencing data has emerged as a new field within genomics, and changes in best practices occur quickly.

RESOURCES FOR INTERPRETING GENOMIC TESTING

A constant feature of current genomic testing is the rapid introduction of new technologies and, along with them, new methods to allow their interpretation. In an ideal setting, close collaboration exists with genetics colleagues who maintain currency with this evolving field. However, appropriate expertise may not be readily available in all of the settings where child neurologists evaluate individuals with neurodevelopmental disorders. A summary of the tools discussed here is found in Table 34-2.

CNVs for which no literature exists to help interpretation can be evaluated using DECIPHER (https://decipher.sanger.ac.uk/), and the Database of Genomic Variants (http://dgv.tcag.ca/dgv/app/home).

Most genomic variants that are causative of neurodevelopmental diseases are rare, not present in the general population, and in the case of relatively common disorders such as autism and epilepsy (Epi4K Consortium), are often but not always due to de novo mutations that are not inherited from the parents. Other disorders are autosomal recessive or X-linked, in which case a disease causing variant may be present in one (usually the mother in the case of X-linked) or both parents (in the case of autosomal recessive). Several online resources provide expert-curated gene-phenotype associations relevant to child neurology (Table 34-5). Finally, the Developmental Brain Disorders Database (DBDB; https://www.dbdb.urmc.rochester.edu/home) provides a repository of genes, phenotypes, and syndromes specifically targeted at neurodevelopmental disorders.

TABLE 34-2 Glossary of Terms Used for Genomic Diagnostic Technologies and the Genomic Variations They Detect

Diagnostic Technology	Genomic Variation Detected
Karyotype	Aneuploidy (trisomy, monosomy), structural rearrangements including balanced translocations, deletions and duplications >5 Mb.
Fluorescence in situ hybridization (FISH)	Specific deletions or duplications.
Methylation studies	Abnormal parental methylation patterns.
Chromosomal microarray (CMA)	Copy number variations (deletions, duplications) >50-100 kb. SNP arrays can detect loss of heterozygosity (regions of homozygosity), uniparental disomy.
Sanger sequencing	Single nucleotide variants, small frameshift indels
Multiplex ligation probe amplification	Exon-level deletions or duplications
Southern blot	Triplet repeat expansions
Next-generation sequencing	Massively parallel detection of single nucleotide variants, small indels in many genes simultaneously across targeted region of interest

Recently a statistical approach was proposed to determine whether or not variants in a given gene are likely to be disease causing based upon the prevalence overall of common variation in that gene, with the hypothesis that some genes are more tolerant of variation whereas others are not. The proposed residual variance intolerance score (RVIS) is derived from the regression of common coding variants in a gene upon all variants in that gene. A value lower than the 25th percentile is taken as a cutoff higher than which a gene is said to "tolerate" variation and therefore is unlikely to be a disease gene; indeed, many known neurodevelopmental disease genes fall lower than this percentile. A difficulty with this approach, however, is that it treats all variation as equal when clearly this is not the case. Null mutations anywhere in a gene may be deleterious, even in a gene with many common sequence variants. Likewise, specific amino acid substitutions at biologically critical loci within a gene (whether or not variations in the gene overall are frequent) can also cause disease.

Although the use of whole-exome sequencing for clinical diagnostics has resulted in the identification of causative mutations in many individuals, the overall diagnostic yield of 25% has not been as impressive as initially hoped. It is suggested that adoption of whole genome sequencing able to identify both CNVs and SNVs will increase the diagnostic yield of next-generation sequencing to over 40%.

Somatic Mosaicism and Challenges of Tissue of Origin for DNA

DNA isolated from patient leukocytes has been the traditional source for diagnostic genetic testing, including in neurologic disorders. However, a spectrum of disorders has been identified in which the causative mutations are present in affected brain tissue in a somatic mosaic manner. This observation began with the identification of "second-hit" somatic mutations in TSC1/2, in neurons of individuals with tuberous sclerosis complex, and in germline mutations in the same gene. Then, mosaic mutations were identified in a spectrum

TABLE 34-5 Summary of Online Tools Involved in Analysis of Genomic Diagnostic Testing

Tool and URL	Use Case
Database of Genomic Variants (DGV) http://dgv.tcag.ca/dgv/app/home	Evaluation of copy number variants
DECIPHER https://decipher.sanger.ac.uk/	Evaluation of copy number variants
Human Gene Mutation Database (HGMD) http://www.hgmd.cf.ac.uk/ac/index.php	Evaluation of known mutations in known disease genes
SIFT http://sift.jcvi.org/	Prediction of effect of amino acid substitution on protein function
PolyPhen http://genetics.bwh.harvard.edu/pph2/	Prediction of effect of amino acid substitution on protein function
Ensembl's Variant Effect Predictor (VEP) http://grch37.ensembl.org/Homo_sapiens/Tools/VEP	Allows batch annotation of genomic variants for SIFT, PolyPhen, dbSNP membership, and other annotations
dbSNP http://www.ncbi.nlm.nih.gov/SNP/	Evaluation of single nucleotide polymorphisms for population frequency
UCSC Genome Browser http://www.genome.ucsc.edu/	Allows visualization of a range of genomic regions of interest and multiple annotations
Eukaryotic Linear Motif server (ELM) http://elm.eu.org/	Evaluation of amino acids within functional protein domains
Exome Variant Server (EVS) http://evs.gs.washington.edu/EVS/	Allows search for variants in >6500 other whole exomes
Exome Aggregate Consortium browser (ExAC) http://exac.broadinstitute.org/	Allows search for variants in >63,000 whole exomes
GeneReviews http://www.ncbi.nlm.nih.gov/books/NBK1116/	Expert curated chapters on well-described single gene syndromes
Online Mendelian Inheritance in Man (OMIM) http://www.ncbi.nlm.nih.gov/omim/	Expert curated information on a broad range of genetic syndromes
Developmental Brain Disorders Database (DBDB) https://www.dbdb.urmc.rochester.edu/home	Expert curated gene-phenotype-syndrome associations specific to neurodevelopmental disorders

of megalencephaly polymicrogyria syndromes, hemimegalencephaly, and focal cortical dysplasia type II, with the mutations documented at varying levels in blood, skin, brain, and saliva-derived DNA. Clearly, blood-derived DNA may not be the most informative in these disorders, an issue now being addressed by diagnostic testing laboratories.

Determining an etiology for a child's developmental delays/intellectual disability or autism spectrum disorders may influence a child's treatment. In a survey of 48 patients with positive chromosomal microarray results, physicians noted a direct effect on the family in 70% of cases. The most beneficial effect to families was the ability to provide recurrence risks, providing access to educational and insurance services, avoiding other tests to determine a diagnosis, and helping target additional medical referrals such as to a cardiologist or ophthalmologist. Failure to diagnose a genetic disease can have negative effects for both the family, including lack of potential treatments, clinical trials, or recurrence risks, and for society as continued genetic testing or therapies increases medical expenditures.

A three-generation family pedigree should be recorded at the initial patient visit and should be periodically updated. There are several methods of gathering family history information, including physician-directed questions or a questionnaire given before the patient's visit. Factors to consider when assessing a family pedigree for patterns of inheritance include the possibilities of variable expressivity, age related penetrance, gonadal mosaicism, and incomplete penetrance.

Next generation sequencing panels and whole-exome sequencing are becoming more popular testing options and increase the complexity of the genetic counseling process.

Pretest counseling for whole-exome sequencing should include a formal consent process by a medical geneticist or genetic counselor and should include the expected outcomes of testing, likelihood and type of incidental findings, and what results will or will not be disclosed (ACMG Board of Directors). Patients should be informed of the possibility that incidental or secondary findings, as defined by the minimum list of incidental findings recommended by the American College of Medical Genetics, that are unrelated to the patient's symptoms, but may influence medical care may be detected on clinical whole-exome sequencing) and the patient should be given the option to opt-in or opt-out of this additional information (Allyse and Michie, 2013). Patients should be counseled regarding alternatives to testing and informed consent should be included with written documentation (ACMG Board of Directors, 2013). Pretest counseling should also include a description of the differences between research and clinical whole-exome sequencing.

It is important for healthcare providers to include the detailed family pedigree, information on physical examination, and previous laboratory tests with the patient's sample to assist with interpretation of results. Results of clinical whole-exome sequencing may include pathogenic variants known to be associated with the phenotype, variants of uncertain significance in genes possibly related to the patient's phenotype, and medically actionable pathogenic variants not related to the patient's phenotype (ACMG Board of Directors, 2013). Interpreting results of whole-exome sequencing should be done in the context of the patient and family history and requires an understanding of a range of inherited conditions. Candidate variants in genes suspected to be related to the patient's phenotype are often identified and require further studies to determine its role in disease, but a variant of uncertain significance should not be used in the patient's medical decision making. It is strongly recommended to include parental sample with the proband to help in interpretation of variants. The majority of variants for autosomal dominant diseases can be ruled out with parental samples if either of the parents carry the same variant and are unaffected. In addition to information directly related to the patient's phenotype, additional information from whole-exome sequencing may include carrier status of a disease that may influence reproductive decisions and disease susceptibility or predisposition.

Standards of Genomic Care

The recent advances in genomic medicine have brought new recommendations about best practices in the evaluation of individuals who may have genomic-mediated disorders. Arriving at a molecular genetic diagnosis may have care related consequences for affected individuals and may include recommendations for surveillance for known complications, in addition to affecting decisions about choice of medications. The difficulty is there are now so many characterized disorders and the spectrum of presenting symptoms can be so varied that any one practitioner is unlikely to be able to rule out a specific genetic syndrome solely on clinical grounds.

Identification of a genetic diagnosis also allows affected individuals to participate in clinical trials and/or natural history studies that may be available for that disorder. An accurate molecular diagnosis is usually an inclusion criterion for participation. Although it should be noted that insurance providers are not in the business of paying for diagnostic testing for the purpose of enabling participation in a clinical trial, it is still within the purview of the physician to provide optimal care to their patients, and this should include making families aware of the availability of clinical trials and/or natural history studies. Funding agencies are unlikely to provide resources to pay for genetic tests that are clinically available. This is one aspect of the current tension surrounding the best practices of care for children with developmental disorders. It should be noted that much of the medical surveillance recommendations for conditions such as MECP2-related disorder come in part from the results of natural history studies. The ability to identify individuals made possible the

recent treatment trials for fragile X syndrome and Duchenne muscular dystrophy.

LOOKING TOWARD THE FUTURE

Genomic medicine as it applies to child neurology has undergone dramatic changes in the past decade. The advent of new molecular diagnostic technologies has meant that children once diagnosed with "developmental delay," "epilepsy," and "intellectual disability" now have access to much more specific molecular diagnoses. In many cases, more specific diagnoses now have specific health surveillance and treatment recommendations. Just one exciting example is the discovery of the molecular basis underlying focal cortical dysplasia and hemimegalencephaly and their associated intractable epilepsy, which means that new avenues of treatments that are based on biological pathways are now investigation.

The technology to assay the human genome will continue to mature, as will the computational algorithms to identify pathogenic variation. New methods are in development to address gaps in next-generation sequencing analysis, in particular structural rearrangements, copy number variants, repeat expansions, and large indels. Many of these mutational classes will be addressed through new targeting chemistries, longer read sequencing, and novel analysis techniques. Still, the current gaps mean that chromosomal microarray, Southern blot, MLPA, Sanger sequencing, as well as karyotype will continue to have their place in clinical diagnosis.

EXAMPLE OF PRINCIPLES IN PRACTICE

Patient AB is a 3-year-old with a history of progressive complex partial seizures. Onset of seizures began approximately 5 weeks ago. Her mother describes AB as "blanking out and staring into space" during a seizure episode. Episodes usually last less than 2 minutes and are not followed by a prolonged postictal period. After diagnosis of her seizures, she was placed on Keppra; however, her seizures continued and changed in nature. Her seizures are now accompanied by lip smacking and stiffening, occurring up to 20 times a day. A brain MRI was normal. EEG activity appeared focal during seizures and best described as complex partial with a tonic component. A microarray was ordered (Fig. 34-9).

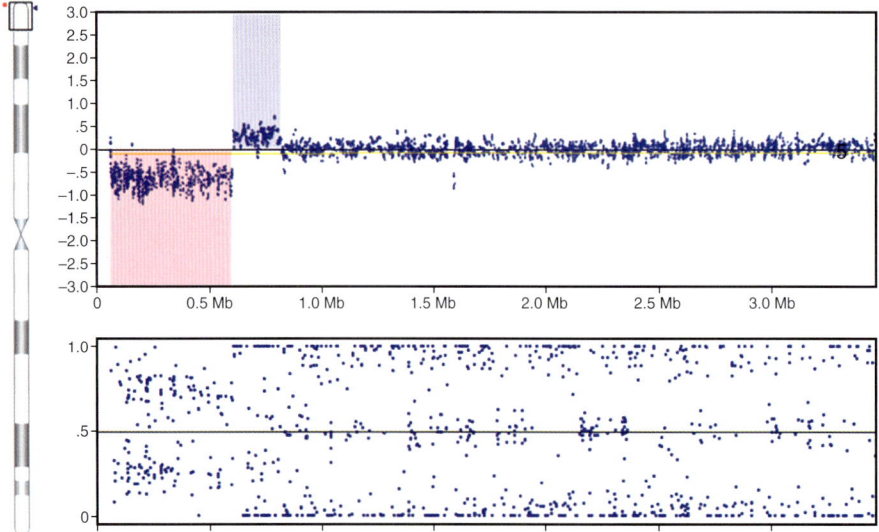

Figure 34-9. CMA result from the short arm of chromosome 20 in the case patient.

Clinical interpretation of CNVs requires knowledge of several factors including:

1. Performance characteristics of the chromosomal microarray being used for testing
2. Frequency of CNV in databases of both control individuals as well as individuals with disease
3. Gene content of the CNV
4. Deletion versus duplication status
5. Inheritance of the phenotype/disease under consideration and disease genes within the CNV
6. De novo or inherited status and cosegregation with disease phenotype in a family

The evaluation of a clinical CMA test begins with knowledge of the microarray platform being used. The ACMG recommends that CMA platforms should be able to detect genome-wide CNVs of at least 400Kb at 99% analytical sensitivity (with a lower limit at the 95% confidence interval greater than 98%) and a false-positive rate of less than 1% (Cooper et al., 2011). This is the minimum standard clinical CMA platforms must meet; however, most clinical laboratories offering CMA today use platforms that allow for the reliable detection of much smaller CNVs—typically on the order of 50 to 100kb. In the above referenced clinical case, the CMA platform used was able to detect CNVs as small as 50kb in size.

The first challenge in interpreting a clinical CMA test is determining which of the myriad of CNVs detected are benign and thus not needing of additional consideration as an underlying cause of disease. Several publically available databases exist to aid in this task, including the Database of Genomic Variants. The Database of Genomic Variants (DGV) is a comprehensive collection of curated structural variation found in the genomes of control individuals from numerous studies and multiple ethnicities. It is important to note that data from control individuals is not precisely the same as data from healthy, "unaffected" individuals. Many of the control individuals with data in DGV were not screened for the myriad of neurodevelopmental or psychiatric conditions that are often times a part of the clinical phenotypic spectrum of patients being evaluated by CMA testing. However, despite this limitation, the copy number variants deposited within DGV have other associated information that makes them suitable for the interpretation of potential pathogenicity. As with SNVs, one of the most consistently used pieces of data is the frequency at which a particular region of the genome is found to be copy number variable in control populations. Different clinical laboratories will often have different frequency thresholds but they are typically in the range of 1% to 5% variant frequency. Furthermore, it is also recommended that, before a CNV be considered benign, it also be found at a relatively high frequency in more than one study deposited in DGV and in studies with a sufficient number of individuals. Lastly, given the rapidly evolving rate of both microarray and sequencing technologies, it is important to place higher confidence on those studies that used a CNV detection platform consistent with the one being used clinically. In addition to DGV, there are other clinical databases that can be used to help interpret the likely pathogenicity of CNVs, including the ClinGen Structural Variant database (formerly the International Standards for Cytogenetic Arrays Consortium, or ISCA) and Database of Chromosomal Imbalance and Phenotype in Humans (DECIPHER) (http://clinicalgenome.org/ and (Zarrei et al., 2015). Lastly, each clinical laboratory should maintain a database of their own to identify both recurrent CNVs that may have disease significance but also those that are seen frequently enough to warrant exclusion as benign.

Once all likely benign CNVs have been removed, it is important to perform additional analysis to interpret those remaining CNVs as either variants of unclear clinical significance or likely pathogenic. If a CNV is detected that is a well-established, disease-associated variant, such as a 22q11.2 deletion and DiGeorge syndrome or a 7q11.23 deletion and Williams syndrome, it can be interpreted fairly quickly and accurately. If, however, a CNV does not fall within one of these well-known disease loci, additional steps are necessary. First, does the CNV contain any genes? If no genes are located within the CNV, interpretation of its potential clinical significance is very difficult. Only 2% to 3% of the genome is known to code for protein and, as such, is the portion of the genome most easily interpreted in a clinical sense. If a CNV contains no genes there is very little confident information that can be conveyed about its potential effect on disease or human phenotypes. Such CNVs are typically not mentioned in clinical reports. Gene content of a CNV, as opposed to simply size, appears to be a larger determinant of phenotypic significance. Additionally, deletions tend to disrupt gene function more often than duplications that, when they do, exert a phenotypic effect can be via several different mechanisms. Deletions naturally cause haploinsufficiency of dosage sensitive genes.

Most importantly, interpretation of the clinical significance of a CNV requires knowledge of any disease-associated genes within the CNV as well as the inheritance pattern of the disease in the family under investigation. A thorough family history and creation of a pedigree is highly recommended before any type of genetic testing is ordered. If the condition being investigated has a clear inheritance pattern, interpretation of CMA results can be much more accurate. The majority of conditions diagnosable by CMA are autosomal dominant or X-linked recessive in nature as the vast majority of lesions identified by CMA are single allele deletions or duplications. Genes known to only cause disease in a recessive fashion are less likely to be of clinical significance in the interpretation of a CNV and typically require sequencing of the other allele to determine the status of the other gene copy. This is not the case, however, if a homozygous deletion is detected. Knowledge of other affected individuals within the family is very important as cosegregation of a CNV with disease can contribute to an interpretation of likely pathogenicity. If a potentially disease-associated CNV is found in a proband and is also found to be inherited from an unaffected parent, the likelihood of that CNV being the sole cause of the proband's condition is greatly reduced. In contrast, if such a CNV is found to be de novo in the proband and not found in either biological parent, then that increases the probability of pathogenicity. Parental testing should be considered to help refine the interpretation of CNVs of unclear clinical significance, however, it is likely to have a higher probability of being meaningful if other features of the CNV suggest pathogenicity (such as gene content, disease-associated genes of appropriate inheritance patterns, deletion status, and absence or rarity in control and/or clinical CNV databases).

In the present case, after benign CNVs have been excluded only two remained that were higher than the size threshold of 50kb. Microarray results showed a 540kb deletion at 20p13 followed by 216kb duplication immediately adjacent. There are no identical or very similar deletions or duplications within the DGV or other clinical databases; however, both ClinGen and DECIPHER do list patients with deletions and/or duplications that cover the region of the genome. The deletion contains 14 genes and the duplication contains four genes. Within the deletion interval there are two disease-associated genes: RBCK1 and TBC1D20. RBCK1 is implicated in polyglucosan body myopathy 1 with or without immunodeficiency, an autosomal recessive condition, and TBC1D20 is implicated

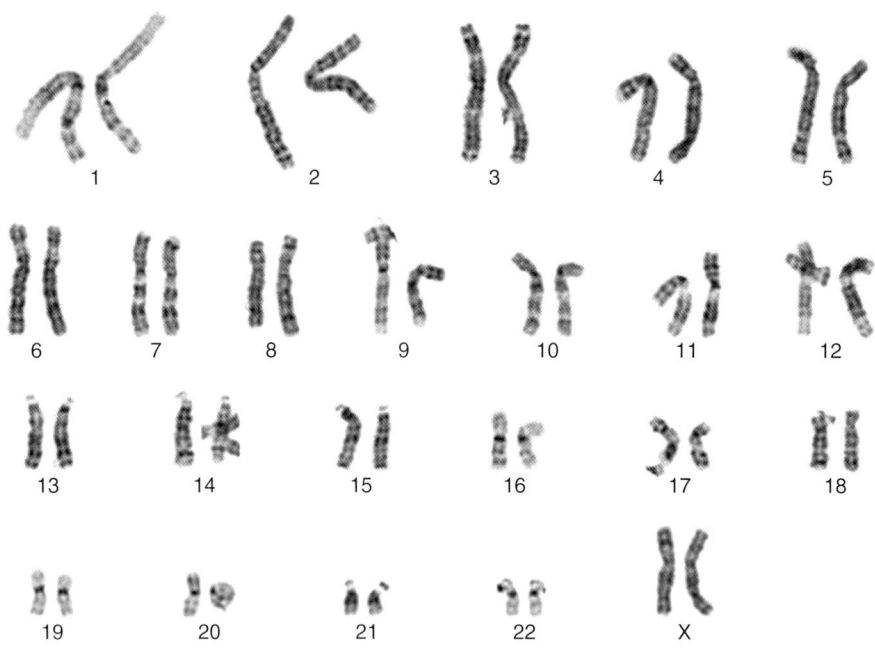

Figure 34-10. Karyotype result exhibiting a ring chromosome 20 in the case patient.

in Warburg micro syndrome 4, also an autosomal recessive syndrome. Neither of these conditions is a good phenotypic fit for the patient under consideration nor would a single copy loss be expected to result in an autosomal recessive phenotype. One gene within the duplication interval is listed as a disease-associated gene with the OMIM database: SLC52A3. This gene is implicated in the conditions Brown-Vialetto-Van Laere syndrome 1 and Fazio-Londe disease. Both of these conditions are autosomal recessive and unlikely to result from a duplication (gain of copy number) of the associated gene. Thus on the basis of the CMA data only, these CNVs would best be classified as variants of unclear clinical significance. However, in this case, convention chromosome analysis was also ordered and a ring chromosome 20 was discovered (Fig. 34-10).

This case illustrates one of the most important limitations of CMA: the inability to detect balanced structural rearrangements. Whereas in this case the formation of the ring chromosome 20 did involve the loss and gain of DNA sequence and was thus detectable by CMA, the true nature of this lesion was only elucidated by chromosome analysis. The ring chromosome 20 syndrome, also referred to as R(20) syndrome, is a rare chromosomal disorder associated with refractory epilepsy. The seizures in this condition are typically partial complex in nature and can be difficult to control. It is interesting and relevant to a discussion of CNVs that, whereas most patients with R(20) syndrome are mosaics with nearly completely balanced chromosomal rearrangements, those patients that are not mosaic, as was the case in Patient AB, typically do have small deletions or duplications identified that are associated with the ring. As is the case with Patient AB, the onset of seizures is typically in childhood and the seizures are typically partial complex in nature. Staring episodes along with automatism and focal motor symptoms are also common. Thus the phenotype described for R(20) syndrome very closely

matches that of Patient AB suggesting the etiology of her seizure conditions has been elucidated.

REFERENCES

The complete list of references for this chapter is available in the e-book at www.expertconsult.com.
    See inside cover for registration details.

SELECTED REFERENCES

ACMG Board of Directors, 2013. Points to consider for informed consent for genome/exome sequencing. Genet Med. 15, 748–749.

Allyse, M., Michie, M., 2013. Not-so-incidental findings: the ACMG recommendations on the reporting of incidental findings in clinical whole genome and whole-exome sequencing. Trends Biotechnol. 31 (8), 439–441.

Cooper, G.M., Coe, B.P., Girirajan, S., et al., 2011. A copy number variation morbidity map of developmental delay. Nat. Genet. 43, 838–846.

Gersen, S.L., Keagle, M.B. (Eds.), 2013. The Principles of Clinical Cytogenetics, 3rd ed. Springer Science+Business Media, New York.

Haines, J.L., Korf, B.R., Morton, C.C., et al. (Eds.), 2012. Current Protocols in Human Genetics. John Wiley & Sons, Inc, Hoboken, NJ.

Kearney, H.M., South, S.T., Wolff, D.J., et al., 2011. Working Group of the American College of Medical Genetics. American College of Medical Genetics recommendations for the design and performance expectations for clinical genomic copy number microarrays intended for use in the postnatal setting for detection of constitutional abnormalities. Genet. Med. 13 (7), 676–679.

Manning, M., Hudgins, L., 2010. Professional Practice and Guidelines Committee. Array-based technology and recommendations for utilization in medical genetics practice for detection of chromosomal abnormalities. Genet. Med. 12 (11), 742–745.

Zarrei, M., MacDonald, J.R., Merico, D., et al., 2015. A copy number variation map of the human genome. Nat. Rev. Genet. 16 (3), 172–183.

⊗ E-ONLY FIGURES AND TABLES

The following figures and tables are available in the e-book at www.expertconsult.com. See inside cover for registration details.

35 Chromosomes and Chromosomal Abnormalities

Maria Descartes, Bruce R. Korf, and Fady M. Mikhail

An expanded version of this chapter is available on www.expertconsult.com. See inside cover for registration details.

The development and maintenance of the human body is directed by an estimated 20,000 genes, consisting of some 3 billion base pairs (bp) of DNA. These genes encode the structure of proteins and noncoding RNAs, which together are responsible for the orderly unfolding of human development, beginning with the fertilized egg (zygote), and for the maintenance of body structure and function. The entire pool of genetic information must be replicated with each cell division and a complete set of information apportioned to the two daughter cells. In addition, the full complement of genes must be transmitted from generation to generation through the germ cells.

Genes do not exist as isolated entities within the cell nucleus but rather are arranged on structural units called chromosomes. Each chromosome contains hundreds or thousands of genes arranged in a linear order. This order is reproducible from cell to cell within an individual organism, and from individual to individual in the population. The normal human chromosome complement consists of 46 chromosomes, including 22 pairs of nonsex chromosomes (autosomes) and either two X chromosomes in females or an X and a Y in males. Each of these chromosomes has a characteristic structure and includes a specific set of genes arranged in a specific order. The chromosomes are units that ensure the orderly distribution of a complete set of genetic information during cell division.

Chromosome number and structure are tightly regulated, and deviations from the norm usually are associated with clinical problems. Multiple genes are simultaneously disrupted as a consequence of chromosomal abnormalities; accordingly, the phenotypic consequences usually are complex. Because of the complexity of the nervous system and its dependence on multiple genes, neurologic problems accompany most of the chromosomal disorders.

This chapter focuses on the approach to chromosomal disorders in pediatric neurology. The various methods of chromosomal analyses are considered first, followed by a description of the various types of chromosomal abnormalities. This discussion is followed by an overview of the clinical approach to chromosomal abnormalities and then a brief clinical description of chromosomal syndromes relevant to the practice of pediatric neurology. The chapter closes with a look at the future of cytogenetic analysis.

METHODS OF CHROMOSOME ANALYSIS
Chromosome Preparation

Chromosome structure is most easily appreciated during mitosis, when the chromatin fiber is condensed and coiled into a characteristic structure. Spontaneously dividing cells are rarely available, except in tumors or chorionic villus tissue used in prenatal diagnosis. Rather, cells are grown in short-term culture. For routine analysis, peripheral blood lymphocytes most commonly are used, although skin fibroblasts also may be cultured and analyzed. Phytohemagglutinin-stimulated peripheral blood usually is grown in culture for 3 days. Blocking the mitotic spindle with a drug such as colchicine leads to accumulation of dividing cells, which then are induced to swell by treatment with hypotonic saline, fixed, and spread on to a microscope slide (Nussbaum, McInnes, and Willard, 2015a).

Chromosome Banding

Until the 1970s chromosomes were identified on the basis of their size and the position of the centromeres. This allowed chromosomes to be classified into groups labeled A to G (A: chromosomes 1-3, B: chromosomes 4-5, C: chromosomes 6-12 and X, D: chromosomes 13-15, E: chromosomes 16–18, F: chromosomes 19–20, G: chromosomes 21–22 and Y), but not unambiguously identified. The introduction of banding techniques finally allowed each chromosome to be identified and permitted the identification of chromosome regions, bands, and subbands. Most laboratories use Giemsa stain banding (G-banding), which involves treatment of the metaphase chromosomes with a protease (i.e., trypsin), followed by Giemsa staining for routine analysis. The advent of chromosome banding stimulated a second wave of discovery of structural chromosomal abnormalities during the 1970s. Chromosomes are displayed as a karyotype, which is prepared by arranging homologous chromosomes in an orderly fashion, starting from chromosome 1 and ending with chromosome 22 and including the sex chromosomes. The resolution of this technique, however, is limited to 3 to 5 million bp (Mb) of DNA, which may include dozens of genes (Nussbaum et al., 2015a).

Molecular Cytogenetics

The gap between light microscope resolution of chromosome structure and the gene was bridged by the introduction of several molecular cytogenetic techniques. Fluorescence in situ hybridization (FISH) involves hybridizing a fluorescently labeled single-stranded DNA probe to denatured chromosomal DNA on a microscope slide preparation of metaphase chromosomes and/or interphase nuclei prepared from the patient's sample. After overnight hybridization, the slide is washed and counterstained with a nucleic acid dye (e.g., DAPI, or 4′,6-diamidino-2-phenylindole), allowing the region where hybridization has occurred to be visualized using a fluorescence microscope. FISH is now widely used for clinical diagnostic purposes. There are different types of FISH probes, including locus-specific probes, centromeric probes, and whole-chromosome paint probes (Nussbaum et al., 2015a).

FISH using locus-specific probes has been extremely useful in the detection of microdeletion syndromes resulting from deletions of multiple contiguous genes (Figure 35-2). These are subtle submicroscopic deletions that are below the resolution of the routine G-banded chromosome analysis. Use of FISH usually requires that the patient either exhibits features consistent with a well-defined syndrome with known chromosomal etiology or demonstrates an abnormal karyotype. This is because single FISH probes reveal rearrangements only of the segments being interrogated and do not provide

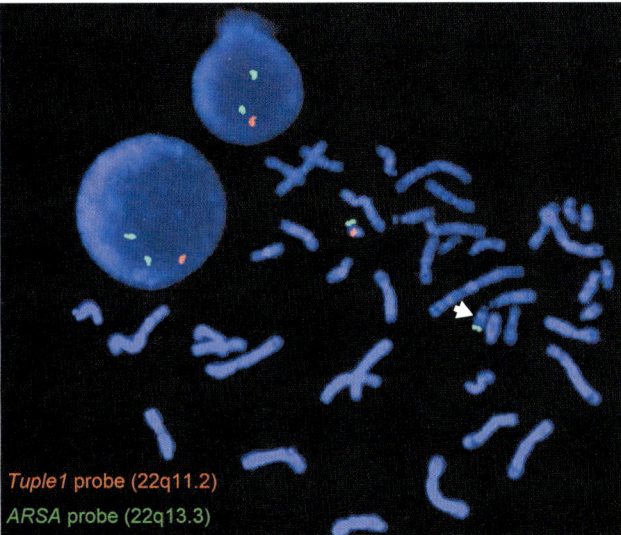

Figure 35-2. Fluorescence in situ hybridization (FISH) analysis using the DiGeorge/velocardiofacial syndrome probe. Note the deleted *Tuple1* (22q11.2) red probe on one chromosome 22 (arrow). The *ARSA* (22q13.3) green probe is included as an internal control.

information about the rest of the genome. Another limitation of FISH is the number of probes that can be applied in a simultaneous assay.

The latest addition to molecular cytogenetic techniques is chromosomal microarray (CMA) technology, including array comparative genomic hybridization (array CGH) and single-nucleotide polymorphism (SNP) arrays (Nussbaum et al., 2015a). Array CGH involves hybridizing a test sample of interest and a control reference sample, each differentially labeled with different colored fluorescent dyes, to an array slide containing thousands of DNA probes. Following hybridization and washing to remove unbound DNA, the array is scanned and analyzed using computer software to measure the relative ratios of fluorescence of the two dyes and detect gains/losses of genomic regions represented on the array (Figure 35-3). High-density SNP arrays can also be used to detect genomic copy-number gains/losses. In these experiments, the patient's DNA is fluorescently labeled with a fluorescent dye and hybridized to a high-density SNP array. Following hybridization and washing, the array is scanned and analyzed using computer software. The deviation from the expected fluorescent intensities of the two alleles of an SNP are compared with previously analyzed control samples spanning several adjacent SNPs to detect genomic copy-number gains/losses. High-resolution CMAs can detect genomic copy-number gains/losses bigger that 50 kb across the euchromatic portion of human genome. In the past few years, high-resolution whole-genome-coverage CMA platforms have been increasingly used in clinical molecular cytogenetic labs (Miller et al., 2010). These provide a relatively quick method of scanning the entire genome for gains/losses with significantly higher resolution and greater clinical abnormality yield than was previously possible. This has led to the identification of novel genomic disorders in patients with autism spectrum disorders (ASDs), developmental delay (DD), intellectual disability (ID), and/or multiple congenital anomalies (MCAs).

CHROMOSOMAL ABNORMALITIES

Most chromosomal abnormalities exert their phenotypic effects by increasing or decreasing the quantity of genetic

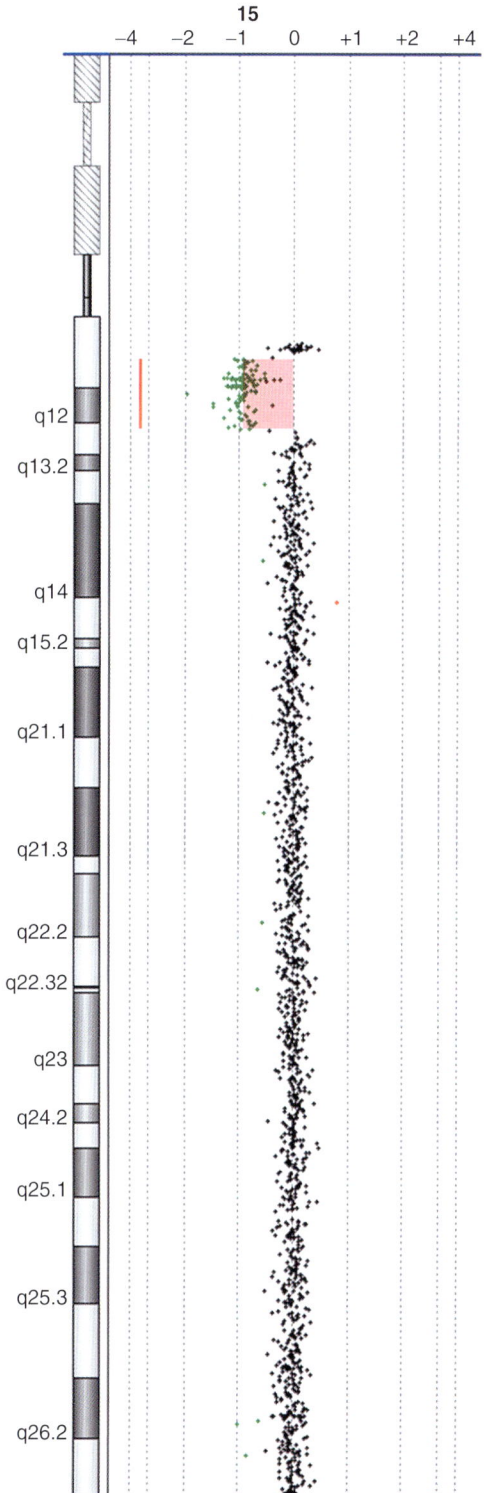

Figure 35-3. Array comparative genomic hybridization (array CGH) analysis using a whole-genome-coverage oligo-array. A chromosome 15 plot is shown with a one-copy loss (heterozygous deletion) in the Prader–Willi/Angelman region at 15q11.2q13.1.

material. Chromosomal abnormalities can be divided into numerical and structural abnormalities (Nussbaum et al., 2015a).

Numerical Abnormalities

The most straightforward of chromosomal abnormalities are alterations of chromosome number. Deviation from the normal diploid complement of 46 chromosomes is referred to as *aneuploidy*; an extra chromosome results in *trisomy*, whereas a missing chromosome results in *monosomy*. Although all the possible chromosomal trisomies have been observed in spontaneous abortions, trisomies 13, 18, and 21 are the only autosomal trisomies to be observed in a nonmosaic state in liveborn infants. All autosomal monosomies are lethal. The only viable monosomy involves the X chromosome (45,X, resulting in Turner syndrome).

Aneuploidy results from an error in cell division referred to as *nondisjunction*, in which two copies of a chromosome go to the same daughter cell during meiosis or mitosis. Nondisjunction occurs most often in the first meiotic division in the maternal germline. Mitotic nondisjunction results in the presence of an aneuploid and a normal cell line, a condition referred to as *mosaicism*. The causes of nondisjunction are unknown. The only well-documented risk factor is advanced maternal age.

The term *polyploidy* refers to presence of a complete extra set of chromosomes; *triploidy* represents three sets with 69 chromosomes, whereas *tetraploidy* represents four sets with 92 chromosomes. Rarely, a triploid fetus will be liveborn, but in general polyploidy is lethal. In a few instances, however, mosaicism for a diploid and a triploid cell line producing congenital anomalies has been compatible with long-term survival.

Structural Abnormalities

Structural chromosomal rearrangements result from chromosome breakage, with subsequent reunion in a different configuration. They can be balanced or unbalanced. In balanced rearrangements the chromosome complement is complete, with no loss or gain of genetic material. Consequently, balanced rearrangements are generally harmless, with the exception of rare cases in which one of the breakpoints disrupts an important functional gene. Carriers of balanced rearrangements are often at risk of having children with an unbalanced chromosome complement. When a chromosome rearrangement is unbalanced, the chromosome complement contains an incorrect amount of genetic material, usually with serious clinical effects.

Deletions and Duplications

A deletion involves loss of part of a chromosome and results in monosomy for that segment of the chromosome, whereas duplication represents the doubling of part of a chromosome, resulting in trisomy for that segment. The result is either decrease (in a deletion) or increase (in a duplication) in gene dosage. In general, duplications appear to be less harmful than deletions. Very large deletions usually are incompatible with survival to term. Deletions or duplications larger than approximately 5 Mb in size can be visualized under the microscope using G-banded chromosome analysis. Clinical syndromes resulting from submicroscopic deletions or duplications (i.e., microdeletions/microduplications) with a size less than 5 Mb have been identified with the help of molecular cytogenetic techniques, including FISH and CMA (Stankiewicz and Lupski, 2010; Vissers and Stankiewicz, 2012).

Translocations

Translocations involve the exchange of genetic material between chromosomes. In a balanced reciprocal translocation the exchange is equal, with no loss or gain of genetic material, although it is possible for a gene to be disrupted at one of the breakpoints. More often, the carrier of a balanced translocation is free of clinical signs or symptoms but is at risk for having offspring with unbalanced chromosomes. The risk for production of unbalanced gametes from a balanced translocation carrier depends on the chromosomes involved, the specific breakpoints of the translocation, and the sex of the carrier. Empirical data are available for some specific translocations. Risks include miscarriage and birth of a liveborn child with congenital anomalies, resulting from chromosome imbalance. The phenotype usually is a complex mixture of the results of loss or gain of at least two chromosome segments and therefore can be difficult to predict.

One specific type of translocation that is relatively common is Robertsonian translocation. This results from a fusion of two acrocentric chromosomes (chromosomes 13, 14, 15, 21, or 22) at the centromere. Carriers of a Robertsonian translocation have 45 chromosomes and are clinically unaffected. The most common clinically significant outcome is trisomy 21, in which a carrier for a Robertsonian translocation involving chromosome 21 produces a gamete with both the translocation chromosome and a normal 21, resulting in trisomy 21 after fertilization.

Inversions

Inversions occur when there are two breaks in a chromosome and the intervening material flips 180 degrees. Inversions that span the centromere are referred to as *pericentric*, whereas those that do not are called *paracentric*. Inversions generally do not result in added or lost genetic material and therefore usually are viewed as neutral changes. Disruption of a gene at one of the breakpoints, however, could change the function of that gene. Also, alteration of gene order at the borders of the inversion could affect the function of blocks of genes that are coordinately regulated (*position effect*). If a crossover occurs in the inverted segment of a pericentric inversion during meiosis, two recombinant chromosomes result, one with duplication of one end and deletion of the other end, and the other having the opposite arrangement. Such a crossover event in a paracentric inversion results in dicentric or acentric chromosomes that tend to be unstable.

Insertions

An insertion occurs when a segment of one chromosome becomes inserted into another chromosome. Because these changes require three chromosomal breakpoints, they are relatively rare. Abnormal segregation in a balanced insertion carrier can produce offspring with either duplication or deletion of the inserted segment, in addition to balanced carriers and normal offspring.

Marker and Ring Chromosomes

A *marker chromosome* is a rearranged chromosome whose genetic origin is unknown based on its G-banded chromosome morphology. Usually, these chromosomes are present in addition to the normal chromosome complement and are thus called supernumerary marker chromosomes (SMCs). The birth prevalence of SMCs is in the range of 2 to 7 per 10,000, and 30% to 50% originate from chromosome 15.

Ring chromosomes are formed when a chromosome undergoes two breaks and the broken ends reunite in a ring structure. Rings encounter difficulties in mitosis and are unstable, resulting in some cells that lose the ring and are therefore monosomic for the chromosome and others that have multiple copies of the ring.

Isochromosomes

An *isochromosome* is a chromosome in which one arm is missing and the other duplicated in a mirror-image fashion. The most probable mechanism for the formation of an isochromosome is the misdivision through the centromere in meiosis II, wherein the centromere divides transversely rather than longitudinally. The most commonly encountered isochromosome is that which consists of two long arms of the X chromosome. This accounts for approximately 15% of all cases of Turner syndrome.

Cytogenetic Nomenclature

By convention, each chromosome arm is divided into regions, and each region is subdivided into bands and subbands, numbered from the centromere outward. Cytogeneticists describe findings of chromosomal analysis using a standardized system of nomenclature (International System for Human Cytogenetic Nomenclature) (Nussbaum et al., 2015a). The normal male karyotype is designated 46,XY, and the normal female karyotype is 46,XX. Any chromosomal abnormality is described after the sex chromosome constitution.

Incidence of Chromosomal Abnormalities

Estimates of the incidence of chromosomal abnormalities vary with the mode of ascertainment and the technology used for chromosome analysis. In general, the incidence falls rapidly from conception to birth. The highest rates have been observed among products of conception from first-trimester spontaneous abortions. Approximately 50% of these spontaneous miscarriages have a chromosomal abnormality. By birth, the rate of chromosomal abnormalities declines to approximately 0.5% to 1% in liveborn infants, although the rate is much higher (5%–10%) in stillborn infants.

CLINICAL INDICATIONS FOR CYTOGENETIC ANALYSIS

Chromosome analysis has been incorporated in the routine battery of tests available to the clinician (Nussbaum et al., 2015a). Some of the more common clinical indications for chromosome analysis include:

1. Problems of early growth and development, including failure to thrive, DD, ID, dysmorphic facies, multiple congenital malformations, short stature, and ambiguous genitalia
2. Fertility problems
3. Family history of known or suspected chromosome abnormality
4. Unexplained stillbirth or neonatal death
5. Prenatal genetic diagnosis
6. Malignant tumor diagnosis and management

SPECIFIC CYTOGENETIC SYNDROMES
Polyploidy

Tetraploidy is an infrequent chromosomal abnormality, but triploidy occurs fairly often. Most triploid embryos miscarry in the first trimester. In approximately 20% of first-trimester spontaneous abortions, the conceptus is found to have a triploid karyotype. Liveborn infants with triploidy exhibit multiple congenital anomalies and rarely survive the newborn period. Those that do usually are mosaics for a diploid and a triploid cell line.

The triploid phenotype is distinct and easily recognized. Polyhydramnios or preeclampsia may complicate the pregnancy. The placenta may be large, and hydatidiform changes may be seen. Birth weight usually is low. Syndactyly involving the third and fourth digits is characteristic. Craniofacial features include low-set and malformed ears, hypertelorism, and micrognathia. Cardiac, renal, and central nervous system malformations are common. Long-term survivors often are mosaics and may have less obvious phenotypic features. Body asymmetry and pigmentary dysplasia may be clues to chromosomal mosaicism in general, including, in some cases, triploidy.

Aneuploidy

Only a minority of aneuploid embryos survive to term; the rest miscarry, usually in the first trimester. Only the most common trisomy and monosomy syndromes compatible with live birth are considered in the following discussion (Nussbaum et al., 2015b).

Trisomy 13 (Patau Syndrome)

Trisomy 13 occurs in approximately 1 in 7000 live births. A majority of affected persons have 47 chromosomes, with an extra copy of chromosome 13. Approximately 5% to 10% have trisomy because of translocation between 13 and another acrocentric chromosome, usually chromosome 14 (Robertsonian translocation). Mosaicism occurs in a small proportion of cases and may ameliorate the phenotype. Duplication of part of chromosome 13 resulting from unbalanced translocation can result in abnormal phenotypic features, although not necessarily similar to those seen in full trisomy 13. Advanced maternal age has been shown to be a factor in the occurrence of this aneuploidy syndrome.

Trisomy 13 is associated with congenital anomalies involving most major organ systems. Holoprosencephaly is the hallmark central nervous system anomaly, occurring in about 80% of cases. Other ocular anomalies include microphthalmia, iris colobomata, cataracts, and retinal dysplasia. Premaxillary agenesis and cleft lip or palate also may be present. Ulcer-like defects in scalp skin (cutis aplasia) occur commonly. Limb anomalies include postaxial polydactyly in two-thirds of patients and rocker-bottom foot. Congenital heart defects, especially ventricular septal defect (VSD), are common, as are renal anomalies, including cystic dysplasia.

Trisomy 18 (Edwards' Syndrome)

Trisomy 18 affects approximately 1 in 4000 live births. It is virtually always associated with a 47-chromosome karyotype, although a small proportion of affected newborns have a mosaic karyotype. Segregation of a parental balanced translocation may result in trisomy for part of the short or long arm of chromosome 18. Advanced maternal age has been shown to be a factor in the occurrence of this aneuploidy syndrome.

Infants with trisomy 18 have low birth weight and microcephaly. Other common features include a prominent occiput, low-set "simple" ears, and a small mouth. Hands usually are tightly clenched in a characteristic configuration, with the fourth and fifth fingers overlapping the first and second.

Trisomy 21 (Down Syndrome)

Trisomy 21 is the most common and widely recognized of the autosomal trisomy syndromes. It occurs in approximately 1 in

800 live births, with a striking increase in frequency with advanced maternal age. Full trisomy 21 occurs in about 95% of cases. Translocation, usually between chromosome 21 and another acrocentric chromosome, most often chromosome 14, is identified in approximately 4%. A parent who carries such a translocation may be at risk for recurrence of Down syndrome. The remaining 1% of affected persons have a mosaic karyotype.

Down syndrome consists of a set of characteristic physical features and developmental impairment. Craniofacial features include upslanted palpebral fissures, epicanthal folds, flat facial profile, and small, low-set ears with narrow ear canals. White speckles (Brushfield spots) may be seen on the iris. A common finding is redundant folds of nuchal skin, which is one of the markers used for prenatal diagnosis by ultrasound examination. Fingers are short, with incurving of the fifth finger (clinodactyly) and, often, a single transverse palmar crease. A wide space between the first and second toes is a frequent finding. The hallmark neurologic feature of Down syndrome is hypotonia. No gross central nervous system malformation is consistently seen, although lack of normal growth of the brain is typical. Impaired neurologic development is a universal feature, but the degree of impairment varies widely. Children with Down syndrome benefit from early intervention, physical therapy, and being reared in a family setting. Linguistic ability may be impaired out of proportion to cognitive impairment. Seizures, including infantile spasms, may be seen with increased frequency. An increased frequency of dementia, associated with pathologic changes of Alzheimer's disease, has been described in patients with Down syndrome. Congenital anomalies commonly associated with Down syndrome include heart and gastrointestinal defects.

Turner Syndrome

Turner syndrome is associated with a 45,X karyotype, with a single X chromosome. Mosaicism is not uncommon, however, with a separate cell line containing either a normal 46,XX or XY karyotype, or 46 chromosomes including a structurally rearranged X or Y. Turner syndrome occurs in about 1 in 4000 female live births worldwide but it is much more common in stillbirths and miscarriages. Unlike other aneuploidy syndromes, the frequency of Turner syndrome does not increase with advancing maternal age.

Patients with Turner syndrome typically have a female phenotype, although those with a cell line including a Y chromosome may have some degree of virilization, often with ambiguous genitalia. At birth, infants may manifest pedal edema or diffuse edema. In older children and adults with Turner syndrome, short stature and webbing of the neck are commonly seen. The thorax is broad, with increased distance between the nipples. Congenital anomalies include abnormalities of the lymphatic system; cardiac defects, especially coarctation of the aorta and bicuspid aortic valve; and renal anomalies.

Although ID is rare, delays in both gross and fine motor development are common in females with Turner syndrome. Some patients display cognitive problems, but difficulties with visuospatial perception are most common. Hearing impairment occurs frequently, and children should be monitored for deficits or progression of impairment.

Klinefelter Syndrome

Klinefelter syndrome occurs in about 1 in 1000 males and is associated with a 47,XXY karyotype. The incidence increases as a function of maternal age in half of the cases. Rare patients may have multiple X chromosomes (e.g., 48,XXXY or 49,XXXXY). Usually the presence of multiple X chromosomes in such persons is associated with more severe cognitive impairment.

The diagnosis of Klinefelter syndrome usually is not suspected at birth. Affected males tend to be tall, with long limbs. They display hypogonadism, and virilization may be incomplete at puberty; gynecomastia develops in some patients. Azoospermia and infertility are characteristic. Breast cancer is 20 times more common in Klinefelter syndrome than in the normal male population. As in Turner syndrome, ID is not a typical feature of Klinefelter syndrome. Learning disabilities, language delay, and behavior problems are reported.

Other Sex Chromosome Aneuploidies

Two other major sex chromosome aneuploidies are 47,XXX and 47,XYY. The XXX aneuploidy is associated with a female phenotype and tall stature; usually other major physical stigmata are absent. XYY is associated with a male phenotype and tall stature but no other physical features. Learning disabilities and neuromotor impairment occur commonly in 47,XXX females. The behavioral phenotype of XYY syndrome has been a source of some controversy because of reports associating the karyotype with criminal behavior. The frequency of learning disabilities and behavioral problems is increased among affected males, although widely ranging cognitive outcomes have been reported.

Structural Abnormalities

Structural abnormalities of chromosomes cause phenotypic effects resulting from loss and/or gain of genetic material. In some cases, these occur sporadically as a result of de novo chromosome rearrangements, whereas in others, they may be inherited as a consequence of segregation of a familial balanced chromosomal rearrangement. Some deletion or duplication syndromes are fairly well characterized in terms of phenotypic effects and may be recognized clinically.

For many years, genomic disorders resulting from microdeletions and microduplications that are clinically recognizable by their typical constellation of clinical features were tested for by FISH using DNA probes specific to these genomic regions. The advances in CMA technologies over the past decade have allowed their widespread use not only in a research setting but also as a clinically diagnostic modality in a wide variety of human diseases. CMA analysis has been very useful in the study of copy-number variants (CNVs), which can be broadly classified as either benign polymorphic CNVs or pathogenic disease-causing CNVs. Between these two ends of the spectrum, many CNVs have uncertain clinical significance, and some of these could potentially be risk factors for human disease.

Clinically relevant CNVs can be either recurrent, with a common size and breakpoint clustering in the flanking segmental duplications, or nonrecurrent, with different sizes and variable breakpoints for each CNV (Stankiewicz and Lupski , 2010). These nonrecurrent CNVs typically share a common genomic region of overlap that encompasses the gene(s) associated with the observed phenotype. These nonrecurrent rearrangements occur at a relatively lower frequency at the individual locus level, but collectively they are as common as recurrent CNVs. Clinically relevant CNVs can encompass multiple contiguous genes, including dosage sensitive genes, with each contributing to the phenotype independently. Others encompass a single gene or just few genes.

Two types of microdeletions and microduplications have been distinguished: the syndromic forms in which the phenotypic features are relatively consistent, and those in which the same CNV can be associated with a diverse set of diagnoses (Girirajan and Eichler, 2010; Cooper et al., 2011; Coe, Girirajan, and Eichler, 2012a, 2012b). The syndromic forms of CNVs were originally described as relatively large microdeletions or microduplications that are highly penetrant, almost always de novo in origin, and usually identified in individuals with ID or MCAs. These are clinically recognizable syndromes that were described well before their genetic causes were known. On the contrary, the more recently described nonsyndromic recurrent CNVs have been reported to have incomplete penetrance and variable expressivity. These have been associated with, but not limited to, DD, ID, autism, seizures, schizophrenia, cardiac and renal anomalies, and other congenital anomalies. Recently it was observed that more than one CNV (the "two-hit" model) can explain the phenotypic variability associated with the nonsyndromic recurrent CNVs (Girirajan and Eichler, 2010; Coe et al., 2012a). Therefore it was proposed that one hit (first CNV) is sufficient to reach a threshold just enough to cause some form of neuropsychiatric disease, whereas a second hit (e.g. second CNV) pushes that individual toward a more severe phenotype with DD and ID. It is worth mentioning that these two hits involve different regions/genes in the human genome as opposed to the two-hit model reported in cancer, which involves both alleles of a tumor-suppressor gene. Variable-expressivity CNVs are much more likely to be inherited from less severely affected parents, which suggests that they are by themselves insufficient to determine the disease outcome. Although the two-hit model was initially applied to large CNVs, it has been proposed that the second hit could also be a smaller CNV or a SNP involving a related gene or a risk allele inherited from a parent.

Approximately 70 microdeletion/microduplication syndromes have been reported to date, as shown in the DECIPHER database (https://decipher.sanger.ac.uk/disorders #syndromes/overview). In the following section, some of the syndromic microdeletions and microduplications that are clinically relevant to the practice of pediatric neurology are discussed.

22q11.2 Deletion Syndrome

The 22q11.2 deletion syndrome includes the phenotypes previously called DiGeorge syndrome (DGS), velocardiofacial syndrome (VCFS, Shprintzen's syndrome), conotruncal anomaly face syndrome, many cases of autosomal-dominant Opitz G/BBB syndrome, and Cayler's cardiofacial syndrome (asymmetric crying facies) (Nussbaum et al., 2015b). The condition is clinically heterogeneous. Congenital heart defects are present in most affected individuals (74%), particularly conotruncal malformation. Additional findings include palatal abnormalities and velopharyngeal incompetence (VPI), learning disabilities, immune deficiencies, hypocalcemia, and characteristic facies. Also reported are hearing loss, seizures without hypocalcemia, speech delays, and behavioral difficulties. The 22q11.2 deletion affects an estimated 1:2000 to 1:4000 live births. Most cases are de novo, but inherited deletions have been reported in 6% to 28% of patients with the syndrome. The inheritance is autosomal dominant.

Prader–Willi and Angelman Syndromes

The recognition of the phenomenon of genomic imprinting has led to the discovery of a new class of genetic disorders associated with aberrations of imprinted genes (Nussbaum et al., 2015b; Kalish, Jiang, and Bartolomei, 2014). The prototype disorders are Prader–Willi and Angelman's syndromes (Nussbaum et al., 2015b). The features of these syndromes are described in Table 35-3. Prader–Willi syndrome (PWS) affects 1:5000 to 1:10,000 individuals. Approximately 70% to 75%

of the individuals with PWS have a deletion of the paternally contributed 15q11.2q13.1 region, whereas in Angelman's syndrome (AS), 70% of affected individuals have a deletion of the maternally contributed 15q11.2q13.1 region. Approximately 1:40,000 children are affected with AS. Most patients with PWS who do not have the 15q11.2q13.1 deletions have uniparental disomy for chromosome 15, with two maternal copies and no paternal copies. Either mechanism—deletion or uniparental disomy—leads to deficiency of a gene or genes on chromosome 15 that are expressed in the paternal but not the maternal homolog. Deletion of a group of small nucleolar RNA (snoRNA) genes, known as the SNORD116 cluster, is thought to play a major role in causing the signs and symptoms of PWS. Paternal uniparental disomy accounts for a low percentage of cases of AS. Mutations in the *UBE3A* gene (a ubiquitin ligase gene involved in early brain development), located at 15q11.2, have been found in some patients with AS. This gene is imprinted in the brain and is the gene responsible for the AS phenotype. A small proportion of patients with PWS or AS may have a small deletion or other mutation that leads to aberrant imprinting of the region.

William–Beuren Syndrome

William–Beuren syndrome (WBS) is a microdeletion syndrome of chromosome 7 at band q11.23 and occurs in 1:10,000 live births. Cardiovascular disease is present in 80% of affected individuals, mostly in the form of supravalvular aortic stenosis (SVAS), peripheral pulmonary stenosis, elastin arteriopathy, and hypertension. The 7q11.23 microdeletion encompasses the elastin gene (*ELN*). Characteristic facial features include periorbital fullness, long philtrum, wide mouth, full lips, full cheeks, and small, wide-spaced teeth. Affected individuals have mild to moderate ID, specific cognitive profile/learning disabilities, and unique or distinctive behavior/personality characteristics. Growth and endocrine abnormalities (hypercalcemia, hypothyroidism, hypercalciuria) and feeding difficulties in infancy are also common.

1p36 Deletion Syndrome

The 1p36 deletion syndrome results from a variable-sized deletion in the terminal end of the short arm of chromosome 1. It is considered to be the most common subtelomeric microdeletion syndrome, with an estimated incidence of 1 in 5000 to 1 in 10,000. It accounts for 0.5% to 1.2% of idiopathic ID. Clinical findings include a characteristic craniofacial appearance: microbrachycephaly, large and late-closing anterior fontanel, straight eyebrows, deep-set eyes, epicanthic folds, broad nasal bridge, midface hypoplasia, abnormally formed low-set ears, and limb and skeletal defects. DD and ID with absent/poor expressive language are constant features. Affected individuals often face serious physical disabilities that include congenital heart defects (70%), cardiomyopathy (25%), brain abnormalities (88%), seizures (44%), and electroencephalogram (EEG) abnormalities (100%). Ocular malformations or vision problems and hearing loss are observed in approximately 50% of affected individuals.

Wolf–Hirschhorn Syndrome

Wolf–Hirschhorn syndrome (WHS) results from a variable-sized deletion in the terminal end of the short arm of chromosome 4. It is characterized by distinctive facial appearance, growth delay, psychomotor retardation, and seizures, and is confirmed by detection of a deletion of the Wolf–Hirschhorn critical region (WHCR) (chromosome 4p16.3). The syndrome has clinical and cytogenetic variability. Characteristic facial

TABLE 35-3 Comparison of Features of Prader–Willi and Angelman's Syndromes

	Prader–Willi Syndrome*	Angelman's Syndrome†
Diagnostic criteria	**Major clinical criteria** Neonatal hypotonia Feeding problems in infancy Rapid weight gain between 1 and 6 years of age Characteristic facies Hypogonadism Developmental delay Hyperphagia **Minor criteria** Decreased fetal movement Characteristic behaviors Sleep disturbances Short stature Small hands Narrow hands Esotropia/myopia Thick, viscous saliva Speech articulation defects Skin picking **Supportive findings** High pain threshold Decreased vomiting	**Consistent features (100%)** Developmental delay Speech impairment Movement disorder (ataxia of gait, tremulous movement of limbs) Behavioral features: frequent laughter or smiling, hand flapping **Frequent features (80%)** Acquired microcephaly Seizures (usually in patients younger than 3 years) Abnormal EEG (high-amplitude 2- to 3-Hz spike-wave discharge) **Associated features (20%–80%)** Flat occiput, occipital groove Protruding tongue Prognathism Wide mouth and widely spaced teeth Drooling, chewing, mouthing movements Strabismus Hypopigmentation Brisk lower limb deep tendon reflexes Sleep disturbance
Cytogenetics	70%–75% paternal 15q11.2q13.1 deletion	70% maternal 15q11.2q13.1 deletion
Uniparental disomy	20%–25% maternal disomy	2% paternal disomy
Imprinting defect	1%–3%	2%–5%
Gene mutation	Unknown	5%–10% UBE3A gene mutation

EEG, electroencephalogram.
*Data from Holm VA, Cassidy SB, Butler MG, et al. Pediatrics 1993;91(8424017):398–402.
†Data from Williams CA, Angelman H, Clayton-Smith J, et al. Am J Med Genet 1995;56(2):237–8.
(Mutation analysis data from Buiting K, Gross S, Lich C, et al. Am J Hum Genet 2003;72(12545427):571–7.; Jiang Y, Lev-Lehman E, Bressler J, et al. Am J Hum Genet 1999;65(10364509):1–6.)

features include the "Greek warrior helmet" appearance of the nose (the broad bridge of the nose continuing to the forehead), high forehead with prominent glabella, ocular hypertelorism, and microcephaly. ID ranges from mild to severe. Other birth defects have been reported in individuals with WHS. One-third of the patients have structural central nervous system defects, and seizures also can occur. In 75% of patients with WHS, the deletion is de novo; in about 13% of patients, the deletion results from the unbalanced segregation of a parental balanced translocation. It is now recognized that WHS and Pitt–Rogers–Danks syndrome (PRDS) represent the clinical spectrum associated with a single syndrome.

Cri du Chat Syndrome

Cri du chat syndrome is a genetic syndrome resulting from a variable-sized deletion in the terminal end of the short arm of chromosome 5. The incidence ranges from 1:15,000 to 1:50,000. A high-pitched, cat-like cry is among the main clinical features in the newborn period; hence the name of the syndrome. Other frequently described features are microcephaly, broad nasal bridge, epicanthic folds, micrognathia, impaired growth, and severe psychomotor and ID. The syndrome has significant clinical and cytogenetic variability. Clinical analysis of affected individuals and detailed molecular cytogenetic analysis suggest the existence of two critical regions, one on 5p15.2 for facial dysmorphism, microcephaly, and ID, and another on 5p15.3 for the typical cry. In affected individuals, 80% of cases are the result of a de novo deletion, and 10% are the result of the unbalanced segregation of a parental balanced translocation.

Chromosome 9q Subtelomeric Deletion

The chromosome 9q subtelomeric deletion represents one of the most common subtelomeric deletions (6%). The syndrome can be caused either by a 9q34.3 microdeletion or by mutations in the EHMT1 gene, which is involved in histone methylation. Affected individuals invariably have severe hypotonia, with speech and gross motor delay. Facial features include micro-/brachycephaly, hypertelorism, synophrys, arched eyebrows, midface hypoplasia, short nose with upturned nares, protruding tongue, everted lower lip, and downturned corners of the mouth. Congenital heart defects have been reported in approximately 50% of affected individuals. Epilepsy and behavior and sleep disturbances have also been reported in some (10%–20%).

Jacobsen Syndrome

Jacobsen syndrome is a contiguous-gene deletion syndrome caused by deletion of the distal portion of the long arm of chromosome 11 (11q23.3qter). Typical features include DD, ID, short stature, congenital heart defects, thrombocytopenia, and characteristic dysmorphic facial features. Some of the facial dysmorphism described includes skull deformities, hypertelorism, epicanthic folds, ptosis, broad nasal bridge, and small ears. Malformation of heart, kidney, gastrointestinal tract, central nervous system, and skeleton is common. The deletion is de novo in 85% of cases, and in the remaining patients it results from the unbalanced segregation of a parental balanced chromosome rearrangement.

Charcot–Marie–Tooth Neuropathy Type 1A and Hereditary Neuropathy With Liability to Pressure Palsies

Charcot–Marie–Tooth neuropathy type 1A (CMT1A) represents 70% to 80% of all CMT1 and results from an approximately 1.5-Mb duplication at 17p12, which encompasses the *PMP22* gene (peripheral myelin protein 22). Reciprocal deletion of the same region results in the milder phenotype of hereditary neuropathy with liability to pressure palsies (HNPP). The duplication is inherited in around two-thirds of individuals and is de novo in the remaining third.

Smith–Magenis Syndrome and Potocki–Lupski Syndrome

Approximately 90% of individuals with Smith–Magenis syndrome (SMS) have a deletion on chromosome 17 at band p11.2 that encompasses the *RAI1* gene. The remaining 5% to 10% of cases carry a mutation in the *RAI1* gene. Physical features include short stature, obesity, craniofacial dysmorphism, and small hands and feet. Behavior disturbances, especially sleep problems and self-injurious behavior, are frequently reported. All affected individuals have mild to severe learning disabilities. The phenotypic features may be subtle in infancy and early childhood.

The reciprocal duplication of this 17p11.2 region has been reported (Potocki–Lupski syndrome). The most frequent features of this syndrome are hypotonia in infancy, DD, language and cognitive impairment, autistic features, poor feeding and failure to thrive in infancy, oral-pharyngeal dysphagia, obstructive and central sleep apnea, structural cardiovascular abnormalities, EEG abnormalities, and hypermetropia. Most have short stature and mild to normal facies. Variability in the phenotype is observed. It is expected that persons with large duplications that encompass the more distal CMT1A region will have a more severe phenotype, including peripheral neuropathy.

Miller–Dieker Syndrome

Miller–Dieker syndrome represents a microdeletion syndrome spanning the *PAFAH1B1* gene (also known as *LIS1*) at 17p13.3, which results in severe lissencephaly with characteristic facial changes, other more variable malformations, and severe neurologic and developmental abnormalities. The facial features consist of high and prominent forehead, bitemporal hollowing, short nose with upturned nares, protuberant upper lip with downturned vermillion border, and small jaw. The reciprocal duplication results in DD, hypotonia, and facial dysmorphism. In contrast to patients with the deletion, those with the duplication have neither gross brain malformations nor lissencephaly.

Neurofibromatosis Type 1

Approximately 5% of patients with neurofibromatosis type 1 (NF1) have deletions of the entire *NF1* gene and contiguous genes at 17q11.2, resulting in the NF1 microdeletion syndrome. NF1 with large deletions is more likely to have dysmorphic features, cardiac anomalies, connective tissue dysplasia, and ID. Patients with reciprocal microduplications have been reported.

X-Linked Ichthyosis Resulting From Steroid Sulphatase Enzyme Deficiency

Males with X-linked ichthyosis resulting from steroid sulphatase enzyme deficiency have generalized scaling that usually starts shortly after birth. In 90% of cases, it is caused by a microdeletion encompassing the *STS* gene (Xp22.31). In 5% of cases, the deletion is extensive enough to involve adjacent genes, resulting in learning disabilities, autism, and epilepsy in some of the affected boys.

Loss of Function of the *MECP2* Gene/Duplication of the *MECP2* Region (Xq28)

Loss-of-function mutations involving the *MECP2* gene at Xq28 result in Rett syndrome, a severe neurodevelopmental disorder that almost always occurs in females. Males with non-Rett mutations in *MECP2* demonstrate a wide variety of phenotypes, including X-linked ID with spasticity and other variable features. Males with Rett mutations in *MECP2* have neonatal severe encephalopathy that is usually lethal. Duplications at Xq28 that span the *MECP2* gene in males are associated with severe X-linked ID and progressive spasticity. These duplications usually also span the *L1CAM* gene.

Finally, some of the nonsyndromic microdeletions and microduplications that present with neurodevelopmental problems are as follows:

Distal 1q21.1 microdeletion and microduplication
2p15p16.1 microdeletion
Terminal deletions of the long arm of chromosome 2 (2q37 microdeletion)
3q29 microdeletion
7q11.23 microduplication
Maternal duplication of the 15q11.2q13.1 region
15q13.3 microdeletion
15q24 microdeletion
16p11.2 microdeletion and microduplication
16p11.2p12.2 microdeletion
16p13.11 microdeletion and microduplication
17q21.31 microdeletion
Distal 22q11.2 microdeletions
22q13 microdeletions (Phelan–McDermid syndrome)

THE FUTURE OF CLINICAL CYTOGENETICS

Clinical cytogenetics began with the cytologic analysis of chromosomes in the 1950s but has steadily moved toward an increasingly molecular approach. This began with the advent of FISH and has accelerated since the introduction of CMA. CMA is moving us toward a whole-genome approach, with no need to know in advance where to look. This is raising questions about whether CMA should be used before a comprehensive dysmorphology evaluation because many of the deletions or duplications detected are not associated with well-delineated syndromes. A caution in use of this approach, however, is that some gene-dosage changes are not known to be associated with an abnormal phenotype and are likely to be benign variants of no clinical significance. Therefore correct interpretation of dosage changes still requires a high level of sophistication and care in counseling the patient/family. The resolution of genomic analysis will continue to increase. Clinical whole-exome or whole-genome DNA sequencing is currently being used to uncover clinically relevant gene mutations with a much higher power than previously possible. Both CMA and whole-exome or whole-genome sequencing will undoubtedly reveal an increasing number of genomic changes that underlie neurologic disorders, leading to an increase in the power and precision of genetic diagnosis.

REFERENCES
The complete list of references for this chapter is available in the e-book at www.expertconsult.com.
   See inside cover for registration details.

SELECTED REFERENCES

Coe, B.P., Girirajan, S., Eichler, E.E., 2012a. A genetic model for neurodevelopmental disease. Curr. Opin. Neurobiol. 22 (5), 829–836.

Coe, B.P., Girirajan, S., Eichler, E.E., 2012b. The genetic variability and commonality of neurodevelopmental disease. Am. J. Med. Genet. C Semin. Med. Genet. 160C (2), 118–129.

Cooper, G.M., Coe, B.P., Girirajan, S., et al., 2011. A copy number variation morbidity map of developmental delay. Nat. Genet. 43 (9), 838–846.

Girirajan, S., Eichler, E.E., 2010. Phenotypic variability and genetic susceptibility to genomic disorders. Hum. Mol. Genet. 19 (R2), R176–R187.

Kalish, J.M., Jiang, C., Bartolomei, M.S., 2014. Epigenetics and imprinting in human disease. Int. J. Dev. Biol. 58 (2–4), 291–298.

Miller, D.T., Adam, M.P., Aradhya, S., et al., 2010. Consensus statement: chromosomal microarray is a first-tier clinical diagnostic test for individuals with developmental disabilities or congenital anomalies. Am. J. Hum. Genet. 86 (5), 749–764.

Nussbaum, R., McInnes, R., Willard, H. (Eds.), 2015a. Thompson & Thompson Genetics in Medicine, eighth ed. Elsevier. (Chapter 5: Principles of Clinical Cytogenetics and Genome Analysis).

Nussbaum, R., McInnes, R., Willard, H. (Eds.), 2015b. Thompson & Thompson Genetics in Medicine, eighth ed. Elsevier. (Chapter 6: The Chromosomal and Genomic Basis of Disease: Disorders of the Autosomes and Sex Chromosomes).

Stankiewicz, P., Lupski, J.R., 2010. Structural variation in the human genome and its role in disease. Annu. Rev. Med. 61, 437–455.

Vissers, L.E., Stankiewicz, P., 2012. Microdeletion and microduplication syndromes. Methods Mol. Biol. 838, 29–75.

E-BOOK FIGURES AND TABLES

The following figures and tables are available in the e-book at www.expertconsult.com. See inside cover for registration details.

36 Approach to the Patient with a Metabolic Disorder

Linda De Meirleir and Lance H. Rodan

An expanded version of this chapter is available on www.expertconsult.com. See inside cover for registration details.

INTRODUCTION

Inborn errors of metabolism (IEMs) are genetic disorders that disrupt biochemical processes in the body by altering enzyme activity, cellular transport, or mitochondrial bioenergetics. Over 600 IEMs have been described to date, and this number is increasing with the more widespread use of whole exome sequencing. Although IEMs are individually rare, their collective incidence is approximately 1 in 1000. The clinical manifestations of IEMS are protean because almost every organ and tissue can be affected. The nervous system is often affected with selective vulnerability given its high bioenergetic demand and its reliance on a delicate balance of complex biochemical processes for normal functioning. It is particularly important for the pediatric neurologist to be familiar with the diagnosis of IEMs because most are associated with neurologic symptoms, and many have effective, disease-specific treatments.

INHERITANCE

The inheritance pattern of most IEMs is autosomal recessive because residual enzyme activity is usually sufficient to preclude the development of disease; however, X-linked and autosomal dominant inheritance are possible (Table 36-1). X-linked recessive disorders can present variably in carrier females based on the pattern of X-inactivation. X-linked dominant disorders are often lethal in males. Disorders of mitochondrial DNA (mtDNA) are maternally inherited and show phenotypic variability based on the percentage and tissue distribution of mutant mtDNA (termed "heteroplasmy"). A detailed three-generation pedigree should be obtained in every patient presenting for evaluation for an IEM. Particular attention should be paid to any history of sudden infant death syndrome (SIDS), siblings with neurologic disorders, including epilepsy and "cerebral palsy," and parental consanguinity.

LABORATORY EVALUATION

Most inborn errors of metabolism can be diagnosed through specialized biochemical testing. This includes measurement of metabolites in body fluids and specific enzyme assays. Molecular testing is clinically available for most disorders, either as single gene tests or next generation targeted gene panels based on disease category. A molecular diagnosis may be useful for predicting prognosis and treatment response (e.g., cofactor responsiveness) and can be used for prenatal testing to reduce recurrence risk. Newborn screening protocols have been instituted in a number of countries that evaluate for some of the treatable IEMS, potentially including organic acidemias, fatty acid oxidation and carnitine disorders, some amino acidopathies, galactosemia, and biotinidase deficiency. The specific disorders included and methodologies vary considerably from country to country and even between states in the United States. Readers are encouraged to contact their local newborn screening laboratory to determine which disorders are included in their screening program. It should be emphasized that this testing represents screening and not diagnostic testing, and both false positive and false negative results are possible. Normal newborn screening does not preclude the possibility of an inborn error of metabolism. Likewise, abnormal newborn screening must be followed by confirmatory diagnostic evaluation by a clinician with expertise in biochemical genetics.

CLASSIFICATION

When evaluating a patient for an inborn error of metabolism, it is necessary to use a systematic and organized approach to maximize the potential for diagnosis. Different approaches to the diagnosis of IEMs have been described. One approach groups IEMs into categories based on the affected metabolic pathway (e.g., urea cycle) or organelle (e.g., lysosome) because most disorders in each grouping share some clinical and biochemical features (see Table 36-2). Another approach, particularly suited for the pediatric neurologist, is a symptoms-based approach focused on neurologic phenotype. This chapter provides a symptoms-based approach that incorporates age of onset and predominant neurologic signs.

Before approaching these aforementioned symptom categories, it is useful for the reader to adopt a broad framework for classifying IEMs based on pathophysiology and general symptomatology. This broad classification divides IEMs into *small molecule disorders, large molecule disorders, disorders of cerebral energy metabolism,* and *miscellaneous IEMs.* This is a modified version of the original classification proposed by Saudebray and associates that is adapted for the pediatric neurologist (Saudubray et al., 2012). This classification will be referred to throughout this chapter.

Small molecule disorders are IEMs affecting intermediary metabolism, including the metabolism of amino acids, organic acids, fatty acids, ketones, and ammonia. These disorders result in intoxication from accumulation of substrate and are often associated with basic and readily detectable biochemical abnormalities such as acidosis, hyperammonemia, or hypoglycemia. These disorders generally present acutely with encephalopathy and may also be accompanied by ataxia, headache, nausea, and respiratory abnormalities. The disease course of these IEMs is often episodic with periods of deterioration provoked by illness, fasting, or other bioenergetics stressors. Most of these disorders are amenable to specific treatments based on dietary modification and/or cofactor supplementation.

Large molecule disorders are IEMs that affect synthesis or catabolism of complex molecules and include disorders of the lysosome and peroxisome, disorders of glycosylation, and disorders of complex lipid metabolism. Large molecule disorders typically follow a chronic course that may be static or gradually progressive. Many of these disorders are associated with congenital malformations or dysmorphic physical features. A number of lysosomal disorders can be treated effectively with enzyme replacement therapy.

Disorders of cerebral energy metabolism include defects impairing mitochondrial bioenergetics, pyruvate metabolism, creatine metabolism, coenzyme Q10 biosynthesis, and the transport of glucose into the CNS. In general, disorders of

TABLE 36-1 Iems With X-Linked and Autosomal Dominant Inheritance

Inheritance	Classification of IEM
X-LINKED RECESSIVE DISORDERS	
Ornithine transcarbamylase deficiency	Urea cycle disorder
Phosphoribosylphosphate synthetase deficiency	Disorder of purine disorder
Lesch Nyhan syndrome	Disorder of purine disorder
Lowe syndrome	Disorder of phospholipid metabolism
Fabry disease	Lysosomal disorder
Hunter syndrome	Lysosomal disorder
X-linked adrenoleukodystrophy	Peroxisomal disorder
Menkes syndrome	Disorder of copper transport
Monoamine oxidase A deficiency	Disorder of neurotransmitter metabolism
X-linked creatine transporter deficiency	Disorder of energy metabolism
X-LINKED DOMINANT DISORDERS	
X-linked chondrodysplasia punctata	Disorder of cholesterol biosynthesis
CHILD syndrome	Disorder of cholesterol biosynthesis
Beta propeller-associated neurodegeneration (X-linked dominant)	Neurodegeneration with brain iron accumulation
AUTOSOMAL DOMINANT DISORDERS	
Cystinuria	Disorder of amino acid metabolism
Glucose transporter 1 deficiency	Disorder of energy metabolism
SLC6A1-related myoclonic astatic epilepsy	Disorder of neurotransmitter metabolism
Autosomal dominant GTP cyclohydrolase deficiency	Disorder of neurotransmitter metabolism
POLG1-related progressive external ophthalmoplegia	Disorder of energy metabolism
HEM skeletal dysplasia	Disorder of cholesterol biosynthesis
Porphobilinogen deaminase deficiency	Disorder of heme biosynthesis

energy metabolism follow a chronically progressive course, often punctuated by episodic exacerbations. Developmental delay and seizures are a common manifestation, and many disorders in this group can also be associated with movement disorders. Several of these disorders have effective treatments: pyruvate dehydrogenase deficiency and glucose transporter 1 deficiency are treated with the ketogenic diet; creatine deficiency syndromes may respond to creatine supplementation; and disorders of coenzyme Q10 biosynthesis are treated with CoQ10 replacement.

Finally, there are a number of IEMs that are not easily classified into these categories, including disorders in the metabolism of *carbohydrates, purines and pyrimidines, vitamins, minerals/heavy metals,* and *biogenic amine neurotransmitters* (Table 36-3).

PART 1: CLINICAL PRESENTATION OF IEMS IN THE NEONATE OR INFANT LESS THAN 2 YEARS OF AGE

As a general rule, the age of presentation and severity of an IEM is proportional to the degree of enzyme deficiency. Although this section describes IEMs that typically present in infancy, the reader should be cognizant that milder forms of many of these disorders may present for the first time in older children and adults.

Acute Encephalopathy

Many inborn errors of metabolism present in early life with acute or subacute encephalopathy, particularly small molecule disorders and disorders of cerebral energy metabolism (Chapters 37 and 42). Many of these disorders present after a well period in the context of metabolic stressors such as prolonged fasting, illness, and some medications. Most small molecule disorders do not present in fetal life because the placenta is capable of removing many toxic metabolites.

IEMS presenting with acute encephalopathy may be accompanied by abnormalities in tone, seizures, ataxia, emesis, and respiratory abnormalities. Basic biochemical abnormalities are common and may suggest a specific disease category. Urine ketones are always abnormal in the neonate due to increased physiologic ketone utilization and suggest an IEM until proven otherwise. *Ketoacidosis with hyperammonemia* suggests an organic acidemia, of which propionic and methylmalonic acidemias are prototypical. Inappropriate ketosis is also a feature of maple syrup urine disease and disorders of ketone degradation (e.g., ketothiolase deficiency).

Hyperammonemia without metabolic acidosis suggests dysfunction of the urea cycle. There may be accompanying respiratory alkalosis (Chapter 38).

Hypoglycemia with insufficient ketosis is the hallmark of the fatty acid oxidation and carnitine disorders, disorders of ketone synthesis (e.g., HMG-CoA lyase deficiency), and hyperinsulinism. *Recurrent ketotic hypoglycemia accompanied by hepatomegaly* suggests a glycogen storage disorder or disorder of gluconeogenesis. Disorders of gluconeogenesis are also associated with fasting-induced blood lactate elevation (Chapter 39).

Persistent elevations of blood lactate in the neonate or infant that is not critically ill, septic, or hypoperfused should raise consideration for a mitochondrial disorder or disorder of pyruvate metabolism (Chapter 42). A normal blood lactate to pyruvate ratio (less than 20 to 25), a marker of cytoplasmic redox status, is seen in pyruvate dehydrogenase deficiency and some forms of pyruvate carboxylase deficiency. Pyruvate carboxylase deficiency may also be associated with hyperammonemia and hypoglycemia.

A number of IEMs can present with *acute liver failure in the neonate or infant* associated with hepatic encephalopathy, including galactosemia, tyrosinemia type 1, hereditary fructose intolerance, and mitochondrial disorders. Concurrent proximal renal tubulopathy may be present in any of these disorders and is a useful diagnostic clue. In addition, a *Reye-like syndrome,* including fulminant liver failure, metabolic acidosis, and cerebral edema, has been reported in fatty acid oxidation and carnitine disorders, organic acidemias, urea cycle disorders, ketogenesis disorders, gluconeogenesis defects, hereditary fructose intolerance, and mitochondrial disorders. This may be provoked by certain medications, including valproic acid and ASA.

In the absence of basic biochemical abnormalities, neuroimaging findings may suggest a specific IEM in the neonate or infant presenting with acute or subacute encephalopathy. *Symmetric signal change in the basal ganglia,* often associated with diffusion restriction, can be seen in organic acidemias, mitochondrial disorders, and biotin-thiamine responsive basal ganglia disease. These findings can mimic a hypoxic-ischemic injury. *Acute white matter injury* with diffusion restriction can be seen in maple syrup urine disease, glycine encephalopathy (nonketotic hyperglycinemia), and sulfite oxidase deficiency/molybdenum cofactor deficiency, although the specific patterns are different. *Stroke or stroke-like lesions* that cross classic vascular territories can be seen in mitochondrial disorders, congenital disorders of glycosylation, and Menkes syndrome (Van der Knaap and Valk, 2005).

TABLE 36-2 Classification of IEMs by Pathway and Organelle

Category	Symptoms	Biochemical Investigations
Urea cycle disorders	Hyperammonemic encephalopathy	Ammonia, plasma amino acids, urine organic acids (orotic acid)
Fatty acid oxidation & carnitine disorders	Hypoketotic hypoglycemia, episodic rhabdomyolysis, cardiomyopathy, hepatopathy, Reye-like syndrome	Plasma acylcarnitines, free/total carnitine
Organic acidemias	Ketoacidosis, hyperammonemia, metabolic stroke, developmental delay	Urine organic acids, plasma acylcarnitines
Aminoacidopathies	Epilepsy, developmental delay, acute CNS events (toxic, ischemic)	Plasma amino acids, additional metabolic studies based on suspected diagnosis
Peroxisomal disorders	Retinopathy, sensorineural hearing loss, brain malformation, dysmorphisms, leukoencephalopathy	Plasma VLCFAs, phytanic acid, pristanic acid, pipecolic acid, RBC plasmalogens, bile acid intermediates in blood and urine
Lysosomal disorders	Hurler phenotype (coarse facial features, dysostosis multiplex, hepatosplenomegaly, corneal opacitiy), leukoencephalopathy, progressive myoclonus epilepsy, cherry red spot, organomegaly, gaze palsy	Enzymology, urine MPS screen, urine oligosaccharides
Disorders of cholesterol biosynthesis	Multiple congenital anomalies, static developmental delay	Measurement of plasma cholesterol precursors
Congenital disorders of glycosylation	Congenital anomalies, hypotonia, abnormal fat pads, abnormal coagulation profile	Plasma transferrin analysis, urine oligosaccharides and free glycans
Biogenic amine disorders	Movement disorder, diurnal fluctuation, dysautonomia, oculogyric crisis	CSF neurotransmitters, CSF/urine pterins, plasma phenylalanine
Mitochondrial disorders	Highly pleiotropic presentations, including CNS, PNS, multiple organs, failure to thrive, retinopathy, hearing loss, ophthalmoparesis, stroke-like events, epilepsy	Elevated lactate in blood or CSF, elevated plasma alanine

MR spectroscopy can occasionally provide additional information beyond structural imaging. Maple syrup urine disease may be associated with a branch-chain ketoacid peak at 0.9 ppm. Mitochondrial disorders, disorders of pyruvate metabolism, and organic acidemias may be associated with lactate elevations in regions of structurally normal brain. The clinician must keep in mind that if regions of brain affected by stroke, infection, or injury are sampled, lactate may be secondarily elevated. Hyperammonemia may be associated with an elevated glutamine peak.

A few small molecule disorders are associated with abnormal urine odor, including the maple syrup odor of urine and ear wax in maple syrup urine disease, the musty odor of urine and sweat in phenylketonuria, and the sweaty feet odor of urine in isovaleric acidemia and glutaric acidemia type 2.

Specific diagnosis requires evaluation of: urine organic acids and plasma acylcarnitines for organic acid disorders; plasma acylcarnitine profile and free/total carnitine for fatty acid oxidation and carnitine disorders; and plasma amino acids for amino acidopathies and urea cycle disorders. A number of urea cycle disorders are also associated with elevations of urine orotic acid. Homocysteinurias require the measurement of total serum homocysteine for biochemical diagnosis, which is not included in standard plasma amino acid analyses. Biochemical abnormalities in some of these disorders may be normal when the child is well, warranting reevaluation at times of illness.

Epilepsy

Epilepsy in the neonate or infant should raise suspicion for an inborn error of metabolism in a number of circumstances, including medically refractory epilepsy, myo-clonic seizures/myoclonus, concurrent nonneurologic manifestations (see Table 36-4), microcephaly, and epileptic encephalopathies, including early myoclonic encephalopathy (Chapter 76).

Seizures beginning in the first weeks of life that do not respond to standard anticonvulsant treatment should always prompt early evaluation for treatable metabolic epilepsies, including vitamin and cofactor responsive epilepsies and small molecule disorders (see Table 36-5). Pyridoxine and pyridoxal-5-phosphate responsive epilepsies may be associated with irritability, grimacing, and abnormal eye movements, a useful clinical clue at the bedside. The neonate with medically refractory epilepsy should be trialed on pyridoxine, pyridoxal-5-phosphate, folinic acid, and biotin pending metabolic test results.

Myoclonus with profound hypotonia, respiratory failure, and persistent hiccups beginning hours to days after birth suggests glycine encephalopathy. This diagnosis is further supported by burst suppression on EEG, and neuroimaging demonstrating agenesis of corpus callosum and diffusion restriction of the actively myelinating structures. MR spectroscopy may demonstrate a glycine peak at 3.55 ppm. CSF and often plasma glycine are elevated with a CSF to plasma ratio greater than 0.08 in the classic form.

Microcephaly is a useful clinical clue when evaluating the neonate or infant with severe epilepsy for an IEM. Congenital microcephaly is a feature of amino acid synthesis disorders, including serine, asparagine, and glutamine synthetase deficiencies. Postnatal microcephaly is common in severe methylene-tetrahydrofolate reductase (MTHFR) deficiency, glucose transporter 1 deficiency, sulfite oxidase deficiency, molybdenum cofactor deficiency, and Menkes syndrome.

In some circumstances, the electroclinical epilepsy syndrome can suggest specific inborn errors of metabolism.

As previously mentioned, early myoclonic encephalopathy should prompt evaluation for glycine encephalopathy but has also been described in sulfite oxidase deficiency/molybdenum cofactor deficiency, organic acidemias, pyridoxine/pyridoxal-5-phosphate dependent epilepsies, Zellweger syndrome, and adenylosuccinate lyase deficiency. Atypical absence epilepsy has been described in glucose transporter 1 deficiency and serine synthesis disorders. Myoclonic-astatic epilepsy has been reported with glucose transporter 1 deficiency and defects in the presynaptic GABA transporter SLC6A1. Malignant migratory focal epilepsy of infancy has been reported in association with defects in the phospholipase C-beta 1 enzyme.

Specific EEG patterns have been described in some IEMs, including a theta frequency waveform resembling mu waves in the central head regions termed "comb waves" in the neonate with maple syrup urine disease and rhythmic high amplitude delta waves with superimposed spikes and polyspikes (RHADS) in the posterior head region in the mitochondrial disorder Alpers syndrome. Progressive attenuation of the EEG has been reported in the infantile form of neuronal ceroid lipofuscinosis, and a photoparoxysmal response at slow flash frequencies is characteristic of the late infantile form.

Any relation of seizures to meals should be determined; fasting induced (normoglycemic) seizures can be seen in glucose transporter 1 deficiency. Postprandial exacerbation of seizures can be seen in disorders of pyruvate metabolism and hyperammonemic disorders.

An atypical response to specific anticonvulsants should also be noted. Phenobarbital may exacerbate seizures in glucose transporter 1 deficiency, and valproic acid can worsen seizures in glycine encephalopathy and urea cycle disorders. Valproic acid can also induce liver failure in POLG1 associated mitochondrial disorders.

Abnormal Development Associated With Congenital Anomalies and/or Dysmorphic Physical Features

The presence of congenital anomalies or dysmorphic physical features in the neonate or infant with abnormal development should alert the clinician to a possible underlying genetic disorder. In addition to chromosomal disorders and monogenic nonmetabolic genetic syndromes, the pediatric neurologist should maintain a high index of suspicion for inborn errors of metabolism—particularly large molecule disorders—because a number of these disorders have specific treatments (Chapter 41).

Static developmental delay associated with congenital microcephaly, craniofacial dysmorphism (ptosis, short and upturned nose, cleft palate), 2 to 3 toe syndactyly, genitourinary and cardiac malformations, and midline brain anomalies, including dysgenesis of corpus callosum and holoprosencephaly are features of Smith-Lemli-Opitz Syndrome (SLOS), a disorder of cholesterol biogenesis. Serum cholesterol levels are often low, but specific measurement of the cholesterol precursor 7-dehydrocholesterol is necessary for biochemical diagnosis. Additional disorders of cholesterol biosynthesis are also associated with developmental delay and may have associated ichthyosis and skeletal abnormalities (Jira, 2013).

Developmental delay and regression associated with craniofacial dysmorphism (high forehead, epicanthal folds, hypoplastic supraorbital ridges), large anterior fontanelle, redundant neck skin, cystic kidneys and liver, proximal limb shortening, and brain malformations, including polymicrogyria, are features of the peroxisomal biogenesis disorders, of which Zellweger syndrome is prototypical. Affected children typically have significant central hypotonia that can mimic a neuromuscular disorder. Epilepsy is also common. There may be accompanying retinopathy and sensorineural hearing loss. In addition to structural brain anomalies, there is progressive white matter injury in the CNS. The biochemical evaluation for a peroxisomal biogenesis disorder includes measurement of plasma very long chain fatty acids for elevated fractions of C26:C22 and C24:C22 fatty acids. In addition, there may be decreased levels of RBC plasmalogens, elevated plasma pipecolic acid, abnormal bile acid intermediates in urine and blood, and elevated plasma phytanic and pristanic acid (NB: phytanic acid is derived entirely from the diet and is not a reliable marker in the neonate) (Chapter 43) (Klouwer et al., 2015).

Moderate to severe developmental delay associated with nonspecific facial dysmorphism, abnormal fat pads, and cerebellar hypoplasia is characteristic of the congenital disorders of glycosylation, particularly the most common type 1a. Affected children are hypotonic, which is typically central in etiology although there may be superimposed neuropathy. There are often associated clotting abnormalities. This group of disorders can be screened for by evaluating the pattern of glycosylated transferrin and measuring urinary oligosaccharides and free glycans (Chapter 40) (Freeze et al., 2012).

Multiple congenital anomalies, including anorectal malformations and shortening of distal phalanges, can be seen in disorders of glycophosphatidylinositol (GPI) anchor biosynthesis, often in association with abnormal alkaline phosphatase levels (high or low) and epilepsy. Seizures may be responsive to supplementation with pyridoxine. This group of disorders can be screened for by evaluating GPI-linked epitopes on granulocytes using flow cystometry.

Progressive developmental regression associated with coarsening of the facial features, skeletal anomalies, corneal opacity or cataracts, hernias, and hepatosplenomegaly are features of many lysosomal storage disorders, including the mucopolysaccharidoses, oligosaccharidoses, and mucolipidoses (Chapter 41). Neuroimaging may demonstrate prominent perivascular spaces with surrounding white matter gliosis; over time, this pattern may become more confluent resembling a leukodystrophy. A skeletal survey may show characteristic features of dysostosis multiplex, including j-shaped sella turcica, beaking of vertebral bodies, and abnormally shaped acetabulum and phalanges. Screening for a lysosomal storage disorder begins with measurement of urine mucopolysacharides to evaluate for mucopolysaccharidoses and urine oligosaccharides to evaluate for oligosaccharidoses. Salla disease/infantile sialic acid storage disease is evaluated by measuring urinary free sialic acid. If a specific disorder is suspected, enzyme activity can be measured blood or fibroblasts (Pastores and Maegawa, 2013).

Developmental regression beginning at several months of age associated with lax-appearing skin, fair complexion, sparse and wiry hair, and progressive microcephaly should suggest Menkes syndrome. There may be associated vascular tortuosity and bladder diverticulae. Epilepsy and autonomic dysfunction are common. There may be subdural collections mimicking nonaccidental injury. Serum copper and ceruloplasmin are low, as is urinary excretion of copper (NB: serum copper and ceruloplasmin are often low in the first month of life in healthy children). There is an elevated HVA to VMA ratio in urine due to secondary dysfunction of the copper dependent enzyme dopamine beta hydroxylase (Chapter 46) (Bandmann et al., 2015).

Less often, small molecule disorders and disorders of energy metabolism are associated with malformations and dysmorphic features. Untreated maternal phenylketonuria is associated with congenital microcephaly and heart defects in the neonate. The congenital form of glutaric acidemia type II is associated with polymicrogyria, renal cysts, anterior abdominal wall defects, and rocker bottom feet. Multicystic dysplastic kidney and neuronal migration abnormalities can also be seen in the congenital form of carnitine palmitoyltransferase 2 (CPT2) deficiency, a disorder of carnitine metabolism. As previously mentioned, glycine encephalopathy is associated with dysgenesis of the corpus callosum. Glutamine synthetase deficiency is associated with complex brain malformations, enteropathy, and necrolytic skin lesions. The most severe presentation of serine synthesis disorders, termed "Neu Laxova syndrome," is associated with multiple congenital anomalies and early lethality. Pyruvate dehydrogenase deficiency is associated with dysgenesis of corpus callosum and large periventricular cysts; individuals may also have facial features reminiscent of fetal alcohol syndrome. Finally, mitochondrial disorders may be associated with brain malformations.

Abnormal Development in the Absence of Congenital Anomalies or Dysmorphic Physical Features

IEMs account for up to 1% to 5% of children with static developmental delay, making IEMs an uncommon cause relative to chromosome disorders and fragile X syndrome. It is even more uncommon for IEMs to cause static developmental delay without additional neurologic or extraneurologic signs or symptoms. Untreated phenylketonuria is an example of an IEM that can rarely present with essentially isolated developmental delay.

In contrast, IEMs are a relatively common cause of developmental regression in childhood and must always be evaluated for in these circumstances. IEMs presenting with progressive developmental regression include disorders of energy metabolism, the chronic presentation of small molecule disorders, some large molecule disorders in the lysosomal and peroxisomal categories, and additional disorders in the miscellaneous category.

Associated Neurologic Symptoms

Epilepsy is a common accompanying feature in IEMs and was covered in the previous section (Chapter 76).

The motor pathways are also frequently affected in IEMs and manifest with abnormalities of tone, ataxia, and/or extrapyramidal symptoms. Spasticity is a relatively nonspecific sign but can be prominent in metabolic leukodystrophies such as Krabbe disease, Canavan disease, and metachromatic leukodystrophy. Spastic diplegia mimicking cerebral palsy is also a notable feature of arginase deficiency and hyperammonemia, hyperornithemia, and homocitrulluria (HHH) syndrome.

Prominent extrapyramidal symptoms, including dystonia, chorea, and parkinsonism, may be seen in the primary disorders of biogenic amine (neurotransmitter) metabolism and transport. Additional useful clinical clues include diurnal fluctuation, oculogyric crises, and dysautonomia. Extrapyramidal symptoms may also be seen in the purine and pyrimidine disorders, mitochondrial disorders, disorders of creatine metabolism, cerebral folate deficiency, glucose transporter 1 deficiency, and in organic acidemias after metabolic basal ganglia injury (Chapter 93).

An exaggerated startle may be seen in GM2 gangliosidosis, hyperekplexia disorders, sulfite oxidase deficiency, and asparagine synthetase deficiency.

The motor findings in IEMs are almost always bilaterally symmetric because metabolic CNS insults affect specific tracts and pathways symmetrically. An exception to this rule is mitochondrial disorders, which may present with asymmetric stroke-like involvement (e.g., MELAS syndrome). In addition, disorders of neurotransmitter metabolism may present with focal dystonia.

Specific behavioral abnormalities may provide a useful clue to the underlying diagnosis. Autistic behavior can be seen in disorders of creatine metabolism, untreated PKU, cerebral folate deficiency, succinic semialdehyde dehydrogenase deficiency, and purine/pyrimidine disorders, including adenylosuccinate lyase deficiency. Autistic features associated with aggressive and hyperactive behavior are seen in Sanfilippo syndrome (MPSIII), a mucopolysacharidosis that is associated with more subtle extraneurologic features. Children with Sanfilippo syndrome may also demonstrate a lack of fear (Kluver-Bucy syndrome). Prominent self-mutilation is a feature of Lesch-Nyhan syndrome, a disorder of purine metabolism.

Associated Nonneurologic Symptoms (Table 36-4)

Nonspecific failure to thrive is a feature of many small molecule disorders and disorders of energy metabolism.

A formal ophthalmology evaluation is an important component in the diagnostic evaluation of the infant with neuroregression. Many of the neuronopathic lysosomal disorders have telltale ophthalmologic stigmata including cherry red macular spot, corneal opacities, and supranuclear gaze palsy. Mitochondrial disorders may be associated with retinopathy, ptosis, ophthalmoparesis, and, rarely, cataracts. Peroxisomal disorders may also be associated with retinopathy and cataracts.

The skin and hair may be affected in IEMs presenting with developmental regression. Menkes disease was mentioned in the previous section. Sparse and fragile hair, the result of trichorrhexis nodosa, is seen in the urea cycle disorder arginosuccinate synthetase deficiency. Skin rash and alopecia are features of biotinidase deficiency and holocarboxylase synthetase deficiency. Eczema is a feature of untreated phenylketonuria.

Developmental regression with hepatosplenomegaly in a nondysmorphic infant should raise the possibility of a neuronopathic lysosomal storage disorder, particularly Niemann-Pick and Gaucher disease.

Neuroimaging

When evaluating an infant for a neurodegenerative metabolic disorder, neuroimaging is often useful to narrow the differential diagnosis. If possible, the clinician should attempt to distinguish between primary white matter disorders (leukodystrophies) and gray matter disorders.

Progressive demyelination is seen in Krabbe leukodystrophy, metachromatic leukodystrophy, multiple sulfatase deficiency, peroxisomal disorders, cerebral organic acidurias (Canavan disease, L2 hydroxyglutaric aciduria), and mitochondrial disorders, particularly involving complex 1 of the respiratory chain. Hypomyelination, or permanently deficient myelination, is a feature of Salla disease/infantile sialic acid storage disease, fucosidosis, and cerebral folate deficiency (Chapter 99) (Schiffmann and van der Knaap, 2009).

Early cerebral cortical atrophy may be seen in GM1 and GM2 gangliosidosis, neuronal ceroid lipofuscinoses, mitochondrial disorders, and disorders of amino acid biosynthesis, including serine and asparagine synthetase deficiencies. The clinician should be aware that early cerebral atrophy may be associated with *secondary dysmyelination*. Significant cerebellar atrophy in an infant can be seen in mitochondrial disorders, disorders of coenzyme Q10 biosynthesis, neuronal ceroid lipofuscinoses, congenital disorders of glycosylation, adenylosuccinate lyase deficiency, and infantile neuroaxonal dystrophy; associated T2 hyperintensity of the cerebellar cortex consistent with gliosis is a feature of infantile neuroaxonal dystrophy, congenital disorders of glycosylation, and mitochondrial disorders.

Abnormalities of the deep gray nuclei may be a useful clue to the underlying diagnosis. Many lysosomal disorders are associated with T2 hypointensity of the thalamus (dark thalamus sign). Symmetric basal ganglia T2 hyperintensity may suggest a mitochondrial disorder, disorder of pyruvate metabolism, biotin-thiamine responsive basal ganglia disease, or an organic acidemia.

MR spectroscopy demonstrates an increased NAA peak in Canavan disease. A decreased or absent creatine peak suggests one of the creatine deficiency syndromes, including X-linked creatine transporter deficiency, guanidinoacetate methyltransferase deficiency, and arginine-glycine amidinotransferase deficiency.

Neuromuscular Weakness

In the course of evaluating the neonate or infant with peripheral hypotonia and weakness, a number of inborn errors of metabolism should be considered (Chapter 150). As always, appropriate localization within the neuraxis is a prerequisite step.

The infantile form of Pompe disease presents in the first months of life with progressive skeletal myopathy with hyper-CKemia, hypertrophic cardiomyopathy, and feeding and respiratory difficulties. Macroglossia is a useful clinical clue. ECG demonstrates very short PR intervals with giant QRS complexes. Biochemical diagnosis is made through enzyme assay of alpha glucosidase. Treatment is available with enzyme replacement therapy.

Barth syndrome, an X-linked recessive disorder of phospholipid metabolism, is associated with infantile-onset skeletal myopathy, dilated cardiomyopathy that may be associated with endocardial fibroelastosis or left ventricular noncompaction, failure to thrive, and neutropenia. Urine levels of 3-methylglutaconic acid are elevated.

Skeletal myopathy is a common presentation of mitochondrial disorders. Involvement of the CNS, cardiomyopathy, hepatic or renal dysfunction, retinopathy, or sensorineural hearing loss are common accompanying features. Laboratory studies may demonstrate elevations of serum lactate and alanine. Muscle biopsy rarely shows ragged red fibers in infants. Electron microscopy may demonstrate dysmorphic mitochondria. Studies of mitochondrial complex enzyme activity, typically normalized to levels of citrate synthase activity, may be decreased. These abnormalities are not specific, and it is important for the clinician to be cognizant of the possibility that these abnormalities represent secondary mitochondrial dysfunction due to a different underlying disease process.

Skeletal myopathy with elevated CPK may be seen in disorders of long chain fatty acid oxidation and carnitine metabolism; however, these abnormalities are often intermittent and provoked by fasting or intercurrent illness. In the neonate or infant, skeletal muscle involvement is often overshadowed by recurrent hypoglycemia, cardiomyopathy, and hepatopathy. Fatty acid oxidation and carnitine disorders causing rhabdomyolysis will be further described in a subsequent section.

Neuropathy developing in the first 2 years of life has been described in mitochondrial disorders, congenital disorders of glycosylation, neonatal adrenoleukodystrophy, disorders of cobalamin metabolism, infantile neuroaxonal dystrophy, Arts syndrome, serine deficiency syndromes, and riboflavin

transporter disorders. A demyelinating neuropathy often accompanies Krabbe and metachromatic leukodystrophies. Lysosomal storage disorders may present with compressive mononeuropathies. Abnormal neuromuscular transmission has been described in DPAGT1 (dolichyl-phosphate N-acetylglucosamine phosphotransferase) deficiency, a congenital disorder of glycosylation.

CLINICAL PRESENTATION OF IEMS IN CHILDHOOD (GREATER THAN 2 YEARS OF AGE) AND ADOLESCENCE

Ataxia

Whereas cerebellar pathway dysfunction can occur in infancy, frank ataxia is more noticeable in the older child who is ambulatory and relies on a high degree of dexterity for activities of daily living. IEMs presenting with ataxia as a predominant feature can be divided into three groups: disorders associated with insidiously progressive ataxia; disorders associated with episodic ataxia; and ataxic disorders associated with myoclonus and epilepsy (progressive myoclonus epilepsies).

IEMs manifesting in childhood or adolescence with chronically progressive ataxia as the presenting feature include ataxia with vitamin E deficiency, abetalipoproteinemia, Refsum disease, cerebrotendinous xanthomatosis, the subacute and chronic forms of GM2 gangliosidosis, Niemann-Pick disease type C, mitochondrial disorders, PHARC (polyneuropathy, hearing loss, ataxia, retinitis pigmentosa, and cataract) syndrome, and disorders of coenzyme Q10 biosynthesis (Lyon et al., 2006). Many of these disorders are also associated with peripheral neuropathy and ophthalmologic signs.

Episodic ataxia has been reported in a number of small molecule disorders and disorders of energy metabolism, including maple syrup urine disease (intermittent form), urea cycle disorders, Hartnup disease, pyruvate dehydrogenase deficiency, pyruvate carboxylase deficiency, biotinidase deficiency, and mitochondrial disorders. Episodes are often provoked by bioenergetic stressors such as infectious illness or by increased protein intake in MSUD and urea cycle disorders. These disorders must be distinguished from episodic ataxia resulting from genetic channelopathies.

The combination of progressive ataxia, myoclonus, epilepsy, and cognitive regression are features of the progressive myoclonus epilepsies. This category includes a number of lysosomal disorders such as the neuronal ceroid lipofuscinoses (NCLs), sialidosis, and a subtype of Gaucher disease type 3; mitochondrial disorders, including myoclonic epilepsy with ragged red fibers (MERRF) syndrome; and Lafora disease. Many of these disorders are associated with vision disturbance, either from retinal disease (NCLs, sialidosis, mitochondrial disease) or occipital seizures in Lafora disease. Progressive myoclonus epilepsy can also be caused by a number of nonmetabolic genetic defects.

Dystonia

Dystonia beginning in childhood or adolescence as a presenting symptom is a feature of a number of IEMs (Chapter 93). Glutaric acidemia type 1 can present with acute metabolic striatal stroke in the first 5 years of life in a previously developmentally normal child, resulting in severe generalized dystonia. Acute basal ganglia injury associated with extrapyramidal signs can also be seen in mitochondrial Leigh syndrome and biotin-thiamine responsive basal ganglia disease. The latter disorder has an excellent response to the combination of thiamine and high dose biotin.

Exercise-induced paroxysmal dystonia is a feature of glucose transporter 1 deficiency. Intermittent dystonia can also be seen in pyruvate dehydrogenase deficiency. Focal dystonia with diurnal variation is a feature of Segawa disease due to dysfunction in one of two enzymes involved in dopamine biosynthesis, GTP cyclohydrolase, or tyrosine hydroxylase. This dystonia has an excellent and sustained response to low dose L-dopa.

Gradually progressive generalized dystonia is a prominent feature of late onset GM1 gangliosidosis. MR brain imaging in this disorder may demonstrate T2 hypointensity of globi pallidi. There may be subtle extraneurologic features, including skeletal anomalies and short stature.

There are a growing number of IEMs associated with progressive brain mineralization and extrapyramidal signs. The classic brain mineralizing disorder is Wilson disease, in which copper accumulates in the liver and brain. Pediatric Wilson disease is usually associated with hepatic disease, but pure neurologic presentations are possible. Dystonia may be accompanied by prominent bulbar dysfunction, parkinsonism, ataxia, psychiatric symptoms, and cognitive regression. Ophthalmologic evaluation demonstrates pathognomonic Kayser-Fleischer rings, copper deposits in Descemet's membrane of the cornea, in 90% of patients with CNS disease. Neuroimaging is characteristic and demonstrates T1 hyperintensity of globus pallidus, T2 hyperintensity thalami and striatum, white matter hyperintensities, and a characteristic pattern of involvement in the midbrain and pons. Serum ceruloplasmin and total copper are decreased, and 24-hour urine copper is increased.

Another category of neurodegenerative disorders with brain mineralization is the disorders of brain iron accumulation (NBIA). The prototypical disorder in this category is pantothenate kinase associated neurodegeneration that in its classic form presents in the first decade with chronically progressive generalized dystonia, pyramidal signs, and retinal degeneration. Neuroimaging demonstrates mineralization of globus pallidus, most evident on susceptibility weighted sequences, with a central region of T2 hyperintensity creating the appearance of an "eye of the tiger." Additional disorders in this category presenting in childhood include: mitochondrial membrane protein-associated neurodegeneration (MPAN); PLAG2-related neurodegeneration (PLAN); Beta-propeller protein-associated neurodegeneration (BPAN); fatty acid hydroxylase-associated neurodegeneration; Kufor-Rakeb syndrome; Woodhouse-Sakati syndrome; and COASY protein-associated neurodegeneration. Each of these disorders is linically distinct and has a specific neuroimaging pattern. Diagnosis is made through molecular studies; multigene panels are available.

In recent years, the first genetic disorder of brain manganese deposition was described due to mutations in the SLC30A10 gene. This disorder presents in childhood with progressive dystonia associated with polycythemia and liver disease. Neuroimaging demonstrates T1 hyperintensity of the globus pallidus. Blood manganese is markedly elevated. This disorder may be amenable to treatment with chelation therapy and iron supplementation.

Recurrent Rhabdomyolysis

Recurrent rhabdomyolysis should prompt evaluation for a metabolic myopathy or channelopathy (Chapters 49 and 150). IEMs associated with rhabdomyolysis include disorders of long chain fatty acid oxidation and carnitine metabolism (e.g., CPT2 deficiency), muscle glycogenoses, lipin-1 deficiency, mitochondrial disorders, and myoadenylate deaminase deficiency. Some of these disorders can be associated with a progressive chronic myopathy between episodes of rhabdomyolysis.

The precipitants for rhabdomyolysis are important in establishing the differential diagnosis. Muscle breakdown in the long chain fatty acid oxidation and carnitine disorders may be precipitated by prolonged moderate intensity exercise, illness, or prolonged fasting (typically longer than 12 hours). Symptoms provoked by exercise typically begin *hours after the exercise.* Associated symptoms include liver dysfunction, cardiomyopathy, cardiac arrhythmia, and hypoketotic hypoglycemia. Carnitine palmitoyltransferase 2 deficiency is the most common of these lipid disorders to present in childhood or adolescence with isolated exercise-induced rhabdomyolysis (Berardo et al., 2010).

Muscle glycogenoses presenting with recurrent rhabdomyolysis include myophosphorylase deficiency (McArdle disease), phosphofructokinase deficiency, adolase A deficiency, lactate dehydrogenase deficiency, phosphoglycerate kinase deficiency, and phosphoglycerate mutase deficiency. Muscle fatigue, weakness, and rhabdomyolysis in these disorders are typically provoked by anaerobic activity, in particular isometric muscle contraction. Symptoms often begin *during* exercise with muscle stiffness and painful cramps. In myophosphorylase deficiency, muscle symptoms may improve after 10 minutes of aerobic activity ("second wind" phenomenon) due to increased utilization of blood-borne glucose and free fatty acids. Phosphofructokinase deficiency, phosphoglycerate kinase deficiency, and aldolase A deficiency are associated with hemolytic anemia, which may be well compensated. Myophosphorylase deficiency is the most common of the muscle glycogenoses and typically presents in the first decade of life.

Lipin-1 deficiency, a disorder of phospholipid metabolism, presents in childhood with severe episodes of rhabdomyolysis provoked by febrile infectious illness.

Myoadenylate deaminase deficiency is a disorder of the purine-nucleotide cycle, an important pathway in muscle for replenishing the citric acid cycle during exercise. Some individuals present with recurrent exercise induced rhabdomyolysis, whereas others remain asymptomatic, which has raised the question of whether this enzyme deficiency alone is sufficient to cause disease.

Vascular Stroke

Classic homocystinuria due to cystathionine beta-synthase deficiency can present in childhood or adolescence with arterial ischemic or venous infarction. Associated features include developmental delay, marfanoid habitus, high myopia, lens dislocation, and osteopenia. Complexion is often pale, and there may be malar flushing or livedo reticularis. Diagnosis is confirmed by the finding of elevated serum total homocysteine.

Fabry disease is an X-linked, semidominant lysosomal disorder with multisystem involvement. Males may present with arterial ischemic stroke in adolescence or early adulthood from large vessel vasculopathy; the posterior circulation is preferentially affected. Over time, affected individuals develop progressive white matter disease from small vessel angiopathy. A classic neuroimaging finding is a T1-weighted bright pulvinar of the thalamus. Associated features in childhood include gastrointestinal symptoms, painful acroparasthesia, hypohidrosis, and skin lesions termed "angiokeratomas." Cardiomyopathy and renal disease may develop in adulthood. Diagnosis in males is accomplished by measuring alpha-galactosidase enzyme activity in nucleated cells; females require molecular testing because enzyme results overlap with the normal range.

Cognitive and Motor Regression

Gradually progressive loss of cognitive faculties as the predominant symptom in the older child or adolescent can be seen in a number of IEMs, including X-linked adrenoleukodystrophy, neuronopathic lysosomal disorders, mitochondrial disorders, and disorders of brain mineralization. All of these disorders are ultimately associated with additional neurologic findings, potentially including ataxia, spasticity, dystonia, and epilepsy with disease progression (Chapter 52).

The childhood cerebral form of X-linked adrenoleukodystrophy typically presents between 4 to 8 years of age with cognitive decline, behavior change, and auditory verbal agnosia. With disease progression, children develop vision loss, spasticity, ataxia and occasionally epilepsy. MR imaging typically demonstrates characteristic white matter abnormalities of periventricular white matter with a posterior predominance associated with a rim of contrast enhancement. Imaging abnormalities typically precede the onset of symptoms. Most boys have associated adrenal insufficiency at the onset of neuroregression. The diagnosis is established by demonstrating elevated levels of plasma very long chain fatty acids (Chapter 99).

The subacute form of GM2 gangliosidosis classically presents between 2 to 10 years with progressive cognitive impairment, spasticity, ataxia, seizures, retinopathy and optic atrophy. A cherry red macular spot is usually absent. The chronic form of GM2 gangliosidosis presents in the first decade with cognitive and motor regression, psychosis, motor neuron disease, and cerebellar atrophy. The diagnosis is made by finding reduced enzyme activity of hexosaminidase A in nucleated cells.

Niemann-Pick Type C classically presents in middle to late childhood with cognitive regression, ataxia, and vertical supranuclear gaze palsy. Children may also develop dystonia and epilepsy. There may be hepatosplenomegaly. A history of gelastic cataplexy is another useful diagnostic clue. Biochemical diagnosis can be made with filipin staining and cholesterol esterification studies of cultured skin fibroblasts. Plasma oxysterols can be used as a screening test.

Psychiatric Symptoms

A number of IEMs can present in childhood or adolescence with psychiatric symptoms as the predominant manifestation. In these circumstances, more common etiologies should first be considered, including drug ingestion, primary psychiatric disease, and inflammatory brain disorders.

Cobalamin C deficiency, a disorder in the metabolism of vitamin B12, can rarely present after a normal early childhood with subacute psychiatric symptoms, often associated with signs of subacute combined degeneration of the spinal cord. Decompensation can be provoked by exposure to nitrous oxide, an inhibitor of the enzyme methionine synthase. The diagnosis is confirmed by elevated serum total homocysteine and plasma or urine methylmalonic acid in the presence of normal plasma vitamin B12 levels.

Milder forms of the urea cycle disorders often associated with some residual enzyme activity can present with episodic psychiatric symptoms. These episodes may be variably associated with alteration of consciousness, headache, emesis, and ataxia. Episodes may be provoked by illness, high protein intake, and some medications such as valproic acid.

Acute intermittent porphyria, a disorder of heme biosynthesis, rarely presents in the pediatric age group with the exception of the very rare, autosomal recessive 5-aminolevulinate (ALA) dehydratase deficiency. The classic presentation of acute intermittent porphyria includes acute episodes of psychosis, peripheral neuropathy, autonomic dysfunction, abdominal pain, and hyponatremia from SIADH. Episodes may be provoked by medications and hormonal factors, including menses. Diagnosis is confirmed by elevated levels of urine ALA, coproporphyrin, and RBC zinc protoporphyrin. Secondary inhibition of ALA dehydratase can also be seen in tyrosinemia type 1 due to accumulating succinylacetone.

As mentioned in the previous sections, Niemann-Pick Type C, the chronic form of GM2 gangliosidosis, and Wilson disease can occasionally present initially with isolated psychiatric symptoms. With progression of disease, cognitive regression and additional focal neurologic signs become apparent.

CONCLUSIONS

Although individually rare, inborn errors of metabolism collectively are not uncommon in the practice of child neurology. Given its high energetic demand, the nervous system is especially vulnerable and is often the sole presenting system of these disorders that may have protean manifestations. Laboratory diagnosis can be made by testing of metabolites, enzymatic function, or single gene or next generation gene sequencing panels. The IEMs can be conceptualized as disorders of small molecules, large molecules, and bioenergetics. Age of onset and severity tend to be related to degree of enzyme insufficiency. Many of the disorders, especially of small molecule and cerebral energy metabolism, present in early life with acute or subacute encephalopathy. Seizures in the first weeks of life that do not respond to standard anticonvulsant treatment should prompt early evaluation for treatable metabolic epilepsies including vitamin and cofactor responsive epilepsies and small molecule disorders. The presence of dysmorphism may suggest a metabolic disorder, especially large molecule disorder, which may have a specific treatment as well. IEMs are an uncommon cause of static developmental delay, compared with chromosome disorders and Fragile X, but a relatively common cause of developmental regression. IEMs in the older child and adolescent may present with ataxia, dystonia, rhabdomyolysis, stroke, cognitive or motor regression, or psychiatric symptoms.

REFERENCES

The complete list of references for this chapter is available in the e-book at www.expertconsult.com.
    See inside cover for registration details.

SELECTED REFERENCES

Bandmann, O., Weiss, K.H., Kaler, S.G., 2015. Wilson's disease and other neurological copper disorders. Lancet Neurol. 14 (1), 103–113.

Berardo, A., DiMauro, S., Hirano, M., 2010. A diagnostic algorithm for metabolic myopathies. Curr. Neurol. Neurosci. Rep. 10 (2), 118–126.

Freeze, H.H., Eklund, E.A., Ng, B.G., et al., 2012. Neurology of inherited glycosylation disorders. Lancet Neurol. 11 (5), 453–466.

Jira, P., 2013. Cholesterol metabolism deficiency. Handb. Clin. Neurol. 113, 1845–1850.

Klouwer, F.C., Berendse, K., Ferdinandusse, S., et al., 2015. Zellweger spectrum disorders: clinical overview and management approach. Orphanet J. Rare Dis. 10, 151.

Lyon, G., Kolodny, E.H., Pastores, G.M. (Eds.), 2006. Neurology of Hereditary Metabolic Disease of Children, third ed. McGraw Hill, U.S.United States, pp. 417–420.

Pastores, G.M., Maegawa, G.H.B., 2013. Neuropathic lysosomal storage disorders. Neurol. Clin. 31 (4), 1051–1071.

Saudubray, J.M., van den Berghe, G., Walter, J.H. (Eds.), 2012. Inborn Metabolic Diseases: Diagnosis and Treatment, vol. 28, fifth ed. Springer Medizin Verlag, Heidelberg, p. 656.

Schiffmann, R., van der Knaap, M., 2009. Invited article: an MRI based approach to the diagnosis of white matter disorders. Neurology 72, 750.

Van der Knaap, M.S., Valk, J. (Eds.), 2005. Magnetic Resonance of Myelination and Myelin Disorders, third ed. Springer-Verlag Berlin, Heidelberg, Germany.

E-BOOK FIGURES AND TABLES

The following figures and tables are available in the e-book at www.expertconsult.com. See inside cover for registration details.

37 Aminoacidemias and Organic Acidemias

Renata C. Gallagher, Gregory M. Enns, Tina M. Cowan, Bryce Mendelsohn, and Seymour Packman

An expanded version of this chapter is available on www.expertconsult.com. See inside cover for registration details.

Approximately 4% of individuals born in the United States have a genetic or partly genetic disorder. Inborn errors of metabolism contribute significantly to this total. Although each disease is individually rare, the aggregate incidence of metabolic disease is relatively high and may be greater than 1 in 1000 newborns. Newborn screening programs using tandem mass spectrometry, which can detect approximately 20 inborn errors of metabolism, typically have reported an incidence of 1 in 2000 to 1 in 4000. Because there are hundreds of known metabolic conditions, the aggregate estimate seems reasonable.

Metabolic diseases infrequently produce symptoms immediately at birth, and they can manifest with slowly progressive encephalopathies. In this setting, histologic or biochemical abnormalities may be present in the fetal central nervous system (CNS) by 4 to 5 months' gestation. Inborn errors of metabolism also can manifest with rapid clinical deterioration in the newborn period or after an interval period of good health. Presenting clinical features are often nonspecific, and they may be misdiagnosed as infection, cardiovascular compromise or other causes of hypoxemia, trauma, primary brain anomalies, or the effects of a toxin. Recognition of patterns of clinical presentation and rapid implementation of laboratory investigations are essential for the initiation of appropriate therapy without delay. If appropriate therapy is not initiated in a timely manner, there is a high risk of morbidity or mortality, regardless of the cause of the acute illness.

This chapter provides an overview of the diagnosis and treatment of two categories of inborn errors: aminoacidopathies and organic acidemias. The general approaches described are broadly applicable to other heritable metabolic disorders, such as disorders of fatty acid oxidation, urea cycle disorders, and lactic acidosis syndromes. Descriptions of selected disorders of amino acid and organic acid metabolism are provided to illustrate and emphasize the approaches to diagnosis, treatment, and genetic counseling in this area of genetic medicine. In this print version of the chapter, we discuss phenylketonuria, followed by representative aminoacidopathies and organic acidemias likely to be encountered by the pediatric neurologist in an acute or critical clinical setting. For a comprehensive and detailed discussion of additional organic acidemias and aminoacidopathies and important general concepts in the diagnosis, treatment, and genetic counseling involved in heritable metabolic disorders, readers are referred to the online version of this chapter.

SIGNS AND SYMPTOMS: GENERAL CONCEPTS

See the online version of the chapter.

PHYSICAL FINDINGS: GENERAL CONCEPTS

See the online version of the chapter.

LABORATORY APPROACHES TO DIAGNOSIS: GENERAL CONCEPTS

See the online version of the chapter.

TREATMENT: GENERAL CONCEPTS

See the online version of the chapter.

INHERITANCE AND GENETIC COUNSELING: GENERAL CONCEPTS

See the online version of the chapter.

AMINOACIDEMIAS
Phenylketonuria

Phenylketonuria (PKU) is an autosomal-recessive disorder caused by deficient activity of phenylalanine hydroxylase (PAH), a hepatic enzyme that converts phenylalanine to tyrosine (Figure 37-1). The biochemical block results in the accumulation of phenylalanine, which is then converted to phenylpyruvic acid and phenyllactic acid, phenylketones that are excreted in the urine. A range of reduced PAH-specific activity correlates broadly with the severity of the phenotype. Tetrahydrobiopterin is a necessary cofactor in the PAH reaction, and elevated phenylalanine levels rarely may be caused by inherited disorders of tetrahydrobiopterin synthesis (see Figure 37-1). Mandatory population newborn screening for PKU, in combination with postnatal presymptomatic therapy, was begun in the 1960s.

Phenylalanine is neurotoxic, and untreated or poorly treated patients with classic phenylketonuria typically have profound intellectual disability. Patients exposed to chronically elevated phenylalanine levels ultimately develop microcephaly, seizures (e.g., tonic-clonic, myoclonic, infantile spasms), tremors, athetosis, and spasticity, and they may be misdiagnosed as having cerebral palsy. Psychiatric and behavior problems, including autistic behavior and attention-deficit hyperactivity disorder, are common. Brain magnetic resonance imaging (MRI) may detect dysmyelination, especially T2 enhancement in the periventricular white matter, a finding that is potentially reversible with the initiation of dietary therapy.

Elevated maternal blood phenylalanine levels can cross the placenta and cause fetal birth defects, including microcephaly, dysmorphic features, and congenital heart defects. Dietary control (phenylalanine levels < 360 µM) should ideally be achieved before 3 months before conception, and mothers with PKU should be monitored carefully by an experienced center throughout pregnancy.

The presymptomatic institution of and continued adherence to specific dietary therapy prevents intellectual disability. However, children and adults with PKU may experience

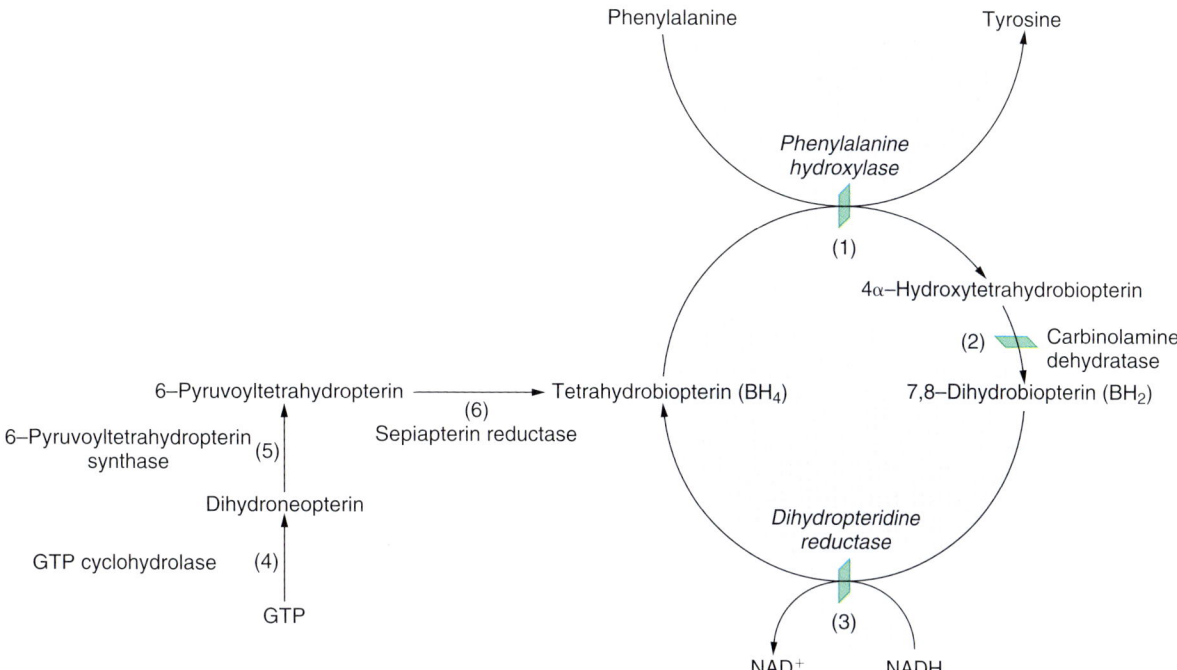

Figure 37-1. Regulation of phenylalanine hydroxylase activity. Phenylalanine is converted to tyrosine (1) by the holoenzyme phenylalanine hydroxylase (PAH). PAH requires tetrahydrobiopterin (BH$_4$) as an active cofactor and is recycled by the sequential actions of carbinolamine dehydratase (2) and dihydropteridine reductase (3). BH$_4$ is synthesized in vivo through a complex series of steps that involve guanosine triphosphate (GTP) cyclohydrolase (4), 6-pyruvoyltetrahydropterin synthase (5), and sepiapterin reductase (6). Genetic defects at any of these steps may be associated with hyperphenylalaninemia. *(From Wilcox WR, Cederbaum SD. Amino acid metabolism. In: Rimoin D, Connor J, Pyeritz R, Korf B, eds. Principles and practice of medical genetics, 4th ed. Philadelphia: Churchill Livingstone, 2002:2406.)*

cognitive symptoms, such as problems in executive functioning, and disturbance in emotional (e.g., depression, anxiety, phobias) and behavioral (e.g., hyperactivity) functioning despite early and continuous treatment. Selective restriction of phenylalanine intake by using phenylalanine-free medical formulas and foods (and tyrosine supplementation), which provides enough additional protein and nutrients to support normal growth, remains the mainstay of PKU therapy. Most clinics in the United States strive to maintain plasma phenylalanine levels between 120 and 360 µM in children younger than 12 years and between 120 and 600 µM in individuals older than 12 years, although there is some evidence to suggest that lowering upper phenylalanine targets even further improves neurocognitive function. An expert, coordinated team approach is clearly the most effective way of managing phenylketonuria; stricter management improves developmental outcome.

In conjunction with dietary therapy, oral administration of tetrahydrobiopterin, the naturally occurring cofactor for the PAH reaction, may be used to control plasma phenylalanine levels. Response to tetrahydrobiopterin is especially robust in mild hyperphenylalaninemia but has also been documented in patients with classic or variant PKU. A trial of tetrahydrobiopterin may be offered to PKU patients of any severity to determine clinical response. Administration of dietary supplementation of large neutral amino acids (LNAAs) is a complementary approach to therapy. LNAAs compete with phenylalanine for transport across the blood–brain barrier by the L-type amino acid carrier and consequently decrease the level of phenylalanine in the central nervous system (CNS) and may increase brain neurotransmitter and essential amino acid concentrations. A novel therapeutic approach currently in clinical trials uses the nonmammalian enzyme phenylalanine ammonia lyase (PAL). This enzyme converts phenylalanine to

transcinnamic acid, a harmless compound, and it has been found to reduce hyperphenylalaninemia in PKU animal models and patients in clinical trials. Other novel therapies are under close investigation, especially given the findings of suboptimal outcomes in phenylketonuria patients who have been continuously treated from the neonatal period. (Enns et al., 2010)

Biopterin Disorders

See the online version of the chapter.

Hepatorenal Tyrosinemia

See the online version of the chapter.

Other Categories of Tyrosinemia

See the online version of the chapter.

Maple Syrup Urine Disease

In 1954, John Menkes and colleagues described four siblings who died in early infancy from a cerebral degenerative disease, with onset occurring when they were 3 to 5 days old. Symptoms included feeding difficulty, irregular respiratory pattern, hypertonia, opisthotonus, and failure to thrive. All had urine with the smell of maple syrup. Soon thereafter, another patient with a similar history was found to have elevated levels of branched-chain amino acids in urine and blood, and the syndrome was initially referred to as maple sugar urine disease. Maple syrup urine disease is caused by mitochondrial branched-chain α-ketoacid dehydrogenase complex deficiency. The enzymatic defect leads to accumulation of branched-chain amino acids and branched-chain α-ketoacids. Five forms of maple syrup urine disease (i.e., classic, intermediate, intermittent, thiamine-responsive, and dihydrolipoyl dehydrogenase [E3] deficiency) have been delineated based on clinical presentation, level of enzyme activity, and response to thiamine administration.

Clinical Manifestations

Classic Maple Syrup Urine Disease. In the classic form, the clinical phenotype is one of severe neonatal encephalopathy, unless presymptomatic therapy is initiated because of abnormal newborn screening, prenatal diagnosis, or positive family history. Untreated neonates typically develop symptoms by the end of the first week of life. Feeding difficulties, alternating hypertonia and hypotonia, opisthotonic posturing, abnormal movements ("fencing" or "bicycling"), and seizures commonly occur. The characteristic urine smell develops on day 5 to 7 of life. Unless an underlying inborn error of metabolism is suspected, affected children may be misdiagnosed as having sepsis and progress to coma and death. Ketosis is often found, and hypoglycemia may occur, but severe metabolic acidosis tends not to occur. Plasma amino acid analysis reveals elevated levels of branched-chain amino acids and the diagnostic presence of alloisoleucine in plasma. Urine organic acid analysis demonstrates excretion of branched-chain α-ketoacids. Hyponatremia and cerebral edema are frequent sequelae during acute metabolic decompensation. Other complications include pseudotumor cerebri, pancreatitis, and eye abnormalities. Ocular findings in untreated or late-diagnosed patients include optic atrophy, gray optic papilla, nystagmus, ophthalmoplegia, strabismus, and cortical blindness. Children who survive the initial metabolic crisis typically have significant neurodevelopmental delays and spasticity. Although motor, visual, and learning deficits may occur, rapid identification of affected infants and careful institution of appropriate therapy can result in normal development.

Neuroimaging studies (Figure 37-3) are typically abnormal in patients with untreated classic maple syrup urine disease (MSUD) who are in crisis. Computed tomographic (CT) scans appear normal in the first few days of life, but they reveal progression to marked generalized cerebral edema if the patient remains untreated. An unusual pattern of edema may occur, characterized by involvement of the cerebellar deep white matter, posterior brainstem, cerebral peduncles, posterior limb of the internal capsule, and posterior aspect of the centrum semiovale. Edema tends to subside in the second month of life. Patients with classic maple syrup urine disease in metabolic crisis with associated hyponatremia demonstrate a prominently increased T2 signal on brain MRI in the brainstem reticular formation, dentate nucleus, red nucleus, globus pallidus, hypothalamus, septal nuclei, and amygdala. One report observed that brain MRI abnormalities were absent or only slight in sick patients with maple syrup urine disease in the absence of hyponatremia. Cranial ultrasonography of neonates in acute metabolic crisis reveals symmetrically increased echogenicity of the periventricular white matter, basal ganglia, and thalami. Chronic changes, including hypomyelination of the cerebral hemispheres, cerebellum, and basal ganglia and cerebral atrophy, may supervene in poorly controlled patients. CT- and MRI-defined abnormalities and the clinical phenotype may improve after implementation of appropriate dietary therapy. Diffusion-weighted imaging and spectroscopy have also documented abnormalities during the acute phase of disease. Markedly restricted proton diffusion, suggestive of cytotoxic or intramyelinic sheath edema, was demonstrated in the brainstem, basal ganglia, thalami, cerebellar and periventricular white matter, and cerebral cortex in six patients with maple syrup urine disease.

MR spectroscopy demonstrated abnormal elevations of branched-chain amino acids, branched-chain α-ketoacids, and lactate in the four patients. All of these changes were reversed after the institution of appropriate nutritional and antibiotic therapy to treat intercurrent illness. However, in a recent study of a cohort of classic MSUD adolescents and adults under dietary control, persistent signal changes were noted in the cerebral hemispheres, internal capsule, brainstem, and central cerebellum (Klee et al., 2013). The authors ascribed the signal alterations to dysmyelination and considered them consonant with clinical studies showing that learning disabilities and variable social, educational, and professional outcomes are present in teenagers and adults with MSUD.

A characteristic comblike electroencephalogram (EEG) pattern may be demonstrated for some patients with classic MSUD between the second and third weeks of life. This unusual rhythm pattern resolves with the institution of dietary therapy.

Intermediate Maple Syrup Urine Disease. Children who have the intermediate form of MSUD do not present in the neonatal period, despite having persistently elevated plasma levels of branched-chain amino acids. Developmental delay and failure to thrive are common. Severe neurologic impairment is absent; episodes of metabolic decompensation may occur, although severe ketoacidosis episodes are variable. These children have a higher tolerance for dietary protein than those who have the classic form. Rarely, patients with intermediate-type MSUD respond to thiamine administration.

Intermittent Maple Syrup Urine Disease. Patients with intermittent MSUD typically come to medical attention when they are 5 months to 2 years old and after stress induced by infection or high protein intake; some have been detected as late as the fifth decade of life. The intermittent form of MSUD can be particularly difficult to diagnose because affected individuals have normal levels of branched-chain amino acids and no odor between episodes of metabolic decompensation. Episodic decompensation is characterized by ataxia, disorientation, and altered behavior, which may progress to seizures, coma, and even death unless therapy is instituted. Early development and intellect are usually normal.

Thiamine-Responsive Maple Syrup Urine Disease. The clinical course of patients with the thiamine-responsive variant of MSUD is similar to that of the intermediate form of the disease. Plasma levels of branched-chain amino acid and urine excretion of branched-chain α-ketoacids decline days to weeks after thiamine administration (10-1000 mg/day) is started. Patients are also treated with nutritional regimens similar to those used in other forms of MSUD. Developmental delay may be present, but normal intelligence has also been documented.

Dihydrolipoyl Dehydrogenase–Deficient Maple Syrup Urine Disease. The dihydrolipoyl dehydrogenase (E3)–deficient form of MSUD is characterized by ketoacidosis crises in infancy. There is also lactic acidemia because the E3 subunit of the branched-chain α-ketoacid dehydrogenase complex is also required for catalytic function of pyruvate dehydrogenase and α-ketoglutarate dehydrogenase. In addition to the typical MSUD metabolites, urine organic acid analysis reveals the presence of lactate, pyruvate, and α-ketoglutarate. The neonatal period is usually uneventful, but progressive neurologic deterioration, characterized by developmental delay, hypotonia or hypertonia, and dystonia, supervenes. Death in early childhood is common. Attempts at therapy had limited success in early reports. However, more recent case reports and studies have identified patients with a wide clinical spectrum, with survival to at least the third decade. In some such patients, and

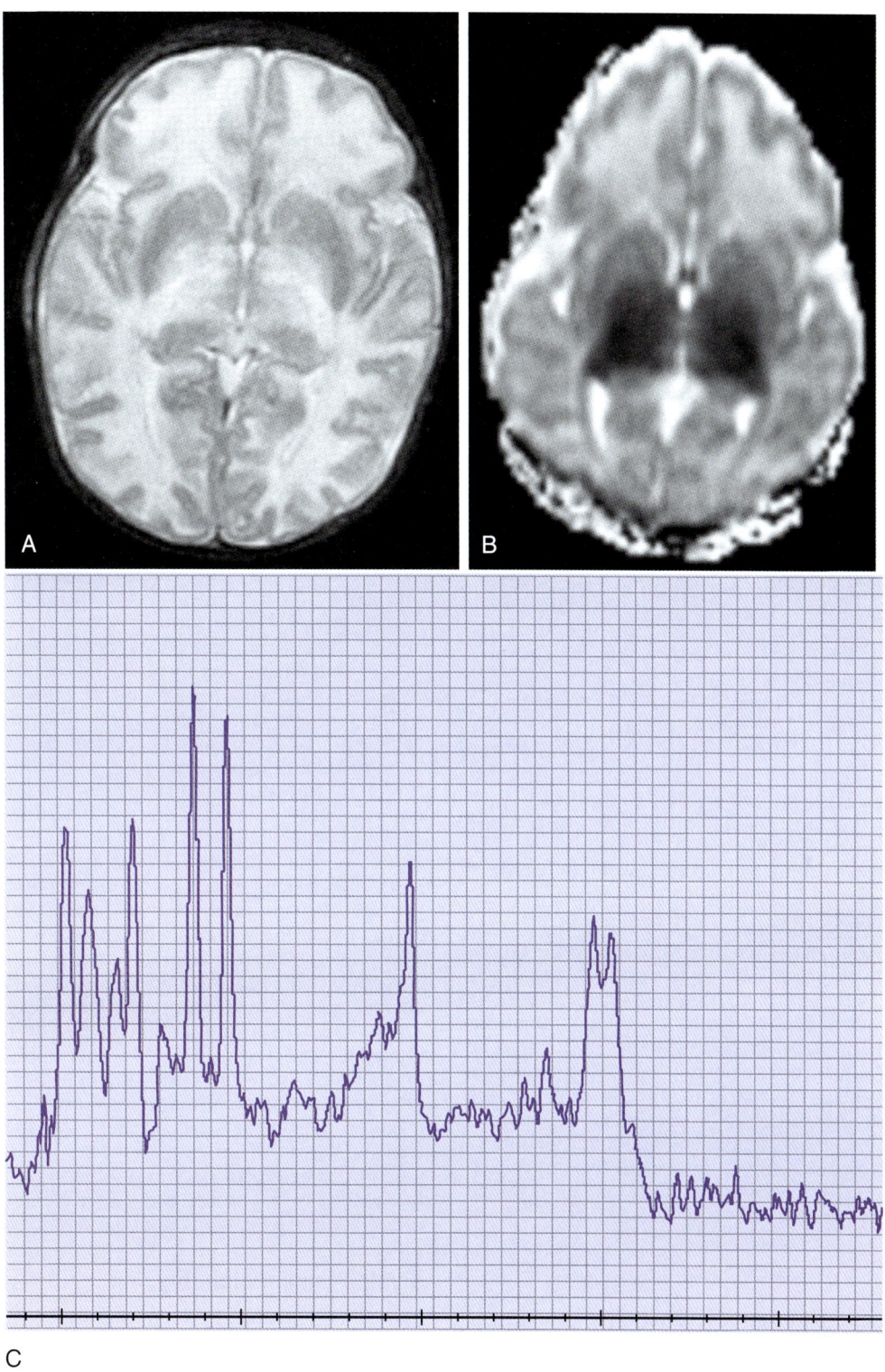

Figure 37-3. Maple syrup urine disease. A, Axial view, T2-weighted image shows edema in the internal capsules, lateral thalami, and globus pallidi. **B,** Axial view, calculated apparent diffusion coefficient image at the same level shows hypointensity, indicated by reduced water diffusion, in the affected areas. **C,** Proton MR spectroscopy (echo time of 26 msec) shows a large peak at 0.9 ppm, believed to represent resonances of methyl protons from branched-chain amino acids and branched-chain α-ketoacids that accumulate as a result of defective oxidative decarboxylation of leucine, isoleucine, and valine. *(Courtesy of Dr. A James Barkovich, University of California, San Francisco, CA.)*

depending on the mutations, there is a positive clinical response to riboflavin, perhaps based on a chaperone-like effect of enzyme stabilization.

Laboratory Tests

MSUD can be detected easily and accurately by tandem mass spectrometry analysis of the newborn blood spot. Plasma amino acid analysis demonstrates elevations of leucine, isoleucine, and valine (5- to 10-fold greater than normal) and the pathognomonic finding of elevated alloisoleucine. Levels of branched-chain amino acids are greatly elevated in urine and cerebrospinal fluid (CSF). The branched-chain α-ketoacids 2-oxoisocaproic acid, 2-oxo-3-methylvaleric acid, and 2-oxoisovaleric acid, derived from the branched-chain amino acids leucine, isoleucine, and valine, respectively, are found to be elevated on urine organic acid analysis during metabolic crises. Branched-chain amino acids levels and excretion of branched-chain α-ketoacids may be normal between episodes of decompensation in the intermittent form of disease.

The branched-chain α-ketoacid dehydrogenase complex consists of three catalytic components—a thiamine pyrophosphate-dependent carboxylase (E1) with an $\alpha_2\beta_2$ structure, a transacylase (E2), and a dehydrogenase (E3)—and two regulatory enzymes (a kinase and a phosphatase). Deficient activity of this complex leads to the accumulation of leucine, isoleucine, and valine and their corresponding α-ketoacids. The decarboxylation activity can be measured in leukocytes, lymphoblasts, or fibroblasts, and it is loosely related to the clinical phenotype: 0% to 2% of normal activity in classic MSUD, 3% to 30% activity in intermediate, 5% to 20% in intermittent, 2% to 40% in thiamine-responsive, and 0% to 25% in E3 deficiency. Because significant overlap exists between measured enzyme activity and clinical phenotype, enzymatic activity cannot be used to predict the clinical course with certainty. In parallel findings on molecular analyses, identified mutations also cannot be correlated with phenotype.

Genetics

MSUD is a pan-ethnic, autosomal-recessive condition that can be caused by mutations in any of the components of the mitochondrial branched-chain α-ketoacid dehydrogenase complex. In a study of 63 individuals, E1β subunit mutations were most common (38%), followed by E1α (33%), and E2 (19%) mutations. Branched-chain α-ketoacid dehydrogenase phosphatase or kinase mutations are also thought to cause MSUD. The overall incidence is approximately 1 case per 150,000 people in the general population, but MSUD is more common in Old Order Mennonites in southeastern Pennsylvania (1 in 176 births). A novel founder mutation in the E1β subunit has been reported in the Ashkenazi Jewish population.

Treatment

Chronic care of the child with MSUD includes regular visits to an integrated metabolic clinic for medical and nutritional assessment. Adequate calories (100-120 kcal/kg per day) and protein (2-3 g/kg per day) are needed for growth. Chronic valine or isoleucine deficiency may cause an exfoliative dermatitis, and supplementation of these amino acids is often needed. Thiamine supplementation is administered to patients with thiamine-responsive forms of MSUD. Because patients on restricted diets are at risk for micronutrient and essential fatty acid deficiencies, patients should be periodically monitored for such deficits and supplementation given as needed.

Acute metabolic decompensation (e.g., fasting or illness severe enough to cause catabolism) is a medical emergency that requires prompt intervention. Initial intervention is aimed at correcting dehydration, starting high-dose intravenous thiamine, and providing adequate calories (approximately 120-140 kcal/kg per day) to prevent further protein catabolism and higher rise in plasma leucine levels. To this end, high-dextrose intravenous fluids (to provide approximately 10 mg/kg per minute) and intralipid are often administered. Branched-chain amino acid–free parenteral nutrition or enteral formula, delivered by continuous nasogastric drip, can also be used. The rate of decrease of leucine is slowed in the face of valine and isoleucine levels inadequate to stimulate protein synthesis. Acute valine and isoleucine deficiency can be avoided by careful supplementation of these amino acids. Leucine is reintroduced to the diet after therapeutic levels are achieved. Hemodialysis and continuous venovenous extracorporeal removal therapies result in more rapid fall in plasma levels of branched-chain amino acids, and this modality is now established as an effective standard-of-care therapy for acute metabolic decompensation.

Liver transplantation has been increasingly performed on large numbers of patients as an essential component of long-term therapy in classic MSUD, even in nonexigent (i.e., elective) clinical circumstances (Strauss et al., 2006). It has become apparent that as patients reach adolescence and adulthood, they show variable intellectual deficits, attention deficits, deficits in executive function, psychological symptoms (e.g., anxiety, depression), and poor social adjustment, even with a history of apparently excellent dietary control and an absence of a history of acute metabolic crises (Strauss et al., 2006). Following transplant, leucine levels either remaining normal or are in a treatment range on an unrestricted protein diet. Long-term clinical evaluations are proceeding, but neuropsychological and patient and family reporting appear to support improvement or stabilization of neurologic status. Three patients who underwent successful transplantation were able to resume normal diets and were no longer at risk for metabolic decompensation. In an important variation of the transplant protocol, domino hepatic transplantation for MSUD has been successfully performed.

A novel treatment approach under investigation takes advantage of the observation that when used in the treatment of urea cycle disorders, Na phenylbutyrate causes a lowering of branched-chain amino acid levels (Burrage, Nagamani, Campeau, and Lee , 2014). Na phenylbutyrate was found to increase the activity of the branched-chain ketoacid dehydrogenase by preventing phosphorylation—and, thereby, inactivation—of the E1α subunit. The increased residual enzyme activity of the branched-chain ketoacid dehydrogenase would be expected to lower branched-chain amino acid levels. Studies are under way using Na phenylbutyrate in cohorts of MSUD patients (Burrage et al., 2014).

Glycine Encephalopathy

Glycine encephalopathy is an autosomal-recessive disorder caused by defective function of the glycine cleavage enzyme system, leading to accumulation of glycine in all body tissues, including the CNS (Figure 37-4). The glycine cleavage enzyme system has four components: glycine decarboxylase, also known as the P protein (it uses pyridoxal-phosphate as a cofactor); aminomethyltransferase, also known as T protein (it is a tetrahydrofolate dependent protein); the glycine cleavage system H protein (a hydrogen carrier protein); and the L protein or lipoamide dehydrogenase (the cofactor is lipoate). Infants with classic disease present in the first week of life with apnea, lethargy, severe hypotonia, and feeding difficulties. Respiratory failure, hiccups, and intractable seizures develop, and many infants die unless assisted ventilatory support is

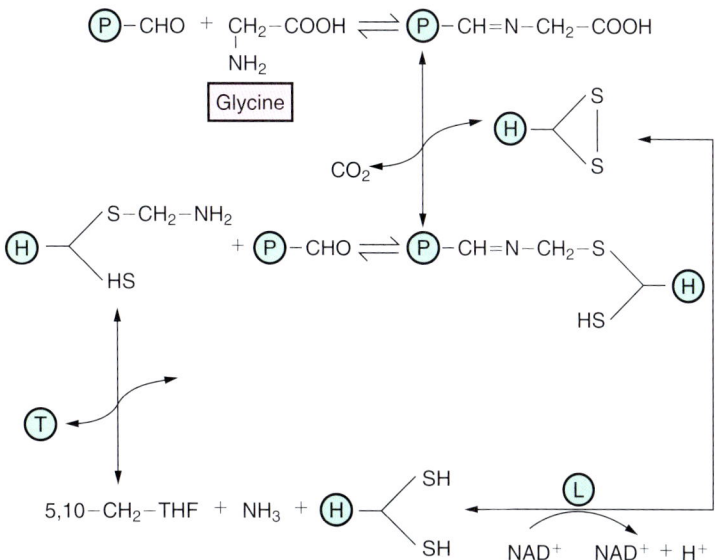

Figure 37-4. The glycine cleavage system. Circles designate proteins with the active group shown. In the presence of P and H proteins, glycine is decarboxylated, and the remaining aminoethyl group binds to the reduced lipoic acid on the H protein. T protein is required to release ammonia and transfer the x carbon of glycine to tetrahydrofolate (THF), forming 5,10-CH_2-THF. The L protein is necessary to regenerate the correct form of the H protein. *(From Scriver C, Beudet A, Sly W, Valle D, eds. The metabolic and molecular basis of inherited disease, 8th ed. New York: McGraw-Hill, 2001:2066, Fig, 90-2. Reprinted with permission from The McGraw-Hill Companies.)*

provided. The EEG commonly has a burst suppression pattern, but hypsarrhythmia has rarely been reported. There are also later-onset forms, including presentation at greater than 4 months of age. A review of 124 patients stratified affected individuals into four categories. Those who could only smile were termed severe. Those who had achieved additional developmental milestones were termed attenuated. Three attenuated forms were delineated, poor, intermediate, and mild; these were defined as a developmental quotient (ratio of developmental age to chronologic age) of less than 20, between 20 and 50, and greater than 50, respectively. Predictors of outcome included age at seizure onset, CSF glycine value, ratio of CSF to plasma glycine, and the presence of severe brain malformations (Swanson et al., 2015). Of presenting neonates, 85% have the severe form of the disease and 15% the attenuated; the proportion for infantile onset is 50% severe and 50% attenuated. In the previously described series of 124 affected individuals, 21% died in the neonatal period, 45% had the severe form, and 34% had an attenuated form (Swanson et al., 2015).

Brain imaging results are normal for about one-half of the neonatal-onset cases. Relatively common brain abnormalities include agenesis of the corpus callosum, progressive atrophy, and delayed myelination.

Mild and transient forms of glycine encephalopathy have been reported. Mild forms manifest in infancy or early childhood after an uneventful pregnancy and neonatal period. Clinical features include seizures (in most cases) and relatively mild developmental delay. Transient glycine encephalopathy is characterized by the same initial clinical and biochemical findings as the classic form, but it has only rarely been reported. In the transient form, elevated CSF and plasma glycine levels partially or completely normalize, and most patients have normal development.

The diagnosis of glycine encephalopathy is established by detecting an elevated CSF glycine concentration, typically 15 to 30 times normal, in association with an increased ratio of CSF to plasma glycine (normal < 0.02). Classic neonatal-onset patients often have ratios higher than 0.2, whereas atypical patients have ratios of approximately 0.09. A ratio higher than

0.08 is usually considered diagnostic of glycine encephalopathy. The plasma and CSF samples should be obtained as closely as possible to one another, and the presence of blood in the CSF invalidates the amino acid results. Other causes of increased CSF glycine levels include valproate therapy, brain trauma, and hypoxic-ischemic encephalopathy. Secondary elevations of plasma glycine, associated with ketosis, are often encountered in organic acidemias (e.g., methylmalonic, propionic, and isovaleric acidemias and β-ketothiolase deficiency; these are the ketotic hyperglycinemias). Because pyridoxine-dependent epilepsy, pyridoxamine 5′-phosphate oxidase deficiency, and cerebral folate deficiency may have presentations similar to that of glycine encephalopathy, concentrations of alpha-aminoadipic semialdehyde, pyridoxal 5′-phosphate, and 5-methyltetrahydrofolate should also be assessed in the CSF. Urine S-sulfocysteine should be sent to test for isolated sulfite oxidase deficiency and molybdenum cofactor deficiency, which may also present with intractable seizures in the newborn period.

Confirmation of the diagnosis may be accomplished by assaying the glycine cleavage system in liver tissue, although, in practice, molecular testing of the genes encoding glycine cleavage system subunits is less invasive and more widely available, and the enzyme defect may be secondary, as described in the following discussion.

Comprehensive mutation analysis in 68 families with glycine encephalopathy detected *GLDC* (P protein gene) or *AMT* (T protein gene) mutations in 68% of neonatal and 60% of infantile types, respectively. No *GCSH* (H protein gene) mutations were identified.

Strikingly, evaluation of patients with abnormal glycine cleavage activity in liver, but without mutations in genes encoding the enzymes of the glycine cleavage system, were identified to have defects in mitochondrial lipoate synthesis]. These defects include those in enzymes involved in lipoate synthesis and transfer and those in iron-sulfur cluster biogenesis because lipoate synthase is a protein that contains iron-sulfur clusters. Importantly, individuals with lipoate synthase defects, sometimes also referred to as variant or atypical glycine encephalopathy, have varied biochemical and clinical presentations. It is important to be aware of these classes of defects and the biochemical and phenotypic overlap of lipoate synthesis defects, which include iron-sulfur cluster biogenesis defects, with glycine encephalopathy.

Treatment of glycine encephalopathy has not improved the overall dismal prognosis in the classic form of disease. Therapy is focused on controlling seizures with antiepileptic drugs, decreasing tissue glycine levels, and administering N-methyl-D-aspartate (NMDA) receptor antagonists to diminish glycine-induced neuronal excitotoxicity. Valproate is contraindicated because it can inhibit the glycine cleavage enzyme system and can cause hyperglycinemia in patients without glycine encephalopathy. Sodium benzoate is given because of its ability to conjugate to glycine to form hippurate, which can then be excreted in the urine. A glycine-specific mitochondrial enzyme, benzoyl-coenzyme A (CoA):glycine acyltransferase, catalyzes the condensation of benzoate and glycine to form hippurate. Sodium benzoate therapy can reduce plasma levels of glycine to the normal range and may have a mild effect on CSF glycine levels, but it does not affect the very poor prognosis. Because high-dose sodium benzoate therapy can result in carnitine deficiency, plasma carnitine levels should be monitored closely and appropriate supplementation provided. Dextromethorphan, an antagonist of the NMDA receptor, is also commonly used in therapy. Treatment with dextromethorphan may lead to improved seizure control and level of interaction in some patients. Rarely, ketamine has been used, but it may provide benefit in controlling seizures and improving overall level of interaction. A low-protein diet has no proven efficacy and may result in severe protein malnutrition, micronutrient deficiency, and exfoliative dermatitis if not monitored carefully.

Sulfur Amino Acid Metabolism and the Homocystinurias

See the online version of the chapter.

Hartnup's Disease

See the online version of the chapter.

Histidinemia

See the online version of the chapter.

ORGANIC ACIDEMIAS
Propionic Acidemia

See the online version of the chapter.

Methylmalonic Acidemias

Multiple genetic defects can lead to methylmalonic acidemia, alone or in combination with elevated homocysteine because both compounds are processed by enzymes that require B_{12}. B_{12} is acquired through dietary sources and must be appropriately transported and modified to participate in methylmalonic acid and homocysteine metabolism. The isolated methylmalonic acidemias and those in combination with elevated homocysteine are caused by deficiencies in the transport or modification of vitamin B_{12} (cobalamin) or by mutations in enzymes requiring a B_{12} cofactor, in addition to several other mechanisms, such as a transcription factor defect that causes combined methylmalonic acidemia and homocystinuria (see Figure 37-6A and B). Because there are a variety of causative defects, this group of conditions has significant clinical heterogeneity and differences in response to therapy. Incidence is estimated at 1 case per 50,000 persons, or greater.

Pathophysiology

The canonical inherited isolated methylmalonic acidemias are caused by defects in the enzyme methylmalonyl-CoA mutase, which requires an adenosylcobalamin cofactor, or in the enzymes that modify B_{12} to adenosylcobalamin. The latter cases are sometimes denoted by the genetic complementation group because the causative genes were identified over time; these are cblA, cblB, and cblD-MMA. Isolated methylmalonic acidemia can also be caused by a defect in methylmalonyl-CoA epimerase (encoded by the *MCEE* gene), which converts D-methylmalonyl-CoA to L-methylmalonyl-CoA; in methylmalonate semialdehyde dehydrogenase (*ALDH6A1*); in a disorder of mitochondrial energy metabolism, succinyl-CoA synthase deficiency (*SUCLA2, SUCLG1*); and in association with mutations in *ACSF3*, in which malonic acid may also be elevated (Pupavac et al., 2016). Elevations of both methylmalonic acid and homocysteine are caused by defects in other genes encoding enzymes, transport proteins, and receptors that affect cobalamin trafficking and modification and can also be caused by dietary deficiency of B_{12} (Pupavac et al., 2016). Methylmalonyl-CoA is derived from propionyl-CoA; both are intermediates in the catabolism of isoleucine, valine, threonine, methionine, thymine, uracil, cholesterol, and odd-chain fatty acids. Methylmalonyl-CoA mutase converts L-methylmalonyl-CoA to succinyl-CoA, which then enters the tricarboxylic acid cycle.

The major causes of isolated methylmalonic acidemia are mutase deficiency (mut^0, mut$^-$), cblA, and cblB. CblD-MMA (formerly described as cblH) is also a cause of isolated methylmalonic acidemia but is more rare. Mutase activity is completely and partially abolished in the mut^0 and mut$^-$ groups, respectively. CblC, cblD-combined, cblF (*LMBRD1*), and cblJ (*ABCD4*) are associated with elevations of both methylmalonic acid and homocysteine, as is cblX, an X-linked defect in *HCFC1*, a transcription factor that affects expression of the gene defective in cblC disease, *MMACHC*. Defective adenosylcobalamin synthesis is responsible for cblA, cblB, and cblD-MMA. CblC and cblD-combined, cblF, and cblJ cause methylmalonic acidemia and homocystinuria because of their effects on both adenosylcobalamin and methylcobalamin biosynthesis (Figure 37-6A and B). CblE (*MTRR*), cblG (*MTR*), and cblD-HC affect methylcobalamin synthesis and therefore homocysteine metabolism alone.

Clinical Manifestations

As with propionic acidemia and other disorders, there are early- and late-onset forms, which likely result, in part, from residual protein function. There is significant variability in presentation of the methylmalonic acidemias, depending on the particular underlying defect. Common features of the canonical isolated methylmalonic acidemias are failure to thrive, developmental delay, megaloblastic anemia, and neurologic dysfunction. Mut^0, cblA, and cblB patients often present in the first days to weeks of life with poor feeding, dehydration, increasing lethargy, emesis, and hypotonia. Metabolic acidosis and secondary hyperammonemia, as with propionic acidemia, may be catastrophic. Mild mut$^-$ or other forms of methylmalonic acidemia may present later in infancy or in childhood with hypoglycemia, acidosis, seizures, and lethargy. A patient with cblC disease can present early in infancy with signs and symptoms of metabolic decompensation, in later childhood, or in adulthood with myopathy, lower-extremity paresthesias, and thrombosis as a result of elevated plasma homocysteine. Other features of cblC

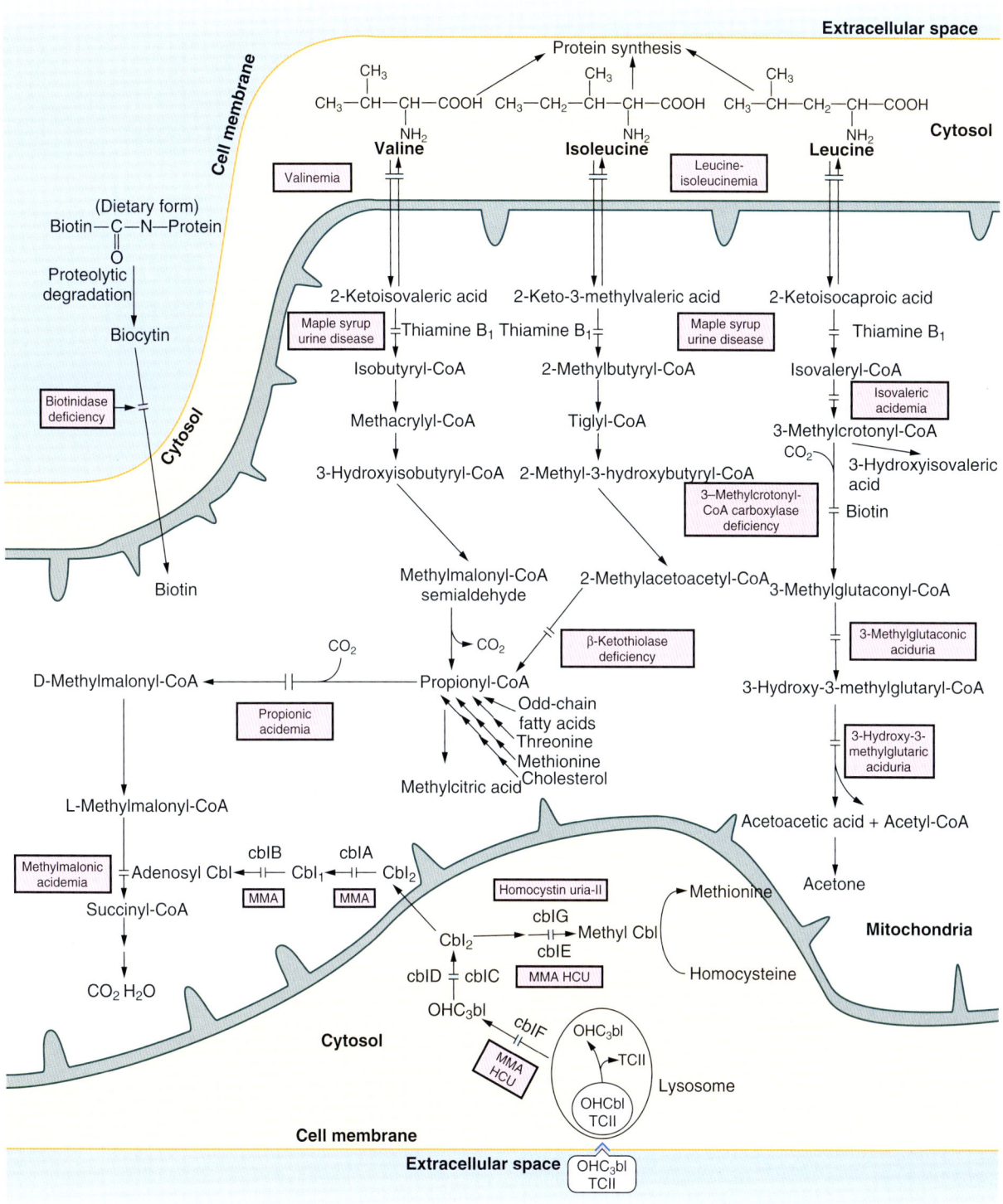

A

Figure 37-6. A, Pathways in the metabolism of the branched-chain amino acids, biotin, and vitamin B_{12} (cobalamin).

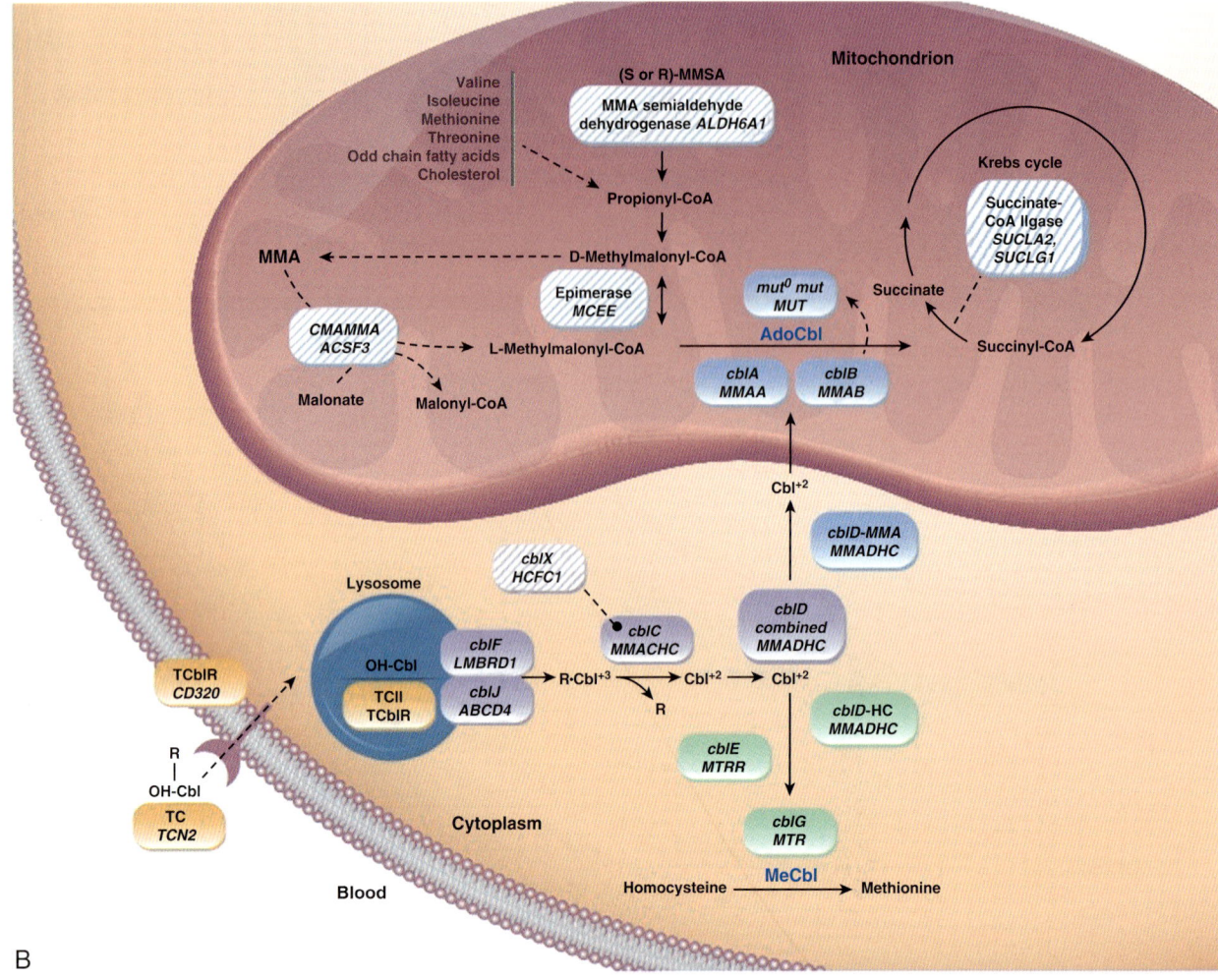

B

Figure 37-6, cont'd B, Updated depiction of cobalamin metabolism. Cbl, cobalamin; cbl, defect in metabolism of cobalamin; HCU, homocystinuria; MMA, methylmalonic acidemia; OHCbl, hydroxocobalamin; TC, transcobalamin. (**A,** *From Rezvani I. Defects in metabolism of amino acids. In: Behrman R, Kliegman R, Jenson H, eds.* Nelson textbook of pediatrics, *16th ed. Philadelphia: WB Saunders, 2000:355.* **B,** *With permission from Pagon RA, Adam MP, Ardinger HH, et al., (eds), Isolated Methylmalonic Acidemi, GeneReviews®, Copyright © 1993-2016, University of Washington, Seattle. All rights reserved, www.genereviews.org.)*

disease include hemolytic-uremic syndrome, cardiomyopathy, subacute combined degeneration of the cord, and psychiatric manifestations such as psychosis. Children with cblC disease can have ocular abnormalities, including optic atrophy, and progressive pigmentary retinopathy with resultant nystagmus, strabismus, and worsening vision (Fischer et al., 2014). They may also exhibit hydrocephalus and microcephaly. Cranial imaging may reveal pathology of the basal ganglia and white matter. The two initial cases reported with cblD presented in later childhood with mental retardation and behavioral problems, although subsequent reports have documented infantile onset with hypotonia and seizures and early childhood presentations with ataxia and gait abnormalities. CblF patients have been reported to have minor facial anomalies and hematologic defects. Transcobalamin II deficiency, a B_{12} transport deficiency, can manifest as failure to thrive in the first months of life, with neurologic disease, hematologic disease, and mental retardation. A benign form of methylmalonic acidemia has been reported in otherwise healthy children; some of these may be caused by mutations in the genes encoding mutase, those encoding epimerase, or in *ACSF3*. There are also reports of individuals with mutations in the receptor for

transcobalamin bound to cobalamin (TCblR); this may be a benign condition.

Laboratory Tests

Methylmalonic acidemia can clinically resemble other organic acidemias, necessitating analysis of urine organic acids for diagnosis. Elevated C3 (propionyl) acylcarnitine identifies methylmalonic acidemia, propionic acidemia, and B_{12} deficiency; therefore, urine organic acid analysis is required after an abnormal newborn screen with elevated C3 acylcarnitine. As with propionic acidemia, some cases are not identified through newborn screening, and some infants will develop clinical symptoms before the newborn screen results are available. Therefore if there is a clinical concern, testing for an organic aciduria should be performed. Ketosis and hyperammonemia are common in the acute neonatal presentation of these conditions, and if these are present, urine organic acids and other biochemical tests should be performed. Urine organic acid analysis reveals large amounts of methylmalonic acid, methylcitrate, propionic acid, and 3-hydroxypropionic acid in mutase deficiency and cblA and cblB disease. Serum amino acids sometimes demonstrate elevation of glycine. When elevated serum or urine methylmalonic acid is identified, it is critical to obtain a total plasma homocysteine as a specific test to assess for defects that cause elevations of both compounds because elevated homocysteine may not be detected through plasma amino acid analysis. Serum B_{12} levels must be assessed to ensure that elevated methylmalonic acid and homocysteine levels, if present, are not the result of a nutritional deficiency of cobalamin. Total plasma homocysteine levels are elevated in cblC, cblD-combined, cblF, cblJ, and CblX diseases. Total and free carnitine levels tend to be low. The cobalamin transport deficiencies are assessed by measuring serum cobalamin levels and absorption by the Schilling test, in addition to DNA testing (Pupavac et al., 2016). Determination of the form of methylmalonic acidemia was often performed through complementation studies in fibroblasts, but this does not identify all causes (Pupavac et al., 2016). DNA mutation analysis is now the appropriate first test. One next-generation sequencing panel includes 24 genes associated with elevated methylmalonic acid (Pupavac et al., 2016).

Treatment

Guidelines for acute and chronic management of methylmalonic acidemia have been developed (Baumgartner et al., 2014). The principles of management are similar to those for propionic acidemia. One critical difference is that some forms of methylmalonic acidemia are responsive to vitamin B_{12}, and hydroxocobalamin (preferred) or cyanocobalamin should be given empirically to a child presenting with hyperammonemia and ketosis. If methylmalonic acidemia is identified, intramuscular or subcutaneous hydroxocobalamin should be continued if the child appears to have a form that is responsive to B_{12} (cblA, mut⁻), which can be difficult to assess. During acute metabolic crises, treatment of known methylmalonic acidemia is directed toward stopping catabolism and restricting protein intake. The usual protein intake is stopped for 12 to 24 hours from last intake, and fat and glucose are given orally or intravenously. Chronic and acute therapy include carnitine; intramuscular, subcutaneous, or intravenous hydroxocobalamin; and metronidazole or neomycin to decrease intestinal propionate production in some cases. Betaine and folate are used if homocysteine is elevated. Treatment of hyperammonemia, which can be marked in the initial presentation, is similar to that for propionic acidemia (Baumgartner et al., 2014). Improved growth and enhanced nutritional status are seen in patients with methylmalonic acidemia fed an elemental medical food. Patients should consume a diet low in the macronutrient precursors proximal to the metabolic block and receive adequate calories and total protein to enable growth. Plasma methylmalonic acid levels are followed for metabolic control. Frequent complications in methylmalonic acidemia include tubulointerstitial nephritis, leading to end-stage renal disease, and basal ganglia stroke, often affecting the globus pallidus. Cardiomyopathy is reported but is less common than in propionic acidemia (Baumgartner et al., 2014). Liver transplantation has been performed but is not curative of the disease. It protects against recurrent metabolic crises but not against metabolic stroke, and it does not lead to a complete clinical or biochemical correction because the pathway is active in other tissues. Kidney transplant, often performed for renal failure, may also protect against metabolic decompensation (Baumgartner et al., 2014), although this is still unclear.

Isovaleric Acidemia

 See the online version of the chapter.

3-Methylcrotonyl-CoA Carboxylase Deficiency

See the online version of the chapter.

Biotinidase Deficiency

See the online version of the chapter.

Holocarboxylase Synthetase Deficiency

See the online version of the chapter.

3-Methylglutaconic Aciduria

See the online version of the chapter.

Beta-Ketothiolase Deficiency

See the online version of the chapter.

Canavan's Disease

See the online version of the chapter.

Glutaric Aciduria Type I

In 1975, glutaric acidemia and aciduria were described in siblings with a neurodegenerative disorder beginning in infancy and characterized by opisthotonus, dystonia, and athetosis. Glutaric acidemia type I, also known as glutaryl-CoA dehydrogenase deficiency, is an autosomal-recessive condition caused by deficiency of glutaryl-CoA dehydrogenase and has an estimated prevalence of approximately 1 case per 100,000 persons. In the United States glutaric acidemia type I is relatively common in the Old Order Amish. Glutaric acidemia type II is also known as multiple acyl-CoA dehydrogenase deficiency (MADD) and is associated with defects in mitochondrial electron transfer flavoprotein or electron transfer flavoprotein dehydrogenase; it is discussed further in Chapter 37. Glutaric aciduria type III is not associated with clinical symptoms and is the result of a deficiency of the enzyme that converts glutarate to glutaryl-CoA. Glutaryl-CoA dehydrogenase is a key enzyme in the degradation pathway of lysine, hydroxylysine, and tryptophan. Deficiency results in accumulation of glutarate and, to a lesser extent, of 3-hydroxyglutarate and glutaconate in body tissues, blood, CSF, and urine (Hedlund, Longo, and Pasquali, 2006).

The classic symptom of glutaric acidemia type I (GAI) is irreversible focal striatal necrosis during an acute illness, most often between the ages of 3 and 18 months. Such an event is termed an encephalopathic crisis. Sequelae of the acute injury to the basal ganglia include irreversible disabling dystonia and, in some cases, dyskinesia, in addition to shortened life expectancy (Kolker et al., 2006). Crucially, newborn screening has changed the natural history of this condition. The combined use of chronic management and emergency management in the treatment of individuals identified presymptomatically greatly reduces neurologic injury (Hedlund et al., 2006; Kolker et al., 2006). Macrocephaly is a feature of GAI and may not be present at birth, but head growth velocity is increased; in some cases progressive macrocephaly has led to the identification of GAI before striatal injury (Kolker et al., 2006). Intraretinal hemorrhages and subdural hematomata caused by the rupture of bridging veins associated with macrocephaly may be present and may be mistaken for nonaccidental injury; this can also lead to the identification of affected individuals before striatal injury. In some cases, striatal injury is not associated with an identified encephalopathic crisis but is insidious, with gradual appearance of symptoms. Systemic manifestations typical of many other organic acidemias, such as pronounced metabolic ketoacidosis, hypoglycemia, and hyperammonemia, generally do not occur (Hedlund et al., 2006). There is a window of neurologic susceptibility to striatal damage during the first years of life. A seminal natural history study of 279 individuals in 37 countries demonstrated that 95% of encephalopathic crises occurred before 2 years of age and that additional basal ganglia injury occurred up to roughly 6 years of age but not beyond (Kolker et al., 2006). Crucially, individuals who are identified presymptomatically and treated according to established guidelines may avoid the devastating neurologic injury in the vulnerable period (Kolker et al., 2006). A late-onset leukodystrophy has been described, and the natural history of this manifestation is unknown.

A characteristic early brain MRI finding is symmetric widening of the sylvian fissure with poor operculization ("bat wing" appearance) caused by frontotemporal atrophy or hypoplasia (Figure 37-8). Other features include basal ganglia injury, subdural hematomata, ventriculomegaly, and delayed myelination (Hedlund et al., 2006). Diffusion-weighted imaging may be more sensitive in demonstrating brain lesions than CT or MRI.

Urine organic acid analysis often documents highly elevated glutaric acid and lesser elevations of 3-hydroxyglutarate and glutaconate, but some children with a classic neurologic phenotype have low or undetectable levels of these metabolites (so-called low excretors). Newborn screening using tandem mass spectrometry has the potential for presymptomatic detection of GAI, although the existence of a low-excretor phenotype can result in missed cases. Roughly one-third of affected individuals have a low excretor phenotype, which is associated with residual enzyme activity of up to 30%. Crucially, these individuals are at no less risk of severe neurologic injury (Kolker et al., 2006).

Increased glutarate and 3-hydroxyglutarate levels in the CNS may induce an imbalance in glutamatergic and GABAergic neurotransmission by inhibiting glutamate decarboxylase, the key enzyme in gamma-aminobutyric acid (GABA) synthesis, or through direct damage to striatal GABAergic neurons. 3-Hydroxyglutarate may mimic the excitatory neurotransmitter glutamate and thereby cause excitotoxic cell damage mediated through activation of NMDA receptors. Glutarate was shown to inhibit synaptosomal uptake of glutamic acid and produce striatal lesions when injected directly into the brain of a rat. Other potential contributors to neurotoxicity include cytokine-induced cell damage, mitochondrial dysfunction, increased production of reactive oxygen species, and production of toxic quinolinic acid, an intermediate in tryptophan metabolism in the brain. Other reports have emphasized the relatively weak neurotoxicity of glutarate and 3-hydroxyglutarate in animal models and primary neuronal cell cultures. The pathogenesis of striatal necrosis and brain lesions in GAI remains the subject of intensive investigation. Animal models may help resolve these conflicting results.

Presymptomatic treatment of GAI includes restriction of dietary lysine intake, carnitine, and sometimes riboflavin; supplementation; and rapid intervention in times of intercurrent illness (Kolker et al., 2006). This therapy is continued in symptomatic patients, who also require symptom management, which includes anticholinergic drugs such as trihexyphenidyl and botulinum toxin to treat generalized or focal dystonia resulting from striatal injury. Stereotactic pallidotomy has been performed, as has deep brain stimulation.

5-Oxoprolinuria

See the online version of the chapter.

Isobutyryl-CoA Dehydrogenase Deficiency

See the online version of the chapter.

3-Hydroxyisobutyric Aciduria

See the online version of the chapter.

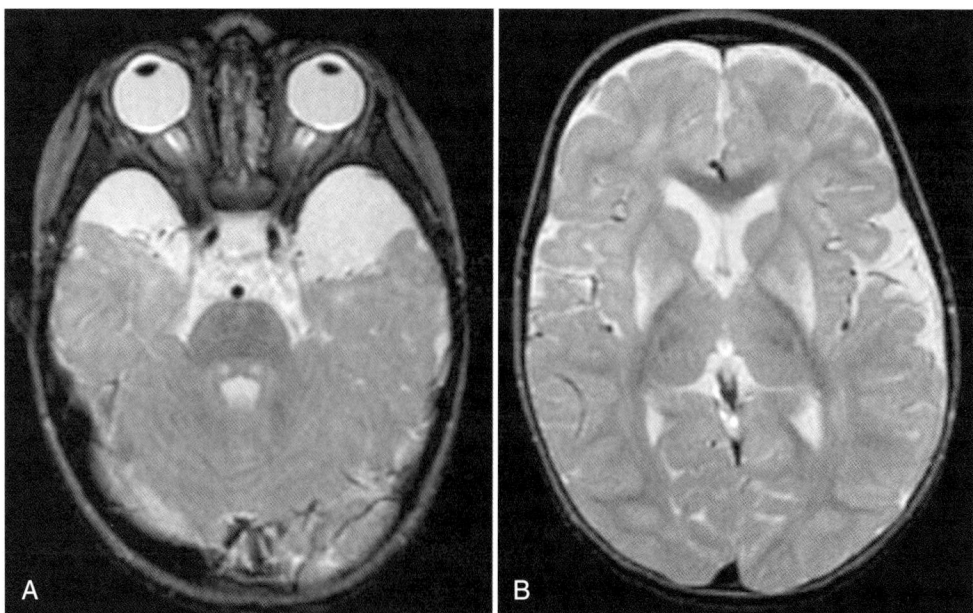

Figure 37-8. Magnetic resonance imaging (MRI) in glutaric acidemia. **A,** Axial view, T2-weighted image shows markedly enlarged sylvian fissures bilaterally and abnormal hyperintensity of the central tegmental tract. **B,** Axial view, T2-weighted image at a slightly higher level shows abnormal hyperintensity of the lentiform nuclei bilaterally. *(Courtesy of Dr. A James Barkovich, University of California, San Francisco.)*

2-Methylbutyryl-CoA Dehydrogenase Deficiency

See the online version of the chapter.

Mevalonate Kinase Deficiency

See the online version of the chapter.

REFERENCES

The complete list of references for this chapter is available in the e-book at www.expertconsult.com.

See inside cover for registration details.

REFERENCES

Baumgartner, M.R., Horster, F., Dionisi-Vici, C., et al., 2014. Proposed guidelines for the diagnosis and management of methylmalonic and propionic acidemia. Orphanet J. Rare Dis. 9, 130.

Burrage, L., Nagamani, S., Campeau, P., et al., 2014. Branched-chain amino acid metabolism: from rare Mendelian diseases to more common disorders. Hum. Mol. Genet. 25, R1R8.

Enns, G.M., Koch, R., Brumm, V., et al., 2010. Suboptimal outcomes in patients with PKU treated early with diet alone: revisiting the evidence. Mol. Genet. Metab. 101, 99.

Fischer, S., Huemer, M., Baumgartner, M., et al., 2014. Clinical presentation and outcome in a series of 88 patients with the cblC defect. J. Inherit. Metab. Dis. 37, 831–840.

Hedlund, G.L., Longo, N., Pasquali, M., 2006. Glutaric Acidemia Type 1. Am. J. Med. Genet. C Semin. Med. Genet. 142C (2), 86–94.

Klee, D., Thimm, E., Wittsack, H.J., et al., 2013. Structuralwhite matter changes in adolescents and yound adults with maple syrup urine disease. J. Inher. Metab. Dis. 36, 945–953.

Kolker, S., Garbade, S.F., Greenberg, C.R., et al., 2006. Natural history, outcome, and treatment efficacy in children and adults with glutaryl-CoA dehydrogenase deficiency. Pediatr. Res. 59, 840–847.

Pupavac, M., Tian, X., Chu, J., et al., 2016. Added value of next generation gene panel analysis for patients with elevated methylmalonic acid and no clinical diagnosis following functional studies of vitamin B_{12} metabolism. Mol. Genet. Metab. 117, 363–368.

Strauss, K., Mazariegos, G., Sindhi, R., et al., 2006. Elective liver transplantation for the treatment of classical maple syrup urine disease. Am. J. Transplant. 6, 557–564.

Swanson, M.A., Coughlin, C.R., Scharer, G.H., et al., 2015. Biochemical and Molecular Predictors for Prognosis in Nonketotic Hyperglycinemia. Ann. Neurol. 78, 606–618.

E-BOOK FIGURES AND TABLES

The following figures and tables are available in the e-book at www.expertconsult.com. See inside cover for registration details.

Fig. 37-2 The tyrosine metabolic pathway.

Fig. 37-5 Abbreviated diagram for the transsulfuration pathway.

Fig. 37-7 Patient with Canavan's disease.

38 Inborn Errors of Urea Synthesis

Sandesh C.S. Nagamani and Uta Lichter-Konecki

An expanded version of this chapter is available on www.expertconsult.com. See inside cover for registration details.

Inherited disorders of the urea cycle represent a group of inborn errors of metabolism that are associated with hyperammonemic encephalopathy and high mortality and morbidity. They comprise deficiencies of a cofactor-synthesizing enzyme, five catalytic enzymes, and amino acid transporters involved in urea synthesis (Fig. 38-1). These disorders are classified as follows (estimated prevalence rates are given in parentheses) (Brusilow and Horwich, 2001; Tuchman et al., 2008; Ah Mew et al., 2003):

- Deficiency of cofactor synthesis
  - *N*-acetylglutamate synthase (NAGS) deficiency (prevalence unknown)
- Deficiency of catalytic enzymes
  - carbamoyl-phosphate synthase 1 (CPS1) deficiency (1 per 62,000)
  - ornithine transcarbamylase (OTC) deficiency (1 per 14,000)
  - argininosuccinate synthase 1 (ASS1) deficiency (citrullinemia) (1 per 57,000)
  - argininosuccinate lyase (ASL) deficiency (argininosuccinic aciduria) (1 per 70,000)
  - arginase 1 (ARG1) deficiency (hyperargininemia) (1 per 353,000)
- Deficiency of transporters
  - citrullinemia type II (mitochondrial aspartate/glutamate carrier [citrin] SLC25A13 deficiency) (1 per 21,000 in Japan; possibly more common in China)
  - hyperornithinemia-hyperammonemia-homocitrullinuria (HHH) syndrome (mitochondrial ornithine transporter, ORNT1 or SLC25A15 deficiency) (prevalence unknown)

All of the urea cycle disorders (UCDs) are inherited as autosomal-recessive traits, except for OTC deficiency, which is X-linked. Other than in ARG1 deficiency, infants with a complete deficiency of any other urea cycle enzyme commonly present in the newborn period with hyperammonemic coma. Universal newborn screening and the availability of drugs and hemodialysis for treatment of hyperammonemia have resulted in improved survival; mortality, however, still remains high, and the majority of survivors have intellectual disability. Patients with late-onset disease may present at any age with hyperammonemic crises that carry a risk of mortality (10%) and intellectual disability.

THE UREA CYCLE

Dietary protein, on average, contains approximately 16% nitrogen. More than 90% of the nitrogen that is not used for anabolic processes is typically metabolized and excreted as urea. Deficiency of one of the enzymes or transporters required for urea synthesis results in accumulation of nitrogen in the form of ammonia, leading to encephalopathy.

One cofactor and its synthesizing enzyme, five catalytic enzymes, and two transporters are necessary for optimal urea cycle activity (see Fig. 38-1). The cofactor *N*-acetylglutamate, which is synthesized by NAGS, activates CPS1, the first enzyme

catalyzing the rate-limiting step of the urea cycle. CPS1 uses ATP, bicarbonate, and glutamine or ammonia to synthesize carbamoyl-phosphate. This reaction is where the first atom of waste nitrogen enters the cycle. OTC, a mitochondrial enzyme, synthesizes citrulline from carbamoyl-phosphate and ornithine. Citrulline is actively transported by the ornithine transporter (ORNT1/SLC25A15) from the mitochondrion to the cytosol, where it is conjugated with aspartate to form argininosuccinic acid by ASS1. Here, the second atom of waste nitrogen is contributed to the cycle by aspartate. ASL cleaves argininosuccinic acid to yield fumarate and arginine. The final step in the urea cycle involves cleavage of arginine by ARG1 to form urea and ornithine. The ornithine is transported back into the mitochondrion by ORNT1/SLC25A15.

Although the complete urea cycle is only present in hepatocytes, other tissues also express some urea cycle enzymes. The intermediates of the urea cycle are linked to the citric acid cycle, the nitric oxide cycle, and possibly other pathways. The enzymes ASS1 and ASL are also required for synthesis of arginine, which is important for generation of nitric oxide (NO), creatine, polyamines, and agmatine. Thus deficiency of urea cycle enzymes may also affect nonureagenic functions, which may contribute to some of the distinct features observed in urea cycle disorders.

CLINICAL DESCRIPTION OF UREA CYCLE DISORDERS

N-Acetylglutamate Synthase Deficiency

Inherited NAGS deficiency leads to hyperammonemia by causing a secondary deficiency of CPS1 activity. NAGS deficiency is characterized by hyperammonemia in the newborn period or later in life that can be fatal or lead to intellectual and developmental disabilities. Plasma amino acid analysis usually demonstrates an increased level of glutamine and reduced or absent levels of citrulline. Urinary orotic acid levels are normal or low. Because enzyme analysis requires large amounts of liver tissue and may not be entirely reliable, analysis of genomic DNA for mutations in the *NAGS* gene is the preferred diagnostic method. Previously, treatment for NAGS deficiency was limited to low-protein diet and use of ammonia scavengers (Table 38-1); however, synthetic cofactor therapy with *N*-carbamyl-L-glutamate is now approved.

Carbamoyl-Phosphate Synthase 1 Deficiency

CPS1 deficiency can manifest with hyperammonemic crises in the newborn period or later in childhood. Biochemically, the principal findings are hyperammonemia, increased glutamine, and reduced or absent citrulline in plasma. Urinary orotic acid levels are normal or low. Patients with neonatal-onset disease generally demonstrate less than 5% of the normal CPS1 activity in liver, whereas those with late-onset disease have higher residual activity. Therapy consists of dialysis and/or intravenous ammonia scavengers during severe hyperammonemic episodes and low-protein diet and oral ammonia scavengers

TABLE 38-1 Long-Term Alternative-Pathway Treatment of Urea Cycle Disorders (UCDs)*

Disorder	L-Citrulline	L-Arginine Free Base	Sodium Phenylbutyrate	N-Carbamylglutamate
NAGS deficiency	—	—	—	~0.10 g/kg/d
CPS1 or OTC deficiency	0.15–0.20 g/kg/d or 3.8 g/m²/d	—	0.45–0.60 g/kg if < 20 kg 9.9–13.0 g/m²/d in larger patients	—
Citrullinemia	—	0.40–0.50 g/kg/d or 8.8–15.4 g/m²/d	0.45–0.60 g/kg if < 20 kg 9.9–13.0 g/m²/d in larger patients	—
Argininosuccinic acidemia	—	0.40–0.50 g/kg/d or 8.8–15.4 g/m²/d	0.45–0.60 g/kg if < 20 kg 9.9–13.0 g/m²/d in larger patients	—
Argininemia	—	—	0.45–0.60 g/kg/d if < 20 kg 9.9–13.0 g/m²/d in larger patients	

*Drugs and dose ranges are those commonly used in patients with UCDs; however, doses can vary and need to be adjusted based on the severity of the disorder and patient response. When using doses at the upper recommended range or above, consideration should be given to increased risk of drug toxicity.
CPS1, carbamoyl-phosphate synthase 1; NAGS, N-acetylglutamate synthase; OTC, ornithine transcarbamylase.

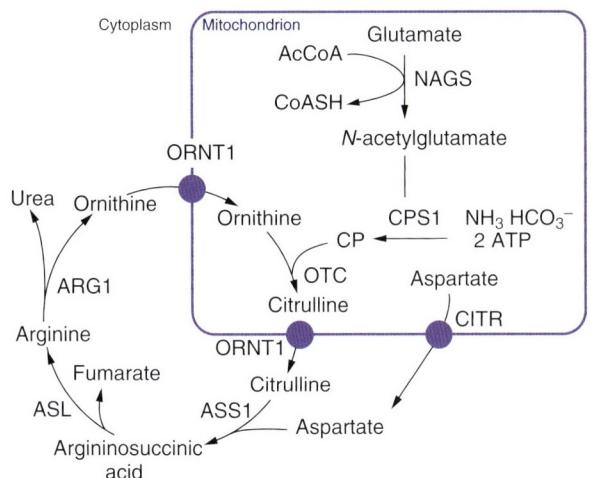

Figure 38-1. The urea cycle. AcCoA, acetyl coenzyme A; ASL, argininosuccinate lyase; ARG1, arginase 1; ASS1, argininosuccinate synthase; CITR, citrin; CoASH, coenzyme A; CPS1, carbamoyl-phosphate synthase 1; NAGS, N-acetylglutamate synthase; ORNT1, ornithine transporter 1; OTC, ornithine transcarbamylase.

for chronic treatment (see Table 38-1). Patients with the neonatal-onset form who survive the initial crisis generally require liver transplantation to have any quality of life.

Ornithine Transcarbamylase Deficiency

OTC deficiency is transmitted as an X-linked recessive disorder and thus is much more severe in males (Lichter-Konecki et al., 2013). The classic presentation of OTC deficiency in hemizygous males is that of a catastrophic illness in the first week of life. In symptomatic female heterozygotes and in males with partial OTC deficiency, symptoms may occur at any time from infancy to adulthood. These patients generally have 5% to 30% of normal OTC activity in the liver. Biochemically, the findings are hyperammonemia, hyperglutaminemia, reduced or absent citrulline in plasma, and increased urinary orotic acid.

More than 340 different point mutations and polymorphisms have been found in the *OTC* gene. Although most families have point mutations, small and large deletions have been identified. When the mutation has been identified, carrier testing and prenatal diagnosis can be offered to the family.

Detection of heterozygous females with OTC deficiency is important for both identifying at-risk family members and prenatal diagnosis. Such detection can be accomplished by either molecular studies or, in cases where no mutation is found, by an allopurinol load. When administered allopurinol (300 mg given orally to adults), in 90% of heterozygotes with OTC deficiency, there is increased excretion of orotic acid. Approximately 15% of OTC-deficient heterozygous females will become symptomatic during their lifetime. Therapy for neonatal-onset OTC deficiency consists of dialysis and intravenous ammonia scavengers, followed by maintenance on a low-protein diet and long-term ammonia scavengers (see Table 38-1). Patients with the neonatal-onset form who survive the initial crisis generally require liver transplantation for prevention of recurrent metabolic crises.

Citrullinemia

Citrullinemia is characterized by marked elevation of citrulline in the blood (Quinonez and Thoene, 2004). Two distinct forms have been reported: neonatal- or childhood-onset citrullinemia (type I; with diminished levels of ASS1 in all organs) and citrullinemia type II or citrin deficiency, an adult-onset citrullinemia that in some but not all cases is preceded by neonatal cholestasis and liver dysfunction.

Biochemically, the principal findings in type I are hyperammonemia, citrullinemia, and citrullinuria. Citrulline levels are elevated 50-fold to 100-fold above normal. Urinary orotic acid levels are also increased. Therapy consists of dialysis during severe hyperammonemic crises, followed by low-protein diet and long-term ammonia-scavenger therapy (see Table 38-1). After the initial crisis, patients are, in general, more stable and easier to manage than patients with more proximal urea cycle defects.

Citrullinemia Type II or Citrin Deficiency

Citrin deficiency is caused by mutations in *SLC25A13*, a gene that encodes citrin, a mitochondrial membrane protein. This carrier enables the exchange of mitochondrial aspartate for cytosolic glutamate across the inner mitochondrial membrane. The lack of aspartate to conjugate with citrulline in this condition leads to a block in urea synthesis. Citrulline levels can be elevated up to 400 μmol/L; plasma ammonia levels are less severely elevated compared with other UCDs.

Citrin deficiency can manifest in adulthood with cyclical bizarre behavior (aggression, irritability, and hyperactivity), dysarthria, seizures, motor weakness, and coma. Treatment generally relies on ammonia scavengers (arginine and phen-ylbutyrate); however, liver transplantation is becoming a more common therapy because of the possible liver complications. More recently, a neonatal-onset form of citrin deficiency has been identified; it is associated with intrahepatic cholestasis. Affected infants have multiple metabolic abnormalities, including aminoacidemia, galactosemia, hypoproteinemia, hypoglycemia, and cholestasis. Treatment usually consists of high-protein/low-carbohydrate diet, and the symptoms often disappear within a year. A few children, however, have a severe form of the disorder with liver damage and tyrosinemia that necessitates liver transplantation. Hyperammonemia is not a major component of this disorder.

Argininosuccinic Aciduria

Argininosuccinic aciduria derives its name from the marked elevation of argininosuccinic acid in the blood and urine of affected persons. In the severe forms, this disorder can present with hyperammonemic coma in the newborn period, whereas those with mild forms have fewer, if any, episodes of symptomatic hyperammonemia (Nagamani, Erez, and Lee, 2011). A specific abnormality of the hair termed *trichorrhexis nodosa* develops in affected children. Some patients develop chronic hepatomegaly. Liver function tests can be abnormal and patients may develop cirrhosis. The reasons as to why some patients with this condition develop cirrhosis, and others do not, are not yet understood. Even individuals with no history of hyperammonemia can have intellectual and learning disabilities, and some develop hypertension that is difficult to control. Biochemically, the principal findings are elevated citrulline level, hyperammonemia, argininosuccinic acidemia, and argininosuccinic aciduria. After the initial hyperammonemic crisis and establishment of the diagnosis, treatment consists of a low-protein diet and L-arginine supplementation (see Table 38-1). Ammonia scavengers may be required in those who have metabolic decompensations. Recent evidence also suggests that ASL is required for synthesis of nitric oxide (NO) and that NO deficiency in this disorder may lead to hypertension.

Argininemia

Argininemia characterized by significant elevations of arginine is caused by a deficiency of ARG1. Argininemia presents differently from all of the other UCDs (Wong, Cederbaum, and Crombez, 2004). Although rarely hyperammonemia can be observed, this condition usually manifests as a progressive neurologic disorder rather than as an acute encephalopathy. The disease runs a chronic course with development of progressive spasticity (diplegia or quadriplegia). Affected children generally do not succumb to hyperammonemic coma and therefore have a longer life span than those affected by proximal UCDs. Patients may also have acute episodes of ataxia, behavioral disturbances, vomiting, lethargy, and seizures precipitated by intercurrent illnesses. The principal biochemical finding is markedly elevated plasma arginine. Urinary excretion of orotic acid and guanidine compounds also is markedly increased. The diagnosis can be confirmed by measuring ARG1 activity in erythrocytes.

The mechanism responsible for the spasticity and cognitive deficits in argininemia is unknown but is unlikely to be the result of the generally moderate hyperammonemia. Arginine, its guanidine metabolites, and altered biogenic amines are candidate neurotoxins. Arginine is the substrate for nitric oxide synthase, so overproduction of NO may play a role in neuropathology. Treatment with ammonia-scavenger therapy and lowering of the arginine level appears to halt the progres-sion of the spasticity, and botulinum toxin (Botox) and surgical tendon release may improve function.

Hyperornithinemia-Hyperammonemia-Homocitrullinuria Syndrome

HHH syndrome is rare, and only about 50 individuals have been reported in the literature. Clinical symptoms are similar to those in other UCDs but rarely develop in infancy. Plasma ornithine concentrations are elevated, ranging from 400 to 600 μmol/L. Plasma lysine level typically is low, and urinary excretion of homocitrulline is increased. HHH syndrome is caused by mutations in the ornithine transporter gene, *ORNT1*, also called *SLC25A15*. The decreased activity of the transporter leads to decreased ornithine levels in mitochondria and secondary impairment of urea synthesis. The expression of *ORNT2*, an intronless gene, encoding a protein about 90% identical to ORNT 1, may explain the milder clinical signs and symptoms compared with those in CPS1 and OTC deficiencies. Treatment of HHH syndrome involves protein restriction, ammonia scavengers, and citrulline supplementation.

COMMON CLINICAL PRESENTATIONS OF UREA CYCLE DISORDERS

The classic presentation of a complete defect in the urea cycle (other than ARG1 deficiency) is that of a catastrophic illness in the first week of life. Clinical manifestations typically appear between 24 and 72 hours of age, starting as a poor suck, hypotonia, vomiting, lethargy, and hyperventilation, with rapid progression to seizures and coma (Ah Mew et al., 2003). The electroencephalogram (EEG) pattern during hyperammonemic coma is one of low voltage with slow waves and asymmetric δ and θ waves. The tracing may demonstrate a burst-suppression pattern, and the duration of the interburst interval may correlate with the peak of ammonia levels. Neuroimaging studies reveal cerebral edema with small ventricles, flattening of cerebral gyri, and diffuse low density of white matter; evidence of intracranial hemorrhage also may be seen.

Partial deficiencies of a urea cycle enzyme have a spectrum of presentations, with hyperammonemic episodes developing in infancy in some, childhood in others, and not until adulthood in still others. Symptoms may be delayed in onset by dietary self-restriction and avoidance of high-protein foods. Signs and symptoms in childhood include anorexia and behavioral abnormalities such as episodes of erratic behavior, acting out of character, irritability, cloudiness to frank changes in mental status and ataxia, nocturnal restlessness, and attention deficit and hyperactivity. In adults, signs and symptoms may mimic those of psychiatric or neurologic disorders and include migraine-like headaches, nausea, dysarthria, ataxia, confusion, hallucinations, and visual impairment (blurred vision, scotomas, vision loss).

Neurologic findings in those with severe manifestations may include increased deep tendon reflexes, papilledema, and decorticate/decerebrate posturing. In metabolic decompensation, seizures generally are a late complication; the seizure episode typically is preceded by alteration in consciousness. There are indications that patients with UCDs may also be prone to seizures outside of hyperammonemic episodes; seizures were observed more often in patients with UCDs than in the general population in one clinic. Analysis of data collected longitudinally from patients with UCDs will allow further investigation of this impression.

In affected individuals, hyperammonemic episodes can be precipitated by any event that induces catabolism, including infections, high-protein meals, medication, trauma, surgery, and childbirth. It is not uncommon for the initial hyperammonemic episode in a child with a partial deficiency to occur after weaning, when low-protein breast milk is replaced by formula or cow's milk. The puerperium in OTC-deficient heterozygotes and valproate therapy in partial CPS1 and ASL deficiencies also have been associated with hyperammonemic crises.

HISTOPATHOLOGIC FEATURES OF UREA CYCLE DISORDERS

Histopathologic examination of the liver in UCDs may be normal but often demonstrates diffuse microvesicular steatosis, marked increased glycogen in periportal cells, and variable portal fibrosis. Cirrhosis has been identified in some patients with argininosuccinic aciduria (ASA), citrullinemia type II, and ARG1 deficiency.

Neuropathologic findings in UCDs are similar to those following the hepatic encephalopathy of acute liver failure. They depend on both the duration of hyperammonemic coma and the interval between coma and death. Neonates who die as a result of hyperammonemic coma have prominent cerebral edema and generalized neuronal cell loss on postmortem examination. Histologically, astrocyte swelling was one of the first observations made in an animal model for hepatic encephalopathy, leading to the hypothesis that swollen astrocytes may be the cellular correlate of the brain edema in acute hyperammonemia. In survivors of prolonged coma, changes observed on neuroimaging studies obtained months after the insult include ventriculomegaly with increased sulcal markings, bilateral symmetric low-density white-matter defects, cystic degeneration, injury to the bilateral lentiform nuclei, and diffuse atrophy with sparing of the cerebellum. Neuropathologic findings in those children who subsequently died were consistent with the neuroimaging findings and included ulegyria, cortical atrophy with ventriculomegaly, prominent cortical neuronal loss, gliosis (often with Alzheimer type II astrocytes), and spongiform changes at the gray–white matter interface and in the basal ganglia and thalamus.

MECHANISM OF NEUROPATHOLOGY

The mechanism of ammonia-induced neuropathology remains unclear. Ammonia normally is detoxified in astrocytes by glutamate dehydrogenase and glutamine synthase. Accumulation of ammonia and glutamine in the brain has a number of potentially toxic effects.

Downregulation of Astrocytic Glutamate Transporters

The downregulation of astrocytic glutamate transporters and elevations of extracellular glutamate observed in hyperammonemia have led to the hypothesis that the brain damage is caused by overstimulation of neurons by elevated extracellular glutamate levels, a mechanism of brain damage called excitotoxicity.

Elevated Glutamine Levels

A negative correlation between the height of brain glutamine levels and brain myoinositol levels has been observed, suggesting depletion of the osmolyte myoinositol by high glutamine levels. High brain glutamine levels may have an osmotic effect and cause brain swelling.

Altered Water Transport

Water transport at blood–brain and brain–cerebrospinal fluid interfaces is facilitated by channel proteins called aquaporins. Aquaporin 4 (AQP4) is the main astrocytic water channel, and altered expression of *Aqp4* has been reported in hyperammonemia.

Altered Glucose Metabolism/Disturbed Energy Metabolism

Ammonia stimulates phosphofructokinase, the key enzyme of glycolysis. The ammonium ion (NH_4^+), under physiologic conditions in vivo, may play a significant role in the regulation of glycolysis in astrocytes. Increased ammonia levels, conversely, inhibit α-ketoglutarate dehydrogenase in the brain. Stimulation of phosphofructokinase and inhibition of α-ketoglutarate dehydrogenase, the key enzyme of the citric acid cycle, cause increased formation of lactate and compromised brain energy metabolism.

Interference With the Normal Flux of Potassium Ions

NH_4^+ can cross cell membranes through ion channels or membrane transporters, and it can replace K^+ on different transporters. Downregulation of the major astrocytic water, gap-junction, and potassium channels during hyperammonemia was described in an animal model for UCDs and led to the conclusion that hyperammonemia may disturb potassium and water homeostasis in the brain.

Oxidative and Nitrosative Stress

An increase in free radical production and nitric oxide synthesis causes oxidative/nitrosative (O/N) stress. Ammonia causes free radical production and a decrease in antioxidant enzyme activity. In addition to oxidative stress, there is also nitrosative stress in hyperammonemic encephalopathy, and increased amounts of NO have been found in animal models of hyperammonemia.

DIFFERENTIAL DIAGNOSIS

In the newborn period, hyperammonemia is similar in presentation to a number of acquired conditions, including sepsis, intracranial hemorrhage, and cardiorespiratory disorders. The measurement of plasma ammonia levels is critical to distinguish between these conditions and hence should be a part of the routine evaluation for serious illnesses in the newborn period. Apart from UCDs, a number of other inborn errors of metabolism can cause hyperammonemia. These include organic acidemias, nonketotic hyperglycinemia, congenital lactic acidoses, lysinuric protein intolerance, and defects in fatty acid oxidation. An algorithm for distinguishing between these disorders is presented in Fig. 38-2. Plasma amino acid patterns also are often distinct in the specific types of UCDs and help narrow the diagnosis (Fig. 38-2). Specific enzymatic or DNA analyses may be required in some instances for diagnosis; however, such testing should not delay the initiation of treatment.

In older children and adults, identification of UCDs resulting from partial deficiencies of enzymes has often been delayed through their misdiagnosis as migraine, cyclical vomiting, viral encephalitis, stroke, Reye's syndrome, drug toxicity, child abuse, psychosis, postpartum depression, seizure disorder, and cerebral palsy. Studies have found a mean delay of 8

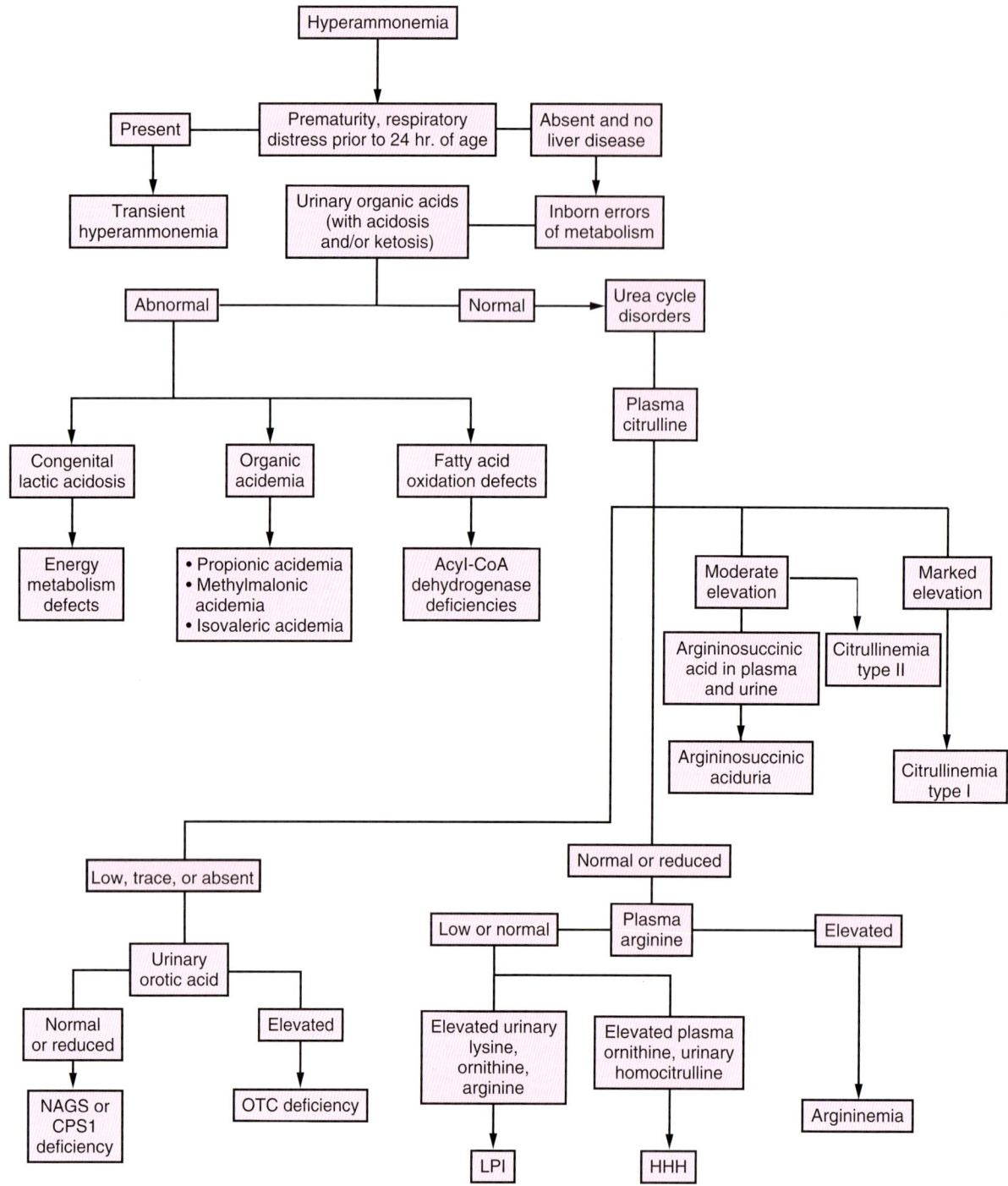

Figure 38-2. Algorithm for differential diagnosis of hyperammonemia. Plasma amino acids, serum lactate, and urinary excretion of orotic acid and organic acids are measured. Acyl-CoA, acyl coenzyme A; CPS1, carbamoyl-phosphate synthase 1; HHH, hyperornithinemia-hyperammonemia-homocitrullinuria syndrome; LPI, lysinuric protein intolerance; NAGS, N-acetylglutamate synthase; OTC, ornithine transcarbamylase.

to 16 months between the onset of symptoms and diagnosis of late-onset UCDs. Plasma ammonia levels may be elevated during symptomatic episodes and normal when the patient is clinically stable.

TREATMENT

Long-term therapy for UCDs consists of dietary modifications, supplementation with urea cycle intermediates (e.g., arginine and citrulline), and use of oral nitrogen-scavenging agents.

Treatment during hyperammonemic crises involves intravenous nitrogen scavengers and hemodialysis. Liver transplantation may be required in individuals who have recurrent metabolic decompensation.

Dietary Therapy

In all UCDs other than citrullinemia type II, a protein-restricted diet should be combined with alternate-pathway therapy unless liver transplantation has been performed. In general, using the minimum daily protein requirement for age is recommended. For neonatal-onset disease, half of the protein is given as an essential amino acid supplement (e.g., Cyclinex, Ross Pharmaceuticals), and the remaining half is provided as natural protein. In children receiving sodium phenylbutyrate, monitoring of branched-chain amino acid levels and supplementation of these as needed has been suggested. Additional calories can be provided via nonprotein formulas, such as Prophree or MJ80056. The diet should be supplemented with vitamins, minerals, and trace elements. Routine monitoring of weight, height, hair, skin, nails, and biochemical indices of nutritional status is recommended.

Alternative-Pathway Therapy

Long-term therapy generally involves protein restriction combined with alternative-pathway therapy (see Table 38-1). Approaches to stimulating alternative pathways of waste nitrogen excretion vary with the site of the enzymatic block. In the case of ASS1 and citrullinemia type II or ASL deficiencies, arginine can stimulate waste nitrogen excretion through enhanced production and excretion of citrulline and argininosuccinic acid, respectively (Batshaw, MacArthur, and Tuchman, 2001). In CPS1 and OTC deficiencies, and in severe deficiencies of ASS1 and ASL, sodium phenylbutyrate has been used to provide an alternative pathway. It initially is converted to sodium phenylacetate, which is then conjugated with glutamine to form phenylacetylglutamine and excreted by the kidney. Sodium phenylbutyrate, although effective, has an unpalatable taste, is a gastric irritant, and has a high sodium load. To circumvent these shortcomings, glycerol phenylbutyrate, a compound that has three molecules of phenylbutyrate attached to a glycerol backbone, was developed. This medication, which is a colorless and odorless oil, was shown to be as efficacious as sodium phenylbutyrate in prevention of hyperammonemia and was recently approved for use in children greater than 2 years of age. ARG1 deficiency typically has been managed with an arginine-restricted diet supplemented with sodium phenylbutyrate when required. Sodium benzoate, a medication that combines with glycine to form hippuric is also used as an alternate-pathway therapy.

N-Carbamyl-L-Glutamate

In NAGS deficiency, administration of *N*-carbamyl-L-glutamate may be an effective therapy because this structural analog of N-acetylglutamate crosses the mitochondrial membrane and activates CPS1. Several patients with NAGS deficiency have been reported to respond clinically to treatment with *N*-carbamyl-L-glutamate.

Liver Transplantation

Long-term treatment of UCDs depends on the severity of the disease. For neonatal-onset severe CPS1 and OTC deficiencies, current clinical guidelines recommend that liver transplantation be considered as a form of enzyme replacement therapy. This procedure usually is performed at 6 to 12 months of age, with use of alternate-pathway therapy before surgery. More recently, and as a result of favorable outcome with liver transplantation, other neonatal-onset and poorly controlled late-onset UCDs also have been considered for this treatment.

The Studies in Pediatric Liver Transplantation (SPLIT) reported on 114 children with UCDs who received a liver transplant between December 1995 and June 2008 (Arnon et al., 2010). The 5-year patient survival rate was 88.7%, and the 5-year graft survival rate was 83.7%. Transplantation corrects most of the metabolic abnormalities in OTC and

CPS1 deficiencies (although citrulline levels remain low) and prevents future hyperammonemic episodes. In terms of morbidity, concerns have included neurodevelopmental delay, and frequent and prolonged hospitalizations for treatment of infections and regulation of immunosuppressive drugs. Overall, however, the reported quality of life has been much improved, with normalization of diet and a decreased frequency of hospital admissions.

Management of Hyperammonemic Crises

In infants with hyperammonemic coma, hemodialysis should be started immediately. In addition, L-arginine HCl (except in hyperargininemia), sodium benzoate, and sodium phenylacetate should be given intravenously.

In children with intercurrent hyperammonemia, treatment involves temporary complete elimination of protein and institution of intravenous administration of sodium benzoate, sodium phenylacetate, and potentially L-arginine. (Caution: Arginine HCl may cause metabolic acidosis, and extravasation may lead to tissue necrosis.) Although these medications are not associated with severe adverse events when they are given at therapeutic doses, severe toxicity and death have resulted from dosing errors. Therefore double-checking of drug administration orders and use of dosing per m² of body surface area in older children and adults are essential. Monitoring of plasma levels of the drug or its metabolites is recommended.

In the event that ammonia levels do not respond to conservative management and biochemical abnormalities or clinical signs and symptoms worsen, hemodialysis or high-flow continuous veno-venous hemofiltration should be initiated. The relative effectiveness of peritoneal dialysis, exchange transfusion, hemodialysis, and continuous arteriovenous hemofiltration has been the subject of some controversy. Yet nitrogen balance studies clearly demonstrate the advantage of hemodialysis, with continuous arterio-venous hemodiafiltration being second best if hemodialysis is unavailable. Hemodialysis or high-flow continuous veno-venous hemofiltration should be continued until ammonia levels fall to 200 μmol/L; continuous hemofiltration should then be used to stabilize the ammonia level and prevent a rebound.

THERAPIES UNDER INVESTIGATION
Hepatocyte Transfer

Infusion of donor hepatocytes into a patient's liver through the portal vein or one of its branches is under investigation as a bridge to liver transplantation in children with severe forms of the disease. This application relies on a proportion of the infused cells to cross the vessel endothelium and to adhere and survive in the liver parenchyma. More studies are required to evaluate the efficacy of this approach. Current research is also exploring biomaterials and induction of liver tissue regeneration as ways to improve engraftment and expansion of the transfused cells. Resection, irradiation, and drug toxicity are being explored as means to induce regeneration.

Gene Therapy

An adeno-associated virus (AAV) vector with the *OTC* cDNA has been created and has been successfully and efficiently delivered to the livers of animal models.

Neuroprotection

A pilot study has assessed the feasibility and safety of whole-body therapeutic hypothermia during rescue treatment for neonatal hyperammonemic coma resulting from metabolic diseases. Further studies are required to assess the efficacy of this procedure in UCDs.

Nitric Oxide Supplementation Therapy

Although there are animal and human data suggesting that NO supplements may be of benefit in ASL deficiency, this has not been evaluated systematically in humans. An ongoing trial is evaluating the effects of short- and long-term NO supplementation on vascular and cognitive features in this disease. (Clinical trials involving UCDs can be found at www.clinicaltrials.gov.)

OUTCOME

Before the development of alternative-pathway therapy, few children with a severe UCD survived infancy. Most died in the newborn period, and the remainder succumbed to intercurrent hyperammonemic episodes or protein malnutrition later in childhood. The mortality and morbidity rates obtained in the 1980s, when the index of suspicion for these disorders was low and a standardized treatment regimen was unavailable, demonstrated 5-year survival rates of approximately 25%; the rate of morbidity (e.g., intellectual disability, seizure disorders) was near universal for infants rescued from hyperammonemic coma. A correlation between intellectual function and duration of hyperammonemic coma rather than the height of the ammonia level was shown. Children in a coma for less than 3 days had a far better outcome than those in a coma for longer periods.

With the general availability of plasma ammonia assays at most hospitals, newborn screening, increased index of suspicion for metabolic disorders, standardized alternative-pathway therapy, and prompt institution of dialysis for neonates at tertiary care centers, the outcome has improved, and it is estimated that 70% of those with neonatal-onset disease and 90% of those with later-onset disease survive their initial crisis. With regard to outcome, the Longitudinal Study of the UCD Consortium recently reported that 66% of children with neonatal-onset UCDs ages 4 years and older and 25% of children with late-onset UCDs have intellectual disability and problems with emotional/behavioral regulation, attention, and executive function (Krivitzky et al., 2009).

SUMMARY

UCDs are inborn errors of hepatic metabolism that can have significant neurologic consequences. Newborn screening programs, a high-degree of suspicion, and a proactive evaluation strategy that routinely incorporates metabolic tests in evaluation of neonates and young children with encephalopathy are critical for appropriate diagnosis. The availability of special diets, medications, dialysis, and hepatic transplantation has improved survival, but long-term intellectual outcomes are far from optimal.

Acknowledgment

Work on which this chapter is based was supported by the following National Institutes of Health (NIH) grants: 5P30HD040677, U54RR019453, M01RR013297. This work was also supported by the Doris Duke Charitable Foundation, Grant #2013095. The project described was supported by Baylor College of Medicine IDDRC Grant Number 1 U54 HD083092 from the Eunice Kennedy Shriver National Institute of Child Health & Human Development. The content is solely the responsibility of the authors and does not necessarily represent the official views of the Eunice Kennedy Shriver National Institute of Child Health & Human Development or the NIH.

REFERENCES

The complete list of references for this chapter is available in the e-book at www.expertconsult.com.
    See inside cover for registration details.

SELECTED REFERENCES

Ah Mew, N., Lanpher, B.C., Gropman, A., et al., 1993–2015. Urea Cycle Disorders Overview. 2003 Apr 29 [Updated 2015 Apr 9]. In: Pagon, R.A., Adam, M.P., Ardinger, H.H., et al. (Eds.), GeneReviews® [Internet]. University of Washington, Seattle, Seattle (WA). Available from: <http://www.ncbi.nlm.nih.gov/books/NBK1217/>.

Arnon, R., et al., 2010. Liver transplantation in children with metabolic diseases: the studies of pediatric liver transplantation experience. Pediatr. Transplant. 14 (6), 796–805.

Batshaw, M.L., MacArthur, R.B., Tuchman, M., 2001. Alternative pathway therapy for urea cycle disorders: twenty years later. J. Pediatr. 138 (1 Suppl.), S46–S54, discussion S54–5.

Brusilow, S., Horwich, A., 2001. The Urea Cycle Enzymes. In: Valle, D., Beaudet, A.L., Vogelstein, B., et al. (Eds.), The Online Metabolic and Molecular Bases of Inherited Disease, eighth ed. The McGraw-Hill Companies. New York McGraw-Hill.

Krivitzky, L., et al., 2009. Intellectual, adaptive, and behavioral functioning in children with urea cycle disorders. Pediatr. Res. 66 (1), 96–101.

Lichter-Konecki, U., Caldovic, L., Morizono, H., et al., 1993–2015. Ornithine Transcarbamylase Deficiency. 2013 Aug 29. In: Pagon, R.A., Adam, M.P., Ardinger, H.H., et al. (Eds.), GeneReviews® [Internet]. University of Washington, Seattle, Seattle (WA). Available from: <http://www.ncbi.nlm.nih.gov/books/NBK154378/>.

Nagamani, S.C.S., Erez, A., Lee, B., 1993–2015. Argininosuccinate Lyase Deficiency. 2011 Feb 3 [Updated 2012 Feb 2]. In: Pagon, R.A., Adam, M.P., Ardinger, H.H., et al. (Eds.), GeneReviews® [Internet]. University of Washington, Seattle, Seattle (WA). Available from: <http://www.ncbi.nlm.nih.gov/books/NBK51784/>.

Quinonez, S.C., Thoene, J.G., 1993–2015. Citrullinemia Type I. 2004 Jul 7 [Updated 2014 Jan 23]. In: Pagon, R.A., Adam, M.P., Ardinger, H.H., et al. (Eds.), GeneReviews® [Internet]. University of Washington, Seattle, Seattle (WA). Available from: <http://www.ncbi.nlm.nih.gov/books/NBK1458/>.

Tuchman, M., et al., 2008. Cross-sectional multicenter study of patients with urea cycle disorders in the United States. Mol. Genet. Metab. 94 (4), 397–402.

Wong, D., Cederbaum, S., Crombez, E.A., 1993–2015. Arginase Deficiency. 2004 Oct 21 [Updated 2014 Aug 28]. In: Pagon, R.A., Adam, M.P., Ardinger, H.H., et al. (Eds.), GeneReviews® [Internet]. University of Washington, Seattle, Seattle (WA). Available from: <http://www.ncbi.nlm.nih.gov/books/NBK1159/>.

39 Diseases Associated with Primary Abnormalities in Carbohydrate Metabolism

Marc C. Patterson

An expanded version of this chapter is available on www.expertconsult.com. See inside cover for registration details.

INTRODUCTION

Carbohydrates are essential elements in the cellular energy economy, and the inability to activate sugars ingested in the diet for use as metabolic fuels (as in the galactosemias), to mobilize glucose from glycogen (as occurs in the glycogen storage diseases), or to oxidize glucose in the glycolytic pathway leads to a variety of phenotypes. The more frequent include symptoms and signs referable to the liver and musculature predominantly and include hepatomegaly, altered volume of skeletal muscle (both increases and decreases), decompensation in the face of stress (manifest as weakness, cramping, and myoglobinuria), and nonspecific manifestations of hypoglycemia. This chapter surveys the primary diseases of carbohydrate metabolism, particularly as they affect the developing nervous system.

ABNORMALITIES OF GALACTOSE METABOLISM
Galactosemia

Galactosemia describes a family of autosomal-recessive disorders characterized by increased blood levels of galactose. Galactose cannot be used directly for glycolysis, and must be converted to glucose-1-phosphate. Five enzymes are involved in this interconversion in most species: galactose mutarotase, galactokinase, galactose-1-phosphate uridyltransferase, uridine diphosphogalactose-4-epimerase, and phosphoglucomutase (Coelho et al., 2015).

Mutations in the *GALK*, *GALT*, and *GALE* genes that encode the second, third, and fourth enzymes, respectively, cause deficiency or absence of these enzymes, with consequent galactosemia (Timson, 2015). These enzymes comprise the Leloir pathway.

Galactose-1-Phosphate Uridyltransferase Deficiency

Galactose-1-phosphate uridyltransferase (GALT) deficiency is by far the most common cause of galactosemia. The incidence of galactosemia in Western Europe varies between 1 in 23,000 and 1 in 44,000. Neonatal screening programs have found population incidence rates as high as 1 in 19,700 in Estonia.

Pathology. The precise link between the metabolic abnormality and the neuropathologic condition remains unknown. Galactose-1-phosphate uridyltransferase is present in the brain in low concentrations. Hypoglycemia may contribute significantly to the pathologic findings in many cases. The toxic effect of galactitol accumulation is not fully understood but is clearly relevant to adverse outcomes in the brain and lens.

Biochemistry. The primary abnormality in galactosemia is the deficiency of activity of galactose-1-phosphate uridyltransferase (Fig. 39-1) that leads to accumulation of galactose-1-phosphate in red blood cells, liver, and brain (Coelho et al., 2015).

Galactose is metabolized through the following four possible pathways:

1. The reduction of galactose to galactitol
2. Oxidation of galactose to galactono-γ-lactone
3. The reaction of galactose-1-phosphate with uridine triphosphate to form uridine diphosphate galactose and eventually glucose-1-phosphate
4. The reaction of galactose-1-phosphate with uridine diphosphate-glucose to form uridine diphosphate-galactose and glucose-1-phosphate

In classic galactosemia, the fourth pathway is obstructed; the other pathways function normally.

The *GALT* locus is at 9p13; various genetic forms of galactosemia result from the presence of inefficient isoenzymes of galactose-1-phosphate uridyltransferase (Table 39-1). Most patients are compound heterozygotes, not true molecular homozygotes.

The isoenzymes are separated and identified by electrophoresis. Transferase activity is absent in homozygous classic galactosemia (Q188R is the most common mutation in the United States). Activity is normal in the Los Angeles variant (L218L). Newborn screening for galactosemia is now performed in every state in the United States, but the detection rate for Duarte galactosemia varies with methodology. The GALT mutation database (http://www.arup.utah.edu/database/galt/GALT_display.php) contained 336 variants when accessed in 2015, most of which were missense mutations.

Clinical Characteristics. Infants usually are normal at birth, except for a slight decrease in birth weight. Symptoms become apparent when milk feedings begin. Jaundice usually develops between 4 and 10 days of age and persists for a longer period than does physiologic jaundice; it may be severe and the hyperbilirubinemia may be indirect, requiring exchange transfusion. Progressive hepatic involvement in the first several weeks causes edema, hepatomegaly, and hypoprothrombinemia. Renal dysfunction is accompanied by generalized aminoaciduria, proteinuria, and acidosis. *Escherichia coli* sepsis is common, and may be the only (and recurrent) feature. Mild hypoglycemia also is common. Cataracts appear between 4 and 8 weeks, reflecting the accumulation of galactose-1-phosphate or galactitol.

Central nervous system impairment is manifested by lethargy and hypotonia, often associated with cerebral edema, which has been correlated with increased brain galactitol on magnetic resonance (MR) spectroscopy. A subgroup of patients may develop marked ataxia and tremor, which does not correlate with cognitive abilities or dietary restriction.

305

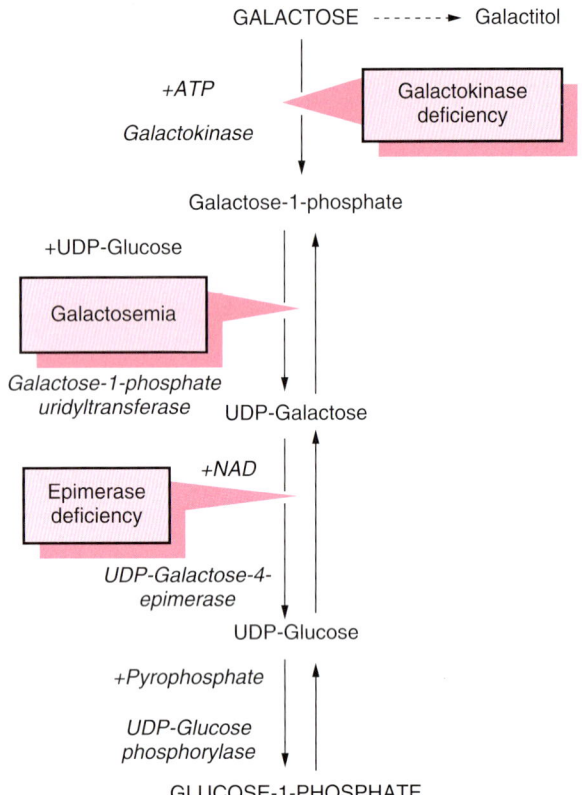

Figure 39-1. Pathway of galactose metabolism depicting sites of metabolic block that lead to galactosemia. ATP, adenosine triphosphate; NAD, nicotinamide adenine dinucleotide; UDP, uridine diphosphate.

TABLE 39-1 Biochemical Criteria for Assigning Phenotypes of Galactosemia*

Galactose-1-Phosphate Uridyltransferase

Activity†	Mobility†	Phenotype	Zygosity
Normal	Normal	Normal	–
Absent	None	Galactosemia (classic form)	Homozygous
Decreased	Duarte (fast)	Duarte variant	Homozygous
Absent	None	African American variant	Homozygous
Decreased	Normal	Galactosemia (classic form)	Heterozygous
Decreased	Slower	Indiana variant	Heterozygous
Much less	Slower	Rennes variant	Heterozygous
Increased	Faster	Los Angeles variant	Heterozygous
Decreased	Fast	Chicago variant	Heterozygous
Decreased	Normal	Munster variant	Heterozygous

*Characteristics of galactose-1-phosphate uridyltransferase.
†Compared with normal.

Galactosemia may prove fatal at any time. Cirrhosis progresses inexorably in patients who do not receive treatment. Gonadal function in women with galactosemia is abnormal and usually manifests as primary ovarian failure.

If treatment is not instituted, moderate to severe intellectual and motor retardation ensue in a majority of cases. Even in patients who are treated adequately, cognitive disability is common.

Clinical Laboratory Tests. Biochemical tests for galactosemia screen for elevated levels of small molecules and directly assay the enzymes in the Leloir pathway.

Bedside urine testing is positive for reducing substances but negative for glucose by the glucose oxidase method. Generalized aminoaciduria, proteinuria, and abnormalities on liver function tests are common.

Magnetic resonance imaging (MRI) shows a variety of findings, including mild cerebral atrophy, cerebellar atrophy, ventriculomegaly, delayed maturation of white matter, and multiple small hyperintense lesions in the cerebral white matter on T2-weighted images.

Management. Because galactose is nonessential, exclusion from the diet is relatively easy. Milk and certain fruits and vegetables contain relatively high concentrations of galactose. Studies of the long-term outcome of therapy have been relatively disappointing, particularly in regard to preservation of central nervous system and ovarian function.

Uridine Diphosphogalactose Epimerase Deficiency

Uridine diphosphogalactose epimerase (GALE) deficiency has conventionally been separated into peripheral and generalized forms. Children previously recognized with generalized (severe) deficiency of GALE (see Fig. 39-1) had manifestations resembling those in classic galactosemia. Most survivors were dysmorphic and deaf. The GALE locus is at 1p36–p35. The patients are either homozygotes or compound heterozygotes for mutations. Three mutations (S81R, T150M, and P293L) have been reported in children with this intermediate form of GALE deficiency. Patients with GALE deficiency require exogenous galactose for the synthesis of glycolipids and glycoproteins.

Galactokinase Deficiency

The birth incidence of galactokinase deficiency varies, ranging from a high of 1 in 52,000 in Bulgaria to 1 in 2,200,000 in Switzerland. Deficiency of galactokinase activity causes a clinical condition similar to that in classic galactosemia. Patients have cataracts and accumulation of galactose. The *GALK1* gene is located at 17q24.

Biochemistry. Galactokinase deficiency causes the accumulation of galactose, which eventually is metabolized to galactitol (see Fig. 39-1). Enzyme activity is reduced rather than absent in erythrocytes. Galactose-1-phosphate does not accumulate.

Clinical Characteristics. In a review of 55 patients, cataract was present in all cases, except for those detected by newborn screening. Thirty-five percent of the patients had other manifestations; only mental retardation and pseudotumor occurred in more than one patient in this series. The mental retardation was thought to be unrelated to the *GALK* deficiency.

Cataracts, the only consistent manifestation of galactokinase deficiency, form in the first months of life.

Management. Treatment consists of elimination of galactose from the diet, as is the case for classic galactosemia.

ABNORMALITIES OF FRUCTOSE METABOLISM
Hereditary Fructose Intolerance

Biochemistry

Fructose is rapidly absorbed from the gut, facilitated by the glucose transporters GLUT 2 and GLUT5, and is metabolized in the liver by the fructokinase pathway, through which it is linked to glycolysis, gluconeogenesis, glycogenolysis, and lipid metabolism. Fructose can also be synthesized endogenously from sorbitol, an important point in management. This condition results from a deficiency of hepatic fructose-1-phosphate aldolase B. The enzyme deficiency is inherited as an autosomal-recessive trait and has an estimated prevalence in central Europe of 1 in 26,100.

Urinary fructose excretion also is present in a harmless metabolic variant resulting from fructokinase deficiency that should not be confused with hereditary fructose intolerance.

Clinical Characteristics and Differential Diagnosis

Patients with hereditary fructose intolerance who ingest fructose experience nausea and vomiting; with continued exposure, weight gain is poor. Hypoglycemia begins immediately and reaches its low point 30 to 90 minutes after ingestion. Subsequent clinical and neuropathologic alterations result primarily from the hypoglycemia.

Neurologic impairment is relatively uncommon but may result from hypoglycemia, cardiovascular collapse, or liver failure. Central nervous system complications include seizures with subsequent epilepsy, increased intracranial pressure, mental retardation, quadriplegia, and deafness.

Clinical Laboratory Tests and Diagnosis

A hydrogen breath test is often employed to screen for HFI but may produce serious adverse effects. Assay of fructose-1-phosphate aldolase B in liver tissue permits definitive diagnosis, but liver biopsy may be avoided by direct genotyping in most patients. Fructosemia causes abnormal glycosylation of transferrin, leading to misdiagnosis of CDG1x on occasion.

Management

Fructose elimination from the diet is accomplished by limited selection of vegetables and cereal products. Sorbitol should also be avoided, as it is an endogenous source of fructose. Dietary counseling is essential for successful therapy.

Fructose-1,6-Diphosphatase Deficiency

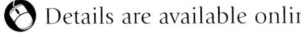 Details are available online.

GLYCOGEN STORAGE DISEASES

The biochemistry of the glycogen storage diseases (GSDs) illustrates the diverse effects of genetically determined enzymatic deficiencies along a single metabolic pathway. In spite of a few inconsistencies and a number of unexplained conditions, a logical approach to these diseases is practical. The GSDs are a family of diseases sui generis, with the exception of at least two disorders that can be included under the rubric of lysosomal diseases—Pompe disease and Danon disease. Indeed, the first lysosomal disease defined as such was Pompe disease. General characteristics of this disease family are discussed in Chapter 41. Patients have also been described who accumulate glycogen in autophagic vacuoles but who do not appear to have an enzymatic deficiency. This phenotype, named Danon disease, is known to result from deficiency of lysosomal-associated membrane protein 2. This X-linked dominant disorder has multisystem effects, most consistently involving the heart and skeletal muscle (Endo et al., 2015).

There is general agreement on the numeric designations of GSDs I to VI, but the nomenclature beyond that is confusing.

For example, GSD types VIII and X were originally considered distinct conditions but are now classified with GSD VI by many authors.

Clinical manifestations of GSD often result from glucose deficiency, with ensuing hypoglycemia occurring separately or in association with increased glycogen storage. The location of the enzymatic block in the pathway determines whether the configuration of the glycogen is normal or abnormal.

GSDs result in the accumulation in various tissues of increased concentrations of glycogen of normal or abnormal configuration (Table 39-2). These diseases result from a deficiency or absence of specific enzyme activity in the metabolic pathway of glycogen.

The glucose molecule is the prime building block in the multistep synthesis of glycogen (Fig. 39-2; see also Table 39-2). Glycogen synthesis occurs in many tissues, predominantly in liver, kidney, and muscle. The details of the metabolic pathway are described online.

Glucose-6-Phosphatase Deficiency (Von Gierke Disease, Glycogen Storage Disease Type I, Hepatorenal Glycogenosis)

Pathology

Patients with von Gierke disease, now known as glycogen storage disease type I, have hepatomegaly and renomegaly. Light microscopy reveals enormous amounts of glycogen in liver cells and in the cells of the renal convoluted tubules. No increase in the concentration of glycogen is found in skeletal muscle, tongue, or heart.

Biochemistry

Two distinct subgroups of glycogen storage disease type I have been identified: those with primary glucose-6-phosphatase deficiency (type Ia) and those phenocopies with additional features of immune impairment (neutropenia and neutrophil adherence defects), now designated as glycogen storage disease type I non-a. Glycogen storage disease type I non-a disorder originally was thought to result from defects in a multicomponent translocase system responsible for transporting glucose-6-phosphatase into microsomes. Cloning of the glucose-6-phosphatase translocase gene (G6PT) demonstrated that the previously proposed subtypes b, c, and d all were associated with mutations in G6PT, producing different kinetic variants. The G6PC gene that codes for glucose-6-phosphatase is located at 17q21.

All forms share common clinical manifestations that are attributable to abnormal metabolism of glucose-6-phosphate. In type Ia, glucose-6-phosphatase deficiency results in storage of glycogen of normal configuration in the liver and kidneys. The enzyme activity is absent or extremely low.

Clinical Characteristics

Hypoglycemia causes much of the morbidity during the first year of life. Seizures are frequent and almost invariably are the presenting complaint of affected children. Hypoglycemia may result in severe, chronic neurologic impairment, including hemiplegia. Hepatomegaly and the failure to thrive syndrome are commonly present. Epilepsy, deafness, and neuroradiologic abnormalities occur far in excess of the rates in the general population or in children with other causes of neonatal hypoglycemia. MRI abnormalities include dilatation of occipital horns and/or hyperintensity of subcortical white matter in the occipital. Subcutaneous fat often is increased, and xanthomas occur over the extensor

TABLE 39-2 Glycogen Storage Diseases (GSDs)

Name*	Clinical Manifestations	Glycogen Structure	Enzyme Defect
1. Glucose-6-phosphatase deficiency (von Gierke disease, Type I GSD)	Enlarged liver and kidneys; hyperlipidemia; hypoglycemia; ketoacidosis; seizures	Normal	Glucose-6-phosphatase
2. Infantile acid α-glucosidase deficiency (Pompe disease, Type II GSD)	Cardiomegaly; death in infancy; progressive hypotonia and weakness; swallowing and respiratory difficulty	Normal	Acid α-Glucosidase
3. Late infantile acid α-glucosidase deficiency, adult acid α-glucosidase deficiency	Atonic anal sphincter; calf muscle hypertrophy; hip weakness (Gowers' sign); slow or regressing motor development, contractures of Achilles tendons	(?)Abnormal—short outer chains	Acid α-Glucosidase
4. Debrancher deficiency (Cori disease; Forbes limit dextrinosis, Type III GSD)	Hepatomegaly; hypoglycemia; late-onset weakness; mild growth failure; early, severe weakness with myopathy rare	Abnormal—short outer chains, increased branch points	Amylo-1,6-glucosidase
5. Brancher deficiency (Andersen's disease, Type IV GSD)	Cirrhosis; growth failure; hepatosplenomegaly; hypotonia; muscle wasting in lower extremities; slow motor development; weakness	Abnormal	Amylo-1,4→1,6-transglucosidase
6. Myophosphorylase deficiency (McArdle disease, Type V GSD)	Atrophy in older patients; myoglobinuria; poor stamina; severe muscle cramps with exercise	Normal	Muscle phosphorylase
7. Hepatophosphorylase deficiency (Hers disease, type VI GSD)	Growth retardation; hepatomegaly; hypoglycemia; mild ketosis	Normal	Liver phosphorylase
8. Phosphorylase kinase deficiency; Type IX GSD (also deficiency of activation sequence including loss of activity of 3′,5′-AMP-dependent kinase in muscle and probably liver); Type IX GSD	Marked hepatomegaly, with glycogen storage; no hypoglycemia; no skeletal muscle disease; normal mental development	Normal	Phosphorylase kinase or 3′,5′-AMP-dependent kinase
9. Phosphoglucomutase deficiency (PGM1-CDG; CDG 1t)	Calf hypertrophy; mild generalized weakness; regression in motor development; toe-walking	Normal	Phosphoglucomutase
10. Phosphohexose isomerase deficiency	Late-onset myopathy; muscle cramps; poor stamina	Normal	Phosphohexose isomerase
11. Phosphofructokinase deficiency (Tarui disease; Type VII GSD) Other defects of terminal glycolysis, including deficiency of phosphoglycerate kinase and lactate dehydrogenase	Similar to those in myophosphorylase deficiency	Normal	Muscle Phosphofructokinase Phosphoglycerate kinase; lactate dehydrogenase
12. Glycogen synthetase deficiency; Type 0 GSD	Hypoglycemia; mental retardation; seizures	Normal	Glycogen synthetase

*The accompanying numerals identify these abnormalities in the pathway of glycogen metabolism shown in Figures 39-2 and 39-3.

surfaces of the limbs and buttocks. Affected children frequently have massive enlargement of the liver. Hepatic adenomas develop in between one-half and three-quarters of adults with glycogen storage disease I; about 10% undergo malignant transformation.

Type I non-a patients typically have recurrent stomatitis, frequent infections, and chronic inflammatory bowel disease secondary to neutropenia and neutrophil dysfunction.

Clinical Laboratory Tests

The diagnosis can be made by assaying the enzyme activity in liver and peripheral white blood cells. Direct assay of hepatic glucose-6-phosphatase activity in liver has been replaced by mutational analysis in most patients.

Severe hypoglycemia frequently occurs because of the failure of glucose formation from glucose-6-phosphate. Severe acidosis is usually associated with lactic acidemia and pyruvic acidemia; hyperuricemia is frequent.

Management

The goal of therapy is to provide sufficient free glucose to maintain a normal blood glucose concentration. Continuous nocturnal intragastric infusion of glucose has been relatively successful, but is challenging for many children. Subsequently, the use of cornstarch suspensions given during the day obviated the need for nocturnal infusion in some children.

Substitution of medium-chain triglycerides for long-chain triglycerides in the diet, along with normal carbohydrate consumption, leads to significant decrease in serum lipid levels, disappearance of eruptive xanthomas, and decrease in liver mass.

Surgical treatment for glucose-6-phosphatase deficiency involves creation of a portacaval shunt, which increases the peripheral blood glucose by allowing portal blood to bypass the liver after absorption of glucose from the gut; excellent metabolic control can be achieved over the long term, and the operation does not preclude subsequent liver transplantation.

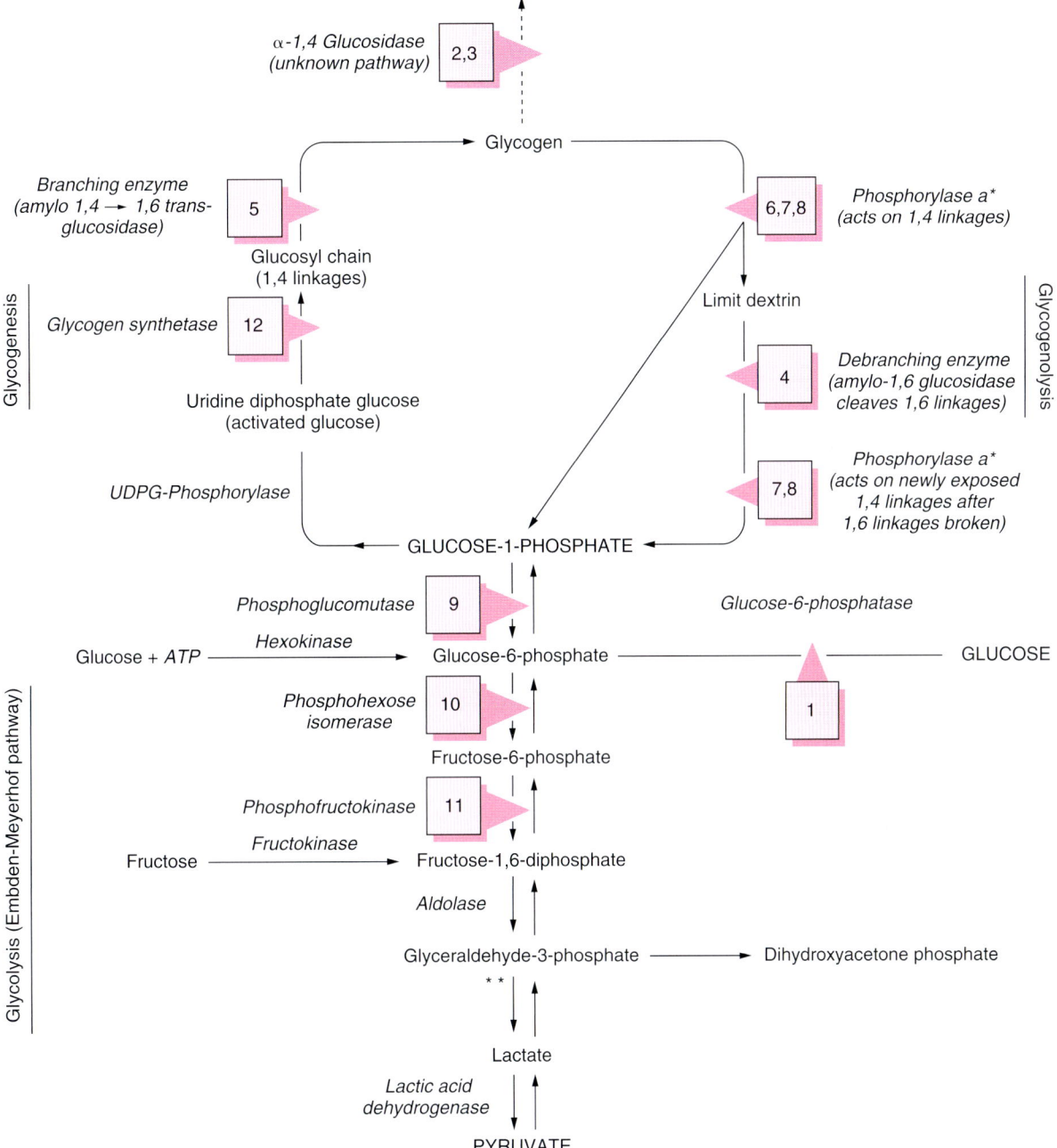

Figure 39-2. Pathways of glycogen metabolism depicting sites of metabolic block that lead to glycogen storage disease. See Table 39-2 for description of abnormalities denoted by Arabic numerals enclosed in boxes. *See Figure 39-3 for phosphorylase activation sequence. **Other defects of terminal glycolysis.

Liver transplantation has been reported to produce beneficial results.

Acid α-Glucosidase (GAA, Acid maltase) Deficiency, Infantile Type (Pompe Disease, Idiopathic Generalized Glycogenosis, Glycogen Storage Disease Type II)

Pathology

Infants with GSD type II have a severe vacuolar myopathy, with accumulation of large amounts of periodic acid–Schiff-positive material within cardiac, skeletal, and smooth muscle fibers and in liver, renal tubules, lymphocytes, glial cells, anterior horn cells, and brainstem nuclei in infantile cases. Storage in later-onset cases is largely restricted to skeletal muscle.

Biochemistry

GSD II is associated with deficient activity of the lysosomal enzyme acid α-glucosidase (α-1,4-glucosidase), located at 17q25.2–q25.3; this is the only enzyme capable of hydrolyzing glycogen to glucose in the acidic environment of the lysosome. Glycogen structure has consistently been normal, and its accumulation is restricted primarily to lysosomes, although lysosomal breakdown and cytoplasmic accumulation with disruption of muscle fibers occur in severe cases. The accumulation of autophagosomes impairs the effectiveness of enzyme replacement therapy by acting as a sink for infused enzyme.

A number of allelic variations have been described and may explain the differences in age at onset. In general, the location and nature of mutations predict the phenotype, but exceptional cases are described in which relatively mild phenotypes occur despite low levels of α-glucosidase expression in cultured fibroblasts.

Clinical Characteristics

Development is usually normal for several weeks to several months; then the affected infant presents with feeding difficulties, weakness, or respiratory impairment (Fig. 39-4). Little spontaneous movement occurs, and the cry is short-lived and weak. Swallowing is grossly limited, and the accessory muscles of respiration are weak. Massive cardiomegaly develops, and a serial echocardiography reveals progressive left ventricular posterior wall diastolic thickening. Hepatomegaly is almost universally present. Subcutaneous fat is sparse, and the muscles are small and firm. The tongue often is enlarged. Deep tendon reflexes are lost by the age of 6 months. Affected infants undergo progressive debilitation, and almost all die by 2 years.

Clinical Laboratory Tests

Acid α-glucosidase (α-1,4-glucosidase) activity can be measured in blood samples or dried blood spots; mutational analysis is increasingly used as a first line diagnostic approach. A urinary glucose tetrasaccharide, Glc-alpha-1,6–Glc-alpha1,4-Glc –alpha-1,4-Glc (Glc4) has proven to be a sensitive biomarker for Pompe disease.

Electromyography (EMG) shows myopathic changes; polyphasic potentials and a reduced interference pattern with low voltage. Unusual high-frequency discharges, best described as myotonic, are very common.

Genetics

GAA deficiency is inherited as an autosomal-recessive trait. The gene for human acid α-glucosidase maps to chromosome 17q25.3; it is approximately 20 kb in length and contains 20 exons. More than 300 mutations have been reported in 2015 and are cataloged online at http://cluster15.erasmusmc.nl/klgn/pompe/mutations.html?lang=en.

Management

Dietary supplementation with L-alanine, designed to reduce the elevated protein turnover characteristic of acid α-glucosidase deficiency, has apparently slowed progression of weakness and even reversed cardiomyopathy in some patients with late infantile and juvenile forms.

In 2006, ERT received Food and Drug Administration (FDA) approval for treatment of acid α-glucosidase deficiency. Infants who received treatment early in the course of their illness demonstrated improved strength and cardiac function, with survival now extending over several years. It has become apparent that ERT is most effective at reversing cardiomyopathy and extending the life span of infants, but that skeletal muscle disease is relatively resistant to this modality (Hahn et al., 2015).

Late Infantile GAA Deficiency

A number of children have been reported who are deficient in acid α-glucosidase activity without the phenotype of Pompe disease. These children are asymptomatic during the first year of life and live beyond the age of 2 years. Most have slowly progressive weakness but no gross signs of overt deposits of glycogen in skeletal or heart muscle or in visceral organs.

Symptoms and signs may mimic those of Duchenne muscular dystrophy (Fig. 39-5). Achilles tendon contractures result in equinus gait. Cardiomegaly is absent, and an intermittent soft, systolic murmur may be heard.

Clinical Laboratory Tests

Light and electron microscopy of muscle biopsy material displays moderate glycogen storage; the glycogen-containing areas appear vacuolated (Fig. 39-6).

EMG documents polyphasic potentials and a reduced, low-voltage interference pattern. The bizarre, myotonic potentials described in early infantile acid α-glucosidase deficiency also occur in the late infantile form.

Biochemistry

Aside from the accumulation of glycogen and its possible abnormal architecture, the most prominent abnormality described is a deficiency of acid α-glucosidase activity.

Management

Attempts to manage patients by dietary means enjoyed modest success after initially disappointing results (see previous mention).

At present, ERT appears to offer the best hope for definitive treatment in this group of patients.

Juvenile and Adult GAA Deficiency

A slowly progressive myopathy characterizes juvenile and adult GAA deficiency. Limb girdle weakness is the most common presentation, but muscle pain is relatively common. Most patients complain of fatigue. Ventilatory failure may be the presenting complaint in as many as one-third of adults, sometimes with predominantly nocturnal symptoms.

Laboratory abnormalities include increased serum enzyme activity of creatine, aspartate aminotransferase, and lactate dehydrogenase. Adult cases cannot be delineated from infantile and late infantile cases on the basis of muscle GAA activity.

Adult patients do not have enlargement of the liver, heart, or tongue.

EMG changes and histologic and electron microscopic findings in muscle biopsy specimens in adult cases are similar to changes in infantile and late infantile cases.

Enzyme replacement therapy tends to slow rather than reverse weakness in late onset cases based on a recent open-label study (Park et al., 2015).

Amylo-1,6-Glucosidase Deficiency (Debrancher Deficiency, Cori Disease, Forbes Disease, Limit Dextrinosis, Glycogen Storage Disease Type III)

Pathology

Electron microscopy of skeletal muscle has demonstrated glycogen deposits just inside the sarcolemmal membrane and between the filaments of the I and A bands, as well as between the myofibrils. These abnormalities are not pathognomonic for this glycogenosis, now classified as glycogen storage disease type III. Glycogen storage in liver is indistinguishable from glycogen storage in other hepatic glycogenoses.

Biochemistry

The human muscle glycogen debranching enzyme (*AGL*) is localized to 1p21. It encodes six isoforms that manifest two distinct functions, both as a debranching enzyme and as a transferase. GSD type III has marked genetic heterogeneity. GSD type IIIa is associated with mutations downstream to exon 3, whereas GSD type IIIb is associated with mutations in exon 3.

Several designated biochemical categories of type III glycogenosis have been identified. In type IIIa deficiency (both transferase and glucosidase deficiency), debranching enzyme activity is either absent or greatly reduced in liver and muscle. When the enzyme activity is deficient in liver alone, the condition is designated type IIIb. Type IIIc patients have deficient glucosidase but not transferase activity.

Myogenic hyperuricemia is common in this condition but is not unique; hyperuricemia also accompanies glycogenosis type V and type VII.

Clinical Characteristics

Infantile Type. Patients with debrancher enzyme deficiency may have muscle or liver involvement, or both. The infantile type usually manifests in the first few months of life and is associated with hypoglycemia, failure to thrive, and hepatomegaly. Affected infants are hypotonic and weak and have poor head control. Glycogen deposition in cardiac muscle is rarely sufficient to create clinical disturbances.

Association of debranching disease with profound cardiac muscle and skeletal muscle involvement accompanied by thyroid insufficiency also has been reported.

Childhood Type. GSD type III presents with exercise intolerance and heart failure. Cardiac and skeletal muscle contains increased stores of glycogen. Branching enzyme deficiency was confirmed with further studies. Hyperlipidemia, hypertriglyceridemia, and reduced bone density may all occur.

Adult Type. Debrancher enzyme deficiency also occurs in older children and adults. Adult patients with GSD type III manifesting as chronic progressive myopathy in middle age have been described; they account for a minority of this population. Progression of muscle disease can be monitored with serial ultrasound examinations. Patients with debrancher deficiency should be monitored for cardiac involvement, although this is usually asymptomatic. Progressive cirrhosis may be more common in adult GSD type III than was previously recognized and, occasionally, is complicated by hepatocellular carcinoma.

Debrancher deficiency is often associated with hypotonia and hepatomegaly. Later in childhood, patients complain of muscle fatigue without tenderness, cramping, or associated hematuria. Persistent diffuse weakness is present, and wasting of the hand and forearm muscles with loss of body weight ensues. Patients may experience recurrent seizures.

Clinical Laboratory Tests

Electromyography and nerve conduction studies show no evidence of peripheral neuropathy, but myopathic discharges are common. Serum creatine kinase activity may increase before and after exercise. Fasting ketotic hypoglycemia is characteristic of GSD, type III; hypertriglyceridemia, hyperlactic acidemia, and hyperuricemia may be observed. Blood lactic acid does not increase on ischemic exercise.

Genetics

GSD type III is inherited as an autosomal-recessive trait. The diagnosis is generally confirmed by gene sequencing.

Management

Patients with growth failure and hepatic dysfunction, including hypoglycemia, appear to benefit from the administration of oral cornstarch, but overtreatment with carbohydrates may be harmful. Cardiomyopathy has been shown to improve with either a high protein or ketogenic/high protein diet.

Amylo-1, 4 →1,6 Transglucosidase Deficiency (Brancher Enzyme Deficiency, Glycogen Storage Disease Type IV)

GSD type IV (Andersen disease) results from a deficiency of glycogen branching enzyme (GBE), leading to the accumulation of abnormal glycogen resembling amylopectin in affected tissues. The reported phenotypes are marked primarily by liver involvement. GSD type IV has been characterized as the most heterogeneous of the glycogen storage diseases (Magoulas and El-Hattab, 1993).

Pathology

Glycogen may accumulate disproportionately in the tongue and diaphragm in comparison with other striated muscles. The characteristic lesion is the polyglucosan body, a periodic acid–Schiff-positive inclusion that also is seen in phosphofructokinase deficiency, Lafora body disease, double athetosis (Bielschowsky bodies), and aging (corpora amylacea).

Biochemistry

The first patient described with deficiency of brancher enzyme activity manifested cirrhosis of the liver and glycogen accumulation, but patients with normal and decreased muscle glycogen concentrations also have been described. These biochemical phenotypes correspond to clinical forms with rapidly progressive cirrhosis through nonprogressive liver disease. Brancher enzyme deficiency results in the synthesis of unbranched glycogen composed of elongated chains of glucose molecules joined together in 1,4 linkages. As a result, the glycogen is composed of long outer chains, has few branch points, and resembles the pattern of starch also known as amylopectin.

Clinical Characteristics

Manifestations of the disease—failure to thrive, hepatosplenomegaly, and liver failure with cirrhosis—usually appear in the first 6 months of life. Affected infants exhibit delayed motor and social development, hypotonia, weakness, and muscle atrophy, accompanied by absent or decreased deep tendon reflexes. Fetal onset with cervical cystic hygroma, akinesia, polyhydramnios and multiple pterygia is the most severe manifestation of GSD IV. A mild, predominantly myopathic variant has been reported in older children and has a highly variable course. Adults with polyglucosan body disease who manifest late-onset pyramidal quadriparesis, micturition difficulties, peripheral neuropathy, and mild cognitive impairment have been described. Jewish families with adults with polyglucosan body disease were homozygous for a Tyr329Ser mutation in *GBE1*. Not all such patients have recognized *GBE* mutations or impaired GBE activity, suggesting both phenotypic and genotypic heterogeneity.

Clinical Laboratory Tests

Diagnosis of brancher deficiency by assay of peripheral white blood cells, skin fibroblasts, and amniotic cell activity is feasible, but diagnosis by mutational analysis is usually preferable.

Genetics

Inheritance is autosomal-recessive. Prenatal testing using cultured amniocytes and chorionic villi is feasible, but has been superseded by molecular analysis when available. The gene encoding brancher enzyme, GBE1, may contain missense, nonsense, intronic donor and acceptor splice-site mutations, small deletion frame shift mutations, small insertion frame shift mutations, or large deletions. Missense mutations are more likely to be associated with milder phenotypes, and truncating mutations or large deletions with severe forms of the disease.

Management

Attempts at enzyme replacement were unsuccessful. Liver transplantation has been successful in a number of patients, but mortality in GSD IV patients may be high.

McArdle Disease (Myophosphorylase Deficiency, Glycogen Storage Disease Type V)

In 1951, McArdle reported a condition characterized by weakness, fatigue, and severe muscle cramping with pain after exercise. He subsequently noted the lack of normal lactate production in the affected muscles after ischemic work. McArdle disease is classified as glycogen storage disease type V (GSD V).

Pathology

Light microscopic studies of muscle reveal moderately increased stores of glycogen beneath the sarcolemmal membrane. Electron microscopy demonstrates disorganization of the I band region and distortion of the myofibrils secondary to glycogen deposition. Quantitative biochemical studies show reduced or absent myophosphorylase activity.

Biochemistry

Glycogen breakdown to lactate begins with the initial disruption of the 1,4 linkage between glucosyl units. The enzyme myophosphorylase facilitates this reaction in skeletal muscle. After this linkage is cleaved, glucose-1-phosphate is freed and metabolized to lactate through the Embden-Meyerhof pathway. The myophosphorylase enzyme is regenerated in a complex reaction involving a number of other enzymes, including phosphorylase kinase (see Fig. 39-3).

Absence of myophosphorylase activity results in decreased glucose-1-phosphate production; as a result, lactic acid is not formed in exercised muscle, and serum lactic acid concentration is not appropriately elevated (Fig. 39-7).

Clinical Characteristics

Affected children have decreased stamina and tire easily. Severe cramping pain after minimal exercise is noted in the involved skeletal muscles. Cardiac symptoms are not usually reported, but cardiac muscle is involved. Myoglobinuria occurs with moderate or strenuous exercise. In adolescence and adulthood, persistent weakness may develop, with moderate loss of muscle bulk. A "second wind" phenomenon has been described. This phenomenon has been attributed to improved energy production when metabolic dependence switches from glycogen stores to blood-borne fuels, including glucose and fatty acids, and is consistently seen in GSD type V but not in GSD type VII, whose phenotype is otherwise indistinguishable. Prolonged or frequent repetitive episodes of myoglobinuria may result in both acute and chronic renal failure.

Onset usually is in childhood; neonatal and adult onset has been reported. A very severe phenotype, lethal in infancy, was reported in a child born to consanguineous parents with mutations in both *PYGM* and *dGK*, the gene encoding deoxyguanosine kinase, whose deficiency causes the hepatic form of mitochondrial depletion syndrome.

Clinical Laboratory Tests

Exercise results in elevated serum creatine kinase activity and increase in activity of other serum enzymes released from muscle, ostensibly a result of loss of sarcolemmal membrane integrity. The ECG may demonstrate an increased QRS amplitude, a prolonged R-S interval, T wave inversion, and bradycardia.

Electromyographic study of contracted muscles after exercise reveals a decreased interference pattern; after ischemic exercise, the contracted muscles may demonstrate no electrical activity.

Ischemic exercise testing is described online.

Genetics

The gene encoding synthesizing myophosphorylase, *PYGM*, is located at 11q13. A number of mutations have been described but do not appear to explain the clinical heterogeneity of GSD type V. A initial study of potential genetic modifiers found a strong association between angiotensin-converting enzyme genotype and clinical phenotype, suggesting that angiotensin-converting enzyme is a modifier of *PYGM*; a further study also found that female gender conferred a more severe phenotype. GSD V is transmitted as an autosomal-recessive trait and may manifest in a heterozygote.

Management

A controlled trial of oral sucrose loading showed improved exercise tolerance and stable glucose levels in 12 adults with GSD type V. Although not suitable for continuous use owing to its tendency to induce weight gain, this regimen, combined with aerobic conditioning, appears likely to be useful in improving performance under stressful conditions and may protect against acute rhabdomyolysis. A review of published trials found that there was low-quality evidence of improvement in some disease measures with creatine, sucrose, ramipril, and a carbohydrate rich diet but no unequivocal evidence of clinical benefit (Quinlivan et al., 2014).

Hepatophosphorylase Deficiency (Hers Disease, Glycogen Storage Disease Type VI)

Biochemistry

GSD type VI was described by Hers in 1959 and is characterized by increased glycogen stores of normal configuration in the liver. Hepatic phosphorylase (hepatophosphorylase) activity is diminished or absent.

Because of the possibility of abnormalities in the complex activating mechanism of hepatophosphorylase, systematic study of enzyme activity in suspected hepatophosphorylase deficiency is necessary to exclude phosphorylase kinase deficiency and other metabolic errors in the activating sequence.

GSD VI could only be diagnosed by enzymology of liver tissue until the *PYGL* gene was identified. A series of eight patients with GSD VI from seven families were studied and found to harbor 11 novel mutations, most of which were missense. The patients' symptoms ranged from hepatomegaly and subclinical hypoglycemia, to severe hepatomegaly with recurrent severe hypoglycemia and postprandial lactic acidosis.

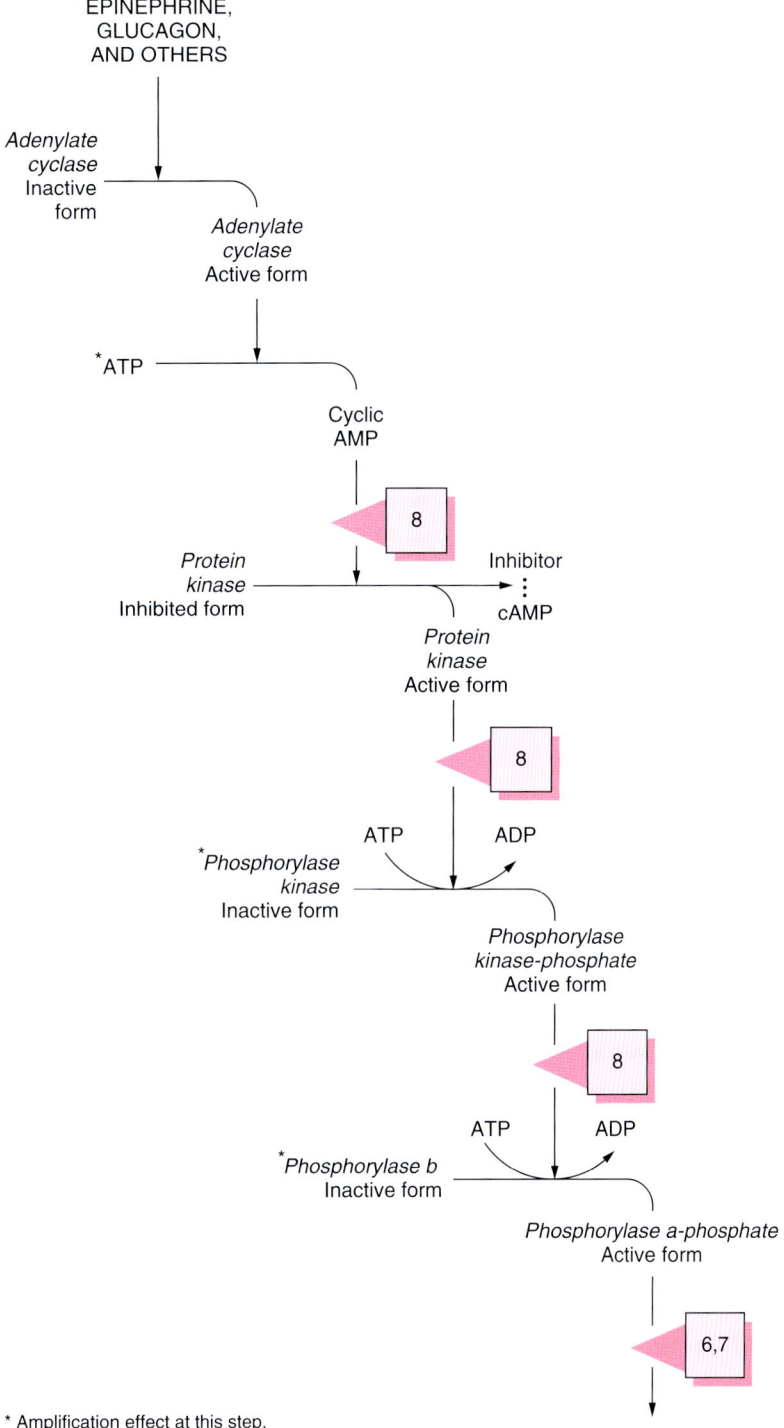

* Amplification effect at this step.

Figure 39-3. Activation sequence of phosphorylase. See Table 39-2 for description of abnormalities denoted by the Arabic numerals enclosed in boxes. ADP, adenosine diphosphate; ATP, adenosine triphosphate; cAMP, cyclic adenosine monophosphate. *(Modified from Goldberg, N.B., 1974. Vigilance against pathogens. Hosp Pract 9, 127.)*

Clinical Characteristics

The patients display various degrees of growth retardation, hypoglycemia, ketosis, and hepatomegaly. Specific neurologic findings are absent. Muscle and cardiovascular tissues are not primarily involved.

Genetics

The gene coding for the enzyme liver glycogen phosphorylase is located on chromosome 14 at 14q21–22. The condition is transmitted as an autosomal-recessive trait. Most mutations are missense; there are no common mutations.

Management

Symptoms can be controlled with frequent small carbohydrate meals. No other forms of therapy have been necessary or recommended.

Muscle Phosphofructokinase Deficiency (Tarui Disease, Glycogen Storage Disease Type VII)

Biochemistry

The enzyme phosphofructokinase transforms fructose-6-phosphate to fructose-1,6-diphosphate. Decreased activity of this enzyme results in increased muscle glycogen stores of normal structure and increased concentration of glucose-6-phosphate and fructose-6-phosphate (Musumeci et al., 2012). Phosphofructokinase exists in five different isoforms with tissue-specific distribution.

Clinical Characteristics

Motor development is normal during the first decade, but patients experience decreased exercise tolerance and easy fatigability during childhood. They complain of muscle stiffness and weakness and, occasionally, muscle cramps. Myoglobinuria may follow moderate to strenuous exercise and has precipitated acute renal failure. The clinical pattern is reminiscent of McArdle disease, except for the absence of a "second wind" phenomenon in GSD type VII.

Physical examination in patients with GSD type VII is unremarkable, except for variable weakness and loss of skeletal muscle bulk.

Clinical Laboratory Tests

After exercise, serum creatine kinase and other serum enzymes released from muscle may be elevated. EMG findings may be normal. Ischemic exercise testing, as described earlier for McArdle disease, results in muscle contracture and decreased lactic acid production. The definitive diagnosis is made by enzymatic assay of muscle tissue.

Genetics

The phosphofructokinase gene (*PFKM*) is encoded at 12q13.3. GSD type VII is prevalent in Ashkenazim; 95% of mutant alleles in this population are accounted for by a splicing mutation in exon 5 (IVS5 + 1 G>A) or a single nucleotide deletion (del C2003).

Hepatic Phosphorylase Kinase Deficiency (Glycogen Storage Disease, type IX) and Activation Abnormalities

Some patients with glycogen storage disease have defects in control of the phosphorylase system at the phosphorylase kinase level, rather than a deficiency of the phosphorylase enzyme (see Fig. 39-3). Although they appear to have hepatic phosphorylase deficiency disease, further studies identify the presence of the enzyme when activation cycle materials are added in vitro.

Phosphorylase kinase has a hexadecameric structure: (α, β, γ, δ) 4. The δ subunit is calmodulin, which interacts with calcium. The α subunit is encoded by *PHKA2* (at Xp22), the β subunit by *PHKB*, and the γ subunit by *PHKG2*. Mutations in these three genes have been associated with phosphorylase kinase deficiency and a GSD phenotype. Current nomenclature subdivides phosphorylase kinase deficiency into four types, GSD IX a through d.

Most cases are grouped together as GSD IXa, X-linked liver glycogenosis, or PHKA2- related phosphorylase kinase deficiency. This relatively mild phenotype most often presents with hepatomegaly in childhood, associated with fasting hypoglycemia, growth and motor delays. Hyperketotic hypoglycemia may be associated with nausea and vomiting; transaminases are often elevated. Some patients experience liver fibrosis or cirrhosis.

GSD IXb affects liver and muscle and is associated with mutations in PHKB. Liver manifestations usually predominate, and weakness is not apparent in some patients. Hypoglycemia and short stature are also encountered.

Phosphorylase kinase deficiency type c (GSD IXc) has a phenotype very similar to types a and b, but generally more severe. The PHKG2 gene is mutated; inheritance is autosomal recessive. Splenomegaly may occur, and the risk of cirrhosis may be greater than in the preceding types.

The least common form of phosphorylase kinase deficiency (GSD IXd) is a pure muscle form, associated with mutatins in PHKA1in which the liver is unaffected. The phenotype is characterized by progressive weakness, cramps, and pain after exercise. Most cases present in adults, although earlier onset has been reported. Some patients with the genetic and biochemical defect may be asymptomatic.

There are no systematic studies of therapy in type IX glycogen storage disease.

Phosphohexose Isomerase Deficiency (Satoyoshi Disease)

Phosphohexose isomerase is also known as glucose phosphate isomerase and phosphoglucose isomerase. This enzyme catalyzes the interconversion of glucose-6-phosphate and fructose-6-phosphate in the Embden-Meyerhof pathway. Most reported cases of deficiency of this enzyme have been manifested as hemolytic anemia, but a few kindreds have been reported with skeletal muscle dysfunction.

Satoyoshi and associates described a family whose members experienced muscle pain and stiffness with exercise beginning in childhood. The symptoms become more prominent in later life. Muscle contractures do not occur after ischemic exercise. Routine examination is normal. Heavy exercise leads to stiffness and tenderness of the muscles without apparent weakness. Lactic acid does not increase during ischemic exercise and serum creatine kinase is increased, but findings on EMG remain normal.

GPI has been assigned to 19cen–q12. It consists of 18 exons and is 40 kb in length. The gene codes for two proteins in addition to hexose phosphate isomerase: neuroleukin, a chemokine, and autocrine motility factor. Antibodies to glucose phosphate isomerase have been shown to sustain a rheumatoid arthritis-like condition in experimental animals and humans. A Japanese report summarized the expanded phenotype of Satoyoshi disease, which includes painful muscle cramps, alopecia, intractable diarrhea, bone and joint deformity, and endocrine disturbances.

Phosphoglucomutase Deficiency (Thomson Disease)

The phosphoglucomutases are a family of enzymes catalyzing the interconversion of glucose-1-phosphate and fructose-1-phosphate. The first recognized case presented in early infancy. This was a boy who experienced numerous episodes of supraventricular tachycardia, requiring digitoxin treatment; development then proceeded normally until the age of 2 years, when he began to walk on his toes. Examination revealed mild weakness and poor muscle development. His calf muscles were bulky and firm, and shortening of the Achilles tendons was noted. No clinical history of exercise intolerance, muscle pain, or myoglobinuria was elicited. Serum enzyme activities, including creatine kinase, aldolase, glutamic-oxaloacetic transaminase, and glutamic-pyruvic transaminase, were elevated. Examination by EMG showed myopathic changes.

In vitro study of biopsy tissue indicated a number of relative enzymatic deficiencies, but phosphoglucomutase deficiency was most pronounced. Glycogen structure appeared normal. Also evident was extensive replacement of muscle tissue by glycogen.

A 35-year-old man with exercise-induced cramps, mild limb girdle weakness, episodes of rhabdomyolysis, normal elevation of lactate, and hyperammonemia on a forearm-exercise test has also been reported. The investigators suggested that this disorder should be designated glycogenosis type XIV, a suggestion which has not been widely accepted, given the already confusing state of glycogenosis nomenclature. A follow up study of this patient, two others identified by an independent group and sixteen new patients, described the findings in a total of 19 patients (Tegtmeyer et al., 2014). Although the phenotypes were highly variable, all had evidence of liver disease, with elevated transaminases, and, in some cases, steatosis or fibrosis. Most had clinical muscle disease, with weakness and exercise intolerance. Five subjects had experienced rhabdomyolysis. Dysmorphic features included cleft palate and bifid uvula. Cardiomyopathy, short stature, and delayed puberty occurred in fewer than half of the subjects. Laboratory abnormalities included elevated creatine kinase and hypoglycemia. This spectrum of findings is highly suggestive of a congenital disorder of glycosylation (see Chapter 40), and these patients were found to have mixed type I and type II patterns of transferrin glycoforms. Oral galactose treatment improved these laboratory abnormalities in some patients, with resolution of hypogonadotropic hypogonadism in two girls. This disorder is now designated PGM1-CDG (CDG 1t using the older nomenclature).

Other Defects of Glycolysis Causing Glycogen Storage

Three enzyme defects affecting the terminal glycolysis pathway have been reported, involving phosphoglycerate kinase, phosphoglycerate mutase, and lactate dehydrogenase. Phosphoglycerate kinase deficiency is an X-linked disorder manifesting with varying combinations of hemolytic anemia, seizures, mental retardation, and exercise intolerance with myoglobinuria. Up to 2007, 26 families had been reported.

Phosphoglycerate mutase deficiency (PGAMD—glycogen storage disease, type X) has been associated in adults with myalgia, cramps, and myoglobinuria after exercise. Twelve well-verified patients had been described by 2009, nine of whom were African American. A patient with PGAMD who experienced muscle cramps on forearm ischemic exercise testing was protected from cramps by dantrolene, suggesting that cramps in this disease reflect excessive calcium release from the sarcoplasmic reticulum relative to calcium reuptake capacity.

Lactate dehydrogenase M subunit deficiency has been reported in three families with exertional myoglobinuria. Additional cases have been identified, and a number of mutations identified in the responsible.

Defects Impairing Glycogen Formation

Muscle glycogen storage disease (glycogen storage disease, type 0) results from deficiency of glycogen synthase 1, encoded by the GYS 1 gene. Glycogen synthase 1 catalyzes the addition of glucose monomers to the glycogen molecule through alpha-1,4-glycoside linkages. Three families have been reported. Clinical manifestations include exercise intolerance and cardiac disease (leading to seizures and sudden death associated with long QT syndrome in the index case), recurrent syncope, weakness, and muscle pain.

Mutations in GYG1, which encodes glycogenin, may also cause muscle glycogen depletion. Glycogenin is required to activate glycogen synthesis; glucose molecules attach to glycogenin to form oligosaccharide chains. The index case was a 27-year-old man who experienced palpitations and dizziness after exercise. He had mild proximal arm, shoulder, and trunk weakness, and an abnormal ECG; an echocardiogram was normal. Skeletal muscle biopsy showed profound depletion of glycogen; endomyocardial biopsy demonstrated hypertrophic cardiomyocytes with enlarged nuclei and central vacuoles. The term glycogen storage disease, type XV was suggested for this entity. Seven adult patients have since been described with a slowly progressive myopathy; in these cases, muscle biopsy demonstrated polyglucosan bodies.

CONCLUSIONS

The disorders of carbohydrate metabolism are a large, heterogeneous group, which are most likely to present to the child neurologist with manifestations of a metabolic myopathy. The presence of cardiac, hepatic, or hematologic abnormalities is often helpful in guiding the practitioner to the correct diagnosis. Although molecular testing is increasingly available to accurately diagnose these disorders (Wang et al., 2013), many still require sophisticated biochemical investigation, electrodiagnostic testing and tissue biopsy—guided, as always, by a complete and accurate history and careful physical examination.

REFERENCES

The complete list of references for this chapter is available in the e-book at www.expertconsult.com.
See inside cover for registration details.

SELECTED REFERENCES

Coelho, A.I., Berry, G.T., et al., 2015. Galactose metabolism and health. Curr. Opin. Clin. Nutr. Metab. Care 18 (4), 422–427.

Endo, Y., Furuta, A., et al., 2015. Danon disease: a phenotypic expression of LAMP-2 deficiency. Acta Neuropathol. 129 (3), 391–398.

Hahn, A., Praetorius, S., et al., 2015. Outcome of patients with classical infantile pompe disease receiving enzyme replacement therapy in Germany. JIMD Reports 20, 65–75.

Magoulas, P.L., El-Hattab, A.W., 1993. Glycogen Storage Disease Type IV. In: Pagon, R.A., Adam, M.P., Ardinger, H.H., et al. (Eds.), GeneReviews. University of Washington, Seattle. Available at: <http://www.ncbi.nlm.nih.gov/pubmed/23285490>.

Musumeci, O., Bruno, C., et al., 2012. Clinical features and new molecular findings in muscle phosphofructokinase deficiency (GSD type VII). Neuromuscul. Disord. 22 (4), 325–330.

Park, J.S., Kim, H.G., et al., 2015. Effect of enzyme replacement therapy in late onset Pompe disease: open pilot study of 48 weeks follow-up. Neurol. Sci. 36 (4), 599–605.

Quinlivan, R., Martinuzzi, A., et al., 2014. Pharmacological and nutritional treatment for McArdle disease (Glycogen Storage Disease type V). Cochrane Database Syst. Rev. (11), CD003458.

Tegtmeyer, L.C., Rust, S., et al., 2014. Multiple phenotypes in phosphoglucomutase 1 deficiency. N. Engl. J. Med. 370 (6), 533–542.

Timson, D.J., 2015. The molecular basis of galactosemia—past, present, and future. Gene doi:10.1016/j.gene.2015.06.077; Jul 2, pii: S0378-1119(15)00801-X.

Wang, J., Cui, H., et al., 2013. Clinical application of massively parallel sequencing in the molecular diagnosis of glycogen storage diseases of genetically heterogeneous origin. Genet. Med. 15 (2), 106–114.

◎ E-BOOK FIGURES AND TABLES

The following figures and tables are available in the e-book at www.expertconsult.com. See inside cover for registration details.

Fig. 39-4 This 8-month-old infant with infantile acid α-glucosidase deficiency (Pompe disease) is profoundly hypotonic and weak.

Fig. 39-5 This 22-month-old child with late infantile acid α-glucosidase deficiency has increased lumbar lordosis, pseudohypertrophy of the calf muscles, and contractures of the Achilles tendons.

Fig. 39-6 Infantile acid α-glucosidase deficiency.

Fig. 39-7 This line graph reflects the failure of increase in blood lactic acid concentration during ischemic exercise of the arm in a patient with McArdle disease.

40 Disorders of Glycosylation

Hudson H. Freeze, Bobby G. Ng, and Marc C. Patterson

An expanded version of this chapter is available on www.expertconsult.com. See inside cover for registration details.

Eukaryotic cells synthesize hundreds of types of sugar chains called glycans, which function within the cell, at the cell surface, and beyond. Within the cell, glycans influence protein folding, stability, turnover, and intracellular trafficking (Varki and Lowe, 2009). At the cell surface, they influence or determine cell-cell binding, receptor-ligand interactions, assembly of signaling complexes, binding to the extracellular matrix, tissue pattern formation, trafficking of lymphocytes, and much more (Varki and Lowe, 2009). The same glycan can function differently on different proteins or in different settings. This three-dimensional complexity makes understanding the roles of glycans challenging, but provides the body with an extraordinarily sensitive fine-tuning mechanism for many physiologic functions. It is not surprising that disrupting normal glycosylation causes moderate to severe pathology in multiple human organ systems.

Well over 100 rare inherited disorders of glycan biosynthesis have been identified. Most of these are called congenital disorders of glycosylation (CDG) (previously called carbohydrate-deficient glycoprotein syndrome). Others such as muscle-eye-brain disease and Walker-Warburg syndrome were well known, but elucidation of their relation to glycosylation has provided new insights into their pathophysiology and opens new therapeutic possibilities.

DEFINING TYPES OF GLYCOSYLATION

Glycan linkage to proteins or lipids defines the biosynthetic pathway. Most CDG defects occur in the N-linked pathway that couples asparagine (Asn) to N-acetylglucosamine (GlcNAc). O-linked glycans occur in many linkages, but mannose (Man) O-Man glycans bound to threonine/serine (Thr/Ser) cause muscle-eye-brain disease and some cases of Walker-Warburg syndrome. A few disorders result from mutations that impair the synthesis of glycosphingolipids, and those deficient in glycophosphatidylinositol (GPI) anchors comprise a rapidly expanding group. Defects in Golgi homeostasis and intracellular trafficking also cause CDG. We focus on glycosylation abnormalities that cause neurologic disorders. Defects in dystroglycan O-Man glycosylation (dystroglycanopathies) are described in Chapter (49).

N-LINKED GLYCOSYLATION
Overview

Sugar chains are added to newly synthesized proteins in the lumen of the endoplasmic reticulum; most are quickly and extensively remodeled there and, later on, in the Golgi apparatus. All eukaryotic cells make a 14-sugar, lipid-linked oligosaccharide in the endoplasmic reticulum membrane that is composed of Man, GlcNAc, and glucose (Glc). This entire chain is transferred to Asn within an Asn-X-Thr/Ser/Cys consensus sequence (X is any amino acid except proline) concurrently or shortly after newly made proteins emerge from the ribosome into the endoplasmic reticulum lumen. Over 50 genes are required to synthesize and transfer this glycan to proteins.

Remodeling begins soon after sugar chain transfer. Up to two-thirds of the original lipid-linked oligosaccharide glycan is discarded, and 6 to 15 other sugar units are then added to create a dazzling array of sugar chains. Why generate this complex process? The initial glycan helps proteins fold and also provides important checkpoints for monitoring proper protein folding in the endoplasmic reticulum. The addition of more sugars in the Golgi usually imparts greater specificity to the sugar chain function.

Biosynthesis

Individual monosaccharides can be synthesized from glucose, derived from the diet, or salvaged from degraded glycans. They must be activated to their nucleotide sugar derivatives to construct glycans. The top of Figure 40-1 depicts the pathway for mannose using standard symbols for the sugar (Varki, et al., 2009). Monosaccharide phosphorylation is the first step, and some pathways interconvert phosphorylated forms such as Man-6-P→Man-1-P. Other routes generate uridine diphosphate (UDP)-GlcNAc, UDP-galactose (Gal), and guanosine diphosphate (GDP)-fucose (Fuc) for adding these sugars. For some types of glycosylation, the nucleotide sugar donates the sugar to a lipid carrier dolichol phosphate (P-Dol). These products include Man-P-Dol and Glc-P-Dol. Dolichol itself is made from polyprenols using a specific reductase.

N-Linked Glycan Biosynthesis

The lipid precursor is built stepwise, adding sugars in specific linkages and in a specific order (Freeze and Elbein, 2009) as shown in Figure 40-1. It begins with P-Dol + UDP-GlcNAc forming GlcNAc-P-P-Dol on the cytosolic face of the endoplasmic reticulum. Another UDP-GlcNAc donates a second GlcNAc using a different GlcNAc transferase, and this is followed by the addition of five Man units derived from GDP-Man. A "flippase" reorients the entire molecule from the cytosolic face into the endoplasmic reticulum lumen in which a series of Man transferases use Man-P-Dol to add four more Man units, to make a three-branched structure. Three glucosyltransferases sequentially add Glc from Glc-P-Dol to one branch to complete the sugar chain. This 14-sugar unit molecule is the optimal substrate for the 8-subunit oligosaccharyl transferase (OST) complex that recognizes the Asn-X-Thr/Ser/Cys consensus sequence on the protein and adds the sugar chain to Asn. Post transfer, the P-P-Dol is converted back to P-Dol and then to Dol for recycling.

Within a few minutes of transfer to protein, the sugar chain is processed (Fig. 40-1) using a set of two glucosidases that remove the Glc units. For some proteins, processing stops here; however, for the majority, a series of α-mannosidases in the endoplasmic reticulum and Golgi remove up to six Man units, and UDP-GlcNAc, UDP-Gal and CMP-Sialic acid (Sia) and GDP-Fuc donate their respective sugars to multiple branches

317

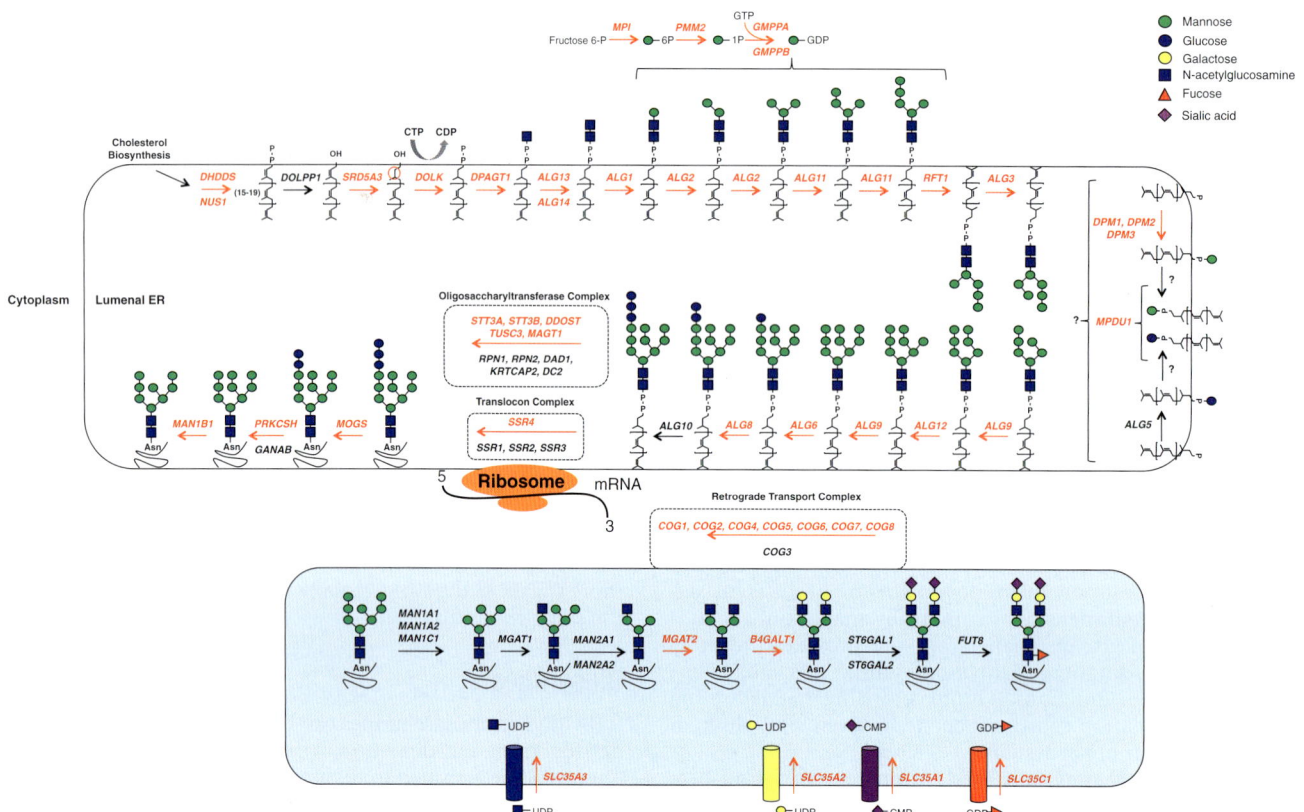

Figure 40-1. N-linked glycan synthesis. The biosynthesis and assembly of the lipid-linked oligosaccharide precursor (LLO), its transfer to protein, and subsequent processing are presented here. The first steps involve the activation and interconversion of monosaccharides such as mannose to form sugar donors, the nucleotide sugars or phosphoryldolichols. Dolichol phosphate serves as the lipid carrier for the sugar chain, which is synthesized in a series of precisely ordered steps that involve addition of N-acetylglucosamine, mannose, and glucose. The completed glycan is transferred to proteins. After transfer to proteins, oligosaccharide processing begins by removing all three glucose units and a mannose unit. Mannose trimming of the protein-bound sugar chains may stop or continue. Addition of a single N-acetylglucosamine or continued mannose trimming next leads to the build-up of sugar chains with two to five branches containing N-acetylglucosamine, galactose, and sialic acid. Fucose may be added to some chains using specific transferases. All of these reactions require delivery of the nucleotide sugar into the Golgi by specific transporters. A series of mutations in seven of the eight COG subunits and a vacuolar H⁺/ATPase disturb N-glycan processing and other biosynthetic pathways by disrupting Golgi homeostasis. Congenital disorders of glycosylation (CDGs) result from defects in some of these steps, indicated by the gene name in red. ER, endoplasmic reticulum; CMP, cytidine monophosphate; GDP, guanosine diphosphate; UDP, uridine diphosphate.

of the chains. Each nucleotide sugar donor must be translocated from its origin in the cytoplasm or nucleus to the Golgi by a substrate-selective transporter. The transferases and transporters recycle through the dynamic Golgi to maintain their correct relationship to the maturing glycoproteins as they pass through the Golgi. Therefore correct trafficking of the biosynthetic machinery is essential for optimal function.

CONGENITAL DISORDERS OF GLYCOSYLATION

Glycosylation is complex, and its disorders defy symptomatic pigeonholing. Congenital disorders of glycosylation (CDG) nomenclature transitioned from a biochemical pathway designation to one based on the mutated gene name. Previously, defects in lipid-linked glycan biosynthesis and transfer to protein defined "group I," and those affecting biosynthesis and processing of the protein-bound sugar chains constituted "group II." Each unique gene disorder carried a lower-case letter (e.g., CDG-Ia, CDG-Ib, CDG-IIa). This nomenclature became too complex, and now the mutated gene name adds a "-CDG" suffix. Both monikers will coexist for some time, but the gene designation is preferred (Jaeken, et al., 2008).

Diagnosis

Most CDG patients were first recognized by abnormal glycoforms of serum transferrin. Commercially available tests include isoelectric focusing, mass spectrometry, zone electrophoresis, and high performance liquid chromatography; however, electrospray ionization-mass spectrometry (ESI-MS) (Babovic-Vuksanovic and O'Brien, 2007) is the most informative because it differentiates absence of entire sugar chains from one or more monosaccharide units. Normal transferrin has two sugar chains, each containing two negatively charged Sia molecules, designated tetrasialotransferrin. Loss of one or two entire chains produces disialotransferrin or asialotransferrin respectively, but this is a misnomer because it is the loss of more than sialic acid. ESI-MS shows losses of 2200 or 4400 mass units, respectively. ESI-MS can also detect loss of single or multiple individual sugars. This distinction helps narrow gene candidates from whole exome or genome sequencing results. ESI-MS is the preferred method (Babovic-Vuksanovic and O'Brien, 2007) and is suitable for routine diagnostics.

Transferrin isoform analysis produces few false-positive results. Uncontrolled fructosemia, galactosemia, and recent heavy alcohol consumption produce a pattern typical of group I disorders. Sometimes, patients with genetically confirmed CDGs develop normal transferrin, and in some patients, previously abnormal patterns normalized in preadolescence. Thus a normal transferrin pattern should not exclude follow-up testing. Healthy neonates sometimes have a slightly abnormal transferrin pattern, which normalizes within a few weeks. Suspicious results in neonates should be repeated.

Some genetic centers and commercial laboratories now offer various CDG gene diagnostic panels (Greenwood Genetic Center, Baylor Medical Genetics, Emory Genetic Laboratory), but falling costs and improved bioinformatics make whole exome sequencing the first choice. However, the proven power of transferrin analysis should always accompany a putative genetic result. Prenatal testing is available for confirmed at-risk families.

General Clinical Features

Over 1000 CDG patients have been identified, most presenting with multiple organ dysfunctions (Haeuptle and Hennet, 2009). Patients with CDGs have protean presentations that, in some cases, may mimic mitochondrial (oxidative phosphorylation) disorders. An informal survey of CDG-affected families indicated that earlier nonspecific diagnoses frequently included a metabolic defect or cerebral palsy. Most patients first present to pediatric neurology or metabolic clinics. They frequently have combinations of liver, gastrointestinal, and coagulation disturbances. The possibility of a CDG should be investigated in any child presenting with developmental delay, seizures, hearing loss or strabismus, particularly if any of these manifestations is accompanied by abnormal coagulation, liver dysfunction, or a gastrointestinal disorder. Most affected children are hypotonic and demonstrate failure to thrive.

SPECIFIC DISORDERS

Table 40-1 summarizes the known glycosylation defects, utilizing the classification scheme published in 2009. This includes the mutated genes and major signs and symptoms. The known defects cover every aspect of the N-linked biosynthetic pathway. Activation or presentation of precursors (PMM2, PMI, DPM1, DPM3 MPDU1 [CDG-Ia, Ib, Ie, If]), glycosyltransferases for lipid-linked oligosaccharide biosynthesis (ALG6, ALG3, ALG12, ALG8, ALG2, DPAGT1, ALG1, ALG9, ALG11, ALG13 [CDG-Ic, Id, Ig, Ih, Ii, Ij, Ik, Il, Ip, Is]), glycosidases that trim the protein-bound sugar chain (MOGS [CDG-IIb], MAN1B1 [MRT15]), Golgi-localized nucleotide sugar transporters (SLC35C1, SLC35A1, SLC35A2 [CDG-IIc, IIf, IIm]), and glycosyltransferases that extend the trimmed chain (MGAT2, B4GALT1 [CDG-IIa and IId]). DOLK (CDG-Im) impair dolichol kinase function and impair the final step of the de novo synthesis of dolichol phosphate. SRD5A3 (CDG-Iq) encodes the α-reductase that converts various polyprenols to dolichols. The conserved, eight-subunit, oligomeric Golgi (COG) complex that binds to the cytoplasmic face of the Golgi is needed for intra-Golgi or Golgi to endoplasmic reticulum retrotrafficking of multiple resident glycosyltransferases and nucleotide sugar transporters. Disorganized trafficking impairs multiple glycosylation pathways. Defects have now been identified in COG7, COG1, COG4, COG8, COG5, COG6, and COG2 [CDG-IIe, IIg, IIj, IIh, IIi, IIl, IIn]. Appreciation of the importance of Golgi homeostasis in glycosylation led to the discovery of another disorder caused by mutations in a subunit of a vacuolar H^+/ATPase that maintains appropriate pH of various organelles within the endocytic and exocytic pathways. The intravesicular pH progressively decreases from the endoplasmic reticulum to Golgi, endosomes, and, finally, lysosomes.

The remainder of this chapter will focus on prominent CDGs with significant neurologic manifestations. Table 40-1 lists those disorders and their common clinical features.

Defects in Protein N-Glycosylation
PMM2-CDG (Ia)

PMM2-CDG (CDG-Ia) is the best-known and most frequently recognized form of CDG, first reported by Jaeken and colleagues in 1980 (Jaeken et al., 1980). The defective gene was identified in 1995 as PMM2, which encodes the phosphomannomutase (PMM) that converts Man-6-P→Man-1-P. This defect results in insufficient production of lipid-linked oligosaccharide, leading to empty glycosylation sites. More than 800 patients are known worldwide, and more than 100 mutations have been cataloged (Haeuptle and Hennet, 2009).

Hagberg and associates described four stages of the typical (severe) phenotype. The first is the infantile phase, marked by various combinations of dysmorphism, abnormal fat distribution (supragluteal and vulval fat pads, focal lipoatrophy), inverted nipples, cryptorchidism, esotropia, recurrent infections, cardiomyopathy or pericardial effusions, coagulopathies, nephrotic syndrome, hypothyroidism, life-threatening episodes of hepatic failure, and unexplained coma. Up to 20% of infants with PMM2-CDG succumb in this phase. In the second phase (comprising the remainder of the first decade), children experience seizures and strokelike episodes, often precipitated by intercurrent infections. The third phase (in the second decade of life) is marked by slowly progressive cerebellar ataxia and limb wasting and by progressive visual loss secondary to pigmentary retinopathy. Adult survivors have moderate intellectual disability with severe ataxia and hypogonadism, with or without skeletal deformities. Presentations are highly variable. In one girl with PMM2-CDG, findings on computed tomography (CT) of the head were normal at 9 months of age, but subsequent imaging studies demonstrated progressive atrophy. The investigators concluded that the cerebellar hypoplasia reported in infancy in most children with CDG-Ia likely reflects atrophy of antenatal onset rather than hypoplasia.

More extensive testing for CDGs has led to the identification of milder PMM2-CDG phenotypes. The patients often have high residual levels of PMM2 activity. Some patients have only borderline cognitive impairment, but strabismus persists in these very mild cases. Few adult CDG-Ia patients are employed. A longitudinal study of eight Spanish patients confirmed the wide range of clinical manifestations, ranging from neonatal hemorrhage, nonimmune hydrops, and death through intellectual disability and motor impairment without acute decompensation in patients in their 20s to one individual with normal development and only gastrointestinal dysfunction in childhood.

The carrier frequency of the most common mutant allele (c.422G>A, p.R141H) is about 1 in 70 in the northern European population. The public Exome Aggregation Consortium (ExAC) database, composed of 60,000 exomes, finds a carrier frequency of 1 in 76. It is lethal in the homozygous state. No effective specific therapy for PMM2-CDG exists. Experiments using patient cells suggested that increasing dietary mannose might improve glycosylation in patients, but clinical trials demonstrated no benefit. Subsequent trials on a few patients did not show any clinical improvement.

Population studies find the risk of having a second child with PMM2-CDG to be close to 1 in 3 rather than the expected Mendelian ratio of 1 in 4, suggesting that reduced glycosylation may have some selective advantage. At-risk couples should be counseled appropriately.

MPI-CDG (Ib)

MPI-CDG (Ib) is caused by mutations in MPI, the gene encoding phosphomannose isomerase, which interconverts Man-6-P and Fructose (Frc)-6-P. This reaction produces most of the mannose for glycoprotein synthesis. About 25 patients have been identified since its discovery in 1998 (de Lonlay and Seta, 2009). This phenotype is not associated with any primary neurologic symptoms. Gastrointestinal and hepatic pathology, with hypoglycemia, coagulopathy, and protein-losing enteropathy, is characteristic. MPI-CDG is unique in that simple dietary mannose therapy corrects the abnormalities, except for liver fibrosis. Liver transplantation proved effective in one patient with severe hepatic fibrosis.

ALG6-CDG (Ic)

Initial cases of ALG6-CDG (Ic) resembled a less severe version of PMM2-CDG, but more severe cases have appeared. It is characterized by moderate psychomotor retardation, hypotonia, esotropia, seizures, and ataxia. Nevertheless, at least five children have died of CDG-related complications. The defect is in a glycosyltransferase hALG6, which results in production of a truncated lipid-linked oligosaccharide sugar chain that is inefficiently transferred to proteins. Patients sometimes experience life-threatening protein-losing enteropathy during bouts of gastroenteritis. Skeletal dysplasia, including a unique form associated with brachytelephalangy, has been described in a compound heterozygote for ALG6. An adult woman has been identified in whom ALG6 deficiency was associated with intellectual disability, skeletal anomalies, virilization, and deep vein thrombosis. ALG6 deficiency was first identified in 1998 and subsequently in over 90 patients, making it one of the most common forms of CDG.

DPAGT1-CDG (Ij)

DPAGT1-CDG (Ij) is caused by a deficiency in UDP-GlcNAc:dolichol phosphate N-acetylglucosamine-1 phosphate transferase (GPT) activity encoded by DPAGT1. Two patients had severe hypotonia, intractable seizures, intellectual disability, microcephaly, and exotropia. Using exome sequencing, Ng and associates have identified an additional seven previously unreported cases of DPAGT1-CDG. In four of the seven cases, the patients were characterized by an extremely severe, multicongenital anomaly phenotype that resulted in death for all four. The remaining individuals have severe hypotonia, intractable seizures, intellectual disability, and microcephaly. Subsequent reports have focused on DPAGT1-CDG as a cause of a myasthenic syndrome characterized by fatigable limb girdle weakness with bulbar sparing, response to cholinesterase inhibitors, and the presence of tubular aggregates on muscle biopsy; there is evidence of both presynaptic and postsynaptic neuromuscular transmission defects.

ALG1-CDG (Ik)

Eighteen patients with ALG1-CDG (Ik) had been described by 2014. Fifty percent had complications during pregnancy, and several had postnatal complications. Eighty percent were hypotonic, and all had at least one seizure, most being intractable; 8 of the 10 were dysmorphic; 7 of the 10 had visual impairment; and 5 of the 10 were microcephalic. Fifty percent had a fatal outcome. Patients with ALG1-CDG are deficient in GDP-Man:GlcNAc$_2$-P-P-dolichol mannosyltransferase, encoded by the *hALG1* gene, which adds the first Man to the lipid-linked oligosaccharide chain.

More recently, Ng and associates identified 39 additional ALG1-CDG cases by various methods, including exome sequencing, targeted gene panels, and traditional Sanger sequencing. It is the largest report of ALG1-CDG cases and triples the number of known cases, making it the third most common CDG in the N-linked pathway. Nearly all the affected had a pronounced neurologic presentation that included developmental delay, hypotonia, seizures/epilepsy, microcephaly, and, for those who could be tested, varying degrees of intellectual disabilities. Other clinical manifestations included facial dysmorphism, coagulopathy, gastrointestinal and skeletal abnormalities. Lethality in the first 5 years occurred in about 45% of the cases.

TUSC3-CDG

Twenty-one patients in six kindreds have been described with TUSC3-CDG. Seven of the original cohort all had nonsyndromic, moderate to severe intellectual disability. Two were siblings from a small French family. TUSC3 encodes a subunit of the oligosaccharyltransferase complex (OST). It is not clear why these patients have no other systemic manifestations of hypoglycosylation, but it is theorized that differential tissue expression of another subunit associated with the OST (IAP) might compensate for TUSC3 deficiency in nonneurologic tissues. About one-third of patients have microcephaly and short stature.

SRD5A3-CDG (Iq)

Nearly twenty cases of SRD5A3-CDG have been described with virtually all being either homozygous or compound heterozygous for complete loss of function mutations (INDEL, premature stop codons, complete gene deletions). No missense mutations have been identified to date. SRD5A3 encodes for a polyprenol reductase that converts polyprenol to dolichol, and unlike SRD5A1 and SRD5A2, does not appear to play a physiologic role in testosterone production. Affected individuals manifest with neurologic deficiencies and nearly always with some form of ocular problems including nystagmus, cataracts, glaucoma and optic nerve atrophy.

NGLY1-CDG

Recently discovered mutations in NGLY1 cause global developmental delay, a movement disorder, hypotonia microcephaly and diminished reflexes, and alacrima by unknown mechanisms (Enns et al., 2014). It shares many symptoms with other typical CDGs. NGLY1 cleaves intact N-glycans from misfolded N-glycosylated proteins that retrotranslocate into the cytoplasm as part of the ERAD pathway, often linked to ER-stress response. It could be considered a highly specific "disorder of de-glycosylation." The liberated N-glycan chains are further degraded by the proteosome the cytoplasm and lysosomes, and the proteins are degraded in the proteasome. Over 40 patients have been identified in less than 3 years since its discovery, mostly due to the outreach efforts of parents of the index patient.

Defects in Protein O-Glycosylation

The most important defects in O-glycosylation are those based in O-mannose pathway, which is covered in Chapter 39. These disorders are listed in Table 40-1.

Defects in Glycosphingolipids (GSL)

The GSL biosynthetic pathway is shown in Figure 40-2. Developmental delay, seizures, and blindness are found in autosomal-recessive Amish infantile epilepsy. A large Amish family was identified with a nonsense mutation in SIAT9 that truncated protein. The presence of abnormal pigmentation that becomes more prominent over time may be a useful diagnostic clue to the presence of this otherwise clinically nonspecific disorder; 20 of 38 affected children were found to have freckled hyperpigmentation on the limbs, with variable hypopigmentation on the limbs and face. SIAT9 is a sialyltransferase needed for synthesis of gangliosides GM3 (Siaα2-3Galβ1-4Glc-ceramide) from lactosylceramide (Galβ1-4Glc-ceramide). Patients accumulate nonsialylated plasma glycosphingolipids such as GM3 and also lack downstream GM3-dependent molecules. Two children with homozygous nonsense mutations in SIAT9 were found to have evidence of secondary respiratory chain dysfunction and apoptosis in their cultured fibroblasts, attributed to accumulation of globosides Gb3 and Gb4.

GalNAc is transferred onto GM3 and GD3 precursors by B4GALNT1 in the biosynthesis of GM2 and GD2 glycosphingolipids and is mutated in hereditary spastic paraplegia subtype 26. Individuals showed developmental delay with varying cognitive impairment and an early onset progressive spasticity due to axonal degeneration.

In twelve affected individuals who had IQ<40, ST3GAL3, mutations were identified that resulted in loss of enzyme activity or mislocalization of ST3GAL3 protein. Furthermore mutations in ST3GAL3 were also identified as an underlying case of West syndrome with developmental delay. Loss of ST3GAL3 function may result in varying clinical presentation because this enzyme has multiple substrates that include both gangliosides as well as N- and O-glycans.

Glycosylphosphatidylinositol Glycosylation

In mammals, hundreds of proteins require a GPI-anchor for proper function. To carry out this essential pathway, at least 27 proteins are required to synthesize and transfer a functional GPI anchor to its target protein (see Fig. 40-3). Several disorders of GPI-anchor synthesis with neurologic features have been described. Mabry syndrome, comprising intellectual disability, hyperphosphatasia, unusual facial features, hypotonia, and seizures, has been associated with mutations in several glycosylphosphatidylinositol synthase genes, including PIGV, PIGO, PIGL, PIGW, PGAP2, and PGAP3; PIGV mutations are found in most cases. The PIGV gene encodes the second mannosyltransferase used for GPI-anchor synthesis. Total surface anchors are reduced, including GPI-anchored alkaline phosphatase, which is instead found at very high levels in the plasma. PIGT mutations have been described in children with encephalopathy, dysmorphism, and hypophosphatasia. PIGL is mutated in the CHIME syndrome (ocular coloboma, heart defects, ichthyosis, mental retardation, and ear anomalies). More recently, a single patient with the hallmarks of Mabry syndrome was also found to have mutations in PIGL. Mutations in PIGA, which have long been known as a cause of paroxysmal nocturnal hemoglobinuria (PNH), can also cause distinct neurologic disorders, including: (1) severe syndromic form of X-linked intellectual disability; (2) early onset epileptic encephalopathies (EOEEs); (3) X-linked syndrome associated with neurodegeneration, cutaneous abnormalities associated with systemic iron overload; and (4) multiple congenital anomalies-hypotonia-seizures syndrome-2. Mutations also occur in PIGN causing multiple congenital anomalies-hypotonia-seizures syndrome-1. Mutations in PIGQ can result in Ohtahara syndrome, whereas defects in PGAP1 cause intellectual disability with encephalopathy (Murakami et al., 2014). The one GPI anchor protein deficiency that has a targeted treatment is

due to mutations in PIGM. In this deficiency, patients carry a promoter mutation resulting in loss of PIGM protein, but treatment with butyrate resulted in increased PIGM expression and correction of both the biochemical defect as well as complete cessation of the child's intractable seizures.

Defects in Multiple Glycosylation and Other Pathways

Several rare disorders are included in this group; they include DPM1-CDG (Ie), DPM2-CDG, DPM3-CDG (Io), MPDU1-CDG (If), B4GALT1-CDG (IId), SLC35A1-CDG (IIf), SLC35A2-CDG, all of which feature varying degrees of intellectual disability, epilepsy (often intractable), dysmorphism, and dystroglycanopathy. Systemic involvement in the form of skeletal, hepatic, and coagulation anomalies is also variable; carbohydrate-deficient transferrin cannot be relied on to make a diagnosis in these forms. A more detailed discussion is available online.

SLC35C1-CDG (IIc)

SLC35C1-CDG (IIc) is one of the few CDG for which disease-modifying therapy is available. It was originally described as leukocyte adhesion deficiency II and is characterized by moderate to severe intellectual disability, rhizomelic short stature, a broad flat nasal bridge, microcephaly, elevated leukocytes, frequent infections, persistent marked neutrophilia, and periodontitis. The disorder is caused by mutations in the GDP-fucose transporter, which limits the synthesis of fucosylated glycans. One of these is sialyl Lewis-X (sLeX), a glycan essential for leukocyte rolling before extravasation. Oral fucose supplements effectively reduced leukocytosis in two patients by allowing synthesis of sufficient sLeX. These patients also lack fucosylated H-antigen, the precursor for the ABO blood group. Fucose supplements have not provoked antigen synthesis or immunologic reactions. Transferrin glycosylation is normal in this type. Patients may present with short stature and developmental delay, without clinical evidence of increased susceptibility to infection.

COG Complex

The COG complex consists of eight (COG1-8) subunits encoded by different genes. Glycosylation disorders have been identified in all except COG3. A wide range of phenotypes has been described; most have an early, severe onset, with intractable epilepsy, profound developmental delay, and early death from infection or multiorgan failure. A detailed discussion of several subtypes is available online.

WHEN TO SUSPECT AND TEST FOR CONGENITAL DISORDERS OF GLYCOSYLATION

CDG should be suspected and tested for in any child presenting with an unexplained syndrome, particularly those characterized by developmental delay, hearing loss, hypotonia, and seizures, especially in combination with lipodystrophy, skeletal dysplasia, or gastrointestinal, hepatic, or coagulation abnormalities. However, nonsyndromic intellectual disability or "pure" neurologic syndromes do occur, including dramatic episodes of regression, apparently provoked by intercurrent illness or immunization. Although transferrin should be done, not all types will show an abnormality; a few confirmed patients even normalized over time. Therefore it is best to test patients early (1 to 18 months of age). Patients with CDGs may have phenotypes resembling mitochondrial disorders, Joubert syndrome, or Dandy-Walker malformation. Abnormal transferrin results still require genetic analysis to identify the defect. Some commercial laboratories now offer various CDG gene panel analyses. Improved technology and decreasing costs of genome or exome sequencing will continue to identify specific defects. However, in many cases the variants may be predicted to be damaging, but additional biochemical and physiologic analysis is required needed to provide certainty as well as hopes for therapeutics.

SUMMARY

Glycosylated molecules are present on the surface and in the interior of all cells. The biosynthesis of glycans is complex, with the potential to produce thousands of different structures at different times and in response to endogenous and exogenous signals. At least 2% of the known genes encode proteins that either synthesize or bind to glycans, often with exquisite specificity. Disrupting glycan biosynthesis leads to a multitude of downstream effects that may involve every aspect of central nervous system's development and function. The analysis of transferrin glycosylation status can point to glycosylation abnormalities in many, but not all, patients. A few patients respond to simple dietary supplements of sugars. Although glycosylation disorders appear to be rare, their recent discovery makes it likely that the true frequency is unknown. As for all inborn errors of metabolism, many patients with mild or atypical manifestations will be found, and new disorders will be recognized as diagnostic testing—particularly whole exome and genome sequencing—becomes more widely available and applied (Freeze et al., 2015).

REFERENCES

The complete list of references for this chapter is available in the e-book at www.expertconsult.com.
See inside cover for registration details.

SELECTED REFERENCES

Babovic-Vuksanovic, D., O'Brien, J.F., 2007. Laboratory diagnosis of congenital disorders of glycosylation type I by analysis of transferrin glycoforms. Mol. Diagn. Ther. 11, 303–311.

de Lonlay, P., Seta, N., 2009. The clinical spectrum of phosphomannose isomerase deficiency, with an evaluation of mannose treatment for CDG-Ib. Biochim. Biophys. Acta 1792, 841–843.

Enns, G.M., Shashi, V., Bainbridge, M., et al., 2014. Mutations in NGLY1 cause an inherited disorder of the endoplasmic reticulum-associated degradation pathway. Genet. Med. 16, 751–758.

Freeze, H.H., Eklund, E.A., Ng, B.G., et al., 2015. Neurological aspects of human glycosylation disorders. Annu. Rev. Neurosci. 38, 105–125.

Freeze, H.H., Elbein, A.D., 2009. Glycosylation Precursors. In: Varki, A., Cummings, R.D., Esko, J.D., et al. (Eds.), Essentials of Glycobiology, 2nd ed. Cold Spring Harbor Laboratory Press, Cold Spring Harbor (NY), pp. 47–62.

Haeuptle, M.A., Hennet, T., 2009. Congenital disorders of glycosylation: an update on defects affecting the biosynthesis of dolichol-linked oligosaccharides. Hum. Mut. 30, 1628–1641.

Jaeken, J., Hennet, T., Freeze, H.H., et al., 2008. On the nomenclature of congenital disorders of glycosylation (CDG). J. Inherit. Metab. Dis. 31, 669–672.

Jaeken, J., Vanderschueren-Lodewyckx, M., Casaer, P., et al., 1980. Familial psychomotor retardation with markedly fluctuating serum prolactin, FSH and GH levels, partial TBG-deficiency, increased serum arylsulphatase A and increased CSF protein: a new syndrome? Pediatr. Res. 14, 179.

Murakami, Y., Tawamie, H., Maeda, Y., et al., 2014. Null mutation in PGAP1 impairing Gpi-anchor maturation in patients with intellectual disability and encephalopathy. PLoS Genet. 10, e1004320.

Varki, A., Cummings, R.D., Esko, J.D., et al., 2009. Symbol nomenclature for glycan representation. Proteomics 9, 5398–5399.

Varki, A., Lowe, J.B., 2009. Biological roles of glycans. In: Varki, A., Cummings, R.D., Esko, J.D., et al. (Eds.), Essentials of Glycobiology, 2nd ed. Cold Spring Harbor Laboratory Press, Cold Spring Harbor (NY), pp. 75–88.

E-BOOK FIGURES AND TABLES

The following figures and tables are available in the e-book at www.expertconsult.com. See inside cover for registration details.

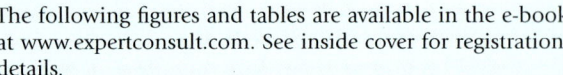

Fig. 40-2 Processing of N-linked glycans in the Golgi membrane.
Fig. 40-3 O-mannose glycan biosynthesis.
Table 40-1 Neurologic and Muscular Features

41 Lysosomal Storage Diseases

Gregory M. Pastores and Raymond Y. Wang

An expanded version of this chapter is available on www.expertconsult.com. See inside cover for registration details.

OVERVIEW AND GENERAL CONCEPTS

The lysosomal storage diseases (LSDs) encompass a heterogeneous group of approximately 50 disorders caused by genetic defects in a lysosomal acid hydrolase, receptor, activator protein, membrane protein, or transporter, causing progressive lysosomal accumulation of undegradable substrates specific to each disorder (Valle et al., 2014). As storage of substrate progresses, derangements of lysosomal function and transport result in deterioration of affected tissues and organs. Many LSDs have central nervous system (CNS) manifestations and other multisystemic pathologies resulting in decreased life span and significant morbidity.

LSDs are often categorized according to the type of substrate stored (i.e., mucopolysaccharidoses, oligosaccharidoses, sphingolipidoses, gangliosidoses, etc.). Although lysosomes and their constituent proteins are usually expressed in cells throughout the body, storage occurs only in those deficient tissues in which relevant substrates are normally turned-over (e.g., G_{M1} ganglioside is present predominantly in the myelin of the CNS; deficiency of β-D-galactosidase, which acts on the G_{M1} ganglioside and can be measured in the blood, causes G_{M1} gangliosidosis, a condition that manifests with neurodegeneration and other systemic signs). In all cases, the diagnosis can be established with biochemical enzymatic assays and/or confirmed by mutational analysis of the gene in question (Wang 2011).

Although each disorder is individually rare, LSDs as a group have an estimated frequency of one in 7000 to 8000 live births. As more countries adopt presymptomatic newborn screening for LSDs, the actual frequency appears to be more common as increasing numbers of infants with attenuated or adult-onset forms of the diseases are being identified. All LSDs are inherited in an autosomal-recessive fashion, except for the X-linked disorders Fabry, Hunter (mucopolysaccharidosis type II [MPS II]), and Danon diseases. Some population groups have higher prevalence rates for certain LSDs (e.g., Gaucher, Tay–Sachs, Niemann–Pick type A, and mucolipidosis IV are more common in Ashkenazi Jews) as a result of ancestral founder mutations. For other LSDs, such as Fabry disease, most kindreds have private mutations.

LSDs can demonstrate locus heterogeneity, where a clinical entity such as Sanfilippo disease (MPS III) is caused by recessive mutations encoding one of four enzymes involved in heparan sulfate catabolism. Conversely, LSDs frequently demonstrate phenotypic heterogeneity, where different mutations in one lysosomal gene result in a spectrum of manifestations depending on the amount of residual enzyme activity and other modifiers. As a general rule, mutations that result in negligible lysosomal enzymatic activity tend to result in more severe, earlier-onset disease with more rapid velocity of disease progression, whereas the mutations that confer residual enzymatic activity tend to manifest with later-onset, more attenuated disease manifestations. However, the age of onset, severity of symptoms, organ systems affected, and CNS manifestations can vary in patients with identical mutations, even those from the same families. Although certain mutations in LSD genes are fairly reliable in predicting clinical outcomes,

for many disorders genotype–phenotype correlations are not completely reliable. For example, patients with Gaucher disease who have the common p.N370S mutation may present in childhood or even be asymptomatic throughout adult life. It is likely there are modifying factors that influence disease expression, but these have not been fully elucidated. For a tabular summary of the LSDs discussed in this chapter, please refer to Table 41-1; for a general algorithm for the diagnosis of LSDs, please refer to Figure 41-1.

Sphingolipidoses

Glycolipids are amphiphilic compounds especially found in CNS cell membranes and are composed of a hydrophobic ceramide attached to polar components, such as saccharide oligomers, phosphocholine, or phosphoethanolamine. The exact nomenclature of a glycolipid depends on its polar moiety: gangliosides contain at least one sialic acid residue; globosides and cerebrosides contain multiple and single hexoses, respectively; and sphingomyelins have either phosphocholine or phosphoethanolamine. Deficiencies of specific degradative enzymes result in lysosomal accumulation of the cognate substrate (Sandhoff, 2013).

G_{M1} Gangliosidosis

GM1 gangliosidosis is allelic to mucopolysaccharidosis IVb and arises from complete deficiency of the β-D-galactosidase enzyme. G_{M1} gangliosidosis often can be recognized in the neonatal period with macrocephaly, frontal bossing, gingival hypertrophy, macroglossia, and edema. The placenta may have a tougher consistency, and pathologic examination often reveals vacuolization of syncytiotrophoblasts. Infants display hypotonia and exaggerated startle to sounds. Development stagnates, and they become deaf, blind, and minimally interactive within the first year of life. Also within the first year, MPS-like symptoms of facial coarsening, hepatosplenomegaly, joint contractures, and vertebral dysplasia arise from accumulation of the keratan sulfate glycosaminoglycan, a polymer of galactose and N-acetyl 6-sulfogalactosamine. As the disease progresses, seizures and macular "cherry-red spots" develop as G_{M1} ganglioside accumulates in the CNS and retina, respectively. Most severely affected children die before their third birthday from aspiration pneumonia. Attenuated cases of G_{M1} gangliosidosis manifest in childhood or adolescence with dystonia, dysarthria, stuttering, and hip dysplasia. There are no currently effective treatments for this disorder, although intracerebroventricular gene therapy is currently being investigated.

G_{M2} Gangliosidoses

Once galactose is cleaved off the G_{M1} molecule, the distal sugar residue on the ganglioside becomes an N-acetyl-D-hexosamine. This sugar is removed by the heterodimeric enzyme hexosaminidase, composed of an A and B subunit encoded by the

TABLE 41-1 The Lysosomal Storage Disorders Classified According to Relevant Substrate Involved

Listing of Known Lysosomal Storage Disorders, Including the Type of Substrate Accumulated in the Disorder, Chromosomal Locus, and Gene Responsible for the Condition

Stored Substrate	Disease	Enzyme/Protein Deficiency	Gene Locus
SPHINGOLIPIDS			
GM_2 gangliosides, glycolipids, globoside oligosaccharides	Tay–Sachs disease GM_2 gangliosidosis (three types)	α Subunit of β-hexosaminidase	*HEXA*, 15q23
	Sandhoff disease GM_2 gangliosidosis	β Subunit of β-hexosaminidase	*HEXB*, 5q13.3
	GM_2 gangliosidosis, AB variant	GM_2 activator	*GM2A*, 5q33.1
GM_1 gangliosides, oligosaccharides, keratan sulfate, glycolipids	GM_1 gangliosidosis (three types)*	β-D-galactosidase	*GLB1*, 3p22.3
Sulfatides	Metachromatic leukodystrophy	Arylsulfatase A (galactose-3-sulfatase)	*ARSA*, 22q13.33
GM_1 gangliosides, sphingomyelin, glycolipids, sulfatide	Metachromatic leukodystrophy variant	Saposin B activator	*PSAP*, 10q22.1
Galactosylceramides	Krabbe disease	Galactocerebrosidase	*GALC*, 14q31.3
α-Galactosylsphingolipids, oligosaccharides	Fabry disease	α-Galactosidase A	*GLA*, Xq22.1
Glucosylceramide, globosides	Gaucher disease (three types)*	β-Glucosidase	*GBA*, 1q22
Glucosylceramide, globosides	Gaucher disease (variant)	Saposin C	*PSAP*, 10q22
Ceramide	Farber disease (seven types)	Acid ceramidase	*ASAH1*, 8p22
Sphingomyelin	Niemann–Pick disease types A and B	Sphingomyelinase	*SMPD1*, 11p15.4
MUCOPOLYSACCHARIDES (GLYCOSAMINOGLYCANS)			
Dermatan sulfate and heparan sulfate	Mucopolysaccharidosis (MPS) I, Hurler–Scheie	α-L-Iduronidase	*IDUA*, 4p16.3
	MPS II, Hunter	Iduronate-2-sulfatase	*IDS*, Xq28
Heparan sulfate	MPS IIIA, Sanfilippo A	Sulfamidase	*SGSH*, 17q25.3
	MPS IIIB, Sanfilippo B	α-N-acetylglucosaminidase	*NAGLU*, 17q21.2
	MPS IIIC, Sanfilippo C	Acetyl-CoA: α-glucosaminide-N-acetyltransferase	*HGSNAT*, 8p11.21
	MPS IIID, Sanfilippo D	N-acetylglucosamine-6-sulfatase	*GNS*, 12q14.3
Keratan sulfate	MPS IVA, Morquio A	Galactosamine-6-sulfatase	*GALNS*, 16q24.3
	MPS IVB, Morquio B	β-D-galactosidase	*GLB1*, 3p22.3
Dermatan sulfate	MPS VI, Maroteaux–Lamy	N-acetylgalactosamine-4-sulfatase	*ARSB*, 5q13–14
Dermatan sulfate and heparan sulfate	MPS VII, Sly	β-D-glucuronidase	*GUSB*, 7q11.21
Hyaluronan	MPS IX, Natowicz	Hyaluronoglucosaminidase	*HYAL1*, 3p21.31
GLYCOGEN			
Glycogen	Pompe disease, glycogen storage disease type IIA	Acid α-D-glucosidase	*GAA*, 17q25.3
Glycogen	Danon disease	Lysosomal associated membrane protein-2 (LAMP-2)	*LAMP2*, Xq24
OLIGOSACCHARIDES/GLYCOPEPTIDES			
α-Mannoside	α-Mannosidosis	α-Mannosidase	*MAN2B1*, 19p13.2
β-Mannoside	β-Mannosidosis	β-Mannosidase	*MANBA*, 4q24
disease type–Fucosides, glycolipids	α-Fucosidosis	α-Fucosidase	*FUCA1*, 1p36.1
disease type–N-acetylgalactosaminide	Schindler–Kanzaki disease	α-N-acetylgalactosaminidase	*NAGA*, 22q13.2
Sialyloligosaccharides	Sialidosis (mucolipidosis I)	α-Neuraminidase	*NEU1*, 6p21.33
Aspartylglucosamine	Aspartylglucosaminuria	Aspartylglucosaminidase	*AGA*, 4q34–35
MULTIPLE ENZYME DEFICIENCIES			
Glycolipids, oligosaccharides	Mucolipidosis II (I-cell disease); mucolipidosis III (pseudo-Hurler polydystrophy) three complementation groups	N-acetylglucosamine-1-phosphotransferase	Mucolipidoses II, IIIA/B: α/β subunit (*GNPTAB*) on 12q23.2; Mucolipidosis IIIC: γ subunit (*GNPTG*) mutations on 16p13.3
Glycolipids, gangliosides, phospholipids	Mucolipidosis IV	Mucolipin-1	(*MCOLN1*), 19p13.2
	Galactosialidosis	Protective protein/cathepsin A	*CTSA*, 20q13.12
Sulfatides, glycolipids, glycosaminoglycans	Multiple sulfatases	Sulfatase-modifying factor 1(SUMF-1)	*SUMF1*, 3p26.1
LIPIDS			
Cholesterol esters	Wolman disease, cholesteryl ester storage disease	Lysosomal acid lipase	*LIPA*, 10q23.2-q23.3
Cholesterol, sphingomyelin	Niemann–Pick disease type C	NPC1; NPC2	(*NPC1*), 18q11.2; (*NPC2*), 14q24.3
MONOSACCHARIDES/AMINO ACID MONOMERS			
Sialic acid, glucuronic acid	Salla disease, infantile free sialic acid storage disease	Sialin	(*SLC17A5*), 6q13
Cystine	Cystinosis	Cystinosin	(*CTNS*), 17p13.2

TABLE 41-1 The Lysosomal Storage Disorders Classified According to Relevant Substrate Involved *(Continued)*

Stored Substrate	Disease	Enzyme/Protein Deficiency	Gene Locus
PEPTIDES			
Bone proteins	Pyknodysostosis	Cathepsin K	*(CTSK)*, 1q21
S-ACYLATED PROTEINS			
Palmitoylated proteins	Infantile neuronal ceroid lipofuscinosis	Palmitoyl-protein thioesterase 1	*(PPT1)*, 1p32
Pepstatin-insensitive lysosomal peptidase	Late infantile neuronal ceroid lipofuscinosis	Tripeptidyl peptidase	*(TPP1)*, 11p15

*Three types imply infantile, childhood, and adulthood presentations.

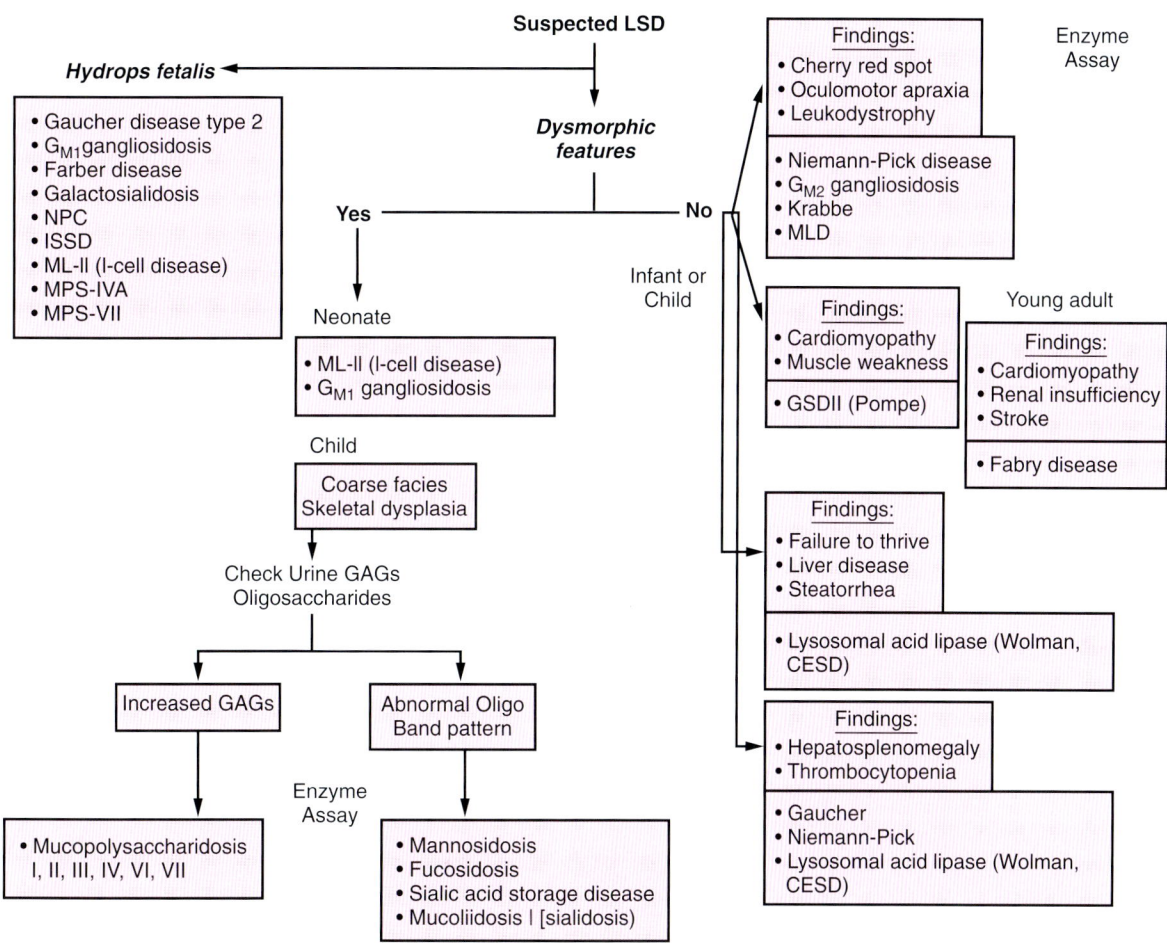

Figure 41-1. General algorithm for the diagnosis of lysosomal storage disorders.

HEXA and *HEXB* genes, respectively. Recessive deficiency in hexosaminidase A results in Tay–Sachs disease, whereas hexosaminidase B deficiency results in Sandhoff disease. Collectively, the two disorders are known as the G_{M2} gangliosidoses because their symptoms are fairly similar and are caused by accumulation of G_{M2} ganglioside. Initial growth and development are normal until 3 to 6 months of age, when hypotonia and exaggerated startle reflex are the usual initial symptoms. As in G_{M1} gangliosidosis, a period of developmental regression ensues in which the child loses all acquired milestones and is minimally interactive, with blindness, deafness, and dysphagia. Seizures develop as gray-matter loss progresses. Cherry-red spot maculae are often visualized, but, importantly, absence of this finding does not rule out the disorder. In

affected children, aspiration pneumonia is the usual reason for death, typically before age 3 years. Intermediate and attenuated forms of these diseases also exist, with disease onset in adolescence or adulthood and manifesting with ataxia, dysarthria, movement disorder, and even isolated psychiatric symptoms such as psychosis or bipolar disease. Although Tay–Sachs disease is well known as a disorder that affects people of European Jewish descent, premarital testing has considerably reduced the prevalence of the disorder in this population; it also occurs with higher frequency in French Canadians of Quebec, Old Order Amish of Pennsylvania, and Cajuns of southern Louisiana. Like G_{M1} gangliosidosis, intracerebroventricular gene therapies are currently being investigated.

α-Galactosidase a deficiency (Fabry Disease)

α-Galactosidase A deficiency (Fabry disease) is an X-linked LSD caused by deficiency in α-galactosidase A, which removes terminal galactose from various galacto-glycolipids, such as globotriaosylceramide (Gal-Gal-Glu-Cer) and blood group B antigen. Typical presenting symptoms are burning pain in the hands and feet, called acroparesthesia, which is often exacerbated by temperature; reduced sweating; gastrointestinal pain; and diarrhea (Rombach et al., 2014). Although hemizygous males tend to have more severe symptoms with onset between the ages of 5 and 10 years, heterozygous females are often equally symptomatic even with random X-inactivation. Progression of systemic glycolipid storage leads to worsening hypertrophic cardiomyopathy, myocardial microvascular ischemia and scarring, increased risk of cerebrovascular ischemia, proteinuria, and loss of renal filtration. Strokes in Fabry disease can be either ischemic or hemorrhagic, involve either the carotid or vertebrobasilar vasculature, and typically affect small vessels. Enzyme replacement therapy with recombinant α-galactosidase (Agalsidase alfa, Shire; Agalsidase beta, Genzyme-Sanofi) can halt or slow loss of creatinine clearance if initiated before onset of significant renal disease; the enzyme can also reduce cardiomyopathy provided it is started before development of cardiac fibrosis. Small molecule therapy to increase endogenous enzymatic activity in patients with specific missense *GLA* mutations is being investigated. Adjunctive therapy for treatment of neuropathic pain, proteinuria, and cardiomyopathy is often required.

β-D-Glucosidase Deficiency (Gaucher Disease)

Gaucher disease, caused by a deficiency in β-D-glucosidase or glucocerebrosidase, was one of the first lysosomal storage conditions to have its enzymatic deficiency elucidated. The enzyme removes glucose from glucosylceramide, the final glycolipid in ganglioside catabolism. Like most lysosomal storage disorders, Gaucher disease manifestations range in severity from an acute "type II" infantile-onset form, to an intermediate "type III" form, to the most common "type I" or "nonneuronopathic" form. Patients with type I disease can present at almost any age, typically with hepatosplenomegaly and thrombocytopenia. Other presentations include osteonecrosis of the femoral head and painful lytic bone lesions. In addition to typical type I symptoms, infants with type II Gaucher disease demonstrate ophthalmoplegia, dysphagia, and other bulbar palsies, whereas type III patients typically have some degree of static cognitive impairment. Type I patients have a higher relative risk of multiple myeloma (5.9×) and hematologic (1.23×) malignancies, although the overall absolute risk of malignancy still remains low. In addition, type I patients and carriers have a higher risk of developing Parkinson's disease (4.7% risk to develop Parkinson's by age 60 for patients, 1.5% for carriers, and 0.7% for noncarriers). Three forms of enzyme replacement therapy (Imiglucerase, Genzyme-Sanofi; Velaglucerase alfa, Shire; and Taliglucerase alfa, Protalix BioTherapeutics) and two forms of substrate reduction therapy (Miglustat, Actelion Pharmaceuticals; Eliglustat, Genzyme-Sanofi) exist for the treatment of nonneurologic manifestations of Gaucher disease.

Sphingomyelinase Deficiency (Niemann–Pick Disease Types a and B)

Lysosomal acid sphingomyelinase deficiency results in types A and B Niemann–Pick disease (NPA and NPB, respectively). Undegraded sphingomyelin accumulates primarily in CNS neurons and reticuloendothelial cells. Collectively, the prevalence of the disorders is 1 in 250,000 live births; NPA is seen more frequently in the Ashkenazi Jewish population, with an incidence of 1:40,000 live births, whereas NPB is more common in individuals of Northern African descent. NPA is characterized by neonatal onset hepatosplenomegaly, thrombocytopenia, neurodegeneration beginning in the first year of life, pulmonary infiltrative disease, and early death before age 3 years. NPB has a more variable presentation, but age of onset is typically in later childhood or adulthood. Primary symptoms are related to hepatosplenomegaly and impaired pulmonary function as a result of accumulation of sphingomyelin in reticuloendothelial and pulmonary tissues. Both disorders may have macular cherry-red spots. Intravenous recombinant human acid sphingomyelinase has been investigated for treatment primarily for NPB, but administration of the enzyme must be closely monitored because ceramide, a degradation product of sphingomyelin, has potent proinflammatory properties.

Niemann–Pick Disease Types C and D

Originally named because affected patients demonstrated hepatosplenomegaly and sphingomyelin accumulation, but were ultimately not linked to the acid sphingomyelinase gene, these two disorders are now known to be caused by deficient lysosomal transport of unesterified cholesterol. Free cholesterol accumulation in lysosomes and cell membranes results in secondary impairment of other lysosomal functions, such as sphingomyelin catabolism. Mutations in the *NPC1* gene are responsible for about 95% of cases, and the remainder result from recessive *NPC2* mutations. Affected individuals of French-Acadian descent from Nova Scotia were termed to have Niemann Pick D (NPD) disease, but eventually found to have *NPC1* mutations. NPC/D clinical manifestations are extremely broad and can present as early as the neonatal period with hepatosplenomegaly and cholestatic jaundice or anytime afterward with a combination of vertical supranuclear gaze palsy, dysarthria, dysphagia, ataxia, dystonia, seizure disorder, or developmental delay. Pulmonary parenchymal disease leading to childhood-onset respiratory failure and death typically affects patients with *NPC2* mutations. The neurologic disease is progressive, and in later stages it is often accompanied by dementia. Miglustat (Actelion Pharmaceuticals), an inhibitor of glycosphingolipid synthesis, may stabilize or slow disease progression, but it is not approved for use in NPC patients in the United States. Therapy with cyclodextrins, circular glucose oligomers that remove cholesterol from cell membranes, is being investigated for NPC disease, as are carbamazepine and histone deacetylase inhibitors.

Acid Ceramidase Deficiency (Farber Disease)

Acid ceramidase deficiency (Farber disease), a lysosomal storage disorder caused by deficiency of acid ceramidase, is classically known for a triad of characteristic subcutaneous lipogranulomas, hoarseness, and swollen, painful arthropathy. Patients with this canonical form also demonstrate hepatosplenomegaly, developmental delay, and pulmonary infiltration. There are also a number of other described "subtypes" of Farber disease, but the very small number of cases in each makes generalizations difficult. However, recessive mutations in the acid ceramidase gene were recently linked to a rare disorder with childhood-onset combined spinal muscular atrophy and progressive myoclonus epilepsy. Affected patients also developed cognitive regression, dysphagia, and difficulty managing airway secretions. Hematopoietic stem cell transplant (HSCT) has been reported as a possible therapy for affected patients without neurologic involvement, and recombinant enzyme replacement therapy is also being developed.

Galactosylceramidase Deficiency (Krabbe Disease)

The galactosylceramidase enzyme functions to remove galactose from galactosylceramide, galactosylsphingosine, and other galactolipids. Both galactosylceramide and galactosylsphingosine have potent proinflammatory effects, and the latter molecule causes oligodendrocyte and Schwann cell death. The symptoms of Krabbe disease correspond to the toxic effects of these lipids. Brain magnetic resonance imaging (MRI) of affected infants demonstrates contrast-enhancing inflammatory demyelination. Peripheral demyelination, delayed conduction velocities, and combined motor and sensory neuropathy are evident on nerve conduction studies even at 1 day of age. Infants with early-onset, severe Krabbe disease are irritable, arching, and even opisthotonic, and they are sometimes misdiagnosed with severe gastroesophageal reflux. Progression of demyelination results in developmental regression. Eventually dysphagia and poor airway clearance lead to aspiration pneumonia. Data regarding treatment are sparse but indicate that HSCT must be performed before 1 month of age to prolong life span, although peripheral neuropathy and posttransplantation gross motor outcomes may continue to worsen in survivors. Transplantation performed following onset of clinically evident symptoms is not effective at preventing central demyelination and regression. Atypical, later-onset variants of Krabbe disease also exist and may be more amenable to treatment with HSCT.

Arylsulfatase a Deficiency (Metachromatic Leukodystrophy)

Metachromatic leukodystrophy (MLD) is an autosomal-recessive disorder caused by insufficient enzymatic activity of arylsulfatase A. This enzymatic defect results in moderate to massive accumulation of sulfated glycolipids, in particular, galactosylceramide-3-O-sulfate (sulfatide), in the brain, peripheral nervous system, and kidneys. Although the age of onset and dynamics of disease progression vary, MLD is primarily characterized by progressive neurodegeneration of the central and peripheral nervous systems. The severe form of the disease presents before the fourth birthday with hypotonia, muscle weakness, areflexia, and peripheral neuropathy. Psychomotor regression is rapid, leading to loss of ambulation, vision, hearing, and swallow ability. Death from aspiration pneumonia typically takes place about 5 years from symptom onset. Symptoms of attenuated, later-onset forms of MLD are characterized by ataxia, gait disturbance, and deterioration of fine motor function. There are also psychiatric presentations of MLD manifesting as personality changes, onset of bizarre behaviors, or frank psychosis. The attenuated forms of MLD also progress toward loss of cognition and function. Early HSCT at a presymptomatic stage for infantile-onset MLD is completely ineffective and is not recommended. When performed for attenuated disease, HSCT before onset of clinical symptoms is able to stabilize cerebral demyelination and arrests or slows disease progression. Peripheral demyelination, however, is not addressed by HSCT, and survivors develop neuropathic motor deficits later on. Intrathecal administration of recombinant human arylsulfatase A enzyme is being investigated as a therapeutic option for MLD.

Mucopolysaccharidoses

The mucopolysaccharidoses (MPSs) are a family of inborn errors of metabolism characterized by deficiencies in enzymes that catabolize glycosaminoglycans (GAGs), highly polar polymers of uronic acid–substituted acetylhexamine disaccharides (Wraith, 2013). Although symptoms of each individual MPS type vary according to the type of GAG accumulated, in general MPS disease manifestations are multisystemic in nature because of the near-ubiquity of GAGs throughout the body. Severe and attenuated forms exist, both of which are associated with similar but varying degrees of somatic involvement, whereas primary neurodegeneration is encountered mainly in severely affected patients. The following discussion summarizes the potential disease symptoms.

Neurologic Manifestations

Patients with certain MPS types have progressive neurocognitive deterioration. Early neurologic signs of disease, manifest as gross motor or speech delay, may be evident in late infancy or later. Patients may initially be suspected to have an autism spectrum disorder. Those with MPS III (Sanfilippo syndrome) and severe forms of MPS I, II, and VII typically develop neurodegeneration. This may be partly attributable to the buildup of heparan sulfate, a GAG localized mostly within the CNS and linked possibly to neuroinflammation. Although the onset and rate of disease progression vary, patients with severe MPS I (Hurler syndrome), who have near complete deficiency of α-L-iduronidase enzyme, and MPS IIIA, who lack sulfoglucosamine sulfohydrolase, have earlier childhood onset and more rapid deterioration. Patients with more attenuated versions of MPS I, II, and VII may have varying degrees of cognitive impairment, which is nonprogressive; this is true as well for some patients with MPS IV and VI.

Secondary neurologic problems may also develop as a consequence of "communicating" hydrocephalus, caused by GAG accumulation in the arachnoid granulations impairing the normal reuptake of cerebrospinal fluid. Additionally, GAG storage in the meninges ("pachymeningitis") and soft tissues surrounding the upper cervical vertebrae can lead to spinal cord compression, typically at the craniocervical junction. Myelopathy may also develop in patients with odontoid hypoplasia at risk for cervical subluxation, and carpal tunnel syndrome is also often encountered.

Ophthalmologic Manifestations

MPS types I, IVA, VI, and VII may develop progressive clouding of the corneas. Early in the disease, this is subtle and appears as a haze that is evident only upon examination with a direct light source. Advanced corneal clouding will disrupt visual acuity and may require corneal transplantation. Glaucoma, as a result of GAG storage in the canals of Schlemm and impaired anterior chamber fluid drainage, develops in older MPS patients.

Otolaryngologic Manifestations

Many affected patients experience recurrent otitis media requiring placement of middle ear drainage tubes. Caregivers often report chronic rhinorrhea and nasal congestion, often predating the diagnosis of MPS. Airway GAG storage, together with macroglossia and abnormal craniocervical bone structure, contribute to the high frequency of obstructive sleep apnea in these patients. Progression of airway compromise, airway floppiness, risk of cervical spinal cord compression with neck hyperextension, and reduced mandibular opening result in very challenging anesthesiologic issues for MPS patients. Intubations are often performed videoscopically and/or nastotracheally by otolaryngologists or anesthesiologists in operating rooms, and patients with severe airway compromise often require tracheostomies.

Cardiovascular Manifestations

Cardiac hypertrophy and progressive valve thickening and dysfunction (typically involving the mitral and aortic valves) are common manifestations of all MPSs. Before treatment, myocardial infarction from coronary artery GAG accumulation and stenosis was a common cause of death for patients with MPS I. Long-term follow-up in the posttreatment era indicates that cardiovascular MPS manifestations continue to progress despite "successful" treatment with either stem cell transplantation or enzyme replacement therapy. MPS patients continue to have arterial storage, as evidenced by increased intimal-medial thickness and severely reduced arterial compliance.

Gastroenterologic Manifestations

GAG storage in the liver and spleen resulting in hepatosplenomegaly is a cardinal sign of nearly all MPS types. Inguinal, umbilical, and hiatal hernias (with resultant gastroesophageal reflux) are extremely common, possibly as a result of increased intraabdominal pressure from enlarged viscera.

Orthopedic Manifestations

Most bones develop from endochondral ossification of growth plate cartilage. Because GAGs are a primary component of cartilage, nearly all patients with MPS develop bony dysplasia ("dysostosis multiplex") of varying severity, as cartilaginous GAG storage impairs chondrocytic proliferation and promotes articular inflammation. The skeletal dysplasia typically is worse in MPS IVA and VI and severe forms of MPS I, II, and VII, and it is most attenuated in MPS III. Indeed, subtle somatic involvement in those with MPS III (Sanfilippo syndrome) may lead to delayed diagnosis. Patients usually have disproportionately short stature, and those with MPS IVA have a short trunk and prominent pectus deformity. Craniofacial structure is altered, resulting in nasal bridge depression and nasopharyngeal airway problems. Vertebral body dysplasia, resulting in platyspondyly (flattened, wafer-like vertebrae) or hook/wedge-shaped vertebrae, often manifests early in infancy or childhood as kyphosis ("gibbus" deformity). Polyarticular joint contractures are extremely common and significantly impair activities of daily living. GAG-induced joint inflammation results in adolescent-onset degenerative joint disease, which is most prominent in the hip and spinal facet joints.

Treatment

Regulatory-approved enzyme replacement therapies currently exist for MPS types I, II, IVA, and VI. As with enzyme-replacement therapy (ERT) for other LSDs, intravenous administration of the cognate exogenous recombinant enzyme relies on cellular uptake via cellular mannose-6-phosphate receptors. HSCT can also be performed for the same MPS types, but it is typically undertaken only for severe MPS I because of the CNS impermeability of intravenous ERT. HSCT has not been shown to alter ultimate neurologic prognosis in patients with MPS II and III, although it continues to be performed primarily in Japan for severe MPS II patients.

Although these treatments usually normalize hepatosplenomegaly and increase patient endurance, each share significant limitations as a result of insufficient access of circulating enzyme to refractory tissues such as bone. Orthopedic disease continues to be extremely common in ERT- and HSCT-treated MPS I patients. Surgeries are often required in treated MPS patients to address carpal tunnel syndrome, degenerative joint disease, and spinal cord compression. It is likely that the avascularity of growth plate and articular cartilage limits enzyme delivery to these tissues. Corneal clouding continues to progress, leading to eventual need for corneal transplant surgery in some patients. Cardiovascular disease also progresses despite treatment, likely because the dense network of connective tissue in the endocardium, heart valves, and vascular intima prevents enzyme access to cardiovascular parenchyma.

Multiple clinical trials for neurologic MPS disease are currently under way to bypass the blood–brain barrier (BBB) completely, through intrathecal ERT in MPS I, II, IIIA, and IIIB, and through protein-tagged enzymes that may allow for intravenous delivery of the enzyme and its subsequent BBB transcytosis and delivery to the CNS in MPS I and II. Clinical trials are also in progress to assess the efficacy of intravenous ERT for MPS VII, and gene therapy is under consideration.

Oligosaccharidoses and Mucolipidoses

Oligosaccharides are short glycan chains released from hydrolysis of glycosylated proteins. Conceptually, oligosaccharidoses are lysosomal storage disorders involving oligosaccharide degradation following detachment from proteins (Figure 41-2), whereas congenital disorders of glycosylation can be thought of as inborn errors of oligosaccharide synthesis, modification, and attachment to proteins.

Mannosidoses

Within the oligosaccharide glycan, there are at least two mannose α-linkages and one β-linkage. Distinct lysosomal enzymes, α-mannosidase and β-mannosidase, are required to hydrolyze the corresponding linkages. Deficiencies of each enzyme result in unique symptoms, despite their closely related functions and substrates.

Individuals with α-mannosidosis have distinct facies notable for macrocephaly, broad prominent forehead, depressed nasal bridge, prognathism, and macroglossia (Govender and Mubaiwa, 2014). Orthopedic manifestations include osteopenia, genu valgum, joint contractures, scoliosis, and hip dysplasia. Neurologic involvement is common because nearly all patients have some degree of moderate to severe intellectual disability and hearing loss, with varying degrees of ataxia, dysarthria, and dysmetria. Depression, anxiety, or hallucinations may occur in response to emotional or physical stressors. In contrast to other LSDs, the natural history of neurologic disease appears to be nonprogressive, although the duration of follow-up is up to 2 years in most reports, and severely affected patients have early childhood mortality. An intravenous ERT is being developed for α-mannosidosis.

There is significant clinical heterogeneity in the clinical manifestations of patients with β-mannosidosis, but most affected patients have intellectual disability and behavioral manifestations such as hyperactivity, aggression, or social withdrawal. They have a higher risk of developing seizures, and many have recurrent respiratory infections. Cutaneous angiokeratomas resembling those of Fabry disease are often seen. Recent exome-based studies have identified β-mannosidase deficiency in patients with "nonclassical" symptoms such as spinocerebellar ataxia and neonatal-onset refractory seizure disorder.

Fucosidosis

Deficiencies of α-L-fucosidase manifest with a broad range of severity. The early-childhood-onset form features neurodegeneration, seizures, extrapyramidal symptoms, hepatosplenomegaly, and bony dysplasia resembling the MPS diseases. Attenuated forms of disease demonstrate mild to moderate developmental delay and coarse facial features. Genotype–phenotype correlations are poor; severe and attenuated siblings have been reported in multiple kindred. Many patients have cutaneous angiokeratomas reminiscent of those seen in Fabry

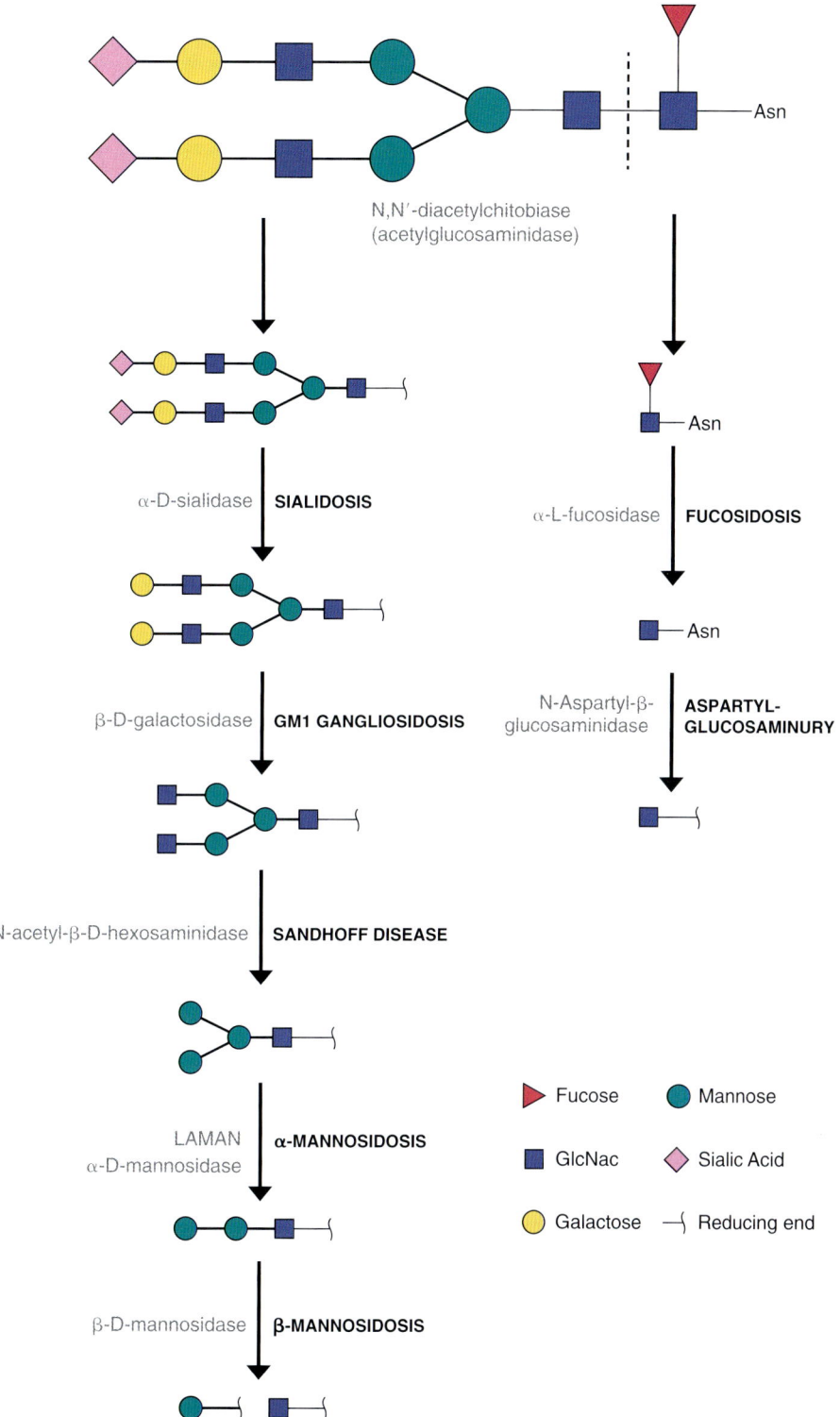

Figure 41-2. Pathway for the catabolism of the N-linked glycan oligosaccharide, enzymes involved, and disorders corresponding with each enzyme deficiency. *(With permission from Bonesso L, Piraud M, Caruba C, et al, Fast urinary screening of oligosaccharidoses by MALDI-TOF/TOF mass spectrometry. Orphanet J Rare Dis. 2014 Feb 6;9:19.)*

disease patients. Brain MRIs of affected patients reveal a very characteristic pattern of T1-weighted hyperintensity and pronounced T2-weighted hypointensity in the globus pallidus, accompanied by generalized subcortical and deep white-matter hypomyelination (Figure 41-3). Presymptomatic HSCT has been performed in a handful of cases. Although cognitive status stabilized posttransplant, it is unclear if this took place as a result of the intervention or, given the intrafamilial variability of the condition, included patients with attenuated disease and a slower disease progression.

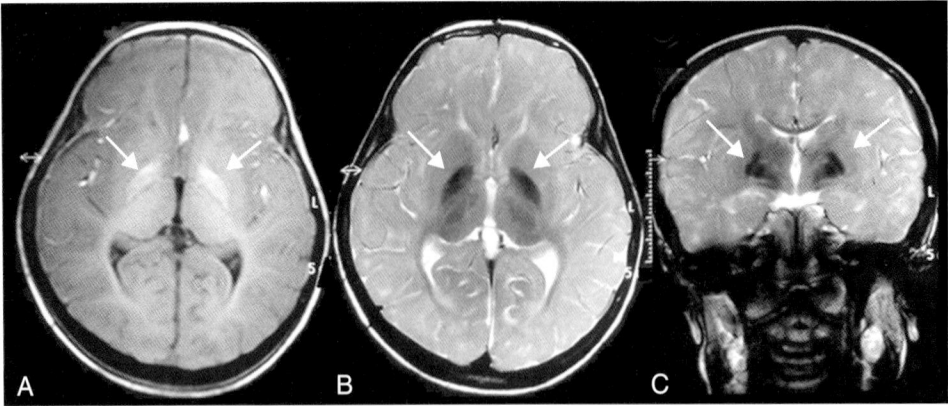

Figure 41-3. Classic MRI findings in fucosidosis. T1-weighted axial (**A**), T2-weighted axial (**B**), and coronal (**C**) MRI of the brain. Bilateral globi pallidi (arrows) show hyperintensity on T1-weighted images and marked hypointensity on T2-weighted images. In addition, there is diffuse symmetric hyperintensity of bilateral subcortical and deep white matter on T2-weighted images with normal appearance on T1-weighted images consistent with hypomyelination. *(With permission from Jain P, Ramesh K, Mohamed A, et al, Neurology. 2012 Jan 31;78[5]:e33.)*

Aspartylglycosaminuria

Deficiency of aspartylglycosaminidase, whose function is to detach the oligosaccharide from the asparagine residue of the glycoprotein, is a disorder more prevalent in Finns that results in slowly progressive intellectual degeneration that begins in childhood and continues throughout adolescence and adulthood. Early symptoms are hypotonia and increased propensity for recurrent acute otitis media and upper and lower respiratory tract infections. Facial features coarsen with time. Adults with this condition are invariably nonverbal and suffer early mortality in their fourth to fifth decade. Brain MRI displays reduced T2 signal intensity in the thalamus, especially the pulvinar region, with poor gray-/white-matter differentiation and atrophy of the cerebrum, cerebellum, and corpus callosum.

Sialidosis (Mucolipidosis I)

Numerous different presentations can be seen in sialidosis, which is also known as neuraminidase deficiency and cherry-red spot myoclonus syndrome. The latter presentation is an attenuated form of the disease that does not significantly affect intelligence or result in early mortality; it presents in adolescence or early adulthood with myoclonus and reduced visual acuity. Affected patients with cherry-red spot myoclonus syndrome eventually lose the ability to ambulate independently because the myoclonus increasingly impairs walking. Sialidosis is also one of the lysosomal storage disorders that causes non-immune hydrops fetalis. This can be severe enough to cause intrauterine death, but even the neonates who survive to be born have severe respiratory distress and hepatosplenomegaly and do not live long. There are also "intermediate" forms of the disease without hydrops, which present in infancy or early childhood with developmental delay, coarse facial features, organomegaly, and skeletal dysplasia. These patients usually develop macular cherry-red spots and myoclonus. Some have developed gram-quantity proteinuria and hypoalbuminemia, with subsequent ascites and peripheral edema. Life expectancy with intermediate sialidoses is also reduced. Currently, there are no treatments available or in preclinical development.

Galactosialidosis

One of the few LSDs whose symptoms reflect a simultaneous dysfunction of two enzymes, galactosialidosis is caused by deficiency of cathepsin A, also known as lysosomal protective protein. Although cathepsin A has lysosomal protease domains, it also forms a complex with neuraminidase and β-D-galactosidase. Without cathepsin A, the latter two enzymes are rapidly degraded, resulting in a disorder that combines features of both sialidosis and G_{M1} gangliosidosis (Caciotti et al., 2013). A neonatal lethal form resembles the severe form of sialidosis, with the development of fetal hydrops, ascites, macular cherry-red spots, and hepatosplenomegaly. A later infantile form develops cherry-red spots, organomegaly, coarse features, sensorineural hearing loss, skeletal dysplasia, and cardiac valvular thickening in the first year of life. Most of the reported patients with the juvenile/adult form are Japanese, and presentation includes intellectual disability, ataxia, myoclonus, very slow neurocognitive decline, and angiokeratomas.

Schindler–Kanzaki Disease

Schindler–Kanzaki disease is a very rare condition, with less than 15 patients identified, and is characterized by oligosaccharidosis, attributed to α-N-acetylgalactosaminidase deficiency. The clinical phenotype is somewhat unclear. The original siblings described with Schindler disease had early onset neurodegeneration, seizure disorder, and hypotonia leading to spastic quadriplegia, cortical blindness, and loss of interaction. Elevated N-acetylgalactosaminyl oligosaccharide excretion and neuroaxonal spheroids were noted. Similar clinicopathologic findings were reported in a second kindred; however, subsequent patients have been identified with neither neurodegeneration nor neuroaxonal dystrophy. Affected patients have a variety of symptoms, including "autism" without facial dysmorphism, neurologic findings, or organomegaly; hepatosplenomegaly; cardiac valvular disease; and infantile death. Some patients have mild psychomotor retardation associated seizures. Because the three original Schindler patients with the infantile neuroaxonal dystrophy form were from two distantly related, consanguineous German kindred, and the gene associated with infantile neuroaxonal dystrophy is immediately proximal to the Schindler–Kanzaki gene, it is possible that the severe expression is a result of the families having two monogenic recessive conditions.

Other Lysosomal Storage Disorders
Mucolipidosis II/III

Two genes, *GNPTAB* and *GNPTG*, encode subunits of the N-acetylglucosamine-1-phosphotransferase enzyme complex, which participates in the formation of the crucial mannose-6-phosphate sugar residue on the glycan complexes of proteins destined for transport to lysosomes. Deficiencies of any subunit result in absent or reduced mannose-6-phosphate, causing lysosomal enzymes to be mistargeted for secretion into plasma. Various substrates accumulate because cells lack the proper intralysosomal hydrolases. Molecular sequencing establishes the diagnosis, but, biochemically, patients have markedly increased plasma levels of lysosomal enzymes (normally measured in leukocytes) and have elevated urinary oligosaccharide excretion.

Mucolipidosis II, historically known as I-cell disease, is the severe form of the disease that resembles rapidly progressive MPS type I. Affected neonates are noticeably coarse with gingival hypertrophy. Spinal kyphosis and other features of dysostosis multiplex are already evident at birth. Growth typically stops by the second birthday. Gross motor development is impaired. Cognitive development, although blighted, allows for the children to interact and have limited communication. Cardiorespiratory failure is the usual cause of death.

Mucolipidosis III, historically known as pseudo-Hurler dystrophy, is an attenuated form of the disease. Age of onset is typically before 3 years, when slowing of growth, joint stiffness, bone pain, and coarsening of facial features becomes evident. Short stature, dysostosis multiplex, bilateral hip dysplasia, and painful ambulation become prominent in the first decade of life. Intelligence ranges from mild impairment to normal. Progressive restrictive lung disease, mitral insufficiency, and aortic regurgitation cause left ventricular enlargement and heart failure, the usual causes of death in early to middle adulthood.

Mucolipidosis IV (ML IV)

Unlike most of the other LSDs, ML IV is not a deficiency of a lysosomal hydrolases. The missing protein, mucolipin-1, is involved in lysosomal substrate transport and exocytosis. Storage granules are evident in skin or conjunctival biopsies. Severe psychomotor delay develops in the first year of life; patients are rarely able to speak or ambulate, and dysphagia is common. Initial neonatal hypotonia eventually evolves into a static, spastic quadriplegia (Wakabayashi et al., 2011). In fact, this condition should be suspected in any child with a cerebral palsy diagnosis, especially if there is concomitant corneal clouding or retinal dystrophy. Ophthalmologic disease is progressive, and by adolescence patients with classical ML IV, most of whom are of Ashkenazi Jewish descent, have severe visual impairment. Achlorhydria, hypergastrinemia, and iron deficiency are common chemical markers of ML IV. No specific treatment exists for this condition.

Cystinosis

Cystinosis is a lysosomal storage disorder like ML IV, but the deficient protein is as transporter rather than a hydrolase. The cystinosin protein transports cystine (the dibasic dimer of the amino acid cysteine) into the cytosol from the lysosome. Intralysosomal cystine crystal storage, caused by cystinosin deficiency, results in a disorder with a range of severity. The classical nephropathic form causes neonatal-onset renal Fanconi syndrome, with resultant hyponatremic, hypokalemic metabolic acidosis, glycosuria, and hypophosphatemic rickets (Ivanova et al., 2014). Consequently, infants have polydipsia, polyuria, and very short stature. Intelligence is not affected. Deposition of cystine crystals in the cornea may result in photophobia and, ultimately, blindness. Untreated, affected children die before the second decade of life because of progressive renal failure. Cystinosis is currently treated with enteral and ophthalmic instillation of cysteamine, which

enables cysteine to exit the lysosome using a different transporter. However, cysteamine is not well tolerated because of its foul odor and side effect of gastrointestinal irritation. Although an enteric-release form has been developed, investigations are under way to determine whether autologous gene-transfer HSCT can effectively treat the condition.

Neuronal Ceroid Lipofuscinoses

The neuronal ceroid lipofuscinoses (NCLs) are a group of lysosomal storage disorders united by their progressive, neurodegenerative course, characterized by visual loss, seizures, and cognitive dysfunction. Despite the overlap in clinical manifestations, there is broad genetic heterogeneity, and the cellular roles of the cognate proteins remain incompletely defined. Interestingly, subcellular localization for the NCL-associated proteins have also been diverse, localized mostly in lysosomes (CLN1, CLN2, CLN3, CLN5, CLN7, CLN10, CLN12, and CLN13) but also in the endoplasmic reticulum (CLN6 and CLN8) or in the cytosol associated with vesicular membranes (CLN4 and CLN14) (Cárcel-Trullols et al., 2015).

Although individual NCL subtypes vary according to age of onset and initial symptoms, the ultimate prognosis for all clinical variants has not changed significantly, and development of treatment and characterization of disease pathogenesis severely lags behind the identification of new gene loci.

Identification of underlying gene defects has not been concordant with prior nomenclature for NCLs, which classified the various subtypes according to age of onset (e.g., infantile-onset NCL [INCL], late-infantile-onset NCL [LINCL], juvenile-onset NCL [JNCL], adult-onset NCL [ANCL]). Currently, there are 14 distinct NCL gene loci, with up to 7 shown to cause LINCL phenotypes. Moreover, four of these seven LINCL loci have also been identified among ANCL cases, whereas three distinct loci have been associated with ANCL phenotypes. This review focuses primarily on the classical NCL gene loci and phenotypes. For information about the more recently described variant loci, please consult the online chapter version.

Ophthalmologic Manifestations

Many of the NCLs demonstrate a characteristic progressive decline in visual acuity. Changes are detected by electroretinography (ERG) before noticeable decline in vision. Depending on the subtype, the first initial observation on ERG may be an abnormal cone/rod downstream signaling in the case of CLN1 (caused by protein palmitoyl thioesterase deficiency [PPT1], previously known as INCL); delayed and reduced cone amplitudes for CLN2 (caused by tripeptidyl peptidase deficiency [TPP], previously known as classical LINCL); or absent rod and reduced cone amplitude responses for CLN3 (caused by Battenin deficiency [CLN3], previously known as classical JNCL).

CLN1 and CLN2 patients typically develop reduced visual attention after onset of neurologic symptoms, whereas CLN3 patients typically manifest first with reduced nighttime visual acuity that then progresses to daytime peripheral vision loss. Eventually, patients with CLN types 1 through 3 become completely blind, with nonresponsive ERGs. Optic nerve pallor, attenuation of retinal vasculature, or pigmentary retinopathy may be visualized on dilated ophthalmologic examination.

Before the availability of genetic testing for NCL, examination of conjunctival biopsies for presence and morphology of cellular inclusion bodies was utilized to identify NCL subtype. With the identification of underlying gene defects, the same morphology of inclusion body was often found in different subtypes. Furthermore, multiple inclusion body types could be found within a single CLN genotype. A summary of these ultrastructural abnormalities, together with causative CLN genes, is presented in Table 41-2.

Neurologic Manifestations

Seizures and neurodegeneration are clinical features shared by nearly all of the NCLs. Affected patients develop mixed generalized tonic-clonic, partial, and absence seizures, with subsequent development of myoclonus. Age of seizure onset overlaps somewhat, but generally follows NCL subtype, with seizures typically beginning in the first 2 years of life for CLN1, 2 to 4 years of life for CLN2, and in the second decade of life for CLN3. Seizures in cathepsin D–deficient NCL have been observed in two neonates, leading to its designation as "neonatal NCL." However, cathepsin D mutations have also been described in two families presenting during school age (8–15 years) with ataxia, cerebellar atrophy, pigmentary retinopathy, and neurodegeneration, highlighting the phenotypic heterogeneity of these disorders.

Most classic patients with the "ANCL" phenotype, manifesting with ataxia, progressive dementia, seizures, and myoclonus after age 30 years (previously referred to as Kufs syndrome), have been shown to have recessive *CLN6* mutations. Recessive mutations in cathepsin F (*CTSF*) have been found in some variant ANCL patients without seizures, but with more prominent behavior abnormalities, movement disorders, and dementia. Mutations that confer residual protein function account for survival past childhood.

Neurodegenerative disease in CLN types 1 through 3 is often preceded by a period of developmental delay or cognitive stagnation. Any cognitive and verbal abilities are pruned and eventually lost, as are ambulation and other motor skills. Dysphagia and difficulty with management of oral secretions leads to cachexia and recurrent aspiration pneumonia. Behavioral abnormalities may be present in CLN3 disease, and they may be more prominent in the CTSF-ANCL phenotype.

Brain MRIs demonstrate progressive loss of cerebral and cerebellar gray and white matter that roughly correlates with progression of seizure severity, neurodegeneration, and ataxia. Pneumonia, sepsis, and seizure-related complications are the usual causes of death for CLN patients.

Diagnostic Testing

Quantitative enzymatic testing can be performed to assay for deficiencies of PPT1 (CLN1), TPP (CLN2), CTSD (CLN10), and CTSF (CLN13). If these enzymatic activities are normal, then targeted or next-generation sequencing of the remaining CLN loci can be performed, depending on the ethnicity of the patient. Neutrophil inclusion bodies can be seen in, but are not specific for, CLN3 disease. Recessive mutations in *CLN5* are responsible for most of the "INCL" presentations in patients of Finnish descent. Another NCL that occurs more frequently in those of Finnish descent is "Northern epilepsy," caused by *CLN8* mutations and characterized by onset of seizures between ages 5 and 10 and followed by intellectual decline, ataxia, and adult-onset vision loss.

Treatment

Currently, there are no effective therapeutic options for any of the NCLs. Supportive care is recommended to reduce the

TABLE 41-2 Neuronal Ceroid Lipofuscinosis

Listing of Neuronal Ceroid Lipofuscinosis Forms, Including Gene Locus, Type of Protein Product, and Morphology of Storage Material Visualized on Electron Microscopy

Clinical Form	Gene	Locus	Gene Product and Localization	Electron Microscopy of Storage Material
Congenital	CLN10 (CTSD)	11p15.5	Cathepsin D	Lysosome
Infantile and juvenile variant	CLN1 (PPT1)	1p34.2	Lysosomal palmitoyl-protein thioesterase	Granular osmiophilic deposits
Classic, late infantile, and juvenile variant	CLN2 (TPP1)	11p15.4	Lysosomal tripeptidyl peptidase	Curvilinear/mixed
Infantile, Finnish variant	CLN5	13q22.3	Novel 407 AA lysosomal membrane protein	Fingerprint, curvilinear, rectilinear complex
Late infantile, Costa Rican variant	CLN6	15q23	Novel 311 AA endoplasmic reticulum membrane protein	Curvilinear, fingerprint, rectilinear
Late infantile, Turkish variant	CLN7 (MFSD8)	4q28.2	Membrane protein	Fingerprint/mixed
Late infantile, rare variant	KCTD7	7q11.21	289 amino acid cytosolic protein connected with ubiquitin ligase complex	Fingerprint, granular osmiophilic deposits, none
Classic, juvenile	CLN3	16p11.2	Lysosomal membrane protein (438 AA)	Fingerprint/mixed
Epilepsy with intellectual disability, Northern epilepsy	CLN8	8p23.3	286 AA endoplasmic reticulum membrane protein	Curvilinear or osmiophilic granular-like
Juvenile variant	CLN1	1p34.2	—	—
Juvenile variant	CLN2	11p15.4	—	—
Juvenile variant	CLN9	?	—	—
Kufs disease (adult variant)	CTSD, PPT1, CLN3, CLN5, CLN6, CTSF, GRN	Multiple	Multiple	Varies

impact of seizures, dysphagia, and aspiration pneumonia. Lamotrigine may be more efficacious with CLN3-associated seizures, but it may worsen CLN2-related seizures and myoclonus. Valproic acid (which can lead to sedation), clonazepam (sialorrhea), and carbamazepine and phenytoin (both associated with seizure exacerbation) are typically not well tolerated by patients with an NCL. HSCT has not been effective, nor was a trial of intracerebroventricular human embryonic stem cell injection. Enteral N-acetylcysteine and cysteamine administration to CLN1 patients prolonged the mean time to isoelectric electroencephalograms and reduced microscopic evidence of storage deposits, but patients continued to demonstrate progressive loss of cognitive and retinal function and failed to acquire developmental milestones. Currently active clinical trials for NCLs include intraventricular delivery of recombinant human TPP enzyme or intracerebral adeno-associated viral gene therapy for CLN2 and immunosuppressive mycophenolate mofetil treatment for CLN3 disease.

REFERENCES

The complete list of references for this chapter is available in the e-book at www.expertconsult.com.
    See inside cover for registration details.

SELECTED REFERENCES

Caciotti, A., Catarzi, S., Tonin, R., et al., 2013. Galactosialidosis: review and analysis of CTSA gene mutations. Orphanet J. Rare Dis. 28, 114.

Cárcel-Trullols, J., Kovács, A.D., Pearce, D.A., 2015. Cell biology of the NCL proteins: What they do and don't do. Biochim. Biophys. Acta 1852 (10 Pt B), 2242–2255.

Govender, R., Mubaiwa, L., 2014. Alpha-mannosidosis: a report of 2 siblings and review of the literature. J. Child Neurol. 29 (1), 131–134.

Ivanova, E., De Leo, M.G., De Matteis, M.A., et al., 2014. Cystinosis: clinical presentation, pathogenesis and treatment. Pediatr. Endocrinol. Rev. 12 (Suppl. 1), 176–184.

Rombach, S.M., Smid, B.E., Linthorst, G.E., et al., 2014. Natural course of Fabry disease and the effectiveness of enzyme replacement therapy: a systematic review and meta-analysis: effectiveness of ERT in different disease stages. J. Inherit. Metab. Dis. 37 (3), 341–352.

Sandhoff, K., 2013. Metabolic and cellular bases of sphingolipidoses. Biochem. Soc. Trans. 41 (6), 1562–1568.

Valle, D., et al. (Eds.), 2014. Part 16: Lysosomal Disorders. In: The Online Metabolic and Molecular Bases of Inherited Disease. McGraw-Hill, New York, NY.

Wakabayashi, K., Gustafson, A.M., Sidransky, E., et al., 2011. Mucolipidosis type IV: an update. Mol. Genet. Metab. 104 (3), 206–213.

Wraith, J.E., 2013. Mucopolysaccharidoses and mucolipidoses. Handb. Clin. Neurol. 113, 1723–1729.

E-BOOK FIGURES AND TABLES

42 Mitochondrial Diseases

Darryl C. De Vivo and Salvatore DiMauro

HISTORY AND MITOCHONDRIAL GENETICS

Mitochondrial diseases represent one of the most exciting chapters of modern medicine. During the last half of the 19th century, scientists gradually recognized the presence of subcellular organelles that were termed *mitochondria* in 1898. The metabolic role of mitochondria in cellular function was defined by a series of observations during the early part of the 20th century: the cytochrome system and oxidation-reduction processes were described, the Krebs cycle was conceptualized, and later the phosphorylation of adenosine diphosphate to adenosine triphosphate was documented, together with the dependence of phosphorylation on oxygen consumption. By the middle of the 20th century, it was clear that the mitochondrion represented the intracellular domain for intermediary metabolism. In 1961 the chemiosmotic theory was proposed to explain the proton-motive force that facilitated the synthesis of adenosine triphosphate. In parallel with these biochemical observations, a series of ultrastructural studies characterized the four components of the organelle, including the outer mitochondrial membrane (OMM), the inner mitochondrial membrane (IMM), the intermembranous space (IMS), and the inner matrix compartment. Subsequent studies have demonstrated that the IMM is largely impermeable to molecules of all sizes, and special adaptive mechanisms are necessary for the translocation of metabolites from the IMS to the matrix. The protein importation process is energy-dependent and requires the macromolecules to be unfolded before traversing the mitochondrial membranes and refolded after entering the mitochondrial matrix.

Two important observations were made in 1963 that were central to the understanding of mitochondrial diseases. The first observation recognized the presence of intramitochondrial fibers with DNA characteristics, documenting DNA in mitochondria (mtDNA). The second observation described ragged-red fibers with abundant mitochondria in biopsied skeletal muscle.

Twenty-five years later, the era of "mitochondrial genetics" opened up with two seminal papers that introduced human diseases due to mutations in mtDNA. As all mtDNA is derived from the ovum, it is inherited exclusively from the mother—hence the terms *mitochondrial inheritance, maternal inheritance,* and *cytoplasmic inheritance.* These interchangeable terms describe a non-Mendelian pattern of inheritance that characterizes human diseases resulting from mtDNA mutations (Schon et al., 2012).

Each mitochondrion contains 2 to 10 copies of the mtDNA genome. Because cells have hundreds or thousands of mitochondria, more than 10,000 copies of mtDNA may exist in each cell. This genome is a small, double-stranded, circular molecule containing 16,569 base pairs; each molecule contains a light strand and a heavy strand, and each strand contains its own origin of replication (Fig. 42-1). Clear differences exist between the mitochondrial genome and the nuclear genome (Table 27-1). The mitochondrial genome contains no introns. The only noncoding region in mtDNA is the displacement loop (D-loop). The D-loop region contains 1000 base pairs and is the site of origin for replication of the heavy strand and the promoter regions for both light and heavy strand transcription. Because the universal genetic code does not apply to mtDNA, the mitochondrial genome requires its own transcriptional and translational factors for synthesis of mitochondrial proteins. The mitochondrial genome contains 37 genes. Thirteen genes encode structural proteins in the respiratory chain. The mitochondrial genome also contains 24 genes for protein synthesis. These genes include two ribosomal RNAs (rRNAs) and 22 transfer RNAs (tRNAS). The mtDNA genes code for 13 messenger RNAs, and all 13 gene products are located in the respiratory chain (Fig. 42-1).

The normal mitochondrial genotype is considered *homoplasmic* if all mtDNA genomes are identical. Conversely, the genotype is *heteroplasmic* if the genomes represent a mixture of wild type and mutated type. The phenotype is determined by the proportion of mutated genomes. When this proportion exceeds a threshold, the biologic behavior of the cell, of the tissue, and of a human individual changes, reflecting the impaired energy state. However, a supersensitive, next-generation sequencing study shows low-level changes (0.2% to 2.0% coexistence of mutated mtDNAs) present in blood and skeletal muscle of clinically unaffected individuals, a phenomenon termed "universal heteroplasmy" (Payne et al., 2013). The *threshold effect* is a relative concept influenced by several factors such as the age of the patient and the energy demands of any specific tissue or organ. For example, brain and muscle cells have high energy demands, as do tissues of the developing child. In these situations, the threshold for phenotypic expression of a pathogenic mutation is lower.

Replicative or *mitotic segregation* is a biologic concept that refers to the stochastic redistribution of the mtDNA genomes during mitochondrial and cell divisions. The random segregation of the mitochondrial genomes during replication influences the oxidative capability of the cellular progeny. The concepts of threshold effect and replicative segregation have provided theoretic explanations for the variable phenotypic expression of maternally transmitted human diseases.

CLASSIFICATION OF MITOCHONDRIAL DISEASES

Several classification schemes of mitochondrial diseases were based on differing criteria. The original classification scheme which attempts to classify mitochondrial diseases by clinical or morphologic criteria was unsatisfactory. The phenotypic heterogeneity of mitochondrial diseases complicated the clinical classification efforts. Similarly, the lack of histopathologic uniformity undermined the morphologic classification efforts.

In 1988, primary mutations of the mitochondrial genome were particularly relevant to respiratory chain defects because this metabolic pathway is under the dual genetic influence of the mitochondrial and nuclear genomes. In recent times, the term "mitochondrial diseases" has been increasingly restricted to defects of one metabolic pathway, the respiratory chain, and further subgrouped as nuclear DNA defects and mtDNA defects.

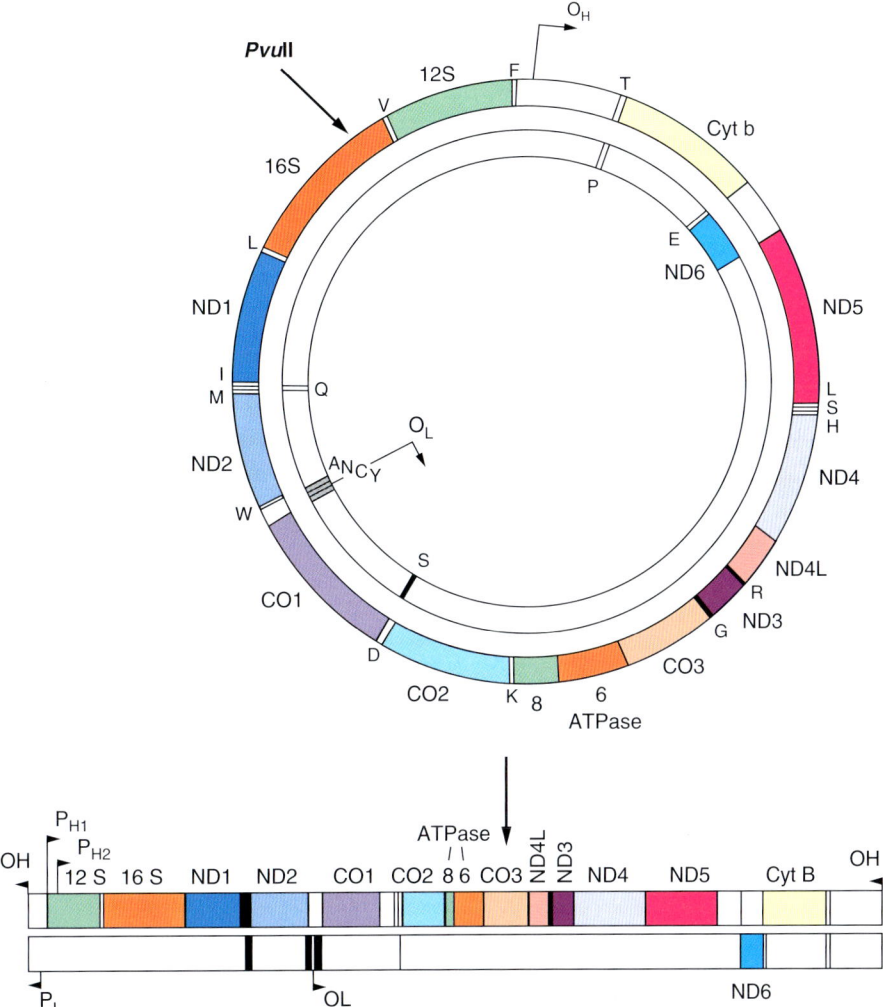

Figure 42-1. The mitochondrial respiratory chain (bottom) and the mitochondrial DNA (top). Genes and corresponding gene products are similarly color-coded. ND denotes the subunits of NADH-CoQ oxidoreductase (complex I); cyt *b* + cytochrome *b;* subunits of cytochrome *c* oxidase (complex IV) are labeled CO in both renditions; A6 and A8 denote subunits 6 and 8 of ATP synthase (complex V). The 22 tRNA genes are identified by one-letter amino acid nomenclature; 12S and 16S denote ribosomal RNAs (rRNAs). O_H and O_L are the origin of heavy- and light-strand replication; HSP and LSP are the promoters of heavy- and light-strand transcription. ADP = adenosine diphosphate; ATP = adenosine triphosphate.Mitochondrial DNA contains 16,569 base pairs and 37 genes. These genes include two ribosomal RNA, 22 transfer RNA, and 13 structural reading frames. Digestion of human mtDNA with a single endonuclease (Pvu II) cleaves the circular molecule in one place and produces a linearized version. *CO,* cytochrome c oxidase; *CYT,* cytochrome; *OL, OH,* origin of replication for L- and H-strands; *ND,* NADH-CoQ reductase; *PH1,2,* primary transcripts of the H-strand starting at H1, H2; *PL,* light (I-strand promoter). *(With permission from DiMauro, S., 2013. Mitochondrial Encephalomyopathies—fifty years on. Neurology 81, 281–291.)*

One of the many exciting features of mitochondrial diseases is the pattern of inheritance of these diverse conditions. The unique dual influence of the nuclear and mitochondrial genomes on respiratory chain function has captivated students of mitochondrial biology. A biochemical defect involving the respiratory chain may be transmitted either by Mendelian or by non-Mendelian patterns. The strictly maternal inheritance of mitochondria determines the pattern of vertical transmission of mtDNA mutations.

Clinical conditions related to mtDNA point mutations are transmitted from the mother to all her male and female progeny, but only the daughters pass the condition to succeeding generations This genetic profile is reminiscent of Mendelian inheritance, including autosomal-dominant and X-linked patterns, but both genders are equally affected, and there is no father-to-child transmission. Expression of the maternally inherited genetic defect is determined by replicative segregation and by the threshold effect. These biologic principles are demonstrated in several neurologic diseases associated with mtDNA mutations, including Leber hereditary optic neuropathy (LHON), MERRF, MELAS, and the syndrome of neuropathy, ataxia, retinitis pigmentosa/maternally inherited Leigh syndrome (NARP/MILS).

Single deletions of mtDNA generally occur sporadically, as with Kearns-Sayre syndrome (KSS), PEO, and Pearson syndrome (PS). A multicenter retrospective study of 226 KSS cases has shown that the risk of a carrier woman to have affected children is very small but finite (1 in 24 births) and disproves the idea that the risk increases with maternal age.

However, the pattern of inheritance for most mitochondrial diseases is not maternal. Rather, classic Mendelian inheritance patterns apply to six main groups of disorders affecting the respiratory chain.

Most subunits of respiratory chain complexes are encoded by nDNA genes directly ("direct hits") or are assembled by nuclear proteins ("indirect hits"). A third dysfunction of the respiratory chain identifies a group of disorders due to altered mtDNA translation. A fourth category includes changes of phospholipid composition of the IMM. A fifth group of mitochondrial diseases is due to altered dynamics (mitochondrial motility, fusion, fission). Interestingly, the sixth disease category (defects of mtDNA maintenance) is due to faulty communication between the two genomes, usually called defects of intergenomic signaling (DiMauro et al., 2013). For example, syndromes of PEO with multiple deletions of mtDNA are inherited as autosomal-dominant or, more rarely, as autosomal-recessive traits. The nuclear gene defects in these cases apparently alter the biologic integrity of the mitochondrial genome and predispose the patient to multiple mtDNA deletions that characterize these clinical syndromes. Another defect of intergenomic signaling is due to a quantitative defect of mtDNA (mtDNA depletion). Syndromes due to mtDNA depletion may affect predominantly one tissue (infantile myopathy or hepatopathy) or multiple tissues (hepatocerebral syndrome) and are due to nuclear gene mutations impairing mtDNA replication.

METABOLIC DISTURBANCES

The principal function of mitochondria is the oxidation of substrates and the synthesis of adenosine triphosphate (ATP) (Fig. 42-2). The primary oxidizable substrates include pyruvate, fatty acids, ketone bodies, and amino acids. Mitochondria also play a role in the intracellular sequestration of calcium and in the detoxification of ammonia in the urea cycle. Biochemical defects involving these pathways are associated with distinctive metabolic disturbances. A biochemical defect altering pyruvate metabolism directly or indirectly leads to an elevation of pyruvic acid. Pyruvate is in equilibrium with lactate and alanine. As a result, there is lactic acidosis proportionate or disproportionate to the elevation of pyruvate, depending on the associated effect of the biochemical defect on the oxidation-reduction potential. If the oxidation-reduction potential is unaffected by the biochemical defect, the lactate and pyruvate elevations are proportional and the lactate/pyruvate ratio is normal (less than 20). In contrast, if the oxidation-reduction potential is disturbed by a primary

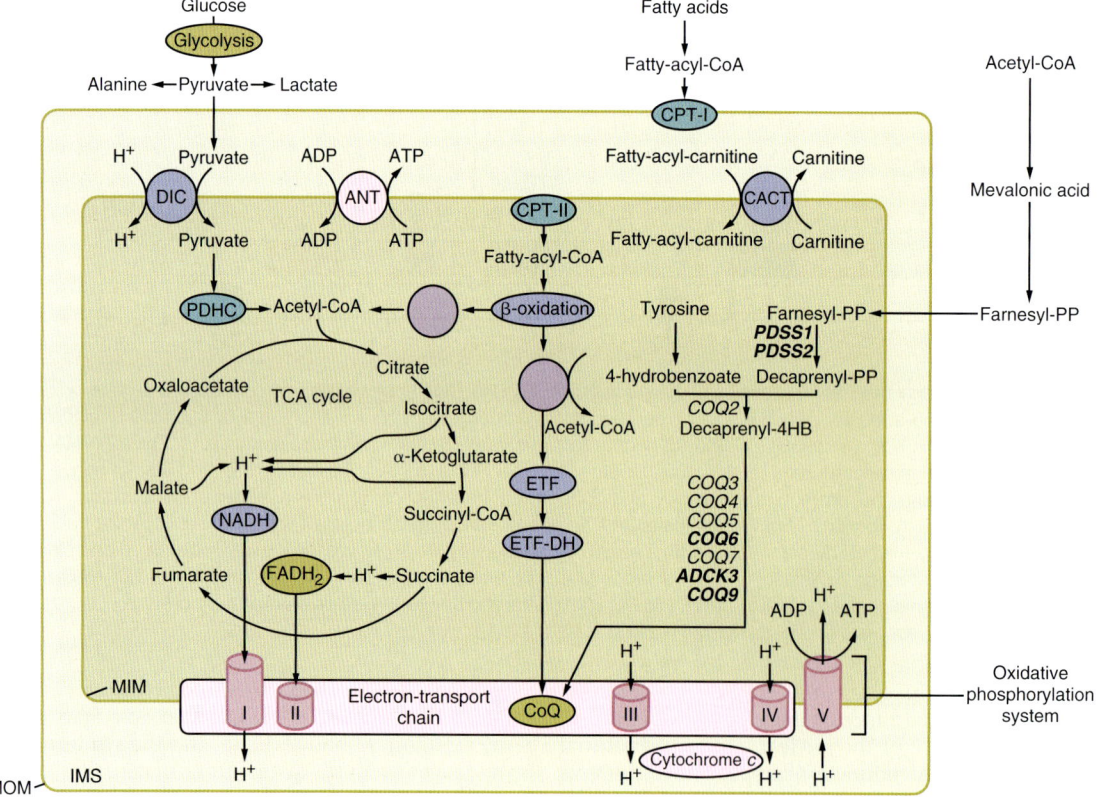

Figure 42-2. Schematic view of mitochondrial metabolism. The respiratory chain is highlighted in red, Electrons from dehydrogenases in the Krebs cycle and in β-oxidation spirals are passed "horizontally" along four protein complexes and two small carriers (the electron-transport chain) that are embedded in the MIM. The electrons travel from complex I (an NADH dehydrogenase) and complex II (a succinate dehydrogenase) to CoQ10 (a small mobile electron carrier also known as ubiquinone), then to complex III (ubiquinone oxidoreductase), cytochrome *c* (another small mobile electron carrier), and complex IV (cytochrome *c* oxidase), ultimately producing water. Concomitant with this horizontal flow of electrons, there is a "vertical" vectorial transport of dehydrogenase-derived protons from the matrix across the MIM into the intermembrane space. This process creates an electrochemical proton gradient across the MIM that is used to drive complex V (F_0F_1 ATP synthase), a tiny "turbine" that converts ADP to ATP. Conventionally, the five complexes comprise the oxidative phosphorylation system. The biosynthetic pathway of CoQ10, beginning with acetyl-CoA, is shown. (Abbreviations: ANT, adenine nucleotide translocator; CACT, carnitine-acylcarnitine translocator; CoA, coenzyme A; CoQ10, coenzyme Q10, CPT, carnitine palmitoyltransferase; DIC, dicarboxylate carrier; ETF, electron-transfer flavoprotein; ETF-DH, ETF dehydrogenase; FAD, flavin adenine dinucleotide; IMS, intermembrane space; MIM, mitochondrial inner membrane; MOM, mitochondrial outer membrane; PDHC, pyruvate dehydrogenase complex; TCA, tricarboxylic acid.) *(With permission from DiMauro, S., 2013. The Clinical Maze of Mitochondrial Neurology. Nat Rev Neurol 9, 429–444.)*

defect involving the respiratory chain, the lactate values are disproportionately elevated and the lactate/pyruvate ratio is increased (greater than 20). Patients with pyruvate dehydrogenase (PDH) deficiency typically have elevated lactate, pyruvate, and alanine concentrations and a normal lactate/pyruvate ratio. In contrast, patients with cytochrome *c* oxidase (COX) deficiency have elevated lactate, pyruvate, and alanine concentrations, but the lactate/pyruvate ratio is increased. These metabolic observations serve as clues to the underlying biochemical defect and may be helpful when all other clinical and metabolic factors are considered simultaneously.

Defects of fatty acid oxidation (FAO) include a variety of mitochondrial defects, but they are considered separately (see Chapter 149) from the more typical mitochondrial encephalomyopathies, which are associated with respiratory chain defects.

HISTOPATHOLOGIC DISTURBANCES

The tissue reactions in mitochondrial diseases may be informative and direct the clinician's attention to the primary metabolic defect, even if they may be modest or absent in some mitochondrial disorders. A muscle biopsy is considered a gold standard for the diagnosis of mitochondrial disease.

Ragged-red fibers (RRF) or, more commonly SDH-intensely positive ("ragged-blue" fibers) and COX-negative fibers have been considered clues to many respiratory chain diseases, including most mtDNA-related disorders. In many nDNA-related disorders, histochemical abnormalities are often seen but not as common or as intense as in mtDNA-related diseases. However, defects of mtDNA maintenance (intergenomic signaling), although unequivocally Mendelian disorders, share many features of mitochondrial genetics, including mtDNA heteroplasmy and the threshold effect. Muscle biopsies often show a checkerboard pattern of ragged-blue and COX-negative fibers.

The brain pathology is distinctive in many mitochondrial diseases. Three patterns are common. The first is a widespread insult to the brain tissue with resulting microcephaly and ventricular dilatation. This pattern is seen in defects of the urea cycle, several defects associated with congenital lactic acidosis, and some of the defects associated with fatty acid metabolism. Malformations also may be seen, including agenesis of the corpus callosum, ectopic displacement of the olivary nuclei, and cystic destruction of the basal ganglia. This pattern is particularly striking in infants with pyruvate dehydrogenase E1 alpha-subunit deficiency. The second pattern is best typified by the neuropathology associated with Leigh syndrome (LS). These patients have a symmetric subcortical distribution of tissue injury with a particular predilection for the basal ganglia, thalamus, brainstem, and cerebellar roof nuclei. Microscopic features include loss of brain cells, proportionate loss of myelin, reactive astrocytosis, and proliferation of the cerebral microvessels. In some patients, particularly those with MELAS, multifocal encephalomalacia develops. This pathologic condition typically is located in the posterior aspect of the cerebral hemisphere. The third pattern is a spongy encephalopathy with loosening and rarefaction of the neuropil. The spongy encephalopathy is the histopathologic counterpart of a defect in cerebral energy metabolism and is commonly seen in patients with KSS. MRI may reflect these patterns of brain tissue injury with a hyperintense signal of the central white matter on the T2-weighted image (Fig. 42-3). Stroke-like lesions in the posterior cerebral hemisphere are typical of MELAS. Signal hyperintensities involving the putamen, globus pallidus, and caudate nuclei are characteristic of Leigh syndrome. A diffuse signal abnormality involving the central white matter is typical of Kearns-Sayre syndrome. Intracranial

calcifications also are seen in these conditions. Basal ganglia calcifications are most commonly associated with KSS and MELAS.

Defects of the Krebs Cycle

Pyruvate is the end product of glycolysis. This metabolite can be reduced to lactate or transaminated to alanine in the cytoplasm. Otherwise, pyruvate is translocated across the mitochondrial membrane (Fig. 42-2). In the mitochondrial matrix, pyruvate is carboxylated to oxaloacetate or decarboxylated and activated to acetyl coenzyme A (acetyl-CoA). The first reaction is catalyzed by pyruvate carboxylase (PC), and the second is catalyzed by the pyruvate dehydrogenase complex (PDHC) (Fig. 42-4). The two reaction products— oxaloacetate and acetyl-CoA—condense to form citrate as the primary reactant in the Krebs cycle. Defects of pyruvate metabolism involve the PDHC, PC, or several enzymes in the Krebs cycle.

Fumarase deficiency is a progressive infantile encephalopathy with failure to thrive, hypotonia, microcephaly, and fumaric aciduria. This condition may be associated with enlarged cerebral ventricles and polyhydramnios in utero.

Succinate dehydrogenase is a critical step in the Krebs cycle and the first component of complex II in the respiratory chain. Before the molecular era, several patients were described with defects of complex II and progressive encephalomyopathy. A mutation in the flavoprotein subunit of succinate dehydrogenase was identified in two sisters with Leigh syndrome, the first example of a nuclear DNA mutation affecting respiratory chain disorder. A few more cases of Leigh syndrome were later associated with mutations in the same gene.

Homozygous mutations in the gene *ACO2*, which encodes the mitochondrial isozyme of aconitase, the Krebs cycle enzyme that interconverts citrate to isocitrate, have been described in infants with a neurodegenerative disorder characterized by optic nerve and retinal atrophy, psychomotor retardation, truncal hypotonia, athetosis, and seizures.

Compound heterozygous *ACO2* mutations can cause either isolated optic neuropathy or syndromic presentations of optic neuropathy plus encephalopathy and cerebellar atrophy.

Combined deficiency of two Krebs cycle enzymes, SDH and aconitase, in skeletal muscle, was described in a young Swedish man with recurrent episodes of exercise-induced myoglobinuria. The etiology of the double enzyme defect is due to the lack of iron-sulfur (Fe-S) cluster proteins, prosthetic groups present in the three complexes (I, II, and III), and in the Krebs cycle enzyme aconitase. Homozygosity mapping revealed a pathogenic mutation in the *ISCU* gene, which encodes iron-sulfur cluster proteins in three Swedish families. Decreased amount of ISCU protein in muscle was associated with decrease of iron regulatory protein (IRP12) and with intramuscular iron overload.

Mendelian Defects of the Respiratory Chain

The respiratory chain contains five functional units or complexes that are embedded in the IMM (see Fig. 42-2). The five complexes contain approximately 80 polypeptides, 13 of which are encoded by mtDNA. Complex II, unlike the other four complexes, is solely under the control of the nuclear genome. The function of the respiratory chain is to transfer electrons from the reduced pyridine nucleotides and flavoproteins to molecular oxygen, with the resulting oxidation of reduced nicotinamide-adenine dinucleotide phosphate and flavin adenine dinucleotide and the production of water. Biochemical defects of the respiratory chain are associated with lactic acidosis. However, unlike defects of pyruvate metabolism, respiratory chain defects are associated with a disturbed

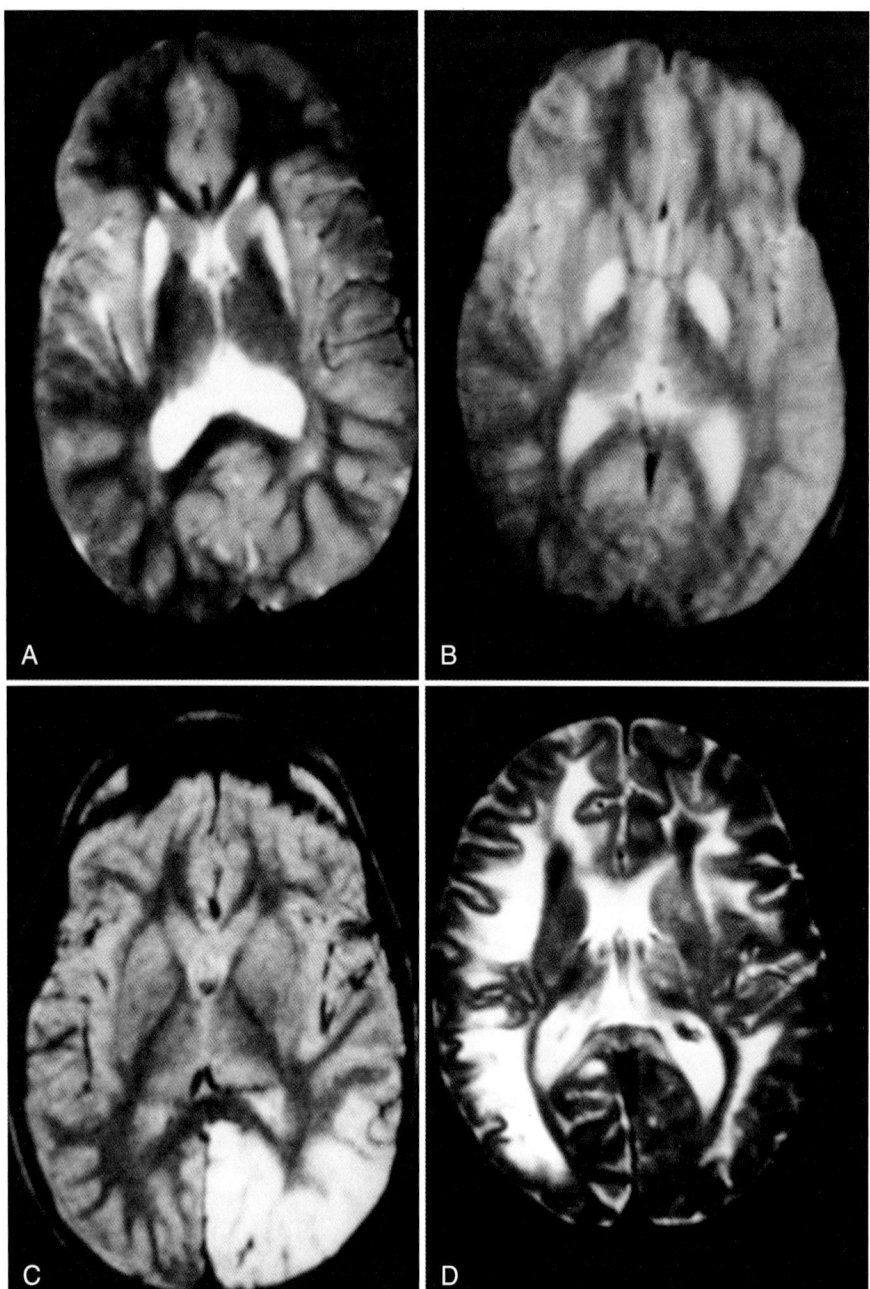

Figure 42-3. Characteristic brain MRI abnormalities in mitochondrial encephalomyopathies. **A,** These T2-weighted images show bilateral putaminal hyperintensities in a child with cytochrome c oxidase (COX)-associated Leigh syndrome; **B,** Bilateral globus pallidus hyperintensities in a child with a familial Leigh syndrome phenotype; **C,** A left posterior cerebral hyperintensity in a child with MELAS; **D,** bilateral white matter hyperintensities in a child with Kearns-Sayre syndrome (KSS). *(With permission from DeVivo, D.C., DiMauro, S., 2011. Mitochondrial diseases. In: Swaiman, K.F., Ashwal, S., Ferriero, D.M., editors. Pediatric Neurology: Principles and Practice, 5th edition. Philadelphia: Mosby Elsevier. p. 452–467.)*

cellular oxidation-reduction potential manifested by an elevated lactate/pyruvate ratio (greater than 20). Respiratory chain defects are complicated by the diversity of clinical presentations. Many patients have neurologic or neuromuscular symptoms and are grouped together in the neurologic literature reports as examples of mitochondrial encephalomyopathies. Others have nonneurologic symptoms, including dysfunction of the liver, heart, kidney, bone marrow, pancreas, and/or gastrointestinal tract. The specific clinical syndromes associated with the six groups of disorders are discussed later in the chapter.

1. Respiratory Chain "Direct Hits"

Pathogenic mutations that directly affect nDNA-encoded respiratory chain subunits have been identified in all five complexes, but more abundantly in the gigantic complex I and relatively rarely in complex II, complex III, complex IV, and complex V. Mendelian direct hits (most of which are recessive) generally manifest at or soon after birth and are severe or lethal in infancy. The most common clinical presentation is Leigh syndrome that reflects the detrimental energy shortage on the developing nervous system. Leigh syndrome is defined

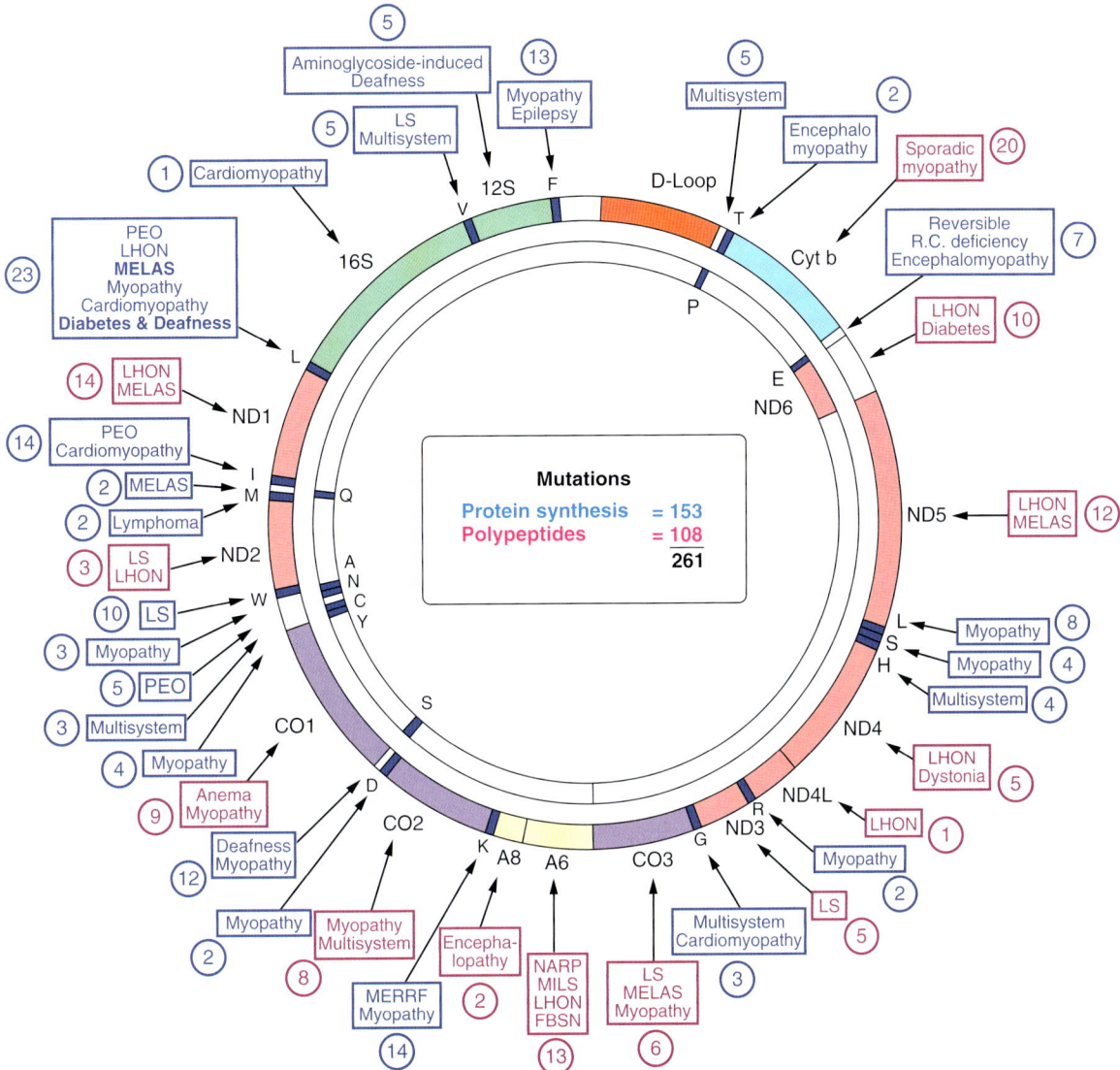

Figure 42-4. Morbidity map of the human mtDNA. Disorders caused by mutations in protein-coding genes are shown in red. Disorders caused by mutations in gene controlling protein synthesis are shown in blue. (FBSN = familial bilateral striatal necrosis; LHON = Leber hereditary optic neuropathy; LS = Leigh syndrome; MELAS = mitochondrial encephalomyopathy lactic acidosis and stroke-like episodes; MERRF, myoclonus epilepsy and ragged-red fibers; MILS = maternally inherited Leigh syndrome; NARP = neuropathy, ataxia, retinitis pigmentosa; PEO = progressive external ophthalmoplegia.) *(With permission from DiMauro, S., 2013. The Clinical Maze of Mitochondrial Neurology. Nat Rev Neurol 9, 281–291.)*

both neuropathologically and neuroradiologically by the presence of symmetric bilateral lesions in the basal ganglia, thalamus, brainstem, and cerebellar roof nuclei (Fig. 42-3). Neuronal loss, demyelination, reactive astrocytosis, and proliferation of cerebral microvessels are shown at the microscopic level. Clinically, children with Leigh syndrome have psychomotor retardation or regression, respiratory abnormalities, hypotonia, failure to thrive, seizures, dystonia, and blindness.

Complex I. Complex I (reduced nicotinamide-adenine dinucleotide phosphate-coenzyme Q reductase) is the largest complex of the respiratory chain, containing about 46 polypeptides. Seven of the polypeptides are encoded by mtDNA, and mutations affecting exclusively the mtDNA genes will be considered separately under the heading of "mitochondrial genetics."

Patients with Mendelian multisystem involvement of complex I deficiency due to direct hits usually present with

Leigh syndrome. In fact, complex I deficiency may be one of the major causes of Leigh syndrome, although it may be overlooked because of the difficulty of documenting the biochemical defect in frozen tissues. This concept seems confirmed by recent studies of nuclear genes, revealing a number of mutations in children with Leigh syndrome or leukodystrophy.

Complex II. Complex II (succinate-coenzyme Q reductase) contains only four polypeptides encoded by the nuclear genome. A few patients with Leigh syndrome and complex II deficiency had mutations in the gene encoding the flavoprotein subunit of the complex II. However, a familial neonatal dilated cardiomyopathy, affecting 15 children of two large consanguineous Bedouin families, was characterized by SDH deficiency in the heart and due to a mutation in the flavoprotein subunit of complex II.

Complex III. Direct hits affecting complex III are infrequent but a deletion in the *UQCRB* gene encoding the ubiquinone-binding protein (QP subunit or subunit VII) was identified in an 8-month-old girl with modest hepatomegaly, hypoglycemia, and lactic acidosis. At age 4 years, the child was normal, although the activity of complex III was decreased in liver, lymphocytes, and fibroblasts. A homozygous mutation of *UQCRB* was associated with a severe encephalomyopathy but was compatible with long survival in 20 members of an Israeli-Bedouin family. They developed psychomotor retardation and extrapyramidal signs, including dystonia, athetoid movements, ataxia, and dementia.

Complex IV. Mutations in the nDNA-encoded 11 subunits of complex IV (COX) are extremely rare, and confined to one subunit, COX6B1. A mutation in *COX6B1* was associated with severe cavitating leukodystrophy in two brothers, one of whom died at 10 years of age: both had failure to thrive but normal psychomotor development until late childhood, when they developed muscle weakness, cognitive impairment, visual problems, and lactic acidosis.

Complex V. Only one patient harbored a direct hit in one complex V subunit, ATP5E. A homozygous mutation in *ATP5E* affected a girl at birth, with poor suck, small size, respiratory distress, lactic acidosis, and 3-methyl-glutaconic aciduria. She had metabolic crises, which improved by 5 to 6 years of age, and she was able to complete school. At age 17 years, she presented with mild ataxia, horizontal nystagmus, exercise intolerance, axonal and demyelinating neuropathy, and mild left ventricular hypertrophy.

2. Respiratory Chain "Indirect Hits"

All nuclear encoded subunits of the respiratory chain have to be translated, imported into mitochondria, and directed to the MIM, where they are then assembled together with their mtDNA- and nuclear DNA-encoded counterparts, acquire prosthetic groups, multimerize, or further assemble into supercomplexes.

Complex I. There are as many indirect as direct hits affecting the assembly of this giant complex, and the encephalopathic phenotypes are similar in the two groups of disorders. Although indirect hits explain many cases of Leigh syndrome, frequently they impair white matter more than gray matter and give rise to leukodystrophies. Cardiomyopathy more commonly is observed in indirect hits, and is often a dominating feature when presenting in infancy or childhood, leading to death or manifesting a fluctuating course (Calvo et al., 2010).

Complex III. A rapidly fatal infantile disorder observed in Finland and termed GRACILE (**g**rowth **r**etardation, **a**minoaciduria, **c**holestasis, **i**ron overload, **l**actic acidosis, and **e**arly death) syndrome was associated with mutations in an assembly protein (BCS1L) needed for the correct synthesis and function of complex III. Mutations in the same nuclear gene (*BCS1L*) have also been found in children with Leigh syndrome.

Coenzyme Q10 Defects. Coenzyme Q (CoQ10) serves as an electron shuttle among complexes I and II and complex III. Coenzyme Q deficiency is associated with three clinical presentations, all autosomal recessive CoQ10 deficiencies. The first presentation, a *myopathic form* first described in 1989 in two sisters, has been reported in three more patients. It is characterized by the triad: (I) myopathy with recurrent myoglobinuria; (II) muscle biopsy with ragged-red fibers (RRF) and lipid storage; and (III) CNS dysfunction, with seizures, ataxia, or mental retardation. The second presentation is an ataxic form dominated by cerebellar ataxia and cerebellar atrophy, inconsistently accompanied by seizures, pyramidal signs, and mental retardation. The third

presentation, an *infantile encephalomyopathic form*, was described in two families with severe brain involvement and renal disease. These syndromes are important to be considered because all patients (especially those with the myopathic and the infantile forms) respond rather dramatically to oral CoQ10 supplementation.

A new group of disorders attributed to deficiency of coenzyme Q10 (CoQ10) can be related to indirect hits, mutations in a cascade of biosynthetic enzymes that result in deficiency of the relatively simple component, CoQ10, which is an integral part of the respirasome, where it shuttles electrons from complex I and complex II to complex III, acts as an antioxidant, and modulates apoptosis. Molecular defects in genes encoding CoQ10 biosynthetic enzymes (*PDSS2* and *COQ2*) were initially discovered in 2006, but mutations in other biosynthetic genes (*PDSS1*, *COQ6*, *ADCK3*, and *COQ9*) followed.

Complex IV. Leigh syndrome was a well known defect of COX activity, and there was a chase to identify direct hit mutations, to no avail, affecting nuclear genes encoding the 11 COX subunits. COX-deficient Leigh patients were clinically asymptomatic during early infancy but systemic and neurologic symptoms developed after age 6 months, and patients died by 4 to 5 years. They had a protracted clinical course associated with deceleration of head growth and peripheral neuropathy with rare seizures. In 1998 the first search for the molecular basis of COX-deficient Leigh syndrome led to simultaneous discovery of a mutant COX assembly gene, *SURF-1*, by two independent groups of investigators. Finding the genetic basis of this condition has greatly improved genetic counseling and has made prenatal diagnosis possible. Mutations in several other ancillary proteins required for COX assembly have been found in children with Leigh-like encephalopathy with involvement often of one other tissue, either liver, heart, or kidney. Thus mutations in the *SCO2* gene cause cardioencephalopathy, when generally the cardiopathy predominates and causes early death, but a few cases presented as spinal muscular atrophy (SMA) with cardiopathy. Mutations in *COX 15* also cause cardioencephalopathy, whereas mutations in *SCO1* cause hepatic encephalopathy, and mutations in *COX 10* cause nephrotic encephalopathy. The reasons for the selective involvement of specific tissues and organs in addition to the brain remain unclear.

Complex V. The first nuclear defect leading to impaired complex V function has been described. It involves a gene (*ATP12*) encoding an assembly protein, which is accompanied by congenital lactic acidosis and a fatal infantile multisystemic disease.

"Indirect hits" in complex V are rather frequently associated with mutations in the gene *TMEM70*, resulting in defective assembly of ATP synthase. Most patients harboring *TMEM70* mutations were severely affected with neonatal hypotonia, apneic spells, psychomotor delay, hypertrophic cardiomyopathy, and profound lactic acidosis; however, a minority presented additionally with infantile-onset cataracts, early onset gastrointestinal dysfunction, and multiple joint contractures.

Defects of Protein Importation

The protein importation process is energy-dependent and requires that proteins be unfolded before traversing mitochondrial membranes and then refolded before reaching their final destination. This requires a complex machinery, involving leader peptides, chaperonins, translocases in the outer and inner membranes, and proteases (Bolender et al., 2008). Relatively few human diseases have been attributed to dysfunction of mitochondrial protein import, possibly because of the devastating consequences that would disrupt the general import machinery. Most of these mutations involve leader peptides. One of these mutations affected methylmalonyl-CoA mutase and accounted for one form of methylmalonic aciduria. A second mutation affected the leader sequence of the E1 alpha-subunit of the pyruvate dehydrogenase complex in a child with PDH deficiency and Leigh syndrome. Two disorders have been associated with mutations in components of the transport machinery. The first is an X-linked disease called *deafness-dystonia syndrome* (Mohr-Tranebjaerg syndrome), characterized by neurosensory hearing loss, dystonia, cortical blindness, and psychiatric symptoms due to mutations in the *TIMM8A* gene, which encodes the deafness-dystonia protein (DDP1), a component of the transport machinery. The second disorder is an autosomal dominant form of hereditary spastic paraplegia due to mutations in the chaperonin HSP60.

3. Defects of mtDNA Translation

The mitochondrial genome is transcribed into 13 mRNAs, which are translated by mitoribosomes into the 13 mtDNA-encoded respiratory chain subunits. As described in a comprehensive review, this process can be divided into two phases: a posttranscriptional phase (involving tRNA modifications, aminoacyl-tRNA synthetases, and processing of ribosomal proteins); and a mtRNA translation phase (initiation, elongation, termination, and recycling). Representative examples of defects of each step of the mitochondrial translation process are briefly highlighted (Pearce et al., 2013).

Abnormal tRNA Modifications. Pseudouridylation is thought to promote stability and conformation of mitochondrial and nuclear tRNAs. Mutations in pseudouridine synthase 1 (*PUS1*) differentially impair nuclear and mitochondrial tRNA maturation causing mitochondrial myopathy, lactic acidosis, and sideroblastic anemia (*MLASA*). Psychiatric symptoms and facial dysmorphism are likely due to abnormal cytosolic protein synthesis.

The mystery of spontaneous improvement in *infantile reversible COX deficient myopathy* (now, more accurately designated reversible infantile respiratory chain deficiency [RIRCD]) was resolved by elucidation of the tRNA modification processes in this disorder. RIRCD is due to homoplasmic mutations in mt-tRNA^{Glu}. Pathogenesis of the disease was noted to be more complex than previously appreciated, when patients in two families were found to harbor mutations in the *TRMU* gene, which modifies a wobble uridine base in mt-tRNA^{Glu}. Skeletal muscle from infants in the initial symptomatic phase showed significantly decreased 2-thiouridylation due to defective TRMU activity, which exacerbated the effect of the mtRNA^{Glu} mutation and triggered the mitochondrial translation defect, thus demonstrating a nDNA modifying effect on the mtDNA mutation.

Mutations of Aminoacyl-tRNA Synthetases. In highly specialized tRNA-charging enzymes, the aminoacyl-tRNA synthetases (ARs), are associated with specific clinical syndromes. Thus pathogenic mutations in the gene *DARS* (encoding aspartyl-tRNA synthetase) cause brainstem and spinal cord involvement and lactate elevation (LBSL). Children from 30 families presented early with cerebellar ataxia, spasticity, dorsal column dysfunction, and mild cognitive decline. Equally severe mutations in the gene *RARS2* (encoding arginyl-tRNA synthetase) have been identified in three patients with severe infantile encephalopathy with *pontocerebellar hypoplasia*. Mutations in *EARS2*, encoding glutamyl-tRNA synthetase, were identified by whole-exome sequencing in a cohort of 11 unrelated cases with symmetric cerebral white matter abnormalities and signal abnormalities of the thalami, midbrain, pons, medulla oblongata, and cerebellar white matter. All patients shared an infantile onset and rapidly progressive disease with severe lactic acidosis. Mutations in *MARS2*, encoding the methionyl-tRNA synthetase, were found to be responsible for autosomal recessive *spastic ataxia with leukoencephalopathy (ARSAL)*, mostly in nine patients from a large French-Canadian family.

Many fewer patients with mutations in *YARS2, HARS2, AARS2, SARS2,* and *FARS2* also have specific clinical phenotypes, including myopathy and sideroblastic anemia (*MLASA*) due to YARS (encoding tyrosyl-tRNA synthetase); a *Perrault syndrome* (characterized by ovarian dysgenesis in females, and sensorineural deafness in both genders) due to HARS (encoding histidyl-tRNA synthetase; a perinatal or infantile hypertrophic cardiomyopathy; a more common presentation with leukoencephalopathy, childhood or adult-onset ataxia, spasticity, and cognitive decline (associated with the gene, AARS2, encoding alanyl-tRNA synthetase); a nonneurologic syndrome dominated by hyperuricemia, pulmonary hypertension, renal failure, and alkalosis in infancy due to SARS2, encoding seryl-tRNA synthetase; a form of hepatocerebral dysfunction simulating closely *Alpers syndrome,* due to FARS2 (encoding phenylalanyl tRNA synthetase). Mutations in *MARS2*, encoding the methionyl-tRNA synthetase, were found responsible for autosomal recessive *spastic ataxia with leukoencephalopathy (ARSAL)*. This was reported in nine patients from a large French-Canadian family.

Defects of Mitoribosomes

These have been associated with complex multisystemic disorders; however, in one family with *MPRL3* mutations, four siblings manifested fatal infantile-onset hypertrophic cardiomyopathy and psychomotor retardation. Similarly, patients with abnormal mitochondrial translational elongation factors typically presented with fatal infantile diseases with early hepatic encephalopathy with *GFM1* (EFG1) mutations and macrocystic leukodystrophy and micropolygyria due to *TUFM* (EF-Tu$_{mt}$) defects.

4. Defects of the IMM Lipid Milieu

Phospholipid metabolism and the lipid composition of the IMM were relatively neglected in the study of mitochondrial diseases, but there was a recent interest in this subject and several new disorders were discovered, thanks in part to whole exome sequencing.

Barth syndrome is due to alterations in cardiolipin, the most abundant phospholipid component of the IMM and due to mutations in the *TAZ* gene that encodes the monolysocardiolipin transacylase (Schlame et al., 2002). Barth syndrome is an X-linked disorder characterized by mitochondrial cardiac and skeletal myopathy, cyclic neutropenia, and growth retardation.

Sengers syndrome, an autosomal recessive disorder was described in 1975 and consisted of congenital cataracts, hypertrophic cardiomyopathy, skeletal myopathy, exercise intolerance, and lactic acidosis. This syndrome was found to be due to mutations in the gene (*AGK*) encoding acylglycerol kinase, which drives the assembly of adenine nucleotide translocator (ANT1) and causes a lack of ANT1 in the IMM. This finding came about through exome sequencing.

A second disorder of the mitochondrial lipid milieu was identified in 15 patients with a *congenital myopathy* characterized by early- onset muscle weakness, mental retardation, and a protracted clinical course (most patients were alive at the time of publication and only four had died between the ages of 2 1/2 and 28 years). The hallmark of the disease was the presence of greatly enlarged mitochondria (megaconial disease) in muscle displaced at the periphery of the fibers. The genetic cause was due to mutations in the gene (*CHKB*) encoding choline kinase beta. A new homozygous *CHKB* mutation was found in an American patient, who also had weakness and psychomotor delay and was alive at 2 years.

A genetic alteration of phospholipid metabolism causes a syndrome characterized by 3-methylglutaconic aciduria (3-methlylglutaconic aciduria type IV, deafness, and Leigh-like encephalopathy, termed *MEGDEL*). This syndrome was caused by mutations in the phospholipid remodeling gene *SERAC1*, a key player in intracellular cholesterol trafficking and a member of the mitochondria-associated ER membranes (MAM).

Some forms of *primary lateral sclerosis* due to defective gene *ERLIN2* and of *juvenile amyotrophic lateral sclerosis* (ALS) due to defective gene *SIGMAR*1 were associated with alterations of the lipid rafts that are part of the MAM.

Another genetic alteration of phospholipid metabolism explained many puzzling cases of recurrent *myoglobinuria in children*. Mutations in the gene (*LPIN1*) encoding the muscle-specific phosphatidic acid phosphatase cause accumulation of phosphatidic acid and lysophospholipids in muscle.

5. Defects of Mitochondrial Dynamics

Mitochondria are dynamic organelles forming complex tubular structures in many cells, which require constant fusion of the mitochondrial tubules, balanced by fission. Also, individual mitochondria move in the cell, sometimes covering considerable distances, as in axons propelled by energy-requiring dynamins along cytoskeletal microtubular rails (Burté et al., 2015).

There are a group of disorders due to numerous mutations in fusion proteins and, less commonly, in fission proteins. Mutations in fusion proteins such as OPA1 result in a dominantly inherited optic atrophy (DOA or Kjer disease), the nDNA-correspondent blindness to the mtDNA-correspondent Leber hereditary optic neuropathy (LHON). Other mutations in fusion proteins such as MFN2 or GADP1 result in Charcot-Marie-Tooth neuropathies (types 2A and 4A).

Two infants with distinct mutations in fission genes (*DRP1* and *MFF*) had shown both mitochondrial and peroxisomal abnormalities, and they were severely affected with rapidly fatal encephalopathy and lactic acidosis.

The role of altered mitochondrial dynamics in neurologic diseases is addressed elsewhere.

6. Defects of mtDNA Maintenance

Here, we consider the main clinical phenotypes associated with mtDNA depletion syndromes (MDS), with multiple mtDNA deletion syndromes (PEO-plus), and finally – with combined appearance of mtDNA depletion and of multiple mtDNA deletions (Fig. 42-5).

mtDNA Depletion Syndromes (MDS)

Myopathic MDS. Patients usually present in the first year of life with failure to thrive, hypotonia, weakness, and occasionally PEO. Patients typically die in childhood due to pulmonary insufficiency, but severity of weakness and survival vary considerably. The myopathic MDS is most commonly due to mutations in the gene (*TK2*) encoding mitochondrial thymidine kinase. About 20 mutations have been reported in as many patients. Notably, mutations in *TK2* can also cause a phenocopy of spinal muscular atrophy (SMA). It is notable, in this respect, that a *TK2* knockin mouse has more severe involvement of the central nervous system than that of muscle.

It is also of practical importance to sequence the *TK2* gene in patients with SMA but without mutations in the *SMN1* gene.

Encephalomyopathic MDS. Two variants of this condition are both due to a defect of succinyl-CoA lyase activity in the Krebs cycle. Mutations in the gene (*SUCLA2*) encoding the ATP-dependent succinyl-CoA lyase (SUCLA2) cause severe psychomotor retardation, muscle hypotonia, hearing loss, generalized seizures, knee and hip contractures, mild ptosis, lactic acidosis and methylmalonic aciduria. There is moderate mtDNA depletion (about 30%) in muscle, and the brain MRI is suggestive of Leigh syndrome.

Mutations in the gene (*SUCLG1*) encoding the GTP-dependent isoform SUCLG1 cause a much more severe and rapidly fatal phenotype with mtDNA depletion in both muscle and liver, characterized clinically by dysmorphic features, congenital lactic acidosis, and methylmalonic aciduria. A less dismal course, similar to the SUCLA2 phenotype, correlates with the degree of residual activity.

Patients with mtDNA depletion may harbor mutations in *RRM2B* (encoding the small subunit, p53R2, of the p53-inducible ribonucleotide reductase protein). Infants are hypotonic, and children are weak. The presentation consists of renal involvement and central nervous system involvement with microcephaly, seizures, and developmental delay.

Hepatocerebral MDS. Mutations in three other genes, *DGUOK*, *MPV17*, and *POLG*, also cause liver and brain involvement. Mutations in *DGUOK*, encoding the mitochondrial deoxyguanosine kinase (dGK), were first reported in 2001, and by 2007, 15 different mutations had been identified in 12 kindreds. Severe mutations cause fatal infantile hepatopathy and brain involvement whereas milder mutations cause isolated liver disease and are compatible with longer survival.

Mutations in *MPV17*, which encodes a small mitochondrial membrane protein of unknown function, cause a rather typical hepatocerebral syndrome in Caucasian children but is associated with a peculiar neurohepatopathy in the Navajo population. Navajo neurohepatopathy (NNH), which has a prevalence of 1 in 1600 live births, was attributed to mtDNA depletion and is due to a homozygous *MPV17* mutation. The clinical features of NNH include peripheral and central nervous system involvement, acral mutilation, corneal scarring or ulceration, liver failure, and immunologic derangement.

Alpers-Huttenlocher syndrome (AHS) is the classical form of hepatocerebral MDS, and it has been attributed to mutations in *POLG*. AHS is defined as a disorder of childhood by the tetrad of refractory seizures, episodic psychomotor regression, cortical blindness, and hepatopathy with micronodular cirrhosis. It is important not to expose these children to the antiepileptic drug valproic acid, which often precipitates fulminant hepatic failure. This interaction of gene and environment contributes to the extreme clinical heterogeneity associated with POLG mutations.

Syndromes Due to Multiple mtDNA Deletions

Mutations in ANT1. Mutations in the gene for one isoform of the adenine nucleotide translocator (*ANT1*) have been identified in patients with autosomal dominant PEO, sometime associated with psychiatric disorders. In a seminal paper, multiple mtDNA deletions were most abundant in brain, followed by cardiac and skeletal muscle. Sporadic PEO also may be due infrequently to mutations in *ANT1*; the association of mitochondrial myopathy and cardiomyopathy, even in patients with recessive inheritance and without PEO, should raise the question of *ANT1* mutations.

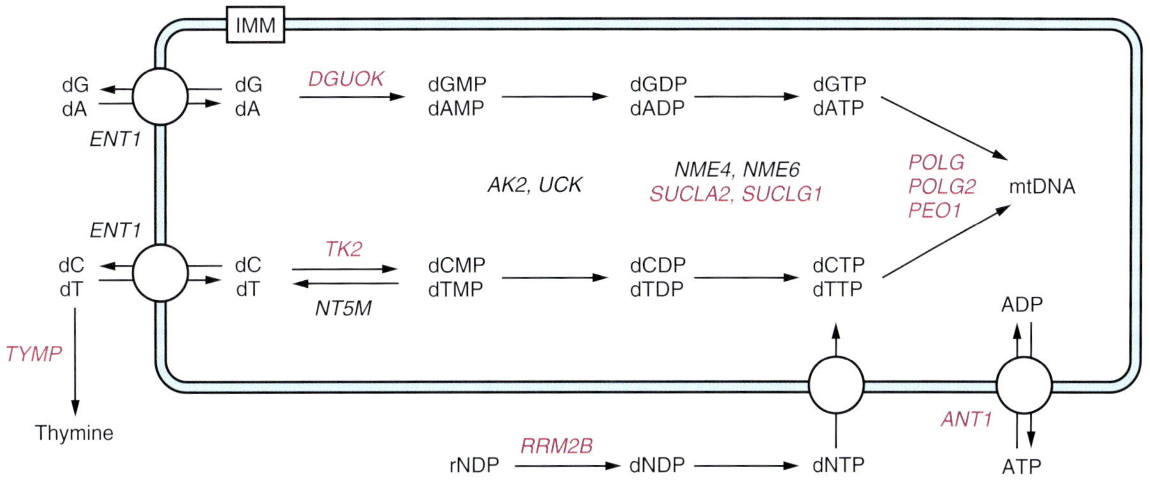

Figure 42-5. Schematic representation of the mitochondrial nucleotide pool, showing the genes whose mutations have been associated with multiple mtDNA deletions, those associated with mtDNA depletion, and those associated with both mtDNA multiple deletions and mtDNA depletion. (dA, deoxyadenosine; dC, deoxycytosine; dT, deoxythymidine; dG, deoxyguanosine; dAMP, deoxyadenosime monophosphate; dCMP, deoxycytosine monophosphate; dGMP, deoxyguanosine monophosphate; dTMP, deoxythymidine monophosphate; dADP, deoxyadenosine diphosphate; dCDP, deoxycytosine diphosphate; dGDP, deoxyguanosine diphosphate; dTDP, deoxythymidine diphosphate; dATP, deoxyguanosine triphosphate; dCTP, deoxycytosine triphosphate; dGTP, deoxyguanosine triphosphate; dTTP, deoxythymidine triphosphate; AK2, adenylate kinase 2; ANT1, adenine translocator 1; dGK (DGUOK) deoxyguanosine kinase; ENT1, equilibrative nucleoside transporter 1; NME4, nucleoside diphosphate kinase D; NME6, nucleoside diphosphate kinase 6; NT5M, 5' nucleotidase, mitochondrial; PEO1, mtDNA helicase; POLG, polymerase gamma, catalytic form; POLG2, polymerase gamma, accessory form; RRM2B, ribonucleoside diphosphate reductase subunit M2 B; TK2, thymidine kinase 2; TYMP, (TP) thymidine phosphorylase; SUCLA2, succinate CoA ligase (ADP forming) beta subunit; SUCLG1, succinate CoA ligase (GDP forming) alpha subunit; UCK, uridine-cytidine kinase.) *(With permission from De Vivo, D.C., Paradas, C., DiMauro, S., 2015. Mitochondrial encephalomyopathies. In: Darras, B.T., Royden Jones Jr., H., Ryan, M.M., De Vivo, D.C., editors. Neuromuscular Disorders in Infancy, Childhood, and Adolescence, A Clinician's Approach, 2nd edition. London: Academic Press of Elsevier. p. 796–823.)*

Mutations in PEO1. In 2001, autosomal dominant PEO with multiple mtDNA deletions was associated with mutations in the gene (*PEO1*), encoding a mitochondrial helicase called Twinkle, an essential factor for mtDNA maintenance and for the regulation of mtDNA copy number. A review of 33 patients from 26 families showed that the most common symptoms were ptosis (97%) and ophthalmoparesis (94%), followed by exercise intolerance (52%) and mild proximal weakness (33%). Central nervous system involvement was infrequent and included visual impairment, migraine, lethargy, hearing loss, and epilepsy. Cardiac problems were noted in 24% of the patients. The relatively benign, long-term progression also was noted in another large family with autosomal dominant PEO.

Mutations in POLG. Mutations in the gene encoding the only mitochondrial polymerase, polymerase γ (*POLG*) have emerged as major causes of a vast array of mitochondrial disorders. Over 150 mutations have been described in all three domains of the gene—exonuclease, linker, and polymerase—and may cause either autosomal dominant or autosomal recessive PEO, a syndrome comprising autosomal recessive sensory ataxic neuropathy, dysarthria, and ophthalmoparesis (SANDO), mitochondrial recessive ataxia syndrome (MIRAS), or parkinsonism with or without PEO.

Mutations in OPA1. One unexpected gene was recently added to those described previously and associated with myopathy and PEO, *OPA1*. Why unexpected? It was unexpected because mutations in *OPA1* were initially associated with a purely ophthalmologic condition, dominant optic atrophy (DOA) or Kjer disease and because the gene product was a mechanoenzyme associated with mitochondrial fusion rather than with mitochondrial maintenance.

However, a syndromic disorder, often termed DOA-plus, has emerged. This condition was characterized more or less sequentially by optic atrophy with visual failure, sensorineural deafness, ataxia, myopathy, axonal sensory-motor polyneuropathy, and PEO. Muscle biopsy in these patients shows scattered ragged-blue, COX-negative fibers and multiple mtDNA deletions are demonstrable by long-range PCR. Interestingly, the proportion of COX-negative fibers is much higher in patients with DOA-plus than in those with nonsyndromic DOA. The relationship between this defect of mitochondrial dynamics and altered mitochondrial maintenance is intriguing. Two explanations have been proposed: decreased ability by the organelles to repair stress-induced mtDNA damage or accelerated accumulation of preexisting age-associated somatic mtDNA mutations.

Coexistence of mtDNA Depletion and mtDNA Multiple Deletions

Mitochondrial Neurogastrointestinal Encephalomyopathy (MNGIE). One of the disorders in which the coexistence of multiple mtDNA deletions and mtDNA depletion was first recognized is MNGIE. This autosomal recessive multisystemic syndrome is characterized by mitochondrial myopathy with ptosis and PEO, peripheral neuropathy, gastrointestinal dysmotility causing severe cachexia, and leukoencephalopathy without cognitive impairment. MNGIE is due to mutations in the gene (*TYMP*) encoding thymidine phosphorylase (TP), resulting in elevated levels of thymidine and deoxyuridine in plasma and tissues. The disease starts in young adults and is relentlessly progressive, with an average age of death at 37 years. Molecular analysis has shown over 50 *TYMP* mutations resulting in mtDNA multiple deletions, depletion, and site-specific somatic mtDNA point mutations in multiple tissues. It has been suggested that the increased levels of thymidine and deoxyuridine lead to imbalance of the mitochondrial deoxynucleotide triphosphate pool, resulting in mtDNA instability.

Infantile onset spinocerebellar ataxia (IOSCA) was described in the 1970s in Finland. Between 9 and 18 months of age, children develop acutely or subacutely ataxia, hypotonia, athetosis, and areflexia; by teenage years, they lose independent ambulation. Additional symptoms include PEO, optic atrophy, sensorineural hearing loss, cognitive impairment, sensory neuropathy, and autonomic nervous system dysfunction. In 2005 this autosomal recessive disorder was attributed to mutations in *PEO1*. MRI revealed cerebellar atrophy. Although no mtDNA alteration was initially identified, it was subsequently found that both brain and liver harbored mtDNA depletion. An early-onset hepatocerebral presentation similar to Alpers-Huttenlocher syndrome has also been associated in two siblings with recessive *PEO1* mutations and mtDNA depletion in liver.

Mutations in *TK2* can also cause adult-onset myopathy with mtDNA depletion and even late-onset PEO with multiple mtDNA deletions rather than mtDNA depletion.

Mutations in *RRM2B* can also be associated with autosomal dominant or recessive PEO and multiple mtDNA deletion. One such case had multisystem involvement mimicking KSS.

Exome sequencing revealed *DGUOK* mutations in five adult patients with PEO and mitochondrial myopathy with multiple mtDNA deletions: only one of these patients had a history of liver problems in childhood.

Mutations in *MPV17* were identified in a 65-year-old man with axonal sensorimotor peripheral neuropathy, PEO and ptosis, diabetes mellitus, exercise intolerance, hepatic steatosis, depression, parkinsonism, and gastrointestinal dysmotility, and with multiple mtDNA deletions in his muscle.

Defects of Oxidation-Phosphorylation Coupling

Luft disease (nonthyroidal hypermetabolism) is the singular example of a defect in this pathway. Only two cases have been reported, both female, sporadic, and with negative family histories. Onset is in adolescence with fever, heat intolerance, profuse perspiration, polyphagia, polydipsia, resting tachycardia, and exercise intolerance. Both women died in middle age. Numerous ragged-red fibers were present in skeletal muscle, but the underlying molecular defect has not yet been elucidated.

Diseases Due to Primary mtDNA Mutations (Fig. 42-4)

Complex 1: Patients with complex I deficiency can be subclassified as examples of a myopathy or a multisystem disorder. The myopathy may develop in childhood or early adult life and is manifested by exercise intolerance and limb weakness. These patients have sporadic "somatic mutations" in mtDNA-encoded genes of complex I—that is, spontaneous *de novo* mutations in the mitochondrial genome occurring in the oocyte or in the embryo but affecting myoblasts after germ-layer differentiation.

Recently, attention has been drawn to mutations in mtDNA-encoded complex I (ND) subunits, especially mutations in the *MTND3* or *MTND5* genes, which appears to be hotspots; these mutations have been associated with maternally inherited Leigh syndrome or with overlap syndromes of Leigh syndrome and MELAS syndrome.

Complex III (coenzyme Q-cytochrome c oxidoreductase): Complex III contains 11 subunits, one of which is encoded by mtDNA (*MTCYB*). Defects involving complex III are subdivided into a generalized multisystem disorder manifested by limb weakness, exercise intolerance, and various neurologic signs or a tissue-specific syndrome manifested either as a pure myopathy with onset in childhood or adolescence or as a pure cardiopathy ("histiocytoid cardiomyopathy") manifesting in early infancy. Some patients with the myopathic phenotype and without apparent maternal inheritance have mutations ("somatic" mutations—see previous mention) in the cytochrome *b* gene (*MTCYB*) of mtDNA.

Complex IV (cytochrome c oxidase): Somatic mutations in mtDNA genes encoding subunits I or III (*MTCOI* or *MTCOIII*) can cause exercise intolerance and recurrent myoglobinuria.

Since 1988, no less than 11 clinical syndromes have been associated with defects of the mitochondrial genome. Three conditions can be subdivided into sporadic disorders associated with single large-scale rearrangements of mtDNA, which include Kearns-Sayre syndrome (KSS), progressive external ophthalmoplegia (PEO), and Pearson syndrome (PS).

KSS

Kearns-Sayre syndrome (KSS) is the prototype of this group of diseases. Males and females are affected in roughly equal number, and there are no documented examples of familial KSS. The dominant clinical features include progressive eye signs such as ptosis, progressive external ophthalmoplegia, and pigmentary retinopathy. Neurologic symptoms include cerebellar ataxia, intellectual disability, and episodic coma. Seizures are infrequent and are usually associated with hypoparathyroidism. Brain MRI shows diffuse white matter hyperintensity. Complete heart block may lead to sudden death and insertion of a pacemaker is lifesaving. Short stature and hearing loss are common. Endocrine disturbances include diabetes mellitus, hypoparathyroidism, and isolated growth hormone deficiency.

Ragged-red fibers (RRF) are found in almost all affected patients. Calcification of the basal ganglia usually occurs in the setting of hypoparathyroidism. The surprisingly rare incomplete forms of KSS demonstrate PEO as an invariant clinical sign. Some cases have unusual clinical presentations such as renal tubular acidosis, whereas others may overlap with clinically distinct syndromes such as MELAS.

Pearson syndrome is a nonneurologic disorder of infancy characterized by pancytopenia, disturbed pancreatic exocrine function, and liver abnormalities. The few survivors of this infantile condition may later develop clinical features of KSS. The phenotypic transformation from Pearson syndrome to KSS is an example of tissue-specific modifications of mitochondrial heteroplasmy (mitotic segregation).

Six clinical conditions are maternally inherited and associated with point mutations in mtDNA protein-coding genes.

Leber hereditary optic neuropathy (LHON) and neuropathy, ataxia, and retinitis pigmentosa (NARP) affect structural genes in the mitochondrial genome. Lactic acidosis is usually absent in LHON and may be absent in NARP. Ragged-red fibers are conspicuously absent in skeletal muscle biopsies from patients with both conditions.

LHON is dominated clinically by the sudden onset of visual loss in a young adult and, more commonly, a man. The peak age of onset is between 20 and 24 years, although children as young as 5 years have reported bilateral visual loss. In most cases, although the condition may first develop in one eye, it is followed by involvement of the second eye in weeks or months. The presentation is a retrobulbar neuropathy, often associated with disc edema and subtle alterations of retinal vessels. The male predominance suggests an X-linked factor that modulates the expression of the mtDNA point mutation, but this remains to be documented. A more likely explanation for the predominant male involvement seems to be an epigenetic factor—that is, a protective effect of estrogens in women.

The condition is relatively static after the subacute visual loss. Other neurologic and psychiatric symptoms have been described in patients and their family members, signifying the global nature of the molecular defect. Variable findings have included hyperreflexia, Babinski sign, incoordination, peripheral neuropathy, and cardiac conduction abnormalities. Three primary mutations are capable of causing LHON alone. All of these genes encode subunits of complex I (m.3460G>A in ND1, m.1178G>A in ND4, and m.14484T>C in ND6).

NARP affecting an mtDNA structural gene results in neuropathy, ataxia, and retinitis pigmentosa (NARP). It was described in four family members of three successive generations with a variable combination of retinitis pigmentosa, ataxia, developmental delay, dementia, seizures, proximal limb weakness, and sensory neuropathy. This maternally transmitted condition was associated with an mtDNA point mutation involving the gene for subunit 6 of mitochondrial ATPase (*MTATP6*). The most severely affected family member was a 3-year-old girl. She had had a history of reduced fetal movement, developmental delay, and a pigmentary retinopathy. Additional features included limb hypertonia, hyperreflexia, bilateral Babinski sign, and generalized ataxia. The m.8993T>G mutation in the ATPase 6 gene of mtDNA has been recognized as one important cause of Leigh syndrome. Curiously, a different mutation at the very same nucleotide (m.8993T>C) causes a milder clinical phenotype and a less severe impairment of ATP synthesis in mitochondria isolated from cultured fibroblasts. Mutations in the ATPase 6 gene of mtDNA appear to be associated with various syndromes characterized by the neuroradiologic features of Leigh syndrome or bilateral striatal necrosis.

There are now more than 250 pathogenic point mutations affecting synthetic genes but only two distinct and frequent clinical conditions that are maternally inherited and associated with mtDNA point mutations affect tRNA genes. These two conditions are MELAS and MERRF.

Mitochondrial encephalopathy with lactic acidosis and stroke-like episodes (MELAS) was first described in 1984 and is the most common mtDNA-related disease. Most patients become symptomatic before age 40 years, and 90% to 100% of patients have normal early development followed by the onset of exercise intolerance, stroke-like episodes, seizures, and dementia. Almost all patients have lactic acidosis and ragged-red fibers in biopsied skeletal muscle. Recurrent migraine-like headaches preceded by nausea and vomiting are common, as is hearing loss, short stature, learning difficulties, hemiparesis, hemianopia, and limb weakness. The cerebrospinal fluid protein concentration is normal in half of the patients and only mildly elevated in the other half. One third of patients have basal ganglia calcifications. Seizures are common and often (or always) precede the stroke-like events. Progressive external ophthalmoparesis was noted in approximately 10% of cases. The m.3243A>G mutation in the tRNA^Leu(UUR) gene (*MTTL*) of mtDNA is responsible for about 80% of MELAS patients worldwide. Several other mutations in the same gene have been associated with MELAS, as well as increasing numbers of mutations in structural genes of mtDNA.

Myoclonic epilepsy and ragged-red fibers (MERRF) was first described in 1980. The major clinical features include cerebellar syndrome, generalized convulsions, myoclonus, dementia, hearing loss, impaired deep sensation, and a positive family history consistent with maternal inheritance. In 1990 Shoffner and colleagues described a point mutation (m.8344A>G) involving the mtDNA gene for tRNA^Lys (*MTTK*). Two more mutations in the same gene (m.8356T>C and m.8363G>A)

are less frequent causes of typical MERRF. One mutation in a different gene (m.611G>A in the tRNA^Phe) gene (MTTF) has been reported to cause typical MERRF.

THERAPY

No panacea for respiratory chain dysfunction and no universal therapy for mitochondrial disorders currently exist. Nevertheless, symptomatic pharmacologic treatments (for example, antiepileptic drugs) and surgical interventions (such as blepharoplasty) are useful in prolonging and improving the lives of patients with these conditions. Exercise therapy has been demonstrated to improve exercise tolerance and quality of life in patients with mitochondrial diseases. Several strategies aimed at curing (or even preventing) mitochondrial diseases have shown promise *in vitro* or in animals, or have produced encouraging preliminary results in humans (Viscomi et al., 2015).

Mitochondrial Replacement Therapy (MRT)

For mtDNA-related diseases, many of which are devastating and undiagnosable prenatally, the ultimate goal is to prevent their occurrence altogether via mitochondrial replacement. In this approach, the nucleus of an oocyte from an mtDNA mutation carrier is transferred to an in vitro-fertilized enucleated oocyte from a normal donor, resulting in the embryo having the nDNA of the biological parents but the mtDNA of a normal mitochondrial donor. In nonhuman primate experiments using oocyte spindle-chromosomal complex transfer, the offspring were healthy and devoid of original maternal mtDNA. The same technique was applied to fertilized and unfertilized but parthenogenically activated human oocytes, and the cells were found to develop into normal blastocysts and containing virtually exclusively donor mtDNA (Paull et al., 2013). Moreover, only donor mtDNA was detected after stem cell lines from blastocysts were differentiated into neurons, cardiomyocytes, and β-cells. Similar results were obtained in the United Kingdom after pronuclear transfer in abnormally fertilized human oocytes developed up to the blastocyst stage. Despite some concerns, the stage appears to be set for approval of this technique for therapeutic application both in the United Kingdom and the United States.

Shifting Heteroplasmy

For mtDNA-related disorders, an obvious but challenging goal is to shift heteroplasmy in patients, thereby lowering the mutation load to subthreshold levels. When deprived of glucose and exposed to ketogenic media, cybrids harbouring single mtDNA deletions shifted their heteroplasmy level and recovered mitochondrial function, probably through selective mitochondrial autophagy (mitophagy). A genetic approach to heteroplasmic shifting involves use of restriction endonucleases to eliminate specific pathogenic mutations.

Enhancement of Respiratory Chain Function

The most obvious therapeutic approach to mitochondrial disorders is to enhance respiratory chain function, thereby mitigating both energy crisis (ATP deficit) and oxidative stress (toxic build-up of ROS). The compound is used almost universally in patients with mitochondrial disease is CoQ10, given the pivotal role of this molecule in electron transport, its antioxidant properties, and its safety even at high doses. Two synthetic analogs of CoQ10—idebenone and parabenzoquinone—seem more promising. Idebenone, a short-chain benzoquinone, has shown positive results in two studies of patients with LHON. The second compound, a parabenzoquinone labeled EPI-743, has so far been tested only in open studies; this compound reversed vision loss in four of five patients with LHON produced clinical improvement in 12 children with various mitochondrial disorders and arrested or reversed disease progression in 13 children with genetically proven Leigh syndrome.

Elimination of Noxious Compounds

The second logical therapeutic approach to mitochondrial disease is to eliminate the noxious compounds that accumulate in these disorders. To decrease brain lactate in patients with MELAS, we used dichloroacetate (DCA), which stabilizes pyruvate dehydrogenase in the active form and favors lactate oxidation. Unfortunately, this agent, DCA, had unacceptable neurotoxicity and treatment had to be discontinued. A more promising "detoxifying therapy" may be allogeneic hematopoietic stem-cell transplantation (AHSCT) aimed at restoring sufficient thymidine phosphorylase activity in patients with MNGIE to normalize the circulating toxic levels of thymidine and deoxyuridine. As of 2012, 9 of 24 patients with MNGIE who had undergone AHSCT were alive and had normal blood thymidine phosphorylase activity, virtually undetectable levels of thymidine and deoxyuridine, and mild clinical improvements. A safety study of AHSCT in patients with MNGIE is under way to assess whether transplants can be performed with low morbidity in mildly to moderately affected individuals.

Alteration of Mitochondrial Dynamics

Mitochondrial dynamics could be exploited therapeutically in two opposing ways. Mitochondrial fission could be enhanced, thereby favoring mitophagy, a natural "quality control" function that sequesters and eliminates dysfunctional mitochondria, perhaps sensing their abnormally low membrane potential. Alternatively, enhancement of mitochondrial fusion and "networking" would allow complementation of "bad" and "good" mitochondria and normalization of overall mitochondrial function.

Although natural mitochondrial proliferation (e.g., RRF) is a futile compensatory mechanism, preliminary studies indicate it may be possible to improve on nature's strategy by enhancing mitochondrial biogenesis through activation of the transcriptional coactivator PGC-1α, AMPK pathway, or Sirtuin1. The advantage over disease-induced mitochondrial proliferation, which appears to favor mutated mtDNAs, is that upregulation of mitochondrial biosynthesis increases numbers of all mtDNAs, allowing wild-type genomes to compensate for mutated ones. Encouraging results have been obtained in four mouse models of COX deficiency.

REFERENCES

The complete list of references for this chapter is available in the e-book at www.expertconsult.com.
    See inside cover for registration details.

SELECTED REFERENCES

Bolender, N., et al., 2008. Multiple pathways for sorting mitochondrial precursor proteins. EMBO J. 9, 42–49.

Burté, F., et al., 2015. Disturbed mitochondrial dynamics and neurodegenerative disorders. Nat. Rev. Neurol. 11, 11–24.

Calvo, S.E., Tucker, E.J., Compton, A.G., et al., 2010. High-throughput, pooled sequencing identifies mutations in NUBPL and FOXRED1 in human complex I deficiency. Nat. Genet. 42, 851–858.

DiMauro, S., et al., 2013. The clinical maze of mitochondrial neurology. Nat. Rev. Neurol. 9, 429–444.

Paull, D., et al., 2013. Nuclear genome transfer in human oocytes eliminates mitochondrial DNA variants. Nature 493, 632–637.

Payne, B.A.J., et al., 2013. Universal heteroplasmy of human mitochondrial DNA. Hum. Mol. Genet. 22, 384–390.

Pearce, S., Nezich, C.L., Spinazzola, A., 2013. Mitochondrial diseases: translation matters. Mol. Cell. Neurosci. 55, 1–12.

Schlame, M., et al., 2002. Deficiency of tetralinoleoyl-cardiolipin in Barth syndrome. Ann. Neurol. 51, 634–637.

Schon, E.A., DiMauro, S., Hirano, M., 2012. Human mitochondrial DNA: roles of inherited and somatic mutations. Nat. Rev. Genet. 13, 878–890.

Viscomi, C., Bottani, E., Zeviani, M., 2015. Emerging concepts in the therapy of mitochondrial disease. Biochim. Biophys. Acta 1847, 544–557.

E-BOOK FIGURES AND TABLES

The following figures and tables are available in the e-book at www.expertconsult.com. See inside cover for registration details.

Table 42-1 Comparison of the Human Nuclear and Mitochondrial Genomes

Table 42-2 Structural (Mit) Gene Products Encoded by Mitochondrial DNA

Box 42-1 Biochemical Genetics Classification of Mitochondrial Diseases

43 Peroxisomal Disorders

Gerald V. Raymond, Kristin W. Barañano, and S. Ali Fatemi

An expanded version of this chapter is available on www.expertconsult.com. See inside cover for registration details.

Disorders of the peroxisome—organelles found in all eukaryotic cells—are characterized by alterations in their unique metabolic functions in the cell and tissues. The pervasive presence of the peroxisome leads to far-reaching consequences of these genetic disorders. Peroxisomal disorders are divided into two major categories. In the first, the organelle fails to develop normally, leading to disruption of multiple peroxisomal enzymes. The second category consists of those disorders in which the peroxisome structure is normal but functioning of a single peroxisomal enzyme is defective. Box 43-1 lists the known peroxisomal disorders; their combined incidence is estimated at 1 in 25,000 or higher. Because peroxisomal disorders are genetically determined with a majority readily identifiable by biochemical means, including prenatal testing, and nearly all affecting the nervous system, knowledge of these diseases is important. As the pathophysiology of these disorders is better understood, novel therapeutic strategies may be developed, which gives new hope for advances not only in the diagnosis but also in the management and outcome of peroxisomal disorders (Vamecq et al., 2014).

STRUCTURE AND FUNCTION OF PEROXISOMES

The peroxisome is bound by a single membrane and contains a fine granular matrix. Histologically, these organelles are identified by the presence of catalase, are present in all human tissues except mature erythrocytes, and demonstrate variation in size and number. They do not contain DNA and appear to be devoid of glycoproteins. The membrane is 6.5 to 7 nm thick and has a trilaminar appearance and a unique protein composition. The peroxisomal membrane contains four ATP binding cassette (ABC) proteins. These proteins have important intracellular roles in transport. As discussed later on, the ABC protein, ABCD1, is defective in X-linked adrenoleukodystrophy, the most prevalent peroxisomal disorder.

The process of peroxisomal biogenesis is highly conserved in all eukaryotic organisms, which has permitted the study of yeast to identify the cellular mechanism for the assembly of the organelle and targeting of proteins to the developing vesicle. Peroxisomal proteins are encoded by nuclear genes, synthesized on free polyribosomes, and discharged into the cytosol in the mature form. Work in yeast has identified more than 20 genes labeled PEX whose products, peroxins, are required for the incorporation of peroxisome membrane proteins and matrix protein importation. Peroxins are required for the proper importation and have roles in receptor docking, stability, and translocation across the membrane.

Targeting information directing matrix proteins into the peroxisomes is inherent in the mature polypeptide. A majority of proteins destined for the peroxisome use peroxisome targeting sequence 1 (PTS1), which consists of a terminal tripeptide of serine-lysine-leucine (-SKL) that is recognized by the soluble receptor Pex5p. Not all matrix proteins contain the carboxyl-terminal PTS1 signal. The peroxisomal enzymes, 3-ketoacyl-coenzyme A (CoA) thiolase and phytanoyl-CoA hydroxylase, have a different peroxisomal targeting sequence (PTS2). PTS2 consists of a nine-residue signal located at the amino terminus. It directs the import of a smaller number of proteins using the soluble receptor Pex7p (Wanders, 2014).

METABOLIC FUNCTION OF PEROXISOMES

Peroxisomes were named for the presence of hydrogen peroxide and catalase, which decomposes the hydrogen peroxide. It is now known that more than 40 enzymatic functions are found in the peroxisome. Some peroxisomal activities such as oxidation of fatty acids and cholesterol synthesis can occur in other cellular compartments as well. Certain reactions, however, occur exclusively in the peroxisome. These reactions include oxidation of very long-chain fatty acids and pipecolic acid and certain steps in the synthesis of plasmalogens and bile acids. These reactions are abnormal in many peroxisomal disorders. The composition of enzymes within the peroxisome varies among species and within tissues in a species, as well as with maturation, metabolic state, and environmental factors.

CLASSIFICATION OF PEROXISOMAL DISORDERS

Peroxisomal disorders may be divided into two categories:

1. Disorders of peroxisome assembly or biogenesis
2. Single-enzyme defects

In the first, the peroxisome fails to form, and abnormalities of multiple peroxisomal functions are present. It is understood that these disorders are defects in protein importation using the PTS1 and PTS2 targeting sequences or membrane incorporation. This group of biogenesis disorders can be further divided by their clinical and biochemical features into the Zellweger spectrum disorders and rhizomelic chondrodysplasia punctata. The second major group consists of a growing number of disorders in which a genetically determined abnormality of a single peroxisomal enzyme is present and peroxisomal structure is intact.

All of these disorders are, in actuality, single-gene and, ultimately, single-protein deficiencies, but the downstream consequences of the first group affect more than one peroxisomal pathway, resulting in multiple diagnostic abnormalities. With the emergence of DNA-based diagnosis, the utility of this division may require reassessment. An overview of diagnostic evaluation of peroxisomal disorders is provided in Figure 43-2.

CONDITIONS RESULTING FROM DEFECTIVE PEROXISOME BIOGENESIS

Conditions resulting from defective peroxisome biogenesis are listed in Box 43-1; Zellweger syndrome and rhizomelic chondrodysplasia punctata are the respective prototypes. Clinical and biochemical variation between these two types of assembly defects still makes it useful to discuss them separately, although it is important to recognize that these disorders were

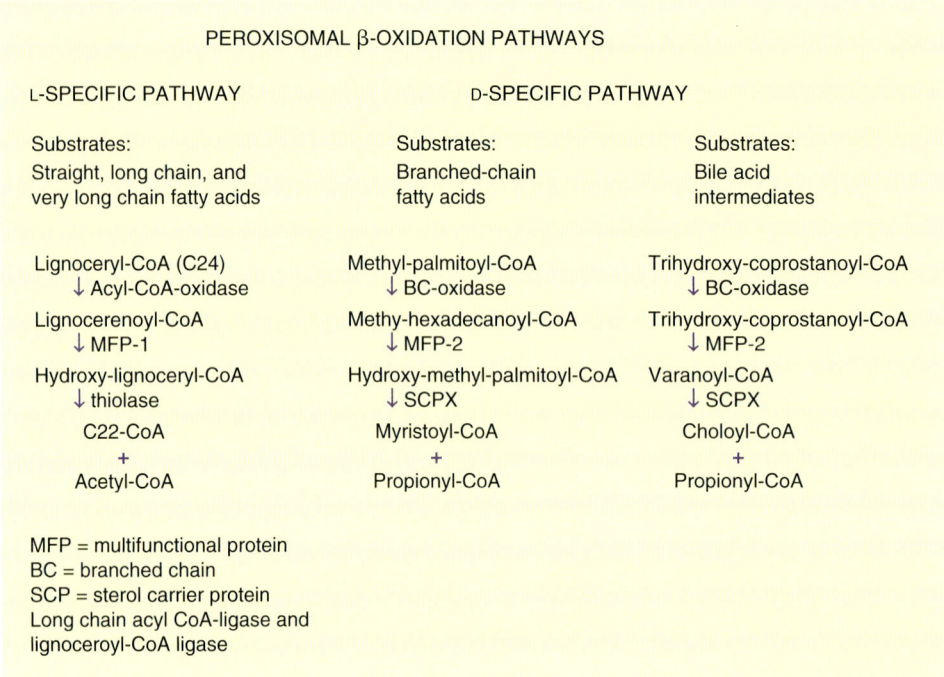

Figure 43-1. Activation and subsequent β-oxidation of very long-chain fatty acids, branched-chain fatty acids, and bile acid intermediates by the l- and d-specific pathways in peroxisomes. CoA, coenzyme A.

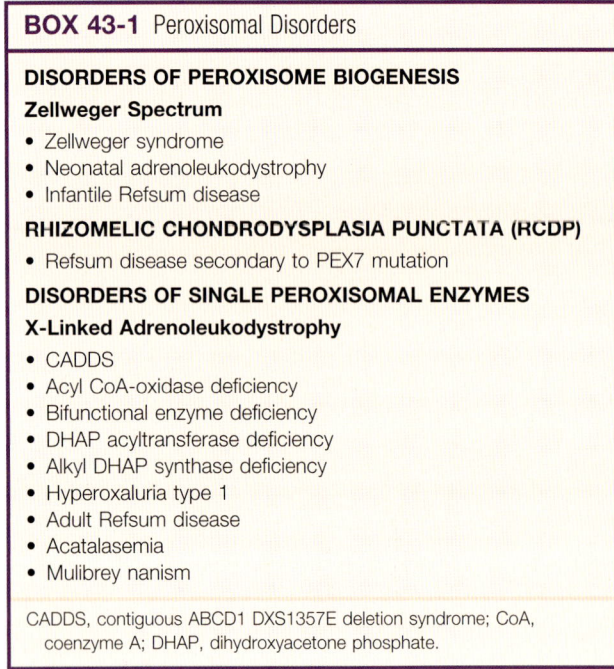

BOX 43-1 Peroxisomal Disorders

DISORDERS OF PEROXISOME BIOGENESIS

Zellweger Spectrum

• Zellweger syndrome
• Neonatal adrenoleukodystrophy
• Infantile Refsum disease

RHIZOMELIC CHONDRODYSPLASIA PUNCTATA (RCDP)

• Refsum disease secondary to PEX7 mutation

DISORDERS OF SINGLE PEROXISOMAL ENZYMES

X-Linked Adrenoleukodystrophy

• CADDS
• Acyl CoA-oxidase deficiency
• Bifunctional enzyme deficiency
• DHAP acyltransferase deficiency
• Alkyl DHAP synthase deficiency
• Hyperoxaluria type 1
• Adult Refsum disease
• Acatalasemia
• Mulibrey nanism

CADDS, contiguous ABCD1 DXS1357E deletion syndrome; CoA, coenzyme A; DHAP, dihydroxyacetone phosphate.

Figure 43-2. Diagnostic evaluation of peroxisomal disorders. Confirmatory genetic or biochemical testing may be required. ALD, adrenoleukodystrophy; RCDP, rhizomelic chondrodysplasia punctata; VLCFA, very long-chain fatty acid.

described on a clinical basis before details of the cell and molecular biology of peroxisomal disorders was known; hence, they were assigned names based on the clinical features, pathologic findings, or biochemical defects that identified them.

MOLECULAR ETIOLOGY OF DISORDERS OF PEROXISOME ASSEMBLY

These disorders result from defects in the PEX genes. A complex interaction of peroxins is necessary for the biogenesis of peroxisomes, and a defect in any of these proteins impairs the process. The final common pathway is peroxisomal dysfunction, with the respective clinical syndromes. Zellweger spectrum disorders are secondary to PTS1-mediated pathways including PEX5, and that rhizomelic chondrodysplasia punctata is secondary to mutations in PEX7, the receptor for PTS2 proteins (Braverman et al., 2013). The most common causes of Zellweger spectrum disorders are mutations in either PEX1 or PEX6, although to date, 13 PEX genes have been identified as potential causes of these disorders. PEX1 and PEX6 encode AAA ATPases. The clinical spectrum is seen in PEX1.

For example, a single base-pair deletion results in a severe phenotype and the common missense mutation G843D allows a milder phenotype (Braverman et al., 2013).

ZELLWEGER SPECTRUM DISORDERS

Zellwegers syndrome (cerebrohepatorenal syndrome) was first described by Bowen and associates. Subsequently, the disorders neonatal adrenoleukodystrophy and infantile Refsum disease were described as separate entities. Although classic Zellweger syndrome is the most severe form with a characteristic phenotype, clinical overlap exists between it and the other forms. All of the Zellweger spectrum disorders share morphologic and biochemical abnormalities, and genetic understanding of the underlying mutations has been obtained in many cases. In view of this overlap, it appears prudent at this time to retain a portion of this clinical nomenclature and refer to the group as Zellweger spectrum disorders.

Clinical and Pathologic Features

Zellweger Syndrome

Zellweger syndrome is a multiple congenital anomaly syndrome characterized by craniofacial abnormalities, eye abnormalities, neuronal migration defects, hepatomegaly, chondrodysplasia punctata, and near-complete absence of peroxisomes. The craniofacial features include a high forehead, hypoplastic supraorbital ridges, epicanthal folds, midface hypoplasia, and a large fontanel (Fig. 43-3). The head circumference usually is normal. Reported ocular abnormalities include cataracts, glaucoma, corneal clouding, Brushfield spots, optic nerve hypoplasia, and pigmentary retinal abnormalities. Severe weakness and hypotonia manifest in the newborn period, often accompanied by seizures and apnea. Most affected infants have oromotor dysfunction and require

tube feeding. Little psychomotor development ensues, and the average life span is limited, with most affected children surviving for 12 to 24 months. The facial appearance, Brushfield spots, and profound hypotonia may lead to a consideration of Down syndrome, although the chromosomal determination will eliminate that as a consideration.

Striking abnormalities of neuronal migration unique to Zellweger syndrome are evident in the cerebral hemispheres as areas of pachygyria or polymicrogyria localized to the opercular region. In the cerebellum, the Purkinje cells form scattered heterotopias throughout the cortex and in the granule cell layer. Laminar discontinuities involving the olivary nucleus are noted, which also are unique to Zellweger syndrome.

Multiple other abnormalities have been reported. The eyes demonstrate loss of retinal ganglion cells and gliosis of the optic nerve. Retinal pigmentary degenerative changes are associated with absent electroretinograms. Hepatomegaly with periportal fibrosis may result in significant cholestasis and jaundice, micronodular cirrhosis, and hypoprothrombinemia. Renal cortical cysts of varied sizes are present in 97% of patients studied pathologically but may be missed by ultrasound analyses. The adrenal gland demonstrates changes similar to those in X-linked adrenoleukodystrophy, with cytoplasmic lamellar inclusions consisting of cholesterol esterified with very long-chain fatty acids. Skeletal abnormalities include clubfoot, thumb rotation, and stippled chondral calcification of the patella and acetabulum in 50% of patients.

Neonatal Adrenoleukodystrophy and Infantile Refsum Disease

We now have a clear understanding that alteration in PEX genes may result in clinical phenotypes that are less severe than in Zellweger syndrome previously termed NALD and IRD. Even in the milder forms, patients generally have

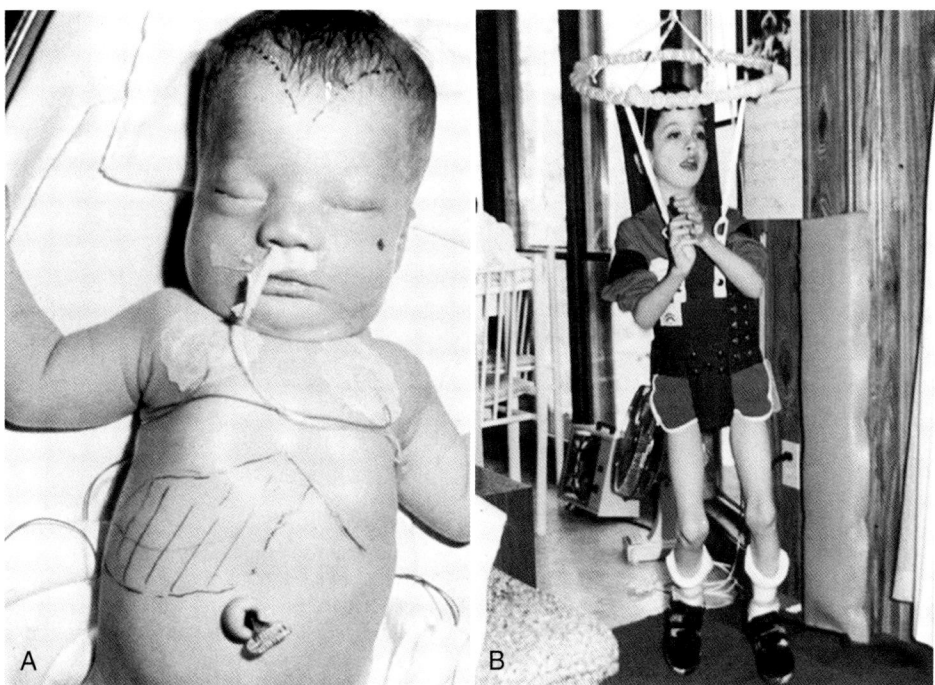

Figure 43-3. Cerebrohepatorenal syndrome of Zellweger. **A,** Note the prominent forehead, large fontanel, hypertelorism, epicanthal folds, hypotonia, and hepatomegaly. **B,** Milder form of generalized peroxisomal disorder: 10-year-old boy with ataxia, significant mental retardation, visual loss secondary to retinitis pigmentosa, absence of speech, and sensorineural hearing loss. Liver biopsy showed micronodular cirrhosis and very few, abnormally small peroxisomes.

intellectual disability, sensorineural hearing loss, retinal degeneration, and motor handicaps. Dysmorphism is less severe than in Zellweger syndrome; renal cysts may be absent, and no radiographic stippling of the cartilage is seen. Although neonatal adrenoleukodystrophy and infantile Refsum disease have in the past been split into distinct clinical presentations, this division can no longer be supported in light of more recent information on the genetic mechanism. This was already apparent from the clear clinical overlap between Zellweger syndrome and neonatal adrenoleukodystrophy and infantile Refsum disease. Attempts to differentiate between these milder phenotypes, either genetically or biochemically, do not reliably predict the clinical course.

Patients with milder forms may present in the neonatal period with mild to moderate dysmorphism, hypotonia, poor feeding, and hepatomegaly. Motor and cognitive development usually is delayed. Even with hypotonia, patients may be able to walk, although gait often is ataxic. Retinal pigmentary degeneration may not become evident until the age of 4 to 6 months and often results in visual loss in the first years of life. Electroretinograms show profound abnormalities in nearly all affected persons and do not correlate well with vision in this population. Sensorineural hearing loss is associated with limited language development. Adrenal dysfunction may develop with age. Liver dysfunction often is present and detectable by persistent elevation of liver enzymes. A bleeding diathesis that responds to vitamin K also may develop; in several children, esophageal varices were observed, consistent with portal hypertension. Optic atrophy and retinitis pigmentosa may be seen in patients. The association of retinal pigmentary degeneration and sensorineural hearing loss has led to misdiagnosis as Usher syndrome.

Life span is variable, and patients have survived to adulthood. All identified patients have been visually impaired, with sensorineural hearing loss.

A progressive leukodystrophy, with variable age at onset, has been reported in a number of patients. This disorder results in loss of previously acquired skills, and, in most cases, progresses to a vegetative state and death. Unlike in X-linked adrenoleukodystrophy, the rate of progression has been more variable.

Clinical recognition of these disorders may present some uncertainty because of nonspecific abnormalities and phenotypic variability. Disorders of peroxisome biogenesis commonly manifest in the neonatal period, and patients come to attention because of hypotonia, seizures, or liver disease. Evaluation appropriately focuses on a search for cytogenetic abnormalities, acute treatable metabolic disorders, and structural liver disease. Later in childhood, patients often are mistakenly diagnosed as having cerebral palsy, X-linked adrenoleukodystrophy, mitochondrial disease, or lysosomal disorders.

All of the disorders in this group are inherited in an autosomal-recessive fashion, so it is important for genetic counseling that an accurate diagnosis is arrived at expeditiously. Carrier detection is possible only by DNA analysis if the molecular defect has been identified in the index case. Carrier detection is not possible by biochemical determination.

Laboratory Diagnosis

The major diagnostic biochemical abnormality is the increased amount of very long-chain fatty acids, which are fatty acids with carbon chains of more than 22. They also are elevated in single-enzyme defects of peroxisomal β-oxidation, so their presence is nonspecific; therefore other studies are required for this diagnosis. Very long-chain fatty acid accumulation here is due to the reduction of peroxisomal β-oxidation, which is greater in Zellweger syndrome than in milder forms (Wanders, 2014). Because the first two steps of plasmalogen synthesis are peroxisomal functions, a reduction of plasmalogen levels is noted in patients with peroxisome biogenesis defects. An age-related increase in the levels of phytanic acid occurs in all of the peroxisome biogenesis disorders.

With broader genetic tools available such as whole exome sequencing (WES) and other DNA-based panels, the older algorithms for diagnosis may be approaching the end of their utility, but because of the ability to rapidly get biochemical information this approach will be warranted where there is appropriate clinical suspicion.

Prenatal Diagnosis

Cultured amniocytes or chorionic villus cells can be used to diagnose all of the disorders of peroxisome biogenesis. A variety of biochemical strategies have been used and focus on the type and degree of biochemical abnormality. Two independent techniques, the measurement of very long-chain fatty acid β-oxidation and plasmalogen synthesis, have demonstrated accurate diagnosis. Molecular genetic techniques may be used in families in which the mutation has been identified and preimplantation genetic diagnosis has been performed.

Therapy

Because many of the abnormalities are already present in the affected fetus, potential for therapy is limited at present and likely to remain so. Treatment is primarily supportive, targeting liver dysfunction with vitamin K for prothrombin deficiency, providing nutrition often with tube feeding, and antiepileptic medication. In the milder phenotypes, rehabilitative approaches, including communication training and physical and occupational therapy, are helpful.

Attempts to normalize some of the biochemical abnormalities include oral ether lipid therapy and dietary restriction of very long-chain fatty acids or phytanic acid have not met with clinical improvement. Therapy with docosahexaenoic acid replaces low levels in plasma and red blood cells of patients with Zellweger spectrum disorder; however, it is ineffective in improving clinical function.

DEFECTS OF SINGLE PEROXISOMAL ENZYMES
Defects of Single Peroxisomal β-Oxidation Enzymes

This is a broad and heterogeneous group of disorders and many are rare. However, this group includes X-linked adrenoleukodystrophy which is the most common peroxisomal disorder and will be discussed here.

Adrenoleukodystrophy

The first clinical cases of what is known as X-linked adrenoleukodystrophy (ALD) were described in 1923 by Siemerling and Creutzfeldt (Moser et al., 2007). The X-linked mode of inheritance was suggested by Fanconi and associates. A key observation of characteristic lamellar lipid-soluble cytoplasmic inclusions in the adrenal cortical cells and brain macrophages of patients with childhood adrenoleukodystrophy was made by Powers and colleagues. Similar inclusions were observed in men with Addison disease and spastic paraparesis, and the related condition was named adrenomyeloneuropathy (AMN). Igarashi and associates defined the biochemical defect by demonstrating that the inclusions in the adrenal cortex and cerebral white matter consisted of cholesterol esters with a striking excess of saturated unbranched fatty acids of 24- to 30-carbon chain length, of which C26:0 and C25:0 were the most abundant. This excess of very long-chain fatty acids in cultured skin fibroblasts, plasma, or red blood cells is the hallmark of the disorder and useful for diagnostic purposes.

Biochemical and Molecular Basis

The peroxisomal β-oxidation pathway consists of four enzymatic steps (as outlined in Fig. 43-1). Before the substrates can enter this pathway, the acyl residues require activation by transfer of a coenzyme A. For very long-chain fatty acids entering the l-specific β-oxidation pathway, lignoceryl-CoA ligase (also referred to as lignoceryl-CoA synthetase) is the activating enzyme. Although this enzyme was originally thought to be the cause, it is known that the genetic basis for X-linked adrenoleukodystrophy is mutations of the ABCD1 gene, which encodes a PMP, an ATP-binding cassette protein; the gene for this protein is located on the X chromosome in the Xq28 region.

The protein is involved in the transport of appropriate fatty acids into the peroxisome and when this path is disrupted they continue to enter the elongation pathway. Multiple mutations in ABCD1 have been identified in patients with X-linked adrenoleukodystrophy, and no phenotype correlation has been identified. Several mouse models of X-linked adrenoleukodystrophy are now available, but to date none of the animals have manifested a cerebral phenotype.

Clinical and Pathologic Features of X-Linked Adrenoleukodystrophy and Adrenomyeloneuropathy

One of the most intriguing aspects of ALD is the variation in presentations depending on age. All affected individuals demonstrate accumulation of very long-chain fatty acid, and molecular studies have confirmed ABCD1 gene mutations. Various phenotypes have been recognized as occurring within the same pedigree, so neither the genetic mutation nor the biochemical abnormality predicts the clinical presentation.

Childhood Cerebral Form of Adrenoleukodystrophy

The childhood cerebral variant is the most common and fulminant form of X-linked adrenoleukodystrophy. Affected boys are normal until 4 to 8 years of age, when they manifest behavior problems and failure in school as a result of rapid regression of auditory discrimination, spatial orientation, speech, and writing. Seizures occur in 30% of patients and, in rare instances, may be the initial sign. The magnetic resonance imaging (MRI) scan reveals parietooccipital white matter lesions (in 85% of patients) or frontal lesions (in 15%) at this stage, with contrast accumulation at the leading edge of the lesion (Fig. 43-5). Rapid clinical deterioration leads to spastic quadriparesis, swallowing difficulty, and visual loss, culminating in a vegetative state usually within 2 years of the initial signs and symptoms. Although males come to medical attention because of the neurologic deficits, impaired adrenal function is seen in the majority of boys at the time of diagnosis.

Adolescent Cerebral Form of Adrenoleukodystrophy

Patients with the adolescent cerebral form of adrenoleukodystrophy manifest signs and symptoms of cerebral involvement, as described previously, between 10 and 21 years of age.

Adult Cerebral Form of Adrenoleukodystrophy

In the adult cerebral form of adrenoleukodystrophy, dementia, psychiatric disturbances, seizures, and spastic paraparesis develop after age 21. Patients may be misdiagnosed as having multiple sclerosis, brain tumor, or schizophrenia and demonstrate rapid deterioration similar to that in the childhood cerebral form. Therefore patients with these clinical presentations and adrenal insufficiency or leukodystrophy should be evaluated by plasma very long-chain fatty acids.

Adrenomyeloneuropathy

The neurologic manifestations of adrenomyeloneuropathy (AMN), an adult form of adrenoleukodystrophy, consist of an insidious onset and slow progression of spastic paraparesis, impaired vibratory sense in the lower extremity, and bladder or bowel dysfunction. Onset is typically in the third decade of life. The primary pathology involves the spinal cord with loss of myelinated axons in the corticospinal tracts, nucleus gracilis, and dorsal spinocerebellar tracts. Sural and peroneal nerves reveal a loss of large and small myelinated fibers.

The development of cerebral demyelination has been seen in approximately 15% to 20% of men with adrenomyeloneuropathy. This pathologic change needs to be differentiated from long tract findings on MRI. Cerebral disease is similar in time course to the childhood form of the disease and leads to dementia, spasticity, blindness, and death. Approximately half of patients with adrenomyeloneuropathy appear to have some degree of cerebral involvement, with mild to moderate abnormalities noted on MRI in 46% (Fig. 43-5). These abnormalities consist most frequently of parietal-occipital white matter and optic radiation involvement.

Primary adrenal insufficiency or Addison disease precedes the onset of neurologic symptoms in 42% of patients; in some, this may occur 3 to 35 years earlier. Serum testosterone levels were abnormally low in 22% of our patients, and early onset sexual dysfunction occurred in one-third.

Addison Disease Only

The diagnosis of adrenoleukodystrophy with Addison disease only includes the patients who have isolated primary adrenal dysfunction disease in the absence of neurologic signs and symptoms and is more common than was previously recognized. This is not surprising because there is no correlation between adrenal and neurologic dysfunction, so males may come to attention in childhood with adrenal insufficiency and develop neurologic issues decades later. Recognition of these patients is vital for genetic counseling and to monitor for the development of adrenomyeloneuropathy or cerebral symptoms later on.

Asymptomatic Patients With the Biochemical Defect of Adrenoleukodystrophy

In asymptomatic patients with the biochemical defect of adrenoleukodystrophy, diagnosis may be accomplished by measurement of plasma very long-chain fatty acids during screening tests of relatives of symptomatic patients. These persons may be of any age and is clearly a function of age. All newborn males are unaffected, and this population appears to decline with age. Whether there are any truly asymptomatic individuals in midadult life is unknown. The elevation of very long-chain fatty acid levels in these males is comparable with that in severely affected family members.

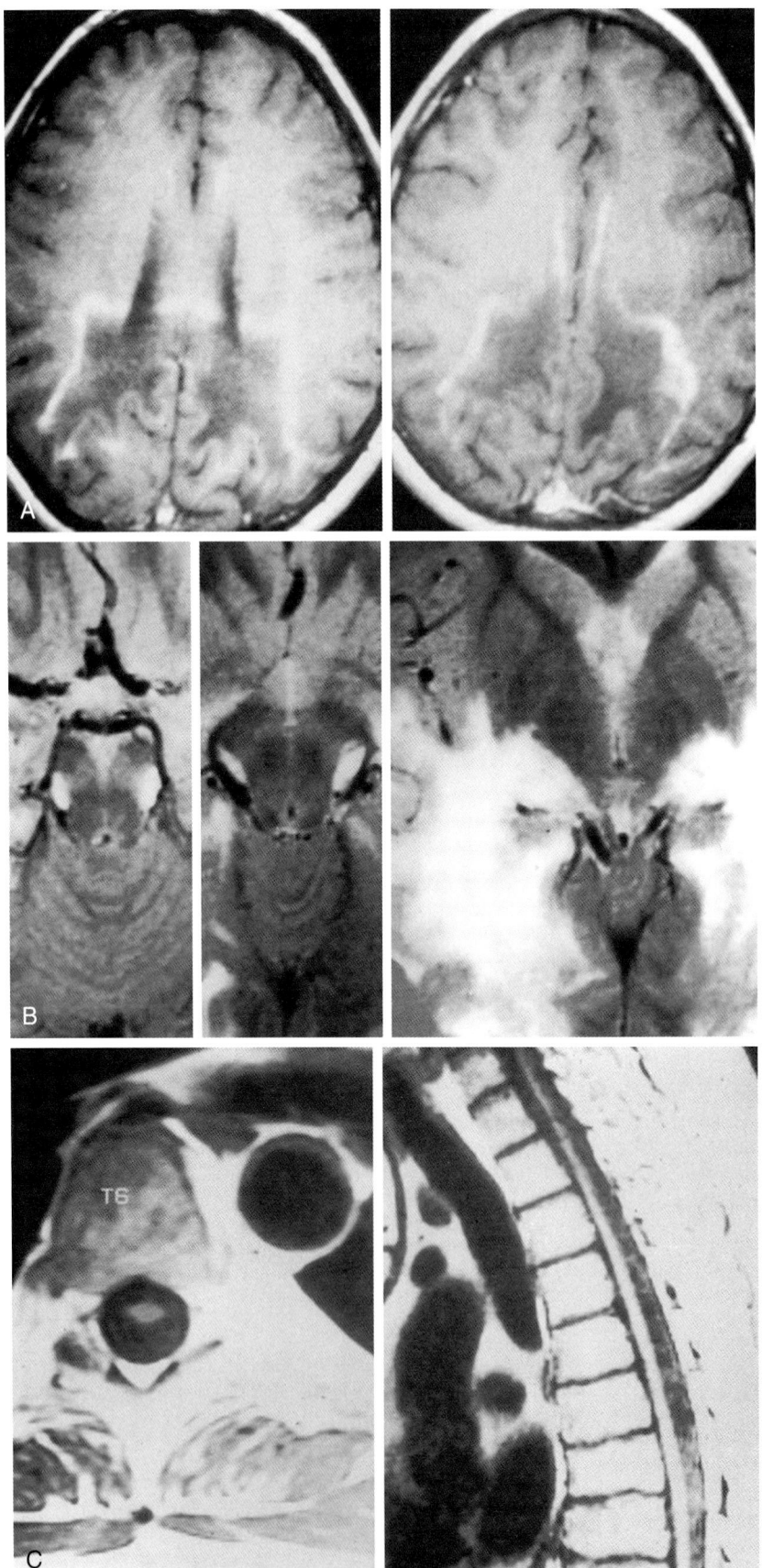

Figure 43-5. Magnetic resonance imaging (MRI) studies in adrenoleukodystrophy. **A,** Typical alteration of the blood–brain barrier at the edge of the demyelinated lesion in childhood adrenoleukostrophy demonstrated on gadolinium-enhanced MRI. **B,** The discrete but continuous auditory pathway involvement from the lateral lemniscus in the pons to the medial geniculate bodies at the midbrain level to the temporal cortex can be seen. MRI permits precise correlation between the location of the lesion and cognitive deficits; the findings may explain the early auditory comprehension deficiency seen in childhood adrenoleukodystrophy. **C,** MRI study of the spine in X-linked adrenoleukodystrophy. Views in axial (left) and lateral (right) planes demonstrate cord atrophy, particularly in the thoracic regions.

Symptomatic Heterozygotes

Between 10% and 20% of the women who are carriers for the adrenoleukodystrophy gene manifest myelopathy resembling that in adrenomyeloneuropathy between the third and fifth decades of life. Long tract signs and diminished vibration sense in the legs are present in two-thirds of the patients, although only 25% complain of symptoms. Approximately 14% have severe spinal involvement requiring assistance with ambulation, and 5% have dementia. In contrast with males, adrenal insufficiency rarely occurs in these women.

In the past, elevation of very long-chain fatty acids in plasma allowed identification of 85% of obligate heterozygotes, but this assay missed 15% of them. Mutation analysis is essential for the accurate identification of females at risk.

Pathogenesis of Adrenoleukodystrophy

The main biochemical defect is the striking excess of very long-chain fatty acids, which accumulate in the cholesterol ester fraction, primarily in the adrenal gland and cerebral white matter. The accumulation of very long-chain fatty acids in X-linked adrenoleukodystrophy is not as severe as in disorders of peroxisome biogenesis or single-peroxisomal β-oxidation enzyme defects. The resultant accumulation does lead to a variety of issues with membrane dysfunction including issues with red blood cell microviscosity, altered response of adrenal cells to adrenocorticotrophic hormone, and other issues with steroid production.

The pathogenesis of the nervous system lesion has been more difficult to discern. It has been presumed that elevation of very long-chain fatty acids results in the axonopathy seen in patients with adrenomyeloneuropathy and in women who are carriers. It is not clear, however, why rapid, inflammatory demyelination affecting the cerebral white matter tracts develops in certain persons. The levels of very long-chain fatty acids in plasma or skin fibroblasts or the capacity to metabolize very long-chain fatty acids in cultured fibroblasts do not differ in males with the childhood form from those in men with adrenomyeloneuropathy or other forms. No correlation exists between severity of the neurologic disease and levels of very long-chain fatty acids. These observations have led to the conclusion that very long-chain fatty acid excess alone is not sufficient to explain cerebral demyelination and that other factors must play a role in the phenotypic variability (Moser et al., 2005).

The presence of the perivascular lymphocytic infiltration in the white matter of the cerebral forms provides evidence of immunologic involvement as one additional factor. This is not seen in the adrenal gland or other leukodystrophies. The pattern seen is that of a cellular immune response in the central nervous system, and the collective evidence implies that an immunologic mechanism contributes to the rapid progression of white matter lesions, possibly in response to the altered lipid composition in brain of patients with adrenoleukodystrophy (Mahmood et al., 2007).

Recent studies have demonstrated a shift in the production of reactive oxygen species, evidence of mitochondrial dysfunction, and activation of low levels of chronic inflammation in all forms of ALD. It has also been shown that at least one inciting factor is the elevation in very long-chain fatty acids. Further studies in this area may identify factors that contribute to the pathogenesis of the nervous system lesions.

Therapy for Adrenoleukodystrophy

Therapy for ALD depends on what manifestations the individual is presenting with; it should also be emphasized that therapy continues to evolve. Adrenal insufficiency should be treated with steroid replacement with increased doses at times of physiologic stress.

The utility of therapies to lower very long-chain fatty acids remains uncertain. Although dietary restriction alone will not lower very long-chain fatty acids, the addition of monounsaturated fatty acids does lower plasma levels of saturated fatty acids. Dietary therapy with the use of glyceryl trierucate, sometimes referred to as Lorenzo's oil, does not alter the course of rapidly progressive childhood cerebral disease. The role in AMN remains unknown, but the results in open studies have not been impressive. In one open study, it was shown that the use of glyceryl trierucate lowered the risk of developing childhood cerebral disease when started in asymptomatic boys (Moser et al., 2005). The usage of this therapy, unfortunately, remains uncertain, and it must be emphasized requires a significant lifestyle change in the subject with unclear benefit.

Bone marrow transplant has been shown to be effective in boys with early cerebral disease as detected by MRI changes (Mahmood et al., 2007). In patients with more advanced disease, transplantation has not resulted in halting the course and may be associated with worsening of the neurologic status immediately after the procedure; therefore this procedure is not advised in those with neurologic findings.

Recently, gene therapy with a lentivirus vector has been successfully used in boys with early cerebral disease. This advancement in the field potentially offers additional avenues of treatment for many individuals who could not previously undergo transplantation.

In patients with advanced cerebral disease, neither dietary therapy nor bone marrow transplantation is effective. A variety of therapies including IVIG, cyclophosphamide immunosuppression, and high dose steroids do not arrest the rapid progression of the illness.

Males at risk for developing the childhood form of ALD (younger than 10 years of age) require appropriate monitoring. MRI should be performed on a yearly basis. Because MRI abnormalities become evident at least 12 months before onset of neurologic symptoms, periodic neurologic examination is not sufficient for monitoring these patients. Timely assessments are especially important because the best outcomes with bone marrow transplantation are in patients identified at an early stage of cerebral disease. Appropriate adrenal monitoring also is indicated in identified patients.

Newborn Screening for XALD

A biochemical assay using tandem mass spectroscopy and the standard newborn blood spot has been developed and has been found to be highly sensitive and specific. This has recently been instituted in New York and may be incorporated in other state panels. If this is subsequently incorporated more broadly into newborn screening programs, it will most likely change the proportion of males coming to attention in the presymptomatic phase and will also improve their care and management.

Current and Future Outlook

With expanding clinical phenotypes, peroxisomal disorders are now included as standard considerations in the differential diagnosis for a variety of neurologic findings in infants, children, and adults. As new peroxisomal functions are being identified, they have provided insight into mechanisms involving biogenesis of the organelle and control of protein import. Their vital role encompassing neuronal migration in fetal brain development through membrane integrity in the axons in adults is being appreciated. All of the disorders can be recognized by noninvasive biochemical and genetic tests, providing valuable information for genetic counseling. These disorders may be severely debilitating or fatal, but therapeutic options are becoming available.

REFERENCES

The complete list of references for this chapter is available online at www.expertconsult.com.

See inside cover for registration details.

SELECTED REFERENCES

Braverman, N.E., D'Agostino, M.D., Maclean, G.E., 2013. Peroxisome biogenesis disorders: biological, clinical and pathophysiological perspectives. Dev Disabil Res Rev 17 (3), 187–196.

Mahmood, A., Raymond, G.V., Dubey, P., et al., 2007. Survival analysis of haematopoietic cell transplantation for childhood cerebral X-linked adrenoleukodystrophy: a comparison study. Lancet Neurol. 6 (8), 687–692.

Moser, H.W., Mahmood, A., Raymond, G.V., 2007. X-linked adrenoleukodystrophy. Nat. Clin. Pract. Neurol. 3 (3), 140–151.

Moser, H.W., Raymond, G.V., Lu, S.E., et al., 2005. Follow-up of 89 asymptomatic patients with adrenoleukodystrophy treated with Lorenzo's oil. Arch. Neurol. 62 (7), 1073–1080.

Vamecq, J., Cherkaoui-Malki, M., Andreoletti, P., et al., 2014. The human peroxisome in health and disease: the story of an oddity becoming a vital organelle. Biochimie 98, 4–15. doi:10.1016/j.biochi.2013.09.019; [Epub@2013 Sep 26:4–15].

Wanders, R.J., 2014. Metabolic functions of peroxisomes in health and disease. Biochimie 98, 36–44. doi:10.1016/j.biochi.2013.08.022; [Epub@2013 Sep 3:36–44].

E-BOOK FIGURES AND TABLES

44 Neurotransmitter-Related Disorders

Kathryn J. Swoboda and Melissa A. Walker

An expanded version of this chapter is available on www.expertconsult.com. See inside cover for registration details.

The term "neurotransmitter disorders" constitutes a broad and increasingly complex spectrum of neurologic conditions associated with defects in the production, transport, release, and reuptake of a variety of chemical compounds involved in neurotransmission. This chapter provides an overview of such disorders, with a primary emphasis on those associated with a dopamine or serotonin deficiency state.

Neurologic symptoms associated with dopamine deficiency are broad and range from extremely mild and subtle alterations in mood or gait to a classic exercise-induced dystonic gait abnormality and an infantile-onset parkinsonism syndrome. In recessive inborn errors of dopamine metabolism associated with tetrahydrobiopterin (BH4) deficiencies, neurologic symptoms are often more severe and accompanied by hyperphenylalaninemia, which can be detected on newborn screening. Associated serotonin deficiency is present in most of these disorders. Even when these disorders are ascertained by newborn screening, repletion of neurotransmitter precursors may not be sufficient, resulting in global developmental impairment, fluctuating tone abnormalities, eye movement abnormalities, encephalopathy, ataxia, and seizures. Diseases related to dysfunction of other neurotransmitter systems (i.e., gamma-aminobutyric acid [GABA], glutamate, and glycine, among others) are more difficult to characterize in humans; however, manifestations of these disorders are equally as diverse as in monoaminergic systems, including seizures, ataxia, hypotonia, oculomotor dyspraxia, and developmental delay.

Screening for neurotransmitter-related disorders occurs primarily by recognition of key neurologic symptoms, though overlap with other disorders with shared features can make accurate identification and diagnosis of these disorders challenging. The routine availability of increasingly more sophisticated diagnostic tools, including cerebrospinal fluid neurotransmitter metabolite studies, cerebrospinal fluid and urine pterin studies, neuroimaging studies, phenylalanine loading studies, enzymatic assays in blood cells or skin fibroblasts, and molecular studies, have facilitated the diagnosis and treatment of patients with monoaminergic neurotransmitter abnormalities.

For ease of classification, neurotransmitter-related disorders can be divided into five groups:

1. Monoaminergic neurotransmitter deficiency states with hyperphenylalaninemia
2. Monoaminergic neurotransmitter deficiency states without hyperphenylalaninemia
3. Amino acid neurotransmitter dysmetabolism
4. Secondary neurotransmitter deficiency states
5. Undefined neurotransmitter deficiency states (Table 44-1)

MONOAMINERGIC NEUROTRANSMITTER DEFICIENCY STATES WITH HYPERPHENYLALANINEMIA

Overview

The neurotransmitter deficiency in infants in this group arises as a result of defects in BH4 metabolism (Fig. 44-1). Patients are usually identified by elevated phenylalanine levels on newborn screening, as BH4 is required for phenylalanine hydroxylation in the liver. The accompanying neurotransmitter deficiency results from the lack of BH4, an obligatory cofactor required for the synthesis of catecholamines and serotonin. Although most academic biochemical genetics clinics that monitor children with phenylketonuria systematically perform the additional studies required to diagnose this group of disorders, children occasionally are not identified until they have progressive neurologic symptoms or clear evidence of developmental delay despite a phenylalanine-restricted diet, prompting the earlier designation of "atypical phenylketonuria." Importantly, newborn screening before an adequate interval of protein intake can lead to a false-negative result. 6-Pyruvoyltetrahydropterinsynthase deficiency results in inadequate BH4 synthesis; dihydropteridine reductase deficiency results in decreased regeneration of BH4 from dihydrobiopterin (see Fig. 44-1). Both are autosomal-recessive disorders in which hyperphenylalaninemia results from a deficiency of BH4. Because of the involvement of BH4 in catecholamine and serotonin synthesis, such infants also have a manifest deficiency of neurotransmitter metabolites in addition to hyperphenylalaninemia. Other conditions in this category include autosomal-recessive guanosine triphosphate cyclohydrolase (GTPCH) deficiency and primapterinuria (Table 44-2).

Role of BH4 in the Central Nervous System

Because BH4 is required for the hydroxylation of aromatic amino acids, its importance in the central nervous system (CNS) becomes immediately apparent, as catecholamine and serotonin synthesis require tyrosine and tryptophan. A BH4-dependent process can be strongly suspected when plasma phenylalanine levels return to normal after BH supplementation. The greater requirement of tyrosine hydroxylase for BH4 in comparison with tryptophan hydroxylase may explain the more severe impairment in the catecholaminergic system compared with the serotonergic system.

6-Pyruvoyltetrahydropterin Synthase Deficiency

6-Pyruvoyltetrahydropterin synthase catalyzes the elimination of inorganic triphosphate from dihydroneopterin triphosphate to form 6-pyruvoyltetrahydropterin. Patients have elevated neopterin to biopterin ratios in urine and plasma. Reduced 6-pyruvoyltetrahydropterin synthase activity can be documented in red blood cells. In the classic form of the disorder, patients have reduced catecholamine and serotonin metabolites and an increased neopterin to biopterin level in cerebrospinal fluid. Patients are usually detected by newborn screening, as with phenylketonurics, and demonstrate progressive neurologic involvement in the first few months of life, including extrapyramidal signs, axial and truncal hypotonia, hypokinesia, feeding difficulties, choreoathetotic or dystonic limb movements, and autonomic symptoms. Many of these patients, despite early diagnosis and supplementation with

TABLE 44-1 Primary Monoaminergic Neurotransmitter Deficiency Disorders

Disorder	Phenotypic Features	Locus	Inheritance
ELEVATED PLASMA PHENYLALANINE			
6-Pyruvoyltetrahydrobiopterin synthase deficiency*	Encephalopathy, dystonia, spasticity, axial hypotonia, autonomic symptoms, oculogyric crises, seizures	11q22.3–23.3	AR
Dihydropteridine reductase deficiency*		4p15.31	AR
GTP cyclohydrolase deficiency*		14q22.1–22.2	AR
Primapterinuria	Benign hyperphenylalaninemia	10q22	AR
NORMAL PLASMA PHENYLALANINE			
GTP cyclohydrolase deficiency*	Exercise-induced dystonia, gait disorder, writer's cramp, restless leg syndrome, tremor	14q22.1–22.2	AD
GTP cyclohydrolase deficiency*	Dystonia, spasticity, torticollis, axial hypotonia, limb rigidity, autonomic symptoms, psychomotor retardation, oculogyric crises	7p11	AR
Sepiapterin reductase deficiency*	Parkinsonian symptoms, psychomotor retardation, behavioral disturbances	2p14p12	AR
Tyrosine hydroxylase deficiency*	Gait disturbance, infantile parkinsonism, dystonia, speech delay	11p15.5	AR
Tryptophan hydroxylase deficiency*	Ataxia, speech delay, hypotonia, psychomotor retardation	11p15.3	AR
Dopamine b-hydroxylase deficiency*	Orthostatic hypotension, lethargy, ptosis	9q34	
Monoamine oxidase A deficiency	Mild mental retardation, tendency to violent or aggressive behavior	Xp11.23	XR
Dopamine Transporter Deficiency*	Hyperkinetic movement disorder progressing to parkinsonism dystonia	5p15.33	AR
Vesicular Monoamine Transporter2 Deficiency*	Mixed hyperkinetic and hypokinetic movement disorder, oculogyric crises, dysautonomia, developmental delay, behavioral and sleep disturbances	10q25.3	AR

*Disorder associated with a dopamine deficiency state.
AD, autosomal-dominant; AR, autosomal-recessive; GTP, guanosine triphosphate; XR, X-linked recessive.

TABLE 44-2 Metabolite Patterns Observed in Urine, Plasma, and Cerebrospinal Fluid in the Inherited Disorders Affecting Dopamine and Serotonin Metabolism

	Phe	BH$_4$	BH$_2$	Neop	Sep	Prim	HVA	5-HIAA	3OMD
GTPCH (Recessive)	↑ (P)	↓ (U, CSF)	N	↓ (U, CSF)	N	N	↓ (CSF)	↓ (CSF)	N
GTPCH (Dominant)	N	↓ (CSF)	N	↓ (CSF)	N	N	↓ (CSF)	± ↓ (CSF)	N
6PTPS	↑ (P)	↓ (U, CSF)	N	(U, CSF)	N	N	↓ (CSF)	(CSF)	N
6PTPS (Mild)	(P)	(U)	N	(U)	N	N	N	N	N
SR	N	(CSF)	(CSF)	N	↑ (CSF)	N	(CSF)	(CSF)	N
PCD	↑ (P)	↓ (U)	N	N	N	(U)	N	N	N
DHPR	(P)	↓ (U) ± ↓ (CSF)	↑ (U, CSF)	N	N	N	↓ (CSF)	↓ (CSF)	N
TH	N	N	N	N	N	N	↓ (CSF)	N	N
AADC	N	N	N	N	N	N	↓ (CSF)	↓ (CSF)	↑ (P, CSF, U)

AADC, aromatic L-amino acid decarboxylase; BH2, 7,8-dihydrobiopterin; DHPR, dihydropteridine reductase; 5-HIAA, 5-hydroxyindoleacetic acid; GTPCH, guanosine triphosphate cyclohydrolase; HVA, homovanillic acid; N, normal; Neop, neopterin; P, plasma; PCD, pterin α-carbinolamine dehydratase; Phe, phenylalanine; Prim, primapterin; Sep, sepiapterin; 6PTPS, 6-pyruvoyltetrahydropterin synthase; SR, sepiapterin reductase; TH, tyrosine hydroxylase; 3OMD, 3-O-methyldopa; U, urine; ↓, decreased; ↑, elevated.
(With permission from Hyland, K., 2007. Inherited disorders affecting dopamine and serotonin: Critical neurotransmitters derived from aromatic amino acids. J Nutr 137, 1568–1572S.)

BH4 and neurotransmitter precursors, continue to manifest delay in development. A "peripheral" form of the disorder is associated with nearly one-third of known mutations with the human PTS gene and is characterized by normal central neurotransmitter levels and less significant or transient hyperphenylalaninemia. Patients with the peripheral form have an excellent prognosis for normal neurologic development, provided the hyperphenylalaninemia is corrected by diet or BH4 administration.

Dihydropteridine Reductase Deficiency

Dihydropteridine reductase deficiency manifests in a variety of phenotypes, all with hyperphenylalaninemia. The clinical presentation is similar to that of central 6-pyruvoyltetrahydropterin synthase deficiency. Without folinic acid to restore methyltetrahydrofolate status in the CNS, these patients can have progressive calcification of the basal ganglia and subcortical regions, despite treatment with BH4 and neurotransmitter precursors. Diagnosis can be confirmed by the pattern of urine pterins and documentation of abnormal dihydropteridine reductase activity in skin fibroblasts. Results of phenylalanine loading tests are abnormal, and phenylalanine status improves or returns to normal with BH4 supplementation. Cerebrospinal fluid neurotransmitter and pterin analysis reveals reduced concentrations of homovanillic acid and 5-hydroxyindoleacetic acid, decreased or normal BH4 levels, and elevated dihydrobiopterin levels.

Autosomal-Recessive Guanosine Triphosphate Cyclohydrolase Deficiency

Patients with the autosomal-recessive form of GTPCH deficiency (in contrast to autosomal-dominant dopa-responsive dystonia) present similarly to patients with dihydropteridine reductase deficiency and 6-pyruvoyltetrahydropterin synthase deficiency with severe global developmental impairment, marked axial hypotonia, eye movement abnormalities, limb hypertonia, convulsions, and autonomic symptoms. GTPCH activity is absent in blood cells, liver, and skin fibroblasts. Cerebrospinal fluid neurotransmitter metabolite analysis reveals low homovanillic acid, 5-hydroxyindoleacetic acid, neopterin, and biopterin levels.

Pterin-4a-Carbinolamine Dehydratase Deficiency (Primapterinuria)

Pterin-4a-carbinolamine dehydratase deficiency, or primapterinuria, causes mild hyperphenylalaninemia these infants are usually identified on newborn screening but generally have a benign course with normal development (Thöny and Blau, 2006).

MONOAMINERGIC NEUROTRANSMITTER DEFICIENCY STATES WITHOUT HYPERPHENYLALANINEMIA
Overview

Neurotransmitter deficiency disorders not associated with hyperphenylalaninemia span a complex clinical spectrum. The lack of newborn screening and increasingly diverse phenotypes make these disorders challenging to recognize. Excepting autosomal-dominant dopa-responsive dystonia and monoamine oxidase a deficiency, these disorders are inherited in an autosomal-recessive fashion. Heterozygous carriers very rarely have a discernible phenotype.

Segawa Disease or Autosomal-Dominant Dopa-Responsive Dystonia

The best-described and most widely identified entity among this group of disorders is autosomal-dominant dopa-responsive dystonia caused by GTPCH deficiency, or Segawa disease. Patients with a classic presentation of exercise-induced dystonia are easily recognized; however, the diagnosis should also be considered in patients with spastic diplegia, particularly with diurnal variation, as well as in more atypical presentations resulting from incomplete penetrance such as writer's cramp, asymmetric limb dystonia, tremor, or restless leg-type symptoms. Patients often benefit greatly from directed treatment of the associated dopamine deficiency state and clinical response to L-DOPA/carbidopa may aid in diagnosis.

Cerebrospinal fluid neurotransmitter metabolite (low homovanillic acid, normal or low 5-hydroxyindoleacetic acid, and reduced BH4) and pterin studies as well as phenylalanine loading can be helpful in confirming the diagnosis in these patients and can help characterize the degree of associated dopamine and serotonin deficiency. GTPCH activity can be measured in skin fibroblasts. Urine biopterin levels are low.

Aromatic L-Amino Acid Decarboxylase or Dopa-Decarboxylase Deficiency

Aromatic L-amino acid decarboxylase is a pyridoxine-dependent enzyme that decarboxylates L-DOPA and 5-hydroxytryptophan to make dopamine and serotonin, respectively. Patients with this disorder typically present in the first few months of life with dystonia or intermittent limb spasticity, axial and truncal hypotonia, oculogyric crises, autonomic symptoms, and ptosis.

Cerebrospinal fluid neurotransmitter metabolites demonstrate a characteristic pattern: low homovanillic acid and 5-hydroxyindoleacetic acid levels; markedly elevated 3-O-methyldopa, 5-hydroxytryptophan, and L-DOPA; and normal biopterin and neopterin levels. Plasma L-DOPA is markedly elevated. Urine catecholamines may be reduced or elevated, specifically with vanillactic acid, despite normal preliminary organic acid results (Fig. 44-2).

Although some children benefit in terms of the underlying movement disorder, treatment is complex, and these patients

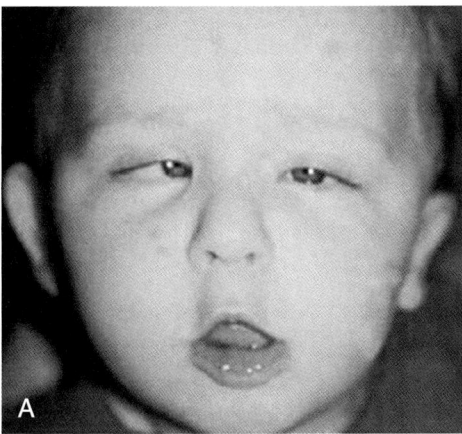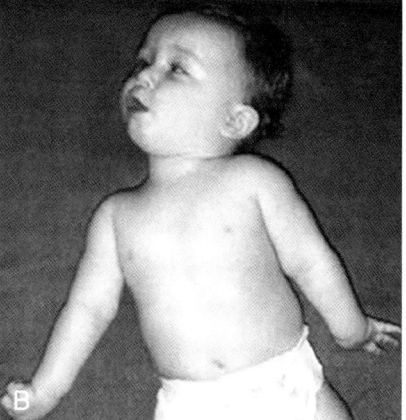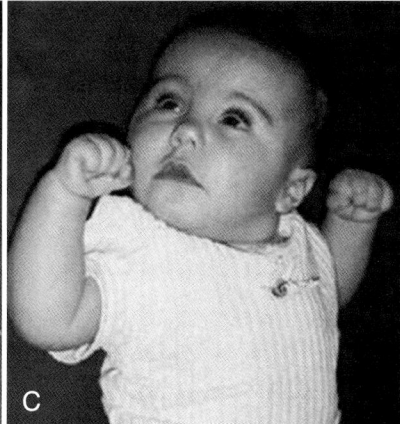

Figure 44-2. Episodic neurologic manifestations in aromatic L-amino acid decarboxylase deficiency. **A,** Ocular convergence spasm, ptosis, and orofacial dystonia. **B,** Torticollis and limb dystonia. **C,** Torticollis and limb rigidity.

are vulnerable to an array of medication-related side effects. Overall clinical outcomes in aromatic L-amino acid decarboxylase deficiency have remained poor, though emerging gene therapies may hold promise.

Sepiapterin Reductase Deficiency

Sepiapterin reductase catalyzes the (NADP) reduction of carbonyl derivatives, including pteridines, and plays an important role in BH4 biosynthesis. It is likely that low dihydrofolate reductase activity in the brain allows accumulation of dihydrobiopterin that inhibits tyrosine and tryptophan hydroxylases and uncouples neuronal nitric oxide synthase, leading to neurotransmitter deficiency and neuronal cell death. Thus identification of low cerebrospinal fluid neurotransmitter levels and the presence of elevated cerebrospinal fluid dihydrobiopterin are essential, and the diagnosis can be confirmed with low skin fibroblast enzyme activity or sequencing of the SPR gene.

Few patients have been described. In the largest published series, motor delay, axial hypotonia, language delay, diurnal fluctuation of symptoms, dystonia, sleep benefit, weakness, oculogyric crises, dysarthria, parkinsonian signs, hyperreflexia, and psychiatric of behavioral signs were observed in more than half of the 38 patients surveyed. Other significant neurologic manifestations included autonomic disturbances, eye movement abnormalities, chorea, ataxia, dysphagia, hyporeflexia, seizures, and myoclonus. In all cases receiving treatment, significant motor improvement resulted from low-dose L-DOPA/carbidopa.

Tyrosine Hydroxylase Deficiency or Autosomal-Recessive Dopa-Responsive Dystonia

Tyrosine hydroxylase deficiency, sometimes referred to as autosomal-recessive Segawa disease, displays diverse phenotypes that can be classified as mild, moderate, or severe. Mild cases may demonstrate clumsy gait, toe-walking, tight heel cords, or abnormal posturing that may worsen at the end of the day and may progress with age. Attention or articulation difficulties are sometimes seen. All children with mild symptoms are readily treated with medication. Moderately affected cases demonstrate an abnormal gait often with dystonic posturing with stressed gait, sometimes accompanied by ataxic, spasticity, speech delay, involuntary eye movement problems (brief upward eye-rolling movements with stress or fatigue), or frank oculogyric crises. Most have an excellent response to treatment, but full benefit may take many months. In the most severe cases, referred to as the infantile Parkinson's disease variant, children are severely disabled and affected from early infancy, demonstrating muscle tightness and rigidity, arching, tremor and poor muscle control, and involuntary eye movements. Ptosis, speech delay, feeding difficulty, and constipation are also common. Less commonly, there are children with generalized low tone, with poor head control and inability to sit unsupported. They often demonstrate torticollis. Dysautonomia can occur, frequently during illness. Severe cases are more difficult to treat, often requiring multiple medications and being unusually vulnerable to side effects of dopaminergic agonists or precursors. Response may be slow, with some continued benefit during months to years. Some cases show persistent mental retardation, encephalopathy, and motor disability despite of treatment.

Cerebrospinal fluid concentration of homovanillic acid is low whereas 5-hydroxyindoleacetic acid, neopterin, and biopterin are normal. Phenylalanine loading studies are normal, and enzymatic assays for confirmation of a suspected diagnosis are not presently available, making confirmation by molecular testing is extremely helpful. A recent analysis has identified mostly missense and compound heterozygous TH mutations, consistent with prior reports of autosomal recessive inheritance.

Patients variably respond to L-DOPA/carbidopa, and some have complete reversal of symptoms. The exception to this is the patient with the severe infantile parkinsonism form, who typically tolerates L-DOPA poorly. Addition of dopamine agonists such as selegiline or anticholinergic agents such as trihexyphenidyl can provide significant benefit and help promote the gradual ongoing attainment of motor skills and ability to ambulate independently, but such achievements may occur over years, rather than months or weeks, in the most severely affected patients (Marecos et al., 2014).

Tryptophan Hydroxylase Deficiency

Tryptophan hydroxylase catalyzes the BH4-dependent hydroxylation of tryptophan to 5-hydroxytryptophan, which is then decarboxylated to form serotonin. Tryptophan hydroxylase expression is limited to certain cells in the CNS and periphery. Although clinically suspected, no confirmed cases have yet been identified.

Dopamine B-Hydroxylase Deficiency

Dopamine b-hydroxylase converts dopamine to norepinephrine. Patients with severe deficiency cannot synthesize norepinephrine, epinephrine, and octopamine in CNS or peripheral autonomic neurons. Dopamine acts as a false neurotransmitter for noradrenergic neurons. Neonates with dopamine b-hydroxylase deficiency can have episodic hypothermia, hypoglycemia, and hypotension, leading to early death. Survivors do fairly well until late childhood, when overwhelming orthostatic hypotension profoundly limits their activities (Robertson et al., 1991).

Most patients have been identified as young adults. Observation of severe orthostatic hypotension in a patient whose plasma norepinephrine/dopamine ratio is much less than 1 supports the diagnosis. Orthostatic hypotension, particularly after exercise, and ptosis are constant features. General lethargy and lassitude improve dramatically, and blood pressure becomes normal with treatment with D,L-threo-dihydroxyphenylserine, a synthetic amino acid that is converted to norepinephrine by aromatic L-amino acid decarboxylase.

Patients may undergo personality change, becoming more "aggressive" with treatment.

Monoamine Oxidase Deficiency

Monoamine oxidase is a mitochondrial enzyme involved in the catabolism of biogenic amines. Monoamine oxidase A, the primary type in fibroblasts, preferentially degrades serotonin and norepinephrine. Monoamine oxidase B, the primary type in platelets and in the brain, preferentially degrades phenylethylamine and benzylamine. These enzymes are critical in the neuronal metabolism of catecholamine and indoleamine neurotransmitters. The genes are closely linked on the X chromosome, near the Norrie's disease locus, and only affected boys have been identified to date.

Monoamine Oxidase A Deficiency

Brunner described a family with an X-linked nondysmorphic mild mental retardation and a tendency to severe aggressive or violent behavior and urine studies consistent with marked disturbance of monoamine metabolism (Brunner et al., 1993). No additional patients have been identified to date.

Monoamine Oxidase B Deficiency

Isolated monoamine oxidase B deficiency has not yet been reported in a patient. Two brothers with a microdeletion, including the Norrie locus and monoamine oxidase B, however, had features consistent with Norrie disease alone. These patients had neither abnormal behavior nor mental retardation, leading the authors to conclude that monoamine oxidase A plays a more significant role than does monoamine oxidase B in the metabolism of biogenic amines, and monoamine oxidase B deficiency alone may have a primarily neurochemical phenotype: that of increased phenylethylamine in urine (Lenders et al., 1996).

Monoamine Oxidase A and B Deficiency

A small number of cases of MAO A and B deficiency (with intact Norrie locus) have been reported, all male. Affected individual's demonstrated episodic hypotonia, intellectual disability and stereotyped movements (Saito et al. 2014).

Dopamine Transporter Deficiency

The presynaptic dopamine transporter (DAT) encoded by SLC6A3 modulates the intensity and duration of dopaminergic signaling by synaptic dopamine reuptake. Individuals with dopamine transporter deficiency syndrome classically present with a hyperkinetic movement disorder of infantile onset that progresses to parkinsonism dystonia and characteristic elevated CSF homovanillic acid to 5-hydroxyindoleacetic acid (HV to 5-HIAA). Inheritance has been consistent with an autosomal recessive pattern. Treatment generally involves ropinirole, L-dopa, and/or selegiline therapy, but most cases are refractory to medical or surgical management (Marecos et al., 2014).

Vesicular Monoamine Transporter 2 Deficiency

A syndrome of mixed hyperkinetic and hypokinetic movement disorder with oculogyric crises, dysautonomia, developmental delay, behavioral and sleep disturbances with no CSF neurotransmitter deficiency has been described in a single family. Affected individuals additionally demonstrate elevated urine 5-HIAA, HVA, and decreased urine norepinephrine and dopamine and were found to carry single family has been described with homozygous missense mutations in SLC18A2, the gene encoding the vesicular monoamine transporter 2. Treatment with pramipexole improved dopamine-related symptoms markedly, and to a lesser extent, other symptoms (Marecos et al., 2014).

DISORDERS OF AMINO ACID NEUROTRANSMITTERS
Overview

Amino acid neurotransmitters are the main inhibitory and excitatory messengers in the nervous system; however, few have been implicated in human disease. GABA and glycine-related disorders are best studied yet incompletely understood. Glycine has ubiquitous function and both excitatory and inhibitory properties. Glycine encephalopathy, formerly referred to as nonketotic hyperglycinemia, will be touched on briefly, as more extensive review occurs elsewhere in this text. Disorders of GABA degradation will also be reviewed (Fig. 44-3), with specific emphasis on succinic semialdehyde dehydrogenase deficiency, the most common and best characterized.

Gamma-Aminobutyric Acid Transaminase Deficiency

GABA is the major inhibitory neurotransmitter of the brain, derived primarily from glutamate, the major excitatory neurotransmitter. The first step of the GABA degradation pathway involves GABA transaminase, which removes an amino group from GABA and adds it to alpha-ketoglutarate, thus replenishing glutamate and reestablishing the closed loop system known as the GABA shunt. GABA transaminase deficiency is a rare, autosomal-recessive disorder characterized by abnormal development, seizures, and high levels of CSF GABA beta-alanine, both of which are also elevated in serum. Cases to date have presented with neonatal seizures, lethargy, hypotonia, hyperreflexia, developmental retardation, and high pitched cry, all with poor outcomes (Definitive diagnosis can be made by measurement enzyme activity in various cell types [Parviz et al., 2014]).

Succinic Semialdehyde Dehydrogenase Deficiency

Succinic semialdehyde dehydrogenase deficiency is an autosomal-recessive inborn error of metabolism associated with a defect in the metabolism of GABA. Phenotypic features range from nonspecific global developmental delay and hypotonia to ataxia, severe mental retardation, visual impairment, and seizures. Somewhat uniquely among neurotransmitter-related disorders, disease course is not intermittent or episodic. Neuropsychiatric symptoms (i.e., sleep disorders, inattention, hyperactivity, obsessive-compulsive disorder, and anxiety) are prominent. MRI is commonly abnormal. Urine organic acid screening to detect elevated 4-hydroxybutyric acid is the most easily available screening strategy, but GABA levels in cerebrospinal fluid and urine are also elevated. Treatment is generally symptomatic and targeted at seizure management (Lapalme-Remis et al., 2015).

Secondary Neurotransmitter Deficiency States

Menkes disease is an X-linked recessive disorder in which multiple copper-dependent enzymes can be secondarily affected, including dopamine b-hydroxylase, leading to secondary autonomic involvement and norepinephrine deficiency (Kaler et al., 2008).

Hyperekplexia, or "startle disease," is a heterogeneous disorder caused by defects in the a1 subunit of the glycine receptor occurring in autosomal-dominant and autosomal-recessive forms, characterized by stimulus-sensitive myoclonus. Transient hypertonia and hypokinesia in infancy in some families with the disorder has led to the designation "stiff baby syndrome." Dubowitz and colleagues described an infant with classic startle disease, with markedly decreased cerebrospinal fluid GABA levels (Dubowitz et al., 1992). Infants with hyperekplexia have higher than expected rates of sudden infant death syndrome. An exaggerated startle response persists throughout life; sudden, acoustic or tactile stimuli can precipitate a brief attack of intense rigidity with falling. Dramatic improvement of symptoms occurs in most patients with clonazepam.

Neurodegenerative disorders are sometimes associated with reduced neurotransmitter metabolites. Such abnormalities have been seen in patients with leukodystrophy and progressive encephalopathy phenotypes in which a primary defect in neurotransmitter or pterin metabolism could not be identified but who still may benefit from directed treatment of the underlying neurotransmitter deficiency.

Periods of hypoxia or ischemia can lead to secondary deficiencies of serotonin and dopamine.

UNDEFINED NEUROTRANSMITTER DEFICIENCY STATES

Increasingly, with more widespread testing of cerebrospinal fluid neurotransmitter metabolites, patients are being identified with documented neurotransmitter deficiency states that do not fit easily into any of the preceding diagnostic categories, and the nature of their underlying defects remains unknown. These include patients with a wide variety of movement disorder phenotypes, encephalopathy, or seizures. Additional studies are needed to determine the precise defects affecting neurotransmitter levels and to ascertain whether they are primary or secondary.

APPROACH TO TREATMENT IN PATIENTS WITH NEUROTRANSMITTER DEFICIENCY STATES

Because patients with neurotransmitter deficiency disorders caused by tyrosine hydroxylase or BH4 deficiency have been deficient for prolonged periods before treatment, they can be extremely sensitive to initiation of neurotransmitter precursors. Starting with extremely conservative dosages, increasing the dosage slowly during weeks or months, and ensuring that peripheral aromatic L-amino acid decarboxylase is fully blocked by providing ample carbidopa can make the transition to treatment much easier. The rate or degree to which children respond depends on a variety of factors, including age at diagnosis, specific disorder and mutation, presence or absence of associated hyperphenylalaninemia, and presence or absence of central BH4 deficiency. In general, optimism about improvement is warranted.

Institution of neurotransmitter precursor treatment may lead to new problems, such as intermittent dyskinesia related to a peak dose effect, changes in appetite, gastroesophageal reflux, diarrhea, and constipation. These problems, greatest in the first few weeks of institution of treatment, tend to improve with time. With regard to replacement of L-DOPA, use of a slow-release form of the medication may theoretically be ideal. However, such formulations are dosed, not for use in children, but for use in adults with Parkinson's disease. In addition, dividing standard dosage forms marketed for adults makes adequate dosing in infants and young children a significant challenge. Thus ideal dosage forms may need to be formulated in compounded preparations, rather than through commercially marketed dosage preparations. Support for parents and children during this often difficult period of transition from initiation of treatment to adjustment of medications is critical because these patients will likely require neurotransmitter precursor replacement throughout their lifetimes.

In a disorder such as aromatic L-amino acid decarboxylase deficiency, in which direct receptor agonists may be indicated, only adult formulations of these often-potent medications are available, making the use of compounding necessary. Giving more frequent and lower doses throughout the day may be necessary in some children.

Although patients with primary neurotransmitter deficiency states are more likely to respond optimally to treatment, patients with secondary neurotransmitter deficiency may have some symptomatic benefit from directed treatment of their underlying neurotransmitter deficiency state.

NEUROLOGIC DISORDERS CHARACTERIZED BY EXCESS NEUROTRANSMITTER LEVELS
Glycine Encephalopathy

Glycine encephalopathy, formerly referred to as nonketotic hyperglycinemia, is a heterogeneous disorder associated with insufficient activity of various components of the mitochondrial glycine cleavage system. The enzyme system for cleavage of glycine is composed of four protein components: P protein, a pyridoxal phosphate-dependent glycine decarboxylase; H protein, a lipoic acid-containing protein; T protein, a tetrahydrofolate-requiring enzyme; and L protein, a lipoamide dehydrogenase. Nonketotic hyperglycinemia may be caused by a defect in any one of these enzymes. It is an autosomal-recessive disorder with several reported phenotypes, including the classic severe neonatal form, an infantile variant, a mild-episodic childhood variant, a late-onset form, and a benign reversible form.

Most patients described to date have the neonatal and most severe phenotype, likely because it is the most distinctive phenotype. These patients present shortly after birth with lethargy, encephalopathy, hypotonia, myoclonic jerks, and apnea. EEG generally reveals a burst-suppression pattern. Those who survive the neonatal period generally develop intractable seizures and profound mental retardation. Patients with the infantile form have seizures and variable cognitive impairment after a short period of apparently normal development. In the mild, episodic form, patients typically present some time after infancy with mild psychomotor retardation and may manifest episodes of delirium, chorea, and vertical gaze palsy during febrile illness. In the late-onset form, children present with progressive spastic diplegia and optic atrophy. They generally do not have seizures, and intellectual function is preserved. Diagnosis is best made by documenting an increased cerebrospinal fluid to plasma glycine ratio. At present, confirmation of diagnosis requires enzyme analysis in liver or transformed lymphoblasts. Treatment with dextromethorphan and sodium benzoate has led to variable improvement in seizure control and behavioral problems in some patients. It is additionally advisable to avoid valproate, as it may increase serum and CSF glycine levels (Hoover-Fong JE et al., 2004).

REFERENCES

The complete list of references for this chapter is available in the e-book at www.expertconsult.com.
   See inside cover for registration details.

SELECTED REFERENCES

Brunner, H.G., Nelen, M., Breakefield, X.O., et al., 1993. Abnormal behavior associated with a point mutation in the structural gene for monoamine oxidase A. Science 62, 578–580.

Dubowitz, L.M., Bouza, H., Hird, M.F., et al., 1992. Low cerebrospinal fluid concentration of free gamma-aminobutyric acid in startle disease. Lancet 340, 80–81.

Hoover-Fong, J.E., Shah, S., Van Hove, J.L., et al., 2004. Natural history of nonketotic hyperglycinemia in 65 patients. Neurology 63, 1847–1853.

Kaler, S.G., Holmes, C.S., Goldstein, D.S., et al., 2008. Neonatal diagnosis and treatment of Menkes disease. N. Engl. J. Med. 358, 605–614.

Lapalme-Remis, S., Lewis, E.C., De Meulemeester, C., et al., 2015. Natural history of succinic semialdehyde dehydrogenase deficiency through adulthood. Neurology 5, 861–865.

Lenders, J.W., Eisenhofer, G., Abeling, N.G., et al., 1996. Specific genetic deficiencies of the A and B isoenzymes of monoamine oxidase are characterized by distinct neurochemical and clinical phenotypes. J. Clin. Invest. 97, 1010–1019.

Marecos, C., Ng, J., Kurian, M.A., 2014. What is new for monoamine neurotransmitter disorders? J. Inherit. Metab. Dis. 37, 619–626.

Parviz, M., Vogel, K., Gibson, K.M., et al., 2014. Disorders of GABA metabolism: SSADH and GABA-transaminase deficiencies. J Pediatr Epilepsy 3, 217–227.

Robertson, D., Haile, V., Perry, S.E., et al., 1991. Dopamine beta-hydroxylase deficiency. A genetic disorder of cardiovascular regulation. Hypertension 18, 1–8.

Saito, M., Yamagata, T., Matsumoto, A., et al., 2014. MAOA/B deletion syndrome in male siblings with severe developmental delay and sudden loss of muscle tonus. Brain Dev. 36, 64–69.

Thöny, B., Blau, N., 2006. Mutations in the BH4-metabolizing genes GTP cyclohydrolase I, 6-pyruvoyl-tetrahydropterin synthase, sepiapterin reductase, carbinolamine-4a-dehydratase, and dihydropteridine reductase. Hum. Mutat. 27, 870–878.

E-BOOK FIGURES AND TABLES

The following figures and tables are available in the e-book at www.expertconsult.com. See inside cover for registration details.

Fig. 44-1 Synthesis and catabolism of catecholamine and indoleamine neurotransmitters.

Fig. 44-3 The gamma-aminobutyric acid metabolism pathway.

45 Phakomatoses and Allied Conditions

Elizabeth A. Thiele and Bruce R. Korf

The disorders referred to as phakomatoses are notable for their dysplastic nature and tendency to form tumors in various organs, particularly the nervous system. Some of these conditions have been referred to as "neurocutaneous disorders" because of the frequent involvement of the skin in addition to the nervous system. Cutaneous features are not present in all phakomatoses, however (e.g., von Hippel-Lindau syndrome), and many include features outside the skin and nervous system (Table 45-1 summarizes the phakomatoses).

THE NEUROFIBROMATOSES

The neurofibromatoses consist of three distinct disorders: NF1 (Ferner and Gutmann, 2013), NF2 (Lloyd and Evans, 2013), and schwannomatosis (Plotkin et al, 2013).

Neurofibromatosis Type 1

Neurofibromatosis type 1 (NF1) is transmitted as an autosomal-dominant trait and is notable for its great variability of expression. It can involve not only the peripheral and central nervous systems, but also the skin, bone, endocrine, gastrointestinal, and vascular systems. Diagnostic criteria for NF1 are presented in Box 45-2.

Clinical Characteristics

In NF1, the usual presenting signs are cutaneous manifestations. Skin changes include café-au-lait macules, cutaneous neurofibromas, nevus anemicus, patchy and diffuse areas of hyperpigmentation, and juvenile xanthogranulomas. Six or more café-au-lait macules measuring at least 5 mm across before puberty or 15 mm after puberty constitute one diagnostic criterion for NF1. Individuals with mutation in the SPRED1 gene may also present with multiple café-au-lait macules, skinfold freckles, and macrocephaly but do not develop neurofibromas or other tumor-related NF1 complications. This condition is referred to as Legius syndrome. Usually the second sign to appear is skinfold freckling. Freckles begin in the inguinal region in children at 3 to 4 years of age and eventually appear in the axillae, at the base of the neck, and in the inframammary region in females.

Cutaneous neurofibromas are a prominent finding in NF1 and are located in or adjacent to the dermis. They are discrete, soft or firm papules, ranging in size from a few millimeters to several centimeters, can be flat, sessile, or pedunculated, and can be readily impressed into the skin below. Neurofibromas can develop at any time and in any location, and may affect any component of the peripheral nervous system, from the dorsal root ganglion to the terminal nerve twigs. Plexiform neurofibromas represent tumors involving a longitudinal section of nerve or multiple branches of a major nerve. Near the surface of the body they can cause thickening and hypertrophy of the skin and soft tissues. They may occur deeper in the body and be detected only by imaging. Tumors of the orbit or limbs can cause major physical deformity. Plexiform neurofibromas can be congenital lesions, often growing rapidly in the early years of life; they then may remain quiescent for long periods of time or grow unpredictably. The tumors are easily visualized by magnetic resonance imaging (MRI), and display a characteristic "target sign." Neurofibromas originating at the dorsal roots may grow in a dumbbell shape and invade the spinal canal, sometimes causing spinal cord compression. The gastrointestinal tract can also be affected by growth of neurofibromas or ganglioneuromas causing intestinal obstruction or bleeding.

Ophthalmologic features of NF1 include Lisch nodules, glaucoma, and optic glioma. Iris Lisch nodules are melanocytic hamartomas that are highly specific to NF1. Optic pathway gliomas are found in approximately 15% of patients. Most are asymptomatic, but these tumors can manifest with decreased visual acuity, visual field defects, or precocious puberty. Visual symptoms do not necessarily correlate with the size or growth of the tumor radiographically. The glioma can involve the optic nerves, chiasm, optic radiations, and hypothalamus; it may manifest rarely as the diencephalic syndrome of infancy or more commonly with precocious puberty. Optic gliomas are pilocytic astrocytomas, but usually are slow-growing.

Aside from optic gliomas, astrocytomas of the cerebrum, brainstem, and cerebellum are the most common intracranial tumors encountered in NF1. Malignant peripheral nerve sheath tumor occurs in 8% to 13% of affected persons. These manifest with pain or sudden growth, usually within a preexisting plexiform neurofibroma. Various other neoplastic disorders occur more frequently in patients with NF1 than in the general population, including leukemia, especially juvenile myelomonocytic leukemia and pheochromocytoma.

Macrocephaly and short stature are common in NF1 and scoliosis has been reported to occur in 10% to 40% of patients. Bowing of the tibia, fibula, and other long bones can be present in early life, with occurrence of spontaneous fractures at the junction of the middle and distal thirds of the bone shaft, resulting in pseudarthrosis. Nonossifying fibromas may occur and can present with pain or fracture.

Children with NF1 manifest an increased frequency of migraine, and these may be associated with features of abdominal pain, nausea, and vomiting. Constipation has also been reported at increased frequency in affected children.

Approximately 50% of patients have learning disabilities, with no specific pattern unique to those with NF1. Both verbal and nonverbal disabilities occur, as well as attention-deficit disorder, hypotonia, and expressive and language problems. Those with attention deficit disorder do tend to respond to stimulant medication. Problems with motor coordination and balance are also seen, and correlate with the presence of other neurocognitive dysfunctions. Children with NF1 may also have problems with sleep. Fewer than 10% have severe intellectual disability, and most of these patients have large deletions of the NF1 gene. There is also an increased frequency of symptoms consistent with autism spectrum disorders.

45

BOX 45-2 Diagnostic Criteria for Neurofibromatosis 1

- Six or more café-au-lait macules more than 5 mm in greatest diameter in prepubertal children, and more than 15 mm in greatest diameter in postpubertal children
- Two or more neurofibromas of any type or one plexiform neuroma
- Freckling in the axillary or inguinal regions
- Optic pathway glioma
- Two or more Lisch nodules (iris hamartomas)
- A distinctive osseous lesion, such as sphenoid dysplasia or thinning of long bone cortex, with or without pseudarthrosis
- Diagnosis of NF1 in a first-degree relative (parent, sibling, or offspring) according to foregoing criteria

(Modified from: Stumpf, D., 1988. Consensus development conference of neurofibromatosis. Arch Neurol 45, 575–578; Gutmann, D.H., et al., 197. The diagnostic evaluation and multidisciplinary management of neurofibromatosis 1 and neurofibromatosis 2. JAMA 278, 51–57.)

Seizures occur in approximately 6–10% of patients, are often focal, and may be associated with structural changes in the brain.

Vascular anomalies in NF1 can occur in peripheral or cerebral vessels and include regions of intimal proliferation and fibromuscular changes in small arteries. Renal artery stenosis can lead to hypertension in children, and involvement of other vessels can cause vascular insufficiency or hemorrhage as a result of arterial wall dissection. Stenosis of the internal carotid artery can lead to moyamoya disease and stroke, although lesions often are asymptomatic. Surgical revascularization has been shown to be effective in prevention of ischemic episodes in instances of internal carotid stenosis.

Pathology

Neurofibromas consist of a mixture of cell types, including Schwann cells, fibroblasts, perineurial cells, and mast cells. In plexiform neurofibromas, the pathologic process extends across multiple nerve fascicles instead of occurring at a focal site in a nerve and may extend across branches of a larger nerve. Malignant peripheral nerve sheath tumor manifests as a malignant tumor of Schwann cell origin, although sometimes rhabdoid elements are present in such tumors. Most, if not all, of these neoplasms arise from preexisting tumors, usually plexiform neurofibromas.

Genetics

NF1, inherited as an autosomal-dominant trait, has an estimated prevalence of 1 in 3000 in all populations; about half of cases are new mutations. The NF1 gene is located at 17q11.2 and encodes a 3818-amino-acid protein referred to as neurofibromin. The protein includes a functional GTPase-activating protein (GAP) domain that regulates conversion of RAS-guanosine triphosphate to Ras-guanosine diphosphate. Neurofibromin functions as a tumor suppressor gene with respect to neurofibroma formation. Transformation to malignancy requires additional genetic changes, such as mutation of p53.

NF1 exhibits a wide range of variability of expression and complete penetrance. Mutations are widely scattered across the gene and include a wide variety of mutational mechanisms. Approximately 50% of cases of NF1 occur sporadically, as a result of a new mutation of the NF1 gene. Because of the high penetrance of the disorder, unaffected parents of a sporadically affected child have a low risk of recurrence, barring the rare instance of germline mosaicism. Somatic mosaicism

for NF1 may manifest with segmental distribution of features. Genetic testing for diagnosis of NF1 is available on a clinical basis. The discovery of mutation in the SPRED1 gene accounting for patients with multiple café-au-lait spots but lacking other features of NF1 (referred to as "Legius syndrome") and provides additional rationale for genetic testing in young children with multiple café-au-lait spots. The majority of mutations in children with multiple café-au-lait spots are found in the NF1 gene, making it cost-effective to begin with NF1 testing, followed by SPRED1 testing if no NF1 mutation is found.

Management

Treatment of patients with neurofibromatosis is symptomatic. Affected persons should be followed on a regular basis by a physician who is familiar with the disorder to recognize treatable complications early and to provide anticipatory guidance and counseling. Genetic counseling should be provided. Controversy surrounds the use of imaging, especially MRI, in screening patients with NF1. Most of the lesions that will be identified are not amenable to treatment, so such testing may create needless anxiety and risks associated with sedation. The value of the "baseline" examination is questionable because most of the lesions of NF1 are slow-growing and will be followed both clinically and by imaging once they come to attention. Current consensus guidelines do not recommend routine imaging, although care should be individualized for specific clinical needs (Gutmann et al., 1997).

Neurofibromas of the peripheral nerves need not be removed unless they are subject to repeated irritation and trauma or develop signs of malignant change. Some plexiform neuromas can be removed for cosmetic reasons, although complete resection is difficult and regrowth is common. Malignant tumors are managed with appropriate surgical measures and often radiation therapy and chemotherapy. Optic gliomas tend to behave in an indolent manner and therefore are followed clinically without treatment in asymptomatic children. Symptomatic tumors most often are treated with chemotherapy; radiation therapy may be associated with second malignant tumors or moyamoya disease. Malignant peripheral nerve sheath tumors tend to be highly malignant, so early diagnosis is essential. Patients with unexplained pain or growth of a neurofibroma should be evaluated, with consideration of biopsy. Positron emission tomography (PET) scanning may be helpful in distinguishing a malignant peripheral nerve sheath tumor from plexiform neurofibroma.

Clinical trials of drugs to treat specific complications are ongoing but no definitive medical therapy has been identified.

Neurofibromatosis Type 2

Clinical Characteristics and Pathology

Diagnostic criteria for NF2 are presented in Box 45-3. The defining feature of NF2 is the occurrence of bilateral vestibular schwannomas. Vestibular schwannomas commonly present with tinnitus and/or hearing loss, and may cause problems with balance. Audiology and auditory brainstem-evoked response testing can be helpful, but definitive diagnosis is based on MRI findings. Schwannomas can occur along any other cranial nerve, the fifth being most common after the eighth. Schwannomas also may occur along spinal nerves, with the potential for causing radiculopathy or cord compression, or along peripheral nerves. In some patients, a polyneuropathy develops as a result of Schwann cell proliferation around peripheral nerves. Dermal schwannomas appear as plaque-like lesions, often with associated hair growth. Café-au-lait macules may occur but are not a reliable indicator of NF2, unlike in NF1. Other central nervous system tumors associated with NF2 are meningiomas and ependymomas. Virtually the entire NF2 phenotype is characterized by proliferative lesions; the one exception is the occurrence of posterior subcapsular cataracts or cortical wedge opacities.

Genetics

NF2 is transmitted as an autosomal-dominant trait with complete penetrance and variable expression. Prevalence is estimated at approximately 1 in 60,000, and birth incidence at 1 in 30,000. Approximately half of cases occur sporadically as a result of new mutation. The NF2 gene was mapped to chromosome 22, and the responsible gene is variously referred to as schwannomin or merlin. Merlin is a cytoskeletal protein that appears to play a role in the control of cell growth in tissues. Schwannomas are clonal tumors, and the NF2 gene acts as a tumor suppressor in formation of these tumors, as well as other NF2-associated tumors. Genetic testing for NF2 is available for diagnostic purposes. Some genotype-phenotype

correlations have been identified; missense or splicing mutations tend to predict milder disease than do mutations that lead to protein truncation. Somatic mosaicism for NF2 mutation may produce localized disease or ameliorate disease severity.

Management

Patients benefit from multidisciplinary care at a center with experience in dealing with the varied manifestations of the disorder. Management of tumors associated with NF2 is primarily surgical. Timing of surgery and the decision to treat one or both vestibular tumors depends on tumor size, degree of hearing loss, and involvement of other cranial nerves or compression of the brainstem. Stereotactic radiosurgery is also used for the treatment of vestibular schwannomas, although there may be an increased risk of malignancy in residual tumor. Use of auditory brainstem implants can be helpful in some patients in restoring some hearing due to tumor progression or surgery.

Treatment with the vascular endothelial growth factor (VEGF) inhibitor bevacizumab have shown promising results in reduction in size of vestibular schwannomas and improvement of hearing. Meningiomas are less likely to respond to bevacizumab treatment. Reduction in tumor size in some patients and improvement in hearing has also been observed with lapatinib treatment.

Schwannomatosis

Schwannomatosis is a more recently recognized entity, characterized only by the occurrence of schwannomas on cranial and spinal nerves other than the vestibular nerve. It often presents with pain or nerve compression. Diagnostic criteria are provided in Box 45-4. Schwannomatosis is transmitted as a dominant trait with incomplete penetrance. About 10% of cases are familial; the remainder are sporadic, presumably due to new mutation or incomplete penetrance. The first gene found to be responsible for the disorder is SMARCB1 and encodes a protein component of a chromatin remodeling complex. It is located on chromosome 22 near the NF2 locus but is distinct from that locus. Although schwannomas are the hallmark feature, meningiomas may also occur in some families with SMARCB1 mutation. Mutation of SMARCB1 do not account for all cases of schwannomatosis. A second gene, LZTR1 has been found to account for some cases of schwannomatosis without germline SMARCB1 mutation. Schwannomas in schwannomatosis patients with germline mutation of either SMARCB1 or LZTR1 have, in addition, mutation of NF2 on the same copy of chromosome 22 and loss of NF2 and either SMARCB1 or LZTR1 on the other chromosome. Not all cases of schwannomatosis are associated with loss of heterozygosity on chromosome 22, indicating that still other genes are involved.

Treatment of schwannomatosis is surgicalt. There is one report of a favorable response to bevacizumab, though no additional studies of the use of this drug have been reported to date.

TUBEROUS SCLEROSIS COMPLEX (TSC)

Tuberous sclerosis complex is a disorder of autosomal-dominant inheritance that affects multiple organ systems, resulting in manifold clinical expressions. TSC is currently recognized as one of the most common single-gene disorders seen in children and adults, with an estimated incidence of 1 in 5800 live births. The first description of tuberous sclerosis complex was by von Recklinghausen, who described a newborn

---

BOX 45-4 Diagnostic Criteria for Schwannomatosis

MOLECULAR DIAGNOSIS:

Two or more pathologically proved schwannomas or meningiomas AND genetic studies of at least two tumors with loss of heterozygosity (LOH) for chromosome 22 and two different NF2 mutations; if there is a common SMARCB1 mutation, this defines SMARCB1-associated schwannomatosis

    Or

    One pathologically proved schwannoma or meningioma AND germline SMARCB1 pathogenic mutation

CLINICAL DIAGNOSIS:

* Two or more nonintradermal schwannomas, one with pathological confirmation, including no bilateral vestibular schwannoma by high-quality MRI (detailed study of internal auditory canal with slices no more than 3mm thick). Recognize that some mosaic NF2 patients will be included in this diagnosis at a young age and that some schwannomatosis patients have been reported to have unilateral vestibular schwannomas or multiple meningiomas.

    * One pathologically confirmed schwannoma or intracranial meningioma AND affected first-degree relative

    * Consider as possible diagnosis if there are two or more nonintradermal tumors but none has been pathologically proven to be a schwannoma; the occurrence of chronic pain in association with the tumor(s) increase the likelihood of schwannomatosis

    Patients with the following characteristics do not fulfill diagnosis for schwannomatosis:

* Germline pathogenic NF2 mutation

* Fulfill diagnostic criteria for NF2

* First-degree relative with NF2

* Schwannomas in previous field of radiation therapy only

(With permission from: Plotkin, et al., 2013. Update from the 2011 International Schwannomatosis Workshop: From genetics to diagnostic criteria.)

BOX 45-5 Diagnostic Criteria for Tuberous Sclerosis Complex

MAJOR FEATURES

- Hypomelanotic macules (≥3, at least 5-mm diameter)
- Angiofibromas (≥3) or fibrous cephalic plaque
- Ungual fibromas (≥2)
- Shagreen patch
- Multiple retinal hamartomas
- Cortical dysplasias*
- Subependymal nodules
- Subependymal giant cell astrocytoma
- Cardiac rhabdomyoma
- Lymphangioleiomyomatosis (LAM)[†]
- Angiomyolipomas (≥2)[†]

MINOR FEATURES

- "Confetti" skin lesions
- Dental enamel pits (>3)
- Intraoral fibromas (≥2)
- Retinal achromic patch
- Multiple renal cysts
- Nonrenal hamartomas

DIAGNOSTIC CERTAINTY CRITERIA

Definite TSC

- 2 major features or
- 1 major feature + 2 or more minor features
- Identification of a known pathogenic mutation in TSC1 or TSC2

Probable TSC

- 1 major feature *or*
- 2 or more minor features

*Includes tubers and cerebral white matter radial migration lines.
†A combination of the two major clinical features (LAM and angiomyolipomas) without other features does not meet criteria for a definite diagnosis.

(With permission from Northrup H, Krueger DA on behalf of the International Tuberous Sclerosis Complex Consensus Group. Tuberous Sclerosis Complex Diagnostic Criteria Update: Recommendations of the 2012 International Tuberous Sclerosis Complex Consensus Conference, Pediatr Neurol. 2013; 49(4): 243–254.)

---

who had died of respiratory distress and was found at postmortem examination to have multiple cardiac tumors and a "great number of cerebral scleroses." Bourneville usually is credited with the first detailed description of the cerebral manifestations of the disease, describing "sclérose tubéreuse," indicating the superficial resemblance of the lesions of a potato. He attached no significance to the facial skin rash of his first patient, calling it acne rosacea, but he and Brissard believed that the renal tumors and cerebral scleroses were associated findings. Facial angiofibromas, previously referred to as adenoma sebaceum, were independently described in several reports, but Vogt emphasized the association of adenoma sebaceum and the cerebral scleroses described by Bourneville. He also described a "classic" triad of clinical features comprising mental retardation, intractable epilepsy, and adenoma sebaceum, which is now known to be present in less than one-third of patients with TSC.

Clinical Characteristics

Diagnostic criteria are provided in Box 45-5. The clinical presentation of TSC depends on the age of the patient, the organs involved, and the severity of involvement. Of importance, both the brain and the skin have more than one major criterion for diagnosis; therefore a diagnosis of definite tuberous sclerosis complex can be based on skin findings alone, or on neuroimaging findings alone.

Epilepsy is the most common presenting symptom in tuberous sclerosis complex and also is the most common medical disorder. In up to 80% to 90% of persons with TSC, seizures will develop during their lifetime, with the onset most frequently in childhood. A majority of children with TSC have the onset of seizures during the first year of life, and approximately one-third develop infantile spasms. Almost all seizure types can be seen in persons with tuberous sclerosis complex, including tonic, clonic, tonic-clonic, atonic, myoclonic, atypical absence, partial, and complex partial. Only "pure" absence seizures are not observed.

Infantile spasms will develop in approximately one-third of children with TSC, although some reports suggest an incidence as high as 75%. TSC is thought to be the most common single cause of infantile spasms, and in some series, 25% of symptomatic infantile spasms are secondary to TSC. Partial complex seizures precede infantile spasms in approximately one-third of patients with tuberous sclerosis complex in whom infantile spasms develop. A strong association between the presence of infantile spasms in tuberous sclerosis complex and subsequent developmental impairment has been noted, although children with tuberous sclerosis complex and infantile spasms can have a normal cognitive outcome.

The electroencephalogram (EEG) in infantile spasms associated with TSC often demonstrates hypsarrhythmia or modified hypsarrhythmia. It is important to realize, however, that the EEG, although usually abnormal, frequently does not have the features of hypsarrhythmia; in some series, up to 70% of children with tuberous sclerosis complex and infantile spasms did not have the characteristics of hypsarrhythmia. Several reports have characterized the EEG patterns of persons with TSC and have found a high incidence of abnormalities, including diffuse slowing and epileptiform features.

TSC is associated with a wide range of cognitive and behavioral manifestations. Approximately one-half of persons with TSC have normal intelligence, whereas the other half have some degree of cognitive impairment, ranging from mild learning disabilities to severe mental retardation. A bimodal distribution of cognitive abilities is evident, with affected persons falling into a severely cognitively impaired group or a group with normal intelligence. Risk factors for cognitive impairment include a history of infantile spasms, intractable epilepsy, and a mutation in the TSC2 gene. Persons with TSC, particularly those with cognitive impairment, also are at high risk for developmental disorders. Autistic spectrum disorders affect up to 50% of persons with tuberous sclerosis complex, and attention-deficit hyperactivity and related disorders also are common, affecting approximately 50% of the patients. During adolescence and adulthood, anxiety disorders, depression, or mood disorders develop in a majority of patients with TSC.

Cutaneous manifestations are found in up to 96% of patients with TSC. Angiofibroma, the skin manifestation initially described in the disorder as adenoma sebaceum, typically appears between the ages of 1 and 4 years and can progress through childhood and adolescence. These lesions typically are pink or red papules that appear in patches or in a butterfly distribution on or about the nose, cheeks, and chin (Fig. 45-10).

Hypopigmented, oval, or leaf-shaped macules, ranging from a few millimeters to several centimeters in length and scattered over the trunk and limbs, are commonly seen. The lesions often are apparent at birth and can appear more prominent during the first several years of life. In fair-skinned persons, visualization of these hypopigmented spots is facilitated by using a Wood's light. At least three types of hypopigmented macules occur: polygonal (similar to a thumbprint) is the most frequent shape (0.5 to 2 cm); an ash leaf-shaped hypopigmented macule is characteristic but is not the most common shape (1 to 12 cm); and a confetti-shaped arrangement of multiple, tiny white macules (1 to 3 mm) (Fig. 45-11). Histologic assessment of the hypopigmented spots usually demonstrates a normal number of melanocytes, and on electron microscopy, a reduction in the number, diameter, and melanization of melanosomes in the melanocytes from the white macule is seen. If hypopigmented macules occur on the scalp, the affected person will have poliosis, or a patch of gray or white hair.

Another skin manifestation currently considered a major criterion for clinical diagnosis of TSC is the shagreen patch, a connective tissue hamartoma that is distributed asymmetrically on the dorsal body surfaces, particularly on the lumbosacral skin (Fig. 45-12). In a majority of the cases, the shagreen patch is characterized by multiple and small areas of connective tissue hamartoma, ranging in size from a few millimeters to 1 cm. Present from birth, the shagreen patch is more easily identified as the child grows. Subungual or periungual fibromas (Koenen tumors) are present in at least 20% of patients and usually first appear during adolescence, although they can be seen earlier. These typically involve the toes more often than the fingers (Fig. 45-13). Oral fibromas or papillomas occur in about 10% of patients and usually are found on the anterior aspect of the gingiva. Dental enamel pits have been found in all adult patients with TSC, compared with 7% of controls.

The kidneys are frequently affected in persons with TSC, and after neurologic manifestations, renal involvement is the most common cause of morbidity and mortality. The two main types of renal lesions are angiomyolipoma and renal cysts. Angiomyolipoma are present in up to 80% of patients with TSC and can develop in either childhood or adulthood. Persons with TSC can have multiple small angiomyolipomas on the surface of the kidneys, throughout the kidney, or one or more larger lesions. The larger lesions are considered to be at greater risk of becoming symptomatic, particularly when they reach 4 to 6 cm in size. They can produce nonspecific complaints such as flank pain, but they also carry a risk of potentially life-threatening hemorrhage from rupture of dysplastic, aneurysmal blood vessels in the angiomyolipoma. Renal cysts are seen in fewer than 20% of persons with tuberous sclerosis complex and are rarely, if ever, symptomatic. Polycystic kidney disease occurs in 3% to 5% of patients with tuberous sclerosis complex and, when present, usually reflects a contiguous gene syndrome, because the polycystic kidney disease gene is adjacent to the TSC2-tuberin gene on chromosome 16.

The cardiac manifestation, rhabdomyoma, is seen in 50% to 60% of persons with TSC. Typically, rhabdomyomas, which can frequently be detected prenatally, are maximal at birth and early childhood and undergo spontaneous regression during the first few years of life. If symptomatic, they result in outflow tract obstruction or valve dysfunction. If the lesions involve the cardiac conduction system, they can predispose the patient to dysrhythmias not only in infancy and childhood, but also throughout life.

Pulmonary involvement in includes lymphangioleiomyomatosis, multifocal micronodular pneumocyte hyperplasia, and pulmonary cysts. Although multifocal micronodular pneumocyte hyperplasia is seen fairly commonly in both men and women with tuberous sclerosis complex, lymphangioleiomyomatosis is thought to occur almost exclusively in women. Although lymphangioleiomyomatosis was once thought to be quite rare, affecting less than 1% of women, recent studies

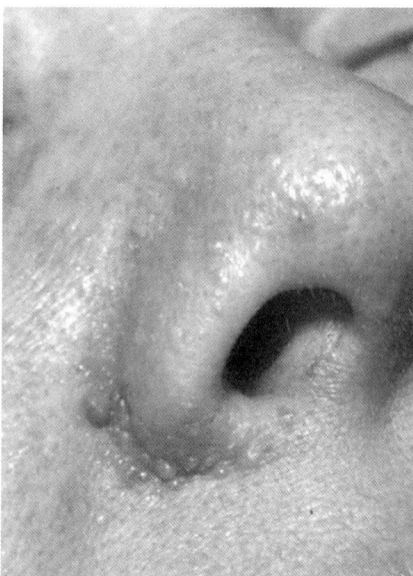

Figure 45-10. Typical angiofibroma in an adult with tuberous sclerosis complex. *(Courtesy of Dr. TN Darling, Uniformed Services University of Health Sciences, Bethesda, MD.)*

have found such abnormalities in up to 40% of women with, many of whom are asymptomatic.

Retinal hamartomas are relatively common, affecting at least 50% of patients, although typically they are not clinically significant. A nodular (mulberry) tumor can be seen on or about the optic nerve head, and round or oval gray-yellow glial patches can be central or peripheral. The large retinal tumors can be cystic. Papilledema is not present, except in those patients with an intracranial mass lesion that obstructs the normal circulation of the cerebrospinal fluid, resulting in increased intracranial pressure.

Hamartomas also can be found in other organ systems, including stomach, intestine, colon, pancreas, and liver. Hepatic angiomyolipoma and cysts have been reported in up to 24% of persons with and are thought to be asymptomatic and nonprogressive. Sclerotic and hypertrophic lesions of bone often can be seen, although these typically are not symptomatic.

Clinical Laboratory Testing

Due to multiorgan involvement in TSC, a variety of clinical testing is recommended both at time of diagnosis and subsequently, to monitor for involvement and allow appropriate intervention (Table 45-2).

MRI and also computed tomography (CT), are important in confirming the diagnosis of TSC, demonstrating cortical tubers, subependymal nodules (Fig. 45-14), and subependymal giant cell tumors (Fig. 45-15). Brain MRI is the preferred imaging modality, because it allows better delineation of cortical tubers and other cortical abnormalities, such as radial migration lines. The imaging characteristics of tubers change with age, related to myelination state. In neonates, tubers appear hyperintense on T1 sequences and hypointense on T2. With increasing age, tubers appear isointense on T1 and hyperintense on T2. In addition to T1-weighted and T2-weighted MRI sequences, fluid-attenuated inversion recovery (FLAIR) sequences appear most useful for identifying tubers and other cortical and subcortical abnormalities. Both CT and MRI can identify subependymal nodules; calcification of the nodules is apparent on CT scan. Development of subependymal nodules into subependymal giant cell tumors occurs in 5% to 10% of persons with TSC; yearly neuroimaging is until the age of 20 years.

Pathology

TSC is a multisystem disorder of cellular migration, proliferation, and differentiation, resulting in the development of hamartias and hamartomas. The major pathologic features in the brain include cortical tubers, subependymal nodules, and subependymal giant cell tumors. Cortical tubers are found in the cortex and subcortical white matter, typically located at the gray-white junction. They vary widely in size and distribution among patients with TSC and may extend centrally in a linear or wedge-shaped zone spanning the full thickness from the ventricular wall to the cortical surface. Histologically, tubers consist of dysplastic, hypomyelinated aggregates of abnormal glial and neural elements, with glia-derived cells and astrocytes predominating. A distinguishing feature of cortical tubers is the giant cell, an enlarged, bizarre-appearing neuron or large cells with both neuronal and glial characteristics. Many children with TSC may experience learning difficulties, as a result of mental retardation or autistic spectrum disorders. Risk factors include early seizure onset, infantile spasms, and an intractable seizure disorder. Correlation between the severity of cognitive deficits and epilepsy with tuber burden is thought

probable, although the data are limited. Distinct from cortical tubers, subependymal nodules do have growth potential and are located around the wall of the lateral ventricle, consisting of astrocytes arising from the subependymal zone and protruding into the ventricles. Subependymal nodules most commonly occur at the caudothalamic groove in the vicinity of the foramen of Monro, and it is thought that they arise from remnants of the germinal matrix in that region.

Genetics

TSC is transmitted as an autosomal-dominant trait with variable penetrance and an estimated incidence of 1 in 5800 live births worldwide. Wide phenotypic variability of clinical manifestations and severity has been noted, even within families having the same mutation. Currently, no known effect of paternal or maternal age or of birth order on disease phenotype has been recognized. Approximately two-thirds of cases are sporadic and the result of apparent spontaneous mutations. Both somatic and germline mosaicism have been described in many patients.

Two genes, TSC1 and TSC2, have been identified for tuberous sclerosis complex. A disease causing mutation in one of these two genes can be identified in approximately 85% of persons with definite tuberous sclerosis complex according to current criteria. TSC1 located at 9q34; it was cloned in 1997, and the protein product, hamartin, was identified and characterized. The TSC2 gene is located on 16p13 and encodes a protein referred to as tuberin.

Tuberin and hamartin interact with one another and function as tumor suppressor molecules. Loss of heterozygosity has been identified in hamartomas from persons with TSC1 and TSC2 mutations, particularly in kidney and lung tissue, but less commonly in cortical tubers or subependymal giant cell astrocytomas. Tuberin has GTPase-activating properties, similar to the NF1 protein product. Hamartin and tuberin are components of the mammalian target of rapamycin (mTOR) pathway, which is involved in many functions, including regulation of cell size. In vivo, it appears that tuberin can be phosphorylated by Akt, at least in part regulating its activity. In normal cells, the tuberin/hamartin complex acts as an inhibitor of mTOR activity. On growth factor stimulation or other stimuli, tuberin is phosphorylated by Akt, which leads to the inactivation of inhibitory activity of TSC1/TSC2 and resultant cell growth. In cells containing mutations affecting the function of hamartin or tuberin, mTOR and S6 kinase activities are significantly increased, and cell growth is no longer regulated by the PI3-kinase-TSC1/TSC2 signaling pathway, which is thought to lead to the development of hamartoma.

Management

TSC affects most organ systems, and management and treatment recommendations vary according to organ manifestations (Table 45-2). Affected persons, both children and adults, should be managed with regular follow-up evaluations by a physician who is familiar with tuberous sclerosis complex, to recognize treatable manifestations early and to provide anticipatory guidance and counseling.

With regard to neurologic manifestations, management focuses on treatment of epilepsy and behavioral disorders and on identification of learning disabilities. Treatment of epilepsy in TSC is similar to that for partial epilepsies resulting from other causes and includes antiepileptic medications, the vagus nerve stimulator, and the ketogenic diet. Vigabatrin is particularly effective in treating infantile spasms in patients with tuberous sclerosis complex. Epilepsy surgery has a very important role in the management of patients who have pharmacoresistant epilepsy.

Rapamycin, an mTOR antagonist, has been shown to reduce the size of subependymal giant cell tumors and renal angiomyolipoma in tuberous sclerosis complex and may also reduce the progression of pulmonary lymphangioleiomyomatosis. In animal models of TSC, rapamycin has also been shown to prevent epilepsy if given prenatally and to improve cognitive deficits. Ongoing multicenter trials are evaluating the role of rapamycin and other mTOR antagonists in the management of TSC. One rapamycin-like drug, everolimus, is FDA approved for treatment of progressive subependyal giant cell astrocytoma or renal angiomyolipoma.

VON HIPPEL-LINDAU DISEASE (VHL)

Von Hippel-Lindau disease is inherited as an autosomal-dominant trait and is characterized by retinal, cerebellar, and spinal hemangioblastomas, cystic tumors of the pancreas, kidney, and epididymis, renal cell carcinoma, endolymphatic sac tumors, and, in some families, pheochromocytoma (Maher et al., 2011).

Clinical Characteristics

Retinal hemangioblastoma is one of the earliest manifestations of the disease. The early retinal lesion has the appearance of an aneurysmal dilatation of a peripheral retinal vessel; typically, tortuous vessels later manifest, with an arteriovenous pair leading to small, elevated retinal lesions. These lesions commonly are located in the retinal periphery and can easily be overlooked unless careful ophthalmoscopy is performed. Fluorescein angiography is helpful in demonstrating the lesion.

Although they usually affect the cerebellum, central nervous system hemangioblastomas sometimes are found in the medulla and spinal cord; they rarely occur in the cerebral hemispheres. The tumor usually is found in patients after the third decade of life but has been reported to occur rarely in children; initial symptoms and signs are those of a space-occupying lesion of the posterior fossa.

A variety of renal lesions has been found in VHL, including benign cysts, hemangiomas, adenomas, and malignant hypernephromas. Cystic lesions vary in size, ranging from a few millimeters to several centimeters across, and, although they can occur unilaterally, these lesions are more often bilateral and multiple. Renal cell carcinoma is a prominent cause of morbidity and mortality, occurring with a frequency next to that of the retinal and cerebellar hemangioblastoma.

Cystic lesions can also occur in the pancreas, adrenal gland, and epididymis. Other organs less commonly affected with cystic changes include the liver, spleen, and lung. Endolymphatic sac tumors associated with VHL can cause hearing loss. Pheochromocytomas occur more often in patients with von VHL than in the general population and tend to cluster in certain families.

The retinal hemangioblastoma diagnosis usually is established by careful ophthalmoscopy with fluorescein retinal angiography, revealing the vascular characteristics of the lesions. Cranial MRI scans demonstrate the cerebellar hemangioblastoma or those tumors affecting the medulla and spinal cord. Intraabdominal cystic lesions can be visualized by CT, MRI, or ultrasonography. Other laboratory studies that can assist in diagnosis include erythrocyte count and hematocrit determination, which can be elevated in patients with cerebellar hemangioblastoma or renal carcinoma because of the increased erythropoietin activity of the cyst fluid.

Pathology

The tumors usually are well circumscribed, can be solid or cystic, and usually are found in the paramedial aspect of the cerebellar cortex. Characteristic microscopic features include large numbers of thin-walled, closely packed blood vessels lined by plump endothelial cells; the cells are separated by large, pale cells and incorporated in the elaborate network of reticulin fibers.

Genetics

VHL disease is inherited as an autosomal-dominant trait. The birth incidence is about 1 in 36,000 persons, and point prevalence has been estimated at 1 in 91,000. Penetrance is nearly complete on careful evaluation. The gene is located on 3p25–26, and encodes a protein that regulates a cellular system that senses and responds to hypoxia. The VHL gene functions as a tumor suppressor; hence, homozygous mutation occurs in tumors, leading to loss of function and constitutive activation of the hypoxia-sensing pathway. Genetic testing is available and has revealed that specific mutations tend to be found in families with von Hippel-Lindau disease associated with pheochromocytoma. VHL disease has been subdivided into type 1, in which all of the manifestations may be present except for pheochromocytoma, and type 2, which includes the full set of features. Type 2 is further divided into 2A (pheochromocytoma and other manifestations, but not renal cell carcinoma), 2B (all features), and 2C (isolated pheochromocytoma).

Management

Affected individuals should be provided a program of surveillance to insure early recognition of treatable complications. Recommendations of the VHL Family Alliance are provided in Table 45-3. Retinal hemangioblastomas should be carefully followed by serial ophthalmologic evaluations when the lesions are small. If, however, visual loss or retinal detachment occurs, the lesions can be treated by either laser photocoagulation or cryocoagulation. Central nervous systems lesions are usually treated surgically or with stereotactic radiation therapy. Medical therapy for the various complications of VHL is currently under investigation.

STURGE-WEBER SYNDROME (ENCEPHALOFACIAL ANGIOMATOSIS) (SWS)

Sturge-Weber syndrome is characterized by presence of a facial angioma (port-wine stain, or nevus flammeus) and an ipsilateral leptomeningeal angioma; it has an incidence currently estimated at 1 case in 20,000 to 50,000 persons. Schirmer initially described a patient with a facial vascular nevus who had associated buphthalmos, but he did not mention the central nervous system lesion. Sturge initially described this syndrome by providing the clinical findings of a 6-year-old girl with a facial nevus who also had angiomas of the lips, gingiva, palate, floor of the mouth, uvula, and pharynx. The child had buphthalmos and was hemiparetic, and Sturge suggested that she had a similar vascular nevus of the underlying brain. Not until 1897, however, did Kalischer perform the first neuropathologic study of a patient with similar findings, demonstrating that Sturge's initial contention of cerebral involvement by vascular nevus was correct. Associated intracranial calcification was later described by Weber.

Clinical Characteristics

SWS, which occurs sporadically, is characterized by angiomas involving the leptomeninges and ipsilateral skin of the face, typically in the ophthalmic (V1) and maxillary (V2) distributions of the trigeminal nerve. It can extend to other facial areas, including the lips, gingiva, palate, tongue, pharynx, and larynx. The neck, trunk, and extremities also can be involved, either ipsilaterally or contralaterally to the facial angioma. The angioma also can involve the nasopharynx, mucous membrane, and ocular choroidal membrane, resulting in glaucoma in approximately 25% of patients (Fig. 45-17). Additional ocular findings include iridic heterochromia, strabismus, optic atrophy, and dilated retinal veins. In the brain, the associated ipsilateral leptomeningeal angioma most commonly involves the parietal and occipital regions, but also may involve the temporal region and, on occasion, can affect both hemispheres. Dimitri reported that these patients had intracranial calcifications observed on the skull radiographs and described the typical serpentine "tram-track sign" of calcific intracranial densities.

Neurologic manifestations vary and depend on location and extent of the leptomeningeal angioma. Seizures occur in 75% to 90% of patients with SWS and may be refractory to treatment. It is hypothesized that the seizure activity results from cortical irritability caused by the leptomeningeal angioma, resulting in regional hypoxia, ischemia, and gliosis, although associated cortical dysgenesis also may be involved. Seizure manifestations are primarily partial motor (40%), although some patients can have primary or secondary generalized tonic-clonic (20%) and both partial and generalized seizures (40%). Other types of seizure activity occur less frequently. Unfortunately, refractory epilepsy develops in a significant number of patients with Sturge-Weber syndrome, ranging in series from 11% to 83%. Surgical procedures, including focal cortical resection, hemispherectomy, and corpus callosotomy, should be considered if seizure activity proves medically intractable.

Persons with SWS also are at risk for hemiparesis contralateral to the leptomeningeal angioma, seen in approximately 33% of patients. The hemiparesis can result from ischemia with venous occlusion and thrombosis due in part to venous congestion resulting from failure of cortical vein development. Transient weakness also may result from seizure activity and may become more severe and less transient with recurrent seizure activity. Leptomeningeal venous angiomas can arise in the absence of any facial angioma; although secondary cerebral signs and symptoms similar to those of SWS can occur, these patients are more appropriately considered to have leptomeningeal angiomatosis.

Persons with SWS also are at risk for developmental delay and mental retardation (50% to 60%) and are more likely in those with bilateral leptomeningeal involvement and in those with a history of seizures. Headaches also are common, occurring in up to 60% of affected persons, and are thought to be secondary to the vascular abnormalities, giving symptoms consistent with migraine. EEG studies document decreased amplitude and frequency of electrocerebral activity over the affected hemisphere. Diffuse, multiple, and independent spike foci commonly are present.

Hemianopsia in young patients also is difficult to determine but is believed to occur in about one-quarter to one-half of patients. About one-third of patients have glaucoma, and approximately half of these have buphthalmos ipsilateral to the facial angioma. Glaucoma can be unilateral or bilateral, regardless of whether the facial angioma is bilateral.

Intracranial calcification is evident on radiographs in 90% of adult patients. Calcifications uncommonly are present at birth but are manifest in virtually all patients by the end of the second decade of life. The intracranial calcifications typically assume a linear, parallel configuration ("tram-track sign"), or a convolutional pattern most commonly seen in the parietal or parietooccipital regions (Fig. 45-18). Cranial CT and MRI scans are complementary in evaluating the cerebral changes of SWS, in that the MRI demonstrates thickened cortex, decreased convolutions, and abnormal white matter, whereas cranial CT scans demonstrate more definitively the characteristic calcification. Cranial MRI scans (T2-weighted images) reveal smaller, nonspecific foci of hypointense signal. Gadolinium enhancement may reveal pial angioma, thereby allowing early diagnosis of SWS before calcification.

Cerebral angiography discloses decreased cerebral venous drainage with dilatation of the deep cerebral veins. Various other vascular abnormalities have been demonstrated in approximately one-third of patients and include thrombotic lesions, dural venous sinus abnormalities, and arteriovenous malformations. PET provides a sensitive measure of the extent of cerebral metabolic impairment. Serial PET scans in children with SWS can be useful and, when used with other neuroimaging studies, document the progression of the disease.

Pathology

SWS is thought to be caused by the presence of residual embryonal blood vessels and their secondary effects on surrounding tissues. During development, a vascular plexus develops around the cephalic portion of the neural tube, under the ectoderm that subsequently becomes facial skin. This plexus forms during the sixth week of gestation and regresses at approximately the ninth week. It is thought that failure of this regression results in residual vascular tissue, subsequently forming the angiomata of the leptomeninges, face, and ipsilateral eye. Neuropathologic studies have demonstrated thickened, hypervascularized leptomeninges that involve the occipital, parietal, or temporoparietal region primarily (Fig. 45-19). These meningeal vessels generally are small and tortuous and rarely enter the underlying brain substance. Calcific deposits are present in the walls of some small cerebral vessels but more commonly are found in the outer pyramidal and molecular cortical layers. Biochemical assays have demonstrated increased calcium content of the gray and white matter, with normal iron content. The pathophysiology of the deposition of intracerebral calcium is not well understood.

Management

Treatment for the neurologic manifestations of SWS includes management of seizure activity and headaches. Approximately 50% of children with seizures achieve control with administration of appropriate antiepileptic drugs. Those patients with seizure disorders refractory to medical treatment should be carefully considered for epilepsy surgery with resection of the affected lobe(s) or hemispherectomy. Rochkind and colleagues reported that seizure control after surgery was better in those patients who received antiepileptic drugs. Aspirin therapy may reduce the incidence of strokelike episodes and is typically used in individuals with either recurrent vascular events or progressive neurologic deficits. Treatment options for the facial angioma include laser therapy using various pulsed-dye lasers, as well as pulsed-light sources, and other laser therapies. The current recommendation is to begin treatment as early as possible; infants have received treatment during the first week of life. Treatment of glaucoma, if present, consists of control of intraocular pressure, to prevent optic nerve injury, by medical or surgical intervention. The management of patients with SWS requires the skill of an attentive physician, psychologist, and social worker.

MAFFUCCI SYNDROME

Maffucci syndrome is a rare congenital disease characterized by multiple enchondromas with secondary hemangiomas, phlebolithiasis, and malformations of bone. Occasionally, associated skin changes, including patches of vitiligo, café-au-lait spots, and other hyperpigmented patches and nevi, are seen. A related disorder, Ollier disease, is characterized by multiple endochondromas without hemangiomas. Both are sporadic and have been found to be due to somatic mosaicism of IDH1 or IDH2 genes. No single treatment plan exists, because each patient must be individually managed.

EPIDERMAL NEVUS SYNDROME

Epidermal nevus syndrome is a heterogeneous group of disorders characterized by patchy cutaneous hamartomatous lesions, central nervous system abnormalities, and various other manifestations (Table 45-4) (Happle, 2010a; Happle, 2010b). Most of these disorders occur sporadically and are highly variable in their presentation. Central nervous system manifestations include unilateral lissencephaly, a paucity of white matter, excessive and heterotopic gray matter, apparent schizencephaly, unilateral colpocephaly, and hemimegalencephaly. Associated neurologic abnormalities include intellectual disability and convulsive disorders. Cortical resection has been helpful in some instances, but no other definitive treatment exists.

The patchy manifestations of these disorders have suggested the possibility that they result from somatic mosaicism; this has been demonstrated in some instances of PTEN hamartoma syndrome, in which mosaicism for PTEN has been found. In the past, these patients were erroneously described as having Proteus syndrome, but it is now known that Proteus syndrome results from mosaic mutations in AKT1.

PARRY-ROMBERG SYNDROME (FACIAL HEMIATROPHY)

Parry-Romberg syndrome, which typically has onset between 5 and 15 years of age, is characterized by a progressive ipsilateral loss of facial soft tissue, cartilage, and bone. This tissue loss usually involves the tissues between the nose and nasolabial fold or above the maxilla, but progresses to affect most of the ipsilateral face during the ensuing years. The tongue, the gums, and the soft palate may also become involved. The eyelashes, eyebrows, and hair on the involved side can be affected, and ipsilateral blanching of the hair or alopecia can occur. Progression of this atrophic process generally lasts between 2 and 10 years and is believed to cease by the end of the second or beginning of the third decade of life. In addition to atrophy of the facial tissues, various other neurologic deficits have been reported, including recurrent headaches, trigeminal neuralgia, ipsilateral Horner syndrome, contralateral partial seizures, and hemiparesis. Moreover, an unusual association of the syndrome with multiple benign tumors has been described. Scleroderma and lipodystrophy must be clinically differentiated from this disease. Cranial imaging can be normal or document cerebral atrophy, encephalomalacia, and abnormal T2 signal intensities. No typical or consistent neuropathologic findings have been reported. No specific treatment for the syndrome exists; however, various reconstructive surgical procedures, often using grafts of autogenous fat after

disease stabilizes, can result in reasonably good cosmetic results.

NEUROCUTANEOUS MELANOSIS

Neurocutaneous melanosis is a rare, nonfamilial, embryonic, neuroectodermal dysplasia characterized by abnormally pigmented cutaneous areas (e.g., giant hairy pigmented nevi, multiple hyperpigmented cutaneous nevi, large congenital melanocytic nevi) and leptomeningeal melanosis (Gerami and Paller, 2013). Diagnosis is usually made in infants and children younger than 2 years of age; however, the condition is present at birth. No gender predilection exists. All patients have areas of abnormal skin hyperpigmentation, the most common pattern of which is multiple giant hairy pigmented nevi. Giant hairy nevi usually have a "bathing suit" or cape-shaped distribution. The presence of multiple satellite lesions, large size, and midline location for pigmented lesions are predictive of neurologic involvement. Mosaicism for specific mutations in the NRAS oncogene have been identified as the underlying cause of this disorder. This suggests the possible use of drugs that block RAS signaling in therapy.

The clinical presentation of neurocutaneous melanosis depends on the location and extent of involvement of this leptomeningeal lesion. Hydrocephalus is commonly encountered because of cerebrospinal fluid pathway obstruction in the basilar cisterns, the arachnoid villi over the cerebral hemispheric convexities, or both, and intraspinal melanotic arachnoid cyst, lipoma, and intraspinal lipoma have been described as obstructed. Association with Dandy-Walker malformation has been reported. Behavioral abnormalities and recurring seizures can occur, as well as cranial nerve dysfunction and signs of spinal cord and root involvement. Attempts to treat hydrocephalus by a shunting procedure are palliative. There is a risk of melanoma.

KLIPPEL-TRÉNAUNAY-WEBER SYNDROME (KTW)

Klippel-Trénaunay-Weber syndrome initially was believed to be characterized only by cutaneous and/or subcutaneous hemangiomas, varicosities, and hypertrophy of the soft tissues and bone of a limb. Additional associated anomalies later recognized included macrocephaly; hydrocephalus; lymphangiomas; hemangiomas of the trunk, intestine, and bladder; and abnormalities of the digits. KTW usually occurs sporadically. Another disorder associated with vascular malformations as well as skeletal anomalies, lipomatous overgrowth, and epidermal nevi, referred to as CLOVES syndrome, is associated with mosaic PIK3CA mutations.

Limb hypertrophy usually is apparent at birth. Lymphedema can be present. An inordinately progressive growth of the affected body part eventually occurs, leading to the development of various other abnormalities. Abnormal growth of one leg, for example, can result in a pelvic tilt and scoliosis, but the patient's overall height is not significantly changed. The legs are affected more commonly than the arms. Additional abnormalities include megalocornea, glaucoma, iridic heterochromia, syndactyly, polydactyly, macrodactyly, and clinodactyly. Hemangiomas of the tongue, pharynx, larynx, and bladder have been described, and labial and scrotal lesions are common. Macrocephaly often is present, and seizures and mental retardation have been reported.

Any treatment plan for these patients must be individualized and requires a multidisciplinary team. Nonsurgical management involves compression of the involved limb. MRI or CT venography can be performed if any vascular surgical procedure is contemplated. Some vascular lesions can be treated with cryotherapy, laser therapy, or sclerotherapy, whereas others can be surgically removed. An osteotomy or epiphyseal stapling procedure can occasionally benefit patients with limb hypertrophy, but limb amputations may be required in others.

INCONTINENTIA PIGMENTI (BLOCH-SULZBERGER SYNDROME)

Incontinentia pigmenti is transmitted as an X-linked dominant trait, predominantly affecting females. Most hemizygous males apparently die in utero. The gene responsible for disorder is IKBKG/NEMO, which regulates nuclear factor kappa b signaling. Most mutations lead to loss of function with the most common, accounting for 78% of cases, an intragenic deletion involving exons 4 to 10. The syndrome is characterized by various hyperpigmented skin lesions that can be apparent at birth and by commonly associated abnormalities involving the central nervous system, eyes, hair, teeth, and bone (Minić et al., 2014).

The skin manifestations have been described as having three stages. The first stage typically is characterized by vesiculobullous lesions present at birth or during the first several weeks of life. These lesions appear in groups or in a linear distribution over the trunk and limbs, following the lines of Blaschko. A preponderance of eosinophils is found in the vesicular fluid, and the peripheral blood also can exhibit an eosinophilia. The lesions rupture, resulting in oozing and crusting, and can persist for months. The second stage is characterized by evolution into verrucous lesions beginning after the sixth week of life. The third stage typically is characterized by hyperpigmented brown or gray-brown macular lesions that follow the lines of Blaschko. These pigmented skin lesions usually become more prominent during the first few years of life and then gradually fade. The decrease of abnormal pigmentation may continue throughout adolescence, and in some patients the pigmentation can completely disappear.

One-third to one-half of patients have symptoms and signs of neurologic abnormalities manifested by developmental disability, corticospinal tract dysfunction, and seizures. Microcephaly and hydrocephaly may occur. Approximately one-third of patients have ocular abnormalities, including optic atrophy, papillitis, abnormal retinal pigmentation, nystagmus, strabismus, and cataracts. Visual loss occurs in about 8% of patients. The most common ocular abnormalities are retinal detachment and a fibrovascular retrolental membrane.

There are often associated ectodermal and skeletal anomalies. Skin changes include atrophic scarring and alopecia, and nails can be flat and thin, commonly with transverse ridges. Skeletal abnormalities include spina bifida, hemivertebrae, accessory ribs, and syndactyly. Delayed dentition, pegged teeth, and abnormal crown formation are also seen. Treatment remains symptomatic and supportive.

INCONTINENTIA PIGMENTI ACHROMIANS (HYPOMELANOSIS OF ITO)

Incontinentia pigmenti achromians has been known as systemic achromic nevus and hypomelanosis of Ito (Pavone et al., 2015). Typical skin changes occur as hypopigmented lesions on any part of the head, trunk, or limbs, either unilaterally or bilaterally. The configuration of the hypopigmented lesions may manifest as linear streaks or whorls of hypopigmentation that follow the lines of Blaschko. The skin lesions are congenital. Multiple associated anomalies are common and can involve the central nervous system or the peripheral

nervous system, eyes, and bone. Common central nervous system abnormalities include mental retardation, language disabilities, seizures, and motor system dysfunction. Ocular abnormalities include strabismus, epicanthic folds, myopia, optic nerve hypoplasia, and hypopigmentation of the fundus; rarely, corneal asymmetry, pannus, and atrophic irides with irregular pupillary margins have been reported. Cataracts and retinal detachments also have been reported.

Characteristic histologic features of skin biopsy specimens include dyskeratosis, increased dermal mastocytes, and pilosebaceous abnormalities.

Hypomelanosis of Ito occurs sporadically and in many cases has been found to be associated with mosaicism for chromosomal abnormalities. The abnormal cells may be confined to the skin lesions and therefore are detected only by cytogenetic analysis of cultured fibroblasts obtained by skin biopsy. No single chromosome abnormality accounts for all cases; rather, it appears that the streaky hypopigmentation associated with the disorder, or sometimes patches of hyperpigmentation following Blaschko's lines, are the cutaneous manifestation of mosaicism for various genes or chromosomal regions.

WYBURN-MASON SYNDROME (RETINOCEPHALIC ANGIOMATOSIS)

Although known as Bonnet-Dechaum-Blanc syndrome in Europe and as Wyburn-Mason syndrome in the United Kingdom and the United States, the condition is more appropriately called a retinocephalic vascular malformation (Fileta et al., 2014). The syndrome is thought to result from an embryonic abnormality in the development of the optic nerve pathway and related vessels from its origin in the mesencephalon all the way to the projection to the retina.

The intracranial vascular malformation usually is deep within the brain substance and can involve the mesencephalon, diencephalon, and basal ganglia, extending to the visual pathways and chiasm. Variable involvement of the cranial nerves occurs, including the third, sixth, seventh, and eighth nerves; nystagmus and Parinaud syndrome have been reported. Corticospinal tract dysfunction can be unilateral or bilateral, and some patients are ataxic. Approximately one-half of patients have vascular malformations that affect the palate, oral mucosa, maxilla, and mandible. Cutaneous lesions also can occur, manifesting as angiomas or punctate erythematous lesions.

The diagnosis of this syndrome is initially considered when the retinal vascular lesion is observed. Cranial CT and MRI scans clearly demonstrate arteriovenous malformation, but only cerebral angiography reliably delineates the extent of the lesion. No beneficial treatment method is currently available for this syndrome. The surgical removal of part or all of the extensive vascular malformation cannot be performed with any practical success, and the use of rigorous radiologic interventional techniques has been unsuccessful.

REFERENCES

The complete list of references for this chapter is available online at www.expertconsult.com.
See inside cover for registration details.

SELECTED REFERENCES

Ferner, R.E., Gutmann, D.H., 2013. Neurofibromatosis type 1 (NF1): diagnosis and management. Handb. Clin. Neurol. 115, 939–955.
Fileta, J.B., Bennett, T.J., Quillen, D.A., 2014. Wyburn-Mason syndrome. JAMA Ophthalmol 132 (7), 805.

Gerami, P., Paller, A.S., 2013. Making a mountain out of a molehill: NRAS, mosaicism, and large congenital nevi. J. Invest. Dermatol. 133 (9), 2127–2130.
Gutmann, D.H., Aylsworth, A., Carey, J.C., et al., 1997. The diagnostic evaluation and multidisciplinary management of neurofibromatosis 1 and neurofibromatosis 2. JAMA 278 (9207339), 51–57.
Happle, R., 2010a. The group of epidermal nevus syndromes Part I. Well defined phenotypes. J. Am. Acad. Dermatol. 63 (1), 1–22, quiz, 23–24.
Happle, R., 2010b. The group of epidermal nevus syndromes Part II. Less well defined phenotypes. J. Am. Acad. Dermatol. 63 (1), 25–30, quiz, 31–32.
Lloyd, S.K.W., Evans, D.G.R., 2013. Neurofibromatosis type 2 (NF2): diagnosis and management. Handb. Clin. Neurol. 115, 957–967.
Maher, E.R., Neumann, H.P., Richard, S., 2011. Von Hippel-Lindau disease: a clinical and scientific review. Eur. J. Hum. Genet. 19, 617–623.
Minić, S., Trpinac, D., Obradović, M., 2014. Incontinentia pigmenti diagnostic criteria update. Clin. Genet. 85 (6), 536–542.
Pavone, P., Praticò, A.D., Ruggieri, M., et al., 2015. Hypomelanosis of Ito: a round on the frequency and type of epileptic complications. Neurol. Sci. 36 (7), 1–8.
Plotkin, S.R., Blakeley, J.O., Evans, D.G., et al. 2013. Update from the 2011 International Schwannomatosis Workshop: From genetics to diagnostic criteria.
Renard, D., Campello, C., Taieb, G., et al., 2013. Neurologic and vascular abnormalities in Klippel-Trénaunay-Weber syndrome. JAMA Neurol 70 (1), 127–128.

E-BOOK FIGURES AND TABLES

The following figures and tables are available in the e-book at www.expertconsult.com. See inside cover for registration details.

46

Disorders of Vitamin Metabolism

Barbara Plecko and Robert Steinfeld

✍ An expanded version of this chapter is available on www.expertconsult.com. See inside cover for registration details.

Vitamins are essential nutritional compounds and work as cofactors of various enzymes. Vitamin deficiency disorders are seen in developing countries and in patients with chronic disease and can affect the central and/or peripheral nervous system, often in the context of a multisystem disease (Kumar, 2010). The vitamin supply of breastfed infants is directly related to maternal nutrition. Hypervitaminoses are seen in faddists and in cases of long-term overdose of vitamin supplements. Nutritional sources, cofactor function, age-dependent daily allowances, signs of deficiency, dosages for treatment of respective vitamin deficiencies, and signs of hypervitaminosis are given in Table 46-1.

In addition to nutritional disorders of vitamin metabolism, there is a growing number of inherited inborn errors of metabolism (IEMs) that affect specific steps of vitamin transport and processing or lead to selective vitamin inactivation. Rapid recognition and treatment of the underlying cause are warranted to avoid irreversible damage.

THIAMINE (VITAMIN B₁)

Thiamine is absorbed in the upper small intestine and is transported across cell membranes by two transporters, encoded by *SLC19A2* and *SLC19A3*. Within the cell, thiamine is phosphorylated to its active form, thiamine pyrophosphate (TPP), and works as a cofactor of the cytosolic transketolase. Another solute carrier, encoded by *SLC25A19*, imports TPP into mitochondria, where it finally acts as a cofactor of the pyruvate dehydrogenase complex, the branched chain keto-thiolase dehydrogenase, and the alpha-ketoglutarate dehydrogenase. Two diseases are linked to vitamin B₁ deficiency: beriberi and the more severe Wernicke's syndrome. Wernicke's disease is still one of the more frequently encountered vitamin deficiency syndromes, and in developed countries, it occurs in patients with severe chronic disorders, malnutrition, or chronic alcohol abuse. In infancy, thiamine deficiency has been reported with breastfeeding by thiamine-deficient mothers and in infants fed with soybean or other formulas in which the thiamine was presumably heat-inactivated during preparation. Infantile thiamine deficiency is characterized by a multisystem presentation, with vomiting, aphonia, abdominal distention, diarrhea, cyanosis, tachycardia, and convulsions. In less fulminant cases, infants have failure to thrive and developmental delay followed by edema, oliguria, constipation, cardiomegaly, and hepatomegaly. Cranial imaging may show signal hyperintensities in T2-weighted images localized in the periventricular gray matter around the third ventricle, sylvian aqueduct, fourth ventricle, and mammillary bodies.

Increased lactate in plasma or cerebrospinal fluid (CSF) and urinary excretion of less than 120 mg of thiamine per gram of creatinine would support the diagnosis. Clinical response to the administration of thiamine is the best confirmatory test. Oral administration of 10 to 50 mg of thiamine daily will reverse clinical symptoms in a few weeks. Serious life-threatening neurologic manifestations or congestive heart failure should be treated with the parenteral administration of 5 to 20 mg of thiamine and may lead to severe long-term sequelae.

Genetic disorders affecting thiamine transport or activation present with surprisingly divergent symptoms and variable age (Brown, 2014).

Rogers Syndrome

Rogers syndrome (Online Inheritance in Man [OMIM] 249270) is caused by autosomal-recessive mutations in the *SLC19A2* transporter and manifests with thiamine-responsive megaloblastic anemia, type 2 diabetes mellitus, and sensorineural deafness. Thiamine levels in plasma are normal, but the presence of sideroblasts in bone marrow suggests the diagnosis. Treatment consists of 25 to 75 mg of oral thiamine per day. Although most manifestations are thiamine responsive, hearing loss may be irreversible.

Biotin- or Thiamine Responsive Basal Ganglia Disease

Biotin- or thiamine-responsive basal ganglia disease (BTBGD; OMIM 607483) is a panethnic, autosomal-recessive disease that is triggered by febrile infections, stress, or trauma. The typical onset is during early childhood, but onset can range from the neonatal period to adulthood. Major symptoms are subacute-onset encephalopathy, confusion, dystonia, ataxia, dysarthria, dysphagia, pyramidal tract signs, external ophthalmoplegia, and partial or generalized seizures. Episodes are followed by slow subtotal recovery and subsequent relapses. If left untreated the disease can lead to coma and, ultimately, death. T2-weighted magnetic resonance imaging (MRI) reveals bilateral signal intensities of the striatum in addition to cortical and subcortical lesions. Chronic changes include atrophy, necrosis, and gliosis (Ortigoza-Escobar et al.., 2014).

BTBGD is caused by mutations in the *SLC19A3* gene, which encodes a thiamine transporter, and a rapidly growing phenotypic spectrum—from neonatal encephalopathy with lactic acidosis to seizures with generalized dystonia—has been described. The partial response to biotin is not fully understood to date. Routine metabolic testing is normal, with the exception of elevated lactic acid during the acute phase, but measurement of free thiamine in CSF may become a valuable diagnostic screening tool. Confirmation is by genetic analysis of the *SLC19A3* gene. Treatment consists of regular oral supplementation of thiamine, 300 to 900 mg/day. During subsequent exacerbation the usual thiamine dose may be doubled and given intravenously. An add-on of biotin, 5 to 10 mg/kg per day, may lead to faster recovery. Antipyretics are essential because fever may trigger decompensation.

Thiamine Pyrophosphokinase Deficiency

Autosomal-recessive thiamine pyrophosphokinase deficiency (OMIM 606370) presents with a late-onset Leigh-like disease and basal ganglia changes on MRI. During acute episodes, elevated blood and CSF lactate and enhanced excretion of α-ketoglutarate are consistent findings. Thiamine pyrophosphate (TPP) concentrations in blood and muscle are reduced, and diagnosis is confirmed by sequencing of the *TPK1* gene. Thiamine supplementation at 100- to 200 mg/day was of limited benefit in symptomatic patients. Earlier intervention with doses around 500 mg/day may be associated with better prognosis.

Amish Lethal Microcephaly and Bilateral Striatal Necrosis Resulting From SLC25A19 Mutations

Amish lethal microcephaly and bilateral striatal necrosis (OMIM 607196) is caused by mutations in the *SLC25A19* gene, which encodes the transport of TPP into the mitochondria. The Amish founder mutation is associated with severe microcephaly at birth and a very short life span. Patients typically show excretion of α-ketoglutarate and lactic acidosis during febrile infections. A few patients with different *SLC25A19* mutations have been described outside the Amish community; these patients presented with associated CNS malformation or bilateral striatal necrosis but a normal head circumference.

In addition to these primary defects in thiamine transport and activation, some enzyme defects may have a favorable response to thiamine administration. Among these are pyruvate dehydrogenase complex and pyruvate carboxylase deficiency and some forms of maple syrup urine disease.

RIBOFLAVIN (VITAMIN B₂)

Riboflavin is the precursor of the metabolically active forms flavin mononucleotide (FMN) and flavin adenine dinucleotide (FAD), which function as cofactors for at least 90 different flavin-dependent proteins (flavoproteins). Flavin-dependent enzymes catalyze oxidation–reduction processes in primary metabolic pathways such as the citric acid cycle, β-oxidation, and degradation of amino acids. Flavin-dependent proteins also play an important role in the biosynthesis or regulation of other essential cofactors and hormones, such as coenzyme A, coenzyme Q, heme, pyridoxal 5′-phosphate, folate, cobalamin, steroids, and thyroxine.

Riboflavin Deficiency

Symptomatic riboflavin deficiency commonly occurs in association with deficiencies of other vitamins. Details are described in Table 46-1.

Riboflavin-Dependent Enzymatic Reactions

At least 50 different deficiencies of flavoproteins have been associated with an inherited human disease. Because a significant proportion of mutations in flavoproteins affect the affinity to their cofactors, a supranormal intake of riboflavin can lead to functional rescue. Disorders that may respond to high riboflavin doses (100-300 mg) include deficiencies of multiple acyl-CoA dehydrogenase, dihydrolipoamide dehydrogenase, and acyl-CoA dehydrogenase-9 (Table 46-2).

DISORDERS OF RIBOFLAVIN TRANSPORT

At least three distinct riboflavin transporters, SLC52A1 through SLC52A3, are involved in riboflavin uptake via the human intestine. The relative contribution and role of these transporters are currently unclear, but deficiency of SLC52A2 and SLC52A3 is associated with genetic neuronopathies.

Riboflavin Deficiency

Haploinsufficiency of the SLC52A1 riboflavin transporter has been reported with mild riboflavin deficiency (OMIM 615026) in a mother whose newborn child developed transient severe symptoms resembling clinical and biochemical features of multiple acyl-CoA dehydrogenase deficiency. Oral supplementation of 100 mg riboflavin per day rapidly normalized the biochemical parameters and clinical condition. The mother was treated with 50 mg of riboflavin per day.

Riboflavin Transporter Deficiency Neuronopathy

Type 1 riboflavin transporter deficiency neuronopathy, also referred to as Brown–Vialetto–Van Laere syndrome-1 (BVVLS1) or Fazio–Londe disease (OMIM 211530), is an autosomal-recessive progressive neurologic disorder that is caused by mutations in the *SLC52A3* gene.

Type 2 riboflavin transporter deficiency neuronopathy, also referred to as Brown–Vialetto–Van Laere syndrome-2 (BVVLS2; OMIM 614707) is an autosomal-recessive progressive neurologic disorder that is caused by mutations in the *SLC52A2* gene.

Both types of riboflavin transporter deficiency neuronopathy are associated with very similar clinical features. More than two-thirds of patients carry pathogenic mutations in the *SLC52A3* gene. Onset of symptoms ranges from a few months of age to the early teenage years and rarely can occur in adulthood. Peripheral nerves are the main site of pathology, manifesting as motor, sensory, and cranial neuronopathy, which can be proven by neurophysiological investigations. Cognition is usually preserved (Foley et al., 2014). The acyl-carnitine profile in blood may show accumulation of short- and medium-chain (and sometimes long-chain) acylcarnitines in some but not all affected individuals.

Oral riboflavin supplementation starting from 10 mg/kg per day, divided into three single doses, is gradually increased to 50 mg/kg per day to establish the optimum individual dose. All treated patients have improved after the initiation of riboflavin therapy.

NIACIN (VITAMIN B₃)

Niacin (also nicotinic acid) and its active forms, the nicotinamides (NAD⁺), function in a variety of oxidation–reduction reactions and serve as main electron donors in the respiratory chain. Niacin deficiency occurs in alcoholics, in adolescents with anorexia nervosa, in individuals following dietary fads, and in patients infected with human immunodeficiency virus, most often confounded with other micronutrient deficiencies. Signs and symptoms of niacin deficiency are outlined in Table 46-1.

NIACIN DEPENDENCY

Hartnup's disease (OMIM 234500) is caused by autosomal-recessive mutations of the neutral amino acid transporter *SLC6A19*. Low tryptophan levels lead to secondary niacin deficiency and Pellagra-like clinical features, which may improve after administration of 50 to 300 mg/day of NAD.

VITAMIN B₆

Vitamin B₆ is derived from the diet in different vitamers as pyridoxine, pyridoxal, or pyridoxamine and their phosphorylated esters (Fig. 46-1). Pyridox(am)ine 5′-phosphate is further oxidized to pyridoxal 5′-phosphate (PLP) by pryidox(am)ine

5'-phosphate oxidase (PNPO). PLP works as the active cofactor for more than 200 enzymatic reactions in amino acid and neurotransmitter synthesis and degradation. It is a cofactor of the glutamate decarboxylase and of the GABA transaminase and the aromatic acid decarboxylase. PLP thus plays a crucial role in brain metabolism. Some drugs (isoniazide, penicillamine, cycloserine, hydralazine, etc.) interact with pyridoxine and warrant preventive pyridoxine supplementation in dosages of 25 to 50 mg/day. Nutritional vitamin B_6 deficiency is rarely seen. Signs and symptoms are outlined in Table 46-1.

Vitamin B_6 Deficiency, Dependency, and Responsiveness

In contrast to nutritional vitamin B_6 deficiency, dependency indicates a lifelong hyperphysiologic demand of pyridoxine or PLP as a result of different IEMs with autosomal-recessive inheritance, which cause reduced availability of PLP by different mechanisms (Table 46-3). In all entities, seizures are a hallmark of the disease. In addition, patients with classical homocystinuria, gyrate atrophy, or X-linked sideroblastic anemia can show pyridoxine response as a result of a chaperone effect. Vitamin B_6 responsiveness has also been described in single individuals with West syndrome or idiopathic epilepsy of unclear genetic background.

Pyridoxine-Dependent Epilepsy

Pyridoxine-dependent epilepsy (PDE; OMIM 266100) is characterized by the onset of neonatal myoclonic or bilateral tonic-clonic seizures that are resistant to antiepileptic drugs and may evolve into status epilepticus. About 30% of patients have encephalopathic signs such as sleeplessness and irritability or show low Apgar scores. Late onset up to 3 years of age has been described. Electroencephalogram (EEG) findings can range from nonspecific slowing and discontinuity to focal discharges or, rarely, burst-suppression patterns. Neuroimaging may be normal or reveal a variety of unspecific changes. About 85% of patients show a prompt cessation of seizures after a single administration of pyridoxine (50-100 mg intravenously), followed by a stepwise normalization of the EEG. The first administration of pyridoxine can lead to prolonged apnea or a comatose state, and thus resuscitation equipment should be at hand. Approximately 15% of patients have an ambiguous clinical response to a single pyridoxine administration.

Therefore a pyridoxine trial with 30 mg/kg per day in two to three standard doses over 3 consecutive days is recommended. Some patients develop systemic signs that resolve upon specific treatment with pyridoxine (Stockler et al., 2011).

In 2006, antiquitin (*ALDH7A1*) deficiency was identified as the major molecular background of PDE (Fig. 46-2). Antiquitin encodes α-aminoadipic semialdehyde dehydrogenase, and its deficiency results in the accumulation of α-aminoadipic semialdehyde (AASA), which is in equilibrium with piperidine 6-carboxylate (P6C). P6C inactivates PLP and leads to a lifelong hyperphysiologic pyridoxine demand. Elevated AASA in urine (plasma or CSF) serves as a reliable biomarker even when on pyridoxine. AASA is also elevated in molybdenum cofactor deficiency (MOCOD) and warrants simultaneous determination of urinary sulfocysteine to avoid false diagnoses. Infants with PDE are supplemented with pyridoxine at dosages of 20 to 30 mg/kg per day in two to three standard doses. Beyond infancy, usual total daily pyridoxine doses vary from 100 mg/day to 300 mg/day. In the case of febrile breakthrough seizures, doubling of the daily pyridoxine dose over 3 to 5 days is recommended in subsequent infections. Long-term pyridoxine dosages above 300 to 500 mg/day can cause (reversible) sensory neuropathy.

Approximately 75% of children with PDE show mild to moderate cognitive impairment. Future trials will show whether reduced formation of α-AASA by a lysine-restricted diet or competitive inhibition of lysine uptake by high-dose arginine supplementation may lead to better outcome. In 2009, folinic acid–responsive seizures, a previously distinct entity of unknown molecular background, was shown to be allelic to antiquitin deficiency. Of note is that no patient on folinic acid monotherapy survived, but an add-on of folinic acid at dosages of 3 to 5 mg/kg per day has been beneficial in neonates with PDE and initial incomplete pyridoxine response.

A minority of PDE cases are caused by etiologies other than antiquitin deficiency, such as pyridoxine-responsive PNPO deficiency, hyperprolinemia type II, and severe neonatal hypophosphatasia. Recently, pyridoxine responsiveness has been described in severe forms of KCNQ2 deficiency.

Pyridox(am)ine 5'-Phosphate Oxidase Deficiency

The clinical presentation of pyridox(am)ine 5'-phosphate oxidase (PNPO) deficiency (OMIM 610090) is indistinguishable from antiquitin deficiency, except for the higher rate of

TABLE 46-3 Biomarkers of Vitamin B_6–Dependent Epilepsies Resulting From Inborn Errors of Metabolism and Their Response to Treatment

IEM- and PLP-related mechanisms	Urine	Plasma	CSF	Response to Vitamin B_6
PNPO deficiency Reduced PLP formation	Vanillactate*	↑ PM and PM/PA	↓ PLP° sek. NT changes*	Mainly to PLP, in certain mutations also pyridoxine
Congenital hypophosphatasia Reduced PLP uptake		↓ AP, ↓ Ph, ↑ Ca		To pyridoxine (or PLP)
Congenital hyperphosphatasia Reduced PLP uptake		↑ AP		Unknown
Antiquitin deficiency (PDE) PLP inactivation	↑ AASA and P6C	↑ AASA and P6C ↑ Pipecolic acid	↑ AASA ↓ PLP° sek. NT changes*	To pyridoxine (or PLP)
Hyperprolinemia II PLP inactivation	↑ Proline, P5C	↑ Proline, P5C		To pyridoxine (or PLP)

AP, alkaline phosphatase; AASA, alpha aminoadipic acid; Ca, calcium; CSF, cerebrospinal fluid; IEM, inborn errors of metabolism; NT, neurotransmitter; PA, pyridoxic acid; PDE, pyridoxine-dependent epilepsy; P5C, pyrrolin-5-carboxylate; Ph, phosphate; PLP, pyridoxal 5'-phosphate; PM, pyridoxamine; PNPO, pyridox(am)ine 5'-phosphate oxidase; P6C, piperideine-6-carboxylate.
*Inconsistent findings.
°Before specific treatment with vitamin B_6.

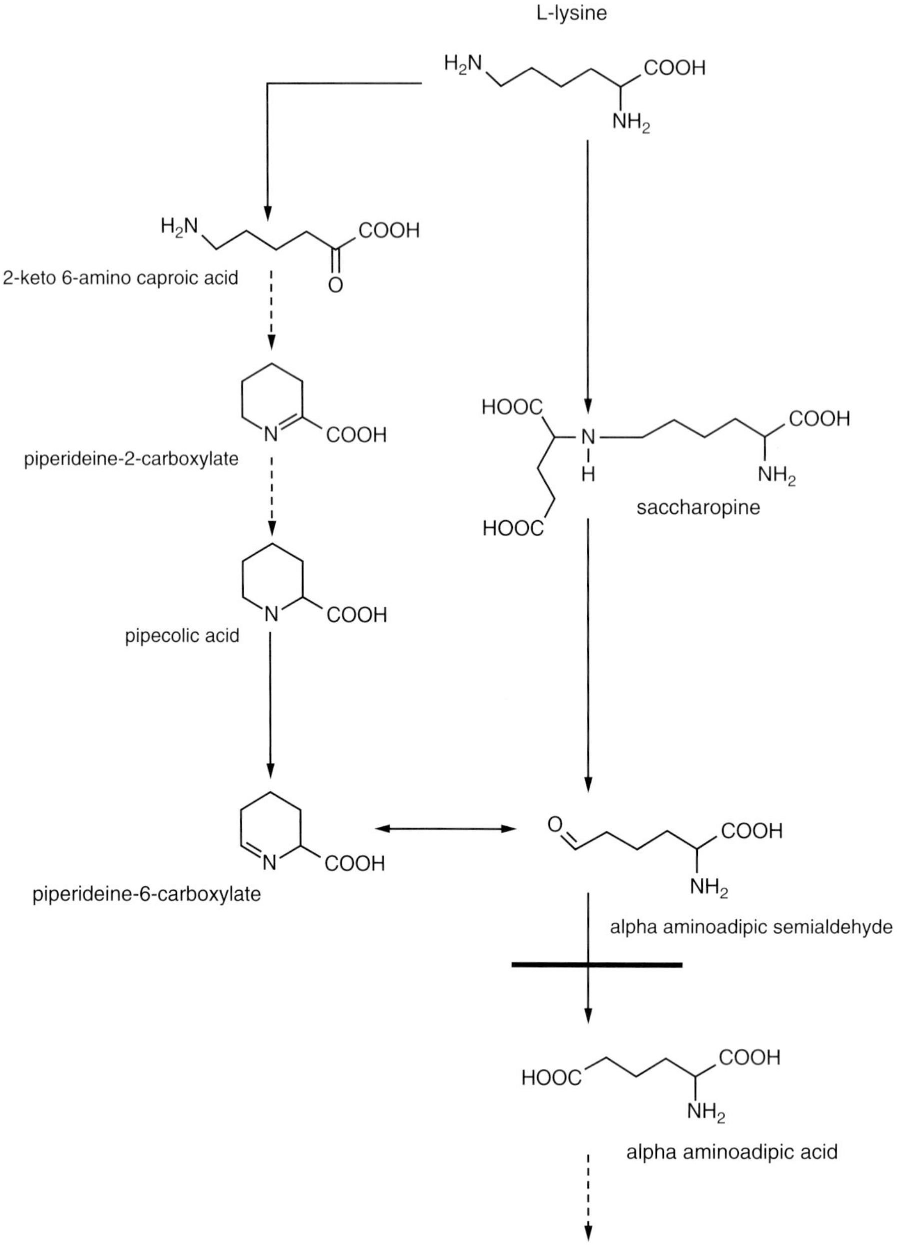

Figure 46-2. Lysine degradation pathway. Antiquitin deficiency causes accumulation of alpha-aminoadipic semialdehyde, which is in a nonenzymatic equilibrium with its cyclic form, Δ1-piperideine-6-carboxylate. Δ1-piperideine-6-carboxylate inactivates PLP by a Knoevenagel condensation.

prematurity observed in 60% of patients. The majority of infants have low Apgar scores and may require intubation. Myoclonic jerks and severe tonic-clonic convulsions are associated with a burst-suppression pattern in about 60% of cases. With the duration of symptoms, brain MRI may reveal white-matter changes and atrophy. In 2005 this disorder was found to be caused by mutations in the *PNPO* gene resulting in reduced PLP formation. Patients were initially characterized as being resistant to pyridoxine but dependent on PLP supplementation, but this paradigm has recently been contradicted by novel pyridoxine-responsive PNPO mutations. Surprisingly, some of these patients showed clear worsening of seizures when pyridoxine was replaced by PLP. In contrast to antiquitin deficiency, PNPO deficiency leads to severe systemic PLP deficiency with anemia and failure to thrive, and most patients die if untreated. Aside from secondary changes of plasma and CSF amino acids and neurotransmitters or inconsistently elevated vanillactate in urine, PNPO lacks a specific biomarker (Mills et al., 2014).

Patients with classical PNPO deficiency need lifelong treatment with PLP (unlicensed outside of Asia), 30 to 60 mg/kg per day in four to six standard doses. To avoid oxidation, PLP should be dissolved immediately before oral administration. The first administration can cause severe apnea and coma, and thus resuscitation equipment should be at hand. Many patients are sensitive to exact dose intervals even during the night, and seizure recurrence is frequent. Because of potential PLP liver toxicity, transaminases should be monitored regularly, and the lowest effective dose should be used. Patients with pyridoxine-responsive *PNPO* mutations may be treated with pyridoxine alone. Residual seizures necessitate a switch to PLP, which can be successful if performed slowly.

Hyperprolinemia Type II

Hyperprolinemia type II (OMIM 239510) is generally considered benign because only 50% of patients present with seizures, which often respond to common anticonvulsants. Hyperprolinemia type II is caused by a deficiency of Δ1-pyrroline-5-carboxylate dehydrogenase leading to the accumulation of Δ1-pyrroline-5-carboxylate (P5C), which inactivates PLP (Fig. 46-2). The diagnosis can be made by marked elevation of plasma proline and the presence of P5C in urine. The action of pyridoxine in this disorders is less clear.

Congenital Hypophosphatasia

Congenital hypophosphatasia (OMIM 241500) is caused by deficient tissue-nonspecific alkaline phosphatase (TNSALP). In addition to its function in bone metabolism, TNSALP is responsible for the cellular uptake of PLP (Fig. 46-1). Patients with severe deficiency may thus present with pyridoxine-responsive neonatal seizures and burst-suppression pattern before recognition of the bone disease. The availability of enzyme replacement therapy will hopefully prevent the osteomalacia and early death associated with severe forms of the disease.

Pyridoxine Versus PLP to Test for Vitamin B₆ Responsiveness

Neonates with seizures of unclear etiology who fail to respond to common anticonvulsants should receive a standardized pyridoxine trial with 30 mg/kg per day over 3 consecutive days. In responders, withdrawal is obsolete and is replaced by molecular workup according to the presence or absence of respective biomarkers. In case of failure, folinic acid, 3 to 5 mg/kg per day, might be added and pyridoxine switched to PLP, with monitoring of liver function tests from day 2. This suggestion is based on the relatively higher frequency of pyridoxine-responsive entities compared with classical PLP-dependent PNPO deficiency, the licensed drug status of pyridoxine in most developed countries, its availability as an IV drug, and the potential liver toxicity of high-dose PLP. Treatment effects have to be observed closely. Confirmation diagnosis in prospectively treated siblings of children affected by antiquitin or PNPO deficiency should be performed as quickly as possible.

VITAMIN B₁₂ (COBALAMINE)

Vitamin B₁₂ (cobalamin; Cbl) is derived from animal food sources only and follows a complex mechanism of absorption, transport, and intracellular modification to finally act as one of the two active cofactors, methylcobalamin (MeCbl) for the recycling of homocysteine to methionine and adenosylcobalamin (AdoCbl) for the conversion of methylmalonyl-CoA to succinyl-CoA.

The estimated daily losses of Cbl are minute compared with body stores. Hence, even in the presence of severe malabsorption, 2 to 5 years may pass before Cbl deficiency develops.

Cobalamin Deficiency

Infants of strictly vegan mothers are at special risk of developing nutritional Cbl deficiency. Rarer causes include intestinal bacterial overgrowth (e.g., *Helicobacter pylori*) or parasites (e.g., *Diphyllobothrium latum*), malabsorption as a result of intestinal disease, and inherited defects affecting absorption and transport. B₁₂ deficiency also has been reported with exposure to anesthesia by nitrous oxide. Megaloblastic anemia and neurologic manifestations are the hallmarks of Cbl deficiency (Table 46-1), but they can occur irrespective of each other. Infants show a consistent pattern of irritability, failure to thrive, and simultaneous growth deceleration, apathy, and anorexia, accompanied by developmental regression. Severe cases may develop acute decompensation with metabolic acidosis, hyperammonemia, and coma. This is clearly distinct from manifestations later in life with glossitis, myelopathy, painful paresthesia, disturbed proprioception, dementia, and neuropsychiatric disorders. CNS symptoms may partly be attributable to secondary disruption of the folate cycle and low methionine levels. In infants, the main MRI abnormality, if present, is delayed myelination or supratentorial atrophy, which may reverse upon treatment.

The diagnosis of Cbl deficiency rests on a thorough history and measurement of biochemical parameters in plasma and urine. Severe deficiency requires injections of hydroxocobalamin (OHCbl), whereas oral treatment with (Cyano) Cbl is sufficient if intestinal absorption is intact. Dietary counseling is of utmost importance, especially in vegan families, and regular Cbl supplementation is the option of choice if dietary habits remain unchanged.

Symptoms of nutritional Cbl deficiency are reversible if recognized early. Treatment delay may result in poor cognitive outcome and microcephaly. Some infants showed a transient movement disorder consisting of tremor and myoclonus, particularly involving the face, tongue, and pharynx, which appeared 48 hours after the initiation of treatment with intramuscular cobalamin.

Cobalamin Dependency

The genetic defects of Cbl metabolism can affect absorption, transport, cellular uptake, or intracellular processing. Hereditary intrinsic factor (IF) deficiency (OMIM 261000) and Imerslund–Graesbeck syndrome (OMIM 261100) lead to reduced intestinal absorption and poor renal reabsorption of Cbl and can manifest from infancy to adulthood with symptoms indistinguishable from those of nutritional Cbl deficiency. TC II deficiency (OMIM 275350) presents with additional symptoms of immunodeficiency and recurrent infections, glossitis, and oral ulcerations. Disorders of absorption lead to reduced Cbl plasma levels, whereas in TC II defects, the Cbl plasma concentrations are normal (Table 46-3). All disorders result in elevated concentrations of homocysteine and methylmalonic acid (MMA) in plasma and urine.

Disorders of intracellular Cbl processing can be classified into combined disorders of metCbl and AdoCbl metabolism, those with isolated metCbl deficiency, also called remethylation defects, and those with isolated adoCbl deficiency. The clinical picture and the presence of elevated homocysteine and MMA, alone or in combination, and the presence of anemia are important biomarkers to guide the molecular workup (Table 46-3).

CblC, CbD-MMA/HC, CbF, and CblJ Deficiency (Combined Defects of Ado- and MetCbl)

The combined defects of Ado- and MetCbl include CblC (OMIM 609831), CbD-MMA/HC (OMIM 77410), CbF (OMIM 277380), and CblJ deficiency; CblC deficiency is by far the most severe and the most common. Most patients have an early onset during infancy, with feeding difficulties, failure to thrive, microcephaly, hypotonia, seizures, ataxia, megaloblastic anemia or pancytopenia, and visual problems such as nystagmus or early-onset retinopathy. Acute symptoms in addition to chronic, such as thromboembolic vasculopathy, renal failure resulting from atypical hemolytic uremic syndrome (HUS), cardiomyopathy, or metabolic crisis with hyperammonemia and ketoacidosis, may occur. MRI reveals delayed myelination and global atrophy or hydrocephalus. Symptom severity seems to correlate with the reduction of methionine levels rather than with MMA or homocysteine concentrations. In late-onset cases, psychiatric problems and myelopathy prevail. The few patients described with CblF deficiency had a milder phenotype but suffered from recurrent infections. Treatment by regular injections of hydroxocobalamin up to 1 mg two to three times weekly, folinic acid 5 to 20 mg/day, betaine at 100 mg/kg per day in four standard doses, and eventually supplementation of methionine improves acute manifestations, but cognitive outcome is often impaired.

CblE, CblG, and CblD-HC Deficiency (Defects of MetCbl; Remethylation Defects)

Most patients with so-called remethylation defects, which include CblE, CblG, and CblD-HC deficiency, manifest in the first year of life with feeding difficulties, hypotonia, developmental delay, and megaloblastic anemia. Infection-related deterioration, thromboembolism, or late-onset disease may occur. Plasma homocysteine is elevated, whereas MMA excretion in urine is normal. Delayed diagnosis can lead to irreversible myelopathy with spastic paraparesis. Anemia may not be present in early phases of the disease. Treatment of isolated MetCbl defects is identical to the treatment of combined deficiencies, and responses can be excellent.

CblA-MMA, CblB-MMA, and CblD-MMA Deficiency (Defects of AdoCbl)

CblA-MMA (OMIM 251100), CblB-MMA (OMIM 251110), and CblD-MMA (OMIM 277410 variant 2) deficiency cause isolated AdoCbl deficiency. Most patients present with acute metabolic decompensation and encephalopathy during early life, often triggered by febrile infections, with metabolic acidosis, variable hyperammonemia, and high MMA excretion but normal homocysteine (Table 46-3). In the acute phase, MRI may show bilateral T2-weighted basal ganglia hyperintensities or metabolic stroke. The neurologic manifestations range from acute extrapyramidal movement disorders or comatose state to more chronic presentations with hypotonia, developmental delay, or optic atrophy. Metabolic crises can lead to irreversible brain damage and need emergency treatment in metabolic centers. A considerable proportion of patients respond to parenteral administration of hydroxocobalamin, 1 mg twice weekly, whereas the remainder will need a protein-restricted diet.

TOCOPHEROL (VITAMIN E)

Vitamin E, including alpha-tocopherol, is the generic term for a group of fat-soluble compounds that function as scavengers of free radicals and protect polyunsaturated fatty acids from oxidation. It is stored predominantly in adipose tissue. Blood levels reflect recent dietary intake and absorption rather than body stores. Nutritional vitamin E deficiency occurs predominantly in disorders associated with either chronic fat malabsorption (e.g., cystic fibrosis, celiac disease, chronic cholestatic hepatobiliary disorders, short bowel syndrome) or a deficiency of plasma lipoproteins (e.g., abetalipoproteinemia, Tangiers disease). Details are described in Table 46-1.

Disorders of Vitamin E Metabolism

Ataxia With Vitamin E Deficiency (= Familial Isolated Vitamin E Deficiency)

Ataxia with vitamin E deficiency (AVED; OMIM 277460) is an autosomal-recessive neurologic disorder that is caused by mutations in the *TTPA* gene coding for the tocopherol transfer protein. Clinical signs comprise progressive spinocerebellar ataxia, areflexia, pyramidal tract lesion, loss of proprioception, retinopathy, ophthalmoplegia, mental retardation, cardiac arrhythmias, xanthelasma, and tendon xanthomas. Laboratory findings include extremely low vitamin E levels and high serum cholesterol, triglycerides, and beta-lipoprotein.

With daily alpha-tocopherol supplementation of 20 to 40 mg/kg po, plasma vitamin E levels will normalize and cognitive function rapidly improves; however, neurologic symptoms often show slow and incomplete recovery.

BIOTIN (VITAMIN H)

Biotin is absorbed through the intestine by active transport mechanisms and serves as a cofactor for five carboxylation enzymes that are involved in carbohydrate, lipid, and amino acid metabolism: pyruvate carboxylase, acetyl-CoA carboxylase (α and β), propionyl-CoA carboxylase, and 3-methylcrotonyl carboxylase. Biotinidase is an important enzyme for the release of protein-bound biotin and for the recycling of biotin from biocytin, which is formed in the degradation of the carboxylases. Nutritional biotin deficiency is extremely rare.

Biotinidase Deficiency

Because of its excellent treatability, biotinidase deficiency (OMIM 253260) is included in most newborn screening programs worldwide. Severe biotinidase deficiency (residual activity [RA] < 10%) presents in the first half year of life with hypotonia; tonic-clonic, myoclonic, and partial seizures or infantile spasms; skin rash; and alopecia. EEG findings vary from normal to burst suppression pattern or hypsarrhythmia. Brainstem auditory-evoked potentials (BAEPs) can show findings consistent with sensorineural hearing loss. MRI can show (reversible) diffuse white-matter changes, edema of the putamen and caudate nuclei, and varying degrees of cerebral atrophy with ventriculomegaly. If untreated, the disease can result in coma or death. Partial biotinidase deficiency (RA 10%-30%) manifests in older children with ataxia or spastic paraparesis, developmental delay, hearing loss, or optic atrophy. Metabolic ketoacidosis with an increased anion gap, elevated lactate, and abnormal analysis of organic acids is present in severely affected patients, whereas attenuated forms may only be detected by measurement of biotinidase activity in serum.

Symptomatic children with biotinidase deficiency improve when supplemented with 5 to 20 mg of oral biotin per day, irrespective of age and weight, and require lifelong treatment. Hearing loss and optic atrophy are usually not reversible.

Biotin-Dependent Holocarboxylase Synthetase Deficiency (Multiple Carboxylase Deficiency)

Multiple carboxylase deficiency (OMIM 253270) is indistinguishable from biotinidase deficiency, but biotinidase activity in serum is normal, whereas the activity of various carboxylases is impaired. Patients are supplemented with higher doses of biotin, approximately 20 mg/day (Baumgartner, 2013).

Biotin-Responsive Basal Ganglia Disease

See the section on thiamine (vitamin B₁).

FOLATE

Folates are essential micronutrients and derivatives of pteridine compounds. Three major folate coenzymes are involved in catalytic one-carbon-transfer reactions: 10-formyl-THF functions as formyl donor in the purine synthesis; 5,10-methylen-THF mediates the methyl transfer to dUMP; and 5-methyl-THF participates in the methylation of homocysteine (Fig. 46-3). The latter reaction is crucial for the synthesis of S-adenosyl-methionine (SAM), which represents the preferred methyl group donor in the majority of methylation pathways. Thus lack of folate coenzymes affects a multitude of metabolic routes and will eventually compromise the synthesis of nucleic acids, amino acids, neurotransmitters, and biomolecules that are essential for myelin formation. The dependency of the brain on the external supply of 5-methyl-THF can be explained by the low concentration of dihydrofolate reductase that is required to regenerate 5-methyl-THF (see Fig. 46-3).

A comparative summary of the characteristic laboratory findings of the folate pathway and transport disorders is illustrated in Table 46-3.

Nutritional Folate Deficiency

Folate deficiency can be encountered along with multivitamin deficiencies or with increased folate requirements such as in pregnancy, lactation, prematurity, or diseases associated with abnormalities of folate absorption, use, or excretion. Drugs such as aminopterin, methotrexate, pyrimethamine, trimethoprim, and triamterene act as folate antagonists and produce folate deficiency by inhibiting dihydrofolate reductase, which is essential for the regeneration of tetrahydrofolate (see Fig. 46-3). Signs of deficiency and treatment are described in Table 46-1.

DISORDERS OF FOLATE METABOLISM
Dihydrofolate Reductase Deficiency

Dihydrofolate Reductase (DHFR) deficiency (OMIM 613839) has an autosomal-recessive inheritance pattern. As a consequence of DHFR deficiency, dihydrofolate accumulates and tetrahydrofolate diminishes, resulting in inhibition of pyrimidine and purine synthesis (see Fig. 46-3). DHFR is a major target of methotrexate, a commonly used chemotherapeutic for leukemias, and thus DHFR deficiency initially affects erythropoiesis and myelopoiesis but eventually may compromise cerebral folate supply and all THF-dependent reactions within the brain.

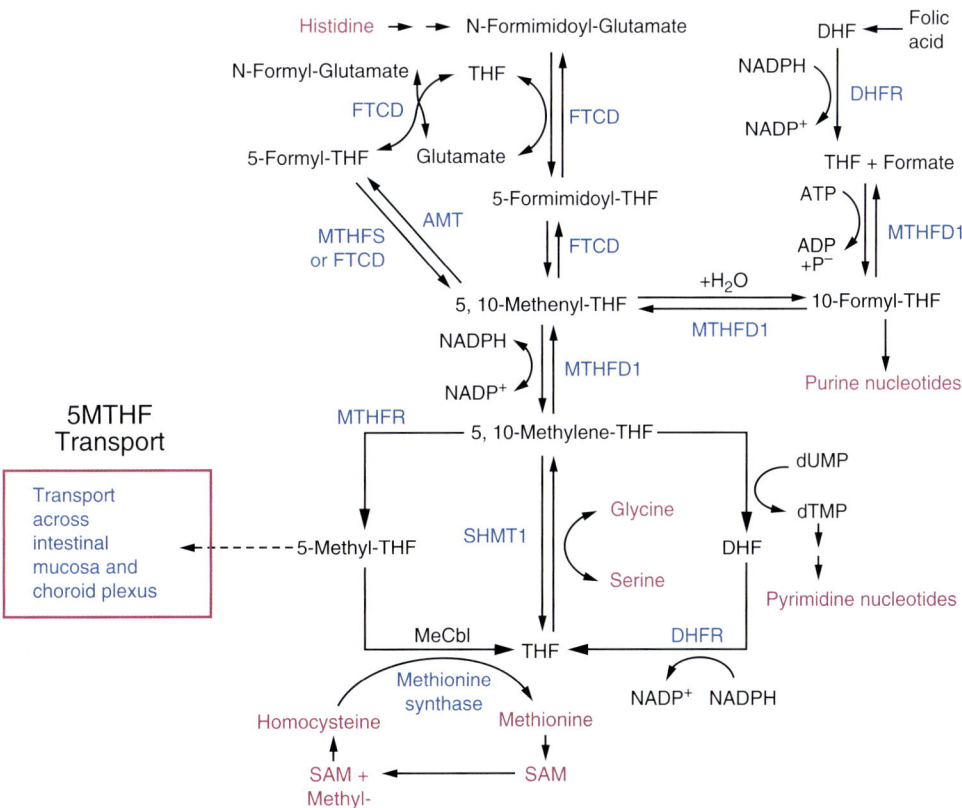

Figure 46-3. Schematic illustration of the folate metabolic pathways. The key metabolites histidine, serine, glycine, homocysteine, and methionine are highlighted in red. Enzymes are depicted in blue. Several enzymes are multifunctional, containing subdomains with distinct enzymatic activities. 5-methyl-THF is the major metabolite that is transported across the mucosa of the small intestine and the choroid plexus. AMT, aminomethyltransferase (EC 2.1.2.10); DHF, dihydrofolate; DHFR, dihydrofolate reductase (EC 1.5.1.3); FTCD, formiminotransferase (bifunctional enzyme, EC 2.1.2.5 + EC 4.3.1.4); MeCbl, methylcobalamin; MTHFD1, 5,10-methylenetetrahydrofolate dehydrogenase (trifunctional enzyme, EC 1.5.1.5 + EC 3.5.4.9 + EC 6.3.4.3); MTHFR, methylenetetrahydrofolate reductase (EC 1.5.1.20); MTHFS, 5,10-methenyltetrahydrofolate synthetase, 5-formyltetrahydrofolate cyclo-ligase (EC 6.3.3.2); SAH, S-adenosyl-homocysteine; SAM, S-adenosyl-methionine; SHMT, serine hydroxymethyltransferase (EC 2.1.2.1); THF, tetrahydrofolate.

All reported patients show infantile onset of symptoms comprising megaloblastic anemia, failure to thrive, and secondary microcephaly. Neurologic symptoms follow shortly and include profound developmental delay, central hypotonia with poor head control, inability to fix and follow, and frequent focal seizures. At later stages, learning difficulties and short episodes of involuntary blinking and winking may develop, eventually with impaired consciousness. The EEG may indicate atypical childhood absence epilepsy with eyelid myoclonia. Brain imaging demonstrates cerebellar and cerebral atrophy, thin corpus callosum, and poor myelination of white matter. Serum folate and plasma homocysteine concentrations are in the normal range (Table 46-4). However, there is a marked depletion of 5-methyl-THF in the CSF and a moderate decrease in tetrahydrobiopterin and neurotransmitter concentrations (homovanillic acid and 5-hydroxyindoleacetic acid) in the CSF.

Folic acid should be avoided in the treatment of DHFR deficiency because DHFR constitutes the only enzyme that catalyzes the conversion of folic acid to dihydrofolate. Infants should be promptly supplemented with 5 to 10 mg/kg body weight of oral folinic acid given daily as a single dose. Dosing for an affected individual should be adjusted to achieve a normal CSF concentration of 5-methyl-THF considering the age-dependent normal range.

Methylenetetrahydrofolate Reductase Deficiency

Methylenetetrahydrofolate reductase (MTHFR) deficiency (OMIM 236250) has an autosomal-recessive inheritance pattern and is the most common inherited disorder of folate metabolism. MTHFR catalyzes the NADPH-dependent reduction of 5,10-methylene-THF to 5-methyl-THF, which in turn is required for the conversion of homocysteine to methionine (Fig. 46-3). The onset and severity of symptoms vary significantly but correlate with the degree of enzyme deficiency. The most common clinical finding in MTHFR deficiency is developmental delay, followed by motor and gait abnormalities, incoordination, cerebral seizures, paresthesias, stroke, muscular weakness, and psychiatric disturbances, including memory deficits. The majority of patients show EEG abnormalities, and about half of them develop microcephaly. In severe early-onset MTHFR deficiency, the infant may present with infantile spasms, developmental regression, and hydrocephalus.

Adult-onset MTHFR deficiency may manifest with the combination of progressive spastic paraparesis and polyneuropathy, variable behavioral changes, cognitive impairment, psychosis, seizures, and leukoencephalopathy. Other clinical signs may be quite variable, for example, marfanoid habitus resembling classical homocystinuria.

Betaine supplementation is the first choice in the treatment of MTHFR deficiency and improves the prognosis of severe MTHFR deficiency when initiated early. Patients should receive daily 100 mg/kg body weight per day (infants up to 250 mg/kg per day and older children up to 20 g/d) of oral betaine, divided in four single dosages. In case of psychomotor regression or epilepsy, the 5-methyl-THF concentrations in CSF should be monitored. Because of the limited folate transport across the blood–CSF barrier and the increased demand of choline for the biosynthesis of myelinated membranes, the concentration of 5-methyl-THF in the CSF is significantly reduced in most early-onset patients and roughly correlates with the severity of the neurologic symptoms in MTHFR deficiency.

In cases where betaine supplementation fails to achieve the aimed therapeutic effect, treatment with folinic acid or MTHF, riboflavin, methionine, pyridoxine, and cobalamin can be tried.

MTHFD1-Encoded Enzyme Deficiency (Methylenetetrahydrofolate Dehydrogenase Deficiency)

The MTHFD1 defect is inherited as an autosomal-recessive trait. In eukaryotes, the MTHFD1 gene encodes a single cytoplasmic protein, a homodimer of 100-kD polypeptides, with three distinct enzymatic activities (Fig. 46-3).

All five reported patients presented with megaloblastic anemia in addition to leukopenia or signs of immune deficiency. Hyperhomocystinuria and mildly decreased synthesis of intracellular methylcobalamin in the presence of exogenous [^{57}Co]cyanocobalamin were common findings. Cobalamin and folate levels in serum were within the normal range.

Three patients were treated with intramuscular hydroxocobalamin, oral folate or folinic acid, and oral betaine or thiamine. In one patient, 5-methyl-THF and methylcobalamin were later empirically added to the regimen at the age of 23 months. One patient had mild mental retardation at the age of 6 years, whereas two other patients had normal cognitive development.

TABLE 46-4 Laboratory and Imaging Findings of Cobalamin or Folate Pathway and Transport Disorders

Disorder	Serum Folate	CSF 5MTHF	Blood Count	Plasma Homocysteine	Brain Imaging
FCTD deficiency	Normal	Low	Normal	Normal	No abnormalities reported
DHFR deficiency	Normal	Low	Macrocytic anemia	Normal	Hypomyelination, thin corpus callosum, brain atrophy
MTHFR deficiency	Normal	Low to normal	Normal	Increased	Periventricular demyelination
MTHFD1 deficiency	Normal	Low	Anemia	Increased	Bilateral small hippocampi, T2 signal changes in lobes
PCFT deficiency	Low	Low	Macrocytic anemia	Increased	Calcifications in the cortex or basal ganglia
CFT deficiency	Normal	Low	Normal	Normal	Hypomyelination, cerebellar (+ cerebral) atrophy
Methylcobalamin deficiency	High to normal	Normal	Macrocytic anemia	Increased	Thin corpus callosum, cortical atrophy, hypomyelination

CFT, cerebral folate transport; CSF, cerebrospinal fluid; DHFR, dihydrofolate reductase; FCTD, formiminotransferase; PCFT, proton-coupled folate transporter; MTHFD1, methylenetetrahydrofolate dehydrogenase-1; MTHFR, methylenetetrahydrofolate reductase.

Formiminotransferase Deficiency

Formiminotransferase (= glutamate formimidoyltransferase, FTCD) deficiency (OMIM 229100) is an autosomal-recessive inherited disorder caused by mutations in the *FCTD* gene. FTCD catalyzes the formation of 5,10-methenyl-THF (Fig. 46-3) in the histidine degradation pathway. The clinical relevance of formiminotransferase deficiency is presently unclear. Patients carrying missense mutations in the *FCTD* gene show developmental or speech delay, muscular hypotonia, and breathing difficulties with late infantile onset. Additional findings are abnormal electroencephalograms and significantly increased urinary excretion of formiminoglutamate (FIGLU).

Because of the poor correlation between clinical phenotype, residual enzymatic activity, and biochemical findings, no specific treatment is currently recommended.

DISORDERS OF FOLATE TRANSPORT
Hereditary Folate Malabsorption

Hereditary folate malabsorption (HFM; OMIM 229050) is an autosomal-recessive inherited trait caused by mutations in the proton-coupled folate transporter (PCFT = SLC46A1), which cotransports folates together with protons. Affected individuals fail to absorb sufficient folates in the small intestine to match the daily requirements of about 0.4 mg. In addition, the frequent failure to correct 5-methyl-THF levels in CSF even under normalized plasma folate concentration indicates impaired folate transport across the blood–CSF barrier in a proportion of patients with HFM.

Patients may show poor feeding and failure to thrive during very early infancy. The folate deficiency results primarily in megaloblastic anemia but may develop into pancytopenia. Anemia may be normocytic in case of poor nutrition and/or concomitant iron deficiency and may be accompanied by diarrhea and/or oral mucositis. Infants with HFM may initially present with profound immunodeficiency, which includes humoral and cellular immunity and mimics severe combined immune deficiency (SCID). Neurologic signs may be part of the initial manifestation of HFM or may develop later and include developmental delay, cognitive and motor impairment, behavioral abnormalities, ataxia and other movement disorders, peripheral neuropathy, and seizures with onset in infancy or early childhood (Zhao et al., 2007). Calcifications in the cortex or basal ganglia have been reported for several individuals with HFM.

Serum folate concentrations are very low or even undetectable. Oral folate supplementation does not result in significant increase in serum folate concentration, and a single oral load of 5-formyl-THF (= folinic acid) shows no or little effect on serum folate concentration over a minimum of 4 hours. CSF 5-methyl-THF concentrations in affected individuals are frequently low (< 5 nM) and remain below the normal range even after correction of the serum folate concentration.

Treatment aims to prevent hematologic and immunologic defects and to optimize the psychomotor development of children (Diekman et al., 2014). Infants should immediately receive 10 to 20 mg/kg body weight of oral folinic acid given daily as a single dose. Dosing should be adjusted to achieve a normal CSF concentration of 5-methyl-THF considering the age-dependent normal range. In case of insufficient response to oral treatment, intramuscular injections of levofolinic acid, either daily 1 mg or 5 mg twice per week or, alternatively, intravenous injection of 50 to 100 mg of levofolinic acid should be tried.

Cerebral Folate Transport Deficiency

Cerebral folate transport deficiency (CFTD; OMIM 613068) is an autosomal-recessive inherited disorder associated with mutations in the *FOLR1* gene, which encodes folate receptor alpha (FRα). CFTD is characterized by the failure of FRα-mediated folate transport in the CSF that differentiates it from other types of cerebral folate deficiency (see Table 46-3). Folic acid possesses a very high affinity for FRα and thus may block 5-methyl-THF transport across the choroid plexus.

The most consistent clinical finding in CFTD is developmental regression, with onset typically before the age of 3 years. Short drop attacks resembling infantile spasms may precede frequent myoclonic epileptic seizures that are often resistant to antiepileptic medication. Ataxia, truncal hypotonia, and lower limb spasticity are frequent neurologic signs. Most patients appear to lose their social contact skills and develop an autistic-like behavior. Some patients present a milder phenotype with developmental delay, ataxia, and autistic features only (Grapp, 2012). Many patients become microcephalic in the course of the disease.

Brain imaging reveals delayed myelination, hypomyelination, and cerebellar and cerebral atrophy. Magnetic resonance (MR) spectroscopy indicates low concentration of inositol and choline in the cerebral white matter. Focal T2 hyperintensities of the white matter can be detected in cranial MR imaging at later stages of the disease. Slow background together with multifocal epileptiform activities are commonly found in the EEG.

Very low CSF concentrations of 5-methyl-THF are the biochemical hallmark of CFTD, and concentrations have been below 5 nM in all patients reported so far. Plasma folate concentrations of untreated patients are measured in the lower normal range, and intraerythrocytic folate concentration is typically normal.

Oral supplementation with 5 to 10 mg/kg of folinic acid results in normalization of cerebral choline and inositol and correction of 5-methyl-THF. In cases of incomplete clinical response, additional intravenous injections of 50 to 100 mg folinic acid once per week should be considered. In selected patients, intrathecal administration of folinic acid may be beneficial. Early treatment is mandatory to achieve complete correction of clinical symptoms.

REFERENCES

The complete list of references for this chapter is available online at www.expertconsult.com.
See inside cover for registration details.

SELECTED REFERENCES

Baumgartner, M.R., 2013. Vitamin-responsive disorders: cobalamin, folate, biotin, vitamins B1 and E. Handb. Clin. Neurol. 113, 1799–1810. Review.

Brown, G., 2014. Defects of thiamine transport and metabolism. J. Inherit. Metab. Dis. 37 (4), 577–585. Review.

Diekman, E.F., de Koning, T.J., Verhoeven-Duif, N.M., et al., 2014. Survival and psychomotor development with early betaine treatment in patients with severe methylenetetrahydrofolate reductase deficiency. JAMA Neurol. 71 (2), 188–194.

Foley, A.R., Menezes, M.P., Pandraud, A., et al., 2014. Treatable childhood neuronopathy caused by mutations in riboflavin transporter RFVT2. Brain 137 (Pt 1), 44–56.

Grapp, M., Just, I.A., Linnankivi, T., et al., 2012. Molecular characterization of folate receptor 1 mutations delineates cerebral folate transport deficiency. Brain 135 (Pt 7), 2022–2031.

Kumar, N., 2010. Neurologic presentations of nutritional deficiencies. Neurol. Clin. 28 (1), 107–170.

Mills, P.B., Camuzeaux, S.S., Footitt, E.J., et al., 2014. Epilepsy due to PNPO mutations: genotype, environment and treatment affect presentation and outcome. Brain 137 (Pt 5), 1350–1360.

Ortigoza-Escobar, J.D., Serrano, M., Molero, M., et al., 2014. Thiamine transporter-2 deficiency: outcome and treatment monitoring. Orphanet J. Rare Dis. 9, 92.

Stockler, S., Plecko, B., Gospe, S.M. Jr., et al., 2011. Pyridoxine dependent epilepsy and antiquitin deficiency: clinical and molecular characteristics and recommendations for diagnosis, treatment and follow-up. Mol. Genet. Metab. 104 (1–2), 48–60. Review.

Zhao, R., Min, S.H., Qiu, A., et al., 2007. The spectrum of mutations in the PCFT gene, coding for an intestinal folate transporter, that are the basis for hereditary folate malabsorption. Blood 110 (4), 1147–1152.

E-BOOK FIGURES AND TABLES

The following figures and tables are available in the e-book at www.expertconsult.com. See inside cover for registration details.

Fig. 46-1 Vitamin B6 is absorbed in different vitamers that are dephosphorylated by intestinal alkaline phosphatases (IPs) and rephosphorylated to their 5'-phosphate esters by phosphate kinase (PK).

Table 46-1 Dietary Reference Allowances of Vitamins

Table 46-2 Riboflavin-Responsive Disorders With Predominantly Neurologic Symptoms

47 Nutrition and the Developing Brain

María Victoria Escolano-Margarit and Cristina Campoy

An expanded version of this chapter is available on www.expertconsult.com. See inside cover for registration details.

The important role that optimal early nutrition has in brain development has been stressed for years. Some authors have stated that nutrition may be the environmental variable with the widest range of effects on brain development. Diet is responsible for both the provision of substrates from which the brain is constructed and the energy required for its function. The central nervous system is most vulnerable to nutritional influence at the periods when growth, development, and plasticity are higher; in the case of human beings this extends from the beginning of the third trimester of pregnancy until 2 years of age. At age 2 years, the volume of the human brain has reached 80% to 90% of adult size (Isaacs, 2013). Between the 24th and 42nd weeks of gestation white- and gray-matter structures undergo a rapid increase in volume, with the cerebellum and cortical gray matter being the structures with highest growth rates. Although the brain initially grows rapidly, its development continues into the teenage years, raising the possibility that the nature of diet at later stages may also be influential.

The effects of malnutrition are based on the timing and magnitude of the nutrient deficit and on the brain's need for the particular nutrient at the time of the deficit. It is important to note that insults early in life when the brain is developing could have long-lasting effects.

PROTEIN-CALORIE MALNUTRITION

Studies based on animal models at the beginning of the last century have demonstrated that undernutrition in early life has dramatic anatomic and biochemical effects on the brain. It seems that the primary effect of protein-calorie deprivation involves replication and growth of cells in those elements most actively proliferating during the insult, rather than cell destruction. Box 47-1 lists major neuropathologic abnormalities resulting from malnutrition described in animal experimental studies. Table 47-1 summarizes the most important nutrients required for brain growth during late fetal and neonatal brain development and the particular brain structure or function that they regulate.

The major aspects of the anatomic and biochemical changes associated with malnutrition in animals have been observed in malnourished children. Malnutrition during brain development leads to reduction in brain cells, number of synapses, dendritic arborization, and myelin production, which result in decreased brain size and macrostructure and alterations in neurotransmitter systems. The structures that are most affected are the hippocampus, cerebellum, and neocortex. All of these alterations are associated with delays in motor and cognitive functions, such as impaired school performance, decreased IQ scores, decreased memory, learning disorders, attention deficit disorders, and reduced social skills (Laus et al., 2011). A combination of intrauterine and extrauterine malnutrition has the greatest effect on brain structure composition and function.

The fetus takes the critical nutrients it needs irrespective of the nutritional status of the mother. This ensures proper delivery of substrates for growth. Only in extreme situations of nutrient deprivation is the placental transfer of nutrients affected. Severe deficiencies in nutrition are widespread in developing countries, and there is evidence that these deficiencies affect brain structural maturation and long-term functioning of the brains of children, resulting in cognitive functional delays and permanent cognitive impairments. Maternal protein-calorie malnutrition can restrict uterine blood flow and growth of the uterus, placenta, and the fetus. Intrauterine growth restriction is associated with many adverse fetal and neonatal outcomes, including delayed neurologic development. After birth, stunting affects one third of children under age 5 years in low-income and middle-income countries. Ninety percent of the worldwide burden of child stunting is attributable to 36 countries. The highest prevalence of stunting occurs in central Africa and south-central Asia, with an approximate prevalence of 40%. Childhood stunting has been linked to poor mental development and school achievements as well as behavioral abnormalities (Laus et al., 2011). Whether some of these effects are reversible remains a matter of debate.

Optimal development of the fetal and infant brain depends on adequate maternal nutritional intake. Stunting early in life has been reported to have lasting effects school performance and IQ scores up to the age of 15 years. Some other authors state that children can recover from an early nutritional insult and improve cognition. Nutrient deficiencies are more likely to occur in disadvantaged environments, which themselves have additional adverse effects on children's behavior and development. An unstimulating home environment could exacerbate the effects of malnutrition on neurologic development. The extent to which nutrition as an independent risk factor influences brain development and its future function is difficult to elucidate (Laus et al., 2011).

Neuroimaging techniques have shown that infants with intrauterine growth restriction that reflects a deficient prenatal nutrition have reduced total brain tissue volumes and reduced cortical gray and hippocampus volumes, compared with children with the same gestational age but appropriate intrauterine growth (Isaacs, 2013). Intrauterine growth restriction has been associated with lower IQ, academic underachievement, reduced social skills, and behavioral problems such as attention deficit and hyperactivity disorder. Although it seems clear that nutrition plays a role in the genesis of brain tissue abnormalities, the effects of other contributing factors, such as dysfunction of fetal-placental perfusion leading to hypoxia and acidosis in fetal circulation, cannot be excluded in these children (Von Beckerath et al., 2013).

Recent advances in perinatal and neonatal intensive care have led to an increase in the survival of preterm extremely low birth weight infants, although undernutrition occurs frequently during hospitalization in these infants. Undernutrition in extremely low birth weight infants is associated with extrauterine growth restriction and other adverse outcomes, such as bronchopulmonary dysplasia, sepsis, and neurodevelopmental impairment. Preterm infants with extremely low birth weight can encounter cognitive problems such as poorer school performance, behavioral and learning problems, and deficits in higher order neurocognitive functions. Studies in preterm infants have shown that those fed high nutrient

383

BOX 47-1 Nutrition and Brain Development

EFFECTS OF MALNUTRITION ON THE DEVELOPING BRAIN

- Reduction in brain volume
- Sparing of cortical neurons
- Increased cell packing
- Disruption of cortical pyramidal cells
- Reduction in cortical dendritic spines
- Decrease in width of cortical neurons
- Decreased dendritic branching in cortex
- Reduced number of cortical glial cells
- Reduced number of cortical synapses
- Reduced number of synaptic reactive zones

EFFECTS OF RESTORING NUTRITION ON REVERSIBILITY OF BRAIN LESIONS

- Increase in brain weight and volume: "catch-up" head growth
- Prolongation of period of mitotic activity
- Prolongation of period of protein synthesis
- Reversal of cell packing
- Reduced cortical glial cell density
- Persistence of reduced number of cortical dendrites and synaptic spines
- Persistence of reduced myelination
- Increase in number of mitochondria in neurons
- Increase in synaptic density

(Modified from Levitsky, D.A., Strupp, B.J., 1995. Malnutrition and the brain: changing concepts, changing concerns. J. Nutr. 125, 2212S.)

---

formulae have larger brain volumes and a better performance in intelligence tests.

The effects of breastfeeding have also been studied. Increasing the percentage of breast milk in the early diet of preterm infants increases the amount of white matter relative to gray and has also been associated with better performance in intelligence tests (Isaacs, 2013; Hsiao et al., 2014). Thus early administration of optimal postnatal nutrition can help to prevent neurodevelopmental impairment in preterm infants, but up to 75% of extremely premature infants do not receive the recommended nutrition and develop extrauterine growth retardation (Hsiao et al., 2014).

The limit of viability for preterm infants is around the 23rd to 24th week of gestation. Thus nutritional deficits in preterm infants will be introduced earlier during development compared with intrauterine growth restricted children. Therefore in preterm infants differences are observed mainly in the white matter, whereas intrauterine growth restricted children tend to show differences in gray matter structures (Isaacs, 2013). White-matter injury is the most common pattern of brain injury after preterm birth.

The third trimester of gestation is critical for brain development, especially for white-matter structures. During this period, preoligodendroglial progenitors differentiate to mature myelin-producing oligodendrocytes, axons develop and form connections, and neurons proliferate and migrate to the cortex and deep nuclear gray-matter structures. The main pathogenic mechanisms of white-matter injury are inflammation and ischemia. Both activate the microglia, which leads to release of free radicals and proinflammatory cytokines,

---

TABLE 47-1 Important Nutrients During Late Fetal and Neonatal Brain Development

Nutrient	Brain Requirement for Nutrient	Described Brain Abnormalities or Disorders
Protein-energy	Cell proliferation, cell differentiation Synaptogenesis Growth factor synthesis	Global Cortex Hippocampus
Iron	Myelin Monoamine synthesis Neuronal and glial energy metabolism	White matter Striatal-frontal Hippocampal-frontal
Zinc	DNA synthesis Neurotransmitter release	Autonomic nervous system Hippocampus, cerebellum
Copper	Neurotransmitter synthesis, neuronal and glial energy metabolism, antioxidant activity	Cerebellum
LC-PUFAs	Synaptogenesis Myelin	Eye Cortex
Choline	Neurotransmitter synthesis DNA methylation Myelin synthesis	Global Hippocampus White matter
Iodine	Cerebral development Cerebellar development	Reduced brain weight, including cerebellum Reduced number of neurons in cerebrum, cerebellum, and brainstem Increased thickness of cerebellar external germinal layer Regional increases in neuronal density in cerebral hemisphere and decreased in synaptic counts visual cortex
Vitamin A	Regulation of gene and protein expression controlling neural growth and differentiation Regulion of patterning of neural tube development Modulion of neurogenesis, neural survival, and synaptic plasticity	Hydrocephalus Microcephaly Retinal and optic nerve defects
Vitamin B_{12}	DNA synthesis Formation and maintenance of myelin sheaths Neurotransmitter synthesis	White-matter degenerative lesions in brain, spinal cord, and peripheral nerves Spinal cord posterior and lateral column involvement

LC-PUFAs, long-chain polyunsaturated fatty acids.
(Adapted from Georgieff, M.K., 2007. Nutrition and the developing brain: nutrient priorities and measurement. Am. J. Clin. Nutr. 85, 614S–620S.)

ultimately resulting in degeneration of preoligodendrocytes. As a consequence there is a failure in the differentiation of preoligodendrocytes into mature myelinating oligodendrocytes, and hypomyelination occurs.

Perinatal infection, which is frequent in preterm infants in intensive care units, has been recognized as an important risk factor for white-matter injury. Infection leads to systemic inflammation, and it is often associated with hemodynamic instability with reduced brain flow, which subsequently potentiates the two main pathogenic mechanisms of white-matter injury previously mentioned. Nutrition in preterm infants not only influences brain growth and maturation, but nutritional supplements that would reduce systemic infections and attenuate inflammation could also protect the brain against injury in this period of high vulnerability. There are some specific nutrients such as glutamine and probiotics that may be of interest as potential neuroprotective agents for preterm infants. Probiotics have shown to improve gut mucosal barrier integrity, regulate adequate bacterial colonization, enhance intestinal innate immune response, and modulate intestinal inflammation, which results in a reduction of necrotizing enterocolitis, bacterial translocation, and inflammation.

Although probiotics have failed to improve neurodevelopmental outcomes, they may attenuate white-matter injury because of a favorable alteration of the immune response, resulting in less inflammation (Hsiao et al., 2014). In addition, they may be able to produce beneficial effects through the recently described microbiome–gut–brain axis. The exact mechanisms by which the gut microbiome modulates brain development are not yet clear, but the immune system seems to play a key role. Glutamine supplementation has also been shown to reduce the risk of serious neonatal infections and systemic inflammation, thereby leading to a reduction of white-matter injury. The mechanism through which glutamine enteral supplementation exerts its effects is yet to be unraveled. The postulated benefits of these nutritional supplements warrant further investigation.

Studies have shown that animals may recover from periods of undernutrition. However, if stunting continues during the entire period of cell replication, there is a persistent reduction in cell numbers, irrespective of the diet subsequently provided. Evidence of recovery in humans is less direct. An adequate calorie and protein intake certainly ends the insult, but it is not clear whether supplements always improve brain function, as genetic and environmental factors play a role in the potential for recovery. Studies evaluating the relationship between nutrition and cognition that took into account the social environment demonstrated that both factors are significantly correlated with cognitive performance. In interventional studies, both treatments, nutrition, or psychosocial stimulation alone seem to improve cognition. Combined treatments are the most effective at preventing large losses of potential cognitive performance, however, with greater effect the earlier the treatment begins. Some authors have stated that malnourished children have less energy to explore their environment and take advantage of opportunities for social contacts and learning processes; thus an unstimulating home environment can exacerbate the effects of malnutrition.

There is evidence that in developing countries clinical deficiencies in nutrition affect the structure and long-term functioning of children's brains. These clinically evident deficiencies are less likely to occur in industrialized countries, where a balanced diet is generally available. In industrialized countries, special attention should be paid to preterm children and those with intrauterine restricted growth who are often nutritionally deprived during critical stages of brain development. Concern should also be focused on those children with malabsorption, metabolic diseases, or increased demands of nutrients caused by underlying pathologies, as well as on those receiving vegan diets.

MICRONUTRIENTS

There is widespread belief that micronutrient intake in industrialized countries is deficient because of changes in nutritional habits. Some studies conclude that in general average intake of nutrients is above reference nutrient intakes, but it is often marginal for some micronutrients, such as iron, folic acid, and vitamins D and B_{12}. Whether such a marginal intake is a matter of concern remains under discussion. In industrialized countries, it is therefore necessary to distinguish those whose diets are deficient from those with minor inadequacies.

All nutrients are important for neuronal growth and development, but certain nutrients have greater effects on brain development than others do. Fetal and neonatal malnutrition can have global or circuit-specific effects on the developing brain given that some nutrients influence a specific brain area preferentially. Each of these nutrients has generated a wide range of research literature examining their relation with the brain.

Minerals

Iron

Iron deficiency is the most prevalent nutritional deficiency in the world. Over 30% of the world's population is anemic, and iron deficiency is the most common cause of anemia. It is prevalent not only in developing countries but also in industrialized countries, and children and women are the most commonly affected. This raises concern, as both isolated iron deficiency and iron deficiency anemia are thought to adversely influence neurodevelopment and behavior. Some of the consequences of developmental delay associated with iron deficiency are decreased motor development, lower IQ, and difficulties with learning and memory. Furthermore, the adverse effects of iron deficiency occurring in the first 6 to 12 months of life are likely to persist even if iron intake is subsequently normalized. In older children, iron deficiency has been related with poorer social-emotional development and problems of sustained attention, which can be reversed by an adequate supply of iron.

Brain tissue is overall rich in iron with concentrations differing according to brain region and stage of development. Some areas—like the cortex, hippocampus, and striatum—are more sensitive to iron deficiency than others. Iron accumulates in the brain during prenatal development. Given the poor bioavailability of iron in human milk, these iron stores in the brain are paramount in the first 6 months of life when infants are unable to regulate iron transport across the blood–brain barrier. Afterward, the brain is able to fully regulate iron entry into the brain even during periods of iron deficiency. The brain's need for and usage of iron does not end during the perinatal period and infancy; the adult brain still requires an adequate supply of iron (Radlowski and Johnson, 2013).

Studies in animals have shown that iron deficiency inhibits neurogenesis in the hippocampus, which provides a basis for behavioral deficits associated with perinatal iron deficiency. Iron homeostasis is critical for the expression of neurotrophic factors that support brain development. These neurotrophic factors influence not only neurogenesis but also neuronal morphology, dendritic outgrowth, and spine density and geometry, which are crucial for cell function. Iron deficiency also affects synaptic plasticity and severely affects myelination (Radlowski and Johnson, 2013). Moreover, iron is essential for neuronal metabolism and the enzymes involved in the synthesis of some neurotransmitters, including serotonin, dopamine, and norepinephrine. Dopamine is important for regulating cognition and emotion, reward and pleasure, movement, and hormone release. Serotonin in highly implicated in neurodevelopmental disorders such as autism, anxiety, and depression (Radlowski and Johnson, 2013).

Although an unequivocal relationship between iron deficiency and neurologic development has yet to be established, it is important to prevent it. Preterm infants and those born to mothers with anemia, diabetes, hypertension with intrauterine growth restriction, and multiple gestations are at risk of developing iron deficiency, as these circumstances lower fetal iron stores. Dietary recommendations for preterm infants are for an elemental iron intake of 2 to 4 mg/kg/day to a maximum of 15 mg/d by 1 month of age and extending through 12 months of age, with the exception of those who received multiple transfusions in which the need of iron supplementation should be assessed. Iron-fortified formulas provide sufficient iron to meet these requirements, but breastfed preterm infants should be supplemented. Healthy term infants usually have sufficient iron stores until 4 to 6 months of age, and the small amount of iron in human milk is enough for exclusively breastfed infants.

Exclusive breastfeeding after the age of 6 months is associated with an increased risk of iron deficiency anemia. Therefore, for exclusively breastfeed term infants, supplementation of 1 mg/kg/day is recommended starting from the fourth month until an appropriate iron intake is achieved with complementary food. Term formula-fed infants do not need any dietary supplementation, as iron requirements can be met for the first 12 months by standard infant formulas containing 12 mg/L iron and the introduction of iron-containing complementary foods at 4 to 6 months. After this age, iron needs can be achieved by consumption of iron-rich foods. Only those children not receiving the recommended iron intake in the diet will require supplementation.

Zinc

Zinc is an essential nutrient with multiple roles. It is involved in the activity of more than 200 enzymes and plays a fundamental role in the synthesis of proteins and nucleic acids. It is involved in gene expression, cellular division and development, and in the growth and function of many organs, including the central nervous system. Severe zinc deficiency during pregnancy has been associated with fetal losses and congenital malformations. Animal studies regarding the central nervous system have shown that zinc deficiency during early development results in adverse effects on brain structure and function. Zinc deficiency alters autonomic nervous system regulation and hippocampal and cerebellar development. There are no conclusive data on humans about the effects of zinc deficiency on neurologic development, but some studies have suggested an association with decreased cognitive and motor function as well as behavioral problems (Gogia and Sachdev, 2012).

Severe zinc deficiency is rare in humans, but mild to moderate depletion appears to be quite prevalent. In the last half of pregnancy when fetal growth is rapid, there is an additional need for 0.6 mg zinc daily. The United Nations International Children's Emergency Fund (UNICEF) recommends that all pregnant women in developing countries use multiple micronutrient supplements that include zinc.

Iodine

Iodine deficiency is the leading preventable cause of mental retardation worldwide. Iodine is essential for the production of thyroid hormones, for normal growth, and for brain development. In chronic severe iodine deficiency, thyroid hormone synthesis is reduced. A severe iodine deficiency during critical periods of brain development will result in irreversible brain damage and is associated with both physical and mental impairments. The most serious consequence of iodine deficiency is cretinism, which is characterized by severe, irreversible alterations in brain development resulting in profound mental retardation and neurologic signs including deafness, impaired language development, abnormal eye movements, and motor disorders.

Iodine deficiency early in life is associated with a loss of 6.9 to 10.2 IQ points in those who do not develop cretinism, which is estimated to be 5% to 15% of those noncretinous children with severe iodine deficiency (Bougma et al., 2013). Thyroid hormone-dependent neurodevelopment begins in the second half of the first trimester, but it is not until the beginning of the second trimester that the fetal thyroid begins to produce hormones. Even then, the reserves of the fetal gland are low, and it does not fully mature until birth. Thus the fetus is dependent on maternal production of thyroid hormones for brain development until birth. It is therefore important to keep an adequate intake of iodine during pregnancy, when a 50% increase in maternal intake is recommended to produce enough thyroid hormones to meet maternal and fetal requirements.

Adequate thyroid hormone for ongoing neurodevelopment remains critical after birth. Newborn intrathyroidal iodine stores are limited to approximately 300 µg, and thyroid hormone requirements for the developing infant are at their highest compared with subsequent growth periods. All this makes newborns and infants particularly vulnerable to iodine deficiency. Prevention of iodine deficiency by iodization of salt has helped to alleviate endemic cretinism, but attention is now turning to the adverse effects of moderate and mild iodine deficiency. In general, it seems that maternal thyroid metabolism can cope with mild iodine deficiency, such that the mother can sufficiently supply the infant with thyroid hormones. Although the developing brain is the most severely affected if iodine is deficient, chronic hypothyroidism also can have effects across all ages. Iodine deficiency has a negative effect on cognitive performance of school-age children, but supplementation of moderately iodine-deficient school children improves cognitive and motor functions, showing that the effects of iodine deficiency later in life are at least partially reversible.

Iodine deficiency is still one of the most common micronutrient deficiencies in the world. Iodine is naturally present in seawater and in the soil, and the iodine content of the soil determines its content in vegetables, milk, and eggs. Fish, seafood, and algae are good sources of iodine. Prevention of iodine deficiency is easily managed by iodization of salt, but it is still present in some regions of the world. Recommended dietary iodine intake in pregnant women is 250 µg/day. Whether routine iodine supplementation should be recommended to pregnant women in areas of mild-to-moderate iodine deficiency remains uncertain. Iodine requirements for newborns have been set at 15 µg/kg/day at term and 30 µg/kg/day for preterm infants. An intake of 130 µg/day is recommended during the second half of the first year of life.

Exclusively breastfed infants rely entirely on maternal iodine intake to meet their requirements. Commercially prepared formulas contain iodine, but its amount varies worldwide. In addition, iodized salt is discouraged in home-prepared complementary foods for infants. International organizations recommend the universal use of iodized salt to prevent iodine deficiency. In countries with severely iodine-deficient populations, single annual doses of iodized oil may be administered to lactating mothers or weaning infants as a strategy for achieving recommended iodine intakes.

Vitamins

Vitamins are organic compounds required by mammals in small amounts to sustain normal metabolism. They must be supplied from exogenous sources because they cannot be synthesized endogenously. Nutritional vitamin deficiency remains a public health problem in developing countries and among the poor worldwide.

Folate

Folic acid is a B vitamin that plays and important role in cell proliferation, brain cell repair, and appropriate epigenetic expression of the genome. Folate is believed to be involved in cell division by means of its influence on nucleic acid synthesis, which is necessary for DNA integrity and replication and amino acids synthesis. During pregnancy the rate of cell division increases dramatically, and folate demand increases beyond maternal requirements. It is therefore essential for growth and necessary for normal development of the fetal spine, brain, and skull, in particular during the first 4 weeks of pregnancy.

There is widespread evidence that both periconceptional folic acid supplementation and high maternal folate concentrations reduce the risk of neural tube defects, including spina bifida and anencephaly. These congenital malformations of the brain and spinal cord result from failure of normal developmental processes involving failure of the neural tube to close properly during the first trimester of gestation, in particular during the third and fourth week of pregnancy (Benton, 2012). The exact mechanism by which folate supplementation prevents neural tube defects remains unknown. Maternal folate levels have also been related to better performance of their children in tests assessing memory, reasoning, attention, and visual–spatial and verbal abilities. Little attention has been given to folate nutritional deficiency later in the course of pregnancy. Folic acid supplementation may also have beneficial effects on cognitive development and preventive effects on neurodevelopmental disorders such as language delay, autism spectrum disorders, and schizophrenia.

The main sources of folate in the diet are vegetables, legumes, and milk. Pregnant women are at risk for folate insufficiency because of the increased need of folate for rapid fetal growth, placental development, and enlargement of the uterus. Generally, reports on average dietary folate intake in pregnant or childbearing women all over the world show low folate intakes compared with the recommendation of 400 µg/day. Neural tube defects occur during the third and fourth week of pregnancy, before a mother becomes aware that she is pregnant. The risk is reduced when women take daily folic acid supplements 3 months before considering pregnancy and continuing up to the sixth week of pregnancy. These recommendations have led some countries to include folic acid food fortification, which has greatly reduced the incidence of spina bifida. Therefore all women of childbearing age are recommended to take a folic acid supplement of 400–800 µg/day, preferably at least a month before conceiving.

Cobalamin (Vitamin B_{12})

Vitamin B_{12} deficiency during pregnancy has been related to adverse fetal and neonatal outcomes such as neural tube defects and delayed defects, delayed myelination, or demyelination. There is evidence that decreased maternal serum levels of vitamin B_{12} in humans are associated with an increased risk of neural tube defects, regardless of folic acid supplementation of the diet.

Most of the data regarding vitamin B_{12} deficiency in infancy are from case studies of infants born to mothers who were not treated for pernicious anemia or infants who were exclusively breastfeed by mothers on vegan or vegetarian diets. The deficiency results in irritability, anorexia, lethargy, and retarded neurodevelopment. Neuroimaging techniques have also shown severe brain atrophy and retarded myelination in vitamin B_{12}-deprived children. After therapy, recovery has been reported to be variable, with recovery of brain structures but brain function remaining delayed in some children. Later in life, poorer measures of intelligence, memory, and frontal lobe function have been reported in adolescents who as children had received vegan diets and who subsequently ate omnivorous or vegetarian diets (Benton, 2012; Black, 2008).

The mechanisms underlying the action of vitamin B_{12} are unclear. Cobalamin deficiency leads to functional folate deficiency because folate cannot be transformed into its active tetrahydrofolate form. Deficiency of folate and cobalamin results in similar biochemical effects; cobalamin deficiency may contribute this way to the development of neural tube defects. It is also involved in fatty acid metabolism and therefore the maintenance of periaxonal myelination, which occurs from midgestation through the second year of life and continues to and during puberty. It influences the speed of nerve conduction and may in this way influence cognitive development. Some other possible mechanisms include its role in the inflammatory process, altering the balance of neurotrophic and neurotoxic cytokines, affecting the S-adenosylmethionine: S-adenosylhomocysteine ratio, and increasing the accumulation of lactate in brain cells (Benton, 2012; Black, 2008).

Provision of vitamin B_{12} is therefore essential for pregnant and breastfeeding mothers and infants. During pregnancy, serum vitamin B_{12} concentrations in the mother decline, and they are concentrated in the placenta and transferred to the fetus down a concentration gradient, with newborn vitamin B_{12} concentrations approximately double those of the mother. The total vitamin B_{12} requirements of the fetus are estimated to be 50 µg, whereas maternal stores in well-nourished women are estimated at greater than 1000 µg. Thus body stores are adequate to meet fetal needs during gestation.

During pregnancy, vitamin B_{12} is stored in the fetal liver, so that infants whose mothers are well supplied with vitamin B_{12} are born with a supply sufficient for the first several months. An increased risk of vitamin B_{12} deficiency is associated with dietary deficiencies with low consumption of animal-source foods, as occurs with strict vegan or vegetarian diets or alternatively with impaired B_{12} vitamin absorption. The recommended dietary allowance (RDA) for vitamin B_{12} in pregnancy is 2.6 µg/day, 0.2 µg/day greater than the RDA for nonpregnant women and adolescents.

Vitamin D

Vitamin D has recently been considered a neurosteroid and is thought to have a role in brain development and function. The role of vitamin D in the brain is not yet known, but research in recent years has yielded considerable evidence supporting this hypothesis. The major metabolites of vitamin D are present in human cerebrospinal fluid, and the enzymes involved in the conversion of vitamin D are present in the brain. In addition, vitamin D receptors are expressed throughout the human brain. All these findings indicate that vitamin D, like other neurosteroids, may play a role in brain function. Vitamin D receptors appear early in the fetal brain and increase in number during gestation, which may indicate that vitamin D is involved in neurologic development (Benton, 2012).

It has been proposed, but not proven, that low levels of vitamin D during pregnancy and infancy could increase the risk of neurodevelopmental disorders and psychiatric problems such as schizophrenia and autism.

Although it is found in some foods, exposure to sunlight is the greatest source of vitamin D. Changes in lifestyle, including less exposure to the sun and obesity, lead to vitamin D insufficiency in industrialized countries. The vitamin D RDA for women, including during pregnancy, has been recently established at 600 IU per day. Breastfed infants are at high risk of vitamin D deficiency because of the low levels of this vitamin in breast milk. Therefore all breastfed infants should receive a daily vitamin D supplement of 400 IU beginning in the first few days of life.

Other Vitamins

Some other vitamins have been related to neurologic development, although evidence is still scarce and the possible mechanisms of action need to be elucidated.

Vitamin A is a member of the family of nuclear steroid transcription regulators, and as such, exerts transcriptional control over genes and proteins in different tissues, including genes that control neural differentiation, and plays an important role in neuromodulation. Retinoic acid is a signaling molecule in the brain of growing and adult animals, and retinoid receptors have been found in the hippocampus of rats, which plays a role in memory. Dietary vitamin A deficiency is globally one of the most common forms of malnutrition, with clinical manifestations including ocular disorders, immunosuppression, and impaired growth. It plays a critical role in visual function, and a deficiency continues to be a major cause of infantile blindness in some developing countries. The role of vitamin A on the human brain is poorly understood, but it has been suggested that it influences memory and sleep and plays a role in depression and Parkinson and Alzheimer diseases. The effects of vitamin A deficiency are more likely to be observed in developing than in industrialized countries, where variations in vitamin intake within the normal range may not have functional implications (Benton, 2012).

Thiamine (vitamin B_1) has an important role in nerve conduction and the synthesis of the neurotransmitter acetylcholine. Studies in animals have noted that thiamine-dependent enzymes play an important role in establishing adult patterns of brain energy metabolism and myelin synthesis. Thiamine requirements are enhanced during pregnancy and lactation, especially in the third trimester when thiamine is preferentially taken up by the fetus. Data from a single study have related thiamine dietary supplementation in children with better intelligence scores, visual acuity, faster reactions times, and better memory. Thiamine deficiency during pregnancy has long-lasting consequences for cognitive development, but this effect has not been demonstrated for subclinical deficiencies (Benton, 2012). Clinical manifestations of dietary thiamine deficiency (beriberi) primarily affect the cardiovascular and nervous systems.

Pyridoxine (vitamin B_6) is a coenzyme necessary for the production of various amino acid neurotransmitters, including serotonin and noradrenaline. Its deficiency has been associated with irritability, seizures, and peripheral neuropathy in children. Infantile seizures caused by dietary B_6 deficiency are rare and may be seen in developing countries. Furthermore, pyridoxine dependency has been recognized in some types of epilepsy and pediatric neurotransmitter diseases. Studies in animals have shown structural and functional impairments in the hippocampus in subjects that are prenatally vitamin B_6 deficient. Some other studies have reported an association between vitamin B_6 and autism, although recent reviews did not have conclusive results. The influence of vitamin B_6 supplementation during pregnancy on neurologic development

has been recently reviewed, but there is insufficient evidence at this time to recommend supplementation (Benton, 2012).

Choline is the precursor of the neurotransmitter acetylcholine, and it is a precursor for phospholipids that are constituents of cell membranes and the methyl donor betaine. Plasma levels of choline are high in the newborn, which suggests an important functional role. During pregnancy it is critical for brain development as it influences stem cell proliferation and apoptosis, thereby altering brain structure and function (Benton, 2012). Although it is accepted that choline plays a role in brain development, there is to date no evidence that adding choline to the diet improves cognitive development.

Long-Chain Polyunsaturated Fatty Acids

The most frequently studied nutrients have been long-chain polyunsaturated fatty acids (LC-PUFA). LC-PUFA have important structural and metabolic functions in the human body. The two major LC-PUFA synthesized in the human body are docosahexaenoic acid (DHA) and arachidonic acid (AA). Mammals are unable to synthesize polyunsaturated fatty acids, thus their precursor essential fatty acids, linoleic acid (LA) and linolenic acid (ALA), must be obtained from the diet. The most abundant fatty acid in cell membranes is DHA. It is present in all organs but it is particularly abundant in neural tissues such as the brain and retina.

Lipids constitute approximately 50% to 60% of human brain dry weight; about 35% of the lipids are polyunsaturated fatty acids, and most of them are LC-PUFA. From the beginning of the third trimester of life to 2 years of postnatal age there is enrichment in the relative content of DHA in the brain. Fatty acids in the brain can either be taken up from the blood as preformed DHA or synthesized from ALA inside the brain. Several hypotheses have been proposed to explain the role of DHA in the brain, which in general can be divided into properties conferred by lipid-bound DHA in the membrane bilayer and those related to unesterified DHA. Changes in membrane DHA content can alter membrane physicochemical properties and also affect the signal transduction pathway and neurotransmission. The high proportion of DHA in neural membranes also raises the possibility that n-3 LC-PUFA deficiency may impair membrane biogenesis, influencing neurogenesis, neuronal migration, and outgrowth. Unesterified DHA has a role in regulating gene expression which is influencing stem cell differentiation to neurons and ion channel activity. It can also be further metabolized to neuroprotective metabolites in the brain, and it has been suggested that it has an important role in neurogenesis. Thus n-3 fatty acid deprivation may affect brain development at multiple levels, with the effects and potential for recovery differing depending on when the deficiency occurs.

The effects of LC-PUFA on neurodevelopment outcome have been widely studied. In premature births, the umbilical transfer of LC-PUFA is interrupted, thus preterm infants have lower LC-PUFA concentrations than full-term infants. The beneficial effects of adding LC-PUFA to preterm formulas have shown conflicting results with regard to neurodevelopment. Several studies have demonstrated improvements in electroretinogram activity, visual acuity, and short-term global developmental outcome, but recent meta-analysis has shown no clear long-term benefits for preterm infants receiving LC-PUFA supplemented formula on pooling results (Campoy et al., 2012).

However, an inappropriate supply of lipids in preterm infants has been reported to lead to biochemical deficiency of essential fatty acids, causing reduced body and brain weight (Hsiao et al., 2014). Meta-analysis of the effects of LC-PUFA in term infants or during pregnancy and early infancy conclude that there is insufficient evidence to affirm that supplementation exerts a clear and consistent benefit (Campoy et al., 2012). Trials are normally conducted in developed countries with relatively healthy infants, thus they should receive adequate DHA transplacentally and in breast milk. The benefits of supplementation on neurodevelopment might be more pronounced in undernourished children. Furthermore, recent evidence shows that n-3 LC-PUFA supplementation is effective for improving behavioral problems such as attention deficit/hyperactivity disorder (Hsiao et al., 2014).

The main natural source of LA and ALA are vegetable oils, particularly safflower and corn oils. AA and DHA are not found in plants, but are synthesized by animals. Only small mammals accumulate a high proportion of them. Meat and eggs are rich sources of AA but not DHA. Marine food is rich in n-3 PUFA as algae are the primary producers of DHA and EPA in the ecosystem. Fish are therefore rich in DHA. Western diets are characterized by low n-3 fatty acids intakes and high amounts of n-6 fatty acids; as a result, EPA and DHA demands are not adequately supplied. The exclusion of fish and meat from the diet can result in very low intakes of DHA. Before birth, DHA is transported to the fetus from the mother across the placenta, and after birth the infant is provided with DHA in breast milk. Therefore pregnant and lactating mothers should receive an average DHA intake of at least 200 mg/day, which means a consumption of two servings of fish weekly.

It is unreasonable to expect that micronutrients examined in isolation will be associated with differences in cognitive functioning. Brain function is the result of millions of metabolic processes in which nutrients act in combination. Furthermore, a diet deficient in one component is also likely to be poor in others. A multivitamin and mineral approach is probably more beneficial in terms of cognitive development.

It is widely accepted that an insufficient intake of calories, proteins, and micronutrients at critical stages of brain development can produce irreversible changes in brain structure and consequently reduce cognitive capacity for life. There is controversy concerning the effects of dietary supplementation in infants who are well fed, however; it is likely that only those children who are poorly nourished respond to nutritional interventions. Further research is necessary to address this question.

REFERENCES

The complete list of references for this chapter is available in the e-book at www.expertconsult.com.
    See inside cover for registration details.

SELECTED REFERENCES

Benton, D., 2012. Vitamins and neural and cognitive developmental outcomes in children. Proc. Nutr. Soc. 71, 14–26.

Black, M.M., 2008. Effects of vitamin B12 and folate deficiency on brain development in children. Food Nutr. Bull. 29, 126S–131S.

Bougma, K., Aboud, F.E., Harding, K.B., et al., 2013. Iodine and mental development of children 5 years old and under: a systematic review and metaanalysis. Nutrients 5, 1384–1416.

Campoy, C., Escolano-Margarit, M.V., Anjos, T., et al., 2012. Omega 3 fatty acids on child growth, visual acuity and neurodevelopment. Br. J. Nutr. 107, 85S–106S.

Gogia, S., Sachdev, H.S., 2012. Zinc supplementation for mental and motor development in children (Review). Cochrane Database Syst. Rev. 12.

Hsiao, C.C., Tsai, M.L., Chen, C.C., et al., 2014. Early optimal nutrition improves neurodevelopmental outcomes for very preterm infants. Nutr. Rev. 72, 532–540.

Isaacs, E.B., 2013. Neuroimaging, a new tool for investigating the effects of early diet on cognitive and brain development. Front. Hum. Neurosci. 7, 445.

Laus, M.F., Vales, L.D., Costa, T.M., et al., 2011. Early postnatal protein-calorie malnutrition and cognition: a review of human and animal studies. Int. J. Environ. Res. Public Health 8, 590–612.

Radlowski, E.C., Johnson, R.W., 2013. Perinatal iron deficiency and neurocognitive development. Front. Hum. Neurosci. 23, 585.

Von Beckerath, A.K., Kollmann, M., Rotky-Fast, C., et al., 2013. Perinatal complications and long-term neurodevelopmental outcome of infants with intrauterine growth restriction. Am. J. Obstet. Gynecol. 208, 130 e1–130 e6.

48 The Neuronal Ceroid Lipofuscinosis Disorders

Joseph Glykys and Katherine B. Sims

An expanded version of this chapter is available on www.expertconsult.com. See inside cover for registration details.

INTRODUCTION

The neuronal ceroid lipofuscinosis (NCL) disorders are a group of genetically inherited lysosomal neurodegenerative diseases characterized by the intracellular accumulation of autofluorescent lipopigment storage material that causes progressive neurologic degeneration in all age groups. The clinical course includes progressive dementia, seizures, progressive visual failure (except in the adult-onset forms), and often movement abnormalities.

Collectively, these disorders are the most common cause of an inherited childhood neurodegenerative disease and are increasingly recognized in late-onset or adult-onset forms. Prevalence is estimated widely from 1.5 to 9 per million, and incidence, which varies among geographic ethnic regions, has been reported from 1.3 to 7 in 100,000 live births. The clinically relevant pathobiology affects primarily the central nervous system and may include, in variant fashion, cognitive failure (dementia, encephalopathy), seizures that often are myoclonic, movement abnormalities that are often ataxic or extrapyramidal in nature, and visual failure. Retinal degeneration and visual failure are rare in the adult forms of these diseases.

This group of genetic disorders has an autosomal recessive inheritance, except the rare autosomal dominant adult-onset disorder. Summaries of NCL disorder mutations and relationship to clinical features have been published.

HISTORICAL CLINICAL CHARACTERIZATION
Nomenclature

Historically, these disorders were characterized by clinical age of onset and pathologic hallmarks of lysosomal deposition. The individual disorders were initially given names honoring those who first identified the clinical spectrum in narrow ethnic populations and in reference to age of onset. The classic clinical distinction was therefore infantile (INCL), late-infantile (LINCL), juvenile (JNCL), and late-onset or adult (ANCL; Kufs). The terminology is confusing because it was established before many clinical variants or disorders were defined and before the identification of the etiologic genes. Classification by age of onset is still useful in clinical evaluation. Atypical forms with variable ages of onset are well described. Distinguishing these disorders by genetic etiology is now currently favored and serves the study of disease-specific pathobiology (Table 48-1).

The term "Batten disease" was originally used to honor the clinician that first recognized this disease in the juvenile-onset form. Although historically incorrect when applied to all the NCL disorders, this designation is a simple and practical one and has been universally adopted and accepted by family groups, private foundations, and U.S. government agencies.

Clinical Description and Characterization

The first clinical description of NCL was that of the juvenile form in a small Norwegian family. This was soon followed by clinical and pathologic descriptions of familial cases within a larger population of so called "amaurotic family idiocy" by Batten, Vogt, Spielmeyer, and Sjögren. A detailed historical summary of the lives and work of these early and seminal clinician researchers has been published.

Significant interfamilial variability in phenotype, in many of the early described NCL cases, gave challenge to a unifying classification. Originally, the NCL disorders were grouped among the sphingolipidosis and the more global clinical characterization as "amaurotic idiocy." The term "neuronal ceroid lipofuscinosis" was introduced by Zeman and Dyken in 1969, referencing primarily the common pathologic feature of these disorders. Earlier investigators had difficulty distinguishing whether these were single disorders or related ones. But by collection, observation, and report of familial cases, five types of NCLs were eventually clinically characterized: congenital, infantile, late infantile, juvenile, and adult onset.

The congenital form was first clinically described by Norman and Wood in 1941 and later associated with cathepsin D deficiency in congenital school-age or adult forms. This NCL has been designated CLN10 (CTSD).

The infantile form (INCL; CLN1; Santavuori-Haltia) was clinically described by Hagberg in 1968 and then by Haltia and Santavuori in 1973. Although originally described as infantile in onset, late-infantile, juvenile, and adult forms have been reported. The underlying cause of CLN1, palmitoyl protein thioesterase 1 deficiency, was identified by linkage and fine molecular mapping.

The classic late-infantile (LINCL; CLN2; Jansky-Bielschowsky) form was originally described in patients by Jansky in 1908 and Bielschowsky in 1913. Cases were reported throughout the 1970s with typical clinical presentation and disease course. The underlying cause of CLN2, tripeptidyl-peptidase deficiency, was identified by protein study. Clinical correlation with genotype has been reported, although the phenotype continues to be expanded. Other nonclassic late-infantile clinical disorders have been described, including variant late-infantile and early-juvenile forms due to defects in the CLN5 gene in patients first described clinically in 1991 and in *CLN6*, CLN7 (MFSD8), and CLN8. A possible CLN9 form has been described that is clinically similar to the juvenile form, although no unique associated genetic locus has been yet identified and the originally reported two sibships have been later shown to have CLN5 disease.

The classic juvenile form (JNCL; CLN3; Batten disease) is the most prevalent and characteristic of the NCL disorders. Juvenile, other than CLN3 disease, and early adult-onset forms have been recently characterized by clinical features and molecular gene identification. The adult-onset disorder, later

TABLE 48-1 NCL Disorders

Disease	Prior Designation	OMIM #	Inherit	Gene	Protein	Usual Age of Onset	Clinical Phenotype	Early Symptoms and Signs [in Order of Usual Appearance]	Usual Survival	EM Inclusions	Imaging	EEG
CLN1	INCL Santovouri-Haltia	256730	AR	*PPT1*	Palmitoyl protein thioesterase 1 [PPT1]	6–24 mo	Classic infantile	Developmental failure, seizures, myoclonus, visual failure	2–9 yr	GROD	Microcephaly; increase periventricular white matter signal. Alter thalamic signal. Cerebral atrophy	Lack of sleep spindles. Absence of attenuation in amplitude when opening eyes by the ages of 16–24 months. Gradual loss of amplitude. EEG isoelectric by around 3 years of age
						2–4 yr	Late-infantile	Developmental regression, seizures, visual failure	5–12 yr +	GROD		
						4–6 yr	Early childhood	Visual failure, seizures, behavioral, dementia	10–20 yr	GROD		
						18 yr +	Juvenile–early adult	Psychiatric, cognitive decline, depression; ataxia, parkinsonism, visual loss	50 yr +	GROD	Cerebral and cerebellar atrophy	
CLN2	cLINCL Jansky-Bielschowsky	204500	AR	*TPP1*	Tripeptidyl peptidase 1 [TPP1]	2–4 yr	Classic late infantile	Malignant seizures, myoclonus, developmental regression, visual failure	6–12 yr +	CL	Cerebral and cerebellar atrophy	Characteristic giant occipital polyspike-spike discharges in response to a single flash of light or to low-frequency, repetitive stimulation
	SCAR7	607998			TPP1 [partial deficiency]	childhood–young adult	Juvenile–adult	Ataxia, cerebellar signs [pyramidal signs] no visual loss	Adulthood	Negative	Cerebellar and pons atrophy	
CLN3	JNCL Spielmeyer-Sjogren	204200	AR	*CLN3*	CLN3	3–8 yr	Classic juvenile	Visual failure, cognitive decline, behavioral and motor difficulties; late seizures	20–40 yr	Vacuolated lymphs, FP (CL, RL)	Cerebral and cerebellar atrophy	Large-amplitude spike and slow-wave complexes by around 9 years
CLN4	Kufs [Parry type]	162350	AD	*DNAJC5*	Cysteine-string protein alpha [CSPα]	teenage–30 yr +	Juvenile–adult	Behavior issues, dementia, seizures, myoclonus, no visual loss	30–40 yr +	GROD (CL, RL, FP)	Cortical atrophy is usually found. Some patients show cerebellar atrophy.	Severely abnormal with generalized or bilateral independent periodic epileptiform discharges
CLN5	fLINCL (1)	256731	AR	*CLN5*	CLN5	3–7 yr	Variant late infantile	Behavior abnormalities, cognitive decline, seizures, visual failure, myoclonus, motor abnormalities	10–30 yr	FP, CL (RL)	Cerebellar atrophy	Posterior spikes to low-frequency photic stimulation
						4–9 yr	Juvenile	Visual failure, motor loss, myoclonus, seizures	Teenage +	FP, CL	‡	
						17 yr	Adult	Motor loss, cognitive regression, visual loss, myoclonus, seizures	Teen–30 yr +	GROD, FP (CL, RL)	‡	

Continued on following page

TABLE 48-1 NCL Disorders *(Continued)*

Disease	Prior Designation	OMIM #	Inherit	Gene	Protein	Usual Age of Onset	Clinical Phenotype	Early Symptoms and Signs [in Order of Usual Appearance]	Usual Survival	EM Inclusions	Imaging	EEG
CLN6	vLINCL(2)	601780	AR	CLN6	CLN6	2–5 yr	Variant late infantile	Seizures, motor and cognitive decline, visual failure, myoclonus	20s	FP, CL, RL	Cerebral and cerebellar atrophy	
	Kufs type A	204300				16–50 yr	Adult-onset	Myoclonic epilepsy, ataxia, dementia, no visual loss	40 yr +	GROD (FP)	‡	
CLN7	vLINCL(3)	610951	AR	MFSD8	MFSD8	18 mo–6 yr	Variant late infantile	Developmental delay, visual failure, seizures, dementia, myoclonus	Teenage +	FP, RL (CL)	Cerebellar atrophy (late)	
						11 yr	Juvenile	Visual failure, motor loss, seizures, ataxia, dementia	40 yr +	?		
CLN8	EPMR	610003	AR	CLN8	CLN8	5–10 yr	Northern epilepsy	Seizures, slow dementia without visual loss	40 yr +	Not reported	Cerebral and cerebellar atrophy	
	vLINCL	600143				2–7 yr	Variant late infantile	Myoclonus->myoclonic seizures, ataxia, cognitive decline, visual loss	Teenage +	FP (CL, GROD)	Cerebral & cerebellar atrophy	
CLN9	reclassified as CLN5**	609055	AR				Juvenile	Classic CLN3 phenotype		CL, FP, GROD		
CLN10	CNCL	610127	AR	CTSD	Cathepsin D	Neonatal	Congenital	Epileptic encephalopathy, microcephaly	< 1 yr	GROD	Microcephaly, general atrophy	
						1st decade	Juvenile-adult	Ataxia, visual loss, regression	Teenage +	GROD	Cerebral & cerebellar atrophy	
CLN11	Kufs type A	614706	AR	GRN	Progranulin	Early 20s	Adult	Visual failure, myclonic seizures, ataxia, dementia	30 +	FP	Cerebellar atrophy	
	FTLD-GRN	607485	AD			35–65 yr	Adult	Myoclonic seizures, ataxia, cognitive decline	50 yr +	TDP-43		
CLN12	Kufor-Rakeb PARK 9	606693	AR	ATP13A2	P-type ATPase	8–12 yr	Juvenile	Parkinsonism, ataxia, dementia no visual loss	30 yr +	FP, vacuolated lymphs	Generalized & brainstem atrophy; Basal ganglia iron accumulation	
CLN13	Kufs type B	615362	AR	CTSF	Cathepsin F	20–30 yr	Adult	Tremor, ataxia, pyramidal/extrapyramidal, dementia, seizures (rare)	40–50 yr 40s–50s	FP [brain]	Diffuse cerebral atrophy	
CLN14	EPM3	611725	AR	KCTD7	K+ channel tetramerization domain-7	8–9 mo	Infantile	Seizures, motor and speech regression, visual failure	Teenage	RL (GROD)	Cerebral & cerebellar atrophy	
		611726	AR			10 mo–3 yr	Late-infantile	Without visual loss	Unknown	None	Cerebral & cerebellar atrophy. Nonspecific white matter lesions	

GROD = granular osmophilic deposits CL = curvilinear bodies
FP = fingerprint profiles RL = rectilinear inclusions
*Kollmann 2013
**Haddad 2012
‡few cases only

1. Variant initially described in Finnish
2. Formally Lake Cavanagh early juvenile NCL variant and Indian-variant late-infantile NCL
3. Formally Turkish variant

termed Kufs disease in honor of the early clinician who recognized this disorder in 1925, is an autosomal recessive form of early-onset dementia with seizures, with or without movement abnormalities, but without vision loss. An autosomal dominant adult-onset form (Kufs, Parry-type) was much later described. Sporadic late-onset cases have since been reported and collectively are grouped as Kufs disease. These include the autosomal dominant form CLN4 associated with DNAJC5, autosomal recessive CLN11 disease, associated with GRN mutations, and with phenotypic overlap with frontotemporal dementia (FTLD-GRN) and CLN12, also termed Kufor-Rakeb or PARK9, associated with mutation in the *ATP13A2* gene. Smith and colleagues also described a late-onset form of NCL, termed CLN13 and associated with mutation in *CTSF*. A late-onset form of CLN6 disease has also been described.

Molecular genetic technologies, studies in families, and sporadic cases eventually have led to a NCL disorder classification based on gene mutation (Table 48-1). Although this allows separation into distinct genotypes, there is much evidence that the NCL genes may participate in interrelated pathways and in an overlapping pathobiology. There is increasing recognition of a broad clinical phenotypic scope of each of these genetic forms, with reports of increased intrafamilial variability and of atypical cases. It is presumed that there are important epigenetic modulators to be identified that directly or indirectly affect clinical expression within any one of these genetically defined disorders.

In addition to observational clinical case and familial reports, formal assessment tools have been developed and validated. Published and utilized in clinical study are those for infantile and late-infantile forms, Hamburg scale, Weil-Cornell scale, and for juvenile CLN3 (UBDRS) scale. These are important instruments for the study of the natural history and for clinical trial efficacy measurements.

Although the classic clinical features, if all present, (encephalopathy/dementia, seizures, visual loss ± movement disorder) clearly point to a NCL disorder, there is broad and important differential diagnosis which needs consideration. This may, in fact, account for the sometimes long delay in diagnosis. There are many NCL masqueraders particularly in the early stages of disease when only a single clinical feature is evident (Table 48-2).

Molecular Genetics

Molecular genetic study of NCL-like patients has allowed for the identification of etiologic genes in clinically identified forms, including congenital, late-infantile, juvenile, and adult-onset. Currently 13 genetic loci are identified in association with human NCL disease (Table 48-1).

The first NCL genes were identified in 1995 for the infantile-onset form (INCL; CLN1), encoding the soluble lysosomal protein palmitoyl protein thioesterase 1 (PPT1) and the *CLN3* gene, responsible for the juvenile form (JNCL) reported by a NCL consortium. This was followed by identification of the late-infantile, classic form (cLINCL; CLN2) gene, encoding the soluble lysosomal protein tripeptidyl peptidase 1 (TPP1) in 1997. Variant late-infantile forms have subsequently been identified and include CLN5, CLN6, CLN7, CLN8, and CLN14 (KCTD7). The later has more commonly been described in association with progressive myoclonic epilepsy without documented NCL-like visual failure or pathologic inclusions. A primarily congenital-onset form CLN10 (CTSD) was identified although later onset cases have been described. The genetic etiology of late adult-onset NCL disorders has been identified among the cohort of both sporadic and familial cases by whole exome sequencing. Genetic loci include one autosomal dominant inherited form CLN4 (DNAJC5) reported simulta-

neously by a number of groups as well as in an autosomal recessive pattern in CLN11, CLN12, and CLN13. As there are cases that, by clinical history and pathologic features, appear to be NCL-like, it is presumed that more genetic loci will be identified in the future. Continued elaboration of a widening phenotypic spectrum, for many of these disorders, is also ongoing.

An updated mutation database of all NCL disorders is maintained at the University College of London by Sara Mole (www.ucl.ac.uk/ncl), and publication of mutation spectrum and phenotypic correlations has expanded our understanding of these disorders.

Pathology

Early pathologic description of storage material in patient tissues documented an autofluorescent, waxy, dusky lipid accumulation in neuronal endosomes, reminiscent of the aging pigment lipofuscin. This led to the term neuronal ceroid lipofuscinosis being applied to these neurodegenerative disorders. By electron microscopy, these pathologic hallmarks are membrane-bound (lysosomal) inclusions most prominently seen in neurons but recognizable in many cell types. Common sites of biopsy and inclusion identification include the skin, conjunctiva, and/or rectal tissues. Inclusions can appear as granular osmophilic deposits (GRODs), curvilinear (CL), rectilinear (RL), or as more crystalline fingerprint bodies (FP) (Fig. 48-1). Unique to juvenile CLN3 disease are the vacuoles seen by EM in circulating lymphocytes. These ultrastructural crystalline structures have remained an important distinguishing feature of the NCL disorders. Identification of this storage material, by biopsy and EM, strongly suggests an NCL diagnosis. Unfortunately, peripheral tissue biopsy may be negative, as is particularly true in the late-onset forms of NCL. In many of these cases, however, central nervous system storage has been demonstrated. Lipopigment accumulation is presumed to alter lysosomal function, lead to autophagy disruption, and/or cellular oxidative damage.

Lysosomal storage of saposins A and D in CLN1 and subunit *c* of the mitochondrial ATP synthase in CLN2, CLN3, and adult-onset forms are most likely epiphenomenon, or secondary markers, and not disease-specific markers of the primary underlying molecular pathology. Neuronal loss in brain, predominantly in cerebral and cerebellar cortices, and retina, is also characteristic of the NCL disorders, although the underlying biology of this cell loss is not yet clear.

Pathobiology

The pathobiologic details are still being elaborated. In the NCL disorders, there is protein deficiency, pathway blockade, and metabolic substrate accumulation, as well as downstream functional deficiencies and potentially detrimental cellular compensatory changes, which may lead to cellular pathobiology and the resultant clinical phenotypes. Active research is ongoing to elucidate the protein functions, the substrates and interacting partners of these proteins, the mechanisms of neuronal death, and the relationships between the various NCL proteins. Affected intracellular pathways involve at least the endosomal-lysosomal autophagy degradation pathways, the synaptic trafficking and function pathways, and the neuroinflammation/immune regulation pathways (Fig. 48-2).

CLN1 and CLN2 are caused by deficiency and metabolic block of the classic soluble lysosomal hydrolases PPT1 and TPP1, respectively. Mitochondrial abnormalities in the NCL disorders have also been described, including abnormal mitochondrial ATP synthase regulation, mitochondrial structural changes, and altered respiratory chain function, as well

TABLE 48-2 NCL Masqueraders

Neuronal Ceroid Lipofuscinosis	Clinical Features	Differential Diagnosis
CLN10 (Congenital)	IUGR In utero seizures Spasticity Central apnea Microcephaly	Infant from untreated PKU mother Hypoxic-ischemic encephalopathy Nonketotic hyperglycinemia Untreated aminoaciduria Untreated organic aciduria Sulfite oxidase deficiency Serine synthesis defects GLUT1 deficiency syndrome Cerebral folate deficiency
CLN1 (INCL)	Head circumference deceleration Rapid progressive loss motor skills, speech loss Vision loss—optic atrophy Involution of retinal vessels, no RP Hyperkinesis Myoclonus Seizures	Sialidosis Cerebral folate deficiency Biopterin defects Peroxisomal disorders Rett syndrome GLUT1 deficiency syndrome Niemann-Pick disease type A and B GM2 gangliosidoses Biotinidase deficiency Pyruvate dehydrogenase complex deficiency Lactate dehydrogenase deficiency Mitochondrial cytopathies Alpers disease 3-methylglutaconic aciduria Neuroaxonal dystrophy Pelizaeus-Merzbacher disease
CLN2 (cLINCL)	Motor decline/clumsiness Seizures, often intractable Myoclonus Axial hypotonia/spasticity	Gangliosidosis (GM1, GM2) Mucopolysaccharidoses (without dysmorphism) Leukoencephalopathies; Leukodystrophies Folate receptor defect Neuroaxonal dystrophy Biotin-responsive basal ganglia disease Mucolipidosis IV Krabbe disease Congenital disorders of glycosylation Schindler disease Myoclonic epilepsy with ragged-red fibers Niemann-Pick type C Sialidosis type 1 3-methylglutaconic aciduria L-2 hydroxyglutamic aciduria Smith-Lemli-Opitz syndrome Succinyl-semialdehyde dehydrogenase deficiency Gaucher disease type III Epileptic encephalopathy vLINCL (CLN5, CLN6, CLN7, CLN8)
CLN3 (JNCL)	Visual failure/RP Behavioral problems Progressive cognitive decline Retinitis pigmentosa Cone-rod dystrophies	Late-onset CLN1, CLN2, CLN10 Pantothenate kinase-associated neurodegeneration; NBAI Niemann-Pick type C Gaucher disease type III Metachromatic leukodystrophy X-Adrenoleukodystrophy MERRF/ETC abnormalities/mito cytopathies Krabbe disease Late-onset GM2, (GM1) Giant axonal neuropathy Cerebrotendinous Xanthomatosis Sanfilippo type A (SGSH; MPSIIIA) Juvenile Huntington disease Neuroferritinopathy Lafora disease Wilson disease Peroxisomal disorders Gyrate atrophy with hyperornithinemia Refsum disease Congenital disorders of glycosylation Cone-rod dystrophy Bardet-Biedl syndrome Joubert syndrome Juvenile nephronopthisis Alström syndrome Spinocerebellar Ataxia type 7 Alport syndrome

TABLE 48-2 NCL Masqueraders *(Continued)*

Neuronal Ceroid Lipofuscinosis	Clinical Features	Differential Diagnosis
CLN11, CLN12, CLN13 (ANCL)	Behavioral disturbances Dementia Ataxia/movement disorder [with or without seizures]	Early onset Alzheimer disease, Parkinson disease Frontotemporal dementia Late-onset lysosomal disorders: GM2, Metachromatic leukodystrophy Early onset Alzheimer disease due to PSEN1 mutations Lafora disease Unverricht-Lundborg myoclonic epilepsy Myoclonic epilepsy with ragged-red fibers (MERRF) Dentatorubral-pallidoluysian atrophy Familial Encephalopathy with neuroserpin inclusions bodies Sanfilippo A (SGSH; MPSIIIA) Niemann-Pick type C Krabbe disease

MERRF: Myoclonic epilepsy with ragged-red fibers
NBIA: Neurodegeneration with brain iron accumulation
ETC: Electron transport chain
MPSIII: Mucopolysaccharidosis type IIIA

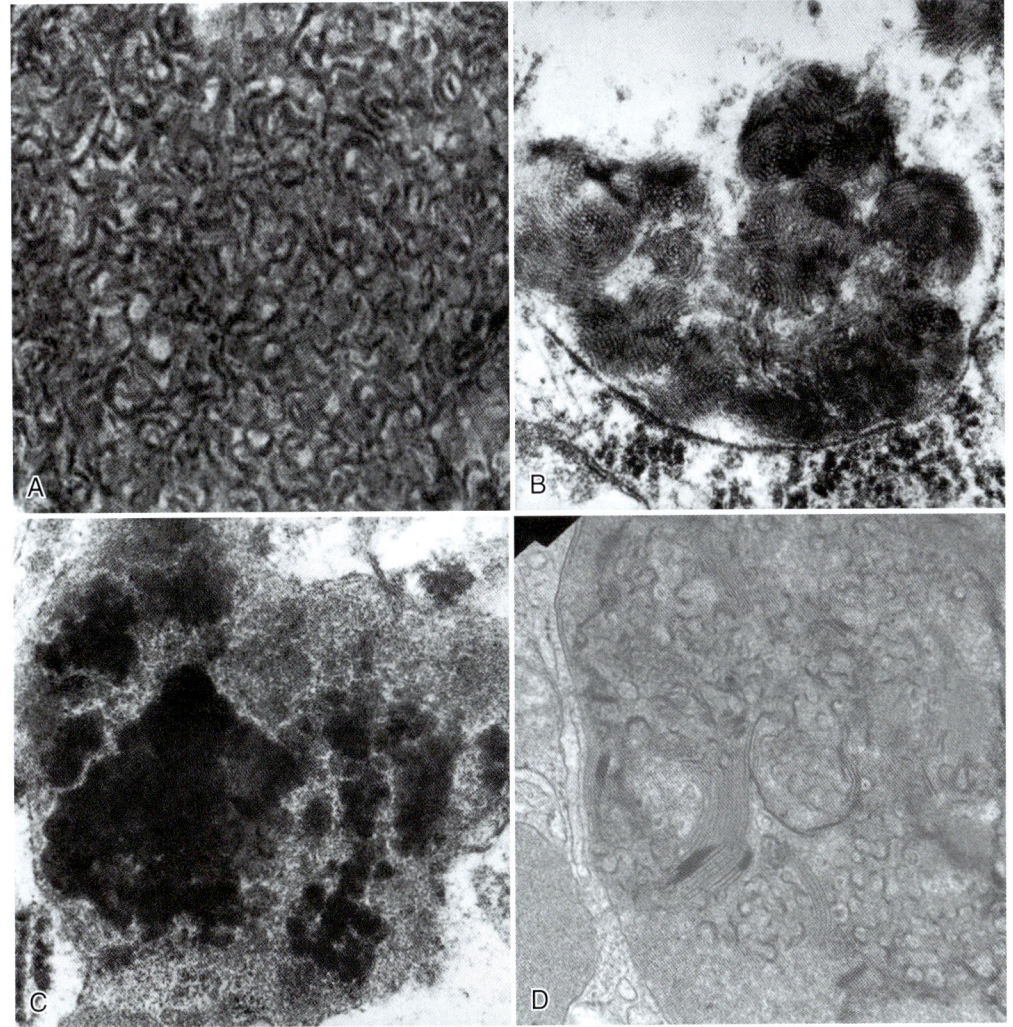

Figure 48-1. EM photomicrographs of typical inclusion patterns. **A,** Curvilinear inclusions. **B,** Fingerprint inclusions. **C,** Granular osmophilic deposits (GRODS). **D,** Rectilinear bodies.

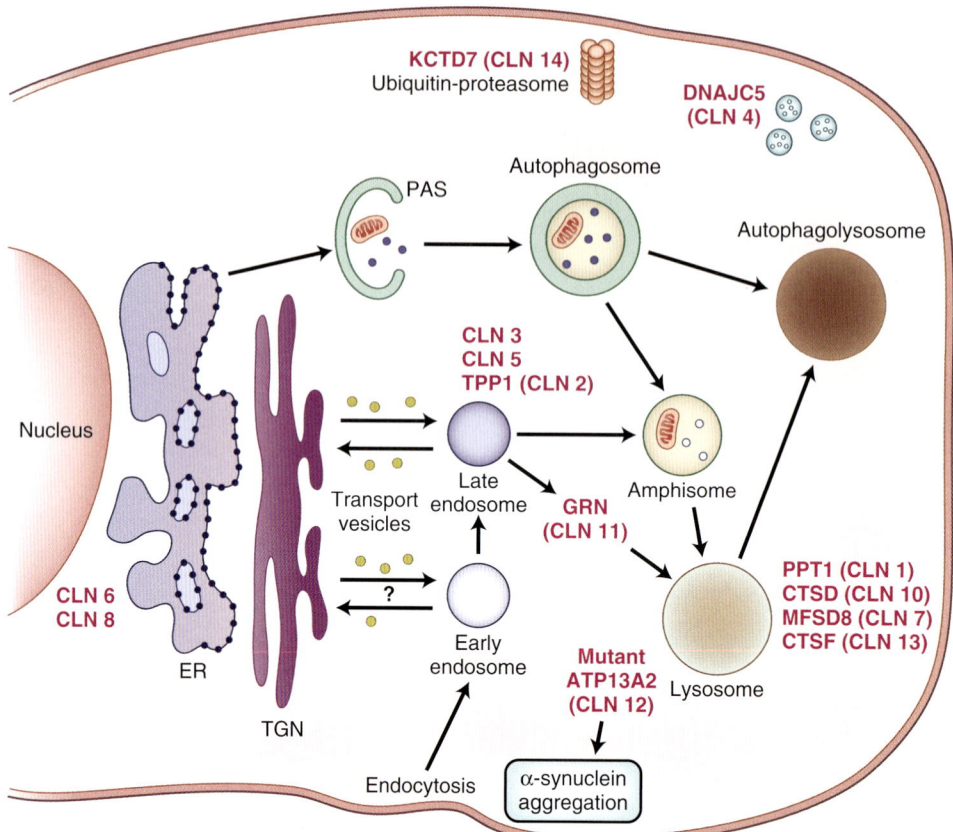

Figure 48-2. NCL protein localization. Endosomal-lysosomal and autophagy-lysosomal pathway convergence. PAS: pre-autophagosomal structure. ER: endoplasmic reticulum. TGN: *trans* Golgi network.

as decreased cellular ATP production and neuronal survival in the context of oxidative stress. Mitochondrial dysfunction appears linked to cytoskeleton-mediated presynaptic inhibition in the homozygous CLN3 knockout mouse. Altered mitophagy as a result of NCL-defective autophagy or increased vulnerability to metabolic stress may play a role in the NCL cellular pathobiology associated with the increased oxidative stress and decreased neuronal survival seen in these disorders. Recently human induced pluripotent stem cells (iPSCs) models of CLN2 and CLN3 have been shown to have mitochondrial structural abnormalities, increase mitochondrial ATPase subunit *c*, in addition to abnormalities in structure and function seen in Golgi, ER, and endosomal-lysosomal compartments.

Altered biometal homeostasis and deregulation has also been noted in the NCL disorders. The cellular mechanisms, which may be a secondary phenomenon in the NCL disorders, have yet to be fully elaborated. CLN5 glycosylation defects have been noted and may be further evidence of the widespread and complex secondary cellular pathobiology. Current studies, focusing on the complex endosomal-lysosomal autophagy pathway, continue to highlight potential network disruptions in these disorders. Specific gene mutations may trigger distinct processes that converge on a common cellular pathway as has been shown in CLN6 and CLN3 murine models. Alternatively, there may be direct and specific interactions between these proteins as has been documented between CLN2, CLN3, and CLN5. These studies speak to the nonindependent nature of these pathways and serve to challenge or models of pathobiology and therapeutic intervention.

NCL Models and Clinical Trials

Animal models, both naturally occurring and those produced by genetic technologies, have been utilized in the pathobiologic study of many of the NCL disorders. The spontaneous models include many large animals (dogs, sheep, cattle, cats, and goats). Even unicellular and simple animals have yielded NCL models, including those in yeast, *C. elegans* and *Drosophila*. The technologies for generating iPSCs lines from human fibroblasts and the techniques being developed that allow for reprogrammed cell-phenotypic differentiation have invaluably changed the ability to make human model systems for these disorders. Recent report of success in generating human iPSCs as models of CLN1 and CLN3 has been reported and allows for study of the endocytic pathway.

Therapeutic approaches to the NCL disorders have included enzyme replacement, gene and stem cell delivery, and pharmacologic therapies.

Diagnosis

The diagnostic approach has changed through the years and will continue to evolve as panels and whole exome/whole genome technologies and bioinformatics improve. One approach to diagnose NCLs, based on the age of presentation, can be found on Figure 48-3. Skin biopsy is still useful when the initial screen for common CLN disorders is negative or when genetic testing is not as readily available as ultramicroscopic techniques. Sequential evaluation of NCL genes based on age of presentation was the common approach. However, the introduction of panels, especially epilepsy panels, makes the latter more time and cost efficient. False negative assay results must be taken into consideration given current next-generation sequencing efficacy. As a general approach, when a patient presents with refractory epilepsy and/or signs/symptoms concerning for a NCL disorder, performing an epilepsy panel that has several NCL genes included is a good strategy. Current epilepsy panels in the United States involve more than 70 genes known to cause epilepsy, including almost all the NCL ones. If successful, this allows an expedited diagnosis of an NCL disorder (avoiding expensive sequential gene testing) or the identification of a non-NCL gene that explains and can guide treatment/counseling of the epilepsy of the patient. Whole exome sequencing (WES) will play an increasingly prominent role in NCL patient identification, particularly in atypical cases.

CLN1 (PPT1; OMIM #256730)
Clinical Description

The typical presentation is of an infantile onset disorder presenting at around 10 to 18 months of age and characterized by profound neurodevelopmental regression with motoric deterioration, seizures, and visual failure. The course of the disease is rapidly progressive and leads to an early vegetative state with prominent spasticity. The children usually die within the first 10 years of life.

There is often microcephaly that may have been evident at birth. Visual impairment can be seen at around 1 year of age and there is blindness by 2 years of age. Optic atrophy, thinned retinal vessels, and a discolored, brownish macula are seen funduscopically. Commonly, myoclonic jerks appear after the first year, and many develop generalized seizures. Hand-knitting movements similar to Rett syndrome are observed early but disappear by 2 years of age. At 3 years of age, children are bedridden, hypotonic, irritable, and spastic. At 5 years of age, severe flexion contractures, acne, hirsutism, and rarely, precocious puberty are observed. Children with CLN1 have hypothermia and bradycardia risk especially during anesthesia. Most children die between the ages of 7 and 13 years.

Other Presentations

- Later presentation similar to the variant late-infantile onset. Onset is between 1.5 and 3 years. The main features are behavioral disturbances and cognitive decline. Myoclonic jerks are the most prominent paroxysmal phenomenon. Neurologic regression was associated with shrinkage of cortical structures.
- Juvenile form is similar to CLN3 but differs as learning problems present initially rather than visual problems and with regression of acquired skills at an earlier age. In a reported case, Behavioral problems followed by vision changes started at 6 years of age and was followed by isolated myoclonic jerks in arms. Seizures appeared at 17 years of age as well as ataxia and intermittent delusions. Another juvenile form presented in an 8-year-old boy with progressive vision loss followed by cognitive and behavior problems. No seizures have been reported.
- An adult presentation, starting after 18 years of age, has been described with mood changes and declining academic performance followed by vision changes (including visual hallucinations). Extrapyramidal syndrome (hypokinesia, bradykinesia, rigidity), an unstable flexed posture, and cerebellar ataxia has also been reported in two French

sisters. Frank seizures have not been reported up to now. Electroencephalography (EEG) showed generalized reduced activity without periodic abnormalities. The progression has been slow.

Genetics and Pathology

The genetic defect is in the palmitoyl protein thioesterase 1 (PPT1) gene, which encodes a soluble lysosomal enzyme (*PPT1*). The function of this lysosomal thioesterase is to remove fatty acids attached in thioester linkages to cysteine residues in proteins. Proteins containing the fatty acylated cysteine residues are usually found at the inner plasma membrane leaflet. PPT1 is located in the lysosome and taken up in a mannose-6 phosphate-dependent manner. PPT1 has also been shown to be localized in synaptic vesicles in neurons. PTT1 deficiency has been implicated in the disruption of the lysosome-endosomal pathway and in other cellular processes, including endocytosis, vesicular trafficking, synaptic function, lipid metabolism, neural specification, and axon connectivity. PPT1 deficiency seems to be involved in cell susceptibility to apoptotic cell death, in abnormalities in the number, intracellular localization, pattern and morphology of mitochondria, as well as defects in the mitochondrial enzyme activities and adaptive energy metabolism. The accumulation of sphingolipid activator proteins A and D (SAPs) in storage cytosomes is probably a secondary phenomenon.

Definitive Diagnosis: PPT1 enzyme analysis with identification of confirmatory *PPT1* mutations. For further details of diagnostic evaluation, see Table 48-1 and Figure 48-3.

CLN2 (TPP1; OMIM #204500)
Clinical Description

CLN2 disease, in its classic form, has an onset between 2 and 4 years of age with epilepsy being the initial symptom in most cases. Seizures can be generalized tonic-clonic, focal, absence, and/or myoclonic (most prominent in the face). Thereafter, there is decline in motor skills, often with ataxia and deterioration of speech and language. Sometimes slowing of developmental milestones is evident before the onset of seizures. Visual loss begins often by the fourth year of life and is slowly progressive. Some patients may retain some visual function during the first decade. An early hypotonia is replaced with severe spasticity with flexion contractures. Autoregulation of vascular tone is lost, resulting in mottled, cold hands and feet and hypothalamic involvement leads to temperature instability. Hyperthermia often leads to unnecessary fever evaluation for infectious cause. Copious secretions and shallow breathing due to poor chest wall excursions often lead to pneumonias. Most children are nonambulatory and mute by 5 years of age, totally dependent of caregivers and need g-tube support when swallowing becomes problematic. Sepsis and uncontrollable seizures are frequently the cause of death at the end of the first decade or in the early teens.

Other Presentations

- An infantile form of CLN2 has been described with onset before the first year of life. In one case, the patient had microcephaly and hypotonia noted at the fourth month of life with impairment of motor and language abilities. By 4 years of life, the patient developed signs and symptoms of progressive myoclonic encephalopathy along with motor and cognitive deterioration.

- A slowly progressive autosomal recessive spinocerebellar ataxia with childhood onset, referred to as SCAR7 (OMIM #609270) has been described.
- A juvenile form of CLN2 disease has been described with disease onset between 6 and 10 years and a protracted phenotype. In one case epilepsy was absent.

Genetics and Pathology

CLN2 is caused by defects in a pepstatin-insensitive lysosomal tripeptidyl peptidase (TPP1) that normally removes tripeptides from the amino terminus of proteins. This protein is a soluble lysosomal hydrolase that is transported to the lysosome by a mannose 6-phosphate receptor mediated pathway. The in vivo substrates of this protein are not fully known, but TTP1 has been reported to initiate degradation of subunit c of the mitochondrial ATPase protein. In CLN2 human disease, the gene mutations are primarily missense ones. They are predicted, based on analysis of the CLN2 protein crystal structure, to disrupt folding and to lead to protein instability and degradation.

Definitive Diagnosis: TPP1 enzyme analysis with identification of confirmatory *TPP1* pathologic mutations. For further details of diagnostic evaluation, see Table 48-1 and Figure 48-3.

CLN3 (CLN3; OMIM #204200)
Clinical Description

The juvenile form of NCL (JNCL), the most common form of this group of neurodegenerative disorders, is associated with mutations in the CLN3 gene. The first sign of the disease is decreased central vision caused by progressive retinal degeneration (retinitis pigmentosa) usually observed between 4 and 6 years of age. Initial clinical difficulties may be attributed to behavioral issues until the visual loss is recognized. These children are usually followed initially by ophthalmologists as normal children with retinitis pigmentosa who show better use of their peripheral vision. Patients become completely blind between 10 and 14 years of age but sometimes even later. Retinal findings can include macular retinal pigment epithelium atrophy, pigment stippling, bull's eye maculopathy, retinitis with the appearance of peripheral bone spicules, and variable disk pallor. Complete blindness is accompanied by a disturbed sleep-wake cycle and insomnia. There is slow cognitive regression that occurs during the initial years of this disorder. A subset of affected children may manifest difficult behavior between the ages of 7 and 9 years. There also can be a variety of behavioral symptoms, including anxiety, aggressive behavior, depression, and visual hallucinations. By at least 10 years of age, cognitive decline is noted. Epilepsy can start as early as 12 years of age, but usually seizures do not occur until 14 years of age. Seizures are primarily generalized tonic-clonic, but patients can also have focal and/or myoclonic seizures. Seizures are relatively easily to control until later stages of the disease. Speech is echolalic with perseveration of speech, and there is dysarthria usually after 15 years of age. Cogwheel rigidity is also present in the limbs, and patients walk with a stooped, shuffling gait reminiscent of patients with Parkinson disease. An intention tremor of variable severity is often observed. Patients generally plateau in their middle teens. A large number of patients become depressed and agitated, and a small number become aggressive and psychotic. Growth and physical maturity are not affected. Late-stage symptoms include drooling, difficulty swallowing, and weight loss. Temperature instability, with episodes of extreme hypothermia down to 92°F, alternating with hyperthermia, points to hypothalamic involvement. Some patients develop a cardiomyopathy or sick sinus syndrome with bradycardia. Most patients succumb in their early to mid-20s to seizures and cardiopulmonary arrest. A small number can survive into the fourth decade of life.

Other Presentations

- Variant forms of CLN3 disease are associated with a slower disease progression. In some cases, there may be a long silent period after initial visual failure, and patients may remain free of additional neurologic deficits even for decades.
- A complex syndrome characterized by autophagic vacuolar myopathy (AVM), hypertrophic cardiomyopathy, pigmentary retinal degeneration, and epilepsy has been described associated with p.Gly165Glu mutation in CLN3.
- Cases of retinitis pigmentosa and cone-rod dystrophy have been associated with CLN3 mutations.

Genetics and Pathology

A common 1.02-kb deletion accounts for 85% of disease alleles in the United States cohort and more than 93% of CLN3 cases carry at least one common 1.02-kb deletion allele. This suggests a founder effect. Deletion alleles are associated with production of prematurely truncated products. Compound heterozygous point mutation cases are rare. More than 60 mutations have been reported in the *CLN3* gene.

CLN3 is an endosomal/lysosomal transmembrane protein that seems to play a pivotal role in the late endosomal/lysosomal membrane transport system. In neuronal cells, a substantial fraction of CLN3 is additionally targeted to neuronal extensions and synaptosomes in which it has been found to reside in early endosomes, presynaptic vesicles, and in so far unidentified vesicles. CLN3 is highly conserved across species. Proposed functions of CLN3 include a possible role in lysosomal acidification, membrane fusion, vesicular transport, autophagy, apoptosis, proteolipid modification, lipid metabolism, mitochondrial abnormalities, and neurotransmission. Furthermore, CLN3 has been shown to interact with CLN5. CLN3 also appears to play a role in the actin/myosin-associated functions and the microtubular system.

Definitive Diagnosis: Molecular testing for the common *CLN3* deletion and, if necessary, full *CLN3* coding region sequence analysis. For further details of diagnostic evaluation, see Table 48-1 and Figure 48-3.

CLN4 (DNAJC5; AUTOSOMAL DOMINANT KUFS; OMIM #162350)

DNAJC5 encodes cysteine-string protein alpha (CSFα) and has been recently identified to cause adult-onset NCL disorder in five kindreds. These familial cases were previously well described with autosomal dominant inheritance.

Clinical Description

Symptoms usually start during the fourth decade with myoclonic seizures, dementia, and movement abnormalities. Visual function is preserved. In the Czechoslovakian proband, onset was at 30 years of age with myoclonic epilepsy, generalized tonic-clonic seizures, progressive dementia associated with depression, and early death at 37 years of age. Brain pathology documented autofluorescent storage material and

GRODS by electron microscopy. Skin biopsy did not evidence storage by ultrastructural examination. In the reported Parry family, the proband carrying the *DNAJC5* mutation (p.L116del) had a clinical history of irritability and obsessive behavior in mid-20s, seizure onset by 32 years of age, followed by gradual loss of memory and an ataxic gait. Normal ophthalmologic examination was noted up to 34 years of age. Other family members were variably affected by a progressive seizure disorder, ataxic gait, and/or progressive dementia, typically starting in the 20 to 30s.

Extended clinical characterization in 19 affected patients from three families was reported. Variable features of generalized of tonic-clonic seizures, myoclonus, ataxia, language dysfunction, and generalized dementia, parkinsonism, and early death were reported.

Genetics and Pathology

Two human *DNAJC5* mutations have been reported to date, p.L115R and p.L116del. These mutations occur in a highly conserved cysteine-string domain of CSFα. By in silico analysis, the identified human *DNAJC5* mutation (p.L116del) has been shown to significantly decrease CSFα membrane binding and lead to intracellular missorting. There is also predicted possible effect on palmitoylation and aggregation propensity. Other studies also support this pathobiology, as the mutants are mistargeted and form palmitoylation-induced membrane-bound aggregates. How these perturbations lead to the neurodegeneration and clinical phenotype seen in CLN4 disease remains unknown.

Definitive Diagnosis: Pathologic mutation identified by molecular sequencing of *DNAJC5*. For further details of diagnostic evaluation, see Table 48-1 and Figure 48-3.

CLN5 (CLN5; OMIM #256731)
Clinical Description

CLN5 disease can present as a variant late-infantile NCL. The usual age of onset is between 3 and 7 years, but juvenile and adult-onset cases have also been reported (see later in this chapter). Patients usually present with slight motor clumsiness and hypotonia followed by learning problems. Visual failure and blindness may also be an early sign and by the age of 7 to 9 years, there is significant optic atrophy. Seizures usually appear about age 9. Myoclonus is frequently observed and can appear earlier and independent of generalized or focal seizures. Behavioral problems seem to be infrequent. Ataxia and athetosis can occur later. Children lose the ability to ambulate by about 10 years of age, and death occurs between the ages of 14 and 32 years.

Other Presentations

- Juvenile onset: visual failure, loss of strength, and tremor in lower limbs starting between 4 and 9 years of age. Disease progression is relatively rapid evidencing behavioral changes, gradual loss of language, myoclonus and seizures, poorly responsive to valproate and clonazepam. There is then rapid progression with blindness and inability to ambulate. Behavioral disturbances and mental deterioration can also be presenting symptoms.
- Adult onset: One patient presented after 17 years of age with cognitive regression, followed by visual deterioration, seizures, and motor difficulties. Two Italian siblings presented in their mid-50s with difficulty walking, dysarthria, and progressive cognitive decline. They carried a homozygous mutation in CLN5.

- A congenital form presenting at 4 months of age has also been described.

Genetics and Pathology

The mutation spectrum is wide but at least 50% of the mutations cause a premature termination codon through small deletions, small insertions, or nonsense changes. There are more than 30 mutations described at this time. Although relatively broad in nature, the clinical phenotype is similar in the different mutation and ethnic groups.

The CLN5 protein is a soluble lysosomal glycoprotein that is targeted to the lysosome after cleavage from a pro form. The *CLN5* gene expression differs between neurons and glia. High expression in microglia and the very early microglial activation in *CLN5* deficient mice suggest a role for CLN5 in microglial function. The function of CLN5 is unknown. It appears to interact with many NCL proteins including PPT1, TPP1, CLN3, CLN6, and CLN8. PPT1 and CLN5 bind F1-ATPase in vitro, suggesting mitochondrial involvement or defects in lipid transport. A defective sphingolipid transport has also been demonstrated in peritoneal macrophages of the *CLN5* knockout mouse. CLN5 is required for the recruitment of Rab7 and subsequently of the retromer complex required for endosome-to-Golgi trafficking.

Definitive Diagnosis: Demonstration of pathologic mutations in *CLN5*. For further details of diagnostic evaluation, see Table 48-1 and Figure 48-3.

CLN6 (CLN6; OMIM #601780)
Clinical Description

CLN6 disease presents as other late-infantile variant forms of NCL. The clinical features are similar to the classic late infantile form of NCL. However, a significant proportion of patients have a slightly later onset and a more protracted course with seizures, ataxia, and myoclonus as the leading symptoms. The age of clinical onset of disease is broad with usual range between 2 to 5 years of age. Initial clinical features include motor delay and cerebellar findings of dysarthria and ataxia. Seizures (including myoclonic jerks) start in more than 50% of patients before 5 years of age. Visual failure occurred early in 50% of patients. This disease is rapidly progressive to a vegetative state.

Other Presentations

- Teenage-onset progressive myoclonus epilepsy: also associated with generalized tonic-clonic seizures and cognitive decline. No report of visual decline, motor weakness, movement disorders.
- Juvenile-onset cerebellar ataxia with seizures: Adolescents presented initially with action tremor, walking difficulty, and ataxia between 7 to 9 years of age. Dysarthria and nystagmus is also present. One patient had generalized tonic-clonic seizures. There was no blindness.
- Adult form: presenting from 16 to 62 years of age with a semiology consistent with Kufs type A or B. Type A patients usually present with seizures (progressive myoclonic and generalized tonic-clonic seizures) followed by dementia. Type B patients often present with dementia or psychosis with ataxia or other movement abnormalities. These patients have no vision changes.

Genetics and Pathology

The *CLN6* gene encodes a nonglycosylated membrane protein that is localized to the ER. Although the gene encodes a protein conserved among vertebrates, no functional or sequence homologies have been identified with other proteins. Biologic function and the human pathobiologic dysfunction are poorly understood. It has been postulated that CLN6 mediates selective transport of proteins or lipids that are essential for lysosomal function and acidification. The intracellular degradation of endocytosed proteins appear to be reduced which might be related to the finding of increased lysosomal pH in CLN6-defective fibroblasts. CLN6 also impairs both maturation and enzymatic activity of lysosomal hydrolases. In CLN6 disease, there is accumulation of autofluorescent lipopigments, subunit *c* of mitochondrial ATP synthase, free cholesterol and phosphosphingolipids and glycosphingolipids in lysosome derived storage bodies. CLN6 protein interacts with other proteins. It binds to CLN5 protein, and it interacts with the collapsing response mediator protein 2 (CRMP-2) that is involved in microtubule assembly and cytoskeletal dynamics during axonal outgrowth. CLN6 also appears to regulate genes involved in cholesterol homeostasis, extracellular matrix remodeling, cell signaling, and the immune/inflammatory responses. There have been more than 70 different mutations reported in the CLN6 gene.

Definitive Diagnosis: Identification of pathologic mutations in *CLN6* gene. For further details of diagnostic evaluation, see Table 48-1 and Figure 48-3.

CLN7 (MFSD8; OMIM #610951)
Clinical Description

This disorder was initially called the Turkish variant of late-infantile NCL as it was described in this ethnic group. It is now recognized to be panethnic as disease cases have been subsequently identified in many countries including Italy, Egypt, India, Croatia, Czech Republic, France, and Greece. This disease is hard to distinguish from other late infantile NCL forms (CLN2, CLN5, CLN6, or CLN8). Its onset is usually between 2 to 7 years of age. Initial symptoms are typically aggressive behavior and severe epilepsy in association with developmental regression. The clinical course is rapidly progressive with the appearance of myoclonus/clonic and nocturnal epilepsy, ataxia, dementia, and blindness. Some cases have presented with onset of visual failure and ataxia. There can be significant personality and behavioral changes as well as sleep disturbances. Rett-like onset and a clinical picture that includes midline stereotypic hands movements have been described. Death usually occurs in late childhood, but some patients survive until the second and third decade. Compared with classical CLN2 disease, CLN7 disease shows a somewhat later onset and a more severe seizure phenotype.

Other Presentations:

- Pure visual presentation: It has been shown that heterozygous missense variant mutation p.Glu336Gln in the *MFSD8* gene is associated with nonsyndromic autosomal recessive macular dystrophy with central cone involvement. Affected individuals showed no other neurologic features typical for variant late-infantile NCL. Age of diagnosis ranged from 27 to 57 years.
- Juvenile: One case has been described. The patient presented with visual failure at age 11 and showed a protracted clinical course. Motor impairment and seizures developed at 24 and 25 years of age, respectively, followed by ataxia at 28 years of age. Mental and speech regression were noticed at 30 and 36 years. Patient was still alive at 43 years of age and wheelchair bound.

Genetics and Pathology

The CLN7 protein is encoded by the *MFSD8* gene, which appears to be evolutionarily conserved. This protein is targeted to the lysosomes. Based on sequence homology analysis, CLN7 belongs to the major facilitator superfamily of transporters proteins and is presumed to function as a lysosomal membrane transporter. Its substrate specificity is not currently known. There have been more than 30 *MFSD8* mutations identified to date. Mutation analysis and biologic study seems to show that the primary consequence of the missense mutations is disturbed functional properties rather than altered subcellular localization.

Definitive Diagnosis: Genetic demonstration of pathologic mutations in *MFSD8*. For further details of diagnostic evaluation, see Tables 48-1 and Figure 48-3.

CLN8 (CLN8; OMIM #600143)
Clinical Description

CLN8 disease was first recognized in the Finnish population in a childhood epilepsy syndrome, designated northern epilepsy (NE) or progressive epilepsy with mental retardation (EPMR), when neuropathologic studies identified cytoplasmic autofluorescent storage typical of a NCL-like disorder. Initial symptoms are short, frequent, and drug resistant generalized tonic-clonic seizures as well as focal seizures, with onset between 5 and 10 years of age, and cognitive decline. Seizures increase until puberty, when epileptic activity starts to decline but does not remit. Cognitive decline starts 2 to 5 years after the onset of seizures. Intellectual decline is most rapid before adulthood leading to mental retardation by the age of 30 at the latest. After 30 years of age, the patients have difficulties with equilibrium, and they walk slowly using broad-based, small steps. The speech becomes dysphasic in some patients. During childhood and puberty almost half of the patients also suffer from behavioral problems such as irritability, restlessness, disobedience, and inattentiveness. Retinal degeneration, a characteristic finding in NCL, has not been reported in EPMR. However, decreased visual acuity has been detected in some EPMR patients without any obvious ocular abnormality. Age at death varies from 17 years to late middle age, but some survive into the fifth decade.

CLN8 disease can present as typical late-infantile variant NCL, showing an earlier onset and more rapidly progressive disease course than EPMR. Symptoms usually start around 2 to 7 years of age with developmental delay (motor and language) and then onset of myoclonic seizures and ataxia. There is rapid disease progression after the onset of disease, and by the age of 8 to 10 years there is severe disability and worsening epilepsy. Focal and generalized seizures as well as absence seizures may evolve, and seizures can become very difficult to control. Frequently, there are behavioral problems. Spasticity, tremors, and extrapyramidal movement abnormalities are common. By 10 years of age, most of the children are wheelchair bound.

Genetics and Pathology

Currently, there are more than 25 mutations in the CLN8 gene. The CLN8 protein is localized in the ER and the ER/Golgi intermediate compartment, and its normal function is unknown. An additional location outside of the ER has been suggested in polarized cells, including neurons. It has been postulated that the CLN8 protein may play a role in sensing, biosynthesis, and metabolism of lipids or protection of proteins from proteolysis as CLN8 is a member of the TLC

(TRAM-LAG1-CLN8) protein family. It is also thought that CLN8 protein may function as a protective sphingolipid sensor and/or in glycosphingolipid trafficking, in the synthesis and transport of lipids, vesicular/membrane trafficking, autophagy, and apoptosis.

Definitive Diagnosis: Identification of pathologic CLN8 mutations. For further details of diagnostic evaluation, see Table 48-1 and Figure 48-3.

CLN10 (CTSD; OMIM #610127)
Clinical Description

CLN10 disease seems, at this point, to be a rare disease. It has been primarily recognized as a congenital form of NCL, although severe late-infantile cases have been described. Clinically, these patients present at birth with microcephaly, respiratory failure, rigidity, and status epilepticus. Death occurs within hours to weeks after birth.

Other Presentations:

• Juvenile presentation: A reported patient first showed neurodegenerative symptoms of ataxia and visual disturbances at early school age. The ocular fundus showed retinitis pigmentosa, and brain MRI revealed cerebral and cerebellar atrophy. The patient developed progressive cognitive decline, loss of speech, retinal atrophy, and loss of motor functions. By 17 years of age, she was wheelchair bound and severely mentally retarded. Another juvenile phenotype (8 to 15 years of age at presentation) was reported in two consanguineous pedigrees. Clinical features included ataxia, retinitis pigmentosa, cognitive decline, and, in one case, cardiomyopathy. All had distinctive muscle pathology (granulovacuolar material in angular atrophic fibers) in addition to GRODs.

Genetics and Pathology

CLN10 disease is caused by CTSD mutations. The CTSD gene encodes the major lysosomal aspartic protease cathepsin D (CTSD). CTSD is transported to the lysosomes via a mannose-6-phosphate receptor-dependent and independent manner. CTSD is a lysosomal endopeptidase implicated in several specific physiologic functions, including proteolytic processing of selected polypeptides (hormones, growth factors, cytokines, and enzymes), presenting brain antigens, degradation of cytoskeletal proteins, regulation of autophagy, and apoptosis. CTSD has over 50 different interaction partners from various cellular compartments, suggesting involvement in multiple cellular functions. A number of substrates have been recognized in vitro, including prosaposin that can be cleaved into saposins A, B, C, and D. Saposins A and D are essential cofactors for some sphingolipid hydrolysis proteins. Currently there have been seven different *CTSD* mutations reported.

Definitive Diagnosis: CTSD enzyme analysis with identification of confirmatory CTSD pathologic mutations. For further details of diagnostic evaluation, see Table 48-1 and Figure 48-3.

CLN11 (GRN; OMIM #614706)
Clinical Description

A report of two siblings with an autosomal recessive late-onset neurodegenerative phenotype, lysosomal NCL-like inclusions, and homozygous progranulin (GRN) mutations established CLN11 as a variant phenotype-genotype from the loss-of-

function heterozygous *GRN* mutations seen in autosomal dominant frontotemporal lobar dementia (FLTD) with TAR DNA-binding protein-43 (TDP-43) inclusions (FTLD-TDP/GRN; OMIM #607485). The identification of NCL cases with GRN homozygous mutations suggests a link between a rare lysosomal disorder and a common late-onset neurodegenerative disease. It also points to potential lysosomal dysfunction in FTLD and highlights the pleiotropic effects of heterozygous/homozygous mutations in a single gene.

The clinical and neurophysiologic features of the CLN11 disorder, as represented by this familial case report and further reported by Canafogliaet and associates include onset in third decade of a retinal dystrophy with optic atrophy, seizures, myoclonus, and ataxia. There was also evidence in some family members in their late 20s of relatively mild cognitive impairment characterized by borderline executive function difficulties and mild depression. Pathologic characteristics of NCL were identified in skin biopsy (vacuoles, fingerprint lysosomal inclusions). Retinal examination showed pigment epithelial dystrophy, vessel attenuation, and optic neuropathy. OCT showed retinal thinning and disruption of retinal pigment epithelium. ERG was absent in one sibling. EEG was abnormal in both siblings with moderate spike and wave discharges predominantly in the posterior regions against a normal background. VEP showed depressed cortical components and distorted waveforms with flash strobe. Brain MRI (age 22 years) showed severe cerebellar atrophy.

Genetics and Pathology

Progranulin (PGRN) is a secreted growth factor involved in the regulation of a number of processes and plays an important role in central nervous system neurodegeneration. PGRN biologic activity is mediated through interactions with a number of proteins. Sortilin is a binding partner for PGRN on the cell surface of cortical neurons. PGRN-sortilin interaction regulates PRGN trafficking as sortilin facilitates endocytosis and delivers PRGN to lysosomes. PGRN is localized to late-endosomes and early lysosomes and appears to have a general role as an activator of lysosomal protein transport and, as such, is important in human pathobiology. PGRN is expressed in motor neurons and seems to promote neuronal survival. It has also been shown to protect against mutant TDP43 induced axonopathy. PGRN may even have an immune-regulatory function.

FTLD Biology/Pathology

The FTLDs are the second most common cause of presenile dementia and, as a group, exhibit variant clinical phenotypes, variable penetrance, selective atrophy of the frontal and temporal brain regions, and variant pathologic characteristics. There is significant overlap with motor neuron disease/amyotrophic lateral sclerosis (FTD-ALS), atypical parkinsonian syndromes, progressive supranuclear palsy, and corticobasal syndromes. These diseases can also be classified by the predominant neuropathological protein that is identified, including FTLD-TDP in which TAR DNA-binding protein-43 is stored. It is within the category of tau- and alpha-synuclein-negative and ubiquitin- and TDP-43-positive cases that those with GRN mutations fall.

FTLD-TDP associated with *GRN* mutations make up about 20% of FTLD-TDP disorders and were first described in autosomal dominant kindreds in association with tau-negative and ubiquitin-positive deposition. *GRN* mutations were identified in two families with primary progressive aphasia. FTLD-TDP/GRN is now considered one of a spectrum of

TDP-43 proteinopathies, and a summary of mutations indicate that all reported to date are confirmed or predicted to lead to loss-of-function. This suggests haploinsufficiency as pathobiologic mechanism.

Clinically GRN-associated FTLD-TDP evidences phenotypic variability with a breadth of features including early behavioral abnormalities and executive function loss, dementia with loss of expressive language, or semantic language comprehension, with or without loss of motoric speech. Clinical features may show an overlap with amyotrophic lateral sclerosis, parkinsonism, or corticobasal syndrome. These cases are grouped into subtypes depending on the associated pathologic protein aggregates.

NCL-FTLD Overlap

FTLD-TDP43/GRN may be a partial deficiency state, with risk of lysosomal dysfunction, whereas in the homozygous state, as seen in CLN11, may represent a more severe pathobiology and include, in addition to the executive dysfunction of FTLD, epilepsy and visual failure. This clinical and pathologic overlap raises the intriguing possibility that lysosomal dysfunction, whether primary or secondary, may be a general feature of neurodegeneration. Further study of the more common human disorder FTLD-TDP/GRN may shed light on the pathobiology of CLN11 and the NCL disorders more broadly.

Definitive Diagnosis: Identification of pathologic mutations in *GRN*. For further details of diagnostic evaluation, see Table 48-1 and Figure 48-3.

CLN 12 (ATP13A2; AUTOSOMAL RECESSIVE KUFS DISEASE; OMIM#610513)
Clinical Description

ATP13A2 mutations were first associated in the very rare autosomal recessive juvenile parkinsonism with dementia phenotype (Kufor-Rakeb syndrome, PARK9, KRS, OMIM #606693) in 2006. After identification of *ATP13A2* (neuronal P-type ATPase gene) mutations in a dog model of late-onset NCL, a Belgian family previously reported as juvenile Parkinson disease (PD) and with typical NCL pathology, was studied by whole exome sequencing and a single homozygous mutation in ATP13A2 was found. In this juvenile PD disorder, the clinical features include pyramidal degeneration, supranuclear gaze palsy, and severe dementia. Putaminal and caudate iron have been demonstrated and complex dystonic features noted in some cases. In the reported CLN12 Belgian family, learning difficulties were noted at about age 8 years. By age 11 to 13 years, there was unsteady gait. Over the next years, myoclonus and worsening ataxia, progressive extrapyramidal features with akinesia, and rigidity and speech difficulties were noted. The proband had severe myoclonus and unintelligible speech and was wheelchair bound by the age of 25 years. In addition to the pyramidal and extrapyramidal dysfunction, there were bulbar signs and evidence of gaze palsy with upgaze restriction. CNS pathologic study showed whorled lamellar inclusions typical of NCL in brain tissue, and there was lipopigment deposition in the retina. Other affected family members showed spinocerebellar ataxia, bulbar signs, extrapyramidal and pyramidal abnormalities, as well as dementia. No visual failure was apparent clinically. A sequence study of ATP13A2 in 28 patients with adult-onset NCL, however, failed to identify pathologic variants. Further pathologic study of KRS patients is needed to confirm that KRS and CLN12 are allelic. This work highlights, however, the potential important parallels between NCL and parkinsonian disorders and suggests that lysosomal pathway disruption may lead to a more general neurodegenerative phenotype.

Genetics and Pathology

ATP13A2 is thought to be a lysosomal type 5 P-type ATPase with 10 predicted transmembrane domains. Lysosomal dysfunction in ATP13A2 defective cells appears to impair α-synuclein degradation and would presumably predispose to α-synuclein accumulation and toxicity. There is a growing literature documenting lysosomal dysfunction in Parkinson disease (PD). A review of P-type transport ATPases in PD summarizes dysfunctional ATP13A2 retention in the ER or other aberrant intracellular localization and function as well as reported evidence of impaired ATPase activity. ATP13A2 has also been shown to maintain zinc homeostasis and promote α-synuclein export via exosome, possibly by regulation of α-synuclein-specific exosome biogenesis and to affect mitochondrial function. In animal models, a loss of ATP13A2 leads to lipofuscin accumulation as seen in NCL disorders and α-synuclein aggregation as seen in PD. A wide variety of ATP13A2 interactors have been delineated, most of which appear to have roles in ER translocation, ER-Golgi trafficking, or vesicular transport. Further study of this interactome may yield additional understanding of the complex interactions in the endosomal-lysosomal pathway broadly important to both NCL and PD pathobiology.

Definitive Diagnosis: Identification of pathologic mutations by sequencing of *ATP13A2*. For further details of diagnostic evaluation, see Table 48-1 and Figure 48-3.

CLN13 (CTSF, OMIM#615362)
Clinical Description

This is, as of yet, a rare identified cause of adult-onset NCL. Two Italian siblings were reported after linkage analysis and whole exome sequencing. Mutation in these siblings identified homozygous mutation in *CTSF* as in one other nonrelated patient. Clinical features were different in the two sisters. Whereas one presented at 20 years of age with cerebellar syndrome characterized by tremor, ataxia and dysarthria, the other patient did not show signs until 32 years of age with onset of a depression and cognitive decline. Seizures were noted in both later, and the younger sister then developed a progressive dementia associated with marked emotional lability and death at 42 years of age. The second sister showed cerebellar signs in later stages as well as pyramidal and extrapyramidal abnormalities and was bedridden by 51 years of age.

A recent familial case with apparent "pseudodominant" transmission has been reported in association with a homozygous *CTSF* splice mutation. Initial apparent autosomal dominant transmission raised question in this Kufs phenotype-expressing patients of possible DNAJC5 (CLN4) disease or PSEN1-related early onset Alzheimer disease. Careful history taking and family residence in a small village prompted consideration of potential autosomal recessive inheritance and molecular analysis that led to diagnosis. Clinical features in all reported family members documented presentation in third decade with tonic-clonic seizures followed by dementia in the third to fourth decade.

CTSF mutations include 4 missense, one splice, and one frame shift mutation. By structural modeling, these *CTSF* mutations were predicted to cause loss of CTSF enzymatic activity. It is less clear how a CTSF deficiency may lead to neurodegeneration and lysosomal storage.

Genetics and Pathology

Human *CTSF* was cloned in 1998 and shown to be a member of a subgroup of the papain family of lysosomal cysteine proteases. CTSF is synthesized as an inactive preproenzyme and has been postulated to be targeted to the endosomal/lysosomal compartment via the mannose 6-phosphate receptor pathway, although original work had suggested that it did not contain the usual cathepsin-related signal sequence for lysosomal targeting and that it might be targeted to the lysosome via an N-terminal signal peptide-independent lysosomal targeting pathway. Recent work also suggests that CTSF may participate in an alternative lysosomal LIMP-2 trafficking pathway.

Definitive Diagnosis: Identification of pathologic mutation in the *CTSF* gene. For further details of diagnostic evaluation, see Table 48-1 and Figure 48-3.

CLN14 (KCTD7; OMIM #611725)
Clinical Description

More than 10 patients have been described to date. Mutations in the *KCTD7* gene are associated with an infantile form of NCL and infantile progressive myoclonus epilepsy.

The NCL form has been reported in two siblings who presented with seizures at 8 and 9 months of age. Seizures were myoclonic, precipitated or worsened by fevers and refractory to multiple anticonvulsive drugs. Normal development was until 18 months of age, followed by motor and speech regression. By 12 and 10 years of age, the patients had microcephaly, were nonverbal, and had no spontaneous motoric function. There was no response to visual threat and diminished pupillary light reflexes. One patient had mild, bilateral, optic atrophy. Brain imaging showed global cortical and cerebellar atrophy, and some loss of subcortical white matter. There was NCL-type storage in fibroblasts, neurons and eccrine secretory epithelial cells, and fingerprint and GRODs in approximately15% of analyzed lymphocytes. Both patients died from complications of progressive disease in their mid teens.

In the infantile progressive myoclonus epilepsy presentation, the disease onset was under 5 years of age (range 10 months to 3 years), presenting with seizures and/or progressive mental and motor impairment with progressive psychomotor regression to severe mental and motor handicap within 2 years (range 1 to 22 months) after onset of seizures. Seizures were myoclonic, atonic, atypical absence, or/and tonic-clonic seizures. Ataxia also developed later and in one case was the presenting symptom. Retinal findings were normal. No lysosomal storage material compatible with NCL was detected in EM analysis of skin biopsies. In the group series of Kousi and colleagues, brain MRI was normal near disease onset in two patients, atrophic changes were seen in one patient, and nonspecific focal lesions were seen in a second patient (only in more advanced disease stages). EEG revealed prominent epileptiform activity with predominance in the posterior region. The patients were still living in 2012.

Other Presentation

- Opsoclonus-myoclonus, ataxia-like syndrome: A patient presented with onset of myoclonus and ataxia by 13 months, and associated with abnormal opsoclonus-like eye movements at 16 months of age. Epileptic activity was seen on EEG 2 years later as well as two episodes of myoclonic seizures. At 4.5 years of age, the patient communicated but did not speak, had limited vocalizations, and understood simple commands. He also had mild truncal ataxia and continuous myoclonus. Brain MRI and ophthalmologic evaluation were normal. A compound heterozygous missense mutation and large deletion in the KCTD7 gene was reported.

Genetics and Pathology

The *KCTD7* gene encodes the potassium channel tetramerization domain-containing protein 7. Currently there are at least eight mutations reported in this gene. *KCTD7* expression in the murine brain is strong in the mitral cells of the olfactory bulb, the dentate gyrus and CA1–CA3 hippocampal cells, the deep layers of the cerebral cortex, and the Purkinje cells of the mouse cerebellum. The KCTD7 protein is located in the cytoplasm, with the highest expression near the nucleus and a partial localization at the plasma membrane. It has been shown that *KCTD7* overexpression in transfected primary cultures of murine neurons hyperpolarizes the cell membrane and reduces the excitability of transfected neurons in patch clamp experiments. Therefore mutations in *KCTD7* are consistent with a depolarizing resting membrane potential and increased excitability. It is hypothesized that KCTD7 is required for the proper permeability of a nongated potassium channel that functions in a voltage range around the resting potential. KCTD7 also associates with Cullin-3, suggesting that KCTD7 could be part of an E3 ubiquitin ligase multiprotein complex.

Definitive Diagnosis: Diagnosis is made by finding mutations in the *KCTD7* gene. For further details of diagnostic evaluation, see Table 48-1 and Figure 48-3.

Management and Treatment of NCL Disorders

Unfortunately, there is no cure for the NCL disorders, and management is mainly symptomatic for the range of clinical problems, including seizures, sleep-related problems, malnutrition, gastroesophageal reflux, pneumonia, sialorrhea, hyperactivity, behavior problems, psychosis, anxiety, spasticity, parkinsonian symptoms, and dystonia. A truthful discussion with the caregivers should include goals of care and when the moment is right code status to avoid sometimes unnecessary suffering for the patient and family. There should be surveillance for swallowing problems and microaspirations due to the risk of pneumonia/sepsis as well as x-ray surveillance of hip joints and spine when there is significant immobility or when the patient is wheelchair bound.

Seizures. It is one of the hallmark manifestations and can cause the most anxiety in the family. There is no single anticonvulsant medication that will work for all the NCL disorders. An anticonvulsant medication should be selected in discussion with the family and based on the stage of the disease, age of the affected individual, and quality of life assessment. A goal of complete control of seizures may be unrealistic in this disorder. A balance between number of seizures and sedation (which is one of the most common side effects of the anticonvulsant medications) should be discussed with the family and patient (if able to communicate).

In a survey of 60 patients with CLN3, one of the largest to date, lamotrigine and valproic acid showed relatively good seizure control in most patients. However, there was no rationale for the choice of these specific anticonvulsive drugs. Importantly, 54% of patients had refractory epilepsy requiring combination therapy by the middle second decade of age. The pathophysiology of epileptogenesis is poorly understood in NCL, and empiric trial of medication is common. Newer anticonvulsive medications may be more beneficial, but there are no studies in this respect for the

NCLs. Levetiracetam and clobazam should be considered (personal experience).

Benzodiazepines may be of benefit for seizures, anxiety, spasticity, and sleep difficulties. However, the main side effect is somnolence; therefore; again, a balance between symptoms and sedation is imperative. Trihexyphenidyl has been used to improve dystonia and sialorrhea. Antidepressants and antipsychotic agents are sometimes indicated for those with severe mood problems and/or aggression.

Unfortunately, most of the patients become bedridden and, because of swallowing dysfunction and aspiration, pneumonia is a risk. Patients with swallowing problems may benefit from placement of a gastric feeding tube.

Children with NCL disorders benefit from school attendance for socialization and stimulation, even late in the disease. This also affords respite for caregivers. Physical therapy, either at home or at school, is important to avoid painful contractures for the longest period of time possible. The use of augmentative therapies as visual failure occurs and even the teaching of Braille may help in education even for temporary benefit in the context of the progressive dementia. Quality of life assessment in these educational interventions is important. The use of digital tools (tablet, speech-assist devices) may help in communication.

Genetic Counseling. (This section is not meant to address all personal, cultural, or ethical issues that individuals may face or to substitute for consultation with genetics professional).

The NCL disorders are autosomal recessive with the exception of one form of adult disease (CLN4) that is autosomal dominant. Once a mutation has been identified in a patient, obtaining parental samples to confirm carrier status is recommended. This will allow family planning for the family as well as discussion with related family members of the risk of inheritance. Siblings of an affected patient have a 25% of being affected, 50% of being an asymptomatic carrier, and 25% of not being a carrier. When the sibling is underage, a discussion with the parents, taking into account current guidelines of national/international genetic associations, is of importance before presymptomatic genetic testing of a minor child. This is particularly controversial and more challenging when the proband has a later onset presentation, and there is a younger sibling. There are genetic guidelines that one should take into account along with the wishes of the family. Patients with infantile NCL, late-infantile NCL, and classic juvenile NCL do not reproduce. Very rarely, individuals with atypical juvenile NCL reproduce, but they are obligate carriers.

An autosomal dominant adult CLN individual has an affected parent. However, an AD adult-onset NCL may have the disorder due to a de novo mutation. Germline mosaicism can also be a cause of not finding a mutation in the parents of an affected individual. Of note, the family history of an affected individual may be negative due to failure to recognize the disorder in a family member, death before onset of symptoms, or late-onset of the disease.

REFERENCES

The complete list of references for this chapter is available in the e-book at www.expertconsult.com.
      See inside cover for registration details.

SELECTED REFERENCES

Anderson, G.W., Goebel, H.H., Simonati, A., 2013. Human pathology in NCL. Biochim. Biophys. Acta 1832 (11), 1807–1826.

Haltia, M., Goebel, H.H., 2013. The neuronal ceroid-lipofuscinoses: A historical introduction. Biochim. Biophys. Acta 1832 (11), 1795–1800.

Jadav, R.H., Sinha, S., Yasha, T.C., et al., 2014. Clinical, electrophysiological, imaging, and ultrastructural description in 68 patients with neuronal ceroid lipofuscinoses and its subtypes. Pediatr. Neurol. 50 (1), 85–93.

Kollmann, K., Uusi-Rauva, K., Scifo, E., et al., 2013. Cell biology and function of neuronal ceroid lipofuscinosis-related proteins. Biochim. Biophys. Acta 1832 (11), 1866–1881.

Kousi, M., Lehesjoki, A.E., Mole, S.E., 2012. Update of the mutation spectrum and clinical correlations in over 360 mutations in eight genes that underlie the neuronal ceroid lipofuscinoses. Hum. Mutat. 33 (1), 42–63.

Lee, J., Giordano, S., Zhang, J., 2012. Autophagy, mitochondria, and oxidative stress: crosstalk and redox signaling. Biochem. J. 441, 523–540.

Mole, S., Williams, R., 2013. Neuronal ceroid-lipofuscinoses. In: Pagon, R.A., Adam, M.P., Ardinger, H.H., et al. (Eds.), GeneReviews. University of Washington, Seattle, Seattle.

Mole, S., Williams, R., Goebel, H.H. (Eds.), 2011. The Neuronal Ceroid Lipofusinoses, second ed. Oxford University Press, Oxford.

E-BOOK FIGURES AND TABLES

The following figures and tables are available in the e-book at www.expertconsult.com. See inside cover for registration details.

Fig. 48-3 NCL diagnostic workup.

49 Channelopathies

Kelly Knupp and Amy R. Brooks-Kayal

An expanded version of this chapter is available on www.expertconsult.com. See inside cover for registration details.

INTRODUCTION

Channelopathies are a group of genetically and phenotypically heterogeneous neurologic disorders that result from genetically determined defects in ion-channel function. These are considered heterogeneous because mutations in the same gene can cause different diseases and mutations in different genes can result in the same disease phenotype. Mutations of ion channels can alter the activation, ion selectivity, or inactivation of the mutated channel. Neurologic manifestations of channelopathies fall into several clinical phenotypes: epilepsy, pain, migraine, ataxia, movement disorders (all covered in this chapter; see Table 49-1), and muscle disorders (myotonia and weakness; covered in Chapter 151).

Ion channels are transmembrane glycoprotein pores that control the excitability of neurons and muscle cells by mediating the flow of charged ions in and out of cells. Channels are typically composed of different protein subunits, each encoded by a different gene. There are two major classes of ion channels: voltage-gated and ligand-gated. Voltage-gated ion channels are activated and inactivated by changes in membrane voltage and are identified according to the principal ion conducted through the channel (e.g., sodium, potassium, calcium, or chloride). Activation and opening of voltage-gated channels have different effects (depolarization, repolarization, or hyperpolarization of the cell membrane), depending on what ion they gate and that ion's charge, the electrochemical gradient for that ion (which determines in which direction the ion flows when the channel is opened), and where the channels are located on the cell. Sodium channel opening results in the generation of the action potential (i.e., depolarization). Opening of potassium channels repolarizes cell membranes after action potential firing and maintains the resting membrane potential. Calcium channels are important for the generation of muscle contraction, neurotransmitter release, and intracellular signaling via second messengers. Opening of voltage-gated chloride channels results in the hyperpolarization of cells.

Ligand-gated channels are heterogeneous complexes composed of multiple protein subunits that are activated by the binding of their respective agonists. Several ligand-gated channels are present in the peripheral and central nervous systems. Gamma-aminobutyric acid (GABA)$_A$ receptors mediate most of the fast synaptic inhibition in the brain beyond the fetal and early neonatal periods. They are anion selective and gate primarily chloride, which flows into the cell, causing hyperpolarization upon GABA$_A$ receptor activation. Glutamate is the primary excitatory neurotransmitter in the central nervous system and binds to three types of ligand-gated, cation-selective receptor channels: N-methyl-d-aspartate (NMDA), α-amino-3-hydroxy-5-methylisoxazole-4-propionic acid (AMPA), and kainate. Glutamate receptors gate either sodium only (most AMPA and all kainate receptors) or sodium and calcium (NMDA receptors and some subtypes of AMPA receptors). Nicotinic acetylcholine receptors are nonselective cation channels permeable to Na$^+$ and K$^+$, and Ca^{2+} in some subtypes; they are located on certain neurons and on the postsynaptic side of the neuromuscular junction. Opening of nicotinic receptors causes depolarization of the plasma membrane and activation of voltage-gated ion channels that can affect the release of neurotransmitters and activate intracellular signaling cascades.

EPILEPSY SYNDROMES

Ion channelopathies, involving sodium, potassium, and calcium channels, have been increasing identified as an etiology of epilepsy. Ligand-gated channels such as GABA receptors and nicotinic receptors have also been implicated. Identifying these syndromes will likely lead to unique treatments for specific syndromes thus entering an era of precision medicine.

Dravet Syndrome

Clinical Features

Dravet syndrome has a classic presentation in most cases. Children begin to have seizures in the first year of life, typically in the setting of fever and characterized by prolonged seizures with hemiconvulsions. Alternating laterality of seizures can occur with each event, and seizures often evolve into status epilepticus. In the second year of life, other seizure types begin to emerge, including absence, myoclonic, and generalized tonic-clonic seizures, and partial seizures that now occur without fever. Tonic seizures are rare and, if they do occur, tend to be brief and nocturnal. Photo-induced seizures occur in some of these children, and self-induced seizures have been reported. Throughout childhood, elevated body temperature and anticonvulsants that are sodium channel blockers (e.g., carbamazepine, phenytoin, fosphenytoin, oxcarbazepine, and lamotrigine) exacerbate seizures. Seizure control is rarely attained. Episodes of status are common, including "obtundation status" (Brunklaus and Zuberi, 2014). The phenotype of the clinical seizure and electrographic correlation may not be congruent, making seizure classification difficult (Kim et al., 2014).

Development of the affected child is universally normal in the first year of life. As seizure types become more varied and more frequent, there is cessation of developmental progress, which can be misinterpreted as developmental regression. Moderate to severe intellectual impairment is present in many children, and the degree of cognitive impairment is somewhat associated with seizure control (Wolff, Casse-Perrot, and Dravet, 2006). Hyperactivity and autistic traits present in the toddler years. As children enter into adolescence, hyperkinetic behavior tends to improve and is replaced with overall slowed behavior.

Not all children with Dravet syndrome present with classic features, as described earlier. Myoclonic seizures need not be present for a diagnosis to be made. These seemingly less affected children continue to be exquisitely sensitive to temperature and sodium channel–blocking anticonvulsants. In some cases these features may suggest the diagnosis. Recently this syndrome was recognized in a large percentage of children

405

TABLE 49-1 Channelopathies Associated with Clinical Syndromes in Pediatric Neurology

Gene Type	Epilepsy	Headache	Ataxia	Pain Syndrome
Sodium	SCN1a SCN1b SCN2a SCN2A1 SCN9a	SCN1A		SCN9A SCN11A SCN10A
Chloride	GABAa CLCN2		CLCN2	
Potassium	KCNQ2 KCNQ3 KCNJ11 KCNJ10 KCNMA1	KCNK18	KCNA1 KCNC3 KCND3	
Calcium	CACNA1A CACNB4	CACN1A	CACN1A	
Ligand-gated channels	GABRG2 GABRB3 GABRD GABRA1 EFHC1 LGI1 CHRNA4 CHRNA7 GRIN2A GPR98 CHRNB2	PRRT2 ATP1A2	ITPR1	

(11 of 14) presenting with seizures and encephalopathy after receiving vaccines (vaccine encephalopathy) (Berkovic et al., 2006).

Genetics/Pathophysiology

Mutations in the sodium channel gene *SCN1A* are found in approximately 80% of children with a clinical diagnosis of Dravet syndrome. Most have a de novo mutation, although some of the families have a higher-than-expected history of febrile seizures.

There remains equipoise regarding how *SCN1A* mutations are predicted to cause a loss of sodium channel function, logically a cause of hypoexcitability of individual neurons, could lead to network hyperexcitability and, consequently, seizures. Some research suggests that this seeming contradiction can be explained by the selective loss of *SCN1A* expression and decreased sodium channel function only in inhibitory interneurons (Yu et al., 2006), causing inhibitory dysfunction and secondary hyperexcitability. Other recent studies suggest that loss of *SCN1A* occurs more broadly and may result in compensatory increases in other sodium channels that produce a net increase in sodium channel currents leading to hyperexcitability (Liu et al., 2013).

Clinical Laboratory Tests

Electroencephalogram (EEG) findings are typically normal in the first year of life, but evolve to demonstrate generalized and multifocal abnormalities. A photoconvulsive response can be seen, and diffuse background slowing can become more prominent as children age. No characteristic pattern is diagnostic of Dravet syndrome, as is seen in Lennox–Gastaut or Doose syndrome; in fact, there can be some overlap between these syndromes and Dravet syndrome, making accurate diagnosis challenging. Magnetic resonance imaging (MRI) in patients with Dravet syndrome is usually without any focal abnormalities (Striano et al., 2007). Genetic testing is appropriate in patients suspected to have Dravet syndrome. Early diagnosis avoids extensive and expensive metabolic testing and inadvertent exacerbation of seizures by certain medications, and provides prognostic information for the family.

Treatment

Seizure control is the primary treatment goal in this disorder. Medications that block the sodium channel exacerbate seizures and should be avoided in most patients (Guerrini et al., 1998). Topiramate, valproic acid, benzodiazepines, and levetiracetam have proven helpful. Combination therapy with stiripentol, clobazam, and either Depakote or topiramate has been reported to be more effective than other combinations of medication (Chiron et al., 2000). Acetazolamide has not been shown to be beneficial. A recent report suggests that verapamil, a calcium channel blocker, may be helpful, but more research is required (Iannetti et al., 2009). Fenfluramine was also successful in a small cohort and requires further study (Ceulemans et al., 2012). Nonpharmacologic treatments, such as vagal nerve stimulation or ketogenic diet, have been useful in some patients. Anecdotal reports in the media suggest that cannabidiol (CBD), a component of marijuana, may reduce seizures in some children, although a retrospective case series found that artisanal CBD oils did not result in a substantial reduction in seizures in most children (Press and Chapman, 2015). Clinical trials of pharmaceutical-grade CBD products are now under way.

Avoidance of hot temperatures, both environmental and elevated body temperature, has been used by many families to reduce seizures. Because of the severity of the cognitive impairment, appropriate support must be initiated for the family. Medications for behavioral issues may also be necessary (see Chapters 59 and 60). Cardiac surveillance may also be indicated, given laboratory models of cardiac dysfunction (Auerbach et al., 2013). Because there is a high rate of sudden unexplained death in this patient population, counseling should be provided.

Generalized Epilepsy with Febrile Seizures Plus

Clinical Features

Generalized epilepsy with febrile seizures plus (GEFS +) is a familial epilepsy syndrome characterized by febrile seizures in childhood in several generations of family members, often with continuation of febrile seizures into adulthood. In addition, afebrile seizures are often present. Seizure types include generalized tonic-clonic, myoclonic, absence, and atonic seizures. There is variable penetrance of seizures in these familial cohorts. Phenotype also varies among family members. Seizure resolution often occurs by age 12. The majority of these patients have normal development and intelligence.

Genetics/Pathophysiology

SCN1B mutations were first reported in a large family cohort (Wallace et al., 1998). Mutations in other sodium channels—*SCN1A* (Escayg et al., 2000) and *SCN2A* (Sugawara et al., 2001)—have been found subsequently. The majority of these have been point mutations. In patients with *SCN1A* mutations, a difference in phenotype from GEFS + and Dravet syndrome can often be predicted, given the location of the mutation (distance from the pore) and alteration in transcription of the gene. Sodium channel mutations do not account for all of the mutations in GEFS +; there also have been reports of mutations identified in two GABA$_A$-receptor subunit genes, *GABRG2* and *GABRD* (gamma 2 and delta subunits) (Harkin et al., 2002).

Treatment

There has been little published discussion of the treatment of these syndromes. For patients with sodium channel mutations, avoidance of sodium channel blockers is wise. Treatment when necessary with broad-spectrum anticonvulsants is thought to be useful. Avoidance of temperature changes and routine use of fever control measures may be of some benefit.

Benign Familial Neonatal Seizures

Clinical Features

Benign familial neonatal seizures are an autosomal-dominant epilepsy presenting with seizures in the first or second week of life, most commonly starting on day of life 2 or 3, resolving within weeks to months. Most seizures have stopped at 4 to 5 months of life. Seizures are usually multifocal clonic seizures or focal seizures. The feature suggesting this entity is the presence of similar seizures in parents and first-degree relatives, occurring at the same age. Development is characteristically normal during this time period, and after seizures stop. Fifteen percent of children will develop epilepsy later in life, usually in childhood or as a young adult. Some children progress to medically refractory epilepsy with encephalopathy (Steinlein, Conrad, and Weidner, 2007).

Genetics/Pathophysiology

Mutations in potassium channels *KCNQ2* (Singh et al., 1998; Biervert et al., 1998) and *KCNQ3* (Charlier et al., 1998) (found on chromosomes 20 and 8, respectively) have been reported in families with benign neonatal seizures. The age specificity of the seizures in this disorder is thought to emanate from brain developmental changes during the neonatal period, when potassium channels play a critical role in inhibition that is rapidly replaced by the action of GABA receptors over the first several months of life.

Clinical Laboratory Tests

EEG generally demonstrates normal interictal features, although at the time of seizure there is an electrographic correlate. MRI is expected to be normal. Other causes of seizures, such as neonatal infection and metabolic abnormalities, should be excluded.

KCNQ2 Encephalopathy

Clinical Features

KCNQ2 encephalopathy presents in the first days of life with poorly controlled seizures, which may resolve within the first year of life, but with residual and often profound intellectual impairment. This syndrome has been increasingly recognized as a severe neonatal encephalopathy and can have an overlapping phenotype with Ohtahara syndrome and West syndrome. Seizures are tonic and focal in nature, with some children having myoclonic seizures and infantile spasms. Autonomic changes can be an associated feature with seizures and may include apnea and bradycardia. Most children have EEG findings of a burst-suppression pattern that resolves and is replaced with diffuse slowing and multifocal epileptiform discharges. MRI findings have been reported in several cohorts, and although not universal, many will have thinning of the corpus callosum, frontal lobe atrophy, and nonspecific white-matter findings.

Seizures often resolve in the first year of life. Varying degrees of intellectual delay are present, ranging from mild to severe (Weckhuysen et al., 2013).

Genetic/Pathophysiology

De novo mutations in *KCNQ2* have been reported. Similar mutations rarely have been present in children with benign familial neonatal seizures. Mutations are present in highly conserved areas, leading to loss of function.

Treatment

Some children have responded to carbamazepine and other sodium (Na) channel blockers. One child is reported to have had cessation of seizures with retigabine (Barrese et al., 2010). This treatment requires more research, but may be promising.

Developmental Delay, Epilepsy, and Neonatal Diabetes

Developmental delay, epilepsy, and neonatal diabetes (DEND) is a rare syndrome, presenting with neonatal diabetes, developmental delay, seizures, and mild dysmorphic features, and has been associated with a mutation in the *KCNJ11* gene that encodes for a subunit of the adenosine triphosphate (ATP)–sensitive potassium channel. This channel is found on pancreatic islet cells and in neurons. Neonates with this disorder usually present with diabetes and subsequently develop seizures and global intellectual impairment. Dysmorphic features, including downturned mouth, bilateral ptosis, prominent metopic suture, and contractures, have also been described (Gloyn et al., 2004). Infantile spasms can present in some children (Bahi-Buisson et al., 2007), in addition to other seizure types, such as tonic-clonic and myoclonic seizures. Seizures have been refractory to traditional antiseizure medications. In contrast, patients are responsive to treatment with sulfonylurea medications, such as glibenclamide, leading to improvement in the effects of diabetes, developmental outcomes, and seizure frequency and effects.

Other Genetic Generalized Epilepsies

Autosomal-Dominant Nocturnal Frontal Lobe Epilepsy

Autosomal-dominant nocturnal frontal lobe epilepsy is a familial epilepsy characterized by frontal lobe seizures that typically occur at night and phenotypically present as arousal from sleep with bizarre hypermotor behaviors, such as spinning, thrashing, and rocking. Seizures can be numerous. Nicotinic receptor mutations have been found in many of these familial cohorts (Steinlein et al., 1995), although there are several families for which no gene mutation has been identified. These ligand-gated receptors allow sodium and potassium to cross the cell membrane. Many patients are responsive to carbamazepine and phenytoin.

Benign Familial Infantile–Neonatal Seizures

Benign familial infantile–neonatal seizures is an epilepsy syndrome that has been described as being similar to benign neonatal seizures, but it occurs at a slightly older age. Mutations have been found in a sodium channel, SCN2A1, in some cohorts (Herlenius et al., 2007).

Childhood Absence Epilepsy

Childhood absence epilepsy has been linked to mutations in GABA receptors (GABRA1 and GABRG2) (Baulac et al., 2001; Wallace et al., 2001) and chloride channels (CLCN2). Mutations have also been described in a calcium channel, CACNA1H. The families with CLCN2 also had members with generalized tonic-clonic seizures on awakening and juvenile myoclonic epilepsy (Baykan et al., 2004).

Juvenile Myoclonic Epilepsy

Juvenile myoclonic epilepsy is a seizure disorder that usually presents in adolescents with myoclonic seizures that are more likely to occur in the early morning after awakening, and generalized tonic-clonic seizures that also tend to occur in the morning hours. Several gene mutations have been found in these patients, although the majority of patients have yet to have an underlying etiology determined. It appears that, similar to childhood absence epilepsy, this is likely a polygenic disorder. Channels that have been identified include GABA receptors (GABRA1 and GABRD) (Cossette et al., 2002), calcium channels (CACNB4) (Escayg et al., 2000), and chloride channels (CLCN2) (Baykan et al., 2004). In addition, a gene that is not a direct channel gene but enhances calcium influx into the cell and can stimulate programmed cell death (EFHC1) (Suzuki et al., 2004) has also been identified as being involved in this epilepsy syndrome.

FAMILIAL PAIN SYNDROMES

Several pain syndromes have been associated with sodium channel mutations. This is not surprising, as sodium channels are located on spinal sensory neurons in the dorsal root ganglion (Bennett and Woods, 2014).

Clinical Features

Inherited Erythromelalgia, Primary Erythermalgia. Inherited erythromelalgia (IEM), or primary erythermalgia, is a pain syndrome characterized by episodes of redness and swelling of the hands and feet, associated with burning pain. These episodes can be triggered by mild warmth or exercise. Erythema can become constant, and edema may be associated (Drenth and Waxman, 2007; Cook-Norris et al., 2012). Age of onset can vary from childhood to adulthood, and can be familial or sporadic (Drenth et al., 2008; Han et al., 2009), with about 15% being familial and having autosomal-dominant inheritance.

Paroxysmal Extreme Pain Disorder. Paroxysmal extreme pain disorder (PEPD), formerly called familial rectal pain, is characterized by episodic severe pain, which commonly occurs in the perirectal region but can also involve the genitals, limbs, and face, especially the periorbital region. Stimulation of the region by bowel movements, contact in the perianal region, eating, or sudden changes in temperature can induce pain episodes. Flushing, harlequin skin changes, pupillary abnormalities, and cardiac abnormalities can occur at the time of the pain episode. Tonic episodes that are nonepileptic in nature can occur with the pain episodes and are secondary to the intense severity of the pain. Weakness has been present with pain in the limbs, lasting up to 24 hours after the pain has resolved. Constipation is a common problem because the episodes are induced by passing stool. Symptoms have been reported as early as at the time of delivery, and occurrence in utero is suspected (Fertleman et al., 2007).

Congenital Indifference to Pain. Congenital indifference to pain (CIP) is a syndrome characterized by insensitivity to pain and, in some cases, loss of smell. A more severe form has been reported that is associated with anhydrosis; intellectual delay and hypotonia may be present in these children. Individuals with anhidrosis can experience episodes of hyperthermia that can be life-threatening if not recognized. Awareness of a stimulus is present, but pain is not experienced in relation to the stimulus. Because of this altered response to pain, fractures, burns, and other significant injuries can go unnoticed. Fractures, foot injuries, and injuries to the fingertips may be present for several days without awareness of injury. Individuals can differentiate between hot and cold, but lack the ability to determine whether a temperature is extreme enough to cause injury. Signs of peripheral neuropathy on clinical examination or neurophysiological testing and autonomic nervous system abnormalities are lacking (Golshani et al., 2014).

Genetics/Pathophysiology

Mutations in SCN9A, a sodium channel, have been associated with IEM, PEPD, and CIP. Mutations thought to lead to hyperexcitability of the sodium channel have been identified in IEM and PEPD. Mutations in IEM allow the channel to be activated by smaller-than-normal depolarizations, and the channel remains open longer after activation (Drenth et al., 2005). Mutations in PEPD lead to prolonged action potentials and repetitive neuronal firing when stimulated (Jarecki et al., 2008). Mutations in this same channel that lead to *loss* of function are associated with CIP (Goldberg et al., 2007; Nilsen et al., 2009). The alteration of function created by the mutation leads to different phenotypes and different pain syndromes.

Treatment

Treatment for IEM, including use of sodium channel blockers, has not been very effective, although there have been reports of some relief with lidocaine, mexiletine (Choi et al., 2009), and carbamazepine (Fischer et al., 2009). Recently a pilot study of an Na channel antagonist demonstrated some benefit, although further studies are needed (Goldberg et al., 2012). Response to medications may vary with different mutations. Carbamazepine has been helpful in treating PEPD, but topiramate and gabapentin have not.

Congenital indifference to pain does not have a specific treatment, but patients need to be observed carefully for occult injuries, including fractures, joint injuries, and burns, in addition to mouth and hand injuries. Establishing a daily routine to monitor for injuries is important.

MIGRAINE AND ATAXIA SYNDROMES
Familial Hemiplegic Migraines
Clinical Features

Familial hemiplegic migraine often presents in the first or second decade of life with severe headache, often unilateral, and is associated with unilateral weakness typically lasting 24 hours or, rarely, several days. Extreme symptoms of prolonged duration (30 days) and coma are rare, as are seizures during hemiplegia. The clinical presentation can be less impressive with unilateral paresthesia and hemianopsia (Roth et al., 2014). Ataxia and dysarthria have been reported between attacks, or for a short duration while recovering from an attack. Family members also have occasionally had a prior diagnosis of benign paroxysmal torticollis of infancy (Giffin et al., 2002), although this is rare, and it is unclear whether this is or is not related to the gene mutation. Diagnostic criteria established by the International Headache Society include migraine with aura with motor weakness and at least one first- or second-degree relative with similar symptoms. Genetic information allows for further subtyping.

Headaches can have features of basilar migraine, including vertigo, visual symptoms, tinnitus, dysarthria, and ataxia. Some patients have been reported to have progressive ataxia later in life (Terwindt et al., 1998). In addition, cognitive impairment has been noted in affected patients (Marchioni et al., 1995).

Genetics/Pathophysiology

Genetic etiology has been linked to a calcium channel mutation (CACNA1A) (Stam et al., 2008); people with mutations of this gene are more likely to have ataxia and coma, and to be more prone to delayed cerebral edema after minor head injury (Terwindt et al., 1998; Kors et al., 2001; Stam et al., 2009). Mutations in CACNA1A (FHM1) also have been reported in patients with alternating hemiplegia of childhood, which phenotypically has some overlap with hemiplegic migraine (de Vries et al., 2008), and in patients with episodic ataxia type 2 (see following discussion) and spinocerebellar ataxia type 6. Mutations in ATP1A2 (FHM2), SCN1A (FHM3), and PRRT2 (Riant et al., 2012) also have been found in some patients with this clinical syndrome (De Fusco et al., 2003; Dichgans and Markus, 2005).

Clinical Laboratory Tests

MRI findings are not pathognomonic, but cerebellar atrophy (Terwindt et al., 1998), particularly in the superior cerebellar vermis, has been reported. Magnetic resonance (MR) spectroscopy of this region has demonstrated metabolic abnormalities consistent with neuron loss (Dichgans and Markus, 2005). EEGs during events can demonstrate slowing in the affected hemisphere, and mild asymmetries with minimal unilateral slowing have been noted on EEGs performed between episodes (Marchioni et al., 1995).

Treatment

Most commonly, patients are treated with acetazolamide, calcium channel blockers such as verapamil, or a trial of other standard migraine prophylactic drugs (tricyclic antidepres-sants, beta blockers). Limited correlation exists between drug response and hemiplegic migraine type. There have been reports of the use of valproic acid and lamotrigine in FHM2 with good response, (Pelzer et al., 2014), and corticosteroids (Sanchez-Albisua et al., 2013); further study is needed.

Episodic Ataxia
Clinical Features

This disorder is characterized by intermittent periods of ataxia (see also Chapter 91). There are two commonly described disorders: episodic ataxia type 1 and type 2. Phenotypic presentation differs slightly in each case, allowing clinical separation.

Episodic ataxia type 1 is characterized by frequent, brief episodes of ataxia, involving ataxic gait and slurred speech, precipitated by strong emotional outbursts, sudden movements, and exercise. Episodes can last several seconds to minutes in duration and can occur several times a day. In addition, there usually is evidence of muscle hyperexcitability manifested by the presence of myokymia, both clinically and electrographically. Some family members have reported seizures and isolated myotonia (Graves et al., 2014).

Episodic ataxia type 2 primarily involves truncal ataxia, with more prolonged periods of ataxia lasting hours to days. Eye movement abnormalities are sometimes present. Episodes can be induced by stress or exercise. Myokymia is rare. Some patients can have subtle, slowly progressive cerebellar features. Cerebellar atrophy has been reported. Migraine symptoms can be present in both types of episodic ataxia, but are more common in type 2; migraine symptoms may have many features consistent with basilar migraine, including vertigo, nausea, and occipital pain (Nachbauer et al., 2014).

Genetics/Pathophysiology

Both disorders are inherited in an autosomal-dominant fashion, with incomplete penetrance. Type 1 has been associated with point mutations in KCNA1 (Lassche et al., 2014; Browne et al., 1994). This is a potassium channel that has no intervening introns. Episodic ataxia type 2 has been linked to mutations in CACNA1A (a calcium channel). Mutations that interfere with splicing or lead to a premature stop have been linked to the episodic ataxia type 2 phenotype (van den Maagdenberg et al., 2002).

Clinical Laboratory Tests

Electromyography (EMG) is helpful with episodic ataxia type 1 in identifying and/or confirming myokymia. MRI also may be useful, especially in episodic ataxia type 2, and should be performed to rule out other underlying etiologies of ataxia. Cerebellar vermis atrophy has been reported in episodic ataxia type 2.

Treatment

Acetazolamide and carbamazepine have both been reported to lead to reduction in the frequency and severity of events.

Spinocerebellar Ataxia
Clinical Features

Several progressive ataxias have been described and reported as resulting from a variety of etiologies (see Chapter 92). Channelopathies are responsible for one subtype, now called spinocerebellar ataxia type 6. This type presents as a slowly progressive cerebellar degeneration, with ataxia, dysmetria, and other cerebellar signs as prominent clinical features. Spasticity and cranial neuropathies are not prominent. There can be some overlap with episodic ataxia type 2, with episodes of truncal ataxia lasting for several hours to days and often precipitated by stress or exertion. There also may be some features associated with basilar migraine or familial hemiplegic migraine.

Genetics/Pathophysiology

Spinocerebellar ataxia type 6 has been reported to be associated with triplet repeats in the *CACNA1A* gene (Zhuchenko et al., 1997). Unlike the gene changes associated with other triplet-repeat disorders, mutations in *SCA6* seem to be relatively stable, and the expansion is smaller than that typically seen in association with an abnormal phenotype. It is unclear if symptoms are related to channel dysfunction or the cytotoxic effects of the repeat, as is seen in other diseases. The overlap between these phenotypes suggests that there is a pathologic role in the abnormal function of the calcium channel. Mutations in this gene also have been reported in cohorts with familial hemiplegic migraine, which usually have point mutations. Cohorts with episodic ataxia type 2 also have been reported to have mutations in this gene that often lead to splicing errors or premature stops.

Clinical Laboratory Tests

MRI is helpful because many patients with symptomatic episodic ataxia will have cerebellar atrophy.

Treatment

Supportive treatment is recommended. Patients with episodes of headaches may be helped by the treatments outlined for the episodic ataxias and familial migraine syndromes.

REFERENCES

The complete list of references for this chapter is available in the e-book at www.expertconsult.com.
    See inside cover for registration details.

SELECTED REFERENCES

Auerbach, D.S., Jones, J., Clawson, B.C., et al., 2013. Altered cardiac electrophysiology and SUDEP in a model of Dravet syndrome. PLoS ONE 8 (10), e77843.

Bahi-Buisson, N., Eisermann, M., Nivot, S., et al., 2007. Infantile spasms as an epileptic feature of DEND syndrome associated with an activating mutation in the potassium adenosine triphosphate (ATP) channel, Kir6.2. J. Child Neurol. 22 (9), 1147–1150.

Barrese, V., Miceli, F., Soldovieri, M.V., et al., 2010. Neuronal potassium channel openers in the management of epilepsy: role and potential of retigabine. Clin. Pharmacol. 2, 225–236.

Baulac, S., Huberfeld, G., Gourfinkel-An, I., et al., 2001. First genetic evidence of GABA(A) receptor dysfunction in epilepsy: a mutation in the gamma2-subunit gene. Nat. Genet. 28 (1), 46–48.

Baykan, B., Madia, F., Bebek, N., et al., 2004. Autosomal recessive idiopathic epilepsy in an inbred family from Turkey: identification of a putative locus on chromosome 9q32-33. Epilepsia 45 (5), 479–487.

Bennett, D.L., Woods, C.G., 2014. Painful and painless channelopathies. Lancet Neurol. 13, 587–599.

Berkovic, S.F., Harkin, L., McMahon, J.M., et al., 2006. De-novo mutations of the sodium channel gene SCN1A in alleged vaccine encephalopathy: a retrospective study. Lancet Neurol. 5 (6), 488–492.

Biervert, C., Schroeder, B.C., Kubisch, C., et al., 1998. A potassium channel mutation in neonatal human epilepsy. Science 279 (5349), 403–406.

Browne, D.L., Gancher, S.T., Nutt, J.G., et al., 1994. Episodic ataxia/myokymia syndrome is associated with point mutations in the

human potassium channel gene, KCNA1. Nat. Genet. 8 (2), 136–140.

Brunklaus, A., Zuberi, S.M., 2014. Dravet syndrome-From epileptic encephalopathy to channelopathy. Epilepsia 55 (7), 979–984.

Ceulemans, B., Boel, M., Leyssens, K., et al., 2012. Successful use of fenfluramine as an add-on treatment for Dravet syndrome. Epilepsia 53 (7), 1131–1139.

Charlier, C., Singh, N.A., Ryan, S.G., et al., 1998. A pore mutation in a novel KQT-like potassium channel gene in an idiopathic epilepsy family. Nat. Genet. 18 (1), 53–55.

Chiron, C., Marchand, M.C., Tran, A., et al., 2000. Stiripentol in severe myoclonic epilepsy in infancy: a randomised placebo-controlled syndrome-dedicated trial. STICLO study group. Lancet 356 (9242), 1638–1642.

Choi, J.S., Zhang, L., Dib-Hajj, S.D., et al., 2009. Mexiletine-responsive erythromelalgia due to a new Na(v)1.7 mutation showing use-dependent current fall-off. Exp. Neurol. 216 (2), 383–389.

Cook-Norris, R.H., Tollefson, M.M., Cruz-Inigo, A.E., et al., 2012. Pediatric erythromelalgia: a retrospective review of 32 cases evaluated at Mayo Clinic over a 37-year period. J. Am. Acad. Dermatol. 66 (3), 416–423.

Cossette, P., Liu, L., Brisebois, K., et al., 2002. Mutation of GABRA1 in an autosomal dominant form of juvenile myoclonic epilepsy. Nat. Genet. 31 (2), 184–189.

De Fusco, M., Marconi, R., Silvestri, L., et al., 2003. Haploinsufficiency of ATP1A2 encoding the Na+/K+ pump alpha2 subunit associated with familial hemiplegic migraine type 2. Nat. Genet. 33 (2), 192–196.

de Vries, B., Stam, A.H., Beker, F., et al., 2008. CACNA1A mutation linking hemiplegic migraine and alternating hemiplegia of childhood. Cephalalgia 28 (8), 887–891.

Dichgans, M., Markus, H.S., 2005. Genetic association studies in stroke: methodological issues and proposed standard criteria. Stroke 36 (9), 2027–2031.

Drenth, J.P., Te Morsche, R.H., Guillet, G., et al., 2005. SCN9A mutations define primary erythermalgia as a neuropathic disorder of voltage gated sodium channels. J. Invest. Dermatol. 124 (6), 1333–1338.

Drenth, J.P., Waxman, S.G., 2007. Mutations in sodium-channel gene SCN9A cause a spectrum of human genetic pain disorders. J. Clin. Invest. 117 (12), 3603–3609.

Drenth, J.P., Te Morsche, R.H., Mansour, S., et al., 2008. Primary erythermalgia as a sodium channelopathy: screening for SCN9A mutations: exclusion of a causal role of SCN10A and SCN11A. Arch. Dermatol. 144 (3), 320–324.

Escayg, A., MacDonald, B.T., Meisler, M.H., et al., 2000. Mutations of SCN1A, encoding a neuronal sodium channel, in two families with GEFS+2. Nat. Genet. 24 (4), 343–345.

Escayg, A., De Waard, M., Lee, D.D., et al., 2000. Coding and noncoding variation of the human calcium-channel beta4-subunit gene CACNB4 in patients with idiopathic generalized epilepsy and episodic ataxia. Am. J. Hum. Genet. 66 (5), 1531–1539.

Fertleman, C.R., Ferrie, C.D., Aicardi, J., et al., 2007. Paroxysmal extreme pain disorder (previously familial rectal pain syndrome). Neurology 69 (6), 586–595.

Fischer, T.Z., Gilmore, E.S., Estacion, M., et al., 2009. A novel Nav1.7 mutation producing carbamazepine-responsive erythromelalgia. Ann. Neurol. 65 (6), 733–741.

Giffin, N.J., Benton, S., Goadsby, P.J., 2002. Benign paroxysmal torticollis of infancy: four new cases and linkage to CACNA1A mutation. Dev. Med. Child Neurol. 44 (7), 490–493.

Goldberg, Y.P., MacFarlane, J., MacDonald, M.L., et al., 2007. Loss-of-function mutations in the Nav1.7 gene underlie congenital indifference to pain in multiple human populations. Clin. Genet. 71 (4), 311–319.

Goldberg, Y.P., Price, N., Namdari, R., et al., 2012. Treatment of Na(v)1.7-mediated pain in inherited erythromelalgia using a novel sodium channel blocker. Pain 153 (1), 80–85.

Gloyn, A.L., Pearson, E.R., Antcliff, J.F., et al., 2004. Activating mutations in the gene encoding the ATP-sensitive potassium-channel subunit Kir6.2 and permanent neonatal diabetes. N. Engl. J. Med. 350 (18), 1838–1849.

Golshani, A.E., Kamdar, A.A., Spence, S.C., et al., 2014. Congenital indifference to pain: an illustrated case report and literature review. J. Radiol. Case Rep. 8 (8), 16–23.

Graves, T.D., Cha, Y.H., Hahn, A.F., et al., 2014. Episodic ataxia type 1: clinical characterization, quality of life and genotype-phenotype correlation. Brain 137 (Pt 4), 1009–1018.

Guerrini, R., Dravet, C., Genton, P., et al., 1998. Lamotrigine and seizure aggravation in severe myoclonic epilepsy. Epilepsia 39 (5), 508–512.

Han, C., Dib-Hajj, S.D., Lin, Z., et al., 2009. Early- and late-onset inherited erythromelalgia: genotype-phenotype correlation. Brain 132 (Pt 7), 1711–1722.

Harkin, L.A., Bowser, D.N., Dibbens, L.M., et al., 2002. Truncation of the GABA(A)-receptor gamma2 subunit in a family with generalized epilepsy with febrile seizures plus. Am. J. Hum. Genet. 70 (2), 530–536.

Herlenius, E., Heron, S.E., Grinton, B.E., et al., 2007. SCN2A mutations and benign familial neonatal-infantile seizures: the phenotypic spectrum. Epilepsia 48 (6), 1138–1142.

Iannetti, P., Parisi, P., Spalice, A., et al., 2009. Addition of verapamil in the treatment of severe myoclonic epilepsy in infancy. Epilepsy Res. 85 (1), 89–95.

Jarecki, B.W., Sheets, P.L., Jackson, J.O., et al., 2008. Paroxysmal extreme pain disorder mutations within the D3/S4-S5 linker of Nav1.7 cause moderate destabilization of fast inactivation. J. Physiol. 586 (Pt 17), 4137–4153.

Kim, S.H., Nordli, D.R. Jr., Berg, A.T., et al., 2014. Ictal ontogeny in Dravet syndrome. Clin. Neurophysiol.

Kors, E.E., Terwindt, G.M., Vermeulen, F.L., et al., 2001. Delayed cerebral edema and fatal coma after minor head trauma: role of the CACNA1A calcium channel subunit gene and relationship with familial hemiplegic migraine. Ann. Neurol. 49 (6), 753–760.

Lassche, S., Lainez, S., Bloem, B.R., et al., 2014. A novel KCNA1 mutation causing episodic ataxia type I. Muscle Nerve 50 (2), 289–291.

Liu, Y., Lopez-Santiago, L.F., Yuan, Y., et al., 2013. Dravet syndrome patient-derived neurons suggest a novel epilepsy mechanism. Ann. Neurol. 74 (1), 128–139.

Marchioni, E., Galimberti, C.A., Soragna, D., et al., 1995. Familial hemiplegic migraine versus migraine with prolonged aura: an uncertain diagnosis in a family report. Neurology 45 (1), 33–37.

Nachbauer, W., Nocker, M., Karner, E., et al., 2014. Episodic ataxia type 2: phenotype characteristics of a novel CACNA1A mutation and review of the literature. J. Neurol. 261 (5), 983–991.

Nilsen, K.B., Nicholas, A.K., Woods, C.G., et al., 2009. Two novel SCN9A mutations causing insensitivity to pain. Pain 143 (1–2), 155–158.

Pelzer, N., Stam, A.H., Carpay, J.A., et al., 2014. Familial hemiplegic migraine treated by sodium valproate and lamotrigine. Cephalalgia 34 (9), 708–711.

Press, C.K.K., Chapman, K., 2015. Parental reporting of response to oral cannabis extracts for treatment of refractory epilepsy. Epilepsy Behav.

Riant, F., Roze, E., Barbance, C., et al., 2012. PRRT2 mutations cause hemiplegic migraine. Neurology 79 (21), 2122–2124.

Roth, C., Freilinger, T., Kirovski, G., et al., 2014. Clinical spectrum in three families with familial hemiplegic migraine type 2 including a novel mutation in the ATP1A2 gene. Cephalalgia 34 (3), 183–190.

Sanchez-Albisua, I., Schoning, M., Jurkat-Rott, K., et al., 2013. Possible effect of corticoids on hemiplegic attacks in severe hemiplegic migraine. Pediatr. Neurol. 49 (4), 286–288.

Singh, N.A., Charlier, C., Stauffer, D., et al., 1998. A novel potassium channel gene, KCNQ2, is mutated in an inherited epilepsy of newborns. Nat. Genet. 18 (1), 25–29.

Stam, A.H., Vanmolkot, K.R., Kremer, H.P., et al., 2008. CACNA1A R1347Q: a frequent recurrent mutation in hemiplegic migraine. Clin. Genet. 74 (5), 481–485.

Stam, A.H., Luijckx, G.J., Poll-The, B.T., et al., 2009. Early seizures and cerebral oedema after trivial head trauma associated with the CACNA1A S218L mutation. J. Neurol. Neurosurg. Psychiatry 80 (10), 1125–1129.

Steinlein, O.K., Conrad, C., Weidner, B., 2007. Benign familial neonatal convulsions: always benign? Epilepsy Res. 73 (3), 245–249.

Steinlein, O.K., Mulley, J.C., Propping, P., et al., 1995. A missense mutation in the neuronal nicotinic acetylcholine receptor alpha 4 subunit is associated with autosomal dominant nocturnal frontal lobe epilepsy. Nat. Genet. 11 (2), 201–203.

Striano, P., Mancardi, M.M., Biancheri, R., et al., 2007. Brain MRI findings in severe myoclonic epilepsy in infancy and genotype-phenotype correlations. Epilepsia 48 (6), 1092–1096.

Sugawara, T., Tsurubuchi, Y., Agarwala, K.L., et al., 2001. A missense mutation of the Na+ channel alpha II subunit gene Na(v)1.2 in a patient with febrile and afebrile seizures causes channel dysfunction. Proc. Natl. Acad. Sci. U.S.A. 98 (11), 6384–6389.

Suzuki, T., Delgado-Escueta, A.V., Aguan, K., et al., 2004. Mutations in EFHC1 cause juvenile myoclonic epilepsy. Nat. Genet. 36 (8), 842–849.

Terwindt, G.M., Ophoff, R.A., Haan, J., et al., 1998. Variable clinical expression of mutations in the P/Q-type calcium channel gene in familial hemiplegic migraine. Dutch Migraine Genetics Research Group. Neurology 50 (4), 1105–1110.

van den Maagdenberg, A.M., Kors, E.E., Brunt, E.R., et al., 2002. Episodic ataxia type 2. Three novel truncating mutations and one novel missense mutation in the CACNA1A gene. J. Neurol. 249 (11), 1515–1519.

Wallace, R.H., Marini, C., Petrou, S., et al., 2001. Mutant GABA(A) receptor gamma2-subunit in childhood absence epilepsy and febrile seizures. Nat. Genet. 28 (1), 49–52.

Wallace, R.H., Wang, D.W., Singh, R., et al., 1998. Febrile seizures and generalized epilepsy associated with a mutation in the Na+-channel beta1 subunit gene SCN1B. Nat. Genet. 19 (4), 366–370.

Weckhuysen, S., Ivanovic, V., Hendrickx, R., et al., 2013. Extending the KCNQ2 encephalopathy spectrum: clinical and neuroimaging findings in 17 patients. Neurology 81 (19), 1697–1703.

Wolff, M., Casse-Perrot, C., Dravet, C., 2006. Severe myoclonic epilepsy of infants (Dravet syndrome): natural history and neuropsychological findings. Epilepsia 47 (Suppl. 2), 45–48.

Yu, F.H., Mantegazza, M., Westenbroek, R.E., et al., 2006. Reduced sodium current in GABAergic interneurons in a mouse model of severe myoclonic epilepsy in infancy. Nat. Neurosci. 9 (9), 1142–1149.

Zhuchenko, O., Bailey, J., Bonnen, P., et al., 1997. Autosomal dominant cerebellar ataxia (SCA6) associated with small polyglutamine expansions in the alpha 1A-voltage-dependent calcium channel. Nat. Genet. 15 (1), 62.

E-BOOK FIGURES AND TABLES

The following figures and tables are available in the e-book at www.expertconsult.com. See inside cover for registration details.

Fig. 49-1 Distribution of mutations in the SCN1A gene.

50 Neurodevelopmental Disabilities: Conceptual Framework

Iris Etzion, Sinan O. Turnacioglu, Karen A. Spencer, and Andrea L. Gropman

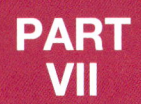 An expanded version of this chapter is available on www.expertconsult.com. See inside cover for registration details.

GENERAL CONCEPTIONS AND CONSIDERATIONS WHEN APPROACHING A CHILD WITH SUSPECTED DEVELOPMENTAL DISABILITIES

Child development, a general term relating to neurologic and psychological growth and development of a human being from birth to adulthood, is a continuum starting in the prenatal period and extending throughout life, with close and inevitable interaction with the environment. Perceiving development as a series of milestones gained in a stepwise fashion in various categories—though practical in the clinical setting—belies the complex concept of its very essence: an integrative process, in which each aspect interacts with all others, leading the individual from utter helplessness to independence, adaptive social skills, and emotional integrity.

The traditional concept of development relates to six domains: gross motor, fine motor, receptive language, expressive language, problem-solving, and social-adaptive skills.

Neuromuscular assessment can be performed as early as 20 weeks of gestation (Ballard et al., 1991). Term newborns already exhibit relation to the environment, and maladaptive patterns of behavior can be identified. Several assessment tools exist (i.e., Brazelton Neonatal Behavioral Assessment Scale) for birth up to 2 months of age. The scale relates to four aspects of early development: regulation of the autonomic system, of the motor system, of the state of alertness in response to various stimuli, and primary communicative skills.

The first 2 years of life are the most striking developmentally. Hence, the various estimation tools used (mentioned in section on approach to the evaluation of a child with NDD) regard development in 3-month intervals. Toddlers are commonly assessed in 6-month intervals and by school age, a yearly evaluation of a neurotypically developing child is customary. By then, focus shifts from the "classical" developmental benchmarks to academic skills as reflected by the child's achievements at school.

Delay refers to a lag in one or more—and occasionally all—aspects of development. *Global developmental delay* (GDD) is a common term used at an early age to describe what might later turn out to be intellectual disability (ID). *Dissociation* regards a discrepancy between different developmental domains. This is typically seen in children with cerebral palsy, who struggle to gain gross motor milestones but do not necessarily display difficulties with language acquisition. Dissociation might be used to describe a difference in the extent of delay in two or more fields, for example, significant language delay along with mild motor delay, as is often seen in children diagnosed with autism spectrum disorder (ASD). *Deviance* is a term used to describe an abnormal sequence of development, usually "skipping" milestones that might indicate a hidden pathology (Accardo et al., 2008). For instance, pushing to stand without crawling might indicate hypertonicity of the lower limbs. The "cocktail-party chatter" typical of William syndrome represents another deviance pattern, in which expressive language appears more elaborate then receptive abilities.

The developmental trajectory observed over time serves as yet another clue to the underlying pathology leading to developmental disabilities. Early delay with later catch-up is typical of preterm infants, with catch-up occasionally continuing into adolescence. On the contrary, normal gain of early milestones with difficulties emerging later on up to possible loss of already acquired skills denotes investigation of a possible metabolic or neurodegenerative disorder. A continuous GDD with a stable yet below age-average learning curve suggests a future ID and might warrant a genetic workup (Moeschler et al., 2014).

Spectrum of Neurodevelopmental Disabilities

In its broadest sense, the term *neurodevelopmental disabilities* can include a wide range of disorders with significant overlap and varying causes (Box 50-1). These include conditions that affect motor, sensory, cognitive, language, and executive functions, and social and behavioral disorders. Typical conditions included within this designation include cerebral palsy, GDD, ID, attention-deficit/hyperactivity disorder (ADHD), ASD, and learning disorders. Neurodevelopmental disabilities are related to abnormalities in central nervous system (CNS) development and may lead to lifelong functional impairment.

They are a heterogeneous group of disorders. They can be defined quantitatively based on results of developmental or neuropsychological assessments, or qualitatively by comparing an individual's developmental profile to that of same-age peers (Shevell, 2010). Socioeconomic, racial, and ethnic factors may affect the timing of diagnosis. In ASD, for example, lower socioeconomic status and Hispanic ethnicity have been associated with a later age at first diagnosis.

The functional implications of neurodevelopmental disabilities are addressed in the World Health Organization's International Classification of Functioning, Disability, and Health, which uses three components—body function and structure, activity, and participation—that help delineate the nature of an individual's disability.

A key aspect of the evaluation of a child suspected of having a neurodevelopmental disability is the approach to establishing diagnoses. Accurate diagnoses help guide further investigation into causality, implementation of necessary services, family counseling, and anticipation of long-term

BOX 50-1 Frequently Encountered Neurodevelopmental Disabilities

Attention-deficit/hyperactivity disorder
Autism spectrum disorder
Cerebral palsy
Communication disorders
Global developmental delay
Epilepsy
Hearing impairment
Intellectual disability
Learning disorders
Leukoencephalopathies
Neurogenetic disorders and inborn errors of metabolism
Neuromuscular disorders
Visual impairment

prognosis. Certain genetic disorders predispose children to neurodevelopmental disorders, as do other predisposing factors, including prematurity, neonatal encephalopathy, and socioeconomic status. It is now well recognized that individual patients can be affected by more than one neurodevelopmental disability.

Overview and Scope of the Problem

These conditions exist at the intersection of the disciplines of neurology, psychiatry, developmental pediatrics, neurodevelopmental disabilities, and psychology, and may be evaluated by specialists in any or all of these fields. Features of neurodevelopmental disabilities highlight the overlap and interaction between the fields of neurology and psychiatry. With growing understanding of the genetics and neurophysiology underlying these conditions, neurologists in the future may be expected to manage conditions previously designated as psychiatric disorders. For example, Rett syndrome was listed as one of the pervasive developmental disorders in American Psychiatric Association's *Diagnostic and Statistical Manual of Mental Disorders—IV* (DSM-IV), but with the identification of MeCP2 as the cause of this syndrome, it has subsequently been considered a neurogenetic disorder and removed from the current edition of the DSM (American Psychiatric Association, 2013).

Neurodevelopmental disabilities can be diagnosed on the basis of practice parameters such as those released by the American Academy of Neurology/Child Neurology Society for Global Developmental Delay (Chapter 51) and ASD (Chapter 57) , or by applying diagnostic criteria as detailed in the DSM-5 (American Psychiatric Association, 2013). In DSM-5, neurodevelopmental disorders are described as "disorders with onset in the developmental period, often before starting school, and that are characterized by a range of developmental deficits that impair normal functioning." They include ID (intellectual developmental disorder), communication disorders (language disorder, speech sound disorder, and childhood-onset fluency disorder), ASD, ADHD, specific learning disorder, and motor disorders (developmental coordination disorder, stereotypic movement disorder, and tic disorders). A formal classification system can be used, for example, with characterization of cerebral palsy by neurologic subtype or by gross motor skills (Chapter 97).

There is a need to consider children's diagnoses in a longitudinal manner. Children with diagnoses of GDD have a high likelihood of experiencing persistent developmental and functional impairments at school age but not necessarily cognitive impairment. These conditions often persist throughout life, and affect adults' health issues as well as have an impact on employment status, social relationships, and activities of daily living.

One way to establish a diagnosis or diagnoses is to refer a child for developmental or neuropsychological evaluation (Chapter 10), which will quantitatively determine the child's level of function related to age expectations or qualitatively establish appropriate DSM diagnoses. Another, not mutually exclusive, approach is a diagnostic workup that may include neuroimaging, metabolic and genetic testing, and neurophysiology studies. Chromosomal microarray has been recommended as a first-line investigation for the etiology of ID and ASD, and ongoing research has explored the yield of more advanced genetic testing, including whole exome sequencing and whole genome sequencing. Identification of a genetic diagnosis for a child with ID or ASD can have a significant impact for a family on the care of the child and may lead to more refined treatments, in the case of dietary treatment and enzyme replacement for metabolic disorders or optimal anticonvulsant treatment in the cases of SCN1A or GLUT1. Recent investigations using animal models now imply that ID can be reversible through pharmacology interventions (Chapter 59) or appropriate learning or retraining paradigms.

The concept that epilepsy itself or the presence of an epilepsy syndrome can contribute to a child's cognitive and behavioral impairments has been explored extensively, and epileptic encephalopathy is addressed in the current classification system for epilepsy. In the absence of clinical evidence that raises concern for epilepsy, current practice parameters advise caution in carrying out electroencephalography in patients with GDD or ASD.

Population-based studies have indicated that 15% of children aged 3 to 17 years have a developmental disability on the basis of parent report. A recently published survey noted that there has been a 21% increase in disabilities related to neurodevelopmental or mental health conditions in the United States in the 2000s.

The breakdown among individual disabilities varies. GDD is estimated to affect 1% to 3% of children, whereas a prevalence rate of 7.66% was found for ID. The Centers for Disease Control (CDC)'s Autism and Developmental Disabilities Monitoring Network noted that the prevalence of cerebral palsy has ranged from 0.31% to 0.36% since 1996. ASD prevalence rates in the most recent CDC surveillance findings were at 1.4% among 8-year-olds. Among learning disorders, reading was reported to have 5.3% to 11.8% cumulative incidence rates, math incidence rates of 5.9% to 13.8%, and writing 6.9% to 14.7% cumulative incidence rates in a population-based birth cohort.

Determinants and Risk Factors

The prime determinants of neurodevelopmental disabilities involve genetic and metabolic abnormalities and aberrant CNS development, prematurity, low birth weight, perinatal complications, chronic physical health conditions, exposure to environmental hazardous substances, compromised family functioning, and low-socioeconomic family background. Families of children with ADHD have been found to have higher rates of alcoholism, other drug abuse, depression, delinquency, and learning disabilities than controls. The concept of the broader autism phenotype addresses the higher incidence of social and communication symptoms and stereotypical behaviors in family members of children with ASD.

Commonalities

Although diagnostic criteria and recommendations for workup and treatment of individual disabilities have been established, a number of common elements are shared among neurodevelopmental disability diagnoses. Individual children can have multiple neurodevelopmental diagnoses, and diagnoses may evolve over time, with the child initially diagnosed with GDD later identified as having a learning disorder.

For conditions that are diagnosed primarily by behavioral manifestations and through application of DSM-5 criteria, there is a notorious lack of biomarkers. Neuroimaging and electroencephalography tend to be unrevealing or nonspecific. The American Academy of Neurology/Child Neurology Society (AAN/CNS) practice parameter recommends neuroimaging as part of the diagnostic evaluation, but indicates that data are insufficient for a recommendation regarding the role of EEG in child with GDD in whom there is no clinical evidence of epilepsy. In ASD, nonspecific EEG abnormalities have been found in most children and there is a lack of evidence to support universal screening EEG without a clinical indication.

Children with neurodevelopmental disabilities are often found to have evidence of neurologic soft or subtle signs, such as mirror movements, synkinesis, clumsy finger movements, difficulties with balance, and motor persistence. These soft signs have been noted in patients with ADHD and ASD and have been followed longitudinally in cohorts of patients.

Beyond treatments for inborn errors of metabolism, medications are typically prescribed to treat specific behaviors in children with neurodevelopmental disabilities, including stimulants and nonstimulants for inattention, hyperactivity, and impulsivity; antipsychotics and nonstimulants for aggression and irritability; and selective serotonin reuptake inhibitors and related medications for anxiety and mood symptomatology. Physical, occupational, language, and educational therapies are prescribed to these children.

Overlap in Neurodevelopment Disorders

Neurodevelopmental conditions are frequently seen in combination in particular patients. Gillberg has proposed the acronym *ESSENCE* (early symptomatic syndromes eliciting neurodevelopmental clinical examinations), to describe the coexistence of impairing symptoms that can be initially identified in the first few years of life. In his classification, the ESSENCE conditions affect general development, communication and language, social interrelatedness, motor coordination, attention, activity, behavior, mood, and sleep. Children who are diagnosed with a particular neurodevelopmental diagnosis at an early age may no longer meet criteria for the specific diagnosis as they age, but may ultimately receive another neurodevelopmental disorder diagnosis (Gillberg, 2010). Children with ASD often have coexisting problems that include ADHD, epilepsy, ID, learning disorder, oppositional defiant disorder, anxiety disorder, mood disorder, and obsessive compulsive disorder.

Recent genetic research has called into question the current categorical diagnostic algorithm used for neurodevelopmental disorders (NDDs) as delineated in DSM-5. Similar genetic findings have been identified in individuals with different neurodevelopmental diagnoses. For example, genetic changes at 16p11.2 that were initially associated with ASD have been found to be associated with developmental delay, ID, communication problems, abnormal head circumference, and psychiatric conditions, including schizophrenia and bipolar disease, and SCN2A mutations have been associated with ASD and epilepsy.

The National Institutes of Mental Health has addressed the difficulty of diagnostic classification by introducing the Research Domain Criteria project as a framework for ongoing research that characterizes psychiatric disorders as neurophysiological disorders with a basis in genetics, electrophysiology, and functional imaging.

Approach to the Evaluation of a Child with Suspected Neurodevelopmental or Intellectual Disability

Many of the principles of evaluating children with a neurodevelopmental disorder are similar to evaluating any child with a neurologic disorder. These principles are covered extensively in Part I: Clinical Evaluation. However, there are few aspects of these that merit special attention for children with neurodevelopmental disorders.

The Developmental History

Ascertaining a child's current developmental milestones is an important part of the evaluation of a child with a neurodevelopmental disorder. Given the limited amount of time during an office visit, it may sometimes be helpful to obtain reports of previous testing that has been performed in other settings, such as school or early intervention.

Another dimension of the developmental assessment is adaptive measures, which refer to the ability to perform activities of daily living. This is an important part of understanding the level of functional disability of a child and is a requirement for the diagnosis of ID in the DSM-5. The Vineland Adaptive Behavior Scale, Second Edition (Vineland-II) is the most commonly used measurement, and can be a helpful tool to identify a child's strengths, as well as areas that require more attention.

Assessing the pattern of a child's development is important in generating a differential diagnosis. Is there a concern for a developmental regression or a loss of developmental milestones? Is one area more affected than another? Children with isolated motor delays raise concern for neuromuscular disorders or cerebral palsy. Children with language delays may have difficulty with hearing or comprehension, or may have autism. Children with abnormal socialization may have autism or Rett syndrome, or may be suffering from the effects of trauma or neglect. Developmental problems that began during the school years can raise concern for ADHD, learning disabilities, or psychiatric issues, including anxiety or depression.

Birth History

Medication and drug exposure during pregnancy may influence the child's development. Information about the child's delivery should include the need for perinatal resuscitation, postnatal respiratory support, or low Apgar scores which may all be indicators of neonatal hypoxic ischemic encephalopathy. Providers should be aware of the newborn hearing screen results and if there was any follow-up.

Social History

Because there is a complex interplay between the family milieu and children with neurodevelopmental disorders, taking a social history is important. Children with neurodevelopmental disorders often require significant financial and emotional support, which places stress on the child as well as the family. Assessing the needs of these families is an important aspect of their care.

Psychosocial stressors in the home can manifest themselves in the child and appear to be consistent with a neurodevelopmental disorder. For example, a child who has suffered from trauma or neglect has abnormal socialization and can present with developmental delay. Exposure to adverse events can make a child more likely to have emotional dysregulation, heightened responses to perceived negative stimuli, and executive dysfunction. These children are at increased risk for developing disorders such as ADHD, anxiety, and depression. Children with neurodevelopmental disorders require a close assessment of their home environment to understand concomitant stressors and adverse exposures so that the child's well-being is preserved.

History should include assessment of the school environment. Children with neurodevelopmental disorders are more likely to have a significant number of missed days at school, have fewer friends than their peers, be bullied at school, and, in the case of children with special healthcare needs who required behavioral services, to bully other children. They participate less in extracurricular activities and are at risk for social isolation. Their happiness and level of inclusion at school should be an important aspect of the social history.

Family History

The family history can give important clues to the etiology of the developmental disorders. ADHD and dyslexia have strong genetic aspects. Children suspected of having fragile X syndrome may have maternal relatives with anxiety or depression, autistic-like features, or ADHD.

Physical Examination

One of the most important aspects of the evaluation of the child is observing his or her behavior in as unstructured an environment as possible, such as providing toys and opportunities for the child to play while the practitioner obtains the medical history from the caregiver. Through this, there are many aspects of a child that may not be apparent through history alone. For example, how does the child interact with the toys? Does the child mouth or lick the toys, or does he or she use them functionally? Does the child share his or her enjoyment with you or the examiner, or does the child prefer to keep to herself? How does the child interact with toys that he or she needs help with? Does the child look to his or her caregivers, or to you, for help, or does the child simply put the toy aside? Or does he or she become inconsolable? Is the child limited in any way by difficulties with coordination or motor functioning? As the examination proceeds, important things to note include the ability of the child to make eye contact and respond to his or her name, to follow directions with and without demonstration, and the level of engagement he or she has with you as the examiner.

For the older child, engaging him or her in conversation during the examination may be more revealing. Is the child able to hold a conversation with you, or does he or she have difficulty? Asking about social life and interests can be an important way to help engage. Adolescents, if developmentally appropriate, may be more easily examined alone, so that they may feel more comfortable sharing information with you.

For a child with neurodevelopmental disorders, special attention is made to the child's appearance to rule out any dysmorphic features, the skin examination to evaluate for neurocutaneous disorders (i.e., neurofibromatosis type I can be associated with learning disabilities and autism), and the eye examination to evaluate for evidence for genetic or metabolic abnormalities.

Testing

Testing children with suspected neurodevelopmental disorder should take a highly individualized approach based on the concern. The initial evaluation will provide clues to the nature of what testing should be pursued. Children with an abnormal neurologic examination finding revealing focal deficits require neuroimaging. Neuroimaging is recommended for children with GDD, per the American Academy of Neurology guidelines.

For many children with neurodevelopmental disorders, the most important testing is a neuropsychological evaluation. For school-aged children, this can occur in the school setting. For children younger than 3 years, they are entitled to a developmental assessment through an early intervention program. Office-based screening tools may be helpful to guide the testing that needs to be done. For example, a Vanderbilt assessment is helpful not only for symptoms of ADHD, but also to screen for any comorbid behavioral difficulties, such as conduct disorder, oppositional defiant disorder, anxiety, and depression. Difficulties in school and activities of daily living are assessed. Identified problems can help guide the provider to refer the child for further testing to address academic performance or for behavioral therapy.

Many children with neurodevelopmental disorders are at risk for having comorbid emotional or behavioral disorders. There are many in-office tools that can be helpful to assess these children's risks. Children who have positive screens for behavioral or emotional disorders should be referred to other providers for further management.

Multidisciplinary Approach to the Care of the Child with a Neurodevelopmental Disorder

Caring for children with neurodevelopmental disorders is often complex and requires a multidisciplinary approach to their care. Families of these children have significant financial stressors and difficulties with coordinating medical care. These patients often have numerous medical providers as well as a team of therapists and educators who are all working to care for them. An attentive medical provider can be instrumental in helping to assure that these children are able to access the care they need to support their disabilities. This section discusses the challenges facing these families.

Children with chronic emotional, behavioral, or developmental problems are more likely to have health conditions that affect their daily activities, as well as be uninsured or underinsured; have unmet healthcare needs; have difficulty obtaining referrals; have more missed days of school; and have at least $1000 per year in out-of-pocket health-related expenses. These families have high levels of financial stress, including decreased levels of employment and high out-of-pocket costs (Kuo et al., 2013). High out-of-pocket costs are associated with the medical severity of the disorder as well as the need for mental health services in addition to medical services. Families of children with autism have the highest reported out-of-pocket costs. Children with special healthcare needs who have functional limitations have more difficulties accessing needed services and getting needed referrals.

Compared with healthy peers, children with neurodevelopmental disorders have significant challenges that can affect their quality of life. Children with ADHD, learning disabilities, and intellectual disabilities are all more likely to have a comorbid psychiatric disorder than their typically developing peers. A study by Klassen et al. reveals that children with ADHD have poorer measures on health-related quality of life than controls, including measures of mental health and self-esteem. Children with ADHD and comorbid psychiatric disorders tend to fare worse on quality-of-life measures (Stein et al., 2011). Children with learning disabilities have an increased risk of comorbid psychiatric disorders and increased social difficulties with peers. Children with intellectual disabilities have a much higher likelihood of having an emotional disorder or psychiatric disorders than typically developing children. Children with autism face social isolation from peers and, as young adults, have a higher likelihood of social isolation than peers with another developmental disorder, including intellectual disabilities. Children with special healthcare needs who have emotional problems or functional limitations have worse school outcomes than children with special healthcare needs who don't have those problems. Families of children with a neurodevelopmental disorder and a comorbid emotional or behavioral disorder tend to fare poorly. A study of children with neurologic conditions and behavioral disorders indicated that families of children with both a neurologic disorder and a behavioral disorder had more unmet needs and reported greater dissatisfaction with care, care coordination, ability to obtain a referral, and to use other services. A study by Nageswaran et al. of children with developmental disabilities with comorbid mental health diagnoses found similar findings (American Academy of Pediatrics, 2005).

REFERENCES

The complete list of references for this chapter is available in the e-book at www.expertconsult.com.

See inside cover for registration details.

SELECTED REFERENCES

Accardo, P.J., Accardo, J.A., Capute, A.J., 2008. A neurodevelopmental perspective on the continuum of developmental disabilities. In: Accardo, P., Accardo, J., Capute, A.J., (Eds.), Capute & Accardo's Neurodevelopmental Disabilities in Infancy and Childhood, third ed. Paul H. Brookes Publishing Co., New York, pp. 3–7.

American Academy of Pediatrics, 2005. Care coordination in the medical home: integrating health and related systems of care for children with special health care needs. Pediatrics 116, 1238–1244.

American Psychiatric Association, 2013. Diagnostic and Statistical Manual of Mental Disorders, fifth ed. APA, Washington, DC.

Ballard, J.L., Khoury, J.C., Wedig, K., et al., 1991. New Ballard Score, expanded to include extremely premature infants. J. Pediatr. 119, 417–423.

Gillberg, C., 2010. The ESSENCE in child psychiatry: early symptomatic syndromes eliciting neurodevelopmental clinical examinations. Res. Dev. Disabil. 31, 1543–1551.

Klassen, A.F., Miller, A., Fine, S., 2004. Health-related quality of life in children and adolescents who have a diagnosis of attention-deficit/hyperactivity disorder. Pediatrics 114 (5), e541–e547. doi:10.1542/peds.2004-0844.

Kuo, D.Z., Goudie, A., Cohe, E., et al., 2013. Inequities in health care needs for children with medical complexity. Health Aff. 33, 2190–2198.

Moeschler, J.B., Shevell, M., Committee on Genetics, 2014. Comprehensive evaluation of the child with intellectual disability or global developmental delays. Pediatrics 134, e903–e918.

Shevell, M.I., 2010. Present conceptualization of early childhood neurodevelopmental disabilities. J. Child Neurol. 25, 120–126.

Stein, D., Blum, N.J., Barbaresi, W.J., 2011. Developmental and behavioral disorders through the life span. Pediatrics 128, 364–373.

E-BOOK FIGURES AND TABLES

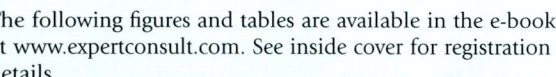

The following figures and tables are available in the e-book at www.expertconsult.com. See inside cover for registration details.

51 Global Developmental Delay and Intellectual Disability

Elliott H. Sherr and Michael I. Shevell

An expanded version of this chapter is available on www.expertconsult.com. See inside cover for registration details.

DEFINITIONS

Global developmental delay (GDD) and intellectual disability (ID) are related, nonsynonymous terms with common and distinctive characteristics. They can be defined as early onset, chronic disorders with disturbance in the acquisition of cognitive, motor, language, or social skills, which has a significant and continuing impact on the developmental progress of an individual (Michelson et al., 2011).

The 2002 consensus definition of the American Association on Mental Retardation (AAMR; now known as the American Association on Intellectual and Developmental Disabilities [AAIDD]) defined ID as "characterized by a significant limitation both in intellectual functioning and in adaptive behavior as expressed in conceptual, social, practical, and adaptive skills." This disability originates before the age of 18 and manifests with severe problems in the capacity to perform (i.e., impairment), ability to perform (i.e., activity limitations), and opportunity to function (i.e., participation restrictions).

For the young child, the term "global developmental delay" has emerged to describe a disturbance across a variety of developmental domains. The latest consensus definition used by the American Academy of Neurology (AAN) and the Child Neurology Society practice parameter statement defines GDD operationally as a significant delay in two or more developmental domains (e.g., gross/fine motor, cognitive, speech/language, personal/social, activities of daily living) (Michelson et al., 2011). Typically, if there is delay in two domains, this often implies delay across all domains.

Thus the definitions of ID and GDD reflect an approach to disability that emphasizes adaptive behaviors and contextual factors as opposed to a single objective measure.

Epidemiology

Assuming a normal distribution of IQ scores (and that adaptive skills correlate closely with these more conventional metrics of intellectual ability), approximately 2.25% of individuals will have an IQ below 70 and a diagnosis of ID. Early population-based studies confirmed this theoretical estimate, documenting an overall rate of ID of 2%, with 1.5% having mild ID (IQ of 50–70) and 0.5% having moderate or severe ID (IQ of less than 50). Although the population studied and the instruments used can influence the rate of mild ID, they seem to have little effect on the rate of severe ID. Thus the prevalence rates for mild ID in 15 subsequent studies varied broadly from 5 to 80 cases per 1000 people, whereas the prevalence of severe ID varied only between 2.5 and 7 per 1000 (Leonard and Wen, 2002).

Many changes that affect the rate of mild ID can affect the overall numbers of persons with ID in the population (e.g., poor education, nutrition, tobacco or alcohol use, environmental toxins such as lead). Additional risk has been associated with low birth weight and maternal age. Paternal smoking also increases the risk of having children with ID. In addition, race and gender disparities have also been reported, with ID overrepresented by as much as 50% among African Americans relative to the Caucasian population (thought to be influenced heavily by social context), and the male-to-female ratio was 1.4 : 1.0.

ID cases are often grouped by prenatal, perinatal, and postnatal causes. Prenatal causes include genetic syndromes and chromosomal disorders, central nervous system malformations, and maternal toxic or infectious causes. Perinatal conditions include birth asphyxia, stroke, and infection. Postnatal conditions include infection, toxins (e.g., lead), and injury, such as nonaccidental trauma. Simple public health measures (e.g., iodized salt, community-wide rubella vaccination, newborn screening) have prevented an estimated 15% of cases of ID in the industrial world. Currently the most common potentially preventable cause of ID in high-resource settings is fetal alcohol syndrome, whereas congenital hypothyroidism caused by maternal dietary iodine deficiency remains the most common preventable cause world-wide.

Using the above framework, over 60% of children with ID do not have identified causes. Among the causes identified, chromosomal defects are common, and Down syndrome is the single most common known chromosomal cause. The increasing widespread availability and application of chromosomal microarray (CMA; also referred to as array comparative genomic hybridization [CGH]) and whole-exome sequencing in the clinical setting will increase the percentage of attributable causes to these subtler genetic disruptions (Sherr et al., 2013).

Many individuals with ID are unable to become productive members of society and require institutionalized or group-home care. The economic costs are substantial, with one study showing the financial burden on society equal to the economic impact of stroke, heart disease, and cancer combined (Meerding et al., 1998). Another analysis estimates lifetime costs of more than $1 million dollars per person with ID, which is more than that for cerebral palsy, hearing loss, or vision impairment.

DIAGNOSIS
Definitions and Testing

Accurate diagnosis of GDD or ID is an essential precondition to proper management and service provision. Accurate diagnosis helps understand the specific medical and psychiatric complications, determine eligibility for service and support provision, aid in family counseling, and confirm legal recognition of disability. Multiple standardized, age-appropriate measures have been normed and validated on typically developing populations to assess intellectual function and adaptive behavioral skills.

Advances in Diagnostic Testing

An approach to the diagnosis of ID/GDD can begin with the AAN practice parameter and evidence report for GDD (Figure 51-1) (Michelson et al., 2011). The recommendations incorporate a combination of broad screening tools and

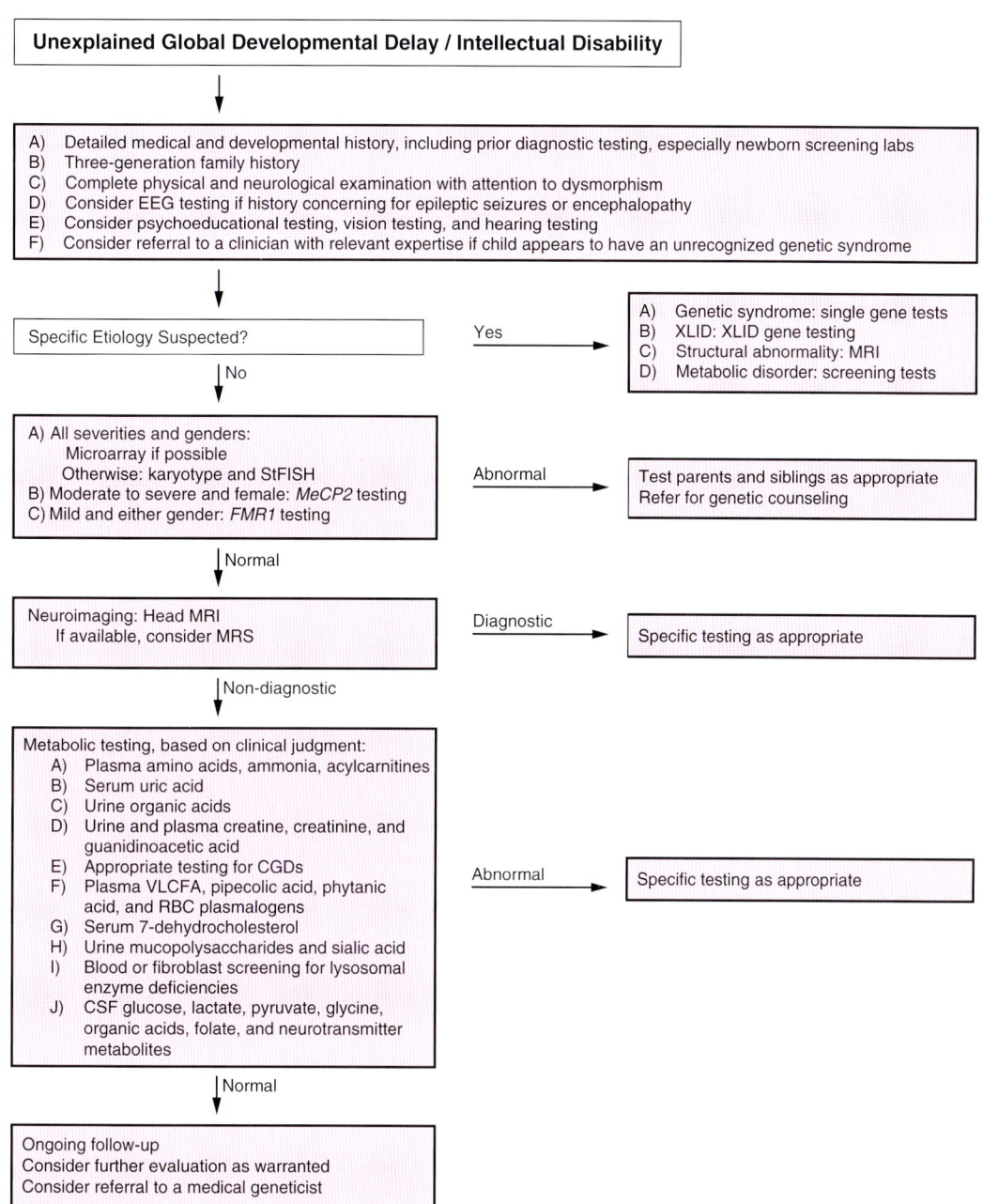

Figure 51-1. Algorithm for the evaluation of the child with unexplained global developmental delay or intellectual disability. A detailed history, a complete physical examination, psychoeducational testing, and screening tests for visual and hearing deficits are recommended for all children with GDD/ID. EEG is recommended when there is concern about seizures or an epileptic encephalopathy. In children with features suggesting a specific etiology, genetic testing, neuroimaging, and metabolic testing may be useful for confirmation. For children without features suggesting a specific etiology, testing can be done in a stepwise or parallel manner for genetic abnormalities, structural brain abnormalities, and metabolic abnormalities. Although an extensive list of metabolic tests is provided in this algorithm, there is insufficient evidence to make specific recommendations as to which testing sequence would have the greatest diagnostic yield. The algorithm is explained in greater detail in the Clinical Context section of this guideline. This algorithm is based on data contained in an evidence-based review on this topic (Michelson et al., 2011). CGD, congenital disorder of glycosylation; CSF, cerebrospinal fluid; EEG, electroencephalogram; GDD, global developmental delay; ID, intellectual disability; MRI, magnetic resonance imaging; MRS, magnetic resonance spectroscopy; RBC, red blood cell; VLCFA, very long chain fatty acids; XLID, X-linked intellectual disability. *(Report of the Quality Standards Subcommittee of the American Academy of Neurology and the Practice Committee of the Child Neurology Society. Neurology 2011.)*

disease-specific testing based on a heightened pretest probability, given identifying clinical features. Correctly applied, *each individual disease-specific test* has a reasonable pretest probability (>1%) of diagnosis, whereas the more recently introduced broad-based genomic screening tools have a high pretest

probability (5% to 25%). The current algorithm begins with a complete clinical assessment. For patients in whom a specific diagnosis is considered, targeted testing is recommended. For the remaining patients a step-wise approach is recommended that begins with CMA followed by chromosomal karyotype if that is negative. This recommendation reflects the capacity of CMA to detect clinically relevant chromosomal changes, and is also recommended by a consortium of clinical genetics laboratories (Miller et al., 2010; Michelson et al., 2011). Fragile X and meCP2 testing are examples of specific gene/syndrome approaches. However, if these tests are unrevealing, the algorithm recommends conducting brain magnetic resonance imaging (MRI; with single-proton spectroscopy, where available). If this approach is not diagnostic, comprehensive metabolic testing is then recommended (see Figure 51-1). As the yield of these diagnostic tools advances (a discussion of some recent advances, such as whole-exome sequencing, are expanded upon below), these algorithms will continue to change to reflect these technical improvements. Regardless, clinical judgment will always be tantamount.

Genomic Microarray

Genomic microarray technology detects copy number changes in the genome, usually with a resolution of 30 kb or less. These platforms identify interstitial copy number variants (CNV). Studies done thus far confirm the importance of CNVs as a cause of neurodevelopmental disabilities, detecting many chromosomal changes not visible with high-resolution karyotyping. Many studies in autism, mental retardation, and cohorts with multiple congenital anomalies (who also have neurodevelopmental disabilities) show that many CNVs occur repetitively with the same chromosomal breakpoints and at a much higher frequency in affected individuals than in controls. Although in some cases the link between CNV and ID is well established, this determination is challenging or not possible when that genetic variation has never been reported previously, or its incidence in cases and controls is not well documented. To address etiology in these variants of unknown significance, the first step is to establish whether a documented copy number change is de novo or familial: determining the size of the CNV, knowing whether it is a deletion or duplication, and knowing the genes (and gene density) in the CNV. The establishment of publicly available and actively updated genotype–phenotype databases aids in the process of establishing pathogenicity of these less common CNV.

Whole-Exome Sequencing: As outlined previously, advances in genetic testing have driven much of the progress in understanding the causes of ID. For example, CMA give positive diagnostic yields of approximately 7% to 8%, above that seen via karyotypes (Sherr et al., 2013). Recent data highlight the diagnostic potential of whole-exome sequencing. Two recent studies from a combined 3000 families demonstrate a diagnostic rate of approximately 25%. When patients with developmental delay were specifically examined, the rate of identification increased to 36% to 40%, exceeding that seen for CMA or karyotypes. Most of these diagnoses resulted from de novo mutations in known genes, and in some cases either homozygous recessive (for consanguineous families) or compound heterozygous inherited mutations were causative. The rate of de novo mutations has been shown to correlate to paternal age and suggests that some of the increased incidence in neurodevelopmental disorders in developed countries can be explained by this societal change in parental age.

Advances in Imaging

High-quality MRI has significantly advanced the ability to detect many brain malformations. Certain studies suggest that structural MRI is useful for detecting abnormalities in up to 50% of children with developmental delay, including the identification of polymicrogyria, pachygyria, lissencephaly, callosal agenesis, and periventricular nodular heterotopia, for

which genes are known to cause these syndromes. Proton MR spectroscopy measures the resonance of molecules in the brain, allowing the measurement of metabolism intermediates and helping in the diagnosis of mitochondrial disorders (lactate and pyruvate) or measuring creatine in disorders of creatine deficiency, potentially treatable forms of ID and GDD.

ETIOLOGY
General Considerations

The known specific causes of ID are too numerous to be listed here. The term "intellectual disability" returns more than 3000 entries in the Online Mendelian Inheritance in Man site alone, and this catalogs only identifiable genetic causes. As mentioned previously, ID usually is classified by prenatal, perinatal, postnatal, and undetermined causes. In most U.S.-based studies, the largest category of known primary causes is genetic or chromosomal (Leonard and Wen, 2002), with up to 75% of the known cases attributable to chromosomal aberrations. In contrast, in some regions of the world, cretinism (stunted physical growth and ID) from severe iodine deficiency occurs in up to 2% to 10% of the population of isolated communities. Mild mental impairment from iodine deficiency occurs five times more frequently than cretinism, making iodine deficiency the most common preventable cause of mental retardation. Treatment during the first trimester has a significant effect on the frequency of cretinism. In regions of mainland China with iodine deficiency, children score on average 10 IQ points less than cohorts in iodine-rich regions. This link between iodine deficiency and mental retardation has a strong genetic component, because alleles of the deiodinase type II gene and the ApoE4 allele confer a significantly greater risk of ID when the pregnant mother is iodine deficient. Despite the tremendous wealth of information about the causes of ID, the cause remains unknown in most individuals. Genetic and epidemiologic approaches likely will continue to make progress toward unraveling and treating these currently unelucidated causes.

Genetic Causes

Both inherited and de novo mutations have been shown to be causative for ID and GDD, and the advances in clinical application of genetic tools have accelerated the rate of discovery of new causes.

Fragile X Syndrome

Fragile X syndrome, caused by inactivation of the *FMR1* gene, has an estimated prevalence of 1 in 3000 males and is the most common inherited causes of ID. Expansion of the trinucleotide sequence CGG to more than 200 copies results in CpG methylation and inactivation of transcription of the *FMR1* gene. Patients have narrow and elongated faces, large protruding ears, macroorchidism in males, and joint hyperlaxity. Up to 50% of patients have ASD and 20% have epilepsy, and most have complex partial seizures. Carrier females and males with somatic mutations have a range of levels of intellectual impairment; studies demonstrate that the amount of the residual FMR protein detected in hair roots correlates well with IQ. Although previous studies suggested that premutation male carriers (55 to 200 repeats) were asymptomatic, later work has demonstrated that a range of symptoms are present in premutation carriers, including migraines, seizures, autism, and ID. Moreover, investigators have identified a progressive neurologic disorder, the fragile X–associated tremor/ataxia syndrome (FXTAS) in premutation carriers. After the age of 50, primarily male patients present with intention tremor and cerebellar ataxia, and cognitive decline. This syndrome, which is unique to these premutation carriers, may result from an increase in expanded repeat *FMR1* mRNA that is consistent with a toxic "gain of function" mechanism. Although treatment still remains symptomatically based, investigators have shown that fragile X syndrome leads to an exaggerated activation through metabotropic glutamate receptors, and early clinical studies have tested compounds that inhibit this signaling. Although the initial results did not demonstrate enhanced outcomes, it is possible that a greater understanding of these mechanisms may lead to targeted therapies.

Other X-Linked ID Conditions

The increased prevalence of ID in males and the relative ease of detecting familial transmission of X-chromosome mutations have led to the discovery of novel ID genes on the X chromosome. Since the early 1990s, more than 120 genes have been identified as causes of X-chromosome-linked syndromic and nonsyndromic ID (Table 51-4).

Mechanistically some of these genes work directly at the level of the synapse. For example, the protein family neuroligin on the postsynaptic membrane (with two X-linked neuroligin genes [*NLGN3* and *NLGN4*]), and its binding partner neurexin on the presynaptic side have been shown to promote synapse formation in vitro. Similarly, multiple genes that participate in signaling at the synapse through the small G protein RHO are mutated in many cases of X-linked ID: *GDI1*, *PAK3*, *OPHN1*, and *ARHGEF6*. There are also many genes without synaptic function that are well-established causes of ID, such as the genes *ARX* and *MECP2*. These genes can cause syndromic ID (as in patients with X-linked lissencephaly with ambiguous genitalia [XLAG] and Rett's syndrome) and nonsyndromic ID, depending on the severity of the mutation. These observations demonstrate the complexity of understanding how genetic alteration causes mental retardation, what form it takes, and how genotype may correlate with phenotype.

DE NOVO DOMINANT GDD AND ID

In addition to inherited cases of ID, there has also been significant strides in identifying genes that cause *de novo* dominant ID. The recent papers to detail the results of clinical exome sequencing report that, of the designated causative genes, nearly 1/3 of these were discovered in the last 18 months. At some point, the community of clinicians and investigators will begin to see a "saturation" for gene discovery, but that is still likely quite a ways off. Thus a specific listing of genes would be unproductive; however, there are many important themes that emerge:

1. The genetics of ID overlaps significantly with other neurodevelopmental disorders. This has been observed clinically, and was recently confirmed in cohorts of patients with de novo mutations demonstrating overlap between ID, ASD, epileptic encephalopathies, and schizophrenia causes.
2. Many genes have both syndromic and nonsyndromic presentations, depending on the severity and penetrance of the mutations.
3. Approximately 5% of patients will actually have two causative genes, suggesting that more complex disorders may be caused by these unexpected combinations.
4. Increasing the risk for de novo mutations by an older population contributes to this disease burden.
5. Postzygotic mutations play a significant role in these disorders in addition to germline mutations.

Other Etiologic Considerations

Several questions arise when considering the causes of mental retardation that guide the clinician in evaluating patients and help the researcher focus on the underlying pathophysiology. What is the prevalence of any genetic cause for ID and how many genes can cause this disorder? Will cases of mild ID be caused by less severe mutations in these same, already-discovered genes or in a completely different subset? How many cases of ID will be found to be caused by genetic factors alone, environmental factors alone, or the interplay between the two, as has been demonstrated for iodine deficiency?

TABLE 51-4 Genes Implicated in X-Linked Intellectual Disability

Gene	Function	Locus	Study
Genes Primarily Implicated in Nonsyndromic Intellectual Disability			
PAK3	P21 (CDKN1A)-activated kinase 3	Xq23	Schulze (2003)
GDI1	Guanosine triphosphate (GTP) dissociation inhibitor 1	Xq28	Ethofer et al. (2004)
IL1RAPL1	Interleukin 1 receptor accessory protein-like 1	Xp21.3	Eichler et al. (2002)
ARHGEF6	Rac/Cdc42 guanine nucleotide exchange factor 6	Xq26.3	Barnea-Goraly et al. (2004)
SLC6A8	Creatine transporter 8	Xq28	Baribeau and Anagnostou (2013)
FACL4	Long-chain fatty acid-coenzyme A ligase 4	Xq23	Fillano et al. (2002)
AGTR2	Angiotensin II receptor, type 2	Xq23	Marin-Garcia et al. (1999)
FTSJ1	S-adenosylmethionine-binding protein	Xp11.23	Lib et al. (2003)
DLG3	Synapse-associated protein 102 (anchoring protein)	Xq13.1	Schulenberg et al. (2004)
NLGN3	Neuroligin 3 (postsynaptic receptor)	Xq13.1	Hou et al. (1998)
NLGN4	Neuroligin 4 (binds neurexin)	Xp22.32	Delange et al. (2001)
PQBP1	Polyglutamine binding protein 1	Xp11.23	Cao et al. (1994)
RPS6KA3	Serine/threonine kinase	Xp22.12	Guo et al. (2004)
ZNF41	Zinc-finger protein involved in chromatin activation	Xp11.3	Wang et al. (2000)
Genes Implicated in Syndromic and Nonsyndromic Intellectual Disability			
OPHN	Rho-GTPase activating protein (cerebellar hypoplasia)	Xq12	Crawford et al. (2001)
ARX	Aristaless-related homeobox (X-linked lissencephaly with ambiguous genitalia [XLAG])	Xp22.11	Willemsen et al. (2004)
MECP2	Methyl-CpG binding protein 2 (Rett's syndrome)	Xq28	Willemsen et al. (2003)

EVALUATION OF THE PATIENT

History

The assessment of a child with suspected GDD or ID begins with a detailed history, including family history, mother's gestational history, perinatal history, birth, and early neonatal history.

The next component of history, history of present illness, includes the age at which the developmental concern became manifested to the caregiver and the timing of developmental milestones determined. The possibility of regression of previously acquired developmental skills should be specifically questioned, as this would mandate a different and more urgent approach to etiologic evaluation and follow-up. Current skill level in developmental domains and the degree of independence in activities of daily living must be documented. For the school-aged child, important points include scholastic history, with special reference to actual school and classroom placement, and the identification of the provision of any supplemental educational resources.

Coexisting medical problems, with particular reference to possible seizure disorders or feeding difficulties, should be questioned. Sleeping and problematic behaviors (e.g., aggressive, inappropriate, or self-injurious) may be particular concerns of the parents and are often underappreciated by health professionals. The medical history, including possible chronic medical conditions, prior hospital admissions, or surgical procedures, should be documented. Past and current medications prescribed, their indications, and their effects (beneficial or deleterious) must be assessed. The current social situation of the child and family must be carefully probed and the examiner must determine whether the patient has access to appropriate rehabilitation services. This approach should provide clear ideas regarding evidence of a static or progressive encephalopathy; the developmental and functional level; the timing of an underlying cause; a prioritized list of etiologic causes; the social or rehabilitation status of the affected child; and the possibility of associated medical or behavioral conditions meriting intervention.

Physical Examination

The physical examination begins with careful observation of the child. The availability of a play area with appropriate toys, including paper, crayons, dolls, and representational toys, may allow for a nonintrusive assessment of developmental skills, behavior, and interaction with the surroundings and others. Much of the neurodevelopmental examination can take place during extended history-taking by observation alone. In the older child, language skills, both spontaneous and responsive, expressive and receptive, should be established, together with an understanding of simple cognitive concepts (i.e., size, shape, analogies, action, commonalities, numbers).

The general physical examination should specifically ascertain possible dysmorphology, hepatosplenomegaly, and markers of neurocutaneous disorders. The spine should be carefully inspected, including the sacral region, to look for dermal sinuses, hair tufts, or other subtle signs of spinal dysraphism. Height, weight, and occipitofrontal circumference should be obtained and plotted. In cases of microcephaly or macrocephaly, the parental occipitofrontal circumferences also should be obtained and plotted. The head shape and status of the anterior and posterior fontanels in the infant, together with the sutures, should be observed. Determination of the presence of any focal or asymmetric neurologic findings is the primary objective of the formal neurologic examination. Careful evaluation of vision, in addition to aiding in a definitive diagnostic process, is indicated to minimize the contribution of potentially correctable visual impairments to the burden of disability. Similarly, this approach applies to evaluating for possible gross auditory impairments in the office setting.

Within the clinical office setting, several test instruments exist for use as objective screening assessments of development during the first years of life (i.e., Denver Developmental Screening Test). These may be supplemented or complemented by the use of parent-based questionnaires (e.g., Child Developmental Inventory and Ages and Stages Questionnaire) that provide an aspect of objective developmental screening.

Laboratory and Other Diagnostic Testing

Laboratory testing is directed at establishing the possible cause of the individual's delay or ID. Laboratory testing is undertaken in the spirit that the potential value of a definitive etiologic diagnosis from individual and familial perspectives may be substantial. Recent work has emphasized the delineation and diagnosis of nearly 90 treatable metabolic diseases associated with GDD or ID. Technologic advances, especially in the domains of genetic testing and neuroimaging, have improved diagnostic yield and precision, and will continue to improve with newer diagnostic tools. Aiding the formulation of a rational approach to laboratory investigations in this clinical population is the AAN practice parameter and updated evidence report (see Figure 51-1) (Michelson et al., 2011).

For the globally or intellectually delayed child without an apparent cause after history and physical examination, current recommendations would include CMA testing, followed, if clinically indicated, by high-resolution MRI. How and with what frequency whole-exome and whole-genome sequencing will be part of the standard clinical evaluation is not completely clear, but given the early success of this tool to aid in diagnosis, it is likely to be quickly incorporated into upcoming practice parameter revisions.

Electrophysiologic studies, such as electroencephalography, should be undertaken only in the situation of a suspected coexisting paroxysmal disorder or evidence of language regression or behavioral abnormalities suggestive of an epilepsy syndrome, such as Landau–Kleffner or electrical status epilepticus during slow-wave sleep. Visual- and auditory-evoked potentials are of use in assessing the integrity of the visual and auditory systems in the young, uncooperative child.

Consultation

Concerns about the developmental and functional patterns highlighted at the time of specialty evaluation should prompt referrals to other health professionals with different but complementary expertise, permitting a multidisciplinary, comprehensive evaluation of the affected child. These health professionals represent genetics, occupational therapy, physical therapy, speech and language pathology, and psychology. Specific care needs, such as tube feeding, respite care, or financial difficulties, may prompt nursing or social service intervention. Vision and hearing screening is important because of the high frequency of potentially correctable primary sensory impairments in this population.

MEDICAL MANAGEMENT OF COEXISTING CONDITIONS

With a greater drive to incorporate intellectually disabled individuals into the community comes a better awareness of the unique and challenging profile of their psychiatric and medical issues, and of how best to optimize their treatment to improve quality of life and outcome for both the individual and family. These disorders, both psychiatric and medical, uniformly occur at a greater frequency in developmentally delayed and intellectually disabled children and youth compared with typically developing or cognitively able children. Psychiatric disorders encountered include anxiety, mood disorders, disruptive behaviors, inattention, and aggression. Medical issues include epilepsy, sleep disorders, sensory impairments, and feeding problems.

OUTCOME AND PROGNOSIS

The vast majority of developmentally delayed or intellectually disabled children presently remain at home with the best caregivers possible—a loving, supportive, and nurturing family.

Longitudinal studies suggest continued intellectual development in those with mild or moderate delay, and the absence of such improvement in those with severe or profound ID. Functional attainment for the child with severe neurodevelopmental disability by age 6 typically represents the functional attainment with respect to ambulation, feeding, toileting, and self-hygiene achieved for the life span. As such, the pragmatic aims for education should be on short-term achievable goals that assist in improving functional capacity.

The transition to adult life can be challenging with issues related to living situations, limited access to entitlements, termination of educational options, sexuality, and employment (sheltered or supported), and the locus of medical care provision (i.e., pediatric to adult). Family involvement in transition planning is essential for the successful adjustment to adult life. Individuals with ID have had higher unemployment rates than the general population and a tendency for placement in segregated (i.e., sheltered) environments. Periodic, ongoing support often has been found to be a necessary precondition for continued employment.

The life expectancy of a child with mild to moderate ID who is in good general health without evidence of cardiorespiratory disease or severe epilepsy can be considered similar to that of the general pediatric population. Significant mobility limitations, lack of functional hand use, and feeding dependency (especially placement of a gastrostomy tube) limit life expectancy. However, a positive trend is evident, with life expectancy improving overall for those with ID, even for the most severely affected individuals.

Acknowledgments

The authors wish to thank Brieana Fregeau for her help with references and Alba Rinaldi for her original secretarial assistance. M.I.S. was supported by the MCH Foundation (Guyda Chair in Pediatrics) during the writing of this chapter.

REFERENCES

The complete list of references for this chapter is available online at www.expertconsult.com.

See inside cover for registration details.

SELECTED REFERENCES

Leonard, H., Wen, X., 2002. The epidemiology of mental retardation: challenges and opportunities in the new millennium. Ment. Retard. Dev. Disabil. Res. Rev. 8, 117–134.

Meerding, W.J., Bonneux, L., Polder, J.J., et al., 1998. Demographic and epidemiological determinants of healthcare costs in Netherlands: cost of illness study. BMJ 317, 111–115.

Michelson, D.J., Shevell, M.I., Sherr, E.H., et al., 2011. Evidence report: genetic and metabolic testing on children with global developmental delay: report of the Quality Standards Subcommittee of the American Academy of Neurology and the Practice Committee of the Child Neurology Society. Neurology 77, 1629–1635.

Miller, D.T., Adam, M.P., Aradhya, S., et al., 2010. Consensus statement: chromosomal microarray is a first-tier clinical diagnostic test for individuals with developmental disabilities or congenital anomalies. Am. J. Hum. Genet. 86, 749–764.

Sherr, E.H., Michelson, D.J., Shevell, M.I., et al., 2013. Neurodevelopmental disorders and genetic testing: current approaches and future advances. Ann. Neurol. 74, 164–170.

E-BOOK FIGURES AND TABLES

52 Cognitive and Motor Regression

Stanford K. Shu, David J. Michelson, and Stephen Ashwal

INTRODUCTION

Progressive encephalopathies (PE) are diseases that cause a gradual decline in cognitive and motor function over time. Toxic, infectious, inflammatory, and neoplastic disorders that can present in a subacute to chronic fashion must be considered in the evaluation of patients presenting with PE. This chapter will focus on the wide array of genetic and metabolic diseases that typically present with PE and pose several diagnostic challenges for clinicians.

One such challenge relates to the etiologies being individually rare and thus generally unfamiliar to clinicians. A second challenge relates to the phenotypic variability of genetic disorders. Many inborn errors of metabolism (IEM) caused by mutations in genes for critical enzymes, for example, have a "classic" and severe presentation related to complete enzyme deficiency (i.e., neonatal encephalopathy with multiorgan failure) but can be milder and even subtle with later presentation (i.e., psychiatric changes in adulthood) owing to increasing degrees of residual enzymatic function.

DEFINITION

There is no accepted definition of the term "progressive encephalopathy," and it has been used interchangeably with such terms as "neurodegenerative disorder," "neurodegenerative encephalopathy," and "progressive intellectual and neurologic deterioration." We use the term PE in this chapter to refer to disorders that cause progressive central nervous system (CNS) injury and loss of function, affecting multiple domains (i.e., cognitive, affective, psychomotor, social, perceptual, and linguistic).

EPIDEMIOLOGY

A few surveillance studies have informed our sense of the overall incidence of PE in various regions of the world. Two studies from Norway reported incidence rates of 0.6 per 1000 person years. Etiologies were most often metabolic (66%) or neurodegenerative (32%), but 20% of cases remained unclassified. A decreasing incidence was seen with age, with cases distributed among neonates (0 to 4 weeks, 32.1%); infants (1 to 12 months, 39.3%); and juveniles (6 to 12 years, 4.8%), with none seen in late juveniles (6 to 12 years, 4.8%) and late juveniles (older than 12 years, 0%). Far more neonatal onset cases were metabolic (46%) than neurodegenerative (7%) in nature.

A related study from the same investigators examined survival rates and prognostic factors for survival among these patients. Overall, 37% of the patients suffered early death, and the cumulative probabilities for survival were 81% at 1 year and 66% at 10 years. Neonatal onset of symptoms and a metabolic versus neurodegenerative etiology were risk factors for mortality. The 10 year survival rate for children with metabolic diseases (58%) was significantly poorer than that of children with neurodegenerative diseases (87.5%). Much of what has been published regarding these disorders has been retrospec-tive and focuses on individual conditions, providing little basis for a discussion of their collective epidemiology.

ETIOLOGY

Most genetic causes of PE are due to either an IEM or a neurodegenerative disorder (ND). Chapters 23, 26, 32, 48, 50, and 99 provide overviews of many of the conditions that can present with PE. Chapters 23, 26, 48, 50, and 99 provide overviews of many of the conditions that can present with a progressive encephalopathy. The IEMs are themselves frequently divided into three groups, based on pathophysiology. In the first group are those disorders in which symptoms of acute or chronic intoxication are caused by the intracellular and extracellular (and thus measurable in blood, urine, and/or cerebrospinal fluid) accumulation of the compounds proximal to the defective enzyme. Examples include errors of amino acid metabolism (e.g., phenylketonuria and maple syrup urine disease), organic acidemias (e.g., methylmalonic aciduria and propionic acidemia), urea cycle disorders (e.g., ornithine transcarbamylase deficiency and argininemia), disorders of carbohydrate metabolism (e.g., galactosemia and hereditary fructose intolerance), disorders of metal transport (e.g., Wilson disease and Menkes disease), and disorders of porphyrin metabolism. Because the placenta acts to maintain homeostasis of small molecules that can cross its capillaries, these disorders are, overall, less likely to cause embryonic toxicity and more likely to present in infancy and childhood after a symptom-free period whose length depends in part on the degree of enzyme deficiency. Other circumstances such as fever, illness, and dietary changes can also influence the timing and severity of symptoms.

The second group of IEMs is comprised of those disorders in which symptoms are due, at least in part, to the inability of the brain and other organs to produce or utilize sufficient energy for normal function. Energy deficiency can result from defective function of the mitochondria, including defects of pyruvate transport and modification, the Krebs cycle enzymes, the fatty acid oxidation enzymes, and the respiratory chain enzymes that allow for aerobic metabolism. Energy deficiency can also result from defects in cytoplasmic enzymes such as those responsible for glycogen synthesis, glycolysis and gluconeogenesis; insulin secretion and responsiveness; creatine synthesis and transport; and the pentose phosphate pathway. It is not uncommon for children with IEMs causing energy defects to present with congenital dysmorphism or cerebral dysgenesis.

Disorders in the third group of IEMs are typically thought of as storage disorders, in which incompletely catabolized complex molecules accumulate within neuronal and extraneuronal tissues and cause progressive neurologic symptoms and somatic changes. Examples include mucopolysaccharidoses, oligosaccharidoses, and lysosomal storage disorders. Some authors expand this third group to include disorders of complex molecule synthesis and breakdown that result in a loss of function without measurably abnormal storage such as peroxisomal disorders, congenital disorders of glycosylation, and disorders of cholesterol biosynthesis.

Nonmetabolic genetic causes of PE associated with progressive neuronal loss, usually demonstrable as atrophy on neuroimaging, are classified as neurodegenerative disorders (ND). The description and recognition of NDs were previously based purely on clinical features. However, the past decades have seen the elucidation of a genetic basis for most and a pathophysiologic basis for many. NDs of as yet unclear pathophysiology are sometimes categorized based on whether they affect the brain homogenously (diffuse encephalopathies) or preferentially affecting the cerebral cortex (poliodystrophies), the cerebral white matter (leukodystrophies), the basal ganglia (corencephalopathies), or the cerebellum, brainstem, and spinal cord (spinocerebellar diseases).

An early study of the incidence of PE at two large academic centers in the United States found 341 pediatric cases with one of more than 50 different CNS disorders among 1218 hospital admissions over the course of 10 years (Table 52-1). Although

72% of the cases were found to have genetic or metabolic disorders, the study also included a significant number of cases with isolated lower motor neuron syndromes and cases attributable to acquired injuries from infections, immunologic disorders, refractory epilepsy, chronic environmental insults, nutritional deficiencies, and iatrogenic factors. Data from another study are summarized in Table 52-2.

After the initial description in 1996 of 10 cases of new variant Creutzfeldt-Jakob disease (nvCJD) affecting young adults in the United Kingdom, several countries instituted prospective surveillance programs to collect data on patients with PE to better identify additional cases of nvCJD. Although these studies have relied on reports from pediatricians and have been unable to describe absolute incidence or prevalence figures, they have reported relative prevalences within their areas. The first report from the surveillance done in the United Kingdom collected and analyzed pediatric cases of progressive intellectual and neurologic deterioration over a 5-year span. Of the 798 cases collected, 577 (72%) had a confirmed

TABLE 52-1 Diagnoses in 341 Cases of PE

Diagnosis	Number (%)	Diagnosis	Number (%)
CORTICAL DISORDERS	**129 (38%)**	Organic acidurias	2
Lysosomal storage disorders	39	Letterer-Siwe disease	2
Hypoxic poliodystrophy	29	Sturge-Weber syndrome	2
Idiopathic poliodystrophy	24	Zellweger syndrome	2
West syndrome	17	Homocystinuria	1
Lennox-Gastaut syndrome	9	Incontinentia pigmenti	1
Metabolic poliodystrophy	4	Sjögren-Larsson syndrome	1
Toxoplasmosis	3	**SPINOCEREBELLAR DISORDERS**	**51 (15%)**
Postvaccine poliodystrophy	3	Spinal muscular atrophy	19
Lowe syndrome	1	Hereditary spastic paraplegia	12
WHITE MATTER DISORDERS	**71 (21%)**	Acute cerebellar ataxia	8
SSPE	26	Infantile polymyoclonus	4
ADEM and MS	17	Charcot-Marie-Tooth disease	2
Adrenoleukodystrophy	8	Friedreich ataxia	2
Metachromatic leukodystrophy	5	Marinesco-Sjögren syndrome	1
Pelizaeus-Merzbacher disease	4	OPCA	1
Krabbe disease	4	Spinocerebellar degeneration	1
Phenylketonuria	2	Refsum disease	1
Cockayne syndrome	2	**BASAL GANGLIA DISORDERS**	**26 (8%)**
Canavan disease	1	Idiopathic corencephalopathy	8
Alexander disease	1	Huntington disease	5
Maple syrup urine disease	1	Mitochondrial disorders	4
DIFFUSE ENCEPHALOPATHIES	**63 (19%)**	Dystonia musculorum deformans	2
Tuberous sclerosis	19	Pantothenate kinase-associated neurodegeneration	2
Idiopathic encephalopathy	17	Ataxia-telangiectasia	1
Hyperammonemic disorders	6	Congenital indifference to pain	1
Mitochondrial disorders	4	Infantile neuroaxonal dystrophy	1
Neurofibromatosis	4	Familial dysautonomia	1
Achondroplasia	2	Wilson disease	1

ADEM, acute disseminated encephalomyelitis; MS, multiple sclerosis; OPCA, olivopontocerebellar atrophy; SSPE, subacute sclerosing panencephalitis.
(Adapted from Dyken, P., Krawiecki, N., 1983. Neurodegenerative diseases of infancy and childhood. Ann Neurol 13, 351–364.)

TABLE 52-2 Diagnoses in 66 Cases of PE

Disease	N (%)
Metachromatic leukodystrophy	14 (21%)
Adrenoleukodystrophy	11 (16%)
Subacute sclerosing panencephalitis (SSPE)	8 (12%)
Wilson disease	6 (9.8%)
Friedreich ataxia	5 (7.5%)
Lipidosis	4 (6%)
Gaucher disease	3 (4.5%)
Alexander disease	2 (3%)
Pantothenate kinase associated neurodegeneration	2 (3%)
Multiple sclerosis	1 (1.5%)
Ataxia telangiectasia	1 (1.5%)
Unknown etiology	6 (9.8%)

(Adapted from Pierre, G., 2013. Neurodegenerative disorders and metabolic disease. Arch Dis Child 98(8), 618–624.)

diagnosis. Higher prevalence rates were seen in populations with higher rates of consanguineous marriage. Updates of the study reported 147 different confirmed diagnoses in 1114 (42%) of the 2636 patients. In total, six of the children were found to have confirmed or probable nvCJD.

A survey-based study conducted in Australia identified 230 cases of childhood PE in a 2-year period, with 134 patients having Rett syndrome, 20 having a lysosomal storage disorder, 16 having a leukodystrophy, and 15 having a mitochondrial disease. The previously described Norwegian study gathered cases of pediatric PE over an 18-year period from the area's single children's hospital and from the national diagnostic laboratory for metabolic diseases. The authors excluded patients with diseases in which cognitive impairment was either atypical (e.g., spinocerebellar ataxia and spinal muscular atrophy) or typically seen only late in the course (multiple sclerosis). In addition, unlike the studies already discussed, this study excluded disorders such as regressive autism and Rett syndrome, in which intellectual deterioration may be seen early in the course but typically stabilizes. As mentioned, the authors reported a total of 84 cases of PE, of which they classified two-thirds as metabolic, one-third as neurodegenerative, and two cases, both due to HIV/AIDS, as infectious. The authors found an increased (seven-fold) risk of PE in children born within communities with higher rates of consanguineous unions. They further estimated that avoidance of consanguineous marriage would decrease the incidence of PE by 30 to 50%.

DIAGNOSTIC EVALUATION

When PE is suspected, a timely evaluation that results in a specific diagnosis can be of great value. It is not uncommon for the child neurologist to uncover clinical features of a progressive process in a patient who is referred for developmental delay or autism. In this regard, a key element in the evaluation of global developmental delay (GDD) or intellectual disability (ID) is a second visit to ensure that the child's condition is nonprogressive. The diagnostic yield for evaluating children with PE is far less well studied than the yield of evaluations of children with GDD or ID. Nevertheless, it is even more urgent that children with PE undergo a comprehensive diagnostic evaluation.

Although specific treatments are available for only a minority of the diseases responsible for PE, an etiologic diagnosis has many other direct benefits (Chapter 59), including the ability to:

1. Relieve caregivers of anxiety and uncertainty when specific information about inheritance and prognosis can be given
2. Empower caregivers to become involved in support groups, advocacy, and research networks
3. Limit further diagnostic testing, which may be costly (in time and money) or invasive
4. Prevent recurrences in family members through carrier screening and prenatal testing, when available
5. Improve understanding of
   a. Available treatments
   b. Long-term prognosis
   c. Associated coexistent conditions
   d. Recurrence risk and mode of inheritance

In all cases, the diagnostic tests employed should be tailored to the presentation of the child and, in most cases, testing should proceed from least to most invasive. Consideration should be given to the early identification or exclusion of all potentially treatable causes of the patient's symptoms.

HISTORY
Developmental History

Every child suspected of having a neurodevelopmental disorder should undergo a thorough clinical evaluation that includes a detailed medical and developmental history, family history, and review of systems and detailed physical and neurologic examinations. The clinical features most suggestive of a PE—the gradual loss of previously acquired skills and the gradual emergence of neurologic signs and symptoms after a period of normal development—are more readily observed when they are of later onset and when they progress more rapidly. In this regard, a key element in the evaluation of GDD or ID is a second visit to ensure that the child's condition is nonprogressive. A combination of late but rapid deterioration is not common to most disorders but can occur. The features of PE are more difficult to recognize when the progression is very slow or when the onset is so early that even initial development is clearly abnormal. A number of children initially given a diagnosis of cerebral palsy (CP) due to a presumed remote brain injury were later found to have an IEM or ND. This experience suggests that children with a diagnosis of CP should undergo further evaluation when there is no definite history of a preceding injury, when there is a family history of neurologic symptoms or of parental consanguinity, or if there is an inadequately explained oculomotor deficit, movement disorder, ataxia, muscle atrophy, or sensory deficit. Unexplained episodes of altered mental status, dietary aversions, vomiting, or abnormal movements should arouse strong suspicion that a child is suffering from an IEM. Conversely, children whose underlying neurologic disease is not itself progressive can nevertheless present with gradual loss of skills and emergence of new neurologic signs and symptoms for a variety of reasons, including medication side effects, intercurrent medical and psychiatric illnesses, and worsening of preexisting hydrocephalus, spasticity, dystonia, or epilepsy. Some epileptic syndromes (e.g., epileptic encephalopathies) and neurodevelopmental disorders (e.g., regressive autism) are associated with a gradual loss of function or developmental arrest during their course but are unlikely to show relentless clinical deterioration, global involvement, or evidence of CNS damage.

The critical elements of the clinical evaluation are the same as have been outlined in detail for children presenting with nonprogressive neurodevelopmental disorders (Chapter 51). To establish the progressive nature of a child's symptoms or clinical findings, however, it can be particularly helpful to review any records of the child's prior appearance and abilities to which caregivers can provide access, including photographs, videos, and examples of the child's writing and drawing. Repeated examinations over months, even years, may be necessary to uncover very subtle regression.

Family History

A family history of developmental delay, intellectual disability, learning disability, early deaths, and seizures can be quite helpful in elucidating the etiology of a child's neurologic issues. A three-generation pedigree should be obtained. Consanguinity varies significantly from one culture to the next. Practitioners should be tactful when asking if the child is the product of a consanguineous union, one in which the parents are second cousins or more closely related.

Maternal History

Chromosomal abnormalities account for 50% to 70% of miscarriages of less than 10 weeks gestation and are found in about 50% of couples with a history of recurrent miscarriages. Previous stillbirths, neonatal deaths, or infant deaths attributed to sudden infant death syndrome (SIDS) may be due to an IEM (Chapter 90). Exposure *in utero* to teratogens have been associated with developmental delay and intellectual disability but not with PE.

Neonatal History

Delivery complications such as hypoxia and early postnatal complications such as hypoglycemia, CNS infection, and seizures may have profound effects on development. Patients with severe perinatal injuries, neuromuscular disorders, and epileptic encephalopathies may be difficult to distinguish from cases of early onset and severe PE given that both groups can show difficulty in reaching even the earliest developmental milestones.

Environmental History

Lead encephalopathy and pica of other toxic substances such as mothballs (paradichlorobenzene) may cause PE. Acute and chronic hydrocarbon exposure has been associated with anxiety, mood disorders, and progressive neuropsychologic changes.

General Medical History

The medical history can be obtained in a systematic fashion by organ systems. A history of complex congenital heart disease (CHD) may cause a progressive encephalopathy due to systemic and cerebral hypoperfusion may can cause permanent cerebrovascular injury and visible hypoplasia or atrophy.

Endocrine disorders such as hypothyroidism and hyperthyroidism have been associated with developmental regression and movement disorders. Hashimoto encephalopathy has presented as a progressive myoclonic epilepsy syndrome. Both Addison disease and Cushing Syndrome are associated with a progressive encephalopathy.

Infections such as Creutzfeldt-Jakob disease (CJD) and subacute sclerosing panencephalitis (SSPE) cause progressive neurologic deterioration that can be drawn out over many years. HIV infection may also be the cause of PE. Current criteria divide patients with HIV-encephalopathy into three groups: those who are asymptomatic, those with a mild neurocognitive disorder, and those with dementia. HIV encephalopathy was previously reported to occur in up to 30% of children with HIV. The use of highly active antiretroviral therapy (HAART) has decreased the incidence to 12%. Additional information on SSPE and HIV are provided in Chapter 115.

Nutritional disorders or vitamin deficiencies (e.g., thiamine, niacin, biotin, folate, and vitamin E) have been associated with PE. Neurologic symptoms due to these conditions are reviewed in Chapters 46 and 47.

Autoimmune encephalopathies with autoantibodies directed against proteins on the neuronal membrane (e.g., NMDA receptors) are increasingly well described and recognized in clinical practice. Symptoms may develop very acutely over the course of days, mimicking infectious meningoencephalitis, or may develop very slowly over the course of weeks to months, with early behavioral and psychiatric changes followed by seizures, dyskinesia, dysautonomia, sleep dysfunction, and an altered level of consciousness. These conditions are discussed in Chapters 118 and 119.

EXAMINATION

The clinicians' ability to recognize clinical patterns and features suggestive of a specific etiology can significantly narrow the diagnostic evaluation of a child with PE (Chapters 1–9). Primary motor and sensory functions are readily assessed by the screening neurologic examination, even in uncooperative children, but higher cortical functions are far more difficult to evaluate. The collective observations of clinicians, parents, and teachers who suspect subtle cognitive decline should be supplemented by those of a neuropsychologist. Chapter 10 reviews the approach to neuropsychological testing in children.

Abnormalities of head size, stature, and facial morphology can suggest specific diagnoses such as Angelman syndrome. Neurocutaneous stigmata may suggest one of the phakomatoses, as with café-au-lait spots (neurofibromatosis); hypomelanotic macules and angiofibromas (tuberous sclerosis); blistering of the skin, swirling macular hyperpigmentation and linear hypopigmentation (incontinentia pigmenti); or a port wine stain on the face and glaucoma (Sturge-Weber syndrome). Hepatosplenomegaly and corneal clouding may suggest one of the mucopolysaccharidoses. Cardiomyopathy may be caused by a mitochondrial disorder. Progressive retinal degeneration has been associated with the neuronal ceroid lipofuscinoses and a cherry red spot is associated with sphingolipid storage disorders, in addition to central retinal artery occlusion, drug toxicity (quinine, dapsone), and toxic exposures (carbon monoxide, methanol).

LABORATORY TESTING

Screening studies that might be done on a regular basis in the evaluation of a child with unexplained PE include those that look for evidence of involvement of non-CNS organ systems and narrow the differential diagnosis. These commonly include a complete blood count (CBC) and comprehensive metabolic profile (CMP). Other tests, often chosen because they can identify treatable causes of PE, include thyroid function tests, serum lead level, and tests of vitamin B_{12} and folate levels. In patients with progressive weakness or hypotonia, a serum creatine kinase level is often done to screen for muscular dystrophies. Other tests are difficult to interpret in cases of PE without highly suggestive and specific clinical and neuroimaging findings and so are rarely included as screening tests.

When it is difficult to decide if a patient has a static or progressive encephalopathy, the diagnostic approach may be the same as for children with global developmental delay or intellectual disability (ID), as is discussed in Chapter 51.

Increasingly microarray studies are being used for initial genetic diagnostic testing. Microarray studies can be used to screen the entire genome for copy number variants (CNVs) that are smaller (0.3 Mb) than can typically be detected by even a high-resolution karyotype (5 Mb). Array comparative genomic hybridization (aCGH) and single nucleotide polymorphism (SNP) arrays are both clinically available and, with reported yields of up to 15% to 20%, are typically used as first-line genetic tests for most children with unexplained ID. Microarrays will not detect mutations other than CNVs such as single nucleotide substitutions within an individual gene or large chromosome rearrangements. A karyotype is still recommended when the child appears dysmorphic or when there is a family history of multiple miscarriages or of similarly affected children. CNVs may be recognizably pathogenic, known to be benign, or may be variants of uncertain significance (VUS). Parental testing may be needed to guide the interpretation of a VUS. If a parent tests positive for the same CNV, it is considered more likely to be benign. However, if neither parent tests positive for the CNV and it appears to be a *de novo* mutation in the child, it is considered more likely to be pathologic.

Although less frequently ordered now, routine cytogenetic testing (G-banded karyotype) has a yield of 3.7% to 10% in patients with mild to moderate developmental delay and is helpful for diagnosing aneuploidy and rearrangements such as translocations and inversions. Fluorescent in situ hybridization (FISH) or multiplex ligation-dependent probe amplification (MLPA) for specific disorders such as velocardiofacial syndrome (22q11 deletion) are done on patients with suggestive clinical features. Subtelomeric FISH studies were previously recommended but such testing for copy number variants (CNV) has been supplanted by the microarray studies with broader genome-wide coverage.

Fragile X is the most commonly inherited cause of ID; however, the family history may be negative, and the dysmorphic features, usually recognizable in older children and adults, may not yet be apparent in young children. Other X-linked disorders such as Rett syndrome are found predominantly in girls. Testing for Rett syndrome (*MeCP2* gene sequencing and MLPA) has been recommended for all girls with unexplained severe ID, particularly those with developmental regression, stereotypic hand movements, deceleration of head growth, and seizures. More than one hundred other genes have been associated with X-linked ID.

Whole exome sequencing (WES), which sequences the protein encoding regions of all genes, has additional diagnostic utility and is increasingly becoming clinically available. The ability to test both parents (forming, along with the child, a trio) is crucial for WES interpretation as this technique regularly identifies hundreds or thousands of benign, inherited mutations. A 2012 study showed a diagnostic yield of 16% for WES in 100 severe ID trios. In the future, sequencing of the entire genome, including noncoding regions, is likely to become available on a clinical basis. Please refer to Chapters 34 and 35 for a more detailed discussion of genetic testing.

The yield from metabolic evaluations of children with global developmental delay and PE is 0.2% to 5%. Some of these disorders are treatable or have symptoms that can be ameliorated with no more than a change in diet. Intrauterine or early diagnosis of some of these disorders may allow affected siblings to be treated at a milder or even asymptomatic stage of the illness. Please see Chapters 36, 50, and 51 as well as the section later in this chapter on the diagnostic approach for additional discussion.

Electroencephalography is a valuable diagnostic tool in the evaluation of children with suspected PE. Epileptic encephalopathies describe a group of disorders in which abnormal CNS electrical activity persistently disturbs neuronal networks involved in cognition. Although the value of EEG is recognized in children with a suspected epileptic encephalopathy, the diagnostic yield in children with cognitive decline without obvious clinical seizures has not been clearly determined. However, it is common practice to acquire an EEG in this subset of patients because clinical seizures may be very subtle and because it is hoped that anticonvulsant use may, in some patients with epileptic encephalopathies, improve cognitive function.

Neuroimaging studies are also an important part of the evaluation of children with PE. Magnetic resonance imaging (MRI) is the investigation of choice for structural abnormalities, neuronal migrational disorders, white matter diseases and posterior fossa structures. Computed tomography (CT) can more readily show intracranial calcifications and cranial bone abnormalities such as craniosynostosis. Specialized applications of MRI as spectroscopy, susceptibility weighted imaging, diffusion weighted imaging, and diffusion tensor imaging can provide additional information about brain structure and function. Up to 40% of patients undergoing evaluation for developmental disability show a structural or biochemical abnormality on neuroimaging. Although the abnormalities are often nonspecific, such as mild global atrophy, there are times when the findings are highly suggestive of a specific disorder (Chapter 12).

A lumbar puncture to quantify cerebrospinal fluid (CSF) amino acids, lactate, and neurotransmitter levels may be considered in patients being evaluated for PE. A recent study reported diagnostic CSF results in 25.8% of 62 patients suspected of having a pediatric neurotransmitter diseases based on their clinical symptoms. See Chapter 44 for further details.

BRAIN BIOPSY

The necessity for brain biopsy for nonneoplastic conditions has substantially diminished over the years as advances in neuroimaging, biochemical, and genetic tests have provided safer and easier means by which to make a diagnosis. However, biopsy may still play an important role in the evaluation of patients with PE that remains unexplained despite extensive noninvasive testing. In some cases, biopsy is the only method by which a particular diagnosis can be confirmed and in others, the biopsy results provide crucial information about therapeutic options and prognosis. See online chapter.

DIAGNOSTIC APPROACH

Professional societies and governmental agencies have produced systematic reviews and evidence-based clinical practice guidelines regarding the evaluation of children with neurodevelopmental disabilities (Miclea et al., 2015; Srour and Shevell, 2014; Dunfield et al., 2014; Michelson et al., 2011; Miller et al, 2010; Moeschler and Shevell, 2006; Curry et al., 1997; Shevell et al., 2003; Valle website). However, these reports were focused on children with nonprogressive symptoms. Studies specifically reviewing the diagnostic workup of children with PE have a variable yield for an etiologic diagnosis depending on the inclusion criteria and which neuroimaging studies, metabolic and genetic testing is done.

Three alternative methods to approach the diagnostic evaluation of children with PE have been described. The first approach, similar to that used to evaluate children with non-progressive developmental disorders, begins with general screening tests that are performed for all such children and then adds additional screening tests for infectious, toxic, endocrinologic, genetic, neoplastic, metabolic, autoimmune, and nutritional disorders based on the child's individual history or initial screening test results (See Table 52-8). This approach is based more on frequency of likely diseases rather than on treatability. Abnormal screening tests will often suggest the need for further neuroimaging with magnetic resonance spectroscopy or diffusion tensor imaging; further electrophysiologic testing with electroretinography or electromyography; or further metabolic or targeted genetic screening tests or tissue biopsies for microscopy or enzyme analysis.

A second approach to the evaluation of PE is to use an interactive database to generate a broad differential diagnosis. SimulConsult (www.simulconsult.com) is a web-based program that is freely available to clinicians and students. As clinical information is entered, the program orders its differential based on likelihood and makes suggestions regarding what additional findings and laboratory tests would most help clarify the diagnosis. A broad differential can help clinicians to avoid cognitive pitfalls that commonly contribute to diagnostic error and delay including the biases of availability and representativeness (favoring familiar diagnoses over less well-known diagnoses or disease variants) and those of framing and premature closure (favoring findings that confirm rather than question a preexisting diagnosis). DiagnosisPro (en.diagnosispro.com) is another web-based database that is not specific to neurology.

A third approach, as proposed by the British Columbia Children's Hospital group, is referred to as the Treatable Intellectual Disability Endeavor (TIDE) algorithm (www.tidebc.org) (Van Karnebeek and Sockler-Ipsiroglu, 2014). The TIDE algorithm emphasizes testing patients for treatable disorders, even when rare, before testing them for more common but untreatable disorders. This protocol is reviewed in Chapter 59. The first tier of testing, to be applied to all children presenting with PE, calls for blood and urine studies that are available at most commercial laboratories at a reasonable price and which are likely to detect up to 60% of the currently known treatable disorders (Table 52-9). Second tier tests are generally more expensive and invasive and are recommended on a more selective basis, based on clinical judgment and suggestions from textbooks, online resources, and other specialists such as metabolic geneticists. Use of the TIDE protocol has the potential to reduce the cost and diagnostic delay involved in identifying patients with treatable IEMs.

The individual disorders causing PE in childhood are too numerous to discuss in detail in this chapter, but they are presented in the online version of the book in tables based on age and symptomatology (i.e., Tables 52-10 to 52-24).

Up-to-date information about the sensitivity and availability of tests for specific genetic disorders is available through the Gene Tests website (www.genetests.org). Some genetic tests can be performed on a research basis through direct communication and cooperation between the clinician and research laboratory.

MANAGEMENT

The specific cause of childhood PE cannot be determined in at least half of the cases (as reported in large epidemiologic surveys). However, because a small number of disorders can be at least ameliorated by medical therapies, pursuit of a diagnostic workup is warranted. Caregivers can be expected to have a great number of questions and concerns that will require a large amount of time, patience, and sensitivity on the part of

TABLE 52-9 Treatable Intellectual Disability Endeavor (TIDE) Diagnostic Protocol

Tier 1: Nontargeted Metabolic Screening to Identify 54 (60%) Treatable IEM:

Blood	Urine
Plasma amino acids	Organic acids
Plasma total homocysteine	Purines and pyrimidines
Acylcarnitine profile	Creatine metabolites
Copper, ceruloplasmin	Oligosaccharides
	Glycosaminoglycans
	Amino acids (when indicated)

Tier 2: Current Practice Adhering to International Guidelines (1 or more of):

Audiology
Ophthalmology
Cytogenetic testing (array CGH)
Thyroid studies
CBC
Lead
Metabolic testing
Brain MRI and 1H spectroscopy
   (where available)
Fragile X
Targeted gene sequencing/
   molecular panel
Other

Low yhreshold for ordering
   tests

Tier 3: Targeted Workup to Identify 35 (40%) Treatable IEM Requiring Specific Testing:

According to patient's aymptomatology and clinician's expertise
Utilization of digital tools (www.treatable-id.org)
Specific biochemical/gene test
Whole blood manganese
Plasma cholestanol
Plasma 7-dehydroxy-cholesterol : cholesterol ratio
Plasma pipecolic acid and urine α-amino adipic semialdehyde (AASA)
Plasma very long chain fatty acids
Plasma vitamin B_{12} and folate
Serum and CSF lactate : pyruvate ratio
Enzyme activities (leukocytes): arylsulfatase A, biotinidase,
   glucocerebrosidase, fatty aldehyde dehydrogenase
Urine deoxypyridonoline
CSF amino acids
CSF neurotransmitters
CSF : plasma glucose ratio
CoQ measurement fibroblasts
Molecular analysis: *CA5A, NPC1, NPC2, SC4MOL, SLC18A2,
   SLC19A3, SLC30A10, SLC52A2, SLC52A3, PDHA1, DLAT, PDHX,
   SPR, TH* genes

(Adapted from Van Karnebeek, C.D., Stockler-Ipsiroglu, S., 2014. Early identification of treatable inborn errors of metabolism in children with intellectual disability: The Treatable Intellectual Disability Endeavor protocol in British Columbia. Paediat Child Health 19(9), 469–471.)

the clinician. Even when disease-specific treatments are not available, the clinician can be of great assistance in maintaining the child's quality of life. Efforts should be made early in the course to direct the child to other sources of supportive care, including rehabilitation specialists, nutritionists, special education instructors, and speech, occupational, and physical therapists. When possible, the child's caregivers should be referred to a social worker who can help them obtain financial support, nursing care, and social support networks and a genetic counselor who can explain the inheritance patterns and aspects of family planning and antenatal diagnostic possibilities, provide talking points to communicate with family members, and help identify support groups and opportunities for advocacy.

FUTURE DIRECTIONS

Earlier diagnosis of conditions causing PE, particularly before devastating neurologic symptoms develop, will improve patient treatment and family planning. Prenatal diagnosis has several advantages but is currently difficult even in families with known risks. Noninvasive prenatal testing (NIPT) can examine a pregnant mother's blood for fetal DNA abnormalities and is currently being offered to mothers at high risk for aneuploidies such as Trisomy 21. This method is likely to expand to screening for CNVs and point mutations as technical and ethical issues are worked out.

Single nucleotide polymorphisms (SNPs) are the most abundant sequence variations in the human genome, with approximately 150 million discovered thus far (www.ncbi .nlm.nih.gov/snp). Current arrays simultaneously genotype thousands of SNPs, providing information about CNVs but also about uniparental disomy and regional homozygosity (which can reflect parental consanguinity). Next generation sequencing (NGS) techniques are faster and less expensive than older sequencing methods and are already providing a greater number of patients with access to large gene panels. It is certain that the future will bring us testing methods for metabolic and genetic disorders that is increasingly personalized, sensitive and specific, cost-efficient, and better able to provide patients with a clear diagnosis with minimal delay.

REFERENCES

The complete list of references for this chapter is available in the e-book at www.expertconsult.com.
See inside cover for registration details.

SELECTED REFERENCES

Curry, C.J., Stevenson, R.E., Aughton, D., et al., 1997. Evaluation of mental retardation: recommendations of a consensus conference. Am. J. Med. Genet. 72, 468–477.

Dunfield, L., Mitra, D., Tonelli, M., et al., 2014. Protocol: screening and treatment for developmental delay in early childhood. Accessed at: <http://canadiantaskforce.ca/>.

Michelson, D.J., Shevell, M.I., Sherr, E.H., et al., 2011. Evidence report: genetic and metabolic testing on children with global developmental delay: report of the Quality Standards Subcommittee of the American Academy of Neurology and the Practice Committee of the Child Neurology Society. Neurology 77 (17), 1629–1635.

Miclea, D., Peca, L., Cuzmici, Z., et al., 2015. Genetic testing in patients with global developmental delay / intellectual disabilities. A review. Clujul Med 88 (3), 288–292.

Miller, D.T., Adam, M.P., Aradya, S., et al., 2010. Consensus statement: chromosomal microarray is a first-tier clinical diagnostic test for individuals with developmental disabilities or congenital anomalies. Am. J. Hum. Genet. 86, 749–764.

Moeschler, J.B., Shevell, M., 2006. Clinical genetic evaluation of the child with mental retardation or developmental delays. Pediatrics 117, 2304–2316.

Shevell, M., Ashwal, S., Donley, D., et al., 2003. Practice parameter: evaluation of the child with global developmental delay: report of the Quality Standards Subcommittee of the American Academy of Neurology and the Practice Committee of the Child Neurology Society. Neurology 60, 367–380.

Srour, M., Shevell, M., 2014. Genetics and the investigation of developmental delay/intellectual disability. Arch. Dis. Child. 99, 386–389.

Valle, D., Vogelstein, B., Kinzler, K.W., et al. The Online Metabolic and Molecular Bases of Inherited Disease. <http://ommbid.mhmedical .com/ommbid-index.aspx>.

Van Karnebeek, C.D., Stockler-Ipsiroglu, S., 2014. Early identification of treatable inborn errors of metabolism in children with intellectual disability: The Treatable Intellectual Disability Endeavor protocol in British Columbia. Paediatr Child Health 19 (9), 469–471.

E-BOOK FIGURES AND TABLES

53 Developmental Language Disorders

Doris A. Trauner and Ruth D. Nass

INTRODUCTION

Developmental language disorders (DLDs) include a number of conditions that adversely affect language development. The most common DLD is specific language impairment (SLI), a neurodevelopmental disorder (NDD) that affects 2% to 11% of the population, making it one of the most common NDDs. The hallmark of SLI is that a child with normal intelligence and hearing fails to develop language in an age-appropriate fashion. SLI is a clinical diagnosis, based on the presence of a normal nonverbal IQ, evidence of expressive and/or receptive language significantly below expected for age and intelligence (SLI is often defined by scoring at least 1.5 standard deviations below the mean for age on standardized, age-appropriate tests of language), and absence of other specific conditions such as autism, global intellectual disability, metabolic or genetic disorders, or severe environmental deprivation. Although this condition is commonly called "specific" language impairment, there is controversy as to how specific the condition is and whether the terminology should be changed to a more generic term, such as language impairment. Despite this controversy, however, at present the terminology remains the same. Other forms of DLD include stuttering, selective mutism, verbal apraxia, and epileptic aphasia. Box 53-1 lists normal language milestones as a baseline for assessing a child's developing language competence.

NEURAL SUBSTRATES OF LANGUAGE

In adults, specific brain regions, primarily in the left hemisphere, are believed to mediate language, based primarily on studies of adults with strokes and more recently on neurophysiological and functional imaging studies. The neural substrates of language during early development are not as clearly defined, and in fact may differ markedly from those that mediate language once it has developed. Children who had a left-hemisphere stroke in early life do not typically demonstrate aphasia, or even a functional language impairment. A classic study by Bates et al. (2001) demonstrated the differences between children with perinatal stroke and adults with late-acquired stroke in the left hemisphere, showing that children performed equally well as their typically developing counterparts on multiple aspects of language, unrelated to the hemispheric side of the lesion, whereas adults who had a later-onset left-hemisphere stroke showed significant impairments on the same tasks. Such findings suggest that language is not "hardwired" into specific brain regions, but that the process of language acquisition requires more widely distributed neural networks. Studies of very early language awareness in the first few months of life indicate that infants learn very early to attend to the linguistic traits that are relevant to the language to which they are exposed. Typically developing children attend more to speech sounds when their attention is directed to auditory rather than visual stimuli, whereas children with SLI are unable to sufficiently attend to speech sounds in the same setting, suggesting that there may be a deficit in auditory attention or in general attentional resources at the basis of SLI. Rapid processing of sensory information, particularly in the auditory modality, may also be a contributing factor to impaired language development. Efficient processing of auditory stimuli has been shown to be impaired in many children with SLI. It is as yet unclear whether the primary deficit is in the ability to focus attention to process auditory information or whether the processing deficit is the principal causal factor. In either event, basic sensory processes are disrupted in SLI, leading to impaired language development.

NEUROANATOMY OF SPECIFIC LANGUAGE IMPAIRMENT

Although SLI has been an important area of research and clinical focus for many years, there have been relatively few studies of brain structure in this condition, and those reported have not been consistent. Clinical neuroimaging scans (magnetic resonance imaging [MRI]) generally yield normal results, although a higher-than-expected incidence of abnormal findings, including ventriculomegaly, central volume loss, and white-matter hyperintensities, has been described, suggestive of possible disruption of normal white-matter structure. Quantitative neuroimaging techniques have focused primarily on the frontal and temporal regions thought to be important for language and have demonstrated abnormal gyrification in the inferior frontal gyrus, the absence of the normal left-right asymmetry of the planum temporale, or atypical right-greater-than-left asymmetry of both anterior and posterior temporal lobes. Arguments for atypical lateralization of the developing brain for language as a cause for SLI have been made based on the differences in brain symmetry observed in some of the imaging studies (Badcock et al., 2012). Functional neuroimaging studies have also demonstrated lack of the expected left lateralization of activation on linguistic tasks.

Diffusion-tensor imaging techniques have demonstrated white-matter structural changes in the superior longitudinal fasciculus (SLF) of adolescents with SLI. The SLF is a major white-matter tract that is thought to be crucial for language processing because it connects the anterior areas of the cortex to the posterior areas and, among other areas, the Broca's area to the Wernicke's area. Differences in SLF structure provide a possible structural explanation for the language-processing problems found in SLI.

Other types of imaging studies have demonstrated functional changes in the brains of children and adults with SLI. Single-photon emission-computed tomography (SPECT) studies have shown reduced cerebral blood flow in the left hemisphere of children with SLI compared with controls. With the use of transcranial ultrasound to examine blood flow to each hemisphere during a word-generation task, aberrant hemispheric blood-flow responses have been demonstrated in adults with SLI. Magnetoencephalography was used to track the spatiotemporal course of brain response to real words and pseudowords in children with SLI compared with typically developing children. Bilateral superior temporal cortex regions

BOX 53-1 Normal Language Milestones

RECEPTIVE

- Some words understood by 9 months
- Follows one-step commands by 12 months without being cued by a gesture

EXPRESSIVE

- Cooing—2 months
- Babbling—6 months
- Variable babble—8 months
- One word other than *dada* and *mama*—12 months
- 10 to 50 words used meaningfully—16–20 months
- Two-word phrases—20–24 months
- Points to at least one body part and to named objects and people on command—20 months
- Vocabulary greater than 200 words—2 years
- Two-word combinations—2 years
- Follows two-part commands—2 years
- Sentences of three to four words—3 years
- Compound and complex sentences—4 years
- Passive voice—6 years

were activated to word and pseudoword presentations, but in contrast to controls, children with SLI showed equally strong activation to both words and pseudowords. Further, children with SLI did not show the typical attenuation of activation the second time the same word was presented, indicating that the linguistic activation that underlies word recognition may be defective in SLI.

FACTORS ASSOCIATED WITH DEVELOPMENTAL LANGUAGE DISORDERS

As with many neurodevelopmental disorders, there is a higher incidence of SLI in males (1.6 : 1 males : females). The cause for the gender differences is not known. Numerous biological and environmental risk factors for SLI have been identified. Low birth weight, prematurity, and prenatal exposure to drugs (e.g., cocaine) and to cigarettes have been reported to adversely affect language development, although no single perinatal complication has been definitively associated with SLI; rather, an aggregate of perinatal complications could contribute to later language impairment.

Although frequent episodes of otitis media have been suggested as causing language impairment, there is little evidence from controlled studies to indicate a causal relationship. Intermittent hearing loss may interfere with language development in at-risk children, but is not likely to cause long-term language issues in otherwise normally developing children.

Language impairment is seen in association with specific neurologic and genetic disorders. For example, perisylvian polymicrogyria (or congenital bilateral perisylvian syndrome) is a disorder of defective neuronal migration that has a spectrum of neurologic impairments that include severe epilepsy and cognitive impairment. In some children with this condition, language impairment is the most prominent feature. Language impairment is also prominent in a number of chromosomal disorders, including Down, Klinefelter, and fragile X syndromes. Epileptic encephalopathies, particularly Landau–Kleffner syndrome (LKS), may have language impairment (often receptive greater than expressive impairment) as an isolated or primary symptom. Rolandic epilepsy, often considered to be "benign," may be complicated by language impairment and learning disabilities.

GENETICS

Heritability rates for SLI run as high as 0.5, but they are variable and are affected by the criteria used to diagnose the disorder (SLI vs. more general DLDs that may be associated with known genetic syndromes) (Bishop and Hayiou-Thomas, 2008). The median incidence rate for language difficulties in the families of children with language impairment is up to 35%, compared with a median incidence rate of 11% in control families. Increased concordance rates in monozygotic versus dizygotic twins indicate that heredity, not just shared environment, is responsible for familial clustering.

Studies using genome-wide scanning have implicated a number of gene loci, but the same loci have not been found in a reproducible fashion (Vernes et al., 2008). Isolated families with specific mutations have been studied. In the three-generation KE family, half the members are affected with a severe speech and language disorder that is transmitted as an autosomal-dominant monogenic trait involving the *FOXP2* forkhead-domain gene. Notably, however, a screening of 270 4-year-olds with SLI was negative for the *FOXP2* mutation.

Recently HLA alleles have been associated with SLI. Maternally but not paternally inherited HLA-B B8 and HLA-DQA1*0501 were associated with impaired receptive language. HLA-A A2 was associated with expressive language ability. HLA-DRB1 was found with greater frequency in individuals with SLI than in controls. In other studies, the calcium-transporting ATPase 2C2 (ATP2C2) gene on chromosome 16 has been considered as a candidate gene for SLI.

It is unlikely that there will be one specific gene whose function would be restricted to forming the genetic basis for language acquisition. It is more likely that there are many genes that contribute to a variety of functions, and that these genes form networks that are recruited in the process of language acquisition. The issue of pleiotropy, or the influence of the same genes on multiple phenotypes, has also been discussed in the literature on SLI, given the substantive overlap in regions of linkage for a variety of developmental disorders, such as speech and sound disorders (SSD) and developmental dyslexia, and SLI and autism. Whether these are true examples of pleiotropy or outcomes of the imprecision of phenotype definitions is yet to be determined.

DIAGNOSIS

SLI is a clinical diagnosis based on a delay in language development for expected age, in the absence of intellectual disability, autism, hearing impairment, or environmental deprivation. In children for whom formal language assessments are conducted, a score of 1.5 or more standard deviations from the normative mean on a standardized test of language is considered diagnostic for SLI.

Box 53-3 lists warning signs that suggest a DLD during the first 3 years. Language delay can be diagnosed very early. The developmental history provides strong evidence for language delay when the child does not meet expressive language milestones, does not seem to understand directions without associated gestures (e.g., "get your ball" without pointing to the ball), or does not point on command. During the examination, similar instructions can be given to the young child, and the child can be asked to point to various body parts or to point to pictures of common objects in a book. If there is a suspicion of language delay, the young child can undergo more formal language testing, such as with the MacArthur-Bates Communicative Development Inventory (normed for 8–30 months) or the Preschool Language Scale–4 (normed for birth to 6 years 11 months), both of which assess receptive and expressive language at young ages.

BOX 53-3 Warning Signs of a Developmental Language Disorder

LIMITATIONS IN EXPRESSIVE LANGUAGE
- Early problems with sucking, swallowing, and chewing
- Excessive drooling
- Failure to vocalize to social stimuli
- Failure to vocalize two syllables at 8 months
- Few or no creative utterances of three words or more by age 3

LIMITATIONS IN VOCABULARY
- Limited repertoire of words understood or used
- Slow or difficult new-word acquisition

LIMITATIONS IN COMPREHENDING LANGUAGE
- Excessive reliance on contextual cues to understand language

LIMITATIONS IN SOCIAL INTERACTION
- Reduced social interaction, except to have needs met

LIMITATIONS IN PLAY
- No symbolic, imaginative play by age 3
- No interactive play with peers

LIMITATIONS IN LEARNING SPEECH
- Numerous articulation errors in expressive speech
- Unintelligible to unfamiliar listeners

LIMITATIONS IN USING STRATEGIES FOR LANGUAGE LEARNING
- Use of unusual or inappropriate strategies for age level, e.g., overuses imitation (echolalia), does not imitate verbalizations of others (dyspraxia), does not use *wh-* questions for learning (*why*, *what*, *where*, etc.)

LIMITATIONS IN ATTENTION FOR LANGUAGE ACTIVITIES
- Little interest in book reading, talking, or communicating with peers

(Modified with permission from Nelson NW. Childhood Language Disorders in Context: Infancy through Adolescence. New York: Macmillan, 1993; Hall N. Semin Pediatr Neurol 1997;4:77–85.)

BOX 53-4 Glossary of Terms Used in Describing Linguistic Functions

Functors	The small words of the language, such as prepositions, conjunctions, and articles; also called closed-class words because they are limited in number
Lexicon	The words in a language; the dictionary of word meanings
Mean length of utterance (MLU)	The number of morphemes per utterance
Morpheme	The smallest meaningful unit in a language, occurring either in a word or as a word. (For example, the compound word *compounding* is made up of three morphemes: *com-pound-ing*.) Prefixes, suffixes, and inflected endings such as *-ed*, *-s*, and *-ly* are also morphemes
Phoneme	A distinct sound unit in a language (In English, there are 46: 9 vowels and 37 consonants.)
Phonology	The rules a speaker follows when combining speech sounds
Pragmatics	The communicative intent of speech rather than its content (e.g., asking a question at the right time and in the right way)
Prosody	The melody of language; the tone of voice used to ask questions, for example, or to show emotion
Semantics	The meaning of words; their definition
Syntax	The grammar of a language; the acceptable relationship between words in a sentence

Before the age of 2 years, delay may not always equal disorder. Research on late-talking toddlers suggests that about 40% of children retained the diagnosis of SLI at ages 3 and 4 years. This is particularly true if the early language delay is primarily expressive. However, many children with early language delay who appear to "catch up" go on to have language-based learning disabilities (e.g., dyslexia). It is therefore important to recommend periodic reassessment of a child's language and academic functioning after an early language delay has been diagnosed.

Children with receptive language impairments are more likely to have a persistent SLI. These children are more likely to have academic and social problems as a result of poor comprehension of language, and in some cases slowed processing of auditory information, which makes it difficult for them to follow a conversation or to follow a spoken lecture. Thus concern for poor language prognosis should be heightened when receptive language deficits are identified.

Speech articulation disorders may be found in isolation or in association with language disorders. Early articulation errors are common and usually mild. However, if there are other features (e.g., excessive drooling or inability to chew food properly) or if a child is not able to be understood virtually 100% of the time by age 4 years, this should raise concern about a more serious condition, such as oral-motor apraxia. A thorough oral-motor examination by the physician will identify apraxia in severe cases. Milder forms may require a more extensive oral-motor assessment by a speech pathologist or pediatric occupational therapist.

NOSOLOGY OF DEVELOPMENTAL LANGUAGE DISORDERS

There is not uniform agreement on the proper nosology of the DLDs. The fifth edition of the *Diagnostic and Statistical Manual of Mental Disorders* (DSM-V) of the American Psychiatric Association (2013) includes DLD under Communication Disorders, and specifies subcategories of language disorder ("language disorder" combines expressive and mixed receptive–expressive language disorders—this is synonymous with SLI in common usage), speech-sound disorder (i.e., phonological disorder), childhood-onset fluency disorder (i.e., stuttering), and social (pragmatic) communication disorder (in the absence of autistic features). These constitute general subtypes of DLDs. A more specific nosology has been proposed by Rapin (1996) based on psycholinguistic features. The subtypes are named for the linguistic areas that are most problematic (see Table 53-1 and the glossary of terms in Box 53-4).

Articulation and Expressive Fluency Disorders
Pure Articulation Disorders

Articulatory skills improve with age, and as with language development, the normal range is considerable. Most children speak intelligibly by age 2 years. Unintelligible speech is the

TABLE 53-1 Subtypes of Developmental Language Disorders

	Receptive Expressive		Expressive		Higher Order	
	Verbal Auditory Agnosia	*Phonological Syntactic*	*Verbal Dyspraxia*	*Phonological Programming*	*Semantic Pragmatic*	*Lexical Syntactic*
Comprehension—Receptive						
Phonology	↓↓	↓				
Syntax	↓↓	↓				
Semantics	↓↓	?			↓↓	↓
Production—Expressive						
Semantics (lexical)	↓↓				↓↓	↓
Syntax	↓↓	↓↓	?	?		↓
Phonology	↓↓	↓↓	↓↓	↓		
Repetition	↓↓	↓	↓		↑	
Fluency	↓↓	↓	N1 or ↓	N1 or ↓	N1 or ↑	↓
Pragmatics	N1 or ↓	N1 or ↓			↓↓	↓

NI = normal; ↓ = impaired; ↓↓ = very impaired; ↑ = atypically enhanced; ? = unknown
(Modified from Nass R, Ross G. Disorders of higher cortical function in the preschooler. In: David R, ed. Child and Adolescent Neurology. St. Louis, MO: Mosby, 1997; Rapin I. Preschool Children with Inadequate Communication. London: Mackeith, 1996.)

exception at age 3 years. However, almost 50% of children at age 4 years still have mild articulation difficulties, primarily defective use of *th* or *r* sounds. At kindergarten entry, one third of children still have minor to mild articulation defects, but speech is unintelligible in less than 5%.

Stuttering and Cluttering

Stuttering is a disorder in the rhythm of speech. The speaker knows what to say but is unable to say it because of an involuntary repetitive prolongation or cessation of a sound. Some degree of dysfluency is common as language skills evolve during the preschool years, particularly as the mean length of utterance (MLU) reaches 6 to 8 words between ages 3 and 4 years. However, stuttering, in contrast to developmental dysfluency, is probably a linguistic disorder (errors occur at grammatically important points in the sentence) and a motor planning problem. Typically, onset of stuttering is between the ages of 3 and 6 years, and reports indicate unassisted recovery rates of 75%. Thus the prevalence of stuttering as a lifetime disorder is much lower than its incidence (0.5%–1% vs. 4%–5%). However, persistence of stuttering may be associated with other aspects of language impairment, such as difficulty with processing of syntactic information.

Stuttering is often a genetic trait. Although the cause of developmental stuttering is unknown, the main theories are anomalous dominance and abnormalities of interhemispheric connections. Cluttering, by contrast, as seen in fragile X syndrome, is characterized by incomplete sentences and short outbursts of two- to three-word phrases, along with echolalia, palilalia (compulsive repetition reiterated with increasing rapidity and decreasing volume), perseveration, poor articulation, and stuttering.

Phonological Programming Disorder

Children with the phonological programming disorder have fluent speech, and their MLU approaches normal. Despite initially poor intelligibility, serviceable speech is expected. Language comprehension is relatively preserved. Most such children show delayed rather than deviant phonology and improve during school years. It is debatable whether this disorder is a severe articulation problem or a mild form of verbal dyspraxia. The fact that patients with phonological programming disorder have more difficulty learning manual signs than do controls supports an association with dyspraxia. A prere-

mediation paired-associate learning task may help select the best remediation method for each child because some are better with symbols and some with signs.

Verbal Dyspraxia

Children with verbal dyspraxia, also called dilapidated speech, are extremely dysfluent. These children are unable to convert an abstract phonological representation into a set of motor commands to the articulators (i.e., there is a deficit in phonology–motor conversion). Utterances are short and laboriously produced. Phonology is impaired and includes inconsistent omissions, substitutions, and distortions of speech sounds. Children with dysarthria make voicing errors that distort, whereas children with dyspraxia make place substitution errors. In conversation, they make phrasal errors. Syntactic skills are difficult to assess in the face of dysfluency. Language comprehension is relatively preserved, but many children have receptive language problems. Children with verbal dyspraxia who do not develop intelligible speech by age 6 years are unlikely to acquire it later. The frequency with which nonverbal praxis deficits—buccal-lingual dyspraxia (e.g., positioning muscles of articulation) and generalized dyspraxia—coexist with verbal dyspraxia is unknown. The presence of a more diffuse disorder of praxis has significant therapeutic implications because children with verbal dyspraxia may depend on signing and writing skills for communication. Developmental coordination disorder (DCD) is commonly comorbid with speech/language learning disabilities. Young children who are in early intervention programs for speech/language delays may have significant coordination difficulties that will become more evident at kindergarten age, when motor deficits begin to affect self-care and academic tasks.

Disorders of Receptive and Expressive Language

Phonological Syntactic Syndrome

Phonological syntactic syndrome (also called mixed receptive expressive disorder, expressive disorder, and nonspecific formulation-repetition deficit) is probably the most common DLD. The phonological disturbances consist of omissions, substitutions, and distortions of consonants and consonant clusters in all word positions. The production of unpredictable and unrecognizable sounds makes speech impossible to understand. The syntactic impairment consists of a lack of functors and an absence of appropriate inflected endings. Plurals, third-person singulars, past tense, the auxiliary verb *be*, *the* and *a*, infinitives (*to*), and case markings on pronouns are particularly vulnerable. Grammatical forms are atypical, not just delayed. Whereas a typically developing young child may say "baby cry" or "a baby crying," children with phonological syntactic syndrome produce deviant constructions, such as "the baby is cry." Telegraphic speech is common. Comprehension is relatively spared. Semantic skills tend to be intact. Repetition, pragmatics, and prosody may be normal. Autistic children with this DLD subtype produce a significant amount of jargon.

Neurologic dysfunction is especially frequent in this subtype. Sucking, swallowing, and chewing difficulties are common, and drooling is often persistent. The neurologic examination may reveal signs of oral motor apraxia, hypertonia, and incoordination.

Verbal Auditory Agnosia

Children with verbal auditory agnosia (VAA) are unable to discern meaning from spoken language, despite intact hearing. VAA may be a developmental condition, apparent from early life, or an acquired disorder, as in Landau–Kleffner syndrome. VAA is common in low-functioning children with autism. The outcome from the developmental form of VAA is generally poor. The outcome from the acquired disorder is somewhat better, with approximately one third of patients having a good outcome with specific treatment.

Higher-Order Language Disorders
Semantic Pragmatic Syndrome

Children with the semantic pragmatic syndrome (also called repetition strength and comprehension deficit, language without cognition, cocktail party syndrome) are fluent and often verbose speakers. Vocabulary is often large and somewhat formal. Parents are often encouraged by the child's sizeable vocabulary, only to find later that the verbosity did not indicate superior cognitive skills. Many children have trouble with meaningful conversation and informative exchange of ideas. Pragmatic skills are lacking. They often show deficits in prosody; their speech has a monotonous, mechanical, or singsong quality. They cannot convey the additional pragmatic intentions that prosody affords, such as speaking with the proper emotion or indicating by tone of voice that they are asking a question. Comprehension may be impaired. Phonological and syntactic skills are generally intact.

Lexical Syntactic Syndrome

Lexical syntactic syndrome (LSS) occurs in approximately 15% of children with DLD. Speech is generally dysfluent, even to the point of stuttering, because of word-finding difficulties and poor syntactic skills. Both literal and semantic paraphasias are common. Most children have delays in word acquisition and less lexical diversity than their age-matched counterparts. Verbs appear to be the most difficult lexical category for them to learn. Syntax is immature but not deviant. Phonology is spared, and speech is intelligible. Repetition is generally better than spontaneous speech. In conversation, idiom use is better than spontaneous speech. In one study, fourth graders with LSS evidenced higher disruption rates at phrase boundaries in narratives than did their age-matched peers, reflecting lexical and syntactic deficits. Pragmatics may be impaired, particularly when this syndrome occurs in autistic children. Comprehension is generally acceptable, although complex questions and other linguistic forms taxing higher-level receptive syntactic skills are often deficient.

OUTCOME OF DEVELOPMENTAL LANGUAGE DISORDERS

Many children with SLI, particularly those with expressive language impairment, appear to improve in their language ability by early school age. Others have persistent language impairment that remains throughout life. There is a high incidence of other problems associated with SLI, including academic, behavioral, social-emotional, and psychiatric issues, and these may occur even when language appears to have reached the normal range.

Attention deficit disorder occurs in about 40% of children with SLI and may cause additional challenges.

Dyslexia is present in approximately 65% of children with SLI. Written composition may also be a challenge for these children. These problems lead to poorer-than-expected school performance and a higher dropout rate.

Adolescents with a history of SLI have a higher likelihood of peer problems, emotional symptoms, and conduct problems (Snowling et al., 2006; Conti-Ramsden et al., 2013). Poor receptive language raises the likelihood of emotional and behavioral difficulties. Anxiety disorder, social phobia, and depression occur at a high rate in children and adolescents (20%–50%) with a history of SLI. Adolescents with SLI have a lower level of academic achievement than their typically developing peers. It is important to note that subtle language and communication problems may persist into adult life in up to 90% of cases and may cause the affected individuals to be shy in social situations and reluctant to enter into conversations with others because of their language problem.

Preschool language skills are the best single predictor of later reading ability and disability. Even children with good receptive skills who speak late may be at risk for continuing subtle language difficulties and later reading- and language-based academic difficulties. Thus both screening and follow-up studies of children with SLI are important. Follow up of 112 individuals with SLI into adult life demonstrated lower levels of functioning in the areas of communication, educational attainment, and occupational status compared with their typical peers. Such studies indicate the need for continued surveillance of individuals with SLI and adequate guidance in terms of academic and career choices (Young et al., 2002; Johnson et al., 2010).

Early intervention, not only with speech/language therapy but also with social skills training and, when indicated, psychological and career counseling, may help to reduce the long-term morbidity of SLI.

EVALUATION OF THE CHILD WITH A SUSPECTED DEVELOPMENTAL LANGUAGE DISORDER

The workup of the child with a DLD (Box 53-6) must include an assessment of hearing and an assessment of overall level of intellectual functioning, in addition to a thorough language assessment that includes both receptive and expressive language components. Other evaluations that may be warranted include tests for auditory processing and neuropsychological assessments for associated problems such as attention deficit disorder.

Certain metabolic disorders can present with isolated language delay, so a metabolic screen is appropriate in some circumstances. Mitochondrial disorders and organic acidemias may have language impairment as their primary feature, particularly in the first few years of life. Numerous other syndromes can present predominantly with language delay.

An electroencephalogram (EEG) should be considered in a child with DLD if there is a history of a language regression or a suspicion from the history that the child might have seizures. Neuroimaging studies are not likely to be helpful unless there are abnormal findings on the neurologic examination.

TREATMENT

Whether intensive early therapy changes the long-term outcome to an appreciable degree remains to be determined. Treatment of language-disordered preschool children varies according to the kind of language impairment and its degree of severity (Warren and Yoder, 2004). Preschool children with moderate to severe language impairment may benefit from a special education preschool for language-impaired children. Mildly impaired children may do well in a regular preschool program combined with individual speech/language therapy. Floor time–based language therapy provides a naturalistic and developmentally appropriate way of working on language skill development. Formal language work typically begins at the phonologic level, involving repetition of sounds and sound sequences to encourage fluency. Treatment of receptive disorders often necessitates the use of visual modalities, such as signs and gesture. Less severe disorders of comprehension are addressed through practiced structuring of conversations with the child. Children with severe comprehension deficits rarely progress as well in treatment as do children with primary expressive disorders.

Children with significant auditory processing disorders may benefit from a systematic computer-based approach to improving the speed of auditory processing, although benefits from this type of intervention remain controversial.

Some classroom accommodations may be necessary for the child with SLI to succeed. Children with SLI may require additional help from a resource specialist or tutor. They may require additional time for giving reports and for taking tests. Whenever possible, presentation of oral information should be accompanied by visual aids. In support of previous research,

children with SLI have problems with inferencing, linking directly observed or stated information to likely outcomes. They also have limited working memory capacity, and they are more likely to make errors related to inattention. Thus children with SLI are likely to be at a disadvantage in classroom situations, particularly for information presented orally and if the information is complex. The use of pictorial aids may help them encode the information. They may also benefit from having information broken into manageable (shorter) units.

When necessary, medications for treatment of attention deficit hyperactivity disorder (ADHD) should be considered. Because there is a high incidence of secondary emotional problems and self-esteem issues associated with SLI, referral for psychological counseling should be considered as soon as these problems become apparent. Families should be informed about their child's condition and be encouraged to provide a positive and supportive environment. A multidisciplinary approach, including physician, speech/language pathologist, teacher, psychologist, and parents, provides the most effective means of helping children with SLI.

REFERENCES

The complete list of references for this chapter is available online at www.expertconsult.com.
See inside cover for registration details.

SELECTED REFERENCES

Badcock, N.A., Bishop, D.V., Hardiman, M.J., et al., 2012. Co-localisation of abnormal brain structure and function in specific language impairment. Brain Lang. 120 (3), 310–320.

Bates, E., Reilly, J.S., Wulfeck, B., et al., 2001. Differential effects of unilateral lesions on language production in children and adults. Brain Lang. 79, 223–265.

Bishop, D.V.M., Hayiou-Thomas, M.E., 2008. Heritability of specific language impairment depends on diagnostic criteria. Genes Brain Behav. 7, 365–372.

Conti-Ramsden, G., Mok, P.L., Pickles, A., et al., 2013. Adolescents with a history of specific language impairment (SLI): strengths and difficulties in social, emotional and behavioral functioning. Res. Dev. Disabil. 34 (11), 4161–4169.

Johnson, C.J., Beitchman, J.H., Brownlie, E.B., 2010. Twenty-year follow-up of children with and without speech-language impairments: Family, educational, occupational, and quality of life outcomes. Am. J. Speech Lang. Pathol. 19 (1), 51–65.

Rapin, I., 1996. Preschool Children With Inadequate Communication. Mackeith Press, London.

Snowling, M.J., Bishop, D.V., Stothard, S.E., et al., 2006. Psychosocial outcomes at 15 years of children with a preschool history of speech-language impairment. J. Child Psychol. Psychiatry 47 (8), 759–765.

Vernes, C., Newbury, D.F., Abrahams, B.S., et al., 2008. A functional genetic link between distinct developmental language disorders. N. Engl. J. Med. 359, 2337–2345.

Warren, S., Yoder, P., 2004. Early intervention for young children with language impairment. In: Verhoeven, L., van Balkom, H. (Eds.), Classification of Developmental Language Disorders. Lawrence Erhbaum, Mahwah, NJ, pp. 367–384.

Young, A.R., Beitchman, J.H., Johnson, C., et al., 2002. Young adult academic outcomes in a longitudinal sample of early identified language impaired and control children. J. Child Psychol. Psychiatry 43, 635–645.

E-BOOK FIGURES AND TABLES

54 Nonverbal Learning Disabilities and Associated Disorders

Margaret Semrud-Clikeman and Doris A. Trauner

 An expanded version of this chapter is available on www.expertconsult.com. See inside cover for registration details.

INTRODUCTION

Nonverbal learning disabilities (NLD) are increasingly being identified by clinicians. NLD generally involve difficulties with visual–spatial reasoning, executive functioning, and mathematics difficulties (Rourke and Tsatsanis, 2000; Davis and Broitman, 2011). For many children with NLD, co-occurring attention and social perception difficulties are present (Mammarella and Cornoldi, 2014; Semrud-Clikeman et al., 2010). Although there is no diagnosis in DSM V or ICD-10, frequently these children may qualify for a diagnosis of a social communication disorder from DSM V.

There are likely two different types of NLD: one with a medical association and one without. Children with non-medical NLD generally are referred to neuropsychological and psychological clinics and only rarely are seen by medical professionals other than pediatricians and physical/occupational therapists. Neurologists and other specialists frequently see children with medically based NLD because of parent concerns about visual–spatial difficulties and social deficits (Ballantyne et al., 2013; Bava et al., 2010; Beaton et al., 2010). Medical conditions frequently associated with NLD include velo-cardio-facial syndrome, some lysosomal storage diseases, and nephropathic cystinosis (Trauner et al., 2007). Neuroimaging findings have indicated differences in the corpus callosum (particularly in the splenial region), anterior cingulate gyrus, and in the parietal white matter volume and gray-matter thickness (Fine et al., 2013; Reiss et al., 1995). Further studies of structural and functional differences are needed, particularly in comparing medically related and nonmedically related cases of NLD.

WHAT ARE NONVERBAL LEARNING DISABILITIES?

The diagnosis of NLD is a fairly new construct first developed by Myklebust and Johnson and further researched by Byron Rourke and colleagues. The incidence of NLD has been estimated to be approximately 5% of the learning disabled population (or around 1% of the general population). These children have been described as having difficulties with visual–spatial processing, mathematics, handwriting, social cognition, and in some cases attention. In contrast to these weaknesses, children with NLD have also been found to be verbally facile and to have good reading recognition skills and rote language abilities.

The definition of NLD has continued to evolve since its original conceptualization, with diagnostic descriptions varying across clinical laboratories. The original conceptualization included difficulties with spatial and temporal perception, handwriting and mathematics weakness, problems with social perception, and a higher verbal than performance IQ. Many studies utilize an approach wherein the child must meet a selection of symptoms from an array of possibilities to qualify for a diagnosis of NLD. Although features of NLD subtypes continue to be refined, NLD is currently characterized by three broad areas of dysfunction: motoric skills, visual/spatial–organizational/memory skills, and social abilities.

Rourke was a pioneer in developing our understanding of NLD. After several decades of clinical research he conceptualized NLD as a set of assets and deficits. These strengths and weaknesses were associated with initial or primary features, which then lead to secondary and tertiary features in many areas of functioning. Using this framework, the social competence difficulties described originally by Myklebust are hypothesized to be the result of problems with visual–spatial processing.

Rourke's conceptualization was similar to that of Johnson in that both developed a neurologic hypothesis for NLD emphasizing white matter involvement. Rourke hypothesized that the myelinated fibers of the brain are related to symptoms of NLD, which subsequently included children with some genetic and medical conditions. For this reason, in addition to children without apparent congenital or acquired neurologic dysfunction, Rourke and associates began to incorporate the several additional neurologic disorders that had some or all of the features of NLD. The overlap with these diagnoses will be discussed in the next section.

Coexistent Issues

One of the controversies in NLD is whether it is a variant or a milder form of autism. Some researchers advocate the use of the NLD phenotype as a heuristic model for understanding autism spectrum disorders (ASD) or Asperger syndrome (AS), whereas others suggest that AS is a more severe form of NLD (Brumback et al., 1996). Still others suggest that these are two separate disorders. In the current version of DSM V, AS is no longer a diagnostic category; rather autism spectrum disorder: high functioning (HFA) is used.

Theoretical models of NLD and HFA both suggest deficits in the developing brain, likely beginning during gestation, that consequently affect the development of normal social interaction. The amygdala is particularly pinpointed as an area of system dysfunction early on that later interferes with the ability to respond to facial expressions due to faulty neural networks involving social understanding. Early experience with social referencing is crucial for the development of empathy, theory of the mind, and social reciprocity. Similarly, Rourke (1995) emphasized difficulties with the connectivity between the limbic structures and the frontal lobe rather than an impairment of specific regions.

Although there are similarities between NLD and AS/HFA in many aspects, there are also many qualitative differences between these groups. It is more common in NLD to find difficulties with mathematics and with visual–spatial processing than in AS/HFA. It is also unusual for children with NLD to show stereotyped behaviors or "bizarre" interests or an emphasis on routine that is frequently seen in individuals with AS/HFA.

Currently there are three comprehensive reviews of NLD that have sought to evaluate the empirical evidence to determine the main characteristics of NLD and to reconcile whether this diagnosis actually exists or is a form of autism. These reviews have generally found that NLD is a complex diagnosis for which there is no consistent criteria for identification. It was also found that many children with NLD showed symptoms of attention deficit hyperactivity disorder (ADHD): predominately inattentive type. The most robust finding was that of visual–spatial deficits, lower mathematics skills compared with reading, and problems with visual–constructive abilities. Moderate support was found for problems with visual memory and social cognition. It has also been suggested by a few authors that social comprehension ability may be evident in a subtype of NLD but not necessarily in all children with NLD. Fewer studies have systematically evaluated executive functioning and/or attentional abilities, so these areas continue to need additional study.

Neuropsychological Findings

Verbal-Performance IQ Split

Several studies have found a difference in the verbal and performance skills on the previous versions of the Wechsler Intelligence Scale for Children. More recent studies also have found this difference for children with NLD, but also for children with AS. In each study, children with NLD showed a larger discrepancy than those with other diagnoses. The discrepancy between verbal and performance abilities alone is not sufficient for a diagnosis of NLD but should be used as one piece of evidence.

It has been found that children with autism with a discrepantly high verbal *or* performance IQ showed significantly more apparent difficulties with social functioning. Others have found that when the nonverbal IQ was higher than the verbal IQ more social difficulties were present. Furthermore a discrepancy between verbal and performance IQ in children with AS was also found with higher verbal scores related to fewer social difficulties in another study. These findings suggest that a significant difference in verbal comprehension and perceptual reasoning on a standardized intelligence measure may be an important marker for NLD. It also is important to recognize that differences of less than 25 points happen in approximately 20% to 25% of the population and therefore are not rare. Furthermore, the discrepancy between perceptual reasoning and verbal comprehension is not in and of itself a sufficient marker for a diagnosis of NLD to be made. Unfortunately, many clinicians continue to diagnose NLD solely on this discrepancy.

Language

Although children with NLD have been found to have relatively good vocabularies, studies evaluating pragmatic language have begun to demonstrate some difficulty in this area. Pragmatic language includes the ability to understand the meaning of what is being said (semantics) and the ability to use language appropriately in social situations (pragmatics). Children with NLD have difficulty understanding the nuances of what is being said or being able to "read between the lines." Studies have found difficulty for children with NLD on measures of pragmatic language, particularly when it involves social referencing. Children with NLD had more difficulty interpreting humor that involved pragmatic language or plays on words (puns) compared with visually oriented slapstick humor.

Achievement

Children with NLD show good single word reading skills with later difficulties found in reading comprehension. Simply reporting facts and information that is contained within the reading selection is generally intact, whereas questions that probe for inferential reasoning are more problematic. In addition, difficulties have been found in mathematics, particularly in mathematical computation. As math demands increase, problems occur ranging from the mechanics of lining up numbers in math problems to comprehending the higher-level abstract concepts required in division, data presentation (charts, graphs), algebra, geometry, and trigonometry. These findings suggest it might not be the academic subject that is most problematic but rather the higher order thinking required to solve a problem.

Writing is an area of particular challenge for children with NLD. For early writers, letter formation, letter spacing, and word spacing may be difficult to manage. An informal assessment of this can be accomplished by simply asking the child to write the alphabet legibly as fast as they can. A child with NLD-based problems might have difficulty physically forming letters that are legible relative to other children their age, even while they work quickly through the letters.

Visual–Spatial and Motor Skills

Studies have found difficulties with visual–spatial skills and visual–motor ability. When children with NLD were compared with children with other disorders on measures of visual–motor organization and visual–spatial skills, the children with NLD scored worse than the other clinical groups and the control group. These findings support Rourke's contention that visual–spatial and perceptual difficulties may underlie the social difficulties frequently found in children with NLD. Motor skills have also been evaluated in children with NLD. Studies found graphomotor difficulties present particularly in younger children. These findings suggest that children with NLD do have more difficulty on tasks which require visual–spatial reasoning as well as visual–motor control and fine motor dexterity. These difficulties are particularly present when tasks are more complex, requiring additional processing for successful completion. It is also important to note that children with disorders such as ADHD and/or AS/ASD can also show difficulties in visual–motor skills, possibly for other reasons than visual–spatial deficits (e.g., impulsivity).

Executive Functioning

Executive functions are a relatively new area being examined in individuals suspected of having NLD. Executive functions that have been identified to be problematic for children with NLD include cause–effect reasoning, learning new material that is complex or novel, and planning and organization. Additional measures of novel problem solving have found difficulty on tasks that are of increasing complexity and that require memory and abstract reasoning skills.

Attention is a related construct to executive functioning. Children with NLD have been found to have more frequent difficulties with attention. Rourke suggested that these attentional problems may be related to visual–spatial deficits rather than to attention. Studies that have examined social perception measures found them to be highly correlated to executive functioning but not strongly related to attention. In contrast the relation between visual–spatial skills and social perception abilities was not found to be significant. A sizable minority of children with NLD show sufficient attentional symptoms for an additional diagnosis of ADHD, which also requires specific targeted treatment. These attentional skill deficits have not been found to be as predictive of social difficulties.

Social Perception and Psychopathology

It has been suggested children with NLD show higher rates of depression and anxiety (Pelletier et al., 2001). Others have not found significantly higher rates of internalizing behaviors when samples are studied that are community based rather than in residential treatment facilities or in psychiatric clinics. Others have found mild symptoms of social withdrawal and sadness in children with NLD, particularly those who are older and in whom peer relations become more important and valued for self-esteem. Measures that require a child with NLD to interpret a social situation that is ambiguous or does not provide verbal cues as to what is occurring have been found to be particularly difficult.

In addition, these children had difficulty perceiving humor (cartoons and nonsequiturs), suggesting that problems with humor comprehension in children with NLD may be more related to social rather than visual–spatial deficits. Further studies have found difficulties with emotional modulation and/or depressed mood to be significantly related to the child's ability to accurately recognize and interpret nonverbal cues in a social situation. If a child has difficulty with nonverbal cues and misidentifies these and acts accordingly to the mistaken perception, it is likely that the child will feel sad and may withdraw from further social interactions, particularly if there is a negative outcome.

Neuroimaging Findings in NLD and AS/ASD

Some have hypothesized that AS/HFA and NLD may be on the same continuum. If this supposition is accurate, then neuro-imaging studies should find similar neuroanatomical differences from typically developing children. Neuroimaging studies have generally focused on autism spectrum disorders (ASD) and/or Asperger syndrome (AS). Findings from neuroimaging studies with ASD have found a larger white matter volume in the temporal and frontal lobes, bilateral amygdala, and hippocampus. It was suggested that these larger structures may be a result of developmental adaptation of the autistic brain caused by a processing overload involving emotional learning experiences. The amygdalar–hippocampal-frontal circuit may be particularly important for mediating emotional perception and regulation and is compromised in children with social reciprocity difficulties. Evidence of enlarged amygdalar regions was not found in the one study of NLD imaging, although the anterior cingulate bilaterally was found to be smaller in the AS and NLD group compared with controls (Table 54-1).

These findings have important implications for our understanding of NLD and of ASD/AS. Previous researchers have suggested that hippocampal enlargement is related to larger amygdaloid volumes. In this theory the reciprocal connections between these structures lead to excitation of both structures through a dense interchange network. Thus a larger amygdala may result in hippocampal enlargement caused by overexcitation in both structures. Supporting this hypothesis is a previous finding that these regions interact strongly when the system is stressed. Children with ASD have a high co-occurrence of anxiety, which may be related or as a result of the enlargement of these regions. In contrast, children with NLD do not evidence the same level of anxiety and show amygdaloid and hippocampal volumes similar to neurotypical children. The smaller volume of the anterior cingulate cortex in children with NLD and ASD implicates the network that is involved in

TABLE 54-1 Major Neuroimaging Findings in ASD and NLD

Study	Patient Groups	Main Findings
STRUCTURAL MRI		
Abell et al. (1999)	ASD, controls	ASD>controls in white matter volume
Groen et al. (2010); Nacewicz et al. (2006)	ASD, controls	ASD>controls in amygdalar volume
Groen et al. (2010)	ASD, controls	ASD>controls on right hippocampus volume ASD>controls in temporal and frontal lobes
Semrud-Clikeman et al. (2013)	NLD, AS, and controls	All groups equal in white and gray matter volumes AS>NLD, controls in amygdala volume; NLD<AS, controls in ACC volume
Fine, Musielak & Semrud-Clikeman (2013)	NLD, ASD, ADHD, controls	Total CC volume equal across groups; NLD<S, ADHD, controls in spenial volume
Semrud-Clikeman & Fine (2011)	NLD, AS, controls	25% of children with NLD showed benign cysts or lesions; 4% of AS and controls
Reiss et al. (1995)	Turner syndrome (TS), controls	TS<controls in gray matter volume of parietal occipital region
LePage et al. (2013)	TS, controls	TS<controls in cortical thickness in parietal occipital regions
FUNCTIONAL MRI		
Happe et al.	Asperger syndrome (AS), controls	AS<controls activation in anterior cingulate
Fine et al. (submitted)	ASD, NLD, controls	Controls more sensitive to emotional valence; ASD or NLD less sensitive to changes in valence of emotional stimuli ASD>activation to negative than positive stimuli
Beaton et al. (2010)	TS, controls	TS<controls in brain activation in parietal regions during visual–spatial tasks
Beaton et al. (2010)	22q11 deletion, controls	22q11>controls in lateral ventricles; brain volumes are similar
Schaer et al. (2006)	22q11 deletion, controls	22q11<controls in gyrification of frontal and parietal lobes
DIFFUSION TENSOR IMAGING		
Yamagata et al. (2012)	TS, controls	TS<controls in white matter integrity
Bava et al. (2010)	Cystinosis, controls	Decreased connectivity in inferior and superior parietal lobules in children with cystinosis; older children with cystinosis showed reduced connectivity and poorer visual–spatial performance

understanding the perspectives of others as well as self. A smaller volume of the anterior cingulate cortex in children with AS or NLD may be related to difficulty in the evaluation and self-monitoring of behavior. An additional study of the corpus callosum found the NLD group to have significantly smaller splenia of the corpus callosum compared with all other groups. Smaller splenia in the NLD group were associated with lower performance but not verbal scores.

fMRI

To further investigate processing of social information in children with ASD and NLD, a functional magnetic imaging study was conducted by the author and colleagues. This study found that not only is face perception affected, but broad regions related to verbal processing were also less sensitive to valence differences. It was also found that the ASD group showed a greater activation to negative than to positive stimuli, whereas typically developing children and those with NLD demonstrated more activation to positive compared with negative stimuli.

Neurologic Aspects of Nonverbal Learning Disabilities

Although NLDs are underrecognized by neurologists, the condition is common and the diagnosis is important in terms of directing appropriate intervention for the child. There are characteristic features both in the medical/neurodevelopmental history and on neurologic examination that may be strongly suggestive of a diagnosis of NLD. On the neurologic examination, common findings include difficulty with pencil control, drawing, and fine motor movements, and problems with staying focused on tasks without focal neurologic deficits.

Turner syndrome results from either a partial or complete absence of one X chromosome. It occurs in approximately 1 in 2500 girls and is associated with short stature, webbed neck, and low hairline. In the partial absence of the X chromosome, there is mosaicism, in which two distinct cell lines exist in the same girl. Many studies have merged the two subtypes of Turner syndrome and have found a consistent cognitive profile. Although most girls with Turner syndrome have normal global intellectual functioning, numerous studies have identified a pattern of neurocognitive deficits that are consistent with NLD. Verbal IQ (VIQ) is typically normal or even above average, whereas Performance IQ (PIQ) is low in comparison with VIQ. Language skills are generally preserved, with the exception of sequencing and syntactic processing. Attention problems are also common in Turner girls. Arithmetic skills are often impaired relative to controls and to other areas of academic functioning. The most consistent cognitive deficit in girls with Turner syndrome is in visual–spatial skills. These deficits are present from early life and show a widening of the gap over time on visual–spatial tasks, indicating that the deficit is not merely a delay in development of visual–spatial skills, but a true deficit.

Quantitative neuroimaging studies have revealed structural and functional differences in the brains of girls with Turner syndrome compared with controls and a difference in the trajectory of brain development. In cross-sectional studies, reductions have been found in the volume of gray matter in the parietal occipital region. Impaired white matter integrity has also been demonstrated using Diffusion Tensor Imaging (DTI). The authors suggest that genetic effects on brain development may produce very disparate pathways associated with cognitive functioning.

Within-group comparisons of brain development over time showed a different trajectory in Turner girls compared with controls. When comparing the same brains at time 1 and time 2 (roughly ages 8 and 9 years), left parietal white matter volume and right parietal cortical thickness were both smaller in TS girls at time 2. The authors suggest that there may be a "critical period" for effective intervention in girls with Turner syndrome based on aberrant developmental trajectories.

22q11 deletion syndrome (Velocardiofacial syndrome, DiGeorge syndrome, Shprintzen syndrome) is common genetic disorder with an estimated prevalence of 1:2000 (Beaton et al., 2010). It is associated with a hemizygous deletion in the long arm of chromosome 22. There are a number of commonly associated features, including heart disease (supravalvular aortic stenosis being the most common type), neonatal hypocalcemia, cleft palate, short stature, facial dysmorphic features, and T-cell immunodeficiency (Robin and Sphrintzen, 2005). One of the names for this syndrome is based on velocardiofacial insufficiency with subsequent hypernasal speech. Intellectual disability is common, as are ASD and attention problems. Although global intellectual functioning is often impaired in individuals with 22q11 deletion syndrome, many studies have identified a relative weakness in visual–spatial ability, mathematics, executive functioning, and attention. Neuroimaging studies have demonstrated somewhat smaller brain volume and an increase in size of the lateral ventricles in 22q11 deletion patients compared with controls, as well as reduced gyrification in the frontal and parietal lobes, indicating that these areas may have a different pattern of brain development that may in turn lead to impaired connectivity and more difficulty with visual–spatial skill formation.

Neurofibromatosis type I (NF1) is the most common neurocutaneous disorder with an autosomal dominant inheritance (on chromosome 17q11.2) and an estimated incidence of 1:3000. Learning disabilities constitute one of the more common problems in NF-1, being recognized in 30% to 40% of children with this disorder. The major commonality among most of the studies has been the presence of visual–spatial deficits in many children with NF-1, as well as attention problems and a lower-than-expected intelligence. Language may be as impaired as visual–spatial skills in some NF-1 patients, whereas others have more prominent nonverbal deficits. The discrepancies are not surprising, however, because neuroimaging shows white-matter lesions in this disorder, but the number, size, and location of these abnormalities may differ from one individual to another, perhaps accounting for some of the differences in cognitive function that have been identified. Despite the variability in results from different studies, it appears that the most prevalent type of cognitive deficit in NF-1 is most consistent with a modified NLD phenotype.

Nephropathic cystinosis is a rare autosomal recessive disorder in which the amino acid cystine accumulates in lysosomes as a result of a cystine transporter protein deficiency. The CTNS gene (on chromosome 17p13) codes for the cystine transporter protein. The incidence of cystinosis is estimated at approximately 1:100,000 individuals worldwide, with a carrier rate estimated at 1:158. This information is important because carriers may be at increased risk for subtle cognitive differences similar to those found in individuals with cystinosis. Individuals with cystinosis have been found to have neurologic and cognitive deficits consistent with NLD. Children with cystinosis have normal verbal intelligence and normal language function, but exhibit problems with visual–spatial skills, spatial memory, visual–motor coordination, mathematics, and subtle social difficulty, similar to NLD. Otherwise asymptomatic carriers of the cystinosis gene have been found to have similar but less prominent visual–motor/visual–spatial deficits. Given the relative frequency of the carrier gene for this recessive condition (1:158), this may prove to be one of the more common associations with NLD.

The studies of cognition in cystinosis have shown that this is one of the few instances in which neuroimaging differences help to explain the cognitive profile. Bava et al., using DTI, found reduced white matter integrity in the parietal regions, and the reduction correlated inversely with visual–spatial performance, suggesting a delay in white matter maturation that may have forced a different approach to neural network development for visual–spatial function.

All of these syndromes are strongly associated both with a clinical profile of NLD and, in most cases, brain structural abnormalities that include either parietal lobe or frontal-parietal developmental differences. Further studies to identify specific genes or gene interactions may help to elucidate the neural mechanisms that underlie normal development of visual–spatial skills and how better to assist in the future those individuals who are found to have NLD.

REFERENCES

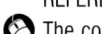 The complete list of references for this chapter is available in the e-book at www.expertconsult.com.

See inside cover for registration details.

SELECTED REFERENCES

Ballantyne, A.O., Spilkin, A.M., Trauner, D.A., 2013. Executive function in nephropathic cystinosis. Cogn. Behav. Neurol. 26, 14–22.

Bava, S., Theilmann, R.J., Sach, M., et al., 2010. Developmental changes in cerebral white matter microstructre in a disorder of lysosomal storage. Cortex 46, 206–216.

Beaton, E.A., Qin, Y.F., Nguyen, V., et al., 2010. Increased incidence and size of cavum septum pellucidum in children with chromosome 22q11.2 deletion syndrome. Psychiatry Res. 181, 108–113.

Brumback, R.A., Harper, C.R., Weinberg, W.A., 1996. Nonverbal learning disabilities, Asperger's syndrome, pervasive developmental disorder - should we care? J. Child. Neurol. 11, 427–429.

Davis, J.M., Broitman, J., 2011. Nonverbal Learning Disabilities in Children: Bridging the Gap Between Science and Practice. Springer, Boston.

Fine, J.G., Musielak, K., Semrud-Clikeman, M., 2013. Functional magnetic resonance findings in children with Asperger disorder, nonverbal learning disabilities, and controls. Child. Neuropsychol doi:10.1080/09297049.2013.854763.

Mammarella, I., Cornoldi, C., 2014. An analysis of the criteria used to diagnose children with Nonverbal Learning Disorder (NLD). Child. Neuropsychol 20, 255–280.

Pelletier, P.M., Ahmad, S.A., Rourke, B.P., 2001. Classification rules for basic phonological processing disabilities and nonverbal learning disabilities: formulation and external validity. Child. Neuropsychol. 7, 84–98.

Reiss, A.L., Mazzocco, M.M.M., Greenlaw, R., et al., 1995. Neurodevelopmental effects of X monosomy: A volumetric imaging study. Ann. Neurol. 38, 731–738.

Robin, N.H., Sphrintzen, R.J., 2005. Defining the clinical spectrum of deletion 22q11.2. J. Pediatr. 147, 90–96.

Rourke, B.P., 1995. The NLD syndrome and the white matter model. In: Rourke, B.P. (Ed.), Syndrome of Nonverbal Learning Disabilities: neurodevelopmental manifestations. Guilford Press, New York.

Rourke, B.P., Tsatsanis, K.D., 2000. Nonverbal learning disabilities. In: Klin, A., Volkmar, F.R.Sparrow, S.S. (Eds.), Asperger Syndrome. Guilford Press, New York.

Semrud-Clikeman, M., Walkowiak, J., Wilkinson, A., et al., 2010. Neuropsychological findings in nonverbal learning disabilities. Dev. Neuropsychol. 35, 582–600.

Trauner, D.A., Spilkin, A.M., Williams, J., et al., 2007. Evidence for an early effect of the cystinosin gene on neural function: Specific cognitive deficits in young children with cystinosis. J. Pediatr. 151, 192–196.

55 Dyslexia

Sally E. Shaywitz and Bennett A. Shaywitz

> An expanded version of this chapter is available on www.expertconsult.com. See inside cover for registration details.

Developmental dyslexia (or specific reading disability) is defined as an unexpected difficulty in accuracy or fluency of reading for an individual's chronologic age, intelligence, level of education, or professional status. Dyslexia is, at its core, a problem with phonological processing: that is, getting to the elemental sounds of spoken language, affecting both spoken and written language. As dyslexic children progress in school, given effective instruction, reading accuracy often improves; however, lack of fluency persists and remains a lifelong problem. As a consequence, individuals who are dyslexic require accommodations for their lack of reading and/or oral fluency. Dyslexia is the most common and most comprehensively studied of the learning disabilities (LD), affecting 80% of all individuals identified as learning-disabled. Although the diagnosis and implications of dyslexia were often uncertain in the past, advances in our knowledge of the epidemiologic, neurobiologic, and cognitive influences on the disorder allow it to be approached within the framework of a traditional medical model. This chapter reviews these advances and their implications for the approach to children and adults with dyslexia.

DYSLEXIA IS SPECIFIC—LEARNING DISABILITIES ARE NOT

Consistent in the original descriptions by the pioneers who described dyslexia, all noted that the reading problem in dyslexic children was *unexpected* in relation to their intelligence. As we review below, the unexpected nature of the reading problem was also the hallmark of what came to be known in the 1960s as LD. In recent testimony before Congress, Dr. Sally Shaywitz emphasized that "Dyslexia differs markedly from all other learning disabilities. Dyslexia is very specific and scientifically validated: we know its prevalence, cognitive and neurobiological origins, symptoms, and effective, evidence-based interventions. Learning disabilities is a general term referring to a range of difficulties which have not yet been delineated or scientifically validated. Learning disabilities are comparable to the term 'infectious' diseases, while dyslexia is akin to being diagnosed with a strep throat—a highly specific disorder in which the causative agent and evidence-based treatment are both known and validated."

Definition of Dyslexia

For over 100 years in the case of dyslexia and over 50 years in the case of LD, the most consistent and enduring core of the definition is the concept of dyslexia (and LD) as *unexpected* underachievement. The most up-to-date, scientifically supported definition of dyslexia is that in the 2015 bipartisan Cassidy-Mikulski Senate Resolution 275: "Dyslexia is defined as an unexpected difficulty in reading in an individual who has the intelligence to be a much better reader; dyslexia reflects a difficulty in getting to the individual sounds of spoken language which typically impacts speaking (word retrieval), reading (accuracy and fluency), spelling, and often, learning a second language."

For the first time there is now empiric data confirming the unexpected nature of dyslexia.

These data come from the Connecticut Longitudinal Study, a sample survey of Connecticut schoolchildren representative of those children entering public kindergarten in Connecticut in 1983. Using the Connecticut Longitudinal Study, Ferrer et al. (2010) demonstrated that, in typical readers, reading and IQ are dynamically linked over time. Not only do reading and IQ track together over time, but they also influence one another. Such mutual interrelationships are not perceptible in dyslexic readers, suggesting that reading and cognition develop more independently in dyslexia (Figure 55-1). These findings provide the long-sought empirical evidence for the seeming paradox involving cognition and reading in dyslexia. Thus, in dyslexia, a highly intelligent person may read at a level above average but below that expected, based on his/her intelligence, age, education, or professional status.

Many confuse the impact of dyslexia with an almost total inability to read. Although that may occur, most commonly and certainly as defined legally and supported by scientific evidence, there is no reading level below which an individual, student or adult, must score to be diagnosed as dyslexic. Rather, the central point is *how* the individual reads, the effort and work that must go into the reading process for him or her to decipher the word accurately and fluently. Think of a motor disability. The question is not whether the person can cross a street, but rather what he or she must do to get to the other side, that is, use a cane or a wheelchair.

EPIDEMIOLOGY AND ETIOLOGY

Epidemiologic data indicate that, like hypertension and obesity, dyslexia fits a dimensional model. Within the population, reading ability and reading disability occur along a continuum, with reading disability representing the lower tail of a normal distribution of reading ability (Shaywitz et al., 1992). Dyslexia is perhaps the most common neurobehavioral disorder affecting children, with prevalence rates ranging from 17.5% to 21% (Shaywitz et al., 1994).

Dyslexia is both familial and heritable. Family history is one of the most important risk factors, with 23% to 65% of children who have a parent with dyslexia reported to have the disorder. Given that dyslexia is familial and heritable, initial hopes that dyslexia would be explained by one or just a few genes have been disappointing. Thus, along with a great many common diseases, genome-wide association studies (GWAS) in dyslexia have so far identified genetic variants that account for only a very small percentage of the risk—less than 1%. Current evidence suggests "that common diseases involve thousands of genes and proteins interacting on complex pathways," and that, similar to experience with other complex disorders (heart disease, diabetes), it is unlikely that a single gene or even a few genes will identify people with dyslexia. Rather, dyslexia is best explained by *multiple* genes, each contributing a *small* amount of the variance.

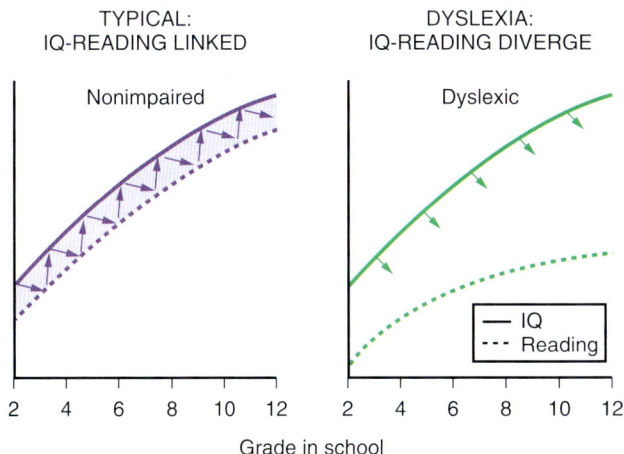

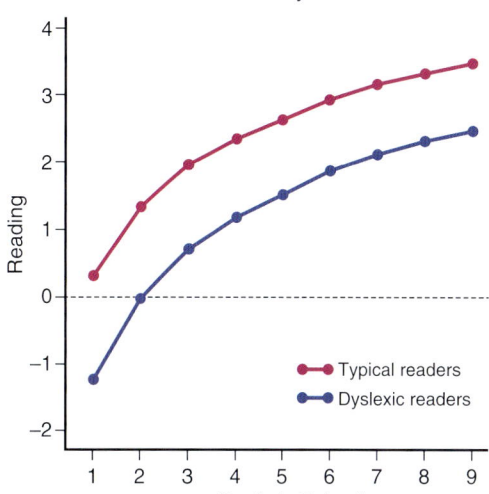

Figure 55-1. Uncoupling of reading and IQ over time: empirical evidence for a definition of dyslexia. Left: In typical readers, reading and IQ development are dynamically linked over time. Right: In contrast, in dyslexic readers, reading and IQ development are dissociated and one does not influence the other. *(Data adapted from Ferrer E, et al. Uncoupling of reading and IQ over time: empirical evidence for a definition of dyslexia. Psychol Sci 2010;21:93–101.)*

Figure 55-2. Reading from grades one to nine in typical and dyslexic readers. The achievement gap between typical and dyslexic readers is evident as early as first grade and persists through adolescence. *(Data adapted from Ferrer et al., Achievement gap in reading is present as early as first grade and persists through adolescence, J Pediatr 2015;167:1121–1125, e2.)*

Recent data indicate that a large achievement gap between dyslexic and typical readers is already present early on (first grade) and persists throughout school. These data make it imperative to identify and provide effective interventions at the start of school. These data indicate that it is no longer acceptable to wait until a child is in third grade or later before undertaking efforts to identify or address dyslexia. Using data from the Connecticut longitudinal study of reading from 1st grade to 12th grade, we found that as early as 1st grade, compared with typical readers, dyslexic readers had lower reading scores and their trajectories over time never converge with those of typical readers. These data demonstrate that such differences are not so much a function of increasing disparities over time but instead reflect marked differences already present in first grade between typical and dyslexic readers. The message is that the achievement gap between typical and dyslexic readers is evident as early as first grade, and this gap persists into adolescence. These findings provide strong evidence and impetus for early identification of and intervention for young children at risk for dyslexia. Implementing effective reading programs as early as kindergarten or even preschool offers the potential to close the achievement gap (Ferrer et al. 2015) (Figure 55-2).

PHONOLOGIC MODEL OF DYSLEXIA

Among investigators in the field, there is a strong consensus supporting the phonologic theory. This theory recognizes that speech is natural and inherent, but that reading is acquired and must be taught. To read, the beginning reader must connect the letters and letter strings (i.e., the orthography) to something that already has inherent meaning—the sounds of spoken language. In the process, a child has to develop the insight that spoken words can be pulled apart into the elemental particles of speech (i.e., phonemes) and that the letters in a written word represent these sounds; such awareness is largely deficient in dyslexic children and adults.

Neurobiological Evidence Supporting Dyslexia
Making a Hidden Disability Visible

Using functional magnetic resonance imaging (fMRI), converging evidence from many laboratories around the world

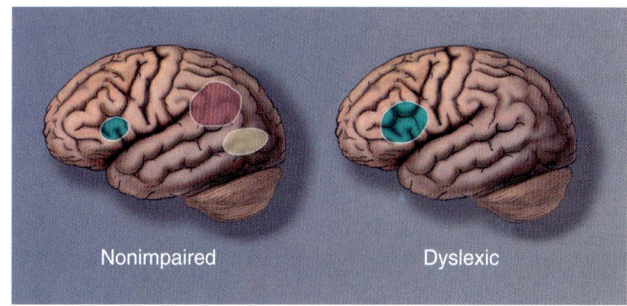

Figure 55-3. Neural signature for dyslexia. A neural signature for dyslexia is illustrated in this schematic view of left hemisphere brain systems in nonimpaired (left) and dyslexic (right) readers. In dyslexic readers, the anterior system is slightly overactivated compared with systems of typical readers; in contrast, the two posterior systems are underactivated. This pattern of underactivation in left posterior reading systems is referred to as the neural signature for dyslexia. *(By W. Hill, copyright © 2003 by S. E. Shaywitz; from Overcoming Dyslexia: a New and Complete Science-based Program for Reading Problems at any Level by Sally Shaywitz, MD. Used by permission of Alfred A. Knopf, an imprint of the Knopf Doubleday Publishing Group, a division of Penguin Random House LLC. All rights reserved.)*

has demonstrated a "neural signature for dyslexia," that is, an inefficient functioning of posterior reading systems during reading real words and pseudowords (Figure 55-3). This evidence from fMRI has for the first time made visible what previously was a hidden disability (Shaywitz et al., 2002). These findings of significantly greater activation in posterior reading systems in typical readers than in readers with dyslexia align with the classic 19th-century reports by Dejerine of acquired alexia caused by left-hemisphere lesions in the parietotemporal areas as well as areas around the fusiform gyrus.

These data from fMRI studies in groups of children with dyslexia have been replicated in reports from many investigators and show a failure of left-hemisphere posterior brain systems to function properly during reading, particularly the systems in the left-hemisphere occipitotemporal region (Richlan et al., 2009). Similar findings have been reported in German (18) and Italian (19) readers with dyslexia. Some studies in Chinese readers with dyslexia show brain abnormalities in left occipitotemporal and anterior frontal regions similar to those found in dyslexia in alphabetic orthographies.

Connectivity analyses of fMRI data represent the most recent evolution in characterizing brain networks in dyslexia. Measures of functional connectivity are designed to detect differences in brain regions with similar magnitudes of activation but whose activity is differentially synchronized with other brain systems across subject groups and/or types of stimuli. Most recently, Finn et al. (2013) have reported that, compared with typical readers, dyslexic readers showed reduced connectivity in the visual word-form area, a part of the left fusiform gyrus specialized for printed words.

Implications of Brain Imaging Studies

The brain imaging studies reviewed above provide neurobiological evidence that illuminates and clarifies current understanding of the nature of dyslexia and its treatment. For example, brain imaging has taken dyslexia from what had previously been considered a hidden disability to one that is visible; the findings of inefficient functioning in posterior reading systems are often referred to as a "neural signature for dyslexia." These findings should eliminate any thoughts of whether dyslexia is real or a "valid" diagnosis; even more so, these cutting-edge converging data from imaging laboratories worldwide should encourage the use of the word "dyslexia," for it has meaning and relevance at levels reaching to the basic neural architecture in reading and its inefficient functioning in struggling readers. These findings too are universal, having been demonstrated in readers of English and other alphabetic scripts with very similar findings in readers of logographic languages as well.

DIAGNOSIS

In *Overcoming Dyslexia* (Shaywitz, 2003), S. Shaywitz conceptualizes dyslexia as a weakness in phonology (getting to the sounds of spoken words) surrounded by a sea of strengths in higher-order thinking. In younger children there is an encapsulated weakness in decoding surrounded by strengths in, for example, problem solving, critical thinking, concept formation, and reasoning. In older children, adolescents, and adults, it may be thought of as an encapsulated weakness in fluent reading surrounded by these strengths in higher-order thinking.

Given that dyslexia is defined on the basis of scientific evidence as an unexpected difficulty in reading in a child or an adult in relation to intelligence, it is not surprising that a measure of intelligence, the Wechsler Intelligence Scale for Children–Fifth Edition (WISC-V) is a critical component of a comprehensive assessment of the child (age 6 to 16 years) with dyslexia. Very often an intelligence test can reveal areas of strength, particularly in areas of abstract thinking and reasoning, which are very reassuring to parents and especially to the child him/herself. They also indicate that the reading difficulty is isolated and not reflective of a general lack of learning ability or intellectual disability.

Kindergarten and first grade teachers are now able to screen for dyslexia with a high degree of accuracy using the brief Shaywitz Dyslexia Screen available from Pearson Publishers. Currently, most children with dyslexia are not diagnosed until they are in third grade or about 9 years old, although it is possible to recognize children at-risk for dyslexia as young as 4 to 5 years of age. As shown in Box 55-1 from S. Shaywitz's

---

BOX 55-1 Clues to Dyslexia Beginning in Second Grade and Beyond

PROBLEMS IN SPEAKING

- Mispronunciation of long or complicated words
- Speech that is not fluent (pausing or hesitating often); lots of "ums"
- Use of imprecise language
- Inability to find the exact word
- Struggle to retrieve words: "It was on the tip of my tongue."
- Need for time to summon an oral response, inability to come up with a verbal response quickly when questioned
- Lack of glibness, especially if put on the spot
- Spoken vocabulary smaller than listening vocabulary; hesitation to say aloud words that might be mispronounced
- Oral presentations often underestimate knowledge of the individual

PROBLEMS IN READING

- Very slow progress in acquiring reading skills
- Lack of a strategy to read new words
- Trouble reading unknown (new or unfamiliar) words that must be sounded out
- The inability to read small "function" words such as *that, an, in*
- Fear of reading out loud
- Oral reading that is choppy and labored
- Disproportionately poor performance on multiple-choice tests
- Inability to finish tests on time
- Disastrous spelling
- Reading that is very slow and tiring
- Messy handwriting but with excellent facility at word processing
- Extreme difficulty learning a foreign language
- Reading whose accuracy improves over time, though it continues to lack fluency and is laborious
- Lowered self-esteem, with pain that is not always visible to others
- Avoidance of reading—gains knowledge from sources other than reading, e.g., audiobooks, discussions, film
- Lack of fluency in reading increases attentional demands—vulnerable to noise, reading tiring
- Comprehension—often higher than word-reading accuracy or fluency
- Sacrifice of social life for studying
- Anxiety around test-taking or reading/speaking aloud
- Noted success, with accommodations, in a range of professions, including writing, science, medicine, architecture, law, journalism
- A history of reading, spelling, and foreign language problems in family members

---

Overcoming Dyslexia, signs and symptoms of children at risk for dyslexia can be observed even before formal reading begins in school.

See Box 55-2, Clues to children at risk for Dyslexia (from © S. Shaywitz, Overcoming Dyslexia (2003) in the e-book.

- Delayed language
- Trouble learning common nursery rhymes such as "Jack and Jill" and "Humpty-Dumpty"
- A lack of appreciation of rhymes

- Mispronounced words; persistent baby talk
- Difficulty in learning (remembering) names of letters and numbers
- Failure to know the letters in his own name

These clues along with a positive family history represent significant risk factors for dyslexia.

The assessment approach we focus on here and elaborated in more detail in Dr. Sally Shaywitz' new edition of *Overcoming Dyslexia* (forthcoming) is an in-depth evaluation of the skills (especially phonologic) known to be related to reading success. We and other researchers have begun to recognize that one source of potentially powerful and highly accessible screening information that has thus far been ignored is the teacher's judgment about the child's reading and reading-related skills. Remarkably, we found that teachers' response to a small subset of questions (Dyslexia Screening Measure [© Sally Shaywitz, 2014] comprising 10 items from the kindergarten and 12 items from the first-grade Multigrade Inventory for Teachers [© Sally Shaywitz, M.D., 1987]) predicts children at high risk for dyslexia with a high degree of accuracy, with good sensitivity and specificity.

Tests Helpful in the Evaluation of Children for Dyslexia

Phonological Processing

Clinicians and researchers often use the Comprehensive Test of Phonological Processing, now in its second edition (CTOPP-2), to test for the full range of phonological skills.

Letter Knowledge

Though not as robust as tests of phonological awareness in predicting whether the young child is at risk for dyslexia, a child's knowledge of letter names and sounds may also serve as a helpful guide to how ready she/he is to read. More formal testing can be obtained by using a reading test that contains a letter-identification section, for example, the letter–word subtest on the Wechsler Individual Achievement Test—Third Edition (WIAT-III); Kaufman Test of Educational Achievement—Third Edition (KTEA-III); or the Woodcock-Johnson IV Tests of Achievement (WJ-IV).

Academic Achievement

Overall, in the school-aged child, reading is assessed by measuring accuracy, fluency, and comprehension. Specifically, in the school-aged child, one important element of the evaluation is how accurately the child can decode words (i.e., read single words). This is measured with standardized tests of single real word and pseudoword reading. Because pseudowords are unfamiliar and cannot be memorized, each nonsense word must be sounded out. Tests of nonsense word reading are referred to as "word attack." Reading fluency, the ability to read accurately, rapidly, and with good prosody, an often overlooked component of reading, is of critical importance because it allows for the automatic, attention-free recognition of words.

The WIAT-III, KTEA-III, and WJ-IV are each reliable, valid, and comprehensive measures of academic achievement. In addition, fluency also may be assessed by asking the child to read *aloud* using the Gray Oral Reading Test—Fifth Edition (GORT-5). In addition to reading passages aloud, single-word reading efficiency may be assessed using, for example, the Test of Word Reading Efficiency, 2nd Edition (TOWRE-2), a test of speeded oral reading of individual real words and pseudowords. Children who struggle with reading often have trouble spelling; spelling may be assessed with the WIAT-III, KTEA-III, or WJ-IV spelling test.

Physical and Neurologic Examination and Laboratory Tests

A general physical examination has a very limited role in the evaluation of individuals with dyslexia. Primary sensory impairments should be ruled out, particularly in young children. The examination should be governed by any non-dyslexic symptoms that indicate specific areas of concern. Results of the routine neurologic examination are usually normal for children who are dyslexic. Laboratory measures, such as imaging studies, electroencephalograms, or chromosome studies, are ordered only if there are specific clinical indications not relating to dyslexia. Functional imaging is currently restricted to research studies of *groups* of typical compared with dyslexic readers, and is not sensitive enough to be used for clinical diagnosis of individual children or adults.

OUTCOME: PHONOLOGIC DEFICIT IN ADOLESCENCE AND ADULT LIFE

Essential Components of Diagnosis in Adolescents and Young Adults

Lack of Automaticity

The failure either to recognize or to measure the lack of automaticity in reading is, along with the failure to assess intelligence, perhaps one of the two most common errors in the diagnosis of dyslexia in older children and in accomplished young adults. Tests relying on the accuracy of word identification alone are inappropriate to use to diagnose dyslexia in accomplished young adults; tests of word identification reveal little to nothing of the child's *struggles* to read. It is important to recognize that, because they assess reading accuracy but not automaticity, the kinds of reading tests commonly used for school-aged children may provide misleading data on bright adolescents and young adults. The most critical tests are those that are timed; they are the most sensitive to a phonological deficit in a bright adult. However, there are very few standardized tests for young adult readers that are administered under timed and untimed conditions; the Nelson-Denny Reading Test represents an exception. Any scores obtained on testing should be considered relative to peers with the same degree of education or professional training. Clinicians and researchers have recognized that in bright young adults a history of phonologically based reading difficulties, requirements for extra time on tests and current slow and effortful reading (i.e., signs of a lack of automaticity in reading), and indications of an unexplained difficulty in reading are the sine qua non of a diagnosis of dyslexia.

Measure of Intelligence

The failure to include a test of intelligence such as the WISC-V represents one of the two most common and harmful errors made in the diagnosis of dyslexia. The demonstration of an unexpected difficulty in reading in relation to intelligence is a key hallmark of dyslexia. Dyslexia is an unexpected difficulty in reading that is best and most reliably and clearly demonstrated by performance on a test of intelligence, on the WISC-V, most often observed using the VCI, though the FS IQ may also be useful.

TREATMENT

(Readers interested in a more detailed account of interventions and approaches to treating dyslexia are referred to *Overcoming Dyslexia* by Sally Shaywitz.)

The management of dyslexia demands a life-span perspective. Early on, the focus is on remediation of the reading problem. As a child matures and enters the more time-demanding setting of secondary school, the emphasis shifts to incorporate the important role of providing accommodations.

Accommodations

An essential component of the management of dyslexia in students in secondary school, college, and graduate school incorporates the provision of accommodations. High-school and college students with a history of childhood dyslexia often present a paradoxical picture; they are similar to their unimpaired peers on measures of word recognition and comprehension, but they continue to suffer from the phonologic deficit that makes reading less automatic, more effortful, and slow. Neurobiologic data provide strong evidence for the necessity of extra time for readers with dyslexia. Whereas readers who are dyslexic improve greatly with additional time, providing additional time to nondyslexic readers results in very minimal to lack of improvement in scores. Although providing extra time for reading is by far the most common accommodation for people with dyslexia, other helpful accommodations include allowing the use of computers for writing essay answers on tests and access to recorded books (from organizations such as Learning Ally and Bookshare) and text-to-voice software from a number of vendors (including Kurzweil) and apps such as Pdf to Speech, Go Read, and many others. Dyslexic students who have difficulty accessing the sound system of their primary language will, almost invariably, have difficulties learning a foreign language. Recognizing this, many colleges and universities offer a partial waiver of the foreign language requirement for students with dyslexia. With such accommodations, many students with dyslexia are successfully completing studies in a range of disciplines, including science, law, medicine, and education.

Acknowledgments

The work described in this chapter was supported by grants from the National Institute of Child Health and Human Development (P50 HD25802, RO1 HD046171, R01 HD057655), by the Yale Center for Dyslexia and Creativity, by Eli Lilly Ltd., and by the Seedlings Foundation.

REFERENCES

The complete list of references for this chapter is available online at www.expertconsult.com.

See inside cover for registration details.

SELECTED REFERENCES

Ferrer, E., Shaywitz, B.A., Holahan, J.M., et al., 2010. Uncoupling of reading and IQ over time: empirical evidence for a definition of dyslexia. Psychol. Sci. 21, 93–101.

Ferrer, E., Shaywitz, B., Holahan, J., et al., 2015. Achievement gap in reading is present as early as first grade and persists through adolescence. J. Pediatr. 167, 1121–1125.e2.

Finn, E., Shen, X., Holahan, J., et al., 2013. Disruption of functional networks in dyslexia: a whole-brain, data-driven approach to fMRI connectivity analysis. Biol. Psychiatry 76, 397–404.

Richlan, F., Kronbichler, M., Wimmer, H., 2009. Functional abnormalities in the dyslexic brain: a quantitative meta-analysis of neuroimaging studies. Hum. Brain Mapp. 30, 3299–3308.

Shaywitz, B.A., Shaywitz, S.E., Pugh, K.R., et al., 2002. Disruption of posterior brain systems for reading in children with developmental dyslexia. Biol. Psychiatry 52, 101–110.

Shaywitz, S., Fletcher, J., Shaywitz, B., 1994. Issues in the definition and classification of attention disorder. Top. Lang. Disabil. 14, 1–25.

Shaywitz, S., 2003. Overcoming Dyslexia: A New and Complete Science-Based Program for Reading Problems at Any Level. Alfred A. Knopf, New York.

Shaywitz, S.E., Escobar, M.D., Shaywitz, B.A., et al., 1992. Evidence that dyslexia may represent the lower tail of a normal distribution of reading ability. N. Engl. J. Med. 326, 145–150.

E-BOOK FIGURES AND TABLES

The following figures and tables are available in the e-book at www.expertconsult.com. See inside cover for registration details.

Box 55-2 Clues to children at risk for dyslexia

56 Attention Deficit–Hyperactivity Disorder

David E. Mandelbaum

An expanded version of this chapter is available on www.expertconsult.com. See inside cover for registration details.

Attention deficit–hyperactivity disorder (ADHD) has been described as the most common neurobehavioral disorder in childhood. Prevailing opinion characterizes ADHD as a disorder of executive function attributable to abnormal dopamine transmission in the frontal lobes and frontostriatal circuitry. In large part, this concept is based on the clinical efficacy of medications affecting catecholamine transmission in these regions.

The first reference to behavior now associated with ADHD was by George Still in 1902, who referred to a deficit of moral control. Within the context of this broad concept, he made the following observation: "A notable feature in many of these cases of moral deficit without general impairment of intellect is a quite abnormal incapacity for sustained attention." Subsequent emphasis on attention and its neurologic substrate, the frontal lobe and frontostriatal circuitry, represents a refinement of the definition of the condition. This extensive history has not prevented some from questioning whether ADHD actually exists.

DIAGNOSIS AND CONTROVERSIES IN THE DIAGNOSIS OF ATTENTION DEFICIT–HYPERACTIVITY DISORDER

ADHD is a clinical diagnosis based on criteria in the fifth edition of the *Diagnostic and Statistical Manual of Mental Disorders* (DSM-5) (American Psychiatric Association [APA], 2013) (Box 56-1). Criteria are divided into two lists of symptoms, one for inattention and another for hyperactive-impulsive behavior. Based on the number of items identified, there are three classifications: ADHD/I (primarily inattentive type), ADHD/HI (primarily hyperactive-impulsive type), and ADHD/C (combined type). A study looking at the trends in the diagnosis of ADHD in the United States found that approximately 2 million more children aged 4 to 17 years were diagnosed with ADHD in 2011 compared with 2003 and that two-thirds of those with a current diagnosis of ADHD were taking medication in 2011. The DSM-5 diagnostic criteria, by reducing the number of symptoms required for a diagnosis from six to five for adolescents 17 and older and adults, will inevitably result in an increased incidence of ADHD in those age groups.

Concern has been raised about the overdiagnosis of ADHD, with the potential influence of pharmaceutical manufacturers and the misdiagnosis of normal behavior as pathologic cited as possible causes (Coon et al. 2014). The use of a stepped diagnosis, which includes five steps of care before making a definite diagnosis, has been proposed to reduce overdiagnosis without risking undertreatment (Thomas et al., 2013) (Box 56-2). One study found a higher rate of diagnoses in high-income households. The authors hypothesize that "higher rates of ADHD observed in affluent, white families likely represent an effort by these highly educated parents to seek help for their children who may not be fulfilling their expectations for schoolwork" (Getahun et al., 2013). Another study comparing the incidence of ADHD diagnoses found a higher frequency of ADHD diagnoses in children from lower socioeconomic levels but a lower rate of medication use in that group. Adding to the problem of possible overdiagnosis, along with the easing of criteria for adolescents and adults, is that malingering ADHD among college students is not easily detected with the current measures used to diagnose ADHD.

The use of the word *often* in the list of symptoms of ADHD lends an element of subjectivity to this diagnostic schema. Symptom rating scales for parents and teachers have been developed to assist in the ascertainment of diagnostic criteria. A comprehensive review of evaluation issues in ADHD concluded that no single test can be used to make the diagnosis and that it is up to the clinician to choose a battery of tests, which, along with the history and exam, a sufficient level of diagnostic certainty. The American Academy of Pediatrics has endorsed the Vanderbilt ADHD rating scales for parents and teachers and has provided a complete "toolkit," including a cover letter to teachers and scoring information, on the Internet (see http://www.nichq.org/childrens-health/adhd/resources) (Visser et al., 2013).

Developmental variability in the presentation of ADHD and the inconsistency of behavior of children with ADHD in different settings and at different times in the same setting add to the diagnostic confusion. Efforts have been made to provide a more objective basis for the diagnosis of ADHD, such as computerized continuous performance tests or tests of variables of attention. However, the correlation of these measures of attention with the behavioral disorder is not sufficient for them to be used as replacements for the behavioral criteria of the DSM.

The DSM-5 clinical criteria for diagnosing ADHD (see Box 56-1) list a number of qualifications that are too often ignored, possibly resulting in an incorrect diagnosis. The text explicitly states that for the symptoms to be diagnostically significant, "There is clear evidence that the symptoms interfere with, or reduce the quality of, social, school, or work functioning" (APA, 2013). Behavior that may not be typical but is not maladaptive does not warrant a diagnosis of ADHD. Similarly, unreasonable expectations of a child at a young age may result in a false diagnosis. The diagnostic criteria are followed by a number of statements regarding the context of the symptoms, for example, "Several symptoms are present in two or more setting, (e.g., at home, school or work; with friends or relatives; in other activities)" (APA, 2013). This qualification allows for the possibility that a child in an inadequate school environment, perhaps with excessive class size, hostile peers, or inexperienced teachers, may present with findings that are unique to that setting and do not represent a disorder of attention. Similarly, a chaotic home environment may explain the child's presentation.

Perhaps most important is the last item, which states: "The symptoms do not happen only during the course of schizophrenia or another psychotic disorder. The symptoms are not better explained by another mental disorder (e.g. Mood Disorder, Anxiety Disorder, Dissociative Disorder, or a Personality Disorder)" (APA, 2013). If a child has symptoms that meet the diagnostic criteria for ADHD in the context of these other

---

BOX 56-1 Diagnostic Criteria for Attention Deficit–Hyperactivity Disorder

DSM-5 CRITERIA FOR ADHD

Attention Deficit–Hyperactivity Disorder

Diagnostic Criteria

A. A persistent pattern of inattention and/or hyperactivity-impulsivity that interferes with functioning or development, as characterized by (1) and/or (2):

1. **Inattention:** Six (or more) of the following symptoms have persisted for at least 6 months to a degree that is inconsistent with developmental level and that negatively and directly affects social and academic/occupational activities:

   Note: The symptoms are not solely a manifestation of oppositional behavior, defiance, hostility, or failure to understand tasks or instructions. For older adolescents and adults (age 17 and older), at least five symptoms are required.

   a. Often fails to give close attention to details or makes careless mistakes in schoolwork, at work, or during other activities (e.g., overlooks or misses details, work is inaccurate).

   b. Often has difficulty sustaining attention in tasks or play activities (e.g., has difficulty remaining focused during lectures, conversations, or lengthy reading).

   c. Often does not seem to listen when spoken to directly (e.g., mind seems elsewhere, even in the absence of any obvious distraction).

   d. Often does not follow through on instructions and fails to finish schoolwork, chores, or duties in the workplace (e.g., starts tasks but quickly loses focus and is easily sidetracked).

   e. Often has difficult organizing tasks and activities (e.g., difficulty managing sequential tasks; difficulty keeping materials and belongings in order; messy, disorganized work; has poor time management; fails to meet deadlines).

   f. Often avoids, dislikes, or is reluctant to engage in tasks that require sustained mental effort (e.g., schoolwork or homework; for older adolescents and adults, preparing reports, completing forms, reviewing lengthy papers).

   g. Often loses things necessary for tasks or activities (e.g., school materials, pencils, books, tools, wallets, keys, paperwork, eyeglasses, mobile telephones).

   h. Is often easily distracted by extraneous stimuli (for older adolescents and adults, may include unrelated thoughts).

   i. Is often forgetful in daily activities (e.g., doing chores, running errands; for older adolescents and adults, returning calls, paying bills, keeping appointments).

2. **Hyperactivity and impulsivity:** Six (or more) of the following symptoms have persisted for at least 6 months to a degree that is inconsistent with developmental level and that negatively and directly affects social and academic/occupational activities:

   Note: The symptoms are not solely a manifestation of oppositional behavior, defiance, hostility, or a failure to understand tasks or instructions. For older adolescents and adults (age 17 and older), at least five symptoms are required.

   a. Often fidgets with or taps hands or feet or squirms in seat.

   b. Often leaves seat in situations when remaining stead is expected (e.g., leaves his or her place in the classroom, in the office or other workplace, or in other situations that require remaining in place).

   c. Often runs about or climbs in situations where it is inappropriate. (**Note:** In adolescents or adults, may be limited to feeling restless.)

   d. Often unable to play or engage in leisure activities quietly.

   e. Is often "on the go," acting as if "driven by a motor" (e.g., is unable to be or uncomfortable being still for extended time, as in restaurants, meetings; may be experienced by others as being restless or difficult to keep up with).

   f. Often talks excessively.

   g. Often blurts out an answer before a question has been completed (e.g., completes people's sentences; cannot wait for turn in conversation).

   h. Often has difficulty waiting his or her turn (e.g., while waiting in line).

   i. Often interrupts or intrudes on others (e.g., butts into conversations, games, or activities; may start using other people's things without asking or receiving permission; for adolescents and adults, may intrude into or take over what others are doing).

B. Several inattentive or hyperactive-impulsive symptoms were present before age 12 years.

C. Several inattentive or hyperactive-impulsive symptoms are present in two or more settings (e.g., at home, school, or work; with friends or relatives; in other activities).

D. There is clear evidence that the symptoms interfere with, or reduce the quality of, social, academic, or occupational functioning.

E. The symptoms do not occur exclusively during the course of schizophrenia or another psychotic disorder and are not better explained by another mental disorder (e.g., mood disorder, anxiety disorder, dissociative disorder, personality disorder, substance intoxication or withdrawal).

(With permission from the Diagnostic and Statistical Manual of Mental Disorders, Fifth Edition, (Copyright ©2013). American Psychiatric Association. All Rights Reserved.)

---

disorders, treatment should be directed at these other conditions before concluding the child has a disorder of attention. Not addressed in the DSM-5 criteria are studies that have demonstrated that children with specific neurologic disorders can present with symptoms that meet criteria for ADHD but are attributable to the neurologic disorder rather than a primary disorder of attention. One study demonstrated symptoms of impaired attention and hyperactivity in children diagnosed with restless leg syndrome; treatment of the sleep disturbance resolved the so-called ADHD symptoms. A subsequent double-blind study of a dopaminergic therapy in 16 children with restless leg syndrome/periodic limb movements in sleep (RLS/PLMS) and ADHD symptoms found that, compared with placebo, L-dopa significantly improved RLS/PLMS but not ADHD symptoms. The authors cautioned that the results may have been influenced by the small sample size and baseline differences in the severity of ADHD symptoms (Subcommittee on Attention-Deficit/Hyperactivity Disorder, 2011).

Disordered breathing during sleep has also been found to manifest with symptoms consistent with ADHD. A study of snoring in 3-year-olds found parent endorsement ("often" or "always") of irritability and hyperactivity to be significantly higher in the habitual snoring group compared with those without habitual snoring. There are reports of children with focal epileptic discharges having symptoms suggestive of ADHD that resolved when the spike activity was suppressed with antiepileptic drugs. Many symptoms of ADHD are prevalent in neurogenetic syndromes as part of the behavioral phenotype.

The recent revision of the DSM criteria for ADHD failed to add neurologic disorders (e.g., sleep disorders, epilepsy, neurogenetic syndromes) to the list of conditions to be excluded before ADHD is diagnosed, which complicates the effort to ascertain the physiologic and genetic underpinnings of ADHD and its optimal treatment.

COEXISTING CONDITIONS

The question of conditions coexisting with ADHD is quite complex. Should a diagnosis of ADHD be reserved for individuals with an isolated disorder of attention, hyperactivity, or impulsivity, with an alternative classification used to describe children who meet DSM-5 criteria for ADHD in the context of other neurodevelopmental problems? The term *pseudo-ADHD* has been to describe children with comorbidities or confounding factors. In a paper describing a father and son both with orbitofrontal epilepsy and associated attention difficulties and hyperactivity, the term *attention-deficit–hyperactivity syndrome* was used to make a distinction from the specific disorder of ADHD, analogous to the distinction between Parkinson's disease and parkinsonism. It has been proposed that ADHD be divided into subgroups based on the patterns of comorbidity.

The presumption that a response to psychostimulant medication indicates that the underlying problem is ADHD can lead to an erroneous diagnosis. Psychostimulant medications can ameliorate depression, chronic fatigue syndrome, and daytime somnolence caused by sleep disorders and enhance normal individuals' cognitive functioning and behavior. A positive response to psychostimulants has no diagnostic significance.

NEUROBIOLOGY OF ATTENTION DEFICIT–HYPERACTIVITY DISORDER

It has been proposed that the core deficit in ADHD is impairment of behavioral inhibition, which leads to the other symptoms of ADHD. This model of impaired behavioral inhibition is limited to ADHD/HI and ADHD/C (i.e., those with hyperactive or impulsive symptoms) and excludes children with ADHD/I (i.e., those with inattention only). Some investigators have proposed that all three ADHD subtypes can be explained as disorders of attention or executive function (other than response inhibition), with symptoms of hyperactivity and impulsivity resulting from these impairments. Others also distinguish ADHD/HI and ADHD/C from ADHD/I, but they posit that the symptoms of hyperactivity and impulsivity can result from poor inhibitory control or differences in motivational style characterized by delay aversion.

A review of the literature regarding the hypothesis that ADHD represents a primary deficit in executive control defined executive function as comprising at least four factors: 1. response inhibition and execution, 2. working memory and updating of memory, 3. set and task shifting, and 4. inference control. The most consistent effects were obtained on measures of response inhibition, vigilance and planning; children with combined and inattentive types of ADHD differed from controls and did not differ from each other, whereas children with hyperactive-impulsive type ADHD had minimal executive function impairment, suggesting that executive function weaknesses are primarily associated with inattention, rather than hyperactivity-impulsivity symptoms. The authors concluded that their findings did not support the hypothesis that executive function deficits alone were the cause of ADHD in all individuals. Rather, it is one of several important deficits comprising the neuropsychological basis for ADHD.

Inhibitory deficits and delay aversion in ADHD can be dissociated by specific types of tasks; either deficit alone is only moderately associated with ADHD, whereas combined these two deficits correctly classify nearly 90% of children with children with ADHD. Thus a formulation was proposed in which executive function (EF) is divided into cognitive aspects associated with the dorsolateral prefrontal cortex ("cool" EF) and affective aspects associated with the orbital and medial prefrontal cortex ("hot" EF). Inattention symptoms were attributed to deficits in cool EF, whereas hyperactivity-impulsivity symptoms reflected hot EF deficits.

An fMRI study found that adolescents with ADHD had difficulty accomplishing a task involving cognitive or cool aspects of executive functions such as working memory, planning, cognitive flexibility, and forethought, as manifest by a significantly greater number of activated brain regions and greater activation of those regions in adolescents with typical development than those with ADHD. The authors also found an unbalance between the high activation of the basal ganglia and cerebellum and the low activation of the prefrontal cortex for the forethought condition in ADHD.

Advances in structural and functional imaging, clinical neurophysiologic techniques, and molecular genetics have been applied to the evaluation of children with ADHD and have provided important insights into this condition. However, inconsistency in the inclusion and exclusion criteria among studies, particularly related to comorbidity, limits comparisons between studies and their conclusions.

Structural Imaging

A study of monozygotic twins discordant for ADHD revealed reduced caudate volume in the affected twin. In another report on twins discordant for ADHD, fathers of twins discordant for ADHD had lower ADHD scores than fathers of ADHD singletons. The rate of breech presentation was greater in affected twins than affected singletons. The data suggest that the discordant twins represented nongenetic instances of ADHD, possibly caused by injury in utero, and that the caudate abnormalities in these individuals might not be pertinent to ADHD that is genetic in nature. A study utilizing large deformation diffeomorphic mapping (LDDMM) found that boys with ADHD had significant shape differences and decreases in overall volume of the basal ganglia compared with controls, whereas girls with ADHD did not have volume or shape differences. Children with comorbidities, including other neuropsychiatric disorders, conduct disorders, mood disorder, generalized anxiety disorder, obsessive compulsive disorder, learning disabilities, or speech and language disorders, were excluded from this analysis.

A study comparing children with ADHD (combined type) who had been on chronic treatment with stimulants to untreated children with ADHD and a control group found that children with ADHD had significantly larger prefrontal regions than the controls, with no effect for medication history; the caudate volumes of the children with ADHD were smaller bilaterally, also with no medication effect. The ADHD/no-Rx group showed smaller anterior cingulate cortex volume on the right compared with the ADHD/Rx and control groups; this was the only finding for a medication difference.

A study highlighting the impact of comorbidities on imaging studies found that when the analysis of cerebral microstructure was restricted to a subgroup of those with no comorbidities (pure-ADHD subgroup), there was more microstructural complexity compared to typically developing children in the frontal and parietal lobes bilaterally, insual, corpus callosum and right external and internal capsules. The authors also found that the pure-ADHD subgroup lacked the normal age-related progression in gray- and white-matter microstructural complexity from the ages of 8 to 18 years. The authors conclude: "our results highlight the shortcomings of including diverse psychiatric comorbidities in the investigation of tissue microstructure in ADHD. Although aberrant findings have been observed with heterogeneous ADHD cohorts, these may lack clinical specificity, as potentially reflected in conflicting results from prior microstructural studies on ADHD."

Functional Imaging

The clinical benefit from medications affecting catecholamine levels has led to a focus on frontostriatal circuitry and dopamine pathways in ADHD. Functional magnetic resonance imaging (fMRI) studies have demonstrated abnormal activation of the frontostriatal regions in children with ADHD. In normal children, maturation is associated with increased activation of the ventral frontostriatal regions and improved inhibitory control. A comparison of children with ADHD with normal control subjects demonstrated greater frontal activation and lower striatal activation during response inhibition in 10 children with ADHD (8 ADHD/C, 2 ADHD/I; children with high comorbidity scores were excluded). Administration of methylphenidate also resulted in improved performance in a test of response inhibition, associated with increased frontal activation in ADHD children and control subjects and increased striatal activation in the children with ADHD.

Untreated adults with ADHD (with no psychiatric comorbidity) have increased striatal dopamine transporter (DAT) levels compared with normal control subjects (as measured by binding to technetium 99m TRODAT-1, the first 99mTc-labeled ligand identified by single-photon emission computed tomography [SPECT] that specifically binds DAT), which decreased after 4 weeks of methylphenidate treatment. This finding, along with increased striatal activity on positron emission tomographic (PET) scanning in adolescents with ADHD compared with normal control subjects, suggests a role for excess dopaminergic activity in striatum or nucleus accumbens in persons with ADHD.

A review and critique of functional imaging studies of ADHD notes that such studies have found multiple loci of abnormalities that are not limited to frontal-striatal circuitry, the regions thought to be most important for executive and motivational function, but also in the parietal, temporal, and motor cortices and the cerebellum. However, it is pointed out that: task specific factors influence activation patterns which may have induced variable performance levels and strategies over the course of development. In the absence of cross-sectional or longitudinal studies, "the developmental origin of differences in activation cannot be inferred." It is concluded that: "current, task-evoked functional imaging provides information about dynamic or state-dependent differences rather than fixed or trait-related differences."

Genetic Studies

Concise reviews of advances in the genetics of ADHD, including findings that may account for the ADHD subtypes, comorbidities, and responses to specific medications, are provided in a commentary and editorial in journal issues devoted to this topic. A summary by D.V. Pauls stated that the evidence was overwheming that ADHD is inherited and that genetic factors play an important role in the manifestation of ADHD. The fact that ADHD is an inherited condition coupled with evidence of dopaminergic involvement led to molecular genetic studies of dopamine transporter and receptor genes. Pursuit of the *DAT* gene (*SLC6A3*, formerly designated *DAT1*) was in part caused by the finding that psychostimulant medications inhibit the activity of DAT. An association between ADHD and the 480 base-pair alleles at a variable-number tandem repeat (VNTR) in *SLC6A3* has been reported. A subsequent study confirmed these findings and demonstrated a significant relation between *SLC6A3* high-risk alleles and the number of hyperactive-impulsive symptoms but not inattentive symptoms. The study involved 117 probands, all but one of whom met criteria for ADHD; the remaining child had oppositional defiant disorder (ODD). Most children with ADHD frequently had symptoms of or were diagnosed with ODD, conduct disorder (CD), and depression or dysthymia. Two subsequent studies, one with a similar rate of coexisting conditions and one with a much lower rate, failed to replicate the association between *SLC6A3* and ADHD.

Studies of DNA from ADHD probands, parents, and healthy controls found a significant association of ADHD with two *NET1* single-nucleotide polymorphisms and two *DRD1* single-nucleotide polymorphisms. There was no association with polymorphisms in 10 other genes previously reported as candidate genes. There were no significant differences in anatomic brain magnetic resonance imaging (MRI) measurements between the children with *NET1* or *DRD1* gene types, nor was there a relationship between the genetic findings and cognitive or behavioral measures. This study represented the first replication of a previously described association between ADHD and polymorphisms in *NET1* and *DRD1* genes.

The Psychiatric Genetics Consortium has published two papers reviewing the findings on genetic relationships between five psychiatric disorders, including ADHD, based on an analysis of genome-wide single-nucleotide polymorphisms (SNPs).

Other Potential Causes of Attention Deficit–Hyperactivity Disorder

Data reported from the National Longitudinal Survey of Youth associated hours of television watched per day at ages 1 and 3 years with parental reports of attentional problems at age 7. The children did not necessarily have clinically diagnosed ADHD; rather, they were scored as having attentional problems by the parents.

A review of the literature on the role of nutritional factors in ADHD, including food additives, sugars, food allergies or sensitivities, and essential fatty acids, concluded: that though a subset of children with behavioral problems are sensitive to one or more food components that my contribute to hyperactivity, there is not a specific food or substance that will precipitate problem behavior in all hyperactive children. There have been many reviews of the literature of food additives, noting major flaws in the methodology of those studies. However, randomized controlled trials have shown that sodium benzoate intake, a common preservative used in soft drinks and fruit juices, contributed to ADHD-like symptoms in young children.

A study looking at the effect of gestational diabetes mellitus (and) socioeconomic status (SES) on ADHD found that "the risk for ADHD increased over 14-fold ($P = .006$) when children were exposed to both GDM and low SES. Neither children exposed to maternal GDM alone nor those exposed to low SES alone had a notable increased risk for ADHD. A study of a sample of 7- to 9-year-old children born extremely prematurely and/or with extremely low birth weight (ELBW) who were making normal progress at school found that biomedical variables such as birth weight and neurobiological risk are associate with aspects of executive function. Specifically, higher birth weights and lower levels of risk predicted better performance. A review of the causes of ADHD concluded that the dichotomy between genetic/biological and environmental factors in ADHD "is incorrect and unhelpful. Indeed, they are complementary rather than competing explanations" (Thapar et al., 2013).

COEXISTING CONDITIONS

Many children who present with symptoms suggestive of ADHD have neurologic or psychiatric conditions that are the cause of those symptoms (e.g., depression, sleep disorders, epilepsy). There are other instances when multiple conditions coexist. The implications for management are significant. Just as correction of a sleep disorder may resolve the symptoms of inattention, hyperactivity, or impulsivity, addressing a child's previously undiagnosed learning disability may resolve these symptoms. Alternatively, a child may have both problems, and remediation of the learning disability may still leave him or her with inattention, hyperactivity, or impulsivity that must be independently addressed. It has been proposed that ADHD be divided into subgroups based on the patterns of comorbidity. ADHD and CD have been posited to be distinct disorders. From a practical standpoint, most studies of children with ADHD and coexisting CD treated with psychostimulants demonstrated a reduction in physical and nonphysical

aggression and had improvement of ADHD symptoms. Antidepressants also reduced symptoms of aggression and ADHD in these children. Anxiety disorder has been shown to be transmitted independently from ADHD in families, suggesting that these two conditions are distinct disorders. Most studies of children with ADHD and coexisting anxiety or depression found a reduced response in ADHD symptoms when treated with psychostimulants compared with children only with ADHD.

It has been proposed, inasmuch as ADHD and mood instability include impulsivity and behavioral problems in their definitions, that both ADHD and mood instability involve impairment in executive function, and given findings of overlapping neuroanatomical abnormalities and treatments, that mood instability be considered a core feature of ADHD rather than a comorbidity. A twin study found a strong genetic association between ADHD symptoms with emotional lability, supporting the idea that emotional lability may be a component of ADHD; this association was stronger in older than younger children.

A review of the overlapping symptoms associated with ADHD and sleep disorders noted that many children with primary sleep disorders have symptoms highly suggestive of ADHD. Conversely, many children with ADHD are reported to have sleep disturbances, which may be primary, attributable to the side effects of medication, or a result of comorbid conditions such as ODD, depression, and/or anxiety disorders. A comorbid sleep disorder may significantly increase the daytime impairment in a child with ADHD. It was recommended that all children presenting with ADHD symptoms be clinically assessed for the presence of sleep problems.

Reading disability and ADHD are two distinct disorders that may occur together. There is evidence of genetic linkage for ADHD and reading disability to the same region on the short arm of chromosome 6. This connection may represent a pleiotropic effect (i.e., the same gene increasing susceptibility to more than one disorder). A survey of audiologists and pediatricians found that although auditory processing disorder and ADHD/I have symptoms in common, there were features that allowed them to be distinguished from each other.

A meta-analysis of the literature reporting on tests of overall cognitive ability in ADHD analyzed data from 137 studies in which full-scale IQ (FSIQ) scores for children with ADHD were compared with those of a healthy control group. The ADHD groups had significantly lower FSIQ scores relative to the control groups, with an average decrement of 9 points in the FSIQ; the verbal and performance IQs were lower in the ADHD group. There was no difference in ADHD subtypes, although the number of children with inattentive-type ADHD was small. The authors concluded that these findings "may indicate that the disorder is characterized by mild global cognitive inefficiencies or by multiple specific deficits affecting several cognitive abilities." They raised the possibility that the decrement could also be attributable to test-taking differences between the groups. The authors expressed surprise at the finding that for only a few of the measures was the effect size for executive functioning tasks significantly larger than effect sizes for the FSIQ. In a comparison of the mean effect size of tests of executive versus nonexecutive functions, there was greater impairment in the tests of executive function. The authors allowed for the possibility that impairment of executive function accounted for differences in overall ability, inasmuch as measures of overall ability are heavily influenced by executive function. The authors commented that achievement measures may be useful for screening for comorbid learning disabilities and characterizing deficits in motivation and behavior that result from executive dysfunction.

DIAGNOSTIC EVALUATION

ADHD is a clinical diagnosis; there are no diagnostic laboratory nor cognitive tests. A child presenting with symptoms suggestive of ADHD should undergo screening for hearing and vision problems, potentially treatable issues that may be mistaken for ADHD. If the child's difficulties are predominantly in the school setting, an evaluation for learning disabilities should be pursued, with educational remediation if problems are identified. Social stressors may also be a significant factor, which may justify intervention by social services agencies. In general, routine diagnostic testing is not needed in the evaluation of a child for ADHD. However, specific testing may be indicated in some circumstances.

Laboratory Studies

Features in the history or on examination may lead to specific tests for disorders manifesting as or coexisting with ADHD, such as hypothyroidism, hyperthyroidism, or phenylketonuria. Reports of an association between lead exposure and ADHD have been inconsistent. Depending on the results of such laboratory studies, therapy targeting the specific condition may be initiated. An uncontrolled study reported improvement in the parents', but not the teachers', Connors Rating Scales scores in children with ADHD treated with iron supplementation, even though they were not iron deficient. Better studies are needed before concluding that routine testing of or supplementation with iron or screening for iron deficiency is advisable.

Electroencephalography

Studies reporting an increased frequency of epileptiform discharges in children with ADHD and reports of ADHD-type symptoms resolving when spike activity was suppressed with antiepileptic drugs have led to proposed guidelines for obtaining an electroencephalogram (EEG). These include a history of clinical events suggesting a seizure (even if only nocturnal or febrile), perinatal stress, head trauma, fluctuating behavioral manifestations, or a family history of epilepsy.

Sleep Studies

A sleep history should be obtained. If the results suggest a diagnosis of a sleep disorder or if there is a strong family history of sleep disorders, a sleep study should be considered.

Imaging Studies

There are few clinical indications for imaging studies in children with ADHD; if the child is clinically stable, the presence of ADHD symptoms does not call for imaging studies beyond those indicated for the primary condition.

TREATMENT
Nonpharmacologic Therapies

Children with ADHD need a classroom environment with minimal distractions and with seating that is somewhat isolated and close to the front of the room in front of the teacher. The setting should be fairly structured with organizational techniques such as checklists and homework assignment pads, and an uncluttered desk at home devoted exclusively to school work.

A multicenter clinical trial of various treatment strategies for ADHD concluded that stimulants were more effective than behavioral therapies for ADHD symptoms. The combination of stimulants and behavioral therapy resulted in improved social skills but did not significantly improve ADHD symptoms over stimulants alone. A review of treatment modalities of children diagnosed with ADHD in the period from 1995 to 1999 found that among children diagnosed with ADHD, 24% also had mental illness. The most frequent treatments were stimulant medication alone (42%), stimulant medication combined with psychotherapy or mental health counseling (32%), and psychotherapy or mental health counseling alone (10.8%). Fifteen percent of children received no treatment other than office visits for initial and follow-up medical care. The percentage of children receiving psychotherapy or mental health counseling alone or in combination with stimulant medication increased with age, and males were more likely than females to receive treatment.

Sleep

A recent study found a positive association between spindle-frequency EEG activity and motor skill learning improvement in children with ADHD (Saletin et al., 2015). This may account, at least in part, for the overlap in symptoms of ADHD and sleep disorders in children. This may also offer an opportunity for nonpharmacologic intervention in children with ADHD. Inasmuch as there is enriched sleep spindle activity in the latter part of sleep, having children with ADHD go to sleep early enough that they wake up spontaneously, rather than have the latter part of their sleep disrupted, might be beneficial to their function.

Biofeedback Programs

Various forms of computerized training programs have been studied in treating children with ADHD. Computerized working memory training improved working memory capacity in children with ADHD and adults without ADHD. Improvement generalized to nonpracticed tasks involving prefrontal cortex, and associated with improvement in working memory was a decrease in head movements in children with ADHD. Children with ADHD trained to modify their slow cortical potentials also showed an increase in contingent negative variation (CNV) during a continuous performance task compared with those who did not receive training. Associated with this electrophysiologic phenomenon were fewer impulsivity errors on the continuous performance task, suggesting that the CNV increase represented a neurophysiologic correlate of improved self-regulatory capabilities. A meta-analysis of studies of nonpharmacologic treatments of ADHD (Hodgson et al., 2014), which was limited to studies of treatment and control groups and excluded studies using within-subjects designs to minimize placebo effects, found that behavior modification was effective in treating ADHD in children, achieving improved function across a number of domains including behavior and test performance. Neurofeedback was found to result in significant improvement in DSM-IV symptoms, test performance and behavior. There was no significant benefit established for school based treatments, parent training, working memory training, self monitoring or multimodal psychosocial treatment interventions in measurements of ADHD functional domains. Psychological treatments for ADHD were more effective among girls than boys and were least effective for children with combined-type ADHD (Martijn et al., 2009).

Use of an EEG biofeedback program was compared with the effectiveness of methylphenidate. After 3 months of the program, both groups had significant improvements in all four subscales on the TOVA and improvement on a behavior rating scale. Changes in the EEG as a result of biofeedback were not monitored in this study. A previous study using biofeedback reported greater improvement on the test of variables of attention (TOVA) in participants with significant EEG changes than in those without changes (although there were improvements in both groups). There was no correlation between behavioral changes reported by the parents and changes in the EEG. This study did not include a control group. A study of EEG biofeedback that used a control group (i.e., association between EEG patterns and feedback to the participants was random) found no benefit from EEG biofeedback.

Pharmacologic Therapy

The American Heart Association recommended that all children placed on stimulant medications for ADHD should have a screening electrocardiogram (ECG); the American Academy of Pediatrics concluded that this is neither necessary nor recommended and, instead, recommended cardiovascular screening based on personal, past, and family histories and the cardiovascular examination.

Stimulant Medications

Stimulant drugs, sympathomimetic agents structurally similar to endogenous catecholamines, act centrally and peripherally by enhancing dopaminergic and noradrenergic transmission. Stimulants have been demonstrated to improve cognitive ability, school performance, and behavior.

The response to methylphenidate in a group of 28 preschoolers (3–5 years old), as measured by behavioral ratings by teachers and parents, documented improvement, with 82% rated as having normal behavior after treatment, higher than the rate generally achieved in older children. With the exception of decreased appetite, there were no adverse side effects. The investigators speculate that the higher normalization rate for preschoolers than elementary-age schoolchildren may be a function of fewer demands placed on the preschooler (e.g., shorter school day, no homework).

The most commonly reported side effects of stimulants include appetite suppression and sleep disturbance. Absorption of stimulant medications is not notably affected when taken with or after meals, which may ameliorate appetite suppression. Insomnia can be a side effect from the medication but may also be caused by a rebound effect as the medication effect subsides. This distinction is important because in the latter situation, a late afternoon or evening dose of stimulant medication may ease falling asleep. Uncommonly, there have been reports of mood disturbances and lethargy after stimulant use. Stimulants may also affect heart rate and blood pressure, but in healthy children, this change is unlikely to have clinical significance. There have been reports of psychostimulants inducing or exacerbating tic disorders, but subsequent studies have not found this to be a universal problem. Although this possibility should be discussed with children and their families, the presence of tics in a child with ADHD or a family history of tics is not an absolute contraindication to the use of psychostimulants. Concerns are often expressed regarding an increased risk of substance abuse in children treated with psychostimulants, but there is no supporting evidence. One study found that pharmacologic treatment for ADHD actually decreased the risk of subsequent substance abuse. However, although the risk of substance abuse in individuals with ADHD appears to be reduced by treatment, it is still higher than in the general population. Inasmuch as illicit substance abuse can manifest with attention difficulties,

hyperactivity, and/or impulsivity, the possibility that substance abuse is accounting for symptoms is to be considered; reevaluation after a period of abstinence may be warranted (Harstad et al., 2014).

One study evaluated the use of methylphenidate in 24 children with at least two epileptic seizures in the previous 6 months and a diagnosis of ADHD and found an improvement in ADHD symptoms for 70.8% of the children, no change in ADHD symptoms for 20.8%, and a worsening of symptoms in 8.3%. Of these 24 children, 22 (71%) showed no increase in seizure frequency; however, there was worsening in two. Santos et al. (2013) found that of 22 children with active epilepsy and ADHD treated for 3 months with methylphenidate, 4 patients reported some increase in seizure frequency, and 1 patient withdrew as a result of increased seizure frequency. There was substantial improvement in ADHD symptoms, such that 16 (73%) of the patients no longer had clinically significant ADHD symptoms. Other studies of children with ADHD and epilepsy or interictal discharges treated with methylphenidate did not find any increase in seizure frequency. Thus, although there is evidence of some risk of seizure exacerbation with stimulant use in children with ADHD and epilepsy, this does not occur in the majority of cases, and there is clear evidence of benefit; the decision to use stimulants in such cases requires an individualized consideration of the risk versus benefit.

A longitudinal study revealed that children treated with medication had a reduced height gain compared with those who were not treated. Growth suppression was still evident during the second year of treatment in the group treated continuously, indicating that this was a persistent effect. The observation that there was less growth suppression in the children who were not treated continuously suggests that interrupting treatment with stimulant medication may limit growth suppression, supporting the concept of drug holidays to address this side effect. However, there have been reports of behavioral deterioration when stimulant medications are abruptly discontinued.

The most commonly used drugs in the stimulant class include methylphenidate, dextroamphetamine, and mixed salts of L-and D-amphetamine. Although in the same class, these drugs have slightly different mechanisms of action, and patients may respond differently to each of them. Failure of one drug does not preclude success with another drug in the same class. A number of these agents are available in short- and long-acting formulations. The results of studies comparing short- and long-acting preparations have been inconsistent, making the choice of formulation an empirical one.

Methylphenidate

Methylphenidate has fewer side effects than amphetamine. In the standard formulation, methylphenidate reaches peak concentrations between 1 and 3 hours after oral intake. It is rapidly and extensively metabolized by nonmicrosomal hydrolytic esterases in liver and other tissues, with an average half-life of 3 hours. A dose in the middle to late afternoon to facilitate completion of homework may also be warranted. Alternatives to multiple daily doses are the long-acting formulations of methylphenidate. These formulations reach peak concentration 6 to 8 hours after oral intake, obviating the need for a midday dose. When using the longer-acting formulations, the entire daily dose is given in the morning. If there is no significant improvement in symptoms at a total daily dose of 1 to 2 mg/kg, alternate medication should be considered. Another sustained-release form of methylphenidate is available as a skin patch that is placed on the skin daily for 9 hours.

Dexmethylphenidate

Dexmethylphenidate is the D-threo-enantiomer of methylphenidate. A positron emission tomography (PET) study found specific binding of the D-enantiomer to a dopamine transporter in the basal ganglia, whereas the L-enantiomer had widespread, nonspecific binding. Studies comparing dexmethylphenidate and methylphenidate have concluded both to be effective in ADHD, but dexmethylphenidate has a longer duration. In children the starting dose of dexmethylphenidate is one-half of the methylphenidate dose (0.15 mg/kg in the morning, rounded to the nearest 2.5-mg tablet). The report of longer clinical efficacy than methylphenidate (despite the similar half-life) may eliminate the need for a midday dose, depending on the clinical response. There is no evidence that giving the D-isomer (dexmethylphenidate) at one-half of the dose of the D,L-enantiomer (methylphenidate) confers any clinical advantage.

Dextroamphetamine

Dextroamphetamine has a time to peak concentration of 60 to 160 minutes and is metabolized in the liver. The average half-life of dextroamphetamine is 10 to 12 hours, but this varies considerably with urinary pH; at a urine pH less than 6.6, more than two-thirds of unmetabolized drug is excreted in the urine, whereas at a urine pH greater than 6.7, it is less than one-half. The initial dose of dextroamphetamine is 0.15 to 0.3 mg/kg (rounded to the nearest 5 mg). Dextroamphetamine's longer half-life compared with methylphenidate may obviate the need for a midday dose. An extended-release preparation of dextroamphetamine eliminates the need for midday dosing.

Adderall is a combination of four amphetamine salts (D-amphetamine saccharate, D- amphetamine sulfate, D,L-amphetamine sulfate, and D,L-amphetamine aspartate), with a 3 : 1 ratio of D-isomer to L-isomer. The time to peak concentration and half-life are similar to those for dextroamphetamine. The initial dose of Adderall is 2.5 or 5 mg, with weekly increments based on the response to a maximum dose of 1.5 mg/kg per day, up to about 40 mg. The half-life of Adderall is such that a midday dose may or may not be necessary. Adderall XR capsules, with one-half of the contents in a delayed-release formulation, eliminate the need for midday dosing; the entire daily dose is given in the morning.

Noradrenergic Potentiation

Atomoxetine

Atomoxetine (Strattera) is a norepinephrine-specific reuptake inhibitor that is effective in the treatment of children with ADHD. In a study comparing atomoxetine to methylphenidate and placebo, the response rate to atomoxetine and methylphenidate was essentially identical, and both were better than placebo. Appetite suppression was somewhat lower in atomoxetine compared with methylphenidate (22% versus 32%), and there was significantly less insomnia on atomoxetine (7% versus 27%). In extensive metabolizers (most patients), atomoxetine half-life is 4 to 5 hours. Substantial decreases in clearance and prolongation of the half-life are seen in poor metabolizers. The starting dose is 0.5 mg/kg per day, with gradual increase to a target dose of 1.2 mg/kg per day. In poor metabolizers (about 7% of the population), the half-life is substantially longer, and the dose requirement may be much lower. Depending on the response, midday dosing may be required for extensive metabolizers. Food does not affect absorption. Because atomoxetine is not a controlled substance

in the United States, prescriptions with multiple refills can be provided, and renewals can be done over the phone, in contrast to the procedures for stimulant medications. In December 2004 the U.S. Food and Drug Administration (FDA) asked the manufacturer to add a bolded warning about severe liver injury to the labeling, indicating that the medication should be discontinued in patients who develop jaundice or laboratory evidence of liver injury. In September 2005 the FDA directed the manufacturer to further revise the labeling to include a boxed warning regarding an increased risk of suicidal thinking in children and adolescents being treated with this drug.

Nonstimulant Medications

It is estimated that at least 30% of children diagnosed with ADHD do not respond to or tolerate stimulant medications. Most studies have reported a reduced rate of response to psychostimulants in children with ADHD and anxiety or depression. The failure to respond to psychostimulants suggests the possibility of an incorrect diagnosis. However, genetic studies have suggested that children with ADHD respond differently to methylphenidate, depending on whether they are homozygous or heterozygous for the 10-repeat allele at dopamine transporter gene *SLC6A3*.

Tricyclic Antidepressants

Other agents found to be effective in the treatment of ADHD include tricyclic antidepressants (TCAs). In one study, comorbidity with conduct disorder, depression, or anxiety or a family history of ADHD did not result in a differential response to desipramine. In studies comparing TCAs with stimulants, TCAs appear to more consistently improve behavioral symptoms rather than cognitive function.

There have been case reports of sudden death in children treated with desipramine. Although a subsequent epidemiologic study did not find greater risk of sudden death with desipramine, it has been suggested that a baseline ECG be obtained before initiating treatment and that serial ECGs be obtained after significant dose increments and periodically during treatment.

Alpha-Adrenergic Agonists

The alpha-adrenergic agents clonidine and guanfacine have been widely used for treatment of ADHD, despite few clinical studies. The success of these agents for Tourette syndrome and other tic disorders has made them especially useful in children with ADHD and tic disorders, particularly if a trial of stimulant medication resulted in exacerbation of tics. Reports of three deaths of children taking a combination of methylphenidate and clonidine prompted reviews that found no evidence of an adverse methylphenidate-clonidine interaction. Nevertheless, if planning to prescribe this combination, a review of this literature and discussion of risks and benefits with the parents is advisable. Guanfacine appears to have an advantage over clonidine because it has a longer half-life and is less sedating. Guanfacine reaches a peak concentration after oral intake in 1 to 4 hours and is metabolized in the liver, with an average half-life of 17 hours. The starting dose is 0.015 mg/kg per day (to the nearest 0.5 mg), with a gradual increase to a maximum of 0.05 mg/kg or 4 mg/day, based on the clinical response. The half-life of guanfacine should allow for once-daily dosing, although in clinical studies it was administered in two to four divided doses. Guanfacine is available in 1- and 2-mg tablets (Tenex). A sustained-release form of guanfacine (Intuniv) is also available; the half-life is 16 hours, and the time to peak serum level is approximately 5 hours. This is effective as a once-a-day dosing schedule in doses of 1 to 4 mg/day. Other agents reported to be effective in ADHD are reviewed in Table 56-1.

A review of prospective trials of medicines used for ADHD in children noted a wide heterogeneity between studies in terms of follow-up duration and the reporting criteria for adverse effects (AEs), limiting the information available on the long-term effects of ADHD treatment. The authors concluded that "drugs for ADHD are generally safe and well tolerated, with decreased appetite, insomnia, headache and abdominal pain being the most common adverse effects (AEs) observed in long-term prospective trials. Tics were reported in all long-term studies of methylphenidate. Emotional lability was reported only with mixed amphetamine salts" (Clavenna and Bonati, 2014). It was noted that although AEs were described as mild or moderate, lack of tolerability resulted in the discontinuation of treatment in 10% to 25% of children, "with most of the AEs and discontinuation cases occurred in the first few months of drug treatment" (Clavenna and Bonati, 2014). The authors added that there was little data available regarding events that occur with a frequency of less than 1%. As a result, "many psychiatric AEs may be missed or underestimated, in particular the more severe ones (e.g., suicide attempts)." The studies available "provided scant information concerning the effect of treatments on growth and on the cardiovascular system" (Clavenna and Bonati, 2014).

A study looking at the effect of aerobic exercise on executive function in children with ADHD found that aerobic exercise

TABLE 56-1 Major Drug Classes Used in the Pharmacotherapy of Attention Deficit–Hyperactivity Disorder*

Drug	Total Daily Dose	Daily Dosage Schedule	Main Indications	Common Adverse Effects/Comments
Stimulants				
Dextroamphetamine	0.3–1.0 mg/kg	2 or 3 times	ADHD	Insomnia, decreased appetite Depression, psychosis (rare, with very high doses) Increased heart rate and blood pressure (mild) Possible growth reduction with long-term use Withdrawal effects and rebound phenomena
Mixed salts of l- and d-amphetamine	0.5–1.5 mg/kg	1 or 2 times	ADHD	Regular form: 6-hour duration of action Extended-release form: 10- to 12-hour duration of action
Lisdexamfetamine	30–70 mg (total)	Daily	ADHD	Less abuse potential than dextroamphetamine
Methylphenidate	1-2 mg/kg	1–3 times	ADHD	Regular forms: 3- to 4-hour duration of action Extended-release forms: 8- to 12-hour duration of action
Methylphenidate patch	10–30 mg/9 hours (total)	Daily	ADHD	
Dexmethylphenidate	0.5–1.0 mg/kg	2 or 3 times	ADHD	
Magnesium pemoline	1.0–2.5 mg/kg	1 or 2 times	ADHD	Associated with rare, serious hepatotoxicity; requires monitoring of liver function tests
Modafinil	200–400 mg (total)	Daily	Narcolepsy	Fewer peripheral sympathomimetic effects than amphetamines
NSRIs				
Atomoxetine	0.5–1.4 mg/kg	1 or 2 times	ADHD ± comorbidity Enuresis (?) Tic disorder (?) Depression/anxiety disorders (?)	Mechanism of action: noradrenergic-specific reuptake inhibitor Mild or moderate appetite depression Gastrointestinal symptoms Mild initial weight loss Mild increase in blood pressure, pulse No ECG conduction or repolarization delays Not abusable
Tricyclic Antidepressants				
Tertiary amines Imipramine Amitriptyline Clomipramine	2.0–5.0† mg/kg 2.0–5.0† mg/kg 2.0–5.0† mg/kg	1 or 2 times 1 or 2 times 1 or 2 times	ADHD Enuresis Tic disorder Anxiety disorders (?) OCD (clomipramine)	Mixed mechanism of action (noradrenergic/serotonergic) Secondary amines more noradrenergic Clomipramine primarily serotonergic Narrow therapeutic index Overdoses can be fatal Anticholinergic effects: dry mouth, constipation, blurred vision Weight loss Mild increase in diastolic blood pressure and ECG conduction parameters with daily doses > 3.5 mg/kg
Secondary amines Desipramine Nortriptyline	2.0–5.0† mg/kg 1.0–3.0† mg/kg	1 or 2 times 1 or 2 times		

Continued on following page

TABLE 56-1 Major Drug Classes Used in the Pharmacotherapy of Attention Deficit–Hyperactivity Disorder* *(Continued)*

Drug	Total Daily Dose	Daily Dosage Schedule	Main Indications	Common Adverse Effects/Comments

MAOIs
Phenelzine
Tranylcypromine
Selegiline
	0.5–1.0 mg/kg
	0.5–1.0 mg/kg
	0.5–1.0 mg/kg
		2 or 3 times
		2 or 3 times
		2 or 3 times
			Atypical depression
			   Treatment-refractory
			   depression
				Difficult medicines to use in juveniles
				Reserved for refractory cases
				Severe dietary restrictions (i.e., high-tyramine foods)
				Drug–drug interactions
				Hypertensive crisis with dietetic transgression or with certain drugs
				Weight gain
				Drowsiness
				Changes in blood pressure
				Insomnia
				Liver toxicity (remote)

Other Antidepressants

Drug	Total Daily Dose	Daily Dosage Schedule	Main Indications	Common Adverse Effects/Comments
SSRIs Fluoxetine Paroxetine Citalopram Sertraline Fluvoxamine	0.3–0.9 mg/kg 0.3–0.9 mg/kg 0.3–0.9 mg/kg 1.5–3.0 mg/kg 1.5–4.5 mg/kg	1 time, in afternoon 1 time, in afternoon 1 time, in afternoon 1 time, in afternoon 1 time, in afternoon	MD, dysthymia OCD Anxiety disorders Eating disorders PTSD (?)	Serotonergic mechanism of action Large margin of safety No cardiovascular effects Irritability Insomnia Gastrointestinal symptoms Headaches Sexual dysfunction Withdrawal symptoms more common with short-acting drugs Potential drug–drug interactions (cytochrome P-450)
Bupropion (SR)	3–6 mg/kg	2 times	ADHD MD Smoking cessation Anticraving effects (?)	Mixed mechanism of action (dopaminergic/noradrenergic) Irritability Insomnia Drug-induced seizures at doses > 6 mg/kg
Venlafaxine (XR)	1–3 mg/kg	1 time	Bipolar depression (?) MD Anxiety disorders ADHD (?) OCD (?)	Contraindicated in bulimics Mixed mechanism of action (serotonergic/noradrenergic) Similar to SSRIs Irritability Insomnia Gastrointestinal symptoms Headaches Potential withdrawal symptoms Blood pressure symptoms
Nefazodone	4–8 mg/kg	1 time	MD Anxiety disorders OCD (?) Bipolar depression (?)	Mixed mechanism of action (serotonergic/noradrenergic) Dizziness Nausea Potential interactions with nonsedating antihistamines, cisapride (cytochrome P-450) Rare, serious hepatotoxicity Less manicogenic (?)
Mirtazapine	0.2–0.9 mg/kg	1 time, in the afternoon	MD Anxiety disorders Stimulant-induced insomnia (?) Bipolar depression (?)	Mixed mechanism of action (serotonergic/noradrenergic) Sedation Weight gain Dizziness Less manicogenic (?)

Noradrenergic Modulators

Drug	Total Daily Dose	Daily Dosage Schedule	Main Indications	Common Adverse Effects/Comments
α2-Agonists Clonidine	0.003–0.010 mg/kg	2 or 3 times	Tourette disorder ADHD Aggression/self-abuse Severe agitation Withdrawal symptoms	Sedation (frequent) Hypotension (rare) Dry mouth Confusion (with high dose) Depression Rebound hypertension Localized irritation with transdermal preparation
Guanfacine (see text for information on long-acting form of Guanfacine)	0.015–0.05 mg/kg	1 or 2 times		Same as clonidine Less sedation, hypotension

TABLE 56-1 Major Drug Classes Used in the Pharmacotherapy of Attention Deficit–Hyperactivity Disorder* *(Continued)*

Drug	Total Daily Dose	Daily Dosage Schedule	Main Indications	Common Adverse Effects/Comments
Guanfacine, extended-release form		1–4 mg/day given once a day		
β-Blockers				
Propranolol	1–7 mg/kg	2 times	Aggression/self-abuse Severe agitation Akathisia	Risk for bradycardia and hypotension (dose-dependent) and rebound hypertension Bronchospasm (contraindicated in asthmatics) Rebound hypertension on abrupt withdrawal

*Doses are general guidelines and must be individualized with appropriate monitoring. Weight-corrected doses are less appropriate for obese children, and adult doses should not be exceeded in older or larger children. When high doses are used, serum levels may be obtained to avoid toxicity.

†Dose adjusted according to serum levels (therapeutic window for nortriptyline).

ADHD, attention deficit–hyperactivity disorder; DR, delayed release; ECG, electrocardiographic; IR, immediate release; MAOIs, monoamine oxidase inhibitors; MD, mood disorder; MR, mental retardation; NSRIs, norepinephrine-specific reuptake inhibitors; OCD, obsessive-compulsive disorder; OROS, oral osmotic; PTSD, posttraumatic stress disorder; SR, sustained release; SSRIs, selective serotonin reuptake inhibitors; XR, extended release.

(Adapted from Biederman J et al. Int J Neuropsychopharmacol 2004;7:77.)

facilitated inhibition and set-shifting, impairments in which are thought to account for executive dysfunctions in ADHD. Another study found that aerobic exercise resulted in smaller theta/alpha ratios in the frontal and central brain regions compared with a control group.

Complementary and Alternative Medications

A survey of parents of children referred for evaluation of ADHD reported that 54% of the parents used complementary and alternative medicine (e.g., acupuncture, nutritional supplements) for the child's ADHD symptoms in the prior year. Only 11% of the parents discussed using such interventions with their child's physician.

OUTCOME

ADHD persists into adulthood. The symptoms of ADHD may be less obvious after the individual is older. The incidence of ADHD in adults depends on diagnostic criteria and whether historical data are obtained from the patients or their parents. As noted in the introduction, the revised criteria in the DSM-5 reduce the number of symptoms required to make a diagnosis in adults and adolescents 17 and older and from six to five, which will inevitably result in an increased incidence of ADHD in those age groups. The finding that adolescents and young adults with ADHD had more car accidents with bodily injuries indicates that this is a serious problem even in older children and adults. A pilot study of 11 adults 55 years or older diagnosed with ADHD found that these patients had the same psychiatric comorbidities as younger adults and at similar rates. Psychiatric comorbidities were pervasive in this group and tended to weaken the effect of stimulant medications on overall functioning while enhancing the effect of medication on impulsivity.

CONCLUSIONS

Study of higher cortical function is inherently complex. Advances in neuroscience have brought new methods to this endeavor. There is still much research required for achieving an understanding of ADHD, not least of which is agreeing on a precise definition so that studies can be compared. Available evidence suggests that there may be value in distinguishing

ADHD/I from ADHD/HI and ADHD/C and in separating cases with comorbidity because these groups have different characteristics and different responses to treatment. A crucial role for the physician assessing a child for the possibility of ADHD is recognizing features in the presentation that suggest alternative diagnoses. Although much remains to be done, substantial advances in the neurobiology, diagnosis, and management of this condition have been made, and the prospect for significant enhancement of the lives of children with ADHD continues to improve.

REFERENCES

The complete list of references for this chapter is available online at www.expertconsult.com.

See inside cover for registration details.

SELECTED REFERENCES

American Psychiatric Association, 2013. Diagnostic Statistical Manual of Mental Disorders, fifth ed. American Psychiatric Press, Washington, DC.

Clavenna, A., Bonati, M., 2014. Safety of medicines used for ADHD in children: a review of published prospective clinical trials. Arch. Dis. Child. 99, 866–872. doi:10.1136/archdischild-2013-304170.

Coon, E.R., Quinonez, R.A., Moyer, V.A., et al., 2014. Overdiagnosis: How Our Compulsion for Diagnosis May Be Harming Children. Pediatrics 134 (5), 1013–1023. doi:10.1542/peds.2014-1778.

Getahun, D., Jacobsen, S.J., Fassett, M.J., et al., 2013. Recent Trends in Childhood Attention-Deficit/Hyperactivity Disorder. JAMA Pediatr. 167 (3), 282–288. doi:10.1001/2013.jamapediatrics.401.

Harstad, E., Levy, S., 2014. and Committee on Substance Abuse. Attention-Deficit/Hyperactivity Disorder and Substance Abuse. Pediatrics 134 (1), e293–e301. doi:10.1542/peds.2014-0992.

Hodgson, K., Hutchinson, A.D., Denson, L., 2014. Nonpharmacological Treatments for ADHD: A Meta-Analytic Review. J. Atten. Disord. 18 (4), 275–282. doi:10.1177/1087054712444732.

Martijn, A.M., de Ridder, S., Ute Strehl, U., et al., 2009. Efficacy of Neurofeedback Treatment in ADHD: The Effects on Inattention, Impulsivity and Hyperactivity: A Meta-Analysis. Clin. EEG Neurosci. 40 (3), 180–189. doi:10.1177/155005940904000311.

Saletin, J.M., Coon, W.C., Carskadon, M.A., 2015. Sleep Spindle-Frequency EEG Activity Is Associated With Overnight Motor Skill Improvement In Children With Attention-Deficit-Hyperactivity-Disorder. Sleep 38 (Suppl. A15).

Santos, K., Palmini, A., Radziuk, A.L., et al., 2013. The impact of methylphenidate on seizure frequency and severity in children with attention-deficit-hyperactivity disorder and difficult-to-treat epilepsies. Dev. Med. Child Neurol. 55, 654–660.

Subcommittee on Attention-Deficit/Hyperactivity Disorder, Steering Committee On Quality Improvement and Management ADHD: Clinical Practice Guideline for the Diagnosis, Evaluation, and Treatment of Attention-Deficit/Hyperactivity Disorder in Children and Adolescents, 2011. Pediatrics doi:10.1542/peds.2011-2654.

Thapar, A., Cooper, M., Eyre, O., et al., 2013. Practitioner Review: What have we learnt about the causes of ADHD? J. Child Psychol. Psychiatry 54 (1), 3–16.

Thomas, R., Geoffrey, K., Mitchell, G.K., et al., 2013. Attention-deficit/ hyperactivity disorder: are we helping or harming? BMJ 347, f6172. doi:10.1136/bmj.f6172.

Visser, S.N., Danielson, M.L., Bitsko, R.H., et al., 2013. Trends in the Parent-Report of Health Care Provider-Diagnosed and Medicated Attention-Deficit/Hyperactivity Disorder: United States, 2003–2011. J. Am. Acad. Child Adolesc. Psychiatry.

57 Autistic Spectrum Disorders

Deborah G. Hirtz, Ann Wagner, Pauline A. Filipek, and Elliott H. Sherr

An expanded version of this chapter is available on www.expertconsult.com. See inside cover for registration details.

The autistic spectrum disorders (ASD) represent a wide continuum of associated cognitive and neurobehavioral deficits, including deficits in socialization and communication, with restricted and repetitive patterns of behaviors. The terms "autism" and "autistic spectrum disorders" are used interchangeably throughout this chapter and refer to the broader umbrella of autism spectrum disorders, as defined by the fifth edition of the *Diagnostic and Statistical Manual of Mental Disorders* (DSM) (APA, 2013) (Box 57-1).

CLINICAL FEATURES OF ASD

All individuals on the autistic spectrum demonstrate deficits in two core domains: social communication/interaction and restricted/repetitive behaviors. There is marked variability in the severity of symptoms across patients, and cognitive function can range from severe intellectual impairment through the superior range. The fifth edition of DSM specifies that in the context of intellectual disability, the social-communication functioning must be more impaired than would be expected on the basis of general developmental level. The symptoms must be sufficient to limit or impair everyday function to warrant a diagnosis of ASD.

Persistent Deficits in Social Communication and Social Interaction

This refers to a *qualitative* impairment in social communication and reciprocal social interactions, which is persistent and observable across multiple contexts. There is not necessarily an absolute lack of social behaviors, but social communication and interactions are clearly atypical for the individual's age and developmental level. Behaviors range from total lack of responsiveness to other people to an oddly stilted interaction style or inappropriate approaches and attempts to interact.

Deficits in social-emotional reciprocity often manifest as the absence of attempts to initiate social interaction and a lack of responsiveness to social overtures. Eye contact is diminished and usually is not responsive to another person's overtures or used to get someone's attention. For school-age children and adolescents with ASD, unfamiliar or unstructured social situations (such as recess and lunch room) are especially challenging due to their difficulty in engaging in a reciprocal interaction and the inability to understand social roles and cues.

Deficits in nonverbal communication behaviors are a hallmark of ASD. Expressive language ranges from essentially nonverbal to verbally fluent. Nonverbal communication deficits can vary from a total lack of facial expressions and nonverbal communication to a lack of integration of gestures (e.g., eye contact, smiling, nodding, shaking the head, shoulder shrugging) with verbal communication. Lack of pretend play or very repetitive "scripted" pretend play is a typical characteristic of children with ASD. The development of friendships is challenging for children with ASD and when formed are usually around a specific shared interest; a lack of social reciprocity is still often apparent. Unfortunately, their social awkwardness often leaves children with ASD vulnerable to teasing and bullying.

Restricted, Repetitive Patterns of Behavior, Interests, or Activities

Restricted, repetitive patterns of behavior, interest, or activities can be manifest in many ways. A common form of repetitive speech is echolalia, which may be immediate or delayed. Immediate echolalia refers to immediate noncommunicative repetition of words or phrases. Delayed echolalia (or scripted speech) refers to the use of highly ritualized phrases that have been memorized, such as from television or overheard conversations. Repetitive questioning and the persistent use of idiosyncratic phrases are other forms of repetitive speech.

Some children have stereotypical movements (e.g., florid hand-clapping or arm-flapping) whenever excited or upset. Running aimlessly, rocking, spinning, bruxism, toe-walking, or other odd postures are also common. Many children with ASD demonstrate the classic behavior of lining up objects or may be preoccupied with repetitive actions, such as opening and closing doors or repetitively flicking pieces of string. Many autistic children are so preoccupied with "sameness" that little can be changed without prompting a tantrum or other expression of distress. Restricted and repetitive behavior may take the form of excessive preoccupation with special interests. The inflexibility and idiosyncratic nature of these preoccupations interfere with the ability to carry on reciprocal conversations or sustain friendships.

Many children with ASD overreact or underreact to sensory input (such as pain or temperature) or may be interested in some sensory aspects of their environment (e.g., lights, patterns, or movement) to an unusual degree. Extreme rigidity or rituals related to the smell, texture, and look of food are common and may result in excessive food restriction.

Onset Patterns in ASD

The onset of ASD may occur early, with abnormalities in social and communication skills becoming apparent in the first year of life, or children appear to develop normally until at least 12 months of age, followed by loss or regression of language and/or social skills. The prevalence of regression in ASD is about 30%.

Dramatic, rapid regression after a period of normal development, particularly after the age of 2 years and involving more than social communication skills, is rare and warrants a thorough medical evaluation. More typical is a "plateauing" or deceleration of development after 6 months of age. This is often accompanied by some loss of social communication skills, typically joint attention, shared affect, and the use of language. During early childhood, some children with ASD

BOX 57-1 Diagnostic Criteria for 299.00 Autism Spectrum Disorder

A. Persistent deficits in social communication and social interaction across multiple contexts, as manifested by the following, currently or by history (examples are illustrative, not exhaustive; see text):
 1. Deficits in social-emotional reciprocity, ranging, for example, from abnormal social approach and failure of normal back-and-forth conversation; to reduced sharing of interests, emotions, or affect; to failure to initiate or respond to social interactions.
 2. Deficits in nonverbal communicative behaviors used for social interaction, ranging, for example, from poorly integrated verbal and nonverbal communication; to abnormalities in eye contact and body language or deficits in understanding and use of gestures; to a total lack of facial expressions and nonverbal communication.
 3. Deficits in developing, maintaining, and understand relationships, ranging, for example, from difficulties adjusting behavior to suit various social contexts; to difficulties in sharing imaginative play or in making friends; to absence of interest in peers.

Specify current severity:
Severity is based on social communication impairments and restricted, repetitive patterns of behavior.

B. Restricted, repetitive patterns of behavior, interests, or activities, as manifested by at least two of the following, currently or by history (examples are illustrative, not exhaustive; see text):
 1. Stereotyped or repetitive motor movements, use of objects, or speech (e.g., simple motor stereotypes, lining up toys or flipping objects, echolalia, idiosyncratic phrases).
 2. Insistence on sameness, inflexible adherence to routines, or ritualized patterns of verbal or nonverbal behavior (e.g., extreme distress at small changes, difficulties with transitions, rigid thinking patterns, greeting rituals, need to take same route or eat same food every day).
 3. Highly restricted, fixated interests that are abnormal in intensity or focus (e.g., strong attachment to or preoccupation with unusual objects, excessively circumscribed or perseverative interests).
 4. Hyper- or hyporeactivity to sensory input or unusual interest in sensory aspects of the environment (e.g. apparent indifference to pain/temperature, adverse response to

specific sounds or textures, excessive smelling or touching of objects, visual fascination with lights or movement).

Specify current severity:
Severity is based on social communication impairments and restricted, repetitive patterns of behavior.

C. Symptoms must be present in the early developmental period (but may not become fully manifest until social demands exceed limited capacities, or may be masked by learned strategies in later life).

D. Symptoms cause clinically significant impairment in social, occupational, or other important areas of current functioning.

E. These disturbances are not better explained by intellectual disability (intellectual developmental disorder) or global developmental delay. Intellectual disability and autism spectrum disorder frequently co-occur; to make comorbid diagnoses of autism spectrum disorder and intellectual disability, social communication should be below that expected for general developmental level.

Note: Individuals with a well-established DSM-IV diagnosis of autistic disorder, Asperger's disorder, or pervasive developmental disorder not otherwise specified should be given the diagnosis of autism spectrum disorder. Individuals who have marked deficits in social communication, but whose symptoms do not otherwise meet criteria for autism spectrum disorder, should be evaluated for social (pragmatic) communication disorder.

Specify if:
With or without accompanying intellectual impairment
With or without accompanying language impairment
Associated with a known medical or genetic condition or environmental factor
(**Coding note:** Use additional code to identify the associated medical or genetic condition.)
Associated with another neurodevelopmental, mental, or behavioral disorder
(**Coding note:** Use additional code[s] to identify the associated neurodevelopmental, mental, or behavioral disorder[s].)
With catatonia (refer to the criteria for catatonia associated with another mental disorder)
(**Coding note:** Use additional code 293.89 catatonia associated with autism spectrum disorder to indicate the presence of the comorbid catatonia.)

(From: American Psychiatric Association. Proposed Revisions to 299.00 Autistic Disorder in DSM-V, 2013. Retrieved February 28, 2013, from http://www.dsm5.org/ProposedRevisions/Pages/proposedrevision.aspx?rid = 94#).

---

continue on a worsening trajectory, others remain stable, and some improve. Currently, there is no reliable way to predict which trajectory will apply to an individual child.

Children who experience a regression with onset of symptoms of autism and an epileptiform EEG are to be differentiated from those with a diagnosis of Landau-Kleffner syndrome, an acquired aphasia associated with an epileptiform EEG, and from those with continuous spike waves during slow wave sleep (CSWS). Although in these conditions there are seizures, regression and epileptiform abnormalities, children with autistic regression have an earlier age of onset and are less likely to have bilateral, temporal EEG patterns, or electrical status during sleep (Table 57-1).

EPIDEMIOLOGY

The prevalence of autism has dramatically increased in the United States from .4 per 1000 before 1991 to 1.2 per 1000

before 2001 and to 14 per 1000, or one in 68 children, in 2010. In the 2010 Autism and Developmental Disabilities (ADDM) cohort, ASD prevalence in children varied based on race: white (1 in 63), black (1 in 81), Hispanic (1 in 93), Asian or Pacific Islander (1 in 81), and overall (1 in 68).

Awareness of autism has been increasing in developing and developed countries, with varying but largely similar prevalence as the U.S. estimates. Several factors contribute to the apparent increase. In the past, autism prevalence was underestimated. Over time, diagnostic criteria have broadened and more recent surveys have included the broadest definitions. There is now codiagnosis with known medical disorders such as Fragile X syndrome, Tourette syndrome (TS), and Down syndrome. There also is increasing public awareness among parents and teachers as well as availability of services. Children earlier diagnosed as mentally retarded may now meet current criteria for autism. Finally, earlier age at diagnosis and population-based screening have also

TABLE 57-1 Landau–Kleffner Syndrome-Continuous Spike Waves during Slow-Wave Sleep versus Autistic Regression with Epileptiform EEG

	Landau–Kleffner Syndrome-Continuous Spike-Waves during Slow-Wave Sleep (LKS-CSWS)	Autistic Regression with Epileptiform EEG (AREE)
Age of regression/ (symptoms)	Usually after 3 years; peak age 3–5 years. In CSWS may be as late as 12 years of age.	Usually before age 2 years with a mean age of regression of 21 months
Seizures	Usually not frequent or intractable. In approximately 25%, seizures are not present.	Seizures are not part of phenotype. In autistic spectrum disorders, when seizures occur, they are usually not frequent and respond well to antiseizure medications.
EEG	Spikes, sharp waves, or spike-and-wave discharges, usually bilateral and occurring predominantly over the temporal regions. They increase during sleep; EEG pattern of electrical status epilepticus during slow-wave sleep is common.	Infrequent spikes, usually centrotemporal. Rarely associated with CSWS. No clear correlation with interictal epileptiform discharges and improvement or worsening of underlying language and social dysfunction.
Treatment	Case reports, mostly with use of steroids, suggest improvement in language. Surgical outcomes with multiple subpial transections are variable. No controlled clinical trials.	No evidence that present medical interventions (antiseizure medications) or surgical interventions are indicated.
Outcome/Comments	Improvement occurs in late childhood/early adolescence. Approximately one third recover. Prognosis for seizure control is excellent but recovery of language is variable and not as good as for seizures.	Improvement seems related to cognitive skills. No data to determine whether interictal discharges combined with regression are markers for worse prognosis.

contributed to the reported increase. The CDC is monitoring the prevalence of autism over time in a number of U.S. sites using consistently applied ascertainment and diagnostic protocols.

The proportion of children with ASDs who had IQs less than or equal to 70 ranged from about 30% to 50% in the CDC's ADDM Network. The mean male to female ratio is about 4 to 1, but as cognitive severity increases, the male to female ratio decreases to 1.3 to 1. Children with an IQ of less than 50 are more likely than those who are high-functioning to be female and to have minor physical anomalies, neuroimaging abnormalities, microcephaly, and epilepsy. Those with specific inherited conditions, such as tuberous sclerosis or phenylketonuria, are likely to be more severely cognitively impaired. In some studies, ASD prevalence increases with increasing socioeconomic status.

Sibling Studies

An autism diagnosis is about 20 times more likely in siblings when one child had autism—about 10.1%, compared with 0.5% prevalence in siblings of controls. The risk is 25% if there are already two siblings with ASD.

Delays in verbal and nonverbal communication have been noted in siblings of those with ASD, beginning at about 12 months of age. However, no consistent specific deficits have emerged as characteristic of Sib-ASD. Response to name at 12 months of age and response to joint attention were predictive of the degree of social impairment and eventual ASD diagnosis at 3 years of age.

Neonatal Intensive Care and Prematurity

There is a higher rate of autism and a much higher rate of positive screening for ASD in infants with extreme prematurity. This increased risk has been associated with perinatal complications such as preeclampsia, intracranial hemorrhage, cerebral edema, low Apgar scores, and seizures. The presence of these risk factors should lead to systematic screening of toddlers and preschoolers who were born prematurely or with neonatal complications.

Parental Age and Other Factors

Risk of ASD is higher with increasing age of mothers, and independently, with increasing age of fathers. Advanced parental age and some other risk factors may act through increasing the risk for de novo mutations. Environment mutagens such as mercury, cadmium, nickel, trichloroethylene, and vinyl chloride may play a role. Air pollution is a risk factor in most but not all studies. Vitamin D deficiency may cause mutations, as vitamin D contributes to repair of DNA damage.

Autoimmune Factors

Autoimmune dysfunction has been associated with autism risk. The presence of maternal thyroid peroxidase antibody (TPOab) increased risk by nearly 80%. Maternal infection requiring hospitalization (but not mild common infectious diseases or febrile episodes) was associated with an increased risk of ASD. Maternal gestational or type 2 diabetes, maternal prenatal stress in the first trimester, and paternal obesity all may increase the risk of ASD. Children born within 1 year of an autistic sibling have an increased risk over those born after longer intervals. A decrease in autism risk has been associated with periconceptual folate intake and may be strongest in those with genetically inefficient folate metabolism.

Vaccines

Resurgence of measles in the United States has focused attention on parents who have refused the measles-mumps-rubella (MMR) vaccination for fear of its causing autism. Five methodologically sound cohort studies involving 1,256,407 children and five case-control studies of 9920 children did not find an increased risk of autism with childhood vaccines or the mercury-containing preservative thimerosol, which has not been used routinely since 2001. Although thimerosal exposure from vaccines was eliminated in Sweden and Denmark by the early 1990s, the incidence of autism was accelerated. Additional data derived from passive surveillance systems also consistently failed to detect an association. There has been no evidence that the incidence of regressive autism has increased after administration of the MMR vaccine. The MMR vaccine has been given at a constant rate since 1979 in the United States, since 1982 in Finland, and since 1998 in the United Kingdom and Denmark, but rates of autism have steadily risen. There is also no causative link with persistent GI problems or the measles virus. Even among children at high risk because of older siblings, there was no harmful association between MMR vaccine and ASD.

Animal Models

One of the most challenging aspects of autism research is the development and validation of animal models. This is discussed in the online version of this chapter.

Neuropathology

The underlying genetic complexity and thus corresponding mechanistic diversity has made study of ASD neuropathology challenging. Brain regions implicated in ASD pathogenesis include the superior temporal sulcus, amygdala, fusiform gyrus, dorsolateral prefrontal cortex, and the cerebellum. Postmortem histopathological studies have shown differences between ASD and matched controls including cortical dysgenesis, such as ectopic gray and white matter and abnormal lamination. Cortical minicolumns have been demonstrated to be more numerous and narrow in ASD brains, and higher prefrontal and midtemporal spine densities in pyramidal neurons have been reported. This increase in spine density as seen in Fragile X and Down syndrome suggests that it is a common morphologic signature in many neurodevelopmental disorders.

Neurotransmitters

Neurotransmitter abnormalities have been described in autism. A study of eight hippocampal neurotransmitter receptors demonstrated a reduction in the GABA-ergic system. Further work has implicated serotonin as central to ASD pathology, including disruption of the 5HT2a receptor binding throughout the cingulate cortex in adults, and altered platelet serotonin levels.

Neuroimaging

Neuroimaging findings in ASD are also variable, demonstrating either decreased or increased cortical white matter volume or microstructure. However, to underscore the complexity, a recent paper demonstrated that the diffusion tensor imaging changes in ASD patients compared with healthy population controls were also seen in their apparently unaffected siblings.

Conducting MRI scans of patients with specific genetic or "syndromic" diagnoses can identify unexpected findings. For example, patients with Williams syndrome have an elevation in fractional anisotropy (FA) in areas associated with language. Other studies have shown that FA levels are altered in Fragile X patients compared with to controls but also to individuals with idiopathic ASD. Phenotypically similar ASD patients have been reported with differing FA levels, white matter and global brain volumes depending on whether a deletion or duplication at the same genetic loci is present. Elevated FA is seen in patients with a deletion at 16p11.2, whereas reduced FA is seen in those with a duplication at the same genetic locus. Because both the deletion and duplication carriers can have ASD and both can have opposing imaging findings, it is not unreasonable to see why imaging assessments of mixed idiopathic ASD groups could result in different or no significant results, depending on the type of genetics that underlie

the ASD patients in any given cohort. This suggests that future imaging for ASD should start from a cohort of patients who have similar or identical genetic or syndromic etiologies.

Genetics of ASD

Perhaps the most significant advance in autism biology over the last decade has been in understanding the genetics of autism. Newly developed powerful genome-wide tools have shown the importance of highly penetrant single de novo genetic events, whether they are copy number variants (CNV) or single nucleotide variants (SNV). CNVs recurrent common loci include deletion or duplication of a 593 kb locus at 16p11.2, duplication at 15q11.2–q13.1 and duplication at the Williams syndrome locus at 7q11.23. Advances in the last 8 to 10 years, through testing many thousands of children with ASD or other neurodevelopmental disorders (NDD), have also proven the pathogenicity of less commonly observed CNVs (Cooper et al., 2011). Guidelines from a consensus statement from the American College of the Medical Genetics and the International Standard Cytogenomic Array (ISCA) consortium states that chromosome microarrays (or any platform that reliably detects chromosomal copy number variants) are a first-line test for determining the cause of autism in affected patients (Kearney et al., 2011).

In addition to CNV, there is now substantial evidence that SNVs play a key role in ASD. With the advent of increasingly less expensive next generation sequencing, it is possible in research and clinical settings to use whole exome sequencing in ASD patients to diagnose more than 25% of cases. This approach of deep sequencing of ASD cohorts (as well as candidate gene sequencing of larger numbers of patients) has identified dozens of new genes that are linked to ASD, using conservative genome-wide statistical thresholds. As with the discovery of CNV, the list of these genes will continue to grow. Currently, one website, https://gene.sfari.org/autdb/Welcome.do, houses genes, CNV, and the supporting data linking these genetic changes to ASD. The frequency of the most common CNVs in an ASD cohort is approximately 0.5% to 1%, for 16p11.2 and 15q11.2–q13.1. For SNVs, (e.g., mutations in genes CHD8, 0.3%; CHD2, 0.2%; ANK2, 0.2%; ARID1B, 0.2%) the rate of de novo mutations is lower, with the most commonly affected genes in the initial exome sequencing cohorts lower than the rate of the most recurrent CNV, such as 16p11.2 deletion/duplication. The Simons Foundation Autism Research Initiative (SFARI) website lists 706 genes associated with ASD, with varying levels of evidence supporting this link.

Both the aforementioned CNV and SNV are principally implicated in ASD because the genetic mutation is de novo, not present in either parent, and likely occurs in the paternal or maternal zygotes. However, there has been substantial evidence linking ASD to a pattern of familial inheritance, with heritability ranging from 55% to 90%. Additionally, ongoing studies confirm that inheritance of common, less penetrant mutations play a key role in ASD biology (Krumm et al., 2015) and that combining findings from both inherited and de novo mutations will better allow development of a model of ASD etiology and pathogenesis.

SCREENING AND DIAGNOSTIC EVALUATION FOR ASD

ASDs can be reliably diagnosed in children in the second year of life, and early intervention has proven to be beneficial to social and communicative function. However, the average age at diagnosis in the United States continues to be high (53 months). Parents often voice concerns months to years before a formal diagnosis is achieved and appropriate intervention initiated.

Age at diagnosis varies as a function of ethnicity and socio-economic status (SES) (Daniels and Mandell, 2013). The mean age at diagnosis in Medicaid-eligible children is 64.9 months, considerably higher than the U.S. average. In addition, Medicaid-eligible African American children were 2.6 times less likely than white children to receive an autism diagnosis on their first specialty care visit, with ADHD being the most common diagnosis.

The 1 in 93 prevalence rate for Hispanic children actually represents a considerable narrowing in the gap relative to white children over the past decade. Although a majority of primary care practicioners (PCPs) offered some form of developmental screening, only 29% offered Spanish ASD screening, and only 10% offered both Spanish general developmental and Spanish ASD screening. Many children, particularly non-English–speaking families with low SES, still are not receiving appropriate early screening and treatment.

The CDC has a website to increase public and professional awareness of autism and other neurodevelopmental disorders, called "Learn the Signs. Act Early," at http://www.cdc.gov/ncbddd/actearly/. The CDC website offers downloadable educational information and screening instruments at http://www.cdc.gov/ncbddd/actearly/hcp/index.html. There also is a developmental pediatric curriculum to improve recognition of ASD that would be appropriate for child neurologists at http://www.cdc.gov/ncbddd/actearly/act/class.html.

The Child Neurology Society and American Academy of Neurology (AAN/CNS) published the initial *Practice Parameter for the Screening and Diagnosis of Autism*. The American Academy of Pediatrics Council of Children with Disabilities subsequently published a set of guidelines on the identification and management of children with ASD; both were reaffirmed in 2010. Risk factors include having a sibling with ASD or whenever there is parental, other caregiver, or pediatrician concern.

Screening Instruments for ASD

"Red flags" for critical delays in social communication development can be recognized or queried and should initiate prompt evaluation for an ASD (Box 57-2). ASD screening tools should be used whenever a concern is raised about an infant's or child's social communication development. ASD screening and diagnostic instruments were reviewed by Charman and Gotham (2013) and Johnson and Myers (2007) (Fig. 57-1).

Diagnostic Instruments for ASD

The combined administration of the semistructured Autism Diagnostic Observation Schedule™—second edition (ADOS-2) and the Autism Diagnostic Interview™—revised (ADI-R) a structured parent interview, are considered the gold standard for the diagnosis of autism in research settings. Many clinical settings use the ADOS-2 independently of the ADI-R. Both instruments are available for purchase (in many languages), and training/ workshop information are available at http://www.wpspublish.com/app/.

Speaking with Parents about a New Diagnosis of ASD

Many parents have known that "something is wrong" for a considerable amount of time and may even come into the evaluation with a chief complaint that "I think my child has autism." However, many parents, although hoping to be vindicated in the diagnosis, also may be hoping that they have been wrong.

BOX 57-2 Red Flags for Social Communication Development

Prompt evaluation should occur for any of the following:

No vocalizations by 6 months

A parent should be able to have a reciprocal "conversation" by this age, consisting of at least several volleys back and forth.

No polysyllabic consonant babbling by 12 months

At least some of these vocalizations should be directed <u>at</u> someone with communicative intent.

No gestures by 12 months

The earliest gesture an infant learns is to raise his/her arms to request to be picked up, usually once sitting independently.

Pointing should be with an isolated index finger, not the whole hand, and should be used "to request" or "to show," not just pointing at pictures in a book or pointing to have an adult label items.

<u>Any</u> use of hand-over-hand by the child, e.g., putting a parent's hand on the cabinet door where the cookies are kept or using the parent's hand to point at pictures in a book, is a hallmark of ASD.

No spontaneous (not echoed) single words by 16 months other than *mama* or *dada*

Spontaneous words must be beyond those used to simply label items and must be used by the child <u>to communicate, to request, to show, or to share</u>.

No spontaneous (not echoed) phrases by 24 months or sentences by 36 months

Spontaneous phrases and sentences must be used by the child <u>to communicate, to request, to show, or to share</u>.

<u>Any</u> loss of social communication abilities, including babbling, single words, phrases, response to name, social engagement, or gestures

If a parent reports their infant has decreased or stopped any social communication milestones, this is usually the hallmark of the onset of regression.

Clinicians should consider incorporating the following points during the evaluation and subsequent counseling. Families should be encouraged to ask questions, offer observations, and provide information. Clinicians should ascertain behaviors seen during the evaluation are typical for this child. Clinicians need to be aware of and address safety issues. The results of the evaluation process should be reviewed, particularly detailing the child's strengths and areas of difficulties. The diagnosis of ASD should be clearly stated, and details of the symptoms of ASD should be described, especially the core deficits of social communication and restricted, repetitive behaviors. The clinician should prioritize the next steps to further evaluate and treat the child and provide the family with contact information to accomplish these steps. It is also important to discuss incorporating ongoing family support as well as providing contact information for external support groups. It is helpful to conclude on a positive note, reminding the parents about the child's and family's strengths.

Recommendations for a Child with Newly Diagnosed ASD

All initial diagnostic evaluations resulting in a diagnosis of ASD should provide the following referrals at a minimum:

1. Evaluation for Individuals with Disabilities Education Act (IDEA) services:
   - Children older than 33 months of age: by the local provider of Early Intervention (EI) services. Many states have

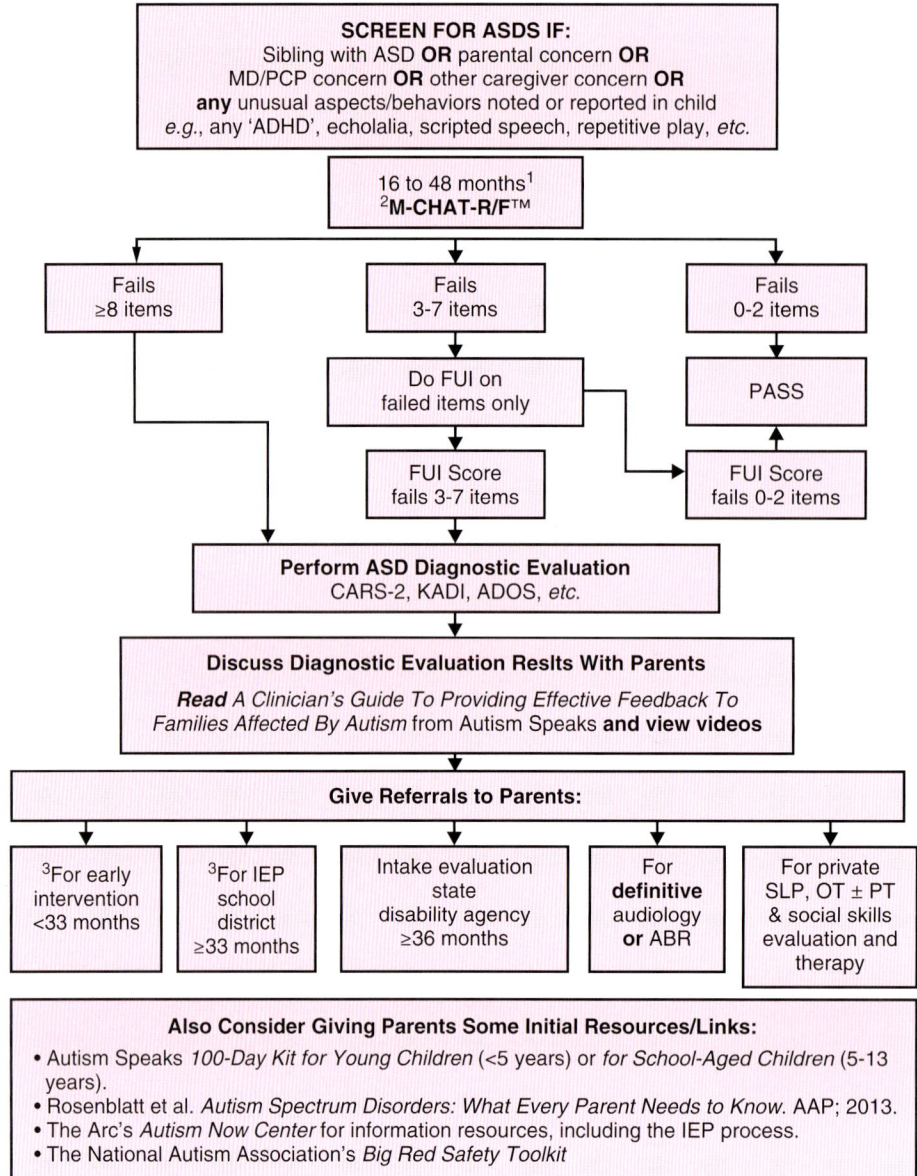

Figure 57-1. Child Neurology "Road Map" for ASD Screening and Diagnosis. *(Courtesy of Pauline A. Filipek MD.)*

a centralized website that provides contact information by zip code or city.

- Children 33 months of age and younger: by the local school district to perform a Full Individual Evaluation (FIE) in order to prepare an Individualized Education Plan (IEP). Parents must make the request for an FIE in writing.
2. Definitive hearing evaluation, either audiology or auditory brainstem responses.
3. Private speech, OT and/or PT evaluations, as indicated.
4. For a child 36 months of age and older, refer the child for an intake evaluation at the state's agency for developmental disabilities.

Safety issues also should be addressed during the initial evaluation. Wandering away from home or school is a significant safety problem in half of all children with ASD, with a substantial number at risk for bodily harm, primarily from traffic injuries (65%) or drowning (24%). Nonverbal or minimally verbal children who wander should wear identification bracelets.

THE NEUROLOGIC EVALUATION IN AUTISM

The neurologic examination in ASD is usually relatively straightforward, with the exception of several possible findings: large head circumference (HC) or frank macrocephaly, somatic overgrowth, motor abnormalities including hypotonia, dyspraxia, stereotypies, and gait disturbances, and/or self-injurious behaviors (SIB).

Large Head Size and Somatic Overgrowth

Many reports have noted that head circumferences in children with ASD are shifted upward, with the mean approximately at the 75th percentile, with correspondingly increased whole brain volume. This is presumed due to an accelerated brain growth rate in infancy, as HC is normal by adolescence and adulthood as is postmortem brain weight. However, many reports are finding either HC within the normal range and comparable to typical controls or large but proportional to somatic overgrowth. Children with ASD, particularly boys, are often taller and heavier than typically developing children of the same age.

Motor Disturbances in Tone, Gait, Praxis, and Stereotypies

Hypotonia is common in children with ASD but not uniquely so. Gait disturbances also have been reported in ASD, localized to abnormal cadence, and hip and ankle kinematics and kinetics; such disturbances may be more pronounced in children with severe rather than with mild ASD symptoms.

Motor dyspraxia, defined as impaired ability to perform skilled gestures, was identified in almost 30% of children with ASD and normal cognitive function, in 75% of children with ASD and intellectual disability (ID), and in 56% of a nonautistic, intellectually delayed control group. Dyspraxia in ASD strongly correlates with the core social, communicative, and behavioral impairments, as measured by the ADOS. Both motor function and visual-motor integration contribute to the dyspraxia.

Motor stereotypies are very common in ASD and have an earlier onset (younger than 3 years) than tics (5 to 7 years) and tend to be consistent and fixed, frequently involving hands, arms, or the entire body. These include hand or finger mannerisms, body rocking, and unusual posturing, Self-injurious behavior (SIB) is reported to occur in varying proportions of individuals with ASD (i.e., 35 to 50%).

Clinical Testing

Definitive Evaluation of Hearing

Many children with ASD are first described by parents as acting "as if deaf." However, most children with autism have normal hearing. Pronounced to profound bilateral hearing loss or deafness was present in 3.5% of all children with ASD, a prevalence greater than that for the general population but similar to the rate for individuals with ID. In contrast, hyperacusis was commonly found, affecting almost 20% of an ASD sample. Definitive audiological evaluation or brainstem auditory-evoked potential testing should be performed in all children with autism so that, if indicated, appropriate referrals can be made.

Lead Level

Children with developmental delay who spend an extended period in the oral-motor stage of play are at increased risk for lead toxicity, which may still be present in certain environments. The prevalence of pica in this group can result in high rates of substantial and often recurrent exposure to lead and other metals. All children with developmental delay or autism should have a periodic lead screen until the pica disappears.

Electroencephalography

There is insufficient evidence to recommend for or against the use of routine screening EEGs in autistic children. Epileptiform EEG abnormalities and interictal discharges (IEDs) have been reported in children with ASD (up to 30%) but do not typically correlate with clinical seizure activity.

Neuroimaging Studies

Routine MRI studies to evaluate a child with autism to determine the etiology is not warranted unless there is neurologic evidence of lateralizing signs or other critical symptomatology. There is a very low prevalence of focal lesions or other abnormalities in ASD, most of which are deemed coincidental. PET and single-photon emission computed tomography (SPECT) are not indicated in the diagnostic evaluation of ASD.

Metabolic Testing

Metabolic screening is indicated only in the presence of suggestive clinical and physical findings (e.g., lethargy, cyclic vomiting, early seizures, dysmorphic or coarse features), ID, questionable newborn screening, or birth outside of the United States.

Tests of Unproven Value

Unsupported claims have led a number of parents to seek various tests in the hope of finding a treatable cause of autism. There is no evidence to support routine clinical testing of undocumented value (e.g., trace elements in the hair, celiac antibodies, immunologic or neurochemical abnormalities, micronutrients such as vitamin levels, intestinal permeability, stool analysis, urinary peptides, and so forth).

COEXISTENT MEDICAL CONDITIONS
Gastrointestinal Problems

Feeding habits and food preferences of children with autism typically are unconventional; however, the majority of children have intakes that meet or exceed dietary standards.

Children with ASD have more GI symptoms than comparison groups, with an overall odds ratio of 4.42, (1.90 to 10.28) (McElhanon et al., 2014). Individuals with ASD should receive the same standard of care in the diagnostic workup and treatment of gastrointestinal concerns as patients without ASD. Available data do not support the use of a casein-free diet, a gluten-free diet, or a combined gluten/casein-free diet as a primary treatment for individuals with ASD, despite anecdotal reports of some benefit.

Sleep Disturbances

The majority of children with autism have sleep problems, often severe, and usually involving extreme sleep latencies, lengthy nighttime awakenings, shortened night sleep, and early morning awakenings. Children with autism also have more unusual and obligatory bedtime routines. These behaviors may lead to memory and learning issues, maladaptive daytime behaviors, and parental stress.

Epilepsy

Epilepsy of all seizure types occur frequently in children with autism. The overall rate, even in idiopathic cases of autism with normal IQ, is higher (13% to 17%) than the risk in the general population (1% to 2%). There is a bimodal distribution of age of onset, with peaks occurring at younger than 5 years and during adolescence and with the rate increased in those with intellectual disability or underlying medical conditions. The prevalence of epilepsy was 21.5% in subjects with ASD and ID compared with 8% in those with ASD and no ID. The presence of cerebral palsy or focal motor findings also increases risk.

The focus of an NIH workshop on autism and epilepsy (Tuchman et al., 2013) was the commonality of possible mechanisms and how we can learn about the pathophysiology of both conditions when they occur together, for example, in disorders such as Fragile X syndrome and Tuberous Sclerosis Complex (TSC). Both abnormal synaptic plasticity and excitatory/inhibitory imbalance can be contributing factors. Changes associated with seizures and epileptogenesis may disrupt normal activity-dependent developmental processes. Changes in functional connectivity determined by EEG are being explored as a biomarker for early identification of ASD. By 12 months of age, high risk infants later diagnosed with ASD showed reduced functional connectivity compared with those who were not later diagnosed.

Seizures in children with autism should be treated as they would be in children without autism, with even more attention than usual paid to the possible behavioral and cognitive side effects of antiseizure drugs. Repetitive and stereotypic behaviors could mimic temporal lobe seizures, and inattention from absence seizures may be construed as autistic behavior.

PHARMACOLOGIC THERAPY

Drug treatment should be one facet of a comprehensive, multidisciplinary approach that includes structured special educational techniques, language or communication interventions, behavior modification, and parent training (Table 57-2). The goal of pharmacologic treatment is to improve specific behaviors such as anxiety, repetitive motor behaviors, obsessive-compulsive symptoms, impulsivity, depression, mood swings, agitation, hyperactivity, aggression, and self-injurious behavior. Although no medication directly influences cognitive impairment, controlling symptoms may allow the child to maximize benefits from educational and behavioral treatments that are directed toward the core impairments. Dosing should start with low amounts and slowly be escalated with careful attention to possible side effects, the most common of which is activation, defined as overactivity, agitation, or emotional lability.

Of the 2853 children enrolled in the Autism Treatment Network, 27% were on psychotropic medication. Use was less common in children age 5 and under and was associated with gastrointestinal symptoms and sleep problems. In children with comorbid diagnoses of ADHD, bipolar disorder, obsessive-compulsive disorder, depression or anxiety, use was 82%, compared with 16% in children without psychiatric comorbidity.

Neuroleptic Agents

Neuroleptics that block dopamine receptors, such as haloperidol, thioridazine, and trifluoperazine, were used until the development of drugs that were more effective in blocking serotonin receptors. Haloperidol decreased motor stereotypies, hyperactivity, withdrawal, and negativism in children with autism, but use is limited by the risk of extrapyramidal symptoms. Weight gain and metabolic changes are common side effects of neuroleptics.

Risperidone and aripiprazole are the only two medications approved by the Federal Drug Administration (FDA) for the treatment of irritability (including aggression, self-injurious behavior, temper tantrums, and mood swings) in school-age children and adolescents with autistic disorder.

These agents have been associated with weight gain, prolactin increases, hyperglycemia, and sedation in some patients. In an 8-week, randomized trial in 101 children with ASD, low dose risperidone (0.5 to 3.5 mg/d) improved irritability, hyperactivity, and stereotypies. Treatment effects were maintained over 16 weeks, and medication discontinuation resulted in return of behavioral symptoms. An 8-week, double-blind, randomized, placebo-controlled trial with aripiprazole in 218 children and adolescents with autistic disorder compared three doses of the drug (5, 10, or 15 mg/d) to placebo. All doses improved irritability, although only the 5 mg/day group reached statistical significance, possibly due to a high placebo response (35%). Improvement was reported within 2 weeks.

Opiate Antagonists

Naltrexone was evaluated in clinical trials with the hypothesis that autism is associated with hypersecretion of brain opioids, including beta-endorphins, and that many symptoms are similar to those induced by opiate administration. In several small studies, 1mg/kg/day decreased hyperactivity and modestly improved behavior, with mild GI side effects and drowsiness.

Serotonin Reuptake Inhibitors (SRIs)

Because of the efficacy of serotonin reuptake inhibitors (e.g., clomipramine, fluoxetine, sertraline, fluvoxamine, and paroxetine) on anxiety and obsessive-compulsive symptoms, and the finding of serotonin abnormalities in individuals with autism, there has been interest in treating disruptive behaviors with these agents. Results of open-label and observational studies as well as double-blind, placebo-controlled, randomized trials have been mixed and suggest that efficacy of SRIs may be moderated by age, with better responsivity in adults than in children. Studies of fluvoxamine and fluoxetine have shown some benefit in autistic adults but not in children.

A large, double-blind, randomized, placebo-controlled trial of 149 children and adolescents with ASD (ages 5 to 17 years) failed to find any effects of citalopram on repetitive behaviors. The most frequently reported side effects were activation, stereotypy, diarrhea, insomnia, dry skin, and pruritus. Two subjects treated with citalopram had seizures. There was a high placebo response rate (34%), which underscores the need for placebo-controlled trials.

The 5HT1A serotonin agonist buspirone was evaluated in a randomized, blinded trial of 166 children ages 2 to 6 years, in doses of 2.5 mg or 5 mg/bid compared with placebo. The primary outcome was the ADOS composite score, which was not affected in either treatment group. Those given the lower dose improved on the repetitive behavior score. This study evaluated pretreatment blood serotonin and regional patterns of metabolism on PET scan. Children with pretreatment elevated blood serotonin and regional patterns of tryptophan on PET scan suggesting brain inflammation were less likely to improve. A Cochrane review of SSRIs did not find overall evidence of benefit in children with ASD, although reduction in anxiety or depressive symptoms in older children may be beneficial (Williams et al., 2013).

In summary, the neuroleptics risperidone and aripiprazole can be used for irritability, aggression, SIBs, and mood swings. SRIs, selective SRIs, and other medications affecting serotonin and dopamine levels can reduce certain symptoms, such as ritualized behaviors, stereotypies, and aggression. Although SRIs appear to be safe, children may be sensitive to the behavioral activation of these drugs. Seizures have

TABLE 57-2 Medications Used to Decrease Specific Symptoms Associated with Autism Spectrum Disorder*

Drug	Dose	Age†	N	Efficacy	Side Effects
Neuroleptic Agents					
Risperidone	0.25–2.5 mg/d <20 kg 0.5–2.5 mg/d 20-45 kg 0.5–3.5 mg/d >45 kg Mean = 2.4 mg/d	5–17	101	Decreased tantrums, aggression, self-injury, hyperactivity	Weight gain; increased appetite; transient sedation
Risperidone	1.2–2.9 mg/d child Mean = 2.0 mg/d 2.4–5.3 mg/d adult Mean = 3.6 mg/d	8–56	36	Decreased irritability, hyperactivity	Increased appetite; weight gain; sedation
Risperidone	.125–.175 vs. 1.25–1.75 vs. placebo	5–17	96	Higher dose improves global function and irritability	Somnolence sedation increased appetite
Risperidone	0.01–0.06 mg/kg/d Mean = 1.17 mg/d	5–12	79	Decreased irritability, hyperactivity, noncompliance, conduct problems	Weight gain; transient somnolence; mildly increased heart rate and blood pressure
Risperidone	0.5–1.5 mg/d Mean = 1.14 mg/d	2.5–6	24	Minimal improvement in global autism severity scores	Weight gain; increased prolactin levels
Risperidone	1.0–10.0 mg/d	18–43	n =?	Reduced repetitive behavior, aggression, self-injury, property destruction	Transient sedation
Aripiprazole	5 mg/d, 10 mg/d, or 15 mg/d	6–17	218	Reduced irritability, hyperactivity, stereotypy at all doses	Sedation, EPS, weight gain
Aripiprazole	2–15 mg/d	6–17	98	Reduced irritability, hyperactivity, stereotypy, inappropriate speech; global improvement	Decreased prolactin level, weight gain, EPS
Aripiprazole	2–15 mg/d Continuation active tx vs. placebo	6–17	85	No difference in time to relapse	
Opiate Antagonists					
Naltrexone	1.0 mg/kg/d	3–8	41	No improvement over placebo in behavior and learning; improved hyperactivity	None greater than placebo
Naltrexone	1.0 mg/kg/d 2 weeks only	3–8	24	No improvement in communication skills	Transient sedation
Naltrexone	40 mg/d Single dose	3–7	23	Decreased hyperactivity, improved attention	Not reported
Naltrexone	1 mg/kg /dose	3–7	23	Decreased hyperactivity and improved attention by teacher, but not parent, report	No side effects
Serotonin Reuptake Inhibitors					
Fluvoxamine	Mean dose = 276.7 mg/d	18-53	n = 30	Reduced repetitive thoughts and behavior, and aggression; improved social communication	Transient nausea and sedation
Buspirone	2.5 mg or 5 mg /d	2–6	166	Improvement in repetitive behaviors not total ADOS	
Clomipramine	5–10 mg/d	8–17	34	No improvement executive fcn	Diarrhea, headache, fatigue
Fluoxetine	4.8–20 mg/d Mean = 10.6 mg/d; 0.38 mg/kg/d	5–17	39	Modest reduction in repetitive behaviors, but no improvement in global functioning	Agitation requiring dose reduction
Citalopram	2.5–20 mg/d Mean = 16.5 mg/d	5–17	149	No improvement in repetitive behavior or global functioning	Increased energy, inattention, impulsivity, hyperactivity, stereotypy, diarrhea, insomnia, dry skin
Stimulants					
Methylphenidate	0.125, 0.25, or 0.5 t.i.d. mg/kg /day	5–14	72	Reduced inattention, distractibility, hyperactivity, and impulsivity	Irritability, decreased appetite, difficulty falling asleep, emotional outbursts
Methylphenedate	.25, .5 mg/kg/dose	5–13	33	Positive efforts on social behavior	None discussed
Methylphenedate	10–40 LA AM, 2.5-10 mg afternoon	7–13	24	Decreased hyperactive and impulsive behavior	Loss of appetite, insomnia
Atomoxetine	20–100 mg/d Mean = 44.2 mg/d	5–15	16	Reduced hyperactivity, impulsivity, social withdrawal	Transient nausea and fatigue

Continued on following page

TABLE 57-2 Medications Used to Decrease Specific Symptoms Associated with Autism Spectrum Disorder* *(Continued)*

Drug	Dose	Age[†]	N	Efficacy	Side Effects
Antiseizure Drugs					
Lamotrigine	Mean = 5.0 mg/kg/d	3–11	28	No improvement greater than placebo in disruptive behavior and autism symptoms	Aggression, insomnia, echolalia
Levetiracetam	20–30 mg/kg/d	5–17	20	No improvement in disruptive behavior or irritability	aggression, agitation
Divalproex sodium	500–1500 mg/d	5–17	13	Reduction in compulsive-type repetitive behavior	Irritability, weight gain, aggression
Divalproex sodium	125 mg QD titrated up to 500 bid	5–17	27	Reduction in irritability	Irritability
Bumetanide	.5mg bid	3–11	60	Improved autistic behaviors and global function	Diarrhea, increased irritability

*Includes only double-blind, randomized, placebo-controlled trials.
†Age in years.
EPS, Extrapyramidal symptoms.

emerged in a few instances, although this is a seizure-prone population, and it is not clear whether the medications were causal. Concern has been raised about possible association of fluoxetine and other selective SRIs with suicidal ideation in depressed children, and the FDA has recommended that children taking these medications be carefully monitored. Evidence for developmentally sensitive altered regulation of serotonin synthesis in autistic children provides a rationale for giving serotonergic drugs to very young autistic children to improve synaptic plasticity during periods of brain development.

Medications to Treat Hyperactivity

Hyperactivity is an important target symptom that can be improved with psychostimulant medication. The Research Units on Pediatric Psychopharmacology (RUPP) Autism Network conducted a randomized, double-blind, placebo-controlled trial of methylphenidate in children with ASDs and high levels of hyperactivity and/or impulsiveness. Doses at the 0.25 and 0.5 mg/kg/day level were effective in reducing hyperactivity and impulsivity but less effective in reducing inattention, at 4 weeks and after 8 weeks. A randomized, crossover study of 24 children ages 7 to 12 showed that extended release MPH improves hyperactivity and impulsivity.

Atomoxetine is a nonstimulant medication for ADHD that inhibits the presynaptic norepinephrine transporter. In a placebo-controlled, double-blind crossover study with 16 children with ASD and ADHD symptoms, atomoxetine was more effective than placebo in reducing hyperactivity. The response rate was similar to that reported for methylphenidate, (mean highest dose was 44.2 [SD = 21.9] mg/d). Side effects, including gastrointestinal symptoms, fatigue, and tachycardia were common but transient. Other trials also demonstrated a beneficial effect of atomoxetine on hyperactivity in children with ASD. Two small placebo-controlled trials found that clonidine, an adrenergic receptor agonist, had some effect in decreasing irritability and hyperactivity in children and adults with autism.

Antiseizure Drugs

Antiseizure drugs have been used for behavioral manifestations of autism, particularly for treating intense rapid mood shifts. Small, randomized trials of lamotrigine and levetiracetam showed no benefits, but sodium divalproex showed some promise for irritability and repetitive behaviors. Bumetanide,

which is currently being evaluated for the treatment of neonatal seizures, was compared with placebo in 60 children (0.5mg bid) and improved both global functioning and some autistic behaviors. Larger placebo controlled trials are needed.

It has been hypothesized that the mechanism of benefit from these medications might be their effect on subclinical seizures. However, there is no evidence or controlled trial investigating whether treatment with anticonvulsants in children with autism, who have epileptiform discharges but no clinical seizures, might improve behavioral or developmental outcomes.

Cholinesterase Inhibitors

Acetylcholine (ACh) plays a significant role in attention and memory performance. Acetylcholinesterase inhibitors (AChE) slow the hydrolysis of ACh. Animal studies have suggested that administration of these agents early in development may enhance learning. A randomized, controlled 6-week trial, conducted in 43 children with autism showed that donepezil (2.5 mg/d), used for the treatment of memory decline, attention, and learning in Alzheimer disease, improved language and reduced overall autistic features. However, the analyses pooled blinded and nonblinded data, leaving the results susceptible to confounders such as placebo effects.

Glutaminergic and Gamma-Aminobutyric Acidergic Agents

On the theory that there is a disturbance of excitatory and inhibitory transmission in ASD, NMDA and GABA receptor modulators have been tried. Memantine and amantadine were not effective, but arabaclofen and oxytocin showed some benefit.

In summary, a number of medications, particularly atypical neuroleptics, psychostimulants, and SRIs, may help decrease specific symptoms associated with autism, such as behavioral outbursts, stereotypic or compulsive behaviors, aggression, anxiety, inattention, and oppositional behavior. Reduction in these behaviors can improve quality of life and promote better opportunities for learning. However, there must be careful attention to matching the medication with the targeted behavior and to possible developmental differences in treatment response. Side effects are common, must be monitored closely and weighed carefully against the drug's benefits.

Complementary and Alternative Medicine

A significant number of families seek complementary or alternative medicine (CAM) treatments, few of which have been studied in well-designed trials. Surveys have estimated that about one third of children were using complementary and alternative medicine. It is reasonable to respect the parents' belief if the complementary medicine is not toxic, but if the treatment is potentially harmful, negotiating a safer replacement practice should be attempted.

Children with autism often have sleep difficulties. Melatonin therapy has been used to treat the sleep disturbances in ASD, based on low plasma levels or urinary excretion of melatonin. Four double-blind, placebo-controlled crossover studies were performed in a total of 70 children with ASD using 3 to 10 mg of regular or controlled-release melatonin. Up to 94% of children derived significant benefits in sleep including sleep duration and latency but not awakenings, without evidence of significant side effects. An open-label melatonin study in 24 ASD children that involved titrating the dose to a maximum of 9 mg showed sleep latency improved at 1 or 3 mg doses. Larger long-term, double-blind, placebo-controlled crossover studies will be needed to document the efficacy of melatonin across the behavioral subtypes of ASD.

Immunoglobulin has been administered intravenously in open trials and not found to be useful. Reported dramatic improvement after the administration of secretin as part of endoscopy in three autistic children led to widespread use by parents. Subsequent blinded, randomized trials did not substantiate its efficacy.

Proponents of chelation therapy suggest that mercury and other heavy metals may be poorly eliminated by children with autism and that this interferes with neurodevelopment through modulation of immune function and other biochemical systems. Despite the lack of scientific evidence of a link between exposure to mercury or other heavy metals and autism, chelation is still used. No placebo-controlled studies have examined the safety or efficacy of chelation for treating autism, and deaths resulting from hypocalcemia have been reported from the inappropriate use of the chelator, edetate disodium (EDTA), including one boy with autism.

Hyperbaric oxygen therapy (HBOT) has been tried on the theory that autism is associated with oxidative stress and neuroinflammation. Although one randomized, controlled trial showed a few differences in outcome between control and HBOT treated groups, there were no differences when replicated, and HBOT carries a risk of barotrauma and exacerbation of pulmonary disease.

In summary, studies are negative or inadequate to recommend nutritional supplements, melatonin, hormones, gluten-free and casein-free diets, immunoglobulins, secretin, vitamin B6, magnesium, dimethylglycine, omega 3 fatty acids, HBOT, and chelation therapy. It is challenging to perform clinical trials enrolling children with autism, but without well-designed, blinded studies, safe and effective therapies cannot be determined. Problems include standardization of diagnoses, heterogeneity of target behaviors, and lack of cooperation of subjects. Whenever feasible, parents should be encouraged to participate in clinical trials to make progress in assessing new therapies. Information about ongoing trials and their locations can be found at www.clinicaltrials.gov.

EDUCATIONAL AND BEHAVIORAL INTERVENTIONS

The core deficits associated with autism affect all aspects of the individual's life, necessitating a comprehensive and multidisciplinary approach. The primary source of intervention for most children with ASD, from birth to age 21, is through the educational system. The Treatment and Education of Autistic and Related Communication Handicapped Children (TEACCH) Program is a structured teaching program founded at the University of North Carolina in the early 1970s. Originally developed as a classroom-based program for school-age children and adults, TEACCH has subsequently been adapted for home-based intervention for young children.

Intervention should be initiated as early as possible. Comprehensive early intervention programs based on basic learning principles for teaching skills and facilitating more appropriate and adaptive behaviors have been tested for their effectiveness in children and adults with autism and other developmental disabilities. Among the most extensively tested programs are Applied Behavioral Analysis (ABA) and Discrete Trial Training (DTT). Improvements in cognitive functioning and language level have been demonstrated at the group level. Improvements in adaptive behavior and autism symptoms have been more variable. Overall, baseline IQ and language skills predict better response to treatment. However, prediction at the individual level is not yet established.

Other comprehensive early education programs also have shown evidence of improving outcomes for children with ASD. Learning Experiences: Alternative Programs for Preschoolers and Parents (LEAP) was developed for implementation in early education classrooms. LEAP integrates behavioral techniques into naturalistic teaching situations, with a focus on integrating children with disabilities into the activities of typically developing children, and has a strong parent education component. Pivotal Response Treatment (PRT) is a naturalistic behavioral program that has been shown in single-subject design studies to be effective for young children with ASD, but has not undergone a randomized, controlled trial. The Denver Model and its adaptation for toddlers, the Early Start Denver Model (ESDM), emphasize the need to establish interpersonal relationships as a foundation to achieving other developmental milestones.

Core deficits in social understanding and social relationships are concerns throughout the life span, and social skills training (SST) is often a component of a treatment plan. Group-based SST programs show promise, but with a few exceptions, they have not been rigorously evaluated. The Joint Attention, Symbolic Play, and Regulation (JASPER) program is a parent-delivered, in-home, manualized treatment program for preschool children that has been shown to improve responsiveness to joint attention and initiation of joint attention, as well as symbolic play. The Children's Friendship Training (CFT) program for school-aged children integrates parents into a group-based social skills program focusing on behaviors critical to initiating and maintaining friendships. It was shown to improve social skills, friendship behaviors, and self-reported loneliness. The Program for the Education and Enrichment of Relational Skills (PEERS) is a group-based intervention for adolescents with ASD that integrates parents into the program to help with generalization of skills into the home and community. Studies demonstrated benefits in social skills and increased frequency of peer socialization.

The PEERS and CFT programs were originally developed for children with ADHD, and adapted for use in autism. Similarly, cognitive behavior therapy (CBT) for children with anxiety disorder has been effectively adapted to treat anxiety in high-functioning ASD. Adapting evidence-based interventions for specific symptom domains and comorbid symptoms in ASD is a reasonable strategy, but there remains a great need for rigorously designed research to demonstrate efficacy.

Although the needs of individuals with ASDs change over time, there is need for lifelong support. In particular, transitions (e.g., to high school, to higher education or vocational training, or to independent or assisted living) are critical periods during which supports already in place may be lost because of changes in eligibility or funding sources.

RESOURCES FOR FAMILIES AND PRACTITIONERS

- Autism Speaks (www.autismspeaks.org) offers numerous services and resources for families on its website. Of particular interest are the 100-Day Kits for parents of newly diagnosed young (https://www.autismspeaks.org/docs/family_services_docs/100day2/100_Day_Kit_Version_2_0.pdf) and for school-aged children 5 years and older (https://www.autismspeaks.org/sites/default/files/docs/100_day_kit_for_school_age_children_final_small.pdf) that are specifically developed to assist parents during the stressful period after diagnosis. There are additional Autism Speaks Tool Kits available addressing other topics, such as advocacy, behavioral health treatments, psychopharmacology and deciding whether to begin medication, toilet training, and sleep tools (https://www.autismspeaks.org/family_services/tool-kits).
- The American Academy of Pediatrics has a useful website (www.healthychildren.org) on which one can search on the topic "autism." The AAP has recently published a book specifically addressing pertinent behavioral and medical advice topics facing parents of children with ASD ranging in age from very young toddlers through adolescence (http://shop.aap.org/Autism-Spectrum-Disorders-What-Every-Parent-Needs-to-Know-Paperback/).
- The Department of Education's Center for Parent Information and Resources (www.parentcenterhub.org) has autism-specific information on special education laws and on educational practices.
- The Arc maintains a website (http://www.thearc.org/page.aspx?pid = 2530) for people with intellectual and developmental disabilities and their families that provides a wealth of information on the special education. The Arc's Autism Now Center provides information resources, including the IEP process (http://autismnow.org/).
- The Organization for Autism Research has several useful brochures and educational publications geared toward families, educators, and other professionals, many of which are in Spanish and English (www.researchautism.org).
- The National Autism Association's Big Red Safety Toolkit (http://nationalautismassociation.org/docs/BigRedSafetyToolkit.pdf) provides information and resources for families on wandering and water safety.
- The National Research Council produced a monograph that evaluated evidence-based interventions for children with ASD aged 8 years and under (http://www.nap.edu/openbook.php?isbn = 0309072697).
- For clinicians, the AAN/CNS Practice Parameter: Screening and Diagnosis of Autism (http://www.childneurologysociety.org/resources/resources-detail-view/practice-parameter-screening-and-diagnosis-of-autism) and the detailed background paper (http://www.childrenslearninginstitute.org/duncan-programs/autism-center/documents/AU2906_241reprint.pdf) continue to be a valuable resource.
- The First Signs program provides resources, including a video glossary of signs of ASD and referral guidelines. The First Signs website (http://firstsigns.org) includes recommendations and information about obtaining autism screening instruments. There are also summaries of evidence-based interventions available to parents and practitioners.
- The Agency for Healthcare Research and Quality provides a summary of the evidence for effectiveness of interventions for children, youth, and adults with ASD (http://effectivehealthcare.ahrq.gov).
- The National Autism Center (www.nationalautismcenter.org) provides resources for parents and professionals including a National Standards Report, which synthesizes research related to the effectiveness of interventions for ASD based on age, diagnostic groups, and intervention targets.
- The National Institutes of Health website (www.nih.gov) can be searched for current research, as can those of specific institutes, including the National Institute of Neurologic Disorders and Stroke (www.ninds.nih.gov), National Institute of Child Health and Human Development (www.nichd.nih.gov), and the National Institute of Mental Health (www.nimh.nih.gov). The CDC's National Center for Birth Defects and Developmental Disabilities has a website (www.cdc.gov/ncbddd/autism/index.html) devoted to providing evidence-based information on ASD and its treatment, including links to resources.
- The National Dissemination Center for Children with Disabilities is now affiliated with the Center for Parent Information and Resources (http://www.parentcenterhub.org/) has information on special education laws and on educational practices, among other timely topics.
- The federal Interagency Autism Coordinating Committee (IACC) website has compiled information about research and Federal activities related to research and service provision for ASD (http://iacc.hhs.gov/index.shtml).

DISCLAIMER

The views expressed in this chapter are those of the authors and do not necessarily reflect the official position of the National Institute of Mental Health, the National Institute of Neurologic Diseases and Stroke, the National Institutes of Health, or any other part of the U.S. Department of Health and Human Services.

REFERENCES

The complete list of references for this chapter is available in the e-book at www.expertconsult.com.
See inside cover for registration details.

SELECTED REFERENCES

American Psychiatric Association (APA), 2013. Diagnostic and Statistical Manual of Mental Disorders, fifth ed. American Psychiatric Association, Washington, DC.

Charman, T., Gotham, K., 2013. Measurement issues: screening and diagnostic instruments for autism spectrum disorders—lessons from research and practice. Child. Adolesc. Ment. Health 18 (1), 52–63.

Cooper, G.M., Coe, B.P., Girirajan, S., et al., 2011. A copy number variation morbidity map of developmental delay. Nat. Genet. 43 (9), 838–846.

Daniels, A.M., Mandell, D.S., 2013. Explaining differences in age at autism spectrum disorder diagnosis: a critical review. Autism 18 (5), 583–597.

Johnson, C.P., Myers, S.M., 2007. Identification and evaluation of children with autism spectrum disorders. Pediatrics 120 (5), 1183–1215; reaffirmed September 2010.

Kearney, H.M., Thorland, E.C., Brown, K.K., et al., 2011. American College of Medical Genetics standards and guidelines for interpretation and reporting of postnatal constitutional copy number variants. Genet. Med. 13 (7), 680–685. doi:10.1097/GIM.0b013e3182217a3a. PubMed PMID: 21681106.

Krumm, N., Turner, T.N., Baker, C., et al., 2015. Excess of rare, inherited truncating mutations in autism. Nat. Genet. 47 (6), 582–588.

McElhanon, B.O., McCracken, C., Karpen, S., et al., 2014. Gastrointestinal symptoms in autism spectrum disorder: a meta-analysis. Pediatrics 133 (5), 872–883. doi:10.1542/peds.2013-3995. PubMed PMID: 24777214.

Tuchman, R., Hirtz, D., Mamounas, L., 2013. NINDS epilepsy and autism spectrum disorders workshop report. Neurology 81, 1630–1636.

Williams, K., Brignell, A., Randall, M., et al., 2013. Selective serotonin reuptake inhibitors for autism spectrum disorders. Cochrane Database Syst. Rev. (8), CD004677.

58 Management of Common Comorbidities Associated with Neurodevelopmental Disorders

Darcy L. Fehlings, Melanie Penner, Elizabeth J. Donner, and Michael I. Shevell

An expanded version of this chapter is available on www.expertconsult.com. See inside cover for registration details.

Neurodevelopmental disorders are associated with health comorbidities and behavioral challenges. Comorbidities discussed in this chapter include hypertonia, musculoskeletal deformities, feeding and gastrointestinal issues, seizures, osteoporosis, sleep disorders, and behavior.

HYPERTONIA

Hypertonia is a resistance to passive stretch of a muscle across a joint and is divided into three subtypes: (i) spasticity, (ii) dystonia, and (iii) rigidity (Sanger et al., 2003). Spasticity is the presence of increasing tone with increasing speed of muscle stretch and the presence of a spastic catch. Dystonia is "a movement disorder in which involuntary sustained or intermittent muscle contractions cause twisting and repetitive movements, abnormal postures or both" (Sanger et al., 2003). Hypertonia is present in cerebral palsy (CP), acquired brain injury, and neurodegenerative or neurometabolic conditions. Spasticity and dystonia are common, and rigidity is rarely seen. Hypertonia contributes to impaired motor control, the development of contractures, pain, and challenges with caregiving.

Assessment

The Hypertonia Assessment Tool (HAT) has been developed to aid in identifying the hypertonia subtypes. Spasticity can be assessed by doing a slow and fast stretch of a muscle, with spasticity diagnosed if a spastic catch and increased tone are elicited with the fast stretch. Dystonia is characterized by fluctuations in tone, in which both tone and involuntary postures can be triggered by a tactile stimulus or a voluntary movement in another body part. Clinicians use the Modified Ashworth Scale and the Modified Tardieu Scale to measure the severity of spasticity. The Modified Ashworth Scale grades the severity of the hypertonia on a 5-point ordinal scale (Table 58-1).

The Modified Tardieu Scale consists of performing a muscle stretch at two velocities, slow and fast, with measurement of the angle of the spastic catch in the fast stretch (defined as R1) and passive range during the slow stretch (defined as R2). The angular difference between R1 and R2 is defined as the dynamic window and represents the therapeutic opportunity for spasticity reduction treatments such as botulinum toxin injections. For dystonia, the Burke-Fahn-Marsden Dystonia Rating Scale and the Barry-Albright Dystonia Scale are used to grade severity.

Interventions

Hypertonia reduction goals include the following:

1. enhanced motor performance,
2. as an adjunct to casting/splinting to increase or maintain range,
3. pain relief, and
4. enhanced caregiver ease of care.

The determination of goals is done with the child's physical abilities in mind. For example, in children with CP, motor abilities are graded using the Gross Motor Function Classification Scale (GMFCS) (Palisano et al., 1997) (Table 58-2).

For children who are ambulatory (GMFCS level of I-III), hypertonia intervention goals focus on enhanced motor performance and maintaining range. For a severe physical disability, goals focus on ease of care and pain relief. Intervention approaches are also based on whether a child has generalized or focal hypertonia. For generalized hypertonia, oral medications or intrathecal baclofen may be good options; for focal hypertonia, botulinum toxin A injections may be a consideration.

Spasticity Interventions

A systematic review of pharmacologic treatment of spasticity in CP identified that for focal spasticity that warrants treatment, botulinum toxin type A should be offered as an effective and generally safe treatment (level A) (Quality Standards Subcommittee of the American Academy of Neurology et al., 2010). For generalized spasticity that warrants treatment, diazepam should be considered for short-term treatment (level B), and tizanidine may be considered (level C). There was insufficient evidence to support or refute the use of dantrolene, oral baclofen, or continuous intrathecal baclofen (level U).

1. Nonpharmacologic Rehabilitation Strategies

All children with hypertonia benefit from rehabilitation consult to consider the following:

- stretching and positioning,
- splinting,
- casting a muscle to provide a prolonged stretch, and
- assessment of specialized equipment needs.

2. Oral Medications for Spasticity

Oral medications are used for generalized hypertonia when the hypertonia significantly affects care or comfort. A conservative approach is undertaken, given the potential for cognitive side effects.

Baclofen is a muscle relaxant that is an agonist for gamma-aminobutyric acid (GABA) B receptors on both presynaptic and postsynaptic neurons in the spinal cord and the brain. Baclofen is the drug of first choice for many clinicians; however, studies show inconsistent evidence. It has a short half-life (4.5 hours) and is given orally 3 to 4 times per day. Dosing recommendations are up to 2 mg/kg/day (80 mg maximal dosage), starting at a lower dosage (e.g., 2.5 mg 3 times a day) and titrating upward. Side effects include drowsiness, which can be minimized by increasing the dosage slowly. The long-term effects on cognitive function are unknown. If baclofen is discontinued, the child should be weaned to avoid withdrawal.

TABLE 58-1 Modified Ashworth Scale

Modified Ashworth Scale Grade	Descriptor
0	No increase in muscle tone
1	Slight increase in muscle tone, manifested by a catch and release or by minimal resistance at the end of the range of motion when the affected part(s) is(are) moved in flexion or extension
1+	Slight increase in muscle tone, manifested by a catch followed by minimal resistance through the remainder of the range of motion, but the affected part(s) is(are) easily moved
2	More marked increase in muscle tone through most of the range of movement, but the affected part(s) is(are) easily moved
3	Considerable increases in muscle tone; passive movement difficult
4	Affected part(s) is(are) rigid in flexion or extension

(Adapted from Mutlu A, Livanelioglu A, Gunel MK. BMC Musculoskelet Disord 2008; 9:44.)

TABLE 58-2 Gross Motor Function Classification System (Children Aged 6–12 Years)

Level I	Walks without restrictions; limitations in more advanced motor skills
Level II	Walks without assistive devices; limitations walking outdoors and in the community
Level III	Walks with assistive mobility devices; limitations walking outdoors and in the community
Level IV	Self-mobility with limitations; children are transported or use power mobility outdoors and in the community
Level V	Self-mobility is extremely limited even with the use of assistive technology

(Adapted from Palisano R, Rosenbaum P, Walter S, et al. Dev Med Child Neurol 1997; 39:214–223.)

Diazepam binds the benzodiazepine-GABA receptor complex presynaptically and postsynaptically and augments GABA-mediated inhibition at the spinal cord. Diazepam is the drug of first choice for muscle spasms following orthopedic surgery. It is given three to four times per day as required, with dosage ranges of 1 to 5 mg per dose for children greater than 5 years of age. Side effects include drowsiness, memory impairment, and respiratory depression.

Tizanidine binds alpha1 adrenergic receptors presynaptically and inhibits the release of excitatory neurotransmitters in the spine. It has been used in adolescents as a second-line medication. Dosing has not been established in pediatrics, with adult dosing being a 2- to 8-mg/dose given 2 to 4 times per day. Side effects include liver dysfunction and sedation.

3. Neurosurgical Procedures

Intrathecal baclofen treatment consists of a pump with a reservoir for liquid baclofen that is inserted into the abdominal wall; the pump is connected to a catheter that is inserted into the intrathecal space, with the tip in the cervical or thoracic region. Baclofen is delivered as an infusion and binds to GABA

B receptors in the dorsal cord, with the dose typically ranging from 300 to 800 micrograms per day. This treatment is often reserved for severe generalized spasticity. Side effects include infections, respiratory depression, and withdrawal, including severe muscle spasms if there is a problem with the drug delivery system.

Selective dorsal rhizotomy involves a partial transection of the dorsal nerve root in the lumbar and sacral nerve roots (L1 to S2), producing a permanent reduction of spasticity in the legs. The evidence for its effectiveness to improve long-term motor outcomes is inconclusive. A critique of the evidence includes small sample sizes with limited power to explore subgroups of children who may respond better than others. Rhizotomies continue to be offered in select clinics, typically to children with bilateral spastic CP–spastic diplegic subtype who are functioning at a GMFCS level of II to III. Current surgical techniques have good safety records with minimal side effects.

4. Botulinum Toxin Injections

Botulinum toxin injections are used for focal management. The toxin creates a reversible neuromuscular blockade, with tone reduction that lasts approximately 2 to 3 months. There is level A evidence for its use to improve short-term motor function in children when paired with therapy as compared with therapy alone (Quality Standards Subcommittee of the American Academy of Neurology et al., 2010). Potential indications are enhanced motor function, improved range in hypertonic muscles when paired with splinting/casting, ease of caregiving, salivary management, and relief of spasms. Side effects include localized weakness and the potential for systemic spread.

Treatment of Dystonia

Dystonia can be treated with many of the options outlined previously, including rehabilitation, oral medications such as baclofen and benzodiazepines (diazepam, lorazepam), intrathecal baclofen, and botulinum toxin injections. In addition, trihexyphenidyl and deep-brain stimulation can be considered.

Trihexyphenidyl inhibits excess cholinergic activity. Many clinicians use this as their drug of first choice, although there is minimal evidence for its effectiveness. Starting dosages are between 0.1 and 0.2 mg/kg/day in 3 to 4 divided doses. The dosage is gradually increased to 0.5 to 0.75 mg/kg/day. Side effects include dry mouth, blurred vision, confusion or sedation, urinary retention, nausea, and chorea.

Deep-brain stimulation involves the stimulation/modulation of the globus pallidus to reduce dystonia. Research has demonstrated some effectiveness for individuals with dystonic CP. This procedure is considered in severe generalized dystonia associated with pain. Potential side effects include complications from insertion of the electrodes, including hemorrhages and infection.

MUSCULOSKELETAL DEFORMITIES

Individuals with spasticity can develop contractures and bony deformities. Musculoskeletal (MSK) deformities in nonhypertonic neurodevelopmental disorders include atlanto-axial instability and scoliosis.

Muscles that are spastic contract as the child grows, putting the child at risk for development of contractures. Strategies to promote flexibility include stretching, positioning, splints, and serial casting. Tendon releases/lengthening can be undertaken.

Children with physical disabilities are at risk for hip subluxation and dislocation (Shore, Spence, and Graham, 2012). For children with hypertonia, hip dislocation can be painful. Hip surveillance is critical and consists of a clinical assessment (e.g., GMFCS level, hip pain, difficulty opening the legs for caregiving) and an anterior-posterior (AP) x-ray with measurement of Reimer's migration percentage. Management includes positioning and bracing to stretch the adductor muscles. Surgical approaches include soft tissue releases and bony reconstruction, including femoral varus derotation osteotomies plus or minus a pelvic osteotomy.

Children with neurologic disorders (e.g., CP, Rett syndrome, Duchenne muscular dystrophy) can develop progressive scoliosis. If present, an AP spine x-ray determines the curvature (defined as the Cobb angle). An orthopedic consult is recommended. Smaller curvatures are managed with customized seating or bracing; however, if the curvature is large and progressive, spinal instrumentation is recommended.

Atlanto-axial instability (AAI) occurs when there is excessive movement between the atlas (C1) and axis (C2), and spinal compression can ensue. It is seen in Down syndrome, osteogenesis imperfecta, and skeletal dysplasias. Clinical symptoms include neck pain, spasticity, and torticollis. If warranted, a lateral cervical x-ray should be performed. AAI is defined as a distance of greater than 5 mm between the odontoid process and the posterior border of the anterior arch of the atlas.

FEEDING AND GASTROINTESTINAL ISSUES

Children with neurodevelopmental disorders are at higher risk for feeding and nutritional problems as compared with their typically developing peers. Over half of children with CP experience difficulties with feeding or nutrition, with a higher risk of these issues in those more severely affected by the disorder. Children with neurodevelopmental disorders may have either increased or decreased resting energy expenditure compared with their typically developing peers (Marchand et al., 2006). Children with autism spectrum disorders (ASD) may have restricted diets because of their insistence on sameness in meals or sensory aversions to certain tastes or textures. Nutritional issues can result in growth failure, overweight, micronutrient deficiencies, and osteopenia, putting the child at risk of further impairment. Successful management of feeding and nutrition issues can result in fewer hospitalizations and a better overall health status for this population.

Assessment of Feeding and Nutrition

Parents commonly experience anxiety about their child's eating habits, and it is best to first elicit the parents' concerns as well as the influence of the family's social and cultural expectations for eating. A thorough medical history should follow and must include a respiratory history to assess for any indication of aspiration leading to respiratory disease, and a gastrointestinal history eliciting symptoms of gastroesophageal reflux (GER), vomiting, or constipation. Medications such as atypical antipsychotics may result in increased appetite, whereas others, such as stimulants used in the treatment of attention-deficit/hyperactivity disorder (ADHD), may lead to decreased appetite. An essential element of the history is a description of the child's developmental skills; this will provide the lens through which to determine expectations for feeding skills. The clinician then obtains a detailed feeding history (Table 58-3).

When possible, age-referenced growth percentiles for height, weight, and body mass index should be monitored using the World Health Organization growth charts (or CDC

TABLE 58-3 Feeding History

MODE OF FEEDING	By mouth, nasogastric tube, gastrostomy tube, gastrojejunal tube
TIMING OF FEEDING	Time of meals and snacks Length of meals Length of feeds for those with feeding tubes (including continuous/overnight feeding)
LOCATION OF FEEDING	Positioning (upright versus supine—may be relevant for gastroesophageal reflux) Seating support (consider gross motor developmental level) Behavioral elements (e.g., at the table versus in front of television)
NUTRITIONAL COMPOSITION AND VARIETY OF FOOD	Food offered at each meal Same or different from what the rest of the family is eating Considerations of food groups, caloric intake, and vitamins/minerals/fiber
CONSISTENCY OF FOOD	The prepared texture of the food Which consistencies cause problems (solids versus thin liquids) Concurrent difficulty managing oral secretions
DESCRIPTION OF THE CHILD DURING FEEDING	Delayed or multiple swallows (indicative of oral-motor coordination difficulties) Gasping/choking (indicative of aspiration) Arching (indicative of gastroesophageal reflux)

(Adapted from Marchand V, Motil KJ, NASPGHAN Nutrition Committee. J Pediatr Gastroenterol Nutr 2006; 43:123–135.)

charts after 2 years of age). For a child whose height is limited by the disorder, it may be necessary to plot weight according to the age at which the child's height represents the 50th percentile. In children with musculoskeletal issues preventing accurate measurement of height, measurements of the upper arm and lower leg can be obtained and compared against reference standards. Other measurements, such as triceps skinfold thickness, can provide information about the child's nutritional status.

A systematic physical examination should follow. The respiratory examination should include auscultation for any signs of chronic lung disease resulting from aspiration. The gastrointestinal examination should include examination of dentition (including signs of enamel erosion from GER) and a full abdominal examination. A fecal mass felt in the abdomen indicates constipation.

Investigations

The most definitive investigation for dysphagia is the video fluoroscopic swallowing study, in which the child is given various textures of food mixed with barium. The progression of the barium from the mouth to the stomach is captured on video to assess for aspiration, dysmotility, and GER.

Management of Common Feeding and Nutritional Issues

Gastroesophageal Reflux

GER is a common comorbidity and can be an important cause of pain. Medical management begins with a proton-pump inhibitor. Medications such as domperidone can be used to promote gastric motility, although there are potentially significant adverse effects associated with these agents, including cardiac conduction abnormalities. If conservative measures fail, a gastrostomy/gastrojejunal feeding tube or surgical fundoplication may be warranted.

Constipation

Constipation is a common condition in children with neurodevelopmental disorders. Polyethylene glycol is a well-tolerated and effective oral agent. Management usually begins with a dose to achieve a "cleanout," with the goal being to completely empty the bowel. After this, polyethylene glycol can be titrated to a dose that results in a daily soft bowel movement.

Need for Gastrostomy Feeding Tubes

Because of difficulties in oral-motor coordination, prolonged feeding time, and the potential for nutritional deficiencies, some children with neurodevelopmental disorders require a feeding tube. Although this is often a difficult decision for parents, gastrostomy tubes are associated with improved weight gain, decreased feeding time, and increased quality of life for caregivers.

SEIZURES IN NEURODEVELOPMENTAL DISORDERS

Seizures and epilepsy, the condition of recurrent unprovoked seizures, affect up to 50% of children with neurodevelopmental disorders (Depositario-Cabacar and Zelleke, 2010). Seizures are more likely in children with more complex neurodevelopmental disabilities (Faulkner and Singh, 2013). Children with CP and intellectual disability or ASD and intellectual disability are more at risk of seizures than those with intellectual disability alone. In contrast to typically developing children, those with neurodevelopmental disorders are also more likely to have both earlier-onset epilepsy and lifelong drug-resistant seizures.

Diagnosis

Diagnosis of seizures in children with neurodevelopmental disorders may be difficult because of the presence of stereotypies and motor and cognitive impairments that mimic seizures. Children with neurodevelopmental disorders often present with nonepileptic events that resemble clinical seizures without an electrographic correlate. When clinical seizures are suspected, a careful history should include an account of clinical events that details semiology, duration, and frequency. If the history is suggestive of seizures, an electroencephalogram (EEG) should be performed.

EEGs may demonstrate both nonepileptiform and epileptiform abnormalities. Nonepileptiform abnormalities, such as focal and/or generalized slowing, are more likely to be identified in children with neurodevelopmental abnormalities and are not necessarily associated with an increased risk of seizures. Epileptiform abnormalities, such as spike and slow-wave discharges, are associated with an increased risk of seizures. With a strong clinical history for seizures and an EEG finding of epileptiform discharges, a presumptive diagnosis of seizures can be made. When clinical events are difficult to characterize, a prolonged video EEG may capture events to clarify diagnosis.

Children with neurodevelopmental disorders may have abnormalities on EEGs, even in the absence of clinical seizures. The contribution of epileptiform discharges to cognitive impairment in children with neurodevelopmental disorders remains controversial. In the syndromes of continuous spike-wave in sleep (CSWS) and Landau–Kleffner syndrome (LKS), typically developing children present with electrical status epilepticus of sleep (ESES) and cognitive regression. Successful treatment and resolution of the ESES is associated with an improvement in cognition, suggesting that the epileptiform discharges, rather than seizures, are responsible for the cognitive regression. However, whether this phenomenon can be generalized to children with cognitive impairment in the context of other neurodevelopmental disorders is not clear.

Treatment

The goal of seizure treatment is the same in all children: freedom from seizures without treatment side effects and optimized quality of life. There are some special considerations when treating seizures in children with neurodevelopmental disorders.

Antiepileptic Drug Adverse Effects

Children with neurodevelopmental disabilities may not be able to clearly communicate the presence of treatment-related adverse effects. It is important to inform caregivers of the potential for specific adverse effects to allow for careful monitoring at home. Children with an intellectual disability may be more sensitive to the sedation associated with some antiepileptic drugs (AEDs). Nonverbal children may demonstrate agitation or aggression in response to certain AEDs. When caregivers report adverse effects, a dose reduction may be sufficient to reduce the effect. When dose adjustments do not result in remission of adverse effects, a change in AED should be undertaken.

Polypharmacy

Children with neurodevelopmental disorders often have multiple seizure types and drug-resistant seizures requiring multiple AEDs. Because polypharmacy is associated with an increased incidence of adverse effects, efforts should be made to minimize polytherapy. This may include reducing the number of AEDs or reducing the dose of each AED when multiple drugs are used in combination. When a single drug fails to control seizures and a second is added with good effect, an effort should be made to reduce the first drug to avoid polypharmacy. When required, the adverse effects of polypharmacy can be limited by selecting drugs that utilize varied mechanisms of action and by considering drug interactions.

Withdrawal of Antiepileptic Drugs

Although many children with seizures and neurodevelopmental disabilities will require lifelong AED therapy, withdrawal of the AED should be *considered* in children who have been seizure-free for 2 years or more. Caregivers should be instructed in the use of a rescue medication, such as rectal, nasal, or buccal benzodiazepines.

Drug-Resistant Epilepsy

Children with neurodevelopmental disorders often present with drug-resistant seizures, defined as failure to achieve seizure freedom with an adequate trial of two appropriate AEDs. These children should be referred to a comprehensive epilepsy program for surgical assessment. For children not deemed to be resection surgery candidates, vagal nerve stimulation and ketogenic diet treatment should be considered.

Treating Seizures in Children with Attention-Deficit/Hyperactivity Disorder

There has been concern that medications used to treat ADHD may lower the seizure threshold in children with and without epilepsy. This is not well supported by evidence, but is frequently listed in information leaflets. An evidence-based review determined that methylphenidate is associated with a low risk of seizures in children with well-controlled epilepsy. There is also emerging evidence that methylphenidate can be used safely in children with difficult-to-treat epilepsy. In clinical practice, ADHD treatments are frequently combined with AEDs. When seizure frequency increases with the addition of an ADHD treatment, an adjustment to AED treatment may be needed.

Treating Seizures in Children with Cerebral Palsy

The sedating effects of some AEDs may particularly affect children with low axial tone, resulting in impaired swallowing and risk of aspiration. Caregivers should be advised to monitor for sedation and changes in airway protection in vulnerable children. Excess sedation may also have an adverse effect on quality of life in children with CP.

FRAGILITY FRACTURES (OSTEOPOROSIS)

Children with physical disabilities can sustain fragility fractures. Decreased weight bearing, poor nutritional status, and medications (e.g., steroids and AEDs) increase risk. An evidence-informed practice guideline recommends preventative strategies of optimizing nutrition and dietary calcium, supplementing vitamin D, and promoting weight-bearing activity (Fehlings et al., 2012). For individuals with a fragility fracture, a bone mineral density test should be undertaken and bisphosphonates considered.

SLEEP DISORDERS

Up to 80% of children with neurodevelopmental disorders experience sleep disorders, including difficulty initiating or maintaining sleep and sleep-disordered breathing, such as obstructive sleep apnea (Simard-Tremblay et al., 2011). Sleep difficulties influence behavior and learning, and create chronic stress for caregivers.

It is important to consider underlying triggers for night awakenings. Children with hypertonia can experience muscle pain, leading to awakenings. Children with severe physical disabilities are not able to reposition themselves and require repositioning. Pain from esophagitis is worsened when the child lies down. Seizures can lead to disrupted sleep.

Behavioral approaches can be considered for difficulty initiating and maintaining sleep, with a focus on establishing a bedtime routine, teaching the child to fall asleep alone, and minimizing positive interactions that happen during the night (e.g., parental contact). Behavioral approaches should be tried before medications (e.g., melatonin or clonazepam). A systematic review of melatonin found it to be "probably effective" at assisting with bedtime settling, but not effective for night awakenings.

BEHAVIOR

Behavioral problems are among the most frequent concerns in children with neurodevelopmental disorders. Many neurodevelopmental disorders have a high co-occurrence with other behavior-based disorders; for instance, the reported frequency of ADHD symptoms in children with ASD ranges from 20% to 78%.

Although there is a biological basis underpinning behavior problems in neurodevelopmental disorders, it is important to remember that behavior is shaped by interactions with the environment. Because of this, it is important not to simply attribute the problem behavior to the diagnosis, as a more in-depth exploration can lead to effective management strategies. It is also essential to base one's behavioral expectations on the child's developmental age, instead of chronologic age.

Assessment of Behavior

The list of medical conditions that can present with a change in behavior covers every bodily system. Individuals with difficulty communicating may have trouble expressing pain, and any change in behavior needs to be met with a thorough review of systems to ensure that no treatable source of pain is missed. Investigations should be based on a differential diagnosis and should be undertaken systematically.

Many behavior experts suggest an ABC approach to evaluating behavior (Antecedent conditions, Behavior, and Consequences). Antecedent conditions are those that directly precede the behavior. One useful question to ask parents and caregivers is, "If I were to offer you a large sum of money to get the child to perform the behavior, what strategy would you try?" This can often help to identify the most successful strategy. Next, the clinician should get a thorough description of the target behavior by asking whether the behavior is directed toward others, property, or the child himself or herself. This can provide clues to the underlying function of the behavior (is there something the child is trying to gain/avoid?), and help to identify significant safety concerns that warrant more intensive intervention. The consequences for behavior powerfully shape the likelihood of using the same behavior in the future. If the child is inadvertently rewarded for the behavior, this may further reinforce it.

Consideration must also be given to the child's social situation. Changes in behavior are a common presenting symptom of nonaccidental injury or neglect, and the clinician must always be attuned to and ready to report any indication of maltreatment. The social situation may also inform the management strategy, because the insight and willingness of families needed to implement behavioral strategies will differ.

General Principles of Management of Behavior Problems

In general, behavioral interventions should be attempted before prescribing psychoactive medications. Behavioral strategies are developed after assessing the function of the behavior using the ABC method and can focus on both antecedent conditions and consequences. Some common strategies to improve antecedent conditions include providing ample warning for transitions, avoiding moving from preferred to nonpreferred activities, and allowing choices between acceptable activities. Basic consequence-based strategies can include a token economy or reward system and redirection to an alternative activity. If simple measures are not effective, consultation with an expert in behavioral management is appropriate.

Psychopharmacology

A full discussion of the use of psychoactive medications is beyond the scope of this chapter. For some neurodevelopmental disorders, such as ADHD, there are various medications with good evidence of effectiveness. For other disorders, such as ASD, there are currently no medications that treat the core symptoms, and instead medications are often prescribed based on co-occurring symptoms, such as ADHD-like symptoms, anxiety, or aggression. When considering prescribing a medication for a child with a neurodevelopmental disorder, it is important to clearly define the target behavior(s) and to determine how any improvement will be demonstrated. Further, psychoactive medications have varying adverse-effect profiles, and it is important to routinely monitor for these. An excellent resource for monitoring for adverse effects of atypical antipsychotics is the 2015 Canadian Alliance for Monitoring Effectiveness and Safety of Antipsychotics in Children (CAMESA) guideline.

REFERENCES

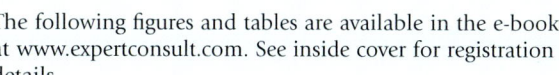
The complete list of references for this chapter is available in the e-book at www.expertconsult.com.

See inside cover for registration details.

SELECTED REFERENCES

Canadian Alliance for Monitoring Effectiveness and Saftey of Antipsychotics in Children (CAMESA). CAMESA guidelines. Available from: <http://camesaguideline.org>. Updated 2015.

Depositario-Cabacar, D.F., Zelleke, T.G., 2010. Treatment of epilepsy in children with developmental disabilities. Dev. Disabil. Res. Rev. 16, 239–247.

Faulkner, M.A., Singh, S.P., 2013. Neurogenetic disorders and treatment of associated seizures. Pharmacotherapy 33, 330–343.

Fehlings, D., Switzer, L., Agarwal, P., et al., 2012. Informing evidence-based clinical practice guidelines for children with cerebral palsy at risk of osteoporosis: a systematic review. Dev. Med. Child Neurol. 54, 106–116.

Marchand, V., Motil, K.J., NASPGHAN Nutrition Committee, 2006. Nutrition support for neurologically impaired children: A clinical report of the north american society for pediatric gastroenterology, hepatology, and nutrition. J. Pediatr. Gastroenterol. Nutr. 43 (1), 123–135.

Palisano, R., Rosenbaum, P., Walter, S., et al., 1997. Development and reliability of a system to classify gross motor function in children with cerebral palsy. Dev. Med. Child Neurol. 39, 214–223.

Quality Standards Subcommittee of the American Academy of Neurology, the Practice Committee of the Child Neurology Society, Delgado, M.R., et al., 2010. Practice parameter: pharmacologic treatment of spasticity in children and adolescents with cerebral palsy (an evidence-based review): report of the Quality Standards Subcommittee of the American Academy of Neurology and the Practice Committee of the Child Neurology Society. Neurology 74, 336–343.

Sanger, T.D., Delgado, M.R., Gaebler-Spira, D., et al., 2003. Classification and definition of disorders causing hypertonia in childhood. Pediatrics 111, e89–e97.

Shore, B., Spence, D., Graham, H., 2012. The role for hip surveillance in children with cerebral palsy. Curr. Rev. Musculoskelet. Med. 5, 126–134.

Simard-Tremblay, E., Constantin, E., Gruber, R., et al., 2011. Sleep in children with cerebral palsy: a review. J. Child Neurol. 26, 1303–1310.

E-BOOK TABLE

The following figures and tables are available in the e-book at www.expertconsult.com. See inside cover for registration details.

Table 58-4 Summary of Common Comorbidities and Treatments

Treatment of Neurodevelopmental Disorders

Clara D.M. van Karnebeek, Elizabeth Berry-Kravis, and Andrea Gropman

INTRODUCTION

This chapter aims to provide an overview of the exciting advances made over the past decades in the development and implementation of "targeted" or "causal" treatments for neurodevelopmental disorders (NDDs), defined as interventions targeting the underlying pathophysiology at a cellular or molecular level. NDDs can be regarded as phenotypes of many genetic conditions with manifestations that include intellectual developmental disability (IDD; defined as intellectual disability with an IQ < 70 at age 5+ years or global developmental delay with deficits in two or more developmental domains at < 5 years), learning disabilities, or autism spectrum disorder (ASD), with or without comorbidities such as epilepsy, cerebral palsy/motor dysfunction, and behavioral disturbances/psychiatric diseases. In this chapter we briefly discuss causal therapies for the following sets of conditions: (1) genetic NDD syndromes, including fragile X syndrome (FXS), Rett syndrome (RS), tuberous sclerosis complex (TSC), and Down syndrome (DS); and (2) inborn errors of metabolism (IEMs) and congenital hypothyroidism (CH). Although NDDs are heterogeneous in etiology, phenotypic presentation, and treatment types, early identification is a prerequisite for initiation of specific intervention to improve outcomes and reduce family burden. Diagnosis is a challenge given the rarity of these conditions, so general awareness and tools (genome-wide sequencing, digital apps) to facilitate diagnosis by clinicians are essential. A systematic approach to the identification of genetic conditions amenable to treatment in children with NDDs shows that collectively these rare diseases account for a significant proportion of cases. The effects, types, and accessibility of treatments vary widely between disorders and patients. Low patient numbers combined with a large heterogeneity in genotypes, phenotypes, and response size and type pose significant challenges to meeting evidence-based standards for treatments. We outline approaches to these challenges and progress in treatment of NDDs.

RETT SYNDROME, DOWN SYNDROME, TUBEROUS SCLEROSIS, AND FRAGILE X SYNDROME

General Concepts Surrounding Treatment for Neurodevelopmental Disorders

Given the impossibility of doing controlled trials for every treatment used in a rare NDD, current medical treatments utilized for NDDs are often employed off-label based on a generalization from other disorders and/or based on symptoms for which there are approved treatments. For only a handful of cases are there specific disease-related treatments approved by the U.S. Food and Drug Administration (FDA) that have demonstrated efficacy in controlled trials. Historically, treatment for NDDs has been almost entirely supportive, designed to support the person to achieve the highest level of adaptive development and function possible and treat co-occurring medical, neurologic, and behavioral symptoms

that may be interfering with function. This could include medical support for control of seizures, sleep management, behavioral modification and/or psychopharmacology for maladaptive behaviors, and special education programs, in addition to cognitive behavioral, occupational, speech/language, and physical therapy. These interventions do not fully treat the disorder and are not directed at the underlying mechanism of disease. Thus there is clearly an unmet need in NDDs, and treatments that modify the underlying disorders would be a tremendous advance.

NDDs have a highly heterogenous etiology with many very-low-incidence but high-impact single-gene or contiguous-gene causes, and even more combinations of common low-impact genetic risk factors operating in concert. Because targeting such a broad array of potential etiologies with specific therapies is virtually incomprehensible, single-gene NDDs, such as TSC, FXS, and RS, have emerged as neurobiological models in which extensive study of the neurobiology and synaptic mechanisms of disease in cellular and animal models has identified compounds that target the underlying disorder. These conditions also serve as clinical models for translation of such targeted treatments to humans. DS, with abnormal gene dose for many genes, is a model for identifying the final common effects of multiple gene defects at a systems level in the brain and then directing treatment to correction of the systems defect. Table 59-1 shows targeted treatments now being explored for genetic NDDs.

Rett Syndrome

RS is primarily caused by loss-of-function mutations in the X-linked *MeCP2* (*methyl-CpG-binding protein 2*) gene (Pozzo-Miller, Pati, and Percy, 2015). Girls are predominantly affected, with variation in the phenotype related to both genotype and X-inactivation. Girls with classical RS have normal early growth and development up to 6 to 18 months, followed by regression with acquired microcephaly, a loss of purposeful hand use, stereotyped movements including hand wringing, gait apraxia and ataxia, tremor, seizures, apnea, hyperventilation, severe IDD, and features of ASD.

MeCP2 codes for a protein that binds to methylated DNA and regulates gene transcription. Genetic correction and restoration of *MeCP2* gene expression in neurons or glia has proven to be sufficient to rescue abnormal behavioral and synaptic phenotypes of the MeCP2 knockout mouse. *MeCP2* appears to regulate insulin-like growth factor-1 (IGF-1) and Akt signaling activity in the MeCP2 knockout mouse, and IGF-1 or its terminal tripeptide restores dendritic spine dynamics and reverses many Rett-like features, including locomotor impairment, breathing abnormalities, and heart-rate irregularities, in MeCP2 knockout mice.

A phase 1 proof-of-concept trial of recombinant human IGF-1 in girls with RS showed good safety and improved apnea, anxiety, and mood scores, along with reversal of right frontal alpha-band asymmetry on electroencephalogram (EEG). A phase 2a double-blind placebo-controlled trial of NNZ-2566 (Neuren Pharmaceuticals), a peptidase-resistant

TABLE 59-1 Targeted Treatments in Clinical Development (2015) for Genetically Defined Neurodevelopmental Disorders*

NDD	Treatment	Target From Animal/Cellular Models	Development Phase
Fragile X syndrome	Lithium	Inhibits excessive GSK3B signaling and PI turnover	1
	AFQ056	mGluR5 NAM—reduces mGluR5-regulated activation of dendritic translation	2b
	RO4917523	mGluR5 NAM—reduces mGluR5-regulated activation of dendritic translation	2b
	Arbaclofen	GABA-B agonist—reduces presynaptic glutamate release	3
	Minocycline	Reduces excessive activity of MMP-9 resulting from dysregulation in absence of FMRP	2
	Ganaxolone	GABA-A agonist—increases deficient GABA signaling	2
	Acamprosate	GABA-A/B agonist	2
	NNZ-2566	Inhibits excessive ERK/Akt signaling	2
	Metadoxine	Inhibits excessive ERK/Akt signaling	2
	Lovastatin	Inhibits ERK pathway	1
Down syndrome	RG1662	GABA-A α5 receptor subunit inverse agonist—reduces excessive GABA signaling	2b
Rett syndrome	Mecasermin (rhIGF-1)	Activation of Akt pathway	1
	NNZ-2566	Akt pathway effects, reversal of LTP/dendritic spine deficits	2
	Fingolimod	Increases BDNF through binding of S1P receptors	1
	Glatiramer Acetate	Increases BDNF	2
Tuberous sclerosis complex	Everolimus	Inhibits excessive mTOR activity	2
Neurofibromatosis	Everolimus	Inhibits excessive mTOR activity	2
	Lovastatin	Inhibits ERK pathway	2
Phelan–McDermid syndrome	IGF-1 (Increlex)	Activation of Akt pathway	2
Angelman syndrome	Minocycline	Increase LTP	2
Prader–Willi syndrome	Oxytocin	Deficit in oxytocin neurons	2

*BDNF, brain-derived neurotrophic factor; GABA, gamma-aminobutyric acid; IGF-1, insulin-like growth factor-1; LTP, long-term potentiation; mTOR, mammalian target of rapamycin; NAM, negative allosteric modulator; NDD, neurodevelopmental disorder.

analog of the IGF-1 terminal tripeptide, in 53 girls with *MeCP2* mutation-confirmed RS showed good safety, improvement in three different efficacy domains, and improvement in a subject-specific efficacy score summing the direction of change in all efficacy outcome measures when compared for NNZ-2566 and placebo. This analysis itself represents a novel solution to the problem of measuring efficacy across multiple domains for a targeted treatment in an NDD.

Down Syndrome

DS (trisomy 21), is the most common genetic cause of IDD (Martinez-Cue et al., 2013). There is high unmet need to develop effective therapies to improve learning, memory, and speech in those with DS, to improve functioning and increase independence. Ts65Dn mice have an extra chromosome 16 in an area analogous to human chromosome 21 and have neuronal morphology similar to that of humans with DS; these mice show deficits in learning and memory, which appear to result from a selective decrease in the number of excitatory synapses and excessive gamma-aminobutyric acid (GABA)-mediated inhibition. Use of GABA-A receptor antagonists, particularly nonconvulsant, nonanxiogenic GABA-A receptor inverse agonists selective for the α5-subtype (α5IA, RO4938581), successfully improved memory and learning deficits, normalized excessive GABAergic synaptic markers, and reversed hippocampal long-term potentiation (LTP) deficits in the Ts65Dn mouse (Martinez-Cue et al., 2013). Based on the preclinical work, RG1662, a selective orally active GABA-A α5 receptor subunit inverse agonist with high selectivity for the GABA-A α5 subunit-containing receptor RG1662, was studied in a phase 2a placebo-controlled safety/pharmacokinetics (PK) trial in DS. RG1662 had a good safety profile and is currently in a placebo-controlled phase 2b efficacy trial targeting

memory, language, and cognition in adults with DS, and a safety/PK trial in adolescents and children with DS.

Tuberous Sclerosis

Tuberous sclerosis complex (TSC) is a genetic multisystem disorder associated with dermatologic findings; growth of benign tumors in the brain, skin, kidneys, heart, liver, and lungs, and less frequently in the retina, gingiva, bones, and gastrointestinal tract; epilepsy; ASD; IDD; and other behavioral problems (Ebrahimi-Fakhari and Sahin, 2015). Magnetic resonance imaging (MRI) of the brain frequently shows cortical tubers (focal malformations of cortical development characterized by disorganized lamination and giant cells expressing markers of neuronal and glial differentiation) and subependymal nodules (SENs), which can evolve into subependymal giant-cell astrocytomas (SEGAs).

TSC is caused by a mutation of either *TSC1* or *TSC2*. TSC1 and TSC2 proteins function as a heterodimeric complex to inhibit mammalian target of rapamycin (mTOR) signaling. mTOR is a kinase that integrates multiple signals to regulate cellular growth, axon growth and specification, synapse development, and synaptic plasticity by modulating translation initiation. Mutations of either *TSC1* or *TSC2* release inhibition of mTOR, resulting in constitutive activation of the mTOR pathway. Rapamycin (sirolimus) inhibits mTOR activity and was shown to improve myelination and cytopathologic architecture, restore normal synaptic function, eliminate epilepsy, prolong survival, and reverse learning and social deficits in TSC mice. Sirolimus (rapamycin) and everolimus (rapamycin analog) were shown to reduce the size of renal angiomyolipomas and SEGAs in patients with TSC. Everolimus is FDA approved for treatment of SEGAs at any age and renal angiomyolipomas in adults with TSC. An open-label trial of everolimus in 20 TSC patients with refractory epilepsy showed reduction of seizure frequency/duration and improved behavior and quality of life. A current randomized placebo-controlled phase 2 study aims to assess the effect of everolimus on neurocognition, seizures, sleep, ASD, behavior, and academic skills.

Fragile X Syndrome

FXS, the most common known inherited cause of IDD and ASD, is caused by a trinucleotide repeat (CGG) expansion mutation of more than 200 CGG repeats (termed the "full mutation") in the promoter region of *FMR1* (*fragile X mental retardation 1*), which results in methylation and transcriptional silencing of FMR1 with consequent loss or significant reduction in expression of FMRP (fragile X mental retardation protein) (Gross, Hoffmann, Bassell, and Berry-Kravis et al., 2015). Females with FXS are more mildly affected than males as a result of production of FMRP from the normal *FMR1* allele in cells expressing the nonmutated X chromosome.

FMRP is an mRNA binding protein that regulates (inhibits) dendritic translation of proteins involved in synaptic plasticity in response to synaptic activation by multiple Gq-linked receptors, including group 1 metabotropic glutamate receptors (mGluR1/mGluR5). Activation of these receptors results in signaling through ERK- and mTOR-dependent pathways, resulting in loss of FMRP repressor function at the ribosome and a pulse of new protein synthesis. FMRP also regulates the activity of some presynaptic and postsynaptic ion channels, such as BK and SLACK channels, through direct protein–protein interactions. These regulatory functions of FMRP are critical for synaptic maturation and plasticity. In the Fmr1 knockout mouse, there is a constitutive elevation of synaptic proteins usually controlled by FMRP and immature elongated morphology of dendritic spines, abnormal spine density, and abnormal synaptic plasticity, including excessive internalization of AMPA receptors; enhanced mGluR-activated hippocampal and cerebellar long-term depression (LTD); impaired LTP in the hippocampus, cortex, and amygdala; impaired circuit physiology; and audiogenic seizures. The morphologic abnormalities and synaptic plasticity deficits found in the Fmr1 knockout mouse are associated with numerous learning, social, and behavioral phenotypes. The *Drosophila* model of FXS shows defects in circadian rhythms, synaptic branching, courtship behavior, and learning.

The abnormalities observed in the Fmr1 knockout mouse have led to treatment targets directed at (1) reduction of excess signaling from group 1 mGluRs or other Gq-linked receptors to the dendritic translational machinery, (2) reduction of excessive activity of individual proteins normally regulated by FMRP, (3) increased activation of surface AMPA receptors, (4) modification of activity of GABA and other systems that regulate glutamate signaling, (5) blocking of excessive translation of FMRP-regulated mRNAs, and (6) correction of abnormal channel activities normally directly regulated by FMRP (Table 59-2). Treatments aimed at all of these types of targets, in particular mGluR5 negative allosteric modulator (NAMs), have resulted in pharmacologic and genetic reversal of a remarkable number of phenotypes in the Fmr1 knockout mouse and dfxr fly models.

The successful preclinical testing in FXS models has led to early proof-of-concept clinical trials and some subsequent larger trials for proposed targeted treatments. Several agents have shown benefits in early-phase or open-label trials in FXS: lithium (mechanism 1 in previous list, reduces phosphatidylinositol [PI] turnover and GSK3B activity) resulted in improvement in behavior, verbal memory, and abnormal ERK phosphorylation rates in lymphocytes; minocycline

(mechanism 2, inhibits MMP9) resulted in mild improvement over placebo in global behavior and reduction of blood MMP-9 levels in responders; arbaclofen (mechanism 4, GABA-B agonist, lowers presynaptic glutamate release) showed improvement over placebo for social withdrawal and parent-nominated problem behaviors; acamprosate (mechanism 4, GABA-A/GABA-B agonist) showed improvement in hyperactivity and social functioning; fenobam (mechanism 1, mGluR5 NAM) showed improvement in abnormal prepulse inhibition (PPI); and AFQ056 (mechanism 1, mGluR5 NAM) suggested improvement in maladaptive behavior over placebo in a posthoc analysis in the subgroup with full methylation of *FMR1*. Larger placebo-controlled trials of arbaclofen, AFQ056, and RO4917523 (mGluR5 NAM) over 3 months in adults and adolescents with FXS have not shown behavioral benefit but have addressed cognitive or learning outcomes. A phase 3 arbaclofen trial in children with FXS showed improved behavior and parenting stress in the highest-dose group relative to placebo, but full analyses are pending. FXS has been an important model to illustrate hurdles in the translation of targeted treatments to NDDs, given problems demonstrating efficacy for behavior in larger trials and ongoing uncertainties about how to optimally demonstrate changes in the disease course in a clinical trial setting. It is clear that issues related to outcome measures, placebo effects, length and timing (age) of treatment, and how to study learning need to be solved to be able to demonstrate the potential benefits of these drugs for synaptic plasticity, as seen in animal models.

Generalization of Treatment From Single-Gene Disorders to NDDs and ASD

RS, TSC, and FXS all show significant clinical and molecular pathway overlaps with ASD and NDDs (Ebrahimi-Fakhari and Sahin, 2015; see Table 59-1). Dysregulated mTOR signaling in TSC results in abnormal dendritic regulation of translation, and other proteins in the mTOR pathway are products of genes associated with ASD and NDDs, including mutations of neurofibromin 1 in neurofibromatosis type 1 (NF-1) and phosphatase and tensin homolog in PTEN-deficiency syndromes. This suggests that dysregulation of the TSC/mTOR pathway predisposes to ASD and that mTOR inhibitors that treat TSC may be effective for a subgroup other NDDs, such as efficacy of sirolimus for growth of plexiform neurofibromas in NF-1.

There is also significant molecular and cellular pathway overlap between FMRP and gene products associated with ASD and NDDs (Figs. 59-1 and 59-2). Like TSC1/TSC2, FMRP is a regulator of mTOR-dependent dendritic translational activation pathways. The Akt pathway is dysregulated in both RS and FXS; this discovery led to a phase 2 clinical trial of NNZ-2566 in FXS that illustrated potential targeted treatment overlap between NDDs sharing dysregulated molecular pathways. Molecular overlap between FXS and other ASD/NDDs is focused on signaling of dendritic translational regulation, which is one of the key pathways onto which gene products associated with autism cluster, and falls roughly into three categories: (1) defects in proteins in the signaling cascade modulating FMRP-regulated translation, (2) defects in proteins regulated directly by FMRP, and (3) defects in proteins involved in the balance of glutamate and GABA systems. Indeed, the FMRP/ASD/NDD pathway overlap has been recently supported by the findings that: (1) FMRP binds about a third of the genes associated with ASD in exome screening studies, (2) genes that code for FMRP target mRNAs are more likely than other genes with similar expression patterns to contribute to ASD, and (3) common variants in genes involved in postsynaptic regulation of FMRP are risk factors for ASD. If targeted treatments directed at molecular pathways, as in TSC, RS, FXS, or other single-gene NDDs, and treatments for circuit dysfunction and glutamate/GABA balance as in DS are ultimately successful (Table 59-1), it is possible that these can be extended to reverse neural defects and clinical manifestations in subgroups of ASD and NDDs with shared pathway deficits.

INBORN ERRORS OF METABOLISM

IEMs constitute a large group of monogenic conditions characterized by impaired chemical intracellular transformations that typically affect the synthesis or breakdown of molecules, leading to the accumulation of toxic molecules, or lack of cell energy or necessary substrates for many important biochemical processes. The majority of these affect the central nervous system (CNS) in the child and thus present as neurodevelopmental disabilities, specifically IDD, epilepsy, cerebral palsy, autism, and behavioral and psychiatric disturbances.

Intellectual Developmental Disabilities

An overview of the 89 IEMs presenting with IDD as the predominant phenotypic feature for which causal therapy was available in 2015 (van Karnebeek and Stockler, 2012; van Karnebeek, Shevell, Zschocke, Moeschler, and Stockler, 2014) is provided in Table 59-3. Nearly all of these conditions are associated with additional phenotypic features. Neurologic features include ataxia, behavioral disturbance, dementia, dystonia, encephalopathic crisis, epilepsy, hearing loss, hypotonia/myopathy, neuroimaging abnormalities (basal ganglia, cerebellum, cerebrum, cysts/dysgenesis, white matter, mixed), neuropathy, ocular movement abnormality, psychiatric disturbance, sensorineural hearing loss, spasticity, stroke, vision loss, and various types and degrees of movement disorders (e.g., spasticity, dyskinesia. and ataxia). However, it is important to note that a significant number of these conditions can present with unspecific IDD as the sole feature (e.g., creatine transporter deficiency). Other presentations vary from neurodegenerative +/– multiorgan involvement to "stable IDD" (i.e., without a history of regression or plateauing; some are characterized by acute decompensations—often in the neonatal or early childhood period—or present with a late-onset form of unspecific or chronic nature. Of note, nonneurologic or systemic features is a prominent phenotype in 57 (64%) of the 89 treatable IDDs listed in Table 59-3.

Diagnostic Approach to Treatable Inborn Errors of Metabolism

To enhance early diagnosis of treatable IEMs in children presenting with IDD, the two-tiered TIDE protocol was designed (Box 59-1). The first tier involves biochemical group tests in blood and urine, which potentially indicate 60% of the currently known treatable conditions. The next step is to apply the 2014 diagnostic practice parameters for IDD, which include chromosome microarray as a first-line test and, in selected cases, fragile X testing, neuroimaging, and other tests, in combination with the second tier of the TIDE algorithm for the identification of the remaining 35 treatable IDs. The latter conditions require a more targeted approach, including single-metabolite or primary molecular analysis, based on a clinical differential diagnosis; these tests often require more invasive sampling procedures and/or extensive funding. A free digital application is available (via www.treatable-ID.org and the Apple App store as the TIDE-BC App) that supports the diagnostic algorithm and provides information on the symptoms, tests, and treatments for these rare diseases.

BOX 59-1 Two-Tiered Algorithm for Diagnosis of Treatable IEMs in IDD*

FIRST TIER: IN ALL PATIENTS WITH UNEXPLAINED ID, NONTARGETED SCREENING TO IDENTIFY 54 (60%) TREATABLE IEMS

Blood:
- Ammonia, lactate
- Plasma amino acids
- Total homocysteine
- Acylcarnitine profile
- Copper, ceruloplasmin

Urine:
- Organic acids
- Purines and pyrimidines
- Creatine metabolites
- Oligosaccharides
- Glycosaminoglycans

SECOND TIER: TARGETED METABOLIC WORKUP TO IDENTIFY 35 (40%) TREATABLE IEMS REQUIRING SPECIFIC TESTING

According to patient's symptomatology and clinician's expertise
Utilization of textbooks and digital resources (e.g., app available at www.treatable-ID.org)
Consider the following biochemical/gene tests:
- Whole-blood manganese
- Plasma cholestanol
- Plasma 7-dehydroxy-cholesterol:cholesterol ratio
- Plasma pipecolic acid and urine alpha-AASA
- Plasma very-long-chain fatty acids
- Plasma vitamin B_{12} and folate
- Serum and CSF lactate:pyruvate ratio
- Enzyme activities (leukocytes): arylsulphatase A, biotinidase, glucocerebrosidase, fatty aldehyde dehydrogenase
- Urine deoxypridonoline
- CSF amino acids
- CSF neurotransmitters
- CSF:plasma glucose ratio
- CoQ measurement fibroblasts
- Molecular analyses: *CA5A, NPC1, NPC2, SC4MOL, SLC18A2, SLC19A3, ALC30A10, SLC52A2, SLC52A3, PDHA1, PDHX, SPR, TH* genes

Note: The first-tier testing comprises group metabolic tests in urine and blood that should be performed in every patient with IDD of unknown cause. Based on the differential diagnosis generated by the patient's signs and symptoms, the second-tier test is ordered individually at a low threshold.
*alpha-AASA, alpha-aminoadipic semialdehyde; CSF, cerebrospinal fluid; IDD, intellectual developmental disability; NDD, neurodevelopmental disability.

Treatments, Outcomes, and Evidence

Treatments include dietary restriction/supplementation, cofactors/coenzymes, vitamins, substrate inhibition, (small molecule) substrate reduction, enzyme replacement, bone marrow and hematopoietic stem cell transplant, and gene therapy (Fig. 59-3) (van Karnebeek and Stockler, 2012). The majority of treatments are affordable, accessible, and safe. Therapeutic effects include improvement in and/or stabilization of psychomotor and cognitive development, behavioral and psychiatric disturbances, seizures, and neurologic and systemic manifestations. As shown in Table 59-3, improvement of cognitive and psychomotor development is only achieved for 20% of IEMs, whereas for the majority of treatable IDDs, related outcomes are positively influenced by therapy. Inherent to small patient numbers in diseases such as these, evidence levels are often limited (most rank at level 4). This is

Text continued on p. 486

TABLE 59-3 Overview of Treatable Inborn Errors of Metabolism Presenting With Intellectual Developmental Disability (*n* = 89 in 2015)

Biochemical Category	Disease Name	MIM #	Major Phenotype	Therapeutic Modality(-ies)	Treatment Effect	Level(s) of Evidence	Clinical Practice
Amino acids	Hyperornithinemia-hyperammonemia-homocitrullinemia (HHH) syndrome	238970	IDD, epilepsy, psych, CP	Dietary protein restriction, ornithine supplement, sodium benzoate, phenylacetate	B, C, D, E, F, G	4	Standard of care
	late-onset (l.o.) Non-ketotic hyperglycinemia	605899	IDD, epilepsy, psych, CP	Glycine restriction; +/–sodium benzoate, NMDA receptor antagonists, other neuromodulating agents	B, D, E, F	4–5	Standard of care
	Phenylketonuria	261600	IDD, epilepsy, psych, CP	Dietary phenylalanine restriction +/– amino-acid supplements [BH4 supplement]	B, D, E [C]	2a (4)	Standard of care [individual basis]
	3-Phosphoglycerate dehydrogenase (3-PHGDH) deficiency	601815	IDD, epilepsy, CP	L-serine and +/– glycine supplements	D, E, F	4	Standard of care
	Phosphoserine aminotransferase (PSAT) deficiency	610992	IDD, epilepsy, CP	L-serine and +/– glycine supplements	D, E, F	4	Standard of care
	Phosphoserine phosphatase (PSPH) deficiency	614023	IDD, epilepsy, CP	L-serine and +/– glycine supplements	D, E, F	4	Standard of care
	Tyrosinemia type II	276600	IDD	Dietary phenylalanine and tyrosine restriction	D, G	4–5	Standard of care
Cholesterol	Sterol-C4-methyl oxidase-like (SC4MOL) deficiency	607545*	IDD	SC4MOL deficiency	B, G	4–5	Standard of care
	Smith–Lemli–Opitz syndrome	270400	IDD	Cholesterol and simvastatin	B, D	4–5	Individual basis
	Cerebrotendinous Xanthomatosis	213700	IDD, psych, CP	Chenodesoxycholic acid, HMG reductase inhibitor	B, D, E, G	4	Standard of care
Creatine	Arginine:glycine amidinotransferase (AGAT) deficiency	612718	IDD, epilepsy, CP	Creatine supplements	A, D, E	4	Standard of care
	Creatine Transporter defect	300352	IDD, epilepsy, psych, CP	Creatine, glycine, arginine supplements	F	4–5	Individual basis
	Guanidinoacetate Methyltransferase (GAMT) deficiency	612736	IDD, epilepsy, psych, CP	Arginine restriction, creatine and ornithine supplements	B, D, E, F	4	Standard of care
Fatty aldehydes	Sjögren–Larsson syndrome	270200	IDD	Diet (low fat, medium chain and essential fatty acid supplements) and zileuton	D, G	5	Individual basis
Glucose transport	GLUT1 deficiency syndrome	606777	IDD, epilepsy, CP	Ketogenic diet	E, F	4	Standard of care
	Hyperinsulinism-Hyperammonemia syndrome	606762	IDD, epilepsy	Diazoxide	D	4–5	Standard of care
Hyperhomocysteinemia	Cobalamin C deficiency	277400	IDD, psych, CP	Hydroxocobalamin	C, D, E, G	4	Standard of care
	Cobalamin D deficiency	277410	IDD, psych, CP	Hydroxocobalamin/cyanocobalamin	C, D, E, G	4	Standard of care
	Cobalamin E deficiency	236270	IDD, psych, CP	Hydroxocobalamin/methylcobalamin, betaine	C, D, G	4	Standard of care

TABLE 59-3 Overview of Treatable Inborn Errors of Metabolism Presenting With Intellectual Developmental Disability (*n* = 89 in 2015) *(Continued)*

Biochemical Category	Disease Name	MIM #	Major Phenotype	Therapeutic Modality(-ies)	Treatment Effect	Level(s) of Evidence	Clinical Practice
	Cobalamin F deficiency	277380	IDD, psych, CP	Hydroxocobalamin	C, D, G	4	Standard of care
	Cobalamin G deficiency	250940	IDD, Psych, CP	Hydroxocobalamin/ methylcobalamin, betaine	C, D, G	4	Standard of care
	Homocystinuria	236200	IDD, psych, CP	Methionine restriction, +/−pyridoxine, +/− betaine	C, D, E, G	2c	Standard of care
	I.o. Methylenetetrahydrofolate reductase (MTHFR) deficiency	236250	IDD, psych, CP	Betaine supplements, +/−folate, carnitine, methionine supplements	C, D, E, G	4	Standard of care
Lysosomes	Aspartylglucosaminuria	208400	IDD	Haematopoietic stem cell transplantation	D	4–5	Individual basis
	Gaucher disease type III	231000	IDD, epilepsy	Haematopoietic stem cell transplantation	D, G	4–5	Individual basis
	Hunter syndrome (MPS II)	309900	IDD	Haematopoietic stem cell transplantation	D, G	4–5	Individual basis
	Hurler syndrome (MPS I)	607014	IDD	Haematopoietic stem cell transplantation	D, G	1c	Standard of care
	I.o. Metachromatic leukodystrophy	250100	IDD, psych, CP	Haematopoietic stem cell transplantation	D, E	4–5	Individual basis
	Niemann–Pick disease type C	257220	IDD, psych, CP	Migalastat	D, E	1b	Standard of care
	Sanfilippo Syndrome A (MPS IIIa)	252900	IDD, psych	Haematopoietic stem cell transplantation	D	4–5	Individual basis
	Sanfilippo syndrome B (MPS IIIb)	252920	IDD, psych	Haematopoietic stem cell transplantation	D	4–5	Individual basis
	Sanfilippo syndrome C (MPS IIIc)	252930	IDD, psych	Haematopoietic stem cell transplantation	D	4–5	Individual basis
	Sanfilippo syndrome D (MPS IIId)	252940	IDD, psych	Haematopoietic stem cell transplantation	D	4–5	Individual basis
	Sly Syndrome (MPS VII)	253220	IDD	Haematopoietic stem cell transplantation	D	4–5	Individual basis
	α-Mannosidosis	248500	IDD	Haematopoietic stem cell transplantation	D	4–5	Individual basis
Metals	Hypermanganesemia with dystonia, polycythemia, and cirrhosis (HMPDC) syndrome	613280	IDD, CP	Iron chelation therapy	D, E, G	4	Individual basis
	Mental retardation, enteropathy, deafness, peripheral neuropathy, ichthyosis, and keratoderma (MEDNIK) syndrome	609313		Zinc acetate	D, E, G	4–5	Standard of care
	Menkes disease / occipital horn syndrome	304150	IDD, epilepsy, CP	Copper histidine	D, E	4	Individual basis
	Wilson disease	277900	IDD, psych, CP	Zinc and tetrathiomolybdate	E, G	1b	Standard of care
	Aceruloplasminemia	604290	IDD, CP	Iron chelation	D, E	4	Standard of care
Mitochondria	Coenzyme Q10 deficiency	607426	IDD, epilepsy, CP	Coenzyme Q10 supplements	E, F	4	Standard of care
	Mitochondrial encephalomyopathy, lactic acidosis, and stroke-like episodes (MELAS)	540000	IDD, epilepsy, psych, CP	Arginine supplements	C, D, E, F	4–5	Standard of care
	Pyruvate dehydrogenase deficiency	312170; 245348; 245349	IDD, epilepsy, CP	Ketogenic diet and thiamine	A, C, D, E	4	Standard of care

Continued on following page

TABLE 59-3 Overview of Treatable Inborn Errors of Metabolism Presenting With Intellectual Developmental Disability (*n* = 89 in 2015) *(Continued)*

Biochemical Category	Disease Name	MIM #	Major Phenotype	Therapeutic Modality(-ies)	Treatment Effect	Level(s) of Evidence	Clinical Practice
Neurotransmission	Aromatic L-amino acid decarboxylase deficiency	608643	IDD, CP	MAO inhibitors, B_6, anticholinergics, dopa agonists	A, D, E, F	4	Standard of care
	Dihydropteridine reductase (DHPR) deficiency	261630	IDD, CP	BH4, diet, amine replacement, folinic acid	A, E	4	Standard of care
	Guanosine triphosphate cyclohydrolase I (GTPCH1) deficiency	261630	IDD, CP	BH4, amine replacement	A, E	4	Standard of care
	Pterin carbinolamine dehydratase (PCD) deficiency	264070	IDD	BH4	A, E	4	Standard of care
	6-pyruvoyl-tetrahydropterin synthase (PTPS) deficiency	261640	IDD, epilepsy, CP	BH4, diet, amine replacement	A, E	4	Standard of care
	Sepiapterin reductase deficiency	612716	IDD, CP	Amine replacement	A, E	4	Standard of care
	Succinic semialdehyde dehydrogenase (SSADH) deficiency	271980	IDD, epilepsy, psych, CP	Vigabatrin	B, E, F	4	Individual basis
	Tyrosine hydroxylase deficiency	605407	IDD, CP	L-dopa substitution	A, E	4	Standard of care
	Vesicular monoamine transporter 2 deficiency	193001*	IDD, CP	Dopamine agonists	A, D, E	4	Standard of care
Organic acids	3-Methylcrotonyl glycinuria type I/II	210200/ 210210	IDD, CP	Dietary protein restriction; carnitine, glycine, biotin supplements; avoid fasting; sick-day management	C, E	5	Standard of care
	3-Methylglutaconic aciduria type I	250950	IDD, CP	Carnitine supplements, avoid fasting, sick-day management	C	5	Standard of care
	Cobalamin A deficiency	251100	IDD, psych, CP	Hydroxocobalamin, protein restriction	C, G	4	Standard of care
	Cobalamin B deficiency	251110	IDD, psych, CP	Hydroxocobalamin, protein restriction	C, G	4	Standard of care
	Ethylmalonic encephalopathy	602473	IDD, CP	N-acetylcysteine, oral metronidazole	E, G	4	Standard of care
	Glutaric acidemia II	231680	IDD, CP	carnitine, riboflavin, β-hydroxybutyrate supplements; sick-day management	C, E, G	5	Standard of care
	HMG-CoA lyase deficiency	246450	IDD, CP	Protein restriction, avoid fasting, sick-day management	C, E	5	Standard of care
	l.o.Glutaric acidemia I	231670	IDD, CP	Lysine restriction, carnitine supplements	C, D, E, G	2c	Standard of care
	l.o. Isovaleic acidemia	243500	IDD, CP	Dietary protein restriction, carnitine supplements, avoid fasting, sick-day management	C, E, G	2c	Standard of care
	l.o. Methylmalonic acidemia	251000	IDD, psych, CP	Dietary protein restriction, carnitine supplements, avoid fasting, sick-day management	C, E, G	2c	Standard of care
	l.o. Propionic acidemia	6065054	IDD, CP	Dietary protein restriction, carnitine supplements, avoid fasting, sick-day management	C, E, G	2c	Standard of care
	Maple syrup urine disease (variant)	248600	IDD, psych, CP	Dietary restriction of branched amino acids, avoid fasting, [liver transplantation]	B, C, D, E [A, C, E]	4 & 4	Standard of care [individual basis]

TABLE 59-3 Overview of Treatable Inborn Errors of Metabolism Presenting With Intellectual Developmental Disability (*n* = 89 in 2015) *(Continued)*

Biochemical Category	Disease Name	MIM #	Major Phenotype	Therapeutic Modality(-ies)	Treatment Effect	Level(s) of Evidence	Clinical Practice
	2-*Methyl*-3-hydroxybutyryl-CoA dehydrogenase (MHBD) deficiency	300438	IDD, CP	Avoid fasting, sick-day management, isoleucine-restricted diet	C, E	5	Standard of care
	mitochondrial 3-hydroxy3-methylglutaryl-coenzyme A (mHMG-CoA) synthase deficiency	605911	IDD, CP	Avoid fasting, sick day management, +/− dietary precursor restriction	C, E	5	Standard of care
	Succinyl-CoA:3-ketoacid CoA transferase (SCOT) deficiency	245050	IDD, CP	Avoid fasting, protein restriction, sick-day management	C, E	5	Standard of care
	β-Ketothiolase deficiency	203750	IDD, CP	Avoid fasting, sick-day management, protein restriction	C, E	5	Standard of care
Peroxisomes	X-linked adrenoleukodystrophy	300100	IDD, epilepsy, psych	Stem cell transplantation [gene therapy]	D, E [D, E]	1c [5]	Individual basis
	Pyrimidine 5-nucleotidase superactivity	GENE OMIM# 606224	IDD, CP	Uridine supplements	A, B, E, F, G	1b	Standard of care
Urea cycle defect	Carbonic anhydrase VA deficiency	615751	IDD	Carglumic acid, sick-day protocol	C	4–5	Standard of care
	Citrullinemia type II	605814	IDD, CP	Dietary protein restriction, arginine supplement, sodium benzoate, phenylbutyrate [liver transplantation]	B, C, D, E, F, G [C]	2b [4]	Standard of care [individual basis]
	l.o. Argininemia	207800	IDD, psych, CP	Dietary protein restriction, arginine supplement, sodium benzoate, phenylbutyrate [liver transplantation]	B, C, D, E, F, G [C]	2b [4]	Standard of care [individual basis]
	l.o. Argininosuccinic aciduria	207900	IDD, psych, CP	Dietary protein restriction, arginine supplement, sodium benzoate, phenylbutyrate [liver transplantation]	B, C, D, E, F, G [C]	2b [4]	Standard of care [individual basis]
	l.o. Carbamoyl phosphate synthetase (CPS) deficiency	237300	IDD, CP	Dietary protein restriction, arginine supplement, sodium benzoate, phenylbutyrate [liver transplantation]	B, C, D, E, F, G [C]	2b [4]	Standard of care [individual basis]
	l.o. Citrullinemia Type I	215700	IDD, psych, CP	Dietary protein restriction, arginine supplement, sodium benzoate, phenylbutyrate [liver transplantation]	B, C, D, E, F, G [C]	2b [4]	Standard of care [individual basis]
	l.o. N-acetylglutamate synthase (NAGS) deficiency	237310	IDD, psych	Dietary protein restriction, arginine supplement, sodium benzoate, phenylbutyrate, carglumic acid [liver transplantation]	B, C, D, E, F, G [C]	2b [4]	Standard of care [individual basis]
	l.o. Ornithine transcarbamylase (OTC) deficiency	311250	IDD, psych, CP	Dietary protein restriction, citrulline and arginine supplement, sodium benzoate, phenylbutyrate [liver transplantation]	B, C, D, E, F, G [C]	2b [4]	Standard of care [individual basis]

Continued on following page

TABLE 59-3 Overview of Treatable Inborn Errors of Metabolism Presenting With Intellectual Developmental Disability (*n* = 89 in 2015) *(Continued)*

Biochemical Category	Disease Name	MIM #	Major Phenotype	Therapeutic Modality(-ies)	Treatment Effect	Level(s) of Evidence	Clinical Practice
Vitamins/cofactors	Biotin-responsive basal ganglia disease	607483	IDD, CP	Biotin supplement	A, E	4	Standard of care
	Biotinidase deficiency	253260	IDD, epilepsy, CP	Biotin supplement	A, E, G	2c	Standard of care
	Brown–Vialetto–van Laere/ Fazio–Londe syndrome	211500	IDD, CP	Riboflavin supplement	A, B, C, D, E	4	Standard of care
	Cerebral folate receptor-α deficiency	613068	IDD, CP	Folinic acid	A, D, E, F	4	Standard of care
	Congenital intrinsic factor deficiency	261000	IDD	Hydroxocobalamin	A, E, G	4	Standard of care
	Dihydrofolate reductase deficiency	613839	IDD, Epilepsy	Folinic acid	A, B, E, F	4	Individual basis
	Holocarboxylase synthetase deficiency	253270	IDD, epilepsy, CP	Biotin supplement	A, E, G	4	Standard of care
	Imerslund–Gräsbeck syndrome	261100	IDD	Hydroxocobalamin	A, E, G	4	Standard of care
	Molybdenum cofactor deficiency type A	252150	IDD, epilepsy, CP	Precursor Z (CPMP)	A, E, F	4	Individual basis
	Pyridoxine-dependent epilepsy	266100	IDD, epilepsy	Pyridoxine	A, F	4	Standard of Care
	Thiamine-responsive encephalopathy	606152	IDD	Thiamin supplement	E	4–5	Standard of care

This table provides an overview of all treatable inborn errors of metabolism (IEMs; with phenotype Mendelian Inheritance in Man number [MIM#]; *indicates the gene) presenting with intellectual developmental disability (IDD) along with the disease's other prominent phenotypic features, the specific therapy(ies) available with relevant level(s) of evidence, therapeutic effect(s) on primary and/or secondary outcomes, and use in clinical practice. For 10 IEMs, two therapies are available; these are listed separately (*in brackets*) with corresponding level of evidence, therapeutic effect(s), and use in clinical practice (*also in brackets*).

<u>Individual basis:</u> The decision to initiate a specific treatment depends on a careful evaluation of the specific patient characteristics, physician's opinion, availability of treatment, and potential side effects.

<u>Levels of evidence</u> (source: http://www.cebm.net): Level 1a = systematic review of randomized controlled trials (RCTs), 1b = individual RCT, 1c = all or none (= [prolongation of] survival with therapy); level 2a = systematic review of cohort studies, 2b = individual cohort study, 2c = outcomes research (focused on end results of therapy for chronic conditions, including functioning and quality of life (source: www.ahrq.gov/clinic.outfact.htm); level 3 = systematic review of case-control studies; level 4 = individual case-control study or case series/report; level 4 to 5 = single case report; level 5 = expert opinion without critical appraisal.

<u>Major phenotypes:</u> Neurodevelopmental disabilities (NDDs) include the following major phenotypes: CP, cerebral palsy; epilepsy; IDD, intellectual developmental disability; psych, psychiatric/behavioral disturbances (including autism).

<u>Sick-day management:</u> Intervention(s) to guarantee sufficient fluid and caloric intake to maintain anabolic state, plus continuation/modification of disease-specific therapy.

<u>Standard of care:</u> Initiation of the specific treatment upon diagnostic confirmation is generally accepted by experts worldwide as "best clinical practice."

<u>Therapeutic effect(s):</u> A, improves psychomotor/cognitive development/IQ; B, improves behavioral/psychiatric disturbance(s); C, prevents acute metabolic decompensation; D, prevents, halts, or slows clinical deterioration; E, improves neurologic manifestations (including neuroimaging); F, improves seizure/epilepsy control; G, improves systemic manifestations.

because of methodological shortcomings other than effect size per se. A prominent example of this is AGAT deficiency, for which treatment comprises oral creatine, which can normalize neurodevelopmental functioning with timely initiation but only has an evidence level of 4. Finally, many treatments with limited evidence levels are considered the standard of care.

Treatable Inborn Errors of Metabolism Presenting With Other Neurodevelopmental Disorder Phenotypes

Epilepsy

Seizures may be the first and the major presenting feature of an IEM or be preceded by other major symptoms (e.g., reduced level of consciousness or loss of skills, progressive weakness, ataxia, and upper motor signs) (Rahman, Footitt, Varadkar, and Clayton, 2013). The common metabolic causes of seizures

vary according to the age at presentation and/or involvement of specific cortical areas of the brain; specific seizure types characteristic of individual IEMs are rare. Features from the history examination, imaging, and first-line biochemical investigations can all provide clues as to which IEM may be involved.

The IEMs with epileptic symptoms that are amenable to metabolic therapy are listed in Table 59-3. The response to targeted metabolic therapy differs among IEMs, and outcomes depend on the manifestation of the disease. In some cases, seizures are a consequence of acute metabolic stress on the CNS (e.g., in the case of hyperammonemia or hypoglycaemia), and treatment of the underlying neurometabolic condition stabilizes seizures. In other treatable IEMs, seizures are the main manifestation, and disease progression can lead to drug-resistant epilepsy (e.g., GAMT deficiency). In a few metabolic disorders, such as phenylketonuria (PKU) and biotinidase deficiency, seizures can be prevented completely if caught early (via newborn screening) and treated (biotin 10–100 mg/

day). However, conventional antiepileptic medications may be needed in addition to metabolic therapy for some IEMs (e.g., glutaric aciduria type 1).

Atypical Cerebral Palsy

A significant number of IEMs (*n* = 67) present as cerebral palsy mimics (i.e., with movement disorders); Table 59-3 lists those amenable to causal therapy (Leach, Shevell, Bowden, Stockler-Ipsiroglu, and van Karnebeek, 2014). An example is Segawa disease, also called GTPCH1-deficient dopa-responsive dystonia (GTPCH1-DRD), characterized by dystonia in childhood that is often misdiagnosed as cerebral palsy (CP). This neurotransmitter disorder can be diagnosed by standard analysis of neurotransmitter metabolites in the cerebrospinal fluid (CSF). Individuals with GTPCH1-DRD benefit from treatment with levodopa/carbidopamine and in some cases 5-hydroxytryptophan and BH4. The majority of treated individuals show rapid clinical improvement in CP-related symptoms (spasticity, dystonia, general tone) and are able to lead "an entirely normal life." Similarly, for 26 (39%) of all IEMs presenting with atypical CP, a treatment is available that targets the primary underlying pathophysiology; for the remaining 41 (61%) IEMs, treatment is available that stabilizes disease or prevents further damage (e.g., fatty acid oxidation disorders; Leach et al., 2014).

The symptoms that should prompt the clinician to search for an underlying IEM or other neurogenetic defect include, but are not limited to, the following "red flags": normal MRI findings on imaging; abnormalities isolated to the globus pallidus; severe symptoms in the absence of a history of perinatal injury; a pattern of familial disease inheritance, or consanguinity; neurodevelopmental regression, or progressively worsening symptomatology; isolated muscular hypotonia; rigidity (as opposed to spasticity) on physician examination; and unexplained paraplegia. Metabolic and molecular testing are required for diagnosis; importantly, lumbar puncture, although invasive, should not be avoided because it allows for CSF neurotransmitter, glucose, and amino acid analysis, which is highly sensitive and often guides the clinician in further diagnostic and therapeutic decisions.

Psychiatric Disease

Psychiatric disease is another frequent phenotype of IEMs and can be divided into three categories: acute, treatable IEMs (urea cycle abnormalities, remethylation disorders, acute intermittent porphyria); chronic, treatable IEMs (Wilson's disease, Niemann–Pick disease type C, homocystinuria resulting from cystathionine beta-synthase deficiency, cerebrotendinous xanthomatosis); and chronic IEMs that are more difficult to treat (lysosomal storage diseases, X-linked adrenoleukodystrophy, creatine deficiency syndromes; Bonnot et al., 2014). Treatments are listed in Table 59-3 for all IEMs with significant psychiatric or behavioral disturbances except acute intermittent porphyria (preventive measures and hemin IV in the acute phase).

The following atypical psychiatric features should trigger a search for IEMs in patients with schizophrenia: first-level features, defined as atypical on their own (confusion, visual hallucinations more prominent than auditory hallucinations, catatonia, progressive cognitive decline, treatment resistance, fluctuating schizophrenia core symptoms), and second-level features, defined as atypical when associated with first-level features (acute onset, early onset, IDD, unusual or severe side effects; Bonnot et al., 2014). Accurate diagnosis is crucial because early symptoms often respond well to treatment.

CONGENITAL HYPOTHYROIDISM

Congenital hypothyroidism (CH), affecting 1 in 2000 to 1 in 4000, is the most common treatable cause of IDD worldwide. Untreated, common symptoms include decreased activity and increased sleep, feeding difficulty, constipation, and prolonged jaundice. On examination, common signs include myxedematous facies, large fontanels, macroglossia, a distended abdomen with umbilical hernia, and hypotonia.

Known genetic conditions etiologic of CH include TSHb mutations, TSH receptor inactivating mutations, thyroid dysgenesis (TTF-2, NKX2.1, or PAX-8 mutations), thyroid dyshormonogenesis (sodium-iodide symporter, hydrogen peroxide, or DUOX2[A] mutations), thyroid peroxidase mutations (Pendred syndrome: Pendred gene, thyroglobulin or deiodinase mutations) or defects in thyroid hormone transport (MCT8 mutation; Rastogi and LaFranchi, 2010). Therapy with levothyroxine is recommended, with the goal of ensuring that these patients are able to have growth and mental development that is as close as possible to their genetic potential. This is achieved by rapidly restoring free thyroxine (T4) and thyroid-stimulating hormone (TSH) to the normal range and then maintaining clinical and biochemical euthyroidism (Rastogi and LaFranchi, 2010). Studies have shown that the timing of therapy (early diagnosis via newborn screening with optimization of treatment within the first 2–3 years) is crucial to neurologic outcome.

CONCLUSIONS AND FUTURE DIRECTIONS

Novel genetic etiologies of NDDs are increasingly identified based on rapid-sequencing methods. It will be important to map disorders onto shared cellular pathways and circuit dysfunctions targetable for novel treatments approaches, including genetic manipulations such as adenoviral-mediated gene therapy, small-molecule therapies targeted to key pathways, receptor or channel ligands that alter signaling in specific neurons or circuits, or microRNAs that can inhibit production of specific key pathway proteins. These could be combined with cellular targeting of therapeutic molecules through linkage to receptor or transporter ligands to encourage transport into the CNS and individuals neurons.

Such novel disease-modifying therapies to reverse the underlying dysfunctional neural mechanisms, combined with the awareness and early diagnosis of the large expanding group of IEMs, makes this an exciting time in the treatment of NDDs, providing hope and relief for families dealing with these challenging conditions.

REFERENCES

The complete list of references for this chapter is available in the e-book at www.expertconsult.com.
See inside cover for registration details.

SELECTED REFERENCES

Bonnot, O., Klunemann, H.H., Sedel, F., et al., 2014. Diagnostic and Treatment Implications of Psychosis Secondary to Treatable Metabolic Disorders in Adults: A Systematic Review. Orphanet J. Rare Dis. 9, 65-1172-9-65.

Ebrahimi-Fakhari, D., Sahin, M., 2015. Autism and the Synapse: Emerging Mechanisms and Mechanism-Based Therapies. Curr. Opin. Neurol. 28 (2), 91–102.

Gross, C., Hoffmann, A., Bassell, G.J., et al., 2015. Therapeutic Strategies in Fragile X Syndrome: From Bench to Bedside and Back. Neurotherapeutics. 12, 584–608.

Leach, E.L., Shevell, M., Bowden, K., et al., 2014. Treatable Inborn Errors of Metabolism Presenting as Cerebral Palsy Mimics: Systematic Literature Review. Orphanet J. Rare Dis. 9, 197-014-0197-2.

Martinez-Cue, C., Martinez, P., Rueda, N., et al., 2013. Reducing GABAA Alpha5 Receptor-Mediated Inhibition Rescues Functional and Neuromorphological Deficits in a Mouse Model of Down Syndrome. J. Neurosci. 33 (9), 3953–3966.

Pozzo-Miller, L., Pati, S., Percy, A.K., 2015. Rett Syndrome: Reaching for Clinical Trials. Neurotherapeutics 12, 631–640.

Rahman, S., Footitt, E.J., Varadkar, S., et al., 2013. Inborn Errors of Metabolism Causing Epilepsy. Dev. Med. Child Neurol. 55 (1), 23–36.

Rastogi, M.V., LaFranchi, S.H., 2010. Congenital Hypothyroidism. Orphanet J. Rare Dis. 5, 17-1172-5-17.

van Karnebeek, C.D., Stockler, S, 2012. Treatable Inborn Errors of Metabolism Causing Intellectual Disability: A Systematic Literature Review. Mol. Genet. Metab. Program and Abstracts for the 2012 Meeting of the Society for Inherited Metabolic Disorders Society for Inherited Metabolic Disorders 105 (3), 368–381.

van Karnebeek, C.D., Shevell, M., Zschocke, J., et al., 2014. The Metabolic Evaluation of the Child with an Intellectual Developmental Disorder: Diagnostic Algorithm for Identification of Treatable Causes and New Digital Resource. Mol. Genet. Metab. 111 (4), 428–438.

E-BOOK FIGURES AND TABLES

The following figures and tables are available in the e-book at www.expertconsult.com. See inside cover for registration details.

Table 59-2 Translation of Targeted Treatments for Fragile X Syndrome: 2002 to 2015

Fig. 59-1. Dendritic translation pathways dysregulated in single-gene NDDs, including fragile X syndrome (FMRP), tuberous sclerosis (TSC) (TSC1/TSC2), Rett syndrome (MeCP2), neurofibromatosis type 1 (NF-1), and autism/macrocephaly (PTEN).

Fig. 59-2. Schematic of how steps in the pathways from Figure 59-1 have been targeted for development of treatments in preclinical studies.

Fig. 59-3. Illustration of the seven different therapeutic strategies for inborn errors of metabolism.

60 Neuropsychopharmacology

Breck Borcherding, Rebecca L. Rendleman, and John T. Walkup

 An expanded version of this chapter is available on www.expertconsult.com. See inside cover for registration details.

INTRODUCTION

With a growing evidence base of tolerable and effective psychotropic medications and more refined targets for treatment, psychopharmacology has become standard practice for many neuropsychiatric disorders, resulting in increased use of medications in children and broadening of the practitioner base for prescribing (see Table 60-1) (AACAP, 2009). There are excellent efficacy and safety data for the short-term treatment of attention deficit hyperactivity disorder (ADHD) with stimulants; of anxiety disorders with selective serotonin reuptake inhibitors (SSRIs); of obsessive-compulsive disorder (OCD) with clomipramine and SSRIs; of depression with SSRIs; and of schizophrenia, bipolar disorder, and irritability and behavioral dysregulation in different pediatric disorders with atypical antipsychotics. In contrast, there remain very little data from placebo-controlled efficacy studies on the short-term benefit of so-called mood stabilizers (e.g., lithium, anticonvulsants) for neuropsychiatric disorders. However, little is known regarding the long-term usefulness of any psychotropic medication, and there is increasing concern about the long-term effects of psychotropic drugs on growth and development. Although medication combinations are commonly used in children, studies of these combinations are also uncommon.

STIMULANTS FOR ADHD

Stimulants for behavioral issues in children have been in clinical use since 1937. Since then, stimulant medications have been consistently found efficacious, leading to comprehensive guidelines for treatment (Pliszka, 2007). Although behavioral treatment may be considered, in head-to-head studies, medication alone has been shown to be more beneficial than behavioral therapy alone in children 5 years of age and older. The combination of medication and behavioral therapy is specifically helpful for oppositional behavior and anxiety in children with ADHD.

The stimulant medications are now used in those with autism spectrum disorders and in preschoolers, although the response rate is less robust than in typically developing older children, and rates of adverse events are higher. These children may experience a worsening of ADHD (e.g., hyperactivity and irritability) or other symptoms (e.g., tics or stereotypies). Parent training and behavioral treatments remain the primary interventions with autistic patients and preschoolers with ADHD.

Despite substantial data supporting the efficacy of stimulants, their use in children remains controversial to the public at large. Concerns have been expressed about the potential for overdiagnosis of ADHD and overuse of stimulant medications in children. Although there is documentation of increases in stimulant use, there is little evidence to support the notion that more children are treated with stimulants than there are cases of ADHD in the population at large. Stimulant medications have also come under public scrutiny because of concerns about safety and side effects. In the context of parental concerns, prudent practice therefore necessitates an evaluation that leads to confidence in the diagnosis, fully informed consent, and use of appropriate doses with close monitoring, combined with effective and available psychosocial treatments.

Identification of co-occurring conditions and risk factors for adverse effects is essential because some medications may be contraindicated, or medication management may require dosing modification or closer monitoring. For stimulant medications, baseline height, weight, family or personal history of a tic disorder, and family or personal history of cardiac disease, including nonvasovagal syncope and sudden death, are also important. The treating clinician, based on physical examination and history, should consider the need for an electrocardiogram (ECG). During the dose-adjustment phase, children often are monitored for side effects, including blood pressure, pulse, height, and weight.

The most common side effects of stimulants are decreased appetite, insomnia, and nervousness. A baseline of sleep and eating patterns, tic symptoms in the patient and family, and anxiety and mood symptoms should be obtained before starting stimulants, to avoid misattribution of such problems to the stimulant treatment. Short-term reductions in weight gain and height have been reported in many studies. The possibility of long-term growth suppression with long-term use of stimulants remains a controversial topic. Tic increases observed after starting stimulants appear to reflect the natural waxing and waning of tic severity. Sudden death may be a very rare side effect of stimulant use in children; however, the risk is quite limited and poorly defined. There is no evidence for increased risk of addiction from appropriate treatment with stimulants for ADHD. Despite their impact on a broad range of ADHD-related symptoms, including irritability, stimulant medications can be associated with undesirable changes in mood and behavior.

After a maintenance dose is achieved, visit intervals can vary from 1 to 3 months or more. Ongoing monitoring of medication efficacy involves assessment of the patient's level of functioning in school, family, community, and peer groups. Data are collected from behavioral observations during office visits and parent and teacher reports and rating scales.

NONSTIMULANT MEDICATIONS FOR ADHD

Atomoxetine is a nonstimulant medication, potentially offering several advantages over stimulant medications: longer duration of action, lower misuse or abuse potential, lower risk of rebound effects, lower risk of precipitating tics or psychosis, and ease of prescribing.

Children should undergo standard psychiatric and medical assessment for ADHD as is done with stimulants. No laboratory screening is required, although obtaining baseline and follow-up liver function studies should be considered in view of reports of rare but severe acute liver dysfunction. Baseline values for weight, heart rate, and blood pressure should be obtained. The effectiveness and tolerability of combining

TABLE 60-1 Labeled and Off-Label Use of Neuropsychopharmacologic Agents in Children and Adolescents

Drug	Labeled Use in Children and Adolescents	Off-Label Use/Clinical Practice in Children and Adolescents
STIMULANTS		
Amphetamine, mixed salts	ADHD (≥3 yrs—IR, ≥ 6 yr—ER, narcolepsy (≥6 yrs, IR only)	
Dextroamphetamine	ADHD (≥6 yrs), narcolepsy (≥6 yrs)	
Lisdexamfetamine	ADHD (≥6 yrs)	
Methylphenidate	ADHD (≥6 yrs), narcolepsy (≥6 yrs)	
Dexmethylphenidate	ADHD (≥6 yrs)	
NON-STIMULANTS		
Atomoxetine	ADHD (≥6 yrs)	
Clonidine	ADHD (≥6 yrs—ER)	Aggression, tic disorders
Guanfacine	ADHD (6-17 yrs—ER)	Aggression, tic disorders
BENZODIAZEPINES		
Clonazepam	None	As a group—agitation, catatonia, short-term anxiety
Lorazepam	Anxiety (≥12 yrs), insomnia (≥12 yrs)	
TRICYCLIC ANTIDEPRESSANTS		
Amitriptyline	Depression (≥12 yrs)	As a group—depression, anxiety disorders, ADHD and pain syndromes
Clomipramine	OCD (>10 yrs)	
Desipramine	None	
Imipramine	Enuresis (≥6 yrs), depression (≥12 yrs)	
Nortriptyline	Depression	
SEROTONIN REUPTAKE INHIBITORS		
Citalopram	None	As a group—depression, anxiety disorders
Escitalopram	Depression (≥12 yrs)	
Fluoxetine	OCD (≥7 yrs), depression (≥8 yrs)	
Fluvoxamine	OCD (≥8 yrs)	
Paroxetine	None	
Sertraline	OCD (≥6 yrs)	
OTHER ANTIDEPRESSANTS		
Bupropion	None	Depression, ADHD
Desvenlafaxine	None	Depression, anxiety disorders
Duloxetine	None	Depression, chronic pain
Venlafaxine	None	Depression, anxiety disorders, ADHD
Mirtazapine	None	Depression, Anxiety disorders
MOOD STABILIZERS		
Lithium	Bipolar Disorder (≥12 yrs)	Aggression
Carbamazepine	Seizure disorders	As a group—bipolar disorder, aggression, mood instability
Gabapentin	Seizure disorders	
Lamotrigine	Seizure disorders	
Topiramate	Seizure disorders	
Valproate	Seizure disorders	
TYPICAL NEUROLEPTICS		
Chlorpromazine	Severe behavioral disturbances	As a group—psychotic disorders
Haloperidol	Psychosis, tics, severe behavioral disturbance	
Pimozide	Tics	
ATYPICAL NEUROLEPTICS		
Aripiprazole	Irritability in autistic disorder (6-17 yrs) Bipolar I disorder (≥10 yrs), schizophrenia (≥13 yrs)	As a group—psychotic disorders, Tourette syndrome, aggression
Clozapine	None	
Olanzapine	Bipolar I disorder (≥13 yrs), schizophrenia (≥13 yrs)	
Quetiapine	Bipolar I disorder (≥10 yrs), schizophrenia (≥13 yrs)	
Risperidone	Irritability in autistic disorder (6-17 yrs), bipolar I disorder (≥10 yrs), schizophrenia (≥13 yrs)	
Ziprasidone	None	

ADHD, attention deficit hyperactivity disorder; IR, immediate release; OCD, obsessive-compulsive disorder; ER, extended release

atomoxetine with methylphenidate in children who have not responded to monotherapy have been reported in a few patients.

Two α2 agonists, clonidine and guanfacine, are prescribed in the treatment of ADHD, Tourette syndrome, aggressive or self-injurious behavior, and the physiologic symptoms of anxiety. Extended-release (ER) guanfacine and ER clonidine have been found effective and are most studied. Before the initiation of clonidine or guanfacine, baseline ECG, heart rate, and blood pressure should be obtained. A history of syncope or cardiovascular disease is a relative contraindication. Heart rate and blood pressure should be monitored regularly during therapy for hypotension and bradycardia.

The most common side effects of clonidine and guanfacine include sedation, dizziness, fatigue, dry mouth and eyes, nausea, hypotension, and constipation. Syncope has been reported in a few children on guanfacine ER. Abrupt discontinuation can lead to rebound hypertension on these agents.

ANTIDEPRESSANTS
Tricyclic Antidepressants

Tricyclic antidepressants are approved for the treatment of depression in adults and adolescents. The use of tricyclic antidepressants for the treatment of depression in children and adolescents has declined because of their equivocal efficacy and safety in this population and the availability of serotonin reuptake inhibitors with a more favorable side-effect profile.

The tricyclic clomipramine has been approved for use in children 10 years of age or older for OCD, but it is also considered second-line treatment in clinical practice, again in part because of a less favorable side-effect profile compared with the SSRIs. Although amitriptyline is still commonly used in neurologic settings for adults, its side-effect profile in doses effective for the treatment of anxiety and depression is often prohibitive—particularly sedation and weight gain. Nortriptyline, the primary metabolite of amitriptyline, is often better tolerated in treatment. Tricyclic antidepressants have been prescribed as third-line treatments for patients with ADHD who have failed adequate trials of other agents. Imipramine appears to be effective in treating enuresis in children who have failed nonmedication interventions and desmopressin.

As with ADHD, assessment for anxiety disorders and depression requires the gathering of information through clinical interview, other informants, and medical evaluation, including laboratory screening (AACAP, 2007). The diagnostic evaluation of children with depression and anxiety should also determine whether other coexisting conditions are present. Risk factors for adverse effects with tricyclic antidepressants should be identified.

A medical evaluation is required before initiating tricyclic antidepressants. A baseline ECG, orthostatic blood pressure and heart rate, complete blood cell count (CBC), electrolyte determination, renal and hepatic function tests, thyroid function tests, and urinalysis should be performed. Other laboratory screening measures may be indicated, based on findings in the history or physical examination. Because of the risk of adverse cardiac effects, serial ECGs are recommended with the use of all tricyclic antidepressants. They should be obtained at baseline, during titration, and at the final dose.

Side effects of tricyclic antidepressants include sedation, weight gain, orthostatic hypotension, and anticholinergic side effects (i.e., dry mouth, constipation, blurred vision, urinary retention, and exacerbation of narrow-angle glaucoma). Although the role of the tricyclic antidepressants is unclear, it has been speculated that the cause of rare reported sudden death on these medications is likely a result of malignant arrhythmias. It is not clear whether the vulnerability to such medication effects can be determined from routine monitoring of cardiac function through regular ECGs.

Behavioral side effects include early and acute increases in anxiety or depression, or manic episodes or rapid cycling in patients. A family history of bipolar disorder may be a risk factor for this effect, but such a history is not an absolute contraindication for the use of antidepressants. A discontinuation syndrome may result from abrupt cessation of antidepressants. The U.S. Food and Drug Administration (FDA) mandated a black-box warning regarding increases in suicidal ideation for all antidepressants.

Selective Serotonin Reuptake Inhibitors

The SSRIs, including citalopram, escitalopram, fluvoxamine, fluoxetine, paroxetine, and sertraline, have FDA approval for a number of mood, anxiety, and eating disorders in adults. In children and adolescents, fluoxetine, fluvoxamine, and sertraline have FDA approval for OCD, fluoxetine also has FDA approval for major depression, and escitalopram has FDA approval for major depression in adolescents (12 years and older). The use of the SSRIs for depression increased significantly through the 1990s. In 2004 the FDA issued a black-box warning for increased risk of suicidal ideation and behavior in children and adolescents using all antidepressants. Since this time, prescriptions of antidepressants in the pediatric population have decreased.

Although some individuals may do better on one SSRI than another, comparative treatment trials suggest similarity in efficacy across all agents in this class. The SSRIs may demonstrate benefit in as little as 1 week, with substantial benefit occurring in 8 to 12 weeks. Improvement may continue at a more gradual rate for up to 6 to 12 months.

The assessment of mood and anxiety disorders before initiation of an SSRI is similar to that described earlier for the tricyclic antidepressants. Risk factors for adverse effects of SSRIs should be identified, and should include a family and personal history of bipolar disorder, history of suicidal ideation or behavior, sensitivity to other SSRIs, concurrent medications that could inhibit or could be inhibited by the SSRI, pregnancy, and hepatic or renal disease. No medical evaluation is required before initiating SSRI treatment, but it may be prudent to clear a child medically by means of a medical history and physical examination.

For all of the SSRIs, treatment usually is initiated with a low dose that is adjusted upward slowly at weekly intervals. Because the time–response pattern for the SSRIs occurs over a minimum of weeks, too aggressive titration often leads to early side effects and may result in early discontinuation of the medication and the need to start again with another medication. Starting low and slowly titrating upward may allow the patient time to develop some tolerance to some of the side effects. However, going too slowly may put the patient at risk for being undertreated.

The adverse-event profiles of SSRIs are similar. In placebo-controlled trials of the SSRIs, a few adverse effects occurred significantly more often on active medication than on placebo. These include gastrointestinal symptoms, insomnia, and anxiety or agitation. Other adverse effects that occur more often on active medication but are less common overall include somnolence, tremor, sweating, sexual dysfunction, epistaxis, and allergic reactions, including rash. The most common causes of medication discontinuation, other than lack of efficacy, are the behavioral or psychiatric side effects, such as anxiety or agitation.

Activation occurs in about 10% to 20% of patients. This activation syndrome (distinct from the mood improvement effects of the antidepressants) can result in a number of complaints, including anxiety, mental restlessness, increased activity level or akathisia, increased impulsivity, and disinhibition. This activation is very similar to but milder than what some children experience when they take diphenhydramine. Activation effects usually appear very early in treatment or after a dose change. Patients do not appear to develop tolerance to these symptoms, but they resolve with dose reduction or discontinuation. Much less common but also serious are manic and hypomanic reactions. In brief clinical trials, manic reactions are much less common (1% to 2%) than activation, occur later in treatment after a period of improvement, do not always go away with dose reduction or discontinuation, and may require medical intervention to control.

Children with anxiety and mood disorders who benefit from SSRI treatment do not always have uniform outcomes. For most, symptom relief is associated with return to normal and appropriate function. However, some children, especially those with behavioral problems or those at risk for other behavioral problems (i.e., poor parental discipline and monitoring), may present with increasing behavior problems after successful treatment of anxiety and depression. Children with anxiety and mood disorders also experience an evolution of symptoms over time. Children first presenting with separation anxiety at age 8 years may evolve into a generalized anxiety disorder or have periods of recurrent depression in their middle to late teens, for example. Half of adequately treated depressed adolescents have a recurring episode within a few years.

The SSRIs have also been reported to induce an apathy syndrome. Although it may manifest early in treatment, those with anxiety and depression may not be sensitive to this subtle medication effect until after a period of recovery.

In general, cardiac side effects from SSRIs are rare. However, citalopram can cause prolongation of the QT interval, and the FDA has issued a safety alert indicating that doses over 40 mg are no longer recommended because this dose potentiates risk for torsades de pointes.

Some individuals do appear to have a discontinuation syndrome with abrupt cessation of therapy that includes flu-like symptoms, such as malaise and gastrointestinal symptoms. Antidepressants with shorter half-lives appear to be more commonly associated with discontinuation syndromes than SSRIs with longer half-lives.

As noted earlier, antidepressants carry warnings in their product labeling regarding the increased risk for suicidal ideation and behavior (i.e., suicidality) in the course of treatment. The mechanism of this effect has never been clear, but it may be attributed to the positive energizing effects of antidepressants outpacing the improvement in baseline low mood and suicidality.

Other Antidepressants

The serotonin–norepinephrine reuptake inhibitors, which include duloxetine, venlafaxine, and desvenlafaxine, have FDA approval for treatment of depression and anxiety disorders in adults, but data are limited for children and adolescents, and the use of serotonin–norepinephrine reuptake inhibitors in children and adolescents is off-label.

Bupropion is approved by the FDA for the treatment of depression, nicotine dependence, and smoking cessation in adults only. Off-label uses of bupropion include monotherapy in the treatment of depression in children and adolescents and as a second-line agent in the treatment of ADHD. Bupropion may improve symptoms of ADHD in prepubertal children, although a study demonstrated that effect sizes of bupropion and placebo differences were smaller than those for standard stimulant medications. Adolescents with ADHD and co-occurring depression may demonstrate improvement with bupropion.

ANXIOLYTICS

Anxiety disorders are one of the most prevalent categories of childhood and adolescent psychopathology. Co-occurring conditions, such as other anxiety disorders, depression, and ADHD, are common. Treatment of anxiety disorders in children and adolescents is multimodal, including psychoeducational and cognitive behavioral therapy, family therapy, school interventions, and pharmacotherapy (Connolly and Bernstein, 2007). Medication choices are multiple, but serotonin reuptake inhibitors are the pharmacologic treatment of choice.

The role of benzodiazepines is limited to the short-term management of anxiety symptoms because data supporting their use in children is sparse. In cases of severe anxiety, they may be added to tricyclic antidepressants or SSRIs for acute management of anxiety symptoms until the therapeutic effects of the antidepressants emerge. Benzodiazepines can be useful for the short-term management of specific anxiety-provoking situations, such as medical procedures, or as short-term adjunctive treatment with SSRIs in the initial treatment of severe anxiety disorders, or in treatment of catatonia.

In considering benzodiazepine therapy for a patient, the clinician should inquire about any possible history of substance abuse. The patient and family should be informed about the risks of tolerance, dependence, and withdrawal effects, in addition to possible effects on cognitive and motor functioning. After the treatment trial is complete, the medication should be tapered slowly because of the potential for withdrawal and rebound anxiety. The most frequent adverse effects in children and adolescents are sedation, drowsiness, and decreased mental acuity. Benzodiazepines may also cause paradoxical agitation, aggression, and hyperactivity. Anterograde amnesia also has been associated with benzodiazepines, particularly high-potency benzodiazepines.

Buspirone is approved for use in the treatment of anxiety disorders in adults, but unpublished, industry-sponsored, randomized controlled trials in children do not demonstrate benefit. The most common adverse effects of buspirone are dizziness, headache, drowsiness, and lightheadedness.

MOOD STABILIZERS

The term *mood stabilizers* refers to medications used to treat severe fluctuating moods, including depression and mania in bipolar disorder. Mood stabilizers have antimanic and antidepressant properties and treat specific mood states without negatively affecting other mood states (e.g., worsening depression when mania is treated, or vice versa). Attempts to mark boundaries between chronic and cyclic irritable mood in children have led to more stringent bipolar diagnostic criteria and the development of the diagnosis of Disruptive Mood Dysregulation Disorder in the *Diagnostic and Statistical Manual of Mental Disorders*, Fifth Edition (APA, 2013).

Mood stabilizers used in clinical practice can be grouped into three categories: lithium, anticonvulsants, and antipsychotics. As with childhood depression, children with bipolar affective disorder are thought to be less responsive to medication compared with adults. Combination of mood stabilizers, or a mood stabilizer with an antipsychotic, is sometimes required to stabilize acute manic symptoms. It appears that second-generation antipsychotics may be more effective for bipolar disorder in children than anticonvulsants or lithium.

Given the complexity of making an accurate diagnosis, the treatment-resistant nature of pediatric bipolar illness, and the complicated regimens of medication sometimes required, the average pediatric neurologist is encouraged to request consultation from a child psychiatrist if faced with a child patient with possible bipolar disorder (McClellan, Kowatch, and Findling, 2007).

Lithium

Lithium is approved by the FDA for use in the treatment of bipolar affective disorder for children 12 years of age and older. It is effective in managing acute manic and depressive episodes, preventing or diminishing the intensity of subsequent episodes in maintenance treatment, and decreasing mood instability between episodes. Data in children and adolescents with bipolar disorder are limited and offer mixed results, but there is concern that lithium is underused compared with other newer mood stabilizers of questionable efficacy.

Before starting lithium therapy, the patient should be screened for pregnancy, renal disease, or diabetes mellitus. A medical evaluation should be completed, including an ECG, laboratory screen for electrolytes, kidney and thyroid function tests, complete blood count (CBC), urinalysis, and urine pregnancy screen. Lithium levels between 0.8 and 1.0 mEq/L may offer the best prophylaxis against mania, whereas lower levels may be adequate for prophylaxis against depression. After mood symptoms are stabilized, lithium levels should be routinely checked every 3 to 6 months.

Side effects of lithium are polydipsia, polyuria or enuresis, gastric distress (i.e., nausea, vomiting, and diarrhea), weight gain, tremor, fatigue, leukocytosis, acne, and mild cognitive impairment. Serious renal side effects are rare but occur. Lithium therapy can induce alterations in thyroid function tests and produce hypothyroidism. Lithium can have rare but serious cardiac side effects. Intrauterine exposure to lithium during the first trimester has been associated with teratogenic effects, most commonly Ebstein's anomaly.

Valproic Acid

The initial support for use of valproic acid in child psychiatric practice came from the adult literature. The evidence for its use in the treatment of juvenile bipolar disorder, however, is limited. Divalproex sodium has also been shown in small studies to benefit children and adolescents with explosive temper and mood lability and for treatment of core symptoms of autism and associated symptoms of affective instability, aggression, and impulsivity.

In addition to the routine psychiatric or neurologic history, patients should be asked about risk factors affecting treatment with valproate, including pregnancy, disorders of metabolism, hepatic or renal disease, concomitant medications, and coagulation disorders. Laboratory screening should include liver function tests and a CBC, and a pregnancy test in females. Families should be educated about potential signs of hepatic or pancreatic toxicity and polycystic ovary disease.

Although therapeutic levels for treating mania have not been established, achieving a plasma concentration of 85 to 110 mg/L is needed to declare a trial adequate for determining outcome in an individual patient. Divalproex ER allows for once-daily dosing. Maintenance involves monitoring of the therapeutic response and side effects and requires laboratory screening. Liver enzymes, CBC, and serum valproic acid levels should be periodically monitored.

Adverse effects include sedation, nausea, vomiting, gastrointestinal upset, increased appetite, weight gain, and hair loss. Rare side effects include thrombocytopenia, platelet dysfunction, prolonged bleeding time, and elevation in liver enzymes, which can occur without clinical symptoms. Children younger than 2 years appear to have an increased risk of hepatotoxicity, and extreme caution should be used in this population.

Carbamazepine

Limited data are available on the efficacy of carbamazepine for the treatment of bipolar disorder children and adolescents. Justification for its use in clinical practice has rested on the adult literature, which is difficult to interpret. Patients should be evaluated for medical conditions that may contraindicate use of carbamazepine, including liver disease, hematologic disorders, immune disorders, cardiac disease, and pregnancy. Laboratory screening should include a urine pregnancy screen, liver function tests, and a CBC. Recommended levels are the same as those for seizure disorder, 4 to 12 mg/ml.

The most common adverse effects are nausea, vomiting, sedation, and ataxia. Carbamazepine can cause mild elevations in liver transaminases; hepatitis, indicated by elevated liver transaminase levels greater than three times normal; and cholestasis, indicated by elevations in bilirubin and alkaline phosphatase. Carbamazepine therapy has been associated with leukopenia in 1% to 2% of patients and agranulocytosis or aplastic anemia in 1 of 250,000 patients. Other adverse effects observed with carbamazepine include cognitive or behavioral disturbance, CNS toxicity, altered cardiac conduction, and life-threatening dermatologic conditions (i.e., exfoliative dermatitis, toxic epidermal necrolysis, and Stevens–Johnson syndrome).

Other Mood Stabilizers

Although lithium and valproate are first-line pharmacologic treatments for bipolar disorder in adults, many children and adolescents do not respond adequately to these medications and cannot tolerate the side effects. In clinical practice, newer anticonvulsants are beginning to be used for the treatment of bipolar disorder. Many of these newer anticonvulsants have a more favorable adverse-effect profile, but use of these medications is more appropriate for patients with bipolar disorder who are unresponsive to traditional therapies or cannot tolerate traditional agents.

Data on lamotrigine in pediatric bipolar disorder are limited to case series and open-label trials but suggest that, in adolescents, lamotrigine may be effective for the treatment of bipolar depression, treatment of mania, and maintenance treatment of bipolar disorder.

Because supporting data are limited in pediatric populations, the use of lamotrigine in children and adolescents for the treatment of bipolar disorder should be reserved for those who have failed alternative treatments and demonstrate persistent disabling symptoms.

A painstaking approach to slow dose adjustment of lamotrigine decreases the risk for rash, including Stevens–Johnson syndrome. Dosing must be adjusted upward for children taking concomitant carbamazepine, phenytoin, phenobarbital, or primidone, which increases lamotrigine clearance, and dosing must be reduced for children taking concomitant valproate, which decreases lamotrigine clearance.

Common adverse effects observed in clinical studies include dizziness, ataxia, somnolence, headache, diplopia, blurred vision, nausea, vomiting, and rash. Lamotrigine has been associated with serious rashes requiring hospitalization and discontinuation of treatment.

Other newer anticonvulsants include topiramate, gabapentin, and oxcarbazepine, all with little empirical data to support their use in young people with mood disorders.

DOPAMINE RECEPTOR ANTAGONISTS: TYPICAL ANTIPSYCHOTICS

Dopamine receptor antagonist is a term used to refer to a medication that is a high-affinity antagonist of dopamine receptors. Other terms used to refer to these drugs include *typical antipsychotics*, *neuroleptics*, and *major tranquilizers*. The antipsychotic effects of these medications are thought to be mediated through the inhibition of dopamine binding at dopamine D_2 receptors, resulting in the reduction of dopaminergic neurotransmission in the central nervous system (CNS). The neurologic side effects appear to be mediated by dopamine antagonism in the nigrostriatal pathway. Other side effects associated with these antipsychotics result from activity at adrenergic, cholinergic, and histaminic receptors.

Dopamine receptor antagonists are distinguished from serotonin–dopamine antagonists, also called novel or atypical antipsychotics or second-generation antipsychotics. In contrast to typical antipsychotics, the serotonin–dopamine antagonists have a higher ratio of serotonin type 2 to dopamine D_2 receptor blockade. Additionally, they appear to have reduced risk of short- and long-term neurologic side effects and to be superior in treating negative symptoms of schizophrenia and acute mania. Unfortunately, as patients and clinicians gained experience with serotonin–dopamine antagonists, other adverse effects, such as weight gain, hyperglycemia, and hyperlipidemia, were recognized. Head-to-head comparisons of first- and second-generation antipsychotics in the treatment of schizophrenia in adult and pediatric populations have revealed no significant difference in efficacy and reinforce the continued role of these earlier medications. Typical antipsychotics continue to be used in certain neuropsychiatric diagnoses, such as Tourette syndrome (Murphy et al., 2013), and when excessive weight gain and metabolic abnormalities result from atypical antipsychotics.

Typical antipsychotics can be classified by their dopamine receptor binding potency. High-potency antipsychotics (e.g., haloperidol, fluphenazine, pimozide) are more likely to cause extrapyramidal symptoms, whereas low-potency antipsychotics (e.g., chlorpromazine, thioridazine) are more likely to cause side effects mediated by cholinergic, α_1-adrenergic, and histaminic receptor activity.

Side effects of dopamine receptor antagonists include orthostatic hypotension, peripheral anticholinergic effects (i.e., dry mouth, blurred vision, constipation, urinary retention), central anticholinergic effects (i.e., agitation, delirium, hallucinations, seizures, and coma), hyperprolactinemia, leukopenia, agranulocytosis, jaundice, photosensitivity, decreased seizure threshold, and weight gain. Thioridazine has been associated with irreversible retinal pigmentation. Chlorpromazine has been associated with skin pigmentation and deposits in the lens and cornea, which usually do not affect vision. Rarely, cardiotoxicity and sudden death have been associated with some typical antipsychotics, especially low-potency antipsychotics and pimozide.

Neurologic side effects of dopamine receptor antagonists include parkinsonism, dystonias, akathisia, and dyskinesias (collectively called extrapyramidal symptoms). Children and adolescents appear to be more sensitive than adults to these side effects. Neuroleptic malignant syndrome is a severe life threatening complication.

ATYPICAL ANTIPSYCHOTICS

Serotonin–dopamine antagonists (also called atypical or second-generation antipsychotics) differ from typical antipsychotics in that they have a higher ratio of serotonin type 2 to dopamine type 2 receptor blockade. Risperidone, olanzapine, quetiapine, ziprasidone, and clozapine are serotonin-dopamine antagonists. Aripiprazole is commonly grouped with the second-generation antipsychotics, but it has a unique mechanism of action as a partial dopamine agonist.

Direct comparisons of serotonin–dopamine antagonists and dopamine receptor antagonists using rigorous methodology in children and adolescents have been limited. When studied, the extrapyramidal symptoms reported by patients on serotonin–dopamine antagonists do not differ substantially from those reported by patients on dopamine receptor antagonists, except for severity. With the exception of clozapine, dyskinesias have been reported with all of the serotonin–dopamine antagonists.

Weight gain has emerged as one of the most common and troubling side effects for children and adolescents on the serotonin–dopamine antagonists. Emerging evidence reveals that serotonin–dopamine antagonists can cause development of metabolic syndrome and diabetes even with short-term treatment. As with typical antipsychotics, elevated prolactin levels can develop with the serotonin–dopamine antagonists. Cardiovascular effects have been noted with the serotonin–dopamine antagonists. Quetiapine and clozapine can cause dizziness and orthostatic hypotension, thought to be mediated by adrenergic blockade. QT prolongation has been observed with ziprasidone and clozapine.

Given the possible adverse effects of all antipsychotics and our limited knowledge of their long-term safety, careful monitoring of pediatric patients is a necessity (Correll, 2008). Recommended baseline measurements include laboratory screening (e.g., CBC, electrolytes, liver and renal function tests, thyroid function test, and fasting glucose and lipid levels), height, weight, and baseline assessment of extrapyramidal symptoms using clinician ratings (e.g., Abnormal Involuntary Movement Scale). A baseline ECG is recommended before initiating ziprasidone or clozapine.

Risperidone

Risperidone is labeled for use in the treatment of schizophrenia and the manic phase of bipolar disorder, either alone or in conjunction with lithium or valproate in adults. In pediatric populations, risperidone is labeled for use in the treatment of schizophrenia (≥13 years), the acute manic phase of bipolar disorder (≥10 years), and irritability associated with autism (5 to 16 years). Risperidone has also been found to be effective in conduct disorder, aggression in children with subaverage IQ, and Tourette syndrome. Risperidone can cause sedation, dizziness, orthostatic hypotension, increased appetite, weight gain, and extrapyramidal symptoms.

Olanzapine

In pediatric populations, olanzapine is labeled for the short-term treatment of schizophrenia and bipolar manic or mixed episodes in adolescents of 13 years of age or older. Additionally, olanzapine has been found useful in the treatment of autism and Tourette syndrome. Compared with the other atypical antipsychotics, olanzapine has consistently had the highest risk for weight gain.

Quetiapine

In pediatric populations, quetiapine is approved for the acute treatment of schizophrenia in adolescents of 13 years or older and treatment of mania associated with bipolar disorder in children and adolescents of 10 years or older. Quetiapine was originally thought to have less risk of weight gain, but quetiapine use in typical clinical practice can increase weight in children and adolescents.

Ziprasidone

In pediatric populations, use of ziprasidone is off-label. Before ziprasidone therapy is initiated, a careful history must be obtained to identify possible cardiac contraindications. Baseline ECG and follow up after reaching final dosage are recommended.

Aripiprazole

Experience with aripiprazole in pediatric populations is growing, and aripiprazole has FDA approval for the acute treatment of schizophrenia in adolescents of 13 years or older, for manic or mixed episodes of acute mania in children and adolescents of 10 years or older, and for irritability associated with autistic disorder in children and adolescents of 6 years or older. As with other mania treatments, combination treatment may be more efficacious than treatment with aripiprazole alone.

Clozapine

Clozapine is off-label for use in pediatric populations, but it has been found effective in the management of treatment-refractory childhood-onset schizophrenia in randomized, double-blind comparison trials. Its use is limited by increased risk of adverse events. Additionally, clozapine is the only antipsychotic for which the risk of tardive dyskinesia is considered minimal. Seizures are reported in 4% of patients, with increasing risk at higher doses. Other adverse events include cardiomyopathy, hepatitis, cerebrovascular accidents, and severe anticholinergic toxicity. Agranulocytosis (absolute neutrophil count [ANC] < 500 mm^3) is a serious and potentially fatal adverse effect of clozapine. The FDA requires painstaking monitoring of the white blood count (WBC) and ANC throughout the course of treatment. Experience with clozapine in the treatment of treatment-refractory childhood-onset schizophrenia has shown that neutropenia is more common in children than in adults and is estimated to occur at a rate of 10% to 13%.

CONCLUSION

Children do benefit from psychiatric medication when treatment is provided in the context of (1) a thorough diagnostic assessment that integrates information from multiple sources, (2) knowledge of the available data for adults and children in the literature, (3) knowledge of standards when prescribing medications off-label, (4) an analysis of the risks and benefits of treatment options, (5) appropriate involvement of the child and parent or guardian in the informed consent process, and (6) close monitoring for adverse effects during therapy. Pediatric neurologists should be prepared to consult child psychiatrists regularly when questions of appropriate diagnosis, of treatment choice of medication versus psychosocial therapies, and of safety and efficacy of medication are outside their scope of practice.

REFERENCES

 The complete list of references for this chapter is available in the e-book at www.expertconsult.com.
See inside cover for registration details.

SELECTED REFERENCES

AACAP, 2007. Practice parameter for the assessment and treatment of children and adolescents with depressive disorders. J. Am. Acad. Child Adolesc. Psychiatry 46 (11), 1503.

AACAP, 2009. Practice parameter on the use of psychotropic medication in children and adolescents. J. Am. Acad. Child Adolesc. Psychiatry 48 (9), 961.

APA, 2013. Diagnostic and Statistical Manual of Mental Disorders, 5th ed. Text Revision. DSM-5. American Psychiatric Association, Washington, D.C.

Connolly, S.D., Bernstein, G.A., 2007. Practice parameter for the assessment and treatment of children and adolescents with anxiety disorders. J. Am. Acad. Child Adolesc. Psychiatry 46 (2), 267.

Correll, C.U., 2008. Antipsychotic use in children and adolescents: minimizing adverse effects to maximize outcomes. J. Am. Acad. Child Adolesc. Psychiatry 47 (1), 9.

McClellan, J., Kowatch, R., Findling, R.L., 2007. Practice parameter for the assessment and treatment of children and adolescents with bipolar disorder. J. Am. Acad. Child Adolesc. Psychiatry 46 (1), 107.

Murphy, T.K., Lewin, A.B., Storch, E.A., et al., 2013. Practice parameter for the assessment and treatment of children and adolescents with tic disorders. J. Am. Acad. Child Adolesc. Psychiatry 52 (12), 1341.

Pliszka, S., 2007. Practice parameter for the assessment and treatment of children and adolescents with attention-deficit/hyperactivity disorder. J. Am. Acad. Child Adolesc. Psychiatry 46 (7), 894.

E-BOOK FIGURES AND TABLES

61 Overview of Seizures and Epilepsy in Children

Phillip L. Pearl

An expanded version of this chapter is available on www.expertconsult.com. See inside cover for registration details.

INTRODUCTION

An estimated 65 million people worldwide live with epilepsy. In the United States, there are approximately 3 million people diagnosed with epilepsy, and 150,000 new cases diagnosed are each year. The annual direct medical cost of epilepsy in the United States is $12.5 billion. Epilepsy is the fourth most common neurologic disease, following migraine, stroke, and Alzheimer-related dementia. There are many gaps in care, including in the areas of access, prevention, education, and stigma. The comorbidities are vast, and include neurologic (e.g., autism), psychiatric (e.g., mood disorders, suicidality), and somatic (e.g., fractures) conditions. The range of outcomes is wide, r from age-restricted conditions and long-term resolution to unemployment or underemployment, poorer overall health status, and increased mortality. Among the population with newly diagnosed epilepsy, children and older adults are the most rapidly growing segments (Hesdorffer et al., 2013). This chapter provides an overview of the changing conceptualization, categorization, and terminology of seizures and epilepsy and introduces the multiple-chapter section that follows.

An Ancient Disease in Modern Times

The term *seizure* derives from a Latin word meaning "attack" or "to take over," and some of its earliest documented usage was as a military term by Thucydides in his description of the Peloponnesian wars, which took place from 431 to 404 BCE. *Epilepsy* derives etymologically from the Greek word *epi-lambanein*, meaning "repeated attacks," and was used as a descriptor of events from wars to diseases. It was known as a sacred disease or the "falling sickness" in ancient times, and physicians of the Hippocratic school, circa 400 BCE, recognized that this was not a supernatural affliction but a physical malady. In particular, they emphasized an important role of heredity in its origin. The more modern understanding of epilepsy as a paroxysmal disorder of brain function, and the notion that a convulsion was but a symptom of epilepsy, began with the writings of Johns Hughlings Jackson (1835–1911) (Temkin, 1971). Today we conceptualize a seizure as a transient event emanating from abnormal excessive neuronal activity in the brain, and epilepsy as an enduring condition whereby an imbalance between excessive neuronal excitation and deficient inhibition leads to a predisposition to recurring seizures (Fisher et al., 2005). The protean manifestations of seizures, recognition of the heterogeneity of epilepsy along with its comorbidities, and new concepts in the definition, categorization, pathophysiology, management, and outcomes derive from these early concepts, but with dramatic recent advancements.

Thus a seizure may be provoked (i.e., situational) or, in contrast, a manifestation of an enduring predisposition to recurrent seizures and thus representative of epilepsy, the preferred term for the anachronistic term *seizure disorder*. A provoked or situational seizure implies that the seizure occurred as an isolated event related to the acute situation (e.g., fever, acute head impact, hypoglycemia, or postsyncopal). In general, after a first unprovoked seizure in childhood, the risk of a recurrence is about 50%, and after the second the risk is about 80%. Seizures are still viewed as unprovoked if they occur with stressors related to personal activity, such as sleep deprivation or severe emotional distress, unless these stresses are extreme. Traditionally, epilepsy had been diagnosed only after a child had at least two unprovoked seizures at least 24 hours apart. The definition of epilepsy, however, has been broadened.

New Conceptual and Practical Definitions

The International League Against Epilepsy (ILAE) has been addressing the core concepts and definitions applicable to seizures and epilepsy, along with changes in classification, since the first publication on classification and terminology in 1960, updated in 1981 for seizures and in 1989 for the epilepsies. Based on advances in basic and clinical neurosciences, and the mandate to incorporate these into clinical practice, the definitions and terminology for both seizures and epilepsy were revised in a special report published in 2010 (Berg et al., 2010), although this revision remains in debate. Generalized seizures are defined as seizures occurring in and rapidly engaging bilaterally distributed networks, and are classified as tonic-clonic, absence, myoclonic, clonic, tonic, and atonic (Table 61-1). Focal seizures are no longer dichotomized as simple versus complex, which was previously based upon whether an alteration of consciousness was present, and furthermore are also no longer called "partial," recognizing that they are no less complete than are generalized seizures. Instead, focal seizures are described according to their manifestations (e.g., focal motor, autonomic, dyscognitive) if there is impairment of consciousness or awareness. Of relevance to child neurologists, neonatal seizures are no longer regarded as unclassified or a separate seizure type, and instead are classified within the proposed scheme. In addition, there is an "unknown category" that includes epileptic spasms, which subsumes infantile spasms and recognizes that these may continue past infancy or even begin after the age of 1 year.

The earlier concepts of idiopathic, symptomatic, and cryptogenic epilepsy have been replaced by genetic, structural-metabolic, and unknown. The three new terms should not be conflated with the three prior terms, despite the rough resemblance. The concept that idiopathic likely represented

TABLE 61-1 Classification of Seizures *(2010 ILAE Classification of Seizures)*

Generalized seizures
  Tonic-clonic (in any combination)
  Absence
    Typical
    Atypical
    Absence with special features
      Myoclonic absence
      Eyelid myoclonia
  Myoclonic
    Myoclonic
    Myoclonic atonic
    Myoclonic tonic
  Clonic
  Tonic
  Atonic

Focal seizures (described by phenomenology)

Unknown
  Epileptic spasms

(Adapted from Berg AT, Berkovic SF, Brodie MJ, et al. Epilepsia 2010; 51:676–685.)

TABLE 61-2 Operational (Practical) Clinical Definition of Epilepsy

Epilepsy is a disease of the brain defined by any of the following:
1. At least two unprovoked (or reflex) seizures occurring > 24 h apart
2. One unprovoked (or reflex) seizure and a probability of further seizures similar to the general recurrence risk (at least 60%) after two unprovoked seizures, occurring over the next 10 years
3. Diagnosis of an epilepsy syndrome

Epilepsy is considered to be *resolved* for the following individuals:
1. Those who had an age-dependent epilepsy syndrome but are now past the applicable age
2. Those who have remained seizure-free for the last 10 years, with no seizure medicines for the last 5 years

(Adapted from Fisher RS, Acevedo C, Arzimanoglou A, et al. Epilepsia 2014; 55: 475–482.)

a pharmacoresponsive disorder with a predictable age-related remission, along with absence of comorbidities, had to be discarded with the realities of the natural history and variety of cognitive and behavioral disorders documented in many patients heretofore diagnosed with idiopathic epilepsy. Only about half of patients with childhood absence epilepsy are seizure-free after treatment with the initial medicine (Glauser et al., 2010). Patients with juvenile myoclonic epilepsy have now been demonstrated to have abnormal structural imaging findings and impaired cognitive development in the first 2 years after diagnosis compared with controls in a prospective trial. In addition, only half of subjects were seizure-free for 1 or more years after 2 years of treatment. The term *structural-metabolic* is intended to distinguish this admittedly heterogeneous group from that of genetic, that is, genetic versus everything else. The "unknown" group is a moving target, especially as new genes are identified, whether coding for channels, receptors, or other structures, or possessing other modifying or regulatory functions.

More recently, a practical clinical definition of epilepsy has been proposed by the ILAE that takes into account the propensity for recurrent seizures even after a single seizure in selected patients, as well the criteria for when epilepsy may be considered to be resolved. The diagnosis of epilepsy may now be applied after a single unprovoked seizure if there is a likelihood of further seizures similar to the general recurrence risk (which is 60% +) after having had two unprovoked seizures over the subsequent 10 years (Table 61-2). Additionally, if the clinical criteria are met to establish the presence of a recognizable epilepsy syndrome even after a single seizure (e.g., juvenile myoclonic epilepsy in the appropriate setting), the diagnosis of epilepsy may be established. Reflex seizures (e.g., following visual patterns or flashes of light) are essentially included in the category of unprovoked seizures in terms of the definition of epilepsy. Epilepsy is considered resolved in the case of an age-dependent epilepsy syndrome in individuals past the applicable age, or in patients who have remained seizure-free for the last 10 years, with no seizure medicines used for the last 5 years (Fisher et al., 2014).

Of particular relevance to pediatric practitioners are the time-honored electroclinical syndromes that identify clusters of characteristics that help to group patients into recognizable cohorts. These designations are meaningful in terms of diagnostic and therapeutic implications and prediction of

outcomes. Clinicians rely on recognizing these patterns to manage and counsel patients and families. Whereas common syndromes such as childhood absence epilepsy and benign rolandic epilepsy previously were classified using the dichotomy of focal versus generalized seizures, this scheme has been abandoned because new gene discoveries have revealed that many of the syndromes overlap these somewhat artificial boundaries. Thus the syndromes have been reorganized based on presentation by age, which is clinically friendly, especially for the developmental approach to disease adapted by pediatric practitioners (Berg et al., 2010) (Table 61-3). Still, the diversity and heterogeneity of etiologies in epilepsy have led to a renaming of this group of disorders as the "epilepsies," and the majority of patients will not fit easily into a defined electroclinical syndrome. The syndromes are in a state of flux because the conditions underlying them have been further elucidated with advances in neuroimaging and gene discovery.

Conceptual Evolution and a New Lexicon for the Epilepsies

The Institute of Medicine (IOM) released a landmark report, "Epilepsy across the Spectrum: Promoting Health and Understanding," that highlighted gaps in the knowledge and management of epilepsy and recommended actions for improving the lives of patients and families (Hesdorffer et al., 2013). The focus on epilepsy has thus enlarged from that of a "seizure disorder" to a wide spectrum including a diversity of seizure types, underlying syndromes, etiologies, comorbidities, and outcomes. The committee responsible for the report was also focused on the longstanding stigma associated with the condition, and suggested that use of the term *epileptic* be discontinued because of its negative connotation. Thus the preferred term is *person with epilepsy*, and the term *antiseizure medications* is preferred over *antiepileptic drugs*. This updated terminology will be employed throughout this text.

EPIDEMIOLOGY

Epidemiologic studies have addressed the incidence and prevalence of epilepsy in children, although differing case ascertainment methods, definitions of epilepsy, age range of subjects, and inclusion of children with febrile seizures make comparison between studies challenging. The newborn period is an additional complicating factor because newborns will have seizures as the result of an acute encephalopathy but without possessing an enduring predisposition to develop ongoing epilepsy. Many incidence/prevalence studies have excluded babies younger than 1 month of age. The issue of whether to include febrile or "illness-related" seizures can also

TABLE 61-3 Epilepsy Syndromes by Age of Onset

NEONATAL

Benign familial neonatal epilepsy
Early myoclonic encephalopathy
Ohtahara syndrome

INFANCY

Epilepsy of infancy with migrating focal seizures
West syndrome (infantile spasms, hypsarrhythmia; to be distinguished
 from benign myoclonus of early infancy, a nonepilepsy)
Myoclonic epilepsy in infancy (benign Dravet variant)
Benign infantile epilepsy
Benign familial infantile epilepsy
Severe myoclonic epilepsy of infancy (classic Dravet syndrome)
Myoclonic encephalopathy in nonprogressive disorders

CHILDHOOD

Genetic epilepsy with febrile seizures plus (GEFS +; can begin in
 infancy)
Panayiotopoulos syndrome
Epilepsy with myoclonic atonic (previously astatic) seizures
Benign epilepsy with centrotemporal spikes (BECTS, or benign
 rolandic epilepsy)
Autosomal-dominant nocturnal frontal lobe epilepsy (ADNFLE)
Late-onset childhood occipital epilepsy (Gastaut syndrome)
Epilepsy with myoclonic absences (Tassinari syndrome)
Lennox–Gastaut syndrome
Epileptic encephalopathy with continuous spike-and-wave during
 sleep (CSWS)
Landau–Kleffner syndrome (LKS)
Childhood absence epilepsy (pyknolepsy)
Generalized epilepsy with eyelid myoclonia (Jeavons syndrome)*

ADOLESCENCE–ADULT

Juvenile absence epilepsy (JAE)
Juvenile myoclonic epilepsy (JME)
Epilepsy with generalized tonic-clonic seizures alone
Progressive myoclonus epilepsies (PME)
Autosomal-dominant epilepsy with auditory features
Other familial temporal lobe epilepsies

LESS SPECIFIC AGE RELATIONSHIP

Familial focal epilepsy with variable foci (childhood to adult)
Reflex epilepsies (e.g., photosensitive, audiogenic, or reading-induced
 seizures; may or may not coexist with spontaneous seizures)

---

*Not listed as a syndrome by the International League Against
 Epilepsy (ILAE) but instead recognized under absence seizures with
 special features.

be confusing, especially when documentation of fever is not always available, children may have a mixture of febrile and afebrile seizures, and seizures associated with acute illness may be difficult to interpret if there is no fever. The age range for febrile seizures is typically given as 6 months to 5 years (basically, to the sixth birthday), although some children older than 5 years will have a seizure with fever but not go on to develop epilepsy.

The average incidence of epilepsy in children across studies is approximately 0.1%. The reported incidence has a wide range, from 41 in 100,000 in all children in Nova Scotia to 187 in 100,000 in children 6 to 9 years of age in Kenya. In developed countries, the incidence has ranged from 33.3 to 82 children less than age 16 years per 100,000 persons per year. The incidence is highest in the first year of life, with a range of 81 in 100,000 in Rochester, Minnesota, in 1945; to 54 to 118 in 100,000 in Nova Scotia, from 1977 to 1985; to 130 in 100,000 in Iceland, from 1995 to 1999. A more recent assessment in Rochester, Minnesota, for 1980 to 2004 showed an incidence of 102 in 100,000 in children up to 12 months of age (Wirrell et al., 2011). The incidence during childhood is about 50 in 100,000, and in adolescence is about 20 in 100,000, similar to

most published rates in adults in developed countries (Wirrell et al., 2011). The incidence is essentially the same in boys and girls.

Despite the previous discussion regarding the new classification of epilepsy syndromes, only about a third of children with epilepsy can be assigned to a specific syndrome, and many of these syndromes are quite rare. Thus incidence data for specific syndromes are inconsistent and overly sensitive to small shifts in the number of reported cases. Yet for a more historically common breakdown of seizure types, studies have shown that focal-onset seizures are more common, occurring in 55% to 60% of children with epilepsy, than are generalized seizures (reported in approximately 40%) (Wirrell et al., 2011), whereas spasms comprise 2% to 5% of pediatric epilepsy.

The prevalence of epilepsy in children is approximately 5 in 1000 in developed countries. As expected, prevalence is higher than incidence because epilepsy is a chronic disorder, although some children will have a flurry of seizures at one time without recurrence. Comparisons between countries can be difficult to interpret, because the proportion of children in the population varies from country to country, with the highest found in developing countries. In underdeveloped countries, the prevalence rates are higher and have a wide range, from 7.5 to 44.3 in 1000 children.

DIAGNOSIS

In clinical practice, the diagnosis of epilepsy rests not only on the traditional definition of two unprovoked seizures and the new definition based on recurrence risk as discussed earlier, but in particular on the differential diagnosis of a seizure versus mimicking events. Misinterpretation and misdiagnosis are not uncommon occurrences. The now widespread use of cellular video and abundant use of video electroencephalogram (EEG) monitoring, whether with inpatient or ambulatory EEG systems, certainly add to the traditional history taking when exploring the underpinnings of paroxysmal clinical events. Still, the details of provoking factors; underlying acute, subacute, and chronic illnesses; and the patient's clinical situation, medical and family history, and environment are mandatory aspects of history taking that go far in constructing the essential differential diagnosis. Parents and observers vary in their capacity to describe these frightening events, and history taking remains an art. Even among neurologists, discordant diagnoses have been reported in 35% of cases of possible first seizures. Additional events may be necessary to establish a diagnosis of epilepsy. Disorders that are frequently confused with epilepsy commonly include syncopal seizures associated with vasodepressor syncope or breath-holding spells. Differential diagnosis of paroxysmal events is described in more detail in the subsequent chapter on seizure management and outcome. The problem of psychogenic nonepileptic seizures is a significant challenge, although there are specific features that incriminate this diagnosis, as is covered in detail in a separate chapter.

The EEG can establish a diagnosis of epilepsy if a seizure is recorded, but interictal EEGs can be problematic because false positives and false negatives occur. Up to 5% of children have epileptiform activity on EEG without having clinical seizures, and up to 40% of children with chronic epilepsy do not demonstrate interictal epileptiform discharges on EEG. EEG findings may confirm syndrome diagnosis but may also change significantly over time, may reveal conflicting findings, and are subject to high interreader variability.

Likewise, the diagnosis of epilepsy cannot be based on brain-imaging studies. The presence of an anomaly on magnetic resonance imaging (MRI) increases the possibility of epilepsy and, depending on the nature of the abnormality, increases the likelihood of a specific seizure type or epilepsy syndrome. For example, lesions typical of tuberous sclerosis in the first year of life increase the risk that a child will have infantile spasms.

OVERVIEW AND SUMMARY

There are many unanswered questions in identifying an accurate description of the incidence, prevalence, comorbidities, and spectrum of the epilepsies, especially given the shifting sands in definitions and classification systems. Overall, it is estimated that the lifetime risk of having a seizure of any kind is 8%, and the lifetime risk for epilepsy is about 1%. About 3% to 4% of all children will have a febrile seizure, although the overall risk of later epilepsy following a febrile seizure is only 2% to 3%. With the exception of febrile seizures, provoked seizures appear to have little risk of recurrence once the provoking factor has resolved, unless there are specific associated risk factors (e.g., the presence of cerebral hemorrhage or penetrating head injury in traumatic brain injury) (Lowenstein, 2009). The advent of modern neurogenetics and increasingly common use of testing for gene microdeletions and microduplications and mutations in nucleotide sequencing in child neurology practice have virtually transformed the practice of pediatric epilepsy, with increasing identification of causes of severe epilepsies and epileptic encephalopathies heretofore poorly understood.

This section begins with a set of chapters covering the fundamentals of the clinical and basic science of epilepsy: principles of management and outcome, neurophysiology, and genetics. Then the broad categories of seizure types, generalized and focal seizures, are covered in addition to the common provoked seizures of childhood, febrile seizures, for which new data and concepts have shed new light on this usually benign but also heterogeneous seizure type. Specific attention is paid to the problems of epileptic spasms and status epilepticus. Then the age-related syndromes, tabulated in this chapter, are expanded as individual chapters, followed by discussions of the acquired and inherited metabolic epilepsies. Each of these topics has important applications to pediatrics. Treatment approaches are then presented in chapters on antiseizure medication therapy, epilepsy surgery, neuromodulation, and dietary therapy. The topics of psychogenic nonepileptic seizures and comorbidities complete the section, with emphases on behavioral and cognitive aspects and a newly added chapter on the problem of mortality. Children with epilepsy are at increased risk for earlier mortality than expected based on age, although this risk is very small, estimated as 1 in 10,000, for patients presenting with a new diagnosis of epilepsy with no neurologic deficit or complicating factors (Callenbach et al., 2001; Camfield, Camfield, and Veugelers, 2002). Early mortality is multifactorial and related to accidents, comorbidities, and complications of seizures and status epilepticus, but sudden unexpected death in epilepsy patients (SUDEP) has emerged as the leading cause. Risk of the latter climbs to approximately 1 in 1000 in patients with medically refractory epilepsy evaluated for surgical candidacy. Thus the spectrum of epilepsy, from its causes to manifestations, comorbidities, and outcomes, is wide in all respects.

Acknowledgment

The author is grateful for the prior version of this chapter and epidemiologic update provided by Peter and Carol Camfield.

REFERENCES

The complete list of references for this chapter is available in the e-book at www.expertconsult.com.
See inside cover for registration details.

SELECTED REFERENCES

Berg, A.T., Berkovic, S.F., Brodie, M.J., et al., 2010. Revised terminology and concepts for organization of seizures and epilepsies: Report of the ILAE Commission on Classification and Terminology, 2005–2009. Epilepsia 51 (4), 676–685.

Callenbach, P.M., Westendorp, R.G., Geerts, A.T., et al., 2001. Mortality risk in children with epilepsy: the Dutch study of epilepsy in childhood. Pediatrics 107 (6), 1259–1263.

Camfield, C.S., Camfield, P.R., Veugelers, P.J., 2002. Death in children with epilepsy: a population-based study. Lancet 359 (9321), 1891–1895.

Fisher, R.S., Acevedo, C., Arzimanoglou, A., et al., 2014. A practical clinical definition of epilepsy. Epilepsia 55, 475–482.

Fisher, R.S., van Emde Boas, W., Blume, W., et al., 2005. Epileptic seizures and epilepsy: definitions proposed by the International League Against Epilepsy (ILAE) and the International Bureau for Epilepsy (IBE). Epilepsia 26 (4), 470–472.

Glauser, T.A., Cnaan, A., Shinnar, S., et al., 2010. Ethosuximide, valproic acid and lamotrigine in childhood absence epilepsy. N. Engl. J. Med. 362 (9), 790–799.

Hesdorffer, D.C., Beck, V., Begley, C.E., et al., 2013. Research implications of the Institute of Medicine Report, Epilepsy Across the Spectrum: Promoting Health and Understanding. Epilepsia 54 (2), 207–216.

Lowenstein, D.H., 2009. Epilepsy after head injury: an overview. Epilepsia 50 (Suppl. 2), 4–9.

Temkin, O., 1971. The Falling Sickness. In: A History of Epilepsy from the Greeks to the Beginnings of Modern Neurology, second ed. The Johns Hopkins Press, Baltimore.

Wirrell, E.C., Grossardt, B.R., Wong-Kisiel, L.C.L., et al., 2011. Incidence and classification of new-onset epilepsy and epilepsy syndromes in children in Olmsted County, Minnesota from 1980 to 2004: A population-based study. Epilepsy Res. 95 (1–2), 110–118.

E-BOOK TABLE

The following figures and tables are available in the e-book at www.expertconsult.com. See inside cover for registration details.

62 Principles of Management and Outcome

Peter R. Camfield and Carol S. Camfield

An expanded version of this chapter is available on www.expertconsult.com. See inside cover for registration details.

The goals of this chapter are to outline when to start antiseizure treatment for children with epilepsy, factors that influence routines of care, when to stop medicines, and how to predict the seizure and social outcomes as children with epilepsy become adults.

STARTING ANTISEIZURE TREATMENT

Antiseizure treatment is usually started when epilepsy is diagnosed but there are exceptions. After a first unprovoked seizure in childhood, the risk of a recurrence is about 50%, and after the second seizure the risk is about 70% to 80%. By convention, epilepsy is diagnosed only after a child has had two or more unprovoked seizures. A recent official report from the International League Against Epilepsy (ILAE) suggests that epilepsy is a disease of the brain defined by any of the following conditions: 1) at least two unprovoked (or reflex) seizures occurring more than 24 hours apart; 2) one unprovoked (or reflex) seizure and a probability of further seizures similar to the general recurrence risk (at least 60%) after two unprovoked seizures, occurring over the next 10 years; 3) diagnosis of an epilepsy syndrome. We doubt that many children should start treatment after a first seizure even if the risk of recurrence is very high, because the direct consequences of a second seizure are typically small. In addition, based on a large randomized Italian study, the chance of a long-term remission is unchanged if antiseizure medicines are started after the first or the second seizure.

The diagnosis of an epilepsy syndrome may also not lead to antiseizure treatment, especially in children with rolandic epilepsy in whom seizures are usually infrequent and mainly nocturnal. Many children with this diagnosis can be managed without treatment. The term "unprovoked" implies that there has been no closely associated concurrent illness, fever, or acute brain injury. Recurrent seizures immediately after a head injury or associated with drug intoxication do not qualify for the diagnosis of epilepsy. Specific provoking factors leading to reflex seizures are permitted, such as seizures provoked by patterns and flashes from video terminals in children with photosensitive epilepsy. Seizures are still viewed as unprovoked if they occur with stresses related to personal activity, such as sleep deprivation or severe emotional distress, unless these stresses are extreme.

Before starting treatment it is imperative that the diagnosis of epilepsy be definite. Box 62-1 lists a number of conditions that may mimic epilepsy. If there is doubt, we are of the opinion that it is better to wait for further similar episodes. Home video may be very valuable. The diagnosis of epilepsy cannot be made from an EEG unless an actual seizure is recorded. Interictal "epileptic" discharges are seen in 3% to 5% of children without seizures. It is also critical that the proposed benefits of treatment are greater than the potential consequences of treatment. For example, a child with infrequent, brief, focal seizures without loss of awareness or motor control may not benefit from treatment, given that all medications have some side effects and that the process of taking daily medicines is intrusive.

The value of treatment is a reduction in recurrent seizures with the hope that associated psychosocial problems, stigma, and injuries will be reduced. There is no evidence that treatment has any effect on the chance of long-term remission, and there is no convincing human evidence that one seizure makes the occurrence of another more likely. Although there is a risk of sudden unexpected death in epilepsy (SUDEP) for anyone with seizures, the risk is tiny in childhood-onset epilepsy. Fear of SUDEP should not be a significant motivation to start treatment. Another reason for starting treatment is to attempt to reduce EEG interictal spike discharges in patients with "epileptic encephalopathy." Here it is postulated that these spike discharges interfere with cognition. Most of these patients have multiple clinical seizures and the decision to start medication is not difficult. Others with epilepsy syndromes such as Landau-Kleffner syndrome or continuous spike–wave in slow wave sleep often have few overt seizures—the potential role of treatment is improved cognition. This issue is dealt with in Chapters 70 to 72. Unfortunately, few conventional antiseizure medicines suppress interictal spikes.

Which Medicine to Start With?

There are very few randomized clinical trials in children with new-onset epilepsy that compare different medicines in "head-to-head" studies. For the most part, clinicians must rely on experience and expert consensus (low forms of evidence). The SANAD study randomized 3158 patients with newly diagnosed epilepsy (mainly adults) to a series of antiseizure medicines and found that, as a first antiseizure medicine, lamotrigine was most effective for focal epilepsy and valproate was best for generalized epilepsy. However, many pediatric epilepsy syndromes were not included in this study. Chapters that follow on individual syndromes outline the "best" first choices for particular syndromes. Factors that should enter the decision of which medication to start first include the specific syndrome, the age of the child, cost, availability of the medication, and ease of administration. There is an unproven but sensible assumption that the best medication should improve rather than exacerbate comorbid problems. For example, lamotrigine or valproate might improve comorbid depression, whereas levetiracetam or clobazam might exacerbate oppositional defiant disorder.

Routines of Care

The "correct" dose of an antiseizure medicine suppresses seizures completely but causes no or minor side effects. This simple concept is not easily applied in clinical practice. Some children have long intervals between seizures, and so it may take many months to be confident that seizures are suppressed. The "rule of threes" may be useful—if there have been no seizures for three times the usual seizure-free interval, then it is likely that the medication is effective. At the beginning of treatment, many children have had too few seizures to estimate the "usual" interval.

BOX 62-1 Disorders That May Mimic Childhood Epilepsy

CONFUSED WITH GENERALIZED TONIC–CLONIC SEIZURES

Pallid syncope (reflex anoxic seizure)
Vasodepressor syncope (reflex anoxic seizure)
Cyanotic breath-holding attacks
Collapsing attacks with cardiac dysrhythmias
Cataplexy

CONFUSED WITH GENERALIZED ABSENCE SEIZURES

Behavioral staring attacks
Complex partial (dyscognitive) seizures
Tic disorder

CONFUSED WITH COMPLEX PARTIAL (DYSCOGNITIVE) SEIZURES

Self-stimulatory behavior, especially in children with autistic spectrum disorders
Sleep walking
Night terrors
Temper tantrums with amnesia for the rage event
Benign paroxysmal vertigo
Migraine-related disorders

CONFUSED WITH EPILEPTIC MYOCLONUS

Physiologic hypnagogic myoclonus
Benign infantile sleep myoclonus
Startle disease

It is often postulated that antiseizure medicines are most likely to be effective if the serum level is in the "therapeutic range." This appealing concept is without scientific proof. Three randomized trials comparing regular blood level monitoring with no monitoring have failed to show any benefit in seizure control. One of the trials showed more clinical toxicity with monitoring than without. The "therapeutic range" for most antiseizure medicines is not based on randomized trials and typically has been developed in a non-evidence-based mode (Camfield and Camfield, 2003).

It is also important to realize that only about 20% of children with epilepsy will have *smooth sailing* epilepsy, which means that they will have no further seizures once the first medicine is introduced (Camfield et al., 1993). Therefore the clinician, patient, and family need to start treatment with the expectation that it may be difficult to find the optimal dose of the optimal drug. The process continues to be characterized by a great deal of trial and error.

Once a drug has been started, monitoring for side effects is important. Based on personal experience, we recommend that patients be seen in person about a month after starting an antiseizure medicine and that the visit focuses on side effects, restrictions, and social aspects. It is surprisingly easy for families and others to lose track of what the child was really like before medications were started. The child may not be able to report a change, and if seizures are controlled, parents may choose to ignore some important behavioral or cognitive effects. Again, there is scant evidence that serum levels "in the therapeutic range" predict a lack of side effects. Side effects may only be recognized when a medicine is changed or discontinued.

There is no evidence that regular monitoring of blood and urine reduces the chance of serious biological reactions to any antiseizure medicine. Minor alterations in these "routine" investigations mean that the tests need to be repeated and may lead to an unnecessary discontinuation of an effective

medicine. For example, a child receiving carbamazepine may develop a viral illness that suppresses the blood neutrophil count, which could lead to the false conclusion of impending bone marrow failure.

There are many ways of enhancing adherence with therapy. Simple measures are to avoid more than twice-daily dosing with medication at breakfast and bedtime. Families need to know what to do if they miss a dose, information that will depend on the specific medication. A 7-day pill dispenser may help some patients. Prescription quantities for many months at a time makes it less likely that families will run out of medication. Most of all, adherence is improved by providing a clear understanding of the rationale for treatment. Issues of adherence should be addressed at every visit. We are of the strong impression that simply asking patients about adherence in a nonaccusative fashion is a more effective technique than multiple blood level determinations.

Injuries resulting from seizures are not uncommon. About 10% of children with epilepsy will eventually have an injury as the result of a seizure that is sufficient to require medical or dental consultation. These injuries usually occur months or years after starting medication, usually occur during normal activities, and cannot be prevented except by complete seizure control. Restrictions to the child's normal activities are usually not warranted, particularly if the seizures appear to be controlled. Drowning in the bathtub is a concern—a shower is a safer alternative.

PREDICATION OF SEIZURE OUTCOME

For many children, epilepsy is transient, and with maturation, the problem seems to vanish. At the time of diagnosis, it is possible to predict that at least 50% to 70% of children will outgrow their disorder and be able to discontinue medication (Berg et al., 2014). The longer the follow-up, the higher the proportion with remission of symptoms. In Rochester, MN, 115 children with epilepsy beginning before age 10 years were followed through the Mayo Clinic record linkage system. Ten years later, 75% had been seizure-free for at least 5 years, and 51% no longer received medication. At the end of a remarkable 30-year follow-up study of children with epilepsy from a population-based sample in Turku, Finland, Sillanpää et al. (1998) found that 76% of survivors had been seizure-free for at least 3 years, although a number of these patients continued with treatment.

Across most studies, factors that predict which children will outgrow their epilepsy have included normal intelligence, normal neurologic examination findings, relatively small numbers of seizures at diagnosis (which means that complex partial or dyscognitive seizures are unlikely to remit), age of seizure onset younger than 1 year of age (unfavorable), age of seizure onset older than 1 year and younger than 12 years (favorable), and absence of a remote symptomatic cause (an identified brain problem that preceded the onset of epilepsy).

A causative lesion on magnetic resonance imaging (MRI) makes remission unlikely; however, two population-based studies have shown that, even with such a lesion, approximately 30% will go on to a seemingly permanent remission (Dhamija et al., 2011). In addition, failure of the first medicine to control seizures in adults is ominous with possibly only a 10% chance of success with subsequent medicines. In children the failure of the first medicine is not as ominous. In the Nova Scotia study, 42% of those who failed their first antiseizure eventually entered remission versus 61% of those who did not fail the first drug. Failure of a second medicine to control seizures is now used as a definition of pharmacoresistant epilepsy and should lead to a careful reevaluation of the

TABLE 62-1 Scoring System for Remission of Childhood Epilepsy at the Time of Diagnosis

Variable	Score*
Age of first seizure (months)	
<12	99
12–144	142
>144	0
Intelligence	
Normal	111
Retardation	0
Previous neonatal seizures	
No	218
Yes	0
Number of seizures before starting medication	
1 or 2	72
3–20	123
>20	0

*Add the scores from this column. If the total score is greater than 495, the child is predicted to have remission of epilepsy.
(Adapted from Sillanpaa M, Camfield PR, Camfield CS. Predicting long term outcome of childhood epilepsy in Nova Scotia, Canada, and Turku: Validation of a simple scoring system. Arch Neurol 1995;52:589.)

diagnosis and consideration of other types of treatments such as surgery or the ketogenic diet.

Based on clinical features present at the time of diagnosis, it is possible to predict the long-term outcome with moderate accuracy. In an 8-year follow-up study of a population-based study of 504 children with epilepsy from Nova Scotia, a predictive scoring system was developed; it is outlined in Table 62-1 (Camfield et al., 1993). Those with a good prognosis had an 80% chance of remission (i.e., seizure-free and no longer receiving medication). For those with one or more of the adverse factors scored, the chance of remission was less but still about 40%. The Dutch Study of Epilepsy in Childhood found comparable predictive variables and supplemented these with the clinical course in the first 6 months of treatment (Wirrall et al., 2011). Rates of correct prediction were similar.

The Dutch and Nova Scotia studies were combined to allow study of 1055 newly diagnosed patients with 5 or more years of follow-up. Multivariate analysis that included clinical factors, syndrome diagnosis, and response to treatment in the first 6 months revealed that, at the time of diagnosis, a prognostic scoring scheme could correctly predict remission or no remission in about 70%. This means that at the time of diagnosis if parents ask, "Will the seizures be outgrown?" the physician will give the wrong answer in about one-third of cases.

Surprisingly, most epilepsy syndromes do not have a definite outcome; however, a few specific syndromes allow an accurate prognosis. Epilepsy is virtually always outgrown in cases of rolandic epilepsy, benign myoclonic epilepsy of infancy, and benign occipital epilepsy, early onset type. Epilepsy is virtually never outgrown in children with Rasmussen syndrome, Lennox-Gastaut syndrome, or Dravet syndrome. Other syndromes have a variable prognosis with some having a permanent remission and others with the same syndrome continuing to require treatment for ongoing seizures. For example, about 65% of children with childhood absence epilepsy will enter a long-term remission, whereas 35% will not.

Intractability

Defining intractable epilepsy is difficult, and many definitions have been suggested (Wirrell, 2013). For a study of 613

children with epilepsy from Connecticut, Berg and Shinnar (1994) defined intractability as a "failure, for lack of seizure control, of more than two first-line antiseizure medications with an average of more than 1 seizure per month for 18 months and no more than three consecutive months seizure free during that interval." There were 60 (10%) intractable cases in the first 24 months after diagnosis. Using the ILAE classification from 1989, the proportions of intractable patients in each major syndrome grouping were as follows: cryptogenic/symptomatic generalized, 34.6%; idiopathic generalized, 2.7%; other localization related, 10.7%; and unclassified, 8.2%. Sillanpää's follow-up study from Turku, Finland, defined intractability as one or more seizures per year in the past 10 years of follow-up. After 20 years of follow-up, 22% of patients met this criterion. Predictors of intractability included poor initial response to medication, remote symptomatic cause, and status epilepticus. The Dutch Study of Childhood Epilepsy (using Berg and Shinnar's definition of intractability), with 453 children followed for 5 years, found that 6% were intractable. For the Nova Scotia study, intractability was defined as "at least one seizure each 3 months for the last year of follow-up, with failure of at least three antiseizure drugs." For those with epilepsies characterized by partial and generalized tonic–clonic seizures, 8% of 511 children became intractable during an average of 8 years of follow-up. After 20 years of follow-up, 51% of 75 patients with childhood-onset symptomatic generalized epilepsy had intractable seizures. In this study, the major predictor of intractability was severe neurologic deficit at the time of diagnosis.

The ILAE's current definition of intractability is failure of two appropriate medications. The definition is most applicable to adults, because some children who meet this definition will still have a permanent remission.

An important issue in the definition of intractability is the length of follow-up, because a number of children with intractable epilepsy eventually become well controlled. For example, in a series of 145 children with intractable seizures (>1 seizure per month for ≥2 years) followed over 18 years, Huttenlocher and Hapke observed that 75% of normally intelligent children and 30% with mental handicap eventually had complete or nearly complete seizure remission (i.e., <1 seizure per year). In contrast, another study retrospectively reviewed the history for adults undergoing a workup for intractable epilepsy. It was common to find long periods of remission during childhood. Apparently, intractable epilepsy in childhood may seem to resolve spontaneously but on rare occasions re-emerges as intractable epilepsy in adulthood.

In summary, intractability for an individual child is difficult to predict before several years of treatment. Intractability appears to decrease with prolonged follow-up, although the burden of this wait-and-see approach may be substantial. Failure of a second medication is an important, but not absolute, risk factor for intractability. As a general rule, consideration for epilepsy surgery should await failure of three appropriate drug treatments. Other factors influence this decision, including seizure etiology, severity, frequency, MRI findings, and the duration of epilepsy.

When to Stop Antiseizure Medicines

About 60% to 70% of children with epilepsy who have become seizure-free for 1 to 2 years can successfully stop medication treatment (Berg and Shinnar, 1994); however, the rate of success is higher if the seizure-free period has been 2 years compared with 1 year. The rate of success is no greater if medication is continued for up to 5 years seizure-free. Factors that predict successful discontinuation of medication include generalized seizures, age of onset before 10 to 12 years, normal neurologic examination, and, in some studies, resolution of interictal EEG spike discharges. Children with no adverse factors have an 80% to 90% success rate. Each factor has an additive effect and those with all of the adverse factors may have only a 10% to 20% success rate.

If an initial discontinuation trial is unsuccessful, medication is usually restarted with a return to seizure freedom. The risk that seizures will not come under control again and become intractable is only about 1%. When medications are restarted, about 50% of children again become seizure-free for sufficient time to try to discontinue medication a second time, with a 70% success rate.

This approach is not applicable to all epilepsy syndromes. For example, the remission rate for juvenile myoclonic epilepsy (JME) is low, although several studies suggest that eventually 40% will no longer require daily medication. Still many experts suggest that medication for juvenile myoclonic epilepsy should be lifelong and that further attempts to discontinue medication after an initial failure are probably not warranted.

The optimal length of treatment has been addressed in several randomized trials. A Scandinavian study randomized 207 children at the time of diagnosis of epilepsy to receive 1 or 3 years of treatment. If the child was seizure-free for the last 6 months of study, medication was discontinued. This practice meant that some of the children in the 1-year treatment group had been seizure-free for only 6 months before medication was stopped. The success rate for those in the short-treatment group was significantly less than for the 3-year group (53% vs. 71%). A Dutch study randomized 161 children with epilepsy that was controlled within 2 months of starting treatment to 6 months or 1 year of treatment. The 6-month group had a higher relapse rate when medication was stopped; however, by 2 years later, the rates of remission were identical. Nonetheless, for a substantial number of children, epilepsy was a short-lived disorder requiring only short-term medication use. Medication treatment for benign rolandic epilepsy often is not needed, and further studies will likely identify other children who do not require drug treatment.

The optimal rate of taper of medication has been subject to a randomized trial—6 weeks versus 9 months. Although the success rate was slightly higher with the slower taper (not statistically significant), we suspect that most clinicians choose a 1- to 3-month schedule. If seizures are to recur after medicine discontinuation, it is nearly always within the first 6 months. Recurrences after 2 years are extremely unlikely.

SOCIAL OUTCOME

Follow-up studies into adulthood have increasingly shown that many adults with childhood-onset epilepsy have unsatisfactory social outcomes. The reasons for this lack of success are unproven but are likely related to four themes. First, varying degrees of cognitive problems are very common in children with epilepsy. These problems are present at the onset of the epilepsy, although they may be exacerbated by medication side effects and frequent seizures. They are very likely to influence academic success, eventual employment, and self-esteem. Second, attention-deficit/hyperactivity disorder, depression, other psychiatric disorders, and behavior disorders are more common in children with epilepsy than controls and are known to have a negative effect on social outcome, especially on personal relationships. Austin and colleagues reported that, at the time of diagnosis, 40% of children were at significant risk of behavior problems, as judged by scores on the Child Behavior Checklist (Austin et al., 2002). Those with multiple recurrent seizures were at even higher risk. Oostrom and colleagues demonstrated greater cognitive and behavioral problems and the need for special educational assistance among 51 outpatient children with idiopathic or cryptogenic epilepsy compared with their classmate controls (Oostrom et al., 2005). Some of these issues are reviewed in more detail in Chapter 82. Third, the diagnosis of epilepsy is associated with considerable stigma in most cultures, which undoubtedly affects social outcome by limiting friendships, activities, and eventual choice of employment. For example, Trostle reported that parents indicate a reluctance to have their normal children play with a child with epilepsy (Trostle, 1988). Less than one third of 20,000 U.S. high school students indicated that they would date a person with epilepsy. Finally, poorly controlled seizures limit many important activities such as driving. Most countries require a year without seizures in order for a person to drive; however, there is considerable variation between locations.

The Nova Scotia epilepsy cohort showed that when children with childhood absence epilepsy became young adults they were much more likely to have a multitude of social difficulties than a chronic disease control group (children with juvenile rheumatoid arthritis). These difficulties included poor education, alcohol abuse, unemployment, and inadvertent pregnancy. Other studies have compared children with epilepsy to those with asthma with similar findings. Therefore social difficulties related to epilepsy are not simply the nonspecific effect of a chronic disease.

In Finland, children with "epilepsy only" were followed into young adulthood and compared with age- and sex-matched controls. "Epilepsy only" meant having normal intelligence and no other neurologic handicaps. About 30% of patients had significant social adjustment problems with decreased rates of stable relationships, marriage, social contacts, job satisfaction, and work achievement. Rates of unemployment or underemployment were high. Social outcome was not clearly related to epilepsy remission. In the Nova Scotia study, seizure-related factors did not predict social outcome. The strongest predictor of poor social outcome in young adulthood was the presence of a learning disorder, although predictive models were inaccurate; the main reasons for the unsatisfactory outcomes were unclear.

Wakamoto and colleagues studied 148 normally intelligent young adults (>20 years old) living in a rural district of Japan who had childhood-onset epilepsy. This population-based study found that 72% attended regular classes (vs. 99% of those without epilepsy), 66% (vs. 97%) entered high school, 67% (vs. 95%) had employment, and 23% (vs. 33%) married.

Few studies have addressed the social outcome of children with specific epilepsy syndromes. Several studies have indicated a favorable outcome for adults with previous benign rolandic epilepsy. The Nova Scotia study has provided population-based data about social outcome 20 to 35 years after diagnosis for a variety of epilepsy types in patients with normal intelligence. Information was gathered by semistructured interviews, and adverse outcomes were defined as failure to complete high school, pregnancy outside of a stable relationship (<6 months), depression or another psychiatric diagnosis, unemployment, living alone, never in a romantic relationship for more than 3 months, and poverty. Table 62-2 shows the percentage of patients with each of these adverse events. We note that, except for rolandic epilepsy, about 75% of each syndrome group had a major indicator of poor social outcome (Camfield and Camfield, 2014).

The social outcome for those with intellectual disability (ID) is perhaps more difficult to study, because of difficulties in assessing social outcome, especially in those with moderate to severe ID. About 20% of children with new-onset epilepsy have ID with more than expected having moderate to severe ID (75%). In the Nova Scotia study after 20 years of

TABLE 62-2 Adult Social Outcome for Epilepsies in Patients with Normal Intelligence: The Nova Scotia Population-Based Study

	Rolandic	Juvenile Myoclonic Epilepsy	Epilepsy with Generalized Tonic–Clonic Seizures Only (IGE-NOS)	Epilepsies Characterized by Complex Partial Seizures	Epilepsies Characterized by Only Focal Seizures with Secondary Generalization
N	32	23	30	108	80
Length of follow-up (years)	29.5 ± 3	25.8 ± 2	22.5 ± 7	28.1 ± 5	27.6 ± 6
Failure to complete high school (%)	22	13	40	33	32
No close friends (%)	3	9	24	29	8
Pregnancy outside a stable relationship (%)	22	48	38	29	21
Psychiatric diagnosis other than ADHD (%)	9	61	27	33	25
Unemployment (%)	3	31	33	33	24
Living alone (%)	16	30	23	19	8
No romantic relationship >3 months (%)	3		24	21	14
Poverty (%)	6	30	50	50	26
≥1 adverse social outcome* (%)	41	76	76	75	62
1 adverse social outcome only (%)	19	26	31	23	26
≥2 adverse social outcomes (%)	22	48	59	52	36

ADHD, attention-deficit/hyperactivity disorder.
*Adverse social outcomes: failure to complete high school, pregnancy outside of a stable relationship (<6 months), depression or another psychiatric
   diagnosis, unemployment, living alone, never in a romantic relationship >3 months, and poverty.

follow-up, almost none of these patients were able to live independently.

If the long-term social outcome of childhood epilepsy is to be improved, physicians must address these issues with equal enthusiasm to medical treatment. Learning problems, sexuality, and socialization should be assessed regularly and appropriate interventions considered. Early referral to both local and Internet sites for an epilepsy support group may also be of benefit.

REFERENCES

 The complete list of references for this chapter is available in the e-book at www.expertconsult.com.
See inside cover for registration details.

SELECTED REFERENCES

Arts, W.F., Arzimanoglou, A., Brouwer, O.F., et al., 2013. Outcome of Childhood Epilepsies. John Libbey Eurotext, Montrouge.

Austin, J.K., Dunn, D.W., Caffrey, H.M., et al., 2002. Recurrent seizures and behavior problems in children with first recognized seizures: a prospective study. Epilepsia 43, 1564–1573.

Berg, A.T., Rychlik, K., Levy, S.R., et al., 2014. Complete remission of childhood-onset epilepsy: stability and prediction over two decades. Brain. 137, 3213–3222.

Berg, A.T., Shinnar, S., 1994. Relapse following discontinuation of antiepileptic drugs: a meta-analysis. Neurology. 44, 601–608.

Camfield, C., Camfield, P., Gordon, K., et al., 1993. Outcome of childhood epilepsy: a population-based study with a simple predictive scoring system for those treated with medication. J. Pediatr. 122, 861–868.

Camfield, C.S., Camfield, P.R., 2014. Rolandic epilepsy has little effect on adult life 30 years later: a population-based study. Neurology. 82, 1162–1166.

Camfield, P., Camfield, C., 2003. Childhood epilepsy: what is the evidence for what we think and what we do? J. Child. Neurol. 18, 272–287.

Dhamija, R., Moseley, B.D., Cascino, G.D., et al., 2011. A population-based study of long-term outcome of epilepsy in childhood with a focal or hemispheric lesion on neuroimaging. Epilepsia. 52, 1522–1526.

Geerts, A., Arts, W.F., Stroink, H., et al., 2010. Course and outcome of childhood epilepsy: a 15-year follow-up of the Dutch Study of Epilepsy in Childhood. Epilepsia. 51, 1189–1197.

Oostrom, K.J., van Teeseling, H., Smeets-Schouten, A., et al., Dutch Study of Epilepsy in Childhood (DuSECh), 2005. Three to four years after diagnosis: cognition and behaviour in children with "epilepsy only." A prospective, controlled study. Brain 128, 1546–1555.

Sillanpää, M., Jalava, M., Kaleva, O., et al., 1998. Long-term prognosis of seizures with onset in childhood. N. Engl. J. Med. 338, 1715–1722.

Trostle, J.A., 1988. Social aspects of epilepsy. In: Hauser, W.A. (Ed.), Current Trends in Epilepsy, Unit 1. Epilepsy Foundation of America, Landover, MD.

Wirrell, E.C., 2013. Predicting pharmacoresistance in pediatric epilepsy. Epilepsia. 54 (Suppl. 2), 19–22.

Wirrell, E.C., Grossardt, B.R., So, E.L., et al., 2011. A population-based study of long-term outcomes of cryptogenic focal epilepsy in childhood: cryptogenic epilepsy is probably not symptomatic epilepsy. Epilepsia 52, 738–745.

63 Neurophysiology of Seizures and Epilepsy

Carl E. Stafstrom and Jong M. Rho

This chapter reviews the cellular basis of seizures and the factors that enhance susceptibility of the immature brain to seizures and epilepsy. We emphasize how dysfunction of ion channels and synaptic transmission can lead to cellular hyperexcitability and hypersynchronous neuronal firing, the hallmark features of seizures. The mechanisms of actions of antiseizure drugs (ASDs) are also summarized.

A seizure is defined as abnormal neuronal firing leading to a clinical alteration of neurologic function (motor, sensory, autonomic, or psychological). A seizure reflects aberrant activity at the level of both single neurons and the neuronal network. Epilepsy is the condition of spontaneous recurrent seizures arising from heightened electrical activity within the brain. Epilepsy is not a singular disease—it is heterogeneous in terms of etiology, clinical features, and pathophysiology. An epilepsy syndrome refers to a constellation of signs and symptoms that often occur together, such as seizure type, age of seizure onset, responsiveness to certain ASDs, and characteristic electroencephalogram (EEG) findings, underlying genetics, and natural history. Epileptogenesis is the process by which neural circuits undergo structural and/or physiologic changes, resulting in an enduring epileptic state.

CLASSIFICATION OF SEIZURES

Seizures are divided into two groups, according to their site of origin and pattern of spread. Focal seizures arise from a localized brain region; the associated clinical manifestations are related to the function ordinarily subserved by that area. Focal discharges can spread locally through synaptic and nonsynaptic mechanisms, distally to subcortical structures, and through commissural pathways that may eventually involve the entire cortex.

Primary generalized seizures begin with abnormal electrical discharges in both hemispheres simultaneously and involve reciprocal thalamocortical connections, manifesting on EEG as bilateral synchronous spike–waves. The manifestations of generalized seizures range from brief impairment of consciousness (e.g., absence seizure) to whole-body convulsion (generalized seizure).

CELLULAR ELECTROPHYSIOLOGY
Excitation–Inhibition Balance

Seizure activity can be conceptualized as a perturbation in the normal balance between neuronal inhibition and excitation, involving a localized region or widespread brain areas (Stafstrom, 2014). This concept is admittedly oversimplified. For example, factors once thought to be solely inhibitory (e.g., γ-aminobutyric acid [GABA]-ergic synaptic transmission) can be excitatory in some instances. Furthermore, synaptic inhibition is critical for certain normal brain rhythms and probably also plays a role in abnormal rhythmic activity, such as spike–wave discharges. The discovery of novel genetic mutations has required expansion of the excitation–inhibition imbalance concept. For example, mutations in genes encoding several proteins involved in both excitatory and inhibitory synapse development and stabilization can lead to epilepsy.

Overview of Ion Channels

Two major types of ion channels—voltage-gated and ligand-gated—are responsible for inhibitory and excitatory activity (Fig. 63-3). Voltage-gated channels include sodium and calcium channels that depolarize the cell membrane toward action potential threshold; potassium channels largely dampen neuronal excitation. Voltage-gated channels are activated by membrane potential changes that alter the conformational state of the channel and allow selective passage of charged ions through a pore. Ligand-gated channels are activated when a neurotransmitter is released from a presynaptic terminal into the synaptic cleft and binds selectively to a recognition site on the receptor localized on the postsynaptic membrane. This binding activates a cascade of events, including a conformational shift to open an ion-permeant pore. Passage of ions across these channels results in depolarization (i.e., inward flux of cations) or hyperpolarization (i.e., inward flux of anions or outward flux of cations). Ion channel mutations underlie several epilepsy syndromes, giving rise to the concept of "epilepsy channelopathies" (Child and Bennaroch, 2014; Steinlein, 2014).

Voltage-Dependent Membrane Conductances
Depolarizing Conductances

A rapidly inactivating inward sodium conductance underlies the depolarizing phase of the action potential. Each sodium channel is composed of a complex of three polypeptide subunits: a major α subunit and two smaller β subunits that influence the kinetic properties of the α subunit. Sodium channel dysfunction can lead to epilepsy and several ASDs work by blocking sodium channels.

Neuronal voltage-dependent calcium channels contribute to the depolarizing phase of the action potential and affect neurotransmitter release, gene expression, and neuronal firing patterns. Calcium currents underlie neuronal burst discharges. Several subtypes of calcium channels are distinguished on the basis of electrophysiological properties, pharmacologic profile, molecular structure, and cellular localization. The molecular structure of voltage-gated calcium channels is similar to that of sodium channels, with a principal pore-forming $\alpha 1$ subunit and one or more smaller subunits that modulate the channel's kinetics.

Hyperpolarizing Conductances

Depolarizing sodium and calcium currents are counterbalanced by an array of voltage-dependent hyperpolarizing (inhibitory) currents, primarily mediated by potassium channels that act by decreasing neuronal excitation. The prototypic voltage-gated potassium channel is composed of four membrane-spanning α subunits and four regulatory β subunits assembled in an octameric complex to form an

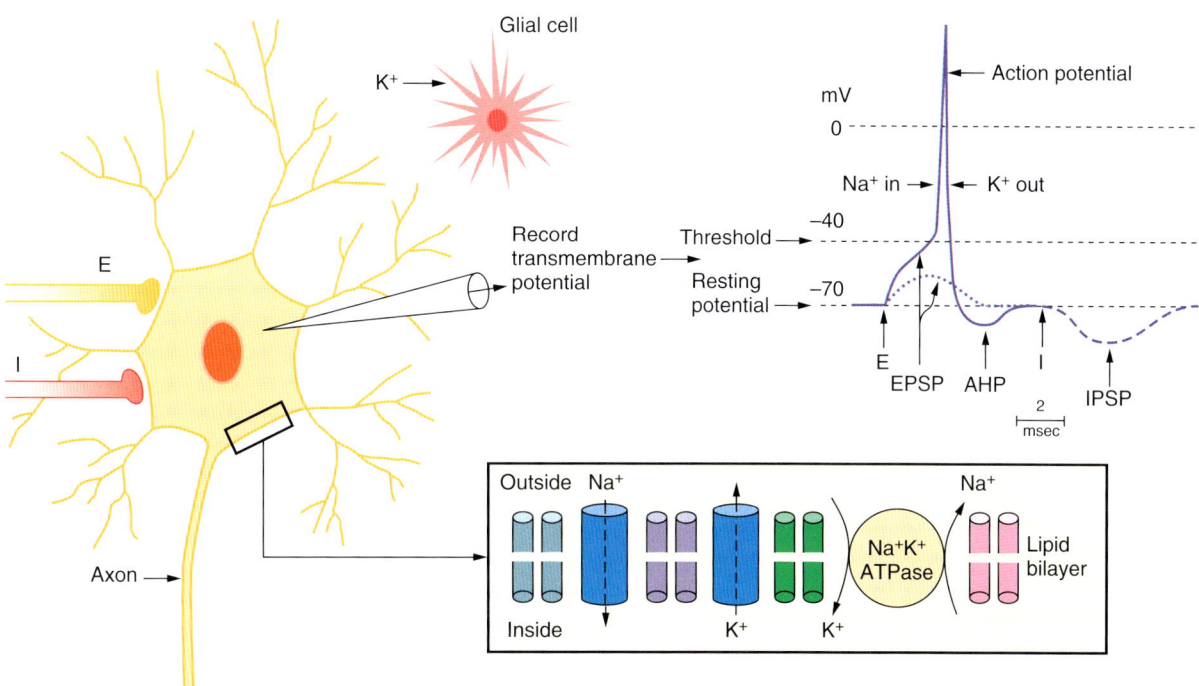

Figure 63-3. Normal neuronal firing. Schematic shows a neuron with one excitatory (E) and one inhibitory (I) input. Right trace shows membrane potential (in millivolts [mV]), beginning at a typical resting potential (–70 mV). Activation of E leads to graded excitatory postsynaptic potentials (EPSPs), the larger of which reaches threshold (approximately –40 mV) for an action potential. The action potential is followed by an after-hyperpolarization (AHP), the magnitude and duration of which determine when the next action potential can occur. Activation of I causes an inhibitory postsynaptic potential (IPSP). The inset shows a magnified portion of the neuronal membrane as a lipid bilayer with interposed voltage-gated Na⁺ and K⁺ channels; the direction of ion fluxes during excitatory activation is indicated. After firing, the membrane-bound Na⁺-K⁺ pump and star-shaped astroglial cells restore ionic balance. *(With permission from Stafstrom, C.E., 2004. An introduction to seizures and epilepsy: cellular mechanisms underlying classification and treatment. In: Stafstrom, C.E., Rho, J.M. (Eds.), Epilepsy and the Ketogenic Diet. Humana Press, Totowa, NJ, pp. 3–29. Reprinted with permission of Springer Science+Business Media.)*

ion-selective pore. Potassium conductances include delayed rectifiers (involved in action potential termination); an A-current (which in part determines the interspike interval and cell firing rate); an M-current (activated by cholinergic muscarinic agonists and which affects resting potential and cell firing rate); and calcium-activated potassium conductances (which are sensitive to intracellular calcium concentration and modulate cell firing rate and interburst interval).

Hyperpolarizing conductances induce antiseizure effects. Some newer ASDs (topiramate, levetiracetam) act in part by modulating potassium channels. Retigabine opens potassium channels and enhances activation of KCNQ2 and KCNQ3 potassium channels. Mutations in KCNQ2 and KCNQ3 have been linked to benign familial neonatal seizures and, in the case of KCNQ2, early onset epileptic encephalopathies.

Synaptic Physiology

Inhibitory Synaptic Transmission

Synaptic inhibition is mediated by two basic circuit configurations—feedback and feedforward. Feedback inhibition occurs when excitatory principal neurons synapse onto inhibitory interneurons, which project back to the principal neurons and inhibit them (negative-feedback loop). Feedforward inhibition occurs when axons synapse directly onto inhibitory interneurons, inhibiting downstream principal neurons.

GABA, the main inhibitory neurotransmitter in the brain, is synthesized from glutamate by the rate-limiting enzyme glutamic acid decarboxylase. GABA released from axon terminals binds to two classes of receptors, GABA$_A$ and GABA$_B$. Dysfunction in either GABA receptor or their subunits can result in epilepsy (Hirose, 2014).

The GABA$_A$ receptor consists of an ion pore and binding sites for agonists and a variety of modulators, such as benzodiazepines and barbiturates, each of which affects the kinetic properties of the receptor. The GABA$_A$ receptor is a heteropentameric complex composed of combinations of polypeptide subunits arranged in topographic fashion to form an ion channel that is selectively permeable to chloride ions. Several types of subunits (α, β, γ, δ, ϵ, π, ρ) have been described. Most functional GABA$_A$ receptors follow the general motif of containing either α and β or α, β, and γ subunits with variable stoichiometry. Subunits may be differentially sensitive to pharmacologic agents, making GABA$_A$ receptors useful targets for new ASDs.

Activation of GABA$_A$ receptors on mature neurons results in influx of chloride ions, generating fast inhibitory postsynaptic potentials, hyperpolarizing the membrane, and inhibiting cell firing. In the immature brain, however, GABA$_A$ receptor activation depolarizes the postsynaptic membrane, because of a reversed chloride electrochemical gradient that is a consequence of the evolving expression of cation chloride cotransporters during development.

Metabotropic GABA$_B$ receptors are located both postsynaptically and presynaptically. GABA$_B$ receptors act through guanosine triphosphate (GTP)-binding proteins to control calcium or potassium conductances. Postsynaptic GABA$_B$ receptors mediate slow, long-lasting inhibitory postsynaptic potentials, primarily in dendrites. Activation of $GABA_B$ receptors on axon terminals reduces the amount of GABA released, resulting in disinhibition. Abnormalities of GABAergic function, including synthesis, synaptic release, receptor composition, trafficking or binding, and metabolism, can each contribute to a hyperexcitable state.

Excitatory Synaptic Transmission

Glutamate is the principal excitatory neurotransmitter of the brain. Glutamatergic activity is critical for normal brain development and activity-dependent synaptic plasticity. There are two broad classes of glutamate receptors—ionotropic and metabotropic. Ionotropic glutamate receptors are divided into N-methyl-D-aspartate (NMDA) and non-NMDA receptors, based on biophysical properties and pharmacologic profiles. Each ionotropic glutamate receptor subtype consists of a heterotetramer that determines its functional properties. An NMDA receptor consists of an obligate GluN1 subunit plus GluN2A, GluN2B, GluN2C, GluN2D, and/or GluN3A and GluN3B subunits.

NMDA receptors contain a binding site for glutamate (or NMDA) and recognition sites for a variety of modulators (glycine, polyamines, MK-801, zinc). NMDA receptors also demonstrate voltage-dependent block by magnesium ions—when the membrane is depolarized and the magnesium block of the NMDA receptor is alleviated, NMDA receptor activation results in influx of calcium and sodium ions. Calcium entry initiates a number of second messenger pathways, such as stimulation of a variety of kinases that subsequently activate signal transduction cascades, leading to changes in transcriptional regulation. NMDA receptor activation leads to generation of relatively slow and long-lasting excitatory postsynaptic potentials. These synaptic events contribute to epileptiform burst discharges.

Non-NMDA ionotropic receptors are divided into α-amino-3-hydroxy-5-methyl-4-isoxazolepropionic acid (AMPA) and kainate (KA) receptors. AMPA receptors are heterotetramers composed of combinations of GluA1, GluA2, GluA3, and/or GluA4 subunits. Kainate receptors are composed of combinations of GluK1, GluK2, GluK3, GluK4, and/or GluK5 subunits. AMPA receptors are responsible for the fast-rising, initial part of the excitatory postsynaptic potential. The depolarization generated by AMPA receptors is necessary to activate NMDA receptors. Non-NMDA receptors typically pass sodium current, but certain subunit combinations endow the receptor with increased calcium permeability, a finding with implications during development as well as for epilepsy.

Metabotropic glutamate receptors ($mGlu_1$ through $mGlu_8$) represent a large, heterogeneous family of G-protein-coupled receptors that subsequently activate various transduction pathways—i.e., phosphoinositide hydrolysis and activation of adenylate cyclase and phospholipases C and D. Metabotropic receptors modulate voltage-dependent potassium and calcium channels, nonselective cation currents, and ligand-gated receptors (i.e., GABA and glutamate receptors), and they can regulate glutamate release. Metabotropic glutamate receptors have been implicated in a wide variety of normal neurologic processes (e.g., long-term potentiation underlying learning and memory) and disease states (e.g., epilepsy).

Abnormal Neuronal Firing

Specific pathophysiological mechanisms mediate each seizure stage, including transition from normal neuronal firing to interictal epileptiform bursts, to ictal activity, and to the postictal state. Intracellular and EEG changes are seen in normal, interictal, and ictal states (Fig. 63-4). When extrapolated to

thousands of synaptic contacts, it can be envisioned how inhibition can "sculpt" cellular responses. For epileptic firing to spread to noninvolved cortical areas, powerful inhibitory influences (inhibitory surround) that normally keep aberrant excitability in check must be overcome. The intracellular correlate of the focal interictal epileptiform discharge on the EEG is the paroxysmal depolarization shift (PDS) (see Fig. 63-4). If PDSs occur in several adjacent neurons, synchronous firing is facilitated.

Synchronizing Mechanisms

The hippocampus normally exhibits several forms of neuronal synchronization, including sharp waves, dentate spikes, theta activity, 40 Hz oscillations, and 200 Hz oscillations. Synchronized neuronal activity is essential for normal hippocampal function, but exaggerated synchrony may generate seizures. Synchronized activity that does not normally trigger seizures may do so in a hippocampus that has undergone selective neuronal loss, synaptic reorganization, or changes in receptor expression.

Recurrent excitatory circuits are another substrate for neuronal synchronization. Recurrent excitatory collaterals are a normal feature of the hippocampal CA3 region. CA3 pyramidal cells form direct, monosynaptic connections with other CA3 pyramidal cells, contributing to the synchronized bursts that characterize this region. In the epileptic temporal lobe, synaptic reorganization and axonal sprouting (termed "mossy fiber sprouting") lead to aberrant recurrent excitation, providing a mechanism to synchronize other regions of the hippocampus and beyond. In the normal hippocampus, for example, dentate granule cells form few or no monosynaptic contacts with neighboring granule cells. However, in the epileptic hippocampus, mossy fiber sprouting results in direct excitatory interactions among granule cells.

Nonsynaptic mechanisms, including gap junctions, electrical field (ephaptic) effects, and changes in extracellular ion concentrations, can also synchronize neuronal firing.

Glial Mechanisms for Modulating Epileptogenicity

Glia play a major role in epilepsy (Hubbard et al., 2013). The ionic balance between the intracellular and extracellular compartments is altered after seizure activity. Astrocytes help to restore ionic homeostasis by regulating (buffering) extracellular potassium levels. A variety of potassium channels mediate potassium uptake into glia; glial end-feet contacting the brain microvasculature provides a convenient "sink" for released potassium. Glia also transport synaptically released glutamate out of the extracellular space through glutamate transporters. Finally, glia modulate excitability by regulating extracellular pH using a proton exchanger and bicarbonate transporter.

Physiology of Absence Epilepsy

Generalized spike–wave discharges accompanying absence seizures reflect a widespread, phase-locked oscillation between excitation (spike) and inhibition (slow-wave) in thalamocortical networks. Pyramidal neurons from neocortical layer VI send excitatory projections to thalamic relay neurons and inhibitory GABAergic neurons of the nucleus reticularis thalami (Fig. 63-7). Excitatory outputs of thalamic relay neurons impinge on apical dendrites of layer VI pyramidal neurons. This reciprocal circuitry is responsible in large part for normal EEG oscillations during wake and sleep states but can become pathologically active and generate the generalized spike–wave discharges that underlie absence seizures.

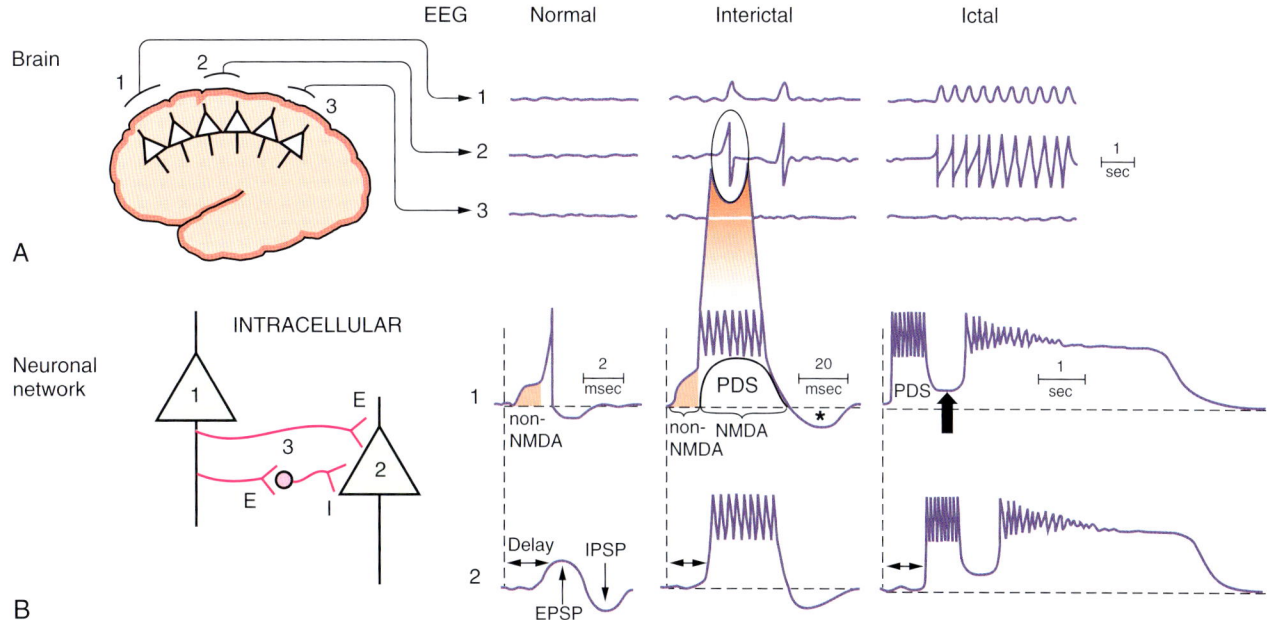

Figure 63-4. Abnormal neuronal firing. Abnormal neuronal firing is shown at the levels of the brain (**A**) and a simplified neuronal network (**B**), consisting of two excitatory neurons (1 and 2) and an inhibitory interneuron (solid circle, 3). Electroencephalogram (EEG; top set of traces) and intracellular recordings (bottom set of traces) are shown for normal (left column), interictal (middle column), and ictal (right column) conditions. Numbered traces refer to like-numbered recording sites. Note the time scale differences in different traces. **A,** Three EEG electrodes record activity from superficial neocortical neurons. In the normal case, activity is low-voltage and desynchronized (i.e., neurons are not firing in synchrony). In the interictal condition, large spikes are seen focally at electrode 2 (and to a lesser extent at electrode 1, where they may be called sharp waves), representing synchronized firing of a large population of hyperexcitable neurons (expanded in time below). The ictal state is characterized by a long run of spikes. **B,** At the neuronal network level, the intracellular correlate of the interictal EEG spike is called the paroxysmal depolarization shift (PDS). The PDS is initiated by a non-NMDA-mediated, fast excitatory postsynaptic potential (EPSP) (shaded area), but it is maintained by a longer, larger, NMDA-mediated EPSP. The post-PDS hyperpolarization (asterisk) temporarily stabilizes the neuron. If this post-PDS hyperpolarization fails (right column, arrow), ictal discharge can occur. The lowest traces, recordings from neuron 2, show activity similar to that recorded in neuron 1, with some delay (double-headed arrow). Activation of inhibitory neuron 3 by firing of neuron 1 prevents neuron 2 from generating an action potential (i.e., the inhibitory postsynaptic potential [IPSP] counters the depolarization caused by the EPSP). If neuron 2 does reach firing threshold, additional neurons will be recruited, leading to an entire network firing synchronously (i.e., a seizure). NMDA, *N*-methyl-D-aspartate. *(With permission from Stafstrom, C.E., 2004. An introduction to seizures and epilepsy: cellular mechanisms underlying classification and treatment. In: Stafstrom, C.E., Rho, J.M. (Eds.), Epilepsy and the Ketogenic Diet. Humana Press, Totowa, NJ, pp. 3–29. Reprinted with kind permission of Springer Science+Business Media.)*

Two ion channels in thalamic relay neurons regulate thalamocortical activity. The low-threshold (T-type) calcium channel is activated by small membrane depolarizations. Calcium influx through these channels triggers low-threshold spikes and activates bursts of action potentials. This burst underlies the spike portion of a generalized spike–wave oscillation. ASDs known to be clinically effective against absence seizures (ethosuximide, valproic acid) block T-type calcium currents.

The second important ion channel involved in regulating thalamocortical rhythmicity is the hyperpolarization-activated cation (HCN) channel. HCN channels are activated by hyperpolarization and produce a depolarizing h-current carried by inward flux of sodium and potassium ions. This depolarization brings the membrane potential toward threshold for activation of T-type calcium channels, producing a calcium spike and action potential burst. Unlike other voltage-gated conductances that are either inhibitory or excitatory, h-currents are both inhibitory and excitatory, possessing an inherent negative-feedback property—hyperpolarization activates HCN channels and leads to depolarization that then deactivates these channels. H-currents tend to stabilize membrane potential around the resting potential, countering hyperpolarizing and depolarizing inputs.

INCREASED SEIZURE SUSCEPTIBILITY OF THE DEVELOPING BRAIN

Seizure incidence is highest during the first decade and especially during the first year of life. Multiple physiologic and developmental factors contribute to the increased susceptibility of the immature brain to seizures (Dulac et al., 2013). The net effect is alteration of excitatory–inhibitory balance in favor of enhanced excitation; developmental changes involve ion channels, neurotransmitters and their receptors, structural changes, and ionic gradients. Seizure propensity in the very young involves a complex interplay between the timing of these cellular and molecular changes, which at times can be opposing, complementary, or synergistic.

Development of Ionic Channels and Membrane Properties

The relative timing of ion channel development plays a major role in the enhanced excitability of the immature brain. Sodium and calcium ion channels develop relatively early. Action potentials are longer in early development and mediate greater calcium current, increasing excitability by enhancing

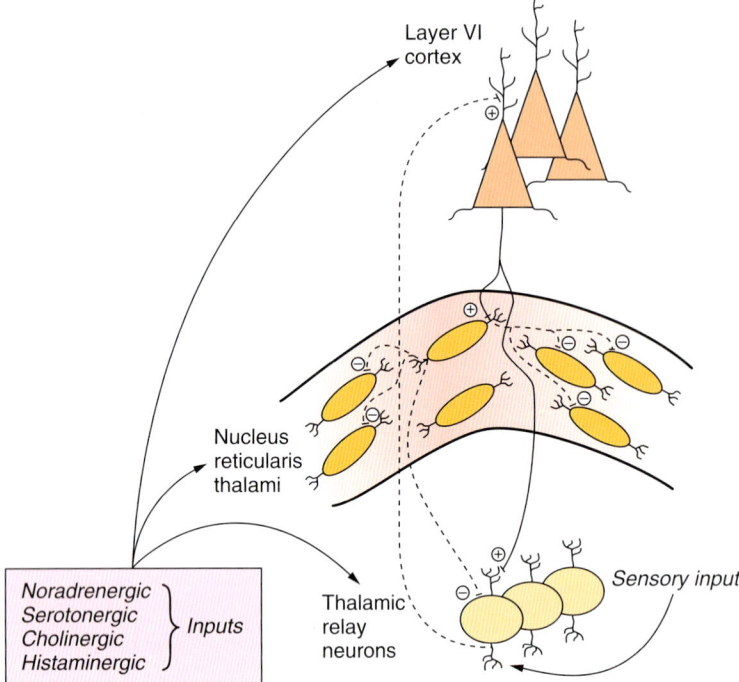

Figure 63-7. Thalamocortical circuitry. Normal oscillatory rhythms, when perturbed, can produce generalized spike–wave discharges seen with absence seizures. This circuitry involves excitatory projections from layer VI neocortical pyramidal neurons onto thalamic relay (TR) neurons and inhibitory neurons comprising the nucleus reticularis thalami (NRT). TR neurons send excitatory axons back to the neocortex. Activation of NRT neurons results in recurrent inhibition of adjacent neurons and TR neurons. The neurotransmitters at the excitatory (+) and inhibitory (–) synapses are thought to be glutamate and gamma-aminobutyric acid (GABA), respectively. Low-threshold (T-type) calcium channels and hyperpolarization-activated cation (HCN) channels in TR and NRT neurons help to regulate intrinsic rhythmicity. Extrinsic modulatory influences on this circuitry include inputs from the forebrain and brainstem nuclei and the sensory inputs from other thalamic nuclei.

neurotransmitter release. However, the brain must achieve a critical balance; activity-driven calcium channel activation is necessary for normal developmental processes such as cellular differentiation, migration, and synaptogenesis, but excessive intracellular calcium can cause neuronal damage and seizures. Mutations of the α1 subunit of the sodium channel are responsible for a spectrum of developmental epilepsies, including genetic epilepsy with febrile seizures plus and Dravet syndrome (severe myoclonic epilepsy of infancy).

A large variety of potassium channels mediate outward currents that counter depolarizing influences and stabilize membrane excitability. Potassium channels develop slightly later than sodium and calcium channels. During a window of early development, the net balance of ion fluxes tilts toward excitation, explaining the increased susceptibility of the immature brain to seizures.

Development of Neurotransmitters, Receptors, and Transporters

Excitatory synapses form before inhibitory synapses. Each glutamate receptor subunit has a distinct ontogenetic profile. For example, NMDA receptors are transiently overexpressed early in postnatal development, when they are needed for critical developmental processes. The early developmental stoichiometry of NMDA receptor subunits favors prolonged depolarizing responses. Early in development, NMDA receptor subunits GluN2A, GluN2B, and GluN3A are elevated and there is decreased sensitivity to blockade by magnesium ions and enhanced calcium influx. All of these physiologic adaptations favor depolarization, seizures, and excitotoxicity. Similarly, the

developmental profile of AMPA receptors consists of subunit stoichiometries that enhance calcium influx. Developmental expression of metabotropic glutamate receptors also favors overall hyperexcitability.

Fast-acting electrical synapses are more prevalent in the developing neocortex and hippocampus than in the mature brain. Electrical transmission facilitates rapid synchrony of the neuronal network and promotes seizure spread.

$GABA_A$ receptor subunits also exhibit a developmental profile and GABA's physiologic action varies during brain maturation (Ben-Ari et al., 2012). Early in development, GABA exerts an excitatory action, rather than an inhibitory action, because of the specific distribution of chloride ions across the cell membrane. Up to about a few months of age in humans, the intracellular chloride concentration is much higher than that in mature neurons. This chloride ion distribution is caused by the presence of a membrane pump, NKCC1, which actively imports chloride ions. Thus, when $GABA_A$ receptors are activated, postsynaptic chloride-permeable channels open and chloride ions exit the neuron down their electrochemical gradient, resulting in decreased intracellular negativity and a depolarizing current that can generate action potentials and activate NMDA receptors.

As development proceeds, the expression and activity of NKCC1 declines and that of another transporter, KCC2, increases. KCC2 has the opposite action—it actively extrudes chloride from the neuron, leaving the extracellular compartment with a higher chloride concentration. Binding of GABA to the $GABA_A$ receptor on a mature neuron results in chloride influx, hyperpolarizing the neuron.

The transition from GABAergic excitation to inhibition is an important physiologic milestone. As glutamatergic synapses develop and begin to mediate their characteristic excitatory action, GABA switches to its mature inhibitory action (via a change in expression of the chloride transporters described above). This time-point also corresponds to other developmental milestones, namely, the appearance of GABA$_B$ inhibitory responses and disappearance of large oscillatory currents known as giant depolarizing potentials (GDPs). GDPs are seen only at early ages, are dependent on both NMDA and depolarizing GABA action, and facilitate the formation of synapses and neuronal circuits. Seizure susceptibility peaks during this time window, when GABA is still excitatory, excitatory glutamate receptors have not yet matured, and GABA$_B$ inhibition is not yet complete. This window of heightened excitability corresponds to approximately term gestation in humans, when neonatal seizures are common.

Phenobarbital, which enhances GABA$_A$ receptor opening, is the most common ASD used to suppress neonatal seizures, but its efficacy is imperfect. Over development, GABA$_A$ receptor sensitivity to benzodiazepines varies. Novel approaches to the management of neonatal seizures are needed. In this regard, bumetanide, a diuretic that blocks NKCC1 and suppresses epileptic activity in brain slices and animal models, might afford clinical utility but this remains to be demonstrated.

Structural Maturation of the Brain and Seizure Susceptibility

In the developing brain, synaptic connections are formed, stabilized, or pruned as a function of neuronal activity. Such changes are referred to as plasticity, a general phenomenon that influences the brain's capacity to learn and respond to the environment. The same properties that govern plasticity may also contribute to increased susceptibility of the epileptic network to synchronize as a result of brain injury. These excessive excitatory connections are later pruned, stabilizing neuronal excitability.

Regulation of the Ionic Environment

The development of several ion transport mechanisms favors excitability early in life. In addition to the developmental profiles of NKCC1 and KCC2, expression of the sodium–potassium pump (Na$^+$,K$^+$-ATPase) also follows a developmental pattern. Extracellular accumulation of potassium after a seizure can further depolarize the neuronal membrane, exacerbating ictal activity. The ability of glial cells to clear extracellular potassium improves with age.

Epileptogenesis in the Developing Brain

The preceding paragraphs emphasize the mechanisms by which the immature brain is susceptible to seizures. The developing brain is also prone to the development of epilepsy, a process called epileptogenesis (Rakhade and Jensen, 2009). Factors playing a role in epileptogenesis are best understood according to a temporal sequence. In the first hours to days after a precipitating brain injury or severe seizure, immediate early genes are activated, leading to transcription of proteins that alter subsequent excitability. After a seizure, many receptors and other proteins involved in excitability are phosphorylated, including potassium channels and GABA$_A$, AMPA, and NMDA receptors. Later, over days to weeks, inflammation occurs. Chronic epileptogenic changes are expressed weeks to months later, including altered neurogenesis and gliosis. Therefore the epileptogenic cascade progresses from changes at the gene level to changes at the structural level. These multifactorial processes provide potential biomarkers to identify which individuals are at risk for the development of epilepsy and optimal ways to circumvent the process.

ANTISEIZURE DRUG MECHANISMS

Most ASDs exert their principal effects on the following molecular targets: GABA$_A$ receptors, glutamate receptors, and voltage-dependent sodium and calcium channels. Several ASDs are thought to possess multiple relevant mechanisms of action (Rogawski and Loscher, 2004; White et al., 2007).

Until recently, the primary drugs for treating focal epilepsy were phenytoin and carbamazepine, both of which block sodium channels in a voltage-, frequency-, and use-dependent manner. Repetitive neuronal firing is limited by both of these agents. Oxcarbazepine, a structural analog of carbamazepine, also blocks sustained repetitive firing and is especially effective against focal seizures. Lamotrigine also blocks sodium channels but has a broader spectrum of activity, with efficacy against both generalized and focal seizures. Lacosamide enhances slow inactivation of sodium channels (whereas older sodium channel-blocking ASDs enhance fast inactivation). Like most sodium channel blockers, rufinamide stabilizes fast sodium channel inactivation.

Binding of benzodiazepines or barbiturates to their respective recognition sites on postsynaptic GABA$_A$ receptors results in enhanced inhibitory current. Vigabatrin is an irreversible inhibitor of the major GABA degradative enzyme, GABA transaminase, and elevates synaptic GABA levels.

Valproic acid is a broad-spectrum ASD that induces a wide variety of biochemical and neurophysiologic changes in multiple neurotransmitter systems. Its precise mechanism of action remains unclear, but recent studies have indicated that valproic acid inhibits histone deacetylases. Valproic acid also elevates brain GABA levels and diminishes repetitive firing, implying an action on voltage-gated sodium channels.

Felbamate is the first pharmacologic agent to potentiate GABA$_A$ receptor-mediated responses and inhibit NMDA receptor-mediated responses within the same drug concentration range. These dual actions may result in synergism with respect to seizure protection. Similarly, topiramate inhibits the AMPA or kainate subtypes of glutamate receptor and augments GABA$_A$-mediated chloride currents.

Zonisamide is a broad-spectrum agent that has a unique mechanistic profile. It reduces repetitive neuronal firing, consistent with actions on sodium channels; it also blocks low-threshold T-type calcium currents, predicting efficacy against generalized spike–wave epilepsies.

Levetiracetam has proven efficacy against partial and generalized seizures. Levetiracetam binds to a specific synaptic vesicle protein, SV2A, which is involved in neurotransmitter release. The exact mechanism by which SV2A binding leads to an antiepileptic action is unknown.

Pregabalin, like gabapentin, binds to the α2δ subunit of voltage-activated calcium channels, reducing presynaptic glutamate release. Retigabine (ezogabine) selectively targets potassium channels and not only can reduce repetitive neuronal firing but also can block action potential propagation at the critical axon hillock. Perampanel suppresses seizure activity by competitively blocking AMPA-type glutamate receptors.

Current ASDs suppress seizures and their spread, but there is no clear evidence that they are antiepileptogenic (i.e., disease-modifying). As underlying mechanisms are better understood, it may be possible to design more specific, rational, age-specific, and epilepsy-specific treatments.

SUMMARY

An epileptic seizure can arise from numerous factors that increase neuronal excitability and synchrony. Unique differences in the ontogeny of ion channels, synapses, and transporters render the immature brain more susceptible to seizures than the adult brain. The concept of excitation–inhibition imbalance is key to understanding the genesis of seizures and epilepsy, yet this concept needs to be expanded to include other cellular mechanisms, particularly in light of recently discovered mutations that underlie rarer forms of epilepsies, such as the epileptic encephalopathies. Ultimately, seizures reflect perturbations of a complex array of cellular and network changes at multiple hierarchical levels of brain structure and function. The major goals of pediatric epilepsy research are to develop pathophysiology- and age-specific treatments, encompassing a more personalized or precision approach to patient care, to reduce seizures and their adverse consequences.

REFERENCES

The complete list of references for this chapter is available in the e-book at www.expertconsult.com.
See inside cover for registration details.

SELECTED REFERENCES

Ben-Ari, Y., Khalilov, I., Kahle, K.T., et al., 2012. The GABA excitatory/inhibitory shift in brain maturation and neurological disorders. Neuroscientist 18, 467–486.

Child, N.D., Bennaroch, E.E., 2014. Differential distribution of voltage-gated ion channels in cortical neurons: implications for epilepsy. Neurology 82, 989–999.

Dulac, O., Milh, M., Holmes, G.L., 2013. Brain maturation and epilepsy. Handb. Clin. Neurol. 111, 441–446.

Hirose, S., 2014. Mutant GABA(A) receptor subunits in genetic (idiopathic) epilepsy. Prog. Brain Res. 213, 55–85.

Hubbard, J.A., Hsu, M.S., Fiacco, T.A., et al., 2013. Glial cell changes in epilepsy: overview of the clinical problem and therapeutic opportunities. Neurochem. Int. 63, 638–651.

Rakhade, S.N., Jensen, F.E., 2009. Epileptogenesis in the immature brain: emerging mechanisms. Nat. Rev. Neurol. 5, 380–391.

Rogawski, M.A., Loscher, W., 2004. The neurobiology of antiepileptic drugs. Nat. Rev. Neurosci. 5, 553–564.

Stafstrom, C.E., 2014. Recognizing seizures and epilepsy: insights from pathophysiology. In: Miller, J.W., Goodkin, H.P. (Eds.), Epilepsy. John Wiley & Sons, Ltd., Chichester, UK, pp. 3–9.

Steinlein, O.K., 2014. Mechanisms underlying epilepsies associated with sodium channel mutations. Prog. Brain Res. 213, 97–111.

White, H.S., Smith, M.D., Wilcox, K.S., 2007. Mechanisms of action of antiepileptic drugs. Int. Rev. Neurobiol. 81, 85–110.

E-BOOK FIGURES AND TABLES

The following figures and tables are available in the e-book at www.expertconsult.com. See inside cover for registration details.

64 Epilepsy Genetics

Maria Roberta Cilio and Tristan T. Sands

An expanded version of this chapter is available on www.expertconsult.com. See inside cover for registration details.

INTRODUCTION

The concept of genetic epilepsy is that the condition is the direct result of a known or presumed genetic defect, and seizures are the core symptom of the disorder. The knowledge regarding the genetic contribution may derive from specific molecular genetic studies that have been well replicated and even become the basis of diagnostic tests. Alternatively, the central role of a genetic component may rely on evidence from appropriately designed family studies. Although the term *genetic* designates the fundamental nature of the disorder, it does not exclude the contribution of environmental factors to the expression of the disease. Genetics has seen a dramatic evolution of information in the past decade, including the definition of rare mendelian epilepsies, which has given insight into broader disease mechanisms and identification of the substrates involved in the more complex inheritance patterns that underlie most genetic epilepsy syndromes. This chapter is intended to provide the most updated information on the genetics of the epilepsies and to introduce newer concepts underlying genotype–phenotype correlation and functional consequences of gene mutations. Some of the most important genetic discoveries in the field have been made possible by a careful definition of the phenotype by epileptologists. On the other hand, epileptogenic gene mutations discovered by molecular biologists have led to recognition of previously unidentified clinical forms of epilepsy (Noebels, 2015). The identification of the genetic basis of epilepsies has improved understanding of the pathophysiology and resulted in targeted therapeutic approaches. Epilepsy syndromes are organized by age at onset: neonatal (<44 weeks' gestational age), infant (<2 years), child (2–12 years), and adolescent (12–18 years).

EPILEPSIES WITH ONSET IN NEONATAL PERIOD
Benign Familial Neonatal Epilepsy

Benign familial neonatal epilepsy (BFNE) is a rare benign autosomal-dominant epilepsy characterized by recurrent seizures from the first few days of life and generally limited to the first months of life. Seizures, lasting 1 to 2 minutes but recurring up to 20 to 30 times daily, are characterized by tonic posturing with shifting laterality, accompanied by autonomic symptoms and progressing to clonic jerks.

The responsible genes, *KCNQ2* (20q13.3) and *KCNQ3* (8q24), encode Kv7.2 and Kv7.3, subunits that coassemble as heteromeric tetramers to form voltage-gated potassium channels (Maljevic and Lerche, 2014). Genetic alteration of *KCNQ2* is 10 times more common as a cause of BFNE compared with *KCNQ3*. Over 50 mutations have been described in *KCNQ2*, and 6 have been identified in *KCNQ3*. Deletions and duplications of *KCNQ2* have also been described.

Pathologic mutations in *KCNQ2/3* cause a loss of function through effects on the channel pore, voltage sensor, and domains important for regulation, assembly, and trafficking, which are induced by a haploinsufficiency mechanism. The functional consequence is a reduction (<20%–30%) in the M-current, a muscarine-regulated, slow, noninactivating subthreshold potassium current that plays a key role in controlling neuronal excitation. *KCNQ2/3* expression increases over the first postnatal weeks in rodents, during which time the M-current may play a predominant role in regulating neuronal excitability. A critical window may determine the age dependence of BFNE. Retigabine is a drug that specifically augments the M-current and suggests the possibility for a targeted therapeutic approach.

KCNQ2 Encephalopathy

De novo *KCNQ2* mutations have been found in patients with severe neonatal-onset epilepsy with intractable seizures and profound psychomotor impairment. The timing of onset and the seizure semiology are similar to those in BFNE, but the interictal electroencephalogram (EEG) is characterized by a burst-suppression pattern or multifocal epileptiform activity. Genetic studies indicate that *KCNQ2* mutation accounts for more than 10% of cases of neonatal epileptic encephalopathy. Although response to retigabine has been described, the best success in treating the seizures appears to be with sodium channel blockers, carbamazepine in particular (Pisano et al., 2015). Sodium channels are bound together with the potassium channels encoded by *KCNQ2/3* in critical locations for action potential generation and maintenance. Modulation of one channel affects the functioning of the entire complex, offering insight into why sodium channel blockers may be particularly effective for a disease caused by potassium channel mutations.

Outcomes remain poor despite seizure control, arguing for additional developmental roles for *KCNQ2*. Compared with mutation associated with BFNE, mutations that cause *KCNQ2* encephalopathy may lead to quantitatively more substantial loss of channel function or to gain of function. Together with reports of occasional poor outcomes in some families with BFNE, it is likely that BFNE and *KCNQ2* encephalopathy likely lie along a phenotypic spectrum determined largely by genotype, but with a significant role for the modifying influences of genetic background.

Ohtahara Syndrome (Early Infantile Epileptic Encephalopathy)

Ohtahara, West, and Lennox–Gastaut syndromes are three age-dependent epileptic encephalopathies, presenting in the neonatal, infantile, and toddler periods, respectively. Each is characterized by frequent seizures of a particular type, a unique and severely abnormal interictal EEG, and poor neurodevelopmental outcomes. The same etiologies may give rise to multiple age-dependent epileptic encephalopathies, and an affected individual may evolve from one syndrome to another with age, suggesting that each condition represents a common final reaction to brain insult determined by developmental period.

Ohtahara syndrome (OS) presents within the first 3 months, with tonic spasms as the main seizure, a burst-suppression pattern on EEG, high mortality, and severe neurodevelopmental impairment. OS is most often associated with gross structural lesions, but nonlesional genetic causes account for up to one-third of cases. The genes mutated in OS tend to be regulators of cortical development and/or synaptic function (Nabbout and Dulac, 2012).

Mutations in the Aristaless-related homeobox (*ARX*) gene, a transcriptional regulator during cortical development, represent an important cause of X-linked cause of OS. However, de novo heterozygous mutation of the gene encoding syntaxin binding protein 1 (*STXBP1*) has been shown to be the most common genetic cause of OS, accounting for approximately one-third of nonstructural causes. *STXBP1* mutation has also been implicated in West syndrome and in cases of mental retardation and nonsyndromic epilepsy. *STXBP1* is a member of the Sec1p/Munc18 family of SNARE (soluble NSF attachment protein receptor) regulators, required for exocytosis. *STXBP1* promotes the formation of fusion complexes via interaction with two N-terminal domains of syntaxin 1a. Causative mutations commonly lead to premature termination, nonexpression, or impaired binding of STXBP1 to syntaxin 1a, leading to dysfunctional neurotransmission through haploinsufficiency.

Loss-of-function mutations in *CASK* (Xp11.4), encoding calcium/calmodulin-dependent serine protein kinase, have been described in males with OS. *CASK* appears to be required for synapse formation and cortical development. De novo missense mutations of *GNAO1* (16q13) encoding the alpha subunit of a heterotrimeric guanine-binding protein (G-protein), a signaling molecule with a role in calcium current inhibition, have been reported to result in a neonatal epileptic encephalopathy and a hyperkinetic movement disorder. Frameshift and missense mutations have been reported in *SLC35A2* (Xp11.23), which encodes a transporter important for galactosylation. Homozygous mutations in *SLC25A22* (11p15.5), which encodes a mitochondrial glutamate transporter, have been described in consanguineous families with OS. Finally, the OS phenotype has been associated with *KCNQ2* and *SCN2A* mutation, although there is increasing evidence that these two genes are associated with unique phenotypes.

Benign Familial Neonatal-Infantile Epilepsy

Benign familial neonatal-infantile epilepsy (BFNIE) is an autosomal-dominant benign epilepsy with a high penetrance. Age of onset ranges from 2 days to 6 months in different family members. Seizures are focal, with eye deviation, apnea, and cyanosis, and they may occur in clusters. Seizures abate by 1 year of life, with a low risk of recurrence.

BFNIE has been shown to be linked to missense mutation causing gain or loss of function in Nav1.2, a sodium channel, encoded by *SCN2A* (2q24.3). Nav1.2 resides at the axon hillock of excitatory neurons, where it is critically poised to influence the firing of these cells. Nav1.2 is supplanted over time by Nav1.6, which may account for the limited temporal expression of benign epilepsy caused by *SCN2A* mutation.

Epileptic Encephalopathy Associated With *SCN2A*

Analogous to the situation with *KCNQ2*, de novo missense or nonsense mutation in the *SCN2A* gene is associated with severe developmental phenotypes in the setting of refractory epilepsy presenting in the neonatal and infantile periods. A hyperkinetic movement disorder may be seen. Mutations associated with the epileptic encephalopathy result in less conservative amino acid substitutions, suggesting more profound effects on channel structure and function.

EPILEPSIES WITH ONSET IN INFANCY
Benign Familial Infantile Epilepsy

Benign familial infantile epilepsy (BFIE) has an autosomal-dominant inheritance pattern and presents with clusters of brief focal seizures with shifting laterality at 4 to 20 months (median 6 months). The disorder has been found mainly associated with mutations in the *PRRT2* gene (16p11.2), which encodes proline-rich transmembrane protein 2, found in presynaptic terminals and implicated in the regulation of neurotransmitter release. Although approximately 80% of BFIE is related to *PRRT2*, mutations in *KCNQ2*, *KCNQ3*, and *SCN2A* have been reported as well (Zara et al., 2013).

Mutation of *PRRT2* is also a cause of a familial form of paroxysmal kinesigenic dyskinesia (PKD), a movement disorder of late childhood through early adulthood characterized by brief attacks of dystonia or choreoathetosis usually triggered by sudden movement, although unprovoked attacks (nonkinesigenic) can also occur (Heron and Dibbens, 2013). BFIE and PKD resulting from *PRRT2* mutation can occur in the same family or even the same patient, and the term *infantile convulsions with choreoathetosis* (ICCA) has been used to refer to this scenario. Seizures tend to be readily responsive to carbamazepine.

The vast majority of the mutations of *PRRT2* leading to BFIE and/or PKD are predicted to cause to protein truncation, leading to haploinsufficiency. Over 80% of cases are the result of a particular frameshift resulting from an insertion of an additional cytosine at c.649 to 650, likely as a result of polymerase slippage at the site, which lies in a poly C tract, predicted to be prone to hairpin secondary structure. De novo mutation of *PRRT2* causes approximately half of sporadic cases of benign infantile epilepsy with the same phenotypic spectrum as the familial form. Homozygous mutation of *PRRT2* is associated with a much more severe phenotype that includes significant cognitive disability.

Epileptic Encephalopathy Associated With Cyclin-Dependent Kinase-Like 5 (*CDKL5*)

Mutation or deletion of *CDKL5*, encoding cyclin-dependent kinase-like 5, causes a unique epileptic encephalopathy presenting with seizures in the first 3 months of life, very often near the end of the neonatal period. The condition is X-linked (Xp22) and is principally seen in girls (12:1 female-to-male ratio). Initially there is hypotonia and poor eye contact. Subsequently, epileptic spasms occur with or without hypsarrhythmia, and a distinctive "hypermotor–tonic–spasms" sequence has been described. Ultimately, children suffer from refractory epilepsy with multiple seizure types, including tonic, myoclonic, and spasms; interictal EEG deteriorates with high-amplitude slowing and bursts of spikes and polyspikes. Developmentally, only about a third of females with the condition learn to walk, and males acquire minimal motor skills. A significant proportion of girls will have a deceleration of head growth and hand stereotypies of some form.

CDKL5 is a serine-threonine kinase capable of signaling to nuclear targets, including the product of *MECP2*, the gene responsible for Rett syndrome. Loss-of-function mutations may cause more severe phenotypes when they affect the catalytic domain of the kinase, but severity is also likely influenced in females by the extent to which the normal gene copy escapes X-inactivation. Predictably, males, who lack a second

X chromosome with a wild-type *CDKL5*, are more severely affected.

A *CDKL5* knockout mouse model replicates behavioral aspects of the human condition, including limb clasping, abnormal eye tracking, and hypoactivity, although not seizures. Pathophysiological correlates include reduced dendritic arborization and altered activity of the mammalian target of rapamycin (mTOR) pathway. Other studies have implicated *CDKL5* in neuronal morphogenesis via *RAC1*-mediated control over the actin cytoskeleton.

Epilepsy of Infancy With Migrating Focal Seizures

Epilepsy of infancy with migrating focal seizures (EIMFS) is a severe electroclinical syndrome, presenting within the first 6 months of life with intractable multifocal seizures that grow increasingly frequent until they are nearly continuous, migrating from one focus to another. Multiple independent seizures can evolve simultaneously. Interictal EEG progresses from normal to disorganized with multifocal epileptiform abnormalities. Neurodevelopmental outcome is typically severe, and there is often acquired microcephaly. Mortality of 28% was reported in the original series.

The most common known cause, accounting for 50% of cases, is de novo mutation in *KCNT1* (9q34.3), a sodium-activated potassium channel. The channel, known as SLACK (sequence like a calcium activated potassium channel), mediates the slow hyperpolarization that accompanies repetitive neuronal firing. Pathologic mutations increase the current amplitude through increased cooperativity between individual channels. Mutation of the same gene account for some cases of autosomal-dominant nocturnal frontal lobe epilepsy, a familial condition that presents in later childhood. The mutations of *KCNT1* resulting in EIMFS have been shown to lead to lower-magnitude increases in conductance, indicating a bimodal genotype–phenotype correlation.

Quinidine has been shown to reverse the increased conductance imparted by the pathologic gain of function mutations in vitro, and a case report has demonstrated efficacy in clinical practice (Bearden et al., 2014). Seizure control has been suggested to improve neurodevelopmental outcomes. However, the C-terminus of SLACK interacts with the fragile X mental retardation protein, raising the possibility that mutation of *KCNT1* could deleteriously affect signaling through important developmental pathways, apart from its effects on cortical excitability. *SCN1A* mutation and *SLC25A22* homozygous mutation represent less frequent causes.

West Syndrome

West syndrome (WS) is an age-dependent epileptic encephalopathy with onset typically around 6 months of age, characterized by epileptic spasms, hypsarrhythmia, and developmental regression. Although the predominant causes are congenital or acquired structural lesions, such as the cortical tubers of tuberous sclerosis complex, associated with *TSC1* and *TSC2* gene mutation, which alone account for more than 7% of cases of WS, there are nonmalformation related genetic etiologies as well. Whereas West syndrome on the one hand represents a common final pathway of many inborn and acquired insults, the underlying etiology creates the context in which the spasms occur, informs their electroclinical manifestation, and determines the treatment approach and outcome (Dulac et al., 2010). As with Ohtahara syndrome, many of the implicated genes are associated with forebrain development and synaptic function.

Mutation of Aristaless-related homeobox (*ARX*) gene (Xp22), encoding a transcription regulator, causes X-linked infantile spasms syndrome (ISSX). *ARX* mutation leads to a wide phenotypic spectrum of X-linked cognitive impairment, including nonsyndromic intellectual disability with or without epilepsy, OS, ISSX, and overt brain malformation. Spasticity and dystonia are additional clinical features. Most of the pathologic mutations in *ARX*, including those giving rise to the ISSX phenotype, cause an expansion in two polyalanine tracts in the *ARX* gene product. Missense mutations or truncations that affect the homeodomain or regions important for transcriptional activation or repression can also cause phenotypes, including ISSX. There is a great deal of pleiotropy within families sharing the same mutation, with some males developing OS, for instance, and others with an ISSX phenotype. Nevertheless, clinical severity has been associated with the length of polyalanine tract expansion, which is thought to interfere with proper localization of *ARX* to the nucleus. A genotype–phenotype correlation also holds in the sense that full loss of function of *ARX* results in the most severe presentation.

In rodents, *ARX* encodes a transcription factor that acts downstream from *Dlx1* and *Dlx2*, transcriptional regulators important in specifying interneuronal fate. *ARX* is required for the migration of populations of interneurons into the cerebral cortex. A mouse knockin of a polyalanine-expanded *ARX* gene causes loss of subpopulations of GABAergic interneurons in the cerebral cortex and deep gray nuclei and causes epileptic spasms in mice during their second and third weeks of life.

A myocyte enhancer factor 2c (*MEF2C*) gene (5q14.3) mutation has been associated with a clinical phenotype that includes intellectual disability with autistic features and a hyperkinetic movement disorder. More than two-thirds of patients develop epilepsy, and the majority have onset in infancy; 20% of patients with *MEF2C* mutation develop infantile spasms. Infants with *MEF2C* mutation are hypotonic, and one-third of patients have myoclonic seizures that may precede epileptic spasms. Complete loss of function mutation is associated with epilepsy. *MEF2C* encodes a transcription factor critically positioned within regulatory networks underlying forebrain development.

Duplication of the region containing the Forkhead box G1 (*FOXG1*) gene, 14q13, or gene mutation results in phenotypes that include epilepsy. Haploinsufficiency of *FOXG1* causes severe intellectual disability with acquired microcephaly, dyskinesia, and epilepsy in two-thirds of patients with onset after infancy. In contrast, 14q13 duplication causes variable developmental delay, prominently affecting language, and more than half of patients develop infantile spasms. The epilepsy usually resolves after the toddler years. *FOXG1* is a transcriptional repressor specific to the brain that is implicated in neuronogenesis.

De novo mutation of *SPTAN1* (9q34.11), encoding alpha-2 spectrin, causes infantile spasms and hypsarrhythmia in association with cerebral hypomyelination, in addition to atrophy of the cerebellum and brainstem. Children suffer from spastic quadriplegia, acquired microcephaly, and severe intellectual disability. There is a high rate of mortality in the first few years of life. Infantile spasms evolve in the majority of patients, with an onset at 3 to 4 months. Responsible mutations in the last two spectrin repeats lead to dominant negative interference with heterodimerization with a beta spectrin. Spectrins are part of the membrane cytoskeleton. Alpha-2 spectrin is necessary for proper myelination in zebrafish.

WS can be caused by de novo mutation of *DNM* (9q34), encoding dynamin-1 and a GTPase specific to the brain that is responsible for synaptic vesicle endocytosis at the presynaptic terminal in response to neuronal activity.

Dravet Syndrome and Genetic Epilepsy With Febrile Seizures Plus

Dravet syndrome (DS) is characterized by seizure onset between 4 and 8 months, with a peak at 6 months of prolonged hemiclonic or generalized seizures, most often triggered by elevated temperature. Later, other seizure types appear, including myoclonic. An early photosensitivity is present in approximately 40%. Children develop neuropsychiatric impairment and ataxia and are at elevated risk of sudden unexplained death in epilepsy (SUDEP). Recent evidence suggests that the severe neurodevelopmental outcome in DS is not related only to seizures, but may be the direct result of the genetic alteration.

The major gene for DS, *SCN1A* (2q24.3), was originally identified in families with genetic epilepsy with febrile seizures plus (GEFS+), an autosomal-dominant epilepsy with incomplete penetrance, in which at least two family members are affected. The most common phenotype is characterized by the association of febrile seizures, at times extending beyond 6 years of age, with afebrile generalized tonic-clonic seizures. GEFS+ is associated with *SCN1A* mutations, generally missense, in roughly 10% of cases. Clinical heterogeneity within families sharing the same mutation is the rule. The discovery of GEFS+ families with family members with DS was followed by discovery of de novo mutations in sporadic cases. De novo *SCN1A* mutation accounts for 70% to 80% of DS and usually arises in the paternal allele.

SCN1A encodes a neuronal sodium channel NaV1.1 alpha subunit, which has four homologous regions, each encoding six transmembrane domains, and a region controlling interactions with the permeable ion (Oliva, Berkovic, and Petrou, 2012). There are over 300 mutations described. More than half of mutations are truncating, with the remainder being largely missense mutations, although deletion and duplication have been reported as well. Truncating mutations seem to contribute to a more severe phenotype. The issue is confounded by genetic and/or environmental modifying factors, as is clear from the variability of phenotypic expression observed in GEFS+ families carrying *SCN1A* mutations. One potential modifying gene is *SCN9A*, encoding a different sodium channel. Mutations of *SCN1B*, *GABRG2*, *GABRA1*, and *STXBP1* have also been reported as associated with DS.

Mice heterozygous for *SCN1A* develop ataxia and age-dependent, temperature-sensitive epilepsy with myoclonic and generalized seizures. These mice have been demonstrated to have reduced sodium currents in cerebellar Purkinje cells, explaining the ataxia. Sodium currents are also reduced in cortical inhibitory interneurons but not in excitatory pyramidal neurons, explaining how loss of function in a sodium channel gene could result in a hyperexcitable cerebral cortex. Additional work has suggested that parvalbumin-positive interneurons, including chandelier and basket cells, with fast-spiking physiology are specifically affected. This explains the observation that sodium channel blockers typically aggravate the condition. The reduced GABAergic tone may explain the therapeutic response to clobazam and stiripentol, which enhance inhibitory GABAergic transmission.

Epileptic Encephalopathy Associated With *SCN8A*

De novo mutation of *SCN8A* (2q24.3), encoding sodium channel Nav1.6, causes 1% of early-onset epileptic encephalopathies, presenting with multiple seizure types during infancy, with a mean age at onset of 4 to 5 months. A strikingly high rate of SUDEP has been observed in patients reported to date (12.5%). Nav1.6 is the most abundant sodium channel in the brain and plays a critical role in regulating neuronal excitability. Pathogenic missense mutations in *SCN8A* are thought to cause a gain-of-function effect, including impaired channel inactivation or shifted voltage dependence of channel activation leading to hyperexcitability. Correspondingly, in contrast to the *SCN1A*-related epilepsies, sodium channel blockers have been found to be among the most useful agents in treating seizures in *SCN8A* epilepsy.

Epilepsy Associated With Protocadherin 19 (*PCDH19*)

PCDH19 mutation causes a "girls-only epilepsy" presenting between 6 and 36 months (median of 10 months), with seizures triggered by elevations in body temperature. There is a characteristic "stormy" ictal pattern with clusters of brief (1- to 5-minute) seizures for several days, with variable periods of quiescence, lasting weeks to months to years. Seizures are most commonly focal tonic, associated with apnea. Interictal EEG may be normal or show slowing and/or focal or multifocal epileptiform discharges. Cognitive outcome—one-third each normal intellect, mild intellectual disability, and moderate-severe intellectual disability—does not seem to be associated with epilepsy severity. *PCDH19* mutations are often de novo, but they can be transmitted with an unusual X-linked inheritance pattern that spares males in the carrier state (Depienne and LeGuern, 2012). Responsible mutations are largely loss of function, with half leading to premature termination. *PCDH19* (Xq22.1) encodes a protocadherin involved in cell–cell adhesion and signaling, and it has been proposed that protocadherin related cell–cell interaction is perturbed by tissue mosaicism present in the disomy X condition (i.e., some cells will express *PCDH19*, whereas some neighboring cells will not. That tissue mosaicism is necessary for the disease is supported by the report of a male patient with a somatic mutation. There is no clear genotype–phenotype correlation, and the phenotypic range in females has been speculated to be caused by the relative skew of X-inactivation.

Other Early-Onset Epilepsies

Novel de novo mutations are being reported at an accelerating pace. *CHD2* (15q26) encodes chromodomain helicase DNA-binding protein 2. De novo mutations have been reported in association with a phenotype manifesting between 1 and 3 years of life, characterized by myoclonic and absence seizures, photosensitivity, and intellectual disability ranging from mild to severe. *SYNGAP1* (6p21.3) encodes synaptic Ras GTPase-activating protein 1. De novo mutations have been reported in association with intellectual disability, autism, and epilepsy characterized by a variety of generalized seizure types with onset between 1 and 3 years of life.

SYNDROMES WITH ONSET IN CHILDHOOD AND ADOLESCENCE

Epilepsy-Aphasia Syndromes

Epilepsy-aphasia syndromes are epileptic encephalopathies that manifest in early childhood with language regression associated with the EEG pattern of continuous spike and wave during slow-wave sleep (CSWS). Landau–Kleffner syndrome affects previously normal children who develop acquired epileptic aphasia, whereas the epileptic encephalopathy associated with CSWS is a condition of more global regression, and in half of cases there is premorbid delay. Mutations in *GRIN2A* (16p13.2), encoding the NMDA receptor alpha-2 subunit, are found in 10% to 20% of children with the epilepsy-aphasia syndromes, opening up the potential for novel therapeutic approaches.

Idiopathic Generalized Epilepsies

Childhood absence epilepsy (CAE), juvenile absence epilepsy (JAE), and juvenile myoclonic epilepsy (JME), are generalized epilepsies with genetic underpinnings. Positive family history is common, but inheritance is not straightforward, and a complex polygenetic etiology has been suggested. When the syndromes occur within GEFS+ families, mutation in *SCN1A*, *SCN1B*, or *GABRG2* may be identified. Mutation of *CACNA1H* at 16p13.3 has been identified as an important cause of primary generalized epilepsies in the Han Chinese population. *CACNA1H* encodes a subunit of the neuronal voltage-gated T-type calcium channel subunit, responsible for the signature 3-Hz spike-and-wave pattern seen in CAE.

An autosomal-dominant form of JME has been described that results from a loss-of-function mutation of the *GABRA1* gene at 5q34. *GABRA1* encodes the alpha-1 subunit of the $GABA_A$ receptor, mutation of which has been associated with CAE as well. Loss-of-function mutations in *EFHC1* are associated with JME in a variety of affected families of differing origin. *EFHC1* at 6p12.3 encodes a protein of unknown function with calcium-binding EF-hand motif, a helix-loop-helix structural domain found in a large family of calcium-binding proteins. There is evidence that the protein modulates apoptotic activity and R-type voltage-dependent calcium channel properties. The complex polygenic inheritance patterns involved in the primary generalized epilepsy syndromes reveal that a single epilepsy phenotype can be generated by combinations of varied mutations, and that, conversely, a given mutation can be associated with more than one phenotype.

Autosomal-Dominant Nocturnal Frontal Lobe Epilepsy

Autosomal-dominant nocturnal frontal lobe epilepsy (ADNFLE) is inherited with near complete penetrance and presents during the first or second decade of life with brief clusters of nocturnal tonic postural or hypermotor seizures. The ictal EEG may show frontally predominant sharp- and slow-wave activity, or it may fail to reveal a definite ictal pattern. *KCNT1*, described previously as the major cause of EIMFS, also causes ADNFLE. Mutations in genes encoding the alpha-4 (*CHRNA4*), beta-2 (*CHRNB2*), and alpha-2 (*CHRNA2*) subunits of the nicotinic acetylcholine receptor have been reported associated with this phenotype in about 10% of patients. The acetylcholine receptor is a pentameric ion channel. The second transmembrane domain of each subunit lines the ion channel pore and is the site for the majority of the mutations that have been described for *CHRNA4* and *CHRNB2*. Functionally, the mutations appear to alter the desensitization kinetics of the receptor, leading to hyperexcitability.

Outcomes for ADNFLE associated with nicotinic receptor subunit mutations are generally good. However, the disease does not typically remit, and the majority of patients require antiepileptic medication, with one-third well controlled on carbamazepine and another third requiring more than one agent. In contrast, *KCNT1* mutation gives a more severe phenotype, in which the seizures may be refractory; half also suffer from behavioral or psychiatric disturbances, and up to a quarter have intellectual disability.

Autosomal-Dominant Focal Epilepsy With Auditory Features

Autosomal-dominant focal epilepsy with auditory features (ADFEAF) has a penetrance of greater than 50% and presents during the second to fourth decades. Seizures are focal at onset, occurring with a frequency from several per month to twice a year. Auditory auras are reported in roughly 50%.

Roughly half of cases of ADFEAF are associated with mutation in *LGI1*, encoding leucine-rich glioma inactivated 1 protein at 10q24. Over 20y mutations have been described, resulting in truncations, deletions, or single amino acid substitutions. Rarely, mutations are associated with idiopathic generalized epilepsy syndromes in some family members as well.

In vitro studies show that mutant LGI1 fails to be secreted, thereby blocking its access to postsynaptic scaffolding proteins, where it plays a role in AMPA receptor-mediated synaptic transmission. Additional studies have found a role for the protein in presynaptic potassium channel assembly, with mutant forms of the protein resulting in changes in the inactivation kinetics of the channel, potentially providing a mechanism for hyperexcitability.

Familial Focal Epilepsy With Variable Foci and *DEPDC5*-Related Epilepsies

Familial focal epilepsy with variable foci (FFEVF) is an autosomal-dominant syndrome with a variable penetrance of 50% to 80%, characterized by focal epilepsy, with age of onset ranging widely from the first weeks of life to fifth or sixth decade (mean of 12 to 13 years). In affected family members, seizure semiology varies according to seizure focus, most often (70%) in the frontal or temporal lobe, which tends to remain consistent throughout life. Seizure frequency and severity are likewise variable. Interictal abnormalities are found in roughly half of recordings and most often reveal epileptiform activity arising from the frontal or temporal regions. The responsible gene, encoding disheveled, Egl-10, and pleckstrin domain-containing protein 5, *DEPDC5* (22q11.3), represents an important genetic cause of both autosomal-dominant familial (including some families with familial temporal lobe epilepsy and ADNFLE) and sporadic focal epilepsies. Mutations are loss of function, often premature truncations or deletions, and are thought to result in disease through a haploinsufficiency mechanism. The *DEPDC5* gene product is a member of the GATOR1 complex, an inhibitory regulator of the mTOR pathway, which plays a critical role in cellular growth and proliferation and in aspects of neuronal development. Components of the mTOR signaling cascade are associated with tuberous sclerosis complex and malformations of cortical development. Indeed, like TSC1/TSC2, the GATOR1 complex regulates GTPases that directly influence mTOR activity. Intriguingly, focal dysplasias—in particular, bottom-of-the-sulcus dysplasias—have been identified in some FFEVF family members but not others.

REFERENCES

The complete list of references for this chapter is available in the e-book at www.expertconsult.com.
   See inside cover for registration details.

SELECTED REFERENCES

Bearden, D., Strong, A., Ehnot, J., et al., 2014. Targeted treatment of migrating partial seizures of infancy with quinidine. Ann. Neurol. 76 (3), 457–461.

Depienne, C., LeGuern, E., 2012. PCDH19-related infantile epileptic encephalopathy: an unusual X-linked inheritance disorder. Hum. Mutat. 33 (4), 627–634.

Dulac, O., Bast, T., Dalla Bernardina, B., et al., 2010. Infantile spasms: toward a selective diagnostic and therapeutic approach. Epilepsia 51 (10), 2218–2219, author reply 21.

Heron, S.E., Dibbens, L.M., 2013. Role of PRRT2 in common paroxysmal neurological disorders: a gene with remarkable pleiotropy. J. Med. Genet. 50 (3), 133–139.

Maljevic, S., Lerche, H., 2014. Potassium channel genes and benign familial neonatal epilepsy. Prog. Brain Res. 213, 17–53.

Nabbout, R., Dulac, O., 2012. Epilepsy. Genetics of early-onset epilepsy with encephalopathy. Nat. Rev. Neurol. 8 (3), 129–130.

Noebels, J., 2015. Pathway-driven discovery of epilepsy genes. Nat. Neurosci. 18 (3), 344–350.

Oliva, M., Berkovic, S.F., Petrou, S., 2012. Sodium channels and the neurobiology of epilepsy. Epilepsia 53 (11), 1849–1859.

Pisano, T., Numis, A.L., Heavin, S.B., et al., 2015. Early and effective treatment of KCNQ2 encephalopathy. Epilepsia 56 (5), 685–691.

Zara, F., Specchio, N., Striano, P., et al., 2013. Genetic testing in benign familial epilepsies of the first year of life: clinical and diagnostic significance. Epilepsia 54 (3), 425–436.

E-BOOK FIGURES AND TABLES

The following figures and tables are available in the e-book at www.expertconsult.com. See inside cover for registration details.

Fig. 64-1 Genes associated with epilepsy by age at presentation.

Table 64-1 Genetic Causes of Epilepsy

65 Febrile Seizures

Syndi Seinfeld and Shlomo Shinnar

An expanded version of this chapter is available on www.expertconsult.com. See inside cover for registration details.

Febrile seizures are a form of acute symptomatic seizures. They occur in 2% to 5% of children and are the most common form of childhood seizures. In the past, it was believed that febrile seizures were associated with a poor prognosis. It is now accepted that the majority of children with febrile seizures do well, but a subgroup of children do experience consequences. Epilepsy will eventually develop in a small minority of children who have had febrile seizures (Nelson and Ellenberg, 1976; Annegers et al., 1979; Berg et al., 1992). This understanding is based on large epidemiologic studies (Nelson and Ellenberg, 1976; Annegers et al., 1979; Berg et al., 1992), as well as on prospective studies from emergency departments not selected for tertiary referral bias. This chapter reviews the current understanding of the prognosis and management of febrile seizures.

DEFINITIONS

A febrile seizure is defined by the International League Against Epilepsy as a seizure occurring in association with a febrile illness, in the absence of a central nervous system infection or acute electrolyte imbalance in children older than 1 month of age without prior afebrile seizures. This definition is similar to the one adopted by the National Institutes of Health (NIH) Consensus Conference, except that the NIH definition described a febrile seizure as an event usually occurring between 3 months and 5 years of age. The febrile illness must include a body temperature of more than 38.3° C, although the increased temperature may not occur until after the seizure.

Febrile seizures are further classified as simple or complex. A febrile seizure is complex if it is focal, prolonged (lasting for more than either 10 minutes (Annegers et al., 1979) or 15 minutes (Nelson and Ellenberg, 1976)), or multiple (occurrence of more than one seizure during the febrile illness). Conversely, it is simple if it is an isolated, brief, generalized seizure. Although neurologically abnormal children are more likely to experience complex febrile seizures and have a higher risk for subsequent afebrile seizures, the child's prior neurologic condition is not used to classify the seizure as simple or complex. When a careful history is obtained, approximately 30% of patients with febrile seizures presenting to the emergency department are found to have complex features.

EPIDEMIOLOGY

Febrile seizures are the most common form of childhood seizures. The peak incidence is at the age of approximately 18 months. In the United States and Western Europe, they occur in 2% to 4% of all children. In Japan, however, 9% to 10% of all children experience at least one febrile seizure, and rates as high as 14% have been reported from the Mariana Islands in Guam. Ninety percent of seizures occur within the first 3 years of life, 4% before 6 months, and 6% after age 3 years. Approximately 50% appear during the second year of life, with a peak incidence between age 18 and 24 months. Children with longer febrile seizures have a younger median age at first febrile seizure (Hesdorffer et al., 2011).

Traditionally, it was thought that febrile seizures most commonly occur as the first sign of a febrile illness. More recent studies, however, found that only 21% of the children experienced their seizure either before or within 1 hour of the onset of the fever, whereas 57% had a seizure after 1 to 24 hours of fever, and 22% experienced their febrile seizure more than 24 hours after the onset of the fever.

Some children are at increased risk of experiencing a febrile seizure. A case–control population-based study (Bethune et al., 1993) examined the risk factors for a first febrile seizure and found that the following four factors were associated with an increased risk of febrile seizures: a history of febrile seizures in a first- or second-degree relative, a neonatal nursery stay of more than 30 days, developmental delay, and attendance at day care. Children with two of these factors had a 28% chance of experiencing at least one febrile seizure.

Another case–control study, using febrile controls matched for age, site of routine pediatric care, and date of visit, examined the issue of which children with a febrile illness were most likely to experience a febrile seizure (Berg et al., 1995). On multivariate analysis, significant independent risk factors were the height of the peak temperature and a history of febrile seizures in an immediate relative. Gastroenteritis as the underlying illness had a significant inverse (i.e., protective) association with febrile seizures. Similar results on the importance of the peak temperature were reported from a hospital-based study.

The majority of febrile seizures are simple seizures. In a study of 428 children with a first febrile seizure, 35% had at least one complex feature, including focality in 16%, multiple seizures in 14%, and prolonged duration (longer than 10 minutes) in 13%. Approximately 6% of children had at least two complex features, and 1% had all three complex features. Of most concern have been prolonged febrile seizures. In that study, 14% of the children had seizures lasting longer than 10 minutes; 9%, longer than 15 minutes; and 5%, longer than 30 minutes, or febrile status epilepticus. Although febrile status epilepticus accounts for only 5% of febrile seizures, it accounts for approximately 25% of all cases of childhood status epilepticus, and for more than two thirds of cases of status epilepticus in the second year of life. The distribution of first febrile seizure duration can be described using a two-population model, one with short seizure duration and the other with long seizure duration, with the cutoff at approximately 10 minutes (Hesdorffer et al., 2011). This suggests that a 10-minute criterion, rather than 15 minutes, is more appropriate for the definition of a complex febrile seizure.

INITIAL EVALUATION

The American Academy of Pediatrics has guidelines for evaluation of a first simple febrile seizure, and states that clinicians should work to identify the source of the fever when a child presents within 12 hours of a simple febrile seizure. In the absence of suspicious findings in the history or on physical examination, routine serum studies are of limited value in the evaluation of a child older than 6 months with a febrile seizure. The labs that are performed should be based on the clinical presentation of the febrile illness.

As reported in several studies, the incidence of meningitis in children with an apparent febrile seizure is between 2% and 5%. In all of the reported series, however, a majority of the children with meningitis had identifiable risk factors. One series reported that the children with meningitis had one of the following four features: a visit for medical care within the previous 48 hours, seizures on arrival to the emergency room, focal seizures, or suspicious findings on physical or neurologic examination. It is well accepted that there is a low yield on routine lumbar puncture in the absence of risk factors. A lumbar puncture is still recommended in children with a prolonged febrile seizure, as well as in any child with persistent lethargy. A lumbar puncture should be strongly considered in a child who has already received prior antibiotic therapy.

The study, Consequences of Prolonged Febrile Seizures (FEBSTAT), recruited 199 children aged 1 month through 5 years who had a febrile seizure that lasted more than 30 minutes. Children recruited most often had focal seizures that were usually their first febrile seizure. Seizure duration in this group was very prolonged, suggesting that the longer the seizure continued, the less likely it was to spontaneously cease. As part of the FEBSTAT study, 136 children had cerebrospinal fluid (CSF) samples from a nontraumatic lumbar puncture done on initial presentation, and it was confirmed that febrile status epilepticus rarely causes CSF pleocytosis (Frank et al., 2012).

Electroencephalograms (EEGs) are of limited value in the evaluation of the child with febrile seizures. EEGs are more likely to be abnormal in the older child with febrile seizures and in children with a family history of febrile seizures, with a complex febrile seizure, or with preexisting neurodevelopmental abnormalities. There is no evidence at this time that an EEG will predict either recurrence of febrile seizures or the development of subsequent epilepsy. EEGs are indicated in the diagnostic evaluation of status epilepticus of all types, including febrile. They may be of particular interest in the child with febrile status epilepticus, as they may have predictive value for the development of subsequent epilepsy. The FEBSTAT study performed baseline EEGs within 72 hours of the episode of febrile status epilepticus. Review of their baseline EEGs showed that there was focal slowing or attenuation in a substantial proportion of children, and the slowing and attenuation were highly associated with MRI evidence of acute hippocampal injury.

PATHOPHYSIOLOGY

The pathophysiology of febrile seizures remains unclear. An age-specific increased susceptibility to seizures induced by fever is likely. Although it was thought that the rate of rise of the temperature was the key factor, more recent data suggest that it is the actual peak temperature (Berg et al., 1995). Gastroenteritis is associated with a lower incidence of febrile seizures. Herpesvirus-6 and herpesvirus-7 infections have had a high reported rate of association with febrile seizures. The FEBSTAT study evaluated children for the presence of human herpes virus (HHV) via HHV-6A, HHV-6B, or HHV-7 DNA and RNA in serum. The study concluded that HHV-6B infection is commonly associated with febrile status epilepticus, and HHV-7 infection is less frequently associated with it. Together, HHV accounted for the infection in one third of the febrile status epilepticus subjects in the study.

RELATED MORBIDITY AND MORTALITY

The mortality associated with febrile seizures is extremely low. No deaths were reported from the National Collaborative Perinatal Project (Nelson and Ellenberg, 1976) or the British Cohort Study. Even in cases of febrile status epilepticus, which represents the extreme end of complex febrile seizures, the mortality rates in recent series are extremely low. Neither the National Perinatal Project nor the British studies found any evidence of permanent motor deficits after febrile seizures. This finding coincides with a recent series of febrile status epilepticus studies.

The cognitive abilities of children with febrile seizures have been extensively studied. No reports describe acute deterioration of cognitive abilities after febrile seizures, even when the studies limited to febrile status epilepticus are included. Cognitive abilities and school performance of children with febrile seizures were found to be similar to those of controls in three large studies. The Collaborative Perinatal Project found no difference in IQ scores or performance on the Wide Range Achievement Test at the age of 7 years between children with febrile seizures and their siblings. The British National Child Development Study reported that children with febrile seizures performed as well in school at 7 and 11 years of age as their peers without a history of febrile seizures. The more recent British Cohort Study also found no difference between 5-year-olds with febrile seizures and 5-year-olds without a history of febrile seizures on a variety of performance tasks.

Even prolonged febrile seizures do not appear to be associated with adverse cognitive outcomes. In the British Cohort Study, no differences were found between 5-year-olds with and those without febrile seizures, even when the analysis was limited to complex febrile seizures. A study of 27 children with febrile convulsions lasting more than 30 minutes found no differences in cognitive function at 7 years of age between them and their siblings.

RECURRENT FEBRILE SEIZURES

Approximately one third of the children with a first febrile seizure will experience a recurrence, and 10% will have three or more febrile seizures (Nelson and Ellenberg, 1976). Factors associated with a differential risk of recurrent febrile seizures are summarized in Table 65-1. The most consistent risk factors reported are a family history of febrile seizures and age at first febrile seizure (before age 18 months) (Nelson and Ellenberg, 1976). This relationship appears to be attributable to the longer period during which a child with a younger age at onset will be in the age group at risk for febrile seizures, rather than to a greater tendency to have seizures with each specific illness.

TABLE 65-1 Risk Factors for Recurrent Febrile Seizures and for Epilepsy After a Febrile Seizure

Recurrent Febrile Seizures	Epilepsy
DEFINITE RISK FACTOR	
Family history of febrile seizures	Neurodevelopmental abnormality
Age less than 18 months	Complex febrile seizure
Height of peak temperature	Family history of epilepsy
Duration of fever	Duration of fever
POSSIBLE RISK FACTOR	
Family history of epilepsy	More than 1 complex feature
NOT A RISK FACTOR	
Neurodevelopmental abnormality	Family history of febrile seizures
Complex febrile seizure	Age at first febrile seizure
More than 1 complex feature	Height of peak temperature
Gender	Gender
Ethnicity	Ethnicity

(Data from multiple sources [see online].)

In studies that examined features of the acute illness, the peak temperature and also the duration of the fever before the seizure were associated with a differential risk of recurrent febrile seizures. Studies by Berg et al. found that patients with a peak temperature of 101° F had a 42% recurrence risk at 1 year, compared with 29% for those with a peak temperature of 103° F and only 12% for those with a peak temperature of 105° F or greater. For those with a febrile seizure within 1 hour of recognized onset of fever, the recurrence risk at 1 year was 46%, compared with 25% for those with prior fever lasting 1 to 24 hours and 15% for those with more than 24 hours of recognized fever before the febrile seizure.

The data regarding a family history of unprovoked seizures or epilepsy are conflicting. A large study in Rochester, MN, found no difference in recurrence risk between children with a family history of epilepsy (25%) and those with no such family history (23%). Other studies have found more equivocal results. However, even those studies that report an increased risk of recurrence in children with a family history of unprovoked seizures found only a modest increase in risk. A complex febrile seizure is not associated with an increased risk of recurrence in most studies. If the initial febrile seizure is prolonged, however, a recurrent febrile seizure also is more likely to be prolonged. The presence of a neurodevelopmental abnormality in the child also has not been demonstrated to be significantly associated with an increased risk of subsequent febrile seizures.

Children with multiple risk factors are at highest risk for recurrence. A child with two or more risk factors has a greater than 30% recurrence risk at 2 years, and the child with three or more risk factors has a greater than 60% recurrence risk. By contrast, the child older than 18 months with no family history of febrile seizures who experiences a first febrile seizure associated with a peak temperature higher than 40° C after a recognized fever longer than 1 hour in duration (i.e., no risk factors) has a 2-year recurrence risk of greater than 15%. No correlation has been identified between duration of the first febrile seizure and duration of the second febrile seizure (Hesdorffer et al., 2011).

FEBRILE SEIZURES AND SUBSEQUENT EPILEPSY

Data from five large cohorts of children with febrile seizures indicate that epilepsy subsequently develops in 2% to 10% of children who experience febrile seizures (Annegers et al., 1979). The higher number comes from the study by Annegers et al., which had the longest follow-up period. In addition, in population- and community-based studies, 15% to 20% of children and adults with epilepsy have a history of prior febrile seizures. In most studies, the risk of developing epilepsy after a single simple febrile seizure is not substantially different from the risk for this disorder in the general population (Annegers et al., 1979).

The risk factors for the development of epilepsy after febrile seizures are summarized in Table 65-1. The presence of a neurodevelopmental abnormality, the occurrence of a family history of epilepsy, and the occurrence of complex febrile seizures are associated with an increased risk of subsequent epilepsy (Annegers et al., 1979). Two studies also have found that the occurrence of multiple febrile seizures was associated with a slightly but statistically significant increased risk of subsequent epilepsy. In addition, in the one study that examined this issue, febrile seizures that occurred within 1 hour of a recognized fever (i.e., at onset) were associated with a higher risk of subsequent epilepsy.

Some controversy exists regarding whether the number of complex features affects the risk of recurrence. Two studies have examined this issue in detail. Both found that prolonged febrile seizures (i.e., febrile status epilepticus) were associated with an increased risk of subsequent epilepsy above that for a complex febrile seizure that was less prolonged. The study by Annegers et al., however, found that the presence of two complex features (e.g., prolonged and focal) further increased the risk of subsequent epilepsy, whereas this association was not found in the study by Berg et al. Note that these two factors are not independent because prolonged febrile seizures are more likely to be focal (Berg et al., 1992, 1997).

Age at first febrile seizure, the height of peak temperature at first seizure, and a family history of febrile seizures, all of which are associated with a differential risk of recurrence for febrile seizures, are not associated with a differential risk of developing epilepsy (see Table 65-1) (Annegers et al., 1979). Duration of fever before the febrile seizure appears to be the only common risk factor for both recurrent febrile seizures and subsequent epilepsy. It may well be a marker for overall seizure susceptibility.

The type of epilepsy that develops after febrile seizures is variable. It has been reported that, in persons with generalized febrile seizures, generalized epilepsies usually develop, whereas focal epilepsies develop in those with focal seizures. This finding suggests that the febrile seizures may be an age-specific expression of seizure susceptibility in patients with an underlying seizure diathesis. Febrile seizures also can be the initial manifestation of specific epilepsy syndromes, such as severe myoclonic epilepsy of infancy. In general, the types of epilepsy that occur in children with prior febrile seizures are varied and not very different from those that occur in children without such a history. The association between prolonged febrile seizures and subsequent epilepsy is being evaluated by the FEBSTAT study that is currently ongoing.

FEBRILE SEIZURES, MESIAL TEMPORAL SCLEROSIS, AND TEMPORAL LOBE EPILEPSY

One of the most controversial issues in epilepsy is whether prolonged febrile seizures cause mesial temporal sclerosis and mesial temporal lobe epilepsy. Prolonged febrile seizures also are usually focal (Hesdorffer et al., 2011). In many cases febrile seizures may be an age-specific marker for future seizure susceptibility.

FEBSTAT and two affiliated studies prospectively recruited 226 children aged 1 month to 6 years with febrile status epilepticus and controls with simple febrile seizures to evaluate hippocampal sclerosis (Lewis et al., 2014). They found that hippocampal T2 hyperintensity after febrile status epilepticus represents acute injury often evolving to a radiologic appearance of hippocampal sclerosis after 1 year. Furthermore, impaired growth of normal-appearing hippocampi after febrile status epilepticus suggests subtle injury even in the absence of T2 hyperintensity. The presence and severity of these acute changes are predictive of subsequent anatomic mesial temporal sclerosis that may occur before the development of clinical seizures. A long-term goal of the prospective FEBSTAT study is to better define the relationship between prolonged febrile seizures, hippocampal sclerosis, and mesial temporal lobe epilepsy. The FEBSTAT study has performed a baseline MRI, with special attention to the hippocampus on 191 of the recruited children. A statistically significant abnormal or equivocally increased hippocampal T2 signal following febrile status epilepticus was observed in 22 children compared with none in the control group. Findings from this study indicate that prolonged febrile seizures are likely to be focal, and are much longer than previously thought. The median duration is an hour, and they usually do not stop on their own but require the administration of a benzodiazepine (Seinfeld et al., 2014).

Developmental abnormalities of the hippocampus were more common in the febrile status epilepticus group, with hippocampal malrotation being the most common finding.

GENETICS

Genetic influences clearly play a major role in febrile seizures. Children with a positive family history of febrile seizures are more likely both to experience a febrile seizure (Bethune et al., 1993; Berg et al., 1995) and to experience recurrent febrile seizures, than children without such a family history. A study of 32 twin pairs and 673 sibling relationship cases reported a concordance rate of 56% in monozygotic twins and 14% in dizygotic twins. Concordance for clinical symptoms, including age at onset and degree of fever, was higher in the twin pairs than in the sibling relationship patients. The results were consistent with a multifactorial mode of inheritance for febrile convulsions in an analysis of the Rochester, MN, dataset. In population-based studies, a majority of children with febrile seizures do not have a first- or second-degree relative with a history of febrile seizures (Bethune et al., 1993).

An autosomal-dominant mode of inheritance has been postulated for a subset of children with febrile seizures, but such cases are relatively rare. Candidate genes in these autosomal-dominant families include both sodium and gamma-aminobutyric acid (GABA) channel mutations. A related syndrome of generalized epilepsy with febrile seizures plus (GEFS +) also has been mapped to several different loci in different families and has been associated with mutations in sodium, potassium, and GABA channels. The phenotype of febrile seizures plus may account for children without a specific epilepsy syndrome who have febrile seizures and then developed generalized epilepsy, with the most severe phenotype of myoclonic-astatic epilepsy. Febrile seizures represent an example of the interplay between genetic susceptibility and environmental factors.

TREATMENT

It is accepted that antipyretic agents do not reduce the risk of a febrile seizure or a seizure recurrence. Prophylactic antiepileptic drug therapy for febrile seizures should be withheld, as the benefits of treatment do not outweigh the risks. There is a concern regarding prolonged febrile seizures. In contrast, brief febrile seizures are not thought to have any long-term consequences. This leads to a therapeutic approach that does not treat brief febrile seizures but focuses on preventing prolonged ones (Subcommittee on Febrile Seizures, 2011).

Febrile seizures often cease by the time a child is examined, but prolonged episodes should be treated similar to seizures of any other etiology. If seizure activity is ongoing when the child arrives at the emergency department, treatment to terminate the seizure is mandatory. All seizures, regardless of etiology, should be treated after 5 minutes. Intravenous (IV) diazepam or lorazepam is known to be an effective treatment option, but treatment should not be delayed because of lack of IV access. In cases in which IV access is difficult, rectal diazepam or diazepam gel, and intramuscular midazolam are appropriate for use. If the seizure activity continues after an adequate dose of a benzodiazepine, then a full status epilepticus treatment protocol should be used.

For either prehospital or in the emergency department management, terminating a prolonged febrile seizure is important to prevent the potential long-term consequences, including mesial temporal sclerosis (Seinfeld et al., 2014). The FEBSTAT study showed that these seizures rarely stop spontaneously and that the time to first drug is highly correlated with the total duration as they are difficult to stop even with medications (Seinfeld et al., 2014). More aggressive early treatment in the ambulance may result in shorter seizure duration.

A majority of febrile seizures are brief, lasting less than 10 minutes, and no intervention is necessary. Rectal diazepam has been demonstrated to be effective in terminating febrile seizures. Rectal diazepam gel is U.S. Food and Drug Administration-approved and readily available in the United States and is an option for treatment of febrile seizures at home. Candidates for this treatment include children at high risk for prolonged or multiple febrile seizures and those who live far from medical care.

Febrile seizures, by definition, occur in the context of a febrile illness. Recommendations for antipyretic therapy should recognize its limitations and avoid creating undue anxiety and feelings of guilt in the parents.

Diazepam, given orally or rectally, at the time of onset of a febrile illness will reduce the probability of a febrile seizure. Although the effect is statistically significant, it is clinically modest. In one large randomized trial comparing placebo with oral diazepam (in a dose of 0.33 mg/kg every 8 hours with fever), seizure recurrence by 36 months was noted in 22% of the diazepam treatment group, compared with 31% of the placebo treatment group. This modest reduction in seizure recurrence must be weighed against the side effects of sedating children every time they have a febrile illness. Intermittent therapy with phenobarbital at the onset of fever is ineffective in reducing the risk of recurrent febrile seizures.

Long-term antiepileptic drug therapy is rarely indicated in the treatment of febrile seizures (Subcommittee on Febrile Seizures, 2011). It will not reduce the risk of subsequent epilepsy. The goal of therapy is to prevent prolonged febrile seizures. Children at risk for prolonged or multiple febrile seizures , or those who live far from medical care, should be prescribed an abortive agent.

COUNSELING AND EDUCATION

In a majority of cases, counseling and education will be the sole treatment. Education is the key to empowering the parents who have just experienced a frightening and traumatic event. The parents' perception of their child's disorder will be an important factor in their later coping and will ultimately affect their perception of quality of life.

Febrile seizures are a common and mostly benign form of childhood seizures. An understanding of the natural history and prognosis will enable the physician to reassure the families of affected children and to provide appropriate counseling and management while avoiding unnecessary diagnostic and therapeutic interventions. Advances in basic science, genetics, and imaging are providing new insights into this common pediatric disorder that continues to be the subject of active research. The next phase will potentially lead to interventional trials that aim at preventing the consequences of very prolonged febrile seizures. But, while focusing on these, it is important to remember that the vast majority of febrile seizures, although very frightening, do not appear to have any long-term sequelae.

Acknowledgments

Supported in part by Grant IR01 NS43209 (S. Shinnar) from the National Institute of Neurologic Disorders and Stroke, Bethesda, MD.

REFERENCES

The complete list of references for this chapter is available in the e-book at www.expertconsult.com.
     See inside cover for registration details.

SELECTED REFERENCES

Annegers, J.F., Hauser, W.A., Elveback, L.R., et al., 1979. The risk of epilepsy following febrile convulsions. Neurology 29, 297.

Berg, A.T., Shinnar, S., Hauser, W.A., et al., 1992. Predictors of recurrent febrile seizures: a prospective study of the circumstances surrounding the initial febrile seizure. N. Engl. J. Med. 327, 1122.

Berg, A.T., Shinnar, S., Shapiro, E.D., et al., 1995. Risk factors for a first febrile seizure: a matched case-control study. Epilepsia 36, 334.

Berg, A.T., Shinnar, S., Darefsky, A.S., et al., 1997. Predictors of recurrent febrile seizures. Arch. Ped. Adolesc. Med. 151, 371.

Bethune, P., Gordon, K.G., Dooley, J.M., et al., 1993. Which child will have a febrile seizure? Am. J. Dis. Child. 147, 35.

Frank, L.M., Shinnar, S., Hesdorffer, D.C., et al., 2012. Cerebrospinal fluid findings in children with fever-associated status epilepticus: results of the consequences of prolonged febrile seizures (FEBSTAT) study. J. Pediatr. 161, 1169–1171.

Hesdorffer, D.C., Benn, E.K., Bagiella, E., et al., 2011. Distribution of febrile seizure duration and associations with development. Ann. Neurol. 70, 93–100.

Lewis, D.V., Shinnar, S., Hesdorffer, D.C., et al., 2014. Hippocampal sclerosis after febrile status epilepticus: the FEBSTAT study. Ann. Neurol. 75, 178–185.

Nelson, K.B., Ellenberg, J.H., 1976. Predictors of epilepsy in children who have experienced febrile seizures. N. Engl. J. Med. 295, 1029.

Seinfeld, S., Shinnar, S., Sun, S., et al., 2014. Emergency management of febrile status epilepticus: results of the FEBSTAT study. Epilepsia 55, 388–395.

Subcommittee on Febrile Seizures; American Academy of Pediatrics, 2011. Clinical practice guideline: febrile seizures: guideline for the neurodiagnostic evaluation of the child with a simple febrile seizure. Pediatrics. 127, 389–394.

66 Generalized Seizures

Gregory L. Holmes

As reviewed in Chapter 61, seizures are classified into two basic groups: focal (previously called partial) and generalized. Generalized seizures are those defined as occurring in bilaterally distributed networks, whereas focal seizures involve networks limited to one hemisphere, with either discretely localized or more widely distributed disturbances. Focal seizures involve only a portion of the brain at the onset but can propagate and become secondarily generalized, evolving to bilateral, convulsive seizures involving tonic, clonic, or tonic and clonic components. Primarily generalized seizures are those in which the first clinical changes indicate initial synchronous involvement of both hemispheres without clinical, electroencephalographic (EEG), or other evidence of focal onset. Impairment of consciousness is usual during generalized seizures, although some seizures, such as myoclonic, may be so brief that the level of consciousness cannot be assessed. The generalized seizures span a wide range of clinical presentations, ranging from the rather benign-appearing absence seizure to the dramatic and frightening generalized tonic-clonic seizure.

In most epidemiologic studies, primarily generalized seizures are reported to be less common than focal seizures. Of the primarily generalized seizures, generalized tonic-clonic are the most common, followed by absence and myoclonic seizures.

These epidemiologic studies may be somewhat misleading. With improvement of diagnostic techniques in recent decades, especially with long-term EEG/video monitoring, it has become clear that the prevalence of primarily generalized tonic-clonic epilepsy has been overestimated. In fact, most generalized tonic-clonic seizures begin as focal seizures and then generalize.

This chapter discusses generalized tonic-clonic seizures and absence, myoclonic, tonic, and atonic seizures. Syndromes in which generalized seizures are prominent are discussed in Chapters 70 to 73.

GENERALIZED TONIC-CLONIC SEIZURES

Some children with generalized tonic-clonic seizures, or their parents, are aware of the impending seizure, hours or days before it occurs. The child may have a headache, insomnia, irritability, or a change in appetite. This prodrome is to be distinguished from an aura, which occurs before generalization of the seizure. Unlike the aura, the prodrome is not associated with any EEG epileptiform activity. Although auras were previously believed to occur only with focal seizures, it is now clear that auras also commonly occur in generalized tonic-clonic seizures. The auras in generalized tonic-clonic seizures may be similar to those occurring with focal seizures, such as déjà vu and epigastric rising, or may be more vague and difficult for the child to describe.

As indicated by the name, generalized tonic-clonic seizures have two distinct phases: tonic and clonic. Loss of consciousness usually occurs simultaneously or shortly after the onset of a generalized stiffening of flexor or extensor muscles—the tonic phase. The loss of consciousness usually is complete, and it is unusual for patients to have awareness of what happened

during the seizure. During the tonic phase, prolonged extension of the back, neck, and all limbs often occurs. The eyes remain open, and a cry or yell is common. The tonic phase typically lasts 10 to 30 seconds and is followed by the clonic phase, which usually starts with a rapid tremor and then slows to massive jerks of the extremities and trunk. A decrescendo pattern to the frequency (although not necessarily the strength) of the jerks is seen as the seizure ceases. The clonic phase typically lasts 30 to 60 seconds.

Cyanosis is common and results from the arrest of ventilation during the tonic phase and insufficient short breaths during the following clonic phase. Pupillary dilation, salivation, sweating, hyperthermia, and incontinence are common.

A postictal state always follows the clonic phase. During the postictal phase the child may have a stertorous respiratory pattern, which is a strong indication that the event was an epileptic seizure rather than nonepileptic event. The duration is quite variable. Some patients, even after a severe and prolonged seizure, respond within a minute or so, whereas other patients may be difficult to arouse for 20 to 30 minutes. Although the postictal phase initially consists of stupor, it may be followed by confusion or agitation.

Some patients have seizures provoked by flickering lights and have a photoparoxysmal response to strobe light on EEG. The photoparoxysmal response is characterized by spike-and-wave and polyspike-and-wave complexes that are bilaterally synchronous, symmetric, and widespread (Fig. 61-1). The photoparoxysmal response may be self-limited and cease during stimulation or continue beyond the stimulation. The most effective frequency of the flash is 10 to 20 Hz.

The seizures evoked by photic stimulation usually are primarily generalized in type: generalized tonic-clonic, absence, or myoclonic seizures. Although patients with focal seizures may have photoparoxysmal responses during an EEG study, it is unusual for a focal seizure to be precipitated by photic stimulation.

Photosensitive epilepsy can be classified into two major groups: (1) pure photosensitive epilepsy, in which clinical seizures occur only when the patient is exposed to the photic stimulus, and (2) photosensitive epilepsy, in which spontaneous seizures occur in addition to those induced by light stimulation. Precipitating stimuli that can produce a seizure include sunlight reflected from water, sunlight viewed through leaves of trees in a breeze or while driving along tree-lined streets, discotheque lighting, faulty fluorescent lamps, television, and video games.

Photoparoxysmal responses in children under the age of 5 years are uncommon, and unlike in older children are more likely to occur at slower frequency trains (1-5 Hz). In young children photoparoxysmal responses are seen in neurogenetic disorders such as Dravet syndrome and the epileptic encephalopathies.

Electroencephalographic Findings

In patients with focal seizures with secondarily generalization, the interictal EEG features are similar to those described for focal seizures. Patients with primarily generalized tonic-clonic seizures typically have either normal interictal EEG activity or bursts of generalized spike-and-wave discharges. As with absence seizures, spike-and-wave or polyspike-and-wave activity can occur with photic stimulation and hyperventilation. Normal interictal EEG activity, however, can be observed in patients with generalized tonic-clonic seizures (Porter et al., 1973).

Initial Evaluation

The initial steps in the evaluation depend to a major degree on the patient's clinical status on first presentation to the physician. For example, the patient who arrives at the emergency department following a generalized seizure with fever and confusion is evaluated differently from the otherwise normal child who presents several hours after a generalized seizure. The former needs an urgent evaluation to look for an infectious etiology, such as meningitis or encephalitis, whereas the latter can be managed less hastily. This chapter deals with the evaluation and treatment indicated for patients with generalized seizures as their only presenting clinical sign.

In all children with their first seizure, a careful history should be obtained, with particular attention to whether the seizure was preceded by an aura or if the seizure had any focal features. A focal onset to the seizures, or Todd's paralysis, would suggest that the seizure was focal rather than generalized. However, primarily generalized tonic-clonic seizures can have lateralized findings such as version of the head or trunk or asymmetric myoclonus. A review of potential precipitating factors, such as sleep deprivation or photic stimulation, may be useful in counseling the patient and the parents. A past medical history of birth asphyxia or trauma, head injury, prolonged febrile seizures, meningitis, or encephalitis may offer etiologic clues indicating that the seizures have a partial onset. A history of other neurologic symptoms should be sought. Headaches, especially those associated with vomiting or occurring at night, should raise the possibility of a structural lesion.

Although neuroimaging appears to have reduced the importance of the neurologic examination, abnormal findings, even if subtle, may provide clues to the location of seizure onset and etiology of the seizures. For example, asymmetries in facial expression or strength may indicate focal deficits, even in the presence of normal neuroimaging findings.

Diagnostic studies ordered depend on findings during the history and neurologic examination. Children with an unremarkable history other than that for the seizures and with normal findings on neurologic examination typically require only an EEG and neuroimaging. An EEG should always be obtained because it may help differentiate focal from generalized seizures. Focal epileptiform activity or slowing would raise the possibility of a structural lesion.

Neuroimaging is recommended in all patients presenting with their first unexplained generalized tonic-clonic seizure, with the recognition that, in patients with normal neurologic examinations, the chance of finding a treatable lesion is quite low. Because generalized tonic-clonic seizures may have a focal onset with subsequent rapid generalization, however, the seizure may be incorrectly diagnosed as primarily generalized in type. In nonemergency settings, the imaging test of choice is a magnetic resonance imaging (MRI) scan. However, in young children, high-quality, artifact-free MRI often requires anesthesia. Although computed tomography (CT) scans can be used in acute situations to determine the presence of a mass lesion and hemorrhage, it does not provide adequate resolution to show subtle malformations of cerebral development.

The need for further diagnostic testing, such as metabolic and genetic screening and cerebrospinal fluid examination, depends on the clinical presentation. In the absence of mental retardation, developmental regression, or abnormalities on neurologic examination, these studies usually are not indicated following the initial seizure.

Comorbidities Associated with Generalized Seizures

Although a major goal in the treatment of epilepsy is stopping the seizures, it is not the only treatment goal. Patients with epilepsy are at risk for a number of comorbidities. Comorbidity refers to the co-occurrence of two supposedly separate conditions that occur together more than by chance (also see Chapter 82). Depression occurs more frequently in patients with epilepsy than in the normal population, and thus epilepsy and depression are comorbidities. Comorbidities are not necessarily causal. For example, because epilepsy and depression are comorbidities does not mean that epilepsy caused the depression or depression caused the epilepsy. Rather, it is possible that both conditions have a common biological substrate or that another independent variable triggers one of the comorbidities. For example, epilepsy often leads to drug therapy, which could cause depression independently of the epilepsy.

Comorbidities associated with epilepsy include depression, suicidality, attention deficit hyperactivity disorder (ADHD), conduct disorders, anxiety, cognitive impairment and learning disabilities, and migraine (Camfield and Camfield, 2009).

Being aware of the comorbidities frequently associated with childhood epilepsy may influence the choice of antiseizure medicine used to treat the epilepsy. For example, lamotrigine and valproate may be helpful in treating both the primarily generalized seizures and mood disturbance. Likewise, topiramate and valproate can treat both seizures and migraine. On the other hand, antiseizure medications may exacerbate the comorbid condition. Topiramate can have adverse cognitive effects, and benzodiazepines and barbiturates can exacerbate ADHD and conduct disorders.

Medical Treatment

The medical treatment of generalized seizures that have a partial onset and secondarily generalize is, in general, the same as the treatment for partial seizures. It is generally assumed that an antiseizure medicine that reduces the likelihood of focal seizures would also prevent focal seizures that secondarily generalize. However, it is possible that there may be a difference in the ability of an antiseizure drug to prevent secondarily generalization following the focal onset.

The major drugs typically used to treat primarily generalized tonic-clonic seizures include valproate, lamotrigine, levetiracetam, and topiramate. Although phenobarbital is effective in the treatment of primarily generalized tonic-clonic seizures, the profile of adverse side effects has reduced its use as initial therapy for primarily generalized tonic-clonic seizures. Although other antiseizure medicines such as lacosamide, zonisamide, perampanel, and clobazam have shown efficacy in primarily generalized seizures in children, additional studies are necessary.

ABSENCE SEIZURES

Absence seizures, formerly termed petit mal seizures, are characterized by an abrupt cessation of activity, change in facial expression, and impairment of consciousness. Absence seizures are not common, accounting for less than 10% of all seizure types. Absence seizures may be the most common seizure type to go undetected. The prevalence of absence seizures is highest during the first 10 years of life and then drops dramatically to a very low level. Absence seizures are more common in girls than in boys. Absence seizures can begin as early as the first year of life.

Absence seizures are classified as typical or atypical in type. Typical absence seizures are short, rarely lasting over 30 seconds; as with other generalized seizures, they are never associated with an aura or postictal impairment. The sudden onset of impaired consciousness, usually associated with a blank facial appearance without other motor or behavioral phenomena, is characteristic. The degree of impairment of consciousness is variable. Some children remember virtually everything that is said during the seizure, whereas for others, the entire duration of the seizure is "time lost."

Although the absence seizure is commonly thought to consist only of staring, in fact the behavioral changes associated with the seizure type usually are more complex. Most absence seizures are accompanied by motor, behavioral, or autonomic phenomena, and seizures characterized by only staring and altered consciousness are unusual. Automatisms, semipurposeful behaviors of which the patient is unaware and subsequently cannot recall, are very common with absence seizures. They either may be perseverative, reflecting continuation of preictal activities, or may arise de novo. Simple behaviors, such as rubbing the face or hands, licking the lips, chewing, grimacing, scratching, or fumbling with clothes, tend to be de novo automatisms. Complex activities, such as dealing cards, moving a chess piece, or handling a toy, are generally perseverative. Speech, if it occurs during the seizure, usually is perseverative and may be slow and slurred, but also may be totally normal. The longer the absence seizure lasts, the more likely automatisms are to occur.

Clonic or myoclonic components are common but may be quite subtle, most frequently consisting of blinking. Clonic activity also may be manifested by nystagmus, rapid jerking or trembling of the arms, or head nods. Alterations in muscle tone may lead to stiffening of the trunk or a fall.

Autonomic phenomena occasionally may be seen with absence seizures and include dilation of the pupils, pallor, flushing, sweating, salivation, and even urinary incontinence.

The frequency of absence seizures varies considerably from day to day and even from hour to hour. The number of absence seizures varies significantly with different environmental situations. Seizures are more likely to occur during periods of inactivity than when the child is busily engaged in a task. Fatigue also may dramatically increase seizure susceptibility.

A majority of children with typical absence seizures have normal findings on neurologic examination, and when neurologic abnormalities are found, they usually are mild and nonprogressive. Most children with typical absence seizures have normal or mildly low intelligence. Compared with age-matched controls, children with absence seizures have lower general cognitive function, with impaired visual-spatial skills and memory disturbances. Children with absence seizures have higher rates of ADHD, behavioral problems, and psychopathology than in the normal population

Typical absence seizures may be associated with generalized tonic-clonic seizures in 40% to 60% of patients. In most children, the generalized tonic-clonic seizures occur after onset of the absence seizures.

Although atypical absence seizures form a separate category of absences, overlap between the two seizure types is considerable, and they appear to represent a clinical continuum. Diminished postural tone, or tonic or myoclonic activity, is significantly more likely to be the initial clinical feature in atypical than in typical absences. Automatisms are less likely in atypical absences than in typical absences. Like typical absences, atypical absences have a distinct onset and ending, without auras or postictal symptoms. Although atypical absences usually are of longer duration than typical absences, a considerable amount of variability exists.

Atypical absences usually begin before the age of 5 years and often are associated with other seizure types and mental retardation. In children who have profound mental retardation, it may be difficult to detect subtle behavioral changes associated with the absence seizures. Many children with atypical absence seizures have Lennox–Gastaut syndrome (Widdess-Walsh et al., 2013).

The primary diagnostic considerations in the child referred because of "staring attacks" include absence seizures, focal seizures, and daydreaming (Table 66-5). Focal seizures are more common than absence seizures and also are manifested by an alteration in consciousness with staring, automatisms, changes in tone, and autonomic symptoms. Complex partial seizures tend to be longer and less frequent, but clinically no absolute distinguishing factor may be present. The presence of an aura or postictal impairment is strongly suggestive of a

TABLE 66-5 Differential Diagnosis of Absence Seizures

Clinical and Laboratory Characteristics	Absence	Focal with Impairment of Consciousness or Awareness (Complex Partial Seizure)	Daydreaming
Frequency/day	Multiple	Rarely > 1–2	Situation-dependent
Duration	Frequently < 10 sec; rarely > 30 sec	Average duration > 1 min; rarely < 10 sec	Seconds to minutes
Aura	Never	Frequent	Never
Clonic component	Common; eye blinking common	Infrequent	Never
Postictal impairment	Never	Frequent	Never
Seizures activated by			
Hyperventilation	Frequent	Rare	Never
Photic stimulation	Frequent	Rare	Never
EEG			
Interictal	Generalized spike wave	Focal spikes, sharp waves	Normal
Ictal	Generalized spike wave	Rhythmic spikes, sharp waves, or slow waves	Normal

EEG, electroencephalogram.

complex partial seizure. In the child not on antiseizure medications, 3 minutes of hyperventilation usually precipitates an absence seizure. It is unusual for focal seizures to be precipitated by hyperventilation. Abnormalities documented on the EEG constitute the best confirmation of either seizure type.

Daydreaming is associated with boredom, can be "broken" with stimulation, and is not associated with motor activity. Absence seizures, however, also can sometimes be terminated with stimulation and tend to increase during periods of relaxation and tiredness. Normal findings on an EEG study that includes several trials of 3 to 5 minutes of hyperventilation virtually rule out absence seizures. Repeated studies or prolonged EEG monitoring occasionally may be necessary when diagnostic confusion persists.

Initial Evaluation

The extent of the diagnostic evaluation required in patients with absence seizures is variable and depends somewhat on findings from the history and physical examination. All patients need a neurologic examination, 3 minutes of hyperventilation, and an EEG with hyperventilation and photic stimulation. Ideally the EEG should include sleep, recognizing this is sometimes difficult to achieve in children. Patients who have normal development, normal findings on neurologic examination, a history suggestive of typical absence seizures, and 2.5- to 4-Hz spike-wave discharges on an otherwise normal-appearing EEG require no further studies. Children with developmental delay, an abnormal neurologic examination, a history suggestive of atypical absences, or an EEG showing slow spike-and-wave (less than 2.5 Hz) discharges, background slowing, or focal epileptiform discharges should have an MRI and possibly more specific tests, such as meta-bolic studies and a lumbar puncture (see Chapter 76). Children with refractory absences, especially if they are associated with developmental delay and a movement disorder, should be tested for glucose transporter type 1 deficiency syndrome, a condition with hypoglycorrhachia with normoglycemia.

Electroencephalographic Findings

The EEG signature of a typical absence seizure is the sudden onset of 3-Hz generalized symmetric spike-and-wave or multiple spike-wave complexes (Fig. 66-2). The voltage of the discharges often is maximal in the frontal-central regions. The frequency tends to be faster, about 4 Hz, at the onset and may slow to 2 Hz toward the end of a discharge lasting longer than 10 seconds. Hyperventilation is a potent activator of typical absence seizures. Failure to induce an absence seizure with several trials of hyperventilation of 3 to 5 minutes' duration in a child not receiving antiseizure medication would make the diagnosis of typical absence seizures unlikely. Photic stimulation also may precipitate seizures, although the frequency of activation does not appear as high as with hyperventilation.

In atypical absences, the ictal EEG is more heterogeneous, showing 1.5- to 2.5-Hz slow spike-and-wave or multiple spike-and-wave discharges that may be irregular or asymmetric (Fig. 66-3). Interictal EEG findings usually are abnormal, with background slowing and multifocal epileptiform features (Holmes et al., 2004; Aghakhani et al., 2004; Crunelli and Leresche, 2002).

Treatment

Medical therapy is recommended for children with absence seizures. Although not life-threatening, absence seizures may

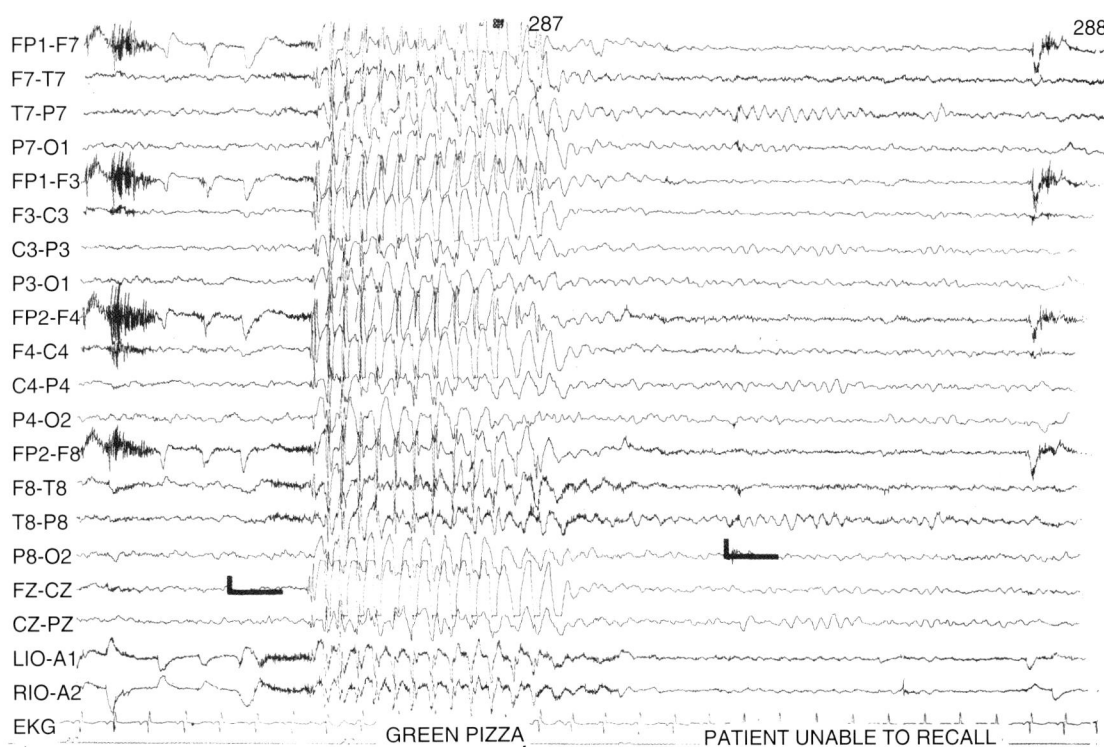

Figure 66-2. EEG from a patient with typical absences. The technician said the phrase "green pizza" during the spike-and-wave discharge. After the absence seizure, the patient did not recall the phrase (calibration: 50 µV, 1 second).

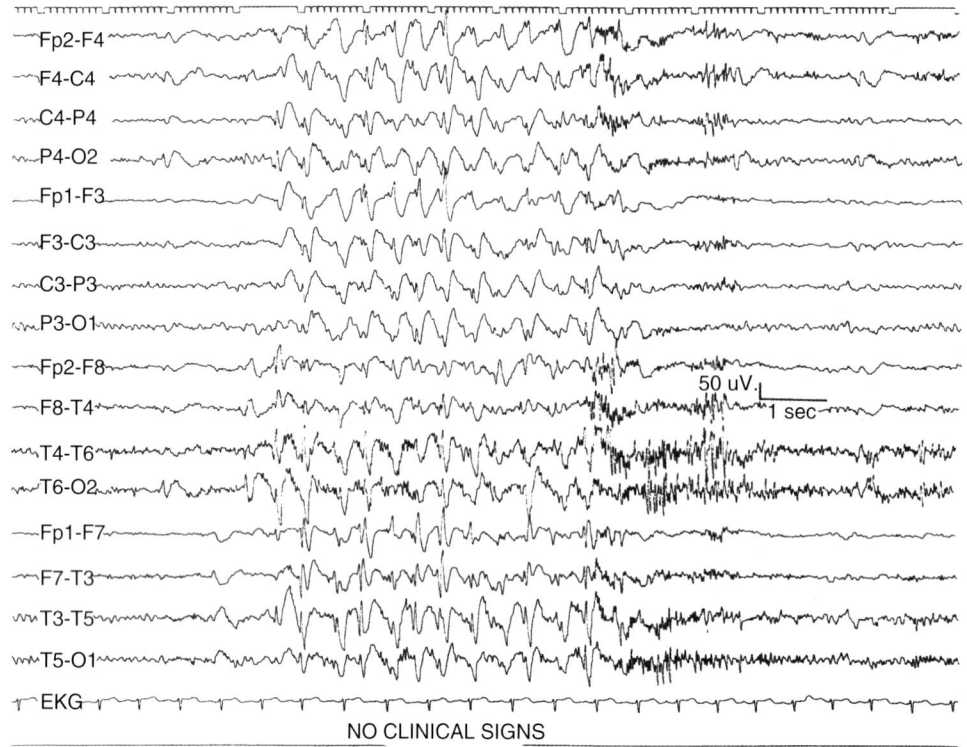

Figure 66-3. Slow, irregular generalized spike-and-wave discharges in a patient with Lennox–Gastaut syndrome and atypical absences (calibration: 50 μV, 1 second).

lead to poor school performance, ridicule, and accidents. Because even brief generalized spike-and-wave discharges can affect cognitive function, it is therefore reasonable to begin drug therapy in most patients once the diagnosis is secure. Drugs of choice in absence seizures are valproate, ethosuximide, and lamotrigine.

Prognosis

Approximately two thirds of children with childhood absence epilepsy can be expected to enter long-term remission (Wirrell et al., 1996; Wirrell, 2003; Berg et al., 2014). Favorable prognostic signs in absence seizures are a negative family history of epilepsy, normal EEG background activity, and normal intelligence. Nearly 90% of children with these characteristics will stop having absence seizures.

Juvenile absence epilepsy may occasionally persist into adulthood, however, and juvenile myoclonic epilepsy does not spontaneously remit. As a general rule, onset of generalized tonic-clonic seizures before absence seizures carries a poorer prognosis than that noted with the reverse order.

MYOCLONIC SEIZURES
Clinical Features

Myoclonic seizures are characterized by sudden, brief (less than 350 μsec), shock-like contractions that may be generalized or confined to the face and trunk, or to one or more extremities, or even to individual muscles or groups of muscles. Myoclonic seizures result in short bursts of synchronized electromyographic (EMG) activity, which often involves simultaneous activation of agonist and antagonist muscles. The contractions of muscles are quicker than the contractions of

clonic seizures. Any group of muscles can be involved in a myoclonic seizure. Myoclonic seizures may be dramatic, causing the patient to fall to the ground, or quite subtle, resembling tremors. Because of the brevity of the seizures, determining whether consciousness is impaired is impossible. Although myoclonic seizures can sometimes be the only seizure type present, they can occur in combination with other seizure types, such as myoclonic-atonic and myoclonic-tonic.

Myoclonic jerks are so brief that they may be missed by parents and physicians. Once seen, diagnosis is usually not difficult. Myoclonic seizures may occasionally be confused with tics. Tics are repetitive, patterned motor activity, often involving multiple groups (see Chapter 98). Unlike seizures, tics can be voluntarily suppressed. Shuddering attacks are common in toddlers and consist of pronounced shivering. Typically, the child keeps the arms flexed and the shoulders adducted. The episodes last from seconds to minutes, and typically occur when the child is excited. Usually, both tics and shuddering attacks can be differentiated from myoclonic seizures. However, in cases in which the diagnosis is in doubt, an EEG can be useful. In both tics and shuddering attacks, the EEG is normal.

It is also important to recognize that myoclonus is not always an epileptic phenomenon. For example, sleep starts or hypnic jerks are normal physiologic events. On the other end of the spectrum, hereditary hyperekplexia and posthypoxic myoclonus are severe conditions not associated with epileptiform activity on the EEG.

Electroencephalographic Findings

Myoclonic seizures are typically associated with generalized spike-and-wave or multiple spike-and-wave discharges on the EEG. Myoclonic seizures are frequently associated with enhanced photosensitivity.

TONIC SEIZURES

Tonic seizures are brief seizures (usually lasting less than 60 seconds) consisting of the sudden onset of increased tone in the extensor muscles. If standing, the patient typically falls to the ground. Electromyographic activity is dramatically increased in tonic seizures.

Impairment of consciousness during the seizure is characteristic, although when seizures are brief, this change may be difficult to detect. Tonic seizures frequently are seen in patients with Lennox–Gastaut syndrome, a disorder consisting of a mixed seizure disorder, mental retardation, and the EEG findings of a slow spike-and-wave pattern (Arzimanoglou et al., 2009). The seizures usually occur more frequently at night.

Tonic seizures frequently begin with a tonic contraction of the neck muscles, leading to fixation of the head in an erect position, widely opened eyes, and jaw clenching or mouth opening. Contraction of the respiratory and abdominal muscles often follows, sometimes leading to a high-pitched cry and brief periods of apnea. The tonic contractions may extend to the proximal musculature of the upper limbs, elevating the shoulders and abducting the arms. Asymmetric tonic seizures vary in severity, ranging from a slight rotation of the head to a tonic contraction of all of the musculature on one side of the body. Eyelid retraction, staring, mydriasis, and apnea also may occur. Occasionally, tonic seizures terminate with a clonic phase. Unlike in generalized tonic-clonic seizures, however, the clonic phase is abbreviated. Postictal impairment, with confusion, tiredness, and headache, is common. The degree of postictal impairment usually is related to the duration of the seizure.

Tonic seizures typically are activated by sleep and may occur repetitively throughout the night. They usually are more frequent during nonrapid eye movement (NREM) sleep than during wakefulness and usually do not occur during rapid eye movement (REM) sleep. Arousal from light sleep may occur after a tonic seizure. Because the child often does not wake up during the seizure, these seizures often go undetected.

Electroencephalographic Findings

The interictal EEG pattern in patients with tonic seizures usually is quite abnormal, consisting of slowing of the background, with multifocal spikes, sharp waves, and bursts of irregular spike-and-wave activity. The EEG ictal manifestations of tonic seizures usually consist of bilateral synchronous spikes of 10 to 25 Hz, of medium to high voltage, with a frontal accentuation. Simple flattening or desynchronization may also occur (Fig. 66-5). Occasional multiple spike-and-wave or diffuse slow-wave activity may occur during a tonic seizure.

ATONIC SEIZURES

Atonic (astatic) seizures, or "drop attacks," are characterized by a sudden loss of muscle tone. They begin suddenly and without warning and cause the patient, if standing, to fall quickly to the floor. Children with atonic seizures are more likely to fall backward than children with tonic seizures. Because muscle tone may be completely absent, the children have little means by which to protect themselves, and injuries often occur. The attack may be fragmentary and manifest as dropping of the head with slackening of the jaw or dropping of a limb.

At times, it may be difficult to distinguish epileptic from nonepileptic head drops. Children with head drops secondary to seizures often have a change in facial expression and subtle myoclonic extremity movements associated with the head drops. Head drops with a rapid head descent, followed by a slow recovery to the upright position, usually represent seizures.

In atonic seizures, a loss of electromyographic activity is characteristic. Consciousness is impaired during the fall, although the patient may regain alertness immediately on hitting the floor. Atonic attacks are sometimes associated with myoclonic jerks, a combination that has been described as myoclonic-astatic seizures.

Electroencephalographic Findings

Atonic seizures usually are associated with rhythmic spike-and-wave complexes varying from slow, 1- to 2-Hz, to more rapid, irregular spikes or multiple spike-and-wave activity. The hallmark of the EEG pattern in Lennox–Gastaut syndrome is the slow spike-and-wave discharge superimposed on an abnormal, slow background. The slow spike-and-wave or sharp-and-slow-wave complexes consist of generalized discharges occurring at a frequency of 1.5 to 2.5 Hz. The morphology, amplitude, and repetition rate may vary both between bursts and during paroxysmal bursts of spike-and-wave activity, and asymmetries of the discharge are frequent. The area of maximum voltage, although variable, usually is frontal or temporal in location. Often, sleep increases the number of epileptiform discharges, but these discharges may slow in frequency and become even more irregular than during the awake state. In REM sleep, the paroxysmal activity decreases markedly. Hyperventilation and photic stimulation rarely activate these discharges.

REFERENCES

The complete list of references for this chapter is available in the e-book at www.expertconsult.com.
 See inside cover for registration details.

SELECTED REFERENCES

Aghakhani, Y., Bagshaw, A.P., Benar, C.G., et al., 2004. fMRI activation during spike and wave discharges in idiopathic generalized epilepsy. Brain 127, 1127–1144.

Arzimanoglou, A., French, J., Blume, W.T., et al., 2009. Lennox-Gastaut syndrome: a consensus approach on diagnosis, assessment, management, and trial methodology. Lancet Neurol. 8, 82–93.

Berg, A.T., Levy, S.R., Testa, F.M., et al., 2014. Long-term seizure remission in childhood absence epilepsy: might initial treatment matter? Epilepsia 55, 551–557.

Camfield, C.S., Camfield, P.R., 2009. Juvenile myoclonic epilepsy 25 years after seizure onset: a population-based study. Neurology 73, 1041–1045, 5-19.

Crunelli, V., Leresche, N., 2002. Childhood absence epilepsy: genes, channels, neurons and networks. Nat. Rev. Neurosci. 3, 371–382.

Holmes, M.D., Brown, M., Tucker, D.M., 2004. Are "generalized" seizures truly generalized? Evidence of localized mesial frontal and frontopolar discharges in absence. Epilepsia 45, 1568–1579.

Porter, R.J., Penry, J.K., Dreifuss, F.E., 1973. Responsiveness at the onset of spike-wave bursts. Electroencephalogr. Clin. Neurophysiol. 34, 239–245.

Widdess-Walsh, P., Dlugos, D., Fahlstrom, R., et al., 2013. Lennox-Gastaut syndrome of unknown cause: phenotypic characteristics of patients in the Epilepsy Phenome/Genome Project. Epilepsia 54, 1898–1904.

Wirrell, E.C., Camfield, C.S., Camfield, P.R., et al., 1996. Long-term prognosis of typical childhood absence epilepsy: remission or progression to juvenile myoclonic epilepsy. Neurology 47, 912–918.

Wirrell, E.C., 2003. Natural history of absence epilepsy in children. Can. J. Neurol. Sci. 30, 184–188.

⊗ E-BOOK FIGURES AND TABLES

The following figures and tables are available in the e-book at www.expertconsult.com. See inside cover for registration details.

67 Focal and Multifocal Seizures

Douglas R. Nordli, Jr.

 An expanded version of this chapter is available on www.expertconsult.com. See inside cover for registration details.

INTRODUCTION

Focal seizures originate in one region of the brain, where they may stay confined or spread to other areas. Focal seizures were previously referred to as *partial*, but this term created confusion when translated into other languages, and the International League Against Epilepsy (ILAE) has recommended that it no longer be used. If a discrete area of eloquent cortex is involved, the first manifestation may be an aura—something that only the patient can describe. If the seizure propagates into bilaterally distributed networks, the patient will likely become unaware of subsequent phases of the seizure. In the past this was referred to as the *complex* phase of the seizure. Other terms, including *dialeptic* and *dyscognitive*, have been used to describe some alteration of awareness and cognition. The simple term *unaware* might also suffice. Further diffuse spread of the ictus can result in secondary generalization with manifestations that are nearly identical to those of a generalized tonic-clonic seizure. When only the last portion of the seizure is witnessed, it may be impossible to discern if the onset was focal or generalized unless the patient can recall early declarative features.

Multifocal seizures arise from multiple locations and are not simply a composite of the individual focal seizures, but may be reflective of different underlying processes and therefore may respond differently to medications. Both focal and multifocal types have been underrecognized in children, but modern epidemiologic studies show that focal epilepsies account for about 60% of all seizure disorders (Berg et al., 1999). The behavioral manifestations of focal seizures relate not only to the region of the brain involved during the ictal discharge, but also to the maturation of the nervous system and the integrity of the pathways necessary for clinical expression.

TYPES OF FOCAL SEIZURES IN CHILDREN

The ILAE Commission on Classification proposed a classification of seizures in 1981 (ILAE, 1981). This scheme was widely used for almost three decades and divided focal seizures into simple partial, complex partial, and partial with secondary generalization. Subsequently, another ILAE commission on classification proposed a substantial revision (Berg et al., 2010; Vendrame et al., 2011). In this revision, the term *focal* replaced the previous term *partial*, and the obligatory separation of partial seizures into simple, complex, and secondary generalized was discarded. This created some consternation, even though the committee proposed that descriptors, albeit slightly wordy, should still be used in the full characterization of seizures.

In adolescents and adults who can communicate normally, it may be useful to subdivide seizures by alteration of awareness. In the ILAE 2010 document, examples of such descriptors were given, including "without impairment of consciousness or awareness," "with impairment of consciousness or awareness," and "evolving to bilateral convulsive seizure." The reader will note that these terms roughly equate to the older terminology delineating simple, complex, and secondary generalized seizures.

Alteration of Consciousness

Classifications that emphasize alteration of consciousness have substantial limitations in pediatrics. It may be very difficult or even impossible to accurately determine alteration of consciousness in the preschool child, even when children have the ability to communicate normally (Nordli, Kuroda, & Hirsch, 2001). In preverbal infants it is all but impossible. Simply because a child does not appear to alert to verbal or visual cues does not necessarily imply alteration of consciousness. Well-known examples are the focal seizures seen in children with rolandic epilepsy. An eye-witness will commonly infer that consciousness was altered in some daytime events because the child did not respond normally, but when one interviews the child, one realizes that awareness was completely preserved throughout the entire event, and the inability to speak was secondary to a selective anarthria. If classification schemes using awareness as the first branch point are widely adopted, another category of "awareness uncertain" may be a convenient way to approach the seizures in younger patients or those with limited ability to communicate.

Semiologic Classification Schemes

Lüders and colleagues (1998) developed a classification system for seizures that has been used in many major epilepsy centers in a wide variety of countries. Others have proposed a similarly simplified semiologic classification system for use in the very young (Nordli et al., 1997). Neither of these schemes has yet been endorsed by the ILAE. Although seizures may sometimes be broadly classified using the most prominent and early feature of the seizure, the various combinations of features, patterns, and time course of the seizure cannot be adequately summarized in a single word or phrase. Nothing can replace a thorough and meticulous description of the seizure. Indeed, the historic narrative of the seizure, as described or observed by parents, is the single most helpful piece of information allowing proper diagnosis of the seizure disorder and should be recorded, as accurately as possible, with few or no editorial comments.

Still, certain features can be identified that increase the likelihood that a described event was a focal seizure, and these same features can be used to characterize the early and prominent features of the majority of pediatric focal seizures. This semiologic approach is simple, demonstrates good interobserver reliability (Nordli et al., 1997), and has a certain degree of sincerity in that it does not infer more than is possible from the clinical manifestations alone. The early manifestations are the most important because they are the closest to the source of the ictus and therefore provide the best localizing information. There is no doubt that the path the ictus takes may have a major influence on the degree of disability induced by the seizure and therefore is not trivial, but the clinical analysis of the complex patterns seen during ictal progression is complicated, and it is important to keep in mind that some features of seizures may not be the direct manifestation of electrical stimulation of the telencephalon, but may be a result of disinhibition of deeper structures or networks. This may be particularly important when evaluating the semiology of frontal lobe seizures. Tassinari and colleagues (2005) make the point that some automatic motor movements may originate from deep structures that are preprogrammed motor movements (central pattern generators), remarkably conserved across species. Recent imaging work has indeed implicated deeper gray-matter and brainstem circuits in the generation of tonic postures, spasms, and atonia. Accordingly, clinical features alone cannot always allow one to correctly diagnose a focal seizure. Rather, "focal seizure" is actually an electroclinical diagnosis. It usually is made following consideration of multiple factors related to the patient and the clinical event, but may require electroencephalogram (EEG) confirmation, particularly in the very young. To summarize, experience using video EEG monitoring suggests that certain clinical features tend to have focal ictal EEG correlates (Figure 67-1), and these may be used as a way to categorize focal seizures in pediatrics, including the very young, although

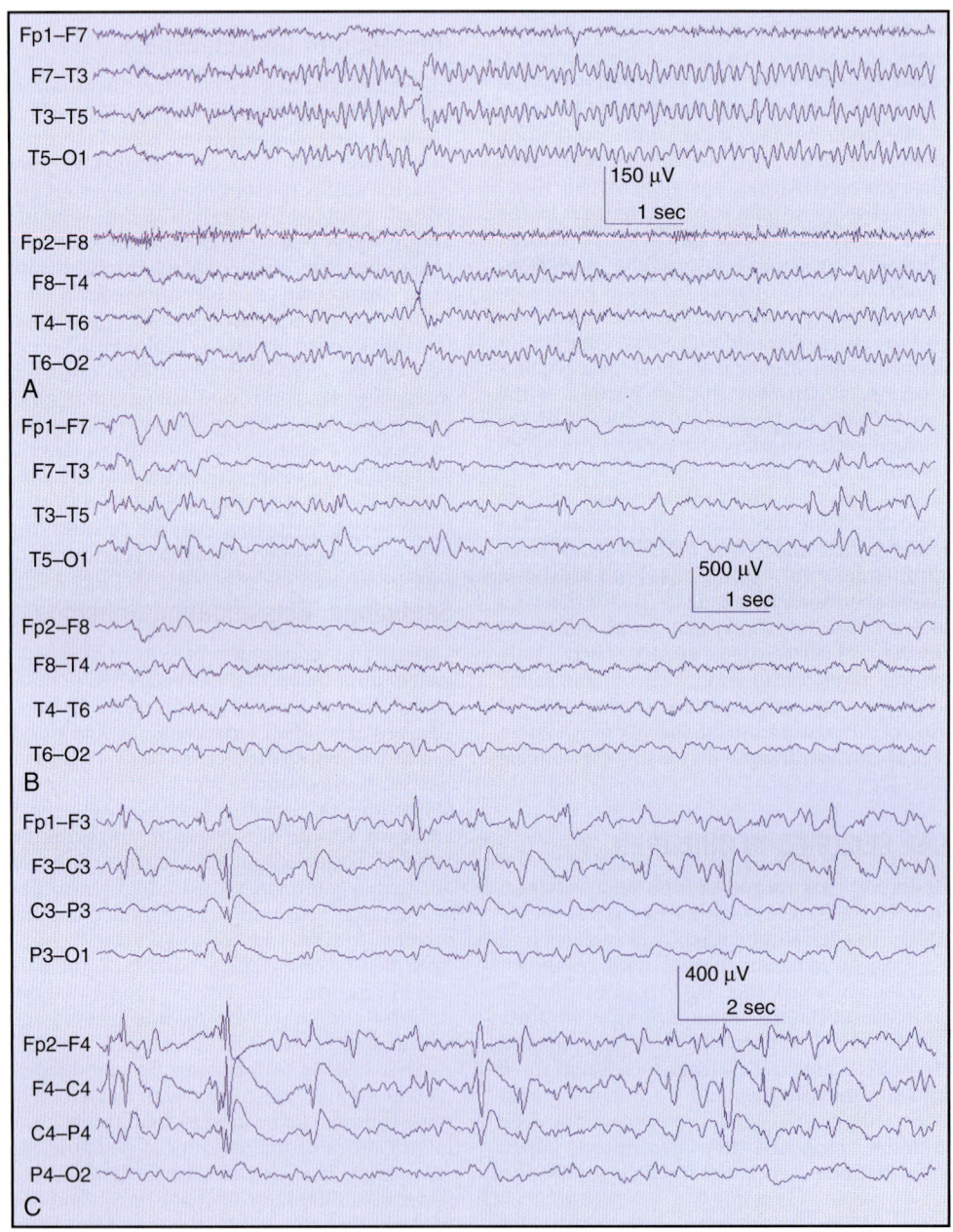

Figure 67-1. Typical interictal findings on electroencephalogram (EEG) in children with focal seizures. **A,** This EEG from a child with benign rolandic epilepsy of childhood (BREC) shows focal stereotypic spikes appearing on a normal background. Notice that each spike closely resembles the others in morphology and location, as is typical of idiopathic localization-related epilepsies. **B,** By contrast, this EEG from a child with an epileptogenic focal structural lesion in the left temporal region demonstrates pleomorphic spikes and background slowing in the same region. **C,** EEGs from children with multifocal seizures often show multifocal interictal epileptiform discharges.

TABLE 67-1 A Simple Semiologic Categorization of Pediatric Seizures

Focal			Generalized
	Aura		Clonic
	Autonomic		Myoclonic
Elementary motor	Focal clonic		Tonic
	Focal myoclonic		Tonic-clonic
	Focal tonic		Epileptic spasms
	Versive		Myoclonic-atonic
Complex motor	Automotor		Myoclonic-tonic
	Epileptic spasms with asymmetry	Negative	Absence
	Gelastic		Atypical absence
	Hypermotor		Myoclonic absence
Negative	Dialeptic/ dyscognitive		Absence with eyelid myoclonia
	Behavioral arrest/ hypomotor		Atonic

confirmation sometimes requires electroencephalographic data (Table 67-1).

Auras

Auras are special sensory or psychogenic phenomena that are perceived only by the patient. They occur in a variety of forms and have important localizing value. Although the concurrent ictal EEG often does not reveal clear electrographic expression in most patients, auras are believed by most authorities to be the manifestation of discrete focal seizures. When a somatosensory aura is specific and an ictal EEG correlate is present, the ictal discharge is often low-voltage fast activity localized over the corresponding region of the sensory homunculus. Other auras arising from limbic structures often are "indescribable," or may have a fearful quality or include a feeling of epigastric discomfort. These discharges arise from subcortical structures, so the EEG may reveal little to no change, other than ipsilateral diffuse delta activity or a rhythmic theta-alpha pattern in the anterior to midtemporal region, particularly when the onset of activity is mesial temporal in location. Auras are supportive of the diagnosis of a focal seizure, especially when having certain clinical characteristics strongly localizing to a particular cortical area, although recent studies have reported the presence of auras in generalized seizures as well.

Autonomic

Rarely, the only manifestation of a focal seizure is through the autonomic nervous system. Some examples include an increase in heart rate, oxygen desaturation, pallor, and piloerection in one region of the body.

Automotor

Limb automatisms are semipurposeful movements, such as rubbing or fumbling of the hands, or picking at the air, that may be seen in focal seizures. Oral automatisms, such as lip smacking, can occur with generalized absence seizures, but unilateral limb automatisms suggest a focal process. Well-developed distal limb automatisms are rarely seen in infants but become more common above age 6 years. When

unilateral, automatisms are another helpful sign, indicating the presence of a focal seizure, and are typically seen ipsilateral to the epileptic focus in older children and adults. Most often automatisms are probably coupled with some alteration of cognition, but this is not invariably the case. In infants and young children rigorous assessment of cognition is sometimes impossible.

Behavioral Arrest or Hypomotor

In some infants and young children, the most conspicuous feature of a focal seizure may be the sudden, abrupt cessation of ongoing activity or a marked change in demeanor, as indicated by subtle but distinct changes in facial expression. Parents easily identify these features because they represent a clear paroxysmal alteration in the child's behavior. Parents are particularly well attuned to the nature of their child's habitual behavior, but these behavioral changes may be challenging for a person unacquainted with the child to identify on videotape. In the preverbal child, and in many children with special needs, it is impossible to ascertain alteration of consciousness reliably. Alteration of consciousness cannot be unambiguously inferred from behavior (e.g., daydreaming in school). To assess consciousness accurately, test items must be given and recall tested after the seizure. In children, this often is not possible, so the simple description of a behavioral arrest is more reliably used, rather than trying to infer if the patient was unaware during the seizure. Behavioral arrest seizures also have been described as hypomotor seizures. This description refers to a sudden reduction in the motor activity of the child. The electrographic ictal accompaniment often emanates from the temporal lobe or posterior quadrant and may be composed of monotonous rhythmic delta or theta-alpha patterns with an electrographic "crescendo" appearance, or low-voltage fast discharges that subsequently evolve to other rhythms (Figure 67-2). In children above age 3 years, behavioral arrest may accompany both focal and generalized seizures (absence seizures), so in isolation it is not a reliable indicator of a focal seizure; however, because absence seizures rarely occur in children less than 2.5 years of age, it is likely to be the correlate of a focal seizure in this age group.

Clonus or Myoclonus—Focal

Hand or arm clonus (clonic seizure) or myoclonus is another reliable feature of focal epilepsy. This activity is easily recognized as ictal by the repetitive nature of the jerking in the case of clonus or the sudden isolated jerk of myoclonus. Clonic seizures can sometimes be distinguished from jitteriness or tremor by the inability to suppress the motion by passive restraint. Clonus is usually accompanied by runs of rhythmic spike discharges in the contralateral rolandic region, and it is a reliable indicator of a focal seizure. The EEG correlate of myoclonias is most often spikes or spike-wave discharges in the contralateral hemisphere.

Dialeptic or Dyscognitive

Dialeptic or dyscognitive seizures are those in which the main manifestation is an alteration of consciousness. The term *dialeptic* was coined as a purely descriptive one, without the need to infer whether the underlying EEG correlate was focal or generalized (Lüders et al., 1998). Another largely synonymous term is *dyscognitive* (Berg et al., 2010), but because there are many aspects to consciousness and cognition, one could argue that a simpler option would be simply to state that the patient was unaware. In the author's personal experience,

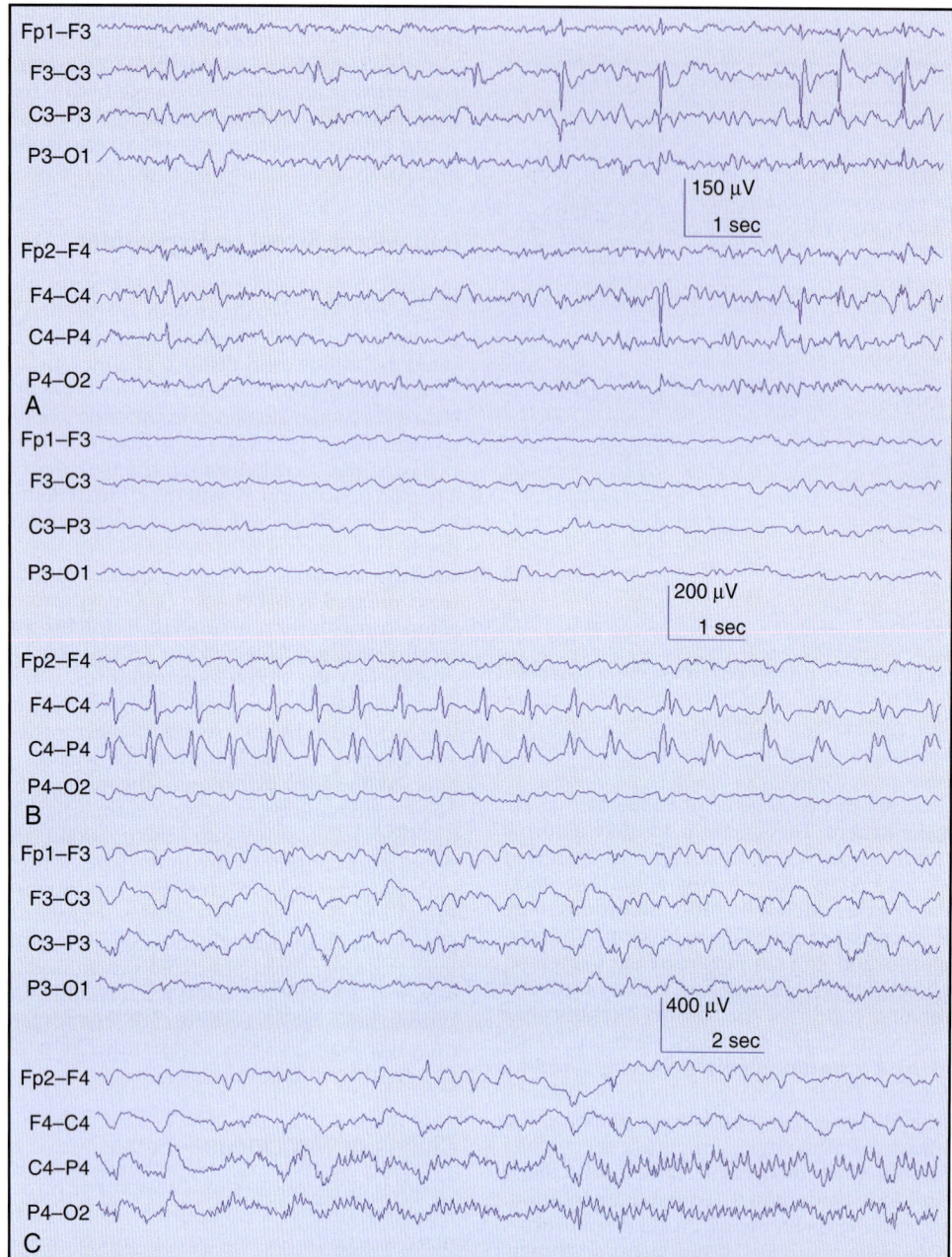

Figure 67-2. Common infantile ictal patterns on electroencephalogram (EEG) in focal seizures. A, EEG during a behavioral arrest seizure shows an ictal discharge in the left temporal region. Notice the rhythmic buildup of fast activity. Ictal discharges usually have an evolution in frequency, amplitude, and spatial distribution (like a crescendo in music). **B,** During a clonic seizure involving the left arm, the EEG demonstrates an ictal correlate consisting of repetitive spikes in the right central region. Notice that the ictal discharge remains very localized. **C,** EEG obtained during a versive seizure with eyes deviating to the right, or the same side as for the ictal discharge, shows a fast ictal pattern superimposed on some rhythmic slowing in the right posterior head region.

it is rare to diagnose pure dialeptic seizures of focal origin in infants and young children. Because consciousness and ongoing cognition are very difficult to assess in the young and because children tend to be more active when awake, the most conspicuous manifestation of a focal seizure with dialeptic features often tends to be an arrest of movement (hypomotor). There are times, however, when there is a constellation of features, including subtle posture, brief body movements, and slight version, that makes it difficult to segregate the seizure into one simple category, and if consciousness can be verified to be abnormal, as is often the case with older children or adolescents, than the terms *dialeptic* or *dyscognitive* can be used.

Epileptic Spasms With Asymmetric Features

Spasms can be recognized by their tendency to recur in clusters, many times in an almost periodic fashion, with a fairly constant interval between successive individual spasms. Spasms have a quick or myoclonic component at the start, followed by a brief sustained posture (tonic phase), followed in turn by a relaxation. Spasms that are asymmetric, that occur in a child with hemiparesis or other focal pathology, or that are associated with marked interhemispheric asymmetries on EEG could be considered to be a form of focal seizures in that they may have a focal telencephalic trigger. In about 25% of patients with spasms, clear electrographic focal seizures can be detected before, during, or after the cluster. The EEG accompaniment of spasms often contains diffuse electrodecrements, even if they are preceded by clear focal seizures.

Gelastic

Gelastic seizures are rarely seen but important to recognize because of their association with hypothalamic hamartomas. They may also be seen with lesions in the frontal lobe. They are characterized by brief epochs of "mirthless" laughter and may have subtle surface EEG correlates.

Hypermotor

Hypermotor seizures usually involve a complex series of large movements, resulting in a violent appearance of the event. Although they have been noted to arise from the mesial frontal supplementary sensorimotor area, or other regions of the frontal lobe in adults, they may also be seen in temporal lobe seizures in children. Temporal lobe seizures in very young infants may show prominent coarse motor manifestations, but these tend to decrease with advancing age (Ray and Kotagal, 2005).

Tonic

Tonic postures, both symmetric and asymmetric, are seen with focal seizures. It is surprising to observe how often symmetric tonic postures can occur as a manifestation of a focal seizure in infants, and also how unreliable asymmetries of tonic postures can be in localizing ictal onsets. It is possible that these tonic postures are generated in deeper brainstem or subcortical structures and are not direct manifestations of the ictal discharges. This finding would explain why some asymmetric tonic postures can be reversed by passive turning of the head during a seizure, in a fashion similar to the tonic neck reflex elicited in the newborn. As the child matures, symmetric tonic postures are seen less frequently as a manifestation of a focal epilepsy. Instead, tonic postures become more asymmetric and show more lateralizing features.

Versive

Pronounced and sustained lateral version of the eyes (as in a so-called versive seizure) is rarely encountered as an ictal manifestation in infants or young children. When present, version is another indicator of a focal seizure. In contrast with older children and adults, in whom the electrographic discharge often is best developed in the contralateral frontotemporal region, the ictal discharge in infants is more often in the ipsilateral occipital lobe.

Ontogeny of Focal Seizures

The clinical expression of focal and multifocal seizures changes with age, in a more or less predictable fashion. Features that occur with more regularity with increasing age include aura, limb automatisms, dystonic posture, secondary generalization, and unresponsiveness. In contrast, the frequency of asymmetric clonus and symmetric tonic posturing decreases with age (Hamer et al., 1999; Acharya et al., 1997)

EVALUATION AND MANAGEMENT

Although it is important to distinguish focal seizures from their generalized counterparts, this simple segregation is not sufficient to guide treatment. A broader understanding of the epilepsy syndrome, category of epilepsy, and etiology is even more important. A good example is Dravet syndrome. Infants with this condition will often have hemiconvulsive events early in their course, even though the EEG features may indicate a more multifocal process (Figure 67-3). If one focused only on the seizure type, one might correctly diagnose focal seizures and be tempted to select drugs that modulate the sodium channel (e.g., carbamazepine or phenytoin), but these medications may actually worsen the underlying sodium channel dysfunction causing the epilepsy and might very well make the patient worse.

If a precise epilepsy syndrome cannot be established, it may be helpful to consider the development of the child and the interictal EEG. If the child is developing normally and the EEG background is normal, then in most circumstances the EEG spikes should be rather stereotyped. If all of this is true for the particular case, it is most likely that one is dealing either with a familial epilepsy or a self-limited epilepsy, such as rolandic epilepsy or Panayiotopoulos syndrome.

If the child shows slowed development and the EEG background is slow, then a diffuse or multifocal encephalopathy needs to be considered. In this case the spikes will usually be multifocal and pleomorphic. A wide variety of conditions may cause this presentation, including metabolic disorders (Chapter 76) and de novo mutations. If these circumstances broader-spectrum agents will usually be more effective. The reader is referred to Chapter 77 focusing on medication.

Finally, if there is focal slowing, attenuation, or both, then a structural lesion needs to be considered. In this case there will often be focal pleomorphic spikes. Imaging should be obtained, and if multiple well-chosen medications have not helped, then a surgical evaluation should be considered (see Chapter 78).

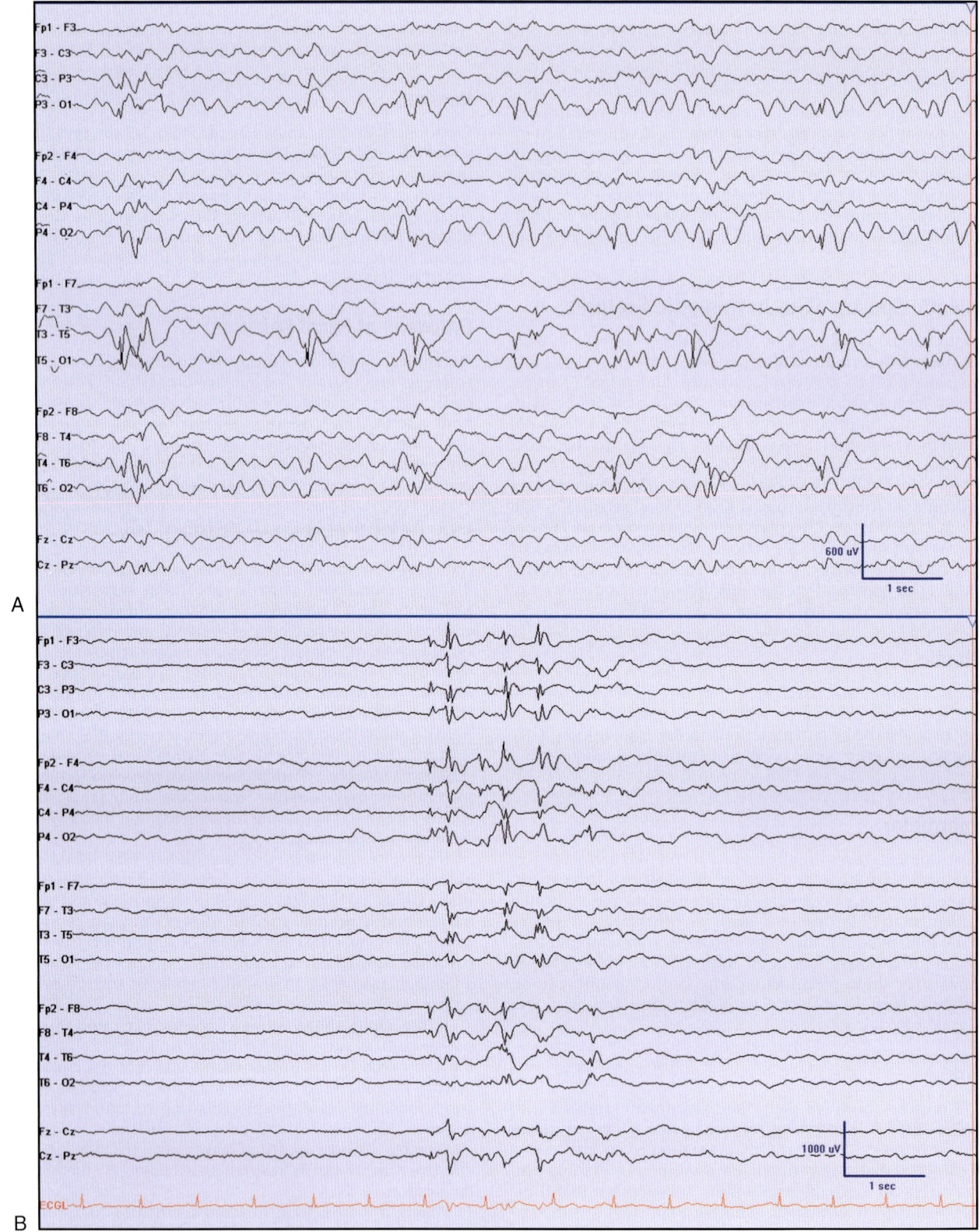

Figure 67-3. Electroencephalogram (EEG) findings in Dravet syndrome in an infant. **A,** In the first year of life EEGs may be normal, although posterior spikes and polyspikes are sometimes seen, as in this child at 10 months. **B,** Later, generalized spike and polyspike-wave discharges are noted. This is the same child 2 years later.

REFERENCES

The complete list of references for this chapter is available in the e-book at www.expertconsult.com.

See inside cover for registration details.

SELECTED REFERENCES

Acharya, J.N., Wyllie, E., Lüders, H.O., et al., 1997. Seizure symptomatology in infants with localization-related epilepsy. Neurology 48, 189.

Berg, A.T., Berkovic, S.F., Brodie, M.J., et al., 2010. Revised terminology and concepts for organization of seizures and epilepsies: report of the ILAE Commission on Classification and Terminology, 2005–2009. Epilepsia 51 (4), 676–685.

Berg, A.T., Shinnar, S., Levy, S.R., et al., 1999. Newly diagnosed epilepsy in children: presentation at diagnosis. Epilepsia 40, 445.

Hamer, H.M., Wyllie, E., Lüders, H.O., et al., 1999. Symptomatology of epileptic seizures in the first three years of life. Epilepsia 40, 837.

International League against Epilepsy, 1981. Proposal for revised clinical and electroencephalographic classification of epileptic seizures. From the Commission on Classification and Terminology of the International League Against Epilepsy. Epilepsia 22, 489.

Lüders, H., Acharya, J., Baumgartner, C., et al., 1998. Semiological Seizure Classification. Epilepsia 39, 1006.

Nordli, D.R., Kuroda, M.M., Hirsch, L.J., 2001. The ontogeny of partial seizures in infants and young children. Epilepsia 42, 986.

Nordli, D.R. Jr., Bazil, C.W., Scheuer, M.L., et al., 1997. Recognition and classification of seizures in infants. Epilepsia 38 (5), 553.

Ray, A., Kotagal, P., 2005. Temporal lobe epilepsy in children: overview of clinical semiology. Epileptic Disord. 7 (4), 299–307.

Tassinari, C.A., Rubboli, G., Gardella, E., et al., 2005. Central pattern generators for a common semiology in fronto-limbic seizures and in parasomnias. A neuroethologic approach. Neurol. Sci. 26 (Suppl. 3), s225–s232. [Epub 2005/12/07].

Vendrame, M., Zarowski, M., Alexopoulos, A.V., et al., 2011. Localization of pediatric seizure semiology. Clin. Neurophysiol. 122, 1924.

E-BOOK FIGURES AND TABLES

The following figures and tables are available in the e-book at www.expertconsult.com. See inside cover for registration details.

Fig. 67-4 This EEG shows the highly stereotyped epileptiform discharges seen in a 3-year-old child with Panayiotopoulos syndrome.

Fig. 67-5 Magnetic resonance image showing left mesial temporal sclerosis in an 8-year-old girl.

Box 67-1 Seizure Semiology Indicating a Focal Seizure

Box 67-2 International Classification of Seizures

Box 67-3 Further Descriptions of Focal Seizures

Box 67-4 Electroclinical Syndromes Categorized by Age at Onset (Eponyms Traditionally Associated with Syndromes Are Provided When Appropriate)

Table 67-2 A Categorization of the Epilepsies Based Upon Prominent EEG Characteristics

Table 67-3 Practical Guide to Antiseizure Medicines

68 Epileptic Spasms and Myoclonic Seizures

Nilika Shah Singhal, Chellamani Harini, and Joseph Sullivan

INTRODUCTION

Myoclonus, myoclonic seizures, and infantile spasms share many common features yet are seen in a wide variety of neurologic conditions. The precise definitions of each of these terms has also been somewhat controversial, but for this chapter we will use the definition proposed by Victor and Adams and define myoclonus simply as a "shocklike irregular jerk" with myoclonic seizures having a similar clinical appearance but also accompanied by neurophysiologic evidence of being cortically generated. The distinction between a cortically generated movement (myoclonic seizure) and a subcortically generated movement (myoclonus) is extremely important, especially when thinking about some of the progressive myoclonic epilepsies as many of these patients can manifest both myoclonus and myoclonic seizures. Infantile spasms, however, should not be confused with either, as the spasm itself is often a more complex constellation of movements with a myoclonic component.

Given this overlap, it is fitting to present myoclonic seizures and infantile spasms together as a continuum of events that occur in a developing nervous system. We will first discuss some of the more common pediatric epilepsy syndromes in which myoclonic seizures are often seen, followed by a more detailed discussion of infantile spasms.

Epilepsy Syndromes With Prominent Myoclonic Seizures

Myoclonic seizures can be seen in a wide variety of pediatric epilepsy syndromes, including Lennox-Gastaut syndrome and childhood absence epilepsy, which are discussed elsewhere in this text. Our focus will be on those syndromes in which myoclonic seizures are a critical feature for the diagnosis. This includes benign myoclonic epilepsy in infants (BME), Dravet Syndrome (SMEI/severe myoclonic epilepsy of infancy), myoclonic-astatic epilepsy (Doose syndrome), and juvenile myoclonic epilepsy (JME).

Benign Myoclonic Epilepsy of Infancy (BMEI)

BMEI was first described by Dravet and Bureau in 1981. The syndrome is characterized by brief, generalized myoclonic seizures with the predominant area of muscle involvement being the proximal upper extremities and usually occurs in children between the ages of 4 months and 3 years. These attacks often occur multiple times per day. Detailed EEG and polygraphic EMG recordings have shown that the myoclonic seizures are often associated with a flexor postural change and approximately 80% of attacks involve the upper limbs. A history of febrile seizures (30%) and a family history of epilepsy (39%) are relatively common.

EEG

The ictal EEG discharge is often a generalized spike wave (GSW) that may be slower than 3Hz. Some infants may exhibit photosensitivity at the onset of the syndrome, and the photic-induced myoclonic seizures are often more prominent than those that occur spontaneously.

Treatment and Outcome

The overall prognosis of myoclonic seizures is excellent, with complete resolution in almost all children usually within 1 to 2 years of diagnosis. The majority of children also have normal neurodevelopmental outcomes, although some studies have reported impaired psychomotor development and behavioral disturbances if the child is not treated or if onset of the syndrome is less than 2 years of age. Those children with a prominent reflex component may have a more favorable neurodevelopmental outcome.

The medication of choice appears to be valproic acid (VPA) with 80% to 90% responding to VPA monotherapy, although high serum levels (greater than 100mg/dl) may be necessary. When VPA monotherapy does not provide complete control, adjunctive use of a benzodiazepine such as clonazepam or clobazam can be helpful.

Dravet Syndrome

First described in 1978 by Charlotte Dravet, and termed severe myoclonic epilepsy of infancy (SMEI) but now more widely known as Dravet Syndrome, this occurs in normally developing children who experience prolonged febrile (longer than 20 minutes) or afebrile seizures, including hemiconvulsions, during the first year of life. Afebrile, mixed seizures follow, and the emergence of myoclonic seizures is common but not necessary for the diagnosis. This syndrome is covered in more detail in Chapter 71.

Myoclonic-Astatic Epilepsy of Doose (MAE)

These children present in early childhood with myoclonic seizures but with a prominent astatic component leading to falls. Although this syndrome does not always have a poor neurodevelopmental outcome, it remains an epileptic encephalopathy and if not appropriately treated can progress and lead to adverse neurodevelopmental sequelae or evolution into Lennox-Gastaut syndrome.

ETIOLOGY

Genetic factors clearly play a role in the pathogenesis of MAE based on the high incidence of seizures (32%) in the siblings and parents in probands with the most common seizure type being absence. SLC2A1 mutations were found in 5%, suggesting genetic testing for GLUT-1 should be strongly considered.

SEIZURE SEMIOLOGY

Onset of MAE is often between the ages of 2 and 6 years, and children are usually developmentally normal. There appears to be a strong male predominance (70% to 90%). These children may begin experiencing unexplained "jerks" and "falls" occurring multiple times per day. These myoclonic seizures can occur in isolation but often are followed by a brief period of atonia, resulting in a dramatic fall in which the child appears to be propelled to the ground.

The atonic falls may be more subtle and the only manifestation of these may be a brief head nod or "head drop," with or without a myoclonic jerk of the upper extremities. Absence seizures are quite common but often are accompanied by more prominent myoclonus of the proximal upper extremities.

EEG

The interictal EEG findings are varied and can be normal. The most common findings are generalized 3 Hz spike-wave discharges as well as rhythmic 4 Hz to 7 Hz biparietal theta activity. Activation of generalized discharges during sleep is common, but generalized fast rhythms such as generalized periodic fast activity (GPFA) are uncommon. Focal EEG findings are uncommon and may suggest a less favorable prognosis.

TREATMENT

The most commonly used and most effective antiseizure medicines have been valproate (VPA), lamotrigine, levetiracetam, topiramate, and benzodiazepines (clonazepam, clobazam, clorazepate). Felbamate is probably underutilized but can be effective against all seizure types. The combination of VPA with ethosuximide may be particularly effective especially if high doses of VPA are used.

The ketogenic diet has been shown to be as effective as other first-line agents in children with MAE and may be considered early in treatment.

Outcome

Cognitive outcomes are highly variable and appear to be somewhat dependent on degree of seizure control, although even with fairly frequent seizures of multiple types there may still be spontaneous remission, usually after approximately 3 years (Oguni et al., 2002). The occurrence of tonic seizures may be a negative prognostic sign, although it remains unclear if these children may actually have an atypical form of Lennox-Gastaut syndrome rather than MAE.

Juvenile Myoclonic Epilepsy (JME)

JME is a generalized epilepsy syndrome characterized by myoclonic seizures, generalized tonic-clonic seizures, and absence seizures. It is common, accounting for 26% of what had been previously considered the idiopathic generalized epilepsies and 10% of all epilepsies. The average age of onset is 15.1 years (7 to 28 years) with a slight female predominance.

Seizure Semiology. In the classic syndrome of JME, myoclonic seizures may precede the first generalized tonic-clonic (GTC) seizure by 6 to 12 months, although GTCs occur as the first seizure type in approximately one-third of patients. Photosensitivity is relatively common, occurring in approximately 30% of patients.

Myoclonic seizures often occur in the early morning hours shortly after awaking. Specific lifestyle features have been commonly associated with breakthrough seizures including sleep deprivation, stress, alcohol, and menses.

EEG. Patients with JME often have abnormal interictal EEGs with the most common finding being generalized 4 Hz to 6 Hz polyspike and wave (61%) or 3 Hz spike and wave discharges (14%). More prolonged (1 to 6 days; average 1 to 2 days) video EEG studies have shown EEG abnormalities of JME in 88% of patients. A photoparoxysmal response in treatment naïve patients is also common and has been seen in as many as 35% of patients.

Treatment. Valproate has long been considered the first-line agent with reports of up to 86% of patients becoming seizure free for 1 year. Valproate has also been shown to be particularly effective in those patients with photosensitivity. Women of childbearing potential must also consider the possible long-term cognitive effects on a fetus. Due to these concerns, many newer antiseizure drugs are also commonly used including lamotrigine, topiramate, zonisamide, and levetiracetam.

Benzodiazepines are widely accepted to have excellent antimyoclonic effects, but in JME only 43% of treated patients become free of GTCs. For this reason, benzodiazepines are not recommended as monotherapy but can be successful as add-on therapy when myoclonic seizures persist.

Outcomes. It has been widely accepted that JME was a life-long condition with a high rate of relapse if weaned off therapy; however, some recent long-term follow-up studies have shown conflicting results, and some patients with JME can successfully discontinue medications. The decision to discontinue medicine should be individualized with every patient, and a detailed discussion with specific attention to the frequency of life-style provoking factors is necessary for a safe and well-informed decision.

Infantile Spasms

Infantile spasms is an age-dependent epilepsy syndrome that presents during infancy and is typically identified by clusters of spasms and an interictal EEG pattern known as hypsarrhythmia. Historically, West syndrome refers to the classic triad of spasms, hypsarrhythmia, and psychomotor arrest or regression. With a worldwide incidence of approximately 1 per 3000 live births, infantile spasms is the most prevalent epilepsy syndrome of infancy, and its emotional and financial costs to society are enormous.

Despite over 150 years of interest in this disorder, various aspects from terminology to treatment remain controversial, in large part because the pathogenesis is unknown.

ELECTROCLINICAL FEATURES

Regardless of etiology, the syndrome manifests during a specific period of brain maturation, most often between 4 and 8 months of life and nearly always before 2 years (Riikonen, 1982).

Spasms

The classic seizure type, referred to as an epileptic spasm, is characterized by symmetric, bilateral, brief contraction of the axial muscle groups. The electromyographic tracing during a spasm reveals an abrupt phasic contraction lasting less than 2 seconds, which may be followed by a less intense tonic contraction lasting from 2 to 10 seconds. Therefore this unique seizure type is longer than a myoclonic jerk and yet shorter than a tonic seizure.

Spasms typically occur in clusters, with a 5-second to 30-second interval between successive spells. The frequency of spasms may vary from only a few to several hundred per day. One common feature to note when taking a history is the common occurrence of spasms upon awakening and their rare occurrence during sleep.

Eye movements, consisting of deviation alone or followed by rhythmic nystagmoid movements, are also commonly seen during spasms. Changes in respiratory rhythm occur in the majority of patients, although alterations in heart rate are rare.

Hypsarrhythmia and the Ictal EEG

The EEG hallmark of infantile spasms is hypsarrhythmia, a disorganized interictal pattern consisting of "random high voltage slow waves and spikes." The spike discharges are usually multifocal, but when generalized, they are never rhythmically repetitive. A state-dependent EEG pattern, hypsarrhythmia is often present during wakefulness and quiet (non-REM) sleep and may be reduced or even absent during active (REM) sleep. Other EEG patterns including modified hypsarrhythmia or multifocal spikes can also be seen in children with infantile spasms.

Children with severe brain abnormalities such as tuberous sclerosis, Aicardi syndrome, and lissencephaly may not usually generate the typical hypsarrhythmic pattern. Asymmetric hypsarrhythmia may indicate the presence of a focal CNS lesion. Regardless of the specific pattern, however, any significant EEG background abnormality in a patient with clinical spasms may contribute to the epileptic encephalopathy, and all patterns should be viewed equally when considering approach to treatment.

The ictal EEG pattern varies, although typically shows a generalized, high-voltage, slow-wave transient followed by an abrupt voltage attenuation. Some children have focal seizures that are temporally related to clusters of spasms, a phenomenon that should raise suspicion for a structural brain abnormality and possibly a focal abnormality with EEG concordance.

CLASSIFICATION

The classification of infantile spasms has been debated for years, though the International League Against Epilepsy (ILAE) Commission on Classification and Terminology published a revised recommendation for terminology and concepts related to infantile spasms and other seizure types (Berg et al., 2010). Spasms are neither generalized nor focal and remain a distinct seizure type.

The following etiologic classification has been recommended: (1) genetic, (2) structural/metabolic, or (3) unknown cause. As many epilepsies related to a structural brain malformation or inborn error of metabolism have an identifiable genetic cause this classification is presently under revision.

ETIOLOGIC FACTORS

Gene mutations in key pathways of central nervous system development have expanded the genetic etiologies of infantile spasms. Examples include genes ARX, CKDL5, FOXG1, GRIN1, GRIN2A, MAGI2, MEF2C, SCL25A22, SPTAN1, and STXBP1 (Paciorkowski et al., 2011). Not every patient with these mutations will develop infantile spasms, but the phenotype is consistent enough to think of these as infantile spasm-associated genes with variable penetrance and expressivity. The early-onset epilepsies may be related to severity of mutation, though more data are needed to demonstrate if this is truly the case.

To evaluate the etiology and yield of investigations, 20 United States pediatric epilepsy centers prospectively enrolled all infants newly diagnosed with infantile spasms in a central database; 251 infants were enrolled. An underlying cause was identified in 64.4% of cases and included genetic causes in 14.4%. Genetic-structural causes were identified in 10%, including tuberous sclerosis, neurofibromatosis, and others. Congenital structural causes were identified in 10.8% and acquired structural causes in 22.4%. Metabolic causes were noted in 4.8% and infectious etiologies in 2.0%. Of note, among those with a defined etiology, the cause was evident on initial clinical assessment or MRI in 85.7%, whereas further genetic and metabolic studies were revealing in the other 14.3%.

DIAGNOSTIC EVALUATION

An approach to the evaluation of infantile spasms is outlined in Figure 68-3. First, in a child with suspected infantile spasms, an EEG is needed to confirm the presence of hypsarrhythmia. Given the state-dependence of hypsarrhythmia, an extended EEG recording that captures at least one full sleep-wake cycle

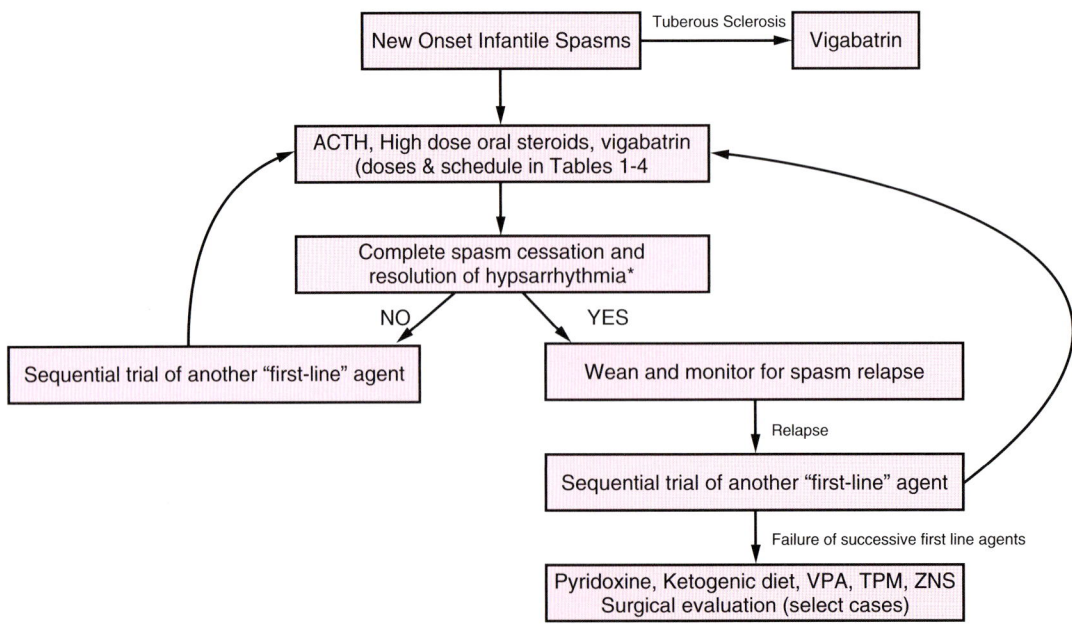

*In cases where clinical spasms have stopped but hypsarrhythmia continues, consider continuing therapy for 1-2 more weeks and then repeat EEG

Figure 68-3. Suggested treatment pathway for new onset IS.

TABLE 68-3 Treatment With Intramuscular (IM) ACTH

Days	Dose—ACTH
1–14	75 U/m² twice daily#
15–17	30 U/m² in the morning
18–20	15 U/m² in the morning
21–23	10 U/m² in the morning
24–29	10 U/m² every other morning (3 total doses)

#If there is no clinical response by day 14, consider alternative treatment.

TABLE 68-5 Treatment With Oral Prednisolone UKISS Protocol

Days	Dose—prednisolone
1–14	10 mg oral 4 times daily*#
15–19	10 mg oral 3 times daily*
20–24	10 mg oral 2 times daily
25–29	10 mg oral daily

*If there is no clinical response after day 7 (i.e., no 24-hour period free of infantile spasms), the dose can be increased to 20 mg three times daily. If done, the taper schedule from day 15 to 19 would be 10 mg 4 times daily and then proceed as in the table beginning on day 20.
#If no clinical response by day 14, consider alternative treatment.

TABLE 68-6 Treatment With Oral Vigabatrin

Days*#	Dose—Vigabatrin
1–3	50 mg/kg/day divided 2 times daily
4–6	100 mg/kg/day divided 2 times daily
>7	150 mg/kg/day divided 2 times daily

*Side effects (e.g., sedation, hypotonia) may necessitate slower titration.
#If no clinical response by day 14, consider alternative treatment.

should be performed in all cases. If the EEG remains normal with no features of hypsarrhythmia or its variants, the EEG should be repeated in 1 to 2 weeks, again capturing at least one full sleep-wake cycle.

COURSE AND PROGNOSIS

Regardless of treatment, however, it appears that clinical spasms and hypsarrhythmia disappear in one-half of children by 2 years of age and in nearly all children by 5 years of age. Approximately 50% of children will develop other seizure types. In many patients who exhibit diffuse or multifocal cerebral dysfunction, the disorder evolves into Lennox-Gastaut syndrome.

Overall, the developmental outcome in infantile spasms is poor (Riikonen, 2010). Children with severe brain malformations tend to have worse prognoses. Early and complete control of spasms has been associated with improved neurodevelopmental outcome even when only evaluating infantile spasms of unknown etiology without confounding underlying diagnoses (O'Callaghan et al., 2011).

Children with infantile spasms due to Down syndrome, neurofibromatosis, and periventricular leukomalacia may have a more benign prognosis. Apart from etiology, the other factors that may translate into better long-term outcome include shorter lag time to treatment and use of hormonal therapy for spasms of unknown cause (Go et al., 2012). Regarding the type of treatment for spasms, developmental outcome, tested at 14 months and 4 years after spasms onset, was better after initial control of IS with hormonal therapy in those without an identified underlying etiology.

It is important to recognize that not all spasms of unknown cause will have a good outcome. In a retrospective series looking at long-term outcome of West syndrome, 50% of the group with no known cause had clear developmental impairment, despite early control of spasms. These adverse outcomes have not changed in several decades

TREATMENT

The goal of treatment is to prevent or ameliorate the encephalopathy by stopping the spasms and improving the EEG background, yet the optimal treatment of infantile spasms has not been clearly defined. The Infantile Spasms Working Group has published a United States consensus report. This group supported ACTH or vigabatrin as the first-line treatments with proven efficacy (Pellock et al., 2010). It did endorse the use of high-dose corticosteroid in the treatment of spasms, but raised concern in that the combination of cessation of spasms as well as resolution of hypsarrhythmia on EEG has not been reported in studies on its use.

A treatment algorithm for infantile spasms based on available evidence of what are considered first line agents is shown in Figure 68-3. Although there remain no comparative effectiveness trials for these agents, sequential use is recommended. (Tables 68-3, 68-5 and 68-6)

Second-line treatments including conventional antiseizure medicines, as well as the ketogenic diet, have been used with variable success when first-line agents fail. Finally, fueled by advances in neuroimaging, surgical resection of focal lesions has emerged as a promising option for patients with medically intractable infantile spasms.

Hormonal Therapy

In 2004, a practice parameter by the AAN and Child Neurology Society deemed ACTH "probably effective," reaffirming the prevailing consensus that ACTH was the gold standard and in 2012, an update to the 2004 practice parameter produced by the American Academy of Neurology and the Child Neurology Society recommended low-dose ACTH, preferred over vigabatrin, particularly in cases in which the underlying cause is not known.

ACTH

Several prospective, randomized trials of ACTH or cosyntropin of varying doses have shown 42% to 87% of patients experienced cessation of spasms within 2 weeks of initiating therapy. Hypsarrhythmia resolved in 20% to 90% of patients, and relapse rates were 15% to 33%. Although there is no agreement about dose or duration of treatment, two randomized controlled trials comparing high-dose ACTH with low-dose ACTH did not show a significant difference in terms of spasm cessation. In a long-term follow-up study, there was no clear benefit of 150 IU/day compared with 40 IU/day. Given no clear consensus on the optimal treatment for infantile spasms and varying doses, the National Infantile Spasms Consortium (NISC), a United States multicenter initiative to improve outcomes through prospective data collection, was started. From 2012 to 2014, 238 infants were enrolled. Initial treatment, including ACTH, oral corticosteroids, vigabatrin, topiramate, levetiracetam, zonisamide, oxcarbazepine, clobazam, phenobarbital, and the ketogenic diet, was documented in 230 cases. Three-month outcome data was available for 205 children. ACTH led to remission in 48%, corticosteroids led to remission in 27%, and vigabatrin led to remission in 38%. Of the other treatments, only 5% achieved remission. This initial study has again motivated the need for a randomized clinical trial to identify best treatment practices.

CORTICOSTEROIDS

The UKISS trial subanalysis showed that oral prednisolone was equivalent to synthetic ACTH (70% versus 76% spasm-free after 14 days, respectively). Although this study was not powered to determine a significant difference between the two groups, it had more subjects than prior studies and represents the only randomized controlled trial evaluating the effectiveness of high-dose oral corticosteroid. Incorporating UKISS results, a 2008 Cochrane review concluded that should oral prednisolone be used, "high dose" is recommended (Hancock et al., 2008).

Vigabatrin

In patients with tuberous sclerosis, vigabatrin has been shown to be particularly effective in the short-term treatment of infantile spasms with more than 90% achieving complete spasm control. In contrast, short-term efficacy rates for all or non-TS infantile spasms range from 35% to 54%. Vigabatrin may be recommended as first-line therapy for patients with infantile spasms due to tuberous sclerosis. In a long-term follow-up study of 180 patients, vigabatrin terminated spasms in 56.9% of patients and did so within 3 to 7 days (mean 5.3 days), again suggesting that if a child does not respond to initial therapy, then rapid sequential therapy is indicated (Djuric et al., 2014).

Surgical Therapy

Facilitated by advances in structural and functional neuroimaging techniques, surgical resection of focal or unilateral CNS lesions has emerged as an effective epilepsy treatment option in select patients with intractable infantile spasms. Epilepsy surgery for infantile spasms was fueled by the observation that positron emission tomography (PET) of glucose metabolism could identify focal cortical lesions localized to epileptogenic regions in infants with infantile spasms of unknown cause whose structural imaging was unrevealing, and that surgical resection was associated with a favorable outcome.

Other Treatments

There are no randomized controlled trials of other antiseizure medications or alternative therapies for the treatment of infantile spasms, although limited evidence suggests that the ketogenic diet, valproate, topiramate, zonisamide, and pyridoxine may provide additional benefit in decreasing spasms and therefore are often used after hormonal therapy and vigabatrin.

The effect of these therapies on neurodevelopmental outcome is unknown. Without strong evidence to support a particular agent, the potential risks of each therapy should influence individual treatment decisions.

LATE ONSET EPILEPTIC SPASMS

Although the focus of most of this chapter has been on infantile spasms that by definition occur during infancy, epileptic spasms can occur in older children though less is known about this clinical presentation. A few studies have described various cohorts from 19 to 54 patients, and there are several features that distinguish late onset spasms from the classical infantile spasms. First, the interictal EEG does not show classical hypsarrhythmia. EEG backgrounds are still very abnormal, often showing both generalized and multifocal spikes with an anterior predominance in the temporal or temporofrontal regions. These cohorts also report a high incidence of asymmetric spasms. Underlying etiologies included tuberous sclerosis, diffuse cortical dysplasia, temporomesial hypoplasia, callosal agenesis, leukoencephalopathy, and hypoxic-ischemic encephalopathy. Response to treatment in these various studies has been variable. The agents that appear to be effective are similar to those used in infantile spasms including ACTH, hydrocortisone, and vigabatrin. In the studies that evaluated developmental outcomes, it is clear that late onset epileptic spasms is still an epileptic encephalopathy with only rare children having normal developmental outcomes.

REFERENCES

The complete list of references for this chapter is available in the e-book at www.expertconsult.com.
 See inside cover for registration details.

SELECTED REFERENCES

Berg, A.T., Berkovic, S.F., Brodie, M.J., et al., 2010. Revised terminology and concepts for organization of seizures and epilepsies: report of the ILAE Commission on Classification and Terminology, 2005–2009. Epilepsia 51 (4), 676–685.

Djuric, M., Kravljanac, R., Tadic, B., et al., 2014. Long-term outcome in children with infantile spasms treated with vigabatrin: a cohort of 180 patients. Epilepsia 55 (12), 1918–1925.

Go, C.Y., Mackay, M.T., Weiss, S.K., et al., 2012. Evidence-based guideline update: medical treatment of infantile spasms. Report of the Guideline Development Subcommittee of the American Academy of Neurology and the Practice Committee of the Child Neurology Society. Neurology 78 (24), 1974–1980.

Hancock, E.C., Osborne, J.P., Edwards, S.W., 2008. Treatment of infantile spasms. Cochrane Database Syst. Rev. (4), CD001770.

O'Callaghan, F.J., Lux, A.L., Darke, K., et al., 2011. The effect of lead time to treatment and of age of onset on developmental outcome at 4 years in infantile spasms: evidence from the United Kingdom Infantile Spasms Study. Epilepsia 52 (7), 1359–1364.

Oguni, H., Tanaka, T., Hayashi, K., et al., 2002. Treatment and long-term prognosis of myoclonic-astatic epilepsy of early childhood. Neuropediatrics 33 (3), 122–132.

Paciorkowski, A.R., Thio, L.L., Dobyns, W.B., 2011. Genetic and biologic classification of infantile spasms. Pediatr. Neurol. 45 (6), 355–367.

Pellock, J.M., Hrachovy, R., Shinnar, S., et al., 2010. Infantile spasms: a U.S. consensus report. Epilepsia 51 (10), 2175–2189.

Riikonen, R., 1982. A long-term follow-up study of 214 children with the syndrome of infantile spasms. Neuropediatrics 13 (1), 14–23.

Riikonen, R.S., 2010. Favorable prognostic factors with infantile spasms. Eur. J. Paediatr. Neurol. 14 (1), 13–18.

E-BOOK FIGURES AND TABLES

The following figures and tables are available in the e-book at www.expertconsult.com. See inside cover for registration details.

Fig. 68-1 Hypsarrthymia with electro decrement
Fig. 68-2 Investigations for new onset IS.
Table 68-1 Common Pediatric Epilepsy Syndromes with Prominent Myoclonic Seizures
Table 68-2 Differentiating Features of PME
Table 68-4 Treatment with Oral Prednisolone UCLA Protocol

69 Status Epilepticus

Iván Sánchez Fernández, Nicholas Scott Abend, and Tobias Loddenkemper

 An expanded version of this chapter is available on www.expertconsult.com. See inside cover for registration details.

Status epilepticus (SE) is one of the most common neurologic emergencies in the pediatric population (Chin, et al., 2006) and is associated with mortality, neurodevelopmental sequelae (DeLorenzo, et al., 1996), and subsequent reductions in quality of life. In this chapter, we will review the epidemiology, clinical presentation, treatment, and outcome of SE. Unless stated otherwise, we will refer to convulsive SE and will only briefly describe nonconvulsive SE.

EPIDEMIOLOGY

Approximately 17 to 23 of 100,000 children experience SE every year with the highest incidence in children less than 1 year of age. In a large series in the UK, the overall incidence was 14.5 of 100,000 (95% CI: 11.5 to 17.6). The incidence was highest in children younger than 1 year (51 of 100,000; 95% CI: 35 to 66), and progressively decreased with increasing age: in children aged 1 to 4 years the incidence was 29 of 100,000 (95% CI: 19 to 35), in children aged 5 to 9 years it was 9 of 100,000 (95% CI: 5 to 11), and in children aged 10 to 15 years the incidence was 2 of 100,000 (95% CI: 0.75 to 3.5). If febrile SE is excluded, the incidence decreases by 25% to 40%. Children with SE have an overall mortality of approximately 0% to 3%. Additionally, a high proportion of children with SE develop subsequent epilepsy and severe cognitive deficits (Raspall-Chaure, et al., 2006).

DEFINITIONS

The essential feature that differentiates SE from other seizures is duration. SE presents as a seizure that lasts longer than expected. The International League Against Epilepsy (ILAE) defines SE as "a seizure that shows no clinical signs of arresting after a duration encompassing the great majority of seizures of that type in most patients or recurrent seizures without interictal resumption of baseline central nervous system function." The ILAE Task Force on Classification of SE proposed the following definition: "SE is a condition resulting either from the failure of the mechanisms responsible for seizure termination or from the initiation of mechanisms which lead to abnormally prolonged seizures (after time point t1). It is a condition that can have long-term consequences (after time point t2), including neuronal death, neuronal injury, and alteration of neuronal networks, depending on the type and duration of seizures." This definition emphasizes the importance of time by defining two time points: t1—the time beyond which the seizure should be considered as "continuous seizure activity"; and t2—the time beyond which there is a risk of long-term consequences. How long a seizure or a cluster of seizures must last to be considered SE is a matter of discussion. The classical definition of established SE requires that seizures (continuous or intermittent without return to baseline mental status) last for a minimum of 30 minutes. However, seizures which last longer than 5 minutes are unlikely to stop spontaneously and may be referred to as impending SE. Management at that time may be indicated to prevent the seizure from lasting 30 minutes at which time it may be producing secondary brain injury.

The classical 30-minute cut-off is based on the fact that approximately after 30 minutes of generalized seizures, the compensatory mechanisms fail against acidosis, hyperthermia, hyperkalemia, and cardiocirculatory collapse. Thus SE-induced irreversible neuronal damage occurs, and seizures become self-sustained and refractory to treatment. The 30-minute cut-off is consistent with epidemiologic studies such as the Richmond SE study, in which mortality for seizures lasting 10 to 29 minutes was 2.6% whereas mortality for seizures lasting longer than 29 minutes was 19%. However, the 30-minute cut-off may miss a window for optimal treatment effectiveness. Treatment in SE should not be delayed until patients reach the established SE stage when neuronal injury and pharmacoresistance have already occurred. The 5-minute cut-off emphasizes this window of opportunity for treatment by identifying seizures with a high risk of progressing to cause neuronal damage and becoming pharmacoresistant at a stage when treatment still can prevent these outcomes.

The 5-minute cut-off for SE is most frequently used in clinical practice as treatment should be initiated after 5 minutes of seizure duration. The 30-minute cut-off is more commonly used in retrospective investigations to study a relatively homogeneous group of patients in whom some degree of neuronal damage and in whom pharmacoresistance has already developed. There are limited studies comparing the clinical characteristics of impending and established SE. A series of 226 patients (135 adults and 91 children) compared seizures lasting 10 to 29 minutes with seizures lasting more than 29 minutes. Demographic characteristics such as gender, race, age, and etiology were similar between the two groups. In the 10- to 29-minute group, seizures stopped spontaneously in 43% of patients whereas in 57% did not. In a series of 445 children aged 1 month to 21 years with seizures lasting more than 5 minutes, a comparison was made between the 296 patients with seizures of 5 to 29 minutes duration and the 149 patients with seizures of 30 or more minutes duration. Patients with seizures of more than 29 minutes duration were younger at the time of seizure onset and were more likely to present with SE. However, there were no differences in seizure frequency, seizure types, presence of developmental delay, and electroencephalographic (EEG) abnormalities at baseline. In a population of 1062 children aged 1 month to 21 years of age with seizures, two different thresholds for SE were used: 5 minutes and 30 minutes. The risk factors for SE were similar when considering the 5-minute or the 30-minute thresholds. In summary, impending and established SE are probably a continuum and the different thresholds are arbitrary cut-offs. What is more, the 5-minute and 30-minute thresholds are essentially derived from studies on generalized seizures. The conceptualization as t1 and t2 emphasizes the need to estimate these times for different seizure types.

TABLE 69-1 Frequency of the Most Common Etiologies of Pediatric Status Epilepticus

	Febrile Seizures	Acute Metabolic Derangement or Central Nervous System Infection	Remote Symptomatic	Acute Symptomatic on Remote Symptomatic	Low Antiepileptic Drug Levels
Chin, et al., 2006 (N = 226)	33%	17%	16%	16%	
De Lorenzo, et al., 1996 (N = 166)	52%*		39%		21%
Singh, et al., 2010 (N = 144)	32%	9%	18%		

*Infections with fever

ETIOLOGY

Most episodes of SE begin in previously healthy children in the out-of-hospital setting. In a large prospective study of 226 children with SE in the United Kingdom, 78% of cases were first-ever episodes of SE. Of those, 56% of patients had normal neurodevelopment at baseline, no history of epilepsy, and no neurologic deficits before the SE episode. The most common etiology of pediatric SE is febrile/infectious followed by other acute symptomatic causes (Table 69-1). Acute symptomatic etiologies are more frequent in younger patients, especially in patients younger than 1 year of age.

A variety of still unknown genetic factors might promote or protect patients from developing prolonged seizures. A study on 8681 twin pairs found a much higher rate of SE concordance in monozygotic than in dizygotic twins (0.38 versus 0). The genetic predisposition to prolonged seizures and SE is probably complex and multifactorial and susceptibility genes are still to be discovered in humans.

CLINICAL PRESENTATION AND INITIAL MANAGEMENT

Any type of seizure may become prolonged and thus evolve into SE. Generalized tonic-clonic SE is the clinically apparent and life-threatening form of SE. Other forms include myoclonic, clonic, tonic, or absence SE. Seizures can be focal or more generalized. Some generalized seizures have a generalized onset whereas others secondarily generalize from initially focal seizures.

Regardless of the etiology and type, SE represents a life-threatening emergency that should be managed rapidly. Generalized tonic-clonic SE is associated with intense muscle activity with the consequent metabolic and cardiovascular demands as well as the risk of multiorgan failure if the needs to sustain intense muscle activity exceed the patient's reserve and if they are sufficiently prolonged. Focal seizures are associated with less metabolic demands but are equally harmful to the brain if sustained in time.

The initial therapy for SE includes maintenance of adequate brain oxygenation and cardiorespiratory function, identification and correction of seizure triggers such as hypoglycemia, electrolyte imbalance, lowered drug levels, infection, and fever, and prevention of systemic complications. In addition to the general management of any pediatric emergency, a main goal of SE treatment is to terminate clinical and electrical seizure as quickly as possible.

TIME TO TREATMENT
Rationale Behind the Need for Rapid Treatment

There are three major determinants of prognosis in SE: age, etiology, and SE duration (Raspall-Chaure, et al., 2006). Age

is a nonmodifiable factor. Etiology is usually not modifiable at least in the short term. In contrast, SE duration might be modified with appropriate and timely treatment management.

The current guidelines and protocols for the treatment of SE recommend rapid administration of antiseizure drugs. These recommendations are based on results from basic and clinical research. Animal models of SE have demonstrated that prolonged seizures cause brain damage independently from the underlying etiology. In addition, several clinical studies have demonstrated that prolonged seizures are associated with worse outcomes. In a study of 182 children with SE, for each minute delay from seizure onset to arrival at the emergency department, there was a 5% cumulative increase in the risk of SE lasting more than 60 minutes. A series of 45 episodes of pediatric SE compared 19 episodes treated with prehospital diazepam with 26 episodes not treated before hospital arrival; the duration of SE was shorter (32 versus 60 minutes) and the risk of recurrent seizures was lower (58% versus 85%) in the 19 episodes treated before hospital arrival. In a series of 157 children with SE, a delay of more than 30 minutes in administering the first antiseizure drug was associated with worse response to treatment (measured as time from the initiation of the treatment to the end of the clinical seizure activity). Another study reported 27 children in whom first line (benzodiazepine) and second-line (phenytoin or phenobarbital) medications were effective in terminating SE in 86% when seizure duration was less than 20 minutes at presentation and only in 15% when seizure duration exceeded 30 minutes. Studies in adults also suggest that a longer duration of SE is associated with a worse prognosis in terms of seizure duration, morbidity, and mortality. These results suggest that an early and appropriate treatment may markedly reduce the duration and improve patient outcomes.

Changes in Neurotransmitter Receptors in the Seizing Brain

As seizures last longer, they become self-sustained and progressively more treatment resistant. The physiologic basis for these processes is only partially understood. In a series of surgical brain samples from three patients with refractory convulsive SE, three patients with electrical status epilepticus in sleep (ESES), and six patients with refractory epilepsy compared with brain samples from four autopsy controls who died without neurologic disorders, subunit composition of neurotransmitter receptors demonstrated the following patterns: elevated GluA1/GluA2 in the alpha-amino-3-hydroxy-5-methyl-4-isoxazolepropionic acid (AMPA) receptors, increased GluN2B/GluN2A ratio in the N-methyl-D-aspartate (NMDA) receptors, and elevated $\alpha2/\alpha1$ in the GABA receptors. These results are concordant with similar results from animal models and other human studies and the elevated ratios are known to promote excitation over inhibition. Further, when the brain is exposed to prolonged seizures, there is a rapid decrease in the number of postsynaptic $GABA_A$ receptors and an increase in the number of functional postsynaptic NMDA receptors. This loss of inhibition and increase in excitation in the brain synapses promote self-sustaining of prolonged seizures and may explain the loss of efficacy of benzodiazepines over time in animal models of SE and the progressive pharmacoresistance to benzodiazepines with prolonged SE.

Time Elapsed From Seizure Onset to Treatment Administration in SE

Whereas these data suggest the importance of rapid antiseizure drug administration in SE, a limited number of studies have evaluated the time elapsed from seizure onset to treatment initiation in SE. Paucity of data can be partially attributed to the fact that most seizures stop after a first medication is administered in the field or are managed in non-referral hospitals. Even in prolonged seizures it is difficult to measure the time elapsed from seizure onset to administration of antiseizure drug.

The few available studies on this topic suggest there are often important delays in treatment administration. In a series of 199 children with febrile SE the median time from seizure onset to administration of the first antiseizure drug was 30 minutes. In a retrospective study of 889 patients (625 adults and 264 children) with SE, approximately 60% of the patients received their first dose after 30 minutes and approximately 25% after 60 minutes. In a retrospective multicenter study of 542 episodes of convulsive seizures of 10 or more minutes duration in children, the median (p_{25} to p_{75}) time from hospital arrival until administration of a nonbenzodiazepine was 24 (15 to 36) minutes. Among 82 adults with SE the time elapsed from seizure onset to administration of nonbenzodiazepine was 180 minutes. The primary outcome in a recent series of 81 children with refractory convulsive SE was the time elapsed from seizure onset to administration of medications. The median (p_{25} to p_{75}) time elapsed from seizure onset to the administration of the first drug was 28 (6 to 67) minutes, to the second was 40 (20 to 85) minutes, and to the third was 59 (30 to 120) minutes. Further, the median (p_{25} to p_{75}) time to administration of the first nonbenzodiazepine was 69 (40 to 120) minutes, and in the 64 patients with out-of-hospital SE onset, 40 (63%) did not receive any antiseizure medicine before hospital arrival.

These data suggest several areas for improvement in the time to treatment of SE including earlier detection and treatment of seizures, more widespread use of home and emergency medical system use of benzodiazepines, and rapid escalation in the administration of medications if seizures persist.

TREATMENT OPTIONS
Treatment Guidelines for SE

Most guidelines and protocols for the treatment of SE recommend a stepwise approach. The first step in the treatment of a seizure, as in any other emergency situation, is to secure the airway, ensure adequate breathing and circulation. Importantly, most seizures resolve spontaneously in less than 5 minutes and will not require rescue medication. However, when seizures last more than 5 minutes, they should be considered as impending SE, and treatment should be initiated immediately. Benzodiazepines are the first-line treatment and, among them, intravenous lorazepam is frequently the preferred option. When intravenous access is not available, intramuscular, rectal, intranasal, or buccal medication applications are potential alternatives. The first dose of benzodiazepines can be repeated if seizures persist. As seizures persist, however, they become progressively more refractory to benzodiazepines. Thus after 10 minutes, rather than administering subsequent doses of benzodiazepines, it may be useful to switch to a nonbenzodiazepine. Among those, the most commonly used antiseizure medication is intravenous fosphenytoin (or phenytoin). If seizures continue, then another nonbenzodiazepine is recommended with phenobarbital as the preferred option. Other nonbenzodiazepine medications that can also be administered intravenously are valproate and levetiracetam. However, once two appropriate doses of nonbenzodiazepine antiseizure drugs have been administered and/or seizure duration is longer than 30 to 60 minutes, initiation of continuous infusions with anesthetic therapy is recommended (Fig. 69-3) (Table 69-2). During this progression, it is important to consider and prepare for the next steps if seizures persist. This will ensure subsequent medications are available at bedside when needed.

Benzodiazepines as First-Line Treatment

Benzodiazepines are typically used as initial treatment for SE because of their wide availability, initial efficacy, and multiple routes of administration. In a double-blind trial, 205 adults with out-of-hospital seizures of at least 5 minutes duration were randomized to receive either intravenous lorazepam, intravenous diazepam, or a placebo. Seizures had been terminated on arrival at the emergency department in more patients treated with lorazepam (59%) or diazepam (43%) (no statistically significant differences in efficacy between lorazepam and diazepam) than in patients treated with placebo (21%). The rates of respiratory or circulatory complications were 11% for lorazepam, 10% for diazepam, and 23% for placebo. This landmark study established that treatment with

TABLE 69-2 Recommended Initial Doses for SE

Drug	Dose	Maximum Dose	Route and Rate
Lorazepam iv	0.1 mg/kg	4 mg	iv push
Diazepam iv	0.3 mg/kg	10 mg	iv push
Diazepam rectally	0.2–0.5 mg/kg	20 mg	Rectal, bolus
Midazolam nasally	0.2–0.3 mg/kg	10 mg	Nasal, bolus
Phenobarbital iv	20 mg/kg	40 mg/kg or 1000 mg	2 mg/kg/min
Fosphenytoin iv	20 mg phenytoin equivalents/kg	300 mg phenytoin equivalents	3 mg phenytoin equivalents/kg/min
Valproate iv	20–40 mg/kg	40 mg/kg	3–6 mg/Kg/min
Levetiracetam iv	30–60 mg/kg	2500 mg	Over 5 min

Legend: iv: intravenous.

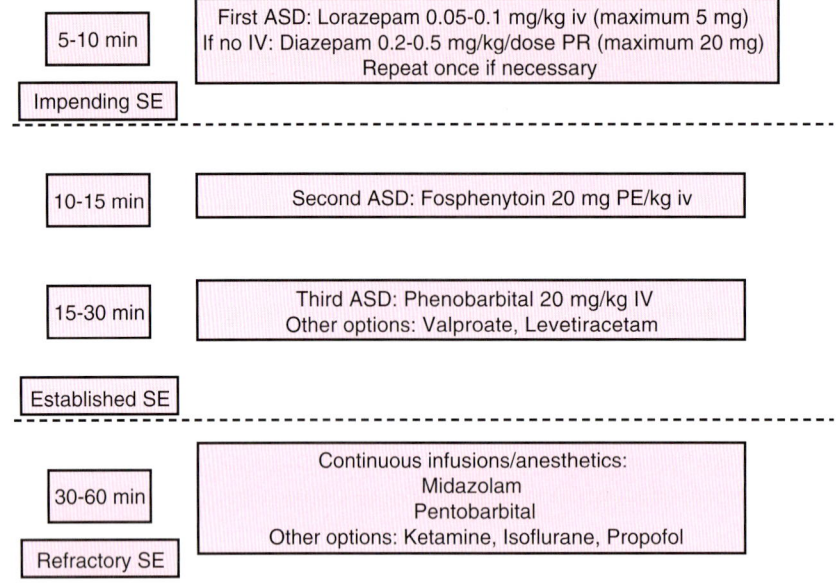

Figure 69-3. Treatment algorithm for status epilepticus. The first-line drug is usually a benzodiazepine (most frequently lorazepam). Sometimes it might be useful to try a second dose of benzodiazepines. However, when seizures last 10 minutes or longer the recommended treatment is fosphenytoin and for seizures of more than 15 to 30 minutes duration a second nonbenzodiazepine antiepileptic drug should be administered. The most commonly used is phenobarbital although other options include valproate or levetiracetam. When seizures last more than 30 to 60 minutes and the patient has not responded to prior medications SE can be considered refractory and switch to continuous infusions of antiepileptic drugs or anesthetic therapies is advised. Legend: ASD—antiseizure drug; iv—intravenous; kg—kilograms; mg—milligrams; min—minutes; PE—fosphenytoin equivalents; PR—per rectum; SE—status epilepticus. (*Reproduced with permission from: Sánchez Fernández I, Loddenkemper T. Therapeutic choices in convulsive status epilepticus. Expert Opin Pharmacother 2015;16:487–500.*)

benzodiazepines was more effective and even safer than not treating impending SE in the out-of-hospital setting. The Veterans Affairs Cooperative Trial—another large double-blind study—randomized 384 adults to receive one of four initial treatments for SE: lorazepam, phenobarbital, phenytoin, and diazepam followed by phenytoin. In this study lorazepam was superior to phenytoin, but in an intention-to-treat analysis, there were no differences among the four treatment groups.

Lorazepam as the Preferred First-Line Drug for SE

Intravenous lorazepam has become widely regarded as the optimal first-line medication for SE. The results of the two previously mentioned studies conducted in adults are frequently extrapolated to children, although neither included children. In pediatrics, the preference of lorazepam as first-line therapy is largely based on the large North London series of 182 children with SE, in which treatment with intravenous lorazepam was associated with a 3.7 (95% CI: 1.7 to 7.9) times greater likelihood of seizure cessation than was treatment with rectal diazepam. However, it is important to note that this study was not only comparing medications (lorazepam versus diazepam) but also routes of administration (intravenous versus rectal) which may have different timeframes in terms of medication administration and absorption.

Multiple studies show the efficacy of benzodiazepines as first-line treatment for SE, but it is not clear if one benzodiazepine or route of administration is superior to the others. In a series of 48 children with prolonged seizures treated in the emergency department, there were no differences in the rate of seizure control between patients treated with intravenous diazepam (65%) and intravenous lorazepam (65%). In a double-blind study, 273 children with SE were randomized to receive intravenous diazepam (N = 140) or intravenous

lorazepam (N = 133). The primary efficacy outcome was cessation of SE by 10 minutes without recurrence within 30 minutes, and the primary safety outcome was the need for assisted ventilation. The rate of SE cessation (72% on diazepam and 73% on lorazepam) and the rate of requiring assisted ventilation (16% on diazepam, 18% on lorazepam) were similar for both medications. In a series of 76 episodes of pediatric seizures of at least 5 minutes duration treated with intravenous midazolam bolus doses of 0.1 to 0.2 mg/kg, seizure control was achieved with the first bolus in 40 of 76 (53%) patients, with a second bolus in 20 of 36 (55%), and with a third bolus in 8 of 16 (50%). The Rapid Anticonvulsant Medication Prior to Arrival Trial (RAMPART) randomized 893 patients (both children and adults) to receive intramuscular midazolam or intravenous lorazepam as a first-line, out-of-hospital treatment (Silbergleit, et al., 2012). Seizure resolution at the time of arrival in the emergency department was 73% in the intramuscular midazolam group, and in 63% in the intravenous lorazepam group (Silbergleit, et al., 2012). In a Cochrane review of three studies that included 264 patients, intravenous lorazepam was slightly superior to intravenous diazepam on cessation of seizures and not different in terms of requirement for ventilator support or other adverse effects. A less frequently considered option is intravenous clonazepam, which controlled SE in 16 of 24 patients in one study and 17 of 17 patients in a second study. In summary, intravenous lorazepam, intravenous midazolam, intravenous diazepam, and intramuscular midazolam have demonstrated similar efficacy and safety (Brophy, et al., 2012).

Alternatives to the Intravenous Route of Administration

Intravenous lorazepam is the current first-line treatment for SE, but requiring intravenous access is a major disadvantage.

Most episodes of SE start in an out-of-hospital setting and, even when medical help is available, obtaining intravenous access in an actively convulsing patient can be challenging. Therefore other nonintravenous first-line treatments are being increasingly considered. A meta-analysis concluded that non-intravenous midazolam was at least as safe and effective as intravenous or nonintravenous diazepam in children and young adults. In a prospective study, 24 children with motor seizures of at least 10 minutes duration were randomized to receive intramuscular midazolam or intravenous diazepam. Patients in the midazolam group received medications sooner (mean: 3.3 versus 7.8 minutes) and had more rapid cessation of their seizures (mean: 7.8 versus 11.2 minutes) than patients randomized to diazepam. A series of 28 children with severe epilepsy at a residential school who presented with seizures of at least 5 minutes duration were randomized to receive buccal midazolam or rectal diazepam. In this series, buccal midazolam was shown to be at least as effective (75% of seizure control) as rectal diazepam (59% of seizure control) with no clinically important adverse events in any of the groups. A prospective randomized study of 92 children compared intranasal midazolam (0.2 mg/kg with a maximum of 10 mg) with rectal diazepam (0.3 to 0.5 mg/kg with a maximum of 20 mg) as home treatment of acute seizures. The median time from medication administration to seizure cessation was 3 minutes in the intranasal midazolam group and 4.3 minutes in the rectal diazepam group. There were no differences in the rate of complications between the two groups. A landmark double-blind noninferiority trial randomized 893 patients (both children and adults) to receive intramuscular midazolam or intravenous lorazepam as a first-line, out-of-hospital treatment (Silbergleit, et al., 2012). The primary outcome was absence of seizures at the time of arrival in the emergency department without the need for rescue therapy. As discussed previously, seizure resolution at the time of arrival in the emergency department was similar in the intramuscular midazolam group and in the intravenous lorazepam group (Silbergleit, et al., 2012). There were no significant differences in the need for endotracheal intubation (14% in both groups) or the proportion of seizure recurrence—11% in both groups. In this study, the time saved using the intramuscular route—1.2 minutes in the intramuscular midazolam group and 4.8 minutes in the intravenous lorazepam group—appears to at least offset the delay in the drug onset of action (3.3 minutes in the intramuscular midazolam group and 1.6 minutes in the intravenous lorazepam group). In summary, there are nonintravenous alternatives to lorazepam which have similar efficacy and are easier and faster to administer. Overall, the exact medication choice may be less important than administering whichever benzodiazepine is available by whatever route can be accessed most quickly.

Nonbenzodiazepine Antiseizure Drugs

If benzodiazepines fail to control SE or SE has lasted for at least 10 minutes—at which point benzodiazepines may be less mechanistically likely to terminate seizures—a switch to non-benzodiazepines is recommended. Although there are several nonbenzodiazepines available, evidence supporting one versus others is weak. Only a few studies have specifically addressed the efficacy of second-line medicines in SE. Their methodology and endpoints vary widely and most of the evidence on preferred nonbenzodiazepines comes from observational and retrospective studies.

At present, phenytoin (or fosphenytoin) is the recommended first option as a nonbenzodiazepine. The most common second option when phenytoin (or fosphenytoin) fails to control SE is phenobarbital. These choices are strongly influenced by tradition as these drugs have been available for much longer than any of the newer antiseizure medicines. Therefore they are time-tested, and there is abundant literature on their efficacy and expected side effects. In the North London series of 182 pediatric patients with SE, treatment with intravenous phenytoin as a second-line therapy was associated with a nine times greater likelihood of seizure cessation compared with treatment with rectal paraldehyde. However, when phenytoin is compared with newer drugs, its position as first-line nonbenzodiazepine is unclear. A retrospective series of 167 adults with SE compared phenytoin, valproate, and levetiracetam as second-line agents (after failure of benzodiazepines as first-line drugs). Valproate failed to control SE in 25% of patients in whom it was prescribed, phenytoin in 41%, and levetiracetam in 48%. After adjustment for SE severity, this study showed that valproate was more effective than levetiracetam (or comparing levetiracetam failure with valproate failure: 2.69, 95% CI: 1.19 to 6.08) whereas there was no difference in the efficacy of phenytoin compared with valproate or phenytoin compared with levetiracetam. In a study of generalized convulsive seizures lasting more than 5 minutes which did not respond to a bolus of intravenous diazepam, patients were randomly assigned to either phenobarbital or valproate. Although differences in this study were not statistically significant, there was a tendency toward a higher rate of seizure cessation with valproate than with phenobarbital (90% versus 77%) with fewer associated clinically significant adverse effects (24% versus 74%). A series on SE randomly assigned 68 patients (including both children and adults) to valproate or phenytoin treatment as initial therapy. Seizures terminated in 66% of the cases in the valproate group and in 42% of the cases in the phenytoin group. As a second choice in refractory patients, valproate was effective in 79% and phenytoin was effective in 25% of the cases. There were no marked differences in adverse effects between the two groups. Considering the previously mentioned studies, newer antiseizure medicines such as valproate or levetiracetam deserve consideration as potential first-line nonbenzodiazepines for SE.

A meta-analysis compared the efficacy of phenytoin, phenobarbital, valproate, levetiracetam, and lacosamide to terminate SE persisting after administration of benzodiazepines. Considering phenytoin, there were eight studies reporting 294 episodes of SE in which phenytoin had a mean efficacy of 50% (95% CI: 43 to 66%). For phenobarbital, there were two studies reporting 42 episodes of SE in which phenobarbital had a mean efficacy of 74% (95% CI: 58 to 85%). For valproate, there were eight studies reporting 250 episodes of SE in which valproate had a mean efficacy of 76% (95%CI: 64 to 85%). For levetiracetam, there were eight studies reporting 204 episodes of SE in which levetiracetam had a mean efficacy of 69% (95% CI: 56 to 79%). There was insufficient detail regarding lacosamide to perform a meta-analysis, although lacosamide shows promising results controlling SE in approximately 45% to 68% of cases in some series.

In summary, multiple studies indicate that new drugs such as valproate and levetiracetam have similar, if not superior, efficacy than phenytoin (or fosphenytoin) and phenobarbital. Additionally, valproate and levetiracetam have potential practical advantages: in general, they can be administered faster than phenytoin (or fosphenytoin), have a better pharmacokinetic profile, and have a lower risk of hypotension and respiratory depression. Importantly, valproate is a generally safe drug in adults and children, but it can lead to serious toxicity in children with underlying metabolic disorders—often still undiagnosed when treatment decisions have to be made—or children under 2 years of age. The Established Status Epilepticus Treatment Trial (ESETT) is a large international randomized trial which aims to determine whether valproate and/or levetiracetam are superior to phenytoin as nonbenzodiazepines for treatment of SE in children and adults. The Pediatric Status Epilepticus Research Group (pSERG) is developing a comparative effectiveness trial of the most efficacious second-line treatments for SE.

Refractory SE

SE is considered refractory when it has not been controlled with appropriate doses of benzodiazepines and 1 or 2 doses of nonbenzodiazepine antiseizure drugs. Once SE is refractory, continuous infusions of antiseizure drugs or anesthetic therapies are often recommended. Initiation of treatment with anesthetic medications such as midazolam or pentobarbital may lead to respiratory depression and hypotension, so close cardiopulmonary monitoring is required and the patient should be in an environment in which intubation, mechanical ventilation, and blood pressure management can be performed if required. The most commonly used continuous infusions are midazolam, pentobarbital, and, less commonly in the pediatric setting, propofol. However, there is insufficient evidence to recommend any one in particular over the others.

One of the most frequently used initial continuous infusions is midazolam. Administration often involves a 0.2 mg/kg loading dose followed by 0.2 to 0.6 mg/kg/h infusion rate. Midazolam infusion may produce respiratory depression and hypotension, although hypotension may be less likely than with pentobarbital infusion. Thus the patient must be managed in a critical care environment with continuous cardiopulmonary monitoring. Tachyphylaxis often develops within 24 to 48 hours, so the infusion dose may need to be increased to maintain a constant pharmacologic action. If seizures persist, the midazolam dosage may be increased. Solely increasing the infusion rate may only very slowly raise midazolam levels, so repeating the bolus in addition to infusion rate increases are generally indicated. In a series of patients with refractory SE, continuous infusion of midazolam with a mean infusion rate of 2 µg/kg/min controlled seizures in 19 of 20 (95%) of children after a mean interval of 0.9 hours from infusion initiation (Sutter, et al., 2013). In another series of children with refractory SE, a continuous infusion of midazolam with a mean infusion rate of 3.1 µg/kg/min controlled seizures in 26 of 27 (96%) cases within 65 minutes of the midazolam infusion initiation.

Another common option is pentobarbital infusion. Administration often involves a 5 mg/kg loading dose followed by 1 to 5 mg/kg/h infusion rate. Pentobarbital may produce respiratory depression and hypotension, so the patient must be managed in a critical care environment with continuous cardiopulmonary monitoring. In a retrospective series of children with refractory SE treated with pentobarbital infusion with a mean loading dose of 5.4 mg/kg followed by an initial infusion of 1.1 mg/kg/h and maximum infusion of 4.8 mg/kg/h, 10 of 30 (33%) achieved sustained burst suppression without relapse during therapy. Of the patients who experienced seizure relapse, 12 of 20 (60%) eventually regained burst suppression. The rate of adverse effects in this series was particularly high, with hypotension requiring inotrope medications in 93% of patients, infection in 66%, metabolic acidosis in 10%, and pancreatitis in 10%. Another limitation of pentobarbital is its long half-life, which may make the weaning process challenging.

A third option for continuous infusion is propofol. Administration often involves a 2 mg/kg loading dose followed by 2 to 5 mg/kg/h infusion rate. Importantly, it may cause propofol infusion syndrome, a very severe and often fatal complication most often seen in critically ill children undergoing long-term propofol infusion at high doses. The mechanism underlying propofol infusion syndrome may be propofol-mediated impairment of free fatty acid utilization and mitochondrial activity. An imbalance between energy demand and utilization is a key pathogenic mechanism that may lead to cardiac and peripheral muscle necrosis. The main clinical features of propofol infusion syndrome are cardiovascular collapse with lactic acidosis, hypertriglyceridemia, and rhabdomyolysis. As this syndrome is frequently lethal, propofol infusions with doses of at least 5 mg/kg/h are not recommended for more than 48 hours, especially in children. In a study of children with refractory SE, propofol infusion controlled 14 of 22 (64%) of episodes. In this series, propofol infusion had to be stopped in four patients: one patient had rhabdomyolysis, and three patients developed hypertriglyceridemia that normalized after stopping propofol.

Super-Refractory SE

When SE continues despite one to two continuous infusions, it is considered super-refractory SE. There is no consensus on when SE should be termed super-refractory, but a proposed definition is "status epilepticus that continues for 24 hours or more after the onset of anesthesia, including those cases in which the SE recurs on the reduction or withdrawal of anesthesia." When patients are in super-refractory SE. several therapeutic approaches should be tried sequentially although evidence on their efficacy is generally limited to case reports or small case series (Table 69-3).

Autoimmune SE and Immune Therapies

Autoimmune encephalitis is a rare etiology of SE. However, it is potentially treatable and should therefore be considered, especially when SE is refractory or super-refractory. Patients of any age who develop rapidly progressing symptoms, including a combination of seizures or SE, behavioral changes, and encephalopathy with no other explanation, should have serum and cerebrospinal fluid autoantibody evaluations. The suspicion or confirmation of autoimmune encephalitis should lead to consideration of treatment with immunotherapy such as steroids, intravenous immunoglobulins, or plasma exchange. The response to these treatments is variable, even when an autoimmune etiology is confirmed.

OUTCOME

Children with SE have an overall mortality of approximately 0% to 3%. Considering only children admitted to pediatric intensive care units, the mortality is approximately 5% to 8%. Further, children surviving SE are at risk of lifelong sequelae, including cognitive and neurodevelopmental impairments, new-onset epilepsy, and recurrent SE. Overall, children with history of SE have a lower quality of life scores than children with similar epilepsy who have not experienced SE, even after correcting for demographic and clinical features known to affect quality of life. In addition to characteristics of the SE itself, other factors such as etiology, age, treatment, or treatment adverse effects have important influences on outcome.

Younger children have the highest rates of morbidity and mortality. In a series of 193 children with SE, neurologic sequelae occurred in 29% of infants younger than 1 year of age, 11% of children with ages between 2 and 3 years, and 6% of children older than 3 years. Given that there was no difference in outcome when these results were stratified by etiology, these data reflect the greater incidence of acute neurologic disease (associated with worse outcome) in younger age groups. Most deaths during hospitalization occur in children with acute or remote symptomatic causes and may not be

TABLE 69-3 Treatment Alternatives for Refractory and Super-Refractory Status Epilepticus

	Comments	Adverse Events
Thiopental	Metabolized to pentobarbital	Hypotension Respiratory depression Cardiac depression
Ketamine	Mechanism of action particularly well-suited to treat refractory and super-refractory SE (NMDA receptor antagonist)	High intracranial pressure Hypotension Hallucinations
Inhaled anesthetics	High rate of complications Needs closed system (gas recovery)	Hypotension Infection Paralytic ileus
Ketogenic diet	Relatively safe (no respiratory and cardiocirculatory instability) Slow onset of action Requires skilled dietician	Gastroesophageal reflux Constipation Acidosis Hypertriglyceridemia
Lidocaine	Minor respiratory depression compared with other drugs	Cardiocirculatory instability Possible induction of seizures
Hypothermia	Only transitory control (cannot be a prolonged therapy)	Hypotension Cardiovascular instability Impaired coagulation (bleeding risks)
Resective surgery	Long-term treatment of seizures Not all patients are eligible	Surgical risks

Legend: NMDA—N-methyl-D-aspartate; SE—status epilepticus.

attributable to SE itself. Long-term mortality data also suggests that the etiology of SE is one of the main predictors for long-term survival. Further supporting the hypothesis that mortality is more likely related to the etiology than to SE itself, febrile SE is associated with a negligible mortality.

SE survivors have an increased risk of subsequent epilepsy, which is reported to occur in 13% to 74% of cases (Raspall-Chaure, et al., 2006). SE recurs in approximately 20% of cases within 4 years of initial presentation, with most recurrences during the first 2 years (Raspall-Chaure, et al., 2006). The occurrence of seizures and the recurrence of SE are influenced by the underlying etiology, with structural or metabolic lesions having the highest risk (Raspall-Chaure, et al., 2006).

Subtle neurocognitive dysfunction—such as focal neurologic deficits, cognitive impairment, and behavioral problems—occurs in patients who have experienced SE, but the contribution of etiology, duration, and other potential confounders has not been clarified.

In summary, SE is associated with substantial mortality and morbidity, including subsequent epilepsy and recurrent SE as well as neurocognitive deficits. The effect of SE itself on these adverse outcomes has not been elucidated, but it is possible that the primary etiology and the comorbidities are the main drivers of these outcomes.

NEONATAL STATUS EPILEPTICUS

Several factors are important to consider in neonatal SE.

First, most neonatal seizures occur secondary to acute neurologic injuries such as hypoxic-ischemic encephalopathy, stroke, or infections. Neonatal epilepsy syndromes are much less common (Table 69-4). Because neonatal seizures typically reflect an underlying functional or structural lesion, the mortality and morbidity burdens are typically higher than in older children. In a series of 89 term newborns with clinical seizures, mortality was 7%, and 28% of the survivors had unfavorable long-term outcome defined as moderate to marked abnormalities in neurologic examination or cognition. In a series of 112 newborns with seizures (33 preterm and 79 term), mortality was 2.7%, and among the survivors, 28% had cerebral

palsy, 36% had epilepsy, and almost half of the patients had delay in at least two domains of development. In both, series etiology was a major predictor of outcome.

Second, diagnosis of neonatal seizures is challenging because many repetitive neonatal movements do not have an ictal EEG correlate and conversely because many electrographic seizures do not have associated clinical manifestations. A series of 20 video clips with repetitive neonatal movements—11 of them being EEG-confirmed seizures and nine being movements with no EEG correlate—were evaluated by 91 doctors and 46 other healthcare neonatal intensive care unit professionals. The average number of correctly identified events was 10 of 20 (50%). Further, clinical identification of neonatal seizures alone substantially underestimates their true incidence because approximately 80% of seizures detected on EEG have no clinical correlate. Further, antiseizure medicines may stop clinical seizures although seizures persist on EEG, a phenomenon termed electroclinical uncoupling. Therefore clinical observation alone may yield false positives (nonictal movement leads to administration and escalation of therapies) and false negatives (EEG seizures go undetected and thus untreated). Based on these data, the guideline of the American Clinical Neurophysiology Society (ACNS) on continuous EEG monitoring in neonates states that "conventional video-EEG monitoring is the gold standard for neonatal seizure identification and quantification and should be used whenever available for seizure identification and differential diagnosis of abnormal appearing, paroxysmal clinical events. It is the ideal tool to measure the exact number and duration of seizures, their site(s) of onset, and spatial patterns of migration."

Finally, the definition of SE in newborns is not as straightforward as in older children or adults. One of the main factors in the SE definition is a prolonged seizure or prolonged cluster of seizures without interictal resumption of baseline central nervous system function between seizures. Most newborns with seizures have some degree of encephalopathy because of the underlying acute disorder producing the seizures, thereby making the evaluation of return to baseline neurologic function challenging. There is no consensus on the definition of SE in newborns although some studies have considered it to

TABLE 69-4 Etiology of Neonatal Seizures in a Series of 112 Newborns (33 Preterm and 79 Full-Term)

Etiology	N (%)
Perinatal asphyxia	32 (28.6)
Intracranial bleeding	19 (17)
Metabolic disease	12 (10.7)
Hypoglycemia	9 (8)
Anomaly of cerebral development	5 (4.5)
Familial epileptic syndrome	5 (4.5)
Hyperbilirubinemia	4 (3.6)
Sepsis	4 (3.6)
Meningitis	4 (3.6)
Hypocalcemia	2 (1.8)
Hypoglycemia + hypocalcemia	2 (1.8)
Pyridoxine dependency	2 (1.8)
Benign neonatal convulsions	1 (0.9)
Attributable to drugs	1 (0.9)
Unknown	10 (8.9)

(Reproduced with permission from: Yildiz, E.P., Tatli, B., Ekici, B., et al., 2012. Evaluation of etiologic and prognostic factors in neonatal convulsions. Pediatr Neurol 47, 186–192.)

be present when more than 50% of a 1-hour EEG epoch contains seizures, which may be a single continuous 30-minute seizure or a series of briefer seizures totaling 30 minutes. Regardless of how SE is defined in newborns, a higher seizure burden is associated with less favorable outcomes—even after controlling for potential confounders. Regarding treatment of neonatal seizures and neonatal SE, phenobarbital and phenytoin remain the preferred choices.

NONCONVULSIVE STATUS EPILEPTICUS

Nonconvulsive status epilepticus (NCSE) broadly refers to prolonged seizure activity in the absence of major motor signs or to a change in behavior and/or mental processes from baseline associated with continuous epileptiform discharges in the EEG. Patients with developmental delay, recurrent seizures on multiple medications, and/or critically ill patients are at high risk for developing NCSE, and in these patients, changes in behavior or cognition can be particularly challenging to detect. The incidence of NCSE has been estimated in approximately 2 to 8 of 100,000, although difficulty in identifying NCSE and heterogeneous diagnostic criteria may yield both underestimation and overestimation. NCSE is a heterogeneous condition that can be broadly classified into subcategories: absence NCSE, complex partial NCSE, and NCSE in coma.

Absence NCSE consists of a prolonged state of drowsiness and confusion in which agitation, violent behavior, and hallucinations can occasionally occur. The EEG shows generalized EEG abnormalities markedly different from the interictal state. Relatively subtle myoclonic movements sometimes occur within this category.

Complex partial NCSE consists of periods of abnormal behavior or abnormal cognitive state including amnesia, aphasia, or hemiparesis in between complex partial seizures. EEG findings are focal with preferential involvement of the temporal and frontal lobes and include spike and wave, polyspikes, and rhythmic slowing.

NCSE in coma consists of prolonged or recurrent electrographic seizures in patients in coma. A multicenter trial in the United States included 550 consecutive pediatric patients (1 month to 21 years) in pediatric intensive care units who underwent EEG monitoring. Electrographic seizures were found in 162 children (30%), of which 59 (36%) had no clinical correlate. In a subset of 98 patients from this study who underwent EEG monitoring after convulsive SE, 11 (11%) patients had electrographic-only seizures after termination of their clinically evident convulsions. A prior diagnosis of epilepsy and/or the presence of interictal epileptiform activity on EEG were identified as risk factors for the occurrence of electrographic seizures. Although risk factors may help identify subpopulations at high risk for seizures, some children with NCSE would have been undetected without EEG monitoring.

SUMMARY

SE is a life-threatening emergency that should be controlled as soon as possible. Although SE is considered established after 30 minutes, the operational definition of impending SE at 5 minutes emphasizes the need of an early treatment. Most episodes of pediatric SE start in the out-of-hospital setting in previously healthy children, and the main etiology is symptomatic SE secondary to fever or systemic infection. Many children have acute symptomatic etiologies for SE, so careful evaluation for precipitating etiologies is essential. The initial management of SE consists of cardiorespiratory stabilization and monitoring followed by antiseizure drug to stop the seizures as soon as possible. Benzodiazepines, and in particular intravenous lorazepam, are the preferred first-line treatment, although other benzodiazepines should be considered when intravenous access is not readily available. If one or two doses of benzodiazepines have not controlled SE or more than 10 minutes have elapsed since seizure onset, administration of nonbenzodiazepine medication is warranted. Fosphenytoin followed, if necessary, by phenobarbital are the traditional initial choices in SE, but other agents such as valproate or levetiracetam have demonstrated at least similar efficacy in nonrandomized studies. Throughout treatment, it is important to anticipate the next needed medication so it can be available at bedside if needed. If SE persists after administration of a benzodiazepine and a second antiseizure drug, the patient is in refractory SE. Continued evaluation for underlying etiologies is essential, and initiation of anesthetic drug infusions is generally warranted, with careful monitoring and management of common cardiopulmonary adverse effects associated with these medications. Overall mortality in pediatric SE is approximately 0% to 3%, and sequelae are common. Although SE etiology is the main predictor of outcome, longer SE may also worsen outcome. Thus efforts to rapidly terminate SE as well as identify and manage any underlying treatable etiology are essential.

REFERENCES

The complete list of references for this chapter is available in the e-book at www.expertconsult.com.
See inside cover for registration details.

SELECTED REFERENCES

Brophy, G.M., Bell, R., Claassen, J., et al., 2012. Guidelines for the evaluation and management of status epilepticus. Neurocrit. Care 17, 3–23.

Chin, R.F., Neville, B.G., Peckham, C., et al., 2006. Incidence, cause, and short-term outcome of convulsive status epilepticus in childhood: prospective population-based study. Lancet 368, 222–229.

DeLorenzo, R.J., Hauser, W.A., Towne, A.R., et al., 1996. A prospective, population-based epidemiologic study of status epilepticus in Richmond, Virginia. Neurology 46, 1029–1035.

Raspall-Chaure, M., Chin, R.F., Neville, B.G., et al., 2006. Outcome of paediatric convulsive status epilepticus: a systematic review. Lancet Neurol. 5, 769–779.

Shinnar, S., Berg, A.T., Moshe, S.L., et al., 2001. How long do new-onset seizures in children last? Ann. Neurol. 49, 659–664.

Silbergleit, R., Durkalski, V., Lowenstein, D., et al., 2012. Intramuscular versus intravenous therapy for prehospital status epilepticus. N. Engl. J. Med. 366, 591–600.

Sutter, R., Kaplan, P.W., Ruegg, S., 2013. Outcome predictors for status epilepticus—what really counts. Nat. Rev. Neurol. 9, 525–534.

Treiman, D.M., Meyers, P.D., Walton, N.Y., et al., 1998. A comparison of four treatments for generalized convulsive status epilepticus. Veterans Affairs Status Epilepticus Cooperative Study Group. N. Engl. J. Med. 339, 792–798.

E-BOOK TABLES AND FIGURES

The following figures and tables are available in the e-book at www.expertconsult.com. See inside cover for registration details.

Figure 69-1. Age-specific distribution of the frequency of SE events, the incidence of SE, and the frequency of SE recurrence per year per 100,000 population in Richmond, Virginia.

Figure 69-2. Schematic cartoon of the changes in neurotransmitter receptor concentration at baseline and during prolonged seizures.

70 Electroclinical Syndromes: Neonatal Onset

Abeer J. Hani and Mohamad A. Mikati

An expanded version of this chapter is available on www.expertconsult.com. See inside cover for registration details.

1.0 INTRODUCTION

The recent rapid advances in bedside video-electroencephalogram (EEG) monitoring, genetic techniques, and imaging modalities have markedly improved the identification and treatment of many epilepsy syndromes and their underlying etiologies. The term "electroclinical syndrome" has been used to designate a set of distinctive and recognizable clinical features, signs, and symptoms that define a specific clinical disorder. Often, this includes a typical age of onset, specific EEG characteristics, seizure types, and other features that permit the diagnosis of the specific syndrome. This is important to further guide management and prognosis. The 2010 revised International League Against Epilepsy (ILAE) classification stratified electroclinical epilepsy syndromes by typical age of onset (Table 70-1). There are four neonatal-onset electroclinical syndromes, two of which are benign: benign neonatal seizures and benign familial neonatal seizures. The other two neonatal epilepsy syndromes are early infantile epileptic encephalopathy and early myoclonic encephalopathy. In this chapter, these neonatal onset electroclinical syndromes will be discussed. For each syndrome, the clinical features, etiology, diagnosis, treatment, and prognosis will be detailed. Most neonatal seizures are often acute and symptomatic in response to a specific etiology such as hypoxic ischemic injury, central nervous system (CNS) infection or trauma, brain infarction, electrolyte disturbances, congenital brain malformations, and inborn errors of metabolism. Seizures due to neonatal-onset electroclinical syndromes are rare compared with acute neonatal seizures; however, prompt identification has implications that often are essential to guide further treatment and prognosis.

2.0 BENIGN NEONATAL SEIZURES

This is a benign electroclinical syndrome that is seen in neonates. It is also referred to as the *fifth day fits* or *benign idiopathic neonatal convulsions*.

2.1 Clinical Features

These seizures occur in term and late preterm infants born after an uneventful pregnancy, labor, and delivery. The prevalence is estimated to be between 4% and 38% of neonatal seizures with males constituting about 62% of the cases. Seizures occur within the first week of life, and 90% of the seizures occur between days 4 and 6 of life. Often, there is no family history of epilepsy, and the neonates are otherwise asymptomatic with normal neurologic examinations between the seizures. The presentation is in the form of repetitive seizures lasting from 1 to 2 minutes, sometimes recurring in clonic status epilepticus that last hours. Seizures may recur during a period of 24 to 48 hours but often do not persist beyond that period. Most frequently, seizures seen are unifocal clonic with rare focal tonic seizures.

2.2 Etiology

The pathogenic mechanism remains unclear with a hypothesis that a causal relationship may exist between rotavirus infections and benign neonatal seizures, but the virus was not identified in cerebrospinal fluid (CSF) (Plouin and Kaminska, 2013). Alternative theories implicate the role of a CSF zinc defect as a possible etiologic mechanism (Plouin and Kaminska, 2013).

2.3 Diagnosis

Diagnosis is based mostly on elements of the history and physical examination that are concordant with the expected clinical features. There is no characteristic ictal EEG pattern, but the interictal EEG may be normal or discontinuous or show multifocal sharp waves. A specific EEG pattern called *theta pointu alternant* is seen in 60% of the cases. This pattern may also be seen in cases with hypocalcemia, neonatal meningitis, and subarachnoid hemorrhage. This rhythm consists of nonreactive, discontinuous focal, rhythmic theta activity that may be mixed with sharp waves. The activity may shift between hemispheres, and this EEG pattern may persist for up to 2 weeks even after resolution of the clinical seizures (Mizrahi and Clancy, 2000).

The following criteria have been proposed for the diagnosis of benign neonatal seizures (Mizrahi and Clancy, 2000):

- Normal pregnancy and delivery
- Full-term gestation
- Appropriate for gestational age birth weight
- Apgar score greater than 7 at 1 minute
- Typical interval between birth and seizure onset (4 to 6 days)
- Normal neurologic examination before seizures and interictally
- Normal laboratory findings (including, but not limited to, metabolic studies, neuroimaging, and lumbar puncture)
- No family history of neonatal seizures or postneonatal epilepsy

2.4 Differential Diagnosis

It is important to differentiate benign neonatal seizures from other nonepileptic phenomena including tremors, benign neonatal myoclonus and hyperekplexia. Also, symptomatic seizures due to various etiologies need to be ruled out (Co, et al., 2007). A family history is important to differentiate this entity from benign familial neonatal seizures.

2.5 Prognosis

The expected outcome of these patients is favorable in terms of neurodevelopment and risk for postneonatal epilepsy, although long-term, follow-up studies are still lacking. Some

TABLE 70-1 Electroclinical Syndromes Arranged by Typical Age of Onset

Age of Onset	Epilepsy Syndromes
Neonatal	Benign neonatal seizures Benign familial neonatal epilepsy (BFNE) Ohtahara syndrome Early myoclonic encephalopathy
Infancy	Febrile seizures; febrile seizures plus Benign infantile epilepsy Benign familial infantile epilepsy West syndrome Dravet syndrome Myoclonic epilepsy in infancy Myoclonic encephalopathy in nonprogressive disorders Epilepsy of infancy with migrating focal seizures
Childhood	Febrile seizures; febrile seizures plus early-onset childhood occipital epilepsy (Panayiotopoulos) Epilepsy with myoclonic atonic seizures Childhood absence epilepsy Benign epilepsy with centrotemporal spikes Autosomal dominant nocturnal frontal lobe epilepsy Late-onset childhood occipital epilepsy (Gastaut type) Epilepsy with myoclonic absences Lennox-Gastaut syndrome Epileptic encephalopathy with continuous spike-and-wave during sleep Landau-Kleffner syndrome
Adolescence—Adult	Juvenile absence epilepsy Juvenile myoclonic epilepsy Epilepsy with generalized tonic-clonic seizures alone Autosomal dominant epilepsy with auditory features Other familial temporal lobe epilepsies
Variable age at onset	Familial focal epilepsy with variable foci (childhood to adult) Progressive myoclonus epilepsies Reflex epilepsies

(Adapted from data in International League Against Epilepsy proposal for Revised Terminology for Organization of Seizures and Epilepsies, 2010. http://www.ilae.org/Commission/Class/documents/ILAE%20HandoutV10.pdf. Accessed March 2015)

studies suggested the presence of minor psychomotor deficits and the possibility of febrile and afebrile seizures.

2.6 Management

The treatment of benign neonatal seizures is controversial. More often, these seizures are treated as acute seizures as the workup is being conducted. Often, phenobarbital is started and then ultimately weaned as the seizures stop and the diagnosis is established. The controversy is that because most of the seizures are brief and self-limited, one may argue that no antiseizure medication may be needed.

3.0 BENIGN FAMILIAL NEONATAL EPILEPSY (BFNE)

This was classically thought of as a benign epilepsy syndrome in the neonatal period and was the first epilepsy syndrome for which the causative genes were identified.

3.1 Clinical Features

This is an autosomal dominant syndrome with a high degree (approximately 85%) of penetrance, the prevalence of which is estimated to be about 14.4 per 100,000. Seizures often start between days 2 and 3 in 80% of the cases in an otherwise healthy term infant, and usually by 1 week of life. Preterm infants may develop seizures later and rarely seizures may occur as late as 3 months (Miles and Holmes, 1990). Seizures are stereotyped starting with hypertonia and brief apnea. This is then followed by autonomic manifestations and oculo-facial and clonic movements of the limbs. Seizures are brief, lasting 1 to 2 minutes, and may be as frequent as 20 to 30 per day. A sample EEG recording of such a seizure is illustrated in Figure 70-1. The seizures may alternatively involve both sides. 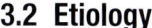 There is no report of myoclonic seizures, spasms, or generalized tonic-clonic seizures with this epilepsy syndrome (Plouin and Kaminska, 2013).

3.2 Etiology

Mutations in genes encoding the subunits of the potassium channels KCNQ2 (on chromosome 20q) and KCNQ3 (on chromosome 8q) are the etiologic factors contributing to benign familial neonatal epilepsy (BFNE). Although it was thought previously that these mutations often result in a benign epilepsy syndrome, recent advances in genetic testing have shown that KCNQ2, and rarely KCNQ3, mutations may result in a picture of severe encephalopathy severe encephalopathy often seen in infancy (Allen et al., 2014). The mutations seen in BFNE are thought to cause a reduction in the current amplitude through the potassium channels, which leads to a transient susceptibility to seizures. The more severe phenotypes of epileptic encephalopathy have been reported to be associated with loss of function as well as with dominant negative and gain of function effects.

3.3 Diagnosis

The brain imaging and metabolic and biochemical screening are usually unremarkable. The interictal EEG may also be normal or discontinuous, or may show focal or multifocal abnormalities. A theta pointu alternant pattern may also be seen. The ictal EEG (Fig. 70-1) often shows onset with bilateral flattening for few seconds coinciding with apnea and tonic activity. This is then followed by asymmetric discharges for 1 to 2 minutes coinciding with the automatisms and clonic activity. The diagnosis of BFNE often is made when there is a normal neurologic examination, family history of neonatal seizures, exclusion of other etiologies of neonatal seizures, and features consistent with seizures expected in BFNE with confirmation on gene testing.

3.4 Differential Diagnosis

BFNE is often a diagnosis of exclusion as a family history of neonatal seizures is needed to establish the diagnosis and is not always available. Similar to benign neonatal seizures, other etiologies need to be excluded including benign neonatal seizures. Genetic testing may also be done and can help confirm the diagnosis. (Table 70-2) compares BFNE and benign neonatal seizures.

3.5 Prognosis

Seizures abate between 1 and 6 months from onset, with about two-thirds remitting in the first 6 weeks. The risk of subsequent epilepsy has been found to be about 16% in some studies. There is no increased risk of intellectual disability or learning difficulties otherwise.

3.6 Management

Seizures usually remit even without treatment but antiseizure medications are often used to shorten or stop recurrent seizures with options including benzodiazepines, phenobarbital, phenytoin, or levetiracetam. Often, it is recommended to stop treatment, if initiated, within 3 to 6 months.

4.0 OHTAHARA SYNDROME

This is also referred to as Early Infantile Epileptic Encephalopathy (EIEE) and is part of the spectrum of severe epileptic encephalopathies that may start in the neonatal period.

4.1 Clinical Features

The onset of Ohtahara syndrome is often within the first 10 days of life in the form of tonic spasms with a characteristic EEG picture of burst suppression. At times, intrauterine onset with increased fetal movements is suspected with onset delayed up to 3 months in some cases. A slight male predominance is present. The prevalence and incidence are not known.

The spasms often consist of tonic forward flexion that lasts 1 to 10 seconds often occurring in clusters 10 to 300 times per day. The spasms may be lateralized and may occur during wakefulness and sleep (Yamamoto et al., 2011). Soon after the onset of the seizures, the infant becomes hypotonic with poor activity, and psychomotor development is arrested with subsequent development of diplegia, spasticity, ataxia, or dystonia.

4.2 Etiology

The most commonly cited etiologic factors of Ohtahara syndrome consist of malformations of brain development. These include hemimegalencephaly, porencephaly, cerebral atrophy, Aicardi syndrome, olivary-dentate dysplasia, agenesis of mammillary bodies, linear sebaceous nevus syndrome, cerebral dysgenesis, and migrational defects (Beal et al., 2012).

Metabolic disorders may be seen in some cases of Ohtahara syndrome (although they are more likely to cause early myoclonic encephalopathy), including glycine encephalopathy (also called nonketotic hyperglycinemia), cytochrome C oxidase deficiency, Leigh encephalopathy, pyridoxine and pyridoxal-5-phosphate dependency, carnitine palmitoyltransferase deficiency, biotinidase deficiency, and mitochondrial respiratory chain complex I deficiency (Beal et al., 2012).

The recent advances in genetic studies have permitted the identification of a wide range of genes that cause EIEE (Table 70-3). Although many of these genetic EIEE present in the infantile period, many present neonatally also:

- EIEE1 caused by gene mutations in ARX—encoding the Aristaless-related homeobox protein involved in cerebral development and patterning—was first discovered as a cause of idiopathic EIEE in patients with early onset seizures in the neonatal or infantile periods with no associated brain malformations. These were due to mutations in the ARX gene outside the homeobox and those with polyalanine expansion mutations. Premature termination mutations and missense mutations within the homeobox of the ARX gene, however, were found to be associated with lissencephaly and abnormal genitalia. This disorder affects males. Females are carriers (X-linked recessive).

- EIEE2 caused by gene mutations in CDKL5—encoding cyclin-dependent kinase like-5 protein involved in regulation of other gene function including MeCP2—has also been described in neonates as early as 10 days of life presenting with generalized convulsions. This disorder predominantly affects females (X-linked dominant).

- EIEE3 caused by gene mutation in SLC25A22—encoding a mitochondrial glutamate carrier—may present in the form of migrating partial clonic seizures within the first 2 weeks of life along with hypotonia and brisk reflexes.

- EIEE4 caused by STXBP1 gene mutation—encoding syntaxin binding protein 1—presents as Ohtahara syndrome often as early as 3 days of age up to 4.5 months of age with tonic or tonic clonic seizures and profound global developmental delay and intellectual disability.

- EIEE7 caused by KCNQ2 mutations have been found to be present in patients with tonic seizures starting in the neonatal period before 2 weeks of age with diagnosis of Ohtahara syndrome.

- EIEE11 caused by SCN2A—encoding the alpha subunit of the voltage-gated sodium channel—may also present in the neonatal period with refractory focal and generalized seizures as early as the first day of life along with neonatal hypotonia.

Mutations of many of these genes and an expanding number of others, such as in the SIK1, CAK, BRAT1, and PIGA genes, may present as neonatal epileptic encephalopathy with classical features of Ohtahara syndrome, or at other times without burst suppression or tonic seizures but with markedly abnormal EEGs, and with drug-resistant seizures of other types, such as focal seizures.

4.3 Diagnosis

The diagnosis often involves identification of the seizures in the neonatal period. The EEG picture often shows a characteristic burst-suppression pattern. The EEG background consists of high voltage (150 to 350 microvolt) slow waves with intermixed multifocal spikes lasting 2 to 3 seconds with periods of suppression lasting for 3 to 5 seconds (Fig. 70-2). This pattern of burst suppression is continuous during wakefulness and sleep; this continuity at times helps distinguish Ohtahara syndrome from early myoclonic encephalopathy (Ohtahara and Yamatogi, 2003). Table 70-4 compares the two syndromes. During a spasm, the activity is more synchronized with a high-voltage slow wave seen followed by generalized fast activity.

The burst-suppression pattern disappears within the first 6 months of life and is often replaced by hypsarrhythmia with progression to West syndrome; it may later progress to a slow-spike wave EEG pattern with Lennox-Gastaut syndrome.

Brain imaging often confirms the presence of an underlying cerebral malformation. Metabolic screening and genetic testing should also be sought to help determine an underlying etiology. Metabolic workup similar to that described for early myoclonic encephalopathy and comprehensive epilepsy gene panels are often used, and whole exome sequencing may be needed in some cases.

4.4 Differential Diagnosis

Ohtahara syndrome is often confused with early myoclonic epilepsy given the similar EEG presentations at times and the overlap between the two syndromes. Table 70-4 shows the differentiating factors between the syndromes. Other differential diagnoses to consider may be early-onset West syndrome or other causes of EIEE. It is also important to differentiate this syndrome from severe neonatal hypoxic-ischemic encephalopathy with burst-suppression pattern.

4.5 Prognosis

Ohtahara syndrome is often associated with high mortality and morbidity. About half of the patients die in infancy and others develop permanent severe mental and neurologic deficits. Often, patients who survive may progress into West syndrome and later into Lennox-Gastaut syndrome with persistent high mortality and severe psychomotor delays.

4.6 Treatment

Often treatment of the seizures proves to be challenging with the absence of effective treatment most of the time. Benzodiazepines, phenobarbital, phenytoin, levetiracetam, and topiramate are often used first. Ketogenic diet, after ruling out metabolic disorders that would contraindicate it, helps at times. Adrenocorticotropic hormone (ACTH) and steroids may be tried but are often of little benefit. Vigabatrin and zonisamide have been used with some success in small case reports. Consideration of surgical workup for cases with focal brain malformations may be worthwhile (Komaki et al., 2001).

Recently the identification of the genetic substrate of some of the syndromes presenting with EIEE has led to consideration of targeted therapy. Such studies are under investigations, including the use of retigabine, a neuronal potassium channel enhancer, in KCNQ2-related severe epileptic encephalopathy (Maljevic and Lerche, 2014) and quinidine in KCNT1 related epilepsies.

5.0 EARLY MYOCLONIC ENCEPHALOPATHY (EME)

This is the second of the severe epileptic encephalopathies that often presents almost exclusively in the neonatal period.

5.1 Clinical Features

Early myoclonic encephalopathy (EME) starts very early on in life often within hours to days after birth. More than 60% start before 10 days of life, with rare cases presenting after the second month. There is no gender preponderance. The prevalence and incidence are not well-defined.

Often, the syndrome presents clinically with a triad of intractable seizures starting with erratic myoclonus followed by focal seizures and later by tonic epileptic infantile spasms. The erratic myoclonic seizures seen at onset are often segmental and fragmentary involving distal limb muscles. The neurologic examination is abnormal at onset in all neonates with encephalopathic picture. There is severe psychomotor arrest and progressive deterioration.

5.2 Etiology

EME is mostly associated with inborn errors of metabolism, namely glycine encephalopathy (nonketotic hyperglycinemia), D-glycemic acidemia, methylmalonic acidemia, propionic acidemia, molybdenum cofactor deficiency, pyridoxine and pyridoxal-5-phosphate dependency, sulfite oxidase deficiency, Menkes disease, Zellweger syndrome, and hyperammonemia due to carbamyl phosphate synthase deficiency (Beal et al., 2012). Some cases are familial and others are considered cryptogenic. No distinct genetic syndromes have been found in association with EME.

5.3 Diagnosis

EME is suspected in patients presenting with erratic myoclonias with encephalopathy and an EEG picture of burst suppression. The burst suppression seen in EME is different from that of Ohtahara syndrome because the burst suppression is more accentuated during sleep and may not occur during wakefulness. Also, this pattern tends to persist throughout infancy. The bursts are often short (1 to 3 seconds) and the periods of suppression last 2 to 10 seconds. There is no associated EEG seizure activity when the erratic myoclonus is present, but seizure activity is recorded with the focal seizures and spasms when these occur subsequently in the course of this disease.

Brain imaging is often normal at the onset of the disease but progressive cortical atrophy may develop. Metabolic testing—particularly plasma and CSF amino acids and urine organic acids to evaluate for increased glycine and CSF to plasma glycine ratio—is often needed. A more extensive metabolic workup is often done to detect other inborn errors of metabolism causing EME. The workup often includes tests for blood amino acids, acyl carnitine profile, carnitine free and total, lactate, pyruvate, ammonia, biotinidase, pipecolic acid, and alpha aminoadipic semialdehyde, as well as urine for organic acids, creatine, guanidino acetate, and sulfocysteine. Magnetic resonance spectroscopy may be needed for lactate and creatine peaks. CSF tests include amino acids, lactate, cells, glucose, neurotransmitter metabolites, 4-hydroxybutyric acid, succinyl adenosine, sialic acid, pyridoxal 5'-phosphate, 5-methyltetrahydrofolate, and alpha aminoadipic semialdehyde. Gene testing can include targeted gene sequencing and deletion/duplication analysis, gene panels, or exome sequencing depending on the case.

5.4 Differential Diagnosis

The differential of EME is similar to that of Ohtahara syndrome. Table 70-4 highlights some clues to differentiate the two syndromes.

5.5 Prognosis

The prognosis is poor for patients with EME with about 50% dying within the first year. Almost all infants show progressive deterioration in their neurologic status and fail to develop milestones.

5.6 Management

The erratic myoclonus often resolves within a few weeks, but the focal seizures are often refractory to treatment. When possible, etiology-specific therapies may be implemented. This may be in the form of sodium benzoate in cases of glycine encephalopathy or pyridoxine and pyridoxal phosphate trials in suspected pyridoxine related epilepsies.

6.0 CONCLUSION

The spectrum of neonatal electroclinical syndromes includes two benign syndromes (benign neonatal seizures [BNS] and benign familial neonatal seizures [BFNS]) and two highly encephalopathic syndromes (Ohtahara syndrome and EME), and potentially yet to be defined syndromes with predominantly focal seizures without burst suppression. Familiarity with the clinical presentation, diagnostic features, and etiologies helps with early and appropriate diagnosis. This, in turn, facilitates prognostication and management. The rapid booming advance in genetic testing has helped uncover many genetic etiologies of these syndromes allowing for investigation of targeted therapies.

REFERENCES

The complete list of references for this chapter is available in the e-book at www.expertconsult.com.

See inside cover for registration details.

SELECTED REFERENCES

Allen, N.M., Mannion, M., Conroy, J., et al., 2014. The variable phenotypes of KCNQ-related epilepsy. Epilepsia 55 (9), e99–e105.

Beal, J.C., Cherian, K., Moshe, S.L., 2012. Early-onset epileptic encephalopathies: Ohtahara syndrome and early myoclonic encephalopathy. Pediatr. Neurol. 47 (5), 317–323.

Co, J.P., Elia, M., Engel, J. Jr., et al., 2007. Proposal of an algorithm for diagnosis and treatment of neonatal seizures in developing countries. Epilepsia 48 (6), 1158–1164.

Komaki, H., Sugai, K., Maehara, T., et al., 2001. Surgical treatment of early-infantile epileptic encephalopathy with suppression-bursts associated with focal cortical dysplasia. Brain Dev. 23 (7), 727–731.

Maljevic, S., Lerche, H., 2014. Potassium channel genes and benign familial neonatal epilepsy. Prog. Brain Res. 213, 17–53.

Miles, D.K., Holmes, G.L., 1990. Benign neonatal seizures. J. Clin. Neurophysiol. 7 (3), 369–379.

Mizrahi, E.M., Clancy, R.R., 2000. Neonatal seizures: early-onset seizure syndromes and their consequences for development. Ment. Retard. Dev. Disabil. Res. Rev. 6 (4), 229–241.

Ohtahara, S., Yamatogi, Y., 2003. Epileptic encephalopathies in early infancy with suppression-burst. J. Clin. Neurophysiol. 20 (6), 398–407.

Plouin, P., Kaminska, A., 2013. Neonatal seizures. Handb. Clin. Neurol. 111, 467–476.

Yamamoto, H., Okumura, A., Fukuda, M., 2011. Epilepsies and epileptic syndromes starting in the neonatal period. Brain Dev. 33 (3), 213–220.

E-BOOK FIGURES AND TABLES

71 Electroclinical Syndromes: Infantile Onset

Elaine C. Wirrell and Katherine C. Nickels

An expanded version of this chapter is available on www.expertconsult.com. See inside cover for registration details.

INTRODUCTION

Epilepsies that begin early in life encompass a broad range of distinct etiologies with vastly different prognoses. Over one third of epilepsies beginning before 3 years of age will be pharmacoresistant, and these may have a devastating influence on cognition. Recognition of a specific electroclinical syndrome often informs decisions regarding therapy, including preferred medications, potential for resective epilepsy surgery, and ketogenic diet, and improves the understanding of the natural history of the seizure disorder.

This chapter will focus on the electroclinical syndromes seen in infants, addressing diagnosis, therapy, and long-term seizure and developmental outcomes.

GENERALIZED SYNDROMES
Myoclonic Epilepsy in Infancy

Myoclonic epilepsy in infancy (MEI) is a rare epilepsy syndrome that presents between 4 months and 3 years of age.

Seizures

MEI presents with brief 1 to 3 second myoclonic seizures during wakefulness and sleep. The myoclonic seizures may be subtle initially but increase in both frequency and intensity, often occurring in daily clusters during drowsiness. In nearly one third of infants, seizures are triggered by tactile, auditory, or photic stimuli, consistent with reflex myoclonus. Although no other seizure types occur at onset, generalized tonic-clonic seizures may occur later in childhood or early adolescence after the myoclonic seizures have resolved.

Other Neurologic Findings

Development and neurologic examination are normal.

Etiology

The etiology is unknown. A history of simple febrile seizures or family history of generalized tonic-clonic seizures may be present.

EEG Findings

The interictal EEG demonstrates a normal background with generalized spike and wave discharges and possible photoparoxysmal response. The ictal recording shows a burst of 3 to 4 Hz generalized discharge, associated with the myoclonic jerk.

Neuroimaging

Neuroimaging is normal.

Other Laboratory Studies

Other metabolic and genetic disorders presenting with infantile myoclonus must be evaluated (Tables 71-1 and 71-2).

Differential Diagnosis

Epileptic spasms must be excluded. Semiology differs in that spasms are brief tonic contractions rather than myoclonic jerks and usually occur in clusters. Additionally, unlike West syndrome, developmental delay and hypsarrhythmia are not present. Both myoclonic-atonic epilepsy and Lennox-Gastaut syndrome include additional seizure types and EEG background slowing. Dravet syndrome should be suspected if there is a history of prolonged or hemiclonic febrile seizures. Nonepileptic myoclonus is not associated with EEG change. Metabolic disorders are typically accompanied by other seizure types, as well as developmental plateauing and regression (Table 71-2).

Treatment

Valproic acid is the preferred treatment, but adverse reactions are more likely to occur in very young children. Therefore other medications, including benzodiazepines or levetiracetam, may be effective as first-line or adjunctive therapy.

Outcome

MEI is usually self-limited and pharmacoresponsive. Occasionally, after resolution of the myoclonic seizures, other seizure types as well as cognitive impairment and behavior disorders may occur.

Myoclonic Encephalopathies in Nonprogressive Disorders

Myoclonic encephalopathy in nonprogressive disorders presents with prolonged myoclonic status epilepticus in cognitively impaired children. This rare epilepsy syndrome has three subgroups based on etiology.

Etiology

The first and most common subgroup is due to genetic etiology (often Angelman or Prader Willi syndrome). The second subgroup is due to malformations of cortical development such as polymicrogyria or is of unknown etiology. Children in the third subgroup have perinatal anoxic injury.

Seizures and EEG

Seizures in the first subgroup occur between 1 month and 4 years of age and present with very frequent absence seizures with periorbital or perioral myoclonias, myoclonic jerks, and myoclonic absence seizures. This status epilepticus can last for years. The EEG shows rhythmic, generalized slow spike and wave discharges initially and then evolves to a quiet period with nearly continuous theta-delta frequency activity and superimposed spikes primarily activated by eye closure.

The second subgroup presents with bilateral positive myoclonic seizures that alternate with prolonged negative myoclonias. The EEG can be difficult to correlate with the positive and negative myoclonias due to subcontinuous, waxing and

Text continued on p. 563

TABLE 71-1 Gene/Genetic Syndromes Associated With Infantile-Onset Epilepsies

Gene or Syndrome	Chromosome	Other Clinical Findings	Seizure Semiology	Interictal EEG Findings	Course
SCN1A	2q24.3	Severe cases: developmental delay, crouched gait, ataxia and pyramidal signs	Severe cases: Dravet syndrome with prolonged hemiconvulsive seizures triggered by fever before 18 months of age. Later on, other generalized and focal seizures Mild cases: GEFS + with febrile seizures and generalized or focal seizures	Generalized or focal/ multifocal discharges Photoparoxysmal response may be seen	Severe cases: medically intractable, lifelong epilepsy Mild cases: Remission
Wolf-Hirschhorn	Partial monosomy 4p	Prenatal growth failure, severe delay, cleft lip or palate, beaked nose, hypertelorism, low-set ears	Focal, myoclonic, generalized tonic-clonic or atypical absence seizures	High voltage spike wave or slow waves or sequences of sharp waves in the centroparietal or occipital regions	Severity decreases with time
HCN1	5p12	Mild to severe intellectual disability, autistic features, behavior disturbances, ataxia	Onset of febrile or afebrile generalized or focal seizures in first year of life, followed by absence and/or myoclonic seizures		Medically intractable
STXBP1	9q34.1	Severe to profound delay, MRI may show hypomyelination, global atrophy or thinning of the corpus callosum	Early-onset tonic seizures, spasms or tonic-clonic seizures	Suppression burst or hypsarrhythmia	Seizures often intractable although rarely remit. Severe to profound developmental delay
SPTAN1	9q33-q34	Progressive microcephaly, spastic quadriplegia, severe intellectual disability, hypomyelination and diffuse brain atrophy on MRI	Spasms, generalized seizures	Hypsarrhythmia	Medically intractable
DNM1	9q34	Hypotonia	Infantile spasms, evolving to Lennox-Gastaut syndrome	Hypsarrhythmia, slow spike wave	Severe to profound intellectual disability, intractable epilepsy
SLC25A22	11p15.5	Hypotonia, microcephaly, abnormal electroretinogram	Myoclonic seizures, spasms	Suppression burst, hypsarrhythmia	Medically intractable
Trisomy 12p	12	Severe delay, short neck, prominent forehead, flat occiput, hypertelorism, micrognathia, low-set ears	Myoclonic or myoclonic absence, generalized tonic-clonic	3 Hz spike and polyspike	Seizures often respond to medications
SCN8A	12q13.1	Movement disorder	Clusters of focal or generalized seizures triggered by fever Spasms	Multifocal or generalized discharges	Often intractable
Ring chromosome 14	14	Severe delay, microcephaly, narrow face, high-arched palate, short palpebral fissures, flat nasal bridge, retrognathia, ocular anomalies	Symptomatic generalized epilepsy with onset in first year of life		
FOXG1	14q11-q13	Severe delay without microcephaly "congenital Rett"	Focal and generalized seizures	Slowing of background, focal and multifocal discharge	Often refractory

TABLE 71-1 Gene/Genetic Syndromes Associated With Infantile-Onset Epilepsies *(Continued)*

Gene or Syndrome	Chromosome	Other Clinical Findings	Seizure Semiology	Interictal EEG Findings	Course
Inversion-duplication 15 syndrome	15	Moderate to severe delay, autism, microcephaly, mild occasional dysmorphic features	Epileptic encephalopathy resembling West or Lennox-Gastaut syndrome, occasional focal seizures	Hypsarrhythmia, slow spike-wave	Often refractory
Angelman	Partial monosomy 15q	Ataxia, tremor, minimal speech, severe delay, happy demeanor	Atypical absence, myoclonic, tonic-clonic, unilateral clonic, Focal dyscognitive	High-amplitude, symmetric, synchronous notched 2 Hz polyphasic slow waves or slow and sharp waves, particularly during slow wave sleep	VPA + BZDs helpful Seizure severity decreases over time
POLG1	15q24	Cerebral atrophy, liver dysfunction	Myoclonic, other focal and generalized seizures	Multifocal discharge with slowing	Refractory
CHD2	15q26	Intellectual disability, may have microcephaly	Fever sensitive generalized tonic-clonic seizures usually after age 1, later with prominent myoclonus and atypical absences	Generalized polyspike and wave discharges initially, later on may see focal or multifocal discharge	Mild–severe intellectual disability
PRRT2	16p11.2	Familial paroxysmal choreoathetosis or kinesigenic dyskinesia	Focal with or without secondarily generalized seizures in neurologically normal infants	Interictal EEG usually normal	Seizures usually pharmacoresponsive and self-limited
Miller-Dieker	17p13.3 deletion	Four layered lissencephaly, microcephaly, bitemporal narrowing, small, anteverted nose, micrognathia, high forehead, cardiac, renal and sacral anomalies	In first weeks to months, massive myoclonus and epileptic spasms are seen. Over time, focal and tonic seizures emerge as predominant seizure types	Prominent fast activity, although slowing is common in the first year of life	Seizures are refractory
KCNQ2	20q13.33	Usually normal infants but rarely may have moderate to profound delay Severe affected infants may have reversible T2 signal changes in the thalami and basal ganglia	Severe cases: early-onset tonic spasms, focal seizures, myoclonic seizures Mild: focal epilepsy in infants	Severe: suppression burst or hypsarrhythmia Mild: normal or focal discharges	Most cases are mild with self-limited seizure disorder and normal development Rarely, may present as early-onset epileptic encephalopathy
Ring chromosome 20	20	Mild–moderate delay, restlessness, aggression, nondysmorphic	Runs of atypical absence or myoclonic status epilepticus	Ictal: high voltage, 2–3 Hz slow activity with superimposed spikes maximal over frontal regions Interictal: normal or mild slowing/sharp waves	Seizures are refractory and don't remit with age
DEPDC5	22q12.3	AD inheritance with incomplete penetrance (50%–82%) May be associated with cortical dysplasias, often bottom-of-the-sulcus	Focal epilepsy (often frontal or temporal)	Focal or multifocal discharges	Heterogeneous—some cases have well-controlled epilepsy, others are intractable Rarely individuals may have intellectual disability, autism, psychiatric features

Continued on following page

TABLE 71-1 Gene/Genetic Syndromes Associated With Infantile-Onset Epilepsies *(Continued)*

Gene or Syndrome	Chromosome	Other Clinical Findings	Seizure Semiology	Interictal EEG Findings	Course
CDKL5	Xp22	More common in girls but seen also in boys Severe developmental delay with hypotonia Acquired microcephaly in some cases. Impaired eye contact and gaze avoidance	Generalized tonic seizures beginning in first 10 wks, followed by spasm, atypical absences and myoclonic seizures	Interictal EEG normal early on, then see slowing of background and modified hypsarrhythmia	Intractable generalized seizures
PCDH19	Xp22.1	Girls only, intellectual disability, autism	Generalized tonic-clonic or focal seizures, typically occurring in clusters with febrile illness	Generalized or focal discharge	Intellectual disability, autism Seizures often medically intractable
Rett Syndrome (MECP2)	X q28	Normal early development followed by acquired microcephaly, autistic features, lack of purposeful hand movement with characteristic hand wringing	Generalized tonic-clonic seizures, other generalized and focal seizures	Slowing of background with multifocal and generalized epileptiform discharge	Often refractory
ARX	Xp22.13	Severe developmental delay and seizures in boys. Often associated cerebral malformations including lissencephaly, agenesis of corpus callosum. May have dystonia, spasticity	Spasms, other generalized seizures	Suppression burst, hypsarrhythmia	Usually refractory
SLC35A2	Xp11.23-p11.22	Moderate to severe intellectual disability, language impairment, early pubertal onset	Spasms, focal epilepsy	Hypsarrhythmia Electrical status epilepticus in slow sleep	Often intractable

TABLE 71-2 Inborn Errors of Metabolism Associated With Infantile-Onset Epilepsies

Metabolic Disorder	Age at Onset	Clinical	Diagnostic Test	Prognosis	Treatment
Pyridoxine dependency	Birth to 1 year	Refractory seizures which may begin in utero, progressive encephalopathy, clinical and EEG response to pyridoxine	Increased AASA in CSF, serum and urine, confirm with ALDH7A1 genetic analysis	Variable, depending on duration of symptoms before supplementation	Pyridoxine 50–200 mg/d
Pyridoxal phosphate dependency	Neonatal	Refractory seizures, often in preterm infant, encephalopathy, clinical and EEG response to pyridoxal phosphate	Low P5P in CSF, confirm with PNPO genetic analysis	Variable, depending on duration of symptoms before supplementation	Pyridoxal-5–phosphate 30 mg/kg/d
Folinic acid responsive seizures	Neonatal	Refractory seizures, encephalopathy, clinical and EEG response to folinic acid, incomplete response to pyridoxal phosphate and pyridoxine	Increased CSF AASA and increased serum pipecolic acid, abnormal peaks on CSF neurotransmitter analysis	Variable, depending on duration of symptoms before supplementation	Folinic acid 3–5 mg/kg/d
Serine deficiency disorders	Neonatal to childhood	Microcephaly, cognitive disability, failure to thrive, spasticity, hypomyelination and brain atrophy on MRI, neonatal or absence seizures	Decreased serine on CSF and plasma amino acids	Variable, depending on duration of symptoms before supplementation	Serine 500–700 mg/kg/d +/– glycine supplementation

TABLE 71-2 Inborn Errors of Metabolism Associated With Infantile-Onset Epilepsies *(Continued)*

Metabolic Disorder	Age at Onset	Clinical	Diagnostic Test	Prognosis	Treatment
Creatine deficiency	Neonatal and infancy	Developmental delay, seizures, autistic features, movement disorder, poor growth	Screen with urine testing for creatine and GAA, followed by definitive genetic testing for AGAT, GAMT or creatine transporter	Poor, majority with moderate to severe mental retardation	Creatine monohydrate 5–20 g/d
Untreated phenylketonuria	Neonatal and infancy	Growth failure, microcephaly, seizures, developmental delay, mousy odor	Increased Phe on plasma amino acids	Good if diagnosed and treated early	Phe restricted diet, consider BH4 trial to rule out tetrahydrobiopterin deficiency
Urea cycle disorders	Neonatal, later if partial enzyme deficiency	Vomiting, lethargy, coma, seizures, developmental delay, protein avoidance, diffuse white matter changes on MRI	Increased serum ammonia, abnormal serum amino acids and urine organic acids	Variable, depending on severity and duration of symptoms	Removal of ammonia with dialysis (if hyperammonemic crisis), sodium benzoate, sodium phenylacetate, arginine supplementation High carbohydrate, low protein diet with provision of essential amino acids
Glycine encephalopathy (Nonketotic hyperglycinemia)	Neonatal or infantile	Lethargy, hypotonia, hiccups, intractable seizures, apnea	Increased CSF and plasma glycine with CSF/plasma glycine >0.08	Poor, death usually within the first year	Benzoate (250–750 mg/kg/d), dextromethorphan Avoid valproate and vigabatrin
GABA transaminase deficiency	Neonatal-infantile	Intractable seizures, lethargy, irritability, severe delay, hypotonia, hyperreflexia, accelerated growth	Increased GABA in serum and CSF	Poor, death usually within the first 5 years	Symptomatic only
Sulfite oxidase deficiency and molybdenum cofactor deficiency	Neonatal or infantile	Intractable seizures, progressive neurocognitive decline, acquired microcephaly, MRI demonstrating leukoencephalomalacia and atrophy. Later onset forms may present with encephalopathy, focal findings and seizures after a febrile illness	Elevate sulfite levels on fresh urine. Low plasma homocysteine. Confirm with specific enzyme analysis of fibroblasts	Poor	Some patients may improve with vigabatrin, dextromethorphan. Some may improve with dietary restriction of methionine
Peroxisomal disorders	Neonatal or infantile	Hepatic disease, developmental delay, retinopathy, deafness, seizures, cortical migration defects	Abnormal very long chain fatty acids and/or phytanic acid	Variable, depending on phenotype	Symptomatic only
Menkes disease	Infancy	Developmental regression, seizures, particularly spasms, hypopigmentation of skin and hair, hypothermia, characteristic "kinky" hair	Low serum copper and ceruloplasmin. Confirm with ATP7A mutation analysis	Poor with progression to death typically within 5 years	Copper histidine supplementation and supportive treatment
Glutaric acidemia type 1	Infancy and childhood	Macrocephaly, acute neurologic decompensation with infection or febrile illness, characterized by hypotonia, opisthotonic posturing, dystonia or dyskinesia, seizures, encephalopathy. MRI shows widening of sylvian fissures	Increased urinary glutaric acid	Poor, although detection and treatment before decompensation may improve outcome	Low protein diet (low lysine and tryptophan) with carnitine supplementation

Continued on following page

TABLE 71-2 Inborn Errors of Metabolism Associated With Infantile-Onset Epilepsies (Continued)

Metabolic Disorder	Age at Onset	Clinical	Diagnostic Test	Prognosis	Treatment
Biotinidase deficiency	Neonatal through childhood	Seizures, hypotonia, developmental delay, ataxia, dermatitis, hair loss, autistic behavior, optic atrophy	Low serum biotinidase	Outcome can be good if diagnosed and treated early	Biotin supplementation (10 mg/day)
Succinic semialdehyde dehydrogenase deficiency	Infancy and childhood	Developmental delay, ataxia, hypotonia, seizures, hyperactivity, behavior problems. Increased T2 signal in globus pallidus, dentate nucleus and subthalamic nucleus with cerebral atrophy	Increased gamma hydroxybutyric acid in urine. Confirm with enzymatic analysis or Aldh5A1 gene sequencing	Variable, treatment targeted at symptoms	Symptomatic
Congenital hyperinsulinism and hyperammonemia	Infancy and childhood	Epilepsy, intellectual disability	Postprandial hypoglycemia, hyperammonemia. Confirm by mutation analysis in glutamate dehydrogenase gene	Outcome can be good if diagnosed and treated early	Protein restriction, diazoxide
Tetrahydrobiopterin deficiencies	2–12 months	Cognitive regression, microcephaly, generalized seizures, irritability, dystonia, rash, basal ganglia calcifications	Elevated Phe on plasma amino acids, abnormal pterions and neurotransmitters in CSF	Outcome can be good if diagnosed and treated early	BH4 supplementation May need additional supplementation with neurotransmitter precursors based on type
Glucose transporter deficiency	Birth to early childhood	Seizures (infantile-onset focal or generalized, or early-onset absence epilepsy), microcephaly, developmental delay, acquired ataxia, paroxysmal dyskinesia	Low CSF/plasma glucose with normal or low lactate Confirm with SCL2A1 genetic testing	Variable, depending on duration of symptoms before treatment with ketogenic diet	Ketogenic diet
Cerebral folate deficiency	Childhood to adolescence	Intractable epilepsy, intellectual disability or regression, microcephaly, dyskinesias, autism	Low CSF methyltetrahydrofolate Further testing requires mutation analysis in FOLR1 gene, assessment for antibodies to folate receptors, and if workup for secondary causes of cerebral folate deficiency	Variable, depending on exact etiology and duration of symptoms before treatment	Folinic acid supplementation (0.5–5 mg/kg/d)
Mitochondrial disorders	Infancy to adulthood	Focal or generalized seizures, spasms, deafness, myopathy, lactic acidosis, ataxia, optic atrophy, hepatic dysfunction,	Elevated plasma and CSF lactate, may have evidence of cardiac, renal or hepatic dysfunction. Elevated lactate peak on MRS. Muscle biopsy, specific genetic analysis	Variable, depending on specific type	Avoid valproate Mitochondrial cocktail (carnitine, coenzyme Q, riboflavin) Ketogenic diet may be helpful in some conditions, e.g. pyruvate dehydrogenase complex deficiency (and contraindicated in others, e.g. pyruvate carboxylase deficiency)
Congenital Disorders of Glycosylation	Infancy to childhood	Developmental delay, hypotonia, failure to thrive, multisystem disease, inverted nipples and/or abnormal fat pads, cerebellar hypoplasia	Abnormalities in carbohydrate deficient transferrin analysis. Confirm with specific genetic analysis	Variable depending on etiology	Symptomatic

waning, multifocal, slow spike and wave discharges. The status epilepticus can become life-threatening, requiring intensive care.

Children in the third subgroup typically have mild neurologic impairment at baseline and experience only focal seizures. The myoclonic status begins between age 7 months to 5 years with rhythmic myoclonic jerking of the face and limbs. The EEG shows nearly continuous generalized or bilateral spike and wave discharges that can have a notched delta appearance. Over days to weeks, there is clinical deterioration with cognitive regression, frequent focal seizures, and movement disorders.

Neuroimaging

Neuroimaging in the first subgroup, of genetic etiology, is normal. In the second subgroup, neuroimaging can be normal (unknown etiology) or show cortical malformations of variable severity. Imaging in the third subgroup is consistent with perinatal anoxic injury. Although there is clinical progression in this third subgroup, the neuroimaging remains unchanged.

Other Neurologic Findings

Development in all children is abnormal at baseline. In the first two subgroups, there is severe neurologic impairment. In the third subgroup, the degree of neurologic impairment at baseline is mild but progresses over days to weeks with movement disorders appearing.

Other Laboratory Studies

A comprehensive genetic evaluation as well as careful neuroimaging with epilepsy protocol to detect malformations of cortical development should be performed (Table 71-1). For those with unknown etiology, a comprehensive metabolic evaluation should be considered (Table 71-2).

Differential Diagnosis

West syndrome can be excluded by differentiating the myoclonic seizures from epileptic spasms and the lack of hypsarrhythmia on EEG. Myoclonic status and similar initial EEG findings can be seen in Lennox-Gastaut syndrome and myoclonic-atonic epilepsy, making them difficult to exclude. However, other seizures typically seen with these syndromes occur much less frequently. Myoclonic seizures are a later occurrence in children with Dravet syndrome.

Identifying the underlying etiology can be helpful in differentiating this syndrome from progressive myoclonic epilepsies.

Treatment

The seizures are pharmacoresistant. Mitochondrial disorders should be excluded before initiating valproic acid. The myoclonic status epilepticus is typically refractory to benzodiazepines and often requires intensive care unit therapy.

Outcome

The myoclonic status epilepticus can resolve, often within 2 to 4 years; however, refractory brief absences and infrequent myoclonic seizures continue. Intellectual disability remains severe. Unfortunately, mortality due to status epilepticus is high in the second subgroup and survivors continue to have status epilepticus into adulthood.

FOCAL SYNDROMES
Epilepsy of Infancy With Migrating Focal Seizures

Epilepsy of infancy with migrating focal seizures is an early-onset epileptic encephalopathy that begins in previously healthy infants after the neonatal period but before the sixth month.

Seizures

Initially, sporadic, focal seizures occur, with semiology suggestive of multifocal onset. Seizures may be accompanied by autonomic signs, including apnea, cyanosis, and flushing (Caraballo, et al., 2008). Seizure frequency and duration increase and frequently culminate in refractory status epilepticus requiring treatment with general anesthesia. After 1 to 5 years, seizures once again become sporadic and easier to control, although seizure clusters and intermittent status epilepticus can still occur.

Other Neurologic Findings

At onset, children have normal neurologic examinations. As the seizures become refractory, hypotonia, loss of motor milestones, and subsequent developmental delay are noted in all infants. Progressive microcephaly, feeding issues, and decreased visual attentiveness are frequent.

Etiology

The etiology is typically unknown with genetic causes found in a minority of children.

EEG Findings

The interictal EEG can initially be normal, but over time, slowing and multifocal epileptiform discharges emerge. The ictal recording demonstrates variable electroclinical patterns (Fig. 71-5).

Neuroimaging

At onset, neuroimaging is normal in all children. Over time, mild to moderate ventricular enlargement and possible mesial temporal sclerosis may evolve.

Other Laboratory Studies

Extensive neurometabolic evaluations and, in most cases, genetic evaluations are normal.

Differential Diagnosis

Structural etiologies such as cortical dysplasia should be ruled out with detailed neuroimaging. Infections such as meningoencephalitis and metabolic disorders can also present with multifocal seizures. Furthermore, both benign infantile epilepsy and benign familial infantile epilepsy can present at a similar age with focal seizures. However, these seizures are pharmacoresponsive and development remains normal in essentially all patients.

Treatment

Although stiripentol, clonazepam, potassium bromides, and levetiracetam may be helpful, seizures are typically refractory to all therapies.

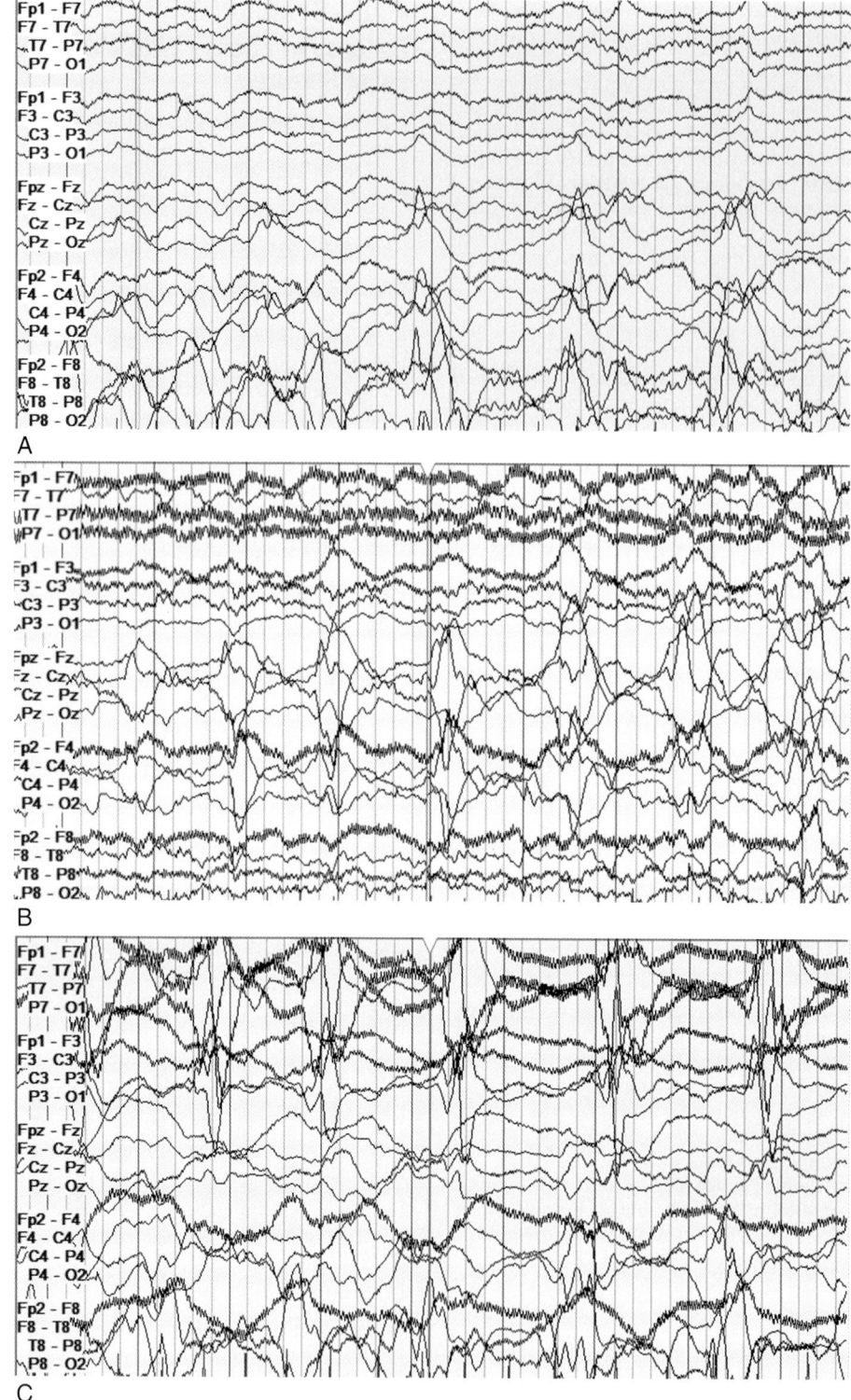

Figure 71-5. EEG during a focal dyscognitive seizure in an infant with epilepsy of infancy with migrating focal seizures demonstrating high amplitude delta frequency sharp waves over the right hemisphere initially (a), followed by involvement of the midline head regions as the right temporal region seizure discharge resolves (b), followed by independent left temporal discharge (c).

Outcome

The outcome is typically poor with severe hypotonia, intellectual disability, refractory seizures, and high mortality, although there may be phenotypic variability.

Benign Epilepsy of Infancy/Benign Familial Infantile Epilepsy

Infants with convulsive seizures and normal neurologic examination, with or without family history of similar seizures, can sometimes follow a benign course. These syndromes have now been termed "benign epilepsy of infancy (BEI)" and "benign familial infantile epilepsy (BFEI)" (Vigevano, 2005). The seizure semiology and outcome are similar for the two syndromes, thus they will be discussed conjointly.

Seizures

The seizures in BEI and BFEI may initially be sporadic, but eventually occur in clusters. Within the cluster, seizures typically occur several hours apart, and the infant returns to baseline in between events. The semiology is variable and includes staring, unresponsiveness, behavioral arrest, eye deviation, head turn, apnea, and automatisms with or without generalized convulsions.

Other Neurologic Findings

Neurologic examination and development are normal. Paroxysmal kinesigenic choreoathetosis and dystonia have been reported to coexist in individuals and families with BFEI. Later development of familial hemiplegic migraine has also been reported.

Etiology

The etiology of BEI is unknown, and the diagnosis can be difficult to make with certainty at onset. Comprehensive metabolic and neuroimaging studies should be done to exclude other causes of early-onset multifocal epilepsy (Tables 71-1 and 71-2).

BFEI has been linked to chromosomes 2, 16 (PRRT2 mutations), and 19 and displays autosomal dominant inheritance with variable penetrance.

EEG Findings

A normal interictal EEG is felt to be one of the characteristics of BEI and BFEI. Ictal EEGs have demonstrated focal onset in all seizures, including those with a generalized tonic-clonic component without focal semiology (Vigevano, 2005).

Neuroimaging

Normal neuroimaging must be present for infants to be diagnosed with either BEI or BFEI. Malformations of cortical development may be difficult to detect on MRI before 2 years of age, so careful clinical follow up is needed to ensure the accuracy of this diagnosis.

Differential Diagnosis

Careful evaluation must be undertaken to assess for malformations of cortical development or other structural causes, as well as potential metabolic disorders. The normal neuroimaging, normal interictal EEG, and normal development throughout the course of this epilepsy are helpful in securing the diagnosis. Furthermore, this is a pharmacoresponsive syndrome, which would not be expected from epilepsy due to structural or metabolic etiology.

Treatment

The seizure clusters are typically several hours apart and can continue for 1 to 3 days. Phenobarbital has been more helpful than benzodiazepines in aborting clusters, although doses higher than 10 mg/kg may be necessary. Multiple preventative medications have been tried and all appear to be beneficial.

Outcome

Children with BEI and BFEI are able to discontinue antiseizure drug therapy by their early preschool years, without recurrence of focal seizures or emergence of new epilepsy syndromes. All children continued to have normal neurologic examinations and normal development. Recurrence of seizures or emergence of learning disorders/intellectual disability should prompt further evaluation.

Hemiconvulsions, Hemiplegia, and Epilepsy Syndrome (HHE)

HHE is a rare condition that usually presents under age 4 years with prolonged unilateral convulsive status epilepticus in the context of a febrile illness followed by hemiplegia. Months to years later, intractable epilepsy emerges.

Seizures

HHE typically presents initially with unilateral, clonic status epilepticus lasting for more than 24 hours. Severe autonomic symptoms can also emerge. The initial seizures are acute symptomatic seizures and, therefore are not epilepsy. This stage is called hemiconvulsions and hemiplegia syndrome (HHS).

Recurrent unprovoked seizures occur in two-thirds to three fourths of children after months to years of seizure freedom, at which point the epilepsy is typically pharmacoresistant. The seizures are focal dyscognitive seizures arising from the temporal regions or from multiple foci within the affected hemisphere.

Other Neurologic Findings

Most children have normal growth and development before onset of the seizure. Hemiplegia ipsilateral to the side of convulsive status epilepticus occurs and must last at least 1 week. Additional neurologic findings such as visual field deficits and aphasia may be seen.

Etiology

The etiology for HHE is unknown. Even in those children with preexisting, structural abnormalities, the cause for the acute-onset, febrile, prolonged hemiconvulsion and subsequent hemiparesis is unclear. The febrile component and mild illness suggest that hyperthermia and inflammation are important contributors to the pathogenesis.

EEG Findings

In the acute phase, EEG is important to ensure complete electrographic cessation of the seizure. The ictal EEG demonstrates rhythmic, high amplitude, 2 to 3 Hz slow wave activity bilaterally but higher over the affected hemisphere and often associated with rhythmic spikes and low amplitude fast activity contralateral to the clonic activity. Postictally, the slowing over the affected hemisphere continues, whereas the unaffected hemisphere has gradual reappearance of normal background activity.

During the chronic phase, presurgical evaluation is often pursued for the intractable epilepsy. The interictal EEG typically shows multifocal spikes and sharp waves, typically most prominent over the affected hemisphere.

Neuroimaging

Neuroimaging is essential for the diagnosis and should be done early. At the time of hemiconvulsive status epilepticus, the MRI reveals edema of the affected hemisphere maximally involving the subcortical white matter. There is hyperintensity on diffusion weighted imaging sequences that corresponds with decreased apparent diffuse coefficient. MRI angiography is normal. These MRI abnormalities are independent of any vascular territory and resolve within 1 month. Hemiatrophy and possible hippocampal sclerosis occur over weeks to months.

Other Laboratory Studies

Additional studies to determine potential metabolic, vascular, infectious, or autoimmune etiology should be completed but are normal in these patients.

Differential Diagnosis

Stroke can be excluded with neuroimaging that does not follow vascular territory, absence of hemorrhage, and normal vascular studies. Metabolic disorders such as mitochondrial cytopathies can present with stroke-like episodes and seizures, especially in the setting of illness. However, seizures due to acute stroke typically present first with motor deficit and then seizure.

Acute traumatic brain injury and neoplasm are also excluded by neuroimaging. The acute edema followed by profound hemiatrophy seen in HHE would make malformation of cortical development unlikely.

Infectious and autoimmune etiologies should be evaluated. Febrile infection-related epilepsy syndrome (FIRES) is characterized by onset of seizures that evolve to refractory status epilepticus in otherwise healthy, school-aged children during or shortly after a nonspecific febrile illness. Unlike HHE, cognitive deficit and pharmacoresistant epilepsy occur at onset.

Finally, Rasmussen's encephalitis typically presents with focal motor seizures and epilepsia partialis continua, but the onset of motor weakness is gradual as is the atrophy on MRI.

Treatment

The treatment in the acute phase is supportive. There is no evidence that initiating chronic treatment with antiseizure drugs will prevent the later onset of unprovoked seizures. Presurgical evaluation should be pursued for pharmacoresistant seizures in the chronic phase.

Outcome

Children with HHE are typically left with variable degrees of permanent motor and cognitive deficits.

The seizures in HHE are usually pharmacoresistant, but seizure control may be obtained through surgical resection. Those with proven temporal lobe onset have excellent seizure outcome after temporal lobectomy, even in the presence of more extensive imaging abnormalities. Multilobar resection or hemispherectomy may be needed in those with extratemporal onset or multiple ictal foci within one hemisphere.

UNDIFFERENTIATED SYNDROMES
West Syndrome

West syndrome is the most common epileptic encephalopathy in infancy, with an estimated incidence of 3 to 4.5 per 10,000 live births. It consists of a triad of: (1) epileptic spasms; (2) hypsarrhythmia on EEG; and (3) arrest or regression of psychomotor development. The onset of epileptic spasms is typically between 3 to 12 months of age.

Seizures

Epileptic spasms involve a sudden flexion, extension, or mixed flexion-extension movement of the proximal and truncal muscles, lasting 1 to 2 seconds, and occur in clusters shortly after waking. Focal seizures may also be seen and suggest an underlying focal pathology.

Other Neurologic Findings

Developmental delay is frequently evident, even before spasm onset. Focal or generalized motor findings, impairments in visual attention, and microcephaly are common. A dermatologic examination using a Wood's lamp should be undertaken to evaluate for neurocutaneous disorders such as tuberous sclerosis. Abnormalities such as organomegaly, unusual odor, or dysmorphic features would suggest the possibility of a metabolic or genetic etiology.

Etiology

An obvious cause of spasms is identified in just over half of cases after initial clinical evaluation and MRI and in up to three fourths of infants after further investigations. Structural etiologies, including malformations of cortical development, tuberous sclerosis, and perinatal brain injury, are most common. Genetic etiologies are increasingly recognized (Paciorkowski, et al., 2011). In contrast, metabolic etiologies are less frequent.

EEG Findings

The classic finding on interictal EEG in West syndrome is hypsarrhythmia, characterized by very high amplitude (often up to 500 microvolts), asynchronous slow waves, and multifocal spikes and polyspikes. Absence of hypsarrhythmia in a child with a suspicious history does not rule out a diagnosis of West syndrome, and a prolonged EEG recording should be considered. Hypsarrhythmia may also be asymmetric in patients with focal lesions.

The typical ictal correlate of an epileptic spasm is a high voltage, often generalized sharp or slow wave followed by an electrodecrement, consisting of low amplitude fast activity.

Neuroimaging

Brain MRI is a necessary test in all cases of West syndrome without known etiology. MRI reveals a cause in 35% to 41% of cases. If the initial MRI is normal and seizures persist, an MRI may be repeated every 6 months and should be redone after age 24 to 30 months, when myelination is more mature, to detect cortical dysplasia (Gaillard, et al., 2009).

Other Laboratory Studies

In children without a clear etiology after imaging, further genetic and metabolic studies should be obtained (Tables 71-1 and 71-2). If imaging is suggestive of an inborn error of metabolism, an extensive metabolic investigation is warranted. In those with normal MRI, genetic testing, including comparative genomic hybridization array, epilepsy gene panel, whole exome sequencing, or mitochondrial genetic studies, should be considered.

Treatment

Hormonal therapy (ACTH or prednisolone) and vigabatrin have been proposed as first-line therapy for infantile spasms. Based on the evidence-based guideline from the American Academy of Neurology, ACTH may have greater short-term efficacy than vigabatrin once infants with tuberous sclerosis are excluded (Go, et al., 2012). Vigabatrin is the treatment of choice in infantile spasms due to tuberous sclerosis, with seizure cessation being seen in 95% of cases and may be effective in spasms due to focal cortical dysplasia. There is insufficient evidence to recommend other medications or the ketogenic diet as first-line agents.

Children with infantile spasms due to focal cortical structural abnormalities not controlled with hormonal therapy and vigabatrin should be expediently referred for possible surgical treatment, even with nonlocalizing EEG.

Outcome

Most children with West syndrome have intellectual disability at follow up and are also at risk for autism (Widjaja, et al., 2015; Riikonen, 2001). The underlying etiology is the most critical predictor of developmental outcome. Additional factors predictive of better outcome include shorter duration from spasm onset to diagnosis, favorable response to initial therapy, absence of other seizures before infantile spasms, and absence of atypical spasms, focal seizures, or asymmetric EEG abnormalities.

Infantile spasms resolve in the majority of children by the early preschool years. However, 50% to 90% of cases develop other seizure types, most commonly either Lennox-Gastaut syndrome (27% to 50%) or focal/multifocal epilepsy.

West syndrome also carries a significant mortality risk. One large study that followed 214 children for a mean of 25 years reported that 31% had died; the most frequent causes of death included infection and complications of therapy (Riikonen, 2001).

Dravet Syndrome

Dravet syndrome is a catastrophic childhood epilepsy syndrome that leads to intellectual disability and motor deficits (Brunklaus, et al., 2012). The estimated incidence is approximately 1 to 2 per 40,000 live births.

Seizures

This epilepsy syndrome begins in the first 18 months of life with prolonged, hemiconvulsive seizures initiated by fever (often associated with vaccines) or hyperthermia. Over the next several months, recurrent febrile and afebrile seizures occur, often switching sides.

In early childhood other seizure types emerge, including myoclonic, atypical absence, and focal seizures. Obtundation status, in which children appear poorly responsive and have erratic myoclonus may also be seen and can persist for hours. Reflex seizures are frequent with the most common provoking factor being hyperthermia. Tonic seizures are unusual in Dravet syndrome.

Other Neurologic Findings

Development is normal at epilepsy onset, but then there is a variable decline in developmental quotient over time. Autistic traits and hyperactivity have also been reported. A greater degree of cognitive and behavioral impairment has been linked to higher frequency of seizures.

The neurologic examination is typically normal at epilepsy onset. However, ataxia and pyramidal signs, as well as crouch gait, may develop.

Etiology

SCN1A mutations (mostly de novo) are found in 80% of patients. However, 5% show familial mutations in which affected relatives are mildly affected with a genetic epilepsy with febrile seizures plus (GEFS +) phenotype. The genetic finding must be correlated to epilepsy phenotype to reach an accurate diagnosis.

EEG Findings

The EEG background is typically normal at epilepsy onset. After 1 to 2 years, patients show diffuse background slowing.

Epileptiform discharges, seen in a minority at onset, are most commonly generalized and may be triggered with photic stimulation. At age 2 to 5 years, an increase in generalized paroxysmal abnormalities, as well as emergence of focal and multifocal discharges, occurs.

Neuroimaging

Neuroimaging studies are normal at presentation, although scans done later in life may show abnormalities, likely due to the prolonged seizures.

Treatment

Dravet syndrome is extremely pharmacoresistant (Chiron, 2011). The goals of treatment are to avoid prolonged status epilepticus, reduce frequency of briefer seizures, and avoid problematic adverse effects of multiple agents used at high doses.

Sodium channel agents should be avoided as they exacerbate seizures. First-line therapy typically involves valproic acid, clobazam, or topiramate. Stiripentol is often considered if first-line therapy is ineffective and has been shown to reduce seizures and status epilepticus. Bromides and ketogenic diet have also been effective.

Isolated case reports and small studies have suggested possible efficacy of fenfluramine, verapamil, fluoxetine, cannabidiol, vagus nerve stimulation, and deep brain stimulation. Careful clinical trials are needed.

Caregivers of children with Dravet syndrome should be taught to administer a home dose of rescue benzodiazepine, and a treatment plan for management of prolonged seizures should be provided.

Outcome

Seizures remain medically refractory. Many seizure types reduce or resolve by early adulthood, with brief, nocturnal, generalized tonic-clonic seizures remaining as the main seizure type. Most patients have moderate to severe disability and cannot live independently as adults.

There is an increased mortality rate in children with Dravet syndrome, with approximately 15% dying by early adulthood, and death is often seizure-related.

Genetic Epilepsy With Febrile Seizures Plus (GEFS +)

GEFS + is a common, familial electroclinical syndrome in which two or more family members have phenotypes consistent with this diagnosis (Scheffer and Berkovic. 1997).

Affected individuals exhibit variable phenotypes. The onset is typically between 6 months and 6 years of age.

Seizures

At the mildest end of the phenotypic spectrum are children with febrile seizures alone, which may be recurrent, prolonged, focal, or occur in clusters. Next most common are those with "febrile seizures plus," in which febrile seizures either continue beyond the age of 6 years, and/or afebrile seizures also occur. At the severe end of the spectrum are individuals with myoclonic-atonic epilepsy or Dravet syndrome. Some individuals may also present with temporal lobe epilepsy, with or without hippocampal sclerosis.

Other Neurologic Findings

With the exception of rare cases on the severe end of the phenotypic spectrum, children with GEFS + are typically neurologically and developmentally normal.

Etiology

GEFS + is usually inherited in an autosomal dominant manner with incomplete penetrance. GEFS + remains a clinical diagnosis, and genetic testing is not required.

EEG Findings

EEG is not indicated in simple febrile convulsions but may be obtained in those with complex features—particularly focal or prolonged febrile seizures. An EEG is typically obtained in children with afebrile seizures, and the findings in GEFS + are heterogenous. The background is typically normal, although diffuse slowing may be seen in individuals with severe phenotypes. In individuals with generalized seizures, the interictal recording typically shows generalized discharge, which can become fragmented in sleep. In those with temporal lobe epilepsy, focal discharge is seen.

Neuroimaging

Neuroimaging is generally not required, particularly with generalized seizures, and is typically normal. Rarely, hippocampal sclerosis can be seen in patients with GEFS + and temporal lobe epilepsy.

Treatment

Simple febrile seizures alone do not require prophylactic drug therapy. If febrile seizures are prolonged or clustered, caregivers should be taught to administer a home dose of rescue benzodiazepine therapy. Prophylactic antiseizure therapy for afebrile seizures should be geared toward the seizure type. Because many mutations in GEFS + may alter sodium channel function, sodium channel blockers may potentially be more problematic.

Children with epileptic encephalopathies such as myoclonic-atonic epilepsy or Dravet syndrome may also benefit from the ketogenic diet.

Outcome

The majority of children with GEFS + have seizures that are easily controlled with medication. Seizures are typically self-limited and resolve at puberty. Rare individuals continue to have generalized seizures into adulthood. Development remains normal.

Children who develop myoclonic-atonic epilepsy are typically pharmacoresistant initially, but many ultimately become seizure free by middle childhood and have remission of their epilepsy.

CONCLUSIONS

Epilepsies that begin in infancy are associated with high rates of pharmacoresistance and are commonly associated with neurocognitive impairment. Recognition of a specific electro-clinical syndrome is imperative to: (1) understand the possible pathogenic mechanisms leading to epilepsy and allow more cost-effective, less invasive, and more streamlined investigations; (2) choose more efficacious therapies to control seizures and prevent associated comorbidities; and (3) better prognosticate long-term development and seizure outcome for families.

REFERENCES

The complete list of references for this chapter is available in the e-book at www.expertconsult.com.
See inside cover for registration details.

SELECTED REFERENCES

Brunklaus, A., Ellis, R., Reavey, E., et al., 2012. Prognostic, clinical, and demographic features in SCN1A mutation-positive Dravet syndrome. Brain 135, 2329–2336.

Caraballo, R., Fontana, E., Darra, F., et al., 2008. Migrating focal seizures in infancy: analysis of the electroclinical patterns in 17 patients. J. Child Neurol. 23 (5), 497–506.

Chiron, C., 2011. Current therapeutic procedures in Dravet syndrome. Dev. Med. Child Neurol. 53 (Suppl. 2), 16–18.

Gaillard, W.D., Chiron, C., Cross, J.H., et al., 2009. Guidelines for imaging infants and children with recent-onset epilepsy. Epilepsia 50, 2147–2153.

Go, C.Y., Mackay, M.T., Weiss, S.K., et al., 2012. Evidence-based guideline update: medical treatment of infantile spasms. Report of the Guideline Development Subcommittee of the American Academy of Neurology and the Practice Committee of the Child Neurology Society. Neurology 78, 1974–1980.

Paciorkowski, A.R., Thio, L.L., Dobyns, W.B., 2011. Genetic and biologic classification of infantile spasms. Pediatr. Neurol. 45, 355–367.

Riikonen, R., 2001. Long-term outcome of patients with West syndrome. Brain Dev. 23, 683–687.

Scheffer, I.E., Berkovic, S.F., 1997. Generalized epilepsy with febrile seizures plus. A genetic disorder with heterogeneous clinical phenotypes. Brain 120 (Pt 3), 479–490.

Vigevano, F., 2005. Benign familial infantile seizures. Brain Dev. 7 (3), 172–177.

Widjaja, E., Go, C., McCoy, B., et al., 2015. Neurodevelopmental outcome of infantile spasms: A a systematic review and meta-analysis. Epilepsy Res. 109, 155–162.

E-BOOK FIGURES AND TABLES

The following figures and tables are available in the e-book at www.expertconsult.com. See inside cover for registration details.

Fig. 71-1 Normal background during wakefulness and sleep.

Fig. 71-2 Generalized atypical spike.

Fig. 71-3 EEG of a 4-month-old infant with benign myoclonus of infancy.

Fig. 71-4 EEG of a 3-year-old boy with intractable epilepsy.

Fig. 71-6 Seizure discharge maximally involving the left temporal region.

Fig. 71-7 Interictal sleep EEG of a 6 month old with epileptic spasms.

Fig. 71-8 Ictal recording of an 8-month-old with a history of West syndrome.

Fig. 71-9 EEG of a 5-year-old girl with Dravet syndrome.

Fig. 71-10 EEG of a 2-year-old boy with a history of two febrile and two afebrile generalized tonic-clonic seizures.

72 Electroclinical Syndromes: Childhood Onset

Jeffrey R. Tenney and Tracy Glauser

An expanded version of this chapter is available on www.expertconsult.com. See inside cover for registration details.

INTRODUCTION

Electroclinical syndromes are important constellations of specific clinical history and electroencephalographic (EEG) findings with onset during a distinct time in brain development. Childhood is a particularly important stage of development in general and epilepsy specifically.

The electroclinical syndromes of childhood can be considered as three distinct categories depending on seizure onset localization. These include childhood generalized epilepsy syndromes, focal epilepsy syndromes of childhood, and a category best described as, "undetermined as to whether focal or generalized."

Making the diagnosis of a specific electroclinical syndrome allows the clinician to provide specific diagnostic and therapeutic recommendations to the family and enhances counseling related to treatment response, remission rates, and potential psychosocial comorbidities.

CHILDHOOD GENERALIZED EPILEPSY SYNDROMES

Childhood Absence Epilepsy (CAE)

Clinical Characteristics

CAE is the most common pediatric epilepsy syndrome comprising 10% to 17% of all childhood onset epilepsies. Females are affected more frequently than males. The International League Against Epilepsy (ILAE) criteria include age of onset between 4 and 10 years that peaks between 5 and 7 years.

The main clinical manifestation of childhood absence seizures is an abrupt impairment of consciousness (without an aura) accompanied by one or more additional features including behavioral arrest, staring, eyelid fluttering, and/or hand automatisms followed by no significant postictal confusion or lethargy. The impairment of consciousness can be assessed at the bedside by asking the child to repeat a code word or perform a continuous motor task such as tapping. Absences can be provoked by hyperventilation. The duration of typical absence seizures has been reported as 9.4 plus or minus 7 seconds but with a range from 1 to 44 seconds. These seizures can be very frequent and occur at least daily but in the most severe cases can occur hundreds of times per day.

The ILAE Report on Terminology and Classification revised in 2010 distinguishes between typical and atypical absence seizures (Berg, et al., 2010). In contrast to typical absence seizures, atypical absences tend to have a less abrupt onset and offset, variable impairment of consciousness, and prolonged duration.

EEG Findings

The characteristic ictal electroencephalogram (EEG) of a typical absence seizure demonstrates generalized, bilaterally synchronous, spike and wave complexes with frontal predominance and repeating at 3 to 4.5 Hz (Fig. 72-1). There is a gradual slowing of the frequency from onset to termination. Often the onset is not truly bilaterally synchronous but rather

with one hemisphere preceding the other by a few milliseconds. A duration of 3 seconds is a clinically reasonable "rule" for distinguishing a burst from a seizure and provides an objective EEG measure when it is difficult to identify a clinical change (Glauser, et al., 2010). Interictal background activity is usually normal in patients with CAE although high voltage occipital intermittent rhythmic delta activity (OIRDA) has been reported in 15% to 38% (Holmes, et al., 1987).

Etiology

CAE is categorized as an idiopathic, and presumed genetic, epilepsy syndrome. Over the past 50 years multiple theories have been proposed to explain the generation of the diffuse spike and wave discharges that characterize absence seizures. Initially, the centrencephalic theory suggested that these rhythms were generated by cells in the midline thalamus that then projected diffusely to the cortex. Similarly, a more recent "thalamic clock" theory implicated the reticular thalamic nucleus as the generator that drives the cortical rhythms seen on EEG. Other investigators have highlighted focal cortical regions as generators for these seizures which then spread diffusely through corticocortical connections. The "corticothalamic" theory of generation highlights the interaction between oscillations in the thalamus and the presence of an excitable cortex that leads to the spike wave discharges. Investigations in animals and humans have highlighted the importance of focal cortical regions that may force larger areas of cortex into a pathologic state, which is then perpetuated by thalamocortical connections.

Genetics has been known to play a role in the development of CAE for over 70 years and recent work has highlighted the genetic complexity of this syndrome. Small populations of affected patients have been shown to have various mutations in genes coding for GABA receptor subunits, nonion channel proteins, and calcium channels.

Treatment

Before 2010 there were only a few, small, randomized, controlled trials completed to assess the most effective monotherapy for children with CAE, and none of them were categorized as Class I or II. These were insufficient for informing routine clinical practice. However, in 2010 a NIH funded double-blind, randomized, multicenter, comparative-effectiveness clinical trial compared ethosuximide, valproic acid, and lamotrigine as initial monotherapy in 446 patients with CAE. Significantly higher freedom from failure rates were seen at the 16 to 20 week visit in patients taking ethosuximide (53%) and valproic acid (58%) than those on lamotrigine (29%; p <0.001). In addition, dysfunctions of attention was seen less in the ethosuximide than valproic acid group (33% versus 49%; p = 0.03). Taking these results together, the authors concluded that ethosuximide is the best initial therapy for CAE. However, this "best" therapy still failed in 47% of subjects (14% due to seizures, 24% due to intolerable side effects, 13% study withdrawal). At the 12-month mark of double-blind therapy, ethosuximide continued to demonstrate superior effectiveness compared with lamotrigine and less attentional toxicity

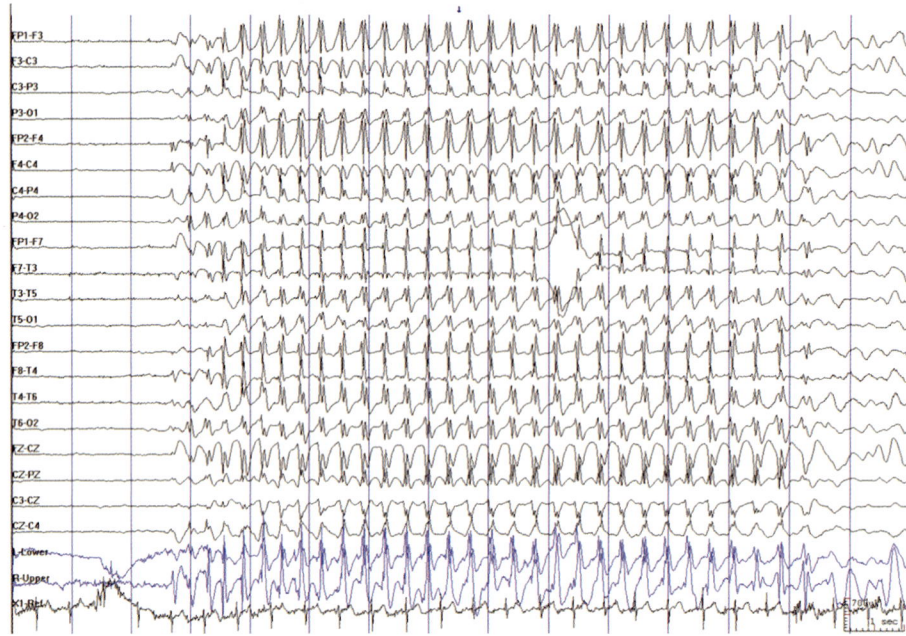

Figure 72-1. Typical absence seizure. EEG showing a typical absence seizure with generalized 3 Hz spike and wave discharges with a bifrontal predominance.

compared with valproic acid, reinforcing it as optimal initial monotherapy for CAE (Glauser, et al., 2013).

Prognosis

Although often considered a "benign" epilepsy syndrome, CAE has a variable clinical course with far lower remission rates than other classic "benign" epilepsies such as benign epilepsy with central temporal spikes. Variable remission rates for CAE have been reported, ranging from 21% to 74%. Multiple prospective cohort studies have reported seizure free rates of 57% to 74% in their patients with CAE.

In those patients without remission of CAE, it has been reported that generalized tonic-clonic seizures (GTCs) develop in approximately 40% (range of 35% to 60%). These tend to occur between 5 and 10 years after the onset of absence seizures, when the children are between 8 and 15 years of age. Long-term follow up (median 7.0 years) of the NIH-funded CAE clinical trial cohort showed only 12% had experienced at least one GTC. Importantly, children who responded to initial ethosuximide monotherapy had a particularly low risk of developing later GTCs.

A consideration for patients with CAE is the possibility of accidental injury. This is a common problem with 20% of patients reported to suffer an injury during an absence seizure. The risk of accidental injury from an absence seizure has been estimated at 3% per person year.

Although clinical seizure outcomes in CAE can be favorable, these children have increased rates of neuropsychiatric comorbidities, including attention problems, depression, anxiety, low self-esteem, and social isolation. The 2010 CAE monotherapy trial reported normal overall cognition in the cohort, but 35% had pretreatment attention deficits that did not resolve, even when seizures were well controlled.

Generalized Epilepsy With Eyelid Myoclonia (Jeavons Syndrome)

Eyelid myoclonia with absences is an epilepsy syndrome characterized by an absence seizure with special features. These seizures consist of prominent jerking of the eyelids with an upward deviation of the eyes, often triggered by eye closure. Eyelid myoclonia with absences can occur as a part of idiopathic (Jeavons syndrome), cryptogenic, or symptomatic epilepsies. The ictal pattern of eyelid myoclonia with absences consists of diffuse 3 to 6 Hz polyspike and wave complexes. A generalized photoparoxysmal response can also be seen on EEG.

This syndrome has a likely genetic etiology given several reports of affected identical twins, but specific gene mutations are unknown. It is commonly thought that this syndrome is resistant to pharmacologic treatments. The most commonly used medications are valproic acid, ethosuximide, benzodiazepines, phenobarbital, and levetiracetam. Patients are counseled to avoid clear seizure triggers, and nonpharmacologic treatments such as wearing glasses with colored filters can be recommended. The long-term outcome of this syndrome is poorly understood but is typically considered lifelong and treatment resistant.

Epilepsy With Myoclonic Absences (Tassinari Syndrome)

These seizures are characterized by absence seizures that are accompanied by severe, rhythmic, and bilateral clonic or tonic activity. Age of onset is 7 years (range of 1 to 12 years). A majority will have additional seizure types, most commonly GTCs and cognitive impairment is present in approximately 50% of patients. The ictal findings are difficult to distinguish from typical absence seizures, but jerks occurring at 3 Hz may be time locked to the spike component.

The cause is unknown but almost 20% have a family history of epilepsy. These seizures are usually considered pharmacoresistant. Medications used include those used to treat typical absence seizures. There is not much data about outcome; it seems a majority will convert to other seizure types over time, and cognitive impairment becomes severe, especially in those patients with frequent GTCs.

Epilepsy With Myoclonic-Atonic (Formerly Astatic) Seizures (EMAS)

This epilepsy syndrome is characterized by multiple seizure types such as myoclonic-atonic, absence, tonic-clonic, and tonic. Episodes of nonconvulsive and myoclonic status epilepticus have been reported. Age at onset has a peak of 3 years (range of 18 months to 5 years). The interictal EEG can be normal, but eventually frequent bursts of generalized spike and polyspike and wave discharges are seen along with central-parietal theta slowing. The EMG just after the jerk is often a brief silent period representing the atonic component.

EMAS is thought to have a predominantly genetic etiology. Studies have shown a relationship between EMAS and genetic epilepsy with febrile seizures plus (GEFS +). Initial pharmacologic treatment of EMAS usually consists of valproic acid, ethosuximide, or benzodiazepines, with those who are drug resistant considered for dietary therapy. If the atonic component is severe, then wearing a helmet should be considered. EMAS spontaneously remits in many (50% to 89%) patients. The remaining minority of patients can have intractable epilepsy with intellectual deficiency.

Lennox-Gastaut Syndrome

Clinical Characteristics

Lennox-Gastaut syndrome (LGS) is characterized by a constellation of symptoms and EEG findings, including: (1) multiple generalized seizure types such as atypical absence, tonic, atonic, and myoclonic; (2) diffuse slow spike and wave interictal pattern; (3) paroxysmal fast activity during sleep; and (4) cognitive abnormalities. Onset is usually by the age of 8 years, with a peak incidence at 3 to 5 years of age and a male pre-dominance. Approximately 20% to 40% of cases have a preceding diagnosis of West syndrome.

Multiple seizure types can occur in LGS (Hancock and Cross, 2013):

1. Tonic seizures are the most common and can be bilaterally symmetric or unilateral.
2. Atypical absence seizures are also commonly seen and can have subtle clinical features with a gradual start and stop.
3. Atonic seizures are less common and are characterized by a rapid loss of muscle tone with symptoms ranging from subtle head drops to violent drops to the ground.
4. Myoclonic seizures have been reported with various incidences in LGS, from rare to up to one-third of patients.
5. Status epilepticus occurs in two-thirds or more of patients with LGS. Status can be either nonconvulsive or convulsive (tonic). Nonconvulsive status will typically consist of almost continuous absence seizures with intermittent tonic seizures that can last from hours to weeks.

EEG Findings

The EEG posterior dominant background is slowed in the majority of patients with LGS and usually correlates with the degree of cognitive impairment. The characteristic interictal pattern is diffuse and slow: 2 to 2.5 Hz spike and wave complexes with a frontal predominance (Fig. 72-3). This most often occurs symmetrically, but a more focal or multifocal appearance can be seen. This interictal pattern may be absent at the time of initial epilepsy diagnosis, and in late childhood the interictal abnormalities may become more infrequent or resolve completely.

Paroxysmal fast activity can often, but not always, be seen during slow wave sleep and has been considered by some to

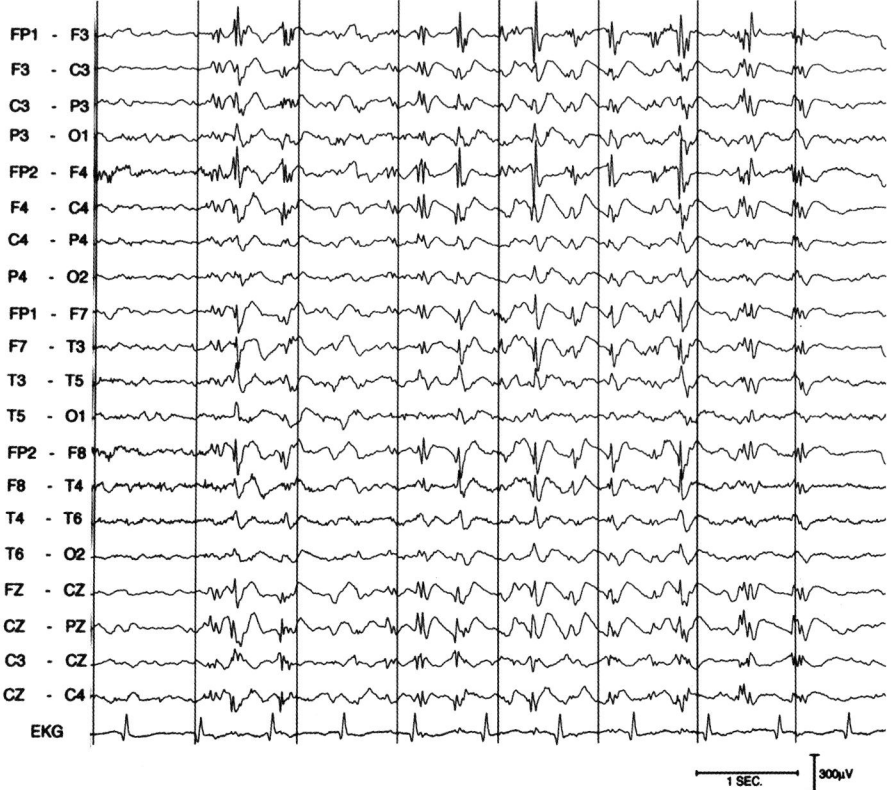

Figure 72-3. Lennox-Gastaut interictal pattern. Interictal EEG of a patient with Lennox-Gastaut syndrome showing slow, generalized 1 to 2Hz spike and wave discharges with a bifrontal predominance.

be a diagnostic feature of LGS. The bursts typically are 10 Hz or faster frequency and are diffusely distributed with an anterior predominance. Careful review of accompanying video may reveal associated subtle clinical tonic symptoms.

The ictal patterns associated with LGS vary with the corresponding seizure types.

Etiology

Up to 30% of patients with LGS have no known etiology, with normal development and brain imaging at the time of diagnosis. In the remaining patients, a presumed etiology can be determined from brain imaging, neurologic examination, genetic analysis, or metabolic testing. The more common etiologies associated with LGS are congenital brain malformations (focal cortical dysplasia, subcortical band heterotopia, perisylvian polymicrogyria, hypothalamic hamartoma), neurocutaneous diseases (tuberous sclerosis, hypomelanosis of Ito), meningitis/encephalitis, hypoxic ischemic encephalopathy, and genetic epilepsies (i.e., GEFS +).

Treatment

Monotherapy with antiseizure medications is typically unsuccessful in patients with LGS and because of this polytherapy is often necessary (Montouris, et al., 2014). Five medications have demonstrated efficacy against the seizures associated with the Lennox-Gastaut syndrome in randomized, double-blind, placebo-controlled, adjunctive therapy trials: felbamate, lamotrigine, topiramate, rufinamide, and clobazam. Despite demonstrated efficacy, all these medications have potential adverse effects or specific practical considerations that need to be considered when selecting a medication. No one specific medication or combination of medications works for all patients with LGS. Finding the optimal combination of medications for LGS patients is a trial and error process. Commonly used medications without randomized double-blind, placebo-controlled, adjunctive therapy clinical trial evidence of efficacy against the seizures associated with LGS include: valproic acid, clonazepam, and zonisamide.

Nonpharmacologic treatments such as the ketogenic diet and vagus nerve stimulator (VNS) can also be effective in these children with treatment resistant seizures. The ketogenic diet has been associated with a greater than 50% reduction of seizures in approximately half of patients with LGS, with some patients having a greater than 90% reduction of seizures. Corpus callosotomy is a palliative treatment that may significantly reduce both atonic seizure frequency and severity.

Prognosis

Prognosis for LGS remains poor despite the availability of new and varied treatments. Most patients have treatment resistant seizures along with significant cognitive deficits which limit their ability to live independently. Persistent daily seizures are present in the majority of patients (60% to 80%) with an early age of seizure onset (before 3 years) as a predictor of poor seizure outcome. Age at seizure onset seems to be a predictor for cognitive development, with earlier onset more likely to be associated with intellectual deficiency.

CHILDHOOD FOCAL EPILEPSY SYNDROMES
Benign Epilepsy With Centrotemporal Spikes (BECTS, or Benign Rolandic Epilepsy)
Clinical Characteristics

Benign epilepsy with centrotemporal spikes (BECTS) is a common pediatric epilepsy syndrome that is thought to

account for 15% to 23% of all childhood epilepsies. Seizures typically begin between 3 and 13 years of age with a peak at 7 to 8 years of age. Although the "typical" form has easily recognizable clinical features, there are many atypical features that can make an accurate diagnosis challenging. Seizures typically occur shortly after the child falls asleep or just before waking. Some patients will have seizures during both wakefulness and sleep, and approximately 25% may have seizures only during the waking state (Beaussart, 1972).

The seizures of BECTS also tend to be infrequent with the majority of patients having only a single seizure with relatively few (less than 10%) being reported to have frequent seizures (Loiseau, et al., 1988). When occurring during the awakened state, the seizure semiology is described as unilateral perioral paresthesias, unilateral jerking of the orofacial muscles, dysarthria, choking/gagging noises, expressive aphasia, and/or excessive drooling. Consciousness can be maintained as these symptoms occur. These symptoms can then self-resolve or evolve into secondary generalized tonic-clonic movements with loss of consciousness. When occurring during sleep, the semiology tends to be either unilateral facial jerking, often with drooling and/or choking/gagging noises, or secondarily generalized tonic-clonic movements. The seizures tend to be brief, lasting seconds to minutes, but there have been rare reports of status epilepticus in those with an atypical semiology. Post ictal Todd's paralysis has been reported in 7% to 16% of children.

Aside from seizures, a wide range of cognitive and behavioral problems have been reported in patients with BECTS. General intellectual functioning (full scale IQ) is in the normal range, but these patients perform worse than age-matched controls on tests of language, visual-spatial skills, nonverbal and verbal memory, and attention. Behavioral problems are also more common in this population. Although the literature suggests that these cognitive problems are prevalent in BECTS, they are also commonly reported in patients with childhood epilepsy in general. The specific cognitive domain may vary, however, raising the possibility that specific epilepsy syndromes may be associated with specific neurocognitive phenotypes.

EEG Findings

The characteristic EEG pattern of BECTS is high voltage, but blunted, spikes in the centrotemporal head regions that can be unilateral or bilateral and become more frequent during drowsiness and non-REM sleep (Fig. 72-6). A horizontal dipole can often be seen with maximal negativity in the centrotemporal region and maximal positivity in the frontal head region. The localization is most often unilateral although bilateral synchronous and asynchronous discharges can be seen. The localization of spikes can vary over time in the same patient. It has been reported that approximately one-third of patients will only have spikes during sleep. There is no known relationship between the frequency of spikes and the number of seizures. The background of the EEG is normal.

It is clear that centrotemporal spikes (CTS) can be seen in a significant percentage (up to 0.7%) of "normal" children with no history of epilepsy. The fraction of children with these EEG findings who then develop BECTS is unclear, but it is thought to be small. For this reason CTS can be considered an incidental finding in children without a clinical history concerning for seizures.

There have been many studies which suggest a possible negative effect of CTS, especially during sleep, on cognition, language, and behavior but none have provided clear proof of a direct relationship.

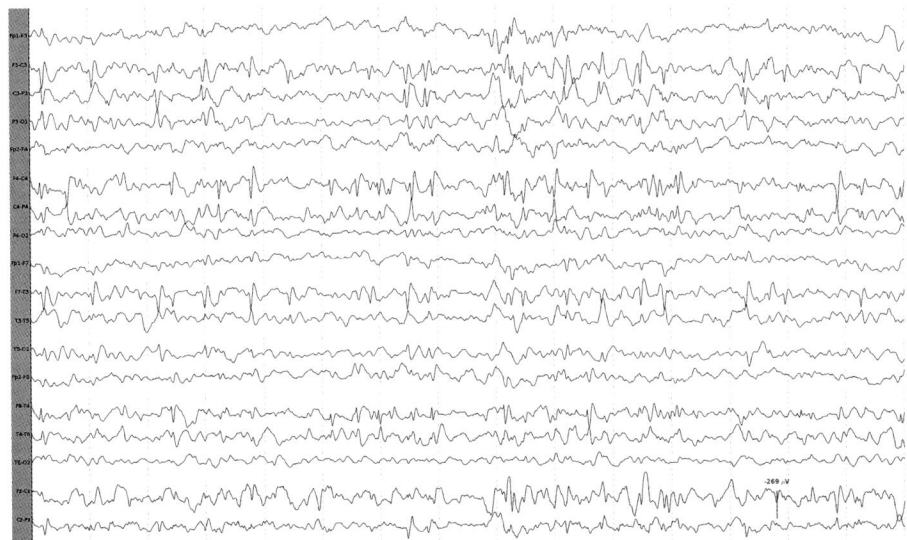

Figure 72-6. Benign epilepsy with centrotemporal spikes. Interictal pattern of a patient with BECTS during stage N2 sleep. Frequent high voltage spikes can be seen independently in the right centrotemporal and left centrotemporal head regions.

Etiology

Typically, BECTS is not associated with any underlying structural brain abnormalities on routine visual analysis, although studies employing quantitative structural analyses have reported a variety of abnormal cortical thickness and atrophy. Genetic studies have suggested that BECTS has a genetic etiology with complex inheritance patterns, although noninherited factors also seem to play a major role. A few chromosomal loci and specific genes have been associated with the syndrome including the glutamate receptor, GRIN2A, as well as mutations in RBFOX1/3 and DEPDC5.

Treatment

Children with BECTS will have remission regardless of treatment, so pharmaceutical treatment can be avoided in many cases. The decision not to treat is based on the fact that the seizures in most are infrequent and tend to occur nocturnally when the children are in a safe location (i.e., in their beds at home). Occasionally, however, seizures are more frequent or occur during the day so that treatment is necessary. When used, medications include carbamazepine, valproate, clobazam, clonazepam, phenytoin, phenobarbital, gabapentin, and sulthiame.

Prognosis

The long-term prognosis for BECTS is thought to be excellent with all patients achieving seizure remission and most by age 13 years. This remission has been reported to occur even when the seizures have been initially resistant to treatment. A recent study of patients 30 years after their onset reported that social outcomes were better for BECTS than other types of childhood onset epilepsy.

Early Onset Childhood Occipital Epilepsy (Panayiotopoulos Syndrome)

The early onset form of benign occipital epilepsy of childhood is referred to as Panayiotopoulos syndrome. Onset is from 1 to 14 years of age with a peak age of onset from 3 to 6 years of age. These seizures, often prolonged and nocturnal, are associated with predominantly autonomic features including nausea, vomiting, and tonic eye deviation, with consciousness usually preserved. In the majority these are followed by impaired consciousness and evolution to secondary generalized tonic-clonic movements. Occipital spikes are seen in approximately 40% of EEG recordings and may activate with sleep.

This syndrome likely has a genetic etiology, but most children lack a family history of epilepsy. Most patients do not require treatment because the seizures are relatively infrequent. Intermittent benzodiazepine use could be considered for those patients with prolonged events. The outcome of Panayiotopoulos syndrome is typically benign with most patients having between one and five lifetime seizures. Remission usually occurs within 1 to 2 years.

Late-Onset Childhood Occipital Epilepsy (Gastaut Syndrome)

This syndrome begins in the later childhood years, with a peak between 8 and 11 years of age. Semiology consists of brief visual symptoms—commonly visual hallucinations in the form of colored circular patterns, lasting seconds to minutes. Brief ictal blindness can occur and consciousness often remains intact. Postictally, a severe headache can occur. In many patients the visual seizures are relatively frequent, occurring daily to monthly, but GTCS are rare. The interictal EEG shows runs of rhythmic biooccipital spikes and sharp waves, especially present upon eye closure and with resolution on eye opening.

Familial late-onset childhood occipital epilepsy is thought to be rare. Most patients require treatment, and carbamazepine can result in good seizure control; however, 40% to 50% may not be seizure free. Fifty percent to 60% of patients may have seizure remission within 2 to 4 years.

CHILDHOOD EPILEPSIES UNDETERMINED WHETHER FOCAL OR GENERALIZED

Epileptic Encephalopathy With Continuous Spike and Wave During Sleep (CSWS)

CSWS is a term that has been used interchangeably with electrical status epilepticus of slow sleep (ESES). This is an epileptic encephalopathy that is a rare cause of childhood epilepsy. The diagnosis is typically made between 5 and 7 years of age. Various seizure types are possible, including GTCs during sleep, atypical absence, atonic, and myoclonic, but are often not the major feature. Global developmental delay or deterioration can often be seen as well as specifically selective regression of language. The hallmark EEG finding of CSWS is spike wave activity occurring during 85% of slow wave sleep.

The etiology is poorly understood with a minority of patients having identifiable structural abnormalities such as cortical dysplasia, polymicrogyria, and thalamic lesions in the neonatal period. Most clinicians agree that the ESES pattern should be treated, and the goal should be normalization of the EEG. Although there is no clear consensus on the optimal treatment, valproate, levetiracetam, high-dose benzodiazepines, and corticosteroids are most commonly used. Ketogenic diet or epilepsy surgery can be considered if these initial treatments fail. The prognosis for seizures in patients with CSWS is usually considered good; however, the prognosis of neurocognitive deficits is not as good. Approximately 50% of patients with have average neuropsychological functioning and are able to live independently.

Acquired Epileptic Aphasia (Landau-Kleffner Syndrome)

This is a rare syndrome of childhood, usually presenting between 3 and 7 years of age. The syndrome is characterized by loss of language skills in children who were previously normal. Attention and behavioral problems are very common.

The majority of children with acquired epileptic aphasia (Landau-Kleffner syndrome; LKS) (70%) also present with seizures of various types. The EEG in the awakened state often has a normal background and epileptiform abnormalities, typically in the central, parietal, and/or temporal head regions. During sleep, there is activation, and a pattern such as ESES can be seen.

It is likely that continuous discharges during sleep, especially in the perisylvian region, disrupt networks involved in normal language processing. It is likely that LKS is on the severe end of spectrum, which also includes BECTS and CSWS. Seizures usually respond well to treatment, and the treatment of choice is valproate with or without and adjunctive benzodiazepine. Corticosteroids or ACTH have been used in an attempt to normalize the EEG and prevent long standing language deficits. The long-term prognosis is unclear, although improvements of language ability seem to be related to the age of onset (prelanguage or postlanguage development), with early onset related to poorer prognosis.

CONCLUSION

The electroclinical syndromes of childhood encompass a diverse collection of epilepsies, from benign to severe (Table 72-1). Childhood is a period of critical brain development, and disruption from seizures and/or electrographic abnormalities could induce lifelong deficits. Early and accurate identification of the electroclinical syndromes of childhood allows clinicians and parents to provide the most effective and appropriate treatments for these children.

TABLE 72-1 Electroclinical Syndromes of Childhood

Syndrome	Age at Onset (peak)	Clinical Manifestations	EEG Findings	Treatment	Prognosis
Childhood Absence Epilepsy (CAE)	4–10 years (5–7 years)	Impaired consciousness Staring Behavioral arrest Automatisms	Diffuse SWDs 3–4.5 Hz	ETX VPA LTG	21–74% remission rate Neuropsychiatric co-morbidities
Jeavons Syndrome	2–14 years (6–8 years)	Eyelid jerking Upward eye deviation Absence seizures	Diffuse polyspike-wave 3–6 Hz Photoparoxysmal response	VPA ETX Benzo LEV PHB	Poorly understood Treatment resistant Low remission rate
Tassinari Syndrome	1–12 years (7 years)	Bilateral tonic/clonic Absence seizures GTCs	Diffuse SWDs 3–4.5 Hz Jerks time locked to spikes	ETX VPA LTG	Poorly understood Treatment resistant Cognitive impairment
Epilepsy with Myoclonic Atonic Seizures (EMAS)	1.5–5 years (3 years)	Multiple seizure types Myoclonus and atonia	Diffuse SWDs Centro-parietal slowing	VPA ETX Benzo KD	Treatment resistant Spontaneous remission possible
Lennox-Gastaut Syndrome	2–8 years (3–5 years)	Multiple seizure types Intellectual deficiency	Diffuse SWDs 2–2.5 Hz Paroxysmal fast activity	LTG FBM TPM RUF CLZ KD VNS CC	Treatment resistant Cognitive impairment
Benign Epilepsy with Centrotemporal Spikes (BECTS)	3–13 years (7–8 years)	Perioral parasthesias Perioral jerking Secondarily GTCs Associated with sleep	Centrotemporal spikes Activation with sleep	None CBZ VPA CLZ	Infrequent seizures 100% remission rate
Early Onset Childhood Occipital Epilepsy	1–14 years (3–6 years)	Autonomic features Prolonged duration Secondarily GTCs	Multifocal IEDs 40% occipital IEDs Activation with sleep	CBZ LEV	Infrequent seizures High remission rate

TABLE 72-1 Electroclinical Syndromes of Childhood *(Continued)*

Syndrome	Age at Onset (peak)	Clinical Manifestations	EEG Findings	Treatment	Prognosis
Late Onset Childhood Occipital Epilepsy	3–15 years (8–11 years)	Visual symptoms Intact consciousness Post-ictal headache	Bioccipital IEDs Fixation off phenomena	CBZ	Frequent seizures Variable remission rate
CSWS	3–7 years	Various seizure types Developmental delay Acquired aphasia Ataxia or dystonia	Diffuse SWDs 1.5–2.5 Hz 85% slow wave sleep	VPA LEV Benzo Steroids KD Surgery	Seizure remission Variable cognitive deficits
Landau-Kleffner Syndrome	2–14 years (3–7 years)	Language regression Various seizure types	Variable IEDs Activation with sleep	VPA Benzo Steroids IVIG	Infrequent seizures Seizure remission Variable language deficits

Benzo, benzodiazepines; CBZ, carbamazepine; CC, corpus callosotomy; CLZ, clobazam; ETX, ethosuximide; FBM, felbamate; GTCs, generalized tonic clonic seizures; IEDs, interictal epileptiform discharges; IVIG, intravenous immunoglobulin; KD, ketogenic diet; LEV, levetiracetam; LTG, lamotrigine; PHB, phenobarbital; RUF, rufinamide; SWDs, spike wave discharges; TPM, topiramate; VNS, vagal nerve stimulator; VPA, valproic acid.

REFERENCES

The complete list of references for this chapter is available in the e-book at www.expertconsult.com.

See inside cover for registration details.

SELECTED REFERENCES

Beaussart, M., 1972. Benign epilepsy of children with Rolandic (centro-temporal) paroxysmal foci. A clinical entity. Study of 221 cases. Epilepsia 13 (6), 795–811.

Berg, A.T., Berkovic, S.F., Brodie, M.J., et al., 2010. Revised terminology and concepts for organization of seizures and epilepsies: report of the ILAE Commission on Classification and Terminology, 2005–2009. Epilepsia 51 (4), 676–685.

Glauser, T.A., Cnaan, A., Shinnar, S., et al., 2010. Ethosuximide, valproic acid, and lamotrigine in childhood absence epilepsy. N. Engl. J. Med. 362 (9), 790–799.

Glauser, T.A., Cnaan, A., Shinnar, S., et al., 2013. Ethosuximide, valproic acid, and lamotrigine in childhood absence epilepsy: initial monotherapy outcomes at 12 months. Epilepsia 54 (1), 141–155.

Hancock, E.C., Cross, J.H., 2013. Treatment of Lennox-Gastaut syndrome. Cochrane Database Syst. Rev. (2), CD003277.

Holmes, G.L., McKeever, M., Adamson, M., 1987. Absence seizures in children: clinical and electroencephalographic features. Ann. Neurol. 21 (3), 268–273.

Loiseau, P., Duché, B., Cordova, S., et al., 1988. Prognosis of benign childhood epilepsy with centrotemporal spikes: a follow-up study of 168 patients. Epilepsia 29 (3), 229–235.

Montouris, G.D., Wheless, J.W., Glauser, T.A., 2014. The efficacy and tolerability of pharmacologic treatment options for Lennox-Gastaut syndrome. Epilepsia 55 (Suppl. 4), 10–20.

E-BOOK FIGURES AND TABLES

The following figures and tables are available in the e-book at www.expertconsult.com. See inside cover for registration details.

Fig. 72-2 Myoclonic-atonic seizure.

Fig. 72-4 Tonic seizure.

Fig. 72-5 Atonic seizure.

73 Electroclinical Syndromes: Adolescent Onset

Andrea M. Harriott and William O. Tatum IV

INTRODUCTION
Ontogenesis and Classification

Adolescence can be a formidable but exciting developmental period. However, when it is complicated by epilepsy it poses a great challenge for both patients and physicians. Adolescent medicine is confronted by immense physical, hormonal, and psychosocial growth occurring between the ages of 10 and 19. Early recognition and treatment of adolescent epilepsy are of paramount importance. The adolescent period also presents a unique set of challenges for seizure control, including medication compliance, pubertal changes, reproductive potential, sleep deprivation, social stressors, and driving (Appleton, 1999).

Adolescent-onset epilepsy can be classified into three broad categories. The first group is the genetic generalized epilepsies (GGEs), which are a heterogeneous group of epilepsy syndromes with substantial genetic influence. This group represents the most common classification of adolescent-onset seizures. The GGEs include juvenile myoclonic epilepsy (JME), juvenile absence epilepsy (JAE), generalized tonic-clonic (GTC) seizures on awakening, and generalized epilepsy with sporadic GTC seizures. The second group is composed of the progressive generalized epilepsies that the result of a structural-metabolic etiology. These include the progressive myoclonus epilepsies and characteristically portend a poorer prognosis compared with the nonprogressive generalized epilepsies. The third group consists of the focal epilepsies. These may be associated with a structural-metabolic pathophysiology, as is the case for temporal lobe epilepsy resulting from hippocampal sclerosis. Genetic and familial causes including mendelian inheritance patterns may also occur, as is the case for autosomal-dominant partial epilepsy with auditory features, autosomal-dominant frontal lobe epilepsy, and familial mesial temporal lobe epilepsy (Wheless and Kim, 2002).

Epidemiology and Psychosocial Implications of Adolescent Epilepsy

Epilepsy syndromes in adolescents create a substantial health and psychosocial burden. In this age group, 4 in 1000 teenagers, representing a prevalence of 1.5% to 2% of the adolescent population, have epilepsy. In fact, it is one of the most common neurologic conditions in adolescence. Adolescent epilepsy contributes to substantial health-care costs and hospitalizations. In the United States, hospitalizations alone account for approximately one-third of the cost associated with epilepsy. Although there are annual changes in the number of epilepsy patients admitted to hospitals, an estimated 100,000 to 120,000 patients under 20 years of age with epilepsy are admitted to hospitals yearly. The majority of these hospitalizations occur in the adolescent age group. Moreover, grave complications, including injury, drowning, and sudden unexpected death in epilepsy (SUDEP), are real consequences faced by young people with epilepsy (Wheless and Kim, 2002).

Seizures may compromise social interaction, personal identity, career choices, relationships, and sexual maturation. Adolescents with epilepsy have greater rates of depression, anxiety, obsessive behaviors, anhedonia, and low self-esteem compared with adolescents who do not have a history of epilepsy. Additionally, when teens with epilepsy and their caregivers are surveyed, they report experiencing lost time from school and emotional instability as a result of their diagnosis, and approximately one-third of adolescents keep their diagnosis of epilepsy a secret. More than one-third of teens reported the expectation that seizures would hinder their lives, including employment and educational opportunities. These quality-of-life measures raise awareness that adolescent epilepsy is far from benign and can have a significant impact on those with epilepsy and their families (Wheless, 2002).

Cognitive, Behavioral, and Compliance Issues

Aside from the real and perceived social stigma, there are additional cognitive implications for adolescent epilepsy. Those diagnosed with a GGE, including JAE or JME, tend to have mild cognitive dysfunction with normal intelligence quotients. In temporal lobe epilepsy, there is a diminution in the expected accumulation of learning and memory skills over time, particularly during the adolescent period, with persistent decreased performance in learning and memory-related tasks. Cognitive impairment is encountered with frontal lobe epilepsy, particularly if radiographic white-matter lesions are identified. A hallmark of progressive myoclonus epilepsy is cumulative neurologic disability with early-onset dementia. Finally, antiseizure drugs (ASDs) can have an independent negative influence on attention, memory, processing speed, and intelligence quotients. However, this is in contradistinction to the presumed benefit that these medications have on cognition if seizures are well controlled.

Compliance with medications can be a challenge when treating adolescent epilepsy. Because the reasons for not adhering to treatment are varied and patient specific, it is important for physicians to ask patients and their families about how they view taking medications to assist in identifying barriers to compliance. Effectively adhering to treatment, particularly early on, may increase the chances of becoming seizure-free. Simplifying ASD dosing and avoiding dosing regimens that require children to take medications during school are simple strategies that can improve compliance and reduce social embarrassment. Other recommended strategies include careful monitoring of ASD levels, patient and parent education, and social support.

Avoiding triggers is just as essential in this age group as medication adherence. In GGE, the recommendation to avoid flashing lights or video games that produce stroboscopic light stimulation is a pragmatic recommendation, especially for patients with photosensitivity. Improving sleep hygiene, addressing emotional and psychological stressors, and emphasizing the impact of substance abuse, including alcohol consumption, are critical. Driving is also a teen-sensitive issue that needs to be addressed. State-specific regulations are available and carry different periods of abstinence for patients with epilepsy. Most careers or jobs are available to people with epilepsy, but employment requiring use of a weapon, such as law enforcement; public transport positions that require a class A or B license; or jobs that require a license to fly, such as airline pilot, should be discouraged. Proactive recommendations are crucial to provide realistic information for career choices.

ADOLESCENT GENERALIZED EPILEPSIES

The genetic generalized epilepsies (GGEs) are the most frequent type of seizures of adolescent onset. The GGEs are polygenic disorders and represent a biologic continuum between epilepsy syndromes (Beghi et al., 2006).

Juvenile Myoclonic Epilepsy

Juvenile myoclonic epilepsy (JME) is the most common GGE, representing 5% to 10% of all epilepsies, with a prevalence of 0.1 per 1000 persons (Wheless and Kim, 2002). The onset of JME occurs during adolescence, commonly between 12 and 18 years of age. It was initially described as "epilepsy with impulsive petit mal." The stereotypical clinical features in all patients with JME consist of myoclonic jerks that often preferentially involve the upper extremities. The jerks involve sudden, irregular, nonrhythmic, lightening-like muscle contractions without loss of awareness, characteristically occurring upon awakening and in the early morning hours. Most individuals with JME exhibit a persistent tendency to manifest seizures as a lifelong condition, with a lower risk of remission (Figure 73-2). Additionally, more than 90% also have generalized tonic-clonic (GTC) seizures, and approximately one-third have absence seizures.

During the interictal period, the routine scalp electroencephalogram (EEG) may be normal. However, 4- to 6-Hz bilateral polyspike- and spike-and-slow-wave discharges are characteristic when observed in repeat or prolonged EEG recordings. Photosensitivity is common, with a photoparoxysmal response observed in 30% of patients. Asymmetric electroclinical features are not uncommonly observed, including lateralized epileptiform discharges. Most abnormalities emerge during sleep and are precipitated by sleep deprivation. Additional triggers include alcohol consumption, menses, photic stimulation, and awakening from sleep. The hallmark features of the ictal EEG in JME include generalized symmetric frontocentral-predominant polyspike-and-wave discharges with a frequency between 10 and 16 Hz or slow-wave discharges between 2 and 5 Hz. The convulsion may occur independently or follow a crescendo increase in myoclonic seizures, with generalized polyspike-and-slow-wave onset transitioning into the usual pattern of generalized fast rhythms seen with GTC seizures.

Juvenile Absence Epilepsy

Juvenile absence epilepsy (JAE) affects approximately 0.1 per 1000 persons and has a prevalence of 0.2% to 2.4% of epilepsy cases. JAE is responsible for 8% to 10% of all GGE cases. The typical age of onset ranges between 10 and 19 years but peaks around age 15. The clinical characteristics of the absence seizures in JAE are similar to those of childhood absence epilepsy (CAE). However, the seizures may be somewhat longer and are characterized by speech and behavioral arrest and loss of awareness. Absences may be accompanied by oral-buccal automatisms and repetitive hand movements and picking behaviors, suggesting temporal lobe involvement. However, the ictal EEG demonstrates a generalized 3- to 4-Hz spike-and-wave or polyspike-and-wave discharge. Similar to other GGEs, seizures may be triggered by sleep deprivation, alcohol consumption, and hyperventilation. Myoclonic jerks and generalized seizures often accompany JAE but are a less prevalent feature.

Genetic Generalized Epilepsies With Convulsions

The GGEs also include those with GTC seizures alone. The syndrome of epilepsy with generalized tonic-clonic seizures on awakening (GTCS-A) may be challenging to separate from epilepsy with sporadic GTC seizures (Figure 73-6). These

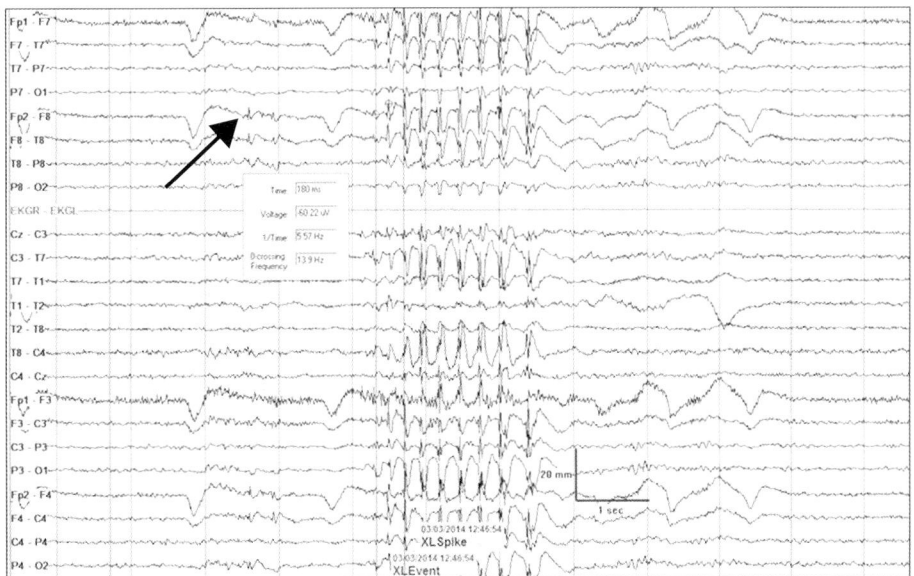

Figure 73-2. Juvenile myoclonic epilepsy (JME) with generalized tonic-clonic seizures and absences. A 17-year-old with JME shows a 2-second burst of "fast" generalized bifrontally predominant spike and waves. Note the fragmented right frontal spike (arrow) and the 5.57-Hz interspike frequency. Longer bursts of greater than 3 seconds were intermittently associated with absence seizures. (*Courtesy of William Tatum.*)

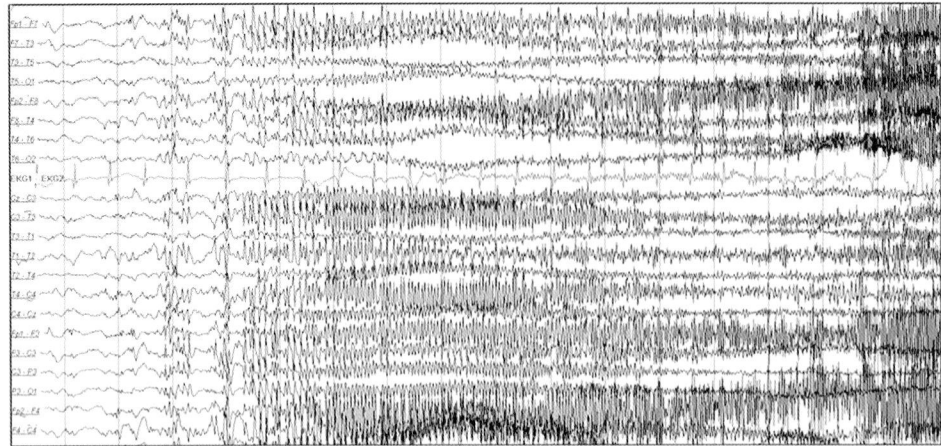

Figure 73-6. Generalized tonic-clonic (GTC) seizures on awakening. Ictal electroencephalogram (EEG) of a generalized tonic-clonic seizure in a 20-year-old with genetic generalized epilepsy (GGE) manifest as recurrent GTC seizures on awakening. Note the single epileptiform complex and then the continuous myogenic artifact that follows the 8- to 10-Hz anterior-predominant activity. *(Courtesy of William Tatum.)*

seizures tend to start in the later adolescent period around age 16. However, the age range is between 6 and 28 years, with frequency estimates between 20% to 30% of GGEs. The seizure semiology involves GTC seizures alone, and in the case of GTCS-A, seizures occur within 1 to 2 hours of awakening from sleep. Some patients will also experience seizures in the evening during relaxation or just before falling asleep. Given the timing of these seizures, there appears to be a considerable circadian influence on seizure threshold. Consistent with an important role of sleep regulation in GTCS-A, alterations in the microstructure of the sleep–wake cycle have been observed in these patients.

The interictal EEG typically demonstrates a 3- to 4-Hz generalized spike-and-slow-wave discharge. First described in the mid-1930s, the presence of bilateral, synchronous, and symmetric generalized spike-and-wave activity is the electrographic hallmark of GGE on the EEG. As in the other GGE subtypes, these may be precipitated by sleep deprivation, photic stimulation, stress, and alcohol consumption. GTCS-A can occur with other seizure types, including "phantom" absences, which are absence seizures that go relatively undetected unless EEG is utilized to identify prolonged bursts of generalized spike-and-slow-wave discharges (Shian and Chi, 1994).

Genetics of Nonmendelian-Inherited Adolescent Epilepsy

The genetics of adolescent-onset epilepsies is an ever-growing topic and has the capacity for providing putative targets for future drug therapies that may be more selective and seizure-subtype specific. JME is regarded as one of several genetic epilepsy syndromes with a complex inheritance pattern. Several gene mutations and loci have been associated with JME. Most of these genes encode for proteins or ion channels that modulate the balance between neuronal excitation and inhibition in cortical and thalamocortical circuits. Mutations in the *GABRA1* gene on chromosome 5 encoding the alpha 1 subunit of the gamma-aminobutyric acid receptor complex (GABA$_A$R) involved in synaptic inhibition were found in a large French Canadian family. Linkage analyses have also revealed an association between JME and genes on chromosome 3q26 encoding voltage-gated potassium and chloride channel subunits. Additional studies have identified associations with loci on chromosome 6 and 18. The *HLA* gene locus (EJM-1) on the short arm of chromosome 6 has been

associated with JME in several studies, although the neurobiological significance of this locus remains unclear. Variants in the *malic enzyme 2* gene located on chromosome 18 that indirectly regulates neuronal GABA synthesis may be involved in JME and other non-JME GGEs. The *CHRNA7* gene encoding the alpha 7 subunit of the nicotinic acetylcholine receptor and the *connexin 36* gene on chromosome 15 may be associated with JME in some families. Finally, a mutation in the *CACNB4* gene encoding the calcium channel beta 4 subunit on chromosome 2 was found in a JME patient. The heterogeneity of these genetic studies reflects the various genotypes involved in the phenotypic syndrome of JME. There is considerable overlap between the genes implicated in JME and those involved in juvenile absence epilepsy (JAE). Linkage analysis has found associations between chromosome 3, 6, and 18 in families and individuals with JAE. Similarly, there appears to be a genetic overlap between JME and GTCS-A, and long-term treatment is typically required. In addition, the seizures associated with GTCS-A can cluster with JME in families, suggesting a common genetic predisposition. In families with both absences and GTCS-A, there appears to be a link between expression of this GGE and the EJM-1 locus on chromosome 6 (Greenberg et al., 1995).

Rare Mendelian-Inherited Progressive Generalized Adolescent Epilepsies

Progressive myoclonus epilepsy (PME) is a rare and heterogenous group of inherited disorders that produce progressive neurologic dysfunction with dementia, ataxia, myoclonic jerks, and GTC seizures. This group accounts for approximately 1% of childhood and adolescent epilepsy syndromes and includes Unverricht–Lundborg disease, Lafora body disease, myoclonic epilepsy with ragged red fibers, neuronal ceroid lipofuscinosis, and others. These syndromes are accompanied by GTC seizures and action or stimulus myoclonus. The EEG pattern typically reveals generalized polyspike-and-wave and spike-and-wave discharges with photosensitivity.

Unverricht–Lundborg disease (ULD) is an autosomal-recessive disorder that presents between the ages of 6 and 16. In Finnish populations, the incidence is 1 in 20,000. Seizures are GTC and myoclonic jerks. The interictal EEG demonstrates progressively slower background activity with generalized anterior-predominant polyspike-and-slow-wave discharges. Dodecamer repeat expansions or point mutations in the cystatin B (CSTB) gene on chromosome 21 result in ULD. The unique histopathologic feature of this disease that distinguishes it from the other forms of PME is the *lack* of abnormal neuronal inclusions or systemic deposits.

Lafora body disease (LBD) is an autosomal-recessive disorder presenting between the ages of 6 and 19; it is characterized histopathologically by polyglucosan intracellular neuronal inclusions, termed Lafora bodies, that stain positive with periodic acid–Schiff stain. Seizures consist of GTC seizures, visual phenomena, and scotomas, progressing to myoclonic jerks. These patients often go on to develop vision loss and a cerebellar syndrome. Mutations in the *NHLRC1* gene encoding laforin, a tyrosine phosphatase, located on chromosome 6q24 are responsible for LBD.

Myoclonic epilepsy with ragged red fibers (MERRF) is a disorder resulting from mutations in mitochondrial DNA that can present in the adolescent period through the second decade of life with myoclonus, generalized seizures, encephalopathy, and ataxia. The histopathology includes ragged red muscle fibers on Gomori trichrome stain with cytochrome c negative fibers. Additional neurologic features include diminished hearing and vision, neuropathy, and myopathy.

Neuronal ceroid lipofuscinosis is a heterogenous lysosomal storage disease that can present in early childhood up to adulthood. Most forms are inherited in an autosomal-recessive pattern and are classified as CLN 1 to 10. Mutations in 13 genes have been identified. Phenotypically, these patients suffer progressive intellectual disability, vision loss, dementia, ataxia, and pyramidal and extrapyramidal dysfunction. The EEG often demonstrates slowed background rhythm, with paroxysmal generalized bursts of spike-and-wave, polyspike-and-wave, or slow-wave discharges. The histopathology includes curvilinear, fingerprint, and granular osmiophilic deposits (Franceschetti et al., 2014; Wheless and Kim, 2002).

ADOLESCENT FOCAL EPILEPSIES

Focal-onset seizures are more common than generalized. Of the focal epilepsy generators, the temporal lobe is the most epileptogenic region of the brain. Accordingly, temporal lobe epilepsy (TLE) is the most common form of localization-related epilepsy in adolescents and adults, accounting for 60% of all patients with epilepsy. Advances in neuroimaging have an immense bearing on the diagnosis of adolescent-onset focal epilepsy.

Mesial Temporal Lobe Epilepsy Resulting From Hippocampal Sclerosis

Mesial temporal lobe epilepsy with hippocampal sclerosis was identified by the International League Against Epilepsy (ILAE) in the new classification system because of its prevalence and homogeneity (Berg et al., 2010). The onset of mesial temporal lobe epilepsy (mTLE) varies, and it can emerge during infancy through the third decade of life. Hippocampal sclerosis (HS) is composed of atrophy and gliosis of the amygdala, hippocampus, parahippocampal gyrus, and enterorhinal cortex. Although HS can be bilateral, it is commonly unilateral, involving the dentate gyrus, CA 1 to 3, and subiculum. It may be easily visualized on qualitative high-resolution brain magnetic resonance imaging (MRI) as mesial temporal sclerosis. Characteristic features include hippocampal formation atrophy (Figure 73-8) and increased signal on coronal fluid-attenuated inversion recovery sequences or T2-weighted images.

mTLE can manifest various auras. Most commonly it presents with psychic and experiential phenomena of déjà vu, jamais vu, and fear. However, other autonomic and abdominal auras, such as rising epigastric sensations, and olfactory and gustatory auras, such as pungent malodorous smells and bizarre tastes, may also occur. The ictal period is also accompanied by a fixed vacant stare with behavioral arrest and impaired consciousness over 30 to 60 seconds. Oral-buccal and bimanual automatisms are common and may consist of repetitive lip-smacking, swallowing, chewing, and picking or fidgeting movements of the hands. Amnesia for the event is typical for left temporal lobe epilepsy, and 30% of the time patients are repeatedly unaware that seizures have occurred. Focal seizures evolving to convulsions are infrequent in mTLE.

The interictal routine scalp EEG may demonstrate anterior temporal spikes or sharp waves occurring in more than 90% of patients during prolonged video-EEG monitoring. In one-third of patients they may appear bitemporally (Figure 73-8), with a regional temporal field that can be augmented by application of additional basal temporal electrodes. Intermittent focal temporal slowing may be seen with localizing value when present as temporal intermittent rhythmic delta activity. The typical ictal tracing demonstrates a unilateral regular rhythmic theta or alpha discharge of 5 to 9 Hz in the anterior temporal head region. When electrophysiological concordance correlates with ipsilateral HS on MRI, this pattern correctly lateralizes seizure onset in more than 95% of patients (Thom, 2014).

Autosomal-Dominant Partial Epilepsy With Auditory Features

The onset of familial lateral temporal lobe epilepsy (flTLE) typically occurs in teenage or early adult life, but it may present earlier or later (range 4-50). The lateral form of familial TLE, also referred to as autosomal-dominant partial epilepsy with auditory features (ADPEAF), is associated with a missense gene mutation in the leucine-rich, glioma-inactivated 1 (*LGI-1*) gene on chromosome 10q22-24. Brain MRI and EEG are often normal. Simple auditory hallucinations are the hallmark of ADPEAF. Typically, simple sounds such as buzzing, clicking, or ringing may occur and are usually referred to the contralateral ear, although they may be bilateral. However, other visual, autonomic, psychic, and olfactory auras can be encountered in addition to more complex features described as singing, whistling, humming, and talking. Infrequently these sensations may progress to focal seizures with impaired consciousness, although they typically occur in isolation. Focal seizures that evolve to convulsions are usually rare and occur during sleep when present. The interictal routine scalp EEG in patients with flTLE is often normal, although it may reveal midtemporal focal slowing. When epileptiform discharges are encountered, they are temporal-occipital spikes or sharp waves. Seizures originate in or propagate into Heschl's gyrus in the primary auditory or auditory association cortices, with left frontotemporal and temporal onset.

Autosomal-Dominant Nocturnal Frontal Lobe Epilepsy

Autosomal-dominant nocturnal frontal lobe epilepsy (ADNFLE) is an uncommon form of familial nonlesional focal epilepsy characterized by focal hypermotor seizures arising from the frontal lobe, classically during sleep. Although the age range for first seizures is between 1 and 30 years old, the mean age is during the early adolescent period around 12 years old. The seizures are brief, often complex, and usually occur in clusters during non-REM sleep, leading

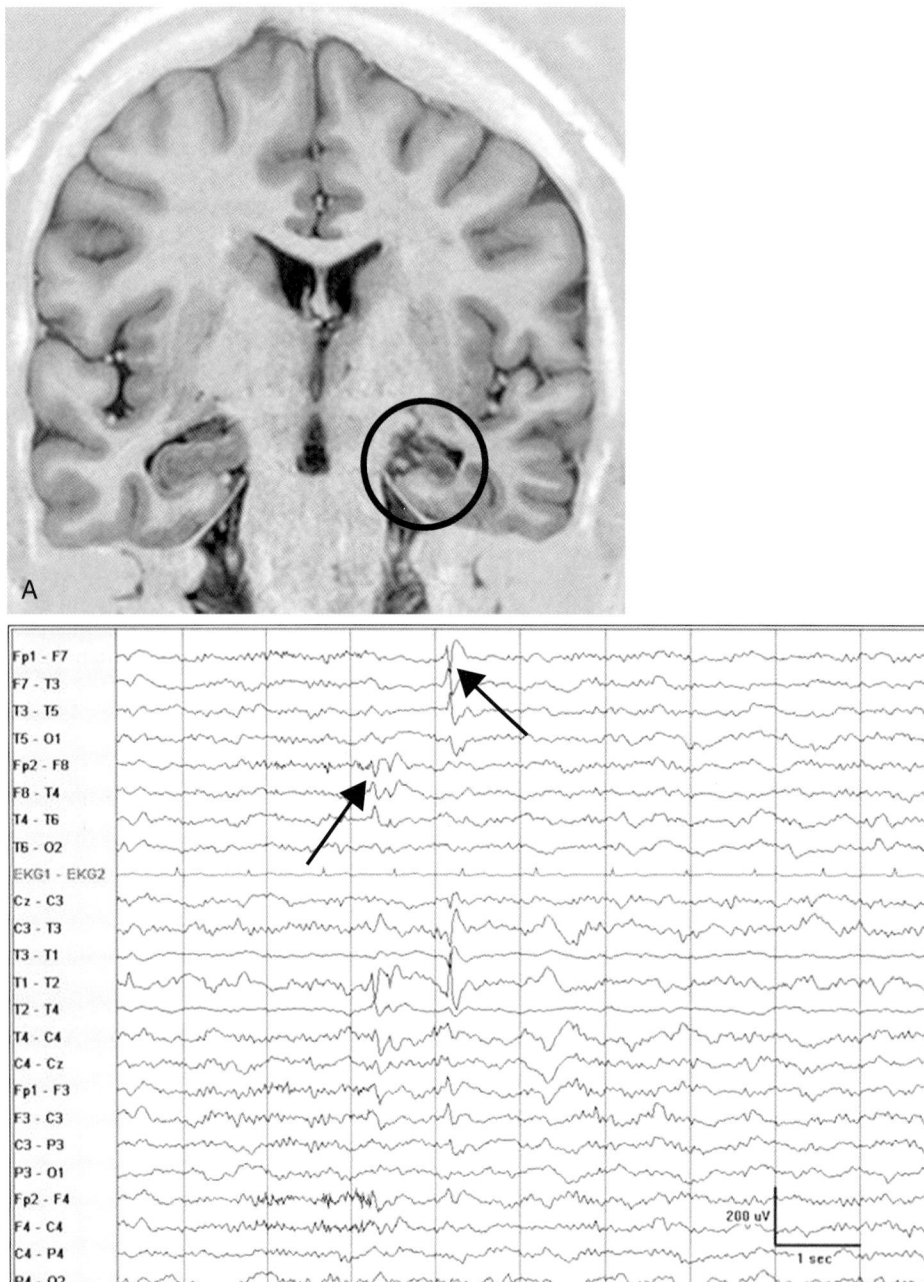

Figure 73-8. Mesial temporal lobe epilepsy resulting from hippocampal sclerosis. A 16-year-old with a history of complex febrile seizure and seizure onset at puberty resistant to multiple antiseizure drugs (ASDs). Note the left hippocampal formation atrophy in 7A (circle) and bitemporal spike-and-wave discharges in 7B (arrows).

to misinterpretation as a parasomnia. Seizures may lead to simple arousals, wandering behavior, or more intense hypermotor movements involving bimanual-bipedal automatism with kicking, bicycling, flailing, or flinging movements. Vocalizations of moaning, crying, or gasping may also occur, simulating nocturnal panic attacks. The brain MRI and interictal routine scalp EEG are frequently normal. Video-EEG may be diagnostic when demonstrating electroclinical seizures of frontal lobe origin. The first gene identified was a missense mutation in a large Australian kindred in the alpha 4 subunit of the neuronal nicotinic acetylcholine (nAch) receptor (*CHRNA4*) located on chromosome 20 (20q13.2-13.3). Mutations of *CHRNA2*, *CHRNB2*, and the sodium-gated

potassium channel gene *KCNT1* have also been associated with ADNFLE.

TREATMENT

Obtaining seizure control is imperative to preventing morbidity and mortality associated with adolescent epilepsy.

Treatment of Genetic Generalized Epilepsies

The majority of JME patients will require continued use of ASDs in adulthood. Carbamazepine, phenytoin, gabapentin, and vigabatrin may exacerbate seizures in JME and produce myoclonic status epilepticus. Therefore these medications should be avoided in JME. Reproductive potential and pregnancy are significant factors in ASD selection. Valproate is a potent teratogen that is strongly associated with major congenital malformations. Therefore it should be avoided in females of childbearing potential. Levetiracetam and lamotrigine have emerged as the ASDs of choice for females with JME, although caution is necessary with lamotrigine because exacerbation of myoclonic jerks may occur. However, valproate is a very effective choice in adolescent males with JME. Treatment with valproate requires careful observation for idiosyncratic adverse effects, including serious rash, hepatopathy, and hemorrhagic pancreatitis. Additional monitoring for chronic changes, such as alopecia, tremor, weight gain, thrombocytopenia, and osteopenia, is important. Despite appropriate use of ASDs, 15% of patients will demonstrate pharmaco-resistant JME requiring multidrug therapy.

Absence seizures respond to treatment with ethosuximide, valproate, or lamotrigine. Ethosuximide targets the T-type calcium channels, thereby decreasing the excitatory drive of thalamocortical networks. If the patient has generalized convulsive seizures in addition to absences, valproate and lamotrigine are better choices. Most patients with JAE are well controlled on monotherapy. However, those refractory to monotherapy may require dual therapy and closer monitoring of ASD level. Valproate increases the serum concentrations of lamotrigine and ethosuximide, giving rise to clinical toxicity if coadministered. The most feared side effect of lamotrigine is Stevens–Johnson syndrome, but other side effects, such as insomnia, headache, incoordination, ataxia, and dizziness, also occur. Importantly, ASDs including phenytoin and carbamazepine in addition to gabapentin, pregabalin, and vigabatrin can aggravate absence seizures and precipitate absence status epilepticus and therefore should be avoided. Finally, adolescents and their parents should be counseled that although JAE can remit, it tends to be life-long, requiring long-term administration of ASDs.

GTC and GTCS-A tend to have a fairly good outcome. Most patients become seizure-free on ASDs. The majority of patients are able to be controlled with ASD monotherapy, but approximately 30% require polytherapy. In contrast, the treatment of PME remains problematic. The reason for this is likely twofold. First, broad-spectrum ASDs that are typically effective in generalized seizures, such ase valproate, lamotrigine, topiramate, levetiracetam, zonisamide, and benzodiazepines, are unfortunately frequently ineffective in PME. Second, the underlying encephalopathy that develops as PME progresses requires supportive care and assistance when sleep, behavior, and mobility become compromised (Panayiotopoulos, 2001; Tatum, 2013).

Treatment of Focal Epilepsies

In regard to treatment of focal seizures such as temporal lobe epilepsy, nearly two-thirds of patients will achieve seizure freedom with ASDs; however, those with HS have the worst prognosis for achieving medical control. Most ASDs are approved for use in patients with focal seizures. Newer ASDs have improved tolerability but provide little benefit once drug resistance becomes evident. Overly aggressive ASD use complicates the risk of serious adverse events and seizure-related morbidity and mortality. Furthermore, health-related quality of life is more difficult to improve over time. When focal seizures remain uncontrolled, epilepsy surgery needs early consideration. Anterior temporal lobectomy and selective amygdalohippocampectomy for refractory patients can be very effective and may improve quality of life. Newer minimally invasive techniques using stereotactic laser ablation are evolving as a reasonable alternative to more invasive surgeries, which may minimize category-related object recognition and naming deficits following standard surgical approaches.

ADDITIONAL DIAGNOSTIC CONSIDERATIONS
Chronobiology

There is a significant influence of circadian periodicity on the timing and threshold for seizures. In adolescence, there are several epilepsies that present with early morning seizures, including JME and GTC seizures on awakening, similar to other seizures, such as those in ADNFLE, that are nocturnal. Additionally, many patients with adolescent-onset epilepsy may be provoked or aggravated by sleep deprivation. This phenomenon may involve light-sensitive neuronal activation of the suprachiasmatic nucleus, which can influence the activity of thalamocortical circuits and other epileptogenic networks, neurotransmitters, and hormones affected by sleep duration and circadian periodicity. Understanding the chronobiology of the epilepsies and the implications of circadian changes in neurotransmitter release and cortical excitation may enhance our understanding of the pathobiology of adolescent epilepsy syndromes. Furthermore, the interplay between sleep deprivation and circadian influences on seizure threshold could uncover targets for therapeutic intervention.

Biomarkers

The advent of biomarker identification is a potentially high-yield area of future research. Structural biomarkers, such as hippocampal sclerosis or focal frontal lobe cortical dysplasia on high-resolution brain MRI, focal hyperperfusion on single-photon emission computed tomography (SPECT), and focal hypometabolism on positron emission tomography (PET), may augment presurgical planning when seizures are drug resistant. Serum and spinal fluid biomarkers such as heat-shock proteins could have the capacity to predict the natural history of epilepsy and treatment outcomes. Additionally, biomarkers may be powerful tools for the generation of newer, more complex animal models in future ASD research. The EEG is an indirect biomarker of epilepsy as well. For example, extending the EEG recording to include frequencies up to 500 Hz or more during invasive EEG required for presurgical evaluations in drug-resistant localization-related epilepsy has revealed high-frequency oscillations with pathophysiologic implications for optimizing resection.

Pharmacogenetics—The Horizon of Epilepsy Treatment

Molecular epilepsy genetics is a dynamic field that is creating a paradigm shift in how we think about epilepsy. Present-day candidate gene testing (e.g., LGI-1 in fITLE), gene panel testing (e.g., autoimmune limbic encephalitis), and array comparative genomic hybridization will probably evolve to whole-exome and whole-genome sequencing, especially when no candidate gene is suspected. These discoveries will expand mechanistic considerations for the many currently unexplained epilepsy syndromes, help identify mechanisms of drug resistance, and lead to more individualized ASD selection to personalize treatment. Perhaps in the future, genetic screening will assist in predicting patients who may respond better to one drug therapy as opposed to another. Finally, although the design of medications used to treat epilepsy has focused on remitting seizures, a more advanced approach to pharmacogenetics in epilepsy should focus on targeting the propensity for seizures and natural history of lifelong or severe epilepsy disorders.

CONCLUSION

There are age-specific electroclinical syndromes that occur in adolescence. In teens, other paroxysmal nonepileptic events, such as syncope, psychogenic nonepileptic seizures, migraine, and recreational drug abuse, that mimic epilepsy must be considered. The potential for misdiagnosis and misuse of ASDs during adolescence may account for morbidity, pseudodrug resistance from incorrect choice of medication, and impaired quality of life. Remaining sensitive to the pressures of this age group and providing information on driving, sexuality, use of drugs and alcohol, and compliance with ASDs is crucial for successful treatment of epilepsy. Many of the GGEs present during this age period and respond to the new-generation ASDs. Focal seizures should be treated aggressively with early surgical evaluation when drug resistance is identified.

REFERENCES

The complete list of references for this chapter is available in the e-book at www.expertconsult.com.

See inside cover for registration details.

SELECTED REFERENCES

Appleton, R.E., Neville, B.G., 1999. Teenagers with epilepsy. Arch. Dis. Child. 81, 76–79.

Beghi, M., Beghi, E., Cornaggia, C.M., et al., 2006. Idiopathic generalized epilepsies of adolescence. Epilepsia 47 (Suppl. 2), 107–110. doi:10.1111/j.1528-1167.2006.00706.x.

Berg, A.T., et al., 2010. Revised terminology and concepts for organization of seizures and epilepsies: report of the ILAE Commission on Classification and Terminology, 2005-2009. Epilepsia 51, 676–685. doi:10.1111/j.1528-1167.2010.02522.x.

Franceschetti, S., et al., 2014. Progressive myoclonic epilepsies: definitive and still undetermined causes. Neurology 82, 405–411. doi:10.1212/WNL.0000000000000077.

Greenberg, D.A., Durner, M., Resor, S., et al., 1995. The genetics of idiopathic generalized epilepsies of adolescent onset: differences between juvenile myoclonic epilepsy and epilepsy with random grand mal and with awakening grand mal. Neurology 45, 942–946.

Panayiotopoulos, C.P., 2001. Treatment of typical absence seizures and related epileptic syndromes. Paediatr. Drugs 3, 379–403.

Shian, W.J., Chi, C.S., 1994. Epilepsy with grand mal on awakening. Zhonghua Yi Xue Za Zhi (Taipei) 53, 106–108.

Tatum, W.O., 2013. Recent and Emerging Anti-seizure Drugs: 2013. Curr. Treat. Options Neurol. 15, 505–518. doi:10.1007/s11940-013-0245-6.

Thom, M., 2014. Review: Hippocampal sclerosis in epilepsy: a neuropathology review. Neuropathol. Appl. Neurobiol. 40, 520–543. doi:10.1111/nan.12150.

Wheless, J.W., Kim, H.L., 2002. Adolescent seizures and epilepsy syndromes. Epilepsia 43 (Suppl. 3), 33–52.

E-BOOK FIGURES AND TABLES

The following figures and tables are available in the e-book at www.expertconsult.com. See inside cover for registration details.

74 Focal Structural Epilepsy

Ghayda M. Mirzaa, Christopher J. Yuskaitis, and Annapurna Poduri

An expanded version of this chapter is available on www.expertconsult.com. See inside cover for registration details.

INTRODUCTION

The role of structural lesions is well recognized in cases of refractory focal epilepsy in children and adults. Although mesial temporal lobe epilepsy with hippocampal sclerosis, a common feature of refractory epilepsy in adults, also plays a role in pediatric epilepsy, there is a notable contribution in pediatric epilepsy from focal cortical malformations, ranging from small heterotopia to large hemispheric malformations, such as hemimegalencephaly. Our recognition of these lesions is likely to increase as neuroimaging continues to become more sophisticated. There are also reports of pathologic evidence of cortical malformation in surgical resections from patients with focal epilepsy without visible lesions on magnetic resonance imaging (MRI) (Sisodiya, 2004). Thus in this chapter we emphasize the role of cortical malformations in pediatric epilepsy and then discuss the more classical focal structural epilepsies associated with mesial temporal lobe epilepsy (MTLE), hypothalamic hamartoma, and Rasmussen encephalitis.

FOCAL STRUCTURAL EPILEPSY WITH FOCAL MALFORMATIONS OF CORTICAL DEVELOPMENT

Focal Cortical Dysplasia

One of the most common causes of focal structural epilepsy is focal cortical dysplasia (FCD). Although FCD is covered in Chapter 28, its prominence in the realm of focal epilepsy warrants discussion in this chapter as well. Neurologists often use the terms *FCD* and *cortical dysplasia* to include a range of abnormalities, from epileptic foci with microscopic cellular abnormalities to large hemispheric lesions visible on MRI. We will use the term *FCD* to refer to the specific malformations with pathologic abnormalities as described in the following section.

Pathology

There are three major types of FCD: type I, with abnormal cortical lamination; type II, with abnormal cortical lamination plus dysmorphic neurons as the key additional feature; and type III, similar to type I but associated with an additional major finding (i.e., dual pathology), such as hippocampal sclerosis, developmental tumor, or vascular malformation. FCD type IIa is distinguished from type IIb based on the presence of enlarged "balloon" cells in the latter.

Imaging Features

FCD is not well seen on computed tomography (CT), and even high-quality MRI may not detect small or subtle FCD. The presence of a focal lesion on MRI may influence the course of treatment of focal epilepsy in that lesional focal epilepsy may be amenable to focal respective surgery. Given the important role of FCD in focal epilepsy, it is necessary to use sensitive MRI techniques to maximize the detection of lesions such as FCD. Additional localizing techniques, including nuclear medicine imaging, may be used when there is a high suspicion of a focal lesion.

The prototypical imaging features of FCD are seen in FCD type II, with blurring of the gray matter–white matter junction, abnormal gyral patterns, increased cortical thickness, and increased T2/FLAIR signal at the base of the lesion and in the underlying white matter, the so-called "T2 tail" that extends down to the ventricular surface. Type I FCDs may appear as blurring of the gray matter–white matter junction and subtle cortical thickening with irregular gyral morphology. These features may be more apparent in FCD type III when they are adjacent to other abnormalities, such as hippocampal sclerosis, although the other abnormalities may be so much more striking that the dysplasia may be initially overlooked.

Clinical Features

In the pediatric epilepsy setting, FCD is most often seen as an isolated focal abnormality. FCD, and the related hemispheric lesion hemimegalencephaly (HMEG), may also be associated with neurocutaneous syndromes, including linear nevus sebaceous syndrome, Sturge–Weber syndrome, PTEN hamartoma tumor (Cowden) syndrome, and hypomelanosis of Ito.

Seizures, typically presenting in infancy or childhood, are often the presenting and chief clinical consequences of FCD. The cases and series in the literature are most often surgical series, reflecting refractory epilepsy. Intellectual disability and focal neurologic abnormalities may also be present, depending on the location and size of the FCD.

Etiology

because the pathologic findings associated with FCD, tuberous sclerosis complex (TSC), and hemimegalencephaly (HMEG) share overlapping features, these disorders have increasingly been considered part of a spectrum, and their causes have been recently identified (Poduri et al., 2013). Indeed, the recently identified genetic causes of FCD support this assertion; genes in the mTOR-PI3K-AKT pathway have been implicated, including germline and somatic mutations in *MTOR*, *PIK3CA*, *AKT3*, *PTEN*, *DEPDC5*, and *NPRL3*. In addition, recessive mutations in the genes *CNTNAP2* and *OCLN* have been identified as genetic causes of FCD.

Management

Treatment of focal epilepsy as a result of FCD begins with antiseizure drugs suitable for focal epilepsy. Although FCD clearly plays a major role in refractory focal epilepsy, it is important to note that not all patients presenting with focal epilepsy attributable to FCD will have refractory epilepsy. Thus the prognosis of a child with focal epilepsy with MRI clearly showing FCD is not always that of refractory epilepsy requiring a surgical approach. Future prospective studies of patients with newly identified FCD are needed to determine the portion of patients with FCD that can be controlled by medication versus those who require surgical consideration.

FCD, particularly smaller and more subtle forms of FCD, may not be recognized on the initial MRI performed as part of the standard focal seizure evaluation. Thus any patient with refractory focal epilepsy with two or more unsuccessful attempts at treatment with antiseizure medications should undergo presurgical evaluation. This should include repeat MRI if no lesion was initially found, if possible using 3T MRI and protocols designed to enhance the detection of epilepsy-related lesions, including both FCD and hippocampal abnormalities.

Presurgical evaluation for patients with FCD follows standard presurgical practice and should include assessment of concordance of localizing features (e.g., seizure semiology, MRI, electroencephalogram [EEG] focality [interictally but more important ictally], nuclear medicine studies, in some cases magnetoencephalography) and assessment of possible deficits that might arise from surgery based on the location and extent of the lesion, neuropsychological evaluation, and in some cases diffusion tensor imaging identifying, for example, corticospinal tracts or arcuate fasciculus with respect to the FCD. Depending on the localization versus the possibility of deficit, invasive monitoring may be required. Furthermore, because the seizure-onset zone in some patients may be located adjacent to rather than directly in a focal malformation, invasive monitoring, such as subdural electrode recording, may be needed to best identify the source of the seizures and achieve the greatest chance of seizure freedom.

Hemimegalencephaly

Hemimegalencephaly (HMEG) is a well-described disorder of abnormal brain development characterized by unilateral enlargement of most of one cerebral hemisphere (Flores-Sarnat, 2002). In its classic form, HMEG is characterized by unilateral cortical malformation, with the involved hemisphere enlarged and characterized by cortical dysgenesis, white-matter hypertrophy, and a dilated and dysmorphic lateral ventricle. The overgrowth and dysplasia may involve an entire hemisphere, part of a hemisphere, and/or part of the contralateral hemisphere as well, with no clear predilection for the right or left side. Various morphologic abnormalities outside the involved cerebral hemisphere have been reported, including ipsilateral cerebral vascular dilatation, ipsilateral and bilateral cerebellar enlargement with dysplastic folia, and ipsilateral olfactory nerve enlargement. Moreover, contralateral volume loss (or hemi-micrencephaly) and white-matter abnormalities have been reported. Neuropathological findings include large neurons, cortical dyslamination with or without dysmorphic and ectopic neurons, heterotopia, balloon cells, and abnormal white matter.

Neurologic Features

Classically, most children with HMEG have early-onset intractable epilepsy, unilateral or focal neurologic signs (such as hemiparesis), tone abnormalities, and severe intellectual disability. Intractable epilepsy usually begins within the first few months of life and is the most frequent and severe neurologic manifestation, occurring in up to 93% of cases. Seizures are typically focal in onset and almost always intractable to medical therapy. Likely because of the early age at presentation, HMEG is associated with infantile spasms in 50% of patients. Intellectual disability (ID) is often early and severe, although in a few cases it can be mild to moderate. Different degrees of hemiparesis are seen contralateral to the hemimegalencephaly. Macrocephaly is usually apparent at birth, and cranial asymmetry dependent on the degree of hemimegalencephaly may be evident. Occipito-frontal circumference

(OFC) may increase rapidly during the first few months, but subsequently the head size diminishes relative to the normal OFC curve, and patients may become normocephalic or microcephalic. Anatomic or functional hemispherectomy may improve both epilepsy and ID in selected patients, albeit with some complications given the often difficult anatomy involved. However, many patients do poorly with hemispheric surgery, possibly as a result of more widespread but asymmetric malformations (Vigevano et al., 1989).

Neuroimaging

The MRI appearance of HMEG includes moderate to severe enlargement of one cerebral hemisphere, with enlargement of the lateral ventricle. In some, enlargement may be localized to the frontal or temporoparietal regions, but in others, it may extend to distinct regions of the contralateral hemisphere. A spectrum of cortical dysplasia is almost uniformly present, ranging from pachygyria to polymicrogyria, with cortical dysplasia often seen in the contralateral hemisphere as well (Barkovich and Chuang, 1990). Gray-matter abnormalities may include areas of thickening and simplification or over-folding, resembling pachygyria or polymicrogyria, respectively. Heterotopias are commonly seen as well. The underlying hemispheric white matter may be increased or decreased, with abnormal signal characteristics in some patients. The ventricular system is enlarged and/or dysplastic in most patients. Figure 74-1 (**B, E, F**) and Figure 28-4 (**B-D**) in Chapter 28 show variable degrees of hemimegalencephaly. EEG abnormalities are often extensive throughout the abnormal hemisphere, and a suppression-burst pattern can be observed in the most severe cases. Predictors of poor outcome are severity of hemiparesis, degree of MRI abnormality, and abnormal EEG activity.

Nonneurologic Features

HMEG can be isolated or associated with somatic features such as focal or segmental body overgrowth and cutaneous vascular malformations, as has been reported in many individuals with Proteus syndrome, Klippel–Trenaunay syndrome (KTS), linear nevus sebaceous syndrome (LNSS), hypomelanosis of Ito, and neurofibromatosis. These associations, combined with recent molecular discoveries identifying mutations in the PI3K-AKT-MTOR pathway in these phenotypes, place HMEG, FCD, and diffuse megalencephaly within a broad spectrum of disorders associated with variable brain and body growth dysregulation.

Etiology

Hemimegalencephaly was classically regarded as the result of an early disturbance in neuronal proliferation and migration. With the advent of next-generation sequencing (NGS), a number of genetic causes of HMEG have been identified. Mosaic (or postzygotic) gain-of-function mutations within key genes of the mammalian target of rapamycin (mTOR)-phosphatidylinositol-3-kinase (PI3K)-v-akt murine thymoma viral oncogene homolog (AKT) pathway have been identified in HMEG. These genes include *PIK3CA*, *AKT3*, *PTEN*, and *MTOR*.

Most of these mutations were detected in abnormal (surgically resected) brain tissue only, and were undetectable in peripheral tissues (such as blood and saliva). Mutations of the same genes have been reported with more focal malformations of cortical development, including FCD and diffuse megalencephaly (as occurs with megalencephaly capillary malformation syndrome and megalencephaly polymicrogyria–polydactyly hydrocephalus syndrome, discussed here and in

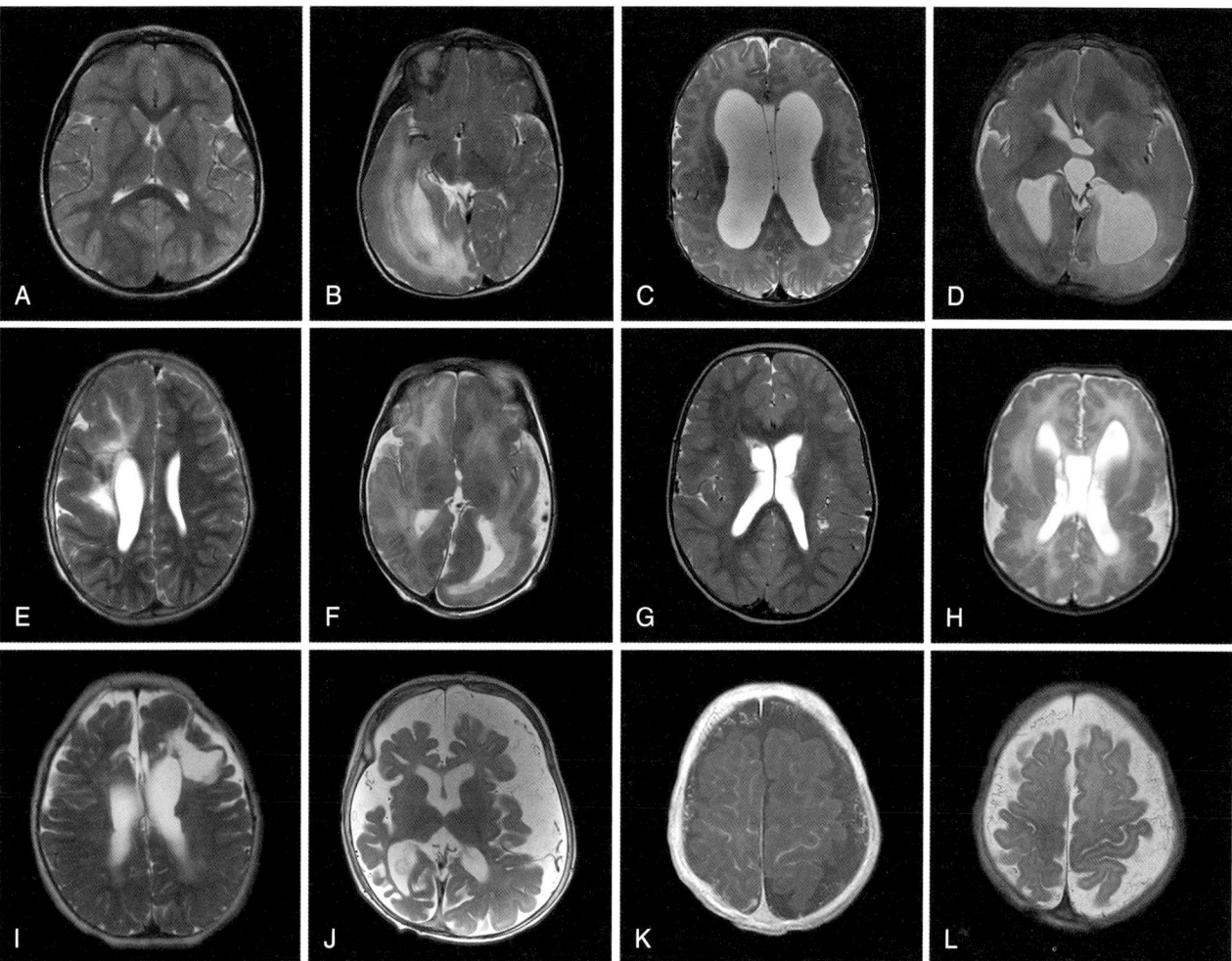

Figure 74-1. Neuroimaging features of focal brain malformations associated with epilepsy. **A,** FCD type 2a resulting from a mosaic mutation of *PIK3CA* (p.H1047R). **B,** Hemimegalencephaly resulting from two mosaic mutations of *PI3KCA* (p.E542K, p.T544N). **C,** MCAP syndrome resulting from a mosaic mutation of *PIK3CA* (p.M1043I). Note also severe ventriculomegaly and megalencephaly. **D,** Bilateral diffuse megalencephaly with cortical dysplasia (i.e., dysplastic megalencephaly) resulting from to a mosaic mutation of *PIK3CA* (p.E545K). Also note bilaterally enlarged and dysplastic ventricles, diffuse white-matter abnormalities, and bilaterally dysplastic basal ganglia. **E,** Hemimegalencephaly resulting from a constitutional (germline) mutation of *PTEN* (p.Y68H). **F,** Hemimegalencephaly resulting from a mosaic mutation of *AKT3* (p.E17K). **G,** Bilateral perisylvian polymicrogyria and mild ventriculomegaly resulting from a mosaic mutation of *PIK3R2* (p.G373R). **H,** Bilateral perisylvian polymicrogyria resulting from a constitutional mutation of *CCND2* (P281S). Also note megalencephaly, ventriculomegaly, and cavum septum pellucidum et vergae (features of MPPH syndrome). **I,** Tuberous sclerosis resulting from a constitutional mutation of *TSC1* (p.Gln301X). Note several subcortical tubers, subependymal nodules, mild ventriculomegaly, and periventricular white-matter T2 signal hyperintensities. This MRI is status following left frontal craniectomy for gross resection of a large left frontal subcortical tuber. **J-L,** Sturge–Weber syndrome (no mutation identified). **J,** T2-weighted axial image showing prominent subarachnoid spaces with diffuse cortical atrophy. **K,** T1-gadolinium (GAD) contrast axial image showing bilateral pial venous angiomatosis with leptomeningeal enhancement. **L,** Matching T2-weighted axial image further showing bilaterally prominent vessels in the subarachnoid spaces. MCAP, megalencephaly capillary malformation syndrome; MPPH, megalencephaly polymicrogyria–polydactyly hydrocephalus syndrome; MRI, magnetic resonance imaging. (*A with permission from Jansen LA, Mirzaa GM, Ishak GE, et al. Brain: a journal of neurology 2015; **B-G** with permission from Poduri A, Evrony GD, Cai X, Walsh CA. Science 2013;341:1237758.)*

Chapter 28). These heterozygous mutations lead to gain of function in pathway activity that regulates several cellular processes, including cell survival, growth, vascular development, and apoptosis (Figure 74-2).

Other less common patterns of focal megalencephaly with cortical dysplasia have been described, and various terms have been used to describe these patterns by distribution, such as total or diffuse HMEG, localized MEG (hemi-hemimegalencephaly), and multilobar cortical dysplasia (Table 74-1).

FOCAL STRUCTURAL EPILEPSY WITH NEUROCUTANEOUS SYNDROMES
Tuberous Sclerosis Complex

TSC, discussed in detail in Chapter 45, is commonly associated with focal epilepsy, with typically refractory epilepsy affecting 80% to 90% of children with TSC, often beginning in infancy in the form of infantile spasms. The majority of patients with TSC have mutations in *TSC1* or *TSC2*, resulting

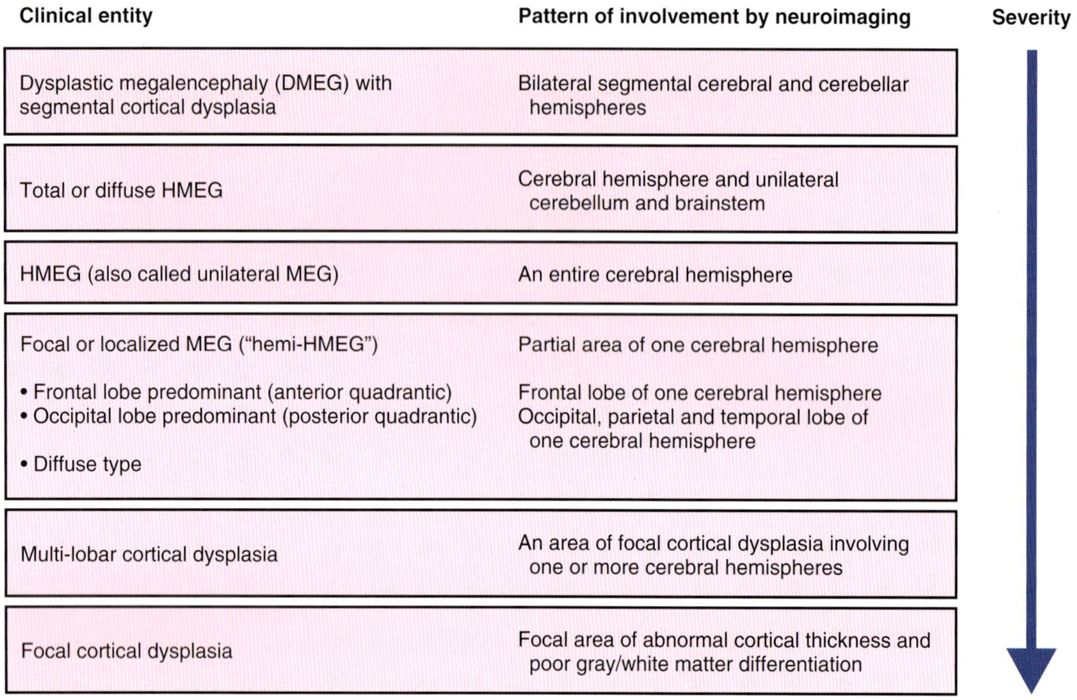

Clinical entity	Pattern of involvement by neuroimaging	Severity
Dysplastic megalencephaly (DMEG) with segmental cortical dysplasia	Bilateral segmental cerebral and cerebellar hemispheres	
Total or diffuse HMEG	Cerebral hemisphere and unilateral cerebellum and brainstem	
HMEG (also called unilateral MEG)	An entire cerebral hemisphere	
Focal or localized MEG ("hemi-HMEG") • Frontal lobe predominant (anterior quadrantic) • Occipital lobe predominant (posterior quadrantic) • Diffuse type	Partial area of one cerebral hemisphere Frontal lobe of one cerebral hemisphere Occipital, parietal and temporal lobe of one cerebral hemisphere	
Multi-lobar cortical dysplasia	An area of focal cortical dysplasia involving one or more cerebral hemispheres	
Focal cortical dysplasia	Focal area of abnormal cortical thickness and poor gray/white matter differentiation	

Figure 74-2. Focal or segmental malformations of cortical development. This figure illustrates the focal brain overgrowth entities described in the literature and their morphologic characteristics based primarily on the extent and distribution of the malformation seen in neuroimaging. These clinical entities include the following (from most diffuse to most localized): dysplastic megalencephaly, total or diffuse hemimegalencephaly, classic hemimegalencephaly, focal or localized hemimegalencephaly (also called hemi-hemimegalencephaly), multilobar cortical dysplasia, and focal cortical dysplasia.

TABLE 74-1 Disorders Associated With Focal Structural Epilepsy, Clinical Features and Causes

Disorder	Neurologic Features	Somatic (Nonneurologic) Features	Cause	Gene	Constitutional Versus Mosaic
With Focal Malformations of Cortical Development					
Focal cortical dysplasia (FCD)	Laminar disorganization, dysmorphic neurons (IIa), balloon cells (IIb)	Typically none	Genetic	*MTOR, DEPDC5, PIK3CA, PTEN*	Mosaic
Hemimegalencephaly (HMEG)	Cortical dysgenesis, white-matter abnormalities, dysmorphic ventricles	Segmental overgrowth, vascular-lymphatic malformations, hypomelanosis of Ito	Genetic	*MTOR, DEPDC5, PIK3CA, PTEN, AKT3*	Mosaic
With Neurocutaneous Syndromes					
Tuberous sclerosis (TSC)	SEN, cortical tubers, hamartomatous lesions, calcifications	Hypopigmented macules, facial angiofibroma, Shagreen patches, subcutaneous nodules, café au lait lesions, subungual fibromas	Genetic	*TSC1, TSC2*	Constitutional, less commonly mosaic
Sturge–Weber syndrome (SWS)	Arachnoid hemangiomata, calcifications	Hemangiomata in the distribution of the trigeminal nerve	Genetic	*GNAQ*	Mosaic
Megalencephaly capillary malformation syndrome (MCAP)	Bilateral perisylvian polymicrogyria	Capillary malformations, somatic overgrowth, digital anomalies (syndactyly, polydactyly)	Genetic	*PIK3CA*	Mosaic
Hypomelanosis of Ito	HMEG or Dysplastic Megalencephaly	Hypomelanosis of Ito	Genetic	*MTOR*	Mosaic

HMEG, hemimegalencephaly; SEN, subependymal nodules.

in overactivation of the mTOR pathway. Given the implication of this pathway in FCD and related disorders, early trials of mTOR inhibition to treat seizures in patients with TSC may extend to the many other mTOR-related forms of focal epilepsy.

Sturge–Weber Syndrome

Sturge–Weber syndrome (SWS) is a neurocutaneous disorder characterized by aberrant vascular development affecting the skin, eyes, and meninges. Classic features include a facial capillary malformation, commonly in the distribution of the trigeminal nerve, sometimes involving the choroid of the eye, with secondary buphthalmos or glaucoma; leptomeningeal angiomatosis; secondary cerebral atrophy; sclerosis; and calcifications. Some affected individuals also develop subdural hematomas.

Neurologic Features

SWS is often associated with severe neurologic sequelae, including epilepsy, intellectual disability, vascular headaches, glaucoma, hemianopia, and hemiparesis. Epilepsy is estimated to occur in 75% to 90% of patients and is most often focal, with onset typically in infancy or early childhood. Further, many individuals with SWS have focal neurologic symptoms such as hemiparesis.

Neuroimaging

Leptomeningeal angiomatosis is unilateral in 75% of cases and bilateral in 25%. Secondary neuroimaging findings include cerebral calcifications, atrophy, and choroidal plexus hypertrophy, among others. Neuropathologic studies have demonstrated various abnormalities, including focal cortical dysplasia and polymicrogyria, some of which were subtle and undetectable on brain MRIs.

Etiology

Recently mutations of the guanine nucleotide binding protein Q polypeptide (*GNAQ*) gene have been identified in SWS. Mutations were mosaic, detected predominantly in affected brain tissue. *GNAQ* encodes a G-class seven-transmembrane domain receptor that activates phospholipase C-beta and has downstream effects on the RAS signaling pathway.

Clinical Management

Epilepsy is often refractory to antiseizure medications in SWS, often necessitating neurosurgical intervention, either hemispherectomy or focal resection. Several studies have shown that early surgery confers better seizure control and developmental outcomes. Some studies have proposed vertical extraventricular functional hemispherectomy to reduce the risk of postoperative hydrocephalus.

Megalencephaly Capillary Malformation Syndrome

Megalencephaly capillary malformation syndrome (MCAP) is a multisystem disorder characterized by diffuse brain overgrowth or megalencephaly, with variable somatic features, including overgrowth and cutaneous vascular malformations. The severity of involvement varies widely, although most affected individuals have congenital-onset megalencephaly and cutaneous capillary malformations. Other somatic features seen in this clinically recognizable syndrome include finger or toe syndactyly (most characteristically two- to three-toe syndactyly), postaxial polydactyly, and connective tissue dysplasia characterized most often by skin and ligamentous laxity.

Neurologic Features

In addition to megalencephaly, approximately 60% to 70% of children with MCAP have cortical dysplasia, most commonly bilateral perisylvian polymicrogyria (BPP), predisposing affected individuals to epilepsy (Mirzaa et al., 2012). The extent of BPP varies widely from focal BPP involving the perisylvian regions only to extensive forms including the frontal and/or occipital poles. Approximately 30% of children with MCAP have seizures, including focal, generalized tonic-clonic, and myoclonic seizures. Epilepsy is usually well controlled on antiseizure medication. A fraction of affected individuals will also have ventriculomegaly predisposing to hydrocephalus, and cerebellar enlargement predisposing to cerebellar tonsillar ectopia. Therefore a fraction of individuals with this disorder undergo neurosurgical intervention for these complications (Mirzaa et al., 2012).

Etiology

Mutations of the *PIK3CA* gene have been identified in the majority of individuals with MCAP (Riviere et al., 2012). Similar to HMEG, most identified mutations are mosaic (postzygotic), with the highest detection rates in affected tissues. There are several PI3K-AKT-MTOR–related pathway disorders that overlap MCAP and are variably associated with focal or generalized epilepsy. Some of these disorders lack vascular malformations and are therefore not neurocutaneous disorders per se.

Megalencephaly polymicrogyria–polydactyly hydrocephalus syndrome (MPPH) is a disorder that partially overlaps MCAP and is characterized by a tetrad of congenital-onset megalencephaly, polymicrogyria (PMG), postaxial polydactyly, and hydrocephalus. The most consistent features of this disorder are MEG and PMG, whereas polydactyly and hydrocephalus are seen less frequently. All reported individuals with this disorder have bilateral perisylvian PMG (BPP), and to date, 100% of reported children have epilepsy, including a subset with infantile spasms (Mirzaa et al., 2012). Mutations in three PI3K-AKT-MTOR pathway genes (*AKT3*, *PIK3R2*, and *CCND2*) have been identified in MPPH. Unlike MCAP and HMEG, most of the identified mutations are constitutional (detected in blood). However, mosaic mutations of *PIK3R2* have been reported in MPPH, and also BPP without megalencephaly.

STRADA (LYK5)–Related Megalencephaly

Recessive mutations in *STRADA* (LYK5) have been identified in children with polyhydramnios, megalencephaly, and symptomatic epilepsy (PMSE) syndrome (Puffenberger et al., 2007). *STRADA* is part of a trimeric complex that phosphorylates and thereby activates the AMP-activated protein kinase (AMPK), which in turn activates the TSC1/TSC2 complex. Recessive mutations of this gene have been predominantly reported in children of Mennonite ancestry. Almost all affected children had early-onset intractable epilepsy, severe intellectual disability, and early death (between 6 months and 6 years of age). Seizures were focal in three children, including one child with epilepsia partialis continua. Two children died of seizure-related complications. Brain MRIs showed subependymal dysplasia, ventriculomegaly, and multiple areas of high diffusion in the subcortical white matter. Neuropathology on one of the deceased children showed enlarged neurons with granular cytoplasm, areas of vacuolization in Purkinje cells and hippocampal neurons, and large dysmorphic cells in the frontal cortex, overlapping some of the histopathological abnormalities seen in FCD. Recently several individuals with PMSE were treated with sirolimus (rapamycin) and were found to have decreased seizure frequency and improvement in receptive language, suggesting that pathway inhibitors may be effective in this spectrum of disorders.

FOCAL STRUCTURAL EPILEPSY WITH OTHER LESIONS

Mesial Temporal Lobe Epilepsy With Hippocampal Sclerosis

Mesial temporal lobe epilepsy with hippocampal sclerosis (MTLE with HS), characterized by seizures involving the limbic structures, is known to have a major role in the pathophysiology of focal epilepsy in adults. MTLE with HS affects children as well, and recognition of this entity in children with refractory epilepsy may lead to earlier intervention with surgery.

Neurologic Features

Patients with focal epilepsy arising from the mesial temporal lobe structures often report auras, including rising epigastric or indescribable sensations or a sense of déjà vu. Alteration of consciousness during seizures and amnesia afterward are also common features. Other clinical features during seizures are oral, verbal, or motor automatisms (e.g., ipsilateral repetitive picking) and contralateral dystonic postures. Some seizures may secondarily generalize, often with contralateral head and eye version followed by contralateral clonus. Characteristically, the interictal EEG shows focal pleomorphic interictal epileptiform discharges in the anterior to midtemporal region.

Neuroimaging

The most common MRI findings are hippocampal atrophy and increased T2 signal in the hippocampus. The hippocampal pathology is best visualized on thin-cut, coronal sequences of an MRI. The entorhinal cortex volume is often decreased in patients with mesial temporal lobe epilepsy; however, this is not a predictor of postoperative seizure recurrence.

Etiology

The features of MTLE-HS are characteristic enough to be considered a specific syndromic diagnostic entity (Wieser, 2004). The typical onset of seizures is in adolescence but ranges between 4 and 16 years. MTLE is more common in adults, but it is seen in 1% to 5% of children and adolescents with epilepsy.

Many individuals have a history of recurrent or prolonged febrile seizures during childhood before the onset of MTLE. Hippocampal sclerosis and impaired growth of normal hippocampi are seen after febrile status epilepticus (Lewis et al., 2014). Genetics may also play a role because sodium channel gene mutations (e.g., *SCN1A*) in humans result in prolonged seizures. Other causes of HS include trauma, hypoxic events, and intracranial infection. The onset of seizures arising from the HS may be several years after the initial insult.

Medical Treatment

Antiseizure medications approved for focal epilepsy are the first-line treatment. Often patients will have periods of seizure remission, but these are often followed by a latency period and subsequent progression to medically intractable seizures.

Surgical Treatment

Temporal lobe surgery is effective for patients with intractable MTLE. Anterior temporal lobectomy yields a worthwhile improvement in 75% to 95% of patients, with approximately two-thirds becoming seizure-free. Up to a third of patients continue to have seizures after surgery. Accurate identification of pathologic features may aid in prognosis after surgical resection.

Gelastic Seizures With Hypothalamic Hamartoma

Although a relatively rare entity, gelastic seizures are characteristic and often the presenting feature of a hypothalamic hamartoma. Gelastic seizures are one of the few seizure types arising from the diencephalon.

Neurologic Features

Gelastic seizures are episodes characterized by brief, frequent, and mechanical bursts of laughter. Facial flushing, pupillary dilation, and at times repetitive complex behaviors may accompany laughing. Additional seizure types, focal or generalized, may develop and are often medically refractory. Cognition remains normal in 35% to 40% of individuals; however, the spectrum of outcomes includes many with deterioration and severe cognitive deficits after the onset of epilepsy. Behavioral problems including aggression, anxiety, and mood disorders are prominent features.

Nonneurologic Features

Approximately 50% of children with hypothalamic hamartomas develop clinically evident precocious puberty. Hypothalamic hamartomas that are pedunculated are more strongly associated with precocious puberty and less likely to develop intractable epilepsy.

Neuroimaging

Hypothalamic hamartomas appear hyperintense in T2-weighted images and hypointense relative to gray matter in T1-weighted images. The size and location of the tumor are important features related to the severity of the syndrome. Intrahypothalamic hamartomas are strongly associated with gelastic seizures, whereas parahypothalamic hypothalamic hamartomas are associated with precocious puberty.

Etiology

Hypothalamic hamartomas can be isolated or part of a syndrome, including Pallister–Hall syndrome, oral-facial-digital syndromes, and Bardet–Biedl syndrome. *GLI3* mutations have been identified in a small proportion of isolated and syndromic causes of hypothalamic hamartomas.

Clinical Management

Although attempts with antiseizure medication are the mainstay of initial treatment, these are often ineffective at controlling gelastic seizures arising from hypothalamic hamartomas. Surgical resection can be curative or reduce seizure burden; thus, this represents a potentially treatable epileptic encephalopathy. Radiosurgery and MRI-guided laser interstitial thermal therapy may be considered effective alternatives to traditional surgical approaches.

Rasmussen Encephalitis

Rasmussen encephalitis—also known as chronic progressive epilepsia partialis continua of childhood—is a rare inflammatory disease characterized by intractable focal epilepsy, progressive hemiplegia, cognitive deterioration, and unilateral inflammation of the cerebral cortex.

Neurologic Features

Median age of onset is 6 years, but it ranges from infancy to adulthood. A prodromal period may occur with mild hemiplegia and infrequent seizures. The acute stage is marked by frequent focal seizures in 50% of patients with epilepsia partialis continua. Untreated, ongoing inflammation occurs resulting in progressive cognitive decline, visual field deficit, and hemiparesis, typically over approximately a 1-year period. The residual stage is characterized by fixed neurologic deficits and often refractory epilepsy. Expressive aphasia can occur when the dominant hemisphere is involved. EEG features are variable in patients with Rasmussen encephalitis. Epileptiform discharges and high-amplitude delta slowing develop in the affected hemisphere. The contralateral hemisphere may also develop interictal discharges in more than half of patients, but these are rarely associated with bilateral disease. A consensus statement concluded the diagnosis of Rasmussen encephalitis can be made without a biopsy if patients display epilepsia partialis continua, unilateral EEG features, and imaging showing progressive atrophy.

Neuroimaging

During the acute stage of disease, T2/FLAIR hyperintense signal and volume loss is often seen initially in the peri-insular region. Ipsilateral atrophy of the head of the caudate nucleus and putamen is often seen early in the disease. Serial MRIs typically show a high rate of progressive atrophy and loss over the cortical and subcortical structures during the acute phase.

Etiology

The exact etiology of Rasmussen encephalitis is unknown, but pathologic studies are consistent with it being an immune-mediated disease. Both the adaptive and innate immune responses play a role in disease progression. Cytotoxic T lymphocytes are a major driver of pathogenicity in Rasmussen encephalitis. The antigen responsible for the T-cell-mediated neurotoxicity is yet to be identified. Antibody-mediated disease may play a role or be causative in a small subset of patients. Anti-GluR3 antibodies were identified in a small cohort of patients, but no autoantibody has been found consistently in patients with Rasmussen encephalitis. Microglia activation is seen in areas of active disease. Unfortunately, it is not known if these findings are causative or secondary to an unknown trigger.

Clinical Management

Antiseizure medications are often ineffective at controlling seizures. Immunomodulatory and immunosuppressive treatments show some promise at slowing down or halting progression of disease, but may delay referral to surgical treatment despite ongoing intractable epilepsy. Surgical hemispherectomy remains the only cure for seizures in Rasmussen encephalitis. Long-term seizure freedom is achieved in 70% to 80% of patients who undergo hemispherectomy. Motor and cognitive improvements have also been reported after surgical disconnection of the affected hemisphere. Homonymous hemianopia and hemiparesis may be present before surgery, but they may be worsened with hemispherectomy.

REFERENCES

The complete list of references for this chapter is available in the e-book at www.expertconsult.com.
   See inside cover for registration details.

REFERENCES

Barkovich, A.J., Chuang, S.H., 1990. Unilateral megalencephaly: correlation of MR imaging and pathologic characteristics. AJNR Am. J. Neuroradiol. 11, 523–531.

Flores-Sarnat, L., 2002. Hemimegalencephaly: part 1. Genetic, clinical, and imaging aspects. J. Child Neurol. 17, 373–384, discussion 84.

Lewis, D.V., Shinnar, S., Hesdorffer, D.C., et al., 2014. Hippocampal sclerosis after febrile status epilepticus: the FEBSTAT study. Ann. Neurol. 75, 178–185.

Mirzaa, G.M., Conway, R.L., Gripp, K.W., et al., 2012. Megalencephaly-capillary malformation (MCAP) and megalencephaly-polydactyly-polymicrogyria-hydrocephalus (MPPH) syndromes: two closely related disorders of brain overgrowth and abnormal brain and body morphogenesis. Am. J. Med. Genet. A 158A, 269–291.

Poduri, A., Evrony, G.D., Cai, X., et al., 2013. Somatic mutation, genomic variation, and neurological disease. Science 341, 1237758.

Puffenberger, E.G., Strauss, K.A., Ramsey, K.E., et al., 2007. Polyhydramnios, megalencephaly and symptomatic epilepsy caused by a homozygous 7-kilobase deletion in LYK5. Brain 130, 1929–1941.

Riviere, J.B., Mirzaa, G.M., O'Roak, B.J., et al., 2012. De novo germline and postzygotic mutations in AKT3, PIK3R2 and PIK3CA cause a spectrum of related megalencephaly syndromes. Nat. Genet. 44, 934–940.

Sisodiya, S.M., 2004. Malformations of cortical development: burdens and insights from important causes of human epilepsy. Lancet Neurol. 3, 29–38.

Vigevano, F., Bertini, E., Boldrini, R., et al., 1989. Hemimegalencephaly and intractable epilepsy: benefits of hemispherectomy. Epilepsia 30, 833–843.

Wieser, H.G., 2004. ILAE Commission Report. Mesial temporal lobe epilepsy with hippocampal sclerosis. Epilepsia 45, 695–714.

75 Other Acquired Epilepsies: Trauma, Stroke, Tumors

Russell C. Bailey, Nicole J. Ullrich, and Howard P. Goodkin

Epilepsy is a spectrum of diseases that share a risk for recurrent, unprovoked seizures. The acquired epilepsies are those that result from either an external (e.g., traumatic brain injury [TBI]) or internal (e.g., stroke, infection, brain tumor) insult to the brain that triggers epileptogenesis, the process by which the "normal" brain is transformed at the molecular, cellular, and network levels, resulting in epilepsy.

The bulk of this chapter focuses on the epilepsies acquired following a TBI, stroke, or brain tumor (Hauser, Annegers, and Kurland, 1993). These three insults are often identified as the etiologies that account for the majority of the acquired epilepsies. It is often stated that neurocysticercosis is the most common cause of acquired epilepsy worldwide. Seizures are often the presenting symptom of neurocysticercosis. The estimated risk of recurrence after a first seizure is approximately 40%, and the risk of recurrence is approximately 70% after a second seizure. However, it has been suggested that the recurrence of seizures in this population is not the result of an epileptogenic process, but simply reflects a recurrence of acute symptomatic seizures provoked by the inflammation and edema created by a degenerating cyst. Further details of the neurologic consequences of neurocysticercosis resulting from an infection with the tapeworm *Taenia solium* can be found in Chapter 116, which outlines fungal, rickettsial, and parasitic diseases of the nervous system.

Another current controversy regarding the acquired epilepsies is the question of whether some cases of mesial temporal lobe epilepsy result from a hippocampal injury sustained during an episode of childhood febrile status epilepticus. Febrile status epilepticus accounts for approximately 25% of all cases of pediatric status epilepticus. Prior epidemiologic studies found a high correlation between a diagnosis of epilepsy and a prior history of febrile seizures; however, such studies could not address whether the febrile status epilepticus directly triggered the epileptogenic process or if the febrile status epilepticus was simply a marker that the epileptogenic process already occurred as a result of a prior insult or congenital abnormality. The question of the relationship between febrile status epilepticus, the infectious agent, prior developmental abnormalities of the hippocampus, hippocampal sclerosis, and the development of temporal lobe epilepsy is currently being addressed by the multicenter FEBSTAT study (Consequences of Prolonged Febrile Seizures in Children), a prospective study of children between 1 month and 5 years of age who experienced a first episode of febrile status epilepticus. The control group is composed of children who have experienced a febrile seizure that was not febrile status epilepticus. Current results include the finding that a developmental abnormality was more likely to be present in the children who had experienced an episode of febrile status epilepticus than in the control group, and, further, that there was electrographic and radiologic evidence of hippocampal injury resulting directly from the febrile status epilepticus in a small proportion of children. Several of these children within the febrile status epilepticus cohort have already developed epilepsy, and continued surveillance of this group is ongoing.

Further details of this landmark study addressing this important question can be found in Chapter 65 on febrile seizures.

Knowledge regarding the role of autoimmunity as a cause of acquired epilepsy is expanding. Antibodies to the voltage-gated potassium channel complex, contactin-associated protein-2 (Caspr2), and the N-methyl-D-aspartate (NMDA) receptor have been identified as causing epilepsy in a small proportion of children. Identification of an autoimmune antibody as the underlying cause of the epilepsy is important because there is a suggestion that these epilepsies may respond poorly to antiseizure medications and require immunotherapy. This developing area of autoimmunity and its links with limbic encephalitis and epilepsy are more completely reviewed in Chapter 119.

An epilepsy presumed to be the result of an infectious or postinfectious autoimmune process is febrile infection-related epilepsy syndrome (FIRES). This epilepsy commences with seizures evolving to status epilepticus in the setting of an intercurrent illness in children between 2 to 15 years with normal psychomotor development. The status epilepticus is typically refractory to standard treatment protocols and immunomodulatory agents, but may respond to the ketogenic diet. Unfortunately, after the status epilepticus is controlled, the child continues to have recurrent seizures refractory to antiseizure medications and has new-onset moderate to severe neurocognitive difficulties. The seizures are often lateralized, with prominent orofacial and limb motor features. The onset of the syndrome during an intercurrent illness led to the hypothesis that the chronic epilepsy is the result of an infectious or postinfectious autoimmune process. However, evaluation for an infectious, inflammatory, metabolic, or genetic etiology is typically negative, which has led to the hypothesis that FIRES is a chronic epilepsy with explosive onset of unknown cause, and not a remote-symptomatic epilepsy with an acute inflammatory antecedent.

POSTTRAUMATIC EPILEPSY

TBI is defined by the presence of an alteration in brain function (e.g., loss of consciousness, confusion/disorientation, amnesia, focal neurologic deficit) or other evidence of brain pathology (e.g., imaging abnormality) that results from an external force. Examples of an external force include the head striking or being struck by an object, the head being subjected to a blast, a rapid acceleration/deceleration of the head that occurs in the absence of a direct force to the head (as may occur in a motor vehicle accident [MVA]), and penetrating injuries to the brain (e.g., gunshot wound). Traditionally, the severity of the TBI is classified as mild (which includes sports concussion), moderate, and severe. The current criteria used to determine the severity are based on a combination of the best available Glasgow Coma Scale (GCS) score within 24 hours of the injury, whether loss of consciousness occurred and its duration, whether posttraumatic amnesia was present and its duration, and the results of head imaging.

TABLE 75-1 Occurrence of Late Posttraumatic Seizures in Children

Study	Cohort	Age (Years)	Follow-Up Period (Years)	N	Late Seizures (%)
Hendrick and Harris, 1968	Admitted	<15	4-12	4,465	1.3
Klonoff et al., 1977	Admitted	2.7-15.9	5	231	4
Appleton and Demellweek, 2002	Pediatric rehabilitation program	1.3-15.2	1.6-7 (median 4 yr)	102	9
Emanuelson and Uvebrant 2009	Population based	<18	10	109	11
Arango et al. 2012	Admitted (severe TBI)	0-17	≤2	270	16.9
Barlow et al., 2005	Admitted (inflicted TBI)	0.1-2.1	4.9 (average)	25	20
Kieslich and Jacobi, 1995	Admitted (substantial head trauma)	0.1-17	>2 (8.75 mean)	318	21.4
Barlow et al., 2000	Admitted (inflicted injury)	0.1-2.8	0.3-18	44	22

TBI, traumatic brain injury.

TBI is the leading cause of neurologic morbidity and mortality. The most common mechanisms of injury in the civilian population include falls, being struck by or against an object, and MVAs. In young children, nonaccidental trauma unfortunately remains a leading cause of severe TBI, whereas MVA and assault are common mechanisms in the adolescent age group.

Early Versus Late Posttraumatic Seizures

Immediately or soon after the TBI, acute symptomatic seizures may be observed that occur in response to the temporary pathophysiological changes of synaptic, axonal, and glial function directly induced by the TBI. These early posttraumatic seizures have been reported in 1.6% to 42.5% of children and typically commence within the first 24 hours after the injury.

Seizures occurring 7 or more days after the injury have been defined as late posttraumatic seizures. In contrast to early posttraumatic seizures, the majority of late posttraumatic seizures are remote symptomatic seizures resulting from the permanent changes of brain function induced as a result of the TBI (i.e., epileptogenesis).

The International League against Epilepsy (ILAE) has recently proposed a new practical clinical definition of epilepsy that defines epilepsy as (1) at least two unprovoked (or reflex) seizures occurring more than 24 hours apart or (2) one unprovoked (or reflex) seizure and a probability of further seizures similar to the general recurrence risk (at least 60%) after two unprovoked seizures, occurring over the next 10 years. Because the recurrence risk of late posttraumatic seizures is greater than 60%, the first occurrence of a late posttraumatic seizure can be considered the onset of the posttraumatic epilepsy.

Epidemiology

The epilepsy that occurs following a TBI is most frequently characterized by seizures of focal onset. Studies performed on adult patients have documented that the seizures most commonly arise from the temporal or frontal lobe. In children, the data are more limited but also support that late posttraumatic seizures are predominantly focal. On occasion, epileptic spasms have been observed in children who are the victims of nonaccidental head injury.

Fortunately, posttraumatic epilepsy develops only in a minority of children who experience a TBI. In those studies in which children with a TBI have been followed for a minimum of 6 months, the occurrence of a late posttraumatic seizure has varied between 1.3% to as high as 21.4% of the study population in those studies in which an unambiguous value could be determined (Table 75-1).

There is frequently a lag between the TBI and the development of the posttraumatic epilepsy. Although the risk for the onset of the epilepsy is highest in the first year after the injury, a small risk may persist for up to 30 years after the injury (Annegers, et al., 1998).

Risk Factors

Severity. Large population-based studies have consistently demonstrated that the risk of developing posttraumatic epilepsy following TBI increases with injury severity. Specific markers of injury severity that have been correlated with an increased risk of developing posttraumatic epilepsy include the duration of loss of consciousness or amnesia at presentation, abnormal findings on head imaging (e.g., presence of a depressed skull fracture, cerebral contusion, subdural or intracerebral hemorrhage, midline shift, uncal herniation), focal abnormalities on neurologic examination, increased intracranial pressure, an acute-stage electroencephalogram (EEG) with focal abnormalities, and the need for multiple intracranial procedures (Christensen et al., 2009).

Age. When comparing children with adults, the risk of developing posttraumatic epilepsy after a TBI is greater in adults than in children. During childhood, the risk of developing posttraumatic epilepsy after a sustained TBI appears to be greater in the very young, which may reflect mechanism and severity of injury.

Early posttraumatic seizures. Early posttraumatic seizures tend to occur more frequently in children under 7 years of age than in adolescents and adults. The published incidence for early posttraumatic seizure in children varies between 1.6% and 42.5%. The high value of 42.5% was from a study performed using continuous EEG within an intensive care unit setting, and the next highest value of 30% was from a study of children with nonaccidental trauma. Risk factors for early posttraumatic seizures include injury severity (low GCS score), nonaccidental trauma, young age (<2 years), intracranial hemorrhage, prolonged loss of consciousness, and depressed or open skull fracture.

An association between the occurrence of early posttraumatic seizures and the later development of posttraumatic epilepsy has been well documented in multiple studies in both children and adults. In children, approximately 20% to 40% of children with early posttraumatic seizures will develop late posttraumatic seizures, compared with less than 5% of children not observed to have an early posttraumatic seizure; therefore, children with early posttraumatic seizures are 3 to 9 times more likely to develop posttraumatic epilepsy.

With respect to early posttraumatic seizures, an important question is whether these seizures exacerbate the TBI and contribute to the epileptogenic process. If this were true, then prevention of these seizures may be expected to prevent or reduce the incidence of posttraumatic epilepsy. The best evidence that early posttraumatic seizures may directly lead to secondary injury comes from a convenience sample of adult patients with a TBI with a GCS score of 3 to 12 who both underwent continuous EEG monitoring at the time of presentation and had early and follow-up volumetric magnetic resonance imaging (MRI) of the brain. The degree of global atrophy was similar between those who did have seizures documented on the continuous EEG and those who did not. However, when the comparison was limited to the hippocampus, there was a greater degree of hippocampal atrophy in those with seizures, which was greater on the side ipsilateral to the seizure focus.

However, to date, only a single study that included both children and adults has demonstrated that prevention of early posttraumatic seizures with phenytoin reduced the risk of posttraumatic epilepsy. Other studies evaluating the prophylactic use of carbamazepine and valproate after TBI have failed to demonstrate a similar finding, and a meta-analysis of the best available studies of prophylactic treatment with either phenobarbital, carbamazepine, or phenytoin concluded that prophylactic antiseizure treatment did reduce the occurrence of early, but not late posttraumatic seizures (Schierhout and Roberts, 2001). Whether newer antiseizure medications, such as levetiracetam, or novel therapies, such as rapamycin, will prove effective is not yet known.

Other. A large population-based study identified family history of epilepsy as a factor that potentially increased the risk of developing posttraumatic epilepsy. Interestingly, single-nucleotide polymorphisms of the gene for glutamic acid decarboxylase type 1 have been linked to an increased risk of developing both early seizures and posttraumatic epilepsy. However, a genetic predisposition to posttraumatic epilepsy has not been demonstrated in all studies.

Natural History and Treatment

The occurrence of late posttraumatic seizures has been associated with poor long-term outcomes. Posttraumatic epilepsy may also increase the risk for mortality. In a study of adults with posttraumatic epilepsy, 27% of the patients with late posttraumatic seizures died 8 to 15 years postinjury, compared with only 10% of those who had not developed posttraumatic seizures.

The optimal treatment and outcome of posttraumatic epilepsy is not well characterized in children. In a study of 50 adult patients (≥16 years) with epilepsy and a history of head trauma, which was not better defined, only approximately 35% of the patients were seizure-free while taking antiseizure medications. In a study of children with nonaccidental trauma, 60% of the children were found to be intractable. When appropriate, epilepsy surgery should be considered because good outcomes for those with posttraumatic epilepsy have been reported.

POSTSTROKE EPILEPSY

Stroke is recognized as an important cause of neurologic morbidity and mortality during childhood. The incidence of childhood stroke is estimated to be 2 to 13 per 100,000 children.

Early Versus Late Poststroke Seizures

In the immediate stroke setting, acute symptomatic seizures, termed early poststroke seizures, may be observed. Early seizures are variably defined as those occurring within 7 days of stroke (Morais, Ranzan, and Riesgo, 2013; Hsu et al., 2014) or those occurring within 14 days of stroke onset. Early poststroke seizures occur in 22.3% to 58% of children who experience stroke, and these seizures frequently occur at the time of initial presentation or within 24 hours of stroke occurrence. In the setting of perinatal arterial stroke, early seizures occur in the neonatal period in 75% to 89% of neonates.

Remote seizures, termed late poststroke seizures, are also variably defined as those occurring 7 days or more after stroke occurrence or as those occurring greater than 14 days following the stroke. Late poststroke seizures are associated with a high risk of seizure recurrence, with 85.7% to 100% of children experiencing at least one seizure recurrence. Therefore, consistent with the ILAE's recent clinical definition of epilepsy, the first occurrence of a late poststroke seizure can be considered the onset of poststroke epilepsy.

Epidemiology

Neonates and older children appear particularly vulnerable to developing poststroke epilepsy. Late poststroke seizures are reported to occur in up to 25% of children with stroke compared with only 3% in adults. Although the risk for developing poststroke epilepsy is greatest in the year following the stroke, the risk persists for many years.

Risk Factors

Risk factors for developing poststroke epilepsy include younger age at the time of the stroke, cortical involvement, and early poststroke seizures. Although several studies have documented the association between the occurrence of early poststroke seizures and later development of poststroke epilepsy, there is no compelling evidence that prophylactic use of antiseizure medications following early seizures reduces the risk of late poststroke seizures (Fox et al., 2013).

Natural History and Treatment

Poststroke epilepsy is frequently refractory to medical management. Several retrospective studies have found that almost 20% of these children will have multiple seizures per month despite treatment with antiseizure medications. Unfortunately, the literature is limited in terms of which antiseizure medications are best used in this setting, with limited head-to-head trials. In a prospective, open-label study evaluating the tolerability and efficacy of lamotrigine versus carbamazepine following a first poststroke seizure in adults, lamotrigine and carbamazepine were found to have equal efficacy, but lamotrigine was better tolerated. Similarly, in a multicenter, prospective, randomized, open-label study comparing the efficacy of levetiracetam versus carbamazepine in the treatment of adult patients with late poststroke seizures, levetiracetam and carbamazepine demonstrated equal efficacy, but levetiracetam was better tolerated because it caused significantly fewer side effects, including less adverse effects on cognitive functions.

When appropriate, epilepsy surgery should be considered because this treatment option has proved effective in treating intractable epilepsy related to perinatal vascular insults, with evidence for favorable long-term functional outcomes including improvements in independence, quality of life, cognitive development and motor skills.

EPILEPSY ASSOCIATED WITH BRAIN TUMORS

Seizures and epilepsy are a frequent complication of pediatric brain tumors and their treatment and constitute a frequent reason for neurologic consultation.

Seizures may herald the initial diagnosis of a brain tumor in childhood or can occur as an acute result of the treatment or as a late treatment-related effect, occurring years after completion of treatment. New onset or recurrence of seizures in known brain tumor patients may raise concern for tumor progression/recurrence or treatment-related brain injury, in addition to other causes, including low antiseizure medication levels and metabolic dyscrasias.

The epilepsy associated with brain tumors likely results from multiple factors, including disruption of the peritumoral environment, altered expression of excitatory and inhibitory neurotransmitter receptors, change in glutamate uptake, tumoral edema, an adjacent scar, local hypoxia, acidosis, or metabolic changes.

Epidemiology

Brain tumors are discovered in 1% to 3% of children with new onset of seizures, and seizures may precede the onset of other symptoms by several years.

Risk Factors

Several factors affect the incidence of seizures, including age, location, histology, and grade of the tumor. Tumor pathology is associated with increased risk of seizures; specifically, slow-growing, infiltrative tumors such as dysembryoplastic neuroepithelial tumors (DNTs) and low-grade gliomas have the highest risk of seizure, with an overall incidence of up to 75% in adults and children. In addition, cortical lesions in the temporal, frontal, and parietal lobes are more often correlated with seizures than tumors in the occipital lobe or posterior fossa (Ullrich et al., 2015).

Causes of seizures related to brain tumor treatment include toxic-metabolic effects of chemotherapy (cyclosporin, asparaginase, imipenem), medication toxicity or withdrawal, radiation injury, renal or liver failure, latent non–central nervous system (CNS) infection, and electrolyte abnormalities (syndrome of inappropriate antidiuretic hormone [SIADH], hypoglycemia, hypomagnesemia, hypo- or hypercalcemia). The strongest association with seizures and chemotherapy has been reported with methotrexate, which is used to treat many pediatric cancers, including acute lymphoblastic leukemia, lymphoma, and sarcomas. Agents known to lower seizure threshold include cisplatin and vincristine because both of these agents can pass through the blood–brain barrier and can induce seizures secondary to electrolyte disturbances from hypocalcemia, hypomagnesemia, or hyponatremia.

Natural History and Treatment

In a child with a brain tumor, the decision to initiate antiseizure medication must be considered with an interdisciplinary approach to determine whether medications are needed. In patients with a brain tumor but no prior history of seizures, the American Academy of Neurology (AAN) task force advised against the use of routine antiseizure medication prophylaxis for individuals with a primary brain tumor, except during the week following surgery (Glantz et al., 2000).

The choice of antiseizure medication is often challenging, particularly because many of the more traditional antiseizure medications, such as phenytoin, carbamazepine, and phenobarbital, can affect metabolism of chemotherapeutic drugs by inducing increased activity of the cytochrome p450 system. This may result in decreased efficacy of antitumor therapy, decreased seizure control, and/or unexpected toxicity. By contrast, some data suggest that the antiseizure medication valproic acid may actually contribute an antitumor effect through action as a histone deacetylase inhibitor. In general, enzyme-inducing or enzyme-inhibiting antiseizure medications are less preferable. Newer medications, especially those without known drug–drug interactions, are becoming accepted as first-line seizure treatment in children who require ongoing seizure treatment (Wells, Gaillard, and Packer, 2012). Another important consideration is that the child with a brain tumor may be more susceptible to side effects of antiseizure medications, with an overall incidence of drug effects as high as 20% to 40%. Lastly, consideration of epilepsy surgery for refractory seizures may be appropriate for uncontrolled seizures in the setting of a brain tumor.

The decision to discontinue antiseizure medications in a child with a brain tumor who has achieved seizure freedom is dependent on several factors, including extent of surgical resection (incomplete resection is associated with higher risk for seizure recurrence), tumor recurrence, tumor location (temporal and cortically based tumors are associated with higher risk), and history of more than one prior tumor resection. Short-term treatment may be adequate during the perioperative period; however, the presence of residual and/or metastatic disease, abnormal EEG, and history of seizure at presentation may suggest the need for longer-term use of anticonvulsants.

REFERENCES

The complete list of references for this chapter is available in the e-book at www.expertconsult.com.
See inside cover for registration details.

SELECTED REFERENCES

Annegers, J.F., Hauser, W.A., Coan, S.P., et al., 1998. A population-based study of seizures after traumatic brain injury. N. Engl. J. Med. 338 (1), 20–24.

Christensen, J., et al., 2009. Long-term risk of epilepsy after traumatic brain injury in children and young adults: a population-based cohort study. Lancet 373 (9669), 1105–1110.

Fox, C.K., et al., 2013. Acute seizures predict epilepsy after childhood stroke. Ann. Neurol. 74 (2), 249–256.

Glantz, M.J., et al., 2000. Practice parameter: anticonvulsant prophylaxis in patients with newly diagnosed brain tumors. Report of the Quality Standards Subcommittee of the American Academy of Neurology. Neurology 54 (10), 1886–1893.

Hauser, W.A., Annegers, J.F., Kurland, L.T., 1993. Incidence of epilepsy and unprovoked seizures in Rochester, Minnesota: 1935–1984. Epilepsia 34 (3), 453–468.

Hsu, C.J., et al., 2014. Early-onset seizures are correlated with late-onset seizures in children with arterial ischemic stroke. Stroke 45 (4), 1161–1163.

Morais, N.M., Ranzan, J., Riesgo, R.S., 2013. Predictors of Epilepsy in Children With Cerebrovascular Disease. J. Child Neurol. 28 (11), 1387–1391.

Schierhout, G., Roberts, I., 2001. Anti-epileptic drugs for preventing seizures following acute traumatic brain injury. Cochrane Database Syst. Rev. (4), CD000173.

Ullrich, N.J., et al., 2015. Incidence, risk factors, and longitudinal outcome of seizures in long-term survivors of pediatric brain tumors. Epilepsia 56 (10), 1599–1604.

Wells, E.M., Gaillard, W.D., Packer, R.J., 2012. Pediatric brain tumors and epilepsy. Semin. Pediatr. Neurol. 19 (1), 3–8.

76 Inherited Metabolic Epilepsies

Phillip L. Pearl

An expanded version of this chapter is available on www.expertconsult.com. See inside cover for registration details.

INTRODUCTION

The inherited metabolic epilepsies are a diverse group of disorders of inborn errors of metabolism in which epilepsy is a clinically significant, if not the presenting or predominant, component. They may be viewed within the rubric of genetic-metabolic epilepsies and bear special emphasis in this section on pediatric epilepsy because of their unique properties. In these disorders, the seizures and associated encephalopathy are generated based on the inborn metabolic error. In some cases, specific therapy directed at the metabolic error can lead to reversal of the epilepsy and encephalopathy, or at least a dramatically improved outcome. Yet prompt diagnosis and targeted intervention, beyond standard and nonspecific anti-seizure medications, are required in order to affect the prognosis in a salutary way.

Although individually rare, metabolic disorders in aggregate represent a substantial clinical problem—and challenge—in child neurology. They may present with various epilepsy phenotypes, including early-onset epileptic encephalopathy (including refractory neonatal seizures, early myoclonic encephalopathy, and early infantile epileptic encephalopathy frequently referred to as Ohtahara syndrome), infantile spasms, or mixed generalized seizure types in infancy, childhood, or even adolescence and occasionally adulthood. Although inborn metabolic diseases are covered elsewhere throughout this text in sections devoted to metabolism, those with special applicability to epilepsy, along with their epileptic aspects, are emphasized here with reference to more comprehensive discussions of single disorders as applicable.

GENERAL PRINCIPLES

The inherited metabolic epilepsies are most likely to occur when seizure onset is in the neonatal, infantile, or early childhood periods (Box 76-3). A typical clinical presentation is that of a newborn with impaired feeding who is noted to ultimately become encephalopathic with hypotonia, lethargy, or respiratory distress. Myoclonic seizures are classic, although apneic episodes, oculofacial movements, grunting, and epileptic spasms are also well described ictal events. EEGs may show discontinuous patterns characterized by burst suppression (or suppression burst, e.g., in early myoclonic encephalopathy), continuous or frequent intermittent generalized sharp or spike wave activity, hypsarrhythmia or modified hypsarrhythmia, and multifocal spike discharges superimposed upon background disorganization, including loss of normal sleep architecture. A family history of consanguinity or a metabolic disorder is a strong contributing historical factor, and poor response to traditional antiepilepsy medication may be an important clue. The absence of a clear diagnosis to explain seizure onset is also helpful, but a suspicion of hypoxic-ischemic newborn encephalopathy, or the presence of structural abnormalities on neuroimaging, should not be taken as evidence of absence of an underlying metabolic disorder. In some cases imaging findings such as callosal dysgenesis in pyruvate dehydrogenase complex deficiency, intraventricular choroid plexus cysts in Zellweger syndrome, and enlarged Sylvian fissures in glutaric aciduria type I are indeed suggestive of a specific underlying metabolic disorder.

These disorders can be classified in several ways. One rational approach is to consider what pathophysiologic mechanisms are likely most responsible for seizure generation such as impaired energy production, accumulation of toxic intermediates, neuronal storage products and cellular dysfunction, absence of vital vitamers (i.e., forms of vitamins that have similar chemical structure and physiologic vitamin activity) or neurotransmitters, or associated structural abnormalities (Box 76-2). On a clinical level, the disorders can be categorized based on typical age of onset, or most likely seizure type. Each of these methods contributes to our understanding of how these disorders may be associated with seizures and lead to an epileptogenic encephalopathy, meaning that the underlying disorder leads to inherent epileptogenesis and an ongoing encephalopathy that would require specific intervention aimed at the metabolic error to reverse or improve the phenotype. EEG is important in the diagnostic assessment and follow-up investigations of these patients but lacks the specificity to obviate investigations with imaging, metabolic profiles including plasma, urine, and CSF analyses, and genetic testing typically involving comparative genomic hybridization, gene sequencing panels relevant to the patient's phenotype, and, in some cases, whole exome sequencing when the earlier studies do not yield a diagnosis. There are, however, some EEG patterns that have a strong association with particular conditions–e.g., comb-like rhythmic waves in maple syrup urine disease, RHADS (repetitive high amplitude delta waves with spikes or polyspikes) in Alper disease associated with POLG mutations (Fig. 76-2), vanishing EEG in infantile type NCL, giant visual evoked potentials and photic responses in Lafora body disease, and certain entities known to present with common patterns such as burst suppression as in glycine encephalopathy and hypsarrhythmia in several of these disorders. One logical and practical approach to categorizing inborn errors of metabolism is to structure them based on whether the primary defect involves small or large molecules.

SMALL MOLECULE DISORDERS
Amino and Organic Acid Disorders

Amino and organic acidopathies present with seizures, typically myoclonic, and cognitive, behavioral, or motor disturbances resulting from the accumulation of toxic intermediaries, or possibly structural damage (Kölker, et al., 2008). Some may induce an epileptic encephalopathy.

EEG findings may include burst suppression, hypsarrhythmia, generalized spike wave discharges, and background slowing. These disorders are covered in detail elsewhere; aspects related to epilepsy are emphasized here.

Methylmalonic Acidemia and Cobalamin Deficiencies. Early myoclonic encephalopathy and epileptic encephalopathy have been associated with these disorders. The most common methylmalonic acidemia involving cobalamin is cobalamin C deficiency; individuals may present in infancy or early childhood with seizures, including status epilepticus and progressive encephalopathy. Treatment with hydroxycobalamin is effective, including prenatal supplementation in affected families but may not reverse existing neurologic injury.

Propionic Acidemia. Epilepsy may present as infantile spasms with hypsarrhythmia or generalized seizures, including myoclonic in infancy or early childhood.

Ethylmalonic Acidemia. Ethylmalonic acidemia is usually lethal in infancy or early childhood and has a severe presentation including seizures, structural brain malformations, and often dermatologic findings, including petechiae and acrocyanosis. EEGs have multifocal spike and slow waves and background disorganization that may progress inexorably over time.

3-Hydroxy-3-Methylglutaric Acidemia. Seizures are linked in most cases to lactic acidemia or hypoglycemia and are associated with multifocal spike wave discharges on EEG. Some presentations show particular association with white matter lesions, dysmyelination, and cerebral atrophy on neuroimaging.

Glutaric Acidemia type I. The phenotype is macrocephaly, increased subarachnoid spaces, and progressive dystonia and athetosis with striatal injury. Seizures can be a presenting sign and are seen during acute encephalopathic events. EEGs show background slowing with generalized spike-and-wave and mixed multifocal discharges. The antiepileptic valproate should be avoided because it is believed to affect acetyl CoA/CoA ratios and may exacerbate metabolic imbalance.

Canavan Disease. Canavan disease, caused by a defect of N-acetylaspartic acid (NAA) catabolism, presents with progressive epileptic encephalopathy with developmental delay, macrocephaly, leukodystrophy, and optic atrophy. Seizures typically begin in the second year of life, and treatment is primarily supportive.

D- and L-2-Hydroxyglutaric Aciduria. Severe cases manifest in the neonatorum with encephalopathy, intractable epilepsy, and cardiomyopathy. MRI findings include abnormal basal ganglia and thalamic signal intensity and agenesis of the corpus callosum.

The enantiomer, L-2-Hydroxyglutaric aciduria, is a disorder of alpha ketoglutarate synthesis. It presents with neurodevelopmental delay, generalized seizures, and progressive ataxia. Multifocal spike waves and burst suppression can be seen on

---

BOX 76-2 Pathophysiologic Mechanisms Invoked in Inherited Metabolic Epilepsies

ENERGY DEFICIENCY

Hypoglycemia, GLUT1-deficiency, respiratory chain defects, creatine deficiency

TOXIC ACCUMULATION

Amino acidopathies, organic acidurias, urea cycle defects

IMPAIRED NEURONAL FUNCTION

Storage disorders

DISTURBANCE OF NEUROTRANSMITTER SYSTEMS

Glycine encephalopathy, GABA transaminase deficiency, SSADH deficiency, creatine synthesis/transport defects, serine synthesis defects, sulfite oxidase/Mb cofactor deficiency

ASSOCIATED BRAIN MALFORMATIONS

Peroxisomal disorders (e.g., Zellweger), O-glycosylation defects

VITAMIN/COFACTOR DEPENDENCY

Biotinidase deficiency, pyridoxine and PLP dependencies, folinic acid dependency, cerebral folate deficiency, Menkes disease

---

BOX 76-3 Metabolic Epilepsies—Examples Based on Age at Onset

NEONATAL

Hypoglycemia, pyridoxine dependency, PNPO deficiency, glycine encephalopathy, organic acidurias, urea cycle defects, neonatal ALD, Zellweger, folinic acid dependency, holocarboxylase synthase/biotinidase deficiency, molybdenum cofactor deficiency, sulfite oxidase deficiency

INFANCY

Hypoglycemia, GLUT1-deficiency, creatine deficiency, biotinidase deficiency, amino acidopathies, organic acidurias, CDG, pyridoxine/P5P dependency, NCL1

TODDLERS

NCL2, mitochondrial disorders, lysosomal storage disorders, thiamine transporter deficiency (biotin-thiamine responsive basal ganglia disease)

SCHOOL AGE

Mitochondrial disorders, NCL3, progressive myoclonus epilepsies, thiamine transporter deficiency

---

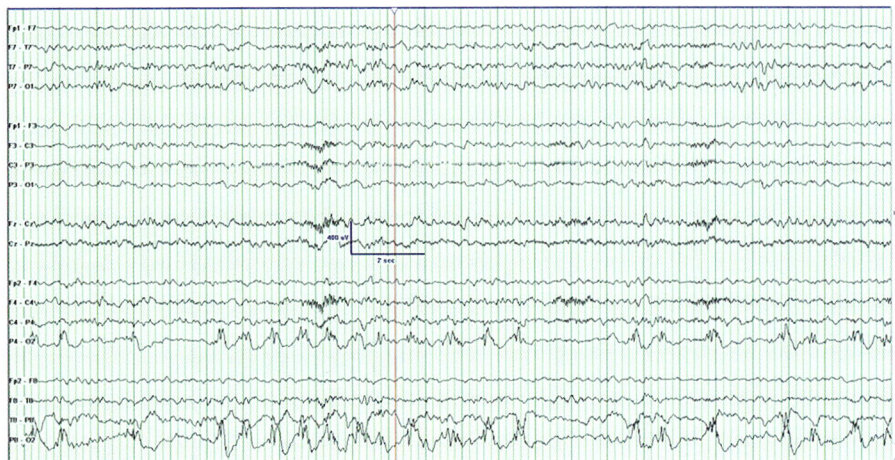

Figure 76-2. EEG shows RHADS, or rhythmic high amplitude delta with (poly)spikes, in 11-month-old girl presenting with status epilepticus, abnormal occipital and thalamic signal on MRI, and compound heterozygosity for two disease-causing POLG1 mutations.

EEGs, and characteristic MRI findings include cerebellar atrophy, subcortical white matter loss, and T2-weighted hyperintensities in the cerebellar dentate nuclei, globus pallidi, and thalami.

Fumaric Aciduria. The disorder can present prenatally with polyhydramnios and cerebral ventriculomegaly and manifests in infancy and early childhood with epilepsy, neurodevelopmental delay, macrocephaly, opisthotonus, and vision loss. Status epilepticus is well reported. Diffuse polymicrogyria, decreased white matter, large ventricles, and open opercula have been identified on neuroimaging.

Maple Syrup Urine Disease (MSUD). Neurologic symptoms present in infancy and include cerebral edema and seizures. The EEG may show a characteristic comb-like rhythm. Treatment focuses on removing leucine from blood with dialysis or by reversing catabolism through feeding.

Serine Synthesis Defects. The clinical phenotype is congenital microcephaly, psychomotor retardation, and refractory seizures including hypsarrhythmia. Juvenile onset has also been reported, with presentation at school age with absence seizures and moderate developmental delay. Supplementation with oral serine and glycine has been reported to improve outcome, including prenatal intervention.

Sulfide Oxidase Deficiency/Molybdenum Cofactor Deficiency. Seizures, primarily myoclonic or tonic-clonic, begin in the first few weeks of life; they can be refractory to therapy and may develop into status epilepticus. EEG findings include burst suppression patterns and multifocal spike wave discharges, and neuroimaging results are usually profoundly abnormal, including diffuse cerebral edema evolving into cystic lesions and brain atrophy within weeks. Low total plasma homocysteinemia is associated with both, and hypouricemia due to secondary xanthine dehydrogenase deficiency can be indicative of Mb cofactor deficiency. Therapy has historically been symptomatic, predominantly with antiseizure medications. There are later-onset forms that can develop a neurodegenerative pattern although recovery and developmental progress can occur. Decreased plasma uric acid can be a diagnostic clue in otherwise unsuspected late cases.

Hyperhomocysteinemias. The spectrum of neurologic dysfunction in homocysteine metabolism disorders is wide, including epilepsy, encephalopathy, peripheral neuropathy, ataxia, microcephaly, and psychiatric disorders. Focal seizures, stroke, neurodevelopmental delay, and cognitive deficiency, as well as psychosis are common neurologic findings. Pyridoxine, cyanocobalamin, folate, and a methionine restricted diet are used in cystathionine beta-synthetase deficiency, whereas high-dose hydroxycobalamin is useful in methionine synthase deficiency.

Autosomal recessively inherited deficiency of *methylene tetrahydrofolate reductase* (MTHFR) may present in early infancy with severe epileptic encephalopathy or infantile spasms, and evolve to Lennox Gastaut syndrome or status epilepticus. The methyl donor betaine may have a therapeutic role.

Creatine Biosynthesis and Transport Deficiencies. Creatine is an organic acid synthesized from L-arginine, glycine, and methionine and is critical in ATP production. Patients with deficiencies in creatine synthesis or transport present with early developmental delay, seizures, neurologic regression, intellectual disability, autistic behavior, hypotonia, and movement disorders. Females with heterozygous mutations of the X-linked creatine transporter gene may be symptomatic with more moderate intellectual disability, learning and behavior problems, and epilepsy. Approximately half of individuals with GAMT deficiency and most males with creatine transporter deficiency develop epilepsy. EEGs demonstrate generalized or multifocal spike discharges and background slowing.

Fatty Acid Oxidation Disorders

Seizures can be a presenting sign of fatty acid oxidation disorders, a large category of diseases that particularly involve the CNS and other organ systems that have high energy demands. Metabolic decompensation can be triggered by physiologic stressors such as fasting, fever, or physical exertion, and symptoms can appear at any age. Acute crises resemble Reye syndrome, with cardiomyopathy and arrhythmia, as well as rhabdomyolysis and hypoketotic hypoglycemia.

Mitochondrial Diseases

Epilepsy is common in mitochondrial disease and includes all seizure types. Myoclonic seizures are the most commonly reported, but epilepsia partialis continua and epileptic encephalopathy occur as well. Seizures are a logical consequence of mitochondrial dysfunction: deficient energy generation disrupts the active maintenance of neuronal membrane potentials, and seizure-induced cellular hyperactivity adds further oxidative stress to already deficient ATP generation. Up to 60% of patients with mitochondrial disease develop seizures, and many of these can be refractory to treatment.

POLG1 Disease. Mutations in the gene POLG1, which facilitates mitochondrial DNA replication, have been linked to a range of disease phenotypes, the most prominent being Alpers-Huttenlocher disease. This is a rapidly progressive encephalopathy with multiple seizure types (Wolf, et al., 2009). The syndrome has been associated with a pattern of Rhythmic High Amplitude Delta with Polyspikes on EEG (RHADS), typically most prominent over the occipital regions (Fig. 2) (Wolf, et al., 2009). Valproate has been associated with liver failure and epilepsia partialis continua in this syndrome.

Myoclonic Epilepsy with Ragged Red Fibers (MERRF). MERRF is a progressive mitochondrial disorder associated with prominent myoclonus, cognitive decline, optic atrophy, hearing loss, and myopathy (DiMauro and Schon, 2008). EEG findings include focal discharges, atypical spike- or sharp- and slow-wave discharges, and suppression of this activity during sleep. MELAS, or myoclonic epilepsy with lactic acidosis and stroke-like episodes, is associated with various forms of focal onset seizures, often occurring during the acute phase of a stroke-like episode, or described as epilepsia partialis continua, hemiclonic status, occipital status, and nonconvulsive status epilepticus.

Leigh Syndrome. Also known as subacute necrotizing encephalomyelopathy, this syndrome manifests with progressive hypotonia, spasticity, and brainstem failure and lesions in the basal ganglia, thalami, midbrain, and brainstem as well as cortical and cerebellar atrophy. Focal and generalized seizures, epilepsia partialis continua, and infantile spasms have all been described. A disorder that may simulate Leigh disease is biotin-thiamine responsive basal ganglia disease, an autosomal recessive disorder due to mutations of the thiamine transporter SLC19A3 gene. Patients present acutely or subacutely with encephalopathy, ataxia, seizures, and a mixed pyramidal and extrapyramidal syndrome, including dystonia, quadriparesis, and hyperreflexia. MRI may show basal ganglia edema acutely and atrophy over time.

Urea Cycle Disorders

The urea cycle, the metabolic mechanism for nitrogen detoxification and removal, is facilitated by six enzymes and a mitochondrial transporter and carrier. In the event of an enzyme or transport defect, the resulting hyperammonemia can lead to overwhelming encephalopathy, often accompanied by seizures that may be exacerbated by metabolic stresses such as fever or infection. EEG monitoring should be initiated early in the course of acute treatment, as seizure activity is thought to be related to hyperammonemic crises or structural damage, and subclinical electrographic seizures are reported. Males with ornithine transcarbamylase deficiency typically present in the neonatorum and with high mortality, whereas female heterozygotes can vary in the severity and timing of presentation depending on hepatic lyonization.

Disorders of Glucose Homeostasis

DEND Syndrome (Developmental Delay, Epilepsy, and Neonatal Diabetes). A syndrome that combines the problems of developmental delay, epilepsy, and neonatal diabetes is an epileptic channelopathy associated with mutations in potassium channel and sulfonylurea receptor genes (Shimomura, et al., 2007). These mutations permanently "lock in" the K channel in an open state, leading to insufficient insulin release and severe hyperglycemia within the first 6 months of life. Clinical manifestations include neurodevelopmental delay, dysmorphic features, hypotonia, and seizures starting as early as the neonatorum. Infantile spasms with hypsarrhythmia, as well as severe tonic-clonic and myoclonic epilepsies, are reported. Sulfonylureas are capable of bypassing the defective regulation of KATP channels and may improve the otherwise poor neurologic outcome (Shimomura, et al., 2007).

Hyperinsulinism-Hyperammonemia (HI-HA). HI-HA is a syndrome of congenital hyperinsulinism and hyperammonemia that has been related to activating mutations that affect GDH (glutamate dehydrogenase), affecting the insulin secretion pathway. These defects cause GDH to become insensitive to inhibition, resulting in excess ammonia production and insulin release and neurologic sequelae from hypoglycemic insults. The clinical constellation of generalized epilepsy, learning disorders, and behavior problems, in the context of hypoglycemia (both postprandial and fasting) and persistent hyperammonemia, is characteristic.

Glucose Transporter 1 Deficiency. Glucose transporter type I (Glut-1) facilitates the passage of glucose across the blood-brain barrier, and its dysfunction in the developing brain leads to the development of a metabolic encephalopathy. CSF shows hypoglycorrhachia associated with normal plasma glucose and low-to-normal CSF lactate, measured in a fasting state. A wide array of phenotypes has been associated with this disorder, but 90% of affected children develop epilepsy (of various types, including absence, focal, generalized myoclonic, clonic, tonic, and nonconvulsive status epilepticus). Microcephaly, ataxia, and psychomotor delay may be present (De Vivo, et al., 1991), but patients may also suffer from epilepsy without any accompanying motor or cognitive deficiencies. EEG findings vary and may be normal but usually include either focal or generalized slowing or attenuation, or spike-and-wave discharges (generalized, focal, or multifocal).

Glucose transporter I deficiency has emerged as the leading metabolic indication for the ketogenic diet, a dietary therapy that replaces glucose with ketone bodies as the primary biochemical energy source. Response is rapid, even in the case of formerly refractory seizures, and treatment should be maintained long term. Additionally, there are certain compounds known to inhibit Glut-1, including phenobarbital, diazepam, methylxanthines (theophylline, caffeine), and alcohol, which should be avoided; valproate is generally avoided as well (Wang, et al., 2015).

Vitamin Dependency States

Pyridoxine, Folinic Acid, and Pyridoxal-5-Phosphate Dependent Epilepsies. There are various epileptic encephalopathies related to vitamin B_6 metabolism, and pyridoxine-dependent epilepsy (PDE) is the prototype, resulting from a loss of the biologically active pyridoxal-5-phosphate (PLP) due to a dysfunction of the protein antiquitin (ALDH7A1) (Mills, et al., 2006). PDE typically presents within the first hours after birth with serial refractory seizures responsive to pyridoxine administration. Improvement is significant and usually rapidly appreciable on EEG. Variants of the disorder that respond to folinic acid instead of, or in addition to, pyridoxine have also been described, as well as atypical cases with long asymptomatic periods or presenting later in infancy (i.e., weeks or months after birth).

PNPO, or pyridoxamine phosphate oxidase, deficiency is due to a defect in the enzyme PNPO, which synthesizes PLP from precursors pyridoxine-P and pyridoxamine-P. This syndrome is more typically associated with premature births and a distinct CSF profile compared with ALDH7 A1 deficiency pyridoxine dependency, although there is considerable overlap between the two including responsiveness to pyridoxine (Plecko, et al., 2014; Mills, et al., 2014).

Cerebral Folate Deficiency (CFD). Known as cerebral folate "deficiency," albeit a dependency state as opposed to a dietary deficiency, CFD can be a common end result of diverse metabolic and genetic conditions. This may be due to one of multiple causes, including loss of function mutations in the folate FR1 receptor, blocking autoantibodies to the folate receptor, or disrupted uptake due to valproic acid. Secondary folate deficiency can also be seen in inborn metabolic diseases such as Rett syndrome, 3-phosphoglycerate dehydrogenase deficiency (a congenital serine biosynthesis disorder), and mitochondrial disorders such as Kearns-Sayre or Alpers disease.

Primary cerebral folate deficiency (CFD) is characterized by normal blood but low CSF levels of 5-methylhydrofolate (5-MTHF), the physiologically active form of folate. The common phenotype includes epilepsy, along with neurodevelopmental delay (or regression) and dyskinesias. In some cases, treatment with high doses of folinic acid (as opposed to folic acid, which has poor blood-brain barrier entry) has been reported to ameliorate seizures and improve neurologic function.

Neurotransmitter Disorders

Disorders of GABA Metabolism. Seizures are an important problem in disorders of the synthesis or degradation of gamma-aminobutyric acid (GABA), the brain's primary inhibitory neurotransmitter. The most common of these is succinic semialdehyde dehydrogenase (SSADH) deficiency, though GABA-transaminase deficiency—although extremely rare—has been more associated with a severe, progressive epileptic encephalopathy (Pearl, et al., 2009).

Glycine Encephalopathy. Glycine encephalopathy is an inherited disorder of glycine degradation resulting from defects in the mitochondrial glycine cleavage system (GCS). The majority of patients present with a severe neonatal-onset form, with primarily myoclonic and intractable seizures, hypotonia, apnea, and coma. Outcomes are generally poor, particularly in the presence of brain malformations such as corpus callosum hypoplasia. There are attenuated forms, lacking congenital malformations, with a better outcome. EEG findings include multifocal epileptiform activity, hypsarrhythmia, and burst-suppression patterns. Treatment with benzoate and a low-protein diet may reduce glycine levels in plasma, and combined antiseizure medical treatment is usually required.

Purine and Pyrimidine Defects

Disorders of purine and pyrimidine metabolism may present with epileptic encephalopathies, including adenylosuccinase (adenylosuccinate lyase) deficiency which has a broad phenotypic spectrum including neonatal seizures. Lesch-Nyhan disease, or X-linked hypoxanthine-guanine phosphoribosyl transferase deficiency, may result in epileptic seizures, but these can be difficult to distinguish from the extrapyramidal manifestations, specifically dystonic spasms, tremor, and myoclonus. Generalized tonic-clonic seizures are the most commonly reported epilepsy type. Treatment with allopurinol is essential for hyperuricemia and may provide some antiepileptic effect. Medication choices must weigh the possibility of exacerbating underlying behavioral irritability with levetiracetam and others. Topiramate and zonisamide are avoided due to the risk of nephrolithiasis.

LARGE MOLECULE DISORDERS
Disorders of Glycosylation

Disorders of protein glycosylation, due to defects in the synthesis of N- and O-linked glycoproteins, are characterized by multiple organ system dysfunction, developmental delay, hypotonia, and epilepsy. Certain of these disorders are associated with severe encephalopathy, particularly those involving alpha-dystroglycan, a protein component of the extracellular matrix, essential to muscle integrity. These are known as dystroglycanopathies. Examples that include frequent seizures are Walker-Warburg syndrome and Fukuyama congenital muscular dystrophy.

Lysosomal Storage Disorders

Lysosomal storage disorders (LSD) involve defects in lysosomal enzyme function, lysosomal biogenesis, activation, trafficking, or membrane transporters. Over two thirds are neurodegenerative and some are associated with epileptic encephalopathy. Specific examples with active associated epilepsy are the neuronal ceroid lipofuscinoses, sphingolipidoses including Gaucher disease (glucocerebrosidase deficiency), and gangliosidoses, including Tay-Sachs disease (hexosaminidase A deficiency).

Peroxisomal Diseases

As a participant in cellular detoxification, lipid metabolism, myelination, neuronal function, migration, and brain development, peroxisomes are essential for neuronal health. Nearly all peroxisomal disorders are known to impair neurologic function, though peroxisomes are present in almost all eukaryotic cells, and consequently the associated diseases will also manifest in multiple organ systems. The disorders may be classified as those of biogenesis, single enzyme deficiencies, or contiguous gene syndromes. Seizures occur particularly in the neonatal period and may be a result of cortical migration defects. Symptomatic treatment using anticonvulsants is the predominant therapy.

Leukodystrophies

Genetic leukoencephalopathies, or inherited white matter disorders, are diseases that primarily affect myelinated structures in the brain and peripheral nervous system. The majority of leukodystrophies primarily feature motor dysfunction rather than encephalopathy, particularly early in the development of the disease. Epilepsy, however, can be a prominent symptom in certain classic leukodystrophies such as Alexander disease. This is associated with defects in the GFAP gene encoding astrocyte intermediate filaments. Early-onset forms of Alexander disease (Type I) frequently feature seizures, particularly associated with fever, that are difficult to control. The clinical course of type I Alexander disease is normally progressive neurodegeneration involving megalencephaly, psychomotor retardation, and spastic paraplegia. Globoid cell leukodystrophy (Krabbe disease), metachromatic leukodystrophy, and hereditary leukodystrophy with spheroids are other examples in which epilepsy may be a prominent component of the phenotype.

CONCLUSION

Epilepsy may be a prominent presenting feature, or major morbidity, of a variety of inborn errors of metabolism. The diagnostic evaluation and oftentimes therapeutic approach, however, are different than what would be considered the classic approach to evaluation and management of epilepsy. Early life onset and epileptic encephalopathies are especially characteristic.

These disorders have various degrees of treatability at present, with some requiring prompt diagnosis and intervention to avert otherwise potentially poor outcomes. Early myoclonic encephalopathy and myoclonic seizures represent a classic epilepsy syndrome and seizure type, respectively, associated with inborn errors of metabolism. Yet the phenotypic spectrum of epilepsy caused by hereditary metabolic disorders is wide and includes refractory neonatal seizures, early infantile epileptic encephalopathy (syndrome of Ohtahara), infantile spasms, and progressive myoclonus epilepsy, as well as syndrome variations such as early-onset absence epilepsy in glucose transporter deficiency. A careful approach to metabolic disorders is helpful to consider the various diseases that may present and develop into a severe epilepsy or epileptic encephalopathy.

The small molecule disorders include amino and organic acidopathies such as maple syrup urine disease, homocysteinemia, multiple organic acid disorders, and cobalamin deficiencies. Dietary intervention is key to preventing encephalopathy in maple syrup urine disease and glutaric aciduria, and hydroxycobalamin has a therapeutic role starting in prenatal intervention in cobalamin C deficiency. Neurotransmitter and fatty acid oxidation disorders may result in epileptic encephalopathies, and mitochondrial disorders present with a range of epilepsy phenotypes, including epilepsia partialis continua in polymerase gamma mutations. Cerebral folate deficiency appears to result from a variety of causes, but primary deficiency, associated with mutations of the folate receptor or blocking antibodies, has a phenotype of intractable generalized seizures in infancy which may respond to folinic acid.

Disorders of serine synthesis may respond to prenatal and postnatal supplementation with serine and glycine. There are several potassium channelopathies involving the pancreas and brain, presenting either with neonatal diabetes or hypoglycemia, with specific therapeutic implications. Glucose transporter deficiency appears to be the prototype of transport defects causing epilepsy and having specific therapy, in this case the ketogenic diet, and the disorders related to the pyridoxine vitamers, specifically pyridoxine and pyridoxal-5-phosphate, require prompt identification and therapy. Autosomal recessively inherited deficiency of MTHFR may be reversible with use of betaine, whereas other small molecule defects causing epileptic encephalopathy, for example, glycine encephalopathy and sulfite oxidase deficiency, have no specific therapy at this time.

Large molecule disorders involve a complex constellation of disorders of glycosylation, lysosomal storage diseases, and peroxisomal disorders. Although epilepsy represents significant gray matter involvement in neurologic disease, seizures can be a prominent aspect of leukodystrophies such as

Alexander disease. These hereditary disorders should be highly considered in the investigation of patients with severe epilepsies and epileptic encephalopathies, leading to specific diagnostic steps and, in some cases, potential therapeutic maneuvers to address the metabolic defect and improve the epilepsy and encephalopathy.

REFERENCES

The complete list of references for this chapter is available in the e-book at www.expertconsult.com.
See inside cover for registration details.

SELECTED REFERENCES

De Vivo, D.C., Trifiletti, R.R., Jacobson, R.I., et al., 1991. Defective glucose transport across the blood-brain barrier as a cause of persistent hypoglycorrhachia, seizures, and developmental delay. N. Engl. J. Med. 325 (10), 703–709.

DiMauro, S., Schon, E.A., 2008. Mitochondrial disorders in the nervous system. Annu. Rev. Neurosci. 31, 91–123.

Kölker, S., Sauer, S.W., Hoffmann, G.F., et al., 2008. Pathogenesis of CNS involvement in disorders of amino and organic acid metabolism. J. Inherit. Metab. Dis. 31 (2), 194–204.

Mills, P.B., Camuzeaux, S.S., Footitt, E.J., et al., 2014. Epilepsy due to PNPO mutations: genotype, environment, and treatment affect presentation and outcome. Brain 137 (Pt 5), 1350–1360.

Mills, P.B., Struys, E., Jakobs, C., et al., 2006. Mutations in antiquitin in individuals with pyridoxine-dependent seizures. Nat. Med. 12 (3), 307–309.

Pearl, P.L., Gibson, K.M., Cortez, M.A., et al., 2009. Succinic semialdehyde dehydrogenase deficiency: lessons from mice and men. J. Inherit. Metab. Dis. 32 (3), 343–352.

Plecko, B., Paul, K., Mills, P., et al., 2014. Pyridoxine responsiveness in novel mutations of the PNPO gene. Neurology 82 (16), 1425–1433.

Shimomura, K., Horster, F., de Wet, H., et al., 2007. A novel mutation causing DEND syndrome: a treatable channelopathy of pancreas and brain. Neurology 69 (13), 1342–1349.

Wang, D., Pascual, J.M., De Vivo, D., 2015. Glucose Transporter Type 1 Deficiency Syndrome. In: Pagon, R.A., Adam, M.P., Ardinger, H.H., et al. (Eds.), GeneReviews® [Internet]. Copyright ©1993–2015. University of Washington, Seattle, Seattle (WA).

Wolf, N.I., Rahman, S., Schmitt, B., et al., 2009. Status epilepticus in children with Alpers disease caused by POLG1 mutations: EEG and MRI features. Epilepsia 50 (6), 1596–1607.

E-BOOK FIGURES AND TABLES

The following figures and tables are available in the e-book at www.expertconsult.com. See inside cover for registration details.

Box 76-1 Clinical Criteria Suggesting Inherited Metabolic Epilepsy.

Box 76-4 Metabolic Epilepsies—Seizure Types.

Box 76-5 Organizational Scheme for Inherited Metabolic Epilepsies.

Table 76-1 Eeg Patterns and Inherited Metabolic Epilepsies.

Fig. 76-1 EEG of 4-day-old infant with MSUD shows comb-like rhythm over the right central (C4) area (sensitivity 7 mcv/mm; HFF 70 Hz; time constant 0.5 sec, 8 sec epoch).

Fig. 76-3 EEG of 3-year-old female with SSADH deficiency. Note diffuse spike wave paroxysm with lead-in over right hemisphere.

Fig. 76-4 EEG of term infant with glycine encephalopathy shows burst-suppression pattern.

77 Antiseizure Drug Therapy in Children

Jeannine M. Conway, Ilo E. Leppik, and Angela K. Birnbaum

An expanded version of this chapter is available on www.expertconsult.com. See inside cover for registration details.

Rational management of antiseizure drug therapy in children requires an understanding of pharmacokinetics, pharmacodynamics, and toxicology of these agents. Pharmacokinetics is the study of drug absorption, distribution, metabolism, and elimination: that is, what the body does to a drug. Pharmacodynamics is the study of a drug's biochemical and physiologic effects: that is, what the drug does to the body. Children, much more than adults, have widely varying abilities to absorb, distribute, metabolize, and eliminate drugs. Evidence also exists that antiseizure drug pharmacodynamics in children differ from those in adults. Application of basic pharmacokinetic and pharmacodynamic principles to antiseizure drug therapy facilitates the attainment and maintenance of targeted serum concentrations, optimization of the clinical response, and control of drug interactions.

Adverse reactions often dictate the choice of an antiseizure drug and subsequent adjustment of therapy. An understanding of these reactions, including their differences and similarities among various antiseizure drugs, and the application of appropriate clinical and laboratory monitoring provide the tools needed for the clinician to prescribe antiseizure drug therapy rationally.

PHARMACOKINETIC PRINCIPLES

Antiseizure drug absorption and elimination varies greatly among patients in the pediatric population, from neonates to teens. Potential sources of variability are numerous, and include drug formulation, behavior (compliance, diet, substance abuse), environment, and physiology. Physiologic variability may be related with the general health of the patient, but also with specific factors such as gender, age, maturation, and, in a few cases, pregnancy. In the management of pediatric patients with seizures, there is a concern with the effects of age and maturation on the pharmacokinetic profile of the antiseizure drugs. A drug's effect on a child's learning and behavior should also be a major determinant influencing the choice of an antiseizure drug. Age has the most influence on antiseizure drug elimination, metabolic pathways, and absorption. Factors such as protein binding and enzyme induction and/or inhibition are similar for children and for adults. Absorption may differ among similar formulations (such as tablets) from various manufacturers (e.g., carbamazepine) or with different formulations from the same manufacturer (immediate vs. extended release). Pharmacokinetic information for the antiseizure drugs is summarized in Table 77-1 and Table 77-3. See online version for more detail (Anderson and Lynn, 2009).

PHARMACODYNAMICS
Dose–Response or Concentration–Response Concept

Substantial evidence exists that both the number of patients experiencing seizure control increases and the degree of seizure control for a given patient improves with higher antiseizure drug concentrations. The minimum effective concentration defines the concentration at which the desired pharmacologic response is first observed and is not always the same in all patients. The intensity of response increases in direct proportion to drug concentration, until a response is maximized defining the maximum pharmacologic effect for that drug. With some drugs, such as phenytoin, further increases in concentration may reduce response (e.g., phenytoin-induced exacerbation of seizures). The incidence and severity of side effects also increase with drug concentration. The concentration at which side effects appear is usually, but not always, greater than the concentrations needed to achieve seizure control. The difference between concentrations that produce desired responses and those that produce toxic responses defines the therapeutic range.

Tolerance

Tolerance is a phenomenon in which pharmacologic or toxicologic effect diminishes with chronic use, even at the same or increasing plasma concentrations. Different mechanisms for the development of tolerance have been recognized. Mechanisms of tolerance can be because of biochemical adaptation (e.g., upregulation or downregulation of receptor sites) or behavioral. For example, the effectiveness of benzodiazepine therapy diminishes over time, necessitating even larger doses. Behavioral tolerance is when patients become progressively insensitive to drug effect without any apparent biochemical change. For example, many patients initiated on phenobarbital or primidone exhibit mild neurotoxicity even at low plasma concentrations but later, at the same concentration, have no symptoms.

Tolerance can produce changes in clinical response that mimic certain drug interactions. For example, loss of seizure control may result from either tolerance, as in the case of clonazepam, or enzyme induction, which decreases concentrations of many antiseizure drugs. Differentiating between these phenomena is important in considering adjustments in drug therapy.

PHYSIOLOGIC FACTORS AFFECTING DRUG DISPOSITION IN CHILDREN
General Considerations

Antiseizure drug pharmacokinetics and dosage requirements are influenced by the changing physiology of children as they age. The physiologic changes associated with maturation produce marked alterations in antiseizure drug pharmacokinetics. The variability with which children reach developmental milestones, along with genetic and environmental factors, causes antiseizure drug pharmacokinetics to vary substantially, even in children of the same age. As a result of the differences between children and adults, children require more frequent and larger doses relative to body size to attain targeted plasma concentrations. Although important age-related, quantitative differences in antiseizure drug pharmacokinetics are recognized, the pattern of drug-specific pharmacokinetics, such as

TABLE 77-1 Formulations, Routes of Administration, and Bioavailability of Antiseizure Drugs

Medication	Available Formulation	Possible Route[*]	T_{max} (hr)	Fraction Absorbed (F)	Special Problems
Acetazolamide	Tablet	PO	1–4	N/a	
	ER capsule	PO	3–6	N/a	
	Injectable	IV, IM	0.25	N/a	
Carbamazepine	Tablet	PO	3–8	0.79	Prolonged absorptive phase with variable T_{max}; induction results in earlier T_{max}.
	Chewable tablet	PO	2	0.79	
	Suspension	PO, PR	0.5–3	0.7–0.9 estimate	Earlier T_{max} results in higher C_{max}, which can produce transient side effects.
	ER tablet	PO	3–12	0.89 relative to susp.	Tablet must be swallowed whole; do not crush or chew.
	ER capsule	PO	4–8	0.79	Capsules may be opened and the beads sprinkled over food, such as a teaspoon of applesauce or other similar food products. Capsules or their contents should not be crushed or chewed.
Clonazepam	Tablet	PO	1–8	0.85	
Clorazepate	Tablet	PO	0.7–1.5	0.91	
Diazepam	Tablet	PO	0.5–2	0.8–1	
	Concentrated oral solution	PO	0.1–0.5	0.8–1	
	Gel	PR	0.75	0.9	
	Injectable	IM, IV	1–1.5	0.8–1	IM absorption is slow and variable.
Ethotoin	Tablet	PO	2	N/a	
Ethosuximide	Syrup	PO	1.5–4	N/a	
	Capsule	PO	3–7	N/a	
Eslicarbazepine Acetate	Tablet	PO	1–4	1 relative to susp	
Ezogabine	Tablet	PO	0.5–2	0.6	Partially active N-acetyl metabolite (NAMR)
Felbamate	Tablet	PO	1–4	N/a	
	Suspension	PO	3.7	N/a	
Fosphenytoin	Injectable	IV, IM	0.5 (IM)	1	Fosphenytoin concentrations after IM administration are lower but more sustained than those after IV administration owing to time required for absorption of fosphenytoin from injection site.
Gabapentin	Capsule	PO	2–4	0.6–0.27	Gabapentin bioavailability decreases as dose increases.
	Tablet	PO	2–4	0.6–0.27	
	Solution	PO	2–4	0.6–0.27	
Lacosamide	Tablet	PO	1–4	1	
	Solution	PO	1–4	1	
	Injectable	IV	End of infusion	1	
Lamotrigine	Compressed tablet	PO	0.5–4	0.98	
	Dispersible tablet	PO, PR	0.5–4	0.98	
Levetiracetam	Tablet	PO	0.3–2	0.95–1	
	Solution	PO	0.3–2	0.95–1	
	Injectable	IV	End of infusion		
Lorazepam	Tablet	PO	1–2.5	0.85–1	
	Injectable	IM, IV, PR	0.75–2	0.85–1	
	Concentrated oral solution	PO	1	0.90	
Methsuximide	Tablet	PO	N/a	N/a	
Oxcarbazepine	Tablet	PO	4.5	1	
	Suspension	PO	6	1	
	ER tablets				

Continued on following page

TABLE 77-1 Formulations, Routes of Administration, and Bioavailability of Antiseizure Drugs *(Continued)*

Medication	Available Formulation	Possible Route*	T_{max} (hr)	Fraction Absorbed (F)	Special Problems
Paraldehyde	Solution	PR, PO	1.5–2 (PR)	N/a	Do not use discolored solution; avoid plastic equipment; withdrawn from U.S. market.
Perampanel	Tablet	PO	0.5–2.5	1.0	Food effect: unchanged AUC, decreased C_{max}, delayed T_{max}
Phenobarbital	Syrup	PO (PR)	1	0.8–1	Unpleasant taste, rejected by many
	Tablet	PO	0.5–8.6	0.8–1	
	Injectable	IM, IV	0.25–1	1	
Phenytoin	Suspension (phenytoin acid)	PO	6–12	0.9–1	Patients should use accurate measuring device; dosing errors possible if suspension not adequately resuspended; strength of suspension must be clearly emphasized when prescribing.
	Chewable tablet (phenytoin acid)	PO	4–8	0.9–1	T_{max} dependent on C_{max}
	Prompt-release capsule (phenytoin sodium)	PO	2–6	0.9–1	
	ER capsule (phenytoin sodium)	PO	2–10	0.9–1	T_{max} dependent on C_{max}
	Injectable (phenytoin sodium)	IV, IM	0.25–0.5	0.9–1	IM injection not recommended; absorption is slow and erratic; injection is painful and must be diluted with normal saline without glucose and slowly administered.
Pregabalin	Capsule	PO	1.3	0.89–1	
	Solution	PO	1.3	0.89–1	
Primidone	Suspension	PO	4–6	N/a	
	Tablet	PO	4–6	N/a	
Rufinamide	Tablet	PO	4–6	<0.85	Rufinamide bioavailability decreases as dose increases.
	Suspension	PO	4–6	<0.85	
Tiagabine	Tablet	PO	0.75–3	0.9	
Topiramate	Tablet	PO, PR	1.4–4.3	0.8	
	Sprinkle capsule	PO	1.4–4.3	0.8	Capsules may be opened and the beads sprinkled over food, such as a teaspoon of applesauce or other similar food products. Capsules or their contents should not be crushed or chewed.
Valproate	Capsule	PO	1–3	0.9–1	Capsule filled with liquid valproic acid; avoid opening.
	Enteric-coated tablet	PO	2–6	0.9–1	Food delays T_{max}
	Sprinkle capsules	PO	4–6	0.9–1	Capsules may be opened and the beads sprinkled over food, such as a teaspoon of applesauce or other similar food products. Capsules or their contents should not be crushed or chewed.
	ER tablet	PO	4–17	0.9	
	Syrup	PO, PR	0.5–1	0.9–1	Valproate has objectionable aftertaste.
	Injectable	IV	1	1	May not give IM.
Vigabatrin	Tablet	PO	1	1	
	Solution	PO	1–2.5	1	
Zonisamide	Capsule	PO	2–6	1	

C_{max}, maximum plasma concentration; ER, extended release; IM, intramuscular; IV, intravascular; N/a, not available; PO, oral; PR, parenteral; T_{max}, time to maximum plasma concentration.
*Primary and alternates.

saturation of absorption, protein binding, metabolism, and enzyme induction, is similar for children and for adults.

A number of physiologic and pathophysiologic processes can alter antiseizure drug pharmacokinetics. Gastrointestinal disorders, particularly those that increase transit time, can alter the endothelial lining and decrease absorption. Antiseizure drugs that are slowly absorbed, such as carbamazepine and phenytoin, are most likely to be affected. Physiologic stress, such as that associated with myocardial infarction, burns, traumatic injury, chronic inflammation, and surgery, increases α_1-acid glycoprotein, resulting in greater binding with carbamazepine and carbamazepine-10,11-epoxide. Febrile illnesses may produce increases in phenytoin clearance that persist for several weeks, resulting in lowering of plasma concentrations by as much as 50%.

Renal failure can affect the excretion of antiseizure drugs for which the kidney is the primary route of elimination. Both clinical response and plasma antiseizure drug concentrations should be carefully assessed in patients with renal disease. Severe liver disease can alter the metabolism of antiseizure drugs, resulting in accumulation of the parent drug. Antiseizure drug metabolism appears to be well preserved in mild to moderate liver disease. Clinical response may vary, depending on the particular antiseizure drug.

Plasma antiseizure drug concentrations can fluctuate over a 24-hour cycle. The mechanism for this alteration is presumed to be a circadian rhythm in clearance (Cloyd, 1991; Italiano and Perucca, 2013).

Neonates

Gastric emptying time is irregular, absorption area is reduced, and biliary function is underdeveloped for several months or more after birth. These factors can contribute to erratic drug absorption. In addition, gastric pH is elevated, which may reduce the absorption of certain drugs, such as clonazepam. In contrast with the oral route, rectal absorption is reliable and efficient. Protein binding is reduced because of lower plasma albumin concentrations, whereas greater extracellular water and less adipose tissue can either increase or decrease volume of distribution (Vd). Reactions mediated by hepatic cytochrome P-450 enzymes reach and then exceed adult values within a few weeks after birth. By contrast, renal elimination of drugs and active metabolites may be lower than that in adults until the age of 6 months.

Infants and Children

Gastric emptying time and intestinal motility are increased as children grow. Absorptive area, microbial flora, and biliary function begin to approach those in the adult. Also, gastrointestinal blood flow is greater than that in adults. These physiologic characteristics contribute to faster absorption of most drugs, resulting in earlier T_{max}. Plasma albumin levels are lower than adult values, particularly in infancy, resulting in an increased free fraction. Infants and children are capable of synthesizing α_1-acid glycoprotein, which will alter the free fraction of drugs bound to this protein. Metabolism remains elevated for the first 2 years of life; in some cases, drug clearances may be 2 to 3 times the values seen in adults. Thereafter, metabolism slowly declines, reaching adult values at puberty. After the first 6 months of life, renal excretion is comparable with that in adults.

DRUG INTERACTIONS

The clinical significance of pharmacokinetic interactions is determined by several factors, including concentration of the

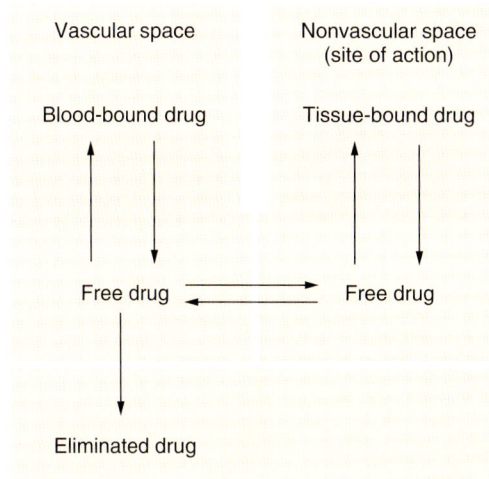

Figure 77-1. Relationship of unbound drug in vascular and nonvascular compartments.

interacting drugs, the patient's seizure control, and presence of toxicity.

Absorption

Concomitant therapy may influence absorption of antiseizure drugs. For example, continuous tube feedings interfere with phenytoin absorption. Calcium- and magnesium-containing antacids appear to complex with phenytoin, decreasing its rate and extent of absorption. They should not be administered concurrently. Gastric pH affects the rate and extent of benzodiazepine absorption; thus, use of antacids and histamine H_2 blockers may decrease the plasma concentration of these drugs.

Protein Binding

In general, only the unbound drug is able to cross the blood–brain barrier and is in equilibrium with brain tissue and spinal fluid (Fig. 77-1; see also Table 77-3). Valproic acid and phenytoin compete for the same binding sites. Concurrent administration may decrease valproic acid and phenytoin binding. When this occurs, unbound concentrations briefly rise, potentially leading to clinical toxicity. Total phenytoin and valproic acid concentrations decrease; however, unbound concentrations rapidly reequilibrate to the original concentration. In general, phenytoin and valproic acid dosing does not have to be adjusted in these circumstances.

Metabolism

Drugs interact in many ways, such as induction and inhibition of liver enzymes. Information on how drugs are metabolized may provide insight into the potential for a drug interaction. For example, if a drug is known to be an inducer or an inhibitor of a particular P-450 isoenzyme, it may be possible to predict if a medication will affect the plasma concentrations of a second drug that is metabolized by that P-450 particular isoenzyme when the drugs are given concomitantly. This approach may be particularly useful in predicting the interaction between the many new antiseizure drugs being developed and other possible concomitant medications.

TABLE 77-3 Pharmacokinetics of Other Antiseizure Drugs

Drug	Age Group*	V_d (L/kg)	Protein Binding (%)	$t_{1/2}$ (hr)	Route of Elimination	Active Metabolites	Initial Maintenance Dose (mg/kg/day)	Comments
Carbamazepine	N	1.1–2.6	65–70	7.2–27	Hepatic	Carbamazepine-10,11-epoxide	5–20	Therapy should be initiated at 30–50% of initial dose and increased as autoinduction occurs.
	C	0.8–2.0	75–85	5–26			15–20	
Clonazepam	C	1.5–4.4	80–90	22–33	Hepatic	None	0.05–0.2	Tolerance to antiseizure effect frequently occurs.
Eslicarbazepine acetate (ESL)	C	0.8–1	40 (A)	6–8	Hepatic	Acetate (ESL) eslicarbazepine	5–30†	
Ethosuximide	N	0.69		32–41	Hepatic	None	15–40	
	C	0.7	<10	15–68				
Ezogabine	A	2–8	80%	7–8	Hepatic	NAMR	No pediatric data, adult dose 600–900 mg/day	
Felbamate	C	0.73–0.82 (A)	30	14–21 (A)	Hepatic 50–55%; renal 45–50%	None	15–45	
Gabapentin	C	0.6–0.8 (A)	0	5–7	Renal	None	10–15	
Lacosamide	A	0.6	<15	13	Renal 40%; hepatic 60%	None	8–12†	
Lamotrigine	1–4 years	0.9–1.4	55	+ ind: 8 + VPA: 45	Hepatic	None	With VPA 1–5 With enzyme inducer 5–15	Slow-dose titration is necessary to lessen incidence of rash; see product information packet for details about titrating.
	5–10 years			+ ind: 7 + VPA: 66 24–31 (A)				
Levetiracetam	C	0.5–0.7	<10	5	Renal	None	10–60	
Oxcarbazepine	C	0.7–0.8	40 (MHD) 4.8–9.3 (MHD)		Hepatic	10-Hydroxy-metabolite (MHD)	8–10	
Perampanel	12–17 years	1.07	95	105	Hepatic	None	Not dosed based on weight, start at 2 mg	Bound to albumin and AAG; blood-to-plasma ratio 0.55–0.59
Phenobarbital	N	0.8–1	32	82–199	Hepatic 50–80%; renal 20–50%	None	3–4	
	I	0.6–0.9		37–73			4–5	
	C	0.7	40–55	21–75			2–3	

TABLE 77-3 Pharmacokinetics of Other Antiseizure Drugs *(Continued)*

Drug	Age Group*	V_d (L/kg)	Protein Binding (%)	$t_{1/2}$ (hr)	Route of Elimination	Active Metabolites	Initial Maintenance Dose (mg/kg/day)	Comments
Phenytoin	N	0.7–1.2	74–90	3–140	95% hepatic; 5% renal	None	4–6	Half-life varies with concentrations.
	C	0.7–0.8	87–93	1.2–60	95% hepatic; 5% renal	None	6–10 in younger children; 4–6 in children older than 10 years	Half-life varies with concentrations.
Pregabalin	A	N/a	0	4.6–6.8	Renal > 90%; hepatic <10%	None	No pediatric data Adult dose 150–600/day	
Primidone	C	0.43–1.1 (A)	20	4.4–11	Hepatic 60–70%; renal 30–40%	Phenobarbital PEMA	10–15	Therapy should be initiated at 30–50% of initial maintenance dose.
Rufinamide	C	0.8–1.2	34	6–10	Hepatic	None	10	
Tiagabine	A	0.74–0.85	96	5–13 Healthy (A)	Hepatic	None	0.375–1.3	
Topiramate	C	0.6–0.8	15	20–30 (A)	Renal >80%; hepatic <20%	None	1–3	
Valproate (valproic acid [VPA])	N	0.28–0.43	68–89	17–40	Hepatic 95%; renal 5%	2-en-VPA, 4-en-VPA, 2, 4-dien-VPA	5–10	
	I	0.2–0.34		6–8			10–20 (monotherapy), 20–30 (induced)	
	C	0.1–0.3	80–95	4–15			10–20 (monotherapy), 20–30 (induced)	
Vigabatrin	I	1.1	0	5.7	Renal	None identified	50–100	Vigabatrin is available as a racemic mixture; the S(+) enantiomer is the active enantiomer.
Zonisamide	A	0.8–1.6 h	40–60 h	63–69	Renal 40–50%; hepatic 50–60%	None	2–12 (C)	

MHD, monohydroxy derivative of oxcarbazepine; PEMA, phenylethyl malonamide; $t_{1/2}$, half-life; V_d, volume of distribution.
*A, adults; C, children; I, infants; N, neonates.
†Being studied, not approved.

DOSAGE FORMULATIONS AND ROUTES OF ADMINISTRATION

Antiseizure drugs are most commonly and conveniently given orally. However, use of an alternative route of administration is necessary. Oral administration is not possible, for example, before and during surgery, with acute severe trauma, when consciousness is impaired, or during gastrointestinal illnesses. Interruption of oral administration occurs in children during frequent bouts of vomiting and diarrhea. In acute emergencies, especially within medical facilities, some antiseizure drugs can be given by intravenous or intramuscular administration. The lack of parenteral formulations, mostly because of their poor solubility in water, creates a significant dilemma

for those persons on maintenance antiseizure therapy when oral administration cannot be continued. The rectal route of administration has been extremely useful for those situations, but water-insoluble antiseizure drugs are generally not well absorbed rectally.

See Table 77-9 and online version for more detail.

MONITORING ANTISEIZURE DRUG THERAPY
Clinical Monitoring of Efficacy

Clinical assessment of patients is of paramount importance in the assessment of the effectiveness of therapy. The ideal response would be the total elimination of seizures without

TABLE 77-9 Antiseizure Drugs Available for Rectal Administration

Drug	Treatment Usefulness	Dose (mg/kg/dose)	Preparation	Pharmacokinetics	Comments
Carbamazepine (CBZ)	Maintenance	Same as oral	Oral suspension (dilute with equal volume of water) Suppository gel (CBZ powder dissolved in 20% alcohol and methylhydroxy cellulose)*	Peak concentration 4–8 hr; 80% absorbed	Definite cathartic effect
Clonazepam	?Acute	0.02–0.1 mg	Suspension	Peak concentration 0.1–2 hr	Onset may be too slow for acute use.
Diazepam	Acute	0.2–0.5 mg	Gel	Peak concentration in ~45 min; concentration >200 ng/mL reached in 15 min	Well tolerated; nordiazepam accumulates with repeated doses.
Lamotrigine	?Maintenance	1.5–2 × oral dose	100-mg tablet crushed and suspended in 10 mL of water		Well tolerated
Lorazepam	Acute	0.05–0.1 mg	Parenteral solution	Peak concentration 0.5–2 hr	Well tolerated
Paraldehyde	Acute	0.3 mL	Oral solution (dilute with equal volume of mineral oil)	Effect in 20 min; peak concentration 2.5 hr	Moderate cathartic effect; use glass syringe
Phenobarbital	?Acute	10–20 mg	Parenteral solution	Peak concentration 4–5 hr; 90% absorbed	Onset may be too slow for acute use.
	Maintenance	Same as oral	Same as acute	Same as for acute	
Secobarbital	Acute	5 mg	Parenteral solution	Peak concentration 0.5–1.5 hr	
Topiramate	?Maintenance	Same as oral	200-mg tablet crushed and suspended with 20 mL of water	Peak concentration 2–3 hr; 95% absorbed	Well tolerated
Valproic acid (VPA)	Acute	5–25 mg	Oral solution (dilute with equal volume of water)	Peak concentration 1–3 hr	Definite cathartic effect
	Maintenance	Same as oral	VPA liquid from capsules mixed into Supocire C lipid base*	Peak concentration 2–4 hr; 80% absorbed	Well tolerated

*Extemporaneously prepared using commercial product; all other preparations are commercial products given rectally.
(Adapted from Graves NM, Kriel RL. Rectal administration of AEDs in children. Pediatric Neurol 1987;3:321; and Garnett WR, Cloyd JC. Dosage from considerations in the treatment of epilepsy. In: Dodson WE, Pellock JM, editors. Pediatric epilepsy: diagnosis and therapy. New York: Demos; 1993. p. 373–85. Additional data from Birnbaum AK, et al. Rectal absorption of lamotrigine compressed tablets. Epilepsia 2000;41:850–3; Birnbaum AK, et al. Relative bioavailability of lamotrigine chewable dispersible tablets administered rectally. Pharmacotherapy 2001;21:158–62; and Conway JM, et al. Relative bioavailability of topiramate administered rectally. Epilepsy Res 2003;54:91–6.)

any adverse effects of therapy. A satisfactory clinical response for many patients, however, might be substantial reduction of seizures with elimination of or decrease in adverse effects. One of the most common clinical errors is the premature interpretation of the clinical response. Assessment of seizure control requires an accurate record of seizure frequency and severity before and during therapy. Seizures may be eliminated, reduced, or increased in frequency, or become more or less severe during therapy. Patients with epilepsy have varying seizure frequency rates before therapy. The length of time required to assess clinical response varies with the frequency of seizures observed before beginning therapy. Patients with infrequent seizures need a longer period of observation on therapy to permit assessment of clinical response. Achievement of steady state with a new drug regimen is necessary to determine whether a medication has been given an adequate trial at any specific dose. The time to achieve a steady state varies considerably from drug to drug, depending on the drug's half-life. In every case, five half-lives must elapse before a steady state is reached.

Interpretation of clinical response in patients in whom polypharmacy is necessary is especially difficult. Clinical improvement or deterioration after the addition of a second antiseizure drug could be attributable to numerous factors. Such factors include the additive or synergistic effect of the two medications, the effect of the second drug alone, and the effect of the second drug on the metabolism and/or displacement of the initial drug. It is important to make clinical conclusions only after a steady state is reached with the new drug regimen. If improvement is obtained after the addition of the second medication, the clinician should attempt to taper and discontinue the first medication, to determine whether the clinical improvement is an effect of synergistic therapy or that of the second medication itself. Finally, it is necessary to remember that withdrawal of comedication might have an effect on the disposition of the remaining drug(s), which could influence clinical response (see Fig. 77-5).

Clinical Monitoring of Adverse Effects

The clinical state of the patient is more important than laboratory testing for the assessment of adverse effects. It is possible to monitor clinical states continuously, whereas laboratory tests generally are obtained at arbitrary times; therefore,

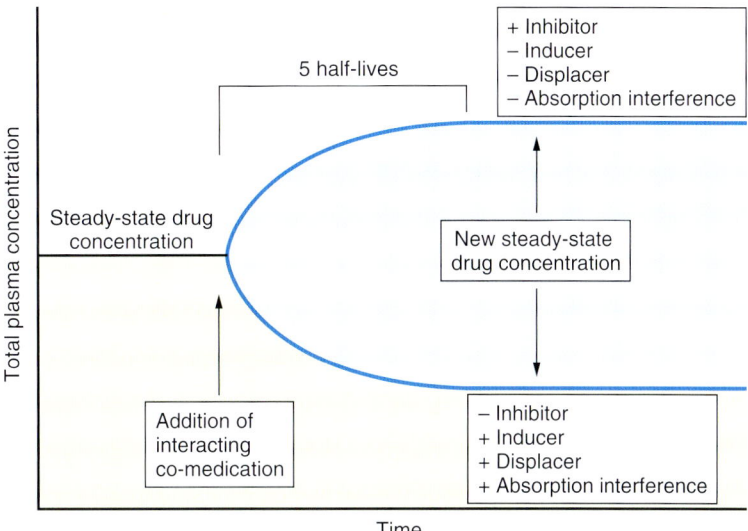

Figure 77-5. Schematic of steady-state plasma concentrations of antiseizure drugs when a particular antiseizure drug is given alone or in combination with other medications.

impending organ dysfunction often may be detected earlier by clinical changes, rather than by laboratory tests. The most frequent adverse effects are dose related and often involve the nervous system. Common manifestations of adverse effects are cognitive changes and drowsiness, impaired attention, incoordination, ataxia, and diplopia. In addition to central nervous system adverse reactions, the liver also may produce signs of toxicity. Early signs of liver failure include anorexia, nausea, vomiting, lethargy, and abdominal pain.

Monitoring of Drug Concentrations

Interpretation of "Optimal Therapeutic Ranges"

Numerous factors should be considered in the interpretation of drug concentrations. Medications that have rapid absorption and clearance have wide fluctuation between dosing intervals. For example, the liquid formulation of valproic acid, especially when given to a child also receiving enzyme-inducing comedications, is rapidly absorbed and eliminated; therefore, a twofold fluctuation during dosing intervals is possible. Recording the time of the blood sample in relation to the last dose is needed to interpret laboratory results properly. Unexpectedly low concentrations are most frequently the result of poor compliance; however, they might be seen after the addition of an enzyme-inducing comedication. Very high drug concentrations are seen with administration of high doses, in persons with genetically low clearance or some disease states, or with use of enzyme-inhibiting comedications such as valproic acid (Perucca et al., 2001).

The terms *optimal drug concentration* and *target range* are preferred over "therapeutic range," for several reasons. First, these terms express the concept that the optimal dose and drug concentration need to be determined for each individual patient to balance seizure control and adverse events. Clinical effects and toxicity of antiseizure drugs correlate better with drug concentrations than with total daily dosage. Published "optimal drug concentrations" are attempts to report ranges of concentrations at which many patients have improved seizure control without significant adverse effects. These ranges generally have not been determined by controlled studies in large populations.

When to Obtain Drug Concentrations

It is useful to measure the antiseizure drug concentration after the patient has reached steady-state dosing and optimal clinical outcome has been obtained. The time after dose of when the sample was drawn should be recorded in order to interpret where the concentration would be on a pharmacokinetic profile. The measured drug concentration could be considered the "optimal drug concentration" or the "target level" for the individual patient. Levels should also be obtained when a breakthrough of the seizure pattern occurs (i.e., a single seizure in a person usually well controlled, or a doubling of the usual seizure rate). If the level is lower than the individual's "target value," one needs to consider nonadherence or alteration in pharmacokinetics. For suspected nonadherence cases, the dose should not be changed, but steps should be taken to increase adherence (pill box, education, and so on) (Gardiner and Dvorkin, 2006). Illnesses affecting absorption or clearance can also be detected by comparing the current value with the "target level." Levels should be measured after changes in comedication once a new steady state has been reached to determine whether any changes in the levels have occurred. If a patient experiences an increase in seizures but the current concentration is at the "target," it is possible that the seizure threshold has changed or was underestimated, and changes in dose may be needed and a new "target level" should be established.

What to Measure

Total drug concentrations generally are measured; however, it also is possible to determine levels of free or unbound drug, as well as of metabolites of the administered drug. Free drug concentrations correlate best with clinical effect and toxicity. In most cases, the ratio of free to bound drug is relatively constant for a particular patient; therefore, total drug concentrations usually are adequate. In certain instances, however, particularly with critically ill patients under intensive care, determination of free drug levels, especially for phenytoin and valproic acid, is essential. In such patients, many drugs are typically administered, increasing the likelihood that antiseizure drugs will be displaced from protein-binding sites. The percentage of unbound valproic acid increases with higher drug concentrations and with comedication, or when valproic acid is rapidly administered. When the bound fraction is doubled, the valproic acid free fraction may be eight times higher.

Occasionally, measurement of antiseizure drug metabolites is useful. With several antiseizure drugs, metabolites are clinically active and contribute to both response and toxicity. Phenobarbital is an active metabolite present during primidone therapy. Carbamazepine-10,11-epoxide is a derivative of carbamazepine and contributes to toxicity. Clinical monitoring of oxcarbazepine and eslicarbazepine acetate treatment is evaluated by measuring their primary metabolites.

Laboratory Tests for Idiosyncratic Reactions

In an effort to identify patients in whom serious or potentially life-threatening adverse effects may develop, obtaining complete blood counts and chemistry profiles at routine intervals has become common practice. It is debatable whether routine laboratory monitoring can actually identify patients at risk for serious reactions or can identify significant adverse events better than clinical monitoring. Identification of life-threatening reactions is rarely made by routine laboratory screening of asymptomatic children. Fulminant or irreversible hepatic failure during valproic acid therapy is not reliably predicted by laboratory monitoring. Many reports, therefore, indicate that routine laboratory screening of asymptomatic patients is of little value. However, obtaining complete blood counts and chemistry profiles before, and then after, initiation of antiseizure drug therapy is reasonable. It is much more effective to caution patients and parents to obtain these tests immediately whenever there are signs of any possible reaction, such as unusual bleeding or bruising, significant loss of appetite, and jaundice. Testing for inborn errors of metabolism may be useful for identifying young children at risk for hepatic dysfunction from valproic acid.

ADVERSE DRUG REACTIONS TO ANTISEIZURE DRUGS

The most frequent adverse drug reactions to antiseizure drugs are dose related, mild, and reversible. Less frequently observed but potentially more serious are the idiosyncratic adverse reactions, which generally are not related to dosage but may be attributable to individual peculiarities of drug metabolism, that is, lack of pathways to process toxic metabolites. Idiosyncratic reactions are almost never seen with antiseizure drugs that are not metabolized.

Central Nervous System Adverse Reactions

The central nervous system adverse reaction profile for children is similar to that for adults. Most of the older antiseizure drugs and their active metabolites have similar side effect profiles, comprising of cognitive impairment, sedation, dizziness, diplopia, ataxia, headaches, and effects on somnolence. The effects of antiseizure drugs on cognitive function generally are concentration and dose dependent. Drug therapy is known to contribute to cognitive deficits, especially treatment with multiple drugs. Removal of antiseizure drugs frequently results in improved cognitive function and motor skills. It is important to recognize that reaction times, disordered attention, and impulsivity, even in untreated children with epilepsy, differ from those in control subjects. The differences in attention and reaction time, however, are small between children with mild, as opposed to severe, seizure disorders.

Side effects frequently occur in children who are given phenobarbital. Phenobarbital has been associated with a significant depression of cognitive function when it is used for treatment of febrile seizures in children. In a randomized, placebo-controlled, prospective study, children had lower mean intelligence quotient (IQ) scores both during and 6 months after stopping therapy with phenobarbital. Clinical tolerance does develop to some degree; however, an unacceptably high frequency of adverse effects from phenobarbital commonly is observed in children. The adverse effects are reminiscent of complaints present in attention-deficit disorders and include overactivity, aggressiveness, inattention, and irritability. The behavioral disorders are observed in 20% to 50% of children receiving phenobarbital for febrile seizures, and result in discontinuation of therapy in 20% to 30% of children. The presence of preexisting behavior problems, especially hyperactivity, is strongly predictive of adverse reactions during phenobarbital therapy. In a study of children receiving phenobarbital for febrile seizures, 80% of those with abnormal behavior before drug therapy reported aggravation of preexisting hyperactive behavior with phenobarbital, versus only 20% for children with normal preseizure behavior. In some cases, these adverse effects may resolve with continuation or with a lower dose of phenobarbital; however, discontinuation of therapy or alternative medication should be considered.

Some antiseizure drugs—gabapentin, felbamate, topiramate, lamotrigine, tiagabine, oxcarbazepine, levetiracetam, vigabatrin, and zonisamide—are thought to have fewer and less severe adverse effects; however, their adverse central nervous system effects are similar to those of the older antiseizure drugs. Although gabapentin has a good safety profile and seems well tolerated in adults, significant behavioral side effects are observed in some children. In other reports, aggression, hyperactivity, temper tantrums, and increased oppositional behavior developed in children taking the drug. Most, but not all, of these children had preexisting cognitive dysfunction, such as mental retardation, autistic features, or behavioral difficulties. The adverse cognitive changes resolved with discontinuation of gabapentin; if administration of the drug was resumed, the adverse cognitive changes tended to recur. In approximately 15% of children, decreased functioning in school, aggression, and other cognitive changes occurred within the first 4 months of initiation of topiramate therapy. A previous history of behavioral changes and concurrent lamotrigine therapy were associated factors. Central nervous system–related adverse effects from topiramate tend to decrease over time. Of greater concern are reports of the development of major depression, schizophrenic-like reactions, and organic psychoses in adults taking vigabatrin. A reversible acute psychosis has been reported in a child taking vigabatrin. Development of hyperkinesia, somnolence, and insomnia in children taking vigabatrin has been reported by a number of investigators.

Gastrointestinal Effects
Weight Gain

A survey in children and adolescents taking valproic acid found the most common side effect to be weight gain; however, for many patients, the weight gain was "beneficial." The incidence of unwanted weight gain was 26% in adults and 15% in children and adolescents. An increase in weight was observed more than twice as frequently in females. Weight increase was independent of dose. Weight gain also was reported in children during therapy with carbamazepine and vigabatrin.

Weight Loss

Sustained weight loss was reported in children on maintenance topiramate therapy. Seventy-five percent of children and adults during clinical research trials reported a loss of appetite and decrease in body weight while taking felbamate. Zonisamide also is associated with weight loss in children.

Gastric Irritation

Signs of gastric irritation, with heartburn and indigestion, are seen with use of some antiseizure drugs. Gastric irritation during valproic acid therapy can be reduced with administration of lower doses or by taking medication with food. Use of enteric-coated preparations of valproic acid will enable most patients who did not tolerate valproic acid because of gastrointestinal symptoms (nausea/vomiting, eructation, heartburn) to resume valproic acid therapy. Aggressive medical intervention with antacids and H_2 receptor antagonists (other than cimetidine) has been helpful for some children with clinical signs of gastritis, allowing valproic acid therapy to continue.

Approximately 20% of patients receiving ethosuximide will demonstrate dose-related adverse effects, primarily gastric distress, vomiting, hiccups, and anorexia. Gastrointestinal disturbances also are encountered in 14% of patients taking carbamazepine, with symptoms of nausea, vomiting, anorexia, and constipation. Nausea and vomiting commonly are observed with felbamate.

Gingival Hyperplasia

Gingival hyperplasia occurs in 10% to 20% of persons treated with phenytoin and is more frequent in young persons. It is observed more frequently in persons taking higher dosages, often appears 2 to 3 months after beginning therapy, and reaches its maximum severity in 12 to 18 months. Gingival hyperplasia generally resolves within 2 to 5 months after discontinuation or a reduction in medication. A vigorous program of good oral hygiene started before and continued during phenytoin therapy can be effective in minimizing gingival enlargement.

Increased Seizures

Some patients, especially those with generalized or absence seizures, may experience an increase in seizure activity when carbamazepine, oxcarbazepine, or phenytoin is added. Vigabatrin also has been reported to increase seizure activity and even lead to status epilepticus. Aggravation of seizures occurred in 3% of children with generalized seizures, most often in those with nonprogressive myoclonic epilepsy, and was extremely unusual in children with partial epilepsies and infantile spasms. Phenytoin and carbamazepine may increase seizures associated with the Lennox–Gastaut syndrome, and gabapentin and pregabalin can increase or induce myoclonic seizures.

Osteomalacia

Osteomalacia (rickets) may occur in patients taking antiseizure drugs. The cause of osteomalacia during antiseizure drug therapy appears to be multifactorial. Many antiseizure drugs presumably enhance hepatic conversion of 25-hydroxyvitamin D to biologically inactive metabolites. Clinically significant rickets seldom develops in ambulatory children on antiseizure drug therapy, or in institutionalized children who are not taking medication. On the other hand,

clinically overt rickets was observed in 10% of institutionalized children on phenobarbital and/or phenytoin. In these patients, sunlight was more important for the maintenance of serum 25-hydroxyvitamin D than were supplements of vitamin D.

In children, no correlation was observed between duration of antiseizure drug therapy and 25-hydroxyvitamin D levels. It was previously thought that older antiseizure drugs resulted in induction of vitamin D metabolism, resulting in decreased bone mineral density; however, the lack of correlation between vitamin D levels and bone mineral density suggests that other mechanisms are operative.

Tremor and Movement Disorders

The benign essential type of tremor seen with valproic acid therapy begins within 1 month of initiating therapy and is dose dependent, occurring in some patients with blood valproic acid levels greater than 40 mg/mL. Reduction of tremor may occur with reduction of dose. Tremor also has been seen with use of lamotrigine and gabapentin.

Other Effects

Hair changes have been associated with antiseizure drug treatment. Hair changes (thinning or wavy hair) are seen in 12% of children during valproic acid therapy. Additional dose-related adverse effects of phenytoin include hirsutism, coarse facial features, and acne, especially in children and teenagers. Pancreatitis has been associated with valproic acid therapy. Visual field changes, which may be irreversible, may occur with vigabatrin treatment. Topiramate has been reported to cause acute myopia and secondary angle closure glaucoma. Patients present with decreased visual acuity and ocular pain. In a majority of cases, immediate discontinuation of topiramate results in a resolution of symptoms. Hyponatremia occasionally is encountered in patients taking carbamazepine and oxcarbazepine. Hyperthermia and oligohydrosis have been reported in several children taking topiramate and zonisamide. Clinical signs included fever, decreased sweating, and exercise intolerance, which resolved in a majority of cases when topiramate or zonisamide was discontinued. Topiramate and zonisamide may cause nephrolithiasis. The risk is increased with topiramate or zonisamide treatment and the ketogenic diet.

Anticonvulsant Hypersensitivity Syndrome in Children
Clinical Features

The hypersensitivity syndrome is characterized by rash, fever, and malaise, generally occurring within the first several months of therapy. Certain types of rash may be particularly alarming, such as those of Stevens–Johnson syndrome or toxic epidermal necrolysis. Often hepatic involvement is part of the syndrome, and the liver is the most frequently involved internal organ. Affected children may present with hepatomegaly and elevations in serum transaminase levels. The involvement may progress to hepatic necrosis. Other systems may be involved, including kidney, lungs, bone marrow, and the lymphatic system.

Pathogenesis

Although the mechanism of the hypersensitivity syndrome is not completely understood, current evidence implicates toxic metabolites (Glauser, 2000). The aromatic AEDs (phenobarbital, phenytoin > carbamazepine > oxcarbazepine), lamotrigine, and felbamate have been more frequently implicated in causing this syndrome. Presumably, accumulation of toxic metabolites, such as reactive aromatic epoxide intermediates, precipitates the syndrome (Glauser, 2000).

Prevention

Routine laboratory monitoring (i.e., with complete blood counts or liver function tests) will not prospectively identify which patients are at high risk for the development of an acute hypersensitivity reaction. Nevertheless, certain factors place some patients at high risk. Clinical profiles that identify patients at high risk for hypersensitivity reactions differ for specific antiseizure drugs (valproic acid, felbamate, and lamotrigine). When one of these drugs is being considered for a patient at high risk, one should proceed with caution. Alternative therapy, if possible, should be considered. Additional laboratory tests to screen for inborn errors of metabolism may be indicated when use of valproic acid is under consideration in children younger than 2 years. Families need to be advised that the child is in a high-risk category and counseled on the early recognition of the syndrome.

Although the identification of a high-risk clinical profile is the most inexpensive and practical way available to reduce the risk of hypersensitivity syndrome, various biomarkers also have been identified (Glauser, 2000). These biomarkers may indicate that some patients have genetic susceptibility to the accumulation of toxic metabolites because of deficient detoxification pathways. Studies in patients of Chinese ancestry indicate a strong association between the risk of developing toxic epidermal necrolysis and Stevens–Johnson Syndrome and the presence of HLA-B* 1502. Clinicians may want to avoid use of carbamazepine in this population.

Managing Adverse Effects

The clinician and the patient are faced with adverse effects approximately 30% of the time when antiseizure drugs are used, especially during initiation of therapy. In many instances, this rate is acceptable, especially when the patient and the physician mutually agree on which problems are most important to avoid. When no urgency exists, many adverse effects can be avoided during initiation of therapy by gradually increasing doses. In general, management of adverse effects depends on the problem. Most adverse effects are concentration dependent, and are less prominent at lower doses and blood concentrations. Seizure control may or may not be maintained at the lower dose; if not, the clinician and the patient need to consider whether a compromise is acceptable with regard to either increased seizures or increased adverse effects, or if alternative medication should be considered.

At times, toxicity is encountered only with high drug concentrations and is seen only at peak times; for these patients, it may be possible to avoid toxicity by more frequent and lower doses or by the use of extended-release formulations. Gastric irritation generally is dose dependent and may be managed in several ways. The amount of drug can be reduced; the effective dose to the gastric mucosa can be lowered by use of enteric-coated formulations, or the patient can be protected by use of H_2 receptor antagonists.

Idiosyncratic reactions pose another problem. Mild, asymptomatic elevations of liver enzymes do not mandate discontinuation of therapy if not in excess of 2 to 3 times normal values. On the other hand, Stevens–Johnson syndrome and toxic epidermal necrolysis, clinically symptomatic hepatotoxicity, pancreatitis, and most rashes are indications for immediate cessation of the responsible medication. If the rash was mild, however, and especially if the patient had an otherwise favorable clinical response to the drug, a cautious rechallenge might be considered. Successful resumption of therapy has been reported in a number of patients, especially with valproic acid after that drug was discontinued, when a more gradual dose escalation was used.

DISCONTINUATION OF ANTISEIZURE DRUG THERAPY

The decision to discontinue antiseizure drug therapy often is as challenging as the decision to initiate and continue long-term drug therapy. Many factors are considered in making these decisions, including the length of the seizure-free interval, drug history, presence of adverse effects, and the neurologic and epilepsy syndrome diagnosis of the patient. Numerous retrospective and prospective investigations are available. Ultimately, the decision to withdraw or to continue antiseizure drug therapy is that of the patient and family, and their perception of acceptable risk of recurrence often differs from that of the treating physician (Camfield and Camfield, 2008).

Benefits of Drug Discontinuation

The potential benefits of drug discontinuation are numerous. Most obvious are the immediate reduction in cost to the family and third-party payer with elimination of drug therapy and usually the reduction in associated expenses incurred by laboratory tests and physician and clinic charges. In addition, in many patients, the adverse, sometimes previously unrecognized, effects of antiseizure drug therapy are reversed. Patients who had been on phenobarbital, phenytoin, valproic acid, and topiramate had subtle improvement in various psychometric tasks, such as memory, vigilance attention, and visual motor performance, and in psychomotor speed, when therapy was discontinued.

Risks of Drug Discontinuation

The obvious risk of stopping antiseizure drug therapy is the recurrence of seizures. In most cases, seizure control can be regained with resumption of the previous drug therapy. Response to therapy after a relapse may be rapid and satisfactory. Chadwick and colleagues observed that approximately 90% of patients who experience seizures after antiseizure drug discontinuation have a 2-year remission after therapy is resumed. Thus control was usually but not always regained despite increasing doses of a previously successful drug regimen. A guideline has been published to assist the physician and the family considering discontinuation of antiseizure drug therapy. The conclusions were based on a MEDLINE search.

Families should discuss withdrawing antiseizure drugs with their neurologist once children have become free of seizures for 1 year or longer while on antiseizure drug therapy. Children whose EEGs have become normal have a somewhat better chance of successful withdrawal of therapy. However, there are critical life transitions when the risk of discontinuing therapy outweighs continuation. These are when children have been seizure-free and are eligible to begin driving, and when they are leaving home and transitioning to college or independent living. Finally, for some patients, withdrawal of antiseizure drugs is rarely successful—for example, those with abnormalities on neurologic examination or with certain seizure syndromes such as juvenile myoclonic epilepsy, Lennox–Gastaut syndrome, or infantile spasms.

REFERENCES

The complete list of references for this chapter is available online at www.expertconsult.com.

See inside cover for registration details.

SELECTED REFERENCES

Anderson, G.D., Lynn, A.M., 2009. Optimizing pediatric dosing: a developmental pharmacologic approach. Pharmacotherapy 29, 680–690.

Anderson, G.D., Saneto, R.P., 2012. Current oral and non-oral routes of antiepileptic drug delivery. Adv. Drug Deliv. Rev. 64, 911–918.

Camfield, P., Camfield, C., 2008. When is it safe to discontinue AED treatment? Epilepsia 49, 25–28.

Cloyd, J.C., 1991. Pharmacokinetic pitfalls of present antiepileptic medications. Epilepsia 32, S53.

Gardiner, P., Dvorkin, L., 2006. Promoting medication adherence in children. Am. Fam. Phys. 74, 793–798.

Glauser, T., Ben-Menachem, E., Bourgeois, B., et al., 2013. Updated ILAE evidence review of antiepileptic drug efficacy and effectiveness as initial monotherapy for epileptic seizures and syndromes. Epilepsia 54, 551–563.

Glauser, T.A., 2000. Idiosyncratic reactions: new methods of identifying high-risk patients. Epilepsia 41, S16–S29.

Italiano, D., Perucca, E., 2013. Clinical pharmacokinetics of new-generation antiepileptic drugs at the extremes of age: an update. Clin. Pharmacokinet. 52, 627–645.

Perucca, E., Dulac, O., Shorvon, S., et al., 2001. Harnessing the clinical potential of antiepileptic drug therapy: dosage optimisation. CNS Drugs 15, 609–621.

E-BOOK FIGURES AND TABLES

The following figures and tables are available in the e-book at www.expertconsult.com. See inside cover for registration details.

Fig. 77-2 Effect of dose on elimination kinetics.

Fig. 77-3 Comparison of serum concentration–time curves after administration of carbamazepine (CBZ) tablets and suspension.

Fig. 77-4 Phenytoin dosing requirements in children.

Box 77-1 Clinical indications for obtaining antiseizure drug concentrations

Box 77-2 Clinical profiles for patients at high risk for idiosyncratic reactions to valproic acid, lamotrigine, and felbamate

Table 77-2 Pharmacokinetics of phenytoin

Table 77-4 Loading doses of antiseizure drugs

Table 77-5 Antiseizure drug involvement with cytochrome P-450 system

Table 77-6 Optimal target ranges for commonly prescribed antiseizure drugs

Table 77-7 Drug disposition at different ages

Table 77-8 Antiseizure drug mechanisms of action

78 Epilepsy Surgery in the Pediatric Population

Mary L. Zupanc, Lily Tran, and Andrew Mower

Epilepsy is one of the most common chronic disorders facing children and adolescents. The overall prevalence of epilepsy has been estimated to be 5 to 8 per 1000. The cumulative risk of developing epilepsy from birth through adolescence is 1%. Unfortunately, only 60% to 70% of patients will achieve seizure freedom with antiseizure medications. The introduction of several new antiepilepsy drugs over the past 15 years has not changed the fact that approximately 30% to 40% of patients with epilepsy will be medically refractory.

The identification of a patient's specific epilepsy syndrome is one of the best determinants of prognosis. Some epilepsy syndromes are genetically determined and may have an excellent prognosis for remission. Other epilepsy syndromes, particularly the lesional epilepsies, are life long chronic disorders. Predictors for low probability of epilepsy remission include the following:

1. The presence of a symptomatic localization-related epilepsy secondary to a remote central nervous system injury
2. Abnormalities on neurologic examination or cognitive/motor delays
3. Persistent epileptiform abnormalities on EEG
4. Older age at onset

The longer epilepsy persists without control, the less likely is the chance of remission. If seizures remain inadequately controlled for longer than 4 years, then the chance of remission decreases to approximately 10%. The presence of multiple seizure types and frequent generalized tonic–clonic seizures also lessens the chance for complete remission. Approximately 60% of these patients will have focal onset seizures. Estimates by several investigators suggest that many of these patients are epilepsy surgery candidates. Currently, however, epilepsy surgery is underutilized in the treatment of intractable epilepsy, as shown by the fact that over the past 15 years, the mean duration of epilepsy before referral to a tertiary care epilepsy center for evaluation for epilepsy surgery was over 20 years.

The developing brain is highly susceptible to recurrent seizures. A growing body of evidence in animal models suggests that early seizures, even if brief and recurrent, can result in demonstrable structural and physiologic changes in the developing brain's circuitry, resulting in aberrant excitation and inhibition. Clinically, these defects may produce spontaneous seizures (epilepsy) and cognitive impairment, with the possibility of missed windows of developmental opportunity. In addition, chronic uncontrolled epilepsy in infants and children poses a significant risk for emotional, behavioral, social, cognitive, and family dysfunction. Population studies have demonstrated that epilepsy reduces life expectancy, and poorly controlled seizures further increase the risk of death in children and adults.

Both location and etiology play roles in determining prognosis of epilepsy surgery. In a meta-analysis of children who have undergone temporal lobectomy, the seizure-free rate overall was 76%, ranging from 52% to 100% depending on etiology (Englot et al., 2013a,b). A meta-analysis was also done for extratemporal lobe resections, with an overall seizure-free rate of 56%.

Several studies have reported on cognitive function after surgery in children who have undergone temporal lobectomy (predominantly older children and adolescents). These studies have generally found that memory and intelligence are unchanged. A study of a small number of children who have undergone temporal and extratemporal resections looked at overall cognitive function pre- and postoperatively and found no differences. In a follow-up study of 24 children operated on before 3 years of age, younger age at surgery was correlated with an improvement in developmental quotient. Retrospective studies that combine temporal and extratemporal cases suggest that a reduction of seizure frequency, not necessarily complete elimination of seizures, resulted in significant improvements in family life, socialization, and behavior, as well as enhanced quality of life and developmental "catch up."

HISTORICAL BACKGROUND

Epilepsy surgery substantially advanced in 1950, when Penfield published his article on 70 cases of temporal lobectomy. His neurosurgical career was devoted to the study of the clinical description of seizures and their correlation with the brain cortex. He used cortical mapping and stimulation in much the same way it is used today. He also recognized the substrates of epilepsy, particularly trauma and infection. His seminal clinical research has been instrumental in guiding the hands of contemporary epileptologists and neurosurgeons interested in the surgical approach to epilepsy.

In the past 30 years, dramatic improvements in brain imaging that identify specific anatomic substrates of epilepsy have sparked renewed interest in surgery for intractable epilepsy. Temporal lobectomy with amygdalohippocampectomy has become the standard of care in adult patients with intractable epilepsy emanating from the temporal lobe. The surgical success rate for a seizure-free outcome in these carefully selected patients approaches 80% to 90%. In a randomized, controlled trial of surgery for temporal lobe epilepsy compared with treatment with antiseizure drugs, 58% of patients demonstrated seizure freedom after 1 year compared with only 8% of patients treated with medications. Unfortunately, surgical success does not necessarily translate to an improved quality of life. The accumulation of years of low self-esteem, loss of independence, poor peer relations, and academic failure, coupled with high financial costs, often without benefit of full insurance coverage, translate to continued lack of employment and depression. The growing recognition of the real costs of epilepsy—medical, psychological, and educational—has led to increased interest in the early identification of children who might benefit from epilepsy surgery.

INDICATIONS FOR EPILEPSY SURGERY

Practice guidelines for temporal lobe and localized neocortical resections for epilepsy have been proposed for adults. Criteria have been proposed for referral and evaluation of children for epilepsy surgery, although there is currently insufficient class I evidence to produce a practice guideline (Cross et al., 2006). In determining whether a child is a candidate for epilepsy surgery, several key issues must be considered. The decision-making task must take into account the following:

- Failure of two or three antiseizure medications in achieving complete seizure control in a child or adolescent.
- Natural history of the epilepsy syndrome. The likelihood of continued intractability usually can be determined on the basis of the identification of a specific epilepsy syndrome.
- Identification of a known epileptogenic substrate. Lesional epilepsy in a young infant should prompt an evaluation for epilepsy surgery, even as the first medication is started. Young infants are particularly vulnerable to deleterious effects of epilepsy in the developing brain.
- Impact of epilepsy on the quality of life, as defined by cognitive and developmental parameters—now and in the future.

The proper classification of seizure type and epilepsy syndrome is crucial in the determination of whether or not a patient is an appropriate epilepsy surgery candidate.

The severe epilepsies of infancy and childhood are recognizable early, and affected patients should be referred to a tertiary epilepsy center for consideration for epilepsy surgery. These epilepsy syndromes are characterized by the tetrad of the following:

1. Multiple daily seizures
2. Medical intractability to standard antiseizure drug therapies
3. Cognitive/developmental stagnation or decline
4. Presumed or known epileptogenic pathology.

The epilepsies of infancy and childhood that have specific surgical indications include the following:

1. Sturge–Weber syndrome: Children with Sturge–Weber syndrome who have frequent, medically refractory seizures should be evaluated promptly for hemispherectomy. Clinical outcome studies indicate that early surgical resection can result in the elimination of seizures, improvement in cognitive abilities, and overall improvement in quality of life despite residual hemiparesis and visual field deficits.
2. Large unilateral or focal malformations of cortical development, such as hemimegalencephaly or unilateral schizencephaly: Hemispherectomy provides relief from seizures (especially in those patients with unilateral epileptiform abnormalities) and improved developmental outcome.
3. Symptomatic infantile spasms with focal malformations of cortical development, typically temporal-parietal-occipital dysplasia. These patients should be considered for early focal cortical resection. Clinical research has documented improvement in seizure control and enhanced developmental gains after epilepsy surgery.
4. Rasmussen syndrome: Rasmussen encephalitis is characterized by intractable focal motor seizures, often evolving into epilepsia partialis continua, cognitive decline, and progressive hemiparesis. The only definitive treatment for Rasmussen encephalitis remains hemispherectomy.

In addition to those with the aforementioned epilepsies of infancy and childhood, children with tumors and concomitant localization-related epilepsy should be considered for early surgical intervention.

Children with other types of lesional, symptomatic, localization-related epilepsy should also be considered as potential epilepsy surgery candidates. Common substrates of epilepsy include encephalomalacia, vascular malformations, tubers, and malformations of cortical development (Harvey et al., 2008).

Patients who have generalized epilepsy syndromes may also be candidates for epilepsy surgery. Children with generalized or multifocal epilepsy should be considered for epilepsy surgery if data suggest an underlying focal generator for the epilepsy (Wyllie et al., 2007). Specifically, in the presence of a lesion on magnetic resonance imaging (MRI), the epilepsy syndrome is most likely to be attributable to symptomatic localization-related epilepsy with rapid secondary bisynchrony. In one study, children who had generalized discharges and focal lesions of early life onset had identical postsurgical seizure-free outcomes (72% seizure-free) to children with similar lesions and ipsilateral focal epileptiform discharges (Wyllie et al., 2007). Patients with tuberous sclerosis and medically refractory, symptomatic, localization-related epilepsy should also be considered for epilepsy surgery. If the presurgical evaluation points to a specific tuber, studies have shown that it can be successfully removed, with a significant improvement in seizure control.

Those children with intractable nonlesional extratemporal localization-related epilepsy represent the biggest challenge to the epileptologist but should still be considered for epilepsy surgery if their seizures remain intractable. The benefits of surgery must be weighed against the risks, especially the risk of neurologic deficits.

PREOPERATIVE EVALUATION

Once a child has been selected as a possible epilepsy surgery candidate, further questions need to be addressed before epilepsy surgery can take place:

1. Can the epileptogenic zone be identified using video EEG, neuroimaging, and other modalities? Is there congruence of the data?
2. Will removal of the epileptogenic zone result in seizure freedom?
3. Can the epileptogenic focus be removed without causing unacceptable neurologic deficits? This requires accurate anatomic localization of eloquent cortex.
4. Will a delay in epilepsy surgery cause loss of developmental plasticity?

A multidisciplinary team is required for addressing the many issues surrounding the prospect of surgery in a child with chronic epilepsy. Epilepsy surgery itself may cure the seizures but will not necessarily address the family's other needs. The family of a child with medically intractable epilepsy has complex and diverse problems—not just medical but also developmental, educational, psychosocial, economic, and relational.

Techniques and Technologies
Seizure Semiology

Seizure semiology can provide insightful clues to the lateralization and localization of the underlying epileptogenic focus. The presence of versive, that is, forced turning, head movements, unilateral motor clonic activity, and eye deviation may constitute critical lateralizing information. Specifically, versive head movements typically indicate that the epileptogenic zone resides in the contralateral hemisphere. Seizures consisting of olfactory or gustatory hallucinations, followed by complex motor automatisms and staring unresponsively, are characteristic of involvement of the temporal lobe. It should be noted, however, that seizures emanating from the temporal lobe in infants and young children commonly are

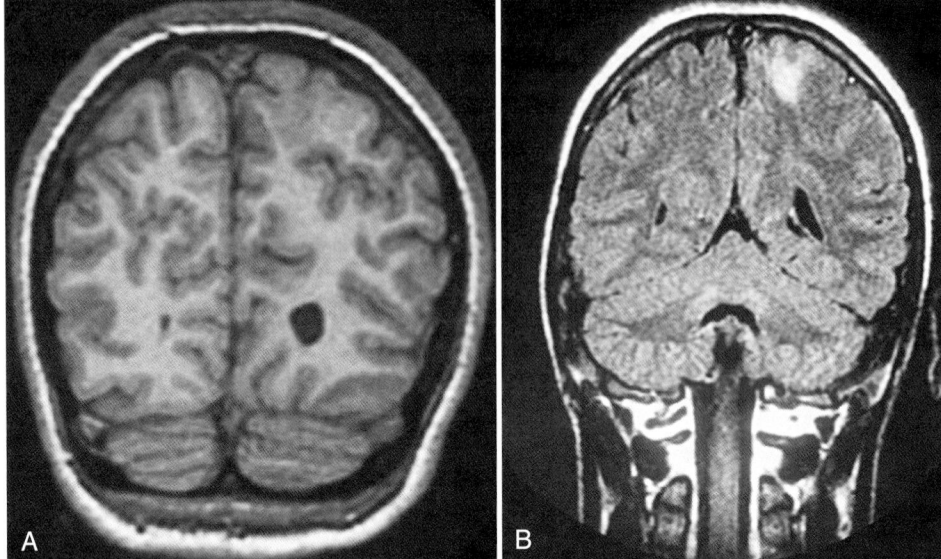

Figure 78-3. Magnetic resonance imaging scans from a patient with focal cortical dysplasia of the posterior left parasagittal region. **A,** With T1-weighted imaging (TR = 24 msec/TE = 9 msec), thickening of the cortex and blurring of the white/gray matter are evident. **B,** The dysplasia is seen more clearly with fluid-attenuated inversion recovery imaging (FLAIR) sequencing (TR = 1100 msec/TE = 142 msec/TI = 2600 msec) (see text). TE, echo time; TI, inversion time; TR, recovery time.

associated with behavioral arrest, motor dystonic posturing, and fewer automatisms.

Frontal lobe seizures may present a challenge, as seizure semiology can vary greatly within the various regions of the frontal lobe (Bonini et al., 2014).

Physical Examination

The physical examination, including attention to dysmorphic or neurocutaneous stigmata, can also provide very valuable lateralizing information. As with seizure onset or its evolution, a focal abnormality on physical examination may point to an underlying focal structural lesion. For example, a child with schizencephaly and focal seizures may have a subtle hemiparesis contralateral to the affected hemisphere.

Electroencephalography

The surface EEG, including continuous video-EEG monitoring, is a critical element in the evaluation of children with epilepsy.

Magnetic Resonance Imaging

- MRI scans have greatly enhanced the ability to detect epileptogenic lesions, especially focal cortical dysplasia. Examples of important new technologies are described below. Thin contiguous cuts of 1.5 to 1.6 mm in multiple sections of the cortex, in combination with a three-dimensional volumetric pulse sequence, provide the necessary resolution to detect small lesions that would be missed with conventional MRI. Quantitative volumetric analysis of the hippocampus allows determination of unilateral or bilateral hippocampal atrophy.
- The fluid-attenuated inversion recovery imaging (FLAIR) technique highlights lesions such as mesial temporal sclerosis and malformations of cortical development. This sequence produces a T2-weighted image that subtracts the cerebrospinal fluid signal (white and bright on T2), but retains the T2 signal in intraparenchymal structures [Fig. 78-3 and Fig. 78-4].

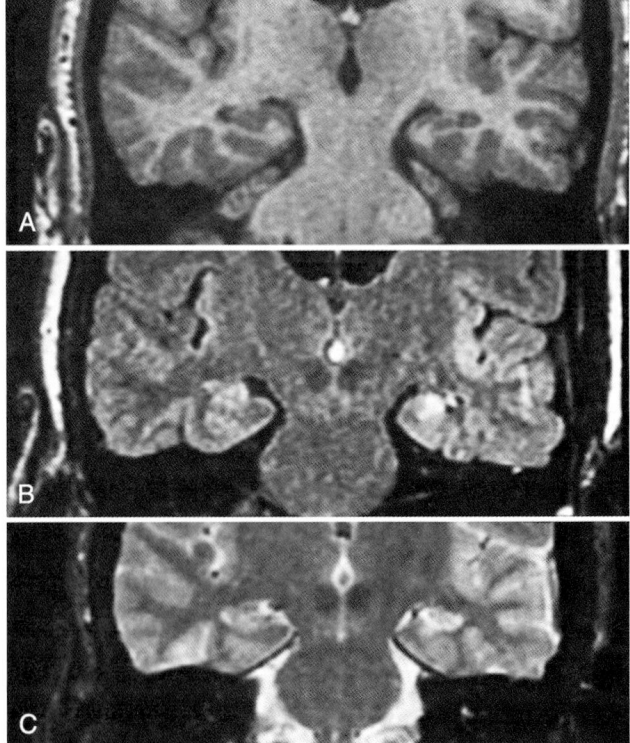

Figure 78-4. Magnetic resonance imaging scans showing coronal cuts through the temporal lobes, from a patient with left temporal hippocampal atrophy. **A,** The atrophy is seen best with T1-weighted imaging (TR = 24 msec/TE = 9 msec). **B,** Concomitant left temporal mesial temporal sclerosis is seen best with fluid-attenuated inversion recovery imaging (FLAIR) sequencing (TR = 1100 msec/TE = 142 msec/TI = 2600 msec). **C,** Middle panel represents the picture created on T2-weighted imaging (TR = 2000 msec/TE = 80 msec).

- Diffusion tensor imaging is an MRI technique that can identify white-matter tracts that may be disrupted in areas of cortical dysplasia and help in surgical planning.
- Multichannel coils (32 phased array and beyond and higher field strengths—3 tesla, 7 tesla, and greater), coupled with newer imaging sequences, including arterial spin labeling and susceptibility-weighted imaging, increase detection of focal cortical dysplasia.

Single-Photon Emission Computed Tomography

SPECT has also enhanced the ability to identify the epileptogenic zone. Penfield and colleagues observed relative hyperperfusion in the epileptogenic zone during a seizure. Interictally, blood flow and metabolism are decreased. SPECT scan technology enables quantification of cerebral blood flow and identification of areas of relative blood flow change. SPECT images are reconstructed from data obtained by recording photon emissions from radiotracers injected intravenously. These radiotracers rapidly cross the blood–brain barrier because of their lipophilic nature and bind within minutes to the brain, producing an instantaneous picture of cerebral blood flow. ^{99m}Tc ethyl cysteinate dimer (i.e., ^{99m}Tc-N,N'(1,2-ethylenediyl)bis-L-cysteine diethyl ester), prepared as technetium ^{99m}Tc bicisate (Neurolite), is the primary radio-isotope for this procedure. Logistically, Neurolite provides distinct advantages for ictal SPECT scans because it is a stable isotope tracer that can be mixed well ahead of the time of injection, as opposed to ^{99m}Tc-HMPAO, which decomposes quickly in vitro and must be used less than 30 minutes after it is reconstituted. For ictal SPECT scans, a technologist or nurse trained in the delivery of these radioisotopes can sit at the bedside and deliver the Neurolite within seconds after the onset of a seizure.

Clinical research indicates that interictal SPECT studies alone have a relatively low sensitivity for identification of the epileptogenic focus in adults with temporal lobe epilepsy and even lower sensitivity with extratemporal epilepsy. Data pooled from several studies yield estimates of interictal SPECT sensitivity of 66% for temporal lobe epilepsy and 60% for extratemporal epilepsy localized by EEG (Knowlton, 2006).

Ictal SPECT scan data, however, have proved valuable with respect to localization of the epileptogenic focus. Ictal SPECT scans typically reveal an area of regional hyperperfusion that corresponds to the underlying epileptogenic focus, as verified by surgical pathology and surface EEG localization. Using data pooled from several centers, the sensitivity of ictal SPECT (as judged by EEG correlation) has been estimated at 90% for temporal and 81% for extratemporal epilepsy, with specificity at 77% and 93%, respectively (Knowlton, 2006).

Several techniques have been developed whereby the ictal and interictal SPECT scan data are coregistered with one another and the interictal image is subtracted from the ictal image, producing the area of true ictal hyperperfusion. This difference image, called a subtraction SPECT scan, is then coregistered with a three-dimensional representation of the MRI scan. Several studies have demonstrated that peri-ictal subtraction SPECT provides useful information for seizure localization in patients with focal malformations of cortical development, even when the MRI study is nonlocalizing (i.e., "nonlesional") (O'Brien et al., 2004). In a large series involving pediatric and adult epilepsy patients, if the site of the surgical resection was concordant with the subtraction SPECT localization (using technology that performs subtraction SPECT and then coregisters the results to a volumetric MRI), postoperative seizure frequency scores were significantly lower and postoperative improvement was greater. In summary,

SPECT scan technology, particularly subtraction SPECT, holds merit for localization of the epileptogenic zone.

Positron Emission Tomography

PET is another imaging modality used for localization of the epileptogenic focus. It uses radiotracers labeled with specific positron-emitting isotopes (^{11}C, 15 O, and 18 F) to measure a variety of biochemical brain functions. Cerebral glucose metabolism is the most commonly measured parameter, using 18F-fluorodeoxyglucose (FDG) (see Fig. 78-9). Other tracers also can be used to measure cerebral blood flow, benzodiazepine and opiate receptors, pH, serotonin metabolism, and amino acid transport.

FDG-PET images are averaged over a 40-minute time interval, suggesting the limited value of this technique for ictal studies. The interictal images, on the other hand, are highly sensitive in focal onset seizures emanating from the temporal lobe. In several studies in adult patients with medically refractory epilepsy of temporal lobe origin, glucose hypometabolism in the temporal lobe correlated highly with localized ictal EEG and MRI abnormalities.

Analysis of nonlesional, extratemporal epilepsy in adult patients undergoing PET scans has provided data that are less definitive. In one recent analysis, the sensitivity and specificity of FDG-PET scans decreased to 40% in MRI-negative extratemporal cases. In children with refractory epilepsy, however, with poor localization on surface EEG and negative findings on MRI, FDG-PET may still provide useful information in identifying an underlying epileptogenic focus. Newer ligands have also been developed. In flumazenil PET scans, the flumazenil binds to benzodiazepine receptors. In the area of the epileptogenic zone, benzodiazepine binding appears to be decreased. In one clinical study, the flumazenil PET scan demonstrated a more restricted area of decreased binding than was apparent on the FDG-PET scan; the resection of this cortical region was associated with good surgical outcome. C-alphamethyl-L-tryptophan (AMT) PET scans have also been studied. AMT is an analog of tryptophan and a precursor for serotonin synthesis. Data suggest that the AMT PET scans may be useful in identifying the most epileptogenic tuber in patients with tuberous sclerosis, multiple tubers, and medically intractable epilepsy. Concordance of the epileptogenic tuber with increased AMT uptake has been observed in PET scans.

Magnetic Resonance Spectroscopy

MR spectroscopy has been used in the study of patients with intractable epilepsy. Specifically, phosphorus MR spectroscopy measures phospholipid metabolism. In the region of the epileptogenic focus, investigators have found abnormal phosphocreatine to inorganic phosphate ratios. Proton MR spectroscopy can also measure regional abnormalities in lactate, N-acetyl-aspartate (NAA), creatine (Cr), and choline (Cho). Lactate levels increase during a seizure and remain elevated for several hours. Abnormal NAA/Cr and NAA/Cho ratios may serve as indices of regional cellular pathology. MR spectroscopy may have a role as an adjunctive noninvasive technique for assisting with the identification of the underlying epileptogenic zone.

Magnetoencephalography

MEG is another technology that has been developed to improve the ability to identify epileptogenic foci. It measures tiny magnetic fields created by the electrical activity of the brain. Most institutions are using 128-channel MEG technology to enhance resolution. MEG offers several advantages over EEG. First, the magnetic fields are not attenuated by the skull, scalp, and skin, in contrast to electrical potentials. Second, MEG is a monopolar measure and does not require a dipolar montage, eliminating the possibility of artifact associated with an "active reference." Third, MEG provides high temporal resolution. Finally, MEG measures postsynaptic intracellular currents in the dendrites of neurons situated tangentially to the skull, whereas the EEG measures extracellular postsynaptic ionic currents.

Clinical research suggests that, although surface interictal EEG spike recordings may indicate multifocal activity, MEG can more precisely localize the underlying epileptogenic focus (Wheless et al., 1999). In this regard, MEG provides complementary data to EEG. MEG has been employed in children with intractable epilepsy to provide spatial information to be used in planning the excision area. MEG spike source clusters have been used to indicate the epileptogenic zone.

Functional Mapping

If an underlying epileptogenic focus is identified, the next question to consider is whether the epileptogenic zone can be removed without causing unacceptable neurologic deficits. In infants and young children, this proves to be less problematic because of brain plasticity.

Classically, in the older child and adolescent, the amobarbital test (Wada test) is used in the preoperative evaluation for the lateralization of speech and language and to determine whether memory can be supported in the contralateral hemisphere. This test involves injecting amobarbital into either the left or the right internal carotid artery, in an attempt to transiently eliminate ipsilateral hemispheric function chemically and to determine which hemisphere is "dominant." It is a time-consuming test that is invasive and provides a broad but nonspecific overview of hemispheric function.

Two other techniques used frequently to identify eloquent cortex are somatosensory-evoked potentials and cortical stimulation mapping. The measurement of somatosensory-evoked potentials has the advantage of being able to be applied successfully regardless of the state of the patient. This modality can be used in the operating room in the anesthetized patient, or in an awake and cooperative patient. Somatosensory-evoked potentials are used primarily to identify the sensorimotor cortex.

Cortical stimulation mapping is a useful, dependable, and safe technique to assess motor, sensory, and speech function. It involves the application of subdural electrodes followed by sequential electrical stimuli between two electrodes at various intensities and durations.

Although cortical stimulation mapping has yielded a tremendous amount of information about the localization of functions, several other emerging techniques are providing valid, noninvasive methods for mapping out functional areas of the brain. These techniques include functional MRI (fMRI) scans, MEG and magnetic source imaging, and transcranial magnetic stimulation.

fMRI is based on the fact that performance of a specific act will activate the anatomically appropriate cortex in the brain. With activation, a concomitant increase in blood flow occurs, resulting in a change in the paramagnetic properties of the affected cortex. This produces a signal that can then be detected by the MRI scanner. fMRI is a technique that is being increasingly used to map out eloquent functions, such as sensorimotor cortex and speech and language centers.

Concept of Congruence

Under ideal conditions, identification of the epileptogenic focus is made by the congruence of data obtained during the preoperative evaluation, with the precise localization based on seizure semiology, physical examination, surface ictal and interictal EEG monitoring, and MRI, along with additional studies as discussed above, that is, ictal and interictal SPECT, interictal PET, MEG, fMRI, MR spectroscopy, and transcranial magnetic stimulation. Each case must be individualized, with various combinations of the above procedures used at different centers.

The most complex cases are those of nonlesional extratemporal epilepsy. In these patients, placement of invasive subdural strips or grids or depth electrodes is generally necessary for precise localization of the epileptogenic focus.

INVASIVE INTRACRANIAL ELECTROENCEPHALOGRAPHY MONITORING

There are noninvasive tools available to help identify the epileptogenic zone, defined as the minimum amount of cortical tissue that must be resected to produce seizure freedom. Defining the epileptogenic zone entails accurate seizure localization, mapping the extent of the epileptogenic zone, and assessing the functional status of the epileptogenic zone. When the noninvasive tools do not accurately achieve the goals of defining this epileptogenic zone in a patient with pharmacoresistant epilepsy, invasive intracranial electroencephalography may identify a clear resective surgical strategy. Indications for invasive monitoring include the following:

- No cortical lesion is detected on MRI.
- Data obtained from noninvasive evaluation are conflicting and do not clearly delineate the borders of the epileptogenic zone.
- There is a suspicion of multifocal epilepsy.
- Noninvasive data identify the epileptogenic zone being in close proximity or involving eloquent cortex.

Invasive monitoring is the placement of subdural grids and strips directly over the cortex. These disk electrodes are 2 to 5 mm in diameter and are embedded in silicon elastometer aligned in a linear fashion separated by 10 mm from center to center. Advantages of using subdural grids/strips include comprehensive spatial cortical coverage, which allows for accurate anatomic and functional mapping over the area of coverage. Limitations include inadequate and/or incomplete coverage of intrasulcal, deep cortical regions, and interhemispheric areas as well as difficulty covering multilobar and large functional networks.

Another invasive monitoring technique is the stereo-electroencephalography (SEEG). Its aim is to produce a three-dimensional spatial-temporal organization of epileptic discharges within the cortical and subcortical brain structures. This method is technically complex, using the Talairach stereotactic frame and the double-grid system in association with teleangiography to place depth electrodes, which are linear probes containing multiple cylindrical contacts (Gonzalez-Martinez et al., 2014). More modern and less complex methods of stereotactic implantation of depth electrodes, using a robotic arm, are emerging to make SEEG more feasible.

SEEG may provide an advantage in cases where the epileptogenic zone is hypothesized to be deep-seated or in a region that may be difficult to be adequate cover using subdural grids/strips. Examples of such regions include mesial temporal, perisylvian opercular, cingulate, orbitofrontal, and insular cortex (Gonzalez-Martinez et al., 2014).

A limitation to SEEG includes restricted ability to perform functional mapping, especially contiguous mapping in eloquent cortex because of the limited number of contacts located on superficial cortex (Gonzalez-Martinez et al., 2014).

Complication rates range from 3% to 6% and include hemorrhage or intraparenchymal hematoma (Gonzalez-Martinez et al., 2014).

TYPES OF SURGERY

Several types of epilepsy surgery are performed in children and adults, depending on the identification of the epileptogenic focus and its location and extent. The most common surgical procedures are as follows:

1. Temporal lobectomy
2. Cortical resection—lobar and multilobar
3. Stereotactic lesionectomy
4. Hemispherectomy—either anatomic or modified
5. Multiple subpial transection
6. Corpus callosotomy
7. Implantation of a vagus nerve stimulator
8. Minimally invasive surgical techniques

Temporal lobectomy is the most common epilepsy surgery performed in adolescents and adults. This procedure is almost exclusively a temporal lobectomy with amygdalohippocampectomy. Removal of the mesial temporal structures is correlated with a 90% chance of becoming seizure free in patients with mesial temporal sclerosis.

Extratemporal cortical resection is more commonly performed in children, often involving extensive lobar or multilobar resections. The extent of the resection is dictated primarily by the extent of the lesion. As the ability to identify focal cortical dysplasias and the concomitant epileptogenic zone improves, epilepsy surgical outcomes may also improve. Focal cortical dysplasias are a common cause of intractable partial epilepsy in children, accounting for 60% of the cases. The best predictive factors in successful surgical outcome in focal cortical dysplasia are completeness of the resection and the presence of an identifiable lesion on MRI brain imaging (Cross et al., 2006).

Stereotactic lesionectomy, performed in highly selected cases in children and adults, has a reported 50% to 60% chance of rendering the patient seizure-free. Outcome is improved if intraoperative electrocorticography is used to remove not only the lesion, but also the surrounding "epileptogenic zone."

Hemispherectomy is performed in young children, including infants. The indications for this type of surgery are medically resistant epilepsies in which the substrate of epilepsy is limited to one hemisphere. Typical indications include Sturge–Weber syndrome, hemimegalencephaly or extensive unilateral cortical dysplasia, Rasmussen encephalitis, and (usually postinfarction) porencephaly.

Multiple subpial transection is a surgical technique that may be used when the epileptogenic zone overlies an area of functional cortex. Multiple subpial transection involves the disruption of connecting horizontal fibers, preserving vertical connections and avoiding resection of tissue. The technique is not as effective as cortical resection.

Corpus callosotomy is a palliative surgery that can reduce the seizure burden in carefully selected patients. It is most commonly used in children with Lennox–Gastaut syndrome, with the goal being reduction of tonic and atonic seizures, and can be highly effective. Although there is no consensus in the published literature, one series comparing anterior versus complete corpus callosotomy showed better seizure control in patients with complete corpus callosotomy. The use of a complete corpus callosotomy, coupled with lateralizing strips, has been demonstrated to be effective in identifying an epileptogenic zone as part of a multistage surgery. Complications of corpus callosotomy include surgical complications, transient mild hemiparesis, and disconnection syndrome (apathy, urinary incontinence, and nondominant hemineglect). The risk for disconnection syndrome is greater in patients with higher cognitive function and older age.

Minimally invasive surgical techniques have emerged as potential alternatives to open epilepsy surgery because of the high costs of resective epilepsy surgery, the reluctance of patients and referring physicians to seek invasive surgery for definitive treatment, and surgical morbidities. These techniques include stereotactic radiosurgery, stereotactic radiofrequency thermocoagulation, and laser-induced thermal therapy (LITT).

Stereotactic radiosurgery involves delivering ionizing radiation to small foci deep within brain tissue while sparing damage to surrounding tissue. This technique has been used to treat lesions that are difficult to access, such as deep brain tumors and arteriovenous malformations. There are a few sources of focal ionizing radiation in clinical use, one of which is the Gamma Knife (Eleckta AB), which consists of approximately 200 separate radioactive cobalt-60 sources housed inside a hemispheric chamber and focused to a single target.

Stereotactic radiofrequency thermocoagulation is a procedure that causes a permanent lesion by heating brain tissue until proteins denature. This technique uses a monopolar needle, inserting it into the surgical target under stereotactic guidance. After the needle is inserted into the desired focus, high-frequency current is injected, resulting in heating tissue at the electrode tip.

LITT, also known as MRI-guided thermal laser ablation, is tissue coagulation accomplished via laser delivery. Studies rigorously evaluating use of this technology are few. Though preliminary data for LITT are promising, use of LITT in epilepsy treatment is limited at this time.

Further surgical options as palliative procedures, namely, vagus nerve stimulation and responsive nerve stimulation, are discussed in the chapter on neuromodulation for epilepsy.

GOALS OF SURGERY

With use of innovative, noninvasive technologies, the ability of the clinician to identify the underlying epileptogenic zone and achieve the elimination of seizures in patients with medically intractable epilepsy through surgery has improved. The goals of epilepsy surgery, however, may vary, depending on the epilepsy syndrome, the underlying pathophysiology, the cognitive and developmental status of the child or adolescent, and the identification and location of an epileptogenic zone.

RESEARCH ISSUES: TRENDS FOR THE FUTURE

There are many unanswered questions that still need to be addressed in the pursuit of helping children with intractable epilepsy.

Future trends for exploration will involve several avenues of research: source localization and predictive EEG patterns for identification of the epileptogenic zone; expanded use of minimally invasive surgical techniques; and implantable devices that can detect predictive EEG patterns before a clinical seizure and deliver antiseizure medication or an electrical stimulus.

REFERENCES

The complete list of references for this chapter is available online at www.expertconsult.com.

See inside cover for registration details.

SELECTED REFERENCES

Bonini, F., McGonigal, A., et al., 2014. Frontal lobe seizure: from clinical semiology to localization. Epilepsia 55, 264–277.

Cross, J.H., Jayakar, P., Nordli, D., et al., 2006. Proposed criteria for referral and evaluation of children for epilepsy surgery: recommendations of the subcommission for pediatric epilepsy surgery. Epilepsia 47, 952.

Englot, D.J., Breshears, J.D., et al., 2013a. Seizure outcomes after respective surgery for extra-temporal lobe epilepsy in pediatric patients. A systematic review. J. Neurosurg. Pediatr. 12, 126–133.

Englot, D.J., Rolston, J.D., et al., 2013b. Seizure outcomes after temporal lobectomy in pediatric patients. A systematic review. J. Neurosurg. Pediatr. 12, 134–141.

Gonzalez-Martinez, J., Mullin, J., et al., 2014. Stereoelectroencephalography in children and adolescents with difficult-to-localize refractory focal epilepsy. Neurosurgery 75, 258–268.

Harvey, H., Cross, J.H., Shinnar, S., et al., 2008. Defining the spectrum of international practice in pediatric epilepsy surgery patients. Epilepsia 49, 146.

Knowlton, R.C., 2006. The role of FDG-PET, ictal SPECT, and MEG in the epilepsy surgery evaluation. Epilepsy Behav. 8, 91–101.

O'Brien, T.J., So, E.L., Cascino, G.D., et al., 2004. Subtraction SPECT coregistered to MRI in focal malformations of cortical development: localization of epileptogenic zone in epilepsy surgery candidates. Epilepsia 45, 367.

Wheless, J.W., Willmore, L.J., Breier, J.I., et al., 1999. A comparison of magnetoencephalography, MRI and V-EEG in patients evaluated for epilepsy surgery. Epilepsia 40, 931.

Wyllie, E., Lachhwani, D.K., Gupta, A., et al., 2007. Successful surgery for epilepsy due to early brain lesions despite generalized EEG findings. Neurology 69, 389–397.

E-BOOK FIGURES AND TABLES

The following figures and tables are available in the e-book at www.expertconsult.com. See inside cover for registration details.

Fig. 78-1 Magnetic resonance imaging scans from a patient with a ganglioglioma of the right temporal lobe.

Fig. 78-2 Magnetic resonance imaging scan from a patient with left temporal hippocampal atrophy.

Fig. 78-5 Magnetic resonance imaging scan from a patient with focal cortical dysplasia of the left frontal region.

Fig. 78-6 Magnetic resonance imaging scan from a patient with unilateral perisylvian dysplasia with polymicrogyria (left hemisphere).

Fig. 78-7 Three-dimensional computed tomography–derived electrode model overlaid on patient-specific postelectrode placement magnetic resonance imaging–derived brain surface used in planning of subsequent resective surgery.

Fig. 78-8 Single-photon emission computed tomography (SPECT) scans.

Fig. 78-9 Fluorodeoxyglucose positron emission tomography (FDG-PET) scan from a 12-year-old girl with focal dyscognitive seizures, showing a focal decrease in glucose metabolism in the left parietal and, to a lesser extent, the left occipital cortex.

Fig. 78-10 Magnetoencephalography (MEG) complements electroencephalography (EEG) data in the presurgical evaluation.

Fig. 78-11 The high temporal resolution of magnetoencephalography (MEG) allows for the dissociation of functional brain activity in different areas, as well as analysis of seizure propagation.

Fig. 78-12 Functional magnetic resonance imaging scan.

79 Neuromodulation in Epilepsy

Sameer C. Dhamne, Harper L. Kaye, and Alexander Rotenberg

An expanded version of this chapter is available on www.expertconsult.com. See inside cover for registration details.

INTRODUCTION

The twenty-first century has seen a rise of interest in neuromodulation, a term that describes the family of brain-stimulation techniques that alter brain function. Neuromodulation is particularly relevant in epilepsy, where seizures are resistant to pharmacotherapy in approximately one-third of all instances, a statistic that has not changed despite the introduction of more than 20 new antiseizure drugs in the late twentieth and early twenty-first centuries (Loscher and Schmidt, 2011). Accordingly, neurostimulation protocols are emerging as potentially valuable tools for seizure control.

Stimulating the nervous system to treat neuropsychiatric symptoms is not new. In the first century AD, the Roman physician Scribonius Largus documented treating headaches by applying electric torpedo fish to the head, and another Roman physician, Pedanius Dioscorides, in 76 AD applied the torpedo fish to a patient with epilepsy. As with brain stimulation in general, neuromodulation for epilepsy has advanced considerably in recent years, particularly as a set of palliative interventions in clinical epilepsy (Krishna et al., 2016). Neurostimulation protocols can be coarsely divided into either invasive or noninvasive. Among the invasive options, those that require surgical placement of a neurostimulation device are vagus nerve stimulation (VNS), deep-brain stimulation (DBS), and responsive neurostimulation (RNS). Noninvasive neuromodulation protocols include transcranial magnetic stimulation (TMS), trigeminal nerve stimulation (TNS), and transcranial direct current stimulation (tDCS). Although the most widely used neuromodulation approach to control seizures remains VNS, other technologies have become viable options for patients with intractable seizures.

VAGUS NERVE STIMULATION

VNS is one of the oldest neuromodulation protocols for epilepsy. As early as 1937, Schweitzer and Wright demonstrated suppression of strychnine-induced convulsions by experimental VNS in cats. The first human patient to undergo VNS via an implanted stimulator became seizure-free in 1988. In 1997 the U.S. Food and Drug Administration (FDA) approved VNS for use in adolescents and adults with intractable focal seizures, and since then VNS has developed as an established adjunctive therapy for medically refractory epilepsy.

VNS involves surgical implantation of a generator beneath the skin of the upper chest. From there, a subcutaneous cable connection is made to the stimulation electrode terminals placed directly on the left vagus nerve. The VNS device has two common stimulation modes: scheduled stimulation with predefined ON and OFF periods and on-demand firing, in which the patient or caretaker can activate the device during a seizure with a magnetic switch. The most recent VNS models also have the capacity to program a threshold heart-rate change such that stimulation will be triggered by tachycardia associated with seizure activity. The VNS surgical procedure carries a relatively low risk. Stimulation-related side effects such as cough, hoarseness, or throat discomfort are typically mild and can be relieved by adjusting the stimulation parameters.

The mechanisms by which VNS suppresses seizures are not fully understood. Anatomically, the vagus nerve carries both parasympathetic efferents to viscera and also visceral afferents that project diffusely to cortex and subcortical structures, particularly the thalamus, via the medial reticular formation, yet how these projections may modify seizure threshold is unknown. VNS may also activate unmyelinated nociceptive C fibers and lead to an arousal-like effect that is also associated with an elevation of seizure threshold. One study indicates reduced medial thalamus metabolic activity during the ON stimulation state in patients with favorable VNS effects, as assessed by single-photon emission computed tomography (SPECT). Results from another study that aimed to measure the effects of VNS on the cortical excitation : inhibition (E : I) ratio indicate that the VNS ON state corresponds to enhanced intracortical inhibition, as measured by paired-pulse transcranial magnetic stimulation (ppTMS; see discussion later in this chapter). A measure of scalp electroencephalogram (EEG) interregion synchrony in patients with successful VNS also identified desynchronization of cortical electrical activity as a possible VNS mechanism.

Overall, VNS results in modest seizure reduction. In adults with intractable seizures, a multicenter randomized controlled trial ($N = 114$) measured seizure suppression after chronic stimulation or on-demand VNS activation by instructing patients to activate the device during a seizure aura. For chronic stimulation, subjects were randomized to one of two conditions: treatment (up to 3 mA, 20–50 Hz, 500-µs pulse width, ON 30–90 sec, OFF 5–10 min) or active control (up to 2.75 mA, 1 Hz, 130-µs pulse width, ON 30 sec, OFF 60–180 min). After 14 weeks of VNS, the treatment group experienced significant mean seizure frequency reduction (24% vs. 6%). In regard to the effectiveness of patient-controlled on-demand VNS activation by a portable magnet switch, there was no significant difference in efficacy between groups assigned to treatment versus control conditions (0-mA output programmed for magnet activation), although most subjects perceived seizure reduction with the on-demand intervention. A subsequent large ($N = 196$) VNS trial with similar study parameters confirmed seizure frequency reduction in the treatment group receiving high stimulation compared with the control group receiving low stimulation (28% with high stimulation vs. 15% with low stimulation), with particular efficacy among patients with complex partial seizures (Handforth et al., 1998).

In pediatrics, the results of VNS trials have been mixed. A double-blind randomized controlled trial measured VNS efficacy in children ($N = 41$) aged 3 to 17 years, 85% with focal epilepsy and 15% with generalized epilepsy. Seizure frequency and severity were monitored by diary and the National Hospital Seizure Severity Scale (NHS3). Participants were randomized to the treatment (0.25 mA, 30 Hz, 500-µs pulse width, ON 30 sec, OFF 5 min) or active control (0.25 mA, 1 Hz, 100-µs pulse width, ON 14 sec, OFF 60 min) groups. After the initial phase, the treatment group received stimulation at the maximum tolerated current (up to 1.75 mA), whereas in the control group, the output current was initially increased during the clinic visit but was then restored to 0.25 mA. Although there was an overall reduction in seizure frequency and severity from baseline, there was no statistical difference in seizure reduction between the two groups.

Results from retrospective and open-label studies in children are more encouraging. One review of records in 69 children who had undergone insertion of VNS for intractable epilepsy identified a satisfactory outcome, as defined by an Engel class I, II, or III rating, in 55.0% of the sample, yet no change in seizures (Engel class IV) in 45%. An additional retrospective study reviewed patient records of 43 children with medically refractory epilepsy, aged 3 to 12 years, 46% with generalized seizures, 19% with focal onset seizures, and 35% with mixed types. The VNS output settings ranged from 0.5 to 2.0 mA, ON 30 sec, OFF 1.1 to 10 min (median 3 min). Postimplant seizure reduction was greater than 50% in 51% of the children. However, there was no relief of medication burden for any of these patients after VNS implantation. Yet another retrospective analysis of antiseizure VNS efficacy in 69 children at a single epilepsy center found an overall seizure frequency reduction of 50% at 6-month follow-up and 40% at 12 months. In this study, patients were classified as either high- or low-baseline seizure frequencies. Seizure frequency decrease in the low-baseline seizure frequency group (≤45 seizures/month for 3 months before implantation) was 25% at 6 months but not significant after 12 months. However, in the subgroup with high-baseline seizure frequency (>45 seizures/month), seizure reduction was significantly higher at 61% after 6 months and 69% at the 12-month follow-up. Taken together, these data indicate plausible VNS efficacy in pediatrics, although without confirmation by a large randomized controlled trial.

ANTERIOR NUCLEUS OF THE THALAMUS DEEP-BRAIN STIMULATION

In the United States, DBS has been approved by the FDA for treatment of movement disorder symptoms such as tremor and dystonia since 1997. Although research into DBS efficacy as an antiseizure therapy dates back to the 1970s, it has yet to be approved by the FDA for seizure suppression. However, one specific form of DBS, in which stimulating electrodes target the anterior nucleus (AN) of the thalamus, is nearing approval. The rationale for AN stimulation is based in part on the AN role as the primary relay nucleus of the limbic system—the AN both receives major projection from the mammillary bodies of the hypothalamus and projects fibers to areas such as the cingulum, amygdala, hippocampus, orbito-frontal cortex, and hypothalamus.

The DBS procedure is similar to VNS in that a generator is implanted beneath the skin in the chest. However, the leads are bilateral and tunneled to connect with two stereotaxically placed intracranial electrodes. As with VNS, the surgical procedure is well tolerated, with few complications.

A favorable outcome with AN stimulation in a patient with intractable seizures was first reported by Upton and Cooper in 1985 and supported by subsequent small-scale studies, the results of which indicated both seizure suppression and an acceptable safety profile of AN DBS in epilepsy. The early AN DBS data then prompted a large multicenter randomized trial, Stimulation of Anterior Nucleus of Thalamus for Epilepsy (SANTE), in patients ($N = 110$) with intractable seizures and baseline median seizure frequency of 19.5 seizures/month (Fisher et al., 2010). One month after DBS implantation,

subjects were randomized to two groups for the blinded phase of the study: treatment, in which the device was turned on at the start, and control, in which the device was turned on only after a 3-month blinded phase. The results from the SANTE trial are encouraging: 40% reduction in seizure frequency was identified in the treatment group, with stimulation parameters 5 V, 145 Hz, 90-μs pulse width, ON 1 min, OFF 5 min, in comparison to 15% decrease in the control group. In a subsequent 12-month open label follow-up, in which stimulation settings could be adjusted to 7.5 V and 185 Hz, an overall 56% reduction in median seizure frequency was found, with 54% of subjects reporting at 50% or greater seizure frequency reduction. Moreover, in subsequent long-term follow-up, 14 patients (13%) were seizure-free for at least 6 months, 8 (7%) were free for 1 year, 4 (3%) for at least 2 years, and 1 (1%) remained seizure-free for more than 4 years (Salanova et al., 2015). AN DBS is approved for the treatment of refractory epilepsy in Europe and Canada but not in the United States at the time of this writing.

AN DBS complications in the SANTE trial cohort included infection (12.7%), hemorrhage (4.5%), status epilepticus (4.5%), and death (4.5%). Of the five deaths that occurred during the SANTE trial period, three were attributed to sudden unexpected death in epilepsy (SUDEP), either in the baseline or follow-up phase. However, no deaths were reported during the first month after surgery (Fisher et al., 2010). Additional adverse events reported during the blinded phase included depression (15%) and memory impairment (13%), which were the most common reported side effects in the active treatment group.

RESPONSIVE NEUROSTIMULATION

Closed-loop responsive electrical brain stimulation is a novel treatment paradigm for epilepsy that involves implantation of subdural or depth electrodes in an epileptogenic brain region. In contrast to open-loop stimulation devices, the RNS electrodes are both stimulating and recording. The RNS electronics are self-contained in a cranial implant. EEG at the target is continuously monitored and recorded by the RNS computer. When electrical activity that signals seizure onset is detected, electrical stimulation with predetermined parameters is delivered via specified lead contacts, with the goal of disrupting the abnormal local electrical activity and either terminating an ongoing seizure or preventing seizure onset. The first implantable RNS device was FDA approved in the United States in 2013 as an adjunctive therapy in adults with medically uncontrolled focal onset seizures localized to one or two epileptogenic foci.

RNS safety and efficacy were established in three clinical trials: a 2-year primarily open-label safety trial ($N = 65$), a 2-year randomized controlled trial ($N = 191$), and a 7-year long-term extension study ($N = 230$). In the pivotal multicenter randomized controlled trial, adults with refractory focal seizures were treated with a responsive neurostimulator connected to either depth or subdural leads at one or two prespecified seizure foci. As in the SANTE trial, subjects were randomized 1 month after surgery into either the control or treatment group and followed for a 12-week blinded observation period, after which all participants entered an 84-week open-label period. During the first postsurgical month, both the control and treatment groups experienced a decrease in mean seizure frequency; notably, a postimplantation seizure reduction was also seen in the postsurgical month follow-up in the SANTE trial. Over the blinded evaluation period, mean seizure frequency fell by 38% in the treatment group compared with a 17% reduction in the control group. Of 102 patients assessed at the 2-year mark of the open-label period, 46% had at least 50% mean seizure frequency reduction. Both control and treatment RNS groups had similar improvements in secondary outcome measures, including quality of life, at the end of the blinded evaluation period. There were no significant differences in adverse events between the groups. The rate of intracranial hemorrhage was 4.7%, and 5.2% of subjects experienced implant site infection. There were 6 deaths in the pivotal 191-subject RNS controlled trial study: 4 attributed to SUDEP, 1 to lymphoma, and 1 patient with a history of depression who committed suicide (Morrell and RNS System in Epilepsy Study Group, 2011). Notably, mortality in this trial did not significantly exceed expected mortality rate in this vulnerable population.

TRIGEMINAL NERVE STIMULATION

TNS (in some texts termed *external trigeminal nerve stimulation*, or eTNS), like VNS, is a means to access the antiepileptic capacity of cranial nerve stimulation. In contrast to VNS, TNS can be delivered noninvasively via cutaneous electrodes that activate branches of the trigeminal nerve, usually in the V_1 distribution, where stimulating electrodes are positioned over the skin of the forehead. The mechanisms by which TNS may suppress seizures are not clear but, as in VNS, may relate to activation of the brainstem reticular formation and C-fiber stimulation that lead to an arousal state. TNS clinical trials were supported by early preclinical data that showed suppression of chemoconvulsant seizures in rats with high-frequency stimulation of the infraorbital nerve. These preclinical data prompted an open-label trial, which produced favorable results in 13 adults with intractable epilepsy. As with other neuromodulation protocols, data from a larger randomized control trial ($N = 42$) were less impressive. In the phase II TNS trial, adults with intractable epilepsy were randomized to receive TNS with a bipolar transcutaneous gel-based electrode designed to stimulate the right and left branches of the ophthalmic and supratrochlear nerves (DeGiorgio et al., 2013). TNS in the treatment group was delivered at 120 Hz and a pulse duration of less than 250 µs. The active control group received TNS at 2 Hz, pulse duration 50 µs, ON 2 sec, OFF 90 sec. Subjects in both groups received stimulation for at least 12 hours per day and were followed for an 18-week trial period, with evaluation at weeks 6, 12, and 18. After 18 weeks of stimulation, 41% of patients who received active stimulation had more than 50% seizure frequency reduction, compared with 16% in the control group. Although an intergroup statistically significant difference was not found, patients in the treatment group had a significant within-group increase in responder rate ($\geq$50% seizure frequency reduction) over time, whereas patients in the control group did not. The TNS side-effect profile is favorable: no major adverse events were reported in the controlled TNS trial, apart from a transient (only at week 6 follow-up) increase in heart rate in the treatment group. At the time of this writing, TNS is approved in Europe and Canada and is under investigation by the FDA for approval in the United States.

REPETITIVE TRANSCRANIAL MAGNETIC STIMULATION FOR SEIZURE SUPPRESSION

Therapeutic noninvasive brain-stimulation in epilepsy has been approached largely with two techniques: TMS and, to a lesser extent, tDCS. TMS is a method for focal noninvasive brain stimulation in which small intracranial electrical currents are induced by a fluctuating extracranial magnetic field that is typically generated by a hand-held electromagnet. Repetitive TMS (rTMS), at a low frequency (0.3–1 Hz) can induce a lasting reduction in cortical excitability and has plausible antiseizure therapeutic utility. As with other forms of brain stimulation, the mechanisms by which rTMS may reduce cortical excitability and suppress seizures are only partially understood, but they likely resemble those of use-dependent long-term depression (LTD) of excitatory synaptic strength that follow electrical low-frequency cortical stimulation.

Encouraging open-label trials show a potential for seizure reduction by rTMS when applied over the epileptogenic region, or even when applied in a neutral scalp location, such as over the vertex. The positive response of some patients to stimulation outside of the epileptogenic zone, and in one series a favorable response of patients with primary generalized seizures to rTMS, raises the possibility that the rTMS antiseizure mechanism is not just local suppression of intracortical excitability, but rather a network effect whereby excitability is modulated at sites distal to the locus of stimulation (Shafi et al., 2015).

In contrast to the open-label data, placebo-controlled rTMS trials have yielded inconsistent results. The first trial, in patients with temporal lobe epilepsy (TLE), did not reveal an antiseizure benefit in patients with TLE. A second trial showed a significant seizure reduction and improvement of the interictal EEG in patients with intractable seizures attributable to cortical dysplasia. The third, which investigated rTMS in a mixed group of patients with either focal or primary generalized seizures, found that rTMS was no better than placebo for seizure reduction but that active treatment significantly reduced interictal EEG epileptiform abnormalities. However, the most recent large, randomized, single-blinded, controlled clinical trial ($N = 60$) reveals a substantial effect: subjects randomized to a 2-week "high-intensity" treatment group (90% resting motor threshold, rMT; threshold to muscle activation) 0.5-Hz rTMS over the epileptogenic focus showed an 80% reduction in mean seizure frequency along with decreased interictal EEG discharges compared with the low-intensity (20% rMT) control group, with a mean seizure reduction of 2%. The antiseizure effects were relatively long-lasting and maintained up to 2 months after treatment.

The rTMS safety profile in the treatment of epilepsy is favorable. A 2007 review of the literature identified a crude per-subject seizure risk approximating 1.4% in patients with epilepsy undergoing rTMS. A subsequent case series also identified that in-session seizures during rTMS were most likely in patients whose seizure frequency exceeded one per day. The events were, in all instances, identical in semiology to a patient's typical seizures and were of either typical duration or shorter than a patient's native seizures. Further, any documented in-session seizures during rTMS thus far have not been correlated with a poor neurologic outcome or the absence of an rTMS response. Seizure exacerbation in patients with epilepsy by rTMS has not been recorded, and there are no instances of rTMS-provoked status epilepticus. The absence of reported seizure exacerbation appears to be a common finding independent of whether rTMS is administered interictally or during an ongoing seizure, as in epilepsia partialis continua (EPC). The incidence of the remaining rTMS-related adverse events (such as headache, neck pain, or tinnitus) is similar in patients with epilepsy to that which is described in healthy volunteers and in other patient populations. Last, rTMS appears to be safe and well tolerated in specialized populations with implanted VNS devices or with titanium skull plates, both of which are relatively prevalent in the population of patients with intractable seizures.

DIAGNOSTIC TRANSCRANIAL MAGNETIC STIMULATION

TMS is unique among the neurostimulation techniques that are used in epilepsy in its potential as either a diagnostic or a therapeutic tool. For instance, neuronavigated TMS (termed *nTMS* in some texts) is an FDA-approved method for noninvasive presurgical mapping of the motor and language cortices. Another TMS protocol, paired-pulse TMS (ppTMS) is a means to measure the cortical E:I ratio and is emerging as a technique to either track disease severity or to measure the therapeutic effect of an intervention.

In presurgical motor cortex mapping, TMS is applied over the motor cortex and coupled with surface electromyography (EMG) such that TMS elicits an evoked muscle contraction in a contralateral limb muscle that is quantified by skin electrodes and the recording of a motor evoked potential (MEP). During presurgical mapping, the TMS operator, guided by a patient's brain magnetic resonance imaging (MRI), can test whether stimulation of a specified brain region evokes an MEP from a specific muscle group. These data are then registered to the patient's MRI to generate a precise motor map where the spatial resolution approximates that which can be obtained by intraoperative monitoring of the MEP. In addition to motor mapping, TMS offers a unique tool for mapping the language cortex. For language mapping, repetitive stimulation is delivered in trains to potential cortical language areas while a subject performs a linguistic task, such as object naming, and the operator then identifies regions where stimulation interrupts the task performance.

In a more experimental diagnostic TMS role, measures of the cortical E:I ratio can be derived from the MEP. Among these is the threshold to muscle activation, or motor threshold (MT). The MT, which is obtained by single-pulse TMS, likely reflects neuronal membrane excitability and is increased by anticonvulsants, such as phenytoin and carbamazepine, that block voltage-gated sodium channels. Other measures can be obtained from ppTMS protocols, where stimuli are delivered as closely-spaced pairs and the cortical response to a single test stimulus is modulated by the preceding conditioning stimulus. With ppTMS, measures of γ-aminobutyric acid (GABA)-mediated cortical inhibition and glutamate-dependent cortical excitability can be quantified. These metrics are affected preferentially by GABA-ergic drugs such as barbiturates and benzodiazepines. Taken together, these TMS measures can detect abnormalities in the E:I ratio in patients with epilepsy. In particular, pathologic suppression of intracortical inhibition as detected by ppTMS appears to be a common finding in patients with epilepsy and may in some instances reflect disease severity. A shift in the E:I ratio toward excess excitation occurs in the preictal period in patients with epilepsy, suggesting prospects for TMS in identifying periods of seizure vulnerability that could allow for prognosticating the timing and likelihood of seizure. Another potentially useful application of TMS may be to measure whether antiseizure drug treatment has shifted the E:I ratio in a favorable direction, and thus predict seizure control (Badawy et al., 2010).

The capacity to probe the E:I ratio by TMS may address an important unmet need for patients undergoing antiseizure therapies for which there are limited biomarkers to guide dosing or to aid in the identification of a favorable therapeutic effect in advance of a change in seizure count. As noted earlier, VNS may lead to an increase in intracortical inhibition that can be detected by ppTMS. TMS-derived intracortical inhibition measures are also enhanced by the ketogenic diet. Although the clinical utility of these findings will have to be determined in controlled trials, these data indicate a potential for diagnostic TMS to guide existing treatments for epilepsy.

TRANSCRANIAL DIRECT CURRENT STIMULATION

tDCS modulates cortical activity by conductance of low-amplitude direct electrical current delivered through scalp electrodes. Applied to the mammalian cerebral cortex, cathodal tDCS induces a durable reduction in cortical excitability, whereas anodal tDCS increases excitability after a single session that typically lasts 20 to 30 minutes. In epilepsy, the capacity of cathodal tDCS to reduce cortical excitability has prompted research into this technique's potential. In contrast to other neurostimulation methods, tDCS amplitudes are insufficient to generate action potentials in the area of stimulated cortex, suggesting a mechanism of action reliant more upon modulation of ongoing neuronal activity than the induction of new neuronal activity.

The relatively low intracranial currents associated with tDCS likely, in part, account for its favorable safety profile. In contrast to other noninvasive neurostimulation techniques such as TMS, seizures have not been associated with tDCS in patients with epilepsy, and the remaining side effects are largely limited to skin irritation at the electrode sites. However, tDCS antiseizure efficacy and overall clinical utility in epilepsy are less established than in the aforementioned techniques.

Clinical tDCS data in epilepsy are limited, but a few reports suggest a realistic role for tDCS in seizure suppression. A randomized controlled study of adults with medically refractory epilepsy ($N = 19$) referable to malformations of cortical development found that interictal epileptiform discharges on EEG were reduced by 64% for 30 days after one 20-min application of 1-mA cathodal tDCS over the seizure focus. In a pediatric study ($N = 36$), children aged 6 to 15 years with refractory focal epilepsy were randomized to active (1-mA cathodal tDCS for 20 minutes) or sham control tDCS, in which current was applied only for 60 secs before the current was turned off. The results indicate that tDCS was well tolerated and corresponded to a significant decrease in the EEG spike frequency for up to 48 hours after stimulation. Clinical seizure reduction in this cohort was small (about 5%) but also statistically significant, supporting continued efforts to test whether multiple tDCS courses will result in a meaningful antiseizure effect.

The incomplete knowledge of the efficacy of human tDCS trials underscores the need for further preclinical studies that will help to inform future clinical tDCS study designs. Published reports using cathodal tDCS in animal epilepsy models show increased seizure threshold in focal electroshock and amygdala seizure kindling models. In an additional study, 7 days of cathodal tDCS treatment 1 day after pilocarpine-induced status epilepticus was shown to have an antiseizure and neuroprotective effect in rat pups. In a more recent experiment, cathodal tDCS was tested in the acute seizure setting that approximates status epilepticus to assess an immediate anticonvulsant effect. Electrographic seizure suppression was seen within minutes of stimulation in a rat pentylenetetrazole status epilepticus model. Of translational relevance for future clinical application, cathodal tDCS in this experiment worked synergistically with lorazepam to suppress seizures. These data indicate an important direction for neuromodulation research toward systematic testing of combination drug–device therapy in epilepsy (Dhamne et al., 2015).

CONCLUSION

Given the incomplete efficacy of pharmacotherapy in epilepsy, the prospects for neuromodulation to play a significant role in patient management are rapidly improving. As with many technologies reliant on electronics, the neuromodulation tools available to patients, physicians, and investigators are growing in abundance and are maturing in sophistication. Among these evolving protocols are established techniques such as VNS, techniques repurposed specifically for epilepsy such as DBS, and emerging technologies such as RNS and noninvasive brain stimulation. Novel neurostimulation tools are likely to be added to this short list in the future.

REFERENCES

The complete list of references for this chapter is available in the e-book at www.expertconsult.com.

See inside cover for registration details.

SELECTED REFERENCES

Badawy, R.A., et al., 2010. Predicting seizure control: cortical excitability and antiepileptic medication. Ann. Neurol. 67 (1), 64–73.

DeGiorgio, C.M., et al., 2013. Randomized controlled trial of trigeminal nerve stimulation for drug-resistant epilepsy. Neurology 80 (9), 786–791.

Dhamne, S.C., et al., 2015. Acute seizure suppression by transcranial direct current stimulation in rats. Ann. Clin. Transl. Neurol. 2 (8), 843–856.

Fisher, R., et al., 2010. Electrical stimulation of the anterior nucleus of thalamus for treatment of refractory epilepsy. Epilepsia 51 (5), 899–908.

Handforth, A., et al., 1998. Vagus nerve stimulation therapy for partial-onset seizures: a randomized active-control trial. Neurology 51 (1), 48–55.

Krishna, V., et al., 2016. Neuromodulation for Epilepsy. Neurosurg. Clin. N. Am. 27 (1), 123–131.

Loscher, W., Schmidt, D., 2011. Modern antiepileptic drug development has failed to deliver: ways out of the current dilemma. Epilepsia 52 (4), 657–678.

Morrell, M.J., R.N.S.S.i.E.S.RNS System in Epilepsy Study Group, 2011. Responsive cortical stimulation for the treatment of medically intractable partial epilepsy. Neurology 77 (13), 1295–1304.

Salanova, V., et al., 2015. Long-term efficacy and safety of thalamic stimulation for drug-resistant partial epilepsy. Neurology 84 (10), 1017–1025.

Shafi, M.M., et al., 2015. Physiological consequences of abnormal connectivity in a developmental epilepsy. Ann. Neurol. 77 (3), 487–503.

80 Ketogenic Diets

James W. Wheless and Eric H. Kossoff

An expanded version of this chapter is available on www.expertconsult.com. See inside cover for registration details.

Antiseizure medicines are the primary treatment modality and provide good seizure control in most children. However, more than 25% of children with epilepsy have either intractable seizures or suffer treatment-limiting adverse medication effects. Only a limited number of these children are candidates for surgical therapy. In addition, uncontrolled seizures pose a variety of risks to children, including higher rates of mortality, accidents, and injuries, as well as a greater incidence of cognitive and psychiatric impairment, poorer self-esteem, higher levels of anxiety and depression, and social stigmatization or isolation.

Thus effective treatment to control seizures is fundamental to improving overall outcome in childhood epilepsy. The ketogenic diet has proven to be an effective treatment for many children (and adults) with epilepsy (Kim and Rho, 2008; Neal et al., 2009; Stafstrom and Rho, 2004). In this chapter, the history of the development of the diet, current understanding of the biochemistry of ketone body formation and its relation to the anticonvulsant effect of the diet, considerations related to patient selection, and diet efficacy, complications, advantages, and disadvantages are reviewed.

HISTORY

For centuries, fasting has been used to treat many diseases, including seizures; it was even used in biblical times (Wheless, 2004). Dr. Russell Wilder at the Mayo Clinic suggested in 1921 that a diet high in fat and low in carbohydrates could maintain ketosis and its accompanying acidosis longer than fasting and be maintained indefinitely. Wilder was also the first to coin the term "ketogenic diet." The beneficial effects of this diet were initially recorded by investigators from Johns Hopkins University, the Mayo Clinic, and Harvard University. Until 1938, the ketogenic diet was one of the few available therapies for epilepsy, but it fell into disfavor when researchers turned their attention to the development of new antiseizure medicines. The ketogenic diet was also perceived as expensive, difficult-to-maintain, and less "modern" in many ways compared with drugs. Use of the ketogenic diet decreased greatly until it received national media attention in the mid-1990s. The creation of the Charlie Foundation (www.charliefoundation .org) in 1994 by a parent of a child with epilepsy successfully treated with the diet has led to significant research and use. The year 2008 was an important one in the history of the ketogenic diet. Two randomized, controlled studies (one double-blinded) were published demonstrating efficacy of this approach. In addition, a consensus statement from 26 dietitians and neurologists at worldwide ketogenic diet centers was published in *Epilepsia* to help guide clinical management of ketogenic diet patients.

EFFICACY
Efficacy of the Classic Ketogenic Diet

Initial reports began to appear in the 1920s and 1930s that documented the efficacy of the ketogenic diet. Over the next 60 to 70 years, many more clinical reports appeared (Lefevre and Aronson, 2000; Levy and Cooper, 2003). About one-half of children appear to have had an excellent response to the diet, defined by cessation or marked reduction (a greater than 50% reduction) in seizure activity. About 15% of children become seizure-free after initiation of the ketogenic diet and typically stop the diet after 2 years. Of those children who become seizure-free, a minority have recurrence after the diet is stopped. Risk factors that increase the likelihood of recurrence are epileptiform abnormalities on electroencephalograms (EEGs) obtained within 12 months of diet discontinuation, a focal abnormality on magnetic resonance imaging (MRI), lower initial seizure frequency, and tuberous sclerosis complex. Younger children as well as adolescents and adults do well on the diet.

In a 2010 single-center report, 104 infants (mean age 1.2 years) were started on the diet for mostly symptomatic and very refractory infantile spasms (mean 3.6 anticonvulsants tried). Nearly two-thirds (64%) had a greater than 50% spasm reduction, including one-third with at least 6 months of spasm freedom and EEG improvement. Those who were older age and had tried fewer anticonvulsants when the diet was started did better.

The diet may also be helpful for Dravet syndrome (severe myoclonic epilepsy of infancy). As part of the Korean multi-centered experience, Kang and associates retrospectively reviewed efficacy in 49 infants treated with the ketogenic diet. Only 1 of 14 children with severe myoclonic epilepsy of infancy was seizure-free at 12 months, but 56% had a greater than 50% seizure reduction. Caraballo and colleagues reported similar results, with 10% seizure-free and 55% achieving a greater than 50% seizure reduction at 12 months.

There have been several large studies demonstrating efficacy with the ketogenic diet. The first multicenter prospective study of the efficacy of the ketogenic diet was based on data collected at seven comprehensive epilepsy centers. All children in this study had intractable epilepsy, averaging 230 seizures per month. It was found that 10% of treated patients were seizure-free at 1 year. A greater than 50% decrease in seizure frequency was observed at 3 months in 54% of patients. This improvement was maintained at 6 months (53% controlled) and 12 months (49% controlled) after initiation of the diet. Patient age, seizure type, and EEG abnormalities were not related to outcome. Approximately 47% remained on the diet for at least 1 year. Reasons for discontinuation included insufficient seizure control, intolerable side effects, concurrent medical illnesses, or inability to tolerate the restrictive nature of the dietary regimen. Although the number of patients was small, the study demonstrated that the diet could be used effectively in different epilepsy centers with different support staff and that children and their families were able to comply with the diet when it was effective.

One of the largest prospective evaluations of the ketogenic diet was conducted in 150 consecutive children aged 1 to 16 years (mean age 5.3 years) (Freeman et al., 1998; Hemingway et al., 2001). The children were followed for a minimum of 1 year, had previously been on an average of 6.24 medications, and were on a mean of 1.97 medications at the diet's initiation. Seventy percent of children had an intelligence or developmental quotient of lower than 69. The children averaged 410 seizures per month before the ketogenic diet. At 6 months, 71% remained on the diet, and 32% had a greater than 90% decrease in seizures. At 1 year, 55% remained on the diet, 7% were seizure-free, and 27% had a greater than 90% decrease in seizure frequency. There was no statistically significant difference in seizure control based on age, sex, or seizure type, although none of the patients had only focal seizures. Most of those discontinuing the diet did so because it was either insufficiently effective or too restrictive.

A randomized controlled trial of the ketogenic diet was performed in children aged 2 to 16 years. Children with various seizure types or epilepsy syndromes experiencing daily seizures were recruited. They were randomly assigned to receive the ketogenic diet immediately (n = 73), or after a 3-month delay, with no other changes in their treatment (n = 72, control group). Children were also randomly assigned to the classic or the MCT ketogenic diet. After 3 months, the percentage of patients with baseline numbers of seizures despite treatment was significantly lower (p <0.0001) in the diet group (62%) than in the controls. The children in the diet group had a mean of 13.3 seizures per day at baseline; after 3 months of treatment, 1 was seizure-free, 28 (38%) had a greater than 50% reduction in seizures, and 5 (7%) had a greater than 90% reduction. Efficacy was the same for symptomatic generalized or symptomatic focal epilepsies. The most common adverse events were constipation, vomiting, lack of energy, and hunger.

The same authors reported on the 1-year follow-up of those children randomized to the classic or MCT versions of the ketogenic diet. Of the 125 children who started the diets, data from 64 were available at 6 months and from 47 at 12 months. At 12 months, there was no significant difference between groups in the number of patients achieving greater than 50% (17.8 versus 22.2%) or 90% (9.6 versus 9.7%) seizure reduction. There was no significant difference in tolerability of the diet, except increased reports of lack of energy after 3 months, and vomiting after 12 months, both in the classical group.

Efficacy of the Ketogenic Diet for Adults

Many early studies and now several recent studies have evaluated use of the ketogenic diet in adults. Some revealed improved seizure control, but several reports have also concluded that the diet is not particularly beneficial in adolescents and adults with epilepsy. Reasons cited for this were poor dietary compliance, types of seizures seen in these age groups, and the developmental differences in the ability of the brain to use ketone bodies. Mady and associates reviewed their experience with 45 adolescents who had been on the ketogenic diet for an average duration of 1.2 years. They found no evidence to support the belief that the diet was not efficacious and was too restrictive in this age group. Adolescents with multiple seizure types did best, and those with simple and complex partial seizures had the poorest response. The retention rate for motivated adolescents on the diet was not significantly different than reports in younger children.

Efficacy of Alternative Ketogenic Diets

In recent years, two alternative diet regimens that are less restrictive and perhaps more palatable have emerged: the modified Atkins diet and a low glycemic index treatment (Fig. 80-1). The modified Atkins diet is similar in fat composition to a 1 to 1 ketogenic ratio (grams of fat to protein and carbohydrate combined) diet, with approximately 65% of the calories from fat sources; it can be started as an outpatient, with guidance from a nutritionist. It is started without a fast or admission, and carbohydrates are limited to 10 to 20 grams per day. Parents and patients are instructed to count carbohydrates (by reading food labels and carb-counting guides) in comparison to the weighing and measuring of foods typically used for the classic ketogenic diet. Protein, calories, and fluids are unlimited.

Subsequent studies in over 450 children, adolescents, and adults reveal that 45% have a 50% to 90% seizure reduction, and slightly over 25% have a greater than 90% seizure reduction (Table 80-5).

The low glycemic index diet includes approximately 20% to 30% of calories from protein and 60% to 70% from fat. Total carbohydrates are gradually decreased to 40 to 60 g/day (about 10% of calories), using foods with a low glycemic index. In a retrospective review of 76 children on the low glycemic index diet, there was a greater than 50% seizure reduction from baseline seizure frequency in 42%, 50%, 54%, 64%, and 66% of the group at follow-up intervals of 1, 3, 6, 9, and 12 months, respectively. Efficacy did not differ between partial onset and generalized seizure types. Increased efficacy was correlated with lower serum glucose levels at the 1-month and 12-month follow-up visits. Side effects were minimal, with only three patients reporting transient lethargy.

MECHANISMS OF ACTION

Although clinical reports support the efficacy of the ketogenic diet, several theories have emerged to explain the diet's mechanism of action. Four major areas have been investigated: cerebral acidosis; water balance; the direct effect of ketones or lipids; and alteration in brain energy substrates. The importance of ketone body formation was recognized early in the search for the mechanism of action of the ketogenic diet. Animal models and human evidence suggest a prominent role of ketonemia. Despite its long history of use and proven value, the exact mechanism of action of the diet remains unknown.

Oxidation of Fatty Acids: Ketogenesis

Ketonemia is essential for the ketogenic diet to work. Ketonemia occurs as a result of fatty acid oxidation during fasting or when on the ketogenic diet. Fatty acid biosynthesis (lipogenesis) takes place in the cytosol, whereas fatty acid oxidation occurs in mitochondria and generates adenosine triphosphate (ATP). The brain does not directly use fatty acids but readily oxidizes ketone bodies. Increased fatty acid oxidation leading to ketone body formation by the liver is characteristic of the ketogenic diet. Glucose, present in small concentrations, is necessary to facilitate ketone body metabolism. Acetoacetate, a ketone body constituent, continually undergoes spontaneous decarboxylation to yield acetone that is volatilized in the lungs and gives the breath a characteristic odor.

The liver is the only organ capable of synthesizing significant quantities of ketone bodies that are released into the blood (see Fig. 80-3). Once formed, acetoacetate cannot be significantly metabolized back to fatty acids in the liver because it lacks the enzyme 3-oxoacid-CoA transferase. This accounts for the net production of ketone bodies by the liver. Ketone bodies are then transported to and oxidized in extrahepatic tissues proportionately to their concentration in the blood. Oxidation and brain influx rates of ketone bodies are proportional to their blood concentration of approximately 12 mmol/L. At this level, the oxidative machinery and uptake mechanisms of the cell are saturated.

Glucose is the principal substrate for brain metabolism. Under certain conditions (e.g., ketogenic diet), the human brain uses ketone bodies for fuel; the movement of ketone bodies into the brain is dependent on a monocarboxylic transport system. Acetoacetate and β-hydroxybutyrate (BHB), the two constituents of ketone bodies, are metabolized primarily in the mitochondrial compartment. In the brain, the main pathway for the conversion of acetoacetate to acetoacetyl-CoA involves succinyl-CoA. Acetoacetyl-CoA is split to acetyl-CoA and oxidized in the tricarboxylic acid cycle. Ketone bodies not only serve as a source of energy but also contribute to the synthesis of the neurotransmitters, glutamate and gamma-aminobutyric acid (GABA), and cerebral metabolic pathways normally dependent on glucose metabolism. Furthermore, fatty acid oxidation increases brain ATP concentration. Elevation of brain ATP concentration has been verified in an animal model of the ketogenic diet, suggesting that the ketogenic diet improves cerebral energetics. Increased alpha-ketoglutarate on the diet may also increase activity of the GABA shunt. Thus improved cerebral energetics, along with decreased excitatory (glutamatergic) and increased inhibitory (GABAergic) neurotransmission, may contribute to the efficacy of the ketogenic diet.

Clinical Studies of Ketosis

Ketonemia is necessary but not sufficient for ketogenic diet-induced seizure control. Urine ketones are commonly measured due to ease of testing and cost (versus fingerstick blood BHB meters) and typically the desired range is 80 to 160 mmol/L (large). Seizure control correlates significantly ($p = 0.03$) with serum BHB levels greater than 4 mmol/L, although urine ketones of 160 mmol/L can be found when blood BHB levels exceed 2 mmol/L. Anecdotally, there are many children with fluctuating or low levels of BHB who maintain excellent seizure control, which has also been noted in studies of the modified Atkins diet and low glycemic index treatment. When using these latter two therapies, ketones may even be completely absent despite seizure control. Freeman and associates evaluated serum BHB levels of 35 children 3 months after diet initiation. There was a significant correlation between higher levels of BHB and seizure control. The mean serum BHB level in patients with greater than 90% seizure control was over 6 mM.

It is also accepted that the classic ketogenic diet produces the most ketone bodies. Ketones from the circulation are transported across the blood-brain barrier by facilitated diffusion, using a monocarboxylate transport system. The efficacy of the diet in childhood and the slightly lower efficacy in older children, and adults may be due to maturational changes in this transport system. A child's ability to extract ketones from the blood into the brain is 4 to 5 times greater than that seen in adults. MR spectroscopy has also been used to study changes in cerebral energetics induced by the ketogenic diet. Alteration of tricarboxylic acid cycle activity by ketosis, resulting in an increased adenosine triphosphate to adenosine diphosphate (ATP to ADP) ratio or greater cerebral energy, has been hypothesized to have an anticonvulsant effect. This hypothesis is supported by recent experiments in patients with Lennox-Gastaut syndrome that used MR spectroscopy (31P) to document improvement in cerebral energy metabolism on the ketogenic diet.

Additionally, during chronic ketosis, adaptive mechanisms are active that increase the cerebral extraction of ketone bodies. These mechanisms may be why ketosis develops promptly within several days after initiation of the diet, but the anticonvulsant effect may be delayed for 1 to 2 weeks. Once ketone bodies are extracted, it is postulated that there is a secondary biochemical change or a cascade of biochemical effects that has some form of anticonvulsant effect.

Experimental Studies of Diets in Animal Models

At the present time, there are several animal models used to study the effects of the ketogenic diet. One of the most effective to demonstrate the diet's antiseizure effects is the 6-Hz model for inducing seizures. In general, these animal models demonstrate that the ketogenic diet provides protection for partial-onset seizures with secondary generalization and generalized myoclonic, tonic, and tonic-clonic seizures. The mechanism appears to be a lowering of neuronal excitability and a raising of seizure threshold.

A limited number of animal studies have investigated the effect of age at diet onset versus efficacy. The diet provides a greater level of seizure protection in younger animals, but older animals also demonstrate an elevated seizure threshold. Although it would seem intuitive that increasing ketonemia would correlate with diet efficacy, experimental studies have not revealed a positive correlation. However, rats that developed higher levels of ketosis also showed higher thresholds for seizure induction. Caloric restriction can significantly influence seizure threshold and augment the effects of the ketogenic diet on seizure control. Animal data support the hypothesis that a ketogenic diet enhances brain metabolism. Several animal models provide evidence that the ketogenic diet can prevent epileptogenesis and mediate neuroprotection. These studies also support the clinical observation that children can be gradually weaned off the ketogenic diet, resume a normal diet, and not experience loss of seizure control.

SELECTION OF CANDIDATES FOR THE DIET

Many seizure types appear to respond to the ketogenic diet, but children with atonic seizures seem to particularly benefit. In general, however, several groups of children are widely accepted as potential candidates for treatment (Kossoff et al., 2009). These include the following groups:

1. Those with medically intractable seizures (failed at least two anticonvulsant drugs)
2. Those with poor tolerance of or significant side effects from antiseizure medicines
3. Those with intractable seizures who are being considered for epilepsy surgery (i.e., callosotomy; nonlesional, extratemporal resections)
4. Those with specific neurometabolic disorders or neurologic syndromes (Box 80-1)

The ketogenic diet is a strictly regulated medical diet. Its success depends on the accuracy and consistency with which the regimen is carried out within the home. Continued support, monitoring, and education by an interdisciplinary team of professionals are necessary.

Approximately 20 years ago, the only metabolic disorders that were indications for use of the ketogenic diet were GLUT-1 deficiency syndrome and PDH (pyruvate dehydrogenase deficiency). Today, there are numerous other "indications" for the diet, and these potential candidates should be referred sooner in the course of their epilepsy. Table 80-1 of the 2009 expert consensus statement lists these conditions.

The ketogenic diet may be the preferred initial therapy in children with seizures and specific metabolic defects or seizures associated with specific neurologic syndromes (see Box 80-1 and Fig. 80-5). These specific metabolic disorders are reviewed in other sections of this book.

For some patients, the ketogenic diet is contraindicated (Box 80-2). When indicated, metabolic screens, including urine amino and organic acids, serum amino acids, lactate,

---

BOX 80-1 Specific Conditions Treated With the Ketogenic Diet

- Glucose transporter deficiency syndrome (GLUT1-DS, *SLC2A1* gene, McKusick 138140)*
- Pyruvate dehydrogenase complex deficiency (McKusick 312170)*
- Infantile spasms
- Myoclonic-astatic epilepsy (Doose syndrome)
- Severe myoclonic epilepsy of infancy (Dravet syndrome)
- Associated with Leigh's syndrome
- Associated with lactic acidosis and cerebral dysgenesis
- Succinic semialdehyde dehydrogenase (SSADH) deficiency†
- Phosphofructokinase deficiency
- Mitochondrial respiratory chain complex defects
- Ketotic hypoglycemia
- Glycogenosis type V (McArdle disease)
- Acquired epileptic aphasia (Landau-Kleffner syndrome)
- Rett syndrome
- Tuberous sclerosis complex

*The ketogenic diet is specifically indicated for these two metabolic disorders.
†Documented improvement in mouse model.

BOX 80-2 Specific Contraindications to the Ketogenic Diet

- Pyruvate carboxylase deficiency
- Organic acidurias
- Selected mitochondrial disease
- Porphyria
- Defects in fatty acid oxidation
  - Short-chain acyl dehydrogenase deficiency (SCAD)
  - Medium-chain acyl dehydrogenase deficiency (MCAD)
  - Long-chain acyl dehydrogenase deficiency (LCAD)
  - Medium-chain 3-hydroxyacyl CoA deficiency
  - Long-chain 3-hydroxyacyl CoA deficiency
- Carnitine deficiency (primary)
- Carnitine palmitoyltransferase (CPT) I or II deficiency
- Carnitine translocase deficiency
- Glutaric aciduria, type II
- Pyruvate dehydrogenase phosphate deficiency

BOX 80-3 Initiation of the Ketogenic Diet (Johns Hopkins Hospital Protocol)

HOSPITALIZATION FOR 3 DAYS

Day 1
- Maintenance fluids without glucose
- Check urine ketones each void
- Check fingerstick blood glucose every 6 hr
- Simplify antiseizure medicine regimen; change to low carbohydrate or carbohydrate-free formulation
- Dietitian consultation
- Education
- After 12 to 24 hour fast, typically 5pm, begin ketogenic diet at half total daily calories using 4 : 1 ratio (3 : 1 in infants), with food as an eggnog or formula

Day 2
- 4 : 1 ratio (3 : 1 in infants), with one-half of total calories using eggnog for additional 2 meals then with dinner advance to full calories and a solid food meal
- Stop fingerstick blood glucose checks
- Continue education

Day 3
- Breakfast and lunch using typical ketogenic diet meals
- Ensure all medication prescriptions are provided and follow-up appointment made
- Discharge home

---

pyruvate, and carnitine profile, should be performed before starting the ketogenic diet. Lastly, children who do not have assured, stable nutrition should not be started on the ketogenic diet due to risk of malnutrition and/or weight loss. In many of these patients, the ketogenic diet is only recommended after a gastrostomy tube has been placed.

Value of the EEG in Ketogenic Diet Prediction

The predictive value of an EEG obtained before, during, or after initiation of the ketogenic diet is unknown. In a cohort of 29 children, 90% of children with normal pretreatment EEGs responded favorably to the diet, compared with only 12% with abnormal pretreatment EEGs.

Many studies have suggested improvement or normalization of the EEG after the diet has been implemented. A recent study showed that improvement in background slowing (described as "encephalopathy") after starting the diet was correlated with a greater than 95% seizure reduction, although surprisingly fewer interictal spikes was not. Kang and associ-

ates showed improvement in generalized epileptiform abnormalities more often than focal epileptiform discharges and a correlation between seizure control and EEG improvement. Caraballo also reported improvement in the EEG epileptiform abnormalities in children responding to the diet. In the randomized, double-blind study of the ketogenic diet, clinical seizure reduction and EEG improvements were quite different, especially for Lennox-Gastaut syndrome.

INITIATION AND MAINTENANCE

A comprehensive book on the evaluation and management of patients being considered for placement on the ketogenic diet has been published and subsequently revised in 2011. In addition, a videotape, "The Ketogenic Diet for Families, Dietitians, Nurses, and Physicians," and other resource material are available from The Charlie Foundation (www.charliefoundation.org). Of importance, the manner in which the ketogenic diet is started can be highly variable, and yet maintain efficacy. The following is a brief overview of how the diet can be implemented.

Prehospital Evaluation

Once a child is considered a candidate for the diet, a screening evaluation by selected members of the team responsible for implementing the diet is initiated (e.g., dietitian, physician, nurse). The purpose of this evaluation is to educate the family and to assess their ability, on many levels, to carry out the rigorous and exacting program necessary to maximize the diet's success. At the same time, the different types of meal plans and foods that the child can eat are discussed, along with their preparation.

Hospitalization

The child is typically scheduled for elective admission to the hospital for initiation of the diet (Box 80-3). However, in recent years, both retrospective and prospective studies have documented the feasibility of initiating the diet as an outpatient. The intense educational process afforded by inpatient initiation may be preferable for some families and ketogenic diet centers; it also may allow the families to have medications carefully reviewed, spend additional time with their treating neurologist familiarizing him/her with the epilepsy, and also to meet other families starting the diet at the same time (if admissions are done in a group). Additionally, inpatient initiation allows observation of the child to gauge the initial response to and the adverse effects of the diet. Parents are told to view this treatment as a 2 to 3 month trial. When effective, the ketogenic diet works quickly, typically within the first 1 to 2 weeks. If there is no seizure reduction after 3 months, the ketogenic diet can be discontinued. During this time, patients must adhere strictly to the diet, with proof of persistent ketosis. The frequency of seizures usually decreases gradually, but reversal of the effect may occur rapidly if the child cheats with carbohydrate-containing foods. If the seizures are improved, this usually is sufficient motivation for the parents to have the child adhere to the diet. If the child might have an underlying metabolic disease that could be exacerbated by the initial fast, an appropriate evaluation should be performed before initiating the diet.

The day before hospital admission, after dinner, the child begins fasting, with only noncaloric, noncaffeinated beverages given. Laboratory studies (complete blood count, platelet count, chemistry panel, fasting lipid profile, and antiseizure medicine levels) are obtained, either preferably a week before or at the time of admission. During this time, the child receives maintenance fluids but no foods (if fasting). Fingerstick glucose levels are checked every 6 hours. The dietitian uses this time for further review of meal plans and the child's food preferences and eating habits with the parents. Recent studies have suggested no improvement in long-term seizure control with initial fasting or fluid restriction, and fewer adverse events with a nonfasting, gradual initiation.

On the first night of admission, the child is started on the ketogenic diet, using a 3 to 1 or 4 to 1 ratio (grams of fat to protein plus carbohydrate), depending on the child's age. A ketogenic eggnog or premade formula (several are in use) is often used for the initial feedings. The child receives three meals at one-half of the total calories on the second day and then is advanced as tolerated to full calories with solid foods on the final day. Before discharge, the parents may prepare their first ketogenic meal for their child under the supervision of the dietitian. At discharge, the parents have several meal plans for their child and are instructed to monitor the urine ketones on a daily basis and record all occurrences of seizures. Individual decisions are made during the hospital stay as to whether the antiseizure medicine regimen will be simplified. The child is given a prescription for sugar-free multivitamin, mineral, and calcium supplementation and instructed to begin this at home. Oral citrates are often prescribed empirically as well. Vitamin B supplements are given to prevent optic nerve dysfunction. Vitamin D supplementation and calcium prevent osteomalacia while on the ketogenic diet. The child is then seen regularly (typically every 3 months) for follow-up (Box 80-4). Special attention should be paid to the serum albumin and total protein concentration to make sure that the diet is providing enough protein. Cholesterol and triglyceride levels typically rise when the diet is started but usually decrease after several months and return to normal. It is not unusual to see minor elevations in the direct bilirubin.

Decisions regarding withdrawal of antiseizure medicines depend on the child's response to the diet and the family's wishes. Early reduction (during diet initiation or the first month afterward) of antiseizure medicines appears to be safe

---

> **BOX 80-4** Ketogenic Diet Maintenance
>
> **1 MONTH**
> - Adjust diet as needed
> - Laboratory tests—complete blood count (CBC), platelets; SMA20; medication level(s); fasting lipid profile, serum lipid and carnitine profiles
> - Clinic appointment with neurologist and dietitian for infants and other children (as necessary)
>
> **3, 6, 9, AND 12 MONTHS**
> - Neurologist, dietitian, nurse
> - Laboratory tests—CBC, platelets, SMA20; fasting lipid profile, serum lipid and carnitine profiles
> - Antiseizure medicine level(s)
> - Discussion about relative risk/benefit of ketogenic diet (consider wean at 1–2 years)

---

and well tolerated; however, it offers no definite advantage compared with a late taper. Benzodiazepines and phenobarbital are associated with a higher risk of seizure recurrence so should be tapered carefully. At follow-up, the dietitian also reviews the parental concerns about implementing the diet and makes adjustments in the meal plan, as necessary, to maintain the child in maximum ketosis. There are other methods to "fine tune" the ketogenic diet including ratio changes, calorie adjustment, fasting, and so forth, although the likelihood of improvement with these diet modifications is approximately 1 in 5.

In children who can be successfully withdrawn from antiseizure medicine therapy and are seizure-free for 2 years on the ketogenic diet (about 10% of treated children), an EEG is repeated and the ketogenic diet is slowly withdrawn. A study of 183 children in whom the diet was discontinued determined that the speed of the wean did not matter: children tapered over several weeks did just as well as those in whom the diet was stopped more slowly. Children in whom there was a good, but not complete, seizure reduction with the diet (50% to 99% seizure reduction) were at highest risk for seizure worsening with the diet discontinuation. Should seizures worsen, many of these families elect to continue a low-carbohydrate diet versus new anticonvulsants.

SIDE EFFECTS

It needs to be emphasized to parents and patients that the diet is a form of medical therapy, and as such, although it is relatively safe, it is not without side effects (Box 80-5). However, only 6% to 17% of patients discontinue the diet due to side effects; the vast majority are either treatable or even preventable. If the child has an unrecognized metabolic defect, a catastrophic event could occur during the fasting phase (see Box 80-2). Other adverse events can occur during the initial hospital stay, and, if recognized, are usually treatable. A number of side effects can occur during the maintenance phase. The most common side effect encountered is constipation. Renal stones have occurred in less than 5% to 10% of patients and can usually be easily managed. The risk of stone formation may be increased in younger patients (younger than 3 years of age) and those with hypercalciuria and low urine volume. Oral potassium citrate as a preventative supplement results in urine alkalization, decreasing the prevalence of kidney stones. Universal potassium citrate supplementation appears to be warranted.

Acetazolamide, topiramate, and zonisamide, as well as all carbonic anhydrase inhibitors, which, when combined with

---

BOX 80-5 Possible Adverse Events During Initiation of the Ketogenic Diet

Adverse Event	Monitoring/Treatment Strategy
• Dehydration	• Encourage fluids (do not limit fluids to less than 75% of maintenance); intravenous fluids if necessary (without dextrose)
• Hypoglycemia	• Check blood sugars every 6 hr until diet is initiated; if symptomatic or blood sugar <30 mg/dl, give small amount (e.g., 1–2 oz) orange juice. Screen for metabolic errors in advance
• Vomiting	• Intravenous fluids; give orange juice

---

the ketogenic diet, predispose to metabolic acidosis. The ketogenic diet can be cautiously initiated in children on these drugs. However, the physician should be aware that, in some children, this may cause worsening of their metabolic acidosis, especially during ketogenic diet initiation and may require adjustments in the drug dose, adjustments in the diet, or the addition of oral citrates.

Fatigue occurs in many children during initiation of the diet but is prolonged in only a small number. The high fat content decreases gastric emptying, which promotes gastroesophageal reflux. This problem usually can be managed medically. Close attention to growth measurements, laboratory data, and medical supervision is indicated in infants on the ketogenic diet. Very young children (0 to 2 years) grew poorly on the diet, whereas older children (7 to 10 years) grew almost normally. A recent study of children who discontinued the diet years prior suggests that growth will catch up once the diet is discontinued.

Several laboratory abnormalities have been reported in children on the ketogenic diet, although none has been found to have clinical significance. Patients on the ketogenic diet are in a chronic acidotic state, putting them at risk for osteopenia. A single longitudinal study has evaluated the effect of the ketogenic diet on bone density, serum hydroxy vitamin D, and parathyroid hormone. A progressive loss of bone mineral content, resulting in osteopenia and osteoporosis, occurred with ketogenic diet treatment, despite improved serum vitamin D concentrations. Supplementation of vitamin D and calcium was not sufficient to prevent bone mineral content loss. Increased supplementation and periodic surveillance with dual energy x-ray absorptiometry may be needed to prevent or treat the loss of bone mineral content in children treated with the ketogenic diet. This compensated metabolic acidosis puts the young child, who becomes ill, at risk of becoming markedly acidotic, ketotic, or dehydrated. This can be addressed by forewarning parents to increase fluid intake during illness. Serum cholesterol and triglycerides may increase, especially during the first 6 months; they tend to plateau by 6 months, then decline and require routine monitoring. Patients on the diet and undergoing surgery should be evaluated for symptoms of bleeding tendency. Changes in the serum carnitine concentrations have also been described. Some believe a carnitine supplement should be given routinely, but this is highly debatable. Carnitine status should be monitored, although most children do not need supplementation. Supplementation with magnesium, zinc, calcium, vitamin D, and B vitamins is recommended to avoid deficiency-related disease states. The ketogenic diet is deficient in several

trace minerals, and if children are maintained on the diet for more than 2 years, these need to be supplemented.

Serious complications of the ketogenic diet are rare and typically have only been described in single case reports, including the occurrence of Fanconi renal tubular acidosis (in cotreatment with valproate), severe hypoproteinemia, marked increase in liver function tests (in cotreatment with valproate), cardiomyopathy, prolonged QTc, acute hemorrhagic pancreatitis, basal ganglia injury, scurvy, lipoid pneumonia, and fatal propofol infusion syndrome. Selenium deficiency has been described with increasing frequency and some advocate for additional supplementation beyond standard multivitamins.

A single retrospective chart review reports maintenance of efficacy and tolerability with long-term use of the ketogenic diet (duration of 6 to 12 years, n = 28). The diet was well-tolerated after 6 years with maintained efficacy and little effect on serum cholesterol values. However, side effects of decreased growth (23 out of 28), kidney stones (7 out of 28), and fractures (6 out of 28) occurred; therefore careful monitoring with strategies to minimize these complications is suggested.

The ketogenic diet field is moving in the direction of adding vitamins and supplements empirically to the regimen of all children on the diet to prevent adverse effects before they occur. Although not mentioned in the 2009 consensus statement, many now advocate for universal treatment with oral citrates, selenium, extra vitamin D, laxatives, and even antacids. Several nutrition companies have created products that are designed for ketogenic diet patients such as NanoVM™ and FruitiVits™. Continued research into preventative supplements is warranted.

ADVANTAGES (AND DISADVANTAGES) COMPARED WITH OTHER TREATMENTS FOR EPILEPSY

Advantages

The ketogenic diet has several advantages compared with other medical therapies. Anecdotal reports have indicated that many of the children who are maintained on the diet are able to have their antiseizure medicines decreased or withdrawn. This usually results in the child being more alert and exhibiting better behavior. However, even children whose medications cannot be substantially lowered or withdrawn may have marked behavioral or cognitive improvements. This has occurred in children who have become seizure-free on the diet and had antiseizure medicines withdrawn, as well as in those whose seizures are only minimally improved and who have not had dramatic changes in their medication regimen.

For many families, the ketogenic diet provides a dramatic change in their role in the treatment of their children's epilepsy. The requirement for preparation and monitoring gives the parents an active role in the treatment of their children and a sense that what they are doing is directly influencing their children's epilepsy and psychosocial well-being. Only if the diet is ineffective can this become a disadvantage.

Disadvantages

The most common reasons cited for discontinuation of the ketogenic diet are lack of efficacy, complications, noncompliance (especially in older children), and caregiver concerns. The ketogenic diet is a strictly regulated medical diet that requires an epilepsy team for success. It requires active participation by the parents and children. The work required on the part of the parents to initiate and maintain this rigorous diet may be considered a disadvantage.

The costs of ketogenic diet foods (especially dairy and meats) may be more expensive than that eaten previously (e.g., rice and grains). This is an issue as the diet is being expanded to developing countries.

Many physicians perceive the diet as unpalatable and difficult to initiate and maintain. However, modern nutritional labeling requirements and the use of computer programs allow the dietitian to construct a palatable diet, keeping the patient's food preferences in mind, and this permits a much more varied meal plan.

THE KETOGENIC DIET IN THE 21ST CENTURY

Nearly a century has passed since the ketogenic diet was initially used, and many more therapies are now available for children with epilepsy. The ketogenic diet compares favorably with other new treatments that have been introduced to treat children with epilepsy. The question that remains unanswered is, "When, in the course of therapy for a child with intractable epilepsy, should the ketogenic diet be used?" For myoclonic-astatic epilepsy (Doose syndrome) and infantile spasms, the diet has been proposed even as a first-line therapy. If the child has an epilepsy syndrome that is often resistant to current therapy and if the seizures are not controlled on medication, the ketogenic diet should be mentioned as an alternative therapy at the time of the initial therapeutic discussions. This is especially true in children who are not good candidates for epilepsy surgery or whose parents do not wish their children to have epilepsy surgery.

Many children who are not seizure-free or who are not able to come off all antiseizure medicines are improved on the ketogenic diet. The improvement in seizure control or behavior and cognitive abilities is such that parents wish to continue the ketogenic diet. The ketogenic diet might be useful in other childhood neurologic disorders such as alternating hemiplegia of childhood or tumors of the nervous system. There is an expanding experimental literature suggesting that the ketogenic diet may treat several neurologic conditions.

As we approach the second century of the ketogenic diet, it is clear that clinical use, research, and parent/patient interest are at all-time highs. Dietary therapy is being used increasingly for adults, nonepilepsy indications, as a first-line therapy, and also for longer durations than in years past (Kossoff et al., 2011). As usage grows, we will continue to learn about this unique therapy and better define its place in the algorithm for treating epilepsy.

REFERENCES

The complete list of references for this chapter is available online at www.expertconsult.com.
See inside cover for registration details.

SELECTED REFERENCES

Freeman, J.M., Kelly, M.T., Freeman, J.B., 1994. The Epilepsy Diet Treatment: An Introduction to the Ketogenic Diet. Demos, New York.

Freeman, J.M., Vining, E.P.G., Pillas, D.J., et al., 1998. The efficacy of the ketogenic diet—1998: a prospective evaluation of intervention in 150 children. Pediatrics 102, 1358.

Hemingway, C., Freeman, J.M., Pillas, D.J., et al., 2001. The ketogenic diet: a 3- to 6-year follow-up of 150 children enrolled prospectively. Pediatrics 108, 898.

Kim, D.Y., Rho, J.M., 2008. The ketogenic diet and epilepsy. Curr. Opin. Clin. Nutr. Metab. Care 11, 113.

Kossoff, E.H., Freeman, J.M., Turner, Z., et al., 2011. Ketogenic Diets: Treatments for Epilepsy and Other Disorders. Demos, New York.

Kossoff, E.H., Zupec-Kania, B.A., Amark, P.E., et al., 2009. Optimal clinical management of children receiving the ketogenic diet: recommendations of the international ketogenic diet study group. Epilepsia 50, 304.

Lefevre, F., Aronson, N., 2000. Ketogenic diet for the treatment of refractory epilepsy in children: a systematic review of efficacy. Pediatrics 105 (4), E46. Available from: <http://www.pediatrics.org/cgi/content/full/105/4/e46>.

Levy, R., Cooper, P., 2003. Ketogenic diet for epilepsy. Cochrane Database Syst. Rev. (3), CD001903.

Neal, E.G., Chaffe, H.M., Schwartz, R.H., et al., 2009. A randomized trial of classical and medium chain triglyceride ketogenic diets in the treatment of childhood epilepsy. Epilepsia 50, 1109.

Stafstrom, C.E., Rho, J.M. (Eds.), 2004. Epilepsy and the Ketogenic Diet. Humana Press, Inc, Totawa, NJ.

Wheless, J.W., 2004. History and origin of the ketogenic diet. In: Stafstrom, C.E., Rho, J.M. (Eds.), Epilepsy and the Ketogenic Diet. Humana Press, Inc, Totawa, NJ, p. 31.

RESOURCES

Kossoff, E.H., Freeman, J.M., Turner, Z., et al., 2011. Ketogenic Diets: Treatments for Epilepsy and Other Disorders. Demos, New York.

Martenz, D.M., Cramp, L., 2012. The Keto Cookbook. Demos, New York.

Neal, E. (Ed.), 2012. Dietary Treatment of Epilepsy: Practical Implementation of Ketogenic Therapy. Wiley-Blackwell, West Sussex.

Snyder, D., 2007. Keto Kid. Demos, New York.

Videotapes on the ketogenic diet for families, dietitians, nurses, and physicians. The Charlie Foundation to Help Cure Pediatric Epilepsy, 501 10th Street, Santa Monica, CA 90402; Fax (310) 393-2347. Available from: <www.charliefoundation.org>.

Whitmer, E., Riether, J.L., 2013. Fighting Back With Fat: A Parent's Guide to Battling Epilepsy Through the Ketogenic Diet and Modified Atkins Diet. Demos, New York.

Zupec-Kania, B.A., 2009. Ketogenic Diet: Parent's Guide. The Charlie Foundation, Santa Monica, CA. Available from: <www.charliefoundation.org>.

WEBSITES

Atkins Diet. <http://www.atkins.com>.

ILAE Ketogenic Diet Task Force Site. <http://www.ilae.org/Commission/medther/keto-index.cfm>.

Keto Calculator. <http://www.ketocalculator.com>.

Keto News. Monthly News Feature. <http://www.epilepsy.com/ketonews>.

Matthew's Friends. <http://www.matthewsfriends.org>.

The Charlie Foundation. <http://www.charliefoundation.org>.

E-BOOK FIGURES AND TABLES

The following figures and tables are available in the e-book at www.expertconsult.com. See inside cover for registration details.

Fig. 80-1 Composition of diets, CHO, carbohydrate.

Fig. 80-2 Initial steps in ketogenesis: lipolysis.

Fig. 80-3 Ketogenesis in the liver.

Fig 80-4 Ket1 body use and oxidation in the brain.

Fig 80-5 Metabolic defects and the ketogenic diet.

Box 80-6 Possible Adverse Events during Maintenance of the Ketogenic Diet

Table 80-1 Efficacy of Fasting (1921–1928)

Table 80-2 Efficacy of the Ketogenic Diet (1921–1976)

Table 80-3 Efficacy of the Ketogenic Diet, Large Series (1989–Present)

Table 80-4 Efficacy of the Classic Ketogenic Diet in Adolescents and Adults

Table 80-5 Efficacy of the Modified Atkins Diet, Large studies (selected)

81 Pediatric Psychogenic Nonepileptic Seizures and Psychiatric Disorders

Sigita Plioplys and W. Curt LaFrance Jr.

An expanded version of this chapter is available on www.expertconsult.com. See inside cover for registration details.

1. OVERVIEW

Pediatric psychogenic nonepileptic seizure (PNES) can be a difficult diagnosis to reach because of its clinical resemblance to epilepsy and prevalent medical and psychiatric comorbidities (Plioplys et al., 2014; Reilly, Menlove, Fenton, and Das, 2013). The patients, their families, and society bear an enormous cost if PNES is not diagnosed and psychiatric care provided in a timely fashion, or if inappropriate neurologic therapy is instituted. Misdiagnosis and mistreatment of PNES as epilepsy costs an estimated $920 million annually in diagnostic evaluations, inappropriate administration of antiseizure drugs, and emergency department utilization. Although PNESs are not responsive to antiepilepsy medications or may even worsen with their use, patients with PNES take double the number of these medicines compared with patients with epilepsy. "Nonepileptic psychogenic status" was reported in 13.5% of youth with PNES who were treated with intravenous antiseizure medicines, received potentially dangerous invasive diagnostic studies, or underwent emergency intubation (Patel, Scott, Dunn, and Garg, 2007).

PNES is less frequent in children than in adults and most commonly found in 15- to 24-year-old individuals, with an incidence of 3.4 per 100,000. In children with suspected epilepsy, the prevalence of PNES ranges from 1% to 9% (Patel et al., 2007).

Clinically, paroxysmal nonepileptic events are either physiologic or psychological in origin. Physiologic nonepileptic events are associated with medical or metabolic issues, but they are not epilepsy. The differential diagnosis of physiologic paroxysmal nonepileptic events in children includes vasovagal or neurocardiogenic syncope, stereotyped movements, daydreaming, sleep myoclonus, hypnic jerks, tonic posturing, parasomnias, and movement disorders (Kotagal, Costa, Wyllie, and Wolgamuth, 2002). PNESs, the focus of this chapter, resemble epileptic seizures and present as a sudden, involuntary, time-limited alteration in behavior, motor activity, autonomic function, consciousness, or sensation. However, unlike epilepsy, PNESs do not result from epileptogenic pathology and are not accompanied by an epileptiform electrographic ictal pattern. PNES comprise 30% of all paroxysmal nonepileptic events in children (Vincentiis et al., 2006).

PNES are classified under DSM-5 diagnoses of Somatoform, Conversion, and Dissociation Disorders (American Psychiatric Association, 2013). A much smaller percentage (<5%) of patients intentionally produce their seizures, and these are classified as Factitious Disorder and Malingering, which are not psychogenic in origin. DSM-5 made changes in the criteria for Conversion Disorder, allowing clinicians to make a positive diagnosis based on symptom presentation. Also, the prior necessary criteria of presence of a psychological stressor and ruling out of intentional production have been modified from diagnostic criteria to a descriptive note, aligning the DSM system with ICD-10 (World Health Organization, 2004).

2. EVALUATION OF THE PATIENT
Risk Factors

There are two main types or "causes" of PNES: posttraumatic and developmental. Posttraumatic PNES are thought to develop in response to acute or chronic exposure to traumatic experience(s), such as violence, severe personal medical illnesses or procedures, and physical, sexual, or psychological abuse. *Developmental PNES* refers to coping difficulties with daily tasks and milestones along the individual's continuum of normal psychosocial development.

The demographic risk factor profile points to female predominance beyond adolescence; however, there is equal sex distribution in younger children (Patel et al., 2007; Reilly et al., 2013). The mean age of PNES onset is 12.9 years (Patel et al., 2007), but it can begin in younger ages. The youngest age of PNES onset described in the literature is 5 years (Reilly et al., 2013).

Youth with PNES have higher rates of medical comorbidities, including epilepsy, and take more medications (prescription and over the counter) than their siblings (Plioplys et al., 2014). In a retrospective chart review study, Patel et al. (2007) reported coexisting neurologic illness in 55% of youth with PNES. Headaches were found in 19%, past head trauma in 10%, and abnormal brain magnetic resonance imaging (MRI) findings in 21% of subjects (Patel et al., 2007). Comorbid epilepsy ranges from 29% to 61%, with higher rates noted in children younger than 12 years (Patel et al., 2007; Plioplys et al., 2014). Focal-onset epilepsy has been identified as the most common type, found in 45% to 80% of patients, with comorbid epilepsy and PNES (Patel et al., 2007).

Psychosocially, the most common risk factors for PNES in children are family discord, school problems, and interpersonal problems (Patel et al., 2007; Plioplys et al., 2014; Vincentiis et al., 2006). In contrast to adults with PNES, physical and sexual abuse are not reported as often in children (Patel et al., 2007; Plioplys et al., 2014; Vincentiis et al., 2006). Compared with their siblings, children with PNES have significantly more lifetime adversities, such as domestic or community violence, bullying, and serious personal illness, surgery, or medical procedures, but not physical or sexual abuse, or loss (Plioplys et al., 2014). It is possible that sexual and physical abuse may be underreported. These data, however, emphasize that common, everyday stressors can be traumatic for vulnerable children. Furthermore, Plioplys et al. (2014) demonstrated that previously described individual risk factors for pediatric PNES are interconnected and thus may have a cumulative effect.

In addition to the child's individual vulnerabilities, family- and school-related factors play a significant role in the conversion process. Parents of children with PNES are often unaware or culturally unable to accept the psychological distress that children experience. As a result, parents do not recognize the early signs of emerging psychopathology and do not provide necessary support and interventions. Moreover, parents of children with PNES may understand and accept physical somatic symptoms better than psychological ones; parents themselves report more somatization than parents of children with epilepsy. Somatization, the process during which physical symptoms are experienced in response to psychological stress, becomes an intergenerational family communication model.

A past history of chronic medical illnesses and treatment or frequent life adversities in a child who has fearful interpretation of physical body sensations, high levels of somatization, and ineffective coping increases the risk for PNES.

History

Obtaining an accurate diagnosis of PNES is the essential first step for instituting proper therapy and avoiding unnecessary and potentially dangerous therapies. Acute neurologic events, such as head trauma, have not been found to be antecedents for PNES in children (Vincentiis et al., 2006). Typically, parents and patients cannot identify any specific triggers for the new onset of PNES, but recognize ongoing stress at school, home, or socially. Sometimes, a specific traumatic experience in the recent past, such as severe illness, medical procedure, abuse, or loss, can be identified.

A description of the events is obtained in assessing semiology. Clinical features of epileptic seizures and PNES overlap, however, and there is no one clinical feature that reliably distinguishes them. Subjective visceral, sensory, or psychic phenomena; alterations in responsiveness; and convulsive motor activity can be present in both disorders. Ictal presentations of PNES range from uncoordinated, disorganized motor activity to unresponsiveness without motor signs. Clinical differentiation between PNES and epilepsy has been based on other identifiers, such as the presence of preictal pseudosleep (where the patient reports being asleep, but electroencephalogram [EEG] shows the patient to be awake), geotropic eye movements (forced downward deviation of the eyes toward the floor, with head turning), eye closure, and postictal whispering with PNES, versus the presence of postictal headache and postictal nose rubbing (usually ipsilateral to the seizure focus) with epilepsy. The use of suggestion to both provoke and stop PNES is documented. With the issue of disclosure and informed consent, provocative procedures (e.g., saline injection, alcohol swab) have raised concern as a potentially unethical intervention, potentially compromising the trust in the physician–patient relationship. These maneuvers, however, have been demonstrated to have high specificity and positive predictive value.

Differential Diagnosis Between Epilepsy and PNES

The distinction between physiologic nonepileptic events and PNES is based on the combination of thorough history, physical examination in the peri-ictal period, and neurophysiological monitoring. Other studies are used as adjuncts to video-electroencephalogram (vEEG), and the sensitivities and specificities for EEG, neuroimaging, and prolactin levels have been reviewed (Cragar, Berry, Fakhoury, Cibula, and Schmitt, 2002).

PNES are not associated with epileptiform discharges on vEEG recordings, the gold standard for diagnosis. Studies of interrater reliability in vEEG show moderate to excellent consistency for PNES diagnosis. Therefore diagnosing PNES without vEEG confirmation should not be practiced, no matter how suggestive the clinical manifestation of a paroxysmal event may be. One study of epileptologists revealed a specificity of only 50% for seizure identification. In another study, prediction of the nature of unusual seizures by the admitting neurologist was accurate in only 67% of cases. When observing these events without accompanying EEG, determination from observations of unit personnel and neurologists was correct in less than 80% of episodes. Of note, PNESs were formerly referred to as pseudoseizures. Use of this term, however, has been discouraged given the negative connotations of "false" it conveys.

EEG abnormalities in patients with PNES do not necessarily confirm the diagnosis of epilepsy. For example, EEGs showing "sharpish waves" or paroxysmal slowing provide little support of epileptic seizures. Normal variants can also be misinterpreted as interictal epileptiform discharges in patients without epilepsy. A positive neurologic history, predominantly characterized as cognitive dysfunction, was present in almost half of children with PNES, and a positive family history of epilepsy was present in 35% of children with PNES (Patel et al., 2007). Although neurologic signs, symptoms, and history are important to note in seizure patients, they are in no way pathognomonic in distinguishing PNES from epileptic seizures. Three criteria in patients with PNES admitted for vEEG yielded a positive predictive value of 85%: (1) *at least two PNES* per week, (2) *refractory to at least two antiseizure medicines*, and (3) *at least two EEGs* without epileptiform activity. Using "the rule of 2s" and documenting seizure frequency, EEG abnormalities, and drug-treatment response before vEEG may help with definitive diagnosis of PNES. A paper commissioned by the International League Against Epilepsy provided diagnostic levels of certainty for PNES based on history, witnessed event semiology, and studies (with vEEG being the gold standard) (LaFrance, Baker, Duncan, Goldstein, and Reuber, 2013).

Multidisciplinary Assessment Including Psychiatric Evaluation

The initial multidisciplinary assessment of PNES must combine both neurologic and psychiatric evaluations. Supplementing the psychiatric evaluation is the vEEG, to establish the diagnosis. Only ictal EEG can be used to differentiate PNES from epileptic seizures definitively at the individual level. After conducting a thorough history, mental status examination, and neurologic examination, a few neurophysiological and neurohumoral tests can be used to assist in the diagnosis of PNES and may include increased ictal prolactin, lower heart rate variability, and decreased oximetry. Neuropsychological and standardized self- and parent-report questionnaires do not distinguish PNES from epileptic seizures but can be used to identify cognitive, educational, emotional, behavioral, and family difficulties. For patients with other comorbid conversion symptoms, such as astasia abasia, tremor, weakness, vision problems, pain, stuttering, or physical/occupational/speech disorders, specialty evaluations may be indicated.

3. PSYCHOPATHOLOGY IN CHILDREN WITH PNES

As discussed earlier, the primary psychiatric diagnosis accounting for PNES is conversion disorder. Exceptionally rarely, children with PNES can have dissociative or factitious disorders when seizure-like episodes result from the dissociative states or sick-role-seeking behaviors. It can be difficult to correctly diagnose conversion disorder in a timely manner because children often deny the underlying emotional conflict and associated distress and may perceive seizure-like symptoms as their primary and only problem. Limitations in recognizing and resolving underlying emotional distress are multifactorial and may be associated with the child's developmental characteristics, such as emotional immaturity and, ineffective problem solving, communication, and coping with stress.

Comorbid psychopathology is reported in 16% to 100% of youth with PNES (Caplan and Plioplys, 2010; Patel et al., 2007; Plioplys et al., 2014; Vincentiis et al., 2006). It is more frequent and severe in adolescents with PNES than in children younger than 13 years (48.6% vs 16%). Literature demonstrates that youth with PNES have significantly more lifetime emotional, behavioral, and learning problems than their siblings (Plioplys et al., 2014).

The most common comorbid psychiatric diagnoses in youth with PNES are mood disorders, such as anxiety (7%-84%), depression (19%-62%), and posttraumatic stress disorder (PTSD) (3%-25%), followed by disruptive behavior disorders, including attention deficit hyperactivity disorder (ADHD)(15%-29%) and oppositional defiant disorder (8%) (ODD) (Caplan et al., 2010; Patel et al., 2007; Plioplys et al., 2014; Vincentiis et al., 2006). A multisite PNES study reported that youth with PNES have significantly higher rates of PTSD than their siblings (25.5 % vs 2.9%), more lifetime adversities, and a higher mean number of adversities (Plioplys et al., 2014). A Turkish study of adolescents with PNES reported suicide attempts in 15% of PNES patients compared with none in a control group of adolescents with epilepsy.

Compared with their siblings, youth with PNES report higher levels of somatization and anxiety sensitivity, a tendency to view anxiety-related bodily sensations as dangerous (Plioplys et al., 2014). Fatigue, sleep problems, headaches, pain, weakness, and abnormal gait or muscle movements are commonly experienced by children with PNES. Secondary somatic symptoms reveal a more severe conversion disorder, and as patients become more functionally impaired, they receive more unnecessary medical investigations and treatments compared with PNES patients without symptomatic transformation. High social anxiety associated with performance fear and the presence of somatic symptoms have been reported in youth with PNES. In addition, adolescents with PNES display significantly lower self-esteem than healthy adolescents and those with epilepsy.

Data on cognitive problems in youth with PNES are inconsistent. Some studies identified cognitive and learning problems in 5% to 14.8% of the PNES subjects, whereas other studies using standard cognitive testing instruments have reported average IQ scores and no cognitive difference compared with siblings. However, clinical learning problems, as reported by patients, are identified in 14% to 67% of youth with PNES. These children demonstrate more school underachievement than patients with epilepsy and healthy control and have more medical and psychiatric illnesses, take more medications, and have more school absenteeism than their siblings (Plioplys et al., 2014). Rather than primary cognitive deficits, school absenteeism, cognitive impairment resulting from underlying medical and psychiatric disorders and treatments, and poor coping with stress may be contributing factors to learning difficulties and school-related stress.

4. MULTIDISCIPLINARY TREATMENT MODEL

Timely PNES diagnosis and psychiatric treatment are associated with better outcomes and resolution of PNES episodes in children. However, PNES treatment can be a challenging process to all clinical services involved because of the heterogeneous PNES presentation, common symptom transformation to other types of somatic symptoms, high medical and psychiatric comorbidities, frequent use of urgent medical services, diagnostic procedures and treatments, and difficulties in obtaining adequate mental health services.

At the present time, there are no randomized, controlled treatment studies of pediatric PNES published. Despite the existence of treatment guidelines for PNES from expert consensus being available (Kerr et al., 2011), treatment of youth with PNES varies between providers. In adults with PNES, several randomized controlled trials provide evidence that cognitive behavioral therapy (CBT) alone (LaFrance et al., 2014) or a combination of CBT-informed psychotherapy and selective serotonin reuptake inhibitors (SSRIs) have been effective in decreasing PNES frequency (LaFrance et al., 2014).

Most importantly, treatment of pediatric PNES should be provided by a multidisciplinary team that includes a mental health professional (psychiatrist, psychologist, or social worker), a pediatric neurologist or epileptologist, and a primary care physician (PCP), with the school staff and family playing an active role. To assure the successful handover of PNES management from neurology to psychiatry, a transition process must be developed by both services. After the patient with PNES is discharged from the EEG monitoring unit to the outpatient setting, the mental health clinician should assume the primary PNES treatment and case management role.

The Role of the Neurologist

The primary role of the neurologist is to conduct a thorough diagnostic evaluation, to provide a sensitive diagnostic feedback to the family, and to discontinue or optimize antiseizure medicines in patients with comorbid epilepsy. Diagnostic feedback should be delivered to the patient and family together, ideally with a mental health clinician. The successful communication of the PNES diagnosis can be considered as the first and one of the most important therapeutic steps in PNES management (Caplan et al., 2010). In adults with PNES, a significant reduction of PNES frequency, visits to the emergency room, and other PNES-related healthcare use has been reported immediately after the PNES diagnosis is communicated and before the initiation of psychiatric treatment.

During the feedback, the neurologist should communicate that the seizures captured on the vEEG are not epilepsy, unambiguously confirm that the events are real and the patient is not faking them, and clearly state that PNES has a psychological origin. Viewing the typical events recorded during the vEEG evaluation can help parents accept this diagnosis, especially when the child also has epilepsy. For patients with PNES and comorbid epilepsy, the diagnostic feedback has to include a careful explanation of the differences between the epileptic seizures, which can respond to antiseizure medicines, and the PNESs that do not respond to antiseizure medicines and require different treatments, including psychiatric interventions with a mental health provider. The neurologist should recommend psychiatric care as the primary treatment modality. The neurologist together with a mental health clinician outlines a multidisciplinary treatment plan that involves changes in antiseizure medicines, behavioral management of the PNES, ongoing psychiatric treatment, and full transition to school and regular life routines.

The secondary role of the neurologist is to provide follow-up care during the antiseizure medicine taper and also after its discontinuation, especially in the transition period to mental healthcare. At the time of the initial PNES diagnosis, 50% to 95% of children take antiseizure medicines. In general, withdrawal from antiseizure medicines is safe; patients use less "rescue" antiseizure medicine treatment and do not have an increase in events. However, the antiseizure medicine discontinuation process can be complex and may be negatively influenced by the clinician's uncertainty about the PNES diagnosis; fear of making a clinical mistake, especially when nonspecific EEG findings are present; limited knowledge and experience with PNES; parental requests to continue antiseizure medicines; and lack of available psychiatric services.

In a recent national survey of 236 pediatric neurology clinicians, 96% were very willing to discontinue antiseizure medicine treatment in patients with PNES without comorbid epileptic seizures. Clinicians with sufficient knowledge of how to diagnose and treat PNES were less concerned about making a potential medical error and were less influenced by patient or parental requests to continue antiseizure medicines. The strength of clinicians' decision to discontinue antiseizure medicines was significantly associated with patients having ongoing psychiatric care.

Continuity of neurologic care during and after antiseizure medicine discontinuation decreases parental anxiety, strengthens acceptance of the diagnosis of conversion disorder, and prevents further "doctor shopping" when seizure-like events linger or change into other somatic symptoms. It also supports patients' transition to psychiatric care, especially during the early treatment, when rapport with the mental health clinician is still evolving and when some parents are still hesitant to accept the PNES diagnosis.

The neurologist or epileptologist also serves as a consultant to the other members of the treatment team because a majority of mental health clinicians and primary care providers have limited experience with PNES and may feel uncomfortable managing patients with dramatic, seizure-like symptoms. Often, mental health clinicians require backup support in communicating a behavioral PNES management plan to schools or athletic programs. To assure that youth with PNES return to regular school, athletic, and social activities, the mental health clinician together with the neurologist must provide letters to the school outlining the behavioral PNES management plan and instructing the school staff not to use the "seizure management plan" of calling paramedics and taking the patient to the emergency room.

Basic Principles of Psychiatric PNES Treatment

Psychiatric treatment consists of the behavioral management of PNES, supporting the patient's return to regular life activities, psychotherapy for conversion disorder, and treatment for comorbid psychiatric disorders using standard evidence-based psychopharmacological and psychotherapeutic modalities along with appropriate educational and family interventions (Caplan et al., 2010).

Treatment of conversion disorder is based on multimodal individual and family therapy because there is no evidence that antiseizure medicines or psychopharmacological agents, specifically antidepressants or antianxiety medications, have been effective. Most youth with PNES receive psychiatric treatment in the outpatient setting. Intensive outpatient treatment programs (day hospital) may be indicated if the child is not able to successfully reintegrate back to school within 2 to 3 weeks after receiving a PNES diagnosis, is not able to stay in school despite provided accommodations, or has severe comorbid psychopathology and nonsuicidal self-injurious behaviors. An inpatient psychiatric admission is recommended when patients are suicidal, are homicidal, have an unsafe family environment, are psychotic, or are undergoing investigation for newly disclosed abuse.

5. OUTCOME

Literature demonstrates that PNES outcomes in youth is more positive than in adults; 35% to 100% of youth achieve a full remission or significant reduction in PNES frequency over up to a 3-year follow up. Although systematic studies of factors associated with PNES remission or reduction in frequency in children are not available, shorter duration of illness, less severe psychopathology, absence of personality disorders, and earlier interventions may be contributing variables to improvement. Epilepsy, on the other hand, was associated with ongoing PNES in youth. Addressing the different psychological mechanisms may lead to symptomatic improvement in children with PNES.

SUMMARY

Pediatric PNES is a high-impact disorder because of diagnostic and treatment difficulties resulting in medical interventions that do not treat the disorder, high economic cost and medical utilization, and the psychosocial burden to the patient and family. Early PNES diagnosis leads to timely psychiatric treatment and improved outcomes. Recent findings demonstrate the importance of screening for the broad range of interrelated risk factors that represent somatopsychiatric and adversity variables.

Manifestations of PNES range from uncoordinated, disorganized motor activity to unresponsiveness without motor signs. Identifiers that are helpful to distinguish PNES from epileptic seizures include the presence of preictal pseudosleep, geotropic eye movements, eye closure, and postictal whispering with PNES, versus the presence of postictal headache or nose rubbing in epilepsy.

The gold standard diagnostic approach includes comprehensive history, psychiatric assessment, and a vEEG recording capturing the event in question without an ictal EEG epileptiform correlate. Additional testing of ictal prolactin, heart variability, oximetry, and cognitive and psychological functioning can be used as supplemental, but not diagnostic, tests. Using the "Rule of 2s" (at least two PNES per week, refractory to at least two antiseizure medicines, and at least two EEGs without epileptiform activity) may help to identify a person who has PNES.

PNES treatment is multidisciplinary, with a mental health clinician taking the primary role, and includes neurologist/epileptologist, primary care physician, school staff, and family. PNES treatment starts while patient is still in the hospital with an accurate diagnosis of conversion disorder and sensitive diagnostic feedback provided by the neurologist together with the mental health clinician. Treatment of patients with PNES and comorbid epilepsy must address both disorders: Adjust the antiseizure medicines for epilepsy, and educate parents about the differences in management of the epileptic seizures and the PNES.

Ongoing neurology involvement beyond antiseizure medicine discontinuation is very important because it can decrease parental anxiety, strengthen acceptance of the diagnosis of conversion disorder, and prevent further "doctor shopping." The neurologist must support patients' involvement in psychiatric treatment and back up mental health clinicians in their work with family and school staff.

REFERENCES

The complete list of references for this chapter is available in the e-book at www.expertconsult.com.

See inside cover for registration details.

SELECTED REFERENCES

American Psychiatric Association, 2013. Diagnostic and statistical manual of mental disorders (DSM-5®). American Psychiatric Pub.

Caplan, R., Plioplys, S., 2010. Psychiatric features and management of children with psychogenic nonepileptic seizures. In: Schachter, S.C., LaFrance, W.C., Jr. (Eds.), Gates and Rowan's Nonepileptic Seizures, third ed. Cambridge University Press, New York, NY, pp. 163–178.

Cragar, D.E., Berry, D.T., Fakhoury, T.A., et al., 2002. A review of diagnostic techniques in the differential diagnosis of epileptic and nonepileptic seizures. Neuropsychol. Rev. 12, 31–64.

Kerr, M.P., Mensah, S., Besag, F., et al., 2011. International consensus clinical practice statements for the treatment of neuropsychiatric conditions associated with epilepsy. Epilepsia 52, 2133–2138.

Kotagal, P., Costa, M., Wyllie, E., et al., 2002. Paroxysmal nonepileptic events in children and adolescents. Pediatrics 110, e46.

LaFrance, W.C. Jr., Baird, G.L., Barry, J.J., et al., 2014. Multicenter pilot treatment trial for psychogenic nonepileptic seizures: a randomized clinical trial. JAMA Psychiatry 71, 997–1005.

LaFrance, W.C. Jr., Baker, G.A., Duncan, R., et al., 2013. Minimum requirements for the diagnosis of psychogenic nonepileptic seizures: a staged approach: a report from the International League Against Epilepsy Nonepileptic Seizures Task Force. Epilepsia 54, 2005–2018.

Patel, H., Scott, E., Dunn, D., et al., 2007. Nonepileptic seizures in children. Epilepsia 48, 2086–2092.

Plioplys, S., Doss, J., Siddarth, P., et al., 2014. A multisite controlled study of risk factors in pediatric psychogenic nonepileptic seizures. Epilepsia 55, 1739–1747.

Reilly, C., Menlove, L., Fenton, V., et al., 2013. Psychogenic nonepileptic seizures in children: a review. Epilepsia 54, 1715–1724.

Vincentiis, S., Valente, K.D., Thome-Souza, S., et al., 2006. Risk factors for psychogenic nonepileptic seizures in children and adolescents with epilepsy. Epilepsy Behav. 8, 294–298.

World Health Organization, 2004. International statistical classification of diseases and health related problems (The) ICD-10. (Doctoral dissertation, World Health Organization).

82 Behavioral, Cognitive, and Social Aspects of Childhood Epilepsy

Wendy G. Mitchell, Michèle Van Hirtum-Das, Jay Desai, and Quyen N. Luc

An expanded version of this chapter is available on www.expertconsult.com. See inside cover for registration details.

Children and adolescents with epilepsy and adults with childhood-onset epilepsy often have poor educational attainment, lower than expected occupational status, poorer perceived health, more behavior problems, and higher rates of social isolation. In most patients, one or more causes of poor functioning may be identified and, at times, remedied. The causes of cognitive and behavioral dysfunction are multifactorial. Underlying neurologic lesions or genetic syndromes such as channelopathies cause epilepsy and cognitive dysfunction. In other disorders, such as benign focal epilepsy of childhood, learning and behavioral disorders are more difficult to explain, and the relationship with seizures is almost certainly not causal.

COGNITIVE AND BEHAVIORAL DISORDERS
Cognitive Disabilities in Children With Epilepsy

Epilepsy is more frequent in intellectually disabled children than in the general population. Population-based studies of children with intellectual disabilities document the prevalence of epilepsy to be 15%–35%. Those with severe intellectual disabilities and cerebral palsy have highest epilepsy rates. Likewise, intellectual disability is more common in children with epilepsy than in children without epilepsy (Berg et al., 2008).

Learning Disabilities and Academic Underachievement

Learning disability is diagnosed when academic performance in one or more areas falls below expectations and cannot be explained by cognitive level, sensory abnormalities, or lack of educational opportunities. Learning disabilities are more frequent in children with epilepsy, even accounting for sociocultural variables. Children with epilepsy are at higher risk for requiring special education services with the need being higher in children with remote structural/metabolic epilepsy and epileptic encephalopathies. However, almost half of neurologically intact children with cryptogenic or genetic epilepsies require special education services. A diagnosis of epilepsy provides sufficient cause to screen children for learning disability.

Academic underachievement in reading, writing, and mathematics has been reported in children with epilepsy, in comparison with their normal peers and children with chronic illnesses (e.g., asthma). It is unclear whether the relationship is a direct one, in which the epilepsy, seizures, or antiseizure medicines cause learning disability, or an indirect one, in which an underlying neurologic condition causes both seizures and abnormalities in perception, memory, and visual–motor skills. Detailed neurocognitive batteries in children with epilepsy demonstrate higher than expected rates of dyslexia, slowed processing speeds, and visual–spatial, attention, executive, and constructional difficulties. However, numerous studies attempting to identify demographic, neurologic, and seizure-related risk factors for academic underachievement have shown inconsistent results. Posited risk factors such as inadequate seizure control, early age of onset, longer duration of epilepsy, and polytherapy are not universally associated with academic underachievement.

Attention Deficit, Impulsivity, and Overactivity

Studies of children with epilepsy demonstrate a higher incidence of inattention, impulsivity, and slowed reaction time. This should not imply that clinical attention deficit hyperactivity disorder is extremely common in children with epilepsy, although the prevalence is probably somewhat higher than in the general population. As with overall cognitive function, simple cause and effect relationships are uncommon. Common neurobiological mechanisms and causative factors may be present in these two disorders. Antiseizure medications may positively and negatively affect attention and impulsivity. In rare instances, frequent seizures affect attention, and improved seizure control may ameliorate this problem. Anticonvulsants are unlikely to improve attention in children who have epileptiform discharges without clinical seizures.

If needed, treatment with stimulants, atomoxetine, or tricyclic antidepressants generally does not compromise seizure control. Bupropion may increase risk of seizures, particularly at high doses. Most pediatric neurologists avoid doses greater than 100 mg per day in these patients.

Autism and Autistic Spectrum Disorders

Autistic spectrum disorders are associated with an increased incidence of epilepsy, but evidence that one causes the other is lacking. The risk for developing seizures in children with autistic spectrum disorders is highest during early childhood, with a second peak occurring in adolescence. Features of autism are common in children with epilepsy, regardless of cognitive ability. A number of syndromes are associated with a high incidence of autistic behavior and epilepsy (e.g., tuberous sclerosis, Angelman syndrome, and Rett syndrome), but the coincidence of seizures and behavioral symptoms is due to the underlying condition. A possible rare exception is the child in whom autistic behavior develops along with language regression, accompanied by an epileptiform EEG (continuous spike-and-wave pattern during sleep). This condition has been considered to be a variant of Landau–Kleffner syndrome. Behavior and language may improve with treatment.

Psychiatric Disorders in Childhood Epilepsy

Little evidence exists to support the notion that severe psychiatric disorders are significantly more common in children with epilepsy. Although major psychiatric illnesses such as schizophrenia, obsessive–compulsive disorder, or affective disorders may coexist with childhood epilepsy, the prevalence is not higher than expected (Dunn, Austin & Perkins 2009). Treatment of coexisting severe psychiatric disorder and epilepsy may be complex. Some antiseizure medications (carbamazepine, valproic acid) are beneficial in treatment of certain psychiatric disorders (e.g., bipolar affective disorders). However, treatment of epilepsy does not usually relieve symptoms of major psychiatric illness.

Mood disturbances are more frequent in adolescents and adults with epilepsy than in healthy peers. Depression and anxiety are common and frequently underdiagnosed and undertreated. Suicidal ideation also is more likely in children and adolescents with epilepsy.

Behavioral Problems, Conduct Disorders, and Delinquency

Behavioral disturbances may be related to family factors and parental anxiety about epilepsy, rather than a primary result of epilepsy or the underlying disorder. Self-esteem is lower and behavioral problems are more frequent than in peers with or without chronic illnesses. Even in children assessed at the time of first seizure diagnosis, behavior problems are frequent, particularly in children who had previously unrecognized seizures. Children with epilepsy also have higher rates of oppositional–defiant disorder and conduct disorder.

Adolescents and young adults with childhood-onset epilepsy have slightly higher than expected rates of delinquency in a population-based Canadian study. It is uncertain whether this propensity is due to underlying brain disease with poor impulse control, stigma, lack of opportunity, or other sociocultural factors. In contrast, a Finnish population-based study failed to find a similar relationship in males up to age 22 years.

Cognitive and Behavioral Outcome of Specific Epilepsy Syndromes

Epileptic Encephalopathy, a Model of System Epilepsy

Advances in metabolic imaging, genetic analysis, and the development of animal models have provided significant understanding of the underlying pathophysiology in epileptic encephalopathies. One hypothesis is that the effects of a focal lesion may be magnified by interactions between cortical and subcortical structures. Disruption of subcortical arousal centers that regulate the early cortical development may lead to altered synaptic connectivity, which may affect cognitive development. Alternately, impairment of global interneuronal functions via genetic alteration of widely distributed potassium or sodium channels may manifest as developmental arrest and/or generalized slowing on EEG. Lastly, prolonged focal epileptic activity in sleep may interfere with local slow wave activity, therefore disrupting plasticity associated with regional learning and memory. Although seizures can contribute to these pathologic processes, they are unlikely to be necessary for development of the encephalopathy. Rather, they may be a symptom of the underlying lesion.

Infantile Spasms

Certain pediatric epilepsy syndromes (e.g., infantile spasms) have been associated with severe cognitive deficits. Many patients exhibit global developmental arrest as well as specific cognitive deficits, delayed speech and impaired visual–spatial function. Thirteen percent of children with cryptogenic infantile spasms exhibit persistent autistic features, and the rate is higher in children with tuberous sclerosis. Effective early treatment may improve cognition and behavior. Other prognostic factors for better cognitive outcomes include sustained seizure control with the first medication, age at onset equal to or greater than 4 months, and absence of atypical spasms and partial seizures (Partikian & Mitchell 2010).

Epileptic Encephalopathies of Infancy

Many neonatal or infantile-onset epileptic encephalopathies (e.g., Dravet syndrome, Ohtahara syndrome, early infantile myoclonic encephalopathy, and migrating partial seizures of infancy) are associated with global developmental delays and regression. Delayed development and behavioral disorders such as autism and hyperactivity generally present by the second year of life.

Lennox–Gastaut Syndrome

Lennox–Gastaut Syndrome (LGS) describes a constellation of seizure types and a characteristic slow spike and wave EEG pattern, but etiologies are multifactorial, including both genetic and secondary symptomatic epilepsies. Intellectual disability is seen in nearly all patients, and behavioral problems including autistic spectrum disorders are frequent. Seizure patterns and EEG may evolve, making diagnosis in later adolescence or adulthood difficult if records from earlier childhood are not available. Long-term follow up reveals ongoing—and at times increasing—intellectual disabilities, deficits in motor speed, apathy, and perseverative behavior.

Electrical Status Epilepticus in Sleep and Landau–Kleffner Syndrome

Electrical status epilepticus in sleep is an EEG pattern associated with specific cognitive and language dysfunction. With continuous spike-and-wave activity in sleep, a typical decrease in the IQ or developmental quotient is noted. Approximately 40%–60% of children with continuous spike-wave sleep exhibit an expressive aphasia, which is in contrast to children with Landau–Kleffner syndrome, who present with verbal or auditory agnosia. In patients with Landau–Kleffner syndrome language may recover spontaneously, partially improve with therapy, or remain permanently affected despite EEG improvement.

Self-Limited Focal Epilepsies of Childhood

The syndrome termed benign childhood epilepsy with centrotemporal spikes (BECTS or benign Rolandic epilepsy) was thought to be benign, but increasing evidence suggests that a subpopulation may have impaired cognitive function and difficulties with visual perception, concentration, and short-term memory, impaired phonologic processing skills, and reading disability. Sleep disturbances are also more frequent than expected. Self-limited childhood epilepsy with occipital paroxysms has been associated with selective dysfunction in perceptive–visual attentional ability, verbal and visual–spatial memory abilities, visual perception, visual–motor integration, some language tasks, and reading, writing, and arithmetic abilities.

Childhood Absence Epilepsy

Cognitive dysfunction detected in childhood absence epilepsy includes deficits in visual sustained attention and execution of visual–motor tasks, verbal and nonverbal memory, and word fluency.

EFFECTS OF ANTISEIZURE MEDICATIONS ON BEHAVIOR, ATTENTION, AND MOOD
General Effects

Cognitive, psychiatric, and behavioral abnormalities in children with epilepsy are often attributed to medications. However abnormalities are commonly multifactorial in origin, with duration of epilepsy, etiology, seizure frequency, and antiseizure medications all affecting cognition and behavior. Most studies examining the impact of antiseizure medications on cognition and behavior are from adults. Randomized, prospective clinical research in children is limited. When applying adult data to children, several factors need to be recognized. Epilepsy occurring in the developing brain is likely to be substantially different from that in the adult in both its quality and response to treatment. In addition, most refractory epilepsies begin in childhood. These severe childhood epilepsies may have cognitive and behavioral abnormalities as a component of these syndromes.

Current research suggests that most medication-related cognitive adverse events are mild or difficult to document objectively, but idiosyncratic adverse behavioral and cognitive responses can occur with any medication. Risk of cognitive and behavioral effects generally increases with rapid titration, higher doses or serum concentrations, and polypharmacy. A few studies have randomized patients at the onset of seizures to monotherapy with an antiseizure medication. Most studies, however, are not randomized and monitor cognitive and behavioral effects when a medication is added or withdrawn (Mandelbaum, Burack & Bhise 2009).

Psychotropic Effects and Adverse Psychiatric Effects

Psychopathology in epilepsy has a multifactorial etiology, and antiseizure medications provide only one of the potentially numerous contributing neurobiological factors. Investigation into the drug-specific adverse interactions is challenging in part because of methodological problems., There have been prior attempts when addressing the psychotropic potential of antiseizure medications to differentiate those that have positive from those that have negative effects.

Drugs that exhibit a *sedating* effect are typically characterized by fatigue and cognitive slowing. Examples include benzodiazepines, phenobarbital, tiagabine, valproate, and vigabatrin, all of which potentiate gamma amino butyric acid (GABA) inhibitory neurotransmission. Alternately, *activating* drugs—often with anxiogenic and antidepressant properties—usually attenuate glutamate excitatory neurotransmission. This rather straightforward model, however, does not address the complicating factors of the underlying epilepsy itself. Issues such as epilepsy severity or the presence of limbic system abnormalities may be important. Some features cannot be ignored, such as forced normalization, postictal psychosis, or release. The psychotropic effects of antiepileptic drugs are most likely related to their direct (e.g., mechanism of action, drug toxicity, drug withdrawal, polytherapy) and indirect mechanisms (e.g., epilepsy-related phenomenon or patient-related factors).

Recently concerns have been raised about potential for suicidal ideation or suicide in children and adults taking antiseizure medications. Most of the medications now contain warnings that suicidal ideation may occur. However, the risk of suicidality in patients who are treated with antiseizure medications for epilepsy is very low compared with use of the same medications for bipolar affective disorder or pain indications (Mula et al. 2013).

Forced Normalization

The first publications regarding the concept of forced normalization date back to the 1950s. Patients with psychotic episodes were reported to have associated improvement or normalization of their EEGs. It was noted that drug withdrawal with subsequent seizure recurrence correlated with resolution of the abnormal mental state. Although several psychological profiles have been associated with forced normalization, psychosis is probably the most common. Anxiety, insomnia, and social withdrawal also have been reported. The exact incidence of forced normalization occurring in pediatric patients is unknown, but probably is very low.

Mood Disorders

Mood disorders—depression in particular—are the most frequent psychiatric comorbidity in epilepsy but are often undiagnosed and therefore untreated. Epilepsy variables associated with depression include seizure type (temporal lobe epilepsy), seizure severity or frequency, and treatment. One study reported on specific features associated with medical therapy and depressive symptoms. These include enhanced GABA neurotransmission, folate deficiency, polytherapy, comorbid presence of hippocampal sclerosis, forced normalization, and a history of mood difficulty. Medications with GABAergic effect all have been linked with depression. There is also quite a substantial body of older literature linking depression and treatment with barbiturates.

Folic acid is an important cofactor for transmethylation reactions and monoamine metabolism within the central nervous system. Patients on polytherapy had low serum, red blood cell, or cerebrospinal fluid folate levels. Even greater deficiencies were found in patients with epilepsy and psychopathology. Antiseizure drugs such as carbamazepine and lamotrigine, which have a well-known positive effect on mood and behavior, have minimal impact on folate levels. On the other hand, barbiturates and phenytoin can depress serum or CSF folate levels.

Psychosis

The reported frequency of psychoses related to treatment is approximately 1% to 2%, all occurring in medically refractory patients on polytherapy. It has been described with felbamate, vigabatrin, zonisamide, topiramate, tiagabine, and levetiracetam, suggesting that this phenomenon is not specific to a particular medication.

Fear of Side Effects and Effective Medication Use

Despite the relative paucity of documentation of sustained adverse cognitive effects of antiseizure medications, parents may be under the erroneous impression that a particular medicine will "make the child retarded," and may blame developmental problems that subsequently emerge on previous administration of antiseizure medications, or may avoid administration of these medications because of fear of disturbing the child's behavior or development.

Behavioral and Cognitive Effects of the Older Versus Newer Antiseizure Medications

Reviews of the adult literature suggest that there is no significant difference in efficacy, tolerability, and long-term retention between older versus new antiseizure medications. New medications approved over the last 30 years have generally undergone at least add-on trials in children, with some studies including behavioral and cognitive assessment. These newer antiseizure medications have been reported to cause both positive and negative behavior changes. Very few have included behavioral or cognitive measures in properly designed, blinded monotherapy studies either in comparison with placebo or another antiseizure medication. This is particularly true for the most recently approved medications. Comparison of antiseizure medications across studies is further hampered by varying criteria for selection of the participants and use of differing neuropsychological tests and study designs.

Phenobarbital

There are double-blind, placebo-controlled, long-term studies of the behavioral effects of monotherapy with phenobarbital for febrile seizures in infants and toddlers. Children on phenobarbital tended to have lower IQs or displayed IQ declines compared with control subjects. This is due in part to decreased processing speed and poorer attention, and the situation improves or reverses after discontinuation. There may be long-term effects on language skills and academic achievement, however. Its continued use as the drug of first choice in neonates has raised significant concerns and debates.

Phenobarbital can cause sustained behavioral difficulties, primarily overactivity, and can cause irritability and disturbed sleep, particularly in infants and toddlers. Estimates of the number of children who do not tolerate phenobarbital because of overactivity range from 5% to 25%. This is more frequent in toddlers and preschool-aged children.

Phenytoin

There are no randomized studies examining behavioral and cognitive outcomes in children on phenytoin. Early reports that phenytoin caused generalized cognitive decline were later disputed when further data analysis and research found that the major effect of phenytoin was on motor speed. Other cognitive functions are relatively spared, if analyzed independent of response speed.

Valproic Acid

In a recent prospective, randomized, blinded study of children with absence epilepsy, valproic acid adversely affected memory more so than ethosuximide or lamotrigine (Glauser et al. 2010). However, smaller earlier studies showed no memory or cognitive impairments. Valproic acid occasionally causes a confused state or psychosis. Hyperammonemia may result in mental slowing and encephalopathy.

Carbamazepine

A recent open-label, prospective, randomized study of children with new onset partial epilepsy showed no decline in neuropsychological performance after 32 weeks on carbamazepine. Performance IQ, perceptual organization, and externalizing behaviors all improved (Eun et al. 2012). In addition, no cognitive impairment from carbamazepine was seen in two studies in children using a withdrawal design. One prospective study reported worsening reaction time and reaction time variability after treatment for 12 months.

Oxcarbazepine

Three prospective, open-label studies have been performed in children on oxcarbazepine monotherapy; all have shown no cognitive impairment over a period of up to 6 months. In one study, cognitive effects were compared with carbamazepine and valproic acid in children ages 6 to 17 years with new onset partial epilepsy. In all treatment groups there was improvement in mental processing speed and no cognitive impairment. Recently a study found statistically significant improvement in some cognitive and behavioral variables after 28 weeks on oxcarbazepine in children with new onset partial epilepsy.

Lamotrigine

Since its introduction the United States in 1994, lamotrigine has received much attention with respect to its potential positive psychotropic effects. In adults with newly diagnosed epilepsy, lamotrigine has been reported to have fewer cognitive effects than carbamazepine, phenytoin, and topiramate. Significant improvements in behavior, cognition, and motor skills (unrelated to seizure control) also have been noted in children.

Felbamate

Felbamate modulates glutamate neurotransmission and is generally "activating" rather than sedating. Sleep disturbances and overactivity have been reported, along with isolated instances of psychosis. Several studies found reduction in daytime drowsiness and increased alertness in children taking felbamate.

Topiramate

Topiramate has been reported to cause significant cognitive difficulties in adult patients, with and without epilepsy, involving primarily word finding and verbal memory, particularly during initial treatment and titration. These adverse effects sometimes dissipate over time, particularly if the dosage is increased slowly. Studies have shown that a gradual introduction of topiramate does not necessarily prevent cognitive effects, and adverse effects on verbal fluency, verbal memory, and cognitive speed may persist until withdrawal of the medication.

Zonisamide

There is one randomized open-label study of children with newly diagnosed epilepsy on zonisamide monotherapy. Children on low doses (3–4 mg/kg/day) showed improvement in several behavioral variables and no cognitive impairment after 28 weeks on zonisamide, whereas children on higher doses (6–8 mg/kg/day) displayed vocabulary impairment. In several observational studies, 26% to 61% of patients reported mild to moderate adverse events, with only a mild development of tolerance. Cognitive dysfunction—specifically attention, memory, and language changes—was reported in 2% to 11%. Reports from Japan suggest that psychotic episodes and behavior changes may occur in children.

Levetiracetam

Prospective studies with adjunctive levetiracetam therapy in children have shown no cognitive impairment; however behavioral or mood abnormalities are common (up to 50% in one study) and often necessitate discontinuation (Schiemann-Delgado et al. 2012). A few anecdotal reports have described improved behavior in children with autism treated with levetiracetam, but in the same population, some children experienced increased aggressive behavior. Pyridoxine is sometimes added to levetiracetam to ameliorate mood-related symptoms based on empirical evidence.

Clobazam

A randomized, double-blind, prospective, multicenter study addressed the cognitive tolerability of clobazam compared with carbamazepine and phenytoin in children with newly diagnosed epilepsy and found no deterioration of intelligence, memory, attention, psychomotor speed, or impulsivity in children on clobazam.

Gabapentin

Gabapentin occasionally has been reported to cause aggressive or agitated behavior. It was noted to cause no significant alteration of psychomotor or memory abilities.

Vigabatrin

Mild and transient drowsiness, dizziness, and irritability are frequently reported with vigabatrin initiation, but do not appear to affect cognition in a strong, adverse way. Both a single review of the cognitive effects of vigabatrin and a monotherapy study comparing it to carbamazepine in adult patients with partial epilepsy showed no cognitive deterioration, and in fact reported improvement in tests of memory, psychomotor speed, and flexibility of mental processing.

Lacosamide

Patients aged 16 to 74 years in a recent open-label lacosamide prospective study exhibited faster information processing reaction times at the second evaluation using a computerized visual searching task.

Perampanel

Cognition was not specifically assessed during the clinical trials of this recently approved selective noncompetitive antagonist of the AMPA receptors. Fatigue, dizziness, irritability, and aggression were reported among the side effects, however. Perampanel carries a black box warning label of serious neuropsychiatric side effects, including homicidal ideation reported in several adult patients.

MANAGEMENT OF COGNITIVE, SOCIAL, ACADEMIC, AND BEHAVIORAL PROBLEMS ASSOCIATED WITH EPILEPSY

Social acceptance and inclusion of children and adolescents with epilepsy is far from satisfactory, even when seizures are infrequent or fully controlled. In some cultural settings, diagnosis of epilepsy is not generally disclosed to friends or extended family. Despite laws guaranteeing disabled and medically impaired children full access to education, some schools discourage attendance by children with frequent seizures. Such prejudices may further impair social and academic function.

Assessment of the developmental, cognitive, academic, and behavioral status of the child and the social functioning of the family must be integrated into the management of a child with epilepsy. Although treatment generally will not alter the underlying cognitive capacity of the child, early intervention and referral to appropriate community and school resources will maximize function. Appropriate counseling may minimize later behavioral and adjustment difficulties.

School Inclusion and Academic Planning

At times, parents report that a child with epilepsy is excluded from school programs, sent home repeatedly, or placed in a more restrictive class setting than is appropriate. The physician may need to intervene if a child is being denied appropriate educational experiences because of concerns about possible seizures. Having a treatment plan for seizures may be useful

in reducing the anxiety of school personnel. Any child with special needs or suspicion of learning disabilities should be thoroughly evaluated by the school, and have an individualized educational plan (IEP or 504 plan in the USA).

Local branches of voluntary organizations, such as the Epilepsy Foundation of America, may be helpful in providing informational programs to schools. In the United States federal law mandates inclusion of children with disabilities and medical conditions in educational programs in the least restrictive environment appropriate for the child's needs.

Behavior Problems and Discipline

Behavioral problems and parent–child interaction should be addressed regularly. Parents may avoid disciplining a child with epilepsy out of fear that causing the child to become angry or upset may trigger seizures. Parents must be reassured that this is not the case. Even in children with well controlled seizures, parental anxiety may impair their ability to allow the child to take on age-appropriate behaviors such as sleeping in their own room, going out with peers, and participating in sports.

Significant abnormalities in behavior, activity, or attention warrant a more detailed evaluation. This may include psychiatric evaluation and/or psychometric testing. Psychometric testing, along with a clinical history gathered from parents, teachers, and patients, may be necessary to differentiate behavioral difficulties associated with coexisting ADHD from those due to family dysfunction, oppositional disorders, inappropriate parental expectations, and other factors.

Peer Relationships, Teasing, and Social Isolation

Social isolation and poor peer relationships are a particular problem in school-aged and adolescent children with epilepsy and are difficult to address therapeutically. Nonverbal learning disabilities comorbid with epilepsy may make the child socially maladroit and target them for teasing by peers. Children may be particularly at risk for teasing and exclusion by peers if they have had seizures at school or are singled out by the need to take medication during school. Therapeutic or educational programs that emphasize social skills and assertiveness training may be helpful.

Social and Occupational Adjustment of Adults With Childhood-Onset Epilepsy

Population-based studies from several countries document that adults who had childhood-onset epilepsy have impaired social functioning compared with their healthy peers. Employment is less frequent and included less skilled occupations; marriage is not as common, and social isolation is more frequent. Differences are more striking when adults have ongoing seizures, but are present even when complete remission or control has been obtained. Even when studies were restricted to adults with childhood-onset absence epilepsy, social functioning continued to be impaired in comparison with peers without epilepsy. Other studies of outcome in adults with childhood-onset epilepsy find substantial maladaptation as well, particularly in social and vocational function (Sillanpaa 1990). A Canadian study of adults evaluated 25 years after a diagnosis of juvenile myoclonic epilepsy documented a high frequency of social isolation, unemployment, and social impulsivity (Camfield & Camfield 2009).

Given these issues, vocational plans, postsecondary education, and appropriate goal setting should be discussed with adolescents who have epilepsy. Adolescents with well-controlled epilepsy may be assured that their epilepsy will not interfere with career goals, with a few exceptions: military service, airlines, and public safety professions generally will exclude applicants with epilepsy, regardless of control. Some states will restrict commercial drivers' licenses, even with good seizure control. Appropriate resources for assessment, training, and placement should be identified in the community. In addition to school-based programs, local Epilepsy Foundation affiliates may be a good resource, as may the state department of vocational rehabilitation.

REFERENCES

The complete list of references for this chapter is available in the e-book at www.expertconsult.com.
  See inside cover for registration details.

SELECTED REFERENCES

Berg, A.T., Langfitt, J.T., Testa, F.M., et al., 2008. Global cognitive function in children with epilepsy: a community-based study. Epilepsia 49, 608–614.

Camfield, C.S., Camfield, P.R., 2009. Juvenile myoclonic epilepsy 25 years after seizure onset: a population-based study. Neurology 73, 1041–1045.

Dunn, D.W., Austin, J.K., Perkins, S.M., 2009. Prevalence of psychopathology in childhood epilepsy: categorical and dimensional measures. Dev. Med. Child Neurol. 51, 364–372.

Eun, S.H., Eun, B.L., Lee, J.S., et al., 2012. Effects of lamotrigine on cognition and behavior compared to carbamazepine as monotherapy for children with partial epilepsy. Brain Dev. 34, 818–823.

Glauser, T.A., Cnaan, A., Shinnar, S., et al., 2010. Childhood Absence Epilepsy Study Group. Ethosuximide, valproic acid and lamotrigine in childhood absence epilepsy. N. Engl. J. Med. 362, 790–799.

Mandelbaum, D.E., Burack, G.D., Bhise, V.V., 2009. Impact of antiepileptic drugs on cognition, behavior, and motor skills in children with new-onset, idiopathic epilepsy. Epilepsy Behav. 16, 341–344.

Mula, M., Kanner, A.M., Schmitz, B., et al., 2013. Antiepileptic drugs and suicidality: an expert consensus statement from the Task Force on Therapeutic Strategies of the ILAE Commission on Neuropsychobiology. Epilepsia 54, 199–203.

Partikian, A., Mitchell, W.G., 2010. Neurodevelopmental and epilepsy outcomes in a North American cohort of patients with infantile spasms. J. Child Neurol. 25, 423–428.

Schiemann-Delgado, J., Yang, H., de la Loge, C., et al., 2012. A long-term open-label extension study assessing cognition and behavior, tolerability, safety, and efficacy of adjunctive levetiracetam in children aged 4 to 16 years with partial-onset seizures. J. Child Neurol. 27, 80–89.

Sillanpaa, M., 1990. Children with epilepsy as adults: outcome after 30 years of follow up. Acta Paediatr. Scand. 368 (Suppl.), 1.

83 Mortality in Children with Epilepsy

Jeffrey Buchalter, Carol S. Camfield, and Peter R. Camfield

INTRODUCTION

The recognition that children with epilepsy can die during seizures is not a new concept. However, the frequency and the circumstances of these tragic deaths have come under relatively recent scrutiny. This is attributable in part to the increased awareness of sudden unexpected death in epilepsy (SUDEP) and a desire to more accurately communicate to families the risks associated with the various types of seizures and epilepsy syndromes. The intent of discussion with the caregivers is to provide full disclosure regarding living with epilepsy and potential preventive measures to avoid mortality. This chapter focuses on mortality in childhood-onset epilepsy with the recognition that much of the literature addresses adults. The causes of premature mortality are divided into those that are directly related to seizures (e.g., status epilepticus) and those that are "comorbid" (e.g., etiology, pneumonia). We attempt to highlight those areas in which mortality in children differs from adults. The "bridging" literature is that which addresses epilepsy that starts in childhood, the consequences of which become apparent in the adult population.

EPIDEMIOLOGY

Five relatively recent prospective cohort studies have defined the risks of mortality for children with epilepsy. Three of these are population-based studies (Nova Scotia; Finland; Rochester, Minnesota), and two are very close to population-based studies (Connecticut, the Netherlands) (Berg et al., 2013; Devinsky, 2011; Sillanpää and Shinnar, 2010).

All five studies have strikingly similar results, except for the findings about SUDEP in Finland (see following discussion). Each of these cohorts includes incidence cases only (new-onset epilepsy), except the Finish cohort, which includes a mixture of incidence and prevalence cases. The *average* length of follow-up after seizure onset for the cohorts is 10 to 15 years, except in the Finland cohort, where the *median* follow-up was 40 years. Details of case findings of all children newly diagnosed with epilepsy and cause of death within these cohorts are summarized in Table 83-1.

The findings from these prospective cohort studies can be considered in five categories. First, children with epilepsy have a markedly increased risk of death. The standard mortality ratio (SMR) compares the death rate in children with epilepsy to that in the general population matched for age and sex and the time period under consideration. SMRs for children with epilepsy in four of the prospective cohorts range from approximately 6 to 8.5 (i.e., the risk of death for children with epilepsy in the next 10–40 years is 6–9 times that of the general population). Children without neurologic deficits and without symptomatic causes for their epilepsy have the same risk of death during follow-up as the general population (Nova Scotia; Connecticut; the Netherlands; Rochester, Minnesota). This remarkable and robust finding should have a major influence on the type of information about death that is shared with patients and families.

Second, the vast majority of deaths in children with epilepsy are not the direct result of seizures or SUDEP. They are the result of associated comorbid neurologic conditions, especially in those with swallowing difficulties resulting in aspiration pneumonia. Children with neurologic deficits sufficient to interfere with activities of daily living are markedly more likely to die than those with epilepsy but without neurologic deficits. Those with neurologic deficits were 22 times more likely to die in the Nova Scotia cohort over 20 years and 23 times more likely in the Connecticut study. In the Nova Scotia cohort, 20% of patients with serious comorbid neurologic conditions were dead within 20 years of seizure onset. Some but not all of the cohort studies included patients with progressive metabolic brain diseases (e.g., Menke's syndrome). Here the epilepsy is a symptom, and the progressive brain disease leads inevitably to death. These patients are uncommon; hence, studies that excluded them come to similar overall conclusions.

Third, deaths directly from seizures are uncommon. Status epilepticus is the most frequent way in which a child may die of a seizure. In the Finland study, four deaths were from status epilepticus compared with one in the Nova Scotia study. The risk of death from status epilepticus may be higher in some epileptic syndromes, reaching 10% to 15% in Dravet syndrome. Accidents resulting from a seizure (e.g., a fall with fatal head injury) are even less common; however, drowning is more common in children with epilepsy than controls. The excess number of drownings presumably is the result of seizure events, although the events are usually not witnessed. In the Finnish study, there were a total of 60 deaths from all causes, and 6 (10%) were from drowning. The most common site of drowning is most likely the bathtub. This observation suggests that a shower might be a safer way of cleansing for people with epilepsy than a bathtub, provided that the shower drain is not easily occluded by someone falling on it. Hot water taps that may be knocked all the way open by a falling person are best avoided; pirouetting (screw-in, screw-out) taps are preferable and less likely to lead to a scalding injury. The degree of direct supervision that is reasonable for a child in the shower or bathtub is unclear and may depend on the child's degree of seizure control. At the very least, it would seem prudent to have someone else in the household aware of when a child with epilepsy is bathing and to avoid locking the bathroom door. In general, most accidents that result from seizures do not appear to be easily preventable.

Drownings in swimming pools, lakes, or the ocean can only be prevented by avoiding swimming when seizures are not well controlled and providing a swimming "buddy" capable of intervening if necessary.

Fourth, suicide in people with childhood-onset epilepsy, although tragic, is not common (two cases in the Nova Scotia study and two in Finland, both cohorts with follow-up to age 36 and 50 years, respectively).

Fifth, SUDEP (see following section for definition) was very uncommon in the cohorts other than the Finnish. The number of SUDEP cases in the four cohorts, as updated by Berg et al.

TABLE 83-1 Details of Methodology and Findings From the Five Cohorts

	Finland	Nova Scotia	Netherlands	Connecticut	Rochester
Methods and patient source	Prospective, population based, mixture of incidence and prevalence	Prospective, population based	Prospective, regional	Prospective, community based	Retrospective, population based
Years of cohort recruitment	1961–1964	1977–1985	1988–1992	1993–1997	1980–2009
Cohort size	245	686	472	613	468
Mean age at last FU or death*	39.5 y	19.2 y	20.7 y	23.3 y	16.7 y
Number of deaths from all causes	60	26	15	13	14
Number of deaths from SUDEP	23 (55%); none under 14 years of age	1 (at age 23 years)	2 possible SUDEP	1	1
Age range at death (years), all causes	0.1–50	0.5–30	2.1–26.9	1.8–28.7	0.2–21.7

*All followed to death or ≥ 5 years after diagnosis.
FU, follow-up; SUDEP, sudden unexpected death in epilepsy.

in 2013, was only 10 out of 2239 children with new-onset epilepsy. These children were followed for more than 30,000 person-years. None of those dying with SUDEP had epilepsy syndromes of childhood absence epilepsy, juvenile absence epilepsy, juvenile myoclonic epilepsy, or rolandic epilepsy.

As mentioned earlier, nearly 40% of the Finnish cohort were prevalence cases, which typically represent patients with more severe epilepsy. The rate of death for incidence cases was 5.3/1000 person-years and for prevalence cases was nearly twice as high at 9.6/1000 person-years. This suggests that the severity of epilepsy in the Finnish cohort may be higher than in the other four cohorts.

In the Finnish cohort there were 18 cases of SUDEP, confirmed by autopsy in 15. The median age of SUDEP was 25 years (range 4–49 years). The overall risk of SUDEP for a child with epilepsy over 40 years of follow-up was 7% and only 5% in those with "cryptogenic or idiopathic" etiology. It is important to note that there were no cases of SUDEP in patients with "cryptogenic or idiopathic" epilepsy who were younger than 14 years of age. Overall, SUDEP was very rare before young adulthood and was strongly associated with uncontrolled seizures. It would appear that persistent uncontrolled childhood-onset epilepsy is associated with an increased risk of SUDEP in adulthood. This important observation finding needs additional confirmation.

SUDDEN UNEXPECTED DEATH IN EPILEPSY

Although the reality that people living with epilepsy died for unknown reasons had been known for some time, attention turned to SUDEP in the 1980s and was expanded in the 1990s after unexpected deaths in new antiseizure drug trials. This interest culminated in two sets of similar, but not identical criteria for SUDEP. The essential features common to both included deaths in people (children and adults) with the following characteristics: (1) known epilepsy, (2) no known other cause of death, (3) unexpected death, (4) death with or without a witnessed seizure (excluding status epilepticus), and (5) postmortem examination required for a definite diagnosis. Criteria were suggested to further classify cases as unlikely, possible, probable, and definite based on the strength of the information surrounding the death. In 2012 the research community recognized that the core criteria needed to be further clarified and expanded with a "unified" definition of SUDEP, which was outlined by Nashef, So, Ryvlin, and Tomson (2012) (Box 83-1). The additional features included specifying 1 hour

---

BOX 83-1 Definition of Sudden Unexpected Death in Epilepsy (SUDEP) and Variants

1. **Definite SUDEP**: A sudden, unexpected, witnessed or unwitnessed, nontraumatic and nondrowning death, occurring in benign circumstances, in an individual with epilepsy, with or without evidence for a seizure and excluding documented status epilepticus (seizure duration > 30 min or seizures without recovery in between), in which postmortem examination does not reveal a cause of death.
2. **Definite SUDEP Plus**: Satisfying the definition of Definite SUDEP, if a concomitant condition other than epilepsy is identified before or after death, if the death may have been a result of the combined effect of both conditions, and if autopsy or direct observations/recordings of terminal event did not prove the concomitant condition to be the cause of death.
3. **Probable SUDEP/Probable SUDEP Plus**: Same as Definite SUDEP but without autopsy. The victim should have died unexpectedly while in a reasonable state of health, during normal activities, and in benign circumstances, without a known structural cause of death.
4. **Possible SUDEP**: A competing cause of death is present.
5. **Near-SUDEP/Near-SUDEP Plus**: A patient with epilepsy survives resuscitation for more than 1 h after a cardiorespiratory arrest that has no structural cause identified after investigation.
6. **Not SUDEP**: A clear cause of death is known.
7. **Unclassified**: Incomplete information available; not possible to classify.

(Adapted from Nashef L, So EL, Ryvlin P, Tomson T. Epilepsia, 2012:53[2]: 227–233.)

---

as the limit in which to consider an event SUDEP after the terminal event and 30 minutes as the duration of status epilepticus to exclude the diagnosis, noting that death associated with drowning not associated with evidence of submersion should be considered "Possible SUDEP," and creating new categories designated as "SUDEP Plus" to allow other possible etiologies of death (e.g., known cardiac disease) when the criteria for SUDEP have been met and "Near-SUDEP" to indicate that resuscitation prevented likely death.

CLINICAL RISK FACTORS FOR SUDDEN UNEXPECTED DEATH IN EPILEPSY

To date it has been difficult to identify powerful risk factors for SUDEP (Tomson et al., 2008). Generalized tonic-clonic or focal seizures with secondary generalization appear to be important, especially if they occur during sleep (Walczak et al., 2001). There is a suggestion that children with comorbid neurologic deficits are at higher risk than those who are otherwise neurologically normal. A major theme has been the duration of epilepsy. As mentioned earlier, the Finland study noted an increasing rate of SUDEP after childhood onset if seizures persisted into adulthood. A review of published cases of SUDEP, noted only three studies with robust methodology, and calculated that the longer the duration of epilepsy, the higher the risk of SUDEP. Walzak et al. studied 4578 patients who had been admitted to several epilepsy monitoring units in the United States. During more than 16,000 person-years of follow-up, there were 10 definite and 10 probable cases of SUDEP. The odds ratio (OR) of SUDEP was 14 for patients with more than 30 years of epilepsy compared with those with less than 15 years.

Coupled with the duration of epilepsy are seizure severity and frequency. The lowest rate of SUDEP is seen in incidence (new-onset) cohorts, followed by prevalence cohorts, and then epilepsy clinics. The highest reported rates are in cohorts of refractory patients, especially those who have had unsuccessful epilepsy surgery.

DISCUSSIONS ABOUT SUDDEN UNEXPECTED DEATH IN EPILEPSY WITH FAMILIES AND PATIENTS

One of the most contentious issues regards the "if, when, and how" relating to disclosure of SUDEP when taking care of people with epilepsy. The issues to be confronted include (1) the patient/family right to full disclosure of potential risks associated with seizures and (2) potential strategies to prevent seizure-related death. Reasons offered to not have this conversation are (1) concern about the psychological effects of this information, (2) inability to affect outcome, and (3) lack of need in low-risk populations (Morton, Richardson, and Duncan, 2006). The current practice of providers has been documented by several survey studies. A questionnaire of 738 British neurologists had a response rate of 52% ($n = 387$) and revealed that only 31% discussed SUDEP with some or all of their patients, adults and children. In contrast, a survey of 250 British nurse specialists in which 58% returned questionnaires revealed that SUDEP education was provided by 50% of nurses. It should be noted that this was in the context of a 2004 national guideline from the National Institute of Clinical Excellence indicating that SUDEP should be discussed as part of the general education of people living with epilepsy. A subsequent study querying the SUDEP disclosure practice of physicians at a British regional epilepsy clinic revealed that this information was provided to 20% of all parents but increased to 63% of parents whose children had intractable epilepsy. In contrast, a questionnaire of these same parents revealed that 91% expected the pediatric neurologist to provide this information, and 67% wanted the information at the first visit (Gayatri et al., 2010). There was a significant disparity in what providers did and what parents wanted. Similar results have been found by focus-group qualitative research with Canadian parents who have children with different severities of epilepsy.

The findings from the epidemiologic and risk-factor studies noted previously suggest several things about the discussion

of SUDEP: (1) the topic should be discussed with the majority of patients/families at the time of diagnosis or soon thereafter, and (2) the risk for each child needs to be presented based on the available literature in children, which indicates that there are at least two types of discussions. The first is for those in the higher-risk population. These are children who have frequent generalized tonic-clonic seizures during sleep, underlying neurologic disorders that predispose to premature mortality, abnormal neurologic examinations, and significant intellectual disability. One of the purposes of the discussion in this group is to encourage adherence with aggressive therapies and to allow families to prepare for the worst of all outcomes. In contrast, the discussion with the lower-risk group (i.e., "benign" epilepsy syndromes, infrequent nonconvulsive seizures) is one of reassurance. These families should not live under the specter of possible death related to seizures that may have been brought to their attention by media or information intended for the higher-risk group.

Mechanisms: During the last decade it has been suggested that the primary "system" failure in SUDEP was either dysfunction of brainstem breathing centers, cardiac dysrhythmias, or "cerebral shutdown," in which a seizure results in flattening of the electroencephalogram (EEG), referred to as postictal generalized EEG suppression, followed by lack of cerebral drive to cardiac and respiratory centers (Massey, Sowers, Dlouhy, and Richerson, 2014). It is acknowledged that the mechanisms underlying SUDEP are likely heterogeneous and that an individual's genotype may predispose to this uncommon, but tragic event. The importance of respiratory dysfunction was highlighted in a recent study of deaths in epilepsy monitoring units in which the majority of deaths were preceded by tachypnea followed by apnea and cardiac arrest. Brainstem serotonergic dysfunction may play a critical role, as suggested by rodent experiments.

PREVENTION OF MORTALITY RELATED TO SEIZURES

Although there are inadequate data specifically in the pediatric population, it is prudent to assume that reducing generalized tonic clonic seizures (GTCs) lowers the risk of SUDEP in children. The most direct evidence comes from a prospective case-controlled study from four epilepsy centers. Patients were all admitted to an epilepsy monitoring unit and then followed. There were no SUDEP cases in children. However, in adults, those who had at least four GTCs in the last year had an increased risk of dying from SUDEP by a factor of 8 compared with those with no GTCs. Another piece of evidence indicates that the most significant potential method of preventing SUDEP is reduction of seizures. This information comes from studies demonstrating decreased risk in a group of patients undergoing epilepsy surgery who were then seizure-free (0 of 199) compared with those who had recurrent seizures after surgery (11 of 194). It should be noted that both of these studies involved patients with more complicated cases than those of the typical community patient, as reflected by receiving their care in epilepsy centers and certainly those with intractable epilepsy requiring surgery.

A key assumption in the purpose of disclosing information regarding the risk of death and SUDEP specifically is that by doing so, the patient/family will be inclined to be more compliant with medications and/or pursue more aggressive therapies such as epilepsy surgery. The results to date have not been conclusive in this regard. One study of 39 parents living with a highly selected group of children with epilepsy indicated that this knowledge resulted in only a 31% increase in monitoring of antiseizure drugs. However, a survey of young adults

(18–20 years old) revealed that although 81% wanted to be informed of SUDEP, they had a fatalistic attitude, with no clear influence regarding therapy or lifestyle changes. This important study indicates that more than just disclosure will be required to change behavior with regard to adherence. At this point there is no direct evidence that increased adherence leads to decreased seizure frequency and decreased rates of SUDEP. Thus the recommendation to be adherent with treatment recommendations as a means of decreasing SUDEP is speculative, but logical.

It has not been proven that detection of seizures during sleep can avert SUDEP, but the results of two studies suggest that supervision during sleep may be protective. The first described 14 people who were enrolled in a residential school for 4 to 18 years and died of SUDEP when they were out of the facility. Because the students had nocturnal supervision (attendant available to respond to an auditory alarm) while at the school, it is possible that the supervision prevented deaths while the students were in the residential facility. The second was a case-control study of 154 individuals with SUDEP in whom an autopsy was performed and in which risk factors were compared with four controls for each case. It was found that nocturnal monitoring by a person 10 years of age or older in same room (odds ratio [OR]: 0.4, 95% confidence interval [CI]: 0.2–0.8) or precautionary measures such as a listening device (OR: 0.1, 95% CI: 0.0–0.3) were protective for SUDEP.

Based on the possibility that intervention might avert SUDEP, a significant amount of research has been directed to seizure-detection devices that could be used in the home (see Ramgopal [2014] for a recent comprehensive review). All of the issues that pertain to any diagnostic test (e.g., sensitivity, specificity) apply to seizure-detection devices and the feasibility of acting on the alarm. In addition to portable EEG systems with seizure-detection algorithms, widely varying devices have been proposed and include the following: accelerometers to detect motion (worn on the wrist, placed under the mattress, present as an app on a smartphone), audio and recording devices, and autonomic function (heart rate, sweat) monitors. Some devices have combined several modalities of detection, and others have utilized modern technologies (e.g., Bluetooth) for alerting someone who could intervene. The ability of dogs to detect seizures has been reported, but the sensitivity, specificity, and utility in the sleeping child have not been established.

To date, there are no definitive studies that establish that any monitoring device can reduce the risk of SUDEP. Based on the experience with sudden infant death syndrome (SIDS), it is likely that monitoring devices have a significant effect on family life and may possibly do more harm than good. Physicians should be cautious about recommending such devices for children with epilepsy.

A recent study has suggested that a preventive measure may be available that does not require a detection device. A systemic analysis of reported SUDEP cases found that 73% of the 253 cases where body position was noted occurred in the prone position; all 11 cases in video EEG reports were in the prone position. In 88 cases body position and basic demographics were available, and when stratified by age, 86% of patients under 20 years of age who died were found in the prone position. Thus an education effort targeted at those living with epilepsy similar to that implemented for SIDS might play a role in preventing SUDEP. However, patients may roll or be tossed from supine to prone during a convulsive seizure, so a "back to sleep" program may not be effective.

PREVENTION OF MORTALITY NOT RELATED TO SEIZURES

As described in the Epidemiology section, the majority of children with epilepsy who suffer premature death die from a cause not related to seizures. Unfortunately, prevention related to an underlying neurodegenerative disorder, frequently of a genetic etiology, is limited to symptomatic care if a specific therapy is not available. Fortunately, suicide is uncommon in this population, but the clinician must be alert to signs of depression, which is the most common antecedent of suicide in people living with epilepsy. In contrast, drowning is preventable by supervision in the bathtub or shower and near bodies of water. Finally, infectious causes of premature mortality such as pneumonia and urinary tract infections are potentially preventable by clinical surveillance (particularly in intellectually disabled individuals) and rapid introduction of antibiotic therapy.

CONCLUSIONS

Death in children with epilepsy is almost always related to the underlying neurologic disorder, not the seizures. Death from status epilepticus is rare but should be preventable. Death from accidents caused by seizures is also rare. SUDEP is fortunately rare in children with epilepsy, but the risk may increase if seizures persist into adulthood. The mechanism of SUDEP is likely multifactorial, and it can only be prevented by completely controlling seizures, especially generalized tonic-clonic seizures. Seizure-detection devices for home use are in development, but they remain of uncertain value. SUDEP should be discussed with families close to the time of epilepsy diagnosis.

REFERENCES

The complete list of references for this chapter is available in the e-book at www.expertconsult.com.

    See inside cover for registration details.

SELECTED REFERENCES

Berg, A.T., Nickels, K., Wirrell, E.C., et al., 2013. Mortality risks in new-onset childhood epilepsy. Pediatrics 132 (1), 124–131.

Devinsky, O., 2011. Sudden, unexpected death in epilepsy. NEJM 365 (19), 1801–1811.

Gayatri, N.A., Morrall, M.C., Jain, V., et al., 2010. Parental and physician beliefs regarding the provision and content of written sudden unexpected death in epilepsy (SUDEP) information. Epilepsia 51 (5), 777–782.

Massey, C.A., Sowers, L.P., Dlouhy, B.J., et al., 2014. Mechanisms of sudden unexpected death in epilepsy: the pathway to prevention. Nat. Rev. Neurol. 10 (5), 271–282.

Morton, B., Richardson, A., Duncan, S., 2006. Sudden unexpected death in epilepsy (SUDEP): don't ask, don't tell? J. Neurol. Neurosurg. Psychiatry 77 (2), 199–202.

Nashef, L., So, E.L., Ryvlin, P., et al., 2012. Unifying the definitions of sudden unexpected death in epilepsy. Epilepsia 53 (2), 227–233.

Ramgopal, S., Thome-Souza, S., Jackson, M., et al., 2014. Seizure detection, seizure prediction, and closed-loop warning systems in epilepsy. Epilepsy Behav. 37, 291–307.

Sillanpää, M., Shinnar, S., 2010. Long-term mortality in childhood-onset epilepsy. NEJM 363, 2522–2529.

Tomson, T., Nashef, L., Ryvlin, P., et al., 2008. Sudden unexpected death in epilepsy: current knowledge and future directions. Lancet Neurol. 7 (11), 1021–1031.

Walczak, T.S., Leppik, I.E., D'Amelio, M., et al., 2001. Incidence and risk factors in sudden unexpected death in epilepsy: a prospective cohort study. Neurology 56 (4), 519–525.

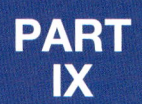

84 Headache in Children and Adolescents

Marielle A. Kabbouche, Joanne Kacperski, Hope L. O'Brien, Scott W. Powers, and Andrew D. Hershey

An expanded version of this chapter is available on www.expertconsult.com. See inside cover for registration details.

INTRODUCTION

Headache is a common complaint among children and adolescents and is a common referral to neurologists, with migraine being one of the top five childhood diseases. However, it is frequently ignored by parents, teachers, and primary care providers as a significant problem, resulting in lost school days and social interactions. It is therefore essential for clinicians to have a thorough and systematic approach to the evaluation of headaches, because proper diagnosis and management can lead to improved outcomes and quality of life (Hershey, 2010).

The most common cause of recurrent, episodic headaches in children is migraine. Primary headache such as migraine and tension-type headaches are intrinsic to the brain, in contrast to secondary headaches caused by something else, such as head trauma, brain tumors, infection, inflammatory diseases or increased intracranial pressure. One of the first steps in the evaluation of headache is to exclude secondary causes. Evaluation begins by obtaining a thorough history, which includes the following elements:

1. Identification of any secondary etiologies
2. Timing, including when the child first began developing headaches, not just "bad" headaches
3. Headache characterization, including quality of the pain and the location, duration, severity, and frequency of the headaches
4. Associated features, signs, and symptoms
5. Warning signs that initiate or aggravate the headaches
6. Family history for headaches and also for medical, neurologic, and psychiatric illnesses

In addition to a complete history, a complete physical, neurologic, and headache examination is necessary. If abnormalities are observed, the cause of the abnormality needs to be determined. The neurologic examination is the most significant determinant if neuroimaging studies are warranted. In most patients, the initial evaluation and examination can be diagnostic and provide reassurance that additional testing is unnecessary. Once the diagnosis is established, a comprehensive treatment plan should be developed that includes a combination of pharmacologic and nonpharmacologic modalities.

CLASSIFICATION

An international standardized set of criteria has been established to diagnose all headache disorders, the International Classification of Headache Disorders (ICHD) third edition (beta; ICHD-3b) (http://www.ihs-classification.org/_downloads/mixed/International-Headache-Classification-III-ICHD-III-2013-Beta.pdf). The ICHD-3b is divided into three major categories: primary headaches, those that are diseases by themselves; secondary headaches, those caused or exacerbated by a secondary factor, and the cranial neuropathies; and other facial pains and headaches. In addition, an appendix contains criteria to be tested. ICHD-3b requires that all headache diagnoses should be included in the diagnostic list for that patient, thus describing the full phenotype.

Migraine Without Aura

Patients can be given the diagnosis of migraine without aura using ICHD-3b criteria if they have had at least five recurrent, episodic headaches over the past year that last 2 to 72 hours untreated (<18 years old; 4-72 hours for adults); have two of the four features of pulsatile quality, unilateral location, worsening with activity or limiting activity, and moderate to severe in intensity; and are associated with either nausea, vomiting, photophobia, or phonophobia (all four symptoms can be present). Not all headaches need to meet all ICHD-3b criteria. They just need enough criteria to establish the diagnosis. There are special comments for children, including that sleep is considered part of the duration, associated symptoms can be inferred by parent or guardian based on the child's action, and location may be bilateral, namely, frontotemporal.

Migraine with Aura

If the patient has a neurologic warning of an oncoming headache, migraine with aura should be considered. To make this diagnosis, ICHD-3b requires at least three headaches over the past year to be associated with an aura. The aura needs to be one of six types, visual, sensory, dysphasic, motor, brainstem, or retinal, that should have two of the following four features: lasting more than 5 minutes but less than 60 minutes (multiple auras can be additive), fully reversible, unilateral (dysphasia or aphasia is defined as unilateral), and the pain of the headache starts within 60 minutes (although it can be simultaneous, and the aura can occur when the patient has pain). What was formerly called basilar or basilar-type migraine is now recognized as a migraine with brainstem aura. Hemiplegic migraine (whether familial or sporadic) is also considered a migraine with aura and has an additional diagnostic hierarchy that can include the genetic identification of the polymorphism causing familial hemiplegic migraine.

Chronic Migraine

When migraines become frequent (15 or more days per month), a diagnosis of chronic migraine can be included.

ICHD-3b requires at least 15 headache days per month for 3 months with at least 5 meeting ICHD-3b criteria and having at least 8 headaches per month that meet the ICHD-3b criteria for migraine that are responsive to migraine-specific medication or in the interpretation of the patient are migraine.

Migraine Variants

Several migraine variants were included under the category of childhood periodic syndromes in earlier ICHD versions. In ICHD-3b, the limitation of childhood was removed, because it has been recognized that adults can learn from the experience of children, and the term has now been changed to *episodic syndromes that may be associated with migraine*. Within this larger category are recurrent gastrointestinal disturbance (cyclic vomiting syndrome and abdominal migraine), benign paroxysmal vertigo, and benign paroxysmal torticollis. In the ICHD-3b appendix, infantile colic, alternating hemiplegia of childhood, and vestibular migraine are included for testing to determine whether they should be included in or eliminated from future revisions. Please refer to the online version of the chapter for additional migraine variants.

Tension-Type Headache

The other common primary headache in children is tension-type headache (TTH), which can be thought of as the opposite of migraine, and when migraine features occur, the ICHD-3b recommends defaulting to making a diagnosis of migraine. TTH can be divided into infrequent (<1/month), frequent (1-14 times per month), and chronic (>15 per month for ≥ 3 months). The ICHD-3b TTH criteria are recurrent headaches with at least 10 episodes in the past year, lasting 30 minutes to 7 days, with two of the following four headache features: nonpulsatile, diffuse in location, not worsened or aggravated by physical activity, and mild to moderate in severity. Clarification was added for differentiating migraine from TTH, and in contrast to the earlier discussion about being inclusive, if the diagnosis of migraine is made, the diagnosis of TTH should not be made.

Trigeminal Autonomic Cephalalgia

The trigeminal autonomic cephalalgias (TACs) represent a group of primary headache disorders associated with excruciating head pain accompanied by autonomic features such as lacrimation, ptosis, rhinorrhea, and vasomotor changes. Cluster headache is an uncommon TAC in children and adolescents. The prevalence of childhood onset of cluster headache is approximately 0.1%. The diagnostic criteria require at least five attacks of severe unilateral orbital, supraorbital, and/or temporal pain, lasting 15 to 180 minutes, with a sense of restless agitation accompanied by ipsilateral conjunctival injection, lacrimation, nasal congestion, rhinorrhea, eyelid edema, forehead sweating, miosis, or ptosis. Cluster headaches may be episodic or chronic, and attacks occur in series that last for weeks or even months. A cluster may be precipitated by alcohol, histamine, or nitroglycerine. Males are three times more likely to be affected than females. Additional TACs include paroxysmal hemicranias and indomethacin-sensitive headaches.

EPIDEMIOLOGY

The prevalence of any complaint of headache ranges from 37% to 51% in 7-year-olds, gradually rising to 57% to 82% by age 15. The prevalence of recurrent migraine is approximately 2.5% to 4.0% in younger children (under age 8 years),

which increases to approximately 10% in 5- to 15-year-olds and continues to increase to adult levels throughout the late-teen years.

The epidemiology of TTH is less well studied, because it is often complicated by a mixed-headache picture with migraine. Patients frequently have diagnoses of mild headaches as TTH and severe headaches as migraine.

For additional information, please see the online chapter.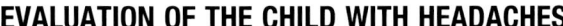

MIGRAINE PATHOPHYSIOLOGY

Migraine is a disorder of neurologic dysfunction with a strong genetic basis. The underlying pathophysiology is likely to be a complex, heterogeneous process, with the ultimate phenotype being a common appearance from multiple pathways. For a more complete review of migraine pathophysiology, please see the online chapter and the review by Goadsby, Charbit, Andreou, Akerman, and Holland (2009).

EVALUATION OF THE CHILD WITH HEADACHES

Evaluation follows the traditional medical model and begins with a thorough medical history and complete physical and neurologic examination. The role of ancillary diagnostic studies, such as laboratory testing, electroencephalography (EEG), and neuroimaging, has been extensively reviewed. The American Academy of Neurology (AAN) Practice Parameter determined that there is inadequate documentation in the literature to support any recommendation as to the appropriateness of routine laboratory studies (e.g., hematology or chemistry panels) or performance of a lumbar puncture or an EEG unless a secondary headache is being evaluated (Lewis et al., 2002). At the end of the clinical evaluation, the clinician should be confident in narrowing the differential diagnosis and deciding whether or not there is a need for further testing.

Neuroimaging

An imaging study is warranted if one or more of the following factors are present during the clinical interview (for a review of recommendations, see the online chapter):

- Subacute headache with rapidly progressive increase in severity
- New-onset headache in the immunosuppressed patient
- Headache of new onset in patients older than 50 years of age
- First or worst headache
- Associated systemic symptoms (e.g., fever or nuchal rigidity)
- Headache with focal neurologic abnormalities on examination

These guidelines apply to the general population. Because of the possibility of specific headache types in children, the following additional factors need to be considered:

- Headache of less than 1 month in duration
- Absence of family history of migraine/primary headache
- Abnormal neurologic examination
- Gait abnormalities
- Seizures
- Sleep-related headaches, vomiting, and confusion (headaches waking the child from sleep or intractable vomiting upon awakening)
- Children younger than 6 years old
- A history consistent with an occipital headache

In 1994, the AAN published its Practice Parameter on the use of neuroimaging in the evaluation of adults with headache with normal neurologic examination and recommended that an imaging study is not warranted in patients older than 6 years with recurrent migraine when there is no change in pattern, no history of seizures, and an absence of other focal neurologic signs.

The recommendations for children were reported in 2002 by the AAN and the Child Neurology Society (CNS):

- Obtaining a neuroimaging study on a routine basis is not indicated in children with recurrent headache and a normal neurologic examination.
- Neuroimaging should be considered in children with an abnormal neurologic examination and in whom there are historical features suggesting recent onset of headache, change in the type of headache, neurologic dysfunction, and occipital location of the headache.

Based on the available current literature, imaging should be considered for the following factors:

1. Abnormal neurologic examination
2. Atypical headache presentation: vertigo, intractable vomiting, or headache waking the child from sleep
3. Headache onset within the last 6 months
4. Child of less than 6 years of age
5. No family history of migraine and/or primary headache
6. Occipital headache
7. Change in headache type
8. Subacute onset and progressive headache severity
9. New-onset headache in an immunosuppressed child
10. First and/or worst headache
11. Systemic symptoms and signs
12. Headache associated with confusion, mental status changes, or focal neurologic complaints

Computed tomography (CT) imaging can be acquired rapidly and is widely available in almost all emergency departments. It is highly sensitive in detecting acute hemorrhage. Magnetic resonance imaging (MRI) is more sensitive in evaluating the posterior fossa, an area of high incidence of pathology in children. MRI is also more sensitive for neoplastic and vascular disorders, ischemia, and infection. One should consider acquiring an MRI scan if an imaging study is considered necessary, unless an acute surgical lesion such as an intracranial hemorrhage is suspected.

Lumbar Puncture

A lumbar puncture is indicated in the evaluation of headache in children as detailed in the AAN/CNS guidelines for headache evaluation when there is a suspected secondary etiology and any of the following features:

1. First and/or worst headache to evaluate for a subarachnoid hemorrhage, especially if suspicion is high and the CT scanning is negative
2. Headache with fever/nuchal rigidity or other signs of meningitis or meningoencephalitis
3. Headache in an immunosuppressed patient
4. Evaluation for increased/decreased intracranial pressure (pseudotumor cerebri/low-pressure headache)

A lumbar puncture is not indicated for routine diagnosis of a primary headache such as migraine or TTH.

Clinical Laboratory Testing

Clinical laboratory studies are not needed in the routine evaluation of primary headache. Routine baseline testing can be of value before initiating preventive headache medications, and in monitoring of prescribed drugs for toxicity and compliance.

Low levels of vitamin B_2 and coenzyme Q10 have been associated with an increased frequency of headache.

Electroencephalogram

Routine electroencephalogram (EEG) is not recommended.

For additional information on evaluation, please see the online chapter.

MANAGEMENT OF PEDIATRIC MIGRAINE

Once the diagnosis of migraine is established and appropriate reassurances have been provided, a balanced and individually tailored treatment plan can be instituted. The first step is to appreciate the degree of disability imposed by the patient's headache. An understanding of the effects of the headache on the patient's quality of life will guide the decisions regarding the most appropriate treatment. Despite often experiencing significant disability, many children do not receive preventive therapy. One third of adolescents meet the criteria for preventive therapy, yet only 10% to 19% are offered treatment. Moreover, controlled clinical trials investigating the use of acute and preventive medications in children have suffered from high placebo response rates. As a result, treatment practices vary widely, even among headache specialists, as a result of the absence of evidence-based guidelines.

An AAN guideline has established the general principles for the management of migraine headache (Silberstein, 2000), which include the following:

1. Reduction of headache frequency, severity, duration, and disability
2. Reduction of reliance on poorly tolerated, ineffective, or unwanted acute pharmacotherapies
3. Improvement in quality of life
4. Avoidance of acute headache medication escalation
5. Education and enablement of patients to manage their disease to enhance personal control of their migraine
6. Reduction of headache-related distress and psychological symptoms

To achieve these goals, it is becoming increasingly clear that a balanced treatment plan must include biobehavioral strategies and nonpharmacologic methods in addition to pharmacologic ones. Biobehavioral treatments include biofeedback, cognitive behavioral therapy, stress management, sleep hygiene, exercise, and dietary modifications.

Biofeedback has shown effectiveness in adults and children in controlled migraine trials. Although the physiologic basis is unclear, data suggest that plasma beta-endorphin levels can be altered. Biofeedback commonly uses electrical devices that provide audio or visual displays to demonstrate a physiologic effect. Thermal biofeedback is the most commonly used technique, wherein children are taught to raise the temperature of one of their fingers. Children can use these methods to manage future headaches, allowing them to feel that they have greater control of their health.

Stress management and relaxation therapies use techniques such as progressive relaxation, self-hypnosis, and guided imagery. Controlled trials have reported relaxation therapies to be equally effective as propranolol in reducing migraine frequency.

Maintenance of healthy habits is an essential component of the treatment plan. Sleep disturbances occur in 25% to 40% of children with migraine. It remains unclear whether sleep disturbances increase the occurrence of migraine, whether frequent and intense migraine leads to sleep disturbances, or whether the two are unrelated. Current practice is to recommend good sleep hygiene (Miller, Palermo, Powers, Scher, and

Hershey, 2003). Exercise also is recommended, and a review of Internet websites serving headache sufferers reveals the common endorsement of regular physical activity. Extensive dietary restriction is not recommended. The once-popular elimination diets are now judged to be excessive, and they generally set the stage for a battleground at home when parents attempt to force a restrictive diet upon an unwilling adolescent. A more reasonable approach is to review the list of foods thought to be linked to migraine and invite the patient to keep a headache diary and see if a temporal relationship exists between ingestion of one or more foods and headache development. In addition to looking at what patients eat, it is important to encourage them to eat regular meals and to drink plenty of fluids. Many teenagers routinely skip breakfast. Missing meals is a common precipitant of migraine and is identified by adolescents as one of the leading triggers.

Caffeine warrants special mention. Caffeine influences headache frequency and may disrupt sleep and/or aggravate mood, both of which may exacerbate headache. Furthermore, caffeine withdrawal headache, which begins 1 to 2 days following cessation of regular caffeine use, can last up to a week.

Pharmacologic Therapies for Migraine Headache

Pharmacologic management has been subjected to thorough review, but controlled data are limited (see the online chapter for a description of treatment studies).

Acute Therapy/Outpatient Abortive Therapy

For the acute treatment of migraine, the most rigorously studied agents are ibuprofen, acetaminophen, and the triptans (Table 84-1), all of which have shown safety and efficacy in controlled trials. Almotriptan and rizatriptan are the only triptans approved by the U.S. Food and Drug Administration (FDA) for use in children and adolescents. Almotriptan has been approved for use in children ages 12 and above. The use of rizatriptan for pediatric migraine was approved for children ages 6 to 17.

In general, a nonsteroidal anti-inflammatory drug (NSAID) such as ibuprofen or naproxen sodium should be used as the first-line acute therapy. If this is not consistently effective, addition of a triptan may be warranted. Care should be taken to avoid overusing these medications, because they may cause medication-overuse headaches (see online chapter).

Emergency Room Management of Migraine Exacerbation

Sometimes the headache continues despite acute outpatient therapy, and if it is disabling, a more aggressive approach may be needed.

Status migrainosus is an acute migraine attack lasting 72 hours or more. It is imperative to break this type of headache before it becomes intractable and unresponsive to acute therapy. The patient should initially be referred to an infusion center or the emergency department (ED) for therapy.

Therapeutic approaches vary because of the lack of guidelines for the treatment of acute refractory headache in children. Available treatments for status migrainosus in an ED include antidopaminergic medications (prochlorperazine and metoclopramide), NSAIDs (e.g., ketorolac), dihydroergotamine (DHE), antiepileptic drugs (e.g., sodium valproate), and triptan compounds.

Antidopaminergic Drugs. Prochlorperazine is very effective in aborting an attack in the ED when given intravenously (IV) with a load of IV fluids (Kabbouche, Vockell, LeCates, Powers, and Hershey, 2001). Results show a 75% improvement with 50% headache freedom at 1 hour and 95% improvement with 60% headache freedom at 3 hours. Prochlorperazine was compared with metoclopramide and a placebo in a well-controlled study; improvement in headache severity was 82% for prochlorperazine, 42% for metoclopramide, and 29% for the placebo.

The average dose of prochlorperazine is 0.15 mg/kg, with a maximum dose of 10 mg. The average dose of metoclopramide is 0.13 to 0.15 mg/kg, with a maximum dose of 10 mg, given intravenously over 15 minutes. These medications are usually well tolerated, but extrapyramidal reactions are more frequent in children. Patients experiencing symptoms or severe irritability and restlessness can be given diphenhydramine to control these side effects. Diphenhydramine does not prevent these side effects when given early.

Nonsteroidal Anti-Inflammatory Drugs. Ketorolac is often used in the ED as monotherapy (0.5 mg/kg, with a maximum of 30 mg) or in combination with other medications. Ketorolac alone results in 55.2% improvement, and the recurrence rate at 24 hours is 30%. When combined with Prochlorperazine, the response rate increases to 93%.

Antiepileptic Drugs. Sodium valproate is given as a bolus of 15 to 20 mg per kg intravenously over 5 minutes that can be

---

TABLE 84-1   Selective Serotonin (5-HT$_1$) Receptor Agonists

Generic Name	Trade Name	Route	Dosage
Almotriptan*	Axert®	Oral	6.25-12.5 mg at onset; may repeat in 2 h; no more than 2 doses in 24 h
Eletriptan	Relpax®	Oral	40 mg at onset; may repeat in 2 h; max 80 mg/d
Frovatriptan	Frova®	Oral	2.5 mg at onset; may repeat in 2 h; no more than 3 doses in 24 h
Naratriptan	Amerge®	Oral	1-2.5 mg at onset; may repeat in 4 h; not to exceed 30 mg/24h
Rizatriptan*	Maxalt® Maxalt-MLT®	Oral Disintegrating tablets	5-10 mg at onset; may repeat in 2 h; not to exceed 30 mg/24h
Sumatriptan	Imitrex®	Oral Subcutaneous Intranasal Suppository	25, 50, 100 mg at onset; may repeat in 2 h, up to 100 mg 6 mg at onset, may repeat dose in 1 h, up to 12 mg/d 20 mg, one spray in one nostril at onset; may repeat within 2-24 h; limited to two sprays/d
Zolmitriptan	Zomig® Zomig-ZMT®	Oral, nasal spray Disintegrating tablets	2.5-5 mg at onset; may repeat in 2 h; not to exceed 10 mg/24h

*Almotriptan and rizatriptan are the only triptans with FDA approval for pediatric and adolescent migraine.

followed by an oral dose (15-20 mg/day) in the 4 hours after the infusion. Patients may benefit from a short-term preventive treatment with an extended-release form after discharge. Sodium valproate is usually well tolerated.

Triptan Compounds. An open-label study showed the effectiveness of subcutaneous sumatriptan. With a dosage of 0.06 mg per kg, overall efficacy was 72% at 30 minutes and 78% at 2 hours, with a recurrence rate of 6%. DHE, if recommended for recurrences, should not be given within 24 hours of triptan use. The triptan can be used in the outpatient setting, and the patient does not need referral to the ED (Table 84-1).

Dihydroergotamine Use in the Emergency Department. Ergots are one of the oldest treatments for migraine. DHE is a parenteral form used for acute exacerbations. Its effect is attributable to 5HT1A-1B-1D-1F receptor agonist affinity and central vasoconstriction. DHE has a greater alpha-adrenergic antagonist activity and is less vasoconstrictive peripherally. Before treatment initiation, a full history and neurologic examination should be performed. Females of childbearing age should be evaluated for any concerns regarding pregnancy. DHE is used as a potent central vasoconstrictor to abort the vascular phase of the attack. One dose can be effective for an acute prolonged headache. Compared with valproate, the response was similar at 1, 2, and 4 hours for both therapies, with 60% improvement in headache severity; however, DHE was still effective in 90% of patients versus 60% for those patients receiving valproate at 24 hours. An additional study in 30 children using DHE for acute treatment showed an 80% response rate. Dosing ranged from 0.1 to 0.5 mg, considerably lower than dosages used for treating adults.

Inpatient Therapy for Severe Debilitating Acute Exacerbation of Primary Headache

Approximately 7% of children and adolescents will fail acute therapy in the ED and will require hospital admission for more intensive therapy. Inpatient treatment for status migrainosus has not been carefully studied, but clinical reports and reviews have been done in pediatric headache facilities, with positive results. These patients are usually admitted for a 3 to 5 days and receive extensive IV treatment. A child should be hospitalized when he or she is in status migrainous that was refractory to outpatient infusion center or ED treatment, or if the patient has an exacerbation of chronic severe headache. The goal is to control a disabling headache that has been unresponsive to other abortive therapies. Treatment protocols include the use of DHE, antiemetic medications, and sodium valproate.

Dihydroergotamine Use in the Inpatient Setting. Patients hospitalized for DHE treatment should be premedicated with 0.13 to 0.15mg/kg of prochlorperazine a half hour before the DHE dose for up to three doses. If the patient continues to have significant nausea, the antidopaminergic medications are replaced by Ondansetron for the remaining treatments. The DHE dose is 0.5 to 1 mg (depending on age and tolerability) and is used every 8 hours until headache freedom. The first dose is halved and given a half hour apart to evaluate tolerability. When the headache ceases, two extra doses are given to prevent recurrence. The response to this protocol results in 97% improvement and 77% headache freedom. Response starts being noticeable by dose 5 and can reach its maximum effect after dose 10. Side effects include nausea, vomiting, abdominal discomfort, flushed face, and transient increases in blood pressure during infusion.

Sodium Valproate. Sodium valproate is used when DHE is contraindicated or has been ineffective. One adult study recommends the use of valproate as follows: bolus with 15 mg per kg followed with 5 mg/kg every 8 hours until headache freedom or up to 10 doses, whichever occurs first. An additional dose can be given after the headache ceases. This protocol was studied in adults with chronic daily headaches and showed an 80% improvement.

Preventive Treatment

Prophylaxis should be limited to those children and adolescents whose headaches occur with sufficient frequency and/or severity to warrant daily medication (Lewis, Diamond, Scott, and Jones, 2004). Treatment goals include reducing headache frequency and progression to chronic headache and lessening associated disability. Most specialists recommend a minimum of one headache per week or three to four headaches per month to consider prevention medication. Preventive treatment should also be considered if acute treatments are ineffective, not well tolerated, contraindicated because of other medical conditions, or overused, or if the patient has infrequent but severely disabling headaches.

The clinician and family must also establish a sense of functional disability before committing the child to a course of daily medication, because therapy should also aim to improve the overall quality of life. All patients warranting prevention should be provided with appropriate education regarding their diagnosis and treatment plan, thus enabling patients to manage their disease and enhance personal control of their headaches. Clinicians should discuss this long-term treatment plan so that families understand that the effort is often a long-term one, and response will not occur rapidly. It should be emphasized that the onset of improvement is often delayed in pediatric patients, and ideally these medications should only be used for a finite period of time. A goal of three or less headaches per month is recommended for a sustained period of 4 to 6 months. The dose of the medication should be titrated slowly to minimize side effects. Once an effective dose is achieved, relief must be sustained for 2 to 3 months before considering an alternative medication. Once these goals are achieved, a plan to slowly wean the child off the agent is also necessary.

A variety of medications are used to prevent migraine attacks, including antidepressants, antiepileptic agents, antihistamines, and antihypertensive agents (Table 84-2). The majority of these medications are extensively prescribed for other conditions, including depression, mood disorders, epilepsy, and other pain disorders, making their side-effect profiles well known. When selecting an agent, the clinician should take into account coexisting conditions. Clear instructions should be given to families regarding the medication's mechanism of action, potential side effects, and the importance of adhering to therapy. Clear titration instructions should be provided. It is important to remind families that it may take time, often several weeks, for the treatment to become effective. Slow titration over a period of 4 to 12 weeks may be necessary to assure that the child tolerates the medication with minimal adverse effects. If improvement is seen, the dose may be increased to achieve optimal control.

For specific details on preventive medications, please see the online chapter. The typical preventive medications are discussed next.

Antidepressants. Antidepressants are the mainstay of migraine prevention in adults; few studies have been performed in children. Yet they remain one of the most widely used medications for both age groups. Amitriptyline is the only tricyclic antidepressant for which studies have provided

TABLE 84-2 Preventive Agents for Childhood and Adolescent Migraine

Agent	Dosing	Available Formulations	Commonly Encountered Adverse Effects
Antidepressants			
Amitriptyline	10-150 mg qhs (max 1 mg/kg/day)	Tablets—10, 25, 50, 75,100, 125, 150 mg	Sedation, dizziness, constipation, decreased GI motility, increased appetite, weight gain, urinary retention
Nortriptyline	10-75mg qhs	Capsules—10, 25, 50, 75 mg Liquid suspension—10 mg/5 ml	Drowsiness, dizziness, constipation, increased appetite, orthostatic hypotension, QT prolongation (regular ECG surveillance necessary)
Antiepileptics			
Topiramate	1-10 mg/kg/day Typical dose 50 mg bid	Tablets—25, 50, 100, 200 mg Sprinkle caps—15, 25 mg	Paresthesias, somnolence, dizziness, anorexia, metabolic acidosis, cognitive/memory dysfunction, abdominal pain
Valproic acid	15-30 mg/kg/day	Tablets DR—125, 250, 500mg Tablets ER—250, 500 mg Sprinkle caps—125 mg Liquid suspension—250 mg/5 ml	Somnolence, nausea/vomiting, thrombocytopenia, tremor, alopecia, increased appetite, weight gain, emotional lability, lymphopenia, hyperammonemia, elevated pancreatic enzymes, PCOS, birth defects
Levetiracetam	500-1500 mg bid	Tablets—250, 500, 750, 1000 mg Liquid suspension—100 mg/ml	Somnolence, fatigue, irritability, mood/behavioral changes
Zonisamide	100-600 mg/day	Tablets—25, 50, 100 mg	Somnolence, dizziness, anorexia, nausea, irritability
Gabapentin	300-1200 mg tid	Tablets—100, 300, 400, 600, 800 mg Liquid suspension—50 mg/ml	Dizziness, sedation, ataxia, fatigue, peripheral edema
Antihistamines			
Cyproheptadine	0.25-1.5 mg/kg/day	Tablets—4 mg Liquid suspension—2 mg/5 ml	Drowsiness, fatigue, increased appetite, weight gain, dizziness
Antihypertensives			
Propranolol	2-4 mg/kg/day	Tablets—10, 20, 40, 60, 80 mg Tablets ER—60, 80, 120, 160 mg Liquid suspension—20, 40/5 ml	Fatigue, dizziness, constipation, hypotension, depression, exercise-induced asthma
Verapamil	4-10 mg/kg/day tid	Tablets—40, 80, 120 mg Tablets ER—120, 180, 240 mg	Constipation, dizziness, nausea, hypotension
Flunarizine*	5-10 mg qhs	Tablets—10 mg	Sedation, weight gain

DR, delayed release; ECG, electrocardiogram; ER, extended release; GI, gastrointestinal; PCOS, polycystic ovary syndrome.
*Not available in the United States.

consistent evidence of benefit in the adult population. In children, most research with amitriptyline has consisted of open-label studies, with no placebo-controlled trials, resulting in unclear dosing guidelines.

Antiepileptic Drugs. Antiepileptic agents are the most widely studied preventive agents for migraine in adults and children and include topiramate, valproic acid, levetiracetam, zonisamide, and gabapentin. Topiramate and valproate are approved by the FDA for headache prevention in adults, and topiramate became the first drug approved for migraine prevention in children ages 12 and over. Multiple retrospective studies have demonstrated a reduction in headache severity with antiepileptic drugs. More prospective studies are needed in children to assess efficacy and tolerability.

Data from several studies suggest that topiramate is effective in the preventive treatment of pediatric migraine, leading to its recent FDA approval. The effective dose in the pediatric population is not known, but a dose of 2 to 4 mg/kg/day is beneficial.

The preventive properties of valproate, levetiracetam, zonisamide, and gabapentin have also been examined, with few studies in children (see the online chapter).

Antihistamines. Cyproheptadine, an antihistamine with antiserotonergic properties, is commonly prescribed for pediatric migraine. It tends to be very well tolerated; its most significant side effects are sedation and weight gain, which specifically limit its tolerability in adolescents. Despite the lack of data, it is often used with target doses of 0.2 to 0.4 mg/kg/day and is considered a first-line option for children less than 6 years of age.

Beta Blockers. Propranolol and atenolol have been approved for the prevention of migraine in adults. Propranolol has long been used in children, but the results of this agent for preventing headache have been conflicting.

Botulinum Toxin. OnabotulinumtoxinA is effective for chronic migraine headaches in adults and was approved by the FDA in 2010. The prevalence of chronic migraines in children and adolescents, defined as at least 15 headache days/month for 3 consecutive months, is between 2% and 3%. The efficacy of OnabotulinumtoxinA in children and adolescents has begun to be evaluated.

Nutraceuticals for Headache Prevention. The use of dietary supplements, known as *nutraceuticals,* has become increasingly popular in the general population for the treatment of migraine and many other medical disorders and is often the preferred choice among parents of children and adolescents during discussions regarding preventive treatment. The decision to try nutraceuticals is based on the notion that they are often well tolerated, and families may view nutraceuticals as "natural" and may feel reluctant to start a conventional medication because of the concern for adverse effects. Also, conventional prophylactic medication may have failed for some patients as a result of ineffectiveness, toxic effects, or intolerable side effects. Furthermore, nutraceuticals are relatively inexpensive, and medical costs have become an increasing concern.

Some of the nutraceuticals that are used for headache prevention include riboflavin (vitamin B_2), coenzyme Q10 (CoQ10), butterbur, *Petasites hybridus,* magnesium, and feverfew (see the online chapter).

Nonpharmacologic Treatment

Patients with frequent headaches should be counseled on the importance of diet and lifestyle modification. Focus should include ensuring adequate sleep, staying hydrated, incorporating regular exercise, and maintaining a well-balanced diet. Cognitive behavioral therapy (CBT) and biofeedback-assisted relaxation training should be implemented early if headaches are disabling. These techniques are typically taught over multiple sessions, although they are also effective in a single session, and the patient is given a single recording for home use. For best results, patients must be motivated, because improvement could take several weeks. Implementation of CBT resulted in a significant reduction of headache days and migraine-related disability in pediatric patients (Powers et al., 2013). CBT has the potential of significant benefit, especially for overall improvement of mood and reduction of stress, without the concern of the negative side effects that often accompany pharmacologic treatments.

SPECIFIC SECONDARY HEADACHE SYNDROMES

One of the keys to diagnosis of primary headaches is the lack of an identifiable etiology. When a secondary cause is suspected, appropriate investigation and treatment must be implemented. Confirmation of the diagnosis of a secondary headache can only be made after successful treatment of the underlying etiology. If treatment is not successful, further investigation is warranted.

Secondary headaches are headaches in which an underlying disorder initiates and perpetuates the headache. These headaches are less likely to be recurrent. When recurrent, it suggests that the underlying etiology has not been successfully managed or that the diagnosis is incorrect.

Principles for diagnosing a secondary headache include the following:

1. A known cause of the secondary headaches has been identified through history, laboratory testing, or neuroimaging.
2. A temporal and causal relationship exists between the identified disorder and the headache.
3. With implementation of effective treatment of the underlying etiology, the headache resolves or significantly improves.
4. Unless the secondary cause is episodic, the episodic headaches are typically primary.

Patients with primary headaches can also develop secondary headaches.

Posttraumatic Headache

Headache following closed head injury (Chapter 102) or neck trauma in children and adolescents is one of the most common secondary headache syndromes, but has not been systematically studied (Kuczynski, Crawford, Bodell, Dewey, and Barlow, 2013). Epidemiologic data are not readily available. Headaches are common after mild traumatic brain injury or concussion and often occur with a constellation of physical, cognitive, emotional, and behavioral signs. The ICHD-3b classifies posttraumatic headaches as acute if lasting less than 3 months and persistent if lasting more than 3 months. This time period is consistent with ICHD-2 diagnostic criteria, although the term *persistent* has been adopted in place of *chronic*. Although the ICHD-3b criteria define posttraumatic headache as beginning within 7 days after injury to the head or after regaining consciousness, this 7-day cutoff is arbitrary, and some experts believe that headaches may develop after a longer interval (see the online chapter).

Acute posttraumatic headache must immediately raise concerns for traumatic brain injury, such as an intracranial hematoma, subarachnoid hemorrhage, cerebral contusion, or skull fracture, and warrants neuroimaging, particularly if associated with alteration of consciousness, seizures, or a Glasgow Coma Scale score of less than 13. If focal neurologic symptoms or signs are present, evaluation for vascular injury (e.g., carotid dissection) may be indicated, and detection may require specific MRI sequences (magnetic resonance angiogram [MRA]). Cerebrospinal fluid (CSF) leaks following meningeal tears can lead to positional, or "ow-pressure, headaches.

Headaches developing after head trauma closely resemble primary headache disorders, most commonly TTH and migraine without aura, although some are referred to as "unclassifiable." Other headaches may resemble neuralgias such as occipital neuralgia, temporomandibular joint dysfunction, and, on rare occasions, cluster headache. Management should be relevant to the type of headache and focused on the clinical needs of the child. Referral for biobehavioral therapy for coping strategies may be necessary. As with primary headaches, adherence to treatment recommendations should be optimized.

Persistent posttraumatic headache may be part of a global postconcussive syndrome, with behavioral changes such as hyperactivity or hypoactivity, dizziness, tinnitus, vertigo, blurred vision, memory changes, sleep disturbance, irritability, and attentional disorders resembling attention deficit disorder (ADD)/attention deficit hyperactivity disorder (ADHD). The duration of symptoms is variable, with some patients having symptoms for more than 6 to 12 months.

Although headache is the most common symptom following concussion, there is a paucity of evidence regarding the safety and efficacy of headache treatments for posttraumatic headaches. These headaches can be difficult to treat, and management requires an appreciation of the degree of disability. There are no established guidelines for the treatment of posttraumatic headaches, and practices vary widely. There are currently no randomized controlled trials evaluating the efficacy of therapies for posttraumatic headaches in children or adults. Most proposed algorithms have been extrapolated from the primary headache literature, small uncontrolled trials, and expert opinion.

Similar to treating a child with a primary headache disorder, the goal of acute treatment should be a consistent response with minimum side effects and a rapid return to normal function. These treatments should be properly dosed and used as quickly as possible, while minimizing the potential for medication overuse. It should be incorporated into the child's life by providing the ability to receive these treatments in school or at home and without missing school or social activities. To avoid the development of medication-overuse headache (MOH), abortive medications should be used no more than 3 days per week. Triptans should be used fewer than nine times per month. From the characteristics of the headache, the clinician should make every effort to classify the headache type, because this may have treatment implications.

Patients with persistent posttraumatic headaches may require frequent analgesics, and although their use may be beneficial in the short term, rebound headaches are common and can complicate treatment and recovery. Because analgesics are commonly recommended, the risk exists that some susceptible patients will develop a medication-overuse pattern that causes a chronic headache syndrome. Several retrospective studies and case reports have addressed medication overuse as a potential cause of persistent posttraumatic headaches.

For persistent posttraumatic headaches, preventive medication may be indicated and typically includes those used for migraine. However, their efficacy has not been well studied.

Idiopathic Intracranial Hypertension

Also known as pseudotumor cerebri, idiopathic intracranial hypertension (IIH) produces a global, daily, pounding headache and is an important consideration in the differential diagnosis of children presenting with a chronic daily headache. The incidence is 1 per 100,000, although the incidence in childhood is unknown. It appears to be more common in females and more common in obese individuals, although it does occur in males and in nonobese individuals. The pathogenesis of IIH is uncertain but may involve impairment of CSF reabsorption or CSF overproduction (see Chapter 105 and the online chapter).

For IIH headaches, there is a direct correspondence to increased intracranial pressure. The ICHD-3b establishes increased pressure as greater than 250 mm CSF measured by lumbar puncture performed in the lateral decubitus position and without sedative medications. The headache is typically relieved by reducing intracranial pressure. Typically, the pain is moderate and chronic and may be progressive. Headaches often resemble migraine or a tension-type headache. Physical activity, including the Valsalva maneuver and postural changes, can aggravate the pain. Neck stiffness and transient visual disturbances may be present.

Once an increase in intracranial pressure has been identified, other etiologies need to be investigated. IIH can be caused by multiple disorders, including endocrinopathies (e.g., hypothyroidism), Addison's disease, oral steroid use, pregnancy, medications (including tetracycline, sulfonamides, lithium, cyclosporine, and oral contraceptive agents), anemia, systemic lupus erythematosus, chronic sinopulmonary infection, and obesity, or may be idiopathic. In children, one should ask about vitamin A intoxication, either from excessive dietary intake or prescriptions, as in the case of adolescents seeking treatment for acne with retinoids.

Lumbar puncture not only provides critical diagnostic information, but also the relief of pressure usually provides a significant decrease in headache symptoms. The volume of CSF to be removed is controversial. Generally, removal of a sufficient volume to lower the pressure to about 200 mm H_2O is beneficial and safe. Care must be taken to limit the risk of postlumbar puncture headache by keeping the patient recumbent for several hours following the procedure.

Acetazolamide can be used to lower CSF pressures, most likely as a result of a diuretic mechanism. Side effects are few but include paresthesias, polyuria, and sedation. The dose is typically 250 mg twice a day up to 1000 mg per day. There is an extended-release once-daily preparation available. Recovery is slow, over weeks or months. If obesity is a contributing factor, a weight-loss program is strongly recommended. If the visual symptoms are severe or progressive, or if there is visual compromise, ophthalmologic intervention may be necessary, with performance of an optic nerve sheath fenestration.

Intracranial Hypotension

Headaches also can be caused by low CSF pressure (Chapter 105). The most typical example of this is headache following a lumbar puncture or other conditions that cause a tear in the dura mater, including penetrating trauma or cranial surgery. The typical clinical presentation is a headache that worsens with positional changes, especially upon standing, after a lumbar puncture. The cardinal clinical feature is orthostatic or positional headache, in which a severe, pounding, nauseating headache occurs immediately upon standing or sitting up from a reclined position. Importantly, symptoms resolve when the patient lies back down. Criteria include neck stiffness, tinnitus, hyperacusia, and photophobia. The CSF opening pressure is about 60 mm H_2O in the sitting position. Although the majority of headaches following a lumbar puncture resolve spontaneously, persistence of disabling symptoms may necessitate consideration of a "blood patch" or other technique to repair the source of the CSF leak; this may take 72 hours to be effective.

Headache Secondary to a Brain Tumor

About two thirds of children with brain tumors will have headache as a presenting symptom. There is, however, no invariable profile for "brain tumor headache." A steady, gradual rise in intracranial pressure produces the chronic progressive pattern. On occasion, an anaplastic tumor or hemorrhage into tumor may cause an acute pattern. Several historic clues suggest space-occupying lesions, such as brain tumors, but such findings also may be present in other expanding masses, such as brain abscess, hematoma, or vascular anomalies. Headaches that awaken the child from sleep are a classic symptom of the dependent edema of intracranial lesions. Likewise, nocturnal or morning emesis, with or without headache, suggests increased intracranial pressure and is a particularly common symptom of tumors arising near the floor of the fourth ventricle. Head pain aggravated by exertion or the Valsalva maneuver suggests a mass lesion. In addition to headache, parents may note behavioral or mood changes, cognitive impairment, or declining school performance.

Accompanying symptoms may suggest localized disturbances of neurologic function. Ocular symptoms are common and include loss of vision (e.g., craniopharyngioma, optic pathway tumor) and diplopia (e.g., brainstem glioma, medulloblastoma). Disorders of coordination, such as truncal ataxia (e.g., medulloblastoma, ependymoma) or dysmetria (e.g., cerebellar astrocytoma), suggest posterior fossa tumors. The presence of seizures indicates cortical disturbances, often localized to the temporal lobes.

Key physical examination signs that indicate brain tumor include papilledema, abnormal eye movements, hemiparesis, ataxia (truncal or appendicular), and abnormal tendon reflexes.

Chiari Malformation

Chiari malformations (type I) are among the most common incidental findings when performing MRI in children with headache, and they are a source of great controversy. Tonsillar ectopia of 5 mm or less is not considered pathologic. When symptomatic, children with Chiari I malformation may complain of occipital headache, neck pain or stiffness, arm weakness, and gait abnormalities. The headache may be aggravated by neck flexion or extension or the Valsalva maneuver. Basal skull abnormalities or scoliosis may be identified. In a retrospective MRI analysis of 49 children with Chiari I malformation, 57% of children were asymptomatic. Headache and neck pain were the most frequent complaints. Syringomyelia was detected in 14% of patients and skull-base abnormalities in 50%. The magnitude of tonsillar ectopia (5-23 mm) correlated with the severity score ($p = 0.04$), but not with other clinical measures. Children with greater amounts of tonsillar ectopia on MRI are more likely to be symptomatic. Extreme care must be exercised before undertaking surgical decompression. MRI with CSF flow studies may help to determine whether suboccipital decompression is necessary.

Metabolic Causes of Headache in Children
MELAS

Mitochondrial encephalopathy, lactic acidosis, and stroke-like episodes (MELAS) constitute a mitochondrial disorder characterized by migraine-like headaches, episodic hemiparesis, development regression/dementia, short stature, seizures, and cortical blindness. The initial presentation is seizures in 28% of patients, recurrent headache in 28%, gastrointestinal symptoms (emesis or anorexia) in 25%, limb weakness in 18%, short stature in 18%, and stroke in 17%. The age of onset is usually younger than 2 years in 8%, 2 to 5 years in 20%, 6 to 10 years in 31%, 11 to 20 years in 17%, 21 to 40 years in 23%, and over age 40 in only 1%.

Diagnosis requires stroke-like episodes, encephalopathy with seizures and/or dementia, mitochondrial myopathy (ragged red fibers on muscle biopsy), lactic acidosis, and clinical features such as recurrent vomiting. The disorder is caused by a point mutation in the mitochondrial DNA *MT-TL1* encoding tRNA^{Leu}. With expanded genetic testing, the phenotype of MELAS is evolving (see Chapter 42).

CADASIL

Cerebral autosomal-dominant arteriopathy with subcortical infarcts and leukoencephalopathy (CADASIL) is a mitochondrial disorder that usually affects young adults but on occasion can be seen in adolescents. It should be considered in adolescents with migraine with aura, in whom neuroimaging discloses subcortical infarcts and/or multifocal T2/fluid-attenuated inversion recovery (FLAIR) hyperintensities in the deep white matter. An autosomal-dominant family history of migraine, early stroke, and/or dementia may be present. The clinical spectrum is variable, but migraine headache occurs in more than one third of patients and may be the only manifestation. A recent case report described a 14-year-old girl with a 3-year history of episodic headaches, three episodes of right hemiparesis, persistent hypertension, negative family history, normal MRI, and a "Notch3" mutation. This report raises the possibility of screening for CADASIL in children with headaches and episodes of hemiplegia (hemiplegic migraine)

using skin biopsy and genetic testing for the Notch3 mutation, even when MRI is normal and family history is negative.

REFERENCES

The complete list of references for this chapter is available in the e-book at www.expertconsult.com.
     See inside cover for registration details.

SELECTED REFERENCES

Goadsby, P.J., Charbit, A.R., Andreou, A.P., et al., 2009. Neurobiology of migraine. Neuroscience 161 (2), 327–341.

Hershey, A.D., 2010. Current approaches to the diagnosis and management of paediatric migraine. Lancet Neurol. 9 (2), 190–204.

Kabbouche, M.A., Vockell, A.L., LeCates, S.L., et al., 2001. Tolerability and effectiveness of prochlorperazine for intractable migraine in children. Pediatrics 107 (4), E62.

Kuczynski, A., Crawford, S., Bodell, L., et al., 2013. Characteristics of post-traumatic headaches in children following mild traumatic brain injury and their response to treatment: a prospective cohort. Dev. Med. Child Neurol. 55 (7), 636–641.

Lewis, D.W., Ashwal, S., Dahl, G., et al., 2002. Practice parameter: evaluation of children and adolescents with recurrent headaches: report of the Quality Standards Subcommittee of the American Academy of Neurology and the Practice Committee of the Child Neurology Society. Neurology 59 (4), 490–498.

Lewis, D.W., Diamond, S., Scott, D., et al., 2004. Prophylactic treatment of pediatric migraine. Headache 44 (3), 230–237.

Miller, V.A., Palermo, T.M., Powers, S.W., et al., 2003. Migraine headaches and sleep disturbances in children. Headache 43 (4), 362–368.

Powers, S.W., Kashikar-Zuck, S.M., Allen, J.R., et al., 2013. Cognitive behavioral therapy plus amitriptyline for chronic migraine in children and adolescents: a randomized clinical trial. JAMA 310 (24), 2622–2630.

Silberstein, S.D., 2000. Practice parameter: evidence-based guidelines for migraine headache (an evidence-based review): report of the Quality Standards Subcommittee of the American Academy of Neurology. Neurology 55 (6), 754–762.

85 Breath-Holding Spells and Reflex Anoxic Seizures

Sarah M. Roddy

Breath-holding spells and reflex anoxic seizures are nonepileptic paroxysmal events. These events are benign, but can be frightening to parents and others observing an episode. It is important to differentiate these episodes from epileptic seizures so that the child is not inappropriately treated with antiepileptic medication.

Possibly the earliest report of breath-holding spells was published in 1737 by Nicholas Culpepper, who gave this description: "There is a disease … in children from anger or grief, when the spirits are much stirred and run from the heart to the diaphragms forcibly, and hinder or stop the breath … but when the passion ceaseth, this symptom ceaseth."

The clinical characteristics of breath-holding spells were well recognized and described in the pediatric literature in the 19th and early 20th centuries. More recent reports have provided a better understanding of the pathophysiology of these events.

BREATH-HOLDING SPELLS
Clinical Features

The term *breath holding* is a misnomer and implies that the child is voluntarily holding his or her breath in a prolonged inspiration. Breath-holding episodes actually occur during expiration and are involuntary. Breath-holding spells are not uncommon, with an incidence of 4.6% to 4.7%. The typical age of onset is between 6 and 18 months, although occasionally the onset may occur in the first few weeks of life. Fewer than 10% of children have an onset after 2 years of age. The frequency of episodes ranges from several times daily to once yearly. The spells are often spaced weeks to months apart at onset and increase in frequency to as many as several per day during the second year of life (Dimario, 2001). Breath-holding spells are classified by the color change manifested in the child during an event. Cyanotic episodes are more common than pallid episodes. In some instances, there are features of both cyanosis and pallor, and these are termed *mixed episodes.*

Cyanotic breath-holding spells are often precipitated by emotional stimuli, such as anger or frustration. The child typically cries vigorously, usually for less than 15 seconds, then becomes silent and holds the breath in expiration. The apnea is associated with the rapid onset of cyanosis. Some episodes may resolve at this point, but there may be a brief loss of consciousness and a period of limpness, followed by opisthotonic posturing. Recovery is usually within 1 minute, with the child having a few gasping respirations and then a return to regular breathing and consciousness.

Pallid breath-holding spells are usually provoked by sudden fright or pain. A fall with a minor injury to the head is frequently the precipitating event. An unexpected event or a surprise seems to play a role in triggering the spell. Sometimes the provoking event is not witnessed, and the child is found already in the midst of an episode. The child may gasp and cry, although it is usually for only a brief period of time. The child then becomes quiet, loses consciousness, and becomes pale. Limpness and diaphoresis are common accompaniments. Clonic movements of the extremities and incontinence may occur with more severe and prolonged episodes. Cyanosis may occur during the episode but is much milder than with cyanotic breath-holding spells. The child typically regains consciousness in less than 1 minute but may sleep for several hours after the episode.

An association between behavior problems, emotional factors, and breath-holding spells has been discussed by many investigators. In the past, breath-holding spells were thought to occur in spoiled children or be a sign of a disturbed parent-child relationship. More recent studies of behavior in children with breath-holding spells compared with controls have found no differences in the behavioral profiles between the two groups, suggesting that breath-holding spells are nonvolitional and cannot be equated with a temperamentally difficult child.

Breath-holding spells generally decrease in frequency during the second year of life. By 4 years of age, 50% of children will no longer have episodes. Almost all will have stopped having episodes by age 7 to 8 years. Syncopal episodes occur in late childhood or adolescence in as many as 30% of patients with prior breath-holding spells.

Serious complications with breath-holding spells are exceedingly rare. There has been a report of a prolonged cardiac arrest in a patient with breath-holding spells. The few reported deaths may have been precipitated by aspiration or occurred in children who were at the severe end of the spectrum of breath-holders, often with structural abnormalities of the respiratory tract or complicated medical histories.

Clinical Laboratory Tests

A detailed history of the event, including the precipitating circumstances, is essential in making the diagnosis of breath-holding spells. If the event was not witnessed from onset, important details may not be available. A video recording by the parents may be helpful in confirming the diagnosis. Usually, no laboratory tests are needed to make the diagnosis. An electroencephalogram (EEG) is usually not indicated, unless the convulsive activity after the breath holding is prolonged or the clinical description is incomplete and epileptic seizures cannot be definitively ruled out by historical features. If ocular compression is performed in patients with pallid breath-holding spells, there may be asystole on cardiac monitoring, and slowing or suppression of voltage on EEG (Lombroso and Lerman, 1967). Long QT syndrome is rare but should be considered as part of the differential diagnosis in a child with breath-holding spells. Patients with Long QT syndrome have episodes of loss of consciousness that may be induced by injury, fright, or excitement. An electrocardiogram should be considered in any patient with breath-holding spells.

Pathophysiology
Cyanotic Spells

The pathophysiology of cyanotic breath-holding spells is complex and not completely understood. Cyanosis occurs early in the episode, which is unusual during voluntary breath holding. In breath-holding spells, the breath is held in full expiration, which also is not typical with voluntary breath holding. An early study of a child during a cyanotic breath-holding episode with cinefluorography showed that the diaphragm was high, as would be seen in full expiration, and motionless during the period of apnea. Spasm of the glottis and respiratory muscles, with increased intrathoracic pressure, occurs during expiration. Increased intrathoracic pressure reduces cardiac output, causing a decrease in cerebral perfusion. Violent crying could lead to hypocapnia, which would also impair cerebral circulation.

Further evaluation of the prolonged expiratory mechanism in nine infants with cyanotic episodes that were usually triggered by noxious stimuli showed that the arterial oxygen saturation fell below 20 mm Hg within 20 seconds of initiation of the noxious stimuli. Loss of consciousness occurred after 30 seconds. Measurements of respiratory movements, airflow, and esophageal pressure, and, in some patients, microlaryngoscopy and chest fluoroscopy were obtained and documented no inspiratory flow during the period of apnea but continued expiratory muscle activity at low lung volumes with partial or complete glottic closure. No intracardiac shunt could be demonstrated. The rapid fall in arterial oxygen saturation was attributed to a lack of ventilation at a maximum expiratory position in the presence of a rapid circulation time. The authors hypothesized that central and peripheral neural respiratory control was functioning normally but was interfered with by a mechanical defect involving lung-volume maintenance. This defect could occur because of an excessively compliant rib cage, allowing alveolar collapse. This collapse, in turn, could lead to stretching of the airways and their stretch receptors, inappropriately simulating maximum lung volumes and thereby inhibiting further inspiration. Evaluations of prolonged expiratory apnea with krypton infusion scans demonstrated krypton outside the lung fields, without evidence of an intracardiac shunt, suggesting that there was intrapulmonary shunting that contributed to the rapid onset and severity of the hypoxemia.

The relation between breath-holding and chemosensitivity has also been investigated. Due to the difficulty of measuring chemosensitivity in toddlers, ventilatory responses to progressive hypercapnia and to progressive hypoxia were measured in subjects aged 11 to 50 who had a history of cyanotic breath-holding spells compared with a control group. The majority of persons with a history of cyanotic breath-holding spells had normal ventilatory responses. However, no one with a history of breath-holding spells had high normal responses to hypercapnia or hypoxia, as did some individuals in the control group. This study raised the possibility that ventilatory chemosensitivity may play a role in breath holding, but the ventilatory chemosensitivity may resolve with maturation.

The relation between breath-holding and cardiorespiratory control was studied in 71 infants with a history of breath-holding spells and age- and gender-matched controls. The median age of infants in the study was 14 weeks, which is younger than the typical age for onset of breath-holding episodes. The infants with breath-holding spells were significantly more often covered with sweat during sleep and wakefulness compared with control infants. One-night sleep studies were obtained in each infant. The infants with breath-holding spells had significantly less nonrapid eye movement (REM) stage III sleep, more indeterminate sleep, more nocturnal arousals, and more sleep-stage changes than the control infants. Airway obstructions during sleep occurred in 41 infants with a history of breath-holding, compared with six in the control group. The obstructions were generally short and not accompanied by significant bradycardia or oxygen desaturation. The researchers concluded that there was a common underlying mechanism resulting in airway obstruction during breath-holding spells and sleep, which possibly involved the autonomic nervous system (ANS) because the ANS controls the patency of the upper airways. Another study of polysomnography in 14 children with cyanotic breath-holding spells showed an abnormal respiratory index in all, and ear, nose, and throat (ENT) examination showed upper airway narrowing. Adenotonsillectomy in this group of patients resulted in marked subsequent improvement in sleep-disordered breathing and resolution of their breath-holding spells.

Polysomnography has also been used to evaluate REM sleep in children with breath-holding spells compared with age-matched controls. The children with breath-holding spells had a significant decrease in ocular activity during REM sleep, especially during the last third of the night, compared with the controls. A relative elevation of cholinergic tone, compared with monoaminergic tone, is considered to be involved in the physiologic increase of REM sleep in the later cycles of the night. The vestibular nucleus and the medioventral caudal pons are believed to be involved in bursts of eye movements during REM sleep. The changes may indicate a functional disturbance in the pons of children with breath-holding spells. The study also suggests that the ANS is involved because of the more pronounced decrease in eye movement in the later cycles of the night, which are regulated by the ANS. Brainstem auditory evoked potentials in children with breath-holding spells have shown that the III-V and I-V interpeak latencies were significantly prolonged compared with controls also suggesting a disturbance in the brainstem.

Noninvasive evaluation of the ANS function in children with cyanotic breath-holding spells has been reported. Compared with controls, the breath holders had a significantly greater increase in pulse rate at 15 seconds of standing after rising from the supine position. Breath-holders also had a greater decrease in diastolic blood pressure without an increase in systolic blood pressure after standing from the supine position. These results suggest that in children with cyanotic breath-holding spells there is parasympathetic excess and subtle sympathetic excess, which mediates vascular resistance, arterial distensibility, and blood flow through the lungs. This sympathetic overactivity could cause the intrapulmonary shunting and subsequent hypoxemia.

There are reports of increased QT dispersion and cardiac repolarization changes in children with breath-holding spells. The significance of these findings is unclear but may also be a reflection of autonomic dysfunction.

Pallid Spells

Excessive vagal tone leading to cerebral hypoperfusion is the underlying cause of pallid breath-holding spells. Observation of children during a typical episode reveals marked bradycardia or asystole. Ocular compression that triggers the oculocardiac reflex has been used to evaluate vagal tone in children with breath-holding. This maneuver results in transmission of afferent signals to the brainstem via the ophthalmic division of the trigeminal nerve and efferent parasympathetic signals via the vagus nerve. In 61% to 78% of children with pallid breath-holding spells, ocular compression resulted in an asystole of 2 seconds or longer, compared with 23% to 26% of children with cyanotic breath-holding spells (Lombroso and Lerman, 1967). Episodes that occurred spontaneously during cardiac monitoring were also associated with asystole. The asystole during spontaneous episodes is believed to be vagally mediated. When asystole is prolonged, a reflex anoxic seizure may eventually occur.

The role of underlying autonomic dysfunction in children with pallid breath-holding spells has been investigated in a small number of patients. Measurements of mean arterial pressures, pulse rates, electrocardiograms, and plasma norepinephrine levels were obtained in patients and controls during changes in position. The breath-holders had a statistically significant decrease in mean arterial pressure and an unsustained increase in pulse rate during the prone to standing maneuver. One child with pallid breath-holding spells had a plasma norepinephrine level that was 60% lower than the mean for both groups. Further evaluation of autonomic function was performed in children with either pallid or cyanotic breath-holding spells. Respiratory sinus arrhythmia, which is an established measure of vagal tone, was measured. There were no significant differences between controls and children with cyanotic breath-holding spells. The children with pallid spells, however, had a marked difference in respiratory sinus dysrhythmia, with less variability compared with controls and those with cyanotic episodes (DiMario et al., 1998). A comparative study of 24-hour Holter monitoring in children with severe breath-holding spells showed a lower mean heart rate and lower mean minimal heart rate compared with controls. Time domain measures of heart rate variability also showed significant changes in patients compared with controls. These studies suggest that there may be an underlying parasympathetic dysregulation in children with pallid breath-holding spells.

The role of anemia in the pathophysiology of breath-holding spells has been studied. Twenty-three percent of 102 children with breath-holding had a hemoglobin level less than 8 g/100 mL, compared with 7% and 2.6% in two control groups. Some studies did not find any significant difference in hemoglobin levels in the breath-holding group, compared with the control group. Asystole during breath-holding spells was prolonged in children with coexisting iron deficiency. There are reports of children with breath-holding spells and concomitant anemia, who had resolution of their spells with the correction of the associated anemia (Mocan et al.,1999; Orii et al., 2002). A child with pallid breath-holding spells associated with transient erythroblastopenia of childhood has been reported. The spells resolved after treatment with iron but before the anemia resolved. The effect of iron therapy on breath-holding spells has been investigated. Treatment and placebo groups were similar with respect to gender, age at onset, and frequency and type of spells, and had similar blood indices, including packed cell volume, mean corpuscular volume, saturation index, total iron binding capacity, and serum iron. At the end of the treatment period, 51.5% of the children treated with ferrous sulfate had complete remission of spells, and an additional 36.4% experienced a greater than 50% reduction. No children in the placebo group had total remission of spells, and only 5.9% had a greater than 50% reduction. As expected, the treatment group experienced significant improvement in the hemoglobin level and total iron-binding capacity. However, some children who were not iron-deficient had a favorable response to iron therapy, and some who were iron-deficient did not respond. Another study suggests that checking serum soluble transferrin receptor levels in children with breath-holding spells may be helpful in assessing iron status. An increase in serum soluble transferrin receptor levels is an early change seen in iron deficiency before anemia develops. Iron deficiency may play a role in the pathophysiology of breath-holding spells because iron is important for catecholamine metabolism and neurotransmitter function.

Other small studies have evaluated the role of the oxidant and antioxidant systems in the pathophysiology of breath-holding. Malondialdehyde, which is an indicator of free radical generation, was significantly higher in children with breath-holding spells than controls. Glutathione peroxidase and superoxide dismutase, which remove oxygen radicals, and selenium, which acts as a cofactor for glutathione, were significantly lower in the patients.

Genetics

In children with breath-holding spells, there is a positive family history of similar episodes in 23% to 38%, suggesting a possible genetic influence (Lombroso and Lerman, 1967). An evaluation of family pedigrees found that 27% of 114 proband parents and 21% of proband siblings had a history of breath-holding. Several families had some members with pallid spells and other members with cyanotic spells. The male to female ratio was 1 : 1.2 and the risk of transmission from parent to child was 50 : 50. There were seven instances of father-to-son transmission, ruling out an X-linked inheritance. Using a regression model for pedigree analysis, the inheritance pattern was consistent with an autosomal-dominant pattern with reduced penetrance.

Treatment

The most important aspect of treatment of breath-holding spells is to reassure the family of the benign nature of the spells. It is important to emphasize that the episodes do not lead to intellectual disability or epilepsy. Although parents are inclined to pick up a child who is having a breath-holding spell, they should be instructed to place the child in a lateral recumbent position so as not to prolong the period of possible cerebral anoxia. Initiation of cardiopulmonary resuscitation should be avoided. Although anger and frustration are often precipitants for breath-holding spells, parents should be encouraged not to alter customary discipline for fear of triggering an episode. Parenting a child with breath-holding spells has been associated with more maternal stress than parenting a child with a convulsive seizure disorder, and parents of children with breath-holding spells are at risk for developing dysfunctional parenting behaviors. Referral of parents to professionals to help with stress and parenting skills should be considered in cases in which parental stress becomes evident (Mattie-Luksic et al, 2000).

Treatment with iron therapy should be initiated in any child who has iron deficiency anemia and should be considered in any child with breath-holding spells because children without anemia may have improvement in their breath-holding spells. The convulsive movements seen during breath-holding spells are reflex anoxic seizures, which are not epileptic and do not require antiepileptic treatment. There have been a few patients who have been reported to have prolonged seizures and even status epilepticus from breath-holding spells (Kuhle et al., 2000). It is presumed that these patients have a lowered seizure threshold and that hypoxia-ischemia triggered the seizures. These episodes have been termed anoxic-epileptic seizures. Treatment with antiepileptic medication may stop the seizure activity but not the breath-holding spells. Atropine (0.01 mg/kg 2 or 3 times daily) is effective for pallid breath-holding spells, but its use is rarely clinically warranted. Piracetam, which has a chemical structure similar to gamma-aminobutyric acid (GABA), has been used to treat children with breath-holding spells. Several studies using doses ranging from 40 mg/kg/day to 100 mg/kg/day have shown significant decreases or complete resolution of episodes compared with controls (Donma, 1998). Piracetam has not received approval from the U.S. Food and Drug Administration and is designated only as an orphan drug for use in refractory myoclonus. Levetiracetam, which is structurally similar to piracetam, did not affect the occurrence of breath-holding spells in a 10 month old child, but after treatment was initiated, the child no longer had asystole or unconsciousness with the episodes. In a retrospective study of six patients treated with fluoxetine, three had resolution of symptoms, and two had decreased frequency of episodes. A toddler with severe pallid breath-holding spells was treated with a combination of glycopyrrolate and theophylline and no longer had loss of consciousness but continued to have breath-holding spells.

REFLEX ANOXIC SEIZURES

Reflex anoxic seizures are nonepileptic events resulting from cardiac asystole of vagal origin. Pain and surprise are common provoking factors for the events. Reflex anoxic seizures may occur with pallid breath-holding spells but also have been reported with minor blows to the occiput, expelling hard stools past an anal fissure, venipuncture, intramuscular injections, and seeing an intravenous scalp drip. Nonepileptic anoxic seizures may also occur after syncope, cyanotic breath-holding spells, or any event that results in a sudden reduction in cerebral perfusion or hypoxia.

Clinical Features

Reflex anoxic seizures occur a few seconds after the provocation and are characterized by loss of muscle tone initially and later by tonic posturing. There may be opisthotonic posturing in some patients. A few jerks at the onset and end of an anoxic seizure may occur and probably represent myoclonic phenomena. A snoring type of inspiration or snort occurring close to the restoration of the cardiac rhythm is often noted. Urinary incontinence happens in approximately 10% of children with anoxic seizures, with bowel incontinence occurring less commonly. Other less common features include adversive head movements, limb quivering or twitching, agitation or fear, vomiting, and tongue biting. The color change seen with an anoxic seizure may be cyanosis or pallor, depending on the mechanism producing loss of consciousness. The duration of unconsciousness is almost always less than 1 minute. Most patients experience a rapid recovery of consciousness, but some will be dazed or disoriented for a short period. Some will be drowsy after an episode and may sleep. Occasionally, patients will have prolonged seizure activity after syncopal spells. These events, termed anoxic-epileptic seizures, are epileptic seizures triggered by hypoxia in patients with a lowered seizure threshold. A positive family history of epilepsy may make some children more prone to anoxic-epileptic seizures (Horrocks et al., 2005).

Pathophysiology

The mechanism of reflex anoxic seizures has been studied by using ocular compression with EEG and cardiac monitoring. Ocular compression induced asystole in susceptible patients. If asystole lasted 3 to 6 seconds, there were no clinical symptoms and the EEG demonstrated only desynchronization. When asystole lasted 7 to 13 seconds, slow waves appeared and were usually associated with altered consciousness. If asystole was prolonged for 14 seconds or more, there were often myoclonic jerks or tonic posturing. The EEG during this time reveals no electrocerebral activity. With return of cardiac activity, there was again high-voltage slow-wave activity on the EEG with return of normal activity over 20 to 30 seconds. At no time during EEG monitoring were epileptiform discharges present. Some patients have had spontaneous episodes or episodes triggered by other stimuli, such as venipuncture during EEG and cardiac monitoring, and have demonstrated similar changes to those seen with ocular compression. Ocular

compression increases vagal tone, with the afferent pathway involving fibers from the trigeminal nerve originating from the cornea, iris, and eyelids. In contrast, episodes induced by exteroceptive stimulation, such as pain and emotion, have afferent fibers in various sensory pathways. In both situations, the vagal reflex centers are located in the brainstem in the nucleus ambiguous. The efferent pathway involves the cardio-inhibitory fibers of the vagus nerve that depresses heart rate.

Clinical Laboratory Tests

Diagnosis of reflex anoxic seizures is usually made by obtaining a history of the episode. Details about the precipitating circumstances and onset are essential. Parents may state that their child had a seizure, and a careful description of the movements and posture, length of the episode, and recovery period will be helpful. Usually, no laboratory tests are needed, although consideration should be given to obtaining an electrocardiogram to evaluate for a cardiac cause if the episodes are not typical. Rarely is it necessary to obtain an EEG. If there are atypical clinical features and an EEG is performed, ocular compression may be helpful in confirming the clinical diagnosis.

Treatment

Treatment of reflex anoxic seizures focuses on explaining the nature of the event to the parents and reassuring them that the episodes are not epileptic seizures and do not need treatment with antiepileptic medication. In more severe cases, atropine, theophylline, and transdermal scopolamine have been helpful. Cardiac pacemaker implantation has also been useful in the rare patient with severe recurrent episodes (Sartori et al., 2015). Children with reflex anoxic seizures are at risk of bradycardia during surgical procedures, and modifications in the anesthesia protocol may be warranted.

REFERENCES

The complete list of references for this chapter is available in the e-book at www.expertconsult.com.
  See inside cover for registration details.

SELECTED REFERENCES

DiMario, F.J. Jr., 2001. Prospective study of children with cyanotic and pallid breath-holding spells. Pediatrics 107 (2), 265–269.

DiMario, F.J. Jr., Bauer, L., Baxter, D., 1998. Respiratory sinus arrhythmia in children with severe cyanotic and pallid breath-holding spells. J. Child Neurol. 13 (9), 440–442.

Donma, M.M., 1998. Clinical efficacy of piracetam in the treatment of breath-holding spells. Pediatr. Neurol. 18 (1), 41–45.

Horrocks, I.A., Nechay, A., Stephenson, J.B., et al., 2005. Anoxic-epileptic seizures: observational study of epileptic seizures induced by syncopes. Arch. Dis. Child. 90 (12), 1283–1287.

Kuhle, S., Tiefenthaler, M., Seidl, R., et al., 2000. Prolonged generalized epileptic seizures triggered by breath-holding spells. Pediatr. Neurol. 23 (3), 271–273.

Lombroso, C.T., Lerman, P., 1967. Breath-holding spells (cyanotic and pallid infantile syncope). Pediatrics 39 (4), 563–581.

Mattie-Luksic, M., Javornisky, G., DiMario, F.J. Jr., 2000. Assessment of stress in mothers of children with severe breath-holding spells. Pediatrics 106 (1 Pt 1), 1–5.

Mocan, H., Yildiran, A., Orhan, F., et al., 1999. Breath-holding spells in 91 children and response to treatment with iron. Arch. Dis. Child. 81 (3), 261–262.

Orii, K.E., Kato, Z., Osamu, F., et al., 2002. Changes of autonomic nervous system function in patients with breath-holding spells treated with iron. J. Child Neurol. 17 (5), 337–340.

Sartori, S., Nosadini, M., Leoni, L., et al., 2015. Pacemaker in complicated and refractory breath-holding spells: when to think about it? Brain Dev. 37 (1), 2–12.

86 Syncope and Postural Orthostatic Tachycardia Syndrome

Manikum Moodley

An expanded version of this chapter is available on www.expertconsult.com. See inside cover for registration details.

Paroxysmal disorders, including epilepsy and syncope, represent one of the most common neurologic problems in the pediatric population. However, autonomic disorders like postural orthostatic tachycardia syndrome are only now becoming recognized in increasing numbers in children and adolescents. Their disease characteristics, diagnostic criteria, and therapies are still evolving and remain largely undefined.

SYNCOPE

Syncope is defined as the temporary loss of consciousness and postural tone resulting from transient and diffuse cerebral hypoperfusion, followed by spontaneous recovery with no neurologic sequelae. In the young patient, syncope often results from a fall in systolic pressure lower than 70 mm Hg or a mean arterial pressure of 30 to 40 mm Hg. The event is typically preceded by a prodrome lasting several seconds to 1 to 2 minutes, with distinctive premonitory features such as nausea, epigastric discomfort, blurred or tunnel vision, muffled hearing, dizziness, lightheadedness, diaphoresis, hyperventilation, palpitations, pallor, cold and clammy skin, and weakness. Although syncope is commonly a benign self-limiting event, it may rarely be the first warning sign of a serious underlying cardiac or noncardiac disease. Furthermore, the term "syncope" may have different meanings to different people; therefore specific questions should be asked to help differentiate cardiac from neurologic, psychogenic, and metabolic conditions.

Epidemiology

Syncope is a common clinical problem affecting 15% to 25% of children and adolescents. Its true incidence, however, remains unknown. According to Sheldon and colleagues, the most common age for a child's first vasovagal syncopal episode is approximately 13 years. The recurrence rate of syncope ranges from 33% to 51% when patients are followed up to 5 years.

Etiology

Syncope may result from cardiovascular or neurologic causes (cardiovascular-mediated or neurally mediated syncope). Each of these categories accounts for about 50% of adult syncope, but, in children, cardiovascular-mediated syncope is less frequent than it is in adults. The differential diagnosis of pediatric syncope is given in Box 86-1.

Cardiovascular-Mediated Syncope

Cardiovascular-mediated syncope has a higher mortality and a higher incidence of sudden death than neurally mediated syncope. It is therefore imperative to distinguish syncope from seizures and to triage patients with syncope due to malignant cardiac causes for urgent and appropriate investigations and management. Risk factors that suggest structural or

conduction heart defects are given in Box 86-2. Cardiovascular causes of syncope in children are given in Box 86-3.

Neurocardiogenic Syncope

Neurocardiogenic syncope, previously known as vasodepressor, vasovagal, or neurally mediated syncope, is the most common cause of syncope and also the type most commonly confused with epilepsy. The history that suggests this type of benign syncope includes triggers such as postural changes, prolonged standing or sitting, obnoxious stimuli (anger, pain, sight of blood), and a positive family history.

Clinical Features

The patient's history, physical examination, and electrocardiography (ECG) have a combined diagnostic yield of about 50%. A prodromal phase of presyncope consists of lightheadedness, blurred vision, epigastric discomfort, nausea, pallor, or diaphoresis. When present, these clinical features help to differentiate syncope from epilepsy. A detailed history usually reveals contributory environmental factors before the loss of consciousness and postural tone. These environmental factors include upright posture, prolonged standing, change in posture (orthostasis), crowding, heat, fatigue, hunger, or a concurrent illness. Emotional or stress factors, such as venipuncture, public speaking, "fight-or-flight" situations, pain, and fear, are also commonly identified (Driscoll et al,, 1997). The loss of consciousness is usually brief, lasting from a few seconds to 1 to 2 minutes, followed by rapid spontaneous recovery without neurologic deficits. During the ictus the patient may have tonic posturing, myoclonic jerking, or a brief clonic seizure rarely associated with incontinence. The postictal period may be accompanied by persistent nausea, pallor, diaphoresis, and a generally "washed-out" appearance. Complete recovery usually evolves in less than an hour.

Distinguishing between neurocardiogenic syncope and seizure is the most common clinical dilemma and a frequent source of diagnostic error. In distinguishing patients with syncope due to cardiac causes, a history or physical signs of cardiac disease can be 95% sensitive for a cardiac etiology. Patients with pseudosyncope and pseudoseizures typically use the events consciously or unconsciously to avoid an unpleasant emotional situation. Most of these patients are young females. A very high number of events, episodes without injury, and florid symptomatology are typical. Furthermore, in these patients, recovery after a syncopal event is often prolonged (10 to 30 minutes), despite a supine posture. In true syncope, consciousness returns within 1 minute of lying down, and unconsciousness for more than 5 minutes is rare.

The evaluation of syncope may therefore result in unnecessary and costly investigations. A complete evaluation would include neuroimaging studies, electroencephalography (EEG), ECG, echocardiography, Holter monitoring, and selected hematologic and metabolic testing. Despite extensive investigations, more than 40% of patients with recurrent syncope do not have a specific diagnosis.

Pathophysiology

There is no consensus concerning the mechanisms underlying the vasovagal reaction, but several theories have been proposed (Grubb and Kosinski, 1996). The ventricular theory (Fig. 86-1) proposes that, among predisposed individuals who experience recurrent syncope, excess peripheral venous pooling on prolonged standing results in diminished venous return. Decreased cardiac ventricular filling activates mechanoreceptors located mainly in the inferoposterior wall of the left ventricle, which send afferent impulses via C-fibers to the dorsal nucleus of the vagus. Arterial baroreceptors and carotid sinus afferent activation may also contribute to the complex pathophysiology of syncope. These inhibitory cardiac and arterial receptors mediate increased parasympathetic activity, and inhibit sympathetic activity that results in bradycardia, vasodilatation, and hypotension (Bezold-Jarisch reflex) (Shen and Gersh, 1993). In individuals susceptible to recurrent syncope, a "paradoxical" reflex bradycardia and peripheral vascular dilatation occur (Grubb and Kosinski, 1996). The previous emphasis on parasympathetic (vagal) output is shifting to sympathetic withdrawal as the main mechanism responsible for the bradycardia or asystole (cardioinhibitory response) and hypotension (vasodepressor response) that accompany neurocardiogenic syncope. Although parasympathetic-mediated

bradycardia remains a contributory factor in syncope, the responsible phenomena are vasodilatation and hypotension.

Diagnostic Evaluation

The patient history is the cornerstone on which the diagnosis of syncope is made. Important historical details to take from patients are given in Box 86-4. On clinical examination, blood pressure and heart rate should be taken in the supine and upright positions, noting any orthostatic hypotension with or without an increase in heart rate. Special attention should be paid to detecting cardiac anomalies. An ECG should be obtained on all patients who present with syncope, especially if it is recurrent or occurs with exercise. All patients with recurrent syncope, family history of syncope, or sudden unexplained death should be referred to cardiology for further evaluation. This may include echocardiography and a Holter or event monitor.

Tilt-Table Testing

Until the mid-1980s, the diagnosis of neurocardiogenic syncope was made primarily by a careful and detailed patient and family history, the physical examination, and an ECG. Tilt-table testing as a potential diagnostic tool for neurocardiogenic syncope was introduced only in 1986 after the groundbreaking report by Kenny and associates. A number of reports have since emerged, attesting to the utility of the test in reproducing syncopal episodes in patients who are predisposed to neurocardiogenic hypotension and bradycardia.

Despite criticisms, the tilt-table test still continues to enjoy popularity as a noninvasive and physiologically appropriate neurophysiologic test for the diagnosis of neurocardiogenic syncope.

The test is done by positioning the patient head upright at an angle of 60 to 80 degrees for 10 to 60 minutes on a tilt table with a supporting footboard. A tilt-table test result is positive when the symptoms of syncope or presyncope are reproduced. To standardize the test, the duration of head-up tilting has been increased to 45 minutes or 2 standard deviations (SD) of the mean time required to reproduce syncope.

Experience with tilt-table test among pediatric populations is limited. Of note, the tilt-table test has been used in children as young as 3 years of age.

In addition to heart rate and blood pressure monitoring during tilt-table testing, concomitant EEG recording may be used to differentiate anoxic from epileptic seizures. More controlled studies and standardization of degree and duration of tilting are necessary to validate the tilt-table test as a safe, practical, and useful diagnostic tool for neurocardiogenic syncope in children.

Treatment

Once a diagnosis of neurocardiogenic syncope is confirmed, treatment requires counseling of the patient and his or her parents. The benign nature of these events should be explained to allay concerns about epilepsy or sudden death. Most patients presenting after a single uncomplicated syncopal event require simple reassurance, education about the disease, and advice on recognizing prodromal symptoms and how to avoid provocative situations—in particular, prolonged standing, sudden postural changes, dehydration, and irregular meal times. If a prodromal phase is consistently present, the patient may be taught to recline or sit to avoid injury from a fall. Supplemental fluids and electrolytes are usually beneficial; up to 2000 to 3000 mls per day are recommended for adolescents. Patients should be instructed to increase dietary salt,

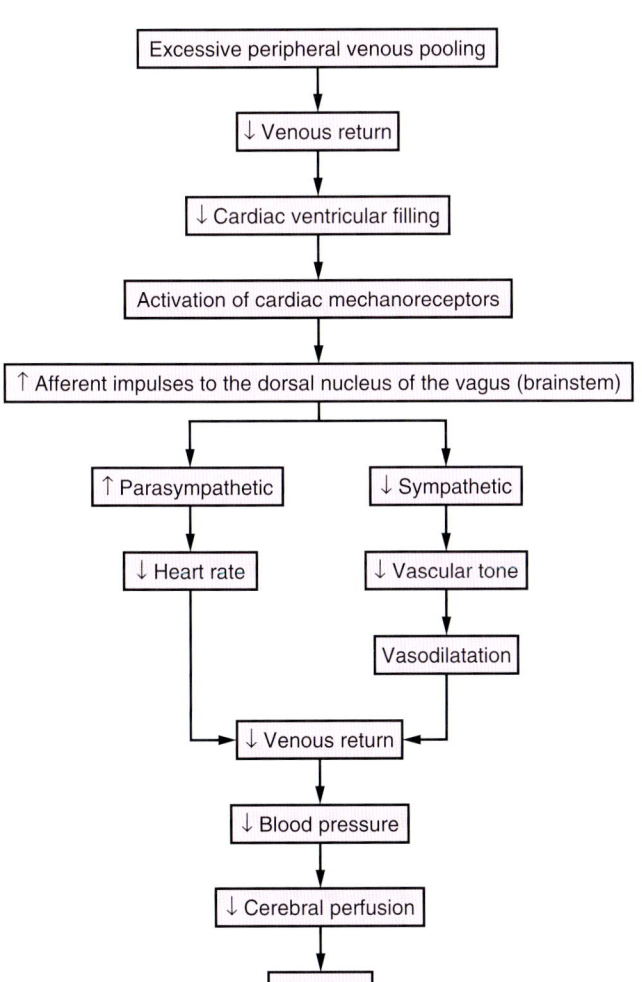

Figure 86-1. The pathophysiology of syncope.

either as salt tablets up to 10 g per day or the liberal use of salt with meals (Box 86-5).

If, despite these conservative measures, the syncopal episodes become refractory, pharmacologic therapy may be tried. Favorable but not consistent response to treatment has been reported with β-adrenergic receptor antagonists, α-adrenergic receptor agonists, anticholinergic agents, theophylline, serotonin reuptake inhibitors, and mineralcorticosteroids (Box 86-6). Beta blockers, fludrocortisone, and midodrine, an α-adrenergic agonist, are often prescribed in children, but none of these agents has shown a consistent therapeutic benefit in clinical trials. Some authorities currently recommend low-dose midodrine as a promising first-line therapy for vasovagal syncope in children (Stewart, 2006). When using fludrocortisone, combine with increased salt intake for an optimal effect.

Prognosis

The prognosis for recovery is excellent in neurocardiogenic syncope. Most patients show spontaneous resolution of their syncope and presyncope within the first year after onset; 5% to 10% will, however, continue to show symptoms over an extended period of time, often up to 5 years.

Convulsive Syncope

A brief tonic or, rarely, a clonic seizure may occasionally accompany syncope. Most convulsions consisted of tonic spasms (65%), characterized by eye rolling, nuchal rigidity, arm flexion, and clenched fists, followed usually by prompt recovery. Other types of convulsions were myoclonic (23%), clonic (6%), and tonic-clonic (6%). Convulsive syncope results from cerebral ischemia and is not indicative of an epileptic predisposition. The EEG reveals diffuse slowing, followed by loss of electrocerebral activity; epileptiform activity is absent. Rarely, an epileptic seizure is triggered by syncope, and in such cases, the EEG reveals epileptiform activity.

Reflex Syncope

Syncope that is triggered by specific factors or events is known as reflex or situational syncope. The most common of these among infants and children is breath-holding spells. These are discussed in greater detail in a chapter elsewhere in this book. Another related but distinctive type of reflex syncope—pallid breath-holding spells or pallid infantile syncope—is frequently confused with breath-holding spells. A simple and more appropriate designation for this type of paroxysm is reflex syncope.

In reflex syncope, the antecedent event is minor trauma before loss of postural tone and consciousness. The rapid or immediate onset of syncope after minor trauma or other unexpected painful stimuli differentiates reflex syncope from breath-holding spells. There is general agreement that reflex syncopal attacks do not represent epileptic seizures, but the mechanism responsible is less clear. Some refer to these events as reflex anoxic seizures.

Situational Syncope

Other triggering factors associated with syncope include cough, deglutition (cold liquids), defecation, diving, micturition, sneezing, trumpet playing, weight lifting, hair grooming, and the Valsalva maneuver. These events are more common in adults than in children and are referred to as situational syncope. Hair-grooming syncope is an uncommon type of situational syncope among adolescent females; hair pulling or scalp stimulation activates the trigeminal nerve and the syncope is often followed by a brief seizure activity.

Hyperventilation Syncope

If the syncope is preceded by paresthesias, lip tingling, and anxiety or panic, consider hyperventilation as the cause. Loss of postural tone and consciousness during hyperventilation is thought to result from cerebral vasoconstriction induced by hypocapnia. This type of syncope is discussed in more detail elsewhere in the book.

Suffocation or Strangulation Syncope

Meadow syndrome (Munchausen by proxy) is a rarely suspected cause of syncope. A caretaker induces loss of consciousness by obstructing the infant's airway using a pillow or by pressing the infant's face against the caretaker's trunk. In other cases, compression of the neck by strangulation results in cerebral hypoxia and, after repeated attempts, brain damage.

Metabolic and Drug-Induced Syncope

When syncopal episodes begin with a slow onset and gradual recovery, consider a toxic or metabolic cause, such as hypoglycemia, alcohol, or drugs (illicit or prescribed). Among the medications that can cause syncope are those that induce ventricular tachycardia or cause hypotension. Cardiovascular medications (vasodilators and antiarrhythmics), psychotropics, diuretics, and glucose-controlling medications are the most common drugs associated with syncope. Alcohol and illicit drugs (cocaine and marijuana) can cause syncope by several mechanisms, including exacerbation of a supraventricular or ventricular tachyarrhythmia. Drug-induced syncope is common among the elderly but rare among children.

However, illicit drug use is increasing significantly in the younger age group. Urine and plasma toxicology screens often provide clues to this diagnosis.

Psychogenic Syncope

One of the most important causes of syncope in pediatric patients, in particular adolescents, is psychogenic syncope. Several features help distinguish psychogenic syncope from neurocardiogenic syncope (Benbadis and Chichkova, 2006):

1. Episodes are extremely frequent (sometimes several episodes per day).
2. The episodes are usually not associated with injury and lack any of the usual precipitating or triggering factors.
3. Patients experience onset of syncope in the supine position.
4. Patients fail to regain consciousness rapidly after a syncopal event (occasionally taking as long as several hours), during which time there are no cardiovascular or neurologic abnormalities, and resumption of the supine posture does not terminate the event.
5. Finally, patients manifest remarkable indifference to their syncope. During tilt-table testing, these patients may suddenly faint without any changes in their heart rate and blood pressure.

A detailed psychosocial history may provide clues about the possible mechanisms involved. Many of these individuals turn out to have conversion reactions, most frequently secondary to sexual abuse. A useful clinical maneuver in the unresponsive patient whose eyes are closed is to touch the eyelashes gently. This touch elicits a blink reflex in the conscious patient and alerts the examiner to the underlying psychopathology. Appropriate referral to a behavioral specialist or pediatric psychiatrist should be made for further evaluation and management.

POSTURAL ORTHOSTATIC TACHYCARDIA SYNDROME
Introduction

Of several autonomic disorders in children the most intriguing is postural orthostatic tachycardia syndrome (POTS), a disorder of unknown etiology in which patients exhibit orthostatic intolerance (OI) associated with significant tachycardia (Moodley, 2013). OI is a constellation of symptoms and signs provoked by standing upright and relieved by recumbence. Symptoms of OI included dizziness, lightheadedness, near syncope, syncope, headache, nausea, vomiting, blurred vision or transient "blackout" or "whiteout" of vision, diminished concentration, hyperpnea, tiredness, and leg weakness (Box 86-4). Symptoms of sympathetic activation include palpitations, chest pain, vasomotor skin changes and warm feeling, tremulousness, increased sweating, anxiety, and occasional sympathetic or autonomic storms.

POTS is one of the most common manifestations of OI and is now being increasingly recognized in children and adolescents. According to current criteria for adults, POTS consists of symptoms of chronic OI and sustained increase in heart rate (HR) of 30 beats per minute (bpm) or more, or an absolute HR of 120 bpm or more, or both within 10 minutes of active standing or head-up tilt. The diagnostic criteria for orthostatic intolerance and POTS in adults are not appropriate for children and adolescents, and new criteria for these disorders in this age group have recently been proposed. A heart rate increment of 40 bpm or more is now considered the required increment for a diagnosis of POTS in children and adolescents (Singer et al., 2012).

Patients with POTS occasionally faint, but unlike OI from autonomic failure, significant orthostatic hypotension is unusual. In fact the blood pressure in POTS may actually increase upon standing secondary to a hyperadrenergic response.

POTS is a multisystem disorder with heterogeneous clinical features and pathophysiology that can be severe and quite disabling with significant effect on the daily quality of life; patients suffer significant functional impairment, yet many of these patients are misdiagnosed as having psychiatric disorders like severe anxiety, panic disorder or depression.

Although POTS has been reported in adults more than a century ago, the condition is rarely reported in children. The first report of POTS in adolescents was in 1999 by Stewart and associates; currently, it affects millions of Americans, particularly young women.

Clinical Features

Patients are typically female with a 5 : 1 female to male ratio and the vast majority of the patients are Caucasian. POTS is relatively uncommon in preadolescent children and more typically affects females between the ages of 15 to 50 and therefore roughly span the ages from menarche to menopause.

Patients with POTS experience chronic and daily symptoms of OI and sympathetic overactivation. These symptoms are commonly exacerbated by heat and exercise. In addition they may experience a myriad of other somatic symptoms including migraine, abdominal pain, cognitive dysfunction, fatigue, sleep disorders, weight loss, and poor exercise tolerance. Moreover, associated anxiety, panic attacks, depression, and other psychiatric disorders add to the complexity of this syndrome and contribute to the disability and poor quality of life in these patients (Jarjour, 2013).

The prevalence of POTS is unknown. In adults, it is estimated to be at least 170 in 100,000, but there are no prevalence data for children.

Early studies suggested that approximately 50% of pediatric patients with POTS have an antecedent illness typically a virus such as infectious mononucleosis, rickettsia, trauma, surgery, or extreme physical activity (Johnson et al., 2010). How these triggers affect the autonomic nervous system is unclear. Many children have severe gastrointestinal dysfunction and chronic debilitating fatigue. Patients complain of poor exercise tolerance and low energy level even at rest, typical of patients who are deconditioned such as in patients who have had prolonged bed rest (Low et al., 2009).

Pathophysiology

POTS represent a syndrome rather than a single disease entity in which no etiology is found despite exhaustive diagnostic testing. Common to all its variants is a final physiologic pathway involving excessively reduced venous return to the heart when in the upright position. The related symptoms of POTS are thought to be secondary to excessive central hypovolemia, and the signature tachycardia may therefore result from related reflex parasympathetic withdrawal and sympathetic activation. The chest pain reported by some patients with POTS and the electrocardiographic wave changes sometimes seen may be secondary to cardiac sympathetic overactivity.

Furthermore factors that reduce compensatory response to decreased thoracic blood volume such as dehydration and hemorrhage can simulate and exacerbate symptoms of POTS.

Additional pathophysiological mechanisms in POTS include defective "skeletal muscle pump," especially in the legs and buttocks. Ambulation is therefore always encouraged for the reduction of POTS symptoms.

Several authors have attempted to classify POTS into one of several phenotypes based on clinical and laboratory testing. A recent study of 152 patients by Thieben and associates described three groups of patients with POTS:

I. Hypovolemic and Deconditioned POTS

This was the most common type confirmed by urinary sodium excretion of less than 100 meq/24 hours. Patients with this type of POTS have decreased plasma volume associated with venous pooling in the legs and mesenteric bed during standing upright or tilt. These patients tend to respond well to increased fluid, salt, and exercise treatment measures (Johnson et al., 2010). Jarjour and collagues found a high prevalence of low iron stores and mild anemia in patients with POTS and neurally mediated syncope, as well as hypovitaminosis D in patients with POTS (Jarjour, 2013). Patients with hypovolemic POTS often complain of extreme fatigue and fibromyalgia-type symptoms with decreased exercise tolerance (Jarjour, 2013). Physical deconditioning is often present in patients with POTS either as the primary etiologic factor or may be secondary to POTS symptoms (Benarroch, 2012).

II. Hyperadrenergic POTS

This type of POTS is characterized by excessive increase of plasma norepinephrine and a rise of blood pressure (BP) on standing. Hyperadrenergic POTS is defined as POTS associated with systolic BP increment of 10 mm Hg or more within 10 minutes of head-up tilt, and an orthostatic plasma norepinephrine of 600 pg/ml or more. The absolute heart rate increment is often 120 beats per minute or more. These patients often have prominent symptoms of sympathetic activation such as palpitations, anxiety, tachycardia, tremulousness, pallor, excessive sweating, migraine type headaches, chest pain, and vasomotor skin changes (Low et al., 2009).

Autonomic or sympathetic storms may occur in a subset of these patients with extreme rise in BP, anxiety, headache, excessive sweating, and other features of sympathetic overactivation (Jarjour, 2013). Secondary hyperadrenergic POTS has been associated with mast cell activation disorders and norepinephrine transporter deficiency. In patients with hyperadrenergic POTS, the possibility of hyperthyroidism or a catecholamine secreting tumor such as pheochromocytoma should be considered (Benarroch, 2012). Laboratory studies should include plasma and urinary metanephrines and, if elevated, imaging studies to rule out pheochromocytoma (Benarroch, 2012).

III. Neuropathic POTS

The term "neuropathic POTS" describes a subgroup of patients who have partial distal autonomic neuropathy, a length-dependent pattern that especially affects larger fibers in the lower limbs (Benarroch, 2012). Distal postganglionic sudomotor denervation can be demonstrated with the quantitative sudomotor axon reflex test and the thermoregulatory sweat test demonstrating sudomotor denervation to the foot and toes (Low et al, 2009).

An acute or subacute autonomic neuropathy may be caused by autoimmunity, as is the case with autonomic ganglionopathy due to antibodies directed against the nicotinic ganglionic acetylcholine receptor. The symptoms come on gradually and involve orthostatic hypotension, significant GI dysfunction, bladder dysfunction, and anhydrosis. This form of POTS is uncommon in children.

Comorbidities in POTS

Many patients with POTS experience chronic symptoms not easily explained by postural intolerance or excessive tachycardia. These associated symptoms include:

I. Visceral Pain and Dysmotility

A significant percentage of patients with POTS experience visceral symptoms referable mainly to the gastrointestinal tract and bladder. Nearly 80% of children with POTS have abdominal pain, and 60% have recurrent nausea and vomiting (Chelimsky and Chelimsky, 2013). Other associated symptoms include bloating, diarrhea, constipation, and bladder symptoms (Benarroch, 2012).

II. Chronicfatigue, Neurocognitive Disorders, Insomnia, and Fibromyalgia

Chronic fatigue, neurocognitive disorders, sleep disturbances, decreased exercise intolerance, and fibromyalgia have been frequently associated with POTS.

III. Nutritional Deficiencies

Several studies have shown that nutritional factors can affect symptoms in patients with dysautonomia. In patients with POTS and neurally mediated syncope, low iron stores and mild anemia were detected, as well as low vitamin D and B12 levels (Jarjour, 2013). The mechanisms by which iron deficiency and hypovitaminosis D and B12 affect autonomic function are unclear (Johnson et al., 2010).

IV. Headache

Moderate to severe headaches with or without migraine features, orthostatic headaches and chronic daily headaches are commonly reported by both adult and pediatric patients with POTS.

V. Ehlers-Danlos Syndrome (EDS)

EDS is a heterogeneous disorder characterized by skin hyperextensibility, joint hypermobility, and connective tissue fragility. Studies have linked joint hypermobility syndromes such as EDS with POTS, but the mechanism of this association remains unclear.

Clinical and Laboratory Evaluation

Patients with POTS require a multidisciplinary evaluation and multimodality treatment (Low et al., 2009). The first and most important step in the evaluation of patients suspected of POTS is to obtain a detailed history followed by a thorough physical examination, including a complete neurologic and cardiac examination in addition to bedside orthostatic measurements.

The physical examination is invariably normal except for the bedside orthostatic measurements that may show excessive postural tachycardia. Examination could also reveal signs

BOX 86-12 Pharmacological Management of POTS

I. β-adrenergic antagonists
  • Atenolol 1–2 mg/kg/d
  • Metoprolol 1–2 mg/kg/d
  • Propranolol 0.5–4 mg/kg/d
  • Nadolol
II. α-adrenergic agonists
  • Midodrine 2.5–10 mg tid
  • Pseudoephedrine 60 mg bid
  • Methylphenidate 5–10 mg tid
III. Mineralocorticolds
  • Fludrocortisone 0.1–0.3 mg/d
IV. Pyridostigmine 30 mg bid
V. Selective serotonin reuptake inhibitors
  • Fluoxetine 10–20 mg/d
  • Sertraline 25–50 mg/d

of venous pooling (edema) or excessive sympathetic activity (such as cold, clammy hands) (Benarroch, 2012). Other clinical signs include hypermobile joints, hypotonia and, tissue-paper-thin skin as seen in EDS. The history and physical examination will guide practitioners in choosing the diagnostic studies that apply to a given patient. Box 86-10 provides details of the laboratory evaluation of suspected POTS.

Treatment

Pediatric POTS is best managed by a multidisciplinary team (neurologist, cardiologist, gastroenterologist, gynecologist, psychologist, geneticist, psychiatrist, and the pain rehabilitation team). The treatment is difficult and based largely on adult studies because of a lack of pediatric specific studies. Patient and family education is a fundamental aspect of POTS management; deconditioning is significant and significantly affects school attendance and education.

Initial treatment includes increasing fluid and salt intake. Most patients require about 2 to 3 L of water per day; and more than 5 g of salt per day. Avoid excessive caffeine intake as it increases diuresis and promotes hypovolemia. Thermotabs may be a substitute if ordinary salt tablets are not well tolerated.

Physical countermaneuvers such as leg crossing or active contraction of abdominal or buttock muscles may produce small increases in mean arterial pressure to maintain an adequate cerebral blood flow (Benarroch, 2012).

In all patients with POTS and physical deconditioning, aerobic exercise and resistance training are exceedingly helpful during their rehabilitation. Patients should be well hydrated before, during, and after exercise (Johnson et al., 2010).

In patients with POTS, blood pooling or standing occurs both in the abdomen and lower limbs. Some patients may therefore benefit from wearing supportive garments such as knee-high, thigh-high, or waist-high tight support stockings with a pressure of 30 to 40 mm Hg. Box 86-11 outlines the nonpharmacologic management of POTS.

If despite these conservative measures the patients continue to have symptoms, pharmacologic therapy may be tried (Box 86-12). Low-dose beta blockers such as metoprolol, labetalol, and propranolol are commonly used, primarily to control heart rate. These medications are reported to be particularly effective in patients with hyperadrenergic POTS.

As inappropriate control of peripheral vascular resistance has been postulated as a cause of POTS the use of α-agonists

(α-1, midodrine hydrochloride, pseudoephedrine α-2, clonidine) can improve orthostatic intolerance, reduce venous pooling, and suppress the related tachycardia. Avoid taking α-agonists within 4 hours of a prolonged supine posture, including sleep, to prevent supine hypertension.

Fludrocortisone (0.1 to 0.3 mg daily) is a mineralocorticoid often used in combination with other medications for the treatment of POTS. Fludrocortisone promotes intravascular volume expansion and at the same time induces potassium excretion; thus serum potassium levels need to be carefully monitored and potassium supplements provided when necessary. Fludrocortisone needs time to work, so 2 or more weeks should be allowed between dose increases.

Other medications have been used in POTS with mixed results and mainly in adults. These include vasopressin (DDAVP); erythropoietin, clonidine, methylphenidate, octreotide, selective serotonin reuptake inhibitors, serotonin norepinephrine reuptake inhibitor (venlafaxine), and pyridostigmine (Johnson et al., 2010). Pyridostigmine is thought to be particularly helpful in patients with hyperadrenergic POTS (Johnson et al., 2010). Starting dose is 30 mg twice daily. Clonidine, an α-receptor agonist, is a useful drug for the treatment of sympathetic storms as it works by inhibiting central venous system sympathetic out flow.

Patients with neuropathic POTS who are seropositive for autoimmune autonomic ganglionopathy or neuropathy may respond well to immunotherapy.

CONCLUSIONS

Systematic studies of autonomic disorders in children and adolescents are relatively new. The disease characteristics, diagnostic criteria, and therapies are evolving and remain largely undefined.

As with all chronic illnesses, psychological and psychiatric comorbidity adds to the difficulty in the optimal management of these patients. Deconditioning is commonly associated with POTS, adding to its disability. In some centers, up to 50% of patients with POTS are placed on SSRIs because of the high burden of psychological and psychiatric comorbidity. Psychological counseling and participation in a chronic pain management program are useful adjuncts in the rehabilitation of patients with POTS. There are limited long-term outcome data for children and adolescents with POTS. Most available studies however, suggest an overall good potential for recovery in newly diagnosed adolescents compared with adults with newly diagnosed postural orthostatic tachycardia syndrome.

REFERENCES

The complete list of references for this chapter is available in the e-book at www.expertconsult.com.
  See inside cover for registration details.

SELECTED REFERENCES

Benarroch, E.E., 2012. Postural tachycardia syndrome: a heterogeneous and multifactorial disorder. Mayo Clin. Proc. 87 (12), 1214–1225.

Benbadis, S.R., Chichkova, R., 2006. Psychogenic pseudosyncope: an underestimated and provable diagnosis. Epilepsy Behav. 9, 106–110.

Chelimsky, G., Chelimsky, T., 2013. Gastrointestinal manifestations of pediatric autonomic disorders. Semin. Pediatr. Neurol. 20 (1), 27–30.

Driscoll, D.J., Jacobsen, S.J., Porter, C.J., et al., 1997. Syncope in children and adolescents. J. Am. Coll. Cardiol. 29, 1039–1045.

Grubb, B.P., Kosinski, D., 1996. Current trends in etiology, diagnosis, and management of neurocardiogenic syncope. Curr. Opin. Cardiol. 11, 32–41.

Jarjour, I.T., 2013. Postural orthostatic tachycardia syndrome in children and adolescents. Semin. Pediatr. Neurol. 20 (1), 18–26.

Johnson, J.N., Mack, K.J., Kuntz, N.L., et al., 2010. Postural orthostatic tachycardia syndrome: a clinical review. Pediatr. Neurol. 42 (2), 77–85.

Low, P.A., Sanddroni, P., Joyner, M., et al., 2009. Postural tachycardia syndrome (POTS). J. Cardiovasc. Electrophysiol. 20, 352–358.

Moodley, M., 2013. Pediatric autonomic disorders. Semin. Pediatr. Neurol. 20 (1), 1–2.

Shen, W.K., Gersh, B.J., 1993. Syncope: mechanisms, approach, and management. In: Low, P.A. (Ed.), Clinical autonomic disorders. Little Brown & Co, Boston, MA.

Singer, W., Sletten, D.M., Opfer-Gehrking, T.L., et al., 2012. Postural tachycardia in children and adolescents: what is abnormal? J. Pediatr. 160 (2), 222–226.

Stewart, J.M., 2006. Midodrine for the treatment of vasovagal syncope (simple faint). J. Pediatr. 149, 740–742.

E-BOOK FIGURES AND TABLES

Nocturnal Paroxysmal Disorders

Sanjeev V. Kothare and Sejal V. Jain

An expanded version of this chapter is available on www.expertconsult.com. See inside cover for registration details.

Many childhood sleep disorders have paroxysmal onset and offset. It is therefore not uncommon that these episodes may be interpreted as parasomnia or seizures. In this chapter, common sleep disorders that may mimic parasomnia and epilepsy are emphasized.

A. PARASOMNIAS

According to the International Classification of Sleep Disorders, third edition (ICSD-3), parasomnias are defined as undesirable physical events or experiences that occur during entry into sleep, during sleep, or during arousals from sleep (American Academy of Sleep Medicine [AASM], 2014). They are classified as (1) disorders of arousals from nonrapid eye movement (NREM) sleep, (2) parasomnias associated with rapid eye movement (REM) sleep, and (3) other parasomnias (AASM, 2014).

Lists of the parasomnias and disorders mimicking parasomnia are provided in Table 87-1 and Table 87-2, respectively.

I. Disorders of Arousal from NREM Sleep

Disorders of arousal from NREM sleep are the most common parasomnias in the pediatric population. Most disorders of arousal occur during slow-wave sleep (SWS) as incomplete transitions into wakefulness, and are characterized by automatic behavior, altered perception of the surrounding environment, and a variable degree of amnesia for the event (Mahowald, Bornemann, and Schenck, 2004). Episodes tend to occur in the first third of the night when SWS is more prominent. Electroencephalograms (EEGs) recorded during such episodes demonstrate a mixture of theta, delta, and alpha frequencies (Fig. 87-1). These disorders are thought to result from a faulty switch that prevents normal sleep-cycle progression. Episodes may be brought on by sleep deprivation, medications, noisy or stimulating environments, stress, and fever. Sleep fragmentation as a result of obstructive sleep apnea (OSA) or periodic limb movements of sleep (PLMS) may also be a precipitating factor. In one study, an association with another sleep disorder was found in 61% of children with parasomnias. In this study, the children who were successfully treated for an associated sleep disorder had resolution of the parasomnia events, whereas untreated children continued to have events (Guilleminault, Palombini, Pelayo, and Chervin, 2003). Additionally, patients with one type of parasomnia may also have other types. Based on a recent study, 41% of children with sleepwalking may also have sleep terrors, and 92% of children with persistent sleep terrors at age 6 years may also have somniloquy. At a later age, sleep terrors may progress to sleepwalking. Bruxism, hypnogogic hallucinations, and nightmares may also be associated conditions. Moreover, several studies suggest a genetic predisposition to some of the arousal parasomnias. In one study, a remarkable 96% of the patients with sleepwalking or night terrors had a positive family history in first- to third-degree relatives.

The clinical history in a child with any parasomnia should include a complete description of the events, time of night when the events happen, frequency of episodes, recollection of the events by the child, and presence of the events during daytime naps. Information regarding whether the movements are rhythmic and stereotypical, associated with eye deviation, and associated with focal tonic-clonic activity may support an epileptic origin to the events. A home video often proves useful for identifying and classifying parasomnias and differentiating them from seizures (Mason and Pack, 2007). Examination should focus on looking for evidence of upper airway obstruction, such as adenotonsillar hypertrophy, midfacial hypoplasia, and retrognathia (Sheldon, 2004). In appropriate cases, a video EEG concurrent with sleep may be indicated to rule out seizures (Fusco and Specchio, 2005). Overnight polysomnography is indicated when there is concern for an intrinsic sleep disorder, such as OSA or PLMS, rather than to document the parasomnia per se.

Management usually includes reassuring parents that parasomnias are common in childhood and that they are benign and self-remitting. Parents should be counseled when appropriate on instituting important safety measures, including securing windows, staircases, and doors, to prevent injuries. They should be educated about appropriate pediatric sleep hygiene, such as avoiding sleep deprivation, maintaining regular sleeping hours, avoiding caffeinated drinks, and avoiding any attempts to restrain or awaken the child during an episode, which may actually be counterproductive. Scheduled or anticipatory awakenings several minutes beforehand have been attempted to abort such events when they happen consistently at particular times, but in general this approach has not been well accepted by families. Treatment of the underlying intrinsic sleep disorder such as OSA with tonsillectomy and adenoidectomy has been shown to result in disappearance of the parasomnia events. Oral iron supplementation for PLMS also has been shown to lead to improvement of parasomnia. Iron is an essential cofactor for synthesis of dopamine via tyrosine hydroxylase. Iron deficiency causes lower dopaminergic activity, which, along with complex interactions with other neurotransmitter systems, may lead to restless leg syndrome (RLS) or PLMS. A ferritin level above 50 ng/mL is the target for treatment of PLMS. Thus iron and ferritin levels should be checked in children with suspected RLS or PLMS. Medications for treatment of parasomnia itself should be reserved for those rare, protracted cases with no associated sleep disorders, with frequent parasomnias, or with a real threat for self-injury. Low-dose clonazepam or tricyclic antidepressants for a short duration have been used with good success in such cases.

Sleepwalking

Sleepwalking occurs in up to 17% of children, is most common in children 12 to 13 years of age, and has no gender

TABLE 87-1 Classification of Parasomnias

NREM	REM	Other Parasomnias	Normal Variants	Other Disorders
Sleepwalking	REM sleep behavior disorders	Nocturnal enuresis	Sleep talking	Catathrenia (classified as a sleep-related breathing disorder)
Confusional arousal	Recurrent isolated sleep paralysis	Exploding head syndrome	Sleep starts	Hypnic headaches
Sleep terrors	Nightmare disorder	Sleep-related hallucinations		Head banging
Sleep-related eating disorder				

NREM, nonrapid eye movement; REM = rapid eye movement.

TABLE 87-2 Differential Diagnosis of Parasomnia

Neurologic/Psychiatric	Cardiopulmonary	Gastrointestinal	Miscellaneous
Headache	Arrhythmias	Gastroesophageal reflux	Muscle cramp
Seizures	Angina pectoris		Tongue bite
Panic attacks	Hiccough		Pruritus
PTSD	Coughing		Night sweats
Dissociative disorders	Choking Asthma		Alternating hemiplegia of childhood in sleep

PTSD, posttraumatic stress disorder.

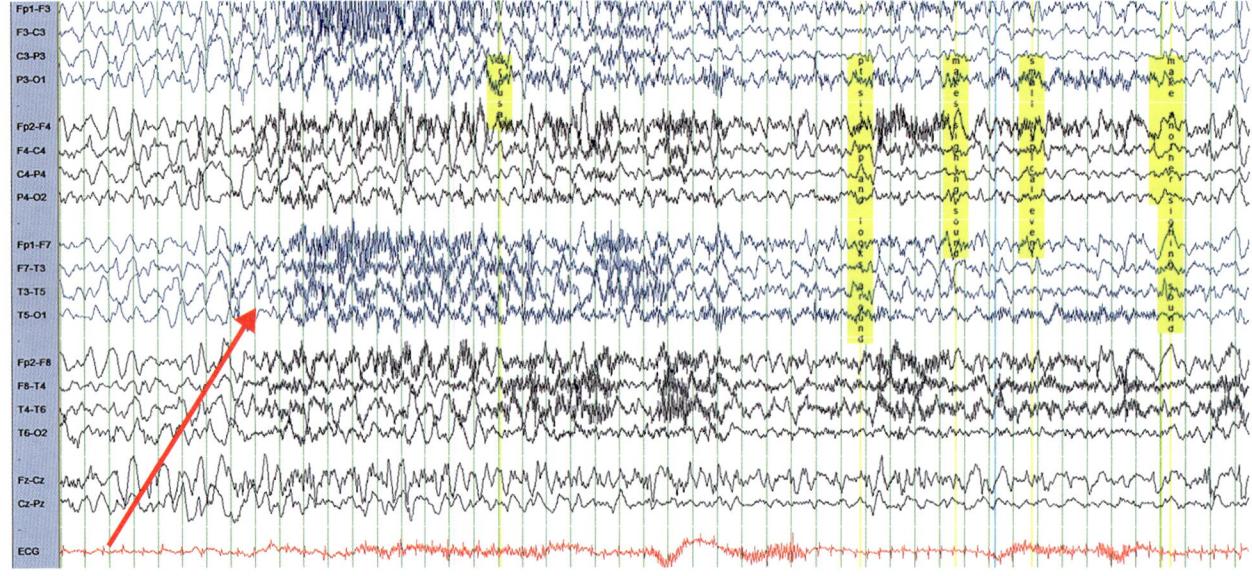

Figure 87-1. EEG showing a parasomnia event from N3. Arrow points to the onset of the event.

predilection. Most of the patients with onset before 10 years of age outgrow the condition, but up to 25% continue to be affected by sleepwalking into adulthood. Teenagers who continue to have sleepwalking episodes often have comorbid psychiatric disorders, including panic disorder, anxiety disorder, alcohol or cigarette use, suicidal ideation, and simple phobia. Sleepwalking episodes are characterized by behaviors such as sitting up in bed and displaying complex motor movements, including changing of body position, turning, playing with sheets, and eventually getting out of the bed. Some children walk around the house, going into different rooms, downstairs, or even outside the house. Sleepwalking can be further classified into calm or agitated subtypes, with the former more common in children. Although children may get agitated if awakened in the middle of an episode, they do not have any recollection of the event in the morning. Because there is altered awareness, the major concern during these benign behaviors is the risk for self-injury from, for example, falling down the stairs, going out of the house, or running into closed doors (Avidan and Kaplish, 2010).

Confusional Arousals

Confusional arousals occur in up to 17.3% of the population, mainly in infants and toddlers. A typical event begins with moaning, evolving to confused and agitated behavior lasting from 5 to 15 minutes. Attempts to fully wake up the child are unsuccessful. Sleep-sex disorder (sexsomnia) is a subtype of this disorder that has been reported in adults, with onset around adolescence in some individuals. Sexsomnia involves inappropriate sexual behavior that occurs during sleep, without the conscious awareness of the individual.

Sleep Terrors

Episodes of sleep terror occur in 1% to 6% of children, with a peak frequency between 4 and 8 years of age; gender differences have not been observed. The child may sit up suddenly and scream with a blood-curdling "battle-cry." There is an expression of intense fear on the child's face, and this is accompanied by apparent autonomic activation, including mydriasis, tachycardia, and diaphoresis. The child may be unresponsive to consoling, and if awakened, confusion and disorientation may occur. Some children may report indistinct recollections of a threat, such as monsters, spiders, or snakes, from which they have to defend themselves. In most cases however, there is no recollection of the event. The event may last from a few minutes up to 20 minutes, but a longer duration may also be seen. Because the amount of time spent in slow-wave sleep decreases with age, most cases go into natural remission by adolescence. In two studies, only 0.9% to 1.2% of affected children continued to have episodes at 7 to 13 years of age.

Sleep-Related Eating Disorder

Usually seen accompanying sleep walking and daytime eating disorder, sleep-related eating disorder is characterized by out-of-control eating binges, predominantly of carbohydrate-containing foods, 2 to 3 hours after sleep onset, with no subsequent recall of the event. Episodes can begin in childhood, but onset is more common in the teenage years and adulthood. These behaviors have recently been described in association with the use of hypnotics such as zolpidem.

Diagnosis

Clinicians must differentiate parasomnias classified as disorders of arousal from NREM sleep from nocturnal seizures. Frontal lobe seizures are especially important to consider, because they occur predominantly in sleep, sometimes many times per night, and are characterized by stereotypical movements, thrashing of the entire body, vocalizations, and dystonic posturing lasting 20 seconds to a few minutes, with minimal postictal drowsiness or confusion. Paroxysmal nocturnal dystonia, which is now considered to be a frontal lobe seizure, is characterized by an arousal from NREM sleep accompanied by dystonic posturing, bizarre movements of the extremities, and vocalizations, with minimal evident EEG correlation as a result of the deep-seated focus of seizure onset in the mesial frontal region. In-patient video EEG monitoring is useful in confirming the diagnosis and differentiating such events from nocturnal panic attacks, fugue states, conversion reactions, and parasomnias such as night terrors, confusional arousals, and sleepwalking.

II. Parasomnias Associated with REM Sleep

Nightmares

Nightmares are a form of parasomnia associated with REM sleep and are characterized by vivid dreams in the second half of the night accompanied by an intense feeling of terror or dread that typically awakens the child from sleep. The child can be easily aroused and has good recollection of the event. Nightmares are frequently seen in children between 3 and 6 years of age. Prevalence ranges from 30% to 90% for occasional episodes and 5% to 30% for frequent episodes. In children, psychiatric disorders are seen more often in those experiencing nightmares than in those without nightmares. Nightmares may also occasionally be a marker for a history of trauma or sexual abuse in children and adolescents.

REM Sleep Behavior Disorder

REM sleep behavior disorder is characterized by the behavioral enactment of unpleasant and combative dreams with complex movements that can be vigorous and violent because of the lack of atonia during REM sleep. This disorder typically occurs in the 60s or 70s in males and may precede the onset of Parkinson disease or a progressive supranuclear palsy (PSP). The disorder is uncommon in children but may be seen in association with the use of selective serotonin reuptake inhibitors (SSRIs) such as fluoxetine, or accompanying narcolepsy and Tourette syndrome. These episodes respond very well to small doses of clonazepam given at bedtime.

Recurrent Isolated Sleep Paralysis

Recurrent isolated sleep paralysis is characterized by a generalized inability to speak or to move the trunk, head, and limbs that occurs during the transitional period between sleep and wakefulness. The episodes are brief and transient but may be accompanied by vivid hallucinations, which often make them very distressing. Although the condition is usually seen with narcolepsy, it may also be seen in isolated form in otherwise healthy individuals and in those with a strong family history.

III. Other Parasomnias

Nocturnal Enuresis

Nocturnal enuresis (bedwetting) refers to the involuntary passage of urine while asleep. It occurs in approximately 15% to 25% of children at 5 years of age, more often in boys, and in 1% to 3% of adolescents. It may be classified as primary (when present from birth) or secondary (with periods of at least 6 months of dryness before the recurrence of enuresis), and as nocturnal (occurring at night) and/or diurnal (occurring during the day). Three major pathologic factors have been considered as possible etiologies: group 1, volume dependent, with polyuria; group 2, detrusor dependent, with involuntary detrusor contractions and a small urinary bladder; group 3, with decreased arousability. There are strong associations of enuresis with genetic and familial factors, and a high prevalence of secondary enuresis in children with OSA. Treatment involves the removal of inciting factors, reassurance, behavioral programs, and the use of nasal desmopressin or oral tricyclic antidepressants such as imipramine.

Exploding Head Syndrome

Exploding head syndrome is a harmless but potentially terrifying situation, usually occurring while a patient is falling asleep, characterized by a terrifying loud noise accompanied by myoclonic jerks or the perception of a flash of light. These episodes are very brief but lead to intense anxiety. There is no headache or pain accompanying these episodes, and they can begin in childhood. No treatment is needed aside from accurate diagnosis and reassurance.

Sleep-Related Hallucinations

Sleep-related hallucinations are characterized as vivid dreams, or perceptions not based in reality, that occur either at sleep onset (hypnagogic hallucinations) or upon awakening (hypnopompic hallucinations). They can occur in otherwise healthy individuals, but are frequently seen as part of the symptoms of narcolepsy. The hallucinations may be visual, tactile, auditory, or kinetic in nature. They are thought to result from the brief intrusion of REM sleep into NREM sleep or wakefulness.

IV. Normal Variants

Sleep Talking

Sleep talking is very common in the general population and has a strong familial and genetic propensity. It can occur in REM or NREM sleep, and the main feature is talking during sleep, with or without comprehension. Arousal from sleep rarely occurs. The individual is rarely aware of it, but the talking disturbs others sharing the room. Sleep talking may be associated with other parasomnias.

Sleep Starts

Also called hypnic jerks, sleep starts are common and involve sudden whole-body jerks experienced during the sleep–wake transition. Variations include sensory, auditory (e.g., exploding tinnitus), and visual sensations, which may occur without motor jerks. No treatment other than reassurance is necessary.

V. Other Disorders

Catathrenia

Also called nocturnal groaning, catathrenia can occur in REM or NREM sleep during expiration in clusters of 2 minutes to an hour. Episodes end with a snort and are accompanied by changes in heart rate. Onset may occur during childhood or adolescence. The exact etiology is unknown, and no specific therapy has been found to be effective.

Hypnic Headaches

Hypnic headaches are characterized by diffuse headaches occurring at a consistent time, usually 4 to 6 hours after sleep onset, lasting 30 to 60 minutes. This condition is most commonly seen in older adults, and is often accompanied with nausea but no other autonomic features. Hypnic headaches are rare in children, but reported cases also show lack of autonomic symptoms; response to melatonin is seen in 40% of affected children.

Head Banging

Also called jactatio capitis nocturna, head banging is now classified as a rhythmic movement disorder of sleep, and is characterized by rhythmic movements of the head and body at sleep onset in infants and toddlers. It is seen more often in children with developmental disabilities and autism, but may be seen in normal children. No specific treatment other than reassurance is indicated.

B. NOCTURNAL PANIC ATTACKS

Nocturnal panic attacks are events in which the individual wakes from sleep in a state of panic, with panic defined as an abrupt and discrete period of intense fear or discomfort that is accompanied by cognitive and physical symptoms of arousal. These symptoms include tachycardia, sweating, shortness of breath, chest pressure, choking sensations, dizziness or lightheadedness, depersonalization or derealization, stomach discomfort, and intense fears of dying or going crazy (Table 87-3). A full panic attack (in contrast to a limited symptom attack) is defined by observation of four or more of these symptoms. The symptom profile of nocturnal panic attacks does not differ significantly from that of panic attacks that occur during wakeful states, although breathlessness and choking are more prominent. A nocturnal panic attack is an abrupt waking from sleep in a state of panic without an obvious trigger. Nocturnal panic attacks are most often experienced by individuals with a daytime panic disorder, an anxiety disorder characterized by unexpected panic attacks, and persistent apprehension regarding the recurrence of panic attacks or changes in lifestyle as a result of their occurrence. Thus most patients with nocturnal panic attacks experience panic attacks during wakeful states as well, although a small subset predominantly or exclusively experiences nocturnal panic attacks (Nakamura, Sugiura, Komada, and Inoue, 2013). The only other anxiety disorder in which nocturnal panic attacks have been documented is posttraumatic stress disorder. Most patients report that nocturnal panic attacks occur between 1 and 3 hours after sleep onset, and only occasionally occur more than once per night. Nocturnal panic attacks typically last from 2 to 8 minutes, and return to sleep is usually difficult. Patients are able to vividly recall their nocturnal panic attacks.

Although epidemiologic studies have not been conducted, surveys of select clinical groups suggest that nocturnal panic attacks are relatively common among patients with a panic disorder, with 44% to 71% reporting having experienced nocturnal panic attacks at least once. In the largest survey to date, 58% of 1166 individuals with definite or probable panic disorder reported having experienced nocturnal panic attacks at least once, and 30% to 45% reported repeated nocturnal panic attacks. Many patients who suffer nocturnal panic attacks frequently become fearful of sleep and attempt to delay sleep onset. Avoidance of sleep may thus result in chronic sleep deprivation, in turn precipitating more nocturnal panic attacks.

Nocturnal panic attacks are an NREM event, usually occurring in late stage II or early stage III of sleep and in the absence of any associated EEG abnormalities. Nocturnal panic attacks are distinct from sleep terrors, which occur mostly during stage IV sleep and are followed by a quick return to sleep, without later recall of the event. The absence of EEG abnormalities distinguishes these attacks from nocturnal seizures. Nocturnal choking episodes may be a predominant symptom of both nocturnal panic attacks and epileptic seizures. Choking is often seen in nocturnal seizures arising from the insula, the mesial frontal cortex, and the supplementary motor area. The major distinction between nightmares and nocturnal panic attacks is the stages of sleep during which they occur; nocturnal panic attacks are an NREM event, whereas nightmares are a REM event. Also, according to EEG data, patients with panic disorder are accurate in their discrimination between dream-induced anxiety and nocturnal panic attacks, even though both are associated with autonomic activation.

TABLE 87-3 Criteria for Nocturnal Panic Attacks

An abrupt and discrete period of intense fear or discomfort, in which four or more of the following symptoms develop out of sleep:

1. Sensation of shortness of breath*
2. Feeling of severe choking*
3. Fear of losing control of breathing*
4. Fear of dying
5. Tachycardia
6. Sweating
7. Chest pain and discomfort
8. Stomach discomfort such as nausea
9. Dizziness or lightheadedness
10. Depersonalization or derealization
11. Hot or cold flashes
12. Trembling or shaking
13. Paresthesias

*Respiratory symptoms are the predominant features in nocturnal panic attacks compared with daytime panic attacks.

Assessment of nocturnal panic attacks focuses on ruling out alternative explanations for these episodes (e.g., seizures, apnea, other emotional disorder). Differential diagnosis is made on the basis of interviews, sleep polysomnography in a sleep laboratory, and ambulatory recordings of sleep in the natural environment.

Psychological treatment for these attacks is based on recent work demonstrating that cognitive factors, such as expectations about arousal during sleep, predict increased distress and panic attacks arising out of sleep. Nocturnal panic attack is thus conceptualized as triggered by interoceptive conditioning, whereby fluctuations in normal bodily sensations that are not consciously recognized because of the sleep state elicit a conditional fear as a result of prior associative pairings with panic. Cognitive behavioral therapy (CBT) targets both daytime and nocturnal panic attacks and the accompanying chronic apprehension over their recurrence, with emphasis on the benign nature of normal physiologic fluctuations during sleep. Breathing retraining is taught as a coping technique, especially for symptoms associated with overbreathing, and patients practice interoceptive inductions tailored to these attacks (e.g., deep relaxation, "buzzer arousal inductions" from a sleeping state). Maladaptive behaviors specific to nocturnal panic attacks (e.g., television watching to facilitate sleep induction) are targeted, as are poor sleep habits, because sleep-onset insomnia often accompanies these attacks and may contribute to its augmented recurrence. Recent evidence suggests that relative to precipitant desensitization, CBT for these attacks led to substantial reductions in the frequency and severity of daytime and nocturnal panic attacks, and these gains persisted at 9-month follow up.

Pharmacologic treatment has not yet been subject to rigorous empirical testing (Craske and Tsao, 2005), although uncontrolled trials suggest that agents typically used to treat daytime panic attacks (e.g., benzodiazepines, antidepressants) can ameliorate nocturnal panic attacks, suggesting the need for future double-blind, placebo-controlled trials to establish the efficacy of these agents. Additional work is also needed to compare treatment outcomes for nocturnal parasomnias treated with CBT in combination with pharmacologic agents versus use of these agents alone.

C. SANDIFER SYNDROME

Gastroesophageal reflux (GER) involves the retrograde movement of gastric contents across the lower esophageal sphincter into the esophagus. Although episodes of GER are often physiologic in nature, the condition can become pathologic in children when episodes are more frequent and persistent. Consequences of GER include esophagitis, esophageal symptoms, and respiratory sequelae (Lehwald et al., 2007). GER afflicts approximately 7% of infants and children. It is seen more commonly in children with neurologic impairment. Named after the neurologist Paul Sandifer, Sandifer syndrome was first reported by Kinsbourne in 1962. It is characterized by gastroesophageal reflux disease (GERD), presenting with spastic torticollis and paroxysmal dystonic head and neck movements, head/eye version, irritability, crying, vomiting, and abdominal pain, with or without hiatus hernia. It is a rare but important symptom complex seen in 1% of children with GER; it usually appears in early infancy or childhood but has been reported to have onset even in adults. It is postulated that the abnormal movements during the reflux are the result of a mechanism to protect the airway passages from reflux or to relieve the pain caused by acid reflux. Sandifer syndrome is often mistaken for seizures, including infantile spasms. A normal EEG, especially during the event, rules out seizures. It is important to be cognizant of this condition because delay in diagnosis can lead to significant morbidity, including aspiration of the stomach acid into the lungs, anemia, and esophageal ulcers. The diagnosis is confirmed with a 24-hour pH probe study, and if necessary an upper gastrointestinal endoscopy. The symptoms of Sandifer syndrome respond very well to medical management with use of a proton pump inhibitor, although rare cases need surgical intervention, especially those involving hiatus hernia.

REFERENCES

The complete list of references for this chapter is available in the e-book at www.expertconsult.com.

    See inside cover for registration details.

SELECTED REFERENCES

American Academy of Sleep Medicine, 2014. International Classification of Sleep Disorders, third ed. American Academy of Sleep Medicine, Darien, IL.

Avidan, A.Y., Kaplish, N., 2010. The parasomnias: Epidemiology, clinical features, and diagnostic approach. Clin. Chest Med. 31 (2), 353–370.

Craske, M.G., Tsao, J.C., 2005. Assessment and treatment of nocturnal panic attacks. Sleep Med. Rev. 9 (3), 173–184.

Fusco, L., Specchio, N., 2005. Non-epileptic paroxysmal manifestations during sleep in infancy and childhood. Neurol. Sci. 26 (Suppl. 3), s205–s209.

Guilleminault, C., Palombini, L., Pelayo, R., et al., 2003. Sleepwalking and sleep terrors in prepubertal children: what triggers them? Pediatrics 111 (1), e17–e25.

Lehwald, N., Krausch, M., Franke, C., et al., 2007. Sandifer syndrome– a multidisciplinary diagnostic and therapeutic challenge. Eur. J. Pediatr. Surg. 17 (3), 203–206.

Mahowald, M.W., Bornemann, M.C., Schenck, C.H., 2004. Parasomnias. Semin. Neurol. 24 (3), 283–292.

Mason, T.B. 2nd, Pack, A.I., 2007. Pediatric parasomnias. Sleep 30 (2), 141–151.

Nakamura, M., Sugiura, T., Nishida, S., et al., 2013. Is nocturnal panic a distinct disease category? Comparison of clinical characteristics among patients with primary nocturnal panic, daytime panic, and coexistence of nocturnal and daytime panic. J. Clin. Sleep Med. 9 (5), 461–467.

Sheldon, S.H., 2004. Parasomnias in childhood. Pediatr. Clin. North Am. 51 (1), 69–88, vi.

88 Disorders of Excessive Sleepiness

Sejal V. Jain and Sanjeev V. Kothare

An expanded version of this chapter is available on www.expertconsult.com. See inside cover for registration details.

Excessive daytime sleepiness (EDS) is not uncommon in children and adolescents, with a prevalence of 4% in preadolescents and almost 20% in high school seniors. EDS is associated with changes in mood, attention, and behavior, as well as poor performance in school and on cognitive tests. Hence, it is important to accurately diagnose and treat disorders of excessive sleepiness.

Etiologies of EDS can be divided into three broad categories—insufficient sleep, fragmented sleep, and an increased need for sleep—that are detailed in Table 88-1. Insufficient sleep could be due to sleep disorders such as primary insomnia or behavioral insomnia in younger children. In adolescents, insufficient sleep is typically multifactorial. In studies, the sleep duration reduced from 9.9 hours to 8 hours in 10- to 16-year-olds. Almost 40% of adolescents showed more than a 2-hour sleep difference between school days and weekends. Additionally, there is physiologic delay in sleep onset in teenagers. This delay in sleep onset combined with the increased use of various electronic media causes sleep disturbances. When combined with earlier school start times, these problems result in EDS.

Fragmented nocturnal sleep can be due to a variety of causes. These include behavioral causes, such as nighttime electronic media exposure, and behaviorally induced insufficient sleep. In younger children fragmented sleep can be caused by behavioral insomnia-sleep-onset association type. Medical disorders also can fragment sleep.

Finally, increased sleep drive or increased sleep need is the most important cause of EDS, which can be temporary or permanent. The temporary causes are physical or emotional trauma, infections, acute illnesses, or other factors. Primary permanent and recurrent hypersomnia are considered central hypersomnias and are discussed in detail in this chapter.

The International Classification of Sleep Disorders-3 (ICSD-3) classifies central hypersomnia as: 1) narcolepsy type 1 (previously narcolepsy with cataplexy); 2) narcolepsy type 2 (previously narcolepsy without cataplexy; 3) idiopathic hypersomnia; 4) Kleine-Levin syndrome (KLS); 5) hypersomnia due to a medical disorder; 6) hypersomnia due to medication or substance abuse; 7) hypersomnia due to a psychiatric disorder; and 8) insufficient sleep syndrome (American Academy of Sleep Medicine, 2014).

ASSESSMENT OF SLEEPINESS

The assessment of EDS is important to differentiate the previously described disorders and central hypersomnias as well as to specify the type of hypersomnia (Kothare and Kaleyias, 2008; Kotagal, 2012). Figure 88-1 shows an algorithm that can be used for the evaluation of EDS.

Clinical Assessment
History

A detailed history is crucial to identify if excessive sleepiness is truly present and assess total sleep time, as well as associated disorders which could cause symptoms of sleepiness, and to determine whether other sleep disorders are present. The history should focus on sleep-wake patterns, including bedtime, rise time, arousals, sleep-onset latency, and the ability to wake up refreshed in the morning. Obtaining additional history pertaining to the duration and timing of naps, planned versus spontaneous naps, factors precipitating spontaneous naps, and feeling refreshed after naps is important. Associated features such as cataplexy, hallucinations, sleep attacks, and sleep paralysis also should be evaluated. To determine whether other sleep disorders are present, questioning should focus on snoring, witnessed apnea, "restless leg" symptoms in the evening and movements of the legs during sleep. A history pertaining to whether or not there is coexistent or underlying neurologic disorders such as epilepsy, migraine, genetic conditions, and head injuries also should be evaluated.

Physical Examination

Obesity, assessed by an elevated age-appropriate body mass index, craniofacial anomalies (micrognathia, midfacial hypoplasia), tonsillar hypertrophy, enlarged tongue base, deviated nasal septum, swollen inferior turbinates, high arched palate, and mouth breathing may all be associated with obstructive sleep apnea (OSA) and should be evaluated. Additionally, the presence of linea nigricans, reflecting insulin resistance, should be assessed. Signs suggestive of other neurologic disorders such as a head injury also should be identified.

Subjective Evaluation Tools

Subjective evaluation tools include questionnaires and sleep logs/diaries. Sleep logs give an estimate of the number, duration, and timing of daily episodes of nocturnal sleep, daytime naps, and wake periods. These can be used to evaluate sleep-wake habits. These may reveal the evidence of chronically insufficient sleep.

To assess sleepiness, questionnaires such as the Stanford Sleepiness Scale (SSS), the Epworth Sleepiness Scale (ESS), and the Pediatric Daytime Sleepiness Scale (PDSS) can be used. SSS and ESS are mainly used in adults, whereas the PDSS was specifically developed to assess sleepiness in school-age children.

Objective Evaluation Tools

Objective evaluation tools are discussed in detail in the online chapter.

Actigraphy

Actigraphs are miniature computerized wristwatch-like devices that measure limb activity, based on which sleep and wake periods can be indirectly calculated. Actigraphs help to determine whether sleep is insufficient and to confirm sleepiness.

Nocturnal Polysomnography

Polysomnography (PSG) is the gold standard for evaluating sleep disorders. As the name suggests, it is an electrophysiological recording of multiple parameters, including an electroencephalogram (EEG), a chin electromyogram (EMG), and an electrooculogram which help to score various sleep stages. Respiratory effort is detected using chest and abdominal belts. Oronasal flow is detected using nasal thermistors and nasal flow pressure transducers. Extremity movements are monitored by EMG leads placed on the legs and sometimes on the arms. Gas exchange is assessed by monitoring oxygen and CO_2 via pulse oximetry and end-tidal/transcutaneous CO_2. Simultaneously, video monitoring is performed.

Multiple Sleep Latency Test (MSLT)

The MSLT is a validated measure of the ability or tendency to fall asleep. The MSLT is performed to assess the degree of sleepiness and the timing of rapid eye movement (REM) sleep onset. The MSLT is performed by allowing five nap opportunities, lasting 20 minutes each, at 2-hour intervals. For each nap opportunity, sleep latency is defined as the time from lights out to N1. Sleep-onset REM periods (SOREMPs) are characterized by onset within 15 minutes of sleep onset. The mean sleep latency (MSL; arithmetical mean of sleep latency of all naps) is an index of the severity of sleepiness. The combination of MSL and the number of SOREMPs help to differentiate various central hypersomnias as seen in Figure 88-1 and discussed later in this chapter.

The Maintenance of Wakefulness Test (MWT)

The MWT is a validated objective measure of the ability to stay awake for a defined time. The MWT assesses the efficacy of treatment for safety issues regarding driving.

TABLE 88-1 Etiologies of Excessive Sleepiness in Children

Insufficient Sleep	Increased Sleep Drive	Fragmented Nocturnal Sleep
Paradoxical insomnia	Central hypersomnias	Primary sleep disorder
Behaviorally induced insufficient sleep syndrome	Traumatic brain injury	GERD
Behavioral insomnia of children—sleep onset association type	Medications	Allergy, eczema
Behavioral insomnia of children—limit setting type	Infections	Asthma
Circadian rhythm sleep disorders	Metabolic disorders	Other medical disorders
Psychophysiological insomnia		Medications
Idiopathic insomnia		Illicit drugs, alcohol

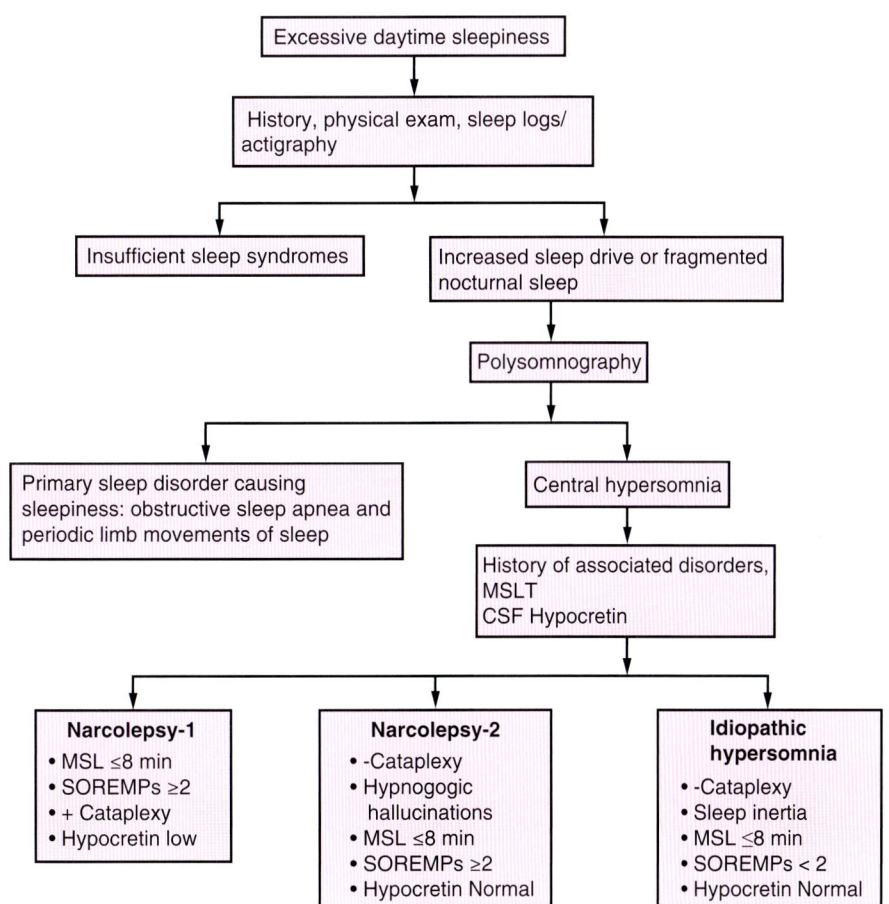

Figure 88-1. Algorithm showing the approach in evaluation of children with excessive daytime sleepiness.

Cerebrospinal Fluid Hypocretin-1 Levels

The levels of CSF hypocretin are diagnostic in narcolepsy type 1 and are a part of the new diagnostic criteria for this disorder. The CSF hypocretin level also help in the diagnosis of narcolepsy type 2. Hypocretin-1 is measured from CSF by radioimmunoassay (RIA), using a polyclonal antibody.

Histocompatibility Antigen (HLA) Subtypes

HLA subtypes are helpful in the differential diagnosis of hypersomnias. HLA DQ1*0602 is positive in 76% to 90% with narcolepsy type 1, 40% to 57% narcolepsy type 2, and 12% to 38% in the normal population.

NARCOLEPSY TYPE 1 (NARCOLEPSY WITH CATAPLEXY)

The ICSD-3 definition of narcolepsy type 1 is: a) daily periods of an irrepressible need to sleep or daytime lapses into sleep occurring over for at least 3 months; b) cataplexy and a MSL of 8 minutes or less and two or more SOREMPs on MSLT (SOREMP within 15 min of sleep onset in nocturnal polysomnography may replace one of the SOREMPs on MSLT); or c) CSF hypocretin level of 110pg/mL or less.

Chronic daytime sleepiness, hypnagogic hallucinations (vivid dreams at sleep onset), sleep-onset paralysis, cataplexy, and fragmented night sleep are the characteristic symptoms of narcolepsy. The incidence of narcolepsy in the United States is 1.37 per 100,000 persons per year (men: 1.72; women: 1.05), which is highest in the second decade, followed by a gradual decline. The prevalence is approximately 56 per 100,000 persons. Recently there was an increase in the incidence after H1N1 infection or after receiving a specific adjuvanted H1N1 vaccine, mostly affecting prepubertal children and adolescents. The onset of narcolepsy type 1 is commonly in childhood, and 34% of all narcolepsy subjects experienced symptoms before the age of 15 years, 16% before the age of 10 years, and 4.5% before age 5 years (Fig. 88-2). Rare cases with the onset during infancy also have been reported. The patients with H1N1 vaccine-related narcolepsy have the onset at a younger age than nonvaccinated cases.

EDS is the most common presenting symptom of narcolepsy type 1 and is seen in over 90% of patients. However, sleepiness may be unrecognized, leading to a delay in the diagnosis. The lack of recognition may be due to parents considering children as "lazy," or unaware that sleepiness in children presents as mood swings, inattentiveness, or hyperactive

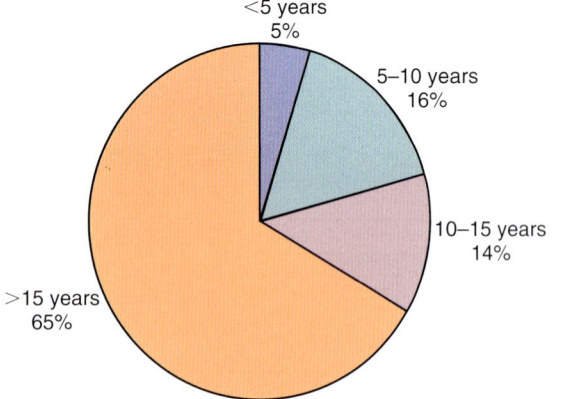

Figure 88-2. Graph depicting the age of onset of narcolepsy. (*Data derived from Challamel, M.J., et al., 1994. Narcolepsy in children. Sleep 17S:17.*)

behavior. Additionally, children may have a chronic waxing and waning of drowsiness with superimposed excessive sleep periods and long, unrefreshing naps (Nevsimalova, 2014). Over time, the sleepiness may improve to a limited degree.

Cataplexy consists of episodes of sudden muscle weakness in all skeletal muscles except the extraocular and respiratory muscles in response to an emotional stimulus—most commonly laughter. It is the most specific symptom of narcolepsy type 1. It may not be present at onset. In large case series, 83% to 100% of patients had cataplexy. Other triggers are emotions such as anger, surprise, or others. The resulting muscle weakness generally lasts for a few seconds to minutes and is associated with muscle atonia, the absence of muscle stretch reflexes, the absence of H- and F-waves on nerve conductions studies, and the full preservation of consciousness. Moreover, at the onset, one third of children may have "cataplectic facies": semipermanent facial weakness leading to droopy eyelids, open mouth, and/or tongue protrusion. Emotion-triggered cataplectic attacks may occur on top of this weakness. Cataplectic facies may later be replaced by typical cataplexy. Additionally, hypotonia and complex motor movements also occur closer to the onset of narcolepsy, more commonly in younger children. Complex motor movements also may resolve later in the disease. Moreover, the children with H1N1 vaccine-related narcolepsy more commonly have cataplexy, hypotonia, and tongue protrusion than the children with sporadically occurring cases.

Hypnogogic hallucinations also are present in children with narcolepsy representing REM dysfunction. In large case series, 32% to 57% of children had such hallucination (Wu, et al., 2014). Contrasting with cataplexy, hallucination is not very specific to narcolepsy. Unlike adults, hallucinations may be in the form of simple visual forms. These occur in relation to sleep and are multisensory as opposed to auditory hallucinations seen in schizophrenia. The hallucinations are frequently associated with sleep paralysis, which also is a phenomenon of REM dysfunction. Sleep paralysis occurs in 19% to 41% of children with narcolepsy, lasts seconds to minutes, and may end spontaneously or by verbal or tactile stimuli.

Fragmented nocturnal sleep also is common in narcolepsy. Fragmentation may be related to the lack of orexin, influencing the on-off sleep/wake switch. Patients with narcolepsy exhibit less circadian clock-dependent alertness during the daytime and sleepiness at night. Moreover, obesity and precocious puberty are seen in up to 74% and 17% respectively of such children, especially in the younger patients. Children with obesity and narcolepsy have an earlier onset of sleepiness and cataplexy and have poorer nocturnal sleep and higher sleep-disordered breathing. The suggested mechanisms for obesity are reduced hypocretin and leptin levels and decreased basal metabolic rate. In addition, obesity could be related to eating disorders. Moreover, weight gain is significantly more common in children with H1N1 vaccine-related narcolepsy than in sporadic cases.

Pathophysiology

The key pathophysiologic event in human narcolepsy-cataplexy is hypocretin ligand deficiency caused by targeted loss of hypocretin-secreting neurons in the hypothalamus. The most likely mechanism of loss is autoimmune (Partinen, et al., 2014), which is discussed in detail in the online version.

Diagnosis

The diagnosis of narcolepsy in children remains challenging with the delay in diagnosis ranging 8 to 22 years. The presence of cataplexy and younger age at onset were associated with earlier diagnosis. With better technologies and improved health professional awareness, the gap between the onset and diagnosis is closing. A careful history examination, relevant questionnaires, and sleep logs/actigraphy are important in excluding other disorders. On actigraphy, increased sleep fragmentation and daytime naps are seen. Nocturnal polysomnography is performed to evaluate for other sleep disorders that fragment sleep and cause daytime sleepiness. Nocturnal polysomnography followed by MSLT remains the gold standard in the diagnosis. The MSLT and nocturnal polysomnography diagnostic criteria are discussed earlier in this chapter. A recent study identified that the specificity of SOREMP in nocturnal polysomnography for detection of narcolepsy with cataplexy was 97%, whereas the sensitivity was 88.5%.

HLA testing also is useful. There is a strong association between narcolepsy and HLA DQ antigens, specifically DQB1*0602, which are present in up to 95% of patients with narcolepsy type 1. HLA DQB1*0602 positive subjects are at a 251-fold increase risk of narcolepsy. Additionally, all subjects with H1N1 vaccine-related narcolepsy have a positive HLA DQB1*0602.

Low CSF hypocretin levels can confirm the diagnosis of narcolepsy type 1. CSF hypocretin levels of less than 110 pg/mL have a greater than 95% specificity in diagnosing narcolepsy type 1. Positive DQB1*0602 and low CSF hypocretin-1 are found in 87.4% of cases of narcolepsy type 1. The hypocretin assay may be most useful when an HLA DQB1*0602-positive patient with suspected narcolepsy-cataplexy is already receiving psychostimulants and in whom discontinuation of these medications is inconvenient or impractical. Additionally, CSF hypocretin levels also may help in the differential diagnosis of hypersomnia as narcolepsy type 1 have low levels, whereas subjects with narcolepsy type 2 and idiopathic hypersomnia patients exhibit normal levels (Fig. 88-3). Furthermore, ASO and anti-DNAse B titers also may assist in establishing the diagnosis.

Treatment

Currently, narcolepsy is an incurable, lifelong disease. Available treatments focus on improving symptoms, which include reducing daytime sleepiness, controlling cataplexy, and correcting nocturnal sleep fragmentation. The management of narcolepsy is difficult in the pediatric population due to lack of data from randomized studies and no FDA-approved

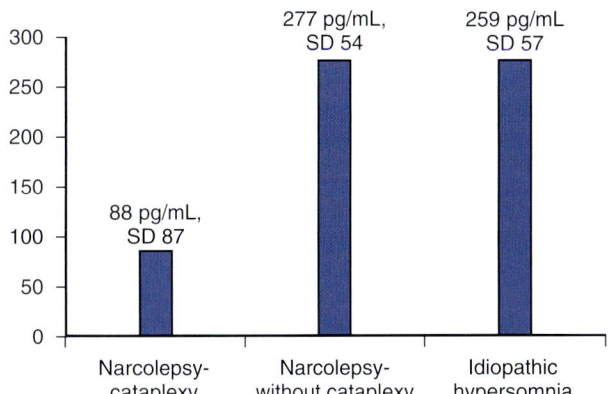

Figure 88-3. Cerebrospinal fluid levels of hypocretin-1 in patients with narcolepsy-cataplexy, narcolepsy without cataplexy, and idiopathic hypersomnia. *(Data derived from Kanbayashi, T., et al., 2002. CSF hypocretin-1 [orexin-A] concentrations in narcolepsy with and without cataplexy and idiopathic hypersomnia. J Sleep Res 11, 91.)*

medical treatments. Lifestyle changes also are a mainstay of management, especially in children. These include increasing nighttime sleep, having a scheduled 20- to 30-minutes nap, and a daily exercise regimen. Teenagers should be counseled against driving and avoiding endangering work and social situations if daytime sleepiness is uncontrolled.

TREATMENT OF DAYTIME SLEEPINESS
Wake-Promoting Agents

Modafinil and its biologically active r-isomer, armodafinil, are approved for treatment of excessive sleepiness in narcolepsy in adults. These agents are believed to be dopamine reuptake inhibitors and affect alpha-adrenergic, serotonergic, and GABA pathways (Dauvilliers, et al., 2007; Mignot, 2012; Lecendreux, 2014). Modafinil is metabolized through cytochrome P450 with a half-life of 13 hours. Armodafinil has a longer half-life than modafinil. In various case series in children and adolescents, modafinil has been efficacious in up to 85% of subjects. Daily doses ranging from 50 to 600 mg have been reported. However, additional benefit is not seen beyond 400 mg daily dosing. The typical starting dose in children is 50 to 100 mg, which should be titrated to achieve the desired control of sleepiness. Common side effects are headache, irritability, and a loss of appetite. It also may cause hepatic dysfunction and severe skin reactions such as Stevens-Johnson syndrome.

Stimulants

Amphetamines and related compounds are simple derivatives of catecholamine and affect the dopaminergic and noradrenergic pathways and possibly the serotonergic systems. Dextroamphetamine and the newer lisdexamfetamine dimesylate, which is a prodrug with a long half-life, may be useful in pediatric narcolepsy. The side effects are tachycardia, hypertension, palpitations, anxiety, irritability, and psychotic reactions. Development of tolerance and dependence also are possible. Due to the effects on the metabolism and endocrine and cardiac function, close monitoring is recommended. Typical starting doses are 2.5 to 5 mg and 20 mg daily for dextroamphetamine and lisdexamfetamine, respectively, with gradual increases based on the patient's response.

Methylphenidate and related compounds are similar to amphetamines but do not completely substitute the catecholamine mechanism of action which is through dopamine reuptake inhibition and dopamine release. Methylphenidate is short acting and hence has a high potential for dependence and tolerance. Various longer acting formulations are available with varying half-life, onset of action, and reduced addiction potential. The side effects are similar to amphetamines, and similar precautions and monitoring are recommended. Methylphenidate preparations also have been used to treat sleepiness in narcolepsy.

Treatment of Cataplexy

Antidepressants have been used in the treatment of cataplexy. The use is off label even in adults. Selective serotonergic reuptake inhibitors (SSRI) such as fluoxetine and dual serotonergic and noradrenergic reuptake inhibitors (SNRI) such as venlafaxine are the most commonly used agents with venlafaxine apparently being the most efficacious. Tricyclic antidepressants such as clomipramine and protriptiline also have been used but are less effective. Common side effects are headache, nausea, agitation, abdominal pain, and diarrhea. A few series describe successful treatment with SSRI/SNRIs for pediatric cataplexy. In one study, venlafaxine was the third most commonly used medication in pediatric narcolepsy. The maximum daily doses ranged from 63 to 95 mg with high continuation rates. The most common side effect was irritability. It did not improve sleepiness, sleep paralysis, and hypnagogic hallucinations significantly.

TREATMENT OF NOCTURNAL SLEEP FRAGMENTATION

The successful treatment of nocturnal sleep fragmentation can improve the daytime sleepiness. Although not specifically studied, longer acting melatonin and other hypnotics may be used to improve fragmentation.

Sodium Oxybate

Sodium oxybate was initially developed as an anesthetic agent but was found to increase N3 and REM and thus was studied in detail in adults with narcolepsy and cataplexy. It is now approved for the treatment of cataplexy and excessive sleepiness in adults with narcolepsy. It was also found to improve nocturnal sleep fragmentation, thus becoming the only drug that treats all symptoms of narcolepsy. The mechanism of action is unclear, but it is believed to activate the GABA-B receptor. The half-life is 30 minutes and the total duration of effect is only 2 to 4 hours. Therefore two doses given 4 hours apart in older children and three divided doses for very young children are required. However, it may take weeks or months to see a clinically meaningful effect on sleepiness and cataplexy. Several case series have reported the use of sodium oxybate in children. Murali and Kotagal reported that 88% showed symptom improvement, including the reduced frequency and severity of cataplexy in a small study in pediatric narcolepsy. Aran and associates reported using doses of 6800 to 7600 mg with side effects of irritability, weight loss, and nausea. These side effects were more common in prepubertal than postpubertal children. Mansukhani and Kotagal reported improved symptoms in 86% of the children in combination with other medications. Increased nightmares, nocturnal awakenings, tremors, and blurred vision were reported as side effects. The doses used ranged from 3 to 7 grams. In another study, efficacy of 85% for daytime sleepiness, 82% for cataplexy, and 95% for nocturnal fragmentation symptom relief have been reported. Headache, nausea, weight loss, irritability, and parasomnias were reported side effects.

Apart from the limited data in children, one of the biggest limiting factors is the safety concern. The street form of sodium oxybate has been used recreationally and as a "date rape" drug. It also can cause respiratory depression at high doses, especially with concomitant use of alcohol, and can precipitate withdrawal symptoms in certain situations. Due to this concern, the availability of the prescription drug is limited through a central pharmacy and training is required. Nevertheless, most studies suggest that it is safe when used at nighttime in patients with narcolepsy. However, psychiatric comorbidity and the need for extensive parental involvement also may be limiting factors for its increased use in children.

Future Treatments

Immunosuppressive agents such as immunoglobulin and natalizumab have been used for the treatment of narcolepsy. Additionally, mazindol, pitolisant (an H3 receptor inverse agonist), and hypocretin replacement therapies also have been used. However, currently there are limited data to recommend their use in children.

NARCOLEPSY TYPE 2

The ICSD-3 definition of narcolepsy type 2 differs from narcolepsy type 1 in that it is not associated with cataplexy and if the CSF hypocretin test is performed, levels greater than 110pg/mL are seen. The definition also requires ruling out other disorders that present with daytime sleepiness. The diagnosis of narcolepsy type 2 is more challenging as cataplexy is absent. The main presenting feature of narcolepsy type 2 is sleepiness, which may be similar to that seen in narcolepsy type 1. Hypnogogic hallucinations, with or without sleep paralysis, can occur in up to 28% of patients. On average, the frequency of hallucination is three episodes per month. These occur with less frequency in the general population, but hallucinations commonly occur in various psychiatric disorders. Hence, frequent sleep paralysis and hallucinations in the absence of psychiatric symptoms may help to diagnose narcolepsy type 2. There is a poorer association with HLA DQB1*0602, which is positive in 40% of subjects. CSF hypocretin levels are low in 24%, borderline in 8%, and normal in 68% of patients. Low CSF hypocretin levels in a narcoleptic child may be predictive of the future development of cataplexy. Additionally, the first SOREMPs in nocturnal polysomnography in narcolepsy type 2 may arise out of N1 or wakefulness and from N1 on MSLT in many subjects, which may help to differentiate this entity from nonnarcoleptic disorders. However, MSLT may be falsely negative. In a study, after the second MSLT, the diagnosis changed in 53% of the subjects with sleepiness. Hence, a second MSLT is often recommended (Baumann, et al., 2014).

KLEINE-LEVIN SYNDROME (KLS)

Kleine-Levin syndrome (KLS) is a rare neuropsychiatric disorder of relapsing-remitting episodes of hypersomnia and behavioral, psychiatric, and cognitive disturbances. The ICSD defines it as at least two recurrent episodes of excessive sleepiness and sleep duration, lasting 2 days to 5 weeks, recurring at least once every 18 months with normal alertness, cognitive function, behavior, and mood between the observed episodes and cognitive dysfunction, altered perception eating disorder, or disinhibited behavior during the episodes that is not better explained by another disorder(s). The onset is in adolescence, with a male predominance. Hypersomnolence is characterized by sleeping 18 to 20 hours per day. Incomplete forms of the syndrome also have been recognized. Hyperphagia may be in the form of binge eating, leading to a 2 to 5 kg increase in body weight. In a recent large study, 45% had birth and developmental abnormalities. In patients with prolonged episodes, the durations of the first episode was on an average of 32 days with longer subsequent episodes and an average 9 years for the disease-course. During the episodes, affected individuals had shorter sleep time, higher levels of anxiety, increased agitation, and more feelings of disembodiment and amnesia than subjects with shorter episodes. Between episodes, individuals with KLS were more tired, needed more naps, fell asleep more rapidly, and had higher anxiety/depression scores. Nocturnal polysomnography during the sleepy period exhibits decreased sleep efficiency (SE), latency to REM, and N3. The MSLT reveals moderately shortened mean sleep latency in the 5- to 10-minute range but lacks the two or more SOREMPs that are typically seen in narcolepsy. The episodic hypersomnia gradually diminishes or evolves into classic depression. A disturbance of hypothalamic function has been hypothesized but not yet definitively established. The association of Kleine-Levin syndrome with HLA DQB1*0201 and the occasional precipitation after systemic infections, as well as the relapsing and remitting nature, are suspicious for an autoimmune etiology. There is no satisfactory treatment, although lithium is somewhat effective. Modafinil may reduce the duration of the symptomatic episodes.

Menstrual-related Kleine-Levin Syndrome (previously menstrual-related hypersomnia), idiopathic hypersomnia (IH) and hypersomnia due to medical disorders, medications, or substance abuse are discussed in detail in the online chapter.

INSUFFICIENT SLEEP SYNDROME (ISS)

The ICSD-3 defines insufficient sleep syndrome as: a) daily periods of irrepressible need to sleep or daytime lapses into sleep or behavioral disturbances in prepubertal children for most days for at least 3 months; b) shorter sleep times on history, sleep logs, or actigraphy; c) longer sleep duration on weekends or vacations; and d) sleepiness not better explained by other disorders. These individuals may have short MSL on MSLT and one in six subjects has multiple SOREMPs. However, most of the SOREMPs in ISS occur after N2 as opposed to N1 in narcolepsy. The additional differentiation from narcolepsy is that longer sleep duration is noted on weekends or holidays compared with weekdays.

In conclusion, EDS in children may be caused by a variety of disorders, which may be difficult to accurately diagnose. As EDS significantly affects overall functioning, these disorders should be assessed and managed appropriately so as to improve overall quality of life.

REFERENCES

The complete list of references for this chapter is available in the e-book at www.expertconsult.com.

See inside cover for registration details.

SELECTED REFERENCES

American Academy of Sleep Medicine, 2014. International Classification of Sleep Disorders. American Academy of Sleep Medicine, Darien, IL.

Baumann, C.R., Mignot, E., et al., 2014. Challenges in diagnosing narcolepsy without cataplexy: a consensus statement. Sleep 37 (6), 1035–1042.

Dauvilliers, Y., Arnulf, I., et al., 2007. Narcolepsy with cataplexy. Lancet 369 (9560), 499–511.

Kotagal, S., 2012. Hypersomnia in children. Sleep Med. Clin. 7 (2), 379–389.

Kothare, S.V., Kaleyias, J., 2008. The clinical and laboratory assessment of the sleepy child. Semin. Pediatr. Neurol. 15 (2), 61–69.

Lecendreux, M., 2014. Pharmacological management of narcolepsy and cataplexy in pediatric patients. Pediatr. Drugs 16 (5), 363–372.

Mignot, E.J.M., 2012. A practical guide to the therapy of narcolepsy and hypersomnia syndromes. Neurother. 9 (4), 739–752.

Nevsimalova, S., 2014. The diagnosis and treatment of pediatric narcolepsy. Curr. Neurol. Neurosci. Rep. 14 (8), 469.

Partinen, M., Kornum, B.R., et al., 2014. Narcolepsy as an autoimmune disease: the role of H1N1 infection and vaccination. Lancet Neurol. 13 (6), 600–613.

Wu, H., Zhuang, J., et al., 2014. Symptoms and occurrences of narcolepsy: a retrospective study of 162 patients during a 10-year period in eastern China. Sleep Med. 15 (6), 607–613.

89 Restless Legs Syndrome and Periodic Limb Movement Disorder in Children and Adolescents

Allison Przekop

An expanded version of this chapter is available on www.expertconsult.com. See inside cover for registration details.

INTRODUCTION

Restless legs syndrome (RLS) is a common neurologic sensorimotor disorder characterized by the complaint of a strong or irresistible urge to move the legs (Simakajornboon et al., 2009). Also known as Willis–Ekbom disease (WED), RLS was first described by Thomas Willis in 1685. However, Swedish neurologist Karl-Axel Ekbom formally described the traits of this disorder in a monograph titled *Restless Legs* written in 1945 (Allen et al., 2014). Later, in his 1960 publication in *Neurology*, Ekbom defined all clinical features, provided diagnostic criteria, and coined the term "restless legs syndrome" (Mitchell, 2011).

Much of the medical literature since the initial descriptions of RLS has focused on adult populations, and it was not until the mid-1990s that detailed reports of RLS affecting children started to appear (Picchietti and Stevens, 2008). Then, in 2003, consensus criteria for the diagnosis of RLS in children and adolescents were published after a workshop meeting by the International Restless Legs Syndrome Study Group (IRLSSG) at the National Institutes of Health (Picchietti and Stevens, 2008). Because of updates being made to the adult RLS diagnostic criteria and the numerous publications regarding pediatric RLS since 2003, the pediatric RLS diagnostic criteria were revised and updated in 2013 (Picchietti et al., 2013).

PREVALENCE

In the United States and Western Europe, RLS is found to occur in 5% to 10% of adults (Picchietti et al., 2007) with about one third affected to a moderate or severe degree (Picchietti and Picchietti, 2008). However, histories obtained from adults who meet criteria for RLS reveal that 40% had initial onset of symptoms before the age of 20 years (Simakajornboon et al., 2009). In 2007 the Peds RLS Epidemiology, Symptoms and Treatment (REST) Study found that criteria for definite RLS were met by 1.9% of 8- to 11-year-olds and 2.0% of 12- to 17-year-olds (Picchietti et al., 2007). These findings suggest that approximately 984,000 school-aged children in the United States are affected by RLS (Picchietti and Picchietti, 2008). One quarter to one half of the affected 8- to 17-year-olds in this population were reported to have moderate to severe symptoms (Picchietti et al., 2009). Unlike adult RLS, in which there is a 2:1 female-to-male ratio, there is no gender bias in pediatric RLS (Picchietti and Picchietti, 2008).

SYMPTOMS

In his 1960 publication providing diagnostic guidelines, Ekbom wrote that "the sensations appear only when the patient is at rest, most often in the evening and early part of the night, and produce an irresistible need to keep the legs moving. Furthermore, the sensations are not felt in the skin but deep down inside the legs" (Ekbom, 1960). Over the years, the diagnostic criteria that evolved placed more emphasis on the urge to move, or akathisia, and less on the uncomfortable sensations, or dysesthesias (Allen et al., 2014). The 2003 consensus statement published by the IRLSSG again included "unpleasant sensations" as part of the diagnostic criteria for RLS (Allen et al., 2014). This allowed the use of leg discomfort as one of the criteria for making the diagnosis of definite RLS in children. Children undergoing evaluation for RLS are encouraged to use terms in their own words, when able, to describe the unpleasant sensations. Terms and phrases such as "oowies," "boo-boo," "tickle," "bugs," "spiders," "ants," "want to run," and "a lot of energy in my legs" have been used by children (Picchietti et al., 2007; Simakajornboon et al., 2009). These symptoms or unpleasant sensations are worse at rest, relieved by movement, and most severe at night (Picchietti and Stevens, 2008). Because of difficulties that children may have in describing their symptoms, the time that elapses between initial sleep consultation and diagnosis of definite RLS is 4.4 years (Simakajornboon et al., 2009). The time between onset of clinical sleep disturbance and diagnosis is even longer at 11.6 years (Simakajornboon et al., 2009).

PRESENTATION

RLS is an underrecognized disorder among children and adolescents. The fact that it is underrecognized, combined with the difficulties young children have in providing a description of their symptoms, makes RLS an underdiagnosed disorder in children (Simakajornboon et al., 2009). Children often present to specialty clinics when family members seek medical advice for moderate to severe symptoms that often result in sleep disturbances (Picchietti et al., 2007). Children and adolescents in the Peds REST Study who met criteria for the diagnosis of definite RLS were more likely to have a history of difficulty falling asleep or staying asleep at night compared with those who did not meet criteria for definite or probable RLS (69.4% vs. 39.6%) (Picchietti et al., 2007). As a consequence, many of these children also present with a history of daytime sleepiness. Other complaints and problems at the time of initial presentation include "growing pains," "school problems," "short attention," and hyperactivity (Picchietti and Stevens, 2008).

DIAGNOSIS

In 2003, the NIH/IRLSSG published diagnostic criteria for RLS that included separate criteria for children and defined definite, probable, and possible pediatric RLS (Allen et al., 2014). Information from new research led to the simplification of the pediatric diagnostic criteria and integration with the newly revised adult RLS criteria in 2013 (Box 89-1) (Allen et al., 2014). Special considerations for the diagnosis of RLS in children were also outlined (Box 89-2), and research criteria for

---

BOX 89-1 International Restless Legs Syndrome Study Group (IRLSSG) Consensus Diagnostic Criteria for Restless Legs Syndrome/Willis–Ekbom Disease (RLS/WED)

RLS/WED, a neurologic sensorimotor disease often profoundly disturbing sleep and quality of life, has variable expression influenced by genetic, environmental, and medical factors. The symptoms vary considerably in frequency from less than once a month or year to daily, and severity from mildly annoying to disabling. Symptoms may also remit for various periods of time. RLS/WED is diagnosed by ascertaining symptom patterns that meet the following five essential criteria, adding clinical specifiers where appropriate.

Essential diagnostic criteria (all must be met):

1. An urge to move the legs usually but not always accompanied by, or felt to be caused by, uncomfortable and unpleasant sensations in the legs.[a,b]
2. The urge to move the legs and any accompanying unpleasant sensations begin or worsen during periods of rest or inactivity such as lying down or sitting.
3. The urge to move the legs and any accompanying unpleasant sensations are partially or totally relieved by movement, such as walking or stretching, at least as long as the activity continues.[c]

4. The urge to move the legs and any accompanying unpleasant sensations during rest or inactivity only occur or are worse in the evening or night than during the day.[d]
5. The occurrence of the above features is not solely accounted for as symptoms primary to another medical or a behavioral condition (e.g., myalgia, venous stasis, leg edema, arthritis, leg cramps, positional discomfort, habitual foot tapping).[e]

Specifiers for clinical course of RLS/WED[f]:

1. Chronic-persistent RLS/WED: symptoms when not treated would occur on average at least twice weekly for the past year.
2. Intermittent RLS/WED: symptoms when not treated would occur on average <2/week for the past year, with at least 5 lifetime events.

Specifier for clinical significance of RLS/WED:
The symptoms of RLS/WED cause significant distress or impairment in social, occupational, educational, or other important areas of functioning by their impact on sleep, energy/vitality, daily activities, behavior, cognition, or mood.

[a]Sometimes the urge to move the legs is present without the uncomfortable sensations, and sometimes the arms or other parts of the body are involved in addition to the legs.
[b]For children, the description of these symptoms should be in the child's own words.
[c]When symptoms are very severe, relief by activity may not be noticeable but must have been previously present.
[d]When symptoms are very severe, the worsening in the evening or night may not be noticeable but must have been previously present.
[e]These conditions, often referred to as "RLS/WED mimics," have been commonly confused with RLS/WED particularly in surveys because they produce symptoms that meet or at least come very close to meeting criteria 1–4. The list here gives some examples that have been noted as particularly significant in epidemiologic studies and clinical practice. RLS/WED may also occur with any of these conditions, but the RLS/WED symptoms will then be more in degree, conditions of expression, or character than those usually occurring as part of the other condition.
[f]The clinical course criteria do not apply for pediatric cases or for some special cases of provoked RLS/WED such as pregnancy or drug-induced RLS/WED, where the frequency may be high but limited to duration of the provocative condition.
(Allen RP, Picchietti DL, Garcia-Borreguero D, et al. Restless legs syndrome/Willis-Ekbom disease diagnostic criteria: updated International Restless Legs Syndrome Study Group (IRLSSG) consensus criteria-history, rationale, description, and significance. Sleep Med 2014;15:860–73.)

BOX 89-2 Special Considerations for the Diagnosis of Pediatric Restless Legs Syndrome

- The child must describe the RLS symptoms in his or her own words.
- The diagnostician should be aware of the typical words children and adolescents use to describe RLS.
- Language and cognitive development determine the applicability of the RLS diagnostic criteria, rather than age.
- It is not known if the adult specifiers for clinical course apply to pediatric RLS.
- As in adults, a significant impact on sleep, mood, cognition, and function is found. However, impairment is manifest more often in behavioral and educational domains.
- Simplified and updated research criteria for probable and possible pediatric RLS are available (Box 89-3).
- Periodic limb movement disorder may precede the diagnosis of RLS in some cases.

(Picchietti DL, Bruni O, de Weerd A, et al. Pediatric restless legs syndrome diagnostic criteria: an update by the International Restless Legs Syndrome Study Group. Sleep Med. 2013;14:1253–9.)

BOX 89-3 Research Diagnostic Criteria for Probable and Possible Pediatric Restless Legs Syndrome

PROBABLE RLS

The child meets all five essential criteria for RLS, except criterion 4 (occurrence only or worsening in the evening or night).

POSSIBLE RLS

The child is observed to have behavior manifestations of lower extremity discomfort when sitting or lying, accompanied by motor movement of the affected limbs. The discomfort is characterized by RLS criteria 2–5 (is worse during rest and inactivity, relieved by movement, worse in the evening or night, and is not solely accounted for as primary to another medical or a behavioral condition).

(Picchietti DL, Bruni O, de Weerd A, et al. Pediatric restless legs syndrome diagnostic criteria: an update by the International Restless Legs Syndrome Study Group. Sleep Med 2013;14:1253–9.)

---

probable and possible pediatric RLS were updated (Box 89-3) (Picchietti et al., 2013). Other conditions that may mimic RLS (Box 89-4) should be ruled out (Picchietti et al., 2013). The common mimics of RLS are often described as pain without the need to move (Picchietti and Picchietti, 2010).

In order to diagnose RLS in children and adolescents, a description of the RLS sensations should be obtained from the patients in their own words. In addition, the presence and nature of any sleep disturbances and a detailed family history should be obtained from the parents, and an investigation of any suspected contributing factors or differential diagnoses should be completed. A physical and neurologic examination

BOX 89-4 Differential Diagnosis of Pediatric Restless Legs Syndrome

COMMON MIMICS

- Positional discomfort
- Sore leg muscles
- Ligament sprain/tendon strain
- Positional ischemia (numbness)
- Dermatitis
- Bruises
- Growing pains

LESS COMMON MIMICS

- Leg cramps
- Arthritis
- Other orthopedic disorders
- Peripheral neuropathy
- Radiculopathy
- Myelopathy
- Myopathy
- Fibromyalgia
- Complex regional pain syndrome
- Drug-induced akathisia
- Sickle cell disease

(Picchietti DL, Bruni O, de Weerd A, et al. Pediatric restless legs syndrome diagnostic criteria: an update by the International Restless Legs Syndrome Study Group. Sleep Med 2013;14:1253–9.)

should be performed, and in some cases, polysomnography may be needed for those children who are unable to provide a description of the unpleasant sensations they may be experiencing because of RLS and in whom periodic limb movement disorder (PLMD) is suspected (Picchietti and Picchietti, 2008; Picchietti and Picchietti, 2010).

One diagnosis that many children and adolescents are given before being diagnosed with RLS is growing pains. In the Peds REST Study, 29.6% of children and 36.8% of adolescents in the study were previously diagnosed with this condition (Picchietti et al., 2007). Growing pains is a common pediatric diagnosis with a conservative estimated prevalence of 4.7%, but unlike RLS, there is no unified definition or diagnostic criteria. There is overlap between the diagnostic criteria for RLS and the accepted or adopted diagnostic criteria for growing pains, but two features or criteria do distinguish the two disorders. The first is that growing pains are thought to be strictly bilateral, whereas RLS can be unilateral or bilateral; the second is that growing pains are strictly painful, whereas RLS can be associated with a variety of discomforts or unpleasant sensations.

Iron Deficiency

Iron plays a role in brain dopamine production and synaptic density, myelin synthesis, energy production, and probably in norepinephrine and serotonin neurotransmitter systems (Picchietti and Picchietti, 2010). Serum ferritin, a measure of body iron stores, has been found to be low in adults and children with RLS, and adult studies have shown that a serum ferritin level below 50 mcg/L is associated with increased severity of RLS (Picchietti and Picchietti, 2008). Low ferritin has been shown to correlate with the occurrence of RLS augmentation. Studies also have shown an increased prevalence of RLS in individuals with iron-deficiency anemia and in blood donors (Picchietti and Picchietti, 2008). Serum ferritin levels have been found to be below 50 mcg/L in 83% to 89% of pediatric cases of RLS and less than median normative

values for age and sex in up to 75% of cases (Picchietti and Picchietti, 2008; Picchietti and Picchietti, 2010). In addition, serum ferritin levels of <12 mcg/L were found in children with RLS and attention deficit hyperactivity disorder (ADHD) compared with children with ADHD alone. Caution should be used when interpreting the results of serum ferritin levels as ferritin is an acute-phase reactant and can be elevated for up to 4 weeks after a febrile illness.

Iron and Neuroimaging

Studies revealing decreased concentrations of iron and ferritin in cerebrospinal fluid (CSF) suggest that RLS is also associated with a low brain iron content. These findings have prompted investigations of iron concentrations in the brain using other diagnostic modalities, including magnetic resonance imaging (MRI). One of the first studies using a 1.5T MRI found decreased iron concentration in the substantia nigra (SN). A subsequent study using a 3T MRI found decreased iron concentration in the SN of RLS patients who had symptom onset before age 45 years. Non-MRI assessments of brain iron concentrations have supported these findings. Postmortem analyses of the brains of RLS patients have shown lower concentrations of iron in the dopaminergic neurons of the SN. B-mode ultrasound imaging of the midbrain also has shown decreased iron in the SN of RLS patients.

Family History and Genetics

In the Peds REST Study, 71.4% of children with definite RLS and 80% of adolescents with definite RLS had at least 1 parent respond who had symptoms suggestive of RLS (Picchietti et al., 2007). A positive history in both parents was found in 17.1% of children and in 16% of adolescents with definite RLS (Picchietti et al., 2007). In both groups, mothers were more likely to have symptoms with a parental female-to-male ratio of 2.4 : 1 in children and 2.2 : 1 in adolescents (Picchietti et al., 2007). In a later study, one or both biological parents had a positive family history of RLS in 77% of individuals, and when both parents were available for interview, 85% of cases had a parent with RLS (Picchietti and Stevens, 2008). Early onset of RLS with symptoms occurring before the age of 35 to 40 years is now recognized as highly familial (Picchietti and Picchietti, 2008), and adult studies of early-onset RLS have shown a 40% to 92% family prevalence (Picchietti and Picchietti, 2010).

In adults, genome-wide studies reported that RLS is associated with gene variants of BTBD9 (on chromosome 6p21.1), MEIS1, and MAP2K5/LBXCOR and possibly associated with PTPRD and A2BP1 (Simakajornboon et al., 2009; Picchietti and Picchietti, 2010). BTBD9 also is associated with periodic limb movements in sleep (PLMS) (Picchietti and Picchietti, 2010). One study of gene variants in pediatric RLS showed that 87% of children in the study had a positive family history of RLS and association with MEIS1 and MAP2K/LBXCOR variants but not BTBD9.

Coexistent Conditions

In addition to sleep disturbances and daytime sleepiness, children with RLS may also experience other problems that are often recognized and diagnosed before the diagnosis of definite RLS is made. These include ADHD, depression, and anxiety (Picchietti et al., 2013). Two earlier studies found a high incidence of PLMS in children diagnosed with ADHD (26% of 69 children in the first study and 64% of 14 children in the second study). More recent findings suggest that approximately 25% of those with RLS have problems with attention, and 13% to 35% of those with the diagnosis of ADHD meet criteria for RLS (Picchietti et al., 2013). In addition to causing difficulties with attention, poor sleep can also affect memory and emotional regulation in childhood and adolescence (Picchietti and Picchietti, 2008). Poor sleep can lead to negative effect and emotional lability, easy frustration, and difficulty controlling impulses (Picchietti and Picchietti, 2008). In adolescents with sleep disturbance, those with RLS symptoms were found to have a lower grade point average. In a recent study, adolescents and young adults between age 12 to 20 years with the diagnosis of RLS and associated difficulty falling asleep were also found to have worse psychosocial health scores and lower health-related quality of life.

Children may also present with a history of frequent parasomnias such as sleepwalking, sleep terrors, and nightmares (Picchietti and Stevens, 2008). In one study, some children were reported to have sleep-related rhythmic movement disorder such as head rolling and body rocking in addition to the parasomnias (Picchietti and Stevens, 2008). The parasomnias resolve after treatment of RLS and PLMD, suggesting that sleep disruption associated with RLS and PLMD may trigger the occurrence of parasomnias.

Sleep-related rhythmic movement disorder should not be confused with PLMS, a common feature in those with RLS. PLMS are brief extremity jerks during sleep lasting 0.5 to 5.0 seconds, occur at 20- to 40-second intervals, are more common in the lower extremities (legs, feet, and toes) than in the upper extremities, and may be accompanied by transient arousals from sleep, cardiac accelerations, spikes in blood pressure, and sleep disruption (Picchietti and Picchietti, 2008; Picchietti and Stevens, 2008). Often, patients with PLMS are unaware of the movements and the associated arousals from sleep (Picchietti and Picchietti, 2008). Up to 26% of children referred for sleep studies were found to have >5/hour PLMS, and in some children and adolescents, sleep disturbance and PLMS may predominate over complaints of leg discomfort leading to a delay in the diagnosis of RLS for up to 11 years after the onset of clinical sleep disturbance (Picchietti and Picchietti, 2008). One study found that PLMS occur more commonly in Caucasian children than in African American children. Approximately 80% to 90% of adults with RLS also have PLMS, which should not be confused with PLMD (Picchietti and Stevens, 2008). The diagnosis of PLMD is made in the absence of other primary sleep disorders, including RLS (Box 89-5) (Picchietti and Picchietti, 2008). In other words, an individual can have RLS with PLMS but not RLS and PLMD (Picchietti and Picchietti, 2010). In young children, a diagnosis of PLMD can precede a diagnosis of RLS because these children are unable to provide a description of the sensory symptoms associated with RLS (Picchietti and Picchietti, 2010).

With an estimated prevalence of 3% to 15%, enuresis is another common pediatric problem that can occur with PLMS and fragmented sleep. One study found that children with nocturnal enuresis (NE) had a significantly higher periodic limb movement index, a higher arousal index, and a higher awakening index on polysomnography compared with controls.

TREATMENT

RLS can be managed with pharmacologic and nonpharmacologic treatments. First, it is important to identify and avoid any exacerbating factors (Box 89-6) (Picchietti and Picchietti, 2010). Two exacerbating factors are related to sleep habits, and establishment of healthy and consistent sleep habits is important in children as these changes alone can eliminate symptoms of RLS in mild cases (Picchietti and Picchietti, 2010). The number of hours of sleep recommended for children between

---

BOX 89-5 Diagnostic Criteria for PLMD

A. Polysomnography shows repetitive, highly stereotyped limb movements that are
- 0.5 to 10 seconds in duration
- minimum amplitude of 8 µV above resting EMG
- in a sequence of 4 or more movements
- separated by an interval of more than 5 seconds (from limb-movement onset to limb-movement onset) and less than 90 seconds (typically there is an interval of 20 to 40 seconds)

B. The PLMS index exceeds 5/hour in pediatric cases and 15/hour in most adult cases.

C. There is clinical sleep disturbance or a complaint of daytime fatigue.

D. The PLMS are not better explained by another current sleep disorder, medical or neurologic disorder, mental disorder, medication use, or substance use disorder (e.g., PLMS at the termination of cyclically occurring apneas should not be counted as true PLMS or PLMD).

(Picchietti MA, Picchietti DL. Restless legs syndrome and periodic limb movement disorder in children and adolescents. Semin Pediatr Neurol 2008;15:91–9.)

BOX 89-6 RLS Exacerbating Factors

- Insufficient sleep for age
- Irregular sleep schedule
- Low body iron stores
- Pain
- Caffeine
- Nicotine
- Alcohol
- Medications

(Picchietti MA, Picchietti DL. Advances in pediatric restless legs syndrome: iron, genetics, diagnosis and treatment. Sleep Med 2010;11:643–51.)

---

age 2 and 10 years is 12 to 10 hours, respectively, and adolescents should get 9 hours of sleep (Picchietti and Picchietti, 2010). Additional nonpharmacologic remedies that have been suggested include mental activity, such as reading, card games or computer work, and physical activity, such as aerobic and lower-body resistance training for 3 days per week (Mitchell, 2011).

Because low serum ferritin levels have been found in a higher percentage of children with RLS and is associated with increased severity of symptoms, iron replacement is recommended when the serum ferritin level is 50 mcg/L or less. Two pediatric trials with oral iron supplementation found improvement with a rise in mean serum ferritin levels from 40.8 to 74.1 mcg/L and from 29.1 to 55.7 mcg/L (Picchietti and Picchietti, 2010). The typical dose of iron recommended for children 6 years of age and older is 50 to 65 mg of elemental iron once or twice daily (Picchietti and Picchietti, 2010). Vitamin C can enhance iron absorption and can be given with the oral iron supplement in the form of fruit juice. However, iron absorption can be reduced when taken with calcium, and so the iron supplement should be given 1 to 2 hours before or after the consumption of dairy products (Picchietti and Picchietti, 2008). Iron studies, including serum ferritin level, should be rechecked 2 to 4 months after initiation of iron supplementation.

For those children who are unable to tolerate oral iron supplementation because of intolerable gastrointestinal side effects or when there is a need for rapid replenishment of iron stores, intravenous infusion of iron formulations (iron dextran, low-molecular-weight iron dextran, ferric carboxymaltose, and iron sucrose) can be provided. One study found improvement in symptoms associated with RLS and PLMD in children when given a one-time infusion of iron sucrose with an average dose of 3.6 mg/kg (range 1.21 to 6.6 mg/kg), and serum ferritin levels were found to increase from a mean pretreatment level of 15.3 mcg/L to a mean postinfusion level of 45.7 mcg/L.

Because studies have shown improvement in RLS after supplementation with iron, therapy with iron is often the first choice for treatment. However, for those who do not respond to iron replacement therapy, other medication options should be considered. Although there are no FDA-approved medications for pediatric sleep disorders, several medications have been used clinically based on efficacy in adults with RLS. In adults, dopaminergic medications are widely used and considered first-line treatment for RLS (Simakajornboon et al., 2009). Carbidopa/levodopa and dopamine agonists (pramipexole and ropinirole) are commonly used, and ropinirole was the first FDA-approved medication for treatment of moderate to severe primary RLS in 2005 followed by pramipexole in 2006 (Simakajornboon et al., 2009). The use of dopaminergic medications is associated with improvement in RLS symptoms and reduction of PLMS and associated arousals from sleep (Simakajornboon et al., 2009). Common side effects of dopaminergic medications include nausea, vomiting, insomnia, daytime drowsiness, hallucinations, obsessive-compulsive behavior, nasal congestion, and fluid retention (Simakajornboon et al., 2009).

Another medication not FDA-approved for the treatment of RLS in children but used clinically is clonidine, an alpha-2 adrenergic receptor agonist used to treat hypertension. Clonidine, given at a dose of 0.2 to 0.4 mg at bedtime, can be helpful for children who have sleep onset problems and also can help manage symptoms of ADHD (Picchietti and Picchietti, 2010). Clonazepam, a benzodiazepine, can be used to reduce the unpleasant sensations associated with RLS and improve quality of sleep (Picchietti and Picchietti, 2008). Gabapentin, which is an anticonvulsant approved by the FDA for treatment of epilepsy in children that blocks voltage-dependent calcium channels and modulates excitatory neurotransmitter release, can also reduce the sensory and motor symptoms of RLS and improve sleep quality (Picchietti and Picchietti, 2010). Temazepam, a benzodiazepine, and zolpidem, which interacts with GABA-benzodiazepine receptor complexes, are used in adults with RLS and may be considered for older children and adolescents with RLS who have severely disturbed sleep (Picchietti and Picchietti, 2010). Intrathecal baclofen has not been shown to be effective in relieving RLS symptoms.

CONCLUSIONS

Studies over the last 20 years have shown that RLS is a common disorder in pediatric populations and should be considered when evaluating a child for sleep difficulties and sleep disturbances. RLS should especially be considered when a child presents with these complaints and has been diagnosed with ADHD or has signs and symptoms of mood disorders such as anxiety and depression. RLS is not a diagnosis that should be overlooked as untreated symptoms can lead to poor school performance and lower quality of life in older children and adolescents.

REFERENCES

The complete list of references for this chapter is available in the e-book at www.expertconsult.com.

See inside cover for registration details.

SELECTED REFERENCES

Allen, R.P., Picchietti, D.L., Garcia-Borreguero, D., et al., 2014. Restless legs syndrome/Willis-Ekbom disease diagnostic criteria: updated International Restless Legs Syndrome Study Group (IRLSSG) consensus criteria—history, rationale, description, and significance. Sleep Med. 15, 860–873.

Ekbom, K.A., 1960. Restless legs syndrome. Neurology 10, 868–873.

Mitchell, U.H., 2011. Nondrug-related aspect of treating Ekbom disease, formerly known as restless legs syndrome. Neuropsychiatr. Dis. Treat. 7, 251–257.

Picchietti, D.L., Allen, R.P., Walters, A.S., et al., 2007. Restless legs syndrome: prevalence and impact in children and adolescents—the Peds REST Study. Pediatrics 120, 253–266.

Picchietti, D.L., Bruni, O., de Weerd, A., et al., 2013. Pediatric restless legs syndrome diagnostic criteria: an update by the International Restless Legs Syndrome Study Group. Sleep Med. 14, 1253–1259.

Picchietti, D.L., Rajendran, R.R., Wilson, M.P., et al., 2009. Pediatric restless legs syndrome and periodic limb movement disorder: parent-child pairs. Sleep Med. 10, 925–931.

Picchietti, D.L., Stevens, H.E., 2008. Early manifestations of restless legs syndrome in childhood and adolescence. Sleep Med. 9, 770–781.

Picchietti, M.A., Picchietti, D.L., 2008. Restless legs syndrome and periodic limb movement disorder in children and adolescents. Semin. Pediatr. Neurol. 15, 91–99.

Picchietti, M.A., Picchietti, D.L., 2010. Advances in pediatric restless legs syndrome: iron, genetics, diagnosis and treatment. Sleep Med. 11, 643–651.

Simakajornboon, N., Kheirandish-Gozal, L., Gozal, D., 2009. Diagnosis and management of restless legs syndrome in children. Sleep Med. Rev. 13, 149–156.

E-BOOK FIGURES AND TABLES

The following figures and tables are available in the e-book at www.expertconsult.com. See inside cover for registration details.

Box 89-7 Pediatric Behavioral Interventions for Better Sleep

90 Apparent Life-Threatening Event and Sudden Infant Death Syndrome

Michael A. Mohan and Kiran P. Maski

 An expanded version of this chapter is available on www.expertconsult.com. See inside cover for registration details.

APPARENT LIFE-THREATENING EVENTS

Introduction

An apparent life-threatening event (ALTE) is an acute, unexpected episode in an infant that is witnessed by and is frightening to a caregiver because of some combination of apnea, color change, change in muscle tone, choking, or gagging. The term may be applied to any of a heterogeneous group of events, and therefore the list of possible underlying etiologies is broad, ranging from benign to severe. Although previous terminology such as "near-miss SIDS" (sudden infant death syndrome) or "aborted crib death" was occasionally applied to such events, research has not borne out the assumption that ALTE may represent a precursor to SIDS. Therefore the relationship between ALTE and SIDS has been rejected. However, in many infants such events represent a manifestation of serious underlying disease. Distinguishing which infants have medically significant events from those that do not poses a significant challenge to the clinician.

Definition

The widely accepted definition of ALTE was established at a consensus conference of the National Institutes of Health in 1986, which defined ALTE as "an episode that is frightening to the observer and that is characterized by some combination of apnea (central or occasionally obstructive), color change (usually cyanotic or pallid but occasionally erythematous or plethoric), marked change in muscle tone (usually marked limpness), choking, or gagging. In some cases, the observer fears the infant has died" (National Institutes of Health, 1987). The term is usually applied only to children younger than 1 year of age. Although in many cases such episodes are aborted through stimulation or resuscitation, note that contrary to the belief of some this is not a requirement to meet the definition, as some ALTEs may self-resolve.

Epidemiology

The incidence of ALTEs ranged from 0.58 to 2.46 per 1000 live births in recent population-based studies in the Netherlands and Austria, respectively, and ALTEs were estimated to account for 0.6% to 0.8% of all emergency department visits by infants in two British studies. The average age of infants with ALTE is 8 weeks, and ALTEs occur in roughly equal frequency between males and females.

Risk Factors

Risk factors for ALTE include a history of prematurity, likely because of immature respiratory center and arousal mechanisms; history of prior ALTE or of episodes of pallor, cyanosis, apnea, or feeding difficulties; common cold or symptoms of upper respiratory infection; and age less than 10 weeks.

Etiology/Differential Diagnosis

The differential diagnosis of ALTE is extremely broad (Box 90-1) and ranges from normal phenomena in infants such as periodic breathing or transient choking and gagging during a feeding to true medical or surgical emergencies. Often the infant appears perfectly healthy by the time he or she presents to medical attention, and in many cases—ranging from roughly 10% to nearly 50% in some studies—no underlying cause of the event is ever identified despite appropriate evaluation. Alternatively, some infants receive more than one diagnosis.

In cases for which a cause is assigned to the event, the three most common diagnoses are gastroesophageal reflux (GER), seizure, and lower respiratory tract infection. Of these, gastroesophageal reflux is the most common diagnosis, accounting for roughly 30% of diagnoses in many case series. However, whether GER is the true etiology of the event is highly uncertain because GER is common in healthy infants and a causal relationship between GER and ALTE is difficult to establish. GER may more likely be the true cause of the ALTE if the event was characterized by choking or gagging during or immediately after a feeding, if it was characterized by obstructive apnea rather than a lack of respiratory effort, or if gastric contents were noted in the infant's mouth or nose during the episode. Furthermore, the clinician should distinguish between GER symptoms and feeding difficulties (poor suck, poor swallowing coordination).

The second most common diagnosis assigned after evaluation for ALTE in many case series is seizure, accounting for approximately 15% to 30% of all cases when febrile seizures are included. Seizures are more commonly the etiology in patients who exhibited a change in muscle tone and no history of choking or gagging during the event. The EEG is often normal immediately after the ALTE. In one cohort of infants with ALTEs who were diagnosed with seizures, only 47% were diagnosed within 1 week of their ALTE presentation and 71% were diagnosed within 1 month (Bonkowsky et al., 2008). Abnormal brain MRI and developmental delay were found only in those patients who went on to develop chronic epilepsy (Bonkowsky et al., 2009).

Lower respiratory tract infections are the third most common diagnosis for ALTE in many studies, accounting for approximately 10% to 20% of all patients. Pertussis was diagnosed in 6% to 9% of patients presenting to the ER with ALTE and RSV in up to 15% in some study series.

Any number of other gastrointestinal, neurologic, respiratory, and infectious conditions as well as pathology of nearly every bodily system can also present as ALTE. ALTE may be the initial presentation of metabolic disorders, including inborn errors of metabolism (2% to 5% of cases), many of which are treatable if recognized in a timely manner. Specific inborn errors of metabolism such as organic acidurias, urea cycle disorders, maple syrup urine disease, and fatty acid oxidation disorders may present with acute life-threatening illness.

BOX 90-1 Differential Diagnosis of an Apparent Life-Threatening Event

Cardiac
Congenital heart disease
Arrythmia (long QT syndrome, WPW)
Myocarditis
Cardiomyopathy

Child abuse
Munchausen syndrome by proxy (suffocation, intentional salt poisoning, medication overdose, physical abuse, head injury)
Smothering (unintentional or intentional)

Gastrointestinal
Gastroesophageal reflux
Volvulus
Intussusception
Laryngeal chemoreflex
Gastroenteritis
Incarcerated hernia

Infectious
Sepsis
Urinary tract infection
Upper respiratory tract infection
Encephalitis/meningitis
Pneumonia

Metabolic
Inborn errors of metabolism
Reye's syndrome
Nesideoblastosis
Hypocalcemia
Hypomagnesemia
Hypoglycemia

Neurologic
Malignancy
Seizure disorder
Febrile seizure
Congenital brain malformations
Craniostenostosis
Hydrocephalus
Central apnea
Ventriculoperitoneal infection
Neuromuscular disorders
CNS bleeding

Other
Developmental delay
Feeding difficulties
Medication
Hypothermia
Anemia
Idiopathic
Anaphylaxis
Food allergy

Respiratory
Anatomic airway obstruction
Infections of the respiratory tract
Periodic breathing
Breath holding spell
Choking episode
Foreign body

(Adapted from DePiero AD. Apparent life-threatening events: an evidence based approach. Pediatric Emergency Medicine Practice; published by EB Practice LLC; 2006.)

BOX 90-2 Key Elements of Patient History After an Apparent Life-Threatening Event

Chief complaint	Setting of the child
History of present illness	Awake or asleep, position of infant, location, type of bedding used
	Activity at time of event: feeding, coughing, gagging, choking, vomiting
	Length of time
	Time to when infant regained normal respiratory effort
	Recent illness or exposure, rash, fever
	Weight loss, poor feeding, spitting up, wet burps
	Irritability, lethargy
Interventions	None
	Gentle stimulation
	Blowing air in face
	Vigorous stimulation
	Mouth-to-mouth breathing
	Cardiopulmonary resuscitation by medically trained person
Medical history	Prior episodes
	Home monitor
	Heart rate or breathing alarms, frequency of alarms, lead placement, reason for monitor
	Gastroesophageal reflux
	Birth history
	Prenatal history
	Accidents
	Previous hospitalizations/surgeries
Family history	SIDS or other unexplained childhood deaths
	Cardiac arrhythmias
	Congenital diseases
Social history	Smoking in the home
	Caretakers
	Medications in the home
Medication	Prescriptions
	Over-the-counter medications
	Herbs, herbal teas, or supplements

(Adapted from Hall KL, Zalman B. Evaluation and management of apparent life-threatening events in children. American Family Physician; published by the American Academy of Family Physicians; 2005.)

Nonaccidental trauma has been shown to be a frequently missed cause of ALTE, and is another important consideration as mortality rates in these patients are extremely high.

EVALUATION

The evaluation of an infant presenting with ALTE consists primarily of a focused history and physical examination with diagnostic testing as indicated based on the results of this assessment.

History

The history should elicit a detailed description of the event. If apnea was present the history should attempt to determine whether it was central or obstructive and the length of the apneic period. Shallow breathing, episodes of central apnea less than 30 seconds, and periodic breathing of the newborn may be normal events if not associated with cardiac instability. If color change was observed, the history should attempt to distinguish central cyanosis, which is more concerning, from acrocyanosis or flushing, which are common in normal infants. The history should assess whether the event was self-resolving, required stimulation for resolution, or required resuscitation. Further elements of patient history relevant to the evaluation of ALTE are shown in Box 90-2.

Physical Examination

The physical examination should begin with a general assessment of appearance and complete vital signs, including blood pressure and blood oxygenation measurements. Height, weight, and head circumference should also be measured and compared with norms. Particular attention should be paid to the neurologic, cardiac, and respiratory systems as well as possible signs of abuse such as bruising or a bulging anterior fontanel.

Diagnostic Testing

There is no widely accepted consensus or algorithm for diagnostic testing in infants presenting with ALTE; instead, it is largely dependent on the individual patient's history and physical examination. In 2009 the Dutch Academy of Pediatrics recommended a minimum initial diagnostic panel for ALTE that includes complete blood count with differential, C-reactive protein, serum glucose level, arterial blood gas determinations, urinalysis, electrocardiography, and assessments for *Bordetella pertussis* and respiratory syncytial virus in season. Some experts believe that serum electrolytes, ammonia, pyruvate and lactate, and urine toxicology screen should also be included in the minimum diagnostic evaluation. Further testing including, but not limited to, chest x-ray, EEG, full septic workup, evaluation for nonaccidental trauma (such as neuroimaging, retinal examination, and skeletal survey), investigations for GER, and polysomnography may be appropriate as dictated by the individual clinical picture. Several excellent reviews discuss the circumstances under which such tests may be merited in further detail (Fu et al., 2012; Tieder et al., 2013).

INPATIENT VERSUS OUTPATIENT MANAGEMENT

Most experts agree that admission for at least 24 hours of in-hospital observation is warranted in most cases of ALTE. In a retrospective study of 625 infants admitted for ALTE, 46 (7.4%) had a subsequent extreme cardiorespiratory event (central apnea >30 seconds, bradycardia >10 seconds, or desaturation >10 seconds with pulse oximetry <80%), usually within 24 hours of admission. Risk factors that increased the likelihood of having subsequent extreme events were postconceptional age less than 43 weeks (5.2-fold increase), premature birth (6.3-fold), and URTI symptoms (11.2-fold) (Al-Kindy et al., 2009). Infants with a history of multiple ALTEs also have been shown to be at especially high risk (approximately fourfold) of requiring significant subsequent medical intervention because of a serious underlying diagnosis. Infants without a previous history of ALTE, who were not born prematurely, who have a normal physical examination, who are greater than 30 days old, and who had a brief self-resolving episode may be reasonable to discharge without admission for observation. In all cases, however, caretakers should be given resources for prompt medical follow up and for basic life support courses. They should also be instructed not to shake their infants as a method of stimulation during an ALTE, a practice that has been found to occur in up to one third of ALTE cases.

HOME MONITORING

The use of home cardiorespiratory monitors that alert caregivers to bradycardia or absence of chest wall movement (and in some cases to blood oxygen desaturation) is controversial. There is no evidence that home monitors prevent SIDS or provide therapeutic benefit after ALTE. However, some experts agree that on a case-by-case basis such monitors may be appropriate for infants with a high risk of apnea, bradycardia, or desaturations because of prematurity or for infants with unstable airways, dysregulated breathing, or chronic lung disease.

RISK OF SIDS

The American Academy of Pediatrics Task Force on SIDS has stated that there is no evidence that ALTE is a precursor to SIDS (Moon, 2011). Although longitudinal studies tracking outcomes of infants who experience ALTE have found elevated death rates in these infants from some etiologies as described below, SIDS has not been found to be one of them. Bolstering the argument that SIDS and ALTE do not lie on the same pathophysiologic continuum is the finding that risk factors for SIDS and ALTE appear to be largely distinct; that ALTEs tend to occur during the day and SIDS at night; that ALTEs peak in the first 2 months of life compared with SIDS between 2 and 4 months of age; and that while SIDS is more common in boys, ALTE occurs equally among genders. Even though SIDS has several modifiable risk factors, particularly the placement of an infant in the prone sleeping position, the same has not been found for ALTEs. In fact, though the 1994 recommendation from the AAP that infants be placed supine for sleep led to a dramatic reduction in SIDS rates (see SIDS section), no reduction in ALTE rates was noted.

RISK OF DEATH

The risk of death in infants presenting with ALTE ranges from roughly 0.5% to 1.1% in 12-month to 5-year follow-up periods in studies that tracked the outcomes of patients presenting with first ALTE. Causes of death included pneumonia, underlying neurologic disorder, child abuse, and SIDS. Risk factors for a serious underlying diagnosis include a history of multiple ALTEs and suspected child maltreatment. Infants with a history of prematurity are at increased risk for subsequent severe events likely because of immature respiratory control, and possibly at increased risk of death, although in some studies this risk appears to return to baseline once the infant reaches between 43 and 48 weeks of postconceptional age.

SUDDEN INFANT DEATH SYNDROME
Introduction

SIDS is characterized by the sudden unexpected death of an infant during sleep. Despite a dramatic decline in recent decades, SIDS remains the leading cause of death in children between 1 month and 1 year of age. Although SIDS has long been enigmatic—perhaps because it likely represents the common result of a heterogeneous set of processes—insight into its pathogenesis continues to evolve. Below are reviewed selected hypotheses regarding the biological basis of SIDS as well as key risk factors—and some protective factors—that appear to make some infants more or less vulnerable to this devastating and still largely mysterious occurrence.

Definition

SIDS is defined as the sudden death of an infant less than 1 year of age that remains unexplained after a thorough case investigation, including a death scene investigation, autopsy, and review of the clinical history. SIDS is a subset of sudden unexpected infant deaths and comprises roughly 80% of such deaths. Approximately 20% of sudden unexpected infant deaths have a clear cause such as unequivocal suffocation or entrapment, infection, ingestions, metabolic diseases, or trauma (accidental or nonaccidental). However, in many cases distinguishing between SIDS and other causes of sudden unexpected infant death, particularly those that seemingly occur during a sleep period, is challenging. Some cases initially classified as SIDS are subsequently found to be attributable to entities such as metabolic disorders or cardiac channelopathies after further investigation.

Pathogenesis

The Triple-Risk Model

The biological basis of SIDS remains an area of active research. However, the improved understanding of risk factors for SIDS, along with the distribution of most deaths between 1 month and 4 months of age, helped lead to the creation of the widely cited triple-risk model for SIDS proposed by Filiano and Kinney in 1994. This model suggests that SIDS occurs in infants when (1) an external stressor or trigger event is encountered, (2) by an infant with an intrinsic vulnerability, and (3) during a critical period of development. External risk factors include prone or side sleeping, airway covering from soft or loose bedding, bed-sharing, overheating, and infections, as discussed below. These represent homeostatic stressors for the infant that may lead to airway obstruction, rebreathing of exhaled gasses, altered cardiorespiratory regulation in response to heat stress, or impaired arousal.

Although an infant would normally be able to overcome such stressors with a compensatory or protective response, in some vulnerable infants these responses fail, particularly when the stressor converges on the infant between 1 and 4 months of age. It is hypothesized that this convergence leads to a failure of homeostatic protective mechanisms such as arousal and head turning or head-up tilt—a failure that is likely potentiated by sleep—resulting in progressively worsening respiratory effort and/or gas exchange, hypoxia, bradycardia, acidosis, hypotension, and death (Fig. 90-1).

The 5-Hydroxytryptamine System

Investigation of what contributes to the intrinsic vulnerability of some infants to SIDS has focused on the brainstem because of its role in arousal and homeostatic functions. The most well-studied brainstem system in relation to SIDS is the medullary 5-hydroxytryptamine (serotonergic) system, which is important for arousal and autonomic control, including responses to hypercarbia and hypoxia. There is evidence that there is decreased 5-HT(1A) receptor binding density in areas of the medulla important for autonomic control in SIDS victims compared with controls as well as in male infants compared with female infants, which could potentially account for the gender discrepancy observed in SIDS rates. Recent studies have also shown decreased levels of serotonin itself and of tryptophan hydroxylase, an enzyme that synthesizes serotonin, in relevant areas of the medulla. Perhaps also supporting the serotonin hypothesis is evidence of decreased medullary 5-HT(1A) receptor immunoreactivity in infants exposed to nicotine in utero, which could potentially contribute to the higher rate of SIDS observed in such infants.

EPIDEMIOLOGY

SIDS is the leading cause of death of infants between 1 month and 1 year of age in the United States, with a rate of 42.6 deaths per 100,000 live births in 2012, accounting for 1679 cases (U.S. Department of Health and Human Services, 2014). Fortunately, SIDS rates have declined dramatically since the discovery in the early 1990s that the prone sleep position dramatically increases the risk of SIDS, which led the American Academy of Pediatrics to issue a recommendation that infants be placed in the nonprone sleep position (the "Back to Sleep" campaign) as a strategy for reducing SIDS rates. Despite minimal change in the years preceding the recommendation, SIDS rates declined by over 50% in the United States in the subsequent decade, with a decrease from 120

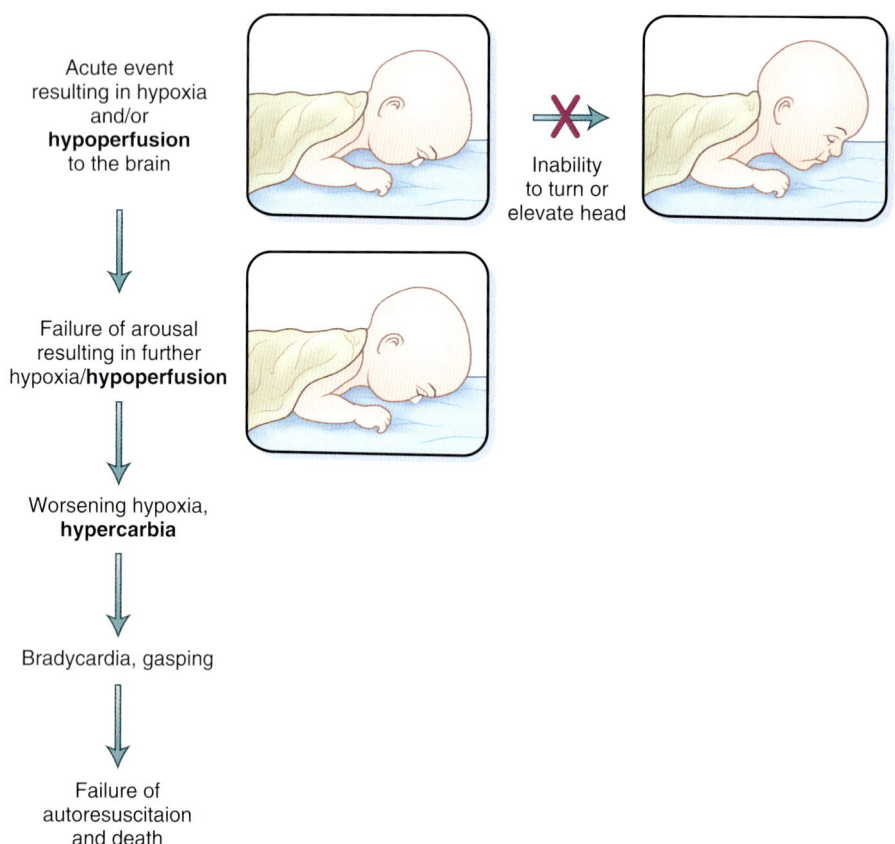

Acute event resulting in hypoxia and/or **hypoperfusion** to the brain

Inability to turn or elevate head

Failure of arousal resulting in further hypoxia/**hypoperfusion**

Worsening hypoxia, **hypercarbia**

Bradycardia, gasping

Failure of autoresuscitaion and death

Figure 90-1. Hypothesized five stages in death from SIDS. *(Adapted from Kinney HC, Thach BT. The sudden infant death syndrome. N Engl J Med 2009;361:795–805.)*

deaths per 100,000 live births in 1992 to 58.1 per 100,000 live births in 2002 as the prevalence of infants placed to sleep in the supine position increased from 13% to 72% (Moon, 2011). The rate of SIDS remains highest in American Indian/ Alaska Native (90.4 per 100,000 live births in 2012) and non-Hispanic black (85.1) infants compared with non-Hispanic white (41.8), Hispanic (22.1), and Asian or Pacific Islander (14.8) infants. This may be because of differences in risk factors for SIDS, most notably prone positioning during sleep, which may differ between racial and ethnic groups. According to the National Infant Sleep Position Study, the rate of supine positioning for black infants was 53%, Hispanic infants 73%, white infants 75%, and Asian infants 80% (National Infant Sleep Position Study, 2015).

SIDS is more common in male than in female infants in a roughly 3:2 ratio for unknown reasons.

Perhaps surprisingly, only approximately 10% of SIDS cases occur in the first month of life. Roughly two thirds of SIDS deaths occur in the second, third, or fourth month of life, with a median age of 11 weeks. Ninety percent occur before the age of 6 months and 98% occur before 9 months of age.

Risk Factors

Hundreds of epidemiologic and case–control studies have examined the risk factors for SIDS, including both environmental and inborn risk factors, and the identification of some of these risk factors has helped lead to a dramatic decline in SIDS rates as discussed above. Below, several of the most widely studied and agreed-upon risk factors are discussed, along with proposed pathophysiologic explanations of why such factors might contribute to SIDS.

Prone and Side Sleep Position

The prone sleep position is the most well-established risk factor for SIDS, with an excess odds ratio compared with supine positioning varying from 2.4 to as high as 13.1 across studies. Prone positioning has been shown to increase the risk of rebreathing expired gases, particularly when soft bedding is used, leading to hypercarbia and hypoxia. Moreover, the prone position is associated with decreased arousals from sleep, even in the face of apnea. Prone positioning may also increase the risk of hyperthermia and even decrease cerebral oxygenation compared with supine positioning. Other studies have found that there is altered cerebrovascular control in infants sleeping in the prone position and that compensatory responses for prone positioning are diminished between 2 and 3 months of age, corresponding to the peak age of SIDS.

Though much less well studied, side positioning of an infant for sleep is also unsafe compared with the supine position, with an elevated risk similar in magnitude to that of prone positioning. This is perhaps because of the high likelihood of rolling prone.

Bed-Sharing

A 2012 meta-analysis of 11 studies investigating the association of bed-sharing and SIDS revealed a summary OR of 2.88 (95% confidence interval [CI]: 1.99–4.18) (Vennemann et al., 2012). The risk was highest for infants of smoking mothers (OR, 6.27; 95% CI, 3.94–9.99) and infants less than 12 weeks old (OR, 10.37; 95% CI, 4.44–24.21). Some argue that this may be confounded by infants who are brought into bed because they are ill. Moreover, deaths from an adult rolling onto an infant during sleep are more properly classified as "accidental suffocation or strangulation in bed" rather than SIDS, but this is often difficult to ascertain. The AAP

recommends that infants share a room with their parents without bed sharing.

Soft Bedding and Bedding Accessories

Soft bedding and bedding accessories such as pillows, quilts, comforters, and sheepskins are associated with an increased risk of SIDS, as they increase the potential of airway covering and rebreathing. In one study of soft bedding there was a 5-fold increased risk regardless of sleep position, which increased to 21-fold when the infant was placed prone with soft bedding (Hauck et al., 2003). The AAP recommends that infants sleep on a firm surface without any soft or loose bedding, with infant sleep clothing used in place of blankets as necessary.

Overheating

Several studies have suggested that thermal stress may increase the risk of SIDS. Although overheating is more likely to occur in infants placed in the prone position, both overheating and prone positioning appears to be independently associated with SIDS. It is less clear, however, if the risk associated with overheating is independent of the increased risk of asphyxia posed by additional clothes or blankets in the sleep environment.

Maternal Smoking

Maternal smoking during pregnancy is thought to be the largest preventable risk factor for SIDS aside from sleep position, with an effect that appears to be dose dependent. The putative pathways through which prenatal nicotine exposure leads to elevated SIDS risk are numerous. Several studies have demonstrated an adverse effect of exposure to tobacco products in utero on infant arousal thresholds in both term and preterm infants; some have also demonstrated impaired responses to hypoxemic and hypercarbic challenges. These phenomena may be related to effects of nicotine exposure on the brainstem serotonergic, as discussed above. Smoke exposure also increases the risk of preterm birth and low birth weight, both of which are additional independent risk factors.

Prematurity

Premature infants are at a roughly fourfold greater risk of SIDS than term infants. This may be because of immature autonomic control systems and the presence of fewer and shorter arousal periods in preterm compared with term infants, particularly in the prone position.

Infection

There is postulated to be a role of infection in some cases of SIDS, as approximately half of infants who die of SIDS have a seemingly trivial infection at the time of death. Some polymorphisms that could contribute to an excessive inflammatory response in response to infection have been found to be more common in SIDS victims than in controls, and microbial isolates in victims of sudden unexpected infant death are more likely to grow some pathogens at autopsy than are those from infants dying of known noninfectious causes such as drowning or congenital heart disease. However, a causal relationship between these pathogens and SIDS is less clear.

Genetics

Although there is no evidence of a strong heritable contribution to SIDS, several genetic polymorphisms have been observed that may increase susceptibility to SIDS in combination with environmental risk factors. These include polymorphisms in genes affecting serotonin transport and autonomic function, which are found more often in SIDS victims than in controls. Mutations in cardiac sodium or potassium channel genes such *SCN5A*, a sodium channel gene that is related to a prolonged QT interval, may be found in 5% to 10% of cases of sudden unexpected infant deaths after molecular testing. Mutations in genes involved in energy metabolism, particularly mutations in the medium-chain acyl-coenzyme A dehydrogenase gene, may be found in approximately 1% of cases of sudden unexpected infant deaths upon metabolic evaluation. If case investigation reveals a "lethal" genetic defect, such as mutations yielding long-QT syndrome or MCAD deficiency, such cases should no longer be classified as SIDS but as explained deaths. In most cases, however, genetic polymorphisms are believed to simply provide a predisposition to SIDS, which may make SIDS more likely when combined with other triggers such as prone sleeping, maternal smoking, infection, or overheating.

PREVENTION

As discussed above, evidence suggests that the risk of SIDS is minimized with supine sleep position, firm sleep surface without loose bedding, avoidance of overheating, and avoidance of tobacco product exposure, among other measures. Additionally, several studies, including a 2011 meta-analysis, have concluded that breastfeeding has a protective effect against SIDS even when accounting for potential confounding factors, with an approximate halving of the risk (Hauck et al., 2011). In addition to providing immune benefits and reducing the rates of infectious illnesses, which are a risk factor for SIDS, breastfed infants have been found to have a lower arousal threshold during sleep, which may contribute to the protective effect.

Pacifier use also appears to have a protective effect against SIDS, reducing risk by twofold or even greater in several studies, including a meta-analysis. Pacifiers may be protective because of alterations in jaw/airway positioning during sleep or through favorable alterations in autonomic tone that persist even after loss of the pacifier during sleep.

There is no evidence that home cardiorespiratory monitors are protective against SIDS, and the AAP recommends against their use for this purpose.

REFERENCES

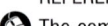 The complete list of references for this chapter is available in the e-book at www.expertconsult.com.

See inside cover for registration details.

SELECTED REFERENCES

Al-Kindy, H.A., Gélinas, J.F., Hatzakis, G., et al., 2009. Risk factors for extreme events in infants hospitalized for apparent life-threatening events. J. Pediatr. 154, 332–337.

Bonkowsky, J.L., Guenther, E., Filloux, F.M., et al., 2008. Death, child abuse, and adverse neurological outcome of infants after an apparent life-threatening event. Pediatrics 122, 125–131.

Bonkowsky, J.L., Guenther, E., Srivastava, R., et al., 2009. Seizures in children following an apparent life-threatening event. J. Child Neurol. 24, 709–713.

Fu, L.Y., et al., 2012. Apparent life-threatening events: an update. Pediatr. Rev. 33 (8), 361–368.

Hauck, F.R., Herman, S.M., Donovan, M., et al., 2003. Sleep environment and the risk of sudden infant death syndrome in an urban population: the Chicago Infant Mortality Study. Pediatrics 111, 1207–1214.

Hauck, F.R., Thompson, J.M., Tanabe, K.O., et al., 2011. Breastfeeding and reduced risk of sudden infant death syndrome: a meta-analysis. Pediatrics 128, 103–110.

Moon, R.Y., Task Force on Sudden Infant Death Syndrome, 2011. SIDS and other sleep-related infant deaths: expansion of recommendations for a safe infant sleeping environment. Pediatrics 128, 1030–1039.

National Institutes of Health, 1987. Consensus Development Conference on Infantile Apnea and Home Monitoring, Sept 29 to Oct 1, 1986. Pediatrics 79, 292–299.

National Infant Sleep Position Study. Available at: <http://slone-web2.bu.edu/ChimeNisp/Main_Nisp.asp> [home page]. Accessed 12 Mar 2015.

Tieder, J.S., et al., 2013. Management of apparent life threatening events in infants: a systematic review. J. Pediatr. Res. 163 (1), 94–99.

U.S. Department of Health and Human Services, Centers for Disease Control and Prevention, National Center for Health Statistics. Compressed Mortality Files 1979–2012 on CDC WONDER Online Database, released October 2014. Available at: <http://wonder.cdc.gov/cmf-icd10.html>. Accessed 15 Dec 2014.

Vennemann, M.M., Hense, H.W., Bajanowski, T., et al., 2012. Bed sharing and the risk of sudden infant death syndrome: can we resolve the debate? J. Pediatr. 160, 44–48.

E-BOOK FIGURES AND TABLES

The following figures and tables are available in the e-book at www.expertconsult.com. See inside cover for registration details.

Box 90-3. Key American Academy of Pediatrics recommendations for SIDS prevention.

91 The Cerebellum and the Hereditary Ataxias

Paymaan Jafar-Nejad, Stephen M. Maricich, and Huda Y. Zoghbi

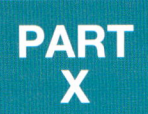 An expanded version of this chapter is available on www.expertconsult.com. See inside cover for registration details.

The cerebellum governs complex motor movements. Disruptions of its inputs or basic structure secondary to developmental anomalies, degenerative diseases, vascular insults, or trauma result in a characteristic spectrum of motor symptoms and signs (Ito, 2002). We will begin by considering these signs and their relation to cerebellar structure; we will then consider the prominent causes of ataxia, with a primary emphasis on the hereditary ataxias. Other conditions associated with cerebellar dysfunction are discussed thoroughly in other sections of this volume.

THE LANGUAGE AND LOGIC OF CEREBELLAR DYSFUNCTION

Cerebellar lesions or dysfunction disturb regulation of muscle tone, motor control, and coordination of movement. A number of studies have also linked the cerebellum to various higher order cognitive processes subserved by the cerebellar hemispheres and the dentate nuclei, such as sensory discrimination, attention, working memory, semantic association, verbal learning and memory, and complex problem solving. The specific constellation of symptoms is sometimes useful for localizing the cerebellar lesion, but often there is considerable overlap (Manni and Petrosini, 2004).

Ataxia is a broad term that refers to a disturbance in the smooth performance of voluntary motor acts. It can be manifested as *abasia* (inability to walk due to spasticity, chorea, or tremor), *asynergia* (lack of coordination between parts that normally act in unison), *dysmetria* (inaccuracy in judging distance or scale, resulting in undershoot or overshoot of intended position of limb or eye), *dysdiadochokinesia* (inability to perform rapid alternating movements, such as pronation and supination of the hand or screwing in a light bulb), and impaired check/excessive rebound responses. Vermal lesions result in truncal ataxia and *titubation* (a faltering, staggering gait when walking and bobbing or swaying of the head and trunk when in a sitting position), whereas hemispheric lesions cause limb ataxia.

Cerebellar (ataxic) dysarthria produces abnormalities in articulation (slurring and inaccuracy in range, force and timing; patients sound as if they are inebriated), phonation (vocal quality can be harsh or uneven), resonation (a nasal quality is common), and prosody (patients tend to place equal and excessive emphasis on each syllable). Other kinds of dysarthria exist: there is, for example, the hypokinetic dysarthria seen in Parkinson disease, in which bradykinesia due to loss of dopaminergic neurons in the substantia nigra tends to produce low volume of speech or hoarseness, reduced pitch variability, palilalia (repetition of syllables), and very slow speech. There is evidence that left cerebellar lesions interfere with speech prosody because of disruptions of interconnections with the right cerebral hemisphere, which mediates this process. *Cerebellar mutism* is sometimes seen after removal of vermian tumors and may result from bilateral involvement of the dentatorubrothalamic tracts.

Hypotonia is a decrease in muscle tone in response to stretch. It is typically seen with acute hemispheric lesions and is often accompanied by hyporeflexia. Hypotonia likely results from decreased fusimotor activity resulting in decreased muscle spindle afferent response. It is usually a transient phenomenon after an acute lesion but can be seen in chronic lesions as well.

Intention tremor can occur after lesions of the dentate nuclei and is manifest only when the individual attempts to make a directed movement. Postural tremor is a rare manifestation of cerebellar damage.

Eye movement abnormalities are also a manifestation of cerebellar disease, predominantly in the form of pathologic nystagmus (smooth pursuit in one direction alternating with saccadic pursuit in the other). They usually occur when the vermis or flocculonodular lobe are affected. *Ocular dysmetria* (conjugate overshoot or undershoot of a visual target accompanied by voluntary saccades) can result from midline or hemispheric lesions.

Nonmotor manifestations of cerebellar disease can also occur. A cerebellar cognitive affective syndrome has been described in patients with isolated cerebellar lesions of a number of different etiologies; executive functions, spatial cognition, personality changes, and language deficits are all present. The postulated neural substrate involves circuits that link prefrontal, posterior parietal, superior temporal, and limbic cortices to the cerebellum.

Disorders that specifically affect different cerebellar subdivisions lead to a characteristic spectrum of motor abnormalities. *Midline cerebellar disease* causes disorders of stance and gait, truncal titubation, rotated postures of the head, and disturbances in eye movements. These can be subdivided into *rostral vermal lesions* that result in abasia or gait ataxia and *caudal* vermal lesions that cause nystagmus in addition. Lesions of the *fastigial nuclei*, which receive their input from the vermis, result in abasia. *Intermediate hemisphere disease* or lesions of the interposed nuclei cause delayed check (rebound) responses, truncal titubation, dysdiadochokinesia, action tremor, oscillation of outstretched extremities, and incoordination on finger-nose-finger and heel-shin maneuvers. Disruption of the *cerebellar hemispheres and dentate nuclei* result in dysarthria, limb ataxia, hypotonia, terminal and intention tremor, and abnormal eye movements.

NONHEREDITARY CAUSES OF ATAXIA

Cerebellar disease can result from a number of underlying conditions, many of which are listed in Box 91-1. The most prevalent causes of acute cerebellar ataxia are viruses (e.g., coxsackievirus, rubeola, varicella), traumatic insults, and toxins (e.g., alcohol, barbiturates, antiepileptic drugs) (see Chapter 92).

Congenital abnormalities of the nervous system, such as Chiari malformation, Dandy-Walker malformation, and basilar impression, can be associated with ataxia. Hemorrhage, infarction, and embolism are unusual causes of selective cerebellar damage. Tumors of the cerebellum (vermal and hemispheric) or the adjacent brainstem, particularly pontine gliomas, are relatively common, but angioblastomas of the cerebellum are rare; von Hippel-Lindau disease, a neurocutaneous condition, is associated with vascular lesions of the cerebellum, as is the PHACE syndrome (**p**osterior fossa malformations, **h**emangiomas, **a**rterial anomalies, **c**oarctation of aorta and **c**ardiac defects, and **e**ye abnormalities).

Numerous metabolic conditions affecting the central and peripheral nervous systems lead to ataxia. Endocrinologic abnormalities, particularly hypothyroidism, may present with ataxia as the predominant manifestation. Autoimmune disorders can cause ataxia, although this is rare in children; detection of antigliadin and antiendomysial antibodies indicates gluten sensitivity, a treatable cerebellar syndrome that can appear even in the absence of gastrointestinal symptoms or malabsorption.

THE HEREDITARY ATAXIAS

The hereditary ataxias can be conceptually divided into two main classes. The first group is ataxias that are caused by enzymatic defects, which are usually inherited in an autosomal recessive manner and typically present in childhood; fortunately, many of these are now treatable. Their basic features and treatments are presented in Table 91-1. The second group, consisting of the progressive degenerative ataxias, can be further categorized based on their mode of inheritance: the autosomal recessive ataxias, of which Friedreich ataxia is by far the most common; the autosomal dominant inherited ataxias (spinocerebellar ataxias, episodic ataxias, and dentatorubropallidoluysian atrophy [DRPLA]); and the very rare X-linked ataxias. The spastic ataxias can be either autosomal recessive or autosomal dominant, and will be considered as their own group. Given the space constraints and clinical focus of this volume, we will devote the greater part of our discussion to the ataxias that are more likely to be encountered in the clinic, particularly those that present in childhood, along with any distinctive features, treatments, and differential diagnoses that should be considered. We refer readers interested in detailed molecular genetics to the online version of this chapter and to the burgeoning literature that each year sheds greater light on pathophysiology.

Autosomal Recessive Inherited Syndromes

The recessive ataxias tend to present earlier than the autosomal dominant syndromes, usually in childhood. Because of the inheritance pattern, many cases will present without a clear family history of progressive ataxia; the clinician must maintain genetic causes high on the list of differential diagnoses. We begin here with Friedreich ataxia and ataxia-telangiectasia, the two most common of this relatively uncommon class of diseases. Other recessive ataxias are considered in light of differential diagnosis.

Friedreich Ataxia (Spinocerebellar Ataxia— MIM 229300)

Friedreich ataxia (FRDA) is the most common autosomal recessive spinocerebellar ataxia, with a prevalence rate of 1 to 2 per 100,000. FRDA shares one notable feature with many of the autosomal dominant ataxias discussed later in this chapter: it is caused by a dynamic mutation—in this case, the expansion of an intronic GAA repeat in the *Frataxin* (FXN) gene (Brigatti et al., 2012). Dynamic mutations are notable for causing clinical variability because shorter expansions produce milder phenotypes whereas longer expansions produce more severe, earlier onset disease. For this reason, although FRDA is

TABLE 91-1 Treatable Causes of Inherited Ataxia

Disorder	Metabolic Abnormality	Distinguishing Clinical Features	Treatment
Ataxia with vitamin E deficiency	Mutation in alpha-tocopherol transfer protein	Ataxia, areflexia, retinopathy	Vitamin E
Bassen-Kornzweig syndrome	Abetalipoproteinemia	Acanthocytosis, retinitis pigmentosa, fat malabsorption	Vitamin E
Hartnup disease	Tryptophan malabsorption	Pellagra rash, intermittent ataxia	Niacin
Familial episodic ataxia type 1 and type 2	Mutations in potassium channel (KCNA1) and a_{1A} voltage-gated calcium channel, respectively	Episodic attacks, worse with pregnancy or birth control pills	Acetazolamide
Mitochondrial complex defects	Complexes I, III, IV	Encephalomyelopathy	Possibly riboflavin, CoQ$_{10}$, dichloroacetate
Multiple carboxylase deficiency	Biotinidase deficiency	Alopecia, recurrent infections, variable organic aciduria	Biotin
Pyruvate dehydrogenase deficiency	Block in E-M and Krebs cycle interface	Lactic acidosis, ataxia	Ketogenic diet, possibly dichloroacetate
Refsum disease	Phytanic acid, alpha-hydroxylase	Retinitis pigmentosa, cardiomyopathy, hypertrophic neuropathy, ichthyosis	Dietary restriction of phytanic acid
Urea cycle defects	Urea cycle enzymes	Hyperammonemia	Protein restriction, arginine, benzoate, alpha-ketoacids

(Modified with permission from Stumpf DA. Pediatr Neurol 1985a; 1:129.)

BOX 91-1 Selected Causes of Ataxia in Childhood

CONGENITAL

Agenesis of vermis of the cerebellum
Aplasia or dysplasia of the cerebellum
Basilar impression
Chiari malformation
Cerebellar dysplasia with microgyria, macrogyria, or agyria
Cervical spinal bifida with herniation of the cerebellum (Chiari malformation, type 3)
Dandy-Walker syndrome
Encephalocele
Hydrocephalus (progressive)
Hypoplasia of the cerebellum

DEGENERATIVE AND/OR GENETIC

Acute intermittent cerebellar ataxia
Ataxia, retinitis pigmentosa, deafness, vestibular abnormality, and intellectual deterioration
Ataxia-telangiectasia
Biemond posterior column ataxia
Cerebellar ataxia with deafness, anosmia, absent caloric responses, nonreactive pupils, and hyporeflexia
Cockayne syndrome
Dentate cerebellar ataxia (dyssynergia cerebellaris progressiva)
Familial ataxia with macular degeneration
Friedreich ataxia
Hereditary cerebellar ataxia, intellectual retardation, choreoathetosis, and eunuchoidism
Hereditary cerebellar ataxia with myotonia and cataracts
Hypertrophic interstitial neuritis
Marie's ataxia
Marinesco-Sjögren syndrome
Pelizaeus-Merzbacher disease
Periodic attacks of vertigo, diplopia, and ataxia—autosomal dominant inheritance
Posterior and lateral column difficulties, nystagmus, and muscle atrophy
Progressive cerebellar ataxia and epilepsy
Ramsay Hunt syndrome (myoclonic seizures and ataxia)
Roussy-Lévy syndrome
Spinocerebellar ataxia (SCAs); olivopontocerebellar ataxias

ENDOCRINOLOGIC

Cretinism
Hypothyroidism

INFECTIOUS OR POSTINFECTIOUS

Acute cerebellar ataxia
Acute disseminated encephalomyelitis
Cerebellar abscess
Coxsackievirus
Diphtheria
Echovirus
Fisher syndrome
Infectious mononucleosis (Epstein-Barr virus infection)
Infectious polyneuropathy
Japanese B encephalitis
Mumps encephalitis
Mycoplasma pneumoniae
Pertussis
Polio
Postbacterial meningitis
Rubeola
Tuberculosis
Typhoid
Varicella

METABOLIC

Abetalipoproteinemia
Argininosuccinic aciduria
Ataxia with vitamin E deficiency (AVED)
GM2 gangliosidosis (late)
Hartnup disease
Hyperalaninemia
Hyperammonemia I and II
Hypoglycemia
Kearns-Sayre syndrome
Leigh disease
Maple syrup urine disease (intermittent)
MERRF (Myoclonic epilepsy with ragged red fibers)
Metachromatic leukodystrophy
Mitochondrial complex defects (I, III, IV)
Multiple carboxylase deficiency (biotinidase deficiency)
Neuronal ceroid-lipofuscinosis
Neuropathy, ataxia, retinitis pigmentosa (NARP)
Niemann-Pick disease (late infantile)
5-Oxoprolinuria
Pyruvate decarboxylase deficiency
Refsum disease
Sialidosis
Triose-phosphate isomerase deficiency
Tryptophanuria
Wernicke encephalopathy

NEOPLASTIC

Frontal lobe tumors
Hemispheric cerebellar tumors
Midline cerebellar tumors
Neuroblastoma
Pontine tumors (primarily gliomas)
Spinal cord tumors

PRIMARY PSYCHOGENIC

Conversion reaction

TOXIC

Alcohol
Benzodiazepines
Carbamazepine
Clonazepam
Lead encephalopathy
Phenobarbital
Phenytoin
Primidone
Tick paralysis poisoning

TRAUMATIC

Acute cerebellar edema
Acute frontal lobe edema

VASCULAR

Angioblastoma of cerebellum
Basilar migraine
Cerebellar embolism
Cerebellar hemorrhage
Cerebellar thrombosis
Posterior cerebellar artery disease
Vasculitis
von Hippel-Lindau disease

typically thought of as manifesting during the early school years, its onset can sometimes be detected as early as 2 years of age or as late as the beginning of the third decade of life. (Dynamic repeats will be discussed in greater detail in the section on autosomal dominant ataxias.)

The first sign of FRDA is usually a progressive gait ataxia, although occasionally electrocardiogram (ECG) abnormalities reveal cardiomyopathy before the ataxia manifests with widening of the base and wavering, which seems to be caused by a loss of proprioception. The poor balance is accentuated when visual input is removed, as in the Romberg test. The gait can be grossly disorganized, with such a marked reeling or lurching quality that it appears contrived. The upper extremities soon become uncoordinated, distal muscles begin to waste, and tremor or choreiform movements may develop in the face and arms. Irregular ocular pursuit is often prominent; dysmetric saccades, square wave jerks, and failure of fixation suppression of the vestibuloocular reflex are common. Cataracts, retinitis pigmentosa, and optic atrophy can also occur. Dysarthria typically develops early in the disease course and the slurring and staccato volume changes are severe enough to quickly render speech ineffectual. Auditory dysfunction is common and may be accompanied by vertigo. Within several years kyphoscoliosis shifts the patient's center of gravity, making walking nearly impossible.

Deep tendon reflexes are lost early on in the disease course, unless the patient had adult onset (usually after age 25). Position and vibration sense are grossly impaired, and pain and temperature sensations are lost in the distal extremities. Clubfoot and pes cavus are nearly always present. Cardiomyopathy occurs in two-thirds of FRDA patients and is progressive. In advanced stages of the disease, patients may experience exertional dyspnea, palpitations, and anginal pain; later in the disease course, arrhythmias (especially atrial fibrillation) and congestive heart failure are frequent. (Cardiac dysfunction is the leading cause of death in FRDA.) Twenty percent of patients show an abnormal glucose tolerance curve due to insulin resistance, which may also affect relatives; another 10% develop diabetes mellitus. Thermal dysregulation, intermittent emesis, and respiratory dysfunction have been reported. The mean age of death is in the middle thirties.

In the minority of patients with shorter GAA expansions (less than 500), the age of onset is between 26 and over 40 years, with the smaller repeats producing later onset and milder symptoms. Disease progression is slower in these patients and they have a lower incidence of secondary skeletal abnormalities. Very rarely, patients homozygous for GAA expansions may present with spastic paraparesis and hyperreflexia but not ataxia.

Differential diagnosis. Children with FRDA who have not yet developed dysarthria or extensor plantar responses may be difficult to distinguish on clinical criteria alone; because one-fourth of FRDA patients display atypical clinical signs, DNA testing is the only means to a definitive diagnosis. FRDA is most frequently confused with *demyelinating hereditary motor and sensory neuropathy type I (HMSNI or CMT1)*, which can present in childhood with clumsiness, areflexia, and minimal distal muscle weakness. Another consideration is *ARSACS (Autosomal Recessive Spastic Ataxia of Charlevoix-Saguenay;* Table 91-2), in which patients are characterized by spasticity, dysarthria, distal muscle wasting, foot deformities, truncal ataxia, absence of sensory potentials in the lower limbs, retinal striations similar to those in Leber optic atrophy, and frequent mitral valve prolapse. *Vitamin E deficiency* causes ataxia with areflexia but is usually distinguishable from FRDA by the greater likelihood of hyperkinesia and titubation, less severe peripheral neuropathy, and the lack of cardiomyopathy. It is obviously important to test for both abetalipoproteinemia and alpha-tocopherol deficiency, because these ataxias can be cured by large doses of Vitamin E. *Friedreich Ataxia 2 (MIM 601992)* has been reported in families with a FRDA phenotype but without point mutations or GAA expansions in the *X25* gene; the biological basis for the phenocopy is not known, but it has been proposed that mutations in genes that lie in the iron metabolism pathway may be responsible.

Treatment. Frataxin is thought to be active in iron/sulfur cluster biosynthesis; the repeat expansion diminishes frataxin levels and leads to increased oxidative stress, which can be mitigated by certain antioxidant treatments. Notably, a high proportion of FRDA patients have decreased serum CoQ10 levels; as CoQ10 deficiency causes mitochondrial dysfunction, low- and high-dose CoQ10/vitamin E therapies have proven effective in improving International Cooperative Ataxia Rating Scale scores. A0001 (α-tocopheryl quinone; EPI-A0001), a potent antioxidant, causes a dose-dependent improvement in neurologic function, as measured by the Friedreich Ataxia Rating Scale (FARS). Therapy with other antioxidants, iron chelators, and/or glutathione peroxidase mimetics has been suggested but not thoroughly tested. Idebenone, a short-chain analog of coenzyme Q10, has been able to improve cardiac function and decreased ventricular mass. In low dose trials, idebenone treatment has no effect on the progression of ataxia, but higher doses (up to 60 mg/kg/day) are well tolerated, provide neurologic benefit, and improve activity of daily life in FRDA patients who are still ambulatory. Symptomatic treatment in the form of antispasticity agents can be helpful to relieve painful muscle spasms, and surgical correction of scoliosis is palliative (Di Prospero et al., 2007).

Ataxia-Telangiectasia (Louis-Bar Syndrome— MIM 208900)

Several ataxia syndromes are caused by defects in DNA repair mechanisms; why the cerebellum is particularly vulnerable to such defects is unknown. Ataxia-telangiectasia (AT), caused by mutations in the DNA repair factor *ataxia-telangiectasia mutated (ATM)*, is one of the most common inherited causes of early childhood-onset ataxia in most countries, with a prevalence of one in 40,000 to 100,000 live births in the United States. Its core neurologic features are ataxia, oculomotor apraxia, and choreoathetosis, but neoplasia and sinopulmonary disease are equally prominent concerns and usually the cause of death by the fourth or fifth decades of life.

Early motor development appears to be normal until around the time that the child starts walking, when ataxia is noted. The ataxia progresses until ambulation is impossible, by the beginning of the second decade. Choreoathetosis and dystonia occur in up to 90% of patients, and these motor findings become more prominent with increasing age. Facial weakness leads to the characteristic impassive faces, as well as drooling and dysarthria. Although strength is initially normal, many patients in their 20s and 30s develop progressive spinal muscular atrophy predominantly affecting the hands and feet. Peripheral neuropathy in the form of diminished deep tendon reflexes and loss of large fiber sensation is also seen. Mental function is well-preserved, although deficits in short-term memory can occur in the third and fourth decades.

Oculomotor apraxia is a distinguishing feature of the disease. The apraxia commonly presents before the appearance of conjunctival telangiectasias and is characterized by defects of initiating voluntary saccades, hypometric voluntary saccades accompanied by compensatory eye-blinking and/or head-thrusting movements, and disrupted smooth pursuit movements. Involuntary saccade initiation and optokinetic nystagmus can be impaired as well, and vestibuloocular reflexes can be increased.

TABLE 91-2 Autosomal Recessive Cerebellar Ataxias

Ataxia	Chromosome	Gene	Gene Product	Mechanism	Age of Onset (Years)
Friedreich ataxia	9q13	X25	Frataxin	GAA repeat	2–51
Friedreich ataxia 2	9p23-p11	Unknown	Unknown	Unknown	5–20
Ataxia with vitamin E deficiency	8q13	TTP1	TTPA	Missense mutation, deletion, insertion	2–52
Ataxia-telangiectasia	11q22.3	ATM	ATM	Missense and deletion mutations	Infancy
Ataxia-telangiectasia–like disorder 1 (ATLD1)	11q21	hMRE11	MRE11A	Missense and deletion mutations	9–48 months
Ataxia-telangiectasia–like disorder 2 (ATLD2)	20p12	PCNA	PCNA	Missense mutation	Infancy
Ataxia-ocular apraxia 1 (AOA1)	9p13.3	APTX	Aprataxin	Frameshift, missense, nonsense mutations	2–18
SCAR1 (AOA2)	9q34	SETX	Senataxin	Frameshift, missense, nonsense mutations	9–22
Ataxia-ocular apraxia 3 (AOA3)	17p13.1	PIK3R5	PIK3R5	Missense mutation	14
SCAR2	9q34-qter	Unknown	Unknown	Unknown	Birth
SCAR3	6p23-p21	Unknown	Unknown	Unknown	3–52
SCAR4	1p36	Unknown	Unknown	Unknown	23–39
SCAR5	15q25.3	ZNF592	ZNF592	Missense mutation	1–10
SCAR6	20q11-q13	Unknown	Unknown	Unknown	Infancy
SCAR7	11p15	TPP1	TPP1	Missense mutation	Childhood
SCAR8	11p15	SYNE1	SYNE1	Splice site mutation, nonsense mutations	17–46
COQ10D4 (SCAR9)	1q41	ADCK3	ADCK3	Splice site mutation, missense, nonsense mutations	3–11
SCAR10	3p22	ANO10	ANO10	Missense, nonsense, frameshift mutations	13–35
SCAR11	1q32	SYT14	SYT14	Missense mutation	Childhood
SCAR12	16q	WWOX	WWOX	Missense mutations	Infancy
SCAR13	6q24	GRM1	GRM1	3 bp deletion, Splice site mutation	Infancy
SCAR14	11q13	SPTBN2	SPTBN2	Nonsense mutations	Childhood
SCAR15	3q29	KIAA0226	SCAR15	Frameshift deletion	Infancy–7
SCAR16	16p13	STUB1	STUB1	Missense mutation	Birth–19
SCAR17	10q24	CWF19L1	CWF19L1	Splice site mutation	Birth
Ataxia, Cayman Type	19q13.3	ATCAY	Caytaxin	Missense mutation	Birth
IOSCA (infantile onset spinocerebellar ataxia)	10q24	C10orf2	Twinkle	Missense, silent mutations	9–24 months
Progressive Myoclonic Epilepsy	21q22.3	CST6	Cystatin B	5′ Dodecamer repeat	6–13
Spastic ataxias					
SPAX2	17p13.2	KIF1C	KIF1C	Missense, nonsense mutation, deletion	1–16
SPAX3	2q33.1	MARS2	MARS2	Complex rearrangements	2–59
SPAX4	10p11.23	MTPAP	MTPAP	Missense mutation	Early childhood
SPAX5	18p11	AFG3L2	AFG3L2	Missense mutation	Early childhood–22
ARSACS	13q12	SACS	Sacsin	Frameshift and nonsense mutations	1–20

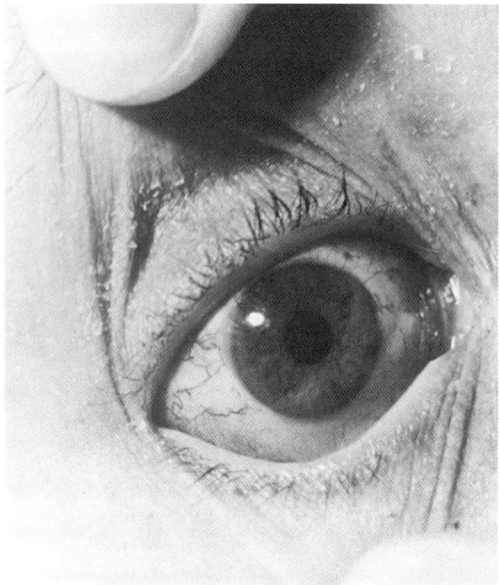

Figure 91-5. Characteristic conjunctival telangiectasis observed in a 12-year-old with ataxia-telangiectasia.

Telangiectasias are usually first observed in patients between the ages of 2 and 4 years, although they can occur as early as birth and as late as 14 years of age (Figure 91-5). In addition to the conjunctivae, they appear on exposed areas of the skin, particularly areas of friction and trauma such as the auricle, nasal bridge, antecubital, and popliteal spaces. Sun exposure enhances their appearance. Premature aging of hair and skin is common, as are skin infections, including chronic blepharitis. Vitiligo and café-au-lait spots can be seen. Rarely, scleroderma-like lesions occur.

Recurrent sinopulmonary infections are common, affecting 90% of patients, and usually result in chronic bronchitis, bronchiectasis, or both. The impairment of cellular immunity is also manifest by abnormally developed or absent adenoids, tonsils, lymphoid tissue, and thymus gland. Patients have impaired delayed hypersensitivity response to skin-sensitizing antigens and a delayed homograft-rejection response. The DNA repair defect puts patients at greater risk than the general population for Hodgkin disease, leukemia, lymphoma, and lymphosarcoma. Other commonly associated neoplasms are brain tumors, gastric adenocarcinomas, ovarian dysgerminomas, gonadoblastomas, cystic adenofibromas, uterine leiomyomas, and thyroid adenomas. Hypogonadism is frequent in both genders, and growth retardation is notable despite normal levels of growth hormone. Insulin-resistant diabetes is also occasionally seen as part of the clinical constellation.

Differential diagnosis. The core triad of ataxia, oculomotor apraxia, and choreoathetosis occurs in several related diseases, usually without the extraneurologic features of AT. One nonclassic presentation of AT includes early onset dystonia. Patients with mild variant forms of classic AT may lack immunodeficiency, telangiectasias, cancer or sinopulmonary infections; these individuals have a later onset and slower progression of neurologic signs, longer lifespans, and somewhat less chromosomal instability and cellular radiosensitivity. Interestingly, atypical AT can be misdiagnosed as FRDA until the natural progression of the disease reveals a greater spectrum of symptoms. *Ataxia-telangiectasia–like disorder 1 (ATLD1; MIM 604391)* patients are almost identical to those with AT except they lack telangiectasias. They do, however, show increased susceptibility to DNA damage because of the underlying defect in DNA repair (the mutated gene, *MRE11*, is part of a complex that senses DNA double-strand breaks and recruits ATM to repair the damage). Approximately 6% of ataxia-telangiectasia patients may in fact have ATLD1. *ATLD2 (MIM 615919)* has been described in several patients from an extended Ohio Amish family with developmental delay, ataxia, and sensorineural hearing loss. Other features include short stature, cutaneous and ocular telangiectasia, and photosensitivity with evidence of predisposition to sun-induced malignancy in one patient. None of the patients had evidence of immunodeficiency. *Early onset ataxia with ocular motor apraxia and hypoalbuminemia (EAOH; also known as ataxia-oculomotor apraxia 1/ AOA1; MIM 208920)* is also clinically similar to AT but without extraneurologic features (see separate entry). *Xeroderma pigmentosum (XP)* and *Cockayne syndrome* (MIM 278760), caused by mutations in the DNA repair factor ERCC4, can also present neurologically, with ataxia, tremor, weakness, nystagmus, and sensorineural hearing loss, though the cutaneous manifestations such as sun sensitivity appear earliest and are very prominent. Interestingly, some XP patients do not develop neurologic signs until midlife.

Laboratory findings. Serum alpha-fetoprotein (AFP) is elevated about 10 ng/mL in greater than 90% of classic AT (but note that serum AFP can remain higher than normal in unaffected children up to around 24 months of age). Carcinoembryonic antigen (CEA) levels are also typically elevated in affected individuals. Most patients have decreased concentrations or absence of immunoglobulin (Ig) A and E; IgM, G1, and G3 concentrations are normal or elevated, and immunoglobulin G2 and G4 concentrations are generally decreased. Although the diagnosis can be made clinically, genetic testing for mutations in the *ATM* gene is recommended, as *ATM* heterozygotes are at an increased risk of cancer.

Treatment. Patients with severe recurrent infections and low IgG levels can receive intravenous Ig; those with chronic bronchiectasis need aggressive pulmonary hygiene. Early and continued physical therapy can minimize contractures and scoliosis. Children must be monitored for early signs of malignancy (bruising, localized pain or swelling, weight loss), but treatment of neoplasms is a delicate proposition because patients are extremely sensitive to radiation and chemotherapy and demonstrate resultant ulcerative dermatitis, severe esophagitis, dysphagia, and deep-tissue necrosis. Conventional doses of cancer therapies are fatal in AT. In fact, patients should avoid exposure to ionizing radiation, such as CT scans. L-DOPA derivatives and anticholinergics may improve basal ganglia dysfunction; amantadine, fluoxetine, or buspirone may help with the loss of balance and impaired speech; tremors can often be controlled by gabapentin, clonazepam, or propanolol (Lavin et al., 2007).

Early Onset Ataxia with Ocular Motor Apraxia and Hypoalbuminemia (Ataxia-Oculomotor Apraxia 1, AOA1—MIM 208920)

EAOH/AOA1 is the most frequent cause of autosomal recessive cerebellar ataxia in Japan, and the second most common cause in Portugal; it accounts for up to 10% of autosomal recessive cerebellar ataxias. Caused by mutations in *ataxin (APTX)*, which is involved in single-strand DNA repair, the disease is clinically similar to AT (see previous section) and should be considered in early onset ataxia when both FRDA and AT have been excluded. A slowly progressive ataxia (mean age of onset 4 years of age; range 2 to 10 years) is followed by dysarthria, upper-limb dysmetria, mild intention tremor, choreoathetosis, and upper limb dystonia. Ocular apraxia typically occurs a few years after symptom onset, progressing to ophthalmoplegia. Areflexia, sensory and motor neuropathy, and retinal/macular lesions seen on fundoscopy are common. Different degrees of cognitive impairment can be observed, but intellect can also be normal. Lifespan is not affected.

Laboratory studies reveal hypoalbuminemia and hypercholesterolemia in the majority of cases as a later manifestation of the disease. An EMG invariably reveals axonal neuropathy. Genetic testing to rule out AT and locate mutations in the gene *APTX* is useful.

Differential diagnosis. A second ataxia-telangiectasia–like disease has been described in families of several different ethnic backgrounds. *Ataxia with Oculomotor Apraxia 2 (AOA2)*, also known as *Spinocerebellar ataxia autosomal recessive 1 (SCAR1)* (MIM 606002), is caused by mutations in the *SETX* gene, which produce gait ataxia, sensory motor neuropathy, and ocular apraxia, the latter occurring about 50% of the time. Although overall cognitive function is normal, subtle changes in executive function can be seen on neuropsychological testing. AOA2 is distinguished from AOA1 by its slightly later age of onset (ages 10 to 22 years), less common ocular apraxia, high levels of serum alpha-fetoprotein (AFP), and normal serum albumin. The functional prognosis is also better in AOA2. Half of the Portuguese families diagnosed with AOA, however, have no mutations in either *APTX* or *SETX* identifiable by mutation scanning; they may have mutations in other genes or mutations not detectable by this method, such as large deletions. Interestingly, other mutations in *SETX* are transmitted in an autosomal dominant manner and cause juvenile amyotrophic lateral sclerosis (ALS4). Some mutations in *APTX* produce an adult-onset ataxia with oculomotor apraxia. Other SCARs (SCAR2 through SCAR17) have each been described in only a handful of individuals in geographically distinct populations (listed in Table 91-2; see online chapter for more information).

Treatment. Muscle coenzyme Q10 (CoQ10) is often low in patients with AOA1, but this deficiency responds to supplementation. Also recommended is a high protein diet to restore serum albumin concentration and prevent edema. It is interesting to note that SCAR9, also known as Coenzyme Q10 Deficiency Primary 4 (COQ10D4—MIM 612016), and SCAR10 also show some clinical improvement with CoQ10 supplementation, suggesting these ataxias involve respiratory chain dysfunction.

Mitocondrial DNA Depletion Syndrome 7 (Hepatocerebral Type) (MTDPS7—MIM 271245); Infantile Onset Spinocerebellar Ataxia

MTDPS7, previously known as infantile onset spinocerebellar ataxia (IOSCA) is the second most common inherited ataxia in Finland, with a population carrier frequency of more than 1 in every 230. That said, it has been described only in Finland, and only a few dozen cases have been thoroughly reported. It is characterized by hypotonia, ophthalmoplegia, sudden onset hearing loss, seizures, and sensory axonal neuropathy. Dysfunction starts usually within the first 2 years of life with clumsiness and difficulty walking or loss of the ability to walk; athetosis, ataxia, ophthalmoplegia, and hearing loss appear by school age, with sensory axonal neuropathy appearing by adolescence. Refractory epilepsy can occur early or late and is the predominant cause of death.

Differential diagnosis. IOSCA disease results from a recessive mutation in C10Orf2 encoding Twinkle (Y508C), a mitochondrial deoxyribonucleic acid (mtDNA)-specific helicase. Different mutations in this same gene cause *autosomal dominant progressive external ophthalmoplegia (adPEO)* with multiple mtDNA deletions (MIM 606075), a neuromuscular disorder

sharing a spectrum of symptoms with MTDPS7. *Progressive myoclonic epilepsy* (MIM 254800) was first described in families from Estonia and eastern Sweden, but Finland has a greater number of affected individuals. The disease typically presents with generalized tonic-clonic seizures and myoclonus, with ataxia seen later in the course. *Ramsay Hunt syndrome* is actually a heterogeneous group of disorders whose clinical hallmarks are progressive ataxia and myoclonus. The presentation, age of onset, and severity are variable, and the differential diagnoses includes *myoclonic epilepsy associated with ragged red fibers* (*MERFF*, MIM 545000) and *sialidosis* (MIM 256550), which are described elsewhere in this text.

Other early onset ataxias that affect the eyes and ears include *Behr syndrome* (MIM 210000), which is an optic atrophy beginning in childhood, in conjunction with ataxia, spasticity, and mental retardation. *Marinesco-Sjögren syndrome* (MIM 248800) is characterized by cataracts, ataxia, myopathy, varying degrees of mental retardation, and short stature.

Autosomal Dominant Inherited Ataxias (Spinocerebellar Ataxias)

The dominantly inherited spinocerebellar ataxias (Table 91-3) are a group of conditions characterized by premature cerebellar neuronal loss, with some types involving additional structures such as the optic nerve, basal ganglia, brainstem, and spinal cord. When the onset is in adulthood, as is typical, the patient may first notice difficulty turning corners or decrements in acquired fine motor control skills, such as those used in sport. Despite the rather circumscribed pathology, these disorders are surprisingly heterogeneous: patients with SCA display various clinical features of progressive ataxia, motor impairment, extrapyramidal symptoms, retinal degeneration, deafness, ophthalmoplegia, dorsal column dysfunction, and peripheral neuropathy. The overall incidence of SCA is 1 to 5 in every 100,000, with an average age of onset in the fourth decade of life.

We should note that the SCAs were earlier designated the *olivopontocerebellar atrophies* (OPCAs) because of the frequent presence of atrophy involving the cerebellum and the pontine and olivary nuclei. They have also been known as autosomal dominant cerebellar ataxias (ADCAs), primarily because of the Harding classification system, which attempted to categorize these disorders by constellation of clinical signs. Type I ADCAs have a cerebellar syndrome plus pyramidal signs, supranuclear ophthalmoplegia, extrapyramidal signs, and dementia. Type II ADCAs show a cerebellar syndrome plus pigmentary maculopathy. Type III ADCAs are "pure" cerebellar syndromes that have mild, if any, pyramidal symptoms (Harding, 1993). Some authors have attempted to keep these clinical categories and assign genetically defined SCAs to them, but the clinical findings are so variable that they are unreliable for precise diagnosis.

Genetic studies over the last 25 years have confirmed that genetic heterogeneity underlies the complex clinical picture (Table 91-3). It is worth noting that a number of these ataxias appear to result from a common mutational mechanism: expansion of a repeat tract, usually a trinucleotide repeat, within the disease-causing gene. The expanded repeats, whether in the coding or noncoding region of the disease gene, are known as *dynamic mutations* because they show repeat instability, with a tendency to expand in germline transmission. Repeat expansions that occur in the noncoding region of the gene underlie Friedreich ataxia (discussed previously) and spinocerebellar ataxias 8 and 12 (Dick et al., 2006). Interestingly, two diseases that share this mutational mechanism, fragile X syndrome and myotonic dystrophy, are not characterized by ataxia—but fragile X syndrome is related

TABLE 91-3 Molecular Genetics and Salient Features of Autosomal Dominant Cerebellar Ataxias

Ataxia	Chromosome	Gene	Gene Product	Mechanism	Age of Onset (Years)	Normal Repeat	Expanded Repeat	Core Features in Addition to Ataxia
POLYQ EXPANSION								
SCA1	6p23	SCA1	Ataxin-1	CAG repeat	6–60	6–44*	39–82*	Ophthalmoparesis, pyramidal and extrapyramidal signs
SCA2	12q24	SCA2	Ataxin-2	CAG repeat	2–65	15–24	35–59	Slow saccades, peripheral neuropathy
SCA3/MJD	14q32.12	ATXN3	Ataxin-3	CAG repeat	11–70	13–47*	45–84*	ophthalmoparesis, pyramidal, extrapyramidal, and amyotrophic signs
SCA6	19q13	CACNA1A	Cav2.1	CAG repeat	16–73	4–20	21–33	Dysarthria, nystagmus, occasional mild proprioceptive deficit
SCA7	3p14.1	SCA7	Ataxin-7	CAG repeat	Birth-53	4–35	37–460	Ophthalmoparesis, retinopathy, pyramidal signs, dementia
SCA17	6q27	SCA17	TBP	CAG repeat	3–48	25–42	45–66	Gait ataxia, extrapyramidal signs, dementia
DRPLA	12p13.31	DRPLA	Atrophin-1	CAG repeat	4–55	7–34	53–93	Choreoathetosis, dystonia, seizures, myoclonus, dementia
NONCODING EXPANSION								
SCA8	13q21	SCA8	SCA8 RNA	CTG repeat in 3' UTR	18–72	2–91*	110–1300*	Gait ataxia, dysarthria, nystagmus, spasticity
SCA10	22q13	SCA10	Ataxin-10	ATTCT repeat in intron 9	14–45	10–29	750–4500	Gait ataxia, dysarthria, nystagmus, spasticity, seizures, neuropathy
SCA12	5q32	SCA12	P2R2B	CAG repeat in 5' UTR	8–55	7–32	51–78	Tremor, dysarthria, hyperreflexia, sometimes dystonia, late dementia
SCA31	16q22.1	BEAN/TK2	BEAN/TK2	TGGAA repeat insertion in intron of BEAN and TK	45–72	Rarely (0.23%) 1.5–2.0 kb	2.5–3.8 kb	Decreased muscle tone, horizontal nystagmus
SCA36	20p13	NOP56	NOP56	GGCCTG repeat in intron 1	>50	4–14	650–2500, rarely short repeats of 25–31	Slowly progressive gait ataxia, ocular abnormalities, upper motor neuron signs, some develop hearing loss
OTHER MUTATIONS								
SCA5	11q13.2	SPTBN2	β-3 spectrin	Deletion, missense mutations	10–68			Pure, slowly progressive cerebellar syndrome (ataxia, dysarthria)
SCA11	15q15.2	TTBK2	TTBK2	Truncation mutation	15–43			Mild, slowly progressive gait and limb ataxia
SCA13	19q13.33	KCNC3	KCNC3	Missense mutations	<1–60			Early onset: motor delay, mental retardation, hyperreflexia
SCA14	19q13.4	PKC-γ	PKC-γ	Missense mutation	0–69			Facial myokymia, hyperreflexia, dystonia, myoclonus; late-onset cases are more pure cerebellar ataxia
SCA15	3p26.1	ITPR1	ITPR1	Deletion, missense mutation	Child-Adult			Slowly progressive pure cerebellar syndrome
SCA16	-	-	-	-				Early reports now merged with SCA15; SCA16 considered "vacant"

TABLE 91-3 Molecular Genetics and Salient Features of Autosomal Dominant Cerebellar Ataxias *(Continued)*

Ataxia	Chromosome	Gene	Gene Product	Mechanism	Age of Onset (Years)	Normal Repeat	Expanded Repeat	Core Features in Addition to Ataxia
SCA19/22	1p13.2	KCND3	KCND3	Missense mutations	10–45			Cognitive impairment, postural tremor, myoclonus in Dutch family; pure cerebellar syndrome in Chinese kindred
SCA20	11q12	260kb duplication	Multiple genes	Duplication	19–64			Palatal tremor, dysphonia; dentate calcification on computed tomography
SCA21	1p36.33	TMEM240	TMEM240	Truncation, missense mutations	6–30			Extrapyramidal signs, severe cognitive impairment
SCA23	20p13	PDYN	PDYN	Missense mutations	43–56			Slowly progressive gait and limb ataxia, hyperreflexia
SCA26	19p13.3	EEF2	EEF2	Missense mutation	26–60			Slowly progressive pure cerebellar syndrome
SCA27	13q34	FGF14	FGF14	Fibroblast growth factor deficiency	5–20			Early onset hand tremor, dyskinesia, slowly progressive ataxia; psychiatric symptoms, cognitive deficits
SCA28	18p11.21	AFG3L2	AFG3L2	Missense mutations	12–36			Slowly progressive; dysarthria, lower limb hyperreflexia
SCA29	3p26.1	ITPR1	ITPR1	Missense mutation	Infant			Motor and mild cognitive delay; very slowly progressive or nonprogressive gait ataxia
SCA34	6q14.1	ELOVL4	ELOVL4	Missense mutation	Early skin lesions, late ataxia			Skin lesions appear after birth, disappear by age 25, then reappear in middle age along with ataxia and decreased tendon reflexes
SCA35	20p13	TGM6	TGM6	Missense mutations	40–48			Gait affected first; upper limbs later; hyperreflexia, tremor, torticollis, ocular dysmetria
SCA38	6p12.1	ELOVL5	ELOVL5	Missense mutations	34–51			Nystagmus, slow saccades
SCA40	14q32.11	CCDC88C	CCDC88C	Missense mutations	42–43			Ocular dysmetria, intention tremor, dysdiadochokinesia, hyper-reflexia
MUTATION UNKNOWN								
SCA4	16q22	Unknown	Unknown	Unknown	19–59			Sensory axonal neuropathy and pyramidal signs
SCA18/SMNA	7q31-q32	Unknown	Unknown	Unknown	12–25			Peripheral neuropathy
SCA25	2p	Unknown	Unknown	Unknown	1.5–39			Severe sensory neuropathy, gastrointestinal symptoms
SCA30	4q34.3-q35.1	Unknown	Unknown	Unknown	45–76			Slowly progressive pure cerebellar syndrome
SCA32	7q32-q33	Unknown	Unknown	Unknown	Broad range of age at onset			Cognitive impairment, infertility
SCA37	1p32	Unknown	Unknown	Unknown	38–64			Dysmetric vertical saccades, some nystagmus

to an ataxia. Whereas the full-blown CGG expansion in the *FMR1* gene that causes fragile X silences the gene, subtle "premutation" expansions cause a late-onset, progressive ataxia with tremor (and sometimes cognitive impairment) known as *Fragile X-associated Tremor/Ataxia Syndrome (FXTAS;* MIM 309550) that occurs in older relatives of children with fragile X. Interestingly, the small expansions characteristic of premutations do not silence the *FMR1* gene, but rather cause a dominant toxic effect at the RNA level. FXTAS could easily be mistaken for a late-onset SCA, though it is usually misdiagnosed either as essential tremor, Parkinson disease, or as Alzheimer disease when it involves dementia. Regardless, different repeat expansions in the same gene can produce dramatically different phenotypes.

There is a particular subclass of repeat diseases caused by a CAG repeat expansion in the coding region of the respective disease genes, where it produces an expanded polyglutamine tract in the resultant protein that encodes for the amino acid glutamine (Zoghbi and Orr, 2000). These "polyglutamine diseases" consist of dentatorubropallidoluysian atrophy (DRPLA), spinocerebellar ataxias (SCAs) 1, 2, 3, 6 and 7, Huntington disease (HD), and spinobulbar muscular atrophy (SBMA). SBMA and HD are not spinocerebellar syndromes, although some patients with HD can present with ataxia. The polyglutamine expansion is usually a few repeats, but this is enough to cause earlier onset ("anticipation") and a progressively more severe phenotype in each subsequent generation. Here, then, is the reason this group of diseases is so clinically heterogeneous. The longer the polyglutamine protein, the greater the neural toxicity, and the greater the number of brain regions that succumb to it (Riess et al., 2008). It is not clear why the threshold for vulnerability to toxicity differs across brain regions, but the cerebellum seems to be especially sensitive in this regard.

One consequence of the dynamic nature of these mutations is that family history can be deceiving. An older relative might develop a slight ataxia at the same time a grandchild is developing changes in mood or behavior and losing vision. Often, older relatives have died before developing clear phenotypes or are misdiagnosed with conditions related to advanced age. The difficulty is most extreme with infantile onset cases, which often look nothing like the adult-onset disease. Adult SCA2, for example, begins with ataxia, but one case of infantile onset SCA2 has been reported to cause apneic episodes and frequent vomiting in the perinatal period progressing to hypotonia, severe developmental delay, blindness, and death by 2 years of age. As mentioned previously, juvenile cases often show pathology in neural tissues quite distinct from those affected by the adult-onset disorders; the retina is neural tissue that appears to have a higher threshold for damage from polyglutamine toxicity than many other brain tissues. In this regard, it is interesting to note that in SCA7 patients with more than 59 repeats, visual impairment is the most common presenting symptom; in individuals with pathologic repeats of less than 59, the presenting symptom is ataxia. This supports the notion that larger expansions are required to elicit ocular symptoms, although there is yet no mechanistic explanation.

In short, the clinical phenotypes of the SCAs are so variable that one cannot reliably diagnose a particular case on clinical grounds alone. This holds even for the SCAs that are caused by nonrepeat mutations, such as SCA5, 13, 14, and 27. Genetic testing has simplified matters in many cases, and Table 91-3 provides a snapshot of the various SCAs and DRPLA according to genotype. These features should help the clinician prioritize gene testing, which is commercially available for the most common SCAs (in fact, screening for SCAs 1, 2, 3, and 6 should identify 50% of familial cases). The curious reader is encouraged to consult the online version of this chapter and other references for a more thorough account.

Episodic Ataxias

There are currently eight episodic ataxias, all of which are rare dominant disorders (see online chapter). They tend to have early onset; the frequency and duration of attacks varies widely, as do the features (Jen et al., 2007). The episodic ataxias (EAs) are summarized in Table 91-4.

TABLE 91-4 The Episodic Ataxias

Episodic Ataxia	Chromosome	Gene	Gene Product	Mechanism	Age of Onset (Years)	Duration of Episodes, Frequency	Features
EA1	12p13	EA1	KCNA1	Channelopathy	Early childhood	Seconds to minutes can be several per day	Ataxia, triggered by exercise, fever, stress, sudden motion
EA2/FHM	19p13	CACNA1A	Cav2.1	Channelopathy: missense and nonsense mutations, deletion	4–30	Minutes to days	Ataxia, migraine, ocular features; interictal nystagmus, ataxia, epilepsy. Responds to acetazolamide
EA3	1q42	Unknown	Unknown	Unknown	1–42	1 min to 6 hours	Vertigo, imbalance, tinnitus, diplopia. Responds to acetazolamide
EA4	Unknown	Unknown	Unknown	Unknown	23–42	Short, can evolve to constant	Vertigo, nausea, tinnitus, horizontal nystagmus, oscillopsia; triggered by sense of visual motion
EA5	2q22-q23	CACNB4	CACNB4	Channelopathy: missense and nonsense mutations	Juvenile	Hours	Ataxia; same mutation in German kindred-produced general epilepsy without ataxia

TABLE 91-4 The Episodic Ataxias *(Continued)*

Episodic Ataxia	Chromosome	Gene	Gene Product	Mechanism	Age of Onset (Years)	Duration of Episodes, Frequency	Features
EA6	5p13	SLC1A3	EAAT1	Missense mutation	5	Hours to days	Progressive ataxia, seizures, hemiplegia
EA7	19q13	Unknown	Unknown	Unknown	<20	Hours to days; once a month to once a year	Weakness, dysarthria
EA8	1p36-p34	Unknown	Unknown	Unknown	2	Minutes to hours; twice a day to twice a month	Ataxia, weakness, dysarthria, persistent intention tremor

TABLE 91-5 The Hereditary Spastic Ataxias

Spastic Ataxia (MIM#)	Gene	Mode of Inheritance	Age of Onset (Years)	Features
SPAX1 (108600)	VAMP1		10–20 yrs	Progressive leg spasticity, dysarthria, ocular movement abnormalities
SPAX2 (611302)	KIF1C		1–16 yrs	Frequent falls, ataxia, head tremor, hyperreflexia, fasciculations
SPAX3/ARSAL (611390)	MARS2	AR	2–59 yrs; mean 15 yrs	Ataxia and spasticity
SPAX4 (613672)	MTPAP	AR	Early childhood	Ataxia, spastic paraparesis, dysarthria, optic atrophy, upper limb hypertonia
SPAX5 (614487)	AFG3L2	AR	Childhood	Spasticity, ataxia, oculomotor apraxia, dystonia, myoclonic epilepsy
SPAX6/SACS/ARCSACS (270660)	SACS	AR	Childhood	Spasticity and ataxia, very slow course, stops progressing after age 20
SPAX7	Unknown	AD	Infancy–20	Symmetric ataxia, dysarthria, pyramidal signs, optic atrophy
SPAR (607565)	Unknown	-	15–35	Later onset: spastic paraplegia early onset: + ataxia, mental retardation

Hereditary Spastic Ataxias

The hereditary spastic ataxias are a heterogeneous group of disorders that combine the features of hereditary spastic paralysis and spinocerebellar ataxia (see online chapter). They typically present first with lower limb spasticity followed by ataxia, dysarthria, impaired ocular movements, and gait disturbance (Table 91-5).

X-LINKED SPINOCEREBELLAR ATAXIAS

Besides Fragile X-associated ataxia syndrome (FXTAS, noted previously), several very rare X-linked ataxias have been described based on the pattern of inheritance in specific kindreds. No genetic localization has yet been established for any of them. The reader is referred to the online version of this chapter for brief descriptions and relevant references.

MANAGEMENT OF CEREBELLAR DYSFUNCTION AND ATAXIA

When ataxia is the result of certain metabolic disorders or toxins, trauma, or neoplasia, specific therapies for the underlying condition can be curative (Table 91-1). Direct neurologic causes of ataxia, however, such as inherited diseases, are for the most part not yet amenable to treatment. The only therapies at present that have proven beneficial to patients, though far from curative, are acetazolamide for certain episodic ataxias (Table 91-4), vitamin E, and coenzyme CoQ10 for the respective deficiencies. The array of genes involved makes the notion

of developing specific therapies for each of these very rare diseases rather daunting, yet ongoing research has turned up promising avenues for therapeutic development, especially for the polyglutamine diseases. The advent of high-throughput screening approaches in cellular and invertebrate models of these diseases is facilitating the search for compounds that reduce polyglutamine toxicity.

In the meantime, it is important to remember that patients benefit from physical and occupational therapy and all the supportive forces that promote health and happiness in any of us; though these approaches will not restore mobility in advanced disease, they nonetheless alleviate other symptoms such as spasticity and greatly improve quality of life.

REFERENCES

The complete list of references for this chapter is available in the e-book at www.expertconsult.com.
 See inside cover for registration details.

SELECTED REFERENCES

Brigatti, K.W., Deutsch, E.C., Lynch, D.R., et al., 2012. Novel diagnostic paradigms for Friedreich ataxia. J. Child Neurol. 27 (9), 1146–1151.

Di Prospero, N.A., Baker, A., Jeffries, N., et al., 2007. Neurological effects of high-dose idebenone in patients with Friedreich's ataxia: a randomised, placebo-controlled trial. Lancet Neurol. 6 (10), 878–886.

Dick, K.A., Margolis, J.M., Day, J.W., et al., 2006. Dominant non-coding repeat expansions in human disease. Genome Dyn. 1, 67–83.

Harding, A.E., 1993. Clinical features and classification of inherited ataxias. Adv. Neurol. 61, 1–14.

Ito, M., 2002. Historical review of the significance of the cerebellum and the role of Purkinje cells in motor learning. Ann. N. Y. Acad. Sci. 978, 273–288.

Jen, J.C., Graves, T.D., Hess, E.J., et al., 2007. Primary episodic ataxias: diagnosis, pathogenesis and treatment. Brain 130 (Pt 10), 2484–2493.

Lavin, M.F., Gueven, N., Bottle, S., et al., 2007. Current and potential therapeutic strategies for the treatment of ataxia-telangiectasia. Br. Med. Bull. 81–82, 129–147.

Manni, E., Petrosini, L., 2004. A century of cerebellar somatotopy: a debated representation. Nat. Rev. Neurosci. 5 (3), 241–249.

Riess, O., Rub, U., Pastore, A., et al., 2008. SCA3: neurological features, pathogenesis and animal models. Cerebellum 7 (2), 125–137.

Zoghbi, H.Y., Orr, H.T., 2000. Glutamine repeats and neurodegeneration. Annu. Rev. Neurosci. 23, 217–247.

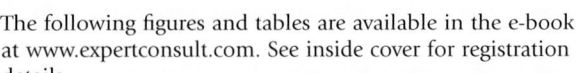

E-BOOK FIGURES AND TABLES

The following figures and tables are available in the e-book at www.expertconsult.com. See inside cover for registration details.

Fig. 91-1 Dorsal view of the human cerebellum.

Fig. 91-2 Major cell types of the cerebellar cortex.

Fig. 91-3 Denver–II Sensorimotor representation in the human cerebellar cortex based on fMRI data.

Fig. 91-4 Friedreich ataxia and moderate scoliosis in a 13-year-old boy who is unable to walk independently.

92 Acute Cerebellar Ataxia

Harry T. Whelan, Gregory S. Aaen, Kumar Sannagowdara, and Megan B. DeMara-Hoth

An expanded version of this chapter is available on www.expertconsult.com. See inside cover for registration details.

The term "cerebellum" is from Latin, meaning "the little brain." It is a part of the hindbrain situated in the posterior cranial fossa. The cerebellum is organized into different regions with specialized functions. The cerebellum integrates massive sensory information from many regions of the brain and spinal cord. This information is used by the cerebellum to smoothly coordinate ongoing movements and to participate in motor planning. Detailed anatomy and physiology of the cerebellum and its pathways are discussed in Chapter 91.

Acute cerebellar ataxia refers to a group of acquired disorders that result in acute dysfunction of the cerebellum. These conditions are usually associated with either intoxication or inflammation of the cerebellum from infectious, postinfectious, or paraneoplastic processes. The cerebellum regulates the coordination of movement, muscle tone, and motor control. The word "ataxia" is derived from the Greek word *ataktos*, which means "lack of order." Acute ataxia is defined as an unsteadiness of walking, coordination, or fine motor movement with duration greater than 72 hours. Acute cerebellar ataxia is the most common cause of childhood ataxia, accounting for about 30% to 50% of all cases, in children less than 6 years of age.

CLINICAL EVALUATION OF ACUTE ATAXIA

Acute cerebellar ataxia typically presents with rapidly progressive symptoms evolving over a few hours but at most over 1 to 2 days. In cases associated with a prodromal illness, the onset of ataxia is usually within 1 to 3 weeks after the onset of the prodromal illness. Although a gait disturbance is the primary or only symptom in most patients, in other patients, a wide range of clinical signs of cerebellar dysfunction could be observed (Box 92-1).

Evaluating a pediatric patient presenting with acute ataxia begins with obtaining a detailed history of the presenting illness, including the onset, timing, and progression of symptoms. This process could be a key component for excluding serious etiologies (Ryan and Engle, 2003). The most commonly reported causes of childhood ataxia include postinfectious, toxin ingestion, and Guillain–Barré syndrome (GBS). A history of fever, antecedent respiratory and gastrointestinal infections, and varicella and Epstein–Barr virus infections are commonly reported in postinfection-mediated cerebellar ataxia. A history of recent vaccinations or an exposure to toxins, alcohol, drugs, or household medications and chemicals commonly provides information suggesting a specific diagnosis. A family or personal history of recurrent ataxic episodes, seizures, or migraine headaches may propose a metabolic or genetic disorder. Recent head or neck trauma can present with ataxia and may be because of vertebrobasilar dissection or intracranial bleeding.

Signs of cerebellar dysfunction (see Video 92-1) could be categorized into the following groups: (1) speech deficits, (2) oculomotor disturbances, (3) limb ataxia, (4) deficits of posture and gait, and (5) cognitive disturbances (Pandolfo and Manto, 2013).

Physical examination may be challenging in significantly ataxic children, especially in cases of altered responsiveness.

Children with postinfectious cerebellar ataxia are normally alert and interactive. Abruptly altered responsiveness suggests toxic ingestion or a severe central nervous system (CNS) disturbance, such as stroke or an acute disseminated encephalomyelitis (ADEM). Therefore it is essential to differentiate poor coordination from weakness. Physical examination should focus on identifying life-threatening conditions that may require immediate intervention. Symptoms such as confusion, hallucinations, or somnolence may indicate toxin ingestion, demyelinating diseases, stroke, or meningoencephalitis (Sivaswamy, 2014). Signs of elevated intracranial pressure such as papilledema should be excluded. Motor examination should focus on eliciting weakness as younger children with hemiparesis or paraparesis may present with ataxia (i.e., "paretic ataxia"). A detailed cerebellar examination should evaluate different components of cerebellar dysfunction. Ataxia caused by pathology of the cerebellum is present even with eyes open and is not or only minimally exacerbated by eye closure; therefore, a Romberg test will be negative. Sensory examination and an examination of deep tendon reflexes should be performed to evaluate peripheral nerves or roots, dysfunction of which may result in a "sensory" ataxia.

Acute cerebellitis presents with a wide range of symptoms varying from subtle gait abnormality to more fulminant forms involving truncal instability, head titubation, intention tremor, dysmetria, and nystagmus. Physical examination may possibly reveal fever or meningismus, which can be indicative of a CNS infection. Pharyngitis, lymphadenopathy, and splenomegaly occur in Epstein–Barr virus infection. Otoscopic and skin (viral exanthema) examination may be useful. In addition, ataxia is a common feature of acute postinfectious demyelinating encephalopathy. Brainstem encephalitis can involve the inflow and outflow tracts of the cerebellum, resulting in ataxia (Ryan and Engle, 2003).

CAUSES OF ACUTE CEREBELLAR ATAXIA

The most common causes of acute cerebellar ataxia are inflammatory cerebellitis and toxin ingestion. Together they constitute nearly 80% of the cases of childhood ataxia (Ryan and Engle, 2003). Other common causes of childhood ataxia are listed in Box 92-2 and discussed in this section.

Inflammatory Cerebellitis
Infectious/Postinfectious

Acute cerebellar ataxia most commonly results either from postinfectious autoimmune-mediated cerebellar inflammation or as a result of direct infection of the cerebellum. This accounts for about 30% to 40% of all cases. A history of antecedent illness 1 to 3 weeks before presentation is obtained in about 70% of patients (Ryan and Engle, 2003). Numerous infectious agents have been implicated (Table 92-1), with varicella being the most common organism associated with cerebellar inflammation (Bozzola et al., 2014). Cerebellar dysfunction can occur before the eruption of the exanthem. When direct infection of cerebellar parenchyma

BOX 92-2 Causes of Acute Cerebellar Ataxia

INFLAMMATORY
- Infectious cerebellitis
- Postinfectious cerebellitis
- Brainstem encephalitis
- Acute disseminated encephalomyelitis
- Multiple sclerosis
- Vasculitis
- Paraneoplastic disorders
- Miller Fisher variant of Guillain–Barré syndrome

INTOXICATION
- Alcohol
- Drugs

BRAIN SPACE OCCUPYING/MASS LESIONS
- Tumors
- Abscesses

VASCULAR
- Vertebrobasilar dissection
- Thromboembolism

CNS TRAUMA
- Contusion
- Hemorrhage
- Postconcussion syndrome

MISCELLANEOUS
- Labyrinthitis
- Basilar migraine
- Benign paroxysmal vertigo
- Epilepsy (nonconvulsive status, minor motor status)

TABLE 92-1 Reported Causes of Infectious/Postinfectious Cerebellitis in Childhood

Direct Infection	Infections Associated with Post- or Parainfectious Cerebellitis	Systemic Infections
• Bacterial meningitis (pneumococcal, meningococcal) • Coxsackie B* • Echovirus type 9 • Varicellar zoster	• Coxsackie A • Echovirus type 6 • Enterovirus type 71 • Epstein–Barr virus* • Hepatitis A • Herpes simplex virus I • Influenza A and B • Japanese B encephalitis • Legionella pneumophila • Malaria • Measles • Mumps • Mycoplasma pneumoniae* • Parvovirus B19 • Poliovirus type 1 • Varicellar zoster*	• Diphtheria • Leptospirosis • Mycoplasma pneumoniae • Scarlet fever • Typhoid fever

*Most commonly reported.

occurs, postinfectious cerebellitis is felt to represent the majority of cases.

Demyelinating

ADEM and multiple sclerosis (MS) are acquired inflammatory demyelinating diseases of the CNS white matter that can involve the cerebellum. ADEM is typically a monophasic condition that usually occurs after a preceding infection. Patients present acutely with multifocal neurologic deficits invariably including encephalopathy. The cerebellum is involved in about half of all cases. Magnetic resonance imaging (MRI) often reveals large, confluent multifocal white matter lesions of the cerebral and cerebellar hemispheres.

MS is a recurrent demyelinating disorder of the CNS that often involves the cerebellum and spinal cord. Approximately 5% of all patients with MS have their first attack before age 18. Cerebellar involvement at MS disease onset is more common in children compared with adults.

Neuromyelitis optica (NMO) is a recurrent demyelinating condition caused by antibodies to aquaporin 4 water channels on astrocytic foot processes. These channels are concentrated in the lining of the cerebrospinal fluid aqueductal system. Given the proximity of the fourth ventricle to the cerebellum, children with aquaporin 4 autoantibodies often have episodic ataxia (EA). Unlike ADEM and MS, Neuromyelitis optica (NMO) relapses are more likely to result in permanent disability.

The Miller Fisher variant of GBS is another inflammatory cause of acute ataxia consisting of ataxia, areflexia, and ophthalmoparesis. These may occur in up to 10% of all children with GBS. It is associated with antibodies to the gangliosides GQ1b, GD3, and GT1a (van Doorn et al., 2008).

Paraneoplastic

The presence of malignancy frequently triggers a complex immunologic response in the affected individual, including activation of cell-mediated and humoral immune systems. As part of the normal humoral response to malignancy, antibodies that cross-react with normal CNS antigens can be produced. Opsoclonus-myoclonus ataxia syndrome (OMAS) is a rare paraneoplastic condition that is associated with neuroblastoma. The condition typically affects toddlers between age 1 and 3 years. It presents with acute onset of ataxia, behavioral disturbance, rapid chaotic movements of the eyes (opsoclonus), and myoclonic jerking of the limbs, leading to common description of the condition as "dancing eye, dancing feet syndrome." This was initially described as "Kinsbourne encephalitis." Ataxia may be the only initial symptom leading to an initial diagnosis of an acute cerebellar ataxia. With time, opsoclonus and myoclonus become prominent. Early behavioral disturbances in a child with acute ataxia should raise suspicion for OMAS. Although the condition is felt to be immune-mediated, no specific antibody has been identified. However, a number of studies have identified autoantibodies to CNS antigens in patients with OMAS. The most commonly reported target is to the cerebellar Purkinje cells. However, anti-Hu antibodies, usually associated with small-cell lung cancers in adults, have also been reported. Neuroblastoma underlies more than half of all cases of OMAS, but only 2% to 3% of patients with neuroblastoma develop OMAS. Detecting the presence of neuroblastoma requires CT or MRI, bone and metaiodobenzylguanidine (MIBG) scans, bone marrow testing, urine catecholamine measurements, and other studies. Studies report strong diagnostic yields of ^{131}I MIBG scintigraphy ranging from 70% to 92% in detecting the primary tumor. Ataxia has also been described as a paraneoplastic phenomenon in isolated pediatric cases of Hodgkin disease, Langerhans cell histiocytosis, and hepatoblastoma.

BOX 92-3 Reported Toxicology Screening for Acute Ataxia

- Alprazolam
- Triazolam and temazepam
- Diazepam and lorazepam
- Benzodiazepine
- Phenytoin
- Phenobarbitone
- Carbamazepine
- Phenothiazine

Intoxication

Accidental poisoning in children aged less than 6 years is the most common form of toxin ingestion. Ataxia may be seen with ingestion of lead, alcohol, anticonvulsants, benzodiazepines, antihistamines, organic chemicals, or heavy metals. A retrospective study reports that 32.5% of acute ataxia in children is caused by ingestion regardless of whether a history of toxin exposure is elicited (Gieron-Korthals et al., 1994). Agents responsible for positive screening are listed in Box 92-3 (Whelan et al., 2013). Several studies have reported benzodiazepines as a common cause of ataxia. Isopropanol (found in rubbing alcohol) ingestion has been reported to cause ataxia in 5% of 91 children younger than 6 years of age. Clinical evidence of toxicity typically develops between 0.5 and 2 hours postingestion.

Mass Lesions

Posterior fossa tumors, including medulloblastoma, pilocytic astrocytoma, and ependymoma, account for approximately 50% of all childhood brain tumors. These usually present with a slowly progressive ataxia and symptoms of increased intracranial pressure such as headache, vision disturbances, and focal deficits on neurologic examination. Cerebellar abscess is an uncommon cause of acute ataxia as symptoms usually develop slowly over a period of days and weeks. Nevertheless, the sudden hemorrhage into a posterior fossa tumor with resultant acute ataxia may be the first evidence of malignancy.

Trauma

Isolated acute ataxia is uncommon from blunt force trauma. Cerebellar contusion or posterior fossa bleeds can cause ataxia, which can be associated with headache. This may be caused by direct axonal injury or because of mass effect.

Vascular

Posterior circulation strokes, although rare in children, can present with acute ataxia. This possibility should be considered especially in children predisposed to thromboembolic disease. Arteriovenous malformations with hemorrhage and traumatic vertebral artery dissection can present with acute ataxia. Cerebral angiography identifies an abnormality mostly in the V2 segment (C1 to C6) of the vertebral artery in dissection.

Metabolic/Genetic

Many inborn errors of metabolism can present with ataxia, which can develop acutely or intermittently because of triggered decompensation (see Table 92-2). The first presentation of such disorders in childhood can mimic an acute cerebellar ataxia. Several inborn errors of metabolism can present with ataxia as an early, prominent symptom. Some examples include glucose transporter-1 deficiency syndrome, pyruvate dehydrogenase deficiency, and biotinidase deficiency. Furthermore, disorders affecting mitochondrial function are also well known to have ataxia as an early and prominent symptom. A recent study found that specific risk factors were helpful in differentiating acquired (i.e., noninherited) from inherited etiologies of subacute or chronic childhood ataxia (Benini et al., 2012). These risk factors included (1) duration of symptoms greater than 2 weeks; (2) consanguinity; (3) a first-degree relative with similar presentation; (4) presenting symptoms of abnormal gait, rash, ichthyosis, or multiorgan abnormalities; and (5) an abnormal examination finding of motor function (gait, tone, strength), deep tendon reflexes, and clonus, dysmetria, pes cavus, or sensory deficits. The presence of these risk factors suggested a greater likelihood of a genetic or metabolic disorder that frequently could be determined by specific testing, including mitochondrial DNA testing, chromosomal microarray, serum lactate, pyruvate, carnitine, acylcarnitine, vitamin E and amino acid determinations, urine organic acid screening, and testing for fragile X syndrome. For more information on hereditary ataxias, see Chapter 91.

Recurrent genetic ataxias (EA type 1 [EA1] to EA7) may mimic acute cerebellar ataxia at first presentation. However, recurrent episodes, a favorable response to acetazolamide, and typical clinical features (see Chapter 91) distinguish these disorders from acute cerebellar ataxia. EA1 (KCN1A) and EA2 (CACNA1A) account for the majority of cases.

Other Neurologic Disorders

Ataxia is common in basilar migraine, in which it can be associated with vertigo and focal neurologic deficits. Focal causes of cerebellar dysfunction have to be ruled out, although positive visual phenomena strongly suggest the migrainous nature of the episode.

Benign paroxysmal vertigo is thought to be a migraine equivalent and is more common than benign paroxysmal positional vertigo, which can also present as acute ataxia. Detailed event description, family history, and the Dix–Hallpike maneuver could be revealing.

Ataxia can be prominent during the ictal or postictal phases of seizures and in nonconvulsive seizures. Glutamic acid decarboxylase (GAD) antibody (GAD-ab) has been implicated in a spectrum of neurologic syndromes. However, there is insufficient presently data regarding the role of GAD-ab in childhood acute ataxia. The role of antimyelin-associated glycoprotein, glutamate receptor delta-2 autoantibody, and post-varicella anticentrosomal antibodies in acute ataxia remains to be clearly delineated.

Sensory ataxia results from loss of sensory input to the cerebellum owing to lesions in the posterior column of the spinal cord or the peripheral nervous system. It is characterized by a positive Romberg sign (ataxia worse on closing eyes) and diminished deep tendon reflexes. Sensory ataxia is present in as many as 15% of pediatric cases of GBS, usually in association with neuropathic weakness and other sensory symptoms (Gieron-Korthals et al., 1994).

Optic ataxia is caused by impaired visual control of the direction of limb-reaching for a visual target. It may be associated with lesions in the superior parietal lobule, which also affects visual-guided saccades and other forms of eye–hand coordination.

Psychogenic

A psychogenic or nonorganic cause of ataxia must be considered when the examination findings are bizarre, inconsistent, or incongruent. Further evaluation should address possible previous psychiatric illness, secondary gain, or a precipitating event. Psychogenic ataxia is a diagnosis of exclusion.

INVESTIGATIONS IN ACUTE ATAXIA

Acute postinfectious cerebellar ataxia is a diagnosis of exclusion. A thorough history and physical examination are far more likely to identify the etiology rather than an extensive workup. The selection of primary laboratory and radiologic investigations should be based on clinical scenario. Serious conditions that may present with ataxia should be excluded. Of all investigations performed in the diagnostic workup of acute cerebellar ataxia, the urine and/or serum drug screen are most likely to prove diagnostic, even where a source of ingestion is not immediately apparent (Gieron-Korthals et al., 1994). Neuroimaging should be obtained if there is concern of a mass lesion. CSF analysis should be done if there is concern for acute CNS infection or the diagnosis is uncertain.

Computed Tomography and Magnetic Resonance Imaging

The diagnostic screening yield of CT and MRI is low; only 5% of children initially being evaluated for ataxia showed any telling abnormalities (Figure 92-1). CT and MRI are more commonly used to rule out a specific diagnosis such as tumor, stroke, ADEM, or the risk of herniation before lumbar puncture (Whelan et al., 2013).

In children with OMAS, MRI or CT of the chest, abdomen, and pelvis, with thin cuts through the adrenals, is recommended. Nuclear scintigraphy is also recommended if conventional imaging is nondiagnostic.

Cerebrospinal Fluid

CSF examination is frequently performed in the evaluation of children with acute ataxia. Data from reported studies of children with acute ataxia found abnormal CSF findings in 43% of children undergoing lumbar puncture (Whelan et al., 2013). CSF studies showed mild pleocytosis and variable elevations of protein. In one study, CSF was analyzed according to the suspected etiology (e.g., viral, vaccine-related, and idiopathic) and no significant differences were noted (Connolly et al., 1994).

Electromyography and Electroencephalography

Electromyography (EMG) and nerve conduction velocity studies should be considered in evaluation of acute-onset ataxia in cases in which clinical diagnosis of the Miller Fisher variant of GBS is suspected (Whelan et al., 2013). Very early (less than 4 days) electromyography assessment in GBS may be nondiagnostic; however, testing multiple motor and sensory nerves (greater than or equal to 3) may detect abnormal findings suggestive of disease. EMG is also useful in confirming the diagnosis of EA1, by showing continuous motor unit activity, most often in the hands.

Studies reported electroencephalographic (EEG) findings in 24 of 57 children with acute ataxia. Data on 24 children with acute ataxia showed nonspecific EEG abnormities in 42%.

Acute ataxia may be present during the ictal or postictal phase of seizures in children (Ryan and Engle, 2003). Nonconvulsive epileptic states have also been referred to as pseudoataxia and may present as ataxia with or without alteration of consciousness. Clinicians can consider obtaining an EEG if there is a history of epilepsy or evidence of an altered mental status or the clinical suspicion of nonconvulsive status epilepticus. Nonconvulsive seizures are usually seen with preexisting seizure disorders and cognitive impairment. This diagnosis is associated with underlying EEG abnormalities with dramatic clinical and electrographic improvement when treated appropriately (Whelan et al., 2013).

Toxicology

Ataxia after ingestion is most frequently caused by medications but less often from exposure to organic chemicals, solvents, and heavy metals. Accidental poisoning in children less than 6 years of age is the most common form of toxin ingestion, with a second peak in adolescence, where intoxication occurs as a result of substance abuse (Gieron-Korthals et al., 1994). A high index of suspicion should always be maintained, because a history of ingestion or exposure might not be forthcoming. After ingestion, ataxia is often accompanied by mental status changes such as lethargy, confusion, inappropriate speech, or unconsciousness. Toxicology screens are therefore of value in the initial evaluation of acute ataxia in children. Other agents associated with ataxia in children include phencyclidine and other recreational drugs, antiepileptic drugs, anticholinergic agents, muscle relaxants, "magic" mushrooms, and cold remedies.

Urinary Catecholamines/Metaiodobenzylguanidine Scintigraphy

Opsoclonus-myoclonus syndrome is a rare autoimmune disorder in which a neuroblastoma is found in at least 50% of affected individuals. Evaluation for an occult neuroblastoma should occur in all children with opsoclonus or myoclonus accompanying the ataxia as well as in children with isolated ataxia whose symptoms do not begin to resolve within 2 weeks (Figure 92-2). On the use of MIBG scintigraphy in patients suspected of having neuroblastoma, studies have reported a sensitivity for tumor detection in the range of 70% to 92% (Brunklaus et al., 2012). One study detected residual, recurrent, or metastatic neuroblastoma in 16 of 20 patients (80%). Another study showed MIBG sensitivity of 70% in detecting abdominal or pelvic neuroblastoma and 83% in detecting thoracic neuroblastoma (Brunklaus et al., 2012). In a third study, sensitivity differences between ^{131}I MIBG and ^{123}I MIBG were not observed. Neuroblastomas frequently spontaneously involute, which may account for the observation that no tumor is found in up to half of all cases of OMAS.

Neuroblastoma may be associated with elevated levels of one or more urinary catecholamine metabolites; vanillylmandelic acid (VMA) and homovanillic acid (HVA) are the most common catecholamines examined. In a reported study, only 37 of 408 (9%) patients had elevated urinary HVA or VMA levels, and neuroblastoma was subsequently diagnosed.

Other Tests

Autoimmune disorders are believed to play an important role in acute ataxia. Testing performed to screen for autoimmune disorders includes examination for the presence of antinuclear antibodies—anti-SS-A/Ro and anti-SSB/ladanticardiolipin antibody, and antiphospholipid antibodies. There are insufficient data regarding the role of GAD-ab in childhood acute ataxia (Whelan et al., 2013). There are insufficient data to draw conclusions regarding the diagnostic yield of screening testing of autoimmune disorders in children presenting with acute ataxia.

Treatment and Prognosis

Acute postinfectious cerebellitis is usually a self-limited condition with most children showing a spontaneous recovery within the first week. Full recovery is expected within 3 months of onset in at least 50% of children, but recovery remains incomplete in a minority of cases. The typical approach to a child with inflammatory cerebellitis is to exclude a primary infectious etiology. After an active infection is ruled out, a trial of immunosuppression is usually warranted. Corticosteroids, such as solumedrol in a daily dose of 20 to 30 mg/kg up to 1000 mg a day, are usually pulsed for 3 to 5 days. If there is no improvement in symptoms, then plasmapheresis or intravenous immunoglobulin is the second-line alternative. Intravenous immunoglobulin (IVIg) is frequently given at 2 g/kg/day. Plasmapherersis is typically done with five exchanges performed every other day. In patients who do not have the resolution of symptoms, the use of rituximab 375 mg/m^2 weekly for 4 weeks has been reported to show benefit.

Children with OMAS frequently require prolonged treatment with IVIg and corticosteroids to prevent relapses. Typical IVIg dosing is 1 to 2 g/kg/day every month or every other month. Pranzatelli and colleagues (Tate et al., 2012) have described symptom improvement using a multimodal approach of adrenocorticotropic hormone in conjunction with IVIg or rituximab for over 1 year.

Children with the Miller Fisher variant of GBS should be admitted to the hospital for careful monitoring of respiratory and autonomic function. Corticosteroids are felt to be contraindicated for GBS, with IVIg or plasmapheresis as the first-line therapy. The recommended dose of immunoglobulin is 2 g/kg over 2 to 5 days. The decision for active treatment depends on status of ambulation and respiratory and bulbar involvement. With or without specific treatment, more than 90% of children with GBS and Miller Fisher syndrome recover completely within 6 to 12 months of disease onset.

Recovery from acute postinfectious demyelinating encephalopathy is typically somewhat slower than that from acute cerebellar ataxia and can be hastened by treatment with corticosteroids. However, a minority of patients were left with significant sequelae. Single relapses can occur in as many as 10% of affected children. Multiple relapses raise the possibility of an underlying diagnosis of MS.

Systemic infections and brainstem encephalitis should be treated with standard antibiotic/antiviral protocols, although outcome in brainstem encephalitis is uncertain.

Treatment of toxic ingestion depends on the nature and amount of the ingested substance. Monitoring the blood concentration of the drug, the liver and kidney functions, and stabilizing vitals while allowing spontaneous elimination of the ingested agent is important. Often times, no specific treatment is available. In some cases, administration of an antidote, chelation, dialysis, or other therapies is required (Ryan and Engle, 2003).

Ataxia related to postconcussion syndrome usually clears by 6 months. Tumors, stroke, and traumatic brain injury are likely to have significant sequelae with incomplete recovery. Vertebrobasilar dissection may need anticoagulation in the short-term followed by a period of antiplatelet therapy. Significant cerebellar bleeds need posterior fossa decompression. Determination of the precipitating stress is important in managing psychogenic ataxia. EA1 may respond to antiepileptic medication. Both EA1 and EA2 respond to daily acetazolamide.

Daily nicotinamide administration (50–300 mg) may reverse neurologic complication in Hartnup disease. Acute ataxia in some cases of maple syrup urine disease may respond to thiamine 1 g and ongoing supplementation (maintenance 100 mg daily). Acetazolamide has been shown to abort acute attacks of ataxia in pyruvate dehydrogenase deficiency.

Basilar artery migraine can be managed the same as other forms of migraine. Migraine prophylaxis is useful when attacks are frequent, as in benign paroxysmal vertigo.

Nonmetastatic neuroblastoma should be removed surgically. If no obvious tumor is detectable at first presentation, periodic surveillance is essential in suspected cases. Adrenocorticotrophic hormone, corticosteroids, and IVIg will improve symptoms in 80% of patients with neuroblastoma. Relapses may occur during course of treatment or after discontinuing therapy. Epileptic ataxia (pseudoataxia) responds to anticonvulsant drugs.

Behavioral or learning difficulties were present in 20% of children during the recovery phase from acute cerebellar ataxia but resolved in most within 6 months (Connolly et al, 1994). Some data suggest that immunosuppression improves developmental outcome in children with OMAS.

REFERENCES

The complete list of references for this chapter is available in the e-book at www.expertconsult.com.
See inside cover for registration details.

SELECTED REFERENCES

Benini, R., Ben Amor, I.M., Shevell, M.I., 2012. Clinical clues to differentiating inherited and noninherited etiologies of childhood ataxias. J. Pediatr. 160 (1), 152–157.

Bozzola, E., Bozzola, M., Tozzi, A.E., et al., 2014. Acute cerebellitis in varicella: a ten year case series and systematic review of the literature. Ital. J. Pediatr. 40, 57.

Brunklaus, A., Pohl, K., Zuberi, S.M., et al., 2012. Investigating neuroblastoma in childhood opsoclonus-myoclonus syndrome. Arch. Dis. Child. 97 (5), 461–463.

Connolly, A.M., Dodson, W.E., Prensky, A.L., et al., 1994. Course and outcome of acute cerebellar ataxia. Ann. Neurol. 35 (6), 673–679.

Gieron-Korthals, M.A., Westberry, K.R., Emmanuel, P.J., 1994. Acute childhood ataxia: 10-year experience. J. Child Neurol. 9 (4), 381–384.

Pandolfo, M., Manto, M., 2013. Cerebellar and afferent ataxias. Continuum. (Minneap. Minn.) 19 (5 Movement Disorders), 1312–1343.

Ryan, M.M., Engle, E.C., 2003. Acute ataxia in childhood. J. Child Neurol. 18 (5), 309–316.

Sivaswamy, L., 2014. Approach to acute ataxia in childhood: diagnosis and evaluation. Pediatr. Ann. 43 (4), 153–159.

Tate, E.D., Pranzatelli, M.R., Verhulst, S.J., et al., 2012. Active comparator-controlled, rater-blinded study of corticotropin-based immunotherapies for opsoclonus-myoclonus syndrome. J. Child Neurol. 27, 875–884.

van Doorn, P.A., Ruts, L., Jacobs, B.C., 2008. Clinical features, pathogenesis, and treatment of Guillain-Barré syndrome. Lancet Neurol. 7 (10), 939–950.

Whelan, H.T., Sumit, V., Guo, Y., et al., 2013. Evaluation of the child with acute ataxia: a systematic review. Pediatr. Neurol. 49 (1), 15–24.

E-BOOK FIGURES AND TABLES

The following figures and tables are available in the e-book at www.expertconsult.com. See inside cover for registration details.

Fig. 92-1 Cerebellitis.
Fig. 92-2 Metaiodobenzylguanidine scintigraphy.
Box 92-1 Signs of cerebellar dysfunction.
Table 92-2 Causes of Acute Episodic Cerebellar Ataxia
Video 92-1 Signs of Ataxia

93 Movement Disorders: An Overview

Jonathan W. Mink and Terence D. Sanger

An expanded version of this chapter is available on www.expertconsult.com. See inside cover for registration details.

INTRODUCTION

Movement disorders are characterized by impaired voluntary movement, the presence of involuntary movements, or both. There may be impaired targeting and velocity of intended movements, abnormal involuntary movements, abnormal postures, or excessive movements that appear normal at inappropriate or unintended times. Movement disorders in children include athetosis, chorea, dystonia, myoclonus, parkinsonism, stereotypies, tics, and tremor (Carducci and Fernandez-Alvarez, 2007; Singer et al., 2016). Movement disorders may be accompanied by weakness, spasticity, hypotonia, ataxia, apraxia, and other motor deficits, although many authors do not include these accompanying deficits.

Movement disorders have been divided into "hyperkinetic" disorders, in which there is excessive movement, and "hypokinetic" disorders, in which there is a paucity of movement. Hyperkinetic disorders consist of abnormal, repetitive involuntary movements and include most of the childhood movement disorders, such as chorea, dystonia, athetosis, myoclonus, stereotypy, tics, and tremor. Hypokinetic movement disorders are primarily akinetic or rigid. The primary syndrome in this category is parkinsonism, occurring most commonly in adulthood as Parkinson disease or one of the many forms of secondary parkinsonism.

Movement disorder terminology has been well defined for adults, but less so for children. Therefore it is likely that movement disorders are underreported in children, and that there is inconsistent terminology. Recently there have been attempts to provide specific definitions of childhood motor disorders. According to these definitions, childhood disorders can be divided into three major categories: hypertonic disorders, hyperkinetic disorders, and negative signs (Sanger et al., 2003; Sanger et al., 2006; Sanger et al., 2010). Hypertonic disorders include spasticity, dystonia, and rigidity. Hyperkinetic disorders include chorea, dystonia, athetosis, myoclonus, tremor, stereotypies, and tics. Negative signs include weakness, reduced selective motor control, ataxia, apraxia, and developmental dyspraxia, although we will not discuss these here. Consensus definitions for these terms have been established, although the list is not intended to be exhaustive and disorders of gait, balance, speech, and eye movement are not included. The prevalence in children of different types of disorders is not known, although there have been studies investigating symptoms in certain populations, including children with cerebral palsy.

In this chapter, general features of pediatric movement disorders will be discussed followed by discussion of many specific movement disorders. Other related disorders are discussed in other chapters in this book, including hereditary ataxias (Chapter 91), acute ataxia (Chapter 92), paroxysmal dyskinesias (Chapter 94), movement disorders of infancy (Chapter 95), drug-induced movement disorders (Chapter 96), cerebral palsy (Chapter 97), and tics (Chapter 98).

CHARACTERISTIC FEATURES OF PEDIATRIC MOVEMENT DISORDERS

Movement disorders in children differ from those in adults in several aspects. Perhaps the most important is that movement disorders in childhood occur in the context of development, and thus manifestations may vary with age and developmental stage. Diagnosis in children may be complicated by the fact that many symptoms have more than one cause, and any particular underlying pathophysiology may lead to a complex combination of symptoms. The diagnostic workup in children is guided by symptoms, but the existence of a large class of diseases that can lead to the same set of symptoms often necessitates a broad etiologic workup. There may be both specific etiologic treatments, as well as symptomatic treatments, both of which may be beneficial in an individual child. In particular, many of the causes of childhood movement disorders do not yet have any specific treatment, yet symptomatic treatment for the resulting movement disorder can be extremely helpful and lead to improvement in quality of life.

DIAGNOSIS OF MOVEMENT DISORDERS

Classification of a movement disorder based upon the spatial and temporal pattern is essential for diagnosis. It is also important to define the context in which the movements occur. Although it is often helpful to list the characteristics of the movements (Table 93-1), the diagnosis relies on pattern recognition, and the clinician must see the movements. If the movements are not apparent during the neurologic examination, repeating the examination at another time or obtaining video recordings of the movements is important to making an accurate diagnosis. The widespread availability of video cameras has substantially improved diagnosis of movement disorders.

When approaching a patient with a movement disorder, it is helpful to address some key questions:

1. Is the number of movements excessive (hyperkinetic) or diminished (hypokinetic)?
2. If hyperkinetic, do the individual movements appear normal or abnormal?
3. Is the movement paroxysmal (sudden onset and offset), continual (repeated again and again), or continuous (without stop)?
4. What is the developmental stage of the child, and has development been normal?
5. How does voluntary movement influence the movement disorder? Are symptoms and signs present at rest (body part supported against gravity), with maintained posture, with action, with approach to a target (intention), or a combination?
6. Has the movement disorder changed over time?

TABLE 93-1 Phenomenological Classification of Movement Disorders

Movement Disorder	Brief Description
Athetosis	Slow, continuous, writhing movements of distal body parts, especially the fingers and hands
Chorea/ballism	Chaotic, randomly triggered, repetitive, brief, purposeless movements or movement fragments of multiple body parts that may overlap in time. Rapid, but not as rapid as myoclonus. When very large in amplitude and affecting proximal joints, choreic limb movements are often called ballism
Dystonia	Repetitive, sustained, abnormal postures and/or movements, worsened by attempted movement or posture. Abnormal postures typically have a twisting quality
Myoclonus	Sudden, brief, shocklike unidirectional movements that may be repetitive or rhythmic
Parkinsonism	Hypokinetic syndrome characterized by a combination of rest tremor, slow movement (bradykinesia), rigidity, and postural instability
Stereotypy	Patterned, purposeless, episodic, rhythmic movements
Tics	Intermittent, discrete, repetitive brief movements or postures, most frequently involving face, head, or upper body
Tremor	Rhythmic oscillation about a central point or position, involving one or more body parts

7. Do environmental stimuli or emotional states precipitate, exacerbate, or alleviate the movement disorder?
8. Is the patient aware of the movements?
9. Can the movements be suppressed voluntarily?
10. Are the movements heralded by a premonitory sensation or urge? (It may be helpful to ask the patient, "Why do you do that?")
11. Does the movement disorder abate with sleep?
12. Are there other findings on the examination suggestive of focal neurologic deficit or systemic disease?
13. Is there a family history of a similar or related condition?

Obtaining a very careful history of the time course of symptoms is often extremely helpful. With careful questioning, it is often possible to distinguish between relentlessly progressive disorders, paroxysmal disorders with intervening periods of normal function, stepwise progressive disorders, or paroxysmal episodes of worsening superimposed on a background of progression. The effect of intercurrent illness should be assessed because many disorders (static or progressive) will have episodic worsening in the context of otherwise minor viral or bacterial illness.

Laboratory tests, imaging, and other diagnostic testing should be based on the specific movement disorder. There is no "movement disorder workup" because the causes are varied and some movement disorders (e.g., tics) are rarely symptomatic of an underlying disease.

Movement disorders may be difficult to characterize, unless other symptoms and behavioral context are taken into account. Chorea can resemble myoclonus. Dystonia can resemble spasticity. Paroxysmal movement disorders, such as dystonia and tics, may resemble seizures. Movements in some situations may be normal and in others may indicate underlying pathology. For example, frequent eye blinking can be perfectly normal and appropriate in one setting (a windy day at the beach) but excessive in another (tics). Movements that raise concern about a degenerative disorder in older children (progressive myoclonus) may be completely normal in an infant (benign neonatal myoclonus). Thus it is important to view the movement disorder in the context of a complete history and neurologic examination.

ETIOLOGY OF MOVEMENT DISORDERS IN CHILDREN

The causes of pediatric movement disorders are extensive. The most common cause of secondary disorders is likely to be cerebral palsy, with a prevalence of 2 per 1000. However, cerebral palsy itself represents a constellation of injuries and symptoms, and there is a wide range of types of injury, localization, and combinations of symptoms. Cerebral palsy can be associated with almost all forms of childhood movement disorders, and despite the lack of an ongoing destructive process, the clinical picture may change during development. The diagnosis and management of cerebral palsy is discussed in Chapter 97.

Specific types of movement disorder may represent dysfunction of particular localized regions of the central nervous system. Ataxia most likely occurs due to dysfunction of the cerebellum or its afferent and efferent pathways. Bradykinesia most likely occurs with dysfunction of the substantia nigra or striatum, leading to presynaptic or postsynaptic failure of dopaminergic transmission. Chorea typically occurs with dysfunction of the striatum or subthalamic nucleus, but it also can occur with widespread cerebral injury (e.g., after encephalitis). Dystonia most likely involves dysfunction of the striatum or globus pallidus, but thalamic, cortical, or cerebellar abnormalities cannot be excluded as contributors. Myoclonus most likely involves cortical, brainstem, or spinal injury to gray matter. Localization of tremor depends on the type, with some forms involving cerebellar or brainstem circuits. Tic disorders probably involve an abnormality of the basal ganglia, but cortical mechanisms may also contribute.

APPROACH TO TREATMENT

Treatment of childhood movement disorders is based primarily on symptomatology, independent of the underlying cause. When a specific treatment for the underlying cause is available, this should be implemented, but in many cases such treatment is only partially effective. The goal of symptomatic treatment is to disrupt the connection between the pathophysiology and the expression of clinical impairment.

It is essential to ask both the child and the parents for the most significant cause of disability. In some cases, the impairment that is most evident to the clinician is not the primary cause of disability. Sometimes, treatment of the functional limitation or direct treatment of a disability is more effective, less time-consuming, and less risky than attempts to treat the underlying pathophysiology, and therefore it is essential to be certain that any treatment addresses the needs and goals of the child and family. In particular, it is usually neither necessary nor possible to treat all symptoms. It is most helpful to pick specific goals and to monitor progress toward those goals. In many cases, a team approach has been found to be helpful, particularly when there are multiple impairments leading to disability, and the team approach allows appropriate focusing and selection of interventions. In some cases, a supportive environment and adaptive equipment are more effective than any medical intervention.

CLASSIFICATION OF CHILDHOOD MOVEMENT DISORDERS

The first step toward diagnosing and treating a movement disorder is to define the disorder (Table 93-1). Individual names of movement disorders can refer to neurologic signs or to neurologic syndromes or diseases, which can cause some confusion.

CHOREA

Chorea describes an apparently random, nonrhythmic, purposeless set of movements of either distal or proximal muscles that appears to flow from one muscle or muscle group to another without any pattern. Chorea occurs at rest and with action and gives the child a "fidgety" appearance and the inability to remain still. It is associated with motor impersistence (e.g., the inability to maintain the tongue extended). Chorea may worsen or improve with voluntary movement, but even very severe chorea may not prevent accurate voluntary movement for some children. Many individuals with chorea will incorporate the involuntary movements into a voluntary movement in order to mask the movements. However, the involuntary movements can lead to significant disability, and some children will injure themselves if they have large amplitude movements.

The causes of chorea in childhood are numerous. A list of important causes of chorea in children is presented in Box 93-1. See the online version of this chapter for a more detailed description of specific entities.

Sydenham Chorea

Sydenham chorea is the most common cause of chorea in children. It has its onset weeks or months after an acute infection with group A beta-hemolytic streptococcus (GABHS) and is one of the major Jones criteria for the diagnosis of rheumatic fever. Symptoms may persist for weeks or months, but chorea almost always resolves spontaneously within 6 months. There have been rare reported cases of continued or recurring symptoms. The chorea typically involves the distal musculature, initially of one hand and then of both, with a "piano-playing" pattern. Other, more severe forms of chorea, including ballism, have been observed. Large, generalized

---

BOX 93-1 Causes of Chorea in Childhood

STATIC INJURY/STRUCTURAL DISORDERS
- Cerebral palsy
- Stroke
- Trauma
- Moyamoya disease
- Vasculitis
- Tumors
- Congenital malformations
- Joubert syndrome

HEREDITARY/DEGENERATIVE DISORDERS
- Ataxia-telangiectasia (A-T), and Ataxia-Telangiectasia-Like Disorder (ATLD)
- Ataxia oculomotor apraxia (AOA) (includes AOA-1, AOA-2, and early onset cerebellar ataxia and hypoalbuminemia [EOCA-HA])
- Fahr disease
- Pantothenate kinase-associated neurodegeneration (PKAN, associated with mutations in *PANK-2*, pantothenate kinase-2 gene), and other causes of Neuronal Brain Iron Accumulation (NBIA)

METABOLIC DISORDERS
- Acyl-coA dehydrogenase deficiencies
- Mitochondrial disorders, including Leigh's syndrome
- GM_1 gangliosidosis
- Lesch-Nyhan disease
- Niemann–Pick type C
- Methylmalonic aciduria
- Nonketotic hyperglycemia
- Kernicterus
- Hypoparathyroidism
- Propionic acidemia
- Hypernatremia
- Hypomagnesemia
- Hypocalcemia
- Hypo- or hyperglycemia
- Vitamin E deficiency or malabsorption
- Bassen-Kornzweig disease
- Complications of cardiac bypass

INFECTIOUS/PARAINFECTIOUS DISEASE
- Encephalitis/postencephalitis

IMMUNE-MEDIATED/DEMYELINATING DISORDERS
- Sydenham chorea
- Lupus erythematosus
- Henoch-Schönlein purpura
- Anticardiolipin or antiphospholipid antibody syndrome
- Anti-NMDA antibody syndrome

DRUGS/TOXINS
- Neuroleptic medications, and neuroleptic-like antiemetics (haloperidol, chlorpromazine, pimozide, prochlorperazine, metoclopramide)
- Calcium channel blockers (flunarizine, cinnarizine)
- Antiseizure medications (phenytoin, carbamazepine, valproate, phenobarbital)
- Anticholinergic medications (trihexyphenidyl, benztropine)
- Antihistamines
- Tricyclic antidepressants
- Clomipramine
- Stimulants (including methylphenidate, dexamphetamine, pemoline, and bronchodilators)
- Clonidine
- l-DOPA
- Cocaine
- Bismuth
- Lithium
- Manganese
- Ethanol
- Carbon monoxide
- Oral contraceptives
- General anesthesia (including propofol)—during induction or emergence

PAROXYSMAL DISORDERS
- Complex migraine
- Alternating hemiplegia of childhood
- Paroxysmal kinesigenic dyskinesia (PKD)
- Paroxysmal nonkinesigenic dyskinesia (PNKD)
- Paroxysmal exercise-induced dyskinesia (PED)

ENDOCRINE DISORDERS
- Hyperthyroidism
- Pheochromocytoma

body movements in some patients previously inspired the term "St. Vitus' dance."

Antibasal ganglia antibodies (ABGA) are found in some children, and it has been hypothesized that production of these antibodies is triggered due to molecular mimicry by streptococcal antigens. ABGA can be detected in the cerebrospinal fluid and antistreptolysin (ASLO) antibodies can be detected in serum. However, the high prevalence of positive ASLO titers in the general population means that both acute and convalescent ASLO titers must be measured in order to probe for an acute infection. The clinical situation often provides a strong indication for the diagnosis, but if other neurologic symptoms are present or there is doubt about the etiology, a more complete workup may be needed, including tests for thyroid function, toxins, metabolic disorders, or encephalitis.

Sydenham chorea usually does not require treatment, although acute streptococcal infection should be treated if present. All children diagnosed with Sydenham chorea, even in cases of isolated chorea, should be treated with penicillin, both acutely for treatment and long term for prophylaxis, according to the American Heart Association guidelines (Gerber et al., 2009). Valproic acid, carbamazepine, or neuroleptics may provide symptomatic benefit for Sydenham chorea. When associated obsessive-compulsive or behavioral symptoms are present, these symptoms are often managed with selective serotonin reuptake inhibitors. Treatment with immune suppressant medication, including corticosteroids or intravenous immunoglobulin preparations, has been studied, but the natural history, with spontaneous resolution of symptoms, makes interpretation of efficacy in open clinical trials difficult. A randomized, blinded, placebo-controlled study showed that a 4-week, 2-mg/kg daily oral dose of prednisone, followed by a taper, reduced duration of chorea and accelerated the reduction in symptoms. Weight gain was substantial by the end of 2 months, and long-term outcome, including recurrence rates, was not different between groups (Paz et al., 2006).

The prognosis for the movement disorder is excellent, and complete resolution occurs in most cases. Recurrence is rare and is sometimes associated with recurrence of other symptoms of rheumatic fever. There appears to be a higher risk of chorea gravidarum in women with a previous history of Sydenham chorea.

Medication-Induced Chorea

Medication-induced chorea can be dose-related or a tardive phenomenon, so evaluation of a child with chorea requires a careful history of past and current medication exposure. Medication-induced chorea is discussed in Chapter 96. Treatment of medication-induced chorea requires elimination of the precipitating agent.

Genetic Chorea

A large number of genetic disorders have chorea as a symptom. For some, such as benign hereditary (familial) chorea, chorea is major or sole manifestation. For others, chorea is accompanied by other neurologic or system symptoms. These disorders are listed in Box 93-1 and are discussed in detail in the online version of this chapter.

Chorea Associated With Systemic Illness and Autoimmune Disorders

Several systemic disorders may have chorea as a major manifestation. Hyperthyroidism can be a cause of chorea,

and any child with unexplained acute or persistent chorea should have serum testing for thyroid function. Autoimmune diseases, including lupus erythematosus, and antiphospholipid antibody syndromes, can be a cause of chorea, and there is increasing recognition of the association of chorea with vasculitis and autoimmune syndromes with antibodies to neuronal membrane channels, including anti-NMDA encephalitis. Other systemic diseases associated with chorea are listed in Box 93-1. Because early treatment can be life-saving, a high level of suspicion for autoimmune disorders in children with acute onset of chorea in conjunction with encephalopathy should be maintained (Chapters 118, 119).

Ballism

Ballism is a high-amplitude, flinging movement, usually due to involuntary movements of proximal joints. Ballism is part of the spectrum of chorea and involves similar pathophysiological mechanisms. When ballism involves one side of the body, it is called hemiballism. Hemiballism is the classical manifestation of hemorrhage or infarction affecting the subthalamic nucleus but can be associated with lesions in other parts of the basal ganglia.

Treatment of Chorea

Chorea is often difficult to treat. Sydenham chorea responds to symptomatic treatment with dopamine D2 receptor antagonists, valproic acid, or carbamazepine. Other forms of chorea are less likely to respond to those medications. Benzodiazepines or dopamine depletors (tetrabenazine, reserpine) may be helpful in some cases. Deep brain stimulation can be considered in severe refractory cases.

DYSTONIA

Dystonia occurs as an isolated phenomenon or in association with other neurologic signs or symptoms. Dystonia is defined as "a movement disorder in which involuntary sustained or intermittent muscle contractions cause twisting and repetitive movements, abnormal postures, or both." Although the term seems to imply an abnormality of tone, dystonia is not primarily a disorder of tone, but rather a disorder of posture and/or movement. When individuals with dystonia are at rest, tone is often diminished, although, in severe dystonia, involuntary contractions persist during attempted rest and tone may be increased. Dystonia can manifest as either hypertonic dystonia with increased stiffness, hyperkinetic dystonia with increased movements, or a combination of the two. Due to the complexity of identifying causes of dystonia, an international classification system has been proposed (Albanese et al., 2013). This system is based on two axes: clinical characteristics and etiology.

Dystonia is commonly triggered or exacerbated by voluntary movement, and it may fluctuate in severity over minutes, weeks, or months. Dystonia can be movement-specific, so that a muscle may exhibit involuntary contraction only during certain voluntary movements and not others. Dystonic contractions resolve during sleep. Individuals with dystonia sometimes discover that touching one part of the body may relieve the dystonic spasms; this phenomenon is called a sensory trick or *geste antagoniste*. Sensory tricks are less common in patients with symptomatic dystonia. Dystonia may be generalized or focal, involving just a single body part. Causes of dystonia in childhood are summarized in Box 93-2.

BOX 93-2 Causes of Dystonia in Childhood

STATIC INJURY/STRUCTURAL DISORDERS

- Cerebral palsy
- Hypoxic-ischemic injury
- Kernicterus
- Head trauma
- Encephalitis
- Tumors
- Stroke in the basal ganglia (which may be due to vascular abnormalities or varicella)
- Congenital malformations affecting basal ganglia

HEREDITARY/DEGENERATIVE DISORDERS

- DYT1 (autosomal dominant, TorsinA)
- DYT2 (autosomal-recessive, Hippocalcin)
- DYT4 (autosomal dominant, β-tubulin 4a)
- DYT5 (autosomal dominant, GTP cyclohydrolase 1)
- DYT6 (autosomal dominant, THAP1)
- DYT8 (autosomal dominant, Myofibrillogenesis regulator 1)
- DYT9 (autosomal dominant, GLUT1)
- DYT10 (autosomal dominant, PRRT2)
- DYT11 (autosomal dominant [maternal imprinting], ε-Sarcoglycan)
- DYT12 (autosomal dominant, Na^+/K^+ ATPase α3 subunit)
- DYT15 (autosomal dominant, unknown)
- DYT16 (autosomal recessive, Protein kinase activator PRKRA)
- Pantothenate kinase-associated neurodegeneration (PKAN; neuronal brain iron accumulation type 1, due to mutations in *PANK2*)
- PLA2G6-associated neurodegeneration (PLAN)
- Huntington disease (Westphal variant, IT15–4p16.3)
- Spinocerebellar ataxias (SCAs, particularly SCA3/Machado–Joseph disease)
- Striatal necrosis
- Leigh syndrome
- Neuroacanthocytosis

- HARP syndrome (hypoprebetalipoproteinemia, acanthocytosis, retinitis pigmentosa, and pallidal degeneration)
- Tay-Sachs disease
- Sandhoff disease
- Niemann–Pick type C

METABOLIC DISEASE

- Glutaric aciduria types 1 and 2
- Acyl-CoA dehydrogenase deficiencies
- Neurotransmitter disorders
- Mitochondrial disorders
- GM_1 gangliosidosis
- Lesch-Nyhan disease
- Wilson disease
- Vitamin E deficiency
- Methylmalonic aciduria
- Tyrosinemia

DRUGS/TOXINS

- Neuroleptic and neuroleptic-like antiemetic medications (haloperidol, chlorpromazine, olanzapine, risperidone, prochlorperazine)
- Calcium channel blockers
- Stimulants (amphetamine, cocaine, ergot alkaloids)
- Anticonvulsants (carbamazepine, phenytoin)
- Thallium
- Manganese
- Carbon monoxide
- Ethylene glycol
- Cyanide
- Methanol

PAROXYSMAL DISORDERS

- Paroxysmal kinesigenic dyskinesia (PKD)
- Paroxysmal nonkinesigenic dyskinesia (PNKD)
- Exercise-induced dyskinesia (PED)

Genetic Dystonias

The tremendous advances in molecular and genetic research and diagnostic tools have led to the identification of specific etiologies of dystonias that were previously considered to be idiopathic. Many genetic forms of dystonia have assigned genetic loci identified as DYTx. The most important forms are discussed here. More detailed and extensive discussion can be found in the online version of this chapter. Paroxysmal dystonias are discussed in Chapter 94.

DYT-1 Dystonia

DYT-1 dystonia is also known as Oppenheim's dystonia, or dystonia musculorum deformans. The median age at onset is 10 years, with a range of 4 years to adulthood. Usually, onset is either in an upper or lower extremity. The general features include a gradually progressive dystonia that eventually involves multiple limbs and progresses to generalized dystonia, often affecting both distal and proximal musculature. However, there is great variation in the progression and severity. DYT-1 dystonia is autosomal-dominant, with reduced penetrance.

DYT-1 dystonia usually does not respond to dopaminergic medication. The mainstay of treatment is anticholinergic medication, but often very high doses are required. Other medications such as benzodiazepines, baclofen, carbamazepine, neuroleptics, or tetrabenazine have been tried with varied

success. Deep brain stimulation is especially effective in patients with DYT-1 dystonia.

DYT-5 Dystonia (Dopa-Responsive Dystonia)

Dopa-responsive dystonia (DYT-5) is also known as Segawa disease after its first description in 1976. The presentation is very similar to DYT-1 dystonia in many patients, although it can have onset at an earlier age. The average age at onset is 6 years, with a range of onset from 1 to 12 years. It frequently starts in a limb in children. In adolescents and adults, it is often accompanied by parkinsonism. The combination of dystonia and parkinsonism is due to decreased but not absent dopamine production. Diurnal variation is present in 77% of children, with milder symptoms in the morning and gradual worsening of symptoms as the day progresses. Untreated, DRD is a progressive disorder and this helps to distinguish it from static disorders such as cerebral palsy. Untreated cases can develop secondary orthopedic deformities, including joint contractures, muscle and tendon shortening, and scoliosis.

DRD is due to mutations in the GTP cyclohydrolase 1 gene. GTP cyclohydrolase is an enzyme that is important for the synthesis of tetrahydrobiopterin, which is a cofactor for the enzyme tyrosine hydroxylase. Tetrahydrobiopterin is also a cofactor for tryptophan hydroxylase and phenylalanine hydroxylase, although reduced function of these enzymes does not seem to be the primary cause of symptoms. Rare cases of homozygosity for GTP cyclohydrolase mutations have been reported, with a more severe phenotype.

Dramatic improvement during a trial with l-DOPA strongly suggests the diagnosis, but a precise diagnosis can be made by quantitative evaluation of cerebrospinal fluid neurotransmitters and pterins or genetic testing (Chapter 44).

DYT11 Dystonia (Myoclonus Dystonia Syndrome)

Myoclonus dystonia syndrome (DYT11) is a disorder with a combination of both symptoms. The major cause for this syndrome is mutation in the epsilon-sarcoglycan gene. Myoclonus involves the neck, trunk, and arms and is often alcohol-responsive. Dystonia occurs in approximately half of patients and may be the only manifestation, usually with torticollis or arm dystonia. Mood disorders and obsessive-compulsive disorder have also been associated with gene mutations. This disorder is autosomal-dominant, although de novo mutations may occur. When the epsilon-sarcoglycan gene is inherited from the father, there is approximately 100% symptomatic expression, but when inherited from the mother, there is only 10% symptomatic expression, suggesting an important role of maternal imprinting. The myoclonus responds to ethanol, and alcoholism may be a problem in adults with myoclonus-dystonia syndrome. Treatment is with benzodiazepines, valproate, or trihexyphenidyl. In severe cases, DBS may be effective.

Dystonias Associated With Neurodegenerative Disorders

Pantothenate Kinase-Associated Neurodegeneration (PKAN)

PKAN is a member of the group of diseases referred to as neurodegeneration with brain iron accumulation (NBIA). The NBIAs are discussed in the online version of this chapter. Symptoms of PKAN include progressive dystonia, dysarthria, rigidity, ballism, choreoathetosis, spasticity, dementia, and pigmentary retinal degeneration. In its later stages, this disorder has characteristic ballistic flinging movements of arms and legs, as well as involuntary and repetitive tongue protrusion. The limb and tongue movements may lead to injury, requiring restraint of the arms and legs, and dental extraction. There is a gradual progression over years, with loss of ambulation within 5 to 15 years of onset. The initial symptoms usually occur in either the childhood or the juvenile years. Dystonia in PKAN usually starts in the leg, but axial dystonia may be prominent. There is often associated bradykinesia. The rate of progression is more rapid with younger onset. An atypical form of PKAN generally starts later, between 10 and 30 years of age with a mean of 13 years. It has slower progression, and retinopathy is rare. The atypical form presents with dysarthria and psychiatric disturbances, which include emotional lability, depression, and sometimes aggressive or violent behavior. There are also freezing episodes similar to those seen in Parkinson disease.

MRI shows a characteristic "eye of the tiger" sign. This sign consists of a dark globus pallidus internus on T2 imaging, with a bright region in the center of the globus pallidus that is thought to be due to central necrosis. The dark signal is due to iron accumulation, although deposition of iron may be secondary to other metabolic deficits rather than the primary cause of symptoms. When the full eye of the tiger sign is present in childhood, 100% of such cases have the *PANK-2* mutation. Children with clinical features of PKAN but without the eye of the tiger sign only have a 50% chance of being positive for the *PANK-2* mutation.

Treatment is symptomatic. Some children receive benefit from benzodiazepines, anticholinergic medications, botulinum toxin, baclofen, or deep brain stimulation. The prognosis is universally poor, with death from medical complications usually within 10 to 20 years of the onset in the typical form. Deep brain stimulation can helpful as a palliative treatment in PKAN.

Lesch-Nyhan Disease

Lesch-Nyhan disease is a progressive neurodegenerative disorder that initially presents with hypotonia and developmental delay in the first year of life. It progresses over several years and can mimic athetotic cerebral palsy with ballism, choreoathetosis, axial dystonia, and spasticity. Dystonia is a prominent neurologic sign in Lesch-Nyhan disease. There is a striking prevalence of self-mutilation behaviors, including tongue-biting, head-banging, biting the fingers and lips, and thrusting of the arms or legs against objects. The behavioral disorder seems to be unique, with adult patients describing compulsions to injure themselves or to behave inappropriately. There is an increase in uric acid in both the blood and the urine, and this leads to symptoms of gout in advanced cases, although gout is less common in children. Both arthritis and renal stones have been reported, but usually in older patients.

Treatment is symptomatic. Allopurinol may alleviate signs of gout and prevent renal calculi. Behavioral programs can be used to reduce self-mutilation. Benzodiazepines, carbamazepine, and possibly selective serotonin reuptake inhibitors can be helpful for the behavior disorder. Tetrabenazine or l-DOPA may be helpful to treat the dystonia. Naltrexone has been used to reduce self-mutilation but with limited success. In some patients, restraint and removal of teeth are required in order to prevent self-mutilation, and patients who can communicate often will request to be placed in restraints in order to reduce self-injury. The prognosis is poor. Most children with the severe childhood-onset form never walk, and there may be progression of symptoms over several years.

Dystonia Associated With Other Metabolic Disorders

Organic Acidemias

Organic acidemias, including methylmalonic aciduria, glutaric aciduria types 1 and 2, biotinidase deficiency, disorders of fatty acid oxidation, and mitochondrial respiratory chain disorders, can lead to dystonia. Many of these disorders do not present until a time of metabolic stress, at which time a rapid decompensation with onset of severe generalized dystonia over a period of hours to days is possible. Once dystonia has occurred, symptoms are often irreversible. Specific treatment is usually needed urgently, and in some cases this requires limitation of intake of specific amino acids, whereas, in other cases, specific medications or metabolites are needed.

Many of these disorders can be detected with newborn screening. For children with new onset of symptoms or rapid progression of symptoms, there needs to be a high index of suspicion in order to detect these disorders, as any delay in treatment usually leads to a significantly worse prognosis. Most of these diseases are autosomal-recessive.

A particularly striking presentation that often occurs in infancy, but which can occur later in childhood, has been referred to as infantile bilateral striatal necrosis (IBSN). This can occur with many metabolic disorders but also seems to occur in the context of acute infections, particularly with mycoplasma, and it has been reported in children with *PANK-2* mutations. Most often, the cause is unknown. There have been some rare familial cases. This disorder is characterized by a rapid onset of dystonia and dyskinesia, sometimes associated with chorea, and the MRI often shows evidence of irreversible striatal and sometimes pallidal injury on diffusion-weighted, T2, or gadolinium-enhanced images. There have been a few reported cases of a biotin-responsive type of striatal necrosis that has been thought to be due to an abnormality of biotin transport, and such cases may have rapid and effective resolution when treated with biotin.

Non-Dopa-Responsive Disorders of Dopamine Synthesis and Metabolism

Aromatic l-amino acid decarboxylase deficiency (ALAD) leads to dopamine agonist-responsive dystonia. In this disorder, conversion of l-DOPA to dopamine is impaired, and therefore administration of l-DOPA will not be helpful. Although this disorder does respond to dopamine agonists, due to the combination of severe autonomic and sleep disturbances, treatment with serotonergic medication is often required as well. Very few cases have been reported. This disorder is detectable by a characteristic pattern of cerebrospinal fluid neurotransmitter metabolites. Symptoms include dysautonomia, sleep disturbances, eye movement disturbances, and severe generalized dystonia, usually with onset in the first year of life. It appears to be autosomal-recessive.

Dopamine-transporter deficiency is a newly reported disorder in which the presynaptic reuptake of dopamine in the striatum is impaired (Kurian et al., 2011). The disorder is due to mutations in the dopamine transporter (*DAT*) gene, and symptoms include severe dystonia, hypotonia, bradykinesia, and developmental delay, with onset in the first year of life. Some children exhibit spontaneous hyperthermic spells associated with rigidity and rhabdomyolysis. Cerebrospinal fluid shows dramatic elevation of homovanillic acid, and serum prolactin levels may be decreased, particularly during hyperthermic episodes. No specific treatment has been found, although some children have responded to tetrabenazine, l-DOPA, dopamine agonists, or a combination.

Dystonia Due to Nonprogressive Disorders
Cerebral Palsy

Cerebral palsy is probably the most common cause of dystonia in childhood. This is due to its relatively high prevalence. Further details about this disorder, including the etiology and details of the symptomatology, can be found in Chapter 97. Dyskinetic cerebral palsy represents between 6% and 15% of all cases of cerebral palsy. In dyskinetic cerebral palsy, dystonia is usually the primary feature. Dystonia occurs frequently as an associated feature in other forms of cerebral palsy, including tetraplegic and hemiplegic cerebral palsy. Although the dystonia in cerebral palsy presumably is due to a static injury, the symptom can worsen over time. In fact, the onset of dystonia may be many years after the initial injury leading to cerebral palsy.

Kernicterus

Kernicterus occurs due to high bilirubin levels in the perinatal period, but the effects are variable and unpredictable. Injury to the globus pallidus is thought to be the etiology of the movement disorder. Symptoms include choreoathetosis, dystonia (which can be progressive), sensorineural hearing loss, and supranuclear gaze palsy. Symptom type and severity may be quite variable across individuals. In the absence of other associated injury, the intellect is usually normal, and the motor disorder is often the single greatest cause of disability.

The most effective treatment is prevention of neonatal hyperbilirubinemia. Treatment of symptomatic cases is often quite difficult. There is only a slight benefit to anticholinergic medications, valproic acid, benzodiazepines, or botulinum toxin. Some children have benefited from intrathecal baclofen. In general, treatment of this disorder is poorly effective. Life span is shortened in severely affected children due to pulmonary complications.

Medication-Induced Dystonias

Medication-induced dystonia can occur as a dose-related, idiosyncratic, or tardive phenomenon, so evaluation of a child with dystonia requires a careful history of past and current medication exposure. This is particular true for acute-onset dystonia. Medication-induced dystonia is discussed in Chapter 96. Treatment of medication-induced dystonia requires elimination of the precipitating agent. Tardive dystonia is rare in children.

Treatment of Dystonia

Because DRD is highly responsive to treatment with l-DOPA, it is recommended that all children with unexplained dystonia be given a trial of l-DOPA. L-DOPA may also be helpful in other forms of dystonia, but the benefits are usually incomplete. The optimal dose of l-DOPA is very low in DRD (typically 50 to 100 mg per day) but may be much higher in other forms of dystonia. Dosages as high as 10 mg/kg/day divided into three doses are sometimes needed. Common side effects of l-DOPA include nausea, vomiting, diarrhea, and more rarely, somnolence. L-DOPA must be combined with a peripheral decarboxylase inhibitor such as carbidopa in order to increase central uptake and decrease peripheral side effects. Commercial preparations with a ratio of l-DOPA to carbidopa of 4 : 1 are typically used.

Anticholinergic medications are the mainstay of treatment in many forms of dystonia. It is often necessary to proceed to very high doses to achieve maximum benefit. The effectiveness may be greater in young children, and speech and hand function seems to improve the most. The dose must be increased gradually, and it may often take 3 to 4 months to achieve an appropriate dosage. The initial dosage is 0.05 to 0.1 mg/kg/day or less and is divided into dosing three times per day. Side effects are similar to those of other anticholinergic medications.

Baclofen has been used and may be effective in some patients, and painful dystonia may respond best to baclofen. As with anticholinergic medications, high doses may be required to provide optimal benefit (120 to 180 mg/day in older children). Intrathecal baclofen may be effective in children with mixed dystonia and spasticity, but evidence for efficacy in isolated dystonia is limited.

When dystonia-related disability is limited to a small number of muscles, botulinum toxin may be effective. Diazepam and other benzodiazepines may be helpful in some individuals.

Deep brain stimulation may be highly effective in some forms of isolated dystonia (e.g., DYT1), and it may be variably helpful in patients with dystonia due to progressive or nonprogressive neurologic disorders.

TREMOR

Tremor has been described as "a rhythmical, involuntary, oscillatory movement of a body part." It can be classified based on the time of greatest severity as rest, postural, action, or intention tremor. Tremor can affect the head, extremities, trunk, voice, or a combination. Estimation of frequency can be useful in categorizing tremor. Tremor associated with parkinsonism is between 4 and 6 Hz, whereas essential tremor is more likely at 6 to 8 Hz, and physiologic tremor has two components at 8 to 12 Hz and at 20 to 25 Hz. In diagnosing tremor, it is important to distinguish it from myoclonus. Myoclonus can be rhythmic, but the rapid shocklike quality distinguishes it from tremor. Causes of tremor in childhood are summarized in Box 93-3.

Primary Tremor Disorders

Essential tremor is an autosomal-dominant disorder with variable penetrance and severity. It can present in childhood and often is slowly progressive over many years. It is rarely

---

BOX 93-3 Causes of Tremor in Childhood

BENIGN DISORDERS
- Enhanced physiologic tremor
- Shaking/shuddering spells

STATIC INJURY/STRUCTURAL DISORDERS
- Stroke (particularly in the midbrain or cerebellum)
- Multiple sclerosis

HEREDITARY/DEGENERATIVE DISORDERS
- Familial essential tremor
- Juvenile parkinsonism
- Pallidonigral degeneration
- Wilson disease

METABOLIC DISORDERS
- Hyperthyroidism
- Hyperadrenergic state (including pheochromocytoma and neuroblastoma)
- Hypomagnesemia
- Hypocalcemia
- Hypoglycemia
- Hepatic encephalopathy
- Vitamin B_{12} deficiency

DRUGS/TOXINS
- Valproate
- Lithium
- Tricyclic antidepressants
- Stimulants (cocaine, amphetamine, caffeine, thyroxine, bronchodilators)
- Neuroleptics
- Cyclosporine
- Toluene
- Mercury
- Thallium
- Amiodarone
- Nicotine
- Lead
- Manganese
- Arsenic
- Cyanide
- Naphthalene
- Ethanol
- Lindane
- Serotonin reuptake inhibitors

OTHER CAUSES OF TREMOR
- Cerebellar disease or malformation
- Anxiety
- Functional tremor

---

disabling in childhood except in extreme cases. Tremor is primarily postural but can also worsen with action. Tremor with holding a cup or handwriting may be some of the earliest complaints, but ultimately the head, trunk, and voice can be affected.

Physiologic tremor is normally present and becomes particularly noticeable when a muscle is exerting high levels of force. The distinguishing characteristic of physiologic tremor is that it occurs or worsens only when the child is carrying a heavy object or otherwise needs to contract the muscle against high resistance. Some children have an enhanced physiologic tremor that can become noticeable but is only rarely bothersome.

Secondary Tremor Disorders

There are a large number of secondary causes of tremor, and many of these are listed in Box 93-3. Tremor may be a side effect of many medications (Chapter 96). It may also accompany a number of systemic disorders that result in increased sympathetic output. Hyperthyroidism also may cause tremor.

In teenagers with new onset of a course tremor, it is important to exclude Wilson disease. This disorder is characterized by a wing-beating tremor that often involves the adductors of the arm and is shown when the child is asked to abduct the arms with elbows bent. The tremor is primarily postural but may occur at rest (Chapter 159). Other forms of tremor may occur in individuals with Wilson disease.

Holmes (rubral) tremor describes a large amplitude, rhythmic, but partly ballistic movement that often affects the arms and can be unilateral. It is associated with attempts at movement and is therefore an action tremor. It can be distinguished from chorea by the triggering or significant worsening with attempted movement. Holmes tremor is associated with lesions in the thalamus, midbrain, pons, or cerebellar peduncles, and not necessarily the red nucleus, despite its name. Holmes tremor is usually nonprogressive but can be severely disabling.

Treatment of Tremor

The first goal in treatment of tremor is to exclude other possible causes of rhythmic movement, including myoclonus, dystonia, seizures, or cerebellar dysfunction. Any underlying metabolic or hormonal cause must be corrected. Tremor-causing medications should be eliminated. Essential tremor is treated with propranolol, primidone, benzodiazepines (clonazepam may be particularly effective), or gabapentin. Tremor due to "stage-fright," social phobia, or panic disorder often responds to propranolol. Holmes tremor is refractory to most interventions, although some cases will respond to l-DOPA, clonazepam, or thalamic deep brain stimulation.

PARKINSONISM

Parkinsonism is defined by the presence of two or more cardinal signs of Parkinson disease. These include tremor at rest, bradykinesia, rigidity, and postural instability. Tremor is much less common in childhood parkinsonism than it is in adult Parkinson disease. Bradykinesia is slowness of movement in the absence of weakness or ataxia. There may also be hypokinesia with paucity of movement, few spontaneous movements, and decreased amplitude of movement. Hypokinesia is often seen as diminished spontaneous facial expression, soft speech (hypophonia), small handwriting (micrographia), and general slowness. Rigidity is increased muscle tone that is equal in all directions of movement and does not have a particular preferred posture. Rigidity may have a "lead-pipe" quality in which the limb can be moved with difficulty into arbitrary postures but, once placed in a posture, will remain there against gravity. If there is superimposed tremor, the rigidity can feel ratchety, like a cogwheel. Postural instability manifests as increased likelihood of falling and is due to dysregulation of postural reflexes. Clinically, it is evaluated with the "pull test," in which the patient stands, facing away from the examiner with feet apart at shoulder width. The examiner gives a gentle pull backward at the shoulders bilaterally (and is prepared to catch the patient to prevent a fall). A normal individual may take a step backward, but an individual with parkinsonian postural instability will take many steps backward (retropulsion) or may fall backward with no attempt to compensate. Etiologies of parkinsonism in children are listed Box 93-4.

Juvenile Parkinson Disease

Juvenile Parkinson disease is rare. The most common cause is due to mutations in the *Parkin* gene (PARK2). This is an autosomal-recessive disorder that typically begins in the second or third decade of life. Other causes for Juvenile Parkinson disease include mutations in the PINK1 and DJ1 genes. Juvenile Parkinson disease progresses over time. Typically these disorders respond to treatment with l-DOPA and dopamine agonists. However, escalating doses are required, and individuals with Juvenile Parkinson disease may develop DOPA-induced dyskinesia early in the course of treatment.

Other genes causing juvenile parkinsonism have been described recently. These disorders have parkinsonism as a prominent feature but are typically accompanied by other signs and symptoms. These genes include ATP13A2, PLA2G6, FBX07, DNAJC6. Pyramidal signs, eye movement abnormalities, and cognitive symptoms are common in these disorders.

Secondary Parkinsonism

There are many causes of secondary parkinsonism, as listed in Box 93-4. One of the more important causes to recognize is Huntington disease. When it starts in childhood, Huntington disease commonly present with parkinsonism as the initial manifestation. In those cases, the parkinsonism may respond to l-DOPA, which may be a source of diagnostic confusion. Several medications are known to cause parkinsonism. These are discussed in Chapter 96.

Treatment of Parkinsonism

Bradykinesia is the primary symptom that is responsive to treatment in childhood parkinsonism. It is usually due to dopamine deficiency and therefore is treated with l-DOPA or dopamine agonists. L-DOPA is combined with a peripheral decarboxylase inhibitor such as carbidopa in order to reduce side effects and increase delivery to the brain. Treatment is often initiated with a single dose of l-DOPA 1 mg/kg (or 50 to 100 mg total) given in the morning to evaluate for potential side effects, including nausea or postural hypotension. If this dose is tolerated for 3 to 4 days, then therapeutic treatment can be initiated three times per day. Dosage can be increased to a maximum of 10 to 15 mg/kg/day (divided into three doses), depending on effectiveness. In addition to nausea, common side effects in patients with parkinsonism can include dystonia, agitation, sleeplessness, and behavior changes. The dosage must be adjusted gradually in order to find the optimal dose, and the optimal dose may change as the child grows. Additional carbidopa may be given to decrease nausea.

BOX 93-4 Causes of Parkinsonism

STATIC INJURY/STRUCTURAL DISORDERS
- Basal ganglia infarcts
- Brain tumor
- Hydrocephalus

HEREDITARY/DEGENERATIVE DISORDERS
- Juvenile Parkinson disease
- Spinocerebellar ataxia
- Huntington disease (Westphal variant)
- Pallidal-pyramidal Disorder
- Neurodegeneration with Brain Iron Accumulation (NBIA)
- Pantothenate kinase-associated neurodegeneration (PKAN)
- Rett syndrome
- Pelizaeus-Merzbacher disease
- Machado-Joseph disease (spinocerebellar ataxia type 3)
- Neuronal ceroid lipofuscinosis
- Neuronal intranuclear inclusion body disease

METABOLIC DISORDERS
- Dopa-responsive dystonia
- Tyrosine hydroxylase deficiency and other abnormalities of bioamine metabolism
- Abnormalities of folate metabolism
- Wilson's disease
- Basal ganglia calcification (Fahr syndrome, hypoparathyroidism)

INFECTIOUS/PARA-INFECTIOUS DISORDERS
- Encephalitis lethargica (Von Economo disease)
- Autoimmune encephalitides, including anti-NMDA receptor associated encephalitis
- Viral encephalitis
- Acute demyelinating encephalomyelitis

DRUGS/TOXINS
- 1-methyl-4-phenyl-1,2,3,6-tetrahydropyridine (MPTP) poisoning
- Rotenone
- Tetrabenazine
- Reserpine
- Methyldopa
- Sedatives
- Neuroleptics
- Antiemetics
- Calcium channel blockers
- Isoniazid
- Serotonin reuptake inhibitors (sertraline, fluoxetine)
- Meperidine

DISORDERS THAT MIMIC PARKINSONISM
- Catatonia
- Spasticity
- Hypothyroidism
- Depression (with psychomotor retardation)

In Juvenile Parkinson disease, long-term treatment with l-DOPA will eventually lead to dyskinesias and freezing episodes that can limit its use. Some authors have advocated "dopamine-sparing" strategies that involve the early use of dopamine agonists such as pergolide, pramipexole, or ropinirole, or of dopamine breakdown inhibitors such as entacapone or selegiline. This approach has not been studied in children.

MYOCLONUS

Myoclonus consists of very brief, abrupt, involuntary, nonsuppressible, jerky contractions (or interruption of contraction), involving a single muscle or muscle group. The rapidity of these movements warrants the descriptor "shocklike," as if an electrical shock had just been applied to the peripheral nerve innervating the muscle. Myoclonus can be rhythmic, in which case it often appears tremor-like. However, in true tremor the movement oscillates with near-equal amplitude around a midpoint, whereas in myoclonus, the movement has more of a "sawtooth" character. It is present in normal (associated with sleep, exercise, or anxiety) and pathologic situations, both epileptic and nonepileptic. Epileptic myoclonus is discussed elsewhere. We limit our focus here to nonepileptic myoclonus.

Classification of Myoclonus

Several different schemes have been used to classify myoclonus, using clinical, anatomic, or etiologic criteria. Perhaps the simplest classification is based upon when the myoclonus occurs. Thus myoclonus may occur at rest, with action, or in response to a sensory stimulus (reflex myoclonus). In adults, it is helpful to classify based on presumed neuroanatomical location (e.g., cerebral cortex, thalamus, brainstem, or spinal cord). The neurophysiology of myoclonus has been reviewed elsewhere. In children, etiologic classification is the most useful, as summarized in Box 93-5.

Physiologic and Developmental Myoclonus

Physiologic myoclonus is that which occurs in normal individuals in specific settings. It includes such entities as hiccups, sleep starts, and sleep myoclonus. Sleep starts, also known as hypnic or hypnagogic myoclonus, occur with sleep initiation. They are often accompanied by a sense of falling. Benign myoclonus may occur in association with specific developmental stages. Benign neonatal sleep myoclonus and benign myoclonus of early infancy are discussed in Chapter 95.

Essential Myoclonus

Essential myoclonus is a relatively mild condition, starting in the first or second decade. It is inherited as an autosomal-dominant trait with incomplete penetrance. It is usually slowly progressive for a few years after onset and then stabilizes. The myoclonus may fluctuate slightly over the years or may show mild spontaneous improvement. Essential myoclonus may be allelic with Myoclonus Dystonia syndrome (DYT11). Essential myoclonus may respond to benzodiazepines, primidone, or propranolol.

Symptomatic Myoclonus

Myoclonus can by symptomatic of many disorders, as listed in Box 93-5. These are discussed in detail in the online version of this chapter. Opsoclonus-Myoclonus-Ataxia syndrome (OMAS) is discussed in detail in Chapter 120.

BOX 93-5 Etiologic Classification of Myoclonus

PHYSIOLOGIC
- Hiccups
- Hypnic jerks (sleep starts)
- Nocturnal (sleep) myoclonus

DEVELOPMENTAL
- Benign neonatal sleep myoclonus
- Benign myoclonus of early infancy
- Myoclonus with fever

ESSENTIAL
- Familial myoclonus dystonia syndrome

FUNCTIONAL
Symptomatic
Storage Diseases
- Juvenile Gaucher disease (type III)
- Sialidosis type 1 (cherry-red spot–myoclonus)
- GM$_1$ gangliosidosis
- Neuronal ceroid-lipofuscinosis (late infantile)

DEGENERATIVE CONDITIONS
- Dentato-rubro-pallido-luysian atrophy (DRPLA)
- Huntington disease
- Progressive myoclonus ataxia
- Ramsay–Hunt syndrome
- Early myoclonic encephalopathy
- Rasmussen encephalitis

DEMENTIAS
- Bovine spongiform encephalopathy
- Creutzfeldt–Jakob disease

INFECTIOUS AND POSTINFECTIOUS
- Meningitis (viral or bacterial)
- Encephalitis
- Epstein–Barr virus (EBV)

- Coxsackie virus
- Influenza
- Human immunodeficiency virus (HIV)
- Acute disseminated encephalomyelitis (ADEM)

METABOLIC
- Uremia
- Hepatic failure
- Electrolyte disturbances
- Hypo- or hyperglycemia
- Aminoacidurias
- Organic acidurias
- Urea cycle disorders
- Myoclonic epilepsy with ragged red fibers (MERRF)
- Mitochondrial encephalomyopathy, lactic acidosis, and strokelike episodes (MELAS)
- Biotinidase deficiency (usually epileptic)
- Cobalamin deficiency (infantile)
- Opsoclonus-myoclonus syndrome (myoclonic encephalopathy of infancy)

TOXIC
- Psychotropic medications (tricyclic antidepressants, lithium, selective serotonin reuptake inhibitors, monoamine oxidase inhibitors, neuroleptics)
- Antibiotics (penicillin, cephalosporins, quinolones)
- Antiepileptics (phenytoin, carbamazepine, lamotrigine, gabapentin, benzodiazepines [in infants], vigabatrin)
- Opioids
- General anesthetics
- Antineoplastic drugs
- Strychnine, toluene, lead, carbon monoxide, mercury

HYPOXIA
- (Lance–Adams syndrome)

Treatment of Myoclonus

Myoclonus is often refractory to medical treatment. Cortical myoclonus may respond to benzodiazepines and is commonly treated with clonazepam. Valproic acid is sometimes helpful, but it must be used with caution due to the ability to cause tremor as a side effect, with consequent confusion of symptoms. Piracetam has been used for many years in the UK and Europe to treat myoclonus, with good efficacy. Levetiracetam is a piracetam analog but does not seem to have equivalent efficacy to piracetam for treatment of myoclonus. There are reports of efficacy with zonisamide in some forms of myoclonus. Posthypoxic myoclonus seems to be particularly responsive to serotonergic medications, including selective serotonin reuptake inhibitors and oral administration of 5-hydroxytryptophan or 5-hydroxytryptamine. Baclofen has been occasionally used, but the mechanism of action is not clear. Carbamazepine can worsen myoclonus.

STEREOTYPY

Motor stereotypies are rhythmic, patterned, repetitive, involuntary movements that can occur in association with specific diseases or in otherwise normal children. Stereotypies may be associated with autism, sensory deficits, or intellectual disabilities, but they are also seen in otherwise normal children. Typical movements include repeated, recurrent raising and lowering of the arms, flapping, waving, wrist rotation, and finger wiggling. They are often accompanied by facial movements or grimacing. Other terms have been used to describe stereotypies, including "rhythmic habit patterns," "gratification phenomena," "self-stimulation," and "motor rhythmias." Physiologic stereotypies may be present in any setting but are most common when the child is excited, mentally engaged, stressed, or bored. They may increase with fatigue. A hallmark of stereotypies is that they usually cease when the child is distracted or engaged in a new activity. Most children appear to be unaware of the stereotypies.

There is no consistently effective pharmacologic treatment for stereotypies. They typically do not bother the patient but can be distressing to the parents. Stereotypies rarely interfere with task performance by the individual but may cause embarrassment or have some other social influence. Behavior therapy has been effective in some cases.

OTHER MOVEMENT DISORDERS
Restless Legs Syndrome and Periodic Leg Movements of Sleep

Restless legs syndrome (RLS) manifests as an uncomfortable sensation in the legs that is typically relieved by movement. The sensation is poorly described by most children, but adults often use the descriptors "crawling," "pulling," or "creeping" in connection with the sensation under the skin. The sensation and movements occur most often at night and usually peak within the first 20 minutes of lying down. Relief is obtained by moving the legs when lying down or by walking. RLS responds to treatment with dopaminergic medication, and dopamine agonists are most often used for adults with this condition. If serum ferritin is low, then iron supplementation may be considered. RLS is associated with Periodic Leg Movements of Sleep (PLMS), usually diagnosed on polysomnography. Treatment for PLMS, when needed, is the same as for RLS. Treatment is not needed in most children unless PLMS interferes with sleep or RLS prevents classroom participation. These disorders are discussed in Chapter 89.

Hyperekplexia

Hyperekplexia, otherwise known as familial startle disease, is an autosomal-dominant disorder characterized by an exaggerated startle reaction in response to sudden, unexpected auditory or tactile stimuli. Symptoms may begin in the neonatal period with profound and potentially fatal paroxysmal hypertonia and opisthotonic extensor posturing. Such episodes often resolve if the examiner flexes the neck, back, and knees of the child. Older children and adults may display nonadapting head retraction in response to nose tapping. The disorder is associated with several different gene mutations, but the classic form is due to mutation in the alpha-1 subunit of the glycine receptor. Symptoms respond well to treatment with clonazepam.

Bobble-Head Doll Syndrome

The bobble-head doll syndrome is a condition in which an infant or child has jerky head movements similar to certain types of toy doll. The movement is a continuous or episodic, involuntary, forward-and-backward or side-to-side movement of the head at the frequency of 2 to 3 Hz. The condition is usually associated with structural abnormalities leading to third ventricular dilatation, including third ventricular cyst, aqueductal stenosis, or tumor. Brain imaging virtually always confirms the presence of a structural abnormality. Surgical treatment is usually beneficial.

REFERENCES

The complete list of references for this chapter is available in the e-book at www.expertconsult.com.
 See inside cover for registration details.

SELECTED REFERENCES

Albanese, A., Bhatia, K., Bressman, S.B., et al., 2013. Phenomenology and classification of dystonia: a consensus update. Mov. Disord. 28, 863–873.

Carducci, N., Fernandez-Alvarez, E. (Eds.), 2007. Movement disorders in children: a clinical update with video recordings. John Libbey Eurotext.

Gerber, M.A., Baltimore, R.S., Eaton, C.B., et al., 2009. Prevention of rheumatic fever and diagnosis and treatment of acute Streptococcal pharyngitis: a scientific statement from the American Heart Association Rheumatic Fever, Endocarditis, and Kawasaki Disease Committee of the Council on Cardiovascular Disease in the Young, the Interdisciplinary Council on Functional Genomics and Translational Biology, and the Interdisciplinary Council on Quality of Care and Outcomes Research: endorsed by the American Academy of Pediatrics. Circulation 119 (11), 1541–1551.

Kurian, M.A., Li, Y., Zhen, J., et al., 2011. Clinical and molecular characterisation of hereditary dopamine transporter deficiency syndrome: an observational cohort and experimental study. Lancet Neurol. 10 (1), 54–62.

Paz, J.A., Silva, C.A., Marques-Dias, M.J., 2006. Randomized double-blind study with prednisone in Sydenham's chorea. Pediatr. Neurol. 34 (4), 264–269.

Sanger, T.D., Chen, D., Delgado, M.R., et al., 2006. Definition and classification of negative motor signs in childhood. Pediatrics 118 (5), 2159–2167.

Sanger, T.D., Chen, D., Fehlings, S.L., et al., 2010. Definition and classification of hyperkinetic movements in childhood. Mov. Disord. 25 (11), 1538–1549.

Sanger, T.D., Delgado, M.R., Gaebler-Spira, D., et al., 2003. Classification and definition of disorders causing hypertonia in childhood. Pediatrics 111 (1), e89–e97.

Singer, H.S., Mink, J.W., Gilbert, D.L., et al., 2016. Movement Disorders in Childhood, second ed. Academic Press, London.

⊗ E-BOOK FIGURES AND TABLES

The following figures and tables are available in the e-book at www.expertconsult.com. See inside cover for registration details.

94 Paroxysmal Dyskinesias

Laura Silveira Moriyama, Thomas T. Warner, and Jonathan W. Mink

INTRODUCTION

Paroxysmal dyskinesias are a relatively rare subset of hyperkinetic movement disorders that are defined by their episodic nature. Patients present with repeated episodes of dyskinesia (dystonia, chorea, or both) that have sudden onset and, after a duration that ranges from seconds to days, remit entirely and subsequently recur in a stereotyped fashion. They may be primary or secondary, and when primary they are often associated with genetic causes.

The clinical syndromes of paroxysmal dyskinesia were characterized throughout the 20th century according to their clinical features, including triggers, duration, and frequency of the episodes. These syndromes were named based on the main triggering factor that promotes the dyskinesia attacks. Paroxysmal kinesigenic dyskinesia (PKD) is triggered by sudden movements, paroxysmal exercise-induced dyskinesia (PED) is triggered by sustained physical effort, and paroxysmal nonkinesigenic dyskinesia (PNKD) is not triggered by movement, but sometimes is provoked by consumption of coffee or alcohol or by stress.

Although classic descriptions delineated clear motor phenotypes, it is now clear that paroxysmal dyskinesias form part of a spectrum of clinical manifestations. These manifestations include movement disorders, other paroxysmal phenomena like epilepsy, ataxia and migraine, and in addition some patients may present cognitive difficulties. Overlapping phenotypes as well as underreported associated features are now being integrated into the decision-making process for treating these conditions.

In the previous decades enormous progress was achieved in discovering gene mutations that underlie these very characteristic phenotypes, and previously overlooked clinical features (like the association with epilepsy, migraine, or other motor phenomena) gained renewed interest. The pathophysiology of these conditions is not entirely clear but some experimental evidence demonstrates increased activity in the basal ganglia corresponding to the dyskinesias. A link with epilepsy was proposed in the past and largely ignored until recently when it became clear that mutations in two of the genes associated with paroxysmal dyskinesias (namely, PRRT2 and SLC2A1) could cause both paroxysmal dyskinesia and epilepsy.

Paroxysmal dyskinesias can also be secondary to varied causes, including structural, metabolic, infectious, and inflammatory damage to the basal ganglia. These include head trauma, cerebral palsy, stroke, multiple sclerosis, moyamoya disease, infection, hypoglycemia, hyperglycemia, thyrotoxicosis, hypoparathyroidism, pseudohypoparathyroidism, maple syrup urine disease, biopterin synthesis defects, and methylphenidate therapy. For a review of secondary causes of paroxysmal dyskinesia (Roze et al., 2015). Management of secondary paroxysmal dyskinesias varies widely and includes the management of the etiologic factors as well as symptomatic treatment. Currently there are no guidelines as to how symptomatic treatment of secondary and primary paroxysmal dyskinesias differs, and so it is reasonable to adopt the more structured approach to treat primary dyskinesias, which are mainly classified by their phenomenology. Therefore a patient with a secondary PKD can be treated like one with primary PKD if the baseline condition does not contraindicate this approach. For instance, for a patient with Wilson disease that presents with PKDs, a trial of carbamazepine is warranted, except if contraindicated. For example, clinical or laboratorial alterations in liver function might preclude the use of carbamazepine. If this is the case, another strategy can be tried.

Paroxysmal dyskinesia may occasionally appear as a secondary phenomenon in various genetic conditions, but the classic idiopathic phenotypes are largely associated with mutations in specific genes reviewed in this chapter. The prevalence of idiopathic paroxysmal dyskinesias is not known, but they are assumed to be rare. Their iconic phenotypes, the possibility of genetic diagnosis, and the often positive response to treatment warrant recognition by any practicing clinician. In this chapter we describe in detail the clinical features of the classic idiopathic paroxysmal dyskinesias and the current management strategies. The online expanded version also includes a review of the historical context and often confusing terminology used to describe paroxysmal dyskinesias over the years, under a section named "Historical context and terminology." An expanded section, "Other phenotypes", elaborates further on the clinical description of rarer atypical forms of genetic paroxysmal dyskinesias as well as the expanded phenotypic spectrum of manifestations of the paroxysmal dyskinesia genes, including episodic ataxias, benign paroxysmal torticollis of childhood, paroxysmal tonic upward gaze and recurring hemiplegia (e.g., hemiplegic migraine and alternating hemiplegia of childhood).

HISTORICAL CONTEXT AND TERMINOLOGY

The variations in terminology used for these basic three forms have been a cause for confusion and are reviewed in the expanded online edition under this section. The current classification is largely based on the one proposed by Demirkiran and Jankovic in 1995. This classification is based primarily on the precipitating triggers, and divides the paroxysmal dyskinesias into kinesigenic, nonkinesigenic, exertion-induced, or hypnogenic (also known as paroxysmal nocturnal dystonia of sleep). After this initial categorization, they proposed a secondary categorization based on duration of the episodes into short (<5 minutes) or long (>5 minutes) and a tertiary classification based on etiology: idiopathic (familial vs. sporadic) and secondary.

CLASSIC PHENOTYPES OF PAROXYSMAL DYSKINESIA

Table 94-1 summarizes the main clinical features that characterize the classic phenotypes of PKD, PNKD, and PED. We now describe in detail the clinical and genetic features of these conditions, along with management strategies, including diagnosis and treatment. A review of more than 500 cases of

TABLE 94-1 Clinical Features of Paroxysmal Dyskinesias

Features	Paroxysmal Nonkinesigenic Dyskinesia (PNKD)	Paroxysmal Exercise-induced Dyskinesia (PED)	Paroxysmal Kinesigenic Dyskinesia (PKD)
Age of onset*	Variable, up to teenage onset	Variable, up to young adult onset	Usually in the first decade of life
Disease course	Improvement in adulthood and with ageing	Variable	Improvement or remission by 4th decade of life
Attacks duration	Minutes to hours	Minutes to hours	Seconds to minutes
Attacks frequency	Multiple attacks per month	Variable	Multiple daily attacks
Triggers	Alcohol, caffeine, emotional stress or excitement, fatigue, sleep deprivation	Prolonged exercise, fasting, emotional stress	Sudden voluntary movements (sprinting, standing up, etc.)
Main gene associated	PNKD	SLC2A1, Parkin, GCH1	PRRT2

GCH1, GTP cyclohydrolase 1; SLC2A1, solute carrier family 2 member 1 (also known as GLUT1).
*For most cases of primary paroxysmal dyskinesia, onset is in childhood.

genetically proven paroxysmal dyskinesia has been recently published (Erro et al., 2014).

Paroxysmal Kinesigenic Dyskinesia

Clinical Features

PKD is often inherited as an autosomal-dominant trait, but one quarter of the cases are sporadic. It is the most common form of primary paroxysmal dyskinesia, and most neurologists are likely to come across a couple of patients throughout their practicing years. Males are affected more often than females. The age of onset is 5 to 15 years in familial cases but may be variable in sporadic cases. The attacks are typically precipitated by startle or making a sudden movement after a period of rest. There is often a refractory period after an episode, during which a sudden movement will not provoke an attack. The attacks may occur up to 100 times per day, but most patients will report a few per day. The duration is typically a few seconds to a few minutes, usually less than a minute, but longer-lasting attacks may occur. The movements may be preceded by an abnormal sensation in the affected limbs, and some patients may only have an abnormal sensation without developing involuntary movements. Most patients have dystonia combined with choreiform movements, but some have a combination of chorea, dystonia, and, rarely, ballism. The attacks may be limited to one side of the body or even one limb. The attacks decrease in frequency during adulthood and usually subside or become very mild by the fourth decade of life. For a series of videos of attacks, see Silveira-Moriyama et al. (2013). The classic trigger is sudden voluntary movement after a period of rest or being still. Examples include quickly standing up from a chair, or quickly running after standing for a period of time. The well-known maneuver of asking the patient to quickly stand up after sitting down for a few minutes might elicit attacks during a clinic visit and is often found to be useful, although not very sensitive. The majority of patients will also report spontaneous nonkinesigenic attacks in association, and so their presence should not discourage the diagnosis of PKD.

Genetics

After the initial clinical descriptions mentioned in the historical background section, it became evident that PKD often had a hereditary nature. In addition, in some of the families with PKD a number of patients presented with infantile seizures similar to benign familial infantile convulsions (also called benign familial infantile seizures, BFIS; OMIM No. 605751), and this association was called infantile convulsions and paroxysmal choreoathetosis (ICCA; OMIM No. 602066). In 1997

ICCA was linked to the pericentromeric region of chromosome 16, and it was observed that individuals homozygous for the disease haplotype in the pericentromeric region of chromosome 16 had earlier age of onset and higher frequency of attacks than heterozygous family members. Later on, PKD without infantile convulsions was also linked to the pericentromeric region of chromosome 16, except for one single family with PKD linked to 16q in another region. It became clear that the ICCA locus was linked to other families with PKD, ICCA, or both. In 2011 mutations in the proline-rich transmembrane protein 2 gene (PRRT2) were identified as the cause of ICCA, BFIS and also PKD linked to chromosome 16. Soon after, the same PRRT2 mutations were found to be associated with hemiplegic migraine, and also one case of benign paroxysmal torticollis and a few of episodic ataxia.

Numerous different pathogenic mutations have been reported in PRRT2, most of which are deletions, nonsense and occasionally missense, suggesting haploinsufficiency. The most commonly reported is an insertion (c.649dupC) that leads to a premature stop codon and a consequently truncated protein. This mutation has been associated with various different phenotypes within the spectrum, posing a challenge to clear-cut genotype–phenotype correlations, except for more severe homozygous cases. The few families in which PRRT2 mutations have been found in homozygosity show a more severe phenotype often involving earlier onset of attacks, coexistence of paroxysmal dyskinesia and episodic ataxia, and cognitive changes, including intellectual disability. Interestingly, a previous study using next-generation sequencing and homozygosity mapping in familial intellectual disability had associated PRRT2 with nonsyndromic intellectual disability in one family. PRRT2 codes for a transmembrane protein that is highly expressed during developmental stages of the animal brain, and although its specific function is not known, protein network studies suggest it is associated with synaptic transmission. The homozygous phenotype emphasizes the role of PRRT2 in brain development. In addition, PKD has also been associated with microdeletions encompassing PRRT2 in a few cases. In these cases, associated features such as speech delay, intellectual disability, and mild dysmorphic features were described and are likely to be related to neighboring genes.

Diagnosis

Bruno et al. (2004) proposed a set of clinical criteria for the diagnosis of PKD, which is often useful in clinical practice and is summarized below:

1. Identified kinesigenic trigger of the attacks
2. Short duration of attacks (<1 minute)
3. No loss of consciousness or pain during attacks

4. Exclusion of other organic diseases and normal neurologic examination
5. Control of attacks with phenytoin or carbamazepine, if tried
6. Age at onset between 1 and 20 years, if no family history of PKD

It is important to note that although PNKD and PED are unlikely to have classic kinesigenic attacks, the opposite is not true: PKD often presents with spontaneous nonkinesigenic attacks, and attacks might be caused by stress or exercise. In a minority of PKD patients, attacks might be elicited during the clinical visit when patients present sudden movements.

The diagnosis of PKD is made on clinical grounds, but investigation is often warranted to exclude other conditions. In cases with recent onset without a clear family history, brain imaging might be needed to investigate structural brain damage associated with secondary paroxysmal dyskinesias. In most cases EEG can be performed either to rule out epilepsy, or to investigate the coexistence of epilepsy.

In classic cases of PKD, genetic testing can confirm the presence of a *PRRT2* mutation in order to provide the appropriate genetic counseling. Because of the expanding phenotypic spectrum, atypical cases might also be tested for *PRRT2* mutations. In many centers worldwide, panels of genes associated with paroxysmal motor phenomena will include *PRRT2* along with other genes described later in this chapter. Microarray analyses to screen for microdeletions encompassing 16p11.2 might be indicated when additional features suggest microdeletions.

Treatment

PKD responds well to anticonvulsants, including phenytoin, carbamazepine, phenobarbital, and levetiracetam. The dose required is usually less than the standard anticonvulsant dosage and familial PKD is exquisitely responsive to carbamazepine. It is possible that PRRT2-related PKD (as opposed to cases in which gene testing is negative) might indicate a better response to low doses of carbamazepine, but gene testing is not needed for therapeutic management. Carbamazepine is usually well tolerated in low doses, but in Asian populations human leukocyte antigen (HLA) testing for haplotypes associated with carbamazepine-induced pharmacodermia may be useful to guide anticonvulsant therapy. With or without treatment, the attacks tend to diminish during adulthood and individuals with the classic phenotype do not have progressive neurologic deficits.

Paroxysmal Nonkinesigenic Dyskinesia

Clinical Features

PNKD is usually inherited as an autosomal-dominant trait. Males are affected more often than females, by a ratio of 2 : 1. The age of onset is usually in early childhood, but attacks may start in the first months of life, or as late as young adulthood. The frequency varies from three per day to two or fewer per year. Typical precipitating factors are alcohol, caffeine, fatigue, and emotional excitement. Alcohol and caffeine are the most consistently reported. Attacks might be preceded by sensory aura (in about half the patients), and an episode usually starts with involuntary movements of a single limb or hemibody, but tends to spread to involve all extremities and the face. The usual duration is minutes to 3 to 4 hours, but shorter and longer episodes have been reported. Attacks may be relieved by sleep. During the attack, the patient may be unable to communicate, but remains conscious and continues to breathe normally. Some individuals have mostly dystonia, whereas others have predominantly chorea but most have a combination of both.

For detailed and systematized clinical information of more than 40 cases of PNKD, see Bruno et al. (2007).

Genetics

In 1997 PNKD was linked to chromosome 2q and in 2004 mutations of the myofibrillogenesis regulator 1 gene (then called the *MR1* gene, and now called the *PNKD* gene) were found to cause the majority of PKND cases. Bruno et al. (2007) compared 8 kindreds with detailed clinical information on 49 subjects harboring PNKD mutations to 6 kindreds without the mutations and found the following criteria to be predictive of positive testing for PNKD mutations:

1. Hyperkinetic involuntary movement attacks, with dystonia, chorea, or combination of these, typically lasting 10 minutes to 1 hour, but up to 4 hours
2. Normal neurologic examination results between attacks, and exclusion of secondary causes
3. Onset of attacks in infancy or early childhood
4. Precipitation of attacks by caffeine and alcohol consumption
5. Family history of movement disorder meeting criteria 1 through 4

PNKD mutation carriers studied by Bruno and colleagues (2007) presented the classic features described by Mount and Reback, had onset in childhood (average 4 years ± 4.6 years), reported frequency up to once a week at least at some point in life, and were likely to respond to benzodiazepines and improve with ageing. Migraine was a frequent comorbidity, but none of 49 patients had epilepsy.

The function of the PNKD protein is not well known. PNKD is expressed in the brain, and pathogenic mutations lead to abnormalities of postprocessing (cleavage and stability) of the PNKD protein affecting the cell gluthatione antioxidant system in animal models. In addition, PNKD might be linked with an enzyme that metabolizes methylglyoxal, which is found in coffee and alcoholic beverages, possibly explaining why they act as triggers in PKND.

In addition to PNKD, another gene has been associated with PNKD in a single family that had PNKD and generalized epilepsy. The locus was therefore named *generalized epilepsy and paroxysmal dyskinesia* (GEPD), and a mutation was found in the gene *KCNMA1* segregating with the phenotype. This gene codes for the pore-forming alpha subunit of a specific potassium channel activated both by intracellular Ca(2+) ions and by membrane. Although this remains a possibility in cases of PED with concomitant generalized epilepsy, there has been only a single description of pathogenic mutation, and therefore screening for *PRRT2* mutations, which can also cause nonkinesigenic episodes as well as epilepsy, might be warranted in most patients.

Diagnosis

The clinical criteria proposed by Bruno et al. (2007) help to make the diagnosis, in particular when associated with videorecordings of attacks, either in telemetry or homemade. PNKD is less prevalent than PKD, and the attacks are very unlikely to be witnessed by the physician. Except for the positive diagnosis of *PNKD* mutations, PNKD is a clinical diagnosis. EEG may be warranted to exclude epileptic seizures. Imaging may be warranted to rule out structural damage to the basal ganglia causing secondary paroxysmal dyskinesia. Metabolic testing might be indicated based on the age and associated features. In older children and teenagers, psychogenic movement disorder is an important differential. Because various genetic causes of paroxysmal dyskinesia can cause nonkinesigenic attacks, in atypical cases genetic testing by a panel can be indicated, although empirical management should be performed regardless.

Treatment

Management of PNKD relies on avoidance of precipitating factors, such as alcohol, caffeine, and stress. Several medications have been used, including clonazepam, haloperidol, oxazepam, acetazolamide, and anticholinergics. Anticonvulsants are ineffective in most cases of PNKD, including those that are mutation negative and positive. In PNKD mutation-positive cases, clonazepam is likely to be helpful, taken as both prophylactic and abortive agent. In Bruno et al (2007) 97% (34/35) of patients who tried benzodiazepines responded. Other medications tried included a variety of anticonvulsants (including carbamazepine and phenytoin) and haloperidol, all without a consistent response. Deep-brain stimulation surgery might be considered in selected cases with significant impairment of quality of life, given that two reports exist of successful treatment of PNKD with this technique.

Prognosis is variable and depends on the underlying cause, but in familial cases, neurologic function between the attacks is normal, even after repeated attacks, and the frequency of attacks decreases with age.

Paroxysmal Exertion-Induced Dyskinesia

Clinical Features

PED is usually inherited in an autosomal-dominant fashion, although sporadic cases have been described. The characteristic feature of PED is the triggering of attacks by sustained exercise (minutes to hours of exercise, as opposed to the sudden movements in PKD). Stress and fasting have also been described as additional triggers in these patients, although their presence as triggers alone does not characterize PED, remitting more to PNKD. The frequency varies from one per day to two per month. The usual duration is 5 to 30 minutes and therefore an intermediate duration between what is expected of PKD (seconds to minutes) and PNKD (minutes to hours). Unlike PKD and PNKD, which are more clinically homogeneous and in which a significant proportion of the cases (more than half) have genetic cause, PED is more likely to be an umbrella phenotype encompassing manifestations of different conditions.

Genetics

Many cases of PED remain idiopathic, although cases of the classic form of PED have been linked to mutations in the *SLC2A1* gene. SLC2A1 codes for a transmembrane protein that facilitates glucose transport, known as GLUT1, and its mutations cause a range of neurologic manifestations, including a well-recognizable form of neonatal epileptic encephalopathy, and various other pleomorphic manifestations, including epilepsy and movement disorders. For a review of SLC2A1 manifestations, see Pearson et al. (2013). De Giorgis and colleagues (2015) observed that in a cohort of 22 patients with GLUT1 deficiency syndrome and confirmed SLC2A1 mutations, at least half presented with PED, making it a common feature for SLC2A1. GLUT1 facilitates transport of glucose across the blood–brain barrier, and mutations usually lead to loss of function causing low glucose levels in the CNS, which can be detected in many patients with GLUT1 deficiency syndrome as hypoglycorrhachia providing a useful diagnostic clue.

In addition to classic PED linked to GLUT1 deficiency syndrome, cases of exercise-induced paroxysmal dyskinesia have also been described in dopamine deficiency syndromes, more specifically in dopa-responsive dystonia caused by mutations in *GCH1* and levodopa-responsive young-onset parkinsonism caused by *PARKIN* mutations. It is likely that the paroxysmal episodes have a different pathophysiology to classic PED and are phenocopies. In favor of this is the fact that the episodes are usually dystonic and localized (although this is also seen in PED), and they are often associated with fatigue, instead of being truly exercise induced. Nevertheless, there is definitely an overlap with classic PED features, and two cases of response to levodopa in PED caused by *SLC2A1* mutations have been described, pointing out a possible pathophysiological overlap between the functions of these three genes.

Diagnosis

Like other paroxysmal dyskinesias, PED must be differentiated from secondary forms of paroxysmal dyskinesia, and brain imaging, EEG, and biochemical studies are often needed. Most cases of PED are still idiopathic, but the positive diagnosis can be made by finding hypoglycorrhachia (which is not sensitive but is specific for *SLC2A1* mutations) and by encountering mutations in *SLC2A1*, *GCH1*, or *PARKIN* on genetic testing. Given that the coexistence of seizures in individuals suffering from SLC2A1-related PED is high, they can also be considered a diagnostic clue. Given the growing availability of diagnostic gene panels and the genetic heterogeneity that marks paroxysmal movement disorders, testing by a gene panel including genes associated with episodic motor phenomena might be warranted.

Treatment

Avoidance of prolonged exercise may help diminish the frequency of attacks and might be recommended given that drug therapy is often ineffective in PED. There are isolated and conflicting reports of response to different strategies, including carbamazepine, acetazolamide, gabapentin and levodopa. In the patients from Di Giorgi and colleagues who were put on a classical 3 : 1 ketogenic ratio diet (i.e., 3 g lipids:1 g carbohydrates + proteins), later reduced to 1.8 : 1 ratio, there was a noticeable response of PED episodes, which disappeared in a few weeks, compatible with previous reports of response of PED to the ketogenic diet found in the literature. Nevertheless, the practical challenges in effectively implementing this diet make it a second-line option in isolated PED. One recent report of four patients with GLUT1 deficiency syndrome suggested the use of a modified Atkins diet, which is more tolerated, as an alternative to ketogenic diet, but further studies are needed. For a review of GLUT1 deficiency syndrome and its phenotypic spectrum, please see Chapter 76.

OTHER PHENOTYPES

Paroxysmal Hypnogenic Dyskinesia

For a review of the current knowledge about paroxysmal hypnogenic dyskinesia, please refer to the online material. This condition, previously thought to be a movement disorder and now mostly believed to be a form of epilepsy, is discussed in detail in the online expanded edition under this same section.

For a brief review of nocturnal frontal lobe epilepsy (NFLE), see Nobili (2007).

Genotype–Phenotype Association in Paroxysmal Dyskinesia

In addition to abnormalities in PRRT2, PNKD, SLC2A1, GCH1, and PARKIN, a series of other genetic disorders can cause paroxysmal episodes of dyskinesia. Usually in these conditions, there are also other features, which can point toward the genetic diagnosis. Alternating hemiplegia of childhood, which is caused by mutations in the ATP1A3 gene, often presents with associated episodes of paroxysmal dyskinesia. This gene also causes rapid-onset dystonia parkinsonism (RDP), a juvenile condition in which dystonia and/or parkinsonism develops acutely over the course of hours or days, and remains stable thereafter. Patients with alternating hemiplegia or childhood or RDP can present with paroxysmal dyskinesia, although these are thought to be rare in RDP. Attacks can be nonkinesigenic or exercise-induced, and although mainly dystonic can also present with choreiform movements.

SLC2A1 mutations can manifest with a wide range of clinical phenotypes, both chronic and paroxysmal, of which PED is a common (and relatively mild) feature. Some patients present with more chronic pyramidal and extrapyramidal disorders (such as spasticity, dystonia, or ataxia) or cognitive decline (a spectrum from clear-cut encephalopathy to varying degrees of cognitive difficulties) in addition to epilepsy, whereas others can have milder phenotypes with isolated PED, or with PED and combined epilepsy. The locus originally reserved for DYT9, called paroxysmal choreoathetosis/spasticity, was later found out to correspond to SLC2A1, and it is now clear that these manifestations fall within the spectrum of SLC2A1 disease.

In addition to genetic heterogeneity and variable expressivity, there is ample phenotypic pleiotropy in the paroxysmal dyskinesia genes. Phenotypic pleiotropy is the name given to the fact that one single gene, or even a single gene mutation, can influence various different phenotypic traits. *PRRT2*, for instance, is a gene with a very wide phenotypic pleiotropy, and can cause isolated PKD, isolated BFIS, combined ICCA, various forms of epilepsy of varied age of onset, hemiplegic migraine, episodic ataxia, benign paroxysmal torticollis, progressive ataxia, and intellectual disability. This particular spectrum of manifestations overlaps largely with that of *CACNA1A*, the gene that is associated with episodic ataxia type 2.

Figure 94-1 shows how various genes can cause paroxysmal episodes of dyskinesia. The overlap in clinical presentations and expression mean that it is reasonable that genetic testing with gene panels with all these genes will be suitable for the investigation of paroxysmal dyskinesia patients.

These overlapping phenotypes between the genes for paroxysmal dyskinesias, episodic ataxias, and some other paroxysmal conditions (such as alternating hemiplegia) have been used as a rationale to justify empirical treatment of paroxysmal dyskinesias with some of the drugs used to treat these other conditions, and reports of successful treatment with rescue therapies are progressively appearing in the literature. It is possible that, in the future, treatment will be guided by the underlying genetic basis of the condition, but for the moment there is not enough evidence to support this as first line. Table 94-2 summarizes the current main treatment strategies used for paroxysmal dyskinesias.

TABLE 94-2 Treatment Strategies for Paroxysmal Dyskinesias

Features	Main Treatment Strategies
Paroxysmal nonkinesigenic dyskinesia (PNKD)	Variable response to treatment. Benzodiazepines can be tried and many report benefit from clonazepam. Unlikely to respond to antiseizure medications. Anecdotal reports of other treatments being successful. Usually improves or disappears with age.
Paroxysmal exercise-induced dyskinesia (PED)	Variable response to pharmacologic treatment, which can include benzodiazepines, acetazolamide, ketogenic diet, antiseizure medications, and levodopa. Variable course can persist into adulthood. When caused by GCH1 and *Parkin* can evolve into dystonia or parkinsonism, which is responsive to levodopa.
Paroxysmal kinesigenic dyskinesia (PKD)	Reassurance. Pharmacotherapy with antiseizure medications. Carbamazepine is the most widely used, and many report successful use of phenytoin. Other antiepileptic drugs can be tried. Usually subsides by 4th decade of life.

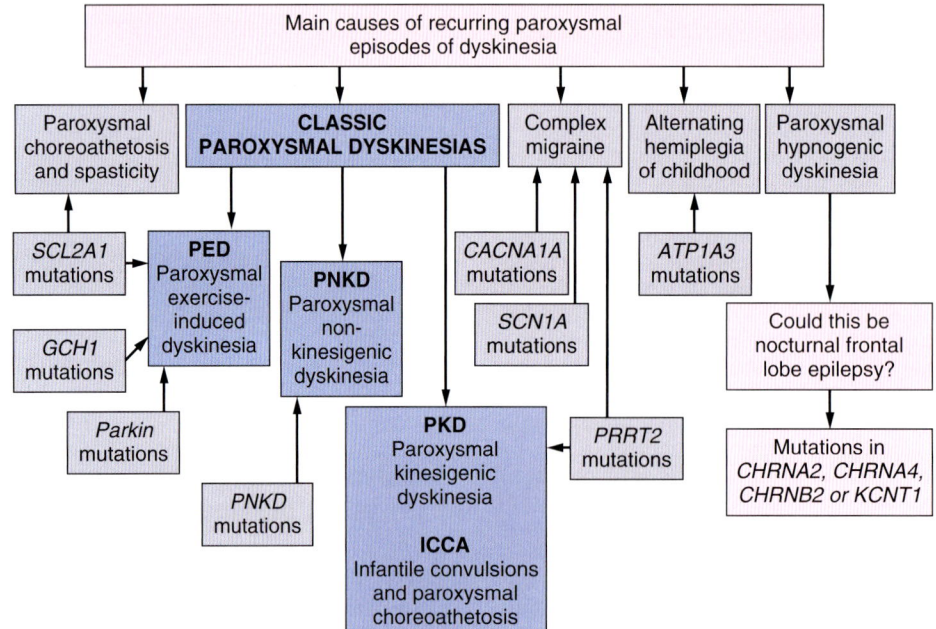

Figure 94-1. Main genetic causes of recurring paroxysmal episodes of dyskinesia. *ATP1A3*, ATPase, Na+/K+ transporting, alpha-3 polypeptide; *CACNA1A*, calcium channel, voltage-dependent, p/q type, alpha-1a subunit; *CHRNA2*, A4 and B2, cholinergic receptor, neuronal nicotinic, polypeptide alpha 2, alpha 4, beta 2; *GCH1*, GTP cyclohydrolase 1; *KCNT1*, potassium channel, subfamily t, member 1; *PRRT2*, proline-rich transmembrane protein 2; *SCN1A*, sodium channel, neuronal type I, alpha subunit; *SLC2A1*, solute carrier family 2 member 1 (also known as *GLUT1*).

Acknowledgments

The authors would like to thank Rafael Carvalho for reference management of the online version, Kathleen Munger for proofreading, and Prof. Emmanuel Roze for useful suggestions about paroxysmal hypnogenic dyskinesia (see extended online version).

REFERENCES

The complete list of references for this chapter is available in the e-book at www.expertconsult.com.

See inside cover for registration details.

SELECTED REFERENCES

Bruno, M.K., Hallett, M., Gwinn-Hardy, K., et al., 2004. Clinical evaluation of idiopathic paroxysmal kinesigenic dyskinesia: new diagnostic criteria. Neurology 63, 2280–2287.

Bruno, M.K., Lee, H.-Y., Auburger, G.W.J., et al., 2007. Genotype-phenotype correlation of paroxysmal nonkinesigenic dyskinesia. Neurology 68, 1782–1789.

De Giorgis, V., Teutonico, F., Cereda, C., et al., 2015. Sporadic and familial glut1ds Italian patients: A wide clinical variability. Seizure Eur. J. Epilepsy 24, 28–32.

Erro, R., Sheerin, U.M., Bhatia, K.P., 2014. Paroxysmal dyskinesias revisited: a review of 500 genetically proven cases and a new classification. Mov. Disord. 29, 1108–1116.

Nobili, E., 2007. Nocturnal frontal lobe epilepsy and non-rapid eye movement sleep parasomnias: differences and similarities. Sleep Med. Rev. 11, 251–254.

Pearson, T.S., Akman, C., Hinton, V.J., et al., 2013. Phenotypic spectrum of glucose transporter type 1 deficiency syndrome (Glut1 DS). Curr. Neurol. Neurosci. Rep. 13, 342.

Roze, E., Meneret, A., Vidailhet, M., 2015. Paroxysmal movement disorders: classification and genetics. In: Ledoux, M.S. (Ed.), Animal Models of Movement Disorders: Genetics and Methods. Academic Press, New York, pp. 767–776.

Silveira-Moriyama, L., Gardiner, A.R., Meyer, E., et al., 2013. Clinical features of childhood-onset paroxysmal kinesigenic dyskinesia with PRRT2 gene mutations. Dev. Med. Child Neurol. 55, 327–334.

95 Movement Disorders of Infancy

Joanna S. Blackburn and Jonathan W. Mink

An expanded version of this chapter is available on www.expertconsult.com. See inside cover for registration details.

The presence of a movement disorder in an infant usually raises concerns about an underlying serious, progressive, degenerative, or metabolic disease. However, many movement disorders are benign and related to normal stages of development. In fact, it may be difficult to justify the term "disorder" in describing many of these movements. The developing nervous system may produce a variety of motor patterns that would be pathologic in older children and adults, but are simply a manifestation of central nervous system immaturity. Like many of the neonatal reflexes (e.g., grasping, rooting, placing, tonic neck reflexes), these motor patterns disappear as neuron connectivity and myelination mature. Examples include the minimal chorea of infants, the mild action dystonia commonly seen in toddlers, and the overflow movements that are seen in young children. Other transient or developmental movement disorders of infancy may be manifestations of abnormal neural function, but do not correlate with serious underlying pathology. These are typically associated with complete resolution of the abnormal movements and, ultimately, normal development and neurologic function. It is important to recognize these transient developmental movement disorders of infancy to distinguish them from more serious disorders, and to be able to provide reassurance when possible. Correct identification of this group of disorders may decrease the need for additional diagnostic testing. Often these disorders can be distinguished from a pathologic movement disorder on the clinical basis alone. The phenomenologies of movement disorders of infancy include myoclonus, stereotypic movements, tremors, and dystonia or posturing (Table 95-1).

Benign Neonatal Sleep Myoclonus

Benign neonatal sleep myoclonus was first described in 1982 and is characterized by repetitive myoclonic jerks occurring during sleep (Maurer, Rizzi, Bianchetti, and Ramelli, 2010). The myoclonic jerks are typically in the distal more than proximal limbs, and more prominent in the upper than the lower extremities. In some cases, jerks of axial or facial muscles can be seen, but involvement of the facial muscles is more rare. The myoclonus can be focal, multifocal, unilateral, or bilateral. The movements can be rhythmic or nonrhythmic. Typically, the movements occur in clusters of jerks at 1 to 5 Hz over a period of several seconds.

The prevalence of benign neonatal sleep myoclonus is 0.8 to 3 cases per 1000 births (Maurer et al., 2010). Benign neonatal sleep myoclonus begins during the first week of life, diminishes in the second month, and is usually gone before 6 months of age, but has been reported to persist as long as 3 years in one patient and 4 years in another patient. The movements are most likely to occur during quiet (non-REM) sleep but have been described in all sleep stages. Waking the baby causes the movements to abruptly cease. The differential diagnosis of benign neonatal sleep myoclonus includes benign neonatal seizures, neonatal status epilepticus, typical hypnic jerks, and jitteriness. Episodes of myoclonus are not associated with eye deviation, oral movements, apnea, color changes, or crying, which can distinguish them from seizures (Maurer et al., 2010). Neurologic examination is normal. Ictal and interictal EEG are typically normal. Episodes of myoclonus can be exacerbated by treatment with benzodiazepines. Episodes of myoclonus have been described to be triggered by rocking motion, tactile stimulation (Maurer et al., 2010), and riding in a car. Benign neonatal sleep myoclonus has been described to occur at a higher incidence in opioid-dependent mothers. Treatment is not required, and neurologic outcome is normal.

Familial cases of benign neonatal sleep myoclonus have been described, with some pedigrees showing an autosomal-dominant inheritance pattern. It was found to be nonallelic to KCNQ2 and KCNQ3, the most common causes of benign familial neonatal seizures, which present at the same age as benign neonatal sleep myoclonus.

Benign Myoclonus of Early Infancy

Benign myoclonus of early infancy was first described in 1977 as a syndrome that was clinically indistinguishable from West syndrome, but these children had normal EEGs and a good prognosis. Benign myoclonus of early infancy is characterized by episodes of myoclonic spasms involving flexion of the trunk, neck, and extremities in a manner resembling the infantile spasms of West syndrome. The myoclonic spasms typically occur in clusters. In some cases, they involve a shuddering movement of the head and shoulders; in others, the movements of the trunk and limbs are extensor. The clinical spectrum of movements has been expanded to include myoclonic jerks, nonepileptic spasms, brief tonic contractions, shuddering or shivering, and nonepileptic atonic events or negative myoclonus, or a combination of these motor phenomena (Caraballo et al., 2009). There is no change in consciousness during the spells.

The onset of these spells is usually between ages 3 and 9 months, but they may begin in the first month of life. The spells usually cease within 2 weeks to 8 months of onset, but may persist for 1 to 2 years. In most cases, the episodes cease during the second year of life (Caraballo et al., 2009). Both ictal and interictal EEGs are normal. The movements occur only in the awake state. There is no known genetic cause, and cases are sporadic.

The differential diagnosis of benign myoclonus of infancy includes West syndrome, myoclonic epilepsy syndromes, shuddering attacks, benign neonatal sleep myoclonus, and hypnic jerks. Unlike benign neonatal sleep myoclonus, the movements in benign myoclonus of early infancy only occur in the waking state. Both ictal and interictal EEGs are normal, distinguishing this entity from infantile spasms and myoclonic epilepsy syndromes. An EEG is usually needed to exclude infantile spasms or infantile myoclonic epilepsy syndromes. Differentiating benign myoclonus of early infancy from epileptic syndromes of infancy is essential to avoid unnecessary extensive diagnostic workup and treatment with

TABLE 95-1 Movement Disorders of Infancy

Disorder	Age at Onset	Age at Resolution	Key Features
Benign neonatal sleep myoclonus	<1 month	6 months	Occurs exclusively in sleep
Benign myoclonus of early infancy	3–9 months	<2 years	Normal ictal and interictal EEG
Jitteriness	<1 week	<6 months	Stimulus sensitive Suppressible
Shuddering	Infancy to early childhood	Variable	Predictable triggers Preserved consciousness
Paroxysmal tonic upgaze	<1 year	1–4 years	Sustained upward or, less often, downward gaze
Spasmus nutans	3–8 months	Within a few months	Triad of head tremor, nystagmus, and torticollis
Head nodding	<3 years	Variable	Occurs while sitting or standing, suppressible
Benign paroxysmal torticollis	<1 year	<5 years	Family history of migraines
Benign idiopathic dystonia of infancy	<5 months	<1 year	Segmental dystonia
Infantile masturbation	<3 years	Variable	Characteristic position, distractible

unneeded, potentially harmful medications, and to provide an accurate prognosis. Treatment of benign myoclonus of early infancy is not needed, and movements are self-limited. Development and neurologic outcomes are normal.

Jitteriness

Jitteriness is the most common movement disorder observed in the neonatal period. Jitteriness manifests as generalized, symmetric, rhythmic oscillatory movements that resemble tremor or clonus. Jitteriness can involve the chin and/or extremities. Jitteriness is highly stimulus sensitive. It can be precipitated by startle and suppressed by gentle passive flexion of the limb. Unlike seizures, there are no associated abnormal eye movements or autonomic changes, and the EEG is normal.

Jitteriness is divided into four categories: no jitteriness if observed in sleep only, mild if only when irritable or crying, moderate if when in the awake state, and extreme if during several behavioral states. Up to 50% of term infants exhibit jitteriness during the first few days of life, especially when stimulated or crying. Jittery movements have been noted to occur in sleep (Shuper et al., 1991). Jitteriness usually disappears shortly after birth, but can persist for months or recur after being gone for several weeks (Shuper et al., 1991). Jitteriness usually resolves by a year of age but may persist until 2 years of age. Those with mild jitteriness outgrow their symptoms earlier than those with more severe jitteriness. Jitteriness has been associated with mildly increased muscle tone, hyperactive deep tendon reflexes, and a low threshold to startle (Shuper et al., 1991). Jitteriness has also been associated with infants who are more difficult to console and who are less visually alert. Persistent jitteriness has been associated with hypoxic-ischemic injury, intracerebral hemorrhage, hypocalcemia, hypoglycemia, hypomagnesaemia, and drug withdrawal, which may produce neuronal hyperirritability. Jitteriness has been described to co-occur with spasmus nutans.

Idiopathic jitteriness may be related to a maturational phenomenon rather than cerebral irritability. Peripheral and central mechanisms may contribute to jitteriness in infancy. There may be an increased sensitivity of the muscle spindle afferent endings that causes a response to a tiny stretch of the muscle, leading to jitteriness. With maturation of the inhibitory tracts in the central nervous system, the jitteriness disappears (Shuper et al., 1991). It has also been suggested that temporarily elevated levels of circulating catecholamines may contribute to jitteriness. Idiopathic jitteriness is usually associated with normal development and neurologic outcome. The outcome of infants with symptomatic jitteriness depends on the underlying cause. There is no treatment needed.

Shuddering

Shuddering episodes are characterized by periods of rapid tremor of the head, shoulders, and arms that resemble shivering (Kanazawa, 2000). Shuddering is often accompanied by facial grimacing. During a spell, there is no change in consciousness or color change. The episodes last several seconds and can occur up to 100 times a day, with high interindividual and intraindividual variability. Spells are often triggered by excitement, frustration, embarrassment, or surprise. They usually occur in the sitting or standing position. Onset is in infancy or early childhood, but can occur as late as 10 years of age. Ictal and interictal EEGs are normal. Shuddering episodes typically abate as the child grows older. The differential diagnosis of shuddering attacks includes benign neonatal sleep myoclonus, jitteriness, epilepsy, benign myoclonus of infancy, and tremor. The preservation of consciousness, predictable triggers, ability to abort an episode when distracted by a parent, and normal EEG distinguish this entity from seizures. However, frontal lobe epilepsy secondary to focal cortical dysplasia has been described to have a similar semiology to shuddering attacks, but onset of spells was at age 6. Similarity to benign myoclonus of early infancy has been suggested (Kanazawa, 2000), but shuddering differs in the phenomenology of the movement and is better classified as tremor than myoclonus. There may be similarity or overlap between shuddering episodes and stereotypies. Stereotypies are rhythmic, patterned, and repetitive involuntary movements. Similar features include the age of onset in infancy and early childhood, rhythmicity, presence of facial grimacing, and precipitating factors. Stereotypies differ in that they tend to last longer (minutes rather than seconds) and persist into later childhood and adulthood. An association with essential tremor has been described, but further studies have not supported this association. The pathophysiology of shuddering attacks is unknown. The prognosis for development and neurologic function is uniformly good. Treatment with propranolol has been described to be effective in a single patient, but treatment is generally not needed.

Paroxysmal Tonic Upgaze of Infancy

Paroxysmal tonic upgaze of infancy is a disorder characterized by repeated episodes of upward gaze deviation first described in 1988 (Ouvrier and Billson, 1988). The gaze deviation can be sustained or intermittent during an episode, sometimes associated with flexion of the neck apparently compensating for abnormal eye position. The typical episode lasts for a few hours but can persist for days. Attempts to look downward are accompanied by down-beating nystagmus. Horizontal eye movements are normal during an episode. Spells may resolve with sleep and be aggravated by fatigue or infection. There is a suggestion that cases with a later onset have a better prognosis. Two infants with paroxysmal down gaze have been described.

In follow up of children with paroxysmal tonic upgaze of infancy, neurologic and ophthalmologic abnormalities have been described. Ocular abnormalities include persistent gaze-evoked nystagmus, hypometric saccades, and strabismus. Neurologic abnormalities include cognitive disorders, structural lesions, epilepsy and ataxia although some infants may only have ataxia during the episodes (Ouvrier and Billson, 1988). Cognitive disorders have been noted in about 50% of children, with the majority having mild deficits. Structural MRI abnormalities include periventricular leukomalacia (Ouvrier and Billson, 1988), hypomyelinating leukoencephalopathy, vein of Galen malformation, and pinealoma. Paroxysmal tonic upgaze of infancy has been described to coexist with absence epilepsy, worsening with valproate treatment in one instance and improving in another, and with to febrile seizures. This suggests the possibility that it can be the marker of an underlying neurologic or developmental abnormality and may not always have a positive outcome.

The pathophysiology may be related to immaturity of the cortico-mesencephalic control of vertical gaze or from a lesion of the mesencephalic region. Familial cases have been described with both autosomal-dominant and autosomal-recessive inheritance. Associations with de novo mutation in CACNA1A and partial tetrasomy of chromosome 15 have been described in case reports. Additional laboratory evaluation is usually unrevealing. There is no specific treatment, but there have been a few reports of improvement with l-DOPA treatment (Ouvrier and Billson, 1988).

Spasmus Nutans

Spasmus nutans is a condition beginning in late infancy (3–8 months) that is characterized by a slow head tremor (approximately 2 Hz) that can be horizontal ("no-no") or vertical ("yes-yes"). The head movements are accompanied by a small-amplitude nystagmus that can be dysconjugate, conjugate, or uniocular. The nystagmus is typically pendular, with high frequencies (up to 15 Hz) and low amplitudes (0.5–3 degrees). When the child is looking at an object, the nodding or nystagmus may increase; if the head is held, the nystagmus typically increases. These observations have led to the suggestion that the head nodding is compensatory for the nystagmus. Torticollis by clinical observation and electrooculography has been shown to dampen the nystagmus, suggesting that this also is compensatory. Spasmus nutans generally resolves within several months, but the majority of patients continue to have a fine subclinical nystagmus until at least 5 to 12 years of age (Gottlob, Wizov, and Reincecke, 1995). Long-term outcome for visual acuity is good.

The differential diagnosis of nystagmus in infancy includes congenital nystagmus, retinal abnormalities, and nystagmus in association with an optic glioma. Spasmus nutans most commonly must be distinguished from congenital nystagmus. Congenital nystagmus usually begins earlier than spasmus nutans, starting in newborn period or before 6 months of age. Congenital nystagmus is usually bilaterally symmetric, whereas spasmus nutans is often asymmetric. Congenital nystagmus

persists beyond a few months. Visual acuity is abnormal in about 90% of children with congenital nystagmus. Although these features are useful in distinguishing congenital nystagmus from spasmus nutans, some children who clinically appear to have spasmus nutans at the time of presentation have been found to have retinal abnormalities on electroretinography (ERG).

Neuroimaging abnormalities, including tumor and aplasia of the cerebellar vermis, have been described in patients with spasmus nutans, but this is a rare association. Children found to have optic nerve gliomas or suprasellar tumors often have additional findings on examination, including a relative afferent pupillary defect, optic atrophy or optic nerve swelling, macrocephaly, café au lait spots, coexistent neurologic dysfunction or emaciation. It has been noted that spasmus nutans resolved spontaneously in a child with a chiasmal glioma. The patient with cerebellar vermis hypoplasia also had oculomotor apraxia. Routine neuroimaging in the absence of other evidence for intracranial pathology has limited yield, but the possibility of a mass lesion or destructive process in the posterior fossa must be considered.

Head Nodding

Head nodding without accompanying nystagmus can occur as paroxysmal events in older infants and toddlers. These head movements can be lateral ("no-no"), vertical ("yes-yes"), or oblique. The episodes may occur several times per day. The frequency (1–2 Hz) is slower than that of shuddering. The movements do not occur when the child is lying down, but can occur in the sitting or standing position. Older children describe an inability to suppress the movement (DiMario, 2000). The movements typically resolve within months, but can persist longer. Some children with head nodding have a prior history of shuddering spells; a few have been noted to have dystonic posturing of the legs when concentrating; others may have a family history of essential tremor (DiMario, 2000). A case of head nodding has been described in an 8-month-old with Down syndrome. Typically, development and neurologic outcomes are unaffected by this condition. Remission is spontaneous and treatment is not needed. The differential diagnosis of head nodding includes spasmus nutans (discussed earlier), stereotypies, and bobble-head syndrome. Stereotypies can persist through adolescence. Bobble-head syndrome is characterized by a forward-backward head nodding in children younger than 5 and is most often caused by a tumor or lesion of the third ventricle, suprasellar arachnoid cyst, or aqueductal stenosis.

Benign Paroxysmal Torticollis

Benign paroxysmal torticollis is an episodic disorder starting in the first year of life. It typically manifests as a head tilt to one side for a few hours or days. Spells can last as little as 10 minutes or as long as 2 months, but this is uncommon. The torticollis may occur without any associated symptoms, or may be accompanied by pallor, vomiting, irritability, or ataxia. Additional findings may include tortipelvis, persistence in sleep, and upper limb dystonia (Rosman, Douglass, Sharif, and Paolini, 2009). Often there is no trigger for the events. Episodes typically recur with some regularity, initially up to twice a month then become less frequent as the child grows older. The spells abate spontaneously, usually by 2 to 3 years of age, but always by age 5. The child is normal between spells. However, gross motor delay and fine motor delay have been noted in these children, which in some cases did resolve (Rosman et al., 2009). Interictal and ictal EEGs are normal. No treatment has been shown to be effective.

It has been suggested that benign paroxysmal torticollis is a migraine variant. There is often a family history of migraine. Some older children complain of headache during a spell, and many children go on to develop typical migraine after they have "outgrown" the paroxysmal torticollis. Children may develop other migraine variants, such as benign paroxysmal vertigo and cyclic vomiting.

Benign paroxysmal torticollis is idiopathic in most cases. It has been described in association with two genetic mutations. Two patients with benign paroxysmal torticollis have been reported from a kindred with familial hemiplegic migraine with ataxia linked to a CACNA1A mutation; an additional CACNA1A mutation was described in another family without a family history of hemiplegic migraine. More recently, mutations in PRRT2 have been associated with benign paroxysmal torticollis. PRRT2 mutations have been associated with other paroxysmal disorders, including paroxysmal dyskinesias, hemiplegic migraine, benign infantile epilepsy, and episodic ataxia. Family members with the same mutation may develop different clinical phenotypes.

The differential diagnosis is broad, and diagnosis of benign paroxysmal torticollis is one of exclusion. Torticollis can be seen as an acute dystonic reaction to medication, as a symptom of a posterior fossa or cervical cord lesion, or as a symptom of cervical vertebral abnormalities, including Klippel–Feil syndrome. It is important to exclude posterior fossa abnormalities, including Chiari syndrome or a mass. In the case of structural lesions, the torticollis tends to be persistent and not paroxysmal. Torticollis can also be a sign of sixth-nerve palsy. Congenital muscular torticollis is another possibility; it is present from birth, is nonparoxysmal, and is associated with palpable tightness or fibrosis of the sternocleidomastoid muscle unilaterally.

Benign Idiopathic Dystonia of Infancy

Benign idiopathic dystonia of infancy is a rare disorder characterized by a segmental dystonia, usually of one upper extremity, that can be intermittent or persistent. The syndrome usually appears before 5 months of age and disappears by 1 year of age. The characteristic posture is of shoulder abduction, pronation of the forearm, and flexion of the wrist. The posture occurs when the infant is at rest and goes away completely with volitional movement. Occasionally, both arms, an arm and leg on one side of the body, or the trunk can be involved. In some infants, the posture is only apparent with relaxation or in certain positions. In others, it may be present during all waking hours. The rest of the neurologic examination is normal, as are the developmental and neurologic outcomes. Exclusion of progressive dystonia, brachial plexus injury, infantile hemiplegia, and orthopedic abnormalities is important.

Posturing during Masturbation

Masturbation is a normal behavior that occurs in the majority of children. Although masturbation occurs at all ages and has even been observed in utero, it is most common at about 4 years of age and during adolescence; it occurs in 90% to 94% of males and 50% to 60% of females at some point in their lives (Yang, Fullwood, Goldstein, and Mink, 2005). Frequency and duration are variable. Masturbation in young children may involve unusual postures or movements (Yang et al,

2005), which may be mistaken for abdominal pain or seizures. Masturbatory movements in boys are usually obvious to the observer because of direct genital manipulation. In girls, they are more subtle. Stereotypic motor manifestations include adduction and rubbing together of the thighs, sitting on a hand or foot and rocking, rocking the body against an object asymmetrically, and stereotyped posture or lower limb scissoring. When the movements are accompanied by posturing of the limbs, they are often mistaken for paroxysmal dystonia. Several characteristic features of masturbating girls who present for diagnosis have been identified: (1) onset after 2 months of age and before 3 years of age; (2) stereotyped posturing with pressure applied to the pubic area; (3) quiet grunting, diaphoresis, or facial flushing; (4) episode duration of less than a minute to several hours; (5) no alteration of consciousness; (6) normal findings on examination; (7) cessation with distraction or engagement of the child in another activity.

Multiple diagnostic tests are often performed before the true nature of the behavior is recognized. No imaging or laboratory evaluation is required if the movements abate when the child is distracted, the movements involve irregular rocking, the child remains interactive, there is some degree of volitional control, direct genital stimulation is involved, and the neurologic and physical examinations are normal. There appears to be no association with sexual thoughts in the child. Instead, it is probably better to view these movements on the spectrum of other self-comforting behaviors, such as thumb sucking or rocking, which have no worrying connotations for the parents. Masturbation is a normal human behavior, so there is no expectation that this behavior will cease as the child grows older. However, the frequency of the behavior usually decreases as the child gets older, and the behavior is less likely to occur under the observation of the parents. Neurologic and developmental outcomes are normal. There is no need for treatment, but parent education and reassurance are important.

REFERENCES

The complete list of references for this chapter is available in the e-book at www.expertconsult.com.
See inside cover for registration details.

SELECTED REFERENCES

Caraballo, R.H., Capovilla, G., Vigevano, F., et al., 2009. The spectrum of benign myoclonus of early infancy: Clinical and neurophysiologic features in 102 patients. Epilepsia 50 (5), 1176–1183.

DiMario, F.J., 2000. Childhood head tremor. J. Child Neurol. 15 (1), 22–25.

Gottlob, I., Wizov, S., Reinecke, R., 1995. Spasmus nutans. A long-term follow-up. Invest. Ophthalmol. Vis. Sci. 36, 2768–2771.

Kanazawa, O., 2000. Shuddering attacks-report of four children. Pediatr. Neurol. 23, 421–424.

Maurer, V., Rizzi, M., Bianchetti, M., et al., 2010. Benign neonatal sleep myoclonus: A review or the literature. Pediatrics 125, e919–e924.

Ouvrier, R., Billson, F., 1988. Benign paroxysmal upgaze of childhood. J. Child Neurol. 3, 177–180.

Rosman, N.P., Douglass, L.M., Sharif, U.M., et al., 2009. The neurology of benign paroxysmal torticollis of infancy. J. Child Neurol. 24 (2), 155–160.

Shuper, A., et al., 1991. Jitteriness beyond the neonatal period: a benign pattern of movement in infancy. J. Child Neurol. 6, 243–245.

Yang, M., Fullwood, E., Goldstein, J., et al., 2005. Masturbation in infancy and early childhood presenting as a movement disorder: 12 cases and a review of the literature. Pediatrics 116 (6), 1427–1432.

An expanded version of this chapter is available on www.expertconsult.com. See inside cover for registration details.

INTRODUCTION AND OVERVIEW

The problem of pediatric drug-induced movement disorders (DIMDs) has received increased attention as the number of children treated with psychotropic medications has increased. Clinical trials and systematic reviews such as those from the Cochrane Collaboration have analyzed recent pediatric data. Naturalistic studies of polypharmacy and epidemiologic studies, particularly those involving children with autism (Spencer et al., 2013) can provide additional insights.

Following most texts and reviews, this chapter is organized by drug class rather than by movement disorder phenomenology. Because dopamine receptor blocking agents, also termed *antipsychotics* or *neuroleptics*, can cause tardive dyskinesia and are widely used in children, these agents require comprehensive discussion.

In recent years, the U.S. Food and Drug Administration (FDA) has approved antipsychotics for several pediatric indications. These include psychiatric symptoms that can be difficult to consistently define, recognize, and diagnose: irritability in autism, schizophrenia in adolescents, manic or mixed episodes of bipolar disorder. It is important to understand that although the newer agents, sometimes referred to as the *atypicals*, were designed to confer lower risks of dopaminergic side effects, this does not indicate the absence of risk.

Fortunately, in the short term, it appears that most DIMDs are reversible in children. It is important to be vigilant for these, however, and to recognize them early.

DEFINITION OF DRUG-INDUCED MOVEMENT DISORDERS

Iatrogenic movement disorders, or **drug-induced movement disorders** (DIMDs), are conditions in which the abnormal movements are related to the use of medication. Several time courses may occur (Singer, Mink, Gilbert, and Jankovic, 2016), as detailed in Table 96-1.

CLINICAL CHARACTERISTICS— PHENOMENOLOGY OF DRUG-INDUCED MOVEMENT DISORDERS IN CHILDREN

The phenomenologies of DIMDs span the spectrum of movement disorders: tremor, hypokinetic/rigid syndrome (parkinsonism), ballism, athetosis, chorea, dystonia, ataxia, tics, stereotypies, and poorly specified dyskinesias. Tremor is one of the most common DIMDs. The case report literature supports clinical experience in that almost any movement disorder may be linked to almost any medication. However, there are certain patterns. Table 96-2 is not exhaustive but presents the more common types of movement disorders seen with the five broad classes of medications emphasized in this chapter. Akathisia may be included in discussions of DIMDs because of the motor phenomenology of restlessness. Akathisia primarily involves uncomfortable sensations of inner restlessness, with compulsion to move secondarily (Table 96-2).

DRUG-INDUCED MOVEMENT DISORDERS

In general, for each drug class, epidemiology, clinical features, pathophysiology, diagnostic approach, treatment, and outcome are discussed.

Drug-Induced Movement Disorders Associated with Dopamine Receptor Blockade: Typical Antipsychotics, Atypical Antipsychotics

Epidemiology

For decades, conventional low- and high-potency neuroleptics have been prescribed in children as antiemetics and for behavioral indications, particularly in children with intellectual impairment and autism. High-potency dopamine receptor blockers, effective for tic suppression in Tourette syndrome, are known to have both high risks of side effects and high discontinuation rates. In addition, the dopamine receptor blockers, such as metoclopramide, have been used in children as antiemetics and for migraine-associated nausea for many years, despite descriptions of DIMDs.

Pharmaco-epidemiologic studies show dramatic increases in the use of antipsychotics for behavior problems in children of all ages (Olfson, Blanco, Liu, Moreno, and Laje, 2006). Conventional neuroleptics are still prescribed because of their effectiveness, relatively lower cost, and concerns about metabolic consequences of the atypical antipsychotics, including weight gain and increased risk of type 2 diabetes.

It is important for neurologists to be aware of situations and groups of patients at risk for DIMDs. Table 96-3 is meant to aid in this process. Because dopamine receptor blocking agents have many short- and long-term uses outside of neurology and psychiatry, Table 96-3 shows the FDA-labeled and non-FDA-labeled indications and specifically pediatric indications. It is important to note that there are other uses besides those listed. Further, although pediatric indications (underlined in Table 96-3) form only a subset of the total uses, it is common for pediatric use to follow adult approval. It is important to consult an updated reference when prescribing any of these medications and particularly to adhere to recommendations regarding electrocardiogram (ECG) monitoring. Dizziness and chest pain are common, and a possible serious side effect of many neuroleptics is a prolonged QT interval. Prescribers need to be aware of the range of complications of these medications (Table 96-3).

With regard to the prevalence of DIMDs, three recent systematic studies with different methods have generated estimates worth considering. The rates reported in two of the studies are remarkably close. Taking the estimates in the context of the study methodologies is informative.

Study 1: Systematic review of clinical trials A recent systematic review identified and analyzed 10 open-label and controlled studies of atypical antipsychotics with duration of 12 months or more, involving 783 children and adolescents. The authors reported an overall prevalence of DIMDs of 16%, with tardive dyskinesia in three patients (two prescribed risperidone and one prescribed olanzapine), or 0.4% of the children in the study (Correll and Kane, 2007).

Study 2: Large, single site cohort In a more naturalistic setting, researchers at the Maryland Psychiatric Research Center studied a cohort of 424 pediatric psychiatry patients over a 3-year period. They reported that 9.3% of children ages 5 to 18 treated for 6 or more months with typical or atypical antipsychotics developed tardive dyskinesia (Wonodi et al., 2007). With regard to generalizability, here are some key points:

- The cohort was ethnically diverse.
- The study had a 90% capture rate of the children in the psychiatric facilities involved.
- Polypharmacy, including exposure to multiple antipsychotics, and multiple concurrent diagnoses were common, as is true in the clinical setting of psychiatry patients referred to child neurologists.
- Although there was no placebo control, the authors did identify two comparator groups: (1) 80 neuroleptic-naïve, age- and gender-matched youths with psychiatric disorders and (2) 35 healthy children with no psychiatric disorders.

TABLE 96-1 Temporal Classification of Drug-Induced Movement Disorders

Temporal Category	Time Course of Appearance and Duration of Movement Disorder
Acute	Onset at treatment onset, within a short time interval of treatment onset, or at the time of a dose increase. Usually reversible/transient.
Chronic	Onset early or insidiously during treatment, persistence for weeks or longer while treatment is ongoing. Reversible.
Tardive	Emergence gradually, after prolonged treatment with the medication. Can be permanent.
Withdrawal	Onset subacutely after dose decreases or discontinuations. May persist for days or weeks. Usually resolves if medication reinitiated.

(Modified from Singer HS, Mink JW, Gilbert DL, Jankovic J. Movement Disorders in Childhood. 2nd ed. Philadelphia, PA: Elsevier, Inc.; 2016.)

- The authors used a structured and validated assessment, the Involuntary Movement Scale.
- The authors trained raters to a high interrater reliability (intraclass correlation coefficient) level of 0.80.
- Raters were blinded to treatment group and diagnosis.

Key findings from this study should inform clinical practice. First, the cohort did not have psychosis. Rather, 80% of the prescriptions of antipsychotics were for youths with mood and other problems, not psychosis. Second, attention deficit hyperactivity disorder (ADHD) was highly comorbid. Third, a total of 9.3% (11 of 118) of the children treated for greater than 6 months with antipsychotics showed tardive DIMDs. This is compared with none in the antipsychotic-naïve group. This tardive dyskinesia risk is much higher than the 0.4% risk estimate from the systematic review of clinical trials (Correll and Kane, 2007) and higher than the 0% incidence reported in a 48-week, open-label extension of risperidone (Findling et al., 2004). Finally, the tardive dyskinesia appeared to be reversible, not permanent. The size of this study allowed for statistical exploration of potential risk factors. Possibly important factors included longer duration, race, medication class, and the effects of polypharmacy.

Study 3: Systematic review of published literature The methodology of the third study involved counting patients in the medical literature from 1953 to 2009 to estimate risks for tardive syndromes in children (Mejia and Jankovic, 2010). After removing the case reports and the Maryland study (so as not to double count), this analysis was able to identify 50 affected children out of 540 exposed to neuroleptics, for a rate of 9.3% for tardive dyskinesia, essentially identical to the rate identified in the Maryland study.

Taken together, these studies should promote clinical caution and vigilance, whether atypical or typicals are prescribed.

Clinical Features of Drug-Induced Movement Disorders Induced by Dopamine Receptor Blocking Agents

Dopamine receptor blocking agents are known to induce parkinsonism, dystonia, tics, tremor, oculogyric movements, orolingual and other dyskinesias, and akathisia from infancy through the teenage years. Symptoms may occur at any time

TABLE 96-2 Common Drug-Induced Movement Disorders and Classes of Medications

DIMD Phenomenology	Dopamine Receptor Blockers	Stimulants	Serotonin Reuptake Inhibitors	Antiseizure Drugs	Chemotherapeutic and Immunosuppressive Agents
Akathisia	X		X		
Ataxia				X	X
Dystonia	X		X		X
Myoclonus			X		
Oculogyric crises	X				
Orolingual dyskinesias	X			X	
Other dyskinesias/chorea	X	X	X	X	X
Parkinsonism/rigidity	X		X		X
Stereotypies	X	X			
Tardive dyskinesia	X		X		
Tics	X	X		X	
Tremor—postural	X	X	X	X	X
Tremor—resting	X	X			X

TABLE 96-3 Selected Dopamine Receptor Blocking Agents: Indications, Approvals, and Risks

Medication	FDA-Labeled Indications*	Non-FDA-Labeled Indications	Common Adverse Events: Neurologic	Serious Adverse Events: Neurologic
TYPICAL NEUROLEPTICS				

Chlorpromazine	Acute intermittent porphyria
	Apprehension, presurgical
	Bipolar disorder
	Hiccoughs, intractable
	Nausea and vomiting
	Problem behavior (severe)
	Schizophrenia
	Tetanus, adjunct
		None	Akathisia Dystonia
			  Parkinsonism Somnolence
			Tremor
				Ineffective thermoregulation
				Heatstroke or hypothermia
				Neuroleptic malignant
				  syndrome
				Seizure
				Tardive dyskinesia

Fluphenazine	Schizophrenia	None	None	None

Haloperidol	Tourette syndrome severe
	  refractory Hyperactive
	  behavior Problematic
	  behavior Schizophrenia
		None	None	Neuroleptic malignant
				  syndrome
				Seizure
				Tardive dyskinesia

Metoclopramide	Chemotherapy-induced
	  nausea/vomiting, prophylaxis
	Diabetic gastroparesis
	Gastroesophageal reflux
	  disease
	Intestinal intubation, small
	  bowel
	Postoperative nausea and
	  vomiting
	Radiography of gastrointestinal
	  tract, adjunct
		Administration of analgesic
		Decreased lactation
		Indigestion
		Nondiabetic gastroparesis
		Pheochromocytoma, diagnosis
		Postoperative atelectasis
		Vomiting of pregnancy
			Asthenia
			Headache
			Somnolence
				Neuroleptic malignant
				  syndrome
				Tardive dyskinesia

Pimozide	Tourette syndrome	Chronic schizophrenia	Akathisia Dizziness Dystonia
			  Parkinsonism Somnolence
			Tremor
				Ineffective
				  thermoregulation,
				  Heatstroke or
				  hypothermia Neuroleptic
				  malignant syndrome
				Seizure
				Tardive dyskinesia

Prochlorperazine	Nausea and vomiting, severe	None	Akathisia Dizziness Dystonia Parkinsonism Somnolence Tremor	Neuroleptic malignant syndrome Tardive dyskinesia
ATYPICAL ANTIPSYCHOTICS				

Aripiprazole	Autistic disorder—agitation
	Bipolar disorder—agitation
	Bipolar I disorder, adjunctive
	Bipolar I disorder, manic or
	  mixed episodes
	Major depressive disorder,
	  adjunctive
	Schizophrenia
	Tourette syndrome
		Borderline personality disorder	Akathisia
			Dystonia Headache
			  Insomnia Somnolence
			Tremor
				Cerebrovascular accident
				Seizure
				Tardive dyskinesia
				Transient ischemic attack

Lurasidone	Bipolar disorder Schizophrenia	None	Akathisia Insomnia Parkinsonism Somnolence	Cerebrovascular accident Dystonia Seizure Tardive Dyskinesia

Olanzapine	Bipolar I disorder—agitation
	Bipolar disorder—manic or
	  mixed episodes;
	  maintenance
	Depressed bipolar I disorder,
	  adjunctive
	Major depressive disorder,
	  adjunctive
	Schizophrenia
		Agitation, acute—dementia
		Anorexia nervosa
		Nausea and vomiting,
		  chemotherapy-induced
		Delirium
		Schizophrenia, refractory
		Severe major depression with
		  psychotic features
			Akathisia
			Asthenia
			Somnolence
			Tremor
				Cerebrovascular disease
				Dystonia
				Seizure
				Status epilepticus

Paliperidone	Schizoaffective disorder Schizophrenia	Bipolar disorder	Akathisia Asthenia Dyskinesia Headache Hyperactivity Parkinsonism Somnolence	Dystonia Seizure Tardive dyskinesia

TABLE 96-3 Selected Dopamine Receptor Blocking Agents: Indications, Approvals, and Risks *(Continued)*

Medication	FDA-Labeled Indications*	Non-FDA-Labeled Indications	Common Adverse Events: Neurologic	Serious Adverse Events: Neurologic
Quetiapine	Bipolar disorder—acute mania, depressed phase, maintenance Major depressive disorder, adjunct Schizophrenia	Bipolar disorder, maintenance Major depressive disorder, monotherapy	Asthenia Dystonia Headache Insomnia Somnolence Tremor	Neuroleptic malignant syndrome Seizure Tardive dyskinesia
Risperidone	Autistic disorder—irritability Bipolar I disorder Schizophrenia	Behavioral syndrome—intellectual disability Tourette syndrome Autism spectrum disorder	Akathisia Parkinsonism Somnolence	Neuroleptic malignant Syndrome Seizure Tardive dyskinesia
Ziprasidone	Bipolar disorder—acute mania, maintenance adjunct Schizophrenia	Schizoaffective disorder	Akathisia Anxiety Dystonia Headache Psychomotor slowing Somnolence Spasmodic movement Tremor	Neuroleptic malignant syndrome Seizure Tardive dyskinesia

*Underlining indicates there is an FDA indication for children. Specifics about age approval may vary (e.g., for risperidone approval the lower age limit for ASD is 5 years, for bipolar is 10 years, and for schizophrenia is 13 years). Consult Micromedex®, DrugPoint®, or other sources for details.

(Modified from Singer HS, Mink JW, Gilbert DL, Jankovic J. Movement Disorders in Childhood. 2nd ed. Philadelphia, PA: Elsevier, Inc.; 2016.)

after treatment onset. Acute DIMDs, especially dystonia, oculogyric crises, and akathisia, are common and present dramatically, often to the emergency department. Chronic DIMDs occur after 3 or more months of treatment and may take the form of more subtle dystonia, tremor, and rigidity. Tardive DIMD phenomenologies include dyskinesias, stereotypies, tics, dystonia, and oculogyric crises. These symptoms may also develop when dopamine receptor blocking agents are withdrawn, tapered down rapidly, or discontinued because of carelessness or neglect (nonadherence). When dyskinetic movements occur in this setting, it is termed the **withdrawal emergent syndrome** (WES).

Pathophysiology

The pathophysiology of DIMDs associated with dopamine receptor blocker use may involve effects on the striatal dopamine receptor blockade and imbalance in the striatum of dopamine and acetylcholine levels. Much remains unknown, however, regarding an individual's vulnerability or susceptibility to DIMDs, so this remains an area of active research.

Clinical experience suggests that the occurrence of DIMDs in childhood is not completely random. It may relate in some basic way to the perturbed circuits underlying the neurodevelopmental or psychiatric symptoms treated with these agents. It is intriguing that tardive DIMDs seem to be so much more common in neuroleptic-treated schizophrenia than in, say, neuroleptic-treated Tourette syndrome. Yet tics, stereotypies, and other movement disorders are more common in children with autistic spectrum disorder (ASD) (Canitano and Vivanti, 2007), and clinically children with ASD seem to be particularly susceptible to DIMDs.

With regard to specific genetic risk factors, much research has been done, but few findings have been replicated. On a cellular basis, mechanisms may include the long-term effects of neuroleptics on dopamine receptor density and function, or damage to striatal GABAergic or cholinergic neurons. Genome-wide association studies may support previously unsuspected pathways as well. Evidence related to dopamine receptor polymorphisms has been mixed. GABAergic pathway genes have also been implicated. Within serotonergic systems, polymorphisms in genes encoding receptors 2A or 2C but not

3A may increase risk. Genetic variation in enzymes handling oxidative stress, such as glutathione-S-transferase, glutathione peroxidase, catalase, and tumor necrosis factor alpha polymorphisms, have not been linked to risk for DIMDs.

Diagnosis of Acute, Chronic, Tardive, and Withdrawal Emergent Syndromes

The acute onset of an involuntary movement disorder in a toddler should raise the diagnostic possibility of ingestion of a dopamine receptor blocking agent. Sources of possible exposure should be sought. Acute onset of dystonia, akathisia, parkinsonism, or other dyskinesias after initiating or raising the dose of a dopamine blocker is also straightforward.

Diagnosis of a chronic or tardive DIMD in children should often be considered when a movement disorder is unusual. For example, unilateral resting tremor, rigidity, and orolingual dyskinesias are all uncommon as idiopathic or genetic presentations but common as drug-induced presentations. Stereotypies and especially tics are less straightforward because they are common, and a tendency to tics may have preceded drug treatment. Thus the emergence of these symptoms later in childhood may be unrelated to medication.

When a new movement disorder occurs at the time of medication tapering or discontinuation, a WES disorder should be considered as a possibility. This is often missed or not considered in the emergency department and even on the inpatient psychiatry service. This phenomenology can also be severe choreic or ballistic movements, among the most severe presentations within the realm of DIMDs. However, if dyskinetic symptoms that have emerged are mild, then the differential diagnosis includes preexisting hyperkinetic movements, emerging after symptoms had been masked by treatment.

Treatment of Drug-Induced Movement Disorders Related to Use of Dopamine Receptor Blocking Agents

Acute Drug-Induced Movement Disorders. For acute DIMDs caused by dopamine receptor blockade, antihistamines and anticholinergic agents, such as diphenhydramine and benztropine, remain the mainstay of treatment. For akathisia, other options include the alpha-2 adrenergic agonist clonidine and beta blockers such as propranolol.

Chronic Drug-Induced Movement Disorders. For chronic DIMDs caused by dopamine receptor blockade, anticholinergics are also used. In chronic and tardive DIMDs, when dyskinesias are mild, withdrawing the offending agent may be sufficient. For functionally impairing tremor or rigidity in situations where withdrawing the dopamine receptor blocking agent is not safe because of aggression or severe mental illness, long-term anticholinergic treatment is reasonable. As an alternative for mood stabilization and aggression, substitution of anticonvulsants as mood stabilizers could be considered.

Tardive Movement Disorders. Vigilance for emergence of DIMDs is critical because of the possibility of permanent tardive dyskinesia. Although the risk is highest in adults with schizophrenia, the risk is nonzero in other groups. It is important not to give the impression that dopamine receptor blockers should be avoided at all costs. Rather, when possible, the treatment duration and dose of these dopamine receptor blocking agents should be limited and alternatives considered. In cases where tardive dyskinesia is diagnosed or strongly suspected, removal of the dopamine receptor blocking drug is recommended whenever possible, via slow taper.

For pharmacologic treatment of tardive dyskinesia or tardive dystonia, there are several options. Alpha-methyl-para-tyrosine (AMPT), reserpine, and tetrabenazine have been recommended. Depression is sometimes noted as a side effect of dopamine depletion. Extensive studies of vitamin E, based on the rationale that oxidative stress may be involved, have yielded negative results. Calcium channel blockers are not currently considered effective.

Neuroleptic Malignant Syndrome

Neuroleptic malignant syndrome (NMS) is rare in children. This most commonly occurs after initiation or dose increases and mainly has been described as occurring after taking antipsychotics (including the atypicals), but occasionally has been reported as occurring after the use of other psychiatric medications. NMS can also occur as a withdrawal phenomenon after chronic dopaminergic therapy. The main manifestations are autonomic (fever, tachycardia/tachypnea, diaphoresis), motoric (rigidity/bradykinesia with elevated rhabdomyolysis and creatine kinase), and cognitive (confusion). This is a life-threatening presentation. Treatment may include withdrawing the offending medication, administration of the dopamine agonist bromocriptine, and administration of the skeletal muscle relaxant dantrolene, in addition to general supportive care (hydration, fever reduction).

The differential diagnosis includes several other serious reactions, including malignant hyperthermia (hyperpyrexia, muscle contractions attributable to general anesthesia) and anticholinergic or sympathomimetic poisoning. In addition, **serotonin syndrome** may occasionally be confused with NMS. In serotonin syndrome, hyperreflexia, clonus, tremor, myoclonus, and shivering occur, but rigidity should be less severe.

Drug-Induced Movement Disorders Associated with Treatment of Attention Deficit Hyperactivity Disorder

Epidemiology of Psychostimulant Use in Children

The prevalence of the ADHD diagnosis and the use of pharmacologic treatment have increased markedly in the last 20 years in the United States. This includes primarily stimulants in an ever-increasing variety of preparations, but also includes atomoxetine, a selective norepinephrine reuptake inhibitor marketed for ADHD treatment, and the alpha-2 adrenergic agonists guanfacine and clonidine.

Clinical Features

Stimulants have been prescribed for decades. When dosed at less than 1.0 mg/kg/day, they only rarely induce clinically significant movement disorders. These medications and, to a less acute degree, the nonstimulants affect dopamine and norepinephrine levels. Therefore the most common DIMDs are hyperkinetic disorders such as tics, stereotypies, chorea, or other dyskinesias. The risk of DIMDs is higher in children who manifest clinical or subthreshold diagnostic features of obsessive-compulsive disorder (OCD) or ASD. Such children may experience new or increased repetitive behaviors, including tics, compulsions, or repetitive picking behaviors. They may also become hyper-focused or have personality changes parents describe as a "zombie" or "robot" effect, in part resulting from increased attention to internal stimuli or thoughts.

A longstanding concern is the clinical observation that stimulants seem in some cases to induce, unmask, or exacerbate tics. Fortunately, rigorous randomized controlled trials support that stimulants reduce ADHD symptoms for most children, irrespective of the presence of a tic disorder, and that should worsening of tics occur, it is usually transient, usually mild, and always reversible. Prospective studies suggest that in most cases tics would have occurred eventually, even in the absence of any exposure to stimulants. The most rigorous clinical assessment of the relationship between stimulants and tics is the Treatment of ADHD in Children with Tics (TACT) study (Group, 2002). In that study, children with comorbid tics and ADHD were randomized to treatment with methylphenidate, clonidine, both, or double placebo. Tics improved by the study's end in all treated groups, even the group treated with methylphenidate alone, compared with the placebo. Even in cases where tics consistently worsen on stimulant medication, some individuals and families choose to continue stimulant medication if the benefits warrant.

Atomoxetine has been reported in a few cases to induce tics and dyskinesias in the context of rapid dose change and polypharmacy. However, in a randomized, placebo-controlled trial of atomoxetine treatment for ADHD in 148 children with tics, atomoxetine tended to reduce tic severity (Allen et al., 2005).

Pathophysiology

The pathophysiology of this susceptibility is unknown. Induced stereotypies and tics, as with idiopathic ones, may be more general markers of perturbed neurodevelopment. A genetic influence on the risk of DIMDs has been suggested through genotyping data from the Preschool ADHD Treatment Study (PATS). In that study, 183 preschoolers were treated with methylphenidate at several doses or placebo. Several modestly statistically significant associations were identified, including polymorphisms in synaptosomal-associated protein 25 (SNAP25) associated with tics, buccal-lingual movements, and irritability and variants of dopamine receptor 4 (DRD4) associated with picking (McGough et al., 2006).

Diagnosis

The diagnosis of a DIMD in a child treated for ADHD should be suspected if the movements have the typical hyperkinetic phenomenology and the onset is within a week or two of treatment onset or a dose increase. Stimulants are short acting and readily discontinued or restarted, allowing for a plan of stopping and restarting medications to clarify cause and effect.

Treatment

It is most often not necessary to discontinue stimulants when mild tics or tremor emerge. If the stimulant dose exceeds 1 mg/kg/day, it is generally beneficial to reduce the dose.

Drug-Induced Movement Disorders Associated with Other Medications

Serotonin Reuptake Inhibitors

Selective serotonin reuptake inhibitors (SSRIs) are widely prescribed in children with mood disorders and OCD and tend to work better in combination with cognitive behavioral therapy. The emergence of movement disorders related to use of SSRIs is well known. Phenomenology can include akathisia most commonly, with parkinsonism, dystonia, acute dystonic reactions, and dyskinesias also described. The most serious complication, rare in childhood, is serotonin syndrome as a result of excess SSRI exposure. This involves neuromuscular excitation (manifest by clonus, hyperreflexia, myoclonus, tremor, shivering), autonomic stimulation (hyperthermia, diarrhea, tachycardia, diaphoresis, tremor, flushing), and changed mental state (anxiety, agitation, confusion). More commonly, treatment with an SSRI results in a mild degree of hyperreflexia and tremor. The emergence of hyperreflexia in a child prescribed an SSRI is an indication that toxicity is more likely if the dose is increased or if other psychiatric agents are prescribed. Lack of awareness of SSRI-induced tremor and hyperreflexia may result in unnecessary medical diagnostic tests such as brain magnetic resonance imaging (MRI). Similarly, failure to observe and document SSRI-induced neurologic symptoms may place patients at risk of developing more severe symptoms with future dose increases. Myoclonus, in distinction to tics, is involuntary, not urge driven.

The identification of SSRI-induced movement disorders in children supports the importance of clinician and patient education. Treatment is dose reduction, elimination of the medication, or selection of alternative interventions or cognitive behavioral therapies.

Antiseizure Medications

Physicians prescribe antiseizure medications for diverse indications, including prevention of seizures and migraines, and sometimes stabilization of mood. Numerous case reports describe acute and chronic DIMDs in children caused by antiseizure medications. The most common acute clinical presentations are acute ataxia and nystagmus. Phenytoin and carbamazepine are most commonly identified. These medications are also prone to cause problems resulting from pharmacokinetics and drug–drug interactions.

Less commonly, antiseizure drugs may produce other hyperkinetic movement disorders. Phenytoin, carbamazepine, and even valproic acid have been reported to produce acute chorea, orofacial dyskinesias, and Tourettism. Lamotrigine has been reported to induce tics. Tremor is also common.

Generally, the treatment plan involves clinical watch and wait, weighing the impairment related to the movement disorder against the benefits of the seizure control, with thoughtful consideration of reduction of dose or changing of medication or formulation if the movement disorder causes much impairment.

Drug-Induced Movement Disorders Associated with Chemotherapeutic, Immunomodulatory, and Anti-infectious Medications

Neurology consult teams seeing oncology patients may encounter DIMDs. Chemotherapeutic agents such as vincristine may cause sensory ataxia, along with dysarthria and tremor. Seizures, stroke-like episodes, and ataxia can occur with intrathecal methotrexate. Acute neurologic symptoms such as headaches, confusion, and seizures, but also associated with tremor, ataxia, dysarthria, and parkinsonism, may occur during bone marrow transplantation.

Seizures, tremor, and acute dystonic reactions have been observed after organ transplantation, sometimes with a leukoencephalopathy syndrome involving headache, confusion, and myoclonus. Metronidazole may rarely cause cerebellar dysfunction.

CONCLUSION

Neurologists should be aware of the wide spectrum of phenomenologies of drug-induced movement disorders that may present acutely or chronically in childhood. Treatment strategies may involve specific antidotes, such as anticholinergics for acute dystonic reactions, or longer-term changes in medical regimens.

REFERENCES

The complete list of references for this chapter is available in the e-book at www.expertconsult.com.
See inside cover for registration details.

SELECTED REFERENCES

Allen, A.J., Kurlan, R.M., Gilbert, D.L., et al., 2005. Atomoxetine treatment in children and adolescents with ADHD and comorbid tic disorders. Neurology 65, 1941–1949.

Canitano, R., Vivanti, G., 2007. Tics and Tourette syndrome in autism spectrum disorders. Autism 11, 19–28.

Correll, C.U., Kane, J.M., 2007. One-year incidence rates of tardive dyskinesia in children and adolescents treated with second-generation antipsychotics: a systematic review. J. Child Adolesc. Psychopharmacol. 17, 647–656.

Findling, R.L., Aman, M.G., Eerdekens, M., et al., 2004. Long-term, open-label study of risperidone in children with severe disruptive behaviors and below-average IQ. Am. J. Psychiatry 161, 677–684.

Group, T.S.S., 2002. Treatment of ADHD in children with tics: a randomized controlled trial. Neurology 58, 527–536.

McGough, J., McCracken, J., Swanson, J., et al., 2006. Pharmacogenetics of methylphenidate response in preschoolers with ADHD. J. Am. Acad. Child Adolesc. Psychiatry 45, 1314–1322.

Mejia, N.I., Jankovic, J., 2010. Tardive dyskinesia and withdrawal emergent syndrome in children. Expert Rev. Neurother. 10, 893–901.

Olfson, M., Blanco, C., Liu, L., et al., 2006. National trends in the outpatient treatment of children and adolescents with antipsychotic drugs. Arch. Gen. Psychiatry 63, 679–685.

Singer, H.S., Mink, J.W., Gilbert, D.L., et al., 2016. Movement Disorders in Childhood. Elsevier, Inc, Philadelphia, PA.

Spencer, D., Marshall, J., Post, B., et al., 2013. Psychotropic medication use and polypharmacy in children with autism spectrum disorders. Pediatrics 132, 833–840.

Wonodi, I., Reeves, G., Carmichael, D., et al., 2007. Tardive dyskinesia in children treated with atypical antipsychotic medications. Mov. Disord. 22, 1777–1782.

97 Cerebral Palsy

Maryam Oskoui, Michael I. Shevell, and Kenneth F. Swaiman

I. INTRODUCTION

Cerebral palsy (CP) is a chronic neurodevelopmental disorder that is heterogeneous in all of its aspects: etiology, presentation, functional severity, comorbidities, treatment options, individual trajectories, and outcomes. It is never the same disease twice. CP is frequently accompanied by a range of conditions that implicate the child neurologist in medical management and in the utilization of an interdisciplinary team for comprehensive management. The chronicity of CP enables the neurologist to form close and enduring bonds with the affected child and family that facilitates the practice of family-centered care that addresses changing challenges as the child matures and that prioritizes these challenges according to the individual and family context. Some children with CP graduate from universities and become health professionals. Other children with CP may be unable to roll or feed and may be entirely dependent for all activities of daily living with a lifespan shortened by decades compared with their chronologic peers. The challenge for healthcare practitioners is to comprehensively and holistically address this entire spectrum of individual care needs.

II. CURRENT DEFINITION

The current definition of CP is the product of an international effort of consensus drawing upon the experience of a diverse interdisciplinary group of recognized experts. The value of CP as a diagnostic entity was affirmed as a clinical descriptor of a group of individuals with a neurodevelopmental disability of diverse etiologies featuring varying presentations, functional limitations and individual life trajectories.

Cerebral palsy (CP) describes a group of permanent disorders of movement and posture, causing activity limitation, that are attributed to nonprogressive disturbances that occurred in the developing fetal or immature brain. The motor disorders of CP are often accompanied by disturbances of sensation, perception, cognition, communication, and behavior, by epilepsy, and by secondary musculoskeletal problems.

The definition fits well into the World Health Organization's International Classification of Functioning, Health, and Disability (ICF) framework by providing as necessary and sufficient conditions for CP both bodily impairment ("disorders of movement and posture") and "activity limitation." Neuromotor impairment, reflecting an alteration in motor control, is the invariable sine qua non of CP, as is the latter's explicit recognition that all individuals with CP have difficulties in executing a motor-dependent task or action. The heterogeneity of CP is captured by the term "group" and the avoidance in the definition of any specification by etiology, presentation, or severity. Transitory processes are eliminated from consideration by the word "permanent," which also emphasizes CP's chronicity over the lifespan and the recognition of its clinical evolution as the individual ages and matures. CP is fundamentally a disruption in the orderly sequential processes of early child development, and this is captured by the words "disorders," "disturbances," and "developing."

Although the clinical manifestations of CP will change over time in a particular individual, the underlying pathology is "nonprogressive." This lesion is the result of either a single event or a discrete series of events that has "run its course" by the time the clinical features of CP are apparent and diagnosable. Pathologic processes that are progressive are excluded from CP. However, the brain injury that underlies CP may occur in the immature brain; it alters the developmental trajectory of the brain and, consequently, produces a clinical picture that changes over time.

A further aspect of the current consensus definition is its specification of CP as an attributable neurobiologic disorder rooted in an abnormality occurring at an early phase in the not-yet-mature brain. Specifically excluded from being considered as CP are early-onset neuromotor disorders with activity limitations that are the result of spinal disorders or neuromuscular processes. A final important and unique aspect of this most recent definition is the notation that CP is "often accompanied" by a range of "comorbid" conditions that include: convulsive disorders, abnormalities in the primary senses, perceptual integrative disorders, intellectual disability, speech-language limitations, behavioral disorders, and orthopedic deformities. Some of these comorbidities may be attributed to the underlying pathologic lesion that does not uniquely respect motor control pathways but may also represent the influence of these motor dysfunctions on complex processes or on skeletal structures.

Although the current definition has been widely accepted, limitations have been recognized. A lack of clarity with regards to the meaning of "nonprogressive" has been highlighted. Syndromes traditionally excluded from categorization as CP are not enumerated as they have been elsewhere in the literature. Similarly, the lower threshold for severity for inclusion as CP is left open, as is an upper age limit for both an acquired pathology and clinical diagnosis. These aspects of imprecision will influence on the operationalization of CP for such traditional epidemiologic processes as determining prevalence and incidence. For most CP registries currently in existence, a pathologic onset and a clinical diagnosis before the age of 2 years have been implemented.

III. PRESENTATION AND DIAGNOSTIC ASSESSMENT

Two distinct cohorts of children present with CP. The first and largest consists of children considered at high risk for CP as an eventual outcome due to evident perinatal adversity. This group includes infants born preterm. The second group includes those born at term experiencing a neonatal encephalopathy, which includes as a subset those with documented intrapartum asphyxia. These "at-risk" newborns are carefully monitored in regional neonatal follow-up programs with rigorous developmental surveillance and screening. The appearance of motor delay and findings on neurologic examination would prompt consideration of a diagnosis of CP. These infants typically have an earlier age of diagnosis and onset of rehabilitation interventions with more severe functional impairments and worse outcomes compared with the second cohort of infants with CP.

The second cohort typically has experienced no evident perinatal adversity. Developmental surveillance provided through a community-based provider may alert to the possibility of motor delay in gross and fine motor domains, prompting referral to a pediatric specialist for evaluation. Some children without prior perinatal adversity may present in a symptomatic manner, either acutely or in a chronic fashion. The former typically involves urgent in-hospital evaluation for a paroxysmal event highly suspicious of a seizure of any type. The chronic mode of presentation may be suggested by the early preferential hand use or the parental observation of "stiffness" or gait disturbances. The diagnosis of this second cohort of children with CP and the implementation of interventions may be delayed beyond the child's second birthday.

In both cohorts, the diagnosis of CP is made on clinical grounds. Documentation on neurologic examination of neuromotor impairment and either observation or report of activity limitation in the affected child are required and sufficient conditions. The neuromotor impairment is grounded in either motor delay or abnormalities in strength, tone, reflexes, or gait. The activity limitation may be readily evident in the office in the execution of a motor-based task or by historical report by parents. An underlying etiology does not need to be identified to satisfy a diagnosis of CP. Spinal dysraphisms, neuromuscular disorders, progressive pathology, and specific syndromic diagnoses need to be excluded to merit a diagnostic assignation of CP. Due to the known occurrence of transitory neuromotor deficits in infancy, there is some reluctance to diagnose CP formally in infants younger than 1 year, unless severely affected. Thus some practitioners speak of "probable" CP before the age of 2 years, and "definite" CP after the age of five.

An evidence-based consensus guideline on the diagnostic assessment of the child with CP was developed by the American Academy of Neurology and Child Neurology Society (Fig. 97-1). CP is a clinical diagnosis, and all children should undergo a detailed history and physical examination that excludes a neurodegenerative disorder and that also classifies the neurologic subtype of CP. Among children with hemiplegic CP and a history of perinatal stroke (Chapter 20), diagnostic testing for a coagulation disorder should be considered (level B). Screening for associated comorbidities (such as epilepsy, cognitive or visual impairments, speech, language or hearing deficits, and oromotor dysfunction) is also recommended (level A). An EEG is recommended only if paroxysmal events suggestive of seizures are present (level A). Neuroimaging is also recommended in all children with CP to establish an etiology, with MRI as the preferred modality done either in the perinatal period or at the time of presentation (level A). Metabolic and genetic studies are not routinely recommended (level B) unless there are atypical features such as normal neuroimaging, episodic decompensation, or the presence of a family history of CP (level C).

IV. EPIDEMIOLOGY

Cerebral palsy is the most common cause of motor disability in childhood, affecting about 2 per 1000 live births in high resource settings. Over the past few decades, there have been major changes and advances in obstetric and neonatal care, with a decline in neonatal mortality. The prevalence of CP has been shown to be constant over time by several studies; however, the at-risk population and subtypes observed appear to have changed. The pooled prevalence of CP across studies from North America, Europe, and Australia is 2.11 per 100 live births (95% CI 1.98–2.25).

Prematurity is one of the largest risk factors for CP, with a well-established inverse relationship between CP prevalence and gestational age. The pooled birth prevalence of CP is highest in children born earlier than 28 weeks' gestation (82.25 per 1000 live births) and lowest in children born at term (1.35 per 1000 live births). Intrauterine growth restriction and low birth weight are also strongly associated with a risk of CP. The pooled prevalence of CP shows a similar inverse relationship to birth weight, affecting 56.64 per 1000 live births in children with a birth weight lower than 1000 grams and 1.33 per 1000 live births in children with a birth weight of 2500 grams or greater.

V. ETIOLOGIC SPECTRUM

Our understanding of the etiologic spectrum of CP has advanced, over the past few decades, yet much of the underlying pathophysiology continues to remain poorly understood. Individual risk factors have been identified across numerous population-based studies, broadly classified as antenatal, perinatal, and postnatal risk factors, which differ among term and preterm born children. However, in each individually affected child, multiple risk factors can be involved and their contribution along causal pathways and timing of injury is complex. Two recent systematic reviews have explored the risk factors for CP in term-born children. Although birth asphyxia was historically considered as a major causal factor in term CP, improved understanding has shown this to be a factor in only a minority of children. Preconceptional antenatal risk factors identified in these systematic reviews include social deprivation (both individual and area-based indicators), prior maternal disease such as epilepsy, thyroid disease, and intellectual disability, and both early and late maternal age (younger than 20 and older than 40 years). Among antenatal risk factors in term-born children, major and minor birth defects and aberrant intrauterine growth both hold a strong association with CP. Other antenatal factors include polyhydramnios or oligohydramnios, multiple gestation, documented genetic abnormalities, second or third trimester bleeding, intrauterine infection, chorioamnionitis, and placental abnormalities. Intrapartum events found to increase the risk of CP across population-based studies include meconium aspiration, breech or nonvertex presentation, and instrumental deliveries. Birth asphyxia associated with a sentinel event (uterine rupture, major placental abruption, or cord prolapse)

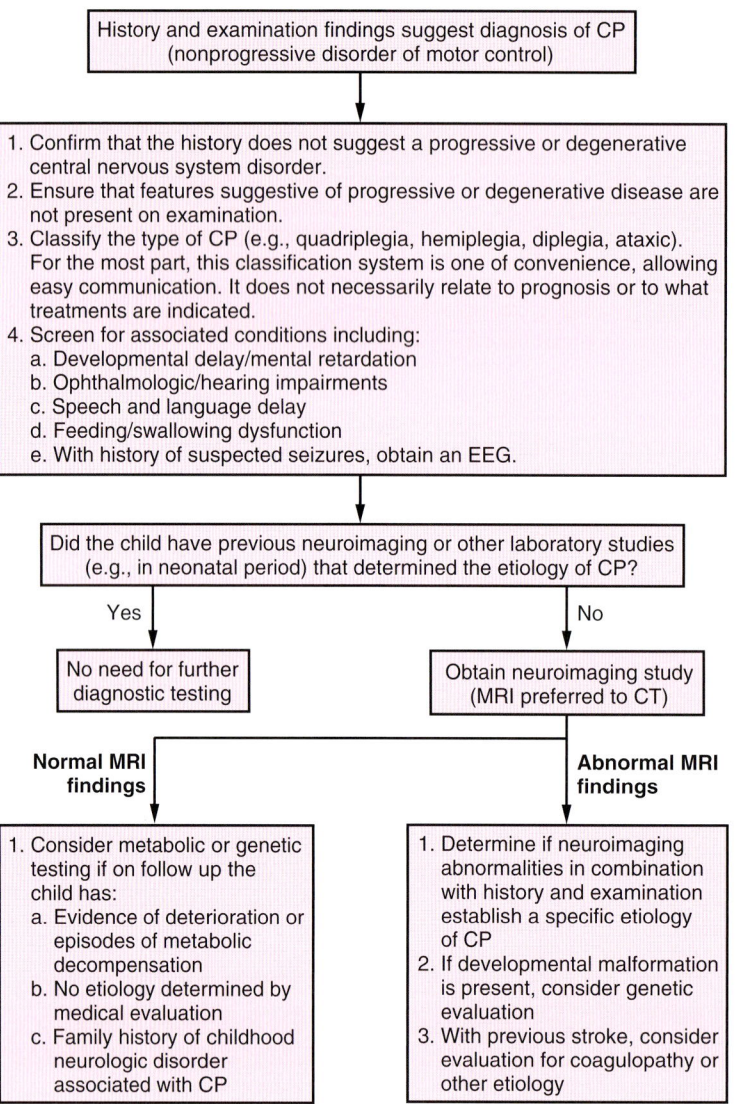

Figure 97-1. Diagnostic assessment of a child with CP. *(With permission from Ashwal, S., Russman, B.S., Blasco, P.A., et al., 2004. Practice parameter: diagnostic assessment of the child with cerebral palsy: report of the Quality Standards Subcommittee of the American Academy of Neurology and the Practice Committee of the Child Neurology Society. Neurology 62, 851–863.)*

was consistently established as a risk factor. Birth asphyxia is variably defined across studies, often in the absence of a true sentinel event. Birth asphyxia, however, cannot be reliably solely defined by clinical indicators such as Apgar scores, cord pH, or presence of a neonatal encephalopathy, all of which are multifactorial. During the neonatal period, presence of seizures is a strong predictor of CP. Neonatal infection, hypoglycemia, hyperbilirubinemia, and respiratory distress syndrome also have been reported as risk factors. Improved management of neonatal hyperbilirubinemia has resulted in a decreased number of affected children who develop CP (typically the athetoid or dystonic subtypes) from kernicterus in developed countries.

Among very preterm infants, the EPIPAGE (étude EPidemi-ologique sur les Petits Âges GEstationnels) population-based cohort study in France identified several risk factors for CP in an unadjusted model, including cystic periventricular leuko-malacia, intraparenchymal hemorrhage, earlier gestational age, male gender, preterm rupture of membranes, respiratory distress syndrome, maternal-fetal infection, acute anemia, and postnatal corticosteroid use. In multiple adjusted models,

male gender and cerebral lesions documented with neuroim-aging were the strongest predictors of CP.

Multiple risk factors are often identified in children with CP, especially in children born preterm, suggesting a sequence of events along a causal pathway. In children with CP born at term, an antenatal or a single risk factor suggests an existing vulnerability, with no specific risk factor identified in up to 30% of individual cases. These risk factors are also believed to have a differential effect across gestational ages. For example, in a population-based study in Norway, preeclampsia was found to increase the risk of CP in offspring, mediated by either preterm birth or being born small for gestational age only in term infants. Among preterm infants, there is emerging robust evidence for a cerebral dysmaturation process. In response to an initial ischemic insult, there is both an expansion of the preoligodendrocyte pool that is blocked from maturation and survival of immature neurons. This leads to dysmaturation of both gray and white matter during a critical period of rapid brain growth and connectivity in which post-natal environmental factors can further enhance or impair brain health. Slower postnatal growth (related to nutrition or other factors) has been associated with delayed cerebral cortical maturation. Brain growth and maturation in preterm infants is also influenced by systemic illness such as postnatal infections, which have been linked to altered development of white matter pathways and impaired neurodevelopmental outcome. Procedural pain and stress exposure in premature newborns in the neonatal intensive care unit have also been linked to altered brain maturation and impaired postnatal growth. Although the consensus definition of CP describes a static injury, this injury occurs in an immature brain thereby altering the course of its developmental maturation. This shift from static to dynamic injury broadens the potential targets for both preventive and disease-modifying interventions.

VI. CLASSIFICATION
A. Common Cerebral Palsy Syndromes

The standardized neurologic examination forms the basis of the classification approach to CP most familiar to child neurologists. This approach utilizes both the topographic distribution of affected limbs and the predominant quality of the observed motor impairment to stratify CP into mutually exclusive subtypes. The quality of the motor impairment has its basis in neuropathology, specifically whether cortical and/or subcortical structures are affected (i.e., basal ganglia, cerebellum) and is divided broadly into pyramidal (i.e., spastic) and

extrapyramidal (i.e., dyskinetic [choreoathetotic, dystonic], ataxic-hypotonic, or mixed [dyskinetic and spastic elements both present]) categories. Further stratification within the spastic (pyramidal) category is based on the observed distribution of affected limbs: a) quadriplegic—all four limbs affected, with an asymmetry between the left and right side permitted (i.e., double hemiplegia); b) hemiplegic—hemibody involvement with asymmetry permitted between the affected upper and lower limb; c) diplegic—involvement of both lower extremities without appreciable upper limb involvement noted; and d) other monoplegic or triplegic limb distribution.

B. Functional Classification

As neuromotor impairment is a core feature of CP, it is not surprising that a functional classification focused on gross motor skills, particular ambulation, was initially formulated (Rosenbaum et al., 2008). The Gross Motor Function Classification System (GMFCS) stratifies individuals with CP into five nonoverlapping categories ranging from most able (level I) to least able (level V). The distinctions between successive levels are clinically and functionally meaningful and are captured quite succinctly in Figure 97-2. Individuals at level I and II can ambulate independently without assistance, varying in terms of their capacity to run, jump, and climb stairs; individuals in level III ambulate independently with assistance

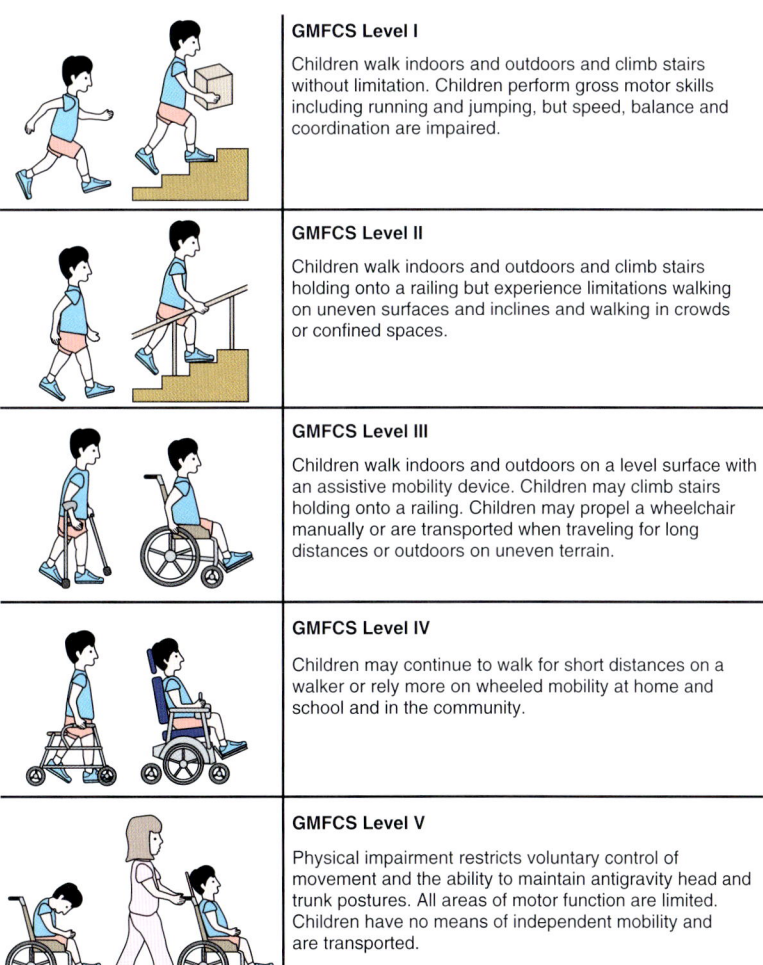

GMFCS Level I

Children walk indoors and outdoors and climb stairs without limitation. Children perform gross motor skills including running and jumping, but speed, balance and coordination are impaired.

GMFCS Level II

Children walk indoors and outdoors and climb stairs holding onto a railing but experience limitations walking on uneven surfaces and inclines and walking in crowds or confined spaces.

GMFCS Level III

Children walk indoors and outdoors on a level surface with an assistive mobility device. Children may climb stairs holding onto a railing. Children may propel a wheelchair manually or are transported when traveling for long distances or outdoors on uneven terrain.

GMFCS Level IV

Children may continue to walk for short distances on a walker or rely more on wheeled mobility at home and school and in the community.

GMFCS Level V

Physical impairment restricts voluntary control of movement and the ability to maintain antigravity head and trunk postures. All areas of motor function are limited. Children have no means of independent mobility and are transported.

Figure 97-2. GMFCS. *(With permission from GMFCS descriptors: Palisano et al. (1997) Dev Med Child Neurol 39:214–23 CanChild: www .canchild.ca. Illustrations Version 2 © Bill Reid, Kate Willoughby, Adrienne Harvey and Kerr Graham, The Royal Children's Hospital Melbourne.)*

(i.e., walker, crutches, leg braces), whereas those at levels IV and V are wheelchair bound, differing in their ability to control the wheelchair themselves. The GMFCS has been extensively validated and shown to be reliable, psychometrically robust, and sensitive to the effects of therapeutic intervention. Introduced in the late 1990s, it is now a standard part of international care provision, rehabilitation, registry inscription, and research in CP.

About three quarters of individuals with CP will have appreciable involvement of an upper extremity. Half of such individuals will have bilateral involvement of the upper limbs. These individuals are thus at risk for functional impairment in bimanual ability (i.e., fine motor skills). Upper limb function is influenced by contextual factors such as physical capability, the immediate environment, social advantage, and personal motivation. Contextual factors may act to produce different function in bimanual ability despite the same objective degree of physical motor impairment. Bimanual ability can be defined as "the capacity to manage daily activities that require the use of the upper limb, with whatever strategies involved, which can be observed from activity or performance in the person's everyday context." The fine motor limitations evident in a subset of children with CP prompted the development of the Manual Ability Classification System (MACS) subsequent to the GMFCS. In a manner analogous to the GMFCS, the MACS stratify individuals with CP into five nonoverlapping categories ranging from most able (level I) to least able (level V). The distinction between the levels is based on the quality and quantity of bimanual performance in "everyday" life and whether there is any requisite need for assistance or adaptation to carry out these tasks (Fig. 97-3). The MACS is also noted to be psychometrically robust with its validity and reliability well-established. It is, however, generally applied consistently to individuals older than the age of 4.

Communication through oral language is dependent on cognitive processes and the complex interplay of oral, pharyngeal, laryngeal, lingual, and diaphragmatic musculature. Communication may also be nonverbal, and this is also dependent on cognitive and voluntary motor control. The underlying lesion responsible for an individual's CP may subtly or dramatically affect each of these components. Within the past decade, the Communication Function Classification System (CFCS) has been developed to stratify everyday communication. All methods of communication are considered for the affected individual's performance as both a sender and receiver of varied communication, including the pace and the effectiveness of communication in the context of either a familiar or unfamiliar conversational partner. Five nonoverlapping categories are utilized ranging from most able (level I) to least able (level V) (Fig. 97-4).

The eventual capacity to ambulate ("Will my child walk?") represents a major concern for parents upon being told the diagnosis of CP if the affected child is not yet ambulatory. Stratification through the GMFCS objectively responds to this explicit concern. Two thirds of individuals with CP will be assigned to GMFCS levels I through III, indicating ambulation with (level III) or without (levels I and II) assistance. Slightly more than half (55%) will be in level I (45%) and level II (10%), and 12% will be in level III. The one third that will be wheelchair bound (levels IV and V) will be equally split between these two assignments. There is a dichotomous correlation observed between neurologic subtype and GMFCS levels. For children with either a diplegic or hemiplegic neurologic variant, more than 95% will be GMFCS levels I through III, whereas for those with a quadriplegic or dyskinetic variant only 25% will be ambulatory with or without assistance (levels I through III).

With respect to bimanual function, roughly 60% of children stratify to MACS levels I (35%) and II (25%), indicating

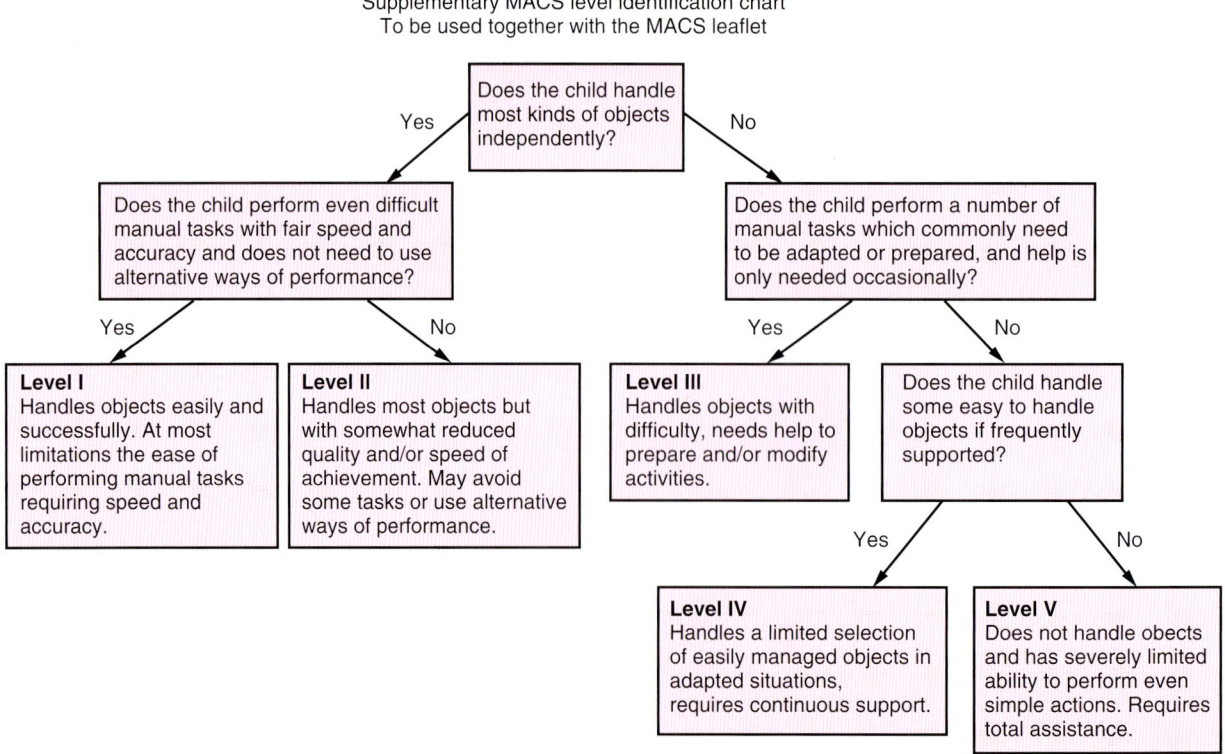

Supplementary MACS level identification chart
To be used together with the MACS leaflet

Does the child handle most kinds of objects independently?

Yes → Does the child perform even difficult manual tasks with fair speed and accuracy and does not need to use alternative ways of performance?

No → Does the child perform a number of manual tasks which commonly need to be adapted or prepared, and help is only needed occasionally?

Yes → **Level I** Handles objects easily and successfully. At most limitations the ease of performing manual tasks requiring speed and accuracy.

No → **Level II** Handles most objects but with somewhat reduced quality and/or speed of achievement. May avoid some tasks or use alternative ways of performance.

Yes → **Level III** Handles objects with difficulty, needs help to prepare and/or modify activities.

No → Does the child handle some easy to handle objects if frequently supported?

Yes → **Level IV** Handles a limited selection of easily managed objects in adapted situations, requires continuous support.

No → **Level V** Does not handle obects and has severely limited ability to perform even simple actions. Requires total assistance.

Field trial version

Figure 97-3. MACS Level Identification Chart. *(With permission from Manual Ability Classification System, 2016. www.macs.nu)*

CFCS Level Identification Chart

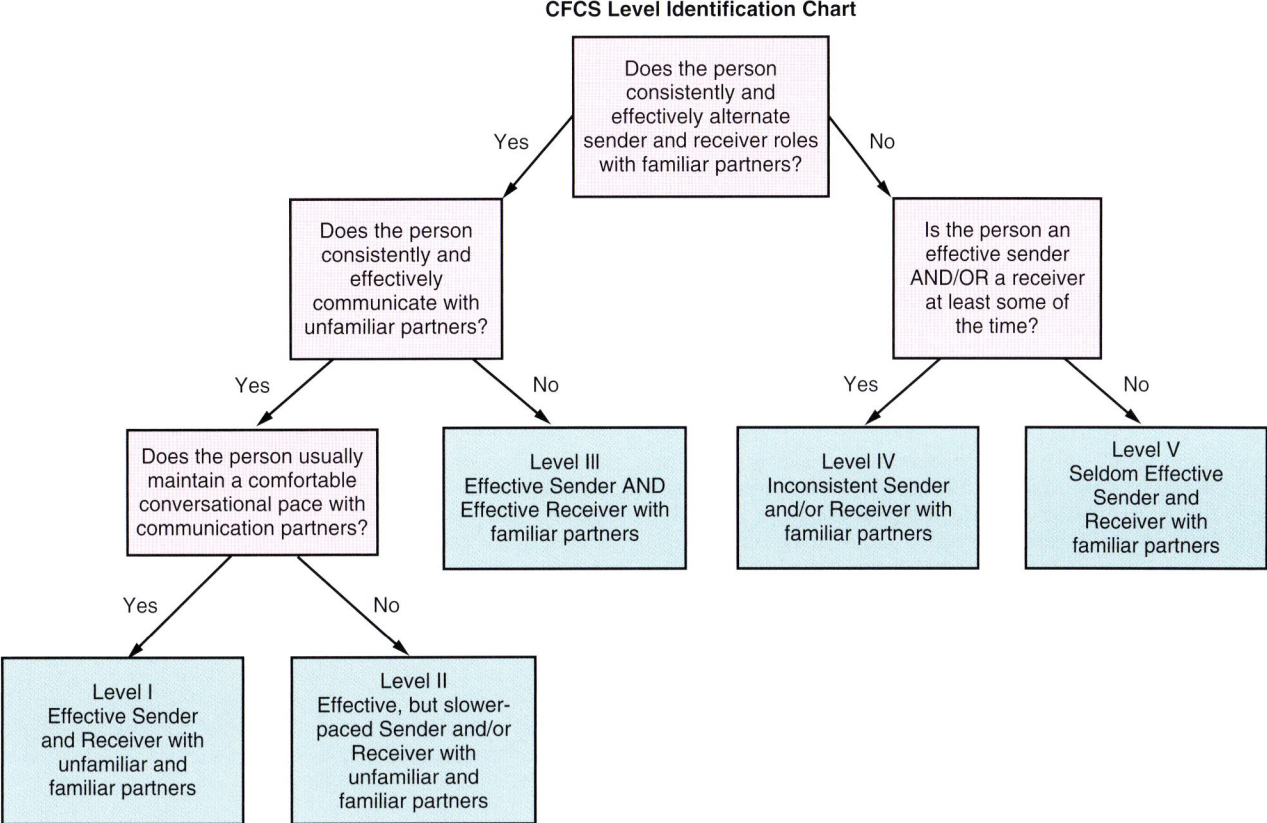

Figure 97-4. CFCS. *(With permission from The Communication Function Classification System, 2016. www.cfcs.us)*

an ability to do bimanual tasks at an age-appropriate level without the need for adaptation or external assistance. For a third of children with CP, no limitations aside from that related to speed and accuracy of handling was noted (level I). One in seven children with CP will have no discernible functional hand use (level V), leading to major task limitations that effectively preclude the eventual attainment of individual autonomy.

The GMFCS and MACS levels are positively correlated, varying by neurologic subtype and cognitive level. The agreement between GMFCS and MACS levels is moderate in quadriplegic or dyskinetic youth, fair in diplegic youth, and poor in hemiplegic youth. Quadriplegic youth tend to have worse ambulatory skills, hemiplegic youth worse bimanual ability, and diplegic youth equivalent skills in both functional domains. The presence of concurrent intellectual disability was noted to strengthen the correlation in gross and fine motor skills.

A similar distribution across levels has been reported for the CFCS measure. Half of children with CP were noted at school entry to be effective communicators as senders and receivers with both familiar and unfamiliar partners (level I: 32%; level II: 22%). One in seven were at level V, indicating a noncommunicative status in both verbal and nonverbal capacities, with one in six at level IV, indicating inconsistent communication skills restricted to familiar communication partners only. Level V status strongly correlated with documentation of greatest impairment (i.e., level V) on the GMFCS and MACS.

VII. COMORBIDITY SPECTRUM

The current consensus definition of CP explicitly recognizes associated conditions in addition to the core neuromotor

impairment. Half of children with CP will experience a comorbid condition with many of these experiencing more than one. Comorbidities occur disproportionately among those with a spastic quadriplegic or dyskinetic variant or those individuals who are nonambulatory. These comorbidities may be the major health burdens that effectively limit activity, participation, and health-related quality of life.

A recent systematic review on co-occurring conditions in CP provides clinical prognostic information. Among children with CP, 3 in 4 were in pain; 1 in 2 had an intellectual disability (IQ lower than 70), and 1 in 3 had a severe intellectual disability (IQ lower than 50); 1 in 3 could not walk, 1 in 6 walked with assistance and 1 in 2 walked independently; 1 in 3 had a hip displacement (migration greater than 30%); 1 in 4 could not talk; 1 in 4 had active epilepsy, and 1 in 3 had epilepsy at some point; 1 in 4 had a behavior disorder; 1 in 4 had bladder-control problems; 1 in 4 had a sleep disorder; 1 in 5 had excessive drooling; 1 in 10 were blind; 1 in 15 were tube-fed; and 1 in 25 were deaf. The highest reported comorbidity in this review was pain, and it affected children and adults with CP regardless of levels of physical disability. In ambulatory patients, pain was reported in the neck, back, and feet, and individuals with contractures were also at increased risk of pain, which appeared to increase in prevalence with age.

In a population-based study in Europe, the prevalence of CP with epilepsy was 0.69 (99% CI, 0.66 to 0.72) per 1000 live births. Of their cohort of children with CP, 35% had a history of epilepsy, which was seen more often in children with a bilateral spastic subtype and associated other comorbidities. Neonatal characteristics independently associated with epilepsy in this cohort were the presence of a brain malformation or a syndrome, a term or moderately preterm birth compared with a very premature birth, and signs of perinatal distress including neonatal seizures, need for neonatal ventilation, and an admission to a neonatal care unit. In a surveillance study of 8-year-old children in the United States, 35% of children with CP had concurrent epilepsy. Among children with CP who were nonambulatory, 70% had a concurrent diagnosis of epilepsy. The proportion of children with CP who have epilepsy has been consistent across several studies, ranging between 30% and 35%.

Receptive and expressive language impairment is one of the most common comorbidities in children with CP. In a longitudinal study, development of an expressive language impairment was most closely related to motor function, with the best developmental trajectory seen in children with unilateral spastic CP. Receptive language development, however, was most closely related to intellectual disability.

Excessive drooling is a common comorbidity in CP, affecting up to 40% of children aged 7 to 14 years. Predictors of drooling include nonspastic (dyskinetic) or spastic quadriplegic subtypes, feeding difficulties, anterior open bite, intellectual disability, poor gross motor function, and the lack of speech. Saliva control improves in some children over time, with benefit from oromotor therapy, botulism toxin injection, or salivary gland duct surgery. In children with dyskinetic CP, poor oromotor coordination and an excessive salivary production from hyperkinetic oral motor activity are believed to cause drooling.

Associated psychiatric comorbidities and behavioral disorders in CP contribute to family stress and quality of life. A behavioral disorder was found in a quarter of children with CP in the previously mentioned systematic review and seen equally across functional severity. Similarly, in a cross-sectional study in school-age children with CP, 39.4% scored in the borderline to clinically abnormal range in the total difficulties score of the Strength and Difficulties questionnaire. These difficulties did not appear to be associated with sociodemographic variables and physical and cognitive characteristics. In a population-based study in Norway, 57% of children with CP had a psychiatric comorbidity, the most common being ADHD/ADD seen in 50% of the children. Communication impairment was the best predictor of psychiatric comorbidity, with no association detected with intellectual disability, clinical subtype, and motor function. In a surveillance study among 8-year-old children in the United States, an autism spectrum disorder was seen in 8% of children with CP.

Limited studies have looked at sleep disorders in CP. In a single European study, 23% of school-aged children with CP had a sleep disorder, including difficulty in initiating and maintaining sleep, sleep-wake transition, and sleep breathing disorders. Active epilepsy was 17 times more likely to be associated with the presence of a sleep disorder, as was being the child of a single-parent family (4 times more likely), sleeping with parents (6 times more likely), having a spastic quadriplegia subtype (13 times more likely) or dyskinetic CP (21 times more likely), and having a severe visual impairment (13 times more likely).

IX. CONCLUSION

Challenges remain in understanding the causal spectrum and mechanisms of CP and providing comprehensive care for these individuals. At present, a subset remains without an apparent underlying etiology and normal neuroimaging despite objective findings of substantive neuroimpairment on examination. Genetic and epigenetic factors are clearly at play, affecting both the predisposition to either congenital or acquired etiologies and modifying interindividual differences in resiliency and the response to acquired injury. These factors remain to be elucidated. Early diagnosis, in both at-risk and community-derived populations, should be a goal as early interventions are thought to improve later functional outcomes. Increasing emphasis on the functional categorization of severity, together with sensitivity to the contextual influences on individual participation and quality of life, should prompt a widening of the lens of care provision and foster partnerships across healthcare professions to optimize individual potential. Policy changes at a health service delivery and societal level, at least in high resource settings, can effectively enable this alteration in approach and improve outcomes. In contrast, low resource settings will need to address fundamental issues of prevention, through improved maternal and obstetric care, and a fairer population-wide distribution of access to healthcare. Through these efforts in a variety of domains, we can foresee a lessening of the incidence of CP and improvements in the quality of life of those affected and their primary caregivers.

REFERENCES

The complete list of references for this chapter is available online at www.expertconsult.com.
See inside cover for registration details.

SELECTED REFERENCES

Back, S.A., Miller, S.P., 2014. Brain injury in premature neonates: a primary cerebral dysmaturation disorder? Ann. Neurol. 75, 469–486.

Coleman, A., Wein, K., Ware, R.S., et al., 2015. Predicting functional communication ability in children with cerebral palsy at school entry. Dev. Med. Child Neurol. 57, 279–285.

Eliasson, A.C., Krumlinde-Sundholm, L., Rosblad, B., et al., 2006. The Manual Ability Classification System (MACS) for children with cerebral palsy: scale development and evidence of validity and reliability. Dev. Med. Child Neurol. 48, 549–554.

Ellenberg, J.H., Nelson, K.B., 2013. The association of cerebral palsy with birth asphyxia: a definitional quagmire. Dev. Med. Child Neurol. 55, 210–216.

Himmelmann, K., Ahlin, K., Jacobsson, B., et al., 2011. Risk factors for cerebral palsy in children born at term. Acta Obstet. Gynecol. Scand. 90, 1070–1081.

McIntyre, S., Taitz, D., Keogh, J., et al., 2013. A systematic review of risk factors for cerebral palsy in children born at term in developed countries. Dev. Med. Child Neurol. 55, 499–508.

Novak, I., Hines, M., Goldsmith, S., et al., 2012. Clinical prognostic messages from a systematic review on cerebral palsy. Pediatrics 130, e1285–e1312.

Oskoui, M., Coutinho, F., Dykeman, J., et al., 2013. An update on the prevalence of cerebral palsy: a systematic review and meta-analysis. Dev. Med. Child Neurol. 55, 509–519.

Rosenbaum, P., Paneth, N., Leviton, A., et al., 2007. A report: the definition and classification of cerebral palsy April 2006. Dev. Med. Child Neurol. 49, 8–14.

Rosenbaum, P.L., Palisano, R.J., Bartlett, D.J., et al., 2008. Development of the Gross Motor Function Classification System for cerebral palsy. Dev. Med. Child Neurol. 50, 249–253.

98 Tics and Tourette Syndrome

Laura Tochen and Harvey S. Singer

An expanded version of this chapter is available on www.expertconsult.com. See inside cover for registration details.

Tourette syndrome is a disorder characterized by chronic motor and vocal tics. It is one of several disorders that have tics as a cardinal feature, and many other psychopathologies can coexist with tic disorders. There is now strong evidence for involvement of genetics and environmental influences in underlying etiology. Cortico-striatal-thalamo-cortical pathways have been implicated, but a precise pathophysiological location remains under investigation. There is no cure for tics, but various behavioral and pharmacologic therapies are currently used for symptom control.

TIC PHENOMENOLOGY

Tics are involuntary, sudden, rapid, abrupt, repetitive, recurrent, and nonrhythmic movements or vocalizations. They have differing degrees of intensity and frequency and have unpredictable durations (Cohen, Leckman, and Bloch, 2013). Because some vocal (phonic) tics are the result of muscle contractions of the diaphragm or oropharynx forcing air across the vocal cords or through the nose and mouth, the formal separation of tics into motor and vocal components has been questioned. Both motor and phonic tics are subdivided into simple and complex categories. Simple motor tics are brief, rapid movements that involve only a single muscle or localized group. Examples include eye blinking, head jerking, nose wrinkling, shoulder shrugging, and abdominal tensing. In contrast, complex motor tics involve either a cluster of simple actions or a more coordinated sequence of movements. Complex motor tics can be nonpurposeful, such as facial or body contortions, have a more prolonged maintenance of a position or dystonic character, or appear purposeful but actually serve no purpose, such as touching, hitting, smelling, jumping, repeating observed movements (echopraxia), or making obscene gestures (copropraxia). Some have subdivided tic movements into additional categories such as clonic (eye blinking, head jerking), tonic (muscle tensing), dystonic (sustained posture), and blocking (prolonged tonic or dystonic tics that interrupt ongoing motor activity). Simple phonations include various sounds and noises, such as grunts, barks, yelps, sniffs, screeches, and throat clearing. Complex vocalizations involve the repetition of words, syllables, phrases, echolalia (repeating other people's words), palilalia (repeating one's own words), or coprolalia (repeating obscene words).

Several common characteristics of tics include their presence in typical locations, a waxing and waning course, the presence of particular factors that exacerbate or reduce tics, a suggestible nature, the report of a premonitory sensation, and suppressibility. Although tics may involve almost any external body part, nearly all TS patients at some time have tics involving the face and head regions. Tics can be exacerbated by periods of anticipation, emotional upset (e.g., stress, anxiety, excitement, anger), or fatigue. Tic reduction often occurs when the affected individual is concentrating, focused, engaged in an activity, emotionally pleased, or during sleep. Patients with tics may occasionally attempt to disguise a tic as a seemingly purposeful behavior.

Premonitory urges are sensory phenomena and can consist of a feeling, urge, impulse, tension, pressure, itch, burning, or tingle that occurs before a motor or phonic tic. These sensations occur in more than 90% of adults with TS but less frequently in young children. The "urge" often immediately disappears following performance of the tic, but recurs. Severity of premonitory sensations has been correlated with tic severity. The ability to briefly suppress tics is relatively common. This active suppression of tics, however, is often associated with an exacerbation of premonitory sensations.

Misdiagnoses are common because, for example, eye-blinking tics may be thought to stem from ophthalmologic problems, ocular tics can be confused with opsoclonus, throat-clearing tics can be thought to result from sinusitis or allergic conditions, involuntary sniffing frequently results in referral to an allergist, and a chronic and persistent cough-like bark could be mistaken for asthma. Nontic movements that should be distinguished from tics include motor stereotypies, drug-induced akathisia, dystonia, and parkinsonism, and those associated with common comorbidities such as obsessive-compulsive disorder (OCD), attention deficit hyperactivity disorder (ADHD), and impulsive and antisocial behaviors.

Tics can be assessed clinically with the use of several scales. The most widely used is the Yale Global Tic Severity Scale (YGTSS), which consists of (1) a total tic score based on number, frequency, intensity, complexity, and interference of tics, and (2) a tic impairment score based on the effects on self-esteem, family life, and social acceptance (Cohen et al., 2013).

TIC DISORDERS

The diagnosis of a tic disorder is based solely on historical features and a clinical examination that confirms their presence and eliminates other conditions. There is no biomarker for the disorder, and thus no blood test, brain scan, or genetic screen is available for diagnostic confirmation. The fifth edition of the *Diagnostic and Statistical Manual of Mental Disorders* (DSM-V) lists six different tic disorders, as shown in Box 98-1.

Provisional tic disorder is the new recommended term established to designate an individual with ongoing fluctuating motor and/or vocal tics that began before age 18 years and have been present for less than 1 year.

Chronic motor or vocal tic disorder requires that fluctuating tics start before age 18, be present for more than 1 year, and individuals have either solely motor or, less commonly, solely vocal tics, but not both.

Tourette syndrome (TS) formal criteria based on the definition provided by the Tourette Syndrome Classification Study Group are very similar to those for Tourette disorder (TD) in the DSM-V. Diagnoses require multiple motor and at least one vocal tic to have been present at some time during the illness, although not necessarily concurrently. Criteria from the TS classification group retain an age of onset before 21 years, rather than the DSM-V's age-of-onset limitation to less than

BOX 98-1 Tic Classifications

DSM-V CLASSIFICATION

Provisional Tic Disorder
Chronic Motor or Vocal Tic Disorder
Tourette Disorder (Tourette Syndrome)
Substance-Induced Tic Disorder
Tic Disorder Due to a General Medical Condition
Tic Disorder, Not Otherwise Specified

18 years. Tics should occur many times a day, nearly every day or intermittently, throughout a period of 1 year.

Substance-induced tic disorder requires evidence that motor and/or vocal tics developed during or within 1 month of substance intoxication or withdrawal, or that substance use is etiologically related to the disturbance. Examples include cocaine-induced tics and tics that developed following the use of neuroleptics. Stimulants used to treat ADHD are not included, because evidence indicates that treatment with stimulants does not exacerbate tics.

Tic disorder due to a generalized medical condition can involve many diagnoses, because tics have been reported in many sporadic, genetic, and neurodegenerative disorders. For example, tics have been associated with neuroacanthocytosis, Huntington disease, neurodegeneration with brain iron accumulation, encephalitis, infection, stroke, and head trauma.

Tic disorder not otherwise specified refers to disorders that do not meet criteria for a specific tic disorder because the movements or vocalizations are atypical in age of onset (i.e., adult onset) or clinical presentation. Tic disorders in adults usually have their onset in childhood, although some have had their onset beyond the age of 21 years. Symptoms with origination in adulthood are often associated with potential environmental triggers, are typically more severe, have a greater social morbidity, and show a poorer response to medications.

COURSE

Motor tics typically begin between the ages of 4 to 8 years with a mean of about 6 to 7 years. The average age of diagnosis is just over 8 years of age. Coprolalia, when present, has a mean age of onset of 14 years. Tics have a waxing and waning course, and fluctuation of symptoms is expected. Fluctuations occur within the course of a day and throughout periods of months or longer. The course of TS can be quite variable, with most patients having a decline in symptoms during the teenage and early adulthood years. Maximum tic severity tends to be between the ages of 10 to 12 years. Long term, most studies support a broad "rule of thirds"—one third of cases disappear, one third are better, and about one third continue—as a reasonable estimate of outcome. Predictors of outcome are controversial, with severity, motor control, and imaging findings having been investigated (Singer, Gilbert, Wolf, Mink, and Kurlan, 2012).

EPIDEMIOLOGY

Epidemiologic studies have shown that about 20% to 27% of children in a regular classroom setting will exhibit tics. Tourette syndrome occurs worldwide, with evidence of common features in all cultures and races. Prevalence is estimated at 0.52%. The disorder is more common in males than in females, with a ratio of about 3 to 4 boys to 1 girl. TS is more common in those with autism spectrum disorders or fragile X syndrome.

COMORBID DISORDERS

Comorbid diagnoses are common in TS, specifically psychiatric diagnoses. Approximately 85% of TS patients qualify for at least one psychiatric diagnosis, most commonly ADHD or OCD (Hirschtritt et al., 2015).

ADHD is characterized by impulsivity, hyperactivity, and a decreased ability to maintain attention. Symptoms begin in early childhood and typically precede the onset of tics. ADHD is reported to affect approximately 50% of patients with TS. ADHD symptoms in TS correlate with increased psychosocial difficulties, disruptive behavior, peer rejection, emotional problems, functional impairment, family conflict, learning disabilities, and school problems. Those with comorbid ADHD may have poorer overall functioning and worse scores on quality-of-life assessments.

OCD is characterized by persistent obsessions (persistent recurrent intrusive, thoughts, images, or impulsions that are unwelcome and intrude upon conscious thought) or compulsions (repetitive seemingly purposeful behaviors usually performed in response to an obsession, in accord with certain rules, or in a stereotyped fashion). Obsessive-compulsive behaviors (OCBs) become a disorder (OCD) when activities are sufficiently severe to cause marked distress, take up more than 1 hour of the day, or have a significant negative effect on normal routine, function, social activities, or relationships. In patients with TS, behaviors usually include a need for order or routine and a requirement for things to be symmetric, involving behaviors such as arranging, ordering, hoarding, touching, tapping, rubbing, counting, checking for errors, or evening up. In contrast, OCD subjects without tics typically have compulsions related to fear of contamination and cleaning. Differentiating OCB from tics may be difficult; however, suggestive features for OCD include a cognitive-based drive and need to perform the action in a particular fashion (e.g., a certain number of times, until it feels "just right," or equally on both sides of the body). OCBs occur in from 20% to 89% of patients with TS, generally emerge several years after the onset of tics, typically become more severe at a later age, and are more likely to persist than tic symptoms.

Anxiety and depression are also commonly diagnosed in TS patients. The high-risk period for development of an anxiety disorder begins around age 4, and for mood disorder around age 7. Children with chronic tic disorders are more likely to have suicidal thoughts or behaviors. Additional non-OCD-related anxiety disorders include separation anxiety, agoraphobia, and panic disorder.

Disruptive behaviors have been noted in some individuals with TS, including significant problems with labile emotion, anger control, and aggression. Episodic outbursts may include screaming, threatening behaviors, stomping, kicking, destroying objects, punching holes in walls, and so forth. Self-inflicted, nonaccidental behaviors (head banging, body punching or slapping, banging oneself against a hard object, poking sharp objects into the body, scratching body parts) also occur in TS. Explosive outbursts are more common in patients with younger age of tic onset, greater tic severity, and ADHD. Conduct disorder and oppositional defiant disorder are also seen in TS, although no evidence exists to suggest that patients with TS are more likely to engage in criminal activities. Other psychopathologies such as personality disorders may also be more frequent in TS.

Despite typically having normal intellectual functioning, poor school performance is common in children with tics. This effect may extend into adulthood; adults with tics can have impairments within the workplace. Potential etiologies for academic problems are multiple and include tic severity, psychosocial problems, ADHD, OCD, learning disabilities, executive dysfunction, and prescribed medication.

Problems associated with sleep have been reported in about 20% to 65% of children and young adults with TS and include difficulties with insomnia, bedtime rituals, dreams, and parasomnias. Restless leg syndrome (RLS) has been reported in up to 10% of patients with TS.

ETIOLOGY

Genetic A genetic or epigenetic basis for TS has long been hypothesized, but despite extensive subsequent investigations, the precise pattern of transmission and the identification of the gene remain elusive. Family studies show a 10- to 100-fold increase in incidence of TS in first-degree relatives. The strongest support for a genetic disorder is based on studies of monozygotic and dizygotic twins; there is 77% to 94% concordance for tic disorders in monozygotic twins versus 23% in dizygotic twins (Paschou, 2013). Linkage analyses identified strong evidence for linkage to markers on chromosome 2p23.2, with suggestive evidence for linkage on chromosomes 5p and 6p. Candidate gene studies, focusing primarily on genes involved in neurotransmitter systems, have found a significant association between TS and a dopamine transporter polymorphism and a serotonin receptor polymorphism. A heterozygous loss-of-function mutation in L-histidine decarboxylase has been identified (Paschou, 2013). A genome-wide association study (GWAS) in TS failed to find any significant loci, but several strong signals were identified, including COL27A1, POLR3B, and the intergenic region between SLITRK1 and SLITRK6. It is possible that no causative gene has been identified as a result of the phenotypic heterogeneity of the disorder. Epigenetic factors and in utero exposures have also been suggested to have a role.

If a mother or father has TS, the likelihood that a son will develop a condition on the TS spectrum is estimated to be about 40% to 45%: the approximate risk for TS is 10% to 15%; for chronic tics 15% to 20%; and for OCB without tics approximately 5% to 10%. The overall risks for a daughter are about 25% to 35%: 3% to 5% for TS; 10% to 15% for chronic tics; and 10% to 20% for OCB without tics. If both parents have TS and/or OCD, based on studies of only small numbers of bilineal families, the offspring's risk for a TS-spectrum problem may be as high as 70% to 90%: for TS 25% to 50%, and for chronic tics 40% to 65%. It is emphasized, however, that although susceptibility risks may be high, most affected individuals have very mild conditions.

Autoimmune Several investigators have proposed that, in a subset of children, tic symptoms are caused by a preceding β-hemolytic streptococcal infection (GABHS). Labeled as pediatric autoimmune neuropsychiatric disorder associated with streptococcal infection (PANDAS), proposed criteria include the presence of OCD and/or tic disorder; prepubertal age at onset; sudden, "explosive" onset of symptoms and/or a course of sudden exacerbations and remissions; a temporal relationship between symptom exacerbations and GABHS; and the presence of neurologic abnormalities, including hyperactivity and choreiform movements. The existence of PANDAS as an etiologic entity remains controversial based on both epidemiologic and autoimmune studies (Elamin et al., 2013). Concerns about individual criterion proposed for the diagnosis include the following: the age of onset does little to separate tic disorders from the PANDAS subgroup; neuropsychological and family genetic studies of PANDAS cases show few differences from what is typically seen in early-onset OCD or TS; the sudden, explosive onset or worsening of tic symptoms occurs frequently in unselected children with tic disorders; studies do not consistently support an epidemiologic

link to GABHS; and clinical findings have shown that exacerbations in PANDAS cases are usually not temporally related to a streptococcal infection. Results of serum antineuronal antibodies and other immune factors in PANDAS have been inconclusive via multiple methodologies. Although the PANDAS diagnosis is controversial, there still remains the clinical entity of an acute or fulminant onset of neuropsychiatric symptoms, which can include tics in some individuals. Updated diagnoses with broader criteria have been proposed: childhood acute-onset neuropsychiatric symptoms (CANS) and pediatric acute-onset neuropsychiatric syndrome (PANS). Diagnostic criteria for PANS include lack of other known medical diagnosis to account for symptoms, abrupt onset of OC symptoms or restrictive food intake, and at least two of the following: anxiety, emotional lability/depression, aggression, developmental regression, school performance deterioration, motor or sensory abnormalities, somatic symptoms. Presence of tics has been deemphasized in newer PANS criteria. The diagnosis of CANS requires the acute onset of symptoms. These diagnoses do not suggest a definite relationship with a specific infectious etiology, such as streptococcal infection, and such dramatic symptom onset should prompt a thorough evaluation for multiple possible underlying causes, such as infectious, metabolic, toxic, and autoimmune etiologies (Singer et al., 2012).

NEUROBIOLOGY OF TIC DISORDERS
Anatomic Abnormalities

A series of parallel cortico-striatal-thalamo-cortical (CSTC) circuits provides a framework for understanding the neurobiological relationships that exist between tic disorders and associated comorbidities. The motor circuit, proposed to be abnormal in the production of tic symptoms, originates primarily from the supplementary motor cortex and projects to the putamen in a somatotopic distribution. The oculomotor circuit, possibly influencing ocular tics, begins principally in the frontal eye fields and connects to the central region of the caudate. The dorsolateral prefrontal circuit links Brodmann's area 9 and 10 with the dorsolateral head of the caudate and appears to be involved with executive functions (flexibility, organization, constructional strategy, verbal and design fluency) and motor planning (sequential and alternating reciprocal motor tasks). The lateral orbitofrontal circuit originates in the inferior lateral prefrontal cortex (area 11 and 12) and projects to the ventral medial caudate. This circuit is associated with obsessive-compulsive behaviors, personality changes, mania, disinhibition, and irritability. Finally, the limbic circuit arises in the cingulate gyrus and projects to the ventral striatum, which also receives input from the amygdala, hippocampus, medial orbitofrontal cortex, and entorhinal and perirhinal cortex. A variety of behavioral problems may be linked with this circuit. Although direct and indirect evidence suggest that components of CSTC circuits are involved in the expression of tic disorders, identification of the primary abnormality (i.e., cortical or striatal) remains an area of active research (Singer, 2005).

The striatum is often implicated in anatomic investigations of TS. Postmortem studies showed a reduction in GABAergic interneurons in the striatum. Multiple volumetric magnetic resonance imaging (MRI) studies have shown abnormalities in the shape or volume of the caudate or lenticular nuclei. One hypothesis suggests a striatal compartment abnormality at the level of striosome-matrix organization based on anatomic, physiologic, and lesion studies (Ganos, Roessner, and Munchau, 2013). The ventral striatum, with its role in sequential learning and habit formation, has also been a focus, and positron emission tomography (PET) studies with ^{11}C-raclopride and amphetamine have also shown robust increases in DA release in the ventral striatum of TS subjects compared with controls. Functional MRI has shown decreased putamen and globus pallidus activity and increased caudate activity during tic suppression, and activation of the putamen before tic onset, and single-photon emission computed tomography (SPECT) imaging demonstrated decreased glucose utilization in the basal ganglia.

Although there is support for striatal involvement, there is also persuasive evidence supportive of primary cortical dysfunction in TS. Children with TS have executive dysfunction, cognitive inhibitory deficits, larger dorsolateral prefrontal regions on volumetric MRI, larger hippocampal regions, increased cortical white matter in the right frontal lobe, and alterations in size of the corpus callosum. Diffusion-tensor MRI studies of the corpus callosum in TS have shown lower fractional anisotropy, suggesting reduced white-matter connectivity in this interhemispheric pathway and in tracts of the CSTC pathway. Imaging has identified frontal and parietal cortical thinning, most prominent in ventral portions of the sensory and motor homunculi. Event-related ^{15}O-H$_2$O PET techniques showed that tics activated sensorimotor, language, executive, and paralimbic regions, and functional MRI studies have shown cortical activation before tic onset.

Neurotransmitter Abnormalities

Dopamine Evidence supporting a dopaminergic abnormality in TS is derived from therapeutic responses to neuroleptics, data from postmortem studies, and a variety of nuclear imaging protocols. An increased release of dopamine has been demonstrated in both striatal and extra-striatal regions following amphetamine stimulation. With some variability, imaging studies of the striatum have shown a slight increase in the binding potential of dopamine receptors. A potentially unifying hypothesis has been proposed involving an abnormality of the phasic release of dopamine. The phasic DA hypothesis is further supported by clinical findings, including (1) the exacerbation of tics by stimulant medications, likely secondary to enhanced dopamine release from the axon terminal; (2) tic exacerbation by environmental stimuli, such as stress, anxiety, and medications, events shown to increase phasic bursts of dopamine; and (3) tic suppression with very low doses of DA agonists, likely attributable to presynaptic reduction of phasic DA release. Although this hypothesis could refer to either the cortex or striatum, a frontal dopaminergic abnormality is favored (Felling and Singer, 2011). Genetically, an association has been identified between a polymorphism of the dopamine transporter gene, DAT Ddel, and TS (Paschou, 2013).

Serotonin Serum studies in TS patients have shown decreased levels of serotonin and tryptophan. [[123I]]βCIT and SPECT studies investigating serotonin transporter binding capacity in TS patients show reduced binding in TS, but these findings are likely associated with the presence of OCD. PET imaging of tryptophan metabolism (alpha-[11C]methyl-L-tryptophan) has demonstrated decreased uptake in the dorsolateral prefrontal cortical regions and increased uptake in the thalamus. Polymorphic variants of tryptophan hydroxylase 2 have been postulated to be associated with TS, as have serotonin transporter gene polymorphisms and receptor gene polymorphisms.

Glutamate Reduced levels of the amino acid glutamate have been identified in the globus pallidus interna, globus pallidus externa, and substantia nigra pars reticulata regions of four TS brains (Felling and Singer, 2011). A large multigenerational family genome scan and a genome scan using sibling pairs and multigenerational families have identified evidence for linkage to 5p13, an area that overlaps with the genomic region for the glial glutamate transporter1 (*SLC1A3* or *EAAT1*) gene (Paschou, 2013). Other factors supporting a potential role for glutamate in TS include its essential role in pathways involved with CSTC circuits, the extensive interaction between the glutamate and dopamine neurotransmitter systems, and reports demonstrating that glutamate-altering medications have a beneficial therapeutic effect on obsessive-compulsive symptoms.

GABA On pathologic examination, brains of TS patients were found to have a decrease in parvalbumin-positive GABAergic interneurons in the caudate and putamen (Felling and Singer, 2011). PET imaging of GABA binding using ^{11}C-flumazenil showed reduced GABA receptor binding within the striatum and other areas. Magnetic resonance spectroscopy has shown increased GABA concentrations in cortical supplementary motor areas. GABA-related gene expression has also been shown to correlate with tic severity.

TREATMENT

Despite advances in understanding TS, there is neither a cure for tics nor an ideal tic-suppressing therapy. It is essential for the treating physician to identify whether tics or associated problems (e.g., ADHD, OCD, school problems, behavioral disorders) represent the greatest handicap. Specific criteria for initiating tic-suppressing therapy include the presence of psychosocial problems (e.g., loss of self-esteem; peer problems; difficulty participating in academic, work, family, social, and after-school activities; disruption of classroom settings) and/or musculoskeletal and physical difficulties. Tics have a natural waxing and waning course, and education is an essential component of the treatment process. The goal of treatment is not complete suppression of tics, but rather their reduction to a level at which they no longer cause significant psychosocial or physical disturbances.

Nonpharmacologic Treatments Classroom strategies include educating teachers and fellow students, providing optional study breaks, and eliminating unnecessary stressful situations. Various behavioral approaches (supportive psychotherapy, conditioning techniques, exposure and response prevention, cognitive behavioral therapy, awareness training, habit reversal, and hypnosis) have been tried in the treatment of tics. Comprehensive Behavioral Intervention for Tics (CBIT), a behavioral therapy that incorporates several approaches (psychoeducation, habit reversal therapy, functional intervention, reward system, and relaxation training), has been shown to be effective in randomized controlled trials of children and adults (Roessner et al., 2013). Alternative diets, supplements, and vitamins have not been validated in controlled trials. Acupuncture and repetitive transcranial magnetic stimulation may be helpful.

Pharmacotherapy Despite the absence of an ideal tic-suppressing medication, numerous medications have been tried, with varying levels of empirical support (Roessner et al., 2013) (see Table 98-1). A two-tiered approach is recommended based on side-effect profiles. For milder tics, non-neuroleptic medications (tier 1) can be used, and for more severe tics, typical and atypical neuroleptics (tier 2) may be needed (McNaught and Mink, 2011). Medications should be prescribed at the lowest effective dosage. The patient should be periodically reassessed and determinations made about the need for continued therapy. General principles include obtaining a ECG before starting neuroleptics, starting all medications at low doses, gradually increasing the dose if tic-induced psychosocial and/or physical difficulties persist, monitoring efficacy and side effects on an ongoing basis, using monotherapy whenever possible, and considering a

TABLE 98-1 Medications

Tier 1		Tier 2		Tier 3	
Drug	*Category*	*Drug*	*Category*	*Drug*	*Category*
Clonidine	A	Pimozide*	A	Dopamine agonists	—
Guanfacine	A	Fluphenazine	B	Pergolide	(B)
Baclofen	C	Risperidone	A	Pramipexole	—
Topiramate	B	Aripiprazole	B	Tetrabenazine	C
Levetiracetam	C	Olanzapine	C	Delta-9-THC	C
Clonazepam	C	Haloperidol*	A	Donepezil	C
		Ziprasidone	B	Botulinum toxin	B
		Quetiapine	C	Sulpiride and tiapride	—

A, good supportive evidence (two randomized, placebo-controlled studies); B, fair (one positive placebo-controlled study); C, minimal (open-label, case reports)
*Drug is FDA approved for the treatment of tics.

gradual medication taper during a nonstressful (e.g., summer vacation) period. Only two medications, pimozide and haloperidol, are approved by the U.S. Food and Drug Administration (FDA) for tic suppression.

Tier 1 Medications. Tier 1 medications include clonidine and guanfacine, among others. Clonidine and guanfacine are preferred in the treatment of comorbid ADHD as well.

Tier 2 Medications. Dopamine receptor antagonists (antipsychotics) are effective tic-suppressing agents, but side effects frequently limit their usefulness. The typical neuroleptics pimozide and fluphenazine are preferred over haloperidol because of fewer side effects. Long-term follow up of patients taking fluphenazine showed tolerability and no incidences of tardive dyskinesia. Atypical neuroleptics (risperidone, aripiprazole, olanzapine, ziprasidone, quetiapine) are characterized by a relatively greater affinity for serotonin receptors than for D2 receptors and a reduced potential for extrapyramidal side effects.

Surgery Deep-brain stimulation (DBS) has had preliminary success in treating tics. Target sites for high-frequency stimulation have included the centromedian-parafascicular complex of the thalamus, the globus pallidus interna, and the anterior limb of the internal capsule, although the ideal target site remains to be determined. DBS can be considered in refractory cases in which therapies such as alpha-adrenergic agents, neuroleptics, behavioral therapy, and additional agents such as tetrabenazine or clonazepam have failed (McNaught and Mink, 2011). The approach should involve a multidisciplinary team, and additional ethical review is recommended for patients under age 18. Comorbidities need to be adequately addressed and managed.

REFERENCES

The complete list of references for this chapter is available in the e-book at www.expertconsult.com.
    See inside cover for registration details.

SELECTED REFERENCES

Cohen, S.C., Leckman, J.F., Bloch, M.H., 2013. Clinical assessment of Tourette syndrome and tic disorders. Neurosci. Biobehav. Rev. 37 (6), 997–1007.

Elamin, I., Edwards, M.J., Martino, D., 2013. Immune dysfunction in Tourette syndrome. Behav. Neurol. 27 (1), 23–32.

Felling, R.J., Singer, H.S., 2011. Neurobiology of tourette syndrome: current status and need for further investigation. J. Neurosci. 31 (35), 12387–12395.

Ganos, C., Roessner, V., Munchau, A., 2013. The functional anatomy of Gilles de la Tourette syndrome. Neurosci. Biobehav. Rev. 37 (6), 1050–1062.

Hirschtritt, M.E., Lee, P.C., Pauls, D.L., et al., 2015. Lifetime prevalence, age of risk, and genetic relationships of comorbid psychiatric disorders in Tourette syndrome. JAMA Psychiatry 72 (4), 325–333.

McNaught, K.S., Mink, J.W., 2011. Advances in understanding and treatment of Tourette syndrome. Nat. Rev. Neurol. 7 (12), 667–676.

Paschou, P., 2013. The genetic basis of Gilles de la Tourette Syndrome. Neurosci. Biobehav. Rev. 37 (6), 1026–1039.

Roessner, V., Schoenefeld, K., Buse, J., et al., 2013. Pharmacological treatment of tic disorders and Tourette Syndrome. Neuropharmacology 68, 143–149.

Singer, H.S., 2005. Tourette's syndrome: from behaviour to biology. Lancet Neurol. 4 (3), 149–159.

Singer, H.S., Gilbert, D.L., Wolf, D.S., et al., 2012. Moving from PANDAS to CANS. J. Pediatr. 160 (5), 725–731.

99   Genetic and Metabolic Disorders of the White Matter

Adeline Vanderver and Nicole I. Wolf

An expanded version of this chapter is available on www.expertconsult.com. See inside cover for registration details.

INTRODUCTION

Over the past several decades, an increasing number of novel heritable disorders affecting the white matter of the brain, or leukodystrophies, have been described, often with identification of a causative gene (Table 99-1). Pathognomonic MRI patterns (Fig. 99-1) or clinical characteristics permitted identification in a number of these disorders, and should guide the clinician's molecular diagnosis for many conditions (see Fig. 99-3 and 99-5 for MRI features). In addition, the recent advent of next generation sequencing approaches has permitted rapid increase in the number of novel diseases identified, as well as improved diagnosis for individual patients.

It remains challenging to distinguish inherited disorders from acquired white matter pathologies such as periventricular leukomalacia, immunologic disorders, toxic or infectious processes. This distinction is critical to patient management and genetic counseling, and acquired etiologies should be excluded by clinical history, examination, and laboratory testing before pursuing differential diagnosis of the heritable white matter disorders. Special consideration should be given to endocrine dysfunction, as both congenital and acquired thyroid and adrenal dysfunction have been associated with white matter abnormalities, as have nutritional factors such as vitamin B12 deficiency.

Although history and clinical examination are critical to excluding acquired leukoencephalopathies or disorders with secondary white matter manifestations, many classic leukodystrophies share clinical manifestations with these other disorders. The hallmarks of CNS white matter disorders are progressive spasticity (often associated with rigidity or ataxia), bulbar symptoms, and relatively preserved cognitive function. Cranial nerve abnormalities such as optic nerve atrophy, strabismus, or nystagmus and hearing loss can be seen. Peripheral nerve function may be impaired depending on the disorder. Seizures are less commonly seen and should alert the clinician to the possibility of an underlying neuronal disorder, as should prominent dementia.

Given the heterogeneity and limited specificity in clinical findings, MRI pattern recognition is the most useful tool for evaluating suspected leukodystrophy patients (Schiffmann and van der Knaap, 2009) (Fig. 99-1). Imaging should be reviewed comprehensively, with attention to changes over time, expected myelin development for the patient's age, and characteristics of T1-weighted and T2-weighted signal abnormalities. Broadly, there are two groups of leukodystrophies. Hypomyelinating leukodystrophies show increased white matter signal on T2 relative to age and often isointense or hyperintense white matter signal on T1. Conversely, demyelinating leukodystrophies show increased white matter signal on T2 relative to

age and hypointense white matter signal on T1. Additional radiologic features should be assessed, such as white matter vacuolization or cysts, best seen on FLAIR or similar imaging paradigms; involvement of the basal ganglia, brainstem, cerebellum, or spinal cord; and abnormalities of cortical gray matter. Finally, findings consistent with calcifications should be noted, and a CT scan or calcium-sensitive MRI sequences should be acquired to exclude the presence of calcifications that might be missed on standard MR imaging. An overview of those features and the disorders exemplifying them can be found at GeneReviews (http://www.ncbi.nlm.nih.gov/books/NBK184570/).

PART I. HYPOMYELINATING WHITE MATTER DISORDERS

White matter disorders with hypomyelination are relatively frequent; hypomyelinating leukodystrophies comprise 20% of leukodystrophies. They are characterized by a significant and permanent deficit of myelin (Pouwels et al., 2014; Schiffmann and van der Knaap, 2009). Even with thorough genetic investigation, at least half of these hypomyelinating disorders lack definitive diagnosis, prognostic information, and potential for prenatal diagnosis. Although most of these disorders show autosomal recessive inheritance, both X-linked inheritance and de novo mutations are possible. Clinical manifestations common to hypomyelinating disorders are ataxia, spasticity, and nystagmus. Other nonneurologic features such as hypodontia in 4H syndrome or cataracts in hypomyelination with congenital cataracts can be valuable in diagnosis.

The diagnosis of hypomyelination may be made if two MRIs at least 6 months apart after the age of 12 months show little or no myelin development. Images in hypomyelinating leukodystrophies demonstrate a diffusely hyperintense signal of the supratentorial white matter in T2-weighted images and an isointense or hyperintense white matter signal on T1-weighted images. Certain areas such as the posterior internal capsule may have more normal-appearing myelin signal. Myelin deposition in infratentorial structures is usually less affected. A definitive diagnosis of hypomyelination is not possible in young infants, as myelination is incomplete. If no myelin deposition is visible on the first MRI of a child older than 24 months, however, hypomyelination is highly probable (Schiffmann and van der Knaap, 2009).

Delayed myelination is sometimes misdiagnosed as hypomyelination. In contrast to hypomyelination, myelination progresses on serial MRI images to near normal myelin development (Fig. 99-2). A typical example of a disease with severely delayed but progressing myelination is the X-linked recessive condition thyroid hormone transporter (MCT8)

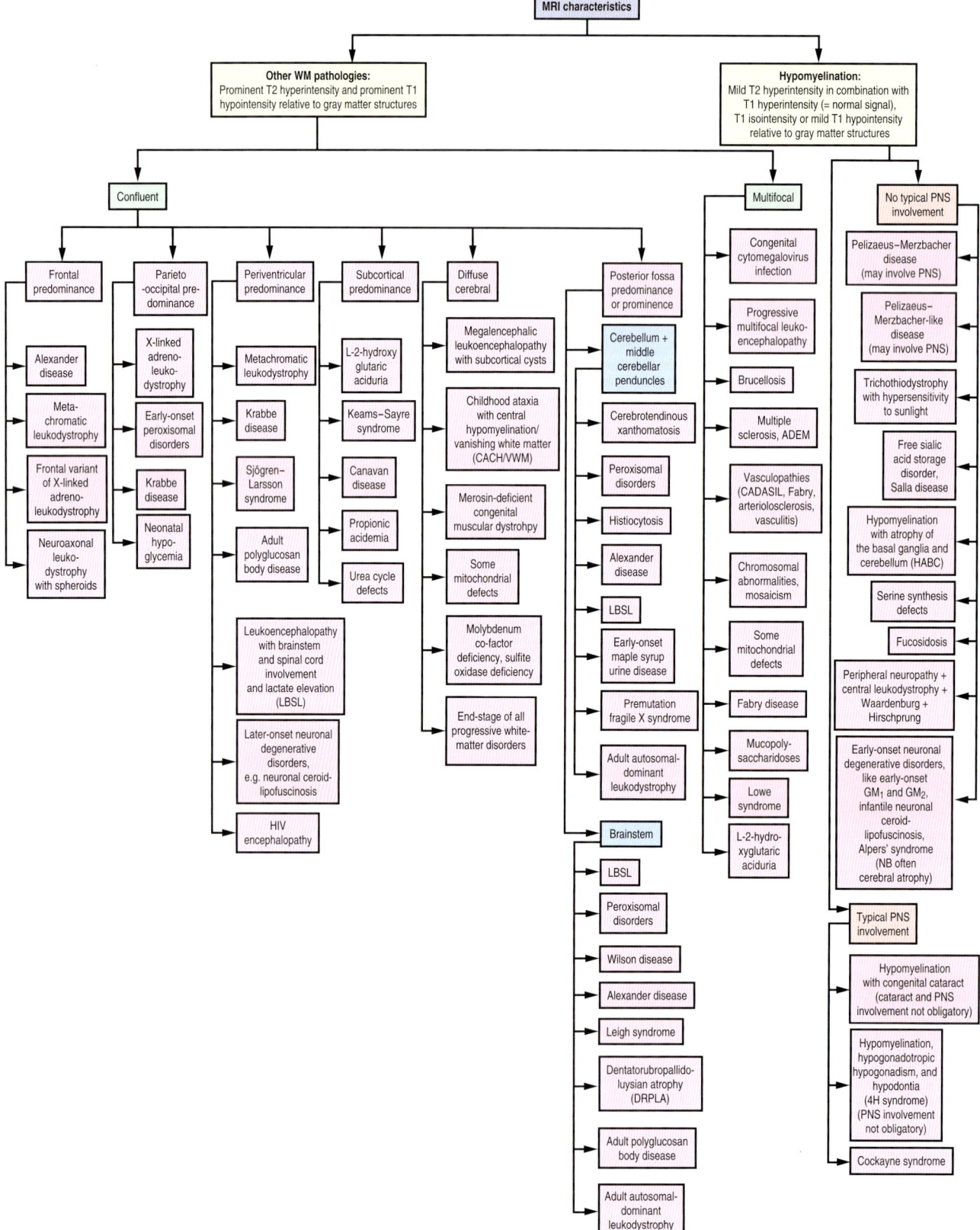

Figure 99-1. Diagnostic algorithm for use in patients with abnormal myelination by MRI. *(With permission from Schiffmann, R., van der Knaap, M.S., 2009. Invited article: an MRI-based approach to the diagnosis of white matter disorders. Neurology 72, 750–759).*

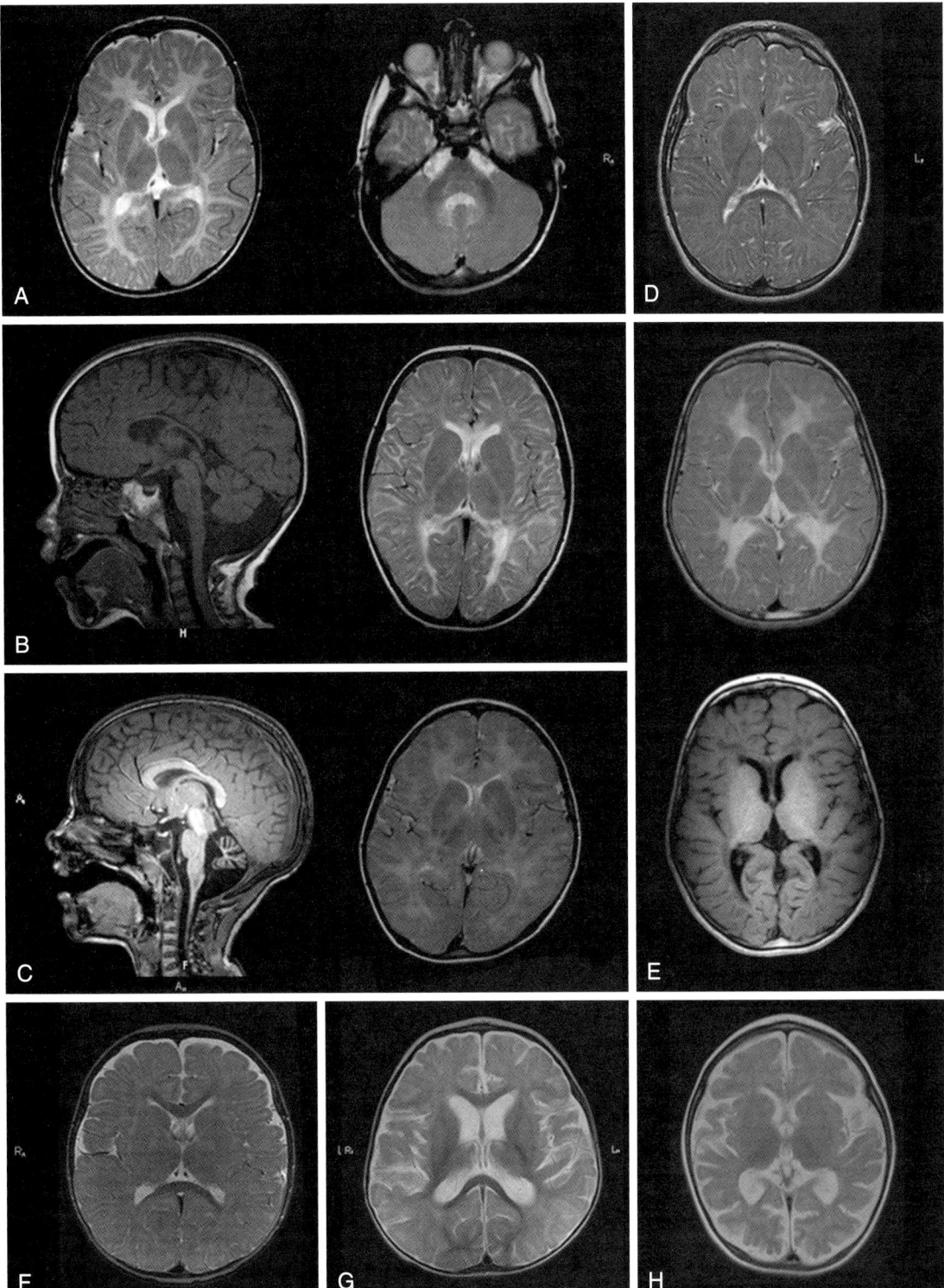

Figure 99-3. Hypomyelinating leukodystrophies and their differential diagnosis. A, MRI of a 23-month-old child with Pelizaeus-Merzbacher disease and a duplication of PLP1. The supratentorial axial T2-weighted images show homogeneous hyperintense white matter signal, indicating profound hypomyelination. There is also lack of myelin in the cerebellum. **B,** MRI of a 5-year-old child with Pelizaeus–Merzbacher-like disease due to a missense mutation in GJC2. The brainstem is less well myelinated, and the signal of the pyramidal tracts is slightly elevated. In the supratentorial structures, signal of the white matter is too high in the T2-weighted image. The sagittal T1-weighted image shows a normal cerebellar volume but a thin corpus callosum. **C,** MRI of a 3-year-old child with 4H syndrome. White matter shows diffusely elevated signal with sparing only of a part of the posterior limb of the internal capsule and of the optic radiation. The coronal and sagittal images demonstrate the cerebellar atrophy. **D,** MRI of an 8-year-old child with Salla disease. Note diffuse increased signal of the supratentorial white matter, with relatively better myelination of the corpus callosum and posterior limb of the internal capsule. **E,** MRI of a child with hypomyelination with congenital cataracts. The white matter signal in the T2-weighted image is slightly higher than in other hypomyelinating disorders. In the corresponding T1-weighted image, there are hypointense areas. Both indicate elevated water content. **F,** MRI of a 20-month-old child with GM1 disease. Note the delayed myelination, accompanied by globus pallidus signal abnormality. **G,** MRI of a 15-month-old child with POLG1 deficiency. Note the delayed myelination and atrophy in this child with a gray matter disorder. **H,** Axial T2-weighted image of a 12-month-old child with infantile neuronal ceroid lipofuscinosis; the signal of the white matter is also elevated compared with healthy children. Note the severe atrophy in the child with this gray matter disease.

deficiency, and thyroid function should be tested in boys with severe myelination delay on MRI, severe cognitive delay, and a pyramidal syndrome. Appropriate testing includes free T3 (which is elevated) and reverse T3 (which is decreased) in the context of either normal or reduced T4 and normal or slightly elevated TSH. Gray matter disorders with early onset often show hypomyelination, presumably a result of defective axonal function. Features such as early atrophy and signal changes of cortex and basal ganglia may help distinguish between primary hypomyelination and hypomyelination secondary to neuronal dysfunction (Fig. 99-3F, G, and H).

1. Pelizaeus-Merzbacher Disease

Pelizaeus-Merzbacher disease (PMD, OMIM 312080) is the prototypic hypomyelinating disorder and is caused by alterations in the proteolipid 1 (PLP1) gene. Located on Xq22.2, this gene encodes the PLP1 protein, which constitutes roughly half of all myelin protein. The most common abnormality is a duplication of the entire gene, found in 60% to 70% of PMD cases and associated with the classic form of the disease. Missense mutations account for 10% to 15% of cases. Deletions are also seen in a smaller number of cases. Triplications or even higher copy numbers are present in 1% to 2% of cases. More complex chromosomal rearrangements involving PLP1 or its promotor region have been described in individual cases. Deletions or null mutations are rare.

2. Pelizaeus–Merzbacher-Like Disease

Pelizaeus–Merzbacher-like disease (PMLD, OMIM 608804) is phenotypically similar to PMD, although its inheritance is autosomal-recessive instead of X-linked. Children with hypomyelination on MRI but without the PMD phenotype are often mischaracterized as PMLD. The primary clinical features include early nystagmus, ataxia, and spasticity. PMLD is a genetically heterogeneous disease. In most cases, no gene has been identified. In a small subset of clinically identified PMLD patients (fewer than 10%), mutations in GJC2 (also called GJA12), coding for Connexin 46.6 (Cx47), have been found (OMIM 608804), and the term PMLD is now mostly used for patients with GJC2 mutations.

3. 4H Syndrome

This recently described leukoencephalopathy (OMIM 607694, 614381) is also characterized by hypomyelination. Its name is derived from its three main clinical findings: hypomyelination, hypodontia, and hypogonadotropic hypogonadism. About 90% of cases are caused by recessive mutations in either POLR3A or POLR3B, encoding the two largest subunits of RNA polymerase III. 4H syndrome is the second most frequent hypomyelinating white matter disorder after PMD.

4. Hypomyelination Related to Cytoplasmic tRNA Synthetase Defects

Recently two hypomyelinating disorders were described due to mutations in DARS or RARS—coding for the cytoplasmic tRNA synthetases for aspartate (OMIM 615281) and arginine (OMIM 616140), respectively. Clinically, both entities are remarkably similar with onset in infancy in most cases, a fine, rapid nystagmus, early severe spasticity, and ataxia. Again, cognition is much less affected than motor abilities, with normal cognitive abilities in a part of the patients with DARS mutations. Two patients with subacute onset in late adolescence and DARS mutations have been reported, mimicking multiple sclerosis, including presumed response to steroids.

5. Oculodentodigital Dysplasia

Oculodentodigital dysplasia is another hypomyelinating disorder characterized by dental abnormalities (ODDD, OMIM 164200). Its inheritance is autosomal dominant. Dominant mutations in another connexin gene on chromosome 6q21-23.2, GJA1 coding for connexin 43 (Cx43), cause ODDD. There is one family described with autosomal recessive mutations leading to the same phenotype. Cx43 is expressed in the developing brain and teeth, as well as in hands and feet.

6. Hypomyelination With Congenital Cataract

Hypomyelination with congenital cataract (HCC, OMIM 610532) is a recently described disorder with CNS hypomyelination reported in five families. The genetic locus of HCC is FAM126A, earlier called DRCTNNB1A, on chromosome 7p15.3. It encodes the hyccin membrane protein. Missense mutations, mutations affecting splice sites, and a deletion of the entire gene have been identified, but its role in myelination remains obscure.

7. Hypomyelination With Atrophy of the Basal Ganglia and Cerebellum

Hypomyelination with atrophy of the basal ganglia and cerebellum (H-ABC, OMIM 612438) is a rare disorder caused by dominant de novo mutations in the gene coding for one of the beta-tubulins, TUBB4A. MRI shows hypomyelination, cerebellar atrophy, and atrophy or absence (in later stages) of the putamen apparent within the first year of life. The caudate is reduced and disappears entirely in some patients. Over time, white matter loss leads to supratentorial atrophy. These MRI features are considered diagnostic. Recently it became obvious that basal ganglia may be normal in this disorder. TUBB4A is therefore an important gene to consider in the differential diagnosis of hypomyelination.

8. Sialic Acid Storage Disorders

Salla disease (OMIM 604369) and infantile sialic acid storage disease (ISSD, OMIM 269920) are both caused by autosomal recessive mutations in SLC17A5 coding for sialin, a lysosomal membrane protein transporting sialic acid from lysosomes. The gene is located on chromosome 6q14/15.

9. Fucosidosis

Fucosidosis is another lysosomal storage disorder characterized by hypomyelination (OMIM 612280). MRI shows hypomyelination. A characteristic imaging feature of fucosidosis is high T1-signal and low T2-signal in globus pallidus, thalamus, and substantia nigra. Cerebral and cerebellar atrophy may be prominent in older patients.

10. Serine Synthesis Defects

Serine is synthesized by a three-step biochemical pathway, and defects in any of the three enzymes in this pathway have been shown to cause serine biosynthesis defects: 3-phosphoglycerate dehydrogenase (OMIM 601815), phosphoserine phosphatase (OMIM 172480), and phosphoserine aminotransferase (OMIM 610992). The biochemical hallmark of these disorders is low serine and glycine concentration in CSF. Supplementation with serine and glycine is effective in seizure management. If treatment is commenced prenatally, head circumference at birth and development are normal. In untreated children, MRI shows hypomyelination and white matter volume loss.

11. Cockayne Syndrome and Trichothiodystrophy

Cockayne syndrome (CS) is a rare disease combining neurologic and nonneurologic features. This disorder and related disorders of DNA repair such as cerebro-oculo-facial syndrome (COFS) and trichothiodystrophy (TTD) are genetically heterogeneous. The classic form, Cockayne syndrome type I, presents in the first year of life with failure to thrive; weight is more affected than length ("cachectic dwarfism"), and there is loss of subcutaneous fat, leading to a "wizened," bird-like, progeroid face. Microcephaly also develops, usually by the end of the second year. Children develop contractures of the large joints, giving them a typical posture. Hands and feet are disproportionally large. Dental caries are prominent. Psychomotor development is also delayed resulting in mild to severe cognitive disability. In Cockayne syndrome type II, the clinical picture is much more severe with growth failure already evident at birth. Loss or even absence of subcutaneous fat is striking. Joint contractures and kyphosis develop rapidly. Hypotonia is prominent initially, followed by development of spastic tetraparesis. MRI of patients with Cockayne syndrome shows hypomyelination. In severe cases with Cockayne syndrome type II, hypoplasia of cerebellum and brainstem are possible. Basal ganglia calcifications are common. Similar features are seen in trichothiodystrophy, although calcifications are less common than in Cockayne syndrome.

12. 18q Minus Syndrome

In this disorder (OMIM 601808), the distal region of the long arm of chromosome 18 is deleted. It occurs de novo most commonly. The contiguous gene deletion usually involves the bands 18q22.3→qter. The gene for myelin basic protein (MBP), a component of healthy myelin, is located within this region. It has been postulated that haploinsuffiency for MBP leads to the myelin abnormalities observed in 18q minus syndrome. Heterogeneity in severity of clinical symptoms and hypomyelination between patients, despite consistent loss MBP, is a focus of ongoing inquiry.

13. SOX10-Associated Disorders

These rare syndromes are caused by mutations in SOX10 on chromosome 22q13, which encodes a transcription factor for various genes, some such as GJB1 (connexin 32) involved in myelin formation and metabolism. They are characterized by a white hair lock and hypomelanotic spots, sensorineural deafness, and Hirschsprung disease. Patients are affected with varying severity, ranging from antenatal onset with congenital arthrogryposis multiplex and severe neurologic abnormalities to more mildly affected patients, lacking neurologic manifestations (Waardenburg-Shah syndrome, WS4, OMIM 277580). Consistent with a neurocristopathy, many features of this disease can be explained by defective differentiation or migration of neural crest cells. In the severe cases, MRI reveals hypomyelination.

PART II. WHITE MATTER DISORDERS WITH DEMYELINATION

If MRI is not consistent with hypomyelination, if there is white matter hypointensity on T1 instead of isointensity or hyperintensity, and if there is hyperintensity on T2, then the imaging pattern fits the demyelinating leukodystrophies. They comprise the leukodystrophies with primary demyelination, leukodystrophies with white matter vacuolization and intramyelinic edema, calcifying leukoencephalopathies, cystic leukoencephalopathies, leukoencephalopathies with brainstem involvement, and most adult-onset leukoencephalopathies. In assessing patients with these leukodystrophies, careful attention should be paid to specific neuroimaging features, including basal ganglia or brainstem signal abnormalities, contrast enhancement, cysts, calcifications, contrast enhancement, or specific FLAIR imaging abnormalities (Figs 99-3 and 99-5) to assist in the differential diagnosis.

A. Primary Demyelinating Leukodystrophies

These conditions comprise several of the "classic" leukodystrophies and include Alexander disease, X-linked adrenoleukodystrophy, metachromatic leukodystrophy, and Krabbe disease, as well as other less common disorders.

1. Alexander Disease

Alexander disease (AxD, OMIM 203450) is associated with mutations in the gene encoding the glial fibrillary acidic protein (GFAP). GFAP mutations are thought to confer gain of function mutations, and a mutation on a single allele is sufficient to cause disease. In most cases, mutations are sporadic, although familial cases are described in adult or juvenile onset cases.

Type I AxD typically presents before the fourth year of life and with typical MRI features (van der Knaap et al., 2001). In very rare cases, patients present in the neonatal period with macrocephaly and delay in milestones, with both cognitive and motor deficits. Patients may present with seizures. Pyramidal and sometimes extrapyramidal features develop and children often lose motor skills in the first decade of life. Bulbar features such as intractable vomiting, swallowing difficulties, and respiratory compromise can be present early on or only develop over time. Hydrocephalus can become a significant clinical issue. Type II AxD (older than 4 years at onset) typically is associated with atypical MRI abnormalities, often sparing the supratentorial white matter and affecting predominantly the brainstem. These patients present with predominant motor dysfunction, often with progressive gait disturbance or fine motor difficulties and clinically evident spasticity. Bulbar symptoms, in particular palatal myoclonus, can be very suggestive of the diagnosis. Over time, dysphonia and dysphagia can become increasingly debilitating. Dysautonomia is frequent. Sleep apnea is a commonly reported problem.

2. X-Linked Adrenoleukodystrophy

X-linked adrenoleukodystrophy (XALD, OMIM 300100) is associated with mutations in the ABCD1 gene encoding a peroxisomal membrane transporter. This disorder follows X-linked inheritance. Differences in disease manifestations are known to occur with identical genotype and even within a sibship, underscoring the likely effect of other genetic factors on clinical presentation.

XALD is characterized by three predominant phenotypes. The best known is the childhood-onset cerebral form (35%

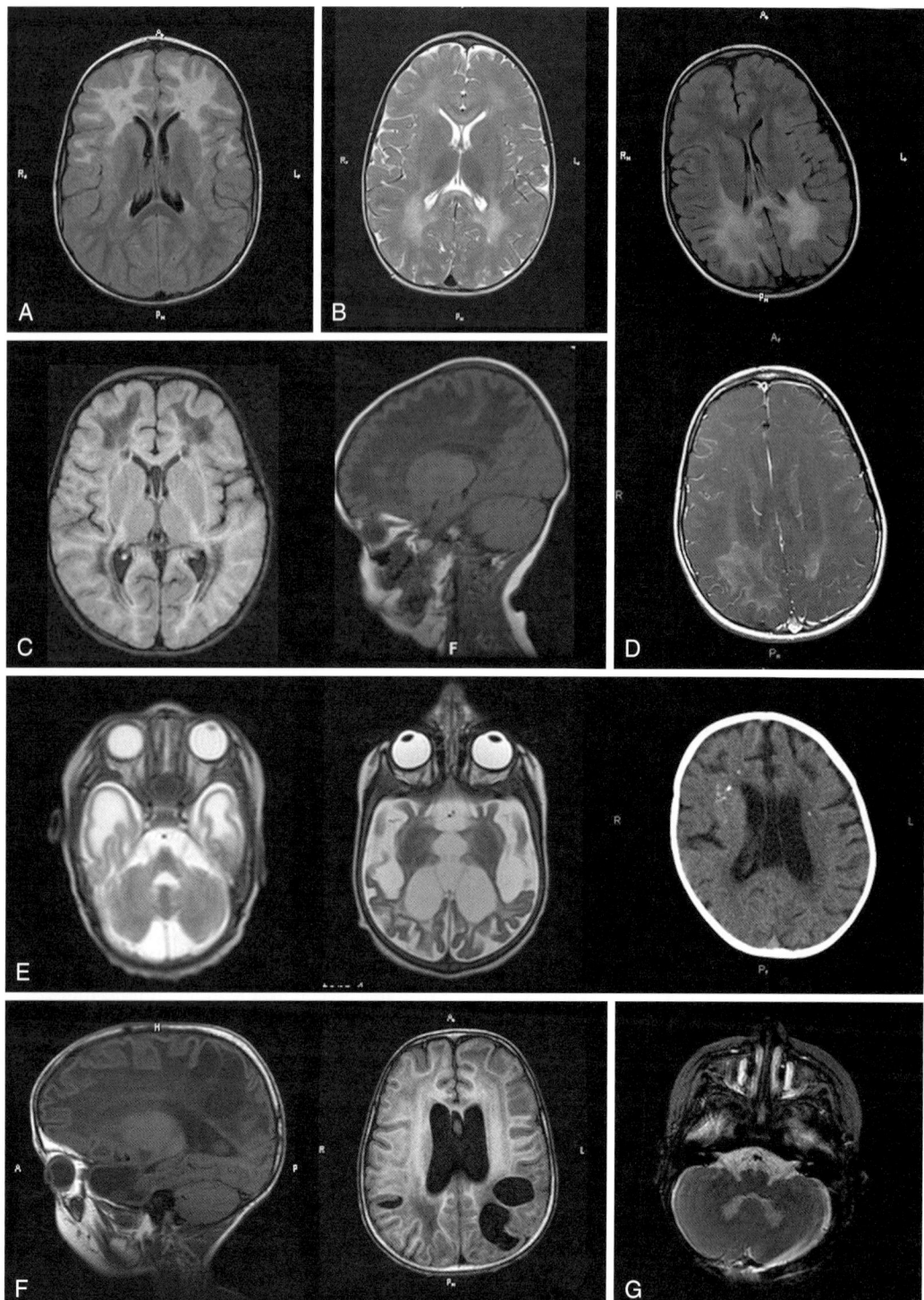

Figure 99-5. Dysmyelinating/Demyelinating leukodystrophies and pathognomonic MRI features, part I. A, MRI of a child with juvenile-onset Alexander disease shows frontal predominance of white matter abnormalities on FLAIR imaging. Other features not demonstrated here include brainstem and basal ganglia abnormalities, contrast enhancement of various intracranial structures, T1 high and T2 low periventricular rim, ventricular garlands, and characteristic capping of the frontal horns of the lateral ventricles. **B,** MRI of a 20-month-old male with metachromatic leukodystrophy shows the butterfly pattern of involvement in the cerebral white matter, sparing the U-fibers. Note the prominent involvement of the corpus callosum. Within the affected white matter the presence of radiating stripes can be seen that are low signal on T2 and high signal on T1. **C,** MRI of a child with eIF2B4 mutations and vanishing white matter, demonstrating (image to the left) rarefaction of affected white matter on FLAIR images, and typical appearance of radiating strips on sagittal T1 images (image to the right). **D,** MRI images of a 10-year-old male with X-linked adrenoleukodystrophy, demonstrating (top image) posterior predominance of white matter involvement and involvement of the corpus callosum on FLAIR images, as well as the pathognomonic contrast enhancement of the border of the demyelinating lesion on post contrast images (lower image). **E,** Neuroimaging from a child with TREX1 mutations resulting in Aicardi-Goutières syndrome. MRI at 2 and 4 months (left and middle images) show the swollen appearance of subcortical white matter, in particular in the temporal lobes, and the rapid atrophy that occurred over a period of weeks. CT imaging of the head shows the sometimes limited calcifications in periventricular white matter, not visualized on standard MR imaging. **F,** MRI of a 3-year-old child with megalencephalic leukoencephalopathy with subcortical cysts. Sagittal T1 weighted images demonstrate subcortical swelling and cystic degeneration of the white matter, in particular in the temporal lobes (image to the left). FLAIR imaging clearly demonstrates cystic degeneration of affected white matter (image to the right). **G,** MRI of a 9-month-old female with Krabbe disease, demonstrating increased signal in the hilus of the dentate. This infant also had thickening of the optic chiasm, and diffuse white matter involvement.

of affected individuals), in which male children of school age (usually 4 to 8 years) present with a prior history of behavioral or cognitive changes. These are often initially misdiagnosed as attention deficit disorder, or hyperactivity. The progressive nature of the symptoms, overlaid with progressive motor difficulties, deteriorating school function and handwriting, altered perception of speech, and worsening behavior problems, usually brings the child to medical attention, and neuroimaging frequently is highly suggestive of the diagnosis. Disease course is variable, but complete symptom development occurs over a range of 6 months to 2 years. Over time, significant motor involvement develops with a spastic quadriplegia. In addition, bulbar dysfunction becomes problematic and often necessitates gastrostomy tube feeding. Adrenal insufficiency is a life-threatening complication of XALD, and studies suggest that a large number of subjects with the childhood-onset cerebral form have adrenal insufficiency at time of diagnosis. Adrenal function should be tested at diagnosis and monitored thereafter to permit symptomatic management.

A second frequent type of presentation is adrenomyeloneuropathy (AMN; 40% to 45% of affected individuals), characterized by onset in young adult males (20s to middle age) of progressive gait abnormalities, sexual dysfunction, and abnormalities of sphincter control. A third type is isolated adrenal insufficiency. On occasion, patients with adrenoleukodystrophy may first present with an Addisonian crisis and no neurologic features or abnormalities on neuroimaging. XALD should be on the differential diagnosis of isolated adrenal insufficiency in a male subject. Female carriers were long thought to be asymptomatic, but recent research demonstrated that the vast majority does develop symptoms and signs by the age of 60 years, especially progressive spastic paraparesis and urinary incontinence.

Diagnosis is based on characteristic clinical presentation and suggestive MRI features. MRI shows a predominance of occipital findings (Fig. 99-5C), although frontal and corpus callosum variants are recognized. The affected white matter appears hyperintense on T2 and hypointense on T1. Characteristically, there is a rim of enhancement around the abnormal tissue that can be very helpful in establishing the diagnosis, as few other leukodystrophies, with the exception of Alexander disease, show significant contrast enhancement. Treatment is possible in early stages of the childhood cerebral form and consists of hematopoietic stem cell transplantation (HSCT). Several children have been successfully treated with gene therapy.

3. Peroxisome Biogenesis Disorders

Peroxisome biogenesis disorders (PBD) are abnormalities of peroxisome biosynthesis caused by mutations in a series of PEX genes (at least 15 in humans) encoding various peroxins. A variety of clinical presentations exist. Rhizomelic chondrodysplasia punctata, characterized by skeletal deformities, facial dysmorphisms, and developmental abnormalities, is associated with hypomyelination or focal white matter signal abnormalities. A second clinical phenotype is characterized by the Zellweger spectrum, in which patients can present at variable ages with facial dysmorphisms, hypotonia, seizures, liver dysfunction, and developmental delay. Neuroimaging can show polymicrogyria and both hypomyelination and demyelination in cerebral and cerebellar white matter (Fig. 99-5F). Single enzyme deficiencies of peroxisomal fatty-acid β-oxidation (acyl-CoA oxidase deficiency (OMIM 264470), D-bifunctional protein deficiency (OMIM 261515), and peroxisomal thiolase deficiency) are clinically and radiologically similar to the peroxisomal biogenesis disorders.

4. Metachromatic Leukodystrophy

Metachromatic leukodystrophy (MLD, OMIM 250100) is caused by recessive mutations in the ARSA gene encoding Arylsulfatase A on chr. 22q13.31 and is inherited in an autosomal recessive manner. It is one of the most prevalent inherited white matter disorders. Homozygous or compound heterozygous ARSA mutations impair arylsulfatase A degradation of sulfatides, causing sulfatide accumulation within the brain and peripheral nervous system. Complete loss of arylsulfatase A activity ("I" or "O" alleles) is typically associated with early infantile MLD. Partial loss of arylsulfatase A activity ("R" or "A" alleles) is typically associated with juvenile or adult-onset MLD. Compound heterozygosity with an I and A allele usually results in juvenile onset MLD.

Additionally, there are common polymorphisms of ARSA (referred to as "PD" alleles), which result in sufficient residual activity to avoid sulfatide accumulation (pseudodeficiency). Enzymatic evidence of low arylsulfatase activity must be accompanied by abnormal urine sulfatides or demonstration of pathogenic ARSA mutations before establishing a diagnosis of MLD.

MLD is characterized by three clinical subtypes, defined primarily by age at presentation. Late-infantile MLD patients usually present by age 30 months, after a period of apparently normal development. Initial clinical manifestations include gait disturbance, ataxia, dysarthria. Initially symptoms may be slowly progressive or plateau, sometimes followed by a rapid loss of motor skills over a few weeks, during which time the diagnosis is commonly made. In the beginning, demyelinating peripheral neuropathy may be prominent, causing misdiagnosis as chronic inflammatory demyelinating polyneuropathy. Tonic spasms with pyramidal and extrapyramidal dysfunction and loss of peripheral reflexes are striking. Eventually, the disease progresses to severe motor impairment with loss of volitional movements, bulbar dysfunction, loss of vision and hearing, and seizures. The time course of deterioration is highly variable, and, with maximal supportive care, death often occurs much later than reported in older texts. The disease, however, is relentlessly progressive after the initial period.

Juvenile MLD patients present between age 30 months and 16 years (12 to 14 years). Patients presenting after this age are classified as having adult-onset MLD. Patients often present with cognitive and behavior difficulties. Younger juvenile-onset patients often show early motor involvement and may also show rapid decline. Clumsiness, gait problems, dysarthria, incontinence, and worsening behavioral problems occur later in the course and often prompt etiologic evaluation and diagnosis. Patients may have seizures, most often complex partial seizures. Progression is similar in juvenile MLD as described in infantile MLD, with a slower course.

Adult-onset MLD patients may present with motor symptoms common to earlier presentation. More commonly, they develop severe neuropsychiatric symptoms, often leading to misdiagnosis until motor features evolve. Patients may initially present with predominant peripheral neuropathy, or with seizures.

MLD diagnosis is often suspected based on clinical manifestations of central motor impairment with a peripheral neuropathy. Typical MRI features include sparing of arcuate fibers and a rim of subcortical white matter with involvement of periventricular and deep white matter in the supratentorial CNS (Fig. 99-5B). Involved white matter takes on the appearance of radiating stripes that can be highly suggestive of the disorder and reflects accumulation of sulfatides in perivascular macrophages. These radiating stripes are also present in other disorders, however, including Krabbe disease.

MLD is the focus of intensive research exploring approaches to restore partial enzymatic activity. HSCT has been performed in patients with MLD, but its success is dependent on the age and stage of disease progression and does not appear to completely halt disease progression. Gene therapy may be an emerging treatment option.

5. Metachromatic Leukodystrophy-Like Variants

In some cases, there is strong clinical suspicion of MLD, including presence of urinary sulfatides, but ARSA sequencing is normal. Two disorders should be considered in this clinical situation: deficiency of arylsulfatase activator protein (Saposin B) (OMIM 249400) and multiple sulfatase deficiency (MSD) (OMIM 272200).

6. Krabbe Disease or Globoid Cell Leukodystrophy

Krabbe disease (OMIM 245200) is caused by autosomal recessive mutations in the gene encoding galactosylceramidase (GALC) on chromosome 14q31(83-87). Two recurring mutations are associated with specific phenotypes. One common 30-kb deletion results in the classic infantile form in the homozygous state or when compound heterozygous with another mutation associated with severe disease. The 809G>A mutation is associated with the late-onset form of Krabbe disease, even when associated with mutations associated with severe disease.

Krabbe disease has two main forms. In the classic infantile form, onset is within the first 6 months, typically after a few months of apparently normal development. Patients present with irritability, hypertonia, and peripheral nerve involvement (stage I). CSF protein is elevated. This stage is followed by rapid deterioration leading to decerebrate posturing and almost opisthotonic positioning of the head and neck (stage II). Optic atrophy develops and pupillary light reflexes are abnormal. Seizures often occur at this stage. This period is often followed by a longer period of slow deterioration in infants in a near vegetative state (stage III). Infants often succumb to respiratory infections in the first years of life, although supportive care has been known to extend life. Late-infantile-onset forms (after 6 months of age) present with symptoms of vision loss, developmental regression, and spasticity. Juvenile (after 4 years of age) and adult-onset cases present with variable symptoms, including gait dysfunction, loss of vision, seizures, or cognitive-behavioral changes. The rapidity of decline appears to correlate with age at onset, with younger patients (late infantile and juvenile) progressing more rapidly than the adult-onset cases.

Diagnosis is suspected based on combined motor and peripheral nerve involvement. Neuroimaging can also guide diagnosis, with CT demonstrating highly suggestive hyperdensity of the thalami, caudate, corona radiata, and, in some cases, cerebellum, and brainstem. MRI is less pathognomonic than in other disorders; however, early involvement of the brainstem and cerebellar white matter, in particular the hilus of the dentate nucleus, can be helpful in establishing the diagnosis (Fig. 99-5G) . If diagnosed early enough, cases with later onset may be treated with HSCT.

7. Saposin A Deficiency

An infant with abnormal myelination resembling Krabbe disease was found to have a mutation in the saposin A region of the prosaposin (PSAP) gene (OMIM 611722). Prosaposin is one of several known sphingolipid activator proteins and interacts with the enzyme GALC to catalyze the hydrolysis of lipids.

8. Sjögren-Larsson Syndrome

Sjögren-Larsson syndrome (OMIM 270200) is an autosomal recessive disorder characterized by ichthyosis, spastic diplegia or tetraplegia, and cognitive disability. The disorder is caused by mutations in the fatty aldehyde dehydrogenase (FALDH) gene, which result in impaired oxidation of long-chain aliphatic aldehydes derived from fatty alcohol metabolism. Neuroimaging reveals white matter disease in most patients with mild periventricular signal abnormalities on T2-weighted images.

B. White Matter Disorders With White Matter Vacuolization and Intramyelinic Edema

Among the specific radiologic features associated with white matter disease, white matter vacuolization is very helpful in the differential diagnosis of leukodystrophies. The disorders most likely to present with white matter vacuolization are Canavan disease and eIF2B-related disorders, also known as vanishing white matter (VWM) and CACH (childhood-onset ataxia and central nervous system hypomyelination), although these disorders are clinically and radiologically distinct. One other disorder, not considered a leukoencephalopathy or leukodystrophy but which may have vacuolization on MRI is Lowe disorder. The oculocerebrorenal syndrome of Lowe (OCRL) is a multisystem disorder with major ocular, cerebral and renal abnormalities. OCRL is an X-linked disorder caused by mutations in OCRL1, encoding a phosphatidylinositol -4,5- bisphosphate 5-phosphatase.

In addition to disorders with white matter vacuolization, a new category of disorders is emerging, related to intramyelogenic edema. These include megalencephalic leukoencephalopathy with subcortical cysts (MLC), which is detailed in the section on cystic leukodystrophies, as well as the mechanistically related ClC-2 chloride channel-related leukoencephalopathy.

1. Canavan Disease

Canavan disease (CD; OMIM 271900) is caused by a deficiency of aspartoacylase, encoded by ASPA. This disorder has been documented since at least the 1950s, but a biochemical marker was not identified until nearly 30 years later. Inheritance is autosomal recessive. Incidence is increased in patients of Ashkenazi Jewish descent, with two common mutations, p.Glu285Ala and p.Tyr231X, responsible for 98% of disease alleles, facilitating carrier screening in this population. In addition, p.Ala305Glu is responsible for 40% to 60% for the disease-causing alleles in non-Jewish populations and is responsible for 1% of disease-causing alleles in the Ashkenazi Jewish population.

Most patients with CD present with the infantile form. These children appear normal until approximately 3 to 6 months of life, when hypotonia with loss of head control, irritability, loss of milestones, and head circumference growth become notable. Over time, spasticity replaces hypotonia, optic atrophy, extrapyramidal movement disorders, seizures, and autonomic disturbances develop. In time, a more chronic vegetative state develops that can evolve over years. Tonic extensor spasms are often described. More rarely, a congenital variant is seen in which poor feeding, irritability, and hypotonia become evident within days after birth, followed by rapid deterioration and death.

Aspartoacylase deficiency results in accumulation of N-acetylaspartic acid (NAA) in the brain, which can be ascertained by proton MR spectroscopy and its excretion in the urine. The synthesis and role of NAA, and the related compound N-acetylaspartylglutamate (NAAG) within the brain remains poorly understood and the subject of active research.

2. eIF2B-Related Disorder (Vanishing White Matter)

The eIF2B-related disorder and its various allelic clinical subtypes (VWM, OMIM 603896 or CACH [Schiffmann et al., 1994], ovarioleukodystrophy, and Cree leukoencephalopathy) are caused by mutations in one of the five genes (EIF2B1-5) encoding a complex, eIF2B (Leegwater et al., 2001). The eIF2B disorder, or eukaryotic translation initiation protein 2B, is the guanine nucleotide exchange factor for eIF2, another critical protein in initiation of translation. The eIF2B-related disorders are inherited in an autosomal recessive manner, with 65% of mutations found on the gene EIF2B5. There is known genotype-phenotype correlation for certain more common genotypes, including homozygous R113H mutation positive subjects, who have an adult onset with milder phenotype, and the homozygous R195H mutation positive subjects, who have a more severe early-onset presentation.

Patients with eIF2B mutations may present with a variety of clinical syndromes. The best-known presentation is the infantile or early childhood presentation with VWM. These children, previously healthy, present with acute neurologic decompensation after events of physiologic stress, including fever, falls, or fright. The precipitating event is usually followed after several hours by acute motor dysfunction, typically hypotonia or ataxia, and even coma. The child may die during the acute event or survive with neurologic sequelae and be vulnerable to future events of decompensation. On occasion, no acute event is noted, but loss of skills is gradual and relentlessly progressive. At opposite ends of the phenotypic spectrum, eIF2B mutations can also present in a connatal form, where neurologic disability is evident from birth (with additional findings such as ovarian dysgenesis, cataract or hepatomegaly) or present in an adult form with progressive spastic paraparesis.

Diagnosis of eIF2B-related disorder is based on appropriate clinical history, neuroimaging and molecular genetics. Common MRI features include diffuse signal abnormality of the supratentorial white matter, with less constant signal abnormalities in the cerebellar white matter, brainstem, thalamus, and globus pallidus. In supratentorial white matter, FLAIR images show low signal intensity, isointense with CSF, and suggestive of white matter rarefaction and cystic degeneration. On sagittal T1-weighted images, a pattern of radiating tissue strands may be seen, compatible on pathology with preserved tissue (Fig. 99-5C). MRI findings of eIF2B-related disorder are nearly pathognomonic, except in very early-onset or late-onset cases.

3. Megalencephalic Leukoencephalopathy With Subcortical Cysts

Megalencephalic leukoencephalopathy with subcortical cysts (MLC, OMIM 604004) is an autosomal recessive disease associated with mutations in the gene encoding MLC1 protein, HEPACAM, encoding GlialCAM. These proteins contribute to water homeostasis in myelin sheath (van der Knaap et al., 2012).

Synonyms for MLC include leukoencephalopathy with swelling and discrepantly mild course, cysts, infantile leukoencephalopathy and megalencephaly, van der Knaap disease, and vacuolating leukoencephalopathy. There is a founder effect in the Agarwal community in India, with a common genotype in MLC1 (p.Cys46LeufsX34), as well as some more common mutations in individual populations, including

persons of Libyan and Turkish Jewish descent and Japanese descent.

Postnatal macrocephaly is the predominant presenting symptom, developing in the first year. This is of diagnostic importance because a number of other disorders can present with temporal lobe subcortical cysts, including AGS, CMV infection, and RNAseT2-deficient leukoencephalopathy, among others. Stabilization of head growth rate often occurs after age 1, up to four to six standard deviations higher than normal. Patients may have normal early development or mild delays in motor and cognitive milestones. Later in life, patients develop a spastic ataxia of variable severity. Epilepsy, often easily controlled, is common. Cognitive deterioration is usually late and mild. Dysarthric speech can be particularly debilitating in MLC. In the dominant forms of HEPACAM mutations, there is a discrepantly mild course, with improvement over time of both the clinical and radiologic manifestations.

4. ClC-2-Related Leukoencephalopathy

ClC-2 chloride channel deficiency results in a leukoencephalopathy (OMIM 615651) associated with cerebellar ataxia, spasticity, chorioretinopathy with visual field defects, optic neuropathy, cognitive defects, and headaches. Patients may present in childhood or adolescence/adulthood. This disorder is characterized by T2-weighted MRI signal abnormalities in the posterior limbs of the internal capsules, midbrain cerebral peduncles, and middle cerebellar peduncles. MRI also shows restricted diffusion, suggesting myelin vacuolation confined to the specified white matter structures in adult patients, and more diffusely involved the brain white matter in children (Depienne et al., 2013).

C. Calcifying Leukoencephalopathies

A series of leukoencephalopathies is distinguished by calcifications on neuroimaging. Although not all of these disorders qualify as classic leukodystrophies, significant white matter abnormalities on MRI may cause confusion unless the calcifications are recognized. Although in some cases the calcifications are large and unlikely to be missed on standard MR images, in other cases the white matter abnormalities may precede or so overshadow visible calcifications that these patients are initially thought to have an unsolved leukodystrophy. Therefore imaging modalities that will detect calcium, CT or MR based, should be considered in patients with unsolved leukoencephalopathies and should be performed serially for patients without specific diagnoses whose status continues to deteriorate. Several heritable disorders that might be confused with leukodystrophies are described here, although a comprehensive list of calcifying brain disorders exceeds the scope of this chapter and includes multiple infectious, immune, and vascular disorders such as congenital CMV, toxoplasmosis or rubella infections, HIV, systemic lupus erythematosus, and radiotherapy or methotrexate leukoencephalopathy. In addition to the classically calcifying leukoencephalopathies, certain leukoencephalopathies mentioned in other sections that may also develop calcifications include Krabbe, Alexander disease, RNase T2-deficient leukoencephalopathy, and mitochondrial cytopathies.

1. Aicardi-Goutières Syndrome

Aicardi Goutières syndrome (AGS; OMIM number[s] 225750 [AGS1], 610181 [AGS2], 610329 [AGS3], and 610333 [AGS4]) is a genetically heterogeneous disorder associated with mutations in a series of genes encoding nucleases or putative nucleases, or resulting in interferon activation. These include TREX1, SAMHD1, RNAseH2 A, B, and C, ADAR1, and IFIH1.

In most cases, AGS appears to be autosomal recessive, although rare cases of heterozygotes with AGS phenotypes are reported. The disorder presents in a fairly homogenous fashion, with a subacute encephalopathy associated with dystonia, spasticity, progressive microcephaly, leukoencephalopathy, and intracranial calcifications. Additionally, rare patients with clinical diagnoses of systemic lupus erythematous have been found to harbor heterozygous mutations in TREX1. In addition, a disorder now referred to as autosomal dominant retinal vasculopathy with cerebral leukodystrophy (RVCL) is allelic with AGS. This disorder has previously been described as cerebroretinal vasculopathy (CRV)/hereditary retinal vasculopathy (HRV)/hereditary endotheliopathy with retinopathy, nephropathy, and stroke (HERNS), associated with linkage to 3p21, and with heterozygous mutations in TREX1. RVCL is a rare disorder with retinal vasculopathy, migraine, Raynaud phenomenon, stroke, and dementia with onset in middle age. Allelic disorders with AGS with an autosomal recessive inheritance include familial chilblain lupus, Cree leukoencephalitis, and TORCH-like disorders.

AGS is characterized by leukoencephalopathy, basal ganglia or white matter calcifications, and elevated CSF alpha interferon, with no detectable infectious etiology. Patients present most often in the neonatal period or in infancy. Early-onset patients may present in the neonatal period with a syndrome that mimics in utero viral infections, including Coombs positive hemolytic anemia and autoimmune thrombocytopenia, elevated transaminases, microcephaly, seizures, vasculitic skin lesions, and cerebral calcifications. This condition may also present in older infants with progressive microcephaly, dystonia, seizures, and developmental delay, as well as sterile pyrexias, lupus-like skin and joint manifestations, progressive intracranial calcifications, chronically elevated CSF lymphocytes, autoantibodies, and elevated CSF pterins. Less common presentations include peripheral neuropathy, striatal necrosis, intracranial large vessel vasculopathy, and spastic paraplegia (Crow et al., 2015).

2. Cerebroretinal Microangiopathy With Calcifications and Cysts

Cerebroretinal microangiopathy with calcifications and cysts (CRMCC, OMIM 612199) is caused by mutations in CTC1, which encodes the CTS telomere maintenance complex component 1. CRMCC is a spectrum of affected patients with presumed microvascular disorders affecting the brain, eyes, liver, intestines, and bones. Prenatal and postnatal growth retardation is common. The patient may develop visual symptoms leading to an ophthalmologic examination before or after the onset of neurologic symptoms. Ophthalmologic evaluation identifies bilateral retinal telangiectasias and retinal exudates. Patients may develop spontaneous fractures of the long bones or skull and have documented osteopenia. Life-threatening intestinal bleeding may occur, and many patients are found to have cirrhosis or portal hypertension. Less often, patients may have dystrophic nails, hyperpigmented skin lesions, and sparse hair with premature graying. Neuroimaging suggests the diagnosis.

3. Leukoencephalopathy With Calcifications and Cysts

Leukoencephalopathy with calcifications and cysts (LCC) is thought to be on a continuum with CRMCC and Coats plus syndrome. An underlying genetic etiology has not been identified, although reports of affected siblings, male and female probands, and children born to consanguineous families suggest an autosomal recessive inheritance pattern. LCC is similar in MRI pattern to CRMCC but the disorder lacks the systemic manifestions of CRMCC and Coats plus.

4. Bandlike Intracranial Calcification With Simplified Gyration and Polymicrogyria

Bandlike intracranial calcification with simplified gyration and polymicrogyria has been found to be caused by mutations in the OCLN gene, encoding occludin, an integral component of tight junctions. Neuropathologic analysis demonstrates calcification predominantly associated with blood vessels. Two series of patients have been characterized by severe postnatal microcephaly, dysmorphic facial features, developmental arrest, and seizures. Neuroimaging demonstrates simplified sulcation, and a large calcified band most often in the frontal white matter and basal ganglia, as well as large central brainstem calcifications.

5. Cockayne Syndrome

Cockayne slyndrome, as discussed previously, is a disorder characterized by cachectic dwarfism, neurologic disability, cutaneous photosensitivity, pigmentary retinopathy, leukodystrophy, and, occasionally, intracranial calcifications. Disorders allelic with Cockayne, including COFS and TTD, are less likely to have significant intracranial calcifications, although these have been described in a restricted number of cases.

6. Spondyloenchondrodysplasia

Spondyloenchondrodysplasia (SPENCD, OMIM 271550) is a disorder with generalized enchondromatosis and platyspondyly that may also develop progressive intracranial calcifications. Its molecular cause is not known, and its inheritance pattern is unclear. The bone abnormalities in these subjects should suggest this diagnosis when cerebral calcifications are present.

7. Cytomegalovirus

Although a number of prenatal and perinatal infections can result in significant brain disorders, cytomegalovirus (CMV) deserves a special mention in this chapter because of its significant white matter injury, leading to frequent concerns of an underlying inherited leukoencephalopathy. In addition, CMV frequently, but not always, results in intracranial calcification. This phenomenon is discussed in the section on cystic leukoencephalopathies. Other infections can cause significant white matter changes and intracranial calcification, including HIV, tuberculosis, and toxoplasmosis, but clinical features should indicate that these are unlikely to be consistent with an inherited leukoencephalopathy.

8. Cerebral Autosomal Dominant Arteriopathy With Subcortical Infarcts and Leukoencephalopathy

Cerebral autosomal dominant arteriopathy with subcortical infarcts and leukoencephalopathy (CADASIL, OMIM 125310) is a primarily cerebral microangiopathy, presenting in adults with a history of migraine headaches, progressive early-onset cerebrovascular disease, and early-onset dementia, with leukoencephalopathy and subcortical infarcts on neuroimaging. Over 90% of individuals have dominant mutations in NOTCH3.

9. Intracranial Calcification Associated With Leukoencephalopathy

Intracranial calcification associated with leukoencephalopathy is also seen in mitochondrial disease, sporadically reported for various disorders, including MELAS.

10. Dihydropterine Reductase Deficiency

Dihydropterine reductase deficiency can be associated with leukoencephalopathy and calcifications.

11. 27-Hydroxylase Deficiency or CTX

CTX or 27-hydroxylase deficiency (OMIM 213700) is an inherited disorder of sterol storage, with accumulation of cholestanol and cholesterol in xanthomas, gall bladder, and brain. Affected patients have encephalopathy, myelopathy, cerebellar ataxia, early atherosclerosis, tendon xanthomas, and cataracts. Diagnosis is based on clinical manifestations and elevations in cholestanol in the serum. Neuroimaging is remarkable for deep white matter changes, and hyperintense lesions seen on T2-weighted images in the dentate nucleus, globus pallidus, substantia nigra, and inferior olive. Affected white matter may become calcified. Patients may be treated successfully using chenodeoxycholic acid.

12. Bilateral Occipital Calcifications With Leukoencephalopathy, Seizures, and Clinical or Subclinical Celiac Disease

This has also been reported as a distinct entity.

13. Familial Hemophagocytic Lymphohistiocytosis

Familial hemophagocytic lymphohistiocytosis (FHLH) is characterized by proliferation and infiltration of hyperactivated macrophages and T-lymphocytes. It can be caused by autosomal recessive mutations in a number of genes, including *PRF1* (FHL2, OMIM 603553), UNC13D (FHL3, OMIM 608898), STX11 (FHL4, OMIM 603552), and Munc-18-2 (FHL5, OMIM 613101), although a number of patients have no identified mutation. FHLH is characterized by acute illness with prolonged fever (longer than 7 days), and features associated with macrophage activating syndrome, including hepatosplenomegaly, cytopenias (anemia, thrombocytopenia, and neutropenia), hypertriglyceridemia and/or hypofibrinogenemia, and bone marrow hemophagocytosis. Neurologic symptoms are highly variable and may include motor deficits and seizures. Onset is usually within the first few months of life. MRI may show hypomyelination or demyelination and also multifocal abnormalities at the gray white matter junction, hemorrhage, atrophy, focal necrosis, and edema. Calcifications can be seen in areas of abnormal brain tissue. Allogeneic HSCT is the only curative therapy.

D. Cystic Leukoencephalopathies

In addition to demyelination, several leukodystrophies and leukoencephalopathies present with cystic lesions. Megalencephalic leukoencephalopathy with subcortical cysts (MLC), caused by mutations in MLC1, is one of several other disorders characterized by cystic changes in abnormal white matter exist. Others include RNAse T2 deficiency, congenital CMV infection, and cerebroretinal microangiopathy with calcifications and cysts, also known as Coats plus syndrome. Cystic changes can less commonly be seen in an array of other leukodystrophies, including Aicardi-Goutières syndrome and Alexander disease. Other disorders beyond the classically defined leukodystrophies include mitochondrial leukoencephalopathies, which can present with cystic leukoencephalopathies in a number of molecularly defined mitochondrial disorders, or COL4A1/2 associated disorder. Mutations in the gene encoding type IV collagen α-chain 1 or 2, COL4A1 and COL4A2, are thought to disrupt the vascular basement membrane. In patients with a history of familial intracranial hemorrhage and stroke, as well as familial intraventricular hemorrhage and porencephalic cysts in neonates, this disorder should be considered as a possible cause of cystic leukoencephalopathy (Gould et al., 2005).

E. Leukoencephalopathies With Brainstem, Cerebellum, and Spinal Cord Involvement

Certain leukoencephalopathopathies present with significant brainstem, cerebellum, and spinal cord involvement. This MRI feature should always be carefully noted and is often useful in differential diagnosis. In addition to the disorders discussed in detail later in this chapter, other disorders, including Alexander disease, peroxisomal disorders, mitochondrial cytopathies, Krabbe, cerebrotendinous xanthomatosis, and familial histiocytosis, may have brainstem or cerebellar involvement. In addition, X-linked Charcot-Marie-Tooth, fragile-X premutation, and dentatorubral-pallidoluysian atrophy (DRPLA), although not considered leukoencephalopathies, may have significant brainstem and cerebellar involvement, occasionally mischaracterized as primary leukoencephalopathies.

1. Leukoencephalopathy With Brainstem and Spinal Cord Involvement and Lactate Elevation

Leukoencephalopathy with brainstem and spinal cord involvement and lactate elevation (LBSL, OMIM 611105) is caused by autosomal recessive mutations in DARS2, encoding mitochondrial aspartyl-tRNA synthetase. Patients, with single exceptions, are compound heterozygous for pathogenic mutations, one of which usually affects splicing in intron 2.

LBSL is characterized by slowly progressive cerebellar and sensory ataxia, spasticity and dorsal column dysfunction. Onset ranges from infancy to adulthood, with childhood onset as most typical variant. Severe infantile presentation is rare. In some patients, gait is never normal, but most patients have initial normal milestones. The predominant presenting feature is spastic ataxia accompanied by distal abnormalities in vibration and proprioceptive sensation. Loss of motor function is slowly progressive and may result in loss of independent ambulation in adulthood. There may be mild cognitive difficulties. A few patients have a paroxysmal and partially reversible neurologic decline associated with physiologic stressors, including febrile infection or minor head trauma (van der Knaap and Valk, 2005).

Classic MRI features include patchy cortical and cerebellar white matter abnormalities with striking tract involvement over the entire length of the central nervous system, including the spinal cord. Initial reports note involvement of the pyramidal tracts from the internal capsule to the spinal cord corticospinal tracts; the sensory tracts including the dorsal column, medial lemniscus, thalamus, and corona radiata; cerebellar peduncles; and the trigeminal nerve and mesenchymal trigeminal tracts. The corpus callosum is involved. Elevated lactate in affected white matter on MRS is often seen, but not always.

2. Alexander Disease (AxD)

As described previously, AxD patients may have significant and sometimes isolated brainstem signal abnormalities, particularly in late-onset cases, in which clinical and radiologic features are primarily related to brainstem structures. Of note, posterior fossa abnormalities are sometimes misdiagnosed as gliomas, only correctly identified by histopathologic evidence of excessive Rosenthal fiber aggregation.

3. Polyglucosan Body Disease (PGBD, OMIM 263570)

PGBD is an adult-onset leukoencephalopathy with upper and lower neuron motor impairment, distal sensory neuropathy, and neurogenic bladder, characterized by polyglucosan body accumulation in nervous structures. GBE1, encoding 1,4-alpha-glucan-branching enzyme, is the only gene known to be associated with APBD.

4. Autosomal Dominant Leukodystrophy With Autonomic Disease (LaminB1)

Autosomal dominant leukodystrophy with autonomic disease (ADLD, OMIM 169500) is an adult-onset leukoencephalopathy caused by duplications in LMNB1, encoding lamin B1. The first neurologic sign is often autonomic dysfunction such as urgency in urination, impotence, constipation, anhidrosis, and postural hypotension. Disease onset is typically in the fourth to sixth decade. These symptoms are followed by pyramidal tract dysfunction and ataxia with slow progression, sometimes over decades. No peripheral neuropathy is reported. Mild cognitive decline may be seen. Notable radiologic features include confluent white matter changes in supratentorial regions, predominantly affecting the deep white matter, with relative sparing of the periventricular white matter and the subcortical fibers. In some cases, predominance in the rolandic regions and pyramidal tracts is seen at onset, evolving over time into diffuse white matter abnormalities. The corpus callosum is relatively spared but can show posterior abnormalities. The posterior limb of the internal capsule is often involved. Abnormal signal is seen in brainstem tracts, and the upper and middle cerebellar peduncles are often involved.

F. Adult-Onset Leukoencephalopathies

A number of leukoencephalopathies that may present in adults have already been discussed previously, including ADLD, PGBD, CTX, adult-onset Krabbe, adult-onset MLD, adult-onset AxD, adult-onset eIF2B-related disorder, ovarioleukodystrophy, and adrenomyeloneuropathy, as well as theoretically almost any of the childhood-onset leukoencephalopathies. Several inborn errors of metabolism can also present in adulthood with leukoencephalopathy, such as Sjögren-Larson disease, Fabry disease, disorders of transsulfuration such as cobalamin disorders, and PKU, to name a few. Additionally, many adult-onset leukoencephalopathies remain unsolved, and the study of these patients is likely to produce new nosologic entities. Neuroaxonal leukodystrophy with spheroids is an important leukoencephalopathy with primarily adult presentation. Leukoencephalopathy due to mutations in AARS2 has recently been identified with nonspecific, mild developmental delay in some patients and rapid deterioration in adolescence or adulthood with cerebellar ataxia, spasticity, and prominent cognitive decline. MRI shows involvement of left-right connections also affecting the corpus callosum and also longitudinal tracts.

PART III. SECONDARY LEUKOENCEPHALOPATHIES TO INBORN ERRORS OF METABOLISM, EXCLUDING THE CLASSICAL LYSOSOMAL AND PEROXISOMAL DISORDERS

Inborn errors of metabolism result in significant disturbances of cellular function, and the resultant disruption in energy metabolism or accumulation of toxic metabolites interferes with a normal function of a number of organs. The brain, specifically glial cells, is sensitive to such disturbances and, as such, secondary abnormalities of cerebral white matter can be seen in a broad range of inborn errors of metabolism. In some cases, such as metachromatic leukodystrophies and Krabbe disease, the phenotype nearly exclusively affects the white matter of the brain, and these disorders have long been classified as leukodystrophies. In a number of other disorders, however, multisystem abnormalities are seen, and white matter involvement is one of many disease symptoms (Table 99-3). In the majority of cases, straightforward biochemical testing will exclude these disorders, and comprehensive testing should be considered in unsolved leukodystrophies because many of these disorders show nonspecific white matter abnormalities (Table 99-2).

Acknowledgments

Special thanks is given to the patients who provided images for this review and to Marjo van der Knaap and Raphael Schiffmann who have provided mentorship and education to the authors. We also thank Marjo van der Knaap for providing some of the MRIs used in this chapter.

REFERENCES

The complete list of references for this chapter is available in the e-book at www.expertconsult.com.
See inside cover for registration details.

SELECTED REFERENCES

Crow, Y.J., Chase, D.S., Lowenstein Schmidt, J., et al., 2015. Characterization of human disease phenotypes associated with mutations in TREX1, RNASEH2A, RNASEH2B, RNASEH2C, SAMHD1, ADAR, and IFIH1. Am. J. Med. Genet. A 167A (2), 296–312.

Depienne, C., Bugiani, M., Dupuits, C., et al., 2013. Brain white matter oedema due to ClC-2 chloride channel deficiency: an observational analytical study. Lancet Neurol. 12 (7), 659–668.

Gould, D.B., Phalan, F.C., Breedveld, G.J., et al., 2005. Mutations in Col4a1 cause perinatal cerebral hemorrhage and porencephaly. Science 308 (5725), 1167–1171.

Leegwater, P.A., Vermeulen, G., Konst, A.A., et al., 2001. Subunits of the translation initiation factor eIF2B are mutant in leukoencephalopathy with vanishing white matter. Nat. Genet. 29 (4), 383–388.

Pouwels, P.J., Vanderver, A., Bernard, G., et al., 2014. Hypomyelinating leukodystrophies: translational research progress and prospects. Ann. Neurol. 76 (1), 5–19.

Schiffmann, R., Moller, J.R., Trapp, B.D., et al., 1994. Childhood ataxia with diffuse central nervous system hypomyelination. Ann. Neurol. 35 (3), 331–340.

Schiffmann, R., van der Knaap, M.S., 2009. Invited article: an MRI-based approach to the diagnosis of white matter disorders. Neurology 72 (8), 750–759.

van der Knaap, M.S., Boor, I., Estevez, R., 2012. Megalencephalic leukoencephalopathy with subcortical cysts: chronic white matter oedema due to a defect in brain ion and water homoeostasis. Lancet Neurol. 11 (11), 973–985.

van der Knaap, M.S., Naidu, S., Breiter, S.N., et al., 2001. Alexander disease: diagnosis with MR imaging. AJNR Am. J. Neuroradiol. 22 (3), 541–552.

van der Knaap, M.S., Valk, J., 2005. Magnetic Resonance of Myelination and Myelin Disorders, third ed. Springer, Berlin.

E-BOOK FIGURES AND TABLES

The following figures and tables are available in the e-book at www.expertconsult.com. See inside cover for registration details.

Fig. 99-2 Sequential MRIs.
Fig. 99-4 Dental phenotype of children with 4H syndrome.
Fig. 99-6 Dysmyelinating/Demyelinating leukodystrophies and pathognomonic MRI features, part II.
Table 99-1 Molecular causes of leukodystrophies
Table 99-2 Metabolic blood, urine, and cerebrospinal fluid testing to consider in the evaluation of a patient with leukoencephalopathy of unknown cause
Table 99-3 Disorders Characterized as Genetic Leukoencephalopathies

100 Acquired Disorders Affecting the White Matter

Naila Makhani, J. Nicholas Brenton, and Brenda Banwell

An expanded version of this chapter is available on www.expertconsult.com. See inside cover for registration details.

Demyelination of the central nervous system (CNS) may occur as a monophasic illness or may represent the first attack of chronic inflammatory diseases such as multiple sclerosis (MS) and neuromyelitis optica (NMO). Herein, we review the clinical and neuroimaging features of childhood acquired CNS demyelinating disorders.

ACUTE CENTRAL NERVOUS SYSTEM DEMYELINATION

Children with an acquired demyelinating syndrome (ADS) may present either with neurologic signs and symptoms attributable to a single CNS location (monofocal ADS) or with signs attributable to multiple CNS sites (polyfocal ADS), with or without encephalopathy (Krupp et al., 2013).

OPTIC NEURITIS

Optic neuritis (ON) should be considered in any child presenting with acute or subacute visual loss (Fig. 100-1). Demyelinating ON is typically clinically characterized by reduced visual acuity, a central visual field deficit, pain with eye movements, and red color desaturation. Optic disc edema is sometimes seen, but may be absent in retrobulbar ON.

Although some studies suggest that childhood ON is more commonly bilateral, others have reported that ON is more commonly unilateral. In one study of 36 children with ON, neuroimaging studies of the optic nerve were abnormal in 55%, and 88% had abnormal visual-evoked potentials (typically a P100 latency delay).

Optical coherence tomography (OCT) utilizes near-infrared light to measure the thickness of the retinal nerve fiber layer (RNFL) and ganglion cell layer (GCL), yielding a quantitative measure of axonal and neuronal loss. RNFL and GCL thinning have been demonstrated in children with isolated ON and MS and may provide quantifiable information about retinal integrity.

Following ON, 80% to 85% of children achieve full visual recovery. Children with ON have a 30% risk of a subsequent MS diagnosis. Magnetic resonance imaging (MRI) evidence of one or more T2-weighted lesions apart from the optic nerve is strongly predictive of MS, with up to 68% of such patients being diagnosed with MS within 2 years. Concurrent or rapidly sequential transverse myelitis, MRI features of brainstem or diencephalic involvement in a pattern atypical for MS, and serum antibodies against aquaporin-4 suggest a diagnosis of NMO.

Transverse Myelitis

Demyelination of the spinal cord is termed transverse myelitis (TM). Typical features of TM include subacute bilateral lower extremity weakness, a spinal sensory level, and impaired bowel/bladder control. L'Hermitte's symptom (pain with forward neck flexion) suggests a cervical cord lesion. Paresis is often initially flaccid with hyporeflexia, and later hyperreflexia develops below the lesion level. These features help distinguish TM from other spinal cord pathologies (Fig. 100-2).

A review of 47 pediatric TM patients reported that, at the time of maximal deficit, 89% either were unable to walk and/or required ventilator assistance. After 3 years, 43% were unable to ambulate more than 30 feet, and 21% required an ambulatory aid; in addition, 68% had residual bladder symptoms. Younger age at TM, complete paraplegia, sphincter dysfunction, and less than 24 hours to maximal deficit are associated with poorer functional outcomes. MS risk following TM is 2% to 8%. Less than 24 hours to symptom nadir and abnormal baseline brain MRI were strong predictors of relapse in one study.

Longitudinally extensive TM (LETM) (≥ 3 spinal segments), recurrent TM, and TM with ON should prompt consideration of NMO.

Polyfocal Demyelination

Neurologic symptoms suggesting multiple CNS areas of involvement may occur +/–encephalopathy (Fig. 100-3). When encephalopathy (behavioral change or alteration in level of consciousness) is present, the clinical syndrome is acute disseminated encephalomyelitis (ADEM). ADEM occurs in younger patients (especially < 10 years). Fever and a recent history of infection are often present.

ADEM generally carries a favorable prognosis, but 11% to 17% of children experience residual motor deficits. Cognitive deficits may also persist.

ADEM is typically monophasic. However, approximately 5% to 29% of children will go on to have additional demyelinating attacks characteristic of MS. Rarely, ADEM represents the first attack of NMO. ADEM may also precede or follow a diagnosis of anti-NMDA receptor encephalitis.

Other Clinical Presentations

Children with ADS may also present with intranuclear ophthalmoplegia (INO), focal motor deficits, sensory loss/paresthesias, or isolated cerebellar deficits.

Investigation of a Child with Acute Demyelination

Laboratory Investigations

Cerebrospinal fluid (CSF) analysis is important for excluding other diseases, including infection and malignancy. CSF leukocyte counts in children with MS are elevated (>4 cells/µL) in 66% (typically < 30 cells/µL). Higher leukocyte counts are more consistent with infection, vasculitis, or NMO. A study of 107 children with MS reported that those younger than 11 years of age had a higher percentage of CSF neutrophils and

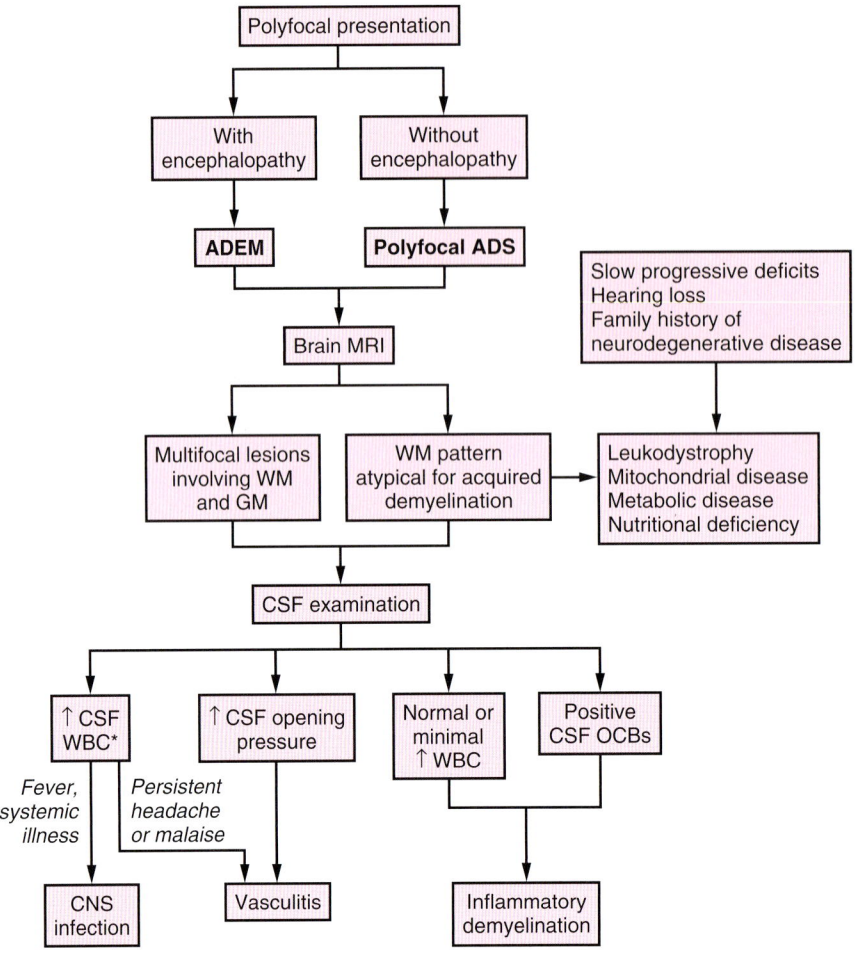

Figure 100-3. Approach to polyfocal neurologic symptoms. ADEM, acute disseminated encephalomyelitis; ADS, acquired demyelinating syndrome; CNS, central nervous system; CSF, cerebrospinal fluid; GM, gray matter; MRI, magnetic resonance imaging; OCBs, oligoclonal bands; WBC, white blood cell count; WM, white matter.

a lower percentage of monocytes and were less likely to have an elevated IgG index than children older than 11 years of age. Elevated protein (typically 100–720 mg/L) may be seen, indicating disruption of the blood–CSF barrier. CSF oligoclonal bands (OCBs) are detected at diagnosis of ADS in up to 90% of children subsequently diagnosed with MS, which is lower than the reported rate of 98% in adult MS. Isoelectric focusing methods have the highest yield for OCB detection. CSF OCBs are detected in less than 10% of children with either ADEM or NMO. CSF immunoglobulin G synthesis can occur later in the disease course, and OCBs may therefore only be detected over time.

Evoked potential testing in the visual-evoked potential, brainstem auditory-evoked potential, and somatosensory-evoked potential pathways is useful for confirming the presence of demyelination and for detecting clinically silent disease. In one study, almost 50% of 85 children with MS demonstrated clinically silent abnormalities in at least one of the evoked potential pathways, most commonly the visual pathway.

Magnetic Resonance Imaging

MRI is a valuable tool to illustrate inflammatory demyelination and to exclude other diagnoses. The MRI appearance of MS in children younger than 10 years of age is similar to that of adults (Figure 100-4). MS lesions are typically ovoid and

are often seen in the periventricular or juxtacortical region, brainstem, and/or spinal cord. Periventricular lesions are often oriented 90 degrees perpendicular to the long axis of the corpus callosum. Infratentorial lesions and large, ill-defined lesions are more common in children than in adults. The presence of one periventricular lesion and one "black hole" (a T1 iso- or hypo-intense lesion relative to cortical gray matter) on imaging obtained at ADS identifies children with MS with 84% sensitivity and 93% specificity.

Large lesions, ill-defined lesions, and lesions in gray and white matter commonly occur in younger children, especially those with ADEM. Lesions located predominantly in the diencephalon or periaqueductal gray matter, longitudinally extensive spinal cord lesions, and bilateral or extensive optic nerve lesions characterize NMO.

Management of Acute Demyelination

Acute demyelination is generally treated with corticosteroids if symptoms are severe enough to interfere with daily functioning (Fig. 100-5). Typically 20 to 30 mg/kg/day of intravenous methylprednisolone (maximum 1 g) is given as a single daily dose for 3 to 5 days. If there is a significant improvement in symptoms, no further treatment is required. If there is an incomplete response to treatment but residual symptoms are relatively mild, a tapering course of oral steroids (starting at

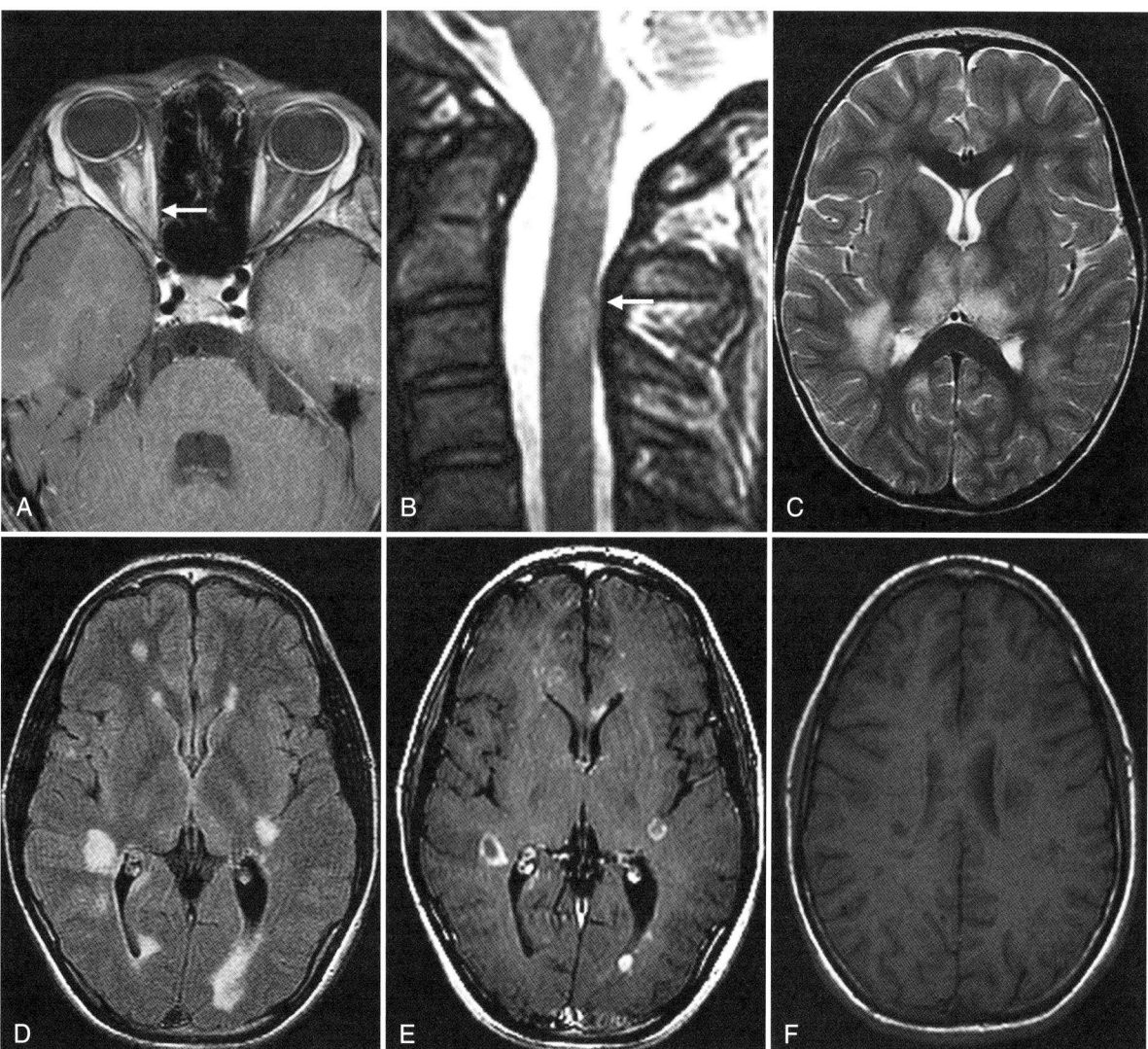

Figure 100-4. MRI in childhood ADS and MS. A, Axial T1-weighted image with gadolinium of a child with optic neuritis shows optic nerve thickening and enhancement *(arrow).* **B,** T2-weighted hyperintense spinal lesion *(arrow)* in a child with transverse myelitis. **C,** Axial fluid-attenuated inversion-recovery (FLAIR) image demonstrates diffuse bilateral deep gray- and white-matter lesions in a child with acute disseminated encephalomyelitis. **D,** Axial FLAIR image demonstrates multiple lesions in a child with multiple sclerosis. **E,** Several of the lesions observed in panel D enhance following gadolinium administration. **F,** Multiple nonenhancing T1 "black holes" are present in the same child, suggesting chronic disease.

1 mg/kg/day and tapering over 14–21 days) is often considered. If children have significant residual symptoms after intravenous steroid treatment, a second 3- to 5-day course may be given. Alternatively, treatment with intravenous immunoglobulin (IVIg; 2 g/kg over 2–5 days) may be of benefit (class IV evidence).

Profound encephalopathy and respiratory depression may occur with brainstem/upper cervical spinal cord involvement and may be a life-threatening condition. Plasma exchange may be useful in this situation (class I evidence in adult-onset MS). A typical regimen of plasma exchange treatment is 5 to 8 exchanges in 10 days.

RELAPSING DEMYELINATING DISORDERS
Multiple Sclerosis

MS, a chronic inflammatory and degenerative disorder of the CNS, is being increasingly diagnosed in children.

Epidemiology of Pediatric Multiple Sclerosis

Childhood-onset MS has been reported in many countries. Although the exact incidence remains unknown, 3% to 10% of MS patients experience their first symptoms at younger than 18 years of age.

Gender differences in pediatric MS are related to age. In children younger than 10 years of age, the female-to-male ratio is approximately 1 : 1. After age 10, this ratio increases to 3 : 1.

A family history of MS is reported in 5% to 15% of children, slightly lower than the 20% to 30% of adult MS patients who report MS in at least one first-degree relative.

Diagnostic Criteria for Pediatric Multiple Sclerosis

MS diagnosis requires demonstration of CNS demyelination separated in both space and in time (Fig. 100-6). A child with two separate characteristic attacks meets the clinical criteria for dissemination in space (DIS) and time (DIT). MRI may

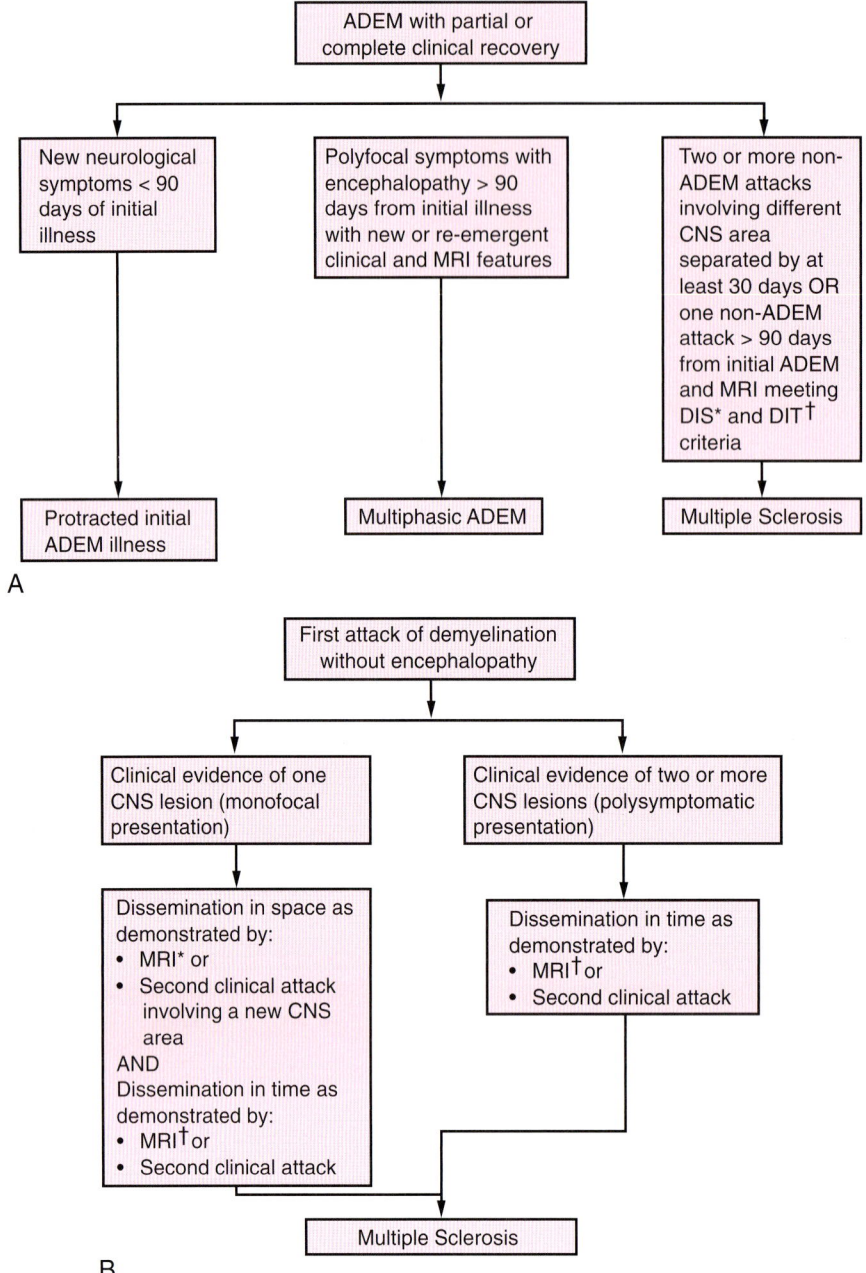

Figure 100-6. **Classification of further attacks of demyelination. A,** Approach to further attacks of demyelination in the child initially presenting with acute disseminated encephalomyelitis (ADEM). **B,** Approach to further attacks of demyelination in the child presenting with a monofocal or polyfocal neurologic syndrome without encephalopathy. *MRI criteria for dissemination in space require the presence of at least one lesion in the following locations: periventricular, juxtacortical, infratentorial, and spinal cord. †MRI criteria for dissemination in time require either new T2 lesions on serial scans or the simultaneous presence of a clinically silent gadolinium-enhancing and nonenhancing lesion on a single baseline scan (Polman, Reingold et al., 2011).

also be used to demonstrate DIS or DIT (Polman et al. 2011). Specifically, MRI evidence of DIS requires at least one T2-hyperintense lesion in two of four CNS areas: periventricular, juxtacortical, infratentorial, and/or spinal cord. MRI DIT criteria require new T2 or gadolinium-enhancing lesions over time (≥30 days from a baseline scan) or at the time of initial presentation, provided the baseline scan shows the simultaneous presence of asymptomatic gadolinium-enhancing and nonenhancing lesions.

McDonald 2010 MS criteria have a positive predictive value of 76% and a negative predictive value of 100% when applied to children with ADS; however, these criteria are less predictive in younger children and cannot be reliably applied in ADEM.

Clinical Course of Pediatric Multiple Sclerosis

MS is relapsing-remitting in more than 95% of children. A study of 21 pediatric and 110 adult patients demonstrated that, compared with adults, children with MS experience more frequent relapses in the first few years following diagnosis (annualized relapse rate of 1.13 versus 0.4, $p < 0.01$). A German study showed that relapse rates decreased between year 1 and year 5 following diagnosis in both patients younger than 11 years of age (relapse rate of 2.1 versus 0.79) and patients between 14 and 16 years of age (1.8 versus 0.42). Secondary disease progression, when accrual of disability occurs in the absence of discrete relapses, typically begins after 15 years of age. Because of their younger age at onset, pediatric MS patients accrue disability approximately 10 years earlier than do adult patients.

Magnetic Resonance Imaging Features of Pediatric Multiple Sclerosis

Imaging studies have shown that pediatric-onset MS is associated with a global reduction in brain volume, especially in the thalami, and a reduction in age-expected head size. Both T1- and T2-weighted lesion volume is higher in pediatric-onset MS patients compared with adults, with a greater lesion burden located infratentorially in children. The long-term effects of this extensive pathology on cognitive, physical, psychiatric, and socioeconomic functioning have yet to be defined.

Complex imaging modalities, including diffusion-tensor imaging (DTI), magnetization transfer ratio (MTR) imaging, and functional MRI (fMRI), hold great promise as tools to link structural and functional parameters.

Pathobiological Insights Into Pediatric Multiple Sclerosis

The greatest genetic contributor to MS risk in children and adults is associated with the HLA DRB1*1501 haplotype. Over 100 non-HLA risk SNPs have been identified as contributors to adult-onset MS risk. Early studies indicate that similar non-HLA risk SNPs also contribute to pediatric-onset MS risk.

Several environmental risk factors have been shown to contribute to pediatric MS risk (reviewed in Waldman et al., 2014), including:

1. Low serum 25-hydroxyvitamin D levels
2. Remote Epstein–Barr virus (EBV) infection
3. Earlier age at menarche
4. Secondhand smoke exposure
5. Increased body mass index (BMI)

Case-control studies suggest that cytomegalovirus infection may be associated with reduced pediatric MS risk.

A Canadian study of children with ADS found a higher risk of later MS diagnosis in children who had (a) low serum 25-hydroxyvitamin D level (<75 nmol/L), (b) evidence of remote EBV infection, and (c) at least one HLA DRB1*1501 allele compared with those children who had none of these risk factors at presentation (hazard ratio [HR] = 5.27, 95% confidence interval [CI] = 1.23–22.6) (Banwell et al., 2011).

Children with demyelination may display antibodies against MOG, aquaporin-4, NMDA receptors, voltage-gated potassium channels, and glycine receptors. Defining the range of autoantibodies present in children with demyelination and their associated clinical phenotypes will be of considerable future interest.

The cerebrospinal fluid (CSF) of children with ADS appears to be enriched in components of the axoglial apparatus, including neurofascin, contactins, and contactin-associated proteins, suggesting that axoglial apparatus disruption may be involved in MS pathobiology.

Altered cellular immune responses are associated with pediatric-onset MS. Both T-cell repertoire (proportions of naïve versus memory T-cells) and functional T-cell responses to myelin and nonmyelin antigens appear to be disrupted in children with MS.

Immunomodulatory Therapy in Pediatric Multiple Sclerosis

Principles of Immunomodulatory Therapy. There are now 12 MS therapies approved by the U.S. Food and Drug Administration (FDA) available in the United States. In children, first-line treatment is usually with interferons (beta 1a or 1b), or glatiramer acetate (GA) (Table 100-1). These agents reduce relapse rates by approximately one third in adult MS patients and also reduce the number of T2 brain MRI lesions. Interferons and GA are generally considered safe and well tolerated in children with MS. Transaminitis is the most frequent laboratory abnormality in children treated with interferons and is possibly reduced by a gradual dose titration starting at one fourth of the usual adult dose. GA is utilized at full dose.

TABLE 100-1 Immunomodulatory Therapies for Pediatric Multiple Sclerosis

Drug	Dosing Regimen	Common Side Effects	Potential Laboratory Abnormalities
Interferon beta 1a (Avonex®)	30 µg IM weekly	Flu-like myalgia and headache Depression	Transaminitis (typically 2- to 3-fold elevation of transaminases) Rarely, fulminant liver failure
Interferon beta 1a (Rebif®)	22–44 µg SC weekly	Flu-like myalgia and headache Injection-site reaction (redness, pain, and induration) Depression	Transaminitis (typically 2- to 3-fold elevation of transaminases) Rarely, fulminant liver failure
Pegylated Interferon beta 1a (Plegridy®)	125 µg SC every 14 days	Flu-like myalgia and headache Injection-site reaction (redness, pain, and induration) Depression	Transaminitis (typically 2- to 3-fold elevation of transaminases) Rarely, fulminant liver failure
Interferon beta 1b (Betaseron®)	0.25 mg SC every 2 days	Flu-like myalgia and headache Injection-site reaction (redness, pain, and induration) Depression	Transaminitis (typically 2- to 3-fold elevation of transaminases) Rarely, fulminant liver failure
Glatiramer acetate (Copaxone®)	20 mg SC daily or 40 mg SC 3 times a week	Injection-site reaction (redness, pain, and induration) Immediate postinjection reaction (flushing, tachycardia, and chest pain)	No significant effect on liver or hematological function

IM, intramuscular; SC, subcutaneous.

White blood cell counts and liver function tests should be monitored monthly for 6 months and then every 3 months thereafter during interferon treatment. Thyroid function should be monitored yearly. Sexually active patients should receive counseling regarding contraceptive use.

Second-Line Therapies. Immunosuppressive therapy is offered when frequent relapses occur despite compliance with interferon or GA. Proposed definitions for inadequate treatment response require full compliance for at least 6 months and at least one of the following: (a) increased or stable relapse rate or new T2- or contrast-enhancing lesions compared with pretreatment baseline or (b) at least two clinical or MRI attacks within 12 months (Chitnis et al., 2012). Therapeutic options for children experiencing an inadequate treatment response include switching between first-line therapies or escalating to a second-line agent. Children with frequent relapses on interferon therapy should be checked for neutralizing antibodies.

Cyclophosphamide, azathioprine, methotrexate, mitoxantrone, and rituximab have all been utilized in isolated cases or small case series of pediatric MS patients. There are increasing numbers of reports of natalizumab use in pediatric-onset MS. A study of 55 children with MS treated with natalizumab reported that the annualized relapse rate (ARR) decreased from 2.4 +/- 1.6 to 0.1 +/- 0.2 ($p < 0.001$). Mild transient hematological abnormalities were observed in 7 out of 55 patients, and no serious adverse events were reported. Natalizumab is associated with increased risk of progressive multifocal leukoencephalopathy, especially in patients seropositive for JC virus (particularly with an index value > 1.5), patients previously treated with other immunosuppressive agents, and those treated for more than 24 months.

Several oral agents (e.g., dimethyl fumarate, fingolimod, and teriflunomide) and infusion-based therapies (e.g., alemtuzumab) are now approved for use in adult-onset MS. Clinical trials for some of these agents are ongoing in pediatric MS, and future trials are expected.

General Care Issues

The care of children with MS requires a multidisciplinary team that often includes a neurologist, nurse, occupational therapist, physiotherapist, psychologist, dietician, and social worker. An MS diagnosis has important implications for social functioning, family functioning, and overall psychosocial well-being.

Multiphasic Acute Disseminated Encephalomyelitis

MS diagnosis in a child with initial ADEM requires either two subsequent non-ADEM attacks or one subsequent clinical attack not accompanied by encephalopathy at least 3 months from the initial ADEM associated with MRI findings meeting current definitions for DIS and DIT (Krupp, Tardieu et al., 2013). Recurrence of ADEM more than 3 months after an initial ADEM episode is termed multiphasic ADEM (Krupp et al., 2013), which is treated in the same manner as an acute demyelinating attack.

Neuromyelitis Optica

NMO is a severe, inflammatory CNS demyelinating disorder with unique clinical, laboratory, and MRI features. The identification of a biomarker for NMO (NMO-IgG) has resulted in improved diagnostic accuracy (Lennon et al., 2004).

Epidemiology of Pediatric Neuromyelitis Optica

The exact incidence of NMO in childhood is unknown. In children and adults, NMO has a marked female predominance, with some studies reporting a female-to-male ratio as high as 9 : 1. There is an overrepresentation of children reporting non-Caucasian ethnicity compared with other demyelinating diseases. In one U.S. study, 42 out of 58 NMO-IgG–seropositive children (73%) with available ethnicity data were non-Caucasian.

Clinical Features of Pediatric Neuromyelitis Optica

NMO is characterized by severe ON (visual acuity typically 20/200 or worse) and TM, occurring either simultaneously or sequentially. When sequential, ON and TM may be separated by months or even years.

Approximately 53% to 100% of pediatric NMO patients experience a relapsing (as opposed to monophasic) course. Predictors of a relapsing course in one study of adult NMO patients included female gender, older age at onset, and evidence of systemic autoimmunity. NMO-IgG–seropositive patients appear more likely to experience a relapsing course compared with seronegative individuals. In a retrospective analysis of 20 children with NMO, mean time to relapse was shorter in seropositive patients compared with seronegative patients (0.76 versus 2.4 years, $p = 0.03$). Serum NMO-IgG titers correlated with disease severity in one study.

NMO is typically characterized by severe attacks with poor recovery, leading to rapid disability accrual. In a study of adults with NMO, 31 out of 66 (47%) were functionally blind (visual acuity of 20/200 or worse) in at least one eye, and 32 out of 71 (45%) exhibited permanent monoplegia or paraplegia, after a mean follow up of 16.9 years in relapsing patients and 7.7 years in monophasic patients. Respiratory failure was observed in one third of relapsing patients. One pediatric study reported that after a median of 12 months of follow up, 54% of NMO patients had permanent visual impairment, and 44% had limb weakness severe enough to affect mobility.

Symptomatic Brain Involvement in Neuromyelitis Optica

Brain MRI lesions in NMO typically follow the distribution of aquaporin-4 water channel expression, including the diencephalon and brainstem periaqueductal gray matter. Brain lesions are symptomatic in 35% to 45% of children. Brainstem involvement may present as hiccups, nausea/vomiting, ophthalmoplegia, and, in severe cases, respiratory failure or death. Symptoms of diencephalic involvement may include hypersomnolence, narcolepsy, inappropriate antidiuretic hormone secretion, or menstrual irregularities. Large multifocal lesions have been associated with encephalopathy and an ADEM-like phenotype.

Diagnostic Criteria for Pediatric Neuromyelitis Optica

Revised pediatric consensus criteria for NMO require the presence of ON and TM with at least two of the following supportive features (Krupp et al., 2013):

1. MRI evidence of a contiguous spinal lesion at least three spinal segments in length
2. Brain MRI not meeting diagnostic criteria for MS
3. NMO-IgG seropositivity

The presence of two of the three supportive criteria has 99% sensitivity and 90% specificity in distinguishing adults with NMO from those with MS (Wingerchuk, Lennon, Pittock,

Lucchinetti, and Weinshenker, 2006). Children may present with recurrent ON or TM associated with serum NMO-IgG; such cases are considered NMO spectrum disorders (Krupp et al., 2013).

Systemic Autoimmunity in Neuromyelitis Optica

There is a high frequency of coexisting systemic autoimmunity in NMO. In one pediatric cohort, 16 out of 38 patients (42%) met the criteria for clinical diagnosis of another auto-immune condition, including systemic lupus erythematosus, type 1 diabetes, juvenile rheumatoid arthritis, and Graves disease. Some children with NMO harbor other autoantibodies without meeting formal diagnostic criteria for another autoimmune disorder. Some children with anti-NMDA receptor encephalitis display NMO-IgG in the absence of clinical NMO symptoms. The relevance of incidentally detected NMO-IgG in children with other CNS autoimmune conditions is unclear.

Laboratory Features of Neuromyelitis Optica

The CSF in NMO patients typically demonstrates a marked pleocytosis (>50 leukocytes/µL), with a neutrophilic or lymphocytic predominance. This is in contrast to the moderate lymphocytic pleocytosis (<25 leukocytes/µL) typical of pediatric MS. One study of lumbar punctures in 89 pediatric and adult NMO patients found that pleocytosis (>5 leukocytes/µL) occurred in 50% of samples, with a median white blood cell count of 15 leukocytes/µL (range = 6–380). The median number of white blood cells and percentage of samples containing neutrophils were higher during relapses compared with periods of clinical quiescence. CSF OCBs are detected in less than 10% of children with NMO. In one pediatric study, OCBs were more commonly detected in seropositive (2/10) compared with seronegative (0/7) NMO patients.

Visual-evoked potentials are frequently abnormal in NMO patients and typically display a prolongation or absence of the P100 response. In adults with NMO, markedly abnormal or absent visual-evoked potential responses at baseline are associated with worse long-term visual outcomes. Delayed P100 responses have been observed in the absence of a clear history of ON, suggesting that optic nerve involvement may be subclinical.

OCT-based studies have demonstrated that RNFL thinning is frequently seen in NMO patients, and that RNFL thinning after an episode of ON is more severe in patients with NMO compared with those with MS.

NMO-IgG is directed against the aquaporin-4 water channel located on astrocytic end feet. This serum biomarker has a sensitivity of 73% and a specificity of 91% in differentiating NMO from other demyelinating disorders, including MS, in adult patients (Lennon et al., 2004) and is detected in up to 78% of children with relapsing NMO. NMO-IgG has also been detected in children with NMO spectrum disorders.

A proportion of individuals with clinical NMO will repeatedly test negative for NMO-IgG, even when sensitive cell-based assays are employed. A subset of these NMO-IgG–seronegative patients displays serum anti-MOG antibodies. Studies suggest that NMO patients with anti-MOG antibodies (without NMO-IgG) have an increased likelihood of being male, are slightly younger, have better recovery from attacks, are less likely to experience a relapsing course, and, in one study, were more likely to present with simultaneous/sequential ON and TM. In three reported children with clinical NMO and anti-MOG antibodies, there was an initial relapsing course, with a beneficial response to longer-term immunotherapy (azathioprine or monthly IVIg). Two children displayed deep gray-matter involvement on MRI.

Magnetic Resonance Imaging in Neuromyelitis Optica

As in MS, MRI during an acute ON attack in NMO typically reveals optic nerve thickening and an increased signal on fat-suppressed T2-weighted images. Fat-suppressed postcontrast T1-weighted images show optic nerve enhancement in 94% of patients. To date, there are no MRI features that reliably distinguish ON in NMO from that in MS, although a trend toward more extensive and greater posterior optic nerve involvement in NMO has been noted.

Brain MRI lesions are common in children with NMO, with 53% to 100% of children demonstrating brain abnormalities distinct from the optic nerves at presentation. In NMO, brain MRI lesions typically occur in areas of aquaporin-4 water channel expression, including (a) lesions surrounding the ventricular system (e.g., diencephalic lesions around the third ventricle, dorsal brainstem lesions adjacent to the fourth ventricle, and peri-ependymal lesions surrounding the lateral ventricles); (b) hemispheric lesions that may be large (>3 cm diameter); (c) lesions involving the corticospinal tracts; and (d) small, nonspecific, deep white-matter lesions (most common lesion type) (Fig. 100-7) (Kim et al., 2015). Enhancing lesions may demonstrate a patchy, diffuse, "cloud-like" enhancement pattern. As discussed earlier, brain lesions may be symptomatic. Lesions that are perpendicular to ventricles, S-shaped U-fiber lesions, lesions along the inferior aspect of the lateral ventricles, temporal lobe lesions, and lesions that have an ovoid or open-ring enhancement pattern are more characteristic of MS (Kim et al., 2015).

Acute spinal MRI in NMO typically reveals lesions spanning at least three contiguous spinal segments that are hyperintense on T2-weighted images (Fig. 100-7A) and hypointense on T1-weighted images. It is important to note, however, that LETM is frequently seen in children with idiopathic TM, in TM with ADEM, and in up to 25% of TM cases associated with an MS attack. NMO patients occasionally present with short-segment spinal lesions. Partial cord lesions in NMO often localize to the cervical and upper thoracic cord. Acutely, lesions typically affect central cord gray and white matter, with diffuse gadolinium uptake within the lesion core. Bilateral and symmetric anterior horn cell signal abnormalities resembling anterior cord infarction have been described. Over time, the development of spinal cord atrophy is associated with an increased likelihood of persistent neurologic deficits.

Treatment of Pediatric Neuromyelitis Optica

Acute attacks are usually treated with intravenous corticosteroids. If symptoms progress despite steroid therapy, IVIg and/or plasmapheresis is usually administered.

Longer-term immunosuppression is generally used to prevent relapses and disability accrual given the aggressive nature of this disease. Azathioprine (+/− oral prednisone), repeated IVIg or plasmapheresis, rituximab, cyclophosphamide, mycophenolate mofetil, and ofatumumab have all been used in children with NMO.

CONCLUSIONS

Acquired demyelination of the CNS, including transient forms and pediatric-onset MS and NMO, is being increasingly recognized and diagnosed worldwide. This has been aided by the development of consensus diagnostic criteria, evolving MRI criteria, and the discovery of the NMO-IgG biomarker. The current and emerging armamentarium of increasingly powerful medications for adult-onset MS will require vigilant and

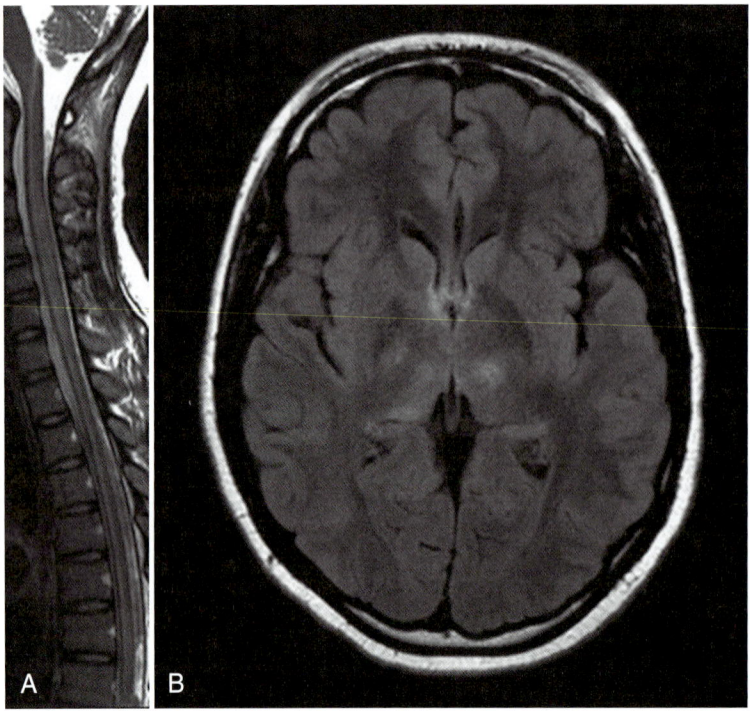

Figure 100-7. MRI in childhood neuromyelitis optica. A, Sagittal T2-weighted MRI image shows a longitudinally extensive intramedullary spinal lesion. **B,** Axial fluid-attenuated inversion-recovery (FLAIR) MRI from a different child shows bilateral hyperintense diencephalic lesions.

thoughtful use in children. Collaboration between clinicians and scientists, such as that fostered by the International Pediatric MS Study Group and other organizations, is essential to optimize care.

REFERENCES

The complete list of references for this chapter is available online at www.expertconsult.com.
   See inside cover for registration details.

RESOURCES

National Multiple Sclerosis Society (United States). <www.nationalmssociety.org>.
Multiple Sclerosis Society of Canada. <www.mssociety.ca>.

SELECTED REFERENCES

Banwell, B., Bar-Or, A., Arnold, D.L., et al., 2011. Clinical, environmental, and genetic determinants of multiple sclerosis in children with acute demyelination: a prospective national cohort study. Lancet Neurol. 10 (5), 436–445.
Chitnis, T., Tenembaum, S., Banwell, B., et al., 2012. Consensus statement: evaluation of new and existing therapeutics for pediatric multiple sclerosis. Mult. Scler. 18 (1), 116–127.
Kim, H.J., Paul, F., Lana-Peixoto, M.A., et al., 2015. MRI characteristics of neuromyelitis optica spectrum disorder: An international update. Neurology.
Krupp, L.B., Tardieu, M., Amato, M.P., et al., 2013. International Pediatric Multiple Sclerosis Study Group criteria for pediatric multiple sclerosis and immune-mediated central nervous system demyelinating disorders: revisions to the 2007 definitions. Mult. Scler.
Lennon, V.A., Wingerchuk, D.M., Kryzer, T.J., et al., 2004. A serum autoantibody marker of neuromyelitis optica: distinction from multiple sclerosis. Lancet 364 (9451), 2106–2112.
Polman, C.H., Reingold, S.C., Banwell, B., et al., 2011. Diagnostic criteria for multiple sclerosis: 2010 revisions to the McDonald criteria. Ann. Neurol. 69 (2), 292–302.
Waldman, A., Ghezzi, A., Bar-Or, A., et al., 2014. Multiple sclerosis in children: an update on clinical diagnosis, therapeutic strategies, and research. Lancet Neurol. 13 (9), 936–948.
Wingerchuk, D.M., Lennon, V.A., Pittock, S.J., et al., 2006. Revised diagnostic criteria for neuromyelitis optica. Neurology 66 (10), 1485–1489.

E-BOOK FIGURES AND TABLES

The following figures and tables are available in the e-book at www.expertconsult.com. See inside cover for registration details.

101 Disorders of Consciousness in Children

Stephen Ashwal

 An expanded version of this chapter is available on www.expertconsult.com. See inside cover for registration details.

Disorders of consciousness (DOCs) in children are usually due to serious nervous system injuries as well as infectious, genetic, and metabolic disorders. Assessment of consciousness remains challenging because of the inherent limitations imposed by the structural and functional developmental level of the neonate, infant, and child and how it affects the ability to evaluate language, cognitive, and behavioral functions. This chapter reviews aspects of the diagnosis, management, and prognosis of DOCs in children as well as recent evolving concepts related to the "neural correlates of consciousness."

HISTORICAL PERSPECTIVE

 Please see online chapter for a discussion of this topic.

Neural Correlates of Consciousness

In the past quarter century, increasing research has focused on the concept of the *neural correlates of consciousness* (NCC), defined "as the minimal neuronal mechanisms jointly sufficient for any one specific conscious percept." Comprehensively reviewing this topic is beyond the scope of this chapter, and the reader is referred to several reviews for further consideration (Giacino et al., 2014; Gosseries et al., 2014).

Consciousness is defined as having two components: awareness and arousal (Di Perri et al., 2014). Arousal, also called wakefulness, refers to the level of alertness (clinically determined by eye opening), whereas awareness refers to the content of consciousness (clinically determined by the obeying of commands or nonreflex motor behavior such as eye tracking or localized responses to pain). Arousal is related to structures in the brain, specifically to the brainstem and hypothalamus, whereas awareness has been shown to be related to a wide fronto-parietal network encompassing associative cortices and the thalamus (Laureys, 2005).

Assessment of awareness remains subjective. One can only determine whether a patient is conscious if he/she is capable of manifesting behavioral or verbal responses. An "unresponsive" patient may be in a locked-in syndrome or have a disorder of consciousness but with a low-level of conscious awareness and be unable to respond because of coexistent conditions such as motor, sensory, or language impairments, complicating medical conditions, subclinical seizures, etc. About 30% to 40% of individuals diagnosed as being in a VS/UWS do manifest conscious behaviors or have neuroimaging or electrophysiological evidence of limited consciousness. The advent of functional imaging and EEG computational methods have provided significant supportive evidence that conscious behavior may be present even in patients who appear

unconscious. Certainty of diagnosis is necessary as it forms the basis of clinical decision making. However, medical centers may not have the facilities and technical and medical staffing/expertise to acquire and interpret such data.

Approaches to Studying the NCC

Several types of experimental paradigms combined with functional neuroimaging and neurophysiological testing are used to explore brain function (Osborne et al., 2015; Di Perri et al., 2014):

Passive stimulation paradigms. Subjects are presented with various stimuli and their brain responses are monitored for characteristic patterns indicative of normal cognitive processing. These paradigms do not require intentional interaction and activation will not appear unless the patient intentionally performs the task.

Active stimulation paradigms. Specific instructions are given to the subject, with or without accompanying stimulation, and brain activation responses are monitored.

Resting state and connectivity studies. Resting state activity using fMRI or EEG to measure regional brain interactions when an individual is not performing specific tasks is based on the concept that even at rest the brain has measurable resting activity. Studies in individuals with disorders of consciousness have identified the default mode network and other NCCs that affect conscious behaviors.

Transcranial magnetic stimulation (TMS). TMS directly perturbs underlying neuronal networks, allowing for the study of effective regional connectivity. In DOC patients, TMS paradigms have shown functional connectivity abnormalities that may correlate with behavioral observations.

Commonly used testing paradigms. Numerous testing paradigms have been used to assess behavioral, imaging, or neurophysiological responses:

a. *Oddball paradigm.* Repetitive audiological or visual stimuli are infrequently interrupted by a deviant stimulus and the responses recorded with event-related potentials (ERPs). Typically detected is an abnormal surface positive P300 response best seen in the parietal regions or with fMRI.

b. *Mismatch negativity.* Similar in concept to the oddball sequence, but the activated response is different. It is a negative frontal response (the N200 response).

c. *Binocular rivalry and flash suppression.* Binocular rivalry is a visual response in which perceptions alternate between different images (e.g. red versus green) presented to each eye. Flash suppression is a form of visual perception in which an image that is presented to one eye is suppressed by a flash of another image to the other eye. Both are used to study visual processing.

  d. *Residual language function.* Many types of language stimuli can be assessed by fMRI or EEG (e.g., the N400 ERP response). Typical stimuli include presentation of narratives that had personally meaningful content and that were read forwards by a familiar voice.

  e. *Visual imagery.* One of the most dramatic tasks in which the "unconscious" patient is asked to visualize is that they are playing tennis, swimming, or navigating about their house, etc. with activation detected in similar regions as control conscious individuals.

  f. *Tactile stimulation/motor movement commands.* Multiple forms of touching or asking the patient to move an extremity have been tried with activation on fMRI interpreted as a sign of consciousness.

Neuroimaging

Positron Emission Tomography (PET) and fMRI studies have been used to study DOC patients (Harrison and Connolly, 2013; Di Perri et al., 2014) and have documented significant (i.e., up to 40%) reductions in cerebral metabolism in patients who were in a VS/UWS. Recovery has been associated with improved connectivity—but not to the degree that PET could be used to differentiate between VS/UWS and MCS. fMRI activation has demonstrated cortical responses in MCS patients resembling those in healthy controls whereas VS/UWS patients showed only low level activation if at all (Fig. 101-1) (Di Perri et al., 2014). Multiple paradigms have been successfully used to detect evidence of brain activation in patients who are deemed unconscious. So far these studies have shown that

only about 20% of unconscious patients will show such activation (Gosseries et al., 2014). Also, almost all studies have been performed in adult patients, and it is uncertain as to whether such studies will be able to be done in pediatric patients. There has been one case report in a pediatric patient who was in a MCS in whom fMRI was acquired.

Neurophysiology

Several reviews have examined the role of EEGs, evoked potentials (EPs), and event-related potentials (ERPs) in patients with DOCs (Harrison and Connolly, 2013). Conventional EEG has limited value and can determine whether a DOC patient is having seizures or if there is evidence of diffuse slowing or suppression. In some patients, changes in sleep/wake EEG patterns correlate with a patient's clinical state.

Evoked potentials (EPs) and event-related potentials (ERPs) have been used in DOC patients to assess brainstem and forebrain integrity. EPs generally reflect sensory processing responses, whereas (ERPs reflect perceptual and cognitive processing and appear more sensitive in detecting functional abnormalities activity. Chapters 102 to 104 describe the different types of EPs for outcome prediction.

Neural Correlates of Consciousness in DOC Patients

Abnormalities in several connectivity networks have been associated with DOCs in adults and include:

Default Mode Network (DMN). The DMN, considered responsible in part for intrinsic awareness, encompasses the posterior and anterior cortical midline structures, with major hubs being located in the posterior cingulate cortex and precuneus, the medial prefrontal cortex, and the angular

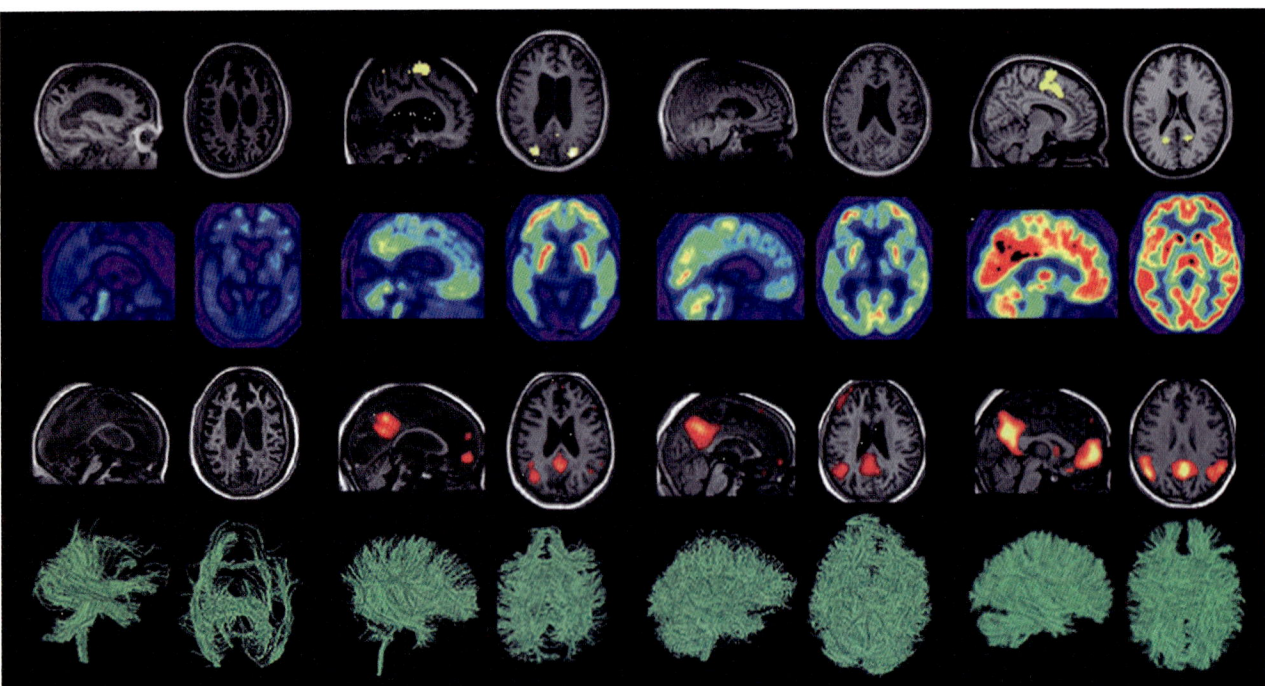

Figure 101-1. fMRI and PET in two Vegetative State (VS)/Unresponsive Wakefulness Syndrome (UWS) patients: one Minimally Conscious State (MCS) patient and one healthy control showing possible dissociations between active and passive paradigms and how they complement each other in the evaluation of patients. fMRI mental imagery tasks (motor imagery on the *left*, navigation imagery on the *right*) show positive results in the control subject and in the second VS/UWS patient. PET and fMRI resting-state results typically show a strong decrease in brain activity and anatomy [here, diffusion tensor imaging (DTI)] in the first VS/UWS patient and show partially preserved brain activity in the second VS/UWS patient as in the MCS patient. Negative responses to active paradigms in MCS patients frequently occur. *(With permission from Gosseries, O., Di, H., Laureys, S., Boly, M., 2014. Measuring consciousness in severely damaged brains. Annu Rev Neurosci 37, 457–478.)*

gyrus (Andrews-Hanna et al., 2014). The DMN shows greater activity during the resting state when an individual is focused internally rather than on the external world or on attention-demanding tasks. Studies have shown that DMN connectivity is reduced in patients with VS/UWS compared with healthy controls. It has been shown that there is limited evidence of the DMN in infancy but that DMN connectivity can be detected in children 9 to 12 years of age, suggesting that the DMN evolves with maturation.

Executive Control Network (ECN). The ECN is considered responsible for extrinsic awareness that regulates executive functions that control and mediate cognitive processes, including working memory, reasoning, flexibility, problem solving, and planning (Qin et al., 2015). Traditionally, ECNs have been considered to be located in prefrontal regions of the frontal lobes (e.g., dorsolateral prefrontal cortex, anterior cingulate cortex, orbitofrontal cortex), but more recent studies suggest that subcortical and brainstem sites participate in network functioning. A previous study has shown altered ECN connectivity in DOC patients compared with controls, but more recent studies have not confirmed such findings (Qin et al., 2015; Demertzi et al., 2014).

Salience Network. The Salience Network (SN) is a large-scale network anchored in the anterior insula and dorsal anterior cingulate cortex and includes three key subcortical structures: the amygdala, the ventral striatum, and the substantia nigra/ventral tegmental area (Menon, 2015). The SN contributes to communication, social behavior, and self-awareness. SN connectivity studies early after injury may differentiate patients in MCS from patients in VS/UWS.

Frontal Mesocircuit Network (FMN). The frontal mesocircuit network consists of hubs in the mesencephalon (pedunculopontine nucleus, PPN), central thalamus, deep anterior frontal lobes, striatum, globus pallidus interna, and regions in the parietal, occipital, and temporal cortex with the major pathways involving thalamocortical, thalamostriatal, and corticostriatal outflow (Giacino et al., 2014). The mesocircuit serves as the basic underlying tonic driver of the forebrain networks and is necessary for supporting consciousness and governing the quality of consciousness.

Other networks include sensorimotor, auditory, cerebellar, and three visual networks in healthy controls and in patients with varying levels of diminished consciousness. Also, as alluded to previously, there is now extensive research examining the development of many of these networks in the pediatric population, particularly in children with neurodevelopmental disabilities.

DEFINITIONS

Along the continuum from normal consciousness to coma or unarousable unconsciousness, many terms are used to describe mental state and reactivity. When there is doubt about the appropriate use of one of these terms, it is far better to describe the state and reactivity of the individual rather than label it. See Table 101-1 and Figure 101-2 that describe the major DOCs and associated conditions.

Clouding of consciousness is the minimal reduction of wakefulness or awareness wherein the main difficulty is attention or vigilance. Clouding of consciousness is distinguished from daydreaming in that the child cannot be easily stimulated to normal consciousness. *Confusion* is the state of impaired ability to think and reason clearly at a developmentally and intellectually appropriate level. Confused children have persistent difficulty with orientation, simple cognitive processing, and acquisition of new memory. Definitions of impairment of consciousness states may be divided into the categories as listed here:

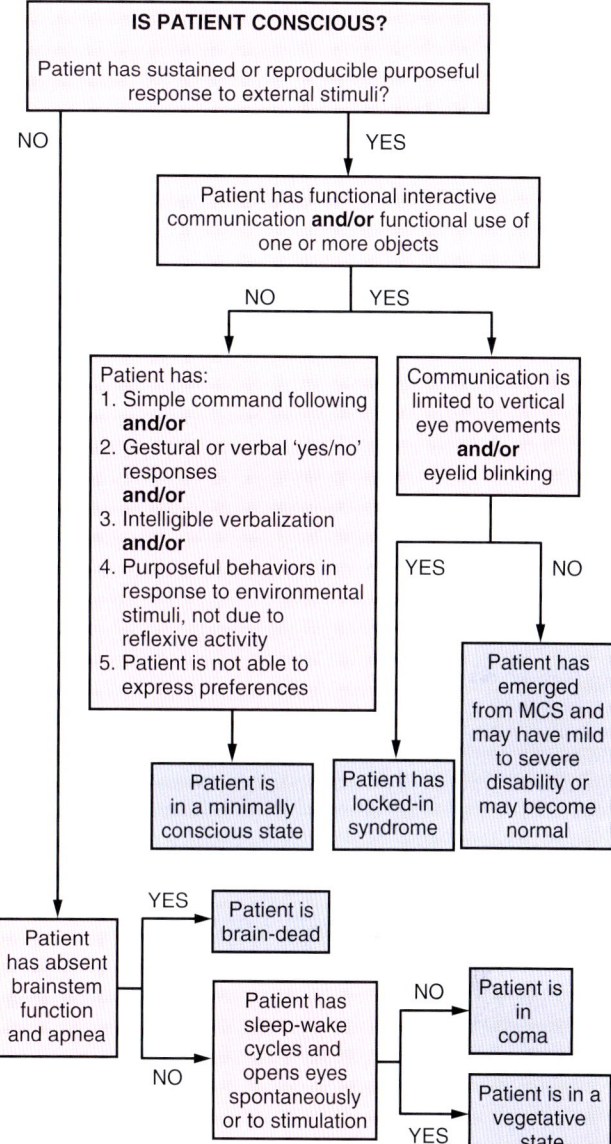

Figure 101-2. An algorithm useful for distinguishing among brain death, vegetative state, locked-in syndrome, and higher-order consciousness. MCS, minimally conscious state. *(With permission from Ashwal, S., Cranford, R., 2002. The minimally conscious state in children. Semin Pediatr Neurol 9, 19.)*

Impairment of Consciousness With Activated Mental State

Hallucinations are perceptions of sensory input that are not present; illusions are misinterpretations of actual sensory stimuli. *Delusions* are incorrect thoughts or beliefs that do not change when challenged by contradictory evidence or logical reason. *Delirium* is an activated mental state that may include disorientation, irritability, fearful responses, and sensory misperception. Common causes include intoxication, infection, fever, metabolic disorders, epilepsy, and might terrors.

Impairment of Consciousness With Reduced Mental State

Obtundation is mild to moderate alertness reduction with decreased interest in the environment and slower than normal

TABLE 101-1 Severe Disorders of Consciousness and Related Conditions

Condition	Self-Awareness	Pain and Suffering	Sleep-Wake Cycles	Motor Function	Respiratory Function	Outcome
Coma	Absent	No	Absent	No purposeful movement	Variably depressed	Evolves to persistent vegetative state, dies, or recovers in 2–4 weeks
Vegetative state	Absent	No	Intact	No purposeful movement	Normal	Depends on etiology
Minimally conscious state	Very limited	Yes	Intact	Severe limitation of movement	Variably depressed	Recovery unknown
Akinetic mutism	Limited	Yes	Intact	Moderate limitation of movement	Normal to variably depressed	Recovery unlikely or limited
Locked-in syndrome	Present	Yes	Intact	Quadriplegia; pseudobulbar palsy; eye movements preserved	Normal to variably depressed	Recovery unlikely; remains quadriplegic
Brain death	Absent	No	Absent	None or only reflex spinal movements	Absent	None

reactivity to stimulation. *Stupor* is a state of unresponsiveness with little or no spontaneous movement, resembling deep sleep from which the patient can only be aroused by vigorous and repeated stimulation.

Coma is a state of deep, unarousable, sustained pathologic unconsciousness with the eyes closed and results from dysfunction of the ascending reticular-activating system in the brainstem or in both cerebral hemispheres. Coma usually requires the period of unconsciousness to persist for at least 1 hour to distinguish coma from syncope, concussion, or other states of transient unconsciousness.

Vegetative State, Minimally Conscious State, and Related Conditions

Table 101-1 lists several of the major neurologic conditions that the clinician must be capable of differentiating from coma. This table was modified from the report issued by the Multi-Society Task Force and more recent work that is defining the concept of the minimally conscious state (see Figure 101-2 algorithm).

Vegetative State/Unresponsive Wakefulness Syndrome

The VS/UWS can be described as a condition of complete unawareness of the self and the environment, accompanied by sleep-wake cycles with either complete or partial preservation of hypothalamic and brainstem autonomic (vegetative) functions (Multisociety Task Force Report, 1994). Recently the term "unresponsive wakefulness syndrome" has been suggested as a better descriptive alternative term (Laureys et al., 2010).

Criteria to diagnose the VS/UWS are listed in Box 101-1. Children in a vegetative state lack evidence of self-awareness or recognition of external stimuli. Rather than being in a state of "eyes-closed" coma, they remain unconscious but have irregular periods of wakefulness alternating with periods of sleeping. Vegetative patients demonstrate a variety of sounds, emotional expressions, and body movements, and they may smile or shed tears. They have inconsistent head- and eye-turning movements to sounds and inconsistent, nonpurposeful trunk and limb movements. The most objective sign is lack of sustained visual fixation or visual tracking.

It is estimated that there are about 4000 to 10,000 children in a vegetative state in the United States and about 100,000

BOX 101-1 Criteria for the Diagnosis of the Vegetative State

No evidence of awareness of themselves or their environment; they are incapable of interacting with others
No evidence of sustained, reproducible, purposeful, or voluntary behavioral responses to visual, auditory, tactile, or noxious stimuli
No evidence of language comprehension or expression
Intermittent wakefulness manifested by the presence of sleep-wake cycles
Sufficiently preserved hypothalamic and brainstem autonomic functions to survive if given medical and nursing care
Bowel and bladder incontinence
Variably preserved cranial nerve (pupillary, oculocephalic, corneal, oculovestibular, gag) and spinal reflexes

(Based on the Multi-Society Task Force on Persistent Vegetative State, 1994. Medical aspects of the persistent vegetative state, Part 1. N Engl J Med 330, 1499–1508.)

worldwide. The etiology of the vegetative state in children can be classified into the following three broad groups of disorders:

1. Acute traumatic and nontraumatic brain injuries
2. Metabolic and degenerative disorders affecting the nervous system
3. Developmental malformations

The most common causes of acute brain injury leading to the vegetative state in children are head trauma and hypoxic-ischemic encephalopathies. The clinical course of evolution to a vegetative state after an acute injury usually begins with eyes-closed coma for several days to weeks, followed by the appearance of sleep-wake cycles.

The progression of many metabolic and degenerative nervous system disorders in children also may result in an irreversible vegetative state and slowly evolves over several months or years. Severe congenital central nervous system (CNS) malformations also can result in a vegetative state. At birth, anencephaly is the only malformation in which an infant can be diagnosed as being in a vegetative state. Other malformations such as hydranencephaly may result in a vegetative state, but because of the limitations of the neurologic examination, it is recommended that such infants not be diagnosed as being vegetative until there is certainty about the diagnosis.

Recovery from the VS/UWS in children depends on the etiology and is reviewed in more detail in the 1994 Multi-Society Task Force Report. In children with severe closed-head injuries who were vegetative 1 month after injury, follow up at 1 year found that 29% remained in a vegetative state, 9% had died, and 62% recovered consciousness.

In contrast, children in a nontraumatic vegetative state have a much poorer prognosis. At 1 year, most children remained in a vegetative state (65%) or died (22%); only 13% demonstrated recovery, usually to a severe disability. It was based on these data and consensus opinion that the Task Force came to the conclusions that, in children (as well as in adults), the vegetative state could be judged permanent 12 months after traumatic brain injury and 3 months after nontraumatic injury. This perspective has received general acceptance, although concerns have been raised about the certainty of diagnosis and whether there is a greater potential for patients to recover than previously realized. In addition, the number of patients in the Task Force report was small and points to the need to do studies with greater numbers of patients.

Children in a vegetative state have a shorter life expectancy. Those younger than 1 year of age had a median survival of 2.6 years; median survival of children aged 2 to 6 years was 5.2 years; and in children 7 to 18 years, the median survival was 7 years.

Minimally Conscious State

The minimally conscious state has been defined as a condition of severely altered consciousness in which the person demonstrates minimal but definite behavioral evidence of self- or environmental awareness. The term minimally conscious state may also be used to describe patients with degenerative disorders who are no longer functionally interactive but are not in the vegetative state. Criteria to diagnose the minimally conscious state are summarized in Box 101-2. Patients show wakefulness and are able to do the following:

1. Follow simple commands
2. Gesture or verbally give "yes" or "no" responses (regardless of accuracy)
3. Verbalize intelligibly
4. Perform movements or affective behaviors, which are not attributable to reflexive activity, in contingent relation to relevant environmental stimuli

Recently the MCS was divided into two subcategories depending on the complexity of behavioral responses: (1) MCS (− minus) in which patients have visual pursuit, can reach for objects, have orientation to noxious stimuli, and show contingent behavior); and (2) MCS (+ plus) in which patients can follow commands, have intentional communication, and intelligible verbalization. A third category, *emergent MCS*, has been defined in which the patients had emerged from a MCS—that is, they were functioning at a higher level and had functional communication (e.g., follow instructions) and functional object use (e.g., use a comb) (Gosseries et al., 2014). It is likely that the terms MCS−, MCS+, and emergent MCS are applicable to children, but there have been no reported studies in children using this terminology.

Based on limited literature on this disorder in adults, it is possible that children in a MCS, depending on the etiology of the insult, may have a better potential for neurologic recovery and a longer life expectancy than children in the vegetative

---

BOX 101-2 Diagnostic Criteria for the Minimally Conscious State

MCS*

Simple command obeying
Gestural or verbal yes-no responses (regardless of accuracy)
Intelligible verbalization

Purposeful behavior, including movements or effective behaviors that occur in contingent relation to relevant environmental stimuli and are not due to reflexive activity. Some behavioral examples of qualifying purposeful behaviors include the following:

- Appropriate smiling or crying in response to the linguistic or visual content of emotional but not to neutral topics or stimuli
- Vocalizations or gestures that occur in direct response to the linguistic content of questions
- Reaching for objects that demonstrates a clear relationship between object location and direction of reach
- Touching or holding objects in a manner that accommodates the size and shape of the object
- Pursuit eye movement or sustained fixation that occurs in direct response to moving or salient stimuli

MCS−

- Have visual pursuit
- Can reach for objects
- Have orientation to noxious stimuli
- Show contingent behavior

MCS+

In addition to what MCS− patients can do, MCS+ patients can also:

- Follow commands
- Have intentional communication and intelligible verbalization

(Adapted from Giacino, J.T. et al., 2002. The minimally conscious state. Definition and diagnostic criteria. Neurology 58, 349.) Criteria for MCS− and MCS+ are from Bruno, M.A., et al., 2012. Functional neuroanatomy underlying the clinical subcategorization of minimally conscious state patients. J Neurol 259(6), 1087–1098.)

---

state. However, studies have shown that mobility may be more important than consciousness in predicting survival.

Locked-in Syndrome

The locked-in syndrome refers to a condition in which patients retain consciousness and cognition but are unable to move or communicate because of severe paralysis. By definition, patients in coma or a vegetative state are unconscious and differ from patients in a locked-in syndrome, who retain awareness, although this difference may be difficult to determine. The locked-in syndrome is quite rare in children.

Akinetic Mutism

Akinetic mutism is a rare condition consisting of pathologically slowed or nearly absent bodily movement, accompanied by a similar loss of speech. It has been reported in children with brain tumors, bacterial and viral CNS infections, hydrocephalus, and occasionally as a postoperative phenomenon. Wakefulness and self-awareness are preserved but the level of mental function is reduced. The condition accompanies gradually developing or subacute, bilateral damage to the paramedian mesencephalon, basal diencephalon, or inferior frontal lobes. The long-term outlook for children with akinetic mutism is unknown.

Brain Death

Please see Chapter 107.

CONSCIOUSNESS RATING SCALES

The best known and most widely used scale is the Glasgow Coma Scale, which yields a score of 3 to 15, based on best response to stimuli in the these three categories: eye opening, verbal response, and motor response (Table 101-2). In its original form, the Glasgow Coma Scale was not developmentally suitable for assessment of newborns, infants, and younger children, and a variety of alternate scales have been proposed. The Pediatric Coma Scale makes minor changes in the verbal scale of the Glasgow Coma Scale and redefines the "best" score based on developmental and age-appropriate norms (Table 101-3). The Children's Coma Scale included pupillary reflexes, extraocular movements, and apnea in its categories, and is therefore substantially different from the Glasgow Coma (Table 101-4). The Glasgow Coma Scale—Modified for Children is also a valuable tool (Table 101-2) as is the Full Outline of UnResponsiveness (FOUR) Score Coma Scale (Table 101-5). The FOUR Score is divided into four categories (eye response, motor response, brainstem reflexes, and respiration) and provides a measure of consciousness. The Coma Recovery Scale-revised (CRS-R) is considered the best tool to use to assess adult patients with a DOC, but it has not been validated in children.

TABLE 101-2 Glasgow Coma Scale and Modification for Children

Glasgow Coma Scale	Score	Glasgow Coma Scale (Infant Modification)	Score
EYE OPENING (E)		EYE OPENING (E)	
Spontaneous	4	Spontaneous	4
To speech (to shout)	3	To speech (to shout)	3
To pain	2	To pain	2
None	1	None	1
VERBAL RESPONSE (V)		VERBAL RESPONSE, MODIFIED FOR INFANTS (V)	
Oriented	5	Babbles, coos appropriately	5
Confused conversation	4	Cries, but consolable	4
Inappropriate words	3	Cries inconsolably	3
Incomprehensible sounds	2	Grunts or moans to pain	2
None	1	None	1
MOTOR RESPONSE (M)		MOTOR RESPONSE (M)	
Obeys commands	6	Purposeful movements	6
Localizes pain	5	Localizes pain	5
Withdraws	4	Withdraws	4
Abnormal flexion	3	Abnormal flexion	3
Extensor response	2	Extensor response	2
None	1	None	1

TABLE 101-3 Pediatric Coma Scale

Response	Score
EYE OPENING	
Spontaneous	4
To speech	3
To pain	2
None	1
BEST VERBAL RESPONSE	
Oriented	5
Words	4
Vocal sounds	3
Cries	2
None	1
BEST MOTOR RESPONSE	
Obeys commands	5
Localizes pain	4
Flexion to pain	3
Extension to pain	2
None	1
NORMAL AGGREGATE SCORE	
Birth to 6 months	9
Less than 6–12 months	11
Less than 1–2 years	12
Less than 2–5 years	13
More than 5 years	14

TABLE 101-4 Children's Coma Scale

Sign	Score
OCULAR RESPONSE	
Pursuit	4
Extraocular movement intact, pupils react appropriately	3
Fixed pupils or extraocular movement impaired	2
Fixed pupils and extraocular movement paralyzed	1
VERBAL RESPONSE	
Cries	3
Spontaneous respiration	2
Apneic	1
MOTOR RESPONSE	
Flexes and extends	4
Withdraws from painful stimuli	3
Hypertonic	2
Flaccid	1
Best Total Score	11

TABLE 101-5 "FOUR" Score Coma Scale

Category and Response	Score
EYE RESPONSE	
Eyelids open or opened, tracking or blinking to command	4
Eyelids open but not tracking	3
Eyelids closed, opens to loud voice, not tracking	2
Eyelids closed, opens to pain, not tracking	1
Eyelids remain closed with pain	0
MOTOR RESPONSE	
Thumbs up, fist, or peace sign to command	4
Localizing to pain	3
Flexion response to pain	2
Extensor posturing	1
No response to pain or generalized myoclonus status epilepticus	0
BRAINSTEM REFLEXES	
Pupil and corneal reflexes present	4
One pupil wide and fixed	3
Pupil or corneal reflexes absent	2
Pupil and corneal reflexes absent	1
Absent pupil, corneal, and cough reflex	0
RESPIRATION	
Not intubated, regular breathing pattern	4
Not intubated, Cheyne–Stokes breathing pattern	3
Not intubated, irregular breathing pattern	2
Breathes higher than ventilator rate	1
Breathes at ventilator rate or apnea	0

(With permission from Wijdicks, E., et al., 2005. Validation of a new Coma Scale: The FOUR Score. Annals of Neurology 58[4], 584–593.)

PATHOPHYSIOLOGY

 See online chapter and also Chapters 102, 103, and 104.

ETIOLOGIES

A more relevant and practical classification for the etiology of impairment of consciousness and coma in children produces three distinct but overlapping categories (Box 101-3):

1. Infectious or inflammatory
2. Structural
3. Metabolic, toxic, or nutritional

Bacterial, viral, rickettsial, or protozoan infections of the CNS may cause conscious alteration by direct involvement of brain parenchyma, interference with blood flow, production of cerebral edema with resulting increased intracranial pressure, and increasing metabolic activity beyond metabolic substrate availability. Viral infections are more likely to involve brain parenchyma (encephalitis). The meningitis produced by bacterial infections may produce injury as a result of large blood vessel occlusion, microvascular inflammation, or disturbance of cerebral autoregulation. Cerebral edema, focal mass or abscess, and hydrocephalus as a result of intracranial infection

may produce injury by reducing cerebral blood flow or leading to herniation.

Structural causes of consciousness impairment or coma include intracranial neoplasm, infectious space-occupying lesion (abscess, tuberculoma), nonaccidental and accidental trauma, cerebral infarction or hemorrhage, and hydrocephalus. These conditions are described in detail in other chapters.

Metabolic and toxic causes of impaired consciousness or coma include hypoxic-ischemic injury (focal or generalized), electrolyte abnormality, endocrinopathy, hepatic or renal failure, and inherited disorders, including organic and aminoacidurias, urea cycle disorders, mitochondrial disorders, and porphyria. Paroxysmal disorders such as uncontrolled seizures, nonconvulsive status epilepticus, or migraine may produce changes in consciousness that may be episodic. The diagnosis, pathophysiology, and treatment of specific disorders are reviewed elsewhere in this book. Children with psychiatric disorders such as conversion, panic, or anxiety disorders may present with neurologic symptoms including genuine or apparent impairment of consciousness. Nutritional causes of alteration of consciousness or coma are relatively uncommon in and are reviewed in Chapters 46 and 47.

EVALUATION

Coma is a medical and neurologic emergency requiring immediate consideration of key issues, including immediate life support, identification of the cause of coma, and institution of specific therapy. These critical issues will be reviewed in sequence. As accidental and nonaccidental traumatic brain injury (Chapters 102, 103), global hypoxic-ischemic injury (Chapter 104) and disorders associated with increased intracranial pressure (Chapter 105) are the most common conditions causing coma in children; the reader is referred to these chapters for additional discussion.

Clinical Evaluation

The ABCs of basic life support (immediate life support—airway, breathing, and circulation) must be evaluated and managed as an emergency (see online chapter).

Identification of Cause

Accurate and rapid identification of the cause of coma is important to direct specific treatment. The history and physical examination are the basis for identification of the cause of coma.

History

Coma may manifest as the progression of a known underlying illness, unpredictable consequence, or complication of a known disease, or it may be the result of a totally unexpected event or illness. Sudden onset of coma suggests convulsions or intracranial hemorrhage. Coma preceded by sleepiness or unsteadiness suggests ingestion of a drug or toxin. Fever is typical when coma is due to an infectious process. A history of headache may suggest elevated intracranial pressure. In patients who were in coma after a traumatic brain injury and in whom CT scanning was normal or could not explain the severity of clinical symptoms, MRI should be performed to evaluate for diffuse axonal injury.

General Physical Examination

See online chapter and Chapters 102 to 104.

BOX 101-3 Etiologies of Impaired Consciousness and Coma

Infectious or Inflammatory
A. Infectious
    Bacterial meningitis
    Viral encephalitis
    Rickettsial infection
    Protozoan infection
    Helminth infestation
B. Inflammatory
    Sepsis-associated encephalopathy
    Vasculitis, collagen vascular disorders
    Demyelination
    Acute disseminated encephalomyelitis
    Multiple sclerosis
Structural
A. Traumatic
    Concussion
    Cerebral contusion
    Epidural hematoma or effusion
    Intracerebral hematoma
    Diffuse axonal injury
    Abusive head trauma
B. Neoplasms
C. Vascular Disease
    Cerebral infarction
    • Thrombosis
    • Embolism
    • Venous sinus thrombosis
    Cerebral hemorrhage
    • Subarachnoid hemorrhage
    • Arteriovenous malformation
    • Aneurysm
    Congenital abnormality or dysplasia of vascular supply
    Trauma to carotid or vertebral arteries in the neck
D. Focal Infection
    Abscess
    Cerebritis
E. Hydrocephalus
Metabolic, Nutritional, or Toxic
A. Hypoxic-Ischemic Encephalopathy
    Shock
    Cardiac or pulmonary failure

Near-drowning
Carbon monoxide poisoning
Cyanide poisoning
Strangulation
B. Metabolic Disorders
    Sarcoidosis
    Hypoglycemia
    Fluid and electrolyte imbalance
    Endocrine disorders
    With acidosis
    • Diabetic ketoacidosis
    • Aminoacidemias
    • Organic acidemias
    With hyperammonemia
    • Hepatic encephalopathy
    • Urea cycle disorders
    • Disorders of fatty acid metabolism
    • Reye's syndrome
    • Valproic acid encephalopathy
    Uremia
    Porphyria
    Mitochondrial disorders
    Leigh's syndrome
C. Nutritional
    Thiamine deficiency
    Niacin or nicotinic acid deficiency
    Pyridoxine dependency
    Folate and B12 deficiency
D. Exogenous Toxins and Poisons
    Alcohol intoxication
    Overthe-counter medications
    Prescription medications (oral and ophthalmic)
    Herbal treatments
    Heavy-metal poisoning
    Mushroom and plant intoxication
    Illegal drugs
    Industrial agents
E. Hypertensive Encephalopathy
F. Burn Encephalopathy

Neurologic Examination

The neurologic examination is of paramount importance in assessing the comatose patient. Examination of the fundi, pupillary size and reactivity, eye movement control, corneal reflexes, motor responses, body posture, and the presence or absence of meningeal signs gives important information. Localization may be aided by detailed understanding of brainstem pathways involved in the eye examination. Funduscopic examination offers important clues about the etiology of coma, including papilledema and retinal hemorrhages. See online chapter and Chapters 102 to 104. Passive resistance to neck flexion suggests meningeal irritation, tonsillar herniation, or craniocervical trauma.

Pupillary reactivity can be elicited by shining a light on the eye or by opening and closing the eyelid. An abnormality of the pupillary light reflex suggests midbrain dysfunction. With unilateral loss of visual acuity, the opposite pupil may dilate when the light is moved from the unaffected to the affected side. This reaction results from a defect in the afferent limb of the reflex arc on the affected side. Most metabolic disorders

and drug ingestions produce symmetrically small pupils that retain some reactivity to light. Severe hypoxic-ischemic injury produces symmetric dilated pupils that may not respond to light. Structural or mass lesions of the cerebral hemispheres typically do not produce pupillary abnormalities unless herniation occurs. Midbrain injuries may interrupt both sympathetic and parasympathetic pupillary innervations, producing midposition unresponsive pupils.

Unilateral stimulation of the frontal gaze center produces conjugate eye deviation to the opposite side and can be produced by seizure activity or other unilateral irritating stimuli. Unilateral injury, destruction, or metabolic exhaustion of the frontal gaze center produces conjugate deviation toward the affected side.

The oculocephalic maneuver is performed by moving the head side to side or vertically and should only be performed when there is certainty that there is no cervical spine injury or abnormality. A positive oculocephalic response consists of conjugate deviation of the eyes in the direction opposite head movement. Absence of a positive oculocephalic response may be seen in structural abnormalities of the brainstem, in which it may be asymmetric, and in metabolic-toxic encephalopathies, in which it is almost always symmetric.

Caloric testing or oculovestibular responses are obtained by irrigating one or both external ear canals with warm and cold water and should only be performed when the external canal is clean and the tympanic membrane intact. The usual protocol for unconscious patients involves cold-water irrigation with the head elevated 30 degrees from the horizontal, which induces convection currents in the endolymphatic fluid of the labyrinth. The resulting vestibular nuclei stimulation affects the ipsilateral paramedian pontine reticular formation-abducens nuclear complex and also the contralateral oculomotor and trochlear nuclei through the medial longitudinal fasciculus. In awake patients, cold-water irrigation produces a lateral nystagmus, with the quick phase away from the stimulated ear. Warm-water stimulation has the opposite effect. This finding gives rise to the mnemonic COWS (cold opposite, warm same). In the unconscious patient, however, the quick phase is lost, and slow tonic deviation is noted toward the irrigated ear. Unilateral or asymmetric caloric responses suggest a brainstem structural abnormality, whereas bilateral absence can be seen in metabolic, as well as structural, abnormalities.

The corneal reflex consists of closure of the eyelid, elicited by gently touching the cornea with a suitable stimulus. An absent response suggests abnormal afferent or trigeminal input or bilateral pontine involvement. A contralateral blink response suggests intact sensory input through the fifth cranial nerve, whereas an abnormal motor limb response on the ipsilateral side is more consistent with an ipsilateral structural abnormality. Metabolic lesions typically produce bilateral loss of the response. Absence of the corneal reflex must be interpreted with caution in the presence of conjunctival edema or injury.

Observation of spontaneous movement and motor responses to stimulation is an important clue in the assessment of coma and localization of the level of injury or lesion. Asymmetric involvement is a hallmark of structural abnormality. Unilateral cortical or subcortical structural lesions may cause contralateral weakness. Bilateral absence of movement or tone (flaccidity) occurs in metabolic-toxic encephalopathies such as drug intoxications and in disruption of brainstem-cortical interconnections higher than the pontomedullary junction. Flaccidity resulting from spinal cord injuries or neuromuscular paralysis is not associated with coma unless other injuries exist.

Posturing may occur spontaneously or in response to stimulation. Decorticate posturing involves flexion of the upper extremities and extension of the lower extremities and usually indicates cortical or subcortical abnormalities with preservation of brainstem function. Decerebrate posturing involves extension of all extremities with internal rotation and may be seen with metabolic-toxic disorders or midbrain compression.

BRAIN HERNIATION

Within the skull are unique dural reflections that divide the intracranial contents into compartments. The falx cerebri lies between the cerebral hemispheres, and the tentorium cerebelli separates anterior fossa structures (cerebral hemispheres and diencephalon) from posterior structures (brainstem and cerebellum). The opening in the tentorium through which the midbrain passes is called the tentorial notch. Focal or generalized lesions, which produce mass effect or increased intracranial pressure, may produce one of the three brain herniation syndromes based on squeezing of brain structures over or through the tentorium or through the foramen magnum.

Historical Perspective

See online chapter.

Herniation Syndromes

Three herniation syndromes are briefly presented and are discussed in detail in Chapter 102.

Uncal Herniation

Uncal herniation refers to the medial displacement of the uncal gyrus of the temporal lobe over the free lateral edge of the tentorium, associated with an asymmetric supratentorial mass or edema. The uncal gyrus (uncus) comes in direct contact with the oculomotor nerve, producing ipsilateral pupillary dilatation and external ophthalmoplegia. Radiologic studies, however, emphasize horizontal shift of the mesencephalon away from the lesion as the cause of early consciousness alteration because the ambient cistern and prepontine cistern are widened ipsilaterally. The ipsilateral pupillary dilation is due to stretch of the oculomotor nerve over the clivus.

There is early ipsilateral pupillary dilation with sluggish reactivity to light because of interruption of parasympathetic innervation to the pupil, producing unopposed sympathetic response (dilatation). Further, horizontal displacement of the upper brainstem may cause the contralateral cerebral peduncle to be pressed against the opposite tentorial edge and produce hemiparesis ipsilateral to the lesion (and ipsilateral to the enlarged pupil). False localization may occur if the uncus compresses the ipsilateral cerebral peduncle, producing contralateral hemiparesis, or if the contralateral oculomotor nerve is caught between the mesencephalon and the edge of the tentorium, producing contralateral pupillary dilation and external ophthalmoplegia. Uncal herniation is often associated with the central or transtentorial downward herniation syndrome.

Central or Transtentorial Downward Herniation

With generalized increases in intracranial pressure, there is gradual downward displacement of the diencephalon (thalamus and hypothalamus) through the tentorium cerebelli, producing progressive compression and ischemia of the brainstem from mesencephalon (rostral brainstem) to medulla (caudal brainstem). In the diencephalic stage, patients do not follow instructions but will localize to noxious stimuli and have small reactive pupils and preserved oculocephalic and oculovestibular reflexes. Respiration may be regular, with yawns or sighs, or Cheyne-Stokes respirations may appear. In the midbrain-upper pons stage, patients have decerebrate rigidity or no movement, midposition pupils that may be irregular in shape and demonstrate no reactivity, and abnormal or absent oculocephalic and oculovestibular reflexes. Patients usually hyperventilate. In the lower pontine-medullary stage, there is no spontaneous motor activity or activity in response to stimuli, midposition fixed pupils, absent oculocephalic and oculovestibular reflexes, and shallow and rapid or slow and irregular (ataxic) respirations. The lower extremities may withdraw to plantar stimulation. Finally, in the medullary stage, there is generalized flaccid tone, absence of pupillary reflexes and ocular movements, further slowing and irregularity of respiration, and ultimately death.

Infratentorial (Cerebellar) Herniation Syndromes

Space-occupying lesions in the posterior fossa can produce upward herniation of brainstem structures through the tentorial notch and may result in obstructive hydrocephalus, brainstem ischemia, and death. Progressive alteration of consciousness or coma, associated with miotic pupils, gaze paresis, decerebrate posturing, and asymmetric or absent caloric response with relative preservation of respiration, suggests upward transtentorial herniation.

Downward herniation of the cerebellum and medulla at the foramen magnum may cause apnea and death because of pressure on medullary respiratory centers. The lesions that cause cerebellar herniation in children are often subacute or chronic and are discovered before herniation as a result of widespread use of neuroimaging.

In children with meningitis, the cerebellar pressure cone effect has been implicated as a cause of death after lumbar puncture, even with a normal CT scan of the head. In cases of suspected bacterial meningitis, lumbar puncture should be avoided if there is evidence of increased intracranial pressure or early coning. When lumbar puncture is performed, measurement of opening pressure is essential to allow early treatment if increased intracranial pressure persists.

DIAGNOSTIC TESTING

All patients with significant impairment of consciousness or coma should have an immediate blood glucose finger stick determination and should have blood drawn for a chemistry profile, complete blood count, and arterial blood gas analysis. The blood chemistry profile should minimally include glucose, sodium, potassium, blood urea nitrogen, calcium, magnesium, and ammonia. When infection is suspected, blood and urine cultures should be obtained.

Lumbar puncture should be performed when there is a suggestion of infection of the CNS, with or without fever. Depending on the clinical findings and evaluation, CT needs to be performed before the lumbar puncture. When medically stable, all patients with impairment of consciousness of undetermined etiology should have a CT performed as rapidly as possible. In children with closed-head injury, CT or preferably MRI may be critical in identifying the specific cause of impaired loss of consciousness.

The EEG is essential to diagnose clinically inapparent status epilepticus. Certain EEG patterns such as periodic lateralized epileptiform discharges may suggest herpes simplex encephalitis. The EEG also is useful in the serial reassessment and evaluation of patients in status epilepticus or persistent coma, as well as in patients requiring pharmacologic paralysis or sedation. See Chapters 102 to 104.

TREATMENT

Treatment requires scrupulous attention to basic principles while definitive diagnostic tests are obtained and therapy initiated. Specific etiologies of many individual causes of disordered consciousness are listed in Box 101-3 and are reviewed by specific diagnostic category in other sections of this book. The following principles of management are similar in most patients and are described here (see Box 101-4):

1. Maintain Airway, Oxygenation. and Ventilation

Maintenance of an adequate airway remains one of the most important principles in the management of children with altered states of consciousness and coma. It is important to ensure that cervical spine injuries are not worsened in the process of managing a patient's respiratory problems. Monitoring adequacy of oxygenation with pulse oximetry and providing supplemental oxygen as needed are important.

2. Maintain Circulation

To maintain cardiovascular function, intravascular access is critical and should be provided. Fluid resuscitation or support with vasoactive drugs may be needed.

3. Administer Glucose

Glucose administration is recommended if the glucose levels reveal an abnormally low value. All other therapies are superfluous when oxygen and glucose are not delivered to neurons and toxic metabolites are not removed.

4. Correct Acid-Base and Electrolyte Imbalance

Electrolyte imbalance is often mediated by inappropriate antidiuretic hormone secretion. Inappropriate administration of fluids may worsen this situation. More commonly, hyponatremia, hypernatremia, hypocalcemia, or hypomagnesemia occur in conjunction with systemic illness and be the cause of coma.

5. Consider Specific Antidotes

Naloxone is available for treatment when an opiate overdose occurs. Physostigmine may reverse CNS and cardiac effects of anticholinergic agents but may cause nonspecific CNS stimulation or seizures. Flumazenil, a benzodiazepine receptor antagonist, may be valuable in such patients.

6. Reduce Increased Intracranial Pressure

See Chapter 105.

7. Stop Seizures

Treatment of status epilepticus and other seizure emergencies is discussed in Chapter 69. It is always important to consider seizures, even when there are no obvious outward seizure manifestations. Continuous bedside EEG monitoring is now commonly used for this purpose.

8. Treat Infection

Underlying infectious processes should be treated if specific treatment is available. When there is concern about focally elevated intracranial pressure, it may be appropriate to start antibiotic therapy for meningitis or antiviral therapy for encephalitis before lumbar puncture.

9. Adjust Body Temperature

Usually, normal body temperature is best for recovery and prevention of acidosis. Patients with fever should have appropriate antipyretic agents administered. The use of hypothermia is being reevaluated as a potential treatment for coma. Recent studies have shown that therapeutic hypothermia improves outcomes in neonates with hypoxic ischemic injury (Chapter 19) but not in older children with traumatic (Chapter 102) or hypoxic-ischemic injuries (Chapter 104).

10. Manage Agitation

Agitation may increase intracranial pressure and make it difficult to control respiration. The decision to sedate may make serial neurologic examination difficult as a measure of change in a patient's status. In these circumstances, EEG may be valuable.

11. Treatment of Chronic Impairments

The previously mentioned management principles relate to the acute care of patients in coma, but many of the principles also apply to patients who do not fully regain consciousness and have long-term functional disabilities. Other chapters in this book review overall principles of neurorehabilitation (Chapter 162) and more specifically management after accidental (Chapter 102) and nonaccidental (Chapter 103) traumatic brain injury and after global hypoxic-ischemic brain injury (Chapter 104).

There are no pharmacologic agents that have undergone appropriate clinical trials and subsequently been approved for use in children with DOCs. In adults, amantadine and zolpidem have been shown to improve awareness. One small case series involving seven children with DOCs has been reported and demonstrated safety but no efficacy. Neuromodulation is another approach gaining increasing interest.

MONITORING OF THE COMATOSE PATIENT

After initiation of treatment, it is necessary to reevaluate serially the patient's condition and effectiveness of intervention. The neurologic examination is the gold standard for evaluation and reevaluation, but often is significantly modified by iatrogenic intervention such as mechanical ventilation, sedation, and paralysis. Many clinical neurophysiology monitors are available to improve critical care monitoring; some are in more widespread use than others.

Traditionally, the EEG has been used to identify presence of or risk for seizures and has additive value in that certain patterns may suggest specific pathology such as triphasic waves in metabolic causes of coma and periodic lateralized epileptiform discharges in focal injury and infection. Continuous EEG monitoring may be very helpful in children.

EEG reactivity to sensory stimulation is considered a favorable sign in coma recovery. EEG has the advantage of ready availability in most centers and is usually definitive in the evaluation for ongoing seizures. These and other issues related to the use of EEG for outcome prediction are discussed in other parts of this book and in the online chapter.

Sensory-evoked potentials allow assessment of the integrity of visual, auditory, and somatosensory pathways in the unconscious patient. Somatosensory-evoked potentials are relatively resistant to sedation effect and are useful in predicting outcome in comatose patients. Visual-evoked potentials have not been as valuable. Brainstem auditory-evoked potentials are valuable for monitoring brainstem function but do not predict cortical function. Middle latency auditory-evoked potentials have cortical representation and have been shown to improve coma outcome prediction in adults.

Measurement of cerebral blood flow is a direct way to determine delivery of essential metabolic substrate to the brain but is not useful for continuous monitoring. Brain-tissue PO_2 measurement, however, is suitable for continuous monitoring. Low brain-tissue PO_2, as a measure of cerebral hypoxia, is predictive of poor neurologic outcome and is an important independent measurement parameter in adults with severe traumatic brain injury. Monitoring of brain tissue PO_2 may also allow early detection of critical and potentially irreversible worsening, and allow measurement of intervention effect on a continuous basis.

Local sampling of energy substrates by microdialysis during ischemia is feasible and allows measurement of glucose, lactate, pyruvate, and glutamate in brain tissue serially over time. Microdialysis measurements have thus far only been applied in children for monitoring of severe traumatic brain injury.

Near-infrared spectroscopy (NIRS) noninvasively monitors brain-tissue oxygenation by measuring the distinct absorption spectra of oxygenated and deoxygenated hemoglobin in the frontal cortex. Cerebral oxygenation measured by NIRS also

has been found to be of some value in pediatric patients being monitored for seizures in the pediatric intensive care unit and in patients being evaluated in the epilepsy monitoring unit, in which it was shown that preictal increases in cerebral oxygenation suggested perfusion-metabolism mismatch during seizure activity. The use of NIRS to monitor brain-tissue oxygenation has not been studied extensively in children, except in surgery for congenital heart defects.

OUTCOME MEASUREMENT

When consciousness is impaired, outcome is related to the etiology of the insult and rapid identification and treatment of the underlying cause. Outcome studies in childhood coma are available for traumatic and nontraumatic causes, and typically emphasize predictive value of signs and symptoms at the time of initial medical intervention. These studies are described in detail in Chapters 102 to 104.

A commonly used and widely accepted measurement of outcome after severe closed-head injury is the Glasgow Outcome Scale. The Glasgow Outcome Scale has the following five broad outcome categories:

1. Death
2. Persistent vegetative state
3. Severe disability (conscious but disabled)
4. Moderate disability (disabled but independent)
5. Good recovery

The Glasgow Outcome Scale heavily emphasizes functional independence in mobility, transportation, and self-care but is limited in its ability to quantify impairments related to social skills and emotional and cognitive dysfunction.

Early studies using the Glasgow Outcome Scale as an outcome measure after closed-head injury reported that patients advance to the highest functional level by 6 months after injury. Meaningful recovery may occur for months to years after injury.

Another scoring system, the Pediatric Cerebral Performance Category Scale is a modified form of the Glasgow Outcome Scale. This six-point outcome scoring system has been validated in children and also been shown to correlate with neuropsychological test scores. The score has six categories and the numbering system is the reverse of the GOS score—that is, a lower number indicates a better functional outcome:

1. Normal—able to perform all age-appropriate activities
2. Mild disability—conscious, alert, and able to interact at an age-appropriate level, but may have a mild neurologic deficit
3. Moderate disability—conscious, sufficient cerebral function for most age-appropriate independent activities
4. Severe disability—conscious, dependent on others for daily support because of impaired brain function
5. Persistent vegetative state
6. Death

Another scoring system is the King's Outcome Scale for Childhood Head Injury (KOSCHI). The KOSCHI expands the five-category Glasgow Outcome Scale to provide increased sensitivity at the milder end of the disability range (Table 101-6). The scale is easy to use and reliable and is very helpful in differentiating children with milder outcomes into subcategories.

The Disability Rating Scale consists of eight items divided into four categories:

1. Arousability and awareness (best eye-opening, verbal, and motor response)
2. Cognitive ability for self-care activities (feeding, toileting, and grooming)

TABLE 101-6 King's Outcome Scale for Childhood Head Injury (KOSCHI)

	Category	Definition
1	Death	
2	Vegetative	The child is breathing spontaneously and may have sleep–wake cycles. He may have nonpurposeful or reflex movements of limbs or eyes. There is no evidence of ability to communicate verbally or nonverbally, or to respond to commands
3	Severe disability	The child is at least intermittently able to move part of the body/eyes to command or make purposeful spontaneous movements; e.g., confused child pulling at nasogastric tube, lashing out at caregivers, rolling over in bed. May be fully conscious and able to communicate but not yet able to carry out any self-care activities, such as feeding Implies a continuing high level of dependency, but the child can assist in daily activities; e.g., can feed self or walk with assistance or help to place items of clothing. Such a child is fully conscious but may still have a degree of posttraumatic amnesia
4	Moderate disability	The child is mostly independent but needs a degree of supervision/actual help for physical or behavioral problems. Such a child has overt problems; e.g., a 12-year-old with moderate hemiplegia and dyspraxia, insecure on stairs or needing help with dressing The child is age-appropriately independent but has residual problems with learning/behavior or neurologic sequelae affecting function. He probably should have special needs assistance but his special needs may not have been recognized/met. Children with symptoms of posttraumatic stress are likely to fall into this category
5	Good recovery	This should only be assigned if the head injury has resulted in a new condition that does not interfere with the child's well-being and/or functioning; e.g., Minor headaches not interfering with social or school functioning Abnormalities on brain scan without any detectable new problem Prophylactic anticonvulsants in the absence of clinical seizures Unsightly scarring of face/head likely to need cosmetic surgery at some stage Mild neurologic asymmetry but no evidence of effect on function of limb. Includes isolated change in hand dominance in young child Implies that the information available is that the child has made a complete recovery with no detectable sequelae from the head injury.

(With permission from Crouchman, M., et al., 2001. A practical outcome scale for pediatric head injury. Arch Dis Child 84, 120–124.)

3. Physical dependence on others
4. Psychosocial adaptability for work or school

The Functional Independence Measure and its pediatric counterpart, the Wee Functional Independence Measure (WeeFIM), further refine outcome assessment using six items and 18 categories. The WeeFIM items and categories are as follows:

1. Self-care (eating, grooming, bathing, dressing—upper body, dressing—lower body, toileting)
2. Sphincter control (bladder and bowel)
3. Mobility/transfer (chair or wheelchair, toilet, tub, shower)
4. Locomotion (walking, wheelchair, crawling, stairs)
5. Communication (auditory and visual comprehension, verbal and nonverbal expression)
6. Social cognition (social interaction, problem solving, memory)

The Pediatric Evaluation of Disabilities Inventory measures both capability and performance of multiple functional activities in three areas:

1. Self-care
2. Mobility
3. Social function

This score is designed for use from 6 months to 7 years of age but is appropriate for older children whose functional level is within the intended age range.

The WeeFIM and the Pediatric Evaluation of Disabilities Inventory are sensitive measures of functional outcome and are suitable for inpatient rehabilitation monitoring and long-term outpatient follow up. They are two of the most commonly used functional outcome measures in children and are superior to the Glasgow Outcome Scale and its pediatric variants.

The School Functional Assessment was developed to measure performance of functional tasks that are important for participation in an elementary school level program. The School Functional Assessment evaluates:

A. Ability to participate in major school activity settings
B. Support necessary to participate effectively in an education program
C. Performance of specific school-related functional activities

The Barthel Index is commonly used as a prognostic indicator in adult clinical stroke trials. It has functional disability categories (Table 101-7) that lend themselves to use in children who are emerging from coma, but it has not been studied in detail.

Neuropsychological assessment in children with acute brain injuries is discussed in more detail in Chapters 10, 162 and 168.

PROGNOSIS
Traumatic Injury

Children who survive traumatic injury have a better prognosis than children who suffer a global hypoxic-ischemic injury. In a study of 127 children said to be in the persistent vegetative state for at least 30 days, 84% of the traumatic brain injury group, but only 55% of the hypoxic-ischemic injury group, improved beyond the vegetative state. Up to 80% to 90% of children with severe traumatic brain injury have good outcomes or recover to a moderate disability, based on studies using the Glasgow Outcome Scale score. See previously mentioned information, the online chapter, and Chapters 102 and 103.

TABLE 101-7 Barthel Score

Activity	Score
Feeding	
0 = unable; 5 = needs help cutting, spreading butter, etc., or requires modified diet; 10 = independent	0, 5, 10
Bathing	
0 = dependent; 5 = independent (or in shower)	0, 5
Grooming	
0 = needs to help with personal care; 5 = independent face/hair/teeth/shaving (implements provided)	0, 5
Dressing	
0 = dependent; 5 = needs help but can do about half unaided; 10 = independent (including buttons, zippers, laces, etc.)	0, 5,10
Bowels	
0 = incontinent (or needs to be given enemas); 5 = occasional accident; 10 = continent	0, 5, 10
Bladder	
0 = incontinent, or catheterized and unable to manage alone; 5 = occasional accident; 10 = continent	0, 5, 10
Toilet use	
0 = dependent; 5 = needs some help, but can do something alone; 10 = independent (on and off, dressing, wiping)	0, 5, 10
Transfers (bed to chair and back)	
0 = unable, no sitting balance; 5 = major help (one or two people, physical), can sit; 10 = minor help (verbal or physical); 15 = independent	0, 5, 10, 15
Mobility (on level surfaces)	
0 = immobile or <50 yards; 5 = wheelchair-independent, including corners, >50 yards; 10 = walks with help of one person (verbal or physical) >50 yards; 15 = independent (but may use any aid; e.g., stick) >50 yards	0, 5, 10, 15
Stairs	
0 = unable; 5 = needs help (verbal, physical, carrying aid); 10 = independent	0, 5
Total (0–100)	

(With permission from Jöhnk, K., et al., 1999. Assessment of sensorimotor functions after traumatic brain injury (TBI) in childhood—methodological aspects. Restor Neurol Neurosci 14(2–3), 143.)

Nontraumatic Injury

Outcome after coma resulting from nontraumatic causes is poor but better than that seen in adults. In a cohort of 104 children ranging in age from 1 month to 17 years with nontraumatic coma, 32% died, 50% were normal, and the remaining 18% had mild to severe handicaps. In another retrospective study of nontraumatic coma (278 children aged 1 month to 16 years), 12-month follow up found that the overall mortality rate was 46%, and the etiology-specific mortality rate varied from 3% (intoxication) to 84% (accident). The overall incidence of moderate to severe disability was 70%. See online chapter and Chapter 104.

Clinical Neurophysiology

In the comatose patient, clinical neurophysiology evaluation (EEG, somatosensory-evoked potential) is the most valuable method for prediction of survival, brain death, and functional recovery. There are, however, a few reports of contrary findings such as normal somatosensory-evoked potentials in a child in a vegetative state after near-drowning. Therefore the neurophysiology assessment is used as an adjunct to the clinical examination and other outcome predictors. Also see Chapters 13 and 102 to 104.

Neuroimaging

MRI has been explored to help evaluate patients with disorders of consciousness and is reviewed in depth in Chapters 12 and 102 to 104. Several studies also have indicated the prognostic value of proton MR spectroscopy, susceptibility-weighted imaging, and diffusion tensor imaging in children with CNS insult or injury.

CONCLUSIONS

Altered states of consciousness in pediatric patients are urgent situations, and coma is a medical emergency requiring rapid and organized intervention. Specific diagnoses must be treated appropriately, but there are key general principles to management of impaired consciousness and coma that apply in all situations.

The outcome for children with coma is better than for adults. Even with the best and most appropriate care, some children die, some survive on mechanical ventilation and become brain-dead, and some survive beyond mechanical ventilation and have minimal consciousness, severe disability, or remain in a vegetative state. Decisions concerning basic life sustenance, type and location of care, and need for rehabilitation should take into consideration the type of injury, time from injury, recovery potential, family wishes, and appropriate ethical guidelines and standards. Application of fMRI and neurophysiological testing will help provide a better understanding of the neural correlates of consciousness and hopefully lead to development of novel strategies to improve outcomes in these severely injured children.

Acknowledgment

This chapter is based on the chapter published in the previous edition that was coauthored by Dr. Donald Taylor.

REFERENCES

The complete list of references for this chapter is available in the e-book at www.expertconsult.com.
   See inside cover for registration details.

SELECTED REFERENCES

Andrews-Hanna, J.R., Smallwood, J., Spreng, R.N., 2014. The default network and self-generated thought: component processes, dynamic control, and clinical relevance. Ann. N. Y. Acad. Sci. 1316, 29–52.

Demertzi, A., Gómez, F., Crone, J.S., et al., 2014. Multiple fMRI system-level baseline connectivity is disrupted in patients with consciousness alterations. Cortex 52, 35–46.

Di Perri, C., Thibaut, A., Heine, L., et al., 2014. Measuring consciousness in coma and related states. World J. Radiol. 6 (8), 589–597.

Giacino, J.T., Fins, J.J., Laureys, S., et al., 2014. Disorders of consciousness after acquired brain injury: the state of the science. Nat. Rev. Neurol. 10 (2), 99–114.

Gosseries, O., Di, H., Laureys, S., et al., 2014. Measuring consciousness in severely damaged brains. Annu. Rev. Neurosci. 37, 457–478.

Harrison, A.H., Connolly, J.F., 2013. Finding a way in: a review and practical evaluation of fMRI and EEG for detection and assessment in disorders of consciousness. Neurosci. Biobehav. Rev. 37 (8), 1403–1419.

Laureys, S., 2005. The neural correlate of (un)awareness: lessons from the vegetative state. Trends Cogn. Sci. 9 (12), 556–559.

Laureys, S., Celesia, G.G., Cohadon, F., et al.; European Task Force on Disorders of Consciousness, 2010. Unresponsive wakefulness syndrome: a new name for the vegetative state or apallic syndrome. BMC Med. 8, 68.

Menon, V., 2015. Salience Network. In: Toga, A.W. (Ed.), Brain Mapping: An Encyclopedic Reference, vol. 2. Academic Press: Elsevier, pp. 597–611.

The Multi-Society Task Force on PVS, 1994. Medical aspects of the persistent vegetative state, Part 1. N. Eng. J. Med. 330, 1499–1508.

The Multi-Society Task Force on PVS, 1994. Medical aspects of the persistent vegetative state, Part 2. N. Eng. J. Med. 330, 1509–1572.

Osborne, N.R., Owen, A.M., Fernández-Espejo, D., 2015. The dissociation between command following and communication in disorders of consciousness: an fMRI study in healthy subjects. Front. Hum. Neurosci. 9, 493.

Qin, P., Wu, X., Huang, Z., et al., 2015. How are different neural networks related to consciousness? Ann. Neurol. 78 (4), 594–605.

E-BOOK FIGURES AND TABLES

The following figures and tables are available in the e-book at www.expertconsult.com. See inside cover for registration details.

Box 101-4 Treatment goals for patients with impaired consciousness and coma.

102 Traumatic Brain Injury in Children

Jason T. Lerner and Christopher C. Giza

 An expanded version of this chapter is available on www.expertconsult.com. See inside cover for registration details.

INTRODUCTION AND BACKGROUND
Epidemiology of Pediatric Traumatic Brain Injury

Traumatic brain injury (TBI) is a major cause of death and disability in the pediatric population and has been identified as a significant public health problem in the United States and worldwide. Age-related incidence rates for TBI in children have been estimated to be as high as 670 per 100,000 when head injuries of all severities are included. In the developing world, TBI as a result of traffic accidents and other causes is predicted to surpass many diseases as a cause of mortality. Overall, TBI is responsible for the majority of trauma-related death and hospitalization. Moderate and severe pediatric TBI has been associated with long-standing impairments, often borne throughout the person's lifetime. Fortunately, the majority of all TBI is considered mild; however, recent studies suggest that even mild pediatric TBI, particularly if repetitive, may have adverse long-term functional consequences. Despite these facts, no specific treatment standards exist for pediatric TBI, either acutely or during recovery. A recent review of guidelines for pediatric TBI management concluded that acute supportive therapies are often administered inconsistently or simply extrapolated from adult TBI protocols, not taking into account the unique physiology of the immature brain (Kochanek et al., 2012).

The peak incidence of pediatric TBI occurs in the adolescent and young adult, with a secondary peak in infancy. The etiology of TBI varies with age (Fig. 102-1). Adolescents sustain most head injuries in motor vehicle accidents, along with sports-related concussions and assaults. Preadolescent children are also frequent victims of motor vehicle accidents, but more often as a pedestrian or while riding a bicycle. Those under the age of 5 years are more prone to falls, whereas infants are particularly vulnerable to repeated severe TBI in the form of abusive head trauma (AHT). TBI is roughly twice as common in boys as in girls, with this gender distinction becoming increasingly evident in the childhood and adolescent years.

Sequelae of TBI include headaches, posttraumatic epilepsy, motor disturbances, learning disabilities, cognitive impairments, and behavioral problems. The vast majority of children suffering TBI, even those surviving moderate or severe injury, fail to receive adequate follow up upon hospital discharge. Given the magnitude of recurrent head trauma as a problem of youth, it is increasingly noted that healthcare providers should take every opportunity to disseminate education to patients and their families, particularly with regard to potential sequelae of repeated injuries and the importance of injury prevention.

Anatomy

To understand the mechanisms and types of TBI, knowledge of the basic anatomy of the brain and its coverings is essential. From outside in, these layers are the scalp, galea, subgaleal space (potential), periosteum, skull, epidural space (potential), dura mater, subdural space, arachnoid, subarachnoid space, and pia mater. The different "spaces" (actual and potential) are areas for traumatic hemorrhage to occur, with different characteristics in each location.

Biomechanics

Trauma is a unique form of brain injury, whereby a biomechanical force (linear or rotational) is imparted to the brain. Because the brain "floats" in the CSF, these forces often result in compression of the brain at the site of contact (termed the "coup" injury). This injury can take the form of local hemorrhage or contusion, accompanied by overlying soft tissue swelling and occasionally skull fracture. As the intracranial contents are shifted toward the point of contact, however, a relatively low-pressure area evolves in a location opposite to the coup injury. Injury in this area is termed "contre-coup," and it can often be larger and more serious than the coup injury.

Because the brain parenchyma is itself soft and deformable, the brain is also prone to injury from rotational forces. The underlying white-matter tracts are subjected to significant shearing forces that can result in stretch injury and microhemorrhages seen clinically and in experimental models, referred to as diffuse axonal injury (DAI). More details about biomechanics are included in the online version of the chapter.

PATHOPHYSIOLOGY OF TRAUMATIC BRAIN INJURY

Multiple factors affecting TBI are distinct in the developing brain. Some of these include biomechanical factors, cerebral metabolism, neurovascular regulation, neurotransmission, and ongoing cerebral maturation. These are covered in greater detail in the online version of the chapter.

The Posttraumatic Neurometabolic Cascade

TBI results in an immediate release of glutamate, widespread ionic changes, fluctuating cerebral glucose metabolism (initially elevated, then reduced), and dynamic changes in blood flow. Later, axonal damage and disconnection, reduced responsiveness to physiologic stimuli, impaired neurotransmission, and apoptosis occur. For an overview of posttraumatic pathophysiology at the cellular level, see Figure 102-4. Specific components of the brain's response to traumatic injury are summarized in the online version of the chapter; these include ionic flux, energy crisis, axonal disconnection, cell death, and impaired plasticity.

PATIENT HISTORY

The clinical approach to pediatric TBI differs based on whether the presentation is acute (emergency) or delayed (clinic). Essential information includes mechanism of injury, protective factors, loss of consciousness, posttraumatic amnesia,

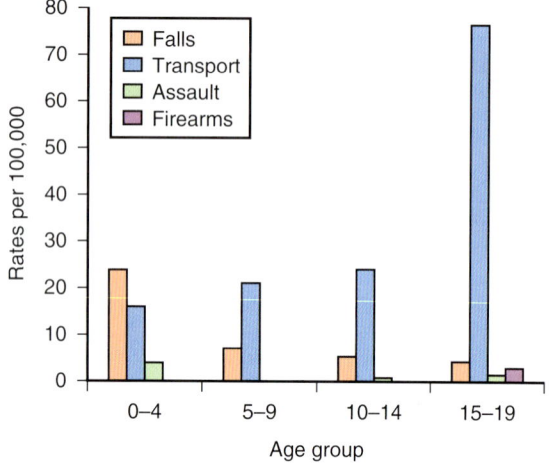

Figure 102-1. Etiology of pediatric traumatic brain injury by age group. *(With permission from Thurman D, for the Centers for Disease Control and Prevention. Traumatic brain injury in the U.S.: Assessing outcomes in children, Appendix B. Available at: http://www.cdc.gov.)*

TABLE 102-1 Glasgow Coma Scale and Modification for Children

Glasgow Coma Scale	Score	Glasgow Coma Scale (Infant Modification)	Score
EYE OPENING (E)		**EYE OPENING (E)**	
Spontaneous	4	Spontaneous	4
To speech (to shout)	3	To speech (to shout)	3
To pain	2	To pain	2
None	1	None	1
VERBAL RESPONSE (V)		**VERBAL RESPONSE, MODIFIED FOR INFANTS (V)**	
Oriented	5	Babbles, coos appropriately	5
Confused conversation	4	Cries, but consolable	4
Inappropriate words	3	Cries inconsolably	3
Incomprehensible sounds	2	Grunts or moans to pain	2
None	1	None	1
MOTOR RESPONSE (M)		**MOTOR RESPONSE (M)**	
Obeys commands	6	Purposeful movements	6
Localizes pain	5	Localizes pain	5
Withdraws	4	Withdraws	4
Abnormal flexion	3	Abnormal flexion	3
Extensor response	2	Extensor response	2
None	1	None	1

seizure activity, current medications, and any persistent neurologic signs. Examination, monitoring for ABCs (airway, breathing, circulation, spine), and initial management are begun simultaneously. Additional relevant history includes premorbid development, prior head injuries, prior neurosurgical procedures, history of epilepsy or other neurologic disorder, and other pertinent medical conditions. In older children or teens, the possibility of drug or alcohol use should be considered. In infants and toddlers, inconsistencies in the history and presence of associated injuries should raise suspicion of child abuse.

For patients presenting in the clinic with persistent neurologic problems after head injury, the same historical information is sought. In addition, the child and parent should be asked about posttraumatic symptoms. The presence of constant symptoms should be ascertained, along with alleviating or exacerbating factors and premorbid conditions such as attention deficit hyperactivity disorder (ADHD), anxiety, and headache. Episodic symptoms should be characterized, including triggers, duration, pattern, and resolution.

EXAMINATION

For the acutely and severely brain-injured child, the physical and neurologic examination must be done expediently, with the aim of identifying immediately life-threatening signs that would direct initial management. Airway and breathing are of paramount importance. Examination of skin color, pulses, blood pressure, capillary refill, and excessive bleeding is essential. In a hypotensive patient, bodily injuries that result in internal bleeding should be identified as soon as possible. In infants, massive scalp hematomas may result in hypotension and shock. Spinal cord or cardiac injury can also result in hypotension.

The Glasgow Coma Scale (GCS) is a quick rating of the severity of the patient's neurologic injury (Table 102-1). There are three components to this score:

1. Eye opening (ranging from 1 to 4)
2. Best verbal response (1 to 5)
3. Best motor response (1 to 6)

Some obvious pediatric limitations to this scale include how to determine verbal score in preverbal children. Several GCS modifications have been proposed for this age group,

and one modified scale is shown in Table 102-1. By convention, mild TBI is defined by a GCS score of 13 to 15, moderate by 9 to 12, and severe by 8 or less. A patient with a GCS score of 13 to 15 but having an intracranial lesion may be classified as having a complicated mild TBI or even a moderate TBI.

Assessment of the patient's mental state should be made, including alertness, orientation, confusion, combativeness, or unresponsiveness. Inspection of the head can reveal lacerations, contusions, and hematomas. Careful examination is warranted to identify foreign bodies, fractures, or penetrating injuries that may underlie more superficial damage. In infants, the open fontanel can be assessed quickly. Periorbital ecchymosis ("raccoon eyes") and/or rhinorrhea raise concern for a fracture of the anterior skull base. Retroauricular ecchymosis ("Battle sign"), hemotympanum, and/or otorrhea are signs indicative of a temporal basilar skull fracture. Ophthalmoscopic examination to detect retinal hemorrhage is very important, particularly in cases of suspected nonaccidental trauma.

Patients rendered unconscious, or those who retained consciousness but report posttraumatic neck pain, should have the cervical spine immobilized until cleared of any significant fracture or dislocation.

The posttrauma neurologic examination is, by necessity, short and directed; it should be performed in just a few minutes. Cranial nerve (CN) testing offers rapid, objective evaluation of brainstem functions. The pupillary response tests integrity of CN II and CN III. Fixed midposition pupils suggest symmetric midbrain dysfunction. A unilateral fixed dilated pupil in conjunction with declining mental status is a sign of impending transtentorial herniation and warrants immediate intervention. Bilateral pinpoint pupils raise the possibility of opiate ingestion or severe pontine injury. Bilateral fixed dilated pupils are evidence of widespread injury, but can also result from the systemic effects of resuscitation drugs. A pupil that fails to constrict under direct light (but does so when light is presented to the opposite eye) is indicative of an afferent pupillary defect (APD), a sign of ipsilateral optic nerve injury resulting from fracture of the orbit.

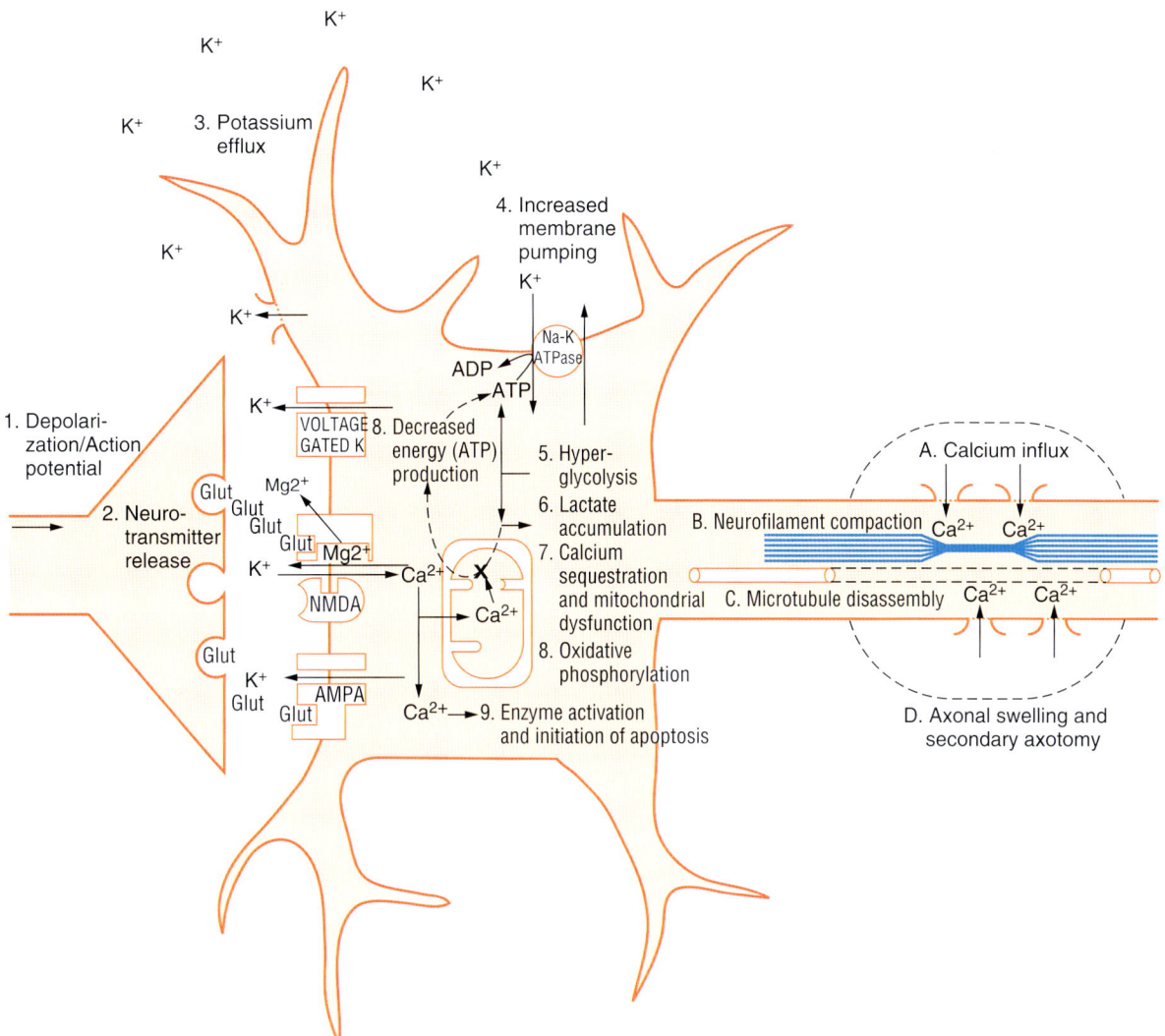

Figure 102-4. Neurometabolic cascade after traumatic injury. Cellular events: **1,** Nonspecific depolarization and initiation of action potentials. **2,** Release of excitatory neurotransmitters. **3,** Massive efflux of potassium. **4,** Increased activity of membrane ionic pumps to restore homeostasis. **5,** Hyperglycolysis to generate more adenosine triphosphate (ATP). **6,** Lactate accumulation. **7,** Calcium influx and sequestration in mitochondria, leading to impaired oxidative metabolism. **8,** Decreased energy (ATP) production. **9,** Calpain activation and initiation of apoptosis. Axonal events: **A,** Axolemmal disruption and calcium influx. **B,** Neurofilament compaction via phosphorylation or sidearm cleavage. **C,** Microtubule disassembly and accumulation of axonally transported organelles. **D,** Axonal swelling and eventual axotomy. ADP, adenosine diphosphate; AMPA, alpha-amino-3-hydroxy-5-methyl-4-isoxazole propionic acid; Glut, glutamate; NMDA, N-methyl-d-aspartate. *(With permission from Giza CC, Hovda DA. J Athl Train 2001;36:230.)*

Integrity of nerves innervating the extraocular muscles (CN III, CN IV, CN VI) and their brainstem connections can be tested by observation of the eyes for spontaneous conjugate movements, the oculocephalic response (doll's-eye maneuver), or the oculovestibular reflex (caloric reflex test).

An intact corneal response demonstrates function of CN V and CN VII. If, upon corneal stimulation, the globe rotates upward but the eye does not close, this suggests an intact afferent limb but impaired motor output. Other evidence of CN VII palsy involves tickling the inside of the nose with a wisp of cotton or administering a noxious stimulus and observing the facial grimace for symmetry.

Sensorimotor examination starts with the best motor response elicited on GCS testing. Limb posture and muscle tone should be examined, and particular note should be made of any asymmetry. If the patient is unable to follow commands, sensorimotor responses may be assessed by a peripheral noxious stimulus (e.g., nail bed pressure). If no response

occurs, the site of noxious stimuli can be moved centrally (e.g., sternal rub, supraorbital pressure) to distinguish between afferent versus efferent impairment. Look for changes in vital signs and whether the child can localize pain. If the child is awake, coordination should be assessed by observation of posture, spontaneous movements, and directed movements. Deep tendon reflexes should be checked for asymmetry, hyperreflexia/clonus or areflexia. Flaccid paresis with no reflexes should immediately raise suspicion of a spinal injury. An outline of the rapid trauma examination is provided in Box 102-1.

In the mildly injured child who is conscious at the time of initial evaluation, the neurologic examination can be conducted less urgently and more completely. Mental status testing can be more extensive, including attention, orientation, language, memory, and behavior. Cranial nerve, motor, coordination, and sensory examinations can include voluntary responses to the examiner's commands and subjective

---

BOX 102-1 Rapid Pediatric Trauma Examination

1. ABCs, brief history—mechanism of injury, loss of consciousness, amnesia, seizure, persistent neurologic symptoms
2. Glasgow Coma Scale score
3. Physical examination, particularly head and neck
   a. Scalp—depressions, stepoffs, fluid collections, lacerations
   b. Other signs of skull fracture—otorrhea, hemotympanum, rhinorrhea, raccoon eyes, Battle sign
   c. Cervical spine—deformity, point tenderness
   d. Associated severe bodily injuries—thoracic, abdominal, long bone
4. Mental status—describe succinctly, avoid ambiguous terms
5. Cranial nerves
   a. Pupillary response (cranial nerve II, III)
   b. Oculocephalic "doll's-eye" response (cranial nerve III, IV, VI)
   c. Oculovestibular "caloric" response (cranial nerve III, IV, VI, VIII)
   d. Corneal response, facial grimacing (cranial nerve V, VII)
   e. Gag response (cranial nerve IX, X)
6. Sensorimotor—asymmetry, abnormal muscle tone, coordination (if possible), movement (spontaneous, to command), movement to pain (withdrawal, decorticate, decerebrate, no movement)
7. Reflexes—asymmetry, areflexia, hyperreflexia/clonus, upgoing toes

---

reports of sensory input. Gait should be observed for signs of unsteadiness or ataxia. Deep tendon reflexes and plantar responses should be normal and symmetric.

In either setting, neurologic reassessment is mandated based on the severity of the injury. Deterioration of the neurologic examination may be a sign of progression of the underlying injury or may represent a new complication and should be evaluated immediately so that appropriate treatment may be instituted.

IMMEDIATE MANAGEMENT

Initial management of the child suffering from moderate or severe TBI centers on implementation of the ABCs and avoidance of secondary insults. Early management will occur concomitantly with initial evaluation and examination. Appropriate noninvasive monitors should be placed. Intubated patients should also have an end tidal CO_2 monitor. Intravenous access must be established immediately and fluid resuscitation begun. Blood should be drawn for serum electrolytes, glucose, renal and hepatic function, complete blood count, prothrombin time (PT)/partial thromboplastin time (PTT), type and cross for blood transfusion, and, if appropriate, alcohol or drug screens.

ACUTE CLINICAL SYNDROMES

Because TBI is a heterogenous disorder with multiple manifestations, acute syndromes may occur in isolation but are often overlapping. Concussion can occur alone or as a repeated injury and is rarely associated with more significant complications.

Herniation Syndromes

Herniation is the displacement of brain tissue from one intracranial compartment to another. The Cushing response is a paradoxical bradycardia with hypertension and slow irregular respiration that can be seen in the setting of elevated intracranial pressure (ICP) and impending herniation. Definitive treatment for herniation requires surgical removal of the offending mass. Nonsurgical measures to control elevated ICP include proper head positioning, sedation, hyperventilation, and hyperosmolar therapy. Ventriculostomy with cerebrospinal fluid (CSF) drainage should be instituted when possible.

In lateral transtentorial (uncal) herniation, a hematoma can displace the medial temporal lobe structures across the tentorial notch and compress the midbrain, resulting in impaired consciousness, ipsilateral pupillary dilation, and contralateral hemiparesis. Occasionally, this type of herniation compresses the posterior cerebral artery, resulting in an ipsilateral occipital lobe cerebral infarction and contralateral homonymous hemianopia.

A unilateral mass can also result in "midline shift," which can be readily seen on an acute computed tomography (CT) scan. When most severe, the cingulate gyrus will herniate under the falx, compress the anterior cerebral artery (or arteries), and infarct the medial frontal lobe(s).

Diffuse bilateral edema or lesions can cause central transtentorial herniation. Examination findings consistent with this syndrome include impaired mental status, fixed midposition pupils, impaired upward gaze, hyperventilation (central neurogenic hyperventilation), and posturing (decorticate followed by decerebrate). In the later stages of central herniation, pupils may become symmetrically constricted and respirations may become irregular.

Cerebellar tonsillar herniation occurs when the posterior fossa contents are pushed down through the foramen magnum. Because the infratentorial compartment is smaller than the supratentorial compartment, critical pressure effects can occur rapidly and with much smaller lesions. Tonsillar herniation can cause head tilt, neck stiffness, and lower cranial neuropathies, or can present relatively abruptly with cardiorespiratory compromise.

All of these herniation syndromes can lead to ischemic and hemorrhagic complications. The final stages of herniation occur as medullary centers are compressed, resulting in apnea, cardiac collapse, and death.

Diffuse Cerebral Swelling

Diffuse cerebral swelling is more common in children, whereas focal cerebral damage, such as contusion, is more common in older adolescents and adults. Diffuse edema can occur as a direct response to trauma, but can also be the result of a post-traumatic secondary insult, such as hypotension or hypoxia. At its extreme, diffuse edema can result in central transtentorial herniation and death.

Diffuse Axonal Injury

Diffuse axonal injury (DAI) is thought to result from shearing and rotational forces on white-matter fiber tracts and is most commonly seen after a high-impact injury.

Clinically, the patient with DAI has a prolonged period of unresponsiveness or coma that is not explained by a mass lesion or diffuse hypoxia. Gradually, the patient recovers some movement and can initially appear to be posturing or restless. Because of brainstem involvement, autonomic symptoms may be prominent.

DAI is rarely seen on CT, and then only if hemorrhage is present. Magnetic resonance imaging (MRI) is much more sensitive in detecting DAI, which can be seen as hypointensity on T2*-weighted gradient recall echo (GRE) imaging. MRI using susceptibility-weighted imaging (SWI) has more clearly demonstrated and allowed quantification of hemorrhagic DAI lesions. In general, patients with DAI will have lasting neurologic impairments, with good outcome at 3 months ranging from 65% of mild DAI patients to only 15% of severely injured.

Paroxysmal Sympathetic Hyperactivity

Autonomic disturbances are well known to accompany CNS injuries, and the term *paroxysmal sympathetic hyperactivity* has been defined as a syndrome after TBI "of simultaneous paroxysmal transient increase in sympathetic and motor activity" (Baguley et al., 2014). Patients with dysautonomia had worse functional outcomes than those without such symptoms, both groups having had comparable injury severities. Interestingly, the average age of patients with dysautonomia tends to be lower in descriptive studies. Treatment to mitigate autonomic disturbances is directed toward minimizing external triggers and pharmacologically reducing hyperactive autonomic neurotransmission.

Abusive Head Trauma

Many different terms, including *nonaccidental trauma, inflicted TBI*, and *shaking impact syndrome*, have been used to describe this clinical entity; however, in 2009 the American Academy of Pediatrics officially adopted the term *abusive head trauma* (AHT).

The clinical presentation is rarely straightforward, and history may be unclear. These infants can present with lethargy, irritability, seizures, or vomiting. Physical signs include a tense or bulging fontanel, split sutures, enlarged head circumference, retinal hemorrhages, and often evidence of other inflicted bodily injuries. CT scanning typically reveals subdural hematomas, contusions, or intracranial hemorrhage. Subdural hematomas of differing ages are particularly suspicious for AHT and are frequently seen over the cerebral convexities or along the falx (Fig. 102-6B). Inconsistencies in the history should lead the physician to suspect child abuse.

Infants with AHT may need vigorous resuscitation, controlled ventilation, anticonvulsant treatment, and intensive care unit (ICU) management. Beyond CT neuroimaging, diagnostic workup may include whole-body x-rays to look for fractures of varying ages, ophthalmoscopic examination to identify retinal hemorrhages, and a careful inspection of the skin for burns or excessive bruising. Laboratory tests should be sent to evaluate for a coagulopathy.

The outcome of infants suffering AHT is exceedingly poor. Mortality rates range from 7% to 30%, and severe neurocognitive sequelae are reported in one-third to one-half. Up to 80% of deaths resulting from trauma in children under the age of 2 years are attributed to nonaccidental injury. Medical care for these children is often delayed, perhaps setting the stage for secondary injuries as a result of hypoperfusion, hypoxia-ischemia, and recurrent seizures.

Subarachnoid Hemorrhage

Subarachnoid hemorrhage (SAH) occurs commonly after TBI. Blood products are irritating to the brain itself and to the cerebral vasculature, which can result in seizures or vasospasm, usually after several days. Vasospasm can be severe enough to cause cerebral ischemia or infarction. SAH is easily seen on CT. Subarachnoid blood in the ventricular system is associated with an increased risk of posttraumatic hydrocephalus.

Subdural Hematoma

Subdural hematomas (SDHs) can be seen after significant head trauma. These hemorrhages can present with a sudden or, more often, gradually progressive focal deficit. Mass effect can lead to neurologic symptoms of depressed mental status and, in severe cases, signs of impending herniation.

The appearance of SDH on CT scan is a crescent-shaped hyperdensity along the inner surface of the skull. Large lesions may track across suture lines (Fig. 102-8). SDHs can also occur over the cerebral convexities, along the falx or tentorium, or, more rarely, in the posterior fossa.

Definitive treatment of an acute symptomatic SDH involves neurosurgical consultation and probable surgical evacuation. If edema is extensive, placement of a ventriculostomy is helpful to monitor ICP and for CSF drainage. Other interventions to control elevated ICP should be instituted if needed. Outcome after SDH is good, with up to 75% of infants developing normally.

Subacute and chronic subdurals will appear as crescent-shaped subdural fluid collections that can be isodense and hypodense, respectively. In infants, a bulging fontanel and an enlarging head size may suggest AHT in an otherwise nonspecific clinical picture of irritability, poor feeding, lethargy, and vomiting. Seizures are frequently seen.

Chronic SDH needs to be distinguished from benign extracerebral collections of childhood (BECCs), which appear hypodense on CT and occur without a history of head trauma. These collections are associated with normal development and spontaneously resolve.

Epidural Hematoma

Epidural hematomas (EDHs) are often the result of temporal skull fracture with tearing of the middle meningeal artery. On CT, an EDH classically appears as a convex lens-shaped hyperdensity adjacent to the skull (Fig. 102-9). EDHs generally are constrained by dural attachment to the skull and do not cross suture lines.

EDHs occur less frequently in children than in adults. In children, EDH from bridging veins or dural sinuses is more likely, and EDHs are thus less commonly associated with skull fracture. Although the majority of EDHs in adults or children are supratentorial, the percentage of posterior fossa EDHs is higher in the pediatric population. Because of the risk of compression of critical brainstem structures and potential cardiorespiratory collapse, surgical removal is preferred.

Mortality as a result of EDHs ranges from 7% to 15%. Prognosis is less certain with infants, whose nonspecific presenting symptoms increase the likelihood of diagnostic delays. If EDHs are recognized and evacuated promptly, recovery is generally good in up to 90% of children.

Cerebral Contusion and Laceration

Cerebral contusion and laceration represent types of direct, focal damage to the brain. These injuries are less common in children than in adults. Contusions tend to be frontal or temporal and appear as a subtle hypodensity on CT. Some contusions evolve into hemorrhagic lesions.

Lacerations are also fairly rare and can be associated with a depressed fracture or penetrating injury. Dura and vascular structures can be similarly torn.

Traumatic Arterial Dissection and Traumatic Aneurysms

There is increasing awareness that traumatic arterial dissection may be a more common cause of acute ischemic stroke in children than previously thought, occurring in approximately 5% of cases, more frequently in boys. There are no evidence-based guidelines for treatment of pediatric craniocerebral dissections. Onset of focal symptoms in the first week after TBI or unexplained subarachnoid hemorrhage later after TBI should prompt additional diagnostic testing. Magnetic resonance (MR) angiography may be the preferred initial diagnostic modality because of its noninvasive nature.

Concussion

Concussion has been defined as any traumatically induced disturbance of neurologic function and mental state, occurring with or without actual loss of consciousness. Concussion is often referred to as mild TBI, and is the most common form of TBI in all age groups, accounting for over 75% to 85% of all head injuries.

Acute symptoms include headache, transient confusion or amnesia, dizziness, unsteadiness, nausea, or vomiting. Signs of concussion include vacant staring, observable confusion, disorientation, memory disturbance, ataxia, incoordination, slurred speech, behavioral disturbances, and any witnessed unconsciousness (less than 10%). The hallmark of concussion is that the acute symptoms are self-limited and occur in the absence of demonstrable structural brain injury (with conventional CT imaging). Because of this, concussive symptoms are often ascribed to neural dysfunction that recovers over time.

Several points regarding concussion are particularly relevant in children. First, there is much concern about the proper evaluation of concussion/mild TBI so as not to miss any associated intracranial injury. Second, a child returning to normal activity before complete physiologic recovery may have subtle deficits that need be considered to integrate the child into his or her preinjury educational settings. Premature return to physical activity, such as contact sports, may place the individual at greater risk for a second injury. Third, studies of a single mild TBI in children showed results different from those of adults with regard to the significance of long-term sequelae. Finally, there is increasing evidence that repeated mild TBI may result in a chronic accumulation of subtle deficits or even an early onset of memory disturbances later in life.

Sports Concussion/Repeated Concussion

Sports concussion is an increasingly common problem in childhood, occurring during team play in contact sports and accidents involving bicycles, rollerblades, skateboards, and scooters. An important opportunity is the possibility of more effective prevention strategies, by using approved protective gear when engaging in these activities, modifying rules to improve safety, and avoiding return to at-risk sports activity until recovery from injury is complete. There are increasing laws and policies that govern sports concussions in youth athletes, and practitioners are advised to be aware of their local regulations.

Epidemiology

It is estimated that over 1.6 to 3.8 million sports-related traumatic brain injuries occur annually in the United States, the majority of them mild. For those who have sustained a concussion, there is a three-fold risk of a subsequent concussion during the same sports season. There is a common mentality among players and coaches that one can "shake it off," which sets the stage for recurrent injuries.

Symptomatology

One consideration with subjective reporting of symptoms in a sports setting is that the player, being motivated to return to play, may attempt to minimize symptoms. Many athletic teams and physicians are utilizing a concussion checklist or computerized neuropsychological test that can be administered by a certified athletic trainer shortly after injury and again during recovery. Interestingly, there is some evidence that recovery from sports concussion is prolonged in high school students compared with college athletes (Williams, Puetz, Giza, and Broglio, 2015). Other studies of pediatric mild TBI showed lower rates of subacute postconcussive headaches or symptoms in younger ages compared with teens (McCrory et al., 2013).

Sequelae

Although the long-term significance of a single mild TBI is uncertain, individuals with multiple previous concussions have shown a significantly longer duration of symptoms and length of recovery.

There are no studies that specifically address long-term cognitive consequences of repeat pediatric concussions; however, evidence-based reviews have demonstrated multiple neurocognitive deficits in professional contact athletes. In amateur athletes, some studies have found impairments and others not, although studies below the high school level are few. A recent study of retired NFL players reported an association between an age at first exposure to tackle football of younger than 12 years and late-life cognitive impairment, but group size was small ($n = 21$), the cutoff age (12 years) was arbitrary, and the age at first exposure could not be separated from a longer duration of exposure. There also are case series of postmortem tau protein deposition in the brains of ex-athletes who had neurobehavioral problems preceding death. This condition has been termed chronic traumatic encephalopathy (CTE), but risk or incidence cannot be calculated from these types of studies. Clearly, further work is needed to delineate the risk of chronic cognitive impairment and its relation to timing, number, and age at injury.

Second-Impact Syndrome

Some controversy surrounds the existence of the so-called "second-impact syndrome" described in circumstances where a mild TBI, usually in a child or adolescent, resulted in catastrophic brain swelling and often death. On some occasions, an earlier head injury was reported, but a careful review of the literature raised concerns regarding poor documentation of a "first impact" in many cases, and the terminology *malignant brain swelling* was proposed.

Skull Fractures

Skull fractures are relatively common in the pediatric TBI population, particularly in the youngest age groups. The main concern about skull fractures is their association with underlying intracranial injury, such as hematomas.

Linear fractures account for 66% to 75% of all pediatric skull fractures. These are most commonly temporoparietal in location, and can be associated with an overlying scalp injury. Although the fractures themselves rarely require intervention, CT scanning should always be performed to determine whether there is underlying pathology.

Depressed skull fractures involve displacement of the bony skull and increase the risk of underlying cerebral contusion or laceration. Indications for surgical repair of depressed

BOX 102-2 Pediatric Traumatic Brain Injury in a Child Greater Than 2 Years Old: Indications for CT Scanning

DEFINITE INDICATIONS

- Glasgow Coma Scale score less than 15 in emergency department
- Altered mental status
- Skull fracture (on x-ray or clinically)
- Focal neurologic signs
- Deteriorating neurologic condition
- Suspected nonaccidental trauma

RELATIVE INDICATIONS

- Loss of consciousness or posttraumatic amnesia
- Seizure
- Known coagulopathy
- Need for anesthesia or prolonged sedation
- Persistent or worsening headache, nausea, or vomiting

BOX 102-3 Pediatric Traumatic Brain Injury in a Child Younger Than 2 Years Old: Indications for CT Scanning

DEFINITE INDICATIONS (HIGH-RISK PATIENT)

- Altered mental status, irritability
- Focal neurologic signs
- Skull fracture (on x-ray or clinically)
- Seizure
- Bulging fontanel
- Vomiting at least 5 times or for more than 6 hours
- Loss of consciousness for at least 1 minute
- Deteriorating neurologic condition
- Suspected nonaccidental trauma

RELATIVE INDICATIONS (INTERMEDIATE-RISK PATIENT)

- Vomiting 3 to 4 times
- Loss of consciousness for less than 1 minute
- Previous irritability or lethargy, now resolved
- Caregivers concerned about patient's current behavior
- High-energy mechanism of injury
- Scalp hematoma, especially if large or nonfrontal
- Known coagulopathy
- Need for anesthesia or prolonged sedation

fractures vary, but treatment is certainly indicated in patients with bony fragments displaced into brain parenchyma, dural tear, an underlying large hematoma, associated focal neurologic deficits or seizures, and overt wound contamination.

Basal skull fractures tend to occur frontally or in the area of the petrous bone. Periorbital or retroauricular ecchymosis (raccoon eyes or Battle sign), rhinorrhea, otorrhea, and hemotympanum all point to a fracture of the skull base. CSF leaks, when present, tend to resolve spontaneously. Persistent leaks may require CSF diversion or surgical repair. Traumatic cranial neuropathies are also associated with these fractures.

Compound or open skull fractures represent a significant risk of infection, and surgical debridement, removal of foreign bodies, repair of any existing dural defects, and prophylactic antibiotics are indicated.

Scalp Lacerations and Hematomas

Scalp injuries are one of the most common types of accidental injury in childhood, and because of their propensity to bleed profusely, they also tend to generate significant parental concern. Most scalp injuries resolve without significant complication.

DIAGNOSTIC EVALUATION

Skull X-Rays

Skull x-rays may be warranted in TBI settings where there is a suspicion of nonaccidental trauma, in infants younger than 1 to 2 years of age with scalp swelling or hematoma, or as a screening tool in older children only if CT scanning is not readily available.

Computed Tomography

Noncontrast CT scanning is the neurodiagnostic test of choice in the evaluation of acute head trauma. Given the high frequency of intracranial lesions in children with moderate or severe TBI, cranial CT is warranted in patients with a GCS score of less than 13. Imaging recommendations are summarized in Box 102-2 and Box 102-3.

The indication for CT is more controversial when only mild-TBI pediatric patients are considered. A recently developed and validated clinical prediction rule is valuable in identifying the subset of children with mild TBI who do not require

CT scanning (Kuppermann et al., 2009); the specifics of this rule are discussed later in the chapter (Fig. 102-14).

Recommendations for CT scanning are even broader when children under the age of 2 years are concerned. In this age group, skull fractures are more common, and neurologic examination is more limited. A well-validated CT rule for children younger than 2 years of age shows very good negative predictive value for clinically significant TBI (Fig. 102-14).

Magnetic Resonance Imaging and Angiography

Although MRI is not currently indicated as the standard of care for evaluation of acute pediatric TBI, it is being used more frequently to identify lesions poorly seen on CT, such as microhemorrhages, isodense hematomas, and posterior fossa lesions. MR spectroscopy performed subacutely (within the first week) in patients with persistent coma has been valuable in predicting outcome and is discussed in the online version of this chapter.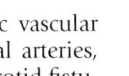

Angiography is useful for diagnosing traumatic vascular lesions, particularly dissections of the great cervical arteries, traumatic intracranial aneurysms, and cavernous carotid fistulas. In some cases, MR angiography is being recommended as a screening test.

Neurophysiological Testing

Electroencephalogram (EEG) is increasingly utilized in the evaluation of patients with TBI. EEG may be very useful in persistently comatose patients whose mental status is altered disproportionately to the documented injury or to monitor patients with more severe injury who are being sedated. In some cases, subclinical seizures may underlie prolonged unresponsiveness after TBI. Continuous EEG (cEEG) monitoring is one method of measuring cerebral function that may play a particularly important role in patients with TBI.

Continuous EEG monitoring may be particularly important in children. It is often quite challenging to assess the mental status in young children, and it is often difficult to determine the cause of paroxysmal events in children. In a recent prospective study of consecutive pediatric admissions

CLINICAL PREDICTION RULE FOR MINOR PEDIATRIC HEAD INJURY

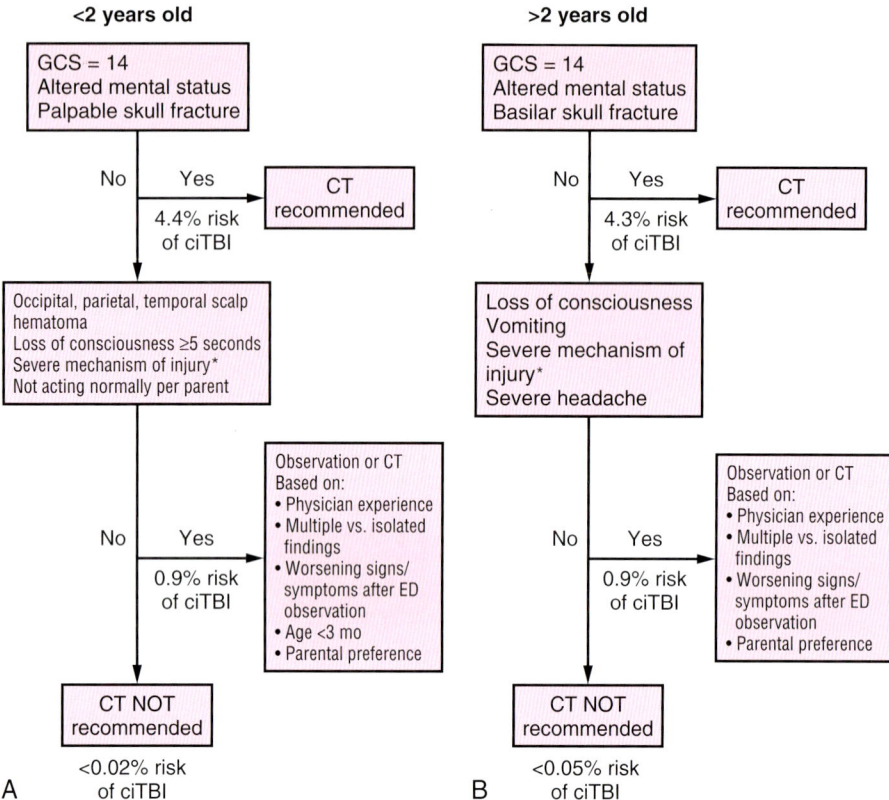

Figure 102-14. Clinical algorithm for CT scanning in children with minor head injury (Glasgow Coma Scale [GCS] score of 14 to 15). **A,** Algorithm for children less than 2 years old. **B,** Algorithm for children over 2 years old. *Includes motor vehicle crash with ejection, death of another passenger, or rollover; pedestrian or bicyclist without helmet struck by motor vehicle; fall greater than 0.9 m (3 ft) for **A,** greater than 1.5 m (5 ft) for **B;** head struck by high-impact object. A clinically important TBI (ciTBI) is one that results in death, neurosurgery, intubation for more than 24 hours for TBI, hospitalization for more than 48 hours for TBI. ED, emergency department. *(With permission from Kuppermann N et al.,* Lancet *2009; 374: 1160–1170.)*

for TBI monitored with cEEG, 43% had seizures, 16% had subclinical seizures, 18% had status epilepticus, and 13% had subclinical status epilepticus (Arndt et al., 2013).

GENERAL MANAGEMENT PRINCIPLES FOR SEVERE PEDIATRIC TBI

An expert review, updated in 2012, summarizes the existing published literature regarding medical management of severe pediatric TBI. The literature did not support any level I recommendations. Four items were listed as level II treatment recommendations:

1. Hypertonic saline should be considered for treatment of intracranial hypertension after severe pediatric TBI.
2. Avoid moderate hypothermia (32 to 33° C) for only 24 hrs duration; consider moderate hypothermia for up to 48 hrs duration. Use slow rewarming (<0.5° C/hr).
3. Use of corticosteroids for severe pediatric TBI is not recommended.
4. The use of an immune-modulating diet to improve outcome is not supported.

Multiple level III treatment options and their rationales were provided, and the following sections summarize these findings and synthesize them with traditional management strategies.

Interestingly, studies have shown that adherence to published guidelines and establishment of neurocritical care management teams are associated with improved outcomes. One study of five regional pediatric trauma centers demonstrated that guideline adherence was associated with improved survival. The same study found favorable outcomes associated with all operating room and ICU cerebral perfusion pressures greater than 40 mm Hg or no surgery. A retrospective study showed that implementation of a pediatric neurocritical care program (PNCP) improved favorable disposition at hospital discharge (from 48% preprogram to 67% postprogram) (Pineda et al., 2012).

Stabilization and Prevention of Secondary Injury

After initial assessment and resuscitation, acute management is aimed primarily at avoiding or preventing secondary injuries until more definitive therapy can be instituted. Airway maintenance and supplemental oxygen are crucial, and intubation and ventilation are often necessary for the more severely injured child. Fluid resuscitation to avoid hypotension is also essential.

Intracranial Pressure Management

The second edition pediatric severe TBI guidelines no longer separate ICP management into "first-tier" and "second-tier" interventions. Previous "first-tier" interventions included sedation/neuromuscular blockade, controlled hyperventilation, hyperosmolar therapy, ICP monitoring and drainage and cerebral perfusion pressure management. Some of the previous "second-tier" strategies involve methods to reduce brain metabolism and activity (barbiturates, hypothermia) or physical opening of the intracranial space to relieve pressure (craniectomy). Furthermore, corticosteroids are associated with increased mortality and not recommended.

Sedation and Neuromuscular Blockade

Sedatives and analgesics may be useful to reduce struggling and exacerbation of elevated ICP, promote optimal ventilation, alleviate pain, and allow for adequate nursing care. Sedation may reduce cerebral metabolic activity and prevent seizures. Potential adverse effects of sedation are hypotension, which can exacerbate poor cerebral perfusion, and obscuration of the neurologic examination.

Neuromuscular blockade may aid in the management of TBI patients by promoting ease of ventilation, reducing ICP, and stopping metabolic demands from skeletal muscle. Complications of neuromuscular blockade include an increased risk of pneumonia, cardiovascular depression, immobilization stress (if used with inadequate sedation), unnoticed seizure activity, and prolonged paralysis/myopathy.

Hyperventilation

Hyperventilation reduces blood and tissue PCO_2 levels, resulting in vasoconstriction, decreased cerebral blood volume, and reduced ICP, often within minutes, making hyperventilation an important tool in managing acute neurologic deterioration. However, the routine use of prophylactic hyperventilation ($PCO_2 < 35$ mm Hg) in severe pediatric TBI is no longer recommended because of the potential for ischemic complications. Controlled hyperventilation (PCO_2 30 to 35 mm Hg) is sometimes useful to control refractory elevated ICP.

Hyperosmolar Therapy

Two agents have been recommended for hyperosmolar therapy in pediatric TBI: 3% saline and mannitol; neither has proven superior to the other in a direct comparative study. Mannitol is administered with a bolus infusion, at 0.25 to 1.5 g/kg up to every 4 hours. Overall, mannitol begins to exert its ICP-reducing effects within 10 to 20 minutes, and these may last for several hours. Dosing of hypertonic (3%) saline was on a sliding scale titrated to ICP and serum sodium, but the infusion rates ranged from 0.1 to 1.0 ml/kg/hr. Potential adverse effects include osmotic rebound and, with 3% saline, central pontine myelinolysis.

Intracranial Pressure Monitoring—Indications and Treatment Threshold

ICP monitoring is recommended in children with a GCS score of 8 or less. In addition, ICP monitoring may be reasonable in selected patients with moderate TBI, particularly those whose clinical examination may be clouded. ICP monitoring may be beneficial in infants, particularly those with severe injuries as a result of abusive head trauma. In general, it is recommended to institute ICP-lowering therapy in pediatric patients whose ICP exceeds 20 mm Hg.

Cerebral perfusion pressure (CPP) is defined as the difference between the mean arterial pressure (MAP) and ICP. Based on the available evidence, maintaining CPP above 40 mm Hg at all times in pediatric TBI patients is recommended, and the range of CPP from 40 to 65 mm Hg most likely represents a spectrum of optimal CPP across the pediatric age range

(Chambers et al., 2006). Use of vasopressor agents may be associated with an increased risk of pulmonary complications.

Cerebrospinal Fluid Drainage

Physical drainage of CSF is the most direct means of reducing ICP and has been done via intraventricular catheters in patients with severe TBI. CSF drainage can be considered a reasonable treatment option to reduce elevated ICP in children.

Barbiturates

The use of barbiturates is an option in patients with intractable elevation of ICP. Proper EEG and cardiovascular monitoring should be used at all times. The use of barbiturate coma in traumatically injured neonates and infants should be approached with caution.

Temperature Control and Hypothermia

Temperature control can be used either to avoid hyperthermia or to institute hypothermia. There is substantial experimental and adult clinical literature suggesting that hyperthermia can exacerbate brain injury. It is recommended that fever/hyperthermia be avoided in brain-injured children. Induced hypothermia for pediatric moderately severe TBI has shown mixed results—for a more thorough discussion, please see the online version of the chapter.

Surgical Management of ICP

Decompressive craniectomy has been used to alleviate intractable intracranial hypertension and malignant cerebral edema. Expert review of the literature suggested that severely injured children with intractably elevated ICP who are more likely to benefit from decompressive craniectomy could be selected on the basis of meeting at least some of the following criteria: (1) diffuse cerebral swelling on CT, (2) less than 48 hours postinjury, (3) no episodes of sustained ICP greater than 40mm Hg, (4) GCS greater than 3 at some point postinjury, (5) secondary clinical deterioration, or (6) evolving herniation syndrome.

Early Posttraumatic Seizures and Seizure Prophylaxis

Posttraumatic seizures are divided into early and late. Early posttraumatic seizures (EPTS) occur within the first week after injury. EPTS are generally reactive seizures in response to an acute or subacute insult but may also act as a secondary injury. The incidence of EPTS is higher in children than in adults, and, following severe pediatric TBI, early seizure rates of 20% to 39% have been reported. This risk is increased with lower GCS and younger age. Most EPTS in children occur within the first 24 hours. Prophylaxis for posttraumatic seizure activity in children should be considered for use in the first week after injury. Fosphenytoin can be administered intravenously more rapidly and has fewer infusion-related side effects than phenytoin. Loading doses of either drug range from 10 to 20 mg/kg, and maintenance doses are typically 5 to 7 mg/kg/day, divided at least into two doses per day. Intravenous lorazepam (0.05 to 1.0 mg/kg/dose) may be administered until fosphenytoin levels become therapeutic. Levetiracetam may also be considered, although a pediatric-specific trial remains to be carried out. An alternative strategy is to monitor for seizures with EEG and only treat when needed.

Despite the effectiveness of early prevention, prospective adult studies have revealed the inability of anticonvulsant prophylaxis to prevent subsequent development of late posttraumatic epilepsy. In addition, there are also substantial animal data demonstrating that the immature brain is particularly vulnerable to apoptosis induced by anticonvulsants and anesthetics. Thus anticonvulsants cannot be recommended routinely for long-term prophylaxis after pediatric TBI. After the acute period, anticonvulsants can be gradually weaned.

Supportive Care

Management of severe TBI includes general supportive measures to prevent complications of ICU hospitalization and potentially prolonged immobilization. This includes aspiration precautions, nutritional support, skin care, deep venous thrombosis prophylaxis, autonomic monitoring, sedation and analgesia (with periodic "wake-ups" to assess neurologic status), and psychosocial support.

GENERAL MANAGEMENT OF MILD TRAUMATIC BRAIN INJURY/CONCUSSION

There are multiple guidelines for management of pediatric mild TBI and concussion; currently the Centers for Disease Control are assembling a formal evidence-based guideline for mild pediatric TBI. There are three major guidelines presented in greater detail in the online chapter and summarized here: (1) American Academy of Pediatrics consensus guidelines for the evaluation and management of the mildly head-injured child, with some added clinical prediction rules for CT scanning; (2) the Concussion in Sport Group guidelines, with ongoing updates; and (3) the American Academy of Neurology strict evidence-based guidelines for sports concussion that incorporate some pediatric/youth recommendations.

Neuroimaging (acute CT) is not generally recommended for concussion, but may be helpful in a setting of persistent alteration of mental status or suspected intracranial hemorrhage or skull fracture. Clinical observation and symptom monitoring may be helpful in most other cases.

When the CT scan and examination are normal, the likelihood of clinically significant late deterioration is very low, so children in this category can be discharged home under parental observation. Preverbal children and infants should be managed more conservatively.

Guidelines for Return to Play Following Sports Concussion

Current sports concussion guidelines have moved away from grading concussion severity and return to activity based on early symptoms. All recent guidelines and updates recognize that acute concussion management, return to school activity, and return to play need to be individualized to the particular patient, and usually proceed in a stepwise fashion (Table 102-3). Optimal management, particularly for chronically symptomatic patients, is best handled in a multidisciplinary clinic.

PROGNOSIS AND OUTCOME

Determining the degree of recovery in children is difficult in the early days following a severe head injury. Despite the overall better prognosis seen in children compared with adults, there are certain characteristics worth considering when discussing outcome with the child's parents. Younger age, particularly infants, greater severity of acute injury, and occurrence of secondary insults (e.g., hypoxia or ischemia) are risk factors for worse long-term outcomes.

Elevations of ICP greater than 20–30 mm Hg have been associated with worse outcomes in children, as have age-specific reductions in cerebral perfusion pressure. Impaired autoregulation (in addition to significant hypotension) was an independent risk factor for a poor 6-month global outcome. For more in-depth discussion of clinical prognostic factors for pediatric TBI outcome, including imaging and electrophysiological measures as well as prognosis after mild TBI, please refer to the online version of the chapter (Ashwal, Tong, Ghosh, Bartnik-Olson, Holshouser, 2014).

LATE CLINICAL SYNDROMES
Vegetative and Minimally Conscious States

Following severe TBI, children can emerge from coma into a vegetative state (VS) (Chapter 101). This condition is characterized by the eyes being open and the presence of intact sleep–wake cycles, but with no self-awareness nor any purposeful movement. At the time of discharge, approximately 12% to 15% of severe-TBI patients were in VS across all age ranges. Two studies found that in post-TBI adolescents still in VS after 3 months, 33% to 43% remained in VS at 1 year.

More recently, a distinct state of consciousness termed the *minimally conscious state* (MCS) has been described and is distinguished from the vegetative state by the presence of self-awareness and some limited purposeful movements, in addition to the potential to experience pain and suffering. Children may enter into an MCS as they emerge from a VS.

TABLE 102-3 Graded Return-to-Play Protocol After Concussion

Rehabilitation Stage	Functional Exercise	Objective
1. No activity	Physical and cognitive rest	Recovery
2. Light aerobic exercise	Moderate-intensity walking, swimming, stationary cycling; no resistance training	Increase heart rate
3. Sport-specific exercise	Skating drills in hockey, running drills in soccer; no head-impact activities	Add sport-specific movement
4. Noncontact training drills	Progression to more complex training drills (passing drills in football and hockey, etc.); start resistance training	Exercise, coordination, and cognitive load
5. Full-contact practice	Following medical clearance, participate in normal training activities	Restore confidence and assess functional skills by coaching staff
6. Return to play	Normal competitive game play	

(With permission from McCrory P et al. Clin J Sport Med 2009;19:185.)

Cognitive Impairment and Behavioral Disorders

Deficits in many cognitive domains have been demonstrated following moderate to severe TBI in children, including impaired executive function, language, memory, visual-motor integration, attention, and speed of thinking. A meta-analysis of recovery from pediatric TBI suggests that injury severity affects the magnitude of deficits and the trajectory of recovery, with more severely injured children unable to "close the gap" with their uninjured peers over time. Factors associated with a positive outcome included preinjury adaptive ability. Lower socioeconomic status has also been associated with poorer outcomes from pediatric TBI in multiple studies. There is growing evidence that younger children are more likely to develop later impairments that become evident when they fail to acquire higher-level functions normally (Anderson et al., 2005; Babikian and Asarnow, 2009).

The presence of lasting cognitive and academic impairments after mild pediatric brain injury is controversial. Several large studies have failed to detect significant neurocognitive impairment in mildly head-injured children. However, subtle overall impairments have been reported that may indicate weak injury effects across a large spectrum of measures, rather than a major effect in a single cognitive domain.

There is also considerable evidence that pediatric TBI is associated with later behavioral disturbances, including problems with impulse control, attention, and social cognition, including recognition of emotions and social problem solving. Some of this may be attributable to premorbid problems, but there is also evidence for new-onset behavioral disturbances after TBI.

Sleep Disorders

A variety of sleep problems have been reported after all severities of TBI, particularly sleep–wake cycle disorders. As in most sleep disorders, behavioral changes and sleep hygiene tend to be the first line of therapy. Polysomnography and evaluation by a sleep specialist may be necessary in some cases.

Spasticity and Motor Impairment

Focal or diffuse injury may injure corticospinal tract pathways, resulting in spasticity, weakness, and loss of dexterity. As a general rule, focal deficits recover better than diffuse ones, and younger age appears to predict better recovery in these circumstances (except perhaps in the earliest age groups). Spasticity can lead to pain and discomfort, contractures, and scoliosis, and it may interfere with bladder and bowel function. Management includes physical and occupational therapy, splints and orthotic devices, assistive devices, and pharmacotherapy (Chapter 162).

Posttraumatic Hydrocephalus

Posttraumatic hydrocephalus can be seen following intraventricular or subarachnoid hemorrhage and may manifest with chronic headache, sometimes with nausea, vomiting, impaired vertical eye movements, and diminished level of consciousness. Shunting may be necessary to alleviate pressure. Ventriculomegaly ex vacuo is perhaps more common but does not warrant shunting.

Posttraumatic Epilepsy

Epilepsy is defined as a disorder of recurrent seizures that are not attributable to an underlying metabolic derangement or other provocation. TBI is responsible for about 5% of all new epilepsy cases annually in the United States. One study showed the risk of developing posttraumatic epilepsy (PTE) across all ages after severe TBI was 7% at 1 year and 11% at 5 years; and after moderate TBI, it was less than 1% at 1 year and 1.6% at 5 years. Strong predictors of posttraumatic seizures/epilepsy include severity of TBI, age, and type of TBI, in particular penetrating head wounds. Other potential risk factors for the development of posttraumatic epilepsy include the presence of early seizures, longer period of unconsciousness, prolonged amnesia, skull fracture, and the presence of intracranial blood on neuroimaging.

Although children are more likely than adults to experience an early posttraumatic seizure, the relation between early and late posttraumatic seizures/PTE in children is unclear.

Posttraumatic epilepsy includes late, recurrent, unprovoked seizures with a significant antecedent history of TBI. When these patients present with their first seizure, they should undergo a thorough history, examination, and EEG. Focal findings on examination or EEG should prompt neuroimaging, with MRI being the modality of choice.

Because the specific type of posttraumatic seizure is usually one of partial onset, medication choice is generally directed toward agents with effectiveness for localization-related epilepsy. Carbamazepine, lamotrigine, valproate, topiramate, oxcarbazepine, gabapentin, and levetiracetam may be useful. Tailoring the choice of agent to take advantage of potentially beneficial side effects (mood stabilization, migraine prevention) is often worthwhile. Surgical resection may be an option in a patient with a focal lesion and seizures refractory to medication. For a more complete discussion of the early and late seizure manifestations after TBI, please see the online version of the chapter.

Subacute and Chronic Subdural Hematoma

Subacute and chronic SDHs may manifest with signs of gradually increasing ICP—recurrent vomiting, macrocrania, papilledema, seizures, slowly progressive motor deficits, and spasticity, and occasionally systemic signs, such as anemia, poor appetite, or fever. Treatment of these hematomas may require drainage. In cases where abusive head trauma is suspected, a careful search for other bodily injuries is warranted, including a whole-body x-ray series (to look for multiple fractures) and skin examination (to look for bruising, burns, or other injuries).

Posttraumatic Headache

Acute posttraumatic headache is usually self-limited. Trauma may also appear to precipitate migraines acutely or chronically. Worsening or progressive headache, particularly associated with nausea and vomiting, should warrant performing a careful history and examination to determine whether there is a delayed progressive intracranial complication (chronic subdural, hydrocephalus). If necessary, a cranial CT may be obtained for further evaluation.

Chronic posttraumatic headaches in children may be of new onset or an exacerbation of a preexisting headache disorder (Choe and Blume, 2015). Management of chronic posttraumatic headaches is directed at the etiology. Chronic daily headaches may be treated with analgesics, nonsteroidal anti-inflammatory agents, or antidepressant (amitriptyline) or anticonvulsant (gabapentin) medication. Narcotics should be avoided.

Migraine, tension headaches, and neuralgias should be treated similarly to nontraumatic headaches. These may best be addressed in a multidisciplinary pediatric concussion or pain clinic and include medications, education, and nonpharmacologic interventions.

Postconcussive Syndrome

The constellation of symptoms seen in postconcussion syndrome (PCS) in children is similar to that in adults, with chronic headache, dizziness, irritability, behavior change, inattention, sleep disturbance, fatigue, and concentration problems being prominent. The causes of PCSs are unknown, and the exact relation between physiologic abnormalities and the patient's symptomatology remains unknown. Other nonphysiologic factors have been implicated in the development of PCSs, including premorbid personality traits, socioeconomic status, educational level, medicolegal compensation, and family dynamics.

Management of PCS in children should focus on a return to normalcy as quickly as possible. Balance is required because prolonged absence from school may take on a life of its own and become clouded with issues of secondary gain and avoidance.

Medical management should be aimed at identifying treatable problems and initiating appropriate interventions. Postconcussive behavior disturbances should be evaluated by a child psychiatrist or psychologist. Although it is uncertain whether mild TBI results in an increased risk of new-onset behavioral problems, it is clear that children with particular behavioral tendencies (ADHD, oppositional behavior) are more prone to mild TBI, and treatment of these underlying problems is often beneficial. Cognitive problems identified after mild TBI may be best addressed by school assessment or neuropsychological testing. Children with pre-existing learning disabilities may have disproportionate cognitive problems after mild TBI.

Late Complications of Skull Fracture

The majority of nondisplaced skull fractures will heal without aggressive management. However, "growing skull fracture," or leptomeningeal cyst, complicates less than 1% of cases, usually after cranial vault fractures in infants. In these circumstances there can be outward herniation of dura and underlying brain matter that require carefully planned surgical correction.

Traumatic cranial neuropathies can also occur following fractures of the skull base, most commonly affecting olfactory, optic, facial, and vestibulocochlear nerves. In cases of basilar skull fracture, particularly with persistent CSF leakage, there is an increased risk of central nervous system infection. Patients with known basilar skull fractures who present with fever, meningismus, seizures, or focal neurologic findings should be evaluated promptly for brain abscess, empyema, or meningitis.

CONCLUSIONS

TBI is a major public health problem in children and is the number one cause of death and acquired disability. No brain-specific therapies exist, and follow up for affected children is limited and often nonexistent. Recently published recommendations for management of severe and mild pediatric TBI provide some direction for practitioners but also point out the lack of firm guidelines available for the effective management of this common clinical problem. Although the majority of children with mild injury make a good recovery, controversy remains as to whether subsequent learning and behavioral complications are more common in these children than in uninjured controls. Severely injured children generally will have partial recovery and persistent deficits. Persistent subjective symptoms can also occur after all levels of severity of pediatric head injury. In addition, posttraumatic medical complications, such as hydrocephalus, epilepsy, infection, CSF leak, spasticity, and growing skull fracture, must be monitored for and treated promptly. The pediatric physician must not lose the opportunity to educate the child and parents about the significance of head injury, particularly with regard to appropriate measures for injury prevention, such as motor vehicle restraints and helmet use during recreational activities at risk for TBI. A balanced discussion of the risks for repeat concussion and the benefits of sports participation is also an important aspect of patient and parent education.

REFERENCES

The complete list of references for this chapter is available online at www.expertconsult.com.
  See inside cover for registration details.

SELECTED REFERENCES

Anderson, V., Catroppa, C., Morse, S., et al., 2005. Functional plasticity or vulnerability after early brain injury? Pediatrics 116, 1374.

Arndt, D.H., Lerner, J., Matsumoto, J., et al., 2013. Subclinical early post-traumatic seizures detected by continuous EEG monitoring in a consecutive pediatric cohort. Epilepsia 54 (10), 1780–1788.

Ashwal, S., Tong, K.A., Ghosh, N., et al., 2014. Application of advanced neuroimaging modalities in pediatric traumatic brain injury. J. Child Neurol. 29 (12), 1704–1717.

Babikian, T., Asarnow, R., 2009. Neurocognitive outcomes and recovery after pediatric TBI: meta-analytic review of the literature. Neuropsychology 23, 283.

Baguley, I.J., Perkes, I.E., Fernandez-Ortega, J.F., et al., for the Consensus Working Group, 2014. Paroxysmal sympathetic hyperactivity after acquired brain injury: concensus on conceptual definition, nomenclature, and diagnostic criteria. J. Neurotrauma. 31, 1515–1520.

Chambers, I.R., Jones, P.A., Lo, T.Y., et al., 2006. Critical thresholds of intracranial pressure and cerebral perfusion pressure related to age in paediatric head injury. J. Neurol. Neurosurg. Psychiatry 77, 234.

Choe, M.C., Blume, H.K., 2016. Pediatric posttraumatic headache: a review. J. Child. Neurol. 31 (1), 76–85.

Kochanek, P., Carney, N.A., et al., 2012. Guidelines for the acute medical management of severe traumatic brain injury in infants, children, and adolescents—Second Edition. Pediatr. Crit. Care Med. 13 (Suppl. 1), S1–S8.

Kuppermann, N., Holmes, J.F., Dayan, P.S., et al., 2009. Identification of children at very low risk of clinically-important brain injuries after head trauma: a prospective cohort study. Lancet 374, 1160.

McCrory, P., Meeuwisse, W., Aubry, M., et al., 2013. Consensus statement on concussion in sport: the 4th International Conference on Concussion in Sport held in Zurich, November 2012. Br. J. Sport Med. 47 (5), 250–258.

Pineda, J., et al., 2012. Effect of implementation of a paediatric neuro-critical care programme on outcomes after severe traumatic brain injury: a retrospective cohort study. Lancet Neurol. 4422 (12), 45–52.

Williams, R.M., Puetz, T.W., Giza, C.C., et al., 2015. Concussion recovery time among high school and collegiate athletes: A systematic review and meta-analysis. Sports Med. 45, 893–903.

🕑 E-BOOK FIGURES AND TABLES

The following figures and tables are available in the e-book at www.expertconsult.com. See inside cover for registration details.

103 Abusive Head Trauma

Elizabeth E. Gilles and Cindy W. Christian

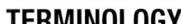 An expanded version of this chapter is available on www.expertconsult.com. See inside cover for registration details.

INTRODUCTION

Abusive head trauma (AHT) is a form of traumatic brain injury (TBI) resulting from assault of typically, but not exclusively, infants and young children less than 3 years of age. It remains a major cause of morbidity and mortality among young children. Infants with abusive head injuries have the most severe illness, the highest mortality risk, and the worst outcome in comparison with other forms of childhood trauma. Of the 1760 child fatalities reported in 2012 by The National Child Abuse and Neglect Data System (20 deaths/100,000), 45% were the result of physical abuse or multiple forms of maltreatment and 44% of victims were infants.

HISTORICAL PERSPECTIVE

In the past 60 years, much has been learned about the differences between TBI from assault sustained by infants and young children and traumatic brain injuries from other etiologies at other ages. Recognizing that the caregiver history was incompatible biomechanically with the range and extent of injuries involving the craniospinal axis led to acknowledging these as caused by physical abuse. (An extensive review of the history of AHT is found online.)

TERMINOLOGY

Abusive head trauma is the preferred term to use when referring to neurotrauma from assault in children (Christian et al., 2009). *Inflicted head injury* or *nonaccidental head injury* are other terms that also have been used. These are inclusive terms encompassing the range of craniospinal injuries sustained by infants and young children as a consequence of violent assault by parents or other caretakers. Unintentional, or accidental, head injury refers to injury sustained by chance and is unrelated to specific deliberate actions of caretakers.

DEVELOPMENTAL DIFFERENCES PREDISPOSING THE IMMATURE NEURAXIS TO INJURY

Structural and functional changes of central and peripheral nervous system organization and function are greatest during the first 2 years of life, when AHT occurs most frequently. The infant's unique biochemical and physiologic makeup renders the immature nervous system more vulnerable (Hagberg et al., 2014). Mitochondria, for instance, are important to far more than cellular energetics. They affect brain susceptibility to injury, alter postinjury cascades, and play a role in recovery as well as in apoptosis (Hagberg et al., 2014). A number of biologic and mechanical factors predispose the infant and young child to injury of the craniospinal axis (Box 103-1).

Mechanical Factors

Important differences from adults biomechanically are that infants and young children have a larger head-to-body ratio,

less muscle development, and thinner, more flexible skull bones that are not yet fused and incomplete myelination.

Biologic Factors

There are many age-related biochemical, microscopic, and macroscopic differences with infants having greater neuronal excitability and synaptic density, and differences in receptor number, structure, and function.

RESPONSES TO INJURY

Injury and repair after a CNS insult are quite different in the immature versus the mature CNS. The infant's unique biochemical and physiologic makeup renders the immature nervous system more vulnerable to injury. Many of the postinjury cascades are affected, including mitochondrial function, inflammatory and excitotoxic mechanisms, impaired autoregulation, oxidative stress, apoptosis, and decreased ischemic and seizure thresholds. The immature gyrencephalic brain (having convolutions) is more resistant to direct cortical deformation and isolated subdural hematoma than the mature brain, but is more sensitive to white-matter strains. These mechanisms are discussed in detail in Part IV of this book as well as in Chapters 102 and 104.

MECHANISMS OF INJURY

Mechanisms of head injury are similar across the age spectrum and are reviewed in Chapter 102. Briefly, injuries occur when applied forces strain the tissue beyond its structural or functional tolerance. Specific patterns of response vary at different ages. The exact type and the magnitude of applied forces determine the severity of injury, with greater applied forces resulting in more severe injuries, regardless of whether the injury was abusive. Primary mechanisms of injury include impact and inertial forces, with impact forces occurring at the surface of the scalp, skull, and brain as a result of contact and inertial forces arising from head deceleration. Most severe primary brain injuries in the clinical world result from head contact. Rotational movement of the head on the neck may be caused by a number of mechanisms, including, but not limited to, shaking. Lateral (side to side) rotational movement is associated with greater brain damage than equivalent anterior–posterior head movements. Primary injury mechanisms are frequently mixed. There are numerous factors affecting severity of injury (Box 103-2).

Contribution of Hypoxia-Ischemia

Infant animals and human children less than 24 months of age are particularly prone to secondary injury from hypoxia-ischemia after severe TBI, the most significant variable contributing to the evolution of parenchymal injury and deleterious outcome. Most infants with severe head injury, abusive or not, experience apnea or altered respiration during or just after injury (Piteau et al., 2012). Apnea and hypotension can also

BOX 103-1 Biologic and Mechanical Features Predisposing the Infant to Head Injury

BIOMECHANICAL FACTORS

- Large head-to-body ratio
- Proportionally heavy head in relation to body mass and neck strength
- Greater skull compliance
- Anatomy of inner skull table (smoother in younger infants)
- More firmly attached dura

NEUROANATOMIC FACTORS

- Immature brain (incomplete myelination)
- Increased brain water content
- Increased excitotoxicity
- Increased synaptic density
- Increased excitatory amino acid receptors
- Decreased inhibitory networks

BOX 103-2 Factors Affecting Severity of Injury

- Types of injury events
  - Biomechanical
  - Deceleration
  - Translational
  - Strangulation
  - Smothering
- Sequence of events
- Single or multiple events
- Other factors
  - Duration of apnea, hypotension
  - Delay in seeking medical care
  - Level of consciousness at the time of the event or events
  - Neuromuscular maturity of the child
  - Antecedent dehydration and/or malnutrition
  - Premorbid brain injury

be a response to smothering or to direct vessel compromise caused by strangulation.

CLINICAL FEATURES
Acute Presentation

The brain's response to mechanical trauma, whether blunt force or angular deceleration, or both, is predictable. Symptoms of brain injury are nonspecific and vary by the severity of injury. Mildly injured infants may exhibit a depressed level of consciousness, irritability, altered behavior, seizures, decreased visual alertness, decreased babbling, feeding difficulties, vomiting, fever, or altered respiration. Acutely, they may not appear ill enough for the perpetrator to seek medical attention and the accompanying caregiver may be unaware that an injury has occurred. Children with moderate injuries may have waxing and waning mental status and variable neurologic findings, and usually have preservation of primitive reflexes such as sucking. Severely injured infants may have varying degrees of altered consciousness and respiratory function and often have lost most the ability to perform coordinated actions such as sucking, eating, sitting, or walking.

Sudden neurologic decompensation of a previously healthy infant, accompanied by severe respiratory distress and flaccidity, with or without seizures or posturing, in the absence of any trauma history is consistent with a major intracranial event (e.g., trauma, herniation, subarachnoid or intraparenchymal bleeding, stroke, uncompensated hydrocephalus).

Early Posttraumatic Seizures

Early posttraumatic seizures (those occurring in the first 72 to 96 hours after trauma) occur in 30% to 80% of infants and young children after AHT and vary in severity and type of seizure depending on the age of the infants (more likely if less than a year of age), severity of injury, and the degree of hypoxia-ischemia.

Subacute and Chronic Presentation

Infants who have sustained less severe brain injury and lack external findings of trauma manifest nonspecific symptoms, not easily ascribed to trauma. Signs and symptoms attributable to hydrocephalus or an accumulating extraaxial fluid collection include progressive macrocephaly, vomiting, seizures, irritability, high-pitched cry, increasing spasticity, regression of motor skills, and loss of upward gaze, when intracranial pressure is increased.

Predictors of Outcome

Clinical predictors of poor outcome after abusive TBI are similar to older children and include the presence of a low Glasgow Coma Scale score, severe brainstem dysfunction, and coma duration of longer than 7 days (Robertson et al., 2002). Other variables helpful in determining that the outcome will be poor include younger age, greater severity of parenchymal injury, early and difficult-to-treat posttraumatic seizures, and the presence of severe retinal hemorrhages.

Laboratory predictors of poor outcome include initial mixed metabolic acidosis plus respiratory acidosis, hematocrit less than 30%, coagulopathy, early and sustained hyperglycemia, hypocortisolemia, and central diabetes insipidus.

Imaging findings on computed tomography (CT) scan associated with worse outcome and greater mortality include the presence of a midline shift of greater than 1 cm, diffuse hypodensities, evidence of herniation, presence of shear injuries, and larger volume of ischemic infarction. The presence of certain magnetic resonance imaging (MRI) abnormalities also correlate with poor outcome. Conventional sequences may demonstrate restricted diffusion and abnormal apparent diffusion coefficient values. Susceptibility-weighted imaging may demonstrate multiple microhemorrhages, and on MR spectroscopy, the presence of reduced N-acetylaspartate levels and increased lactate are associated with a poor outcome.

Mortality Predictors. Ten percent to 30% of children die of their injuries. Infants and young children admitted with hypotension, coma with severely abnormal brainstem reflexes, marked autonomic dysfunction, and retinal findings are more likely to die. Children with disseminated intravascular coagulation, severe sustained hyperglycemia, and severe endocrine derangements. Imaging signs, including reversal sign (brainstem compression) or other signs of herniation, also portend an earlier demise.

SEQUELAE OF ABUSIVE HEAD TRAUMA

In contrast to the majority of children with severe unintentional head injury, infants who were abused have significant sequelae. Microcephaly develops as a function of evolving cerebral atrophy.

Posttraumatic Epilepsy

Posttraumatic epilepsy develops in 20% to 30% of young children after AHT, compared with children with unintentional injury or adults after closed head injury where the incidence is less than 2%.

Cognitive and Executive Function

More than 50% of survivors have severe developmental disabilities, with a sizeable proportion completely dependent on caretakers for daily care. Cognitive and executive functions are often severely impaired, particularly attention and emotional regulation.

Behavioral Sequelae

Behavioral problems are common, ranging from perseveration to oppositional behavior. Temper tantrums are frequent and may begin to manifest as the child reaches a functional age of 2 years. There are no systematic studies as to the most effective interventions for these behavioral disorders.

Visual Sequelae

A large percentage (32% to 90%) of children with AHI have visual sequelae. Cortical visual impairment, most frequently a homonymous hemianopia, is more common than visual impairment from retinal hemorrhages. Persistent hemorrhages overlying the macula may affect central vision permanently.

Motor Sequelae

Over 50% of survivors of early life AHT have motor deficits. Findings range from spastic hemiparesis or quadriparesis, typically with truncal hypotonia to mixed tone with elements of dystonia or choreoathetosis. Severe extensor posturing is not uncommon.

Neuropathology

Neuropathologic findings of infants dying a period of months to years after injury include diffuse and focal cortical atrophy with multicystic encephalomalacia, microgyria and ulegyria, attenuated white matter, border-zone and arterial infarcts, and evidence of previous subdural hematomas.

PATHOLOGIC FEATURES

Many physical findings are associated with AHT, but not all injuries must be present to make the diagnosis. No individual markers are pathognomonic of abusive injury. The major markers of injury are outlined in Box 103-3.

Extracranial Injuries

Scalp. The most common extracranial impact injuries after AHT are scalp bruising, soft-tissue swelling, cephalohematoma, and subgaleal hematoma (Fig. 103-1).

Skull Fractures. Skull fractures are found in 25% to 74% of infants and children with abusive neurotrauma. Simple linear fractures of the parietal and occipital regions are most common. Fractures that are complicated (bilateral, comminuted, multiple, or that cross suture lines) may be more likely in abused children, although, on occasion, these complicated fractures occur after falls.

BOX 103-3 Abusive Head Injury: Markers of Injury

INTRACRANIAL
- Extraaxial fluid collections
  - Subdural hematoma
  - Subarachnoid hemorrhage
  - Subdural effusions
- Brain injury
  - Brain swelling
  - Infarction syndromes
  - White-matter contusional tears
  - Evidence of shearing injury
  - Diffuse axonal injury
- Skull fractures

EXTRACRANIAL
- Scalp and soft tissues
  - Subgaleal hematoma
  - Cephalohematoma
  - Soft tissue swelling
  - Hair loss
  - Bruising
- Ear
  - Pinna bruising
  - Hemotympanum
  - Ruptured ear drum
- Ocular
  - Periorbital edema and ecchymosis
  - Retinal hemorrhages
  - Peripapillary intrascleral hemorrhages
  - Retinal folds
  - Retinoschisis
  - Retinal detachment
  - Hyphema
  - Lens dislocation
- Mouth
  - Lip injury
  - Frenulum tear
  - Soft palate petechiae
  - Dental injury
- Other
  - Pattern bruising (e.g., from strangulation)
  - Long bone and rib fractures
  - Liver, kidney, or genital injury
  - Dehydration
  - Malnutrition
  - Burns
  - Excessive scarring

Intracranial Injuries

In most severely injured children, neuroimaging reveals intracranial abnormalities, most often acute subdural hematoma, cerebral hypodensity, and, less commonly, intraparenchymal hemorrhage (Figs. 103-2, 103-3, 103-4, 103-5A, 103-6, and 103-9).

Subdural Hematoma. Subdural hematomas are the most common intracranial pathologic abnormality found in AHT. They are typically interhemispheric and unilateral or bilateral over the convexities.

Mixed-Density or "Hyperacute" Subdural Hematoma. Mixed-density subdural hematomas on CT are frequently misdiagnosed as "acute on chronic" subdural hematomas. The mixed-density subdural collection in an abused infant more commonly results from rapidly accumulating blood in the potential subdural space, with fresh nonclotted blood found at surgery and no evidence of an organizing membrane.

Chronic Subdural Hematoma. Chronic subdural hematomas develop when an acute subdural hematoma fails to organize. There is a predictable sequence in their growth, the development of a membrane around the liquefying clot, and neovascularization, and finally ossification.

Chronic Subdural Effusions. Development of a chronic subdural collection (hygroma or effusion) may be associated with tears in the arachnoid and may not have the classic membrane structure. These subdural hygromas either resolve with time or persist because of evolving secondary atrophy.

Subarachnoid Hemorrhage. Subarachnoid hemorrhage develops after direct surface trauma to the brain, or from leakage of blood from injured cerebral vessels within the subarachnoid space. In the context of AHT, subarachnoid hemorrhage is not generally significant. On occasion, lesions that appear to be acute subdural hematomas resolve rapidly in 1 to 2 days.

Epidural Hematomas. Epidural hematomas are uncommon after AHT. The majority of arterial epidural hematomas develop from damage to the middle meningeal artery associated with skull fracture. Symptom progression parallels the rate of epidural blood accumulation. Lucid intervals are more common. These children generally have an excellent clinical outcome compared with abused infants consistent with their mechanism of injury.

Brain Injuries

Brain swelling. Younger infants present more often with diffuse brain swelling, whereas older infants and children present with focal or hemispheric brain swelling subjacent to an acute convexity subdural hematoma (Figs 103-4, 103-5, 103-8, and 103-9). None of the patterns of focal brain swelling are specific for abusive TBI.

Hemispheric swelling. One third of abused infants and young children present with hemispheric hypodensities subjacent to an acute subdural hematoma. Several mechanisms have been proposed, but the etiology remains poorly understood.

Cerebral infarction. Posttraumatic cerebral infarction after TBI is usually caused by vascular compression. Patterns include posterior cerebral artery and branch anterior cerebral artery distribution and lenticulostriate–thalamoperforator distribution infarctions (Figs 103-7 and 103-9). Hemispheric necrosis and border zone infarction also occur frequently (Fig. 103-9).

Diffuse axonal injury. Diffuse axonal shear injury (DAI) or traumatic axonal injury (TAI) is a common feature of severe TBI in older children and adults. Its frequency is not established in infants after TBI, and there is conflicting evidence about the precise pathogenesis of axonal injury identified in AHT. Major angular deceleration forces are required for the development of widespread TAI. It occurs at the moment of injury and, when severe, is associated with loss of consciousness at the moment of impact. Imaging findings of shear injuries include punctate hemorrhages, particularly at the gray–white matter junction, and tearing of the corpus callosum (Fig. 103-8).

Cerebral contusions. An infant younger than 8 months is much less likely to develop cortical contusions in coup or contrecoup locations than an older child or adult. The incidence of contrecoup injuries increases rapidly from later

infancy to 3 years of age, when it approximates that of the adults.

White-matter contusional tears. White-matter gliding contusions or contusional tears occur where shear strain is greatest, namely deep to the gray–white matter junction most often in the frontal and temporal lobes (Figs 103-12 and 103-13). They range from 1 to 3 cm in length. They are most easily visualized on follow-up imaging studies (Fig. 103-12).

Ocular Pathology

Retinal Hemorrhages (Table 103-1). Retinal and optic nerve sheath hemorrhages are the most common injuries to the globe, optic nerve, and surrounding tissues with a frequency of 47% to 100% depending on inclusion criteria. Explanations of the possible mechanism leading to retinal hemorrhages are discussed in the online chapter. Retinal hemorrhages in children with AHT have variable appearance and distribution (Figs 103-14 and 103-15). Younger age and greater hypoxic-ischemic injury correlate with more severe hemorrhages. Resolution rates of retinal hemorrhages after AHT have not been systematically studied but typically resolve within 10 days. Other documented findings include retinoschisis, retinal folds, retinal detachment, peripapillary intrascleral hemorrhages, periorbital edema and ecchymosis, subconjunctival hemorrhages, hyphema, and cataracts.

Optic Nerve Sheath Hemorrhage. Optic nerve sheath hemorrhages are found in the subdural and the potential subarachnoid space and tending to be more predominate in the distal optic nerve. They are found in 70% to 100% of abused children at postmortem examination.

Spinal Injuries

Spinal trauma, whether ligamentous or bony, needs to be distinguished from clinically significant spinal cord injury. It is increasingly recognized that spinal trauma, particularly in the cervical cord, is commonly associated with AHT, and the majority of injuries are ligamentous and identified primarily with MRI. Clinically significant spinal cord injury in children who have sustained AHT has rarely been reported and predominantly involves the cervical cord.

DIFFERENTIAL DIAGNOSIS

The range of clinical and physical findings in abusive neurotrauma is unique. It is extremely uncommon for infants to suffer severe brain injuries from unintentional mechanisms (falls and birth trauma) (Kuppermann et al., 2009). In establishing the likelihood that the injuries resulted from abusive versus unintentional mechanisms, the alternatives for each marker must be considered along with the patterns of injury to the craniospinal axis as well as other organ systems, along with the history of injury.

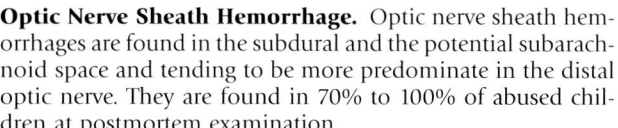

TABLE 103-1 Terminology for Retinal Hemorrhages

Name	Location
Vitreal	Vitreous
Subhyaloid (sublaminar or boat)	Preretinal
Intraretinal	
Flame or splinter	Nerve fiber layer
Dot (dot and blot)	Inner retinal layers (including bipolar)

Unintentional Injury

Falls. Fall data overwhelmingly support the conclusion that children younger than 2 years of age are extremely unlikely to sustain severe TBI and severe retinal hemorrhages in uncomplicated short falls (Kuppermann et al., 2009). Fall data should be interpreted cautiously. The majority of published data were collected retrospectively without consistent evaluation protocols. Routine neuroimaging is generally not performed in children who are not clinically symptomatic. Intracranial injuries, such as small, insignificant subdural hematoma, thus would be missed (Kuppermann et al., 2009). It is exceedingly unlikely that an infant presenting with a Glasgow Coma Score of 14 to 15 has significant brain injury.

Short falls. Short falls are generally low-impact, low-velocity injuries. The most common findings are concussions, scalp contusions, some fractures, an occasional epidural hematoma, and an occasional focal subarachnoid hemorrhage. In falls of less than 2 feet, clavicle fractures predominate; skull fractures are more common in falls of 2 to 4 feet. Similarly, household free falls from furniture of less than 3 feet do not generally result in significant brain injuries. The exception are epidural hematomas, which can be a life-threatening injury if not treated promptly.

Skull fractures that result from falls of 2 to 4 feet onto a hard surface, such as pavement, cement, linoleum, and wood, generally cause simple fractures. Rarely, complicated skull fractures occur in infants younger than 6 months of age. In very rare cases, a complicated short fall, usually with impact to the occiput, results in a more severe injury.

Walker and stroller falls. Walkers continue to be widely used in the United States despite the substantial amount of data detailing their risks. The majority of cases are because of falls down stairs, but tipping over is another mechanism. Most injuries include extremity bruises, skull and other skeletal fractures, and minor concussions. Rarely, infants sustain more significant intracranial injuries, including subdural hemorrhages and growing fractures.

Falls down stairs. Children falling down stairs (or infants dropped while being carried down stairs) typically do not sustain injury, although some falls may result in skull or skeletal injury. More severe injuries are occasionally seen when an adult falls on top of the child. Stairway falls usually are less serious than free falls of the same vertical distance regardless of the number of steps.

Falls from heights. Children falling from heights incur extremity injuries more than head injuries, and overall, recover better than adults. The brain and skull accelerate at the same rate in a high free fall. The brain may escape major injury, but the skull may shatter with impact because the skull absorbs much of the translational energy and there is little rotational component. A comminuted skull fracture with surface brain contusion, subarachnoid hemorrhage, or both in older children is consistent with a history of a high free fall.

Birth Trauma

Symptomatic injuries arising from the birth process are uncommon. Extracranial injuries predominate (caput succedaneum, cephalohematomas, and subgaleal hematomas). Skull fractures are generally either linear or depressed. Complicated skull fractures usually herald serious intracranial pathologic processes such as epidural and subdural hematomas, subarachnoid hemorrhage, and intracerebral hemorrhage. Small, generally asymptomatic subdural hematomas may occur after a difficult delivery or when an infant is large for gestational age. Eleven percent to 50% of full-term newborns have retinal hemorrhages after vaginal delivery. These hemorrhages are more frequent after complicated (vacuum extraction, protracted labor, premature, or traumatic) births. Although the types of hemorrhages are similar to those in infants with abusive injuries (flame, dot and blot, subhyaloid), they are rarely severe. Most of these hemorrhages are small and disappear within several days to 2 weeks.

Infants injured through the birth process exhibit symptoms perinatally. Review of the maternal and infant birth records, as well as any pediatric records, is exceedingly helpful. This review can firmly establish if birth-related complications or other conditions were or were not factors contributing to the acute clinical presentation.

Neurometabolic Disease

There are rare case reports of infants with metabolic disease presenting with signs and symptoms suggestive of abusive injury. Children with metabolic disease do not typically present with the range of findings found in abused infants. Specific findings on the history, physical examination, and imaging characteristics usually suggest the possibility of a metabolic disease. The organic aciduria, glutaric aciduria type 1, has been found most frequently. The most common finding is ocular involvement including intraretinal hemorrhages, cataracts, pigmentary retinopathy, and gaze palsies. Infants with glutaric aciduria type 1 may present with encephalopathic crises, macrocephaly, retinal hemorrhages, chronic subdural effusions, and spasticity.

The neurologic crises are typically precipitated by an infectious illness to which the brain responds with swelling, metabolic depression, and necrosis of basal ganglia gray matter. These infants have microencephalic macrocephaly from birth. Other neuroimaging features include widened operculae, alterations of signal intensity in the basal ganglia, subdural effusions, and dilated transarachnoid vascular plexuses.

Menkes's disease is a rare, x-linked recessive neurodegenerative disorder of copper transport. Vascular abnormalities predispose these infants to spontaneous intracranial hemorrhage. Infants, typically less than a year of age, present with subdural fluid collections, seizures, and developmental delay. C2 posterior arch defects have been found in 11% of infants.

On rare occasions, osteogenesis imperfecta type I has been reported to present with subdural hematoma, with and without retinal hemorrhages after minor trauma.

Metabolic screening tests should be considered in infants presenting with somnolence, vomiting, seizures, dystonia, or dyskinesia and extraaxial fluid collections (either subdural effusion or subdural hematoma), particularly if ketoacidosis or basal ganglia involvement are present.

DIFFERENTIAL OF SPECIFIC FINDINGS
Retinal and Optic Nerve Sheath Hemorrhages

Whereas retinal hemorrhages are very common after AHT, they are reported rarely after accidental head injury and in association with epidural hematoma. In this case they are usually mild, small, and scattered. In these instances, they are typically superficial and confined to the posterior pole.

Retinal and optic nerve sheath hemorrhages are found in numerous disorders. They have been reported in newborns but also in children who are critically ill and have vascular malformations, coagulopathies, anemia, leukemia, meningitis, bacterial endocarditis, hypertension, infections, and papilledema. Vitreous hemorrhages and epidural hematomas have been reported with hypofibrinogenemia. Retinal hemorrhages are not associated with seizures, coughing, or vomiting.

In the presence of papilledema, retinal hemorrhages cannot be causally related to abusive head injury. Retinal hemorrhages are rare in the context of acute life-threatening events, sometimes heralding a diagnosis of trauma.

Optic nerve sheath hemorrhages are not specific to abusive injury, having been reported secondary to sudden or prolonged increases in intracranial pressure (e.g., extensive subarachnoid hemorrhage) and, in rare cases, with unintentional head injury.

Extensive Subarachnoid Hemorrhage

Extensive subarachnoid hemorrhage can be seen in several conditions aside from AHT. These include vascular malformations, birth trauma, coagulopathy, meningitis, and unintentional trauma. These are uncommon causes of subarachnoid hemorrhage, and, in the presence of extensive subarachnoid bleeding, a vascular malformation is the most likely etiology. Vascular malformations (arteriovenous malformations, dural fistulas, and aneurysms) are exceedingly rare in young children (Chapter 111).

CLINICAL ASSESSMENT
General Examination

A detailed history of the injury and a timeline of the infant's behavior for a minimum of the 72 hours preceding the injury is invaluable. This history should be documented in a legible summary, with quotations from caregivers where possible. Histories of minor injury should be closely examined, and any available caretakers should be questioned independently if possible. The biomechanical history of the fall should include details such as the specific surface on to which the child fell, the location and type or types of injury, and the presence of corroborative witnesses. It is also useful to ask about exactly what happened after the event—"What did the child look like?" "What position was he or she in?" "What did he or she do next?" "What happened then?"—and so on. The age of the child and their developmental level should be documented. Documentation of inconsistencies in histories obtained from caregivers and family members is especially important, as are inconsistencies between the historical record and the clinicopathological findings (Christian et al., 2015).

General Examination

After initial coma scale scoring and resuscitative efforts, an extensive physical examination should be completed. Serial vital signs, including temperature (rectal preferred), can be helpful in developing a postinjury timeline. Growth parameters, including head circumference, state of hydration, and any obvious signs of neglect, need to be documented. The examiner should palpate and inspect all skin surfaces, particularly the cranium, behind the ears, and the occiput. Battle's sign (bruising over the mastoid) and "raccoon eyes" (periorbital ecchymoses) are suggestive of a basilar skull fracture. Hemotympanum can result either from direct impact over the ear or from a basilar fracture. The examiner should inspect the frenula and the palate for tears and petechiae; forced feeding, smothering, and gagging can cause these injuries. Any unusual pattern of injuries should be documented, including both a complete written record of the examiner's involvement with the child, and appropriate photographic documentation. Serial photographs are also very helpful. These should be taken with a color bar and a ruler in the photograph.

Classic features of asphyxia are facial cyanosis, petechial hemorrhages of the eyes and face, foam in the nose and mouth, and prominent bulging eyes. Some or all of these features may be present, depending on the amount of force applied to the neck, its rate and duration, and the surface area involved. Decreased carotid pulsations ipsilateral to neck bruising are suggestive of carotid injury. The neck should also be inspected closely, particularly along the mandible, to assess for subtle signs of strangulation.

The examiner should note the location and extent of any skin lesions, including bruises or bite marks. Bruises involving skin surfaces that are fairly protected, such as inner arms and other flexor surfaces, torso, ears, or neck, are of particular concern. A history of a simple fall is incongruous when there are multiple bruises of the same or different age, or if the bruises are on multiple and different body planes.

Neurologic Examination

Serial neurologic examinations, including the level of coma, should be documented (Chapter 101). Repeated funduscopic examinations are useful for documenting retinal hemorrhage development. Particular attention needs to be given to identifying and documenting asymmetries on the examination. The presence of a neurogenic bladder or bowel, or other findings that suggest a spinal level, should raise suspicion of spinal injury.

Autonomic and Neuroendocrine Responses

Endocrine and autonomic reactions to TBI are reviewed in detail in the online chapter. Briefly, TBI and other critical illnesses are potent activators of the hypothalamic–pituitary–adrenal axis and the sympathetic efferent pathways. There is a significant correlation between injury severity and loss of adaptive negative feedback control mechanisms.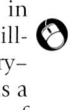

Within the first day after severe TBI, increased cortisol and adrenocorticotropin hormone may occur. Endocrinopathies develop in many survivors of AHT, and some are seen shortly after injury. Gonadotropin deficiency is common (up to 80%), as is vasopressin abnormalities (up to 40%), leading to diabetes insipidus or syndrome of inappropriate antidiuretic hormone release (SIADH), and corticotrophin and cortisol deficiencies.

Factors predictive of endocrine dysfunction include injury severity and the presence of skull fractures. Lower cortisol levels correlate with younger age, hypotension, hypoxia, anemia, and injury severity. In pediatric patients, adrenal insufficiency is more severe when intracranial hypertension is present. Acute adrenal insufficiency and central diabetes insipidus are predictive of mortality. During the acute hospitalization, many of these alterations are transient with cortisol and ACTH levels returning toward normal in the majority of patients.

Thirty to fifty percent of children have persistent evidence of hypopituitarism even up to 5 years after injury. Growth hormone deficiency and disturbances in puberty are the most common endocrine deficiencies, but children can also experience ACTH deficiency, diabetes insipidus, central hypothyroidism, and elevated prolactin levels. Every hormonal axis can be affected, although growth hormone deficiency and alterations in puberty are the most common (Personnier et al., 2014).

To date, there have been three studies examining hypothalamic–pituitary–adrenal function in infants after AHT (Personnier et al., 2014). In the only prospective study of 87 infants and children after accidental ($n = 73$) or abusive ($n = 14$) TBI, 30% of patients had persistently low growth hormone peak levels, with 15 meeting criteria for growth hormone deficiency and 5 had severe growth hormone deficiency. By 1 year after injury, pituitary dysfunction only was detected in 8% of patients (Personnier et al., 2014). All children admitted with TBI should be assessed for endocrine dysfunction. If the basal cortisol level is less than 15 mg/dL or increases by over 9 mg/dL after stimulation, treatment should be considered. Intravenous hydrocortisone at 50 to 100 mg every 8 hours or by continuous infusion is usually sufficient but may be supplemented with a mineralocorticoid if hyponatremia persists. All patients sustaining severe TBI should be tested for abnormal endocrine function (adrenal, thyroid, and growth hormone) at 3 and 12 months after injury. Although many abnormalities will slowly improve, a significant subpopulation has persistent abnormalities that require long-term treatment.

Autonomic cardiac control in children with TBI can be altered depending on injury. When efferent sympathetic pathways are completely interrupted (i.e., autonomic failure), heart rate variability is lost and low-frequency heart-rate power decreases; these findings are highly correlated with brain death in children and adults.

LABORATORY AND RADIOGRAPHIC EVALUATION
Laboratory Evaluation

Infants who have sustained abusive head injuries are frequently anemic and acidotic when hospitalized. Leukocytosis is not uncommon. As in adults, hyperglycemia has been associated with a more severe head injury and a poorer prognosis and is also suggestive of more recent injury. The combination of lower GCS scores, lower hemoglobin levels, and increased glucose levels are associated with a greater risk of developing a coagulopathy. As in other TBI populations, secondary consumptive coagulopathy is associated with a higher mortality rate and more severe brain injury (Peiniger et al., 2012). These abnormalities do not appear to reflect preexisting coagulation abnormalities. In situations in which a clinical index of suspicion arises or an alternative diagnosis has been proposed, such as an inherited metabolic disease, additional studies or consultation with a metabolic geneticist may be useful.

Biochemical Markers. There is a remarkable body of literature evolving that is studying the acute-phase changes of numerous "biomarkers" after pediatric TBI as a means toward identifying therapeutic targets (Kochanek et al., 2013). This is reviewed in detail in the online chapter. Although many protein degradation products, S-100B, neuron-specific enolase, inflammatory mediators, soluble intracellular adhesion molecule, L-selectin, and endothelin, increase acutely after TBI, these changes have not differentiated abusive from unintentional injuries (Kochanek et al., 2013).

Neuroimaging and Radiographic Evaluation

In symptomatic infants and children, the initial neuroimaging study of choice is a noncontrast CT scan with bone windows. A CT scan may miss skull fractures within the plane of the section, and so skull films should be included as part of the skeletal survey. A full skeletal survey should be obtained in any child younger than 2 years of age, or in any older child with multiple traumatic injuries suspected to be caused by abuse. In instances where there is a suspicion of fracture, repeating the survey 2 to 3 weeks after presentation may establish conclusively that a fracture occurred. A bone scan may be indicated in equivocal or negative cases in which there is a high level of suspicion of injury. If carotid or vertebral injury is suspected, cerebral angiography may be helpful.

MRI is more sensitive and accurate than CT scanning in defining the extent and age of extraaxial collections, hemorrhagic and nonhemorrhagic injury, and evolution of ischemic changes, and in demonstrating infarctions. Repeat or serial imaging is often helpful in establishing the extent of injury.

Advanced imaging techniques (susceptibility-weighted imaging, diffusion-weighted imaging, MR spectroscopy, and diffusion tensor imaging) in addition to CT and standard MRI improve sensitivity in defining the extent of parenchymal injury and total injury volume as well as improving outcome prediction in young children with TBI. More detail about imaging techniques is discussed in the online chapter. A review of advanced neuroimaging modalities after TBI was published in 2014 (Ashwal et al., 2014).

There is considerable variability in the radiologic interpretation of neuroimaging data. Few clinicopathological studies have been published, and caution should be exercised in relying only on imaging to establish timing of injury. It is strongly recommended that clinicians review the neuroimaging studies themselves, and if possible with a neuroradiologist.

POSTMORTEM EXAMINATION

A full postmortem examination, including examination of the eyes and testing for metabolic disease, is mandatory for any child with an unexplained death, as these findings frequently assist in establishing an unintentional or abusive etiology. This is particularly true in infants younger than 1 year of age, in whom the incidence of sudden infant death syndrome is higher than that of abusive head injury. At postmortem examination, evaluation of the reflected scalp allows for identification of galeal hemorrhage and impact sites (periosteal hemorrhages). The temporalis muscle and posterior cervical muscles are additional sites where internal soft tissue injury may be found. Small patchy areas of subarachnoid hemorrhages are almost universally found at postmortem examination in infants who die of abusive injury.

Aside from greatly assisting in documenting the full extent of injuries, the postmortem examination provides additional information about the pathologic timing of injury events. The presence of intraalveolar siderophages, for instance, is suggestive of previously imposed suffocation. Confirmation of specific findings, such as subdural neomembranes and positive retinal staining for hemosiderin and iron, can further assist in the timing of injuries (Figs 103-14, 103-18, and 103-19). However, in instances in which the infant has been kept alive while a brain death determination is being made and in which resultant necrosis evolves, clinical timing of injury is frequently more precise than timing based on pathologic findings.

MAKING THE DIAGNOSIS OF ABUSIVE HEAD INJURY
General Considerations

Child abuse is rarely premeditated. It occurs when caregivers lose control, often when trying to stop certain behaviors (such as crying) or when punishing perceived transgressions (such as toileting accidents). Abusive injuries may be one-time events, or repeated and complex scenarios occurring in 1 day, over days, weeks, or months. The sequence of injury events is highly variable. Events can include shaking, throwing, hitting, slapping, gagging, strangling, and smothering. Only children with injuries severe enough to frighten the caregiver are likely to be brought to medical attention. Resuscitation delay, while a potentially important factor, does not occur uniformly, and is not unique to abuse.

> **BOX 103-4** Key Questions in the Evaluation of the Child With Suspected Abusive Head Injury
>
> - What is the distribution of injuries?
> - Are the injuries confined to the head?
> - Are the brain injuries focal, diffuse, or both?
> - What is the clinical timing of the injury?
> - Are there injuries that suggest a specific injury mechanism (slap mark, strangulation bruising, etc.)?
> - Are there other suspicious patterns of injury (e.g., rib fractures)?
> - What forces were necessary to cause such injuries?
> - Is the history congruent with the physical injuries?
> - Is there an accidental mechanism that would explain these injuries?
> - Is there a nonaccidental mechanism that would explain these injuries?
> - Is there evidence of injuries of varying ages (e.g., old bite marks)?
> - Was there a delay in seeking medical attention?
> - Was the injury witnessed?
> - Are there more than one history for the injury or injuries? Changing histories?
> - If there is suspicion of a nonaccidental etiology, has the child been reported to the hospital child abuse team and to the local child protective services?

> **BOX 103-5** Factors Associated With an Abusive Etiology
>
> - Age less than 1 year
> - Greater severity of illness
> - Unexplained injuries
> - A biomechanically inconsistent history
> - A changing history or one inconsistent with the child's developmental level
> - A delay in seeking medical attention
> - Parental risk factors
> - History of past abuse and neglect
> - Alcohol and drug use
> - Previous social service intervention

Evidence of previous maltreatment or neglect does not necessarily assist in identification of the perpetrator, unless he or she is the only caregiver.

Evaluating the History

Histories given by perpetrators typically minimize actual injury events. Often, there is a history of minor trauma (such as a short fall with no neurologic symptoms) or no history at all. Changing histories, either by the same caregiver or by multiple caregivers, should raise concerns. In many situations, perpetrator admissions are not straightforward and event sequences are quite variable. Typically, the actual injury and timeline of the events are understated, whereas descriptions of the clinical behaviors of the infant are accurate. There are a number of clues that suggest an abusive etiology (Box 103-5).

Timing

The timing of injury events in the still-living child can usually be estimated by using a combination of clinical course, physical findings, and imaging data, although best estimates may be insufficiently precise to eliminate all possible perpetrators. Children who sustain moderate to severe TBI are almost always immediately symptomatic, and often demonstrate an immediate apneustic response to mechanical events, whether abused or not. Persistence of coma, apnea or respiratory distress, irritability, seizures, hypotonia, and vomiting reflects the severity of injury and evolving secondary pathophysiologic cascades. Early posttraumatic seizures should not be used to time injury events.

Lucid Interval

The lucid interval occurs after an initial loss of consciousness after a head injury consisting of a period of clinical improvement, not necessarily normalcy, followed by neurologic deterioration within minutes to hours. Lucid intervals occur in less than 3% of children after moderate to severe TBI of all etiologies, and generally result in a nonlethal injury if prompt care can be delivered. Periods of improved consciousness have been reported in children with GCS scores of less than 8 after initial unconsciousness followed by rapid secondary deterioration within minutes to hours.

Dating by Neuroimaging

Dating of parenchymal injuries by neuroimaging is confounded by variability in the rate of brain swelling, from within 20 to 30 minutes to several hours. In general, evolution

Establishing the diagnosis of abusive trauma is frequently problematic and requires a high index of suspicion. The fewer markers of injury and the more nonspecific the history, the more difficult it is to distinguish abusive from unintentional injury. The less severe the injury, the less pronounced the postconcussive syndrome. Findings indicating more significant force generation include injuries to the neck and rostral spine, contusions/lacerations of the olfactory system, partial or complete transection of the corpus callosum, tearing of the septum pellucidum, and evidence of diffuse axonal injury.

Children interface with the medical system at all points along their response curve after brain injury. It is unrealistic to expect findings in all children to be similar. Certain key questions should be asked and answered (Box 103-4). The physical findings, in conjunction with inconsistent historical features, usually point to trauma as the most likely etiology. Obvious cases are those with clear and convincing findings in the absence of an injury mechanism that accounts for the findings. The combination of acute serious brain injury, retinal hemorrhages, and posterior interhemispheric subdural hematomas appear to have greater specificity for an abusive etiology, but are not unique to abusive injury.

Evidence of impact is helpful in establishing abusive injury when caregivers have specifically denied trauma. Multiple impact injuries are not consistent with a history of a simple short fall, especially if the alleged fall did not occur the same day. On the other hand, complicated short falls do occur. In the infant who survives, however, the absence of external scalp bruising, soft-tissue swelling, or skull fracture does not conclusively exclude blunt-force trauma, as evidence of impact may be found only at the time of the postmortem examination.

Particular patterns of injury are more supportive of abusive injury, such as accompanying rib or long bone fractures, or pulmonary or liver contusions. Neck bruising and hyoid injury indicate that strangulation has occurred. Bruising in unusual regions (such as the neck, ears, abdomen, or buttocks), human bites, and acute genitoanal trauma may be evidence of abuse and is supportive of an abusive etiology.

of cerebral parenchymal abnormalities occurs rapidly after injury in adults and similarly have been documented within 1 to 3 hours in abusive and accidental childhood TBI.

Dating of subdural hematomas by CT imaging is difficult because of differences in interpretation of signal densities, variability in development and resolution of findings, and influence of confounding variables. In general, hyperintense subdural collections on noncontrast CT imaging are less than 7 days old; isointense collections, 7 to 14 days old; and hypointense collections, more than 14 days old. In 43 abused infants with specific times of injury, the first hypointense component within the subdural hematoma appeared 0.3 to 16 days after injury and the last hyperdense component disappeared from 2 to 40 days after injury.

Attempts have been made to standardize dating estimation with some success. However, subdural hematomas may appear hypodense in the very anemic infant or if there is a mixture of cerebrospinal fluid with subdural blood or arterial blood contributes to the subdural collection. Subdural neomembranes, visualized with contrast CT scans, begin to develop between 7 and 10 days after injury. Mixed-density subdural collections on CT imaging should not be diagnosed as acute on chronic bleeding without confirmation of neomembranes (either at surgery or necropsy).

MRI, like CT, cannot date injuries precisely, and the finding of blood of different intensities does not always mean that there has been repeated trauma, in as much as blood in various compartments may have different signal characteristics. Without pathologic correlation, definitive dating of extra-axial blood collections by standard neuroimaging should be made cautiously.

Medicolegal Issues

Child abuse and neglect were defined by the Federal Child Abuse Prevention and Treatment Act (CAPTA) 42 U.S.C.A. §5106g, and most recently amended in 2010.

Key elements of this definition are as follows:

- Any recent act or failure to act on the part of a parent or caretaker that results in death, serious physical or emotional harm, sexual abuse, or exploitation
- An act or failure to act that presents an imminent risk of serious harm

Assault of infants and children has specific medicolegal consequences and implications that accidental injuries do not have. As mandated reporters, when we report a suspected case of abuse or neglect, there are often concurrent civil and criminal investigations that cross jurisdictional lines. This is often confusing for medical professionals. Taking an infant off life-support may mean that the alleged perpetrator is charged with second-degree murder, rather than felony child abuse (this varies by state). Lastly, because both abusive and accidental injuries occur with a spectrum of findings and via a variety of mechanisms, more general terminology is helpful to avoid trying to fit all cases into narrow semantic and conceptual descriptors.

Mandated reporting laws require physicians and other healthcare professionals to report for investigation, patterns of injuries, and behavior when reasonable suspicion of abuse or neglect arises. Reasonable suspicion does not mean that the clinician must be certain of the diagnosis; it means only that the clinical picture warrants full investigation and possible protection of the injured child and any siblings. Healthcare providers actually fail to diagnose or misdiagnose about one third of abusive head injuries in infants and children during initial examinations, especially when injuries are not severe.

The law protects the physician if suspicion should prove erroneous but was made in good faith. Conversely, failure to report suspected abuse is actionable and places children at significant risk for further harm if they are returned to the setting in which they were injured. Although there is a cross-reporting mandate between social service and law enforcement officials, it may not happen immediately. When serious physical injury is suspected to have resulted from assault, notification of both law enforcement and social services is recommended.

Translating and interpreting complex information from the medical to the legal arena is a critical component of the evaluation of suspected abusive head injury for the protection of the child, other siblings, and the alleged perpetrator. This process begins with adequate written, photographic, and schematic documentation, and extends through communication with Child Protective Services, law enforcement agencies, legal counsel, and the judicial system. Documentation of inconsistencies in the histories obtained from various family members is especially important, as is inconsistencies between the historical record and the clinicopathological findings (Christian et al., 2015).

Investigating agencies want treating clinicians to know whether the injuries were abusive or not, but the clinician is sometimes unable to say more than that the injuries are clearly traumatic in origin. If there is uncertainty about the significance or timing of particular findings, an expert opinion, usually from a child abuse team physician, neurosurgeon, child neurologist, or forensic neuropathologist with expertise in this area, is often helpful. Ultimately, the diagnosis of abusive injury relies on the constellation of physical findings, a history of injury that is not biomechanically feasible, and the timing of injury. It is imperative to have either the services worker or law enforcement complete a scene investigation and obtain photographs, again with tape measures, as soon as a fall history is given. Optimally, these data will be reviewed by the clinicians who are determining whether the clinical and radiologic findings are consistent or inconsistent with the given history.

CONCLUSIONS

Abusive childhood neurotrauma is a complicated form of traumatic injury with a well-defined continuum of injury findings. There is much that remains to be learned about early life TBI, regardless of whether injury occurred by assault or unintentional mechanisms. Systematic research studies using consistent definitions and methodology are the next step in elucidating mechanisms of injury and defining evidence-based practice.

REFERENCES

The complete list of references for this chapter is available in the e-book at www.expertconsult.com.

See inside cover for registration details.

SELECTED REFERENCES

Ashwal, S., Tong, K.A., Ghosh, N., et al., 2014. Application of advanced neuroimaging modalities in pediatric traumatic brain injury. J. Child Neurol. 29, 1704–1717.

Christian, C.W., Block, R., Committee on Child Abuse and Neglect; American Academy of Pediatrics, 2009. Abusive head trauma in infants and children. Pediatrics 123, 1409–1411.

Christian, C.W., Committee On Child Abuse and Neglect, 2015. The evaluation of suspected child physical abuse. Pediatrics 135, e1337–e1354.

Hagberg, H., Mallard, C., Rousset, C.I., et al., 2014. Mitochondria: hub of injury responses in the developing brain. Lancet Neurol. 13, 217–232.

Kochanek, P.M., Berger, R.P., Fink, E.L., et al., 2013. The potential for bio-mediators and biomarkers in pediatric traumatic brain injury and neurocritical care. Front Neurol. 4, 40.

Kuppermann, N., Holmes, J.F., Dayan, P.S., et al., 2009. Identification of children at very low risk of clinically-important brain injuries after head trauma: a prospective cohort study. Lancet 374, 1160–1170.

Peiniger, S., Nienaber, U., Lefering, R., et al., 2012. Glasgow Coma Scale as a predictor for hemocoagulative disorders after blunt pediatric traumatic brain injury. Pediatr. Crit. Care Med. 13, 455–460.

Personnier, C., Crosnier, H., Meyer, P., et al., 2014. Prevalence of pituitary dysfunction after severe traumatic brain injury in children and adolescents: a large prospective study. J. Clin. Endocrinol. Metab. 99, 2052–2060.

Piteau, S.J., Ward, M.G., Barrowman, N.J., et al., 2012. Clinical and radiographic characteristics associated with abusive and nonabusive head trauma: a systematic review. Pediatrics 130, 315–323.

Robertson, C.M., Joffe, A.R., Moore, A.J., et al., 2002. Neurodevelopmental outcome of young pediatric intensive care survivors of serious brain injury. Pediatr. Crit. Care Med. 3, 345–350.

⊘ E-BOOK FIGURES AND TABLES

The following figures and tables are available in the e-book at www.expertconsult.com. See inside cover for registration details.

Fig. 103-1 Occipital skull fracture extending into the foramen magnum in a 6-month-old infant.

Fig. 103-2 Nonenhanced computed tomographic scan of an 11-month-old infant admitted with acute loss of consciousness and apnea with no history of trauma.

Fig. 103-3 Nonenhanced computed tomographic scan of an acute interhemispheric subdural hematoma.

Fig. 103-4 Nonenhanced computed tomographic scan with an acute mixed-density right subdural hematoma.

Fig. 103-5 Evolution of hypoxic-ischemic injury.

Fig. 103-6 Nonenhanced computed tomographic scan of a 9-month-old infant admitted with macrocrania, seizures, and irritability.

Fig. 103-7 Nonenhanced computed tomographic scan obtained 2 weeks after admission with seizures, apnea, and left hemiparesis.

Fig. 103-8 Images of a 3-month-old presenting with a growing head and with rib fractures.

Fig. 103-9 Images of a 4-year-old who was picked up, strangled, and thrown, hitting the occiput on a marble coffee-table edge.

Fig. 103-10 Strangulation injuries in a 4-year-old child.

Fig. 103-11 Three-year-old child injured because of a toileting accident.

Fig. 103-12 Computed tomographic appearance of healed white-matter tears in the bifrontal regions.

Fig. 103-13 Gross specimens from a 2-month-old infant with multiple acute white-matter contusions of the left hemisphere. One contusion is marked.

Fig. 103-14 Hematoxylin and eosin stain photomicrograph of retina, revealing prominent hemosiderin-laden macrophages (center).

Fig. 103-15 Nerve fiber layer and intraretinal layer retinal hemorrhages.

Fig. 103-16 Extensive sublaminar and intraretinal layer retinal hemorrhages.

Fig. 103-17 Seventeen-month-old child who fell from an unprotected 8-foot high porch on to a 2 × 4 feet piece of wood and suffered immediate sustained loss of consciousness and posturing.

Fig. 103-18 Gross photograph of an unstained section of retina, revealing a prominent sublaminar hemorrhage and multiple intraretinal hemorrhages.

Fig. 103-19 Retinal section stained for iron.

104 Hypoxic-Ischemic Encephalopathy in Infants and Older Children

Craig M. Smith, Mark S. Wainwright, and Stephen Ashwal

CARDIAC ARREST: ETIOLOGY, SURVIVAL, AND NEUROLOGIC OUTCOME

In the majority of cases, pediatric cardiac arrest results from asphyxia, in contrast with adult cardiac arrest, which is predominantly the result of ventricular fibrillation (VF). The morphologic pattern of brain damage is different in asphyxial and VF cardiac arrest because of the differences in patterns of cerebral blood flow (CBF). Cardiac arrests in children generally result from progressive tissue hypoxia and acidosis resulting from respiratory failure, circulatory shock, or both. Electrocardiographic rhythms of cardiac arrests in children usually progress through bradyarrhythmias to asystole or pulseless electrical activity rather than to VF. Although the outcomes from cardiac arrhythmias or shock in children are generally good, the outcomes from pulseless cardiac arrests in children are poor.

A multicenter study of children who had a sustained return of circulation after in-hospital cardiac arrest showed a rate of survival to hospital discharge of 48.7%. Of those who survived to discharge, 76.7% had a good neurologic outcome. In contrast, survival following out-of-hospital arrest ranges between 6% and 10%. Survival following cardiac arrest in the emergency department in a study of 16,782 patients over 10 years in the Get with the Guidelines—Resuscitation database found that survival to discharge was not different (23% vs. 20%) between children and adults, and there was no effect of age on outcome. A prospective international study of 502 children with in-hospital cardiac arrest found that only 9% survived to hospital discharge, but of these patients, 88 had good neurologic function at 1 year (Del Castillo et al., 2015), which is consistent with the results of a single-center study of recovery following in- and out-of-hospital arrest. A comparison of these two groups is presented in Table 104-1 and Table 104-2.

The incidence of cardiac arrest in infants approaches that of adults and is higher compared with that of children and adolescents. Outcomes have been improving, mainly because of increased understanding of the pathophysiology, expansion of resuscitation training programs, and improvement in resuscitation techniques. Postarrest care has evolved, and substantial attention has been paid to focused central nervous system (CNS) resuscitation and support because neurologic injury is one of the most significant complications of cardiac arrest (Donoghue et al., 2015).

POSTCARDIAC-ARREST SYNDROME

Postcardiac-arrest syndrome includes brain injury, myocardial dysfunction, and systemic ischemia and reperfusion injury (Galland and Elder, 2014). The four phases of resuscitation in cardiac arrest are *prearrest* (events leading to cardiac arrest, i.e., hypoxia, bradycardia, hypovolemia, arrhythmia), *arrest* (no flow), *resuscitation* (chest compressions: low or no flow, and assisted ventilation), and *recovery after resuscitation*. The term *postcardiac-arrest syndrome* was proposed in a scientific state-

ment by the International Liaison Committee on Resuscitation, and four phases of this syndrome were described:

1. Immediate postarrest phase (first 20 minutes after return of spontaneous circulation)
2. Early postarrest phase (20 minutes to 6–12 hours)
3. Intermediate phase (6–12 hours to 72 hours)
4. Recovery phase (beyond 3 days)

Therapy targeting each of these phases has a defined goal; interventions in the early phases focus on limiting further injury and vital support, whereas those in the later phases focus on prognostication and then rehabilitation.

RESPONSE TO INADEQUATE OXYGEN DELIVERY: MECHANISMS OF BRAIN INJURY

Asphyxia produces a state of hypoxemic, hypotensive perfusion before cardiac arrest. During ischemia, energy stores of the brain are depleted, and toxic metabolites accumulate (lactate and hydrogen ion). Upon reperfusion, injury to the brain is caused by excitotoxicity, calcium accumulation, protease activation, and formation of reactive oxygen and nitrogen species. The mechanism of neuronal damage after cardiac arrest is a combination of necrosis, apoptosis, autophagy, and inflammation. Necrosis is a process characterized by immediate mitochondrial and energy failure, leading to cellular swelling, loss of cell membrane integrity, and a prominent inflammatory response in surrounding tissue. Apoptosis is an energy-requiring process necessitating new protein synthesis. Enzymatic degradation of cytoskeletal proteins results in cell soma and nuclear shrinkage, and DNA is characteristically fragmented via endonucleases. In contrast to necrosis, apoptosis produces minimal inflammation and autophagy. Autophagy is an adaptive response to starvation and results in autodigestion of cellular proteins and organelles to feed the cell. Triggering of autophagy after acute insults may be beneficial or detrimental, likely depending on the degree or duration of injury.

Brain Energy Failure

Because of its high metabolic demands, limited energy stores, and reliance on oxidative metabolism, the brain depends on large amounts of exogenous substrates (oxygen and glucose). Cellular energy depletion is postulated to be the triggering event that initiates the cascade of injury that occur during ischemia. Under normal conditions, this function accounts for nearly 50% of total cellular expenditure. Interruption of CBF results in loss of consciousness and reductions in electroencephalographic (EEG) activity within seconds. Within 5 to 7 minutes, complete energy failure occurs, accompanied by disturbances of neuronal and glial ion homeostasis, including sodium and water influx and efflux of potassium (Figure 104-1). When the extracellular potassium concentration reaches a critical threshold, voltage-gated channels undergo depolarization, precipitating extracellular calcium influx. If flow remains inadequate and energy failure persists, calcium-mediated events, including phospholipase and protease activation, can lead to irreversible cellular injury and necrosis, as well as cerebral acidosis with elevated lactate levels and decreased hydrogen ion concentration (pH). If blood flow is restored, recovery of basal cellular metabolism (adenosine 5-triphosphate [ATP] levels, protein synthesis, oxygen consumption) and normal pH occurs if the ischemic injury is of limited duration. For an excellent recent review of cell death

mechanisms, see Tovar, Penagos-Puig, and Ramirez-Jarquin (2015).

Cell necrosis results from progressive reduction in cellular ATP content and involves a series of morphologic alterations, including swelling of cells and organelles, development of subsurface cellular blebs, amorphous deposits in mitochondria, condensation of nuclear chromatin, and breaks in plasma and cell organelle membranes. Cell death after hypoxic-ischemic insults can also occur by apoptosis. Apoptosis is an energy- and substrate-dependent process. The development of apoptosis involves new protein synthesis and the activation of endonucleases, with a resultant characteristic cleavage of DNA at linkage regions between nucleosomes to form fragments of

TABLE 104-1 Comparison of the Etiology of Cardiac Arrest for In-Hospital and Out-of-Hospital Cohorts*[†]

	In-Hospital Overall ($n = 353$), n (%)	Out-of-Hospital Overall ($n = 138$), n (%)	p
Cardiac (not congenital heart disease)	124 (36)	20 (15)	<0.01
Congenital heart disease	130 (37)	6 (4)	<0.01
Respiratory	145 (42)	98 (72)	<0.01
Neurologic	8 (2)	5 (4)	0.53
Drug overdose/ ingestion	3 (1)	4 (3)	0.1
Trauma	22 (6)	15 (11)	0.09
Electrolyte imbalance	30 (9)	4 (3)	0.03
Terminal condition	12 (3)	1 (1)	0.12

*Patients could have multiple categories identified for etiology of arrest.
[†]Chi-square or Fisher's exact test was used for comparison between in-hospital and out-of-hospital arrests.
(Modified from Moler FW et al. Crit Care Med 2009;37:2259–2267.)

TABLE 104-2 Characteristics of Successfully Resuscitated Pediatric Patients with In-Hospital or Out-of-Hospital Cardiac Arrest

	Out-of-Hospital Cardiac Arrest	In-Hospital Cardiac Arrest
Initial rhythm (%)	Asystolic (46) Bradycardia (10) VF/VT (7)	Bradycardia (49) Asystole (16) VF/VT (10)
CPR duration (median, min)	31	9
Cause (%)	Respiratory (72)	Cardiac (73)
Preexisting chronic condition	49	88
Good neurologic outcome	24	47
Mortality rate (%)	62	51
Neurologic injury as the cause of mortality	69	20

CPR, cardiopulmonary resuscitation; VF, ventricular fibrillation; VT, ventricular tachycardia.
(Modified from Moler FW et al. Crit Care Med 2009;37:2259–2267.)

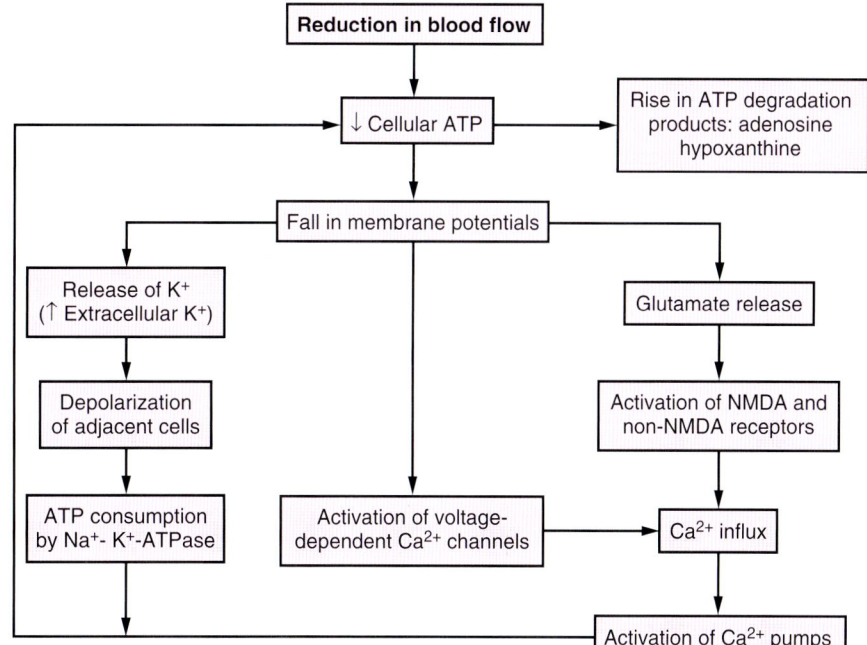

Figure 104-1. Global ischemia results in a cascade of events. These include reduction in adenosine triphosphate (ATP), loss of cellular ionic gradients, increases in extracellular K^+ concentration, glutamate release with activation of N-methyl-D-aspartate (NMDA) and non-NMDA receptors, calcium influx and release of intracellular calcium, and activation of secondary messenger systems and a variety of destructive enzymatic processes.

double-stranded DNA. The stimuli triggering apoptosis are not clearly defined, although protease activation or oxidant injury to DNA has been proposed. After a global ischemic insult, DNA fragmentation is most pronounced in neurons of the CA1 region of the hippocampus, which suggests that apoptosis may play a role in both selective neuronal necrosis and delayed neuronal death. Apoptosis is also seen in penumbral regions around evolving cerebral infarctions. Because apoptosis occurs in stages, there exist several potential strategies for reducing cell death.

Calcium-Mediated Injury

Calcium plays a critical role in the regulation of many cellular metabolic processes; therefore the concentration of cytosolic free calcium is tightly controlled. Hypoxic-ischemic injury interrupts intracellular calcium homeostasis, which results in massive increases in the intracellular concentration of calcium. This calcium accumulation is believed to promote irreversible cellular injury (Figure 104-2). Transient calcium accumulation occurs in all cells during ischemia, but secondary irreversible accumulation occurs in the selectively vulnerable zones many hours later.

The disturbance of intracellular calcium homeostasis is recognized as a final common pathway of neuronal death, either necrotic or apoptotic. These conditions, in concert with excessive release of calcium-dependent excitatory neurotransmitters (glutamate, aspartate), lead to uncontrolled excitotoxicity and cell death.

Excitotoxic Injury

During hypoxic-ischemic damage, pathologically prolonged membrane depolarization occurs and, in certain neuronal populations, leads to excessive release of neurotransmitters into the synaptic cleft. The effect of these neurotransmitters is prolonged by failure of the ATP-dependent presynaptic reuptake mechanisms. Glutamate and aspartate are the major excitatory amino acid neurotransmitters in the mammalian CNS.

Activation of Intracellular Enzymes

The marked increase in intracellular calcium concentration activates a number of important enzymes. Phospholipases break down the lipid cellular membrane, releasing arachidonic acid that generates prostaglandins and free radicals. Protein kinases activate enzymes in an unordered manner, including nitric oxide synthase and xanthine oxidase, which are also generators of free radicals. Proteases begin the uninhibited breakdown of the cytoskeleton, and endonucleases initiate DNA fragmentation.

Phospholipase Release of Free Fatty Acids

Free fatty acids are released from neuronal membranes during ischemia and have potential detrimental effects through at least three mechanisms (Figure 104-3). First, free fatty acid metabolism via the cyclo-oxygenase pathway contributes to oxygen radical production during reperfusion. Second, free fatty acid and diacylglycerol directly increase membrane fluidity, inhibit ATPases, increase neurotransmitter release, promote brain edema, and uncouple oxidative phosphorylation. Third, enzymatic oxidation of arachidonic acid during reperfusion by cyclo-oxygenase, lipoxygenase, or cytochrome P-450 produces a large number of bioactive lipids (prostaglandins, thromboxanes, leukotrienes, and hydroxyl acids), many of which have detrimental effects.

Activation of Nitric Oxide Synthesis

Nitric oxide plays a multifaceted role in the brain as a neurotransmitter and a regulator of CBF. Sites of nitric oxide

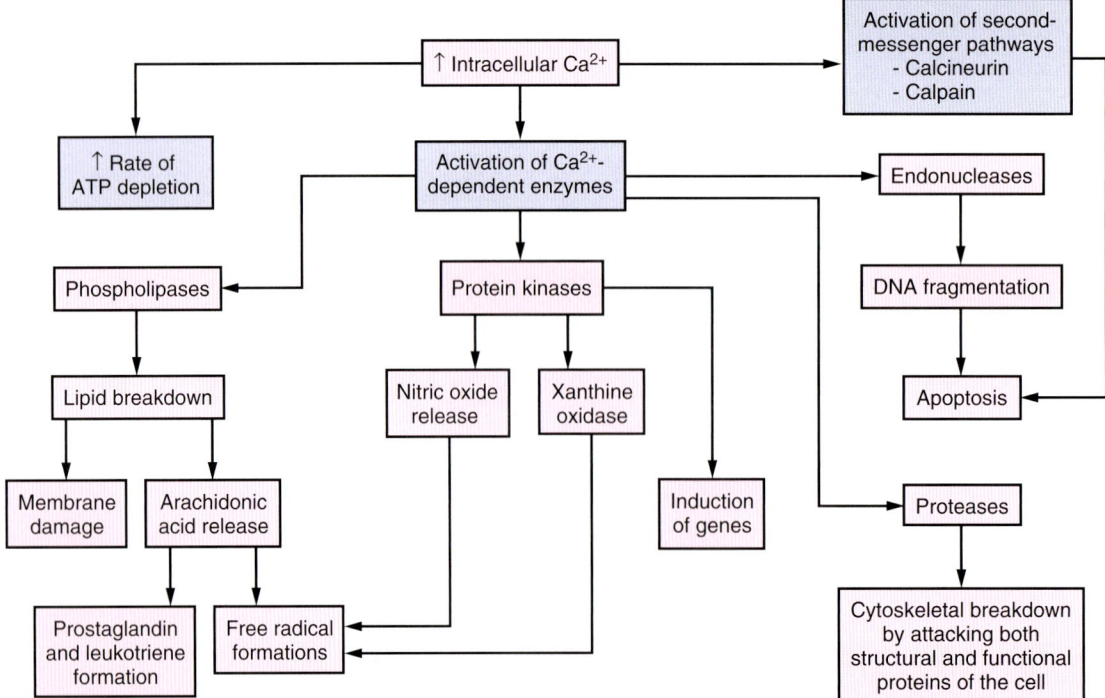

Figure 104-2. Increases in intracellular Ca^{2+} mediate several enzymatic pathways that cause cell injury. These include pathways of protein kinases, proteases, phospholipases, nitric oxide synthase, other free radical synthesis, and endonucleases, and other second-messenger systems. The net effect is related to the severity and duration of ischemia and a series of complex events that results in cell necrosis and apoptosis, and other forms of partial injury that remain poorly understood. ATP, adenosine triphosphate.

production include neurons, vascular endothelium, perivascular neurons, and astrocytes (Figure 104-4). If present in abnormally high concentrations, nitric oxide may exert neurotoxic effects.

Nitric oxide is produced in a reaction catalyzed by nitric oxide synthase, in which oxygen and L-arginine are converted into L-citrulline and nitric oxide. Neurons containing nitric oxide synthase are present throughout the brain, with the highest concentration in the cerebellum and the lowest concentration in the medulla.

As part of the excitotoxic cascade of injury, glutamate release activates both endothelial and neuronal nitric oxide synthase, which increase nitric oxide production during focal and global ischemia. Nitric oxide produced under conditions of ischemia contributes to the cytotoxicity of glutamate, presumably through hydroxyl radical production (Figure 104-4). Nitric oxide and superoxide radical react to form peroxynitrite, which then decomposes to yield nitrogen dioxide and the

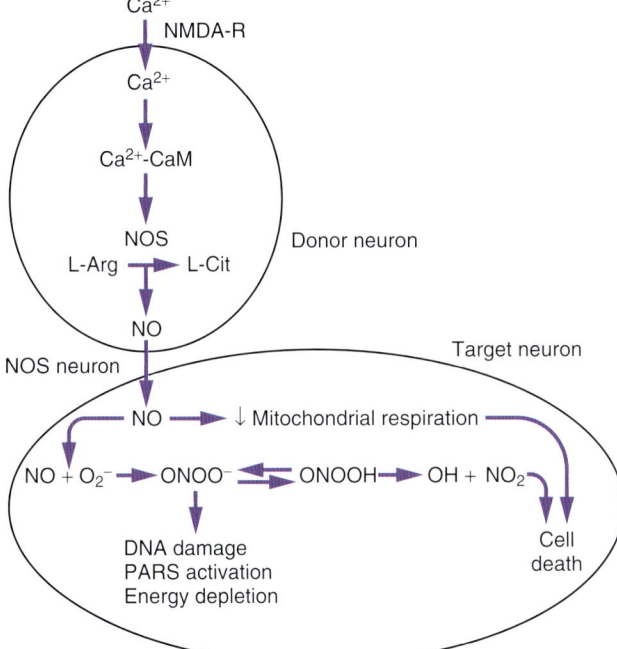

Figure 104-4. Excessive nitric oxide is formed on sustained glutamate stimulation of *N*-methyl-D-aspartate receptors (NMDA-Rs). Nitric oxide (NO) freely diffuses to adjacent target neurons, in which it combines with the superoxide anion (O2⁻), produced by mitochondria and xanthine oxidase, to yield the peroxynitrite anion (ONOO⁻), which is an extremely potent oxidant. ONOO⁻ also is protonated and decomposes to the hydroxyl (OH) free radical and the nitrogen dioxide (NO₂) free radical, which are potent activators of lipid peroxidation. Damaged DNA activates the nuclear enzyme poly-adenosine diphosphate (ADP)-ribose synthetase (PARS). PARS transfers ADP-ribose units to nuclear proteins by using nicotinamide adenine dinucleotide (NAD) as the source of ADP-ribose. For every mole of NAD consumed in this reaction, it takes four energy equivalents of adenosine triphosphate to regenerate NAD from nicotinamide. PARS can transfer more than 100 ADP-ribose units/protein in a matter of seconds. This rapid consumption of energy can deplete a cell of its energy stores. It is hypothesized that if there is sufficient DNA damage and free radical production, the activation of PARS initiates a futile cycle, resulting in the complete depletion of cellular energy stores, impairment of the ability to regenerate those energy stores, and, subsequently, cell death. CaM, calmodulin; L-arg, L-arginine; L-cit, L-citrulline; NOS, nitric oxide synthase; ONOOH, peroxynitrous acid.

toxic hydroxyl radicals. An established pathway of nitric oxide–mediated neuronal cell death is nitric oxide activation of the nuclear enzyme poly-adenosine diphosphate (ADP)-ribose-synthetase (PARS). Nitric oxide activates PARS by damaging DNA. (Nitric oxide synthase isoforms are shown in Table 104-3).

Depending on its source, nitric oxide may be toxic or protective in the brain under ischemic conditions. Overproduction of nitric oxide from either neuronal or inducible nitric oxide synthase leads to neurotoxicity; however, nitric oxide production from endothelial nitric oxide synthase protects brain tissue by maintaining regional CBF.

Formation of Oxygen Radicals

Toxic oxygen radical species, produced during postischemic reperfusion, are important contributors to reperfusion injury and delayed cell death. Oxygen free radicals are formed during ischemia when oxygen becomes unavailable as the terminal electron acceptor in the electron transport chain (Figure 104-5).

The brain may be particularly vulnerable to free radical injury for several reasons. One is the high concentration of polyunsaturated fatty acids, especially arachidonic acid. As noted previously, free fatty acids are released throughout ischemia. On exposure to oxygen radical species, these free fatty acids are vulnerable to lipid peroxidation. Lipid membranes are a natural target of free radicals, especially in the brain, because they are abundant, and their polyunsaturated nature makes them easy to oxidize. The effects of free radicals on membranes include changes in membrane fluidity and alteration of ion channels and transport proteins. In addition to disruption of the cell membrane, fragmentation of the mitochondrial membrane results in a decrease in cellular energy production.

The ability of the cell to defend itself against free radicals is limited, and free radical–scavenging enzymes, such as superoxide dismutase and catalase, may be overwhelmed after an ischemic area is reperfused. Surprisingly, restoration of blood flow to hypoxic-ischemic areas is potentially detrimental because the influx of oxygen can be used as a source of oxygen free radicals through the processes noted previously. Stimulated by high tissue carbon dioxide tension, low oxygen tension, and low pH, restored blood flow to an ischemic area is often increased above normal (luxury perfusion).

Neuroinflammation, Glia, and the Neurovascular Unit

Numerous studies have implicated activation of astrocytes and microglia and formation of the "inflammasome" after global hypoxia-ischemia. The release of proinflammatory cytokines and activation of complement contributes to recruitment of microglia and breakdown of the blood–brain barrier. Failure of normal astrocyte function results in increased synaptic excitation associated with increase in extracellular potassium (as a result of downregulation of Kir4.1 inward rectifying potassium channels), an increase in glutamate (as a result of downregulation of astrocyte glutamate transporters), and cerebral edema (through compromise of aquaporin-4 transporters). The neurovascular unit (comprising neurons, astrocytes, endothelial cells of blood–brain barrier, myocytes, pericytes, and extracellular matrix components) regulates CBF. By regulating cerebral blood vessel diameter, astrocytes play a central role in neurovascular coupling, a mechanism by which CBF is directly coupled to the fluctuating metabolic requirements of neurons. The functioning of the neurovascular unit is disrupted by focal or global ischemic insult. Compromise of neurovascular coupling may contribute to long-term symptoms following cerebral hypoxia-ischemia, as has been shown for traumatic brain injury (TBI).

Genetic Damage and Regulation

Ischemia and reperfusion can induce gene damage in the CNS. Reactive oxygen species generated by cerebral oxidative stress interact with nucleic acids and cause the formation of oxidative DNA and RNA lesions that result from DNA base modifications or single-stranded breaks in neurons or astrocytes. Oxidative DNA lesions cause a change in coding properties during DNA and RNA synthesis (replication and transcription) or may terminate chain elongation during transcription and translation. Either process can affect protein synthesis.

Autophagy

Autophagy is a normal homeostatic mechanism that allows cells to recycle intracellular proteins, lipids, and damaged organelles into their constituent molecules (amino acids, fatty acids). Autophagy is essential for the normal function of neurons and the brain. Under normal conditions, this process is constant, energy dependent, tightly regulated, and it occurs at a low level. Defects in autophagy may result in a cell's inability to eliminate toxic macromolecules that result from a variety of normal cellular processes or are synthesized in response to a stress. Following hypoxic-ischemic insults, autophagy may cause cellular injury by intracellular accumulation of toxic substances.

CLINICAL PATHOPHYSIOLOGY
Cerebral Blood Flow and Metabolism After Resuscitation

A pattern of early transient postischemic hyperemia and subsequent delayed postischemic hypoperfusion has been observed almost universally in global cerebral ischemia models, including asphyxia-induced cardiac arrest. The level of hyperemia and subsequent hypoperfusion varies in relation to the duration of the insult. Although these phases of increased and decreased CBF characterize the net global effect, regional CBF is often heterogeneous, particularly during postischemic hypoperfusion, when areas of decreased and increased perfusion may coexist. Metabolism, as assessed by the cerebral metabolic rate for oxygen, is reduced during the early postischemic period and then progressively recovers to a level that varies depending on the model used and the duration of ischemia

The concept of "no reflow" was suggested by Ames and colleagues in 1968. These investigators noted that, after a period of global cerebral ischemia, flow could not be reestablished. At a microscopic level, areas of "no reflow" are interspersed with areas of restored blood flow and microinfarcts. Brain regions that are selectively vulnerable include the thalamus, amygdala, hippocampus, and striatum. Vasospasm, perivascular edema, and increased blood viscosity have been proposed as potential mechanisms. The second phase of the CBF response to global hypoxia-ischemia is characterized by increased global CBF and is often referred to as the "hyperemic" phase.

In summary, immediately after cardiac arrest accompanied by restoration of systemic hemodynamic stability, transient global brain hyperemia occurs and is followed by a period of patchy hypoperfusion. The magnitude and duration of these CBF alterations appear to be related to the duration of the insult. In patients with good outcomes, global CBF recovers over a subsequent 24 to 72 hours, and CO_2 reactivity remains intact. In patients who do not regain consciousness or progress to brain death, CBF is reduced, and autoregulation of CBF is compromised or lost.

MAJOR DISORDERS CAUSING CARDIAC ARREST

Table 104-4 lists common causes, by category, of pediatric cardiorespiratory arrest taken from major published pediatric cardiac arrest series. Common specific disease entities resulting in cardiac arrest include nonaccidental trauma, drowning, sudden infant death syndrome, strangulation, and lightning/electrical injury.

Abusive Head Trauma

Please see Chapter 103 for a discussion of this topic.

Sudden Infant Death Syndrome

Sudden infant death syndrome (SIDS) is defined as the sudden death of an infant younger than 1 year that remains unexplained after a thorough case investigation, including performance of a complete postmortem examination, examination of the death scene, and review of the medical history. The diagnosis remains one of exclusion. This topic also is discussed in Chapter 90.

Drowning (Submersion Injury)

Drowning is defined as the process resulting in respiratory impairment from submersion or immersion in a liquid medium. In the United States drowning is the second leading cause of unintentional injury death for children and accounts for more than 1000 deaths per year. Pediatric hospitalization rates for drowning have been increasing over the past 19 years (Bowman, Aitken, Robbins, and Baker, 2012).

Epidemiology

In the United States submersion accidents remain the second most common cause of injury and death in children 1 to 4 years of age. Children younger than 5 years have the highest drowning mortality rates. Annually, about 1100 drowning deaths occur in the United States in children younger than 19 years. Approximately 75% of these victims are children of the ages of 1 to 4 years. Just over one-half of these drowning deaths occur in residential pools. The distribution of submersion accidents by age follows a well-defined bimodal pattern. Children younger than age 5 years represent the first peak, which is followed by a second peak at ages 16 to 24 years.

Management. Rapid application of cardiopulmonary resuscitation (CPR) provides the best chance for neurologic perfusion and recovery after a drowning event. Table 104-2 lists factors associated with successful resuscitation for in- and out-of-hospital arrest. In the event of respiratory arrest without cardiac arrest, rescue breathing alone, with reestablishment of ventilation and oxygenation, may be sufficient to ensure good neurologic recovery. In the setting of drowning, reestablishment of ventilation and oxygenation via rescue breathing is, along with chest compressions, essential to effective resuscitation.

As with other forms of acute brain injury and resuscitation, hypoxemia should be identified and corrected as soon as possible, preferably in the field. Airway management and mechanical ventilation are often required to maintain oxygenation and ventilation. Drowning victims present with concomitant respiratory and metabolic acidosis and hypoxemia; efforts to repair these metabolic conditions should begin with initiation of resuscitation. Similarly, hypotension may have a negative effect on the recovery of the ischemic brain and should be identified and reversed as soon as possible.

Strangulation Injury

Strangulation injuries result from external compression of the neck. Several forms have been described according to the method of application of compression, including hanging, postural strangulation, manual strangulation, and ligature strangulation. Children who are pulseless when discovered after hanging are at significantly higher risk for death or disability, with one study finding an 84% mortality rate (Davies, Lang, and Watts, 2011).

Lightning and Electrical Injuries

Lightning is an uncommon form of electrical injury. Only 150 to 300 people die each year in the United States of injury secondary to lightning strike; the death rate is highest in adolescents. Nearly two-thirds of people struck by lightning survive, although many have significant sequelae.

The primary effect of lightning results from a massive direct-current insult to the entire myocardium and CNS, which is highly sensitive to electrical injury. Myocardial injury may result in secondary CNS anoxic insult. The pathophysiologic mechanism of CNS injury includes coagulation in the cortex, formation of epidural or subdural hematomas, paralysis of the respiratory center, and intraventricular hemorrhage. Symptoms of CNS injury include loss of consciousness, confusion, transient disorientation, seizures, restlessness, retrograde amnesia, and varying degrees of transient paralysis. Coma and symptoms of cerebral edema are not unusual. Lightning strikes may also cause transient autonomic dysfunction, which may result in fixed and dilated pupils, mydriasis, anisocoria, loss of the red reflex, and Horner's syndrome. Pupillary responses cannot be used reliably as an indicator of brainstem function.

Electrical Shock

Electrical shock is associated with a fatality rate of 0.5 per 100,000 per year in the United States and accounts for approximately 1000 deaths annually. Cardiopulmonary arrest is the primary cause of immediate death from electrical injury. Respiratory arrest may occur immediately after electrical shock. Electrical injuries cause an additional 5000 patients to require emergency treatment and constitute 4% to 7% of burn center admissions. More than 20% of all electrical injuries occur in children. Risk-taking behavior among adolescent boys can expose them to high-tension electrical sources. The inquisitive nature of toddlers and their habit of exploring their environment with their mouths contribute directly to the most common electrical injury in childhood, the perioral burn, which affects 4000 children per year.

Sudden Cardiac Arrest in Children and Adolescents

Sudden cardiac arrest is the sudden cessation of cardiac activity, so that the victim becomes unresponsive, with no normal breathing and no signs of circulation. Without immediate CPR and other treatments to restore normal cardiac activity, the victim will die. Although the precise incidence of sudden cardiac arrest in children is unknown, it is not a leading cause of death.

When sudden cardiac arrest does occur in children and adolescents, it may be precipitated by ventricular fibrillation or rapid ventricular tachycardia (pulseless ventricular tachycardia). Ventricular fibrillation occurs in 5% to 15% of all pediatric victims of out-of-hospital cardiac arrest and is reported in up to 20% of pediatric in-hospital arrests at some point during resuscitation. The incidence increases with age. These abnormal heart rhythms in children are typically caused by inherited or congenital cardiac conditions or by acute medical problems that cause inflammation of the heart. Examples of such conditions include long QT syndrome, hypertrophic cardiomyopathy, abnormal development of the coronary arteries, aortic dissection, myocarditis, coronary artery aneurysm associated with Kawasaki's disease, and congenital aortic stenosis. If a child develops sudden cardiac arrest caused by ventricular fibrillation or pulseless ventricular tachycardia, immediate CPR by a bystander and early defibrillation are needed.

NEUROLOGIC COMPLICATIONS AFTER CARDIAC ARREST

There is now an accepted role for the use of continuous (cEEG) monitoring in adults and children for the detection of secondary injuries, including seizures and ischemia, in critically ill patients with altered mental status, and for prognostication after cardiac arrest (Herman et al., 2015). This recommendation also applies to neonates. In a study of 90 term neonates treated with therapeutic hypothermia for HIE who underwent cEEG monitoring on day of life 1, 48% had electrographic seizures, of which 9 (10%) had electrographic status ellipticus. Importantly, only the initial EEG background, but not any clinical variables, was predictive of the occurrence of seizures.

Delayed Posthypoxic Injury

Delayed posthypoxic injury may occur 24 to 48 hours after the initial recovery of consciousness after coma. In children, this injury occurs most frequently after near-drowning accidents or cardiac surgery in which profound hypothermia and either low-flow bypass or circulatory arrest were used. Magnetic resonance imaging (MRI) studies may reveal evidence suggestive of edema or demyelination, which may be postanoxic or osmotic in etiology. In addition, diffusion-weighted imaging may reveal restricted diffusion, typically in the basal ganglia, cerebellum, and cortex. These changes are seen initially in gray matter and later in white matter.

Postischemic Seizures

The use of EEG as a prognostic tool in critically ill patients has been limited by a lack of consensus on EEG classification systems. However, in a study of 35 children treated with therapeutic hypothermia (TH) after cardiac arrest who underwent cEEG monitoring, a simple classification system (continuous and reactive; continuous but unreactive; any degree of discontinuity, burst suppression, or lack of cerebral activity) was predictive of short-term outcome (Pediatric Cerebral Performance Category Score scale at hospital discharge). At present, despite the progress still needed for uniform definitions of EEG abnormalities, it is reasonable to conclude that mild slowing and rapid improvement of the EEG are predictive of good outcome, whereas lack of reactivity, attenuation, or burst suppression are not. Another prospective study of all children admitted to a pediatric and cardiac intensive care unit has provided some of the best evidence that electrographic seizure burden independently is associated with a poorer outcome.

Whether treatment of such seizures improves outcome will require additional studies.

Delayed Postanoxic Myoclonic Seizures

Myoclonus usually appears within the first 24 to 48 hours after cardiac arrest and is generalized, involving all voluntary muscles. The EEG is usually abnormal, with generalized synchronous spike discharges or burst-suppression activity. The presence of postanoxic myoclonus is usually indicative of a high risk for long-term neurologic sequelae.

In one study of comatose adult patients after cardiac resuscitation, myoclonic seizures developed in 37%, and all of those patients died. The authors concluded that myoclonic status epilepticus in comatose survivors after cardiac resuscitation indicates devastating anoxic brain injury (Table 104-5).

Paroxysmal Sympathetic Hyperactivity

Disturbance in autonomic nervous system function may present after any brain injury, and a brain suffering from global ischemia, as in cardiac arrest, is particularly susceptible. Historical reports estimate that up to 8% to 33% of patients suffering TBI and 6% to 29% of patients with global anoxic injuries may exhibit paroxysmal sympathetic hyperactivity (PSH). PSH is characterized by sudden, paroxysmal changes in vital signs manifest as hyperthermia, tachycardia, hypertension, and/or tachypnea. Associated findings on examination may include pupillary dilatation and diaphoresis. Patients suffering from PSH may exhibit agitation and hypertonia with extensor posturing during events.

A recent retrospective analysis examined the medical records of 249 children admitted to an intensive care unit with acute brain injuries (TBI, global ischemia, focal ischemia, CNS infection) over a 7-year period. Overall, 13% of patients had treatment for dysautonomia. Most individuals with PSH manifest symptoms over a week after the initial CNS insult.

The timing of onset of symptoms of PSH is variable, and identification of PSH requires a high index of suspicion. To establish the diagnosis the clinician should assess for other events that might cause similar physiologic derangements, including narcotic or other drug withdrawal, pain in response to an occult injury (fracture, dislocation), urinary retention or ileus, seizure, and occult infections. Treatment of acute bouts of PSH includes administration of medications aimed at providing symptomatic relief and reducing sympathetic tone, including propranolol or clonidine, narcotics (morphine), benzodiazepines (lorazepam), and antipyretic agents (acetaminophen or ibuprofen). No single drug has proven effective, but combinations of long-acting benzodiazepines, gabapentin, and baclofen are often used.

NEUROLOGIC PROGNOSIS AFTER CARDIAC ARREST

Currently, the most powerful individual predictor of neurologic outcome after cardiorespiratory arrest is the neurologic examination. Sequential observations of a patient's breathing pattern, eye movements, body posture, and reflexes provide essential information to help predict outcome. A study involving 109 comatose children with hypoxic-ischemic encephalopathy documented that the absence of a motor response on the third day after admission was associated with an unfavorable outcome. Nevertheless, in 23% of the children, clinical evaluation was difficult because of neuromuscular paralysis or heavy sedation. This reinforces the importance of other early prognostic factors, such as electrophysiological data.

The absence of a pupillary reaction to light suggests a poor prognosis but has unclear specificity when assessed early after a cardiac arrest. Early after an arrest the pupillary reflex might be absent; however, studies have demonstrated that persistence of pupillary dysfunction at day 3 after cardiac arrest can reliably predict a poor outcome. After review of existing evidence in adults in coma, the American Academy of Neurology stated that outcome is invariably poor when there is absent pupillary light reflex, absent corneal reflex, and no or only extensor motor response to pain 3 days after cardiac arrest.

Electroencephalography Following Cardiac Arrest

There is now a specific recommendation for the use of cEEG monitoring for the detection of nonconvulsive seizures and to aid in prognosis after supratentorial brain injury, including cardiac arrest, in children and adults (Herman et al., 2015). Specific EEG patterns can be used to predict outcome. Background EEG features such as continuity, spontaneous variability, reactivity, and sleep patterns suggest good outcome, whereas an isoelectric EEG or burst suppression increases the likelihood for an unfavorable outcome.

Somatosensory- and Auditory-Evoked Potentials

Evoked potential monitoring has been used in an attempt to provide early prognostic outcome information after CPR (Figure 104-6). Evoked potentials can be obtained within the intensive care unit; their advantages over EEG are that the responses are not affected by sedative medication and they are insensitive to environmental electrical noise. In a study of sensory-evoked potentials (SEPs) in 441 adults after successful resuscitation from cardiac arrest, 20% of the patients had no N_{20} response. The presence or absence or the prolongation of the cortical N_{20} peak reliably differentiated between poor versus favorable outcome with 100% predictive ability. A preserved N_{20} peak was not useful for discriminating whether an individual patient would survive. Testing was performed within 48 hours of resuscitation, which is a clinically relevant time frame. In a single-center study of 56 unconscious children and adults (age range 10–73 yr), the presence of an N_{20} response was an independent predictor of recovery of awareness up to 1 year after injury.

Brainstem auditory-evoked testing has been used in children who experienced cardiac arrest after submersion accidents. Normal evoked responses were observed in all children who recovered neurologically intact. Children who recovered with significant handicaps demonstrated reduction in wave V amplitude over time and prolonged wave I through V interpeak latencies.

Neuroimaging

Please see the online version of this chapter as well as Chapter 12 for an overview of this topic as it relates to neuroimaging findings after hypoxic-ischemic injury (HII), Chapter 19 on neonatal HII because the findings in older children are similar to those in newborn, and Chapter 103 on post-TBI imaging findings because frequently there is a component of HII in this patient population.

The majority of the data using diffusion-weighted imaging (DWI) and apparent diffusion coefficient (ADC) MRI sequences are from adult studies of cardiac arrest outcomes. Reduction in ADC values is highly predictive for poor outcome after cardiac arrest in adults. Reports in children also suggest that cortical and/or basal ganglia lesions detected with DWI/ADC, FLAIR, or T2-weighted imaging are associated with poor outcomes. An example of the differences in MRI findings between a good and poor outcome following cardiac arrest is shown in Figure 104-7. Overall, the available neuroimaging data suggest that the regional patterns of brain injury and changes in magnetic resonance spectroscopy produced by global hypoxic-ischemic insults are similar in adults and children, although many of these studies are limited by the lack of long-term outcomes.

Issues that require further study for children include the optimal time to acquire MRI for the purpose of predicting long-term outcome, whether regional versus whole-brain data are more sensitive/specific, and whether such imaging data can provide more granular information regarding the degree of disability that are superior to currently used measures such as the Glasgow Outcome Scale (GOS) or Pediatric Cerebral Performance Category Scale score.

TREATMENT

Treatment of children with global hypoxic-ischemic brain injuries involves multiple specialties and a systematic approach to providing emergency care in the field, emergency department, and intensive care unit (Donoghue, et al., 2015). Urgent neuroimaging studies and early neurologic evaluation are helpful in the initial evaluation to determine the presence of a neurosurgical condition that necessitates immediate treatment, the etiology of injury, and the appropriate course of treatment specific to each of the four phases of cardiac arrest (Table 104-6).

Temperature Control

The effect of hypothermia on the injured brain is complex. For each 1°C decrease in temperature, the cerebral metabolic rate for oxygen decreases by 6% to 7%. However, hypothermia's main beneficial effect is to provide protection against numerous deleterious biochemical mechanisms as described previously.

Despite the great promise of therapeutic hypothermia, enthusiasm for the clinical application for treatment of out-of-hospital cardiac arrest has waned following the first results from the THAPCA study (Moler et al., 2015). The THAPCA trials included two multicenter, randomized controlled trials in which patients were assigned to either a controlled normothermia (36.8°C) protocol or a moderate hypothermia (33.0°C) protocol. Results of the out-of-hospital cardiac arrest study showed no treatment benefit with TH. In this study, 295 patients were enrolled and randomized, and 1-year survival and neurologic outcome analysis demonstrated no statistically significant difference in good neurologic outcome (20% in hypothermia vs. 12% in normothermia; 95% confidence interval [CI], 0.86–2.76; P = 0.14). or survival (38% in hypothermia vs. 29% in normothermia; 95% CI, 0.93–1.79; P = 0.13). A concurrent trial is examining the effects of TH on neurologic outcome and survival of pediatric patients suffering cardiac arrest while admitted to the hospital. These results have not yet been published. Hyperthermia is common after cardiac arrest in children and is associated with poor neurologic outcome. This may represent either noxious effects of hyperthermia on the injured brain or a worse insult overall with multiorgan system failure and impaired autonomic control of thermoregulation. As little as 1°C of hyperthermia appears to be important (Bowman et al., 2012). Therefore, postcardiac-arrest temperature elevations should be actively prevented and treated. Indeed, patients in the control group in the THAPCA study were maintained within a narrow temperature range, preventing hyperthermia, and this itself was likely neuroprotective.

Resuscitation

For pediatric cardiac arrests in the prehospital setting, CPR and advanced life support from emergency medical service providers may be applied late, after prolonged hypoxia and hypoperfusion of vital organs. Animal and human data both show that basic life support delivered early is more important than advanced life support delivered late. Prompt action by a citizen bystander in the prehospital setting is generally more effective than late heroic efforts in the intensive care unit. On-scene time spent resuscitating the patient is critical. A study of 2244 children using the Resuscitation Outcomes Consortium cardiac arrest database from 11 North American regions from 2005 to 2012 showed the highest survival (10.2%) among those with a duration of resuscitation of 10 to 35 minutes and those who received fluid resuscitation.

Intracranial Pressure Monitoring and Control

See Chapter 105 for a discussion of this topic.

Glucose Homeostasis

Observations in animals and humans have suggested that an elevated serum glucose level at or about the time of an ischemic insult is associated with enhanced postischemic damage of cerebral tissue. Preexisting hyperglycemia worsens the outcome from global hypoxic-ischemic injury in adult and juvenile animals. Outcome from out-of-hospital cardiac arrest is worse in adults with elevated glucose concentrations at admission and in hyperglycemic children after submersion injury.

The optimal level of either low or elevated blood glucose determinations after resuscitation from either a global or focal hypoxic-ischemic event has not been determined. From a practical standpoint, it seems wise to avoid hypoglycemia in a neonate with hypoxic-ischemic injury and to avoid hyperglycemia (i.e., > 300 mg/dL) in older patients.

Cardiovascular Support

Persistent circulatory insufficiency is common in the postarrest state when there is return of spontaneous circulation. Arterial hypotension can result from a combination of factors, including myocardial stunning, neurally mediated cardiac dysfunction, relative adrenal insufficiency, and a profound proinflammatory response related to global ischemia and reperfusion injury that induces a sepsis-like state. Although the optimal cerebral perfusion pattern for neuronal recovery remains to be defined, blood pressure fluctuations adversely affect outcome. The phase of therapy following return of spontaneous circulation is a critical window of opportunity to influence survival and neurologic function after cardiac arrest.

A recent retrospective observational study examining blood pressure in adults after in-hospital cardiac arrest demonstrated that maintaining mean arterial pressures within a predefined range during the immediate postresuscitation phase was associated with survival and good neurologic function. Among the 319 adult arrest victims, 56 survived with a favorable neurologic outcome; the mean arterial pressure (MAP) in this group was 95 mm Hg, and favorable outcome was statistically correlated with postresuscitation MAP greater than 85 mm Hg. Subphysiologic and supraphysiologic blood pressures both trended toward nonsurvival and poor functional survival. This study did not control for preexisting hypertension, but these results suggest that extremes of blood pressure after cardiac arrest are important contributors to neurologic recovery.

Extracorporeal Membrane Oxygenation-Cardiopulmonary Resuscitation

Perhaps the ultimate technology to control postresuscitation temperature and hemodynamic parameters is extracorporeal membrane oxygenation (ECMO). In addition, the concomitant administration of heparin may optimize microcirculatory flow. The use of venoarterial ECMO to reestablish circulation and provide controlled reperfusion following cardiac arrest has been published, but prospective, controlled studies are lacking. See the online chapter for additional discussion.

Postcardiac-Arrest Brain Injury—Potential Therapies

Despite validation of numerous therapeutic targets in preclinical studies, none of the interventions tested thus far in prospective clinical trails has improved outcomes after out-of-hospital cardiac arrest. The gap between compelling preclinical data and translation to effective clinical therapy is common to other forms of acute CNS injury. For example, the PROTECT investigators examined the effects of early progesterone administration in the setting of severe TBI in adults. This therapy, for which convincing animal evidence demonstrating improved recovery and neuroprotection had been obtained, demonstrated no benefit over placebo when administered in adult humans.

Other evidence from pediatric neurotrauma suggest that expertise with a particular condition and adherence to evidence-based guidelines can result in improved survival and functional outcome. In addition, the development of formal pediatric multidisciplinary neurocritical care clinical programs may have some effect on improved outcomes after critical CNS injury. Introduction of such a team for the treatment of severe TBI resulted in a decrease in mortality from 52% to 33%. Collectively, these studies suggest that in the absence of new cellular or molecular therapeutics, we may still be able to improve outcomes with available care and monitoring strategies for cardiac arrest. A meta-analysis of more than 18,000 episodes in 16 data sets of children with cardiopulmonary arrest who received an attempt at resuscitation suggested that the lack of consistent outcome reporting and short-term neurologic outcome measures limit conclusions about recovery from cardiac arrest in children (Phillips, et al., 2015). This underscores the need for caution in conclusions about success or failure of therapies such as therapeutic hypothermia.

DILEMMA OF NEUROLOGIC MORBIDITY

Although young children are considered more likely than adults to survive anoxic-ischemic events, much of this pediatric survival appears to result from brainstem recovery. Thus after prolonged ventilatory support, a child may be more likely to recover the ability to breathe and survive, but there will be little or no return of cortical functions. Indeed, survival following cardiac arrest has significantly improved over the last decade (Table 104-5). Physicians are often faced with decisions about the degree of continued medical support to be given to patients who do not awaken after cardiac arrest and, to a lesser degree, with decisions about specific treatment modalities. The degree of medical support that a patient needs after cardiac arrest is straightforward and is based on medical indications. Certain treatment modalities, such as mechanical ventilation, pharmacologic support of the heart, and intravenous nutrition, however, may be considered heroic or futile by the physician or the family. Brain damage in these severely injured survivors is typically profound, and long-term improvement is limited.

Children in such situations require long-term intensive care, which is financially expensive, whether they are supported at home or in long-term care facilities. In addition to issues of the child's well-being and the financial burden, the effect on the family's quality of life is profound, although difficult to quantify. Some of these issues are reviewed in Chapter 164 on ethical issues in child neurology.

REFERENCES

The complete list of references for this chapter is available in the e-book at www.expertconsult.com.
See inside cover for registration details.

SELECTED REFERENCES

Ames, A.I., Wright, R.L., Kowada, M., et al., 1968. Cerebral ischemia II. The no-reflow phenomenon. Am. J. Pathol. 52, 437.

Bowman, S.M., Aitken, M.E., Robbins, J.M., et al., 2012. Trends in US pediatric drowning hospitalizations, 1993–2008. Pediatrics 129 (2), 275–281.

Davies, D., Lang, M., Watts, R., 2011. Paediatric hanging and strangulation injuries: A 10-year retrospective description of clinical factors and outcomes. Paediatr. Child Health 16 (10), e78–e81.

Del Castillo, J., Lopez-Herce, J., Matamoros, M., et al., 2015. Long-term evolution after in-hospital cardiac arrest in children: Prospective multicenter multinational study. Resuscitation 96, 126–134.

Donoghue, A.J., Abella, B.S., Merchant, R., et al., 2015. Cardiopulmonary resuscitation for in-hospital events in the emergency department: A comparison of adult and pediatric outcomes and care processes. Resuscitation 92, 94–100.

Galland, B.C., Elder, D.E., 2014. Sudden unexpected death in infancy: biological mechanisms. Paediatr. Respir. Rev. 15 (4), 287–292.

Herman, S.T., Abend, N.S., Bleck, T.P., et al., 2015. Consensus Statement on Continuous EEG in Critically Ill Adults and Children, Part I: Indications. J. Clin. Neurophysiol. 32, 87–95.

Moler, F.W., Silverstein, F.S., Holubkov, R., et al., 2015. Therapeutic hypothermia after out-of-hospital cardiac arrest in children. N. Engl. J. Med. 372 (20), 1898–1908.

Phillips, R.S., Scott, B., Carter, S.J., et al., 2015. Systematic review and meta-analysis of outcomes after cardiopulmonary arrest in childhood. PLoS ONE 10, e0130327.

Tovar-Y-Romero, L.B., Penagos-Puig, A., Ramirez-Jarquin, J.O., 2015. Endogenous recovery after brain damage: molecular mechanisms that balance neuronal life/death fate. J. Neurochem.

E-BOOK FIGURES AND TABLES

105 Disorders of Intracranial Pressure

Mark S. Wainwright

INTRODUCTION

The most robust evidence for the contribution of intracranial hypertension (IIH) to neurologic injury in children is provided by studies of outcomes after severe traumatic brain injury (TBI). Numerous studies involving pediatric patients have demonstrated an association between IIH and neurologic morbidity or survival. Since the last edition of this textbook, new studies have called into question the benefit of intracranial pressure (ICP) monitoring (Chesnut et al., 2012), published updated recommendations for the management of severe TBI (Kochanek et al., 2012), and provided evidence that adherence to these guidelines, including maintaining cerebral perfusion pressure (CPP), improved outcome (Vavilala et al., 2014).

The online version of this chapter contains more extended discussion of the following topics: (1) age dependence of cerebral blood flow (CBF) and normal ICP; (2) noninvasive approaches to ICP monitoring; (3) evidence for pathologic "doses" of increased ICP and abnormal CPP; (4) ICP-directed therapy in nontraumatic causes of increased ICP; (5) clinical manifestations of increased ICP; (6) evaluation and management of intracranial hypotension and idiopathic IIH; (7) effects of gender on ICP; and (8) cellular mechanisms regulating CBF, including the glymphatic system (Iliff et al., 2012).

PATHOPHYSIOLOGY OF RAISED INTRACRANIAL PRESSURE

The skull is a rigid cavity and its contents are relatively noncompressible, consisting of the brain parenchyma, intravascular blood, and CSF. Expansion in the volume of one component can be offset by a decrease in the volume of the others (Monro–Kellie doctrine). When the reserve of each compartment to accommodate increases in volume is exhausted, the slope of the pressure–volume relationship becomes hyperbolic, and small increases in volumes cause large increases in ICP (Figure 105-1 and Box 105-1).

Compliance and Cerebral Blood Flow Changes with Age

The pressure–volume relationships in the brain are expressed by the equation $C \sim dV/dp$, where C represents compliance and dV represents the change in volume that accompanies a change in pressure (dp). As ICP rises, compliance decreases. In the healthy brain, compliance is along the horizontal segment of the curve, whereas in a damaged, swollen brain, compliance is located along the vertical segment of the curve. The overall slope of the pressure–volume curve is steeper in infancy than in older children (Figure 105-2). An increase in intracranial volume by 10 mL is not likely to cause as much of an increase in ICP in an adolescent as in an infant.

CBF decreases from age 3 years (approximately 60 mL/100 g/min) to 18 years (approximately 50 mL/100 g/min) after a transient increase at age 6 years (approximately 70 mL/100 g/min). The relationship between ICP and blood flow is a function of changes in systolic (S) and diastolic (D) arterial pressure (AP) expressed as follows: CPP = MAP − ICP, or CPP = [(SAP + 2DAP)/3] − ICP (CPP, cerebral perfusion pressure; MAP, mean arterial pressure).

Cerebral Autoregulation

CPP reflects the vascular pressure gradient across the cerebral beds, and is determined by both the CPP and cerebrovascular resistance (CVR), according to the formula CBF = CPP/CVR. Under normal conditions, CBF can be maintained as a constant of approximately 50 mL/100 g/min over a wide range (60–150 mm Hg in the healthy brain) of CPP (Figure 105-3). When autoregulation is preserved, increasing blood pressure leads to a progressive compensatory decrease in the caliber of cerebral resistance, thereby maintaining a constant CBF by increasing CVR. As CVR increases, cerebral blood volume decreases and ICP falls if autoregulation is intact. When CPP falls below the lower limit of autoregulation (LLA) (40–50 mm Hg), CBF decreases as the autoregulatory reserve is exhausted, and the system becomes pressure-passive. The severity of the resulting ischemic injury will depend on the degree and duration of decreased CBF, with ischemic injury beginning at approximately 18 to 20 mL/100 g/min. Conversely, when compliance is impaired and shifted to the steep segment of the pressure–volume curve, autoregulation is also impaired, and even minor increases in CBF can lead to hyperemia and significant rises in ICP.

Effects of Intracranial Hypertension on Autoregulation

Autoregulation of CBF in healthy adults is constant, between a CPP of 50 and 150 mm Hg or a MAP of 60 and 160 mm Hg. Under these conditions, changes in CPP or MAP have little effect on CBF. Autoregulation is compromised after TBI, and maintaining adequate CPP to overcome the effects of increased ICP is a cornerstone of medical management in the algorithms for treatment of TBI in adults. In children, the incidence of impaired cerebral autoregulation increased with the severity of injury, and ranges from 17% after mild injuries up to 42% after severe injuries. After TBI, autoregulation may be compromised without radiographic evidence of injury. Dysfunction of autoregulation may worsen over 9 days after severe TBI.

The LLA of CBF is the CPP at which vascular reactivity fails and CBF cannot be maintained despite arterial hypotension (see Figure 105-3). As CPP decreases below the LLA, the relation of CBF to CPP is passive and CBF falls linearly with CPP. The relationship of ICP to changes in the LLA is not well understood. Evidence from a piglet model of controlled cortical impact suggests that the upper limit of CBF autoregulation is decreased as ICP increases.

If this relation is shown to occur in children with IIH, this implies that (1) monitoring autoregulation should be included in the management of these patients; (2) treating acute increases in ICP with an equal increase in arterial blood pressure may be insufficient to maintain CBF as the LLA increases with increased ICP; and (3) the zone of autoregulation narrows

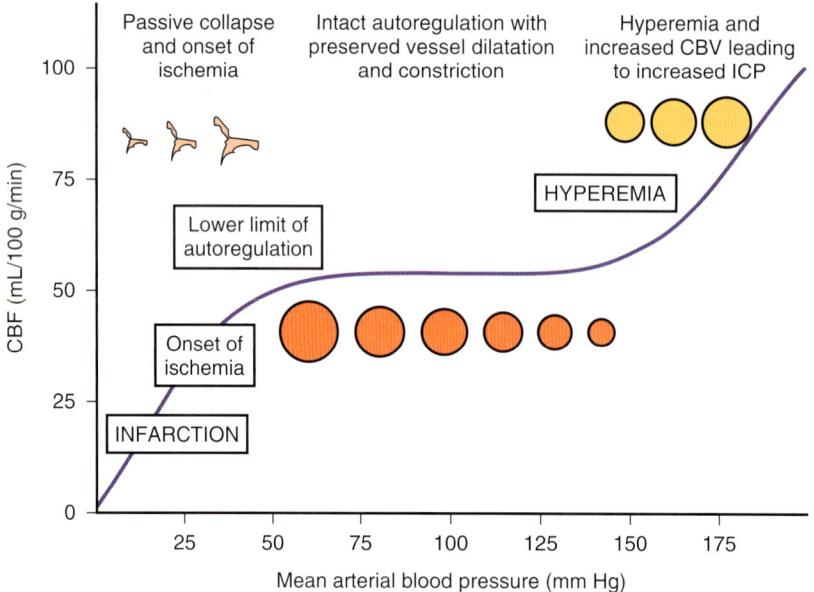

Figure 105-3. Schema of cerebral autoregulation. When mean arterial pressure (MAP) and cerebral perfusion pressure (CPP) are maintained in the normal range for age, cerebral blood flow (CBF) is constant. When pressure falls below the lower limit of autoregulation, or autoregulation is compromised by either increased intracranial pressure (ICP) or other metabolic derangements, the resulting fall in CBF causes ischemia and then infarction. Conversely, when MAP or CPP becomes too high, autoregulation fails and CBF becomes pressure-passive, resulting in hyperemia, increased cerebral blood volume (CBV), loss of compliance, increased ICP, and cerebral tamponade.

as ICP increases requiring meticulous control of blood pressure to preserve optimal CPP.

Regulation of Cerebral Blood Flow

CBF is mostly regulated at the level of precapillary cerebral resistance by a combination of glial, neurogenic, myogenic, and metabolic processes, which maintain CBF over a wide range of arterial pressures. Astrocytes play a pivotal role in neurovascular coupling, another mechanism by which cerebral blood vessel diameter is directly coupled to the fluctuating metabolic requirements of neurons. Compromise of neurovascular coupling may contribute to long-term symptoms after TBI.

INTRACRANIAL PRESSURE MONITORING
History

ICP measurements were first reported in patients with a variety of intracranial lesions by Guillaume and Janny in 1951, using an electromagnetic transducer to measure ventricular fluid pressure signals. Subsequently, Lundberg in 1960 laid the foundation for modern ICP monitoring by providing a method for ventricular cannulation that had a low risk of infection and leakage, enabled continuous recording of ICP, and was minimally traumatic. Lundberg described the following three basic patterns of physiologic changes in ICP:

- Plateau or A waves: increases of ICP in the range of 540 to 650 mm H_2O (40–50 mm Hg) that are sustained for 2 to 10 minutes
- B waves: brief elevations of a moderate degree (range of 272–408 mm H_2O [20–30 mm Hg]); related to fluctuations in respiration and also indicative of decreased compliance
- C waves: small-amplitude fluctuations related to intracranial transmission of arterial pulses

Methods of Intracranial Pressure Monitoring

ICP monitors are classified both anatomically (ventricular, parenchymal, subdural, or extradural) and by mechanism (fluid-coupled or non–fluid-coupled). The external ventricular drain remains the gold standard for reliable and accurate ICP monitoring. This is a fluid-coupled system that provides real-time measurement of ICP, allows CSF drainage to control ICP, and can be recalibrated in situ.

Noninvasive Approaches to Intracranial Pressure Monitoring

Noninvasive approaches to the measurement of ICP, including tonometry, tympanic membrane displacement, and optic nerve sheath diameter, have been reviewed and critiqued for their lack of accuracy or availability for continuous monitoring. Several such methods have been proposed, including transcranial Doppler (TCD), changes in optic nerve sheath diameter, estimated middle-ear endolymph pressure, and visual-evoked potentials. None of these approaches is in routine clinical use. TCDs can be used in children to estimate ICP, CBF, and CPP and to measure autoregulation.

THRESHOLDS AND DOSES OF RAISED INTRACRANIAL PRESSURE

The concept of a specific threshold for ICP from which to guide the clinical management of children at risk for increased ICP may be an oversimplification of the pathophysiological processes involved. It is reasonable to think that there are age-dependent differences in the limits of ICP and CPP that may be compatible with survival after acute brain injuries. A number of pediatric studies have sought to determine age-specific changes, and thresholds associated with good outcome, and to develop methods to assess the effects of amplitude and duration of increased ICP.

Using age-specific values, Jones and colleagues examined the relation between the "dose" of abnormal CPP (duration of exposure to abnormal pressure) and favorable or unfavorable outcome. The percentage duration of low CPP, but not raised ICP, was significantly associated both with mortality and the likelihood of poor (nonindependent) outcome.

As part of a larger prospective study of CPP and ICP thresholds affecting outcome after severe TBI, Chambers and colleagues recorded ICP and CPP, acquiring data between 6.3 and 173 hours in 84 children (age 3 months to 16 years) every 2 minutes, and assessed outcome at 6 months using the Glasgow Outcome Scale score (Chambers et al., 2005). Over each 1-hour interval, they calculated the maximum ICP and minimum CPP as a summary measure. They calculated receiver operating characteristic curves for ICP_{max} and CPP_{min}, and dichotomized outcome to independent (good recovery or moderate disability) and dependent (severely disabled, vegetative, or dead). These results suggested that the ICP_{max} threshold for independent outcome was 35 mm Hg, and for CPP_{min} 43 to 45 mm Hg.

Evidence Supporting Age-Dependent Physiologic Thresholds

The lack of age-specific CPP thresholds was addressed in a study using an online Internet database, TBI-trac, containing data from 22 of the 46 designated trauma centers in New York State (Allen et al., 2014). In this study of 317 children, they measured the survival rates and relative risks of mortality for patients with severe TBI based on predefined age-specific higher and low CPP thresholds (60 and 50 mm Hg for 12 years old or older, 50 and 35 mm Hg for 6–11 years, and 40 and 30 mm Hg for 0–5 years). Based on the significant decrease in survival found in groups with CPP below the goal threshold, this analysis supported age-specific CPP targets above 50 or 60 mm Hg in adults, above 50 mm Hg in 6- to 17-year-olds, and above 40 mm Hg in 0- to 5-year-olds.

This study supported other evidence that a CPP below 35 mm Hg might be a minimal threshold to aim for, as it is associated with reduced mortality. The authors assumed that the zero point for the ICP and blood pressure transducer was uniform across institutions and both set at the level of the foramen of Monro. Since these data were not collected, some patients may have had the head of bed elevated and this may have led to variability in the calculation of CPP. In addition, the authors derived the threshold for increased mortality based on the lowest CPP a patient experienced. Thus a comparison with the "dose" of abnormal ICP or CPP as proposed by other investigators is not possible.

These data suggest that there are age-dependent differences in ICP and CPP after TBI, and that these differences are associated with outcome. Nevertheless, these data do not indicate whether treating ICP or CPP improves outcome, or what the optimal strategies for such management should be.

Lessons and Limitations of These Studies

Collectively, these data show that elevated ICP and low CPP are associated with poor outcome. Treatment should aim to maintain ICP below 20 mm Hg and CPP above a minimum of 40 mm Hg. There appear to be age-dependent thresholds of ICP, although these thresholds require validation in larger, prospective studies. In general, ICP above 40 mm Hg and CPP below 49 mm Hg are associated with unfavorable outcomes, and CPP may be a superior predictor of outcome. Overall, the interpretation of these pediatric studies is limited by their mostly retrospective design, relatively short durations of recovery, variable outcome measures, small sample sizes, varying indications for ICP monitoring, and limited data on medical management and therapies to treat IIH.

INTRACRANIAL HYPERTENSION RELATED TO COMPROMISE OF AUTOREGULATION

Ideally, therapy would be individualized to select the optimal CPP and ICP for each patient. A number of studies have sought to determine the age-dependent thresholds for outcomes associated with abnormal ICP and CPP after TBI, and to calculate the "dose" of physiologic derangement predictive of outcome.

Calculation of Cerebrovascular Reactivity

Other pressures can also be derived from measurement of ICP and CPP. These include the correlation coefficient between slow waves of the ICP and arterial blood pressure, defined as the pressure reactivity index (PRx). This index reflects the changes in the vasoreactivity of the cerebral vasculature associated with the perturbation of physiologic vascular responses to changes in arterial blood pressure, and is expressed as the correlation coefficient of the linear regression of arterial blood pressure and ICP signals. Under normal conditions, when autoregulation is preserved, a fall in MAP leads to cerebral vasodilatation, and an increase in cerebral blood volume. As MAP falls and cerebral blood volume increases, subject to cerebral compliance, this will lead to an increase in ICP. Conversely, as MAP increases, cerebral vessels vasoconstrict, leading to a decrease in cerebral blood volume and ICP. Thus when the cerebral vascular bed is reactive and autoregulation is preserved, slow waves of arterial blood pressure and ICP values are inversely related and PRx is negative. When pressure reactivity is compromised, slow waves of arterial blood pressure and the ICP change in concert and PRx is positive.

Autoregulation-Directed Therapy in Pediatric Neurotrauma

In the first study to monitor PRx in pediatric patients with TBI, Brady and colleagues (2009) prospectively studied 21 children with severe TBI to test the hypothesis that intact pressure reactivity would be associated with survival. The average ICP in the survivors (11 ± 4 mm Hg) was significantly lower than that in nonsurvivors (73 ± 17 mm Hg, $p = 0.0005$). There was a significant association of PRx with survival. In the survivors (n = 15), the mean PRx (0.08 ± 0.19) was significantly lower than that in nonsurvivors (0.69 ± 0.21, $p = 0.0009$). Notably, PRx was dependent on CPP with greater reactivity at higher CPP values, particularly, above 40 mm Hg. These data suggest that measurement of pressure reactivity using PRx can be used in pediatric TBI to identify optimal and harmful CPP ranges. Indeed a feasibility study of 36 children using autocorrelation of NIRS and MAP to determine the optimal MAP for preservation of cerebrovascular reactivity autoregulation after cardiac arrest suggests great promise for this approach (Lee et al., 2014). Whether autoregulation-directed therapy for IIH after pediatric TBI will improve functional outcome will require further study.

Linking Intracranial Pressure and Cerebral Metabolism

Combining precise control of cerebral metabolism and cerebral perfusion may be more effective at reducing neurologic

TABLE 105-2 Clinical Manifestations of Increased Intracranial Pressure

Signs and Symptoms	Mechanism	Clinical Findings
Headache	Traction on dura with pain mediated by trigeminal nerve	Exacerbated by coughing, bending, sneezing Worse when recumbent
Diplopia	Traction on abducens nerve	Uni- or bilateral paresis. Binocular diplopia, worse in direction of gaze of paretic muscle. False localizing sign because not caused by intrinsic lesion in pons
Decreased sensorium or change in personality	Compression of edematous hemisphere by other hemisphere, or compression of reticular activating system	Symptoms begin in adults when ICP reaches 15–40 mm Hg. No comparable pediatric data. May be subtle, ranging from irritability or poor attention to stupor
Impaired upgaze	Pressure over pretectal region of midbrain	Mild retraction of eyelids caused by sympathetic overactivity. Prominent eyes with downgaze in infants (sunset sign)
Increased head size	Chronic or acute mass effect	Tense anterior fontanel, bulging scalp veins, splitting of sutures, acceleration of head growth
Papilledema	Edema in nerve fiber layer of retina caused by impaired retinal venous return	Early: loss of venous pulsations Later: elevation of disk margins, tortuous retinal veins. Visual acuity is normal until late stages
Cushing response	Compression of brainstem	Slowing of respiratory rate, bradycardia, and increased blood pressure. Triad is variable, with tachycardia also seen with increased ICP. Triad present only in up to one third of cases in intracranial hypertension

ICP, intracranial pressure.

injury than ICP- or CPP-directed therapy alone. Experience with multimodality monitoring in conditions with abnormal ICP is increasing (Padayachy et al., 2012). Children with severe TBI underwent continuous brain tissue oxygen (PbtO$_2$) monitoring in the uninjured frontal cortex. For these 46 children, CPP was the only factor that was independently associated with a favorable outcome at 6 months. Indeed, the authors found some cases in which PbtO$_2$ was preserved in the goal range but outcome was poor. This may reflect loss of autoregulation and uncoupling of the neurovascular unit. Differences in the site for probe placement and the thresholds selected for treatment make comparisons between all studies using this technology impractical. More generally, the interpretation of PbtO$_2$ values is limited because they do not solely reflect the presence of ischemia and may be influenced by other factors such as arterial partial pressure of oxygen, and are a measure of local tissue conditions but may miss hypoxic-ischemic insults in other brain regions.

Utility of Measurement of Intracranial Pressure

An important multicenter controlled trial of 324 patients aged 13 years or older with severe TBI was carried out in Bolivia and Ecuador (Chesnut et al., 2012). These patients were randomly assigned either to guidelines-based management using a protocol for monitoring ICP or to a protocol in which treatment was based on imaging and clinical examination. There was no significant difference either in the primary outcome (a composite measure of functional and cognitive status) or in 6-month mortality. The external validity of this study with respect to practice in Europe and North America is limited in part by the differences in postdischarge care as none of the subjects received any rehabilitative therapy or extensive medical care after hospital discharge.

It is clear that ICP values associated with many types of CNS injuries cannot adequately be interpreted in the absence of data on cerebral perfusion, autoregulation, metabolism, and metabolic demand. This approach to multimodal brain monitoring has not been investigated in children. Precedent from adult neurotrauma in a study of severe TBI suggests that specific CPP targets can be set for individual patients using real-time monitoring of a combination of cerebral oximetry, CBF, and ICP to measure autoregulation (PRx) and define an optimal CPP.

CLINICAL MANIFESTATIONS OF RAISED INTRACRANIAL PRESSURE

Physical Examination Findings

The clinical signs of increased ICP range from subtle changes in higher cognitive function to stupor and focal neurologic findings (Table 105-3). Brain imaging may be normal in the early stages of increased ICP. Each herniation syndrome has a specific clinical correlate (Table 105-2). See Chapters 101, 102, and 104 for further discussion of herniation syndromes.

MANAGEMENT OF ACUTELY ELEVATED INTRACRANIAL PRESSURE

A guideline for the treatment of IIH in the management of severe TBI has been published (Kochanek, 2012). An algorithm for the evaluation and management of a child with suspected increased ICP is shown in Figure 105-4.

Initial Assessment, Imaging, and Surgical Intervention

The first key steps in management are to establish a baseline neurologic examination and to identify and, if possible, reverse the primary cause of increased ICP. The medical management proceeds in a tiered approach, but if the initial imaging study shows a surgically operable lesion (e.g., epidural or subdural hematoma), unilateral edema with mass effect, or hydrocephalus caused by obstructed CSF outflow, the first intervention is neurosurgical.

General Principles of Medical Management

Therapies are directed at minimizing extremes of blood pressure, temperature, oxygenation, glucose, and Pco$_2$, with the

TABLE 105-3 Brain Herniation Syndromes

Type	Mechanism	Clinical Findings
Transtentorial	Medial and caudal displacement of uncal portion of temporal lobe with entrapment in the tentorial notch. Compression of the ipsilateral third cranial nerve, midbrain, cerebral peduncle, and posterior cerebral artery	Ipsilateral dilated pupil (compression of pupilloconstrictor fibers); progressive decline in consciousness; loss of oculocephalic reflexes; decorticate posturing; ipsilateral hemiparesis (pressure on contralateral cerebral peduncle)
Central	Swelling of both hemispheres, leading to compression of diencephalon and midbrain	Early: decline in consciousness, constricted pupils (sympathetic dysfunction), Cheyne–Stokes respiration Late: loss of oculocephalic reflexes, central neurogenic hyperventilation, decerebrate posturing
Tonsillar	Cerebellar tonsils affected in the foramen magnum, leading to compression of medulla and upper cervical spinal cord. Most common with posterior fossa mass lesions	Abrupt loss of consciousness, opisthotonic posturing, stiff neck, irregular respiration, apnea
Cingulate	Displacement of edematous cingulate gyrus under the free edge of the falx cerebri. Compression of ipsilateral or bilateral anterior cerebral arteries and internal cerebral vein	Variable symptoms. Often a precursor to other herniation syndromes, commonly associated with uncal herniation
Late stages	Later stages of uncal, central, and tonsillar herniation manifest as coma, flaccid limbs, midsize unresponsive pupils, loss of corneal and oculocephalic reflexes, and irreversible apnea	

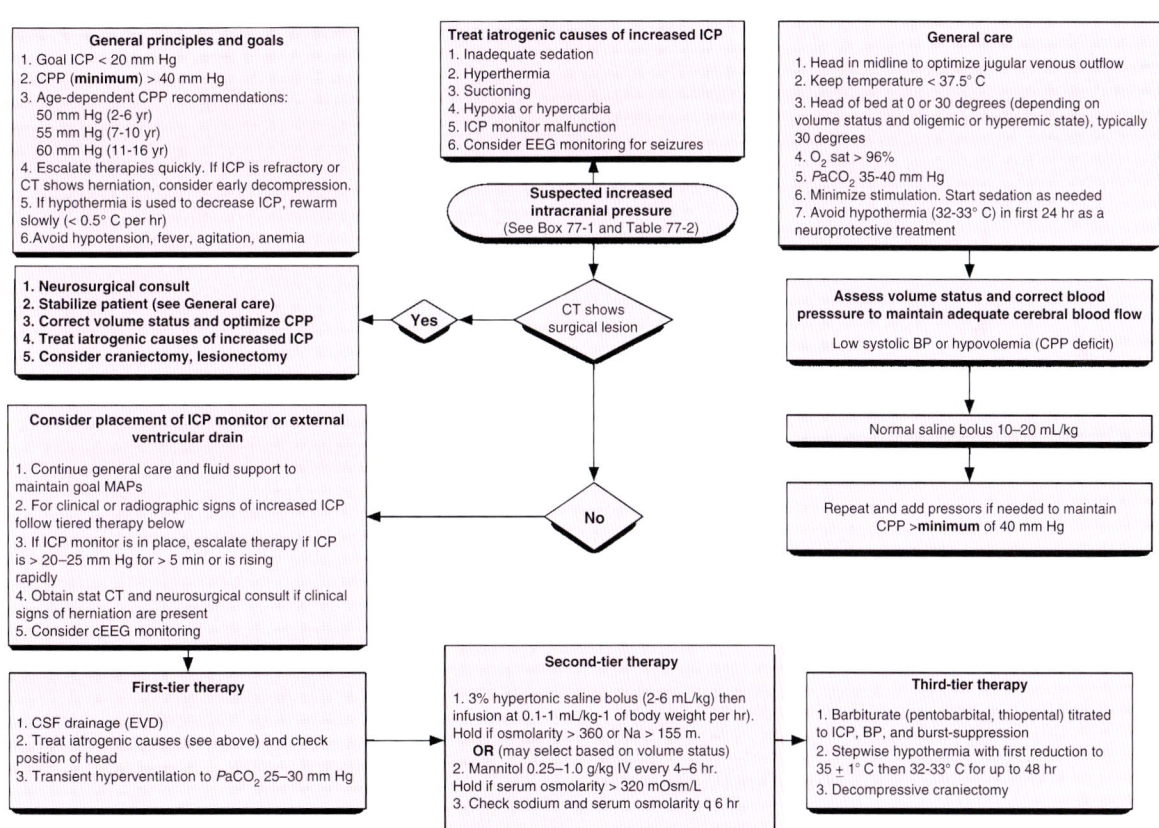

Figure 105-4. Approach to the evaluation and management of the child with suspected increased intracranial pressure. BP, blood pressure; CPP, cerebral perfusion pressure; CSF, cerebrospinal fluid; CT, computed tomography; EEG, electroencephalogram; EVD, external ventricular drain; ICP, intracranial pressure; IV, intravenous; MAP, mean arterial pressure. For an example of these approaches, see Hutchinson et al. (2010).

goal of preventing secondary injury, and to maintain ICP less than 20–25 mm Hg, CPP greater than 50 mm Hg, and systolic blood pressure within age-dependent limits. This may require sedation. Interventions (suctioning, line placement) that may increase ICP should be minimized. If the child is normovolemic, elevation of the head of the bed to 30 degrees will reduce ICP. The head is secured in a neutral position to optimize CSF

outflow via the jugular veins. The lowest ICP is usually, but not invariably, achieved by the highest bed elevation. Although this relation is usually linear, it is dependent on the patient's height, which determines the difference in distance between the foramen of Monro (ICP) and the right atrium (MAP). Thus a given bed elevation may have less impact on ICP in younger (shorter) patients.

Evidence in Support of Guideline-Directed Management of Intracranial Pressure

The extent of adherence to the 2003 Brain Trauma Foundation Guidelines and the impact of adherence on outcome for children with severe TBI were measured in a retrospective study from 5 academic U.S. centers (Vavilala et al., 2014). The overall adherence rate was 72.8%. In the prehospital setting, absence of hypoxia was associated with lower mortality. In the intensive care unit and operating room, maintaining CPP greater than 40 mm Hg was associated with a favorable discharge Glasgow Outcome Score. Overall, the results of this study showed that a 1% increase in adherence was associated with a 1% decrease in the change of poor functional outcome among survivors. This is the first study to provide evidence in support of the benefit of guideline-based acute care in these children and further supports a minimum goal CPP in the first 72 hours after TBI in children. In this context, ICP monitoring may be beneficial to ensure that CPP is preserved about this minimum value.

Intracranial Pressure-Directed Therapy

If there is clinical, radiographic, or monitoring evidence of elevated ICP, a series of stepwise maneuvers are undertaken. In practice, for many pediatric disorders other than TBI, this management is undertaken without an ICP monitor in place because of the lack of evidence that such monitoring improves outcome and concerns over the complications of placement. If ICP is elevated, despite appropriate temperature control, oxygenation, P_{CO_2} 35 to 40 mm Hg, and sedation, the next intervention comprises hypertonic (3%) saline beginning with a bolus of 2 to 6 mL/kg and followed by continuous infusion range between 0.1 and 1 mL/kg/hr. Mannitol (0.25–1 g/kg of body weight, repeated every 4–6 hours as required, up to serum osmolarity of 320) is commonly used but no studies in support of this practice met criteria for inclusion in the Brain Trauma Injury Guidelines. Selection of one agent over the other may need to be guided by the patient's volume status, as mannitol is a diuretic. Brief hyperventilation (P_{CO_2} less than 35 mm Hg) may be effective; however, for each 1 mm decrease in P_{CO_2}, there is a 3% drop in CBF, and so this is only a short-term option. If the patient is hemodynamically stable, high-dose barbiturate therapy may be used for treatment of refractory IIH.

The third tier of interventions for refractory increased ICP includes decompressive craniotomy or moderate hypothermia (32–34°C). Importantly, the decision for decompression should be made before irreversible neurologic injury occurs, although this is clearly a challenging assessment in the intubated, sedated patient. Hypothermia is effective in reducing ICP. Three major clinical trials of therapeutic hypothermia in pediatric TBI have failed to show improvement in outcome (Adelson et al., 2013), or have shown increased mortality in the hypothermia group. The slower rate of rewarming than the 24 hours used in this study may be needed, and accompanied by meticulous use of volume and pressors to maintain CPP (Hutchinson et al., 2010).

The experience with therapeutic hypothermia for severe TBI in children suggests that early hypothermia, irrespective of ICP, does not improve outcome and may increase the risk of death. If hypothermia is used in the management of severe TBI, the 2012 Brain Trauma Foundation Guidelines recommend continuing for less than 24 hours. Importantly, rewarming should carried out at a rate slower than 0.5°C every 2 hours. Hypothermia may still be considered for the treatment of refractory IIH when other therapies have failed. This intervention should be undertaken only in centers with expertise in its use, particularly with experience in the controlled rewarming after hypothermic therapy.

SPONTANEOUS INTRACRANIAL HYPOTENSION

Spontaneous intracranial hypotension is rare, compared with the occurrence of elevated ICP after trauma. However, the clinical manifestations of low pressure, including persistent daily headaches in young adults, may be easily overlooked and result in a delay in diagnosis (Table 105-4). Spontaneous intracranial hypotension is believed to result from development of a spontaneous CSF leak after minor trauma. Postural headache is the distinctive symptom of low-pressure headaches, but other headache patterns (nonpositional, exertional) occur as well. Other associated symptoms may include neck stiffness, vomiting, vague auditory symptoms, and even coma likely caused by deformation of the diencephalon. A connective tissue disorder should be considered in these patients.

CHRONIC INTRACRANIAL HYPERTENSION
Idiopathic Intracranial Hypertension

Primary idiopathic IIH (previously termed pseudotumor cerebri) may develop at almost any age. IIH has an annual

---

TABLE 105-4 Clinical Features of, Diagnostic Criteria for, and Conditions Associated with Intracranial Hypotension

Clinical Features	Diagnostic Criteria for Headache Caused by Spontaneous CSF Leak and Intracranial Hypotension	Differential Diagnosis for Low-Pressure Headache Symptoms
Orthostatic headache	1. Diffuse and/or dull headache worsening within 15 min of sitting or standing and ≥ 1 of a. Tinnitus b. Nausea c. Photophobia d. Neck stiffness e. Hyperacusia	Primary headache disorder Chronic daily headache
Worsens in upright position		Secondary headache Spontaneous intracranial hypotension Carotid or vertebral dissection
Improves when lying down	2. At least one of a. CSF opening pressure < 60 mm H₂O in sitting position b. Evidence of CSF leakage by myelography c. MRI evidence of low CSF pressure	Cerebral sinovenous thrombosis Benign intracranial hypertension Posttraumatic headache
Typically occipital	3. No history of dural puncture 4. Headache resolves within 72 hr of epidural blood patching	Meningitis

CSF, cerebrospinal fluid; MRI, magnetic resonance imaging.

incidence of 0.9/100,000 persons and 3.5/100,000 in women aged 15 to 44 years. To some extent, it is a diagnosis of exclusion, dependent on excluding identifiable causes of raised ICP. IIH presents subacutely, with daily headache that is made worse by maneuvers that raise ICP, such as coughing and bending. Infants may manifest irritability, the sunset sign, and a bulging anterior fontanel. Cranial nerve VI paresis from traction on the nerve caused by raised ICP may lead to diplopia that worsens with lateral gaze. Other manifestations include pulsatile tinnitus, transient visual obscuration, photopsia, retrobulbar pain, vertigo, and decreased visual acuity. Adolescents with IIH may be obese.

The differential diagnosis for IIH should include evaluation for cerebral sinovenous thrombosis that may also present with these symptoms and requires MR or CT venogram to establish the diagnosis.

The major morbidity associated with IIH is vision loss, and management is directed at preventing this complication. Bedside and formal visual field testing may demonstrate enlargement of the blind spot but, in general, only in advanced stages. Snellen acuity and visual-evoked potential testing are insensitive measures to follow vision loss in patients with IIH. These patients should be followed with perimetry. MRI, MR venography, and CT studies usually yield normal results. Infrequently, the ventricles may appear slit-like. Lumbar puncture is needed to establish a definitive diagnosis. It reveals significantly raised opening and closing pressures and normal white blood cell count, protein, and glucose. Disorders associated with secondary IIH are listed in Box 105-2.

Treatment of Idiopathic Intracranial Hypertension

Any contributing factors (weight, diet, drugs) should be eliminated. The treatment of IIH depends on whether visual function is compromised. In patients with unimpaired visual function, the treatment consists of agents that decrease the formation of CSF (acetazolamide, 20 mg/kg/day in 2 divided doses) or diuretics, such as furosemide (1 mg/kg/day in 2 divided doses). There are no evidence-based data for this therapy. Patients receiving acetazolamide should be monitored for the following side effects: drowsiness, anorexia, nausea, numbness of the hands and feet, and signs of dehydration.

Serial lumbar punctures, carried out every 5 to 7 days, with drainage of 20 to 25 mL of CSF on each tap, are also helpful in lowering the closing pressure below 200 mm Hg. Although common, this approach is controversial because CSF pressure returns to prelumbar puncture levels within 82 minutes. Visual acuity and formal visual field assessment should be performed every 1 to 3 months. Patients who demonstrate compromise of visual function, despite medical therapy, may need optic nerve sheath fenestration, a surgical procedure that reduces pressure around the nerve. A number of series have reported good outcome with this procedure.

CONCLUSIONS

Increased ICP is a major determinant of neurologic morbidity after TBI and other neurologic insults common to children, including CNS infections, metabolic disorders, acute liver failure, stroke, cardiac arrest, and diabetic ketoacidosis. The cumulative evidence now supports a minimum CPP of 40 mm Hg for the management of severe TBI. The benefits of ICP-directed therapy in other disorders, including acute liver failure (ALF) and diabetic ketoacidosis (DKA), are at present unproven. The emergence of noninvasive ICP monitoring approaches is promising, but there remains a need to link data on pressure, tissue perfusion, and cerebral metabolism in order to optimize neuroprotection strategies. There is great

potential for the automated, high-frequency collection of these data, and integration with other physiologic measures. Progress in ICP-directed care will require real-time integration and analysis of multiple physiologic variables and must demonstrate that ICP-, CPP-, and autoregulation-directed therapy improves long-term functional neurologic outcome in pediatric neurocritical care.

REFERENCES

The complete list of references for this chapter is available in the e-book at www.expertconsult.com.
 See inside cover for registration details.

SELECTED REFERENCES

Adelson, P.D., Wisniewski, S.R., Beca, J., et al., 2013. Comparison of hypothermia and normothermia after severe traumatic brain injury in children (Cool Kids): a phase 3, randomised controlled trial. Lancet Neurol. 12 (6), 546–553.

Allen, B., Chiu, Y., Gerber, L., et al., 2014. Age-specific cerebral perfusion pressure thresholds and survival in children and adolescents with severe traumatic brain injury. Pediatr. Crit. Care Med. 15 (1), 62–70.

Brady, K., et al., 2009. Continuous monitoring of cerebrovascular pressure reactivity after traumatic brain injury in children. Pediatrics 124, 1205–1212.

Chambers, I., Stobbart, L., Jones, P., et al., 2005. Age-related differences in intracranial pressure and cerebral perfusion pressure in the first 6 hours of monitoring after children's head injury: association with outcome. Childs Nerv. Syst. 21 (3), 195–199.

Chesnut, R., Temkin, N., Carney, N., et al., 2012. A trial of intracranial-pressure monitoring in traumatic brain injury. N. Engl. J. Med. 367 (26), 2471–2481.

Hutchinson, J., Frndova, H., Lo, T., et al. (for the Hypothermia Pediatric Head Injury Trial Investigators and Canadian Critical Care Trials Group), 2010. Impact of hypotension and low cerebral perfusion pressure on outcomes in children treated with hypothermia therapy following severe traumatic brain injury: a post hoc analysis of the hypothermia pediatric head injury trial. Dev. Neurosci. 32 (5–6), 406–412.

Iliff, J.J., Wang, M., Liao, Y., et al., 2012. A paravascular pathway facilitates CSF flow through the brain parenchyma and the clearance of interstitial solutes, including amyloid β. Sci. Transl. Med. 4 (147), 147ra111.

Kochanek, P., Carney, N., Adelson, P., et al., 2012. Guidelines for the acute medical management of severe traumatic brain injury in infants, children, and adolescents—second addition. Pediatr. Crit. Care Med. 13 (Suppl. 1), S1–S82.

Lee, J.K., Brady, K.M., Chung, S.E., et al., 2014. A pilot study of cerebrovascular reactivity autoregulation after pediatric cardiac arrest. Resuscitation 85 (10), 1387–1393.

Padayachy, L.C., Rohlwink, U., Zwane, E., et al., 2012. The frequency of cerebral ischemia/hypoxia in pediatric severe traumatic brain injury. Childs Nerv. Syst. 28 (11), 1911–1918.

Vavilala, M., Kernic, M., Wang, J., et al., 2014. Acute care clinical Iindicators associated with discharge outcomes in children with severe traumatic brain injury. Crit. Care Med. 42 (10), 2258–2266.

E-BOOK FIGURES AND TABLES

The following figures and tables are available in the e-book at www.expertconsult.com. See inside cover for registration details.

106 Spinal Cord Injury

Chellamani Harini and N. Paul Rosman

⊘ An expanded version of this chapter is available on www.expertconsult.com. See inside cover for registration details.

EPIDEMIOLOGY

Acute spinal cord injury occurs worldwide, with an annual incidence of 5 to 40 cases per million. Most pediatric spinal injuries occur in conjunction with motor vehicle accidents (52%), followed by sports-related injuries (27%), falls (15%), child abuse (3%), and other less frequent accidents (Huisman et al., 2015). For 2012, the estimated annual incidence in the United States was ~12,000 new cases per year. Spine fractures constitute 3% to 5% of all pediatric fractures. Approximately 55% of injuries involve the cervical spine, 30% involve the thoracic spine, and 15% involve the lumbar spine. Determinants of injury severity include the following: (1) nature, direction, and degree of the insult; (2) site of injury; (3) presence of preexisting spine anomalies; (4) extent of tissue damage; (5) degree of vascular compromise; and (6) rapidity ⊘ and efficacy of treatment. See online chapter for additional information.

ANATOMY

Figure 106-1 demonstrates the anatomy of the spinal cord showing the spinal cord root levels in relation to the vertebral bodies. For discussion of the anatomy and blood supply of the bony spine, ligaments and spinal cord, please see the ⊘ online chapter.

PATHOGENESIS: MECHANISMS OF SPINAL CORD INJURY

The pediatric cervical spine is more flexible than the adult cervical spine. It is therefore possible to injure the spinal cord without suffering an obvious injury to the bony spine, resulting in *spinal cord injury without radiographic abnormality* (SCIWORA).

There are five major ways in which spinal trauma results in cord injury: forward flexion, lateral flexion, rotation, axial compression, and hyperextension (Chilton and Dagi, 1985). The forces generated by these movements can result in vertebral distraction, dislocation, fracture, and disk herniation. Often several forces act at the same time (Glasser and Fessler, 1996).

Vertebral fractures are less frequent in young children than in adults. By contrast, dislocations, ligamentous injuries, epiphyseal detachments, and lesions of the ossification centers are more frequent. The pediatric craniocervical junction and upper cervical spine are particularly vulnerable to sudden acceleration and deceleration forces and trauma-related injuries. Most pediatric spinal traumas occur in the cervical spine (80%). In children younger than 8 years, primarily the first three cervical segments are involved. With progressive age, the fulcrum of flexion gradually shifts caudally from C2/3 to C5/6. In older children and young adults, the lower cervical spine is more frequently affected. The thoracic spine is less frequently affected than the cervical spine because of the stabilizing effects of the adjacent rib cage. The lumbar spine is more mobile (Huisman et al., 2015). As children approach the age of 9 years, the vertebrae start to mature and

ossify. Anteriorly, the wedge-shaped vertebral body becomes more rectangular, the orientation of the facets becomes less horizontal and more vertical, and the uncinate processes begin to protrude. These features predispose older children to lower spine injury similar to that found in the adult population.

Forward flexion can lead to wedge or teardrop fractures, which usually begin at or near the intervertebral disk (Figure 106-2). These fractures are often encountered in motor ⊘ vehicle accidents in passengers not wearing seat and shoulder belts, but also can be seen in children wearing ill-fitting adult types of lap-sash belts (cervical seat-belt syndrome). Excessive lateral flexion of the cervical spine is always accompanied by ⊘ rotation and can cause a unilateral locked facet (Figure 106-3).

Axial compression occurs in diving accidents, falls, and sports injuries and can result in a burst fracture in which the vertebral end plate is injured, allowing the intervertebral disk to rupture into the vertebral body, which then bursts. In the Jefferson fracture, a direct blow to the top of the head, for example from diving into shallow water, results in axial compression that is transmitted through the occipital condyles to the atlas, the arch of which bursts, allowing fragments to be ⊘ displaced outward (Figure 106-4). Severe hyperextension is often encountered in rear-end motor vehicle accidents (whiplash injury) and in the head-shaking injury of child abuse. This hyperextension can result in transverse fractures of the neural arches of the cervical spine, usually accompanied by tearing of the anterior longitudinal ligament. The so-called hangman's fracture occurs from a hyperextension injury through the synchondrosis between the odontoid and the arch of C2. Because the vertebral arteries lie in the transverse processes of these vertebrae, they can be torn or thrombosed after such injuries with resultant ischemia to the anterior two thirds of the spinal cord. Such injuries have been reported after neck hyperextension in football games and in infants with C1-C2 instability. Displacement of the vertebrae during spinal trauma can compress the arteries of the spinal cord, resulting in ischemic injury, often without radiographic abnormalities. A *Chance fracture* is a compression injury to an anterior portion of a vertebral body, with a transverse fracture through its posterior elements. It is caused by violent forward flexion. The most common site is midlumbar in children. These were often seen in children restrained in automobiles by lap seat belts alone, but since shoulder belts were added, they have become much less common.

CLINICAL ASSESSMENT

History

A detailed history should obtain details concerning the mechanism of injury, the activity of the child, and the use of restraining devices as well as the possible presence of any genetic disorders or blood dyscrasias (e.g., hemophilia) that may render a child more vulnerable.

General Physical Examination

Particular attention should be directed to the child's respiratory and cardiovascular status, looking for a traumatic

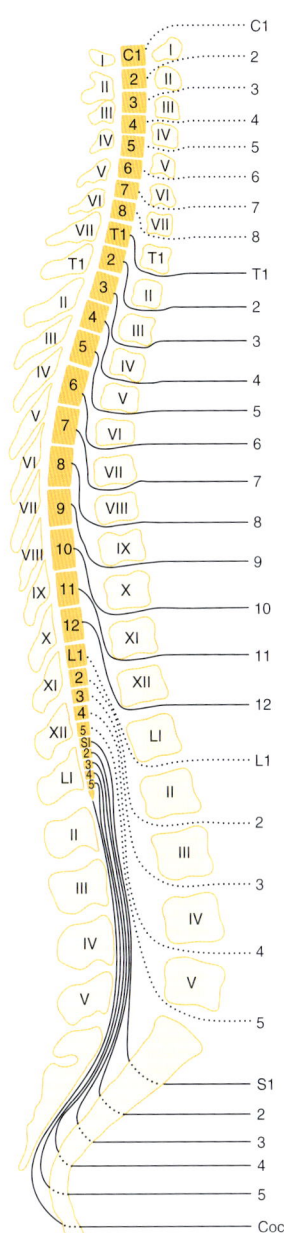

Figure 106-1. Spinal cord root levels in relation to the vertebral bodies. *(With permission from Haymaker W, Woodhall B. Peripheral nerve injuries, 2nd ed. Philadelphia: WB Saunders, 1953.)*

pneumothorax or diaphragmatic paralysis. Hypotension with tachycardia may result from intraabdominal bleeding from a ruptured spleen. The entire spine should be palpated for any point tenderness, deformities, crepitus, or muscle spasm.

Neurologic Examination

Patients with spinal cord injury can present with any combination of the following symptoms and signs: neck or back pain, weakness, sensory loss, decrease in deep tendon reflexes, loss of bladder or bowel control, autonomic dysfunction, and meningismus. Such symptoms may be: acute, subacute, chronic, intermittent, delayed or late, or progressive. After the initial neurologic deficit in acute spinal cord injury, secondary deterioration is sometimes seen. This can be (1) early (<24 hours) (e.g., from spinal immobilization and traction), (2)

A. Complete: No motor or sensory function is preserved in sacral segments S4 to S5.
B. Incomplete: Sensory but not motor function is preserved below the neurologic level and includes sacral segments S4 to S5.
C. Incomplete: Motor function is preserved below the neurologic level, and more than half of key muscles below the neurologic level have a muscle grade less than 3.
D. Incomplete: Motor function is preserved below the neurologic level, and at least half of key muscles below the neurologic level have a muscle grade of 3 or more.
E. Normal: Motor and sensory function is normal.

*This scale distinguishes complete spinal cord injury and three degrees of incomplete injury from an absence of injury with normal motor and sensory function.
ASIA, American Spinal Injury Association; IMSOP, International Medical Society of Paraplegia.

delayed (1–7 days) (e.g., from hypotension complicating fracture-dislocation, or (3) late (>7 days) (e.g., from vertebral artery injury). Signs of spinal cord injury usually include impairment of motor and sensory function. The degree of motor involvement can vary from subtle weakness to complete quadriplegia. Loss of sensation is often ascertainable at an obvious dermatomal level. In 1992 the American Spinal Injury Association (ASIA) and the International Medical Society of Paraplegia (IMSOP) published a Standard Neurologic Classification of Spinal Cord Injury. The seventh edition of the International Standards for Neurologic Classification of Spinal Cord Injury (ISNCSCI) provided some clarifications and revisions and a modest update of the accompanying worksheet (Figure 106-5). This classification systematically documents motor, sensory, and sphincter function in acute spinal cord injuries. Ten key muscle groups are tested for motor function (using the Medical Research Council 0-to-5 muscle grading) and sensation (tested over 28 dermatomes on both sides of the body). The neurologic levels and completeness or incompleteness (partial preservation) of spinal cord injury are documented (Kirshblum et al., 2011).

The ASIA/IMSOP Spinal Cord Impairment Scale (Box 106-1), differentiates *complete* and *incomplete* spinal cord deficits. *Complete* injury is defined as loss of all motor and sensory function in all segments below the neurologic level, including the sacral dermatomes (S4-S5). The anorectal examination, a frequent determinant of completeness of injury, is less reliable in young children than in adults. With preservation of any sensory or motor function below the neurologic level, the injury is classified as *incomplete* (Figure 106-5). The examiner identifies the most caudal spinal cord segment with normal sensory and motor function on both sides. The zone of partial preservation is defined as the dermatomes caudal to the neurologic level with partial preservation of function in an otherwise complete injury. This zone implies injury of multiple spinal cord segments, whereas its absence implies injury at only one level. An abbreviated sensory examination (16 dermatomes) was recently developed to replace the 56 dermatome examination, and the shortened version was found to correlate well with the longer one.

After injury to the spinal cord, the deep tendon reflexes are depressed or absent, with this lack of response persisting until spinal shock has resolved (1–12 weeks). Thereafter, hyperreflexia and extensor posturing are evident below the level of the lesion, with autonomic dysfunction a frequent accompaniment.

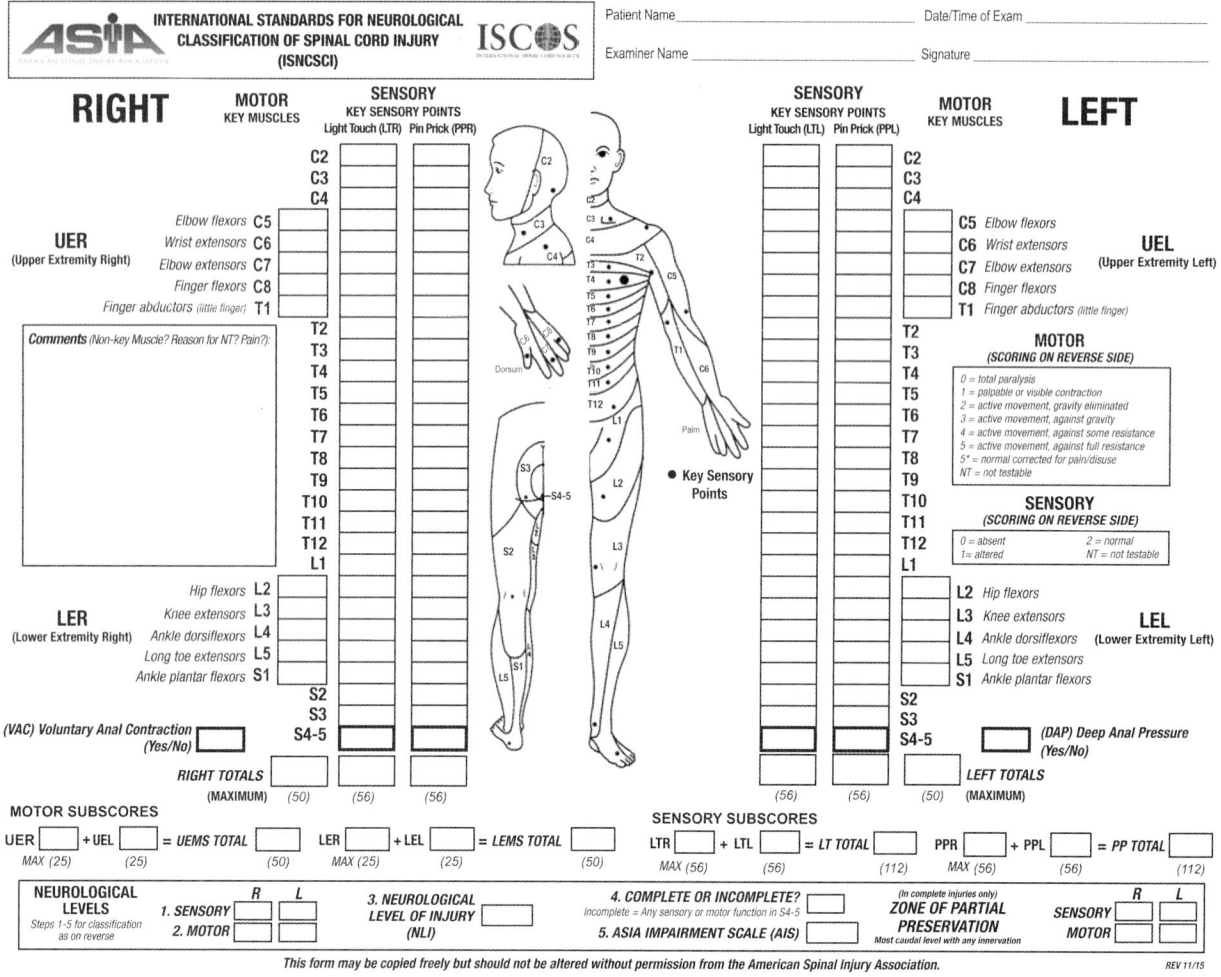

Figure 106-5. American Spinal Injury Association: International Standards for Neurologic Classification of Spinal Cord Injury. American Spinal Injury Association (ASIA) and International Medical Society of Paraplegia (IMSOP) Standard Neurologic Classification of Spinal Cord Injury. This classification provides quantitative assessment of motor, sensory, and sphincter function; neurologic level of dysfunction; and whether any loss is complete or incomplete. *(American Spinal Injury Association: International Standards for Neurological Classification of Spinal Cord Injury, revised 2011; Atlanta, GA, Revised 2011, Updated 2015.)*

Laboratory Studies

Radiographic Evaluation

This should begin in the emergency department with plain films of the entire spine to look for unstable fractures or vertebral dislocations that may require emergency surgery. It is crucial to obtain anteroposterior, lateral, and oblique views of the spine (Huisman et al., 2015; Klein, 2015). Care must be taken not to misinterpret normal variations in cervical spine anatomy, such as pseudosubluxation of C2 on C3, and the synchrondrosis between the dens and body of C2 (often mistaken for a fracture). Also, the physiologic anterior wedging seen in young vertebral bodies might be misinterpreted as compression fractures. In patients who cannot be assessed adequately by plain radiography, early CT or MRI may be needed (Figure 106-6).

In children, spondylolisthesis (malposition of one vertebral body over another) is most often caused by spondylosis, and is seen most often in the lower lumbar spine, especially following repetitive trauma.

In spine-injured children, the upper cervical spine is especially susceptible to injury. Specific injuries to this region include (1) occipitoaxial dislocations, (2) atlantoaxial instability, (3) fractures of the atlas (C1) (Jefferson fracture), (4) odontoid fractures, and (5) fractures of the axis (C2) (hangman's fracture).

Further limitations of plain radiographs of the spine include 40% false-positive and 20% false-negative interpretations. Plain radiographs may miss 20% to 40% of cervical spine fractures. Also, significant spinal cord injury frequently occurs in children without radiographic abnormality (SCIWORA) (e.g., vertebral fracture or dislocation), with this discrepancy observed in 15% to 70% of all pediatric spinal cord injuries. SCIWORA is seen most frequently in infants and young children and most often affects the cervical spine, typically producing signs of a central cord syndrome. The finding of fracture, subluxation or abnormal intersegmental motion excludes SCIWORA as a diagnosis. With MRI, many such cases show radiologic evidence of injury to the spinal cord or spinal cord ligaments.

Klein has recently summarized imaging modalities, sequences, and appearance of different structures seen in spine imaging (Figure 106-7).

Electrophysiologic Evaluation

For discussion, please see the online chapter.

Lumbar Puncture

 For discussion, please see the online chapter.

CLINICAL SYNDROMES

A recent review has summarized many of these clinical syndromes (Cho, 2015).

Intraspinal Intramedullary Injuries

Intraspinal intramedullary injuries can cause complete or incomplete loss of spinal cord function. With complete loss, there is absence of all motor, sensory, and reflex function below the level of injury. With incomplete loss, some motor, sensory, and reflex function persists (Box 106-1).

Complete Spinal Cord Injuries

Complete loss of spinal cord function, can be physiologic or pathologic. In physiologic loss, there is no morphologic alteration of the spinal cord, which becomes dysfunctional after impact. This dysfunction can occur with transient compression of the cord by a dislocated vertebra. With more sustained cord compression, anatomic disruption may result, with accompanying pathologic loss of function. The frequency of complete spinal cord injury in pediatric patients ranges from 20% to 95%.

The initial phase of complete loss of spinal cord function is characterized by spinal shock. The truncal and extremity muscles below the level of the lesion are flaccid, deep tendon and superficial reflexes are depressed or lost, plantar responses are absent, anesthesia to all modalities is present, and autonomic dysfunction (hypotension and bradycardia) is seen. The mechanism of spinal shock is unknown, but its physiologic effects must be differentiated from the more permanent pathologic effects of spinal cord injury. Motor and sensory deficits resulting from spinal shock alone resolve within 1 hour. Persistence of motor and sensory deficits beyond 1 hour implies that more permanent injury has occurred. After 6 to 13 weeks in adults and within 1 week in children, tendon reflexes return, and muscle tone improves. The reflexes later become pathologically active, spasticity ensues if the injury is more permanent, and there usually is no significant return of motor or sensory function. A four-phase model of the sequential changes seen in spinal shock and the neuronal mechanisms that may underlie these changes have been described: phase 1 (0–1 day), areflexia/hyporeflexia (from loss of descending facilitation); phase 2 (1–3 days), initial reflex return (from denervation supersensitivity); phase 3 (1–4 weeks), initial hyperreflexia (from axon-supported synapse growth); and phase 4 (1–2 months), final hyerreflexia (from soma-supported synapse growth).

Autonomic dysfunction can persist for weeks to months. Ventilation may be compromised if the intercostal muscles are involved. Flaccid paralysis of the bladder can develop, with urinary retention and overflow incontinence. The gastrointestinal tract can be atonic. Vasomotor dysfunction can develop, with orthostatic hypotension, impaired shivering, sweating, and disturbances in temperature regulation persisting for weeks to months, and at times years. After complete injury of the cervical or upper thoracic spinal cord, an acute syndrome of bradycardia, hypotension, and hypothermia can occur, probably because of disturbed sympathetic outflow at the cervical and upper thoracic levels; most patients with quadriplegia after spinal cord injury have chronic hypothermia with poor temperature control related to loss of sympathetic peripheral vascular control. Recovery from complete cord injury is rare, for less than 2% of patients recover some distal cord function. More encouraging was a comprehensive review of several large series of patients with complete spinal cord injury that found that 2% of the patients became ambulatory.

Incomplete Spinal Cord Injuries

Incomplete spinal cord injuries warrant special attention because the children often show significant functional recovery. These include cervical nerve root/brachial plexus neuropraxia, cervical cord neuropraxia, the cervicomedullary syndrome, central spinal syndrome, syndromes of the anterior spinal cord and posterior spinal cord, Brown-Séquard syndrome, and conus medullaris syndrome.

Cervical Nerve Root/Brachial Plexus Neuropraxia

American football, a high energy contact sport, places players at particularly risk for cervical neuropraxic injuries. The relatively common "stinger" is a reversible peripheral injury resulting from neuropraxia of cervical nerve root(s) or brachial plexus causing a temporary physiologic block in nerve conduction. It is characterized by unilateral burning pain radiating from the neck down the arm to the hand, usually lasting seconds to hours. There may be associated weakness of the deltoid and/or supra/infra spinatus muscles that resolves within 24 hours to 6 weeks. Less often, such injuries can involve one or both lower limbs. The most common mechanism of injury is hyperextension, often with lateral flexion of the neck and an axial load, resulting in cervical nerve root compression caused by intervertebral foraminal narrowing. Additional injury mechanisms are traction or stretching of the brachial plexus and direct trauma to the brachial plexus. Radiographs are usually normal. Cervical stenosis is a predisposing cause. Most patients are managed with 2 weeks of cervical immobilization with a hard collar.

Cervical Cord Neuropraxia

Less common and more serious is cervical cord neuropraxia, due to hyperextension, hyperflexion, or axial loading of the cervical spine. Clinically, it is characterized by burning pain, paresthesias and loss of sensation and/or weakness (ranging from no weakness to complete paralysis) in more than one limb, with rapid and complete resolution of symptoms within 10 minutes to 48 hours. Mechanically, the posterior-inferior margin of the vertebral body above and the anterior-superior portion of the lamina of the vertebra below combine to produce spinal cord compression (Penning's pincer mechanism) with local anoxia and an increase in intracellular calcium temporarily disrupting spinal cord function. Radiographs often show congenital abnormalities such as cervical stenosis and Klippel-Feil syndrome. Cervical cord neuropraxia occurs in 0.2 per 100,000 participants at the high school level and 2 per 100,000 at the collegiate level.

Cervicomedullary Syndrome

With upper cervical injury, there is often injury to the medulla, causing diaphragmatic weakness, respiratory failure, hypotension, quadriparesis, and facial and upper cervical (C1 to C4) anesthesia. Obstruction of CSF outflow at the foramen magnum may lead to downbeat nystagmus and papilledema. The facial anesthesia is of an 'onion skin' or Dejerine type. It is important that facial sensation be tested carefully in all patients with spinal cord injury. As in the central spinal cord syndrome, there can be selective weakness in the arms, with little if any weakness in the legs. This pattern is due to the crossing of fibers subserving the arms in the pyramidal decussation so that they come to be located more centrally than the leg fibers, which cross at a lower level. Several authors have challenged this concept, pointing to evidence that the fibers of the corticospinal tract may not be layered but are intermingled and that pathologically there is little evidence of central necrosis or hydromyelia in such patients. An "around the clock" pattern of weakness can be seen because upper extremity pyramidal fibers cross more rostral to lower extremity pyramidal fibers and the fibers for one side frequently cross completely before those from the other side, resulting in weakness that spreads from ipsilateral upper limb, to ipsilateral lower limb, to contralateral lower limb, to contralateral upper limb (Cho, 2015). The mechanisms of injury causing cervicomedullary syndrome include atlantoaxial dislocation, atlantooccipital dislocation, odontoid fracture, burst fracture of C1, and a ruptured C1 to C2 disk.

Central Spinal Cord Syndrome

Central spinal syndrome can complicate hyperextension injury, particularly when there is a preexisting spinal abnormality, such as spinal canal stenosis, disk herniation, bony spurs, or compression by an abnormal ligamentum flavum. Conversely, this syndrome often can occur, particularly in young children, without an accompanying radiographic abnormality. Here the central portion of the cord (usually cervical) is damaged, probably from ischemia because the central cord is perfused by end arteries from the anterior spinal artery, making it vulnerable to states of low perfusion. As these lesions commonly affect the lower cervical and upper thoracic cord, the sensory loss is classically seen in a "cape" or "vest" distribution across the neck and shoulders or trunk. Initial quadriplegia evolves into a more prominent upper extremity weakness with relative sparing of the lower extremities. Neurologically, the motor and sensory deficits are partial, with the greatest impairment in the distal upper limbs. The resulting distribution of deficits is referred to as the "man-in-the-barrel" syndrome. Bowel and bladder function can be lost early, but usually return. Patients are generally ambulatory with a spastic gait; painful arm dysesthesias may persist for years. There is still debate whether early surgery is warranted because many patients recover spontaneously.

Anterior Spinal Cord Syndrome

Anterior spinal cord syndrome, which can follow hyperflexion spinal injury, is characterized by paresis with loss of pain and temperature sensation below the level of the lesion, with preservation of proprioception, light touch, and vibration. Bladder control is impaired. This condition is usually caused by direct compression of the anterior and lateral white matter tracts by a herniated disk or by a fractured vertebra with posterior dislocation. The posterior columns are spared. There is no evidence for compression of the anterior spinal artery in this disorder. Early surgery is probably warranted in all cases.

Posterior Spinal Cord Syndrome

Posterior spinal cord syndrome is an extremely rare disorder (some doubt its existence), characterized by major damage to the posterior spinal cord, resulting in loss of vibration sense and proprioception below the level of the lesion. This results in a pronounced sensory ataxia and a "stomping" gait, with residual anterior cord function, with retained perception of pain and temperature.

Brown-Séquard Syndrome

Brown-Séquard syndrome is caused by injury of the lateral half of the spinal cord (usually cervical) and is characterized by ipsilateral motor paralysis, ipsilateral loss of vibration sense, proprioception and touch, and contralateral loss of pain and temperature sensation below the level of the lesion. Because the involvement of the descending autonomic pathways is unilateral, bladder dysfunction does not occur. Although this syndrome is often caused by penetrating trauma to the spine, cases also have been caused by hyperextension injury, compression fractures, and disk herniation. Blunt trauma with central cord injury sometimes can result in asymmetric pareses and sensory impairment that can mimic the true syndrome. Recovery is variable.

Conus Medullaris Syndrome

Conus medullaris syndrome causes early flaccid bladder and bowel dysfunction, late and mild pain, and symmetric sensory impairment in a saddle distribution, often with sacral sparing. Motor impairment is relatively mild and symmetric. This syndrome can be impossible to differentiate from cauda equina syndrome on clinical grounds. The lumbar cord is positioned opposite the T12 vertebra, and the sacral cord is opposite L1. Dislocation, displaced fractures, and disk herniation of T12 and L1 can produce this injury. Prognosis for recovery is poor.

Intraspinal Extramedullary Injuries

Intraspinal extramedullary injuries include hemorrhage into the epidural, subdural, and subarachnoid spaces; spinal epidural abscess; spinal arachnoid cysts; spinal epidural tumor; herniation of the nucleus pulposus; cauda equina injuries and catastrophic spinal cord injuries.

Spinal Epidural Hematoma

Spinal epidural hematoma can occur with substantial trauma to a normal spine, particularly in a newborn after breech delivery, or with mild trauma to the spine in a patient with a bleeding diathesis, with a spinal epidural hemangioma, or after multiple lumbar punctures. In contrast to most intracranial epidural hematomas, spinal epidural hemorrhage is of venous (not arterial) origin. The main venous structure within the spinal epidural space lies ventrolateral to the cord and comprises a "rope ladder" plexus of thin-walled veins lacking true valves. This internal plexus connects with an external plexus of veins around the spinal column, with segmental spinal veins draining into the inferior vena cava, and with intracranial dural sinuses. Signs of spinal epidural hematoma can be acute, chronic, or intermittent. A newborn with acute spinal epidural hematoma typically manifests respiratory depression, hypotonia, areflexia, and other signs of spinal shock. The occurrence of clinically significant traumatic spinal epidural bleeding is uncommon after infancy. When it occurs in older children (as with minor trauma complicating a blood dyscrasia), there is usually severe neck or back pain that is worsened by pressure over the spine, neck flexion, or the Valsalva maneuver. Over the ensuing hours to weeks, signs of spinal cord compression usually develop.

Spinal Subdural Hematoma

Spinal subdural hematoma occurs much less commonly; the source of bleeding in this hematoma is unclear. Similar to spinal epidural hematoma, it occurs mainly in the neonatal period, although occasionally it is observed in children and adolescents with bleeding diatheses who sustain an otherwise insignificant injury to the spine, such as that occurring at the time of lumbar puncture. It also has been reported in a

4-month-old infant following nonaccidental trauma. Clinical features include back and radicular pain. In 18 infants with abusive head injury, 8/18 (44%) had accompanying spinal subdural hematomas; in all eight, there were accompanying intracranial (supratentorial and infratentorial) subdural hematomas; all eight of the spinal subdural hematomas were clinically occult. This suggests that in many of these cases the spinal subdural hemorrhage developed consequent to a tracking downward of intracranial subdural blood. In a retrospective study of 252 children with *abusive* head trauma, there was complete clinical and radiologic data in 67. A spinal subdural bleed was found in 31/67 cases (46%). Of 29 children with evaluable cervical imaging results, 7/29 (24%) had cervical subdural hemorrhage; of 38 children with evaluable thoracolumbar imaging results, 24/38 (63%) had thoracolumbar subdural hemorrhage. By contrast, in 70 children with *accidental* injury and complete clinical and radiologic data, there was only 1 case of spinal subdural hemorrhage, thoracolumbar in location. Proposed mechanisms for the occurrence of subdural blood in abusive head injury include: (1) tracking downward of intracranial subdural blood into the spinal canal; (2) direct injury to intradural vessels around the spinal cord; (3) spinal vessel rupture from hyperflexion of the spine and/or increased intraabdominal pressure; (4) increased intracranial pressure causing shearing intraspinal injury with bleeding from the inner dural layer of the spine. Surgical evacuation of spinal subdural hematomas is generally reserved only for those cases with evidence of spinal cord compression.

Spinal Subarachnoid Hemorrhage

Traumatic subarachnoid hemorrhage caused by injury to the spine is uncommon. This hemorrhage can occur after penetrating injury, but most often occurs after birth trauma (often with accompanying epidural, subdural, or intraspinal hemorrhage). The amount of blood that accumulates is usually not great, and significant compression of the cord is rare. Signs of spinal subarachnoid hemorrhage are difficult to distinguish from signs of other spinal hemorrhages (e.g., epidural) that often coexist. Spinal subarachnoid hemorrhage should be suspected when back pain, meningismus, or fever occurs. The diagnosis is indicated by the presence of blood in the spinal fluid or by cerebrospinal fluid xanthochromia. Occasionally, blood obstructs the subarachnoid space, resulting in a "dry tap." Spinal subarachnoid hemorrhage must be differentiated from subarachnoid bleeding of intracranial origin and from blood caused by a traumatic lumbar puncture. As spinal subarachnoid hemorrhage mixes with CSF, it does not show any distinct margins on MRI. When bleeding is acute, spinal hemorrhage, as with intracranial hemorrhage, is usually isointense on T1 sequence and hypointense on T2. When subacute, blood becomes hyperintense on T1 and T2 MRI sequences (Figure 106-8).

Spinal Epidural Abscess

Infections of the skin overlying the spine or of the bony spine itself (osteomyelitis) can occur after spinal trauma and may result in a spinal epidural abscess. Staphylococcus aureus is the organism most often responsible for such infections. The signs and symptoms of spinal epidural abscess are difficult to differentiate from the signs and symptoms of spinal epidural hematoma. Usually, other signs of inflammation and local infection of the overlying skin or bone can be identified. Spinal epidural abscesses are potentially increasing in incidence consequent to an increase in risk factors, including spine trauma, skin infection, intravenous drug use and immunodeficiency. Also, enhancement of imaging studies has allowed for increased detection.

Spinal Arachnoid Cysts

Spinal arachnoid cysts are rare. They can be congenital or acquired, and extradural or intradural in location. The lesions reflect an outward bulging of arachnoid tissue through a congenital or acquired defect in the dura; acquired defects are usually traumatic in etiology. The most common symptoms are limb weakness, sensory loss and radicular pain. In an extensive literature review, of 21 pediatric cases of idiopathic intradural spinal arachnoid cysts, most of the anterior cysts were cervical in location, while most of the posterior ones were thoracic or thoracolumbar. Most children presented with motor deficits. In many of the reports there was a history of trauma; in some, there were associated neural tube defects. Open microscopic surgical fenestration was the treament of choice, with favorable outcomes and a low recurrence rate.

Spinal Epidermoid Tumor

Intraspinal epidermoid tumors can be congenital or acquired. Acquired epidermoid tumors are extremely rare. About 40% occur as infrequent, late complications of lumbar puncture, resulting in implantation of epidermal and subcutaneous tissues into the spinal subarachnoid space. Other causes include spinal trauma, spinal anesthesia, surgery, bullet wounds and myelography. The clinical symptoms are slowly progressive and include leg weakness, muscle atrophy, limited straight leg raising, sensory loss, back pain, and gait abnormalities. These tumors can develop 1 to 20 or more years after a lumbar puncture.

Herniation of Nucleus Pulposus

Herniation of the nucleus pulposus (protrusion of central intervertebral disk tissue) can result from severe flexion/compression of the spine and can cause compression of the underlying spinal cord. Symptoms may include low back pain, sciatica, spinal rigidity, sensory loss, weakness and impaired reflexes.

Cauda Equina Injuries

A special category of extramedullary injury comprises injury involving the cauda equina, which is technically not a spinal cord injury. The level of spinal column and ligament displacement in these injuries varies with age, depending at which vertebral level the spinal cord terminates. When any of the extramedullary pathologies are localized below the spinal cord, they can cause injury to the cauda equina. Because of involvement of lumbosacral nerve roots, these injuries are typically heralded by radicular pain in one or both lower limbs. There is accompanying asymmetric sensory loss to all modalities in the lumbosacral dermatomes, with bladder and bowel dysfunction later in the course, compared with the conus medullaris syndrome, where bladder and bowel dysfunction is early. Weakness is generally more marked and asymmetric than with the conus medullaris syndrome, where it is relatively mild and symmetric. The prognosis in cauda equina injury is better than in spinal cord injury because the lower motor neuron apparently has a greater capacity to recover than the upper motor neuron.

Catastrophic Spinal Cord Injuries

Although quite rare, catastrophic neurologic injury refers to a complication of a cervical spinal cord injury, most often caused by a neck injury suffered while playing tackle football, resulting in permanent neurologic injury or death. The incidence of this injury is 0.5 per 100,000 participants at a high school level and 1.5 per 100,000 at the collegiate level. The mechanism of injury is most often forced hyperflexion, as occurs with "spear tackling," in which the player initiates contact with the crown of his helmet, with his neck in a slightly flexed position, resulting in an axial force applied to the helmet being transmitted to the cervical spine, with fracture and/or subluxation or dislocation of the subaxial spine. Of the permanent neurologic injuries that occur in football, 70% occur in defensive players, usually while tackling or blocking.

Supraspinal Changes

For discussion, please see the online chapter.

MANAGEMENT

Medical management of spinal cord injury includes measures aimed at treating the acute cord injury and more long-term management.

Short-Term Management

Spine Immobilization and Supportive Care

Treatment acutely must include stabilization of the spine to prevent further injury, in addition to maintenance of vital signs. At the scene of the accident, the child should be placed on a rigid stretcher or firm backboard and the head fixed by sandbags or towel rolls with tape over the forehead to prevent movement of the head on the spine. Because the high cervical region is the most likely level of injury, neck flexion is particularly dangerous. Flexion can be avoided with a special board with a recess for the occiput, allowing the head to rest in line with the body, or by placing something under the child's shoulders to elevate the neck in line with the head. A spine board eases transfer of the patient to and from an ambulance stretcher. Because the head is proportionately larger than the body in children, children under age 8 years require a mean of 2.5 cm of thoracic elevation with respect to the occiput to achieve a neutral position. When the patient arrives at the hospital, a hard cervical collar and a firm mattress adequately immobilize the patient before application of traction or definitive stabilization.

A patent airway must be established, which may necessitate endotracheal intubation, which is frequently required in complete cervical cord injury (with impairment of diaphragmatic and intercostal muscle function). Intubation should be accomplished by chin lift without or with minimal neck extension. Cardiac rate and rhythm should be monitored, and intravenous, central venous and arterial lines should be placed. Cervical spinal cord trauma is often associated with significant hemodynamic deficits, including hypotension. In addition, injury to other organs (e.g., a ruptured liver or spleen) can cause significant blood loss and hypotension, which must be treated promptly with intravenous crystalloid or blood. Intravenous norepinephrine or dopamine may be needed to maintain normal blood pressure after volume depletion is corrected. Hypotension is treated with a combination of volume resuscitation and the use of vasopressors with chronotropic properties (norepinephrine, dopamine). Vasopressors, such as dopamine, which functions as both an $\alpha 1$ and $\beta 1$ agonist, can be used to treat symptomatic hypotension with associated bradycardia seen in neurogenic shock. Persistent bradycardia may require atropine. Aggressive treatment of hypotension after spinal cord injury may significantly improve outcome. The stomach should be emptied by a nasogastric tube. With urinary retention, the bladder should be catheterized. Radiologic studies usually should be performed. With cervical spine trauma, if the child is alert and interactive and has no neurologic deficits, no midline cervical tenderness, no painful distracting injury, and no evidence of intoxication, cervical spine films are probably not needed. Spinal alignment is an important next step that usually can be accomplished with skeletal traction (see section on Long-Term Management).

Completed Randomized Controlled Clinical Trials

Methylprednisolone, Naloxone, and Tirilazad

Steroids have often been used in the treatment of acute spinal cord injury in an attempt to reduce cord swelling and limit central cord necrosis.

The National Acute Spinal Cord Injury Study (NASCIS 1,2,3) had studied the use of intravenous methylprednisolone in SCI. NASCIS 1(no placebo group) compared high-dose methylprednisolone to standard-dose and found no significant differences in recovery of motor or sensory function at 1 year. NASCIS 2, a randomized controlled study, compared methylprednisolone with naloxone and placebo. Methylprednisolone given within 8 hours of injury was associated with a significant improvement in motor function and sensation at a 6-month follow up. At 1-year follow-up, the methylprednisolone group still exhibited significantly improved motor scores, but there were no significant differences in sensory scores among the three groups. NASCIS 3 (no placebo) compared methylprednisolone given for 24 or 48 hours or tirilazad, a 21-amino steroid lipid peroxidation inhibitor, given for 48 hours.

Among patients who started treatment with methylprednisolone between 3 and 8 hours of injury, those given 48 hours of methylprednisolone recovered significantly more motor function at 6 weeks and 6 months than those given 24 hours of methylprednisolone. Patients treated with tirilazad for 48 hours showed motor recovery rates equivalent to patients who received methylprednisolone for 24 hours.

Currently in adults, new recommendations (2013) of the American Association of Neurologic Surgeons (AANS) and the Congress of Neurologic Surgeons (CNS) concluded that methylprednisolone should not be given for the treatment of acute spinal cord injury because of its associated harmful side effects, including infection, sepsis, gastrointestinal bleeding, poor wound healing, psychiatric side effects, and death (Hurlbert et al., 2013). Yet some controversy continues to exist regarding steroid use in acute spinal cord injury. Some authorities feel that although high-dose methylprednisolone cannot be recommended as a standard of care, it remains an option until supplanted by future evidence-based therapies.

A review of high dose methylprednisolone in children with acute spinal cord injuries highlighted the lack of evidence to support its use, noting that the majority of pediatric spinal cord trauma patients are managed on the basis of evidence extrapolated from adult studies. They recommended that steroids in acute spinal cord injuries in children should be reserved for research purposes until better evidence of its efficacy has been found (Pettiford et al., 2012).

Please see the online chapter for discussion of:

1. additional randomized controlled clinical trials with agents that did not result in long term benefits (*GM1 Ganglioside, Nimodipine, Lithium*);
2. additional pharmacologic clinical trials (*Minocycline, Riluzole, Erythropoietin [EPO]*),
3. nonpharmacologic clinical trials (*Hypothermia, Oscillating Field Stimulation [OFS]*);

4. molecular mechanisms and therapeutic approaches (*myelin-associated Inhibitors, glial scar-associated Inhibitors*);

5. *cell transplantaton therapies* (*activated autologous macrophages* [*AAM*], *schwann cells, olfactory ensheathing cells* [*OECs*], *stem cell therapy,* and *bone marrow stromal cells;*

6. therapeutic approaches currently undergoing human investigation (*nogo, rho pathway antagonists*), gene therapy for spinal cord injury and the "Future and Concerns" section.

ADDITIONAL BENEFICIAL TREATMENTS
Long-Term Management

Cervical Spine Immobilization

In childhood spine and spinal cord injuries, the main imperatives are to decompress the neural elements and to stabilize the spine to prevent further injury (Proctor, 2002). A rigid collar combined with supplemental devices that partially enclose the head (e.g., Kendrick Extrication Device®) and tape provide the best prehospital immobilization of the pediatric cervical spine. Cervical collars can lead to supraphysiologic distraction and neurologic injury in the presence of occipitoatlantal dislocation. Sandbags and tape should be used in this situation.

There are five low-risk criteria for clearing the cervical spine put forth by the National Emergency X-Radiography Utilization Study (NEXUS). These include: (1) no posterior midline cervical spine tenderness; (2) no evidence of intoxication; (3) normal alertness (score of 15 on the Glasgow Coma Scale score); (4) no focal neurologic deficits; (5) no painful distracting injuries. If all five criteria are met, there is no obvious need for cervical spine radiography; with fewer than five, radiography should be done. The Canadian C-Spine (cervical-spine) Rule (CCR), includes five low-risk and three high-risk criteria and made note of the patient's ability to rotate his/her head actively. In the presence of any high-risk criterion, or with an inability to rotate the neck actively, cervical spine radiography should be done. Some authorities have added the ability for appropriate verbal communication before the cervical spine can be cleared.

Cervical traction serves to immobilize the spine and reduce fractures. Reduction of fractures or subluxation must be undertaken with care in young patients because overdistraction can worsen the patient's neurologic dysfunction. Manual positioning under fluoroscopy often is required in cases of cervical ligamentous injury. Crown halo rings can be applied in younger patients. In older patients, cervical traction can be used with relative safety. Many spine-injured children can be managed with external stabilization without a need for later surgery (Proctor, 2002). Various devices can be used, depending on the level and severity of injury, including the Philadelphia cervical collar, Yale braces, SOMI braces, four-poster braces, halo rests, crown halo rings, and thoracolumbar orthoses. When such devices are used, frequent radiographic reevaluations are needed to ensure continuing proper alignment of spinal elements because adequate external (and internal) fixation can be difficult to achieve in a young child (Proctor, 2002).

Supportive Medical Care

After cervical spine injury, respiratory, cardiovascular, and neurologic failure are frequently found, while renal, hepatic, and hematologic failures are uncommon. Patients with acute cervical cord injury frequently develop hypotension, hypoxemia, cardiovascular instability and pulmonary dysfunction, often despite being initially stable. Although patients with midcervical cord injuries initially may have adequate spontaneous ventilation, their ventilatory ability may deteriorate within several days consequent to ascending spinal cord edema. Children with high cervical lesions who are ventilator dependent may be candidates for phrenic nerve pacing.

Both the ASIA motor score and the AIS correlate with development of organ dysfunction and failure. Tracheostomy is often needed after cervical cord injury. Lower ASIA motor scores and "complete" cervical spinal cord injury are significantly associated with the need for tracheostomy, but the anatomic level of cervical spinal cord injury was not.

Complications are not limited to patients with complete spinal cord injury. Transient life-threatening cardiovascular instability and respiratory insufficiency may be seen and may recur in the first 7 to 10 days after injury. Patients with spinal cord lesions above T7 requiring long-term management have decreased cardiac output, hypotension, and problems with temperature regulation, limiting adaption to exercise.

Retrospective studies consistently report that volume expansion and blood pressure augmentation, in an ICU setting, are linked to improved ASIA scores in patients with acute spinal cord injury compared with historical controls. Class III evidence suggests that maintenance of mean arterial pressure (MAP) at 85 to 90 mm Hg after acute spinal cord injury for a duration of 7 days is safe and may improve cord perfusion and neurologic outcome.

Nutritional support to meet caloric and nitrogen needs, not to achieve nitrogen balance, is safe and may reduce the deleterious effects of catabolic, nitrogen wasting that occurs after acute spinal cord injury. Early enteral nutrition (initiated within 72 hours) is safe, but has not been shown to affect neurologic outcome, the length of hospital stay, or the incidence of complications.

Nasogastric tube feeding after restoration of normal intestinal activity, antacids, hyperalimentation when bowel atonia persists, and rectal digital stimulation, especially in young children, may be needed. In some children, gentle disimpaction is indicated. The use of enema continence catheters for bowel dysfunction after spinal cord trauma may significantly facilitate bowel care. Intermittent catheterization of the bladder is preferred to placement of an indwelling catheter to reduce the risk of urinary tract infection and renal failure.

Renal and urologic problems can occur after spinal cord injury. Anticholinergic and botulinum toxin therapy can reduce the effects of detrusor hyperreflexia (neurogenic bladder), present in approximately 60% of patients rendered quadriparetic from spinal cord injuries. Renal failure is a major cause of mortality in patients with chronic spinal cord injury.

Autonomic dysreflexia (AD) is a well-known clinical emergency in subjects who have had a spinal cord injury, especially at T6 or above. It is defined as "an increase in systolic blood pressure of at least 20% associated with a change in heart rate (and either tachycardia or bradycardia) and is accompanied by at least one of the following signs (sweating, piloerection, facial flushing) or symptoms (headache, blurred vision, anxiety, stuffy nose). Profuse sweating, flushing and piloerection occur above the level of injury and dry and pale skin below the injury. The higher the injury level, the more severe is the AD.

Untreated episodes of AD can have serious consequences, including intracranial hemorrhage, retinal detachment, seizures, and death. Physiologically, AD is caused by massive sympathetic discharge, triggered by either a noxious or nonnoxious stimulus, originating below the level of the spinal cord injury. The more complete the spinal injury, the more likely is AD to occur. The most frequent triggers are irritation of the urinary bladder or colon. Symptoms usually are short-lived, although there have been reports of AD sustained for days to weeks. It is usually evident a month or more postinjury, although cases has been reported after 1 week. Management of an episode of AD includes placing the patient upright, loosening tight clothing, eliminating any precipitating stimulus (bladder distention or bowel impaction in 85% of cases) and antihypertensive drugs in the presence of sustained hypertension.

Other general measures include chest physiotherapy to prevent pneumonia, frequent repositioning of the patient and the use of spinal beds (Stryker frame RotaBed) to avoid decubiti, and the use of Jobst stockings to minimize the risk of deep vein thromboses complicating pulmonary emboli. Occasionally, ventilation-perfusion scanning and pulmonary angiography are needed to establish the diagnosis of pulmonary emboli. The use of miniheparin treatment (continuous infusion) or intermittent low-dose heparin therapy may reduce the risk of pulmonary embolism. The risk of deep vein thrombosis in children younger than 12 years is low enough that chemoprophylaxis is not routinely recommended, unless other significant risk factors are present. Spine or spinal cord injury are at high risk for venous thromboembolism, with more severely injured patients at higher risk. Additional factors impacting on that risk are injury type and the presence of a central venous catheter. Vena cava filters are not recommended as a routine prophylactic measure, but are recommended for selected patients who fail anticoagulation or who are not candidates for anticoagulation and/or mechanical devices.

The healing of decubitus ulcers is aided by treatment with vitamin C (15–20 mg/kg/day). Muscle relaxants, such as diazepam, baclofen, cyclobenzaprine, and intravenous orphenadrine citrate may be helpful in the long-term management of spasticity after spinal cord injury. Additional antispasmodic treatments include intrathecal baclofen and tizanidine. Progressive spinal deformity is common in children after spinal cord injury, particularly after laminectomy. Chronic pain is also common, and its management can be difficult, necessitating intervention by pain management specialists and pediatric orthopedists. In patients in whom there is delayed deterioration of neurologic functioning, the presence of a syrinx should be sought; if one is found, the syrinx may need to be shunted (Proctor, 2002).

Physical Therapy

Physical therapy is an important component of the long-term care of all patients with spinal cord injury. It should begin early and continue indefinitely. Proper limb positioning and passive muscle stretching can be instituted when the patient is medically and surgically stable. Later, after spinal shock has resolved, and early spasticity is evident, inhibitive casting can be used to minimize the development of limb contractures. Despite such measures, many patients later require botulinum toxin injections, phenol blocks, tendon lengthenings, and tendon transfers.

Functional Electrical Stimulation (FES)

FES involves using electrical current to activate muscles through the stimulation of intact peripheral motor nerves to promote functional activities. By using FES across a certain sequence of muscle groups, a cycling motion can be produced, so-called FES cycling (FESC). FESC demonstrates limited yet encouraging results improving maximum volume of oxygen utilized in 1 minute (VO2) compared with passive cycling and quadriceps strengthening.

Despite spectacular videos in selected patients, FES has not yet fulfilled expectations with respect to achievable gait function. To date, there remains an absence of randomized clinical trials to access the true efficacy of FES to improve walking.

Gait Training

In the early 1990s, treadmill training with partial body weight support was used for patients with incomplete spinal cord injuries. Numerous open studies have suggested efficacy of body-weight supported treadmill training in improving gait ability and function in spinal cord injury patients. FES and gait training have often been used together. Treadmill training can induce significant improvement in walking speed, endurance, mobility and specific activities of daily life in incomplete spinal cord injury patients, whereas overground locomotor training can result in greater improvements in functional walking capacity.

Individuals with incomplete motor spinal cord injuries have demonstrated gains from locomotor training during the acute phase (up to 12 months post injury) as well as in the chronic phase (over 12 months post injury) of rehabilitation. The use of locomotor training in individuals with complete spinal cord injury has not produced gains in walking ability. For this population, the benefits of locomotor training may be limited to the advantages of exercise, such as a reduction of secondary complications of spinal cord injury (e.g., bone loss, muscle atrophy, impaired circulation, pressure sores, weight gain, diabetes) and improvements in quality of life (Filli and Schwab, 2012). Optimal onset and amount of training are still under active investigation but are not strictly standardized among centers, often complicating the interpretation and comparison of treatment effects between different treatment sites (Filli and Schwab, 2012).

Gradual mobilization out of bed should include increased sitting tolerance, with proper weight shifts and pressure relief techniques; ambulation should be instituted early. Early initiation of the rehabilitation process is considered fundamental to enhance plasticity, but the best timing of treatment interventions is not known. Locomotor training with practiced walking might improve a person's ability to walk, but there are many additional helpful strategies as well, including treadmill training, body weight support, robotic-assisted gait training and electrical stimulation. A very comprehensive overview of therapies used to regain ambulatory function can be found in SCIRE 2006, a user-friendly, online neurotrauma research evidence resource (http://www.scireproject.com).

In a systematic review comparing different locomotor therapies for adults with incomplete spinal cord injury, it was not possible to identify the superiority of one locomotor treatment over another. A Cochrane review had similar conclusions citing insufficient evidence from randomized controlled trials. Additionally, the effects of robotic-assisted locomotor training are not clear.

Adaptive Technology

While in bed, patients who are unable to mobilize their ankle dorsi- or plantar flexors should wear pressure relieving ankle-foot orthoses to prevent muscle shortening of the gastrocsoleus complex and to prevent pressure injury of the heels. Molded wrist-hand orthoses can help to maintain a functional position and prevent flexion contractures of the digits in those with flexor spasticity. FES can be used along with adaptive technology. A power-assisted wheelchair for those who are able to use their hands can facilitate functional independence. The use of strollers should be limited to infants and toddlers. Children, as young as 1 year of age, should be encouraged to utilize a powered or manual wheelchair to facilitate independence. An ankle-foot orthosis provides ankle and foot support for the user who has sufficient hip and knee strength to control the knee during stance and swing. For incomplete motor spinal cord injury (AIS C and AIS D), the decision to use an orthosis and ambulation potential are determined by the strength and function of individual lower limb muscle groups, as well as biomechanical alignment, proprioception, and range of motion, in addition to upper extremity strength. For children without cognitive disabilities, power mobility training can be started within the first year of life. It is natural for children with spinal cord injury to progress to different orthotics, different assistive devices, and ultimately to a wheelchair, Progression to increased reliance on a wheelchair must be viewed as a natural process and not as a failure.

Future directions in assistive device technology include brain-based command integration for the manipulation of neuroprostheses or other assistive devices as shown by a person with chronic tetraplegia performing consistent, natural, and complex movements with an anthropomorphic robotic arm to regain clinically significant function.

Psychological Therapy

For discussion, please see the online chapter.

The Multidisciplinary Needs of the Child With a Spinal Cord Injury

The spectrum of possible needs of a child who has suffered a spinal cord injury is vast, as is the spectrum of available services. Children do best when a team of health care professionals work together, with one member the "quarterback" of the team. Depending on the severity/complexity of the case, health professionals who could be helpfully involved include: *physicians* (cardiologist, gastroenterologist, generalist, intensivist, nephrologist, neurologist, neurosurgeon, orthopedist, pain specialist, pediatrician, physiatrist, pulmonologist, urologist;) *nurses and nurse practitioners; nutritionists; therapists* (physical; occupational; speech/language); mental health specialists (social worker, psychologist); educators (teacher, tutor); job coaches; home health aides.

Surgical Management

The Surgical Timing in Acute Spinal Cord Injury Study (STASCIS), a multicenter prospective cohort study in adult patients with cervical cord injury compared early surgery (mean 14.2 hours) and late surgery (mean 48.3 hours). Decompression within 24 hours of injury was associated with improved neurologic outcome, defined as at least a two-grade improvement on the ASIA scale at 6-month follow up. This study reflects a growing consensus among spine surgeons favoring early surgery.

One reasonable approach might be to limit surgery to patients with partial cord injuries and a progressing neurologic deficit and patients with bilaterally locked facets, an unstable fracture and/or dislocation; surgery in the latter group would minimize the risk of later development of curvature of the spine. Additional indications for surgery might include: (1) inadequate reduction of a spinal fracture by traction alone, (2) epidural hematoma, (3) traumatic disk herniation, and (4) spinal cord compression by bony fragments (Figure 106-9).

A recent review assessing management of pediatric cervical spine and spinal cord injuries reported difficulty in collecting criteria for operative intervention in children with such injuries. From the available literature, the following guidelines were provided, based on class III evidence: (1) For odontoid injuries in children younger than 7 years of age, closed reduction and halo immobilization; (2) For acute atlantoaxial

rotatory fixation (AARF) (< 4 weeks duration) that does not reduce spontaneously, reduction with manipulation or Halter traction; (3) For chronic AARF (> 4 weeks duration), reduction with Halter traction or tong/halo traction; (4) Internal fixation and fusion for patients with recurrent and/or irreducible AARF.

Primarily ligamentous injuries of the cervical spine in children may heal with external immobilization alone, but these injuries are associated with a relatively high rate of persistent or progressive deformity when treated nonoperatively. Therefore operative treatment should also be considered for primary ligamentous injury, particularly when accompanied by unstable or irreducible fractures/dislocations associated with deformity. (class III evidence).

About 7.5–30 % of patients with thoracolumbar fractures need operative treatment. In one prospective study of children with thoracolumbar vertebral fractures, indications for surgery included: unstable fractures, fracture dislocations, fractures with more than 20° kyphosis, canal compromise of more than 50% with neurologic deficits. Spinal fusion and instrumentation were reported to have a favorable radiologic and functional outcome. Minimally invasive spinal (MIS) surgery techniques have been used sporadically in thoracolumbar junction spinal trauma cases for the past 5 years, and have been used successfully in select cases of burst fractures.

PROGNOSIS

Mortality rates in pediatric patients with cervical spine injuries ranges from 16% to 18%, with morbidity and mortality especially high in children with an upper cervical spine injury or atlantooccipital dislocation (Huisman et al., 2015). In-hospital mortality in the infant/toddler group (ages 0–3 y), where cervical spine injuries, particularly of the upper spine, were much more common than in the younger group (4–9 y), was significantly greater in the infant/toddler group (25% vs 9%). Two-year survival rates were better in younger patients (16–30 years old) than in older ones (61–86 years old), 95% versus 59%.

In the past, renal failure was the leading cause of death. More recently, it has been replaced by sepsis, pneumonia and respiratory failure. Age, level and severity of injury are important factors affecting prognosis including mortality. Most motor recovery occurs within the first 2 months of rehabilitation. Recovery depends on the severity of injury, segment of the spinal cord where the injury occurs and which nerve fibers are damaged (NINDS, 2006). An important outcome predictor is the amount of damage to the sensory pathways. If sensory function is spared, the motor outcomes appear to be better. For patients with incomplete sensory lesions (AIS: B), with preserved sacral sensitivity to pin, often more than 50% of individuals become ambulatory; for patients with incomplete motor lesions (AIS: C) 75% will recover community ambulation.

In a review of the role of MRI in acute spinal cord injury, patients were stratified by the AIS scale and the MRI findings on T2 weighted images into: normal cord, single level edema, diffuse edema, and hemorrhage. Patients with hemorrhage are initially ASIA A about 95% of the time and improved one ASIA grade about 5% of the time. Single-level edema patients showed an improvement of about two grades in ASIA score, compared with an improvement of one grade for patients with diffuse edema. Based on Delphi discussions, it is strongly recommended, based on moderate evidence, that an MRI (sagittal T2 MRI sequence) be done in the acute period following a spinal cord injury to assist with prognostication.

In a study looking at complications of spinal cord injury in 159 children 5 years or younger, 96% developed scoliosis,

57% had hip dysplasia, and 7% had latex allergy. Thirty-four percent with injuries at or above T6 experienced autonomic dysreflexia, 41% developed pressure ulcers, and 61% experienced spasticity. Of those without bowel or bladder control, 82% were on intermittent catheterization and 69% were on a bowel program. Median age of initiating wheelchair use was 3 years 4 months (range 1y 2mo to 12y 5mo). Twenty-four were community ambulators, and were more likely to have AIS D lesions. Using manual or powered mobility, 98% of participants in this study were capable of independent wheelchair propulsion.

PREVENTION

Spinal cord injuries are devastating at any age, but are especially tragic and expensive in children. Preventing these injuries is probably the greatest challenge in dealing with spinal cord injuries. Continued investment in educational programs, with ongoing efforts to heighten public awareness of the risks and consequences of spinal cord injuries, is crucial. Highway driving speed limits should be strictly enforced. People who drink alcohol should not drive. Risk-taking behavior must be minimized, particularly in people taking sedating medications, alcohol or illicit drugs. The need for protective helmets, in sports such as baseball, skiing, snowboarding, soccer and bicycling, cannot be overstressed. Diving into unfamiliar waters, particularly if shallow, must be avoided. Certain sports, particularly tackle football, carry with them a substantial risk of spinal injury, and this needs to be recognized. Other sports placing the child at potential risk for spinal cord injury include hockey, gymnastics, skiing, snowboarding, lacrosse, rugby and mountain biking. Appropriate use of rear-facing car seats, forward-facing car seats and booster seats, until the child is old/large enough to be secured by seat belts, saves lives and prevents spinal and accompanying injuries. Airbags also save lives and neurologic function, particularly since side airbags have been added to motor vehicles previously equipped with only frontal airbags. Further, any efforts that can result in reduction of societal violence, particularly involving guns and knives, can be expected to result in a corresponding reduction in spinal cord injuries.

REFERENCES

The complete list of references for this chapter is available in the e-book at www.expertconsult.com.
   See inside cover for registration details.

SUGGESTED REFERENCES

Chilton, J., Dagi, T.F., 1985. Acute cervical spinal cord injury. Am. J. Emerg. Med. 3, 340.

Cho, T.A., 2015. Spinal cord functional anatomy. Continuum (Minneap Minn) 21 (1 Spinal Cord Disorders), 13–35.

Glasser, R.S., Fessler, R.G., 1996. Biomechanics of cervical spine trauma. In: Narayan, R.K., Wilberger, J.E., Povlishock, J.T. (Eds.), Neurotrauma. McGraw-Hill, New York.

Filli, L., Schwab, M.E., 2012. The rocky road to translation in spinal cord repair. Ann. Neurol. 72 (4), 491–501.

Huisman, T.A., Wagner, M.W., Bosemani, T., et al., 2015. Pediatric spinal trauma. J. Neuroimaging 25 (3), 337–353.

Hurlbert, R.J., Hadley, M.N., Walters, B.C., et al., 2013. Pharmacological therapy for acute spinal cord injury. Neurosurgery 72 (Suppl. 2), 93–105.

Kirshblum, S.C., Burns, S.P., Biering-Sorensen, F., et al., 2011. International standards for neurological classification of spinal cord injury (revised 2011). J. Spinal Cord Med. 34 (6), 535–546.

Klein, J.P., 2015. A practical approach to spine imaging. Continuum (Minneap Minn) 21 (1 Spinal Cord Disorders), 36–51.

Pettiford, J.N., Bikhchandani, J., Ostlie, D.J., et al., 2012. A review: the role of high dose methylprednisolone in spinal cord trauma in children. Pediatr. Surg. Int. 28 (3), 287–294.

Proctor, M.R., 2002. Spinal cord injury. Crit. Care Med. 30 (Suppl.), S489.

E-BOOK FIGURES AND TABLES

107 Determination of Brain Death in Infants and Children

Mudit Mathur and Stephen Ashwal

 An expanded version of this chapter is available on www.expertconsult.com. See inside cover for registration details.

The diagnosis of brain death in infants and children is made after careful review of the medical history and performance of a detailed neurologic examination establishing irreversible cessation of brain function. In the United States and most other countries, the 1987 pediatric guidelines of the American Academy of Pediatrics (AAP) provided the basis for brain death determination in children (AAP Task Force on Brain Death in Children, 1987). These guidelines were revised in 2011 (Nakagawa et al., 2011). Revisions include updates related to the initial waiting period before conducting the first brain death examination, who should conduct the examination, the number of examinations, the interexamination interval, the number of apnea tests, partial pressure of carbon dioxide ($PaCO_2$) thresholds during apnea testing, and when an ancillary test may be used to reduce the interexamination observation interval or assist with the diagnosis of brain death (Nakagawa et al., 2011). Further clarification is provided regarding the determination of brain death in newborns. A checklist is included to assist clinicians with consistent performance and documentation of examination elements and ancillary testing (see Fig. A-2 in Appendix A).

HISTORICAL PERSPECTIVE

A state beyond coma, or coma dépassé, was proposed in 1959 by Mollaret and Goulon to describe a premorbid clinical condition with loss of sensation, motor activity, consciousness, and vegetative functions, and in 1968 an ad hoc committee of the Harvard Medical School faculty recommended clinical guidelines that subsequently shaped the development of brain death concepts. Failure of improvement over 24 hours established a diagnosis of brain death in a normothermic patient, with drugs capable of maintaining coma excluded. Two iso-electric electroencephalograms (EEGs) performed 24 hours apart were considered confirmatory, but not essential, in the declaration of brain death. Reports in the 1970s from the Medical Royal College and Faculties in the United Kingdom recommended that brainstem death be considered death, and in 1980 the National Institute of Neurologic and Communicative Disorders and Stroke (NINCDS) Collaborative Study of Brain Death emphasized that the combination of loss of the pupillary light reflex, corneal reflex, oculocephalic reflex (doll eye phenomenon), and oculovestibular reflex (caloric eye deviation) was highly predictive of death. Apnea, coma, and absence of brainstem reflexes, combined with an electrocerebral silent EEG, were highly associated with pathology in a brain that had experienced long-term ventilator exposure. The report concluded that drug screening and EEG monitoring were mandatory before declaring brain death. Subsequent reports in adults and children documented that EEG activity could persist in unequivocally brain dead patients.

In 1981, a U.S. presidential commission established brain death guidelines based on the irreversible cessation of function of the entire brain and noted that adult criteria might not be applicable to children younger than 5 years of age. The American Academy of Neurology (AAN) published adult (i.e.,

individuals older than 18 years of age) brain death guidelines in 1995 and revised them in 2010, with the more recent guidelines recommending that only one examination be required, that ancillary testing is not necessary, and that the diagnosis could be made solely on clinical criteria. Box 107-1 summarizes the recommendations section of the 2010 American Academy of Neurology (AAN) parameter that provides practical (non–evidence-based) guidance for determination of brain death in adults.

It was suggested that if the examination is equivocal, additional neurodiagnostic testing could be done (Wijdicks et al., 2010). As noted, the first pediatric brain-death guidelines were published in 1987 by the AAP (AAP Task Force on Brain Death in Children, 1987) and substantially revised in 2011 (Nakagawa et al., 2011); these guidelines are summarized in Boxes 107-2 and 107-3.

LEGAL DEFINITION OF BRAIN DEATH

The American Medical Association and the American Bar Association supported enactment of the Uniform Determination of Death Act (UDDA) of 1980, which defined death, stating that "an individual who has sustained either (1) irreversible cessation of circulatory and respiratory functions; or (2) irreversible cessation of all functions of the brain including the brainstem is dead." Brain death is legally accepted as death under the UDDA in almost all states and recognized in the rest through judicial opinion.

EPIDEMIOLOGY
Incidence of Brain Death

It is estimated that approximately 1800 children in the United States are declared brain-dead every year (Figure 107-1). Studies from pediatric intensive care units in the 1990s reported that the incidence of brain death in older infants and children ranged from 0.65% to 1.2% of admissions. A recent case series reported that brain death occurred in 16% of 192 patients who died, with withholding or withdrawal of life support being the predominant mode of death (in 70%). The length of stay for 80% of the patients declared brain-dead was less than 7 days (median of 2.9 days). In some pediatric intensive care units, the percentage of patients diagnosed as brain-dead has been reported to be up to 38% of all deaths.

Etiologies of Brain Death

Brain death most commonly occurs in adolescents and less so in infants younger than 1 year of age (see Table 107-1). Closed head injury is the most common clinical presentation leading to brain death (50%), followed by intracranial hemorrhage and stroke (12%). Asphyxial injury usually occurs as a complication of septic or hemorrhagic shock, with unexplained out-of-hospital cardiac arrest, or from strangulation or suffocation. Sudden infant death syndrome is a rare cause of brain

---

BOX 107-2 Summary Recommendations for the Diagnosis of Brain Death in Neonates, Infants, and Children from the 2011 Pediatric Guidelines

1. DETERMINATION OF BRAIN DEATH

- Determination of brain death in neonates, infants, and children relies on a clinical diagnosis that is based on the absence of neurologic function with a known irreversible cause of coma. Coma and apnea must coexist to diagnose brain death. This diagnosis should be made by physicians who have evaluated the history and completed the neurologic examinations.

2. PREREQUISITES FOR INITIATING A BRAIN DEATH EVALUATION

1. Hypotension, hypothermia, and metabolic disturbances that could affect the neurologic examination must be corrected before examination for brain death.
2. Sedatives, analgesics, neuromuscular blockers, and anticonvulsant agents should be discontinued for a reasonable time period, based on elimination half-life of the pharmacologic agent, to ensure that they do not affect the neurologic examination. Knowledge of the total amount of each agent (mg/kg) administered since hospital admission may provide useful information concerning the risk of continued medication effects. Blood or plasma levels to confirm that high or supratherapeutic levels of anticonvulsants with sedative effects are not present should be obtained (if available), and repeated as needed or until the levels are in the low to middle therapeutic range.
3. The diagnosis of brain death based on neurologic examination alone should not be made if supratherapeutic or high therapeutic levels of sedative agents are present. When levels are in the low to middle therapeutic range, medication effects sufficient to affect the results of the neurologic examination are unlikely. If uncertainty remains, an ancillary study should be performed.
4. Assessment of neurologic function may be unreliable immediately following cardiopulmonary resuscitation or other severe acute brain injuries, and evaluation for brain death should be deferred for 24 to 48 hours or longer if there are concerns or inconsistencies in the examination.

3. NUMBER OF EXAMINATIONS, EXAMINERS, AND OBSERVATION PERIODS

1. Two examinations, including apnea testing, with each examination separated by an observation period, are required.
2. The examinations should be performed by different attending physicians involved in the care of the child. The apnea test may be performed by the same physician, preferably the attending physician who is managing ventilator care of the child.
3. Recommended observation periods are as follows:
   a. 24 hours for neonates (37 weeks' gestation to term infants 30 days of age)
   b. 12 hours for infants and children (>30 days to 18 years)
4. The first examination determines that the child has met neurologic examination criteria for brain death. The second examination, performed by a different attending physician, confirms that the child has fulfilled criteria for brain death.
5. Assessment of neurologic function may be unreliable immediately following cardiopulmonary resuscitation or other severe acute brain injuries, and evaluation for brain death should be deferred for 24 to 48 hours or longer if there are concerns or inconsistencies in the examination.

4. APNEA TESTING

1. Apnea testing must be performed safely and requires documentation of an arterial $PaCO_2$ 20 mm Hg above the

baseline $PaCO_2$ and $\geq$ 60 mm Hg, with no respiratory effort during the testing period, to support the diagnosis of brain death. Some infants and children with chronic respiratory disease or insufficiency may only be responsive to supranormal $PaCO_2$ levels. In this instance the $PaCO_2$ level should increase to $\geq$ 20 mm Hg above the baseline $PaCO_2$ level.

2. If the apnea test cannot be performed because of a medical contraindication or cannot be completed because of hemodynamic instability, desaturation to < 85%, or an inability to reach a $PaCO_2$ of 60 mm Hg or greater, an ancillary study should be performed.

5. ANCILLARY STUDIES

1. Ancillary studies (electroencephalogram and radionuclide cerebral blood flow) are not required to establish brain death, unless the clinical examination or apnea test cannot be completed.
2. Ancillary studies are not a substitute for the neurologic examination.
3. For all age groups, ancillary studies can be used to assist the clinician in making the diagnosis of brain death to reduce the observation period, or in the following situations:
   a. When components of the examination or apnea testing cannot be completed safely because of the underlying medical condition of the patient.
   b. When there is uncertainty about the results of the neurologic examination.
   c. When medication effect may interfere with evaluation of the patient.
   If the ancillary study supports the diagnosis, the second examination and apnea testing can then be performed. When an ancillary study is used to reduce the observation period, all aspects of the examination and apnea testing should be completed and documented.
4. When an ancillary study is used because there are inherent examination limitations (i.e., i–iii), the components of the examination done initially should be completed and documented.
5. If the ancillary study is equivocal or if there is concern about the validity of the ancillary study, the patient cannot be pronounced dead. The patient should continue to be observed until brain death can be declared on clinical examination criteria and apnea testing, or a follow-up ancillary study can be performed to assist with the determination of brain death. A waiting period of 24 hours is recommended before further clinical reevaluation or a repeat ancillary study is performed. Supportive patient care should continue during this time period.

6. DECLARATION OF DEATH

1. Death is declared after confirmation and completion of the second clinical examination and apnea test.
2. When ancillary studies are used, documentation of components from the second clinical examination that can be completed must remain consistent with brain death. All aspects of the clinical examination, including the apnea test, or ancillary studies must be appropriately documented.
3. The clinical examination should be carried out by experienced clinicians who are familiar with infants and children and have specific training in neurocritical care.

(Adapted from Nakagawa TA et al. Crit Care Med 2011 Sep;3[9]:2139–55.)

1. Coma: The patient must exhibit complete loss of consciousness, vocalization, and volitional activity.
2. Apnea: The patient must have a complete absence of documented respiratory effort (if feasible) by formal apnea testing demonstrating a $PaCO_2 \geq 60$ mm Hg and ≥ 20 mm Hg increase above baseline.
3. Loss of all brainstem reflexes, including the following:
   - Midposition or fully dilated pupils that do not respond to light
   - Absence of movement of bulbar musculature, including facial and oropharyngeal muscles
   - Absent gag, cough, sucking, and rooting reflexes
   - Absent corneal reflexes
   - Absent oculovestibular reflexes.
4. Flaccid tone and absence of spontaneous or induced movements: excluding spinal cord events, such as reflex withdrawal or spinal myoclonus.
5. Reversible conditions or conditions that can interfere with the neurologic examination: must be excluded before brain death testing.

death, as are meningitis, rare metabolic diseases, perioperative insults, acute hydrocephalus, and other rare disorders that affect the brain.

Outcome after Diagnosis of Brain Death

Most children are removed from life support or undergo organ donation within a 2-day time period after the diagnosis of brain death is confirmed. Some children are continued on ventilator support until cardiac arrest occurs, and their "survival" has averaged about 17 days. In rare cases, children have been maintained on ventilator support for 6 months to 5 years.

NEUROLOGIC EVALUATION

Variability exists in the diagnosis of brain death in children, including the use of apnea testing. Issues involved in this variability include lack of documentation of the history and examination findings, insufficient knowledge of brain death criteria, inappropriate use of ancillary testing, failure to perform serial examination, and lack of awareness that brain death can be diagnosed without ancillary testing in children older than 1 year of age. The 2011 guidelines update (Nakagawa et al., 2011) facilitates completeness of the neurologic evaluation and seeks to reduce practice variability by providing a checklist for the determination and documentation of brain death (see Fig. A-1 in Appendix A).

Clinical Examination
Cerebral Unresponsiveness

Clinicians should first identify an underlying etiology for coma and exclude potentially reversible diagnoses. The initial period of stabilization and diagnostic workup before clinical evaluation for brain death may be 24 hours or longer following severe acute brain injuries. Normalizing body temperature (core temperature greater than or equal to 95° F [35° C]) and

blood pressure, correcting severe metabolic disturbances, and ensuring that sedative or neuromuscular blocking agents have had adequate time to be metabolized are important prerequisites. Assessment for cerebral unresponsivity, loss of cranial nerve function, and determination of apnea (tested with a hypercapnic stimulus) must then be performed and documented. Cerebral unresponsivity or coma can be quantified using the Glasgow Coma Scale score (Chapter 101). In young children, recovery may occur after unresponsiveness has occurred for prolonged periods, and even when serious structural nervous system abnormalities are present. If the neurologic evaluation is uncertain or inconsistent, the examination may be repeated to exclude reversible or changing neurologic function; alternatively, supportive ancillary tests may be considered.

Brainstem Examination

Cessation of brainstem reflexes is generally accepted as the hallmark of brain failure. The NINCDS report indicated that although the combination of the loss of the pupillary light response and oculocephalic and oculovestibular reflexes had the greatest specificity, this combination included 4% of patients who retained other brainstem reflexes. The 2011 pediatric guidelines (Nakagawa et al., 2011) recommend that doing cold caloric testing is sufficient and that oculocephalic testing (which involves turning the patient's head) is not necessary; the guidelines also state that because some individuals could have spinal cord injury, such testing might pose additional risk. Box 107-4 in the online chapter outlines the procedures used to assess the cold caloric (oculovestibular) response. Premature infants of less than 32 weeks' conceptual age do not have completely developed cranial nerve function. Clinicians examining these infants should be aware of the development of the different cranial nerve reflexes during gestation (see Table 107-2). Newborns often present obstacles to examination. Ear canals are frequently small and may be plugged, pupils are small, adhesive tape obscures the face and extremities, and neuromuscular blocking agents alter the examination. The 2011 pediatric guidelines (Nakagawa et al., 2011) include recommendations for term infants from 37 weeks' gestation. Recommendations for preterm infants younger than 37 weeks were not included because of insufficient evidence. Brain death rarely occurs in preterm infants, so clinicians will likely not have to confront the issue of trying to diagnose brain death in this population.

Number of Examinations, Examiners, and Observation Periods

Number of Examinations and Examiners. The 2011 guidelines (Nakagawa et al., 2011) recommend performance of two examinations separated by an observation period and that the best interests of the child and family would be served if at least two different attending physicians participate in diagnosing brain death to ensure that (1) the diagnosis is based on currently established criteria, (2) there are no conflicts of interest in establishing the diagnosis, and (3) there is consensus of at least two physicians involved in the care of the child that brain death criteria are met. The 2011 guidelines also note that because the apnea test is an objective test, it may be performed by the same physician, preferably the attending physician who is managing ventilator care of the child. The recommendation for two complete clinical examinations has been criticized for making the diagnosis of brain death in children unnecessarily complicated and creating delays in the possibility of organ donation. The opinion of the committee members who drafted the 2011 guidelines was based on the fact that cases with "improvement" and apparently reversible brain death days after brain injury often have diagnostic errors when critically reexamined.

Duration of Observation Periods. A literature review of 171 children diagnosed as brain-dead found that 47% had ventilator support withdrawn, on average, 1.7 days after the diagnosis of brain death was made (Ashwal and Schneider, 1987). Of those continued on ventilator support, 46% suffered a cardiac arrest an average of 22.7 days later. These data and the reports of more recent studies suggest that there is likely no biological justification for using different durations of observation to diagnose brain death in infants greater than 1 month of age. Although some authors have reported apparent reversibility of brain death, review of these cases reveals that these children would not have fulfilled currently used criteria.

Based on the data just noted, current literature, and clinical experience, the 2011 guidelines recommend that the observation period between examinations should be 24 hours for neonates (37 weeks up to 30 days) and 12 hours for infants and children (>30 days to 18 years). The first examination determines that the child has met neurologic examination criteria for brain death. The second examination confirms brain death, based on an unchanged and irreversible condition.

Apnea Testing

Documentation of apnea is the most important determination in the clinical evaluation of brain death. Virtually all protocols recommend a period without assisted ventilation. The normal physiologic apneic threshold (minimum PCO_2 at which respiration begins) depends on many factors, and can be altered by anesthetic agents, narcotics, sedatives, and certain disease states. The maximal PCO_2 apneic threshold in children is probably similar to that in adults (60 mm Hg); the data from previous pediatric studies is summarized in Table 107-3 in the online chapter. Apnea testing of patients who are hypothermic or receiving medications that suppress respiration is not valid for documenting brainstem failure. It still can be performed, however, because the presence of respiratory effort would eliminate brain death as a diagnosis. Several case reports involving only a few patients have raised related issues concerning apnea testing in young infants and children that also apply to newborns. These cases were associated with compressive brainstem lesions and the return of ineffective minimal respiratory effort, but are too few in number to draw any conclusions.

Technique for Performing Apnea Testing. An apnea test should be performed with each brain death examination unless a medical contraindication (e.g., high cervical spine injury) exists. Recommendations for performing apnea testing in term newborns, infants, and children are provided in the 2011 pediatric brain death guidelines (Nakagawa et al., 2011; see Box 107-5). This includes normalization of the pH and $PaCO_2$, measured by arterial blood gas analysis, maintenance of core temperature greater than 35° C (95° F), normalization of blood pressure appropriate for the age of the child, and correction of factors that could affect respiratory effort as a prerequisite to testing. The patient must be preoxygenated, using 100% oxygen, before initiating this test. Intermittent mandatory mechanical ventilation should be discontinued once the patient is well oxygenated and a normal $PaCO_2$ has been achieved. The patient can then be changed to a T piece attached to the endotracheal tube (ETT), or a self-inflating bag-valve system. Tracheal insufflation of oxygen using a catheter inserted through the ETT has also been used; however, caution is warranted to ensure adequate gas excursion and to prevent barotrauma. High gas-flow rates with tracheal insufflation may also promote CO_2 washout, preventing adequate $PaCO_2$ rise during apnea testing. Physicians performing apnea

testing should continuously monitor the patient's heart rate, blood pressure, and oxygen saturation while observing for spontaneous respiratory effort. If no respiratory effort is observed from the initiation of the apnea test to the time the measured $PaCO_2$ is greater than or equal to 60 mm Hg *and* greater than or equal to 20 mm Hg above the baseline level, the apnea test is consistent with brain death. The patient should be placed back on mechanical ventilator support and medical management should continue until the second neurologic examination and apnea test confirming brain death is completed. If oxygen saturations fall below 85%, hemodynamic instability limits completion of apnea testing, or a $PaCO_2$ level of greater than or equal to 60 mm Hg cannot be achieved, the patient should be placed back on ventilator support with appropriate treatment to restore normal oxygen saturations, normocarbia, and hemodynamic parameters. Another attempt to test for apnea may be performed later, or an ancillary study may be pursued to assist with determination of brain death. Evidence of any respiratory effort is inconsistent with brain death, and the apnea test should be terminated and the patient placed back on ventilatory support.

ANCILLARY NEURODIAGNOSTIC STUDIES

Virtually all guidelines have stressed that the historical events leading to coma, when combined with the clinical triad of coma, absence of brainstem reflexes, and a failed apnea challenge, are fundamental to brain death diagnosis. Many physicians have sought an absolute laboratory test to confirm brain death. The combination of clinical evaluation and pertinent diagnostic studies (EEG, cerebral blood flow [CBF] studies) can yield a sound clinical decision. However, data acquired over the past two decades have clearly shown that some patients may have EEG activity or demonstrable CBF when they meet clinical criteria for irreversible brain death. Because of such observations and general consensus, the 2011 pediatric guidelines (Nakagawa et al., 2011) note that ancillary studies are not required to establish brain death and should not be viewed as a substitute for the neurologic examination. The guidelines (Nakagawa et al., 2011) recommend ancillary studies to assist the clinician in making the diagnosis of brain death in the following situations:

1. When components of the examination or apnea testing cannot be completed safely because of the underlying medical condition of the patient;
2. If there is uncertainty about the results of the neurologic examination;
3. If a medication effect may be present;
4. To reduce the interexamination observation period.

The 2011 guidelines also recommended that, similar to the neurologic examination, hemodynamic and temperature parameters should be normalized before obtaining EEG or CBF studies. Pharmacologic agents that could affect the results of testing should be discontinued and levels determined as clinically indicated (see Table 107-4). The 2011 guidelines note that therapeutic levels of barbiturates in the low to middle range should not preclude the use of EEG testing, and that a CBF study could be used in patients with high-dose barbiturate therapy to demonstrate absence of CBF.

Electroencephalogram

Despite limitations of the EEG, many physicians tend to equate an isoelectric EEG (electrocerebral silence [ECS]) with brain death. An isoelectric EEG, combined with the clinical triad of coma, absent brainstem reflexes, and apnea, remains a common method to determine brain death. The American

Electroencephalographic Society (1994) developed criteria for brain-death recordings. According to these guidelines, the recording should be isoelectric for a minimum of 30 minutes and show no electrical activity beyond 2 μV at a sensitivity of 2 μV/mm, with filter settings at 0.1 or 0.3 second at 70 Hz.

Electroencephalogram in Pediatric Brain Death

Pediatric patients present unique difficulties in interpretation of the EEG because of shorter interelectrode distances, greater electrocardiogram contamination, reduced cortical potentials in premature infants, and delayed metabolism of barbiturates. Reversible ECS may occur with the use of drugs that depress the activity of the central nervous system, hypothermia, cardiovascular shock, or metabolic encephalopathies. In children, the most common medications causing the reversible loss of brain electrocortical activity include barbiturates, benzodiazepines, narcotics, and certain intravenous and inhalation anesthetics.

A core temperature greater than 32.2° C (>90° F) has been regarded as a prerequisite for reliably determining brain death by EEG. In children, suppression of EEG activity does not appear until 24° C (75.2° F), and complete loss of EEG activity does not occur until the temperature is less than 18° C (<64.4° F). The average temperature when EEGs are obtained for confirmation of brain death is 36.2 ± 0.8° C (97.3° F ± 1.4° F). Reversible ECS may occur soon after a child has had a cardiac arrest.

Although not well documented, electrolyte, acid-base, and blood-gas abnormalities; severe hepatic and renal dysfunction; and certain inborn errors of metabolism all have been considered capable of decreasing brain electrocortical activity to the point of causing complete cortical inactivity. In selected children in whom the etiology of brain death is uncertain, evaluation for metabolic diseases should be considered.

Extensive literature exists documenting persistent EEG activity in brain-dead infants, children, and adults. Table 107-5 in the online chapter and Table 107-8 summarize data from the 2011 guidelines (Nakagawa et al., 2011). The data show that 76% of all children who were evaluated with EEG for brain death had ECS on the first EEG. Multiple EEGs increased the yield to 89%. For those children who had ECS on the first EEG, 97% had ECS on a follow-up EEG. Of those patients with EEG activity on the first EEG, 55% had a subsequent EEG that showed ECS. The remaining 45% either had persistent EEG activity or additional EEGs were not performed. All died (spontaneously or by withdrawal of support).

Since a 1972 report of two infants who displayed the return of some EEG activity after an initial ECS recording, there have only been a few reports of additional infants in whom EEG activity returned. A previous report, based on these cases, estimated that the return of EEG activity when the initial study was isoelectric was approximately 0.02% (Ashwal, 1997). Concerns about the return of EEG activity have been overemphasized. If one considers issues related to subsequent clinical status of the patients in whom EEG activity returned, no patients have made significant clinical recoveries.

Measurements of Cerebral Perfusion

Several technologies are available for estimating or measuring CBF (see Table 107-6).

Cerebral Angiography

Direct visualization of the cerebral circulation with angiography that shows the complete cessation of CBF was long accepted as the standard for comparing all other neuroimaging modalities for brain-death confirmation. This technique has multiple limitations and is no longer used for documenting cessation of CBF in children.

Radionuclide Imaging

Several radionuclide techniques have been used in brain-dead patients to determine noninvasively whether there has been cessation of cerebral circulation. Circulation can be assessed during an early "dynamic" phase and later by examining static images for cerebral uptake of the specific radionuclide (technetium-99m pertechnetate, technetium-99m glucoheptonate, or technetium-99m diethylene-triamine-pentaacetate [DTPA]) (see Figure 107-2). During the dynamic phase, a radionuclide bolus is injected rapidly, and isotopic cranial images are obtained similar to those of carotid arteriograms. In the arterial phase, cerebral activity is detectable within several seconds, followed by sagittal sinus activity within 6 to 8 seconds. If activity is not detectable in this early phase, CBF is considered absent, resulting from either low cardiac output or very high intracranial pressure. Because most tracers have a half-life of several hours, the static phase of a radionuclide imaging study usually is done later, to look for the absence or presence of diffuse parenchymal isotopic uptake. Most centers use single-photon emission computed tomography scanning and technetium-99m hexamethylpropylene amine oxime (HMPAO) as the isotopic agent.

Multiple studies have documented radionuclide imaging to be accurate, reproducible, and similar to other methods of CBF detection. This technique is particularly useful when hypothermia or elevated barbiturate levels preclude valid EEG interpretation. Premature and full-term newborns, despite having extremely reduced CBF compared with older children, can be evaluated using radionuclide measurements.

The 2011 guidelines (Nakagawa et al., 2011) summarize CBF data from 12 studies in 681 suspected brain-dead children (see Table 107-7). Absent CBF was found in 86% of clinically brain-dead children, and the yield did not significantly change if more than one CBF study was done (89%). It was found that 92% of patients who initially had absent CBF also had no flow on follow-up studies. The two exceptions, in whom flow developed later, were newborns. In those patients with preserved CBF on the first CBF study, 26% had a second CBF study that showed no flow. The remaining 74% had preserved flow or no further CBF studies were done, and all but one patient died (either spontaneously or after withdrawal of support).

Computed Tomographic Angiography and Perfusion

The computed tomographic angiography (CT-a) and perfusion (CTP) techniques combine conventional CT with rapid bolus infusion of a contrast agent to examine the vascular structure and flow of any organ system. Several recent studies have examined their use in adults who met brain death criteria; these studies report very good sensitivity and specificity. There have been several case reports documenting that CT-a may not show findings confirming the absence of CBF. CT-a is a promising method for use in determining the absence of intracranial circulation, but studies in pediatric brain-dead patients have not yet been published.

Magnetic Resonance Imaging and Magnetic Resonance Angiography

Magnetic resonance imaging (MRI) and magnetic resonance (MR) angiography also have been used to evaluate cerebral circulation in brain dead adults. Characteristic features include transtentorial and foramen magnum herniation, absent intracranial vascular flow void, poor gray–white matter differentiation, no intracranial contrast enhancement, carotid artery enhancement (intravascular enhancement sign), and prominent nasal and scalp enhancement. Presumably, similar neuroimaging findings would be present in children, but this has not yet been well established.

Transcranial Doppler Ultrasonography

Transcranial Doppler ultrasonography has advocates because of its obvious portability, noninvasiveness, and isolette accessibility. Recent studies document a high rate of false-negative test results and lower levels of specificity and sensitivity, which suggest sufficient limitations in the use of this technique for brain-death confirmation.

Digital Subtraction Angiography

Digital subtraction angiography can be used to assess the intracranial circulation. A small amount of nonionic contrast material is injected intravenously or intraarterially while digital subtraction imaging of the cerebral vasculature is completed. This procedure allows visualization of contrast within the major intracranial vessels; lack of such visualization indicates absence of CBF. There are few reports of use of this technique in children and only one case report in a neonate diagnosed with brain death.

Xenon Computed Tomography

Stable xenon CT and 133-xenon CT are examples of reliable and well-documented tests that are seldom available because of cost and limited personnel, and these methods are seldom if ever used in children being evaluated for brain death. Xenon CT allows quantitative and regional measurement of CBF, and previous studies have documented marked CBF reductions in brain-dead adults and children compared with comatose patients.

Positron Emission Tomography

The results of positron emission tomography (Chapter 12) have been reported for only a few brain-dead patients. Because of limited availability, cost, and lack of comparison studies, positron emission tomography offers no advantages over the more standardized techniques and is not used for confirmation of brain death.

Magnetic Resonance Spectroscopy

In the 1980s and 1990s, phosphorus (^{31}P) and proton (^{1}H) MR spectroscopy were used to measure aspects of brain metabolic activity noninvasively (Chapter 12). Studies in neonates, older infants, and children have reported significant abnormalities, with loss of metabolic activity associated with severe acute central nervous system insults and with poor long-term outcomes. The advantage of spectroscopy is that it can be done in conjunction with MRI, which allows acquisition of anatomic and metabolic data. There are no published case reports concerning proton MR spectroscopy and brain death in children. At Loma Linda University Children's Hospital, 10 brain-dead children were studied with proton MR spectroscopy. All spectra were markedly abnormal but were similar to spectra from patients who became vegetative or severely disabled, suggesting that the specificity for brain death determination of MR spectroscopy is insufficient.

Comparison of Electroencephalogram and Cerebral Blood Flow Studies

Table 107-8 summarizes the comparative diagnostic yield of EEG versus CBF determinations in children who had both

TABLE 107-8 Electroencephalogram and Cerebral Blood Flow Diagnostic Screening Yield by Age Groups

	ECS	EEG+	Total	Diagnostic Screening Yield
ALL CHILDREN (N = 149)				
No CBF	86	18	104	% patients with ECS = 70%
CBF+	19	26	45	% patients with no CBF = 70%
Total	105	44	149	
NEWBORNS ONLY (<1 MONTH OF AGE; n = 30)				
No CBF	8	11	19	% patients with ECS = 40%
CBF+	4	7	11	% patients with no CBF = 63%
Total	12	18	30	
CHILDREN (>1 MONTH OF AGE; n = 119)				
No CBF	78	7	85	% patients with ECS = 78%
CBF+	15	19	34	% patients with no CBF = 71%
Total	93	26	119	

CBF, cerebral blood flow; CBF+, cerebral blood flow present; ECS, electrocerebral silence; EEG+, activity on electroencephalogram. (Adapted from Nakagawa TA et al. Crit Care Med, 2011;3 [9]:2139–55.)

studies done as part of the initial brain death evaluation. Data from the studies cited in Table 107-5 and 107-7 in the online chapter were stratified by three age groups: all children, newborns, and children greater than 1 month in age to 18 years. The data in Table 107-8 for the all-children group show that when both studies were initially performed, the diagnostic yield was the same (70% had ECS; 70% showed absent CBF). The diagnostic yield for children greater than 1 month of age was similar for both tests (EEG with ECS, 78%; no CBF, 71%). For newborns, EEG with ECS was less sensitive (40%) than absence of CBF (63%) when confirming the diagnosis of brain death, but even in the CBF group, the yield was low.

Evoked Potentials

Brainstem auditory evoked potentials and somatosensory evoked potentials have been studied extensively as ancillary tests for brain death. The portability, rapidity, and noninvasiveness seem ideal, but multiple studies have raised significant doubts as to their reliability. Most clinicians do not rely on evoked potential studies as an ancillary test for brain death; rather, such testing remains useful as a prognostic indicator in children who survive catastrophic brain injury.

Brain Tissue Oxygenation

The brain tissue oxygenation technique uses invasive monitors to directly assess brain tissue oxygenation in an attempt to optimize neurocritical care therapy in patients with elevated intracranial pressure. Incidentally, it was observed that brain tissue oxygenation decreased to zero in five children who progressed to brain death, and remained above this threshold in 80 other children who did not. Comparative data are needed to evaluate the utility of this potential ancillary test against established modalities.

BRAIN DEATH IN NEWBORNS

The revised 2011 pediatric brain-death guidelines (Nakagawa et al., 2011) state that brain death can be diagnosed in term infants of more than 37 weeks' gestation, provided the physician is aware of the limitations of the clinical examination and ancillary studies in this age group. Recommendations for preterm neonates of less than 37 weeks' gestation were not included in the guidelines because of insufficient data.

Preterm and term infants of less than 7 days of age were excluded from the 1987 pediatric brain-death guidelines (AAP Task Force on Brain Death in Children, 1987). Several years after the publication of these guidelines, data on 18 brain-dead neonates were published, and it was suggested that brain death could be diagnosed in full-term newborn infants and preterm infants of more than 34 weeks' gestational age within the first week of life (Ashwal, 1997). Because a newborn has patent sutures and an open fontanel, increases in intracranial pressure after acute injury are not as significant as in older patients. These observations may account for the relatively large proportion of clinically brain-dead newborns who have detectible EEG activity and CBF. The use of whole-brain death criteria might not be appropriate in a newborn. It might be more medically justifiable to use brainstem death as the major criterion for brain death in newborns. In many situations, the issue of whether a neonate is brain-dead or just catastrophically and irreversibly brain-injured is resolved by the decision of physicians caring for the neonate with the understanding and agreement of the family to withdraw ventilator support and redirect to compassionate care.

Epidemiology

It has been estimated that there are about 550 newborns diagnosed each year as brain-dead out of a total of 3,900,089 live births (Ashwal, 1997). Etiologies of neonatal brain death include hypoxic-ischemic encephalopathy, birth trauma, central nervous system malformations, central nervous system hemorrhage, infection, sudden infant death syndrome, nonaccidental trauma, and metabolic disorders.

Clinical Examination

Examination of preterm infants of less than 37 weeks' gestation to determine whether they meet brain-death criteria may be difficult because some brainstem reflexes may not be completely developed (see Table 107-2) and because it is difficult to assess the level of consciousness in a critically ill, sedated, and intubated neonate. The revised 2011 guidelines (Nakagawa et al., 2011) emphasize the importance of carefully and repeatedly examining term newborns, with particular attention to examination of brainstem reflexes and apnea testing. As with older children, assessment might be unreliable immediately following an acute injury; therefore, a period of 24 hours or longer is recommended before evaluating the term newborn for brain death.

Duration of Observation

The consensus-based recommendations in the 2011 guidelines recommend a 24-hour observation period between the two neurologic examinations for term infants (>37 weeks' gestation). Data from 87 newborns allowed an estimation of the duration of coma after the insult until brain death was initially diagnosed (37 hours), duration of time before brain-death confirmation (75 hours), and duration of time to transplantation (20 hours) (Ashwal, 1997).The average duration of brain death in these patients was about 95 hours (i.e., 4 days). Recovery of brainstem function was not observed in any patients, despite a variety of EEG and CBF results. Other studies in neonates undergoing cardiac transplantation reported that the total duration of brain death (including time to transplantation) averaged 2.8 days in neonates less than 7 days of age and 5.2 days in neonates 1 to 3 weeks old. The data suggest that a 24- to 48-hour observation period in neonates less than 7 days of age should be sufficient to confirm the diagnosis of brain death.

Apnea Testing

Neonatal studies reviewing $PaCO_2$ thresholds for apnea are limited. Data from 35 neonates who were determined to be brain-dead revealed a mean $PaCO_2$ of 65 mm Hg, suggesting that the threshold of 60 mm Hg is also valid in the newborn.

Ancillary Studies

EEG and radionuclide imaging techniques remain the most commonly used ancillary studies to confirm the diagnosis of neonatal brain death. Ancillary studies are less sensitive in detecting the presence or absence of brain electrical activity or CBF than in older children (Table 107-8). Of the two studies, detection of absence of CBF (63%) was more sensitive than demonstration of ECS (40%); however, even in the CBF study group, the sensitivity was low. Previous studies also have reported that about one-third of neonates with ECS showed evidence of CBF, and 58% with absent CBF had evidence of EEG activity. These data suggest that, in neonates, clinical rather than laboratory data may be more appropriate, provided that a sufficient period of observation is allowed. Because of these data, the 2011 guidelines (Nakagawa et al., 2011) emphasize that the diagnosis should be made clinically and based on repeated examinations over longer periods of observation rather than relying exclusively on ancillary studies.

Determination of Brain Death in the Comatose Pediatric Patient

An algorithmic approach to the evaluation of a comatose child to determine whether the child is brain-dead is presented in Figure 107-3. The question of whether a comatose child is brain-dead arises within the first days of hospitalization. Occasionally, this issue occurs later because the long-term use of sedative and paralytic agents does not permit the necessary screening to assess for the presence of coma and loss of brainstem function. Assessment may also be delayed in patients receiving therapeutic hypothermia. Assessment must include determination of the proximate cause of coma, with review of all neuroimaging, neurophysiologic, metabolic, and toxicology screening studies that were performed. Serum and urine studies should include toxicology screens and serum electrolytes, glucose, calcium, urea nitrogen, creatinine, liver enzymes, lactate, pyruvate, and ammonia determinations. If the history suggests a metabolic disorder, serum amino acid and urine organic acid studies should be considered. Neuromuscular blocking agents and all sedative agents also should be discontinued for several elimination half-lives to exclude medication effect as a confounding variable. Clearance of neuromuscular blocking agents can be established at the bedside with the use of a nerve stimulator.

It is necessary to ensure that the core body temperature and blood pressure are within the normal range. The presence of purposeful movements in response to external stimuli or spontaneous (not spinal-related) movements, posturing, or occurrence of seizures would obviate the diagnosis of brain death. A careful examination and documentation of the absence of brainstem reflexes is crucial and may be difficult to perform. Generally, parents should be allowed to observe the process, and nursing and respiratory therapy staff should be informed of the findings if they are not present at the bedside during the clinical examination.

The duration of observation between examinations to confirm the diagnosis of brain death depends on the child's

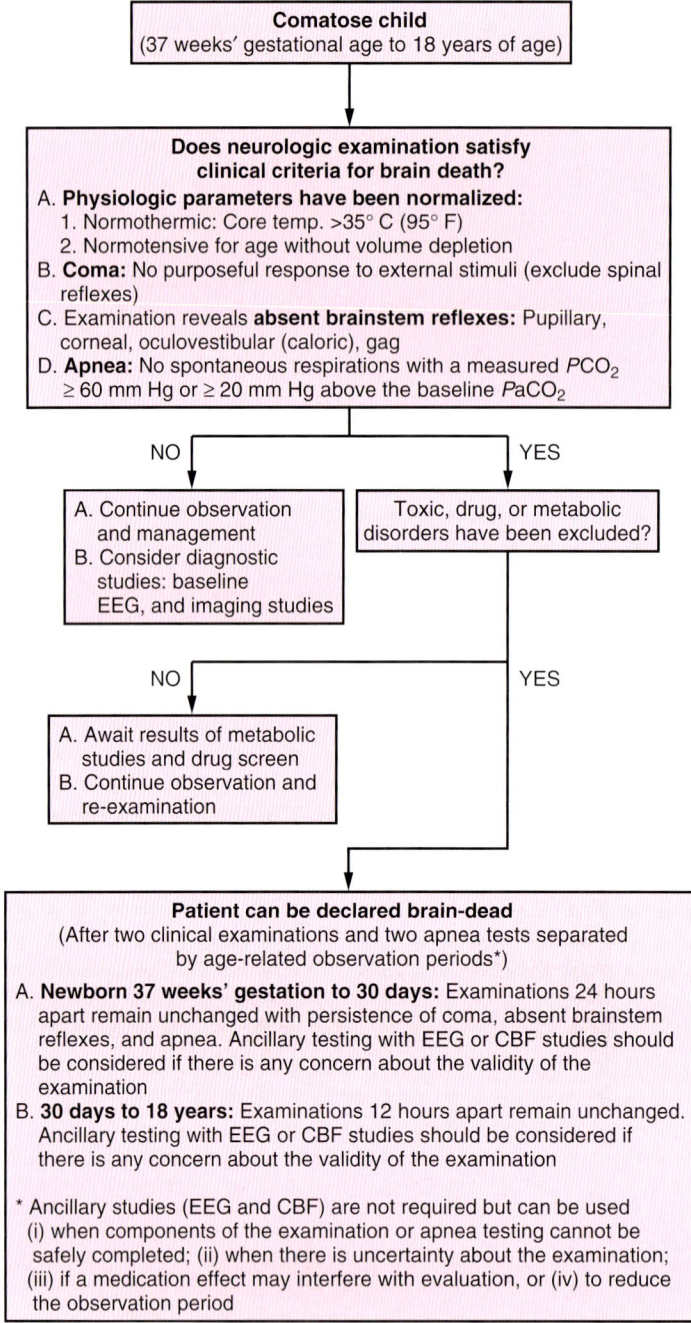

Figure 107-3. Algorithm for the evaluation for brain death in a comatose child. It is assumed that patients have had an extensive clinical and laboratory evaluation to determine the etiology of coma, including toxicology testing and, if indicated, evaluation for structural, infectious, and metabolic diseases. This algorithm suggests the process for confirmation of brain death in patients in whom this condition is suspected. CBF, cerebral blood flow; EEG, electroencephalogram. *(This algorithm is based on Nakagawa TA, Ashwal S, Mathur M, et al. Crit Care Med. 2011 Sep;39[9]:2139–55.)*

age, as do recommendations for ancillary testing (Boxes 107-2 and 107-3). Ancillary studies, depending on the child's age, are recommended as outlined in Box 107-2. Results of these tests provide physicians with an opportunity to discuss with the child's family the concept of brain death and the loss of electrocortical activity and CBF. The time of the second brain death examination (including apnea test and ancillary study if needed) is the legal time of death.

Discussions with Family Members and Staff

Most pediatric brain-death determinations are done on children who were healthy just hours or days before the injury, and even after extensive discussions with family members, the concept of brain death remains unclear for many. Grieving parents may not understand the futility of continued ventilator support. Without being confrontational, physicians caring for the child should discuss the prognosis with parents. A conference with family members involving various members of the healthcare team is helpful in educating the family members and assuring them that the healthcare professionals are in agreement with the diagnosis and recommendations.

Organ Donation

The National Organ Transplant Act of 1987 requires that every hospital in the United States develop a protocol for requesting organ donation. Most hospitals have formulated protocols stipulating that trained personnel from the regional Organ Procurement Organization (OPO) are the designated requestors. "Uncoupling" the request for donation from the pronouncement of death, early referral to the OPO, and a trained requestor making the request improve overall consent rates. Refusal from parents with whom donation has been explored should be respected. If the family declines organ donation, ventilator support can be discontinued.

Strategies for stabilization of consented donors and retrieval of organs should be in place in the pediatric intensive care unit. Brain-dead child abuse victims represent a significant percentage of brain-death diagnoses and, as such, require medicolegal evaluation before organ donation can proceed. Maintenance of brain-dead patients requires careful management in anticipation of organ donation (Lutz-Dettinger et al., 2001). Maintenance of temperature and provision of adequate fluids and supplemental oxygen to achieve satisfactory perfusion are necessary, as is consideration for hormone replacement with corticosteroids, vasopressin, and thyroxine. Diabetes insipidus, hypernatremia, hyperglycemia, and coagulopathies commonly occur in brain-dead children and require special management if transplantation is being considered (Lutz-Dettinger et al., 2001). Anticipatory and protocol-driven donor management improve donor stability and increase organ yield (Rosendale et al., 2003). Optimal donor management has the potential to help thousands of potential recipients waitlisted for solid organ transplantation.

REFERENCES

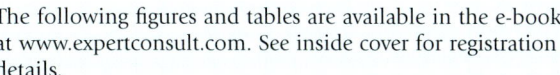 The complete list of references for this chapter is available in the e-book at www.expertconsult.com.
See inside cover for registration details.

SELECTED REFERENCES

American Academy of Pediatrics Task Force on Brain Death in Children, 1987. Report of special task force. Guidelines for the determination of brain death in children. Pediatrics 80 (2), 298–300.
American Electroencephalographic Society, 1994. Guideline three: minimum technical standards for EEG recording in suspected cerebral death. J. Clin. Neurophysiol. 11 (1), 10–13.
Ashwal, S., 1997. Brain death in the newborn. Current perspectives. Clin. Perinatol. 24, 859–862.
Ashwal, S., Schneider, S., 1987. Brain death in children: part I. Pediatr. Neurol. 3 (1), 5–11. Part II, Pediatr Neurol 1987;3(2):69–77.
Lutz-Dettinger, N., de Jaeger, A., Kerremans, I., 2001. Care of the potential pediatric organ donor. Pediatr. Clin. North Am. 48 (3), 715–749.
Nakagawa, T.A., Ashwal, S., Mathur, M., et al., 2011. Guidelines for the determination of brain death in infants and children: an update of the 1987 Task Force recommendations. Crit. Care Med. 39 (9), 2139–2155.
Rosendale, J.D., Kauffman, H.M., McBride, M.A., et al., 2003. Aggressive pharmacologic donor management results in more transplanted organs. Transplantation 75 (4), 482–487.
Wijdicks, E.F., Varelas, P.N., Gronseth, G.S., et al., 2010. Evidence-based guideline update: determining brain death in adults: report of the Quality Standards Subcommittee of the American Academy of Neurology. Neurology 74 (23), 1911–1918.

E-BOOK FIGURES AND TABLES

The following figures and tables are available in the e-book at www.expertconsult.com. See inside cover for registration details.

Fig. 107-1 Number of children declared brain-dead by age in the United States.
Fig. 107-2 Technetium cerebral blood flow study.
Box 107-1 American Academy of Neurology 2010 Recommendations for the Diagnosis of Brain Death in Adults
Box 107-4 Cold Water Caloric Tympanic Membrane Stimulation
Box 107-5 Procedure for Carrying Out Apnea Challenge Testing
Table 107-1 Age Distribution and Etiologies of Brain Death in Children
Table 107-2 Reflex Development in Preterm Infants
Table 107-3 Apnea Testing in Pediatric Brain Death
Table 107-4 Medications Administered to Critically Ill Pediatric Patients and Recommendations for Time Interval to Testing after Discontinuation
Table 107-5 Electroencephalogram in Pediatric Brain Death: Diagnostic Yield from First versus Any Study
Table 107-6 Principal Methods of Assessing Cerebral Blood Flow in Brain-Dead Patients
Table 107-7 Cerebral Blood Flow in Pediatric Brain Death: Diagnostic Yield from First versus Any Study
Appendix A: Fig. A-1 Checklist for documentation of brain death examination in infants and children.

108 Development and Function of the Cerebrovascular System

William J. Pearce

An expanded version of this chapter is available on www.expertconsult.com. See inside cover for registration details.

INTRODUCTION

Since the beginning of the 20th century, the fetal cerebral circulation has attracted the research interests of a broad variety of investigators using methods of ever increasing sophistication. The earliest studies focused on fetal cerebrovascular anatomy, and by the 1960s the first studies of fetal cerebral blood flow and oxygen consumption were reported. Since those early beginnings, the development of high resolution analytical tools for the detailed study of cellular and molecular biology have expanded dramatically our ability to probe the dynamic relations between structure and function in the developing fetal and neonatal cerebral circulation. This chapter summarizes some of the recent advances in this field, which are presented in three main sections: 1) brain vascular formation and differentiation; 2) fetal and neonatal cerebral artery contractility; and 3) fetal and neonatal whole brain cerebrovascular reactivity.

BRAIN VASCULAR FORMATION AND DIFFERENTIATION

The processes that govern cerebral vessel development are highly dynamic and plastic. Even in the adult brain, cerebral arteries continuously undergo angiogenesis, differentiation, and even dedifferentiation in response to stress or injury. These adult processes, however, depend directly on modulation of existing vasculature that is formed during embryonic vasculogenesis.

Vasculogenesis and Angiogenesis

Brain vasculature begins as a leptomeningeal plexus at 24 days that develops into distinct arteries, veins, and capillaries by 28 days. This plexus undergoes waves of differentiation that begin at the base of the brain and spread toward the midbrain convexity. By day 44, the internal carotid artery has formed from a merger of sections from the first and third aortic arch and the dorsal aorta. At this time, the Circle of Willis is also recognizable. Thereafter, an extensive leptomeningeal vascular bed arborizes to supply vasculature to the developing cortex. This vascularization process is not complete at birth and continues through the third postnatal month at which time the number of leptomeningeal anastomoses declines. In tandem is a progressive expansion of capillary density that is near complete at term in telencephalic white matter but can continue to expand in cerebral gray matter well beyond the third or fourth year of life. This time course demonstrates the highly dynamic nature of fetal cerebral vasculogenesis and emphasizes the fragility and vulnerability of the fetal and neonatal vasculature to metabolic and mechanical injury.

Whereas vasculogenesis is driven by the proliferation and migration of mesodermal angioblasts that differentiate into endothelial cells to form the initial vascular structures, these vessels subsequently give rise to new branches through angiogenesis (Lee, et al., 2009), which exquisitely matches vessel density to local metabolic activity. When increased metabolic activity or decreased oxygen delivery produce local tissue hypoxia, multiple parenchymal cell types produce the transcription factor hypoxia inducible factor-1α, which translocates to the nucleus where it combines with its coactivator HIF-1β. The resulting complex promotes transcription of multiple genes that promote angiogenesis, including vascular endothelial growth factor and erythropoietin (Semenza, 2000). The influences of these factors integrate with those of other angiogenic factors, including angiopoietin, transforming growth factor-β and Wnts to determine the extent of new vessel growth. In turn, the direction and pattern of new vessel growth is governed by a variety of dual-purpose axon guidance cues, including ephrins and semaphorins, along with locally produced neurotrophins such as nerve growth factor, brain-derived neurotrophic factor, and NT-3 (Lee, et al., 2009). The diversity of mechanisms regulating angiogenesis might suggest a delicate system with many vulnerable components, but in actuality it is a highly robust system with multiple redundancies that assure a tight matching of vascular density to local metabolic demand. This highly dynamic system is essential to support the rapid growth and expansion of the fetal and neonatal brain.

Smooth Muscle Differentiation

Recent advances in genomic biology have elucidated numerous molecular factors that govern smooth muscle proliferation and differentiation (Owens, et al., 2004). Smooth muscle was first categorized as either synthetic or contractile based largely on morphologic characteristics. Increased availability of immunologic tools capable of detecting subtle changes in contractile protein abundance and distribution, together with major improvements in high resolution confocal microscopy, has established that smooth muscle exists not in just two phenotypes but in a continuum of different cell types that include broad variations in the capacity for migration, proliferation, secretion, and contraction (Owens, et al., 2004) (Fig. 108-1). In turn, the transformation of one smooth muscle phenotype into another is governed by a large family of growth factors, including fibroblast growth factors, platelet-derived

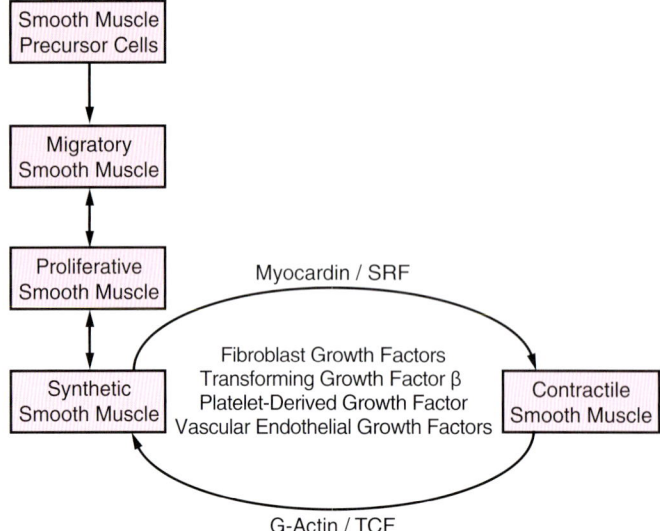

Figure 108-1. Smooth Muscle Differentiation. Smooth muscle cells arise from mesodermal precursor cells, of which several cell types have been proposed, including fibroblasts, myofibroblasts, pericytes, and bone marrow-derived cells. These precursor cells progressively acquire smooth muscle characteristics, the first of which is expression of smooth muscle alpha actin. With further differentiation in response to growth factors, chemical factors, and mechanical influences, the smooth muscle cells sequentially exhibit the capacity for migration, proliferation, and synthesis followed by secretion of extracellular matrix proteins. The synthetic phenotype also sequentially expresses virtually all the contractile proteins, pumps, ion channels, and receptors required for contractile function. The pace and pattern of this synthetic activity is regulated by the integrated influence of multiple growth factors, as well as mechanical, chemical, and metabolic factors unique to each vascular bed. At the molecular level, stimuli that increase the cytosolic availability of the transcription factor myocardin, along with its coactivator serum response factor (SRF), promote contractile differentiation. Conversely, factors such as injury or stress that increase cytoskeletal depolymerization and increased cytosolic concentrations of monomeric G-actin, and/or increased availability of ternary complex factor (TCF), promote dedifferentiation of contractile smooth muscle back into a synthetic phenotype. Importantly, the interconversion between synthetic and contractile smooth muscle is highly plastic and dynamic, particularly in immature neonatal arteries.

growth factor, vascular endothelial growth factors, and many others. The receptors for these growth factors include both receptor tyrosine kinases and G-protein coupled receptors that regulate multiple signaling pathways within the vascular smooth muscle cytoplasm. The majority of these cytosolic pathways influence the phosphorylation and/or nuclear translocation of key transcription factors including serum response factor, ternary complex factor, elk-1, and myocardin (Parmacek, 2007). Together, these mechanisms determine the exact characteristics of every smooth muscle cell in cerebral arteries and thereby determine smooth muscle structure and function.

Smooth muscle cells in the immature artery wall are phenotypically very heterogeneous. Numerous smooth muscle cells in fetal cranial arteries express nonmuscle myosin heavy chain, which is a marker for synthetic smooth muscle. With advancing postnatal age, the nonmuscle myosin heavy chain isoform gradually disappears to be replaced by smooth muscle myosin heavy chain, a marker of complete contractile differentiation. Because of incomplete contractile differentiation, fetal cerebral arteries exhibit higher secretory activity and reduced contractility, compared with fully mature adult cerebral arteries.

An important feature of smooth muscle phenotype in neonatal cerebral arteries is that, just as Yamanaka's Nobel-winning work demonstrated with fibroblasts (Takahashi and Yamanaka, 2006), the phenotypic characteristics of smooth muscle cells are reversible. In the event of injury, contractile smooth muscle can dedifferentiate into synthetic, proliferative, or even migratory phenotypes. This reversibility demonstrates that smooth muscle is never "terminally differentiated" and instead remains somewhat plastic in regards to smooth muscle phenotype. Correspondingly, phenotypic transitions,

whether induced physiologically by growth factors or pathophysiologically by injury, ultimately determine the contractile characteristics of cerebral arteries not only in the fetus and neonate, but also in the adult.

Endothelial Differentiation and the Blood-brain Barrier

The vascular endothelium serves four main functions, including: 1) initiation of angiogenesis; 2) hemostasis; 3) barrier function; and 4) release of vasoactive factors (Fig. 108-2). Each of these functions matures at slightly different rates. The ability of the vascular endothelium to initiate angiogenesis is one of the first endothelial functions to develop fully in the fetus. The fetal vascular endothelium is highly active and can release multiple proangiogenic factors, including platelet-derived growth factor, basic fibroblast growth factor, insulin-like growth factor 1, and thrombospondin. The fetal vascular endothelium also can release growth-inhibiting factors including heparin, heparan sulfate, transforming growth factor β, nitric oxide, and prostacyclin. The ability of the fetal vascular endothelium to support high rates of angiogenesis is essential for the rapid expansion of the cerebral vasculature characteristic of the neonatal period.

The hemostatic functions of the vascular endothelium also appear well-developed at term. Fetal endothelial cells contain tissue factor (also known as thromboplastin), platelet activating factor, factor V, factor X, and von Willebrand Factor (Andrew, et al., 1990). These factors can be released upon endothelial injury to promote hemostasis. Conversely, intact fetal endothelium continuously releases nitric oxide and prostacyclin, which inhibit initiation of hemostasis (Andrew,

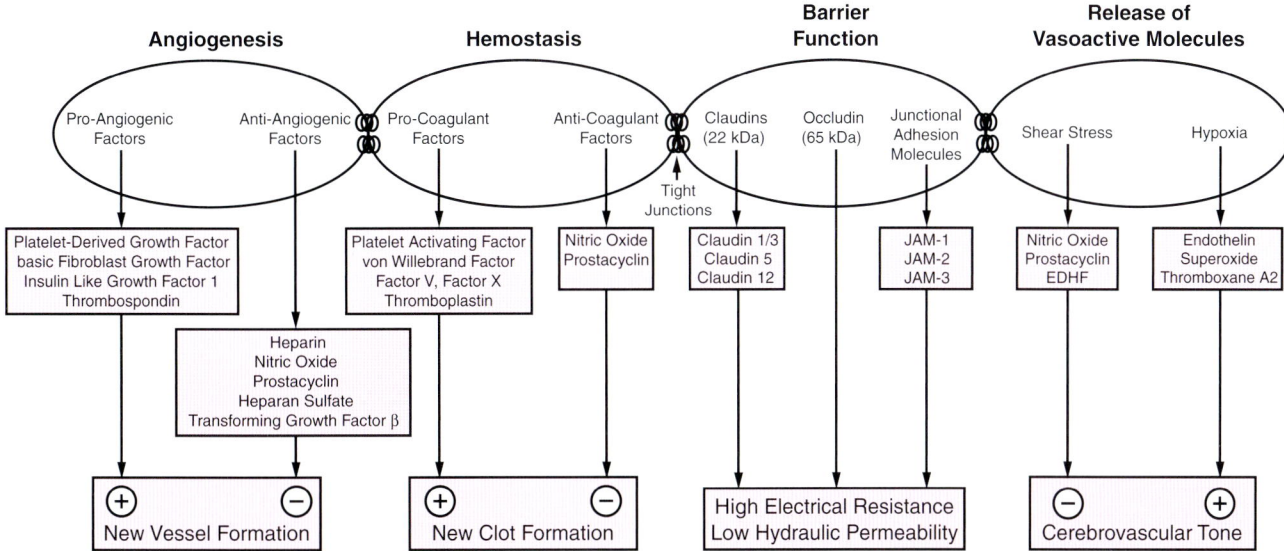

Figure 108-2. Endothelial Functions. Summarized in this diagram are the four main functions of the vascular endothelium. In response to either locally released or circulating growth factors, the endothelium can release a variety of proangiogenic factors that stimulate new vessel formation (angiogenesis). Some stimuli also promote the release of antiangiogenic factors that help control the rate of angiogenesis. Intact endothelial cells also continuously release anticoagulant factors, but injured endothelial cells release multiple procoagulant factors that rapidly facilitate local clot formation. In the cerebrovasculature, endothelial cells are connected by tight junctions, including claudins, occludin, and junctional adhesion molecules; together these proteins confer high electrical resistance and low hydraulic permeability. Endothelial cells also contain other proteins important for barrier formation including zona occludens, cingulin, and cadherens. Finally, in response to shear stress caused by blood flow, endothelial cells continuously release multiple vasoactive factors that promote vasodilation. Under some conditions, including hypoxia, endothelial cells can also release factors that stimulate vasoconstriction and reduced local blood flow. All four functions of the vascular endothelium change with developmental age; see text for details.

et al., 1990). Although the relative abundances of many endothelial components of the hemostatic cascade change during fetal and postnatal maturation, it is clear that the fetal vascular endothelium is functionally mature in relation to its role in hemostasis.

Endothelial barrier function is uniquely important in the cerebral circulation, in which the endothelium constitutes a "blood-brain barrier" that efficiently restricts the movement of most blood-borne constituents into the brain parenchyma. This barrier function is the consequence of tight junctions between adjacent endothelial cells and is due in large part to the presence of the integral membrane protein occludin, which spans the intracellular gap between adjacent endothelial cells and effectively binds the cells together. Another family of intercellular proteins present in the blood-brain barrier is the claudins, which further bind adjacent endothelial cells together and help increase hydraulic and electrical resistance across the endothelial cell layer. Other cell adhesion proteins also appear to be present in the tight junctions that are characteristic of the blood-brain barrier (Lee, et al., 2009).

At birth, the blood-brain barrier is not fully developed and continues to tighten with advancing postnatal age. This delayed tightening of the blood-brain barrier is a consequence of the high rates of new vessel formation in the fetal brain and the time required to synthesize, secrete, and position the main barrier proteins. In addition, astrocytes also play a major role in the development of the blood-brain barrier by virtue of their direct contact with capillary endothelial cells. Astrocyte maturation, however, is not complete at birth and continues throughout early postnatal life, which may contribute to the slow development of complete blood-brain barrier function in the neonate. Pericyte proliferation and maturation are also closely coupled with the development of the blood-brain barrier and may further influence the timing of blood-brain barrier tightening (Lee, et al., 2009). Overall, this pattern of development reinforces the view that the blood-brain barrier is functional but vulnerable throughout the neonatal period.

The fourth function of the cerebrovascular endothelium is the release of factors that influence local vascular tone, such as nitric oxide, which can diffuse into adjacent vascular smooth muscle in which it activates synthesis of the vasodilator compound cyclic GMP (Moncada, et al., 1991). The immature endothelium is less responsive to shear stress and produces less NO than the mature endothelium. In contrast, the mechanisms mediating endothelial release of the vasodilator prostacyclin appear fully functional in the immature cerebral endothelium of human infants. Another important vasodilator released from the endothelium is endothelium-derived hyperpolarizing factor, but the importance of this molecule has yet to be examined in the immature cerebral circulation. Conversely, the cerebral endothelium also can release several constricting factors including superoxide, thromboxane A2, and endothelin, but endothelial synthesis and release of these compounds has yet to be demonstrated in fetal or neonatal cerebrovascular endothelium. Consistent with the developmental delay in NO synthesis and release and the gradual development of blood-brain barrier tightening, it is reasonable to expect that endothelial release of most vasoactive molecules also is attenuated relative to adult cerebrovascular endothelium. This hypothesis awaits further investigation.

FETAL AND NEONATAL CEREBROVASCULAR CONTRACTILITY

Compared with adult cerebral arteries, fetal cerebral arteries have greater water content, smaller smooth muscle cells, a larger extracellular space, and reduced stiffness (Pearce, et al., 1991). During early postnatal maturation, hydration decreases, wall thickness increases, and stiffness increases due to the secretion and increasing organization of extracellular matrix proteins. As maturation proceeds, remodeling of the extracellular matrix continues with the production of relatively more type III and less type I collagen and increases in the collagen to elastin ratio that are greatest in the largest cerebral arteries.

Accompanying postnatal changes in cerebral artery composition and stiffness are major changes in contractility and vascular reactivity. These shifts are due to progressive changes in smooth muscle phenotype that, in turn, are driven by major changes in circulating levels of growth factors and hormones during the early postnatal period. In the fetus and neonate, for example, plasma levels of adenosine, arginine vasopressin, T3, and T4 are all higher than in adults. Increased circulating levels of neonatal glucocorticoids also can induce major changes in vascular differentiation and maturation. Together, these influences drive a continuous transformation of fetal vascular and cerebrovascular contractility during the early postnatal period.

Calcium Handling and the Contractile Apparatus

A main determinant of contractility in all vessel types is the cytosolic calcium concentration (Horowitz, et al., 1996). In fetal cerebral arteries, the internal stores of releasable calcium are small, and contraction is more dependent on calcium influx compared with adult arteries. Correspondingly, the density of the L-type calcium channel is greater in fetal than in adult cerebral arteries. The reduced ability to release intracellular calcium is due in part to the presence of low-affinity inositol triphosphate (IP3) receptors, which are more abundant in immature than in mature arteries. In response to receptor activation, fetal arteries tend to synthesize and mobilize greater concentrations of IP3, but these increased IP3 responses do not fully offset the reduced affinity of fetal IP3 receptors. The net result is that receptor-induced increases in cytosolic calcium are generally much smaller in fetal than adult arteries.

For any vascular contraction, the magnitude of the force produced is the product of the cytosolic calcium concentration and the myofilament calcium sensitivity (Horowitz, et al., 1996). In fetal and neonatal cerebral arteries, their reduced ability to increase cytosolic calcium is offset by increased myofilament sensitivity. This is another major theme of cerebrovascular development: with advancing postnatal age, cerebral artery contractions depend less on calcium influx, less on myofilament sensitization, and more on intracellular calcium release. Increases in myofilament calcium sensitivity are mediated by receptor-mediated activation of rho-kinase, and these g-protein dependent effects are more pronounced in fetal than adult cerebral arteries.

Ion Pumps and Channels

In tandem with calcium influx and intracellular release, the calcium pumps that extrude or sequester calcium, and the numerous proteins that bind and buffer calcium (Horowitz, et al., 1996) are also major determinants of cytosolic calcium concentrations but remain largely unstudied in the immature cerebrovasculature. In contrast, ion channels have received greater attention, due in large part to the critical influence of the membrane potential on calcium entry through the potential dependent L-type calcium channels. Smooth muscle cells tend to be less polarized in fetal than in adult cerebral arteries,

and this is coincident with greater outward current through calcium-dependent potassium channels (BK channels) in fetal compared with adult cerebral arteries. Despite the greater BK channel activity, calcium spark activity is depressed in immature compared with mature cerebral arteries. As a result, truncation of contraction and initiation of relaxation are more poorly developed in immature arteries. Similarly, ATP-sensitive potassium channels, which couple metabolic activity to membrane hyperpolarization, are also less sensitive in immature compared with mature cerebral arteries, and voltage-dependent potassium channels are more functional in adult than fetal arteries. Overall, these results demonstrate that electrophysiological contractile regulation is not fully functional in immature compared with adult cerebral arteries. This feature of immature cerebral arteries, again, is due to the high proportion of synthetic, noncontractile smooth muscle cells, which regulate membrane potential and calcium movements differently than smooth muscle in the contractile phenotype.

Vasoactive Ligands and Receptors

The outer plasma membrane of all smooth muscle cells is populated with numerous receptor subtypes, and fetal smooth muscle is no exception to this general rule. In turn, the smooth muscle response to any receptor ligand is primarily determined by three factors: 1) ligand concentration; 2) receptor density; and 3) coupling of the receptor to intracellular signal transduction pathways. All three factors undergo major developmental changes, but in a highly receptor-dependent manner. For contractile amines, sensitivity to norepinephrine and serotonin are upregulated in immature compared with mature cerebral arteries, and this effect is largely attributable to increased receptor density. Coupling of adrenergic and serotonergic receptors to the contractile apparatus appears fully developed at birth and changes little during postnatal maturation. In contrast, cerebral artery reactivity to the contractile peptide endothelin-1 increases postnatally, due to increases in ET-B receptor vascular expression. For the potent vasodilator adenosine, cerebral production is lower in the immature compared with the adult brain and increases with postnatal age. Conversely, cerebrovascular reactivity to adenosine appears fully developed at birth, which allows the neonatal cerebrovasculature to dilate in response to any perturbation, such as hypoxia or hypoglycemia, which increases the local adenosine concentration. These patterns of reactivity emphasize that the neonatal cerebral circulation is fully capable of responding to changes in circulating and locally produced vasoactive agents that mediate cerebrovascular homeostasis. More importantly, the cerebrovascular capacity to respond to these vasoactive agents develops in advance of the ability of cerebral tissues to produce these agents. The overall capacity to produce vasoactive molecules such as adenosine, endothelin, and amines increases steadily throughout postnatal maturation.

Prostaglandins are another category of receptor-dependent vasoactive compounds that are particularly important in the immature circulation. Prostaglandins, which are derived from the precursor arachidonic acid by the action of cyclooxygenases, maintain the patency of the ductus arteriosus before birth and, throughout the perinatal period, regulate hydraulic resistance in multiple vascular beds. Total prostaglandin concentrations are higher in cerebrospinal fluid taken from the cortex than from the cisterna magna or from the arterial blood, suggesting that the cerebral cortex is an active site of neonatal prostaglandin synthesis. Given that indomethacin, an inhibitor of prostaglandin synthesis, increases cerebrovascular resistance and decreases cerebral perfusion, prostaglandins appear to exert an overall vasodilating effect in the immature cerebral circulation.

One of the most important prostaglandins for neonates is PGE2. Both plasma concentrations and the cerebrovascular vasodilator potency of PGE2 are greater in fetuses and neonates than in adults, suggesting that PGE2 contributes to the low cerebrovascular resistance characteristic of the immature cerebral circulation. PGE1 is also an effective dilator that is somewhat selective for the cerebral circulation, and similar to PGE2, its potency is greatest in the neonate and diminishes over time. Prostacyclin (PGI2) is another important vasodilator in the immature cerebral circulation, but this prostanoid retains its vasodilator potency throughout postnatal maturation and is an effective vasodilator is most vascular beds regardless of postnatal age. At very low concentrations, the prostaglandin PGF2α can dilate neonatal cerebral arteries, but at higher concentrations PGF2α is a strong vasoconstrictor in immature and mature cerebral arteries. Many other derivatives of arachidonic acid, including multiple members of the leukotriene and thromboxane families, are potent vasoconstrictors in the immature cerebral circulation.

In a more general sense, the importance of prostaglandins and other eicosanoids in the newborn is a natural consequence of heightened lipid metabolism characteristic of the developing brain. The free fatty acid metabolism necessary to support myelination is very active during the peripartum period, and some of the same phospholipids needed for myelination also can give rise to arachidonic acid through the action of phospholipases. The arachidonic acid thus liberated can fuel the synthesis and release of numerous prostanoids and eicosanoids, as determined by local enzyme activity. This high level of arachidonic acid availability and metabolism explains why prostanoids and eicosanoids act as both primary signal molecules and secondary paracrine signals in so many vascular and metabolic responses of the immature cerebral circulation.

FETAL AND NEONATAL WHOLE BRAIN CEREBROVASCULAR REACTIVITY

When considering whole brain patterns of cerebrovascular reactivity, it is critically important to bear in mind another main theme of the immature brain: heterogeneity. Different regions of the brain vasculature, such as pial arteries, brainstem arteries, parenchymal arteries, and arteries of the Circle of Willis, all have distinct characteristics in terms of smooth muscle phenotype, innervation, receptor expression patterns, and others. In addition, all cerebral arteries exhibit developmental heterogeneity such that their structure and reactivity change with age and at very different rates. Finally, there is chronologic heterogeneity, which is the change in vasoreactivity over relatively short time periods due to an artery's local contractile and metabolic history. This diversity in regional, developmental, and chronologic heterogeneity can complicate recognition of global patterns of cerebrovascular regulation but is also the fundamental feature that enables the immature brain to dynamically maintain cerebrovascular homeostasis under constantly changing conditions. Among these changing conditions, one of the most universally important is local cerebral metabolic rate.

Flow-Metabolism Coupling

In all vascular beds, close coupling between blood flow and tissue metabolic rate is a fundamental requirement for cardiovascular homeostasis. Because of the unique reliance of cerebral metabolism on glucose, flow-metabolism coupling in the brain normally manifests as a three-way coupling between rates of glucose oxidation, oxygen consumption, and cerebral blood flow. In human neonates, cerebral blood flow and total cerebral metabolic rate are low at birth, and both variables increase steadily through the first 6 years of life, after which cerebral flow and metabolism gradually decline throughout the remainder of life. Throughout fetal and postnatal development, oxygen consumption and cerebral blood flow appear tightly coupled not just in human neonates (Pryds, et al., 1990) but in other mammalian newborns as well.

The molecular mediators of flow-metabolism coupling have been intensively investigated for many years, and this work reveals that one of the most important mediators is adenosine, which is released from cells when the oxygen supply to demand ratio falls. The metabolic pathways for the synthesis, release, and degradation of adenosine are well developed in the fetus and neonate, and free adenosine under resting conditions increases with postnatal age. In parallel, the A2a receptors that bind adenosine and promote cerebral vasodilation are expressed early in brain development and persist throughout adult life. Given these characteristics, adenosine may exert feedback regulation that matches oxygen delivery to oxygen demand in the immature brain. This regulation is particularly important in the neonate due to the transition from fetal hemoglobin to adult hemoglobin, which gradually increases the amount of tissue extractable oxygen per unit of blood flow as maturation proceeds.

Hypercapnic Vasodilation

Carbon dioxide is one of the oldest known cerebral vasodilators and can increase cerebral perfusion in preterm and newborn (Pryds, et al., 1990) human infants. The magnitude of hypercapnic vasodilation increases with postnatal age, an effect that may be a consequence of reduced reactivity to acidosis in immature cerebral arteries. Age-related changes in hematocrit also might play a role, given that in newborn baboons, the hematocrit is inversely proportional to cerebral CO_2 reactivity. In some species, neonatal vasodilator prostaglandins mediate up to half of cerebrovascular responses to hypercapnia, although the importance of these pathways for human neonatal responses to CO_2 remains unclear. On the other hand, neonatal hypercapnic cerebral vasodilation does not involve reflex changes in sympathetic vascular tone or effects on cerebral metabolic rate.

Hypoxic Vasodilation

Because of the inaccessibility of the human fetal cerebral circulation to investigation, understanding of cerebrovascular responses to acute hypoxia has arisen mainly from studies in animal models. In neonates of virtually all mammalian species, acute hypoxia elicits potent cerebral vasodilation. Limited studies in premature human infants have yielded similar results. In general, the brain regions with the highest metabolic rates, such as the brainstem, demonstrate the most robust responses to acute hypoxia. Mild hypoxia produces a graded increase in cerebral perfusion that maintains the oxygen supply to demand ratio with little initial change in the oxygen extraction fraction. Worsening severities of hypoxia can gradually increase the oxygen extraction fraction and once extraction is maximal, cerebral oxygen consumption decreases with attendant increases in anaerobic glycolysis and lactic acidosis. In many respects, the cerebrovasodilation produced by hypoxia is an extended response mediated by the same mechanisms responsible for flow-metabolism coupling. Adenosine release plays a major role in neonatal hypoxic cerebral vasodilation in most species. Acute hypoxia also can promote the release of vasodilator prostaglandins. Finally, hypoxia can exert direct vasodilating effects on the vascular smooth muscle and endothelium of immature cerebral arteries through mechanisms that are developmentally regulated. This rich mechanistic redundancy assures that neonatal cerebral blood flow and metabolism are well coupled under all but the most severe conditions.

Autoregulation

Another important component of cerebrovascular regulation is blood flow autoregulation (Fig. 108-3), which is defined as the maintenance of near constant blood flow independent of changes in cerebral perfusion pressure. In the cerebral circulation, perfusion pressure is defined as the difference between arterial pressure and either cerebral venous pressure or intracranial pressure, whichever is greater. This is a particularly important consideration for cases of intracranial hypertension, which can dramatically reduce overall cerebral perfusion. In most mammalian species, including humans (Pryds, et al., 1990), cerebral autoregulation is fully functional at birth. Cerebral autoregulation in the immature brain is effective until perfusion pressure falls lower than approximately 30 to 40 mm Hg, which is the lower limit of cerebral autoregulation in most mammalian neonates, including human infants. The upper limit of cerebral autoregulation typically ranges from 70 to 100 mm Hg, but this relatively low upper limit renders the immature brain vulnerable to vessel leakage and rupture secondary to hypertensive transients that exceed this upper limit. As average arterial pressures rise progressively during postnatal maturation, so too do the upper and lower limits of cerebral autoregulation. In the adult brain, the lower and upper limits of cerebral autoregulation usually range from 50 to 60 mm Hg and from 140 to 150 mm Hg, respectively.

The cellular mechanisms responsible for cerebral autoregulation have been actively investigated since autoregulation was first discovered in the 1930s. The model of autoregulation that has emerged from this work portrays autoregulation as a composite response that integrates myogenic, metabolic, and neurogenic mechanisms. The myogenic component is perhaps the most fundamental because it operates at the level of individual arteries and can be demonstrated in vitro. At the level of individual smooth muscle cells, stretch mobilizes intracellular calcium, and many mechanisms have been proposed to explain this response including activation of integrins and TRP calcium channels. Acting in concert with myogenic mechanisms are metabolic mechanisms that establish the level of blood flow that is protected. Thus autoregulation can be observed at many different levels of metabolic activity, each with its appropriate level of blood flow, once oxygen supply and demand become balanced. Consistent with this view, decreases in perfusion pressure in neonates increase adenosine, prostanoids, and opioids. In addition, sympathetic autonomic mechanisms extend the upper limit of autoregulation in neonates as in adults. The complex composite nature of cerebral autoregulation helps explain why this response is highly vulnerable to numerous neonatal insults including metabolic acidosis, severe hypoxia, asphyxia, cerebral ischemia, and intracranial hemorrhage.

Neurovascular Mechanisms

Adult cerebral arteries are innervated by adrenergic, cholinergic, and peptidergic perivascular nerves. Each of these nerve types exhibit three phases of development, including the outgrowth of new axons, the development of transmitter synthesis and storage, and the differentiation of nerve varicosities. In general, the postsynaptic receptors that communicate the effects of neurotransmitter release become functional before the perivascular nerves fully mature. Consistent with the fundamental concept of heterogeneity, the time course of functional development for each neurotransmitter system varies uniquely with brain region and chronologic age.

The adrenergic sympathetic innervation is the best-understood category of perivascular nerves that innervate neonatal cerebral arteries. Sympathetic nerves develop first in the most rostral regions of the human fetal brain and appear with varicosities between 19 and 23 weeks of gestational age. Exogenous norepinephrine elicits contractile responses in neonatal cerebral arteries through activation of $\alpha 1$ adrenergic receptors in resistance arteries and $\alpha 2$ adrenergic receptors in pial arterioles. The action of norepinephrine on postsynaptic adrenergic receptors can stimulate the release of PGE2, which in turn can limit the vasoconstrictor response to norepinephrine. Electrical stimulation of cerebrovascular sympathetic innervation can decrease cerebral blood flow up to 25%, depending on age and region. Interestingly, cerebrovascular contractile reactivity to norepinephrine is greatest in the fetus and diminishes with postnatal age, emphasizing that adrenergic neurovascular mechanisms are uniquely important in the immature cerebral circulation.

Cholinergic perivascular nerves appear at the adventitia-medial junction of fetal human cerebral arteries between 19 and 23 weeks of gestational age but become fully functional near term. Unlike adult cerebral arteries, neonatal cerebral arteries contract in response to high concentrations of acetylcholine and dilate only at very low acetylcholine concentrations. Contractile responses to acetylcholine in neonatal cerebral arteries can be blocked by indomethacin, suggesting

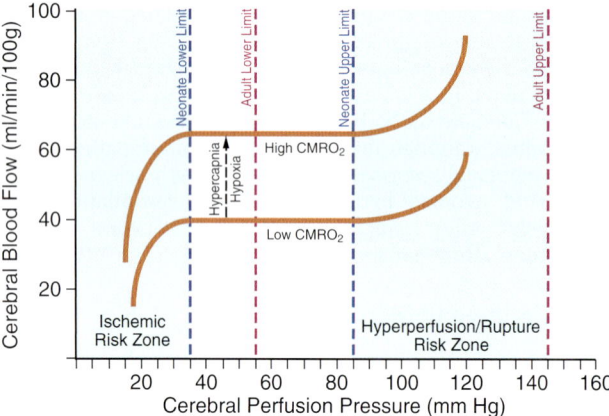

Figure 108-3. Cerebral Autoregulation As in adults, neonates exhibit cerebral autoregulation, although over a lower range of cerebral perfusion pressures. In neonates, the lower limit of cerebral autoregulation is a perfusion pressure of approximately 30 to 40 mm Hg, and lower than this threshold the neonatal brain is at risk for ischemic injury. The upper limit of cerebral autoregulation in neonates ranges from 70 to 100 mm Hg, and higher than this threshold the neonatal cerebrovasculature is at risk for hyperperfusion, possible small vessel rupture, and hemorrhage. The lower (50 to 60 mm Hg) and upper (140 to 150 mm Hg) limits for cerebral autoregulation are proportionately higher in adults than in neonates and correspond with resting levels of mean arterial pressure. Cerebral perfusion pressure is defined as mean arterial pressure less either cerebral venous pressure or intracranial pressure, whichever is greatest. At any given level of cerebral perfusion pressure, the level of cerebral blood flow that is "autoregulated" is determined by cerebral metabolic activity ($CMRO_2$); higher metabolic activity shifts the autoregulated level of cerebral flow to a higher level, as does either hypercapnia or hypoxia. Autoregulation is a complex, multifactorial behavior that integrates myogenic, metabolic, and neurogenic mechanisms.

that vasoconstricting prostaglandins such as PGF2α or thromboxane A2 mediate these responses.

Perivascular nerves containing neuropeptide-Y and vasoactive intestinal polypeptide also innervate human fetal cerebral arteries. These nerves are most prominent in the major arteries of the Circle of Willis and the large pial arteries. Fetal cerebral arteries can also be innervated by sensory fibers from the trigeminal ganglion that synthesize and release substance-P, vasoactive intestinal polypeptide, cholecystokinin, somatostatin, and calcitonin gene-related peptide. Although the vasodilating effects of these peptides have been well characterized in adult cerebral arteries, their uncertain roles in cerebrovascular regulation in the immature cerebral circulation remain a topic of active investigation.

CONCLUSIONS

The principles of cerebrovascular developmental physiology, anatomy and biochemistry outlined in this chapter represent many of the fundamental concepts needed to understand mechanisms involved in the cerebrovascular disorders described in later chapters. Hopefully, these fundamentals also will facilitate interpretation of results obtained with advanced, noninvasive, bedside methods for imaging and monitoring multiple cerebrovascular variables in neonates, infants, and children. The advent of new analytical tools, together with deep understanding of the physiological and pathophysiological processes involved, offers unprecedented promise to advance understanding of both the normal and injured immature brain and will ultimately help improve age-related strategies for the clinical management of neonatal and pediatric patients with cerebrovascular disorders.

REFERENCES

The complete list of references for this chapter is available in the e-book at www.expertconsult.com.
See inside cover for registration details.

SELECTED REFERENCES

Andrew, M., Paes, B., Johnston, M., 1990. Development of the hemostatic system in the neonate and young infant. Am. J. Pediatr. Hematol. Oncol 12 (1), 95–104. [Epub 1990/01/01].

Horowitz, A., Menice, C.B., Laporte, R., et al., 1996. Mechanisms of smooth muscle contraction. Physiol. Rev. 76 (4), 967–1003.

Lee, H.S., Han, J., Bai, H.J., et al., 2009. Brain angiogenesis in developmental and pathological processes: regulation, molecular and cellular communication at the neurovascular interface. FEBS J. 276 (17), 4622–4635. [Epub 2009/08/12].

Moncada, S., Palmer, R.M., Higgs, E.A., 1991. Nitric oxide: physiology, pathophysiology, and pharmacology. Pharmacol. Rev. 43 (2), 109–142. [Epub 1991/06/01].

Owens, G.K., Kumar, M.S., Wamhoff, B.R., 2004. Molecular regulation of vascular smooth muscle cell differentiation in development and disease. Physiol. Rev. 84 (3), 767–801.

Parmacek, M.S., 2007. Myocardin-related transcription factors: critical coactivators regulating cardiovascular development and adaptation. Circ. Res. 100 (5), 633–644.

Pearce, W.J., Hull, A.D., Long, D.M., et al., 1991. Developmental changes in ovine cerebral artery composition and reactivity. Am. J. Physiol. 261 (2 Pt 2), R458–R465.

Pryds, O., Andersen, G.E., Friis-Hansen, B., 1990. Cerebral blood flow reactivity in spontaneously breathing, preterm infants shortly after birth. Acta Paediatr. Scand. 79 (4), 391–396. [Epub 1990/04/01].

Semenza, G.L., 2000. Expression of hypoxia-inducible factor 1: mechanisms and consequences. Biochem. Pharmacol. 59 (1), 47–53.

Takahashi, K., Yamanaka, S., 2006. Induction of pluripotent stem cells from mouse embryonic and adult fibroblast cultures by defined factors. Cell 126 (4), 663–676. [Epub 2006/08/15].

109 Arterial Ischemic Stroke in Infants and Children

Mark Mackay, Adam Kirton, and Gabrielle deVeber

 An expanded version of this chapter is available on www.expertconsult.com. See inside cover for registration details.

OVERVIEW AND DEFINITIONS

Ischemic stroke is defined as sudden, focal infarction of brain tissue on neuroimaging or autopsy. Imaging findings typically correspond to an acute neurologic deficit but occasionally can be "silent" as seen in children with sickle cell disease. Arterial ischemic stroke (AIS) occurs when there is sudden occlusion of cerebral arteries, usually because of thromboembolism. In children, fundamental biological differences from adults create unique issues in the pathophysiology, risk factors, clinical presentations, diagnosis, treatment, and outcomes of AIS.

This chapter provides a clinically focused review of AIS in infants and children based on the best available evidence through February 2015. Chapter 20 reviews AIS in newborns.

Epidemiology, Mortality, and Burden of Pediatric Stroke

Multiple population-based studies report incidence rates of 1.3 to 1.8/100,000 children/year for childhood AIS (Mallick and O'Callaghan, 2010; Mallick et al., 2014). Increasing incidence rates reflect more sensitive diagnostic tests, particularly magnetic resonance imaging (MRI), and increased survival in previously lethal pediatric diseases predisposing to stroke such as congenital heart disease, sickle cell disease, and childhood malignancies. Incidence rates are increased in infants, and in black and Asian populations. Childhood stroke has a mortality of 5% to 10% and is among the top 10 causes of death in children but may be declining. Childhood stroke is associated with significant economic and social burden as survivors face many years of living with disability. Health care costs vary by age at onset, associated risk factors, and stroke subtype.

Pathophysiology

Arterial Circulation: Anatomy and Vascular Patterns of AIS

The brain receives arterial blood via the "anterior" circulation, consisting of the paired internal carotid arteries, and the "posterior" circulation, consisting of the paired vertebral arteries that join to form the basilar artery ("vertebrobasilar system"). The major cerebral arteries arise from the Circle of Willis as the paired anterior, middle, and posterior cerebral arteries. Small "perforating arteries" arise from these major cerebral arteries to supply the deep brain regions, including basal ganglia, thalamus, and midline brainstem structures, whereas the lateral brainstem and cerebellum receive blood via the larger circumferential arteries (posterior inferior, anterior inferior, and superior cerebellar arteries). Collateral flow via the Circle of Willis and distal smaller leptomeningeal anastomoses can enhance brain perfusion during vaso-occlusive stroke. Peripheral wedge-shaped lesions involving cortex and white matter are characteristic of infarction caused by occlusion of large-caliber arteries. Most AIS involves the middle cerebral artery (MCA) (see Figure 109-8), in recognizable vascular patterns based on the site of arterial occlusion, including 1) proximal M1 occlusion (entire MCA infarcted), 2) distal M1 (basal ganglia spared), 3) anterior or posterior trunk M2 occlusion (frontal or parietal/temporal respectively), and 4) lenticulostriate only (basal ganglia and deep white matter only) (see Figure 109-8). Specific topographic patterns help predict the underlying etiology with lenticulostriate AIS commonly associated with focal arteriopathy.

Topographic patterns within the posterior circulation include P1 (proximal PCA) infarction in occipital and mesial temporal lobes and perforator thalamic infarcts. Basilar artery thrombosis often combines multiple infarcts involving brainstem perforators, cerebellar branches, and the PCA. Diffuse hypoperfusion can cause apparently focal ischemic lesions within "watershed zones" at arterial borders.

Diffuse hypoperfusion can cause apparently focal ischemic lesions within "external" watershed zones at arterial borders. Although typically bilateral, they can also be asymmetric in the setting of proximal arterial steno-occlusive disease. In Moyamoya syndrome, low-flow infarcts may appear as a "string of pearls" within periventricular white matter "internal" watershed zones.

Mechanisms of Thromboembolism

Thrombotic occlusion of a cerebral artery is the principal mechanism underlying AIS. Thrombus may develop locally within arteries or travel there from an embolic source. Thrombosis is a product of both the coagulation (fibrin-forming) and the platelet hemostatic systems (Chapter 113). The balance of which system predominates varies with flow rate, shear stresses, endothelial integrity, concentrations of circulating anticoagulants, and other factors. In situations of blood stasis or slow blood flow, the coagulation system may predominate but the relative balance depends on the specific disease. Exposure of blood to arterial wall inflammation (e.g., vasculitis) or disruption of the endothelium with exposure to collagen and tissue factor (e.g., dissection) activates both platelets and fibrin formation. Maturational changes to coagulation and platelets across childhood are also likely important.

In AIS with large-artery occlusion, thrombi usually arrive as an embolus from the heart or another proximal artery. Venous thromboemboli can also reach the cerebral arteries via paradoxical right-to-left intracardiac shunting across a patent foramen ovale, atrial septal defect, or complex congenital heart lesions. Embolism of infectious material (in endocarditis), fat, air, and inert surgical matter can also cause AIS.

Mechanisms of Infarction

In AIS, severity of cerebral tissue damage is a function of multiple factors, including 1) duration and extent of ischemia and timing of reperfusion, 2) availability of collateral arterial blood supply, 3) volume and functional components of brain structures affected, 4) maturational status of the brain, and 5) concurrent disease processes and metabolic demands of the ischemic brain tissue.

Initial ischemic neuronal dysfunction evolves to irreversible infarction with increasing duration and/or degree of ischemia, or increased rates of neuronal metabolic activity. Transient ischemic attacks (TIAs) have no permanent parenchymal lesion on MRI. In AIS a central core zone of decreased perfusion results in irreversibly damaged brain. Surrounding this core is an unstable "penumbral zone" where collateral perfusion may sustain neuronal viability. In the penumbra, factors that increase the discrepancy between metabolic rate and the delivery of oxygen and glucose may result in additional tissue injury and cell death. Secondary insults include seizures and alterations in temperature, blood pressure, and serum glucose. The primary objective of acute neuroprotective stroke treatment is to rescue this "at-risk" penumbral tissue to salvage functional brain.

Risk Factors

Multiple factors have been described in association with childhood AIS (Mackay et al., 2011; Mallick et al., 2014). There is increasing evidence for causality of AIS by vasculopathy, infection, trauma, and cardiac and hematological disorders from case–control and population-based studies. Contrasting with adults, atherosclerosis is a rare cause for childhood AIS. Chronic diseases of childhood frequently underlie childhood AIS; however, approximately half of children are previously healthy. Multiple risk factors converge in >50% of children with AIS. At least 10% remain idiopathic. A comprehensive list of potential risk factors for childhood AIS is included in Table 109-1. It is critical to determine all active AIS mechanisms and implement appropriate corrective treatments.

Infection

Fever and recent infectious symptoms are frequent in children with AIS. Population-based case–control studies have confirmed that recent infection is associated with a fourfold increased odds of stroke. Emerging data from the Vascular Effects of Infection in Pediatric Stroke (VIPS), an international multicenter case–control study, implicate herpes group viruses as a major contributor to pediatric stroke. Arterial or venous stroke has been identified in 5% to 12% of children and 75% of infants with bacterial meningitis. Tuberculous meningitis is an important cause of childhood AIS in developing countries. AIS has also been associated with mycoplasma, toxoplasmosis, rocky mountain spotted fever, Lyme disease, cryptococcus, Japanese encephalitis, coxsackie B4 and A9, influenza A, enterovirus, parvovirus B19, HIV, and chlamydia.

Arteriopathies

Diseases that directly affect the craniocervical arteries supplying the brain have emerged as the leading cause of childhood AIS and are the most important predictor of recurrence and poor outcome. Arteriopathy is present in >50% of children with AIS (Amlie-Lefond et al., 2009). Vascular imaging is essential for accurate initial identification and classification of arteriopathy. Given the progressive nature of some arteriopathies, ongoing

surveillance with vascular imaging is also important and may dictate specific treatment. Important arteriopathy categories are 1) focal or transient cerebral arteriopathy (Figure 109-4), 2) primary angiitis of the central nervous system, 3) arterial dissection, 4) moyamoya syndrome (Figure 109-7), and 5) congenital or genetic arteriopathies.

Focal or Transient Cerebral Arteriopathy. Focal cerebral arteriopathy (FCA), also termed "transient cerebral arteriopathy" (TCA), is associated with 1) unilateral intracranial arteriopathy affecting distal internal carotid and proximal middle or anterior cerebral arteries; 2) lenticulostriate infarcts within basal ganglia; 3) narrowing, banding, striae, or stenosis of the affected vessel wall; and 4) serial arterial imaging often showing instability in the initial 3 to 6 months, followed by

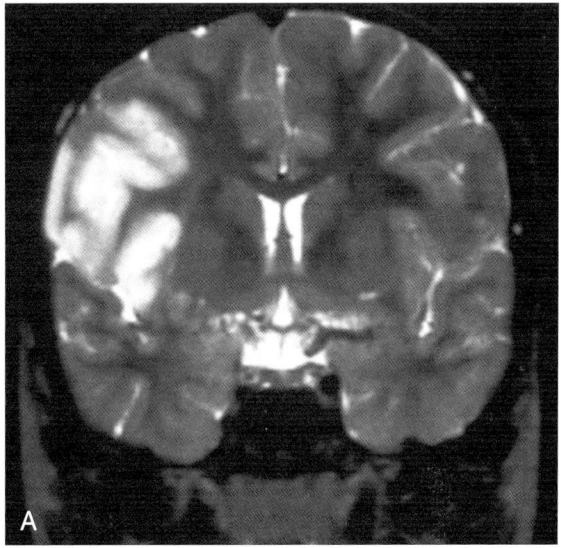
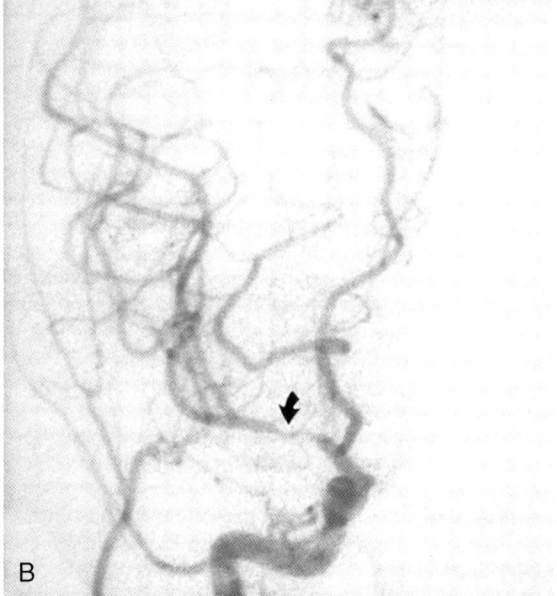

Figure 109-4. Large-vessel arterial infarct in the right middle cerebral artery territory associated with "transient cerebral arteriopathy" of childhood in an 11-year-old female presenting with hemiparesis. **A,** T2-weighted magnetic resonance imaging shows right middle cerebral artery infarct maximally involving the cortex. **B,** Conventional angiogram shows irregular stenosis in the proximal right middle cerebral artery. (**B,** *Courtesy of Division of Neuroradiology, Hospital for Sick Children, Toronto, Ontario, Canada.*)

TABLE 109-1 Potential Risk Factors for Childhood AIS

Category	Common	Uncommon
Arteriopathy	**Inflammatory/parainfectious** Childhood primary angiitis of CNS (cPACNS; nonprogressive or progressive; large vessel or small vessel) Transient cerebral arteriopathy (TCA) Focal cerebral arteriopathy (FCA) Postvaricella angiopathy (PVA) **Infectious** Bacterial and tuberculous meningitis HIV **Dissection** Internal carotid artery Vertebral artery Intracranial arteries **Moyamoya** disease (idiopathic) Moyamoya syndrome Neurofibromatosis-1, trisomy 21	Secondary CNS vasculitis SLE, PAN, IBD Takayasu arteritis Infectious: mycoplasma, toxoplasmosis, RMSF, Lyme disease, cryptococcus, chlamydia, Japanese encephalitis, coxsackie B4 and A9, influenza A, enterovirus, parvovirus B19 Postradiation vasculopathy Reversible segmental cerebral vasospasm (RSCV, Call-Flemming syndrome) Genetic: COL4A1 CT disease (Marfans, Ehler's-Danlos) Pseudoxanthoma elasticum Congenital: PHACES, progeria, Alagille, dwarfism (MOPDII), fibromuscular dysplasias
Cardiac	**Complex congenital heart disease** Cardiac surgery (e.g., Fontan) Cardiac catheterization (e.g., BAS) **Other cardiac conditions** Bacterial endocarditis Atrial septal aneurysm Atrial septal defect* Patent foramen ovale* Venous thrombosis + right-to-left shunt	Cardiomyopathy, myocarditis Aortic coarctation Severe ventricular dysfunction Atrial myxoma Valvular disease (e.g., rheumatic fever) Arrhythmia (atrial fibrillation) ECMO Cerebral angiography Embolism (air, fat, amniotic fluid)
Prothrombotic	Factor V Leiden Prothrombin gene 20210A Elevated lipoprotein (a) Protein C deficiency Lupus anticoagulant Anticardiolipin antibodies	MTHFR, hyperhomocysteinemia Protein S deficiency Antithrombin III deficiency Factor VII/IX/XI* Plasminogen deficiency* Dysfibrinogenemia* Sticky platelet syndrome Pregnancy, puerperium
Hematological	Sickle cell disease Iron deficiency anemia	Leukemia Thalassemias* Thrombocytosis* Polycythemia* Hemolytic uremic syndrome Immune thrombocytopenic purpura Thrombotic thrombocytopenic purpura
Medications/drugs	Oral contraceptives Chemotherapy (L-aspariginase)	Cocaine, methamphetamine, ecstasy Ergots, triptans
Other	Migraine Inborn errors of metabolism: Fabry disease, homocystinuria, mitochondrial	Metabolic syndrome: hypertension, diabetes, insulin resistance, dyslipidemia, atherosclerosis Cigarette smoking, second-hand smoke

*Uncertain.
BAS, balloon atrial septostomy; CT, connective tissue disease; CNS, central nervous system; ECMO, extracorporeal membrane oxygenation; HIV, human immunodeficiency virus; IBD, inflammatory bowel disease; MPODII, Majewski osteodysplastic primordial dwarfism II; MTHFR, methylene tetrahydrofolate reductase; PAN, polyarteritis nodosum; PHACES, posterior fossa malformations–hemangiomas–arterial anomalies–cardiac defects–eye abnormalities–sternal cleft and supraumbilical raphe syndrome; RMSF, Rocky Mountain spotted fever; RSCV, reversible segmental cerebral vasoconstriction; SLE, systemic lupus erythematosus.

stabilization or improvement. Early descriptions of this condition used the term "transient cerebral arteriopathy" (TCA), and subsequent studies have confirmed the nonprogressive nature of the disorder in over 90% of children. An example of the angiographic appearance of TCA is shown in Figure 109-4. The pathophysiology of this arteriopathy remains undetermined but an association between infection and TCA/FCA arteriopathy is well recognized. However, it is yet to be established whether TCA represents an inflammatory arteriopathy and, if so, whether it is provoked by active viral infection, postviral inflammation, or "idiopathic" inflammation.

Postvaricella angiopathy (PVA) provides some evidence for an association between infection and arteriopathy. PVA shares imaging features with TCA with the main difference being a history of clinical varicella infection within 12 months. Proposed mechanisms include viral reactivation from trigeminal ganglion with spread to proximal cerebral arteries. Rare histopathological studies have revealed viral particles or antigens in cerebral artery smooth muscle cells. Naturally occurring PVA is expected to decrease with varicella vaccination becoming routine and there is no known association between varicella vaccine and childhood stroke.

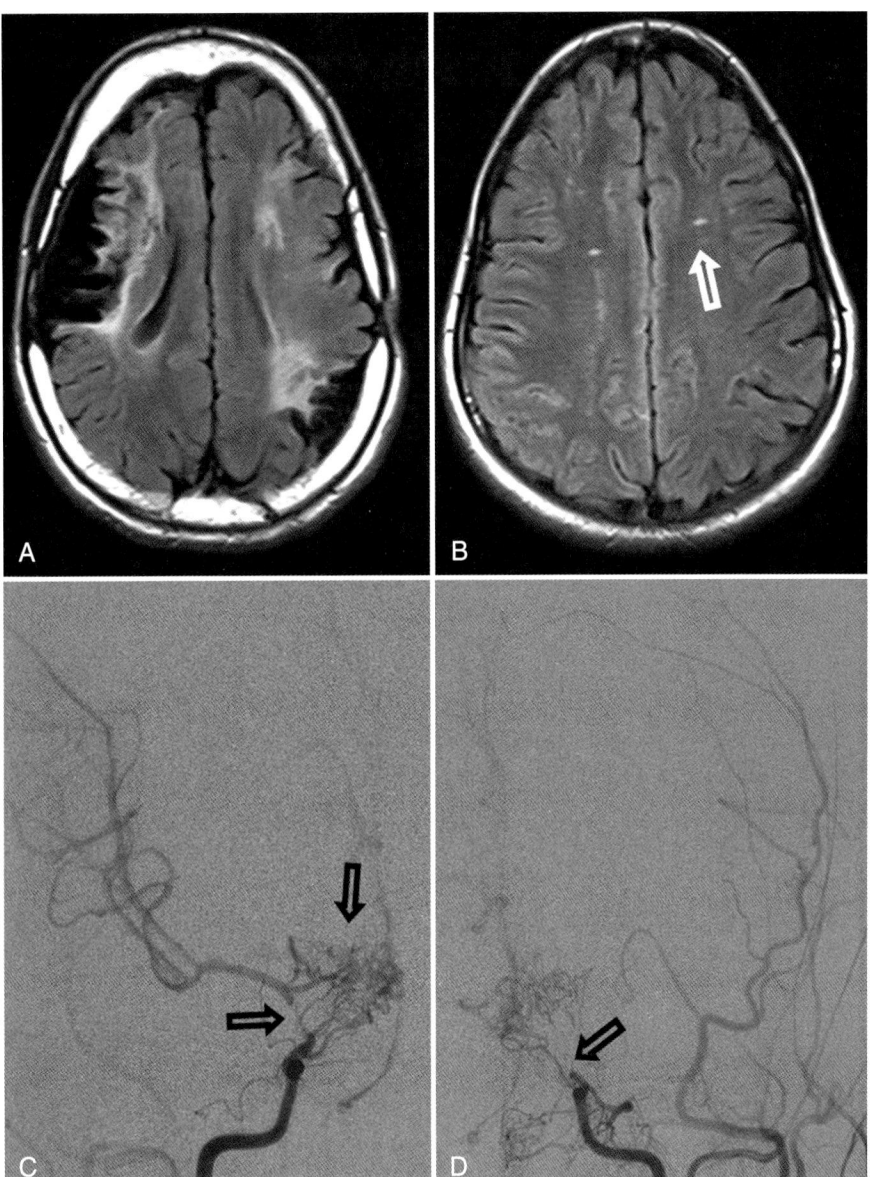

Figure 109-7. Moyamoya disease. An 8-year-old boy presented with acute-onset left hemiplegia after 10 months of transient alternating hemiplegia related to hyperventilation. **A**, A large-arterial ischemic stroke of the right frontal lobe is accompanied by additional large-vessel and watershed lesions bilaterally. The patient has severe motor disability bilaterally, with cognitive delays, and is nonverbal. **B**, His 15-year-old sister mentioned having headaches at her brother's follow-up visit and was imaged. She has several small ischemic lesions in the periventricular white matter (arrow), but is an honors student with normal examination findings. Both children have moyamoya. **C** and **D**, The girl's angiogram (antero-posterior view) shows severe narrowing **(C)** and occlusion **(D)** of the distal internal carotid arteries, with abnormal collateral development (arrows). Both patients have been asymptomatic after bilateral revascularization surgery.

Primary Angiitis of the Central Nervous System and Other Conditions Associated with Cerebral Arteriopathy. Noninfectious arterial inflammation or vasculitis is referred to as childhood primary angiitis of CNS (cPACNS). Unilateral large-vessel versions are interchangeable with TCA terminology but bilateral large- and small-vessel varieties tend to be progressive. For the latter, aggressive anti-inflammatory treatment may be required to prevent rapid deterioration and multifocal strokes. cPACNS limited to distal, small cerebral arteries ("angiogram-negative") typically presents with insidious symptoms, including headaches, seizures, cognitive decline, and behavioral or personality change, and MRI demonstrating multifocal enhancing lesions. Conventional angiography is

indicated but may be negative, and brain biopsy is often required for definitive diagnosis.

Systemic vasculitides and connective tissue diseases occasionally involving cerebral arteries include Kawasaki disease, Henoch–Schohnlein purpura, polyarteritis nodosa, Wegener granulomatosis, systemic lupus erythematosus, Behcet syndrome, mixed connective tissue disease, Sjogren syndrome, and inflammatory bowel diseases. These conditions are reviewed in Chapter 121.

The range of infectious/inflammatory arteriopathies must be a primary consideration in all children with AIS with important implications for investigation, treatment, and risk of recurrence and poor outcome. Diagnostic investigations should be clinically tailored but may include screening for specific infections (serology, virology, PCR) in addition to routine hematological blood work, and inflammatory (ESR, CRP) and vasculitic (ANA, extractable nuclear antigens, complement, etc.) markers and cerebrospinal fluid analysis. Treatment trials for the infectious/inflammatory cerebral arteriopathies are lacking in children but antivirals and corticosteroids may be considered. Other immunosuppressive agents such as cyclophosphamide, azathioprine, and mycophenolate are indicated in progressive cPACNS.

Dissection and Other Physical Injury. Craniocervical dissection causes intraluminal thrombosis or wall hematoma with frequent artery-to-artery thromboembolism. Dissection accounts for up to 20% of childhood. Extracranial arterial dissection occurs at predictable locations, including proximal ICA and the vertebral arteries at C1–C2 level. Intracranial dissection also occurs, and carries a theoretical added risk of secondary subarachnoid hemorrhage. It is may be difficult to distinguish intracranial dissection from TCA on vascular imaging. Dissection may result from trauma to the neck, spine, or retropharyngeal area but many cases occur spontaneously. Symptoms and signs of dissection include head or neck pain, ipsilateral Horner's syndrome, and cervical bruit, and stroke onset may be delayed by 7 to 10 days. Stroke recurrence rates are estimated at 20% or higher.

The medical management of dissections is controversial with no randomized controlled trials. Current guidelines suggest consideration of anticoagulation in children with stroke because of extra cranial dissection but adult meta-analyses have found no difference in outcomes between anticoagulation and antiplatelet therapy. Intracranial dissection may be a relative contraindication to anticoagulation due to the risk of subarachnoid hemorrhage.

Moyamoya Disease and Moyamoya Syndrome. Moyamoya is characterized by progressive occlusion of distal internal carotid arteries (ICAs) and branches of the Circle of Willis. Compensatory angiogenesis forms collateral vessels resulting in an abnormal network termed "moyamoya" (Japanese for "puff of smoke") (see Figure 109-7). Moyamoya *disease*, the idiopathic form, is an important cause of childhood stroke, particularly in Asians in whom mutations in the ring finger 213 gene (*RNF213*) are common. Moyamoya *syndrome* is associated with systemic conditions, including sickle cell disease (Sickle Cell Disease), Down syndrome, neurofibromatosis type 1, postradiation vasculopathy, and congenital arteriopathies. Moyamoya is therefore a syndrome and not a single disease.

In contrast to other forms of AIS, an important mechanism for moyamoya-associated infarction is hypoperfusion, which often affects watershed zones. Impaired cerebrovascular autoregulation in chronically underperfused territories appears to predict infarction. Stroke or TIA symptoms may be precipitated by alterations in Pco_2 such as during hyperventilation (cerebral vasoconstriction) or breath-holding (cerebral vasodilatation with "steal"). Moyamoya progresses slowly over time, causing accumulating injury and poor neurologic outcomes. In addition, artery-to-artery occlusion of larger cerebral arterial branches can result in more typical AIS. Hemorrhagic stroke can also occur from the compensatory basal collateral vessels (*rete mirable*) and risk increases in early adulthood. Headaches, often with migrainous features and hypertension, are common in moyamoya.

MRI findings include multifocal infarcts (see Figure 109-7) particularly affecting subcortical white matter, vascular flow voids in the basal ganglia, and the "ivy sign" on FLAIR imaging, which correlates with impaired autoregulation. MR

angiography (MRA) is sensitive at detecting moyamoya arteriopathy but conventional angiography is required to confirm collaterals, characterize disease extent, and determine options for revascularization surgery (see Figure 109-7).

Treatment of moyamoya is complex. Antiplatelet therapy with ASA is often employed and is likely safe. Carbonic anhydrase inhibitors, including acetazolamide, may shift acid–base balance to favor vasodilation but may also cause a steal phenomenon with risk of stroke. Use of antihypertensives in children with moyamoya must be avoided or carefully titrated as even small decreases in cerebral perfusion can lead to infarction. Surgical revascularization procedures are highly successful at improving perfusion in children with moyamoya. Direct revascularization connects extracranial blood vessels such as the superficial temporal artery to distal portions of intracranial vessels, usually the middle cerebral artery. These are technically difficult in small children and carry some risk of reocclusion. Indirect procedures are more often employed in children, in whom extracranial vessels are approximated to the cortical surface overlying areas of decreased perfusion. Studies comparing the different surgical approaches are lacking. Perioperative infarctions occur in <10% of patients.

Congenital or Genetic Arteriopathies. An increasing number of congenital or genetic cerebral arteriopathies are recognized. NF1, ACTA2, COL4A1, Alagille syndrome, CADASIL, CARASIL, and possibly fibromuscular dysplasia are examples each with unique imaging characteristics.

Cardiac

Cardiac disorders are associated with 10% to 31% of infants and children with AIS (Figure 109-8) (Sinclair et al., 2015). Congenital heart defects account for the majority of cases with a 19-fold increased stroke risk. Cardiac surgery carries a 1 : 185 risk, and cardiac catheterization a 1 : 600 to 700 risk of symptomatic AIS with increased risk for interventional catheterization. High-risk procedures include Fontan and balloon atrial septostomy.

Atrial septal defects (ASD) and patent foramen ovale (PFO) remain controversial risk factors for stroke in young adults that have not been well studied in children. Associations between PFO and cryptogenic stroke have been demonstrated in young adults but randomized trials do not support surgical closure of uncomplicated PFO over medical treatment.

Infective endocarditis predisposes to AIS and intracerebral hemorrhage and is suggested by subacute constitutional symptoms, fever, Janeway lesions, and Roth spots. Anticoagulation is relatively contraindicated because of bleeding risk from mycotic aneurysms. Other acquired cardiac defects include infectious or metabolic cardiomyopathy, valvular heart disease (e.g., rheumatic fever, artificial valves), dysrhythmias, atrial myxoma, extracorporeal membrane oxygenation (ECMO), and ventricular assist devices.

Multifocal infarcts across different vascular territories and hemorrhagic transformation may suggest a cardiac source. Children with cryptogenic AIS should undergo prompt cardiac evaluation, including an electrocardiogram and echocardiography. Agitated saline "bubble studies" can help exclude PFO and atrial septal defects. Screening for prothrombotic states is recommended. Recurrent strokes are not uncommon in children with congenital heart disease and associated with mechanical valves, prothrombotic states, acute infection, and lack of antithrombotic treatment.

Consensus-based pediatric stroke guidelines suggest anticoagulant treatment over antiplatelet therapy for cardiogenic AIS. A randomized controlled secondary prevention trial in children undergoing the Fontan procedure found no difference between anticoagulant or antiplatelet therapy but did not

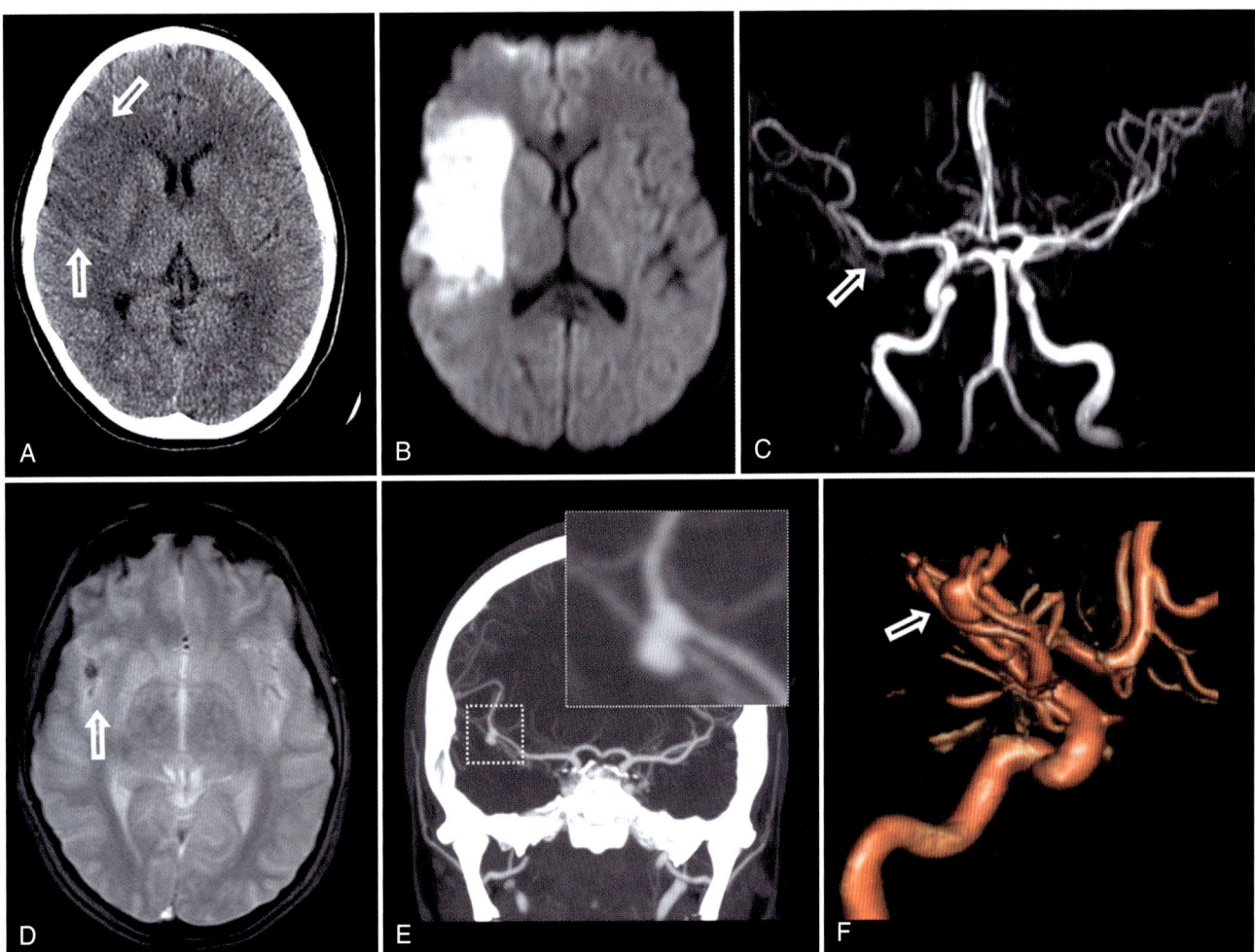

Figure 109-8. Acute cardioembolic arterial ischemic stroke. An 11-year-old girl presented with weeks of fatigue, low-grade fever, and skin lesions. She suddenly developed left-sided hemiplegia in hospital. **A,** Computed tomography (CT) scan at 90 minutes shows hypodensity (arrows) and loss of cortical ribbon in the right frontal lobe. She did not receive thrombolysis because of suspicion of endocarditis. Diffusion-weighted magnetic resonance imaging (MRI; **B**) and magnetic resonance angiography **(C)** confirm arterial ischemic stroke secondary to occlusion (arrow, **C**). The patient subsequently grew streptococcus and required aortic valve replacement. **D,** Follow-up imaging at 6 months included gradient ECHO MRI, which demonstrated hypodensity in the area of previous occlusion (arrow). **E** and **F,** CT angiography confirmed a mycotic aneurysm (arrow, **F**), which grew over the next month and was clipped surgically with success.

address asymptomatic cerebrovascular events. Bacterial endocarditis requires urgent antibiotic treatment and investigation for mycotic aneurysm. Specific guidelines for prevention and treatment of thrombosis for children with congenital heart disease are available. Chapter 157 also discusses the neurologic disorders associated with cardiac disease.

Prothrombotic and Hematological Disorders

Prothrombotic disorders refer to abnormalities of the coagulation, fibrinolytic, and platelet systems that predispose to pathologic thrombus formation. Inherited or acquired coagulation disorders have been identified in 20% to 50% of children with AIS but interpretation of the data is limited by inconsistent testing and variability in laboratory methods. Meta-analyses have demonstrated a predisposing role for prothrombotic disorders in childhood AIS, with frequent coexistent "triggering" risk factors (Kenet et al., 2010). Genetic prothrombotic factors associated with childhood AIS include Factor V Leiden (odds ratio 3.7 to 4.3), prothrombin G20210A (odds ratio 2.6 to 3.5), lipoprotein (a) (odds ratio 6.5), and protein C deficiency (odds ratio 6.5 to 11.0). Protein S and

antithrombin III may also be associated with increased risk of stroke. Acquired prothrombotic factors include antiphospholipid antibodies and lupus anticoagulant (odds ratio 6.95). Coexistent multiple prothrombotic factors are associated with the highest risk (combined odds ratio 11.9). Coagulation testing should be performed in all children with AIS, even in the presence of other risk factors, because prothrombotic disorders may be associated with increased recurrence. Children with stroke and a significant prothrombotic disorder should be counseled in prevention strategies such as the avoidance of dehydration and possible prophylactic dosing of anticoagulation in high-risk situations. These conditions are discussed further in Chapter 113.

Sickle Cell Disease

SCD is the most common hematological disorder associated with cerebrovascular disease in children and increases ischemic stroke risk 400-fold. About 25% of SCD children develop cerebrovascular complications, with risk being highest during acute sickle crises. Stroke is responsible for 10% of SCD mortality. There are two main mechanisms for AIS in SCD:

1) a progressive internal carotid (large vessel) Moyamoya arteriopathy and 2) occlusion of small cerebral end arteries. Extracranial carotid disease, anemia, hypertension, and proinflammatory genetic polymorphisms may also contribute to cerebrovascular disease.

Transcranial Doppler (TCD) studies are a noninvasive means of following flow rates related to large-vessel vasculopathy with flows >200 cm/s, predicting increased stroke risk. The STOP randomized controlled trial demonstrated that regular transfusion therapy (hemoglobin S <20% to 30%) produced a 90% relative risk reduction in initial stroke in children with elevated velocities. Recurrent stroke rates were also reduced. A follow-up study showed that stroke risk returns with discontinuation of transfusions. MRI surveillance can detect silent infarcts secondary to small-vessel disease, large-vessel disease, and possible Moyamoya syndrome. In children with radiologic evidence of silent cerebral infarction, regular transfusions also confer protection against cerebrovascular events but the relative risk–benefit ratio is not well defined (DeBaun et al., 2014). Additional stroke prevention strategies under evaluation include hydroxyurea and nocturnal oxygen supplementation. Antithrombotic therapy has not been studied but aspirin should be considered, especially in cases with large-vessel vasculopathy, prothrombotic abnormalities, or recurrent stroke.

Additional Considerations

A comprehensive list of additional conditions associated with childhood AIS is in Table 109-2. Iron deficiency anemia is an important and treatable risk factor, present in up to 40% of childhood AIS but the underlying pathophysiology has not been established. Migrainous infarction is rare in children, and preventative treatment with ASA and flunarizine is indicated, and vasoconstrictor agents such as triptans and sympathomimetics should be avoided. Reversible cerebral vasoconstriction syndrome, another rare vasospastic condition, occurs in children and may respond to similar interventions. Use of medications and illicit drugs should be determined. Inborn errors of metabolism predisposing to AIS include homocystinuria and Fabry disease, and mitochondrial disorders can mimic AIS. The role of other genetic factors in stroke and cerebral vasculopathies is complex, ranging from single-gene disorders imparting a high risk to complex, multigene polymorphisms influencing additional risk factors.

Clinical Features and Diagnostic Delays

Prompt diagnosis is essential to enable emergent neuroprotective management, and interventions to promote recanalization and prevent early recurrence. Unfortunately, multiple studies confirm long diagnostic delays, often beyond 24 hours from symptom onset. Physician recognition and quick availability of sensitive imaging are probably important contributors to delayed diagnosis.

The acute onset of focal neurologic deficits in childhood is a stroke until proven otherwise. Hemiparesis is a common presenting deficit that may be erroneously attributed to stroke mimics, including migraine, Todd's paresis, encephalitis/meningitis, demyelination, or tumors. Other focal deficits include dysarthria, dysphasia, facial weakness, vertigo, abnormal eye movements, sensory disturbance, ataxia, and neglect (Mallick et al., 2014). The frequent occurrence of seizures in childhood AIS is a notable difference to adults. Nonfocal neurologic signs such as headache, irritability, and altered mental state are also common, particularly in infants. Stroke-induced deficits usually begin suddenly and severity is maximal at the onset, aiding differentiation from mimics such as migraine

and demyelination. However, fluctuating or stuttering onset of symptoms can occur, and may be clues to specific etiologies such as arteriopathies.

Specific historical and examination findings may provide clues to the stroke mechanism and etiology. History of infection is important, including varicella within 12 months. Head or neck trauma, including chiropractic neck manipulation within the preceding weeks, may suggest dissection. Previous TIA is important and symptoms switching sides suggest a proximal embolic source or bilateral arteriopathy (e.g., Moyamoya syndrome). Migraine history in the child and family may be relevant. Previous head or neck irradiation and medication history including oral contraceptives, chemotherapy, sympathomimetics, or illicit drugs should be sought. Family history should screen for early onset thrombotic events, cardiovascular disease, and genetic disorders. Important elements of the physical examination include cardiovascular examination with blood pressure, peripheral pulses, and auscultation of the head and neck for bruits. Ophthalmologic examination may suggest arteriopathic diseases or increased intracranial pressure. Skin lesions may suggest neurofibromatosis, Fabry disease, or PHACES syndrome (posterior fossa abnormalities, hemangiomas, arterial cervicocerebral anomalies, cardiac defects, eye anomalies, sternal defects, and/or supraumbilical raphe).

Diagnosis: Neuroimaging

Appropriate and timely neuroimaging is essential to confirm the diagnosis of AIS, exclude stroke mimics, and guide initial management decisions. Computed tomography (CT) can exclude intracranial hemorrhage but has low detection rates for acute brain ischemia, ranging from 16% to 56% in pediatric studies. Therefore magnetic resonance imaging (MRI) is the neuroimaging investigation of choice. Diffusion-weighted MRI (DWI) reliably detects early brain ischemia characterized by combined DWI hyperintensity (see Figure 109-8) and apparent diffusion coefficient (ADC) map hypointensity. This pattern normalizes over 1 to 2 weeks. Abnormalities appear on T2-weighted and FLAIR sequences within several hours and persist. Susceptibility-weighted methods can detect blood. Perfusion-weighted imaging demonstrates regional brain perfusion abnormalities but pediatric studies have been limited.

Vascular imaging of the intracranial and neck vessels should be performed simultaneously. Time-of-flight MRA can image the major first- and second-order cerebral arteries but because it relies on flow signal, signal dropout artifact can mimic occlusion in areas of turbulent flow or stenosis. An abrupt arterial "cutoff" suggests embolic stroke, whereas stenosis or irregularity favors arteriopathy. Gadolinium-enhanced MR angiography has better resolution and specificity than time-of-flight imaging. MRI "wall imaging" may demonstrate concentric vessel wall enhancement suggesting inflammation, a potentially valuable marker in pediatric arteriopathies.

Conventional angiography (CA) remains the gold standard for cerebrovascular imaging (see Figures 109-4 and 109-7). Specific arteriopathies may only be diagnosed by CA, including "string," "double lumen" or intimal flap signs in dissection, "string of beads" in vasculitis, and arteriopathies limited to smaller-caliber arteries. CA should be performed in children with AIS in whom a specific etiology remains undetermined after initial MRA or CTA and considered in others to better characterize probable arteriopathies.

Treatment

Current treatment of pediatric stroke is informed by multiple consensus-based guidelines, generated from panels of child neurologists, thrombosis experts, and others experienced in pediatric stroke (Roach et al., 2008; Monagle et al., 2012). These guidelines are concordant for major treatment recommendations although they differ in certain areas because of the paucity of data from randomized controlled trials.

Stroke Unit Care and Neuroprotection

There is substantial evidence in adults of the benefits of stroke units in reducing length of hospital stay, morbidity, and mortality. The general principles of specialized teams providing stroke care can be applied at pediatric centers meeting key infrastructural requirements. Therefore children with stroke should be rapidly transferred to centers with expertise in management of cerebrovascular disorders after stroke diagnosis.

Immediate measures to prevent secondary brain injury are a crucial, easily overlooked aspect of emergency stroke care in children. Neuroprotective therapy is aimed at optimizing perfusion, delivering oxygen and glucose to penumbral tissue, and reducing neuronal metabolic demand through control of fever and seizures. Hypertension is associated with increased mortality and hypotension compromises perfusion of penumbral tissue. Although ideal blood pressure parameters for treatment of hypertension in acute childhood stroke are unknown maintenance of blood pressure up to 15% above the 90% percentile seems reasonable for most patients. Maintenance of normal blood oxygen and carbon dioxide levels is also prudent in the face of tenuous cerebral perfusion and acute alterations in autoregulation.

Both hyper- and hypoglycemia are associated with poorer neurologic outcomes in adult stroke and critically ill children but there are no specific data in pediatric stroke. Ischemic brain injury is clearly exacerbated by hyperthermia in animal models and adult stroke and guidelines recommend temperature control. Therapeutic hypothermia has not been studied in childhood AIS but results are predominantly negative in childhood traumatic brain injury and adult stroke. Acute seizures are common in childhood AIS, likely worsen ischemic brain injury, and should be monitored for and treated with anticonvulsant medications.

Thrombolysis and Thrombectomy

There is a paucity of efficacy and safety data for tissue plasminogen activator (tPA) or thrombectomy in children because of exclusion of subjects <18 years from clinical trials. As a consequence, pediatric stroke guidelines do not recommend these approaches in children. The following discussion is presented to educate the reader and does not represent a recommendation for such interventions.

Thrombolytic agents such as tPA promote the conversion of plasminogen into plasmin to dissolve thrombi. Meta-analyses of published adult trials demonstrate a time-dependent benefit for tPA outweighing early risks of intracranial hemorrhage within 4.5 hours of onset. The safety and efficacy of thrombolysis in children remains poorly studied. Developmental differences in the fibrinolytic system, including decreased plasminogen and free tissue plasminogen levels and higher plasminogen activator inhibitor-1 (PAI-1) levels, may substantially alter both the benefits and anticipated risks of thrombolysis. Off-label usage of tPA is reported in up to 2% of children in large multicenter data sets often beyond recommended time windows and with higher rates of symptomatic intracranial hemorrhage. Up to 10% of children may be eligible for thrombolysis using adult selection criteria but several obstacles exist, including paucity of age-appropriate safety data and long diagnostic delays. Tools allowing identification of children with the worst prognosis such as the Pediatric NIH Stroke Scale are available. Emerging

evidence in adults suggests that mechanical thrombectomy may be the most effective means of achieving recanalization but only anecdotal data are available for children. Therefore the role of mechanical thrombectomy is unclear in children.

Antithrombotic Therapies

Managing childhood AIS without antithrombotic agents is no longer considered appropriate in most cases because of the high risk of early recurrence and the availability of safety data for these agents in acute childhood stroke. However, choosing between antiplatelet and anticoagulation treatments in the acute setting is not well informed by evidence, reflected by discordant practices among pediatric stroke experts and differing recommendations across consensus guidelines. Prompt initiation of antithrombotic therapy aims to prevent thrombus propagation or reembolization and promote early recanalization. The first option is anticoagulant treatment with agents including heparin, low-molecular-weight heparins (LMWH), or warfarin. Anticoagulants may be theoretically favored in certain circumstances such as cardiogenic embolism, paradoxical venous embolism, slow flow with severe stenosis, a major prothrombotic disorder, and possibly dissection. The second option is antiplatelet treatment with aspirin, which may be more appropriate in the arteriopathies in which high flow thrombus formation theoretically favors platelet-rich thrombi. These treatment approaches are not mutually exclusive and their indications may vary across acute, subacute, and chronic timeframes as the cause of a child's stroke becomes more evident.

Anticoagulation. The decision to employ acute anticoagulation therapy (ACT) in childhood AIS rests on balancing the potential benefit of reducing thrombus extension or recurrence with risk of hemorrhage. Decisions should be based on suspicion of pathologic fibrin clot formation (coagulation system) playing a dominant role. Evidence suggests that clinically significant hemorrhagic transformation of childhood AIS is rare and not significantly increased with anticoagulation. Large adult clinical trials across different stroke populations have shown only modestly improved efficacy of heparin over ASA that is generally negated by an increased risk of hemorrhagic complications. Post hoc analysis of the Warfarin Aspirin Recurrent Stroke Study (WARSS) found a 30% risk reduction for recurrent stroke with warfarin over aspirin among adults with cryptogenic strokes, which may be relevant to children. Acute anticoagulation has an established role in certain adult stroke situations where there is high risk of thrombus extension or embolic recurrence, such as nonvalvular atrial fibrillation. Relative ACT contraindications include intracranial hemorrhage, uncontrollable hypertension, or bleeding diathesis.

Although there are no large-scale clinical trials of anticoagulation therapies in children with AIS, extensive pediatric experience has established safety. The American College of Chest Physicians and AHA guidelines support the initial use of anticoagulation in childhood AIS, after diagnosis, pending further investigations, whereas the UK guidelines favor initial use in only selected circumstances such as cardiogenic stroke. Dosing guidelines for anticoagulant treatment in children with AIS are available.

Unfractionated heparin (UFH) potentiates antithrombin's inactivation of thrombin and other enzymes. Children require lower doses than adults. Dose monitoring includes activated partial thromboplastin times (APTT) and heparin levels. Rapid and complete reversal of the anticoagulation effects of heparin with protamine confers a potential advantage in situations of higher bleeding risk or impending surgery. *Low-molecular-weight heparins (LMWH)* are molecular subcomponents of unfractionated heparin. Advantages of LMWH include more reproducible pharmacokinetics, subcutaneous injection, less frequent monitoring, and modestly increased safety profiles. Antifactor Xa levels are used to monitor treatment. LMWH carries a low risk of thrombocytopenia. Oral anticoagulation with *warfarin* is generally reserved for children requiring long-term anticoagulation, such as those with complex congenital heart diseases or severe prothrombotic disorders. Warfarin antagonizes the activity of vitamin K–dependent coagulation factors in a dose-dependent manner. A target INR (international normalized ratio) of 2.0 to 3.0 is appropriate for most children (2.5 to 3.5 for mechanical heart valves). Relative contraindications include infants or children with unpredictable vitamin K levels, gastrointestinal disorders, and older children unwilling to forgo contact sports.

Antiplatelet Therapy. Management guidelines recommend antiplatelet agents as secondary prevention for non cardioembolic AIS. *Aspirin* is the primary antiplatelet agent for children with a well-established safety profile and inhibits platelet aggregation by decreasing thromboxane A2 production. Reye syndrome is likely related to rare inborn errors in metabolism and has never been reported in pediatric stroke but some physicians recommend reduction of therapy during a febrile illness and annual influenza vaccination. Alternative antiplatelet agents include clopidogrel, extended release dipyramidol, ticlopidine, or the glycoprotein IIb-IIIa antagonists.

Malignant Cerebral Edema

Poststroke cerebral edema is a life-threatening early complication of childhood AIS. Malignant MCA syndromes, large hemorrhagic transformations and cerebellar infarcts carry the highest risk of brain herniation. Urgent imaging should be performed for any neurologic deterioration within the first 72 hours, especially decreased level of consciousness or unilateral pupillary dilatation. Medical management includes measures to reduce increased intracranial pressure, including sedation, paralysis, manipulation of P_{CO_2}, and osmotic therapy. Decompressive hemicraniectomy is lifesaving.

Outcomes and Chronic Management

Sequelae of AIS

More than 50% of childhood stroke survivors have long-term moderate to severe neurologic impairments or epilepsy (deVeber et al., 2000). Rehabilitation must target the physical, occupational, language, cognitive/behavioral, and psychosocial consequences of stroke for the child and their family. Compared with adults with stroke, children have improved potential for recovery; however, among children, younger age at time of injury is associated with higher risk of long-term impairment. Stroke in adults results in loss of function, whereas similar injury in children results in both loss of function and reduced ability to acquire new abilities. Therefore pediatric rehabilitation treatments must incorporate knowledge of normal age-related developmental skills, trying to distinguish differences between relearning a brain function versus acquiring it for the first time.

Hemiparesis and motor disabilities are common sequelae of childhood stroke. Hemidystonia can emerge months after basal ganglia stroke. Neuroimaging may facilitate early prediction of poor motor outcomes in childhood AIS, possibly identifying those in need of aggressive rehabilitation. Rehabilitation programs that combine strength and aerobic conditioning, task-specific training, and assistive devices are generally recommended in children. Constraint induced movement therapy (CIMT) is a therapeutic approach to promote

functional use of an impaired limb after stroke. The results from pediatric CIMT studies in children with perinatal stroke and hemiplegic cerebral palsy are encouraging but clinical trials are required in childhood stroke. Bimanual therapy approaches, focusing on function of the unaffected extremity may complement CIMT. Noninvasive neuromodulation such as repetitive transcranial magnetic stimulation (TMS) has been shown to improve motor functions in chronic adult stroke, and preliminary data suggest that it may also have a role in childhood stroke. Peripheral electrical stimulation, robot-assisted rehabilitation, and virtual reality training strategies being explored in adult stroke are yet to be tested in children.

Assistive devices, including ankle-foot orthoses and Lycra hand splints, may facilitate joint positioning and function, and are supported by evidence in adult stroke. Spasticity interventions must include comprehensive, objective, and blinded pre- and postinterventional outcome measures of efficacy. Botulinum toxin may alleviate increased tone though effects on motor function and quality of life in children have been questioned. Careful selection criteria and better evidence of efficacy are also required for surgical interventions such as tendon-lengthening procedures. Physical growth asymmetries with resultant leg length discrepancy and scoliosis may require orthopedic intervention.

Neuropsychological impairments are common in children with stroke, limiting academic, social, and independent functional success. On average, childhood stroke survivors exhibit mildly compromised global intellectual function. Younger age at stroke does not appear to predict better cognitive outcomes. Language function, verbal learning, and memory are also often impaired, usually related to dominant hemisphere injury. Comprehensive, serial testing of cognitive, language, and other higher brain functions by pediatric neuropsychologists using standardized measures is important because defects in higher brain function often emerge over time in young children. Emotional, behavioral, and socialization problems after childhood stroke may occur and potentially affect all aspects of quality of life. Bilateral lesions may increase the risk of emotional or behavioral problems.

Remote symptomatic epilepsy complicates childhood AIS in approximately 15% to 20% of cases Predictors of childhood epilepsy include large cortical lesions, acute seizures, and younger age at presentation. Treatment usually consists of anticonvulsants but some children with medically refractory poststroke epilepsy may require epilepsy surgery. Headache disorders are also common after stroke, occurring in 33% of individuals with risk factors including preexisting conditions (e.g., migraine), the underlying disease (e.g., Moyamoya syndrome), and psychosocial stressors. Most established pharmacologic interventions are safe in children with AIS with the exception of vasoconstricting agents, including triptans.

Psychosocial and social support of families is essential. Adverse effects of stroke on quality of life are frequent. A family-centered treatment approach should consider the individual child's lifestyle, goals, and level of functioning and be well-integrated into the school and home environments. Alleviation of parental guilt may also provide substantial benefit. Parents also require guidance in the interpretation of a growing number of therapeutic options, including those with legitimate potential such as stem cells and "pseudo therapies" such as hyperbaric oxygen, which are unfairly marketed to families, offering incredible but unsubstantiated claims of efficacy. The treating physician must therefore guide families to make informed decisions, respecting their motivations to help their children, while advocating on their behalf for responsible and equal regulation of all therapies offered to children with disabilities.

Stroke Recurrence

Stroke recurrence is significant, mandating a thorough approach to secondary stroke prevention over the long-term. Stroke and TIA recurrence risks range from 7% to 35%, with population-based data suggesting 5-year recurrence rates approaching 50%. Presence of arteriopathy is the most important risk factor for recurrence with rates >65%. With no randomized trials, the relative efficacy of various secondary stroke prevention interventions is unknown. Antiplatelet therapy is the mainstay of long-term secondary stroke prevention in childhood AIS. Certain cardiac and prothrombotic conditions may require long-term anticoagulation with warfarin. Additional treatments may include immunosuppression for inflammatory vasculitis, transfusions for SCD, and revascularization surgery for Moyamoya syndrome. Attention to arterial health with balanced diet, exercise, avoidance of smoking and drugs, and surveillance for hypertension, dyslipidemia, or insulin resistance may also help prevent recurrence over the long-term.

REFERENCES

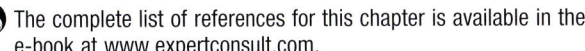 The complete list of references for this chapter is available in the e-book at www.expertconsult.com.

See inside cover for registration details.

REFERENCES

Amlie-Lefond, C., Bernard, T.J., Sebire, G., et al., 2009. Predictors of cerebral arteriopathy in children with arterial ischemic stroke: results of the International Pediatric Stroke Study. Circulation 119, 1417–1423.

DeBaun, M.R., Gordon, M., McKinstry, R.C., et al., 2014. Controlled trial of transfusions for silent cerebral infarcts in sickle cell anemia. N. Engl. J. Med. 371, 699–710.

deVeber, G.A., MacGregor, D., Curtis, R., et al., 2000. Neurologic outcome in survivors of childhood arterial ischemic stroke and sinovenous thrombosis. J. Child Neurol. 15, 316–324.

Kenet, G., Lutkhoff, L.K., Albisetti, M., et al., 2010. Impact of thrombophilia on risk of arterial ischemic stroke or cerebral sinovenous thrombosis in neonates and children: a systematic review and meta-analysis of observational studies. Circulation 121, 1838–1847.

Mackay, M.T., Wiznitzer, M., Benedict, S.L., et al., 2011. Arterial ischemic stroke risk factors: the International Pediatric Stroke Study. Ann. Neurol. 69, 130–140.

Mallick, A.A., Ganesan, V., Kirkham, F.J., et al., 2014. Childhood arterial ischaemic stroke incidence, presenting features, and risk factors: a prospective population-based study. Lancet Neurol. 13, 35–43.

Mallick, A.A., O'Callaghan, F.J., 2010. The epidemiology of childhood stroke. Eur. J. Paediatr. Neurol. 14, 197–205.

Monagle, P., Chan, A.K., Goldenberg, N.A., et al., 2012. Antithrombotic therapy in neonates and children: Antithrombotic Therapy and Prevention of Thrombosis, 9th ed: American College of Chest Physicians Evidence-Based Clinical Practice Guidelines. Chest 141, e737S–e801S.

Roach, E.S., Golomb, M.R., Adams, R., et al., 2008. Management of stroke in infants and children: a scientific statement from a Special Writing Group of the American Heart Association Stroke Council and the Council on Cardiovascular Disease in the Young. Stroke 39, 2644–2691.

Sinclair, A.J., Fox, C.K., Ichord, R.N., et al., 2015. Stroke in children with cardiac disease: report from the International Pediatric Stroke Study Group Symposium. Pediatr. Neurol. 52, 5–15.

E-BOOK FIGURES AND TABLES

The following figures and tables are available in the e-book at www.expertconsult.com. See inside cover for registration details.

Fig. 109-1 Lateral view of the cerebral arteries detailing the branches of the anterior and middle cerebral arteries.

Fig. 109-2 Anteroposterior view of the cerebral arteries. Anterior circulation only.

Fig. 109-3 The vertebral-basilar posterior circulation artery system.

Fig. 109-5 Postvaricella angiopathy in a 4-year-old male presenting with hemiparesis and speech loss 3 months after chickenpox.

Fig. 109-6 Childhood primary angiitis of the central nervous system.

Table 109-2. Differential diagnosis of stroke-like episodes in children

An expanded version of this chapter is available on www.expertconsult.com. See inside cover for registration details.

INTRODUCTION

Cerebral sinovenous thrombosis (CSVT) is included under the "ischemic stroke" category in children. In CSVT, brain dysfunction occurs due to thrombotic occlusion of cerebral veins and/or dural venous sinuses. CSVT is rare but remains underrecognised children due to nonspecific presentation, resulting in delayed or missed diagnosis. CSVT is distinct from arterial ischemic stroke (AIS) even though there is an overlap in predisposing conditions. Although randomized controlled trials (RCTs) have established the usefulness of anticoagulation therapy (ACT) in adults, pediatric data are limited to observational and cohort studies. Timely diagnosis and management is essential as CSVT is a potentially life-threatening condition. This chapter will focus on CSVT in infants (older than 28 days) and older children. Neonatal CSVT is comprehensively reviewed in Chapter 20.

EPIDEMIOLOGY

CSVT includes all children with thrombosis of the structures of the intracranial venous system with or without radiologically evident parenchymal lesions. Isolated thrombosis of the internal jugular vein (IJV) is not included under CSVT. Published epidemiologic studies suggest an incidence of 0.25 to 0.67 per 100,000 children per year. The ratio of pediatric CSVT to AIS cases is estimated at 1:4 annually. Like AIS, CSVT occurs more frequently in neonates and in males. Awareness of CSVT has increased in the last decade after the seminal population-based study of pediatric CSVT from Canada (deVeber and Andrew, 2001). Several large case series, cohort studies (Moharir et al., 2010; Grunt et al., 2010), and multicenter registry studies (Ichord et al., 2015) have now been published.

PATHOGENESIS

Sinovenous Circulation: Anatomy and Vascular Patterns

Cerebral venous drainage occurs through a network of veins and sinuses that comprise broadly the superficial and deep venous systems (Fig. 110-1). In the superficial venous system (SVS), cortical veins drain cortical and subcortical white matter (WM) from both hemispheres medially toward the superior sagittal sinus (SSS), which remains the largest conduit for venous drainage. The deep venous system (DVS) includes internal cerebral (ICV), medullary, thalamic, and choroidal veins that converge centrally at the vein of Galen (VOG), which drains into straight sinus (STRS). The DVS predominantly drains basal ganglia, thalami, and deep WM. The SVS and DVS unite posteriorly at the torcula. Bilateral, often asymmetric, transverse sinuses (TS) then drain laterally into sigmoid sinus (SIGS), which connects to the IJVs. The SVS usually drains into larger right TS whereas DVS drains into the smaller left TS. Additional venous drainage pathways connect with this system at recognizable locations including the cavernous and petrosal

sinuses and large superficial cerebral veins (e.g. Trolard, Labbé). Although the IJVs are the major exit for cerebral venous drainage, extrajugular pathways such as vertebral venous plexus (VVP) appear to be active, but poorly understood.

Adult and more recent pediatric data suggest that patterns of parenchymal brain lesions following CSVT may have some predictability (Fig. 110-2). Bilateral, parasagittal lesions, with or without hemorrhage are associated with SSS thrombosis. DVS thrombosis involving ICV, STRS and/or VOG produces lesions of deep WM, basal ganglia, and thalamus. Hemorrhagic lesions close to the ventricles can result in intraventricular hemorrhage (IVH) in young infants.

Intracranial Venous Physiology

The cerebral sinovenous system lacks valves and is a low-pressure, slow-velocity circuit. The dura of venous sinuses is rigid and noncollapsible, resulting in passive drainage of blood to the heart. The flow in sinuses is gravity- and respiration-dependent and can be bidirectional depending on the venous pressure gradient. The IJV appears to drain blood primarily in the supine position whereas the VVP appears to drain blood mainly in the upright position in humans. Reduction in systemic blood pressure can lead to stasis or reversal of blood flow. Venous sinus caliber is probably unresponsive to changes in systemic blood pressure. As the SSS and TS are main sites for CSF reabsorption through arachnoid granulations into the venous circulation, thrombosis or hypertension of these structures can cause communicating hydrocephalus. In supine infants with open fontanelles, mechanical compression of SSS by occipital bone may compromise venous drainage causing stasis and increased thrombosis risk.

Mechanisms of Thrombosis

CSVT essentially results from a "hypercoagulable" state secondary to Virchow's triad: abnormalities of blood (prothrombotic state), blood flow (stasis), and blood vessel (veins/sinuses). As in systemic venous thrombosis, but in contrast to most AIS, the role of the coagulation cascade and thrombin-rich thrombosis predominates. Platelets appear to play a minor role, hence antiplatelet therapy like aspirin is not considered in CSVT treatment. Inherited/acquired coagulation abnormalities play a prominent role in pathogenesis. A relative thrombomodulin deficiency in the cerebral venous endothelium may increase thrombotic tendency. In septic CSVT, infection within or immediately adjacent to venous structures directly provokes thrombophlebitis. In many cases, the exact mechanism of thrombosis is not evident. Slower, passive venous flow may favor initial formation and subsequent propagation of thrombosis. Dehydration, a potent risk factor for CSVT, may result in hemoconcentration and impaired laminar flow. Mechanical compression or injury (trauma, neurosurgery, venous catheter insertion, compressive masses, and occipital bone compression in supine infants) of venous structures may result in both venous stasis and/or endothelial

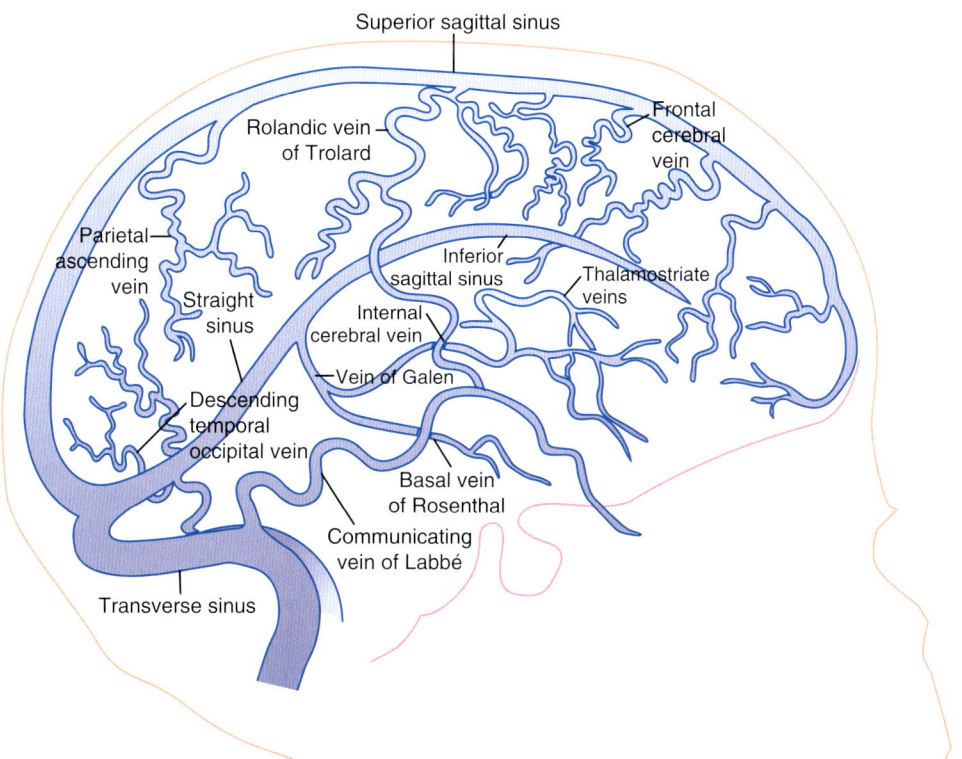

Figure 110-1. Cerebral venous anatomy.

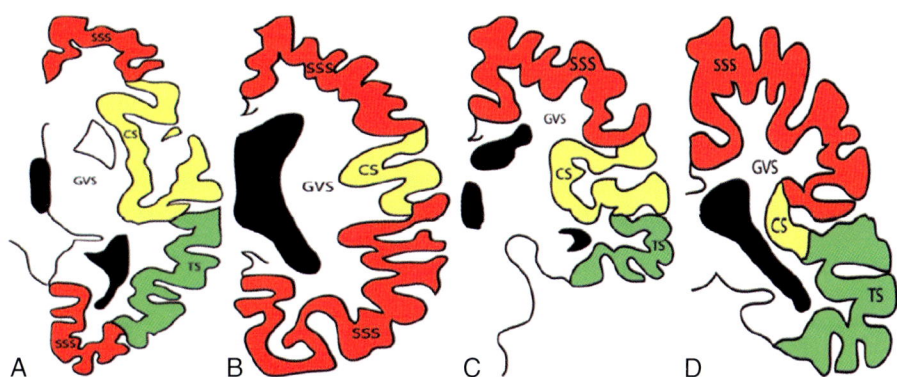

Figure 110-2. Intracranial venous drainage patterns. Diagram of cerebral venous drainage territories. Axial section at the level of the basal ganglia **(A)** and corona radiata **(B)**. Coronal section at the level of the basal ganglia **(C)** and thalamus **(D).** The venous drainage of the intracranial venous structures is depicted; superior sagittal sinus (SSS), transverse sinus (TS), cavernous sinus (CS), and galenic venous system (GVS). *(With permission from Teksam, M., Moharir, M., deVeber, G., Shroff, M., 2008. Frequency and topographic distribution of brain lesions in pediatric cerebral venous thrombosis. Am J Neuroradiol 29, 1961–1965.)*

damage. In essence, CSVT results from a net imbalance between "procoagulant" forces (excess) and intrinsic "fibrinolytic" mechanisms (relative deficiency).

Mechanisms of Brain Injury

Thrombosis within the venous system results in outflow obstruction and decreased venous drainage. This causes retrograde venous pressure elevation. It may occur locally in a single venous territory resulting in local/regional effect or globally when major venous sinuses are involved resulting in diffusely elevated intracranial pressure (ICP). This in turn causes elevated local capillary hydrostatic pressure resulting in fluid transudation across capillary channels. Hemorrhage can result from diapedesis of red cells through leaky capillaries. This explains the high rate of spontaneous hemorrhage in CSVT. Hemorrhage occurs mainly in intraparenchymal and intraventricular (IVH) compartments and more frequently in younger infants. Initially, the increased hydrostatic pressure may produce only parenchymal edema and neuronal dysfunction resulting in symptoms without infarction. Further rise in regional tissue pressure may eventually exceed the arterial inflow pressure causing critically low cerebral perfusion and permanent infarction. Alternative venous drainage can develop but this may require time. Therefore total and rapid thrombotic occlusion carries the highest risk of infarction and permanent damage. The severity and duration of clinical symptoms associated with CSVT depend on the involved anatomic site(s), thrombosis acuity and collateral drainage. If collateral venous circulation develops adequately and rapidly, significant venous obstruction is tolerable without decompensation. Embryonic venous collaterals can sometimes develop even in older children as a compensatory mechanism.

CLINICAL FEATURES

Clinical diagnosis of childhood CSVT is challenging due to the nonspecific nature of presenting neurologic symptoms and signs that can develop gradually over many hours, days, or even weeks. Abrupt onset can also occur. Diffuse neurologic signs and seizures are more common. Headache, lethargy, nausea and vomiting, and signs of raised ICP including papilledema and sixth nerve palsy are seen frequently. These are clinically indistinguishable from idiopathic intracranial hypertension (IIH); hence, CSVT must be ruled out in all children with suspected IIH. Acute symptomatic seizures are more common than in AIS ranging from 23% to 90%. Altered mental status ranging from isolated lethargy and irritability on the milder end of the spectrum, to frank coma on the severe end, may occur. However, frank coma can also occur. The clinical features of associated risk factors (see following section) are usually present at diagnosis. Given the nonspecific clinical manifestations of childhood CSVT, a low index of suspicion is essential in any child with unexplained raised ICP, seizures and encephalopathy.

RISK FACTORS

Risk factors readily are identifiable in most children. Multiple risk factors may co-exist in the same child and a broad range of investigations should be considered. Head and neck infections occur in nearly one in every three preschool children whereas other associations like systemic disease and trauma are clustered in older children.

Infection

Infection is a major risk factor for childhood CSVT reported in 24% to 62% of published cohorts. "Septic" CSVT is defined as thrombosis of venous sinuses associated with head and neck infections like otitis media, mastoiditis, sinusitis, meningitis, and, less frequently, intracranial abscess. Although the relative proportion of septic to nonseptic CSVT has decreased in general, infection remains an important and treatable cause of CSVT. Mechanisms include direct extension of infection from structures adjacent to venous sinuses causing thrombophlebitis. The infectious state per se also increases the risk of dehydration and a transient systemic prothrombotic state. Given the frequency of septic CSVT, thorough infectious disease history, physical examination, and diagnostic investigations must be sought in childhood CSVT.

Anemia

Anemia is reported in 10% to 20% of children with CSVT, though the pathophysiologic mechanism of CSVT is unclear. Iron-deficiency anemia (IDA) (Fig. 110-3) is most commonly reported in pediatric cohorts, though chronic anemias secondary to hemolysis, thalassemia, and sickle cell disease, have also been reported. Screening for anemia in CSVT is recommended though diagnosis may be difficult due to hemoconcentration in dehydrated children and the dilutional effect of parenteral rehydration.

Prothrombotic Disorders

Prothrombotic disorders are reported in 20% to 80% of children with CSVT; their pathogenic role remains uncertain. These figures exceed adult CSVT estimates (15% to 20%). Several case-control studies have reviewed the role of prothrombotic risk factors in CSVT. In a recent pediatric meta-analysis, thrombophilia increased the risk of AIS or CSVT, particularly when more than one abnormality was detected (Kenet et al., 2010). The detection of specific prothrombotic disorders has varied across studies due to lack of systematic and variable testing methods and normative ranges across different laboratories. These include genetic thrombophilias such as mutations in Factor V Leiden and Prothrombin G20210A genes, and deficiencies of protein C, protein S, and antithrombin. Prothrombin gene mutation significantly increases recurrent thromboembolism risk in children older than 2 years, especially in the setting of additional risk factors. Other disorders include anticardiolipin antibodies, elevated lipoprotein (a), hyperhomocysteinemia, and MTHFR homozygosity. Elevated D-dimer may be present in CSVT, but its clinical utility in children has not been determined. Most children with CSVT undergo prothrombotic testing, but the cost-effectiveness and yield of comprehensive testing is unknown.

Acute Systemic Conditions

Dehydration is the most common acute risk factor for CSVT. History and physical examination should screen for decreased fluid intake, excessive sensible and insensible volume losses, potential fluid shifts and third-spacing in systemic disease, urinary output, and physical signs of dehydration. Isolated emesis without diarrhea should not be presumed to be secondary to gastroenteritis. It may, especially when accompanied by headache, be one of the first clinical indicators of increased ICP. Nausea and emesis from increased ICP can compound preexistent dehydration and place the child at higher risk of thrombus propagation and venous infarction. Head trauma or cranial surgery may also lead to CSVT. Head injury-associated CSVT may result from a mechanical shearing injury of the venous endothelium and extrinsic compression of dural sinuses causing stasis. Head injury, as an associated risk factor in pediatric CSVT cohorts, ranges from 6% to 9% (Xavier et al., 2014). It is also important to consider CSVT in the differential diagnosis of infants with suspected nonaccidental head trauma due to overlapping radiologic features.

Chronic Systemic Conditions

Several chronic systemic diseases increase CSVT risk. Childhood cancers and their treatments carry potential risks including chemotherapy-related hypercoagulable states (L-asparaginase), antithrombin deficiency, infections secondary to compromised immunity, direct CNS involvement of cancer, cranial surgery, and neck venous catheters. CSVT occurs at a rate of 1 in 50 to 200 cases of acute lymphoblastic leukemia. In inflammatory bowel disease (IBD), systemic inflammation may combine with gastrointestinal disease factors such as dehydration, medications, and IDA. Conditions that lose protein (enteropathies, nephropathies, liver failure) may lead to relative deficiencies in antithrombin-III. Systemic lupus erythematosus is associated with procoagulants like lupus anticoagulant and antiphospholipid antibodies. Cardiac disease increases CSVT risk probably due to decreased venous return (cerebral venous hypertension) or treatments (jugular lines, ECMO, etc.). CSVT is also reported in association with steroid and estrogen-containing contraceptive use in teenagers (Fig. 110-3).

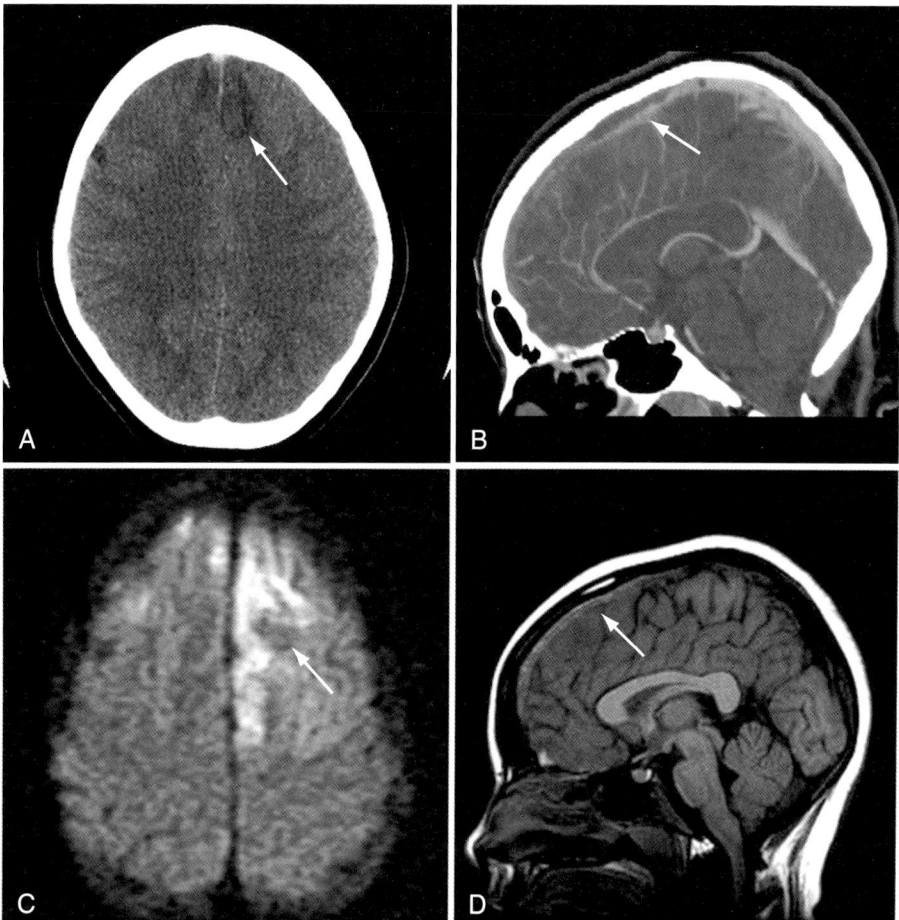

Figure 110-3. Iron deficiency anemia and birth control pill related CSVT in a teenager. A 14-year-old girl presented with increasing headache and new-onset focal seizures. She was being treated with iron supplements for iron deficiency anemia secondary to heavy menstrual bleeding. She was also on the birth control pill to regulate her periods. **A**, Axial plain head CT scan showing area of bilateral frontal parenchymal hypodensities. **B**, Sagittal CT venogram. **C**, Axial Diffusion-weighted imaging showing diffusion restriction of the frontal parenchymal lesions that eventually completely reversed on follow-up imaging. She was treated with low-molecular-weight heparin for 6 months with full recanalization of the thrombus. **D**, Sagittal T1-weighted MRI showing an occlusive thrombus in the anterior half of superior sagittal sinus. CT, computed tomography. MRI, magnetic resonance imaging.

DIAGNOSIS: NEUROIMAGING

Radiologic diagnosis of childhood CSVT poses some challenges. Awareness of pitfalls and limitations of imaging modalities and knowledge of variations in intracranial venous anatomy is needed to prevent misdiagnosis. The goals of imaging include direct visualization of the thrombus and parenchymal brain injury. Noninvasive modalities include cranial ultrasound (cUS) (applicable in newborns), computed tomography (CT), and magnetic resonance imaging (MRI). Each imaging modality has its own advantages and disadvantages. Imaging in pediatric CSVT has been extensively reviewed (Shroff and deVeber, 2003).

Computed Tomography

Plain CT (noncontrast) with estimated sensitivity of only 40% to 60% is not adequate to exclude CSVT. It can miss early edema or infarction and may underestimate as well as overestimate thrombosis extent. Caution is required to avoid false positive results, particularly in young infants with higher hematocrit, slower venous flow, and unmyelinated brain that may create an illusion of sinus hyperdensity. Subdural hemorrhage layering along the tentorium can mimic TS thrombosis.

Plain CT may be quite sensitive for deep system CSVT where there is STRS hyperdensity along with thalamic hypodensity or hemorrhage into thalamus or ventricles. Contrast-enhanced CT venography (CTV) is highly sensitive and specific for childhood CSVT diagnosis. Thrombus is represented by a filling defect in the vein/sinus in which contrast flows through a narrowed channel or bypass via venous collaterals. The empty triangle or "empty delta" sign is an example, seen with occlusion of the larger dural sinuses like SSS and TS. The "empty delta" refers to the shape of the enhancing dura encompassing the nonenhancing intraluminal clot on axial CT slice. A multislice contrast-enhanced CT with submillimeter slices and multiplanar reformations for axial, coronal, and sagittal views have significantly improved yield of CSVT. As CTV requires additional radiation exposure and most children will require serial scanning, age-adjusted radiation dosages must be considered.

Magnetic Resonance Imaging

MRI is the diagnostic modality of choice for pediatric CSVT. MRI lacks radiation and provides additional details of both brain parenchyma and the venous system. The need for sedation remains a drawback in young children. Combining MRI modalities sensitive to vasogenic edema (e.g., fluid-attenuated inversion recovery [FLAIR]), cytotoxic edema and infarction (e.g., diffusion-weighted imaging [DWI]) and blood products (e.g., susceptibility-weighted imaging [SWI]) can both confirm and characterize CSVT-related parenchymal changes. MRI can also image the thrombosis itself, providing more information on both the age and nature of the lesion. Subacute thrombus often appears hyperintense on T1/T2-weighted images. This can be helpful in cortical vein thrombosis in which filling defects are hard to visualize amid numerous artifactual mimics. Approximation of the age of the thrombus can be attempted on MR pulse sequences, but ultimately, this is difficult due to poor correlation between age of thrombus and its signal characteristics. Diffusion-weighted imaging (DWI) can be helpful in investigating the location and extent of associated parenchymal abnormalities, including edema and infarction. However, lesions with diffusion restriction must be interpreted with caution as many resolve on follow-up imaging. Restricted diffusion may also be directly observed within a thrombus and has been reported to predict incomplete recanalization in adults. An SWI is exquisitely sensitive to blood products and is very sensitive to detect hemorrhage and thrombus in smaller venous channels.

MR-venography (MRV) can employ time-of-flight (TOF-MRV), phase-contrast (PC-MRV) or contrast-enhanced methods to image the venous system in a comparable fashion to CTV. The TOF-MRV depends on flow signal characteristics and vessel orientation and is therefore subject to artifacts. As such, apparent "filling defects" on TOF-MRV are not equivalent to those observed with CTV and must be interpreted with caution. Expert interpretation is essential and confirmatory CTV may be required if abnormalities on TOF-MRV are equivocal. Contrast-enhanced MRV appears superior to TOF-MRV in adults but is less studied in children. The effects of flow turbulence are less than what is observed with TOF-MRV and contrast-enhanced MRV is better at delineating smaller veins and collaterals. The PC-MRV can overcome the limitations of TOF-MRV to a large extent, but has not been widely adopted yet in children.

Catheter Angiography

CA is rarely employed for CSVT diagnosis nowadays due to vastly improved CT and MRI. CA is typically performed only when thrombolytic or endovascular intervention is being considered. It adds dynamic information regarding the presence of collateral veins, delayed venous emptying, reversal of normal venous flow, or anatomic venous abnormalities.

TREATMENT

The three pillars of management of CSVT in children include: (1) antithrombotic therapy, and nonantithrombotic strategies such as (2) neuroprotection and (3) treatment of associated risk factor.

ANTITHROMBOTIC THERAPY
Anticoagulation Therapy

The role of anticoagulation therapy (ACT) in childhood CSVT is supported by adult clinical trials and pediatric cohort studies and ACT experience in systemic thrombosis. The goal of ACT is to maintain sinovenous system patency by preventing thrombus propagation and new thrombosis. The exact frequency with which children are anticoagulated is unknown as practice patterns vary even among pediatric stroke experts. Factors influencing treatment decisions include the child's age,

thrombus extent/location, CSVT propagation, ICH, reversibility of associated risk factors, and capacity to monitor ACT.

Randomized controlled trials in adults, although relatively small in sample-size, and large cohort studies have demonstrated improved survival and outcome in patients treated with ACT. Metaanalysis of adult data suggests good safety and a trend for efficacy, as well reduction in death and disability. In children, ACT safety is supported by recent cohort studies (Moharir et al., 2010; Grunt et al., 2010) though randomized controlled trials are lacking. In a single-center prospective study of 79 children, among 56 (71%) who received ACT only 3 (5%) had significant, but nonfatal, ICH due to ACT (Moharir et al., 2010). The study was underpowered to determine the effect of hemorrhagic complication on outcome. Two consensus-based pediatric-specific guidelines for AIS and CSVT management have been published by the American Heart Association (AHA) (Roach et al., 2008) and the American College of Chest Physicians (ACCP) (Monagle et al., 2012). These address the safety and efficacy of antithrombotic therapies in children and generally agree on the indications, contraindications, and duration of ACT for CSVT. More recently, specific guidelines for adult and pediatric CSVT have been published (Saposnik et al., 2011) that relatively contraindicate ACT only in the presence of "major" intracerebral/systemic bleeding. If ACT is not initiated at diagnosis, early repeat venous imaging (5 to 7 days) is indicated to exclude thrombus propagation and/or new venous infarction. It is important to note that one third of children with CSVT who are not treated with ACT will propagate their thrombus in the first week after diagnosis and 40% of these will develop additional parenchymal infarction and worse outcome (Moharir et al., 2010). A recent retrospective review of head injury-associated CSVT in 14 of 20 children anticoagulated in the subacute phase post-injury did not find any fatality or major hemorrhagic complication even with significant ICH (Xavier et al., 2014).

ACT options include intravenous (IV) unfractionated heparin (UFH), subcutaneous low-molecular-weight heparin (LMWH), and oral warfarin. LMWH is considered first-line in many centers. Intravenous UFH may be used initially when there is concern for increased hemorrhage risk, as UFH may be more easily reversed than LMWH. Warfarin is a reasonable alternative although there are challenges to maintain a satisfactory international normalized ratio (INR), particularly in young children. ACT needs close monitoring by periodic assessment of activated partial thromboplastin time (APTT), anti-Xa level, and INR. The duration of ACT typically follows common adult practice and is planned for 3 to 6 months (Moharir et al., 2010). Repeat venous imaging is performed at 3 to 6 months. If complete recanalization has occurred and none of the provoking risk factors remain, ACT can be discontinued. Longer-term ACT is required only if there are persistent risk factors for CSVT is expected or severe inherited/acquired prothrombotic states.

Endovascular Treatment and Thrombolysis

Neither the AHA nor ACCP guidelines endorse use of recombinant tissue plasminogen activator (tPA) or other thrombolytic therapies for pediatric CSVT given the lack of safety and efficacy data. Thrombolysis is usually reserved for cases in which there is a high risk of mortality (extensive CSVT, multifocal/diffuse infarction) or clinical deterioration despite adequate ACT during acute/subacute stage of CSVT. The decision to initiate this therapy must be carefully weighed using a multidisciplinary consensus approach. There is some adult data suggesting possible efficacy of thrombolytics/endovascular interventions in select circumstances. Publications in children are even more limited and include small case series only. Success has been reported with local catheter-mediated thrombolysis tissue plasminogen activator (tPA), mechanical thrombectomy, and agents like abciximab.

Nonantithrombotic Therapies

In addition to ACT, supportive and neuroprotective care is vital in CSVT treatment. Simple measures, such as maintenance of normal blood pressure, blood volume, glucose, and temperature, have been shown in adults to limit the extent of brain injury and are recommended in infants and children with CSVT (AHA Class 1, level of evidence C) (Roach et al., 2008; Saposnik et al., 2011). Head elevation to 30 degrees is also suggested.

Increased Intracranial Pressure

Screening, recognition, surveillance, and management of raised ICP are of paramount importance. Malignant ICP and resulting ischemic optic neuropathy can occur acutely or over the long term and be secondary to thrombosis, narrowed venous sinuses, or communicating hydrocephalus. Baseline fundoscopy at diagnosis and regular follow-up are required given that many children are not able to reliably report changes in vision. At-risk patients require repeat visual field testing and imaging. Treatment options include the temporary use of carbonic anhydrase inhibitors (acetazolamide, topiramate) or furosemide to lower CSF production, serial lumbar punctures, and, in resistant cases, lumboperitoneal shunting or optic nerve fenestration. Decompressive craniectomy in children with severely raised ICP secondary to ICH and impending herniation has been employed on a case by case basis, but there is no published data to guide the clinician at the bedside.

Seizures

Given the high incidence of acute symptomatic seizures during presentation, particularly in presence of parenchymal lesions (deVeber and Andrew, 2001), a low threshold for anticonvulsants is necessary. Timely recognition and treatment of seizures with standard anticonvulsants is warranted to prevent added brain injury. Consideration may be given for routine and/or continuous electroencephalogram (EEG) monitoring in selected cases. There is no evidence to support prophylactic use of anticonvulsants.

Steroids

Adult evidence suggests that steroids are not beneficial and may be harmful and/or a risk factor for CSVT. Therefore, routine pediatric use is not supported. However, this needs to be balanced for children with systemic inflammatory diseases such as irritable bowel syndrome (IBD), nephropathy, or malignancy.

Risk Factor Management

Judicious treatment of CSVT-associated infection in consultation with an infectious disease expert is essential. Surgical approaches may be necessary for localized infections in selected patients. Dehydration should be corrected and iron replacement considered in patients with IDA. Treatment of other systemic diseases that provoked CSVT is important. Other modifiable risk factors include removing jugular venous lines, altering chemotherapy protocols, or possibly replacing depleted anticoagulation factors.

OUTCOME

Outcome data are available in pediatric CSVT, although few studies have employed standardized outcome measures. Long-term follow-up is required to account for the full spectrum of morbidity after childhood brain injury. Consistent with this, 25% of children with CSVT followed in the CPISR showed increased severity of their neurologic deficits over time (deVeber and Andrew, 2001). Several large studies have shown that only 10% to 15% of adult CSVT patients have adverse neurologic outcomes. By contrast, the range of adverse outcomes reported in children ranges from 25% to 74%, implying heterogeneity in outcome measures and worse prognosis. Neurologic deficits range from mild to severe sensorimotor impairments, developmental delay, cognitive and behavioral difficulties as well as remote symptomatic seizures and epilepsy. The largest population-based, prospective cohort study of childhood CSVT (mean follow-up: 1.6 years) reported favorable outcomes in 48% only, including 35% with neurologic deficit and 20% with epilepsy (deVeber and Andrew, 2001). Mortality rates (comparatively higher in neonates) range from 4% to 25%, though the primary causes of death are often not described (deVeber and Andrew, 2001).

Adult predictors of poor outcome include presentation with coma, ICH, and DVS involvement. Predictors of poor outcome in children include comorbid neurologic conditions, ICH, and longer follow-up duration (Moharir et al., 2010). Of note, radiologic recanalization *beyond* the acute period after diagnosis does not seem to have any effect on the clinical outcome, but recanalization *rate in* the acute period may influence prognosis and thrombus propagation may potentially affect it adversely (Moharir et al., 2010).

In adults, recanalization rates appear maximal after 4 months of ACT, whereas in children maximal recanalization is achieved by 6 months (Moharir et al., 2010).

Persistent intracranial hypertension, communicating hydrocephalus, and visual sequelae have been reported in one of every three children. Twenty percent develop recurrent cerebral or systemic thrombosis (deVeber and Andrew, 2001). Fifty percent of these recurrences are systemic. These rates are comparable to adults (CSVT—12%; pulmonary embolism—11%). Recurrences are less common in children younger than 2 years of age at diagnosis.

REFERENCES

The complete list of references for this chapter is available in the e-book at www.expertconsult.com.
    See inside cover for registration details.

SELECTED REFERENCES

deVeber, G., Andrew, M., Adams, C., et al., 2001. Canadian Pediatric Ischemic Stroke Study Group. Cerebral sinovenous thrombosis in children. N. Engl. J. Med. 345 (6), 417–423.

Grunt, S., Wingeier, K., Wehrli, E., et al., 2010. Swiss Neuropaediatric Stroke Registry. Cerebral sinus venous thrombosis in Swiss children. Dev. Med. Child Neurol. 52 (12), 1145–1150.

Ichord, R.N., Benedict, S.L., Chan, A.K., et al. for the International Paediatric Stroke Study Group, 2015. Paediatric cerebral sinovenous thrombosis: findings of the International Paediatric Stroke Study. Arch. Dis. Child. 100 (2), 174–179.

Kenet, G., Lutkhoff, L.K., Albisetti, M., et al., 2010. Impact of thrombophilia on risk of arterial ischemic stroke or cerebral sinovenous thrombosis in neonates and children: a systematic review and meta-analysis of observational studies. Circulation 121 (16), 1838–1847.

Moharir, M.D., Shroff, M., Stephens, D., et al., 2010. Anticoagulants in pediatric cerebral sinovenous thrombosis: a safety and outcome study. Ann. Neurol. 67 (5), 590–599.

Monagle, P., Chan, A., Goldenberg, N., et al., 2012. Antithrombotic therapy in neonates and children: American College of Chest Physicians Evidence-Based Clinical Practice Guidelines (9th Edition). Chest 141 (2 Suppl.), e737s–801s.

Roach, E.S., Golomb, M.R., Adams, R., et al., 2008. Management of stroke in infants and children: a scientific statement from a Special Writing Group of the American Heart Association Stroke Council and the Council on Cardiovascular Disease in the Young. Stroke 39, 2644–2691.

Saposnik, G., Barinagarrementeria, F., Brown, R.D., et al., 2011. Diagnosis and management of cerebral venous thrombosis: a statement for healthcare professionals from the American Heart Association/American Stroke Association. Stroke 42, 1158–1192.

Shroff, M., deVeber, G., 2003. Sinovenous thrombosis in children. Neuroimaging Clin. N. Am. 13, 115–138.

Xavier, F., Komvilaisak, P., Williams, S., et al., 2014. Anticoagulation therapy in head injury-associated cerebral sinovenous thrombosis in children. Pediatr. Blood Cancer 61 (11), 2037–2042.

E-BOOK FIGURES AND TABLES

The following figures and tables are available in the e-book at www.expertconsult.com. See inside cover for registration details.

111 Vascular Malformations, Intracerebral Hemorrhage, and Subarachnoid Hemorrhage in Infants and Children

Lauren A. Beslow, Lori Jordan, and Edward Smith

 An expanded version of this chapter is available on www.expertconsult.com. See inside cover for registration details.

INTRODUCTION AND EPIDEMIOLOGY

Intracerebral hemorrhage (ICH) refers to bleeding into the brain parenchyma and/or ventricles, whereas subarachnoid hemorrhage (SAH) refers to bleeding into the subarachnoid space. Approximately half of childhood stroke is ICH and SAH. Incidences of ICH and SAH in pediatric patients obtained from a California-wide discharge database are 0.8/100,000/year and 0.4/100,000/year, respectively (Fullerton et al., 2003). This chapter focuses on nontraumatic or spontaneous ICH and SAH caused by ruptured vascular malformations.

Most childhood spontaneous ICH and SAH are caused by secondary causes such as ruptured vascular malformations, tumors, cerebral infections, or hematological abnormalities (Beslow et al., 2010). Even after a complete workup, 9% to 23% of childhood ICH/SAH remains idiopathic. Depending on the series, vascular malformations are responsible for approximately 17.5% to 73.5% of pediatric ICH; arteriovenous malformations are more common than cavernous malformations (cavernomas or cavernous angiomas) or aneurysms. Presentation and indicated studies will be included under each subtype and discussed in full online.

INITIAL MANAGEMENT

Stabilization of the patient and minimizing secondary brain injury are the goals of acute management. A neurosurgeon should be consulted promptly upon diagnosis of ICH or SAH. Basic management includes frequent neurologic examinations to assess for deterioration, keeping the head of bed elevated to at least 30 degrees to facilitate venous drainage, isotonic fluids, and maintenance of normoglycemia and normothermia. Children with seizures should be treated with an antiseizure medication.

There are no data from clinical trials regarding medical treatment in children with ICH. It may be a reasonable goal to lower blood pressure to the 95th percentile for age and sex. Elevated blood pressure in the setting of ICH can be an autoregulatory mechanism to maintain cerebral perfusion. Therefore caution must be utilized when lowering blood pressure in a child with ICH so that secondary ischemia is not caused, and ICP monitoring should be considered.

ACUTE MEDICAL AND SURGICAL MONITORING AND MANAGEMENT

Increased Intracranial Pressure: Signs, Symptoms, and Monitoring

Increased ICP can occur as a result of direct mass effect from an ICH or from intraventricular hemorrhage and hydrocephalus that can occur with ICH or SAH. Monitoring for increased ICP should be considered in any pediatric patient with ICH or SAH with abnormal or deteriorating mental status.

An intraventricular catheter (IVC), also called an extraventricular drain (EVD), is often the monitoring tool of choice because it can measure ICP and manage ICP via drainage of cerebrospinal fluid or intraventricular blood. A subdural bolt can be used to measure ICP if an IVC is not an option.

Increased ICP: Medical Management

Medical management for reducing ICP acutely is typically temporizing and includes hyperventilation to PCO_2 of 25 to 30 mm Hg, maintaining the patient's head midline and at least 30 degrees to facilitate venous drainage, and hyperosmolar therapy with either hypertonic saline or mannitol. Sedation is sometimes used. Corticosteroids have not been helpful in adult trials.

Increased ICP: Surgical Management
Intraparenchymal Hemorrhage Evacuation

Emergent supratentorial hematoma evacuation did not improve outcome in adults with spontaneous ICH in the Surgical Trial in Intracerebral Hemorrhage, but few young adults were enrolled. The 2010 adult ICH guidelines state that patients with cerebellar hemorrhage, with clinical deterioration, with brainstem compression, or with obstructive hydrocephalus from compression of the ventricles should undergo surgical hemorrhage evacuation. Children are less likely to have cerebral atrophy than older adults, and typically have lobar hemorrhages rather than deep hemorrhages. Urgent hematoma evacuation may be required to reduce mass effect and to prevent or relieve herniation syndromes.

Hemicraniectomy

Decompressive craniectomy may be both life-saving and function-sparing when there is rapid deterioration in the setting of a large arterial ischemic stroke or ICH in adult trials. In a series of 10 children with malignant MCA infarction, 7 underwent hemicraniectomy and all survived and had moderately good recovery. In a pediatric prospective cohort, 3 of 22 children with ICH had decompressive craniectomy; all were functionally independent (Beslow et al., 2010).

Seizures: Monitoring and Treatment

Seizures are a common presenting symptom and sequela of ICH and SAH. In a prospective cohort, over 40% of children with ICH presented with a seizure. For those who have seizures it is reasonable to treat with an antiseizure medication, at least in the acute period. The American Heart Association pediatric stroke guidelines recommend against prophylactic anticonvulsant use in the setting of ischemic stroke and do not make recommendations in ICH.

Continuous EEG monitoring should be considered in children who have 1) persistently altered mental status, or 2) movements or vital sign changes that are suggestive of seizure that cannot be captured on a routine EEG. Although continuous EEG has been used in children in the setting of SAH to detect vasospasm, there are no studies to demonstrate its utility for this indication in children.

RECURRENT HEMORRHAGE

In a population-based cohort of 116 children with ICH, 11 (9.5%) had recurrent ICH at a median of 3.1 months from the initial hemorrhage. Nine of 11 recurrences were in children with vascular malformations, 6 of which were not treated. The two children with medical etiologies of ICH recurred within 1 week of the incident hemorrhage.

OUTCOMES

Estimates of mortality after childhood ICH range from 5% to 54%. Predictors of mortality in one study included Hispanic ethnicity, older age at presentation (11 to 18 years vs. 1 to 10 years), coagulopathy, and coma. Poorer outcomes have been associated with ICH volume, altered mental status within 6 hours of presentation, infratentorial location, Glasgow Coma Score (GCS) less than or equal to 7 at admission, aneurysmal cause of hemorrhage, age younger than 3 years at the time of ICH, and underlying hematological disorders. In one prospective cohort of 72 children and neonates with ICH, 1- and 2-year seizure-free survival rates were 82% and 67%, respectively.

HIGH FLOW LESIONS
Arteriovenous Malformations

Cerebral arteriovenous malformations (AVMs) are characterized by abnormal connections of arteries and veins in the brain without intervening capillaries. Epidemiology and pathogenesis are discussed online.

Evaluation

Magnetic resonance angiography (MRA) or computed tomography arteriogram (CTA) can diagnose or suggest AVM in many cases. Conventional catheter angiogram (CCA) is more sensitive and should be considered when an underlying vascular malformation is not seen on MRI. Even when MRA or CTA diagnosis of AVM is made, a CCA should still be performed to characterize the lesion better and to assess for associated aneurysms, which may influence treatment. When a CCA is negative acutely after a hemorrhage, a follow-up CCA should be considered because a compressed AVM might become evident when the hematoma has resolved.

Treatment indications: The risk of hemorrhage from a cerebral AVM in children has been estimated at 2% per year (Fullerton et al., 2005), so most should be evaluated for treatment. Some AVMs may not be treatable because of their location or size. In a patient who presents with hemorrhage and is stable, it may be reasonable to wait a month or more for the hematoma to regress before definitive AVM treatment. In a comatose or deteriorating patient with an AVM, acute treatment may be required. The timing of AVM treatment after a hemorrhage is often dependent on the interventionalist and surgeon. The Spetzler–Martin system grades AVMs based on their characteristics in order to predict surgical risk of morbidity. AVMs are graded on size, adjacent eloquent cortex, and

venous drainage. Total score ranges from 1 to 5 points, with higher scores conferring greater risk. One study found that children have better outcomes than adults after microsurgical resection of AVMs, which is not explained by hemorrhage rates or AVM characteristics (Sanchez-Mejia et al., 2006). Therefore, surgical resection should be carefully considered in each pediatric case.

Treatment

Treatment options include surgical resection, embolization, stereotactic radiosurgery, or a combination (Fig. 111-1). Embolization rarely obliterates AVMs, and is more often used as an adjunct therapy to surgical resection or radiosurgery. Some pediatric data suggest that embolization alone may increase the rate of posttreatment hemorrhage relative to the natural history. Embolization before operative resection reduces flow to the AVM, thereby reducing the bleeding risk during surgery. Moreover, preoperative embolization in high-flow lesions may provide a staged reduction in blood flow over 24 to 48 hours, potentially reducing the risk of intraparenchymal hemorrhage. Embolization may also facilitate subsequent radiosurgery by reducing the nidus volume and immediately addresses the risks related to AVM-associated intranidal and extranidal aneurysms.

Surgical approach (microsurgery vs. radiosurgery) is typically based on both AVM location and anatomy. In children, evidence supports use of surgical resection (with or without embolization) as a first-line therapy in the majority of low- to moderate-risk AVMs contrary to the more controversial data in adult patients from the ARUBA trial.

Outcome/follow up: In a small series, intraoperative CCA was helpful because it detected residual AVM in 4/18 children who underwent intraoperative CCA, which resulted in immediate repeat resections. In this series, recurrent AVMs were found in 4/28 children with a recurrence risk of 0.08 per person-year. Recurrence was associated with diffuse AVMs. A second series demonstrated that intraoperative catheter angiography reduced postoperative residual/recurrent AVM rates from 14% to 0% in a cohort of 117 patients and that 1- and 5-year follow-up data indicated an overall annual hemorrhage rate of 0.3% and a recurrence rate of 0.9%. Therefore, although the duration and interval of long-term follow up for pediatric AVMs is not clear, data suggest that at least 5 years of imaging surveillance may be justified. Compared with adults, outcome after AVM resection seems to be more favorable in children.

Arteriovenous Fistulas
Definition

Arteriovenous fistulas (AVF) represent the least structurally complex variation of arteriovenous malformations, consisting of direct arterial-to-venous connections without intervening capillaries, occurring in the cerebral hemispheres, brainstem, and spinal cord. Connections can be single or multiple between an artery and vein. They differ from AVMs by the absence of a discrete nidus between the arterial feeder and draining vein. Two subtypes of AVF exist, defined by their location: pial or dural. Pathogenesis, epidemiology, and associated conditions are discussed online.

Presentation

AVFs pose a high risk of hemorrhage in addition to brain and spine injury secondary to high flow. Dural AVFs may also present with hemorrhagic venous infarctions secondary to venous outlet restriction. Overall, risk of hemorrhage has been reported at 1.5% annually, with specific risk factors, including fistulas at the vein of Galen, petrosal or straight sinus, venous

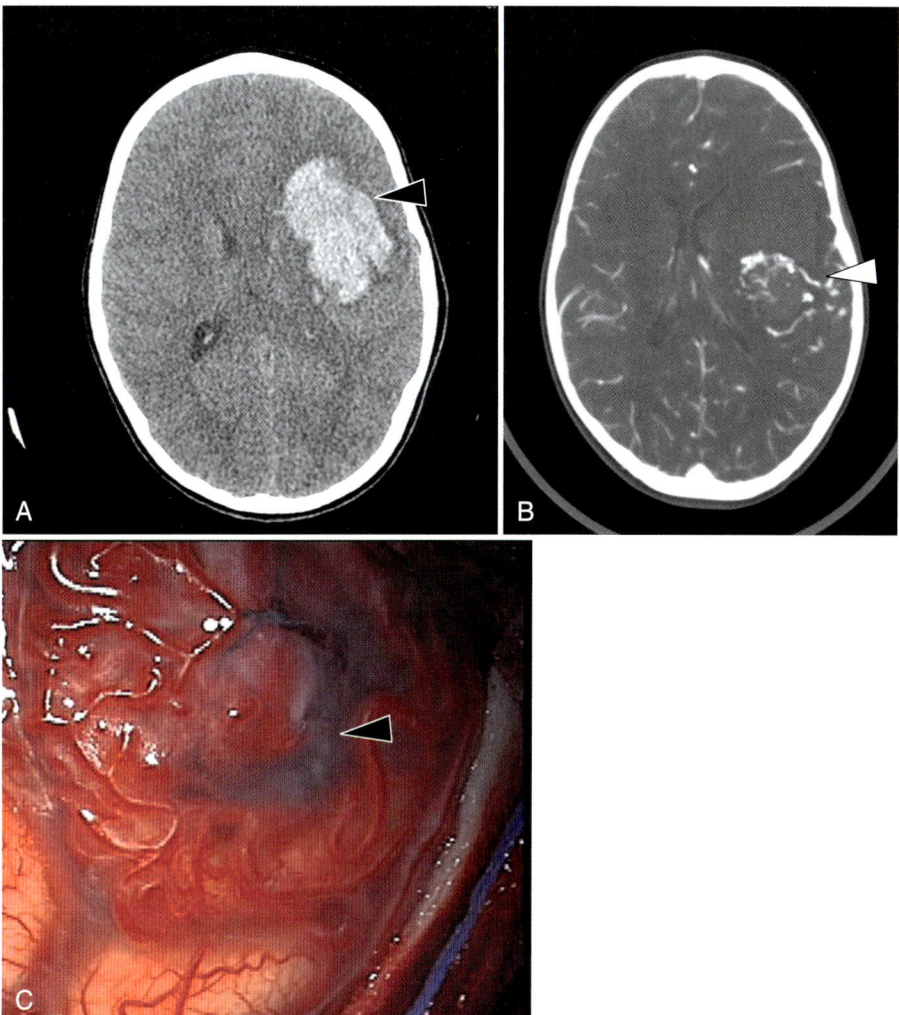

Figure 111-1. Left frontal arteriovenous malformation with hemorrhage. **A**, Noncontrast axial computerized tomography (CT) scan with left frontal intraparenchymal clot (black arrowhead). **B**, CT angiogram (CTA) in axial plane showing nidus of vessels at posterior aspect of clot, representing arteriovenous malformation (AVM; white arrowhead). **C**, Intraoperative view of cortical surface with AVM present; dark area (black arrowhead) represents visible intraarterial embolic agent (Onyx).

varices (especially with aneurysmal dilatation), and extensive cortical venous drainage. Specific to the pediatric population, AVFs may present with high-output cardiac failure, developmental delay, cognitive impairment, macrocrania, seizures, or with focal neurologic deficits from large venous varices exerting mass effect. Venous congestion may impair CSF absorption, leading to hydrocephalus. On physical examination in the case of carotid-cavernous fistulas (CCF), proptosis, chemosis, and loss of cranial nerve function in II–VI may be present.

Evaluation

Catheter angiography remains the gold standard for evaluation of AVFs. Seminal to the diagnosis is evidence of arteriovenous shunting directly into a dural sinus from meningeal branches of the external and internal carotid and vertebral arteries or a direct connection into a pial vein.

MRI is useful in the evaluation of AVF, but has limitations. Cross-sectional imaging may be nondiagnostic or may show only sinus thrombosis or dilated vessels. Cortical venous reflux may manifest as engorged cortical vessels without a clear fistulous connection. Cerebral venous hypertension may produce other findings, such as cerebral edema, hydrocephalus, and ischemic atrophy or infarction.

Treatment

Indications for treatment and recommendations for timing of treatment have evolved with development of novel technologies. Any symptomatic, high-flow lesion should be considered for treatment (Weon et al., 2005).

Dural AVFs involving the cavernous sinus (CCF) and transverse sinuses are distinct groups of AVFs relative to indications for treatment. Slow-flow, smaller lesions with minimal or absent symptoms may be followed with observation, as there is a possibility of spontaneous closure. However, high-flow lesions, or CCFs with symptoms—particularly visual deterioration—are high risk and warrant aggressive treatment.

Successful treatment of pediatric AVFs requires a team approach. AVF treatment involves endovascular or microsurgical techniques to close the fistulous connection (with isolated reports of radiation therapy for some cases). Recent data from pediatric AVF series suggest that dural AVFs have a higher likelihood of successful treatment using solely endovascular techniques (85%), whereas pial AVFs have a greater probability of combined endovascular-open surgical approaches (71%).

Outcome

Outcomes for children with AVFs are strongly related to age at time of treatment. For those older than 2 years, 72% had a good clinical outcome, whereas children under age 2 had higher complication rates and more frequently needed multiple procedures. Current reports of AVF treatment suggest high rates of lesional obliteration (86%), with age-appropriate outcome scores at an average of 16 months of follow up.

The risk of catastrophic complications from treatment is about 3% for adults, but the risk seems much higher in children, with procedural complication rates of up to 60% and major complications (and death) in the range of 10% to 12%. These risks are related most strongly to age, with children under 1 year having very high complication rates (up to 85%), and children older than 2 years having much lower complication rates (closer to 33%).

After treatment of AVFs, patients should be monitored for development of hydrocephalus, which may be a result of venous thrombosis, altered venous outflow, or deranged CSF dynamics.

Vein of Galen Malformations

Definition

Vein of Galen malformations (VOGM) are an AVF type.

Pathogenesis: There is abnormal development of cerebral midline venous structures. The choroidal arteries drain into a dilated vein, the median prosencephalic vein of Markowski, the embryonic precursor of the vein of Galen. Normally, this vein is present from 8 to 11 weeks of gestation, and then the anterior two thirds of this vein regress and the posterior one third persists as the normal vein of Galen. This regression does not occur in VOGM. Instead, arteriovenous shunts are present and the anterior segment of the median prosencephalic vein does not regress and instead progressively enlarges. Therefore a VOGM is a cluster of AVFs draining into a persistent and dilated median prosencephalic vein of Markowski. There are two types of VOGM, choroidal and mural. The choroidal type involves multiple feeders, including thalamoperforating, choroidal, and pericallosal arteries that are located in the subarachnoid space in the choroidal fissure. These vessels converge on a fistula site at the anterior aspect of the median prosencephalic vein and have little outflow restriction. This type of direct fistula has multiple shunts and tends to be seen in neonates with severe symptoms. The mural type corresponds to interposition of an arterial network between the arterial feeders and the venous structure. The fistulas may be single or, more often, multiple and converge into a single venous chamber or into multiple venous pouches. Presentation of the mural type is often with macrocephaly and is less severe. Combined or mixed types exist. Epidemiology is discussed online.

Evaluation

Ultrasonography is helpful for monitoring VOGM flow in an ill neonate. MRI assesses brain parenchyma; cerebral atrophy and ischemia may be present before treatment as a result of steal of cerebral blood flow by the VOGM. An echocardiogram assesses cardiac function.

Treatment

Urgent treatment in the neonatal period is necessary when a child has heart failure that cannot be managed medically. In neonates, high-output cardiac failure can lead to renal insufficiency, hepatic insufficiency, and rarely myocardial ischemia. In infants and older children, treatment is to prevent cerebral atrophy and cognitive delays.

Treatment: Endovascular treatment is the treatment of choice. The endovascular approach is typically staged. In the modern era, transarterial embolization is preferred at most centers, reserving transvenous embolization for instances in which transarterial embolization has been exhausted (Lasjaunias et al., 2006). In the neonate, the goal of treatment is to reduce flow through the VOGM so that heart failure can be medically managed. If the patient is stable, additional treatment is typically completed after 5 months of age. Hydrocephalus can be treated with CSF diversion. However, hydrocephalus can significantly improve with embolization of the VOGM, and therefore embolization should precede hydrocephalus treatment if possible. In rare cases of transtorcular embolization, a surgical window is created to provide venous access. Primary surgical repair of VOGM is not indicated.

Outcome

In a series of 27 children treated at a single center, outcome was worse for those with choroidal VOGM than for those with mural VOGM. Features associated with worse outcome were perinatal presentation, presence of CHF, and choroidal angioarchitecture. In a series of 233 patients with VOGM treated with embolization, overall mortality was 10.6%. Young age is a risk factor for death. Notably, 74% of surviving children were neurologically normal.

LOW FLOW LESIONS

Cavernous Malformations

Definition

Cavernous malformations (CMs) consist of dilated sinusoidal vessels lined by endothelium without intervening neural parenchyma (Gross et al., 2011, 2013). They are low-flow lesions that can range in size from submillimeter to several centimeters in diameter. Pathogenesis, epidemiology, and associated genetics are discussed online.

Presentation

CMs can occur anywhere in the central nervous system, with symptomatic lesions most commonly presenting with hemorrhage, seizure, or focal neurologic deficits. New seizure rates after the diagnosis of CM range from 1.5% to 4.3% per patient/year, and a history of previous seizure increases this rate to 5.5% per patient/year.

Evaluation

Evaluation of CMs usually begins with CT or MRI. CMs are generally poorly visualized with angiography. MRI studies are distinctive—typically, a "popcorn" appearance with an associated "bloom" on susceptibility imaging, suggesting hemosiderin deposition. If multiple CMs are seen on imaging, a familial or postradiation etiology should be considered. Developmental venous anomalies (DVA) are often found in association with CMs, approaching 100% in some series.

In patients presenting with acute hemorrhage, it may be difficult to ascertain the diagnosis. In children presenting with cystic or calcified lesions, the differential diagnosis may include tumors. Susceptibility imaging may aid in identifying evidence of previous hemorrhage or other CMs.

Treatment

Even though there are no evidence-based guidelines delineating indications for treatment in children with CMs, data generally support surgical excision of symptomatic lesions (seizure, focal headache, neurologic deficits), lesions with recurrent hemorrhage, or lesions with high risk of neurologic deficits (such as large lesions or those located in the posterior fossa). There has been debate regarding the utility of extirpation of asymptomatic lesions. The decision to intervene is especially difficult in the patient who presents with symptoms and has multiple lesions. If the symptoms can be localized to a single lesion, which is amenable to surgical resection, then that lesion should generally be removed.

Treatment

If treatment is planned for a CM, surgical resection is the preferred option. Radiation therapy is controversial and generally reserved for surgically inaccessible lesions with a demonstrated malignant natural history.

Outcome

Surgical outcomes have been remarkably good, with most series reporting a near 0% mortality rate and a 4% to 5% rate of new permanent deficits. Surgical resection of the most common type of CM in children, supratentorial lobar lesions, provides high rates of symptomatic improvement. With nearly 5 years of follow up, one large series demonstrated a 98% resection rate, no rebleeding in completely resected lesions, and abrogation of seizures in 96% of patients, with a 5% complication rate.

Close follow up is indicated in patients who have undergone surgical resection of a CM. CMs can recur if not excised *in toto,* and generation of new lesions has been documented, particularly in the setting of radiation-induced lesions and in familial cases. The length and frequency of monitoring with imaging remains a topic of debate; many institutions perform annual MRI studies for the first 3 to 5 years after surgery and then at greater intervals thereafter.

Aneurysms

Definition

Aneurysms are one of the most common vascular anomalies of the central nervous system, but are far less common in children than in adults. These structurally abnormal areas of arterial wall can cause bleeding, compression of adjacent structures, and concomitant loss of neurologic function. Pathogenesis, epidemiology, and genetic conditions associated are discussed online.

Presentation

Most aneurysms are asymptomatic and often are never detected. For those that are found because of symptoms, headache is most common (80%), followed by loss of consciousness (25%), seizure (20%), focal neurologic deficits (20%), and visual changes (10%). Children with SAH from aneurysm often present with less severe symptoms compared with adults.

Evaluation

Up to 80% of all nontraumatic SAH in children results from a structural lesion. A CTA can be a means of identifying the presence of an aneurysm. Patterns of hemorrhage in pediatric aneurysm CT studies include SAH (60%), intraventricular hemorrhage (10% to 15%), IPH (10% to 15%), and subdural (1% to 3%).

MRI is also useful in the diagnosis and delineation of the three-dimensional anatomy of an aneurysm, particularly with MRA. Use of catheter-based digital subtraction angiography

(DSA)—the "gold standard" of imaging in aneurysm—was able to identify lesional pathology in 97% of patients, versus 80% of the time without DSA. Three-dimensional angiography with computer-generated reconstruction is increasingly employed to depict lesional anatomy.

If the aneurysm is fusiform, the segment of vessel involved, delineation of normal borders, and involvement of perforators are important.

Treatment

If treatment is planned, success is predicated on removing the lesion from circulation while preserving normal blood flow. This can be achieved by open surgery, endovascular techniques, or a combination.

The advent of endovascular therapy has revolutionized the treatment of pediatric aneurysms. There is a great deal of evolution of this field, limiting long-term outcome data. Consequently, it is important, when possible, to have cases reviewed at institutions that offer both endovascular and open techniques in order to provide a balanced approach to formulating care plans (Hetts et al., 2009).

In general, aneurysms that have ruptured or that demonstrate enlargement over time or symptomatic lesions should be considered for treatment. Depending on location and patient status, it may be reasonable to treat aneurysms greater than 3 mm in size, particularly given the long expected lifespan of children. Mycotic aneurysms sometimes will regress with effective antibiotic therapy. In addition, flow-related aneurysms located proximal to a lesion like an AVM may regress after definitive treatment of the primary lesion, demonstrating another scenario when direct aneurysm treatment might not be required.

Although debatable, lesions 2 mm or smaller in size and those located outside the subarachnoid space are sometimes followed.

Outcome

Overall treatment morbidity and mortality vary widely dependent on age, aneurysm type, and presentation. Recent series describe average mortality rates of 1% to 3% and morbidity rates of 8% to 14% (Hetts et al., 2009; Kakarla et al., 2010). However, it is important to note that treatment of aneurysms often includes management of the posttreatment and posthemorrhage issues. These can include stroke, hydrocephalus, vasospasm, and electrolyte derangements.

Most patients spend a period of time after treatment in the intensive care unit. For patients with SAH, the first week or so after ictus is the key period for developing hydrocephalus, vasospasm, and cerebral salt wasting. Some patients may benefit from "triple-H" therapy—hypertension, hypervolemia, and hemodilution—in order to reduce the risk of vasospasm (only after aneurysm treatment). The benefit of calcium channel-blocking agents, such as nimodipine, is unclear in children.

There is a wide range of reported outcomes for pediatric aneurysms, with "good" posttreatment outcomes ranging from 13% to 95% and treatment-related mortality ranging from 3% to 100%. Shunting will be required for 14% of patients with hydrocephalus after SAH. Of patients who survive treatment, 91% (with a mean of 25 years of follow up) go on to enjoy independent living, with high rates of university graduation and employment. In one study of 59 patients with aneurysms treated in childhood and an average follow up of 34 years, 41% developed recurrent or de novo aneurysms after treatment. The annual rate of hemorrhage was 0.4%, with 4 deaths. The only identified risk factor for recurrent or de novo aneurysm development was smoking.

In addition to the periprocedural angiogram to confirm obliteration of the aneurysm, MRI and MRA at 6 months may be helpful as a baseline study, to then be compared with subsequent annual MRIs and MRAs. Imaging is performed annually for 5 years if feasible, with some centers suggesting lifetime imaging every 3 to 5 years thereafter. An angiogram is often performed 1 year postoperatively to confirm cure.

REFERENCES

The complete list of references for this chapter is available in the e-book at www.expertconsult.com.

See inside cover for registration details.

SELECTED REFERENCES

Beslow, L.A., Licht, D.J., Smith, S.E., et al., 2010. Predictors of outcome in childhood intracerebral hemorrhage: a prospective consecutive cohort study. Stroke 41, 313–318.

Fullerton, H.J., Achrol, A.S., Johnston, S.C., et al., 2005. Long-term hemorrhage risk in children versus adults with brain arteriovenous malformations. Stroke 36, 2099–2104.

Fullerton, H.J., Wu, Y.W., Zhao, S., et al., 2003. Risk of stroke in children: ethnic and gender disparities. Neurology 61, 189–194.

Gross, B.A., Lin, N., Du, R., et al., 2011. The natural history of intracranial cavernous malformations. Neurosurg. Focus 30, E24.

Gross, B.A., Smith, E.R., Goumnerova, L., et al., 2013. Resection of supratentorial lobar cavernous malformations in children: clinical article. J. Neurosurg. Pediatr. 12, 367–373.

Hetts, S.W., Narvid, J., Sanai, N., et al., 2009. Intracranial aneurysms in childhood: 27-year single-institution experience. AJNR Am. J. Neuroradiol. 30, 1315–1324.

Kakarla, U.K., Beres, E.J., Ponce, F.A., et al., 2010. Microsurgical treatment of pediatric intracranial aneurysms: long-term angiographic and clinical outcomes. Neurosurgery 67, 237–249, discussion 250.

Lasjaunias, P.L., Chng, S.M., Sachet, M., et al., 2006. The management of vein of Galen aneurysmal malformations. Neurosurgery 59, S184–S194, discussion S3–S13.

Sanchez-Mejia, R.O., Chennupati, S.K., Gupta, N., et al., 2006. Superior outcomes in children compared with adults after microsurgical resection of brain arteriovenous malformations. J. Neurosurg. 105, 82–87.

Weon, Y.C., Yoshida, Y., Sachet, M., et al., 2005. Supratentorial cerebral arteriovenous fistulas (avfs) in children: review of 41 cases with 63 non choroidal single-hole avfs. Acta Neurochir. (Wien) 147, 17–31, discussion 31.

E-BOOK FIGURES AND TABLES

The following figures and tables are available in the e-book at www.expertconsult.com. See inside cover for registration details.

Fig. 111-2 Vein of Galen malformation (VOGM).

Fig. 111-3 Cavernous malformation.

Table 111-1: Genetic disorders associated with cerebral cavernous malformations, AVM/AVFs, and aneurysms

Box 111-1: Hunt–Hess subarachnoid hemorrhage classification

112 Cerebral Arteriopathies in Children

Catherine Amlie-Lefond and Dennis W. Shaw

An expanded version of this chapter is available on www.expertconsult.com. See inside cover for registration details.

CEREBRAL ARTERIOPATHIES IN CHILDREN

The importance of cerebral arteriopathy in childhood stroke cannot be overestimated. The reported incidence of cerebral arteriopathy is 18% to 68% in children presenting with acute stroke, reflecting variable vascular imaging practices and challenges in diagnosis. More recently, in the Vascular Effects of Infection in Pediatric Stroke (VIPS) (Wintermark et al., 2014) study, vascular imaging on 355 children with arterial ischemic stroke (AIS) revealed definite arteriopathy in 36% and possible arteriopathy in 9.6% of patients. The incidence of arteriopathy among the 184 previously healthy children enrolled in the VIPS study was 42% with definite arteriopathy, 13% with possible arteriopathy, and 45% with no arteriopathy.

Recognition of cerebral arteriopathy is critical because it is a significant risk factor for primary and recurrent stroke in childhood. In addition, acute cerebral arteriopathy is a risk factor for poor outcome after stroke. Importantly, cerebral arteriopathy has been found in children in whom traditionally stroke has been ascribed to cardioembolic phenomenon, such as those with congenital heart disease. Despite increasing appreciation of the importance of arteriopathy in childhood stroke, diagnosis and management remain challenging.

Cerebral arteriopathy can be classified by etiology: genetic, traumatic, infectious, and inflammatory causes; and by pattern of vessel involvement: focal vs. multifocal, large vs. small vessel, anterior vs. posterior circulation. Sébire and colleagues have grouped arteriopathies into inflammatory vs noninflammatory (Sébire et al., 2004). These types of categorizations are confounded by the multiple and overlapping risk factors and etiologies. Multiple etiologies can result in a common pattern on arterial imaging. For example, the moyamoya pattern can be associated with underlying genetic syndromes, follow trauma such as radiation, or be idiopathic.

Arteriopathies traditionally considered noninflammatory—such as focal or transient cerebral arteriopathy and moyamoya—may have an inflammatory component to them. The picture is further hindered by the fact that the natural history of childhood cerebral arteriopathies is not well known, although arteriopathy often progresses after stroke in childhood. In addition, in children with AIS and cerebral arteriopathy, the risk of recurrent stroke is three times higher in children with progressive arteriopathy than those without progression (Danchaivijitr et al., 2006). Current classifications will need to evolve to incorporate these overlapping etiologic, radiographic, and pathophysiologic features.

FOCAL CEREBRAL ARTERIOPATHY/TRANSIENT CEREBRAL ARTERIOPATHY

Focal cerebral arteriopathy (FCA), characterized by focal intracranial arterial stenosis, accounts for approximately one fourth of arteriopathies in childhood AIS. A viral or inflammatory trigger has been proposed. FCA typically involves large and medium-sized arteries and is usually well visualized on MRA. Infarction of the basal ganglia is frequently seen, whereas associated cortical infarction is less common. FCA has been well associated with varicella zoster virus infection. Focal cerebral artery stenosis occurring within a year of primary varicella infection has also been called post-varicella arteriopathy.

A subset of FCA is classified as transient cerebral arteriopathy (TCA), defined as lack of progression or improvement of FCA at 6 months. In TCA, arterial narrowing will most commonly be seen unilaterally in the proximal middle cerebral artery (MCA). Similar to other FCA, TCA is believed to be likely a large and medium vessel acute vasculitis that occurs as a sequela of infection, most likely viral, and/or inflammatory (Figs 112-1, *A* and 112-1, *B*). If arteriopathy is stable at 6 months, it is most likely to represent TCA, but follow-up vascular imaging is a consideration because later progression can occur.

MOYAMOYA ARTERIOPATHY

In the setting of progressive FCA, there is often development of basal collateral vascularization representing moyamoya arteriopathy. Moyamoya is a progressive steno-occlusive disease typically involving the distal internal carotid artery (ICA), proximal MCA bilaterally, and not infrequently the anterior cerebral arteries (ACA). This arterial steno-occlusive disease is associated with development of extensive collaterals at the base of the brain, most commonly enlargement of lenticulostriate vessels producing the "moyamoya" (Japanese for "puff of smoke") configuration seen on catheter cerebral angiogram (Fig. 112-2, *A-C*). Basal collaterals are absent in both FCA and stage 6 moyamoya, but moyamoya will demonstrate external carotid collaterals.

Although the diagnostic criteria for moyamoya do not address the posterior circulation, steno-occlusive disease of the posterior cerebral arteries is present in approximately one fourth of cases. In addition, moyamoya can also occur unilaterally, or markedly asymmetrically, particularly moyamoya syndrome (discussed later). Involvement or progression of arteriopathy in the less affected hemisphere can occur over time in some cases.

Moyamoya has a bimodal incidence with a peak at 5 years and a smaller peak in the fourth decade. Moyamoya usually presents with bland ischemic stroke in childhood, whereas adults frequently present with hemorrhagic stroke. Moyamoya is often not diagnosed until stroke occurs. Acute stroke heralds the diagnosis of moyamoya in approximately half of all children with the disease, despite a history of transient ischemic attacks (TIAs) in many patients. The clinical picture can be unappreciated because TIAs are difficult to detect, particularly in very young children, who are most at risk of an aggressive course and poor outcome.

Children with moyamoya may present with headache and TIAs. TIAs frequently precede a sentinel stroke, which is confirmed by imaging. Signs of anterior circulation ischemia are often seen, including aphasia, dysarthria, hemiparesis, and seizures, but less common presentations, such as syncope, visual changes, and chorea can occur. Symptoms are often

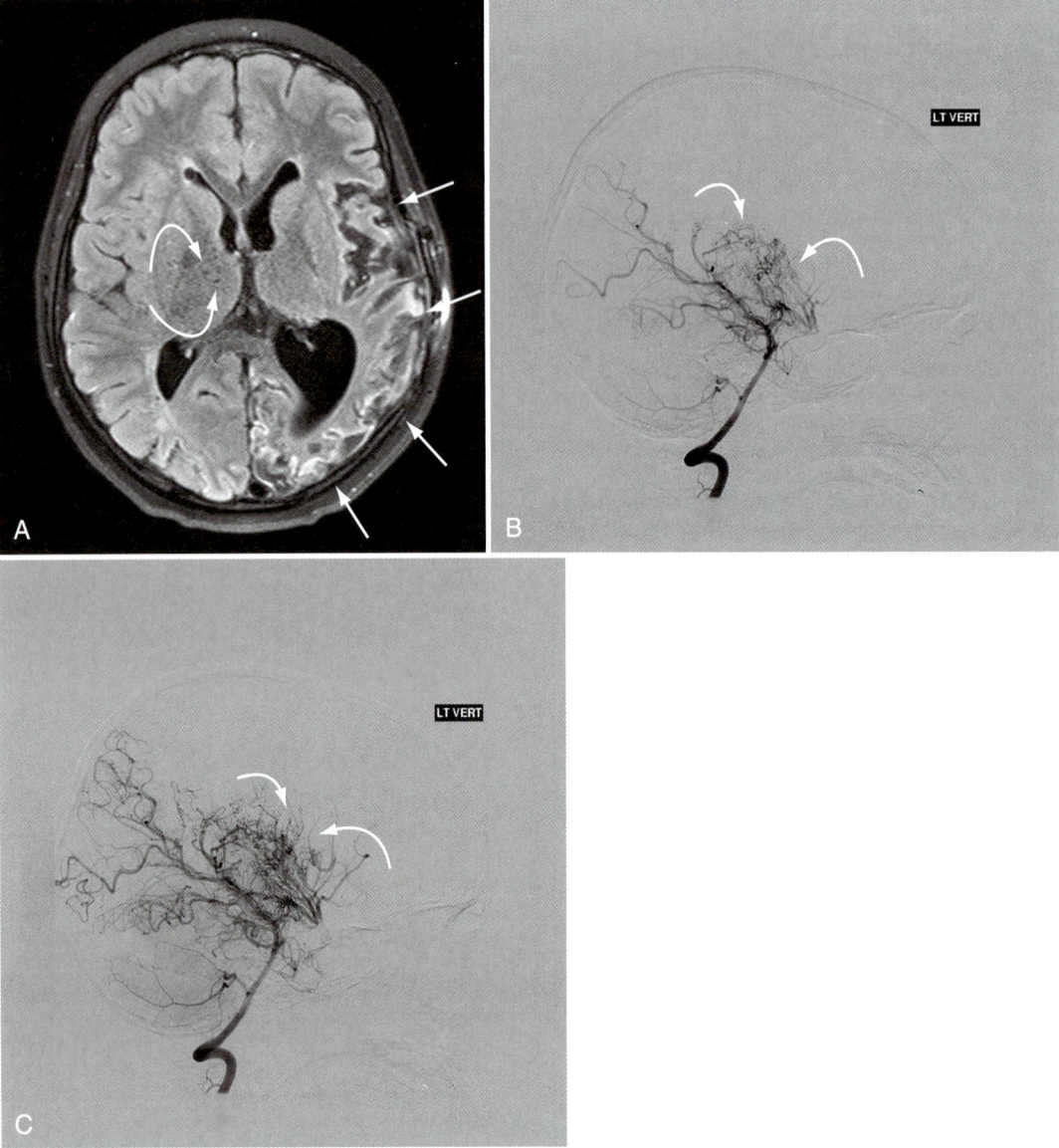

Figure 112-2. Moyamoya arteriopathy. A 10 year old boy with moyamoya and developmental delay presenting with TIAs then developing acute right hemiparesis and aphasia. Axial FLAIR image **(A)** demonstrates prior large left MCA stroke *(straight arrows)* and flow voids resulting from enlarged lenticulostriate collaterals *(curved arrows)*. Vertebral injection on a catheter angiogram in early **(B)** and mid **(C)** arterial phases demonstrate extensive central collaterals *(curved arrows)*, corresponding to flow voids on MR FLAIR, which provide delayed supply to the right MCA distribution.

provoked by hyperventilation, for example with crying or exercise, as a result of hypocarbia-induced vasoconstriction.

Moyamoya may be idiopathic ("moyamoya disease") or occur in association with syndromes ("moyamoya syndrome"), such as sickle cell disease and trisomy 21 or as the sequela of injury. The term "moyamoya disease," however, is often used more loosely to include both moyamoya disease and syndrome (Scott & Smith, 2009). Moyamoya is associated with many underlying genetic disorders, including sickle cell disease, trisomy 21, Noonan syndrome and neurofibromatosis type 1 (Table 112-1. See conditions associated with moyamoya online.)

Moyamoya disease is likely a genetic disease, most probably polygenic, based on the high prevalence of moyamoya in Asia and familial aggregation in 5% to 10% of cases. Approximately 15% of patients with nonsyndromic moyamoya (moyamoya disease) have a family history of moyamoya. The mode

TABLE 112-1 Conditions Associated With Moyamoya Arteriopathy

Genetic Syndromes	Trisomy 21
	Noonan syndrome
	Alagille syndrome
	Williams syndrome
Neurocutaneous	Neurofibromatosis Type 1
	Hypomelanosis of Ito
Hemoglobinopathy	Sickle cell disease
Metabolic	Glycogen storage disease type 1a
Trauma	Radiation injury
Infection	Tuberculous meningitis
	Human immunodeficiency syndrome
Autoimmune	Hyperthyroidism
	Antiphospholipid syndrome
Cardiovascular Disease	Coarctation of the aorta
	Pulmonary stenosis

of inheritance appears to be autosomal dominant with incomplete penetrance. Familial moyamoya in the Asian population has been linked to a susceptibility region on 17.q25.3, a ring finger domain containing protein 213 or RNF213.

Given the high risk of stroke in moyamoya, revascularization surgery is recommended for symptomatic patients to decrease the risk of further TIAs and ischemic and hemorrhagic stroke, as well as asymptomatic patients who are at risk of progression. Revascularization can be performed by direct or indirect measures. Direct revascularization most commonly employs anastomosing the superficial temporal artery to the middle cerebral artery. Indirect revascularization usually involves pial synangiosis where the superficial temporal artery is place on the surface of the brain. Direct revascularization has the advantage of immediate improvement in flow but is technically demanding, requiring a minimal artery size and therefore is not an option in very young children. Indirect revascularization has the advantage of not being limited to a particular arterial territory but requires months to show benefit as collaterals take time to develop. In children, direct and indirect revascularization appears equally efficacious with most centers preferring indirect revascularization due to lower surgical morbidity.

A 2005 review of the revascularization of pediatric moyamoya reported in the literature found that symptomatic benefit was independent of whether indirect or direct/combined approach was used. Revascularization not only reduces the incidence of ischemic stroke in childhood, but appears to decrease the risk of hemorrhagic stroke in adulthood as well. Revascularization should be pursued promptly in eligible children, particularly very young children, in whom the disease can be more aggressive with poor outcome.

ARTERIOPATHY OF SICKLE CELL DISEASE

Patients with sickle cell disease (SCD) are at an increased risk of stroke, including silent stroke. The Cooperative Study of Sickle Cell Disease (CSSCD) found that the incidence of ischemic stroke peaks in children between 2 and 10 years and again in adults older than 30 years. Without treatment, 11% will have stroke by 20 years of age and 37% will have silent strokes by age 14 years. The risk of recurrent stroke is decreased by regular red blood cell transfusions, or if this is not possible, hydroxyurea therapy. The risk of a recurrent stroke is approximately 20% even with the use of chronic red blood cell transfusion.

Approximately 25% of patients with SCD have cerebral arteriopathy, which is a risk factor for primary stroke, silent stroke, and recurrent stroke. In addition, SCD-associated arteriopathy often progresses despite red blood cell transfusions. Large vessel moyamoya-pattern arteriopathy vasculopathy is well described in SCD.

Elevated transcranial Doppler (TCD) velocity in the middle cerebral artery is strongly associated with stroke risk in SCD, and the incidence of first overt stroke is markedly decreased by regular red blood cell transfusions in children with increased velocities (Lee et al. 2006). Routine TCD monitoring is recommended for children age 2 to 16 years with SCD, although abnormal TCDs can be seen in children younger than 2 years. Reversion of elevated to normal TCD velocities with regular transfusions is well documented, as is subsequent reversion of normalized TCD velocities to elevated TCD velocities with cessation of transfusion.

Although chronic transfusions prevent development of stenosing arteriopathy in vessels with increased velocities, once arteriopathy is present, it can progress with resultant stroke despite use of regular transfusions. Similar to other types of moyamoya syndrome as well as moyamoya disease, once

arterial steno-occlusive disease is present, the only effective treatment for this moyamoya cerebral arteriopathy is indirect and/or direct surgical revascularization, which has been performed in patients with SCD and appears to be a safe and effective treatment.

CERVICOCEPHALIC ARTERIAL DISSECTION

Cervicocephalic arterial dissection (CCAD) has been reported to account for 7.5% to 20% of childhood AIS. CCAD involves the anterior cerebral circulation more often than the posterior circulation, and is more common in boys than girls in both the anterior and posterior circulation. CCAD can be posttraumatic or spontaneous. Spontaneous dissection may be more common in children than adults, although the history of trauma may be difficult to obtain in children. In addition, trauma may only be a trigger in a susceptible individual. For example, dissection is more likely to occur in the setting of infection or connective tissue disorder (Table 112-2. Risk factors for cervical artery dissection in childhood are available online only). Headache and neck pain are often present at diagnosis but this is not universal. Vertebral dissection may present with ataxia and vomiting. Diagnosis of dissection is important because these children are at significant risk for recurrent stroke, subarachnoid hemorrhage due to aneurysmal dilation, and recurrent dissection.

Dissection of the cervical carotid arteries most often occurs 2 to 3 cm above the carotid bulb. Dissections of the vertebral arteries most frequently involve the V2/V3 portion of the vertebral artery as it passes around the C1-C2 lateral masses and through the transverse foramina. In the anterior circulation, intracranial dissection is more common than extracranial dissection, whereas extracranial dissection is more common in the posterior circulation. Subarachnoid hemorrhage can occur due to vessel leakage or rupture of pseudoaneurysm formation. The risk of arterial rupture is higher following dissection of intracranial than extracranial arteries.

The diagnosis of arterial dissection is now most often made on magnetic resonance imaging/magnetic resonance angiography (MRI/MRA) (Fig. 112-3). Imaging should include the head and neck extending to the aortic arch and incorporate the use of T1W fat saturation or PD sequences to allow for visualization of intramural hematomas (methemoglobin) in a false lumen, which is usually seen in cervical arterial dissections. Narrowing of the true lumen, analogous to that demonstrated on catheter angiogram (CA), is usually seen on MRA, although subtle dissections, such as the C1-C2 level of the vertebral arteries, may be missed particularly in areas of turbulent flow.

Intimal flaps and dissecting aneurysm are diagnostic for dissection, as mentioned earlier, however, subtle lesions can be missed on MRI/MRA, or mistaken for other arteriopathies such as TCA. If the MRA/MRI is negative and there is still

TABLE 112-2 Risk Factors for Cervical Artery Dissection in Childhood

Trauma	
Infection	
Connective Tissue Disease	Ehlers–Danlos syndrome
	Marfan syndrome
	Loeys–Dietz syndrome
	Arterial tortuosity syndrome
Cervical abnormalities	Abnormalities of odontoid process
	Klippel–Fiel syndrome

significant clinical concern, cerebral catheter angiogram (CA) generally remains the most sensitive test for detecting subtle lesions. The findings on CA indicating CCAD are intimal flap and arterial stenosis and in more severe cases tapered occlusion and aneurysm formation. With advances in MR vessel wall imaging this approach may change because CA will not directly demonstrate arterial wall hematoma or inflammation.

Although computed tomography (CT) angiogram is often pursued in adults before pursuing a cerebral CA, not infrequently the cerebral CA is still required to confirm the diagnosis of a subtle dissection. In children, if there is still high suspicion for dissection after MRI, even with a normal or equivocal MRA, moving directly to cerebral CA is usually recommended as CTA requires significant radiation and may not be diagnostic. In a child with acute trauma or who is medically unstable, CTA may be the preferred study. Follow-up vascular imaging is indicated to assess for complications such as extension of dissection or formation of aneurysm. This can usually be accomplished with MRI/MRA.

The possibility of connective tissue disease, such as Ehlers–Danlos syndrome, Marfan syndrome, Loeys–Dietz syndrome, or arterial tortuosity syndrome, needs to be considered in patients presenting with dissection (Vanakker, Hemelsoet & De Paepe, 2011). In children with dissection who have hyperflexibility or other stigmata of possible connective tissue disease, evaluation including echocardiogram and genetics evaluation is indicated.

Vertebral artery dissection occurs more often in boys than girls and is often associated with head or neck trauma. Vertebral dissection most commonly involves the V2/V3 segment. Presenting symptoms often include abnormal eye movements, ataxia, nausea and emesis, and headache, although, in contrast to adults, neck pain uncommon. Vertebral artery dissection has been reported with cervical bony abnormalities in children, most commonly abnormalities of the odontoid process.

In adults, dissection is treated with antiplatelet therapy or anticoagulant therapy. Anticoagulant therapy is recommend for stroke due to dissection in childhood, with treatment duration based on follow-up imaging. Late complications after vertebral artery dissection, including pseudoaneurysm formation and recurrent stroke, have been reported. Recurrent dissection occurs in approximately 10% of patients. After cervical artery dissection, avoidance of potential triggering events such as contact sports, roller coasters, and chiropractic manipulation is recommended.

CENTRAL NERVOUS SYSTEM VASCULITIS

Central nervous system (CNS) vasculitis is an inflammatory arteriopathy that can be primary or idiopathic or secondary to a systemic cause, most commonly systemic rheumatologic disease or infection. CNS vasculitis can have protean manifestations that make diagnosis challenging, but early diagnosis and treatment are critical to prevent progressive encephalopathy.

Primary Central Nervous System Vasculitis

In childhood primary angiitis of the central nervous system (cPACNS), inflammation is limited to the arteries of the central nervous system (Moharir, Shroff & Benseler, 2013). cPACNS can be divided into large-medium vessel disease, in which arteriopathy can be detected on cerebral catheter angiogram, and small vessel cPACNS, in which it is not visible on a catheter angiogram. In large-medium vessel cPACNS, catheter angiogram shows irregularities, often described as beading,

most often involving the middle cerebral artery, anterior cerebral artery, and distal internal carotid arteries. In large-medium vessel cPACNS, brain parenchymal lesions involving these vascular territories may be detected on head MRI. Vessel wall thickening and inflammation may also be seen on MRI and MRA, particularly with use of vessel wall imaging.

Large-medium vessel cPACNS typically present hemiparesis, hemisensory dysfunction, or aphasia. Stuttering onset of ischemic symptoms, including TIAs, is common and may herald stroke. Inflammatory markers are frequently uninformative in large-medium angiitis. Only one third of children with large-medium vessel cPACNS will have CSF pleocytosis or elevated CSF protein. Treatment of progressive large-medium vessel cPACNS requires immunosuppression, including consideration of plasmapheresis in refractory cases. Anticoagulation or antiplatelet treatment may decrease the risk of artery to artery embolus in both progressive and nonprogressive large-medium cPACNS.

Small vessel cPACNS is particularly challenging to diagnose because the cerebral catheter angiogram is by definition unrevealing. The brain on MRI is usually abnormal, but findings are nonspecific. White- and gray-matter lesions can be seen, more often in the anterior than posterior circulation, with frequent involvement of the basal ganglia. Acute and subacute lesions may show DWI and ADC abnormalities consistent with ischemic stroke.

Patients often present with diffuse neurologic deficits and headache. Many patients have elevated inflammatory markers, including CRP, ESR, and CBC findings of leukocytosis, anemia, and thrombocytosis, but all can be normal in other patients. Analysis of the CSF may show mild predominantly lymphocytic pleocytosis and mildly elevated protein. In patients with suggestive neuroimaging and clinical findings, brain biopsy is critical to diagnose small vessel CNS vasculitis but may miss the diagnosis in a significant number of patients. High index of suspicion and prompt diagnosis is critical because treatment with immunosuppressants may prevent devastating injury.

Secondary Vasculitis

Secondary CNS vasculitis can be associated with multiple etiologies, including underlying systemic inflammatory or infectious disease, and malignancy. The arteriopathy associated with secondary CNS vasculitis often involves multiple sized vessels. MRA and CTA arterial imaging does not have the resolution to show abnormalities in small vessel vasculitis, but in medium and large artery vasculitis, irregular lumen and vascular stenosis may be seen on MRA and CTA. Cerebral catheter angiogram has greater sensitivity for luminal abnormalities but does not directly visualize vessel walls. In some cases, gadolinium enhancement of thickened arterial walls may be seen on MRA. Inflammatory markers such as erythrocyte sedimentation rate and C-reactive protein may be elevated, but are unreliable.

Takayasu arteritis (TA) is a chronic, granulomatous arteritis involving the aorta and its branches. Twenty percent of cases of TA present in childhood. Stroke frequently occurs due to vessel wall inflammation, thickening, and segmental stenosis, with thrombus formation, as well as aneurysm (Fig. 112-4). Corticosteroids and other immunosuppressants markedly improved outcome, but recurrent stroke and death from complications are not uncommon despite treatment. Polyarteritis nodosa (PAN) can be associated with arteritis, typically involving large-medium arteries but small arteries can be involved as well.

Systemic lupus erythematosus (SLE) can be associated with cerebrovascular disease, including ischemic infarct, TIA, and hemorrhage. Diagnosis is challenging because neuroimaging, including brain MRI, lacks sensitivity and specificity. Mechanisms of NPSLE arteriopathy include frank vasculitis, but noninflammatory microangiopathy with vascular hyalinization, endothelial proliferation and fibrinoid necrosis is the most common pathology.

Multiple infections have been reported in association with secondary CNS vasculitis, including Epstein–Barr virus, human immunodeficiency virus, parvovirus, *Mycoplasma* pneumonia, *Mycobacterium* tuberculosis, and acute bacterial meningitis. Heparin and aspirin have been used to prevent recurrent stroke in childhood bacterial meningitis.

Primary infection and reactivation of varicella zoster virus are both well reported associations with stroke in children and adults. Direct viral replication within the arterial wall by VZV is likely responsible for VZV vasculopathy. Confirmation of diagnosis of VZV vasculopathy requires virological confirmation either by the detection of VZV DNA by PCR in CSF or by the detection of anti-VZV IgG antibody in CSF, or both. Nagel and colleagues have shown that the diagnostic value of detecting anti-VZV antibodies in CSF is greater than that of detecting VZV (Nagel et al., 2008). Early diagnosis of VZV vasculopathy is critical because untreated it results in significant morbidity and death, and antiviral treatment can halt progression of disease or be curative. Treatment with both acyclovir and corticosteroids is recommended.

The VZV vaccine, recommended by the American Academy of Pediatrics in 1995, is not associated with childhood ischemic stroke, thus it is expected that it will result in a decrease in VZV-associated stroke in childhood as well as in adults.

The optimal use of antiplatelet and anticoagulant medication in CNS vasculitis is unknown, although most patients with secondary noninfectious CNS vasculitis are started on antithrombotic medication. Large vessel involvement or visible thrombus may be indications for anticoagulation. Although antithrombotic treatment has been used in small vessel arteriopathy, concerns about the risk of hemorrhage often outweigh concerns about thrombosis, particularly as it is not clear how effective antithrombotic medication is in preventing injury due to small vessel CNS vasculitis.

Fibromuscular Dysplasia

Fibromuscular dysplasia (FMD) is a noninflammatory arteriopathy of unknown etiology primarily affecting women age 20 to 60, but which can occur in children, with associated ischemic and hemorrhagic stroke in childhood. Typically, irregular narrowing ("string of beads") on angiography of the internal carotid and renal arteries is seen. The string-of-beads sign can be seen in other childhood arteriopathies, and most patients with pathologically proven FMD have less specific angiographic abnormalities including focal and segmental stenosis and occlusion, with a string-of-beads sign in only one fourth of patients. Diagnosis of FMD is important because these patients are at increased risk of stroke, TIA, dissection, and aneurysms. In addition, patients require screening for systemic arteriopathy, particularly patients with hypertension who may have renal arteriopathy.

DIAGNOSIS OF CEREBRAL ARTERIOPATHY

Prompt diagnosis is essential in the child presenting with possible cerebral arteriopathy, so that strategies to limit injury and prevent overt stroke or recurrent stroke can be instituted. Children with cerebral arteriopathy may present with TIAs or stuttering onset of stroke symptoms. Therefore cerebral arterial imaging is indicated in children presenting with an unex-

plained history of localized neurologic dysfunction, particularly with recurrent episodes.

Head CT is often the initial imaging study because it is widely available and can be done quickly and usually without sedation. This will identify acute hemorrhage but has limited sensitivity for the detection of acute ischemia. Confirmation of AIS usually requires MRI, as will evaluation of stroke mimics; therefore MR imaging should be pursued first, unless it is contraindicated. The MRI should include DWI early in the order of sequences; this will answer the question of whether an acute stroke is present because normal DWI excludes acute infarct with rare exception. This in turn will direct the choice of subsequent imaging sequences, although TIA may not have associated DWI changes. In suspected cerebral arteriopathy, whether or not acute stroke is present, arterial imaging with TOF MRA is warranted and may alter immediate management. A dedicated MRA (with arterial vessel wall imaging if available) may not always be feasible in the acute setting, but should be pursued as soon as possible.

MRA can be insensitive to subtle vessel irregularity especially in cases of dissection in areas of poor resolution, particularly given the propensity for dissection in areas with complex flow. If the brain MRI shows multiple infarcts attributable to a single vessel, imaging of the neck for evidence of dissection should be pursued. In cases with high imaging suspicion for dissection despite normal MRA findings, catheter angiogram is indicated.

Once the presence of cerebral arteriopathy has been confirmed, etiologic investigation is crucial. The medical history may suggest etiologies for specific syndromes, particularly in the case of moyamoya arteriopathy or secondary vasculitis. Physical examination may show features of connective tissue disease or collagen vascular disease. Systemic inflammatory markers may be informative in inflammatory or infectious arteriopathies. CSF evaluation for inflammatory markers or infection should be considered in children with arteriopathy of unknown etiology.

FOLLOW UP

Children with cerebral arteriopathy require close monitoring for progression of their arteriopathy and management of underlying associated conditions. In some cases, cerebral arteriopathy may herald systemic conditions. In addition, children with cerebral arteriopathy are at increased risk of renovascular disease with elevated blood pressures. Although blood pressure monitoring can be challenging in the very young or developmentally delayed child, it is an important aspect of the care of these children.

CONCLUSION

Cerebral arteriopathy is the most commonly identified etiology of stroke in childhood and is associated with poor outcome including recurrent stroke. Despite its importance, the underlying mechanism in many cases is elusive. It is likely that inflammation plays a significant role, even in arteriopathies not typically classified as "inflammatory." In this regard, the field of pediatric stroke is moving toward a model that incorporates radiographic, etiologic, and pathophysiologic features of underlying cerebral arteriopathies.

REFERENCES

The complete list of references for this chapter is available in the e-book at www.expertconsult.com.

   See inside cover for registration details.

SELECTED REFERENCES

Danchaivijitr, N., Cox, T.C., Saunders, D.E., et al., 2006. Evolution of cerebral arteriopathies in childhood arterial ischemic stroke. Ann. Neurol. 59, 620–626.

Lee, M.T., Piomelli, S., Granger, S., et al., 2006. Stroke Prevention Trial in Sickle Cell Disease (STOP): extended follow-up and final results. Blood 108, 847–852.

Moharir, M., Shroff, M., Benseler, S.M., 2013. Childhood central nervous system vasculitis. Neuroimaging Clin. N. Am. 23, 293–308.

Nagel, M.A., Forghani, B., Mahalingam, R., et al., 2008. The varicella zoster virus vasculopathies: clinical, CSF, imaging, and virologic features. Neurology 70, 853–860.

Scott, R.M., Smith, E.R., 2009. Moyamoya disease and moyamoya syndrome. N. Engl. J. Med. 360, 1226–1237.

Sébire, G., Fullerton, H., Riou, E., et al., 2004. Toward the definition of cerebral arteriopathies of childhood. Curr. Opin. Pediatr. 16, 617–622.

Vanakker, O.M., Hemelsoet, D., De Paepe, A., 2011. Hereditary connective tissue diseases in young adult stroke: a comprehensive synthesis. Stroke Res Treat 712903.

Wintermark, M., Hills, N.K., deVeber, G.A., et al., 2014. Arteriopathy diagnosis in childhood arterial ischemic stroke: results of the Vascular Effects of Infection in Pediatric Stroke Study. Stroke 45, 597–3605.

E-BOOK FIGURES AND TABLES

The following figures and tables are available in the e-book at www.expertconsult.com. See inside cover for registration details.

Fig. 112-1 A and **B,** Transient cerebral arteriopathy.
Fig. 112-3 Cervical dissection.
Fig. 112-4 Takayasu arteritis.

113 Coagulation Disorders and Cerebrovascular Disease in Children

Timothy J. Bernard, Sharon Poisson, Brian R. Branchford, and Ulrike Nowak-Göttl

 An expanded version of this chapter is available on www.expertconsult.com. See inside cover for registration details.

INTRODUCTION

Cerebrovascular disease in pediatrics is typically divided into three separate categories (Fig. 113-1): arterial ischemic stroke (AIS; Fig. 113-2), cerebrosinovenous thrombosis (CSVT; Fig. 113-3), and hemorrhagic stroke (Fig. 113-4). Within these separate classifications, disease in neonates (age from birth to 28 days) is usually considered separately from the childhood form (age 29 days to 18 years). This distinction originates from the different risk factors seen in childhood and neonatal disease, including coagulation disorders. As previously described (Chapter 20), neonatal stroke is further subdivided into perinatal AIS (PAIS) and presumed perinatal stroke (PPS), depending on whether the presentation is acute seizures and encephalopathy in the first few days of life, as seen in PAIS, or a chronic evolving hemiparesis at 4 to 8 months of life as seen in PPS (see Fig. 113-1). Coagulation disorders play a unique role in the etiology of each subset of pediatric cerebrovascular disease—AIS, CSVT, and hemorrhagic stroke—requiring tailored evaluation and management of each disease.

The purpose of this chapter is to review disorders of both excessive thrombosis and deficient hemostasis in the context of pediatric cerebrovascular disease. In addition to describing the specific evidence supporting the role of each coagulation abnormality within pediatric cerebrovascular disease, the authors describe the application of these data in clinical practice. The identification of coagulation disorders in pediatric cerebrovascular disease is essential to proper management of the disease, and may have implications for secondary prevention of cerebrovascular disease in these children and their similarly affected family members.

Thrombophilia, or a hypercoagulable state, is a general description of several inherited (lipoprotein (a), or deficiencies of natural anticoagulants [protein C, protein S, antithrombin], prothrombin gene mutation, or factor V Leiden) or acquired (elevated factor VIII, or antiphospholipid antibodies [APAs; lupus anticoagulant [LA], anticardiolipin [aCL] antibodies, or anti-β_2 glycoprotein Ib antibodies]) prothrombotic abnormalities (Table 113-1).

COAGULATION DISORDERS IN PEDIATRIC ARTERIAL ISCHEMIC STROKE

Acquired Thrombophilia (Bernard et al., 2011)

Presentation

Acquired thrombophilia in pediatric AIS is mostly studied in childhood AIS, although acquired thrombophilia may also play a role in PAIS and PPS. APAs are the most common acquired thrombophilia investigated in clinical practice in childhood AIS. Of particular concern are those patients who develop APA syndrome, defined outside of pregnancy as

vascular thrombus and positive APA (LA, aCL, or anti-β_2 glycoprotein-I [anti-β_2 GP]) present on two or more occasions, at least 12 weeks apart (Miyakis et al., 2006). Children with AIS and APA syndrome may present with stroke as the solitary clinical feature, although a history of previous venous thrombosis, thrombocytopenia, or livedo reticularis is highly suggestive. More rare presentations in children include ischemic bone fractures, or renal and celiac artery stenosis.

In childhood AIS, the role of APAs is also uncertain. Acutely, conventional APAs (LA, anti-β_2 GP, aCL) are elevated in 7% to 14% of cases, and increase to 25% of cases when including novel APAs (anti-protein S, anti-protein C, anti-prothrombin) (Poisson S, unpublished data). The incidence of APA syndrome in childhood stroke remains uncertain. A meta-analysis performed by Kenet and colleagues determined that there is a significant association between positive APAs and childhood stroke and neonatal stroke (Table 113-2; OR 6.95; CI 3.67–13.14) (Kenet et al., 2010), but influence upon recurrent risk remains uncertain. Finally, although APA syndrome may occur in neonatal stroke, preliminary evidence about the risk of recurrent events in these children suggests that the risk may be low, although further data are clearly needed. As a result of these preliminary studies in adults, the American Heart Association (AHA) recommends evaluating adults with idiopathic stroke for APA syndrome.

In addition to traditionally acquired thrombophilia, such as APA syndrome, other transient abnormalities of coagulation and the hematologic system have recently been investigated in childhood AIS. Iron deficiency anemia may be an independent risk factor for childhood AIS, occurring in over 50% of children (compared with 9% of controls). Transient elevations of factor VIII, D-dimer, von Willebrand factor (vWF), and PAI-1 have been observed in children with AIS, but the significance of these elevated prothrombotic factors remains uncertain. Future prospective studies in childhood and neonatal AIS are needed to evaluate the significance of these coagulation abnormalities.

Evaluation

In childhood AIS, the minimal evaluation for acquired thrombophilia should include conventional APA testing for anti-β_2 GP IgG/IgM, aCL antibodies IgG/IgM, and dilute Russell's viper venom time (dRVVT) (see Fig. 113-1). If these tests are positive in the acute setting, repeat testing should occur just beyond 12 weeks postischemia. Testing of neonates with isolated AIS and/or PPAIS remains controversial, as the treatment of APA syndrome in this setting is unclear. In the context of a positive family history of thrombosis or multiple thrombosis, APA testing for neonates is clearly indicated, but the extent of testing in isolated neonatal AIS remains uncertain.

In childhood and neonatal AIS, testing should also include evaluation of complete blood count (CBC) to assess for hallmarks of iron deficiency anemia (low mean cell volume and

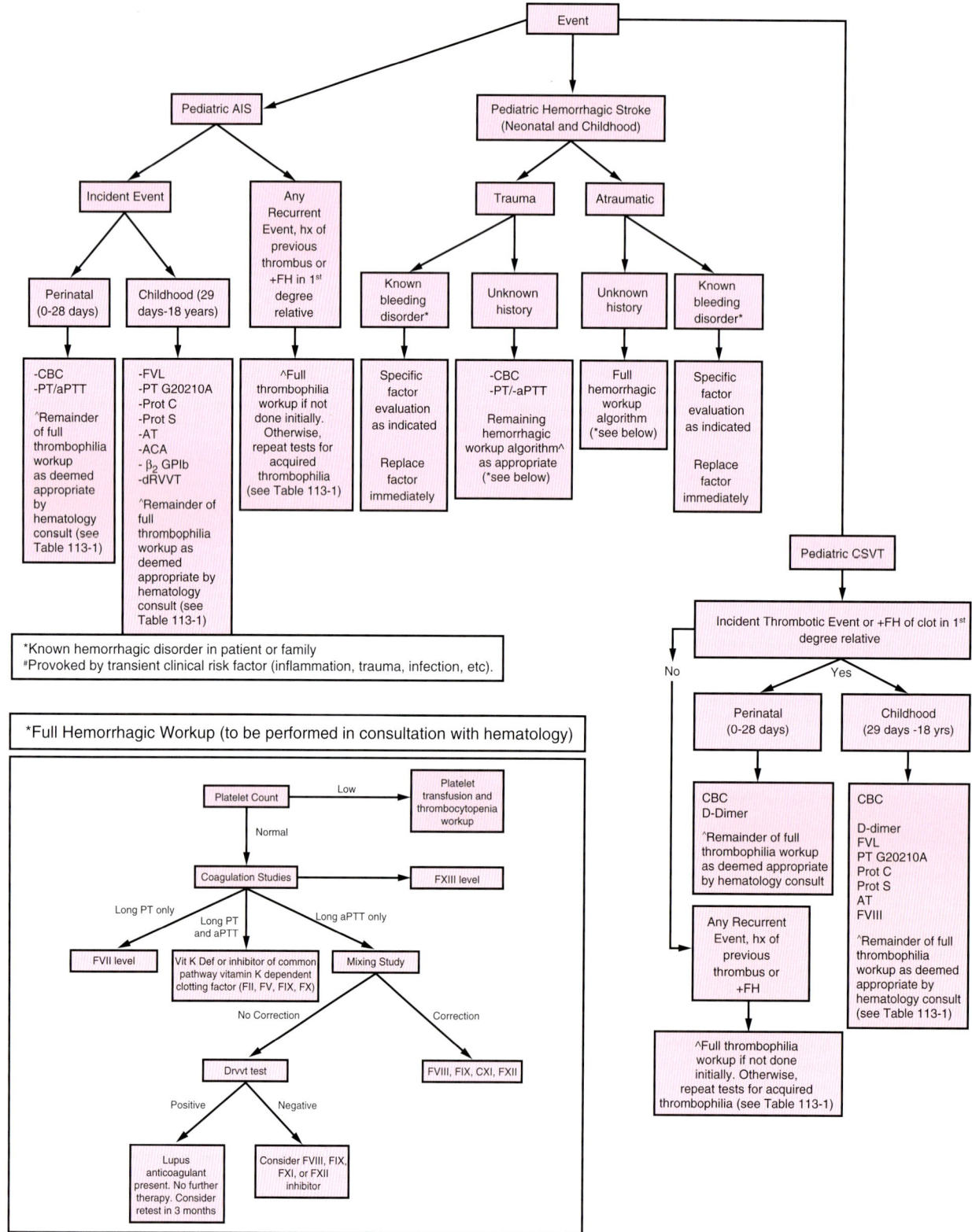

Figure 113-1. Guideline for thrombophilia evaluation and management in pediatric cerebrovascular disease.

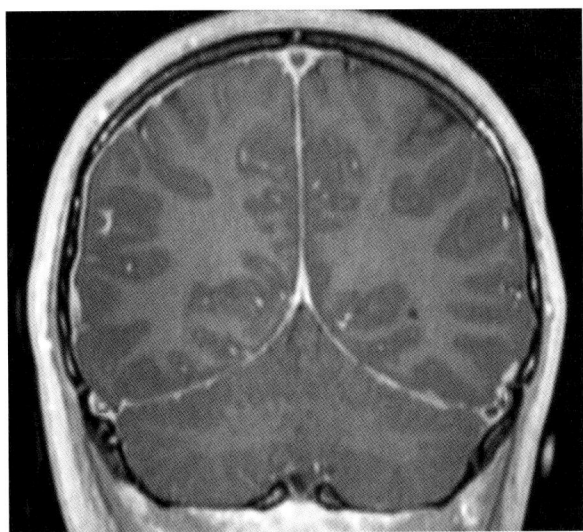

Figure 113-3. Contrast-enhanced coronal T1-weighted MR image illustrates the "empty delta" sign within the superior sagittal sinus in a child with cerebrosinovenous thrombosis (CSVT).

TABLE 113-1 Extensive Thrombophilia Evaluation to Consider in Pediatric AIS and CSVT

	Mild	Severe
Inherited	FVL heterozygous	FVL homozygous
	PT G20210A heterozygous	PT G20210A
	Prot C mild deficiency	homozygous
	Prot S mild deficiency	Prot C severe
	AT mild deficiency	deficiency
	Second Tier:	Prot S severe
	Lipoprotein (a)	deficiency
	MTHFR mutation	AT severe deficiency
	Hgb Electrophoresis	
Acquired	Lupus anticoagulant (dRVVT)	Lupus anticoagulant
	aCL IgG/IgM >40 MPL	(dRVVT)
	Anti-β_2 GPIb IgG/IgM	aCL IgG/IgM >99th
	>40 MPL	percentile
	Second Tier:	Anti-β_2 GPIb IgG/IgM
	FVIII level	>99th percentile

aCL, Anticardiolipin Antibodies; Anti-β_2 GPIb, Anti–β_2-glycoprotein Ib antibodies; dRVVT, Dilute Russell's viper venom time; FVIII, Factor VIII; FVL, Factor V Leiden; Hgb, Hemoglobin; MTHFR, methylenetetrahydrofolate; PT, Prothrombin; Prot, Protein reductase.

high red cell distribution width), while testing of factor VIII, D-dimer, vWF, and PAI-1 is likely practitioner dependent.

Treatment

Treatment of APA syndrome in neonatal and childhood AIS remains indeterminate, secondary to the lack of pertinent randomized trials. The AHA recommends treatment of adults who suffer AIS associated with transient APAs and AIS with antiplatelet therapy. Similarly, it recommends treatment of APA syndrome and stroke with antiplatelet therapy, while acknowledging the lack of consensus surrounding this recommendation. Indeed, the13th International Congress on Antiphospholipid antibodies recommends treatment of APA syndrome in adult AIS with anticoagulation alone, or combined with aspirin in more severe cases. It is the clinical practice of these authors to treat APA syndrome in childhood AIS with anticoagulation (usually warfarin or LMWH) while

the antibodies persist, but this approach remains largely unstudied. In neonates, treatment decisions may be influenced by degree of APA positivity, family history of clotting, and additional thrombosis. Given the lack of data about acquired thrombophilia in pediatric AIS, optimal treatment will likely include a multidisciplinary team of practitioners experienced in the treatment of stroke in children.

Genetic Thrombophilia (Bernard et al., 2011)

Presentation

Genetic thrombophilias vary greatly in their severity, with some abnormalities such as heterozygous prothrombin gene mutations or factor V Leiden only mildly increasing thrombotic risk, whereas others such as severe protein C or S deficiency significantly increasing the lifelong risk of clotting (see Fig. 113-1). Therefore genetic counseling surrounding these traits is best performed by a hematologist and/or genetic counselor who is familiar with these traits. In pediatric stroke, the prevalence of each of these genetic abnormalities is almost uniformly increased compared with matched controls (see Table 113-2), suggesting that thrombophilia, even when mild, may play an important role in pediatric AIS of all subtypes. Indeed, inherited thrombophilias have been associated with risk of stroke in multiple subtypes.

Some inherited thrombophilias, such as severe protein S or protein C deficiency, may be the underlying cause for childhood or neonatal AIS. Protein C deficiency is a well-established risk factor for childhood and neonatal AIS (see Table 113-2) and, when present, is likely to increase recurrence risk. Similarly, protein S is a risk factor for incident AIS that is often inherited. The risk of stroke recurrence with protein S deficiency has not been studied in a large cohort of childhood stroke. Some milder thrombotic traits, such as prothrombin G20210A, factor V Leiden mutations, antithrombin deficiency, and MTHFR C677T mutation have all been associated with incident childhood AIS (see Table 113-2) but their association with recurrence risk remains uncertain. The association between lipoprotein (a), another heritable mild thrombotic trait, and recurrent childhood AIS is of particular interest. Two separate studies have demonstrated an elevated risk of recurrent AIS in children with elevated lipoprotein (a) (RR = 4.4, 95% CI = 1.9–10.5).

Evaluation

Although the majority of genetic thrombophilia traits are established as independent risk factors for pediatric AIS, data supporting significant prognostic impact on recurrence risk exist only for a few individual traits such as elevated lipoprotein (a), protein C deficiency, and the presence of multiple risk factors. AHA pediatric stroke guidelines recommend that, "although the risk of stroke from most prothrombotic states is relatively low, the risk tends to increase when prothrombotic disorder occurs in children with other risk factors. Thus, it is reasonable to evaluate for the more common prothrombotic states even when another stroke risk factor has been identified" (Roach et al., 2008). Without an adequately powered study to detect the impact of genetic thombophilia on recurrence risk in pediatric AIS, definite recommendations about evaluation remain challenging (Manco-Johnson et al., 2002).

Treatment

In childhood AIS, patients should be treated with antithrombotic therapy from the onset of stroke, regardless of thrombophilia traits, unless a contraindication exists. The AHA and CHEST guidelines suggest acute treatment with aspirin (2 to

5 mg/kg) in most cases, reserving anticoagulation (typically LMWH or coumadin) in cases of dissection or cardioembolism (Monagle et al., 2012). The presence of a severe genetic thrombophilia or multitrait thrombophilia requires consideration of more aggressive treatment, such as anticoagulation in the chronic phase of secondary prevention, especially during times of increased clotting risk, such as prolonged immobility after surgery or trauma. Treatment decisions surrounding childhood stroke in the setting of multiple thrombophilia and/or genetic thrombophilia are best made by a multidisciplinary stroke team that includes a pediatric hematologist familiar with the multiple thrombophilia states and their implications across the human lifespan.

Sickle Cell Disease

Presentation

Sickle cell disease (SCD), particularly the hemoglobin SS variant, results in both small vessel infarctions and large vessel AIS because of moyamoya syndrome. SCD is the best studied hematological abnormality in childhood stroke, and presents one of the rare opportunities for primary prevention of stroke in children. The importance of stroke in children with SCD has been known for decades with an incidence of stroke in 285 per 100,000 per year in children with SCD. However, the great importance of silent infarcts upon cognition and outcomes has only been more recently recognized. Although children with SCD present with similar symptoms of stroke as those without AIS when infarcts are large, silent infarcts typically present with cognitive issues, including plateau and/or decline.

Evaluation and Treatment

Typically, stroke is not the presenting symptom for children with SCD, although a screening CBC with blood smear review and hemoglobin electrophoresis should be considered in any child with new-onset AIS. For acute AIS in the setting of SCD, both AHA and American College of Chest Physicians (ACCP) guidelines recommend urgent erythrocyte exchange transfusion to reduce hemoglobin S levels to less than 30% of total hemoglobin. In addition, primary prevention of stroke in children with SCD is possible through transcranial Doppler (TCD) screening for intracranial artery stenosis (Monagle et al., 2012 and Roach et al., 2008). In the multicenter randomized controlled STOP trial, 130 children with elevated velocity (>170 to 200 cm/s) of intracranial arterial blood flow as measured by TCD were randomized to regular exchange transfusion program intended to reduce Hgb S to less than 30% of total Hgb versus no intervention. In the untreated group, the yearly stroke risk remained over 10%, whereas in the transfused group the stroke risk was reduced to 1% per year (Adams et al., 1998). Therefore RCP and ACCP guidelines also recommend that children older than 2 years who have SCD be screened yearly with TCD and placed on a chronic transfusion regimen if found to have elevated TCD velocities. Unfortunately, the real-world impact of this finding has been imperfect, as many children with SCD remain unscreened or underscreened for arterial narrowing. Chronic transfusions should also be considered in children with silent infarcts in addition to those with abnormal TCD screening.

COAGULATION DISORDERS IN PEDIATRIC CEREBRAL SINOVENOUS THROMBOSIS

CSVT in children and neonates is a rare disorder, even compared with pediatric AIS, with an incidence of 0.67 per 100,000 children per year (DeVeber, 2001). Many risk factors outside of overt thrombophilias are associated with CSVT. In neonates, some other factors include birth trauma, delivery-related stress on the venous circulation, infection, and underdeveloped hemostatic systems. In children, trauma, dehydration, surgery, and infection are among the more common risk factors for CSVT. In addition, chronic systemic diseases, including inflammatory/rheumatologic disease, renal disease, and cardiac disease may contribute to CSVT risk. Among neonates with CSVT, prothrombotic states are found in about 20% and in children, estimates range from 24% to 64%.

Prothrombotic states may be the sole risk factor for CSVT or in combination with other risk factors. Previous studies demonstrated an elevated incidence of CSVT when a genetic or acquired hypercoagulable state is combined with a concomitant clinical risk factor for thrombosis. Interestingly, the prevalence of thrombophilias is higher in children with "idiopathic" CSVT (up to 85%) than in children with a CSVT provoked by a known clinical risk factor. In addition, the finding of multiple different genetic or acquired thrombophilias likely increases the risk of CSVT.

The role of prothrombotic factors likely differs between CSVT and AIS, as fibrin-rich thrombi are common in the low-flow system venous system, compared with platelet-rich thrombi as seen commonly in the high-flow arterial vascular system. Therefore workup and management of thrombophilias in patients with CSVT may differ from the management in children and neonates with AIS.

Acquired Thrombophilia

Presentation

In the neonatal and childhood period, the most common acquired thrombophilias are secondary to underlying medical illnesses. As example in children, cyanotic heart disease can lead to polycythemia, dehydration, cancer, or an endogenous hypercoagulable state. Similarly, infection is a well-known acquired cause of CSVT in neonates, with 23% to 73% of neonates and children with CSVT with a comorbid infection. Children with malignancies have a hypercoagulable state, which is most common in acute lymphoblastic leukemia (likely associated with L-asparaginase), followed by sarcoma and lymphoma. In addition, nephrotic syndrome in children is frequently associated with thromboembolism, occurring in up to 9%. Anemia is common in children with CSVT, most commonly iron deficiency anemia, although its role in the formation of thrombus is not clear.

Few studies have quantified the incidence of APA syndrome in childhood CSVT. Multicenter studies have reported the incidence or elevated RVVT is elevated in children with CSVT (4% to 11%), compared with controls. Among children with known APA syndrome, venous thrombotic events are common, occurring in up to 60%. However, only about 7% present with CSVT. In neonates, transplacental passage of maternal APAs from a mother with APA syndrome or systemic lupus is an uncommon cause of venous thrombosis. In several series of infants with perinatal thrombosis born to mothers with APA syndrome, only 10% to 20% had venous thrombosis, and all in the peripheral circulation. Neonatal APA-related CSVT has been described rarely, however. Several reports have documented APA-negative maternal testing, suggesting that there are some cases of de novo fetal production of APA's associated with CSVT.

Evaluation

As in AIS, evaluation for APA in children and neonates with CSVT is uncertain. In children or neonates with a history of multiple-site thrombosis or repeat CSVT, testing should include conventional APA testing for β2GP IgG/IgM, ACA antibodies IgG/IgM, and a dRVVT assay for LA (see Fig. 113-2). This same evaluation should be undertaken in children with idiopathic CSVT, or in those with other symptoms of APA syndrome. As in AIS, children who are found to have APAs in the acute setting should have repeat testing at least 12 weeks later to evaluate for true APA syndrome (Miyakis et al., 2006). When to test for APAs in neonates with CSVT and no other systemic thrombi is uncertain and somewhat controversial. Guidelines recommend that all neonates and children with CSVT should have a complete blood count to evaluate for anemia.

Treatment

Guidelines suggest treating childhood CSVT acutely with anti-coagulation unless there is a contraindication, continuing for 6 weeks to 6 months regardless of the etiology. In neonates with CSVT, anticoagulation is more controversial. Variability in treatment strategies for neonates exists across geographic regions, with some areas utilizing anticoagulation in almost all patients and others only initiating anticoagulation if clot propagation is seen on a 5- to 7-day scan. In childhood CSVT, however, anticoagulation is almost uniformly suggested at onset of CSVT, unless a contraindication exists. For children with CSVT without significant hemorrhage, CHEST guidelines suggest initiating anticoagulation. For children with CSVT and significant hemorrhage, CHEST guidelines suggest initiation of anticoagulation *or* radiologic monitoring of the thrombosis at 5 to 7 days and anticoagulation for thrombus extension (Monagle et al., 2012). APA syndrome has been found among adults with first ever idiopathic DVT or pulmonary embolism to increase the risk of recurrence by 4- to 7-fold, and so adult guidelines recommend anticoagulation for the duration of APA syndrome. As previously mentioned, these authors use a similar approach. There are no clear guidelines on the long-term treatment of neonates with CSVT and APA syndrome.

Genetic Thrombophilia

Presentation

Many inherited procoagulant disorders have also been found to be risk factors for venous thromboembolism in adults and children. In several systematic reviews, protein C deficiency, protein S deficiency, antithrombin deficiency, factor V Leiden mutation, prothrombin G20210A mutation, and lipoprotein (a) have been found significantly associated with first venous thromboembolism in children. Fewer data are specifically available regarding inherited thrombophilias in CSVT in children, though in a meta-analysis of the existing studies, all of these factors except prothrombin G20210A mutation remained significantly associated (Table 113-3). Although the prothrombin G20210A mutation is rare, it is the only inherited thrombophilia with evidence supporting its role in CSVT recurrence (OR 5.5). The role of inherited thrombophilias is even less clear in neonates. In fact, one prospective multicenter study of children and neonates with CSVT found no recurrence of venous thromboembolism in children under the age of two at onset of CSVT.

Diagnosis

Children with CSVT, especially those with no clear provoking factor, should have an evaluation for inherited prothrombotic conditions. The most important thrombophilias to evaluate are prothrombin G20210A mutation, factor V Leiden mutation, protein C, protein S, and antithrombin III. The utility of evaluation of other abnormalities such as lipoprotein (a), hyperhomocysteinemia and factor VIII is less clear, and interpretation and management of results is difficult. D-dimer may be drawn as a marker of clot formation and lysis to follow during therapy. In neonates, the utility of these studies is unclear. Because most children with CSVT are treated initially with anticoagulation, it is important to note that protein C, protein S, and antithrombin III levels can be falsely depressed if checked during the acute phase. Therefore it is critical to check these studies using serum from before the start of anticoagulation or 2 to 4 weeks after anticoagulation is discontinued.

Treatment

As discussed above, guidelines and standard practice suggest treating childhood CSVT in the acute period with anticoagulation in children and possibly neonates. As in genetic thrombophilia and pediatric AIS, the treatment team should include an experienced hematologist and/or genetic counselor who is familiar with clotting disorders in children. Given the current relative lack of data, it is reasonable to follow adult guidelines, which suggest consideration of long-term anticoagulation in patients with severe inherited thrombophilias, such as *homozygous* prothrombin G20210A or factor V Leiden mutations, or severe deficiencies of protein C, protein S, or antithrombin III. Long-term treatment should also be considered in those who have multiple genetic or acquired thrombophilias or recurrent events.

COAGULATION DISORDERS IN PEDIATRIC HEMORRHAGIC STROKE

Introduction

Hemophilia is the most prevalent coagulation disorder in pediatric hemorrhagic stroke. Hemophilia A and B, caused by deficiency of clotting factors VIII and IX, respectively, are X-linked bleeding disorders known for joint and soft tissue hemorrhages, but are also associated with intracranial hemorrhage (ICH) in 3% to 12% of patients with hemophilia that may cause disability and long-term neurologic sequelae. Morbidity in these cases is high, with neurologic deficit in 60% to 75% of the cases, and death in up to 20%. Patients with hemophilia are 20 to 50 times more likely to develop ICH than those without, particularly in the newborn period (4% rate compared with 0.1%), likely due in part to germinal matrix immaturity. Outside the neonatal period, the risk of ICH is approximately 300 to 800 per 10^5 patient years. The next sections will consider the different evaluation, management, and prevention approaches for patients with known disorders of hemostasis and those children who present with a priori ICH.

Evaluation

In any case of known or suspected ICH, emergent imaging is imperative, but the sequence of events differs based on the underlying diagnosis. If a known coagulation factor deficiency exists, that defect must be corrected immediately even as imaging is being arranged. If, however, the child has no known bleeding disorder, then the priority becomes imaging (rapid noncontrast CT unless MRI is immediately available, in which case it is preferred) and expert consultation with neurology, hematology, and neurosurgery to determine the next steps in what may be the result of either an accident in a healthy child or the first manifestation of a congenital or acquired bleeding diathesis. In this case once the child is stabilized, the focus should turn to the workup to rule out an undiagnosed underlying bleeding disorder or alternative cause of hemorrhage, including full history, physical examination, and a stepwise series of laboratory evaluations (see Fig. 113-1).

Treatment

The standard treatments for general ICH are limited, consisting of close observation, standard medical management, and consideration of neurosurgical intervention. In the particular setting of hemophilia, clotting factor replacement (or inhibitor bypass strategies if necessary) is an essential first therapeutic step. Treatment for known or suspected ICH in a patient with hemophilia must include immediate clotting factor replacement to the 100% level (with goal of trough level of 50% or greater), even at the same time the clinician arranges for diagnostic imaging. Expert consultation from pediatric hematology, neurology, and neurosurgery should also be sought. High levels of factor replacement should be continued for approximately 7 days and then taper to goal of 30% to 50% factor trough to complete 2 to 3 weeks, depending on the nature of the inciting event (if any) and interim clinical progression. Additionally, the use of antifibrinolytic agents may reduce the risk of rebleeding in subarachnoid hemorrhage and has been recommended as adjunctive therapy for hemophiliacs who suffer ICH. Patients with specific clotting factor inhibitors present a special challenge and may require the use of rFVIIa or prothrombin complex concentrates. If the hemorrhage is spontaneous, strong consideration should be given to subsequent prophylactic clotting factor infusion to prevent another event, because the rate of rebleeding after initial ICH may be as high as 26%. Primary prevention strategies for patients with known bleeding disorders begin with frank discussions at initial diagnosis about the dangers of head injury (as well as the possibility of spontaneous ICH in patients with severe disease) and continued reinforcement at subsequent clinic visits.

Regarding the perinatal period specifically, it is important to avoid instrumental delivery (vacuum extraction, forceps, etc.) and fetal scalp monitors if possible. Screening of other potential hazards, such as cephalopelvic disproportion, is also recommended. It is essential to avoid complication by superimposed hemorrhagic disease of the newborn with standard newborn vitamin K supplementation.

Secondary prevention is the focus in any child who suffers an ICH, especially those with an idiopathic presentation. It is imperative that the child with idiopathic ICH be worked up appropriately to determine the underlying coagulation disorder (see Fig. 113-1) and subsequently take appropriate preventative measures to decrease the likelihood of a recurrence. In cases with a known nonhematologic etiology such as traumatic brain injury or vascular malformation, children should be screened with a PT/PTT/INR, and further evaluation considered if the hemorrhage is out of proportion to what is expected from the inciting cause.

Other Rare Bleeding Disorders

ICH has also been described with other rare bleeding disorders, including neonates with vitamin K deficiency as well as severe deficiencies of factor II, factor V, and factor VII. ICH is also particularly common in factor X (up to 20% of affected individuals) and factor XIII (30% of affected) deficiencies, which are often also associated with umbilical cord bleeding. Specific diagnosis is important because it may change the therapeutic approach such as using factor XIII concentrate, for example. Physiologic concentrations of vWF and the proportion of high-molecular-weight multimers are increased in the neonatal period, likely secondary to the physiologic stress of the birth process, severe/type 3 form (complete vWF deficiency) may be apparent in the newborn period. ICH in the context of vWF requires much of the same management above, but the factor replacement product must also contain vWF.

REFERENCES

The complete list of references for this chapter is available in the e-book at www.expertconsult.com.
See inside cover for registration details.

SELECTED REFERENCES

Adams, R.J., McKie, V.C., Hsu, L., et al., 1998. Prevention of a first stroke by transfusions in children with sickle cell anemia and abnormal results on transcranial Doppler ultrasonography. N. Engl. J. Med. 339, 5–11.

Bernard, T.J., Manco-Johnson, M.J., Goldenberg, N.A., 2011. The roles of anatomic factors, thrombophilia, and antithrombotic therapies in childhood-onset arterial ischemic stroke. Thromb. Res. 127, 6–12.

DeVeber, G., Andrew, M., Adams, C., et al., 2001. Cerebral sinovenous thrombosis in children. N. Engl. J. Med. 345, 417–423.

Kenet, G., Lutkhoff, L.K., Albisetti, M., et al., 2010. Impact of thrombophilia on risk of arterial ischemic stroke or cerebral sinovenous thrombosis in neonates and children: a systematic review and meta-analysis of observational studies. Circulation 121, 1838–1847.

Manco-Johnson, M.J., Grabowski, E.F., Hellgreen, M., et al., 2002. Laboratory testing for thrombophilia in pediatric patients. On behalf of the Subcommittee for Perinatal and Pediatric Thrombosis of the Scientific and Standardization Committee of the International Society of Thrombosis and Haemostasis (ISTH). Thromb. Haemost. 88, 155–156.

Miyakis, S., Lockshin, M.D., Atsumi, T., et al., 2006. International consensus statement on an update of the classification criteria for definite antiphospholipid syndrome (APS). J. Thromb. Haemost. 4, 295–306.

Monagle, P., Chan, A.K., Goldenberg, N.A., et al., 2012. Antithrombotic therapy in neonates and children: Antithrombotic Therapy and Prevention of Thrombosis, 9th ed: American College of Chest Physicians Evidence-Based Clinical Practice Guidelines. Chest 141, e737S–e801S.

Roach, E.S., Golomb, M.R., Adams, R., et al., 2008. Management of stroke in infants and children: a scientific statement from a Special Writing Group of the American Heart Association Stroke Council and the Council on Cardiovascular Disease in the Young. Stroke 39, 2644–2691.

E-BOOK FIGURES AND TABLES

114 Bacterial Infections of the Nervous System

*Geoffrey A. Weinberg and Robert Thompson-Stone**

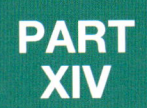 An expanded version of this chapter is available on www.expertconsult.com. See inside cover for registration details.

The brain is normally a sterile site that is protected from infection by specialized barriers, including the bony skull and the blood–brain barrier. Consequently, infections of the central nervous system (CNS) are comparatively rare, but they remain potentially devastating medical emergencies that can lead to death or severe neurologic sequelae. Injury to the brain from meningitis is a consequence of both the invasion by the particular pathogens and the host's ensuing overwhelming inflammatory response. The impact on mortality varies greatly by patient age, global location, and the causative organism, with high-risk patients including neonates and children in lower-income countries.

ACUTE BACTERIAL MENINGITIS

Bacterial meningitis involves inflammation of the leptomeninges, triggered by the presence of bacteria in the subarachnoid space. Prevention, prompt diagnosis, and aggressive management of acute bacterial meningitis remain the critical goals to prevent children from dying or suffering permanent neurologic sequelae (Brouwer, Thwaites, Tunkel, and van de Beek, 2012; Brouwer, Tunkel, and van de Beek, 2010; Kim, 2010).

Epidemiology

The epidemiology of bacterial meningitis in children and adults in the United States and elsewhere has changed drastically over the last 25 years with the global spread of conjugate vaccine initiatives, first significantly affecting infection with *Haemophilus influenzae* type b and then, later, *Streptococcus pneumoniae* and *Neisseria meningitidis*. In the United States, the median age at diagnosis of bacterial meningitis is now 25 years rather than 15 months as a result of the 99% reduction of *H. influenzae* type b meningitis incidence in children after initiation of routine conjugate vaccination.

In newborns, the most common causative organism for early-onset neonatal sepsis and/or meningitis (defined as occurring within the first 7 days of life) is *Streptococcus agalactiae* (group B beta-hemolytic streptococcus), followed by *Escherichia coli* and *Listeria monocytogenes*. With the use of intrapartum maternal antimicrobial prophylaxis for women found to be carriers of group B streptococcus, the incidence of group B streptococcus early-onset disease declined from 2 in 1000 live births in 1990 to 0.3 in 1000 live births in 2004 (Thigpen et al., 2011).

*The authors acknowledge work performed by Dr. M. Täuber and Dr. U. B. Schaad, the authors of this chapter in previous editions.

Pathogenesis

Most cases of bacterial meningitis likely arise from bacteremia, which is caused by invasion of the bloodstream by the pathogen after colonization of the nasopharyngeal mucosa. From the nasopharyngeal surface, encapsulated organisms adhere to, colonize, and cross the epithelial cell layer and invade blood vessels. Viral coinfection of the respiratory tract also may promote invasive disease, possibly by increasing epithelial invasion. After surviving host defenses in the bloodstream, the "successful" meningeal pathogen must cross the blood–brain barrier either transcellularly or paracellularly. In neonates, however, colonization or transmission may occur vertically during birth, or from bacteremia associated with intravenous lines or mechanical ventilation. However, not all bacterial infections of the CNS are the result of bacteremia. Nonhematogenous invasion of the cerebrospinal fluid (CSF) by bacteria occurs in situations of compromised integrity of the barriers surrounding the brain (e.g., otitis media, mastoiditis, and sinusitis). Bacteria also can reach the CSF as a complication of neurosurgery, spinal anesthesia, cochlear implantation, or ventriculostomy placement.

Clinical Manifestations

The cardinal manifestations of bacterial meningitis are fever, nuchal rigidity, toxicity, and alteration of consciousness (Box 114-1). However, the presentation differs based on age of onset and causative organism. Other focal neurologic signs sometimes can develop, including cranial nerve dysfunction. In particular, CNV III can be affected, leading to deafness and/or vestibular dysfunction. Seizures will develop in approximately one-third of patients either before or within the first few symptomatic days.

Children may demonstrate more nonspecific findings than do adults. The majority of children greater than 1 year of age (≥80%) exhibit fever, vomiting, and meningismus and toxicity on examination. Signs of meningeal irritation on examination include Kernig's and Brudzinski's signs. Kernig's sign is elicited by flexing the patient's hip and extending the knee to approximately 135 degrees in the supine position. The test is positive if the movement leads to pain in the hamstring and back (although in an ill or preverbal child, resistance of extension of the knee is considered positive). Brudzinski's sign is elicited by flexing the patient's neck in the supine position, and the test is positive if the patient involuntarily flexes the hips and knees. In contrast, the absence of meningeal signs does not exclude a diagnosis of bacterial meningitis, especially in infants younger than 12 months of age, who often do not exhibit nuchal rigidity with bacterial meningitis.

- Fever
- Nuchal rigidity
- Alteration of consciousness
- Irritability, photophobia, headache
- Vomiting, anorexia
- Kernig's sign
- Brudzinski's sign
- Seizures, focal neurologic deficits

Clinical Presentations of Neonatal Meningitis

In neonates and infants, the clinical features of bacterial
meningitis can be quite subtle, which necessitates a higher
index of suspicion. Meningitis in neonates is classified as
early-onset infection (within the first 72 hours of life) and
late-onset infection (from 1 week to 3 months of life). Those
with early onset may be more likely to be associated with risk
factors related to pregnancy and delivery, and more frequently
exhibit nonneurologic, nonspecific signs, mostly related to
sepsis and respiratory distress. Late-onset neonatal meningitis
is more likely to present with neurologic features in addition
to the nonspecific signs, including seizures (approximately
50%), focal neurologic signs (e.g., weakness), extensor rigidity,
and cranial neuropathies. A bulging or full fontanel is present
in one-third to one-half of cases and confers a 3.5 times
greater likelihood of bacterial meningitis.

Infection of Implantable Devices

Infections of CNS shunts may occur in as many as 5% to 10%
of patients, usually within 1 to 2 months of surgical insertion.
Most of these infections are a result of coagulase-negative
Staphylococcus or *Staphylococcus aureus;* however, a variety of
other organisms, including gram-negative bacteria and other
skin flora, can be causative. Clinical manifestations of CNS
shunt infection usually include low-grade fever, vomiting,
irritability or lethargy, and other signs of increased intracranial
pressure. The onset is often insidious but can be more acute,
particularly if shunt malfunction also is present. Neck stiffness
is uncommon. Shunt infection should be suspected in any
child with an indwelling CNS drainage system and fever. Some
children with CNS shunt infection may present with abdominal pain or even peritonitis, resulting from infected CSF
draining into the abdomen. Cochlear implants (neural stimu-
lators whose electrode is placed surgically in the lumen of
the cochlea) for severe to profound sensorineural hearing
loss can also predispose children to develop bacterial meningitis, especially that caused by *S. pneumoniae* (~80%) and *H.
influenzae* (~16%, both type b and nontypeable strains). Infectious complications from cochlear implantation are unusual,
but the incidence of *S. pneumoniae* meningitis in children with
cochlear implants is as much as 30-fold that of the greater U.S.
pediatric population.

Diagnostic Evaluation

The differential diagnosis of bacterial meningitis includes
viral meningitis, encephalitis, brain abscess, febrile seizure,
head trauma, subarachnoid hemorrhage, and leptomeningeal
neoplastic disease. In addition, unusual infectious agents,
such as fungi, rickettsia, *Toxoplasma gondii,* or *Mycobacterium
tuberculosis,* should be considered in selected patients.
Many other conditions may cause nuchal rigidity, including

chemical meningitis (from idiopathic reactions to oral
trimethoprim-sulfamethoxazole, nonsteroidal antiinflammatory drugs, intravenous immune globulin, and certain injected
monoclonal antibody therapeutics), ingestion of heavy metals,
infection of internal neck and throat structures, cervical
lymphadenitis, and Kawasaki disease.

The diagnosis of bacterial meningitis is based on examination of CSF, together with the clinical context of the patient.
Minimizing sequelae of bacterial meningitis depends on the
prompt initiation of effective antibiotic therapy, which therefore demands consideration of lumbar puncture early in the
evaluation and diagnosis of ill children.

Lumbar puncture for CSF examination is typically a safe
procedure and should therefore be performed whenever there
is even low clinical suspicion of meningitis. Four reasons
for delaying lumbar puncture exist: (1) clinically important
cardiorespiratory compromise; (2) signs of significantly and
focally increased intracranial pressure; (3) infection in the
skin, soft tissues, or epidural area at the site of lumbar puncture; or (4) suspicion or history of bleeding disorders. In these
circumstances, blood cultures should be obtained, and antibiotics are provided empirically. Even 12 to 24 hours after initiation of antimicrobial therapy, the interpretation of CSF white
blood cell (WBC) counts and protein and glucose concentrations is helpful in making a diagnosis. The CSF can sterilize
as early as 2 to 4 hours after initiation of intravenous antibiotics, and the chance of obtaining a positive CSF culture can
decline by one-third to one-half after 24 hours of therapy.

Neuroimaging studies are neither necessary nor adequate
for the diagnosis of bacterial meningitis, but may be undertaken for patients when there is concern for impending
herniation or intracranial mass lesions (e.g., subdural
empyema, abscess, stroke). It must be noted that many patients
with meningitis have some degree of increased intracranial
pressure by virtue of the disease process; the level of concern
among providers regarding herniation is typically out of
proportion to its likelihood, which is only 1% to 4% or less.
Herniation of the brain on removal of a small amount of CSF
is rare in meningitis. Thus performing computed tomography
(CT) scans routinely before lumbar puncture is *not* necessary
in all patients with suspected meningitis. Nevertheless, lumbar
puncture should be performed cautiously if significantly
increased intracranial pressure is suspected, especially if the
examination is difficult and the patient cannot be adequately
evaluated for focal signs. Obtaining CT scans before lumbar
puncture in *selected* patients is reasonable, especially for those
children or adults with a history of immunosuppression,
hydrocephalus, ventricular shunts, or head trauma, and in
those who have focal neurologic signs or who have signs of
greatly increased intracranial pressure.

Cerebrospinal Fluid Analysis and Other Laboratory Testing

The CSF opening pressure in children varies slightly with
body mass index (BMI) and level of sedation, but should
generally be less than 25 cm of water (with the 98 percentile
in children of 28 cm water) (Avery et al., 2010). The CSF
should be sent promptly to the laboratory for Gram stain,
bacterial culture, cell count and differential, and protein and
glucose concentrations. The Gram stain and bacterial culture
are very useful in confirming bacterial meningitis and identifying a causative organism early in the disease course. The Gram
stain is positive in approximately 70% to 90% of cases resulting from *S. pneumoniae, N. meningitidis,* gram-negative bacilli,
and *H. influenzae* type b, but it is positive in only 33% of cases
resulting from *L. monocytogenes.* Generally, bacterial cultures
will be positive within 2 days if pathogens are present.

TABLE 114-1 Characteristic Cerebrospinal Fluid (CSF) Findings in Children With and Without Meningitis

CSF Findings	Normal	Bacterial	Viral	Fungal or Tuberculous
LEUKOCYTES/µL				
Usual	<5	>500	<500	50–750
Range	0–10	10–20,000	0–1000	10–1500
POLYMORPHONUCLEAR NEUTROPHILS (% OF LEUKOCYTES)				
Usual	2	>80	<50	<50
Range	0–20	20–100	0–100	0–80
GLUCOSE, mg/dl				
Usual	60	<40	>40	<40
Range	45–65	0–65	30–65	5–50
Usual CSF/blood (%)	≥60	<30	30–60	<40
PROTEIN, mg/dl				
Usual	≤30	>100	<100	50–200
Range	0–40	40–500	20–200	40–1500
OTHER POSITIVE TESTS	None	Gram stain, antigen detection	Polymerase chain reaction	Cryptococcal antigen, acid-fast stain

(From Weinberg GA, Buchanan AM. Meningitis. In: McInerny TK, Adam HM, Cambell DE, Kamat DM, Kelleher KJ (eds). American Academy of Pediatrics Textbook of Pediatric Care, 2nd Edition. Elk Grove Village, IL: American Academy of Pediatrics; 2017. p. 2295–309).

TABLE 114-2 Representative Cerebrospinal Fluid (CSF) Findings in Neonates Without Meningitis

CSF Finding	Full-Term Neonates, Mean (Range)		Preterm Neonates, Mean (Range)	
	0–7 Days	*8–28 Days*	*0–7 Days*	*8–28 Days*
Leukocytes/µL	8 (1–30)	6 (0–18)	4 (1–10)	7 (0–44)
Polymorphonuclear neutrophils (% of leukocytes)	5	3	7	9
Protein (mg/dl)	81	64	150 (85–222)	148 (54–370)
Glucose (mg/dl)	46	51	72 (4–96)	64 (33–217)
CSF/blood glucose (%)	0.73	0.62	Not reported	Not reported

(From Weinberg GA, Buchanan AM. Meningitis. In: McInerny TK, Adam HM, Cambell DE, Kamat DM, Kelleher KJ (eds). American Academy of Pediatrics Textbook of Pediatric Care, 2nd Edition. Elk Grove Village, IL: American Academy of Pediatrics; 2017. p. 2295–309).

The majority (>90%) of cases of bacterial meningitis will have a CSF WBC count greater than 500 cells/µL, and polymorphonuclear leukocytes (PMNs) will predominate (>80% of the total count) (see Table 114-1). The CSF protein is elevated in the vast majority of cases of bacterial meningitis, and conversely, the CSF glucose is low (Table 114-1). When considering CSF WBC counts in neonates, one needs to reference the common normative values in that population (see Table 114-2). Other diagnostic tests on the CSF, such as polymerase chain reaction (PCR) amplification tests for microbial nucleic acid detection, may be used as an adjunct diagnostic study to the CSF bacterial culture. When available, these tests are quite sensitive.

The main ancillary study that aids in the diagnosis of bacterial meningitis is blood culture, which can be especially helpful if antibiotics need to be started before lumbar puncture. Blood culture can identify the causative organism in up to 80% of cases. Various prediction models based on CSF characteristics have been developed in an attempt to help identify children at very low risk for bacterial meningitis, who might then be managed outside of the hospital. However, such models are most valuable in excluding the diagnosis of bacterial meningitis, rather than establishing it (i.e., "rules out," but does not "rule in").

Neuroimaging

As discussed previously, neuroimaging studies are neither necessary nor sufficient to diagnose bacterial meningitis. However, neuroimaging may be very useful in the following situations: (1) assessing the safety of lumbar puncture when signs of focal neurologic dysfunction and/or raised intracranial pressure are present; (2) defining unusual anatomic causes of persistent seizures, fever, or focal neurologic dysfunction after treatment has been started (e.g., infected subdural effusion, brain abscess); (3) assessing neurologic deterioration; and (4) assessing for secondary complications (e.g., hydrocephalus, venous or arterial infarctions, ventriculitis).

Complications

Pathophysiologic Changes

The permeability of the blood–brain barrier increases in meningitis, and this increase contributes to vasogenic brain edema. Brain edema contributes substantially to the acute fatal outcome of bacterial meningitis. The major dangers of extensive brain edema during meningitis are herniation of brain tissue and compression of the brainstem secondary to focally increased intracranial pressure, which can cause complete cessation of cerebral circulation.

Patients with acute meningitis often present with hypovolemia secondary to dehydration, and some develop hyponatremia. Syndrome of inappropriate antidiuretic hormone secretion (SIADH), with fluid retention and hypotonicity of the extracellular fluid, has been reported to be present in 29% to 88% of patients with bacterial meningitis. However, differences in definitions of whether ADH secretion is "inappropriate" for the degree of dehydration may be a factor in the wide ranges of the estimates of SIADH prevalence. It appears that the overall risk of worsened clinical outcome as a result of SIADH is small and does not justify routine fluid restrictions in patients with meningitis and hyponatremia.

Increased intracranial pressure is present early in most patients with bacterial meningitis, yet in general, it neither contraindicates lumbar puncture nor leads to severe sequelae. The symptoms of massively increased intracranial pressure in meningitis are seizures and coma. In very advanced disease, signs of critical impairment of cerebral blood flow or impending herniation, such as unresponsive pupils, decorticate or decerebrate posturing, abnormal respiratory patterns, bradycardia, elevated blood pressure, and irregular vital signs, are observed.

In the early phase of bacterial meningitis, an increase in cerebral blood flow is observed, but as the disease progresses, cerebral blood flow reductions are observed globally and focally. Focal ischemia is the result of vascular involvement of cerebral arteries and veins caused by inflammation of the subarachnoid space, and ischemia is likely an important mediator of brain damage in meningitis.

Seizures

Seizures complicate 20% to 30% of cases of childhood bacterial meningitis. They occur most frequently 2 to 3 days into the illness and cease 1 to 3 days later. Seizures may be focal or generalized, and the electroencephalogram (EEG) may be normal or may show generalized or focal epileptiform abnormalities, focal slowing, or only background slowing. Chronic seizures after recovery from meningitis are several-fold more common in patients than in age-matched control children.

Deafness and Cranial Nerve Damage

Deafness is the most frequent neurologic sequela of bacterial meningitis. Of patients with pneumococcal bacterial meningitis, 31% develop hearing loss; with meningococcal meningitis, 10%; and with *Haemophilus influenzae* b meningitis, 6%. Some children exhibit fluctuating degrees of hearing impairment after meningitis, with eventual improvement, but much of the loss is severe, permanent, and may be bilateral. Hearing should be assessed in children with bacterial meningitis before discharge.

Neuronal Damage

The neurologic sequelae after meningitis, in addition to hearing loss, include infarction, focal sensorimotor deficits, developmental delay, seizure disorders, and cortical blindness, which may occur in 15% to 25% of survivors.

Hydrocephalus

Meningitis leads to disturbances of CSF homeostasis, with increased CSF production and reduced CSF absorption across the sagittal sinus–arachnoid villi system. In the acute phase, these disturbances can lead to transient ventriculomegaly associated with intracranial hypertension. Chronic hydrocephalus may occur as a long-term sequela of bacterial meningitis, particularly in infants but also in children. Chronic internal shunting with internal drainage is necessary in patients with persistent obstructive hydrocephalus.

Septic Shock and Disseminated Intravascular Coagulation

Bacterial meningitis can be complicated by sepsis and septic shock, independent of the infecting organism. The association of sepsis and extensive disseminated intravascular coagulation suggests infection caused by *N. meningitidis,* and patients present with rapidly progressive signs of severe illness, rigors, severe muscular pain, and skin lesions that progress from an early maculopapular rash to petechiae to enlarging purpuric lesions. Signs and symptoms of meningitis often are not prominent in patients with disseminated meningococcemia.

Extraaxial Fluid Collections

The subdural space is a potential intracranial space situated between the arachnoid and dura. Fluid can collect in the subdural space and in the subarachnoid space. Because imaging often cannot distinguish between a fluid collection and a widened subarachnoid space, the fluid collection as seen on imaging is referred to as an extraaxial fluid collection. Extraaxial fluid collections are found in 20% to 50% of children with bacterial meningitis who have cranial CT performed. In general, clinical management is not influenced by the diagnosis of extraaxial fluid collections. Subdural empyema, however, is most commonly a complication of sinusitis or otitis media, and requires emergent treatment (as is discussed later in this chapter).

Brain Abscess

The development of brain abscess is extremely rare, perhaps surprisingly so, after bacterial meningitis, given the pyogenic infection of the meninges. Brain abscess formation following bacterial meningitis is nearly exclusively seen only among neonates who have meningitis caused by *Citrobacter* or certain *Cronobacter* (formerly *Enterobacter)* species, in whom abscesses occur in approximately 80%.

Pathology

The inflammation of the subarachnoid space in bacterial meningitis appears as a grayish yellow to green exudate covering the base and convexities of the brain (see Figure 114-4). Histologic examination indicates that the exudate in acute bacterial meningitis consists predominantly of granulocytes; there is a mixture of lymphocytes, macrophages, and granulocytes in subacute to chronic forms of meningitis. Cerebral arteries and veins have focal infiltration of the vessel walls by the inflammatory cells. The inflammation of the vessel wall may be associated with thrombosis and vascular occlusion. Damage to the brain parenchyma in fatal cases of meningitis is manifested by signs of brain edema and by areas of cerebral infarction resulting from ischemia; neuronal loss associated with a marked reaction of astrocytes and microglia, and sometimes cerebral herniation, have been reported.

Treatment
General Care

Antimicrobial therapy, fluid management, and possibly antiinflammatory adjunctive treatments are crucial for all patients who have bacterial meningitis. Acute bacterial meningitis is always a medical emergency, and all infants and children who have an altered state of consciousness should be observed closely and the need for intensive care anticipated.

As soon as bacterial meningitis is diagnosed, intravenous access should be secured and appropriate antimicrobial agents (and possibly antiinflammatory agents, see following discussion) provided. Management of the child who is awake and has stable cardiorespiratory vital signs consists primarily of administering antimicrobial agents and fluids and careful

TABLE 114-3 Antimicrobial Therapy of Bacterial Meningitis

Part A. Empirical Therapy Pending Culture and Susceptibility Data		
Age	Likely Pathogens	Antimicrobial Agent
0–1 mo	Streptococcus agalactiae, Escherichia coli, Listeria monocytogenes	Ampicillin + cefotaxime or Ampicillin + aminoglycoside
1–3 mo	S. agalactiae, L. monocytogenes, Streptococcus pneumoniae, Neisseria meningitidis, Haemophilus influenzae b	Ampicillin + (cefotaxime or ceftriaxone) plus vancomycin (see text)
3 mo–21 yr	S. pneumoniae, N. meningitidis (H. influenzae b if not vaccinated)	(Ceftriaxone or cefotaxime) plus vancomycin (see text)

Part B. Specific Therapy	
Pathogen	Therapy
Streptococcus agalactiae	Ampicillin or penicillin G for 14–21 days; first 3 days, add gentamicin; cefotaxime also acceptable
Listeria monocytogenes	Ampicillin for 14–21 days; first 3 days, add gentamicin
Streptococcus pneumoniae	Penicillin MIC < 0.1 µg/ml and ceftriaxone or cefotaxime MIC ≤ 0.5 µg/ml: penicillin G or ampicillin for 10–14 days; ceftriaxone or cefotaxime also acceptable Penicillin MIC ≥ 0.1 µg/ml and ceftriaxone or cefotaxime MIC ≤ 0.5 µg/ml: ceftriaxone or cefotaxime for 10–14 days Penicillin MIC ≥ 0.1 µg/ml and ceftriaxone or cefotaxime MIC 1.0 µg/ml: (ceftriaxone or cefotaxime) + vancomycin for 10–14 days Penicillin MIC ≥ 0.1 µg/ml and ceftriaxone or cefotaxime MIC ≥ 2.0 µg/ml: (ceftriaxone or cefotaxime) + vancomycin ± rifampin for 10–14 days
Neisseria meningitidis	Penicillin G for 7 days; alternatives: ampicillin, ceftriaxone, cefotaxime
Haemophilus influenzae b	Ceftriaxone or cefotaxime for 10 days; alternative: ampicillin if isolate is susceptible

Part C. Antimicrobial Dosage			
	Dose (mg/kg Per Day)		
Agent	Age 0–7 Days	Age 8–28 Days	Infants and Children
Ampicillin	150–200 divided every 8 hr	200–300 divided every 6 hr	200–300 divided every 6 hr
Cefotaxime	100 divided every 12 hr	200 divided every 8 hr	200–300 divided every 6 hr
Ceftriaxone	Not recommended	80–100 divided every 12–24 hr	80–100 divided every 12–24 hr
Gentamicin	5 divided every 12 hr	7.5 divided every 8 hr	7.5 divided every 8 hr
Penicillin G	100,000–150,000 Units divided every 12 hr	150,000–200,000 Units divided every 6 hr	300,000–400,000 Units divided every 4–6 hr
Rifampin	10 divided every 12 hr	20 divided every 12 hr	20 divided every 12 hr
Vancomycin	20 divided every 12 hr	30 divided every 8 hr	40–60 divided every 6 hr

MIC, Minimum inhibitory concentration.
(From Weinberg GA, Buchanan AM. Meningitis. In: McInerny TK, Adam HM, Cambell DE, Kamat DM, Kelleher KJ (eds). American Academy of Pediatrics Textbook of Pediatric Care, 2nd Edition. Elk Grove Village, IL: American Academy of Pediatrics; 2017. p. 2295–309).

monitoring for changes in level of consciousness, development of seizures, changes in vital signs, and development of SIADH. If high intracranial pressure is a major clinical concern and treatment has been initiated or is anticipated, then a neurosurgeon should be consulted and placement of an intracranial pressure monitoring device considered.

Antibiotics

Effective eradication of the infecting pathogen generally requires antibiotics that are both bactericidal and able to penetrate well through the blood–brain barrier into the CSF. CSF concentrations of antibiotics, even with inflamed meninges, are only a fraction of the simultaneous serum concentration (~5% to 25%), such that antibiotic therapy for meningitis involves greater dosages than those used for most other infections.

Empiric therapy should be instituted rapidly in all children with suspected bacterial meningitis. In practice, the appropriate sequence of obtaining CSF and blood for cultures and other tests, instituting antibiotics, and possibly obtaining

imaging studies to exclude mass lesions and other pathologies needs to be adapted to the individual patient. The sicker the patient and the more rapidly progressive the disease, the more urgent is the start of antibiotic therapy. Antibiotic therapy should not be delayed by more than approximately 15 minutes in critically ill patients for an attempt to obtain CSF or blood. The choice of empiric antibiotics depends on the pathogens suspected to be causative, which in turn depends in part on the age and immunization status of the child, in addition to the local geographic epidemiology of pathogen frequency and antibiotic susceptibility. Recommended empiric treatment regimens adequate for patients without additional risk factors are shown in Table 114-3.

Disease caused by *N. meningitidis* is treated reliably with penicillin G at high doses or, alternatively, either by ampicillin or a third-generation cephalosporin; there has been no clinically significant antibiotic resistance among meningococci in the United States or Europe. Meningitis caused by *H. influenzae* type b may be treated reliably with either ceftriaxone or cefotaxime; ampicillin may be used only if the isolate is known to be susceptible.

Currently, up to 40% of *S. pneumoniae* strains may be resistant to penicillin at some level, and many also are resistant to the third-generation cephalosporins. Therefore infants and children suspected of having bacterial meningitis caused by pneumococci (i.e., gram-positive cocci in pairs seen on a Gram stain of the CSF) should receive vancomycin in addition to either ceftriaxone or cefotaxime. Because dexamethasone (see following discussion) can decrease the CSF penetrance (and thus the activity) of vancomycin, some experts advise that either dexamethasone should be omitted or rifampin plus vancomycin plus a third-generation cephalosporin should be used when dexamethasone is provided. As soon as the antimicrobial susceptibility of an isolate is known, vancomycin should be discontinued if the isolate is susceptible to penicillin or if it is not susceptible to penicillin but still s usceptible to the third-generation cephalosporins. Vancomycin is continued with ceftriaxone or cefotaxime for those isolates found not to be susceptible to both penicillin and the third-generation cephalosporins (and rifampin is added to the combination in some circumstances) (Table 114-3). Consultation with an infectious diseases subspecialist is suggested.

In areas with a low prevalence of penicillin-nonsusceptible pneumococci, especially when examination of the CSF Gram stain shows the absence of gram-positive cocci, providing a third-generation cephalosporin alone (without vancomycin) for empiric therapy is reasonable because such therapy will empirically treat *H. influenzae* type b, meningococci, and pneumococci (Table 114-3).

The principles of antimicrobial therapy for neonatal meningitis are the same as those for infants and children, but because the organisms are different, the antimicrobial selection must be adjusted. The ideal antimicrobial agent(s) would be potent against the most common organisms that cause neonatal meningitis (i.e., *E. coli* and other enteric organisms) and against group B beta-hemolytic streptococci and other gram-positive organisms. The combination of parenteral ampicillin plus gentamicin is a time-tested regimen for neonatal meningitis, although development of antimicrobial resistance has limited its utility. Cefotaxime and ceftriaxone, two third-generation cephalosporins, are extremely active against the organisms that usually cause neonatal meningitis, but they have poor activity against *L. monocytogenes* (which is best treated by ampicillin). Although ceftriaxone exhibits a much longer serum half-life than cefotaxime, ceftriaxone is highly protein bound and can displace unconjugated bilirubin from albumin, so its use in premature infants at risk for kernicterus or in term infants who have hyperbilirubinemia is restricted. Thus the combination of parenteral cefotaxime plus ampicillin (the latter to empirically treat *Listeria*) should be used to treat suspected neonatal meningitis (i.e., suspected disease plus abnormal CSF). Dosages and characteristics of the antimicrobials used most often to treat neonatal meningitis are listed in Table 114-3.

When culture results are available, modifications to treatment are made to provide definitive antibiotic therapy (Table 114-3). For susceptible pathogens, ampicillin, cefotaxime, or ceftriaxone are the usual choices. Group B beta-hemolytic streptococci and *L. monocytogenes* are thought to undergo quicker and more effective killing by beta lactam antibiotics if an aminoglycoside such as gentamicin is given concurrently for several days (Table 114-3).

Meningitis caused by *N. meningitidis* is usually treated for 7 days, that caused by *H. influenzae* type b for 10 days, and that caused by *S. pneumoniae* for 10 to 14 days, although the duration of therapy is not strictly defined by randomized trials. Neonatal meningitis caused by group B beta-hemolytic streptococci or *L. monocytogenes* is usually treated for 14 to 21 days, and that caused by Enterobacteriaceae for 21 to 28 days.

Antiinflammatory Therapy

The use of glucocorticoids as adjunctive therapy to reduce neurologic damage in patients who have bacterial meningitis has been studied for decades, yet it continues to be controversial. There appear to be differences in benefit in studies of adults as opposed to children and in the industrialized world as opposed to the developing world. At present, it can be said that dexamethasone likely improves the hearing outcomes of children in the industrialized world who have bacterial meningitis caused by *H. influenzae* type b, but its usefulness in other forms of meningitis (pneumococcal, meningococcal, and gram-negative enteric or group B streptococcal neonatal disease) remains unproven. In addition, dexamethasone does not appear to benefit children or adults with bacterial meningitis in developing nations. In the United States, dexamethasone should be administered before or within 1 hour of the first dose of antimicrobial agents to children 6 weeks of age or older who have *H. influenzae* type b meningitis and considered for children who have pneumococcal meningitis; it has no role in cases of neonatal meningitis or aseptic meningitis. If given, dexamethasone is generally administered parenterally shortly before or simultaneously with the first antibiotic dose, at a dosage of 0.15 mg/kg every 6 hours for 4 days.

Fluid Therapy

Maintenance fluids are necessary to perfuse, oxygenate, and deliver host defenses to the CNS, and although SIADH occurs in bacterial meningitis, no firm evidence has been found that fluid restriction prevents it. Thus obvious fluid deficits should be rapidly corrected, and serum sodium concentrations should be closely monitored several times during the first 24 hours of therapy, along with measurements of urine specific gravity. If the serum sodium concentration drops below 125 mEq/L, the test should be repeated as soon as possible. If the serum sodium is still below 125 mEq/L, fluids should be restricted to keep the vein open until the serum electrolyte concentrations have been corrected. Otherwise, for the child with bacterial meningitis, providing routine maintenance fluids (such as 0.2% saline with added potassium and dextrose) at approximately 80% of the maintenance rate after fluid repletion and advancing to full maintenance rates as the serum sodium increases beyond 135 mEq/L would appear to be appropriate. The period of fluid restriction likely only needs to be 1 day or less.

Prognosis

Despite the appropriate use of bactericidal antibiotics, the modern mortality rate for bacterial meningitis remains at 5% to 10%. Approximately 15% to 25% of survivors will have long-term morbidity, including developmental delay and lower educational achievement, seizure disorder, spasticity, and hearing loss. Predicting long-term sequelae for an individual child is difficult at the time of discharge from the hospital because some who appear normal at discharge will have hearing or learning deficits subsequently diagnosed, and occasionally children with marked defects at discharge may improve over time.

Hearing loss is the most common sequela of bacterial meningitis; it appears to occur soon after infection. Hearing should be tested formally before discharge from the hospital because most sensorineural hearing loss can be detected at this time. The rate of persistent bilateral or unilateral sensorineural hearing loss is 31% after pneumococcal meningitis, 10.5% after meningococcal meningitis, and 6% after *H. influenzae* type b meningitis.

The complications of neonatal meningitis are similar to those seen among older infants and children, but are more frequently encountered. These include hearing loss, hydrocephalus, and blindness. The modern case-fatality rate ranges from 5% to 25%. Approximately 65% of survivors of coliform meningitis are normal 3 to 7 years after the illness, approximately 15% to 30% have mild to moderate neurologic sequelae, and 5% to 10% have major sequelae. Approximately 55% of cases of group B beta-hemolytic streptococcal meningitis survivors are normal, 25% have mild to moderate sequelae, and 20% have major sequelae (i.e., blindness, bilateral sensorineural hearing loss, cerebral palsy, profound developmental delay). As with older infants and children, all infants recovering from meningitis should have careful audiologic testing and close evaluation for attainment of developmental milestones.

Prevention

Prevention of bacterial meningitis may be subdivided into immunization against meningeal pathogens and antibiotic chemoprophylaxis of contacts of meningitis cases.

Immunization

As noted earlier (under "Epidemiology"), the widespread use of H. influenzae type b and pneumococcal conjugate vaccines has resulted in dramatic declines in the incidence of both invasive H. influenzae type b and pneumococcal infection. Similar changes have been noted in the United Kingdom with meningococcal serogroup C conjugates.

H. influenzae type b conjugate vaccines are routinely provided to U.S. infants beginning at 2 months of age. Pneumococcal conjugate vaccine (currently containing 13 serotype products, i.e., 13-valent) is recommended for routine universal administration to infants and children younger than 2 years of age, in a similar fashion to H. influenzae type b conjugate vaccines. The pneumococcal conjugate vaccine is also suggested for high-risk children 2 to 5 years of age, including children who have sickle-cell disease, functional or anatomic asplenia, cancer, immunosuppression, chronic renal disease, chronic cardiopulmonary disease, CSF leaks, and diabetes. At present, a tetravalent (serogroups A, C, Y, and W-135) meningococcal polysaccharide conjugate vaccine is routinely used for children and adults at higher risk of disease and for young adolescents 11 to 12 years of age (with a booster dose in late adolescence). Two new meningococcal serogroup B vaccines have recently been licensed in the United States and are available for use in interrupting epidemics and protecting children and adults at high risk of meningococcal group B disease; their role in the routine infant immunization schedule is not yet clear.

Chemoprophylaxis

Many studies have documented an increased risk of disease in close contacts of any age of index patients with invasive disease caused by N. meningitidis *and* in unimmunized or underimmunized young children who are contacts of those with H. influenzae type b infection. The risk for the latter is age dependent, and disease among unvaccinated household contacts younger than 4 years old is increased. The spread of such strains is a particular concern in daycare centers.

Chemoprophylactic regimens are aimed at eradicating nasopharyngeal carriage of potentially invasive bacteria, and the preferred drug is rifampin (20 mg/kg per day, once daily, maximum daily dose 600 mg) for 4 days (H. influenzae b). For contacts of invasive N. meningitidis disease, the preferred drug also is rifampin, but in a different dosage (10 mg/kg per dose every 12 hours, maximum daily dose 1200 mg) for 2 days. Alternatives for the elimination of nasopharyngeal carriage of N. meningitidis include single doses of either ciprofloxacin or ceftriaxone. Because treatment for bacterial meningitis with ampicillin or penicillin does not eradicate either meningococci or H. influenzae from the nasopharynx, chemoprophylaxis also is recommended for the index patient before discharge—unless the index patient was treated with cefotaxime or ceftriaxone, drugs that do eradicate colonization.

Numerous studies also have found that maternal intrapartum chemoprophylaxis can prevent maternal febrile morbidity and early-onset neonatal group B streptococcal disease, including early-onset meningitis, but, notably, not late-onset meningitis. Women who are found to be carriers of group B streptococci, based on cultures taken at 35 to 37 weeks of gestation; women who have had a previous child with group B streptococcal disease; women who have had group B streptococcal bacteriuria or urinary tract infection; and women whose group B streptococcal status is unknown at onset of labor or rupture of membranes and who have a gestation less than 37 weeks, membrane rupture greater than or equal to 18 hours, or an intrapartum temperature of greater than or equal to 38.0° C are given intravenous penicillin (or ampicillin) until delivery.

RECURRENT ACUTE BACTERIAL MENINGITIS

Recurrent bacterial meningitis is rare and must prompt a careful evaluation for either an anatomic defect facilitating access of bacteria to the CSF space or an immunologic deficit. Anatomic defects can be acquired or developmental, and they typically lead to meningitis caused by S. pneumoniae or, less often, H. influenzae (especially nontypeable or non-b-type encapsulated isolates). Defects may involve the temporal bone or the anterior skull base and are not always associated with CSF rhinorrhea or otorrhea. Contrast-enhanced high-resolution CT, magnetic resonance imaging (MRI) cisternography, and search for CSF leakage into the nose or middle ear can help identify an anatomic defect. If such a defect is found, surgical correction usually is indicated.

Among the immunologic conditions predisposing to recurrent meningitis, deficiencies of the latter components of the complement pathway (C5 through C9) or properdin (alternative pathway) have been associated with recurrent infections caused by N. meningitidis. Functional or anatomic asplenia, agammaglobulinemia, and deficiencies of the early components of complement (C1 through C3) have been associated with recurrent episodes of meningitis caused by S. pneumoniae, H. influenzae, and N. meningitidis. Commonly, children with congenital immunodeficiencies have a history of frequent infections other than meningitis.

Nonbacterial causes of recurrent meningitis are more common in adults than in children. These include Behçet's syndrome, sarcoidosis, and Mollaret's meningitis associated with recurrent herpes simplex infection. Repeated episodes of aseptic meningitis may also result from an allergic reaction to drugs (e.g., trimethoprim-sulfamethoxazole, nonsteroidal antiinflammatory drugs, and intravenous immunoglobulin).

CHRONIC (SUBACUTE) BACTERIAL MENINGITIS

Chronic or subacute bacterial meningitis evolves over days to weeks. Patients complain of headaches, often associated with constitutional signs of infection (fever, anorexia). Many forms of chronic meningitis involve the base of the brain and lead to cranial nerve palsies through direct inflammation or increased intracranial pressure. As the syndrome progresses, signs of brain involvement, with seizures, mental status changes such as confusion or hallucinations, and focal neurologic deficits, may develop, along with hydrocephalus and increased intracranial pressure.

The bacterial causes of chronic or subacute meningitis include tuberculosis, Lyme borreliosis, syphilis, and leptospirosis; these are discussed in the following sections. Nonbacterial causes of chronic or subacute meningitis include fungal infections, such as *Cryptococcus neoformans, Histoplasma capsulatum,* or *Coccidioides immitis,* and viral infections such as cytomegalovirus and human immunodeficiency virus. Noninfectious causes of chronic or subacute meningitis include metastatic neoplastic disease and sarcoidosis.

Tuberculous Meningitis

Epidemiology and Pathogenesis

Tuberculosis (TB) remains one of the most common prevalent infections worldwide. *Mycobacterium tuberculosis* is transmitted by respiratory aerosols and frequently infects infants and children, particularly in developing countries. CNS involvement is a life-threatening extrapulmonary manifestation of tuberculosis, and 1% to 2% of children with untreated tuberculosis develop meningitis. The mean age at diagnosis of TB meningitis in a 20-year retrospective cohort study of 554 South African children was 37 months, with a median age of 28 months. A history of close contact with a known case of tuberculosis is often found in children with CNS tuberculosis.

The meninges are not directly invaded from the bloodstream; rather, a subcortical or meningeal caseous granuloma discharges organisms into the subarachnoid space. Multiplying organisms induce an inflammatory basilar meningitis and focal parenchymal infections (tuberculomas).

Clinical Characteristics

Tuberculous meningitis usually evolves over several days to a few weeks, and initial symptoms include generally poor weight gain or weight loss, irritability, and apathy. In young infants, fever, cough, altered consciousness, bulging anterior fontanel, and generalized tonic-clonic seizures may be presenting symptoms. In older children, fever, nausea, vomiting, and headache are common. As the infection progresses, unilateral or bilateral cranial nerve deficits result from the basilar meningitis, along with neuro-ophthalmologic changes, impaired consciousness, and motor defects.

Diagnosis

Head CT and MRI document findings similar to those of bacterial meningitis, especially around the base of the brain, and may reveal parenchymal lesions, infarction, and tuberculomas. Some degree of hydrocephalus is found in most children with TB meningitis. In addition, tuberculosis may affect the vertebral bodies (Pott's disease) and the spinal cord; MRI of the spine is indicated in a child with suspected tuberculosis and neurologic signs of cord involvement. Chest radiographs are commonly but not universally abnormal (~70%), with lymphadenopathy or pulmonary infiltrates; a miliary pattern is only seen in approximately 10%. The CSF opening pressure is often very elevated in TB meningitis. The CSF seldom contains more than 500 cells/μL, most of which are lymphocytes; protein content is elevated (>80 mg/dl); and CSF glucose concentration is low in relation to that of the blood glucose. Detection of the infecting organism in CSF is notoriously difficult. Large quantities of CSF (10 ml, if possible) should be collected and examined for acid-fast bacilli.

Treatment

The increase in multidrug-resistant (MDR) TB is an increasing problem in several areas of the world. Isoniazid, rifampicin, ethambutol, pyrazinamide, ethionamide, and, to a lesser extent, streptomycin, remain the first-line drugs for the treatment of TB meningitis. Initial therapy for TB meningitis is started with four drugs for 2 months (isoniazid, rifampicin, pyrazinamide, and ethionamide or streptomycin). After 2 months, treatment is reduced to two active drugs, based on susceptibility testing, with rifampicin and isoniazid as first choices. Pyridoxine is recommended in malnourished children to prevent isoniazid-induced peripheral neuropathy. Response to antituberculous treatment usually is evident within 2 weeks. Therapy should be continued for at least 9 to 12 months. The use of corticosteroids for TB meningitis is strongly advocated (as opposed to the weaker support for typical bacterial meningitis), particularly in patients with a decreased level of consciousness, papilledema, focal deficits, or tuberculomas. A course of prednisone or dexamethasone for 6 weeks, with subsequent tapering over several weeks, is the most common regimen recommended.

The mortality rate of tuberculous meningitis remains 10% to 20%, and among survivors, 50% to 80% will have CNS sequelae, including vision or hearing loss, motor deficits, and, in children, developmental delay.

Syphilis

Epidemiology and Pathogenesis

Syphilis, caused by the spirochete *Treponema pallidum,* remains an important and prevalent sexually transmitted disease worldwide. In developed countries, syphilis in children is rare, but it is disproportionately frequent in underprivileged segments of the population and in the settings of HIV infection and substance abuse. In resource-poor countries, congenital syphilis remains an important health issue. Maternal syphilis acquired early in pregnancy is less often transmitted to the fetus, but if transmitted, it is more likely to result in fetal resorption in utero or spontaneous abortion. Maternal syphilis acquired later in pregnancy is more likely to be transmitted across the placenta, especially after the fifth month of gestation, and may lead to either symptomatic or asymptomatic neonatal infection.

Clinical Characteristics

Congenital syphilis is associated with stillbirth or perinatal death in half of the cases. Early congenital syphilis manifests at birth or within the first weeks of life. Early signs include prematurity and low birth weight, skin and mucous membrane lesions, hepatosplenomegaly, and skeletal abnormalities (osteochondritis), which can be painful and prevent the child from moving affected limbs. Snuffles consist of a thick nasal discharge rich with spirochetes. The eyes (chorioretinitis, uveitis) and CNS (meningitis, meningovascular syphilis, hydrocephalus) are commonly involved, but clinical signs of neurosyphilis are rare in neonates.

In late congenital syphilis, clinical findings do not appear until several years of age. Interstitial keratitis (commonly bilateral) occurs typically in the second decade. Bone lesions result in destruction of the palate and nasal septum, with depression of the nose (saddle nose); also the tibia may become bowed (saber shins), and the knee joint can be affected with hydrarthrosis (Clutton's joints). Scars appear around the mouth from earlier fissures (rhagades). The permanent dentition is abnormal, especially the upper central incisors, which are dwarfed and notched (Hutchinson's teeth), and the first lower molars, which have poorly developed cusps (mulberry molars).

CNS syphilis may present with various defects. Meningovascular syphilis leads to findings of chronic meningoencephalitis, such as intellectual decline (juvenile paresis), which may begin by 4 to 5 years of age, headache, seizures, blindness, cranial nerve VIII deafness, other cranial nerve involvement, hemiparesis, and hydrocephalus. Sensorineural hearing loss is one part of the diagnostic Hutchinson's triad, along with the presence of Hutchinson's teeth and interstitial keratitis.

Acquired (noncongenital) syphilis can occur in children and adolescents; it resembles the disease in adults. The primary stage with chancre appears 2 to 4 weeks after exposure, followed by cutaneous eruptions of the second stage within 2 months, and can be associated with mucous membrane patches, condylomata lata, and patchy alopecia. Rarely, secondary syphilis is associated with meningitis, leading to headache, meningismus, nausea, and vomiting. If the condition is not treated, the tertiary stage of neurosyphilis (tabes dorsalis) may develop after an asymptomatic period of many years (thus it is extremely rare in pediatric patients).

Diagnosis

The diagnosis of syphilis relies mainly on clinical suspicion and serologic testing, rather than stains or culture. Serologic testing relies on two different categories of assays: nontreponemal (i.e., the rapid plasma reagin [RPR] antibody test and Venereal Disease Research Laboratory [VDRL] antibody test) and treponemal tests (*T. pallidum* particle agglutination, microhemagglutination, and fluorescent treponemal antibody absorption tests [TPPA, TP-MHA, and FTA-ABS, respectively]). Traditionally, nontreponemal tests have been used as the first diagnostic test to yield relatively high sensitivity screening for syphilis; positive tests are then confirmed with the more specific treponemal test (e.g., RPR screening, confirmed by FTA-ABS or TPPA). Recently this order of testing has been inverted by the "reverse algorithm" of syphilis testing, made possible by the development of even more sensitive (and easily automated by mechanized laboratory equipment) treponemal enzyme-linked immunosorbent assay (EIA) antibody tests. In reverse algorithm testing, a positive treponemal antibody screen is followed by both a nontreponemal test (to stage the infection and provide a baseline for possible treatment) and by a different, confirmatory, treponemal test. This algorithm appears to have boosted both sensitivity and specificity for the diagnosis of syphilis, and it is expected to become the diagnostic gold standard in the near future. Possible congenital syphilis should be investigated by serologic testing of both the mother and child; acquired syphilis is diagnosed using serologic testing of the child, and if positive, the possibility of sexual abuse must be investigated.

Laboratory diagnosis of CNS syphilis depends on examination of the CSF. CNS involvement is assumed if CSF pleocytosis or elevated protein is present; CSF should also be submitted for testing by the VDRL assay (which is the only assay standardized on CSF, unlike the situation in blood, in which the RPR is superior to the VDRL as a nontreponemal test).

Treatment

Penicillin remains the treatment of choice for all clinical forms of syphilis. For early stages of acquired syphilis, one injection of benzathine penicillin is sufficient. For neurosyphilis and congenital syphilis, high-dose treatment with intravenous penicillin G is recommended.

Lyme Disease (Lyme Neuroborreliosis)
Clinical Characteristics

Lyme disease is caused by the spirochete *Borrelia burgdorferi* (sensu lato), which includes *B. burgdorferi* (sensu stricto) in the United States and *B. afzelii* and *B. garinii* in Europe and Asia. The major manifestations of Lyme borreliosis are very similar, but not identical, in disease caused by the three species, with *B. burgdorferi* being more arthritogenic, *B. afzelii* causing chronic cutaneous disease, and *B. garinii* being neurotropic. Lyme borreliosis is transmitted in endemic areas by the bite of *Ixodes* ticks during the warm season, and children frequently are affected. The disease occurs in three stages: early localized disease, characterized by the rash of erythema migrans; early disseminated disease, characterized by extracutaneous CNS or cardiac signs and symptoms; and late disease, as manifested by Lyme arthritis.

Neurologic manifestations of Lyme disease are observed in 10% of infected patients and become apparent during the early disseminated phase. These manifestations include lymphocytic meningitis, radiculitis, neuritis, and, in rare cases, encephalomyelitis and subtle encephalopathic syndromes with memory and cognitive dysfunction. Neurologic symptoms develop within weeks to months after onset of erythema migrans and tend to be more frequent and severe in Europe than in the United States, likely as a result of the increased neurotropism of *B. garinii*. Infection with *B. garinii* is associated with a painful meningoradiculitis known as Bannwarth's syndrome; this is rare with U.S. Lyme disease caused by *B. burgdorferi* (Mygland et al., 2010). In children, fatigue, peripheral palsy of cranial nerve VII, loss of appetite, and fever are all common manifestations of CNS early disseminated Lyme disease.

Diagnosis

The diagnosis of erythema migrans (i.e., early Lyme disease) is based solely on epidemiologic and clinical grounds and does not require laboratory confirmation. Serologic tests are used to diagnose early and late disseminated Lyme disease. EIAs with high sensitivity serve as screening tests in patients with symptoms compatible with Lyme disease; positive or equivocal tests must be confirmed by more specific Western blot tests (for both IgM and IgG antibodies) or, more recently, by a different EIA directed at the C6 peptide epitope of the variable surface protein of the *Borrelia* spirochete. Neurologic involvement is diagnosed based on suggestive symptoms combined with CSF signs of inflammation (lymphocytic pleocytosis, increased protein concentrations) (Halperin et al., 2008; Shapiro, 2014). Antibodies (IgM, IgG, and IgA) can be detected in the CSF as a result of intrathecal antibody production. Direct demonstration of spirochetes in the CSF is not feasible in most cases, even by PCR amplification.

Treatment and Outcome

In early stages of the disease, doxycycline or amoxicillin is recommended. The latter is preferred in children younger than 8 years old. Doxycycline and ceftriaxone are equally effective for CNS disease in adults, and are both used in children with CNS symptoms; recent experience favors outpatient therapy with doxycycline in Lyme neuroborreliosis unless symptoms are severe. The prognosis is generally excellent for children and adults with CNS Lyme disease who are treated with appropriate antimicrobial agents, but in up to 10% of children with facial nerve palsy, recovery is not full after 6 months.

Leptospirosis

Leptospirosis, caused by spirochetes of the *Leptospira* spp., is an uncommonly diagnosed cause of meningitis; it is typically acquired through abraded skin or the conjunctivae coming into contact with water contaminated by rodent (rat) urine, but it also can be transmitted to children by contact with dog urine (rats and dogs commonly have leptospiruria). A typical case scenario would be a child with high fever and constitutional symptoms, headaches, gastrointestinal symptoms, myalgia, and conjunctival suffusion who appears to recover, only to have a second, immunologically mediated phase of illness occur, with liver, kidney, and nervous system involvement. Nervous system involvement typically takes the form of aseptic meningitis and may be more common in children than in adults. Severe leptospirosis may present as Weil's disease, with jaundice, renal failure, and hemorrhage; this manifestation of leptospirosis appears to be more common in adults. The diagnosis of leptospirosis is difficult to definitively establish; serologic techniques are most common but are not widely available outside of reference laboratories. Visualization of the organism in urine is difficult and requires dark-field microscopy; culture is slow and insensitive and is rarely available. In the future, PCR amplification tests may facilitate diagnosis, but they are not yet standardized. Penicillin, ceftriaxone, and doxycycline are among the antibiotics effective for the treatment of leptospirosis, although most disease is self-limiting, and there is controversy about which patients require antibiotic therapy.

ASEPTIC MENINGITIS

Aseptic meningitis is most strictly defined as meningitis in which the gram-stained CSF does not reveal organisms. The term is often used to indicate enteroviral meningitis, which is the most common cause of aseptic meningitis; however, many pathogens, including bacteria, may cause aseptic meningitis (see Table 114-4). Discussion of all of the causes of aseptic meningitis is beyond the scope of this chapter.

OTHER BACTERIAL INFECTIONS OF THE NERVOUS SYSTEM
Bartonella

Bartonella spp. are small, fastidiously growing, gram-negative bacteria that are the major cause of cat scratch disease (CSD), a regional lymphadenopathy/lymphadenitis that is uncommonly associated with CNS disease. CSD is a mildly febrile or afebrile illness, typically transmitted to children by the scratch or bite of an infected kitten or young adult cat or, more rarely, through infected cat fleas. CNS involvement from *B. henselae* infection is found in about 2% to 5% of infected healthy hosts, with the major manifestations being encephalopathy and neuroretinitis.

CSD encephalopathy typically presents as acute generalized tonic-clonic seizures, combativeness, and even coma approximately 1 to 6 weeks following the development of the skin papule (which itself may not have been noticed or may have been long forgotten). The encephalopathy may be accompanied by regional lymphadenopathy, a finding that should increase the diagnostic consideration of CSD encephalopathy in a child with acute onset of encephalopathy or seizures. The CSF profile is most commonly normal, but a slight lymphocytic pleocytosis is sometimes observed; neuroimaging studies are often unremarkable. Recovery from CSD encephalopathy tends to be rapid, over days to weeks, with few sequelae. Diagnosis of CSD is typically made serologically, by demonstrating IgM and IgG antibodies in the blood. Antibiotic therapy of uncomplicated CSD lymphadenitis is generally not undertaken because the infection is self-limiting, and antibiot-

ics have not been demonstrated to have more than a minimal clinical effect on its resolution.

CSD neuroretinitis occurs in children and young adults. It typically includes anterior optic neuropathy with papillitis, short-segment retrobulbar inflammation of the optic nerve (as demonstrated by MRI), and, often, development of a macular star—a stellate exudate in the macular region caused by neuroglial ingestion of lipids. Clinically, the disease presents as a subacute to acute progressive loss of vision, which slowly resolves over weeks to months. CNS neuroretinitis and macular star formation from CSD neuroretinitis appear to be the cause of the stellate maculopathy of Leber, described in 1916 and previously thought to be idiopathic.

Mycoplasma pneumoniae

Mycoplasma pneumonia has been implicated in diseases affecting the CNS (either by neurotropic invasion or immune-mediated disease). It is estimated that up to 5% to 10% of cases of pediatric encephalitis are attributable to *M. pneumoniae* infection. However, the diagnosis of CNS involvement secondary to *M. pneumoniae* is difficult, and its exact role in causing CNS disease is unclear because serologic tests for *M. pneumoniae* are fraught with false positives, and they remain positive long after unrelated episodes of infection preceding the presumed CNS illness. CNS disease attributed to *M. pneumoniae* includes a variety of neurologic syndromes, including meningoencephalitis, acute disseminated encephalomyelitis, and an ascending paralysis similar to Guillain–Barré syndrome. PCR amplification of respiratory secretions (or if available, CSF) is likely a more accurate diagnostic method and is useful in confirming *M. pneumoniae* serologic studies in children with CNS disease, alongside concurrent evaluation of other potential pathogens (e.g., enterovirus, arbovirus, or herpes simplex virus). In suspected cases of *M. pneumoniae* CNS disease, antimicrobial therapy with drugs that penetrate into the CNS and have in vitro activity against *M. pneumoniae* (e.g., doxycycline, quinolones, azithromycin) should be instituted, despite the lack of firm evidence of a beneficial effect.

Leprosy (Hansen's Disease)

Despite increasing efforts to control leprosy (Hansen's disease), it is still prevalent in some countries of Asia, Africa, and South America, and it is one of the most common treatable causes of peripheral neuropathy. The disease should be considered in patients with persistent skin lesions and peripheral neuropathy who have lived in countries with warm climates and limited resources. The most common neurologic manifestations of leprosy are peripheral mononeuritis, mononeuritis multiplex, polyneuropathy, and cranial neuropathy (trigeminal and facial nerves). The disease often affects peripheral nerve trunks in fibro-osseous tunnels (e.g., ulnar, median, lateral popliteal, and posterior tibial nerves) and small dermal nerves. This results in sensory and motor loss, hypesthesia, and anhidrosis. The diagnosis of leprosy is made clinically, based on the presence of hypopigmented or reddish patches of skin with reduced sensation, thickening of peripheral nerves, or infiltrative skin lesions with the presence of acid-fast bacilli on skin smears or biopsy material. *M. leprae* may be cultured from skin biopsies, or the nucleic acid may be amplified by PCR methods. Treatment depends on the form of disease and uses multidrug approaches, consisting of combinations of dapsone, clofazimine, rifampicin, ofloxacin, and minocycline. Guidelines from the U.S. National Hansen's Disease Center should be consulted, and consultation with

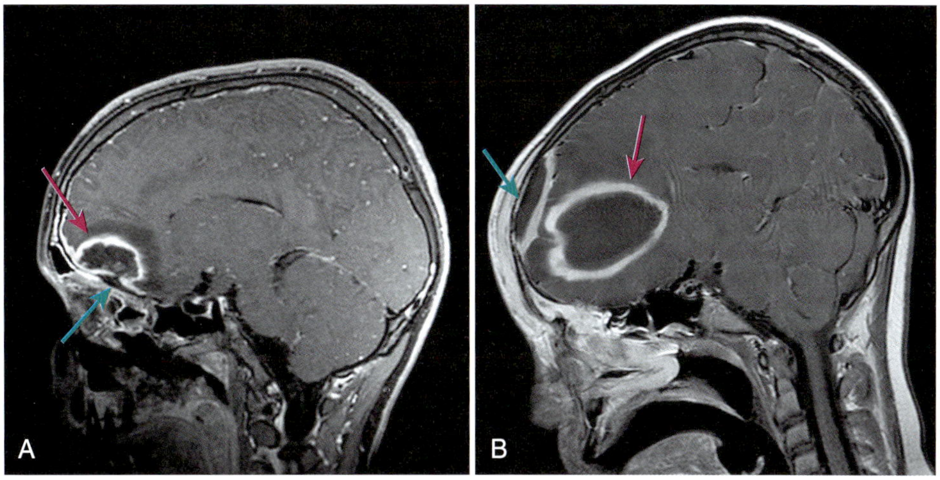

Figure 114-5. Magnetic resonance sagittal T1-weighted images with gadolinium contrast, from two different patients with cerebral abscess (red arrows). Each abscess has a hypointense core with a rim of contrast enhancement. In addition, each patient exhibits an epidural empyema (green arrow), developing from a contiguous area between the abscess and epidural space.

infectious diseases specialists with experience treating leprosy is advised.

CENTRAL NERVOUS SYSTEM ABSCESS

Abscesses are focal infections consisting of an encapsulated collection of pus, pyogenic bacteria, and, less commonly, mycobacteria, fungi, protozoa, or helminths. Abscesses may be found in various sites of the nervous system, including the brain parenchyma, cranial epidural space, and spinal epidural space. All are rare in children.

Brain Abscess
Epidemiology and Pathogenesis

The incidence of bacterial brain abscesses in the general population is 0.5 to 0.9 per 100,000 population, although the number is likely significantly lower in children (Brouwer, Tunkel, McKhann, and van de Beek, 2014). Predisposing factors are found in the majority (~80%) of cases; these include contiguous focus of infection (50%; including otitis media, mastoiditis, sinusitis), conditions associated with bacteremia (30%; including cyanotic congenital heart disease and odontogenic or pulmonary infection), or the presence of an immunosuppressive condition or a disruption of the body's natural barriers (e.g., neurosurgical procedure or head trauma). The most common causative organisms in patients with trauma or surgical procedures are *S. aureus,* coagulase-negative staphylococci, or gram-negative bacilli. The most common causative organisms from contiguous spread from the middle ear or sinuses are *Streptococcus* spp., including *S. pneumoniae.* Anaerobic and microaerophilic bacteria (e.g., *Bacteroides fragilis, Eikenella corrodens, Abiotrophia* and *Granulicatella* spp.) are found in many brain abscesses, and over 25% of such abscesses are polymicrobial. Bacterial meningitis in the older child or adult is very rarely associated with brain abscess. However, neonatal meningitis is more often associated with development of one or more abscesses, especially if the meningitis is caused by *Citrobacter* spp. (which leads to the development of ≥ 1 brain abscess in 85% of infected babies) or *Cronobacter* (formerly *Enterobacter*) *sakazakii.*

Clinical Manifestations and Diagnosis

Only ~20% of patients with brain abscess will present with the "classic triad" of fever, headache, and focal neurologic deficits. The most common symptom of a brain abscess is headache (70%), with fever and focal neurologic deficits occurring in about half of patients. About 25% of individuals will develop seizures. Papilledema, a distinctly uncommon finding with bacterial meningitis, occurs with brain abscesses in older children and adults.

The most important study for initial diagnosis of brain abscess is cranial imaging, with either MRI or CT with contrast. Early cerebritis will be suggested by hypodense areas on CT and focal edema on MRI. With a more mature abscess, classic ring-enhancing lesions with a necrotic center and surrounding edema can be documented with intravenous contrast (Figure 114-5; see also Figure 114-6).

Lumbar puncture should not be performed in patients with a suspected brain abscess because of the risk of herniation secondary to elevated intracranial pressure; in addition, it is uncommon to have a positive CSF culture in this situation. Identification of the causative organism is best attempted by obtaining Gram stain and culture information on material obtained through stereotactic aspiration of the abscess. Blood cultures can identify the causative organism in one-third of cases.

Neurosurgical Management and Antimicrobial Therapy

Neurosurgical intervention is generally undertaken in the majority of cases, with stereotactic aspiration, for both etiologic diagnosis and reduction of lesion size, being the most common indication. In stable patients with multiple abscesses, none of which are greater than 2.5 cm in diameter, nonsurgical management with antibiotic therapy has had success in some reports. Intravenous antimicrobial therapy should be given without delay to patients with brain abscess. For cases likely to be caused by continuous spread from the middle ear or sinuses, a third- or fourth-generation cephalosporin plus metronidazole is used (with the addition of vancomycin if methicillin-resistant *S. aureus* [MRSA] is suspected). If head trauma or a neurosurgical procedure is thought to be a factor, vancomycin plus metronidazole plus a third- or fourth-generation cephalosporin may be indicated. The duration of intravenous antibiotic therapy is typically 6 to 8 weeks, although some experts advocate shorter intravenous courses (e.g., 2 weeks) followed by oral therapy for several weeks in selected patients. Serial CT or MRI should be used to determine when medical therapy is failing. Corticosteroids may be useful to reduce edema in symptomatic patients, but they are only used in about 50% of cases because the effect of this therapy on antimicrobial penetration is unclear. Both case-fatality and morbidity rates have declined substantially over the last 6 decades as a result of improvements in cranial imaging, neurosurgical techniques, and antimicrobial therapy.

EPIDURAL ABSCESSES
Spinal Epidural Abscess

Spinal epidural abscess is a rare diagnosis, but it is one that requires emergent identification and management for optimal outcome. The abscess typically is attributable to a hematogenous source in healthy children (as opposed to adults, who generally have predisposing conditions). Spinal epidural abscesses tend to extend over three to four vertebral segments, and they are most common posteriorly (where the epidural space is largest, with a fat pad containing a venous plexus) and in the thoracolumbar segments. *S. aureus* (including MRSA) is the most common organism recovered (60% to 70%). Presentation is typically back pain (75%) and fever (50% to 66%) accompanied by neurologic symptoms (30%) referable to the spinal cord. The "classic triad" of pain, fever, and spinal cord neurologic symptoms is seen only in the minority of children at the onset of infection (Darouiche, 2006).

With a suspicion of spinal epidural abscess, emergent MRI with gadolinium contrast is indicated, whereas lumbar puncture is contraindicated. Surgical treatment involves either incision and drainage with laminectomy or CT-guided needle drainage. Patients also require appropriate intravenous antibiotic coverage for *S. aureus,* including MRSA, and other bacteria (e.g., vancomycin and a third- or fourth-generation cephalosporin); treatment is often given parenterally for 6 to 8 weeks. In cases known to be caused by methicillin-sensitive *S. aureus,* nafcillin or cefazolin is preferred. The factors that most significantly affect outcome include length of time before initiation of treatment and severity of neurologic deficits at presentation.

REFERENCES

The complete list of references for this chapter is available in the e-book at www.expertconsult.com.
See inside cover for registration details.

SELECTED REFERENCES

Avery, R.A., Shah, S.S., Licht, D.J., et al., 2010. Reference range for cerebrospinal fluid opening pressure in children. N. Engl. J. Med. 363, 891–893. PMID: 20818852.

Brouwer, M.C., Thwaites, G.E., Tunkel, A.R., et al., 2012. Dilemmas in the diagnosis of acute community-acquired bacterial meningitis. Lancet 380, 1684–1692. PMID: 23141617.

Brouwer, M.C., Tunkel, A.R., McKhann, G.M., et al., 2014. Brain Abscess. N. Engl. J. Med. 371, 447–456.

Brouwer, M.C., Tunkel, A.R., van de Beek, D., 2010. Epidemiology, diagnosis, and antimicrobial treatment of acute bacterial meningitis. Clin. Microbiol. Rev. 23, 467–492. PMID: 20610819.

Darouiche, R.O., 2006. Spinal epidural abscess. N. Engl. J. Med. 355, 2012–2020.

Halperin, J.J., Shapiro, E.D., Logigian, E., et al., 2007. Practice parameter: treatment of nervous system Lyme disease (an evidence-based review): report of the Quality Standards Subcommittee of the American Academy of Neurology. Neurology 69, 91–102. Erratum in: Neurology. 2008;70:1223. PubMed PMID: 17522387.

Kim, K.S., 2010. Acute bacterial meningitis in infants and children. Lancet Infect. Dis. 10, 32–42. PMID: 20129147.

Mygland, A., Ljøstad, U., Fingerle, V., et al., 2010. European Federation of Neurological Societies (EFNS) guidelines on the diagnosis and management of European Lyme neuroborreliosis. Eur. J. Neurol. 17, 8–16, e1-4. PubMed PMID: 19930447.

Shapiro, E.D., 2014. Clinical practice. Lyme disease. N. Engl. J. Med. 370, 1724–1731. PubMed PMID: 24785207.

Thigpen, M.C., Whitney, C.G., Messonnier, N.E., et al., 2011. Emerging Infections Programs Network. Bacterial meningitis in the United States, 1998-2007. N. Engl. J. Med. 364, 2016–2025. PMID: 21612470.

E-BOOK FIGURES AND TABLES

The following figures and tables are available in the e-book at www.expertconsult.com. See inside cover for registration details.

Fig. 114-1. Magnetic resonance axial T1-weighted image with contrast in a patient with bacterial meningitis.

Fig. 114-2. Magnetic resonance axial T1-weighted image with contrast in a patient with bacterial meningitis.

Fig. 114-3. Magnetic resonance axial diffusion-weighted image, purulent meningitis.

Fig. 114-4. Acute bacterial meningitis.

Fig. 114-6. Magnetic resonance axial diffusion-weighted images of a cerebral abscess.

Table 114-4. Selected Causes of Aseptic Meningitis

115 Viral Infections of the Nervous System

Daniel J. Bonthius and James F. Bale, Jr.

An expanded version of this chapter is available on www.expertconsult.com. See inside cover for registration details.

More than 100 virus species have been associated directly or indirectly with disorders of the human central or peripheral nervous system (Box 115-1) (Johnson, 1998). Although infections with several viruses have become infrequent because of immunization programs or less severe because of antiviral therapies, may others remain potential threats to children worldwide (Pickering et al., 2012). This chapter describes virus-induced neurologic disorders, emphasizing the epidemiology, clinical manifestations, treatment, and prevention.

GENERAL CONSIDERATIONS

The pathogenesis of a virus-induced neurologic disorder reflects the complex interactions of the viral pathogen and the host (Reiss, 2008). Because the majority of viral neurologic disorders begin with virus entry and replication in the skin or cells lining the respiratory or gastrointestinal tracts, several host factors, including the integrity of skin or mucosal barriers and the innate immune response of the host, determine whether viruses successfully invade human tissues and cause neurologic disease. Most viruses reach the central nervous system (CNS) hematogenously and enter the brain via the choroid plexus or directly through the vascular endothelium (Johnson, 1998). Rabies virus and a few others reach the CNS via neural routes. Rabies virus, a negative-strand RNA virus, infects neuromuscular junctions, enters motor nerve endings, travels via retrograde transport to the neurons of the spinal cord, and then ascends to the brain. Neural pathways can also participate during infections with the herpes simplex virus (HSV) and the varicella zoster virus.

Viruses can cause neurologic disease directly by infecting and damaging neural cells or indirectly by stimulating immune responses that alter host cell function (Johnson, 1998). Several factors, including neuroinvasiveness (the ability of viruses to enter the nervous system), neurotropism (the capacity of viruses to infect certain neural cell types), neurovirulence (the capacity of viruses to induce neurologic disease), and the immune responses of the infected host, determine the spectrum and severity of virus-induced neurologic signs and symptoms. Certain viruses, such as the herpes simplex viruses, produce lytic infection of neural cells and induce necrosis of infected cells, whereas other viruses, such as La Crosse encephalitis, produce minimal neural cell damage despite direct infection. Other viruses, such as the childhood respiratory viruses, may not infect neural cells directly, but may induce neurologic disease through secondary, immune-mediated mechanisms, such as the events that lead to acute disseminated encephalomyelitis, a disorder that accounts for a substantial proportion of "viral" encephalitis in young children.

Cellular and humoral immune responses, including those mediated by small molecules such as interferons and inflammatory cytokines, have major roles in inhibiting viral CNS infections. Toll or toll-like receptors participate in host responses to viruses, and in certain instances, mutations in the human genes encoding such proteins can determine the risk of acquiring herpes simplex virus (HSV) encephalitis. Mutations in RANBP2, a gene encoding a nuclear pore protein, can influence whether children have acute necrotizing encephalomyelitis, a potentially life-threatening disorder triggered by several common viral infections. Host immune responses can provoke several neurologic disorders, including Guillain-Barré syndrome (GBS), Bell palsy, transverse myelitis, or acute disseminated encephalomyelitis (ADEM). The latter disorders can complicate infections with several viruses that commonly infect young children.

EPIDEMIOLOGY OF VIRAL INFECTIONS

During the past fifty years, the epidemiology of virus-induced neurologic disease has changed dramatically due to the development of vaccines and the implementation of vaccination programs. Poliomyelitis, the consequence of infection with polioviruses types 1 to 3, has been eliminated in nearly all regions of the world, and subacute sclerosing panencephalitis (SSPE), the consequence of latent measles virus infection, is exceptionally rare in nations with widespread measles-mumps-rubella (MMR) vaccination coverage (Johnson, 1998).

Many neurologic disorders, including meningitis or encephalitis caused by several different viruses, cannot be prevented by vaccination. The herpesviruses (especially herpes simplex viruses), tick- or mosquito-borne viruses (arboviruses), and nonpolio enteroviruses account for the majority of encephalitis cases among children in many regions of the world. Some of these, especially the nonpolio enteroviruses, cause many cases of viral, or aseptic, meningitis in young children. The incidence rates of viral encephalitis in the pediatric population range from 3 to 30 or more per 100,000 persons of all ages annually. However, rates of viral CNS infections are likely higher, because current surveillance systems fail to capture all cases of viral encephalitis and meningitis.

Major outbreaks of viral infections appear periodically in human populations. In 1999, West Nile virus (WNV) emerged in the United States, and by the end of 2003, the Centers for Disease Control and Prevention (CDC) had recorded approximately 14,000 cases of human WNV infections in the United States and 6000 cases of WNV neuroinvasive disease. Approximately 260,000 hospitalizations due to all causes of encephalitis occurred between 1998 and 2010 in the United States, corresponding to slightly more than 20,000 children and adults with encephalitis annually or approximately 6 cases of encephalitis per 100,000 persons/year. Herpes simplex encephalitis affects approximately 1 in every 250,000 to 500,000 persons. Human rabies affects 1 in 100,000 to 1 million inhabitants annually in Africa and India, causing several thousand deaths annually in Africa.

Neurologic disorders caused by environmentally derived pathogens, such as the tick- or mosquito-borne encephalitis viruses, occur when vectors are active, typically late spring through fall, and display characteristic epidemiologic patterns

---

BOX 115-1 Selected Viruses Associated with Neurologic Disease in Pediatric Populations

DNA VIRUSES

Adenoviruses

Adenovirus—several types

Herpesviruses

Herpes simplex viruses types 1 and 2
Cytomegalovirus
Varicella zoster virus
Epstein-Barr virus
Human herpesviruses 6 and 7

RNA VIRUSES

Arenaviruses

Lymphocytic choriomeningitis virus

Picornaviruses

Polioviruses types 1-3
Nonpolio enteroviruses
Parechoviruses

Bunyaviruses

La Crosse encephalitis virus
California encephalitis virus

Reoviruses

Colorado tick fever virus
Rotavirus

Flaviviruses

Japanese encephalitis virus
St. Louis encephalitis virus
Rabies virus
Tick-borne encephalitis viruses
West Nile virus
Dengue virus
Zika virus

Retroviruses

Human immunodeficiency viruses types 1 and 2
Human T-cell lymphotropic virus type 1

Orthomyxoviruses

Influenza virus

Rhabdoviruses

Rabies virus

Paramyxoviruses

Mumps virus
Measles virus
Nipah virus

Togaviruses

Eastern equine encephalitis virus
Western equine encephalitis virus
Venezuelan equine encephalitis virus
Chikungunya virus
Rubella virus

(Fig. 115-2). La Crosse encephalitis, a common arthropod-borne disorder in the United States, typically affects children who reside in the Eastern and Midwestern United States, prime habitat for the *Aedes triseriatus*, the principal mosquito vector. Cases occur from June to October, reflecting peak activity of the vector, and frequently involve boys 5 to 15 years of age who live near or enter wooded areas.

Transmission of several viruses, including the herpesviruses and nonpolio enteroviruses, requires direct contact with infected humans or with fomites harboring virus-infected human secretions. Infections with these viruses can occur throughout the year, although some, such as measles and chickenpox, peak in the late winter or early spring, whereas others, such as the nonpolio enteroviruses, peak during the summer and fall.

CLINICAL FEATURES OF VIRUS-INDUCED NEUROLOGIC DISORDERS
Meningitis

Viral, or aseptic, meningitis, the most frequent virus-induced neurologic disorder, produces malaise, headache, vomiting, irritability, stiff neck, and neck or back pain (Bonthius

and Karacay, 2002). Children and adolescents with viral meningitis appear moderately ill with signs of meningeal irritation, including the Kernig sign (involuntary spasm of the hamstring muscle evoked by knee extension in a supine patient) or Brudzinski sign (flexion of the knees provoked by forced flexion of the patient's neck). However, meningeal signs may be subtle or absent in young infants, indicating that the clinician must maintain a high index of suspicion when considering CNS viral infections in the neonate.

Systemic features in pediatric patients with aseptic meningitis sometimes provide useful etiologic clues. The nonpolio enteroviruses, agents frequently associated with aseptic meningitis, commonly produce gastrointestinal symptoms and an evanescent, erythematous rash or oral lesions of the hand-foot-mouth syndrome. Diarrhea and an erythematous, truncal exanthem can also accompany or precede neuroinvasive disease due to WNV. Hepatomegaly or prominent lymphadenopathy can suggest infection with the Epstein-Barr virus (EBV), cytomegalovirus or, possibly, human immunodeficiency virus (HIV).

Encephalitis

In addition to headache, fever, and vomiting, important features of viral meningitis, viral encephalitis produces symptoms or signs of cerebral dysfunction, including seizures, focal neurologic dysfunction, and altered alertness, ranging from somnolence to deep coma (Johnson, 1998). Because the clinical features of meningitis often accompany those of encephalitis, the term *meningoencephalitis* is sometimes used to describe encephalitis. Seizures, focal or generalized, affect 10% to 50% or more of patients with encephalitis, and when focal, can suggest serious conditions, such as HSV encephalitis, or relatively benign conditions, such as La Crosse virus encephalitis. The neurologic examination of pediatric patients with encephalitis can reveal cognitive dysfunction, ataxia, hyperreflexia, diffuse weakness, movement disorders, and focal deficits, such as aphasia or hemiparesis. Severe encephalitis can be associated with coma and signs of cerebral edema and central or uncal herniation.

Other Disorders

Guillain-Barré syndrome (GBS), myelitis, Bell palsy, acute cerebellar ataxia, and poliomyelitis-like disorders are additional neurologic conditions that can result from viral infections. GBS and myelitis, frequently called transverse myelitis, commonly begin with weakness or vague sensory symptoms that can evolve rapidly to severe, flaccid paralysis. Marked sensory dysfunction, such as sensory loss corresponding to a spinal level, indicates myelitis, whereas facial paralysis, either unilateral or bilateral, suggests GBS. Autonomic nervous system dysfunction, a potential feature of the latter disorder, can produce hypertension, hypotension, or life-threatening cardiac arrhythmias. Myelitis or GBS can result from infections with numerous viruses, including the nonpolio enteroviruses, EBV, varicella zoster virus, and cytomegalovirus (CMV). Several viruses, including WNV and the nonpolio enteroviruses (EV) 70 and 71, can damage anterior horn cells and produce a poliomyelitis-like disorder with flaccid paralysis and areflexia in the affected extremities.

Acute cerebellar ataxia, a potential complication of several viral infections, can produce vomiting, headache, behavioral dysfunction, and truncal or appendicular ataxia. Chickenpox-associated ataxia, a disorder that has become uncommon in regions with widespread varicella vaccine coverage, typically begins 5 to 14 days after the onset of the varicella rash, although occasional cases can begin during the preeruptive

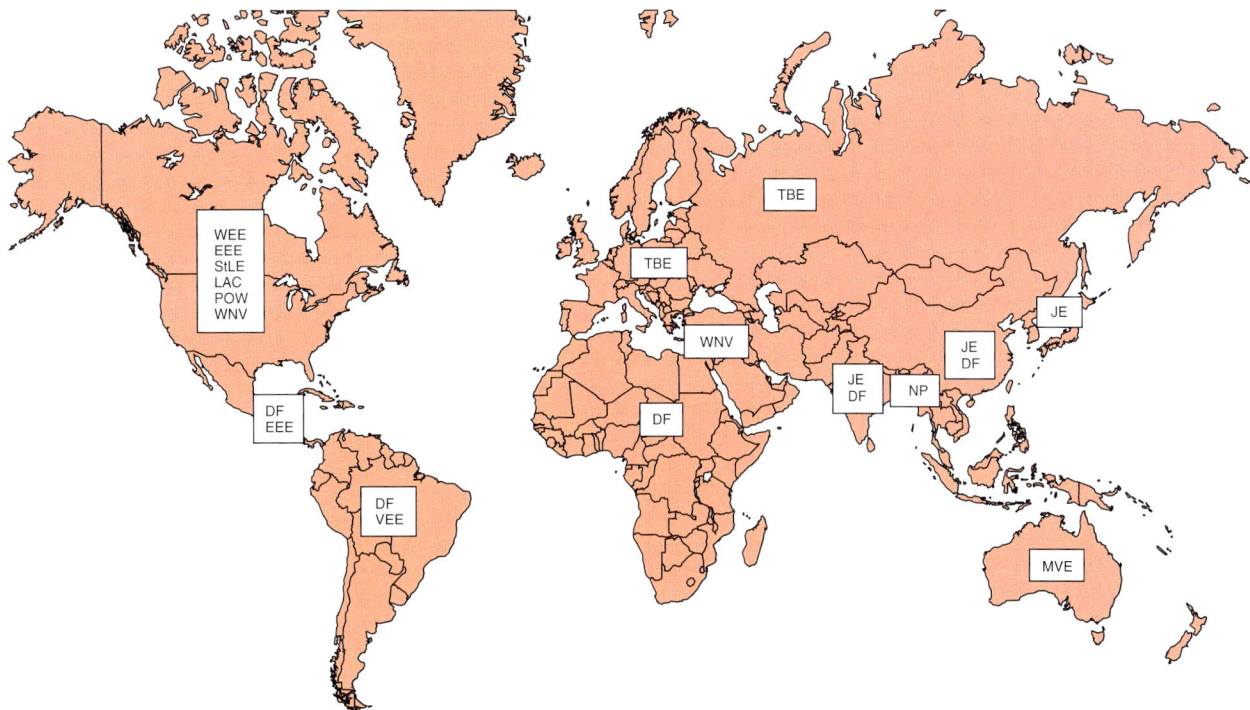

DF: Dengue fever
EEE: Eastern equine encephalitis
JE: Japanese encephalitis
LAC: La Crosse encephalitis
MVE: Murray Valley encephalitis
NP: Nipah encephalitis

POW: Powassan encephalitis
StLE: St. Louis encephalitis
TBE: Tick-borne encephalitis
VEE: Venezuelan equine encephalitis
WEE: Western equine encephalitis
WNV: West Nile encephalitis

Figure 115-2. Map showing the worldwide geographic distribution of encephalitis caused by arthropod-borne viruses (the "arboviruses").

Abbreviations
EEG: Eastern equine encephalitis
DF: Dengue Fever
JE: Japanese encephalitis
LAC: La Crosse encephalitis
MVE: Murray Valley encephalitis
POW: Powassan encephalitis

StLE: St. Louis encephalitis
NP: Nipah encephalitis
TBE: Tick-borne encephalitis
VEE: Venezuelan equine encephalitis
WEE: Western equine encephalitis
WNV: West Nile encephalitis

phase of chickenpox. Virus-induced ataxia and the associated behavioral dysfunction peak by 1 to 2 weeks and gradually resolve, usually completely, in 4 to 8 weeks.

Intrauterine Viral Infections

Intrauterine or congenital infections with a small number of viruses, as well as nonviral pathogens, can cause microcephaly, hydrocephalus, intracranial calcifications, schizencephaly, porencephaly, lissencephaly, and other brain malformations (Bale 2009). Linked conceptually by the acronym TORCH (Toxoplasmosis, Rubella, Cytomegalovirus, Herpes simplex virus), these infectious pathogens produce similar systemic manifestations, including intrauterine growth retardation, hepatomegaly, splenomegaly, jaundice, and skin lesions. Neurologic manifestations include microcephaly, macrocephaly, seizures, sensorineural hearing loss, chorioretinitis, cataracts, and hypotonia. Although the TORCH acronym reminds clinicians that these agents produce similar clinical features in infected infants, some TORCH agents produce unique, distinguishing abnormalities. Rubella virus can produce congenital

heart lesions, whereas varicella-zoster virus can cause a cicatrix, a dermatomal pattern of skin scarring. Lymphocytic choriomeningitis virus (LCMV), a rodent-borne arenavirus, can induce postnatal hydrocephalus through infection of ependymal cells and aqueductal obstruction.

Because congenital infections begin with maternal viral infection, the outcome relates to the maternal immune status and the timing of infection. Vaccination with the MMR vaccine protects women and their fetuses from rubella virus infection; women who are seropositive for CMV are less likely than seronegative women to deliver infants with congenital CMV disease. Maternal infections during the first half of pregnancy tend to be associated with more severe fetal consequences (Bale, 2009). During the first 8 to 12 weeks of gestation, maternal rubella may lead to cataracts or optic atrophy and congenital heart lesions, such as patent ductus arteriosus or atrial septal defect. By contrast, maternal rubella after week 20 of gestation, although producing sensorineural hearing loss in some infants, rarely causes neurologic sequelae. Similarly, the outcome of LCMV is closely linked to the timing of maternal infection, a conclusion supported by animal studies.

DIAGNOSIS

Cerebrospinal Fluid

The cerebrospinal fluid (CSF) in viral meningitis or encephalitis typically has a lymphocytic pleocytosis (5 to 500 cells/mL), mildly elevated protein content (50 to 200 mg/dL), and normal or slightly low glucose content. Normal CSF examination does not eliminate the possibility of a serious viral CNS infection. As many as 15% of patients with HSV encephalitis have an entirely normal initial CSF profile, and 10% or more of children with La Crosse virus encephalitis have normal CSF findings throughout their infection.

Early in the course of many viral CNS infections, neutrophils predominate in the CSF thus suggesting bacterial disease, but the profile typically shifts to a lymphocytic predominance over time. CSF protein in viral meningitis and encephalitis tends to be mildly abnormal, and the glucose content, although modestly depressed to levels of 30 to 50 mg/dL in some instances, rarely reaches the low levels (10 mg/dL or lower) associated with bacterial disease. However, occasional viral infections, such as eastern equine encephalitis, a rare but serious disorder, are associated with CSF profiles that appear more bacterial than viral.

The CSF profiles in other virus-induced neurologic disorders vary widely. The CSF in viral myelitis can be normal or similar to that of aseptic meningitis (lymphocytic or mixed pleocytosis, mildly elevated protein content, and normal glucose content), and the CSF in ADEM, a condition that accounts for at least 15% of cases of viral encephalitis in children, often mimics that of viral encephalitis or meningitis. Children with GBS can have normal CSF during the early course of the disorder, but by 7 to 14 days, most display the characteristic albuminocytologic dissociation (elevated protein with few or no leukocytes).

Neuroimaging

Computed tomography (CT) and magnetic resonance imaging (MRI) have considerable utility in evaluating pediatric patients with suspected CNS viral infections, especially when encephalitis is being considered. The sensitivity of brain MRI exceeds that of CT, especially in patients with HSV encephalitis or ADEM. The brain MRI in nonneonatal HSV encephalitis usually identifies T2 hyperintensities in the medial temporal lobe, orbitofrontal region, or cingulate gyrus; cortical enhancement in these regions, especially in the insular cortex (Fig. 115-3), supports the diagnosis of HSV encephalitis. However, atypical features can be observed in HSV encephalitis in young children, including abnormal diffusion-weighted imaging and diffuse or parietooccipital localization of T2 hyperintensities. The MRI in ADEM characteristically demonstrates multiple areas of T2 hyperintensity involving the white matter of the cerebrum, cerebellum, or brainstem. The CT or MRI in neonatal HSV encephalitis commonly shows diffuse abnormalities, consisting of brain edema, cortical enhancement and neuronal necrosis.

The brain MRI in other forms of virus encephalitis can be normal or characteristically abnormal. Children with Japanese or EBV virus encephalitis, for example, often have focal abnormalities of the thalamus and/or basal ganglia, seen best on T2-weighted or fluid-attenuated inversion recovery (FLAIR) sequences, and patients with neuroinvasive WNV infection can have MRI abnormalities of the thalamus, basal ganglia, brainstem, or spinal cord. Nipah virus produces focal lesions of the gray matter and subcortical white matter. Mild encephalitis with reversible lesions of the splenium of the corpus callosum (mild encephalitis) has been associated with several common viral and nonviral infections of childhood. In severe

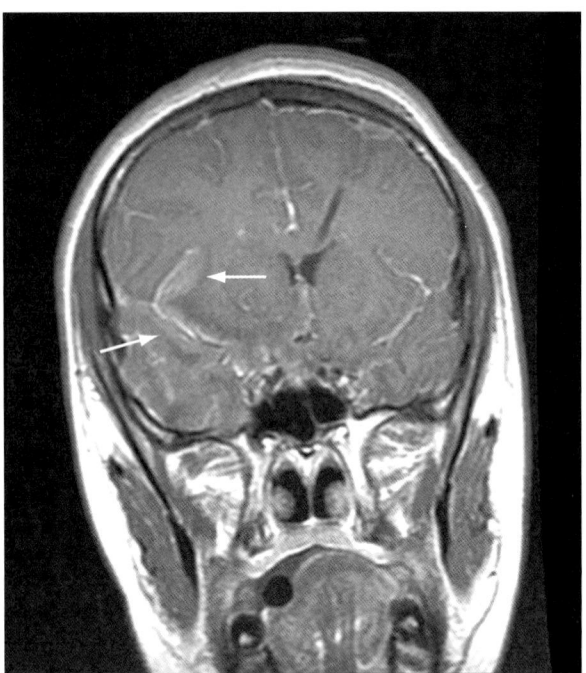

Figure 115-3. Gadolinium-enhanced, T1-weighted brain magnetic resonance imaging in a teenager with herpes simplex virus encephalitis. The scan shows gadolinium enhancement in the right insular cortex (arrows).

cases of encephalitis, CT or MRI can reveal cerebral edema with uncal or central herniation.

Children with viral myelitis frequently have MRI abnormalities of the spinal cord, especially on T2-weighted or fluid-attenuated inversion recovery sequences, consisting of signal hyperintensities, spinal cord edema or gadolinium-enhancing lesions. These lesions may extend for several cord segments and can occasionally be hemorrhagic. The syndrome of acute flaccid paralysis, once the characteristic feature of childhood poliomyelitis, can be associated with lesions of the central cord. Patients with GBS commonly have evidence of nerve root inflammation, seen best on T1-weighted, gadolinium-enhanced sagittal MRI of the spinal cord. Pediatric patients with viral meningitis, on the other hand, typically have normal neuroimaging studies.

Cranial ultrasound, a useful, bedside study in unstable infants, detects hydrocephalus, periventricular calcifications or cystic lesions in infants with congenital viral infections. The CT effectively detects small intracranial calcifications (Fig. 115-5), although calcifications can be detected by newer, more sensitive MRI sequences, such as susceptibility-weighted imaging. MRI has greater sensitivity than either CT or cranial ultrasonography in detecting cortical abnormalities, such as lissencephaly, polymicrogyria (Fig. 115-6), or cortical clefting, that can be present in infants with intrauterine viral infections.

Microbiological Evaluation

Serology, cell culture, immunohistochemistry, and nucleic acid amplification techniques, such as the polymerase chain reaction (PCR), are available to detect specific etiologic pathogens in cases of suspected viral neurologic infections (Glaser et al., 2003) (Table 115-1). Serologic studies remain the principal means of diagnosing infections with the Epstein-Barr virus, LCMV, and WNV. Immunoglobulin M (IgM) capture antibody assays remain the standard diagnostic methods for children with suspected infections with several

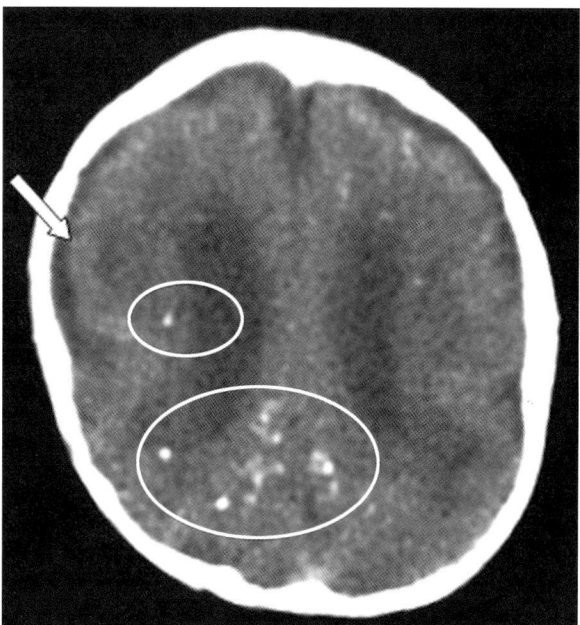

Figure 115-5. Unenhanced computed tomography scan of an infant with symptomatic congenital cytomegalovirus infection. The scan shows multiple calcifications *(circles)* and a smooth appearance to the cerebral cortex *(arrow).*

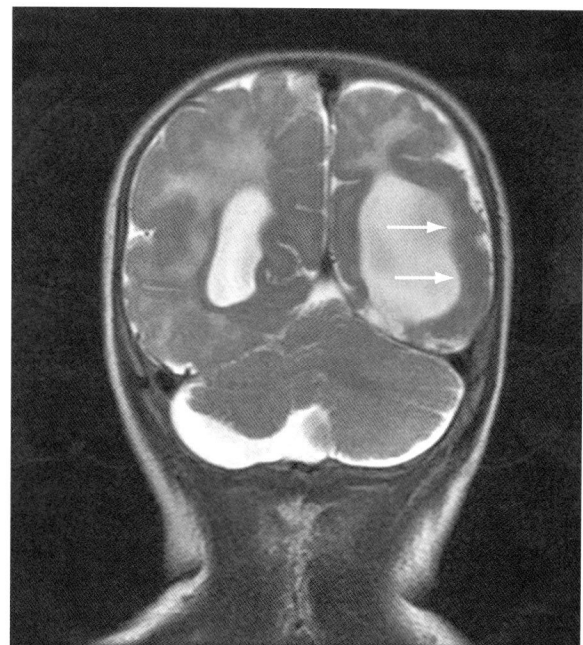

Figure 115-6. A coronal T2-weighted magnetic resonance image in a child with congenital cytomegalovirus infection. The image shows ventriculomegaly, cerebellar hypoplasia, and cortical dysplasia *(arrows).*

Table 115-1 Cerebrospinal Fluid Profiles in Central Nervous System Infections

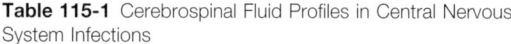

	Organism			
Parameter	*Virus*	*Bacterium*	*Mycobacterium*	*Fungus*
Cell number*	n to ↑↑	↑ to ↑↑↑	↑ to ↑↑	n to ↑↑
Cell type†	Lymph	PMN	Lymph	Mixed
Protein content‡	n to ↑	↑ to ↑↑↑	n to ↑↑	n to ↑↑
Glucose content§	n to ↓	↓ to ↓↓↓	n to ↓	n to ↓

*Cell number: n, <5; ↑, 10–100/mm³; ↑↑, 100–1000/mm³; ↑↑↑, >1000/mm³.

†Dominant cell type: Lymph, lymphocyte; PMN, polymorphonuclear leukocyte; Mixed, variable mix of PMNs and lymphocytes, depending on the organism. PMNs can be the dominant cerebrospinal fluid leukocyte during the early phase of viral CNS infections, and meningitis with certain bacteria, notably *Listeria monocytogenes,* can be associated with a predominance of lymphocytes. Eosinophils occasionally can be observed in viral, fungal, or parasitic CNS infections.

‡Protein content: n, <50 mg/dL; ↑, 50–100 mg/dL; ↑↑, 100–500 mg/dL; ↑↑↑, >500 mg/dL.

§Glucose content: n, cerebrospinal fluid to serum ratio of >0.6; ↓, cerebrospinal fluid to serum ratio of <0.4; ↓↓↓, 0. Virus-associated reductions in the cerebrospinal fluid glucose content are usually modest, with levels ranging from 25 to 50 mg/dL in herpes simplex, lymphocytic choriomeningitis, and mumps viruses.

arthropod-borne viruses, including La Crosse, eastern equine, western equine, and Japanese encephalitis viruses (Baron et al., 2013).

Because of enhanced sensitivity compared with cell culture, PCR has become the preferred method ("Gold Standard") for the diagnosis of HSV encephalitis at all ages. PCR also facilitates the diagnosis of neurologic infections with CMV, varicella-zoster virus, human herpesvirus (HHV)-6 and HHV-7, rabies virus, and the nonpolio EVs (Baron, 2013). The specificity of PCR approaches 100% for most viral pathogens, although the clinical sensitivity of PCR may vary considerably depending on the virus and the clinical setting. PCR analysis of CSF in suspected HSV encephalitis has approximately 75% sensitivity in the newborn and approximately 95% in children and adolescents. Coupling PCR with brain MRI enhances the predictive value of both studies in cases of suspected HSV encephalitis; a negative CSF HSV PCR and a normal brain MRI, for example, make HSV encephalitis exceedingly unlikely at any age. Because the clinical sensitivity of PCR in other neurologic infections of presumed viral etiology has not been determined completely, clinicians must use sound clinical judgment when managing patients with negative PCR results. In some instances, repeating the CSF examination and PCR analysis may be necessary to establish or exclude viral infections, particularly in cases of HSV encephalitis.

Treatment

Supportive Care

Therapy for CNS viral infections must be tailored to the severity of the illness and the availability of specific antiviral therapy (Johnson, 1998). Although numerous viruses cause neurologic disease, relatively few can be treated effectively with antiviral medications. Consequently, clinicians must carefully monitor pediatric patients for seizures, increased intracranial pressure, or respiratory compromise. Pediatric patients with severe infection-related neurologic disorders require hospitalization in nursing units, such as pediatric or neonatal intensive care units, that are experienced in managing such patients. The outcome of viral infections varies according to the pathogen, the availability of specific antiviral therapy, and the management of potential complications.

Specific Medications

HSV encephalitis, varicella zoster virus encephalitis or myelitis, systemic or CNS HIV infections, and congenital or invasive cytomegalovirus infections can be treated with specific antiviral drugs. Although the mechanisms of action vary according to the drugs, the goal of drug therapy is to inhibit effective viral replication and reduce or prevent virus-induced neural cell damage. Survival from symptomatic human rabies has been associated in two cases in the United States with pharmacologically induced coma and antiviral therapy (Willoughby et al., 2005). Corticosteroids, intravenous immunoglobulin, and immunomodulators, such as rituximab or cyclophosphamide, can be effective in selected conditions, including GBS and myelitis, as well as ADEM and anti-N-methyl-D-aspartate receptor antibody encephalitis, conditions that mimic viral encephalitis and account for a substantial proportion of encephalitis of nonviral etiology.

SELECTED VIRAL INFECTIONS

Herpesviruses

The human herpesviruses, a family of large DNA viruses, can produce neurologic disorders during intrauterine, perinatal, or postnatal infections. Important members of this family are HSV-1, a major cause of focal encephalitis in children and adults; HSV-2, an important cause of neonatal infection, CMV, the most common cause of congenital infection; Epstein-Barr virus (EBV), a cause of the GBS; human HHV-6 and HHV-7, the agents of roseola and frequent causes of febrile seizures; and varicella zoster virus (VZV), a pathogen often associated with acute cerebellar ataxia in unimmunized children. Other neurologic disorders associated with the HHVs include aseptic meningitis, myelitis, optic neuritis, Bell palsy and postinfectious neuritis.

Herpes Simplex Viruses Types 1 and 2

Clinical Manifestations

Most humans acquire HSV-1 by oral transmission during childhood. Some children experience gingivostomatitis, a condition associated with fever, diminished oral intake, drooling, and herpetic lesions of the throat, oral mucosa, and face. Primary infection with HSV-2, usually acquired during sexual contact, is frequently asymptomatic; genital lesions associated with HSV-2 can appear during primary or reactivated infections. HSV-associated neurologic disorders in children can be the results of either primary or reactivated infections.

Neonatal HSV infections, more often due to HSV-2, are categorized as: (1) skin, eyes, mouth disease, affecting 43% of HSV-infected neonates; (2) disseminated disease, affecting 23% of HSV-infected neonates; or (3) encephalitis, affecting 34% of HSV-infected neonates. Neonatal HSV disease begins nonspecifically with poor oral intake, somnolence, irritability, or low-grade fever as early as the first day of life, but more often during the second or third week. Neonatal HSV encephalitis, due to HSV-1 or HSV-2, can produce focal or generalized seizures, apnea, lethargy, or coma and can be accompanied by hepatitis, pneumonia, or disseminated intravascular coagulopathy. Approximately two thirds of infants with HSV encephalitis have vesicular rashes. Neonatal HSV encephalitis can be rapidly fatal due to multiorgan system failure or be indolent with apnea, bulbar dysfunction, and frequent seizures. Approximately 5% of HSV-infected infants acquire HSV in utero and display a relatively characteristic congenital syndrome with microcephaly, cataracts, intrauterine growth retardation and intracranial calcifications.

HSV encephalitis in children or adolescents, typically due to HSV-1, begins nonspecifically with headache, fever, malaise, vomiting, and somnolence. Focal or generalized seizures and focal neurologic signs, such as aphasia, visual field defects, or paralysis, appear subsequently in most infected patients (Whitley and Kimberlin, 2005). Focal abnormalities reflect the predilection of HSV to infect the frontotemporal brain regions, but other areas can be affected, especially in young children. The course of HSV encephalitis can be rapidly progressive, with intractable seizures, coma, and increased intracranial pressure, or be indolent with behavioral disturbances, memory loss, and focal seizures. HSV infections in pediatric populations have also been linked to Bell palsy, primary or recurrent aseptic meningitis (Mollaret meningitis), and myelitis.

Diagnosis

Neonates with HSV-1 or HSV-2 can have elevated serum transaminases, direct hyperbilirubinemia, or features of disseminated intravascular coagulopathy. The CSF in neonatal HSV encephalitis contains a lymphocytic pleocytosis and elevations of the protein content; CSF glucose can be normal or mildly low. An MRI and CT usually reveal diffuse cerebral edema and cortical enhancement in the acute stages of infection, and atrophy, cystic encephalomalacia, or passive ventriculomegaly later. EEGs frequently show diffuse slowing or epileptiform discharges that can be periodic. HSV infection of the newborn can be confirmed by detecting HSV DNA in serum, CSF, or vesicular lesions using the nucleic acid amplification techniques, particularly PCR (Baron, 2013). In infants with confirmed HSV infection, PCR detected HSV DNA in the CSF of 93% of the infants with disseminated infections, 76% of the infants with encephalitis, and 24% of the infants with skin-eye-mouth disease.

In older children and adolescents with suspected HSV-1 encephalitis, MRI frequently demonstrates signal abnormalities of the temporal lobe(s) or insular cortex and gadolinium enhancement of the same areas (Fig. 115-3). Focal abnormalities can be detected in other cortical regions, including the occipital and parietal lobes, particularly during atypical infections in young children. Electroencephalograms (EEGs), abnormal in approximately 80% or more of pediatric patients with HSV encephalitis, show focal or diffuse slowing and focal epileptiform features that can be lateralized and periodic. The sensitivity and specificity of current PCR methods for detecting HSV DNA in the CSF of pediatric patients with HSV encephalitis is approximately 95% (Baron, 2013). Some of the negative results can be attributed to the timing of CSF analysis; CSF analysis in children or adolescents with suspected HSV encephalitis is most sensitive 3 to 5 days after the onset of CNS symptoms. Consequently, clinicians must interpret negative CSF PCR results for HSV cautiously. However, a negative CSF HSV-1 PCR and normal brain MRI in a patient with signs of encephalitis make HSV-1 encephalitis very unlikely.

Treatment and Outcome

Neonates with skin-eye-mouth infections should receive acyclovir for 14 days; those with disseminated infections or encephalitis should receive the drug for 21 days (Pickering et al., 2012). Infants with neonatal encephalitis, disseminated disease, or skin-eye-mouth infections should receive suppressive therapy for 6 months thereafter. Children with HSV-1 encephalitis should also receive acyclovir every 8 hours for 21 days; because of potential nephrotoxicity, children 12 years of age and older should receive a reduced dose of acyclovir.

All acyclovir-treated infants with skin-eye-mouth HSV infections survive with no long-term sequelae, other than the propensity to have recurrent herpetic skin lesions. Cutaneous recurrences and potential systemic dissemination of HSV during recurrences can be reduced by suppressive therapy with acyclovir. Prolonged courses of acyclovir can be associated with neutropenia and occasionally with the emergence of acyclovir-resistant HSV strains, although the risk of inducing resistance appears to be low. As many as 30% of infants with disseminated HSV infections die despite therapy, and approximately 30% of the survivors have neurologic sequelae, ranging from mild (speech or motor delay) to severe (cerebral palsy, global developmental delay, or epilepsy). Approximately 10% of neonates with HSV encephalitis die despite therapy, and 20% to 30% or more have severe neurodevelopmental sequelae, including cerebral palsy, bulbar palsy, and epilepsy. A prolonged course of acyclovir is associated with improved developmental outcome. Infants with congenital HSV infections generally have poor prognoses. The vast majority of children and adolescents with HSV-1 encephalitis survive when treated with acyclovir (Whitley, 2005). However, 40% or more have permanent sequelae with developmental delay/cognitive impairment, behavioral abnormalities, memory deficits, motor dysfunction, and epilepsy (Whitley, 2005).

Signs or symptoms of HSV encephalitis, manifesting as fever, headache, lethargy, and movement disorders, can recur in infants, children, or adolescents who have received acyclovir and appropriate supportive care. Children with suspected relapse should undergo repeat CSF analysis and MRI. If CSF PCR is positive for HSV, a repeat course of acyclovir for 21 days should be provided. If MRI suggests ADEM, high-dose methylprednisolone should be given intravenously. Some cases of relapse may be the result of the emergence of anti-N-methyl-D-aspartate (NMDA) receptor antibodies, indicating that serum and CSF should be analyzed for these antibodies (Peery et al., 2013). When anti-NMDA receptor antibodies are detected, methylprednisolone should be administered; intravenous immunoglobulin (IVIg) and/or rituximab may be required in such patients should methylprednisolone not provide benefit. Recovery from anti-NMDA receptor encephalitis can be protracted (Peery, 2013).

CYTOMEGALOVIRUS
Clinical Manifestations

CMV infections have been associated with several neurologic conditions, including congenital infection, infantile spasms, GBS, myelitis, and encephalitis. Some conditions, such as infantile spasms and GBS, occur in immune competent hosts, whereas others, such as encephalitis and myelitis, occur more often in immunocompromised hosts, especially those with HIV/AIDS. Approximately 1% of infants shed CMV at birth, indicating congenital infection. Humans acquire CMV steadily thereafter throughout life such that, by late adulthood, the majority of persons have been infected with CMV, most often without recognizable symptoms.

Approximately 10% of CMV-infected newborns have signs of congenital infection, including intrauterine growth retardation, microcephaly, hepatomegaly, splenomegaly, jaundice, petechiae, purpura, or chorioretinitis. CMV has been linked to infantile spasms, predominantly in infants with symptomatic congenital CMV infections. CMV-infected, immunocompetent children or adolescents may have GBS or a mild, self-limited encephalitis, associated with seizures and altered consciousness. Patients immunocompromised by HIV/AIDS, malignancy, transplantation, or immunosuppressive therapy are at risk of severe, invasive CMV-induced disease, including hepatitis, colitis, retinitis, encephalitis, myelitis, and GBS-like disorders.

Diagnosis

Intrauterine CMV infections can be confirmed by assaying saliva or urine using cell culture or PCR methods. Newborn blood spot analysis can be used to establish the diagnosis of congenital CMV infection retrospectively. CMV infection in older children or adults can be established by detecting CMV in urine, saliva, serum, or CSF using PCR. Head CT detects intracranial calcifications in 25% to 50% of symptomatic infants with congenital CMV infection. Many other abnormalities seen in congenitally infected infants, such as hydranencephaly, lissencephaly, schizencephaly, white matter lesions, and cerebral or cerebellar atrophy, can be identified better by MRI (Fig. 115-6). CT or MRI in children with acquired CMV infections can detect abnormalities of the brain or spinal cord including demyelination, edema or inflammation.

Treatment and Outcome

Infants and children who survive symptomatic congenital CMV infection have high rates of permanent neurodevelopmental disorders including cognitive impairment, cerebral palsy, visual impairment, sensorineural hearing loss, and epilepsy. Approximately 35% to 50% of infants with symptomatic congenital CMV infections have sensorineural hearing loss. Infants with asymptomatic congenital CMV infections have an 8% to 10% risk of sensorineural hearing loss that can be evident at birth or appear later in childhood, usually by age 8 years. Infants with abnormal head CT or MRI studies have higher rates of adverse neurodevelopmental outcomes.

Prolonged treatment with ganciclovir can improve hearing and neurodevelopmental outcomes in infants with symptomatic congenital CMV infections. Bone marrow suppression and nephrotoxicity are potential side effects. Although studies of a human vaccine based on glycoprotein B, the major immunogenic protein of CMV, were encouraging, no vaccine is currently available to prevent congenital CMV infection. Immunocompromised children with invasive CMV disease, especially retinitis or CNS infections, should also receive ganciclovir. Children or adolescents with CMV-associated GBS require therapy with intravenous immunoglobulin using standard doses.

EPSTEIN-BARR VIRUS
Clinical Manifestations

Encephalitis caused by the EBV accounts for approximately 5% of encephalitis cases in childhood and produces fever, headache, altered consciousness, and seizures, including acute status epilepticus. The Alice-in-Wonderland syndrome, which can accompany mild cases of EBV encephalitis, causes personality changes and illusions or hallucinations of distorted size, shape, or distance ("metamorphopsia").

Diagnosis, Treatment, and Outcome

Acute or recent infection is suggested by the presence of EBV viral capsid antigen (VCA) IgM or IgG and the absence of EBV nuclear antigen (EBNA) IgG. The presence of EBNA IgG indicates past infection. A positive serum heterophile antibody response supports acute or recent EBV infection, although young children frequently have false negative results. An EBV infection also can be established by using PCR to detect EBV DNA in CSF, although this assay can be negative in EBV encephalitis (Baron et al., 2013). Pediatric patients with EBV infection also frequently have elevated serum transaminases or hematological abnormalities consisting of thrombocytopenia, leukopenia and atypical lymphocytosis.

During acute EBV encephalitis or the Alice-in-Wonderland syndrome, EEGs may show slowing or epileptiform discharges. Neuroimaging studies can occasionally be abnormal, showing features similar to acute disseminated encephalomyelitis. Although most children with EBV encephalitis recover completely with supportive care, some have permanent neurologic sequelae. Anecdotal reports suggest that therapy with acyclovir or ganciclovir may be beneficial in severe, invasive EBV infections, although no controlled studies have been conducted to assess efficacy. The prognosis for other EBV-associated neurologic conditions, such as GBS, Bell palsy, ataxia, or chorea, is generally favorable.

FLAVIVIRUSES
West Nile Virus

In 1999, WNV encephalitis, linked to a virus strain closely related to a strain identified in Israel in 1998, caused seven deaths among adults in the New York City metropolitan area, marking the first appearance of WNV in the Western Hemisphere. By 2000, WNV was detected in 12 states surrounding New York (210). WNV spread rapidly among North American birds and mosquitoes thereafter, leading to a massive human outbreak in 2003 that affected nearly 10,000 persons from New York to California. WNV activity has persisted, making WNV the most common neuroinvasive arboviral disease in the United States.

WNV is maintained in a bird–mosquito cycle, involving rural and urban wild birds and Culex and Aedes mosquitoes in several areas of the world (Fig. 115-2). Humans typically acquire WNV from mosquito bites, although human-to-human transmission by organ transplantation and blood transfusion can occur. Neuroinvasive disease, including meningitis, encephalitis, myelitis, and polio-like illness, affects approximately 1 of every 150 infected persons, and adults comprise the majority of cases.

Clinical Features

After an incubation period of 2 to 14 days, systemic symptoms of fever, malaise, headache, nausea, and vomiting occur in symptomatic infections. Of symptomatic patients, 50% have a maculopapular rash and lymphadenopathy. Encephalitis, affecting approximately 60% of persons with WNV neuroinvasive disease, manifests as altered mental status, coma, diffuse muscle weakness (proximal greater than distal), respiratory paralysis, and hyporeflexia. Tremor, myoclonus, and parkinsonian features are additional components of the acute illness. Less common neurologic manifestations of WNV infection include aseptic meningitis, myelitis, optic neuritis, and GBS. Involvement of the anterior horn cells can lead to a poliomyelitis-like disorder with asymmetric paralysis of the upper or lower extremities. A single report suggests that WNV can cause intrauterine CNS infection.

Diagnosis, Treatment, and Outcome

The CSF of WNV encephalitis has a mild, lymphocytic pleocytosis (30 to 100 cells/μL), elevated protein content (80 to 100 mg/dL), and normal glucose content. Cranial CT is normal, whereas MRI can reveal leptomeningeal enhancement, periventricular inflammation, or abnormalities of the spinal cord. The diagnosis of WNV infection can be confirmed by detecting neutralizing antibodies to the virus in acute or convalescent serum samples or WNV-specific IgM in serum or CSF. WNV-specific IgM persists in serum for at least 16 months in more than half of infected persons. Infected patients experience brief periods of viremia, but infectious virus is rarely isolated from serum or CSF; reverse transcription PCR can sometimes detect WNV in clinical samples. A CDC protocol guides the evaluation of infants with potential intrauterine WNV infection.

Therapy for the neurologic complications of WNV infection currently consists of supportive care, with close observation for respiratory decompensation. The mortality rate for WNV neuroinvasive disease is approximately 5%, and most deaths occur among the elderly. Approximately one third of survivors of neuroinvasive disease have permanent sequelae affecting cognition, behavior, or motor function. Patients with limb paralysis usually have permanent deficits.

PARAMYXOVIRUSES
Measles and Subacute Sclerosing Panencephalitis

Before vaccine availability, measles typically caused disease in infants and young children during the winter and spring. Symptoms of measles include fever, cough, coryza, and conjunctivitis, beginning approximately 12 days after exposure in susceptible persons. The characteristic morbilliform, maculopapular exanthem appears on the face and spreads centrifugally to involve the trunk and extremities.

Clinical Features

Approximately 1 of every 1000 measles virus-infected children experienced measles encephalitis, either from direct brain infection or immune-mediated mechanisms. SSPE, a neurodegenerative disease caused by persistent infection of the brain by a mutated form of the measles virus, results from a complex and poorly understood interaction between the host's immune system and the measles virus. The risk of SSPE correlates with age; the prevalence of SSPE is nearly 20 per 100,000 when measles occurs under 1 year of age versus 1 per 100,000 for infections after 5 years of age. The disorder displays relatively stereotyped clinical stages, beginning with insidious declines in behavior and cognition mimicking a psychiatric disorder. Myoclonus, a prominent component of the next phase of disease, involves the extremities, trunk, or head. Generalized or focal seizures may begin concurrently. As the disorder progresses, speech and intellectual function deteriorate; myoclonus intensifies; and other neurologic abnormalities, such as choreoathetosis, bradykinesia, or rigidity, appear. Approximately half of patients have chorioretinitis and visual impairment. The disorder typically ends in debility, coma, and death. SSPE is rare in the United States and other regions with mandatory vaccination programs.

Diagnosis

Children with measles encephalitis can have CSF pleocytosis and elevated protein content. Patients with SSPE have elevated CSF immunoglobulin levels, oligoclonal bands, and increased IgG synthesis rates, indicating dramatic production of measles-specific IgG. High CSF titers of measles-specific IgG establish the diagnosis of SSPE, and measles virus RNA can be detected in CSF or plasma by reverse transcription PCR. EEGs show bilaterally synchronous spike-wave or slow-wave bursts with regular periodicity that eventually assume a suppression-burst pattern, and MRI commonly exhibits T2 prolongation of subcortical and periventricular white matter and eventually cortical atrophy (Fig. 115-14).

Treatment and Outcome

Unfortunately, SSPE cannot be effectively treated. Antiviral agents, including isoprinosine and ribavirin, immunoglobulin

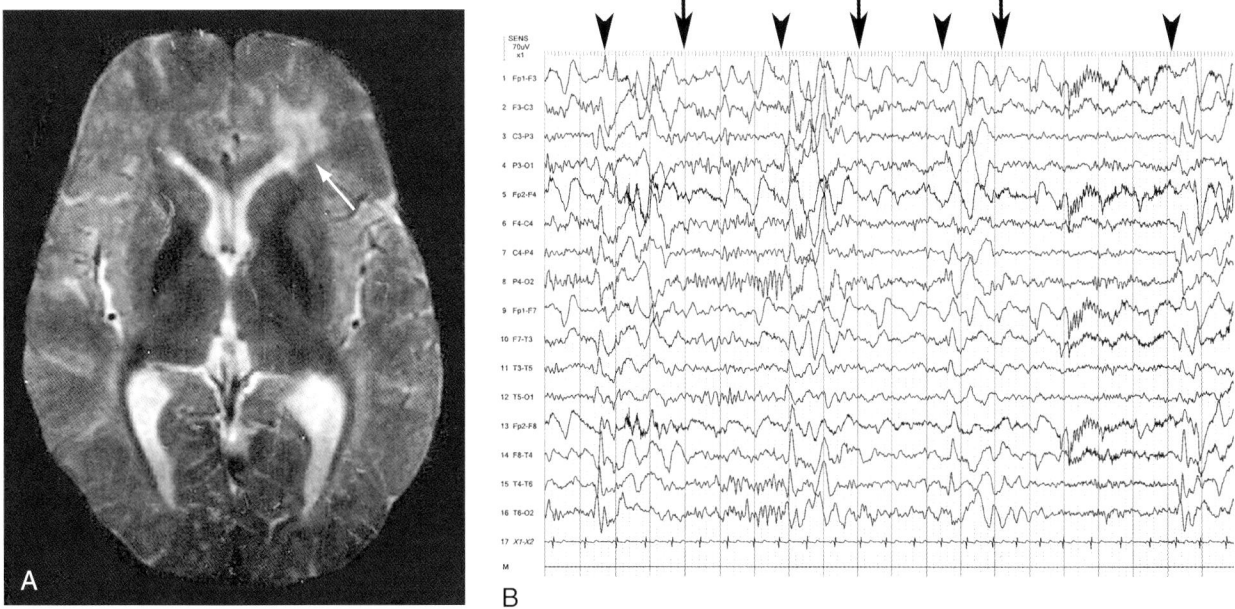

Figure 115-14. Magnetic resonance imaging (MRI) scan and electroencephalogram from a 13-year-old boy with subacute sclerosing panencephalitis (SSPE). **A**, T2-weighted MRI scan demonstrates a hyperintense signal abnormality in the white matter of the left frontal lobe *(arrow)*. **B**, EEG shows periodic bursts of high amplitude slow wave complexes *(onset marked by arrowheads; offset marked by arrows)*, a pattern characteristic of SSPE.

therapy, interferons, and H2 receptor blockers, have been tried, alone and in combination, with little or no effect on the disease course. Divalproex sodium, clonazepam, or levetiracetam may provide some relief for SSPE-associated myoclonus.

RHABDOVIRUSES
Rabies Virus
Clinical Features

Rabies poses a threat to individuals in many regions of the world, especially in the developing countries of Africa and Asia, where the incidence of 1 in 100,000 to 1 million inhabitants corresponds to 25,000 to 50,000 deaths annually. In these regions, unvaccinated domestic dogs transmit rabies virus to humans, and children constitute most human rabies cases. By contrast, human rabies is rare in the US and has been eradicated in a few regions as a result of quarantine and vaccination of domestic animals (Johnson, 1998). Most recently, domestically acquired human rabies cases in the US have been linked to strains carried by bats, often the insectivorous silver-haired and Brazilian free-tailed bats.

After a variable incubation period, averaging 20 to 60 days, human rabies begins with chills, fever, headache, sore throat, malaise, nausea, or abdominal pain (Johnson, 1998; Willoughby, 2005). Pain or itching corresponding to the site of inoculation is common. Neurologic symptoms and signs begin thereafter; symptoms and signs are cerebral in 80% and GBS-like in the remainder. Patients with cerebral symptoms have agitation, hypersalivation, delirium, opisthotonic posturing, and seizures. Hydrophobia, present in 20% to 50%, produces spasms of the laryngeal muscles, diaphragm, and accessory respiratory muscles, and leads to respiratory arrest and death. Patients with rabies encephalitis eventually lapse into a fatal coma. Paralytic rabies induces a GBS-like disorder with muscle paralysis, bulbar dysfunction, cardiac arrhythmias, coma, respiratory arrest, and death (Johnson, 1998).

Diagnosis

Human rabies, often unsuspected during the early, nonspecific phase, is identified most often at postmortem examination. Premortem diagnosis can be established by immunofluorescence examination of skin from the nape of the neck, detection of rabies virus antibody in CSF or serum (assuming the patient was not vaccinated previously), or isolation of rabies virus from saliva or CSF (Johnson, 1998). Reverse transcription PCR can be used to detect rabies virus and determine the molecular profile and origin of the virus strain. The CSF may be normal or reveal a mixed or lymphocytic pleocytosis and mild protein elevation (Johnson, 1998). The CT is normal; MRI can demonstrate signal abnormalities of the basal ganglia or thalami.

Treatment and Outcome

In the United States, where almost all domestic cats and dogs are vaccinated, people must avoid contact with wild animals, especially bats. However, caution must also be exerted around unfamiliar cats and dogs, as unvaccinated free-roaming cats and dogs remain sources of rabies in the United States. In many developing countries, rabies remains prevalent among wild and domesticated dogs. Consequently, rabies is a major concern for travelers to India, the Philippines, Mexico, Morocco, and Algeria. Risk factors include young age and tourism. Therefore travelers should avoid animals and immediately cleanse and disinfect any animal-related injuries.

Virtually 100% of humans with symptomatic rabies die despite supportive care, and only a handful of survivors have been reported in the medical literature over the past four decades (Willoughby, 2005). Children with suspected or possible rabies exposures, including anyone with exposure to live or dead bats, should receive postexposure prophylaxis in accordance with public health guidelines, taking into account the animal species and the nature of the exposure. All postexposure treatment should begin with immediate and thorough cleansing of the wound with soap and water (Johnson, 1998).

Human-to-human transmission of rabies virus has been reported after corneal and organ transplantation, but transmission by body fluids has not been described. Nonetheless, persons with suspected rabies should be maintained in strict isolation to minimize contact with rabies virus-contaminated fluids and to reduce the number of health-care workers who require postexposure prophylaxis.

ARENAVIRUSES
Lymphocytic Choriomeningitis Virus

Most human infections with LCMV are transmitted by the common house mouse, *Mus musculus*, but human disease has also been linked to hamsters and laboratory mice. Postnatal infections are relatively minor, although those of prenatal infections are usually severe. Acquired LCMV infection can produce a nonspecific, influenza-like disorder, with fever, headache, myalgia, nausea, vomiting, backache, and cough. Virtually all infants with congenital LCMV infections have chorioretinitis, and most also have microcephaly and periventricular calcifications. Other infants have porencephaly, neuronal migration defects, hydrocephalus, or cerebellar hypoplasia. LCMV rarely damages the systemic organs of congenitally infected infants. The diagnosis of congenital LCMV infection can be established by detecting LCMV-specific antibodies in CSF or serum, and potentially by detecting LCMV RNA in CSF with reverse transcription PCR. Current antiviral drugs do not possess clinically useful anti-LCMV activity. Cognitive impairment, vision loss, epilepsy, cerebral palsy, and ataxia are commonly present in congenitally infected infants.

INFLUENZA VIRUSES

Although primarily causing disease of the respiratory system, influenza viruses can occasionally induce CNS disease. Encephalitis lethargica, associated with the influenza A pandemic of 1918, caused ophthalmoplegia, vomiting, vertigo, stupor, and coma. In the 1960s, Reye syndrome, a disorder of the liver and brain most frequently associated with influenza B infections, produced intractable vomiting, lethargy, coma, hyperammonemia, and other signs of liver dysfunction. Pernicious cerebral edema led to coma, decorticate posturing, and death. After peaking in the 1970s, the prevalence of Reye syndrome declined dramatically, largely due to the avoidance of aspirin in children with influenza-like symptoms or varicella, another triggering infection.

Influenza encephalopathy, currently the most common neurologic complication of influenza virus infection, begins within a few days of the onset of respiratory symptoms and produces confusion, delirium, and sometimes seizures, including status epilepticus refractory to anticonvulsant therapy. Children under the age of 6 years are at highest risk. The CSF usually contains no leukocytes and has normal glucose and protein concentrations, and although the brain MRI is often normal, diffuse cerebral edema can be identified. Most patients with uncomplicated influenza encephalopathy have favorable outcomes.

Children with acute necrotizing encephalopathy (ANE), a more severe CNS condition associated with the influenza viruses, are critically ill with coma and markedly abnormal neuroimaging; death occurs in more than 30%. Children under the age of 6 years are at highest risk, but older children and adults have been affected, as well. The CSF usually has an elevated opening pressure, lacks pleocytosis, and usually has normal glucose and protein concentrations. MRI often demonstrates areas of T2-weighted hyperintensity in the thalami, basal ganglia, brainstem, and cerebral white matter. No effective therapy has been identified, and approximately 50% of the survivors have permanent neurodevelopmental sequelae. Although the pathogenesis of sporadic ANE is poorly understood, mutations in the nuclear pore gene *RANBP2* contribute to familial and recurrent cases of ANE.

RETROVIRUSES

The HIV type 1 (HIV-1), HIV type 2 (HIV-2), and human T-cell lymphotropic virus type 1 (HTLV-1) are human retroviruses that were linked in the 1980s to HIV/AIDS and progressive myelopathy, respectively. Maintained in human reservoirs and transmitted via virus-contaminated human fluids or blood products, the retroviruses produce neurologic disease during primary infection or virus reactivation. Cures or vaccines to prevent these infections have not yet been identified.

Human Immunodeficiency Virus
Clinical Features

Early cases of AIDS in children were linked to blood transfusions, hemophilia requiring factor replacement, or having a parent with AIDS or an AIDS-related condition. Most HIV-1 infections in infants and children are now the result of vertically transmitted HIV-1 via the placenta, during delivery, or via breast milk. The offspring of untreated, HIV-1-infected women have a 20% to 45% risk of infection. With current combination antiretroviral treatment and management strategies, the risk of vertical transmission of HIV can be reduced to 2% or less. HIV-1 infection remains a major threat to the world's population; approximately 35 million people are living with HIV/AIDS worldwide and approximately 3.4 million of these are children. More than 1.5 million people die of AIDS each year, and nearly 40 million people have died from AIDS since the first cases were identified.

Infants infected vertically with HIV-1 can become symptomatic after the third month of life, manifesting hepatomegaly, lymphadenopathy, failure to thrive, interstitial pneumonitis, opportunistic infections (especially with *Pneumocystis jiroveci* [formerly, *Pneumocystis carinii*] or cytomegalovirus), or neurologic disease. In some children HIV-1 infection can remain dormant, however, and 10 or more years may lapse before the symptoms of HIV-1 infection appear. Before current combination antiretroviral therapies, a child infected vertically with HIV-1 had a 50% probability of HIV/AIDS-related disease by age 5 years.

Before the initiation of antiretroviral therapy, infants and children with HIV-1 can display global developmental delay, seizures, attention-deficit/hyperactivity disorder, behavioral problems, or school failure. Neurologic findings attributable to the direct CNS effects of HIV-1 include microcephaly and spastic diplegia. HIV-1 invades the CNS early after intrauterine or postnatal infection and displays tropism for microglia/macrophages and astrocytes; microglia and macrophages are the principal reservoirs of HIV-1 infection within the CNS.

Diagnosis

Passive transfer of maternal antibody complicates the diagnosis of HIV-1 infection during the first 18 months of life. Consequently, detection of HIV-1 nucleic acids (DNA or RNA) by the PCR is necessary to identify HIV-1 infections in young infants. HIV-1 infection in exposed infants (i.e., infants with positive antibody tests shortly after birth or infants born to HIV-1–seropositive mothers) can be confirmed by serial serum PCR assays, with the first test in the immediate newborn period, a second test during the first or second month of life, and a third test at 4 to 6 months of age. If two samples are positive for HIV-1, the infant is considered infected; two successive negative tests indicate that infection is unlikely. In children and adolescents, serologic studies using enzyme-linked immunosorbent assay and Western blotting can identify HIV-1 infection.

The CSF is usually normal in HIV-1-associated progressive encephalopathy, whereas the EEG may exhibit diffuse slowing. Neuroimaging studies reveal cortical atrophy in vertically or horizontally acquired infections. Calcifications of the basal ganglia or frontal white matter—best detected by CT—and nonspecific abnormalities of white or gray matter—most evident by MRI—occur in vertically acquired HIV infections.

Treatment and Outcome

With currently available medications, the risk of death from AIDS has declined dramatically. Current strategies use combinations of at least three different antiretroviral drugs from the classes of nucleoside analog reverse transcriptase inhibitors, protease inhibitors, and nonnucleoside reverse transcriptase inhibitors. Because treatment of HIV/AIDS continues to evolve, individuals and centers experienced in HIV/AIDS treatment should be consulted regarding current therapeutic approaches. For updated, downloadable information regarding the available antiretroviral therapies and current evaluation and treatment guidelines for pediatric HIV/AIDS, see www.aidsinfo.nih.gov.

EMERGING VIRAL INFECTIONS
Nipah Virus

In the fall of 1998, an outbreak of severe encephalitis appeared in Malaysia due to a paramyxovirus, named Nipah virus after the Malaysian village in which the virus was first detected. The clinical features included fever, headache, vomiting, cough, cerebellar signs, pupillary abnormalities, seizures, autonomic dysfunction, and coma. The initial outbreak of Nipah encephalitis resulted from contact with pigs or with pig excrement, and after slaughter and disposal of pigs, the initial outbreak ended. Fruit bats (genus *Pteropus*) serve as a natural reservoir of the virus, and during recent outbreaks, person-to-person spread, as well as foodborne transmission, has been documented. The disease remains highly fatal; cognitive impairment is common among survivors.

Dengue Virus

Dengue virus, spread by the bites of *Aedes aegypti* or *Aedes albopictus* mosquitoes, commonly causes "breakbone fever," a self-limited disorder associated with high fever, headache, myalgia, bone pain, rash, and easy bruising. The more severe form of infection, dengue hemorrhagic fever, produces severe abdominal pain, dyspnea, and persistent vomiting, and deaths can result from shock or congestive heart failure. Dengue virus infections in adults and children have been associated rarely with encephalitis manifesting with fever, seizures, weakness, or alterations in consciousness. Neurodiagnostic features consist of CSF pleocytosis, EEG slowing, and cerebral edema or focal areas of T2 hyperintensity on MRI. The diagnosis is established by detecting virus in clinical samples, serologic responses using IgM antibody capture enzyme-linked immunosorbent assay (MAC-ELISA), or viral nucleic acids in serum or CSF using real time, reverse transcription PCR. At present, treatment consists of fluid replacement, supportive care, and avoidance of medications, such as aspirin, that potentiate the hemorrhagic complications.

Parechoviruses

The human parechoviruses (HPeVs), members of the picornavirus family, have been linked to neonatal encephalitis and injury to cerebral white matter. Infected infants have sepsis-like illnesses, accompanied by rash, irritability, and seizures. Although CSF should be obtained to exclude other conditions, including neonatal HSV infections, CSF pleocytosis is uncommon. Parechovirus infection can be confirmed by reverse transcription PCR analysis of blood or CSF, or by culturing the virus from CSF, stool, or nasopharyngeal secretions. Given the propensity of HPeVs to damage the white matter, infants with confirmed infections should undergo serial examination by MRI. There is no effective antiviral treatment for infection with HPeVs.

Chikungunya Virus

Chikungunya virus, an alphavirus of the *Togaviridae* family, is transmitted to humans and other amplifying hosts by Aedes mosquitoes. In December 2013, chikungunya virus first appeared in the Western Hemisphere and within 7 months, the virus caused more than 400,000 cases of disease in more than 20 countries in the Caribbean and in Central and South America. The term *chikungunya* translates as "disease that bends up the joints," reflecting the severe pains affecting the wrists, hands, knees, and ankles. In some patients, chikungunya virus causes encephalitis with altered mental status, seizures, coma, and, occasionally, death. Newborns who acquire chikungunya virus perinatally can develop a severe encephalopathy, with high rates of morbidity and mortality. Children who survive perinatal chikungunya infection frequently have microcephaly, global developmental delay, and cerebral palsy. Thus far, few cases of chikungunya virus have been acquired in the continental United States.

Zika Virus

First isolated from a rhesus monkey infected with a previously unknown virus in the Zika Forest of Uganda in the late 1940s, Zika virus belongs to the *flaviviridae*, a family of RNA viruses transmitted to humans by arthropod vectors (Hayes, 2009). Zika virus, related to St. Louis encephalitis and yellow fever viruses, naturally circulates among primates and Aedes species mosquitoes, particularly *Aedes africanus*, in endemic regions of Africa and Asia. Until recently, Zika virus infrequently caused human disease.

In 2007, Zika virus appeared in Micronesia, and in the fall of 2013 the virus caused a massive human outbreak in French Polynesia, eventually affecting nearly 30,000 persons or more than 10% of the population (Musso et al., 2014). Most infected persons had a mild viral syndrome with low-grade fever, conjunctivitis, arthalgias, and a maculopapular rash, but some experienced Guillain-Barré syndrome approximately 1 week after Zika virus infection (Oehler et al., 2013). The virus continued its eastward trajectory and in early 2015, cases of Zika virus began to appear in Brazil, most likely transmitted to humans by *Aedes aegypti*, a mosquito species prevalent throughout the Americas.

As with prior outbreaks, the majority of human infections (~80%) in Brazil occurred asymptomatically; when symptoms occurred, they mirrored those of the French Polynesia outbreak. In contrast to the Polynesian outbreak, however, the Brazilian epidemic was associated with a marked increase in the numbers of infants born with microcephaly and intracranial calcifications, suggesting intrauterine transmission of Zika virus and damage to the developing central nervous system (Mlakar et al., 2016). Zika virus infection of the fetus was confirmed by isolation of the virus from placenta, amniotic fluid and brain tissue. In addition to the apparent effects of Zika virus on the brain, congenital Zika virus infections have been associated with optic nerve hypoplasia and abnormalities of the retinal pigment (Ventura et al., 2016).

Zika virus infection should be suspected in infants with microcephaly, intracranial calcifications and ophthalmological abnormalities in the absence of microbiological evidence for the agents typically associated with congenital infection, including CMV, lymphocytic choriomeningitis virus, rubella virus, *Toxoplasma gondii*, *Treponema pallidum*, herpes simplex virus, herpes zoster virus, and *Trypanosoma cruzi*. The diagnosis of Zika virus infection can be established by serologic testing of mothers and infants for Zika virus-specific IgM or neutralizing antibodies and RT-PCR testing of the infant's serum and CSF for Zika virus RNA (Staples et al., 2016). At time of this writing many questions regarding maternal-fetal transmission, the clinical spectrum, and the neuropathogenesis of congenital Zika virus infection remain unanswered. The virus represents an ominous, potential threat to pregnant women visiting or residing within the host range of *Aedes aegypti* mosquitos, including the United States.

REFERENCES

The complete list of references for this chapter is available in the e-book at www.expertconsult.com.
    See inside cover for registration details.

SELECTED REFERENCES

Bale, J.F. Jr., 2009. Fetal infections and brain development. Clin. Perinatol. 36 (3), 639–653.
Baron, E.J., Miller, J.M., Weinstein, M.P., et al., 2013. A guide to utilization of the microbiology laboratory for diagnosis of infectious diseases: 2013 recommendations by the Infectious Diseases Society of America (IDSA) and the American Society for Microbiology (ASM). Clin. Infect. Dis. 57, e22–e121.
Bonthius, D.J., Karacay, B.K., 2002. Meningitis and encephalitis in children. An update. Neurol. Clin. 20 (4), 1013–1038.
Glaser, C.A., Gilliam, S., Schurr, D., et al., 2003. In search of encephalitis etiologies: diagnostic challenges in the California Encephalitis Project, 1998–2000. Clin. Infect. Dis. 36 (6), 731–742.
Hayes, E.B., 2009. Zika virus outside Africa. Emerg. Infect. Dis. 15, 1347–1350.
Johnson, R.T., 1998. Viral Infections of the Nervous System, second ed. Lippincott Raven, Philadelphia.
Mlakar, J., Korva, M., Tul, N., et al., 2016. Zika virus associated with microcephaly. N. Engl. J. Med. 374 (10), 951–958.
Musso, D., Nilles, E.J., Cao-Lormeau, V.M., 2014. Rapid spread of emerging Zika virus in the Pacific area. Clin. Microbiol. Infect. 20, 595–596.
Oehler, E., Watrin, L., Larre, P., et al., 2014. Zika virus infection complicated by Guillain-Barré syndrome-case report, French Polynesia, December 2013. Euro. Surveill. 19, 2720.
Peery, H.E., Day, G.S., Doja, A., et al., 2013. Anti-NMDA receptor encephalitis in children: the disorder, its diagnosis, and treatment. Hand. Clin. Neurol. 119, 1229–1233.
Pickering, L.K., Baker, C.J., Kimberlin, D.W., et al. (Eds.), 2012. Red Book: 2012 Report of the Committee on Infectious Diseases, twenty-ninth ed. American Academy of Pediatrics, Elk Grove Village, IL.
Reiss, C.S. (Ed.), 2008. Neurotropic Viral Infections. Cambridge University Press, Cambridge, UK.
Staples, J.E., Dzuiban, E.J., Fischer, M., et al., 2016. Interim guidelines for the evaluation and testing of infants with possible congenital Zika virus infection-United States 2016. MMWR. 65 (3), 63–67.
Ventura, C.V., Maia, M., Ventura, B.V., et al., 2016. Ophthalmological findings in infants with microcephaly and presumable intra-uterus Zika virus infection. Arq. Bras. Oftalmol. 79 (1), 1–3.
Whitley, R.J., Kimberlin, D.W., 2005. Herpes simplex encephalitis: children and adolescents. Semin. Pediatr. Infect. Dis. 16 (1), 17–23.
Willoughby, R.E., Tieves, K.S., Hoffman, G.M., et al., 2005. Survival after treatment of rabies with induction of coma. N. Engl. J. Med. 352 (24), 2508–2514.

E-BOOK FIGURES AND TABLES

The following figures and tables are available in the e-book at www.expertconsult.com. See inside cover for registration details.

Fig. 115-1 Data for paralytic poliomyelitis in the United States from 1960 to 1994.
Fig. 115-4 Axial T2-weighted spine magnetic resonance image.
Fig. 115-7 Unenhanced computed tomography scan of an infant with congenital herpes simplex virus infection.
Fig. 115-8 Unenhanced computed tomography scan of a young child who survived herpes simplex virus encephalitis.
Fig. 115-9 T2-weighted magnetic resonance image from a child with Epstein-Barr virus encephalitis.
Fig. 115-10 T1-weighted magnetic resonance image from a child with Epstein-Barr virus encephalitis.
Fig. 115-11 Axial, T2-weighted magnetic resonance image from a child with agammaglobulinemia and presumed progressive nonpolio enterovirus encephalopathy.
Fig. 115-12 Data regarding the incidence of rubella and congenital rubella syndrome in the United States from 1966 to 1992.
Fig. 115-13 A map of the United States showing data regarding West Nile virus infections in 2003, the peak year of West Nile virus activity in the country.
Fig. 115-15 Unenhanced head computed tomography scan of a 1-year-old child with congenital lymphocytic choriomeningitis infection demonstrating ventriculomegaly and periventricular calcifications (arrows).
Fig. 115-16 An acquired immune deficiency syndrome mural on a school building in rural Namibia.
Fig. 115-17 Unenhanced computed tomography scan in a child with hemophilia and progressive human immunodeficiency virus encephalopathy.
Box 115-2 Viruses Associated with Aseptic Meningitis and Encephalitis in Children
Box 115-3 Viruses Associated with Myelopathy, Guillain–Barré Syndrome, Acute Cerebellar Ataxia, and Intrauterine Infection
Table 115-2 Diagnostic Methods for Selected Viruses Causing Encephalitis in Infants and Children
Table 115-3 Outcome of Selected Viral Central Nervous System Disorders

116 Fungal, Rickettsial, and Parasitic Diseases of the Nervous System

Alexander L. Greninger and Carol A. Glaser

 An expanded version of this chapter is available on www.expertconsult.com. See inside cover for registration details.

FUNGAL DISEASES

The importance of invasive fungal infections, including those of the central nervous system (CNS), has risen as the population of immunologically compromised patients, including preterm infants, has grown. Patients with congenital immunological deficiencies, aplastic anemia, poorly controlled human immunodeficiency virus (HIV) infection, patients receiving chemotherapy as well as transplant recipients are susceptible. The normal host can also develop invasive fungal infection but does so less often and to a smaller spectrum of organisms.

Fungal diseases involving the brain are usually spread via the bloodstream after a systemic or pulmonary focus is established. Alternatively, these pathogens invade the CNS via direct extension from adjacent sinuses, the cranial vault, orbits, or the spine. With exceptions such as *Candida* spp. meningitis in premature neonates and *Aspergillus* spp. brain abscess in the highly compromised host, CNS fungal infections in children are rare. Table 116-1 provides a more extensive list of risk factors, syndromes, and treatments for fungal infections of the nervous system. Because clinical manifestations of CNS fungal infections can be subtle and not specific to individual pathogens, errors and delays in diagnosis occur. Fungi may cause a variety of clinical syndromes, including meningitis, brain abscesses, granulomas, and invasion of the vasculature, further complicating clinical presentation and treatment.

Cryptococcosis

Cryptococcosis is globally distributed and is most commonly seen in patients with acquired immunodeficiency syndrome (AIDS) and in those receiving systemic corticosteroids; infection also occurs in those without apparent predisposition but at a lower frequency. Infants have contracted the disease, and vertical transmission has been reported from a mother with advanced AIDS. The mode of entry in humans is probably through inhalation or ingestion, and dissemination to the nervous system can follow. The most common cause, *Cryptococcus neoformans,* is encapsulated yeast found widely in the environment, particularly in bird feces and soil (Fig. 116-1). Infection with *Cryptococcus gattii* is emerging in humans in British Columbia and the northwestern United States. Notably, *C. gattii* most often affects immunocompetent individuals.

Cryptococcus most often causes a meningoencephalitis but can also cause brain abscess and cryptococcomas. Typical meningitis features such as nausea, vomiting, headache, and fever are often present. Caution is urged in ruling out the diagnosis based on history and physical examination alone because presenting symptoms may be nonspecific and a substantial number of patients are afebrile and lack meningeal signs. In AIDS patients, CNS *Cryptococcus* tends to be acute, with fever and headache in 70%; meningismus, photophobia, or mental status changes in 20% to 25%; and focal deficits in a small percentage. A substantial minority of these patients may have initially normal CSF cell counts, glucose, and protein.

When *C. neoformans* causes mass lesions, it can result in papilledema, cranial neuropathies, and hemiparesis. Brain abscess and cyptococcomas may begin with an indolent course, but hydrocephalus occurs and often necessitates shunting; if untreated, the mortality is high. *Cryptococcus* can be identified by culturing CSF on Sabouraud agar, but large volume culture on more than one occasion may be needed. Latex agglutination detection of cryptococcal antigen is a rapid and useful adjunct test for both serum and CSF specimens. The Infectious Disease Society of America (IDSA) recently published treatment guidelines and recommends an initial combination of amphotericin B and flucytosine for cryptococcal CNS disease in all age groups, regardless of HIV status (Perfect et al., 2010).

Coccidioidomycosis

Coccidioidomycosis is caused by the fungus *Coccidioides immitis*. Disease caused by *C. immitis* most commonly occurs in the southwestern United States, northern Mexico, and portions of Central and South America. Coccidioidomycosis is acquired by inhalation of spore-laden dust or transcutaneously after skin abrasion. Only 40% of acutely infected normal hosts experience acute respiratory symptoms, typically within 3 weeks after exposure and accompanied by fever, chills, night sweats, cough, anorexia, and weight loss. Dissemination of the infection from the pulmonary focus to distant sites usually occurs 1 to 6 months after primary infection in approximately 0.5% of cases; half of these are meningitis. Other sites of dissemination include skin, lymph nodes, bones, and joints. The risk of dissemination is highest in patients of Filipino, African American, and Hispanic backgrounds and in immunocompromised individuals.

The clinical characteristics of coccidioidal meningitis are nonspecific and prompt diagnosis can be difficult. The most prevalent manifestations are headache, fever, malaise, and weight loss; meningismus may be absent (Saitoh et al., 2000). Findings can include confusion, personality changes, focal neurologic deficits, ataxia, obtundation, and coma. Brain and spinal cord abscesses can occur with or without concurrent meningitis. Spinal cord symptoms may also occur in conjunction with coccidioidal osteomyelitis of the cervical vertebrae. CSF abnormalities include mononuclear pleocytosis, increased protein content, increased chloride concentration, and normal or decreased glucose concentration. Diagnosis can be confirmed by either direct microscopy or culture of the CSF (Fig. 116-2). Unfortunately, CSF cultures and microscopy are often negative in *C. immitis* meningitis, requiring other testing. Complement fixation and precipitin tests provide accurate diagnosis in more than 99% of patients with disseminated infection.

The 2008 IDSA guidelines for treatment of coccidioidal meningitis recommend oral fluconazole or itraconazole for all patients; intrathecal amphotericin was recommended by some clinicians but was graded C-III (poor evidence) by the IDSA.

North American Blastomycosis

Blastomycosis is caused by inhalation of airborne spores from *Blastomycosis dermatitidis*, a dimorphic fungus found in soil. The endemic area includes the midwestern, southeastern, and south central United States, and the Canadian provinces near the Great Lakes and the St. Lawrence Seaway. The spectrum of clinical manifestations in adults includes pulmonary disease, acute and chronic skin disease, and disseminated disease involving the bones, the genitourinary tract, or the CNS. The three major CNS clinical manifestations are meningitis, intracranial mass, and spinal mass. Children are infrequently affected but suffer a similar spectrum of illness as adults.

In pulmonary disease, the organism can be identified on microscopy and culture of respiratory tract specimens. For CNS disease, ventricular and cisternal fluid may have a higher yield than lumbar CSF, which is rarely positive. Amphotericin B for 4 to 6 weeks is recommended for moderate to severe disease, followed by prolonged treatment with oral fluconazole, itraconazole, or voriconazole.

South American Blastomycosis

South American blastomycosis is caused by the fungus *Paracoccidioides brasiliensis*. Acquisition of disease is restricted to people living in latitudes between Mexico and Argentina, with most patients reported from Brazil. CNS involvement may follow disseminated infection. The most common findings of CNS infections included seizures, hemiparesis, cerebellar signs, and hydrocephalus. CNS infection usually causes single or multiple mass lesions that appear hypodense and enhance on CT scan; MRI may show contrast-enhancing brain lesions with occasional meningeal involvement.

CSF findings are typically normal, except for slightly elevated protein, and CSF cultures are often negative. The diagnosis of South American blastomycosis is best suggested by simultaneous involvement of several organs or by characteristic oral and skin lesions in patients who reside in endemic areas. Brazilian guidelines on treatment are available in Portuguese and recommend that CNS infection be treated with trimethoprim-sulfamethoxazole for prolonged periods.

Histoplasmosis

Histoplasmosis is globally distributed; *Histoplasma capsulatum* is found in the Americas (the Mississippi River basin, Mexico, and Central and South America), and *Histoplasma duboisii* is found in Africa. In most cases, infection is self-limited, but an estimated 10% of those infected with *Histoplasma capsulatum* develop pulmonary symptoms to a degree prompting medical evaluation; those younger than 2 years, the elderly, and those with immunocompromising conditions are more likely to be symptomatic. Only a small subset of individuals with primary histoplasmosis develops disseminated disease, and an even smaller group develops a CNS infection. *Histoplasma* can remain quiescent in the lungs or the adrenal glands for more than 40 years before dissemination.

Most children with respiratory infection are asymptomatic. Fever, chills, and a productive cough can occur, and initial chest radiographs may document a nodular or diffuse infiltrate. Years later, chest radiographs demonstrate characteristic calcification in the central lymph nodes and peripheral lung fields.

Signs and symptoms associated with CNS involvement in children include memory impairment, confusion, seizures, ataxia, cranial nerve palsies, and urinary incontinence. Neuroimaging may show evidence of hydrocephalus. Diagnosis is made via a four-fold rise in complement fixation titers between acute and convalescent specimens; a single elevated titer in the correct clinical setting is diagnostic. The organism can be directly detected through culture of CSF, blood, and bone marrow, and through biopsy of liver, bone marrow, and lymph nodes.

CNS infection in children should be treated with amphotericin B followed by itraconazole, according to the 2007 IDSA guidelines.

Nocardia

Nocardia spp., gram-positive, branching, filamentous bacteria, are ubiquitous in the environment; *Nocardia asteroides, Nocardia farcinica*, and *Nocardia brasiliensis* are the species most often responsible for clinical disease. Risk factors for pediatric CNS infections include malignancy, chronic granulomatous disease, lupus, HIV infection, organ transplantation, and surgery.

Brain abscess is the most frequently reported CNS manifestation of nocardial infection, but meningitis can occur, typically after rupture of an abscess or, more rarely, as the primary presentation.

Diagnosis of *Nocardia* brain abscess may require a drainage procedure to obtain an adequate specimen for prolonged laboratory incubation to ensure growth on culture. Treatment and management of nocardial CNS infection requires multiple agents for prolonged periods and susceptibility testing should be done at a reference laboratory.

Actinomycosis

Actinomyces spp. are anaerobic or microaerophilic, gram-positive, nonspore forming, branching bacilli that normally colonize the mouth, intestine, and female genital tract. CNS disease in young children has not been reported, but risk factors for CNS disease in older children and adults include untreated focal infections, immunosuppression, and congenital heart disease with right-to-left shunts.

Actinomycosis is a chronic, slow-growing, inflammatory mass, most frequently affecting the lungs, cervicofacial region, abdomen, and pelvis (in association with intrauterine devices). Cerebral involvement is rare and manifested as an abscess (solitary or multiple) and, less commonly, meningitis. CNS *Actinomyces* may be difficult to recover on culture. The etiology of CNS disease may be inferred if *Actinomyces* spp. are isolated at another site. Standard recommended treatment for CNS disease is penicillin for at least 6 months. Recently, successful shorter courses of treatment with drugs other than penicillin for CNS disease have been reported. Surgical drainage may also be needed.

Aspergillosis

Aspergillus spp. comprise a variety of highly aerobic, asexual molds that initially gain entrance to the lung by inhalation. Aspergillosis of the CNS was rare until the population of immunocompromised hosts increased during the past two decades. Among compromised hosts, the highest frequency of invasive aspergillosis is in heart and lung transplant recipients (19% to 26%), followed by those with chronic granulomatous disease (24% to 40%), acute leukemia (5% to 24%), bone marrow or hematopoietic stem cell recipients (0.5%

to 9%), AIDS (0 to 12%), and solid organ transplant recipients (0.5% to 10%). CNS disease complicates 10% to 20% of invasive disease.

Clinical Characteristics, Clinical Laboratory Tests, and Diagnosis

Three types of clinical presentation have been reported with CNS aspergillosis:

1. An intracranial form, the most common, presenting like a space-occupying lesion
2. A rhinocerebral form, with primary involvement of the sinuses and secondary involvement of the skull base, cranial nerves, and brain
3. A vascular form with stroke-like symptoms

Other less common manifestations include meningitis, meningoencephalitis, hemorrhagic or ischemic necrosis, solitary granulomas, and invasive fungal arteritis. Neuroimaging may reveal sinus invasion, enhancing or nonenhancing hypodense brain lesions indicative of abscess, or prominent ischemic lesions in the basal ganglia; concurrent chest radiography or CT scan usually shows multiple nodular lesions.

Definitive diagnosis of invasive *Aspergillus* is made by smear and culture of biopsy material. A presumptive diagnosis of CNS infection can be made if *Aspergillus* is identified from another site at the same time that neuroimaging shows multiple mass lesions. A positive serum galactomannan test supports the diagnosis. The 2009 IDSA guidelines for *Aspergillus* spp. infection of the CNS recommend voriconazole as the primary medical therapy, with itraconazole, posaconazole, and liposomal formulations of amphotericin B as alternatives in cases of intolerance.

Candidiasis

Candida spp. are the most common invasive fungal infections in infants and children. Cerebral candidiasis is a rare sequela of disseminated disease in debilitated patients. Risk factors include prematurity, prolonged broad-spectrum antibiotics, total parenteral nutrition, central venous catheterization, immunosuppression, immunodeficiency (congenital or acquired), chronic renal disease, diabetes, neutropenia, and ventriculoperitoneal shunts. Meningitis is the most common manifestation of candidal CNS disease, but abscesses and granulomas occur independently and in combination with meningitis. When brain abscesses occur, they are typically multiple in number, illustrating the consequence of hematogenous dissemination. Arterial and venous involvement can lead to the development of intracranial mycotic aneurysms.

Diagnosis can be confirmed by identification of the organism in spinal fluid or infected neural tissue. Pleocytosis or reduced CSF glucose occurs in only about half of the patients who are culture-positive. Recent IDSA guidelines for adults for *C. albicans* infection in the CNS recommend amphotericin, with or without 5-flucytosine followed by fluconazole.

Zygomycosis

Zygomycetes are ubiquitous, broad, irregularly branched fungi found in soil and decaying matter. The classic progression to the syndrome known as rhinocerebral zygomycosis begins with a nasopharyngeal or sinus focus, followed by direct invasion into the CNS. This invasive infection rarely, if ever, occurs in the normal host. Risk factors include diabetes mellitus, intravenous drug use, solid organ or bone marrow transplantation, and other immunocompromising conditions. Fever, facial and ocular pain, or CNS symptoms may herald the

onset, and a black eschar-like plaque may be seen in the oropharynx or nasopharynx. Etiology of CNS disease seen on neuroimaging can be inferred from biopsy of nasopharyngeal or sinus specimens. Hyphae can be found in biopsy material. Amphotericin and posaconazole are the most commonly used therapies.

Scedosporium spp. Infection

Two species of *Scedosporium* environmental molds, *prolificans* and *apiospermum* (sexual state known as *Pseudallescheria boydii*), can cause a wide variety of human disease, including CNS infection. Risk groups include compromised hosts and survivors of near drowning.

Scedosporium spp. can cause skin, lung, bone, joint, ocular, and bloodstream and CNS infections. Brain abscess is the typical CNS manifestation and can be solitary or multiple. Definitive diagnosis is through brain biopsy, although culture from a nonsterile site can support the diagnosis. The principles of therapy are similar to those for aspergillosis and zygomycosis, and include surgical resection of accessible brain abscesses, reduction or reversal of immunosuppression, and the use of antifungal agents.

RICKETTSIAL DISEASES

Rickettsiae are pleomorphic coccobacilli that are obligate intracellular bacteria whose arthropod vectors include ticks, mites, fleas, or lice. Rickettsial diseases include the spotted fevers, typhus fevers, scrub typhus, Q fever, and ehrlichioses. Rickettsial infections often have an accompanying skin eruption. *Coxiella burnetii*, the rickettsia causing Q fever, differs from the other organisms because it does not require a vector and rarely causes a skin rash.

The clinical and pathologic response of the CNS to different infections caused by *Rickettsia* spp. is generally similar and differs only in severity. Headache is often the earliest and most frequent symptom in all rickettsial infections.

Diagnostic testing is also similar for most rickettsial infections. Serology is the most generally available and widely used method. The indirect fluorescent antibody assay is considered the gold standard. However, because most patients with rickettsial diseases do not develop antibodies reactive in the first week of illness, serologic tests are often negative early in illness. Evaluation of paired serum specimens collected during the acute and convalescent phases of the illness for a four-fold or greater change in antibody titer confirms the diagnosis. Extensive crossreactivity exists among antigens of the spotted fever group rickettsiae (e.g., *Rickettsia rickettsii*, *Rickettsia akari*, and *Rickettsia conorii*), and among antigens in the typhus group (*Rickettsia prowazekii* and *Rickettsia typhi*). In this context, most indirect fluorescent antibody assays are group-specific rather than species-specific tests for rickettsial infection.

Doxycycline is the drug of choice for Rocky Mountain spotted fever and other rickettsia in all age groups (except for pregnant women). Empiric treatment with doxycycline should be initiated early in the course if clinical and epidemiologic findings are suggestive of a rickettsial infection because delays in treatment can lead to adverse outcomes.

Rocky Mountain spotted fever is the prototypic condition for these infections and is discussed in the next section. The epidemiology, clinical, and laboratory features of other Rickettsia infection are outlined in Table 116-2.

Rocky Mountain Spotted Fever

Rocky Mountain spotted fever (RMSF) is caused by *Rickettsia rickettsii* and is the most common fatal tick-borne illness in the United States.

RMSF has been reported throughout the United States, with the exception of Hawaii and Vermont. The states with the highest incidence of RMSF are Oklahoma and North Carolina. In the United States the number of RMSF cases has increased in recent years, averaging over 2000 cases a year reported between 2005 and 2010—the highest recorded levels in more than 80 years (Walker et al., 2008). Children are at a higher risk of infection (half of the cases are under 19 years of age) as are Native Americans (Buckingham et al., 2007). The incubation period ranges from 2 to 14 days (mean 7 days) after a tick bite. Symptoms of RMSF vary in severity from mild to severe; the course may rapidly lead to death. RMSF is characterized by the classic triad of fever, headache, and rash particularly in the setting of a recent tick bite. Most patients with RMSF, however, do not present with the classic triad. Additionally, many patients are unaware of tick bite. Initial symptoms are nonspecific and include fever, malaise, lethargy, and headache. The headache is usually intense and refractory to most analgesics. Progressive restlessness, irritability, confusion, and delirium may also occur. By day 5 of the illness, 85% of patients develop a rash. The rash often begins with a maculopapular appearance and becomes more defined as petechiae as the rash evolves. The rash often begins around the ankles or wrists and then spreads to other parts of the body. Acute renal failure, coagulopathy, and cerebral edema are well-recognized complications. Edema, usually periorbital at first and then generalized, is characteristic of and may suggest the diagnosis. Hepatosplenomegaly and liver dysfunction, including coagulation defects, may also be present. Skin necrosis and gangrene can be a late complication. Ophthalmic features in all rickettsial disorders are virtually identical, and may include photophobia, conjunctivitis, petechiae on the bulbar conjunctiva, exudates and retinal venous engorgement, papilledema, and ocular palsies.

The differential diagnosis of RMSF includes meningococcemia, enteroviral infection, scarlet fever, toxic shock syndrome, Kawasaki disease, Epstein-Barr virus, syphilis, typhoid, rat-bite fever, and other tick-borne diseases. Spinal fluid may demonstrate a lymphocytic pleocytosis, and the protein is elevated in about 30% to 50% of patients. Direct immunofluorescence antibody studies can be performed on skin biopsy, and PCR for *R. rickettsii* DNA can be done on serum, whole blood, or tissue specimens but is available only at specialized research laboratories.

PARASITIC DISEASES

Human parasitic infestation occurs worldwide in tropical, temperate, and cold climates. Parasitic infections impair the CNS by a variety of mechanisms, including the following:

1. Direct invasion from the circulation or lymphatic system may cause local changes, such as inflammation and edema.
2. Granuloma development may result in disturbances associated with mass lesions.
3. Remote effects associated with nutrient deprivation of the CNS may cause diffuse or focal CNS symptomatology.
4. Immunologic or hypersensitivity effects may develop.

Changes in society have spread what were once exotic diseases largely restricted to developing countries into the developed world. Ease and frequency of travel require that all clinicians have general familiarity with these infections when considering differential diagnoses. Population shifts, whether due to immigration or social unrest, have brought unfamiliar parasitic infections into urban and other areas of the world. Please see Table 116-3 for a complete list of parasites that can affect the CNS.

PROTOZOAL INFECTIONS OF THE CENTRAL NERVOUS SYSTEM

Amebic Infections of the Central Nervous System

For information on *Entamoeba histolytica* and *Microsporidia* sp., see Table 116-3 and the online version of this chapter.

Primary Amebic Meningoencephalitis: *Naegleria fowleri*

Primary amebic meningoencephalitis (PAM) is a fulminant disease occurring in children and young adults caused by *Naegleria fowleri*. *N. fowleri* is a free-living, facultative parasite that can be found in water, soil, sewage, or other decaying organic material where there is a bacterial food source. Of an estimated 200 cases since the first descriptions of PAM, more than 90% of the patients have died. The disease has been reported primarily from the United States, Australia and Europe but cases occur worldwide.

Typically, infection with *N. fowleri* occurs when swimming, or washing in warm, fresh water containing the amebas such as ponds, man-made lakes, hot springs, wading pools, irrigation canals, thermally polluted streams, and inadequately chlorinated swimming pools. Those affected are previously healthy children or young adults. Most infections have been associated with diving and underwater swimming, but sinus irrigation has been recently associated with PAM.

The onset of PAM is usually within 2 to 3 days after exposure. Amebas enter the nasal passages and gain access to the nervous system by penetrating the olfactory mucosa, entering the submucosal nervous plexus, migrating along the olfactory nerves, and traversing the cribriform plate.

The most common manifestations of PAM are severe headache, stiff neck, nausea, vomiting, fever, behavioral changes, change in smell, seizures, diplopia, and coma. Spinal fluid typically has a decreased glucose concentration, increased protein content (75 to 970 mg/dl), and innumerable white blood cells (300 to 24,600/mm³) with a predominance of polymorphonuclear cells and erythrocytes.

A CSF wet mount can aid in the diagnosis—the amebas can be recognized by their relatively swift movement with an anterior, eruptive pseudopod. A multiplex, real-time polymerase chain reaction has recently been developed with the ability to detect *Naegleria*, *Balamuthia*, and *Acanthamoeba* simulatenously (Qvarnstrom et al., 2006). There is a high mortality associated with PAM; however, occasional favorable outcomes have been achieved with a combination of various therapies (Linam et al., 2015). Miletfosine has recently been recommended for PAM and is available as an investigational drug from the CDC.

Granulomatous Amebic Encephalitis: Acanthamoeba spp. and Balamuthia mandrillaris

Two different, closely related amebas cause granulomatous encephalitis: *Acanthamoeba* spp. and *Balamuthia mandrillaris*. Acanthamoeba granulomatous encephalitis is an opportunistic, chronic disease that may have a prodromal period of weeks to months, with most patients being immunocompromised. A small number of *Acanthamoeba* granulomatous encephalitis cases have been described in immunocompetent children.

Acanthamoeba is commonly found in soil. *Acanthamoeba* is also found in the home in aquariums, flower pot soil, humidifiers, sink taps, and drains and has been isolated from hot tubs, hydrotherapy baths, dental irrigation equipment, and laboratory eye wash stations. Infection may take place through breaks in the skin that are contaminated with soil, or by inhalation of airborne ameba cysts originating from soil.

In addition to encephalitis, *Acanthamoeba* can cause nasopharyngeal, cutaneous, and disseminated infections. Nasopharyngeal and cutaneous infections can be precursors to disseminated amebiasis or encephalitis, as amebas spread from their initial portal of entry. The CNS becomes infected by hematogenous transport of amebas, either from the lungs or from cutaneous lesions.

Clinical features typically have a subacute to chronic presentation, with fever, headache, seizures, personality change, lethargy, or confusion. Children with *Acanthamoeba* exhibit headache, stiff neck, vomiting, abnormal behavior, fever, ataxia, and tonic-clonic seizures. CSF protein is elevated (range 31 to 500 mg/dl), as is the white blood cell count (14 to 750 cells/µL) and glucose level (17 to 240 mg/dl); among the white blood cells are lymphocytes (19% to 100%) and polymorphonuclear leukocytes (2% to 70%). Neuroimaging may show punctate focal lesions in the cerebellar hemispheres or in the corpus callosum or hydrocephalus. Sequential MRIs may resemble a rapidly expanding brain mass. *Acanthamoeba* can sometimes be seen on CSF wet-mount slide preparations. A multiplex, real-time polymerase chain reaction has recently been developed with the ability to detect *Balamuthia, Acanthamoeba,* and *Naegleria* simultaneously (Qvarnstrom et al., 2006).

Acanthamoeba infections of the CNS are usually fatal, although some reports of successful antimicrobial treatment are described. Most recoveries result from successful treatment with combinations of different antimicrobials as outlined in online version of this chapter. In vitro studies suggest that miltefosine and voriconazole have activity against *Acanthamoeba.*

Granulomatous Amebic Encephalitis:
Balamuthia mandrillaris

Balamuthia granulomatous encephalitis was initially described in immunocompromised humans, but more recent cases have occurred in immunocompetent adults and children. The importance of *Balamuthia* as a CNS pathogen is increasingly recognized (Schuster et al., 2009). Most cases are reported in the United States and South America but cases are now recognized across the globe. Like *Acanthamoeba,* it is likely to enter the body by inhalation of cysts in windblown soil or through breaks in the skin contaminated by soil, followed by hematogenous spread. Signs and symptoms of *Balamuthia* granulomatous encephalitis include fever, headache, vomiting, ataxia, hemiparesis, tonic-clonic seizures, cranial nerve palsies (particularly third and sixth cranial nerves), and consequent diplopia. Areas of the brain that are typically infected are the basal ganglia, midbrain, brainstem, and cerebral hemispheres. CSF may have mild to markedly elevated protein and leukocyte levels, and normal or slightly decreased glucose.

Neuroimaging reveals single or multiple space-occupying or ring-enhancing lesions, enlarged ventricles, atypical demyelinating lesions, or ring-enhancing lesions with surrounding edema or hydrocephalus. A multiplex, real-time polymerase chain reaction has recently been developed with the ability to detect *Balamuthia, Acanthamoeba,* and *Naegleria* simultaneously (Qvarnstrom et al., 2006).

Of the approximately 200 recognized *Balamuthia* cases, successful outcomes have been reported in 10 individuals, including four pediatric patients, using various combinations of antimicrobials. Miltefosine is currently available through the CDC as an investigational new drug and available for treatment of the free-living amoeba.

Toxoplasmosis

Toxoplasma gondii is found worldwide in a variety of mammals and birds and is a public health problem in both developed and developing countries. Approximately 20% to 40% of the adult population in the United States is seropositive. The cat is the definitive host of the parasite and excretes oocysts in the feces. Ingestion of the oocyst by animals and humans continues the life cycle of the parasite.

Humans are infected by ingestion of raw or inadequately cooked meat containing tissue or by ingestion of oocysts shed in cat feces. Reactivation of a latent infection can be triggered by the host becoming immunodeficient or immunocompromised.

Intrauterine or congenital toxoplasmosis may develop in the fetus when the mother is infected during pregnancy. The incidences of maternal and fetal infection in the United States are 6 and 2 per 1000, respectively. The risk of fetal infection increases as the pregnancy progresses: 25% in the first trimester, 54% in the second trimester, and 65% in the third trimester. Severity of infection is inversely related to when infection occurs during pregnancy. When disseminated, acquired toxoplasmosis produces systemic manifestations consisting of multiple organ infection, including the brain.

Clinical manifestations of congenital infection are extremely variable. The well-known clinical constellation of hydrocephalus, cerebral calcifications, and chorioretinitis is variably present in affected infants. The approximate incidence of abnormalities in 180 cases of intrauterine toxoplasmosis included microcephaly (20%), hydrocephalus (25%), microphthalmia (35%), seizures (40%), psychomotor retardation (45%), cerebral calcification (60%), and chorioretinitis (95%). Although the manifestations of some cases have been similar to those of congenital cytomegalic inclusion disease, CNS involvement is usually more common and extensive in toxoplasmosis. Skull radiographs and ultrasound demonstrate punctate, scattered calcifications and separated cranial sutures. Delayed onset of seizures, chorioretinitis, and cognitive impairment can also occur. Even in those infants with toxoplasmosis who are asymptomatic at birth, up to 85% may develop chorioretinitis or serious neurologic disability by 8.3 years.

Outside the newborn period, the infection is often asymptomatic in the immunocompetent host. In contrast, immunosuppressed individuals can develop a life-threatening illness either from acute infection or through reactivation. The acquired form of toxoplasmosis causes meningoencephalitis, and long-term sequelae are common.

Immunologic diagnosis of toxoplasmosis relies on the Sabin-Feldman dye test (which detects live parasites), the direct hemagglutination test, the double-sandwich enzyme-linked immunosorbent assay, the immunosorbent agglutination assay, the complement fixation test, the evaluation of immunoglobulin M levels, and the indirect fluorescent antibody test. Diagnosis of congenital toxoplasmosis can be especially challenging—consultation and testing with a laboratory experienced with toxoplasmosis diagnostics is warranted.

Early treatment with spiramycin for the mother and sulfadiazine, pyrimethamine, and folinic acid for the infant is beneficial and 70% effective (Montoya and Liesenfeld, 2004). Outside the newborn period, treatment is usually not required, except in immunocompromised hosts. There are recommended treatment protocols for children infected with HIV and CNS toxoplasmosis.

Malaria

Malaria is one of the most common tropical infectious diseases. In 2013 the WHO estimated that there were 198 million cases worldwide. Malaria is caused by the protozoal parasites of the genus *Plasmodium,* with life cycle stages alternating between the mosquito and a variety of mammals and birds. The definitive host and vector for malaria is the female *Anopheles* mosquito. Several species of *Plasmodium* cause disease in humans—*Plasmodium falciparum, Plasmodium vivax, Plasmodium malariae,* and the recently discovered *Plasmodium knowlesi.* However, *P. falciparum* and *P. vivax* are the only members of the genus that have been well documented as affecting the CNS in humans.

In endemic areas, neonates are protected from infection by maternal (transplacental) antibody, in part, from the vestigial presence of fetal hemoglobin. This protection lasts for about 1 year, after which the infant becomes susceptible to disease. The child of 1 to 4 years of age is the most vulnerable to infection and the development of severe malaria, with a mortality of about 5%. Malaria acquired by recipients of blood transfusions from infected but asymptomatic carriers is also a major problem in endemic regions of the world. Because of more frequent international travel, increasing numbers of cases in adults and children are being recognized in the United States.

The clinical features of malaria are notoriously nonspecific, especially in children. Initial symptoms can include influenza-like illness with fever, chills, rigors, headache, and myalgia. These vague prodromal symptoms precede the development of acute paroxysms of high fever and chills, with the classically described periodic fever patterns observed after several days of untreated illness. Gastrointestinal and respiratory symptoms are also common.

Cerebral malaria is most often heralded by mental deterioration, particularly confusion or delirium, followed by progression to stupor and coma that transpires over the next 1 to 3 days. In children, cerebral involvement can be more fulminant, with most patients becoming comatose within 2 days. New-onset seizures may be confused with febrile seizures in young children. Extensor plantar responses, cerebellar impairment, abnormal movements, and psychosis may also occur. Children with severe illness exhibit evidence of transtentorial herniation. Papilledema and extramacular retinal edema are markers of a poor prognosis.

In patients with impaired consciousness, a lumbar puncture should be performed to assess for concurrent meningitis. Caution, however, should be exercised due to the potential for focal gradients of elevated intracranial pressure. Acutely, MRIs may demonstrate multifocal T2-enhancing lesions indicative of capillary occlusion and cerebral edema or increased brain volume.

The current gold standard for diagnosis of *P. falciparum* infection remains the study of thick and thin peripheral Giemsa-stained blood films. If antimalarial therapy was started before preparation of blood smears, the smears may be negative. Although examination of Giemsa-stained blood films remains the gold standard, rapid diagnostic tests also play an important role in diagnostics.

In 2010, the World Health Organization published updated guidelines for the treatment of malaria (WHO, 2010). The new guidelines emphasize the importance of parasitologic confirmation of diagnosis before initiation of antimalaria treatment. Artemisinin derivatives are the most rapidly acting of all antimalarial drugs and have transformed current treatment strategies. In the United States artemisinin-based drugs are available under investigational use only, and can be obtained by contacting the CDC directly at the CDC Malaria Hotline [(770) 488-7788 or (770) 488-7100].

Trypanosomal Infections of the Nervous System

The trypanosomes are a group of flagellated protozoa that infect a variety of vertebrates, but the clinically important species for humans are *Trypanosoma cruzi* (Chagas disease or American trypanosomiasis) and *Trypanosoma brucei* (African sleeping sickness). Both species are transmitted to humans by insect vectors.

Chagas Disease

Chagas disease (American trypanosomiasis) affects 15 to 16 million people in Latin America and extends from Argentina to the Mexican border with the United States (mostly in southern tier). The vector, the triatomine bug or "kissing bug" (*Triatoma* spp.), lives in thatched walls and roofs of houses and primarily affects those living in poor housing conditions. At the time the triatomine bug bites a human, it defecates on the skin surface, leaving a drop containing parasites. The parasite penetrates the broken skin when the presumptive host scratches or rubs the deposited fecal matter into the site of the insect bite or when fecal matter is transferred by fingers on to the corneal surface of the eye or mucous membranes.

The disease can also be passed by transplacental infection, breastfeeding, and blood transfusions. Intrauterine Chagas disease occurs in 2% to 4% of infants born to mothers who have acute or chronic infection with *T. cruzi.* Such infants are usually born prematurely and are small for gestational age. When meningoencephalitis occurs, seizures, hypotonia, and a weak suck are characteristically present. Almost half the infants who acquire infection in utero die by age 4 months.

When Chagas disease is acquired from an insect vector, it can manifest in two phases: acute and chronic. The acute phase begins about a week after infection, and is often asymptomatic, subclinical, and undiagnosed in 66% to 99% of cases, most of whom are babies or young children (Pittella, 2009). The acute phase is characterized by mild, nonspecific symptoms and signs (e.g., fever, vomiting, diarrhea, and hepatosplenomegaly). Inflammation develops at the portal of entry of the trypanosomes, producing a nodule (chagoma) and causing swelling of proximal lymph nodes. The Romaña sign (unilateral palpebral and periocular swelling) may occur as a result of conjunctiva contamination with the vector's feces. A small percentage of acutely infected patients develop cardiac symptoms suggestive of myocarditis or signs of meningoencephalitis.

After the latent asymptomatic phase of 10 to 25 years, chronic Chagas disease may represent in young adulthood. Most symptoms are due to severe cardiac or gastrointestinal involvement. Reactivated chronic Chagas disease is also observed in immunosuppressed patients, most commonly those with AIDS (75% to 80% of cases) and less frequently in patients after organ transplant or with chronic use of immunosuppressive medications.

In children with acute meningoencephalitis due to Chagas disease, CSF reveals a mild to moderate pleocytosis (less than 100 cells/mm^3), predominantly of lymphocytes, and protein elevation. Neuroimaging studies may reveal nonspecific ring-enhancing lesions. The diagnosis of CNS Chagas disease is often made by direct examination of the CSF, which will reveal *T. cruzi* trypomastigotes.

Nifurtimox and benznidazole are the only approved drugs with trypanocidal activity and are only available in the United States by contacting the CDC.

African Sleeping Sickness

Human African trypanosomiasis, or sleeping sickness, is prevalent in many sub-Saharan countries and is transmitted by the bite of an insect vector, the tsetse fly. Tryptophol, the 3-indole ethanol formed by the parasite, produces the characteristic sleep. Only two subspecies of the parasite are infectious to humans: *Trypanosoma brucei gambiense* in West and Central Africa, and *Trypanosoma brucei rhodesiense* in East and Southern Africa (Fig. 116-18).

Approximately 60 million people are at risk for infection; disease transmission occurs during activities such as farming, hunting, fishing, or washing clothes in remote rural areas.

Between 5 and 15 days after the bite, a painful skin lesion (chancre) may develop at the site of the bite. The parasites spread in the bloodstream 1 to 3 weeks after the initial bite, invading lymph nodes, liver, spleen, heart, endocrine system, and eye (hemolymphatic stage).

The typical symptoms and signs can be divided into two stages, although with *T. b. rhodesiense* infection there may be no clear distinction between the first and second stages. The early, first stage, symptoms include chronic and intermittent fever, regional lymphadenitis around the bite site, malaise, headache, arthralgia, erythematous and edematous cutaneous eruption, hepatosplenomegaly, and generalized lymphadenopathy, particularly in the posterior cervical nodes (Winterbottom sign).

The second stage is characterized by parasite invasion of the CNS. In *T. b. rhodesiense* disease, CNS involvement occurs early after infection, usually within 3 to 4 weeks of the bite. In contrast, in *T. b. gambiense* disease, CNS invasion can be delayed until many months or even years after infection. Signs of neurologic involvement include irritability, lack of concentration, personality changes, seizures, muscle fasciculation, and, in some cases, paralysis, hyperesthesia, anesthesia, or intense itching, and a variety of sleep disturbances such as daytime somnolence accompanied by night-time insomnia. As the disease progresses to the final stage, untreated patients become difficult to rouse and eventually progress to coma and death (Brun et al., 2009).

The clinical presentation is very different in travelers compared with African patients and is similar for both *T. b. gambiense* and *T. b. rhodesiense* infections. Patients frequently present with acute febrile illness, a chancre at the inoculation site, and a trypanosomal rash. These cases may manifest severe hematological disorders, impaired kidney function, electrolyte disturbances, and elevated liver enzymes.

The diagnosis and staging of disease rely on laboratory examination, given the nonspecific symptoms and signs. Correct staging is critical because the treatment is dependent on the stage of illness. Criteria for diagnosis of trypanosomiasis are the presence of flagellates in the CSF, elevated CSF leukocyte levels and the presence of intrathecal immunoglobulin M, as shown by the card agglutination trypanosomiasis test.

Suramin is recommended for patients with *T. b. rhodesiense* disease in early stages but avoided in western and central Africa because, where *Onchocerca* spp. are also present, its high activity against these parasites can cause severe allergic reactions. Pentamidine is the treatment of choice for first-stage disease caused by *T. b. gambiense*. In contrast, pentamidine treatment in intermediate-stage disease does not appear to be effective, and is not generally recommended. In late stages of the disease, melarsoprol is recommended.

HELMINTHS

For information on Toxocara and Trichinella species, see Table 116-3 and the online version of this chapter.

Baylisascaris Procyonis Infection

Baylisascaris procyonis is a roundworm of raccoons and causes rapidly fatal eosinophilic encephalitis in humans. Raccoons are the definitive host, and humans are considered an accidental intermediate host. *B. procyonis* infection in raccoons is usually asymptomatic and occurs in North America, Europe, and parts of Asia (Gavin et al., 2005). Infected humans may have classical visceral larva migrans with fever, leukocytosis, eosinophilia, hepatomegaly, and pneumonitis. If larvae reach the CNS, they produce damage and inflammation, resulting in progressive CNS disease, and the severity is often dose-related. Presenting CNS symptoms include lethargy, irritability, loss of muscle coordination, ataxia, nystagmus, loss of spontaneous movement, and extensor rigidity, and ultimately, the illness culminates in coma and death.

Ocular larva migrans usually involves children 7 years of age and older, with no history of pica and without marked eosinophilia. Laboratory findings of persistent eosinophilia in the blood and spinal fluid are typical findings. Early in the course of illness, neuroradiologic studies may demonstrate periventricular white-matter disease. Atrophy occurs in later stages of illness. Larvae can sometimes be visualized in histopathology or biopsy of brain tissue. In ocular larva migrans, migration tracks or live larvae are sometimes observed by funduscopic examination. Serologic testing is available in a limited number of laboratories throughout the world.

Treatment with antiparasitic agents and steroids has been attempted with variable success (Pai et al., 2007).

Angiostrongylus Infection

Angiostrongylus cantonensis, the rat lungworm, is the principal cause of human eosinophilic meningitis worldwide. Rodents are the definitive host of the parasite and mollusks are the intermediate host. Humans are an incidental host and become infected by ingestion of the third-stage larvae in the molluscan intermediate host (e.g., snails, crabs, freshwater prawns) or contaminated vegetables. The larvae penetrate the intestinal wall and reach the CNS via the bloodstream after ingestion.

The infection is most common in tropical climates, especially in Southeast Asia, the South Pacific, and Taiwan. Cases have also been reported in Africa, Polynesia, and eastern Australia. In the United States *Angiostrongylus* is endemic to Hawaii. Other countries in the Western Hemisphere where cases have occurred include Puerto Rico, Cuba, Jamaica, and the Dominican Republic.

The onset of CNS symptoms occurs 1 to 35 days after ingestion of the infective larvae. *A. cantonensis* larvae often invade leptomeninges and brain parenchyma, although a minority of larvae may invade the lungs and cause eosinophilic pneumonitis. When the larvae reach the CNS, the worms die in the meninges, brain, or eyes. Upon death of the worm, intense inflammation occurs. The resultant clinical forms, sometimes overlapping, include meningitis, encephalitis, or ocular forms. Severe headache, photophobia, meningeal signs, hyperesthesia, and paresthesia are common. Migratory sensory symptoms are sometimes described as "pain under the surface" or "like a sunburn," and affected individuals often experience discomfort wearing clothes. Individuals with the encephalitis form are severely ill, with paralysis of extremities or coma. Neuroimaging findings include meningeal enhancement, abnormalities in the brainstem, spinal cord, and basal ganglia. Crescent-shaped or stick-shaped linear enhancements in the parenchyma are particularly suggestive of neuroangiostrongylus.

Conjunctivitis, periorbital swelling, retinal hemorrhage, retinal detachment, or blindness may occur if the eye is infected. In most cases, recovery occurs approximately 4 weeks after onset but may take several months. In some cases involving very young children, progressive deterioration of CNS function has been described. Severity is likely related to the number of larvae ingested.

Eosinophilic pleocytosis, peripheral eosinophilia and elevated immunoglobulin E levels may be seen. The eosinophilia may persist for months. The diagnostic gold standard is identification of larvae in the CSF but is only found in 2% to 12% of cases (Ramirez-Avila et al., 2009). Serologic and molecular tests are available in a few specialized laboratories. Treatment with antihelmintics has been attempted, but efficacy is questionable. Sequential lumbar punctures, steroids, and analgesics may improve symptoms.

Gnathostomiasis

Gnathostomiasis, most commonly caused by the nematode *Gnathostoma spinigerum*, is the cause of eosinophilic myeloencephalitis. Most cases are associated with the ingestion of raw or undercooked fish, frogs, snakes, chickens, or ducks. The disease is well-established in Southeast Asia, particularly Thailand and Japan, and is emerging as a public health problem in Peru, Ecuador, and Mexico (Moore et al., 2003). The median time from ingestion of infected food to onset of symptoms may be several months.

Infection can be grouped into cutaneous, visceral, and CNS forms. Common symptoms include intermittent episodes of cutaneous larva migrans ("creeping eruption") with localized pain and pruritus. These lesions may recur for several years. Visceral symptoms occur if larvae migrate to deep tissues.

CNS involvement is rare and occurs more frequently in adults, but occasional cases occur in older children. CNS findings include the sudden onset of radicular pain or headache. Paralysis of the extremities and loss of bladder control typically follow. Acute eosinophilic meningitis, encephalitis, and cranial nerve abnormalities are also described. Neuroimaging of the spinal cord may reveal enlargement and diffuse high-signal intensity of the gray and white matter. Hemorrhagic tracts and scattered deep intracerebral hemorrhages are seen in the brain parenchyma. CT scans may demonstrate subarachnoid or intracerebral hemorrhage. Occasionally, parasite tracts can be visualized and appear as diffuse, fussy, high-intensity signals in the white matter.

Intermittent symptoms can occur for 10 to 15 years because the larvae are long-lived. Deaths are usually due to direct involvement of the brainstem or to secondary complications of pneumonia or sepsis. Ocular involvement can result in iris holes, anterior uveitis, and subretinal hemorrhages. Serologic (enzyme-linked immunosorbent assay and Western blot) tests have been developed but are not widely available.

Patients with gnathostomiasis will often have pronounced eosinophilia. In cases with CNS involvement, spinal fluid analysis shows eosinophilic pleocytosis. If there is ocular involvement, worms can sometimes be visualized by an eye examination.

Treatment recommendations include albendazole or ivermectin for dermal and subcutaneous gnathostomiasis. The role of steroids and antihelmintics for CNS involvement is undefined. Surgical removal is often needed if larvae are identified in the eye.

Cestodes

For information on *Diphyllobothrium latum*, see Table 116-3 and the online version of this chapter.

Sparganosis

Sparganosis is caused by a larval cestode of the genus *Spirometra sparganum*, which can invade the CNS. Humans typically acquire the infection via ingestion of raw frogs, snakes, or freshwater fish that are infected with *Spirometra sparganum*. Most cases have been reported in Southeast Asia, China, Japan, and Korea. Larvae migrate to the subcutaneous tissue or muscle but can also migrate to the genitourinary tract, pleural or abdominal cavity, scrotum, spinal cord, or brain. The clinical and radiologic presentation of cerebral sparganosis can resemble a tumor or tuberculoma. Neurologic manifestations may occur as many as 20 years after infection and include headache, seizure, or hemiparesis. Abnormalities seen on neuroimaging include unilateral ventricular dilation, cortical atrophy, irregular or nodular enhancing lesions, and punctate calcifications. Migratory lesions (also known as "wandering lesions"), the "tunnel sign" and "string-knots" sign are particularly suggestive of this infection. Surgical excision may be both diagnostic and curative. Praziquantel and steroids have been successful in some individuals.

Echinococcosis

Echinococcosis, commonly referred to as hydatid disease, has a worldwide distribution. The two major species of *Echinococcus* that are of public health and medical importance are *Echinococcus granulosus* and *Echinococcus multilocularis*. *E. granulosus* disease is characterized by cystic lesions found primarily in the liver and lungs and is known as cystic hydatid disease. *E. multilocularis* disease is less common but is a more malignant form than that caused by *E. granulosus*. *E. multilocularis* infection is characterized by tumor-like collections of vesicular parasites found primarily in the liver and is known as alveolar hydatid disease.

Certain activities, such as the widespread rural practice of feeding dogs the viscera of home-butchered sheep, facilitate transmission to dogs and, consequently, raise the risk of humans becoming infected for *E. granulosus*. The disease is often acquired in childhood, with latency periods lasting as long as 20 years. During the initial stage of the infection, humans are asymptomatic. In cases of *E. granulosus*, cysts grow slowly and may ultimately contain several liters of fluid. Symptoms are frequently caused by pressure induced by the expanding cysts in adults; only 10% to 20% of cases are diagnosed in patients younger than 16 years (Moro and Schantz, 2009). The majority of hydatid cysts occur in the liver (75%) or lungs (15%). Less common sites include the bone, pelvis, spleen, and CNS.

E. granulosus infection of the CNS occurs in 2% to 5% of cases and may be primary or secondary when lesions occur in the CNS. CNS disease is more common in children than in adults. Most cysts are singular, intraparenchymal, and in the region of the middle cerebral artery. Patients with *E. granulosus* lesions in the CNS typically present with signs of increased intracranial pressure. Symptoms of *E. multilocularis* infection are almost always limited to adults and characterized by invasive growth of larvae in the liver, with occasional metastasis. When metastasis to the brain occurs, the patient often presents with a mass lesion.

Neuroimaging is extremely helpful in the diagnosis of CNS hydatid disease. In cases of *E. granulosus,* neuroimaging often demonstrates oval or spherical, homogeneous, sharply demarcated cystic lesions with smooth borders. If the protoscolex, referred to as "hydatid sand," is seen in the image, it is considered diagnostic. In CNS *E. multilocularis* infections, cysts may appear as an ill-defined mass. A cauliflower-like contrast enhancement pattern on MRI is sometimes described. Eosinophilia is present in less than 25% of cases. Liver involvement is almost always present in these cases and ultrasound or other imaging of the abdomen may be helpful.

Serology can be helpful in cases that have unclear neuroimaging studies. Enzyme-linked immunosorbent assay or indirect hemagglutination is available for screening, and immunoblot assay can help confirm the diagnosis.

Surgical removal and an antiparasitic drug are usually the recommended treatments for CNS disease. In cases of *E. granulosus,* meticulous care must be taken during surgery to prevent spillage of the contents of the cysts. For *E. multilocularis,* CNS involvement is usually a consequence of advanced disease. Surgery and prolonged antiparasitic medications are generally recommended.

Cysticercosis

Cysticercosis, an infection caused by the larval form of the pork tapeworm *Taenia solium,* is the most common parasitic infection of the CNS worldwide. The WHO estimates that over 50,000 deaths due to cysticercosis occur annually. Cysticercosis is found in areas with poor sanitation, especially in places in which pigs have access to human feces. It is especially prevalent in Central and South America, sub-Saharan Africa, and Southeast Asia.

Neurocysticercosis is characterized by pleomorphic clinical manifestations and depends on location of parasites (brain parenchyma, subarachnoid space, ventricular system or spinal cord), number of lesions, and the intensity of the host's immune response. Spinal fluid analysis is abnormal in 50% of cases and may show moderate pleocytosis, a normal glucose level (although hypoglycorrhachia is seen in 12% to 18%), and a moderately increased CSF protein (range 50 to 300 mg/dl). CSF eosinophilia is variably present. In severe forms of neurocysticercosis (e.g., location of cysts in the subarachnoid space at the base of the brain or in the ventricular system), CSF cell counts may exceed 1000 cells/mm^3. Neuroimaging typically shows cystic lesions, single or multiple ringlike or nodular enhancing lesions, and parenchymal brain calcifications. If a cystic lesion with an associated scolex is seen, this is considered pathognomonic for cysticercosis.

The immunoelectrotransfer blot (EITB) assay generally has both high sensitivity and specificity; however, approximately 30% of cases with a single brain lesion may test negative. In the United States the EITB assay is available at the CDC.

Treatment of the adult tapeworm is routinely recommended. Praziquantel and niclosamide are highly effective for the eradication of the adult tapeworm. Niclosamide is not absorbed from the intestine. Considerable controversy exists about the role of antiparasitic treatment of neurocysticercosis and reviewed in the online version of this chapter.

Coenurosis

For information on Coenurosis, see Table 116-3 and the online version of this chapter.

Schistosomiasis

Schistosomiasis is a neglected tropic disease that ranks second only to malaria as the most devastating parasitic disease worldwide in terms of human suffering and economic influence. It is caused by the blood-dwelling fluke worms of the genus *Schistosoma;* snails are the intermediate hosts. Many species of Schistosoma exist, but only a few are responsible for human infection—primarily *Schistosoma haematobium, Schistosoma mansoni,* and *Schistosoma japonicum.*

Over the past few decades man-made reservoirs and irrigation systems have contributed to the spread with stagnant or slow-flowing water bodies enhancing the survival of the intermediate hosts, snails. Children and adolescents are most commonly infected particularly because they are more likely to play in contaminated water. *S. mansoni* is endemic in Africa, South America, and the Caribbean Islands. *S. haematobium,* the organism that causes classic urinary tract bilharziasis, is found in Asia, from Bombay to the Suez Canal, and in Africa. *S. japonicum* causes illness in the Far East, including China, Japan, Indochina, the Philippines, and Indonesia.

Two types of CNS lesions occur. One consists of isolated granulomatous masses that contain ova and can be surgically excised. The other type consists of diffuse small lesions that are located in both white and gray matter, and are often asymptomatic. Space-occupying lesions, known as bilharziomas, are apparent on MRI and CT scans. Adult worms, which can remain viable for 10 to 25 years, have also been reported in ectopic locations such as brain tissue.

S. japonicum infections are more likely to involve the brain and meninges, whereas *S. mansoni* and *S. haematobium* usually affect the spinal cord. Lesions from *S. mansoni* are usually located at the level of T6 or lower, coinciding with the more frequent anastomosis of the Batson venous plexus with the portal venous system at this region.

Clinical symptoms occur in three phases, the first being associated with cutaneous penetration and migration of the *Schistosoma* that result in an active dermatitis ("swimmer's itch"). The second phase (Katayama fever) occurs 6 to 8 weeks later and consists of a wide variety of symptoms, including chills, headache, fever, fatigue, hepatosplenomegaly, lymphadenopathy, eosinophilia, urticaria, and gastrointestinal distress. For *S. haematobium,* the beginning of egg output in the urine may be accompanied by dysuria and nocturia. Hematuria is the most important finding. In *S. mansoni* infection, patients may be asymptomatic, or they may present with chronic or intermittent abdominal pain, loss of appetite, and diarrhea alternating with slimy, blood-tinged stools; these symptoms and signs indicate the beginning of egg excretion in the descending colon, sigmoid, and rectum. About 10% of children in endemic areas progress to the third stage, with hepatosplenic involvement and liver fibrosis, usually 5 to 15 years after acute infection. The hallmark presentation is a healthy-looking child with preferential enlargement of the left liver lobe and an enlarged spleen. The progression to liver fibrosis can be more rapid in *S. japonicum* infection, in some cases with little or no interval between acute and chronic disease. In these cases, hematemesis from gastroesophageal varices, anemia, cachexia, and growth retardation may be seen.

Symptoms of neuroschistosomiases are directly caused by inflammation around ectopic worms or eggs in the cerebral or spinal venous plexus, which can progress to fibrotic scars.

S. japonicum, and rarely *S. haematobium* and *S. mansoni,* can be associated with cerebral granulomatous lesions. Headache, seizures, nausea, vomiting, visual abnormalities, speech disturbances, ataxia, vertigo, sensory impairment, and hemiparesis have all been reported, depending on location of the lesion. Growth retardation in children, associated with depressed function of the pars anterior of the pituitary gland, can occur. Cognitive and memory impairment have also been reported. Duration of the symptoms varies from a few weeks to more than a year, but most present within 3 months.

Ectopic *S. mansoni* and *S. haematobium* infections are associated mainly with spinal pathology with myelitis, myeloradiculopathy, or a granulomatous form. The most frequent initial complaint is lower back pain radiating to lower limbs or nonspecific pain in the lower limbs. Spinal neuroschistosomiasis can mimic a neoplastic process. Lower limb weakness, progressing to paraplegia, urinary retention, and paresthesia of the limbs, is a common presentation in pediatric patients.

CSF examination may reveal pleocytosis, eosinophilia, and elevated protein with oligoclonal bands. Brain neuroimaging studies may reveal edema, multifocal lucencies, and atrophy in later stages of the disease, whereas investigation of spinal cord schistosomiasis may reveal myelitis, swelling at the base of the cord (conus medullaris), or cord compression. A characteristic MRI pattern can be seen in cerebral schistosomiasis and consists of multiple intensely enhancing nodules with areas of linear enhancement. Spinal cord involvement is characterized by swelling of the cord with ill-defined regions of hyper intensity on T-2 weighted images. The conus medullaris and cauda equine are the most common sites of involvement.

Ova have not been found in CSF but can be found in urine, feces, and tissue and are diagnostic; concentration of the specimen may be necessary (Kato technique). In chronic schistosomiasis, however, eggs may not be passed, and serial stool examinations may be negative; in this situation, rectal biopsy can increase sensitivity to 95% to 100%. Several other tests are available, including an intradermal skin test, a complement fixation test, a cholesterol-lecithin cercarial slide flocculation test, and a bentonite flocculation test.

Praziquantel is the drug of choice for *S. haematobium*, *S. mansoni*, and *S. intercalatum* infections. Most experts recommend that CNS disease merits treatment with praziquantel in conjunction with steroids.

Paragonimiasis

Paragonimiasis, a neurologic and neurosurgical condition, has a high incidence in certain areas of Asia (China, Korea, Japan, and Taiwan), and occurs less frequently in some regions of Africa and South America. Human paragonimiasis results from the ingestion of freshwater crayfish or crabs containing the metacercarial form of the parasite. After humans ingest infected raw or poorly cooked crab or crayfish, the metacercariae excyst in the small intestine and pierce the intestinal wall as larvae, embedding in the abdominal wall. After several days, the larvae reenter the abdominal cavity and migrate to the diaphragm, pleural cavity, and lungs to mature into adult flukes. The lungs are the primary habitat in the human host, and adult worms are reported to live for 10 to 20 years. Lung disease, including pleurisy, pneumothorax, and hemoptysis, constitutes the cardinal clinical feature of human paragonimiasis.

Cerebral infection occurs in approximately 0.8% of patients; spinal cord involvement is even less common. Headache, nausea, vomiting, visual impairment, hemiplegia, and mental deterioration often occur early in the course of the illness. Neurologic evaluation frequently reveals dementia, homonymous hemianopia, optic atrophy, diminished visual acuity, hemiparesis, hemihypesthesia, and meningismus. The most common location of spinal involvement is in the lower thoracic area. An extradural mass may cause spastic paraplegia. Individuals with cerebral paragonimiasis may have history of a seizure disorder with onset during childhood, but the diagnosis may not be made until several decades later. Cerebral

paragonimiasis has been reported to lie dormant for 30 years before becoming symptomatic.

Characteristic neuroimaging during the acute phase includes multiple, ring-enhancing lesions referred to as "grape clusters," whereas the chronic phase reveals multiple, round or oval-shaped calcification. In the pediatric age group, irregular hemorrhages are common findings, although multiple and conglomerated enhanced lesions and migratory tracks of adult worms are sometimes seen.

Peripheral blood eosinophilia is often present. Pleocytosis (approximately equal numbers of polymorphonuclear cells and mononuclear cells), decreased glucose concentration, and increased protein content are frequent spinal fluid findings. The definitive diagnosis of paragonimiasis requires finding the operculated eggs in sputum or feces. Serologic assays are available and both are sensitive and specific. Praziquantel is the drug of choice for paragonimiasis, although surgical removal of the parasite may also be necessary in some cases.

REFERENCES

The complete list of references for this chapter is available online at www.expertconsult.com.
   See inside cover for registration details.

SELECTED REFERENCES

Brun, R., Blum, J., Chappuis, F., et al., 2010. Human African trypanosomiasis. Lancet 375 (9709), 148–159. [Epub 2009 Oct 14].

Buckingham, S.C., Marshall, G.S., Schutze, G.E., et al., Tick-borne Infections in Children Study Group, 2007. Clinical and laboratory features, hospital course, and outcome of Rocky Mountain spotted fever in children. J. Pediatr. 150 (2), 180–184, 184.e1.

Gavin, P.J., Kazacos, K.R., Shulman, S.T., 2005. Baylisascariasis. Clin. Microbiol. Rev. 18 (4), 703–718.

Linam, W.M., Ahmed, M., Cope, J.R., et al., 2015. Successful treatment of an adolescent with Naegleria fowleri primary amebic meningoencephalitis. Pediatrics 135 (3), e744–e748.

Montoya, J.G., Liesenfeld, O., 2004. Toxoplasmosis. Lancet 363 (9425), 1965–1976.

Moore, D.A., McCroddan, J., Dekumyoy, P., et al., 2003. Gnathostomiasis: an emerging imported disease. Emerg. Infect. Dis. 9 (6), 647–650.

Moro, P., Schantz, P.M., 2009. Echinococcosis: a review. Int. J. Infect. Dis. 13 (2), 125–133. [Epub 2008 Oct 19].

Pai, P.J., Blackburn, B.G., Kazacos, K.R., et al., 2007. Full recovery from Baylisascaris procyonis eosinophilic meningitis. Emerg. Infect. Dis. 13 (6), 928–930.

Perfect, J.R., Dismukes, W.E., Dromer, F., et al., 2010. Clinical practice guidelines for the management of cryptococcal disease: 2010 update by the infectious diseases society of America. Clin. Infect. Dis. 50 (3), 291–322.

Pittella, J.E., 2009. Central nervous system involvement in Chagas disease: a hundred-year-old history. Trans. R. Soc. Trop. Med. Hyg. 103 (10), 973–978. [Epub 2009 May 19].

Qvarnstrom, Y., Visvesvara, G.S., Sriram, R., et al., 2006. Multiplex real-time PCR assay for simultaneous detection of Acanthamoeba spp., Balamuthia mandrillaris, and Naegleria fowleri. J. Clin. Microbiol. 44 (10), 3589–3595.

Ramirez-Avila, L., Slome, S., Schuster, F.L., et al., 2009. Eosinophilic meningitis due to Angiostrongylus and Gnathostoma species. Clin. Infect. Dis. 48 (3), 322–327.

Saitoh, A., Homans, J., Kovacs, A., 2000. Fluconazole treatment of coccidioidal meningitis in children: two case reports and a review of the literature. Pediatr. Infect. Dis. J. 19 (12), 1204.

Schuster, F.L., Yagi, S., Gavali, S., et al., 2009. Under the radar: balamuthia amebic encephalitis. Clin. Infect. Dis. 48 (7), 879–887.

Walker, D.H., Paddock, C.D., Dumler, J.S., 2008. Emerging and re-emerging tick-transmitted rickettsial and ehrlichial infections. Med. Clin. North Am. 92 (6), 1345–1361.

World Health Organization, 2010. Guidelines for the Treatment of Malaria. WHO, Geneva. <http://www.who.int/malaria/publications/atoz/9789241549127/en/>.

❖ E-BOOK FIGURES AND TABLES

The following figures and tables are available in the e-book at www.expertconsult.com. See inside cover for registration details.

Fig. 116-1 Capsulated budding yeast cells of *Cryptococcus neoformans* mounted in India ink.

Fig. 116-2 Infectious fragmentation spores of *Coccidioides immitis*.

Fig. 116-3 Spore heads of *Aspergillus fumigatus* in culture.

Fig. 116-4 Candida infection.

Fig. 116-5 *Dermacentor andersoni,* the tick responsible for transmission of Rocky Mountain spotted fever in western regions of the United States.

Fig. 116-6 Petechial rash of Rocky Mountain spotted fever involving the ankle.

Fig. 116-7 Necrosis and gangrene of digits is a late complication of Rocky Mountain spotted fever.

Fig. 116-8 Eschar seen in scrub typhus.

Fig. 116-9 Intracytoplasmic inclusion (morulae) of *Ehrlichia* morula seen in the white blood cells from a bone marrow aspirate.

Fig. 116-10 Section through cerebral cortex of an individual with primary amebic meningoencephalitis.

Fig. 116-11 *Naegleria* ameba from culture in wet mount.

Fig. 116-12 Indirect immunofluorescent antibody-stained section of the brain of a 3-year-old child with *Balamuthia* granulomatous encephalitis.

Fig. 116-13 Magnetic resonance image of the brain of a 2-year-old with *Balamuthia* amebic encephalitis.

Fig. 116-14 Toxoplasmosis. A radiograph of the infant skull demonstrates fine intracranial calcifications.

Fig. 116-15 Hydrocephalus in congenital toxoplasmosis.

Fig. 116-16 Cerebral malaria. Petechial hemorrhages are scattered throughout the brain.

Fig. 116-17 Blood film showing human erythrocytes, some of which are infected with *Babesia*.

Fig. 116-18 *Trypanosoma gambiense* in peripheral blood (Leishman stain.)

Fig. 116-19 Magnetic resonance image (axial T2 image) showing abnormal hyperintensity in the periventricular white matter.

Fig. 116-20 Pork infected with the larval form of *Taenia solium*, also known as "measly pork."

Fig. 116-21 Cerebral cysticercosis revealed on computed tomography scan.

Table 116-1 Fungal Infections

Table 116-2 Rickettsial Infections

Table 116-3 Parasite Infections

117 Neurologic Complications of Immunization

Claudia A. Chiriboga

Immunization programs are undoubtedly cost-effective public health measures that protect against infectious disease. Recommendations on immunization schedules are made by the Advisory Committee on Immunization Practices (ACIP) of the Centers for Disease Control and Prevention (CDC) to the Surgeon General. New recommendations of the ACIP are published in *Morbidity and Mortality Weekly Report*, and they are the standard of care for immunization practices (Table 117-1). Vaccination programs have proved successful in eradicating diseases worldwide, best exemplified by smallpox, which was eradicated in 1980.

Despite these early successes in the United States and other industrialized nations, such programs are currently threatened. As more parents choose vaccine exemptions for their children, an erosion of herd immunity has ensued. This has resulted in a 3-fold increased rate of pertussis and a 10-fold increased rate of measles in the United States. The reason for the increase in antivaccine sentiments in industrialized countries is not known but would appear to be fueled by ignorance, celebrity endorsement, lack of scientific scrutiny of the Internet, anecdotal reports, and frustration among parents relating to the lack of well-defined causes to explain neurologic or developmental disorders (e.g., autism) that may coincide temporally with vaccination.

ASSESSING CAUSALITY

Events that are associated temporally are not necessarily linked causally. Determining causal relationships between vaccinations and specific disorders with certainty is difficult. Among existing methods, the least helpful in assessing causality are the anecdotal and case report, which rely on simple temporal associations that may easily have occurred by coincidence. Such chance associations can be expected to occur and often do when the outcomes are common (e.g., developmental disorders) and do not denote causality.

Clinical trials and epidemiologic population-based studies are more robust in assessing links between vaccines and adverse outcomes. Clinical trials are valid, but they are limited by their relatively small sample size, which precludes the identification of associations with rare outcomes. Population-based studies are useful, especially if large, because they can assess even rare outcomes. However, causality cannot be determined with certainty, only suspected, unless there is a biologic marker. Further complicating the assigning of causality is the administration of several vaccines at one time.

The U.S. Institute of Medicine (IOM) was charged with undertaking the first reviews of vaccine-related complications, and it continues to review vaccine safety. Because absence of proof is not proof of absence, the IOM takes into account level of proof and does not make determinations based on lack of evidence. In 2011 the IOM committee revised its methodology and established a new framework by which two lines of evidence (epidemiologic weight of evidence and mechanistic factors) influence determinations of causality based on a revised classification (Institute of Medicine, 2011):

- Evidence convincingly supports a causal relationship.
- Evidence favors acceptance of a causal relationship.
- Evidence is inadequate to accept or reject a causal relationship.
- Evidence favors rejection of a causal relationship.

The weight of epidemiologic data was classified as high, moderate, limited, or insufficient based on the number of studies with negligible methodological limitations. In determining causality, biologic mechanisms were also taken into account. The committee considered whether the vaccine had been linked to a specific condition in one or more individuals (high or moderate weight of evidence), whether there was an appropriate latency of the exposure, and whether there was a plausible mechanism by which the vaccine could cause the complication or disease in question based on human, animal, or in vitro studies.

VACCINE INJURY COMPENSATION PROGRAM

The U.S. Vaccine Injury Compensation Program (VICP), effective since 1988, is a federal no-fault system designed to compensate individuals or families of individuals who have been injured by childhood vaccines. The list of vaccines and covered complications are shown in Table 117-2. Vaccines are covered, whether administered individually or in combination. VICP further includes a provision to cover any new vaccine recommended by the CDC for routine administration to children, after publication by the Secretary of the Department of Health and Human Services of a notice of coverage.

TYPES OF VACCINES
Vaccines Composed of Whole-Killed Organisms

Vaccines composed of whole-killed organisms were the first laboratory-produced vaccines. They provoke an antibody response that provides temporary immunity. Some vaccines made from whole-killed organisms may cause immune-mediated disorders.

Inactivated Polio Vaccine

Sabin's oral poliovirus vaccine (OPV) was replaced in the United States in 2000 by an enhanced-potency trivalent polio vaccine (eIPV) that is not associated with vaccine-associated poliomyelitis (see section Vaccines composed of live-attenuated viruses).

Influenza Virus Vaccine

Epidemic human influenza illness is caused by influenza A and B. Influenza A viruses are categorized into subtypes, based on two surface antigens: hemagglutinin (H) and neuraminidase (N). These two surface antigens of the influenza A viruses vary over time through the process of drift and shift. Influenza B viruses are separated into two distinct genetic lineages (Yamagata and Victoria). Antigenic drift is caused by point mutations arising during viral replication in hemagglutinin

TABLE 117-1 Schedule of Routine Immunization of Healthy Infants and Children

Recommended Age	Immunizations
Birth	HBV
2 months	HBV, DTaP, Hib, eIPV, PCV, RV
4 months	DTaP, Hib, eIPV, PCV, RV
6 months	HBV, DTaP, Hib, PCV, RV
12–15 months	DTaP, Hib, MMR, eIPV, Var, PCV, influenza (yearly), HepA (2 doses)
4–6 years	DTaP, eIPV, MMR, Var
11–12 years	DT, MMR, MCV4, HPV (3 doses), and Var if not given at or after 12 months

DT, diphtheria–tetanus; DTaP, pertussis vaccine combined with diphtheria and tetanus toxoids; eIPV, enhanced-potency trivalent inactivated polio vaccine; HBV, hepatitis B virus; HepA, hepatitis A virus; Hib, *Haemophilus influenzae* type b; HPV, human papillomavirus; MCV4, meningococcal conjugate vaccine; MMR, measles, mumps, and rubella vaccine; OPV, oral polio vaccine; PCV, pneumococcal conjugated vaccine; Var, live-attenuated varicella vaccine; RV, rotavirus.

(HA) and neuraminidase (NA), whereas antigenic shift involves major changes in RNA caused by replacement of the gene segment. New influenza virus variants result from antigenic drift, whereas antigenic shift may facilitate cross-species infection and fuel pandemics.

Every year, a new influenza vaccine is developed to protect against the prevalent virus strains that are expected to appear in the United States the following winter. Each vaccine contains three influenza viruses: one A (H3N2) virus, another A (H1N1) virus, and one B. Two types of flu vaccines are available: the inactivated flu vaccine (discussed later) and the nasal-spray flu vaccine (i.e., live-attenuated influenza vaccine [LAIV]). The LAIV is prepared from live-attenuated flu viruses that do not cause disease in humans and is approved for use in healthy people 5 to 49 years of age who are not pregnant. The CDC recommends treating with LAIV within 48 hours of symptoms onset in high-risk individuals. A recent Cochrane review (2014) suggests that LAIV does not reduce the risk of serious influenza complications (pneumonia, hospitalization, or death).

The "flu shot" vaccine is prepared from inactivated flu virus and is approved for use yearly in all high-risk groups (young children, the elderly, and people with chronic diseases). There are two types of inactive vaccine: the trivalent flu vaccine that contains three influenza viruses (one A [H3N2] virus, one A [H1N1] virus, and one B virus), and the new quadrivalent flu vaccine that includes four different flu viruses (two influenza A viruses and two influenza B viruses). The CDC does not endorse any specific inactive flu vaccine.

Guillain–Barré Syndrome. Increased rates of Guillain–Barré syndrome (GBS) ranging from 8 to 13 per million were reported to be associated with the swine vaccine of 1976 [Institute of Medicine, 2003]. After 1976, no influenza season has shown a significant increase risk of GBS after influenza vaccination, including the 2009 H1N1 vaccine (Baxter et al., 2013). Rates of GBS are elevated 16-fold within 30 days of an influenza-like illness, compared with influenza vaccination.

Multiple Sclerosis. Although early studies suggested an association with multiple sclerosis relapse, numerous studies show no evidence of increases in the risk of multiple sclerosis (MS) relapse after influenza vaccination (Langer-Gould et al., 2014). As with GBS, the rate of MS relapse after an influenza-like illness was significantly higher (33%) than after vaccination (5%). There is consensus that influenza vaccination does not induce MS relapse and should be used in affected individuals when indicated, based on risk factors (Institute of Medicine, 2003).

Acute Disseminated Encephalomyelitis. Influenza infection is a known risk factor for acute disseminated encephalomyelitis (ADEM) occurring at a rate of about 0.4 cases per 100,000 children. Case reports and passive surveillance studies have described a temporal, though not causal, link between influenza vaccinations and ADEM (Institute of Medicine, 2011). In population studies, such associations are very rare, about 1 case per 10 million vaccines.

Bell's Palsy. Higher rates of Bell's palsy were reported after intranasal vaccination with inactivated influenza virus in a case–control study in Switzerland. Such reports have not been replicated elsewhere.

Narcolepsy. An increased risk of narcolepsy, including a 10-fold elevated risk in children, was noted in Europe after vaccination with a monovalent 2009 H1N1 influenza vaccine during the H1N1 influenza pandemic (Miller et al., 2013). This vaccine uses an adjuvant, ASO3, that likely contributed to findings. No adjuvanted influenza vaccines have been used in the United States during any influenza season. A recent detailed study found no association between influenza vaccinations in the United States and narcolepsy (Duffy et al., 2014).

Rabies Vaccine

The early rabies vaccine was developed in the central nervous system of animals and contained myelin basic protein. These vaccines (Semple vaccine), still in use in developing countries, were linked to high rates of ADEM (0.15%), polyradiculitis, and polyneuritis. The rabies vaccine licensed for use in the United States is prepared from rabies virus grown on human diploid cells, and it has an excellent safety record. Rare cases of demyelinating reactions have been reported, usually during the administration of the vaccine series or 1 week after completion, including atypical GBS and ADEM.

Whole-Cell Pertussis Vaccine

Whole-cell pertussis vaccine, routinely combined with diphtheria and tetanus toxoids (DwPT), was replaced in 1992 by the acellular pertussis vaccine (see section Component vaccines below). The endotoxin contained in the whole-cell vaccine causes fever and pain at the injection site. DwPT was associated with febrile seizures within a day of vaccination and hypotonic hyporesponsiveness in about 1 case per 1750 doses, and with a rare (0–10.5 cases per 1 million doses administered) acute encephalopathy, characterized by persistent crying. The IOM review in 1994 concluded that the evidence was consistent with a causal relationship between DwPT and an acute encephalopathy in the children who experience a serious acute neurologic illness within 7 days after receiving DwPT vaccine. There is no evidence to support a causal relationship between DwPT and chronic nervous dysfunction.

Hepatitis A Vaccine

Hepatitis A vaccine, licensed for use in 1995, is composed of an inactivated whole-virus vaccine that is derived from an attenuated strain of hepatitis A virus grown in human diploid cell lines. It has been recommended since 2006 for use in all children aged 1 year or older. No adverse neurologic events have been attributed to hepatitis A vaccine.

TABLE 117-2 Vaccine Injury*

Vaccine	Adverse Event	Time of First Onset
I. Tetanus toxoid–containing vaccines (DTaP, Tdap, DTP-Hib, DT, Td, TT)	A. Anaphylaxis or anaphylactic shock B. Brachial neuritis C. Any acute complication or sequela (including death) of above events within time period prescribed	4 hours 2–28 days Not applicable
II. Pertussis antigen–containing vaccines (DTaP, Tdap, DTP, P, DTP-Hib)	A. Anaphylaxis or anaphylactic shock B. Encephalopathy (or encephalitis) C. Any acute complication or sequela (including death) of above events within time period prescribed	4 hours 72 hours Not applicable
III. Measles, mumps, and rubella virus–containing vaccines in any combination (MMR, MR, M, R)	A. Anaphylaxis or anaphylactic shock B. Encephalopathy (or encephalitis) C. Any acute complication or sequela (including death) of above events within time period prescribed	4 hours 5–15 days No <5 or >15 days Not applicable
IV. Rubella virus–containing vaccines (MMR, MR, R)	A. Chronic arthritis B. Any acute complication or sequela (including death) of above event	7–42 days Not applicable
V. Measles virus–containing vaccines (MMR, MR, M)	A. Thrombocytopenic purpura B. Vaccine-strain measles viral infection in an immunodeficient recipient C. Any acute complication or sequela (including death) of above events within time period prescribed	7–30 days 6 months Not applicable
VI. Polio live virus–containing vaccines (OPV)	A. Paralytic polio In a nonimmunodeficient recipient In an immunodeficient recipient In a vaccine-associated community case B. Vaccine-strain polio viral infection In a nonimmunodeficient recipient In an immunodeficient recipient In a vaccine-associated community case C. Any acute complication or sequela (including death) of above events within time period prescribed	 30 days 6 months Not applicable 30 days 6 months Not applicable Not applicable
VII. Polio inactivated-virus–containing vaccines (e.g., IPV)	A. Anaphylaxis or anaphylactic shock B. Any acute complication or sequela (including death) of above event	4 hours Not applicable
VIII. Hepatitis B antigen–containing vaccines	A. Anaphylaxis or anaphylactic shock B. Any acute complication or sequela (including death) of above event within time period prescribed	4 hours Not applicable

Information effective as of March 6, 2015.

*Based on data from http://www.hrsa.gov/vaccinecompensation/vaccinetable.html (see original table for full definition of each adverse event). No condition specified for compensation for the following vaccines: *Haemophilus influenzae* type b, varicella, rotavirus, pneumococcal, hepatitis A, trivalent and tetravalent influenza, meningoccal tetravalent, and human papillomavirus.

DT, diphtheria–tetanus vaccine; DTaP, acellular pertussis vaccine combined with diphtheria and tetanus toxoids; DTP-Hib, diptheria, tetanus pertussis, and hemophilus influenza type b; Hib, *Haemophilus influenzae* type b; IPV, inactivated polio vaccine; MMR, measles, mumps, and rubella vaccine; MR, mumps and rubella vaccine; OPV, oral polio vaccine; P, pertussis; Td, tetanus and diphtheria toxoid; Tdap, tetanus and reduced dose of diptheria and pertussis (for older children aged >11 years); TT, tetanus toxoid.

Vaccines Composed of Live-Attenuated Viruses

Live-attenuated virus vaccines are intended to cause an asymptomatic infection. However, properly constituted vaccines can cause symptomatic infection and the expected complications of the natural disease. The immunity provided by live-attenuated virus vaccines is similar to that from natural diseases, and it may persist for life.

Measles: Rubeola

Measles vaccinations have been in use since 1963. As of 2000, measles is no longer endemic in the United States. The measles epidemic of 2014 saw a 10-fold increase in rates in the United States. Measles cases in the United States are imported from Europe and Asia and spread readily because of the increasing number of unvaccinated children in the community and concomitant loss of herd immunity. Infants who are not vaccinated until after age 12 months are most vulnerable to infection because of other children's vaccine exemptions.

The licensed measles vaccine uses the Edmonton B measles virus, attenuated by prolonged passage in chick embryo cell culture, and is combined with mumps and rubella vaccines (MMR). Children who receive live-attenuated measles vaccines are expected to develop an asymptomatic case of measles. Children with vaccine-induced measles can develop any of the known complications of natural infection, except for subacute sclerosing panencephalitis (SSPE). Some children develop fever, rash, and conjunctivitis in the second week after immunization (i.e., the incubation period is at least 5 days). The main neurologic complication of measles immunization is a 2- to 6-fold elevated risk of febrile seizures, often complex, in the second week after immunization (Ward et al., 2007). Measles vaccine is not associated with increased risk of afebrile seizures or epilepsy, even among high-risk children. Cases of SSPE among measles-vaccinated children, when studied, are found to be caused by wild-type measles infection. Rare cases of measles encephalitis have been linked temporally, but not causally, to the vaccine. Measles inclusion body encephalitis has been causally linked (Institute of Medicine, 2011) to MMR in immunocompromised children.

Mumps

The mumps vaccine is administered with MMR vaccination. It is prepared by passage of the Jeryl Lynn strain of mumps virus in chick embryo cell culture. No adverse neurologic events are associated with the mumps vaccine used in the United States. Aseptic meningitis has been linked to the mumps vaccine used in other countries that use a different viral strain, but not the Jeryl Lynn strain. Unilateral sensorineural deafness has been linked temporally, but not causally, to immunization with MMR on passive surveillance, for an estimated rate of 1 case for each of 4 to 6 million vaccines. The rate of hearing loss linked to mumps is 1 in 20,000 cases.

Rubella

The rubella vaccine used in the United States has been prepared since 1979 from human diploid cells. The immunologic response it produces parallels that of the natural infection. Up to 25% of people receiving the current rubella vaccine may develop transient arthralgias and paresthesias. In children, a controlled study found a 3.6 elevated risk of arthralgias between 6 to 14 days after MMR vaccination. In 2011 the IOM review concluded that the evidence supported a causal relationship between MMR and transient arthralgias, but not chronic arthralgias. Rubella virus vaccine has been highly successful in eradicating endemic rubella and congenital rubella in the United States. Inadvertent rubella vaccination of pregnant women has not resulted in any case of congenital rubella syndrome.

Oral Polio Vaccine

Sabin's OPV, introduced in 1963, was successful in eradicating polio in the United States. However, because the greatest risk of contracting polio in the United States was vaccine associated (i.e., the risk of wild polio is nil), OPV was replaced by eIPV. The overall risk for vaccine-associated paralytic poliomyelitis (VAPP) after OPV administration was 1 case per 2.4 million doses distributed, with 82% of cases occurring after the first vaccination. Risk of VAPP is greatest among immunodeficient patients: 3200- to 6800-fold greater than the risk for immunocompetent OPV recipients. There is no evidence that administration of OPV or IPV increases the risk for GBS.

Varicella

A live-attenuated varicella virus (Oka strain) vaccine was licensed in 1995 in the United States, and is currently recommended for routine immunization of children between 12 and 24 months of age. It is safe and effective in normal and mild to moderately immunocompromised children (e.g. with leukemia and HIV infection), but not recommended in severely immunocompromised children. The vaccine produces a mild case of chickenpox, resulting in any of the neurologic complications linked to the wild-type varicella infection, but at lower rates. For acute cerebellar ataxia (ACA), the vaccine-associated rate is 33-fold lower than ACA linked to varicella; for herpes zoster (HZ), rates are 4.7-fold lower than among unvaccinated children (van der Maas et al., 2009). About half of HZ cases among vaccine recipients are attributable to wild-type reactivation. Zoster complications with Oka virus, compared with wild-type VZV, tend to occur in younger children (about 2 years of age) and have a shorter onset after vaccination (318 vs. 588 days) (Wen and Liu, 2015). The zoster eruption correlated with the site of the vaccination in 46% of cases. The rate of zoster among varicella vaccinees aged 10 to

23 years and followed for 10 years was 1 case per 1000 person-years, which is comparable to zoster rates described after wild-type VZV infection. The IOM identifies an association between meningitis or encephalitis and reactivated Oka strain months to years after varicella vaccination with causal implications. Varicella vaccine–associated stroke from Oka virus vasculopathy has not been reported in a study that reviewed over 3 million vaccinees. No major neurologic adverse effects were reported as being associated with Oka virus 42 or more days after varicella vaccination.

Smallpox

The smallpox vaccine eradicated the disease in 1980. Smallpox reemerged as a potential risk in the wake of terrorist events because of its potential use as a biologic weapon. Smallpox is prepared from vaccinia, a live poxvirus that causes mild disease, including rash, fever, and aches. The main neurologic complication of smallpox vaccination is postvaccinal encephalomyelitis. Among the 1.2 million U.S. operational forces and health care workers vaccinated with smallpox after a 2002 U.S. Presidential directive, the rate of encephalitis was about 2 cases per million and there were 40 cases of myopericarditis that showed good recovery. In data collected before 1970, the mortality rate among patients with postvaccinial encephalomyelitis was 29%; the highest risk for developing postvaccinial encephalomyelitis was among infants younger than 1 year (risk ratio = 2.80, compared with vaccinees 1 year or older). These risks were significantly reduced among revaccinees.

The smallpox vaccine currently is recommended only for high-risk personnel (i.e., laboratory workers and at-risk military personnel), and is contraindicated for children and individuals with cutaneous disorders and immune suppression. In case of an outbreak, individuals of all ages would be vaccinated. Clinical trials with a recombinant smallpox vaccine, designed to be safer, are being carried out. Compensation for smallpox vaccination complications is part of the vaccine compensation program.

Rotavirus

Rotavirus (RV) vaccine is composed of a live, attenuated human G1P RV. No adverse neurologic side effects have been attributed to RV vaccine.

Component Vaccines

Acellular pertussis vaccine, *Haemophilus influenzae* type b vaccine, and meningococcal conjugate tetravalent vaccine are made from components of the bacteria. Human papillomavirus is made of noninfectious virus–like particles (VLPs). Toxoids are composed of denatured bacterial toxins. Toxoids prevent disease but not infection.

Acellular Pertussis Vaccine

Since 1997, acellular pertussis vaccines have been recommended for initial vaccination of children, beginning at 6 weeks of age. Acellular pertussis vaccines contain substantially fewer proteins (five) and less endotoxin than whole-cell pertussis vaccines. Acellular pertussis vaccination is associated with fewer local adverse events and systemic adverse events compared with DwPT, including lower rates of febrile seizures and hypotonic unresponsive events. No cases of encephalopathy have been identified that could be attributable to acellular pertussis after the administration of millions of doses of vaccines. A handful of vaccine-associated encephalopathy patients were found to have an SCN1A mutation thought to explain the encephalopathy.

Meningococcal Conjugate Vaccine

Meningococcal conjugate vaccine (MCV4) is a tetravalent vaccine constituted by capsular polysaccharide of serotype A, C, Y, or W135. It was licensed for use in January 2005 and is recommended for routine administration in adolescents 11 to 18 years of age. In October 2005, five cases of GBS among recipients of MCV4 reported to VAERS, first raising the possibility of an increased risk of GBS in association with MCV4 (within 42 days of vaccination). Subsequently, 2 population-based studies and a multicenter, retrospective cohort study assessed the occurrence of GBS in more than 10 million adolescents between 11 to 19 years of age. No study has found a relationship between MCV4 and GBS.

Haemophilus Influenzae Type b

Haemophilus influenzae type b (Hib) vaccines in use in the United States are based on Hib polysaccharide (PRP) conjugated to a protein carrier. The conjugation of PRP to the protein induces a T-cell-dependent immune response to the Hib polysaccharide. The vaccine is administered in the United States during infancy concomitantly with diphtheria–tetanus–acellular pertussis vaccine (DTaP) as repeated doses. Hypersensitivity to the vaccine components is the only contraindication to its administration. No neurologic adverse events have been attributed to the vaccine in the United States.

Pneumococcal Conjugated Vaccine

The first conjugate pneumococcal vaccine was licensed in the United States in 2000. It is composed of purified capsular polysaccharide of seven serotypes of streptococcal pneumonia, conjugated to a nontoxic strain of diphtheria toxoid. Pneumococcal conjugated vaccine is indicated for routine vaccination of children younger than 2 years. The vaccine produces local side effects, fever, and myalgias. No serious neurologic side effects have been attributed to pneumococcal conjugated vaccine.

Human Papillomavirus Vaccine

Human papillomavirus vaccine (HPV) is recommended for routine vaccination of children aged 11–12 years. It is composed of VLPs of the major capsid L1 protein of HPV types 6, 11, 16, and 18. It has been found to be effective in preventing cervical, vulvar, and vaginal dysplasia, genital warts, and cervical cancer caused by these specific HPV types. In the United States, HPV vaccine–associated adverse effects reported to VAERS were nonserious. Ninety-three percent of side effects related to arm pain at the injection site and syncope, including convulsive syncope. Increased risk of venous thrombotic disease has been temporally linked to HPV, but the IOM has concluded that these cases had other thromboembolic risk factors. Rates of GBS and CNS demyelination after HPV vaccination are no greater than those encountered in the general population. Vaccination is contraindicated in individuals with yeast allergies.

Tetanus and Diphtheria

Tetanus and diphtheria are toxoids that are produced by formalin inactivation of the toxins elaborated by the two organisms. Both have low rates of complications. Tetanus toxoid is given alone to children and adults after injury or burn exposure. The only contraindication for either toxoid is a history of a neurologic or severe hypersensitivity reaction after a previous dose.

GBS has been temporally, though not causally, associated with tetanus toxoid in two children and one adult. Controlled studies have noted no association between diphtheria–tetanus vaccine (DT) and GBS. Two cases of brachial neuritis were reported temporally associated with DTP immunization, and in such cases, the tetanus toxoid has been implicated. The IOM concluded that a causal relationship exists between tetanus toxoid and brachial neuritis (Institute of Medicine, 2011).

Recombinant Vaccines

Recombinant vaccines are genetically engineered vaccines. Hepatitis B is the only recombinant vaccine in use.

Hepatitis B Vaccine

Hepatitis B vaccine is prepared by introducing DNA coding for the hepatitis B surface antigen into yeasts for cloning. The original plasma-derived vaccine is also safe and effective, and it is still used elsewhere in the world. Multiple sclerosis initially was associated temporally with hepatitis B vaccine in France after hepatitis B immunization became mandatory for health-care workers in that country. Controlled studies, however, have not noted an association between hepatitis B vaccine with new-onset multiple sclerosis in adults or adolescents. The IOM has determined that the evidence is insufficient to support a cause-and-effect association.

COMBINATION VACCINES AND ADDITIVES

Most vaccination preparations involve combination vaccines. Concerns have been raised that combination vaccines (e.g., MMR) or vaccine additives (e.g., thimerosal) could elicit specific developmental disorders of childhood.

Mumps, Measles, and Rubella Vaccine and Autism

A major debate arose after Wakefield's publication of a small gastroenterology study in 1998 in Britain claiming a causal link between the MMR vaccine and autism. The study was subsequently retracted, deemed fraudulent, and Wakefield disciplined by the U.K. General Medical Council, but not before causing broad repercussions throughout Britain and the United States. Subsequently, numerous studies around the globe have found no association between MMR and pervasive developmental delay or autistic regression. The IOM has concluded, after a careful review of existing studies, that data do not support a causal relationship between MMR and autism (Institute of Medicine, 2004).

Thimerosal-Containing Vaccines and Developmental Disorders of Childhood

Thimerosal is an organic mercury compound preservative that has been in use since the 1930s. It was contained in more than 30 vaccines licensed and marketed in the United States, including some of the vaccines administered to infants (DTP, HIB, hepatitis B). Theoretical concerns were raised that cumulative exposure to ethylmercury, a metabolite of thimerosal and known neurotoxin, could have developmental side effects. In 1999 thimerosal was removed from vaccines to trace amounts (<3 μg). Several studies have found no association between thimerosal-containing vaccines and autism. Ecologic studies reported that, after discontinuation of thimerosal-containing vaccines, rates of autism remained unchanged or increased. Other studies targeting development and cognition have failed to identify thimerosol-associated impairments. The IOM has concluded that thimerosal-containing vaccines are not associated with neurodevelopmental disorders, including autism, attention deficit hyperactivity disorder, and developmental delay.

VACCINE INJECTION–RELATED OUTCOMES

Bursitis and syncope are vaccine-associated outcomes that can occur independently of vaccine type.

Deltoid Bursitis

Deltoid bursitis can develop after vaccine injection, not only from inadvertent introduction into the bursa, but also by the injection itself. The IOM has concluded that the evidence convincingly supports a causal association between injection of a vaccine and deltoid bursitis.

Syncope

Increased rates of syncope are reported to be temporally linked to vaccination and about 50% occur within 15 minutes of administration. The IOM concluded that the evidence convincingly supports a causal relationship between the injection of a vaccine and syncope. Vaccine recipients should be observed for 15 minutes after vaccination to prevent syncope.

REFERENCES

 The complete list of references for this chapter is available in the e-book at www.expertconsult.com.
See inside cover for registration details.

SELECTED REFERENCES

Baxter, R., Bakshi, N., Fireman, B., et al., 2013. Lack of association of Guillain-Barré syndrome with vaccinations. Clin. Infect. Dis. 57, 197–204.

Duffy, J., Weintraub, E., Vellozzi, C., et al., Vaccine Safety Datalink, 2014. Narcolepsy and influenza A (H1N1) pandemic 2009 vaccination in the United States. Neurology 83, 1823–1830.

Institute of Medicine, 2003. Immunization Safety Review: Influenza Vaccine and Neurological Complications. National Academy Press, Washington, DC.

Institute of Medicine, 2004. Immunization Safety Review: Vaccine and Autism. National Academy Press, Washington, DC.

Institute of Medicine, 2011. Adverse Effects of Vaccines: Evidence and Causality. The National Academies Press, Washington, DC.

Langer-Gould, A., Qian, L., Tartof, S.Y., et al., 2014. Vaccines and the risk of multiple sclerosis and other central nervous system demyelinating diseases. JAMA Neurol. 71, 1506–1513.

Miller, E., Andrews, N., Stellitano, L., et al., 2013. Risk of narcolepsy in children receiving an AS03 adjuvanted AH1N1 (2009) influenza vaccine in England. Br. Med. J. 346, f794.

van der Maas, N.A., Bondt, P.E., de Melker, H., et al., 2009. Acute cerebellar ataxia in the Netherlands: A study on the association with vaccinations and varicella zoster infection. Vaccine 27, 1970–1973.

Ward, K.N., Bryant, N.J., Andrews, N.J., et al., 2007. Risk of serious neurologic disease after immunization of young children in Britain and Ireland. Pediatrics 120, 314–321.

Wen, S.Y., Liu, W.L., 2015. Epidemiology of pediatric herpes zoster after varicella infection: A population-based study. Pediatrics 135, e565–e571.

E-BOOK TABLE

The following figures and tables are available in the e-book at www.expertconsult.com. See inside cover for registration details.

Table 117-3. Types of vaccines

118   Paraneoplastic Neurologic Syndromes

Adrienne Boire and Yasmin Khakoo

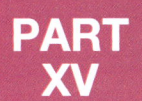 An expanded version of this chapter is available on www.expertconsult.com. See inside cover for registration details.

INTRODUCTION

Paraneoplastic neurologic syndromes (PNS) are the result of indirect effects of malignancy on the nervous system. These syndromes represent a diagnostic challenge because of both their rarity and protean neurologic presentations. Indeed, these syndromes may present at any time during the course of malignancy and may occur virtually anywhere along the neuraxis. Furthermore, select PNS may masquerade as direct effects of the primary tumor and/or metastases, or even as treatment-related complications. Importantly, in the setting of appropriate and timely therapy, PNS may respond to therapy, with regain of neurologic function. The aim of this chapter, therefore, is to provide the neurologist with an understanding of the scope of the most common PNS and their diagnosis and management.

HISTORY OF PARANEOPLASTIC SYNDROMES

Broadly defined, paraneoplastic syndromes encompass any indirect effect of cancer on the organism. Identifying the relationship between cancer and thrombosis, Armand Trousseau described the first paraneoplastic syndrome in 1865. From a neurologic perspective, Derek Denny-Brown identified two patients with sensory neuronopathy and lung cancer in 1948; the first case of encephalomyelitis and carcinoma was described in 1965.

The term "paraneoplastic syndrome" was first employed in 1956 by Cabanne and colleagues, who described three patients with paraneoplastic polyneuritis in the setting of cancer. The first antibody associated with paraneoplastic syndrome was formally identified in 1985 by Graus and colleagues. Since then, 16 identifiable syndromes and more than 20 paraneoplastic antibodies have been described. Neuroblastoma-associated opsoclonus-myoclonus-ataxia (OMA) syndrome was the first paraneoplastic syndrome identified in children in 1968 by Solomon and Chutorian. More recently, anti-N-methyl-D-aspartate antibodies have been associated with an encephalomyelitis that may be paraneoplastic in adults but is only rarely associated with an identifiable neoplasm in pediatric patients. Overall, PNS affect fewer than 0.01% of cancer patients.

DEFINITION

PNS are antibody-associated disorders of the nervous system in which antibody directed against a tumor antigen cross-reacts with antigen in the nervous system. These "onconeural antibodies" mediate autoimmune neuronal damage and resulting neurologic dysfunction. PNS may be divided into three major categories: classical PNS, which strongly suggest an associated malignancy; nonclassical PNS, which are only occasionally associated with malignancy; and autoimmune encephalitis, which is strongly associated with malignancy in adults, but rarely in children (Table 118-1). These divisions reflect known pathophysiologic mechanisms and provide insight into therapeutic options and prognosis. The antibodies responsible for classical PNS target intracellular neuronal antigens, and the associated tissue damage is mediated by cytotoxic T-cell responses. Following from this, classical PNS have a limited response to treatment. They are exemplified by Lambert–Eaton myasthenic syndrome (LEMS), OMA syndrome, and sensory neuronopathy. The neurologic symptoms of classical PNS typically, but not always, present before the tumor is diagnosed.

In contrast, the nonclassical PNS are associated with antibodies against intracellular synaptic proteins cyclically expressed on the cell surface through synaptic recycling. These antibodies may or may not be associated with malignancy. Unlike classical PNS, tissue damage may occur as a result of both B- and T-cell responses, and these syndromes display a heterogeneous response to treatment. These syndromes include cerebellar ataxia and the stiff-person syndrome.

Finally, the autoimmune encephalitides, including NMDA receptor encephalitis associated with antibodies against neuronal cell surface or synaptic receptors, are mediated by B-cell responses, and may respond to treatment with substantial neurologic recovery. These syndromes have been the subject of intense investigation in the recent past, and occur more frequently in the pediatric population.

DIAGNOSIS

Perhaps the most critical component in the diagnosis of PNS is clinical suspicion on the part of the medical team. PNS may cause injury anywhere along the neuraxis: autoimmune encephalitis can affect the supratentorial compartment of the brain, whereas the cerebellum is involved in paraneoplastic cerebellar degeneration (PCD) and OMA syndrome. The visual pathway is affected in cancer-associated retinopathy (CAR), whereas the spinal cord can be injured in subacute motor neuronopathy. Sensory neuronopathy involves the sensory nerves and, in LEMS, the neuromuscular junction is the target. Finally, inflammatory myopathies, including dermatomyositis, polymyositis, and inclusion body myositis, are PNS that affect the muscle. Once the neurologic targets of autoimmune attack are identified, laboratory-based screening of the relevant neuroanatomic compartment for autoantibodies should follow (Table 118-2). Paraneoplastic antibodies may be detected in serum and spinal fluid (Table 118-3). An array of paraneoplastic antibodies may be obtained. However, the judicious clinician should bear in mind that these

TABLE 118-1 Paraneoplastic Syndromes of the Nervous System

CLASSICAL

Limbic encephalitis
Encephalomyelitis
Cerebellar degeneration
Opsoclonus-myoclonus
Sensory neuronopathy
Gastrointestinal pseudoobstruction/autonomic neuropathy
Lambert–Eaton myasthenic syndrome
Inflammatory myopathy

NONCLASSICAL

Brainstem encephalitis
Stiff-person syndrome
Motor neuron disease
Necrotizing myelopathy
Optic neuropathy/retinopathy
Acute sensorimotor neuropathy
Chronic sensorimotor neuropathy
Myasthenia gravis

AUTOIMMUNE ENCEPHALITIDES

NMDAR encephalitis
AMPAR encephalitis

AMPAR, alpha-amino-3-hydroxy-5-methyl-4-isoxazolepropionic acid receptor; NMDAR, anti-N-methyl-D-aspartate receptor.

TABLE 118-2 Diagnostic Criteria for Paraneoplastic Neurologic Syndromes

DEFINITE PARANEOPLASTIC NEUROLOGIC SYNDROMES

1. A classical syndrome and cancer that develops within 5 years of the diagnosis of the neurologic disorder
2. A nonclassical syndrome that resolves significantly after cancer treatment without concomitant immunotherapy provided that the syndrome is not susceptible to spontaneous remission
3. A nonclassical syndrome with onconeural antibodies (well characterized or not) and cancer that develops within 5 years of the diagnosis of the neurologic disorder
4. A neurologic syndrome (classical or not) with well-characterized onconeural antibodies (anti-Hu, Yo, CV2, Ri, Ma2, or amphiphysin) and no cancer

POSSIBLE PARANEOPLASTIC NEUROLOGIC SYNDROMES

1. A classical syndrome, no onconeural antibodies, no cancer, but at high risk to have an underlying tumor
2. A neurologic syndrome (classical or not) with partially characterized onconeural antibodies and no cancer
3. A nonclassical syndrome, no onconeural antibodies, and cancer present within 2 years of diagnosis

TABLE 118-3 Paraneoplastic Syndromes and Associated Tumors and Antibodies

Clinical Syndrome	Associated Tumors	Associated Antibodies
Limbic encephalitis	SCLC, testicular cancer, thymoma, teratoma, Hodgkin disease, non-SCLC	**Anti-Hu**(ANNA-1), **anti-Yo**(PCA-1), **anti-Ri**(ANNA-2), ANNA-3, anti-Ma1, **anti-Ma2**(Ta), **antiamphiphysin**, **anti-CRMP5**(CV2), PCA-2, anti-CRMP3,4, anti-NR2B,* NR2A,* neuropil antibodies,* **GABA**B, **AMPAR**
Cerebellar degeneration	Breast cancer, ovarian cancer, SCLC, Hodgkin disease	**Anti-Yo**(PCA-1), **anti-Hu**(ANNA-1), anti-Tr, **anti-Ri**(ANNA-2), antimGluR1, anti-VGCC, anti-Ma1, **anti-RMP5**(CV2), anti-Zic4
Opsoclonus-myoclonus	Neuroblastoma, SCLC, breast	**Anti-Ri**(ANNA-2), **anti-Yo**(PCA-1), **anti-Hu**(ANNA-1),* anti-Ma1, **anti-Ma2**(Ta), **antiamphiphysin**, **anti-CRMP5**(CV2)
Stiff-person syndrome	Breast cancer, SCLC, Hodgkin disease	**Antiamphiphysin**, **anti-GAD**, **anti-Ri**(ANNA-2), antigephyrin
Retinopathies	SCLC, melanoma, breast cancer	**Antirecoverin**, antienolase, anti-TULP1, anti-PTB-like protein, antiphotoreceptor cell-specific nuclear receptor, **anti-CRMP5**(CV2)
Motor neuron disease	Lymphoproliferative disorders, SCLC, breast cancer, ovarian cancer	**Anti-Hu**(ANNA-1), **anti-Yo**(PCA-1), anti-MAG, anti-SGPS, antigangliosides GM1, GM2, GD1a, GD1b
Peripheral neuropathy	SCLC, thymoma, lymphoproliferative disorders	**Anti-Hu**(ANNA-1), **anti-CRMP5**(CV2), anti-MAG, anti-SGPS, antigangliosides GM1, GM2, GD1a, GD1b
Neuromyotonia	Thymoma, Hodgkin disease, SCLC	Anti-VGKC, **anti-Hu**(ANNA-1)
Lambert–Eaton syndrome	SCLC	Anti-P/Q VGCC
Myasthenia gravis	Thymoma	Anti-AChR, **antititin**, antiryanodine
Inflammatory myopathies	Non-Hodgkin lymphoma, ovarian cancer, lung cancer, gastric cancer, pancreatic cancer, bladder cancer	Anti-Jo-1, anti-JO, anti-Mi-2, antip155

Well-characterized onconeural antibodies are in bold.

AMPAR, alpha-amino-3-hydroxy-5-methyl-4-isoxazolepropionic acid receptor; ANNA, antineuronal nuclear antibody; CRMP, collapsin response mediator protein; GABA$_B$, γ-aminobutyric acid type B receptors; GAD, glutamic acid decarboxylase; MAG, myelin-associated glycoprotein; NR, NMDA(N-methyl-D-aspartate) receptor; PCA, Purkinje cell autoantibody; PTB, polypyrimidine-tract binding; SCLC, small-cell lung cancer; SGPS, sulfated glucuronic acid paragloboside; TULP1, tubby-like protein 1; VGCC, voltage-gated calcium channels; VGKP, voltage-gated potassium channel; voltage-gated calcium channels.

*Pediatric cases reported.

(Adapted with permission from Toothaker and Rubin, 2009.)

"paraneoplastic panels" represent only the most commonly encountered paraneoplastic antibodies, and do not encompass the full range of possible onconeural antibodies. In the patient with a well-described PNS such as PCD and elevated anti-Yo paraneoplastic antibody titer, a diligent search for malignancy, including body PET and abdominal and chest imaging, is appropriate. In patients for whom the paraneoplastic panel is unrevealing, demonstration of intrathecal clonal antibody production and/or the presence of a clonal population of antibodies provides supportive evidence. If the serum is reactive against both the patient's own tumor and the relevant neuroanatomic compartment, that is, the dorsal root ganglia in sensory neuronopathy, a paraneoplastic process may be diagnosed despite the absence of a previously described onconeural antibody. These formal principles of PNS diagnosis are of particular use to the clinician presented with a neurologic syndrome not previously described (see Table 118-2).

TREATMENT

The general principles of treatment in PNS reflect the current pathophysiologic understanding of these syndromes. Generation of onconeural antibodies must be suppressed if not arrested by treatment (surgical, radiotherapeutic, or chemotherapeutic) of the underlying malignancy. Antibody load must be reduced to reduce insult to the nervous system. The pace of this treatment process is dictated by the pace of the illness itself, and by the particular nervous structures involved: a slowly progressive LEMS may be initially managed on an outpatient basis with intravenous immunoglobulin (IVIg) infusions, with screening for malignancy. In contrast, a patient with rapidly progressive encephalitis, such as NMDA-receptor encephalitis, may require ICU-level neuromonitoring, airway management, and aggressive immunosuppression concurrent with surgical resection of suspected tumor mass.

There are few trials focused on PNS treatment strategies. Treatments are therefore largely empiric and based on extension of observations from other autoimmune diseases. In practice, initial treatments with corticosteroids, IVIg, plasma exchange, and/or rituximab may be followed by more aggressive immunosuppression with cyclophosphamide, tacrolimus, or cyclosporine in the setting of precipitous neurologic decline. There are no standard dosing regimens for PNS; the interested reader is directed to a recent excellent review on this topic (Rosenfeld and Dalmau, 2013).

These general principles of diagnosis and treatment will be applied to several PNS and will serve to illustrate the wide range of clinical presentations, relevant diagnostic and treatment strategies, as well as outcomes in these fascinating autoimmune syndromes.

CLASSICAL PNDS
Lambert–Eaton Myasthenic Syndrome

Several neurologic paraneoplastic disorders may affect the neuromuscular junction: LEMS, myasthenia gravis (MG), and neuromyotonia. MG and neuromyotonia are well-covered elsewhere in this volume (Chapters 136 and 137). LEMS is a disorder of presynaptic neuromuscular transmission, in contradistinction to the postsynaptic disorder MG.

Clinical features: Diffuse weakness and fatigue are the typical initial complaints, followed by sleepiness, evidence of autonomic dysfunction, muscle weakness on confrontational testing, and diminished deep tendon reflexes. Consistent with their distinct neuroanatomical localization, LEMS and MG display distinct electromyographic responses: patients with LEMS have an incremental response to repetitive muscle stimulation, whereas those with MG have a decremental response. Forty percent to 60% of patients with LEMS harbor a malignancy and neurologic symptoms often precede tumor diagnosis.

Antibodies: The onconeural antibodies associated with LEMS are antivoltage-gated calcium channel antibodies (VGCC, V/Q type). The most common malignancy associated with LEMS is small-cell lung cancer (SCLC). However, this relationship is complex: Payne and colleagues examined 63 patients with the diagnosis of SCLC and found that 5 (8%) had high titers of anti-VGCC antibodies present in the serum, with only 2 (3%) exhibiting clinical and electrophysiologic evidence of LEMS (Payne et al., 2010). Moreover, though classically associated with SCLC, LEMS may occur in other malignancies: there have been several reports of neuroblastoma-associated LEMS in pediatric patients.

Prognosis: The disease course is exceedingly variable; outcome prediction is made more complex by concurrent malignancy. In a retrospective analysis of LEMS associated *without* SCLC, mean antibody titers declined after prolonged immunosuppression, and most patients improved clinically and electromyographically. However, long-term disability was high with over 25% of patients requiring the use of a wheelchair at final follow-up (on average 3 to 4 years after diagnosis).

Treatment: Corticosteroids, IVIg, plasmapheresis, and azathioprine are all commonly employed in the management of this PNS. Although less common, dysphagia and attendant aspiration risk are important sources of morbidity and mortality in this neuromuscular syndrome. Therefore nonpharmacologic measures, including speech and swallow therapies, are also key treatments in the management of these patients.

OPSOCLONUS MYOCLONUS ATAXIA SYNDROME

OMA syndrome (also called "dancing eyes, dancing feet syndrome," myoclonic encephalopathy of infancy, or Kinsbourne syndrome) is a paraneoplastic syndrome associated with neuroblastoma in children and breast cancer in adults.

Case 1: MS is a previously healthy 18-month-old girl who developed sudden onset of ataxia, chaotic rapid eye movements and irritability. MRI of the brain was normal and metaiodo–benzyl-guanidine (MIBG) revealed uptake in the left adrenal gland (Fig. 118-1). Thin-cut contrast-enhanced CT of the chest/abdomen/pelvis confirmed a homogeneously enhancing mass in the left adrenal gland. Tumor was resected and found to be consistent with favorable histology, non-*MYCN*-amplified neuroblastoma. The patient did not require further therapy for neuroblastoma; however, for treatment of refractory OMA syndrome, she received monthly IVIg for 2 years, intramuscular ACTH for 14 months, and a 4-week course of rituximab. Motor symptoms of OMA completely resolved after 24 months of therapy. The patient is now 6 years old and "mainstreamed" for education; gross motor symptoms have resolved and she receives weekly occupational and speech therapy. Her neuroblastoma has been in remission since surgery.

History: Orzechowski first coined the term in 1913 based on the Greek term "opso" meaning eye and "clonus" meaning violent, nonpurposive motion. "… the ocular globes are in a state of continuous agitation, being shaken and increasingly displaced by very rapid unequal movements, which generally take place in the horizontal plane." In 1927, he noted the association between opsoclonus and myoclonus. Kinsbourne described a syndrome of myoclonic encephalopathy in 1962 and finally in 1968, Solomon and Chutorian described the association between neuroblastoma and OMA syndrome.

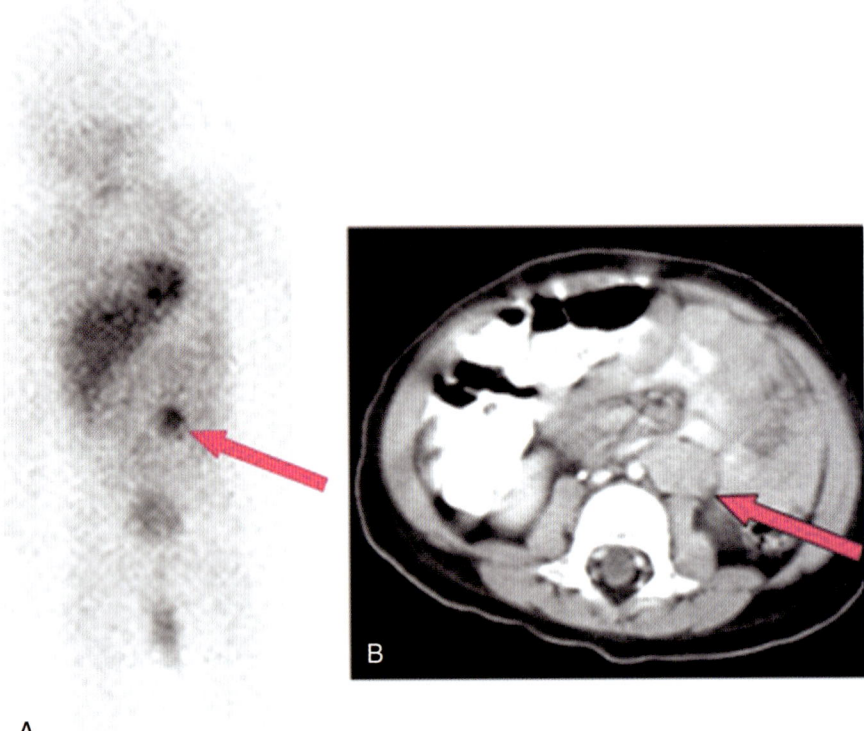

Figure 118-1. Images of the patient in case 1. Metaiodo–benzyl-guanidine (MIBG) showing uptake in the left adrenal gland. Thin-cut contrast-enhanced CT scan of the abdomen confirmed a homogeneously enhancing mass in the left adrenal gland.

Incidence: The incidence of OMA syndrome is estimated at 1 in 10 million, occurring in 2% to 3% of all neuroblastoma patients. Up to 50% of children with OMA harbor a neuroblastoma; some researchers speculate that the incidence of neuroblastoma in children with OMA is actually higher but a cellular and/or antibody-mediated response destroys the tumor before detection. OMA in children has been reported in infections, including EBV, mumps, West Nile virus, salmonellosis, and *Mycoplasma pneumoniae*. OMA is paraneoplastic in 20% of adults. Typically, patients have breast or gynecologic cancers.

Clinical features: Patients with OMA typically have rapid, involuntary, irregular but conjugate eye movements; myoclonic jerking of the limbs, trunk, and head; truncal ataxia; and irritability with rage attacks and other behavioral disturbances. Patients tend to keep their eyes closed, as they experience oscillopsia.

Antibodies: The most common antibody associated with OMA in adults is the anti-Ri antibody that binds to Nova, an RNA-binding protein important in regulating inhibitory neurotransmitters in the brainstem. Despite multiple attempts to isolate a specific antibody in pediatric patients with OMA, to date one has not been identified. Approximately 75% of neuroblastomas express anti-Hu antigen, but only 5% to 15% of serum samples contain the anti-Hu antibody. Classically, the OMA precedes the diagnosis of neuroblastoma. Kurian and colleagues described a 23-year-old woman with OMA syndrome plus other neurologic abnormalities (facial paresis, frontal lobe-type disinhibition behavior). Extensive evaluation for malignancy was negative but the patient did have anti-NMDA receptor antibodies present in the CSF. Morales-Briceño reported a case of OMA that developed in a patient 5 days after an upper respiratory infection. GQ1b antibodies were detected in CSF and patient improved shortly after IVIg.

Evaluation and treatment: MRI of the brain is typically normal at the onset of OMA although it may reveal cerebellar atrophy at a later time. Lumbar puncture early in the course of the illness may reveal normal to slightly elevated protein with no cells or predominantly B-cell lymphocytes. If the patient has already been diagnosed with neuroblastoma, LP should be avoided in patients with known bone marrow disease, as there are data to suggest that LP in these patients may potentially seed the CNS.

Children with OMA should have an MIBG scan in an effort to identify the neuroblastoma. Thin-cut CT through the area of increased uptake will help identify the tumor. Patients usually have lower stage/grade neuroblastoma with favorable histology and unamplified *MYCN*. Treatment of the OMA begins with surgical resection of the tumor and is typically followed by immunomodulation. For 2 days perioperatively, IVIg is administered at a dose of 1 g/kg, as surgery may transiently increase symptoms. There are numerous protocols for immune suppression thereafter, but clearly immunomodulation is the next treatment of choice. In 1997 Russo and colleagues suggested that children with OMA-associated neuroblastoma had better neurologic outcome if they received cyclophosphamide chemotherapy as part of the treatment for neuroblastoma. Pranzatelli and colleagues at the National Pediatric Myoclonus Center have advocated the use of ACTH as follows: within 1 week of surgery, patients are started on ACTH 75 IU/m^2/day intramuscularly twice daily. The ACTH is tapered quickly in the first month and then more slowly over the next 11 months. If OMA recurs, the previous dose of ACTH is reinstituted. High-dose pulse dexamethasone has been successfully used with lower cost of treatment and fewer long-term side effects of ACTH. Pranzatelli and colleagues identified B-cell expansions in the CSF of many of these patients and found that a short course of rituximab (375 mg/m^2/week for 4 consecutive weeks) improves symptoms. If a prominent T-cell population is noted in the CSF of refractory patients, then cyclophosphamide is recommended at a dose of 750 mg/m^2/day monthly for 3 to 6 months. Ofatumumab has also been successfully used: in one patient who developed an allergy to rituximab and in a patient in combination with methotrexate (Ketterl et al., 2013). Patients with OMA should not receive immunizations as any stimulus to the immune system may exacerbate the symptoms.

Prognosis: Patients with neuroblastoma-associated OMA typically have a better overall survival than patients without OMA (Rudnick et al., 2001). Their neurologic and cognitive outcomes, however, are generally not as good. I Catsman-Berrevoets identified 9 children with OMA (4 with neuroblastoma) who were followed for a median of 11 years. Despite severe motor deficits initially, patients actually recovered these functions quite well; in 7/9 patients, however, severe cognitive and behavioral impairments persisted. Hasegawa and colleagues identified 23 patients with OMA from 2005 to 2010 in Japan. They reported 44% with identified neuroblastoma, 40% with infection, and 9% related to immunizations. They also reported a high rate of intellectual impairment (74%) and the most severely affected patients were those whose treatment was delayed (Hasegawa et al., 2014).

Pathophysiology: As yet, the pathophysiology of OMA is poorly understood. In 2003 Helmchen and colleagues performed fMRI in two adults with OMA syndrome and demonstrated disinhibition of the fastigial nucleus in the cerebellum. As mentioned above, unlike adults, children with OMA do not have a specific antibody present in the CSF and serum. The initial suggestion that the syndrome is humorally mediated is being challenged as more evidence supports a cellular etiology. Though the neuroblasts of OMA-associated neuroblastomas appear histologically identical to those tumors in patients without OMA, the tumors themselves are quite distinctive. Patients with OMA-associated neuroblastoma have large lymphocytic infiltrates present in the tumor specimens. In a study by Cooper and colleagues, the pathologist could identify which patients had OMA simply by looking at the tumors in 92% of cases.

Saccades are normally prevented by inhibitory pontine pause cells. Inappropriate timing of pause cell inhibition or excessive firing of burst cells may lead to "saccadomania" (e.g., opsoclonus).

SUBACUTE SENSORY NEURONOPATHY

PNS can affect peripheral nerves, neuromuscular junction, or muscle. In one series, 9% of patients referred to a center for evaluation of a peripheral neuropathy had cancer as the underlying cause. The neuropathy may be axonal or demyelinating, or in the case of a pure sensory neuropathy, a dorsal root ganglionopathy. In patients older than 50 years, particularly smokers and those with acutely developing purely sensory neuropathy, a PNS is likely.

History: In 1948, Denny-Brown described two patients with a rapidly developing and debilitating sensory neuronopathy. Pathologic evaluation revealed inflammatory infiltrates within the dorsal root ganglia and degeneration of the posterior columns of the spinal cord. In 1985 Graus and colleagues identified an antibody called anti-Hu associated with patients who have SCLC and SSN.

Clinical features: Anti-Hu patients typically have sensory loss and paresthesias, which may affect the extremities initially, but may also include the neck and trunk and can occasionally be asymmetric. All sensory modalities are involved, but proprioceptive loss can severely impair gait and use of the hands. In 1992 Dalmau and colleagues identified 71 patients with paraneoplastic encephalomyelitis syndrome/SSN in association with the presence of anti-Hu antibodies. Seventy-eight percent had SCLC. In 9 patients no tumor was detected. In the others, tumors included prostate cancer (2), adenocarcinoma of the lung (1), chondromyxosarcoma (1), and, interestingly, neuroblastoma (1).

Antibody: Anti-Hu antibody is a 35 to 40 kDa protein that immunoreacts with the nuclei of neurons. The antigen is expressed in the nuclei of most neurons in the CNS, including those in the dorsal root ganglia, explaining why the anti-Hu neurologic paraneoplastic syndrome may cause encephalomyelitis and/or SSN in the same patient. In addition, most SCLCs express the antigen as well.

Treatment and prognosis: Detection of the anti-Hu antibody in patients with SCLC is associated with response to cancer treatment and improved survival. However, a retrospective review of 71 patients with anti-Hu syndromes (59% of whom demonstrated sensory neuropathy) revealed that treatment of the primary tumor with surgery, chemotherapy, or radiation did not improve the neurologic symptoms in any patient.

NONCLASSICAL PNS
Paraneoplastic Cerebellar Degeneration

PCD is a paraneoplastic syndrome of pan-cerebellar dysfunction most commonly associated with SCLC, ovarian, and breast malignancies.

History: PCD was actually the first paraneoplastic syndrome to be described and as such is the most well described and easily recognized. In 1919 Brouwer described a patient with rapid onset of a cerebellar syndrome. At autopsy the patient had Purkinje cell loss in the cerebellum and a pelvic tumor, most likely ovarian carcinoma. In 1938 Brouwer postulated the association between PCD and cancer. PCD may occur in isolation but may be associated with other PNS, including limbic encephalitis (LE) and LEMS.

Clinical features: PCD is most commonly associated with SCLC, gynecologic cancers, and Hodgkin lymphoma. Symptoms often begin precipitously with dizziness, nausea, and vomiting. Patients may develop diplopia and subsequently both truncal and appendicular ataxia, and dysarthria and dysphagia: a veritable pan-cerebellar syndrome. Though not necessary to make the diagnosis, the CSF may display mild pleocytosis and MRI may reveal cerebellar edema. There is evidence of clonal antibody production in the CSF, classically anti-Yo. About 50% of patients with SCLC and PCD do not harbor currently identified onconeural antibodies.

PCD clinical manifestations are diverse: patients with SCLC and PCD may also develop LEMS because of the presence of antibodies to VGCC that may cause both syndromes. Sabater and colleagues described a PCD ZIC variant (associated with zinc fingers in the cerebellum) in which MRI is initially normal, but as the disease progresses, cerebellar atrophy may become more prominent. The diversity of PCD clinical presentation suggests that PCD does not represent a single syndrome, but rather a collection of several, similar nonclassical PNS with onconeural antibodies directed against Purkinje cell antigen.

Antibodies: Onconeural antibodies in PCD, such as anti-Yo, are directed against a cytosolic Purkinje cell antigen, cDR2 (cerebellar degeneration-related protein). The resulting cytotoxic T-cell response results in massive Purkinje cell destruction visible on histopathology at autopsy. The anti-Yo antibody is the most frequently detected antibody in patients with PCD and ovarian or breast cancer. Patients with gynecologic cancers who develop PCD invariably harbor anti-Yo antibodies. Interestingly, approximately 60% of patients with ovarian cancer who do not have PCD express cDR2 on their tumor cells. All patients with PCD-associated breast and ovarian cancer express cDR2 antigens on their tumor cells.

Treatment and prognosis: Treatment of PCD has generally consisted of corticosteroid, plasmapheresis, or IVIg; there is scant evidence to support one of these regimens over another. Prognostication response to treatment is challenging, particularly in the setting of active malignancy. However, a small retrospective analysis suggests that modest to substantial functional improvement can occur with inpatient rehabilitation after initial treatment for PCD. In addition, though anti-Yo PCD was formally diagnosed in 34 women, only 63% of these women were eventually diagnosed with malignancy after more than 4 years of follow up.

STIFF-PERSON SYNDROME

History: Moersch and Woltman first described the "stiff-man syndrome" (SMS) in a series of 14 patients with fluctuating truncal and limb rigidity in 1956. This syndrome became notable for distinctive hyperexcitability of spinal motor neurons, as well as marked therapeutic benefit with diazepam treatment. In 1988 Solimena and colleagues demonstrated the autoimmune nature of the disease and first linked glutamic acid decarboxylase antibodies to the syndrome, providing a pathophysiologic mechanism to account for decreased GABAergic tone in these patients.

Clinical manifestations: There are three recognized phenotypes of SMS: classic, variant, and progressive encephalomyelitis with rigidity and myoclonus (PERM). Classic SMS presents with stiffness and spasms of the lumbar region and lower extremities. Variant SMS is characterized by stiffness limited to a single limb or the trunk. Entire-body stiffness in conjunction with encephalomyelitis is the hallmark of PERM syndrome. In all phenotypes, examination of the symptomatic region is notable for rigidity with continuous muscle activity despite attempted relaxation.

Although more common in women than in men, in the pediatric population SMS is evenly distributed between boys and girls (Clardy et al., 2013). A recent retrospective review over a 29-year period at the Mayo clinic found that 5% of SMS cases were diagnosed in patients less than 18 years of age. Importantly, all pediatric cases had positive antiglutamic acid decarboxylase (GAD) serology, 5/8 of the patients had a coexisting immune disorder, and cancer was not identified in any of the pediatric patients.

Brainstem and spinal hyperexcitability are hallmarks of SMS. These are demonstrated by exaggerated and poorly habituating acoustic startle reflex, exaggerated exteroceptive reflexes (tactile, thermal, visual, acoustic, and pain reflexes), and/or continuous paraspinal motor unit activity. In a recent retrospective review, 61% of patients with classic and 45% of patients with variant SMS demonstrated spinal hyperexcitability. Consistent with the poor GABAergic tone in these patients, psychiatric comorbidities, including anxiety and specific phobias, may complicate diagnosis in SMS. The differential diagnosis of these patients includes hereditary spastic paraplegia, hereditary hyperekplexia, and spastic dystonias.

Antibodies: 80% of SMS will have positive serology for GAD65 (glutamic acid decarboxylase, the rate-limiting enzyme for the production of $GABA_A$). Other antibodies associated with SMS include glycine receptor alpha 1 subunit (GlyRα1), accounting for about 10% of SMS. Antiamphiphysin antibodies are also implicated in SMS, most commonly associated with breast adenocarcinoma and SCLC in adults.

Treatment and prognosis: Treatment attempts to increase GABAergic tone, both pharmacologically and immunotherapeutically. Diazepam and baclofen are both commonly employed to improve stiffness and spasms. IVIg, plasmapheresis, prednisone, and rituximab have all been shown to improve symptoms as well. The bulk of clinical improvement was apparent after the first year of treatment, and though stiffness and spasms were improved with immunotherapy, mobility changes because of therapy were infrequent.

LIMBIC ENCEPHALITIS

Limbic encephalitis (LE) is a paraneoplastic syndrome characterized by onconeural antibodies reactive against the limbic regions of the brain. In LE, the presentation is generally abrupt (days to weeks) with onset of personality/behavior changes, seizures, and alteration of consciousness.

History: Paraneoplastic LE was first described in 1968 by Corsellis and colleagues, who published a clinicopathologic series of patients with carcinoma and neurologic symptoms consisting of seizures and memory loss. Since then, two distinct clinical syndromes have emerged: those that result from antibodies directed against cell surface antigens (the autoimmune encephalitides; discussed below), and those like LE that result from antibodies directed against intracellular antigens.

Clinical features: Acute and persistent memory loss with behavioral changes may be the first presenting symptom of malignancies such as SCLC. When these symptoms occur in a previously well person, LE, either paraneoplastic or nonparaneoplastic (autoimmune), must be considered.

Brain MRI may show FLAIR and T2-weighted hyperintensity; imaging changes in the medial temporal lobes are frequently mistaken for herpes simplex. However, the inflammatory process may involve the hippocampi, amygdalae, and, less frequently, frontobasal and insular regions. CSF may reveal lymphocytic pleocytosis, oligoclonal bands, and elevated protein. EEG may show generalized slowing and epileptiform activity primarily in the temporal lobes. LE is associated with SCLC in 50% to 60% of patients, with testicular germ cell tumors in 20% of patients, and breast cancer approximately 8% of patients. If no paraneoplastic antibodies are found and PCR rules out herpes simplex encephalitis, one must search for cancer, usually by body PET imaging.

In addition to symptoms from LE, patients with antibodies directed against intracytoplasmic targets also present with other neurologic symptoms. For example, sensory neuronopathy or encephalomyelitis is frequently present in LE with anti-Hu antibodies.

Antibodies: The anti-Hu antibody is present in 60% of cases in which an antibody is detected; presence of anti-Hu antibody in patients with paraneoplastic LE confers a 94% chance of having SCLC. More than 95% of patients with antibodies against intracytoplasmic targets have cancer, and the outcome is poor with limited response to treatment.

CANCER-ASSOCIATED RETINOPATHY

Paraneoplastic visual disorders are rare. Among these, CAR and melanoma-associated retinopathy are the most common syndromes. CAR was first reported in 1976 by Sawyer and colleagues who evaluated three women with visual loss before or after the diagnosis of cancer was made. In 50% of patients, CAR precedes the diagnosis of cancer, typically SCLC and gynecologic cancers.

Patients complain of painless visual loss that may begin with night blindness. On physical examination the retina may initially appear normal but later is mottled with optic disc pallor and retinal artery narrowing. CAR affects rods and cones and histologically shows loss of both inner and outer layers with occasional inflammation. Vitreous and CSF may contain inflammatory cells. Several antibodies have been identified, but most commonly, antirecoverin is found.

Recoverin is a member of a family of calcium-binding proteins involved in the transduction of light by photoreceptors. Recoverin has been found to be expressed in the lung tumor of a CAR patient but not in similar tumors obtained from individuals without the associated retinopathy.

AUTOIMMUNE ENCEPHALITIDES

The paraneoplastic encephalitides are defined by onconeural antibodies to neuronal cell-surface or synaptic receptors (Dalmau and Rosenfeld, 2014). These encephalitides are the result of onconeural antibodies directed against the AMPA receptor, GABAB receptor, LGI1, Caspr2, GABAA receptor, DPPX, glycine receptor, mGluR1, mGluR5, dopamine-2 receptor, and, most commonly, the NMDA receptor.

ANTI-*N*-METHYL-D-ASPARTATE RECEPTOR ENCEPHALITIS

Case 2: D.F. is a 6-year-old boy who developed a change in behavior followed by focal seizures and gait disturbance. EEG revealed nonconvulsive status epilepticus requiring induction of burst suppression with phenobarbital and levetiracetam. Contrast-enhanced MRI of the brain, lumbar puncture, and CNS PET scan were normal. CSF, however, revealed the presence of anti-N-methyl-D-aspartate receptor (NMDAR) antibodies. He was treated with IV steroids and IVIg. Further oncologic evaluation included a total body PET scan, a CT scan of the chest/abdomen/pelvis, and scrotal ultrasound, all of which were normal. He was weaned off all medications over several months and achieved a complete recovery.

History: In 1997, Nokura and colleagues reported a case of a 19-year-old woman with psychosis and confusion who was found to have an ovarian teratoma. Once the teratoma was removed the patient made a partial recovery. At that time, no clear paraneoplastic antibody was identified. Other similar cases were subsequently described but the first antibody was not identified until 2005 when Vitaliani and colleagues reported four young women with ovarian teratoma with acute behavioral and psychiatric changes, neurologic deterioration, seizures, orofacial dyskinesias, and central hypoventilation. CSF and serum revealed a novel antibody against EFA6A, a protein expressed in the cytoplasm of hippocampal neurons. In 2007 Dalmau and colleagues further characterized these antibodies as being against the NR1 subunit of the NR1/NR2 heteromers of the NMDAR, also expressed on the tumors.

Clinical features: In 2008, the same group analyzed 100 cases of patients with anti-NMDAR encephalitis. Ninety-one percent of patients were women; 59% had tumors (primarily ovarian teratomas), although one man had SCLC. Twenty-two aged 18 years or less, and 55% of these patients had an underlying tumor. Severe neurologic deficits, including poor responsiveness, catatonia, abnormal movements, and central hypoventilation, were present in 93 patients. Ninety-two percent of patients had abnormal EEGs; 95% had abnormal CSF profiles and 55% had FLAIR or T2 signal abnormalities on MRI. Adang and colleagues reviewed 29 cases of nononcologic anti-NMDAR encephalitis and noted that in 78% of cases symptoms began in warm weather months, suggesting a seasonal trigger. Nosadini and colleagues identified four pediatric patients with anti-NMDAR encephalitis and reported 4 distinct phases of EEG findings: 1) early phase, during the behavioral and orofacial/limb dyskinesias where the EEG is essentially normal; 2) florid phase, when consciousness is impaired, stereotyped movements occur, and the EEG shows rhythmic delta/theta that is not responsive to stimuli or antiepileptic medications; 3) recovery phase, when rhythmic sequences decrease; and 4) normalization phase, when EEG is back to baseline usually 2 to 5 months after onset of the disease.

The current view in the pediatric population is that if no tumor is detected during the initial evaluation, further oncologic evaluation is not warranted unless symptoms recur (Dalmau, personal communication, 2010).

Prognosis: Despite severe neurologic deficits, 75% of patients made a complete recovery whereas 25% had severe deficits or died. In 2009 Florance and colleagues reported 81 patients with NMDAR encephalitis from several institutions (Florance et al., 2009). Thirty-two patients were 18 years old or younger. Seventy-seven percent of pediatric patients had seizures; 84% had movement disorders and 60% had personality or behavioral changes. Teratomas were identified in 25% of patients, all of whom were adults. As mentioned above, Kurian et al. reported about a 23-year-old woman with OMA syndrome plus features of LE who was diagnosed with NMDAR encephalitis. A tumor was not identified in this patient and although she made a significant recovery with immunotherapy, she had persistent frontal lobe behavioral abnormalities 5 months after diagnosis. In 2009 at the European Paediatric Neurologic Society meeting, multiple groups reported about individual children with and pediatric patient case series of NMDAR encephalitis, none of whom had evidence of malignancy and most of them had favorable neurologic outcome.

CHAPTER SUMMARY AND FUTURE PERSPECTIVE

Among neurologic complications of cancer, PNS represent a significant challenge in both diagnosis and treatment. These problems loom larger as systemic cancers respond better to treatment leading to longer survival. Discovery of new paraneoplastic antibodies and other diagnostic techniques, particularly advances in imaging (MRI and PET), have allowed for earlier cancer diagnosis. Further work is necessary to understand the exact role of different antibodies in PNS. Many new antibodies against neuronal cell-surface antigens will probably be described in the future. Factors hampering clinical research include methodological difficulties in study design and patient accrual in uncommon entities. A regularly updated classification of PNS and its subtypes, according to autoantibodies and the roles these antibodies have, is needed. It is hoped that understanding pathophysiology, identifying subtypes, and development of newer immunosuppressive agents will lead to improved prognoses in PNS.

REFERENCES

The complete list of references for this chapter is available in the e-book at www.expertconsult.com.
    See inside cover for registration details.

SELECTED REFERENCES

Clardy, S.L., et al., 2013. Childhood onset of stiff-man syndrome. JAMA Neurol. 70, 1531–1536.

Dalmau, J., Rosenfeld, M.R., 2014. Autoimmune encephalitis update. Neuro Oncol. 16, 771–778.

Florance, N.R., et al., 2009. Anti-N-methyl-D-aspartate receptor (NMDAR) encephalitis in children and adolescents. Ann. Neurol. 66, 11–18.

Hasegawa, S., et al., 2014. A nationwide survey of opsoclonus-myoclonus syndrome in Japanese children. Brain Dev. 37, 656–660.

Ketterl, T.G., et al., 2013. Ofatumumab for refractory opsoclonus-myoclonus syndrome following treatment of neuroblastoma. Pediatr. Blood Cancer 60, E163–E165.

Payne, M., et al., 2010. Prospective study into the incidence of Lambert Eaton myasthenic syndrome in small cell lung cancer. J. Thorac. Oncol. 5, 34–38.

Rosenfeld, M.R., Dalmau, J., 2013. Diagnosis and management of paraneoplastic neurologic disorders. Curr. Treat. Options Oncol. 14, 528–538.

Rudnick, E., et al., 2001. Opsoclonus-myoclonus-ataxia syndrome in neuroblastoma: clinical outcome and antineuronal antibodies-a report from the Children's Cancer Group Study. Med. Pediatr. Oncol. 36, 612–622.

Toothaker, T.B., Rubin, M., 2009. Paraneoplastic neurological syndromes: a review. Neurologist 15, 21–33.

119 Immune-Mediated Epilepsy, Movement Disorders, and Hashimoto's Encephalopathy in Children

Russell C. Dale

 An expanded version of this chapter is available on www.expertconsult.com. See inside cover for registration details.

INTRODUCTION
Background
Definitions: Immune Activation, Immune Mediation, Autoimmune

Immunologic activity in the central nervous system (CNS) can take many forms. There is a low rate of immune surveillance of the CNS under normal resting conditions. However, if the acquired immune system is activated peripherally, activated lymphocytes or autoantibodies can access the CNS, which may recognize autoantigens and cause secondary activation of the immune system. A number of other variables are also likely to be important, such as disruption of the blood–brain barrier secondary to infection. There is also no doubt that some people are predisposed to autoimmunity; different populations appear vulnerable to certain autoimmune CNS disorders. Therefore autoimmune CNS disorders are undoubtedly complex, involving genetic vulnerability, environmental factors (e.g., infection), and the acquired and innate immune systems. However, the immune system and its role in the CNS is complex, and for this reason we start with some simple definitions:

Autoimmune: Autoimmune disorders usually result from a loss of immune tolerance or abnormal activation of the acquired immune system. Autoimmunity is typically dominated either by T-cell mechanisms or humoral mechanisms (B cells and autoantibody), or often both. Autoimmune disorders often respond to immune-suppressive therapies.

Immune mediation: This is a more ambiguous term that is typically used when the immune system is clearly driving the inflammatory response in the CNS, although the exact mechanism by which this is occurring is unclear. For example, this term is used in disorders such as acute disseminated encephalomyelitis, which is clearly an inflammatory brain condition, but the exact immune mechanisms are likely complex and incompletely understood.

Immune activation: This term is more typically used when there is activation of the immune system secondary to neurologic damage, such as in stroke, neurodegeneration, metabolic processes, or trauma. This immune response could theoretically be damaging or protective. The benefit of immune suppression in this context is less clear.

Autoantibody: The Cell-Surface Paradigm

Antibodies are part of the body's defense system against infection. Autoantibodies are antibodies that attack the host and are associated with a broad spectrum of acquired autoimmune disorders. Some of these autoantibodies are diagnostic biomarkers but probably do not play a pathogenic role in disease. However, other autoantibodies are both diagnostic biomarkers and pathogenic in the disease process. Even in disorders

that are clearly mediated by autoantibodies, the autoantibody rarely acts in isolation, and the autoimmune process is complex, involving autoantibodies, T cells, and sometimes other immune cells or immune molecules.

Paraneoplastic autoantibodies, such as anti-Hu and anti-Yo antibodies, are autoantibodies that are strongly associated with tumors and almost exclusively described in adults. These autoantibodies are important biomarkers of disease but are not pathogenic autoantibodies, because they bind to intracellular proteins. These autoantibodies will not be described further in this chapter, and their relevance to pediatric neurology is minimal.

In the last decade, increasing examples of cell-surface autoantibodies that are involved in autoimmune CNS disease have been found. This cell-surface paradigm involves the principle that autoantibodies that are pathogenic bind to cell-surface epitopes of neurologic proteins involved in neurotransmission or cell function (Irani et al., 2014). The best examples of this paradigm are antibodies that bind to important neuronal receptors such as the N-methyl-D-aspartate (NMDA) receptor, the gamma-aminobutyric acid (GABA) receptors, or the glycine receptor. Other cell-surface proteins include synaptic proteins such as LGI-1 and CASPR2, which are part of the voltage-gated potassium channel complex. These autoantibodies typically bind to the extracellular domains of these receptors or proteins. For example, the dominant epitope involved in NMDA receptor autoantibody binding is the extracellular amino terminus domain of the NR1 subunit of the NMDA receptor.

Autoantibody Methodology

There are many different methods to detect autoantibodies. However, each of these methodologies can affect the way the protein is presented to the autoantibody. For example, tissue homogenization results in destruction of cells and consequent release of intracellular and membrane proteins. The use of this method will therefore result in detection of autoantibodies against proteins that may not be physiologically relevant. For this reason, to measure cell-surface autoantibodies, it is necessary to present the protein of interest (such as a receptor) in its conformational state on the surface of a representative cell. These cell-based assays have become the classic method to define autoantibodies against cell-surface antigens.

Autoantibody Pathogenic Mechanisms

An autoantibody can have multiple mechanisms of action. For example, an autoantibody can bind to a protein, triggering complement or natural-killer binding with resultant secondary cytotoxicity and cell death. As described earlier, some autoantibody-associated diseases are now recognized to involve additional T-cell mechanisms and engagement of neutrophils and eosinophils, such as in neuromyelitis optica. However, sometimes the autoantibody binding alone results in direct alteration of the antigen. For example, autoantibodies that bind to the NMDA receptor result in alteration of the receptor function, followed by internalization of the receptor away from the cell surface, ultimately resulting in NMDAR receptor hypofunction. A similar mechanism of action has been described for many of the cell-surface autoantibodies. This direct pathogenic process is generally considered to be reversible if the autoantibody is removed.

IMMUNE-MEDIATED EPILEPSY
Autoimmune Encephalitis Syndromes

Before we discuss the different causes of autoimmune epilepsy or movement disorders, we will first consider the different diagnostic categories, which are as follows:

Encephalitis: Encephalitis is inflammation of the brain. Pathologically, there is typically inflammatory infiltrate of the brain parenchyma surrounding the blood vessels. Encephalitis can result from infections, including those caused by viruses and bacteria, but also autoimmune and immune-mediated mechanisms. Encephalitis is a clinical syndrome, and to improve diagnostic classifications, international criteria have been proposed. In brief, encephalitis is diagnosed when there is acute or subacute neurologic dysfunction in association with encephalopathy, plus evidence of brain inflammation evidence on magnetic resonance imaging (MRI) or cerebrospinal fluid (CSF) examination. Although many of the autoimmune CNS disorders result in encephalitis, some of the autoimmune processes result in a focal neurologic deficit without overt encephalopathy, examples being autoimmune cerebellar ataxia and Sydenham chorea.

Limbic encephalitis (autoimmune or paraneoplastic): Limbic encephalitis is encephalitis affecting the limbic region, which classically includes the mesial temporal lobe, the hippocampus, and the amygdala. Typically this results in cognitive dysfunction, personality change, confusion, and temporal lobe seizures, although more diffuse signs are sometimes evident. Limbic encephalitis can result from an autoimmune process, a paraneoplastic process, or, alternatively, infections with certain pathogens, such as HHV-6 infection in immune-suppressed individuals.

Pan-encephalitis: The best example of a pan-encephalitis is anti-NMDA receptor encephalitis. Since its original descriptions, it has been clear that this autoimmune encephalitis particularly affects young people from infancy to middle age. Females are more commonly affected in adulthood, but males and females are nearly equally affected in children under 10 years of age. A diagnosis is made by finding the presence of autoantibodies against NMDA receptor in the CSF and/or sera. CSF NMDA receptor antibodies are more specific than serum antibodies (Dalmau et al., 2011). The syndrome is paraneoplastic and associated with ovarian teratoma in a minority of female adolescents. More commonly the encephalitis is unexplained, or occasionally may follow a well-defined infection. Recently, some cases of anti-NMDAR encephalitis following confirmed herpes simplex encephalitis have been described, providing an example of post-viral autoimmune encephalitis. The clinical syndrome in its full form is very recognizable, with psychosis, agitation, and dyskinesias being typical and characteristic. Encephalopathy, aphasia, seizures, and dysautonomia may also occur, but these features are less helpful in the differentiation from other encephalitis syndromes. MRI results are normal in approximately half of patients, although MRI may show limbic encephalitis or nonspecific white-matter or cortical changes. CSF pleocytosis occurs in two-thirds of children affected by anti-NMDAR encephalitis, and oligoclonal bands may be present in established disease. There is increasing evidence that immune therapy improves outcomes, reduces relapses, and reduces the risk of mortality. First-line immune therapy is with corticosteroids, intravenous immunoglobulin, or plasma exchange, and if this is inadequate, second-line therapy with rituximab or cyclophosphamide, or both, can be used for rescue therapy. Relapses occur in less than 10%, tend to be less severe, and have decreased in incidence since the original descriptions, possibly in relation to the increased use of early immune therapies (Titulaer et al., 2013).

Autoantibody Associations with Epilepsy

The recognition of autoimmune encephalitis has resulted in increased interest in autoimmune and inflammatory causes of seizures and epilepsy (Suleiman and Dale, 2015). Table 119-1 describes autoantibodies associated with seizures and epilepsy in the context of autoimmune encephalitis. The table describes the seizure association and the other features associated with the respective autoantibodies. Many of the syndromes are characterized by movement disorders or other localizing features. Indeed, a recent large study of all types of encephalitis in children noted that the presence of movement disorders was significantly associated with the chance of the encephalitis being autoantibody associated (Pillai et al., 2015). For example, dyskinesias are common in anti-NMDAR encephalitis, and subcortical myoclonus or rigidity occurs in glycine receptor antibody–associated encephalitis.

Autoimmune encephalitis associated with autoantibodies present with acute or subacute change in neurologic function, including encephalopathy, cognitive alteration, and psychiatric features. Seizures occur in a significant proportion and can be refractory, particularly in anti-GABA-A receptor autoimmune encephalitis.

These descriptions have resulted in the hypothesis that some patients with unexplained new-onset epilepsy may have an autoimmune etiology. There are now a number of research cohorts demonstrating autoantibodies in a minority of epilepsy patients (5%–10%). The patients who were positive for autoantibodies tended to have otherwise "unexplained" epilepsy (i.e., no clear genetic or structural causes of epilepsy), were more likely to have focal epilepsy, and often had normal MRI neuroimaging.

Guidelines for Identification of Autoimmune Epilepsy

The recognition of autoimmune causes of seizures and epilepsy has resulted in the generation of guidelines to help identify these patients (Suleiman et al., 2013). In general, the level of evidence for an autoimmune etiology has been grouped into the three categories of *confirmed*, in which autoantibodies are found in the CSF; *probable*, in which the autoantibody is found in serum; and *possible*, in which the autoantibody is absent or not tested, but the patient has a beneficial response to immune therapy and has other features of an autoimmune etiology. This hierarchical approach to diagnosis of autoimmune encephalitis and autoimmune epilepsy needs to be assessed in larger cohorts.

As is true for encephalitis in general, features of an autoimmune epilepsy include the presence of acute or subacute onset of seizures, typically in the context of other features of encephalopathy or neurologic disturbance, plus evidence of inflammation using neuroimaging, CSF examination, or

TABLE 119-1 Neuronal Antibodies Associated with Encephalitis Complicated by Seizures That Have Been Reported in Children*

Antibody Type	Encephalitis Association in Adults	Encephalitis Association in Children	Seizure Types (Adults and Children)	Typical Associated Features	MRI Features
VGKC-complex	Limbic encephalitis Morvan's syndrome	Limbic encephalitis Encephalitis with status epilepticus	Focal (or multifocal) seizures (mostly temporal lobe) Mixed seizure types Faciobrachial dystonic seizures (LGI-1 antibodies)	Fever Encephalopathy Behavioral changes Memory and cognitive impairment	Normal High signal in medial temporal lobes White-matter signal abnormalities, high signal in basal ganglia
NMDAR	Encephalitis with movement disorder, psychiatric disturbances, aphasia, autonomic dysfunction, seizures	Encephalitis with movement disorder, psychiatric disturbances, aphasia, autonomic dysfunction, seizures	Focal seizures (motor and dyscognitive), mostly extratemporal Mixed seizure types Status epilepticus/EPC	Encephalopathy Movement disorder Psychiatric disturbance Autonomic instability	Normal High signal in medial temporal lobes and other regions
GABA$_B$R	Limbic encephalitis	Limbic encephalitis	Focal seizures (temporal lobe) Generalized seizures (primary and secondary) Status epilepticus	Memory disturbance Movement disorder (dystonia, chorea), opsoclonus, ataxia	Normal High signal in medial temporal lobes and other regions
GABA$_A$R	Encephalitis with seizures or status epilepticus (multifocal encephalitis)	Encephalitis with seizures or status epilepticus (multifocal encephalitis)	Focal seizures (temporal and extratemporal) Mixed seizure types Status epilepticus/EPC	Memory and cognitive impairment Behavioral changes, psychosis Movement disorder (dystonia chorea) Other autoimmune disorders	Cortical-subcortical lesions (multifocal) High signal in temporal lobes
GlyR	Other spinal and brainstem disorders (stiff person syndrome, PERM) Limbic encephalitis	PERM Focal encephalitis with seizures	Myoclonic jerks (cortical or subcortical) Hyperekplexia Temporal lobe seizures and status epilepticus	Rigidity (startle induced) Cognitive impairments	Normal
GAD	Limbic encephalitis Stiff person syndrome	Limbic encephalitis	Focal seizures (mostly temporal) Secondary generalized seizures EPC (multifocal)	Memory, cognitive impairment, ataxia Autoimmune disorders or immune deficiency	Normal Lesions in hippocampus, cortex, or cerebellum

EPC, epilepsia partialis continua; GABA, gamma-aminobutyric acid, GAD, glutamic acid decarboxylase; GlyR, glycine receptor; NMDAR, N-methyl D-aspartate receptor; PERM, progressive encephalomyelitis with rigidity and myoclonus; VGKC, voltage-gated potassium channel.
*Although tumors are reported in association with some of these antibodies in adults, these syndromes are rarely paraneoplastic in children. LGI-1, CASPR2, and AMPA-R antibodies associated with epilepsy in children have not been described and so are not presented here.
(Adapted from Suleiman J, Dale RC. Dev Med Child Neurol. May 2015;57[5]:431–440.)

electroencephalogram (EEG) (Box 119-1). Although further studies are required to test these guidelines, it is important for clinicians to be aware of inflammatory causes of epilepsy, because early immune therapy may improve outcomes. For this reason, it is reassuring that an inflammatory subgroup has now been added to the causes of epilepsy in the International League Against Epilepsy (ILAE) classification.

AUTOIMMUNE MOVEMENT DISORDERS
Background

Movement disorders are classically considered to be generated secondary to dysfunction of the basal ganglia, although any disruption of the corticostriatal circuits can produce abnormal or involuntary movements. The classic autoimmune movement disorder is Sydenham chorea, which has been described since the seventeenth century, although more recently the discovery of autoantibodies has helped define other autoimmune movement-disorder syndromes (Mohammad et al., 2013).

Autoimmune Encephalitis Associated with Movement Disorders (Table 119-2)

Anti-NMDAR encephalitis: As described earlier, autoimmune encephalitis associated with NMDA receptor antibodies results in a diffuse pan-encephalitis. Abnormal movements are a common feature in children with this disorder. The movement disorders are very variable but typically are hyperkinetic, with flailing stereotypical movements, often with perseverative characteristics. Perseverative stereotypical movements may include self-injurious movements, repetitive purposeless movements, cycling movements, or catatonic postures of the

---

BOX 119-1 Clinical and Investigative Features Suggestive of Autoimmune Encephalitis in Patients with Seizures

1. **Clinical features**

   Focal seizures, particularly focal motor and focal dyscognitive, secondary generalized seizures

   Seizure clusters—status epilepticus

   Seizures and epilepsy of "unknown" cause

   Refractory seizures

   Associated features: encephalopathy, movement disorders, neuropsychiatric symptoms, cognitive or memory impairment

   History of other autoimmune diseases (personal or family history)

2. **Imaging and other investigations**

   Positive CSF findings suggestive of inflammation (pleocytosis, elevated neopterin, oligoclonal bands)

   Inflammatory MRI changes of high T2 or FLAIR signal in medial temporal structures, cortical or subcortical areas, and cerebellum and basal ganglia

   Focal (or multifocal) electrographic changes including slowing and/or epileptiform activity, particularly involving temporal lobe (s)

   Histopathologic findings compatible with inflammation (such as lymphocytic infiltrates) on biopsy

   Positive cell-surface neuronal autoantibodies (serum or CSF)

3. **Treatment response**

   Resistance to conventional AEDs

   Response to immunotherapy (including steroids, immunoglobulin and immunosuppressive agents)

4. **No other explanation**

AEDs, antiepileptic drugs; CSF, cerebrospinal fluid; FLAIR, fluid-attenuated inversion recovery; MRI, magnetic resonance imaging.

(Adapted from Suleiman J, Dale RC. Dev Med Child Neurol. May 2015;57[5]:431–440.)

---

limbs. Children can also exhibit dystonia, chorea, and other hyperkinetic movements. In the latter phase the child can become akinetic. Typically, the movement disorder is accompanied by agitation, psychiatric features, encephalopathy, and aphasia. The movement disorders are typically refractory to conventional treatment, and the child often requires sedation for treatment of the symptoms.

Basal ganglia encephalitis: Basal ganglia encephalitis is rarer than anti-NMDAR encephalitis, has been described in young children, and is characterized by selective inflammatory changes involving the basal ganglia structures, specifically the caudate putamen, globus pallidus, and substantia nigra. The child typically presents with an extrapyramidal movement disorder, particularly parkinsonism and dystonia, often with emotional psychiatric features such as anxiety or depression. Often there are inflammatory changes selectively involving the basal ganglia, but CSF pleocytosis is less likely than in anti-NMDA receptor encephalitis, although there may be oligoclonal bands or other markers of CSF inflammation. Autoantibodies against dopamine-2 receptor have been found in the serum of patients, although the pathogenic properties of these antibodies have yet to be demonstrated. If the diagnosis is recognized early, patients often respond to corticosteroids or intravenous immunoglobulins and can make a complete recovery, although striatal gliosis or atrophy is recognized as an outcome in some children with residual dystonia or cognitive features (Dale et al., 2012).

Glycine receptor antibody encephalitis: Glycine receptor antibody encephalitis is more commonly described in adults but also can affect children. The disease process is considered to dominantly involve the brainstem and spine, and the classic movement disorder phenotype is myoclonus, or hyperekplexia with a stimulus-induced startle response. Patients often additionally have rigidity, and in the full form, the syndrome is referred to as progressive encephalomyelitis with rigidity and myoclonus (PERM). As with other autoimmune encephalitis syndromes, immune therapy appears to improve outcomes (Carvajal-Gonzalez et al., 2014).

Other autoimmune encephalitis: Movement disorders have been associated with other autoantibodies in a few patients, such as opsoclonus in patients with GABA-B receptor encephalitis and dyskinesias in patients with GABA-A receptor encephalitis.

Sydenham Chorea

Sydenham chorea (SC) is the classic postinfectious autoimmune movement disorder and is the commonest cause of acute chorea worldwide. Occurring after beta-hemolytic streptococcal infections, SC is the neurologic manifestation of rheumatic fever. SC typically occurs in adolescent females, although it can occur in males and younger children. Certain populations appear to be particularly vulnerable, such as indigenous populations of Australia or Brazil. SC typically causes a pure chorea and is typically generalized, although it can result in hemi-chorea. There may be associated emotional symptoms, such as anxiety, obsessive-compulsive symptoms, or depression. Other major changes in neurologic function, such as seizures or pyramidal signs, are rare, other than dysarthria. Magnetic resonance neuroimaging is typically normal. Investigation should focus on proving the presence of previous streptococcal infection with the use of throat swabs and serology, in addition to investigation for associated rheumatic fever involvement such as carditis. Treatment should focus on preventing further heart involvement with the use of antibiotic prophylaxis until 21 years of age; monthly penicillin injections are probably more effective than oral penicillin administration. There is increasing evidence to suggest that SC can result in residual and permanent neurologic or psychiatric problems. For example, 50% of patients may have some residual mild chorea 2 years after illness, and there is an increased rate of neuropsychiatric symptoms after recovery of SC. For this reason, some experts have advocated more aggressive treatment of SC during the acute phase with immune therapy such as steroids or intravenous immunoglobulins (IVIg). A recent study from South Africa found that patients treated with IVIg had better outcomes than those given symptomatic treatment only. Symptomatic management of SC includes the use of sodium valproate, carbamazepine, or antipsychotics.

PANDAS, PANS, and Tourette Syndrome

In the 1990s, a number of investigators noted some similarities between Sydenham chorea and other acute-onset neuropsychiatric syndromes that followed infectious illnesses. Some of these illnesses were *termed pediatric autoimmune neuropsychiatric disorders associated with streptococcal infection* (PANDAS). Patients with PANDAS typically present after a sore throat with acute-onset anxiety, separation anxiety, obsessive-compulsive symptoms, and sometimes tics. Although these symptoms were initially associated with streptococcal infections, more recently observers have noted that these acute neuropsychiatric symptoms can occur after a number of other infections, but still with an acute explosive onset, which has been termed *pediatric acute onset neuropsychiatric syndrome* (PANS). Although

TABLE 119-2 Autoimmune Movement Disorders

Group	Syndrome	Movement Disorder	Other Features	Diagnostic Features
Autoimmune encephalitis with movement disorders	NMDAR antibody encephalitis	Stereotypical hyperkinetic movements, perseverative movements, chorea, dystonia, rigidity	Encephalopathy, agitation and psychosis, aphasia, seizures, dysautonomia, sleep dysregulation	CSF and serum NMDAR antibodies
	Basal ganglia encephalitis	Dystonia, akinesia, chorea	Emotional disorders	MRI basal ganglia lesions, serum D2R antibodies
	Glycine receptor antibody encephalitis (PERM)	Myoclonus, rigidity, hyperekplexia	Encephalopathy, seizures	Serum (and CSF) glycine receptor antibodies
Autoimmune movement disorders	Sydenham chorea	Chorea	Emotional disorder	Recent streptococcal infection, rheumatic carditis
	Opsoclonus myoclonus ataxia	Opsoclonus, myoclonus, ataxia	Sleep disturbance, irritability	Clinical syndrome, neural crest tumor
Infection-associated movement disorders	PANDAS and PANS	Infection-associated relapsing remitting tics	Emotional lability, obsessive-compulsive disorder	Clinical syndrome
Movement disorders associated with systemic autoimmune disease	Neuropsychiatric systemic lupus erythematosus	Chorea, parkinsonism	Emotional disorder, psychosis, cognitive deficits, seizures	Lupus autoantibodies, antiphospholipid antibodies
	Antiphospholipid syndrome	Chorea	Emotional disorder, psychosis, cognitive deficits, seizures	Antiphospholipid antibodies
	Hashimoto encephalopathy	Chorea, dystonia, ataxia	Encephalopathy, psychiatric features, seizures	Antithyroid antibodies, likely cell-surface antibodies (NMDAR antibodies)

CSF, cerebrospinal fluid; MRI, magnetic resonance imaging; NMDAR, N-methyl D-aspartate receptor; PANDAS, pediatric autoimmune neuropsychiatric disorders associated with streptococcal infection; PANS, pediatric acute neuropsychiatric syndrome; PERM, progressive encephalomyelitis with rigidity and myoclonus; VGKC, voltage-gated potassium channel.

(Adapted from Mohammad SS, Ramanathan S, Brilot F, Dale RC. Neuropediatrics. Dec 2013;44[6]:336–345.)

tics remain a key component of this entity, the dominant features tend to be emotional alteration, particularly anxiety and obsessive-compulsive symptoms, and some patients also appear to develop changes in cognitive function, enuresis, and altered eating behavior. Unfortunately, there is no robust biomarker of this entity, and for this reason diagnosis is dependent on the clinical phenomenology. A number of different autoantibodies have been proposed to be important in these patients, but these findings have not been confidently reproduced. It is indeed possible that PANS is not an autoimmune disorder but some other immune-mediated phenomenon. For this reason, the treatment of PANS lacks a convincing evidence base, although antibiotics can be helpful in the acute phase, and other investigators have used steroids or intravenous immunoglobulin.

There is an expanding literature on the role of the immune system in neuropsychiatric disorders such as Tourette's syndrome, and it is probable that the immune system is involved either in a primary causal fashion or, alternatively, in a modifying secondary fashion in genetically predisposed individuals. Large-scale longitudinal studies are required to unravel the complexity of immune involvement in Tourette syndrome.

HASHIMOTO ENCEPHALOPATHY OR SREAT
Background

Hashimoto encephalopathy is a rare entity of acute neurologic dysfunction in patients with confirmed autoimmune thyroid disease. This neurologic syndrome occurs classically in patients with antithyroid antibodies, particularly antithyroid peroxidase antibodies, although it also may occur in patients with Graves' disease. Despite the presence of antithyroid antibod-ies, patients are often clinically and biochemically hypothyroid. Hashimoto encephalopathy has also been termed *steroid responsive encephalopathy associated with thyroid autoantibodies* (SREAT), and many investigators prefer this descriptive term (Castillo et al., 2006). The discovery of cell-surface autoantibodies in the last decade has led to a reconsideration of the etiology of Hashimoto encephalopathy.

Clinical Syndrome

Most of the literature regarding Hashimoto encephalopathy consists of single case reports or small case series. The clinical phenomenology is relatively broad, possibly related to the fact that Hashimoto encephalopathy is not a single entity but a heterogenous group of conditions associated with autoimmune thyroid disease. Children and adults are affected, and females are more commonly affected. All patients have in common an acute or subacute neurologic syndrome, typically with encephalopathy and behavioral change such as psychosis or emotional dysregulation. Seizures are also common, affecting ~60%. Aphasia and movement disorders (myoclonus and tremor) are also commonly described. Magnetic resonance neuroimaging is typically normal, and CSF may show pleocytosis or other markers of inflammation. The presence of thyroid autoantibodies is a requirement of the diagnosis, particularly antithyroid peroxidase antibodies. Part of the challenge with the diagnosis is the fact that a significant proportion of the general population can have antithyroid antibodies, and thyroid autoantibodies may sometimes represent a familial predisposition to autoimmunity, without the presence of biochemical or clinical hypothyroidism. For this reason, isolated antithyroid antibodies can result in false positive issues in the context of acute neurologic disturbance.

Etiology

It had been originally proposed that the thyroid autoantibodies directly affected the brain, resulting in neurologic dysfunction. However, recently, most observers have suggested that the antithyroid antibodies are simply a manifestation of an autoimmune predisposition, and in fact patients with Hashimoto encephalopathy are more likely to harbor cell-surface antibodies, but the antithyroid antibodies themselves are not causing the neurologic disease. There are a number of recent reports demonstrating a higher rate of antithyroid antibodies in patients with anti-NMDA receptor encephalitis. Indeed, the clinical features of historical cohorts of Hashimoto encephalopathy (SREAT) have many similarities with those of anti-NMDAR encephalitis and other autoimmune encephalitis syndromes (as described earlier). There are also many examples in the medical literature of overlapping autoimmune disorders. For example, patients with systemic lupus erythematosus or Sjögren's disease are more likely to develop neuromyelitis optica. Therefore, testing for a broad panel of cell-surface autoantibodies is recommended when the diagnosis of Hashimoto encephalopathy is considered. As the alternative name SREAT suggests, Hashimoto encephalopathy is an immune-responsive condition, and patients typically respond well to steroids or additional immune therapies, and only a minority of patients will experience relapse.

TREATMENT OF AUTOIMMUNE CNS DISEASE AND THERAPEUTIC DECISION MAKING

Therapeutic decision making for patients with autoimmune CNS disease is complex. The discovery of autoantibody biomarkers has empowered the clinician to treat patients with inflammatory brain diseases; however, the therapies have side effects, and the drugs pose potential risk to the patient. Therefore it is essential for the clinician to balance the potential benefit of the therapies with the potential risk. Anti-NMDA receptor encephalitis is a severe disorder, with a 7% risk of mortality and a 50% risk of morbidity. Thus it is possible to rationalize the use of stronger immune therapies in this condition. However, other conditions such as Sydenham chorea, have less risk of permanent disability; in these milder conditions it would be much harder to rationalize potent immune suppression with agents such as rituximab or cyclophosphamide.

First-line immune therapy generally consists of intravenous corticosteroids, sometimes followed by an oral corticosteroid taper. Alternative or additional first-line immune therapies include intravenous immunoglobulins, typically at a dose of 2 g per kilogram over 2 to 5 days. Plasma exchange can be used and is preferred by some centers. There is no clear evidence to suggest which of these first-line therapies is more efficacious; however, corticosteroids are usually used by most physicians. When first-line immune therapies do not produce adequate response, second-line immune therapies can be considered. It is easier to rationalize the use of second-line immune therapies when the diagnosis is clear and undoubted. There are many instances when the diagnosis is less clear, such as for suspected seronegative autoimmune encephalitis; however, these seronegative patients may also respond to immune therapy.

For patients who do not respond to first-line therapy, rescue therapy with rituximab (which depletes B cells for 6 months) or cyclophosphamide is considered. Both rituximab and cyclophosphamide produce immune effects within 1 to 2 weeks, and therefore represent useful rescue therapies.

However, both agents carry the risk of infections induced by immune suppression, such as viral reactivation syndromes or progressive multifocal leukoencephalopathy.

In disorders that are steroid responsive and prone to relapse, such as neuromyelitis optica, steroid-sparing immunosuppressants, such as mycophenolate mofetil or azathioprine, can be considered. However, both of these agents take a few months before they produce adequate immune suppression, and therefore prolonged corticosteroid taper is often required.

REFERENCES

The complete list of references for this chapter is available in the e-book at www.expertconsult.com.
See inside cover for registration details.

SELECTED REFERENCES

Carvajal-Gonzalez, A., Leite, M.I., Waters, P., et al., 2014. Glycine receptor antibodies in PERM and related syndromes: characteristics, clinical features and outcomes. Brain 137 (Pt 8), 2178–2192.

Castillo, P., Woodruff, B., Caselli, R., et al., 2006. Steroid-responsive encephalopathy associated with autoimmune thyroiditis. Arch. Neurol. 63 (2), 197–202.

Dale, R.C., Merheb, V., Pillai, S., et al., 2012. Antibodies to surface dopamine-2 receptor in autoimmune movement and psychiatric disorders. Brain 135 (Pt 11), 3453–3468.

Dalmau, J., Lancaster, E., Martinez-Hernandez, E., et al., 2011. Clinical experience and laboratory investigations in patients with anti-NMDAR encephalitis. Lancet Neurol. 10 (1), 63–74.

Irani, S.R., Gelfand, J.M., Al-Diwani, A., et al., 2014. Cell-surface central nervous system autoantibodies: clinical relevance and emerging paradigms. Ann. Neurol. 76 (2), 168–184.

Mohammad, S.S., Ramanathan, S., Brilot, F., et al., 2013. Autoantibody-associated movement disorders. Neuropediatrics 44 (6), 336–345.

Pillai, S.C., Hacohen, Y., Tantsis, E., et al., 2015. Infectious and Autoantibody-Associated Encephalitis: Clinical Features and Long-term Outcome. Pediatrics 135 (4), e974–e984.

Suleiman, J., Brilot, F., Lang, B., et al., 2013. Autoimmune epilepsy in children: case series and proposed guidelines for identification. Epilepsia 54 (6), 1036–1045.

Suleiman, J., Dale, R.C., 2015. The recognition and treatment of autoimmune epilepsy in children. Dev. Med. Child Neurol. 57 (5), 431–440.

Titulaer, M.J., McCracken, L., Gabilondo, I., et al., 2013. Treatment and prognostic factors for long-term outcome in patients with anti-NMDA receptor encephalitis: an observational cohort study. Lancet Neurol. 12 (2), 157–165.

E-BOOK FIGURES AND TABLES

The following figures and tables are available in the e-book at www.expertconsult.com. See inside cover for registration details.

Fig. 119-1. MRI axial view in limbic encephalitis showing increased T2 signal in the mesial temporal lobe bilaterally, right greater than left. The patient had temporal lobe seizures, confusion, and behavioral change.

Fig. 119-2. Magnetic resonance neuroimaging in basal ganglia encephalitis showing inflammatory changes selectively involving the basal ganglia structures—the caudate, putamen, globus pallidus, and substantia nigra. **A,** Axial MRI T2 sequence showing inflammatory changes in caudate, putamen, globus pallidus. **B,** Coronal MRI T2 sequence showing inflammatory change in caudate and substantia nigra neuroimaging in basal ganglia encephalitis.

120 Opsoclonus Myoclonus Syndrome

Michael R. Pranzatelli and Elizabeth D. Tate

 An expanded version of this chapter is available on www.expertconsult.com. See inside cover for registration details.

INTRODUCTION

Opsoclonus-myoclonus syndrome (OMS) affects an estimated one in a million children worldwide. Although it also occurs in adults, reference only to pediatric OMS is made herein. Recent advances in the neuroimmunology of OMS, prefigured by transformational developments in understanding human autoimmune disorders of the nervous system, have revivified the field. This chapter aims to guide clinical decision making through the authors' 25-year clinical experience from operating the National Pediatric Myoclonus Center (NPMC), now an international specialist center for OMS; a review of the medical literature and practices from the past decade; and recent translational research in the field. Citations to the earlier literature can be found in the authors' previous reviews of the topic (Pranzatelli and Tate, 2010), and the reviews and perspectives of other authors also are available. The broad categories covered are as follows:

1. Clinical aspects
2. Immunopathogenesis
3. Treatment
4. Management of relapse and progression
5. Future directions

CLINICAL ASPECTS
Presentation and Course

Both the clinical presentation and course of OMS are multifarious (Figure 120-1). In typical OMS, the symptom cluster appears acutely and intensifies over days to weeks. After teetering for weeks, OMS may appear to improve or worsen. Motor aspects of OMS include the triad of opsoclonus, myoclonus, and ataxia (see Video 120-1). Opsoclonus must have a random or chaotic multidirectional element in contradistinction from nystagmus (Wong, 2007). Because eye movement disorders can be complex, video-documentation for later consulting should be standard. The subcortical myoclonus is exacerbated by action and contravenes fine motor activity. In the beginning, there is gait ataxia; later, limb dysmetria may emerge. The level of dysfunction ranges from an ambulatory child who is a little shaky or wobbly to a hospitalized, nonverbal, nonambulatory child on a feeding tube, with copious drooling, choking, limpness, and loss of purposeful function. Presence of a Horner syndrome or signs of spinal cord compression signals nonparaneoplastic manifestations of neuroblastic tumors.

Nonmotor comorbidities of OMS affect the quality of life both of children and their parents. Irritability is an early and disruptive characteristic. The OMS sleep disorder comprises prolonged sleep-latency, fragmented sleep, reduced total sleep time, and nonrestorative sleep with excessive daytime fatigue. Wakefulness compromises learning and behavior. Rage "meltdowns" or intermittent explosive disorder may occur several times a day. The child's aggression often targets the mother, who may be bitten or slapped. The "velcro child" is another common phenomenon, clinging to one parent or both

throughout the day. Normal siblings sometimes become angry and depressed at being assailed by the affected child or marginalized by parental focus on the affected child's sick role. Eroded by sleep loss, stress, depression, and anxiety, the family dynamic suffers. In chronic OMS, children display prominent deficits in executive, attentional, and behavioral regulatory skill development. Affective dysregulation, disruptive behavior, impulsivity, and inattention are among the psychiatric symptoms, as are obsessions/compulsions and oppositional defiant behavior.

Differential Diagnosis

Establishing an accurate diagnosis is requisite for treatment. Presence of opsoclonus excludes the diagnosis of acute cerebellar ataxia, with which early OMS is so often confused, when gait ataxia is the presenting or predominant feature (Desai and Mitchell, 2012). Ataxia may be the only neurologic sign in neuroblastoma. Hence, OMS should be considered in all cases of nonexanthematous acute cerebellar ataxia, especially when spontaneous improvement has not occurred within a few weeks.

The term "atypical OMS" or "OMS variant" applies when either the amount of opsoclonus, myoclonus, and ataxia is greatly disproportionate, or when opsoclonus is absent but the rest of the history and examination are compatible with OMS. Isolated opsoclonus or mixed ocular movement abnormalities with predominant nystagmus in infants younger than 6 months of age seldom presage OMS. Although children with OMS may develop strabismus, OMS is not associated with loss of vision or acquired microcephaly. Bone fide seizures (not severe myoclonic jerks imitating seizures), especially if pharmacotherapy resistant, and epileptiform EEG abnormalities should redirect the differential diagnosis. If neuroblastoma is present, consider anti-Hu (ANNA-1) and anti-Ma2 and anti-CV2/CRM5 paraneoplastic syndrome.

Genetics

There are no reported cases of twins in one family both having OMS or more than one family member having OMS across generations. A higher incidence of autoimmune disorders in the parents suggests shared genetic susceptibility to other autoimmune conditions. Infrequently, children with OMS or their parents develop another autoimmune disorder years later; a second paraneoplastic syndrome is rare.

Etiology

In 105 children with OMS, neural crest tumors, such as neuroblastoma, ganglioneuroblastoma, and ganglioneuroma, were found in about 50%, though OMS occurs in only a few percent of patients with neuroblastoma (Tate et al., 2005). Neuroblastoma is an embryonal malignancy of the sympathetic nervous system arising from pluripotent sympathetic cells (neuroblasts). Tumor location frequency is mostly abdominal and thoracic, less often pelvic or cervical. Patients with tumor are not distinguishable by prodromal symptoms, OMS age of onset or severity, relapse rate, or geographic distribution. The relationship of incidence of OMS to patient age does not differ depending on whether neuroblastoma is present or absent. A uniform paraneoplastic classification of OMS etiology has been proposed, but is currently untestable.

When a tumor is not detected, the question arises: Are there two distinct etiologic paths to OMS or two different proximal approaches that converge on the same final common pathway? "Viral," "para-infectious," or "postinfectious" etiologies have been posited. Various microbiologically documented infections are reported, but cause and effect has not been established. Confusion arises because the OMS viral-like prodrome, which can include vomiting, differs little between children with or without a tumor. OMS related to Epstein–Barr virus does not preclude an occult neuroblastic tumor. Designation as "idiopathic" is probably more prudent.

Epidemiology

The OMS onset age spectrum is a bell-shaped curve from 0.5 to 5 years, with outliers in younger infants and elementary-school-aged children (Tate et al., 2005). Whereas neuroblastoma can present in neonates, OMS does not. There is a slight female preponderance. All races and ethnicities are affected. Cases are geographically distributed in keeping with population densities in the United States. The mean OMS onset age is 1.6 ± 0.7 years, with a 3-month average delay to correct diagnosis. Similar observations based on smaller surveys have been made in other countries (Brunklaus et al., 2011). OMS sometimes follows vaccination.

Diagnostic Testing

The main purpose of diagnostic testing is fourfold: 1) find the tumor if there is one; 2) reveal neuroinflammation through state-of-the-art commercially available immunologic tools; 3) rule out other plausible neurologic etiologies; and 4) establish the pretreatment health of the immune system (Figure 120-2).

Tumor Detection

Neuroblastoma may be more difficult to detect in children with than without OMS because of the relative maturity and low metabolic activity of their tumors. A 24-hour collection for urinary catecholamines (VMA, HVA) is a suggestive indicator that is helpful only if positive; false negatives are common in OMS. CT/MRI imaging was found superior to metaiodobenzyl guanidine (MIBG) and urine catecholamines for neuroblastoma detection. The newer MIBG tracer (^{131}I replaced by ^{123}I) is the main functional imaging tracer for neuroblastoma detection. [18F] FDG PET/CT is an alternative for tumors with little or no MIBG uptake. Because neuroblastoma may be discovered several years after OMS onset, patients require continued surveillance in tumor-negative cases.

Neuroinflammation Detection

Neuroinflammation in OMS cannot be detected through blood testing; lumbar puncture is necessary. Improved methods of detecting neuroinflammation should be applied. Cerebrospinal fluid (CSF) *oligoclonal* bands that are not found in a parallel serum sample by isoelectric focusing with immunofixation are indicative of an intrathecal humoral immune response. Lymphocyte subset analysis is practicable at the hospital clinical flow cytometry laboratory. Paraneoplastic autoantibody trawling by commercial laboratories is not cost-effective for typical OMS and best reserved for atypical cases. When sedation is required for children with acute OMS undergoing procedures, the usual sedatives do not work, cause paradoxical excitation, or exacerbate OMS for hours to days. The anesthetics propofol and sevoflurane are tolerated.

Ancillary Testing

To exclude neuroinfectious diseases, an encephalitis panel is routine. Head MRI scanning rules out cerebellitis or a posterior fossa mass. EEG slowing can be seen in OMS, but epileptiform EEGs should raise suspicion.

Pretreatment Immune Health

The pretreatment health of the immune system should be verified by serum quantitative immunoglobulins, blood lymphocyte subset analysis, and serum 25-hydroxyvitamin D levels. IgA deficiency is more frequent in the presence of autoimmune diseases. Vitamin D insufficiency, even deficiency, is not uncommon in OMS, and should be corrected.

ACTH or Dexamethasone Challenge Test

In pursuing the diagnosis of OMS variant, further ancillary tests may clarify the issue, but sometimes a 1-month therapeutic challenge of high-dose ACTH or dexamethasone is necessary when faced with a diagnostic dilemma (Figure 120-3). The unparalleled initial response rate of OMS to ACTH makes the 1-month "ACTH challenge test" clinically useful.

Standard of Care and Quality of Life

The acceptable standard of care for OMS is to rapidly put the child into a durable neurologic remission, and to reverse or prevent relapse and secondary progression. In human terms, it is nothing less than to return children to their lives with the future capability of living independently, holding jobs, and having friends and loved ones. Best practice should be applied in a timely and uniform fashion for all children with OMS. The standard of care at centers seeing larger numbers of children with OMS has improved, and there have been positive changes in practice styles in the United States, but the standard is not uniform and varies across the globe. Denied access to care and inadequate health-care resources are significant barriers.

IMMUNOPATHOGENESIS

Although an autoimmune causation for OMS has not been proven, the evidence for the theory is becoming quite compelling (Pranzatelli and Tate, 2010). The culprit may be ectopic expression of a neuronal antigen in the periphery, engaging the adaptive immune subsystem and transmigration of activated lymphocytes into the CNS. However, despite much searching, the antigen or antigens remain at large. The theater of operations includes the posterior fossa (cerebellum and brainstem), especially the cerebellar vermis, and possibly supratentorial structures (cerebral cortex) (Anand et al., 2015). There are both brainstem and cerebellar hypotheses of opsoclonus (Wong, 2007). A simplistic schema of possible pathophysiologic events in OMS is shown in Figure 120-4.

Tumor Immunology

Neuroblastoma in OMS is more highly infiltrated with lymphocytes than in the absence of OMS. Tumor survival is much greater in the presence of OMS. In the absence of OMS, the frequency of neuroblastoma in the youngest children is higher. Neuroblastomas in OMS exhibit lymphoneogenesis, a feature of chronic inflammatory brain disease as well.

CNS Inflammatory Mediators

Immune Dysregulation. The first putative biomarker of disease activity in untreated OMS was the increased frequency of mature B cells in CSF; the second was CSF oligoclonal bands (OCB). Multiple types of activated B and T cells are involved in abnormal trafficking into the CNS. After encountering self-antigen, dysregulated B-cell signaling can drive autoimmunity.

Inflammatory Proteins. *Chemokines* are *chemo*attractant *cyto*kines and the predominant human cytokines and inflammatory mediators. Recent evidence indicates upregulated production of various inflammatory chemokines in four different chemokine/receptor systems. Of these, CSF CXCL13, a major B-cell chemoattractant acting at the CXCR5 receptor, is a putative biomarker of disease activity and treatment biomarker in OMS (Pranzatelli et al., 2012). The net effect of these abnormalities is to allow autoaggressive B and T cells to permeate the CNS.

The CSF concentration of the cytokine B-cell-activating factor (BAFF) is elevated in untreated OMS. It is lower in patients treated with corticosteroids or ACTH, but not with IVIg, and correlates with the concentration of antibodies to cerebellar granule cells and OMS severity category. Higher CSF BAFF correlates with CSF oligoclonal bands and a higher concentration of inflammatory chemokines in CSF. BAFF may be a bridge between neuroblastoma and OMS (Raffaghello et al., 2013).

Brain-Related Proteins. Recent biochemical data suggest neuronal/axonal injury in a subpopulation of children with OMS. From a panel of seven established markers of neuronal/axonal and astroglial injury, only CSF neurofilament light chain was elevated in untreated OMS versus controls. No significant differences were found for glial fibrillary acidic acid protein or S-100 beta, which are primarily glial markers.

The Effect of Immunotherapy on Brain Inflammation. Some, but not all, immunotherapies decrease concentrations of inflammatory mediators in OMS. The argument can be made that corticotropin and corticosteroids shut down production of inflammatory cell products with clinical benefit. However, the cells, unless reregulated or killed, are ready to start producing again once steroids are tapered (hence relapse).

Autoantibodies. Activated B cells may produce antibodies, but memory B cells, plasmablasts, and plasma cells do so at a faster rate. Using flow cytometry, surface-binding subclass autoantibodies to cerebellar granule neurons were detected. Mostly of the IgG3 subclass, they possessed antiproliferative and apoptosis effects on neuroblastoma cell lines. No antigen was identified. The results await independent confirmation. Detection of other antibodies in OMS has been discussed elsewhere.

TREATMENT
Treatment Strategy

To facilitate the reestablishment of tolerance, neuroinflammation must be expunged. The challenge is how to best deploy the available therapeutics. Unlike relentlessly progressive multiple sclerosis or neuropsychiatric lupus, the brain usually needs protection in OMS for just the few years it is beset with this disorder, and so it will not be left damaged after neuroinflammation's dénouement. The argument hinges not on

whether to use "aggressive" versus "nonaggressive" therapy, but rather on using *sufficient* therapy to achieve full recovery, implementing disease-modifying agents, continually reassessing adequate treatment response, and being mindful of the changeable risk/benefit ratio. Likewise, the contrast of "conventional" versus "unconventional" agents is also fading with the changing practice patterns in OMS. Our semantic lexicon needs to be expanded to include *disease-modifying targeted biotherapies*, use of *biomarker-assisted therapy*, and *personalized medicine* instead. These remarks are prefatory to a discussion of a trenchant division in the initial approach to OMS (Table 120-1).

The Front-Loaded Approach. In the "front-loaded" or "front-end" approach, multiple immunotherapeutic modalities are initiated together for *neuroprotection* as a *medical emergency*. Rituximab or cyclophosphamide is utilized early. Increased immunosuppression with ACTH, IVIg, and rituximab or cyclophosphamide has been associated with improved cognitive and other outcomes. Also, the pathologic B-cell-related chain of events in the CNS occurs early in OMS and cannot be broken by steroids/ACTH or IVIg alone. Early anti-B-cell therapy may prevent autoreactive B cells from differentiating into long-lasting plasma cells and the formation of ectopic lymphoid follicles in the brain. The front-loaded approach is exemplified by *FLAIR* therapy, an acronym for front-loaded ACTH, IVIg, and rituximab. *DEXIR*, also coined by the NPMC, refers to the combination of high-dose pulse dexamethasone, IVIg, and rituximab.

The Staggered Approach. In the "staggered" approach, also termed "escalation treatment" and "treatment intensification," steroids or IVIg are used first, but chemotherapy and anti-B-cell agents are held in reserve. Proponents of this approach disagree about the urgency of OMS and the timing of therapy, and also subscribe to different views as to when to shift strategy from reduplication of initial efforts to nouveau therapies. The choice of preferred steroids has shifted from prednisone, prednisolone, and methylprednisolone to pulse dose dexamethasone. The concern is that unchecked disease activity early in the course of OMS may prevent remission and propagate disease progression. Because of brain developmental vulnerabilities, it is not possible to recapture lost time once the critical window for intervention has closed. Though opinions are polarized, the long-running clinical debate can only be informed by more immunologic and outcome data.

Integrating Neuroinflammation with Clinical Assessment. Biofluid testing for neuroinflammation can be used to inform treatment decisions, which focus on OMS severity and duration (Box 120-1). It is a particularly powerful tool not only for initial evaluation, but also in assessing partial or complete treatment failures, in which concurrent drugs may be masking clinical signs of underlying neuroinflammation. The use of the percentage and numbers of B cells and oligoclonal bands is a step toward biomarker-assisted individualized medicine and a step away from determining the level of treatment on purely clinical grounds. It prevents the delay inherent in the "wait-and-see" approach because the impact of the level of neuroinflammation can be anticipated and helps prevent patient misclassification. The more informed the treatment decision is, the greater the likelihood it will be effective.

Antitumor Therapy

Successful treatment of the tumor usually does not improve OMS. The treatment for neuroblastoma in infants less than 6 months of age is transitioning to expectant observation. With spontaneous tumor regression, many are spared surgery.

BOX 120-1 Factoring Clinical and Neuroinflammatory Severity in Patient Assessments*

SEVERE

Clinical Criteria (Score 25 to 36)

The patient is unable to get to a standing position independently; is unstable with feet apart; cannot stand with feet together; cannot sit without falling forward; cannot target or grasp objects with hands, no finger pincer; eyes cannot track because of frequent opsoclonic intrusions; and dysarthria/anarthria. The nonmotor aspects often include rage, sleeplessness, and encephalopathic appearance.

Immunologic Criteria

Cerebrospinal fluid (CSF) B-cell frequency is >2% and may be as high as 10% to 20%. CD4/CD8 ratio is usually low at <1. Highest frequency of CSF oligoclonal bands. May be mild CSF leukocytosis, 4 to 100 cells.

Treatment Considerations

The consensus among several opsoclonus-myoclonus syndrome (OMS) experts is that three-agent multimodal combination immunotherapy is advised in severe OMS. Which is the best combination of agents can be debated. ACTH (ACTH option 1), the most potent induction agent, is usually given with IVIg, and the third agent is either rituximab or cyclophosphamide. Sole reliance on steroids/ACTH or IVIg in the face of partial response, relapse, or progression is now considered below the standard of care.

MODERATE

Clinical Criteria (Score 13 to 24)

Patient may be ambulatory, but gait is wide-based with front-to-back and side-to-side imbalance; achieves standing with self-support; able to sit; reaches target with moderate to severe jerks; grasps object with two hands, but has difficulty holding it; eyes have frequent/large-amplitude jerks with tracking; and moderate dysarthria. When a patient exhibits mixed levels of severities for OMS components, they may be designated as "moderate-to-severe" or "mild-to-moderate," as the case may be.

Immunologic Criteria

CSF B-cell frequency is >2%. CD4/CD8 T-cell ratio is variable, often 1 to 1.5. CSF oligoclonal bands are often elevated but may be normal.

Treatment Considerations

Moderate-severity OMS carries the same potential risks as severe OMS for neurologic sequelae and long-term prognosis. It is not currently possible to predict which of the moderate cases will have a poor outcome. Therefore the authors recommend three-agent multimodal combination immunotherapy, but may use a shorter course of ACTH (ACTH option 2 or 3), or substitute dexamethasone for ACTH on a case-by-case basis. Treatment delay, an important risk factor for poor outcome, ratchets the level of immunotherapy one notch.

MILD

Clinical Criteria (Score 1 to 12)

Can stand without support, but may exhibit side- or back-stepping; walks with slight wide base and instability; sits with no or minimal support; targets with minimal tremulousness; able to grasp objects with thumb and digit, but hold may be unstable; infrequent or small-amplitude eye jerks may not be present both on fixation and at random; and mild dysarthria.

Immunologic Criteria

CSF B-cell frequency may be 1% to 2% (intermediate range). CD4/CD8 ratio is usually 1.5 to 2.5. CSF oligoclonal bands are often negative.

Treatment Considerations

The management of mild OMS is controversial for lack of long-term data as to whether steroids and IVIg immunotherapies are sufficiently protective. The authors typically combine IVIg and pulse-dose dexamethasone and carefully monitor response, but if B-cell expansion is present, they add rituximab. Others may choose oral glucocorticoids instead of dexamethasone. Mild cases are more often monophasic, but can escalate in severity and relapse.

*The authors base this categorization on their clinical experience and literature review. The clinical and immunologic designations are evidence-based; the therapeutic recommendations are not. Motor severity levels in OMS can be defined by the OMS Evaluation Scale, which was designed and validated as a method to score videotapes of patient response. It is a 12-item scale, scored 0 to 3 in severity, generating a summated total score, which indicates clinical severity. The patient's age may affect these criteria.

Thereafter, the treatment of stage I and stage IIA neuroblastoma is usually surgical excision alone. Neuroblastoma surgery may increase the hematogenous antigenic load in OMS, and so, as not to delay treatment for OMS, giving IVIg *before* (and perhaps *after*) tumor resection is advisable. For higher stage tumors, oncologists apply chemotherapeutic regimens.

Immunotherapy

There are many agents in the OMS armamentarium to optimize therapy (Table 120-2). Oncologists recommend IV ports in infants and toddlers who will receive ongoing IV agents and blood testing for compassionate reasons and poor venous access. The following are practical guidelines on administration.

IVIg. Intravenous immunoglobulin (IVIg or IgV) consists of polyclonal IgG pooled from the serum of thousands of blood donors. Possessing both antiinflammatory and immunomodulatory properties, it has been used to treat children with autoimmune diseases for 30 or more years. Administration of a higher dose for induction is based on better clinical response

and scientific evidence of greater suppressive effect on the provocative dendritic immune cell. In an unpublished NPMC-sponsored open-label trial of IVIg in OMS (BB-IND #5389), the 1 to 2 g/kg dose now used had the best efficacy, with fewer side effects than higher doses.

Corticosteroids. Glucocorticoids act through a multiplicity of mechanisms and targets. They differ in relative antiinflammatory potency: dexamethasone (20 to 30×), methylprednisolone (5×), prednisolone = prednisone (4×), hydrocortisone (1×). High-dose dexamethasone pulse therapy is an attractive alternative to prednisone/prednisolone/methylprednisolone because of its longer duration of action, short-term course, and greater relative antiinflammatory potency (Ertle et al., 2008).

ACTH 1-39. ACTH 1-39 is an agonist at each of the melanocortin receptors 1 to 5, and releases cortisol, which acts through adrenal glucocorticoid receptors. It remains the most potent induction agent for OMS. Clinical response to ACTH is the litmus test for determining steroid responsiveness. One-half of patients with nonprogressive OMS who fail or partially

TABLE 120-2 Immunotherapeutics and Prophylactic Safety Medications

Agent	Dose and Administration
Immunotherapeutics	
IVIg[a]	*Induction:* 2 g/kg (1 g/kg/day × 2 consecutive days), then 1 g/kg single monthly infusion for course of therapy. *Tapering:* sequentially lengthen intervals between infusions from 5, 6, 7, then 8 weeks.
Dexamethasone[b]	*Induction:* 20 mg/m^2/day divided TID. Give for 3 to 4 consecutive days/month. *Tapering:* sequentially lengthen intervals between pulse doses.
ACTH	
ACTH1-39[c]	
Option 1 (for severe onset)[d]	*Induction*: 75 mg/m^2 IM or SC BID × 1 week, then daily × 3 weeks. If child not in remission, continue daily 2 to 4 more weeks if tolerated. *Tapering*: QOD dosing × 1 month at the same dose, then taper over 7 to 9 months. Monitor blood pressure, weight, CBC, BMP, U/A, ECG, and ECHO. Check for adrenal insufficiency when concluded.
Option 2 (for moderate onset)[d]	*Induction*: 75 mg/m^2 IM or SC BID × 1 week, daily for1 week, then QOD for 2 weeks. *Tapering*: If child in remission, go to every other day dosing at 70 mg/m^2 for 1 month, then taper over 4 to 7 months.
Option 3 (for relapsers)	Add monthly 3-day dexamethasone pulses about two-thirds of the way through the ACTH tapering schedule for either option 1 or 2. Continue pulses for 3 to 6 months after ACTH discontinuation.
ACTH1-24[e]	*Induction*: IM M-W-F × 1 week. Usually about 25 IU in infants/toddlers, 50 IU in preschool ages, and 100 IU in school-aged children. *Tapering*: M-Th over several months based on response. Can widen intervals between doses if Cushingoid. Monitor as for ACTH1-39.
Rituximab[f]	300 to 375 mg/m^2/infusion once weekly × 4 consecutive weeks for induction. Monitor for allergic reactions during infusions. Follow serum q Ig and blood LSA.
Cyclophosphamide[g]	750 mg/m^2 IV once monthly × 3 to 6 cycles. Monitor for neutropenia at 21 days and per oncologist.
Methotrexate[h]	Oral, once a week, 5 to 10 mg/m^2 induction, titrate slowly to 15 to 20 mg/m^2 as needed and tolerated. Monitor CBC, LFTs, annual CXR.
Prophylactic Indications, Agents, and Measures	
Trimethoprim/sulfamethoxazole[i] (*Pneumocystis jirovecii*, formerly called *Pneumocystis carinii*)	150 mg/m^2/day // 750 mg/m^2/day twice a day on 3 days/week
Ranitidine HCl (or omeprazole) (GERD/GI bleeding)	2 to 4 mg/kg/day
Calcium with vitamin D supplement (osteopenia/osteoporosis)	800 to 1000 mg/day // 400 IU/day. Obtain annual DEXA scan
Low-sodium diet; no salty treats (Cushingoid syndrome)	Restrict to 1 to 2 g/day

[a,b,c,e]Supported by case series and reports.

[b]A dose of 21 mg/m^2/day can be used instead: 7 mg/m^2 T.I.D. × 3 consecutive days.

[c]Acthar Gel, 80 IU/mL.

[d]See Box 120-1 for differentiation of severe versus moderate opsoclonus-myoclonus syndrome (OMS). Regardless of ACTH option used, tapering should not begin unless the patient is remitting. Children with severe acute OMS may not tolerate tapering ("brittle").

[e]Tetracosactin (Synacthen, Cosyntropin), 100 IU/mL.

[f]Supported by phase I clinical trial, case series, and reports.

[a,f]Pretreatment for IVIg or rituximab: acetaminophen (15 mg/kg), diphenhydramine (1.5 mg/kg, maximum dose 25 mg), and dexamethasone (1 mg). Ceterizine may be substituted for diphenhydramine in case of paradoxical reactions.

[g]Supported by case series and reports (used in unpublished COG phase III clinical trial since 2004).

[h]Based on the experience of the authors, not on evidence-based medicine.

[i]If not tolerated, IV pentamidine can be given at time of IVIg infusions per oncologist.

BMP, basic metabolic panel; CBC, complete blood count; CXR, chest-ray; ECHO, echocardiogram; ECG, electrocardiogram; LFTs, liver function tests; LSA, lymphocyte subset analysis; q Ig, quantitative immunoglobulins; U/A, urinalysis.

Disclaimer: There are no FDA-approved treatments for OMS. All the above agents are used off-label. Although every attempt has been made to verify doses and dosing schedules, the authors cannot assume any responsibility for the accuracy. All treatment decisions need to be made together by treating physicians and the parents.

respond to steroids will respond to ACTH. There are several options when using ACTH (Table 120-2). ACTH 1-24 was available in Europe until recently.

Monoclonal Antibody Therapy. Rituximab was the first targeted immunotherapy for OMS. It is prototypical for first-generation anti-B-cell monoclonal antibodies directed to the B-cell-specific antigen CD20. Besides a clinical trial, there are several small case series or reports on the beneficial clinical response to adding rituximab to steroids or IVIg in OMS (Mitchell et al., 2015). Ofatumumab, a second-generation fully human anti-CD20 monoclonal antibody, has been used successfully to treat two rituximab-allergic children with OMS.

Cyclophosphamide. Cyclophosphamide plus steroids with or without IVIg is used by some oncologists for paraneoplastic OMS since 2004, based on an unpublished clinical trial (COG-ANBL00P3, NCT00033293). Its potential bladder and infertility side effects are well known, but the antiimmune dosage is well below antitumor dosage. Cyclophosphamide and dexamethasone have also been combined as "salvage therapy" in OMS.

Steroid Sparers. Various agents, such as azathioprine, 6-mercaptopurine (6-MP), and mycophenolate mofetil (MMF), have been administered adjunctively to reduce steroid dose in OMS based on utility in various other pediatric inflammatory diseases. Their open-label use in OMS is empiric, not evidence-based. The agents do not appear to normalize CSF B-cell percentage. Two no-responders to cyclosporine were reported.

Methotrexate. In the authors' experience, weekly oral methotrexate has a role in the treatment of chronic relapsing OMS that has not responded to rituximab and cyclophosphamide. The application to OMS is not evidence based, but derives from its longstanding use in pediatric rheumatological disorders. It takes several weeks to safely titrate the dose, and so the clinical effect will be delayed and will persist for weeks after the drug is discontinued.

Plasmapheresis. The therapeutic use of plasma exchange in combination with steroids for OMS remains anecdotal. In very young children, the large-bore catheter placed in the neck is infeasible, especially if there is cognitive impairment. In older symptomatic children, it is an option. There has been no clinical study.

Inadequate Response

"Inadequate response" is defined as failure to achieve a full neurologic remission within a reasonable timeframe. A child who is nonambulatory because of OMS should be able to walk by 4 to 6 weeks after starting multimodal immunotherapy. Three months after beginning treatment, improvements in development should be apparent. By 6 months, the clinical picture should look quite good. Identifying inadequate response is essential to making midcourse corrections to the trajectory of improvement (Figure 120-5).

Potential Side Effects and Safety Monitoring

Most deleterious effects of immunotherapy can be anticipated. Safety monitoring is essential for a favorable treatment risk/benefit ratio (Table 120-2). Prophylactic medications and measures should be scrupulously applied to prevent Cushingoid syndrome, opportunistic infections, osteopenia or osteoporosis, gastroesophageal inflammation, and hemorrhage. Rituximab can cause prolonged or permanent B-cell lymphopenia and hypo/agammaglobulinemia. In an effort to reduce the risk, the NPMC has lowered the rituximab dose to $300 \text{ mg/m}^2 \times 4$. Patients who develop this complication should receive "rescue" IVIg and should not be exposed to any further B-cell-depleting drugs. Fatal reactions to any of these agents are rare but can occur. Given the gravity of OMS and lack of equally effective agents with fewer side effects, the use of these immunotherapies seems justified.

Supportive Therapy

Evaluation and intervention by a behavioral therapist can be crucial for family well-being through modification of maladaptive responses. Children with dysarthria require years of therapy for speech articulation and language development. A child psychiatrist should manage rage, depression, and mood disorder. Attention-deficit disorder is so common in chronic OMS that the threshold for testing should be low. Finding or creating a fitting academic environment requires cooperation of the schools and an individualized education plan.

MANAGEMENT OF RELAPSE AND PROGRESSION
Relapse

Central nervous system relapse is the single biggest clinical stumbling block in OMS (Box 120-2). It may occur at any time in the course of OMS. The first principle of relapse is to treat

---

BOX 120-2 Management of OMS Relapse

TREAT UNDERLYING TRIGGER

Infection Induced

The intercurrent illness may be blatant or occult, and need not be febrile; relapse may precede its appearance. In an immunosuppressed child, opportunistic as well as common infections may be at play, requiring appropriate screening.

Steroid/ACTH Tapering Induced

Relapse occurring during drug tapering requires dose escalation and/or more frequent dosing. It is seldom reversed merely by going back to the dose just before the relapse. A return to 25 IU/m^2 (sometimes 40 IU/m^2) and to daily rather than alternate-day dosing may be required for ACTH. If the ACTH dose at relapse was very low, monthly high-dose pulse dose dexamethasone may obviate the need to restart ACTH.

ADJUST IMMUNOTHERAPY PLAN

If the above measures are insufficient or more than one relapse has occurred, flexibility and empiricism are required. In changing to combination multimechanistic and multitargeted therapy, a disease-modifying agent should be added.

REEVALUATE FOR NEUROINFLAMMATION

Initial cerebrospinal fluid lymphocyte subset analysis (LSA) and oligoclonal bands (OCB) testing are highly recommended to inform clinical decision making. Reevaluation in chronic opsoclonus-myoclonus syndrome (OMS) can also help differentiate active inflammatory disease from "burned out" OMS with permanent sequelae. It is essential to interpret immunologic results in the clinical context.

LOOK FOR NEUROBLASTOMA

Imaging studies for neuroblastoma in so-called tumor-negative cases should be repeated in the setting of incomplete response to immunotherapy or relapses. Multiple types of tests, if done originally, may not be necessary.

---

the underlying trigger when possible. "Corticosteroid- or ACTH-dependency" indicates ongoing autoimmune disease. No patient should be allowed to repeatedly relapse on IVIg and steroids/ACTH alone. In chronic relapsing OMS, the risk of eventual cognitive impairment escalates, and previously used immunotherapeutics are no longer as effective. After multiple medications have failed, empirical approaches are necessary to prevent conversion to progressive OMS.

Progression

OMS sometimes progresses to an implacable chronic state with reduced sensitivity or unresponsiveness to immunotherapy ("treatment resistance") and irreversible cognitive regression. This eventuality can blindside treating physicians and come as a heartbreak to parents, who should be counseled about the possibility. Disease progression occurs more often in children who fail to go into neurologic remission or have multiple relapses despite prolonged immunosuppressive regimens. At some point, the treatment risk/benefit ratio becomes unfavorable. For now, the best treatment for progressive OMS is to prevent it.

Immunization Issues

During the acute phase of OMS, immunizations may trigger disease exacerbation or relapse. The conservative recommendation of the NPMC has been to withhold immunizations for 2 years after cessation of immunotherapy and relapse, and then cautiously reintroduce as singlet vaccinations of killed virus at 6-month intervals. Antibody titer testing can help by checking for immunity to various viruses. For patients on high, immunosuppressive doses of steroids or ACTH, no live-virus vaccines should be given. Live-virus vaccines are generally contraindicated when there is B-cell suppression. Immunization is unlikely to be successful while a child is receiving IVIg and for up to a year after discontinuation. Immunization with attenuated live virus in the aftermath of OMS should be considered on a case-by-case basis.

Future Directions

A cure for OMS might also reveal one for neuroblastoma, the flip side of the same coin. Once the OMS antigen is identified, an animal model can be created, autoimmune causation can be proven, and hindrances caused by disease rarity and lack of brain tissue can be offset. Exploring new therapeutic targets and strategies is essential to improve OMS treatment. Meanwhile, one can expect incremental improvements in multimodal therapy and neuroprotective strategies. The rarity of OMS and ethics issues undermine the standard randomized, controlled trial study design and encourage use of available alternate designs. Based on what is known about neuroinflammation in OMS, all clinical trials in OMS should include biomarker measurement protocols. As new biomarkers are discovered, biomarker-assisted therapy is the emerging treatment paradigm. The past 10 years have brought many exciting developments, but there are still wide gaps in our knowledge. Much work remains to be done.

REFERENCES

 The complete list of references for this chapter is available in the e-book at www.expertconsult.com.
See inside cover for registration details.

SELECTED REFERENCES

Anand, G., Bridge, H., Rackstraw, P., et al., 2015. Cerebellar and cortical abnormalities in paediatric opsoclonus-myoclonus syndrome. Dev. Med. Child Neurol. 57, 265–272.

Brunklaus, A., Pohl, K., Zuberi, S.M., et al., 2011. Outcome and prognostic features in opsoclonus-myoclonus syndrome from infancy to adult life. Pediatrics 128, e388–e394.

Desai, J., Mitchell, W.G., 2012. Acute cerebellar ataxia, acute cerebellitis, and opsoclonus-myoclonus syndrome. J. Child Neurol. 27, 1482–1488.

Ertle, F., Behnisch, W., Al Mulla, N.A., et al., 2008. Treatment of neuroblastoma-related opsoclonus-myoclonus-ataxia syndrome with high-dose dexamethasone pulses. Pediatr. Blood Cancer 50, 683–687.

Mitchell, W.G., Wooten, A.A., O'Neil, S.H., et al., 2015. Effect of increased immunosuppression on developmental outcome of opsoclonus myoclonus syndrome (OMS). J. Child Neurol. 30, 976–982.

Pranzatelli, M.R., Tate, E.D., 2010. Opsoclonus-myoclonus syndrome. In: Russell, C.D., Vincent, A. (Eds.), Clinics in Developmental Medicine No. 184–185, Inflammatory and Autoimmune Disorders of the Nervous System in Children. Chapter 10. Mac Keith Press, London, pp. 152–173.

Pranzatelli, M.R., Tate, E.D., McGee, N.R., et al., 2012. Key role of CXCL13/CXCR5 axis for cerebrospinal fluid B cell recruitment in pediatric OMS. J. Neuroimmunol. 243, 81–88.

Raffaghello, L., Fuhlhuber, V., Bianchi, G., et al., 2013. Role of BAFF in opsoclonus-myoclonus syndrome, a bridge between cancer and autoimmunity. J. Leukoc. Biol. 94, 183–191.

Tate, E.D., Allison, T.J., Pranzatelli, M.R., et al., 2005. Neuroepidemiologic trends in 105 cases of pediatric opsoclonus-myoclonus syndrome. J. Pediatr. Oncol. Nurs. 22, 8–19.

Wong, A., 2007. An update on opsoclonus. Curr. Opin. Neurol. 20, 25–31.

E-BOOK FIGURES AND TABLES

121 Neurologic Manifestations of Rheumatic Disorders of Childhood

Nina Felice Schor, Emily von Scheven, and Stephen Ashwal

An expanded version of this chapter is available on www.expertconsult.com. See inside cover for registration details.

The rheumatic disorders of childhood include conditions ranging from isolated arthritis to complex multisystem autoimmune diseases. The presence and the degree of nervous system impairment varies, and manifestations may precede the onset of other symptoms. The current classification of the chronic rheumatic disorders is shown in Box 121-1 (Dannecker and Quartier, 2009). Examples of autoantibodies found in rheumatic diseases are given in Table 121-1.

Neurologic manifestations arise in primary and secondary fashion (Benseler and Schneider, 2004). Antibodies or cellular immune elements can directly affect nerves, muscle, brain, spinal cord, and sensory organs. Alternatively, innocent bystander (e.g., vascular inflammation and immune complex deposition) or medication effects can impair the nervous system. Rheumatic disease should be considered in evaluating unexplained childhood neurologic syndromes such as persistent fever, weight loss, myalgias, arthralgias, meningeal signs, or multiple nonanatomically contiguous neurologic deficits.

JUVENILE IDIOPATHIC ARTHRITIS (CHRONIC ARTHROPATHIES)

The key neurologic and laboratory findings in chronic arthropathies are summarized in Table 121-2(A). Neurologic manifestations of juvenile idiopathic arthritis (JIA; previously described as juvenile rheumatoid arthritis) vary with the arthritis subtype. Children with pauciarticular or polyarticular JIA rarely have central nervous system (CNS) disease, but approximately 6% with systemic-onset JIA develop CNS involvement.

Neurologic Manifestations

Systemic Juvenile Idiopathic Arthritis

Acute Encephalopathy. The most common form of acute encephalopathy is macrophage activation syndrome (MAS), a complex syndrome with similarities to hemophagocytic lymphohistiocytosis. Symptoms include unremitting fever, rash, hepatic dysfunction, metabolic alterations, lymphadenopathy, as well as cardiac, pulmonary, and renal failure. Neurologic symptoms include seizures, acute encephalopathy, and intracranial hemorrhage.

Laboratory studies demonstrate cytopenia, low albumin, and elevated D-dimer, ferritin, and lactate dehydrogenase, liver enzymes, serum triglycerides as well as cerebrospinal fluid protein and cell counts. Generalized electroencephalographic (EEG) slowing is seen. MAS can occur after use of acetylsalicylic acid, indomethacin, gold, nonsteroidal antiinflammatory drugs (including sulfasalazine), or spontaneously. Immediate corticosteroid treatment is associated with resolution. In resistant disease, cyclosporine A and biologic agents are effective.

Neuropathies. Peripheral motor and sensory neuropathies are associated with epineural vasculitis and axonal neuropathy with demyelination due to occlusion of the vasa nervorum.

Mood Disturbances. Anxiety, a decreased sense of well-being, and depression occur in children with JIA. Premorbid family dynamics, maternal depression, and drug interactions may contribute to psychological disorders.

Myositis. One third of children have mild elevations of creatine kinase without weakness. Proximal weakness and biopsy-confirmed myositis are rare; intermittent myalgias are common.

Polyarticular Juvenile Idiopathic Arthritis (Poly JIA)

Myelopathy. Many children with polyarticular or systemic-onset JIA develop neck stiffness secondary to cervical arthritis. Cervical myelopathy associated with atlantoaxial dislocation is highly unusual.

Pauciarticular Juvenile Idiopathic Arthritis (Pauci JIA)

Iridocyclitis and Uveitis. The incidence of iridocyclitis and uveitis is now similar in children with pauci JIA and poly JIA. In girls, the incidence increases with age and disease duration.

Psoriatic, Enthesitis-Related, and Undifferentiated Syndromes

Approximately 3% of children with inflammatory bowel disease (IBD) have neurologic involvement including myasthenia gravis, myopathy, peripheral or cranial neuropathy, cerebral sinovenous thrombosis, recurrent strokes, myelopathy, seizures, headache, confusional states, meningitis, and syncope. About 5% of patients with enthesitis-related arthritides develop uveitis with eye redness, pain, photophobia, and blurred vision.

Neuropathology

Neuropathologic studies are discussed in the online chapter.

Management

Treatment of JIA has been transformed by the development of biologic agents and varies by disease subtype. Pauci JIA is managed with nonsteroidal antiinflammatory drugs such as naproxen and tolmetin sodium or with intraarticular steroid injection. Iridocyclitis responds to topical ophthalmic corticosteroids. Polyarticular JIA is treated with nonsteroidal antiinflammatory drugs; however, agents such as methotrexate and tumor necrosis factor (TNF)-α inhibitors, such as etanercept or infliximab may be required. Systemic JIA is managed with

BOX 121-1 Classification of the Rheumatic Disorders of Childhood

JUVENILE IDIOPATHIC ARTHRITIS (CHRONIC ARTHROPATHIES)

Systemic arthritis (systemic-onset JIA)
Oligoarthritis, persistent or extended (pauciarticular-onset JIA)
Polyarthritis, rheumatoid factor-negative or factor-positive (polyarticular-onset JIA)
Psoriatic arthritis (not previously classified as JRA)
Enthesitis-related arthritis (previously classified as spondyloarthritis)
Undifferentiated arthritis

PERIODIC FEVER SYNDROMES

NOMID/CINCA
Familial Mediterranean fever
Periodic fever, aphthous stomatitis, pharyngitis, adenitis syndrome
Hyper-IgG syndrome

ARTHRITIS ASSOCIATED WITH INFECTIOUS AGENTS

Acute rheumatic fever
Lyme disease
Reactive arthritis

CONNECTIVE TISSUE DISORDERS

Systemic lupus erythematosus
Juvenile dermatomyositis
Scleroderma
Mixed connective tissue disease
Sjögren syndrome

PRIMARY VASCULITIC DISORDERS

Necrotizing Vasculitis

Polyarteritis nodosa
Kawasaki disease
Microscopic polyangiitis
Cogan syndrome

Leukocytoclastic Vasculitis

Henoch-Schönlein purpura
Hypersensitivity vasculitis

Granulomatous Vasculitis

Churg-Strauss syndrome
Granulomatosis with polyangiitis
Primary angiitis of the central nervous system
Necrotizing sarcoid granulomatosis
Sarcoidosis

Giant Cell Arteritis

Temporal arteritis
Takayasu arteritis

Miscellaneous Vasculitic Disorders

Behçet disease

Miscellaneous Disorders

Thrombotic thrombocytopenic purpura
Erythromelalgia
Antiphospholipid antibody syndrome
CINCA, chronic infantile neurologic cutaneous and articular syndrome; NOMID, neonatal-onset multisystem inflammatory disease; JRA, juvenile rheumatoid arthritis.

(Modified from: Cassidy JT, Petty RE. Textbook of pediatric rheumatology, 4th edition. Philadelphia, WB Saunders; 2001.)

TABLE 121-1 Autoantibodies in Pediatric Rheumatic Diseases

Antibody	Clinical Finding
ANA	97% SLE, but also positive in MCTD, SSc, 10–85% JDMS, 20–88% JRA, SS, and 2%–5% of controls
Antids-DNA	30%–70% SLE, rarely in other CTDs
Anti-Sm	30% SLE
Anti-RNP	MCTD, also in SLE
Anti-SSA/Ro	25% SLE, 75% SS
Anti-SSB/La	10% SLE, 40% SS
Antihistone	50% SLE, >90% DILS
Anticentromere	44%–98% CREST syndrome
Anti-Scl-70	27% SSc
Antic-ANCA	>90% Granulomatosis with polyangiitis
Antip-ANCA	10% Granulomatosis with polyangiitis, 70% CSS, 75% UC, 20% Crohn's disease, 30% SLE
Anti-NR2 NMDAR	10% SLE
RF A	20% polyarticular JRA, 50% SS; 10%–30% SLE, MCTD
LAC	Correlates with thromboembolic risk in SLE
aCL	Correlates with thromboembolic risk in SLE, malignancy; variable in many other diseases

aCL, anticardiolipin antibody; ANA, antinuclear antibody; c-ANCA, cytoplasmic staining antineutrophil cytoplasmic antibody; CREST, calcinosis, Raynaud's, esophageal dysmotility, sclerodactyly, telangiectasia; CSS, Churg–Strauss syndrome; CTD, connective tissue disease; DILS, drug-induced lupus syndrome; ds-DNA, double-stranded (native) DNA; JDMS, juvenile dermatomyositis; JRA, juvenile rheumatoid arthritis; LAC, lupus anticoagulant; MCTD, mixed connective tissue disease; NMDAR, N-methyl-D-aspartate receptor; p-ANCA, perinuclear staining antineutrophil cytoplasmic antibody; RF A, rheumatoid factor A; RNP, ribonucleoprotein; SLE, systemic lupus erythematosus; Sm, Smith; SS, Sjögren's syndrome; SSc, systemic scleroderma; UC, ulcerative colitis.

(Adapted from: Okano, Y., 1996. Antinuclear antibody in systemic sclerosis [scleroderma]. Rheum Dis Clin North Am 22, 709; Moder, K.G., 1996. Use and interpretation of rheumatologic tests: A guide for clinicians. Mayo Clin Proc 71, 391; Bylund, D.J., McCallum, R.M.. Vasculitis. In: Henry JB, editor: Clinical diagnosis and management by laboratory methods. Philadelphia, WB Saunders; 1996.)

nonsteroidal antiinflammatory drugs but often requires steroids, methotrexate, or biologic agents. Etanercept or infliximab is used in resistant cases. High-dose methylprednisolone, intravenous immunoglobulin, and cyclophosphamide are helpful; newer agents that block IL-1 and IL-6 have shown benefit. Some children develop psychological problems; counseling and physical and occupational therapy are beneficial.

PERIODIC FEVER SYNDROMES

Neonatal-Onset Multisystem Inflammatory Disease or Chronic Infantile Neurologic Cutaneous and Articular Syndrome

Neonatal-onset multisystem inflammatory disease (NOMID) or chronic infantile neurologic cutaneous and articular (CINCA) syndrome is an unusual autosomal dominant disorder (NLRP3 gene mutation) that mimics systemic JIA. It occurs

TABLE 121-2 Key Neurologic and Laboratory Findings in the Rheumatic Disorders

A. Chronic and Reactive Arthropathies

Disease	Neurologic Findings	Laboratory Findings
Systemic juvenile idiopathic arthritis	Encephalopathy, seizures, macrophage activation syndrome (Reye-like syndrome), neuropathies	Elevated WBC and ESR, anemia, DIC, elevated CSF protein and cell count, marked increase in ferritin and LDH
Inflammatory bowel disease	Myasthenia gravis, myopathy, neuropathy, seizures, cognitive changes	Elevated ESR, microcytic anemia, melena
Acute rheumatic fever	Chorea, personality changes, seizures	Positive ASO titers, elevated ESR and CRP, abnormal ECG
Lyme disease	Early infection: aseptic meningitis, headache, chorea, cranial nerve palsies, late neuroborreliosis myelitis, MS-like symptoms, subtle encephalopathy, radiculopathy, mononeuritis multiplex	Positive IgG Lyme titer by ELISA, protein by Western blot in serum, positive PCR in CSF

ASO, antistreptolysin O; CRP, C-reactive protein; CSF, cerebrospinal fluid; DIC, disseminated intravascular coagulation; ECG, electrocardiogram; ELISA, enzyme-linked immunosorbent assay; ESR, erythrocyte sedimentation rate; IgG, immunoglobulin G; LDH, lactate dehydrogenase; MS, multiple sclerosis; PCR, polymerase chain reaction; WBC, white blood cell count.

B. Connective Tissue Diseases

Disease	Neurologic Findings	Laboratory Findings
SLE	Encephalopathy, chorea, seizures, aseptic meningitis, psychosis, behavioral or cognitive dysfunction, headaches, strokes, neuropathy, myelitis	Elevated ANA, low C3 and C4, pancytopenia, hematuria, proteinuria, autoantibodies, LAC, elevated aCL
Scleroderma: coup-de-sabre deformity	Seizures, blurred vision, bulbar palsy, optic neuritis, trigeminal neuropathy	Elevated ANA and rheumatoid factor
Mixed connective tissue disease	Same as SLE	Same as SLE plus elevated anti-RNP, elevated CK
Sjögren's syndrome	Encephalopathy, optic neuritis, aseptic meningitis, recurrent paresis, myelopathy, neuropathy, autonomic dysfunction	Positive ANA, rheumatoid factor, antibodies to SSA/Ro and SSB/La

aCL, anticardiolipin antibody; ANA, antinuclear antibody; C3, third component of complement; C4, fourth component of complement; CK, creatine kinase; LAC, lupus anticoagulant; RNP, ribonucleoprotein; SLE, systemic lupus erythematosus.

C. Childhood Vasculitides

Disease	Neurologic Findings	Laboratory Findings
Polyarteritis nodosa	Headache, encephalopathy, stroke, seizures, neuropathies	Elevated WBC, ESR, positive HBsAg and c-ANCA
Kawasaki disease	Aseptic meningitis, focal neurologic findings	Coronary aneurysms, thrombocytosis
Cogan syndrome	Neurosensory hearing loss	None
Henoch-Schönlein purpura	Encephalopathy	Elevated IgA in 50%, hematuria, melena
Churg-Strauss syndrome	Headache, encephalopathy, stroke, seizures, various peripheral neuropathies, coma, intracranial hemorrhage	Eosinophilia, eosinophils on skin biopsy, p-ANCA
Granulomatosis with polyangiitis	Encephalopathy, intracranial hemorrhage, meningitis	c-ANCA
Primary angiitis of the CNS	Headache, encephalopathy, seizures, stroke, myelopathy	Elevated ESR
Sarcoidosis	Obstructive hydrocephalus, seventh nerve palsy, meningitis, seizures, peripheral neuropathies	Noncaseating granuloma
Temporal arteritis	Blindness, encephalopathy, headache	Elevated ESR
Takayasu arteritis	Headache, stroke, syncope, visual loss	Elevated ESR and factor VIII-related antigen
Behçet disease	Headache, meningitis, psychiatric disorders, encephalopathy, pseudotumor cerebri, brainstem signs	Elevated ESR

c-ANCA, cytoplasmic staining antineutrophil cytoplasmic antibody; CNS, central nervous system; ESR, erythrocyte sedimentation rate; HBsAg, hepatitis B surface antigen; IgA, immunoglobulin A; p-ANCA, perinuclear staining antineutrophil cytoplasmic antibody; WBC, white blood cell count.

during the first year of life. Manifestations include hectic fever, intermittent rash, lymphadenopathy, hepatosplenomegaly, uveitis, cognitive and developmental delay, chronic meningitis, hydrocephalus, seizures, hemiplegia, papilledema, optic neuritis, uveitis, and deforming arthropathy with periosteal changes and bony overgrowth. Seventy-five percent of patients develop progressive sensorineural deafness. Long-term prognosis is poor.

Familial Mediterranean Fever

Familial Mediterranean fever is an autosomal-recessive disorder due to mutations in the MEFV gene. Symptoms include fever, abdominal pain, peritonitis, pleuritis, and arthritis. Myalgias after exertion are common. Headache, febrile seizures, aseptic meningitis, and posterior reversible leukoencephalopathy occur, as has progressive sensorineural deafness.

Periodic Fever, Aphthous Stomatitis, Pharyngitis, and Adenitis Syndrome

Periodic fever, aphthous stomatitis, pharyngitis, and adenitis (PFAPA) syndrome has an unclear etiology. It is characterized by febrile episodes persisting for 4 to 6 days, separated by afebrile periods lasting 4 weeks to 4 months. Headaches occur during febrile episodes. Recurrent aseptic meningitis accompanied by seizures has been described.

Hyper-IgG (Autoimmune Lymphoproliferative) Syndrome

This genetic syndrome presents with splenomegaly, skin rashes, enlarged lymph nodes, and autoimmune hemolytic anemia. Neurologic symptoms are associated with other autoimmune phenomena, including Guillain-Barré syndrome.

ARTHRITIS ASSOCIATED WITH INFECTIOUS AGENTS

Acute Rheumatic Fever

Acute rheumatic fever (ARF) is an inflammatory illness that follows a group A beta-hemolytic streptococcal pharyngitis. Manifestations include migratory polyarthritis, fever, carditis, and, less frequently, Sydenham chorea, subcutaneous nodules, and erythema marginatum. The modified 1992 Jones criteria are used to confirm the diagnosis (two major and one minor criteria; or one major and two minor criteria), as well as antibody evidence of preceding streptococcal infection (Box 121-2). In the case of isolated Sydenham chorea, demonstration of streptococcal infection may not be possible and is not a requirement for diagnosis (Dajani, et al., 1992).

Neurologic Manifestations

Sydenham Chorea

Clinical Manifestations. Sydenham chorea is characterized by involuntary, distal, purposeless, rapid movements; hypotonia; and emotional lability. It may be associated with other ARF manifestations or as the sole manifestation. Isolated chorea represents 20% to 30% of acute rheumatic fever cases and occurs long after the pharyngitis has resolved. Laboratory evidence of preceding streptococcal infection may not be demonstrable in up to 35% of children. Onset may be explosive or insidious. Chorea may be misdiagnosed as an emotional disorder, tics, decreased attention span, or a degenerative process.

Choreiform movements involve the face, hands, and feet. Facial movements include grimacing, frowning, grinning, and pouting. Children commonly are unable to sustain prolonged hand contraction ("milkmaid" sign). Emotional lability, personality changes, restlessness, and irritability may herald the onset of chorea. Occasionally, "spooning" with hyperextension of the hands is observed. In adolescents, chorea occurs almost exclusively in females and may be associated with hemichorea or hemiparesis. Choreiform movements subside in 2 to 4 months but can persist. Chorea and arthritis usually do not accompany each other; however, carditis frequently develops as the chorea is improving.

Laboratory Findings. Laboratory studies include documentation of antecedent streptococcal infection with an antistreptolysin-O titer, demonstration of a prolonged PR interval on electrocardiogram, elevated C-reactive protein or erythrocyte sedimentation rate, and leukocytosis. Although throat culture may show group A beta-hemolytic streptococci, an elevated or increasing antistreptolysin-O titer is required. An elevated anti-DNase-B increases the sensitivity of an antistreptolysin-O titer alone. To exclude other choreiform conditions, patients may need additional studies (serum ceruloplasmin, thyroxine, calcium, and antinuclear antibody titers). EEGs may demonstrate diffuse paroxysmal features and generalized slowing. Cerebrospinal fluid (CSF) examination and neuroimaging are rarely necessary. Of interest is the finding of antineuronal antibodies in the CSF of patients with chorea. The specificity of these antibodies is unknown, and they are frequently documented in patients with CNS lupus.

> **BOX 121-2** Jones Criteria for Diagnosis of Acute Rheumatic Fever (Revised 1992)
>
> **MAJOR***
>
> **Carditis**
>
> Murmur consistent with aortic regurgitation or mitral insufficiency; echocardiogram findings without significant auscultatory findings are not adequate
>
> **Chorea**
>
> May be the only manifestation; proof of prior streptococcal infection in only 80%
>
> **Erythema Marginatum**
>
> Rare manifestation; never on the face; transient and migratory
>
> **Migratory Polyarthritis**
>
> Almost always migratory, involving larger joints, responds within 48 hours to aspirin and usually resolves in 1 month
>
> **Subcutaneous Nodules**
>
> Rare manifestation; nontender, on extensor surfaces, usually over elbows, wrists, knees, occipital region, or spinous processes
>
> **MINOR**
>
> **Fever**
>
> Usually greater than 39°C
>
> **Arthralgia**
>
> Consider if arthritis not present
>
> **Prolonged PR Interval**
>
> Does not correlate with the development of carditis
>
> **Elevated Erythrocyte Sedimentation Rate or C-Reactive Protein**
>
> Acute phase reactants
>
> *Prior episodes of acute rheumatic fever are not criteria; if a patient has had a prior attack of acute rheumatic fever, a new attack may be difficult to diagnose on the basis of changing carditis. In this setting, proof of recent streptococcal infection and either one major or one minor criterion may allow a presumptive diagnosis. Proof of recent streptococcal infection is necessary, except for isolated chorea.
>
> (Adapted from: Dajani, et al. and The Special Writing Group, 1992. Guidelines for the diagnosis of rheumatic fever. Jones Criteria, 1992 update. JAMA 268, 2069.)

MRI abnormalities include cystic changes, restricted diffusion in the caudate and putamen, and multiple subcortical and peripheral white matter signal intensity abnormalities.

Neuropathology

Findings in ARF are rare and include small cortical and meningeal endarteritis with spotty patches of gray-matter degeneration.

Treatment

All patients, including those only with chorea, should receive a 10-day course of penicillin or erythromycin. Prophylaxis with penicillin or sulfadiazine should be started immediately and continued until adulthood because of the risk of reinfection and of rheumatic heart disease. When residual valvular disease exists, prophylaxis should continue for at least 10 years after the last episode and at least until age 40. If there is no residual valvular disease, the duration of treatment beyond 10 years or into adulthood is uncertain. When Sydenham chorea is diagnosed and there is no valvular disease, the duration of prophylaxis should be at least 5 years or until age 21, whichever is longer. Children who develop chorea as the sole manifestation of ARF have a 50% risk of developing rheumatic heart disease.

Sydenham chorea has been treated with chlorpromazine, haloperidol, phenobarbital, diazepam, valproic acid, cyproheptadine, and prednisone. Clonidine, pimozide, and pulsed intravenous methylprednisolone followed by an oral taper, intravenous immunoglobulin, or plasma exchange may be beneficial in refractory cases. Recovery can be expected within 2 to 6 months, although some children have residual manifestations.

Postinfectious Tourette Syndrome and PANDAS

Chorea, obsessive-compulsive disorder, tic disorder, and Tourette syndrome may all have a common autoimmune pathway. Some children with chorea have obsessive-compulsive disorder that resolves before or simultaneously with the resolution of the chorea. An increased prevalence of obsessive-compulsive disorder occurs in children with tics and Tourette syndrome; an increased prevalence of antineuronal antibodies, as well as increased levels of antistreptococcal antibodies, occurs in all four of these conditions. The acronym PANDAS (pediatric autoimmune neuropsychiatric disorders associated with streptococcal infections) has been suggested when there is a combination of behavioral problems, obsessive-compulsive behavior, and tics when associated with a group A beta-hemolytic streptococcal infection.

Other Central Nervous System Manifestations

About 3% to 5% of patients with ARF develop other neurologic problems including meningoencephalitis, encephalitis, seizures, pseudotumor cerebri, papilledema, diplopia, central retinal occlusion, transient intellectual loss, and acute psychosis.

Lyme Disease

Lyme disease is an important cause of neurologic symptoms in children (Bingham, et al., 1995). The illness follows a tick bite and occurs in endemic areas during the summer. The early stage begins with a flu-like illness and the appearance of an oval, expanding rash. Systemic infection with *Borrelia burgdorferi* may be documented by culture. Within several weeks, the patient develops neurologic manifestations, with facial nerve palsy, aseptic meningitis, other cranial neuropathies transverse myelitis, and sometimes direct invasion of the organism into CSF. Acute sinovenous thrombosis with consequent pseudotumor cerebri can occur. The illness resolves spontaneously but may be hastened by antibiotic treatment (amoxicillin or erythromycin in children younger than 9 years old; tetracycline in children age 9 years or older, either for 10 to 30 days).

Weeks to months later, untreated patients may develop episodic arthritis of the large joints. The knee becomes acutely effused but not particularly tender or hot. Joint swelling lasts for several days and resolves but returns repeatedly if treatment with antibiotics is not started. Diagnosis may be confirmed after the first few weeks with a positive serum IgG titer against *B. burgdorferi*. Western blotting from blood or polymerase chain reaction (PCR) amplification of the *B. burgdorferi* genome in the CSF is available.

Some patients develop neuroborreliosis years later. This rare complication manifests as a subtle encephalopathy with stuttering and memory disturbances. The diagnosis is confirmed by demonstration of an elevated intrathecal IgG titer compared with serum titers. Treatment with intravenous ceftriaxone for 1 month is indicated, but the response is variable.

Reactive Arthritis (formerly called Reiter Syndrome)

Reactive arthritis is characterized by arthritis, uveitis, and urethritis. Progressive myelopathy, cerebral vasculitis, axonal polyneuropathy, and seizures have been reported as rare neurologic complications in adults.

CONNECTIVE TISSUE DISORDERS

The key neurologic and laboratory findings in connective tissue disorders are summarized in Table 121-2(B).

Systemic Lupus Erythematosus

Revised criteria for diagnosing SLE (2012) (Box 121-3) call for having at least 4 of 17 criteria (at least 1 clinical and 1

BOX 121-3 Revised Criteria for the Classification of Systemic Lupus Erythematosus (2012)

Diagnosis requires at least 4 criteria (at least 1 clinical and 1 immunologic) OR biopsy-proven lupus nephritis with positive antinuclear or anti-DNA antibodies.

CLINICAL CRITERIA

Acute cutaneous lupus: lupus malar rash (not discoid), bullous lupus, toxic epidermal necrolysis variant of lupus, maculopapular lupus rash, photosensitive lupus rash (in the absence of dermatomyositis), nonindurated psoriaform and/or annular polycyclic lesions that resolve without scarring

Chronic cutaneous lupus: classic discoid rash, hypertrophic (verrucous) lupus, lupus panniculitis (profundus), mucosal lupus, lupus erythematosus tumidus, chillblains lupus, discoid lupus/lichen planus overlap

Oral or nasal ulcers: in the absence of a cause other than lupus

Nonscarring alopecia: diffuse thinning or fragility of hair with visible broken hairs in the absence of a cause other than lupus

Arthritis: synovitis involving 2 or more joints

Serositis: pleural or pericardial inflammation, effusions, or rub in the absence of a cause other than lupus

Renal: urine protein–to-creatinine ratio (or 24 h urine protein) representing 500 mg protein/24 h or red blood cell casts

Neurologic: seizures, psychosis, mononeuritis multiplex, myelitis, peripheral or cranial neuropathy, or acute confusional state in the absence of a cause other than lupus

Hemolytic anemia

Leukopenia: leukopenia $<4000/mm^3$ or lymphopenia $<1000/mm^3$

Thrombocytopenia: $<100,000/mm^3$

IMMUNOLOGIC CRITERIA

Antinuclear antibody
Anti-DNA antibody
Anti-Smith antibody
Antiphospholipid antibody
Low serum complement (C3, C4, CH50)
Direct Coombs' test positive in the absence of hemolytic anemia

(Modified from: Petri M, Orbai AM, Alarcón GS, et al. Derivation and validation of the Systemic Lupus International Collaborating Clinics classification criteria for systemic lupus erythematosus. Arthritis Rheum 2012;64:2677–2686.)

immunologic) or biopsy-proven nephritis and a positive antinuclear or anti-DNA antibody. Arthritis, arthralgia, fever, and photosensitive rash are the most common initial complaints, with renal, cardiac, and neurologic involvement responsible for chronic disability. Lymphadenopathy, hepatosplenomegaly, pleural and pericardial effusions, pulmonary infiltrates, pericarditis, abdominal pain, and peritonitis may be present at presentation. Renal disease (nephrotic syndrome, acute or chronic glomerulonephritis) occurs in 60% to 80% of children. Laboratory findings include an abnormal urinalysis, low serum complement levels, high antibodies to double-stranded DNA, a decreased glomerular filtration rate, and abnormal renal biopsy. Management is highly individualized. The prognosis for children with SLE has improved dramatically, with 10-year survival of 85%.

Neurologic Manifestations

Nervous system involvement is common in children, and now the outcome is more favorable, with most recovering (Muscal and Brey, 2010).

Seizures. Up to 50% of children develop seizures, usually during the first year of illness. Interictal EEGs show multifocal paroxysmal sharp-wave or slow-wave activity. Seizures can be secondary to hypertension, uremia, electrolyte disturbances, immunosuppressive treatment, opportunistic CNS infections, or cerebral edema (Appenzeller, et al., 2004).

Neuropsychiatric Lupus. Neuropsychiatric complications range from 22% to 95%. Nineteen neuropsychiatric SLE (NPSLE) syndromes have been defined for adults. Neurologic manifestations in children include headache (72%), mood disorders (57%), cognitive dysfunction (55%), seizures (51%), acute confusional state (35%), peripheral nervous system dysfunction (15%), psychosis (12%), and stroke (12%). Neuropsychiatric manifestations are classified as primary (direct SLE brain involvement) or secondary (related to disease/treatment complications). About 70% of children manifest neuropsychiatric symptoms within the first year; in the remaining 30%, symptoms may be latent. The majority of affected children have more than one neuropsychiatric symptom. Onset may be acute or indolent and may appear as the only presenting symptom. Numerous autoantibodies are associated with NPSLE, including antineuronal antibodies, antiphospholipid antibodies, anti-NR2 N-methyl-D-aspartate (NMDA) receptor antibody, and antiribosomal P antibody. The wide availability of newer MRI sequences is improving the likelihood of identifying brain abnormalities. These abnormalities are not specific for NPSLE; they can also reflect postictal or postischemic phenomena. Some patients with NPSLE have TREX1 mutations that code for the DNA repair enzyme, DNase III.

Headache. Headaches are common, usually occuring during disease exacerbation and in association with other neurologic symptoms. The diagnostic workup may yield few abnormalities; evaluation for a hypertensive encephalopathy or posterior reversible encephalopathy syndrome should be considered. Most patients respond to increasing corticosteroids.

Chorea. Chorea occurs in approximately 5% of children and is the initial nervous system symptom in 25% to 30% of patients. SLE symptoms occur within 1 year of chorea onset; rarely, a prolonged latent interval may ensue. Approximately 50% of children with chorea develop other CNS manifestations. Chorea also is associated with thromboembolic disease and elevated anticardiolipin antibody.

Reye-like Syndrome. A Reye-like syndrome associated with acetylsalicylic acid treatment of SLE has been recognized. This syndrome has not been seen with other nonsteroidal antiinflammatory agents.

Cerebrovascular Disease. Approximately 3% of children develop cerebrovascular occlusive disease usually with serious renal, cardiac, pulmonary, hematologic disease, hypertension or thrombocytopenia. Antiphospholipid antibody has been associated with thrombosis, especially when lupus anticoagulant is present. Microemboli, thrombotic, or thromboembolic disease due to a vasculopathy with or without atheromatous disease, valvular disease, or vasculitis may contribute to stroke occurrence.

Patchy areas of altered MRI signal intensity have been interpreted as acute vascular lesions associated with pulse steroid therapy in patients with SLE. This syndrome responds well to substitution of cyclophosphamide for pulse methylprednisolone.

Hypertensive Encephalopathy. Headache, seizures, coma, and focal ischemic injury can be manifestations of hypertensive encephalopathy with or without posterior reversible leukoencephalopathy in patients with nephritis. Controlling blood pressure and treatment with intravenous corticosteroids improves outcome.

Cranial Nerve, Brainstem, and Spinal Cord Dysfunction. Ophthalmoplegia, ptosis, diplopia, facial numbness, vertigo, sensorineural hearing loss, vocal cord paralysis, and ataxia occur. Approximately 6% of children manifest visual symptoms (e.g., blurred vision, sudden blindness, visual field loss). Retinal hemorrhages, cotton wool exudates, papilledema, optic neuritis, cytoid bodies, and retinal artery occlusion have been reported. Papilledema is associated with pseudotumor cerebri caused by the disease or corticosteroid therapy. Patients with retinal artery occlusion or papilledema should be treated with high dose intravenous corticosteroids after diagnostic elimination of structural or occlusive cerebrovascular disease. Transverse myelopathy and Devic disease with neuromyelitis optica (NMO) antibody seropositivity can occur. High doses of intravenous corticosteroids, alone or in combination with cyclophosphamide or rituximab, show variable improvement.

Central Nervous System Infections. CNS infection is rare. Bacterial meningitis, opportunistic bacterial infection, and fungal meningitis (aspergillosis, nocardiosis, and cryptococcosis) occur. Brain abscess may be difficult to differentiate from a multifocal vasculitis, but differentiation may be facilitated by serial neuroimaging.

Lupus Aseptic Meningitis. Lupus aseptic meningitis, accompanied by a sterile CSF lymphocytic pleocytosis, may be manifested by nuchal rigidity, fever, and headache and can occur in association with nonsteroidal antiinflammatory drugs and trimethoprim-sulfamethoxazole use. Manifestations and CSF abnormalities persist for several weeks before resolving spontaneously. Therapy with intravenous corticosteroids may improve this condition.

Peripheral Nervous System Involvement. Peripheral nervous system involvement occurs in 5% of children. Peripheral neuropathies are relatively mild. Severe forms of lumbosacral plexopathies have been reported as has mononeuritis multiplex. Polyradiculoneuropathy may mimic Guillain-Barré syndrome but is rare.

Myopathy. Myositis is rare, although myalgias and generalized weakness are common. Myasthenia gravis has been reported. Although children with myasthenia gravis may have circulating serum antinuclear antibodies, clinical SLE is unusual.

Drug-Induced Lupus Syndrome. Many drugs can induce a lupus-like syndrome. Arthritis, pneumonitis, and pericarditis are common, whereas rashes and alopecia are less frequent. Hepatosplenomegaly, lymphadenopathy, and acute pancreatitis occur in some patients; renal disease appears less often. Procainamide, hydralazine, and isoniazid most commonly induce this syndrome. Antiepileptic drugs (e.g., carbamazepine, ethosuximide, phenytoin, primidone, trimethadione, valproate, zonisamide, clobazam), clonidine, and phenothiazines all have been associated with this syndrome. Recurrent seizures in patients whose initial seizures were well controlled suggest a drug-induced, lupus-like syndrome. Although antinuclear antibodies are positive in systemic and drug-induced SLE, specific antihistone antibodies are associated with drug-induced disease, whereas antidouble-stranded DNA is elevated in SLE. Discontinuing the drug or substituting other antiepileptic drugs may reduce seizure activity. Only rarely will corticosteroids be necessary.

Laboratory Findings

Laboratory features include a positive antinuclear antibody titer, low C3 and C4 levels, leukopenia, direct Coombs-positive hemolytic anemia, hematuria, and proteinuria. Abnormal autoantibodies include antibodies to double-stranded DNA, Sm (Smith), RNP (ribonucleoprotein), Ro (or SSA), La (or SSB), and anticardiolipin. Some correlation between disease and antiphospholipid antibodies has been demonstrated. Elevated lupus anticoagulant (LAC) confers an increased risk of arterial or venous thrombosis. The pathogenic mechanisms causing CNS lupus are reviewed in the online chapter.

Neuroimaging Evaluation

Neuroimaging may show cortical or cerebellar atrophy (Fig. 121-1), infarction (Fig. 121-2), low-density lesions in the cerebral white matter (Fig. 121-3), or hemorrhage. Perfusion-weighted and diffusion-tensor imaging and MR spectroscopy are increasingly used to identify areas of hypoperfusion in NPSLE. MR angiography or venography may detect sinovenous thrombosis. Cerebral angiography may be helpful in further differentiating arterial thrombotic from embolic disease. Single-photon emission computed tomography (SPECT) is sensitive for demonstrating perfusion abnormalities (Fig. 121-4).

Treatment of Neurologic Manifestations

Treatment requires controlling the underlying inflammatory disorder, correcting metabolic or systemic abnormalities, and administering symptom-directed medications such as antiepileptic drugs, analgesic medications, antidepressants, sedatives, antipsychotic agents, and dopamine-blocking agents for chorea. Although phenobarbital, phenytoin, diazepam, lorazepam, valproate, and carbamazepine have been used for the treatment of seizures, newer antiepileptic drugs may afford a more favorable risk profile. Discontinuation of antiepileptic drugs should be considered when the primary disease is well controlled. In moderate doses, corticosteroids have beneficial effects in adults with NPSLE. Treatment of CNS infection depends on the infectious agent and may necessitate reducing immunosuppressive therapy until the infection is controlled.

Anticoagulation may be considered in patients with cerebral ischemia; evaluation and treatment of arterial ischemic stroke and sinovenous thrombosis are discussed in selected chapters in Part XIII of this book.

Immunosuppressive therapy with corticosteroids is used for patients with NPSLE, vasculitis, coma, seizures, chorea, and transverse myelitis. Cytotoxic agents such as mycophenolate or cyclophosphamide are used in patients with serious renal or neurologic disease. Candidates for such treatment include those with diffuse proliferative glomerulonephritis, CNS lupus, or myelopathy who are refractory to intravenous corticosteroids.

Neuropathology

Neuropathologic studies of childhood and adult SLE are rare and discussed in the online chapter.

Scleroderma

Scleroderma in children occurs in two distinct forms: localized and systemic. Localized scleroderma is further subdivided into morphea, generalized morphea, linear scleroderma, and coup-de-sabre lesions. Coup-de-sabre lesions present as linear sclerodermatous changes of the head or oral cavity. Although there may be CNS involvement, this form of scleroderma is an important finding. Systemic scleroderma is subdivided into progressive systemic sclerosis and a generally milder syndrome termed CREST (calcinosis, Raynaud's phenomenon, esophageal dysmotility, sclerodactyly, and telangiectasia). Progressive systemic sclerosis manifests with progressive hardening of the skin and subcutaneous tissues, with involvement of the gastrointestinal tract, joints, heart, lungs, and kidneys. Raynaud's phenomenon, severe cardiac and pulmonary disease with congestive heart failure, pulmonary interstitial fibrosis, pulmonary vascular sclerosis, and renal sclerosis with acute renal failure contribute to mortality. Skin biopsy is diagnostic, demonstrating increased thickness of the dermal collagen, perivascular mononuclear cell infiltrates without immune complex deposition. Radiographic assessment demonstrates subcutaneous calcinosis, joint effusions, and diminished esophageal peristalsis. Decreased lung diffusion, pulmonary hypertension, and pericardial effusion also occur.

Neurologic Manifestations

Children with the coup-de-sabre localized scleroderma develop intractable partial seizures, pseudopapilledema, strabismus, hemiparesis contralateral to the facial lesions, and developmental regression (Murray and Laxer, 2002). Periarticular muscle atrophy, common in children with systemic scleroderma, is due to disuse and subtle myopathic involvement. Creatine kinase activity is elevated and MRI may localize muscle disease. Children with progressive systemic sclerosis generally do not have primary CNS involvement.

Laboratory Findings

Laboratory evaluation should include determination of antinuclear antibody titers, immunoglobulins, erythrocyte sedimentation rate, rheumatoid factor, and creatine kinase activity. Patients with progressive systemic sclerosis may have antibodies to DNA topoisomerase 1 (Scl-70) or RNA polymerase I, II, or III.

Treatment

Treatment of progressive systemic scleroderma is supportive and is often unsuccessful. Initial management includes oral corticosteroids to improve myopathic weakness. There has been anecdotal support for steroids combined with methotrexate for linear scleroderma. Raynaud's phenomenon should be treated with calcium channel blockers. Occupational and physical therapy to maintain and improve joint mobility is important.

Mixed Connective Tissue Disease

This disorder is characterized by signs and symptoms of SLE, scleroderma, and dermatomyositis or polymyositis. Antibodies reactive to the ribonuclease-sensitive component of extractable nuclear antigen (anti-RNP) are seen, with a speckled pattern antinuclear antibody.

Features include Raynaud's phenomenon, polyarthritis, fever, rash, thickening of subcutaneous tissues, hepatosplenomegaly, myositis, and cardiomyopathy. Secondary Sjögren syndrome may produce parotitis and keratoconjunctivitis sicca (dry eyes). Evaluation may demonstrate elevated erythrocyte sedimentation rate and rheumatoid factor, decreased esophageal motility, diminished tear production, keratoconjunctivitis, abnormal parotid sialography, pulmonary effusion, and abnormal pulmonary function tests.

Neurologic Manifestations

Proximal muscle weakness, increased creatine kinase activity, myopathic electromyograms, and muscle biopsy are consistent with inflammatory myositis. Seizures, headache, increased CSF protein content, aseptic meningitis, stroke, and intracranial hemorrhage have been reported.

Treatment

With mild organ involvement, hydroxychloroquine may be adequate. For more severe involvement or myositis, oral or intravenous corticosteroids may be necessary. Methotrexate, azathioprine, mycophenolate mofetil, rituximab, and cyclophosphamide have been used, similar to therapy for SLE.

Sjögren Syndrome

Sjögren syndrome is a chronic autoimmune disorder in which lymphocytic infiltration of the salivary, lacrimal, and other exocrine glands leads to keratoconjunctivitis sicca, xerostomia, and recurrent salivary gland inflammation. Primary Sjögren syndrome is rare in children, but the secondary form—preceding, accompanying, or after SLE, JIA, mixed connective tissue disease, juvenile dermatomyositis, or scleroderma—is more frequent.

Neurologic Manifestations

Children with primary Sjögren syndrome may develop optic neuritis, aseptic meningitis, cerebrovascular occlusive disease, and recurrent paresis associated with cerebral or spinal cord white matter involvement. Manifestations in adults include seizures, cognitive and behavioral disorders, acute encephalopathy, aseptic meningitis, progressive myelopathies, motor and sensory neuropathies, and carpal tunnel syndrome.

Laboratory Findings

Findings include hypergammaglobulinemia, positive antinuclear antibody, anti-SSA, anti-SSB, and classic rheumatoid factor. Diagnostic confirmation is obtained by labial salivary gland biopsy, demonstrating periductal lymphocytic infiltration. The Schirmer test, sialogram, and salivary scintiphotography support the diagnosis. In adults, CSF abnormalities include increased protein content, pleocytosis, elevated IgG levels, elevated IgG index, increased oligoclonal bands, and abnormal CSF to serum glucose ratios.

Treatment

Hydroxychloroquine and supportive care are used for non-neurologic manifestations. Corticosteroids are needed for significant neurologic manifestations, and if progressive, cyclophosphamide is added.

PRIMARY VASCULITIC DISEASES

Vasculitis may be primary or secondary to a multisystem disorder (Iannetti, et al., 2012). In Box 121-1, the vasculitides are organized by pathologic type. Size and location of affected vessels or, alternatively, distinct clinical patterns with specific laboratory tests may identify a specific disorder. The pathogenesis of vasculitides is discussed in the online chapter. The key neurologic findings are listed in Table 121-2(C).

Necrotizing Vasculitis

These disorders include polyarteritis nodosa, microscopic polyangiitis, Kawasaki disease, and Cogan syndrome. They are characterized by fibrinoid necrosis of small-sized and medium-sized muscular arteries.

Polyarteritis Nodosa

Polyarteritis nodosa (PAN) occurs in older children and adolescents with unexplained fever, arthralgias, calf discomfort, abdominal pain, recurrent pulmonary infection, renal disease, hypertension, fatigability, weight loss, malar rash, and purpura. Severe renal impairment and marked hypertension occur. Renal biopsy shows diffuse glomerulonephritis or necrotizing arteritis. Mesenteric arteritis and bowel wall infarction may lead to gastrointestinal hemorrhage. Histopathology demonstrates necrotizing vasculitis, and angiography shows aneurysms, stenosis, or occlusion of medium or small arteries. Corticosteroid and cytotoxic agent use has dramatically reduced mortality and morbidity. Exacerbations occur despite aggressive immune suppression. Infliximab has been used in refractory disease.

Neurologic Manifestations. Approximately half the patients demonstrate neurologic manifestations including seizures, headache, disturbances of higher cortical function, and affective disorders. Less common symptoms include visual field defects, hemiparesis, increased intracranial pressure, nystagmus, ophthalmoplegia, ataxia, and aseptic meningitis. Neuropsychiatric symptoms (psychosis, encephalopathy) can occur in PAN. The sudden onset of stroke requires MRI and MR angiography, followed by cerebral angiography in selected patients. Evidence of segmental arterial narrowing or microaneurysmal dilatation may be demonstrated (Fig. 121-5B).

Diffuse myalgias can occur. Myositis, although rare, may reveal necrotizing arteritis with fibrinoid necrosis and perivascular inflammation. Sensorimotor neuropathies and mononeuritis multiplex are treated with corticosteroids. Myelopathy occurs rarely and usually only in patients with chronic disease.

Laboratory Findings. Laboratory evaluation reveals leukocytosis, anemia, increased sedimentation rate, abnormal urinalysis, and evidence of nephrosis and nephritis, in the absence of complement consumption, antinuclear antibodies, and rheumatoid factor. Patients may have circulating antineutrophil cytoplasmic antibodies, elevated factor VIII-related antigen, positive serology for hepatitis B surface antigen, and evidence of a preceding streptococcal infection. CSF is usually normal; the presence of blood strongly suggests a ruptured microaneurysm. Angiography may demonstrate aneurysmal dilatation of the medium-sized mesenteric, celiac, or renal arteries (Fig. 121-5A).

Neuropathology. Postmortem studies of pediatric patients with arteritis demonstrate necrotizing angiitis accompanied by polymorphonuclear infiltration of small-sized and medium-sized arteries.

Treatment. Corticosteroids are the mainstay of treatment. Aggressive treatment with high-dose intravenous corticosteroids and cyclophosphamide should be considered for patients with significant multisystem or CNS disease. Plasmapheresis is not beneficial. Overall, 5-year survival has improved substantially.

Kawasaki Disease

Kawasaki disease is characterized by aneurysms that are limited primarily to the coronary arteries. It is diagnosed by the presence of fever of at least 5 days' duration with four of these five criteria:

1. Bilateral nonpurulent conjunctival injection
2. Mucosal involvement of the oropharynx (injected or dry, fissured lips, or strawberry tongue)
3. Changes in the peripheral extremities, including edema, erythema of hands and feet, and desquamation
4. Rash, which may be polymorphous but not vesicular
5. Unilateral cervical lymphadenopathy

Prognosis has been excellent since the use of intravenous immunoglobulin and acetylsalicylic acid. However, myocardial infarction, dysrhythmias, and sudden death may occur.

Neurologic Manifestations. Pronounced irritability, lethargy, and aseptic meningitis are common, but other neurologic manifestations are rare. Cerebral artery involvement including aneurysm development is rare in contrast to PAN.

Neuropathology. Little cerebrovascular involvement has been documented. Major findings have included leptomeningeal thickening, mild endarteritis, and periarteritis.

Treatment. Treatment consists of acetylsalicylic acid, 80 to 100 mg/kg per day in four divided doses, until the patient has been afebrile for 3 to 7 days, followed by 3 to 5 mg/kg per day in a single dose and continued until inflammatory markers return to normal, the thrombocytosis has resolved, and no coronary artery disease exists on follow-up echocardiogram at 4 to 6 weeks. Acutely, intravenous immunoglobulin, 2 g/kg as a single dose over 12 hours, is recommended preferably before the 10th day. In children who have failed this therapy, corticosteroids, other immunosuppressives, and biologic agents have been used.

Cogan Syndrome

Cogan syndrome rarely occurs in children. Features include vertigo, deafness, photophobia, interstitial keratitis, aortitis, aortic valve insufficiency, arthralgia, myalgia, anorexia, episcleritis and/or uveitis, and fever.

Leukocytoclastic Vasculitis

Leukocytoclastic vasculitis is a necrotizing vasculitis with polymorphonuclear leukocytic infiltration and necrosis in the walls of small arteries. These changes are seen most commonly in Henoch-Schönlein purpura, SLE, and hypersensitivity vasculitis.

Henoch-Schönlein Purpura

This disorder is characterized by palpable purpura, petechiae, or ecchymotic rash, typically found over the buttocks and the lower extremities. It is often associated with large-joint arthritis, cramping abdominal pain, fever, peripheral edema, and renal involvement. The illness lasts about 1 to 3 months, and

recurrences occur. Microscopic hematuria, guaiac-positive stools, and elevated IgA levels are found. Skin, renal, and gastrointestinal biopsies demonstrate leukocytoclastic vasculitis with IgA, complement, and properdin deposition.

Neurologic Characteristics. CNS complications occur in 8% of children due to hypertension, renal failure, and vasculitis (Garzoni, et al., 2009). Headache, seizures, encephalopathy with or without hypertension, cerebral vasculitis, intracranial hemorrhage, spastic paralysis, and chorea may occur. Peripheral nervous system complications include lesions of the femoral, sciatic, and facial nerves, Guillain-Barré syndrome, and mononeuritis multiplex.

Treatment. Arthritis is managed with nonsteroidal antiinflammatory drugs, and painful cutaneous edema is managed with steroids. Supportive care is required when massive gastrointestinal bleeding, dehydration, or hypertension occurs. High-dose steroids and plasmapheresis have been used for severe CNS disease.

Hypersensitivity Angiitis

Hypersensitivity, or allergic, angiitis is an acute necrotizing inflammation of blood vessels similar to Henoch-Schönlein purpura. The disorder may be acute and rapidly fatal and may be caused by a hypersensitivity reaction to various drugs or infections. Decreased serum complement and cryoglobulinemia occur. Neurologic complications are rare as cerebral vessels tend to be spared.

Granulomatous Angiitis

Granulomatous angiitis represents a category of systemic necrotizing arteritis manifested by extravascular granulomatous nodules, which consist of a central area of fibrinoid degeneration with surrounding eosinophils and epithelioid and giant cells.

Churg-Strauss Syndrome

Churg-Strauss syndrome, also known as allergic granulomatosis, is associated with asthma, fever, eosinophilia, cardiac failure, renal damage, and peripheral neuropathy. The incidence in children is unknown. Established criteria require the presence of four of the following seven findings:

1. Asthma
2. Eosinophilia
3. History of allergy
4. Mononeuropathy or polyneuropathy
5. Pulmonary infiltrates that are migratory
6. Paranasal sinus abnormality
7. Extravascular eosinophils on biopsy

Neurologic Manifestations. Neurologic involvement is seen in more than half the children and includes mononeuritis multiplex, symmetric polyneuropathy, cranial neuropathies, optic neuritis, stroke, and chorea.

Treatment. Treatment is similar to that for PAN; most patients respond to corticosteroids. Azathioprine is also used. Cyclophosphamide, methotrexate, and omalizumab may be beneficial, whereas the therapeutic effects of etanercept, plasma exchange, and intravenous immunoglobulin therapy are controversial.

Granulomatosis with Polyangiitis (formerly called Wegener's Granulomatosis)

Granulomatosis with polyangiitis is characterized by a necrotizing granulomatous vasculitis of the small vessels in the upper and lower respiratory tract and the kidneys. Symptoms include fever, malaise, rhinorrhea, epistaxis, chronic sinusitis, nasal obstruction, pharyngeal ulcers, parenchymal pulmonary lesions, and chronic glomerulonephritis. The most common laboratory abnormality is a cytoplasmic staining antineutrophil cytoplasmic antibody due to anti-PR3 antibodies. Children are rarely affected.

Neurologic Manifestations. Fourteen to 25% of children have CNS symptoms including myalgias, cranial nerve palsies, seizures, cerebral vasculitis, keratitis, optic nerve granuloma, proptosis, orbital pseudotumor, laryngitis with accompanying aphonia, spasticity, and proximal muscle weakness.

Treatment. Prednisone and daily oral cyclophosphamide have improved the survival rate to greater than 90%. Pulse cyclophosphamide, intravenous immunoglobulin, trimethoprim-sulfamethoxazole, cyclosporine A, methotrexate, and the biologic agents also have variable success in inducing remission.

Primary Angiitis of the Central Nervous System

Primary angiitis of the CNS, also called granulomatous angiitis, is characterized by granulomas in 80% of individuals. Clinical criteria require a history or finding of an acquired neurologic deficit associated with angiographic or histopathologic demonstration of vasculitic changes, exclusion of other etiologies, and no evidence of systemic disease (Calabrese, 1995). It may occur in young children and has an equal gender distribution. Clinical features include headache, confusion, nausea, altered mental status, focal neurologic deficits, and progressive intellectual deterioration.

Neurologic Manifestations. Clinical manifestations correlate with the size of the affected vessels. Patients with small-vessel disease present with headache, focal seizures, or progressive behavioral or multifocal neurologic impairment. Patients with medium-vessel or large-vessel disease present with acute ischemic stroke or transient ischemic attacks. In both groups, cranial nerve abnormalities, hemiparesis, language disorders, seizures, spinal cord abnormalities, cerebral hemorrhage, fever, and weight loss have been reported. Symptoms of this broad spectrum disorder fluctuate, and the prognosis is better for patients with small-vessel disease. A subgroup of patients has "benign angiopathy of the CNS." These patients tend to be young women with sudden onset of symptoms and near-normal CSF studies, and the disease often remits after a monophasic benign course. This condition has been described in children (Calabrese, 1995).

Laboratory Findings. Laboratory studies reveal elevated erythrocyte sedimentation rate, elevated CSF protein concentration, and moderate monocytosis with increased pressure. Cerebral angiography documents small-sized and medium-sized vessel occlusion or segmental narrowing with saccular aneurysms and areas of infarction. Patients with small-vessel disease demonstrate multifocal, hyperintense lesions on T2-weighted MRI with normal CSF, erythrocyte sedimentation rate, and cerebral angiograms. Those with medium-vessel or large-vessel disease demonstrate infarcts and are more likely to have abnormal CSF studies, erythrocyte sedimentation rates, and angiograms (Fig. 121-6).

Treatment. Therapeutic use of corticosteroids, with or without cyclophosphamide, is indicated.

Necrotizing Sarcoid Granulomatosis

This condition is intermediate between sarcoidosis and granulomatosis with polyangiitis. It can cause multifocal neurologic disease and retinal angiitis, responds to corticosteroids, and does not require cytotoxic therapy.

Sarcoidosis

Sarcoidosis is a chronic, multisystem granulomatous disease of unknown etiology that is rare in children. Younger children (younger than 4 years) tend to have different clinical manifestations than older children or adults, characterized by relatively painless, boggy polyarthritis with well-preserved range of motion. Uveitis and cutaneous sarcoid lesions are present; pulmonary involvement is rare. Older children present with pulmonary symptoms, fatigue, weight loss, anorexia, headache, fever, parotid enlargement, hypercalciuria, leukopenia, eosinophilia, hilar and paratracheal adenopathy with interstitial infiltrates, elevated erythrocyte sedimentation rate, and elevated serum immunoglobulins. Pulmonary function is abnormal, and mediastinal or peripheral lymph node biopsies show noncaseating granulomas. Musculoskeletal findings include joint pain, effusions, and noncaseating granulomatous palpable muscle masses.

Neurologic Manifestations. Neurologic findings include obstructive hydrocephalus with noncaseating granulomas, transient cranial nerve VII palsies, and myelopathy. There are reports of optic nerve and orbital involvement, pituitary and hypothalamic lesions, meningitis, and seizures.

About 5% of adult patients have neurologic involvement including meningeal, parameningeal, hypothalamic, pituitary, and intramedullary spinal cord sarcoid infiltration. Peripheral and cranial neuropathies occur. Neurologic symptoms in children include seizures, cranial nerve palsy, CNS mass lesions, hypothalamic dysfunction, and uveitis.

Treatment. Treatment of the early-onset form is with corticosteroids, azathioprine, methotrexate, or, occasionally, cyclophosphamide. Therapy of late-onset or adult-type sarcoidosis depends on whether the arthritis is acute, chronic, or relapsing. Nonsteroidal antiinflammatory drugs have been used. More painful episodes have been managed with colchicine. Attacks unresponsive to colchicine often respond to corticosteroids or methotrexate.

Giant Cell Arteritis
Temporal Arteritis

Classic giant cell arteritis (temporal arteritis) most often affects men older than 50 years of age. A report of biopsy-proven temporal arteritis in a 9-year-old girl with sensorineural hearing loss, monocular blindness, a tortuous superficial temporal artery, and systemic illness with encephalopathy makes it clear that this disorder can occur in childhood. Headache, scalp tenderness, visual disturbances, and jaw claudication appearing in association with an elevated sedimentation rate suggest the diagnosis. Superficial temporal artery biopsy reveals giant cell perivascular inflammatory infiltrates. Optic neuritis, hemiparesis, vertigo, hearing loss, brainstem strokes, seizures, oculomotor disorders, and peripheral neuropathies have been reported. The superficial temporal, vertebral, ophthalmic, and posterior ciliary arteries are involved.

Takayasu Arteritis

Takayasu arteritis involves the aorta and its branches and has been reported in infants and children. In children, the abdominal aorta and its branches are more commonly affected than the aortic arch. In the prepulseless stage, nonspecific symptoms of fever, fatigue, dyspnea, anorexia, and arthralgia occur. The obstructive phase is characterized by aneurysmal dilation and stenosis of the aorta or pulmonary arteries. With abdominal aortic involvement, initial symptoms include abdominal pain or mass, congestive heart failure, and occlusive vascular disease of the abdominal organs or lower extremities. Neurologic symptoms are quite rare and include headache, hypertensive encephalopathy, seizures, and hemiplegia. Treatment with corticosteroids improves the long-term prognosis; most immunosuppressive drugs provide little improvement over corticosteroids.

Miscellaneous Vasculitic Disorders

About one third of vasculitic disorders are categorized as idiopathic or "polyangiitis overlap syndrome." Other diseases, such as Behçet syndrome, do not fit any of these categories.

Behçet Disease

Behçet disease is rare in children, usually with onset in the second decade of life, suggesting that juvenile Behçet disease may differ from that in adults. Diagnosis is based on the presence of recurrent aphthous stomatitis and two of the following: recurrent genital ulcers, uveitis or retinal vasculitis, erythema nodosum, or pustules or pathergy (the appearance of a pustular skin lesion after skin puncture).

Neurologic Manifestations. Three forms of CNS involvement occur:

1. Diffuse involvement associated with an acute meningoencephalitis, psychosis, or dementia
2. Brainstem or spinal cord involvement, with cranial nerve palsies, hemiparesis, and ataxia
3. Intracranial sinovenous thrombosis with signs of intracranial hypertension

Lymphocytic meningitis, vasculitis with perivascular cuffing, and thrombosis of arterioles, venules, veins, and dural venous sinuses are found and associated with cerebral hypoperfusion detectable with neuroimaging.

Treatment. High dose corticosteroids appear beneficial. Thalidomide has been used in steroid resistant patients as has colchicine and various chemotherapeutic agents. Heparinization may be beneficial when sinovenous thrombosis is present. Disease-modifying therapies should be considered for CNS relapse or steroid-refractory disease and include azathioprine, mycophenolate mofetil, methotrexate, and cyclophosphamide. Infliximab, adalimumab, etanercept, or interferon alpha has been used for aggressive neurologic or systemic complications.

Miscellaneous Disorders

Thrombotic Thrombocytopenic Purpura

Rapid onset of thrombocytopenia, severe microangiopathic hemolytic anemia, renal disease, widespread microvascular thrombosis, neurologic symptoms, and fever characterizes this disorder.

Neurologic Manifestations. Neurologic involvement includes headache, confusion, seizures, retinal hemorrhages, and occasionally focal deficits. Thrombotic occlusion may involve the CNS, peripheral nervous system, or skeletal muscles. CSF examination is usually normal and EEG changes are nonspecific. MRI and cerebral angiography may include evidence of arterial ischemic injury, sometimes with hemorrhagic transformation or involving the posterior cerebral artery territory, reversible posterior leukoencephalopathy, or edema.

Laboratory Findings. Decreased levels of protease activity with the presence of von Willebrand factor-cleaving protease inhibitors contribute to the bleeding diathesis. Affected individuals have a deficiency of ADAMTS13, a von Willebrand factor-cleaving metalloprotease. Although often resulting from

ADAMTS13 gene mutations, individuals may develop this syndrome as the result of autoimmune inhibitors against ADAMTS13. Pathologically, amorphous hyaline material occluding small cerebral arteries is seen, and cerebral gray matter contains vascular ischemic lesions.

Treatment. Previously, only 10% of children with this disorder survived for more than 1 year. Plasma exchange transfusion has been beneficial by removing pathogenic substances and supplying other factors that may be deficient. Rituximab has been used successfully.

Antiphospholipid Antibody Syndrome

Antiphospholipid (aPL) antibody syndrome is a multisystem, autoimmune disorder characterized by recurrent thrombosis, pregnancy loss, or thrombocytopenia. The aPL antibodies include lupus anticoagulants (LAC), anticardiolipin antibodies (aCL), antibodies to β_2 glycoprotein-I (β_2GPI), and antibodies directed against prothrombin, annexin V, phosphatidylserine, and phosphatidylinositol. LAC is a group of antibodies directed against plasma proteins (e.g., β_2GPI, prothrombin, and annexin V).

Diagnosis requires specific clinical manifestations in addition to antibody detection. Strict diagnostic criteria for "definite" aPL antibody syndrome have been developed. Individuals must meet at least one clinical and one laboratory criterion including either:

1. Evidence of arterial, venous, or small vessel thrombosis; or
2. Pregnancy morbidity, which can include either one or more unexplained deaths of a morphologically normal fetus; one or more premature births of a morphologically normal neonate before the 34th week of gestation from eclampsia or placental insufficiency; or three or more unexplained consecutive spontaneous abortions before the 10th week of gestation. One of the following three laboratory criteria must be met: (1) the presence of a LAC; (2) medium or high serum or plasma IgG or IgM aCL antibodies; or (3) high serum or plasma IgG or IgM aCL anti-β2GPI antibody. These antibodies must be detected on two or more occasions at least 12 weeks apart.

Patients with aPL antibody syndrome are usually classified as having "primary aPL antibody syndrome" if there is no evidence for another underlying autoimmune disorder or "secondary aPL antibody syndrome" if another autoimmune disorder is present.

Treatment focuses on preventing vascular occlusion and resulting ischemic injury. Low-dose aspirin therapy has been used for preventive treatment. Interventions aimed at inflammatory and immune mechanisms include hydroxychloroquine and avoidance of its fetal toxicity during pregnancy, rituximab and other anti-B cell agents, and eculizumab and other inhibitors of complement.

Erythromelalgia and Erythermalgia

Erythromelalgia and erythermalgia consist of episodes of intense, asymmetric burning sensations with associated erythema and elevated temperature in the extremities, must be distinguished from Raynaud's phenomenon and reflex sympathetic dystrophy, and is discussed in the online chapter.

REFERENCES

The complete list of references for this chapter is available in the e-book at www.expertconsult.com.
    See inside cover for registration details.

SELECTED REFERENCES

Appenzeller, S., Montenegro, M.A., Dertkigil, S.S., et al., 2004. Neuroimaging findings in scleroderma en coup de sabre. Neurology 62, 1585–1589.

Benseler, S., Schneider, R., 2004. Central nervous system vasculitis in children. Curr. Opin. Rheumatol. 16, 43–50.

Bingham, P.M., Galetta, S.L., Arthreya, B., et al., 1995. Neurologic manifestations in children with Lyme disease. Pediatrics 96, 1053–1056.

Calabrese, L.H., 1995. Vasculitis of the central nervous system. Rheum. Dis. Clin. North Am. 21, 1059–1076.

Dannecker, G.E., Quartier, P., 2009. Juvenile idiopathic arthritis: classification, clinical presentation and current treatments. Horm. Res. 72 (Suppl. 1), 4–12.

Dajani, A.S., Ayoub, E., Bierman, F.Z., et al., 1992. Guidelines for the diagnosis of rheumatic fever. Jones Criteria, 1992 update. Special Writing Group of the Committee on Rheumatic Fever, Endocarditis, and Kawasaki Disease of the Council on Cardiovascular Disease in the Young of the American Heart Association. JAMA 268, 2069–2073.

Garzoni, L., Vanoni, F., Rizzi, M., et al., 2009. Nervous system dysfunction in Henoch-Schonlein syndrome: systematic review of the literature. Rheumatology (Oxford) 48, 524–529.

Iannetti, L., Zito, R., Bruschi, S., et al., 2012. Recent understanding on diagnosis and management of central nervous system vasculitis in children. Clin. Dev. Immunol. 2012, 698327.

Murray, K.J., Laxer, R.M., 2002. Scleroderma in children and adolescents. Rheum. Dis. Clin. North Am. 28, 603–624.

Muscal, E., Brey, R.L., 2010. Neurologic manifestations of systemic lupus erythematosus in children and adults. Neurol. Clin. 28 (1), 61–73.

E-BOOK FIGURES AND TABLES

The following figures and tables are available in the e-book at www.expertconsult.com. See inside cover for registration details.

Fig. 121-1 Brain imaging in systemic lupus erythematosus.

Fig. 121-2 Magnetic resonance image of a 15-year-old female with systemic lupus erythematosus, who developed seizures, depression, generalized weakness, and severe membranous nephritis.

Fig. 121-3 Magnetic resonance image of a 9-year-old female with systemic lupus erythematosus, who had fever, leukopenia, abdominal pain, worsening headache, and cardiomyopathy.

Fig. 121-4 Representative single-photon emission computed tomographic study of a 14-year-old male with systemic lupus erythematosus and acute onset of optic neuritis and transverse myelitis.

Fig. 121-5 Angiography in polyarteritis nodosa.

Fig. 121-6 A 4-year-old male with primary angiitis of the central nervous system who had a 2-month history of seizures, chorea, left hemiparesis, and dysarthria.

122 Pediatric Neuro-oncology: An Overview

Roger J. Packer

An expanded version of this chapter is available on www.expertconsult.com. See inside cover for registration details.

INTRODUCTION

Primary central nervous system (CNS) tumors are the second most common form of childhood cancer, exceeded in incidence only by the leukemias, and constitute approximately one quarter of all childhood neoplasms (Louis et al., 2007). In the United States, between 3000 and 4000 children are diagnosed with a primary CNS tumor each year. Concepts and management of pediatric brain tumors are constantly evolving (Pomeroy et al., 2002). The classification of these neoplasms, on which treatment is increasingly based, is changing even more rapidly, primarily as a result of the incorporation of molecular diagnostics (Pomeroy et al., 2002).

For decades, childhood brain tumors were treated with surgery followed by radiotherapy for subtotally resected and/or malignant neoplasms. The need for aggressive surgery and "total" resections, although undeniable in some subtypes of neoplasms, is being increasingly scrutinized because of the risk for permanent surgery-related sequelae. Radiotherapy has been recognized as being crucial for the control of most forms of childhood malignant tumors but is also associated with devastating sequelae. Chemotherapy is now a standard form of adjuvant postsurgical treatment and in some situations is employed to delay, if not obviate, the need for radiotherapy. Molecularly targeted therapy is just beginning to be incorporated into management and holds the promise of radically altering approaches and improving outcome.

Advances and refinements in therapy, to date, have resulted in a modest improvement in overall survival rate (Smith et al., 2014). Given the relative infrequency of specific subtypes of childhood brain tumors, for progress to be made expeditiously, prospective, multicentered, cooperative, group-based trials are optimal. National and, in selected cases, international investigation protocols have become the standard of care of modern management of childhood brain tumors.

INCIDENCE

The incidence rates of brain tumors for patients between 0 and 19 years of age ranges from 3.3 to 4.5 cases per 100,000 person years (see Fig. 122-1). Among the major histologic groupings, rates are highest for tumors of the neuroepithelial tissue, with pilocytic astrocytomas and medulloblastomas being the most common individual subtypes of tumors. Embryonal tumors, including medulloblastoma, comprise 15% to 20% of all tumors in children between 0 and 14 years of age, occurring in approximately 5% of those between the ages of 15 and 19 (see Fig. 122-2).

Primary CNS tumors are more common in the first decade of life. The reported incidence of brain tumors is higher in whites (4.7 per 100,000 person years) than in other racial

groups (3.0 per 100,000 person years). The overall incidence for all brain tumors is highest among those between 0 and 4 years of age (5.2 per 100,000 person years) and lowest among those between 10 and 14 years of age (4.1 per 100,000 person years). However, incidence varies depending on tumor type, with ependymomas and medulloblastomas decreasing with age, and pilocytic astrocytomas peaking at 5 to 9 years of age.

ETIOLOGY

The cause of the majority of all childhood brain tumors is unknown. Despite this, there are genetic conditions and, to a lesser extent, environmental exposures that predispose to the development of tumors. Genetic syndromes related to increased development of specific tumor types have provided molecular genetic insights into childhood brain tumors that have been partially translatable to the study of tumors not apparently of genetic origin. The known syndromes that are associated with the development of childhood brain tumors usually have an autosomal-dominant pattern of inheritance (see Table 122-1).

Of the environmental exposures that predispose to the development of brain tumors, the best documented is ionizing radiation. Secondary brain tumors have been reported after cranial irradiation for leukemia, head and neck tumors, and primary brain tumors. The most common form of malignant brain tumor occurring after radiation is malignant gliomas, which tend to appear 5 to 15 years after radiation and are highly resistant to therapy. Meningiomas are the most common radiation-induced tumors, increase in frequency with time after radiotherapy, and do not begin to peak until 10 years after exposure.

The effects of a multitude of environmental exposures, including maternal diet, on the occurrence of childhood brain tumors have not been conclusively shown. Initial studies suggested an association between significant exposure to electromagnetic waves or the use of cell phones in the development of gliomas, but other studies have not been able to confirm this relationship. Immunosuppression, either because of an underlying disorder of the immune system or after treatment with chronic immunosuppressive agents in situations such as organ transplantation, has been associated with an increased incidence of CNS lymphoma.

PATHOLOGY AND CLASSIFICATION

The World Health Organization (WHO) utilizes a grading scheme that is basically a malignancy scale. Although the WHO classification is applicable to pediatrics, the congenital nature of many tumors, often with elements that seem to show mixed lineage, such as neuronal and glial elements, can make classification difficult. In addition, in the pediatric modifications, tumor location is also a component of classification. Molecular genetic findings, to date, have not been incorporated into the classification system.

Probably the most controversial aspect of the classification of pediatric brain tumors has been the nomenclature utilized for CNS embryonal tumors (Pomeroy et al., 2002). The introduction of immunohistochemical techniques demonstrated the variable cell types that occur in embryonal tumors, although the majority of cells are small, hyperchromatic

round or oval cells (small blue cells). Molecular genetic analysis has demonstrated that primitive embryonal tumors occurring in the cerebellum, pineal region, and cortex are molecularly distinct. Furthermore, it is now clear that even in the posterior fossa, medulloblastoma is comprised of at least four, and likely more, different biologic subtypes, with different propensities to disseminate throughout the nervous system, responsivities to therapies, and prognosis (Kool et al., 2012). CNS primitive neuroectodermal tumors (PNETs) are similarly composed of different tumor subtypes.

By convention, childhood CNS gliomas are often grouped by location, and cerebellar astrocytomas, intrinsic brainstem gliomas, and visual pathway gliomas, especially optic nerve and/or chiasmatic tumors, are considered relatively distinct entities. Biologic information has given some credence to such separation (Jones et al., 2013). The majority, possibly all, pilocytic astrocytomas have aberrations in the RAS-MAPK signaling pathway, although the type of abnormality and prognosis may vary between site (Pfister et al., 2008). Over 90% of cerebellar tumors have an activating BRAF-fusion mutation, whereas 50% or less of chiasmatic gliomas have similar mutations. Abnormality in histone chromatin remodeling genes has been found to be the common molecular abnormality in some, but not all, pediatric higher-grade gliomas, although the incidence of the type of mutation varies, dependent on site of the tumor (Paugh et al., 2010). Midline (brainstem, thalamic tumors) high-grade gliomas harbor a different mutation than cortical tumors. Childhood high-grade gliomas also differ molecularly from those arising in adulthood (Paugh et al., 2010). Ependymomas arising in the posterior fossa and cortex are biologically different, and even within these two regions, molecularly distinct lesions exist.

STAGING AND STRATIFICATION

Pre- and postoperative staging are the cornerstone of therapy for most embryonal childhood CNS tumors and, to a lesser extent, glial neoplasms. The utility of staging for both determination of prognosis and decisions concerning most appropriate therapy has been best shown for medulloblastoma; staging has been an accepted component of management since the mid-1980s. All schemas share the property of being based on degree of surgical resection or, more specifically, the amount of tumor left after surgery and the extent of tumor

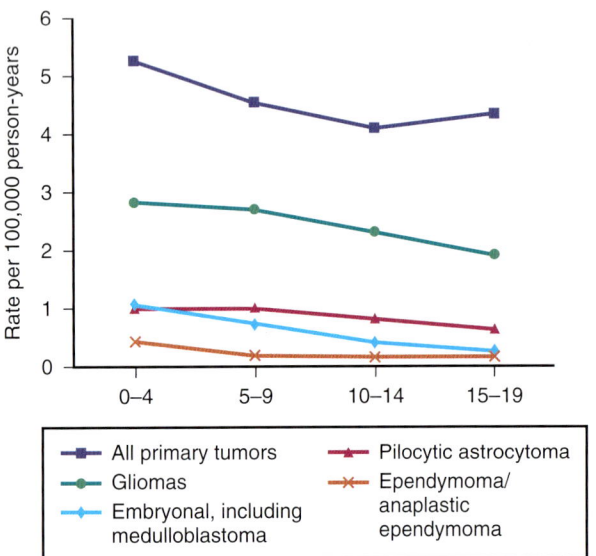

AGE-SPECIFIC INCIDENCE OF CHILDHOOD PRIMARY BRAIN AND CNS TUMORS BY SELECTED HISTOLOGIES CB TRUS 2000–2004

Legend:
- All primary tumors
- Gliomas
- Embryonal, including medulloblastoma
- Pilocytic astrocytoma
- Ependymoma/ anaplastic ependymoma

Figure 122-2. Distribution of childhood primary brain tumors by histology. CBTRUS, Central Brain Tumor Registry of the United States; NOS, not otherwise specified; NPCR, National Program of Cancer Registries; SEER, National Cancer Institute's Surveillance Epidemiology and End Results.

TABLE 122-1 Genetic Syndromes Associated with Pediatric Brain Tumors

Syndrome	Inheritance	Molecular/Genetic Abnormality	Predominant Tumor Types
Neurofibromatosis type 1	Autosomal dominant	NF1 gene (Chr. 17); increased RAS/MAPK signaling	Pilocytic astrocytomas; visual pathway > brainstem > cortical
Tuberous sclerosis	Autosomal dominant	TSC1 (Chr. 9); TSC2 (Chr. 16); increased RAS/MAPK signaling	Giant cell astrocytomas
Cowden's	Autosomal dominant	Germ line PTEN	Cerebellar gangliocytoma
Von Hippel-Landau	Autosomal dominant	VHL gene	Hemangioblastomas in cerebellum, spinal cord, and retina
Li-Fraumeni	Autosomal dominant	Germ line mutation TP 53	High- and low-grade gliomas; medulloblastoma, choroid plexus carcinomas
Gorlin's	Autosomal dominant	Germ line mutation PATCHED 1 (Chr.9); increased SHH signaling	Medulloblastoma
Turcot's (type 1)	Autosomal dominant	DNA mismatch repair	Gliomas
Turcot's (type 2)	Autosomal dominant	APC gene; WNT signaling	Medulloblastoma
Atypical teratoid/Rhabdoid tumor predisposition syndrome	Autosomal dominant	Germ line mutation SMARC1/h SNF5/INI1 (Chr. 22)	AT/RT tumors of brain; rhabdoid tumors of kidney

spread outside the primary tumor site. The latter is determined by a combination of results from magnetic resonance imaging (MRI) of the entire brain and spine and cerebrospinal fluid cytologic examination, preferably from the lumbar space, if deemed medically safe. Embryonal tumors and glial neoplasms rarely spread to nonneural sites; thus, evaluation for disease outside the CNS, at the time of diagnosis, is usually not indicated. The classical tumor, nodes, metastasis (TNM) staging system used for non-CNS tumors is replaced by a TM system for brain and spine tumors. Although the need for lumbar cerebrospinal fluid cytologic examination has been debated, studies have shown that it provides complementary information to imaging results.

Histology has been incorporated into risk stratification for many tumor types. For embryonal tumors, such as medulloblastoma, histologic features, including desmoplasia/ nodularity in infants and anaplasia in infants and older children, are now increasingly accepted as important components of risk-stratification classifications. For glial tumors or ependymomas, histologic features that have been translated into grades are an accepted component of classification and are used for risk stratification.

CLINICAL PRESENTATION

The clinical presentation of childhood CNS tumors is dependent not only on the location of the tumor in the nervous system, but also on the age of the patient and the rapidity and pattern of growth of the tumor (see Tables 122-2 and 122-3). With the wider availability of computed tomography (CT) and, more recently, MRI capabilities, especially in developed countries, the time between onset of symptoms and diagnosis, especially for malignant tumors, has decreased. Longer periods before diagnosis have not been associated with poorer outcomes. Although this may be somewhat counterintuitive, it suggests that more aggressive tumors may result in more severe neurologic symptoms and localizing signs earlier in the course of illness, compared with slower-growing neoplasms that are more likely to have longer, less specific symptomatology.

The greatest delay in diagnosis usually occurs in infants and young children, for a variety of reasons, including the relative rarity of childhood brain tumors, the nonspecific nature of presentation, and the difficulty of evaluating such young patients. Because of age and the presence of open fontanels and sutures, head pain may not be apparent, despite the presence of a very large tumor. In those patients with hydrocephalus, detection of papilledema, which, once again, can be difficult to discern in a young child, is obviously helpful. However, in longstanding increased intracranial pressure, especially in those patients with a slow-growing tumor in the suprasellar region, optic pallor, rather than papilledema, is more likely to be present. Another symptom of increased intracranial pressure in infants is the "setting sun" sign, manifested by impaired upgaze and seemingly enforced downward deviation of the eyes. This is caused by dilation of the third ventricle with resultant tectal pressure as a result of obstructive hydrocephalus.

Large neoplasms in infants may present with developmental delay early in the course of illness, followed by regression of developmental milestones. Tumors of the hypothalamus are notoriously difficult to diagnose early in life, especially in infants. The diencephalic syndrome is a constellation of symptoms and signs, including failure to thrive and emaciation in an otherwise normal child who has seemingly adequate appetite and gastrointestinal function and no focal neurologic or ophthalmologic deficits. Although some children do present in this way, detailed neurologic and neuro-ophthalmologic examination often discloses abnormalities, including unilateral or bilateral nystagmus, optic pallor, some degree of loss of visual acuity or field, and subtle motor dysfunction. Although initial reports suggested that these children seemed happy or "euphoric," children with this syndrome, who predominantly harbor infiltrative gliomas of the hypothalamus,

TABLE 122-2 Differential Diagnosis: Supratentorial Tumors

Tumor Type	Incidence	Peak Age	Common Symptoms	Common Signs	Common Neuroimaging Features
Cortical low-grade glioma	50%	Infancy through childhood	Seizures Headaches Unilateral weakness	Seizures Hemiparesis Hemisensory loss Hemianopsia	Enhancing mass with cyst (juvenile pilocytic tumors) or nonenhancing mass, usually little edema (grade II)
Cortical high-grade glioma	20%	Later childhood through adolescence	Headaches Weakness Seizures	Focal neurologic deficits Hemiparesis Hemisensory loss Hemianopsia Aphasia Papilledema	Mass with edema Variable enhancement
Craniopharyngioma	10%	Throughout childhood, 5–15 years peak	Headaches Personality change Decreased vision Weight loss Slowing of growth School difficulties	Visual field loss Bitemporal hemianopsia ↓ Visual acuity Papilledema Optic atrophy	Cystic, calcified mass in the suprasellar region
Diencephalic low-grade glioma	10%	0–3 years of age	Visual difficulties Weight loss Anorexia	↓ Visual acuity Nystagmus, hemiparesis (if thalamic) Papilledema or optic atrophy Visual field loss Hemiparesis (if thalamic) Stigmata of neurofibromatosis type 1	Ill-defined, at times enhancing if juvenile pilocytic astrocytoma with/without optic nerve or pathway involvement; associated cyst

TABLE 122-3 Differential Diagnosis: Infratentorial Tumors

Tumor Type	Incidence of all Posterior Fossa Tumors	Peak Age	Common Symptoms	Common Signs	Common Neuroimaging Features
Medulloblastoma	40%	1–4 years 7–10 years	Headache Vomiting Unsteadiness	Papilledema 6th-nerve palsy Truncal ataxia Dysmetria	Enhancing mass filling 4th ventricle Hydrocephalus
Cerebellar astrocytoma	40%	5–15 years	Headaches Unilateral dysmetria, early	Appendicular truncal unsteadiness Papilledema late	Cystic mass with enhancing smaller (mural) module
Ependymoma	10%–20%	1–4 years	Double vision Facial weakness Headaches	6th-, 7th-, and 8th-nerve paresis Unilateral and bilateral dysmetria	Solid, at times, laterally placed mass
Brainstem glioma	10%–20%	5–15 years	Double vision Facial weakness Unilateral weakness Unsteadiness Swallowing difficulties	Multiple cranial nerve palsies Ataxia Dysmetria Crossed hemiparesis	Diffusely enlarged, often nonenhancing mass
Atypical teratoid/ rhabdoid tumor	10%–20% of infants	Infancy to 3 years	Vomiting Head pain Unsteadiness	6th- and 7th-nerve palsies Ataxia Dysmetria	Heterogeneously enhancing mass, often laterally placed

more commonly are quite irritable and have significant developmental delay.

GENERAL ASPECTS OF TREATMENT
Surgery

Surgery remains the initial step in the treatment for the overwhelming majority of childhood CNS tumors, and the degree of resection, even for malignant neoplasms that require other forms of adjuvant therapy, is often an important factor in determining outcome (Wisoff et al., 2011). Attainment of a representative portion of the neoplasm for histologic and, increasingly, biological analysis is crucial. Exceptions to the need for tissue for diagnosis include neuroradiographically characteristic diffuse intrinsic brainstem tumors; chiasmatic/hypothalamic infiltrating gliomas in children with neurofibromatosis type 1, and possibly for those without; and germ cell tumors, predominantly mixed germ cell tumors, which secrete diagnostic proteins into cerebrospinal fluid and blood.

Morbidity secondary to surgery in critical brain regions, especially those that subserve motor function, is at times essentially unavoidable, especially secondary to postoperative edema. Such postoperative impairment may be transient. Surgery in the suprasellar area is frequently associated with increased postoperative visual impairments, which may include decreases in visual acuity and increased deficits in visual fields. Hypothalamic abnormalities and significant hormonal deficits secondary to disruption of the hypothalamic–pituitary axis also frequently occur. In large tumors that extend to the subfrontal area, such as craniopharyngiomas, removal of the tumor may cause additional damage and both early and late emotional/personality changes. Such damage can exacerbate hypothalamic injury, which in itself causes abnormalities of satiety control and excessive weight gain.

Surgery for posterior fossa tumors may result in direct brainstem damage, with resultant cranial nerve deficits and damage to the cerebellum or cerebellar peduncles, with increased ataxia and dysmetria. Such direct brainstem damage should be distinguishable from the increasingly recognized posterior fossa mutism syndrome, which is a constellation of the delayed onset of mutism (characteristically, a few hours to a day after surgery), hypotonia, cerebellar deficits, supranuclear palsies, emotional lability, and severe irritability. Seen primarily, but not exclusively, after medulloblastoma resection, it is thought to be secondary to unilateral or bilateral cerebellar dentate nuclei damage and/or disruption of critical pathways between the dentate nuclei and the cortex, especially the premotor and supplementary motor cortices. This syndrome results in permanent sequelae in approximately 50% of initially symptomatic patients, including persistent abnormalities in tone, coordination, speech, and cognitive abilities.

Radiation Therapy

Radiation therapy is an integral component of treatment for many forms of childhood brain tumors. For children with benign tumors, its use is usually limited to those tumors that are not amenable to gross total resections. For children with more aggressive or malignant tumors, radiation therapy has been the backbone of most curative and palliative therapies, even in those patients whose tumors are totally resected (Packer et al., 2006). Craniospinal radiotherapy has been associated with improved survival, but also significant long-term endocrinologic growth, and cognitive sequelae. In very young children, especially infants, radiotherapy may result in even more severe sequelae, and attempts have been made to delay, if not obviate, the need for radiotherapy. Radiotherapy usually utilizes photon particles, delivered in different fractions and by different means (see Table 122-4). Recently proton particles (proton beam) have been increasingly used to decrease "scatter" radiation to nonaffected parts of brain and surrounding organs.

The determination of the optimal, often maximal, safe dose and volume of radiotherapy that can be used is dependent on the tumor type and the radiosensitivity of structures in the CNS, tempered by the age of the child. Younger children are more sensitive to the detrimental effects of radiation on the brain. In general, larger daily-dose fractions cause more acute and possibly long-term neurologic toxicity; standard fractionation is 150 to 180 cGy daily. Preoperative conditions, such as hydrocephalus and preexisting brain injury, affect the tolerance of the developing brain to radiotherapy. Even in children of similar ages with similar diseases, there can be significant differences in how radiotherapy can be tolerated, suggesting that there are molecular genetic differences that affect host vulnerability (see Table 122-5).

Irradiation of the hypothalamic–pituitary axis often is unavoidable because of location of the tumor, and can result in permanent endocrinologic damage. Growth hormone secretion is usually the most sensitive to the effects of radiotherapy, followed, in order of degree of sensitivity, by thyroid-stimulating hormone, follicle-stimulating hormone–luteinizing hormone (FSH-LH), and adrenocorticotropic hormone (ACTH). There is a dose relationship to such damage, with significant impairment of growth hormone secretion occurring more commonly after 2400 cGy, especially in doses greater than 2900 cGy, to the hypothalamus.

The severity of neurocognitive sequelae secondary to whole-brain radiotherapy is dependent on dose, age of the child, poorly understood host vulnerabilities, and probably preexisting brain injury. Craniospinal radiation therapy, especially in children less than 7 years of age, and particularly in those less than 5 years of age, results in a demonstrable drop in overall intelligence and a host of selective learning, attentional, and executive disabilities. In older children, depending on dose, decreases in overall intelligence may not occur, but selective learning disabilities and problems with executive function are common. Another long-term sequela of radiotherapy is development of secondary neoplasms.

Chemotherapy

Within the last decade, chemotherapy has gained an expanded role in the treatment of childhood brain tumors. The most common chemotherapeutic agents utilized for pediatric CNS tumors are in the class of DNA alkylators, such as cisplatin, carboplatin, lomustine, cyclophosphamide, and ifosfamide, which typically serve as the backbone for treatment of medulloblastoma, low-grade glioma, ependymoma, and germ cell tumors (Rutkowski et al., 2005) (see Table 122-6). Plant alkaloids, such as the mitotic inhibitors vincristine and vinblastine or the topoisomerase inhibitor etoposide, are also commonly employed as part of combination regimens (Packer et al., 2006). The overall success of chemotherapy for pediatric CNS tumors has remained somewhat limited. Two major reasons for this limitation are impediments to drug delivery across the blood–brain barrier and resistance to chemotherapy. Means to improve the efficacy of chemotherapy include the use of high-dose systematic chemotherapy with stem cell rescue; regional delivery approaches, including intrathecal and intraventricular drug instillation; convection delivery; and the use of agents to overcome drug resistance.

Biologic Therapy, Immunotherapy, Vaccines, and Gene Therapy

Therapy that specifically targets tumor biology has gained widespread attention due to its potential for greater antitumor efficacy while sparing normal cells from toxic side effects. In contrast to traditional chemotherapy, biologic therapy is more likely to be cytostatic rather than cytotoxic. Examples of this strategy include use of drugs that cause differentiation of tumor cells, receptor tyrosine kinase inhibitors, cellular pathway inhibitors, and antiangiogenesis agents.

Immunotherapy

Immunotherapeutic approaches have great appeal and are increasingly being explored. The CNS is a relatively privileged site immunologically because of its lack of lymphatic drainage and its blood–brain barrier, but there is evidence that, to some degree, peripheral T-cell activity may be carried into the CNS. A variety of different approaches have been utilized in the immunotherapy of CNS tumors, primarily in adults but also, to some degree, in pediatrics. These include administration of cytokines such as interleukin and interferon, expansion of tumor-specific T cells, and the use of monoclonal antibodies, checkpoint inhibitors, and tumor vaccines.

Gene Therapy

Introduced with great enthusiasm over 20 years ago, gene transfer therapy has yet to show efficacy in the majority of adults or children with CNS tumors. It is a process in which genetic material is transferred into cells and carries with it the information either to stop or to slow the ability of these cells to multiply. Gene therapy may also utilize genetic information that, after the tumor cells take up the gene material, makes them sensitive to other forms of treatment. Almost all of the gene transfer therapies have utilized a virus-mediated delivery system.

PROGNOSIS

The specific prognosis of individual tumor types is discussed in subsequent chapters. In general, survival rates have slowly risen over the past twenty years, primarily in the most common embryonal tumor, medulloblastoma. There has been no appreciable improvement in survival for pediatric high-grade glial tumors. Quality of life for survivors remains a major concern, as intellectual, psychological, and neurologic sequelae, often progressive over time, remain common. Alterations in treatment, including more judicious use of surgery, reductions in the dose of craniospinal radiotherapy and volume of focal radiotherapy, and avoidance or at least delay of radiation therapy in infants, have seemed to decrease complications. However, the use of chemotherapy has resulted in other sequelae, such as cisplatin-induced hearing loss, vincristine-related neuropathy, and possibly alkylator-associated secondary tumors. Treatment remains a delicate balance between the need to control tumor growth and potential treatment-related sequelae. Molecularly targeted therapies and other approaches, such as immunotherapy, are being explored to try to improve outcomes with the hope of less neurologic compromise.

REFERENCES

The complete list of references for this chapter is available in the e-book at www.expertconsult.com.
    See inside cover for registration details.

SELECTED REFERENCES

Jones, D.T., Hutter, B., Jager, N., et al., 2013. Recurrent somatic alterations of FGFR1 and NTRK2 in pilocytic astrocytoma. Nat. Genet. 45 (8), 927–932.

Kool, M., Korshunov, A., Remke, M., et al., 2012. Molecular subgroups of medulloblastoma: an international meta-analysis of transcriptome, genetic aberrations, and clinical data of WNT, SHH, Group 3, and Group 4 medulloblastomas. Acta Neuropathol. 123 (4), 473–484.

Louis, D.N., Ohgaki, H., Wiestler, O.D., et al., 2007. The 2007 WHO classification of tumours of the central nervous system. Acta Neuropathol. 114 (2), 97–109.

Packer, R.J., Gajjar, A., Vezina, G., et al., 2006. Phase III study of craniospinal radiation therapy followed by adjuvant chemotherapy for newly diagnosed average risk medulloblastoma. J. Clin. Oncol. 24 (25), 4202–4208.

Paugh, B.S., Qu, C., Jones, C., et al., 2010. Integrated molecular genetic profiling of pediatric high grade gliomas reveals key differences with the adult disease. J. Clin. Oncol. 28 (18), 3061–3068.

Pfister, S., Janzarik, W.G., Remke, M., et al., 2008. BRAF gene duplication constitutes a mechanism of MAPK pathway activation in low grade astrocytomas. J. Clin. Invest. 118 (5), 1739–1749.

Pomeroy, S.L., Tamayo, P., Gaasenbeek, M., et al., 2002. Prediction of central nervous system embryonal tumour outcome based on gene expression. Nature 415 (6870), 436–442.

Rutkowski, S., Bode, U., Deinlein, F., et al., 2005. Treatment of early childhood medulloblastoma by postoperative chemotherapy alone. N. Engl. J. Med. 352 (10), 978–986.

Smith, M.A., Altekruse, S.F., Adamson, P.C., et al., 2014. Declining childhood and adolescent cancer mortality. Cancer 120 (16), 2497–2506.

Wisoff, J.H., Sanford, R.A., Heier, L.A., et al., 2011. Primary neurosurgery for pediatric low grade gliomas: a prospective multi-institutional study from the Children's Oncology Group. Neurosurgery 68 (6), 1548–1554, discussion 1554-5.

E-BOOK FIGURES AND TABLES

The following figures and tables are available in the e-book at www.expertconsult.com. See inside cover for registration details.

123 Medulloblastoma

Roger J. Packer and Stefan M. Pfister

 An expanded version of this chapter is available on www.expertconsult.com. See inside cover for registration details.

INTRODUCTION

Medulloblastoma, which is defined by the World Health Organization (WHO) as an embryonal tumor of the cerebellum, is the single most common form of malignant brain tumor of childhood. Medulloblastomas are highly cellular tumors with deeply basophilic pleomorphic nuclei, little cytoplasm, and abundant mitoses. The WHO classification further subdivides medulloblastoma into histologic subtypes. Integrative molecular analysis has extended these distinctions, dramatically altering concepts of medulloblastoma classification and risk stratification, with at least four distinct molecular subtypes of medulloblastoma having been identified.

As a whole, medulloblastoma constitutes 20% of all primary central nervous system (CNS) tumors and has a bimodal incidence peak, arising most commonly in children between 3 and 4 years of age and then again in those between 7 and 10 years of age. Between 15% and 20% of all medulloblastomas are diagnosed in the first 2 years of life. There is also a male predominance in specific molecular subtypes of the tumor.

With current means of treatment, the majority of children with medulloblastoma can be expected to survive 5 years after diagnosis, and many of these children are cured. Increasing emphasis has been placed on the quality of life of survivors and on potential means to reduce treatment-related sequelae without decreasing the likelihood of survival.

ETIOLOGY

Although the etiology of medulloblastoma is unknown for the majority of patients, several familial syndromes have been associated with increased risk of developing medulloblastoma, generating important insights into tumor pathogenesis. Gorlin's syndrome is present in less than 2% of patients with medulloblastoma, but its recognition led to the understanding that abnormalities of the sonic hedgehog (SHH) pathway may result in medulloblastoma. Also known as nevoid basal cell carcinoma syndrome, diagnosed by characteristic dermatologic and skeletal features, including multiple basal cell carcinomas, odontogenic keratocysts of the jaw, and rib abnormalities, it is caused by an inherited germ line mutation of the PATCHED 1 gene on chromosome 9, a gene that encodes SHH receptor PATCHED 1 and suppresses pathway signaling. Up to 25% of patients with medulloblastoma, especially infants and adults, will have SHH-pathway mutations. The diagnosis of Gorlin's syndrome early in life is difficult, but the presence of bifid or fused ribs, macrocephaly, or early calcification of the falx cerebri is helpful.

Turcot's syndrome (type 2) has also been associated with medulloblastoma. Caused by mutations of the adenomatous polyposis gene, it is marked by colorectal adenomas and a variety of extracolonic manifestations. Patients with type 2 Turcot' disease are at increased risk of developing medulloblastoma as a result of aberrant WNT pathway signaling. WNT abnormalities, not related to Turcot's syndrome, have been noted in between 10% and 15% of children with medulloblastoma, primarily in those with tumors arising in late childhood and adolescence.

Li Fraumeni syndrome, caused by germ line mutations in the TP53 gene, is also associated with medulloblastoma. Medulloblastoma has also been reported in rarer syndromes, including Rubenstein-Taybi and Fanconi's syndromes.

Other than radiation exposure, there are no clear-cut environmental factors that have been linked with medulloblastoma. Preliminary studies suggested a relationship with SV40 virus exposure, predominately as a contaminant of measles vaccination; however, subsequent studies have not confirmed this association.

BIOLOGY

Medulloblastoma is believed to arise from stem cells and neuron progenitor cells in and around the cerebellum, including the ventricular zone (adjacent to the fourth ventricle), the external granular layer of the cerebellum, and the dorsal brainstem (Wang and Wechsler-Reya, 2014). SHH-associated medulloblastomas are believed to primarily arise from the granular neuron precursors present in the external granular layer of the cerebellum. There is increasing evidence that WNT-associated tumors arise from progenitor cells in the dorsal brainstem rather than the cerebellum. Other medulloblastoma tumors likely arise from stem cells, and in some cases, granular neuronal precursors arising from the ventricular zone. Giving even greater credence to the now well-accepted concept that medulloblastoma is biologically comprised of different tumor types is the multitude of recent molecular studies investigating medulloblastoma tumor samples (see Table 123-2). These subtypes have been classified as WNT, SHH, Group 3, and Group 4, with each group having relatively distinct demographics and associated clinical characteristics, including disease course (Taylor et al., 2012).

On the basis of molecular subgroups, it was possible for the first time to put frequently observed genetic changes into context. Examples for genetic lesions specifically enriched in WNT tumors include quasidefining CTNNB1 mutations in exon 3, which are never observed in any other subgroup. For the SHH subgroup, in addition to the age-specific mutations in the tumor-driving SHH pathway, SHH signaling appears to cooperate with PI3K signaling, especially in adult SHH tumors, and with a plethora of different chromatin modifiers. For Group 3 tumors, it has long been established that MYC amplification is a hallmark genetic lesion (including PVT1-MYC fusion), but it is only present in about 30% of cases.

963

TABLE 123-2 Molecular Subgrouping of Medulloblastoma

	WNT	SHH	Group 3	Group 4
Age	Late childhood; Adolescence	Infants, adults > childhood	Infant, childhood	All
Gender	F>M	F = M	M>F	M>F
Molecular findings	Intranuclear β-catenin Staining; Monosomy 6; CTNNB1 mutation	SHH pathway mutations; PTCH1/SMO SUFU/GLI1; Occasional TP53 Mutation	MYC amplification; i179; GFI1; GFI1B	CDKG amplification SNCAIP
Genetic Expression	WNT signaling; MYC +	SHH signaling MYCN +	MYC +++	MYC↓
Histology	Classical, LCA	Desmoplastic; Desmoplastic/nodular	Classical; LCA	Classical/LCA
Mets	Occasional	Occasional	Very frequent	Frequent
Prognosis	Excellent	Good in infants, Adults; poor if MYCN + or TP53 mutation (primarily childhood)	Poor if M + or MYC +; Average otherwise	Average

Recent integrative genomic and epigenomic analyses have identified GFI1 and GFI1B as additional highly recurrent driver genes for Group 3 medulloblastoma. For Group 4 medulloblastoma, in addition to known overrepresentation of CDK6 and MYCN amplifications, inactivating mutations in the histone3 lysine 27-specific histone demethylase KDM6A (located on the X chromosome) and ZMYM3 have been repeatedly identified. Duplication of a region on chromosome 5 around the SNCAIP gene represents another frequent genetic event.

CLINICAL PRESENTATION AND DIAGNOSIS
Clinical Features

Medulloblastoma most commonly presents with nonspecific findings of vomiting and headache, which occur in 80% of patients by the time of diagnosis. This is usually associated with obstruction of cerebrospinal fluid flow at either the third or fourth ventricular outlets, and hydrocephalus. Symptom duration is classically 1 to 3 months before diagnosis; patients with metastatic disease are more likely to be diagnosed earlier and have a poorer prognosis. Usually, by diagnosis, the headache has transformed into one more classically associated with increased intracranial pressure, occurring upon wakening and accompanied by morning nausea and vomiting. Unsteadiness is noted in 50% to 80% of patients at diagnosis and is usually truncal, with significant gait abnormalities.

Medulloblastoma may present acutely with a severe alteration in consciousness and even coma. This is usually a result of macroscopic hemorrhage into the tumor and rapid tumor expansion with acute hydrocephalus and/or compression of the brainstem.

Although diagnosis can be difficult in infants, symptoms such as unexplained macrocephaly, intermittent lethargy, vomiting, and head tilt are noted in most infants by the time of diagnosis. The classical "setting sun" sign, with downward deviation of the eyes as a result of tectal pressure, is seen in only a minority of infants.

Medulloblastomas may be disseminated to other regions of the CNS at diagnosis. In the majority, there are no symptoms associated with dissemination.

Radiographic Features

Medulloblastomas are usually radiographically distinguishable from other posterior fossa tumors because they tend to be relatively well-defined masses arising in the medullary velum or roof of the fourth ventricle, often with some invasion of the middle cerebellar peduncle and compression or invasion of the brainstem. The tumor is hyperdense compared with normal cerebellum on computed tomography (CT), which distinguishes it from juvenile pilocytic astrocytoma. Calcifications may be present in up to 20% of cases, but are usually not conspicuous. On magnetic resonance imaging (MRI), medulloblastomas tend to be homogenous with iso- to hypointense signal on T1-weighted images and hypointense signal on T2-weighted images (Fig. 123-2). The majority of medulloblastomas enhance with contrast agent, although 5% to 10% do not enhance. In infancy, medulloblastoma with extensive nodularity may occur and display discrete contrasting-enhancing masses with an almost grapelike, clustered appearance.

Because between 15% and 30% of medulloblastomas are disseminated to other regions of the nervous system before diagnosis, neuroradiographic evaluation of the entire neuraxis is indicated, if possible, before surgery. Evaluation of dissemination can be difficult after surgery because of changes caused by postoperative blood. Pitfalls in the evaluation of extent of disease include nonenhancing dissemination, especially in patients with initially nonenhancing primary-site tumors, and spinal cord vascularity being interpreted as leptomeningeal disease.

MANAGEMENT AND OUTCOME

The treatment of children with medulloblastoma is multidisciplinary and multimodality, requiring surgery, radiation, and chemotherapy. Treatment is also dependent on the age of the child, predominantly because of the potential neurotoxic effects of radiotherapy, and disease stratification.

Surgery

Surgery is the initial step in management, to relieve hydrocephalus if present and to remove as much of the tumor as possible. Although temporary external ventricular drainage might be necessary, removal of the tumor results in avoidance of permanent ventricular-peritoneal shunting in 50% of cases. In some children with persistent hydrocephalus, third ventriculostomy is another option to avoid ventricular-peritoneal shunting. In nondisseminated patients, who comprise 70% to 80% of all patients with medulloblastoma, multiple studies have demonstrated that the extent of surgical resection is prognostic of outcome, with those patients undergoing more

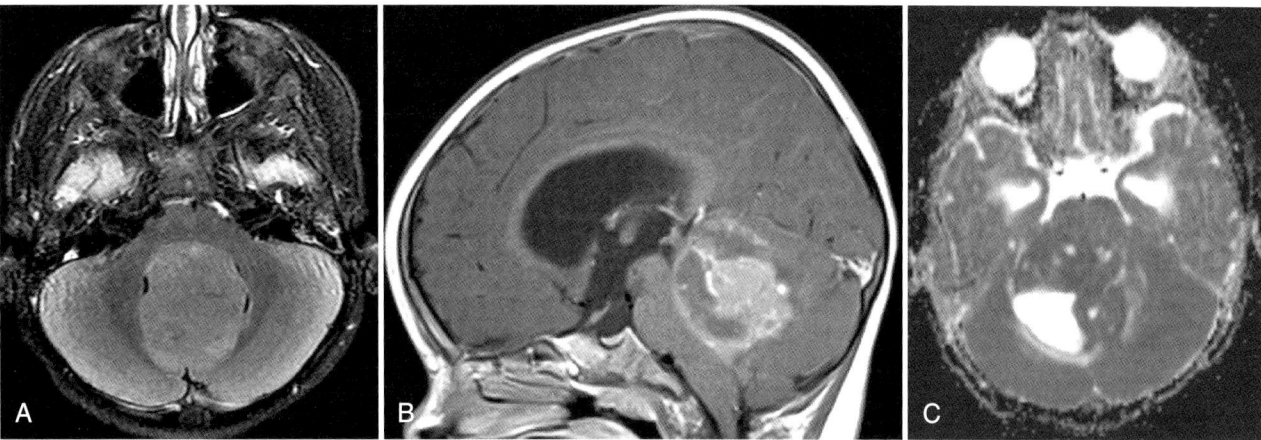

Figure 123-2. **Panel of MRIs of medulloblastoma. A,** Axial FLAIR image demonstrating somewhat hyperintense mass filling the fourth ventricle. **B,** Sagittal T-weighted image, after gadolinium enhancement, demonstrating inhomogeneous enhancement. **C,** Axial ADC image demonstrating diffuse restriction (dark area) within tumor.

complete or near-total resections having better outcome than patients whose tumors were subtotally resected. Arbitrarily, patients with greater than 1.5 cm^2 of residual disease after surgery are considered to have subtotally resected tumors. In older series, children with nondisseminated disease and greater than 1.5 cm^2 of residual disease fared less well than those with less measurable disease. With current means of adjuvant therapy, there is no clear-cut statistical difference in outcome between patients who undergo a total resection and those undergoing a near-total resection. Patients who undergo a minimal resection or biopsy have an extremely poor prognosis. In those with disseminated disease, the degree of surgical resection has never been shown to have independent significance.

Although the goal of surgery is to remove all of the tumor, tumor resections (be they partial or complete) can be associated with significant immediate or delayed postoperative complications (Wells et al., 2010). Direct brainstem and cerebellar damage has been noted in 5% to 10% of patients. Increasingly, posterior fossa mutism syndrome has been recognized. This syndrome can be clinically difficult to separate from postoperative direct damage to the brainstem and is a delayed constellation of mutism, which characteristically is first recognized between 6 and 48 hours after surgery. Mutism is usually associated with hypotonia, cerebellar deficits, supranuclear palsies, emotional lability, and severe irritability. The irritability and personality change may be so predominant that they overshadow the other clinical findings. Likely a form of cerebellar affective disorder, posterior fossa mutism syndrome is believed to be secondary to unilateral (primarily right-sided) or bilateral cerebellar dentate nuclei damage and/or disruption of critical pathways between the cerebellum and cortex. Subsequent MRIs, especially those performed 1 year or later after diagnosis, will frequently disclose cerebellar atrophy. Nearly 25% of patients in one recent North American trial had the syndrome, initially thought to be a rare entity, and one half of all patients with this syndrome had sequelae 1 year later. Over 50% of patients with posterior fossa mutism have impaired neurocognitive outcomes.

Staging and Stratification

Following surgery, patients with medulloblastoma have been traditionally staged by the amount of residual tumor after surgery, extent of dissemination assessed on both neuroimaging evaluation of the entire neuraxis and cerebrospinal fluid cytologic examination, and, in some classification schemes, histology. Historically, children with medulloblastomas who are 3 years of age or older at diagnosis have been classified as having either average-risk or poor-risk disease (see Table 123-2). Patients with average-risk disease are those with nondisseminated, totally or near-totally resected tumors, with a nonanaplastic histology. All other patients are considered to have poor-risk disease. This stratification system has not incorporated biologic data.

In younger children, separation into major risk groups on the basis of similar criteria is also accepted. Young children, usually less than 3 years of age, with extensively nodular/desmoplastic medulloblastoma, presumably whose tumors are driven by signaling of the SHH pathway, have a better prognosis.

Molecular studies that have identified the four stable molecular subgroups are being incorporated into stratification schema. It is now feasible to perform molecular subgrouping from very small amounts of formalin-fixed and paraffin-embedded tissue. These subgroups have distinct demographics and associated clinical variables, including disease course, and demonstrate enrichment for histopathological subtypes (e.g., desmoplastic and extensive-nodular medulloblastomas almost exclusively fall in the SHH subgroup, and Group 3 is strongly enriched for large-cell and anaplastic histiotypes).

As demonstrated in several independent studies, WNT-driven medulloblastoma (probably even when associated with microscopic metastases, i.e., M1) has a favorable clinical course. Recent evidence suggests that nuclear beta-catenin accumulation as assessed by immunohistochemistry alone is not specific enough to define this population. Thus the currently accepted recommendation is that any of two independent methods have to indicate the presence of a WNT-subgroup medulloblastoma to qualify for reduction of therapy intensity. These methods include CTNNB1 immunohistochemistry, sequencing of CTNNB1 exon 3, gene-expression profiling, and DNA methylation profiling.

SHH-driven medulloblastomas show a remarkable age distribution, with one peak in infants and a second peak in adults. Infant SHH disease is largely overlapping with infant desmoplastic or extensive nodular histology and associated with favorable prognosis. Most children with this subgroup can be cured by adjuvant chemotherapy alone. Because hereditary TP53 germline mutations (i.e., Li Fraumeni syndrome) are almost entirely restricted to SHH medulloblastoma, mainly in older children, p53 immunohistochemistry is required in all SHH subgroup patients as a screening measure. In case of evidence for the presence of a TP53 mutation, TP53 should be sequenced in the tumor. SHH-driven medulloblastomas in adults (which in this age group comprise about two thirds of cases, with tumors often located in the cerebellar hemispheres rather than in the vermis) demonstrate good outcomes. In infants, downstream SUFU mutations are quite prevalent in addition to PATCHED 1, whereas in older children with TP53 mutations, downstream amplifications of MYCN and GLI2 are prototypic (Kool et al., 2014).

Within Group 3, an additional marker to identify very-high-risk patients is high-level focal MYC amplification. As for CTNNB1, the detection method and definition of MYC amplification is crucial to identify this very-high-risk population.

Medulloblastoma risk categorization (see Table 123-2 and Fig. 123-4) is still a work in progress and has not been uniformly incorporated into national/international multicenter studies. However, the combination of molecular and clinical parameters (age and extent of dissemination at diagnosis) results in the clearest separations and opens the best possibility for more personalized therapies. The significance of extent of resection is unclear within this framework, although patients undergoing biopsy alone or a minimal resection likely have a poorer prognosis.

Postsurgical Management

Standard treatment for children with average-risk disease, over 3 years of age, includes radiation and chemotherapy. Survival rates improved dramatically when craniospinal irradiation therapy became a standard component of medulloblastoma treatment, independent of whether there was evidence on staging studies of dissemination. Initial doses of craniospinal radiation were chosen arbitrarily; conventionally, following surgery, average-risk patients were treated with 3600 cGy of craniospinal radiation and 1800 to 1960 cGy of boost radiotherapy to the primary tumor site, which, in most patients, included the entire posterior fossa (local tumor dose 5400-5580 cGy). With such treatment, 5-year progression-free survival rates were between 55% and 65%, with some, but not all, 5-year survivors being cured of their disease. Attempts to reduce the craniospinal dose of radiation therapy to 2340 cGy were considered unsuccessful because there was an increased early incidence of leptomeningeal disease failure; however, long-term follow up of the cohort of patients treated in a randomized study comparing 3600 cGy to 2340 cGy did not show a statistical difference in 8-year survival in patients treated with lower-dose radiotherapy compared with those who received higher-dose treatment.

Chemotherapy has improved survival for children with average-risk medulloblastomas (Packer et al., 2006; Gajjar

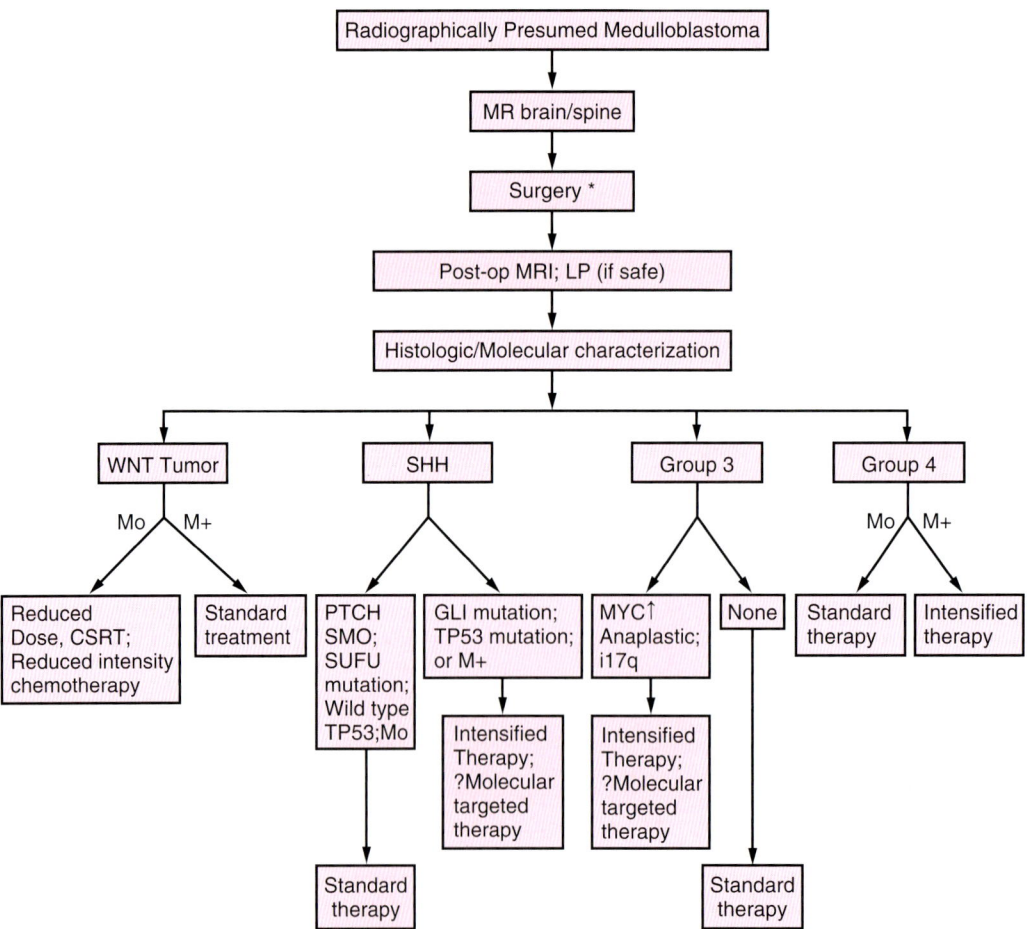

* Patients who are biopsied alone or undergo subtotal resections likely should be considered high risk and are candidates for re-resections or more intensified therapies.

Figure 123-4. Algorithm for medulloblastoma, children 3 years of age or older.

et al., 2006). Treatment with craniospinal radiation therapy and chemotherapy, given during and after radiation therapy and utilizing various multiagent drug regimens, which included vincristine (given during radiation therapy) and CCNU, cisplatin, cyclophosphamide, and vincristine post radiotherapy, has demonstrated progression-free survival rates at 5 years in the 80% to 85% range in children greater than 3 years of age without disseminated disease, with few patients relapsing after 5 years. The sequencing of radiation and chemotherapy seems critical; studies that have delayed radiation by the use of preradiation chemotherapy have demonstrated poorer survival rates.

The addition of chemotherapy has allowed a reduction of the dose of craniospinal radiation therapy to 2340 cGy without any apparent deterioration in overall disease control in children with average-risk disease. This reduction was undertaken to reduce radiation-associated sequelae, and ongoing prospective randomized studies are reducing the dose of craniospinal radiation therapy even further, to 1800 cGy. An important caveat with these studies is that the staging of patients is of extreme importance. Upon central review in two international studies, approximately 20% of patients were judged to have been inappropriately entered into these studies as a result of either misinterpretation of tumor extent or inadequate imaging. Patients who were placed on these reduced-dose craniospinal radiation studies with inadequate imaging or errors in interpretation had a significantly poorer outcome.

It has become clear that the molecular subtype of the tumor dramatically affects the likelihood of successful therapy (Gajjar et al., 2014). WNT-driven tumors have nearly a 100% survival rate after treatment with radiotherapy and chemotherapy. In this subset of patients, studies are already under way to further reduce the amount of craniospinal radiotherapy and/or chemotherapy utilized. For SHH-driven tumors, although infants and adults tend to fare well, children often harbor tumors with TP53 abnormalities and/or downstream SHH pathway mutations; such patients carry a poorer prognosis, which is less than 30% surviving with current therapies, and should not be considered "average risk." Within the Group 3 tumors, a subgroup with MYC-amplified or possibly overexpressed tumors will do poorly, even if identified by other criteria as "average risk," and will require alternative approaches.

For children with poor-risk medulloblastoma, survival after craniospinal and local boost radiotherapy alone is only in the 30% to 40% range at 5 years. Within the poor-risk group, there are mis-stratified children who carry a favorable diagnosis, such as those with WNT-subclass tumors with metastatic disease. Studies that have added chemotherapy, once again primarily either during and/or after radiation therapy, have demonstrated survival rates ranging between 50% and 70%. A variety of different chemotherapeutic approaches have been utilized and are still being studied, including the use of radiosensitizing agents, such as carboplatin, during radiation therapy, and a variety of drugs after radiation therapy, in various combinations, including cisplatin, CCNU, cyclophosphamide, vincristine, and etoposide.

For infants and young children with medulloblastoma, treatment remains quite problematic. Because of concerns regarding the detrimental long-term effects of craniospinal radiation therapy, chemotherapeutic approaches have been used to delay, if not completely obviate, the need for radiotherapy. Approximately 20% of infants can be treated with chemotherapy alone, with a variety of different regimens. These approaches have now evolved into the use of postoperative chemotherapy and, for those patients who remain in remission or respond to the initial chemotherapy, consolidation with even higher doses of chemotherapy supported by autologous bone marrow transplantation or peripheral stem cell rescue. Another approach to augment the efficacy of chemotherapy is to add methotrexate, in some studies intravenously at high dose and in other trials both intravenously and intrathecally/intraventricularly, to improve survival and avoid the need for radiation. It is likely the variable survival rates are a result of previously unappreciated differences in biologic subtypes. The infants most likely to survive are those with the nodular/desmoplastic form of the disease (Rutkowski et al., 2005). Survival for children with nonnodular/desmoplastic (SHH-driven) disease is not as favorable, but some (perhaps 30%) of these children do survive after treatment with chemotherapy alone. Treatment for infants and young children with disseminated disease remains suboptimal. Chemotherapeutic approaches alone have cured only a small group of these patients.

Relapsed Medulloblastoma

Another extremely problematic group of patients to treat for medulloblastoma are those with relapsed disease. Although late relapses, 5 or more years after diagnosis, are reported, it is likely that many of such relapses are secondary, treatment-induced tumors. The majority are high-grade gliomas and resistant to therapy. Histologic confirmation of the type of tumor present at relapse is required in late relapse or in patients with unusual patterns of recurrence, such as intrinsic brainstem disease or cortical infiltrative disease. Because of the nearly universal use of chemotherapy as a part of initial treatment, extraneural relapse is rare.

Given that the majority of older patients are now treated with both radiation therapy and multiagent chemotherapy at time of initial diagnosis, most children over 3 years of age with relapsed disease are highly resistant to further therapy. Furthermore, approximately two thirds of patients with medulloblastoma, be they high-risk, low-risk, or falling in the infant and young child category, will relapse with at least some component of disease outside the primary tumor site. Patients with SHH-driven tumors are more likely to have only primary-site relapse and may respond better to retrieval therapies such as reirradiation at the primary tumor site.

For patients with disseminated disease at relapse, there are no proven effective retrieval regimens. For children who have relapsed only at the primary tumor site, possibly because they are biologically different, retrieval strategies have been somewhat more successful and have included attempts at reresection followed by chemotherapy, followed by local radiotherapy. This approach has been most successful in young children who have not received prior radiation therapy.

Future Therapy

Newer approaches are clearly needed for both older children and infants with disseminated tumors, and possibly, in the future, for those with unfavorable prognostic molecular indicators. Biologic agents are slowly being incorporated into therapeutic trials using drugs such as retinoic acid as maturation agents and specific inhibitors of aberrant cellular signaling pathways, such as SHH pathway inhibitors. Adult SHH patients probably comprise the best cohort for adjuvant or even neo-adjuvant administration of targeted Smoothened inhibitors, because in this age group, SHH mutations upstream of Smoothened (mainly in Patched or Smoothened itself) are most prevalent.

Sequelae in Medulloblastoma Survivors

As more children survive medulloblastoma, it has become clearer that their quality of life is far from optimal. Although the dose of craniospinal radiation therapy has been reduced by almost one-third for patients with nondisseminated disease, it is yet unclear how beneficial such reductions are. At the same time, although the radiotherapy dose has been decreased, there has been an increased use of chemotherapy, which carries its own inherent short- and long-term side effects. In addition, the presence of posterior fossa mutism syndrome negatively affects outcome.

Neurocognitive sequelae are frequently seen in children of all ages treated for medulloblastoma. It has been well documented that the majority of infant survivors are neurocognitively impaired at the time of diagnosis, probably as a result of multiple factors, including the tumor, associated hydrocephalus, and possibly the sequelae of surgery. Although radiation therapy has been avoided in some infants who survived medulloblastoma, follow-up testing demonstrates that the majority remain developmentally and, ultimately, neurocognitively impaired. The addition of potentially neurotoxic drugs, such as methotrexate, to the treatment of these children or the early use of focal radiotherapy may further cause neurocognitive issues.

In children with medulloblastoma who are between 3 and 7 years of age at the time of treatment, significant declines in overall intelligence have been demonstrated after 3600 cGy of craniospinal radiation (Ris et al., 2001). This drop in intelligence can be seen as early as 1 year posttreatment, is progressive, and may not plateau over time. Decline in intelligence in those children treated at full-dose radiation therapy (3600 cGy) has ranged between 20 and 30 IQ points within 3 years of treatment. Preliminary results suggest a lesser decrease in overall intelligence in younger children who are treated with reduced doses (2340 cGy) of craniospinal radiation, but still a 10- to 20-point overall drop in global intelligence is likely. Older children have not demonstrated as severe a drop in global intelligence; however, these patients often have selective learning and attentional difficulties. Global intelligence is a crude estimate of intellectual function, and patients of all ages have been noted, in follow up, to have selective sequelae, including memory difficulties, processing dysfunction, executive functioning abnormalities, visual-spatial difficulties, and attentional disorders. The attentional problems are often overlooked because of the lack of associated hyperactivity. Many of these children are hypoactive, and studies are under way to determine whether the use of stimulants or other agents will decrease fatigue and lethargy and improve attention.

Endocrinologic sequelae are the second most common long-term consequence of medulloblastoma treatment. Growth hormone production is most commonly affected, but over time there can also be deficits in thyroid function, follicle-stimulating hormone–luteinizing hormone (FSH-LH) production, and adrenocortical function. Although there is hesitancy to utilize growth hormone replacement in children with cancer, studies in children with medulloblastoma have not shown an increased incidence of tumor relapse associated with its use. Growth hormone insufficiency is exacerbated by the direct effects of radiation on vertebral growth, and many long-term survivors have disproportionate growth, with a decrease in truncal growth compared with extremity growth. The effects on growth are also exacerbated by associated obesity, which is more common in long-term survivors (Packer et al., 2003).

Increasingly, secondary tumors have been reported in children who have survived brain tumors, including medulloblastomas. In a recent prospective Children's Oncology Group study of 379 children, 14 secondary malignancies occurred within 8 years of follow up, including multiple malignant gliomas. Because this patient population was less than 10 years from diagnosis at the time of the study, it is likely there will be an even greater rate of secondary tumor occurrence, especially the development of meningiomas, over time.

REFERENCES

The complete list of references for this chapter is available in the e-book at www.expertconsult.com.
See inside cover for registration details.

SELECTED REFERENCES

Gajjar, A., Chintagumpala, M., Ashley, D., et al., 2006. Risk-adapted craniospinal radiotherapy followed by high-dose chemotherapy and stem-cell rescue in children with newly diagnosed medulloblastoma (St Jude Medulloblastoma-96): long-term results from a prospective, multicentre trial. Lancet Oncol. 7 (10), 813.

Gajjar, A., Pfister, S.M., Taylor, M.D., et al., 2014. Molecular insights into pediatric brain tumors have the potential to transform therapy. Clin. Cancer Res. 20 (22), 5630.

Kool, M., Jones, D.T., Jager, N., et al., 2014. Genome sequencing of SHH medulloblastoma predicts genotype related response to smoothened inhibition. Cancer Cell 393.

Packer, R.J., Gajjar, A., Vezina, G., et al., 2006. Phase III study of craniospinal radiation therapy followed by adjuvant chemotherapy for newly diagnosed average-risk medulloblastoma. J. Clin. Oncol. 24 (25), 4202.

Packer, R.J., Gurney, J.G., Punyko, J.A., et al., 2003. Long-term neurologic and neurosensory sequelae in adult survivors of a childhood brain tumor: childhood cancer survivor study. J. Clin. Oncol. 21 (17), 3255.

Ris, M.D., Packer, R., Goldwein, J., et al., 2001. Intellectual outcome after reduced-dose radiation therapy plus adjuvant chemotherapy for medulloblastoma: a Children's Cancer Group study. J. Clin. Oncol. 19 (15), 3470.

Rutkowski, S., Bode, U., Deinlein, F., et al., 2005. Treatment of early childhood medulloblastoma by postoperative chemotherapy alone. N. Engl. J. Med. 352 (10), 978.

Taylor, M., Kool, M., Korshunov, A., et al., 2012. Molecular subgroups of medulloblastoma: the current consensus. Acta Neuropathol. 123 (4), 465–472.

Wang, J., Wechsler-Reya, R.J., 2014. The role of stem cells and progenitors in the genesis of medulloblastoma. Exp. Neuro. 260, 69–73.

Wells, E.M., Khademian, Z.P., Walsh, K.S., et al., 2010. Post-operative cerebellar mutism syndrome following treatment of medulloblastoma: Neuroradiographic features and etiology. J of Neurosurgery, Pediatric 5, 329.

E-BOOK FIGURES AND TABLES

The following figures and tables are available in the e-book at www.expertconsult.com. See inside cover for registration details.

Box 123-1 WHO classification of medulloblastoma.
Table 123-1 Stratification of Children over 3 Years of Age with Medulloblastoma
Fig. 123-1 Photomicrographs of medulloblastoma.
Fig. 123-3 MRI of medulloblastoma with dissemination.
Fig. 123-5 Improving survival rates for children with "average-risk" medulloblastoma treated in international, prospective randomized treatment trials by the Children's Cancer Group (CCG, now merged with POG to form the Children's Oncology Group) over past 24 years.

124 Other Embryonal and Pineal Malignancies of the Central Nervous System

Emily Gertsch, Yoon-Jae Cho, and Scott L. Pomeroy

 An expanded version of this chapter is available on www.expertconsult.com. See inside cover for registration details.

INTRODUCTION

Embryonal tumors of the central nervous system (CNS) are recognized as the most common types of malignant pediatric brain tumors. As a group, they are poorly differentiated, highly cellular tumors with aggressive growth behaviors (Li et al., 2009). They include medulloblastomas and atypical teratoid rhabdoid tumors (ATRTs), which are discussed in detail in their own chapters, and an evolving group of tumors formerly classified as primitive neuroectodermal tumors (PNETs). The PNET classification is being phased out; more recently these tumors have been reclassified as CNS embryonal tumors. These other CNS embryonal tumors include embryonal tumors with multilayered rosettes (ETMRs), medulloepithelioma, CNS neuroblastoma, CNS ganglioneuroblastoma, and CNS embryonal tumor Not Otherwise Specified (NOS). These types of CNS embryonal tumors are rare, accounting for approximately 3% of childhood brain tumors. Their rarity combined with their substantial heterogeneity has resulted in a poor understanding of these tumors. However, classification of these tumors is rapidly evolving based on molecular profiling studies, and the mechanisms driving tumorigenesis of these CNS embryonal tumors are just beginning to be recognized.

Historically, CNS embryonal tumors have been treated with protocols used to treat medulloblastoma, perhaps a by-product of these tumors' similar histologic appearances. However, outcomes for patients with CNS embryonal tumors other than medulloblastomas have remained uniformly poor. This has led to the appreciation that these tumors respond poorly to medulloblastoma-based therapies and highlights the need for a better definition of the clinical, histologic, and genetic characteristics of these tumors to appropriately tailor effective therapies for patients.

CLINICAL PRESENTATION

CNS embryonal tumors generally involve the frontal, temporal, and parietal lobes, more so than the deep or posterior fossa structures, and clinical manifestations are dependent on the site of tumor origin. Most children present with nonspecific complaints such as headache, nausea, vomiting, and problems with balance, all of which are manifestations of increased intracranial pressure (ICP). Complications of increased ICP include herniation, and care should be taken to approach lumbar puncture with extreme caution (or avoid completely) if an intracranial lesion is suspected. Other clinical manifestations of a supratentorial tumor might include motor deficits, alteration of consciousness, and seizures. Deeper-seated tumors such as those involving the pineal region may present with Parinaud's syndrome from compression of the pretectal region. Tumors in the suprasellar region may result in visual disturbances and/or endocrine abnormalities. Posterior fossa tumors may present with ataxia, cranial nerve deficits, and signs and symptoms of increased ICP.

TYPES OF CNS EMBRYONAL TUMORS

Embryonal Tumors with Multilayered Rosettes

Embryonal tumors with multilayered rosettes (ETMRs) were first identified in 2000 by Eberhart et al. as a distinct type of supratentorial embryonal tumor. Ependymoblastoma, formerly classified as a distinct entity, has been reclassified as being within the category of ETMR. These tumors, which also are known as embryonal tumors with abundant neuropil and true rosettes (ETANTRs), are rare CNS embryonal tumors that typically arise in the cerebrum but are occasionally seen in the cerebellum and brainstem. They occur in very young children (Ryzhova et al., 2011) and have a slightly higher predominance in girls than in boys (Gessi et al., 2009). Neuroimaging of an ETMR shows a large, well-delineated, solid mass with heterogeneous contrast enhancement (Gessi et al., 2009). Some tumors demonstrate a cystic component (Figure 124-1).

Their histologic characteristics are very distinctive and include focal high cellularity with abundant bands of neoplastic neuropil and the presence of both true rosettes and pseudorosettes (Louis et al., 2007) (Figure 124-2). These tumors are distinguished by high-frequency focal amplification at chromosome locus 19q13.42 of the *C19MC* oncogenic microRNA cluster, often associated with high levels of expression of LIN28 (Li et al., 2009; Ceccom et al., 2014). It has recently been shown that *C19MC* amplification occurs as a fusion of *C19MC* with the promoter of *TTYH1*, a brain-specific gene that encodes a chloride channel. The *TTYH1* promoter is highly active, driving high levels of *C19MC* expression, which in turn activates *DNMT3B*, a DNA methyl transferase that modulates the cells to induce a state of dedifferentiation and, ultimately, tumorigenesis (Kleinman et al., 2014). Thus the high-level amplicon activates a primitive developmental mechanism as part of the oncogenic mechanism (Archer and Pomeroy, 2014).

The prognosis of ETMR is exceptionally poor, with median survival of less than 1 year despite aggressive treatment.

Medulloepithelioma

The most common site of origin for medulloepitheliomas is the periventricular region in the cerebrum. These tumors are typically quite large in size and may involve multiple lobes in one or both cerebral hemispheres. They sometimes occur intraventricularly and can be seen in sellar, infratentorial, and spinal regions, and in the optic nerve.

Their histologic features include neural tube formation, including papillary, tubular, or trabecular arrangements of neoplastic neuroepithelium. These rare malignant tumors are seen primarily in young children between the ages of 6 months and 5 years, and half occur in children less than 2 years old (Louis et al., 2007). There is an equal distribution between males and females.

Medulloepitheliomas have variable neuroimaging characteristics. They are generally well circumscribed and may be isodense or mildly hypodense on computed tomography (CT). Magnetic resonance imaging (MRI) shows hypointense or isointense lesions on T1-weighted sequences and hyperintense lesions on T2-weighted sequences. The tumors may not enhance with intravenous contrast on initial presentation but tend to enhance later as disease progresses (Figure 124-3). Calcifications and cysts are not typical features but have been reported. Medulloepitheliomas are often well circumscribed and have hemorrhagic and necrotic areas. They are frequently diffusely infiltrative in advanced disease.

These tumors have distinctive histopathologic features mimicking the embryonic neural tube, with pseudostratified epithelium arranged in papillary, tubular, or trabecular patterns. They may contain elements of glial, neural, and mesenchymal cell lines. The mitotic index is high, with a high rate of cellular proliferation, and both ependymoblastomatous and ependymal rosettes may be seen.

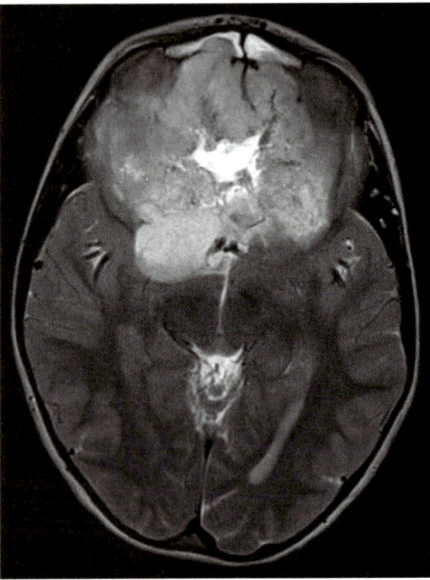

Figure 124-1. Axial T2-weighted MRI of ETANTR showing a large, well-circumscribed heterogeneous-appearing bifrontal mass. Note that the tumor extends into the frontal sinuses, an aggressive feature.

The prognosis of medulloepithelioma is very poor. Cerebrospinal dissemination is common at the time of death, which most often occurs within 1 year of diagnosis.

CNS Embryonal Tumors Not Otherwise Specified

CNS embryonal tumors NOS are highly heterogeneous and may be difficult to distinguish from other high-grade tumors by histology alone (Picard et al., 2012). They may arise in the suprasellar region and deep structures, although they are most commonly found in the cerebrum. The mean age of patients with CNS embryonal tumor NOS is 5.5 years, with a range of 4 weeks to 20 years, and there is a slight male predominance (1.2 : 1) (Louis et al., 2007).

CNS embryonal tumors NOS appear isodense or hyperdense on CT. They may have cystic or necrotic areas, and many of these tumors have calcifications. On MRI, cystic and necrotic areas appear hyperintense on T2-weighted imaging, whereas solid portions of the tumor appear hypointense relative to gray matter on both T1- and T2-weighted imaging (Figure 124-4). The tumors typically enhance with gadolinium contrast. Cerebrospinal dissemination occurs in up to one-third of patients, and metastasis to extraneural sites, including bone, liver, and cervical lymph nodes, has been infrequently reported (Louis et al., 2007).

On histologic examination, these tumors are poorly differentiated, with Homer Wright rosettes often found in varying frequency, and with undifferentiated small anaplastic cells with minimal differentiation of the cell body. GFAP expression is occasionally detected by immunohistochemical techniques. Proliferation as measured by Ki-67 is typically high but may vary extensively. At times the tumors are difficult to distinguish histologically from other malignant supratentorial tumors, including CNS neuroblastomas, which have neuronal differentiation, or CNS ganglioneuroblastomas, which are poorly differentiated tumors that additionally contain differentiated neuronal cells.

The molecular features of CNS embryonal tumors NOS are poorly understood, and molecular profiling studies have revealed that many tumors initially diagnosed as CNS embryonal tumors NOS by histology are actually ETMRs/ETANTRs, glioblastomas, or ATRTs (Picard et al., 2012). Nevertheless, despite this molecular heterogeneity, all of these diagnoses share a poor clinical prognosis even with aggressive treatment, including neurosurgical resection, external beam radiation, and prolonged multidrug chemotherapy. Children less than 2

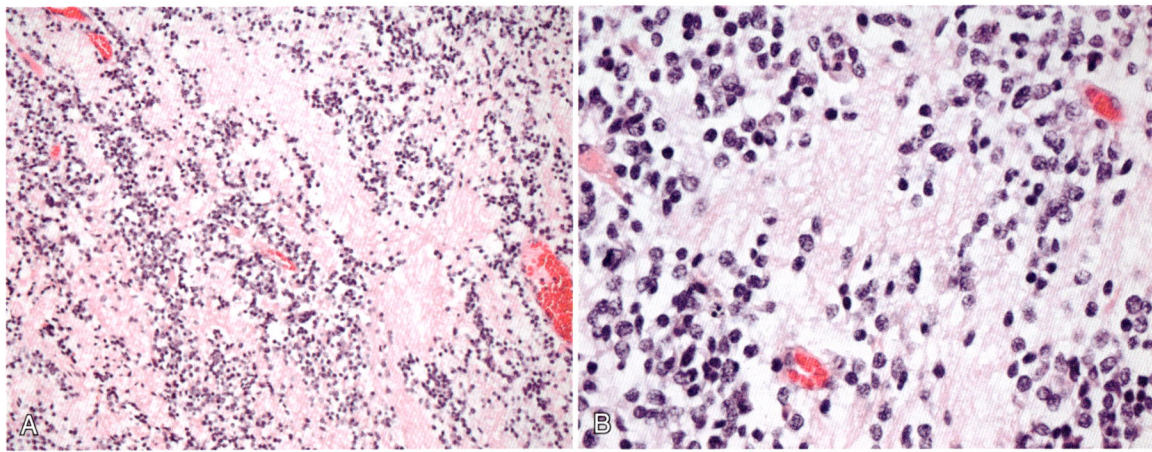

Figure 124-2. Histopathologic features of ETANTR showing abundant bands of neuropil with rosettes and pseudorosettes.

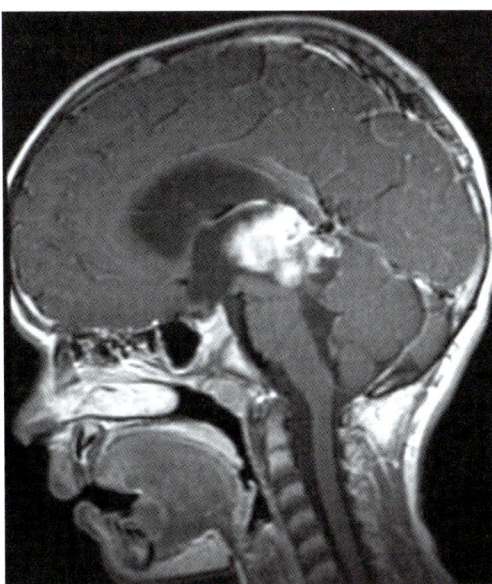

Figure 124-3. Sagittal T1-weighted postcontrast image of a pineal-region medulloepithelioma. Compression of the aqueduct causes the obstructive hydrocephalus.

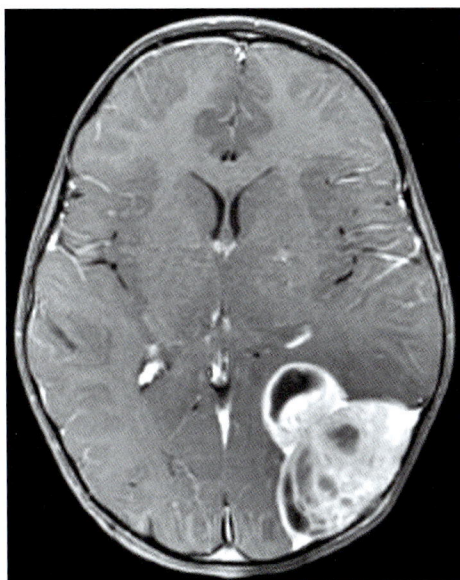

Figure 124-4. Axial T1-weighted postcontrast MRI of a left parieto-occipital CNS embryonal tumor showing heterogeneous enhancement. Note that the tumor involves both cortex and white matter and extends through the skull into the subperiosteal space.

years of age at the time of diagnosis have worse clinical outcomes compared with older children.

TREATMENT AND OUTCOMES

Treatment is typically multimodal and includes surgical resection, followed by irradiation appropriate for age and risk stratification, and chemotherapy (McGovern et al., 2014), although standard treatment regimens have not been established. Generally, gross total resection is a common feature of long-term survivors. One study showed good disease outcomes for a small cohort of young patients less than 5 years of age with CNS embryonal tumor NOS who received

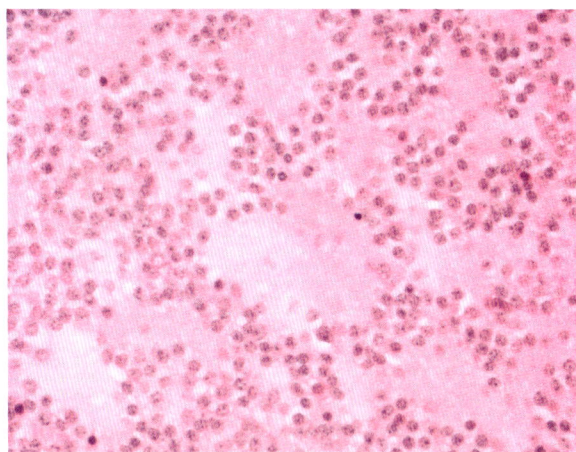

Figure 124-5. Histopathologic features of pineocytoma showing small, well-differentiated cells with low mitotic index.

chemotherapy followed by proton radiation (Jimenez et al., 2013). Overall, however, patients with supratentorial embryonal tumors have very poor clinical outcomes and low survival rates.

PINEAL TUMORS

Pineal tumors are tumors of pineal parenchymal origin that arise in the region of the pineal gland. They are relatively rare and heterogeneous. The two primary types of pineal tumors are pineocytomas and pineoblastomas.

Pineocytomas

Pineocytomas are tumors of pineal parenchymal lineage histologically classified as World Health Organization (WHO) grade I tumors. They are primarily seen in adults and rarely occur in children. Pineocytomas typically arise in the pineal area. They may extend into the posterior third ventricle and compress adjacent structures.

Pineocytomas appear as hypodense, globular, well-defined masses, with occasional cystic components, peripheral calcifications, or hemorrhagic foci seen on CT. MRI shows a well-circumscribed mass that is isointense on T1-weighted sequences and hyperintense on T2-weighted sequences. Tumors demonstrate homogeneous contrast enhancement.

Histopathologic features of pineocytomas include small, well-differentiated cells reminiscent of pineocytes that grow in sheets or lobules (Figure 124-5). In addition, large pineocytomatous rosettes are often seen. Mitotic index is usually low, and microcalcifications are sometimes present.

Pineoblastoma

Pineoblastomas are rare aggressive tumors of pineal parenchymal origin classified as WHO grade IV tumors based on histologic features. They more commonly occur in children, with the majority of pineoblastomas diagnosed in the first two decades of life (Louis et al., 2007). There is equal distribution between males and females.

Pineoblastomas appear as contrast-enhancing, large, ill-defined, lobulated masses on CT. Masses are hypointense or isointense on T1-weighted MRI. Cystic changes and calcifications are infrequently seen (Figure 124-6).

Cerebrospinal and leptomeningeal dissemination, and local infiltration, are common for these poorly delineated tumors. They are comprised of highly cellular small cells that

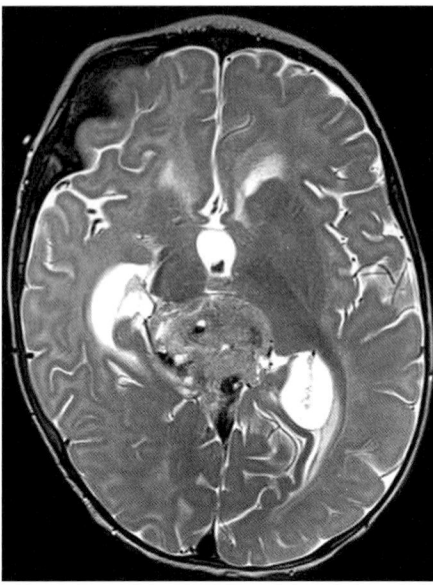

Figure 124-6. T2-weighted axial image of a pineoblastoma showing a hypointense lesion, indicating hypercellularity, with intralesional hemorrhage.

are compactly arranged. Pineocytomatous rosettes are absent, whereas Flexner-Wintersteiner rosettes and Homer Wright rosettes are more typically seen. Tumors tend to exhibit necrosis and high mitotic activity.

Trilateral retinoblastoma syndrome describes the occasional presence of pineoblastoma in patients with bilateral retinoblastoma. Prognosis in patients who have aberrations in the *RB1* gene is even less favorable than that for patients with sporadic occurrence. Pineoblastoma has also been reported to occur in patients with familial adenomatous polyposis (Louis et al., 2007).

TREATMENT AND OUTCOMES

Treatment of pineal tumors typically includes a combination of surgical resection, irradiation, and chemotherapy. Given the location of these tumors, it is also important to manage the hydrocephalus commonly associated with pineal tumors.

The clinical prognosis of patients with pineocytoma is generally quite favorable. Pineocytomas are not known to metastasize. Five-year survival ranges from 86% to 100%, and there have been no relapses reported for patients who undergo a gross total resection (Louis et al., 2007).

In contrast, pineoblastomas are extremely aggressive tumors associated with poor clinical outcomes, particularly when seen in trilateral retinoblastoma syndrome. Craniospinal dissemination is common, as is leptomeningeal seeding, and metastasis to extracranial sites can occur. Survival largely depends on extent of disease at diagnosis and the extent of resection and radiation therapy. Patients with familial and sporadic trilateral retinoblastoma rarely survive beyond 1 year

after diagnosis, and patients who develop recurrent disease have an especially poor prognosis (Farnia et al., 2014).

SUMMARY

In conclusion, embryonal tumors found in the supratentorial compartment represent, for the most part, histologically similar yet molecularly heterogeneous groups of tumors whose classification (and nomenclature) is rapidly evolving. Despite their molecular heterogeneity, they share in common an aggressive clinical course that is generally refractory to conventional chemotherapy and radiotherapy schedules. As our understanding of the genetic underpinnings of these diseases rapidly evolves, so too will our ability to more effectively treat them.

REFERENCES

The complete list of references for this chapter is available in the e-book at www.expertconsult.com.
   See inside cover for registration details.

SELECTED REFERENCES

Archer, T.C., Pomeroy, S.L., 2014. A developmental program drives aggressive embryonal brain tumors. Nat. Genet. 46 (1), 2–3.

Ceccom, J., Bourdeaut, F., Loukh, N., et al., 2014. Embryonal tumor with multilayered rosettes: diagnostic tools update and review of the literature. Clin. Neuropathol. 33 (1), 15–22.

Eberhart, C.G., Brat, D.J., Cohen, K.J., et al., 2000. Pediatric neuroblastic brain tumors containing abundant neuropil and true rosettes. Pediatr. Dev. Pathol. 3 (4), 346–352.

Farnia, B., Allen, P.K., Brown, P.D., et al., 2014. Clinical outcomes and patterns of failure in pineoblastoma: a 30-year, single-institution retrospective review. World Neurosurg. 82 (6), 1232–1241.

Gessi, M., Giangaspero, F., Lauriola, L., et al., 2009. Embryonal tumors with abundant neuropil and true rosettes: a distinctive CNS primitive neuroectodermal tumor. Am. J. Surg. Pathol. 33 (2), 211–217.

Jimenez, R.B., Sethi, R., Depauw, N., et al., 2013. Proton radiation therapy for pediatric medulloblastoma and supratentorial primitive neuroectodermal tumors: outcomes for very young children treated with upfront chemotherapy. Int. J. Radiat. Oncol. Biol. Phys. 87 (1), 120–126.

Kleinman, C.L., Gerges, N., Papillon-Cavanagh, S., et al., 2014. Fusion of TTYH1 with the C19MC microRNA cluster drives expression of a brain-specific DNMT3B isoform in the embryonal brain tumor ETMR. Nat. Genet. 46 (1), 39–44.

Li, M., Lee, K.F., Lu, Y., et al., 2009. Frequent amplification of a chr19q13.41 microRNA polycistron in aggressive primitive neuroectodermal brain tumors. Cancer Cell 16 (6), 533–546.

Louis, D.N., Ohgaki, H., Wiestler, O.D., et al., 2007. WHO Classification of Tumours of the Central Nervous System, fourth ed. International Agency for Research on Cancer (IARC), Lyon, France, p. 312.

McGovern, S.L., Grosshans, D., Mahajan, A., 2014. Embryonal brain tumors. Cancer J. 20 (6), 397–402.

Picard, D., Miller, S., Hawkins, C.E., et al., 2012. Markers of survival and metastatic potential in childhood CNS primitive neuroectodermal brain tumours: an integrative genomic analysis. Lancet Oncol. 13 (8), 838–848.

Ryzhova, M.V., Zheludkova, O.G., Ozerov, S.S., et al., 2011. A new entity in WHO classification of tumors of the central nervous system–embryonic tumor with abundant neuropil and true rosettes: case report and review of literature. Zh Vopr Neirokhir Im N N Burdenko 75 (4), 25–33, discussion.

125 Ependymoma

Richard Grundy and Nicholas K. Foreman

 An expanded version of this chapter is available on www.expertconsult.com. See inside cover for registration details.

INTRODUCTION

Ependymomas are enigmatic tumors, and despite advances in neurosurgery, neuroimaging, and postoperative adjuvant therapy, their clinical management remains one of the more difficult in pediatric neuro-oncology.

INCIDENCE AND EPIDEMIOLOGY

Ependymomas are the second commonest malignant brain tumor occurring in children, accounting for approximately 10% of all such tumors. They have a predilection for young age at onset; indeed, over half of intracranial ependymomas arise in children under 5 years of age. There is slight male preponderance. Children with ependymoma have a worse outcome than adults.

Childhood ependymomas predominantly arise in the intracranial compartment, in contradistinction to the situation for adults, in whom spinal origin predominates. Approximately two-thirds of childhood intracranial tumors arise in the posterior fossa, where they are intimately associated with the fourth ventricle. Signs and symptoms at presentation are consequent on obstruction of cerebrospinal fluid (CSF) movement. The most common presentation is nonspecific with raised intracranial pressure, but patients may present with cerebellar or lower cranial nerve dysfunction. In very young children, irritability and lethargy may be the only presenting symptoms. The duration of these symptoms before presentation varies greatly depending on site and may be prolonged, particularly in spinal tumors (Box 125-1).

LOCATION

Ependymomas probably arise from the ependymal lining of the ventricles and lining of the central canal. However, ependymomas may arise anywhere in the neuraxis, and supratentorial tumors are frequently not related to ventricular cavity. Dissemination via CSF is reported in 7% to 22% of cases. Spinal ependymomas may occur as intramedullary or as intradural extramedullary tumors. The latter arise predominantly of the caudal region (filum terminale) and are usually of the myxopapillary histologic subtype (Box 125-2).

PATHOLOGY

The World Health Organization (WHO) 2016 (Ellison et al., 2016) classification defines grades I through III, with classic ependymoma (grade II) and anaplastic ependymoma (grade III) being prevalent (Box 125-2). A new entity of supratentorial ependymoma a has been added defined by the presence of a RELA-fusion gene, comprising 80% of supratentorial ependymomas. Consistent histologic differentiation of ependymoma between Grade II and grade III has proven difficult because a spectrum of pathologic features exists (Wiestler et al., 2000). It is likely that grade will be determined by a combined morphologic and molecular profile in the near future.

DIAGNOSTIC EVALUATION
Imaging Studies

The imaging of intracranial ependymoma is challenging. On magnetic resonance imaging (MRI), ependymomas typically display iso- to hypointensity on T1-weighted images and hyperintensity on T2-weighted images. They usually enhance heterogeneously with gadolinium. Fourth-ventricle ependymomas can often be distinguished from medulloblastoma radiographically by their tendency to "squeeze" through the foramina of Luschka and Magendie. Complete neuraxis imaging is essential to exclude leptomeningeal disease, even in spinal tumors because these occasionally metastasize to the brain. An unresolved issue is exactly what surveillance protocol is optimal for children with ependymomas to maximize detection of recurrence without unduly wasting resources. The detection of asymptomatic recurrences through routine surveillance does appear to confer some benefit. A widely accepted strategy is acquiring an MRI every 3 to 4 months for up to 2 to 3 years and less frequently until age 6 to 7 years. MRI-visible spinal metastatic disease in the absence of intracranial metastases is uncommon.

PROGNOSTIC FACTORS

Although a number of prognostic factors have been identified, these tend to be based on single-institution retrospective series involving limited numbers of patients accrued over a time span covering many different approaches to both the diagnosis and treatment of ependymoma.

However, the most widely accepted prognostic factor is the degree of surgical resection. Axiomatically, gross total resection is associated with a better prognosis.

Older children (above 3 years of age) appear to have a better prognosis, with a 5-year survival rate of 55% to 83% compared with 12% to 48% for children under 3 years of age. In this regard, factors likely to be important include surgical accessibility and a general reluctance to irradiate very young children. However, it is possible this difference is based on biology, with molecular stratification into two distinct subtypes of ependymoma, groups A and B, with a poorer outcome in group A, more commonly seen in the very young (Witt et al., 2011).

Supratentorial location is thought more favorable despite these tumors often being extensive at diagnosis. Based on small numbers, there is a possibility that completely resected grade II supratentorial ependymomas have a particularly favorable outlook. Recent work suggests that in supratentorial tumors, the presence or absence of *RELA* gene fusions may have prognostic significance (Parker et al., 2014).

Tumor Grade

Despite a number of studies, the relationship between histologic grading and tumor outcome is unclear. Some studies have found that the presence of anaplasia carries a worse

BOX 125-1 Symptoms and Signs of Intracranial Ependymoma

Headache
Nausea and vomiting
Lethargy
Behavioral changes
Slurred speech/visual disturbance
Papilledema
Cranial nerve palsies
Ataxia
Cerebellar signs
Torticollis

SYMPTOMS AND SIGNS OF SPINAL EPENDYMOMA

Pain: localized (backache) and radicular (sciatica)
Gait disturbance
Weakness
Sensory change
Bladder/bowel dysfunction
Spastic paraparesis
Hyperreflexia
Suspended sensory level
Scoliosis

BOX 125-2 World Health Organization (2016) Classification of Ependymal Tumors

WHO GRADE II AND III

Ependymoma
  papillary ependymoma
  clear-cell ependymoma
  tanycytic ependymoma
RELA fusion Positive
Anaplastic ependymoma

WHO GRADE I

Myxopapillary ependymoma
Subependymoma

With permission from Ellison DW, McLendon R, Wiestler OD, Kros JM, Korshunov A, Ng H-K, Witt H, Hirose T. Ependymoma. In: Louis DN, Ohgaki H, Wiestler OD, Cavanee WK, eds. WHO Classification of Tumours of the Central Nervous System, 4th Edition. Lyon, France: IARC Press, 2016

TABLE 125-1 Examples of Genetic Heterogeneity Between Spinal and Intracranial Ependymomas

Intracranial	Spinal
Up-regulation of RAF-1	Up-regulation of PLA2GS, ITIH2, and members of HOX family
Altered expression of Protein 4.1 members	Altered expression of Protein 4.1 members
CDKN2A down-regulated (see Table 125-2)	CDKN2A up-regulated
Loss of chromosomes 22, 3, 6q, 9p, 10q, 13q, and 16q	Loss of chromosomes 1, 2, 10, and 22q12
Gain of chromosomes 1q, 7, and 9q	Gain of chromosomes 7, 9, 11, 18, and 20
Tenascin C, NELL, and LAMMA	Somatic NF2 mutations (adult and spinal tumors only)

TABLE 125-2 Genetic and Epigenetic Heterogeneity Between Ependymoma From Different Intracranial Locations

Supratentorial	Posterior Fossa
Overexpression of EPHB-EPHRIN, Notch cell signaling pathways, and genes involved in the cell cycle	Loss of chromosomes 22, 6, and 17q
Genomic loss of 9p more common, resulting in loss of TSG CDKN2A (p14ARF) and P16^{INK4A}.	High degree of epigenetic silencing of the 17p tumor-suppressor gene HIC-1
C11orf95-RELA (types 1-7) fusion C11orf95-YAP1 fusion	Loss of chromosome 6q CPG island methylator phenotype positive and negative

structural tumors showed few, mainly partial, imbalances. A second numerical group showed 13 or more chromosome imbalances, with a nonrandom pattern of whole chromosome gains and losses that are also highly associated with adult ependymoma. The third group showed a balanced genetic profile that was significantly associated with a younger age at diagnosis, suggesting that ependymomas arising in infants are biologically distinct from those occurring in older children (Kilday et al., 2009). There is a correlation between the structural group and group A, as identified by array technology.

Overall, pediatric ependymomas most frequently demonstrate gain of chromosomes 1q, 7, and 9 and loss of chromosomes 22, 3, 9p, 13q, 6q, 1p, 17, and 6, whereas the commonest genomic aberrations in adult ependymomas are gain of chromosomes 7, 9, 12, 5, 18, X, and 2 and loss of 22/22q, 10, 13q, 6, and 14q (Table 125-1).

One of the most striking differences between the two age groups analyzed by CGH is the genomic gain of 1q seen in over 20% of pediatric ependymomas but in only 8% of adults. Importantly, the genomic imbalances found in adult and spinal ependymomas regularly involve whole chromosomal rearrangements; in contrast, partial and complex imbalances are frequently seen in pediatric cases. Indeed, a recent meta-analysis of pediatric and adult ependymoma revealed marked differences, underscoring the point that these should be considered separate conditions (Kilday et al., 2009).

Comparing childhood intracranial ependymomas from different locations has revealed significant genetic diversity. It has also been suggested that posterior fossa ependymomas can be subdivided based on their gene expression profiles (Witt et al., 2011) (Table 125-2).

prognosis, whereas others have found no difference. The lack of uniformity in the grading system used across series makes it difficult to conclude which histologic features are prognostic.

GENETICS

It has been postulated that embryonic neural stem cells (NSCs) arising from different parts of the central nervous system are transformed by different gene mutations, thereby giving rise to biologically distinct types of ependymoma. For example, *RELA* gene fusions are common in supratentorial ependymomas but virtually absent in fourth-ventricle tumors (Parker et al., 2014). Radial glia-like cancer stem cells have been proposed as the candidate cell of origin for supratentorial and spinal ependymoma.

Cytogenetics

Comparative genomic hybridization (CGH) studies have identified three broad groups of tumors. The first group of

Whole-genome sequencing of supratentorial and posterior fossa ependymomas, with the aim of identifying driver mutations of these tumors, has recently been performed (Parker et al., 2014; Mack et al., 2014). Both studies found very few single-nucleotide variations (SNVs), insertion/deletions, or focal (<5 genes) copy-number variations in ependymomas. The paucity of SNVs in ependymoma led to scrutiny of the epigenome in ependymoma.

Epigenetic Phenomena

There is growing evidence that epigenetic deregulation is involved in pediatric cancers, and recent research has suggested this may be important in ependymoma. The DNA methylation profile can be used to segregate ependymomas according to anatomic location, and supratentorial and spinal tumors display a more hypermethylated phenotype. A more recent study using higher-resolution DNA methylation analysis has identified two distinct groups of posterior ependymomas: group A, which have a much greater extent of CpG island methylation and Group B. Group A tumours predominantly have stable genomes and present predominantly in in very young children and have a poor outcome. The methylated genes in PFA-CIMP converge on genes that are silenced in embryonic stem cells by the Polycomb repressive complex 2 (PRC2) (Mack et al., 2014).

These data suggest that drugs that target DNA CpG methylation, PRC2/EZH2, and/or histone deacetylase inhibitors could represent a rational strategy for treatment of PFA-CIMP ependymoma.

In summary, there is a pressing need to identify robust biomarkers in ependymomas to define biologically relevant subclasses that will, in turn, help to stratify patient management.

Biomarkers

Difficulty in predicting tumor behavior from clinical and histologic factors has shifted the focus to the molecular and cellular biology of ependymoma to identify new correlates of disease outcome and potentially novel therapeutic targets. Several candidate biomarkers have been proposed. However, markers showing reproducible results in prospective and sizeable groups of young ependymoma patients treated in a consistent way within clinical trials are still required (Kilday et al., 2012). Indeed, several purported biologic prognostic markers have lost significance when assessed across clinical trial cohorts, highlighting the importance of analyzing any prospective marker in standardized therapeutic groups (Kilday et al., 2012). To date, only two biomarkers (1q gain [Kilday et al., 2012] and Tenascin C [TNC]) have been evaluated in retrospective national clinical trial cohorts of childhood ependymoma.

It is clearly unlikely that a single biomarker will represent the complex biology and varied clinical presentation of ependymoma, and defining the molecular determinants of the clinical biology of this intriguing disease is the next major task.

TREATMENT OF EPENDYMOMA

Once the acute presentation has been stabilized, it is widely accepted that surgical resection should be the initial treatment, with the aim of gross total resection; a second surgical procedure may be warranted to achieve a gross total resection, albeit mindful of surgical morbidity. However, ependymomas arising in the fourth ventricle have the propensity to adhere to and invade the brainstem and to extend through the foramen of Luschka, enveloping the lower cranial nerves and making complete surgical resection without morbidity difficult. The extent of surgery must be assessed postoperatively by MRI; if there is still residual tumor, referral to a major center to evaluate the need for further surgery should be undertaken—such is the importance of complete resection.

It is now widely accepted that adjuvant therapy is required in most patients with ependymoma and probably all patients with fourth-ventricle tumors. Research is ongoing to define which patients may be spared further treatment. The closed large trial (ACNS 0121) from the Children's Oncology Group will soon answer important questions related to the role of observation after gross total resection for grade II supratentorial ependymoma.

Concerns over the late effects of cranial irradiation in very young children have led a number of national groups to use adjuvant chemotherapy to avoid or delay radiation. There has been divergence between Europe and North America in the age at which focal radiation is considered acceptable, being as young as 1 year of age in North America but generally being over the age 3 in Europe. The large but unreported Children's Oncology Group trial ACNS 0121 radiated focally down to 1 year of age, but long-term toxicity data are not available for this trial.

ACNS 0121 accrued more than 350 patients between August 2003 and September 2007. It explored the role of chemotherapy to achieve complete resection at second surgery after initial subtotal resection. However, for initially completely resected, nonmetastatic ependymomas, this study used radiation without chemotherapy.

Chemotherapy

Chemotherapy has a role in the management of ependymoma, although this remains a controversial area. There is increasing evidence that a proportion of ependymomas are chemoresponsive, but debate exists over the degree of response, and a convincing role for chemotherapy has still to be demonstrated. This in part reflects the difficulties in interpretation of postchemotherapy imaging, and more sophisticated imaging studies are now needed. Early studies from the Pediatric Oncology Group (POG) reported a response rate of 48% in infants using a combination of vincristine and cyclophosphamide. However, this finding was based on computed tomography (CT) imaging. More recently, the Children's Cancer Group (CCG) study 9942 was reported, which used chemotherapy in children with initial incomplete resections before radiation and showed a 57% complete or partial response to this therapy. The outcomes for those treated with chemotherapy for incompletely resected tumor were equivalent to outcomes for those with completely resected tumors who did not receive adjuvant chemotherapy. This benefit was restricted to those who had at least 90% of the tumor resected.

The question of whether chemotherapy is of benefit to children with completely resected tumors postradiation has not been answered, but this is being explored in the Children's Oncology Group (COG) study ACNS 0831 and the international SIOP Ependymoma II study.

Furthermore, it is now clear that a proportion of infants can be cured following adjuvant chemotherapy without the use of radiotherapy (Geyer et al., 2005; Grundy et al., 2007; Strother et al., 2014). Similar results were reported from the U.S. children's CCG (CCG-9921) and the POG, with both reporting "radiotherapy" event-free survival of over 40% (Geyer et al., 2005). although, at least in the CCG data, the extent of resection was a very significant contributor to overall cure and survival for nonmetastatic patients. An important observation was the beneficial effect of dose intensity on event-free survival.

A recent study by the Head Start group, which used myeloablative therapy in newly diagnosed ependymoma to avoid radiotherapy, did not demonstrate outcomes superior to reported chemotherapeutic strategies.

Chemotherapy may improve outcome by enabling second-look surgery. Prospective studies to confirm or refute this are awaited.

In summary, there is increasing evidence that in a proportion of cases, ependymomas are chemo-responsive and chemo-curable. The systematic analysis of tumor specimens may provide useful information as to which tumors would benefit from chemotherapy, which from radiotherapy alone, and perhaps even which can be observed.

Current recommendations for chemotherapy in ependymoma include the following: (i) infants when the aim is to delay or avoid radiotherapy because of concerns about neurocognitive outcomes, particularly those under 12 to 18 months of age, and (ii) patients with residual tumor after initial surgery. Importantly, it remains necessary to define which drugs are active in ependymoma; this might be best achieved through phase II window studies in patients with residual disease postsurgery, as proposed in the new European study (SIOP Ependymoma). Another important question to be addressed is whether the addition of chemotherapy to radiotherapy improves the cure rate, as has been demonstrated in medulloblastoma. Defining which patients are likely to benefit from chemotherapy, which from radiation therapy, and which from both is clearly an important goal, albeit a significant challenge as well.

Radiation Therapy

Postoperative radiation therapy to the tumor bed is an important component in the treatment of localized ependymoma, and its role in the treatment of very young children is changing. Newer radiotherapy methods that incorporate three-dimensional imaging have improved treatment. Only two decades ago, ependymoma was treated with surgery and postoperative craniospinal irradiation with or without chemotherapy. The long-term event-free survival was less than 40%, and most patients experienced primary site progression because a high proportion had a residual tumor at the time of irradiation. Because of concerns about neuraxis dissemination, especially in patients with high-grade tumors, 36Gy craniospinal irradiation was administered to many patients, and 54Gy was prescribed to the primary tumor site using conventional techniques that irradiated large volumes of normal tissue. Survivors treated with craniospinal irradiation experienced debilitating side effects. Craniospinal irradiation was abandoned when investigators learned that neuraxis dissemination at the time of diagnosis was uncommon, and tumor grade was no longer used to determine the treatment volume.

The ability of newer treatment methods to limit the highest dose to the tumor bed and spare normal tissues has been objectively demonstrated in a recent prospective trial (Merchant et al., 2009). Eighty-eight children with ependymoma, including 48 children under the age of 3 years at the time of irradiation, were treated at St. Jude Children's Research Hospital with conformal radiation therapy to 54 to 59.4 Gy using a 1-cm clinical target volume margin surrounding the postoperatively defined tumor bed. Preliminary results reveal a 3-year progression-free survival of 75% ±6% (Merchant et al., 2009). Patients were serially evaluated using objective measures of cognitive function that included testing of IQ, memory, academic achievement, and adaptive behavior. No decline in cognitive function was observed among these patients. However, a subsequent study by the same group suggested attention and school problems in these children postradiation and that these were associated with age at diagnosis and at administration of conformal radiation (Willard et al., 2014). It is essential to obtain long-term data about the effects of radiation on academic and behavioral function and cognition into early adulthood.

A spectrum of complications with various levels of severity has been observed for patients treated with radiation therapy, including cognitive decline, hearing loss, endocrine deficits, and abnormalities in growth and development. Rare but devastating complications such as symptomatic vasculopathy, brain and spinal cord necrosis, and secondary malignancies have been reported. Although functional outcomes after radiation therapy are directly related to the age of the patient at the time of irradiation and morbidity associated with the tumor and surgical intervention, there is a statistically significant relationship between cognitive function after radiation therapy and dosimetry to the supratentorial brain.

Cranio-spinal irradiation is reserved for the treatment of patients with obvious neuraxis dissemination from intracranial or spinal primary tumors. Although the curability of patients with metastatic ependymoma has never been convincingly demonstrated, long-term survivors have been reported. The effectiveness of craniospinal irradiation is likely to be related to the extent and bulk of neuraxis dissemination, ranging from cytologic involvement of CSF to isolated ventricular or spinal metastases to bulky tumor filling the subarachnoid spaces.

Spinal cord ependymomas in children are rare; when completely resected, they do not require radiation therapy. In the setting of incomplete or piecemeal resection, radiation therapy is most often indicated. Treatment of spinal cord ependymoma is challenging and requires detailed neuraxis staging and delineation of the extent of disease. The known association of NF2 and ependymoma should prompt evaluation for suspected metastatic or multifocal disease.

Experimental Therapy

It is possible that the success of targeted therapeutic agents has been limited, in part, as a result of the focus of early-phase clinical trials on molecular aberrations in primary ependymoma, with little understanding of the biology of relapsed disease. A better understanding of the biology at relapse is needed to improve therapy at this critical event.

The use of immunotherapy is being studied in ependymoma. This has some rationale given the potential influence of the difference in the immune microenvironment on prognosis. There is currently a study using vaccination with tumor antigen peptides for ependymoma ongoing in Pittsburgh, but it is too early to know its results.

Recurrence and Patterns of Failure

The majority of recurrences occur as a result of the failure of local tumor control and are identified between 9 and 24 months after therapy. However, an increasing number of distant failures are being recorded in patients treated with conformal radiotherapy to the primary site. The prognosis for relapse is relatively poor; overall, only 25% of children survive first or subsequent relapses (Messahel et al., 2009). Survival at first relapse may be better if it is local only with complete excision of the recurrence and reirradiation, but this needs longer follow-up to be certain.

Relapsed ependymoma presents distinct challenges. Increasingly, children are experiencing multiple relapses and treatments before finally succumbing to the disease. Although children may be salvaged a number of times, the law of diminishing returns applies, and there are few long-term survivors of multiple relapses. Importantly, ependymomas may recur several years after seemingly successful therapy, and long follow-up of 10 to 15 years is essential.

Treatment options following relapse depend on initial treatment. Surgery should always be considered in patients with local recurrence, as should irradiation for infants in whom radiotherapy was not given as part of the primary treatment. The role of chemotherapy in relapse remains uncertain, and international studies are now required.

In the absence of effective salvage therapy, reirradiation in various forms has been considered for patients who relapse after their initial course of radiation therapy. Single-dose radiosurgery and fractionated external-beam reirradiation have both been employed successfully in patients with local recurrence after radiation therapy. The indications for reirradiation and the selection of the best modality are generally based on the feasibility of performing additional surgery at the time of relapse, the presence or absence of residual disease, and the perceived tolerance of the tissues to be encompassed within the reirradiated volume. There have been studies showing prolonged remissions, and potentially cures, after complete surgery and reirradiation for locally recurrent tumor. For unexplained reasons, time to second remission after reirradiation was longer than time to first progression. The benefit of reirradiation may, however, be dependent partly on the biology of tumor, with much better outcomes for children with group B tumors than younger ones with group A disease. Unpublished experience (NKF) would suggest that reirradiation is of very limited benefit when there is substantial residual mass; when it is done within 1 year from prior radiation, it may have unacceptable morbidity.

More challenging is the use of reirradiation in patients who fail with disseminated disease after prior focal irradiation. The options for these patients range from single or multifocal radiosurgery to craniospinal irradiation. In patients with limited metastatic burden and for whom metastasectomy can be performed, craniospinal irradiation with overlap of the primary site is preferred. Shielding of the previously irradiated spinal cord may be indicated.

SUMMARY

Important issues remain to be addressed in childhood ependymoma. Importantly, we need to reach an international consensus on whether, and which, biological characteristics of this tumor determine outcomes and whether there are distinct biological subgroups, as was previously done for medulloblastoma. This has been rendered difficult by very the different median age of patients in large studies. The relationship of biology to traditionally important prognostic factors such as extent of surgery and tumor grade needs more definition. We need to investigate novel imaging methods for assessing chemosensitivity, investigate active chemotherapy or biological agents, and assess the long-term outcomes and side effects of conformal radiotherapy through multicenter studies (Box 125-4).

Significant challenges for the years ahead include defining the place for chemotherapy in completely resected ependymoma and in the very young. New agents need to be developed, using the insights obtained from biological discovery, and then rapidly tested in relapsed cohorts of patients.

There is a clear need to better understand the underlying biology of this disease to improve the therapeutic options and outcomes.

BOX 125-4 Ongoing Issues in Ependymoma

Improving duration of response and reducing local failure
Defining prognostic factors
Understanding Biology
Defining Biomarkers for treatment stratification
Assessing chemosensitivity—role of new imaging techniques
Surgical issues
Role chemotherapy—Which patients/ which agents / dose intensity
Role of radiotherapy—Proton versus Photon and age
Neuropsychological outcome—
Treatment of relapse—International agreement on relapse strategy

---

REFERENCES

The complete list of references for this chapter is available in the e-book at www.expertconsult.com.

   See inside cover for registration details.

SELECTED REFERENCES

Ellison, D.W., McLendon, R., Wiestler, O.D., et al., 2016. Ependymoma. In: Louis, D.N., Ohgaki, H., Wiestler, O.D. (Eds.), WHO Classification of Tumours of the Central Nervous System, fourth ed. IARC Press, Lyon, France.

Geyer, J.R., Sposto, R., Jennings, M., et al., 2005. Multiagent chemotherapy and deferred radiotherapy in infants with malignant brain tumors: a report from the Children's Cancer Group. J. Clin. Oncol. 23 (30), 7621–7631. PubMed PMID: 16234523.

Grundy, R.G., Wilne, S.A., Weston, C.L., et al., 2007. Primary postoperative chemotherapy without radiotherapy for intracranial ependymoma in children: the UKCCSG/SIOP prospective study. Lancet Oncol. 8 (8), 696–705. PubMed PMID: 17644039. eng.

Kilday, J.P., Mitra, B., Domerg, C., et al., 2012. Copy number gain of 1q25 predicts poor progression-free survival for pediatric intracranial ependymomas and enables patient risk stratification: a prospective European clinical trial cohort analysis on behalf of the Children's Cancer Leukaemia Group (CCLG), Societe Francaise d'Oncologie Pediatrique (SFOP), and International Society for Pediatric Oncology (SIOP). Clin. Cancer Res. 18 (7), 2001–2011. PubMed PMID: 22338015.

Kilday, J.P., Rahman, R., Dyer, S., et al., 2009. Pediatric ependymoma: biological perspectives. Mol. Cancer Res. 7 (6), 765–786. PubMed PMID: 19531565. [Epub 2009/06/18]. eng.

Mack, S.C., Witt, H., Piro, R.M., et al., 2014. Epigenomic alterations define lethal CIMP-positive ependymomas of infancy. Nature 506 (7489), 445–450. PubMed PMID: 24553142.

Merchant, T.E., Li, C., Xiong, X., et al., 2009. Conformal radiotherapy after surgery for paediatric ependymoma: a prospective study. Lancet Oncol. 10 (3), 258–266. PubMed PMID: 19274783. [Epub 2009/03/11]. eng.

Messahel, B., Ashley, S., Saran, F., et al., 2009. Relapsed intracranial ependymoma in children in the UK: patterns of relapse, survival and therapeutic outcome. Eur. J. Cancer 45 (10), 1815–1823. PubMed PMID: 19427780. [Epub 2009/05/12]. eng.

Parker, M., Mohankumar, K.M., Punchihewa, C., et al., 2014. C11orf95-RELA fusions drive oncogenic NF-kappaB signalling in ependymoma. Nature 506 (7489), 451–455. PubMed PMID: 24553141.

Strother, D.R., Lafay-Cousin, L., Boyett, J.M., et al., 2014. Benefit from prolonged dose-intensive chemotherapy for infants with malignant brain tumors is restricted to patients with ependymoma: a report of the Pediatric Oncology Group randomized controlled trial 9233/34. Neuro Oncol. 16 (3), 457–465. PubMed PMID: 24335695. Pubmed Central PMCID: 3922508.

Willard, V.W., Conklin, H.M., Boop, F.A., et al., 2014. Emotional and behavioral functioning after conformal radiation therapy for pediatric ependymoma. Int. J. Radiat. Oncol. Biol. Phys. 88 (4), 814–821. PubMed PMID: 24462384. Pubmed Central PMCID: 4261227.

Witt, H., Mack, S.C., Ryzhova, M., et al., 2011. Delineation of two clinically and molecularly distinct subgroups of posterior fossa ependymoma. Cancer Cell 20 (2), 143–157. PubMed PMID: 21840481.

⊗ E-BOOK FIGURES AND TABLES

The following figures and tables are available in the e-book at www.expertconsult.com. See inside cover for registration details.

Fig. 125-1: Proposed staging system for posterior fossa ependymoma.

Fig. 125-2: Transverse T2-weighted magnetic resonance image of fourth-ventricle ependymoma.

Fig. 125-3: Transverse T2-weighted and postcontrast T1-weighted magnetic resonance images of left hemispheric ependymoma.

Table 125-3: Putative oncogenes and tumor suppressor genes involved ependymoma development

Box 125-3 Magnetic Resonance Imaging Features

126 Pediatric Brain Tumors – High-Grade Glioma

Sabine Mueller and Matthias A. Karajannis

An expanded version of this chapter is available on www.expertconsult.com. See inside cover for registration details.

INTRODUCTION

Gliomas are tumors of the central nervous system (CNS) that arise from glial precursors and most commonly are differentiated along the astrocytic or oligodendroglial lineages. Gliomas may occur at all ages and throughout the entire neuraxis. Traditionally, gliomas have been grouped into two main categories according to histologic features: low-grade gliomas (LGGs) and high-grade gliomas (HGGs). This is also reflected in the current World Health Organization (WHO) classification, which distinguishes low-grade (WHO grade I/II) and high-grade (WHO grade III and IV) gliomas. The current WHO classification of HGGs is summarized in Table 126-1.

HGGs are relatively rare in children and comprise approximately 4% of all brain tumors diagnosed in children aged 0 to 14 years and up to 14% in children aged 10 to 19 years. Histologically, the vast majority of pediatric HGGs are either anaplastic astrocytomas (WHO grade III) or glioblastomas (WHO grade IV).

A unifying feature of HGGs is the diffusely infiltrative nature of the disease, representing a major therapeutic challenge. Diffuse intrinsic gliomas (DIPGs) are HGGs arising in the brainstem, and they are discussed in detail in Chapter 129. The molecular features and dismal clinical outcome of DIPGs are highly similar to those of other pediatric HGGs arising in other anatomic midline structures of the CNS, such as thalamic or spinal cord HGGs. As a result, these "midline pediatric HGGs" can be viewed as comprising a spectrum within a single clinico-pathologic entity.

A number of inheritable tumor predisposition syndromes have been found to be associated with HGGs. Patients with Li–Fraumeni syndrome (LFS), an autosomal-dominant condition caused by mutations in the tumor suppressor p53, have an increased risk of developing HGGs (Schwartzentruber et al., 2012). Patients with the autosomal-recessive constitutional mismatch repair deficiency syndrome (CMMR-D) frequently have café-au-lait macules similar to neurofibromatosis type 1 (NF1), resulting in occasional misdiagnosis. CMMR-D is caused by germline biallelic (homozygous or compound heterozygous) mutations in one of the DNA mismatch repair (MMR) genes MLH1, MSH2, MSH6, and PMS2. Germline monoallelic mutations in MMR genes are also found in hereditary nonpolyposis colon cancer, Lynch syndrome, and brain tumor polyposis syndrome type 1 (BTPS1 or Turcot type 1). Patients with CMMR-D are at increased risk for development of HGGs and other brain tumors, typically within the first 2 decades of life.

CLINICAL PRESENTATION

The initial clinical presentation of children with HGGs greatly depends on the anatomic location of the tumor and the age of the patient. The clinical history is typically short, with signs or symptoms of focal neurologic dysfunction, such as weakness or seizures.

DIAGNOSIS AND INITIAL MANAGEMENT

In patients with imaging features consistent with an HGG, maximum safe surgical resection most often is the initial therapeutic step. Depending on location, resection might not be feasible, and a biopsy is performed to establish the diagnosis. It is important to recognize that small biopsy samples may not be fully representative of the entire tumor. Postoperative imaging should be performed within 24 hours after surgery. Leptomeningeal dissemination in pediatric HGGs is rare (approximately 3%) at presentation, but later on occurs in over 20% of patients. Therefore, imaging of the entire neuraxis should be performed either routinely or at least in patients with a clinical suspicion of spinal involvement.

Histopathology and Molecular Pathology

Neuropathology of pediatric brain tumors has changed significantly as a result of deeper understanding of molecular biology. Although the most recent 2007 WHO classification is still based predominantly on histopathology alone and pediatric HGGs are embedded within the adult HGGs, the molecular data indicate that adult and pediatric HGGs are biologically distinct.

In children, two main histopathological and clinical variants of HGGs are recognized. Whereas supratentorial glioblastoma multiforme (GBM) is histologically, albeit not molecularly, similar to its adult counterpart, DIPGs can range in histologic features from diffuse astrocytoma, WHO grade II, to GBM, WHO grade IV, despite aggressive behavior across all grades. Histologic criteria show little, if any, correlation with clinical outcome.

Most pediatric HGGs develop as a result of somatic mutations. The number of somatic mutations in children is relatively low compared with adult GBM (61 mutations per sample); however, it is higher than in many other pediatric cancers, with a median of 15 nonsynonymous coding mutations per sample in both DIPGs and noninfant HGGs. The genomic complexity of pediatric HGGs spans a wide range, with infant HGGs showing extremely low numbers of mutations, with a median of 2. On the opposite side of the spectrum are HGGs from patients with mismatch repair abnormalities, which show the highest mutational burden of all tumors, with a median of 6810 nonsynonymous coding mutations per sample (Jones and Baker, 2014).

Pediatric HGGs show genetic alterations in the same canonical cancer pathways that are affected in adult GBM, including the PI3K pathway, the TP53 pathway, and the RB pathway; however, there are specific differences in what part of the pathway may be affected. For example, PI3K mutations are found in both pediatric and adult tumors. Loss of PTEN function via deletion and/or mutation is rare in pediatric HGGs. The BRAF-V600E mutation is found in approximately 10% of pediatric supratentorial HGGs but is rare in adult gliomas.

TABLE 126-1 World Health Organization Classification of High-Grade Glial Tumors

Astrocytic Tumors	Oligodendroglial and Oligoastrocytic Tumors
Anaplastic Astrocytoma (III)	Anaplastic oligodendroglioma (III) Anaplastic oligoastrocytoma (III) Pleomorphic xanthoastrocytoma with anaplastic features (III)
Glioblastoma (IV), including giant-cell glioblastoma and gliosarcoma	

(Adapted from Luis, D.N. Ohgaki, H. Wiestler, O.D., et al. [Eds.], 2007. WHO Classification of Tumors of the Central Nervous System, 4th ed. Lyon, France: International Agency for Research on Cancer.)

Up to 50% of HGGs in children show some DNA structural abnormalities. The copy-number-variation landscape in pediatric HGGs is highly variable and can range from stable genomes to simple rearrangements and complicated multifocal abnormalities caused by chromothripsis. In addition to the previously mentioned BRAF tandem duplication, NTRK1, 2, and 3 fusions are typically involved and can be the sole molecular aberration, particularly in infant HGGs.

Receptor tyrosine kinases (RTKs) are the most commonly amplified genes both in pediatric and adult HGGs. Whereas EGFR is the most common RTK amplified in adult primary GBM (up to 40% of cases), it is rare in pediatric gliomas. Only 10% to 15% of cases of adult GBM show amplifications and/or mutations of PDGFRa, whereas it is the most commonly mutated RTK in pediatric HGGs, with approximately 30% of pediatric diffuse gliomas showing amplification and/or mutation (Paugh et al., 2013). Amplification of MET and IGF1R and mutations in FGFR1 were also found in pediatric HGGs (Wu et al., 2014). Mosaic heterogeneity described in adult GBM (Snuderl et al., 2011), in which different RTK genes are amplified in a mutually exclusive fashion, has also been described in pediatric gliomas, with coexisting glioma subclones harboring either PDGFRa or MET amplification.

Approximately 55% of pediatric HGGs harbor mutations of the TP53 gene. Up to 20% of DIPGs and midline HGGs carry mutations in PPM1D, which functions downstream of p53 (Taylor et al., 2014). Mutations of TP53 and PPM1D are mutually exclusive in HGGs.

The RB pathway is less commonly affected in pediatric HGGs compared with adult HGGs. Homozygous deletions of CDKN2A are found in approximately 25% of supratentorial HGGs, although they are rare in DIPGs. Amplification of the components of the cyclin–CDK complex were identified across all the subgroups of HGGs from all brain regions. Homozygous loss of function in RB is extremely rare in pediatric HGGs; however, loss of chromosome 13q is found in approximately one third of pediatric HGGs, regardless of location.

In striking contrast to adult gliomas, the most prevalent molecular alterations of pediatric HGGs involve recurrent alterations of genes regulating epigenetic modifications of the genome (Schwartzentruber et al., 2012). Genome-wide studies identified recurrent hotspot mutations in H3 histone, family 3A (H3F3A) and histone cluster 1, H3b (HIST1H3B), which encode the histone H3 variants H3.3 and H3.1, respectively. This was the first example of a human tumor or other disease driven by direct mutation of histones. Point mutations of H3F3A and HIST1H3B genes occur at hotspots, either at amino acid residue 27, resulting in a lysine-to-methionine (K27M) amino acid change, or 34, resulting in either a

glycine-to-arginine (G34R) or glycine-to-valine (G34V) amino acid change. Mutations lead to marked changes of the epigenome, resulting in distinct methylation signatures. The H3.3 mutations are mutually exclusive with IDH1/2 mutations, which are most commonly observed in diffuse gliomas of young adults. Interestingly, both IDH1/2 and H3.3 mutations seem to drive oncogenesis via genome-wide epigenomic changes. The different H3 histone mutations present at different ages, with a median of 6 to 7 years for K27M mutants and a median of 13 to 14 years for G34R/V mutants. Furthermore, survival seems to be different as well. The median survival of patients with the G34R/V mutation is 24 months, whereas K27M-mutated tumors are associated with worse survival, with a median of 12 months. Although these mutations are characteristic of pediatric HGGs, H3 variant mutations can be present in young adult gliomas as well.

In addition to the mutations in the genes encoding the histone variants, other chromatin regulators can also be mutated in pediatric HGGs. Although more prevalent in adult low-grade diffuse gliomas and secondary GBM, the ATRX or DAXX genes are mutated in approximately 20% of pediatric HGGs, often with concurrent G34 mutations (Schwartzentruber et al., 2012; Wu et al., 2014). ATRX and DAXX mutant tumors are strongly associated with a telomerase-independent alternative lengthening of telomeres in pediatric HGGs (Schwartzentruber et al., 2012). Mutations of the telomerase reverse transcriptase TERT promoter, which represent different mechanisms to lengthen telomeres and are typically found in primary adult GBM, are rare in pediatric HGGs. Additional mechanisms to alter the epigenome found in pediatric HGGs include mutations in variety of genes, such as SETD2, MLL, and CHD, further stressing the complexity of epigenetic interactions in these tumors (Wu et al., 2014).

The association between certain molecular aberrations and tumor site has long been appreciated, and points to developmental rather than carcinogenic origins of pediatric HGGs. Whereas histone H3.3 G34R or G34V mutations and BRAF-V600E mutations are predominantly found in supratentorial hemispheric tumors, histone H3 K27M mutations are found in midline tumors, including tumors of the thalamus and brainstem, with the highest frequency in DIPGs. In midline tumors, FGFR1 mutations are found in thalamic HGGs, whereas ACVR1 mutations are restricted to DIPGs. Furthermore, PIK3CA and PIK3R1 mutations, as well as FGF1R and MET amplifications, are prevalent in DIPGs, whereas loss of CDKN2A and NF1 aberrations are more prevalent in supratentorial GBM. In contrast to adult GBM, loss of PTEN is not common in pediatric HGGs, and IDH1/2 mutations are most common in the frontal lobes, whereas H3.3 G34R or G34V are most common in other lobes (Jones and Baker, 2014).

The previously mentioned molecular findings present challenges both for diagnosis and clinical management. Given the molecular heterogeneity of pediatric HGGs, genome-wide and in situ methods are necessary to assess the molecular profile for prognostic and predictive markers. Technically, this stratification can be best achieved by a combination of genome-wide DNA methylation profiling and targeted methods such as sequencing or immunohistochemistry for verification. In situ hybridization methods should also be used for assessment of focal gene amplifications and tumor heterogeneity.

Imaging

Magnetic resonance imaging (MRI) is an essential tool in the diagnosis and treatment of brain tumors, and is considered the current imaging standard for any child with a brain tumor. A complete series should include the following sequences: T1-weighted axial and coronal (both before and after gadolinium), T2-weighted axial and coronal, and fluid-attenuated inversion recovery (FLAIR). In addition, sagittal plane sequences are helpful in defining the anatomy of suprasellar and midline tumors. Other sequences, such as fat suppression and magnetic resonance (MR) angiography, may also be required in specific situations. Contrast-enhanced neuro-imaging of the entire neuraxis should be considered as baseline evaluation for any child with a brain tumor. On T1-weighted images, HGGs often demonstrate central areas of low density corresponding to necrosis and are typically poorly circumscribed. The peritumoral edema surrounding most HGGs appears as a hyperintense region of signal abnormality on T2-weighted images. Most centers also include diffusion-weighted images in their standard imaging protocol, and evidence exists that in addition to enhancement and presence of necrosis, a low apparent diffusion coefficient is a predictor for HGG.

Metabolic Imaging

Proton MR spectroscopy (MRS) is a powerful and sensitive technique that can be added to any standard MR study and allows the measurement of the relative composition of different metabolites, including N-acetyl-aspartate (NAA), choline, creatine, lipid, and lactate. MRS can be useful to differentiate tumor from normal tissue, to help stratify neoplasms as high- or low-grade tumors, and to distinguish between treatment injury and recurrent neoplasm. An HGG is often associated with lower levels of NAA and creatine and higher levels of choline and lactate (see Fig. 126-1). Further, MRS spectra of childhood brain tumors at first relapse do not differ

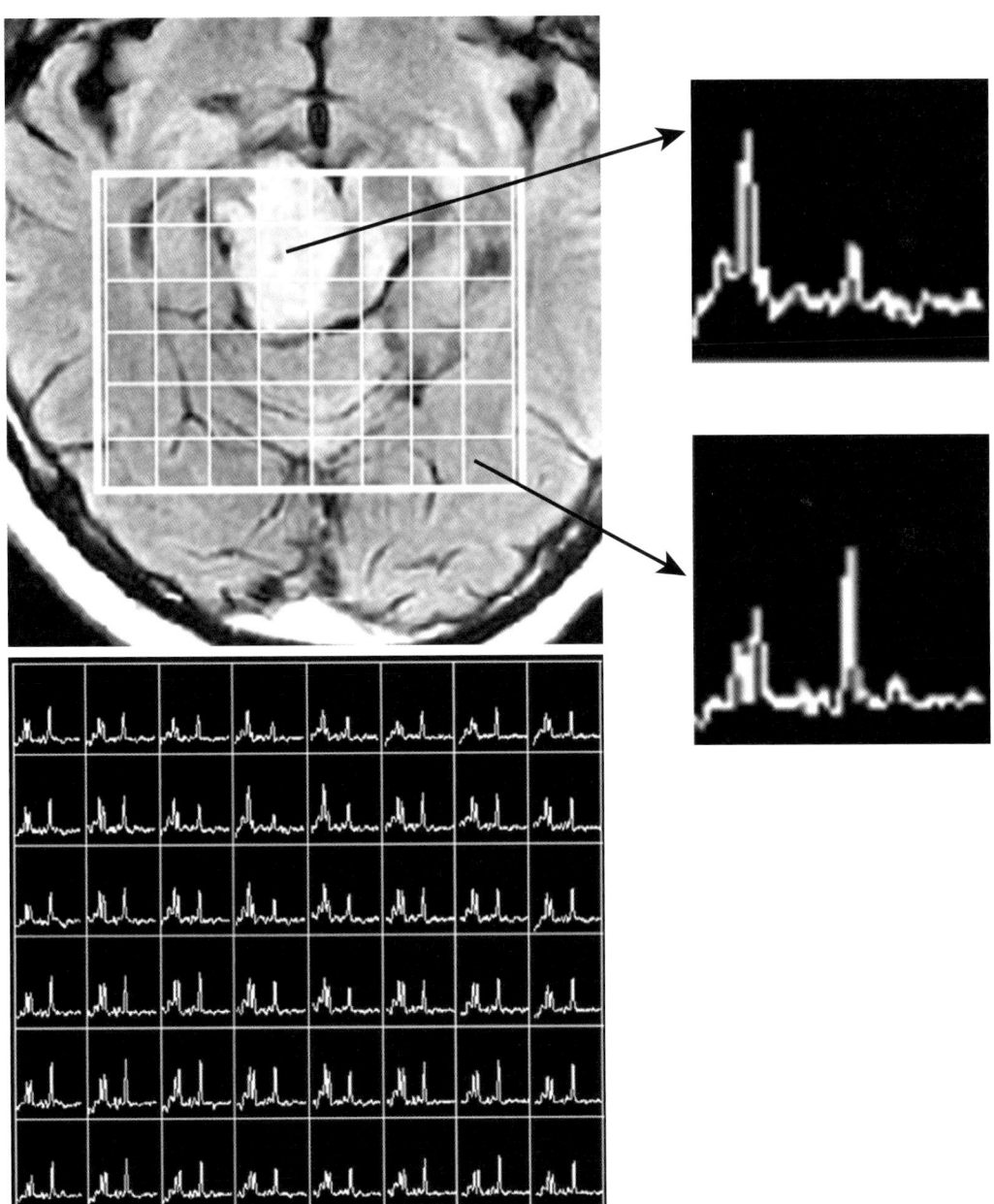

Figure 126-1. Axial fluid-attenuated inversion recovery (FLAIR) image and magnetic resonance spectroscopy (MRS) from an 18-year-old child with infiltrative glioma. The locations for which spectra are reconstructed are shown by the grid. **(A)** shows a typical MRS pattern of tumor with high choline (Cho) and creatine (CR) and low N-acetyl-aspartate (NAA), in contrast to **(B),** which depicts a typical MRS pattern from a normal brain with low Cho/CR and high NAA peak.

significantly from those at initial diagnosis, making MRS effective in helping to distinguish between tumor recurrence versus treatment-related changes. In most centers MRS is now a standard part of the initial evaluation of a lesion concerning for a primary brain tumor and often is added if there is ambiguity of tumor recurrence versus treatment-related changes.

Future directions include novel metabolic imaging using hyperpolarized ^{13}C MR metabolic imaging. Hyperpolarized ^{13}C MR metabolic imaging is a promising new technology that offers an exciting method of assessing in vivo metabolism, with a greater than 10,000-fold signal enhancement over conventional ^{13}C MR methods. Preclinical studies of GBM xenograft tumors demonstrated that pyruvate can be used to monitor the rate and magnitude of conversion to lactate, which is elevated in tumors as a result of increased activity of the enzyme lactate dehydrogenase (LDH). Of particular interest is that reductions in the ratio of lactate/pyruvate can be observed in as little as 1 to 2 days after treatment with temozolomide (Park et al., 2014). This novel technology has been successfully applied to adult patients with prostate cancer, and is currently being evaluated in adult patients with glioblastoma.

Perfusion Magnetic Resonance Imaging

Perfusion MRI is a relatively new technology that provides information on cerebral hemodynamic parameters such as relative cerebral blood volume (rCBV) and cerebral blood flow (CBF). Perfusion MR studies can be obtained using either endogenous (arterial water) or exogenous (gadolinium) contrast agents (Cha et al., 2002). Imaging with dynamic susceptibility contrast (DSC) perfusion MRI is based on the principles of tracer kinetic modeling to determine the cerebral microvasculature and is one of the most commonly used techniques for perfusion quantification. The basic principle of perfusion MRI exploits the signal changes during bolus passage of a contrast agent through the cerebral vessels, and these values are then used to generate perfusion maps of various hemodynamic parameters.

Clinical applications for DSC perfusion MRI include grading of brain tumors, guiding biopsies, distinguishing therapy-related brain injury from residual or recurrent tumor, and predicting clinical outcome. Recently, perfusion MRI technology has also been assessed to predict survival in response to antiangiogenic therapy. Dedicated pediatric studies have shown that this technique can be successfully applied to children with high-grade tumors. However, DSC perfusion MRI results should be interpreted with caution in heterogeneous tumors because cCBV can vary depending on the location. A region of interest placed in an area of necrosis or more benign portion of the brain tumor could erroneously underestimate rCBV and result in undergrading of tumor. Alternatively, cortically based neoplasms that are contiguous with the brain surface vessels may be falsely given a higher grade as a result of a high rCBV from a region of interest placed over vessels.

THERAPY
Current Therapy

Despite many efforts, the outcome for children with HGGs is dismal and has remained virtually unchanged over recent decades. Age younger than 3 years, radical resection, WHO grade III histology, and presence of IDH1 mutations are factors associated with longer survival. External beam radiation therapy (RT) remains the mainstay of adjuvant therapy for HGGs. Currently, three-dimensional conformal radiotherapy (3D-CRT) or intensity-modulated radiation therapy (IMRT) is used at most centers, with 5400 to 594 cGy administered in approximately 30 fractions.

Single-agent temozolomide, considered the standard of care (SOC) for adult GBM, did not improve outcome for children with HGGs compared with historical controls (study ACNS0126). The most recent Children's Oncology Group HGG study, ACNS0822, compared two combined-modality experimental arms that included either vorinostat or bevacizumab with "standard" therapy (i.e., combined modality that included temozolomide). This study was recently closed after interim analysis showed that the predefined endpoint (i.e., improved 1-year event-free survival compared with standard therapy) could not be met (M. Fouladi, personal communication). In the setting of the recent disappointing results of upfront therapy with bevacizumab in adults and the lack of efficacy of bevacizumab-containing regimens in children with recurrent HGGs, bevacizumab is unlikely to play a substantial role in future pediatric HGG trials.

Because no studies have compared RT alone versus RT and chemotherapy in a randomized fashion in pediatric HGGs, it remains unproven whether adding adjuvant chemotherapy of any type is superior to RT alone in this population. Nevertheless, given the lack of proven superiority of any one chemotherapy regimen, most practitioners currently treat pediatric patients with newly diagnosed nonbrainstem HGGs with adjuvant temozolomide.

Given the histologic and biologic heterogeneity of pediatric HGGs, and in some cases the difficulty in differentiating HGGs from other entities on a histologic basis alone, the lack of molecular profiling data in all of the published prospective pediatric HGG studies to date leaves significant uncertainty surrounding the "long-term survivors" and the biology of their disease.

A recently published, and clinically well-annotated, study of a uniformly treated retrospective cohort of pediatric patients with tumors that met histologic criteria of GBM has provided key insights into the molecular heterogeneity of pediatric GBM and striking differences in outcome among them. Patients younger than 3 years of age were treated according to the "Baby-POG" chemotherapy protocol, whereas older patients received chemotherapy and RT, including temozolomide. Based on genome-wide methylation profiling signatures, major subgroups with highly divergent outcome emerged: (1) "LGG-like" tumors and "IDH" mutant tumors with favorable outcome (3-year overall survival [OS] of 91% and 90%, respectively), "PXA-like" tumors with intermediate outcome (3-year OS of 70%), and "GBM" with poor outcome (3-year OS < 20%). Among the GBM subgroup, a high-risk population was identified that included patients whose tumors harbored either K27M mutations or any amplifications of known oncogenes, such as EGFR, PDGFRA, and MYCN. Interestingly, patients in the subset of "long-term survivors" (OS > 36 months) were highly enriched in IDH mutant tumors and G34 mutant tumors without oncogene amplification. K27M mutant GBM had a dismal outcome nearly identical to that of DIPGs, and the fact that nearly all tumors were MGMT promoter nonmethylated provides a biologic explanation for the failure of temozolomide and other alkylator-based chemotherapy in prior DIPG trials. The G34 mutant subset had frequent MGMT promoter methylation, which may explain the more favorable outcome with alkylator-based therapy.

FUTURE DIRECTIONS
Targeted Therapies for Children With High-Grade Gliomas

As outlined previously, current treatment strategies do not lead to acceptable clinical outcomes for children with HGGs, and with the exceptions of surgical resection and focal radiation therapy, there is currently no established SOC. Children with HGGs are usually enrolled in an investigational trial as first-line therapy. Many of the agents being evaluated in clinical trials are chosen empirically, and, not surprisingly, there has been little progress in improving outcomes over the last decades. Presently, there is no validated mechanism to prioritize treatment recommendations for an individual patient with pediatric HGG. We now understand that there are significant biologic differences between adult and pediatric malignant gliomas and differences based on tumor location (Wu et al., 2014). These findings highlight that treatment needs to be tailored to each individual child's tumor.

Individualized treatment based on single-gene expression or mutation has proven to be an effective strategy in multiple cancer types. For children with HGGs, recent studies have shown that approximately 10% to 15% carry the BRAF-V600E mutation, a genetic alteration that is also shared with other tumor types, such as melanoma, thyroid cancer, and colon cancer. There are now several specific BRAF-V600E inhibitors in clinical use, and individual case reports are encouraging regarding the clinical response of pediatric BRAF-V600E-mutated tumors to such targeted therapy. The Pacific Pediatric Neuro-Oncology Consortium (PNOC) is currently conducting a phase I clinical trial of the specific BRAF-V600E inhibitor vemurafenib in children with BRAF-V600E-mutated gliomas.

With advances in bioinformatics and molecular technologies, such as shortened turnaround times for whole-genome sequencing (WGS), combined with our expanding knowledge of molecular networks and mechanisms of action of the existing pharmacopeia (drugs approved by the U.S. Food and Drug Administration [FDA]), strategies using more in-depth profiling of the tumor to guide therapy are slowly entering the clinic, including for children with HGGs (clinical trials NCT02274987, NCT02060890, and NCT02162732). Molecular profiling has provided clinical benefit for patients with various advanced adult cancers, but the clinical benefit derived from such analyses remains unknown in the pediatric population. One of the major challenges in the application of precision medicine remains the classification and prioritization of identified variants by genomic analyses and possible association with drug response. But despite the ongoing challenges, this strategy opens an exciting new area for the treating neurooncologist when therapy is informed by the individual characteristics of the child's tumor. Results of these ongoing precision medicine trials will be critical to inform how this approach can be integrated in the care of children with HGGs.

CNS-Directed Delivery Strategies

A fundamental limitation in the treatment of children with HGGs is that most therapeutic agents do not cross the blood–brain barrier (BBB) and blood–tumor barrier (BTB), and therefore never reach the tumor target. Several delivery strategies have been explored to overcome the BBB and BTB, of which convection-enhanced delivery (CED) and intranasal delivery show promise and have already entered the clinic.

Convection-Enhanced Delivery

CED improves chemotherapeutic delivery to brain tumors intraparenchymally by utilizing bulk flow, or fluid convection, established as a result of a pressure gradient, rather than a concentration gradient. The advantages of CED over diffusion based delivery include (1) an expanded volume of distribution (Vd), (2) a uniform concentration of the infused therapeutic within the target Vd, and (3) the delivery of the vast majority of the infused therapeutic within the target volume. Additionally, CED obviates the challenges of systemic agents

crossing the BBB and BTB while minimizing systemic exposure and toxicity. A major advance in the safe and potentially efficacious use of CED in neurosurgery has been the development of real-time convective delivery (RCD), which utilizes MRI to visualize the CED process with the aid of coconvected contrast agents (Krauze et al., 2008). The use of RCD allows physicians to directly monitor the distribution of therapeutics within the brain. Thus, reflux along the CED catheter or leakage outside the target area, especially at higher flow rates, can be monitored and corrective steps taken, such as retargeting the catheter or altering the rate of infusion.

CED of carmustine has shown to prolong survival in mice with brainstem tumors, and other studies have shown that CED of nanoliposomal irinotecan is superior compared with intravenous administration in an orthotopic model of HGG. A feasibility study using coinfused imaging tracers with interleukin-13-*Pseudomaonas* exotoxin in children with DIPGs has shown that with use of CED, clinically relevant distributions of agents can be achieved in humans. An ongoing clinical trial is currently investigating the feasibility of CED of ^{124}I-8H9, a radiolabeled antibody, in children with DIPGs (NCT01502917).

Intranasal Delivery

Intranasal delivery is a noninvasive method of bypassing the BBB and BTB, and studies have shown that intranasal delivery of an antisense oligonucleotide-targeting telomerase (GRN163) inhibits orthotopic brain tumor growth and significantly prolongs survival in vivo (Hashizume et al., 2008). Other studies have supported intranasal delivery strategies in animal studies using different agents, such as insulin-like growth factor 1, interferon beta, and methotrexate. Intranasal delivery strategies have already entered the clinic for patients with neurodegenerative diseases and have been tested in adult patients with recurrent GBM. For example, intranasal administration of perillyl alcohol in adult patients with recurrent GBM showed good tolerability and regression of tumor size in some patients. Intranasal delivery is an attractive delivery strategy for long-term administration of therapeutics and is especially well suited for children because of the noninvasive nature of the procedure.

REFERENCES

The complete list of references for this chapter is available in the e-book at www.expertconsult.com.
    See inside cover for registration details.

SELECTED REFERENCES

Cha, S., Knopp, E.A., Johnson, G., et al., 2002. Intracranial mass lesions: dynamic contrast-enhanced susceptibility-weighted echo-planar perfusion MR imaging. Radiology 223 (1), 11–29. [Epub 2002/04/04]; eng.

Hashizume, R., Ozawa, T., Gryaznov, S.M., et al., 2008. New therapeutic approach for brain tumors: Intranasal delivery of telomerase inhibitor GRN163. Neuro Oncol. 10 (2), 112–120.

Jones, C., Baker, S.J., 2014. Unique genetic and epigenetic mechanisms driving paediatric diffuse high-grade glioma. Nat. Rev. Cancer 14 (10), [Epub 2014/09/19]; eng.

Krauze, M.T., Vandenberg, S.R., Yamashita, Y., et al., 2008. Safety of real-time convection-enhanced delivery of liposomes to primate brain: a long-term retrospective. Exp. Neurol. 210 (2), 638–644.

Park, I., Mukherjee, J., Ito, M., et al., 2014. Changes in pyruvate metabolism detected by magnetic resonance imaging are linked to DNA damage and serve as a sensor of temozolomide response in glioblastoma cells. Cancer Res. 74 (23), 7115–7124.

Paugh, B.S., Zhu, X., Qu, C., et al., 2013. Novel oncogenic PDGFRA mutations in pediatric high-grade gliomas. Cancer Res. 73 (20), 6219–6229.

Schwartzentruber, J., Korshunov, A., Liu, X.Y., et al., 2012. Driver mutations in histone H3.3 and chromatin remodelling genes in paediatric glioblastoma. Nature 482 (7384), 226–231. [Epub 2012/01/31]; eng.

Snuderl, M., Fazlollahi, L., Le, L.P., et al., 2011. Mosaic amplification of multiple receptor tyrosine kinase genes in glioblastoma. Cancer Cell 20 (6), 810–817. [Epub 2011/12/06]; eng.

Taylor, K.R., Vinci, M., Bullock, A.N., et al., 2014. ACVR1 mutations in DIPG: lessons learned from FOP. Cancer Res. 74 (17), 4565–4570. [Epub 2014/08/20]; eng.

Wu, G., Diaz, A.K., Paugh, B.S., et al., 2014. The genomic landscape of diffuse intrinsic pontine glioma and pediatric non-brainstem high-grade glioma. Nat. Genet. 46 (5), 444–450. [Epub 2014/04/08]; eng.

127 Pediatric Low-Grade Glioma

Nicole J. Ullrich and Bruce H. Cohen

INTRODUCTION

Pediatric low-grade glioma (PLGG) represents the most common brain tumor in childhood and constitutes more than 20% of primary brain tumors in children. Most PLGGs occur in the cerebellum, visual pathways, and diencephalon and comprise a histologically diverse and biologically heterogeneous group of neoplasms. Many low-grade gliomas (LGGs) have defined borders and are amenable to complete surgical resection, with excellent overall survival when treated with surgery alone. However, some LGGs are either invasive to critical structures or located in inaccessible regions, and are thus not amenable to surgical resection. Historically, these tumors were treated with radiotherapy, but in the last three decades, chemotherapy has become increasingly common as the initial postsurgical intervention. The goal of chemotherapy is to both to overcome residual or recurrent disease, and to minimize the toxicity associated with radiation therapy. Although radiation therapy may ultimately be necessary, the current practice among physicians who treat children with brain tumors generally aims to delay cranial irradiation until multiple attempts at other therapies have failed. There have been significant advances in our understanding of the molecular underpinnings of LGGs, which provide compelling preclinical evidence that targeted treatments directed at critical points along the molecular signaling pathways may be a successful approach to management. This chapter reviews the classification, clinical and pathologic features, molecular biology, and current standard and experimental therapeutic strategies for these tumors.

The incidence of LGGs in the United States approximates 2 per 100,000 persons aged 0 to 19 years of age (SEER Program, 2012; Ostrom et al., 2014). The majority of PLGGs arise sporadically; however, they can be associated with an underlying familial cancer predisposition syndrome or neurocutaneous syndromes. For example, children with a diagnosis of neurofibromatosis type 1 (NF1) are at increased risk to develop an LGG involving the visual pathway, which is found in 15% to 20% of children with NF1 and children with tuberous sclerosis complex (TSC) have a higher incidence of subependymal giant cell astrocytoma (SEGA), a subtype of LGG (Listernick et al., 1997; Gutmann, 2014).

CLINICAL PRESENTATION

PLGGs typically are slow-growing tumors, and the clinical presentation depends largely on the tumor location and age of the patient. Symptoms result because of either invasion into the surrounding brain parenchyma, local compression of brain tissue, or generalized increased intracranial pressure (ICP). Children can present with focal or diffuse signs and/or symptoms, or a combination of both (Table 127-1). Generalized increased ICP can result in headaches, vomiting, irritability, and behavioral symptoms that are very different from a child's usual demeanor. Tumors in eloquent regions of the brain often produce focal neurologic signs and symptoms reflecting the anatomic function of the involvement. Older children aware of their visual and motor function are more likely to communicate these symptoms. For example, cerebellar tumors will present with progressive gait changes, ataxia, and/or nystagmus. Tumors within the optic pathway often present with loss of visual acuity, changes in visual fields, hormonal abnormalities, and/or behavioral changes. Lesions within the brainstem typically cause the combination of progressive cranial nerve palsies such as bulbar dysfunction, upper motor neuron signs such as contralateral hyperreflexia or weakness, and ipsilateral ataxia. Supratentorial hemispheric lesions often present with localizing signs that include hemiparesis or seizures. Seizures are more common with tumors involving the temporal lobe, especially mesial structures and the frontal lobe. Seizures with LGG typically have a focal onset but may quickly generalize and thus appear as a generalized seizure from onset. Last, tumors in the region of the pineal gland, including the posterior third ventricle, or with mass effect compressing the nearby tectal plate, may lead to Parinaud syndrome, which is the triad of upgaze paresis, pupillary dilatation with poor or absent response to light, and retraction convergence nystagmus.

Slow-growing, space-occupying lesions often result in poorly localizable symptoms. In general, these symptoms are a result of increased ICP caused by disruption of CSF pathways and resulting hydrocephalus, and lead to a combination of headaches, lethargy, and vomiting. Nausea resulting from increased ICP is often position sensitive and is accompanied by other neurologic symptoms. At times, persistent increased ICP can produce irritability, uncharacteristic behavioral changes, and progressive cognitive dysfunction. In young infants with an open fontanelle, increased head circumference may be the first manifestation of hydrocephalus. Infants may also demonstrate stagnation of development, irritability, failure to thrive, and the "sun-setting sign," where the gaze is in a near-fixed downward position, and so the sclera above the iris is visible.

CLASSIFICATION AND HISTOLOGIC FEATURES

Gliomas are among the most diverse histologic group of brain tumors affecting children and the term LGGs refer to those tumors classified by the World Health Organization (WHO) system as grade I or II gliomas, and can be divided into several distinct entities based on both the dominant cell type observed histologically and by location (Table 127-2). Approximately 15% to 25% of all pediatric brain tumors are grade I juvenile pilocytic astrocytomas of the cerebellum, followed by grade II LGG of the cerebrum (10% to 15%), deep midline structures (10% to 15%), and grade I and II LGGs of the optic nerves and visual pathways (5%) (Bandopadhayay et al., 2014).

Pilocytic Astrocytoma (WHO Grade I)

Pilocytic astrocytomas are the second most common brain tumors, with the embryonal neoplasms (primarily medulloblastomas) the most common brain tumor in children. These tumors are considered histologically benign. Histologic

TABLE 127-1 Clinical Presentation of Primary Brain Tumors in Children

Focal Symptoms	Diffuse Symptoms
Seizures	Headache
Ataxia	Neck stiffness
Hemiparesis or weakness	
Nystagmus	Vomiting
Cranial nerve palsies	Lethargy
Focal sensory changes	Cognitive deterioration
Decreased visual acuity/visual fields	Behavior change
Parinaud syndrome	
Diabetes insipidus	Seizure
Growth retardation	Irritability
Aphasia	Infants: increased head circumference, split sutures, Bulging fontanelle, "setting-sun" sign

TABLE 127-2 Classification of Pediatric Low-Grade Glioma (Based on World Health Organization 2007 Central Nervous System Classification)

Tumor Subtype	Tumor Grade
Astrocytic tumors	
Subependymal giant cell astrocytoma	I
Pilocytic astrocytoma	I
Pilomyxoid astrocytoma	II
Diffuse astrocytoma	II
Pleomorphic xanthoastrocytoma	II
Protoplasmic astrocytoma	II
Oligodendroglial and oliogoastrocytic tumors	
Oligodendroglioma	II
Oligoastrocytoma	II
Neuronal and mixed neuronal-glial	
Ganglioglioma	I
Desmoplastic infantile ganglioglioma	I
Dysembryoplastic neuroepithelial tumor	I
Central neurocytoma	II

characteristics include well-differentiated astrocytes, with Rosenthal fibers and eosinophilic granular bodies as the characteristic findings in these tumors, but usually without any cellular atypia. Cystic formations are common, and in some cases, the majority of the tumor volume is a cyst. The goal of surgery is complete resection, typically with minimal or no sequale. Survival with this histology is excellent overall, with 1-year and 10-year survival of 98.6% and 95.8%, respectively.

Pilomyxoid Astrocytoma (WHO Grade II)

Pilomyxoid astrocytomas are grade II neoplasms most often located in the hypothalamic and nearby midline regions, and occur in younger children (typically less than 1 year old). Pathologically, these tumors are closely related to pilocytic astrocytoma with bipolar cells within a myxoid matrix, but

lack the Rosenthal fibers and eosinophilic grandular bodies. A less favorable subset is represented by young children who present with *hypothalamic syndrome*, also known as *diencephalic syndrome*, a distinct clinical phenotype that includes normal or excessive food consumption with failure to gain weight. There is a worse overall prognosis in this tumor subtype, and in one report, the 1-year progression-free survival was only 37.8%; of the total cohort, 6/18 patients had died.

Dysembryoplastic Neuroepithelial Tumor (WHO Grade I)

Dysembryoplastic neuroepithelial tumors are usually cortical tumors that usually present with refractory seizures, often without other neurologic signs. Pathologically, this neoplasm is composed of glial nodules, with associated cortical dysplasia and glioneuronal elements. In many cases these tumors are small and are amenable to complete surgical resection, which often effectively treats the epilepsy. Because of the cortical location, however, gross total resection (GTR) may be challenging. In general, these tumors have a low recurrence rate after surgery and despite incomplete resection, sometimes the remaining tumor does not grow.

Ganglioglioma (WHO Grade I)

The ganglioglioma is a grade II neoplasm consisting of mixed neuronal and glial elements with mature ganglion cells and abnormal glial cells. These are most frequently located in the temporal lobes, present around 10 years of age, and typically present with seizures. As with DNETs, these tumors are most often completely resectable with a favorable prognosis.

Pleomorphic Xanthroastrocytoma (WHO Grade II)

Pleomorphic xanthroastrocytomas occurs most commonly in teenagers and young adults, and usually involves the cortex, especially the temporal lobes. These tumors were once classified as a giant cell glioblastoma. They are cellular tumors with more nuclear atypia than other LGGs, and can be misdiagnosed as high-grade gliomas. Many of these tumors have clear borders and are amenable to gross-total resection, with a favorable prognosis.

Diffuse Fibrillary Astrocytoma

Diffuse fibrillary astrocytomas are a WHO grade II neoplasm and can be morphologically similar to their adult counterparts. They occur most commonly in the supratentorial space, deep midline structures, and lower brainstem. Microscopically, they are characterized by modest cellularity, lack of significant mitoses, and presence of both fine and course neuroglial fibrils that form a matrix between the cells. These tumors, because of their infiltrating nature, are more difficult to resect completely and have a less favorable outcome than pilocytic astrocytoma. Over time, these tumors can transform into malignant gliomas. Recent data suggest that these tumors are similar to their adult counterparts in terms of pathologic appearance, but have distinct genetic molecular alterations.

Pediatric Low-Grade Glioma; Not Otherwise Specified

As many as one quarter of PLGGs may not fit into a particular WHO LGG subtype classification and are designated as pediatric LGG; not otherwise specified (PLGG, NOS). This category includes tumors that have not been biopsied and then are designated also by the site of origin, such as the optic glioma, which accounts for 3% to 5% of all childhood brain tumors. These tumors can be located anywhere along the visual pathway, including the optic nerve, optic chiasm, optic tract, and optic radiations and often involve the hypothalamus, and the terms *visual pathway glioma, optic pathway glioma,* or *hypothalamic-chiasmatic glioma* may be more fitting. Approximately 15% to 20% of children with NF1 have an optic glioma as seen on imaging, although only one fifth of these children require treatment; this treatment is typically initiated when a change in visual acuity or change in visual function occurs, and not because of incremental growth of the mass. Because of the distinct clinical phenotype and tumor location, a surgical biopsy is typically not required to make the diagnosis. In general, in the absence of any signs of progressive neurologic dysfunction or vision loss (e.g., absence of optic nerve pallor, loss of visual acuity, or visual fields), clinical observation with serial ophthalmologic assessments and neuroimaging studies is generally recommended.

EVALUATION, DIAGNOSIS, AND MANAGEMENT

The diagnosis of an LGG is likely when characteristic neuroimaging findings are seen during the evaluation of a neurologic disturbance such as a seizure or motor dysfunction. PLGGs tend to be isodense or hyperdense on CT, with varying degrees of cystic changes and contrast enhancement. The solid portion of pilocytic astrocytoma enhances vividly with contrast, which should not be mistaken as a sign of a malignant or high-grade nature. Less malignant tumors tend to have a more focal appearance with variable enhancement, with the lowest grade neoplasms demonstrating more confluent enhancement patterns or no enhancement at all. In contrast to higher grade tumors, PLGGs are not typically accompanied by mass effect, edema, or restricted diffusivity. Pilocytic astrocytomas may demonstrate a classical cyst with a mural nodule. The mural nodule may be quite small, and in some instances only the wall of the cyst demonstrates enhancement. Postoperative MRI is suggested, preferably within a day or so from the time of initial surgical resection, to adequately assess extent of surgical resection. After a GTR, these tumors seldom recur, with a survival approaching 100% at 5 years in many series. If the tumor does recur, subsequent attempts at GTR are usually attempted. Some of these tumors may extend into the brainstem and are therefore less amenable to surgical resection. Although these are typically considered "benign" tumors, they may be accompanied by metastatic foci of tumor; this is particularly true for suprasellar tumors in infants and young children.

Depending on the tumor location, other assessments may be needed. An ophthalmologic evaluation and testing of endocrine function are needed for tumors located along the visual pathway and hypothalamic region. Children should be examined for neurocutaneous stigmata of NF1 and TSC. Electroencephalogram may be helpful at diagnosis or any time if there is a question of seizures. Because many of these tumors will affect higher cortical function, including those located in the posterior fossa, all children should have a neuropsychological assessment near the beginning of their illness, at the conclusion of primary therapy and at points post-therapy if educational, social, or employment issues arise.

DIFFERENTIAL DIAGNOSIS

LGGs must be distinguished from other lesions, such as (1) "high-grade" gliomas, including anaplastic astrocytoma, glioblastoma multiforme, and anaplastic oligodendroglioma; (2) other brain neoplasms; (3) nonneoplastic lesions, including infarction; (4) inflammation; and (5) cerebritis/encephalitis, acute demyelinating encephalitis, and antibody-mediated encephalitis (such as NMDA-receptor encephalitis). Occasionally, a large area of focal demyelination can demonstrate mass effect and resemble a glioma. Tumorifactive multiple sclerosis is an aggressive form of multiple sclerosis in which the lesion mimics a brain neoplasm, often accompanied by mass effect and contrast enhancement. None of these entities has a pathognomonic clinical or radiographic presentation, and so histologic, antibody, or other biomarker diagnosis is required.

PATHOGENESIS

Intensive efforts to elucidate the genetic underpinnings of PLGGs are in progress. The gene *BRAF*, which is an oncogene linked to melanoma and some carcinomas, functions to upregulate the RAS/RAR/MEK pathway. Genetic rearrangements, typically duplications and rearrangements, are the most common genetic finding in sporadic PLGGs, and are found in 50% to 100% of pediatric pilocytic astrocytoma. These duplications, however, are not typically identified in NF1-associated LGGs or other PLGGs, which, by contrast, often demonstrate an abnormal gain of function or duplication in the MAP-kinase signaling pathway, with the implication that targeted therapies could be developed along this pathway. Investigation as to environmental impact on LGG occurrence has not been informative.

TREATMENT

Because of the excellent overall prognosis of PLGGs, the goals of therapy must take into account the dual aims of tumor control and reduction of treatment/tumor-associated morbidity. In some children, especially in NF1, PLGGs are found incidentally and may not be causing any acute symptoms, and do not require tumor-directed therapy. In general, treatment approaches include observation, surgery, chemotherapy, and cranial irradiation.

Surgery

Surgery is the mainstay of treatment for many PLGGs. Surgery provides tissue for histopathologic interpretation and molecular characterization. When possible, a gross total or complete resection should be considered, as this is often curative. When a GTR is not safe to perform, removal of some or most of the tumor often provides a therapeutic benefit. The tumor location typically determines the extent of surgical resection; tumors in surgically accessible areas such as the cerebellum or noneloquent cortex can often be excised without sequela. A report from a large cooperative group supported the postulate that the extent of tumor resection is the most significant factor associated with favorable outcome. In children with LGGs who had undergone GTR, the 5-year progression-free survival is about 90%, whereas more than half of children with subtotal resection had disease recurrence during that interval (Wisoff et al., 2011). However, progressive disease or relapse is not indicative of an overall poor prognosis. An analysis of over 4000 children with PLGG showed no overall survival advantage in those children with an initial GTR compared with children not having a complete resection. The 20-year overall survival in this subset of patients was $87\% \pm 0.8\%$, with deaths attributable to the glioma at $12\% \pm 0.8\%$. The risks of permanent surgical morbidity need to be considered when approaching the goal of complete resection, and if the risk is above minimal, the prognostic data for overall survival favor a less aggressive surgical approach.

Chemotherapy

Many LGGs, especially those located in the optic pathway, brainstem, and other cerebral midline structures may not be amenable to surgery or GTR, and adjuvant therapy is used to achieve tumor control and prolong survival. The successful use of chemotherapy before radiotherapy, both at initial diagnosis and recurrence, demonstrated the efficacy of chemotherapy, which can delay or completely avoid the need for subsequent cranial irradiation. Studies conducted since the 1980s have demonstrated that chemotherapy is an effective mode of treatment to achieve disease stability, either when GTR is not possible or cannot be safely achieved, or when these tumors become symptomatic with regrowth (Ater et al., 2012). Standard chemotherapy is administered for approximately 1 year; however, chemotherapy can be halted a cycle or two after maximum therapeutic effect is confirmed by imaging or when dose-limiting toxicity occurs. Some patients may progress during or after completion of chemotherapy, and require one or more additional treatment regimens at time of tumor recurrence (Figs. 127-1 and 127-2). Although there is no standard of care, most pediatric neuro-oncologists advise using several chemotherapy regimens before proceeding with radiotherapy. Progression-free survival for most chemotherapeutic regimens tested is typically in the range of 30% to 40% at 5 years.

There are several chemotherapy regimens used to treat PLGG. The combination of vincristine and carboplatin (CV), administered weekly, has been used since the late 1980s, as well as the combination of thioguanine, procarbazine, dibromodulcitol, lomustine, and vincristine (referred to as TPDCV),

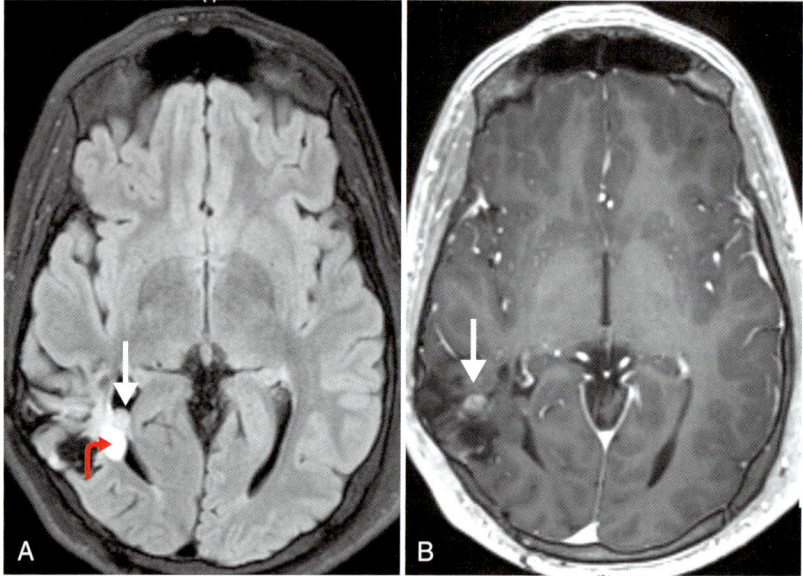

Figure 127-1. a, b, FLAIR *(left)* and T1 gadolinium-enhanced *(right)* images from a 19-year-old male who was diagnosed initially at 11 months of life after a single seizure with a low-grade astrocytoma. After a gross-total resection he was stable for 4 years and experienced subsequent tumor progression. Follow-up treatments included reresection and three different chemotherapeutic regimens. After cystic progression, his imaging has remained stable at 5 years. FLAIR imaging demonstrates multiple cysts (*curved red arc* shows one hyperintense cyst). After administration of gadolinium, multiple solid enhancing nodules are visible (one is marked by an *arrow* on both images). He is currently a college student with a normal neurologic exam.

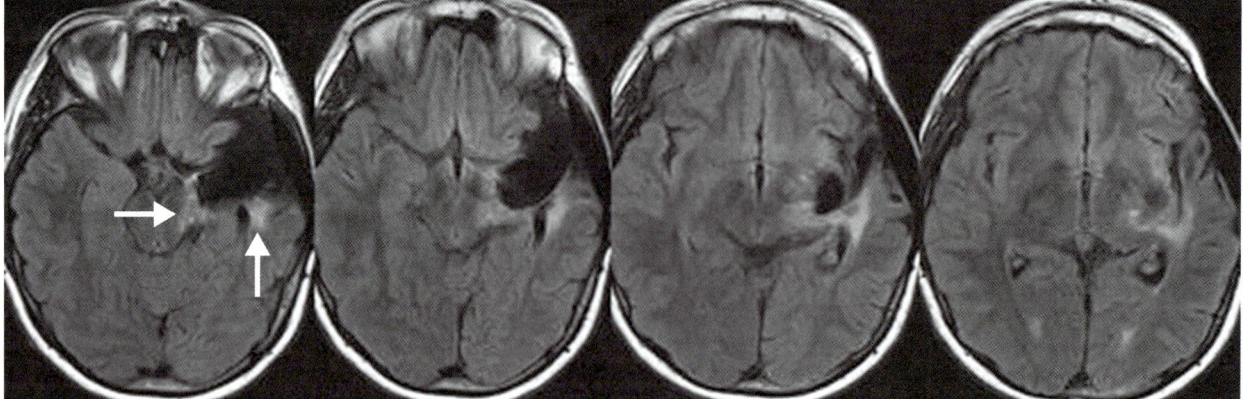

Figure 127-2. A 20-year-old man diagnosed at age 6 years with a left temporal lobe astrocytoma. He has experienced nine recurrences, and treated with two additional surgeries, cranial irradiation, and five different chemotherapy regimens at time of relapse or progression. He developed severe myelodysplastic syndrome preventing further treatment with cytotoxic agents. FLAIR image demonstrates increased signal surrounding tumor resection bed (shown only in left image with *arrows*). The corresponding gadolinium-enhanced images demonstrate several small enhancing nodules (not shown). His examination demonstrates mild cognitive impairment with speech difficulties and a mild right hemiparesis.

and when dibromodulcitol became unavailable, TPCV. A randomized study comparing these two regimens was conducted through the Children's Oncology Group in 274 children with newly diagnosed grade 1 or grade 2 LGG having less than a 95% resection, residual tumor measuring more than 1.5 cm², or radiographically progressing tumors after surgery. There were 137 children in each treatment arm and overall results in the combined groups showed a 45% ± 3.2% 5-year event-free survival and a 86% ± 2.2% 5-year overall survival. The difference in the two treatment arms was not significant (stratified log-rank $p = 0.1$). The 5-year event-free survival in those treated with TPCV was 52% ± 5% and in those treated with carboplatin–vincristine, 39% ± 4%. The 5-year overall survival was essentially identical showing 86% ± 3% for those treated with CV and 87% ± 7% for those treated with TPCV (log-rank $p = 0.52$). This report added several details that add clarity to the understanding of how location, pathology, and extent of resection affect outcome. The 5-year event-free survival (and overall survival) for pilocytic astrocytoma was 49% ± 6% (88% ± 4%), for hypothalamic/optic chiasmal tumors was 44% ± 5% (87% ± 3%), and for fibrillary astrocytoma was 34% ± 10% (79% ± 8%). The relative risk for progression or relapse was 0.65 times lower (95% CI, 0.44–0.97) in children with tumor volume (after surgery is performed) of less than 3.0 cm² than in patients with a residual tumor of greater than or equal to 3.0 cm². Independent factors associated with overall survival included age at diagnosis, tumor site, and amount of residual tumor. The risk of secondary neoplasm caused by the use of the alkylating agents in the TPCV treatment arm has been a source of ongoing concern, but in this trial only one patient developed leukemia. The issue of secondary neoplasms caused by alkylating therapy remains a concern, especially in children with NF1, who have an underlying tumor suppressor inactivating syndrome and a higher risk for development of leukemia and who therefore should avoid the use of alkylating agents.

A number of other chemotherapy-based treatments have been explored, including vinblastine; tamoxifen and carboplatin; cisplatin and etoposide; temozolomide; bevacizumab and irinotecan; carboplatin, vincristine, and temozolomide; and procarbazine, carboplatin, vincristine, etoposide, cisplatin, and cyclophosphamide. Some of these regimens have been studied primarily in the immediate postoperative period, but have not demonstrated added therapeutic advantages over the more conventional initial therapies such as CV or TPCV. These treatment regimens, however, are an important part of the armamentarium, as they are useful in the setting of the multiply relapsed patient (see Figs. 127-1 and 127-2).

Progression or relapse after any initial treatment is common, and additional therapy is required. This treatment may include surgery aimed at further debulking of the recurrent tumor or to drain tumor-associated cysts. In most circumstances, when a child has been treated with chemotherapy, s/he will be treated with a subsequent, typically different, chemotherapy regimen. This approach to treatment with several different chemotherapy regimens will be repeated until the child is free of progressive disease or until such a decision is made to proceed with radiation.

Radiation Therapy

Although radiotherapy was the earliest treatment approach used after incomplete resection or at the time of tumor recurrence, the data supporting its use as an immediate postsurgical treatment for residual disease are not clear, with conflicting data regarding any benefit for progression-free survival. Radiotherapy has not been shown to improve overall survival. Currently irradiation is typically reserved for those children who have no remaining surgical or chemotherapeutic options. Irradiation is generally avoided in young children because of concern for the long-term risks of cognitive effects, secondary radiation-related tumors, vasculopathy, and endocrine dysfunction (Ullrich, 2009; Armstrong et al., 2011).

The duration of disease control after radiation therapy is similar to that of chemotherapy. Because controlled trials randomizing children to receive radiotherapy versus chemotherapy (or observation) after maximal surgery have not been performed, and initial treatment paradigms have not stratified randomized treatments to GTR versus subtotal surgical resections, it is not possible to draw any definitive conclusions about the comparative efficacy of radiotherapy or chemotherapy.

The use of newer radiotherapy techniques permits delivery of the ionizing radiation to a smaller brain volume, which can often avoid or lessen the injury to eloquent brain regions. These techniques include three-dimensional conformal techniques, the use of nonparallel rotating photon arcs, intensity-modulated radiotherapy, and proton beam irradiation.

SUPPORTIVE CARE
Seizures

Seizures follow headache as the most common presenting symptom in supratentorial tumors in childhood and the prevalence may be as high as 75% in children with LGG. The wide variation is in part that some centers have concentrated efforts in the surgical management of epilepsy, and therefore there is a referral bias in the evaluation of patients with both seizure and brain tumor.

GENETIC FEATURES OF PEDIATRIC LOW-GRADE GLIOMA

Years before there was any clear understanding of the molecular genetics of brain tumors, the observation was made that visual pathway gliomas occurred in NF1 at a rate of about 4000-fold greater than in the general population. The most common findings are a gain of chromosome 7 (most true for pilocytic astrocytomas), followed by gains of chromosomes 4, 5, 6, 8, and 11, and deletion of 17p or 1.q. This is quite different from adult LGGs such as oligodendroglioma, where the loss of 19q and 1p is most common. Mutations in *IDH1* and *IDH2*, common in adult gliomas, are rare in childhood gliomas. The mitogen-activated protein kinases (MAPK) and mTOR pathways were found to be activated in NF1, and known to be the major contributory pathway to the formation of LGG in NF1. Similarly, the mTOR pathway is dysregulated in tuberous sclerosis (Berghold et al., 2015).

CURRENT CLINICAL TRIALS
Targeting the RAS/MAP-Kinase Pathway

The majority of PLGGs have alterations of the RAS/MAP-kinase pathway. In NF1-associated LGG, this pathway is constitutively activated because of loss or altered function of neurofibromin. In non-NF1-associated PLGG, the most common alteration is a fusion and tandem duplication of BRAF with KIAA1659. This fusion results in a constitutively active BRAF. A group of diffuse astrocytomas has activating mutations of the *MYB or MYBL1* transcription factors and resulting MAP-kinase activation that is equivalent to that observed in BRAF-driven tumors. This suggests that MAP-kinase may also be a driver pathway in PLGG. The presence of common mutations provides a rational treatment target.

The BRAF inhibitor dabrafenib has been used in melanoma and is currently being investigated in a national pediatric phase I/II trial in patients with known BRAF tumors (NCT01677741). Development of more defined MAP-kinase pathway inhibitors has led to successful preclinical testing and currently a clinical trial of one such inhibitor, selumetinib, which appears to inhibit ERK phosphorylation, in patients with LGG (NCT01089101).

mTOR Pathway Inhibition

Increased activation of the mTOR pathway has been well-defined in PLGGs as demonstrated by the success of rapamycin trials in treating subependymal giant cell astrocytomas. These results suggested that mTOR inhibitors might have activity in other PLGGs. A trial of everolimus in refractory/recurrent PLGG has recently completed enrollment (NCT00782626) as has a second phase II trial with larger numbers of patients (NCT01734512). Last, a separate study using everolimus in children with NF1-associated LGG has recently completed enrollment (NCT01158651).

Antiangiogenic Therapy

There is increased expression of vascular growth factors in PLGG, suggesting that neovascularization may be a crucial step for continued growth stimulation in these tumors. The use of the VEGF inhibitor bevacizumab along with irinotecan resulted in radiologic and clinical responses in small numbers of children. Monotherapy with bevacizumab has also led to tumor regression and disease stability in some patients.

Immunomodulatory Therapy

PLGGs contain characteristic mutations that are not found in nontumor cells, which raises the possibility of using these abnormal peptides as a target for therapy. Lenalidomide alters the immune environment and antiangiogenesis, with direct antitumor effects. Results from a phase I trial using lenalidomide demonstrated decreased tumor progression in PLGG. A phase II study is currently underway comparing two dose levels of lenalidomide (NCT01553149).

OUTCOME

PLGGs are clinically and genetically different from LGGs in adulthood. One of the biggest distinctions is the response to chemotherapy and overall excellent overall survival. Results from the Surveillance, Epidemiology and End Results (SEER) database have provided important prognostic information about PLGGs.

Prognosis for children is excellent, with an overall survival at 30 years of 87%. This favorable survival is not intuitively expected because of the high rate of progressive disease, 5-year progression-free survival of 45%. Although the pilocytic astrocytoma is truly a benign neoplasm that can often be surgically cured with minimal surgical morbidity, this is not universally the case. Because of their location, tumors along the midline diencephalon with a similar histologic appearance often are not amenable to surgical resection. Patients with tumors in these locations often require multiple surgical interventions, repeated courses of chemotherapy, and, occasionally, irradiation. Children with tumors in these locations can experience significant tumor morbidity from the tumor and its treatments; therefore, although they are histologically consistent with LGG, they do not necessarily behave in a *benign* manner and patients can experience severe morbidity and/or mortality.

Ultimately, the genetic features of the tumor itself may direct therapy and correlate with outcome, but this hypothesis will be tested in future trials.

CONCLUSIONS

PLGGs encompass several histologic subgroups of tumors. Most children with an LGG present with specific neurologic signs and symptoms, such as seizure or headaches. Optimal management is often guided by tumor location, size, and clinical presentation. Current management for most PLGGs includes consideration and attempt of a GTR. Survival in PLGG is generally very good, though this is influenced by degree of resection, age, and histologic classification. Current management of PLGGs continues to evolve, with advances in neurosurgical techniques, targeted chemotherapy, tailored radiation, and molecular biology discoveries, which will hopefully improve the overall quality of life and survival.

REFERENCES

The complete list of references for this chapter is available online at www.expertconsult.com.
See inside cover for registration details.

SELECTED REFERENCES

Armstrong, G.T., Conklin, H.M., Huang, S., et al., 2011. Survival and long-term health and cognitive outcomes after low-grade glioma. Neuro Oncol. 13, 223–234.

Ater, J.L., Zhou, T., Holmes, E., et al., 2012. Randomized study of two chemotherapy regimens for treatment of low-grade glioma in young children: a report from the Children's Oncology Group. J. Clin. Oncol. 30, 2641–2647.

Bandopadhayay, P., Bergthold, G., London, W.B., et al., 2014. Long-term outcome of 4,040 children diagnosed with pediatric low-grade gliomas: an analysis of the Surveillance Epidemiology and End Results (SEER) database. Pediatr. Blood Cancer 61, 1173–1179.

Bergthold, G., Bandopadhayay, P., Hoshida, Y., et al., 2015. Expression profiles of 151 pediatric low-grade gliomas reveal molecular differences associated with location and histological subtype. Neuro Oncol. 17, 1486–1496.

Gutmann, D.H., 2014. Eliminating barriers to personalized medicine: learning from neurofibromatosis type 1. Neurology 83, 463–471.

Listernick, R., Louis, D.N., Packer, R.J., et al., 1997. Optic pathway gliomas in children with neurofibromatosis 1: consensus statement from the NF1 Optic Pathway Glioma Task Force. Ann. Neurol. 41, 143–149.

Ostrom, Q.T., Gittleman, H., Liao, P., et al., 2014. CBTRUS statistical report: primary brain and central nervous system tumors diagnosed in the United States in 2007–2011. Neuro Oncol. 16 (4), iv1–iv63.

SEER Program. SEER Cancer Statistics Review 1975–2012, Childhood Cancer by the ICCC, Age-Adjusted and Age-Specific SEER Cancer Incidence Rates, 2008–2012. <http://seer.cancer.gov/> accessed 8/18/15.

Ullrich, N.J., 2009. Neurologic sequelae of brain tumors in children. J. Child Neurol. 24, 1446–1454.

Wisoff, J.H., Sanford, R.A., Heier, L.A., et al., 2011. Primary neurosurgery for pediatric low-grade gliomas: a prospective multi-institutional study from the Children's Oncology Group. Neurosurgery 68, 1548–1554, discussion 1554–1555.

E-BOOK FIGURES AND TABLES

The following figures and tables are available in the e-book at www.expertconsult.com. See inside cover for registration details.

Fig. 127-3 T1 gadolinium-enhanced images from a 10-year-old boy.

128 Diffuse Intrinsic Pontine Glioma

Nicholas A. Vitanza, Paul G. Fisher, and Michelle Monje Deisseroth

 An expanded version of this chapter is available on www.expertconsult.com. See inside cover for registration details.

BACKGROUND

Since the initial report by Wilfred Harris and W.D. Newcomb nearly a century ago, the clinical outcome for children with diffuse intrinsic pontine gliomas (DIPG) has changed very little, and the 2-year overall survival remains less than 10%. As a biopsy was previously suspected to carry a significant morbidity, diagnosis over the past 2 decades has been made by magnetic resonance imaging (MRI), such that laboratory investigation has been hampered by a lack of surgical specimens. Although radiation therapy and oral steroids provide symptomatic relief and modestly prolong survival, the majority of patients survive less than a year from their onset of symptoms. However, armed with new molecular findings, made possible now through an increasing trend toward biopsy, autopsy tissue collection, and international collaboration to share these precious tissue resources, advances finally are being made against the most fatal childhood brain tumor.

EPIDEMIOLOGY

DIPG affect 200 to 400 children in the United States each year, comprising approximately 10% to 15% of all pediatric central nervous system (CNS) tumors and 80% of brainstem gliomas. Peak incidence of DIPG occurs in middle childhood, with median age of diagnosis around age 7 years. Occasional cases have been reported in patients as young as 1 year or as old as 26 years, with an equal distribution between males and females.

PRESENTATION AND DIAGNOSIS

The median duration of symptoms before diagnosis of a DIPG is 1 month and, although these can last for greater than a year in atypical cases, prodromes almost universally last for less than 6 months. On presentation, patients often display a classic triad of symptoms comprised of ataxia, cranial nerve palsies, and pyramidal tract signs. An abducens palsy, reflected in dysconjugate gaze and diplopia, is typically the first symptom, the most common symptom, and associated with a worse outcome. Facial nerve palsies, characterized by facial muscle weakness and asymmetry, are not uncommon. Patients with DIPG experience pyramidal tract dysfunction, resulting in weakness and hyperreflexia and can also experience dysuria, consistent with the location of the pontine micturition center. Pathologic laughter (pseudobulbar affect) can also be a symptom of patients with DIPG, including laughter as the presenting symptom, even during sleep. As these tumors frequently extend into the cerebellum at time of progression, patients often experience ataxia, dysarthria, or dysmetria. Less than 10% of patients also present with obstructive hydrocephalus due to dorsal extension of disease.

Until recently, DIPG were not routinely biopsied, and diagnosis relied upon neuroimaging. Zimmerman provided the initial radiologic description of brainstem gliomas and, although this has been built upon, there remains no formal radiologic classification. However, DIPG share some typical characteristics on magnetic resonance imaging (MRI), including infiltration of the majority of the pons, hypointense to isointense signal on T1-weighted imaging, and hyperintensity on T2-weighted imaging and fluid-attenuated inversion recovery (FLAIR) (Fig. 128-1). Unlike pilocytic astrocytomas, DIPG are generally tumors that do not enhance with gadolinium contrast, except for areas of necrosis, and frequently engulf the basilar artery, which is a poor prognostic finding.

A history of symptoms greater than 6 months or atypical radiographic features should prompt evaluation of a broader differential, which would include pilocytic astrocytomas, primitive neuroectodermal tumors (PNET), or much less commonly demyelinating or vascular diseases of the brainstem. On MRI, the exophytic appearance, definitive boarders, frequent mural nodule and cyst formation, and contrast enhancement can distinguish a pilocytic astrocytoma from a DIPG. The location is most frequently pontomidbrain, pontomedullary, or, less commonly, at the cervicomedullary junction and often present more indolently and have a higher association with neurofibromatosis type 1 (NF1). Histologically, pilocytic astrocytomas (WHO grade I) may display vascular proliferation and even several mitotic figures but will lack necrosis and invasion. PNET (WHO grade IV) on MRI is frequently heterogeneously enhancing with significant peritumoral edema. In up to 22% of cases, the postmortem diagnosis of PNET is made in tumors previously thought to be DIPG, though this percentage is certainly dropping with greater diagnostic techniques and better understanding of the distinct malignancies of the brainstem. Diffuse tensor imaging (DTI) fiber tracking can be used to differentiate between brainstem malignancies and demyelinating processes.

PROGNOSIS

The natural course of a DIPG is swift and devastating, with a median survival of 4 months if radiation therapy is not delivered. With the advent of focal irradiation the progression free survival (PFS) has improved to 5 to 9 months with a median overall survival (OS) of only 8 to 11 months. A small subset of patients, constituting only 2% to 3%, are reported to achieve long-term survival and, though difficult to predict, may share atypical radiologic features. Otherwise, only approximately 30% of children survive beyond 1 year and less than 10% survive beyond 2 years.

HISTOPATHOLOGY

The WHO grading system of diffuse, or fibrillary, astrocytomas fails to distinguish clinically significant subgroups in DIPG, which can be diffuse astrocytomas (WHO grade II), anaplastic astrocytomas (WHO grade III), or glioblastomas (WHO grade IV). In fact, WHO grading is not consistent between primary lesions and metastases, and it remains unknown if the grade II or III lesions for which later histology suggests grade IV underwent evolution or if there is simply an unreconciled

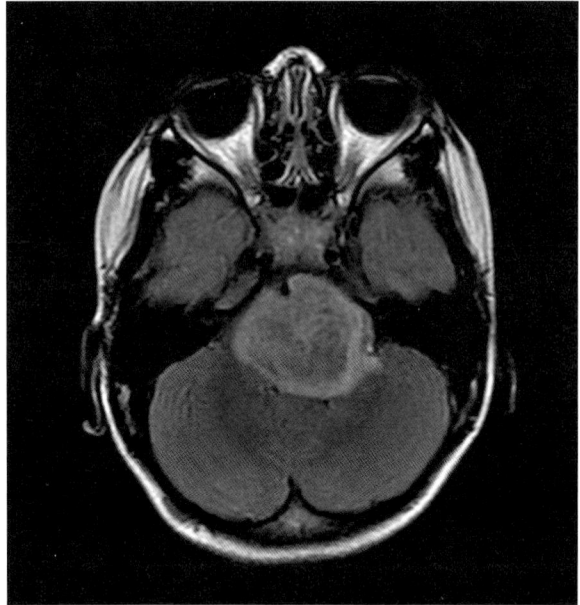

Figure 128-1. Diffuse Intrinsic Pontine Glioma (DIPG). Axial fluid-attenuated inversion recovery (FLAIR) MRI.

degree of tumor heterogeneity that breeds sampling error. There does, however, seem to be a correlation between increasing histologic grade and increasing age, although this has not been confirmed to be a truly developmental phenomenon. Regardless of grade II, III or IV histology, DIPG portends incredibly high mortality.

EXTENT OF SPREAD

DIPGs can infiltrate beyond the pons, commonly extending into the middle cerebellar peduncles, thalami, basal ganglia, or directly into the supratentorium. Metastatic disease is also common; one recent series identified neuraxis dissemination detected by neuroimaging in 17.3% of patients, with a median time of 15 months to the development of metastases. Metastatic disease is likely to be even more common, as a recent autopsy series of patients with DIPG revealed 63% had developed extension into their midbrain and medulla, 63% in the subventricular zone of the lateral ventricles, 56% in the thalamus and/or cerebellum, and 25% in the frontal cortex (Caretti, et al., 2014). As chemotherapy is not curative for DIPG, assessing the tumor size and its change on serial MRI scans is highly important in clinical trials with any therapeutic agents. Although their poorly defined borders often lead to interobserver variability, both FLAIR sequences and volumetric methods based on region of interest (ROI) currently provide the greatest agreement between observers. Specific MRI sequences may also be useful in disease stratification, as both increased enhancement and decreased apparent diffusion coefficient (ADC) values, derived from diffusion-weighted imaging, may coincide with more aggressive disease. Although currently not routine, fluorodeoxyglucose positron emission (FDG-PET) uptake of greater than 50% at the primary site correlated with a decreased PFS and OS, and the majority of DIPG metastases are also FDG-PET positive.

Surgery had been generally deferred due to the impossibility of a gross total or meaningful subtotal resection of a lesion diffusely affecting the pons, potential morbidity associated with a biopsy, and the lack of clinical benefit to the patient in the majority of cases. Coinciding with the molecular revolution in childhood CNS tumors, there is a renewed interest in

obtaining tissue for laboratory investigation and for clinical testing of novel therapeutic agents. Advances in neurosurgery have allowed for relatively safe biopsy of DIPGs, even in typical-appearing cases, and in skilled hands the morbidities are most often transient though reported in 3.9% to 20% of patients. Biopsies are increasingly performed in the setting of clinical trials at specialized medical centers and should be performed to confirm diagnosis if features are nonclassical, such as a prodrome lasting greater than 6 months and/or atypical radiologic features. The greatest immediate clinical influence of doing a biopsy to the patient would be revealing a pilocytic astrocytoma (WHO grade I) or a nonastrocytic lesion, such as PNET, which alters both the treatment and the prognosis.

DEVELOPMENTAL CONTEXT OF DIPG

The region-specific and age-specific nature of brainstem gliomas suggests that the underlying pathophysiology involves dysregulation of a postnatal neurodevelopmental process. Examination of normal human brainstem samples from all three brainstem regions—midbrain, pons, and medulla—in subjects aged 1 day to 19 years revealed a population of neural precursor cells, expressing the oligodendroglial lineage marker Olig2, restricted to the ventral brainstem. This precursor cell type, characterized by immunostaining for the primitive neural cell markers nestin, vimentin, and Olig2 and by a distinct morphology with long thin processes in a bipolar arrangement, is present in the ventral brainstem during infancy and then wanes by 2 years of age. In the human pons, this cell type again increases in density in middle childhood, peaking around age 6 (Monje, et al., 2011). This second peak in the ventral pontine precursor cell population corresponds strikingly with the incidence of DIPG, suggesting a candidate Olig2 + cell of origin for DIPG in the oligodendroglial lineage. In contrast, this cell type is conspicuously absent from the childhood midbrain, a region in which high-grade gliomas essentially never occur (Monje, et al., 2011). In a recent study incorporating MRI-based morphometric and histologic analyses, robust proliferation of Olig2 + progenitors and increased myelination of white matter tracts were found to accompany a striking postnatal volume expansion of the ventral pons observed from birth to middle childhood. A putative oligodendroglial lineage precursor cell of origin for DIPG fits well with observations of PDGFRA expression and signaling in DIPG cells (Monje, et al., 2011). Also consistent with the idea that DIPG originate from an Olig2 + neural precursor cell, analysis of postmortem DIPG specimens reveal that most express the markers Olig2 and/or Sox2 (Monje, et al., 2011; Ballester, et al., 2013).

MOLECULAR CHARACTERISTICS OF DIPG

The molecular investigation of DIPG has been limited historically by the paucity of tissues samples; however, as more specimens have become available for molecular analyses, it has become clear that DIPGs and other pediatric high-grade glioma (HGG) are genomically distinct from adult HGG. The most revolutionary insight gleaned from whole exome and whole genome sequencing studies has been the recognition of specific mutations affecting genes encoding for histone H3 in pediatric HGG, with midline HGG (i.e., DIPG and thalamic HGG) exhibiting H3K27M mutations affecting the genes encoding either H3.3 or H3.1, and cortical HGG exhibiting H3K34R/V mutations (Khuong-Quang, et al., 2012; Wu, et al., 2012). In DIPG, about 80% of tumors exhibit this K27M mutation. H3.3K27M mutations tend to occur in conjunction with p53 aberrations, whereas H3.1K27M tends to coincide with *ACVR1* activating mutations and occurs in patients who tend to be younger females (Taylor, et al., 2014). The substitution of methionine for lysine at position 27 of the histone 3 N-terminal tail results in pan-hypomethylation of K27 in all histone H3 variants, despite the fact that heterozygous mutation in one copy of a histone H3 gene (H3F3A for H3.3 or Hist1H3B for H3.1) accounts for only approximately 10% of total cellular histone H3 (Lewis, et al., 2013). This dominant effect of the mutant histone is due to "poisoning" of the EZH2 methyltransferase by the methionine residue, which binds to EZH2 and sequesters it at the mutant histone and suppresses the polycomb repressive complex 2 (PRC2), an epigenetic gene silencer. As a result of pancellular histone H3 hypomethylation, broad epigenetic dysregulation of gene expression occurs, resulting in a "K27M" gene expression signature exhibiting dysregulation of numerous oncogenic pathways (Chan, et al., 2013).

In terms of other genomic aberrations, DIPGs frequently display chromosomal aberrations with the most common gain being of 1q in 13% to 43% of cases and the most common loss being of 16q in about 25% of cases. Other common chromosomal gains include 2p, 2q, 8q, and 9q, while other common losses include 14q, 17p, and 20p. DIPG also exhibits inactivating mutations of p53 (40% to 77%) and PTEN (10% to 54%), which are associated with a worse prognosis in pediatric HGG (Khuong-Quang, et al., 2012). Unlike adult HGG, DIPG does not harbor deletions of CDKN2A/B, but 30% will have gains in other cell-cycle regulatory components, such as CDK4, CDK6, of D-type cyclins. As noted previously, 24% of patients with DIPG harbor mutations in ACVR1, the gene encoding the receptor serine/threonine kinase ALK2, which occurs twice as commonly in female patients, is associated with a better overall survival, and occurs in the setting of histone H3.1 mutations (Fontebasso, et al., 2014; Taylor, et al., 2014; Wu, et al., 2014). Although EGFR amplifications appear infrequent, several series have shown a majority of pediatric DIPG exhibit immunopositivity for EGFR, though this may be tempered by the fact that EGFR expression can be induced by irradiation, which many of these patients received. Radiation treatment has been shown to correlate with PDGFRA expression, possibly explaining the variable frequency of PDGFRA expression, ranging from 15% to the majority of patients in varying studies (Khuong-Quang, et al., 2012). Interestingly, amplifications of PDGFRA and loss of PTEN appear mutually exclusive from PI3KCA mutations, although PDGFRA amplifications occur entirely in the setting of histone H3.3 mutations (Khuong-Quang, et al., 2012).

Aurora B, a cell-cycle regulatory kinase, has been shown to be overexpressed in two-thirds of DIPG. Aurora kinase B acts both by recruitment of checkpoint protein complexes and by phosphorylation of mitotic centromere-associated kinesin (MCAK), a controller of spindle microtubule-kinetochore attachments during mitosis. Furthermore, aurora kinases also phosphorylate histone H3, offering a layer of epigenetic control. Therefore as a high percentage of DIPG have cell-cycle dysregulation, either through deletion of p53 or aberrant expression of other cell-cycle kinases or cyclins; the overexpression of aurora kinase B may contribute to either DIPG tumorigenesis or tumor maintenance. Several proteins have also been associated with DIPG, most interestingly clusterin, encoded by CLU, and talin 1, encoded by TLN1. Clusterin is a secreted chaperone protein associated with apoptosis and malignant transformation. Talin 1 is an actin binding protein, already suspected to promote cell migration and adhesion in gliomas, which is a proposed biomarker for colon cancer and whose loss of function increases chemotherapy sensitivity in resistant breast cancer.

Ultimately, DIPG likely are comprised of distinct molecular subgroups, differentiated by predominant molecular pathways, though current subgrouping proposals have limited power due to small numbers of samples (Buczkowicz, et al., 2014). There may be separate MYCN oncogene and hedgehog pathway groups, which form distinct clusters through mRNA expression profiling and can be regularly separated by immunohistochemistry as hedgehog pathway lesions demonstrate PTCH1 positivity and GLI1 nuclear expression. DIPG may also be divided into groups characterized by two smaller subgroups of MYCN overexpression and genetically stable lesions, as well as a third larger group with histone H3K27 mutations (Buczkowicz, et al., 2014). Interestingly, other midline gliomas, especially thalamic gliomas and WHO grade III and IV spinal cord gliomas, also display mutations in histone H3, suggesting potential benefit to classifying together as "diffuse midline gliomas, H3-K27M mutants" (Shankar, et al., 2016).

CURRENT TREATMENT

The only treatment modality that has consistently prolonged survival in DIPG is radiation therapy (RT), most frequently delivered conformally to the tumor at 54 Gy divided in 1.8 Gy daily fractions over 6 weeks. Hyperfractionated RT at doses as high as 7800 cGy has been attempted with no improvement in survival and likely prolongation of steroid requirement. Hypofractionated RT of 39 Gy delivered over 13 fractions, however, appears to have comparable results to standard dosing and significantly decreased burden on patients and families, especially in the patient's requiring sedation for their treatments. However, a further hypofractionated approach with an elevated daily dose of 5 Gy for 5 days increased necrosis and possibly shortened overall survival. Although many studies have examined the benefit of cytotoxic and myeloablative chemotherapy for patients with DIPG, no standard regimen extends overall survival. Chemotherapy during radiation therapy has not provided a clear benefit, as Pediatric Oncology Group's POG 9239 trial of cisplatin during RT showed an unexpected worsening of outcome and radiosensitizing agents failed to prolong survival. The Istituto Nazionale dei Tumori in Milan, Italy, attempted multiple, ambitious treatment plans including: etoposide, cytarabine, ifosfamide, cisplatin, and dactinomycin given with RT in study 1; cisplatin, etoposide, vincristine, cyclophosphamide, high-dose methotrexate, and then autologous stem cell transplant after thiotepa, followed by RT and maintenance with vincristine and lomustine in study 2; cisplatin and vincristine along with isotretinoin and RT in study 3; and vinorelbine during RT in study 4. The 1- and 2-year OS were 43% and 21%, respectively, with no differences amongst studies and with the two long-term survivors never having biopsy confirmation. German trials using oral trofosfamide and etoposide (HIT-GBM-A), intravenous (IV) carboplatin, etoposide, and ifosfamide (HIT-GBM-B), and IV carboplatin, etoposide, ifosfamide, and vincristine (HIT-GBM-C) resulted in a 1- and 2-year OS of 39.9% and 9.2%, respectively. Intensive chemotherapy with tamoxifen, carmustine, cisplatin, and high-dose methotrexate with radiation given at time of progression had the greatest 1-year OS of 70% but showed no difference in long-term OS, and the average length of stay for chemotherapy and/or complications was 43 days. Temozolomide also has not improved outcomes in either conventional or metronomic dosing. Several phase I studies utilizing more targeted agents, including imatinib, erlotinib, tipifarnib, and vandetanib, have been completed and patients enrolled in a phase II study of gefitinib, an EGFR-inhibitor, by the Pediatric Brain Tumor Consortium (PBTC) had 1- and 2-year OS of 56.4% and 19.6% OS, respectively.

EMERGING THERAPEUTIC STRATEGIES

Although the aberrant genetic signature produced by histone H3 mutations—also found in other pediatric HGG and a subgroup of posterior fossa ependymomas (PFA-CIMP +)—may share some of the responsibility for radiation resistance and poor prognosis, it may also provide actionable targets with epigenetic agents. JMJD3 and UTX, two histone H3K27 demethylases, may also be targeted in order to restore methylation to H3K27 to the nonmutant histones in the cell. GSKJ4, a selective histone demethylase inhibitor, has already been shown to inhibit JMJD3, increase H3K27me3 levels, and subsequently extend survival in H3K27M-mutant orthotopic xenograft brainstem tumor models. Therapies targeted at molecular anomalies specific to the development of this tumor afford hope for some improvement in the course or survival of this challenging cancer.

Acknowledgment

Kristen Yeom, MD, Assistant Professor of Radiology, Department of Radiology, Pediatric Radiology, Stanford University School of Medicine, provided the MRI photographs comprising Figure 128-2.

REFERENCES

The complete list of references for this chapter is available in the e-book at www.expertconsult.com.

See inside cover for registration details.

SELECTED REFERENCES

Ballester, L.Y., Wang, Z., Shandilya, S., et al., 2013. Morphologic characteristics and immunohistochemical profile of diffuse intrinsic pontine gliomas. Am. J. Surg. Pathol. 37 (9), 1357–1364.

Buczkowicz, P., Hoeman, C., Rakopoulos, P., et al., 2014. Genomic analysis of diffuse intrinsic pontine gliomas identifies three molecular subgroups and recurrent activating ACVR1 mutations. Nat. Genet. 46, 451–456.

Caretti, V., Bugiani, M., Freret, M., et al., 2014. Subventricular spread of diffuse intrinsic pontine glioma. Acta Neuropathol. 128, 605–607.

Chan, K.M., Fang, D., Gan, H., et al., 2013. The histone H3.3K27M mutation in pediatric glioma reprograms H3K27 methylation and gene expression. Genes Dev. 27, 985–990.

Fontebasso, A.M., Papillon-Cavanagh, S., Schwartzentruber, J., et al., 2014. Recurrent somatic mutations in ACVR1 in pediatric midline high-grade astrocytoma. Nat. Genet. 46, 462–466.

Khuong-Quang, D.A., Buczkowicz, P., Rakopoulos, P., et al., 2012. K27M mutation in histone H3.3 defines clinically and biologically distinct subgroups of pediatric diffuse intrinsic pontine gliomas. Acta Neuropathol. 124, 439–447.

Lewis, P.W., Muller, M.M., Koletsky, M.S., et al., 2013. Inhibition of PRC2 activity by a gain-of-function H3 mutation found in pediatric glioblastoma. Science 340, 857–861.

Monje, M., Mitra, S.S., Freret, M.E., et al., 2011. Hedgehog-responsive candidate cell of origin for diffuse intrinsic pontine glioma. Proc. Natl. Acad. Sci. U.S.A. 108, 4453–4458.

Shankar, G.M., Lelic, N., Gill, C.M., et al., 2016. BRAF alteration status and the histone H3F3A gene K27M mutation segregate spinal cord astrocytoma histology. Acta Neuropathol. 131, 147–150.

Taylor, K.R., Mackay, A., Truffaux, N., et al., 2014. Recurrent activating ACVR1 mutations in diffuse intrinsic pontine glioma. Nat. Genet. 46, 457–461.

Wu, G., Broniscer, A., Mceachron, T.A., et al., 2012. Somatic histone H3 alterations in pediatric diffuse intrinsic pontine gliomas and non-brainstem glioblastomas. Nat. Genet. 44, 251–253.

Wu, G., Diaz, A.K., Paugh, B.S., et al., 2014. The genomic landscape of diffuse intrinsic pontine glioma and pediatric nonbrainstem high-grade glioma. Nat. Genet. 46, 444–450.

E-BOOK FIGURES AND TABLES

The following figures and tables are available in the e-book at www.expertconsult.com. See inside cover for registration details.

Fig. 128-2 MRI imaging of pediatric pontine lesions that were not DIPG. Dysplasia seen on (A) axial T2 FLAIR and (B) axial T1 with contrast. Pilocytic astrocytoma on (C) axial T2 FLAIR and (D) sagittal T2. Ganglioglioma seen on (E) axial and (F) sagittal T1. Leukodystrophy secondary to metabolic disease seen on (G) axial T2 and (H) sagittal T2 FLAIR. (Courtesy of Kristen Yeom, MD, Assistant Professor of Radiology, Department of Radiology, Pediatric Radiology, Stanford University School of Medicine.)

129 Atypical Teratoid/Rhabdoid Tumors

Alyssa T. Reddy, Susan N. Chi, and Jaclyn A. Biegel

 An expanded version of this chapter is available on www.expertconsult.com. See inside cover for registration details.

INTRODUCTION

Atypical teratoid/rhabdoid tumor (AT/RT) is a highly malignant central nervous system tumor that occurs predominantly in very young children. The tumor was first described in 1987 by Lucy Rorke and colleagues and officially recognized by the World Health Organization as a WHO grade IV neoplasm in 1993 (Rorke, et al., 1995). Before this distinct recognition, the tumor was often misdiagnosed as medulloblastoma or another embryonal tumor. AT/RT is the first pediatric brain tumor with a consistent known genetic alteration. In recent years, identification of AT/RT has been dramatically simplified with an immunohistochemical assay for the SMARCB1 (also referred to as INI1, hSNF5, BAF47) gene product, the aberrant tumor suppressor gene found in the majority of AT/RTs (Judkins, et al., 2004). Early accounts of the disease reported it to be rapidly fatal in all but a very small minority of patients. Recent prospective studies that incorporated intensified multimodal therapy have reported improved long-term survival rates approaching 50% (Chi, et al., 2009). Although these results are encouraging, much work remains to be done to understand why durable disease control is not obtained for roughly half of the patients with current therapies and to also identify therapies with less toxicity. A better understanding of the function of the SMARCB1 gene will hopefully improve our understanding of the disease and lead to specific targeted treatment.

HISTORICAL BACKGROUND AND INCIDENCE

In the late 1980s, a distinctive brain neoplasm characterized by diverse histologic components was identified and termed atypical teratoid tumor of infancy. The tumor contained mixed elements and had a rapidly fatal course. It took careful inspection of multiple fields to separate this tumor from other embryonal tumors. As more cases were recognized, it was noted that the tumors contained areas of rhabdoid cells in addition to areas of primitive neuroectodermal, mesenchymal, or epithelial cells. The tumor was subsequently renamed atypical teratoid/rhabdoid tumor (AT/RT) in the mid-1990s (Rorke, et al., 1995) and given its own distinction by the World Health Organization as a Grade IV embryonal neoplasm in 1993. Before being recognized as a distinct tumor, AT/RT was often misdiagnosed as medulloblastoma, primitive neuroectodermal tumor, or choroid plexus carcinoma. A heightened awareness of AT/RT led neuropathologists to more extensively examine embryonal tumors in young patients to look for mixed cellular histology and common immunophenotypic patterns, even in the absence of a clear rhabdoid component. The first patients reported with AT/RT all died from their disease within a year of diagnosis despite surgery and chemotherapy. Most patients were initially treated either on or according to protocols that treated a variety of malignant brain tumors. It was not until the 2000s that prospective clinical trials specific to AT/RT were initiated.

AT/RT was initially thought to be extraordinarily rare. With the increased clinical awareness of this tumor and the utility of the immunohistochemistry assay for SMARCB1, it is now estimated that AT/RT accounts for at least 3% of brain tumors in children. All published series report a peak incidence in very young children, less than 3 years of age. Based on prior Pediatric Oncology Group and Pediatric Brain Tumor Consortium studies, approximately 15% of children less than 36 months with malignant brain tumors have AT/RT. In one series the ratio of AT/RT to primitive neuroectodermal tumors was found to be 1 to 3.8 (26%) among patients younger than 3 years of age. A recent Austrian study of 311 newly diagnosed patients demonstrated that AT/RT was the sixth most common entity (6.1%). The number of reported patients with AT/RT has increased 5.5-fold in an analysis of the National Cancer Institute's Surveillance, Epidemiology, and End Results (SEER) data from 1992 to 2008, likely reflecting greater awareness and improved diagnostic techniques (Buscariollo, et al., 2012). Although it is much less common in older children and adults, AT/RT has been reported with increasing frequency in these populations as well.

There are several names given to the mutated gene in AT/RT. It is referred to throughout this chapter as SMARCB1 as that is its official Human Genome Organization (HUGO) name (Kim and Roberts, 2014). Other names that have been used for the gene are SPF5, INI1, and BAF47.

CLINICAL PRESENTATION AND RADIOGRAPHIC FINDINGS

Due to the aggressive nature of AT/RT, the vast majority of patients present with very short histories of progressive symptoms that can be measured in days to weeks. Because AT/RT can arise anywhere in the nervous system, neurologic signs and symptoms are nonspecific and referable to the tumor location. About half the patients have tumors that arise in the posterior fossa, and they often present with symptoms related to hydrocephalus, particularly early morning headaches, vomiting, and lethargy. Ambulatory children may have ataxia and other cerebellar dysfunction. Nonspecific symptoms such as lethargy, regression of milestones, and seizures are often seen in very young children with cortical tumors. Focal weakness may also be seen especially in a child who is old enough to cooperate with the examination. Because infants have open sutures and fairly pliable skulls, a rapidly enlarging head size should alert the clinician to evaluate the patient for a brain tumor as this may be the only sign at presentation. Rarely, AT/RT can arise primarily in the spinal cord, and those patients can present with back pain, diplegia, or bowel and bladder dysfunction.

Imaging characteristics are helpful but also nonspecific for AT/RT. All patients with suspected AT/RT should undergo MRI imaging of brain and spine before surgery unless emergent resection is medically necessary. On T1-weighted MRI, the tumor mass is typically isointense with frequent hyperintense foci secondary to intratumoral hemorrhage. On postgadolinium images, AT/RT does vividly take up contrast but in a heterogeneous pattern (Fig. 129-1). On T2-weighted and flair MRI, the tumor appears heterogeneous as a result of the

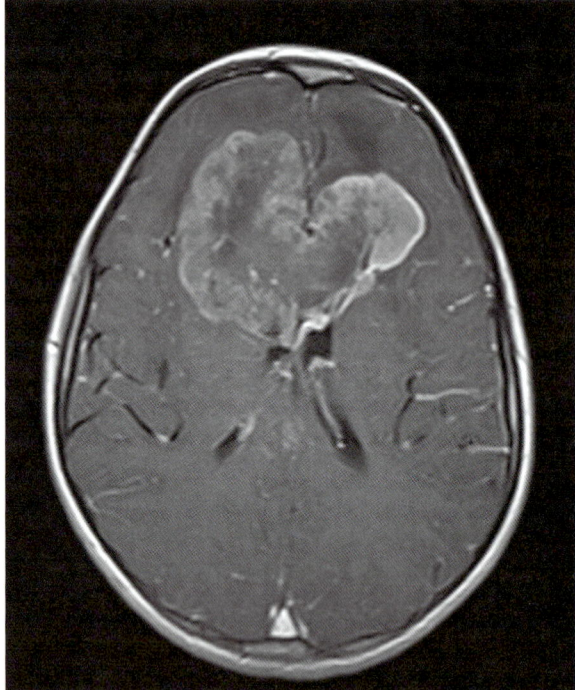

Figure 129-1. Axial gadolinium enhanced T1 brain MRI of a 12-year-old patient with bifrontal AT/RT. The mass has a heterogeneous pattern with more enhancement around the margins and central hypovascularity suggesting necrosis. The patient presented with 1-month history of progressive headaches, morning vomiting, and personality changes.

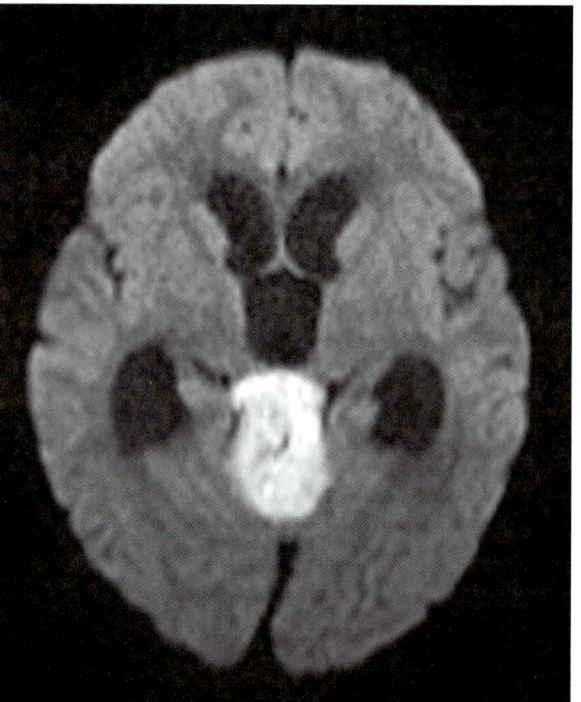

Figure 129-4. Axial diffusion-weighted image (DWI) of an 18-month-old patient with posterior fossa AT/RT. The image demonstrates increased signal intensity (restricted diffusion) within the tumor, related to increased cell density of the AT/RT.

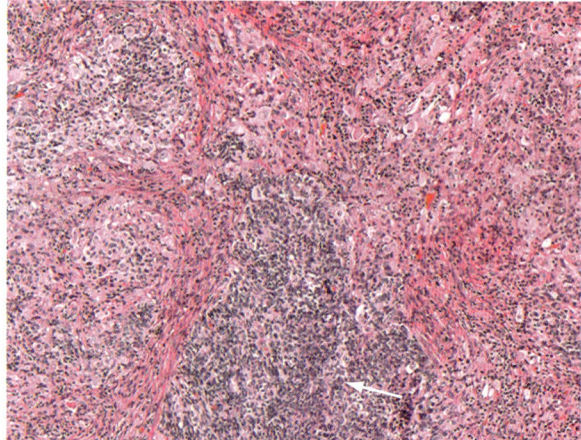

Figure 129-5. Hematoxylin and eosin (H and E) stain of AT/RT demonstrates densely packed rhabdoid cells intermixed with areas of primitive neuroectodermal cells. There is a clump of primitive neuroectodermal cells, so called "small blue cells" in the middle of the picture (arrow).

mixture of tumor cellularity, hemorrhage, necrosis, and cysts (Fig. 129-2). There is often significant peritumoral edema due to rapid growth and high cellular turnover. The tumors often invade into brain parenchyma. The CT appearance is typically that of a large hyperdense mass that enhances intensely with contrast. Dissemination throughout the neuraxis at diagnosis is not uncommon and occurs in approximately 25% of cases (Fig. 129-3) (Packer, et al., 2002). MR spectroscopy is similar to primitive neuroectodermal tumors with marked elevation of choline and low or absent N-acetyl-aspartate and creatine. Other MR sequences such as diffusion weighted imaging (DWI) may augment the suspicion that a tumor is highly cellular. Densely cellular neoplasms have a greater restriction of water diffusion than less dense tissues and therefore give rise to increased signal on DWI (Fig. 129-4).

HISTOPATHOLOGY

As previously mentioned, the pathologic diagnosis of AT/RT requires careful histologic examination of multiple fields of tumor and application of a panel of immunohistochemical markers. Whereas some tumors are composed almost entirely of rhabdoid cells, the more typical finding is that of sheets of rhabdoid cells adjacent to areas of primitive neuroectodermal cells, mesenchymal cells, and/or epithelial cells, as shown in the hematoxylin and eosin (H and E) stained section in Figure 129-5. Immunohistochemical features can help to identify the disease but vary depending on the cellular composition of the tumor. Rhabdoid cells express vimentin, epithelial membrane antigen (EMA), and smooth muscle actin (SMA). The primitive neuroectodermal cells variably express neurofilament protein (NFP), glial fibrillary acidic protein (GFAP), keratin, or desmin. MIB-1 is a marker of cellular proliferation. Not surprisingly, MIB-1 is extremely high in AT/RT with labeling

indices of 50% to 100% (Fig. 129-6). Development of an immunohistochemical stain with a SMARCB1 (BAF47) antibody has greatly assisted the identification of AT/RT (Judkins, et al., 2004). There should be no staining with the antibody in the nuclei of tumor cells due to homozygous inactivation of the gene product (Fig. 129-7).

GENETICS OF AT/RT

Cytogenetic studies of AT/RT demonstrate simple karyotypes, with loss of all or part of chromosome 22 as the primary and often solitary finding. The deletions target the SMARCB1 gene

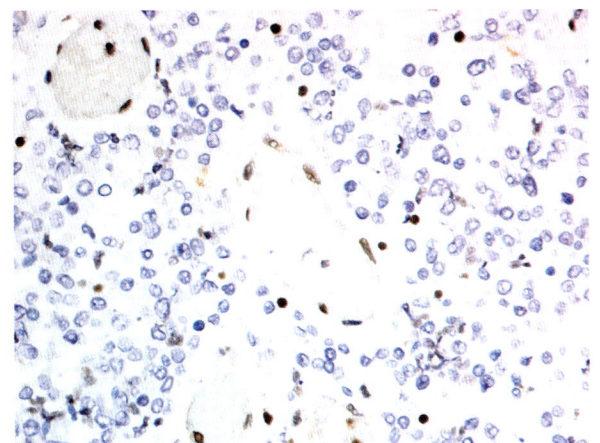

Figure 129-7. Immunohistochemical staining for the SMARCB1 protein is absent in AT/RT tumor nuclei. Nonneoplastic tissue including blood vessels and inflammatory cells serve as positive internal control (dark brown) with retained nuclear reactivity. *(Photo courtesy of Rong Li, MD.)*

in chromosome band 22q11.2, which demonstrates biallelic mutations, deletions, or intragenic duplications in up to 98% of AT/RTs (Biegel, et al., 1999). The homozygous inactivation of the gene leads to loss of expression of the protein, which is the basis for the diagnostic immunohistochemistry assay noted previously, showing loss of nuclear expression of SMARCB1 in the tumor cells. Loss of SMARCB1 expression has now been reported in a variety of CNS malignancies, such as cribriform neuroepithelial tumor; therefore the assay must be performed in the setting of careful histologic evaluation and assessment of other clinical presenting features.

The most common alterations of SMARCB1 are homozygous losses, due to monosomy 22 and/or partial 22q deletions; loss of one copy of SMARCB1 and a mutation in the remaining allele; and deletion or mutation followed by a copy number loss of heterozygosity event such as loss of the normal chromosome 22 and duplication of the remaining homologue. Biallelic mutations, however, are very uncommon. Whole exome sequencing studies of primary rhabdoid tumors have shown that this group of tumors has the lowest total number of mutations among all tumors examined to date. Based on the genomic analyses, loss of SMARCB1 alone appears to be sufficient for tumorigenesis.

SMARCB1 functions as a classic tumor suppressor gene in AT/RT. A germline mutation or copy number alteration is present in up to 35% of patients, which predisposes individuals to rhabdoid tumors of the kidney or soft tissues, as well as AT/RT. Loss of the remaining SMARCB1 allele is a somatic, or acquired, event. Patients may present with multiple primary tumors at diagnosis, strongly implicating the presence of a germline alteration. Careful staging workups for all patients with newly diagnosed AT/RT must therefore include abdominal ultrasound or whole body imaging. Germline mutations, as well as intragenic gains or losses of one or more exons of the gene, may be inherited, often from an unaffected carrier, whereas whole gene deletions are typically de novo, thus reducing the risk to other family members. Germline mutations may be mosaic, affecting only certain cells in the body, and gonadal mosaicism may lead to the development of rhabdoid tumors in siblings even when neither parent appears to be a carrier. Genetic counseling for all families in which a child has presented with a rhabdoid tumor is therefore highly recommended. Germline mutations in SMARCB1, as well as

other members of the SWI/SNF complex, may also predispose carriers to schwannomatosis, and in fact two-thirds of patients with familial schwannomatosis have germline mutations in SMARCB1. Of note, whole gene deletions of SMARCB1, or 22q11.2 deletions that include SMARCB1, appear to be restricted to patients with rhabdoid tumors. There are families in which a carrier parent had one or more schwannomas, but the offspring had AT/RT, suggesting that there is a window in development in which the risk of rhabdoid tumor is high, which diminishes with age. Long-term survivors of AT/RT may therefore be at risk for additional primary rhabdoid tumors, as well as schwannomas and other malignant tumors. The latency for second tumors may be as long as 15 or more years. SMARCB1 is a member of the SWI/SNF chromatin-remodeling complex, which acts in an ATP-dependent manner to remodel nucleosomes, thus allowing or restricting transcription factor and other protein complexes to bind to the regulatory regions of target genes. The specific function of SMARCB1 as it relates to malignant transformation, however, is still unknown. Numerous cell-signaling pathways are altered in primary rhabdoid tumors, thus providing a variety of potential biologic targets for therapy (Kim and Roberts, 2014).

STAGING AND THERAPEUTIC INTERVENTIONS

The initial staging evaluation for all patients should include an MRI of the brain unless emergent surgery is necessary. Preoperative MRI with and without contrast is important to assess the extent of disease both at primary and distant sites. A postoperative MRI should be done within 48 hours of surgery to confirm extent of resection. MRI of the whole spine should also be done preoperatively or within 48 hours of surgical resection. These scans will help the neurooncologist and radiation oncologist formulate treatment plans and are critically important to the care of the patient. A lumbar puncture to obtain cerebrospinal fluid should be obtained 7 to 10 days after surgery to look for disease dissemination, unless medically contraindicated. Molecular genetic analysis of the primary tumor and blood to look for a germline SMARCB1 alteration and abdominal ultrasound or full body imaging are recommended at diagnosis given the risk of concurrent rhabdoid tumors in patients with germline mutations.

There is general consensus that aggressive multimodal therapy is necessary to treat AT/RT, but standard-of-care guidelines have not been established. Published series and case-reports include a variety of multifaceted approaches that include combinations of surgery, conventional and high-dose chemotherapy, and radiation. Neurosurgical tumor resection is usually the first intervention for patients and is necessary to establish the diagnosis. In some cases, the tumor may be so vascular or located in a very eloquent area of brain that only a biopsy is feasible. A prospective clinical trial and retrospective data available from the AT/RT registry demonstrate that patients who have had a gross total resection (GTR) have a longer disease-free and overall survival (Chi, et al., 2009; Hilden, et al., 2004). The Canadian Pediatric Brain Tumor Consortium reported in their population-based registry that patients who achieved a GTR had a better survival with a 2-year overall survival of 60% compared with 21.7% for patients who underwent less than GTR ($p = 0.03$) (Lafay-Cousins, et al., 2012). However, only a third of these patients had a GTR. Due to the invasive nature of AT/RT, complete resection may not be possible, as it may present unacceptable risk to the patient. It has been estimated that less than one-third of patients have tumors that are amenable to complete resection. A less invasive tumor may be biologically different and influence outcome. The goal of surgery should be to remove as much tumor as is deemed safely possible by the surgeon. In the case of a highly vascular tumor that cannot be safely resected at diagnosis, treatment with chemotherapy may decrease vascularity and improve the surgeon's ability to safely resect the tumor. Consideration of "second look surgery" should be given in cases in which complete resection is not possible at the time of diagnosis. Surgery also provides tumor tissue for diagnostic and research purposes. It is highly recommended that fresh frozen tissue be obtained as evolving sequencing of tumors is likely to yield both prognostic and therapeutic information in the future.

CHEMOTHERAPY

Given the very young age of most patients with AT/RT, chemotherapy has been a mainstay of postsurgical therapy. Because of the historical misdiagnosis of AT/RT, in the earliest reports, treatment regimens designed for other CNS neoplasms were utilized in patients with AT/RT. Most commonly, these were regimens designed for embryonal tumors (e.g., medulloblastoma, supratentorial primitive neuroectodermal tumor). Even once AT/RT was more readily recognized, the regimens employed were designed with chemotherapy to delay or exclude radiotherapy altogether (i.e., "baby brain" protocols) because of the young age at which most children with AT/RT were diagnosed. The overall results of many "baby brain" chemotherapy protocols, however, were generally disappointing, although the ability to defer radiation therapy in subsets of patients was an important advance. Consequently, the generally accepted outcome for patients with AT/RT treated with standard chemotherapy regimens is dismal with median survival time reported between 6 to 11 months.

Information presented at a National Cancer Institute Workshop in 2002 incorporating data from a national rhabdoid tumor registry demonstrated a median survival of approximately 8.5 months (Packer, et al., 2002). In a review of 32 infants and children treated for CNS AT/RT, treatment was highly variable but typically included multimodality treatment, including surgery, radiation, and chemotherapy (Hilden, et al., 2004). Median survival in this analysis was 6.5 months. A similar retrospective study of 31 children treated at St. Jude Children's Research Hospital reported equally dismal outcomes for children under the age of 3 years, with 2-year event-free (EFS) and overall survival (OS) of 11% and 17%, respectively (Tekautz, et al., 2005). For children older than 3 years, survival outcomes were much more encouraging, likely due to the inclusion of radiation therapy and high-dose alkylator chemotherapy agents.

In two case series, several patients with newly diagnosed AT/RT achieved prolonged remission after surgery, radiation therapy, and chemotherapy based upon a protocol for children with rhabdomyosarcoma with parameningeal extension (Intergroup Rhabdomyosarcoma Study-III or IRS-III, Regimen 36). Since these initial reports, several investigators have shown that multiagent chemotherapy containing the anthracycline doxorubicin, the backbone chemotherapeutic agent for IRS-III, can be efficacious. Because AT/RT often shows leptomeningeal dissemination, intrathecal chemotherapy has been employed as a method of delivering local treatment to these areas. The first prospective clinical trial for children with newly diagnosed AT/RT using an intensive multimodality approach, systemic and intrathecal chemotherapy, and age-adapted radiation therapy, based on the IRS-III regimen, demonstrated the highest event-free and overall survivals to date, with 2-year progression-free survival (PFS) and overall survival (OS) at 53% and 70%, respectively (Chi, et al., 2009). Long-term survival outcomes have remained encouraging.

High-dose chemotherapy (HDC) with stem cell rescue is a strategy that allows higher doses of cytotoxic agents to be given, and this approach has also shown efficacy in treating AT/RT. The "head start" chemotherapy protocols used high-dose methotrexate as a key component to its chemotherapy backbone before its consolidation stem-cell rescue. Several investigators have shown that long-term survival is achievable using this approach. The Canadian Pediatric Brain Tumor Consortium reported that 9 of the 18 patients who received various HDC regimens were alive at a median follow up time of 40.8 months (10 to 90) from diagnosis (Lafay-Cousin, et al., 2012). HDC was associated with a significant survival benefit with a 2-year overall survival of 47.9% (plus or minus 12.1) versus 27.3% (plus or minus 9.5) for the conventional chemotherapy group ($p = 0.036$). The Children's Oncology Group (COG) conducted a pilot study, 99703, to treat a variety of malignant brain tumors, including AT/RT, which incorporated three cycles of conventional chemotherapy with cyclophosphamide, etoposide, vincristine, and cisplatin, followed by three high dose cycles of carboplatin and dose escalation of thiotepa with stem cell transplants (Cohen et al., 2015). This study demonstrated feasibility of this approach and improved survival. The current national Children's Oncology Group phase III study (ACNS0333) utilizes the chemotherapeutic backbone of 99703 with the additional of high-dose methotrexate during induction and conformal field radiation therapy. The study accrued 70 patients and is currently in analysis. For 55 patients treated on the study who were younger than 36 months at diagnosis, the 2 year event free and overall survival are 39% and 48% respectively. For 11 patients greater than 3 years of age, the 2 year event free and overall survival are 60% and 80% (Reddy et al., 2016). Given the very young age of these patients, these results are also very encouraging.

RADIATION

The vast majority of AT/RT survivors in the literature have received some form of radiation therapy as a component of their treatment and its positive effect on long-term survival has been reported in several series (Hilden, et al., 2004; Tekautz, et al., 2005; Chi, et al., 2009). The most recent compelling evidence comes from analysis of the National Cancer Institute's SEER database, which identified 144 patients with AT/RT from 1973 to 2008 (Buscariollo, et al., 2012). As expected, the majority of patients (82%) were less than age 3 years and approximately one-third of patients received radiation. The median overall survival (OS) of patients who did not receive radiation therapy was 6 months. For those who had received some form of radiation as part of their primary therapy, the mean overall survival had not been reached at the time patients were reported. There was an increased use of radiation in young children after 2005. Both the IRSIII and COG trials, ACNS0333, mentioned in the previous section, both included conformal radiation for all patients. There are some long-term survivors of AT/RT reported in the literature who were treated with HDC but did not receive radiation. Until we are better able to risk-stratify patients, there is good evidence that focal radiation coupled with intensive chemotherapy provides the best chance at durable control of AT/RT.

TOXICITY OF THERAPY

The intensive therapeutic regimens carry potential morbidity, and a few deaths due to treatment toxicity have been reported. It is very well established that craniospinal radiation has significant deleterious effects on the developing nervous system, and its use in young children gives many clinicians great angst. Advanced radiation techniques, specifically 3D conformal therapy and the wider availability of proton beam radiation, are showing decreased long-term neurologic sequelae and less effect on cognitive function. Chemotherapy, surgery, and the tumor itself also contribute to the long-term neurologic sequelae. Intensive chemotherapy also has significant long-term systemic sequelae and the risk of major organ dysfunction. As more patients are long-term survivors of AT/RT, their long-term cognitive, neurologic, endocrine, and systemic function will need to be monitored. Early and ongoing intervention from psychologists, teachers, and therapists is highly important to help patients maximize their potential. Although treatment will likely continue to be refined, the importance of these posttreatment interventions cannot be overemphasized.

FUTURE DIRECTIONS

As current treatment regimens are highly intensive and consequently highly toxic, further improvements in outcome will require improved understanding of the biology of this tumor and targeting of therapy to the tumor. Extensive laboratory investigations have been carried out to better understand the tumorigenesis of AT/RT as well as to identify potential therapeutic targets. Preclinical testing of rhabdoid cell lines and xenografts has shown data that are provocative with regard to the chemo-responsiveness of AT/RT. These have given biologic rationale to early experimental clinical trials with small molecule inhibitors, for example, targeting HDAC, Aurora a kinase, CDK, and EZH2. What remains a limitation, however, is the lack of genetically engineered or orthotopic CNS AT/RT animal models that reflect the human condition. Current modern technologies, including whole exome and genome sequencing and epigenetic assays, have propelled our understanding of AT/RT but will require validation. Undoubtedly, future clinical studies will incorporate targeted approaches based on an improved biological understanding of these tumors.

CONCLUSIONS

Since first being recognized as a distinct tumor in the late 1980s, significant strides have been made in understanding the biology and treatment of AT/RT. It is the first pediatric brain tumor for which a common genetic abnormality has been identified. Immunohistochemical antibody staining for the SMARCB1 gene product has simplified identification of the tumor. Although the function of SMARCB1 is not yet known, modern and evolving technologies will likely help identify targeted therapies. Once a disease that was considered to be universally fatal, recent intensive multimodal regimens have improved long-term overall survival for patients with AT/RT to approximately 50%. Genetic sequencing of tumors in recent trials may also help identify prognostic factors. There is optimism that targeted therapy can be combined with more traditional modalities to improve survival rates. Ideally, targeted therapies will also allow for reduction of more conventional therapies for at least some patients. Although much work remains to be done, continued multidisciplinary collaboration of preclinical and clinical researchers will likely continue to unravel this high aggressive tumor.

REFERENCES

The complete list of references for this chapter is available online at www.expertconsult.com.

   See inside cover for registration details.

SELECTED REFERENCES

Biegel, J.A., Zhou, J.Y., Rorke, L.B., et al., 1999. Germ-line and acquired mutations of INI1 in atypical teratoid and rhabdoid tumors. Cancer Res. 59 (1), 74–79.

Buscariollo, D.L., Park, H.S., Roberts, K.B., et al., 2012. Survival outcomes in atypical teratoid rhabdoid tumor for patients undergoing radiotherapy in a surveillance, epidemiology, and end results analysis. Cancer 118 (17), 4212–4219.

Chi, S.N., Zimmerman, M.A., Yao, X., et al., 2009. Intensive multimodality treatment for children with newly diagnosed CNS atypical teratoid rhabdoid tumor. J. Clin. Oncol. 27 (3), 385–389.

Cohen, B.H., Geyer, J.R., Miller, D.C., et al., 2015. Pilot Study of Intensive Chemotherapy With Peripheral Hematopoietic Cell Support for Children Less Than 3 Years of Age With Malignant Brain Tumors, the CCG-99703 Phase I/II Study. A Report From the Children's Oncology Group. Pediatr. Neurol. 53 (1), 31–46.

Hilden, J.M., Meerbaum, S., Burger, P., et al., 2004. Central nervous system atypical teratoid/rhabdoid tumor: results of therapy in children enrolled in a registry. J. Clin. Oncol. 22 (14), 2877–2884.

Judkins, A.R., Mauger, J., Ht, A., et al., 2004. Immunohistochemical analysis of hSNF5/INI1 in pediatric CNS neoplasms. Am. J. Surg. Pathol. 28 (5), 644–650.

Kim, K.H., Roberts, C.W., 2014. Mechanisms by which SMARCB1 loss drives rhabdoid tumor growth. Cancer Genet. 207 (9), 365–372.

Lafay-Cousin, L., Hawkins, C., Carret, A.S., et al., 2012. Central nervous system atypical teratoid rhabdoid tumours: the Canadian Pediatric Brain Tumor Consortium experience. Eur. J. Cancer 48 (3), 353–359.

Packer, R.J., Biegel, J.A., Blaney, S., et al., 2002. Atypical teratoid/rhabdoid tumor of the central nervous system: report on workshop. J. Pediatr. Hematol. Oncol 24 (5), 337–342.

Reddy, A.T., Strother, D., Judkins, A., et al., 2016. Treatment of Atypical Teratoid Rhabdoid Tumors (ATRT) of the Central Nervous System with Surgery, Intensive Chemotherapy, and 3-D Conformal Radiation (ACNS0333). A Report from the Children's Oncology Group. Abstracts from the 17th International Symposium on Pediatric Neuro-Oncology, Liverpool, UK. Neuro. Oncol.

Rorke, L.B., Packer, R., Biegel, J., 1995. Central nervous system atypical teratoid/rhabdoid tumors of infancy and childhood. J. Neurooncol. 24 (1), 21–28.

Tekautz, T.M., Fuller, C.E., Blaney, S., et al., 2005. Atypical teratoid/rhabdoid tumors (ATRT): improved survival in children 3 years of age and older with radiation therapy and high-dose alkylator-based chemotherapy. J. Clin. Oncol. 23 (7), 1491–1499.

E-BOOK FIGURES AND TABLES

130 Central Nervous System Germinoma and Other Germ Cell Tumors

Jeffrey C. Allen and Ute K. Bartels

An expanded version of this chapter is available on www.expertconsult.com. See inside cover for registration details.

INTRODUCTION

Germ cell tumors (GCTs) of the central nervous system (CNS) are a heterogeneous group of benign and malignant tumors currently classified as germinoma, teratoma (mature, immature, and teratoma with malignant transformation), and nongerminomatous germ cell tumors (NGGCTs). NGGCTs can include either a single tumor type or combinations of embryonal carcinoma, yolk sac tumors (or endodermal sinus tumors), choriocarcinoma, teratoma, and Germinoma. The term NGGCT is considered inaccurate, and efforts are ongoing to seek consensus for a new terminology (Finlay et al., 2008).

The management of this group of rare CNS tumors has been the recent focus of prospective clinical trials throughout Asia, the Americas, and Europe, and the clinical approach to these tumors is undergoing continuous modification. Because of their rarity, most of the research is conducted in large cooperative groups. Most encouraging is the recent exploration of the biologic basis of CNS GCTs, an effort that will likely lead to more targeted, safer therapies. Insight into the biology and management of CNS GCTs has been obtained from experience with these tumors outside the CNS, where they are of highest incidence in the gonads, mediastinum, and retroperitoneum.

From a biologic perspective, unusual features of CNS GCTs include their demographics (males > females, especially in the pineal region; higher incidence in people from Asia); onset primarily during adolescence and early adulthood; midline, extraaxial location in the CNS (pineal region, suprasellar region/neurohypophyseal); unique patterns of presentation in particular locations (bifocal pineal/suprasellar, basal ganglia); histologic distinctions by age and location (germinoma in pineal and bifocal locations; NGGCTs more common in females in suprasellar location; immature teratoma more common in infants); the ability to use tumor markers (alpha fetoprotein and human chorionic gonadotropin) in serum and cerebrospinal fluid (CSF) to diagnose and monitor response to treatment; and association with various genetic syndromes such as trisomy 21, Klinefelter syndrome, and Noonan syndrome. Pure germinomas may produce very low levels of human chorionic gonadotropin (hCG), but never alpha fetoprotein (AFP), in either CSF or serum, whereas NGGCT can produce any combination of both tumor markers.

In general, CNS GCTs often require multimodality therapy for optimum care. With the exception of low-grade variants such as mature or immature teratoma, where a gross total resection may be curative, combinations of chemotherapy and radiation therapy are necessary for most patients. Germinomas are very responsive to chemotherapy, and radiation and current clinical research is aimed at minimizing treatment and its consequences while preserving a high cure rate (5-year overall survival [OS] > 85%). For NGGCTs, more intensive preradiation chemotherapy combined with maximum surgical debulking of the tumor followed by radiation therapy appears to have dramatically improved survival (5-year OS > 70%).

EPIDEMIOLOGY

In a population-based study in Canada using data from a tumor registry, the mean annual incidence of CNS GCT was reported to be 1.06 per million children (0–18 years of age). In this study, the annual incidence of germinoma was approximately twice that of NGGCT. Whereas other Western countries estimate similar incidence rates, with CNS GCTs accounting for up to 3.6% of all pediatric intracranial CNS tumors, the rates appear higher in Japan and the Far East, accounting for up to 15.3% of all pediatric intracranial CNS tumors (Report of Brain Tumor Registry of Japan, 2003). The reasons for these variations in incidence remain elusive, but genetic predisposition and geographic or environmental factors may contribute.

The peak incidence of CNS GCT is in the second decade of life, and male gender increases the likelihood of this diagnosis. The male predominance is striking in GCTs arising in the pineal area, with a male:female ratio as high as 15:1. In contrast, girls are slightly more affected by GCTs arising in the suprasellar region.

PATHOLOGY AND ETIOLOGY OF GERM CELL TUMORS

CNS GCTs are immunophenotypic and morphologic homologues of GCTs arising in extracranial locations, but the distribution of histologic subtypes appears to differ by site of origin. Mature and immature teratomas mimic elements of all three embryonic germ layers: endoderm, mesoderm, and ectoderm. Uncertainty remains regarding the cells of origin of other subtypes, such as choriocarcinoma, germinoma, yolk sac tumors, and embryonal carcinoma. The primordial stem cells that give rise to normal and abnormal germ cell components are totipotent and capable of differentiation along several pathways. As such, the primary occurrence of GCTs in gonadal tissue is not surprising, but they also arise in several unique "midline" locations in the body and CNS, related to either aberrant migratory behavior and eventual neoplastic transformation or the failure of migratory stem cells in the embryo to undergo spontaneous apoptosis. That this aberrant ontogeny is under genetic control is suggested by the occurrence of multiple first-degree relatives affected by primary GCTs, both in the body and CNS, and the occurrence of GCTs in certain genetic syndromes such as Noonan syndrome and trisomy 21. Gonadotropins may also have a role in the etiology of GCTs, as suggested by their midline location, the "neighborhood" of diencephalic centers that regulate gonadotropins, and the increased prevalence in children of peripubertal age and in boys affected by Klinefelter syndrome (47 XXY).

GERMINOMA

The predominant type of CNS GCT is a germinoma, accounting for approximately 60% to 70% of intracranial GCTs (Report of Brain Tumor Registry of Japan, 2003; Calaminus et al., 2013). This section focuses primarily on its clinical management. Most germinomas develop in the suprasellar/neurohypophyseal and pineal regions. Occurrences outside the midline and in the basal ganglia are rare. Progression-free survival (PFS) in germinomas is excellent, with 5-year OS exceeding 90% in retrospective and prospective series.

Clinical Presentation

The clinical presentation is determined by the location of the germinoma. Protracted courses, up to years, of symptoms before diagnosis are not uncommon. Diabetes insipidus, a symptom of the vast majority of patients with suprasellar and bifocal germinoma, can remain clinically compensated for a prolonged time period. Hence diligent history taking and review for polyuria and polydipsia are important. Symptoms of increased fluid intake, nocturia, weight loss, and personality changes are common. New onset of diabetes insipidus should prompt a diagnostic workup, including a referral to a pediatric endocrinologist and brain magnetic resonance imaging (MRI) without and with contrast and with attention to the suprasellar region. Sometimes the initial MRI is nondiagnostic or may show slight infundibular thickening. In the case of documented pituitary stalk thickening, a careful clinical and imaging follow up is recommended because about 15% to 25% of affected individuals may eventually develop germinoma. Other symptoms associated with suprasellar germinoma location are visual disturbances, as a result of the close proximity to the optic chiasm and optic nerves, and endocrinopathies.

The most common symptoms of a pineal germinoma are those related to increased intracranial pressure resulting from obstruction of the aqueduct and, if the mass is large enough, Parinaud syndrome. This syndrome consists of vertical gaze impairment, convergence nystagmus, and pupils that respond to accommodation but not to light. It is a classical sign of tectal compression.

Rare off-midline germinomas, arising in the basal ganglia, thalamus, or internal capsule, are often characterized by insidious (i.e., over 1–4.5 years) onset of cognitive or motor symptoms. They can occur in isolation or synchronously in multiple locations. Affected patients may present with symptoms related to corticospinal tract or extrapyramidal dysfunction, such as hemiparesis and/or choreoathetotic movements, personality changes, and speech disturbances.

Radiology

Classical imaging characteristics of suprasellar and pineal (or bifocal) germinoma are homogenous isointense or hypointense lesions on T1-weighted MRI and isointense or hyperintense lesions on T2-weighted MRI (isodense or hyperdense on computed tomography [CT]), with avid enhancement after contrast administration. However, the tumor may also heterogeneously enhance and include cystic components and intratumoral calcifications. Subependymal ventricular dissemination is common and usually characterized by linear or nodular enhancement along the ependymal ventricular lining of the lateral or third ventricles, especially in the frontal horns. Large tumors may be surrounded by a 2- to 3-cm penumbra of FLAIR signal abnormality suggestive of either edema or infiltration. Basal ganglia germinomas may lack this avid enhancement and sometimes

show little or no mass effect, especially in the early stages of the disease. Ipsilateral cerebral and/or brainstem atrophy (Wallerian degeneration) is present in one third of patients with basal ganglia germinoma. Infiltrative disease appears to exert an anatomic and, most likely, physiologic "toxic" effect on brain parenchyma. After treatment, the tumor bed and surrounding tissue usually become atrophic, with calcium deposition.

Tumor Markers

Intracranial GCTs can secrete tumor markers into the bloodstream and/or CSF. For some tumor markers, such as hCG, there appears to be a CNS/systemic gradient, and lumbar assay values are usually higher. For others, such as AFP, the serum and CSF values are often similar. Germinomas do not secrete AFP but may secrete low levels of hCG and hCGβ either into serum and/or into CSF, possibly as a result of the presence of a small component of syncytiotrophoblastic giant cells (STGCs). Retrospective and prospective analyses found elevated hCG levels in serum and/or CSF in up to 42% of germinoma patients (Allen et al., 2012). The majority of cases have mild elevations of hCG levels solely in CSF; however, the presence of both or an elevated concentration in serum with a normal concentration in CSF have been described. Different timing of the sampling of hCG in serum and CSF (because of the short half-life of hCG [1.5 days]) and different units and kits may contribute to some of the variability in these findings.

Some authors have suggested a different prognosis for germinoma with elevated levels of hCG, but many studies do not specify the site of hCG measurement, and a recent publication suggests that serum hCG is an insensitive screening tool and that lumbar, but not ventricular, CSF is much more sensitive. Nonetheless, tumor marker analysis is currently being used in lieu of biopsy to diagnose germinoma and to distinguish germinoma from NGGCT. Patients with typical midline tumors and modest elevations of hCG are treated as cases of germinoma, and patients with any elevation of AFP are treated as cases of NGGCT in the Children's Oncology Group (COG) Germ Cell Tumor study (ACNS1123) protocol. For patients with normal tumor markers, biopsy is required.

S-Kit in Germinoma

Immunohistochemical studies have shown that c-kit, a protooncogene and transmembrane tyrosine receptor, is highly expressed in germinoma cells. S-kit is its soluble equivalent and can be measured in CSF. S-kit values in CSF are usually higher in germinoma compared with NGGCT patients, and levels correlate with treatment response and relapse (Miyanohara et al., 2002). These data suggest that CSF s-kit may represent a valuable tumor marker of germinomatous components, but currently the assay is used mostly for research purposes in Japan.

Staging

As with malignant childhood brain tumors in general, MRI of the entire CNS at the time of initial diagnosis is essential for staging. Should surgery be required as a result of obstructive hydrocephalus, MRI of the brain and spine should be obtained within a 48- to 72-hour window after the surgical intervention. This minimizes misinterpretation of the contrast enhancement that occurs between 72 hours and 6 weeks after surgery as a result of disruption of the blood–brain barrier. Tumor marker determinations in serum and CSF should be included in the staging. In the case of uncontrolled raised intracranial pressure or a lesion with mass effect, performance of a lumbar puncture is contraindicated. In most cases, however, lumbar CSF for cytology and marker analysis can safely be obtained following either an endoscopic third ventriculostomy (ETV) or placement of a ventriculoperitoneal (VP) shunt. To date, there are insufficient data on the significance and reliability of ventricular CSF tumor or cytology assays. The International Society of Pediatric Oncology (SIOP-CNS-GCT) trial allowed enrollment of patients if CSF cytology was undertaken via either the ventricular route or lumbar puncture. Interestingly, the Japanese working group dismisses CSF cytology because it is not taken into consideration for treatment decisions. Data from prospective studies suggest that 15% to 20% of germinoma patients have disseminated disease at diagnosis either on imaging (M+) or on CSF investigation (M1). Although bifocal involvement is considered metasynchronous but not metastatic disease, there is some controversy about whether observed studding on endoscopic inspection, which is invisible on MRI, or diffuse basal ganglia involvement are should be classified as M0 or M+.

Treatment

Role of Radiation and Chemotherapy

Historically, craniospinal irradiation has been the gold standard of treatment for CNS germinoma. Because of concerns about the long-term sequelae of both large-volume and high-dose radiation, there has been a concerted effort to either completely substitute intensive chemotherapy for radiation therapy or reduce both volume and dose in select cohorts of patients based on response to preradiotherapy chemotherapy. The outcome measures by which success will be gauged include maintenance of high survival rates with decreased long-term negative effects on cognitive and endocrine function and quality of life. Given the rarity of this disease and paucity of cooperative group phase III clinical trials, documentation of the achievement of these goals may be difficult. The current state-of-the-art treatment therapies are reviewed here, with the expectation that changes may emerge as clinical trials progress.

Radiation Therapy. Although reduction of craniospinal irradiation to whole-ventricular (WV) or whole-brain (WB) irradiation in completely staged, M0, primary germinoma appears relatively safe from the standpoint of tumor eradication and has evolved as an accepted practice throughout the world, the safety of elimination of WV irradiation and substitution with involved field (IF) irradiation has been questioned since the observation of increased numbers of ventricular relapses. Currently WV radiation is utilized by the Japanese, French, SIOP, and COG working groups in combination with chemotherapy as the standard of care for nonmetastatic suprasellar and pineal-region germinoma. The relative contributions of chemotherapy and irradiation remain a topic of debate.

Rogers, Mosleh-Shirazi, and Saran (2005) conducted a meta-analysis of radiation therapy for germinoma patients and found a recurrence rate of 7.6% after WB or WV radiation and a rate of 3.8% after craniospinal irradiation (CSI). No predilection for isolated spinal metastasis was found when CSI was omitted (2.9% versus 1.2%). The authors concluded that reduced-volume irradiation should replace craniospinal irradiation (Rogers et al., 2005). Ogawa et al.'s (2004) retrospective review of the Japanese experience concurs with a low risk of spinal relapse, reporting an incidence of 4% (2/56) for patients treated with CSI and 3% (2/70) for patients treated without spinal radiation. Excellent PFS rates for localized

germinomas with the use of either WB or WV irradiation have been reported by several institutions. Nevertheless, the volume of radiation should cover all areas of measurable disease identified at the initial MRI staging.

In addition to the controversies surrounding the optimum volume of radiation therapy, there has also been controversy about the optimum dose to both the primary tumor and any prophylactic field. Small retrospective experiences suggest that radiation doses can be reduced to 36 and 30 Gy WV irradiation, respectively, without preirradiation chemotherapy. However, the use of radiation therapy alone has been associated with the risk of extra-CNS relapses. Several clinical trials have proposed that preradiation chemotherapy may be used to triage patients who can more safely be treated with both volume and dose reductions of radiation, thereby reducing radiation-related long-term sequelae.

Chemotherapy. Germinomas are highly sensitive to radiation therapy and chemotherapy. Platinum compounds and cyclophosphamide are particularly efficacious chemotherapeutic agents in treating germinomas. The largest "chemotherapy-only" experience in newly diagnosed patients is reported in the First, Second, and Third International CNS Germ Cell Tumor Studies. In the first study, chemotherapy consisted of four cycles of carboplatin (500 mg/m^2/day, days 1 and 2), etoposide (150 mg/m^2/day, day 3), and bleomycin (15 mg/m^2/day, day 3). Patients with complete radiologic and tumor marker response proceeded to two more identical cycles, whereas cyclophosphamide (65 mg/kg) was added to the three-drug regimen for those with incomplete response. Of the CNS germinoma patients, 22 of 45 eventually relapsed. Although most relapsed patients were salvageable with high doses and volumes of radiation therapy, the 2-year OS in this study was only 84%. Nineteen germinoma patients were enrolled in the second study using an intensified cisplatin- and cyclophosphamide-based chemotherapy induction. Despite proof of effectiveness with a high rate of complete remission, the 5-year event-free survival (EFS) and OS rates were unsatisfactory at 47% ± 2.3% and 68% ± 2.2%, respectively. Moreover, chemotherapy was associated with unacceptable morbidity and mortality (4 deaths), predominantly in patients with diabetes insipidus. The third study included 25 patients and confirmed the inferior outcome of this strategy, with a 6-year EFS of 45.6% when avoiding radiation. In conclusion, "chemotherapy-only" strategies have not matched the long-term survival rates obtained with either radiation therapy alone or combined chemotherapy and radiation therapy. Chemotherapy should therefore not be used in isolation in patients with germinoma unless new targeted agents or new molecular markers for tumor responsiveness afford the hope of better outcomes.

Combined Chemotherapy and Radiation Therapy. One of the first trials of single-agent, neoadjuvant chemotherapy with carboplatin followed by response-dependent reductions in radiation volume and fields in biopsy-proven CNS germinoma observed a high complete response rate (7/11) and favorable outcome, with 10 of 11 patients experiencing long-term survival (Allen, Kim, and Packer, 1987). Preirradiation chemotherapy with carboplatin, etoposide, and ifosfamide followed by focal irradiation (40 Gy) has been studied in the SIOP-CNS-GCT-96 protocol for patients with nonmetastatic germinomas. Physicians had the option to use this approach or craniospinal irradiation without chemotherapy. This prospective multinational study included 190 patients with localized germinoma. The 5-year EFS and OS rates for patients treated with preirradiation chemotherapy ($n = 65$) were 88% ± 0.4% and 96% ± 0.3%, respectively, whereas the 5-year EFS and OS rates of patients treated with craniospinal radiation

($n = 125$) were 94% ± 0.2% and 95% ± 0.2%. Whereas relapses (4/125) only occurred locally in the CSI group, six of seven relapses occurred in the ventricular area in the chemotherapy/focal radiation treatment group. As a consequence, the current open SIOP trial combines preirradiation chemotherapy with ventricular irradiation (24 Gy) with an additional boost of 16 Gy to the primary tumor bed in patients with localized disease. Metastatic germinoma patients will continue to be treated with CSI only at the doses outlined previously without chemotherapy, as the 45 metastatic patients included in the aforementioned study showed an excellent 5-year EFS and OS of 98% ± 0.2%.

The risk of ventricular recurrence in patients treated with chemotherapy and focal radiation has also been well documented by the French and Japanese working groups. Alapetite et al. (2010) reported the SFOP (Societé Française d'Oncologie Pédiatrique) experience, which included 60 patients treated for CNS germinoma with a combination of carboplatin, etoposide, and ifosfamide followed by focal radiation (40 Gy). The 5-year EFS and OS rates were 84.2% and 98.2%, respectively. Ten of 60 patients relapsed at a median time of 32 months (range: 10–121 months), with the majority ($n = 8$) of relapses occurring within the ventricular system (Alapetite et al., 2010). The second trial of the Japanese GCT study group consisted of three cycles of carboplatin (450 mg/m^2/day, day 1) and etoposide (150 mg/m^2/day, days 1–3) chemotherapy followed by local irradiation (24 Gy). The 5-year OS rate was 98%. However, 13% of the patients (16/123) developed recurrence. In an interim analysis, a high incidence of ventricular/locoregional relapses was reported. As a consequence, current treatment in Japan, Europe, and North America combines chemotherapy with WV irradiation. Although the dose of WV irradiation is 24 Gy in Europe and Japan, the current Children's Oncology Group GCT trial evaluates the efficacy of a reduced dose of 18-Gy WV irradiation (plus boost to tumor bed to a total of 30 Gy) in chemotherapy-responsive germinoma patients with localized disease.

The vast majority of patients with suprasellar germinoma suffer from diabetes insipidus. Cisplatin- or ifosfamide-based chemotherapy requires hyperhydration, which significantly increases the risk for electrolyte imbalances and subsequent complications such as seizures (Afzal et al., 2008). A combination of carboplatin and etoposide chemotherapy is currently employed by the Japanese and North American working groups. This offers the advantage of easier outpatient administration and reduced risk of hyperhydration associated metabolic complications. Interestingly, whereas carboplatin alone has been proven effective (Allen, DaRoso, Donahue, and Nirenberg, 1994), etoposide has never been evaluated as an active single agent in the treatment of germinoma.

Role of Surgery

The Need for Biopsy and Second-Look Surgery

Currently, it is not sufficient to treat patients with isolated pineal or suprasellar tumors as cases of germinoma without biopsy confirmation or demonstration of hCG elevation. There are several types of tumors that arise in these locations, including those with low-grade and malignant histologies. In the era when the risks of operating on a patient with a pineal-region tumor were high, the practice was to use a radiographic response to 2 weeks of radiation therapy to confirm the assumption that a germinoma was involved. However, this practice is no longer viable because tumor types such as pineoblastomas or ependymomas may also briefly respond but would require very different doses and volumes of radiation for potential cure. Second, low-grade tumors such as

pineocytomas or teratomas would be irradiated needlessly when surgery could be curative. Currently, the risks of surgery in this area of the CNS are greatly reduced with the use of modern operating techniques and equipment and steroids. In addition, endoscopic procedures often provide very useful diagnostic information and serve to relieve intracranial hypertension via third ventriculostomy (ETV).

Thus it is the gold standard to establish the histologic presence of a GCT by either open or endoscopic biopsy if the tumor markers are normal. The choice of technique (stereotactic, endoscopic, open craniotomy) and the goal of surgery (tissue diagnosis versus tumor resection) are complex and largely determined by the anatomy of the lesion (size, accessibility through the ventricle, etc.) and the presence and extent of ventriculomegaly. If the tumor is confirmed to be a germinoma, the general goal of surgical intervention (apart from hydrocephalus management) is tissue diagnosis rather than tumor resection, because germinoma is so responsive to medical therapy. Symptomatic obstructive hydrocephalus may necessitate an emergent intervention such as placement of an external ventricular drain (EVD) and/or an ETV. At the time of ETV, many groups favor attempted tumor biopsy to confirm the histology.

The need for tissue biopsy in patients with a bifocal lesion, considered metasynchronous and not metastatic, is debatable. In accordance with the current SFOP, SIOP, and North American approach, a biopsy is not required if the clinical presentation, imaging characteristics, and tumor marker profile (AFP negative, no or mild elevation of hCG) are consistent with a bifocal germinoma. With very rare exceptions, bifocal lesions associated with negative serum and CSF tumor markers are almost always pure germinoma. However, some very rare cases of different pathologies have been reported.

The current North American GCT trial does not mandate a biopsy for suprasellar, pineal, or unifocal ventricular lesions (radiologically consistent with germinoma) if AFP is negative and if serum and/or CSF hCG is elevated but is less than or equal to 50 IU/L. However, in this protocol, a biopsy is required for patients with hCG values above 50 IU/L to a maximum of 100 IU/L. The Japanese approach has been surgical removal of lesions whenever feasible, and subsequent treatment is based on the final pathology result.

Germinomas are highly chemosensitive, and response to treatment is often obvious within days after the first cycle. At the Hospital for Sick Children in Toronto, a transient EVD is favored over a permanent shunt in patients with obstructive hydrocephalus likely caused by a germinoma in whom an ETV is not possible. After the diagnosis of a germinoma is confirmed, one cycle of chemotherapy is administered, and if the patient tolerates clamping of the drain, it is removed before the child becomes neutropenic.

The presence of residual disease at the end of treatment is not predictive of worse outcome, and patients with residual MRI abnormality following chemotherapy and radiation therapy fare as well as those without, as long as the tumor markers remain normal in serum and CSF (Calaminus et al., 2013). Lack of responsiveness to chemotherapy in either an hCG-positive or a biopsy-proven germinoma raises concerns of a potential mixed GCT, especially if there is persistence of or increase in the tumor markers; hence the current Children's Oncology Group GCT trial mandates second surgery at the end of chemotherapy in case of incomplete response if the residual suprasellar or pineal lesion is larger than 1 cm^2 and 1.5 cm^2, respectively, or the tumor markers do not normalize. The "growing teratoma" syndrome has been described primarily in patients with NGGCTs undergoing resection of a residual or enlarging primary tumor whose tumor markers are normal. The histology reflects a mature or immature teratoma.

Prognosis and Summary

The overall survival in germinoma exceeds 90%, with either radiation alone or with combinations of chemotherapy and radiation. Current treatment strategies include preradiation chemotherapy to reduce radiation doses and minimize long-term sequelae. Current evidence suggests that extent of resection does not contribute to superior outcome but may add morbidity. Hence, surgery should be limited to a biopsy or avoided where possible. There are many advances to be made, such as in the search for more specific and sensitive tumor markers, studies of whether responses to neoadjuvant chemotherapy justify radiation dose reductions, determination of the optimum dose and volume of radiation therapy, and determination of whether current efforts to further reduce radiation dose and volume justify the potential avoidance of late effects. Only through cooperative group trials and international collaboration around this rare disease can we make clinical progress. The exploration of the molecular basis of the origin and treatment sensitivity of GCTs deserves further effort, but currently the rate-limiting step is the paucity of tumor tissue given the small size of a biopsy specimen. With improvements in technology, more research will be possible and smaller amounts of tissue and CSF may be required, allowing some of these critical questions to be addressed.

REFERENCES

The complete list of references for this chapter is available in the e-book at www.expertconsult.com.
  See inside cover for registration details.

SELECTED REFERENCES

Afzal, S., Wherrett, D., Bartels, U., et al., 2008. Challenges and difficulties in management of patients with intracranial germ cell tumor having diabetes insipidus treated with cisplatin- and/or ifosfamide-based chemotherapy. Neuro Oncol. 10 (3), 417.

Alapetite, C., Brisse, H., Patte, C., et al., 2010. Pattern of relapse and outcome of non-metastatic germinoma patients treated with chemotherapy and limited field radiation: the SFOP experience. Neuro Oncol. 12 (12), 1318–1325.

Allen, J.C., Kim, J.H., Packer, R.J., 1987. Neoadjuvant chemotherapy for newly diagnosed germ-cell tumors of the central nervous system. J. Neurosurg. 67 (1), 65–70.

Allen, J.C., DaRoso, R.C., Donahue, B., et al., 1994. Aphase II trial of preirradiation carboplatin in newly diagnose germinoma of the central nervous system. Cancer 74 (3), 940–944.

Allen, J., Chacko, J., Donahue, B., et al., 2012. Diagnostic sensitivity of serum and lumbar CSF bHCG in newly diagnosed CNS germinoma. Pediatr. Blood Cancer 59 (7), 1180–1182.

Calaminus, G., Kortmann, R., Worch, J., et al., 2013. SIOP CNS GCT 96: final report of outcome of a prospective, multinational nonrandomized trial for children and adults with intracranial germinoma, comparing craniospinal irradiation alone with chemotherapy followed by focal primary site irradiation for patients with localized disease. Neuro Oncol. 15 (6), 788–796.

Finlay, J., da Silva, N.S., Lavey, R., et al., 2008. The management of patients with primary central nervous system (CNS) germinoma: current controversies requiring resolutions. Pediatr. Blood Cancer 51 (2), 313–316.

Miyanohara, O., Takeshima, H., Kaji, M., et al., 2002. Diagnostic significance of soluble c-kit in the cerebrospinal fluid of patients with germ cell tumors. J. Neurosurg. 97 (1), 177–183.

Ogawa, K., Shikama, N., Toita, T., et al., 2004. Long-term results of radiotherapy for intracranial germinoma: a multi-institutional retrospective review of 126 patients. Int. J. Radiat. Oncol. Biol. Phys. 58 (3), 705–713.

Report of Brain Tumor Registry of Japan (1969–1996). 2003. Neurol Med. Chir. (Tokyo) 43 (Suppl. (11th edition)), 1–111.

Rogers, S.J., Mosleh-Shirazi, M.A., Saran, F.H., 2005. Radiotherapy of localised intracranial germinoma: time to sever historical ties? Lancet Oncol. 6 (7), 509–519.

131 Craniopharyngioma, Meningiomas, and Schwannomas

Michelle Lauren Feinberg, Jeffrey H. Wisoff, and Robert Keating

 An expanded version of this chapter is available on www.expertconsult.com. See inside cover for registration details.

Craniopharyngiomas, meningiomas, and schwannomas are less common than other childhood brain tumors, frequently present insidiously over months to years, and often are amenable to successful surgical and medical intervention. The advent of improved neuroimaging has allowed earlier diagnosis, targeted treatment, and the ability to noninvasively and serially monitor patients. This chapter reviews the epidemiology, clinical presentation, neuroimaging findings, histology, genetics, surgical and medical management, and outcomes of these three tumors as they occur in the pediatric population.

CRANIOPHARYNGIOMAS

Few topics in neurosurgery inspire more controversy than the optimal treatment of craniopharyngiomas. The benign histology of these tumors often belies their malignant clinical course, particularly in children. The location of craniopharyngiomas, and specifically their intimate association with the visual pathways, pituitary, hypothalamus, and limbic system, predisposes patients to severe visual, endocrine, and cognitive deficits, both at presentation and as a result of treatment. Although most children can compensate for neurologic deficits and endocrinologic deficiencies, the cognitive and psychosocial sequelae can be functionally devastating, interfering with education, limiting independence, and adversely affecting the quality of life as these children approach adulthood.

Epidemiology

The Central Brain Tumor Registry found craniopharyngiomas to comprise 4.2% of all tumors in children aged 0 to 14 years (Ostrom et al., 2015). Craniopharyngiomas have a bimodal age distribution with a peak in the pediatric population between age 5 and 14 years and another peak in the adult population between age 50 and 74 years (McCrea et al., 2015). Thirty-three percent to 54% of all craniopharyngiomas occur in children, accounting for 6% to 9% of all pediatric brain tumors. These tumors are the most common nonglial tumors of childhood.

Although there does not appear to be any racial or ethnic predilection for craniopharyngiomas, the influence of gender is not as clear. Considering the available data, craniopharyngiomas may occur slightly more often in males than in females.

Clinical Presentation

The slow growth of craniopharyngiomas often results in a delay between onset of symptoms and diagnosis, with a typical prodrome of 1 to 2 years. The main presenting signs and symptoms of craniopharyngiomas are secondary to pressure upon adjacent neural structures. Headaches from raised intracranial pressure are the most common complaint, occurring in 60% to 75% of patients.

Visual impairment, caused by compression of optic pathway structures, is the presenting complaint in approximately 50% of children. On preoperative neuroophthalmo-logic testing, 70% to 80% of children have abnormal visual acuity or visual fields. The specific deficits are a reflection of the direction of tumor growth and its compression of various portions of the visual apparatus. Prechiasmatic extension will compress optic nerves with loss of visual acuity, whereas posterior tumors cause chiasmatic compression with complex visual field defects. Papilledema is present in approximately 20% of children (Fig. 131-1).

Hypothalamic and endocrine dysfunction, including growth failure (short stature), delayed sexual maturation, excessive weight gain, and diabetes insipidus, is present in 20% to 50% of children at the time of diagnosis, but is less commonly the symptom that brings the child to medical attention. At the time of presentation, less than one third of children are endocrinologically normal, making preoperative endocrine assessment mandatory.

Neuroimaging

The role of neuroimaging is to establish a preoperative diagnosis and then define the location and extent of the cystic, solid, and calcified portions of the tumor and its relation to the distorted normal anatomy. Radiographic evaluation includes computed tomography (CT), magnetic resonance imaging (MRI), magnetic resonance angiography (MRA), and, where available, magnetic resonance spectroscopy (MRS). Vascular anatomy can be well demonstrated by MRI and MRA obviating the need for invasive cerebral angiography.

The noncontrast CT usually demonstrates a suprasellar and often intrasellar mass with calcifications as well as hypodense solid and cystic components (Fig. 131-2). The low-density component usually has an attenuation greater than that of CSF. A small percentage of craniopharyngiomas may be of high density. CT shows secondary changes in the skull base such as enlargement of the sella turcica and/or erosion of the dorsum sella.

MRI provides invaluable information regarding the relation of the tumor to the surrounding critical structures, including the visual pathway, hypothalamus, blood vessels of the circle of Willis, and ventricles (Fig. 131-3). The appearance of a normal pituitary gland helps to make the correct diagnosis. Administration of gadolinium demonstrates the avidly enhancing cystic capsule and solid tumor. The appearance of the cyst fluid is uniformly hyperintense on T2-weighted sequences, but can vary in intensity on T1-weighted sequences based on its biochemical composition (Fig. 131-4).

Solid craniopharyngiomas without calcifications can be difficult to differentiate from other pediatric suprasellar tumors. In these instances, MR spectroscopy can provide additional findings that may help to establish a specific diagnosis. Craniopharyngiomas exhibit an elevated lactate peak and only trace amounts of other spectral metabolites. This is in contrast to gliomas that demonstrate an increased choline–to–N-acetylaspartate ratio compared with normal brain. Pituitary adenomas will exhibit either a choline peak or no abnormal metabolite peaks.

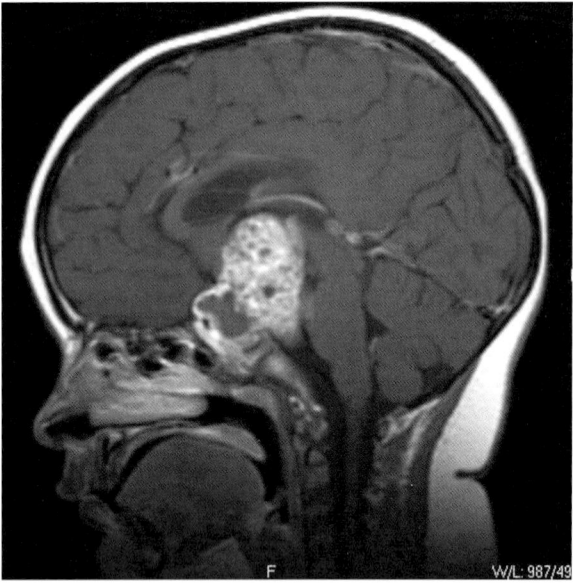

Figure 131-3. Craniopharyngioma. Magnetic resonance imaging (MRI)—Note the heterogeneous nature (solid > cystic) of this cranio-pharyngioma on MRI with significant suprasellar extension. Despite its location, potentially obstructing the foramen of Monro(s), there was no hydrocephalus.

Histopathology

Craniopharyngiomas develop from epithelial nests that are embryonic remnants of Rathke's pouch located along an axis extending from the sella turcica along the pituitary stalk to the hypothalamus and the floor of the third ventricle. The tumors gradually enlarge as partially calcified, heterogeneous solid, and cystic masses predominantly in the suprasellar region. They extend along the path of least resistance into the basal cisterns or invaginate into the third ventricle. Hydrocephalus can result from continued growth superiorly into the third ventricle.

Craniopharyngiomas have two basic patterns of cellular growth—adamantinomatous and papillary. Mixed tumors with both adamantinomatous and squamous papillary components or combinations of craniopharyngioma and Rathke's cleft cysts can occur.

Adamantinomatous tumors are the more common variant. They resemble the epithelium of tooth-forming tumors containing three distinct components: a basal layer of small cells; an intermediate layer of variable thickness with loose, stellate cells; and a top layer facing the cystic lumen where the cells are abruptly enlarged, flattened, and keratinized. At the cyst surface, desquamated epithelial cells are present either singly or in characteristic stacked clusters (keratin nodules). These nodules may undergo mineralization with accumulation of calcium salts, which, in rare instances, progress to metaplastic bone formation. The cysts in these tumors usually contain an oily liquid composed of this desquamated epithelium, rich in cholesterol, keratin, and occasionally calcium (Fig. 131-5).

Squamous papillary tumors occur nearly exclusively in adults and often involve the third ventricle. They consist of solid epithelium, without loose stellate zones, in a papillary architecture that resembles metaplastic respiratory epithelium. They are predominantly solid and rarely undergo mineralization. When cysts occur, the fluid is less oily and dark than in adamantinomatous tumors. As a result of the absence of calcification and minimal cyst formation, complete curative

surgical resection may be obtained more often in these tumors than in adamantinomatous or mixed craniopharyngiomas (Fig. 131-6).

Microscopic islets or "fingers" of adamantinomatous tumor embedded in densely gliotic parenchyma are frequently seen when this tumor arises in the region of the tuber cinereum, hypothalamus, and floor of the third ventricle. The gliotic reaction of Rosenthal fibers and fibrillary astrocytes, varying between several hundred micrometers to millimeters in thickness, effectively separates the tumor from the brain, thus providing a safe plane for surgical dissection. The presence of this gliotic tissue on surgical pathology is associated with a decreased risk of recurrence after gross total tumor resection.

Treatment

The treatment goal for craniopharyngiomas in the pediatric population is permanent tumor control or cure. However, the optimal treatment strategy remains controversial, with the debate centered on the extent of tumor resection, the role of radiation therapy, and the utilization of intracystic therapies, including radionuclides, baclofen, and interferon. The philosophy of curative treatment of craniopharyngiomas is predicated on children and their families having unimpeded access to long-term medical care and the personal or societal financial resources for the costs of lifetime hormone replacement therapy.

A multidisciplinary team including pediatric endocrinology, neuropsychology, pediatric neurosurgery, pediatric oncology, radiation oncology, and pediatric neurology is essential. Primary irradiation without resection, intracystic therapies, and palliative strategies may be more appropriate in those settings in which resources are limited or multidisciplinary expertise is lacking. Although partial resection without adjuvant radiation or cyst aspiration alone may provide temporary relief from symptoms, progressive solid and cystic tumor growth is inevitable. The management of craniopharyngiomas that have failed primary therapy is associated with significantly increased morbidity and mortality.

Radical Surgical Resection

Many pediatric neurosurgeons in North America and Europe favor complete microsurgical resection as the treatment of choice for newly diagnosed craniopharyngiomas (Fig. 131-7). The feasibility and success of such radical resection is dependent on the size and extent of the tumor, whether the tumor is primary or recurrent, the availability of surgical expertise and postoperative endocrinologic support, as well as the presence of societal resources to cope with potential postoperative deficits. If the socioeconomic conditions applicable to an individual patient do not provide appropriate long-term neurologic care and endocrinologic support, functional morbidity may overshadow the merits of curative resection. Proponents of radical surgical resection argue that the advances of microsurgical techniques have facilitated treatment of these tumors and substitutive therapy can ameliorate endocrinologic sequelae secondary to hypothalamic injury. The greater immediate morbidity of this approach may be mitigated by the fact that radiation therapy carries the risk of unpredictable late neurologic, vascular, and oncogenic side effects as well as long-term development of neuropsychologic deficits in children.

Radiographically confirmed total resection can be accomplished in 60% to 100% of primary tumors in children with mortality rates of 0% to 4%. Recurrence rates after total resection range from 0% to 20%, and most recurrences occur within 2 to 3 years after surgery.

The philosophy and experience of the surgeon significantly affect the likelihood of achieving a curative total resection with a low mortality and without disabling morbidity. Centers performing fewer than 2 radical resections per year had a good outcome in only 52% of patients, whereas institutions that performed radical resections more often had a good outcome in 87% of patients. Factors such as tumor size, severity of preoperative deficits, and the presence of hydrocephalus all play a role in postoperative morbidity but not in disease control.

Subtotal Resection With Irradiation

Craniopharyngiomas are radiosensitive tumors. To reduce the morbidity associated with radical surgery, particularly when there is significant involvement of the hypothalamus, subtotal resection with adjuvant irradiation may provide similar disease control and less endocrinologic morbidity compared with radical resection alone. The addition of postoperative radiotherapy in the setting of gross residual disease can decrease the recurrence rate to 15% to 20%, whereas subtotal resection alone results in progression rates of 55% to 85%. Although radiation therapy has significantly improved progression-free outcomes, it does carry its own set of risks. The adjacent critical structures surrounding the tumor bed can be injured as a result of radiation treatment, with risks of visual problems, endocrine derangements, or cognitive changes.

Several radiation modalities have been used in treatment of craniopharyngiomas, including conventional external beam radiation, intensity-modulated radiation, single-fraction stereotactic radiosurgery, fractionated stereotactic radiotherapy, and proton beam radiotherapy. With improvements in neuroimaging and radiation modalities, radiation treatment has become more accurate, resulting in decreased complication rates and improved survival (Lee et al., 2014; Kim et al., 2015). At this time, there is no standard of care regarding radiation for craniopharyngiomas although fractionated external beam radiation with a dose of 54 to 55.8 Gy in 1.8 Gy fractions is commonly used.

Recently a large case series of patients treated for residual tumor or tumor regrowth with single-dose gamma knife radiosurgery was published. In this series, progression-free survival was 70% at 5 years and 43.8% at 10 years, with an overall survival rate of 83.9% at 10-year follow-up. Most of the patients who developed new neurologic or endocrine disturbances demonstrated tumor regrowth; however, a total 10.9% of patients were thought to develop complications as a result of radiosurgery (Kim et al., 2015).

Aspiration

Simple stereotactic aspiration of tumor cysts or placement of an Ommaya reservoir into the cyst for serial aspirations is never indicated as primary therapy in children and should be reserved for palliation when all other treatment modalities have failed. Frequent aspirations tend to stimulate cyst fluid production, leading to progressively shorter symptom-free intervals. Solid tumor growth is unimpeded and may extend into areas of the decompressed cysts. Aspiration may be required to control cyst volume while waiting for the therapeutic effects of intracavitary irradiation (Fig. 131-8).

Intracystic Therapy

Intracystic therapy with bleomycin, interferon, or radionuclide can also be delivered through an Ommaya catheter.

Intracavitary Irradiation. Local treatment of cystic craniopharyngiomas with intracavitary beta irradiation was first described by Leksell and Liden in the 1950s. The procedure is performed by using a fine needle to puncture the cyst or cysts under stereotactic guidance. The amount of radionuclide to be delivered is calculated using a standard formula based on the cyst's volume. This calculation can be difficult in very small cysts. An equivalent volume of cyst fluid is first aspirated before the radionuclide is injected into the cysts. It is important not to alter the size and shape of the cysts, as this ensures even distribution of the radioisotope over the entire internal cyst wall without wall collapse or "wrinkling."

Cyst regression after intracavitary irradiation occurs gradually over several months. It does not control solid tumor growth, nor does it prevent the development of new cysts. Intracystic irradiation is generally well tolerated. Cyst leakage can occur in up to 10% of patients, with no subsequent sequelae. It can often be used in combination with stereotactic radiosurgery in patients with tumors that have a larger cystic component and a smaller residual solid component (Kim et al., 2015).

Intracystic Bleomycin. Bleomycin inhibits DNA production and has shown clinical efficacy in the treatment of analogous epithelial tumors. The cell cycle kinetics and spatial distribution of S-phase proliferative cells in the squamous epithelium of craniopharyngioma cysts provide a rationale for the use of antineoplastic agents.

An Ommaya catheter is placed into the cyst either stereotactically or at the time of craniotomy. Several days after placement, a contrast injection and CT are performed to verify no leakage of cyst contents. Between 1.5 and 10 mg of bleomycin is injected at 1- to 2-day intervals depending on the cyst volume. Repeat injections are performed over a 10- to 21-day period for average total dose of 60 to 80 mg. Similar to intracystic irradiation, involution of cysts occurs slowly over several months. Although the total number of patients treated remains small, the reported series demonstrate reduction in cyst volume in almost all patients, with up to 50% of patients showing complete disappearance of the cyst and indefinite remission.

Despite proper positing of the catheter, bleomycin has been reported to leak into normal surrounding brain with significant complications of hypothalamic injury, seizures, hemiparesis, panhypopituitarism, blindness, and, rarely, death.

Intracystic Interferon. Interferon-alpha has been advocated as a safer alternative to bleomycin. Interferon-alpha is a cytokine with established antitumoral activity with the advantage of not having any neurotoxicity. Interferon-alpha has been used as both systemic and intracavitary therapy for primary craniopharyngiomas. In one of the initial studies, all 19 patients receiving intracystic interferon-alpha showed reduction in tumor size with a mean initial volume 33.50 cm^3 and mean final tumor volume of 3.10 cm^3. Cavalheiro et al. reported an international multiinstitutional open-label trial of intracavitary interferon-alpha in 60 children. This study demonstrated a greater than 50% reduction in cyst size in 78% of children; however, with relatively short follow-up, 22% showed disease progression requiring repeat surgery. Three of the responders had previously experienced tumor progression after bleomycin but were salvaged with interferon. There was no information on long-term outcome or durability of disease control. Side effects in both studies included fatigue and headache with no development of new hormonal deficits or need to stop treatment because of side effects.

Outcomes and Quality of Life

Hypothalamic dysfunction is a unique complication of craniopharyngiomas and can be life-threatening. Symptoms can include obesity, hyperphagia, memory deficits, thermoregulatory abnormalities, labile behavior, and sleep-wake cycle abnormalities. Severe obesity with a body mass index defined as greater than three standard deviations above average has been reported in up to 44% of children after surgical resection (Müller, 2015).

Overview

Craniopharyngiomas are histologically benign epithelial neoplasms that arise in the sellar and suprasellar region. Their intimate relationship with the optic chiasm, pituitary, hypothalamus, and cerebral vasculature leads a unique set of challenges in both treatment and management. There is no current consensus on optimal management strategies with outcomes supporting similar survival rates between gross total resection and subtotal resection followed by radiation. After treatment, patients must be followed with frequent imaging studies for early detection of recurrent tumors.

MENINGIOMAS

Meningiomas are benign tumors that arise from the arachnoid cap cells of the meninges. Although meningiomas are the most common primary brain tumor diagnosed in adults, they are rare in the pediatric population, comprising only 2.6% of pediatric brain tumors. Because of their relatively low frequency, there are little data published regarding pediatric meningiomas. Much of the treatment strategies and management options are based on extrapolations from the adult literature despite significant differences being found between the two groups. In general, pediatric meningiomas are most often related to a pre-existing genetic condition (e.g., neurofibromatosis-2, NF-2), a history of radiation, or arise *de novo*.

Epidemiology

The central brain tumor registry of the United States reported that meningiomas comprise 2.6% of all pediatric brain tumors with a similar rate of 2.4% reported in a recent meta-analysis of all published cases of pediatric meningiomas. A previous diagnosis of NF-2 was found in 10.2% of patients. In contrast to the female predilection seen in adult meningiomas, differing series in children have reported equal gender distributions or a slight male predominance (Stanuszek et al., 2014).

Being derived from arachnoid cells, meningiomas can develop in any location where meninges are present. In approximately 90% of patients, meningiomas are supratentorial and are usually found at the convexity. However, atypical lesions such as intraventricular or locations without obvious dural attachments can be seen in children at higher rates than seen in adults (Stanuszek et al., 2014). For example, intraventricular meningiomas comprise only 0.5% to 2% of tumors in adults, in contrast to 11% in children (Stanuszek et al., 2014). Additionally, tumors that lack dural attachment have been reported to be as high as 30% in children (Stanuszek et al., 2014).

Clinical Presentation

As with any intracranial lesion, the presenting signs and symptoms depend on the size and location of the lesion. Compared with adults, pediatric meningiomas tend to be larger at the time of presentation and thus children often present with signs of increased intracranial pressure such as headache, nausea, vomiting, increased head circumference, or frontal bossing. Seizures have been the presenting symptom in up to 30% of pediatric patients with meningiomas. Based

TABLE 131-1 Presenting Symptoms and Signs of Pediatric Meningiomas

Seizures	33%
Headache	13%
Ataxia	10%
Hemiparesis	10%
Scalp mass	3%
Surveillance	3%
Incidental	1%

(Data from Rushing et al. Central nervous system meningiomas in the first two decades of life: a clinicopathological analysis of 87 patients. J Neurosurg 2005;103:489–95.)

on published series, children present most commonly with headaches, followed by seizures, and least commonly with neurologic deficits (Table 131-1).

Molecular Genetics

Much of the knowledge regarding molecular genetics of meningiomas is due to studies in the adult meningioma population but which has not been further extended to assessment of children. The precipitating cytogenetic event resulting in meningioma development is thought to be caused by a deletion on chromosome 22, close to the *NF-2* gene. Deletions in both *1p* and *14q* have also been found in pediatric meningiomas and are associated with higher rates of tumor recurrence.

Meningiomas and Genetic Conditions

In the pediatric population, meningiomas are commonly associated with several disorders, including NF-2, Gorlin syndrome, Rubenstein-Taybi syndrome, and Castleman disease.

Pediatric meningiomas are most frequently seen in patients with NF-2. It is estimated that 20% to 40% of all pediatric meningiomas are in patients with NF-2 and 53% of patients with NF-2 will develop meningiomas (Stanuszek et al., 2014). The Wishart variant of NF-2 has meningioma rates as high as 83% (Stanuszek et al., 2014). Patients with NF-2 have a much higher risk of being diagnosed with multifocal meningiomas. Children presenting with an isolated meningioma have a 20% risk of developing NF-2 and evaluation for the disease should be undertaken at diagnosis (Stanuszek et al., 2014).

The disease course of NF-2 meningiomas can vary greatly from that of sporadic meningiomas. The location of NF-2–associated meningiomas are different from that in the general population, with higher rates in the spinal canal and optic nerve sheath. Although sporadic meningiomas tend to invade brain tissue causing a poorer short-term prognosis, NF-2 meningiomas have less of a tendency for brain invasion, offering a more favorable short-term prognosis. However, because of multiple tumors that tend to develop in NF-2, the overall long-term prognosis is less favorable than that seen for the general population (Stanuszek et al., 2014). NF-2–associated meningiomas also have been calculated to grow at faster rates than sporadic meningiomas with growth rates of 0.01 to 6.7 cm^3/year and 0.2 to 2.5 cm^3/year, respectively.

Treatment of patients with NF-2 meningiomas differs compared with the regular pediatric population. Because of the frequency of meningiomas and other associated tumors, management of NF-2 focuses on quality of life and conservation of neurologic function (Stanuszek et al., 2014). For these reasons, it is recommended to operate only on lesions that are causing progressive symptoms and not necessarily for radiographic progression alone (Stanuszek et al., 2014). NF-2 meningiomas have been reported to be less sensitive to stereotactic radiosurgery compared with sporadic tumors (Stanuszek et al., 2014).

Radiation-Induced Meningiomas

Radiation therapy for treatment of other malignancies is a well-documented cause for meningioma development. The interval between initial radiation exposure and development of meningiomas is dependent on the intensity of radiation received, with the earliest reports of meningioma occurrence at 2 years after treatment to as late as 63 years after radiation therapy. Meningiomas caused by radiation damage often will show complex structural chromosomal abnormalities as a result of DNA damage. Because of the increased risk of meningioma development, all children who received prior cranial radiation should be followed with serial surveillance MRI screenings into adulthood.

Neuroimaging

Imaging characteristics of meningiomas are similar in both pediatric and adult tumors. Typical findings on CT are isodense or hypodense lesions with surrounding edema. Additionally, hyperostosis of the surrounding bone is a common finding. On MRI, meningiomas appear as hypointense on T1-weighted imaging and hyperintense on T2-weighted imaging (Fig. 131-9). With contrast administration, meningiomas show avid and homogenous enhancement. A dural tail is characteristic of meningiomas but not pathognomonic. Calcifications and cystic transformation can be seen more commonly in children.

As opposed to adults, any patient with a newly diagnosed meningioma should undergo imaging of the complete neuroaxis to evaluate for either multiple lesions or metastatic lesions.

Histopathology

The revised WHO classification divides meningiomas into grade I (benign), grade II (atypical), and, grade III (anaplastic). Based on histopathologic characteristics, meningiomas can be further subdivided into 13 variants. Although this classification scheme is based on adult meningiomas, all variants have been described in pediatric meningiomas as well (Fig. 131-10).

As with adults, WHO grade I meningiomas are most common, with transitional, meningiothelial, and fibrous histopathologic types occurring most frequently (Stanuszek et al., 2014) (Table 131-2). However, in contrast to adults, there are higher rates of atypical histopathology in children,

especially with the clear cell and papillary variants. In the adult population, the incidence of WHO grade II and III meningiomas is 1 to 2.8% whereas in children the incidence reaches 4.7% to 7.2% (Stanuszek et al., 2014). Although histologic grade usually does influence treatment, 15-year survival was not influenced in children and adolescents (Stanuszek et al., 2014). Unlike adults, the behavior of childhood meningiomas can be very difficult to predict based on the WHO grade. There is, however, a tendency for WHO grade III meningiomas to behave in a more aggressive manner, as seen in smaller case series.

The risk of developing recurrent disease in pediatric patients has been shown to be linked to the WHO grade. WHO grade I tumors have a 92% 10-year event-free survival, whereas 10-year event-free survival for WHO grade II and III tumors is 70% and 33%, respectively.

Treatment

Because of the largely benign nature of the disease, treatment options for meningiomas can be either conservative (observation) or via surgical intervention. Because of the rare nature of the disease and often atypical imaging findings, the need for a tissue diagnosis may necessitate operative intervention. Radiation therapy has been shown to be an effective adjuvant treatment, although the risks of radiation in the pediatric brain must be considered, especially with the possibility of malignant transformation. To date, chemotherapy has not been found to be efficacious in the management of meningiomas and is not a reasonable treatment option.

Observation

Conservative management via observation is a potential option in the pediatric population; however, the potential for long-term complications must be taken into account. Characteristics of the lesion, such as size, location, and symptomology, should be evaluated before deciding on conservative management. Observation is a common strategy in incidentally found meningiomas in adults. Studies of the adult population have shown that over 90% of meningiomas managed with observation grew over time with tumors larger than 2.5 cm tending to grow at more significant rates. With the long life expectancy of children, patients and parents should appropriately be counseled on the likely need for future surgical intervention. If conservative management is chosen, patients should be closely monitored with serial MRI every 6 to 12 months. If at any point there is radiographic evidence of tumor growth or if tumor-related symptoms develop, surgical intervention is strongly recommended.

Surgery

The definitive treatment for meningiomas is complete surgical resection, and the extent of surgical resection has been shown to be the most important prognostic factor for survival across all WHO tumor grades. Subtotal resection is associated with disease progression and the potential for malignant transformation. Surgical planning, including patient positioning, approach, and technique, is specifically dependent on tumor location, vascular supply, and patient-related factors. In the pediatric population, where blood loss is a major concern, staged procedures may also be an option in order to achieve gross total resection. Because of the large size of tumors at presentation and small blood volumes in pediatric patients, surgical mortality is estimated to be as high as 3% with a postoperative morbidity of as high as 40%.

As meningiomas tend to be vascular tumors, preoperative angiograms for tumor embolization are commonly employed

TABLE 131-2 Pathologic Classification of Pediatric Meningiomas

Grade I	Typical (<4 mit/10hpf)	Meningothelial fibrous, transitional, psammomatous, angiomatous
Grade II	Atypical (4–20 mit/10hpf)	Chordoid, clear cell
Grade III	Anaplastic (>20 mit/10hpf)	Papillary, rhabdoid

(Adapted from Louis et al. World Health Organization classification of tumors. Pathology and genetics of tumors. Lyon: IARC Press; 2000. p. 176–84.)

in adults (Stanuszek et al., 2014). Evidence has shown that selective embolization of feeding vessels has reduced operative blood loss and the length of surgery. However, because of the small-caliber vessels in children, there may be a significant risk of procedural complications, and treatment decisions must be made on an individual basis (Stanuszek et al., 2014). If preoperative embolization is not undertaken, attempts should be made to access and disrupt the major vascular supply (usually extradural) of the tumor early during surgery. This technique reduces intraoperative blood loss and also may make the tumor softer and more amenable to resection (Fig. 131-11).

For the most part, low-grade meningiomas maintain an arachnoid plane between the tumor and surrounding brain. In cases of atypical or malignant meningiomas, tumors are more likely to violate the arachnoid barrier and invade brain tissue, dura, and vessels. For these reasons, compete resection becomes considerably more difficult. If dura or bone appears to be invaded by tumor, it should be resected as much as possible. Small tumors may be able to be removed *en bloc*; however, larger tumors may require piecemeal resection.

The greatest difficulties arise when a patent's venous sinus is invaded by the tumor. In such cases, it may be prudent to leave a small portion of the tumor behind, rather than sacrificing an open dural sinus. Even in the anterior third of the sagittal sinus, sacrifice of this portion of the vessel cannot always be done with impunity. Close observation, even allowing the affected dural sinus to occlude slowly over time, will often permit an additional attempt at total tumor extirpation. Stereotactic radiosurgery may also be considered a therapeutic option, although the risk of malignant transformation cannot be discounted.

Recurrence rates of meningiomas are largely based on data obtained from the adult literature. With complete resection, recurrence rates of up to 20% within 25 years have been reported. In patients with subtotal resections, recurrence rates may be as high as 80% to 90%. These data necessitate long-term follow-up of children with meningiomas into adulthood.

Radiation

Data regarding adjuvant radiation to childhood meningiomas are limited; however, radiation therapy has been proven to be effective as an adjuvant to surgery in adults. The National Institute for Health and Clinical Excellence recommends radiation treatment for adult patients with WHO grade 2/3 tumors, presence of adjacent brain or local invasion, tumor relapse, or if there is a contraindication to initial surgical resection. With conventional fractionated radiotherapy, doses of 50 to 55 Gy with dose increases to 60 Gy only considered in exceptional circumstances. Progression-free survival was shown to improve from 50% to 80% in adults with subtotal resection after radiation. In the pediatric population, the long-term neurocognitive sequelae must also be taken into account before delivering radiation.

Overview

Meningiomas in the pediatric population manifest significant differences from their adult counterparts with a much lower incidence. Tumors in children are highly associated with genetic syndromes, especially NF-2, and evaluation for such conditions should be done at the time of diagnosis. Although conservative management with close observation is an option, complete surgical resection portends the best long-term outcome of patients.

SCHWANNOMAS

Although intracranial schwannomas are the most common tumor of the cerebellopontine angle in adults, they are exceedingly rare in children. Only 0.7% of all schwannomas develop in the pediatric population and account for 2% of posterior fossa tumors in children. Schwannomas can arise from any cranial nerve and have been reported to grown from nerves III, V, VII, VIII, IX, X, XI, and XII. As in adults, vestibular schwannomas are the most common form and are typically associated with NF-2. Although these are benign lesions, their size and location can make these tumors particularly challenging to treat (Fig. 131-12).

Clinical Presentation

The clinical presentation of intracranial schwannomas is quite varied. As with all mass lesions, common presentation includes signs of increased intracranial pressure with accelerations in head growth, developmental delay, papilledema, headaches, or vomiting. Tumors arising in the cerebellopontine angle can result in obstructive hydrocephalus from mass effect on the fourth ventricle, cerebral aqueduct, or fourth ventricular outflow pathways. As the tumors enlarge, cerebellar symptoms may also develop.

Schwannomas are tumors of the nerve sheath rather than the nerves themselves. For this reason, tumors will grow centripetally outward from the nerve. Cranial nerve palsies will occur only if tumor growth is restricted, usually by local bony anatomy.

Schwannomas and Genetic Conditions

The development of intracranial schwannomas is associated with both NF2 and schwannomatosis. These conditions are a result of genetic mutations in the merlin gene on chromosome 22q12 (Hilton and Hanemann, 2014). In cases of sporadic schwannomas, the majority have also shown loss of the chromosome 22q as well.

Bilateral vestibular schwannomas are pathognomonic for the diagnosis of NF-2, and the presence of a unilateral vestibular schwannoma in patients aged under 30 years should prompt an evaluation for NF-2.

Schwannomatosis is a relatively newly reported clinically distinct form of neurofibromatosis. It is characterized by the development of multiple spinal peripheral, and cranial nerve schwannomas as well as rhabdoid tumors. However, these patients lack vestibular schwannomas and the other diagnostic criteria of NF-2 (Hilton and Hanemann, 2014). In 2007, it was first identified that a mutation in the SMARCB1 tumor suppressor gene is responsible for this condition.

Neuroimaging

Intracranial schwannomas are typically found in the cerebellopontine angle. Noncontrast CT imaging shows isodense lesions to normal brain. On cranial bone imaging, tumors may have expansion of the porus acusticus, jugular foramen, or any other bony foramina. MRI generally shows a T1-weighted isointense lesion to gray matter and homogenous enhancement with contrast delivery.

Histopathology

Schwannomas are benign tumors of Schwann cell origin and are classified by the World Health Organization as a grade I benign nerve sheath tumor. They can originate from any peripheral, cranial, or autonomic nerve (Agarwal, 2015).

Classically, schwannomas are composed of two distinct cellular patterns. *Antoni A* fibers are compact cellular structures with spindle-shaped cells. These cells can palisade to form Verocay bodies. Contrarily, *Antoni B* fibers are less compact with a loose microcystic matrix. They are relatively hypocellular but rich in collagen fibers and macrophages.

Often pediatric schwannomas lack the biphasic histology of adult schwannomas. Rather, they are more uniformly hypercellular with the presence of Verocay bodies. Other features unique to pediatric schwannomas include hemosiderin deposits and reactive vascular changes. Although mitotic figures are not seen in adult schwannomas, they may be present in their pediatric counterparts.

Treatment

Because of the rare nature of pediatric schwannomas, treatment options are extrapolated from the adult literature. Management includes three strategies: observation, radiosurgery, or microsurgery (Zygourakis et al., 2014). Tumor size and symptomatology as well as patient and family preferences dictate the best course of treatment. Complete surgical resection is curative for schwannomas, and symptomatic lesions should be surgically resected when possible. Surgical approaches vary based on tumor location, with the retrosigmoid approach being commonly used. If tumors appear to be highly vascular, preoperative embolization is an option to reduce blood loss.

Overview

Schwannomas are rare in childhood. They occur more frequently in patients with NF-2 but, even then, are seen more commonly in adults than in children. When possible, complete surgical resection is indicated and curative.

SELECTED REFERENCES

Agarwal, A., 2015. Intracranial trigeminal schwannoma. Neuroradiol. J. 28, 36–41.

Hilton, D.A., Hanemann, C.O., 2014. Schwannomas and their pathogenesis. Brain Pathol. 24, 205–220.

Kim, I., Shekhtman, E., Wisoff, J.H., et al., 2015. Stereotactic radiosurgery as part of multimodality craniopharyngioma management. In: Evans, J.J., Kenning, T.J. (Eds.), Craniopharyngiomas: Comprehensive Diagnosis, Treatment and Outcome. Elsevier, New York, pp. 327–334.

Lee, C.C., Yang, H.C., Chen, C.J., et al., 2014. Gamma knife surgery for craniopharyngioma: report on a 20-year experience. J. Neurosurg. 121 (Suppl.), 167–178.

McCrea, H.J., George, E., Settler, A., et al., 2015. Pediatric suprasellar tumors. J. Child Neurol. 2015. [Epub ahead of print].

Müller, H.L., 2015. Craniopharyngioma: long-term consequences of a chronic disease. Expert Rev. Neurother. 15, 1241–1244.

Ostrom, Q.T., Gittleman, H., Fulop, J., et al., 2015. CBTRUS statistical report: primary brain and central nervous system tumors diagnosed in the United States in 2008–2012. Neuro Oncol. 17 (Suppl. 4), iv1–iv62.

Stanuszek, A., Piatek, P., Kwiatkowski, S., et al., 2014. Multiple faces of children and juvenile meningiomas: a report of single-center experience and review of literature. Clin. Neurol. Neurosurg. 118, 69–75.

Zygourakis, C., Oh, T., Sun, M., et al., 2014. Surgery is cost effective treatment of young patients with vestibular schwannomas: decision tree modeling of surgery, radiation, and observation. Neurosurg. Focus 37, E8.

E-BOOK FIGURES

132 Pediatric Intradural Spinal Cord Tumors

Ben Shofty, Ori Barzilai, Zvi Lidar, Eugene Hwang, and Shlomi Constantini

INTRODUCTION

Intradural spinal cord tumors (SCTs) are composed of a heterogeneous group of neoplasms, accounting for approximately 10% of pediatric central nervous system tumors (Russell & Rubinstein 1989). Over the past five decades, the overall mortality and morbidity caused by these tumors has been reduced dramatically. The advantages of early diagnosis via modern imaging and modern neurosurgical tools such as intraoperative electrophysiological monitoring, the surgical microscope, and the ultrasonic aspirator have led to improvements in surgical morbidity and in general prognosis. Today, the standard of care of SCTs is complete surgical resection when possible, although adjuvant therapy provides benefit in selected cases.

This chapter focuses on the diagnosis and management of common intradural (extramedullary and intramedullary) primary pediatric SCTs.

EPIDEMIOLOGY

There is little population-based data available on pediatric primary SCTs. Many of the existing statistics are not current, having often been obtained from outdated surgical series. Intradural spinal tumors as a whole are believed to occur with an incidence that ranges from 0.7 to 1.1 cases per 100,000 persons. Intramedullary spinal cord tumors (IMSCTs) account for approximately 2% to 4% of all CNS tumors in the general population.

It has been estimated that approximately 30% of SCTs in the pediatric population are intramedullary, 24% are extramedullary, 35% are extradural (and not included in this chapter), and 10% are of other types. Astroglial tumors are the most common type of intramedullary tumors, accounting for around 90% of all pediatric IMSCTs, with a mean presentation age of 5 to 10 years and 60% in adolescence. Neurofibromatosis (NF) 1 and 2 are associated with IMSCTs, with as many as 19% of patients suffering from such tumors. Among NF1 patients, astrocytomas are more common. In NF2, ependymomas are more frequent. NF1 and NF2 are also known for their hallmark extramedullary nerve-sheath tumors (NSTs): neurofibromas and schwannomas, respectively.

PRESENTATION

Reported clinical manifestations of SCTs have changed since the beginning of the magnetic resonance imaging (MRI era), potentially due to earlier diagnosis. Yet even today the primary physician, neurologist, and orthopedist must have a high index of suspicion of primary sensory complaints such as dysesthesia and localized back pain to make an early diagnosis before permanent damage occurs.

In the pediatric age group, it is common for parents to become aware of a problem before any objective signs are apparent on the neurologic examination. In many of these patients the onset of symptoms is attributed to an apparently trivial injury. Occasionally, parents describe symptomatic exacerbations and remissions. For both children and adults,

the most common early symptom is local pain along the spinal axis that is usually most acute in the bony segment directly over the tumor. Typically pain is worse in the recumbent position because venous congestion further distends the dural tube, resulting in characteristic night pain.

Other symptoms include motor disturbances, radicular pain (occurring in about 10% of patients, usually limited to one or two dermatomes), paresthesias, painful dysesthesia (hot or cold painful sensations), and rarely, sphincter dysfunction. Weakness of the lower limbs is usually first manifested as an alteration in normal gait. This is often very subtle and may only be evident initially to a watchful parent who notes more frequent falling and/or walking on heels or toes. In young children there is often a history of being a "late walker," and in very young children (under 3 years) there is often a history of motor regression.

IMSCTs usually present with myelopathic symptoms of insidious onset. Localized pain and upper extremity paresthesias are the initial symptoms in 50% to 90% of patients with cervical lesions. Thoracic lesions may present with lower limb sensory losses and with upper motor neuron signs. Sphincter dysfunction is present in up to 40% of patients. In the pediatric population, pain is less often a presenting symptom, but is present in approximately 50% of patients. Symptoms usually last for months or even years before diagnosis.

Different SCT subtypes may present with slightly different clinical pictures. For rare malignant astrocytomas, the clinical presentation will include a more rapid decline in gait and pain of increasing intensity. Cervical ependymomas characteristically present with bilateral, symmetric dysesthesias.

The anatomic location of the tumor usually correlates with the clinical presentation. Cervical tumors may present with torticollis. Scoliosis is the most common early sign of an intramedullary thoracic cord tumor. Sphincter laxity is considered a late sign except in tumors that originate in the conus/cauda equina area. Higher tumors present less commonly with sphincter abnormalities, even with cystic components extending into the conus, Spinal cord compression is more common at presentation of EMSCTs than IMSCTs.

Hydrocephalus due to protein secretion into the cerebrospinal fluid is a common presentation of IMSCTs in infants. Torticollis and progressive kyphoscoliosis are also common (Box 132-1).

DIAGNOSIS

Once an SCT is suspected, spinal MRI (preferably of the entire neuroaxis) is the imaging method of choice. The MRI protocol should always be carefully planned according to the clinical symptoms and neurologic signs in conjunction with a neuroradiologist. It should consist of unenhanced T1- and T2-weighted images and contrast-enhanced T1-weighted images. Gadolinium may enhance the solid component of the tumor and help delineate it from surrounding edema. Ependymomas, meningiomas, and NSTs typically contrast-enhance brightly after gadolinium injection. Astrocytomas have a

TABLE 132-1 Tumor Characteristics, Treatment Recommendations, and Average Prognosis

Tumor	MR Appearance	Typical Location	Treatment	Prognosis
EXTRAMEDULLARY				
Meningioma	T1-hypo T2-hyper Contrast enhancing	Thoracic region Dural based	CR	Generally good Beware of anteriorly located tumors
Schwannoma and Neurofibroma	Solid T1-iso T2-hyper Contrast enhancing	Sometimes dumbbell shaped Extending toward the foramen	Resection	Generally good
Ependymoma of cauda equina (Myxopapillary)	Expansile T2-hyper Contrast enhancing	Filum/Conus/Cauda	Resection RT	Good Beware of infiltration into the conus
INTRAMEDULLARY				
Astrocytoma	Expansile T2-hyper Heterogeneous enhancement Cyst and/or syrinx	Cervical/thoracic	Aggressive resection RT/CT	Good
Malignant Glioma	T2-hyper Contrast enhancing	Cervical/thoracic	Resection RT/CT	Poor
Hemangioblastoma	Syringobulbia Syringomyelia Highly vascular Cord edema	Cervical/thoracic	Resection	Good
Ependymoma	Expansile T2-hyper Contrast enhancing Cyst and/or syrinx	Cervical	Resection RT reserved for special cases	Very good

CR, Complete resection; *CT,* chemotherapy; *MR,* magnetic resonance; *RT,* radiotherapy *T1-hypo,* T1 hypointense; *T2-hyper,* T2 hyperintense.

BOX 132-1 When to Obtain an MRI on a Patient
With Scoliosis

1. Documented rapid progression
2. Atypical curve
3. Age: early onset (<8 years)
4. Any neurologic/urologic sign
5. Vertebral and midline anomalies
6. Persistent pain (especially at night)
7. Screening in all dysraphic children

---

variable enhancement pattern and may give the cord a lumpy appearance. These images should be acquired in both sagittal and axial planes. Anesthesia is sometimes needed in pediatric patients. Table 132-1 describes the radiologic characteristics, recommended treatment method, and overall prognosis of the different SCTs.

Plain films and computed tomography (CT) are not sensitive enough to effectively evaluate patients with suspected intradural—and especially intramedullary—lesions. Secondary bony changes, such as pedicle erosion, scalloping, or foraminal widening, are better demonstrated with CT. Plain films are better for diagnosis of instability and quantification of scoliotic and kyphotic deformities, however. Bladder ultrasound with an examination after emptying is an important baseline study to be done before surgery.

TUMOR SUBTYPES
Extramedullary Spinal Cord Tumors

The most common primary extramedullary spinal cord tumors (EMSCTs) are derived from sheath cells covering the spinal nerve roots (neurofibromas and schwannomas) or the endothelial lining of the meninges (meningiomas). Myxopapillary

ependymomas are glial EMSCTs arising from the conus medullaris or the filum terminale. Other lesion types, such as lipomas and epidermoid/dermoid cysts, are less common but should be considered in the differential diagnosis.

EMSCTs generally cause chronic, slowly progressive compression of the cord. Symptomatology is due to the displacement and compression of the cord and adjacent nerve roots and secondary venous engorgement. Most patients will be symptomatic at the time of diagnosis; symptom onset can precede diagnosis by months to years. Due to the chronic, slow course of these tumors, the cord often looks atrophic, yet neurologic function may be preserved. The most common clinical presentation of EMSCTs is with back pain that may be indistinguishable from that seen with non-neoplastic causes. This pain is often described as aching, pressing, and dull, and is usually more severe at night. Radicular pain is uncommon with meningiomas but is common with NSTs. Paresthesias and numbness are common symptoms, and hypoesthesia or anesthesia at and below the level of the tumor is often evident on clinical examination. Patterns of sensory deficit such as posterior cord syndrome can suggest tumor localization. Upper motor neuron injury manifested as spastic paraparesis is common, too, and is usually first evident when the patient climbs stairs and tries to use proximal muscle groups. High cervical tumors may cause quadriparesis. When the tumor or the associated cyst extends rostrally into the brainstem, low cranial nerve involvement, dysphagia, and respiratory disturbances can occur.

Spinal Meningiomas

Spinal meningiomas are extremely rare in the pediatric population and are almost always associated with NF2. More than 90% of meningiomas are intradural, and more than 95% are benign tumors arising from the endothelium that lines the leptomeningeal spaces (arachnoid cap cells). Most meningiomas arise in the thoracic region (80%). Less common is involvement of the cervical (15%) or lumbar (5%) regions. Intradural meningiomas are usually located laterally or posteriorly to the spinal cord; anterior location is less common.

On MRI, spinal meningiomas appear hypointense to isointense on T1 and hyperintense on T2. They often display homogenous enhancement with gadolinium contrast, but calcifications are common and may preclude gadolinium enhancement.

Spinal meningiomas are managed by surgery. Even with the technical challenges of anteriorly located tumors, gross total removal (GTR; defined as over 99%) of meningiomas is attainable in more than 90% of patients. Tumor recurrence rate is between 3% and 7%. Radiotherapy could be considered after subtotal removal (STR) or recurrence, but is seldom needed and may not add significant therapeutic efficacy. Neurologic morbidity of the surgical procedure is directly related to preoperative neurologic status. Patients with little or no disability are at little risk of sustaining an injury, whereas patients with more advanced neurologic dysfunction have a greater risk of impairment. With modern use of electrophysiological monitoring, perioperative complications are usually limited to wound healing and cerebrospinal fluid fistulas. Long-term recovery is usually excellent. Anteriorly located spinal meningiomas require a very lateral approach, with special care to avoid injury to the pyramidal tracts and to the anterior spinal artery. These cases may be more challenging, carrying a potential risk of spinal cord damage. The use of the ultrasonic aspirator to internally debulk the tumor allows better manipulation of the capsule and careful microsurgical separation from the spinal cord without the need for cord retraction.

Peripheral Nerve Tumors (Neurofibromas, Schwannomas)

NSTs are World Health Organization (WHO) grade I tumors. They usually present as solitary lesions, typically in the fourth or fifth decade of life. Earlier presentation or multiple lesions are usually associated with genetic syndromes such as neurofibromatosis I, II, and schwannomatosis. These syndromes are respectively associated with multiple neurofibromas, spinal meningiomas, and schwannomas. Schwannomas are more common than neurofibromas. Approximately 60% to 80% of NSTs arise from nerve roots before leaving the dural sac, usually affecting the lumbosacral region. Anatomically, schwannomas tend to arise from the dorsal nerve root, whereas neurofibromas are more common on the ventral root. Other than this difference, schwannomas and neurofibromas are indistinguishable on MRI. NSTs have an isointense signal on T1 and a hyperintense signal on T2. Their characteristic pattern on fluid-sensitive sequences has been described as "target lesion." Tumor enhancement varies, ranging from homogenous to a peripheral ring-like enhancement. Schwannoma pathology usually contains neoplastic Schwann cells, whereas neurofibromas more frequently invade the nerve root and contain Schwann cells, nerve fibers, and fibroblasts.

NST management depends on the patient's clinical presentation and radiologic follow up. A clinically and radiologically stable tumor needs only close follow up with MRI and physical examination. Surgical intervention is warranted if the tumor causes additional symptoms or displays imaging progression at presentation or during follow up. In NF, when many such tumors are present and the clinical presentation is often vague and complicated, the threshold for surgery is higher. GTR is the definitive treatment of such lesions, resulting in only a 5% recurrence rate.

To achieve total resection, the ventral or dorsal roots are commonly sacrificed. This, however, is usually not associated with pronounced postoperative motor or sensory deficit. Resection of schwannomas is usually safer because of their typical location on the dorsal root and the fact that they are less invasive than neurofibromas. Subtotal resection may be preferable if the tumor is attached to the spinal cord, if the origin of the tumor is an important ventral rootlet, or if the tumor exhibits extradural components closely associated with vital structures.

EPENDYMOMAS OF THE CONUS-CAUDA REGION

These tumors are usually extradural myxopapillary ependymomas, which account for approximately 40% to 50% of spinal ependymomas. They are more common in young adults. Patients usually present with a long history of back pain, lower sensorimotor deficit, and sphincter dysfunction.

On MRI they are often seen as well-circumscribed masses with hypointense signal on T1 and hyperintense signal on T2. Gadolinium enhancement is usually homogenous.

Complete resection is the treatment of choice and is generally feasible if nerve roots are not entrapped by the tumor. STR is reserved for cases with severe encasement of cauda equina nerve roots, especially low sacral S2–S4 innervation. Radiotherapy after complete or subtotal resection is still controversial. Recurrence after complete resection is less rare than previously thought and may be associated with poor outcome.

INTRAMEDULLARY SPINAL CORD TUMORS (IMSCTS)

A comprehensive discussion of these tumors can be found in Sloof (1964) (Figure 132-1).

Glial Tumors

Although IMSCTs make up only about 20% of all adult SCTs, at least 35% of pediatric SCTs are intramedullary. The vast majority of IMSCTs are members of the glioma family. Among 164 pediatric patients with IMSCTs operated on by Dr. Fred Epstein between 1980 and 1994 (Constantini et al. 2000):

1. 48% presented with astrocytomas
   * 76% low-grade
   * 24% high-grade
2. 26% presented with gangliogliomas
3. 11% presented with ependymomas
4. 6% presented with mixed gliomas
5. 9% presented with other lesions, such as hemangioblastomas, primitive neuroectodermal tumors (PNETs), lipomas, and ganglioneurocytomas

Intramedullary ependymomas almost never appear in the first decade. Note that within the spectrum of low-grade glial tumors, significant differences are found in reported series in the rates of different tumor subtypes such as low-grade astrocytomas, juvenile pilocytic astrocytomas, gangliogliomas, oligodendrogliomas, and others. Maximal surgical resection is considered the optimal treatment for nonastrocytic neuroglial tumors, and adjuvant radiotherapy is usually not indicated.

Intramedullary Ependymomas

Ependymomas are very rare in children, constituting only 11% to 35% of IMSCTs in the pediatric population. Categorization of ependymomas, both spinal and cranial, is based on histologic properties. Classical (WHO grade II and III) cellular ependymomas arise from the spinal canal and usually occupy

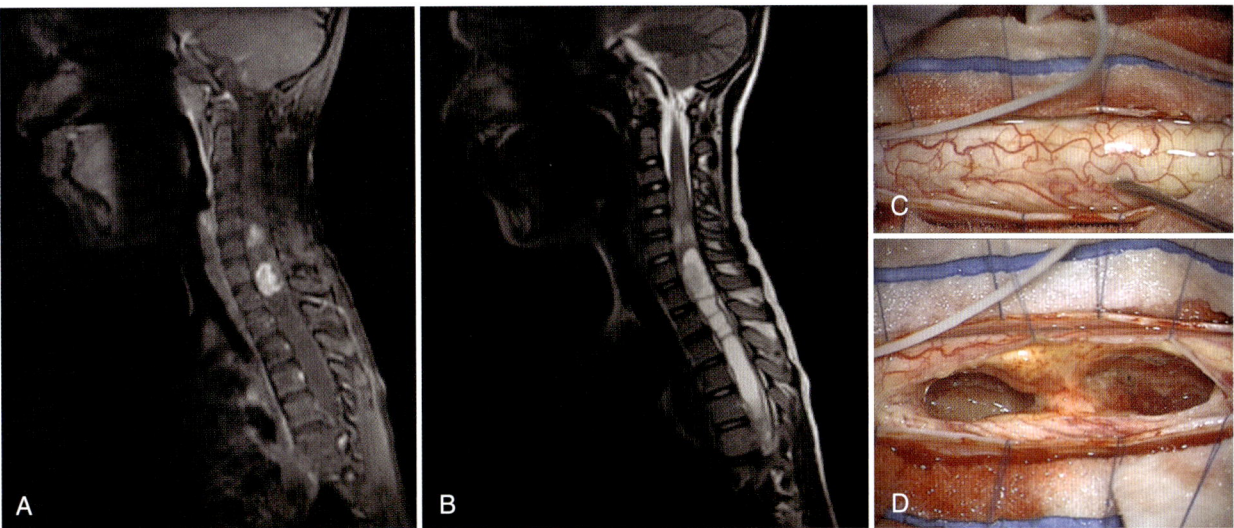

Figure 132-1. An 11-year-old basketball player, presenting with 2 weeks of focal back pain and bilateral hand pain, especially at night. Physical examination was normal beside alert, brisk reflexes, and mild weakness of left hand. MRI revealed intramedullary space-occupying lesion, spanning from C5 to T1 with a large cystic component, receiving inhomogeneous enhancement on T1 with gadolinium **(A)**, and a large cystic component and T2 changes **(B)**. Resection under electrophysiological monitoring was decided upon. Intraoperatively, following C5-T1 laminotomy, a bulky cord rotated to the left was evident **(C)**. A gross total resection was achieved via a left DREZ approach **(D)**, and the child was discharged a few days later with no neurologic deficit.

the cervical and thoracic regions. Myxopapillary (WHO grade I) ependymomas arise from the filum terminale, occupy the conus medullaris almost exclusively, and are usually extradural. Most ependymomas are WHO low-grade tumors (class I and II) (Hsu et al. 2009). Malignant subtype anaplastic ependymomas are rarely encountered in the spine.

On MRI, these tumors appear hypointense on T1 and hyperintense in T2. Ependymomas display homogenous enhancement. Although usually not encapsulated, there is often a clear plane evident between the tumor and the cord. Cysts, syrinx, and hemorrhage may also be evident.

Management of ependymomas is aggressive resection in most cases. Complete resection with the aid of intraoperative electrophysiological monitoring yields local control in 90% to 100% of patients. In partial resections of grade II and III tumors, the addition of adjuvant radiotherapy may be warranted but is still debatable. It is important to remember that adjuvant radiotherapy may make future surgical intervention more difficult and increases postoperative neurologic morbidity. The role of adjuvant chemotherapy is unclear at this time. Spinal intramedullary ependymomas generally have a good prognosis, with an average progression-free survival (PFS) of 82 months and an average overall survival of 180 months.

Low-Grade Astrocytomas

(Figure 132-2)

On MRI, these lesions appear as a fusiform expansion of the cord, sometimes including a cystic component. Syrinx is seen in approximately 40% of patients, and edema is often present. This tumor is hypointense or isointense on T1 image, and hyperintense on T2 and FLAIR, displaying partial enhancement. It is very difficult to differentiate astrocytomas from ependymomas based on MRI alone.

Management of intramedullary astrocytomas is based on maximal safe resection followed by observation. Because of the infiltrative nature of these tumors, complete resection is highly dependent on the surgeon's experience, mostly to identify a change in color (interphase) between the tumor and the normal white matter around it.

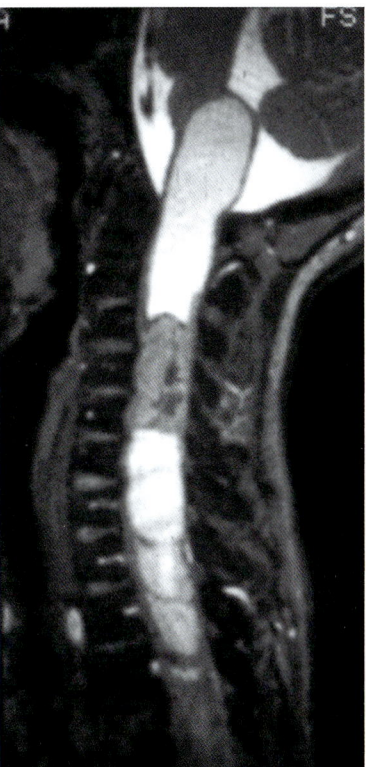

Figure 132-2. An MRI of a 10-year-old boy who presented with drooling and neck pain. The intramedullary low-grade astrocytoma spans from C3–C6.

In the pediatric population, adjuvant oncological treatment is usually reserved for those with multifocal disease, patients who have progressive disease without an adequate surgical option, or children who are at a high risk of developing plegia after a second, or even third, operation. The standard gentle chemotherapy used for low-grade astrocytomas in the brain has been shown to be effective in selected cases of intramedullary astrocytomas, especially in infants (Constantini et al. 1996). Radiation should be avoided in children younger than 5 years because of the detrimental effects on the immature central nervous system (Duffner et al. 1993). Susceptibility to the destructive effects of radiation on the spinal cord increases with the extent of cord irradiation and with the total dose. Therapeutic irradiation in substantial doses over extensive segments of spinal cord may result in myelitis. In addition, irradiation subsequent to spinal surgery predisposes to kyphosis and subluxation. Finally, irradiation may trigger development of a second malignant tumor.

Because there is no clear evidence that radiation or chemotherapy has a significant impact on the outcome for patients presenting with IMSCTs, especially astrocytomas, the role of surgery upon presentation remains substantial. If a pediatric patient with a low-grade IMSCT astrocytoma is treated with radical excision, long-term progression-free survival generally ensues without the need for adjuvant treatment. In many cases, pediatric intramedullary tumors are a "surgical disease."

Malignant Spinal Gliomas

High-grade gliomas of the spinal cord represent approximately 25% of intramedullary gliomas in adults and less than 10% in the pediatric population. These tumors are associated with poor prognosis and almost 100% recurrence. On MRI they display malignant characteristics such as heterogeneous enhancement caused by the presence of intramural cysts, necrosis, and surrounding edema. High-grade astroglial IMSCTs, especially glioblastomas, invariably progress. The optimal treatment for this entity has yet to be determined. Despite aggressive adjuvant therapy, patients with malignant IMSCTs have a postoperative median survival of up to 12 months. This is usually because of progressive infiltration of the tumor within the cord and through its pial banks, resulting in paraplegia, quadriplegia, and eventually death. A patient with a high-grade spinal astrocytoma has an average life expectancy of 15 months.

REFERENCES

The complete list of references for this chapter is available in the e-book at www.expertconsult.com.
    See inside cover for registration details.

SELECTED REFERENCES

Constantini, S., Houten, J., Miller, D.C., et al., 1996. Intramedullary spinal cord tumors in children under the age of 3 years. J. Neurosurg. 85, 1036–1043.

Constantini, S., Miller, D.C., Allen, J.C., et al., 2000. Radical excision of intramedullary spinal cord tumors: surgical morbidity and long-term follow-up evaluation in 164 children and young adults. J. Neurosurg. 93 (2 Suppl), 183–193.

Duffner, P.K., Horowitz, M.E., Krischer, J.P., et al., 1993. Postoperative chemotherapy and delayed radiation in children less than three years of age with malignant brain tumors. N. Engl. J. Med. 328 (24), 1725–1731.

Hsu, W., Pradilla, G., Constantini, S., et al., 2009. Surgical considerations of spinal ependymomas in the pediatric population. Childs Nerv. Syst. 25, 1253–1259.

Russell, D.S., Rubinstein, L.J., 1989. Pathology of Tumours of the Nervous System. Williams & Wilkins, Baltimore.

Slooff, J.L., Kernohan, J.W., MacCarty, C.S., 1964. Primary Intramedullary Tumors of the Spinal Cord and Filum Terminale. WB Saunders, Philadelphia.

E-BOOK FIGURES AND TABLES

The following figures and tables are available in the e-book at www.expertconsult.com. See inside cover for registration details.

Box 132-2 Principles of Intraoperative Neurophysiology in SCT Surgery
Box 132-3 Complications of SCT Surgery

133 System Cancer and the Central Nervous System Involvement

Sharyu Hanmantgad and Yasmin Khakoo

An expanded version of this chapter is available on www.expertconsult.com. See inside cover for registration details.

Children with systemic cancer may develop neurologic symptoms/complications from either metastatic disease or the side effects of treatment. Although primary central nervous system (CNS) tumors are the most common solid tumors of childhood, metastasis of systemic tumors to the CNS is rare. Adults with systemic malignancies develop CNS metastases 20% to 40% of the time, whereas less than 10% of children with systemic malignancies are so affected. In one series of almost 4000 children diagnosed with systemic solid tumors between 1990 and 2012, only 1.4% had brain metastases. In contrast, 3% to 5% of all children with acute lymphoblastic leukemia develop a CNS relapse, and 20% to 40% of children in relapse have CNS disease. Additionally, treatment of systemic malignancy, including surgery, radiation, and chemotherapy, may cause neurologic symptoms. This chapter discusses CNS involvement in systemic childhood cancer (Suki et al., 2014).

Central Nervous System Leukemia

CNS leukemia occurs in approximately 4% of children with leukemia. All children with acute lymphocytic leukemia (ALL) receive routine lumbar punctures at the time of diagnosis and, for the majority, such involvement, if present, is asymptomatic. The leukemic cells found in the cerebrospinal fluid (CSF) are cytogenetically identical to those found in the bone marrow. Protein expression profiles may define subsets of leukemic B cells that are more likely to metastasize to the CNS, and signaling of the cytokine CCL19 through its receptor, CCR7, is required for CNS infiltration by leukemic T cells (Jin et al., 2016).

Leukemic lymphocytes appear to metastasize to the CNS by hematogenous spread with extravasation that depends in animal models on myosin-IIA, or through the CNS lymphatics near the dural sinuses.

Although rare, neurologic symptoms associated with CNS leukemia include headaches (17%), nausea and vomiting (14%), lethargy, and irritability. Symptoms were present in half of patients with greater than or equal to 5 leukocytes/µL with blasts in the CSF or signs of CNS involvement on neurologic examination, and only 20% of patients with less than 5 leukocytes/µL CSF had signs or symptoms whether or not the CSF contained blasts. On examination, there may be nuchal rigidity and papilledema. Cranial nerve involvement is less common but may include seventh, third, fourth, and sixth nerve impairment. Infiltration of the optic nerve can also be seen. Hypothalamic obesity caused by direct infiltration of the hypothalamus is a rare syndrome. Spinal cord involvement has been reported but is quite uncommon. Rarely, patients develop chloromas, distinct masses of leukemic cells, in the CNS.

The presence of CNS leukemia has important implications for treatment and prognosis. Before the common understanding of the likelihood of the CNS acting as a sanctuary for leukemic cells, relapse in the CNS was seen frequently. Leukemic relapse was difficult to eradicate and required aggressive, neurotoxic treatment. To prevent CNS relapse, upfront cranial irradiation was widely employed. Patients experienced neurotoxicities, including cognitive decline, intractable seizures, strokes, and secondary CNS malignancies (e.g., meningiomas). Neurologic sequelae of cranial irradiation, including impaired working memory capacity, inhibition, cognitive flexibility, executive visuomotor control, and attentional fluctuations, may persist into adulthood. Over time, in an effort to reduce the use of prophylactic radiation therapy, intrathecal chemotherapies, such as methotrexate and Ara-C, replaced prophylactic radiation affording similar survival curves but less neurotoxicity. Recent studies of stem cell therapy for childhood ALL suggest that neither additional prophylactic craniospinal irradiation nor intrathecal chemotherapy enhances prognosis beyond that seen in patients treated with a pretransplantation ablative regimen alone.

With the use of methotrexate, intravenously at high doses, orally at lower doses, and intrathecally at any dose, 23% of patients developed leukoencephalopathy. Patients with symptomatic leukoencephalopathy may have generalized or partial seizures, stroke-like episodes, and ataxia. Twenty percent of children receiving methotrexate demonstrate MRI changes consistent with leukoencephalopathy regardless of symptoms. A genome-wide association study revealed enrichment in polymorphisms in genes known to play a role in neurodevelopmental pathways, raising the possibility that the products of these genes contribute to propensity of a given patient to develop methotrexate neurotoxicity. Those patients with high-risk leukemia with CNS involvement may require radiation plus chemotherapy. Neurocognitive outcomes, including measures of intelligence and executive function, were negatively correlated with the cumulative dose of craniospinal irradiation and intrathecally administered methotrexate.

Another neurologic complication observed in children undergoing treatment for leukemia has been the development of arterial and venous strokes, including dural sinus thrombosis. Dural sinus thrombosis may develop secondary to leukemic infiltration of the dural sinus (Fig. 133-1). Both arterial and venous strokes have been more often related to the use of L-asparaginase, which causes deficiencies of antithrombin, plasminogen, fibrinogen, and factors IX and XI. L-Asparaginase is utilized in the induction therapy of children with leukemia, and is associated with an initial hypocoagulable state, followed by a presumed rebound hypercoagulable state, which may result in thrombosis. L-Asparaginase-associated thrombotic strokes tend to occur at the end of induction, characteristically 7 to 10 days after completion of induction, and may result in seizures, focal neurologic deficit, or, less frequently, coma. Arterial strokes have also been reported with intrathecal administration of cytosine arabinoside. Other factors that can cause strokes in children with leukemia include dehydration with secondary venous thrombosis, CNS infection, and later radiation vasculopathy (Levinsen et al., 2014).

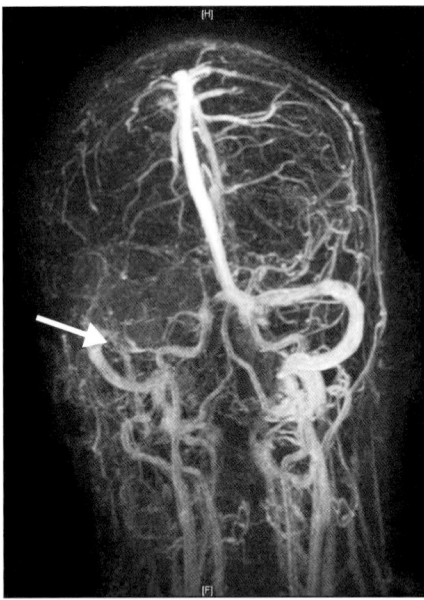

Figure 133-1. Postcontrast magnetic resonance venography (MRV) demonstrating right transverse sinus filling defect secondary to clot formation from L-asparaginase.

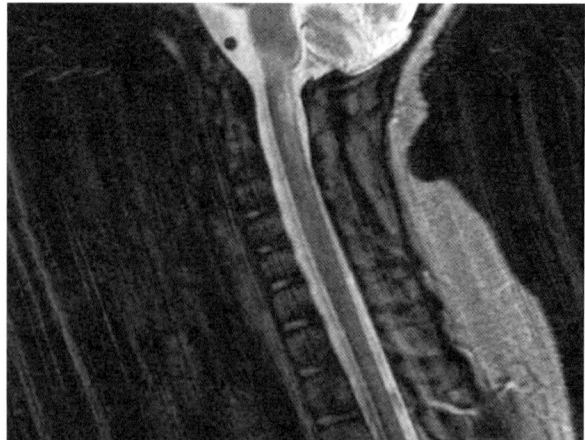

Figure 133-2. Sagittal T2 spine magnetic resonance imaging demonstrating radiation myelitis.

CNS involvement is less frequent in children with acute myelogenous leukemia, but still has been reported to be as high as 20%, and some form of CNS prophylaxis is employed in all patients. Chloromas may occur and may result in focal neurologic deficits, including cranial nerve or spinal cord compression.

A rarer form of leukemia—acute promyelocytic leukemia—can be associated with neurologic complications, especially intracranial hemorrhage and stroke, at presentation or early during treatment in children and adults. This is thought to result from acute tumor lysis and release of procoagulants from the large leukemic granular cells. An intracranial disseminated intravenous coagulation picture can be seen.

CNS infection, especially with fungal organisms, may complicate the course of leukemia, particularly in patients who are immunosuppressed for long periods and in patients from low- and middle-income countries. Similarly, in patients with prolonged immunosuppression, brain abscesses occur because of a variety of organisms. Abscesses are usually associated with pulmonary lesions and may be caused by bacterial involvement with either aerobic or anaerobic bacteria, or by fungal infections, including *Aspergillus, Mucor,* and *Candida.* Encephalitis may also occur, especially after hematopoietic stem cell transplantation, and is caused by viruses, including herpes simplex, varicella zoster, and human herpes virus 6. Progressive multifocal leukoencephalopathy is a rare complication of prolonged immunosuppression, especially with agents such as rituximab.

Recently, chimeric antigen receptor T cells (CAR T cells) have been used with moderate success in treatment of refractory hematologic malignancies in children and adults. Unfortunately, the toxicities associated with this treatment can be life-threatening, affecting many organ systems. Although the cells target tumor-associated antigens, they may also cross react with normal tissue. The mechanism of action is thought to be a cytokine release syndrome that causes a massive inflammatory response leading to potentially irreversible end-organ damage. Neurologic toxicity includes encephalopathy and intractable seizures. There appears to be no correlation with CNS leukemia. The mainstay of therapy is supportive care with anticonvulsants and correction of metabolic abnormalities as

well as interleukin-6 receptor blockade using tocilizumab. Steroid administration is considered a last resort in some instances because of concern of diminishing efficacy of the CAR T cells. As CAR T-cell therapy gains acceptance for treatment of other malignancies as well as nononcologic disorders, neurologic adverse events may increase in prevalence, requiring the practitioner to become familiar with the treatment of these secondary effects (Brudno and Kochenderfer, 2016).

Lymphoma

Primary CNS lymphoma, a subtype of non-Hodgkin lymphoma, is rare in children and is seen primarily in severely immunosuppressed patients, such as those with HIV infection, those who have undergone transplant and require chronic immunosuppression, and those with hemophagocytic disorders. Patients who have undergone bone marrow transplant for other disorders may also develop Epstein-Barr virus (EBV)–associated CNS lymphoma. Cytotoxic T-cell therapy has successfully treated many such patients.

Treatment is challenging; because of the rarity of the illness and the immunosuppressed nature of the patients, patients are often treated with B-cell lymphoma protocols with or without the use of focal, more extensive radiation therapy.

Systemic lymphoma can metastasize directly to the CNS, to the vertebral bodies with secondary spinal cord compression (Hauser et al., 2005), and to the leptomeninges. Non-Hodgkin lymphoma affects the CNS of children and adolescents in approximately 10% of cases.

Mantle radiation therapy, a mainstay of treatment for Hodgkin lymphoma, may cause radiation myelitis in a small subset of patients (Fig. 133-2). Neurologic manifestations include Lhermitte's sign with upper extremity weakness and sensory changes. Treatments have included steroids and hyperbaric oxygen.

Histiocytosis

Langerhans cell histiocytosis (LCH) may involve the CNS in as many as 20% of patients. Diabetes insipidus secondary to posterior pituitary infiltration is the most common presenting symptom. Less commonly, granulomas may develop within the neuroaxis. LCH may be difficult to distinguish clinically from primary CNS tumors (Imashuku and Arceci, 2015).

Years after initial, apparently successful treatment of LCH, subtle neurologic deficits, which may be progressive, can occur. Depending on the area of involvement of the CNS, symptoms include ataxia, vertigo, dysarthria, nystagmus, tremor, and focal motor impairments. Lesions may arise anywhere within the CNS, but they tend to predominate in the hypothalamic-pituitary axis, pineal gland, gray matter of the dentate nucleus and basal ganglia, and in the deep white matter of the pons and hippocampus. There may or may not be associated infiltration by histiocytes. Such lesions may be progressive or static over time. It is unclear whether they represent a paraneoplastic syndrome or direct infiltration of histiocytosis into the brain. Treatments have included 2-chlorodeoxyadenosine, retinoic acid, and intravenous immunoglobulins (with or without antineoplastic chemotherapy), and have had variable success.

Neuroblastoma

Neuroblastoma is a tumor that originates from the sympathetic ganglia and typically occurs in younger children. Neuroblastoma may invade through neural foramina into the spinal canal (classically with a dumbbell shape) and cause cord compression. In addition, neuroblastoma can spread to other extra- and intracranial sites—most notoriously, to the torcula with resultant dural venous thrombosis that can precipitate severe neurologic compromise, including seizures and coma. Recent advances in therapies include the use of radio-labeled anti-GD2 antibodies that target gangliosides specifically expressed on tumors of neural crest origin. With the widespread use of antibody therapy, the long-term survival rate for patients with stage 4 neuroblastoma has risen significantly. However, these intravenously administered antibodies do not cross the blood-brain barrier, and result in a relative increase in the number of patients with CNS neuroblastoma. Treatment of these patients with CNS metastasis includes surgery followed by low-dose external beam craniospinal radiation with a boost to the primary site followed by administration of intrathecal radiolabeled anti-GD2 antibodies ([131]I 3F8 or 8H9). A recent report has shown that 17/21 patients were alive at a median of 33 months from diagnosis of CNS neuroblastoma. Future research will involve attempts to identify which patients are at risk for seeding the CNS, followed by targeted attempts to prophylactically treat these individuals. A recent report suggested that traumatic lumbar puncture in patients with active stage 4 neuroblastoma may increase the risk of CNS seeding, but this observation requires further investigation. Neurologic sequelae of intravenous anti-GD2 antibodies include Horner syndrome, neuropathic pain, and posterior reversible leukoencephalopathy syndrome (PRES).

Spinal cord compression may be acute and cause the rapid onset of motor deficits, including quadriplegia or paraplegia. Conus or cauda equina involvement may result in early bowel and bladder dysfunction. Management of such compression requires immediate commencement of chemotherapy, with surgical decompression generally reserved for benign variants (e.g., ganglioneuroma) (Fawzy et al., 2015).

Neuroblastoma also has been associated with a unique paraneoplastic syndrome, opsoclonus-myoclonus. (See Chapter 118 for a discussion of this syndrome.)

An unusual form of neuroblastoma is esthesioneuroblastoma—neuroblastoma that occurs in the nasopharynx or paranasal sinuses. It accounts for less than 3% of tumors of childhood and adolescence. Radiotherapy is effective in adults with esthesioneuroblastoma, but the scarcity of data in children with this tumor and the significant morbidity of radiation therapy to the head and neck of children have fueled attempts to treat with newer, perhaps safer modalities. One study employing proton beam radiotherapy appeared to demonstrate locoregional control of intracranial and leptomeningeal metastases and tolerable toxicity, but ultimate survival was limited by disease in these sites (Lucas et al., 2015).

Sarcoma

In a study reviewing 12 years of data on pediatric cancer patients, 3950 patients had a solid non-CNS primary cancer. Of those patients, 1.4% had metastases to the brain. Of the primary solid pediatric cancers associated with metastases, sarcomas constituted 54%, whereas melanomas, the next most common tumor, accounted for only 15%. Children between the age of 10 and 15 years are at highest risk. In a postmortem report of 139 pediatric patients with primary solid tumors, 18 patients were found to have CNS metastases. Osteogenic sarcoma and rhabdomyosarcoma were the most frequently reported primary cancers to cause CNS metastases in patients under the age of 15 years.

Pulmonary metastases were found in over 90% of patients with CNS involvement, suggesting that the metastases arise hematogenously from the lungs. In general, primary solid tumors with associated CNS metastases are associated with rapid clinical deterioration (Porto et al., 2010). Patients with brain metastases presented with headache, nausea/vomiting, and seizures as the most common chief complaints. The primary tumor and brain metastasis present synchronously in 15% of patients, and in these patients, other extracranial metastases are also present. The remaining 85% of patients are diagnosed with brain metastasis after treatment of the primary disease has been initiated, with a median presentation interval of 17 months after primary cancer diagnosis.

Treatment of pediatric sarcoma may also result in neurologic compromise. Intravenous ifosfamide, a commonly used alkylating chemotherapeutic agent, causes encephalopathy, asterixis, and seizures during infusion in 2% to 5% of children without CNS tumors. Symptoms may begin during drug infusion or hours to days later. The encephalopathy results from breakdown of ifosfamide to chloroacetaldehyde and subsequent inhibition of the mitochondrial respiratory chain. Treatment includes longer infusion time of ifosfamide; administration of methylene blue and/or thiamine; or switching from ifosfamide to cyclophosphamide. The neurologic outcome is generally good. Other toxicities include vincristine neuropathy.

OSTEOSARCOMA

Osteosarcoma is the most frequently occurring malignant primary bone tumor and most common bone cancer in children. Spread of osteosarcoma is typically hematogenous, primarily reaching the lungs and other bones. Although rare, brain metastases are hypothesized to develop when lung tumor emboli invade the brain; however, there are occasional reports of patients with metastases who have no detectable lung involvement. Dissemination to the brain typically targets the dura and skull and spares the parenchyma (Fig. 133-3). Brain involvement is associated with metastatic disease at diagnosis or with relapse within 12 months of diagnosis.

EWING'S SARCOMA

Ewing's sarcoma comprises about 10% of primary malignant bone tumors and is commonly seen in young adults with a male predominance. Metastases to the lung and other skeletal tissues are common and up to 80% of patients have metastases at the time of diagnosis. In contrast to osteosarcoma, Ewing's sarcoma is frequently associated with CNS involvement because of direct bony extension, rather than by hematogenous spread. Brain metastases usually occur with lung involvement in over 85% of individuals and as a part of systemic disease involvement. Overall, the presence of brain involvement suggests a poor prognosis in patients with Ewing's sarcoma;

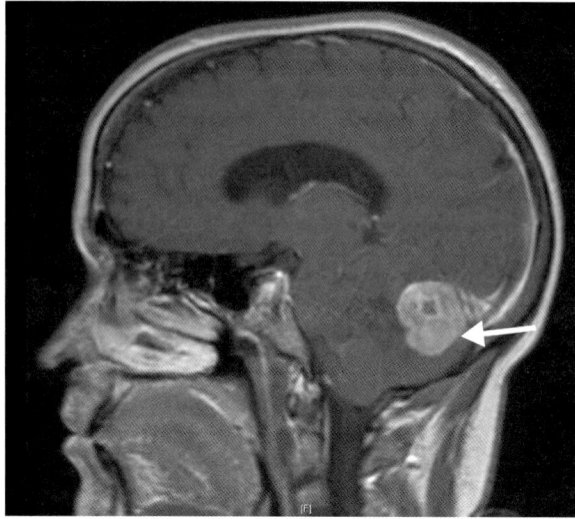

Figure 133-3. Sagittal postcontrast magnetic resonance imaging of brain demonstrating dural-based osteosarcoma metastasis.

however, it is difficult to determine whether this is a function of the systemic disease or the brain involvement.

RHABDOMYOSARCOMA

Rhabdomyosarcoma is the most common soft tissue sarcoma in childhood. Twenty percent of cases arise in the parameningeal area, including the middle ear, nasal cavity and paranasal sinuses, nasopharynx, infratemporal fossa/pterygopalatine, and parapharyngeal area, whereas the remaining cases typically occur in the genitourinary system and the extremities. Parameningeal rhabdomyosarcoma requires more aggressive treatment as its proximity to critical anatomic structures allows for more frequent invasion into the CNS. Systemic dissemination of rhabdomyosarcoma occurs hematogenously or through lymphatics with common metastatic sites in the lungs, pancreas, and bone. Although brain metastases are uncommon, there has been an association with pulmonary metastases and history of recurrent metastasis.

Conclusions

Both systemic cancer and its therapy contribute to the neurologic morbidity in pediatric cancer patients (Khan et al., 2014). Prevention depends on pretreatment identification of children at risk, and treatment of neurologic sequelae requires development of agents that will not compromise anticancer treatment efficacy. There is no standard therapy for CNS metastases of systemic solid tumors in children and adolescents. The relative rarity of CNS metastases of systemic cancer in children has meant that, despite the difference in the primary tumors from which these metastases come, their treatment has been guided by standard clinical practice in adults. Proton beam radiotherapy holds the promise of less toxic radiotherapy for intracranial metastases. In addition, prophylactic cognitive interventions may allow conventional craniospinal radiotherapy to be used without significant deterioration in IQ, memory, or executive function.

Acknowledgment

The authors would like to thank Joseph Olechnowicz for editorial assistance.

REFERENCES

The complete list of references for this chapter is available in the e-book at www.expertconsult.com.
    See inside cover for registration details.

SELECTED REFERENCES

Brudno, J.N., Kochenderfer, J.N., 2016. Toxicities of chimeric antigen receptor T cells: recognition and management. Blood. 127 (26), 3321–3330.

Fawzy, M., El-Beltagy, M., Shafei, M.E., et al., 2015. Intraspinal neuroblastoma: treatment options and neurological outcome of spinal cord compression. Oncol. Lett. 9, 907–911.

Hauser, P., Jakab, Z., Láng, O., et al., 2005. Incidence and survival of central nervous system involvement in childhood malignancies: Hungarian experience. J. Pediatr. Hematol. Oncol 27, 125–128.

Imashuku, S., Arceci, R.J., 2015. Strategies for the prevention of central nervous system complications in patients with Langerhans cell histiocytosis: the problem of neurodegenerative syndrome. Hematol. Oncol. Clin. North Am. 29, 875–893.

Jin, M., An, Q., Xu, S., 2016. Central nervous system disease in childhood acute lymphoblastic leukaemia—a review. Minerva Pediatr, Mar 18 e-pub before print.

Khan, R.B., Hudson, M.M., Ledet, D.S., et al., 2014. Neurologic morbidity and quality of life in survivors of childhood acute lymphoblastic leukemia: a prospective cross-sectional study. J. Cancer Surviv. 8, 688–696.

Levinsen, M., Taskinen, M., Abrahamsson, J., et al., 2014. Clinical features and early treatment response of central nervous system involvement in childhood acute lymphoblastic leukemia. Pediatr. Blood Cancer 61, 1416–1421.

Lucas, J.T., Ladra, M.M., MacDonald, S.M., et al., 2015. Proton therapy for pediatric and adolescent esthesioneuroblastoma. Pediatr. Blood Cancer 62, 1523–1528.

Porto, L., Jarisch, A., Zanella, F., et al., 2010. The role of magnetic resonance imaging in children with hematogenous brain metastases from primary solid tumors. Pediatr. Hematol. Oncol. 27, 103–111.

Suki, D., Khoury Abdulla, R., Ding, M., et al., 2014. Brain metastases in patients diagnosed with a solid primary cancer during childhood: experience from a single referral cancer center. J. Neurosurg. Pediatr. 14, 372–385.

134 Posttreatment Neurologic Sequelae of Pediatric Central Nervous System Tumors

Elizabeth M. Wells and Colin R. Kennedy

 An expanded version of this chapter is available on www.expertconsult.com. See inside cover for registration details.

INTRODUCTION

As more children and adolescents with cancer are becoming long-term survivors as a result of improved multimodal and risk-based therapy, there is increased recognition of long-term consequences. Childhood cancer and its treatment predispose survivors to a variety of chronic conditions that may impair function, limit participatory activity, and reduce quality of life. Central nervous system (CNS) tumors and their treatment may cause acute and chronic adverse effects, including neurologic and neurosensory deficits, seizures, headaches, cognitive impairment, neuroendocrine dysfunction, neurovascular abnormalities, and secondary malignancies. Variation in the incidence of presenting neurologic features by tumor region within the brain is summarized in Figure 134-1. Increased recognition of late effects has prompted organized attempts to prevent and mitigate neurologic sequelae from CNS tumor treatment through risk-stratified treatment and increased surveillance of survivors.

Treatment-related injury may appear early or late and may be transient or permanent. Distinguishing direct tumor effects from treatment effects requires assessment of the timing of symptoms in relation to tumor diagnosis and treatment, whether there is radiographic growth or stability, evidence of posttreatment magnetic resonance imaging (MRI) change, and the location of the tumor and radiation portal if applicable. Sequelae that develop or persist long after tumor diagnosis are referred to as *late effects*. The milestone of 5 years from diagnosis is often used in epidemiologic studies and for survivorship screening guidelines. However, with more children receiving sequential therapies for progressive or recurrent disease and more children remaining on biologic therapies for extended periods of time, the term *posttreatment sequelae* has a broader definition. This chapter takes a symptom-based approach to discussing early and late neurologic sequelae, including epidemiology, risk factors, and management.

MORTALITY IN LONG-TERM TUMOR SURVIVORS

Childhood CNS tumor survivors experience high rates of mortality, subsequent cancers, and other chronic medical conditions. Despite reaching the 5-year survivorship milestone, 25% percent of Childhood Cancer Survivor Study (CCSS) participants treated between 1970 and 1986 died within 30 years of their diagnosis. The cohort experienced a nearly 13-fold increased risk of death compared with their peers as a result of recurrent disease, secondary malignant neoplasms, and cerebrovascular and cardiovascular events (Box 134-1) (Armstrong et al., 2014).

CENTRAL NERVOUS SYSTEM POSTTREATMENT SEQUELAE

Weakness

Patients with CNS tumors may experience weakness in various anatomic distributions depending on the tumor location and type of treatment. The incidence of motor or coordination problems is highest at presentation and during initial treatment. In the acute posttreatment period, upper motor neuron weakness may result from intraoperative injury or swelling, radiation injury, or cerebrovascular infarct. Recovery from these insults depends on patient age and mechanism of injury (e.g., immediate postsurgical weakness often improves) (Escalas et al., 2015). Some patients experience new focal weakness years after therapy as a result of new intracranial events, such as strokes, seizures, or hemorrhage. Weakness that localizes to the spinal cord may result from myelopathy from spinal radiation therapy or chemotherapy, particularly if intrathecal, and may be accompanied by bowel or bladder dysfunction and sensory deficits.

Seizures

Seizures are a common complication of pediatric brain tumors and their treatment, appearing at presentation in 24% of patients and ongoing in about 15% (Ullrich et al., 2015). Although the subject is still debated, a 2000 American Academy of Neurology (AAN) practice parameter advised against prophylactic antiepileptic medications in patients of all ages. New onset or worsening of seizures posttreatment may signify tumor progression or recurrence, treatment-related neurotoxicity, and other causes, including metabolic disturbances.

Careful selection of antiepileptic medication is needed for patients with a CNS tumor. Nonenzyme-inducing antiepileptic drugs are preferred to avoid interactions with chemotherapy (Ruggiero et al., 2010), and monitoring for leukopenia or thrombocytopenia is needed. The antitumoral properties of valproic acid as a histone deacetylase inhibitor have been explored but are unproven and therefore not a reason to start valproic acid over other antiepileptic medications. Patients with CNS tumors may be more sensitive to sedating effects.

Initial tumor surgery, termed lesionectomy, cures more than 75% to 80% of cases of pediatric tumor-associated seizures, and there have been no controlled studies assessing the role of electrocorticography (ECog) during initial surgery. Factors predicting epilepsy cure after brain tumor resection include gross-total resection, preoperative seizure control, duration of seizures of 1 year or less, and semiology, with simple partial seizures having the worst prognosis. Medications may be

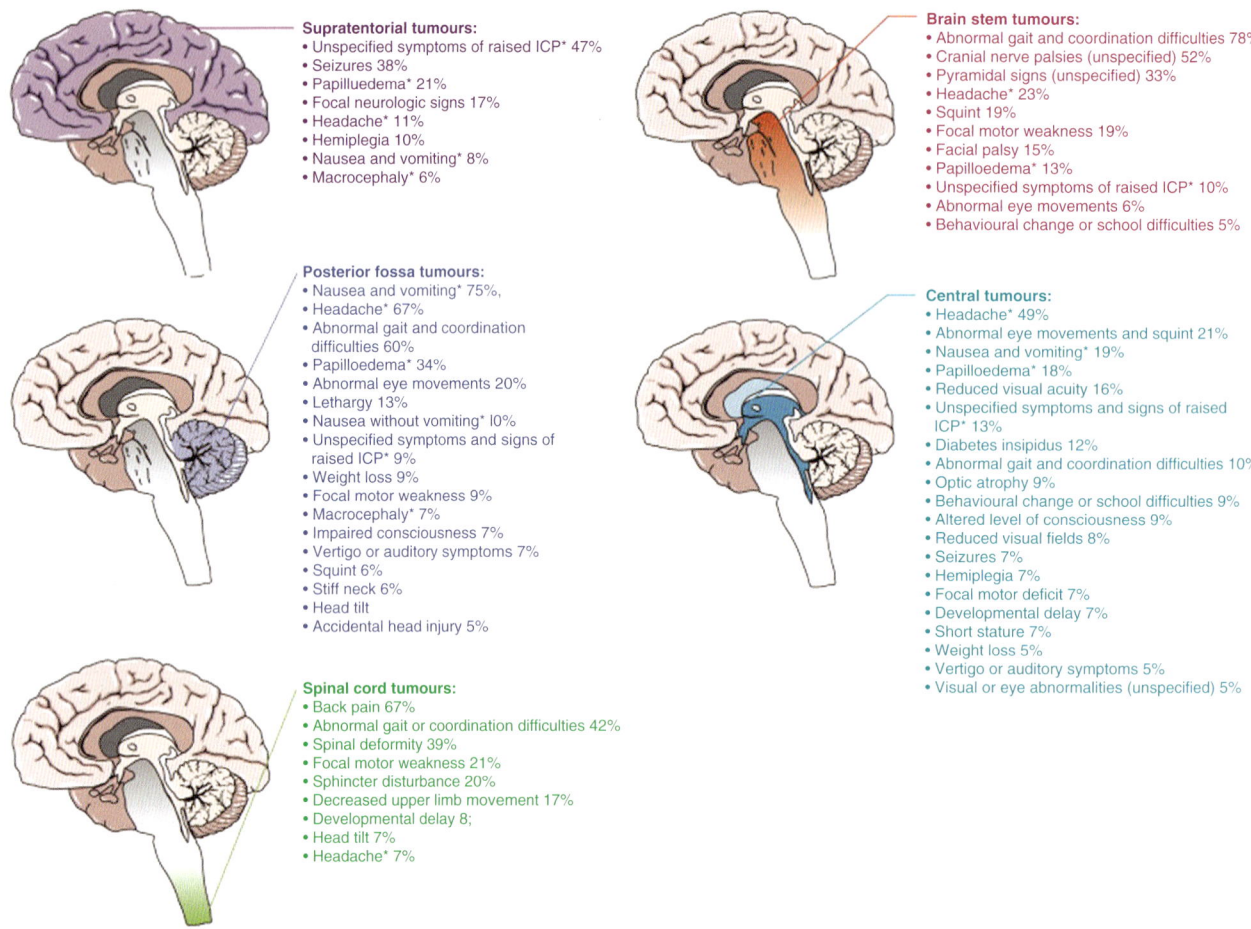

Supratentorial tumours:
• Unspecified symptoms of raised ICP* 47%
• Seizures 38%
• Papilloedema* 21%
• Focal neurologic signs 17%
• Headache* 11%
• Hemiplegia 10%
• Nausea and vomiting* 8%
• Macrocephaly* 6%

Posterior fossa tumours:
• Nausea and vomiting* 75%,
• Headache* 67%
• Abnormal gait and coordination
  difficulties 60%
• Papilloedema* 34%
• Abnormal eye movements 20%
• Lethargy 13%
• Nausea without vomiting* 10%
• Unspecified symptoms and signs of
  raised ICP* 9%
• Weight loss 9%
• Focal motor weakness 9%
• Macrocephaly* 7%
• Impaired consciousness 7%
• Vertigo or auditory symptoms 7%
• Squint 6%
• Stiff neck 6%
• Head tilt
• Accidental head injury 5%

Spinal cord tumours:
• Back pain 67%
• Abnormal gait or coordination difficulties 42%
• Spinal deformity 39%
• Focal motor weakness 21%
• Sphincter disturbance 20%
• Decreased upper limb movement 17%
• Developmental delay 8;
• Head tilt 7%
• Headache* 7%

Brain stem tumours:
• Abnormal gait and coordination difficulties 78%
• Cranial nerve palsies (unspecified) 52%
• Pyramidal signs (unspecified) 33%
• Headache* 23%
• Squint 19%
• Focal motor weakness 19%
• Facial palsy 15%
• Papilloedema* 13%
• Unspecified symptoms of raised ICP* 10%
• Abnormal eye movements 6%
• Behavioural change or school difficulties 5%

Central tumours:
• Headache* 49%
• Abnormal eye movements and squint 21%
• Nausea and vomiting* 19%
• Papilloedema* 18%
• Reduced visual acuity 16%
• Unspecified symptoms and signs of raised
  ICP* 13%
• Diabetes insipidus 12%
• Abnormal gait and coordination difficulties 10%
• Optic atrophy 9%
• Behavioural change or school difficulties 9%
• Altered level of consciousness 9%
• Reduced visual fields 8%
• Seizures 7%
• Hemiplegia 7%
• Focal motor deficit 7%
• Developmental delay 7%
• Short stature 7%
• Weight loss 5%
• Vertigo or auditory symptoms 5%
• Visual or eye abnormalities (unspecified) 5%

Figure 134-1. Incidence of neurologic features by tumor location. *(With permission from Wilne S., et al. Lancet Oncol. 2007 Aug;8(8):685-95.)*

BOX 134-1 Causes of Acute-Onset Neurologic
Impairment in Tumor Survivors

Cerebrovascular event
Metabolic abnormality
Posterior reversible encephalopathy syndrome (PRES)
Radiation injury or necrosis
Shunt failure/increased intracranial pressure
Secondary malignancy
Seizure
Sinus venous thrombosis
Stroke-like migraine after radiation therapy (SMART) syndrome
Tumor recurrence

---

discontinued soon after surgery for children who present with epilepsy and have no seizures following surgical resection. Twenty percent of patients with epilepsy associated with brain tumors have refractory seizures, and additional surgery may be needed to resect epileptogenic tissue surrounding the original lesion. When epilepsy follows treatment of a brain tumor, a trial off medication may be attempted after a patient has been seizure-free for 2 to 3 years. Research is limited, but one study found a recurrence rate of 27% in patients who were weaned off antiepileptic medication. Higher risk was associated with

having more than one tumor resection or whole-brain radiation; spikes or slow waves on electroencephalogram (EEG) before withdrawal did not correlate with recurrence.

Posttreatment Encephalopathy With Neurologic Impairment

Posterior Reversible Encephalopathy

Posterior reversible encephalopathy syndrome (PRES) has been reported in association with cisplatin, cytarabine, cyclosporins, cyclophosphamide, methotrexate, rituximab, paclitaxel, and other chemotherapies. (Fig. 134-2A and B) Presenting symptoms consist of headache, visual disturbances, seizures that may be intractable and require aggressive acute therapy, nausea and vomiting, altered mental status, and possibly focal deficits (McCoy et al., 2010). PRES is usually associated with hypertension or hypotension, sometimes in association with metabolic abnormalities; symptoms and neurologic deficit are usually reversible upon regulation of blood pressure and withdrawal of chemotherapy. Chemotherapy is often resumed after blood pressure control is attained, although this has not been studied, and therefore the risk is unknown. Chemotherapeutic agents such as high-dose arabinosylcytosine (Ara-C), ifosfamide, and methotrexate are also known to cause subacute neurotoxicity, with headaches, seizures, auditory and visual hallucinations, visual disturbances, pseudobulbar palsy, extrapyramidal signs, and paresis.

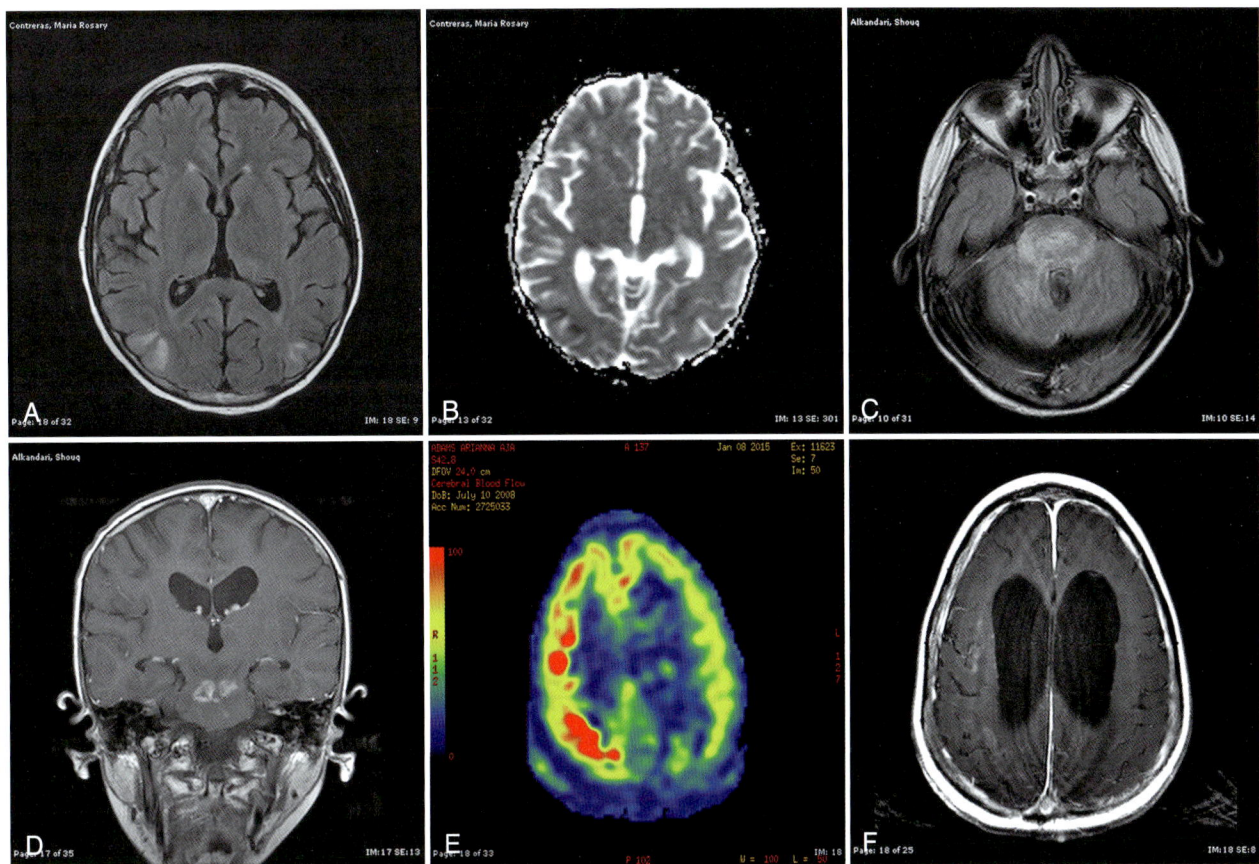

Figure 134-2. Cases of posttreatment syndromes with encephalopathy. A, Magnetic resonance imaging (MRI) of stroke-like migraine after radiation therapy (SMART) syndrome with T2 multifocal patchy enhancement of the cortex involving the right frontal, parietal, and temporal lobes. **B,** Corresponding hyperperfusion. **C,** MRI of posterior reversible encephalopathy syndrome (PRES) with numerous cortical/subcortical white-matter areas of increased T2 signal. **D,** Diffusion restriction raised concern for irreversible methotrexate toxicity, although this ultimately resolved. **E,** MRI of acute postradiation injury with abnormal T2 prolongation involving the pons and cerebral peduncles, medulla, right cerebellar peduncle, and anteromedial right cerebellar hemisphere. **F,** Patchy heterogeneous enhancement, predominantly in the pons.

Pseudoprogression

Another cause of encephalopathy with multifocal neurologic deficits is tumor pseudoprogression from cerebral necrosis, which may present as progressive neurologic deterioration with cerebral edema on imaging, typically 6 weeks to 3 months after radiation therapy (Fig. 134-2C and D). Concurrent treatment with chemotherapy may be a risk factor. When symptomatic, the condition is treated with high-dose corticosteroids, and bevacizumab is increasingly employed for patients who experience rapid deterioration despite corticoid therapy and/or intolerable steroid side effects.

Cerebrovascular Events

Cerebrovascular complications in childhood CNS tumor survivors include stroke, moyamoya, mineralizing microangiopathy, cavernomas and other vascular malformations, and stroke-like migraines. The incidence of neurovascular events in childhood brain tumor survivors has been found to be 100-fold higher than that in the general pediatric population (Campen et al., 2012). Cranial irradiation, particularly to the circle of Willis, is an important dose-dependent risk factor for stroke and cerebrovascular abnormalities (Mueller et al., 2013). Chemotherapy, including methotrexate, anthracyclines, mitomycins, asparaginase (especially venous sinus thrombosis), or antivascular endothelial growth factor (VEGF) may also increase risk (Di Giannatale et al., 2014).

Asymptomatic radiographic findings include microbleeds and superficial siderosis. Radiation-induced cavernous malformations (RICMs) may occur within the radiation field on average 12 years after radiation treatment and may cause symptomatic hemorrhage.

There are no standardized guidelines for posttreatment imaging surveillance for cerebrovascular disease. Magnetic resonance (MR) angiography may not necessarily identify stroke risk because many CNS tumor survivors have small vessel disease. An annual neurologic evaluation is recommended by the Children's Oncology Group (COG). The pathophysiology of vascular damage from radiation is complex and dependent on the targeted blood vessels, and possibly upregulation of proinflammatory and hypoxia-related genes. Moyamoya may occur, and patients with neurofibromatosis type I should not receive radiation therapy because of their very high risk of stroke and high risk of secondary malignancies. The use of antiplatelet agents in asymptomatic individuals has not been systematically studied (Murphy et al., 2015).

Stroke-like migraine after radiation therapy (SMART) syndrome causes acute or subacute focal impairment, often accompanied by encephalopathy and headache. It may be associated with hypointensities on susceptibility-weighted imaging (SWI) and gyriform enhancement on T1-weighted MRI (Fig. 134-2E and F). SWI may help distinguish SMART from other conditions that may have a similar postcontrast MRI appearance. Treatment includes the use of hydration and neuroprotective measures, including avoidance of hypotension, and prophylactic complex migraine treatment for recurrent or prolonged episodes.

Postoperative Cerebellar Mutism Syndrome

Postoperative cerebellar mutism syndrome, also called *posterior fossa syndrome*, was originally described in 1984 and was reported with increased frequency in the late 1990s and early 2000s in association with more aggressive surgery to resect posterior fossa tumors, particularly, but not exclusively, medulloblastoma (Robertson et al., 2006). A multicenter study by the COG found that 107/450 patients with medulloblastoma (24%) manifested the syndrome. It is characterized by development of mutism in the perioperative period, often associated with neurobehavioral abnormalities that may include personality change, emotional lability, decreased initiation of voluntary movements, swallowing dysfunction, ataxia, axial hypotonia, and weakness. Although the mutism is transient, patients have more significant neurologic and cognitive deficits at 1 year and more cerebellar atrophy than those without cerebellar mutism syndrome. Brainstem invasiveness of the tumor appears to be a risk factor, and recent studies have identified postoperative abnormalities in efferent cerebellar pathways, including the dentate-thalamo-cortical outflow tracts, on diffusion-tensor MRI.

Chronic Leukoencephalopathy

Leukoencephalopathy in childhood cancer survivors is a demyelinating process commonly seen after radiotherapy and some chemotherapy, including intravenous or intrathecal methotrexate. A grading system proposed by Zimmerman et al. (1986) is still in use. MR spectroscopic evidence of neuro-axonal damage in normal-appearing white and gray matter associated with radiation and chemotherapy have also been described, and white-matter tract volume and anisotropy have been linked to cognitive and motor function in pediatric posterior fossa tumor survivors (Mabbott et al., 2008; Rueckriegel et al., 2015).

Cognitive Impairment

Definition and Measurement of Neurocognitive Effects

A neurocognitive deficit is a reduction or impairment of cognitive function, particularly when a definable physical change has occurred in the brain, as is the case after a brain tumor. Assessment tools validated in the fields of oncology, neurology, and cognition are used with increasing standardization across studies. A degree of consensus has been achieved in both Europe (Limond et al., 2015) and North America that assessing quality of survival, including health-related quality of life, should involve administration of not only questionnaires for parents and patients (Packer et al., 2003) (e.g., NIH toolbox and Patient Reported Outcome Measurement Information System—PROMIS) but also short batteries of direct psychometric assessments (e.g., IQ, CANTAB and CogState). Intelligence quotient (IQ) testing using the Wechsler Intelligence Scales (WISC) has been the most common means to measure neurocognitive deficits in children treated for brain tumors. Limitations of studies using IQ alone include missing subtle but important deficits in selective attention and executive function, failing to capture important aspects of quality of survival, such as ability to live independently, and questionable generalizability as a result of sample bias from centers where direct assessment is available.

Risk Factors for Neurocognitive Deficits

Risks of neurocognitive impairment in children treated for brain tumors are substantial, and there is a progressive decline in IQ over time, particularly associated with, but not entirely attributable to, craniospinal irradiation (CSI). Three main conclusions can be drawn from a growing body of research in this field. First, longitudinal studies of children treated with CSI for medulloblastoma have consistently found a decline in IQ over time. Second, cross-sectional comparative studies have found that children treated either for ependymoma with postoperative radiation to the posterior fossa alone or treated for low-grade astrocytoma with surgery alone demonstrate less severe deficits in IQ than those treated for medulloblastoma with CSI. Third, younger age at time of treatment increases the risk of decline in IQ. The three cardinal risk factors for neurocognitive deficits are age at diagnosis, neuroanatomical tumor- or surgery-related damage, and adjuvant treatment with radiotherapy and chemotherapy.

1. **Age**: Infants diagnosed in the first year are at high risk of neurologic and cognitive deficits sufficient to interfere with school function, social functioning, choice of occupation, and ability to live independently. Younger children are more vulnerable to surgical insult to the brain than older children even in the absence of additional treatments. In one study, over 70% of young children treated with CSI evaluated at least 5 years postdiagnosis had IQs of less than 70, which represents learning disability. For medulloblastoma, the most common malignant tumor of the posterior fossa, children treated with CSI had lower verbal, nonverbal, and overall IQ scores and lower scores for spelling, reading, and mathematics than those expected for age. The greatest rates of decline have been observed in children younger than 7 years old and appear to be a result of failure to acquire new skills at the expected rate rather than loss of existing skills. Some studies have shown preservation of cognition in children less than 3 years of age at diagnosis treated with systemic chemotherapy without radiation, although young children who receive intraventricular methotrexate may have lower IQ scores.

2. **Radiotherapy and chemotherapy**: Dose, fractionation, volume, and location of radiotherapy (RT) and the combination of RT with chemotherapy are significant risk factors in the neurocognitive effects of treatment. Compared with those receiving CSI, children who have received radiation to the posterior fossa alone may have fewer deficits and may avoid the decline over time. Information about the potentiating effect on the long-term toxicity of adding chemotherapy to cranial or craniospinal irradiation is very limited. Because risk-based strategies are implemented according to the new molecular stratification of medulloblastoma, more information may be gleaned about relative treatment effects.

The neuroanatomical substrate of IQ decline following RT is not clearly understood and may be attributed to volume loss in the cerebral cortex or hippocampus or a reduction in white matter. Newer imaging methods have uncovered associations between structural and functional white-matter connectivity and cognitive outcomes. Specific areas of the brain receiving the same dose of RT are affected differently, with frontal lobes showing a greater deterioration in white matter than parietal lobes. Patients with hemispheric tumors have a significantly greater decline in IQ than those with midline tumors. There is a strong correlation between overall white-matter loss and IQ and between volume of white-matter loss in specific areas (cingulate gyrus, frontal and prefrontal lobes) and attention. Large areas of the supratentorial hemispheres and white matter are spared with local posterior fossa RT, which may partially explain why a moderate reduction in IQ is seen but, in contrast to those treated with CSI, no decline in IQ over time.

3. Neuroanatomical damage—tumor location and surgery: Many tumors always occur in one intracranial location (e.g., craniopharyngioma in the suprasellar region, medulloblastoma in the posterior fossa), but others occur in several locations, enabling examination of the effect of site. Survivors of pilocytic astrocytomas, assessed at least 3 years after diagnosis, were compared with respect to cognitive deficits by tumor location. Those with supratentorial midline tumors did not have tumor- or surgery-ascribable deficits, excepting some language and verbal memory problems in the subgroup with dorsally placed (thalamic) tumors; those with supratentorial hemispheric tumors had problems with selective attention and executive function; and those with infratentorial tumors had deficits in verbal intelligence, visual-spatial memory, executive function, and naming. All groups had problems with sustained attention and processing speed.

Patients with cerebellar tumors typically exhibit neurocognitive deficits, including impaired executive functioning. These deficits have also been observed in the absence of RT and chemotherapy in children treated with surgery alone for benign low grade astrocytoma in the cerebellum (Bull et al., 2014). The combination of these deficits with behavioral and emotional regulation was first described as the cognitive affective syndrome. It is thought that the severing of cerebral–cerebellar connections during surgery leads to a disruption of access to the cognitive control systems in the frontal lobes. In particular, cerebellar mutism syndrome (described earlier in the chapter) is strongly associated with decreased IQ scores. Damage to the dentate nuclei and inferior vermis has also been related to poor neurologic and cognitive outcomes in children treated for posterior fossa tumors, irrespective of RT schedule, age of patient, and pre- and postoperative complications (Puget et al., 2009).

Greater perioperative and short-term medical complications contribute to lower IQ scores. A study showed that the diminished postoperative IQ scores of children with cerebellar astrocytomas typically recover and normalize, in contrast to the IQ scores of children treated for medulloblastomas, indicating additive effects from RT and chemotherapy (Bull et al., 2014).

4. Other factors: Shunted hydrocephalus has been implicated as a possible additional contributor to poorer cognitive functioning, including lower overall IQ, performance IQ, perceptual organization, and visual-motor functioning. Shunt infections and meningitis have been associated with a reduction of overall IQ and verbal IQ and with neurologic deficits such as compromised dexterity, oculomotor deficits, and cerebellar mutism. Gender, attributional style, maternal depression, income, and intensity of targeted rehabilitation, including pharmacotherapy, have been shown to influence neurocognitive outcome. Some of the variability in outcome is likely genetic as a result of allelic variation in recovery following acquired brain injury, either through effects on brain repair mechanisms or through genetic variation in pharmacologic handling of tumoricidal or rehabilitative treatments.

The effect of intellectual decline on academic functioning is evident, and underlies, for example, poor reading, writing, and mathematical skills. Neurocognitive deficits are important to the child's academic, social, and psychological well-being because the effect of poor academic skills on the quality of life of the child is most apparent in school, the main setting in which children socialize with their peers. These deficits have far-reaching consequences not only for a child's academic achievements but also for the child's psychological and social development and ability to be self-sufficient. The effects of early brain damage on development become evident as progressively more functions are expected to mature. Thus many survivors of CNS tumors can be expected to "grow into deficits." Surveillance for detection of deficits is required because the deficits may only become apparent over time, and learning support is an essential prerequisite for successful transition to independent adult life.

NEUROSENSORY DEFICITS
Visual Impairment

More than half of all children with brain tumors develop visual difficulties in the symptom interval between onset of the first symptom and diagnosis, and as a group, children presenting with visual difficulties have a longer-than-average symptom interval. Among children with a brain tumor and a diagnosis of neurofibromatosis (NF1), 41% have impaired visual acuity at diagnosis, 15% have optic atrophy, and 16% have exophthalmos. Hydrocephalus can be chronic or acute and present with lethargy or with asymptomatic papilledema, which may lead to with progressive visual impairment of which the child does not complain. Monocular visual loss is rarely noticed by the patient. Regular assessment of visual function and eye movements is key both to early diagnosis of brain tumors and to early detection of late-onset hydrocephalus, shunt malfunction, or tumor progression. A low threshold for requesting formal visual field testing is prudent because bedside testing may be unreliable.

Visual impairment is often a dramatic part of PRES but fortunately is often largely reversible in that context. It may also feature in SMART and as symptomatic small strokes arising from postradiation cavernous hemangiomas. The management of visual deficits seen in association with centrally placed tumors, especially germinomas, craniopharyngiomas, hypothalamic tumors, and optic pathway gliomas, is beyond the scope of this chapter.

Hearing Loss

A degree of hearing loss after treatment for a brain tumor in childhood is common. The causes may be multifactorial but include tumor location, surgery, RT, and chemotherapy. Ototoxic chemotherapy drugs include the platinum compounds (cisplatin is much more ototoxic than carboplatin) and ifosfamide. Cisplatin causes sensorineural high-frequency hearing loss (with or without tinnitus) by direct injury to the outer hair cells in the organ of Corti or indirectly through biochemical factors affecting the cochlea. Hypomagnesemia during cisplatin treatment may contribute because magnesium is important for maintaining blood flow to the cochlea, hair cell permeability, and the ionic concentration of the endolymph and perilymph in the stria vascularis. Carboplatin affects the ear in a similar way but is less ototoxic than cisplatin. Ototoxicity is dose dependent, occurring with higher doses, and worsened with high cumulative exposure. The high-frequency hearing loss induced by the platinum agents is permanent, although in young children apparent improvement may occur as a result of an increasing ability to cooperate with hearing tests.

High-frequency hearing loss results in difficulty understanding speech and discriminating between words because high-frequency consonants are lost. This may cause educational, social, and educational adaptation difficulties; an increased sense of isolation; and an overall decrease in quality of life. High-frequency hearing loss may become apparent years after the last dose of cisplatin, and it is important to monitor hearing for some time after completion of treatment.

PERIPHERAL NERVOUS SYSTEM IMPAIRMENT

Lower motor neuron weakness may result from toxicity from chemotherapy, in particular, vinca alkaloids (vincristine), platinum drugs (cisplatin, oxaliplatin, carboplatin), methotrexate, and some biologic agents, including those with anti-angiogenic properties. Chemotherapy-induced peripheral neuropathy may be purely sensory (e.g., diminished temperature and vibratory sensation, burning paresthesias, jaw pain), predominantly motor (e.g., foot drop), and/or have an autonomic component, including constipation and orthostatic hypotension. Symptoms are nerve-length dependent and drug-dose dependent, and severity varies, with manifestations ranging from subclinical findings to mild discomfort to severely debilitating symptoms. Neuropathy is often worse in individuals of older age. Attempts to prevent or treat chemotherapy-associated neuropathies have failed, with the exception of medications for hyperesthesia and pain control. The dose for chemotherapy may be reduced when neuropathy is severe. Recent research has focused on molecular genetic predictors such as alterations in CYP5a enzymes, with goals of facilitating risk-adjusted dosing and better prevention of hearing loss.

GROWTH AND OTHER SEQUELAE WITH A NEUROENDOCRINE COMPONENT

Posttreatment neuroendocrine effects are common. In the Childhood Cancer Survivor study, 43% of survivors reported one or more endocrine conditions, and compared with siblings, survivors had a significantly increased risk of late-onset hypothyroidism, growth hormone deficiency, the need for medications to induce puberty, and osteoporosis (Armstrong et al., 2009). Radiation dosimetry, tumor location, and tumor type are predictors of neuroendocrinopathies. COG guidelines recommend annual evaluation for endocrinopathies in survivors who have received cranial radiation. Children with craniopharyngioma show a high rate of endocrine deterioration (e.g., persistent diabetes insipidus and panhypopituitarism). Long-term management of neuroendocrinopathies includes regular monitoring and replacement of hormones as needed, including temporary increase in cortisol dose during intercurrent infection or other physiologic stress of cortisol. Concerns about secondary malignancies from growth hormone have not been supported by research studies.

Fertility in childhood cancer survivors is a major concern. A survey of 1110 childhood cancer survivors found that female survivors receiving 30 Gy or more to the pituitary gland reported fewer pregnancies and higher frequency of permanent amenorrhea compared with patients receiving lower doses of radiation. Chemotherapeutic agents, in particular, high-dose alkylating agents, have been associated with decreased fertility. Recovery from fertility impairment is possible in some patients. Research in this field is increasing, risk counseling is becoming standard, and fertility preservation methods may be offered to eligible patients before treatment (Vargo et al., 2011).

CONCLUSIONS

Survivors of childhood CNS tumors experiences posttreatment sequelae, including high rates of neurologic and neurocognitive impairment and other medical conditions that affect quality of life and put them at risk for early mortality. Little is known about the exact mechanisms of injury from brain tumor treatment. It is understood that in addition to killing target tissues, surgery, cranial irradiation, and chemotherapy may induce damage to adjacent healthy tissues, leading to neurologic damage for which there are few treatments of any efficacy; endogenous healing within the CNS is supported by generic neurorehabilitation to promote the processes whereby healing or undamaged areas recover the ability to perform impaired functions.

Increased recognition of treatment effects has affected tumor treatment and led to efforts to prevent neurologic and neurocognitive impairment. Multicenter cooperative clinical trials involve risk stratification, such that more aggressive therapy is given to patients with higher-risk disease and less aggressive treatment to patients with lower-risk disease. Reductions in radiation have been incremental because risks of adverse sequelae must be balanced against the need for cure. Patients require continued follow-up to monitor disease status and late effects. The high incidence of posttreatment sequelae, often with an insidious and delayed onset, necessitates ongoing monitoring for years and probably throughout the survivor's lifespan. Future research will address whether epidemiology has changed with modern therapies. Increased awareness of risk factors in patients and providers, promotion of healthy lifestyles, and prompt response to new symptoms may reduce and prevent morbidity and mortality from late effects.

REFERENCES

The complete list of references for this chapter is available online at www.expertconsult.com.
  See inside cover for registration details.

SELECTED REFERENCES

Armstrong, A.E., Gillan, E., DiMario, F.J. Jr., 2014. SMART syndrome (stroke-like migraine attacks after radiation therapy) in adult and pediatric patients. J. Child Neurol. 29 (3), 336–341. doi:10.1177/0883073812474843; [Epub 2013 Jan 29]; PMID: 23364656.

Armstrong, G.T., Liu, Q., Yasui, Y., et al., 2009. Long-term outcomes among adult survivors of childhood central nervous system malignancies in the Childhood Cancer Survivor Study. J. Natl. Cancer Inst. 101 (13), 946–958. doi:10.1093/jnci/djp148; [Epub 2009 Jun 17].

Bull, K., Liossi, C., Culliford, D., et al. on behalf of the Children's Cancer and Leukaemia Group (CCLG), 2014. Child-related characteristics predicting subsequent health-related quality of life in 8 to 14 year old children with and without cerebellar tumors: a prospective longitudinal study. Neurooncol Pract 1, 114–122. doi:10.1093/nop/npu016.

Campen, C.J., Kranick, S.M., Kasner, S.E., et al., 2012. Cranial irradiation increases risk of stroke in pediatric brain tumor survivors. Stroke 43 (11), 3035–3040. PMID:22968468.

Di Giannatale, A., Morana, G., Rossi, A., et al., 2014. Natural history of cavernous malformations in children with brain tumors treated with radiotherapy and chemotherapy. J. Neurooncol. 117 (2), 311–320. PMID: 24515423.

Escalas, C., Bourdet, C., Fayech, C., et al., 2015. Long-term effects of radiation on the spine - Results of a cohort of symptomatic survivors of childhood and review of the literature]. Bull. Cancer 102 (7–8), 684–690. doi:10.1016/j.bulcan.2015.03.008; [Epub 2015 Apr 11]; PMID: 25869.

Limond, J.A., Bull, K.S., Calaminus, G., et al. on behalf of the Brain Tumour Quality of Survival Group, International Society of Paediatric Oncology (Europe) (SIOP-E), 2015. Quality of Survival Assessment in European Childhood Brain Tumour Trials, for Children Aged 5 years and Over. Eur. J. Paediatr. Neurol. 19 (2), 202–210. doi:10.1016/j.ejpn.2014.12.003.

Mabbott, D.J., Penkman, L., Witol, A., et al., 2008. Core neurocognitive functions in children treated for posterior fossa tumors. Neuropsychol 22, 159–168.

McCoy, B., King, M., Gill, D., et al., 2011. Childhood posterior reversible encephalopathy syndrome. Eur. J. Paediatr. Neurol. 15 (2), 91–94. [Epub 2010 Nov 11]; PMID: 21074464.

Mueller, S., Fullerton, H.J., Stratton, K., et al., 2013. Radiation, atherosclerotic risk factors, and stroke risk in survivors of pediatric cancer:

a report from the Childhood Cancer Survivor Study. Int. J. Radiat. Oncol. Biol. Phys. 86 (4), 649–655. PMID: 23680033.

Murphy, E.S., Xie, H., Merchant, T.E., et al., 2015. Review of cranial radiotherapy-induced vasculopathy. J. Neurooncol. 122 (3), 421–429. doi:10.1007/s11060-015-1732-2; [Epub 2015 Feb 12]; PMID:25670390.

Packer, R.J., Gurney, J.G., Punyko, J.A., et al., 2003. Long-term neurologic and neurosensory sequelae in adult survivors of a childhood brain tumor: Childhood Cancer Survivor Study. J. Clin. Oncol. 21, 3255–3261.

Puget, S., Boddaert, N., Viguier, D., et al., 2009. Injuries to inferior vermis and dentate nuclei predict poor neurological and neuropsychological outcome in children with malignant posterior fossa tumors. Cancer 115, 1338–1347.

Robertson, P.L., Muraszko, K.M., Holmes, E.J., et al., 2006. Incidence and severity of postoperative cerebellar mutism syndrome in children with medulloblastoma: a prospective study by the Children'sOncology Group. J. Neurosurg. 105 (6 Suppl.), 444–451.

Rueckriegel, S.M., Bruhn, H., Thomale, U.W., et al., 2015. Cerebral white matter fractional anisotropy and tract volume as measured by MR imaging are associated with impaired cognitive and motor function in pediatric posterior fossa tumor survivors. Pediatr. Blood Cancer 62 (7), 1252–1258.

Ruggiero, A., Rizzo, D., Mastrangelo, S., et al., 2010. Interactions between antiepileptic and chemotherapeutic drugs in children with brain tumors: is it time to change treatment? Pediatr. Blood Cancer 54 (2), 193–198. doi:10.1002/pbc.22276; PMID: 19731334.

Ullrich, N.J., Pomeroy, S.L., Kapur, K., et al., 2015. Incidence, risk factors, and longitudinal outcome of seizures in long-term survivors of pediatric brain tumors. Epilepsia 56 (10), 1599–1604. PMID:26332282.

Vargo, M., 2011. Brain tumor rehabilitation. Am. J. Phys. Med. Rehabil. 90 (5 Suppl 1), S50–S62.

Zimmerman, R.D., Fleming, C.A., Lee, B.C.P., et al., 1986. Periventricular hyperintensity as see by magnetic resonance: prevalence and significance. Am J Neuroradiolo 7, 13–20.

E-BOOK FIGURES AND TABLES

The following figures and tables are available in the e-book at www.expertconsult.com. See inside cover for registration details.

Fig. 134-3 Clusters of decreased fractional anisotropy (FA) in medulloblastoma patients.

Fig. 134-4 Fronto-cerebellar fiber tracking: a volume delineated by the frontal cerebral pole

Fig. 134-5 Scatterplot and Spearman correlations between fronto-cerebellar tract volumes

Table 134-1 Imaging Features and Zimmerman Grading System for Leukoencephalopathy

135 Muscle and Nerve Development in Health and Disease

Jeremy K. Deisch

 An expanded version of this chapter is available on www.expertconsult.com. See inside cover for registration details.

One of the most important functions of the central nervous system and the primary outwardly visible manifestation of brain function is movement. Despite the apparent simplicity of achieving purposeful movement, a dizzyingly complex series of electrochemical signals and biochemical transitions is required for completion of even the simplest of motions. The appropriate neural pathways leading from neurons in the brain and terminating on the often remote target skeletal muscle fibers must be intact, the junctions between the nervous system and the muscle fibers (neuromuscular junctions) properly formed and maintained, and the target muscle fibers functional and supplied with metabolic substrates. Defects in any of these components result in weakness. This chapter reviews the embryology, anatomy, and function of the peripheral nervous and skeletal muscle systems. (Also see recent texts by Dubowitz et al., 2013; Goebel et al., 2013; Carpenter and Karpati, 2001.) Subsequent chapters address clinical and laboratory investigations into diseases of skeletal muscle, as well as the diverse array of diseases resulting from both intrinsic and acquired defects.

EMBRYOLOGY AND DEVELOPMENT
Skeletal Muscle

Premyoblasts, the primitive cells that form skeletal muscle, arise from condensations of paraxial mesoderm called somites, structures that lie adjacent to the neural tube and notochord. As these structures mature, dermomyotomes and myotomes are formed, eventually forming the musculature of the body walls and extremities. Craniofacial muscles derive from mesoderm rostral to the first somite, and axial muscles arise from more rostral somites; the limb muscles derive from condensations in the region of the limb buds. The migration of myocytes is not haphazard but rather is guided by preformed mesodermal structures. In the developing limb buds, the proximal tendon primordium is a mesodermal condensation that guides migration of myogenic precursors and serves as an early scaffold for muscle formation. During the process of myogenesis, groups of cells split and recombine, resulting in contributions from several adjacent myotomes in an individual muscle. In the limb bud, the cells coalesce into dorsal and ventral masses (the epimere and hypomeres, respectively).

Orchestration of muscle development is under the guidance of a complex array of genetically determined growth and transcription factors. Premyoblasts express the paired box transcription factors, Pax-3 and Pax-7. Bone morphogenetic protein 4 (BMP4), released from adjacent neural tube and lateral plate mesoderm, inhibits gene expression of myogenic transcription factors, MyoD and Myf-5. Wnt and sonic hedgehog (SHH) signals from adjacent notochord, neural tube, and surface ectoderm activate muscle specific genes Myf-5 and MyoD in premyoblasts. Scatter factor, a growth factor secreted by the lateral plate mesoderm, acts as a chemoattractant by promoting myocyte migration. The transition from the premyoblast to myoblast stage of muscle maturation is marked by the cessation of DNA synthesis. Postmitotic myoblasts elongate and begin attachment and fusion with other myoblasts, end to end, to form a long and slender primary myotube. Secondary and tertiary myotubes are formed from side-to-side fusion of myoblasts to existing myotubes. In the absence of innervation, maturation beyond primary myotubes does not occur, and the muscle develops abnormally. Myofilaments begin to polymerize at 4 weeks gestation, forming recognizable myofibrils with characteristic striations at around 5 weeks gestation. At this stage, the nuclei are located with the center of the muscle fiber. Muscle contraction and fetal movements commences with the onset of muscle innervation at around 8 weeks gestation. At around 16 weeks, the nuclei migrate superficially to adult-type subsarcolemmal position, although a few fibers with centrally located nuclei may persist into adulthood.

Distinctive fiber types do not appear until muscle innervation. Undifferentiated primitive fibers (type IIc) are the precursors of mature fibers. Type I fibers appear at about 18 weeks gestation. Type IIa and IIb fibers appear during the last month of gestation. Only a small percentage of type IIc fibers persist after birth. Differentiation into distinct fiber types depends on neural influences, resulting into the biochemical and physiologic diversity of mature muscle fibers. The neural determination of fiber subtype is modulated by calcineurin, a Ca^{2+}-calmodulin-regulated phosphatase. Firing of motor neurons and the resultant sarcolemmal depolarization results in an increase in sarcoplasmic Ca^{2+}, which in turn activates calcineurin, an indirect activation of the slow myosin heavy chain 2 gene (slow MyHC2) promoter. Fast fibers result from motor neurons with infrequent firing, resulting in sarcoplasmic calcium concentrations that are insufficient to maintain calcineurin activation.

Satellite cells, abundant in fetal muscle, are mononuclear muscle cells that lie beneath the basement membrane of mature muscle fibers. During embryogenesis, satellite cells migrate from the dorsal somites to dermatomyotomes. Transcription factor Pax-7 is a key protein involved in myogenic determination of satellite cells. Transcription factor Pax-3 is required for the migration of these cells from the dorsal somite; Pax-7 is required for the transition to mature muscle cells. Satellite cells are the primary stem cell and are capable of forming individual muscle fibers as well as complete muscle fascicles.

The growth and strength of muscle postnatally is dependent on functional demands, gender, age, training, and other factors. Physiologic enlargement of a muscle body results from hypertrophy of muscle fibers rather than from growth of new fibers. Training and disuse can increase and decrease the cross-sectional diameter of muscle fibers. Muscle atrophy associated with aging is caused by loss of muscle fibers, rather than by fiber atrophy, and a decrease in satellite cells.

Peripheral Nerve

The peripheral nervous system arises from the neural plate, a dorsal thickening of the embryonic ectoderm. Progressive maturation of the neural plate is influenced by a complex milieu of transcription factors, including members of the PAX, MSX, bone morphogenic protein (BMP), and sonic hedgehog (SHH) families. The neural plate invaginates, with eventual fusion of the edges forming an open neural tube. Primitive cells from the apices of the folds form the primitive neural crest, from which cells destined for various sites throughout the body arise, including constituents of the peripheral nervous system such as neurons within the dorsal root ganglia. The neural tube, in addition to forming the brain and spinal cord, is also the origin of the majority of the peripheral nervous system. The motoneural system arises from the basal plates, ventral thickenings in the neuroblastic layer of the neural tube. Thickenings on the dorsal surface, the alar plates, form the sensorineural system. Outgrowths of motoneurons from the basal plate penetrate the developing ventral cord, in which they form in the fourth week of development, after the preceding migrating muscle precursors. SHH, expressed early during spinal cord development, specifies motor neurons in the developing neural tube. The developing axons are guided to their appropriate motor compartments by differential expression of a variety of transcription factors, including Hb9, Mnx1, Lhx3/4 (Sharma and Izpisúa Belmonte, 2001). Myelination proceeds after formation of the peripheral nerve, beginning in the fourth month of development. In the central nervous system, multiple axons are myelinated by oligodendroglia, cells of glioblastic origin. In the peripheral nervous system, Schwann cells arise from the neural crest, migrate to the developing peripheral nerves, and associate with axons of varying caliber. The numeric relationship between Schwann cells varies based upon myelination status of the axons; larger caliber, myelinated axons are ensheathed by a single Schwann cell in a given segment, whereas groups of several smaller unmyelinated axons lie within the processes of a single Schwann cell, resulting in a structure called a Remak bundle.

Attainment of proper myelinated axonal structure is under the control of several factors. Mutations in the genes encoding these factors result in abnormal structure of myelinated axons and in delayed nerve conduction velocity and resultant clinical manifestations. Neuregulin 1 (Nrg1), secreted by axons, regulates myelin thickness. The protein Periaxin regulates myelin internode length. Periaxin mutations result in decreased nerve conduction velocity and, in humans, recessive periaxin gene mutations result in a subtype of Charcot-Marie-Tooth disease (CMT4F). Axonal diameter is regulated by neurofilament light chain expression; mutations in the neurofilament light subunit (NEFL) gene result in early onset CMT disease. Proper myelin compaction and maintenance is regulated by peripheral myelin protein-22 (PMP22); mutations in the PMP22 gene result in the autosomal dominant inherited disorder hereditary neuropathy with liability to pressure palsies (HNPP).

Neuromuscular Junction

During the transition from embryonic to fetal myogenesis, developing peripheral nerve bundles contact the developing musculature, resulting in formation of specialized neuromuscular junctions. Before innervation, acetylcholine receptors are present diffusely throughout the membrane in relatively low numbers. In a process known as prepatterning, clusters of acetylcholine receptors begin to form in the central region of the aneural muscle fiber. Shortly thereafter, motor nerve axons reach the muscle fiber and overlap the prepatterned areas, beginning the process of neuromuscular junction formation. In the areas of overlap, the innervated clusters progressively enlarge while the nonoverlapped clusters disappear (Yang et al., 2001). It is through this process that neuromuscular junction formation progresses in an organized fashion, resulting in rows of neuromuscular junctions innervating the central region of a myofiber and forming a linear end plate. The molecular signaling pathway resulting in acetylcholine receptor accumulation in the neuromuscular junction is regulated by the agrin/lipoprotein receptor-related protein 4 (Lrp4)/muscle-specific tyrosine kinas (MuSK) pathway. The synthesis of agrin by motor neurons, subsequent axonal transport, and influence of neuromuscular junction formation is a prime example of how the nervous system profoundly influences the muscle development (Lin et al., 2001). Agrin serves to activate the postsynaptic membrane tyrosine kinase receptor MuSK through the coreceptor Lrp4. Both Lrp4 and MuSK are necessary for prepatterning and for proper neuromuscular junction formation. Once activated, MuSK activates docking protein-7 (DOK-7), a downstream regulator of neuromuscular junction assembly. Acetylcholine receptors are restricted to the postsynaptic membrane via the interaction with rapsyn, a membrane-bound protein that interacts with cytoskeletal proteins and anchors acetylcholine receptors; proper rapsyn functioning is necessary for prepatterning. These pathways are factors that promote acetylcholine receptor formation and neuromuscular junction formation. Inhibition of acetylcholine receptor formation away from the neuromuscular junction results from acetylcholine-induced sarcolemmal depolarization, resulting in dispersion and decreased stability of acetylcholine receptors through activation of regulatory factors and suppression of AChR gene transcription via inactivation of the myogenin gene (Sanes and Lichtman, 2001). Initially, individual mammalian muscle fibers are multiply innervated. Between 16 and 25 weeks gestation and in association with secondary myotubular formation, all but one synapse is eliminated. Other mammalian species differ in the timing of this process. For example, polyneuronal innervation persists postnatally in the mouse and is an important concept to remember when comparing animal models to human neuromuscular disorders. There is constant denervation and reinnervation as neuromuscular interactions forms physiologic innervations of the motor units. Multiple motor neurons compete for innervation. Competition weakens some synapses and strengthens others so that, ultimately, a single input prevails.

GENERAL ANATOMY AND STRUCTURE OF SKELETAL MUSCLE
Morphology

Muscle as an organ comprises all the individual muscles in the body. Each muscle has an origin and an insertion site on the skeleton and bridges one or more bony articulations; contraction across the articulation results in movement of the joint. The muscle is enclosed within the epimysium, a thick sheath of fibrous connective tissue that is contiguous with the muscle tendon. The muscle is subdivided into individual fascicles by the perimysium, fibrous septae that are contiguous with the epimysium. Within the perimysium are the blood vessels, intramuscular nerves, and muscle spindles (Fig. 135-3). The

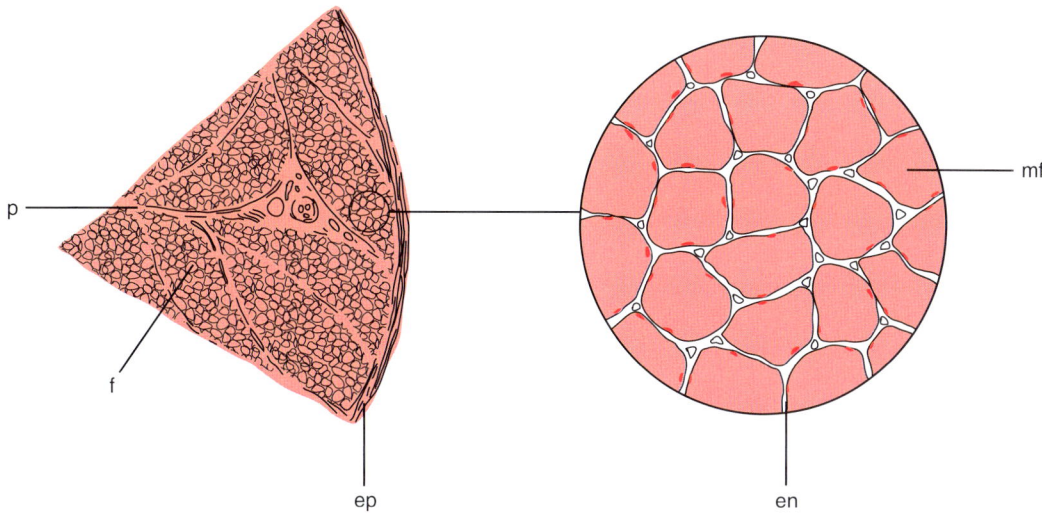

Figure 135-3. Cross-sectional anatomy of skeletal muscle. en, endomysium; ep, epimysium; f, fascicle; mf, muscle fiber; p, perimysium.

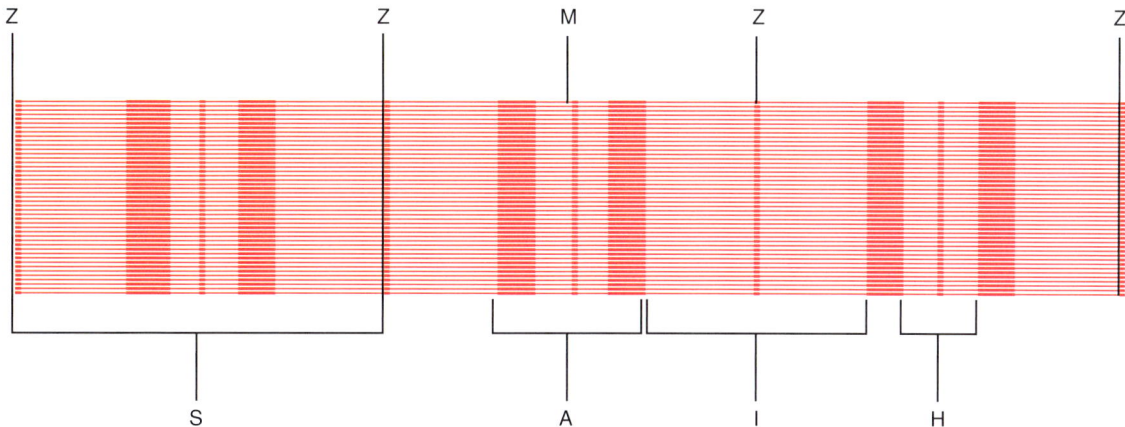

Figure 135-4. Sarcomeric structure. Schematic showing the structure of the sarcomere, which occupies the space between two adjacent Z lines. The M line occupies the midportion of the A band, and is the point of crosslinking of the myosin filaments. The A (anisotropic) band is the portion of the sarcomere occupied by myosin filaments, partially overlapped by actin. The H band is the region of thick filaments not overlapped by actin filaments. The I (isotropic) band comprises thin filaments without superimposed myosin filaments.

muscle fascicle, which is bounded by perimysial connective tissue, is a wedge-shaped structure comprising numerous individual muscle fibers. Surrounding each muscle fiber is a network of fine connective tissue, called the endomysium. The terminal axons and a rich capillary network reside within the endomysium. Individual muscle cells, myofibers, are multi-nucleated, elongated tubular structures that vary in diameter from 10 to 20 μm in the infant to about 50 to 70 μm in the adult.

Sarcomere

The most striking feature of skeletal muscle seen on microscopic examination is the characteristic striations ("striated" muscle) seen under polarized light. Striations are linear bands resulting from the differences in the refractive index of the contractile proteins that are in phase with each other. A repeating unit is called a sarcomere, comprising interdigitating myofilaments and bound on either end by the Z line (Fig. 135-4). The Z disk anchors the thin filaments of actin that extend into each adjacent sarcomere and are located in the I band. The M line bisects the sarcomere and divides the A band, which is formed by an array of thick filaments composed

of myosin. The area within the A band in which the thin and thick filaments do not overlap is called the H band.

Contractile and Sarcomeric Proteins

The two major proteins involved in muscle contraction are actin and myosin, which form the thin and thick filaments and jointly interact to convert chemical energy to mechanical work. Thin filaments are composed of two chains of actin molecules arranged in a double helix. Alpha-actinin is a major component of the Z disk and plays a role in the binding of actin to other cytoskeletal structures. Mutation in the α-actin gene, ACTA1, has been associated with congenital myopathy with actin filament aggregate myopathies, nemaline myopathy, cap myopathy, congenital fiber type disproportion myopathy, intranuclear rod myopathy, and hypertrophic and dilated cardiomyopathies.

Myosin molecules form the thick filaments. The contractile properties of a muscle fiber are due to the mechanochemical properties of myosin. Myosin heavy chain isoforms vary in different fiber types; the different myosin isoforms are determined by neural influences (see previous mention); variation in the myosin isoforms influences the physiologic properties of the muscle fibers. Mutations in myosin gene MYH7 cause hyaline body myopathy with or without cardiomyopathy or familial cardiomyoneuromyopathy. Respiratory failure occurs with mutations in exons 37 and 38 of the MYH7 gene.

Actin and myosin have an inherent affinity for each other; this affinity is influenced by sarcoplasmic calcium ion concentrations and regulated by troponin and tropomyosin. Tropomyosin exists as a helical structure, comprising two long filaments that reside within the groove of the actin chains. One tropomyosin molecule binds one troponin complex, positioning the troponin molecules regularly along the actin filament. The troponin complex holds tropomyosin in an "off" or "on" position on the actin helix, depending on the level of calcium. There are at least two isoforms of tropomyosin. Fast-twitch skeletal muscle contains both α- and β-isoforms; slow-twitch muscle contains only β-tropomyosin. The troponin molecules are located periodically along tropomyosin and comprise three subunits. Troponin T anchors troponin to tropomyosin. Troponin C binds calcium, which induces a conformational change of the protein and results in activation of actomyosin adenosine triphosphatase and muscle contraction. Troponin I inhibits actomyosin adenosine triphosphatase. Thus the contraction of striated muscle is regulated by the troponin complex, which acts as a Ca^{2+} sensor. Ca^{2+} binding to the regulatory sites of troponin C strengthens the interaction with troponin I, weakening the inhibitory activity of troponin I for actin and the affinity of troponin T for tropomyosin (Tm). Tropomyosin then moves toward the groove of the helical actin filament, switching on the myosin active site and resulting in muscle contraction. Troponin binds to actin-tropomyosin in the absence of Ca^{2+}, and the changes in interactions among these thin filament components in the presence of Ca^{2+} promote strong binding of myosin to actin. Mutations of the troponin T1 and tropomyosin genes may cause nemaline myopathy and/or cardiomyopathies.

Titin, the largest known protein of about 3 to 3.7 megadaltons, constitutes about 10% of myofibrillary proteins and is important for maintaining tension during stretch and recentering the sarcomere after relaxation. Titin spans the sarcomere, binding to the Z-disc and anchoring myosin, interconnecting actin and myosin, and providing elasticity to the sarcomere. Titin plays a major role in myofibrillogenesis, and abnormal expression of titin leads to disruption of assembly of the Z disk and sarcomere. Mutations in the titin gene cause familial dilated cardiomyopathy.

Nebulin, another large sarcomeric protein, closely associates with actin and binds to titin, myopalladin, and the actin-capping protein. Nebulin regulates the length of thin filaments in sarcomeres. Nebulin functions to stabilize the thin filaments at a determined length and is critical for generation of optimal force. Nebulin mutations cause nemaline and distal myopathy.

Obscurin is the most recently discovered member of a family of giant proteins involved in maintaining the structure of the sarcomere. Obscurin is localized at the M line and Z disk in skeletal and cardiac muscle. Obscurin binds and interacts with numerous muscle proteins, including titin, ankyrin, calmodulin, and myomesin. Obscurin functions in promoting lateral alignment and fusion of myofibrils into larger bundles. It also has an important part in assembly and stabilization of A bands and M bands in the sarcomere. Mutations of the obscurin gene produce hypertrophic cardiomyopathy by causing loss of binding with titin.

Sarcotubular System

The sarcolemma is the plasma membrane of the muscle cell and is surrounded by basement membrane and endomysial connective tissue. The sarcolemma is an excitable membrane and shares many properties with the neuronal cell membrane. T-tubules are invaginations of the sarcolemma, extending into the interior of the muscle fiber as the sarcotubular system. Depolarization of the sarcolemma is propagated throughout the interior of the muscle fiber through this system. The T tubules project into the interior of the muscle fibers in the area of the junction of the A and I bands, where they come into immediate contact with a second tubular system within the sarcoplasm, the sarcoplasmic reticulum. The close apposition of one T-tubule, bound on either side by the sarcoplasmic reticulum, is referred to as a "triad." The sarcoplasmic reticulum forms a fine plexus around the myofibrils. Excitation of the sarcolemma and T tubules causes Ca^{2+} release from the sarcoplasmic reticulum and initiation of contraction by the myofilaments.

Several important proteins are localized to the triads. The voltage sensors of the T-tubule calcium channels are regulated by dihydropyridine receptors. Ryanodine receptors mediate the calcium release of the sarcoplasmic reticulum during muscle activation. Calcium adenosine triphosphatase pumps calcium back into the sarcoplasmic reticulum during relaxation. Calsequestrin is a calcium-binding protein that increases the storage capacity of calcium in the sarcoplasmic reticulum. Some patients with myasthenia gravis, especially associated with thymoma, have autoantibodies directed against the ryanodine receptor antigens, as well as to titin. Autosomal-dominant and autosomal-recessive mutations of the ryanodine receptor gene (RYR) cause central core disease, myopathy with type 1 fiber dominance, and malignant hyperthermia.

Other features seen on ultrastructural examination of muscle fibers are nuclei and the sarcoplasm and its organelles. A typical muscle fiber has thousands of nuclei located beneath the sarcolemma throughout the length of the fiber. The sarcoplasm contains many of the elements found in the cytoplasm of other tissues. Most important are the mitochondria, which are located primarily in the intermyofibrillary space near the Z line and adjacent to the A bands. Numerous unbound glycogen granules and small fat droplets are present within the sarcoplasm.

Cytoskeletal Proteins

The structural integrity of the muscle is maintained against the physical forces of contraction exerted on the sarcolemma by an intricate system of cytoskeletal and sarcolemmal proteins. These proteins, through a complex pattern of arrangement, anchor the internal structure of the muscle to the basement membrane and extracellular matrix. Abnormalities in many of these proteins have been identified as causing a number of different types of myopathies (Table 135-1).

Dystrophin

Dystrophin is a 427 kilodalton protein that constitutes 0.01% of total muscle protein and 5% of the sarcolemmal cytoskeletal proteins. Dystrophin is localized in the inner aspect of the sarcolemma, and is abundant at the myotendinous junction and at the postsynaptic membrane of the neuromuscular junction. Dystrophin forms an integral part of a muscle's cytoskeleton and links the contractile apparatus to the sarcolemma. The N-terminus is the actin-binding domain, and the carboxy-terminal domain interacts with β-dystroglycan as well as dystrobrevin and the syntrophin. The central rod domain comprises the majority of the mass of the dystrophin molecule, forming a flexible, rod-shaped structure. The fourth cysteine rich domain also binds to β-dystroglycan.

TABLE 135-1 Muscle Proteins and Human Genetic Disease

Protein	Location	Disease	Protein	Location	Disease
PLASMA MEMBRANE			POMGnT1	1p34.1	MDDGA3-C3
Dystrophin	Xp21	BMD, DMD	Fukutin	9q31.2	MDDGA4-C4
α-Sarcoglycan (SGCA)	17q21.33	LGMD-2D	FKRP	19q1	MDDGA5-C6
β-Sarcoglycan (SGCB)	4q12	LGMD-2E	LARGE	22q12.3	MDDGA6, MDDGB6
γ-Sarcoglycan (SGCG)	13q12.12	LGMD-2C	ISPD	7q21.2	MDDGA7, MDDGC7
δ-Sarcoglycan (SGCD)	5q33.2–33.3	LGMD-2F	DAG1	3p21.31	MDDGA9, MDDGC9
Dysferlin	2p13	LGMD-2B, Miyoshi myopathy, DMAT	**SARCOMERIC PROTEINS**		
Caveolin-3	3p25	LGMD-1C, Rippling muscle disease	Titin	2q31.2	LGMD-2J
			Myotilin	5q31.2	LGMD-1A, myotilinopathy
α-Dystroglycan	3p21	Muscular dystrophy-dystroglycanopathy (secondary to abnormal protein glycosylation)	TCAP	17q12	LGMD-2G
			Actin (ACTA1)	1q42	Nemaline myopathy 3, congenital myopathy with cores
EXTRACELLULAR MATRIX			Tropomyosin-3	1q21.3	Nemaline myopathy 1, congenital myopathy with fiber-type disproportion, cap myopathy 1
α₂-Laminin	6q2	Merosin-deficient CMD			
Collagen VI	21q22	Ullrich CMD, Bethlem myopathy	Tropomyosin-2	9p13	Nemaline myopathy 4, cap myopathy 2
SARCOPLASMIC			Nebulin	2q23.3	Nemaline myopathy 2
Calpain-3	15q15.1	LGMD-2A	Slow troponin T	19q13	Nemaline myopathy 5, Amish type
TRIM32	9q31–34	LGMD-2H			
Myotubularin	Xq28	Myotubular myopathy	Ryanodine receptor (RYR1)	19q13.1	Central core disease, minicore myopathy, malignant hyperthermia susceptibility 1
Desmin	2q35	Desmin-related myopathy			
Plectin	8q24.3	Epidermolysis bullosa simplex with late-onset muscular dystrophy	Myosin heavy chain (MyH 7)	14q12	Myosin storage myopathy, cardiomyopathy, left ventricular noncompaction
Dok-7	4p16.3	Congenital myasthenic syndrome	**NUCLEAR PROTEINS**		
REGULATION OF SARCOGLYCAN GLYCOSYLATION			Emerin	Xq28	Emery-Dreifuss muscular dystrophy 1
POMT1	9q34	MDDGA1-C1	LMNA	1q22	Emery-Dreifuss muscular dystrophy 2, LGMD-1B
POMT2	14q24.3	MDDGA2-C2			

BMD, Becker muscular dystrophy; CMD, congenital muscular dystrophy; DMD, Duchenne muscular dystrophy; LGMD, limb-girdle muscular dystrophy. MDDG, muscular dystrophy-dystroglycanopathy.

(Adapted from Vainzof, M., Zatz, M., 2003.. Protein defects in neuromuscular diseases. Braz J Med Biol Res 36, 543–555. Updates from Online Mendelian Inheritance in Man—www.omim.org.)

The dystrophin-glycoprotein complex consists of numerous proteins, including dystroglycans (α and β), sarcoglycans (α, β,γ,δ,ε), sarcospan, syntrophin, and dystrobrevin. The peripheral members of the complex include neuronal nitric oxide synthase, caveolin, laminin, and merosin.

The DMD gene coding for the protein dystrophin is located on the short arm of the X chromosome near the region Xp21. The dystrophin gene is the largest gene identified so far, covering more than 2.5 megabases (Mb), and contains at least 79 exons; the high spontaneous mutation rate is a reflection of the large gene size. Dystrophin is primarily expressed in skeletal, cardiac, and smooth muscle cells, with smaller amounts expressed in the brain and retina. Isoforms of dystrophin, which are smaller in size, are expressed in nearly all tissues examined. Dystrophin in the brain is important in synapse maintenance; deficiency of the brain isoform of dystrophin is associated with cognitive deficits seen in patients with dystrophin mutations. Deletions or abnormalities of the dystrophin gene cause an absence or deficiency of dystrophin, resulting in the X-linked Duchenne and Becker muscular dystrophies (Chapter 146).

Dystrophin-Glycoprotein Complex

The dystrophin-glycoprotein complex is a sophisticated linkage that spans the sarcolemma and links the sarcoplasmic contractile apparatus to laminins in the extracellular matrix, serving to transfer the force of muscle contraction between the myofibrils and surrounding connective tissues. This dystrophin-glycoprotein complex consists of cytoskeletal, transmembrane, and extracellular components and is composed of two subgroups of protein complexes: the dystroglycans and sarcoglycans.

Dystroglycan consists of a transmembrane and an extracellular component encoded by a single messenger RNA and subsequently processed to α- and β-dystroglycan molecules. The α-dystroglycan protein undergoes extensive posttranslational glycosylation and is located on the extracellular side of the sarcolemmal membrane. The size and molecular weight of the dystroglycan molecule expressed in various tissues varies based upon differential glycosylation patterns in those tissues. The glycosylation is mediated by several glycosyl transferases; mutations in these enzymes cause myopathies and brain and eye malformations, as the dystroglycan complex also plays an important role in normal migration of neurons in the cerebral neocortex (Chapter 147).

Primary mutations in the dystroglycans have not yet been identified in human disease. Defective glycosylation, however, results in a spectrum of disorders, in which a limb-girdle muscle dystrophy (type 2-I, due to FKRP mutation) is the mildest manifestation, and structural brain and ocular abnormalities comprise the most severe end of the spectrum in the congenital muscular dystrophies. In the past, these conditions were referred to as Walker-Warburg syndrome, muscle-eye-brain disease, and a subtype of limb-girdle muscular dystrophy. Currently, given the improved understanding of the shared underlying pathogenesis of defective glycosylation of dystroglycan, the conditions are now referred to as muscular dystrophy-dystroglycanopathies (MDDG) (Chapter 147). Table 135-1 lists the genes involved with isolated muscular dystrophy resulting from abnormal glycosylation of dystroglycan.

Sarcoglycans

The sarcoglycan complex consists of α-, β-, γ-, and δ-sarcoglycan, and is integral to the dystrophin-associated glycoprotein complex, conferring structural stability to the sarcolemma and protecting muscle fibers from mechanical stress during muscle contraction. Alpha-sarcoglycan is present only in cardiac and skeletal muscles; the other sarcoglycans are also found in smooth muscle. Gamma-sarcoglycan binds to dystrophin, and δ-sarcoglycan binds to β-dystroglycan. Mutations in any of the sarcoglycan genes cause destabilization of the complex, resulting in different forms of limb-girdle muscular dystrophy (Chapter 147). In muscle biopsies from sarcoglycanopathy patients, this primary loss or reduction of expression of one sarcoglycan, due to a mutation in that gene, is frequently associated with secondary loss of other sarcoglycans. Mutations in the sarcoglycan genes result in limb-girdle muscular dystrophies types LGMD-2C through LGMD2F (Table 135-1).

Utrophin

Utrophin is an autosomally encoded protein that is smaller in size than dystrophin and is localized to the sarcolemmal postsynaptic membrane at the neuromuscular junction and myotendinous junction in the mature muscle fiber. At the neuromuscular junction, it is preferentially concentrated at the acetylcholine receptor-rich crests. Utrophin production is regulated by growth factors released from the neurite such as heregulin, resulting in gene transcription occurring preferentially in the nuclei close to the neuromuscular junction. In animal models, induced utrophin expression has been shown to partially compensate for dystrophin deficiency and attenuate the resultant myopathy. Muscle biopsies from humans with Duchenne muscular dystrophy characteristically demonstrate upregulation of utrophin, with diffuse distribution of this protein along muscle fibers. This feature helps distinguish a primary dystrophinopathy from those with secondary dystrophin reduction. This alternative pathway provides a possible therapeutic target for patients with dystrophinopathies.

Dysferlin

Dysferlin is a sarcolemmal protein expressed in skeletal muscle, cardiac muscle, placenta, and brain tissue. Dysferlin does not directly associate with the dystrophin-glycoprotein complex but rather is peripheral, interacting with multiple proteins including caveolin-3. Dysferlin functions in membrane trafficking and repair of sarcolemmal defects. Defects in dysferlin result in limb-girdle muscular dystrophy type 2B and Miyoshi myopathy.

Caveolin

Caveolin, a family of membrane associated proteins expressed in fibroblasts, adipocytes, endothelium, and muscle cells, regulates caveolae formation. Caveolae are flask-shaped membrane invaginations that function in membrane trafficking, transport, and signal transduction. Mutations in the muscle isoform, caveolin-3, result in limb-girdle muscular dystrophy type 1C, rippling muscle disease, familial hypertrophic cardiomyopathy, and long QT syndrome and have been associated with sudden infant death syndrome.

Merosin (Laminin-α_2)

Laminin-α_2 is a major component of laminin in the basal lamina of postnatal muscle and cardiac muscle and is also expressed in mesenchymal tissue in other organs. Laminin interacts with the sarcolemma through the dystrophin-glycoprotein and vinculin-integrin complexes. Mutations of laminin-α_2 manifest as congenital muscular dystrophy, complete absence of muscle merosin, and abnormalities of cerebral deep white matter. Prenatal diagnosis can be made by merosin immunostaining of chorionic villus biopsy samples.

Intermediate Filaments

Intermediate filaments are cytoskeletal proteins with a diameter intermediate between the thin and thick myofibrils, measuring between 10 and 12 nm in diameter. Intermediate filaments are seen in cells of ectodermal, mesodermal, and endodermal derivation. Desmin, vimentin, nestin, lamin, and plectin are intermediate filaments expressed in muscle.

Desmin is the major intermediate filament in skeletal muscle, cardiac, and smooth muscle. Desmin is located at the Z band beneath the sarcolemma and is denser at the myotendinous junction. Desmin is involved with the alignment of sarcomeres with one another and the plasma membrane by forming a three-dimensional scaffold around the Z disks. Mutations of the desmin gene result in the desmin-related myopathies, also known as myofibrillar myopathies, and cardiomyopathies.

Vimentin is an additional intermediate filament that is expressed in immature muscle cells during myogenesis. After the postnatal period, its expression in muscle is primarily in regenerating and immature cells.

Nestin is a protein that is coexpressed with desmin in developing muscle cells. Postnatally, nestin is found with desmin in regenerating muscle fibers in patients with dystrophic and inflammatory myopathies.

Plectin is a large protein of more than 500 kilodaltons that serves as a cytoskeletal linking protein for desmin and keratin organization. The carboxy-terminus binds intermediate filaments, and the amino terminus binds actin. Plectin provides mechanical strength to tolerate the forces of physical stress. Deficiency of plectin has been identified as the cause of recessive epidermolysis bullosa with congenital muscular dystrophy.

Nuclear Membrane Proteins

Emerin, a 254 amino acid protein encoded by a gene on the X chromosome, is a protein associated with the inner nuclear membrane. Emerin is important in the organization of nuclear membrane during cell division. Mutation of the emerin gene causes X-linked Emery-Dreifuss muscular dystrophy.

Lamins are major components of the nuclear lamina, which is the major structural framework of nuclei in eukaryotic cells. In humans, two forms of type A (A and C) and B (B1 and B2) are present. Lamins interact with themselves, lamin-associated proteins, and chromatin and play a role in DNA replication, chromatin organization, spatial arrangement of nuclear pores, nuclear growth, and mechanical stability of the nucleus. Mutations in the lamin A gene result in increased susceptibility to nuclear injury in response to mechanical stress. Mutations in the lamin A/C gene cause autosomal-dominant Emery-Dreifuss muscular dystrophy, Charcot-Marie-Tooth disease type 2, dilated cardiomyopathy with conduction defects, Dunnigan-type familial partial lipodystrophy, mandibuloacral dysplasia type B, Hutchinson-Gilford progeria syndrome, and restrictive dermopathy.

Muscle Fiber Types

Clinical use commonly divides human muscle fibers into types I and II. Type I fibers have slow-twitch characteristics, are resistant to fatigue, and are rich in mitochondria and substrates for aerobic (oxidative) metabolism, imparting a red appearance ("red muscle"). They are slightly smaller than type II fibers and have a less well-developed sarcoplasmic reticulum and T-tubule systems. Type II fibers, grossly pale in appearance, have fast-twitch characteristics, are susceptible to fatigue, and are rich in glycogen and other substrates and enzymes needed for anaerobic (glycolytic) metabolism. Type II fibers can be subdivided into type IIa and IIb fibers. Type IIb fibers are the prototype for the type II fibers, whereas type IIa fibers are intermediate, with both oxidative and glycolytic properties. Type I fibers are generally found in muscles needed for sustained tonic contraction such as the antigravity muscles of the limbs and trunk. Type II fibers are usually found in muscles concerned with rapid, forceful movement such as those found in the extraocular muscles. The division of muscle fibers into three basic types is an oversimplification, as in reality there is a continuum of physiologic properties of skeletal muscle fibers.

All muscle fibers of a motor unit are of a single type. The physiologic, metabolic, and morphologic properties of the muscle fiber depend on innervation from the anterior horn cell. Small α motor neurons innervate type I fibers, and large α motor neurons innervate type II fibers. Given this determination of fiber type by the type of innervating motor neuron, sprouting and reinnervation from adjacent unaffected motor axons after muscle fiber denervation often results in fiber-type switching. The clinical significance of this phenomenon is fiber-type grouping, in which the normal random "mosaic pattern" distribution of muscle fiber types is lost, and abnormal grouping of myofibers is apparent by electromyography and enzyme histochemistry.

GENERAL ANATOMY AND STRUCTURE OF PERIPHERAL NERVES

Although the functional components of peripheral nerves vary greatly (i.e., compound versus pure sensory, motor, autonomic, etc.), the cellular structure of nerves is quite homogeneous. In the motor nervous system, the motor neuron soma lies within the anterior horn of the spinal cord or from motor brainstem nuclei. In sensory nerves, the neuronal cell bodies lie within the dorsal root ganglia. Axons then exit via the cranial nerves or nerve roots and travel along peripheral nerves. The juncture between the central and peripheral nervous system is delineated by the Redlich-Obersteiner zone, the point at which peripheral nerves join with the spinal cord or brainstem. In this zone, differences in myelin staining mark where oligodendrial myelination transitions to the myelin of Schwann cell origin in the peripheral nervous system. Pulsatile vascular compression in this region may be responsible for the clinical manifestations of trigeminal neuralgia and other localized cranial neuralgias.

To the naked eye, peripheral nerves are smooth, firm white plump structures. In the atrophic state, nerves are smaller in diameter and take on a dull gray color. When viewed by routine light microscopy, the cross-sectional organization of peripheral nerve bundles mirrors that seen in skeletal muscle. In the nerve, individual axons lie within the endoneurium, along with endoneurial capillaries, collagen, fibroblasts, and

Schwann cells. The endoneurial compartment is ensheathed by a layer of specialized perineurial cells and their associated basement membranes into rounded nerve bundles. In this region, tight junctions and adherens junctions between adjacent perineurial cells result in a protective microenvironment, the "blood-nerve barrier" (Peltonen et al., 2013). Finally, the entire peripheral nerve is surrounded by a fibroblast and collagen-rich layer, the epineurium. The longitudinal anatomy of peripheral nerves varies by axonal myelination status. The large myelinated axons demonstrate a one-to-one relationship with Schwann cells, so that a single Schwann cell wraps around a segment of the axon, with multiple layers of Schwann cell cytoplasmic membrane forming the myelin sheath. Between each myelinated segment, gaps of unmyelinated axon are present, the nodes of Ranvier. The segment of axon myelinated by a single Schwann cell is termed the myelin internode. Figure 135-9 demonstrates the longitudinal anatomy of a typical myelinated axon. Unmyelinated small caliber axons lie in groups within the processes of Schwann cells, albeit without the previously-described one-to-one relationship and surrounding myelin sheath. The properties of myelinated axons with periodic unmyelinated nodes of Ranvier allow for saltatory nerve conduction, resulting in a dramatic increase in nerve conduction velocity and minimizing the energy required for nodal repolarization. Factors that result in faster conduction velocity include thicker diameter of the myelin sheath, larger axon caliber, and longer internodal length such that the axons with fastest nerve conduction have larger axon caliber, thicker myelin sheaths, and longer myelin internodes. Pathologic processes that diminish any of these characteristics will result in slowed nerve conduction velocity, detectable on clinical nerve conduction velocity studies.

NEURAL CONTROL OF MOVEMENT

Contraction of a muscle fiber is initiated by depolarization of its anterior horn cell, which is the final common pathway for all cortical and spinal influences that affect movement. The axonal processes of these cells innervate varying numbers of muscle fibers (the "motor unit") via a specialized neuromuscular junction. In the normal state, the muscle fibers within the motor unit are scattered randomly within a segment of muscle When the anterior horn cell discharges, all the muscle fibers innervated by that anterior horn cell contract nearly simultaneously, the variability ("jitter") due to factors of transmission at the neuromuscular junction. The finer and more coordinated the movement of a muscle, the fewer the fibers in the motor unit such that extraocular muscles and some hand muscles may have 30 to 50 fibers per motor unit, whereas larger muscles such as paraspinal muscles may have hundreds of fiber per unit. The nervous system regulates the force of muscle contraction by recruiting motor units in an orderly fashion; increasingly larger motor units are recruited for larger amounts of generated force. During the process of recruitment, slower-twitch motor units are recruited first, followed by fast twitch as demands increase. The rate of discharge of motor neurons also influences the amount of force generated.

The neuromuscular junction is a specialized region of the axon terminus and sarcolemma, separated by a synaptic cleft (Fig. 135-10). The area on the muscle is the end plate and is located near the center of the muscle. The synaptic knob is the unmyelinated terminal dilatation of the nerve axon and contains synaptic vesicles of acetylcholine. Depolarization of the nerve terminus opens voltage-gated calcium channels at the synaptic knob, inducing a calcium-mediated exocytosis of acetylcholine-containing vesicles. The Lambert-Eaton myasthenic syndrome results from autoantibodies directed against

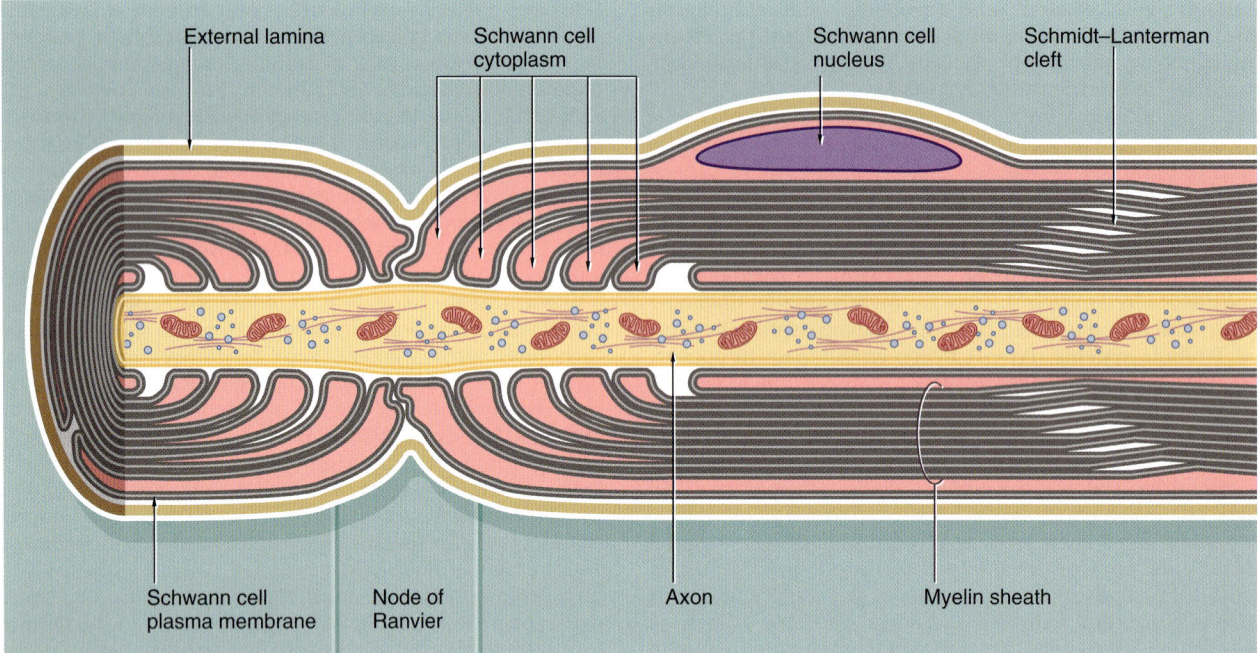

Figure 135-9. Longitudinal anatomy of the myelinated axon. A contiguous axon is surrounded by Schwann cell basal lamina, cell membrane, and cytoplasm; tightly packed concentric layers of Schwan cell membrane comprise the myelin sheath. Pockets of residual Schwann cell cytoplasm are present within the internode, the Schmidt-Lanterman cleft. In the node of Ranvier, the myelin sheath is interrupted, allowing for saltatory nerve conduction.

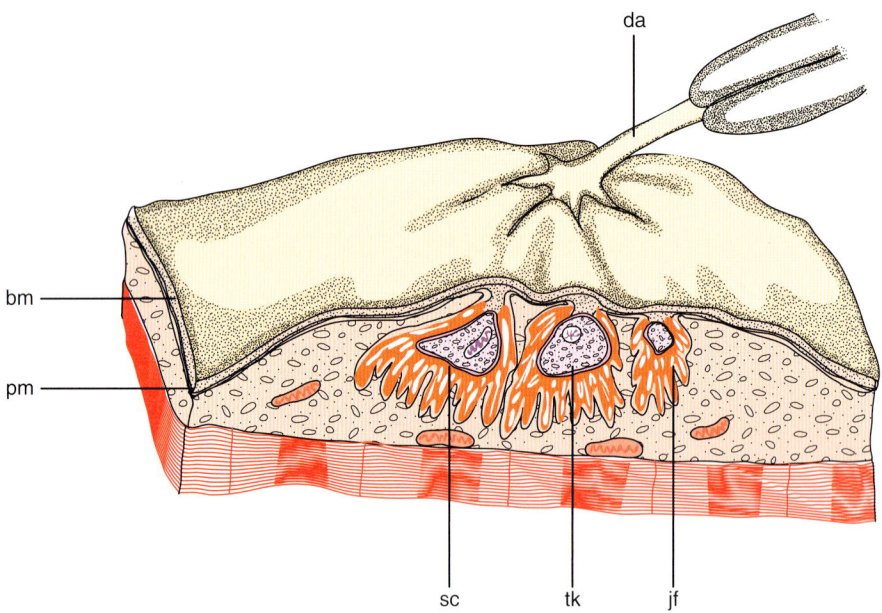

Figure 135-10. Neuromuscular junction. bm, basement membrane; da, distal axon; jf, junctional folds; pm, plasma membrane; sc, synaptic cleft; tk, terminal knob.

these voltage-gated calcium channels (Chapter 145). Acetylcholine is synthesized from acetyl coenzyme A and choline and is stored in a reserve compartment. The process of vesicle formation, fusion, and release is a complex system involving many proteins (Martyn et al., 2009).

Acetylcholine combines with acetylcholine receptors concentrated on the tops of the junctional folds of the postsynaptic membrane of the muscle sarcolemma. The acetylcholine receptor is a transmembrane glycoprotein, composed of four subunits: fetal α, β, δ, and γ; postnatally the γ isoform is replaced by ε. The acetylcholine receptor monomer contains two acetylcholine-binding sites and the cation-specific channel, whose opening is regulated. The acetylcholine receptors are anchored to dystrophin-related protein complexes and connected to the cytoskeleton by dystrophoglycans and sarcoglycan protein complexes. Congenital myasthenic syndromes (CMS) are a heterogeneous group of disorders in which inherited defects in the neuromuscular junction result in pathologic muscle fatigability (Chapter 144). The majority of these syndromes result from postsynaptic defects, most commonly involving abnormalities of the acetylcholine receptor. Myasthenia gravis is caused by antibodies to receptor proteins. Fetal akinesia (Escobar syndrome) can occur from maternal antibodies directed against the fetal γ subunit. Binding of two acetylcholine molecules with the α subunits of the receptor causes a conformational change, opening the center of the receptor for a few milliseconds and increasing the permeability of the sarcolemma to sodium and potassium and localized membrane depolarization. Numerous depolarization events (miniature end-plate potentials) are required to reach the threshold for a propagated sarcolemmal depolarization and resultant myofiber contraction. Interference with the release of acetylcholine or a reduction in the number of receptors lessens the likelihood of successful neuromuscular transmission.

REFERENCES

The complete list of references for this chapter is available in the e-book at www.expertconsult.com.

See inside cover for registration details.

SELECTED REFERENCES

Carpenter, S., Karpati, G., 2001. Pathology of Skeletal Muscle, second ed. Oxford University Press, Oxford.

Dubowitz, V., Sewry, C.A., Oldfors, A., 2013. Muscle Biopsy: A Practical Approach. Elsevier, St. Louis.

Goebel, H.H., Sewry, C.A., Weller, R.O., 2013. Muscle Disease: Pathology and Genetics, second ed. Wiley Blackwell, Chichester.

Lin, W., Burgess, R.W., Dominguez, B., et al., 2001. Distinct roles of nerve and muscle in postsynaptic differentiation of the neuromuscular synapse. Nature 410 (6832), 1057–1064.

Martyn, J.A., Fagerlund, M.J., Eriksson, L.I., 2009. Basic principles of neuromuscular transmission. Anaesthesia 64 (Suppl. 1), 1–9.

Peltonen, S., Alanne, M., Peltonen, J., 2013. Barriers of the peripheral nerve. Tissue Barriers 1 (3), e24956.

Sanes, J.R., Lichtman, J.W., 2001. Induction, assembly, maturation, and maintenance of a postsynaptic apparatus. Nat. Rev. Neurosci. 2 (11), 791–805.

Sharma, K., Izpisúa Belmonte, J.C., 2001. Development of the limb neuromuscular system. Curr. Opin. Cell Biol. 13 (2), 204–210.

Yang, X., Arber, S., William, C., et al., 2001. Patterning of muscle acetylcholine receptor gene expression in the absence of motor innervation. Neuron 30 (2), 399–410.

E-BOOK FIGURES AND TABLES

The following figures and tables are available in the e-book at www.expertconsult.com. See inside cover for registration details.

136 Laboratory Assessment of the Child with Suspected Neuromuscular Disorders

Peter B. Kang and Eugenio Mercuri

INTRODUCTION

Knowledge of pediatric neuromuscular disease through the nineteenth century was largely limited to observations of cohorts of children with similar clinical histories and physical examination findings. The most famous of these observations are the descriptions of the disease that became known as Duchenne muscular dystrophy, with lumbar lordosis, calf pseudohypertrophy, toe-walking, a waddling gait, and the Gowers sign. In retrospect, reports from the first half of the nineteenth century, predating Guillaume-Benjamin-Amand Duchenne's and William Gowers's famous papers, describe the same disease. Duchenne is credited with developing the first muscle biopsy technique in the late nineteenth century; this testing modality has been refined since then, with respect to both acquisition of samples and muscle specimen analysis.

The first half of the twentieth century was marked by the development of clinical electromyography testing, using an oscilloscope, along with nerve conduction studies. Reliable laboratory testing to delineate neuromuscular diseases arose in the mid-twentieth century when the muscle enzymes creatine kinase and aldolase were found to be consistently and dramatically elevated in Duchenne muscular dystrophy.

The cloning of dystrophin as the causative gene for Duchenne muscular dystrophy in 1986 (Monaco et al., 1986) and the identification of the corresponding protein the following year marked the beginning of a revolution in neuromuscular disease and the broader fields of clinical medicine and biomedical science. A steady stream of genetic discoveries for a broad array of inherited neuromuscular diseases followed, transforming the care of diseases such as muscular dystrophy, congenital myopathy, myotonic dystrophy, metabolic myopathies, congenital myasthenic syndrome, Charcot-Marie-Tooth disease, and spinal muscular atrophy. Multiple causative genes have been identified for all of these diseases, revealing an astounding richness in their genetic landscape. In 2001 the full human genome was sequenced for the first time, leading to an explosion of novel approaches to genetic sequencing and upending diagnostic algorithms for pediatric neuromuscular disease. Tests that may be useful for neuromuscular diagnostic evaluations vary significantly depending on the age of the patient (Table 136-1).

LABORATORY CHEMISTRIES AND SEROLOGIES

A routine blood test to screen for muscular dystrophy was not available until the middle of the twentieth century when serum creatine kinase (CK) levels were found to be consistently elevated in patients with clinical diagnoses of muscular dystrophy. Serum aldolase levels were similarly described to be elevated in such individuals and were described first, although CK is more specific for muscle tissue and is currently the most widely used serum biomarker to screen for a variety of neuromuscular diseases (Table 136-2). Serum CK levels may decrease over time in patients with Duchenne muscular dystrophy as muscle tissue is progressively replaced by connective tissue. It is not as well known that three serum transaminases most commonly associated with the liver, alanine aminotransferase (ALT), aspartate aminotransferase (AST), and lactate dehydrogenase (LDH), are also found in smaller amounts in skeletal muscle tissue. In muscle disease, elevations of serum CK and aldolase are typically much more elevated than those of ALT, AST, and LDH. The differences are consistent enough that mathematical formulas have been generated to describe ratios among some of these laboratory values in Duchenne and Becker muscular dystrophy (McMillan, Gregas, Darras, and Kang, 2011). Some patients with muscular dystrophy, especially milder forms such as Becker muscular dystrophy, are initially ascertained by mild elevations of the transaminases, and unfortunately, a small number of these children undergo extensive hepatic evaluations, including liver biopsy, before the possibility of muscular dystrophy is considered. In some cases where transaminases are more dramatically elevated than the serum CK level, the possibility of a glycogenosis should be considered. It is important to remind general pediatricians and pediatric subspecialists, especially pediatric gastroenterologists, of this association to shorten the diagnostic odyssey that some of these children encounter. In juvenile dermatomyositis, the LDH may be elevated when the CK and aldolase are normal.

The interpretation of serum CK levels can be confusing. Elevations in Duchenne muscular dystrophy are not subtle, typically rising above 10,000 U/L (normal values vary by laboratory and are generally less than 240 U/L), and on occasion may exceed 100,000 U/L. As a rule of thumb, CK levels are grossly elevated in muscular dystrophies, whereas congenital myopathies display mild or no elevations. There are exceptions to this rule because serum CK levels may be normal or only mildly elevated in muscle diseases such as facioscapulohumeral muscular dystrophy (FSHD) and certain forms of congenital muscular dystrophy, such as Ullrich congenital muscular dystrophy or SEPN1-related myopathies. Mild elevations of serum CK levels may also be found in nonmuscle diseases, the most prominent example being spinal muscular atrophy, which has been associated with normal levels and elevations as high as 1000 U/L. Mild elevations may also be incidental findings that cannot be tied to objective evidence for a neuromuscular disease.

The diagnostic uncertainty surrounding mild elevations in serum CK levels has implications for newborn screening for neuromuscular disease, an active topic of research, pilot studies, and implementation in some states, including New York and Ohio. Serum CK levels can be checked in dried blood spot samples. Newborn screening now has practical implications for a number of inherited neuromuscular diseases as potential therapeutic compounds are in human clinical trials, and the first new treatment for Duchenne muscular dystrophy was approved by the U.S. Food and

TABLE 136-1 Workup to Be Considered for Suspected Neuromuscular Disease in Various Age Groups

	Neonate	Infant	Child	Adolescent
Systemic evaluation	Sepsis, HIE		Lead	
Basic laboratory	CK, Mg++, thyroid	CK, thyroid, vitamin B$_6$, B$_{12}$, E		
Specialized laboratory	AChR antibodies	Botulinum toxin		
Radiographs	CXR for thin ribs			
Imaging	Muscle U/S (brain MRI)	Muscle U/S, muscle MRI (brain MRI)		
EMG, NCS	+	+	+	+
Edrophonium test	+	+	+	+
Muscle biopsy	+	+	+	+
Genetic testing	Targeted genetic tests and NMD genetic testing panels (targeted genetic tests may include those for Prader-Willi syndrome, myotonic dystrophy, and SMA)	Targeted genetic tests and NMD genetic testing panels		

Neonates are typically defined as those individuals in the first month of life, infants as being those in the first year of life, children as being older than infants but prepubertal, and adolescents as being peri- and postpubertal. Not all tests apply to all circumstances. For example, brain MRI would only be applicable in circumstances, such as suspected cases of certain subtypes of congenital muscular dystrophy.

AChR, acetylcholine receptor; CK, creatine kinase; CXR, chest x-ray; EMG, electromyogram; HIE, hypoxic-ischemic encephalopathy; MRI, magnetic resonance imaging; NMD, neuromuscular disease; SMA, spinal muscular atrophy; U/S, ultrasound.

TABLE 136-2 Serum CK Levels Typically Found in Pediatric Neuromuscular Diseases

Disease	CK level	Limb-girdle muscular dystrophy type 2 (autosomal recessive)	
		LGMD2A (*CAPN3*)	6 to 84x ULN
Spinal muscular atrophy	Normal to 5x ULN, rarely 9x ULN	LGMD2B (*DYSF*)	2 to 150x ULN
		LGMD2C (*SGCG*)	8 to 150x ULN
Charcot-Marie-Tooth disease	Normal	LGMD2D (*SGCA*)	4 to 100x ULN
		LGMD2E (*SGCB*)	3 to 209x ULN
Guillain-Barré syndrome	Normal	LGMD2F (*SGCD*)	5 to 60x ULN
		LGMD2G (*TCAP*)	1.2 to 17.5x ULN
CIDP	Normal	LGMD2H (*TRIM32*)	1.4 to 24.5x ULN
		LGMD2I (*FKRP*)	3 to 60x ULN
Congenital myasthenic syndrome	Normal	LGMD2J (*TTN*)	1.5 to 17x ULN
		LGMD2K (*POMT1*)	20 to 40x ULN
Neonatal myasthenia gravis	Normal	LGMD2L (*ANO5*)	6 to 57x ULN
		LGMD2M (*FKTN*)	6.7 to 343x ULN
Juvenile myasthenia gravis	Normal	LGMD2N (*POMT2*)	8.6 to 22x ULN
		LGMD2O (*POMGNT1*)	28 to 68x ULN
Dystrophinopathy		LGMD2Q (*PLEC*)	19 to 29x ULN
Duchenne muscular dystrophy (DMD)	28 to 350x ULN and above (< 10 years) Normal to 40x ULN (> 10 years)		
		FSHD1	Normal to 3.8x ULN
Becker muscular dystrophy (BMD)	6 to 115x ULN	FSHD2	3 to 4x ULN
Congenital muscular dystrophy		Congenital myopathy	Values typically normal (see following entries)
Collagenopathy			
Ullrich CMD	Normal to 2x ULN	Myotubular myopathy	Normal to 9x ULN
Bethlem myopathy	Normal to 7x ULN	Centronuclear myopathy (*DNM2*)	Normal to moderately elevated
Merosinopathy (*LAMA2* deficiency)	Normal to 125x ULN	Nemaline myopathy	Normal to mildly elevated
Dystroglycanopathy		Central core disease	Normal to 8x ULN
Walker-Warburg syndrome	4 to 260x ULN	Congenital fiber type disproportion	Normal to mildly elevated
Muscle–eye–brain disease	4 to 28x ULN		
Fukuyama CMD	Normal to 15x ULN	Pompe disease	Normal to 15x ULN
Limb-girdle muscular dystrophy type 1 (autosomal dominant)		Myotonic dystrophy type 1 (DM1)	Normal to 4x ULN
LGMD1A (*MYOT*)	1.6 to 9x ULN	Juvenile dermatomyositis	Normal to 100x ULN
LGMD1B (*LMNA*)	Normal to moderately elevated		
LGMD1C (*CAV3*)	4 to 25x ULN	Juvenile polymyositis	Normal to 35x ULN
LGMD1D (*DNAJB6*)	Normal to 10x ULN	Viral myositis	Normal to 59x ULN
LGMD1E (*DES*)	Normal to 2x ULN		
LGMD1F (*TNPO3*)	Normal to 20x ULN		

CIDP, chronic inflammatory demyelinating polyradiculoneuropathy; CMD, congenital muscular dystrophy; FSHD, facioscapulohumeral muscular dystrophy; LGMD, limb-girdle muscular dystrophy; ULN, upper limit of normal.

Drug Administration (FDA) in 2016. The potential false-positive rate and difficulties interpreting mild serum CK levels should be considered as newborn screening programs are rolled out because pediatric neurologists will begin seeing infants with positive screening results. A pilot study of newborn screening in DMD demonstrated high sensitivity and low false-positive rates when the serum CK was over 2000 U/L (Mendell et al., 2012).

Screening serum and urine tests are also available for some metabolic muscle diseases. These include lactate and pyruvate for mitochondrial disease and the serum carnitine panel, serum acylcarnitine panel, and urine acylglycine panel for other metabolic myopathies. The measurement and interpretation of lactate and pyruvate are often difficult. Serum lactate levels may be artifactually elevated if a child is upset during phlebotomy or if a tourniquet is used, and thus mild to moderate elevations do not necessarily indicate the presence of a mitochondrial disorder. Lactate and pyruvate levels measured in cerebrospinal fluid tend to be more reliable but are more invasive to obtain. A third means of quantifying lactate levels is magnetic resonance spectroscopy (MRS), which can detect elevated lactate in selected regions of the brain.

Serum chemistries and serologies may be useful in several acquired neuromuscular disorders, including inflammatory myopathies. If a child is suspected of having dermatomyositis or polymyositis, serum testing for general inflammatory markers and more specific antibody titers may contribute to the diagnostic evaluation. A serum antibody that is specific for dermatomyositis is Jo-1. This topic is discussed in more detail in Chapter 150.

Antibody titers can be very helpful in the diagnostic evaluation of a child with suspected neonatal or juvenile myasthenia gravis (Chiang, Darras, and Kang, 2009). The classic and most commonly elevated antibody titers for myasthenia gravis in both children and adults are the acetylcholine binding, blocking, and modulating antibodies, which are found in about half of children with ocular myasthenia and the majority of children with generalized myasthenia (Liew et al., 2014). Binding antibodies attach to portions of the receptor aside from the acetylcholine binding site, blocking antibodies prevent attachment of acetylcholine to the receptor, and modulating antibodies cross-link acetylcholine receptors with subsequent degradation. Because acetylcholine receptor antibodies were the first to be identified in association with myasthenia and are so commonly found, patients without these laboratory abnormalities are referred to as having "sero-negative" myasthenia gravis. This is to some extent a misnomer because this patient subpopulation is also likely to harbor elevated antibody titers of various types. The most well known of these is the muscle-specific kinase (MuSK) antibody, which is often detected in seronegative adult myasthenia gravis and less frequently in seronegative juvenile myasthenia gravis (Liew et al., 2014). Important therapeutic considerations in MuSK antibody–positive myasthenia gravis are that this subtype of disease tends to be less responsive to cholinesterase inhibitors, which are often first-line therapies for myasthenia gravis, and that the literature regarding the efficacy of thymectomy, although to some extent supportive, is somewhat more conflicted than for acetylcholine receptor antibody–positive cases. A third category of antibody for myasthenia gravis is the antistriated muscle or antititin antibody. In adults, elevations of this antibody are usually seen in conjunction with elevations of acetylcholine receptor antibodies and are associated with a higher incidence of thymoma. In children, elevated antistriated muscle/antititin antibody titers may be found in isolation and do not seem to be associated as consistently with thymoma (Liew et al., 2014). This topic is discussed further in Chapter 145.

With respect to inflammatory neuropathies, serum antiganglioside antibodies are useful for selected subtypes. Anti-GQ1b antibodies may be elevated in the Miller-Fisher variant of Guillain-Barré syndrome, whereas anti-GM1 antibodies are sometimes elevated in chronic inflammatory demyelinating polyradiculoneuropathy (CIDP). However, antibody elevations are less consistently recorded in affected children, especially those with CIDP.

Cerebrospinal fluid analysis is useful in selected situations, most prominently for the evaluation of suspected inflammatory neuropathies such as Guillain-Barré syndrome and chronic inflammatory demyelinating polyradiculoneuropathy (CIDP). The classic finding of cytoalbuminologic dissociation (elevated protein without pleocytosis) supports the diagnosis of an inflammatory neuropathy and is likely caused by the radicular involvement that is often seen in these disorders. However, it is important to remember that cytoalbuminologic dissociation may also be seen in inherited neuropathies, which may be an important consideration for more chronic and indolent presentations.

NERVE CONDUCTION STUDIES AND ELECTROMYOGRAPHY

Peripheral electrodiagnostic testing, consisting of nerve conduction studies and electromyography, was first developed in the 1940s. It continues to be an important test modality for the diagnosis of certain types of peripheral nervous system disorders in the pediatric population (Karakis, Liew, Darras, Jones, and Kang, 2014). Diagnostic categories that may be characterized in this manner include anterior horn cell diseases (spinal muscular atrophy, polio), neuropathies (Charcot-Marie-Tooth disease, inflammatory neuropathies), disorders of the neuromuscular junction (myasthenia gravis, congenital myasthenic syndrome, botulism), and myopathies (congenital myopathies, dystrophies, myotonias and myositis). The one major neuromuscular disease category for which electrodiagnostic testing is typically no longer useful is muscular dystrophy because significantly elevated serum CK levels, especially if associated with abnormal results on muscle ultrasound, will nowadays justify immediate genetic testing. However, electrodiagnostic testing remains useful even in some cases of muscular dystrophy because some subtypes do not yield dramatic elevations of serum CK levels and present differently than other forms. Facioscapulohumeral muscular dystrophy is one example.

Technical considerations abound in the conduct of pediatric nerve conduction studies and electromyography, ranging from potential distress to the patient to electrode placement to differences in normal values. When performed by an electromyographer who is experienced and comfortable with children, these studies are often surprisingly well tolerated by the majority of children without the use of analgesia, conscious sedation, or general anesthesia. Toddlers are typically the most challenging and are more likely than infants or older children to require conscious sedation or general anesthesia. One important practical consideration when general anesthesia is used is that certain drugs, especially propofol, obliterate F-wave responses, and thus these factors should be taken into account when planning and interpreting electrodiagnostic testing in such settings. Electrode placement may be more challenging in infants and younger children because of the smaller extremity sizes. Surface electrodes may need to be trimmed in certain situations, and smaller-sized ring electrodes may be helpful for some sensory studies. Standard distances are impractical for infants and younger children. One specific consideration is that sural sensory responses are typically difficult to record in infants; the medial plantar response is more consistently obtainable in this age group. Normal ranges for latencies, amplitudes, and conduction velocities vary by age. Two general rules are helpful to remember: newborn nerve conduction velocities are typically half the values of those found in older children and adults, and nerve conduction study parameters reach adult values by the age of 3 to 5 years.

The electrodiagnostic approach to disorders of the neuromuscular junction merits particular attention. Repetitive stimulation testing, a variant of a motor nerve conduction study, is as useful in children as in adults, but it is often more difficult for young children to remain still for this delicate test than adults. If there is a high index of suspicion for a disorder of the neuromuscular junction and the child has difficulty with this testing modality, conscious sedation or general anesthesia may be justified depending on what other supportive data are available. Single-fiber electromyography is a specialized form of electromyography that is especially useful in diagnosing disorders of the neuromuscular junction. The core measurement in single-fiber electromyography is the difference in latencies between the potentials generated by two different muscle fibers from the same motor unit. In disorders of the neuromuscular junction, the latencies are more volatile, leading to increased "jitter." Traditional single-fiber electromyography requires that the patient be extremely compliant with the gentle activation of the muscle being tested; ideally, only a single motor unit would be activated at a time. As one can imagine, this degree of subtle motor control cannot realistically be expected of many children. Thus a variant of this test, called stimulated single-fiber electromyography, was developed, and it is especially useful in children (Tidswell and Pitt, 2007; Pitt, 2008). Instead of requiring voluntary motor activation, this variant makes use of a monopolar stimulating electrode to activate individual motor units with small electrical currents. Accurate recordings are possible with ordinary concentric electrodes. In skilled hands, this test has a high degree of accuracy.

MOTOR UNIT NUMBER ESTIMATION

One of the great difficulties in assessing motor neuron disease is the impracticality of sampling motor neurons, either via biopsy or imaging techniques, to measure the progression of these disease processes in clinical and research settings. Functional motor testing is a key component of such assessments, but there is a need for complementary neurophysiological measures. The motor unit number estimate is an approach developed in the 1970s that makes use of a variant of nerve conduction studies to stimulate and estimate the size and number of individual motor units in a given peripheral nerve. The currents used are much lower than in traditional motor nerve conduction studies, and the motor unit amplitudes are measured in µV rather than mV, on the same scale as sensory nerve action potentials. Several specific techniques have been developed to collect relevant data and calculate the motor unit size. Motor unit number estimation was initially applied to the study of amyotrophic lateral sclerosis, polio, and Duchenne muscular dystrophy. In recent years, it has gained increased attention as a potential outcome measure for spinal muscular atrophy in children. Several clinical studies have validated its longitudinal reliability in this setting, and intriguing observations were made in a natural history study that involved this modality. Motor unit number estimation is currently used primarily as a biomarker to track outcomes in longitudinal clinical studies, but it may have future diagnostic applications.

ELECTRICAL IMPEDANCE MYOGRAPHY

Electrical impedance myography is an emerging technique that shows a great deal of promise as a tool to assess the severity of various neuromuscular disorders. It is likely to play a role as an outcome measure for human clinical trials and may eventually have diagnostic applications as well. Its chief virtues are that it is noninvasive and painless, making use of high-frequency, low-intensity electrical currents that are not perceptible by humans; thus, this approach could be especially useful in the pediatric population. As in traditional nerve conduction studies, current is administered, and voltage is measured using surface electrodes. One study demonstrated that electrical impedance myography could distinguish between spinal muscular atrophy types 2 and 3 and between individuals affected and unaffected by spinal muscular atrophy in general, indicating that this tool has a high potential to serve as an outcome measure for spinal muscular atrophy clinical trials. Electrical impedance myography and skeletal muscle ultrasound also appear to be complementary measures that could be used in clinical trial settings.

IMAGING STUDIES

Skeletal muscle imaging via ultrasonography and magnetic resonance imaging (MRI) techniques has become increasingly sophisticated over the years. Both technologies have advantages in various circumstances. Ultrasound technology was first applied to monitoring for cardiac complications in Duchenne muscular dystrophy in the 1970s. The possibility of using sonographic studies of skeletal muscle for primary diagnostic purposes in muscular dystrophy, congenital myopathy, myotonic dystrophy, and spinal muscular atrophy was subsequently examined in the 1980s. Muscle ultrasound was also explored as a means of carrier detection for Duchenne muscular dystrophy and Becker muscular dystrophy. One of the great advantages of muscle ultrasound is that it is a noninvasive technique that can be easily used in infants and children, providing evidence for muscle disease, seen as increased echogenicity with scarce or no visualization of the underlying bone structures. This information can be very useful at the time of deciding on further diagnostic evaluations in children with minimal clinical signs or mildly elevated CK levels without any weakness. The increased echogenicity pattern differs from the one observed in spinal muscular atrophy, which displays a denervation pattern characterized by an increased ratio between subcutaneous tissue and the muscle belly and often a granular pattern in the muscle. As investigators and clinicians gained greater experience with this testing modality, they were able to associate different ultrasound patterns with specific neuromuscular diseases, including congenital muscular dystrophy.

During much of the 1990s, as causative genes for various type of neuromuscular diseases were discovered in rapid succession, skeletal muscle ultrasound was given less attention as a diagnostic modality. However, in the 2000s, it became clear that genetic analysis in isolation would often not be sufficient to clarify the diagnosis for various neuromuscular disorders, especially as genotype–phenotype correlations became more complicated than initially expected. As a result, ultrasonography of skeletal muscles as a diagnostic tool underwent a renaissance, and reference ranges for children were established in greater detail. Currently, skeletal muscle ultrasound is used in a number of centers as a diagnostic tool that helps narrow the differential diagnosis for neuromuscular disorders in children. By examining several muscles, one can assess which are involved and those that are relatively spared. Collectively, this montage can suggest a specific disorder, for example, sparing of the rectus femoris in *RYR1*-related central core myopathy. This technique can be implemented with minimal training. Some studies suggest that skeletal muscle ultrasound may hold promise as a longitudinal outcome measure for human clinical trials.

The potential of applying MRI techniques to the study of skeletal muscle began to be explored in the 1980s, initially for Duchenne muscular dystrophy, followed by other diseases. As in other tissues, this testing modality has the capacity to show even greater morphologic detail than ultrasound in skeletal muscle, allowing for an analysis of the extent and type of involvement of individual muscles. Thus with skeletal muscle MRI studies, detailed portfolios of patterns of muscle involvement may be constructed. A number of disease-specific patterns have been identified in neuromuscular disorders such as myotonic dystrophy, Emery-Dreifuss muscular dystrophy, Ullrich congenital muscular dystrophy, facioscapulohumeral muscular dystrophy, Miyoshi myopathy, and Becker and limb-girdle muscular dystrophies. This has proven to be important to guide genetic testing, especially for muscle disorders with overlapping clinical phenotypes, such as muscular dystrophies with rigidity of the spine (Mercuri et al., 2010) and congenital myopathy subtypes that are associated with mutations in several genes. Short scanner protocols help make this testing modality more accessible to children. MRI findings correlate well with muscle histologic abnormalities. Skeletal muscle MRI is showing increasing promise as a noninvasive outcome measure in clinical trials of new therapies for muscular dystrophy. Longitudinal changes in fat content, for example, are correlated with muscle function changes in boys with DMD.

The use of nerve imaging to aid in the diagnosis of neuropathies has gained more attention recently. Nerve ultrasound data and magnetic resonance neurography can help with the diagnosis of chronic inflammatory demyelinating polyradiculoneuropathy (CIDP) and aid in the detection of nerve entrapment.

Brain imaging does not typically contribute to the diagnostic evaluation of many neuromuscular disorders. The most prominent exceptions to this rule lie among several subtypes of congenital muscular dystrophy. Merosin-deficient congenital muscular dystrophy is classically accompanied by diffuse, symmetric white-matter lesions on MRI. The classic dystroglycanopathies are usually accompanied by striking structural brain abnormalities that overlap among subtypes. These range from isolated cerebellar structural abnormalities that often include hypoplasia or cysts to prominent supratentorial abnormalities that include cortical pachygyria, polymicrogyria, and hypoplasia of the corpus callosum, as observed in Fukuyama congenital muscular dystrophy or muscle–eye–brain disease. One of the most severe cortical malformations, lissencephaly, is a classic finding in Walker-Warburg syndrome.

GENETIC TESTING

The inherited basis of many neuromuscular diseases was strongly suspected for many years, but the tools to investigate such connections did not exist until the late twentieth century. The invention of DNA sequencing in 1970s and the polymerase chain reaction in the 1980s paved the way for the landmark cloning of the dystrophin gene in 1986 and the identification of the dystrophin protein in 1987. Since then, dozens of causative genes for muscular dystrophy and other inherited neuromuscular diseases have been identified. The potential for improved diagnosis is vast, and has been augmented further by the sequencing of the complete human genome at the turn of the millennium and the subsequent development of high-throughput next-generation sequencing technologies. The most widely used next-generation sequencing technique

for clinical applications currently is targeted sequence capture, in which a selection of genes is sequenced based on the putative disease phenotype. Next-generation sequencing can be especially helpful in diagnosing disease categories in which the number of causative genes is especially abundant, such as limb-girdle muscular dystrophy, congenital muscular dystrophy, and congenital myopathy. This technique has also helped with the identification of novel muscle disease genes such as *MEGF10* and its newly identified phenotype, EMARDD, and the identification of novel genotype–phenotype correlations for previously described disease genes. Whole-exome sequencing is offered by some test facilities for clinical use; whole-genome sequencing currently is primarily used in research settings, but it may have greater clinical applicability in the future.

However, the proliferation of causative genes and genetic test modalities has generated increasing confusion among physicians and other health-care providers regarding the best approach to genetic diagnosis in children with neuromuscular diseases. It is important to remember that newer technologies such as next-generation sequencing are currently most accurate with respect to detecting single-nucleotide changes and small insertions and deletions (called "indels") up to about 10 nucleotides in length. Larger mutations may sometimes be detected but not with the consistency that is seen with some of the older genetic technologies. Some of the most common inherited neuromuscular disorders may be missed by next-generation sequencing in its current forms because of the nature of the mutations involved. Examples of such diseases include Charcot-Marie-Tooth disease type 1A (duplication of the *PMP22* gene), Duchenne muscular dystrophy and Becker muscular dystrophy (frequently caused by single- or multiple-exon deletions), facioscapulohumeral muscular dystrophy type 1 (caused in part by contraction of the D4Z4 macrosatellite region on 4q35), and myotonic dystrophy types 1 and 2 (caused by trinucleotide repeat expansions in *DMPK* and quadruplet repeat expansions in *ZNF9*, respectively). All of these neuromuscular diseases are caused by large genetic mutations. Many of the older genetic test modalities will retain pockets of applicability for some time to come.

The delivery and accessibility of genetic testing are also changing rapidly. For example, 23andMe has gained a great deal of attention with its efforts to market its genetic testing products directly to consumers. After extensive discussions and what turned out to be a temporary cease and desist order, the U.S. Food and Drug Administration recently approved the use of 23andMe's product to screen for Bloom syndrome. This is certainly a harbinger of a time to come when many individuals will obtain genetic testing of various types and then come to the physician with a report in hand, requesting an interpretation.

CONCLUSIONS

Major advances in the diagnosis of neuromuscular disease were separated by long intervals in the nineteenth century and the first half of the twentieth century. The pace of discovery has accelerated since then and shows no signs of slowing down. The early years of the 21st century have brought a wealth of diagnostic tools that are being applied to neuromuscular disorders, including increasingly sophisticated genetic testing and noninvasive muscle imaging and electrophysiological techniques. These complement an array of established diagnostic test modalities that still play an important role in the diagnostic evaluation of children with suspected neuromuscular disease. As a result, the test options available have become abundant and sometimes confusing. There is, unfortunately, no single diagnostic test that can provide subtype- and mutation-specific information for all, or even the majority, of such patients. Thus a good history and physical examination remain central to the evaluation of these children, and a basic working knowledge of the information provided by old and new diagnostic tests will be critical to navigating the diagnostic odyssey in the future.

REFERENCES

The complete list of references for this chapter is available online at www.expertconsult.com.

See inside cover for registration details.

SELECTED REFERENCES

Chiang, L.M., Darras, B.T., Kang, P.B., 2009. Juvenile myasthenia gravis. Muscle Nerve 39, 423–431.

Karakis, I., Liew, W., Darras, B.T., et al., 2014. Referral and diagnostic trends in pediatric electromyography in the molecular era. Muscle Nerve 50, 244–249.

Liew, W.K., Powell, C.A., Sloan, S.R., et al., 2014. Comparison of plasmapheresis and intravenous immunoglobulin as maintenance therapies for juvenile myasthenia gravis. JAMA Neurol. 71, 575–580.

McMillan, H.J., Gregas, M., Darras, B.T., et al., 2011. Serum transaminase levels in boys with Duchenne and Becker muscular dystrophy. Pediatrics 127, e132–e136.

Mendell, J.R., Shilling, C., Leslie, N.D., et al., 2012. Evidence-based path to newborn screening for Duchenne muscular dystrophy. Ann. Neurol. 71, 304–313.

Mercuri, E., Clements, E., Offiah, A., et al., 2010. Muscle magnetic resonance imaging involvement in muscular dystrophies with rigidity of the spine. Ann. Neurol. 67, 201–208.

Monaco, A.P., Neve, R.L., Colletti-Feener, C., et al., 1986. Isolation of candidate cDNAs for portions of the Duchenne muscular dystrophy gene. Nature 323, 646–650.

Pitt, M., 2008. Neurophysiological strategies for the diagnosis of disorders of the neuromuscular junction in children. Dev. Med. Child Neurol. 50, 328–333.

Tidswell, T., Pitt, M.C., 2007. A new analytical method to diagnose congenital myasthenia with stimulated single-fiber electromyography. Muscle Nerve 35, 107–110.

E-BOOK FIGURES AND TABLES

The following figures and tables are available in the e-book at www.expertconsult.com. See inside cover for registration details.

Box 136-1. Useful Neuromuscular Websites with Genetic Information

137 Clinical Assessment of Pediatric Neuromuscular Disorders

Richard S. Finkel

 An expanded version of this chapter is available on www.expertconsult.com. See inside cover for registration details.

Pediatric neuromuscular disorders are common and present significant diagnostic and therapeutic challenges for physicians responsible for their care. In addition, the families of affected children are confronted with much uncertainty about their child's condition and how to optimize their child's potential. The combined efforts of multiple specialists are often required to evaluate and manage such children to optimize their potential and quality of life.

This chapter presents an overview of the clinical assessment of the neonate, infant, child, and adolescent with a suspected or known neuromuscular disorder. Other chapters review the general principles of the neurologic examination (Chapters 1 to 5), muscle and nerve development (Chapter 135), laboratory assessment of neuromuscular disorders (Chapter 136), disease-specific information (Chapters 138 to 151), and management of children with neuromuscular disorders (Chapter 153).

DEFINITION, CLASSIFICATION, AND EPIDEMIOLOGY OF PEDIATRIC NEUROMUSCULAR DISORDERS

Definition. Neuromuscular disorders are characterized by the anatomic localization of the pathology within the motor unit, which consists of the motor neuron within the ventral horn of the spinal cord and brainstem motor nuclei, peripheral nerve, neuromuscular junction and muscle. Peripheral neuropathies are further characterized as involving the motor, sensory, and/or autonomic modalities, and by their distribution into focal, multifocal or generalized disorders. Muscle disorders are subdivided into six categories based upon histopathology:

1. Dystrophies (degenerative disorders of the muscle fiber)
2. Congenital myopathies (structural abnormality of the muscle fiber or extracellular collagen matrix)
3. Metabolic disorders affecting muscle (storage diseases, energy processing disorders)
4. Mitochondrial diseases (disordered energy generation or utilization)
5. Inflammatory myopathies (idiopathic)
6. Infectious myositis (bacterial, viral, protozoan)

Myopathies and dystrophies are genetically based disorders that can be further characterized by the subcellular localization of a mutant protein within the contractile apparatus, dystrophin-associated complex in the sarcolemmal membrane, nuclear envelope, or the extracellular matrix. Myotonic disorders are characterized by clinical features and the related abnormal ion channel. Table 137-1 lists the more common pediatric neuromuscular disorders and is organized based upon these anatomic, pathophysiologic, and genetic principles. A more comprehensive compendium, Gene Table of Neuromuscular Disorders, can be accessed online at http://www.musclegenetable.fr.

Epidemiology. The combined prevalence of neuromuscular disorders among children and adults was initially estimated in 1991 at 1 in 3500 individuals and 1 in 3000 in children. See the Table 137-2 for additional information.

The most commonly encountered pediatric neuromuscular disorders, in descending order of prevalence, are Duchenne muscular dystrophy, Charcot-Marie-Tooth disease (i.e., hereditary motor and sensory neuropathies), congenital myopathies, myotonic dystrophy, other myopathies, spinal muscular atrophies, mitochondrial encephalomyopathies, congenital muscular dystrophies, nondystrophic myotonias, unclassifiable disorders, Becker muscular dystrophy, and metabolic myopathies. Remaining disorders all have much lower prevalence.

EVALUATION OF THE CHILD WITH A SUSPECTED NEUROMUSCULAR DISORDER

As clinicians, we endeavor to establish a diagnosis in the neuromuscular patient similar to how we approach other neurologic patients. Sometimes, the diagnosis is obvious and needs only confirmation with a definitive test—for example, the classic infant with spinal muscular atrophy or the boy with Duchenne muscular dystrophy. More often a structured approach is needed to work through the diagnostic process. One such approach is described here and focuses specifically on the more common neuromuscular disorders in the pediatric population.

The clinician needs to address several aspects based upon the history and physical examination findings: presenting symptoms, age at symptom onset, gender, rate of progression, other organ system involvement, and family history. Collectively, these clinical features will enable the clinician to localize the lesion within the neuraxis, develop a differential diagnosis, and strategize a plan for further evaluation. Figure 137-1 presents an algorithmic approach to diagnosing pediatric patients with a suspected neuromuscular disorder. Details on laboratory diagnostic testing can be found in Chapter 136. The www.genetests.org website is a compendium of genetic testing laboratories where testing for specific disorders or gene panels can be obtained.

Localization and Classification

Neuromuscular disorders in each of the four domains of the motor unit can result from genetic or acquired etiologies. The differential diagnosis is often extensive. Having a structured approach sharpens the focus and reduces the diagnostic odyssey for the patient and family.

A fundamental goal of the history and physical examination in the neuromuscular patient is to localize the primary site of dysfunction within the motor unit. Table 137-3 summarizes aspects of the examination that help localize the lesion. This, along with the age of onset, rate of progression, and relevant

TABLE 137-1 Classification of Pediatric Neuromuscular Disorders

This schema is based upon localization within the motor unit with consideration of salient clinical features, electrophysiological findings (for peripheral nerve and neuromuscular junction disorders), muscle biopsy features, and genetic aspects for heritable disorders. The more commonly encountered pediatric disorders are listed here. A full listing of genetic neuromuscular disorders can be accessed on the http://www.musclegenetable.fr. Abbreviations used here are listed at the end of the chapter.

	Disorder	Features	Gene	Protein
Acquired Etiology		**Genetic Etiology**		
Motor Neuron				
Infection:	SMA		*SMN1*	Survival of motor neuron 1
Polio	SMA with respiratory distress (SMARD)		*IGHMBP2*	Immunoglobulin mu binding protein 2
West Nile virus	SMA, X-linked		*UBA1*	Ubiquitin-activating enzyme 1
Enterovirus	SMA, lower extremity predominant		*TRPV4*	Transient receptor potential cation channel, subfamily V, member 4
Peripheral Nerve				
AIDP (Guillain-Barre syndrome)	CMT type 1, AD, demyelinating	6 main types e.g. CMT1A	13 genes e.g. *PMP22*	Peripheral myelin protein 22
CIDP	CMT type 2, AD, axonal	22 subtypes e.g. CMT 2A	22 genes e.g. MFN2	Mitofusin 2
Infection: Tick paralysis Lyme disease	CMT type 4, AR CMT, X-linked	6 types e.g. CMTX1	13 genes *GJB1*	Gap junction protein beta 1
Neuromuscular Junction				
Infantile botulism	CMS, slow channel	4 subtypes 3 subtypes	4 genes 3 genes	
Myasthenia gravis	CMS, fast channel			
Neonatal myasthenia gravis	CMS, acetylcholine receptor deficiency	3 subtypes	3 genes	
	Other specific phenotypes	17 subtypes	*RAPSYN, CHAT, CHRNE, DOK7, COLQ, MUSK, AGRN,* others	
Muscle	**Muscular Dystrophy**	DMD/BMD EDD	*DMD EMD FHL1 LMNA*	Dystrophin Emerin 4 ½ LIM domain 1 lamin A/C
		FSHD LGMDs	*DUX4* 22AR and 8 AD forms	Double homeobox 4
	Congenital Muscular Dystrophy	Merosin deficient Ullrich/Bethlem Rigid spine	*LAMA2 COL6A1, A2* and *A3 SEPN1 ACTA1*	Laminin alpha 2 chain of merosin Collagen type VI A1, A2, A3 Selenoprotein N1 Alpha actin
		Defective glycosylation disorders	18 genes	e.g. FKRP
	Congenital Myopathy	Nemaline Congenital fiber type disproportion	10 genes 5 genes	
		Myotubular Centronuclear Central core	*MTM1* 5 genes RYR1 (also malignant hyperthermia gene)	Myotubularin Ryanodine receptor 1
		Distal Myopathy e.g. Miyoshi	*DYSF*	Dysferlin
	Myotonic Disorders	Myotonic dystrophy type 1	*DMPK*	Myotonic dystrophy protein kinase
		Myotonic dystrophy type 2	*CNBP*	Cellular nucleic acid binding protein
		Myotonia congenita	*CLCN1* (Thompson = AD, Becker = AR)	Chloride channel 1
		Paramyotonia congenita	*SCN4A* (also periodic paralysis)	Sodium channel, voltage-gated, type IV, alpha
		Schwartz-Jampel syndrome	*HSPG2*	Perlecan

Continued on following page

TABLE 137-1 Classification of Pediatric Neuromuscular Disorders *(Continued)*

	Disorder	Features	Gene	Protein
Acquired Etiology			**Genetic Etiology**	
	Metabolic Myopathy	Glycogen storage e.g. GSD type II (Pompe disease)	10 genes *GAA*	Alpha-glucosidase
		Glycolytic pathway e.g. GSD type V (McArdle disease)	4 genes *PYGM*	Muscle phosphorylase
		Lipid metabolism e.g. CPT type 2	12 genes *CPT2*	Carnitine palmitoyl-transferase II
Idiopathic Inflammatory Myopathy				
Dermatomyositis Polymyositis				
Infectious Myositis				
Viral Bacterial Protozoal				

medical and family history, aids in generating a differential diagnosis and plan for further assessment.

Neuromuscular disorders present with distinctive and age-related developmental features. Weakness is the cardinal feature of most neuromuscular disorders but may not be the initial or predominant symptom. Fixed weakness and related impairment need to be distinguished from fluctuating or intermittent weakness. Age at onset varies and may help to limit possible diagnoses.

Acquired disorders generally present with an acute or subacute onset and may progress rapidly, with loss of strength and decline in motor function, although genetically based disorders tend to present with a more indolent onset and subtle influence. Exceptions certainly occur; for example, spinal muscular atrophy (SMA) type 1 can present acutely similar to infantile botulism and chronic inflammatory demyelinating polyneuropathy (CIDP) may present in a chronic manner similar to Charcot-Marie-Tooth (CMT) inherited neuropathies. Motor impairment may be complicated by respiratory, cardiac, musculoskeletal, and nutritional compromise, with resultant morbidity, impaired independent functioning, and effect on survival.

History

The history needs to capture aspects of the patient's onset of symptoms and signs, tempo of progression, effect on motor development, presence or absence of muscle pain or cramps, increased or decreased sensory symptoms, and coordination and balance issues. Related respiratory, cardiac, feeding/growth, and musculoskeletal issues need to be assessed carefully. It is important to inquire about the effect on the patient's independent functioning at home, at school, and in the community. A careful family history should always be explored. The review of systems should search for features of a systemic or genetic disease (Table 137-4 and Box 137-1). Abnormal laboratory chemistry findings (AST and ALT) may incidentally lead to a neuromuscular diagnosis. Measuring the gamma-glutamyl transferase (GGT) helps in eliminating a hepatic component.

Findings in the neonate that indicate prenatal onset include congenital torticollis, scoliosis, or multiple joint contractures. These findings are not specific for a neuromuscular disorder and may be seen in many conditions, including genetic syndromes and skeletal dysplasias. Some neonates

with congenital myopathies may have characteristic facies and ophthalmoplegia.

Signs and symptoms in the infant include hypotonia ("floppy baby"; see Chapter 138), delayed acquisition of motor milestones, dysphagia, failure to thrive, hypoventilation, and cardiomyopathy.

The child with a neuromuscular disorder typically presents with a plateau or slowing of progression in motor development. For example, the boy with Duchenne muscular dystrophy (DMD) may walk at a normal age or be slightly delayed but does not typically come to attention until abnormal running, difficulty climbing stairs, and poor jumping are recognized at age 3 to 4 years. Similarly, the child with SMA type 2 achieves sitting at a normal age and may achieve standing but fails to ambulate independently. An alert parent with CMT may identify the early signs of foot drop or cavus deformity in their similarly affected child.

Initial symptoms in the adolescent often include muscle fatigue and activity-related myalgias rather than weakness or a decline in motor function. Muscle stiffness or cramping should prompt consideration of a myotonic disorder or a metabolic disease. Although aching discomfort is common, frank pain is not typical in most neuromuscular disorders. Exceptions include myotonic dystrophy type 2 and the acute sensory presentation of Guillain-Barre syndrome.

Fluctuating or intermittent weakness is characteristic of disorders of neuromuscular transmission (e.g., myasthenia gravis), the congenital myasthenic syndromes, and different subtypes of periodic paralysis. Patients with primary orthopedic, arthritic, or chronic pain syndromes may present with intermittent deficits in motor function, especially impaired gait.

Examination

The examination can be done in a structured manner to provide maximum information. It includes the following components and is discussed in depth in the online chapter.

Inspection. Assess posture, spontaneous motor activity, respiratory effort, and feeding,

Muscle bulk and quality. Examine for atrophy, hypertrophy, and fasciculation.

Joint mobility and tone. Examine for hypotonia or hypertonia and joint contractures. Joint hyperlaxity can be characterized using the Beighton score (Table 137-5A).

PRESENTATION
Evaluate the history and examination for the following; refer to Table 137-4 and Box 137-1 for additional details

Age of onset: congenital, infancy, childhood, adolescence
Gender: male/female
Clinical symptoms: hypotonia, weakness, motor delay, fasiculations, myotonia, cramping, pain, sensory loss, etc
Rate of progression: acute, subacute, chronic, chronic with acute presentation
Other organ involvement: cardiac, pulmonary, gastrointestinal, hepatic, renal, musculoskeletal, brain
Localization: motor neuron, peripheral nerve, neuromuscular junction, muscle
Personal and family history: Do they suggest a genetic disorder?

ESTABLISH INITIAL DIFFERENTIAL DIAGNOSIS
Genetic or acquired conditions to consider. See glossary for abbreviations

	Motor Neuron	**Peripheral nerve**	**NM junction**	**Muscle**
Congenital	SMA type 0 *In utero toxin, HIE*	CMT variants *In utero toxin*	CMS *Neonatal MG*	Congenital DM1, CM, CMD
Infancy	SMA types 1 and 2 *Enterovirus/polio, WNV*	CMT variants *GBS, toxic, MN*	CMS *Botulism, MG*	CM, DM1, CMD, MM, MiM, DMD, LGMD *EM, IM*
Childhood	SMA type 3 *Enterovirus/polio, WNV*	CMT variants *GBS/CIDP,tick, toxic, IN, MN*	CMS *MG, toxin*	DMD/BMD, CM, LGMD, DM1, CMD, MM, MiM *DM/PM, IM, EM*
Adolescence	Juvenile ALS *Enterovirus/polio, WNV*	CMT variants *GBS/CIDP, tick, toxic, IN, MN*	CMS *MG, toxin*	BMD, LGMD, DM1, DM2, MM, MiM *DM/PM, IM, EM*

PERFORM NON-INVASIVE FIRST-TIER AND, IF NEEDED, INVASIVE SECOND-TIER TESTING TO DETERMINE IF:
1. Neuropathic (motor neuron or peripheral nerve), neuromuscular junction or muscle disorder
2. Genetic or acquired condition

	Motor Neuron and Peripheral Neuropathy	**Neuromuscular Junction**	**Myopathy**
FIRST TIER			
Muscle Enzyme (Creatinine Kinase)	Normal or slightly elevated	Normal	Normal to marked elevation
Other blood tests	*Viral and antiganglioside antibody studies for acquired neuropathy *Heavy metal screen	Acetylcholine receptor antibody titer	Lactate/pyruvate, carnitine, acylcarnitine; K+ for periodic paralysis; aldolase, LDH, ESR and ANA for DM/PM
Muscle imaging	Muscle ultrasound	normal	*Ultrasound for CM and MD *MRI for MD, DM/PM
Brain or other organ imaging	MRI brain for leukodystrophy or mitochondrial features MRI for nerve root enhancement in GBS	Mediastinal MRI or CT for MG associated thymoma	MRI for CMD
SECOND TIER			
Electrophysiology Nerve conduction velocity and electromyography	*NCV: for axonal and demyelinating motor/sensory neuropathy – genetic and acquired *EMG: for motor neuron and axonal motor neuropathy	Repetitive nerve stimulation testing for MG, botulism, or NMJ poisoning	EMG for myopathic features and to exclude a neuropathy
Muscle and Nerve pathology	Nerve biopsy for inflammation or storage, EM for mitochondrial changes	EM of NMJ	Define disease specific myopathology (Chapter 135)
Lumbar Puncture	CSF profile for GBS/CIDP or metabolic neuropathy	N/A	N/A

1. Create 'final' differential diagnosis and if acquired condition complete diagnostic evaluation.
2. If genetic, do disease specific testing, gene panel for neuromuscular disorder subtype or whole genome or exome sequencing (Chapter 136 and elsewhere in this section). The www.genetests.org website provides current information on genetic testing laboratories worldwide that offer this testing.

Figure 137-1. This algorithm presents a suggested pathway for the assessment of the pediatric patient with a suspected neuromuscular disorder. Please refer to Tables 137-1, 137-3, 137-4, Box 137-1 and Figure 137-2 for additional information.

Assessment of muscle strength and weakness. *Weakness* can be identified by formal testing of strength and by indirect assessment of motor impairment on functional testing. *Strength* is a composite of several physiologic elements of motor function: the magnitude, duration, velocity, and torque of muscle contraction.

Peak torque strength is most commonly evaluated using manual muscle testing (MMT). The British Medical Research Council (1941, revised 1943) developed the 0 to 5 "MRC" scale, which has since been expanded into a fuller 10-point version (1976) that is now commonly used by neurologists. Table 137-6 describes the MRC scale and two others in common use. It is generally agreed that grade 5– should not be used; the examiner should make a decision that the muscle is normally strong (5) or mildly weak (4+). Proper position is important for administering MMT correctly by assessing the patient in the following positions:

Sitting: shoulder abduction, elbow flexion and extension, wrist flexion and extension, fingers and thumb, hip flexion, knee extension, ankle dorsiflexion
Supine: neck flexion
Prone: neck extension, hip extension, knee flexion, ankle plantar flexion
Side-lying: hip abduction

The MRC scale focuses upon muscle groups that perform a particular joint motion (e.g., elbow flexion). The MRC scale is nonlinear. For example, on the MRC scale, there is a significant difference in power between a grade 5 (normal; "against strong pressure") and grade 4+ (mildest grade of weakness, "against moderate to strong pressure"); however, little change in power is noted among grades 3 "against gravity," 3+ ("against slight pressure"), and grade 4– ("against slight to moderate pressure.)" None of the MMT methods specify the length of time required to achieve a particular grade. As such, only brief peak torque is typically measured.

Testing in children requires more subjective judgment as to what is normal for age and gender and usually can be assessed reliably by age 5 years. Testing in DMD has been shown to be reliable but more recently has been largely replaced by myometry and motor function testing, particularly in clinical trials. Myometry testing of strength has the benefit of being a linear scale and is typically used in a research setting. The most commonly used method is hand-held dynamometry of isometric strength.

After carefully examining the child for specific areas of weakness, it is important to consider the overall distribution in more general terms of proximal versus distal, and whether there is associated ptosis, ophthalmoparesis, facial, bulbar, neck, or trunk weakness (Fig. 137-2).

Motor function testing. This provides insight into the degree of functional motor impairment in addition to indicating indirectly the extent of weakness and fatigue. These tests need to be developmentally appropriate and should be performed quickly and without requiring special equipment.

(a) *Neonates and infants:* It is important to consider developmental features and distribution of hypotonia and weakness. A healthy premature infant will normally have low tone and limited strength, whereas similar findings in a 6-month-old infant are abnormal. It is useful to use a neonatal scoring scale such as the Hammersmith Infant Neurologic Examination, which can be serially administered.

It is helpful to note the infant's posture and degree of antigravity limb activity and breathing pattern in the supine position and to elicit further activity by stroking the limb or tickling the foot. Next, one should examine for torticollis and

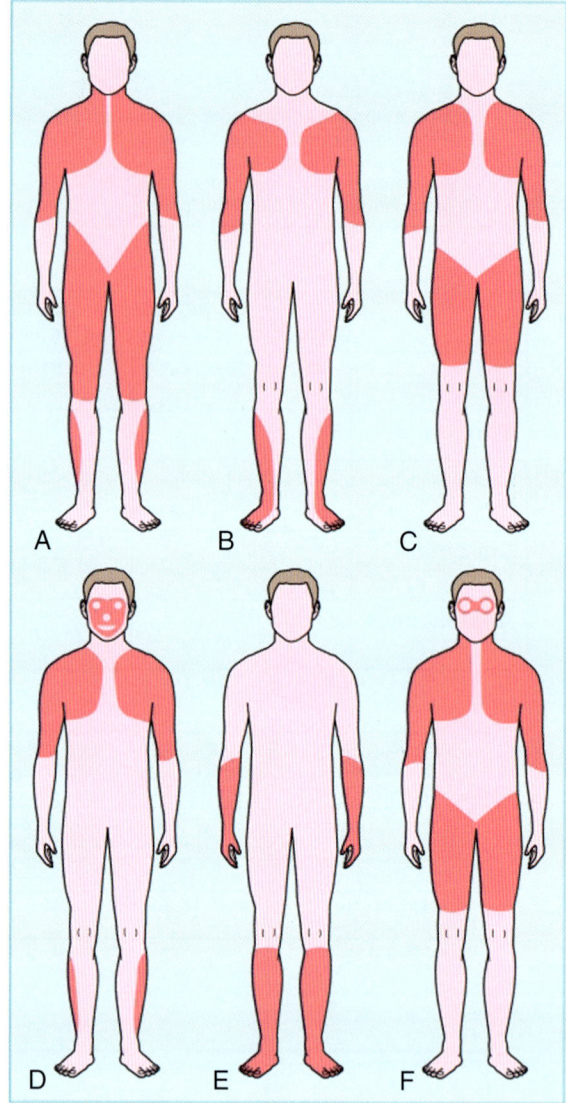

Figure 137-2. Distribution of predominant muscle weakness in different types of muscular dystrophy. **A,** Duchenne and Becker. **B,** Emery-Dreifuss. **C,** Limb-girdle. **D,** Facioscapulohumeral. **E,** Distal. **F,** Oculopharyngeal. Shaded = affected areas. *(With permission from Emery, AEH. Fortnightly review: The muscular dystrophies. BMJ 1998; 317:991–5.)*

limb contractures and palpate the muscles for bulk and consistency. It also is helpful to examine whether the patient is capable of performing the following postural and elicited responses and note if there is related weakness, asymmetry, or fatigue during the maneuver (Table 137-7).

1. Perform the traction test with a slow pull to sit while holding the infant's hands; note neck flexion, shoulder fixation, elbow flexion, and hand grip.
2. Observe for the degree of head and neck control in sitting while supporting the infant at the upper thorax under the arms. The spine can also be examined for excessive kyphosis, scoliosis, or rigidity.
3. Next lift the infant upright and check for "slip-through" at the shoulder girdle.
4. Test for weight-bearing capacity in the lower extremities while the infant is held vertically in one hand by placing the other hand on the plantar surface of the feet and pushing up gently to elicit a hip and knee extension reflex.

5. This is followed by tipping the infant from a vertical to horizontal posture while holding the infant at the thorax and determining whether there is active neck extension. This can also be elicited by the Landau or Galant maneuvers (see online text).

6. In the infant over 9 months of age the parachute reflex should be performed—first to see if the arms extend and the open hands symmetrically extend and "plant" onto the examination table, followed by checking for the ability of the infant to support his/her full upper body weight, then to "wheelbarrow" along the examination table.

A variety of developmental and motor function scales have been used in weak infants and are summarized in the online chapter.

(b) **Child and adolescent**: In the older child and adolescent, clinical symptoms may develop more slowly and findings may be more subtle so a careful and systematic examination can be helpful in detecting motor or sensory abnormalities.

1. **Standing**: Can the child stand securely? Is there a wide-based stance? Encourage the child to squat to pick up a toy and see if she/he can recover upright posture or needs to push off the thigh to do so (Gowers assist). Can a full squat and recovery then be accomplished? Ask the child to stand with feet together and with eyes closed (Romberg test). How well can the child jump?

2. **Gait**: Using the hallway is often useful. The toddler who recently achieved ambulation will walk with a flat-footed stance phase gait but, within a few months, should develop into a more mature heel strike-stance-toe push-off cadence. Watch for toe walking and, if present, examine the Achilles tendons for tightness or knee for hyperextension, crouched gait, hip waddle, exaggerated lumbar lordosis, or if any asymmetries are present. Then encourage walking on toes and heels and running and making a turn. Finally, evaluate a brief jog and then full run.

3. **Supine-to-stand test (Gowers maneuver)**: Have the child lay supine and then ask to him/her to stand up quickly. By age 3 to 4 years, the normal child will do a sit up, push off the floor with one hand, then pop upright quickly. A child with proximal lower extremity weakness will roll over into the prone position, push up onto both hands and knees (quadruped), spread the legs apart, and lift up the buttocks before thrusting the trunk upright to standing posture. With more advanced weakness of the trunk and hip extensors, the child will push off the anterior thigh with one or both hands to achieve an upright position.

4. **Climbing stairs**: Toddlers climb stairs initially marking time (both feet on one step) and use one or both handrails. A normally developing child will climb stairs with a handrail by age 20 months and will alternate feet without a handrail ascending by age 44 months and descending by 68 months.

General Motor Function Scales. In patients with known weakness, upper limb function is often characterized using the Brooke scale and lower limb function with the Vignos scale (Table 137-9).

Many neuromuscular physicians semiquantify how the child runs, arises from supine to stand, and climbs stairs (Table 137-10). This allows for comparison to determine subtle changes and adaptation over time. This can be done informally or in a more structured way that is part of the timed testing (e.g., the North Star Ambulatory Assessment functional scale as described later in this chapter).

Timed testing of motor function is a practical and useful exercise that can be readily incorporated into the routine clinic evaluation of ambulatory children with neuromuscular disorder. The same three tests described previously are commonly employed: 10-meter run/walk, supine-to-stand time (Gowers maneuver), and the four-step climb. When performed serially at each clinic visit, timed tests provide a perspective that complements the patient's, the parents', the physical therapist's, and the physician's bedside assessment of strength. Changes in these timed tests are particularly useful in demonstrating a relative decline in function when no skill has actually been lost, referred to as the "plateau phase." This phase is important to capture in DMD as it is commonly used as the time when initiation of glucocorticosteroid medication should be considered. These timed tests are also predictive of future loss of function. For example, greater than 7 seconds on the supine-to-stand test had an 80% predictive value for loss of ambulation within the next year.

The *6-minute walk test distance (6MWT)* was developed as a test for adults with cardiac and pulmonary disease. The 6MWT segued into the neuromuscular area initially in the study of adults with myotonic dystrophy and with late-onset Pompe disease, based upon the premise that it summates skeletal muscle, cardiac and respiratory aspects of motor disability. A 30-meter difference has been generally accepted to be clinically meaningful and has been used as the basis for determining a therapeutic response to an intervention in ambulant patients with neuromuscular disorders. As such, the 6MWT has been used as a primary outcome measure in several neuromuscular trials.

Additional motor function scales. These scales for older children and adolescents focus largely on lower extremity function (Table 137-11).

Muscle stretch reflexes. These "deep tendon reflexes" (DTRs) can be a challenge to obtain in infants and squirmy children. It is important to have the patient relaxed and to place the joint being testing under slight tension, to load the muscle spindles. This can be difficult in the child with hyperlaxity or who is resisting the examination. Distraction with toys or placing the child on the parent's lap is often useful. It is usually helpful to delay testing reflexes until near the end of the examination, as the child may become upset with the testing and make additional assessment more problematic. Asymmetry in limb tone and reflexes may occur in an infant with an active tonic neck reflex. Thus assessment should be performed with the head midline.

Reduced reflexes are typical of a neuromuscular disorder but are not a necessary finding early in the course of a myopathic or neuropathic disorder. In general, reflexes are reduced or absent in myopathies or dystrophies proportionate to the extent of weakness at that site. For example, the patellar reflex is reduced when there is quadriceps weakness. Similarly, acquired neuropathies such as chronic inflammatory demyelinating polyneuropathy (CIDP) will typically have a reduced Achilles tendon reflex when there is plantar flexion weakness. Generalized reduced or absent reflexes are typical of generalized myopathies/dystrophies or inherited neuropathies. Conditions such as myotonia congenita or periodic disorders without fixed weakness such as hypokalemic periodic paralysis will typically have normal reflexes.

Increased reflexes are usually indicative of an upper motor neuron disorder. One notable exception is acute motor axonal neuropathy (AMAN), a subtype of CIDP, in which lower limb hyperreflexia is often noted. A few beats of ankle clonus is normal in infants; significant asymmetry, however, may prompt a brain or spinal cord imaging study.

Sensory testing. This can be performed in the infant informally by tickle or gentle pinch to the toes. Applying a cool tuning fork to the foot and observing for withdrawal from the stimulus works as well as a pin, and the parents will be less alarmed. More detailed testing is sometimes necessary such as when mapping out any dermatomal loss of sensation in an infant with brachial plexus palsy. The sharp end of a wooden cotton tipped ear swab snapped in half works well. Large fiber modalities are important to check when a peripheral neuropathy is suspected—for example, inherited and inflammatory neuropathies. Joint position and vibration sense involve the same size sensory nerves and share the same central pathway in the dorsal columns. The sensory findings, however, may be divergent in these patients, and both modalities should be evaluated. In the child and adolescent, the Romberg test, standing with feet together and eyes closed, is more reliable, quicker, and more engaging than joint position testing. Semiquantitative testing of vibration sensitivity can be performed using a Rydel tuning fork. When sensory deficits are identified distally, it is then necessary to evaluate the lower extremity more proximally and then to compare to the upper extremity. It also is important to search for asymmetry. In this way a length-dependent neuropathy can be characterized.

Quality of Life and Disability Scales

Patient reported outcome (PRO) and Quality of Life (QOL) instruments serve an important role in identifying the effect of a disease and, potentially, an intervention to treat that disease. Ideally this is from the direct perspective of the patients. For younger children the parents complete a proxy for their child. Age specific questionnaires have been validated and include the PedsQL, a generic QOL scale that has been incorporated into pediatric neuromuscular trials to address aspects particular to children with DMD and SMA.

Abbreviations used in this chapter:
AIDP: Acute inflammatory demyelinating polyneuropathy (Guillain-Barre syndrome)
ALS: Amyotrophic lateral sclerosis
BMD: Becker muscular dystrophy
CIDP: Chronic inflammatory demyelinating polyneuropathy
CM: Congenital myopathy
CMD: Congenital muscular dystrophy
CMT: Charcot-Marie-Tooth inherited neuropathies
CMS: Congenital myasthenic syndrome
DM: Dermatomyositis
DM1: Myotonic dystrophy type 1
DM2: Myotonic dystrophy type 2
DMD: Duchenne muscular dystrophy
EDD: Emery-Dreifuss muscular dystrophy
EM: Endocrine-related myopathy, e.g., thyroid-related
FSHD: Facioscapulohumeral muscular dystrophy
GBS: Guillain-Barre Syndrome
IN: Infection-related neuropathyp e.g., Lyme disease
IM: Infection-related myopathy; e.g., influenza
LGMD: Limb-girdle muscular dystrophy
MiM: Mitochondrial myopathy
MD: Muscular dystrophy
MG: Myasthenia gravis
MM: Metabolic myopathy, e.g. Pompe disease
MN: Metabolic neuropathy, e.g. metachromatic leukodystrophy
PM: Polymyositis
SMA: Spinal muscular atrophy
WNV: West Nile virus

REFERENCES

The complete list of references for this chapter is available in the e-book at www.expertconsult.com.
See inside cover for registration details.

SELECTED REFERENCES

Bushby, K., Finkel, R., Birnkrant, D.J., et al., 2010. Diagnosis and management of Duchenne muscular dystrophy, part 1: diagnosis, and pharmacological and psychosocial management. Lancet Neurol. 9 (1), 77–93.
Bushby, K., Finkel, R., Birnkrant, D.J., et al., 2010. Diagnosis and management of Duchenne muscular dystrophy, part 2: implementation of multidisciplinary care. Lancet Neurol. 9 (2), 177–189.
Darras, B.T., Jones, H.R. Jr., Ryan, M.M., et al., 2015. Neuromuscular Disorders of Infancy, Childhood, and Adolescence: A Clinician's Approach, 2nd ed. Elsevier, London.
Dubowitz, V., 1995. Muscle Disorders in Childhood, 2nd ed. W. B. Saunders, London.
Engel, A.G., Franzini-Armstrong, C., 2004. Myology: Basic and Clinical, 3rd ed. McGraw-Hill, New York.
England, J.D., Asbury, A.K., 2004. Peripheral neuropathy. Lancet 363 (9427), 2151–2161.
McDonald, C.M., Henricson, E.K., Abresch, R.T., et al., 2013. The 6-minute walk test and other clinical endpoints in duchenne muscular dystrophy: reliability, concurrent validity, and minimal clinically important differences from a multicenter study. Muscle Nerve 48 (3), 357–368.
Narayanaswami, P., Weiss, M., Selcen, D., et al., 2014. Evidence-based guideline summary: diagnosis and treatment of limb-girdle and distal dystrophies: report of the guideline development subcommittee of the American Academy of Neurology and the practice issues review panel of the American Association of Neuromuscular and Electrodiagnostic Medicine. Neurology 83 (16), 1453–1463.
Saporta, A.S., Sottile, S.L., Miller, L.J., et al., 2011. Charcot-Marie-Tooth disease subtypes and genetic testing strategies. Ann. Neurol. 69 (1), 22–33.
Wang, C.H., Finkel, R.S., Bertini, E.S., et al., 2007. Consensus statement for standard of care in spinal muscular atrophy. J. Child Neurol. 22 (8), 1027–1049.

E-BOOK BOX AND TABLES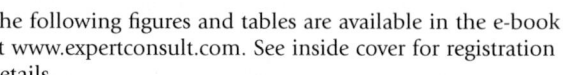

138 The Floppy Infant

Graeme A.M. Nimmo and Ronald D. Cohn

An expanded version of this chapter is available on www.expertconsult.com. See inside cover for registration details.

DEFINING HYPOTONIA

"The floppy infant" is an informal term for generalized hypotonia and is a presenting feature for a wide range of both systemic and neurologic disease. The pediatric neurologist is regularly requested to evaluate an infant with hypotonia, and it poses a particular diagnostic challenge owing to the extensive differential diagnosis. The list of disorders with presenting features, including hypotonia, has expanded rapidly in the genomic era and continues to grow. Although at present most of the conditions have few disease modifying treatments, diagnosis is essential as it provides both families and physicians with prognostic information and screening strategies for associated pathologies. It may also expose certain risks associated with known diagnosis; for example, individuals with RYR1 mutations may be at increased risk for malignant hyperthermia (Brislin and Therous, 2013). Furthermore, many of the diagnoses are genetic and have implications for living family members or future family planning.

Severe hypotonia usually presents in the neonatal period, but milder or slowly progressive pathologies may not come to a physician's attention until the child fails to attain milestones in the latter part of the first or second years. In the neonatal period, the differential diagnosis must include hypoxic-ischemic injury, intraventricular hemorrhage, and systemic disease such as hypoglycemia, sepsis, and heart failure; these diagnoses are not discussed here. For the most part, the remaining conditions presenting in this period have an underlying genetic origin, but acquired causes that present in this age group are also discussed. Chapter 137 provides an approach to the older child with suspected neuromuscular disease.

Muscle Tone

Muscle tone is defined as a skeletal muscle's inherent resistance to passive movement. It is particularly important to differentiate this from muscle strength, which is a muscle's maximum voluntary resistance to movement. Tone is controlled by the peripheral fusimotor system with input from the central nervous system (CNS). The afferent fibers detect muscle spindle stretch and subsequently direct the motor unit system to cause muscle contraction; this is reviewed in detail in Chapter 5. Failure of any component of the motor unit, from the anterior horn cell, motor neuron, neuromuscular junction, or the muscle itself, will result in hypotonia. Supraspinal input from the motor cortex, basal ganglia, striatum, red nucleus, and cerebellum is predominantly inhibitory in its interaction with fusimotor system. In older children and adults, disturbance of inhibitory pathways results in increased excitatory output with hypertonia and hyperreflexia. In contrast, disturbance to these pathways in infancy often presents with decreased muscle tone; but importantly, the reflex arc is the preserved. Hypotonia in infancy, therefore, may be caused by disorders affecting any level of the nervous system.

Some diagnoses may be established directly from history and examination, and confirmation with further testing, often in the form of genetic testing, can be carried out immediately. On the other hand, many of the neuromuscular diagnoses may be more difficult to distinguish based on the initial clinical evaluation alone and require preliminary investigations to better characterize the disease and define a group of diagnoses. The first step in the determination of the cause of hypotonia is to localize the pathology.

LOCALIZATION OF HYPOTONIA

As with other types of neurologic presentation, the first step in the approach to diagnosis is to localize the clinical findings to the site of pathology. Conditions that affect the central nervous system, and therefore supraspinal pathways, cause a clinical picture referred to as central hypotonia. The term peripheral hypotonia is used to describe the clinical features of an infant that presents with pathology affecting the motor neuron unit. The key differentiating feature is the presence or absence of weakness (Dubowitz, 1980).

Infants with a central cause for their hypotonia may present with other findings suggesting disorders involving the CNS: dysmorphic features, decreased level of consciousness, seizures, and may have evidence of brisk reflexes and clonus (Table 138-1). In an older child, there may be a history of developmental delay affecting both cognitive and motor domains.

Infants with peripheral hypotonia, in contrast, have a paucity of antigravity movements and may have myopathic facies but are generally alert and reach cognitive milestones appropriately. Fasciculations, muscle atrophy, and diminished reflexes are characteristic of this group. There are some exceptions in these divisions. Infants with myotonic dystrophy and congenital myopathies often do not have profound weakness. Many of the findings thought to be present in central hypotonia such as seizures and dysmorphic features are found in considerable proportions in both divisions. Nevertheless, the constellation of findings generally allows correct classification an estimated 80% of the time. It is also useful to think of a third group of pathologies that have both central and peripheral features and are referred to here as combined hypotonia. A practical algorithm guiding the approach to a neonate or infant with hypotonia is shown in Figure 138-1.

HISTORY

Key components of the clinical examination confirm the presence of hypotonia, localizes its origins, and narrows the differential diagnosis. A careful and complete history is essential.

The pregnancy history should include corrected gestational age as infants may present with hypotonia secondary to premature gestational age alone. A history of maternal illnesses (particularly myasthenia gravis) and exposure to medications, drugs, and infection should be sought. Results of antenatal ultrasounds, specifically polyhydramnios and paucity of fetal movements, are characteristically seen in peripheral

TABLE 138-1 Features Differentiating Central and Peripheral Hypotonia

Central	Peripheral
Developmental delay	Weakness with paucity of spontaneous movement
Normal CK[a]	Raised (or normal) CK
Decreased LOC	Alert
Increased DTRs, clonus	Decreased DTRs[c]
Seizures[b]	Muscle fasiculations
Dysmorphic facial features	Myopathic facies[d]
Microcephaly	Ophthalmaplegia Ptosis Bulbar dysfunction
Apneas, irregular respiration	Prolonged breathing difficulties, ventilator dependence
High pitched/unusual cry	Fatigable or weak cry
Multiple congenital abnormalities	History of polyhydramnios

[a]CK may be normally raised in the early neonatal period. [b]Seizures are common in patients with LAMA2-related congenital muscular dystrophy. [c]DTRs may be normal in patients with disorders affecting the neuromuscular junction. [d]Tented upper lip, dolichocephaly, long face, and high arched palate. CK, creatinine kinase; DTRs, deep tendon reflexes.

hypotonia, whereas evidence of congenital malformations may be more in line with a multisystem syndrome and a cause of central hypotonia.

Delivery history may uncover risk factors for hypoxic-ischemic injury (HIE), including maternal hypotension, breech extraction, cord prolapse, or placental abruption. HIE must be excluded as it is the most common cause for central hypotonia. Apgar scores and details surrounding resuscitation, if required, may be useful in order to further exclude birth asphyxia. Infants with HIE often present with an altered level of consciousness that gradually improves in the neonatal period. It is also not uncommon for the tone to improve over the first several months of life with evolution to hypertonia and spasticity within the first 2 to 3 months of life. Asphyxia has been observed in peripheral disorders. Details of resuscitation may be required to differentiate between these infants and those with severe diaphragmatic or bulbar muscle weakness of neuromuscular origin that may require early respiratory support.

Onset and progression of the hypotonia should be elucidated. Central hypotonia tends to improve with time, whereas peripheral hypotonia remains stable or progresses gradually. Rapid progression after an uncomplicated pregnancy, delivery, and neonatal course suggests an inborn error of metabolism. Infantile botulism may also present with progressive weakness and history of constipation, after an otherwise unremarkable neonatal course. It is important to exclude the consumption of honey or corn syrup if this diagnosis is suspected. Fluctuation in symptoms may be seen with congenital myasthenia syndromes or in LAMA2-related muscular dystrophy. Many infants with hypotonia will require respiratory support owing to the more complicated delivery, presence of apneas, bulbar dysfunction, or respiratory muscle weakness. However, prolonged intubation, defined by a length greater than 5 days, is more commonly seen in infants with peripheral causes. A feeding history may also be reveal bulbar dysfunction, resulting in choking or aspiration often seen—although not

exclusively—with peripheral hypotonia. Fatigue with feeding may be observed with myasthenic syndromes. Seizures have been traditionally associated with central causes, although have been reported in peripheral disorders particularly in LAMA2-related muscular dystrophies.

Developmental history should be obtained if the infant is of an appropriate age. Motor delay will often result secondary to the hypotonia, but cognitive delay is more common with central causes and myotonic dystrophy.

A detailed family history is essential. Certain conditions are more common in particular ethnicities; Ashkenazi Jews have a high carrier rate for familial dysautonomia and Canavan disease. The presence of consanguinity increases the likelihood of any recessive disease and is commonly reported with inborn errors of metabolism. Familial or maternal history of recurrent miscarriages points to a multisystem, and perhaps syndromic, disorder. Positive family history and details of known skeletal muscle disease, congenital abnormalities, developmental delay, and intellectual disability may also narrow the differential considerably. History of malignant hyperthermia may suggest a congenital myopathy. Maternal features of myotonic dystrophy should also be elicited, as these stable symptoms commonly go unrecognized: distal muscle weakness, intellectual disability, insulin resistance, cataracts, cardiomyopathy, and arrhythmias (Thornton, 2014). If a diagnosis of mitochondrial disease is being considered a positive history of less severe manifestations of exercise intolerance, migraine headache, diabetes mellitus, retinitis pigmentosum, and sensorineural hearing loss may be elicited, and may demonstrate a maternal inheritance pattern (DiMauro, 2013).

EXAMINATION

Identifying an infant as hypotonic is typically difficult for an inexperienced examiner, and a number of unaffected infant examinations may need to be performed before more subtle decrease in tone can be appreciated. Reliable determination of hypotonia, particularly in the NICU setting, is often complicated because tone may be influenced by systemic illness, medication, level of alertness, and gestational age. The examiner will often need to perform serial examinations or defer an examination to a time when the infant is not acutely unwell.

The assumption of unusual postures by the hypotonic infant is often the first indication of decreased tone. Instead of the contracted posture of a healthy term infant, infants with hypotonia typically have flaccid extension of the arms and abduction of the legs of described as "frog-leg." There are several maneuvers that are particularity useful for assessing tone in infants:

1. The **pull-to-sit** (or traction) test may be used to assess both axial tone and upper limb weakness. The supine infant is pulled by the hands to the sitting position with the examiner observing for head lag. Term neonates, until about 2 months, should have only mild head-lag. Infants usually resist this movement with flexion at the shoulder and elbow; this also gives the examiner an opportunity to assess strength in the upper limb.
2. The **scarf-sign** provides a measure of appendicular tone in the upper limb. To elicit this sign the supine infant's hand is pulled toward the opposite shoulder and around the neck. The sign is positive for hypotonia if the elbow can be pulled across the midline.
3. Measurement of the **popliteal angle** is a more objective way to measure tone in the lower limb. In the supine position, the infant's hip is flexed to the torso and the knee

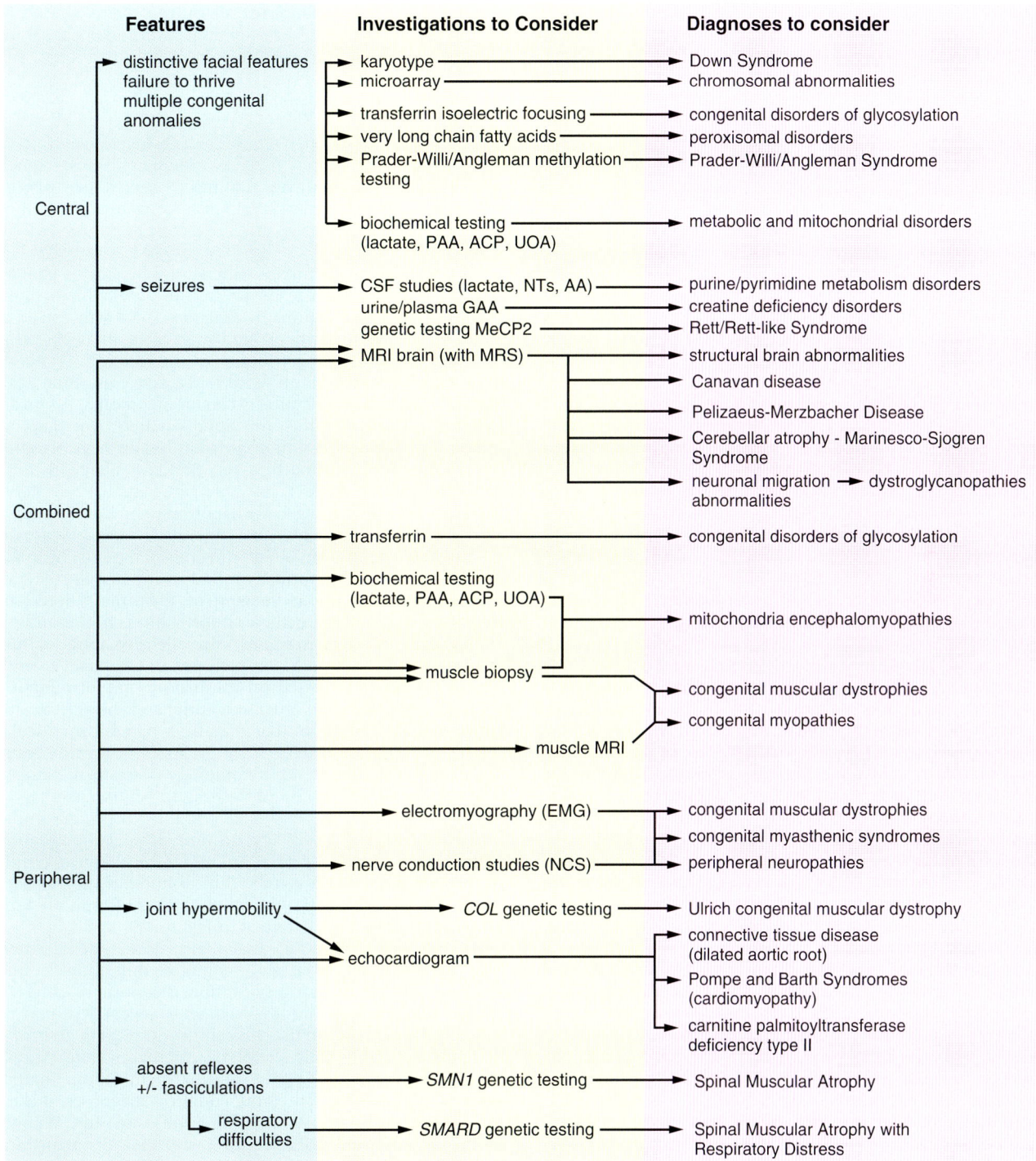

Features

Investigations to Consider

Diagnoses to consider

Central

distinctive facial features
failure to thrive
multiple congenital
anomalies

karyotype ——————————→ Down Syndrome
microarray ——————————→ chromosomal abnormalities

transferrin isoelectric focusing ———→ congenital disorders of glycosylation
very long chain fatty acids ————→ peroxisomal disorders
Prader-Willi/Angleman methylation —→ Prader-Willi/Angleman Syndrome
testing

biochemical testing ——————————→ metabolic and mitochondrial disorders
(lactate, PAA, ACP, UOA)

seizures ——————————→ CSF studies (lactate, NTs, AA) ———→ purine/pyrimidine metabolism disorders
urine/plasma GAA ————————→ creatine deficiency disorders
genetic testing MeCP2 ————————→ Rett/Rett-like Syndrome

Combined

MRI brain (with MRS) ——————→ structural brain abnormalities
                            ——→ Canavan disease
                            ——→ Pelizaeus-Merzbacher Disease
                            ——→ Cerebellar atrophy - Marinesco-Sjogren
                                Syndrome
                            ——→ neuronal migration → dystroglycanopathies
                                abnormalities

transferrin ——————————→ congenital disorders of glycosylation

biochemical testing
(lactate, PAA, ACP, UOA)
                            ——→ mitochondria encephalomyopathies

muscle biopsy ——————————→ congenital muscular dystrophies
                            ——→ congenital myopathies
muscle MRI

Peripheral

electromyography (EMG) ————→ congenital muscular dystrophies
                            ——→ congenital myasthenic syndromes
nerve conduction studies (NCS) ——→ peripheral neuropathies

joint hypermobility ——————→ *COL* genetic testing ————→ Ulrich congenital muscular dystrophy

echocardiogram ——————————→ connective tissue disease
                                (dilated aortic root)
                            ——→ Pompe and Barth Syndromes
                                (cardiomyopathy)
                            ——→ carnitine palmitoyltransferase
                                deficiency type II

absent reflexes
+/- fasciculations ——————→ *SMN1* genetic testing ————→ Spinal Muscular Atrophy

respiratory
difficulties ——————————→ *SMARD* genetic testing ————→ Spinal Muscular Atrophy with
                                                            Respiratory Distress

Legend:
PAA, plasma amino acids
ACP, acylcarnitine profile
UOA, urine organic acids
NTs, neurotransmitters
AA, amino acids

Figure 138-1. Hypotonia algorithm *(Adapted from Lisi, E.C., Cohn, R.D.,2011. Genetic evaluation of the pediatric patient with hypotonia: perspective from a hypotonia specialty clinic and review of the literature. Dev Med Child Neurol 53(7), 586–599.)*

extended as far as possible. The angle between the thigh and the leg is the popliteal angle and should be less than 90 degrees in the term infant.

4. **Shoulder suspension** or vertical suspension test in which the infant is held under the shoulders in the vertical position assesses appendicular tone. A term neonate resists falling through the hands of the examiner.

5. For the **ventral suspension** test, the examiner holds the infant by the torso in a supine position. An infant with adequate tone is able to maintain both upper and lower limbs in flexed posture and, at least transiently, be able to hold their head higher than the horizontal.

The examiner should also get a subjective appreciation of appendicular tone as described in Chapter 5. Axial hypotonia with the relative preservation of peripheral tone should prompt consideration of metabolic disease. This particular pattern is also seen in the LMNA1 congenital muscular dystrophy and SPEN1-congenital myopathy (Bonnemann et al., 2014; North et al., 2014). The most common causes of severe hypotonia are Down syndrome, Prader-Willi syndrome, and centronuclear congenital myopathies.

Once the determination of hypotonia is confirmed, most of the useful information for this age group can be gathered by observation alone. Severe weakness that impairs an infant's spontaneous antigravity movement and appropriate withdrawal response is most likely secondary to a peripheral pathology. The presence or absence of weakness is the most reliable distinguishing feature between central and peripheral causes.

Particular attention should be placed on examining the infant's facial features. Distinctive features may point toward a specific syndromic diagnosis such as Down syndrome, Prader-Willi syndrome, Williams syndrome, or DiGeorge syndrome. Myopathic facies with marked facial weakness, open mouth, tended upper lip with additional dysmorphic features of dolichocephaly, long faces, and high arched palate suggest a severe form of congenital myopathy, myotonic dystrophy, or congenital myasthenic syndrome. Findings of ptosis and ophthalmoplegia should be noted as they are commonly seen in patients with congenital myopathies and congenital myasthenic syndromes. Isolated ophthalmoplegia is rare in neonates but may be associated with disorders of the mitochondrial respiratory chain.

Diaphragmatic breathing is common in the neonatal period; however, respiratory distress with in-drawing of the sternum may indicate intercostal muscle weakness of neuromuscular origin. Weak cry is also a consequence of respiratory muscle weakness, although high pitched or unusual cries are more in keeping with central etiologies. A fatigable cry is associated with myasthenia.

Joint contractures may also be observed in the context of weakness secondary to prolonged periods of decreased movement. Arthrogryposis may be present after fetal akinesia and are most commonly associated with congenital myopathies, congenital myasthenia, and spinal muscular atrophy (Wang et al., 2007). More localized contractures, including talipes equinovarus, may present with any of lower motor neuron etiologies but tend to be proximal in Collagen-VI-related congenital muscular dystrophy and distal in LAMA2-related congenital myopathy.

Reflexes are often unreliable in the newborn period, as they are often brisk or may be normally absent. In older infants, reflexes may be brisk in upper motor neuron lesions and absent or reduced in lower motor neuron lesions. Clonus, if present, may indicate an upper motor neuron lesion, but it must be kept in mind that up to six beats of clonus may be normal in neonates.

Finally, full examination of all other systems should be performed in order to identify any additional congenital abnormalities that may indicate a syndromic diagnosis.

CENTRAL HYPOTONIA

Hypotonia in the absence of weakness is suggestive of disorders affecting the central nervous system. This suspicion is often further supported with findings of altered level of consciousness, dysmorphic features, major congenital anomalies, and/or the presence of seizures. The creatine kinase (CK) is normal.

The approach to an infant with central hypotonia should, as in all areas of medicine, be directed at identifying the most life-threatening and actionable diagnoses first with consideration of the most common etiologies next. It is therefore imperative that the general health of the infant be a part of the initial assessment. Both sepsis and severe congenital heart disease can cause a picture of central hypotonia. Hypoxic-ischemic injury accounts for approximately one-third of infants with hypotonia. Intraventricular hemorrhage accounts for a significant proportion of preterm neonates with hypotonia.

All infants presenting with hypotonia should have a CK level measured. Creatine kinase is not raised with CNS disease, but care must be taken in interpreting this in the early neonatal period as CK may be normally raised in the first few days of life. Magnetic resonance imaging of the brain should be obtained to identify structural abnormalities. Importantly, a cranial ultrasound or MRI may also identify abnormalities characteristic of HIE or IVH as reviewed in Chapter 19. Additional investigations based on the history and examination should be considered in order to identify and characterize any congenital abnormalities that may be a part of a particular syndrome. Further testing may include echocardiogram, abdominal ultrasound, ophthalmology assessment, and/or hearing testing. Biochemical testing for inborn errors of metabolism should be considered and include plasma amino acids, urine organic acids, acylcarnitine profile, glycosylation patterns, and lactate/pyruvate. Additional biochemical testing may be warranted with specific clinical findings suggestive of peroxisomal disorders, Smith-Lemli-Opitz syndrome, or in the presence of seizures as outlined in Figure 138-1.

The findings of multiple congenital abnormalities, dysmorphic facial features, or delay in cognitive milestones should prompt consideration of a syndromic diagnosis or chromosomal abnormalities, and involvement of a geneticist may be valuable. Depending on the clinical context, genetic tests may be indicated and include karyotype, microarray, fluorescence in situ hybridization (FISH), and/or methylation analysis (Watson et al., 2014). The more common diagnoses, including Down syndrome, Prader-Willi syndrome, and William syndrome, are listed in Table 138-2 with their distinguishing features.

PERIPHERAL HYPOTONIA

Hypotonia with weakness suggests a disorder affecting the lower motor neuron. These infants are generally alert, and there are no signs of CNS involvement, although motor development may be delayed in older infants. Creatine kinase may or may not be raised.

Peripheral hypotonia is less common than that of central origin, accounting for approximately 20% of diagnosis in infants with hypotonia in the NICU. The most common causes are spinal muscular atrophy, myotonic dystrophy, and the congenital myopathies. Table 138-3 lists the most common disorders causing peripheral hypotonia and the associated

TABLE 138-2 Distinguishing Features of Common Causes of Central Hypotonia

Diagnosis	Features Suggestive of Diagnosis
Chromosomal abnormalities	Dysmorphic facial features, multiple congenital abnormalities, microcephaly, macrocephaly, failure to thrive, delay in cognitive milestones, advanced maternal age, history of recurrent miscarriages, abnormal aneuploidy screening
Down syndrome	Flat facial profile, up slanting palpebral fissures, epicanthal folds, anomalous ears, transverse palmar crease, and fifth finger clinodactyly, endocardial cushion defects, duodenal atresia
Prader-Willi syndrome	Global developmental delay, distinctive facial features (bitemporal narrowing, almond shaped eyes, strabismus, thin upper lip, downturned upper lip), short stature, genital hypoplasia, failure to thrive in infancy with hyperphagia after 1 year if age
Angelman syndrome	Global developmental delay, acquired microcephaly, seizures, prognathism, skin hypopigmentation
MeCP2-Spectrum disorders	Acquired microcephaly, seizures, repetitive hand movements, regression, female predominant
Williams syndrome	Distinctive facial features (periorbital fullness, hypertelorism, long philtrum, wide mouth, think vermilion boarder, micrognathia), supravalvular aortic stenosis, hypercalcemia
Peroxisomal disorders	Liver dysfunction, seizures, cataracts, retinal dystrophy, hearing loss, chondrodysplasia punctata, large anterior fontanelle, flat facial profile
Smith-Lemli-Opitz	Growth delay, global developmental delay, Y-shaped 2–3 toe syndactyly, cleft palate, cataracts, cardiac abnormalities, downs plating palpebral fissures, prominent epicanthal folds, anteverted nares
Creatine Deficiency disorders	Global developmental delay, seizures, delayed myelination

TABLE 138-3 Distinguishing Features for Common Causes of Peripheral Hypotonia

Diagnosis	Features Suggestive of Diagnosis
Spinal muscular atrophy	Predominantly proximal weakness with relative preservation of facial movements, contractures, absent deep tendon reflexes, tongue fasciculations. SMARD presents with diaphragmatic and intercostal muscle weakness
Congenital Myotonic dystrophy	Facial diplegia with inverted-V shaped upper lip, weak cry, poor suck, maternal history of weakness, cataracts, type 2 diabetes, and contraction myotonia
Congenital muscular dystrophies	
LAMA2-CMD	Kyphoscoliosis, joint contractures, increased signal intensity of white matter with MRI
Collagen VI-deficient CMD (Ullrich CMD)	Distal hypermobility, proximal contractures, scoliosis
Dystroglycanopathies	Combined hypotonia, cobblestone lissencephaly, neuronal migration abnormalities, various ocular abnormalities
SEPN1-related CMD	Axial hypotonia, progressive spinal rigidity, and scoliosis
LMNA-related CMD	Weakness and contractures afecting the proximal upper limb and distal lower limb, cardiomyopathy
Congenital myopathies	Facial weakness with myopathic facies (ptosis, tented upper lip), dolichocephaly, long face, high arched palate, absent DTRs, family history of malignant hyperthermia, cardiomyopathy, orthopedic complications
Centronuclear myopathy	X-linked, severe weakness (no spontaneous movement, respiratory insufficiency), joint contractures, macrocephaly, arachnodactyly, cryptorchidism
Congenital myasthenic syndromes	Weak cry, poor suck, ptosis, facial weakness, occasional arthrogryposis, fatigable weakness, exclude maternal history of myasthenia gravis
Carnitine palmitoyltransferase deficiency type II	Liver failure, cardiomyopathy, neuronal migration abnormalities, hypoketotic hypoglycemia
Pompe disease	Severe hypotonia, hypertrophic cardiomyopathy, hepatomegaly, shortened P-R interval on ECG
Barth syndrome	Cardiomyopathy, neutropenia, growth delay
Polyneuropathies	Distal weakness, sensory loss, decreased DTRs
Guillain-Barré syndrome	Progressive weakness after antecedent illness, DTRs reduced, elevated CSF protein, nerve root enhancement on MRI

Continued on following page

TABLE 138-3 Distinguishing Features for Common Causes of Peripheral Hypotonia *(Continued)*

Hereditary motor and sensory neuropathies/ Charcot-Marie-Tooth disease spectrum	Wide range of presentation. Severe: arthrogryposis, respiratory distress, swallowing difficulties. slow nerve conduction velocities
Familial dysautonomia	Distinguishing features present later, high carrier frequency in Ashkenazi and Eastern European Jewish population
Infantile neuroaxonal dystrophy	Axial hypotonia, developmental regression, seizures, nystagmus, optic atrophy
Infant botulism	Hyporeflexia, constipation, respiratory distress, eye movement abnormalities, history of pica or honey
Connective tissue disorders	Mild hypotonia, hypermobility, aortic root dilitation
Marfan syndrome	scoliosis, pectus deformity, arachnodactyly, dolichostenomelia
Loeys-Dietz syndrome	Craniosynostosis, hypertelorism, cleft palate or bifid uvula, tortuous blood vessels
Congenital disorders of glycosylation	Central hypotonia and weakness, global developmental delay, dysmorphic features, inverted nipples, abnormal fat distribution
Canavan disease	Global developmental delay, macrocephaly, optic atrophy, seizures, spongy appearance of white matter, Ashkenazi Jewish ethnicity
Marinesco-Sjögren syndrome	Global developmental delay, cerebellar atrophy, ataxia, cataracts
Mitochondrial respiratory chain diseases	Central hypotonia or myopathy, exercise intolerance, seizures, migraines, ataxia, cardiomyopathy, ophthalmaplegia, sensorineural hearing loss, optic atrophy, hypothyroidism, diabetes mellitus, maternal family history of above
Pelizaeus-Merzbacher disease	X-linked, progressive peripheral and central hypotonia with evolution to spasticity, ataxia

features. Given the large number of etiologies and overlapping presentation, it may be impossible to make a diagnosis on clinical findings alone, and electromyography, nerve conduction studies, and/or muscle biopsy are often required. In the case in which maternal history of myotonic dystrophy or family history of specific neuromuscular disorder is present, it may be possible to avoid specific neuromuscular investigations and arrange for genetic testing in order to confirm the diagnosis. Certainly, some features, when present, are highly suggestive of specific diagnoses: tongue fasciculations in anterior horn cell disease, joint hypermobility in connective tissue disease or collagen VI–related CMD, and cardiac involvement in metabolic myopathies.

Raised serum creatine kinase (CK) suggests hypotonia of a peripheral origin; further supports hypotonia of peripheral origin; the most marked CK elevations are observed in patients with congenital muscular dystrophies. It is important to note that in all forms of peripheral pathologies, CK may be normal; therefore it is not possible to rule out peripheral hypotonia based on CK results alone. EMG and NCS may identify slowed conduction velocities seen in peripheral nerve pathologies, characteristic response to repetitive stimulation in congenital myasthenic syndromes, denervation consistent with an anterior horn cell disorder, myopathic features with muscle irritability suggesting Pompe disease, or myopathic changes with primary muscle disease. Muscle imaging by ultrasound or MRI, particularly of the thigh muscle, is an emerging modality for identification of specific patterns of muscle involvement observed in the congenital myopathies and congenital muscular dystrophies. Finally, biopsy is often required in order to demonstrate the characteristic histologic findings of congenital myopathies or dystrophic changes in the muscular dystrophies. When selecting a biopsy site, It is important to target muscles that are affected by weakness; information from EMG, ultrasound, and MRI are often useful for selecting a biopsy site involving affected muscle.

Information from the clinical presentation, family history, and investigations allows prioritization of genetic testing to confirm a specific diagnosis. Because there is generally greater accessibility to genetic testing that is less invasive, muscle biopsy is sometimes bypassed, particularly if features of specific myopathy are present from the clinical examination or MRI findings. The route to direct genetic diagnosis with genetic testing does have some drawbacks. The first is the prolonged time required for the result to become available, which can be particularly problematic for families with a severe and unexpected presentation. Second, interpretation of genetic test results may be more complicated if precise diagnosis is unknown, particularly if the pathogenicity of the variant is not obvious or not consistent with the expected pattern of inheritance.

REFERENCES

The complete list of references for this chapter is available in the e-book at www.expertconsult.com.

  See inside cover for registration details.

SELECTED REFERENCES

Bonnemann, C.G., et al., 2014. Diagnostic approach to the congenital muscular dystrophies. Neuromuscul. Disord. 24 (4), 289–311.

Brislin, R.P., Theroux, M.C., 2013. Core myopathies and malignant hyperthermia susceptibility: a review. Paediatr. Anaesth. 23 (9), 834–841.

DiMauro, S., et al., 2013. The clinical maze of mitochondrial neurology. Nat. Rev. Neurol. 9 (8), 429–444.

Dubowitz, V., 1980. The Floppy Infant. JB Lippincott, Philadelphia, PA.

North, K.N., et al., 2014. Approach to the diagnosis of congenital myopathies. Neuromuscul. Disord. 24 (2), 97–116.

Thornton, C.A., 2014. Myotonic dystrophy. Neurol. Clin. 32 (3), 705–719, viii.

Wang, C.H., et al., 2007. Consensus statement for standard of care in spinal muscular atrophy. J. Child Neurol. 22 (8), 1027–1049.

Watson, C.T., et al., 2014. The genetics of microdeletion and microduplication syndromes: an update. Annu. Rev. Genomics Hum. Genet. 15, 215–244.

139 Genetic Disorders Affecting the Motor Neuron: Spinal Muscular Atrophy

Basil T. Darras, Umrao R. Monani, and Darryl C. De Vivo

An expanded version of this chapter is available on www.expertconsult.com. See inside cover for registration details.

In the early 1890s, the Austrian clinician Guido Werdnig at the University of Graz, Austria, and the German physician Johann Hoffmann in Heidelberg, Germany, described a neuromuscular disorder causing progressive muscular weakness associated with the loss of anterior horn cells in the spinal cord, with onset in infancy and early death. Together, their reports provide the first complete description of the severe form of spinal muscular atrophy (SMA), originally named Werdnig-Hoffmann disease. The SMAs have since been defined as a group of genetic disorders characterized by progressive muscle weakness and atrophy, associated with degeneration of spinal and, in the most severely affected patients, lower bulbar motor neurons. The most common of these forms, as well as the leading cause of infant mortality, is classic proximal SMA, which seems to be found in practically all populations but is diagnosed more frequently in infants and children, rather than in adults.

Genetic studies have found that classic SMA results from homozygous deletions or mutations involving the "survival of motor neuron" *(SMN)* gene. Two copies of the *SMN* gene, designated *SMN1* and *SMN2*, are present on each chromosome 5, forming an inverted duplication at locus 5q13 (Figure 139-1). The duplicated *SMN2* gene is differentiated from *SMN1* by 5 nucleotide changes that do not change amino acids. A single-nucleotide change in *SMN2* creates an exonic splicing suppressor in exon 7, leading to exclusion of exon 7 in most transcripts (Monani et al., 1999) and thus diminished production of the functional SMN protein. Patients with 5q proximal SMA harbor homozygous deletions or mutations involving exon 7 of the *SMN1* gene, but maintain at least 1 copy of *SMN2*.

EPIDEMIOLOGY

The incidence of SMA has been estimated at 1 in 6000 to 11,000 live births or about 7.8 to 10 per 100,000 live births and at 4.1 per 100,000 live births for SMA type I. The estimated pan-ethnic disease frequency is approximately 1 in 11,000. The carrier frequency for mutations in the *SMN1* gene has been estimated from 1:38 to 1:70. It should be noted that, despite the high carrier frequency, the incidence of SMA is lower than expected. It has been postulated that this may reflect that some fetuses have a 0/0 *SMN1/SMN2* genotype (i.e., no SMN protein is present at all), which is known in other species to be embryonically lethal.

CLINICAL CHARACTERISTICS

Though most patients with SMA have deletions or mutations involving the *SMN1* gene, a range of phenotypic severity permits division into four broad clinical subtypes. It is recognized that the subtypes represent a phenotypic continuum extending from the very severe, with onset *in utero*, to the very mild, with onset during adulthood; there is also a spectrum of severity within each of these groups (Table 139-1). For the

purposes of clinical classification, or of guidelines developed for standards of care, the "maximal functional status achieved" approach, which classifies type I patients as "nonsitters," type II patients as "sitters," and type III patients as "walkers," has been used (Wang et al., 2007). Patients with a mild phenotype and onset during middle or late age are classified as type IV. The age at onset is also considered in the classification but because of potential overlap between subtypes and the difficulty in accurately determining the onset of symptoms, it has not been considered as the sole determinant of disease subtype.

Type I SMA

After the initial description of infantile SMA by Werdnig and Hoffmann in the early 1890s and further descriptions made by Sylvestre in 1899 and Beevor in 1903, infantile or type I SMA was described again in detail, both clinically and pathologically, by Randolph Byers and Betty Banker at Boston Children's Hospital in 1961. Patients with type I SMA, also known as Werdnig-Hoffmann disease, present between birth and 6 months of age. SMA type I has been further subdivided into 3 groups: type IA (or type 0 in certain reports) with onset *in utero* and presentation at birth, type IB with onset of symptoms before 3 months of age, and type IC with onset between 3 and 6 months of age. Infants with SMA type I have progressive proximal weakness that affects the legs more than the arms. They have poor head control, hypotonia that causes them to assume a "frog-leg" posture when lying and to "slip through" on vertical suspension, and areflexia. They are never able to sit ("nonsitters") or roll over independently (see Table 139-1). There is also weakness of the intercostal muscles with relative sparing of the diaphragm, producing a bell-shaped chest and a pattern of paradoxical or "belly"-breathing. Infants with type I SMA also classically exhibit tongue fasciculations and eventually have difficulty swallowing, with failure to thrive and a risk for aspiration. Other cranial nerves are not as affected, although facial weakness does occur at later stages of the disease. Cognition is apparently normal, and they are often noted at diagnosis to have a bright, alert expression that contrasts with their generalized weakness. Infants with type I SMA usually develop respiratory failure by age 2 years, or much earlier, and in the past most did not survive past 2 years; however, there has been some increase in survival in recent years with the use of assisted ventilation (to be described in more detail in later sections) and other interventions (Darras et al., 2015). Prior natural history studies have reported shortened life span, with 68% mortality within 2 years and 82% by 4 years of age. The application of nutritional and respiratory interventions has reduced the mortality to approximately 30% at 2 years, but about half of the survivors are fully dependent on noninvasive ventilation. In a recent observational study, the median age at reaching the combined endpoint of requiring at least 16 hours/day of noninvasive ventilation or death was 13.5 months. Infants with two SMN2 copies had

1057

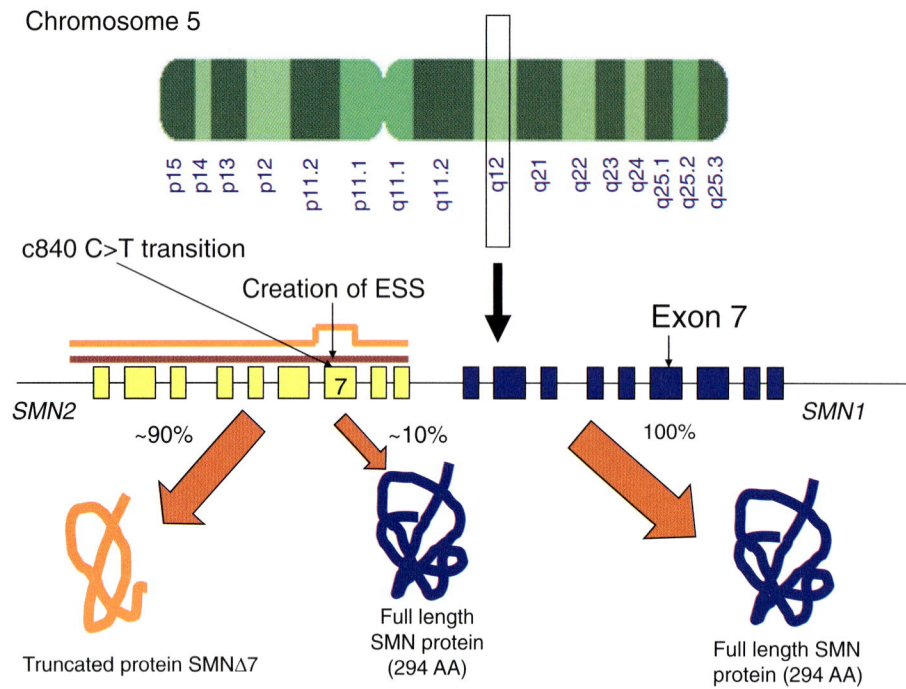

Figure 139-1. **Schematic diagram of human *SMN1* and *SMN2* genes on chromosome 5.** Patients with spinal muscular atrophy have deletions or mutations in both copies of *SMN1*. A C-to-T transition at position 840 of *SMN2* creates an exonic splicing suppressor (ESS) that leads to skipping of exon 7 during transcription and production of the truncated, nonfunctional SMN protein. However, a small amount (~10%) of full-length messenger RNA is produced from the *SMN2* gene, resulting in the functional, full-length SMN protein. *AA*, amino acids. *(With permission of Elsevier: Darras BT et al., editors. Neuromuscular disorders of infancy, childhood, and adolescence: a clinician's approach, 2nd edition. San Diego: Academic Press; 2015.)*

TABLE 139-1 Clinical Classification of Spinal Muscular Atrophy

SMA Type	Other Names	Age at Onset	Life Span	Highest Motor Milestone Achieved	Other Features	Proportion of Total SMA (%)
Type IA	Prenatal (type 0), congenital SMA, Werdnig-Hoffmann disease	Prenatal	<6 months	Mostly unable to achieve motor milestones	• Severe weakness at birth • Profound hypotonia • Facial diplegia • Areflexia • Early respiratory failure • Joint contractures	
Type IB Type IC	Werdnig-Hoffmann disease, severe SMA ("nonsitters")	Type IB (0–3 months) Type IC (3–6 months)	<2 years without respiratory support	Never sits unsupported	• Weakness • "Frog leg" posture, hypotonia • Tongue fasciculations • Hyporeflexia, areflexia • Suck and swallow difficulties • Respiratory failure	60*
Type II	Intermediate SMA ("sitters"), Dubowitz disease	6–18 months	>2 years ~70% alive at 25 years of age	Sits independently, never walks independently	• Proximal weakness, hypotonia • Postural hand tremor • Hyporeflexia • Average or above average intellectual skills by adolescence • Scoliosis	27
Type III	Kugelberg-Welander disease, mild SMA ("walkers")	>18 months Type IIIA (before 3 years) Type IIIB (after 3 years)	Almost normal	Stands and walks	• May have hand tremor • Resembles muscular dystrophy • CK often elevated 2-5X	12
Type IV	Adult SMA	>21 years	Normal	Normal		1

*Spinal muscular atrophy (SMA) types I, IA, IB, and IC all have a 60% proportion of total SMA.
(Modified with permission of Markowitz JA, Singh P, Darras BT. Spinal muscular atrophy: a clinical and research update. Pediatr Neurol 2012;46:1–12.)

greater morbidity and mortality than those with three copies. The need for nutritional support preceded that for ventilation support (Finkel et al., 2014).

It was previously believed that SMA is a purely motor neuron disorder. However, recent studies have shown that severe type I SMA can result in various organ manifestations, apart from spinal cord motor neurons such as brain, cardiac, vascular, and even sensory nerve involvement. Recent autopsy studies have shown increasing evidence of congenital heart disorders in severe SMA, with the most common association being hypoplastic left heart syndrome; however, this finding has not been confirmed and a chance of association has not been firmly excluded. Studies done on various mouse models have also found that severe SMN protein deficiency might present as vasculopathy. This was also noted in the case reports of two unrelated patients with severe SMA type I. Both these infants developed ulcerations and necroses of the fingers and toes. Autonomic dysfunction is thought to be the primary cause of this vasculopathy.

Type II SMA

This intermediate form of SMA was first reported in 1893 at the University of Edinburgh, United Kingdom, and described again by Byers and Banker in 1961 and in detail by Dubowitz in 1964. Patients with type II SMA, also known as intermediate SMA or Dubowitz disease, are able to sit unsupported at some point ("sitters"), but are never able to stand alone or walk independently (see Table 139-1). The onset of symptoms is typically between 6 and 18 months of age. They have progressive proximal weakness affecting legs more than arms, hypotonia, and areflexia. They also develop progressive scoliosis, which, in combination with intercostal muscle weakness, results in significant restrictive lung disease as they grow older. They develop joint contractures and can have ankylosis of the mandible. They exhibit tremor, or polyminimyoclonus, of the hands (Darras et al., 2015). Although their body mass index may be low (at the third percentile or less compared with normal children), this likely represents reduced muscle mass as the high-functioning, nonambulatory patients have a higher relative fat mass index and are at risk of becoming overweight. Cognition is normal and verbal intelligence may be above average. In a study done on 240 type II patients, survival rates were found to be 98.5% at 5 years and 68.5% at 25 years. Patients may live into the third decade, but life expectancy is shortened because of the risk of respiratory compromise (Darras et al., 2015).

Type III SMA

In 1956, Kugelberg and Welander described a much milder form of SMA characterized by prolonged ambulation. Patients with type III SMA, also known as Kugelberg-Welander disease, are able to stand alone and walk at some point ("walkers"). The onset of symptoms occurs after the age of 18 months; it has further been subdivided into type IIIA (onset between 18 months and 3 years) and type IIIB (onset after 3 years). They have progressive proximal weakness affecting legs more than arms and may ultimately need to use a wheelchair, especially the IIIA group, but they generally develop little to no respiratory muscle weakness or severe scoliosis. Loss of ambulation increases the risk of these complications. They may have tremor or polyminimyoclonus of the hands. Sometimes, the calves of these patients can be prominent and hence type III SMA can be confused with Becker muscular dystrophy. Creatine kinase levels are often elevated, usually no more than fivefold, and may lead to an erroneous evaluation for myopathy. EMG and nerve conduction testing is useful in this setting to indicate a neurogenic versus myopathic disorder and focus

appropriate further testing. Life expectancy is not significantly different compared with the normal population (see Table 139-1) (Darras et al., 2015).

There has been much debate about the appropriate classification of patients into these three types of SMA because, as mentioned, there are patients who within these categories exhibit phenotypes of differing severities. A classification system based on a continuous rather than discrete variable (e.g., SMA "Type 1.8" in the case of a less severely affected type I patient) has been proposed to better capture the clinical spectrum of these patients.

Outliers

There are also patients who are outliers on either end of the phenotypic spectrum. As discussed above, an SMA "type IA" has been used to describe neonates who present with severe weakness and profound hypotonia, probably of prenatal onset, as well as with a history of decreased fetal movements. At the severe end of the type 1A subgroup are infants born with severe contractures and no movements. Patients with this severe presentation, known as type 0, require ventilation support and do not attain any motor milestones. Other findings include areflexia, facial diplegia, atrial septal defects, and joint contractures. In SMA type IA, respiratory failure forms an important cause of morbidity and mortality, requiring noninvasive ventilation and endotracheal intubation at birth. Life expectancy is reduced and most of them are unable to survive beyond 6 months of age (see Table 139-1). Furthermore, arthrogryposis multiplex congenita (congenital joint contractures involving at least two regions of body) has been noted in SMA patients with *SMN1* gene deletions, and congenital axonal neuropathy involving motor and sensory nerves in conjunction with facial weakness, joint contractures, ophthalmoplegia, and respiratory failure at birth has been reported in three newborn siblings with deletions in the SMA chromosomal region.

A milder adult-onset SMA, or type IV SMA, has also been described with onset of symptoms after age 21 years and essentially normal life span. Most patients with the SMA type IA and IV phenotypes have homozygous deletions of exon 7 in *SMN1*, but as it will be discussed in the Genetics section, the *SMN2* copy number is usually only 1 in SMA type IA and 4 to 5 in SMA type IV.

Other "Spinal Muscular Atrophies"

The non-5q13–associated spinal muscular atrophies are a heterogeneous group of motor neuron diseases associated with mutations in a variety of different genes (e.g., X-linked and autosomal-dominant or autosomal-recessive spinal muscular atrophies), distal or segmental spinal muscular atrophies or distal hereditary motor neuropathies. Patients with these disorders generally have some clinical characteristics that can help differentiate them from those with 5q13-associated or classic SMA.

GENETICS
The *SMN* Gene

Linkage analysis studies showed that all three forms of SMA map to chromosome 5q11.1-13.3. In 1995 Lefebvre et al. identified the *SMN* (survival of motor neuron) gene within this region, which was absent or interrupted in 98.6% of the patients in their group. The structure of this region is complex, with a large inverted duplication of a 500-kb element. This contains the *SMN1* gene, which is deleted or interrupted in patients with SMA and is evolutionarily older, in the telomeric portion of the region, and the *SMN2* gene, a duplication of

SMN1 that differs from it by only five nucleotides, in the centromeric portion (see Figure 139-1). The critical difference between *SMN1* and *SMN2* is a C-to-T transition that creates an exon splicing suppressor in exon 7 of *SMN2*. Although this splice modulator change is translationally silent (i.e., it does not change the amino acid sequence), it affects the alternative splicing of the gene, so that exon 7 is spliced out of or excluded from most *SMN2* mRNA transcripts. This altered mRNA results in production of a truncated version of the SMN protein, which does not oligomerize efficiently and is degraded. Because exon 7 is not always spliced out of all *SMN2* mRNA, a small amount of full-length transcript and hence functional protein is produced by *SMN2*, but it yields only on average about 10% as much as that produced by *SMN1*. In patients with SMA both copies of the *SMN1* gene are deleted or disrupted, so the individual is left with only the small amount of SMN protein produced by the remaining copies of *SMN2*. The amount of the SMN protein is inversely correlated with the severity of disease.

About 95% to 98% of patients with SMA harbor deletions of the telomeric *SMN1* gene. The remainder have small intragenic mutations or have undergone gene conversions from *SMN1* to *SMN2*. De novo mutations occur at a rate of about 2%, which is relatively high, and explained by the fact that this region of chromosome 5 is unstable, containing not only the inverted repeat of *SMN1* and *SMN2*, but other surrounding low-copy-number repeats.

The number of copies of *SMN2* per chromosome 5 varies among normal individuals, and 10% to 15% of the population possess no copies of *SMN2*. Among patients with SMA, a clear correlation has been established between *SMN2* copy number and phenotypic severity. Feldkotter et al. in 2002 found that in their series 80% of patients with type I SMA had 1 or 2 copies of *SMN2*, 82% of patients with type II had 3 copies of *SMN2*, and 96% of patients with type III had 3 or 4 *SMN2* copies (Figure 139-2). Studies by Mailman et al. in 2002 and Arkblad et al. in 2009 found similar results (95% to 100% of type I patients had 1 or 2 copies of *SMN2*, and all type III patients had at least 3 copies of *SMN2*). However, this correlation is not so perfect as to permit the absolute prediction of clinical severity based on *SMN2* copy number, especially in the intermediate forms of the disease where there is some overlap (patients with three copies of *SMN2* have been described with all three phenotypes). One reason for the overlap is that not all copies of *SMN2* gene are equal; in terms of full-length SMN protein production, some copies probably produce less and some more than 10% functional protein. In general, though, it can be said that a patient with 1 or 2 copies of *SMN2* is highly likely to present with SMA type IA, IB, or IC. Interestingly, unaffected family members with homozygous *SMN1* deletions and five copies of *SMN2* have been described, which suggests that *SMN2* copy number alone cannot be the sole modifying factor in disease severity, because there are patients with type III SMA who also have five copies of *SMN2*.

Genetic Diagnosis

Genetic testing for SMA can be performed with PCR-based targeted mutation analysis using a restriction enzyme that digests exon 7. However, multiplex ligation probe amplification (MLPA) methodology is currently applied in most DNA diagnostic laboratories for deletion analysis of exon 7 of the *SMN1* gene in potential probands and carriers. This type of targeted mutation testing in conjunction with sequence analysis can also detect individuals who are compound heterozygotes with a deletion of exon 7 in 1 *SMN1* allele and an intragenic point mutation in the other allele. In such a case (approximately 2% to 5% of individuals with clinical diagnosis of SMA), sequence analysis of the *SMN* gene will detect the mutation; this sequence testing, however, will not detect exonic deletions or duplications (Prior and Russman, 1993). and will not determine whether the point mutation is in the *SMN1* gene or *SMN2* gene (if one of these genes is not deleted). Fortunately, certain point mutations have been described in more than 1 SMA patient already, and thus the detection of a previously reported mutation supports its pathogenicity and its location in the *SMN1* gene.

Carrier testing is feasible and accurate in the parents of patients with homozygous deletions of exon 7 or compound heterozygosity using a PCR-based dosage assay, known as "*SMN* gene dosage analysis." It can also be performed using other techniques such as long-range PCR, MLPA, and chromosomal microarray (CMA) that includes this gene segment. Sequencing of the *SMN* gene will detect point mutations in nondeletion carriers. Rarely, carriers may have two copies of *SMN1* on one chromosome (both copies in *cis* orientation on one allele, a so-called "2 + 0 carrier"); the incidence of this genotype is about 4% of the general population. In the "2 + 0 carriers," the SMA dosage carrier test will be falsely normal and thus one may need to pursue other methods such as family linkage analysis to identify the disease-associated

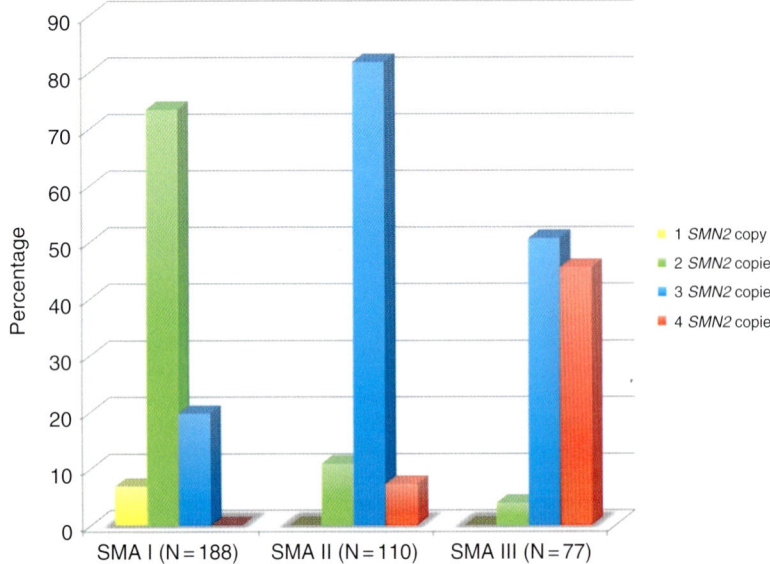

Figure 139-2. Frequency of patients with SMA types I, II, and III and *SMN2* copy numbers. In SMA type I, 80% of patients had 1 or 2 copies of *SMN2*, 82% of patients with type II had 3 copies of *SMN2*, and 96% of patients with type III carried 3 or 4 *SMN2* copies. (Modified with permission. This image was published in American Journal of Human Genetics, *Volume 70, Feldkotter M et al., Quantitative analyses of SMN1 and SMN2 based on based on real-time lightCycler PCR: fast and highly reliable carrier testing and prediction of severity of spinal muscular atrophy, pages 358–368, copyright Elsevier [2002].)*

genotype in families in which a deletion mutation has been transmitted more than once from a parent with two copies of the *SMN1* gene on gene dosage testing. Because of the occurrence of de novo mutations in 2% of patients with SMA, one of the parents may not be a carrier (Prior and Russman, 1993). So, in approximately 6% of parents of a child with SMA secondary to a homozygous *SMN1* deletion, *SMN1* gene dosage testing will be normal.

As mentioned in the introduction, a general correlation has been found between *SMN2* copy number and disease severity, and it is relatively straightforward to determine *SMN2* copy number in individual patients using various methodologies. However, this correlation is not so strict that the severity or type of disease can be reliably predicted based on copy number, and it is hence not advisable to offer families prognostic information based on *SMN2* copy number assays.

Newborn Screening

The potential for newborn screening for SMA has been of great interest because the ideal time to initiate therapy would be before the initial degeneration of motor neurons, and newborn screening may help to identify presymptomatic individuals before the period of greatest motor neuron loss. A few pilot programs have been initiated in the United States.

OTHER DIAGNOSTIC TESTS

In patients with SMA the serum creatine kinase may be 2- to 4-fold elevated, but not more than 10 times normal (Darras et al., 2015). Nerve conduction studies demonstrate normal sensory potentials, but may show diminished compound motor action potential amplitudes. Needle EMG in type II/III patients demonstrates a neurogenic pattern with high-amplitude, long-duration motor unit potentials with reduced recruitment pattern, indicating chronic partial reinnervation. Needle EMG in type I patients shows denervation changes but may not show evidence of reinnervation, as there may not have been enough SMN protein and/or time for this to occur yet. As will be discussed in more detail in the Pathology section, muscle biopsy in all types of SMA demonstrates a neurogenic pattern, with grouped atrophy; the small atrophic fibers are of both types (type 1 and type 2), whereas the large ones are always type 1 fibers. Although EMG continues to be used in the diagnosis of SMA in selected atypical cases, the use of muscle biopsy has become essentially obsolete.

MOLECULAR FUNCTION OF SMN

SMN is a 38-kDa protein found in all cells, located in both the cytoplasm and in the nucleus, where it localizes to structures known as Gemini of Cajal bodies, or simply "gems"; therefore, its expression is ubiquitous. In patient fibroblasts, the number of gems correlates with SMA severity. SMN is also localized in motor neuron axons. The SMN protein in conjunction with several Gemin proteins forms an SMN complex whose chaperone function facilitates the assembly of spliceosomal small nuclear ribonucleoprotein particles (snRNPs), essential components of the spliceosome complex, and hence plays a critical role in pre-mRNA splicing. The SMN protein may also be essential in assisting arginine methylation of some splicing-related proteins, transporting axonal mRNAs in motor neurons and perhaps in other processes in muscle and neuromuscular junction. The role of the SMN protein in axonal mRNA trafficking and mRNA splicing may explain the selective vulnerability of spinal cord motor neurons to decreased SMN protein; although not the only ones, these neurons have long axons and many targets, particularly in large muscles, and thus may be very dependent on axonal

mRNA transport. Further, they may be extremely vulnerable to the mRNA splicing defect. Nevertheless, it continues to be unclear whether a splicing defect caused by SMN protein deficiency, disruption of an additional axonal SMN function, perturbation of an unknown function, or a combination of the above is responsible for the pathogenesis of SMA. The complete absence of the SMN protein in cells is embryonic lethal in mice and other organisms. The reason why motor neurons are specifically vulnerable to partial SMN deficiency is unclear.

Patients with SMA also appear to have structural and physiologic abnormalities of the neuromuscular junction. Kong et al. showed that in severely affected SMA mice, before anterior horn cell death and/or axonal degeneration there is synaptic dysfunction at the neuromuscular junction in the form of decreased synaptic vesicle density at motor terminals, reduced quantal content, and slowed maturation of the acetylcholine receptor with prolonged retention of fetal characteristics. Kariya et al. also demonstrated structural and functional abnormalities at the level of the neuromuscular junction that precede overt symptoms in mice, as well as structural abnormalities in the neuromuscular junctions of humans with SMA, and hence proposed that SMA may be a "synaptopathy" (Kariya et al., 2008). Based on this concept and the electrophysiologic data suggesting dysfunction of the neuromuscular junction in patients with SMA types II and III, treatment approaches directed toward enhancing neuromuscular transmission may also be beneficial to patients with SMA.

DIFFERENTIAL DIAGNOSIS

The differential diagnosis of 5q SMA is listed in Box 139-1. This box also lists the non-5q SMAs, which are discussed in further detail in Chapter 140.

THE PATHOLOGY OF SMA

SMA is characterized by spinal motor neuron loss and skeletal muscle atrophy. However, a precise understanding of how the cellular pathology of the disease evolves over its course continues to be handicapped by a paucity of suitable patient material. Our current appreciation of SMA pathophysiology stems largely from analyses of autopsy material, reflecting pathology at the end of the disease. Analyses of early disease pathology have relied mostly on murine models. Still, from the current studies, certain key findings emerge. These, almost invariably, include a profound loss of the large anterior horn cells of the spinal cord. More infrequently, motor neurons are found mispositioned. Anterior horn motor neurons that remain often appear swollen or chromatolytic, containing phosphorylated neurofilaments, ribosomes, and vesicles.

Considering the degeneration of the spinal motor neurons, an expected pathologic characteristic is neurogenic atrophy of the skeletal muscles. Muscle from severely (type I) affected patients typically consists of a sea of small, rounded, atrophic fibers within which are sometimes seen islands of one or more large hypertrophic cells. In some instances, the atrophic fibers also appear immature with centrally rather than peripherally located nuclei, giving the appearance of a myopathic condition.

Even though SMA has historically been described as a disease characterized by motor neuron cell body loss, more recent data suggest that the earliest pathologic effects of reduced SMN are observed distally, at the neuromuscular junctions (Kariya et al., 2008). This early pathology that affects the pre- and postsynapse was first observed in mouse models of the disease and has now been confirmed in human samples as well (Kariya et al., 2008).

TABLE 139-4 Status of Therapeutics Development in Spinal Muscular Atrophy

Therapeutic Targets	Approaches	Clinical Trials
Increase SMN transcript	• Histone deacetylase inhibitors • Nonhistone deacetylase inhibitors • Quinazoline • Prolactin	• Valproic acid, sodium 4-phenylbutyrate • Hydroxyurea • Repligen RG3039
SMN2 exon 7 inclusion	• Antisense oligonucleotides • Small molecules	• Nusinersen • Roche RG7916 • Novartis LMI070
Stabilization of the SMN protein	• Aminoglycoside • Proteasome inhibitors • Indoprofen	
Neuroprotection	• Neurotrophic factors	• Riluzole • Gabapentin • Olesoxime (TRO19622)
Cell therapy	• Stem cells	
Replacement of *SMN1*	• Gene therapy	• AveXis scAAV9. CB.SMN
Muscle sarcomere	Troponin activator	Cytokinetics (CK-2127107)

(With permission of Lippincott Williams and Wilkins/Wolters Kluwer Health: Singh P, Liew WK, Darras BT. Current advances in drug development in spinal muscular atrophy. Curr Opin Pediatr 2013;25:682–688.)

directed toward finding pharmaceutical compounds that can upregulate *SMN2* expression or affect other modifying genes to produce more functional SMN protein.

Agents That Upregulate *SMN2* Gene Expression and Promote Exon 7 Inclusion

Small Molecules

A class of drugs known as histone deacetylase inhibitors (HDACIs) has been investigated extensively as potential therapeutic agents in SMA (Singh et al., 2013; Darras et al., 2015). Histones, which are core proteins in chromatin, play a role in epigenetic regulation of gene expression via their acetylation status. Several compounds that are HDACIs have been shown to increase full-length *SMN2* transcript levels in cell lines from patients, usually by activating the human *SMN2* promoter, enhancing transcription, and correcting the splicing pattern. Clinical trials of HDACIs, phenylbutyrate, and valproic acid have shown no difference in motor function scores compared with the placebo group in a nonambulatory cohort of type II SMA.

A proprietary small molecule developed by PTC Therapeutics, Inc., extends the life expectancy of the SMNΔ7 severe mouse model from 14 days to more than 6 months. Along with the quinazoline derivatives, this compound is further developed for clinical trials in humans. The distinct advantage of these small molecules is that they can cross the blood-brain barrier (BBB).

The FDA-approved drug hydroxyurea, a non-HDACI, was identified in the course of drug screens using cell lines from SMA patients to increase the amount of full-length *SMN*

TREATMENT

Currently, there is no cure for SMA. However, despite the presence of homozygous deletions of *SMN1* in the majority of patients with SMA, the unique structure of the 5q11.1-13.3 inverted duplication provides potential therapeutic targets. There has been great interest in identifying agents that can increase the amount of the full-length SMN protein by upregulating expression of the *SMN2* gene or promoting inclusion of exon 7. Researchers are also actively exploring several other approaches to treatment.

Clinical Trials in SMA: Therapeutics

SMA is a unique "translational" disease because of the presence of the *SMN2* gene, which is a well-validated target for therapeutic interventions. The status of therapeutics development is shown in Table 139-4. The effort on therapeutics is transcript and protein in vitro. However, a small pilot study of hydroxyurea at 3 different doses for 8 weeks in 33 type II and III patients showed no statistically significant benefit. A randomized, double-blind, placebo-controlled trial failed to show any improvement over an 18-month period.

Albuterol, a beta-adrenergic agonist, was evaluated in a pilot study of 13 SMA type II and III patients because of its reported positive effect on muscle strength in healthy individuals. At 6 months a significant improvement was noted in myometry, FVC, and DEXA scores, but there was no significant change in Medical Research Council strength score. Another pilot study of 23 SMA type II patients treated with salbutamol (a form of albuterol) for 12 months showed improved functional scores on the HFMS after 6 and 12 months, but this was not a placebo-controlled study and must be interpreted with caution (Pane et al., 2008). On an in vitro level, salbutamol has been shown to increase full-length SMN mRNA, SMN protein, and gem numbers by promoting inclusion of exon 7. The response was directly proportional to *SMN2* gene copy number. This finding prompts further interest in exploring the effects of beta agonists on SMA with randomized controlled trials.

Neuroprotective, SMN Protein Stabilization Agents
Other Small Molecules

Riluzole and gabapentin, "the neuroprotective agents," were studied to assess the effect on motor performance in SMA. Unfortunately, the results were not found encouraging or the studies were not adequate to show efficacy.

Olesoxime (TRO19622), a novel neuroprotective compound, has been tested in a randomized, multicenter, parallel-group, double-blind, placebo-controlled trial conducted in Europe. Preliminary results seem encouraging.

CK-2127107, a selective skeletal fast troponin activator slows down the rate of calcium release from troponin C and thus increases fast skeletal muscle contractility; a phase 2/3 study (CY 5021) in Type II and III SMA patients is currently in progress.

Other Approaches
SMN2 Splicing Modifiers

Drugs have been developed to modify splicing of the SMN2 gene to include exon 7 and increase the amount of full-length transcript and, consequently, the amount of normal SMN protein.

Antisense Oligonucleotides. Antisense oligonucleotides (ASOs) have been developed that block an intronic splicing suppressor element, which in turn prevents skipping of exon 7 (Burghes and McGovern, 2010). Hua et al. in their work on transgenic mice found these intronic splicing suppressors to be located in intron 7 as tandem motifs, namely, hnRNP A1/A2. Blocking of these motifs by ASOs enhanced exon 7 inclusion in the SMA mouse model. Similar work by Singh et al. demonstrated enhanced production of full-length SMN mRNA in fibroblasts from patients treated by ASOs. Periodic intracerebroventricular deliveries of ASOs in SMA mice models have been found to improve the motor phenotype. Phase I/II clinical trials and two randomized, double-blind, sham procedure controlled phase III trials demonstrated the safety, tolerability and clinical efficacy of multiple doses of ASO (nusinersen), which is delivered intrathecally into the subarachnoid space of SMA type I and type II patients. Spinraza (nusinersen) was approved by the US FDA in December, 2016, for treatment of all types of SMA and all ages. It is the first approved drug treatment for SMA.

Small Molecule Drugs. Orally delivered small molecule drugs that modulate splicing and promote inclusion of exon 7 are in early phase of clinical development: LMI070 and RG7916. These are listed in Table 139-4.

Stem Cells

Interest in the use of stem cells also continues, both as potential treatment for SMA and for use in constructing model systems for therapeutics development. During the last few years, pluripotent stem cells with the capacity to differentiate into motor neurons that lacked *SMN1* expression were induced from a type 1 SMA patient and his mother; this could serve as an important model system for testing of new compounds and eventually for stem cell approaches to the treatment of SMA.

Gene Therapy

Among other therapeutic targets, gene therapy has shown potential in animal models. Foust et al. demonstrated that self-complementary adeno-associated virus 9 (scAAV9) could cross the BBB and infect approximately 60% of motor neurons when injected intravenously into neonatal mice. When injected systemically with scAAV9 engineered to carry the wild-type *SMN* gene expressed high levels of protein in multiple tissues, these mice derived remarkable therapeutic benefit, surviving in some instances to 12 months or more with no evidence of muscle weakness. Considering proof-of-concept studies demonstrating the ability of scAAV9 to penetrate the mature BBB and infect adult motor neurons, an SMN replacement clinical trial to treat SMA type I is currently underway at Nationwide Children's Hospital and The Ohio State University, United States.

CARE OF THE PATIENT WITH SMA

Patients with SMA and their families benefit greatly from a multidisciplinary approach to care. This approach involves members from neurology/neuromuscular medicine, orthopedics, physical and occupational therapy, pulmonology, nutrition, and gastroenterology. For severely affected patients with type I SMA, early involvement of the pediatric advanced care or palliative care team can provide parents with support and assistance in making decisions that are consonant with their values and help to maximize their child's quality of life. In 2007 a Consensus Statement for Standard of Care in Spinal Muscular Atrophy was released by a multidisciplinary team regarding the current best recommendations for management of patients with SMA (Wang et al., 2007).

Pulmonary

Respiratory failure is the major cause of mortality in patients at the more severe end of the disease spectrum, namely types I and II SMA. Infants with type I SMA have weak intercostal muscles with relatively preserved diaphragm strength, resulting in a bell-shaped chest, pectus excavatum, and in some cases underdevelopment of the lungs. Patients with type II SMA have weak intercostal muscles with scoliosis contributing to progressive restrictive lung disease. The restrictive lung disease results in insidious onset of sleep hypoventilation. Proper use of BiPAP, with correct pressure adjustments and mask placement, has no significant side effects on patient hemodynamics. There should also be a low threshold for the use of antibiotics during acute illnesses in these patients, because of the risk of pneumonia (Wang et al., 2007). Patients should be followed regularly by a pulmonologist experienced in caring for patients with neuromuscular diseases, with home visits by a home ventilation team if available.

Gastrointestinal

Patients with type I SMA are extremely weak and hence tire during feedings, which can lead to failure to thrive and aspiration with recurrent respiratory infections. In a small retrospective study, Durkin et al. found that early laparoscopic Nissen fundoplication and gastrostomy in patients with type I SMA was associated with improved nutritional status in these patients, and also perhaps with a trend toward fewer long-term aspiration events. Lastly, patients with SMA are at risk of constipation, which can, if severe (especially in young type I patients), worsen reflux or even respiratory symptoms.

Nutrition

Failure to thrive or growth failure is common in infants with type I SMA and in some severely affected type II patients. However, though many type II patients plot as having a "normal" body mass index (often as low as third percentile for a healthy child of their age), they may actually have excessive fat mass relative to their muscle mass. Clinically high functioning nonambulatory SMA patients (Hammersmith score ≥12) are at risk of becoming overweight. Hence close attention must be paid to nutritional status in patients with all types of SMA, and consultation with a dietician who is aware of these special concerns is vital.

Orthopedic

Patients with SMA at the severe end of the disease spectrum require close orthopedic follow-up for the development of scoliosis and contractures. Surgical intervention for scoliosis is often required, and careful coordination of perioperative respiratory and nutritional support can help to minimize complications (Wang et al., 2007). With the advent of improved surgical techniques such as growing rods, the interventions are currently considered earlier in life. Fractures and hip subluxation are commonly seen in milder type II and type III SMA patients. Distal femur is the commonest fracture site followed by lower leg, ankle, and upper arm. Most of the fractures can be treated conservatively.

Fatigue

Physiologic fatigue is a common complaint in milder SMA patients and can be measured by the decrement in distance walked from the first to sixth minute of the six-minute walk test (Montes et al., 2010). The mechanism(s) underlying fatigue in SMA remains to be elucidated, but it may be related at least in part to the neuromuscular junction defects described earlier. Anecdotal evidence suggests that albuterol PO in usual pediatric doses is an effective agent in the treatment of fatigue in SMA patients and thus it is frequently used; however, fatigue has not been studied directly in the conducted albuterol pilot studies that showed improvement in motor function (Pane et al., 2008).

CONCLUSIONS

SMA is a chronic, inherited motor neuron disease for which there is no established treatment. Yet there is cause for optimism, as it is an area of active research, and knowledge about the molecular genetics and pathogenesis of SMA is ever increasing. Several groups are actively exploring pharmacologic treatments, whether through the use of approved drugs, identification of new agents via high-throughput screens, or development of novel pharmaceutical compounds. Standards of care have also been developed to optimize the long-term multidisciplinary management of patients with SMA. Although it may seem at times that a treatment for SMA is far in the future, the advances made since the gene was identified in 1995 permit a modicum of hope to patients, their families, and those with the privilege to care for SMA patients.

Acknowledgments

This chapter was funded in part by NINDS R01 NS057482 and by the SMA Foundation (New York, NY).

REFERENCES

The complete list of references for this chapter is available in the e-book at www.expertconsult.com.
  See inside cover for registration details.

SELECTED REFERENCES

Burghes, A.H., McGovern, V.L., 2010. Antisense oligonucleotides and spinal muscular atrophy: skipping along. Genes Dev. 24, 1574–1579.

Darras, B.T., Markowitz, J.A., Monani, U.R., et al., 2015. Spinal muscular atrophies. In: Darras, B.T., Jones, H.R., Jr., Ryan, M.M., et al. (Eds.), Neuromuscular Disorders of Infancy, Childhood, and Adolescence: A Clinician's Approach, second ed. Academic Press, San Diego, pp. 117–145.

Finkel, R.S., McDermott, M.P., Kaufmann, P., et al., 2014. Observational study of spinal muscular atrophy type I and implications for clinical trials. Neurology 83, 810–817.

Kariya, S., Park, G.H., Maeno-Hikichi, Y., et al., 2008. Reduced SMN protein impairs maturation of the neuromuscular junctions in mouse models of spinal muscular atrophy. Hum. Mol. Genet. 17, 2552–2569.

Monani, U.R., Lorson, C.L., Parsons, D.W., et al., 1999. A single nucleotide difference that alters splicing patterns distinguishes the SMA gene SMN1 from the copy gene SMN2. Hum. Mol. Genet. 8, 1177–1183.

Montes, J., McDermott, M.P., Martens, W.B., et al., 2010. Six-Minute Walk Test demonstrates motor fatigue in spinal muscular atrophy. Neurology 74, 833–838.

Pane, M., Staccioli, S., Messina, S., et al., 2008. Daily salbutamol in young patients with SMA type II. Neuromuscul. Disord. 18, 536–540.

Prior, T.W., Russman, B.S., 1993. Spinal muscular atrophy. In: Pagon, R.A., Bird, T.C., Dolan, C.R., et al. (Eds.), GeneReviews [Internet]. University of Washington, Seattle, WA; 1993–2000 Feb 24 [updated 2013 Nov 14].

Singh, P., Liew, W.K., Darras, B.T., 2013. Current advances in drug development in spinal muscular atrophy. Curr. Opin. Pediatr. 25, 682–688.

Wang, C.H., Finkel, R.S., Bertini, E.S., et al., 2007. Consensus statement for standard of care in spinal muscular atrophy. J. Child Neurol. 22, 1027–1049.

E-BOOK FIGURES AND TABLES

140 Other Motor Neuron Diseases of Childhood

Michele L. Yang and Anne M. Connolly

 An expanded version of this chapter is available on www.expertconsult.com. See inside cover for registration details.

ANATOMY: THE ANTERIOR HORN CELLS OF THE SPINAL CORD

Anterior horn cells (α-motor neurons), located in the anterior gray matter of the spinal cord, are found at every segment and are concentrated in the cervical and lumbosacral enlargements. Morphologic differentiation of the anterior horn cells is most evident from 12 to 14 weeks' gestation. There is a period of normal differentiation, followed by programmed cell death. Anterior horn cells are clustered into medial and lateral cell divisions (Figure 140-1). The medial group is subdivided into ventromedial and dorsomedial components. The ventromedial component innervates the superficial larger muscles, and the dorsomedial component innervates the small, deep muscles adjacent to the spine. The lateral cell mass is also subdivided into groups. The ventrolateral group innervates extensor muscles, and the centrodorsal group innervates flexor muscles. These groups of neurons are located in a relatively small region; therefore deleterious influences harm cells from more than one group and weakness may be widespread.

Motor neurons in the nuclei of brainstem cranial nerves are homologous to spinal cord anterior horn cells. Therefore pathologic mechanisms that compromise the cranial motor neurons may initiate symptoms and signs that mimic anterior horn cell dysfunction in the spinal cord. Muscular atrophy, severe weakness, and fasciculations without sensory deficit are signs of anterior horn cell disease. When sensory function is impaired in conjunction with anterior horn cell disease, dysfunction of adjacent tracts of the spinal cord or the peripheral nerves may be present.

DIAGNOSTIC WORKUP

Disorders of the motor neuron typically result in flaccid weakness, hypotonia, and decreased reflexes, with varying degrees of atrophy depending on the chronicity of the disorder. Fasciculations may be present as well. Dysfunction of the motor neurons can result from acquired or hereditary etiologies. Therefore in any patient in whom this is a consideration, a thorough medical and family history, and detailed neurologic examination are crucial. If the child's history and physical suggest a motor neuron disorder, multiple tests can be performed for confirmation, including serum creatine kinase (CK) and electrophysiologic testing (electromyography and nerve conduction study [EMG/NCS]). The serum CK can be normal or mildly elevated, usually not more than three times the upper limit of normal, about 600 mg/dl. Electrodiagnostic studies show normal or near-normal sensory responses and normal motor conduction velocities, often with reduction in amplitudes of compound motor action potentials. Chronic and/or acute denervation may be recognized by electromyography. Motor unit number estimate is a more of a research tool that is reduced in disorders of affecting the motor neuron.

HEREDITARY DISEASES AFFECTING SPINAL MOTOR NEURONS

Inherited motor neuron disease in childhood is most commonly caused by mutations of the *SMN1* gene on chromosome 5q13 (see Chapter 139). However, a small proportion (4%) of patients do not have a mutation or deletion of *SMN1*. The clinical and genetic heterogeneity of this group of disorders can be overwhelming, particularly as the number of new genes identified increases yearly (Table 140-1) (Pestronk, 2003; Peeters et al., 2014). Classifying them by distribution of weakness (proximal, distal, bulbar), inheritance pattern (autosomal dominant, autosomal recessive, or X-linked), and other associated manifestations can guide the diagnostic workup. A simplified algorithm to the approach to the diagnosis of motor neuron disease is presented in Figure 140-2 by distribution of weakness, that is, proximal (Figure 140-2A) or distal (Figure 140-2B) (Finsterer and Burgunder, 2014).

SMA-like Motor Neuron Disorders

Children with SMA-like motor neuron disorders present with symmetric proximal muscle weakness, affecting legs more than arms. This pattern of weakness is similar to those with 5q-associated SMA. Weakness typically is rapidly progressive, with respiratory insufficiency usually resulting in the need for mechanical ventilation, followed by death.

Respiratory insufficiency may be the first clinical feature in patients with spinal muscular atrophy with respiratory distress (SMARD). In SMARD1, patients may have diaphragmatic paralysis with eventration of the diaphragm; the intercostal muscles are spared. Weakness and contractures occur first in the distal extremities. SMARD1 is caused by mutations of *IGHMBP2*. A new phenotype of SMARD2 with a similar clinical presentation has been associated with mutations of *LAS1L*.

As in 5q-associated SMA, the main features of early onset scapuloperoneal SMA include progressive weakness of the extremities beginning at birth or early childhood. A characteristic feature of this subtype of SMA is vocal cord weakness with hoarseness and respiratory stridor. If this feature is present, mutations of *TRPV4* should be considered.

Arthrogryposis is an early feature in boys with X-linked SMA and arthrogryposis (XL-SMA, *UBA1* gene) but otherwise the presentation is similar to that of 5q-associated SMA. Contractures typically occur in the proximal joints and fingers. Respiratory insufficiency also occurs early and is progressive, with death occurring in most patients before the age of 2 years because of respiratory failure.

Motor Neuron Disease With Central Nervous System Manifestations

The presence of predominant central nervous system (CNS) findings such as spasticity, movement disorders, and intellectual disability is unusual in 5q-associated SMA. Cerebellar findings such as ataxia, nystagmus, or oculomotor apraxia in infants with motor neuron disease should prompt an

TABLE 140-1 Motor Neuron Disease Plus Syndromes

Clinical Patterns	Disease	Symptoms	Genes	Inheritance	Diagnostic Testing
SMA-like With proximal muscle weakness	DSMA1 Distal infantile SMA with diaphragm paralysis (DSMA1 or SMARD1)	Onset birth to 2 months Diaphragmatic paralysis with sparing of intercostal muscles Death or respiratory failure less than 3 months Severe distal weakness Distal SMA weakness at age 1 year with progression but variable onset of respiratory failure Occasional mild contractures of the knee and ankle	Immunoglobulin μ-binding protein 2 (IGHMBP2); 11q13.3	AR	Normal CK Eventration of diaphragm on chest x-ray Sural nerve: myelinated axon loss
	SMA with respiratory failure 2 (SMARD2)	Single patient Distal weakness at birth Early respiratory failure Fasciculations of tongue Mild contractures of fingers and toes	LAS1L; Xq12	X-linked recessive	EMG localized to motor neuron
	SMA: scapuloperoneal	Onset: congenital childhood Legs only Proximal and distal contractures Nonprogressive Vocal cord paralysis in some	TRPV4; 12q24.11	AD	Mildly elevated CK EMG/NC: normal CMAP and SNAPs; giant motor units on EMG
	X-linked SMA with arthrogryposis (XL-SMA, SMAX2)	Onset at birth or infancy Pattern of weakness similar to classic SMA Proximal and finger contractures Myopathic facies Respiratory insufficiency Dysmorphic features Death less than 2 years of age	UBE1; Xp11.3	X-linked recessive	
With CNS manifestations Cerebellar hypoplasia	Pontocerebellar hypoplasia (PCH) type 1A	Onset birth to 6 months Hypotonia, weakness, distal symmetric polyneuropathy Ataxia, nystagmus Mild to severe contractures Microcephaly	VRK1; 14q32	AR	Normal CK MRI brain: cerebellar hypoplasia or absence EMG/NCS: axonal sensorimotor polyneuropathy
	PCH2	Onset birth Progressive microcephaly Distal contractures Oculomotor apraxia	EXOSC3; 9p13.2	AR	MRI brain: cerebellar atrophy, small brainstem and cortex EMG/NCS: axonal sensorimotor polyneuropathy
	PCH1C	Onset 2–4 months Severe weakness Spasticity Vision and hearing impairment Stepwise decline with illnesses	EXOSC8; 13q13.3	AR	MRI brain: cerebellar hypoplasia Hypomyelination of lateral descending tracts
Movement disorders Dystonia	Leukoencephalopathy with dystonia and motor neuropathy	Onset: childhood to teens Dystonia Hypergonadotropic hypogonadism Azoospermia Saccadic eye movements Brisk reflexes in arms, diminished in legs Intention tremor, ataxia Hyposmia	SCP2; 1p32.3	AR	MRI brain: hyperintensities in thalamus, "butterfly-like" lesions in pons, lesions in occipital regions
	Hexosaminidase A deficiency (Tay-Sachs disease), juvenile form	Onset: late teens to early adulthood Muscle atrophy, muscle cramping, fasciculations, proximal great than distal weakness Ataxia, dystonia, dysarthria	HEXA; 15q23	AR	MRI brain: cerebellar atrophy EMG/NCS: axonal sensorimotor polyneuropathy, CRDs

TABLE 140-1 Motor Neuron Disease Plus Syndromes *(Continued)*

Clinical Patterns	Disease	Symptoms	Genes	Inheritance	Diagnostic Testing
	Mitochondrial membrane protein associated neurodegeneration (MPAN; NBIA4)	Onset: 3–39 years Dysarthria Spasticity Dystonia, parkinsonism Progressive distal great than proximal weakness Optic atrophy, slow saccades Cognitive decline Psychiatric manifestations	*C19orf12;* 19q12	AR	EMG/NCS: motor neuropathy Serum CK: high MRI: hypointensity of globus pallidus and substantia nigra; cerebellar atrophy
Spasticity	Achalasia-addisonism-alacrima (AAA) syndrome (Allgrove syndrome)	Onset: childhood GI: achalasia, feeding difficulties, xerostomia, fissured tongue Endocrine: adrenal insufficiency Skin: hyperpigmentation, excessive creases on palms and soles, hyperkeratosis Long thin face, long philtrum Eyes: alacrimia, optic atrophy, pupillary abnormalities Intellectual disability Autonomic dysfunction Spasticity	*AAAS;* 12q13.13	AR	EMG/NCS: predominantly axonal motor neuropathy
Seizures	SMA with myoclonic epilepsy	Onset 3–5 years SMA-like with proximal weakness first in legs and then in arms Respiratory failure occurs later in course	*ASAH1;* 8q22	AR	Normal CK EEG: subcortical myoclonic epileptiform activity, sensitive to hyperventilation EMG: chronic denervation
Bulbar involvement	Brown-Vialetto-Van Laere (BVVL)	Onset 8–20 years Pontobulbar palsy Sensorineural hearing loss Ataxia caused by sensory neuropathy	*SLC52A2* and *SLC52A3*	AR, rarely AD	EMG/NCS: motor neuropathy with upper limbs more affected than lower Brain MRI: normal Sural nerve biopsy: severe chronic axonal neuropathy affecting large fibers predominantly, no regeneration seen
	Fazio-Londe disease (FL)	Onset in childhood, usually less than 12 years Respiratory insufficiency Pontobulbar palsy Ataxia caused by sensory neuropathy No hearing loss	*SLC52A2* and *SLC52A3*	AR or AD	EMG/NCS: motor neuropathy with upper limbs more affected than lower Brain MRI: normal Sural nerve biopsy: severe chronic axonal neuropathy affecting large fibers predominantly, no regeneration seen
	Nathalie syndrome	Onset 4–5 years Hearing loss Spinal muscular atrophy Cataract Dilated cardiomyopathy Delayed growth and sexual development	Unknown	AR	ECHO: dilated cardiomyopathy Autopsy: loss of cochlear neurons, atrophy of organ of Corti, atrophy of atria vascularis
	BVVL-like	Juvenile onset bulbar weakness Vocal cord paralysis ± sensorineural hearing loss	*UBQLN1*	AR	
	Spinal and bulbar muscular atrophy (Kennedy's disease)	Exercise-induced muscle cramping Tremors Gynecomastia Facial fasciculations	*hAR;* X	Dominant X-linked	Mildly elevated CK EMG/NCS shows motor neuronopathy

Continued on following page

TABLE 140-1 Motor Neuron Disease Plus Syndromes *(Continued)*

Clinical Patterns	Disease	Symptoms	Genes	Inheritance	Diagnostic Testing
Arthrogryposis	LCCS1	Onset: in utero Hydrops fetalis, arthrogryposis multiplex congenita Pulmonary hypoplasia Fractures Chest wall deformities	*GLE1*; 9q34	AR	
	LCCS2	Onset: birth Multiple joint contractures Markedly distended bladder Single family of Israeli-Bedouin origin	*ERBB3*;12q13	AR	Anterior horn cell atrophy on autopsy
	SMA-LED	Onset: birth Contractures	*DYNC1H1*; 14q32.31	AD	
	X-linked SMA with arthrogryposis (XL-SMA, SMAX2)	Onset at birth or infancy Pattern of weakness similar to classic SMA Proximal and finger contractures Myopathic facies Respiratory insufficiency Dysmorphic features Death less than 2 years of age	*UBE1*; Xp11.3	X-linked recessive	

AD, autosomal-dominant; *AR*, autosomal-recessive; *CK*, creatine kinase; *CMAP*, compound muscle action potential; *CRDs*, complex repetitive discharges on EMG; *EMG/NCS*, electromyography and nerve conduction study; *LCCS*, lethal congenital contracture syndrome; *SMA*, spinal muscular atrophy; *SMARD*, spinal muscular atrophy with respiratory distress; *SNAP*, sensory nerve action potential.

evaluation for pontocerebellar hypoplasia (PCH). Three types of PCH have been associated with an SMA-like phenotype: PCH1A (*VRK1*), PCH1B (*EXOSC3*), and PCH1C (*EXOSC8*). Children generally present at birth or in infancy with variable contractures and cerebellar hypoplasia. An MRI of the brain will identify cerebellar abnormalities. Electrophysiologic testing can demonstrate the presence of an axonal sensorimotor polyneuropathy.

A few of the genetic motor neuron disorders can have associated movement disorders. Patients with leukoencephalopathy with dystonia and motor neuropathy can present in childhood with progressive distal weakness as well as cerebellar and extrapyramidal symptoms. Whereas the infantile form of hexosaminidase A deficiency is primarily characterized by CNS manifestations, the juvenile onset form may have an associated progressive motor neuropathy characterized by muscle atrophy with fasciculations, muscle cramping, and proximal greater than distal weakness in addition to a movement disorder with ataxia, dysarthria, and dystonia. Patients with achalasia-addisonism-alacrima syndrome (triple A syndrome) may present in childhood with intellectual disability, developmental delay, spasticity, and a progressive axonal motor neuropathy. The associated gastrointestinal, endocrine, skin, and autonomic dysfunction makes identification relatively straightforward.

There are few genetic motor neuron disorders associated with seizures. When myoclonic seizures are present in a patient with suspected motor neuron disease, mutations of *ASAH1* should be sought. Symptoms typically are seen between 3 and 5 years of age with progressive weakness of the legs, arms, and then respiratory muscles.

Motor Neuron Diseases With Predominant Bulbar Weakness

Bulbar symptoms are often part of the presentation of many neurodegenerative disorders. However, when dysphagia, dysphonia, and dysarthria are the dominant presenting features, childhood progressive bulbar syndromes should be considered. Brown-Vialetto-Van Laere (BVVL) disease and Fazio-Londe (FL) disease are two distinct clinical entities

recognized to be allelic conditions and present along a phenotypic spectrum. The major features of BVVL disease are pontobulbar palsy, neuronopathy, respiratory insufficiency, and sensorineural hearing loss, presenting in the first or second decade of life. The course is generally progressive, but may appear episodic with worsening with illness. In contrast, FL disease is not associated with hearing loss, and onset is in the first to third decades of life. Patients may present initially with repeated respiratory infections and stridor, with progression to weakness, wasting, hypotonia, and decreased reflexes. In both BVVL and FL, patients often die of respiratory failure. The identification of biochemical abnormalities suggested a multiple acyl-CoA dehydrogenase deficiency (MADD)–like disorder and the finding of decreased plasma flavin levels in these patients indicated that riboflavin transporters could play a role. Subsequently, two genes were identified in patients with BVVL and FL. Solute carrier family 52, riboflavin transporter, member 3 (*SLC52A3*, previously known as *C20orf52*) encodes intestinal human riboflavin transporter 3, which is necessary for riboflavin absorption, and *SLC52A2* (previously G protein-coupled receptor 172A) encodes human riboflavin transporter 2 (RFVT2, previously human riboflavin transporter 3 [hRFT3]). Although with both mutations a MADD-like biochemical profile is seen, plasma flavin levels are normal in patients with *SLC52A2* mutations, likely because the encoded transporter is responsible for transport of riboflavin from blood into target cells. Because the *SLC52A3*-encoded transporter is responsible for uptake of riboflavin from food, flavin levels are low. Therefore acylcarnitine levels taken at birth should be interpreted with these differences in mind if BVVL or FL is suspected.

Recognition that riboflavin transport is affected in these patients is an important advance in the management of these children. Treatment with high-dose riboflavin (10 mg/kg per day) appears to result in significant and sustained clinical and biochemical improvements. The recommendation is for treatment early in the disease course in suspected cases to maximize response.

Spinal and bulbar muscular atrophy (SBMA, or Kennedy's disease) is an X-linked motor neuron disease typically presenting in adult men in the 3rd to 5th decades. The classic presentation is of slow progression of proximal weakness, bulbar weakness including asymmetric or symmetric facial weakness, and gynecomastia. However, some patients may complain of exercise-induced muscle cramps and hand tremors several years before weakness develops, as early as the second decade of life. Weakness and atrophy of the bulbar musculature is striking and may include an atrophied, furrowed tongue and atrophy of the face and jaw. Facial fasciculations around the mouth and chin are striking clinical features best elicited by having the patient whistle or blow out the cheeks. There are no signs of spinal cortical tract dysfunction, and deep tendon reflexes are diminished or normal. EMG/NCS findings and an unusually elevated CK are supportive findings, and should prompt testing for expanded CAG trinucleotide repeats in the androgen receptor gene (*hAR*).

Motor Neuron Disease With Arthrogryposis

Arthrogryposis at birth can occur because of many causes, but in the context of motor neuron disease, this finding indicates severe and early motor neuron dysfunction. Lethal arthrogryposis with anterior horn cell disease (LAAHD) and X-linked spinal muscular atrophy (SMAX2) are the most severe forms of motor neuron disease. The clinical phenotype includes severely decreased fetal movements, severe multiple contractures at birth, hypotonia, chest wall deformities, pulmonary hypoplasia, and bony fractures. In both LAAHD and SMAX2, patients have severe respiratory insufficiency and die by age 2 years. LCCS2 is a rare disorder described in one family, presenting with multiple contractures at birth and markedly distended bladders. Spinal muscular atrophy with lower extremity predominance (SMA-LED) associated with *DYNC1H1* mutations typically presents in early childhood, but has been associated with contractures at birth, from mild talipes to severe generalized arthrogryposis.

Motor Neuron Disease With Distal Weakness

The diagnosis of a distal motor neuropathy or neuronopathy can be difficult, particularly if the presentation occurs later in adulthood (Drew et al., 2011). The phenotypic spectrum is wide and varies from a CMT-like presentation to juvenile amyotrophic lateral sclerosis (ALS) and hereditary spastic paraparesis with associated mild sensory abnormalities and upper motor neuron signs, respectively (Table 140-2). Electrophysiologic studies are one of the most helpful means of distinguishing between these diagnostic possibilities. This section will focus on those disorders presenting with lower motor neuron disease in childhood. They are characterized by a slowly progressive length-dependent weakness, starting in the first 2 decades of life, with distal weakness and atrophy, absent reflexes, and electrophysiologic findings of chronic distal denervation. Bulbar involvement, with the exception of vocal cord weakness, is unusual.

The phenotypic variability of these disorders can complicate diagnostic workup of these disorders. The simplest method to approach the diagnosis is by organization by inheritance pattern and by the dominant weakness (Figure 140-2B). However, even with this approach, the diagnostic yield is low, with genotypic characterization in 20% of patients. Of these disorders, SMA with lower extremity predominance (SMA-LED) type 1 caused by *DYNC1H1* mutations can be easily recognized by the unusual waddling gait and disproportionate weakness of the legs compared with the arms. Patients may present at birth with multiple contractures, but many of the patients present with delayed walking in childhood and a slowly progressive weakness and gait abnormality. Intellectual disability and migrational abnormalities have been noted in some patients as well. Interestingly, mutations of *BICD2*, which functions as an adaptor of the dynein molecular motor,

result in SMA-LED2 with similar weakness and gait abnormalities as SMA-LED1. In both, obtaining a complete family history is important in identifying other affected family members and the autosomal-dominant inheritance pattern.

Although mutations of *TRPV4* can present with leg-predominant weakness, a distinguishing feature that can identify the presence of this gene mutation is a hoarse voice resulting from vocal cord paralysis. Mutations of *DCNT1* can also cause vocal cord paralysis, but the clinical picture is more variable. The lower motor neuron phenotype is more suggestive of ALS or SMA than a length-dependent neuropathy. Symptoms typically begin in adulthood with face-arm weakness first, with leg weakness presenting later. Some patients can present with pyramidal signs, as can patients with mutations of *BSCL2* and *HSPB1*.

Amyotrophic Lateral Sclerosis With Onset in the First Two Decades of Life

ALS represents a spectrum of motor system degeneration involving the corticospinal and corticobulbar pathways and motor neurons associated with the cranial nerves and anterior horn cells of the spinal cord. Onset may be as early as early childhood, although the majority present after the fourth decade of life. Dysfunction of upper and lower motor neurons produces clinical manifestations of both spasticity and muscular atrophy.

To date, more than 25 genes have been associated with ALS or ALS associated with frontotemporal dementia (http://neuromuscular.wustl.edu/synmot.html#Hereditaryals). The first causative gene described for ALS in adults (ALS1 is *SOD*, a gene that encodes a cytosolic Cu/Zn-binding superoxide dismutase, is causative in ALS1.

There are six recognized ALS syndromes with onset in the first two decades of life (Table 140-3). First, ALS 2 is an autosomal-recessive disease caused by mutations in the *Alsin* gene. *Alsin* is a member of the guanine nucleotide exchange factors for the small guanosine triphosphatase, RAB5, and plays a role in endosomal trafficking. Children present in the first decade of life with spasticity involving face and limbs, and may develop pseudobulbar affects. Symptoms are very slowly progressive, with difficulty walking after age 40. Two allelic conditions, infantile-onset ascending paralysis and primary juvenile lateral sclerosis (OMIM 606353) are well recognized. More recently, another allelic variant with ALS and generalized dystonia was described. *Alsin*-deficient mice experience progressive axonal degeneration in the lateral spinal cord but lower motor neurons were preserved.

The second juvenile-onset form of ALS is ALS 4, an autosomal-dominantly inherited distal motor neuronopathy with pyramidal symptoms. ALS 4 is allelic to recessively inherited oculomotor apraxia type 2 (AOA2). Symptoms of ALS 4 begin in the second decade of life with difficulty walking, and examination indicates both upper and lower motor neuron involvement. Bulbar symptoms are infrequent. Electrophysiology confirms localization to the anterior horn cell. The clinical course is slowly progressive, with use of wheelchair by fifth or sixth decade and a normal life span. The senataxin protein plays an essential role with DNA damage response.

The third form of ALS with childhood onset is ALS 5. ALS 5 is recessively inherited and is caused by mutations in the *SPG11* gene, which encodes spatacsin and is allelic with SPG11. The age of onset is 7 to 23 years, with a mean age of 16 years. Spasticity of limbs, face, and bulbar is present with amyotrophy and weakness. The course is slowly progressive with survival duration of 27 to 40 years.

To date, three other genetic forms of juvenile ALS have been determined by small, informative families. They include ALS6 secondary to FUS, ALS 16 secondary to sigma-1 receptor, and

TABLE 140-2 Distal Forms of SMA

Disease	Symptoms	Genes	Inheritance	Diagnostic Testing
Distal SMA, X-linked 3 (SMAX3)	Onset: 1–61 years Early weakness of legs with slow progression; remain ambulatory Pes cavus Temperature sensitivity with worsening in cold Variable reflexes	ATP7A; Xp21.1	X-linked recessive	CK normal EMG/NCS: reduced or absent CMAP, normal SNAPs; widespread denervation on EMG
DSMA1 Distal infantile SMA with diaphragm paralysis SMARD1 (HMN6)	Distal SMA weakness at age 1 year with progression but variable onset of respiratory failure	IGHMBP2; 11Q13.3	AR	
DSMA 2 Jerash type	Onset 6–10 years Distal weakness in legs and then arms within 2 years Atrophy of hands and feet Brisk reflexes at knees, absent at ankles	9p21.1-p12	AR	EMG/NCS: small CMAPs, normal SNAPs Normal CK
DSMA 3	Onset age 9 months to early adulthood Weakness of feet great than hands Diaphragmatic weakness with childhood onset	11q13.3	AR	EMG/NCS: normal nerve conduction studies; denervation on EMG
DSMA 4	Onset 2–11 years Proximal = distal weakness Scapular winging Progressive respiratory failure Contractures of the hips, elbows, hands Hyperlordosis Allelic with CMTR1C	PLEKHG5; 1p36.31	AR	EMG/NCS normal nerve conduction studies; denervation on EMG
DSMA 5 (distal motor neuropathy with young adult onset)	Onset age 16–23 years Foot drop Legs great than hands Absent reflexes Edema in legs Progressive to wheelchair Allelic with CMT 2T	DNAJB2; 2q35	AR	EMG/NCS: small CMAP, especially in legs, normal SNAPs
SMA, lower extremity predominant 1 (SMA-LED)	Onset: birth to early childhood Late walking Slowly progressive Weakness legs great than arms, quadriceps, psoas, and hip abductors typically weak out of proportion to rest of muscles Waddling gait	DYNC1H1; 14q32.31	AD	MRI legs: early involvement of the vastus lateralis and sartorius MRI brain: occasionally see polymicrogyria, cobblestoning
SMA, lower extremity predominant 2	Onset: in utero, infancy, young adulthood Delayed walking Weakness of legs great than arms, like in SMA-LED1 Contractures of ankles, knees Sleep disordered breathing Slow progression Normal sensation, bulbar function, and cognition	BICD2; 9q22.31	AD	MRI legs: early involvement of vastus lateralis and intermedius, rectus femoris; spares semitendinosus, medial adductors EMG/NCS: chronic denervation on EMG
DSMA-calf predominant (HMN2D)	Onset 13–48 years Presentation with difficulty standing or walking Weak calves Triceps also weak Fasciculations present	FBXO38; 5p31.1	AD	EMG/NCS: reduced amplitudes of CMAPs, normal SNAPs, fibrillation potentials
SMA, congenital nonprogressive of the lower limbs	Onset: congenital Weakness of legs only, proximal and distal Nonprogressive Some with vocal cord paralysis Contractures of knees and ankles	TRPV4; 12q24.11	AD	Mildly elevated CK EMG/NCS: giant motor units; normal motor and sensory NCSs
DSMA: upper extremity predominance (HMN5C)	Onset: 15 years (2–40 years) Weak hands (thenar great than first dorsal interosseous) Foot deformities Peroneal weakness Brisk DTRs Decrease vibration in legs	BSCL2; 11q12.3	AD	EMG/NCS: small CMAPs, normal or mildly decreased motor NCVs; large MUPs on EMG
DSMA: upper extremity predominance (HMN5A, SMAD1)	Onset: second decade Weakness of thumb and first dorsal interosseous Lower extremity involvement in 50% in 2 years Slow progression Rare pyramidal involvement	GARS; 7p14.3	AD	

TABLE 140-3 Genetic Forms of ALS Associated With Presentation in Childhood

Name	Inheritance Gene; Loci	Protein	Onset (Years)	Inheritance	OMIM
ALS 2	AR *ALS2;* 2q33	Alsin	1–3	AR	#20511
ALS 4	AD *SETX;* 9q34	Senataxin	6–21	AD	#602433
ALS 5	AR *ALS5;* 15q21	Spatacsin	5–23	AR	#610844
ALS 6 variant	Sporadic *FUS;* 16p11	Fusion	17–22	Sporadic	#608030
ALS 6–21	AR 6p 25; 21q22	Unknown	4–10	AR	
ALS 16	AR *SIGMAR1;* 9p13	Sigma-1 receptor	1–2	AR	#614373

AD, autosomal-dominant; *ALS*, amyotrophic lateral sclerosis; *AR*, autosomal-recessive; #, OMIM gene identified.

a third form currently linked to 6p25 and 32q22. ALS6 is autosomal recessive, is caused by heterozygous mutations in the *FUS* gene, and can present with or without frontotemporal dementia. Although most present in the third and fourth decade, a juvenile form has been reported with onset between age 17 and 22 and may have rapid progression. It is allelic with familial essential tremor-4 caused by heterozygous mutations (*ETM4*). A single family has been found to have autosomal-recessive childhood ALS (ALS16) with onset at age 1 to 2 years because of sigma-1 receptor mutations (SIGMAR1). Progression in 2 of the 6 children led to wheelchair use by age 20 but no respiratory or bulbar weakness. Finally, another single family with four affected children has been shown to have autosomal-recessive ALS linked to 6p25 and 21q22.

OTHER ATYPICAL AND ACQUIRED MOTOR NEURON DISORDERS

If weakness occurs acutely, acquired causes of motor neuron disease should be diagnostic considerations. Infectious, para-infectious, autoimmune, vascular, and traumatic etiologies can result in acute muscle weakness without sensory changes.

INFECTIONS

With the introduction of the polio vaccine, poliovirus as an infectious cause of acute flaccid weakness has virtually been eradicated. However, recent resurgences of children with flaccid weakness remind us that viruses remain an important etiology to consider when suspecting an acquired cause of motor neuron disease.

Poliovirus was one of the most common causes of acquired motor neuron disease. Typically acquired via the fecal-oral route, the virus is stable in the gastrointestinal tract, and can be detected in the throat and stool before the onset of illness. Less than 1% of all polio infections result in flaccid paralysis. Onset is usually indicated by upper respiratory tract symptoms with accompanying malaise, muscle pain, and stiffness. The patient may experience some degree of nuchal rigidity and a low-grade fever as the disease progresses. Paralytic symptoms generally begin 1 to 10 days after prodromal symptoms and progress for 2 to 3 days. Poliomyelitis is characterized by a triad of fever, nuchal rigidity, and spasm of the back, and may be mistaken for typical meningitis. Typically once the temperature normalizes, no further paralysis occurs. Patients with more rapid progression have more severe involvement, typically with respiratory and bulbar weakness. The weakness

is typically asymmetric, associated with decreased reflexes, and reaches a plateau without change for days to weeks. There is no accompanying sensory loss or changes in cognition. Although some persons with paralytic poliomyelitis recover completely, those with weakness present after 12 months will have permanent weakness.

Cerebrospinal fluid (CSF) pleocytosis with mononuclear cells and a normal or slightly elevated protein concentration supports this diagnosis. Complete blood cell count show that polymorphonuclear cells may predominant early in the course. Poliovirus may be recovered from the stool or pharynx. Isolation of the virus from the CSF is diagnostic, but it is rarely found. Treatment is supportive, and typically requires prolonged rehabilitation as some degree of motor deficits persists after the acute infection. Postpolio syndrome may begin two or more decades after the illness, with progressive loss of strength and atrophy of an already affected limb.

Through widespread use of the polio vaccine, the incidence had been drastically reduced in most parts of the world. Most sporadic cases of a polio-like syndrome are no longer associated with the poliovirus but are the results of other viral infections, including Epstein-Barr, enterovirus 71, enterovirus D68, echo 4 virus, and coxsackie virus (Solomon et al., 2014).

Vascular Etiologies

The anterior spinal artery originates from where the vertebral arteries meet and traverses the anterior median sulcus over the entire course of the spinal cord. The radicular arteries are divided into anterior and posterior radicular arteries. Blood from the anterior radicular arteries that enter with the nerve roots between the third cervical and third lumbar segments flows into the anterior spinal artery (Figure 140-5). The anterior spinal artery is then separated further into several sulcal branches that pierce the central gray matter, perfuse the anterior horn cells, and form numerous small penetrating vessels that supply the white matter of the anterior and lateral columns. The anterior spinal artery is vulnerable between the T4 and T8 regions because the radicular artery that supplies it (artery of Adamkiewcz) has poor anastomoses and is effectively an end artery. The anatomic relationship between the two posterior spinal arteries provides a very different vascular pattern for the posterior cord compared with the anterior spinal arteries do for the anterior cord. The posterior circulation enjoys a more extensive collateral system. Therefore occlusion of the posterior spinal arteries usually does not cause severe clinical dysfunction.

Occlusion or hypoperfusion of the anterior spinal artery results in weakness below the level of occlusion, loss of pain, and temperature at or below the level because of involvement of the lateral spinothalamic tracts, and autonomic dysfunction such as loss of bowel and bladder function. The posterior columns mediating proprioception and vibratory sense remain intact. Patients often complain of a diffuse, radicular, or girdle-like pain. Occasionally a partial syndrome is seen in which the gray matter of the spinal cord is preferentially affected, with preserved sensation and bowel and bladder control. In children, the most common etiology is iatrogenic, caused by aortic surgery such as during repair of a coarctation of the aorta. Other causes can include anemia, polycythemia, sickle cell disease, paradoxical embolism from a patent foramen ovale, atlantooccipital dislocation, cervical spondylosis, cervical spinal trauma or sprain, cocaine use, or infections such as tuberculosis.

Although arteriovenous malformations of the spinal cord are rare, they should be considered in a child with acute, subacute, or chronic symptoms of back or radicular pain, sensorimotor changes, or bowel or bladder dysfunction. The most common presentation of a vascular malformation in the spinal cord in children is with weakness. Sudden focal pain may occur with an acute hemorrhage, whereas subacute symptoms that worsen and then improve with gradual deterioration over time may indicate alterations in blood flow because of venous hypertension or repeated hemorrhages. Typically, however, sensory changes are also present, as are changes in bowel and bladder function, suggesting a diagnosis other than primary motor neuron dysfunction. Over time, the acute flaccid paralysis evolves into spasticity. Imaging is key to the diagnosis, and conventional angiography may be required to adequately visualize the malformation to develop a surgical plan. Surgical options include microsurgical exclusion and/or endovascular embolization, but the neurologist should be aware that transient neurologic deficits can occur postoperatively.

Trauma

There are rare case reports of adults and children who develop a delayed upper and lower motor neuron syndrome after exposure to an electrical injury or lightning. In children, electrical injuries typically occur in the household from putting electrical cords in the mouth or from wall outlets. Transient neurologic deficits immediately after an electrical shock are well described and usually recover after hours to several days. A persistent and progressive motor neuron syndrome has been described, developing at variable time intervals after the initial injury, but the relationship between electrical injury and a motor neuron syndrome is controversial.

Trauma to the spinal cord may follow birth trauma, falls, motor vehicle accidents, or blows to the spinal column, resulting in incomplete or total transection of the spinal cord. However, impairment localized only to the anterior horn cells is unlikely unless the anterior spinal arteries are primarily affected.

Unknown Etiologies

Monomelic amyotrophy is a rare form of motor neuron disease with clinical deficits limited to a restricted number of myotomes. Most cases are sporadic though a familial form has been reported and susceptibility genes have been identified. Many names have been used for this disorder, including juvenile muscular atrophy of a unilateral upper extremity, benign focal amyotrophy, juvenile segmental muscular atrophy, and Hirayama's disease. Symptoms typically present in the second or third decade of life, with a male

preponderance of 5:1 to 10:1, male-to-female ratio. Most cases are limited to the arm, with insidious, painless weakness and atrophy of the hand muscles that progresses to the forearm. Of note, the brachioradialis and extensor carpi radialis are usually spared. No preceding injury or infection is typically identified. Progression is typically slow, over 1 to 3 years, and there may be atrophy of the other arm, though it is typically less marked and more confined to isolated muscles. The etiology of the disorder is unknown.

TREATMENT

Other than the potentially riboflavin-responsive BVVL and FL, there are no specific treatments for either the inherited or the acquired motor neuron disorders. The mainstays of treatment remain physical therapy, orthotic support, and orthopedic procedures to protect joints and maximize mobility. Orthopedic procedures performed on patients with arthrogryposis often provided sufficient alignment and stability of the legs to allow independent ambulation. Talectomy before walking ability is acquired may prove beneficial. Scoliosis may be a prominent problem and may require surgical correction. Some improvement in arm and hand function is usually possible with physical therapy and exercise. Anesthesia for these patients requires special consideration. Otolaryngologic management may be necessary for poor suck reflex, omega-shaped epiglottis, airway compromise, achalasia, and micrognathia.

REFERENCES

The complete list of references for this chapter is available in the e-book at www.expertconsult.com.
　　See inside cover for registration details.

SELECTED REFERENCES

Drew, A.P., Blair, I.P., Nicholson, G.A., 2011. Molecular genetics and mechanisms of disease in distal hereditary motor neuropathies: insights directing future genetic studies. Curr. Mol. Med. 11, 650–665.

Finsterer, J., Burgunder, J.M., 2014. Recent progress in the genetics of motor neuron disease. Eur. J. Med. Genet. 57, 103–112.

Peeters, K., Chamova, T., Jordanova, A., 2014. Clinical and genetic diversity of SMN1-negative proximal spinal muscular atrophies. Brain 137, 2879–2896.

Pestronk, A., 2003. Neuromuscular Disease Center. <http://neuromuscular.wustl.edu/>.

Solomon, B.D., Baker, L.A., Bear, K.A., et al., 2014. An approach to the identification of anomalies and etiologies in neonates with identified or suspected VACTERL (vertebral defects, anal atresia, tracheoesophageal fistula with esophageal atresia, cardiac anomalies, renal anomalies, and limb anomalies) association. J. Pediatr. 164, 451–457, e451.

E-BOOK FIGURES AND TABLE

The following figures and tables are available in the e-book at www.expertconsult.com. See inside cover for registration details.

Fig. 140-1. Alpha-motor neurons located in the anterior horn of the spinal cord (anterior horn cells) are clustered in a specific pattern.

Fig. 140-2. A simplified algorithm for diagnosis of distal and proximal predominant motor neuron disease.

Fig. 140-3. This 6-month-old boy has the neurogenic form of arthrogryposis.

Fig. 140-4. A patient with Möbius's syndrome who has bilateral weakness of cranial nerves VI and VII.

Fig. 140-5. Arterial blood supply to the spinal cord.

Fig. 140-6. Deformity of the cervical cord during flexion of the neck in patients with Hirayama's disease.

Table 140-4. Genetic forms of Möbius's syndrome

141 Genetic Peripheral Neuropathies

Kathryn M. Brennan and Michael E. Shy

An expanded version of this chapter is available on www.expertconsult.com. See inside cover for registration details.

DEFINITION

This chapter focuses on those hereditary neuropathies present in the pediatric population. Inherited neuropathies are often referred to collectively as Charcot-Marie-Tooth (CMT) disease, an eponym used in recognition of the three men who initially described the disorder. CMT is, however, an umbrella term that encompasses a wide variety of inherited sensory and/or motor neuropathies. These inherited neuropathies also include other closely related neuropathies such as hereditary neuropathy with liability to pressure palsy (HNPP); distal hereditary motor neuropathy (dHMN), also known as distal spinal muscular atrophy (dSMA); and hereditary sensory neuropathy (HSN). HSN is sometimes referred to as hereditary sensory and autonomic neuropathy (HSAN). Collectively, CMT represents the commonest group of inherited neuropathies observed in the pediatric population and therefore is the main focus of this chapter.

PREVALENCE AND CLASSIFICATION

CMT is the most common inherited neurologic condition, with a prevalence of around 1 : 2500. It is divided into subtypes based on the pattern of inheritance and by neurophysiological studies. Subtypes include AD demyelinating (CMT 1), AD axonal (CMT 2), AR (CMT 4) and X-linked (CMTX) (Harding, 1980a). CMT 1 typically has slow nerve conduction velocities (less than 38 m/s in the upper extremities) and pathologic evidence of a hypertrophic demyelinating neuropathy whereas CMT 2 has relatively normal nerve conduction velocities with evidence of axonal degeneration (Harding and Thomas, 1980b). Because most forms of CMT have both motor and sensory involvement, CMT 1 and 2 are often known as hereditary motor and sensory neuropathy (HMSN) type I or II. Another subtype has emerged, known as CMT Intermediate, with nerve conduction demonstrating intermediate velocities (less than and greater than 38 m/s).

Each type of CMT is now subdivided according to the specific genetic cause of the neuropathy (see Table 141-2). For example, the most common form of CMT1, termed CMT1A, is caused by a duplication of a fragment of chromosome 17 containing the peripheral myelin protein 22-kD (*PMP22*) gene, whereas CMT1B is caused by mutations in the myelin protein zero (*MPZ*) gene. Currently, mutations in more than 80 genes have been identified as causes of CMT neuropathies.

CLINICAL SEQUELAE OF INHERITED NEUROPATHY

Symptoms of inherited peripheral neuropathy include weakness, sensory loss, abnormal balance, and autonomic dysfunction. Weakness is often said to be "length dependent" (i.e., distal and more severe in the legs than the arms). Deep and superficial muscles that are innervated by the peroneal nerve often cause more symptoms than muscles innervated by the tibial nerve, such as the gastrocnemius. As a result, tripping on a carpet or curb and ankle sprains are frequent symptoms. Foot drop can ensue over time. In the hands, symptoms typically involve fine movements, such as using buttons or zippers and inserting and turning keys in locks. Cramping, the painful knotting of a muscle, frequently occurs with motor or sensorimotor neuropathies.

The sensory symptoms of neuropathy reflect disease of small, thinly myelinated or nonmyelinated fibers serving in pain and temperature sensation and large myelinated fibers serving in position sense. Common symptoms of small-fiber sensory neuropathy include feeling as though the feet are "walking on pebbles" or "ice cold" and difficulty determining whether bath water is hot or cold with the foot. Painful dysesthesias are also associated with small-fiber abnormalities. Large-fiber sensory loss usually impairs balance, which may be worse at night when vision cannot overcome the loss of proprioception. Loss of proprioception is also frequently length dependent, so a patient may improve balance by lightly touching a wall with the hand to improve proprioceptive input to the brain.

Autonomic symptoms may occur in the HSN group and various metabolic neuropathies. Symptoms include postural hypotension, cardiovascular incompetence, impaired sweating, urinary retention or incontinence, impotence, and constipation alternating with diarrhea. Often patients will not volunteer autonomic symptoms because they are not aware these symptoms could originate from a neuropathy, and so these particular symptoms need to be specifically addressed when assessing patients.

Despite phenotypic variability, the typical clinical course of CMT1 and CMT2 patients includes normal development before weakness and sensory loss appear gradually within the first 2 decades of life. This is often referred to as the *classical phenotype*. This term is based on the original description by Harding and Thomas. Affected children are often slow runners and have difficulty with activities that require balance (e.g., skating, walking along a log across a stream) but have usually walked on time (i.e., before 15 months). Ankle-foot orthotics (AFOs) are frequently required by the third decade. Generally, hands are rarely as affected as the feet. Most patients remain ambulatory throughout life and have a normal lifespan.

Patients with distal hereditary motor neuropathies (dHMNs) sometimes have mild sensory abnormalities, and patients with hereditary sensory neuropathies (HSNs) usually have some weakness. Indeed, the same mutation in the same gene can cause both CMT and dHMN within the same family (e.g., glycyl-tRNA synthetase or *GARS* mutations can cause both CMT2D and hereditary motor neuropathy type V).

PATHOPHYSIOLOGY

Most of the genes mutated in CMT are involved in maintaining the structure or function of the peripheral nervous system. The first genes identified to cause CMT express proteins that are essential for compact (peripheral myelin protein 22

[PMP22] and myelin protein zero [MPZ]) and noncompact (gap junction protein beta 1 [GJβ1]) myelin, and their altered expressions cause demyelination or dysmyelination. Gene-protein dosage has been shown to be important in some forms of CMT; too much PMP22 (i.e., with a duplication) causes CMT1A; too little (as seen with a deletion) causes HNPP. Abnormal expression of MPZ also causes demyelination, although in this case it is usually a result of point mutations in the MPZ gene.

At a pathologic level, dysmyelination, demyelination, remyelination, and axonal loss are characteristic features of the various demyelinating forms of CMT1. In Dejerine-Sottas neuropathy, myelin may never have formed normally, which is referred to as dysmyelination. In CMT1, onion bulbs of concentric Schwann cell lamellae are usually present on nerve biopsies, with loss of both small- and large-diameter myelinated fibers and sometimes axons. Focal, sausage-like thickenings of the myelin sheath (tomaculae) are characteristic of hereditary neuropathy with liability to pressure palsies (HNPP) but may also be found in other forms of CMT1, particularly CMT1B.

NEUROPHYSIOLOGY

Nerve conduction velocity (NCV) testing will differentiate between demyelinating and axonal neuropathies. In clinical practice, approximately 60% of CMT patients have CMT1, and approximately 20% have CMT2 (Saporta et al., 2011). Neurophysiology is also useful to detect sensory involvement that often is unreported by patients. It can also aid in the classification of axonal inherited neuropathies further into mixed motor and sensory axonal neuropathy (CMT2), pure motor axonal neuropathy (dHMN), and pure sensory axonal neuropathy (HSN/HSAN).

Most CMT1 patients, particularly those with CMT1A, have a uniformly slow nerve conduction velocity of about 20 m/sec. However, asymmetric slowing, which is characteristic of hereditary neuropathy with liability to pressure palsies, may be found in patients with missense mutations in PMP22, MPZ, EGR2, and, particularly in females, GJβ1. CMT1X, caused by mutations in GJβ1, comprises about 15% of all CMT patients. Males with CMT1X usually have NCVs in the "intermediate" range of 30 to 45 m/s. NCVs in women with CMT1X are often normal.

Virtually all forms of CMT1 have axonal loss and demyelination. In cases where the motor and sensory responses are absent, it is worthwhile looking at proximal nerve conduction (e.g., axillary nerve latency) to fully investigate the possibility of a severe demyelinating rather than an axonal pathology.

GENETIC TESTING AND DIAGNOSTIC STRATEGIES

Molecular testing—performed after the family history, neurologic examination, and neurophysiologic testing have suggested the probable candidate genes—is the "gold standard" for the diagnosis of inherited neuropathies. Strategies for focused genetic testing based on inheritance and clinical phenotype are in common use, with the choice of genes tested reflecting the specific population tested. For example, in Northern European and Northern American populations, most patients have dominant inheritance even if the cases are sporadic. Autosomal-recessive (AR) CMT is observed in less than 10% of these cases. However, in populations with high rates of consanguinity AR-CMT is likely to be much more common, even reaching levels of 40%.

An algorithm based on the North American population utilizes neurophysiological data, clinical information, and inheritance patterns to guide testing. Flow charts incorporating the clinical phenotype and electrophysiology findings, illustrated in Figures 141-2 and 141-3, guide the clinician on selection of appropriate testing strategies. With the use of such tools, most CMT clinics will reach a genetic diagnosis in approximately two-thirds of their total CMT population (Murphy et al., 2011). Approximately 90% of patients found to have a genetic diagnosis will have mutations in one of only four genes: PMP22, GJβ1, MPZ, and MFN2. Therefore, the flow charts emphasize the need for considering these particular genes first. Mutations that alter the amino acid sequence of PMP22, GJβ1, and MPZ almost always cause clinical neuropathy, whereas MFN2 and most other CMT genes can also have benign mutations in which the coding sequences are altered without causing disability. This is important to consider when interpreting genetic testing results. Once genetic testing has been done in a proband, other family members do not usually merit genetic testing and instead are identified by clinical evaluation and neurophysiology.

The landscape of genetic testing is rapidly changing with the introduction of next-generation sequencing (NGS) into clinical practice in some areas, which enables sequencing of either the entire genome or exome (only the protein coding sequences) in days. However advanced genetic interrogation will require careful interpretation. Many genes, such as periaxin and MFN2, have a high number of polymorphisms that are not pathogenic. Currently, genetic testing is in a transition phase with both traditional Sanger sequencing and NGS (whole-genome sequencing/whole-exome sequencing [WGS/WES]) technology being used by most dedicated CMT clinics.

SPECIFIC FORMS OF CMT
CMT1: Autosomal-Dominant Demyelinating Neuropathies

CMT1 is the most common subtype of CMT and is caused primarily by mutations in four genes: PMP22, MPZ, LITAF, and EGR2. These genes are essential to formation of the myelin sheath and also Schwann cell function.

CMT1A

CMT1A is the most common form of CMT in most populations, affecting 55% of genetically determined CMT and 36% of all CMT. It accounts for 80% to 90% of CMT1 cases. Patients usually present with the "classical CMT phenotype." Patients usually will walk on time. Lifespan is not affected. Although patients frequently require ankle-foot orthotics, they rarely require wheelchairs for ambulation. Conduction velocities from the median and ulnar nerves are below 38 m/s and are typically in the 20s. The sensory action potentials are either reduced or absent. Nerve biopsy is not required but if performed reveals demyelination and onion bulb formation. Because there is a de novo mutation rate of 10%, children and adolescents without a family history with ulnar motor nerve conduction velocities (MNCVs) less than 35 m/s should first be screened for CMT1A before proceeding with other genetic testing. CMT1A is caused by a 1.4-Mb duplication on chromosome 17p11.2 in the region that carries the PMP22 gene.

CMT1B

CMT1B is the fourth most common type of CMT and clinically is associated with three distinct phenotypes: (1) an early-infantile-onset severe phenotype with delayed walking and NCV less than 10 m/s, often referred to as Dejerine-Sottas

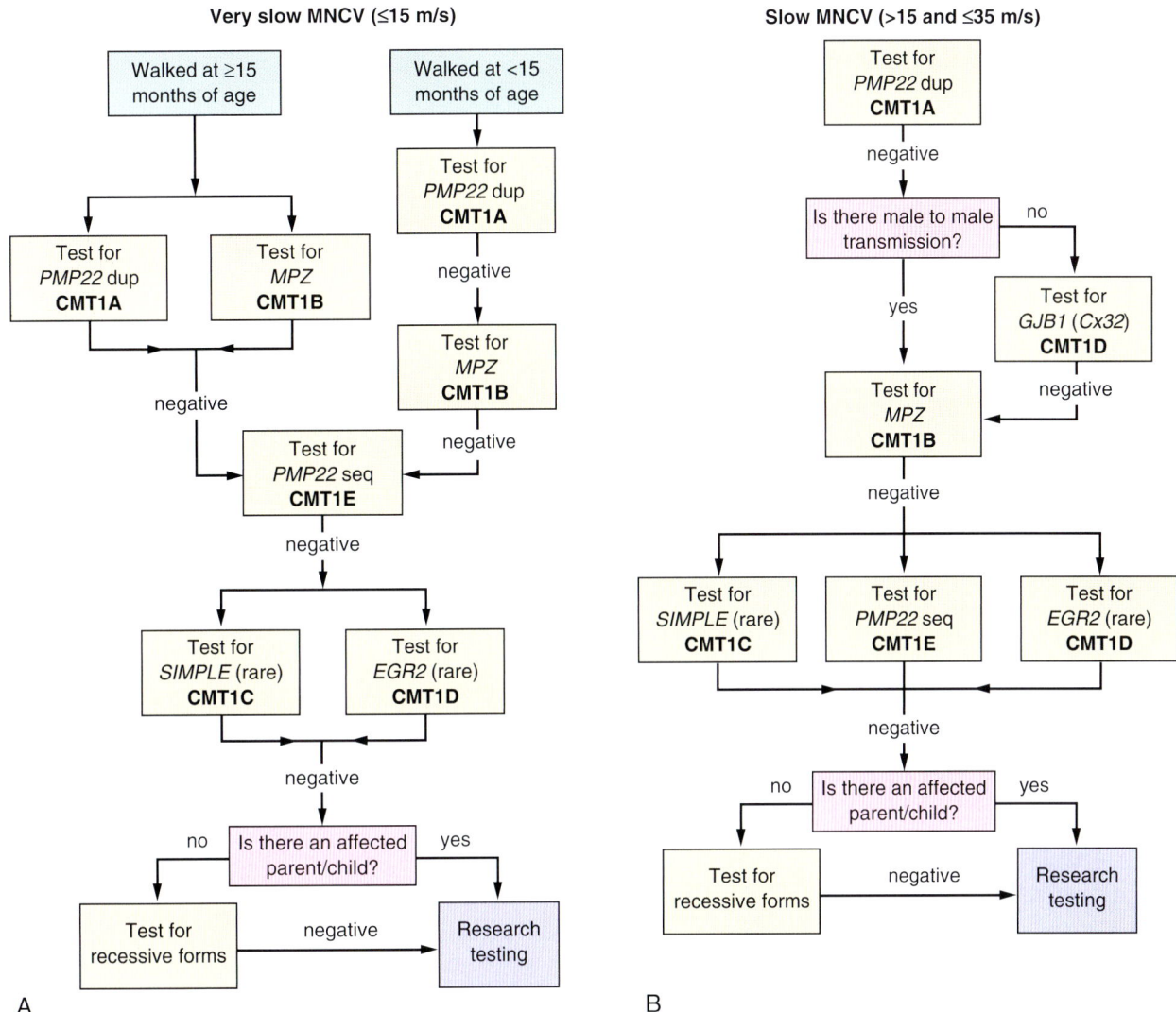

Figure 141-2. Algorithm for the genetic diagnosis of patients with Charcot-Marie-Tooth disease and very slow (**A**) or slow (**B**) upper extremity motor nerve conduction velocities. Dup, duplication; Seq, sequencing. *(With permission from Saporta AS et al. Ann Neurol 2011; 69 [1]: 22-33.)*

disease; (2) less commonly, a classic phenotype as described for CMT1A with normal early milestones but progression throughout the first 2 decades of life; and (3) a much later, milder phenotype with onset at around age 40 and NCV of around 40 m/s. CMT1B is caused by point mutations in the *MPZ* gene.

CMT1C

CMT1C is clinically indistinguishable from CMT1A, presenting in the second decade with the classical phenotype. It is a rare cause of CMT, accounting for less than 1% of the CMT population.

CMT1D

The CMT1D phenotype is severe, with patients typically presenting in infancy with possible hypomyelination (hypotonia), delayed motor milestones, and MNCV less than 10 m/s. In addition, scoliosis and cranial nerve involvement may be features. This is a rare phenotype of CMT and is caused by mutations in *EGR2*, a member of the early growth response family. Autosomal-recessive inheritance has also

been described, with *EGR2* mutations (known as CMT4E) causing a very similar clinical phenotype.

CMT1E

CMT1E is caused by point mutations in the *PMP22* gene. Often these patients have an earlier onset with a more severe phenotype, sometimes associated with deafness, compared with CMT1A patients. Onset within the first 2 years of life with a delay in walking is not uncommon; however, the clinical phenotype is variable, and onset may be later. The disease severity depends on the particular *PMP22* mutation, and some cases can be very mild or even resemble HNPP.

HNPP

HNPP is the third most common type of CMT and is an autosomal-dominant disorder, with patients typically presenting with recurrent neuropathies occurring at sites of entrapments. The age of onset is similar to that in CMT1A, although one larger study suggests that over half of HNPP cases have an earlier onset, typically presenting with delay in walking. The literature suggests a wide range of onset, from early childhood

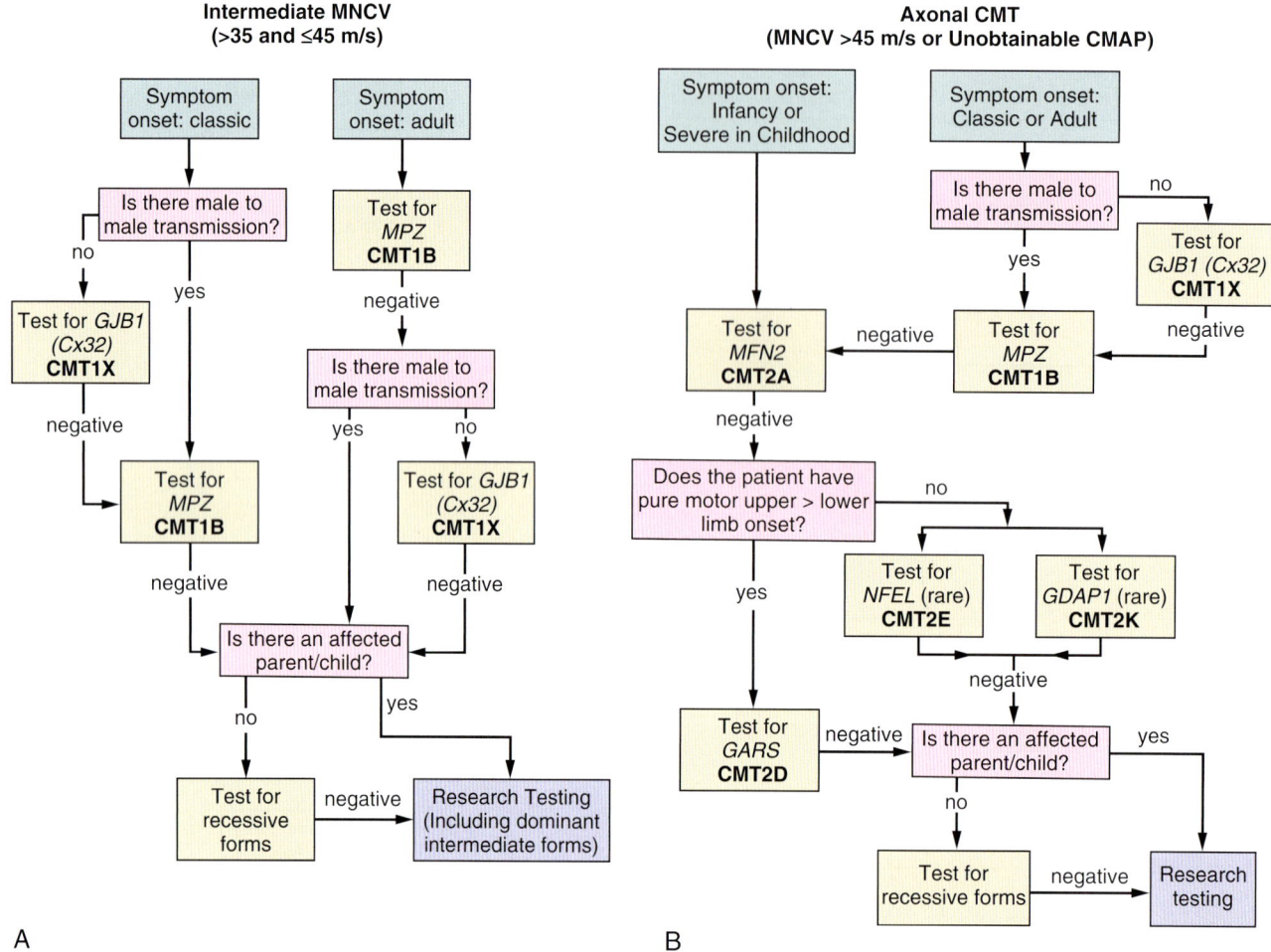

Figure 141-3. Algorithm for the genetic diagnosis of patients with Charcot-Marie-Tooth disease and intermediate (**A**) or normal (**B**) upper extremity motor nerve conduction velocities. *(With permission from Saporta AS et al. Ann Neurol 2011; 69[1]): 22-33.)*

through adulthood. Motor NCVs can be normal but are usually slowed around sites of entrapment such as the fibular head, carpal tunnel, and medial epicondyle. Usually, there is a history of recurrent focal mononeuropathies that are transient, lasting from hours to days or weeks and occasionally longer. HNPP is usually caused by a deletion of *PMP22* or, less commonly, by point mutations in the *PMP22* gene.

CMTX: X-Linked CMT

CMT1X is the main X-linked form of CMT and is caused by mutations in *GJβ1* gene, which encodes the protein connexin32 (Cx32) (Ouvrier, Geevasingha, and Ryan, 2007). This is the second most common form of CMT accounting, for approximately 10% to 15% of CMT. Despite the fact that there are a huge number of mutations described in *GJβ1*, the phenotype in males is virtually the same in all affected males, including those with entire gene deletions, suggesting that mutations lead to a loss of function of the protein. The majority of males will start to have symptoms in childhood, but approximately 20% will have a later onset.

Males are typically more severely affected and tend to have marked atrophy of the intrinsic hand muscles and all compartments of the calf muscles. Males with CMT1X often display a "split hand syndrome," with the abductor pollicis brevis being weaker and more wasted than the first dorsal interosseus. Females with *GJβ1* will usually have abnormalities on neuro-

logic examination or nerve conduction testing. Typically, males with CMTX have MNCVs between 25 and 45 m/s, whereas women have MNCVs in the normal or nearly normal range. Therefore, the presence of nearly normal to intermediate MNCVs in females and slow to intermediate MNCVs in males in families with an absence of male-to-male transmission should prompt the clinician to consider CMT1X.

CMT2: Autosomal-Dominant Axonal Neuropathies

CMT2 is suggested by neurophysiology demonstrating NCVs of greater than 38 m/s in the context of small motor and/or sensory amplitudes. Clinical and electrophysiological data should enable axonal neuropathies to be classified further into pure or predominant sensory form (HSN/HSAN), the mixed motor and sensory form (CMT2), or the pure motor form (dHMN). It is more challenging to obtain a genetic diagnosis in CMT2 because there are many genes known to cause axonal CMT (see http://www.molgen.ua.ac/cmtmutations/), with each gene accountable for only a very small proportion of cases, with the notable exception of *MFN2*. Because disease-causing CMT genes account for the minority of CMT2 patients (around 35%), most CMT2 patients still await an exact genetic diagnosis. Because the number of patients with CMT2 with a genetic diagnosis is, as yet, small, it is difficult to be accurate about exact genotype–phenotype correlations, in particular with regard to age of onset. However, with the advent of improved molecular techniques, it is likely that the number of genetic causes of CMT2 will significantly increase over the next few years. We will discuss only CMT2A, the most common subtype seen. For descriptions of other subtypes, the reader is referred to the online version of this chapter.

CMT2A

CMT2A is the most common type of CMT2, accounting for approximately 20% to 25% of patients with CMT2. This is mostly severe, with onset in infancy or early childhood and with many patients requiring a wheelchair to ambulate by the age of 20. CMT2A is caused by mutations in the nuclear-encoded *MFN2* gene. Often these patients have unrecordable CMAP amplitudes and nerve conduction studies (NCSs) even in the upper extremities, leading to the suggestion to test for *MFN2* mutations as the initial genetic test in such patients. There are a high number of polymorphisms encountered in *MFN2* genetic testing, so care must be taken when ascertaining whether the patient has disease-causing mutations. Most disease-causing mutations are in the GTP-ase domain, coiled-coil domains, or in other evolutionarily conserved regions of the protein. Rarely, some patients present later in life (during childhood, adolescence, or even adulthood) with a milder phenotype.

CMT4: Autosomal-Recessive Neuropathies

CMT4 includes all forms of autosomal-recessive CMT. Typically, demyelinating conduction velocities are seen, although axonal forms of CMT4 exist. CMT4 mostly presents in infancy and should be considered when multiple family members in one generation are affected or if there is a history of consanguinity. We discuss the demyelinating forms first.

CMT4A

CMT4A is caused by mutations in the *GDAP1* gene. This is a severe early-childhood-onset neuropathy with weakness starting in the distal lower extremities and affecting the distal upper extremities within the first decade of life. Progression to wheelchair use is not uncommon, and there may be additional clinical features, such as vocal cord paralysis or hoarseness.

CMT4B1/B2/B3

CMT4B1 neuropathy is characterized by an onset in early childhood with symmetric weakness in all four limbs, with patients typically becoming wheelchair dependent by adulthood (Parman et al., 2004). Additional clinical features of scoliosis and diaphragmatic and facial weakness may be present. CMT4B2 is a similar form with a slightly later age of onset, but symptoms typically begin by age 5 with NCVs around or below 20 m/s. CMT4B1 and CMT4B2 are caused by mutations in myotubularin-related proteins 2 (*MTMR2*) and 13 (*MTMR13*), respectively. *MTMR13* is also called set-binding factor (*SBF-2*). CMT4B3 is caused by AR mutations in *SBF1* and also has a similar phenotype, including focally misfolded myelin, a pathologic feature of all the CMT4Bs.

CMT4C

CMT4C is a recessive neuropathy of slightly later onset, with childhood-adolescent onsets reported. Scoliosis is a particularly common feature and may precede other findings. Occasional additional clinical findings include movement disorders (ataxia and tremors), facial and bulbar weakness, sensorineural deafness, and respiratory insufficiency. Caused by mutations

in the SH3 domain and tetratricopeptide repeat domain 2 (*SH3TC2*) gene, it is the most common of the AR-CMTs in North American and Northern European populations.

CMT4F

CMT4F is caused by mutations in the periaxin gene. Characteristically, patients have demyelinating conductions with a severe early onset neuropathy. Often patients have predominant sensory findings on examination, including sensory ataxia. As with *MFN*, there are a large number of polymorphisms in periaxin, and care should be taken to ensure that mutations segregate with the neuropathy in a family and that the phenotype is appropriate before concluding that mutations are disease causing.

CMT4: Autosomal-Recessive Axonal Neuropathies (Also Known as AR-CMT2). A small number of genes have been found to cause axonal forms of CMT4, also known as AR-CMT2.

Distal Hereditary Motor Neuropathies. The dHMNs are very similar to CMT in that they are inherited length-dependent and slowly progressive neuropathies with onset usually starting in the first 2 decades (Rossor, Kalmar, Greensmith, and Reilly, 2012). They are defined by being exclusively motor in nature. However, many forms have minor sensory abnormalities, and there is a degree of overlap between CMT2 and dHMN in that the same mutation in the same gene can cause both phenotypes within a family, which can be defined as being either CMT or dHMN. Bulbar involvement in dHMN apart from the recurrent laryngeal nerve is rare. Clinical examination confirms distal weakness and wasting with reduced or absent reflexes. Neurophysiology testing reveals reduced motor amplitude potentials with no sensory abnormalities, and electromyography (EMG) testing may reveal a predominantly distal pattern of denervation. Table 141-3 outlines this group of disorders. For many of the dHMNs, the exact genetic mutation remains to be elucidated. The reader is referred to the online version of the chapter for further details of this group of neuropathies.

Hereditary Sensory Neuropathies. The hereditary sensory neuropathies (HSNs) group includes hereditary neuropathies primarily affecting sensory neurons and includes the subtypes of hereditary sensory and motor neuropathies and hereditary sensory and autonomic neuropathies. With HSN, the sensory loss can range from distal numbness with or without loss of proprioception to a complete inability to experience pain and subsequent risk of painless injuries and foot ulcerations. The more severe sensory neuropathies associated with loss of pain can lead to an abnormal mechanical loading in the distal weight-bearing joints; consequent to that, there is significant risk of neuropathic arthropathy and spontaneous fractures. Despite the name of this subtype of neuropathy, motor involvement is commonly observed in patients. The hereditary sensory neuropathies are classified according to their genetic cause and clinical phenotype; however, the majority of these remain genetically unresolved. Table 141-4 summarizes this group of neuropathies. The reader is referred to the online version of the chapter for further details of this group of neuropathies. It is noteworthy that because some of these subtypes (e.g., HSN IV-VII) are both newly described and rare, the range of clinical phenotypes observed in some particular subtypes is unknown (Auer-Grumbach, 2008).

Neuropathies Associated With Inherited Metabolic Disease. It is important to be aware that neuropathies can present as part of a more complex disorder as a result of an inherited metabolic deficit. These conditions are generally

TABLE 141-3 Classification of the Distal Hereditary Motor Neuropathies (HMNs)

Type	Inheritance	Gene/Locus	Specific Phenotype
HMN I	AD	*HSPB1/HSPB8/GARS/DYNCIH1*	Juvenile-onset (2-20 years) dHMN
HMN II	AD	*HSPB1/HSPB8*	Adult-onset typical dHMN/CMT2F or dHMN/CMT2L
HMN III	AR	11q13	Early onset (2-10 years), slowly progressive
HMN IV	AR	11q13	Juvenile onset (months to 20 years), diaphragmatic involvement
HMN V	AD	*GARS*	Juvenile onset (5-20 years), upper limb onset, slowly progressive/CMT2D
HMN V	AD	*BSCL2*	Upper limb onset, +/2 spasticity lower limbs/Silver syndrome
HMN VI	AR	*IGHMBP2*	Spinal muscle atrophy with respiratory distress (SMARD1), infantile-onset respiratory distress
HMN VIIA	AD	2q14	Adult onset, vocal cord paralysis
HMN VIIB	AD	*DCTN1/TRPV4*	Adult onset, vocal cord paralysis, facial weakness
HMN/ALS4	AD	*SETX*	Early onset, pyramidal signs
HMN-J	AR	9p21.1-p12	Juvenile onset, pyramidal features, Jerash origin
Congenital distal SMA	AD	*TRPV4*	Antenatal onset, arthrogryposis

AD, autosomal dominant; AR, autosomal recessive; *HSPB1*, heat-shock protein B1; *HSPB8*, heat-shock protein B8; *GARS*, glycyl-tRNA synthetase; *BSCL2*, Berardinelli-Seip congenital lipodystrophy 2 (Seipin); *DYNC1H1*, cytoplasmic dynein heavy-chain 1; *IGHMBP2*, immunoglobulin mu binding protein 2; *DCTN1*, dynactin1; *TRPV4*, transient receptor vallanoid 4; *SETX*, sentaxin; *SMA*, spinal muscular atrophy.
(Adapted from Reilly MM, Shy ME. J Neurol Neurosurg Psychiatry 2009 80 (12) 1304-14. Copyright 2009. From BMJ Publishing Group Ltd)

much rarer than the more common "umbrella" group of CMT. The neurologic examination needs to be extensive, and the clinician must search extensively for additional neurologic signs, such as ataxia and pyramidal and extrapyramidal deficits. Ophthalmologic involvement and deafness should be specifically investigated. In addition, a good systemic general examination should be performed to look for cutaneous involvement and organomegaly. If a metabolic disorder is suspected, then brain magnetic resonance imaging (MRI) should be done to ascertain if there is brain involvement.

The history is also important. If there are recurrent episodes of neurologic deficit, then specific diagnoses can be considered (e.g., recurrent ataxia with axonal neuropathy in pyruvate dehydrogenase deficiency and acute axonal neuropathy or pure motor neuropathy in porphyria). The main metabolic neuropathies associated with neuropathy are outlined in Table 141-5. These metabolic disorders are discussed more extensively in Chapters 41 through 43. Other genetic neuropathies, such as giant axonal neuropathy and neuroaxonal dystrophy, are discussed in the online version of this chapter.

Differential Diagnosis. Inherited neuropathies must be distinguished from acquired neuropathies (see Chapter 142). Additionally, genetic disorders of the central nervous system (CNS), such as hereditary spastic paraplegia, may mimic inherited neuropathies by causing length-dependent weakness, sensory loss, and foot deformities such as pes cavus; these patients will frequently have upper motor neuron signs, such as increased reflexes or Babinski's signs and do not have neurophysiologic evidence of neuropathy. Neuropathies may present as part of a more multisystem metabolic disorder, such as the leukoencephalopathies, or as part of a more widespread neurologic disorder, such as Friedrich's ataxia or the spinocerebellar ataxias. Hence, the importance of accuracy in clinical phenotyping is paramount.

Treatment Strategies. Despite the great improvement in our biologic understanding of inherited neuropathies, there is still no treatment available for any type of CMT. Physical therapy, occupational therapy, and a few orthopedic procedures are still the cornerstone of all inherited neuropathy treatment. A detailed family history and often examination of family members will be required for prognosis and genetic counseling.

A dedicated multidisciplinary rehabilitation team can significantly contribute to the management of patients with inherited neuropathy and improve functionality and quality of life. Physical therapy strategies to maintain muscle strength and tone, prevent muscle contractures, and improve balance are a common need for most patients. Orthotic aids are an important component of treating these patients, providing support and improving balance for ambulation. Occupational therapy focused on developing tools and strategies to help patients with activities of daily living will benefit patients with inherited neuropathy, especially those with hand weakness. Tendon lengthening and tendon transfers can benefit a subset of patients with muscle contractures and tendon shortening and patients with significant weakness in functionally relevant muscles, respectively; however, the optimal timing of such procedures is still controversial. Foot surgery is sometimes offered to correct inverted feet, pes cavus, and hammertoes. This surgical intervention may improve walking, alleviate pain over pressure points, and prevent plantar ulcers. However, foot surgery is generally unnecessary and does not improve weakness and sensory loss.

Two new technologies recently developed hold huge potential in the search for compounds to treat inherited neuropathy: cellular reprogramming and high-throughput drug screening. Cellular reprogramming is a technique that allows the generation of specific cell types (including stem cell–like cells, neurons, and glia) by genetically modifying readily available somatic cells such as fibroblasts or lymphocytes to generate patient-specific cell lines. These patient-specific cells lines will be particularly useful when combined with high-throughput screening of drug libraries containing thousands of compounds. In these highly automated platforms, the process of identifying compounds capable of correcting certain disease-related cell phenotypes is streamlined, allowing for a faster target selection of compounds to be tested in phase I animal studies.

TABLE 141-5 Inherited Metabolic Disorders Associated With Neuropathy

Category	Disease	Stored Material	Age of Onset	Neurophysiology	Neuropathic Features
1. Lysosomal					
• Mucopolysaccharidoses	Hurler	Dermatan/heparan sulfate	Infantile	Slowing at entrapment sites	Entrapment neuropathy
	Hunter	Dermatan/heparan sulfate	Infantile	Slowing at entrapment sites	Entrapment neuropathy
	Sanfilippo A-D	Heparan sulfate	Infantile	Slowing at entrapment sites	Entrapment neuropathy
• Sphingolipidoses	Krabbe disease	Galactosylceramide	Infantile to adult	NCVs < 10 in young onset	Schwann cell inclusions and segmental demyelination
	Fabry disease	Trihexosylceramide	Adolescence	Small-fiber function abnormal	Lamellar inclusions (perineural cells) and axonal loss
	Metachromatic leukodystrophy	Sulfatide	Late infancy>adolescence	NCVs < 10	Schwann cell ↑ sulfatide and segmental demyelination
• Glycoproteinoses	Fucosidosis	Oligosaccharides	Infantile	Slowing at entrapment sites	Entrapment neuropathy
	α and β mannosidosis	Oligosaccharides	Infantile to adolescence	Slowing at entrapment sites	Axonal inclusion
	Sialidosis I and II	Oligosaccharides	I = juvenile; II = infantile	II = Slowing at entrapment sites	Schwann cell vacuoles and axonal inclusions
	Schindler disease	Oligosaccharides	Infantile	Marked axonopathy	Axonal spheroids
2. Peroxisomal	Adrenomyeloneuropathy	VLCFA	Variable: childhood-adult	Axonal or demyelinating	Schwann cell inclusions and segmental demyelination
	Refsum disease	Phytanic acid	Childhood/adolescence	Slow NCVs	Schwann cell inclusions, onion bulbs and segmental demyelination
	Hyperoxaluria	Calcium oxalate	<5 years	Axonal or demyelinating	Axonal degeneration and segmental demyelination
3. Lipid disorders	Cerebrotendinous xanthomatosis	Cholestanol	Late childhood/adolescence	Clinical symptoms mild; slow NCVs	Axonal loss and Schwann cell vacuoles
	Tangier disease	Cholesterol esters	Childhood/adolescence	Sensory neuropathy; slow NCVs	Axonal loss and Schwann cell vacuoles
	Abetalipoproteinemia		Birth but neuropathy develops in childhood	Sensory neuropathy; sensory CVs prolonged	Axonal degeneration and segmental demyelination
4. Mitochondrial	LCHAD	3-Hydroxy dicarboxylic aciduria	Early infancy	Axonal or demyelinating	Axonal loss and segmental demyelination
	Leigh	Lactate/pyruvate	Early infancy/childhood	Slow NCVs	Segmental demyelination
	NARP	Lactate/pyruvate	Usually adolescence	Sensory demyelinating neuropathy	Segmental demyelination
5. Other	Acute intermittent porphyria	δ = aminolevulinic acid	Usually after puberty	Can be a pure motor axonal picture	Axonal degeneration and segmental demyelination

LCHAD, long-chain 3-hydroxyacyl-CoA dehydrogenase deficiency; NARP = neuropathy, ataxia and retinitis pigmentosa; NCVs = nerve conduction velocities; VLCFA = very-long-chain fatty acids.

Vital to clinical trials in inherited neuropathy is the establishment of solid outcome measures. This can be challenging with neuropathies that progress slowly over many years. To this end, a validated scoring system based on symptoms, signs, and neurophysiological data has been developed for adults that has excellent inter- and intraobserver correlations and can detect changes over 1 year. A more sensitive pediatric scoring system exists for those patients between the ages of 3 and 21, which takes into account growth-related changes and should prove useful in future clinical trials. Sequential yearly MRI of limb muscles looking at progressive replacement of muscle with fatty tissue may also prove to be a valuable outcome measurement and is currently under investigation in a cohort of CMT1A patients.

CONCLUSION

We have entered an exciting period in the study of inherited neuropathy. Investigating CMT has led to the description of several key genes and proteins together with the functional relevance of many others, leading to a better understanding of normal peripheral nerve function and the development of treatment strategies in some of the more common demyelinating inherited neuropathies. Significant challenges remain to be overcome, however, to develop and test treatments to modify disease progression in this heterogenous group of genetic neuropathies.

REFERENCES

 The complete list of references for this chapter is available in the e-book at www.expertconsult.com.

See inside cover for registration details.

SELECTED REFERENCES

Auer-Grumbach, M., 2008. Hereditary sensory neuropathy type I. Orphanet J. Rare Dis. 3 (1).

Harding, A.E., Thomas, P.K., 1980a. Genetic aspects of hereditary motor and sensory neuropathy (types I and II). J. Med. Genet. 17 (5), 329–336.

Harding, A.E., Thomas, P.K., 1980b. The clinical features of hereditary motor and sensory neuropathy types I and II. Brain 103, 259.

Murphy, S.M., Herrmann, D.N., McDermott, M.P., et al. 2011. Reliability of the CMT neuropathy score (second version) in Charcot-Marie-Tooth disease. J. Peripher. Nerv. Syst. 16 (3), 191–198.

Murphy, S.M., Laura, M., Fawcett, K., et al., 2012. Charcot-Marie-Tooth disease: frequency of genetic subtypes and guidelines for genetic testing. J. Neurol. Neurosurg. Psychiatry 83, 706.

Ouvrier, R., Geevasingha, N., Ryan, M.M., 2007. Autosomal-recessive and X-linked forms of hereditary motor and sensory neuropathy in childhood. Muscle Nerve 36 (2), 131–143.

Parman, Y., Battaloglu, E., Baris, I., et al., 2004. Clinicopathological and genetic study of early-onset demyelinating neuropathy. Brain 127, 2540.

Reilly, M.M., Shy, M.E., 2009. Diagnosis and new treatments in genetic neuropathies. J. Neurol. Neurosurg. Psychiatry 80 (12), 1304–1314.

Rossor, A.M., Kalmar, B., Greensmith, L., et al., 2012. The distal hereditary motor neuropathies. J. Neurol. Neurosurg. Psychiatry 83, 6.

Saporta, A.S., Sottile, S.L., Miller, L.J., et al., 2011. Charcot-Marie-Tooth disease subtypes and genetic testing strategies. Ann. Neurol. 69, 22.

E-BOOK FIGURES AND TABLES

The following figures and tables are available in the e-book at www.expertconsult.com. See inside cover for registration details.

142 Acquired Peripheral Neuropathies

Stephen A. Smith

Acquired peripheral neuropathies are caused by a number of infectious, toxic, or metabolic conditions. They may be acute or chronic and classified by the type of peripheral nerve involved—primarily motor, sensory, or autonomic. Pathologically, neuropathies are demyelinating or axonal, depending on whether the main disruption involves the axon or the myelin sheath supported by the Schwann cell. This chapter discusses acquired toxic and metabolic neuropathies occurring in children.

ANATOMY

The peripheral nervous system consists of cranial nerves III through XII, the spinal roots, the nerve plexuses, the peripheral nerves, and the autonomic ganglia. Neuronal cell bodies subserving the nerves in the peripheral nervous system reside in the brainstem; anterior horn cells of the spinal cord; intermediolateral cell column, where the autonomic system originates; and the dorsal root ganglia for afferent sensory function. Peripheral nerves innervate all skeletal muscles via large myelinated nerve fibers. Sensory input from skin, joints, and muscles is transmitted via a combination of unmyelinated and myelinated nerve fibers from the periphery to the central nervous system (CNS).

Evaluation of peripheral nerve diseases includes obtaining a clear history of the distribution and rate of progression of the condition; conducting an appropriate examination; obtaining an electromyogram with nerve conduction velocities, amplitudes, and latencies plus indicated muscle needle electrode study; and, in some instances, performing a sural nerve biopsy. A search for toxins, such as heavy metals, or doing diagnostic tests for metabolic conditions may be indicated. Acquired peripheral neuropathies are not familial or inherited.

FACIAL NERVE PARALYSIS (BELL'S PALSY)

Acute dysfunction of cranial nerve VII, caused by lesions of the facial nerve nucleus in the pons or axial or extraaxial facial nerve, is called Bell's palsy. The result is partial or complete paralysis of the upper and lower facial muscles. Bell's palsy most often results from edema and inflammation of the nerve as it traverses the facial canal within the temporal bone. Lesions involving the facial nerve nucleus or nerve distal to the nucleus result in paralysis of upper (forehead) and lower facial muscles.

Clinical Features

The incidence of Bell's palsy is 2.7 per 100,000 below the age of 10 years, and 10.1 per 100,000 during the second decade of life. Female and male incidence is equal. Ear pain near the mastoid process is the first manifestation of impending facial nerve involvement half of the time. Unilateral inability to close the eyelid and maintain normal facial movement is the initial indication of motor involvement. Facial weakness develops rapidly over several hours to 3 days, resulting in paresis to complete paralysis. Bell's palsy commonly follows an upper respiratory tract infection, indicating possible postinfectious demyelination. Drinking and eating are impaired because of the inability to close the mouth on the involved side.

The differential diagnosis of facial paralysis includes infections, both acute and chronic infections of the inner ear (Özkale et al., 2015), herpes simplex infection, herpes zoster (Ramsay Hunt syndrome), *Mycoplasma pneumoniae* infection, Epstein-Barr virus infection, and Lyme disease (*Borrelia* spp. infection), tumor, acute myeloid leukemia, chemotherapy toxicity, trauma, hypertension, and hypertension secondary to Guillain-Barré syndrome.

Bilateral, congenital facial paralysis, usually in conjunction with ophthalmoplegia involving cranial nerve VI, presents in the newborn as Möbius's syndrome. The condition is the result of aplasia or hypoplasia of cranial nerves and nuclei VI and VII.

Simple asymmetry of facial expression when infants and children are crying is common. The majority of children with asymmetric crying facies are normal.

Laboratory Findings

Uncomplicated facial palsy that resolves relatively quickly does not need detailed evaluation. Palsy that persists or seems atypical requires study. Magnetic resonance imaging (MRI) often reveals gadolinium enhancement of the facial nerve in typical cases of Bell's palsy. MRI can be used in children to find rare tumors invading or compressing the facial nerve.

Treatment and Prognosis

The prognosis for recovery in children is good. Most children do not need drug therapy. A number of drugs have been used, particularly steroids of limited, if any, benefit. Surgical decompression has been recommended in some patients when progressive paralysis and nerve degeneration occur, but benefit is difficult to prove (Zandian et al., 2014). Prednisone is the most widely used drug; it is given in high dosage for 1 week, followed by slow withdrawal of the drug in the second week. The degree to which steroid therapy can alter the natural history of Bell's palsy is unknown, although it appears to be more helpful in completely paralyzed than paretic individuals. Most children recover completely without treatment. Recovery usually begins within 2 to 4 weeks, reaching its maximum within 6 to 12 months and most within 3 months. In meta-analyses comparing steroids to antiviral treatment, usually acyclovir, there is no added advantage in adding antiviral treatment to steroid treatment.

BRACHIAL PLEXUS

Nerve roots from the fifth cervical through the first thoracic nerves form the three primary trunks of the brachial plexus. Once formed, they divide promptly into anterior and posterior divisions. The posterior divisions join to form the posterior cord, which gives rise to the upper and lower subscapular, thoracodorsal, axillary, and radial nerves. The anterior divisions of the fifth, sixth, and seventh nerves form the lateral cord, and the anterior divisions of the eighth cervical and first thoracic nerves form the medial cord. The lateral cord subsequently gives rise to the musculocutaneous nerve and a branch to the coracobrachialis. The medial cord gives rise to the ulnar, medial antebrachial cutaneous, and medial brachial cutaneous nerves. Additional branches from the lateral and medial cords unite to form the median nerve.

METABOLIC NEUROPATHIES
Diabetes Mellitus

It has been known for a long time that up to 10% of children with insulin-dependent diabetes mellitus have symptoms and signs caused by peripheral neuropathy associated with diabetes. These bilaterally symmetric changes, especially in the lower extremities, include mild distal weakness, loss of touch and pain sensation, and decreased ankle tendon reflexes. Despite good management of diabetes, impaired nerve function occurs.

Subclinical diabetic neuropathy is now estimated to occur in half of all children with type 1 diabetes after 5 years of known disease. Reduced motor nerve excitability determined by compound muscle action potential (CMAP) measurements is reduced early in type 1 diabetes mellitus, probably before irreversible axonal damage occurs.

It is clear that careful clinical and electrophysiologic follow-up is required to monitor altered peripheral and autonomic nerve function in childhood-onset diabetes mellitus (Höliner et al., 2013). Blood sugar control, as measured by hemoglobin A1c, and duration of diabetes are significant in the causation of diabetic peripheral neuropathy. The importance of strict metabolic control is helpful in slowing the development and progression of diabetic neuropathy. Peripheral neuropathy is common in young, insulin-dependent diabetics.

Uremic Neuropathy

Uremic neuropathy is rarely diagnosed in children. When recognized, it is characterized by burning sensations in the feet and a symmetric motor sensory neuropathy with progressive muscle weakness. Motor nerve and sensory nerve conduction velocities are decreased early in the course of the disease, often before clinical symptoms appear. Electrophysiologic findings in an adolescent showed a primary axonal sensorimotor polyneuropathy. Sural nerve biopsy showed focal loss of myelinated axons along with axonal degeneration. The facial nerve is a sensitive indicator of uremic neuropathy.

Acute Intermittent Porphyria

This rare inborn error of metabolism, inherited on an autosomal-dominant basis, is caused by mutations in the hydroxymethylbilane synthase (*HMBS*) gene on chromosome 11q23.3. Acute intermittent porphyria (AIP) is diagnosed on the basis of characteristic clinical symptoms, elevated levels of urinary porphyrin precursors aminolevulinic acid (ALA) and porphobilinogen (PBG), and a decreased erythrocytic HMBS activity, although an identifiable HMBS mutation provides the ultimate proof for AIP. Gene carriers are at risk of developing potentially fatal neurogenic attacks if exposed to precipitating factors, including certain medications like tricyclic antidepressants, barbiturates, halothane, valproic acid, sulfonamides, estrogens, and alcohol. Axonal damage, observed on both

sural nerve biopsy and autopsy evaluation, suggests that the neuropathy is primarily axonal. The neuropathy is predominantly motor, with associated abdominal pain, dysautonomia, and CNS involvement. It has been made worse with exposure to antiepilepsy medications, phenytoin and carbamazepine, but not clonazepam.

Acute, severe, colicky abdominal pain is a typical manifestation of an acute episode, accompanied by CNS and peripheral nervous system impairment. Peripherally, motor weakness is most striking, but sensory impairment may also occur.

Vitamin Deficiency

Classic thiamine deficiency in children causes peripheral neuropathy, encephalopathy, and high-output cardiac failure. Infantile beriberi disease has been described in infants born to mothers with thiamine deficiency (Renthal et al., 2014).

Thiamine deficiency can develop secondary to anorexia nervosa in adolescents producing a peripheral neuropathy and Wernicke encephalopathy.

Vitamin E (alpha-tocopherol) deficiency may be associated with peripheral neuropathy and ataxia. It may also occur in children with cystic fibrosis, chronic cholestasis, abetalipoproteinemia, short bowel syndrome, and intestinal malabsorption states.

Congenital Pernicious Anemia

Two forms of pernicious anemia in children are associated with peripheral neuropathy. One occurs as a congenital or early onset disease in children. Congenital pernicious anemia occurs before age 5 years as a result of a vitamin B_{12} deficiency caused by isolated absence of gastric intrinsic factor that may produce a severe and irreversible neuropathy (Dobrozsi et al., 2014). A later-onset form of pernicious anemia resembles that seen in adults. This is histamine-fast achlorhydria associated with gastric mucosal atrophy and the presence of antibodies to parietal cells and intrinsic factor in the serum. These children may experience a variety of endocrinologic disorders. Pathologic changes develop in spinal cord and, less commonly, in peripheral nerve and brain.

Infants who are breastfed by strictly vegetarian mothers or who have undiagnosed pernicious anemia are at risk for developing a megaloblastic anemia because of a deficiency of vitamin B_{12}.

Abetalipoproteinemia

Abetalipoproteinemia, known as Bassen-Kornzweig syndrome, is a rare condition characterized by progressive ataxic neuropathy, retinitis pigmentosa, steatorrhea, hypolipidemia, deficiency of fat-soluble vitamins, failure to thrive, and acanthocytosis. The disease results from mutations in the gene encoding microsomal triglyceride transfer protein (*MTTP*) located on chromosome 4q24. Affected individuals are unable to make beta-lipoproteins to carry fats, cholesterol, and fat-soluble vitamins A, D, E, and K in the blood, and therefore fat absorption is impaired. Sufficient levels of fats, cholesterol, and vitamins are necessary for normal growth and development. Nerve cells and the retina are particularly vulnerable.

Pathology

Degeneration of posterior columns, spinal cerebellar pathways, and cerebellum, caused by vitamin E deficiency, is the major pathologic change. Loss of anterior horn cells is found in the spinal cord. Posterior column degeneration leads to abnormal somatosensory-evoked potentials. Sural nerve biopsy shows decreased numbers of large myelinated fibers and clusters of regenerating fibers. The posterior fundus of the eye shows a loss of photoreceptors, loss or attenuation of pigment epithelium, and preservation of submacular pigment epithelium, with an excessive accumulation of lipofuscin. Macrophage-like pigmented cells invade the retina.

Clinical Characteristics

The most significant neurologic finding is a progressive ataxia that may be present as early as 2 years of age but certainly by age 6. Generalized weakness, ptosis, and extraocular muscle weakness develop. The lower cranial nerves may be involved, with facial and tongue weakness plus twitching movements. A progressive peripheral sensory neuropathy causing hypesthesia, hypalgesia, and proprioceptive loss is associated with absent tendon reflexes. Generalized muscle weakness and wasting may be severe. Intestinal malabsorption produces bulky, foul stools and leads to a delay in normal growth.

Alpha-Lipoprotein Deficiency (Tangier Disease)

Tangier disease is an uncommon autosomal recessive disorder of lipoprotein metabolism, notable for the absence of normal high-density lipoprotein (HDL) from plasma and the accumulation of cholesterol esters in multiple organs. Extremely low plasma cholesterol levels are present. Physical examination shows patches of yellow-orange lymphoid tissue in the tonsils and pharynx, and hepatosplenomegaly. Yellow patches are present on the surface of the liver, and liver biopsy specimens contain cholesterol esters. Fiberscopic rectal examination shows orange-brown spots present throughout the rectum. Foam cells are present in lymphoid tissues. . Onset is between age 2 and 67 years. Sural nerve biopsy shows a reduction of smaller myelinated and unmyelinated fibers, and abnormalities in the paranodal regions. There is lipid deposition, redundant myelin foldings, myelin splitting and vesiculation, and small tomacula. Abnormal lipid storage is found in Schwann cells of unmyelinated fibers. Conduction block is present on electrophysiologic nerve study.

Clinical Characteristics

Recurrent neuropathy occurs in children with fluctuating asymmetric sensory involvement, mostly in the lower extremities, sometimes accompanied by progressive development of weakness of both distal and proximal muscles. Complaints of numbness and tingling in the distal extremities are early symptoms, followed by signs of the neuropathy and weakness. A dissociated loss of pain and temperature sensation may occur.

Krabbe's Disease (Globoid Cell Leukodystrophy)

Galactosylceramide lipidosis, known as Krabbe's disease or globoid cell leukodystrophy, is an autosomal-recessive neurodegenerative disorder that presents most often in infants of 3 to 5 months of age. The clinical profile is a highly irritable infant with spasticity, optic atrophy, intellectual delay, and polyneuropathy, which may be the initial presentation. Children have gross motor delay, absent tendon reflexes, elevated CSF protein levels, and delayed motor nerve conduction velocities before neurodegenerative disease is evident.

Metachromatic Leukodystrophy

Metachromatic leukodystrophy is a recessively inherited disease affecting children and adults caused by mutations in the *ARSA* or *PSAP* genes resulting in a failure of the catabolism of sulfatide, the sulfate ester of galactose cerebroside. Infants may present with cranial neuropathy and multiple cranial nerve enhancement on MRI.

Clinically, in the infantile form of metachromatic leukodystrophy, the infant acquires normal milestones until 1 to 2 years of age and then begins to show signs of the disease. An unsteady gait is an early sign, accompanied by loss of language, intellectual deterioration, and, later, spasticity. Spinal fluid protein is elevated, and nerve conduction velocities are slowed. The juvenile form of the disease occurs after several years of age, again with gait disturbance followed by intellectual deterioration.

Refsum's Disease (Heredopathia Atactica Polyneuritiformis) and Peroxisome Biogenesis Disorders

Refsum's disease is a recessively inherited condition caused by a deficiency of phytanoyl-coenzyme A hydroxylase allowing the accumulation of phytanic acid in body tissues. Retinitis pigmentosa and anosmia are early signs of the disease that is carried on chromosome 10 as a result of *PHYH* gene mutations.

Refsum's disease is one of the peroxisomal disorders, Zellweger's syndrome and neonatal adrenoleukodystrophy being the other two. They are characterized by absence of catalase-positive peroxisomes and general impairment of peroxisomal functions. Presentations include anorexia, ataxia, ichthyosis, and sensorineural hearing loss with malabsorption and steatorrhea presenting early on. Clinical characteristics can be divided into three groups: congenital abnormalities, such as skeletal deformities; retinitis pigmentosa, which develops slowly; and lesions, including neuropathy, rash, and cardiac arrhythmias, which can deteriorate or improve according to plasma phytanic acid level.

Phytanic acid, a branched chain fatty acid, is present in a wide range of foodstuffs, including dairy produce, meat, and fish. There is toxic accumulation of phytanic acid in blood, fat, and neurons. Normally, phytanic acid levels are virtually undetectable in plasma. However, patients with Refsum's disease have extremely high levels with phytanic acid accounting for 5% to 30% of their total fatty acids.

TOXIC NEUROPATHIES
Diphtheria

Diphtheria is an uncommon disease in the Western Hemisphere because most individuals are immunized with diphtheria-pertussis-tetanus vaccine. The disease occurs in unimmunized children and in adults who have lost immunity. An exotoxin produced by *Corynebacterium diphtheriae* infection in the throat produces cardiomyopathy and neuropathy. A systemic radiculoneuropathy may develop, with onset 1 to 16 weeks after infection and marked by sensory loss.

Neuropathy of Serum Sickness

Serum sickness is a systemic illness resulting from hypersensitivity to an injected foreign protein, such as tetanus or diphtheria antisera, producing encephalomyelitis, neuropathy, or brachial plexus neuropathies. Fever, joint swelling, abdominal pain, diarrhea, and cutaneous eruptions develop within days of receiving foreign protein. Deposition of antigen-antibody complexes is associated with disease.

Antibiotic-Induced Neuropathy

A number of antibiotic, antifungal, and antituberculous drugs have been known to cause peripheral neuropathy in a small percentage of cases. For example, chloramphenicol can cause mild, primarily sensory, peripheral neuropathy after long-term use at relatively high doses. Nitrofurantoin may produce a polyneuropathy of sudden onset on rare occasion. Isoniazid causes an axonal neuropathy responsive to pyridoxine therapy in 1% to 2% of patients. The primarily sensory neuropathy begins with paresthesias.

There have been a number of reports of peripheral neuropathy, mainly in adults, associated with the use of fluoroquinolones, ciprofloxacin and levofloxacin , ofloxacin, lomefloxacin, and trovafloxacin.

Pyridoxine-Induced Polyneuropathy

Pyridoxine is an essential cofactor in the metabolism of proteins, carbohydrates, fatty acids, and brain amines. Pyridoxine taken in large doses can cause a sensory neuropathy, with paresthesias, diffuse sensory loss, sensory ataxia, and autonomic dysfunction. Prescribing 50 mg/day or greater amounts for prolonged periods is discouraged.

Pyridoxine deficiency causes a sensory neuropathy, unless severe when motor nerve fibers may also be involved along with CNS dysfunction. Treatment is straight forward with increased dietary pyridoxine intake from foods high in pyridoxine such as vegetables, potatoes, eggs, and dairy products.

Nitrous Oxide–Induced Polyneuropathy

Severe myeloneuropathy and macrocytic anemia associated with a low vitamin B_{12} level are reported after prolonged exposure to nitrous oxide. B_{12} supplementation alone does not result in improvement, but the addition of methionine does arrest the progression of neuropathy. Chronic nitrous oxide exposure inhibits methionine synthetase activity, which remains suppressed after nitrous oxide exposure has ended, underscoring the need for treatment with methionine. Continuous exposure to nitrous oxide for longer than 3 hours causes neuropathy, especially in B_{12}-deficient individuals (Richardson, 2010).

Chemotherapeutic Agent–Induced Neuropathy

Peripheral neuropathy may develop after the use of chemotherapeutic agents to treat neoplasms. Painful sensorimotor peripheral neuropathy may develop after high-dose cytosine arabinoside therapy, and is manifested pathologically by axonal degeneration and scattered destruction of myelin sheaths. The neuropathy is marked by dysesthesias, muscle aching, and progressive weakness. Cytosine arabinoside neuropathic pain may respond to carbamazepine.

Vincristine is often used in children to treat acute lymphoblastic leukemia and may cause acute axonal sensorimotor neuropathy. Less commonly, it may cause autonomic and cranial nerve neuropathy.

Vaccine-Induced Polyneuropathy

The diphtheria-pertussis-tetanus vaccine may rarely produce segmental demyelination and axonal neuropathy from the tetanus toxoid component. Although very rare, demyelinating symmetric neuropathy, when it does occur, responds to immunomodulatory therapy. Rare transient postvaccination polyneuropathy has been reported with complete recovery. CDC (http://www.cdc.gov/flu) recommendations for people who should receive influenza vaccinations are as follows:

Children aged 6 months and older.
Pregnant women
People 50 years of age and older
People of any age with certain chronic medical conditions such as chronic lung, heart, liver, or kidney diseases; blood disorders; and diabetes mellitus
People who live in nursing homes and other long-term care facilities
People who live with or care for those at high risk for complications from influenza
   Healthcare workers
   Household contacts of persons at high risk for complications from influenza
Household contacts and out-of-home caregivers of children less than 6 months of age. Hepatitis B vaccination has been associated with neuropathy in case reports from adults. Acute sensory neuropathy has been reported in a 13-year-old after bacille Calmette-Guérin (BCG) vaccination.

Heavy Metal Neuropathy

Excessive exposure to various forms of lead, both organic and inorganic, produces an axonal neuropathy. It is rare in children but presents typically with foot drop but also with weakness of wrist and finger extensors.

Arsenic is a metalloid element, and high-dose exposure can cause severe systemic toxicity and death. The *NALP2* polymorphism is associated with increased risk of tissue and chromosomal damage from arsenic exposure. Arsenic is an essential ultratrace element in animals. Rare instances of arsenic poisoning, often intentional, have been reported, producing an axonal, sensory-predominant neuropathy.

One source of toxic methylmercury (MeHg) is from the consumption of marine fish and mammals. There is concern for potential neurodevelopmental effects from early life exposure to low levels of MeHg. Continuing exposure may include development of peripheral neuropathy. The European project DEMOCOPHES analyzed mercury (Hg) in hair in 1799 mother-child pairs from 17 European countries comparing results to marine fish and seafood consumption. Eating marine fish and seafood once per week had mercury levels well below health-based limit values established by USA-EPA and WHO. Concern is raised for higher exposures given the presence of mercury in the environment for many years to come and the bioaccumulation in aquatic food chains. The study recommends continuing monitoring of methylmercury exposure (Bora et al., 2014).

VASCULITIC NEUROPATHIES

Cryoglobulinemia may present with a sensory neuropathy and painful dysesthesia because of small-fiber axonal involvement usually in adults, and often in the context of hepatitis C. Rare instances of cryoglobulinemia are reported in children. One child had lower-extremity and one-hand vasculitis, non–hepatitis C, M-spike disease with presumed nerve involvement responsive to steroids. Fever is more common in children with cryoglobulinemia than in adults. Demyelinating neuropathy after vaccination is a rare event with distally predominant sensory symptoms with no or mild distal weakness. Immunomodulatory therapy is effective for treatment. In a study in infants to investigate immune responses to influenza vaccine after two doses of trivalent inactivated influenza vaccine 4 weeks apart, no findings for neuropathy were reported (Hwang et al., 2014).

Organophosphorus pesticides are used as insecticides in agriculture and as eradication agents for termites around homes. Organophosphate intoxication causes cholinergic symptoms early and subsequently a neuropathy with axonal degeneration producing muscle cramping and calf pain along with tingling and burning sensations in the feet. Distal muscle weakness may develop. Neuropsychological assessment of healthy school-aged children exposed to organophosphate pesticides has demonstrated cognitive impairment.

REFERENCES

The complete list of references for this chapter is available in the e-book at www.expertconsult.com.

See inside cover for registration details.

SELECTED REFERENCES

Bora, B., Pino, A., Alimonti, A., et al., 2014. Toxic metals contained in cosmetics: a status report. Regul. Toxicol. Pharmacol. 68, 447.

Dobrozsi, S., Flood, V.H., Panepinto, J., et al., 2014. Vitamin B12 deficiency: the great masquerader. Pediatr. Blood Cancer 61, 753.

Höliner, I., Haslinger, V., Lütschg, J., et al., 2013. Validity of the neurological examination in diagnosing diabetic peripheral neuropathy. Pediatr. Neurol. 49, 171.

Hwang, K.P., Hsu, Y.L., Hsieh, T.H., et al., 2014. Immunogenicity and safety of a trivalent inactivated 2010–2011 influenza vaccine in Taiwan infants aged 6–12 months. Vaccine 32, 2469.

Özkale, Y., Erol, I., Saygi, S., et al., 2015. Overview of pediatric peripheral facial nerve paralysis: analysis of 40 patients. J. Child Neurol. 30, 193.

Renthal, W., Marin-Valencia, I., Evans, P.A., 2014. Thiamine deficiency secondary to anorexia nervosa: an uncommon cause of peripheral neuropathy and Wernicke encephalopathy in adolescence. Pediatr. Neurol. 51, 100.

Richardson, P.G., 2010. Peripheral neuropathy following nitrous oxide abuse. Emerg. Med. Australas. 22, 88.

Zandian, A., Osiro, S., Hudson, R., et al., 2014. The neurologist's dilemma: a comprehensive clinical review of Bell's palsy, with emphasis on current management trends. Med. Sci. Monit. 20, 83.

E-BOOK FIGURES AND TABLES

The following figures and tables are available in the e-book at www.expertconsult.com. See inside cover for registration details.

Fig. 142-1 Normal sural nerve in an infant.

Fig. 142-2 Schematic pathway of the facial nerve (cranial nerve VII).

Fig. 142-3 Relationship of the brachial plexus to peripheral nerves of the shoulder and arm.

Box 142-1 Facial weakness in childhood

Table 142-1 Clinical localization of facial nerve lesions

143 Inflammatory Neuropathies

Malcolm Rabie, Stephen Ashwal, and Yoram Nevo

⊗ An expanded version of this chapter is available on www.expertconsult.com. See inside cover for registration details.

Inflammatory neuropathies are important causes of peripheral nerve disease in childhood because of their relative frequency and response to treatment. Their main etiologies in childhood are acute and chronic immune-mediated polyradiculoneuropathies. Other etiologies such as collagen vascular diseases, rheumatoid arthritis, systemic lupus erythematosus, or mixed connective tissue disease are rare in children.

Acute and chronic immune-mediated polyradiculoneuropathies are acquired autoimmune-mediated disorders in which peripheral nerves become inflamed leading to **varying degrees of weakness**. They are not exclusively demyelinating; axonal forms responding favorably to immunotherapy also occur. Current data suggest that loss of immunologic tolerance to myelin or axonal antigens trigger autoreactive T-cells and circulating autoantibodies (cellular and humoral factors) either independently or in concert with each other, which then play a fundamental role in the cause of these immune-mediated neuropathies (Dalakas, 2015). Nodal, paranodal, and juxtaparanodal regions of the node of Ranvier may present antigenic targets in some of these disorders, causing nerve conduction failure and rapid recovery (Dalakas, 2015).

Acute onset immune-mediated polyradiculoneuropathy or Guillain-Barré syndrome (GBS) is the most common acquired immune-mediated peripheral neuropathy, and the most frequent cause of acute flaccid paralysis worldwide, constituting one of the serious neurologic emergencies (Yuki and Hartung, 2012). However, GBS is an uncommon disorder and is less frequent among children than in adults. GBS typically has been linked to inflammatory destruction of myelin sheaths in peripheral nerves and roots, termed *acute inflammatory demyelinating polyradiculoneuropathy* (AIDP). The categorization of GBS has evolved. For many years GBS was considered synonymous with AIDP, the demyelinating form most commonly encountered in the Western world, until axonal forms were defined in 1986 and in the 1990s in East Asia (northern China and Japan). In 2001 this led to the division of GBS based on whether motor or sensory nerve fibers are involved and whether myelin sheaths or axons are predominantly affected. Four main subtypes are described: (1) acute inflammatory demyelinating polyradiculoneuropathy (AIDP) (motor and sensory nerve fibers involved); (2) acute motor axonal neuropathy (AMAN); (3) acute motor and sensory axonal neuropathy (AMSAN); and (4) Miller Fisher syndrome (MFS/FS). Additional GBS variants with atypical features are rare (Table 143-3) (Yuki and Hartung, 2012).

Chronic inflammatory demyelinating polyradiculoneuropathy (CIDP), although rare in childhood, is the second most common cause of chronic sensorimotor peripheral neuropathy in children. This slow onset immune-mediated disorder presents with either a monophasic subacute course that later relapses, or a slowly progressive course. CIDP patients have proximal and distal symmetric weakness, paresthesias, and hyporeflexia or areflexia. In both GBS and CIDP, high CSF protein with a normal cell count is present.

Evidence-based data regarding the efficacy of GBS and CIDP immunotherapy in children are lacking, relying on retrospective data, open-label studies on small numbers of children, and data derived primarily from adult trials. Immunotherapy (intravenous human immunoglobulin [IVIg] or plasma exchange [PE]) shorten GBS recovery time with most children recovering completely. Childhood CIDP usually responds to corticosteroids, IVIg, and PE. CIDP children who become resistant to corticosteroids or IVIg, or who become steroid dependent, present a therapeutic challenge. Childhood CIDP prognosis is mostly favorable.

GUILLAIN-BARRÉ SYNDROME

GBS is a descriptive clinical entity, presenting as a monophasic, nonfebrile, postinfectious illness characterized by acute or subacute progression lasting up to 28 days, a variable plateau phase, and then recovery over weeks to months or in some cases over a more prolonged period. Weakness beginning distally in the legs; ascending rapidly, progressively, and symmetrically to the arms, face, and muscles of respiration, with or without sensory disturbances, hyporeflexia, or areflexia; and a high cerebrospinal fluid (CSF) protein with normal cell count (albuminocytologic dissociation) are the hallmarks for its diagnosis in children and adults. GBS usually remits spontaneously. The spectrum of GBS presents either typically (classic GBS) or atypically (Figure 143-1), with prominent ⊗ differences in geographic distribution (Asbury, 2000).

Epidemiology

GBS incidence worldwide is reported as 0.16 to 4/100,000/year. A systematic literature review estimated overall GBS incidence in children aged 0 to 15 years as 0.34 to 1.34/100,000/year from Latin America, Middle East, USA, Finland and Taiwan. It affects all ages, genders, and races, and is rare in children younger than age 2 years or in adults greater than age 80 years. Men are about 1.5 times more likely to be affected than woman (Hughes and Cornblath, 2005). AIDP is the most common GBS subtype in North America, Europe, and Australia affecting all ages (Asbury, 2000). In northern China, Japan, Asia, Latin America, and the developing world, axonal forms occur more frequently (Hughes and Cornblath, 2005; Yuki and Hartung, 2012). Atypical cases such as polyneuritis cranialis and MFS are much less common.

Antecedent Events

Initial GBS symptoms usually present 1 to 6 weeks after antecedent respiratory or gastrointestinal infections, or vaccinations in about 26% to 85% of children and approximately 60% of adults, suggesting that a range of bacteria and viruses trigger the syndrome (Box 143-1) (Hughes and Cornblath, ⊗ 2005; Korinthenberg, 2013). *Campylobacter jejuni* infection may be followed by any subtype of GBS but is more frequent with axonal forms (Hughes and Cornblath, 2005).

GBS declined with USA influenza vaccination campaigns between 1990 and 2003; however, a very small increased risk of GBS (1 per million above background incidence) occurred with influenza vaccinations between 1992 and 1994. Rabies

TABLE 143-3 Guillain-Barré Syndrome Subtypes and Rare Variants Described in Childhood

	Relative Frequency	Associated IgG-Antiganglioside Antibodies
SUBTYPES		
Acute inflammatory demyelinating polyradiculoneuropathy (AIDP)	Common (more in Western world)	None/GM1 (~10%)
Acute motor axonal neuropathy (AMAN)	Common (more in developing countries)	GM1, GD1a
Acute motor and sensory axonal neuropathy (AMSAN)	Rare	GM1, GM1b, GD1a
Miller Fisher syndrome (MFS/FS)	Uncommon	GQ1b, GT1a
VARIANTS		
Bickerstaff brainstem encephalitis (BBE)	Rare	GQ1b, GT1a
Polyneuritis cranialis (PC)	Rare	GQ1b, GT1a
Pharyngeal-cervical-brachial variant (PCB)	Rare	GT1a > GQ1b ≫ GD1a
Acute sensory neuropathy	Very rare	GQ1b, GT1a
Acute pandysautonomia	Very rare	
Acute opthalmoparesis	Very rare	GQ1b, GT1a
Paraparesis	Very rare	

vaccine has a GBS risk of about 1 in 1000 individuals. The risk of GBS or CIDP relapse after immunization is low. However, precaution is required when there is a history of GBS or CIDP, and specifically if they occurred within 6 weeks after a vaccination. For specific vaccination guidelines after immune-mediated neuropathies, the *Red Book* published by the American Academy of Pediatrics should be consulted. Rarely, GBS can be the presenting manifestation or develop during the course of lymphoma or systemic lupus erythematosus.

Clinical Features of AIDP (GBS)

AIDP appears similar in children and adults, except children recover faster with fewer residua. The main presenting feature is initial rapid bilateral relatively symmetric ascending weakness beginning in the legs and progressing to the arms, face, and respiratory muscles within ≤4 weeks before a plateau is reached. Eighty percent of children reach maximum severity with inability to walk unaided within 2 weeks after onset, and 90% to 98% of children and adults reach maximum severity by 4 weeks (Hughes and Cornblath, 2005). Early generalized hyporeflexia or areflexia is typical. Cranial nerve involvement occurs early in about 30% of children, and later on in nearly 50%. The facial nerve is the most common cranial nerve affected, often bilaterally. After 7 to 10 days about 60% of children and adults are unable to walk, and respiratory compromise occurs in about 17% to 30% of adults (Hughes and Cornblath, 2005) and about 15% (4.4% to 24%) of children. Respiratory insufficiency and need for artificial ventilation correlate with severe upper limb involvement, degree of disability at nadir (disease peak), and dysautonomias in childhood GBS (Korinthenberg, 2013). Pain is a very prominent early complaint in about 50% to 79% of children and adults at the peak of the disease, and precedes the weakness in some children. In preschool children, weakness and pain often present with gait disturbances or refusal to walk (Asbury, 2000).

Transient dysautonomias, including arrhythmias and labile blood pressure, may be life-threatening and are reported in about 20% of adults and 3.7% to 77% of children with GBS. Transient bladder dysfunction occurs in 15% to 19.5% of childhood GBS. Children with a more severe acute phase may need catheterization and bladder decompression. Impaired swallowing, gastroesophageal dysmotility, pseudoobstruction, hypotension, urinary incontinence/retention, bowel incontinence/constipation, hyperhidrosis, and vasomotor instability may occur in GBS. Rarely cardiac arrest secondary to autonomic dysfunction is described in children. Box 143-2 outlines the classic GBS clinical presentation in children.

BOX 143-2 Classic Guillain-Barré Syndrome Presentation in Children

- Symmetric ascending paralysis
- Diminished or absent reflexes
- Often severe pain—may lead to a delay in diagnosis

Acute Motor Axonal Neuropathy

Initially AMAN described a summer epidemic of acute ascending paralysis in children in northern China, strongly associated with prior *Campylobacter jejuni* infections (Asbury, 2000). Compared with AIDP, AMAN patients less frequently have cranial nerve involvement and generally have pure motor neuropathy involving only motor axons with sparing of the sensory axons. Around 10% of patients with AMAN have normal or exaggerated tendon reflexes throughout the disease, which could cause a diagnostic delay (Yuki and Hartung, 2012). AMAN patients have little or no dysautonomias, more rapid progression, and an earlier disease peak than AIDP (Hughes and Cornblath, 2005; Yuki and Hartung, 2012). Differences between AIDP and AMAN in childhood are outlined in Table 143-4.

Other Subtypes and Variants of GBS

Several clinical subtypes of GBS have been characterized and are discussed online (Table 143-3) (Yuki and Hartung, 2013).

Diagnostic Challenges of GBS in Childhood

Pain and walking difficulties may cause misdiagnosis of this potentially life-threatening disease in children. Presentation early in life may be less classic, with acute severe hypotonia, and may raise concerns of an encephalopathic process with meningismus, vomiting, and headache. Back pain and Babinski sign in an uncooperative child early on in GBS make differentiation from a spinal cord process difficult. Less commonly, weakness starting proximally may be confused with muscle disease. Occasionally botulism with weakness in the face and arms may cause diagnostic confusion.

GBS Diagnostic Criteria

GBS diagnostic criteria and exclusionary features (Asbury, 2000) are outlined in Box 143-3.

BOX 143-3 Clinical and Laboratory Features in the Diagnosis of Guillain-Barré Syndrome

I. REQUIRED FOR DIAGNOSIS
- Progressive motor weakness of more than one limb
- Areflexia—loss of ankle-jerk reflex and diminished knee and biceps reflexes suffice, if other features are consistent with the diagnosis

II. STRONGLY SUPPORTIVE OF THE DIAGNOSIS
- Progression—weakness may develop rapidly but cease to progress after 4 weeks; roughly 50% will plateau within 2 weeks, 80% by 3 weeks, and 90% after 4 weeks
- Relative symmetry
- Mild sensory symptoms or signs
- Cranial nerve involvement; facial weakness develops in about half of patients
- Autonomic dysfunction
- Absence of fever at the onset of neurologic symptoms
- Recovery—usually recovery begins 2 to 4 weeks after progression ceases; it may be delayed for months
- Variants
  - Fever at onset of symptoms
  - Severe sensory loss with pain
  - Progressive phase longer than 4 weeks
  - Lack of recovery or major permanent residual deficit
- Sphincter dysfunction—sphincters are usually spared, although transient bladder paralysis may occur
- CNS involvement

III. FEATURES CASTING DOUBT ON THE DIAGNOSIS
- Marked persistent asymmetry in motor function
- Persistent bowel or bladder dysfunction
- Bowel or bladder dysfunction at onset of symptoms
- Discrete sensory level

IV. FEATURES THAT EXCLUDE THE DIAGNOSIS
- History of recent hexacarbon abuse
- Evidence of porphyria
- Recent diphtheria
- Features consistent with lead neuropathy and evidence of lead intoxication
- A pure sensory syndrome
- Definite diagnosis of an alternate paralytic disorder

(With permission of Asbury AK, Cornblath DR. Assessment of current diagnostic criteria for Guillain-Barré syndrome. Ann Neurol 1990;27:S21.)

BOX 143-4 Differential Diagnosis of Guillain-Barré Syndrome

CEREBRAL
- Bilateral strokes
- Hysteria

CEREBELLAR
- Acute cerebellar ataxia syndrome (multiple etiologies)
- Posterior fossa structural lesion

SPINAL
- Poliomyelitis
- Compressive myelopathy
- Transverse myelitis
- Anterior spinal artery syndrome

PERIPHERAL NERVE
- CIDP
- Toxic neuropathy:
  - *Drugs:* amitriptyline, dapsone, glutethimide, hydralazine, isoniazid, nitrofurantoin, nitrous oxide, incrusting
  - *Toxins:* acrylamide, glue sniffing, fish toxins, heavy metals (lead, arsenic, mercury, thallium), insecticides, N-hexane and other solvents, organophosphates, snake venom
- Critical illness neuropathy
- Vasculitis
- Diphtheria
- Tick paralysis
- Porphyria

NEUROMUSCULAR JUNCTION
- Botulism
- Myasthenia gravis
- Neuromuscular-blocking agents

MUSCLE DISEASES
- Acute viral myositis
- Acute inflammatory myopathies (polymyositis, dermatomyositis)
- Metabolic myopathies (multiple types)
- Periodic paralysis
- Hypo- or hyperkalemia
- Critical illness myopathy

Differential Diagnosis

A variety of other peripheral and occasional CNS disorders can be confused with GBS. These are outlined in Box 143-4 and the reader is referred to the specific chapters discussing these conditions.

Laboratory Findings Supportive of GBS

Cerebrospinal Fluid

Characteristically the CSF has albuminocytologic dissociation, with a raised protein and no significant evidence of inflammation (<10 mononuclear cells/mm³) (Asbury, 2000; Yuki and Hartung, 2012). Protein elevation is present in <50% of patients during the first week of illness, increasing to 75% in the third week (Yuki and Hartung, 2012). Significant CSF pleocytosis (>50 mononuclear cells/mm³) or polymorphonuclear leukocytes raise doubt about the diagnosis. In a pediatric series, CSF protein levels range from 80 to 200 mg/dl (normal <40 mg/dl).

Electrodiagnosis

In the vast majority of children with GBS in the Western world, nerve conduction studies (NCS) show demyelinating features such as conduction slowing (prolonged distal latencies, slowed conduction velocities, prolonged F-wave minimal latencies, prolonged H-reflex minimal latencies) or conduction block over focal nerve segments (Figure 143-2, *A* and *B*). The electrophysiologic criteria outlined by the 88th European Neuromuscular Center (ENMC) for childhood CIDP (Box 143-5) (Nevo and Topaloglu, 2002) can be used to diagnose demyelination in childhood GBS. With more advanced disease, there may also be low-amplitude compound muscle action potentials (CMAPs). NCS performed early in the course or in mild cases may be nonspecific. In Asia, primary axonal subtypes of GBS show low-amplitude CMAPs in AMAN, and low-amplitude CMAPs and sensory nerve action potentials in AMSAN. Mild nerve conduction slowing secondary to axonal damage may occur.

Magnetic Resonance Imaging

Gadolinium lumbosacral MRI is sensitive but not specific for acute demyelinating GBS, showing cauda equina root enhancement in 95% of adults and adolescents 13 days (mean) after onset. This was confirmed in 95% of Turkish pediatric GBS cases.

GBS Pathogenesis

 This is discussed online.

GBS Treatment

Supportive Care

The potential mortality rate of <5% in children and 4% to 15% in adults necessitates hospitalization and regular monitoring for dysautonomias and respiratory compromise until maximal disability is reached. With supportive care alone, recovery usually starts within 2 to 4 weeks after the weakness stops progressing (Asbury, 2000).

Rapid progression, inability to flex the arms or head, bulbar weakness, inability to cough, dysautonomia, or children with a CSF protein >800 mg/dl are more likely to require mechanical ventilation. Indications for intubation are impending respiratory failure, oropharyngeal paresis, and severe dysautonomia. Respiratory failure in children is characterized by paradoxical breathing, lethargy, reduced alertness (hypoxemia until proven otherwise), or hypoxemia diagnosed by pulse oximetry or arterial blood gases. Infants and children with severe respiratory muscle weakness may lack the classical clinical signs of rapid respiratory effort and retractions, having only anxiety and tachycardia. In adults, vital capacity <20 ml/kg warns of imminent respiratory arrest. Weaning from the ventilator should be guided by improved strength, pulse oximetry, or serial arterial blood gases.

Dysautonomias, including arrhythmias and labile blood pressure, may be life-threatening and should be sought. Endotracheal suction or medications may trigger autonomic dysfunction. Adynamic ileus, urinary retention, and hyponatremia must be regularly sought and treated.

Early management involves nasogastric tube feeding for significant dysphagia to avoid aspiration, nutritional support, and positioning the child to avoid pressure palsies and aid pulmonary drainage. Nonsteroidal antiinflammatory drugs, carbamazepine and gabapentin, are useful in pain control. Opioids provide pain relief but may aggravate autonomic bowel dysmotility. Attention for complications such as immobilization hypercalcemia, infections, and gastrointestinal hemorrhage/dysfunction is required. The adult GBS risk of deep vein thrombosis is low in children (Korinthenberg, 2013).

GBS Immunotherapy

Intravenous immunoglobulin (IVIg) and PE are treatment options in severe childhood GBS. Started promptly within the first 2 weeks, IVIg/PE in adults reduces median time to independent walking from 83 to 43 days (PE) and to 51 to 55 days (IVIg). A Cochrane review (Hughes RA, Swan AV, van Doorn PA. 2014. Intravenous immunoglobulin for Guillain-Barré syndrome. Cochrane Database Syst Rev;9:CD002063) of adults and children showed moderate evidence that IVIg started within two weeks from severe GBS onset, hastens recovery as much as PE. In children, IVIg probably hastens recovery compared with supportive care alone (low quality evidence). Small trials in children show a trend towards more improvement with high-dose compared with low-dose IVIg,

and no significant difference when the standard dose was given over two days rather than five days. IVIg is preferred in childhood because of less invasiveness and rarer complications than PE. Combined IVIg and PE is not more effective than either alone. Relapse rates (about 10%) within the first 3 weeks are similar for IVIg and PE, responding to retreatment. PE improved time to independent walking from 60 to 24 days in one small pediatric study, confirmed by other small series. Three randomized pediatric GBS trials compared IVIg with supportive treatment or placebo, suggesting IVIg significantly hastens recovery compared with supportive care. Of these, Korinthenberg et al. (2005) (randomized open study) had two groups: (1) early treatment of mild GBS (walk 5 m unaided) in 21 children—half the usual dose of IVIg (0.5 g/kg/day over 2 days) had significantly faster improvement (median 8 days) compared with supportive treatment (median 32 days); (2) severe GBS (unable to walk 5 m unaided) in 51 children (all treated with IVIg). In this treated cohort no side effect difference or significant differences in primary or secondary outcome measures were found between IVIg 1 g/kg/day over 2 days versus 0.4 g/kg/day over 5 days (median time to unaided walking: 19 days vs. 13 days), except for more early relapses (21.7%) after the 2-day regimen ($p = 0.049$). IVIg side effects are discussed elsewhere. IVIg treatment should be started promptly according to clinical indications. However, IVIg is contraindicated where there is hypersensitivity to human immunoglobulin, severe renal, or severe cardiovascular disease. In patients with IgA deficiency (prevalence about 1:1000), IgA-poor IVIg or alternative therapies may be used to prevent anaphylaxis; however, the risk of anaphylaxis is not completely eliminated with IgA-poor preparations. Avoid PE with marked dysautonomia.

Corticosteroids in GBS

Corticosteroids alone should not be used in GBS treatment. A minor synergistic effect of intravenous methylprednisolone with IVIg on short-term outcome cannot be excluded.

Potential GBS Therapies

These are discussed online.

Childhood GBS Outcome

About 90% to 95% of children with GBS recover completely within 6 to 12 months independent of therapeutic intervention (Asbury, 2000) compared with 20% of adults who have persistent disability. Mean maximal Hughes GBS disability scale of hospitalized children is grade 3.5 (walk 5 m with support) to 4 (bed/chair bound). After IVIg therapy childhood AMAN and AMSAN recover slower than AIDP. All have favorable outcomes at 12 months except for a worse prognosis in some AMAN and AMSAN cases. AMAN does not have the same long-term consequences in children as it does in adults (Korinthenberg, 2013). Children not recovering completely are usually functionally independent with minor residua. Long-term symptoms (paresthesias, pain, severe fatigue) possibly leading to psychosocial/school problems later in life occurred in a Dutch childhood GBS study.

Factors predictive of delayed recovery and long term weakness in children following GBS, include young age, maximum disability score at presentation, quadriplegia at day 10, need for ventilator support, cranial nerve involvement, and absent or unexcitable motor nerve responses on nerve conduction testing (Korinthenberg, 2013). Poor adult prognosis occurs with advanced age, severe GBS, rapid onset, need for assisted ventilation, other serious medical conditions, *C. jejuni* enteritis, recent cytomegalovirus infection, anti-GM1 antibodies, and marked reduction of compound motor action potentials when first measured (Asbury, 2000; Hughes and Cornblath, 2005). A small percentage of children go on to develop CIDP (Korinthenberg, 2013).

CHRONIC INFLAMMATORY DEMYELINATING POLYRADICULONEUROPATHY
Epidemiology

The estimated prevalence is 0.48 per 100,000 children compared with 1 to 1.9 per 100,000 adults, with a male preponderance in children and adults. Onset occurs from birth, with most childhood cases occurring before 10 years of age (Hughes and Cornblath, 2005).

Antecedent Events

These occur in 23% to 53% of children, including infection or immunization during the month before CIDP onset (Nevo, 1998).

Diagnostic Criteria and Clinical Features

The 88th ENMC consortium on childhood CIDP research mandatory clinical criteria are (1) progression of proximal and distal weakness of upper and lower extremities >4 weeks, or rapid progression (GBS-like presentation) followed by relapsing or protracted course (>1 year), and (2) areflexia or hyporeflexia (Box 143-5) (Nevo, 2002). ENMC "confirmed CIDP" criterion require mandatory clinical plus both electrodiagnostic and CSF features. The "Confirmed CIDP" criterion does not require nerve biopsy. "Possible CIDP" requires mandatory clinical plus only one of three laboratory findings (electrophysiologic, CSF, or nerve biopsy). Children with CIDP present mainly with lower limb weakness and/or ataxia, and younger children, with developmental delay. Proximal and distal weakness occurs in most patients. A minority of children have sensory symptoms on presentation, but sensory findings occur in most patients during the disease course (touch and vibration deficits being the most common). Facial weakness occurs in 20% to 33% of children and other cranial nerve dysfunction is uncommon. Deep tendon reflexes are either absent or decreased. Pes cavus and enlarged nerves has been noted in several childhood CIDP cases and tremor is infrequent. In general, the pattern and distribution of weakness and the presence of sensory symptoms are similar to adults. Subacute onset and relapses are more common in childhood. Presentation may be monophasic with complete recovery, relapsing remitting, slowly progressive, or stepwise progressive, and should be distinguished from acute immune neuropathies and hereditary motor and sensory neuropathies (Box 143-6).

ENMC childhood CIDP mandatory research criteria were revised to include progressive muscle weakness over at least 4 weeks (instead of 8 weeks) defining a shorter progression time, as childhood onset is more often acute/subacute than adults, evolving over 2 to 3 months, or in the case of rapid progression (i.e., GBS-like presentation) followed by relapse or protracted course >1 year (Nevo, 2002).

In adults subacute inflammatory demyelinating polyneuropathy (SIDP) is intermediate between GBS and CIDP, reaching nadir between 4 and 8 weeks with no relapse. SIDP has more antecedent infections than CIDP, a high rate of full recovery (64% to 100%), and is set apart from GBS by steroid responsiveness. SIDP cases have been described in children. However, because childhood CIDP is defined as starting from >4 weeks, SIDP is therefore included in CIDP in childhood.

CIDP Laboratory Evaluation
Cerebrospinal Fluid and Electrodiagnosis

Most children and adults with CIDP have an elevated CSF protein with <5 cells/mm³. Electrophysiologic criteria for childhood CIDP are outlined by the 88th ENMC international workshop on childhood chronic inflammatory demyelinating polyneuropathy (Box 143-5) (Nevo, 2002).

CIDP Pathology and Pathogenesis

Reviewed online.

CIDP Magnetic Resonance Imaging

Spinal MRI may show intrathecal and intraforaminal root, and brachial or lumbosacral plexus enhancement or enlargement (Ware et al., 2014).

Childhood CIDP Immunotherapy

In practice, CIDP should be diagnosed clinically, and appropriate therapy should be started as soon as the diagnosis is made even if research diagnostic criteria are not entirely fulfilled. CIDP usually responds to corticosteroids within approximately 2 months; however, there is considerable variability. Starting with either daily oral prednisone or high-dose pulse corticosteroids or IVIg is effective in both children and adults. First-line choice depends on cost, side effects, and personal preference. Resistance to therapy and steroid dependence present a therapeutic challenge. Newer agents offer second-line therapy for treatment-resistant cases.

First-Line CIDP Treatments

Corticosteroids. Corticosteroids induced short-term improvement in 65% to 95% of adults and 71% to 100% of children in small series (Nevo, 1998; Connolly, 2001). The best regimen in children is not known. Initially 1 to 2 mg/kg/day oral prednisone (maximum 60 to 80 mg) usually results in improvement within 1 to 4 weeks. Slow tapering is begun after significant improvement, but not before 4 to 6 weeks. Relapses are frequent with rapid tapering; therefore, a slow reduction by 5 mg every 2 weeks in adults and equivalent slow tapering in children is recommended after a clinical response (Nevo, 1998). Deterioration may occur within days of starting corticosteroids. Intermittent pulse intravenous methylprednisolone may have less corticosteroid side effects over the longer-term than oral corticosteroids.

Intravenous Immunoglobulin. IVIg showed good efficacy in 50% to 88% of pediatric CIDP cases, improving disability for 2 to 12 weeks and may be used as initial therapy because of paucity of side effects (Connolly, 2001). A proportion of patients need recurrent treatments (months to years) to maintain improvement. IVIg improves adult CIDP disability for at least 2 to 6 weeks (possibly for 24 to 48 weeks) compared with placebo, with similar efficacy to PE, oral prednisolone, and intravenous methylprednisolone.

Plasmaphereis/Plasma exchange (PE). PE, usually a temporary measure, showed good short-term improvement in 50% to 100% of children in small CIDP series (Connolly, 2001). Efficacy lasts for 7 to 14 days (up to 8 weeks). PE should be reduced gradually, repeated, and occasionally used with immunosuppressives because of possible rebound worsening.

Potential Second-Line Immunosuppressants for Treatment Resistant CIDP

Cytotoxic drugs may improve the therapeutic response in resistant adult CIDP patients and have a corticosteroid sparing effect or reduce the need for IVIg and PE. However, current evidence for their efficacy is insufficient or does not show significant benefit. These agents are discussed in detail online.

Current Practice in Childhood CIDP Immunotherapy. Current practice in childhood CIDP immunotherapy as described in case reports and series is as follows: (1) *First-line therapy:* either IVIg 0.4g/kg/day for 5 days repeated every 3 to 4 weeks, or corticosteroids (oral prednisone) 1 to 2 mg/kg/day for 4 to 6 weeks and then slow tapering. (2) *Second-line therapy:* azathioprine 1 to 3 mg/kg/day. (3) *Always consider:* combining therapies, individual adjustments of treatment strategy, and alternative therapies (PE, methotrexate, cyclosporine A, mycophenolate mofetil, cyclophosphamide, monoclonal antibodies, IFN-α).

Differentiating Abrupt-Onset CIDP From GBS Fluctuations. There may be difficulty differentiating monophasic GBS with transient fluctuations from CIDP patients with abrupt symptom onset (McMillan et al., 2013). This is further discussed online.

Clinical Variants Not Meeting CIDP Research Criteria. There are clinical variants in which CIDP research criteria cannot be met, but respond to immune-modulating therapy. Infants with CD59 deficiency and chronic hemolysis were reported with a relapsing immune-mediated polyneuropathy mimicking CIDP.

This is discussed online.

Childhood CIDP Outcome

CIDP has complete remission in about 70% to 100% of children compared with adult response rates of 65% to 70% with more severe residua. Simmons et al. (1997), Korinthenberg (1999), and Rossignol et al. (2007) showed very good outcomes in 83% to 85%, with no correlation between rapid onset and outcome. McMillan et al. (2013) found that 87% of CIDP children had a favorable long-term outcome; however, on long-term follow-up some had minimal focal weakness, and 1 child had restricted activity. Nevo et al. (1996) described two outcome groups: short progression (1 to 3 months) with complete resolution in 75%, and mild residua in 25%. Children with longer progression (>3 months) had mild residua in 78%, and severe residua in 22%. Hattori et al. (1998) showed the above short- and long-progression groups. Ryan et al. (2000) identified two populations with very good long-term outcome in general, and mild persistent deficit in cases with progressive deterioration.

OTHER CAUSES OF IMMUNE-MEDIATED NEUROPATHIES IN CHILDREN

These rare causes of inflammatory neuropathy in childhood are discussed online.

REFERENCES

The complete list of references for this chapter is available in the e-book at www.expertconsult.com.
See inside cover for registration details.

SELECTED REFERENCES

Asbury, A.K., 2000. New concepts of Guillain-Barré syndrome. J. Child Neurol. 15, 183–191.

Connolly, A.M., 2001. Chronic inflammatory demyelinating polyneuropathy in childhood. Pediatr. Neurol. 24, 177–182.

Dalakas, M.C., 2015. Pathogenesis of immune-mediated neuropathies. Biochim. Biophys. Acta 1852, 658–666.

Hattori, N., Ichimura, M., Aoki, S., et al., 1998. Clinicopathological features of chronic inflammatory demyelinating polyradiculoneuropathy in childhood. J Neurol Sci 154, 66–71.

Hughes, R.A., Cornblath, D.R., 2005. Guillain-Barré syndrome. Lancet 366, 1653–1666.

Korinthenberg, R., 1999. Chronic inflammatory demyelinating polyradiculoneuropathy in children and their response to treatment. Neuropediatrics 30, 190–6.

Korinthenberg, R., 2013. Acute polyradiculoneuritis: Guillain-Barré syndrome. Handb. Clin. Neurol. 112, 1157–1162.

McMillan, H.J., Kang, P.B., Jones, H.R., et al., 2013. Childhood chronic inflammatory demyelinating polyradiculoneuropathy: combined analysis of a large cohort and eleven published series. Neuromuscul. Disord. 23, 103–111.

Nevo, Y., Pestronk, A., Kornberg, A.J., et al., 1996. Childhood chronic inflammatory demyelinating neuropathies: clinical course and long-term follow-up. Neurology 47, 98–102.

Nevo, Y., 1998. Childhood chronic inflammatory demyelinating polyneuropathy. Eur. J. Paediatr. Neurol. 2, 169–177.

Nevo, Y., Topaloglu, H., 2002. 88th ENMC international workshop: childhood chronic inflammatory demyelinating polyneuropathy (including revised diagnostic criteria), Naarden, The Netherlands, December 8–10, 2000. Neuromuscul. Disord. 12, 195–200.

Rossignol, E., D'Anjou, G., Lapointe, N., et al., 2007. Evolution and treatment of childhood chronic inflammatory polyneuropathy. Pediatr Neurol 36, 88–94.

Ryan, M.M., Grattan-Smith, P.J., Procopis, P.G., et al., 2000. Childhood chronic inflammatory demyelinating polyneuropathy: clinical course long-term outcome. Neuromuscul Disord 10, 398–406.

Simmons, Z., Wald, J.J., Albers, J.W., 1997. Chronic inflammatory demyelinating polyradiculoneuropathy in children: I. Presentation, electrodiagnostic studies, and initial clinical course, with comparison to adults. Muscle Nerve 20, 1008–1015.

Ware, T.L., Kornberg, A.J., Rodriguez-Casero, M.V., et al., 2014. Childhood chronic inflammatory demyelinating polyneuropathy: an overview of 10 cases in the modern era. J. Child Neurol. 29, 43–48.

Yuki, N., Hartung, H.P., 2012. Guillain-Barré syndrome. N. Engl. J. Med. 366, 2294–2304.

E-BOOK FIGURES AND TABLES

The following figures and tables are available in the e-book at www.expertconsult.com. See inside cover for registration details.

Fig. 143-1 Presentations of Guillain-Barré syndrome subtypes and variants.

Fig. 143-2 Nerve conduction studies in Guillain-Barré syndrome.

Fig. 143-3 Cross section through a sciatic nerve from a Lewis rat during the acute phase of experimental allergic neuritis.

Fig. 143-4 Teased fiber preparation of osmicated axons.

Table 143-1 Etiologies of neuropathy in 249 Children (1980 to 1992)

Table 143-2 Causes of inflammatory and immune neuropathy in 112 children

Table 143-4 Distinguishing AIDP and AMAN in Children

Box 143-1 Infectious agents associated with Guillain-Barré syndrome

Box 143-5 Revised diagnostic criteria for childhood CIDP

Box 143-6 Clinical pointers in chronic demyelinating neuropathies

144 Congenital Myasthenic Syndromes

Duygu Selcen and Andrew G. Engel

An expanded version of this chapter is available on www.expertconsult.com. See inside cover for registration details.

INTRODUCTION

Congenital myasthenic syndromes (CMS) are inherited disorders of neuromuscular transmission associated with abnormal weakness and fatigability on exertion. CMS were described as early as 1937 but received little attention until the autoimmune origin of acquired myasthenia gravis in the late 1970s and of the Lambert-Eaton syndrome in the 1980s were described. Then it became apparent that myasthenic disorders occurring in a familial or congenital setting must have a different etiology. By the first decade of this century, clinical, ultrastructural, in vitro microelectrode, and molecular genetic studies of CMS patients revealed a phenotypically and genetically heterogeneous group of disorders.

CLINICAL MANIFESTATIONS

Some patients with CMS can present as early as in fetal life by decreased motility. Patients harboring mutations in rapsyn (Ohno et al., 2002), in the AChR delta subunit, in the fetal AChR gamma subunit (Hoffmann et al., 2006), in ChAT, or in SNAP25B (Shen et al., 2014) can have multiple joint contractures at birth. In the neonatal period, most patients are hypotonic with a weak cry, poor suck, and symmetric eyelid ptosis; they may also have stridor, choking spells, respiratory insufficiency, or apneic episodes. The symptoms are worsened by crying or activity and increase by the end of the day. Motor milestones are delayed, and most patients never learn to run or climb stairs well. They fatigue abnormally on exertion and cannot keep up with their peers in sports. Many have impaired eye movements. Small muscle bulk and spinal deformities can become apparent in later life but in some patients, severe scoliosis is present in infancy. The slow-channel CMS and the CMS caused by mutations in DOK7, GFPT1, and DPAGT1 are slowly progressive and can lead to severe disability in later life. Low-expressor mutations in nonepsilon AChR subunits are associated with a severe clinical phenotype; by contrast, most low-expressor mutations in the AChR epsilon subunit have a mild and static course because expression of the fetal gamma subunit can partially substitute for the defect in the epsilon subunit. The mildest forms of CMS present with fatigable oculobulbar or limb muscle weakness later in life.

The edrophonium or neostigmine test can be positive in some but not in all CMS such as in endplate acetylcholinesterase deficiency, in some cases of the slow-channel syndrome, or in Dok-7 myasthenia. Box 144-1 lists generic and specific clinical features of the various CMS.

DIAGNOSIS

A generic diagnosis of CMS can be made on the basis of classical clinical manifestations, a positive family history, and a decremental electromyographic response. The differential diagnosis of CMS is broad and includes various neuromuscular conditions.

The physical examination should include detailed manual muscle testing as well as tests for fatigable weakness such as measuring the arm and leg elevation time, the number of times a patient can rise from squatting or from a low stool, whether eyelid ptosis increases with sustained upward gaze, and the number of steps the patient can climb or the distance the patient can walk before having to rest. Respiratory muscle strength can be evaluated by measuring the maximal inspiratory and expiratory pressures and the vital capacity.

The EMG examination should include repetitive stimulation of nerves at 2 to 3 Hz in search of a decrease of the amplitude or area of the fourth, compared with the first, evoked compound motor action potential in multiple muscles, and especially in muscles that are significantly weak. The repetitive compound muscle action potential (CMAP) typical in the slow-channel syndrome and endplate acetylcholinesterase deficiency is detected by a repetitive CMAP elicited by a single nerve stimulus. A decremental EMG response is frequently present in facial and trapezius muscles when it cannot be detected in other muscles. If repetitive nerve stimulation studies fail to show a decremental response, then single fiber EMG (SFEMG) is needed to exclude a defect of neuromuscular transmission. However, the SFEMG can also be abnormal in patients with myopathies.

Antiacetylcholine receptor, antimuscle specific tyrosine kinase (MuSK), and antivoltage-gated P/Q type calcium channel antibodies should be searched in sporadic patients whose symptoms present after the age of 1 year, and anti-AChR antibodies should be searched both in mother and the infant with arthrogryposis and weakness to exclude autoimmune myasthenia. Infantile botulism may need to be excluded if the clinical features suggest acute- or subacute-onset fatigable weakness, ptosis, dry mouth, dilated pupils, and loss of light reflex and accommodation.

The genetic diagnosis of a specific CMS is important as it guides the therapy. Identification of the culprit gene is greatly facilitated when clinical and EMG studies point to a candidate gene (Box 144-3).

Testing for CMS mutations in previously identified CMS genes is now commercially available and offered as a panel of tests. In recent years, whole exome sequencing has also been used to identify CMS mutations. If a novel CMS disease gene is discovered, then expression studies with the genetically engineered mutant protein should be used to confirm its pathogenicity.

Deeper insights into disease mechanisms and clues to etiology can be obtained by in vitro analysis of neuromuscular transmission and structural studies of the neuromuscular junction. They are important for identifying direct effects of the mutations on neuromuscular transmission, characterizing novel CMS, and providing clues for therapy.

PRESYNAPTIC CONGENITAL MYASTHENIC SYNDROMES

1. Endplate Choline Acetyltransferase (ChAT) Deficiency

ChAT catalyzes the resynthesis of ACh by transfer of an acetyl group from acetyl-CoA to choline in cholinergic neurons.

BOX 144-1 Generic Clinical Features of the Congenital Myasthenic Syndromes

GENERIC FEATURES

- Fatigable weakness involving ocular, bulbar, and limb muscles since infancy or early childhood
- Similarly affected relative
- Decremental EMG response at 2–3 Hz stimulation
- Negative tests for anti-AChR antibodies, MuSK, and P/Q type calcium channels

EXCEPTIONS AND CAVEATS

- In some congenital myasthenic syndromes, the onset is delayed
- There may be no similarly affected relatives
- The symptoms can be episodic
- EMG abnormalities may not be present in all muscles, or are present only intermittently
- Weakness may not involve cranial muscles

BOX 144-3 Clinical Clues Pointing to a Specific Congenital Myasthenic Syndrome or Disease Protein

- Dominant inheritance: slow-channel CMS, SNAP25 and synaptotagmin
- Refractory or worsened by AChE inhibitors: ColQ, Dok-7, MuSK, Agrin, LRP4, plectin, and laminin-β2
- Repetitive compound muscle action potential (CMAP) evoked by single nerve stimuli: slow-channel CMS and ColQ deficiency
- Delayed pupillary light response: some patients with ColQ deficiency
- Congenital contractures: rapsyn, AChR δ or γ subunit, ChAT, SNAP 25
- Greater than 50% decrease of CMAP amplitude after subtetanic stimulation at 10 Hz for 5 min followed by slow recovery over 5–10 minutes: ChAT deficiency
- Sudden apneic episodes provoked by fever or stress: ChAT, rapsyn, sodium channel myasthenia
- Limb-girdle and axial distribution of weakness: Dok7, GFPT1, DPAGT1, ALG2, ALG14, LRP4, and occasionally rapsyn and ColQ
- Selectively severe weakness and atrophy of distal limb muscle: slow-channel syndrome and in some patients with agrin deficiency
- Tubular aggregates of the sarcoplasmic reticulum in muscle fibers: GFPT1, DPAGT1, ALG2
- Autophagic myopathy: GFPT1 and DPAGT1
- Stridor and vocal cord paralysis in neonates or infants: Dok-7
- Nephrotic syndrome and ocular malformations (Pierson syndrome): laminin-β2
- Association with seizures or intellectual disability: DPAGT1
- Intellectual disability and cerebellar ataxia: SNAP25
- Developmental anomalies of eye, brain, and heart: mitochondrial citrate carrier deficiency
- Association with epidermolysis bullosa simplex: plectin deficiency

Pathogenic mutations, alone or in combination, alter the expression, catalytic efficiency, or structural stability of the enzyme (Ohno et al., 2001). When neuronal impulse flow is increased as during exercise, the decreased rate of ACh resynthesis progressively depletes the ACh content of the synaptic vesicles, which decreases the amplitude of the EPP and of the CMAP.

Some patients present with hypotonia, bulbar paralysis, and apnea at birth. Others are normal at birth and develop apneic attacks during infancy or childhood precipitated by infection, excitement, or no apparent cause. In some children an acute attack is followed by respiratory insufficiency that lasts for weeks. Few patients are apneic, ventilator dependent, and paralyzed since birth, and some develop cerebral atrophy after episodes of hypoxemia. Others improve with age but still have variable ptosis, ophthalmoparesis, fatigable weakness, and recurrent cyanotic episodes; some complain only of mild to moderately severe fatigable weakness. The symptoms are worsened by exposure to cold because this further reduces the catalytic efficiency of the mutant enzyme.

A useful clinical test is to monitor the EMG decrement and the CMAP amplitude during 10 Hz stimulation over 5 minutes and for 10 to 15 minutes after stimulation. A decrease lower than 50% of the potential from the baseline followed by return to the baseline in 2 to 3 minutes is a nonspecific finding that occurs in different CMS. In contrast, in patients with ChAT deficiency the recovery occurs slowly over 5 to 15 minutes.

Treatment consists of prophylactic therapy with pyridostigmine, which increases the number of AChRs activated by each quantum. The parents should be provided with an inflatable rescue bag and a fitted mask, should be instructed in the intramuscular injection of neostigmine methylsulfate, and are advised to have an apnea monitor.

2. SNAP25B Myasthenia

SNAP25B is one of the three essential SNARE proteins required for synaptic vesicle exocytosis. A patient with severe CMS associated with cortical hyperexcitability, ataxia, multiple joint contractures at birth, and intellectual disability harbored a dominant negative mutation in SNAP25B. Treatment with 3,4-diaminopyridine (3,4-DAP), which increases the number of ACh quanta released by nerve impulse, improved the patient's weakness but not her ataxia or intellectual disability.

3. Synaptotagmin-2 Myasthenia

Synaptotagmin 2 is a synaptic vesicle-associated calcium sensor. In two kinships, dominant mutations in this gene caused a Lambert-Eaton syndrome-like disorder with lower limb predominant weakness, areflexia, and a motor neuronopathy. They had low amplitude CMAP that were greatly facilitated by exercise (Herrmann et al., 2014).

SYNAPTIC BASAL LAMINA ASSOCIATED CONGENITAL MYASTHENIC SYNDROMES

1. Endplate Acetylcholinesterase Deficiency

The EP species of acetylcholinesterase (AChE) is an asymmetric enzyme composed of catalytic subunits encoded by $ACHE_T$ and a collagenic structural subunit encoded by COLQ that anchors the enzyme in the synaptic basal lamina.

The clinical course of patients with EP AChE deficiency is variable. Patients typically present in the neonatal period or infancy with apnea and generalized weakness that persist through life. In some patients, the ocular ductions are spared and in some the pupillary light reflex is delayed. Milder cases may present later in childhood with limb-girdle weakness. Absence of AChE from the EP prolongs the lifetime of ACh in the synaptic cleft because each ACh binds multiple AChRs before leaving the synaptic space by diffusion. This prolongs the duration of the MEPP and EPP, and when the EPP outlasts the absolute refractory period of the muscle fiber, it generates a second (or repetitive) muscle fiber action potential, reflected by a repetitive CMAP that is unaffected by edrophonium (Ohno et al., 1998).

Therapy is still unsatisfactory, but ephedrine and albuterol (Liewluck et al., 2011) were noted to have a gradually developing beneficial effect.

2. Congenital Myasthenic Syndrome Associated With β2-Laminin Deficiency

β2-Laminin, encoded by LAMB2, is a component of the basal lamina of different tissues and is highly expressed in kidney, eye, and the neuromuscular junction. Synaptic β2-laminin governs the appropriate alignment of the axon terminal with the postsynaptic region and, hence presynaptic and postsynaptic trophic interactions. Defects in β2-laminin result in Pierson syndrome with renal and ocular malformations. In a single report, a patient carrying two heteroallelic frameshift mutations in LAMB2 had Pierson syndrome associated with ocular, respiratory, and proximal limb muscle weakness. The renal defect was corrected by renal transplant at age 15 months.

A trial with a cholinesterase inhibitor resulted in profound weakness requiring hospitalization and ventilatory support. The patient responded to treatment with ephedrine but still had significant weakness.

POSTSYNAPTIC CONGENITAL MYASTHENIC SYNDROMES

Most postsynaptic CMS stem from molecular defects in the muscle form of the nicotinic AChR. The muscle form of nicotinic AChR is a pentameric transmembrane macromolecule with a subunit composition of $\alpha2\beta\delta\varepsilon$ at adult EPs, and $\alpha2\beta\delta\gamma$ at fetal EPs and extrajunctional sites. The genes encoding the α (CHNRA1), δ (CHRND), and γ (CHRNG) subunits are located in chromosome 2q, and those encoding the β (CHRNB) and ε (CHRNE) subunits are on chromosome 17p. At the human EP, AChR is concentrated on the crests of the junctional folds.

1. Primary Acetylcholine Receptor Deficiency

The clinical phenotypes vary from mild to severe. Patients with recessive mutations in the ε subunit are generally less affected than those with mutations in other subunits because compensatory expression of the fetal γ subunit can partially substitute for the defective ε subunit. The sickest patients have severe ocular, bulbar, and respiratory muscle weakness from birth and survive only with respiratory support and tube feeding. They may be weaned from a ventilator and begin to tolerate oral feedings during the first year of life but have bouts of aspiration pneumonia; they may need intermittent respiratory support during childhood and adult life. Motor milestones are severely delayed; they seldom learn to negotiate steps and can walk for only a short distance. Older patients close their mouth by supporting the jaw with the hand and elevate their eyelids with their fingers. Facial deformities, prognathism, malocclusion, and scoliosis or kyphoscoliosis become noticeable during the second decade. Muscle bulk is reduced. The tendon reflexes are normal or hypoactive.

The least affected patients pass their motor milestones with slight or no delay and show only mild ptosis and limited ocular ductions. They are often clumsy in sports, and fatigue easily. In some instances, a myasthenic disorder is suspected

only when the patient develops prolonged respiratory arrest on exposure to a curariform drug during a surgical procedure.

Patients with intermediate clinical phenotypes experience moderate physical handicaps from early childhood. Ocular palsies and eyelid ptosis become apparent during infancy. They fatigue easily, walk and negotiate stairs with difficulty, cannot keep up with their peers in sports, but can perform most activities of daily living.

Most patients respond favorably but incompletely to AChE inhibitors. The additional use of 3,4-DAP results in further improvement but the limited ocular ductions, pronounced in most patients with AChR deficiency, are typically refractory to therapy. Recently, albuterol was found to benefit patients responding poorly to pyridostigmine and 3,4-DAP.

2. Kinetic Defects in Acetylcholine Receptor

2.1 Slow-channel Myasthenia

The slow channel myasthenia is caused by dominant gain of function mutations that either enhances the affinity or the gating efficiency of AChR (Engel et al., 2003). Either mechanism prolongs the duration of the EP potentials and currents. As in EP AChE deficiency, when the length of the EPP exceeds the absolute refractory period of the muscle fiber, it triggers a repetitive CMAP; however, unlike in AChE deficiency, the repetitive response is enhanced by edrophonium.

The onset of symptoms ranges from infancy to early adult life. There is severe selective involvement of the cervical, scapular, and the wrist and finger extensor muscles.

The slow-channel syndromes are refractory to, or are worsened by, cholinergic agonists but are improved by long-lived open-channel blockers of the AChR, such as quinine or quinidine, or by fluoxetine (Harper et al., 2003).

2.2 Fast-channel Myasthenia

They are recessively inherited disorders caused by either decreased affinity for ACh or reduced gating efficiency, or by destabilization of the channel kinetics, or by a combination of these mechanisms; they leave no anatomic foot prints. Each of these derangements results in abnormally brief channel openings reflected by an abnormally fast decay of the EP potentials and currents. They are thus physiologic and structural opposites of the slow-channel syndromes.

A fast-channel mutation dominates the clinical phenotype when the second allele harbors a null mutation or if it occurs at homozygosity. The clinical consequences vary from mild to severe; no clinical clues point to the diagnosis of fast-channel myasthenia.

Most patients respond to a combination of 3,4-DAP and pyridostigmine, but some are refractory to therapy.

3. Prenatal Congenital Myasthenic Syndrome Caused by Mutations in Acetylcholine Receptor Subunits and Other Endplate Specific Proteins

The first identified prenatal myasthenic syndrome was traced to mutations in the fetal AChR γ subunit. In humans, AChR harboring the fetal γ subunit appears on myotubes around the ninth developmental week and becomes concentrated at nascent nerve-muscle junctions around the sixteenth developmental week. Subsequently, the γ subunit is replaced by the adult ε subunit and is no longer present at fetal EPs after the thirty-first developmental week. Thus pathogenic mutations of the γ-subunit result in hypomotility in utero during the 16th and 31st developmental week. The clinical consequences at birth are multiple joint contractures, small muscle bulk, multiple pterygia (webbing of the neck, axilla, elbows, fingers, or popliteal fossa), fixed flexion contractures of the fingers (camptodactyly), rocker-bottom feet with prominent heels, and characteristic facies with mild ptosis and a small mouth with downturned corners. Myasthenic symptoms are absent after birth because by then the normal adult ε subunit is expressed at the EPs.

A lethal fetal akinesia syndrome is caused by biallelic null mutations in the AChR α, β, and δ subunits as well as in rapsyn, Dok-7, and MuSK.

4. Sodium-channel Myasthenia

Thus far, only one patient with this syndrome has been identified. The patient had abrupt attacks of respiratory and bulbar paralysis since birth, lasting from 3 to 30 minutes, and was normokalemic. Intracellular microelectrode studies of neuromuscular transmission revealed that suprathreshold EPPs failed to generate muscle action potentials pointing to Nav1.4, encoded by SCN4A, as the culprit. After the defect in Nav1.4 was established, the patient was treated with pyridostigmine, which improved her endurance, and with acetazolamide, which prevented further attacks of respiratory and bulbar weakness.

5. Congenital Myasthenic Syndrome Caused by Plectin Deficiency

Plectin, encoded by PLEC, is a highly conserved and ubiquitously expressed intermediate filament-linking protein. By virtue of its tissue and organelle-specific isoforms, it links cytoskeletal filaments to target organelles in different tissues. Mutations in plectin result in epidermolysis bullosa simplex (EBS), a progressive muscular dystrophy in many patients and a myasthenic syndrome in some. In two patients investigated by the authors, microelectrode studies of intercostal muscle EPs showed low-amplitude MEPPs. Morphologic studies revealed clustering of nuclei, endomysial fibrosis, and focal calcium accumulation in some fibers, as in Duchenne dystrophy. Electron microscopy studies showed degeneration and disarray of muscle fiber organelles, plasma membrane defects accounting for calcium accumulation in the muscle fibers, and extensive degeneration of the junctional folds all attributable to lack of cytoskeletal support. Both patients were refractory to pyridostigmine.

CONGENITAL MYASTHENIC SYNDROMES CAUSED BY DEFECTS IN ENDPLATE DEVELOPMENT OR MAINTENANCE

To date, mutations in proteins essential for EP development and maintenance have been detected in MuSK, neural agrin, LRP4, Dok-7. Agrin, secreted into the synaptic space by the nerve terminal, binds to the lipoprotein-related protein LRP4 in the postsynaptic membrane. The Agrin-LRP4 complex binds to and activates MuSK. This enhances MuSK phosphorylation and leads to clustering of LRP4 and MuSK. Activated MuSK in concert with postsynaptic Dok-7 and other postsynaptic proteins acts on rapsyn to concentrate AChR in the postsynaptic membrane, enhances synapse specific gene expression by postsynaptic nuclei, and promotes postsynaptic differentiation. Clustered LRP4, in turn, promotes differentiation of motor axons. The agrin-LRP4-MuSK-Dok-7 signaling system is also essential for maintaining the structure of the adult neuromuscular junction.

1. Agrin Myasthenia

Patients with mutations in agrin can present with mild to severe muscle weakness with eyelid ptosis and facial weakness. One patient responded partially to pyridostigmine, but the other two patients did not respond to pyridostigmine or 3,4-DAP.

In one report five patients in three kinships had a distinct phenotype associated with wasting that first affected the lower and later the upper distal limbs, sparing of the axial and cranial muscles, and slowly progressive weakness. The patients responded to albuterol or ephedrine but not to pyridostigmine.

2. LRP4 Myasthenia

The first reported patient was 17-year-old girl with moderately severe fatigable limb-girdle weakness, dysplastic synaptic contacts, and borderline EP AChR deficiency. The patient has two heterozygous missense mutations in the third β-propeller domain of LRP4. Subsequently, two sisters with moderately severe LRP4 myasthenia and a homozygous mutation in LRP4 were found to have structurally and functionally abnormal EPs and EP AChR deficiency. Expression studies revealed that the mutation hinders LRP4 from binding to, activating, and phosphorylating MuSK. Both patients respond partially to albuterol.

3. MuSK Myasthenia

The patients with mutations in MuSK present at birth or early life with eyelid ptosis or respiratory distress. Subsequently, the ocular, facial and proximal limb muscles, and sometimes the bulbar muscles are affected. Pyridostigmine therapy is ineffective or worsens the disease (personal observation). A program of 3,4-DAP therapy improved symptoms in one patient. Importantly, a recent report indicates that therapy with albuterol has been highly effective in two brothers. No clear genotype-phenotype correlations have emerged.

4. Dok-7 Myasthenia

Patients with mutations in DOK7 have limb-girdle weakness with lesser facial and cervical muscle involvement, but a few have severe bulbar weakness and significant oculoparesis (Beeson et al., 2006). Some are initially misdiagnosed as having limb-girdle muscular dystrophy. The clinical course is mild to severe. Type 1 fiber preponderance, type 2 fiber atrophy, mild myopathic changes, and target formations are associated features. Importantly, this CMS is rapidly worsened by pyridostigmine but responds well over a period of time to ephedrine or albuterol.

5. Rapsyn Myasthenia

Most patients with mutations in RAPSN present in the first year and a few later in life. Arthrogryposis at birth and other congenital malformations occur in close to one third of patients. Intercurrent infections or fever can trigger respiratory crises and can cause anoxic encephalopathy. The ocular ductions are intact in most patients. Most patients respond well to pyridostigmine; some derive additional benefit from 3,4-DAP, and some benefit from the added use of ephedrine or albuterol.

There are no genotype-phenotype correlations except that near-Eastern Jewish patients with a homozygous E-box mutation (c.-38A>G) have a mild phenotype with ptosis, prognathism, severe masticatory and facial muscle weakness, and hypernasal speech.

CONGENITAL MYASTHENIC SYNDROMES ASSOCIATED WITH CONGENITAL DEFECTS OF GLYCOSYLATION

Glycosylation increases the solubility, folding, stability, assembly, and intracellular transport of nascent peptides. O-glycosylation occurs in the Golgi apparatus with addition of sugar residues to hydroxyl groups of serine and threonine; N-glycosylation occurs in the endoplasmic reticulum in sequential reactions that decorate the amino group of asparagine with a core glycan composed of 2 glucose, 9 mannose and 2 N-acetylglucosamine (GlcNAc). To date, defects in four enzymes subserving glycosylation have been found to cause CMS: GFPT1 (glutamine fructose-6-phosphate transaminase); DPAGT1 (dolichyl-phosphate [UDP-N-acetylglucosamine] N-acetylglucosaminephosphotransferase 1); ALG2 (alpha-1,3/1,6-mannosyltransferase); and ALG14 (UDP-N-acetylglucosaminyltransferase subunit). Tubular aggregates of the sarcoplasmic reticulum (SR) in muscle fibers are a phenotypic clue to the diagnosis but are not present in all patients. Because glycosylated proteins are present at all EP sites, the safety margin of neuromuscular transmission is compromised by a combination of presynaptic and postsynaptic abnormalities.

1. GFPT1 Myasthenia

GFPT1 controls the flux of glucose into the hexosamine pathway, and, thus, the formation of hexosamine products and the availability of precursors for N- and O-linked glycosylation of proteins. A defect in GFPT1 predicts hypoglycosylation and, hence, defective function of several endplate-associated proteins. Most patients present in the first decade. As in Dok-7 myasthenia, the weakness affects mainly the limb-girdle muscles. Only a few patients have respiratory complications. The course is relatively benign in most, but one patient whose mutations abrogated expression of the muscle-specific exon of GFPT1 had severe facial, bulbar, and respiratory muscle weakness, and has been quadriplegic since birth. This patient has an autophagic vacuolar myopathy, reduced evoked quantal release, and low MEPP amplitude. Most patients respond to pyridostigmine. Some patients derive additional benefit from albuterol and 3,4-DAP.

2. DPAGT1 Myasthenia

DPAGT1 catalyzes the first committed step of N-linked protein glycosylation. DPAGT1 deficiency predicts impaired asparagine glycosylation of multiple proteins distributed throughout the organism, but in the first five patients harboring DPAGT1 mutations only neuromuscular transmission was adversely affected; this was attributed to reduced AChR expression at the EP, but the patient EPs were not examined. As in GFPT1 deficiency, muscle fibers harbor tubular aggregates, and the weakness tends to spare the craniobulbar muscles. A subsequent study of two siblings and of a third patient extended the phenotypic spectrum of the disease. These patients have moderately severe to severe weakness and are intellectually disabled. The siblings respond poorly to pyridostigmine and 3,4-DAP; the third patient responds partially to pyridostigmine and albuterol. Intercostal muscle studies showed fiber type disproportion, small tubular aggregates, and an autophagic vacuolar myopathy.

3. ALG2 and ALG14 Myasthenia

ALG2 catalyzes the second and third committed steps of N-glycosylation. ALG14 forms a multiglycosyltransferase complex with ALG13 and DPAGT1 and catalyzes the first committed step of N-glycosylation. These defects are predicted to cause endplate AChR deficiency. Two siblings with mutations in ALG14 have fatigable limb-girdle muscle weakness with sparing of ocular muscles. Both patients benefit from pyridostigmine. Four siblings with mutations in ALG2 presented in infancy or less than age 2 years with hypotonia and delayed motor milestones and never achieved ambulation, one other patient presented at age 4 years with limb-girdle weakness, and responded to pyridostigmine.

OTHER MYASTHENIC SYNDROMES

1. PREPL Deletion Syndrome

The hypotonia-cystinuria syndrome is caused by recessive deletions involving the contiguous genes SLC3A1 and PREPL at chromosome 2p21. The major clinical features are type A cystinuria, growth hormone deficiency, muscle weakness, ptosis, and feeding problems. A patient with isolated PREPL deficiency had myasthenic symptoms since birth, including marked hypotonia, ptosis and facial and bulbar muscle weakness. She had growth hormone deficiency but no cystinuria and responded transiently to pyridostigmine during infancy. She harbors a paternally inherited nonsense mutation in PREPL and a maternally inherited deletion involving both PREPL and SLC3A1; therefore the PREPL deficiency determines the phenotype. PREPL expression was absent from the patient's muscle and EPs.

2. Myasthenic Syndrome Associated With Defects in the Mitochondrial Citrate Carrier SLC25A1

The mitochondrial SLC25A1 mediates the exchange of mitochondrial citrate/isocitrate with cytosolic maleate that is cleaved into acetyl-CoA and oxaloacetate by ATP-citrate lyase. Mutations of SLC25A1 were shown to interfere with brain, eye, and psychomotor development. Exome sequencing of two siblings born to consanguineous parents with CMS and intellectual disability revealed homozygous missense mutation in SLC25A1. Another patient harboring two missense mutations in SLC25A1 had hypotonia, severe intellectual disability, epilepsy, postnatal microcephaly, as well hypoplastic optical nerves, agenesis of the corpus callosum, sensorineural deafness and 2-hydroxyglutaric aciduria. At 18 months of age the patient had no spontaneous voluntary movements and was shown to have neuromuscular transmission defect.

3. Myasthenic Syndromes Associated With Congenital Myopathies

Eyelid ptosis, ophthalmoparesis, weakness of facial muscles, exercise intolerance, a decremental EMG, and response to pyridostigmine have been documented in patients with centronuclear myopathies caused by mutations in amphiphysin, myotubularin, and dynamin 2, as well as in patients with no identified mutations. Two patients with congenital fiber type disproportion caused by mutation in tropomyosin 3 had mild abnormalities in single fiber EMG, suggesting CMS. Finally, two siblings harboring mutations in ryanodine receptor 1 had fatigable ptosis and facial and generalized weakness, and responded partially to pyridostigmine.

TABLE 144-2 Treatment of Congenital Myasthenic Syndromes

Type of Congenital Myasthenia	Therapy Options
Choline acetyltransferase deficiency	Pyridostigmine; parental neostigmine sulfate for apneic episodes
SNAP25B-myasthenia	3,4-DAP*
Acetylcholine esterase deficiency	Albuterol or ephedrine
Laminin β2 deficiency	Partial response to ephedrine
Primary AChR deficiency	Pyridostigmine, 3,4-DAP, albuterol can have additional benefit in severe cases
Slow-channel syndrome	Quinine, quinidine, or fluoxetine
Fast-channel syndrome	Pyridostigmine and 3,4-DAP
Agrin-myasthenia	Partial response to ephedrine or albuterol; one patient with partial response to pyridostigmine
LRP4-myasthenia	Partial response to albuterol in two patients
MuSK-myasthenia	Variable response to 3,4-DAP, good response to albuterol in one patient
Dok-7 myasthenia	Albuterol or ephedrine
Rapsyn myasthenia	Pyridostigmine, 3,4-DAP, albuterol
GFPT1, DPAGT1, ALG2, and ALG4 associated myasthenia	Pyridostigmine, 3,4-DAP additional benefit, albuterol in one patient
PREPL deletion syndrome	Pyridostigmine beneficial in infancy
Plectin deficiency	Refractory to pyridostigmine and 3,4-DAP
Na-channel myasthenia	Pyridostigmine and acetazolamide
CMS associated with congenital myopathies	Pyridostigmine with some response

*3,4-DAP = 3,4-diaminopyridine

TREATMENT

Current therapies for CMS include cholinergic agonists, namely pyridostigmine and 3,4-DAP, long-lived open-channel blockers of the acetylcholine receptor ion channel such as fluoxetine and quinidine, and adrenergic agonists such as salbutamol and ephedrine. Some agents that can be beneficial in one type of CMS can be harmful in another type. Hence a specific diagnosis is essential for the treatment of these patients. Table 144-2 summarizes the pharmacotherapy of the recognized CMS.

REFERENCES

The complete list of references for this chapter is available in the e-book at www.expertconsult.com.
See inside cover for registration details.

SELECTED REFERENCES

Beeson, D., Higuchi, O., Palace, J., et al., 2006. Dok-7 mutations underlie a neuromuscular junction synaptopathy. Science 313, 1975–1978.

Engel, A.G., Ohno, K., Sine, S.M., 2003. Sleuthing molecular targets for neurological diseases at the neuromuscular junction. Nat. Rev. Neurosci. 4, 339–352.

Harper, C.M., Fukodome, T., Engel, A.G., 2003. Treatment of slow-channel congenital myasthenic syndrome with fluoxetine. Neurology 60, 1710–1713.

Herrmann, D.N., Horvath, R., Sowden, J.E., et al., 2014. Synaptotagmin 2 mutations cause an autosomal-dominant form of Lambert-Eaton myasthenic syndrome and nonprogressive motor neuropathy. Am. J. Hum. Genet. 95, 332–339.

Hoffmann, K., Muller, J.S., Stricker, S., et al., 2006. Escobar syndrome is a prenatal myasthenia caused by disruption of the acetylcholine receptor fetal gamma subunit. Am. J. Hum. Genet. 79, 303–312.

Liewluck, T., Selcen, D., Engel, A.G., 2011. Beneficial effects of albuterol in congenital endplate acetylcholinesterase deficiency and Dok-7 myasthenia. Muscle Nerve 44, 789–794.

Ohno, K., Brengman, J., Tsujino, A., et al., 1998. Human endplate acetylcholinesterase deficiency caused by mutations in the collagen-like tail subunit (ColQ) of the asymmetric enzyme. Proc. Natl. Acad. Sci. U.S.A. 95, 9654–9659.

Ohno, K., Engel, A.G., Shen, X.M., et al., 2002. Rapsyn mutations in humans cause endplate acetylcholine-receptor deficiency and myasthenic syndrome. Am. J. Hum. Genet. 70 (4), 875–885.

Ohno, K., Tsujino, A., Brengman, J.M., et al., 2001. Choline acetyltransferase mutations cause myasthenic syndrome associated with episodic apnea in humans. Proc. Natl. Acad. Sci. U.S.A. 98, 2017–2022.

Shen, X.M., Selcen, D., Brengman, J., et al., 2014. Mutant SNAP25B causes myasthenia, cortical hyperexcitability, ataxia, and intellectual disability. Neurology 83, 2247–2255.

E-BOOK FIGURES AND TABLES

145 Acquired Disorders of the Neuromuscular Junction

Nicholas J. Silvestri, Richard J. Barohn, and Gil I. Wolfe

ACQUIRED DISEASES OF THE NEUROMUSCULAR JUNCTION

Both acquired and inherited disorders of the neuromuscular junction (NMJ) are seen in childhood. As with adults, the most common NMJ disorders are autoimmune and respond to immunosuppressive therapy. These include myasthenia gravis (MG) and, rarely, Lambert–Eaton myasthenic syndrome (LEMS). Botulism, a toxin-mediated disorder of the NMJ, most commonly occurs in infancy. All NMJ disorders have the ability to produce generalized weakness and fatigability, with a propensity for oculobulbar involvement. Electrophysiological studies will detect an impairment of neuromuscular transmission in most of these disorders. Fortunately, most of these disorders are treatable.

AUTOIMMUNE MYASTHENIA GRAVIS

MG, the best understood autoimmune disease of the nervous system, is most commonly caused by antibodies to acetylcholine receptor (AChRs). Circulating IgG antibodies directed against AChRs bind to the postsynaptic membrane and activate the terminal complement sequence (C5b-9), resulting in lysis of the AChR with complement-mediated muscle endplate degeneration.

AChR-antibody formation has also been shown to block neuromuscular transmission and accelerate turnover of AChR cross-linked by IgG. As a result of these processes, the postsynaptic membrane becomes simplified, with decreased junctional folds.

The process that initiates the immune-mediated NMJ dysfunction is still unknown. The thymus gland may play a role; 75% of MG patients who undergo thymectomy have thymic pathologic findings, with 15% being tumors of the thymus, and the remainder consisting of lymphoid hyperplasia. There may be a hereditary predisposition to develop MG because there is an increased incidence of certain HLA antigens in various MG populations (Meriggioli and Sanders, 2009).

CLINICAL FEATURES

MG has a prevalence of approximately 125 cases per million population. Approximately 11% to 24% of all MG patients have disease onset in childhood or adolescence (Millichap and Dodge, 1960). Overall, there is a slight female predominance of 3:2, although males predominate in older age groups. The disease can arise at any age, but peaks are observed in the third and sixth decades (Grob et al., 2008).

MG is characterized by weakness and fatigability of ocular, bulbar, and extremity striated muscles. The ocular manifestations are ptosis and diplopia, whereas the bulbar manifestations are dysarthria, dysphagia, dysphonia, and dyspnea. Masticatory weakness presents with jaw fatigue and jaw-closure weakness. Proximal limb and axial muscles tend to be weaker than distal extremity muscles. Symptoms of MG tend to worsen with stress, with illness, with exertion, and as the day progresses. These temporal symptoms, however, may be difficult to elicit in many patients. Myasthenic crisis, characterized by respiratory weakness and the inability to handle secretions or swallow, may punctuate a more stable clinical course in some children.

CATEGORIES OF MYASTHENIA GRAVIS IN CHILDHOOD

Autoimmune MG in children is most commonly divided into neonatal transient and juvenile types.

Neonatal transient MG occurs in infants of myasthenic mothers. Placental transfer of AChR-antibody or immunocytes results in transient impairment of neuromuscular transmission in the neonate. Findings such as a weak suck or cry, ptosis, dysphagia, generalized weakness, decreased spontaneous movement, or respiratory distress are usually present in the first few hours of life but may not be evident until the third day (Millichap and Dodge, 1960). The majority of infants have hypotonia or transient weakness, and a very small proportion present with arthrogryposis multiplex congenita. The hypotonia and transient weakness usually resolve in the first 4 weeks but may persist for months and even lead to persistent facial and bulbar manifestations. The severity of the disorder in the infant does not correlate with the degree of maternal involvement, but there is evidence that a higher maternal antibody titer may predict severity. A prior history of neonatal MG in a sibling is the only predictive factor. Fortunately, only 10% to 15% of infants born to myasthenic mothers develop the disorder. Prior thymectomy or remission of disease in the mother does not prevent development of neonatal transient MG but has decreased its likelihood. In terms of treatment, if there is no significant respiratory or swallowing impairment, medications are not necessary. In more severe cases, oral pyridostigmine is given in syrup form (60 mg/5 ml) at an initial dose of 0.5 to 1 mg/kg every 4 to 6 hours. Treatment for 4 to 6 weeks is usually all that is required.

Careful monitoring of pregnant women with MG is critical because there is a 40% chance of disease exacerbation during pregnancy and a 30% risk in the puerperium. Perinatal mortality is approximately 68 per 1000 births, 5 times the risk in uncomplicated pregnancies.

Juvenile MG represents the childhood onset of autoimmune MG seen in adults, but there are differences in the presentation (Chiang, Darras, and Kang, 2009). Onset is usually after 10 years of age, and disease manifestations appear before puberty in half the cases. Onset before 1 year of age is exceptional. Pubertal status might affect the clinical presentation, with higher incidence of ocular MG in prepubertal patients and generalized MG in postpubertal patients. Female predominance was observed only after the age of 10 years.

As with adults, ptosis is the most common clinical finding, frequently accompanied by ophthalmoparesis (Figure 145-2). Ptosis was unilateral at onset in one-third of juvenile MG patients but subsequently spread to the other eye in nearly

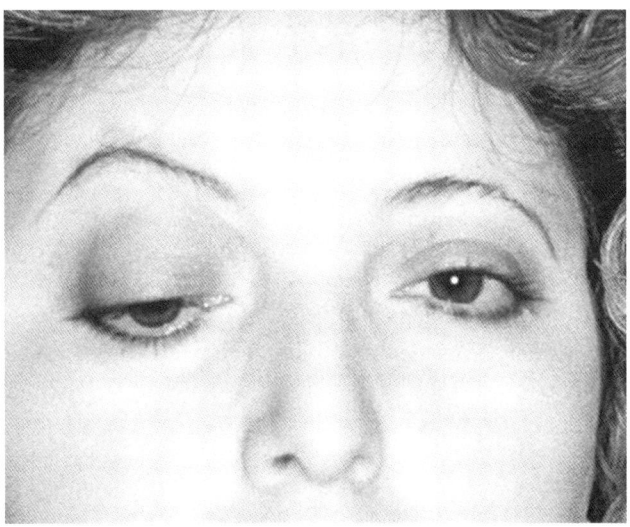

Figure 145-2. Ptosis of the right eyelid in a young woman with juvenile MG. Hypertropia of the left eye is also present.

90% of cases (Afifi and Bell, 1993). Evidence for ptosis and restriction of eye movement can often be found on careful examination. Facial and oropharyngeal weakness are other common findings, producing dysarthria, dysphagia, and difficulty chewing. Facial weakness without ocular involvement is an unusual but recognized presentation of juvenile MG. Extremity weakness can occur and is usually most prominent proximally. Bulbar weakness characterized by slow chewing, dysphagia, nasal dysarthria, and weak cough develops in up to 75% of patients (Rodriguez et al., 1983). Respiratory failure from either diaphragmatic or intercostal muscle weakness or airway compromise related to bulbar dysfunction produces myasthenic crisis, an exacerbation severe enough to endanger life. As in adults, the disease may be generalized at onset, but isolated ocular involvement is a more common presentation, followed by generalization at a later time. However, children with ocular MG appear more likely than adults to remain with purely ocular disease. As many as 85% of adults with ocular MG later go on to develop generalized disease. In children this percentage is closer to 50% to 75% (Afifi and Bell, 1993; Castro et al., 2013).

CLINICAL AND LABORATORY TESTS

In most instances the clinician can be confident about the diagnosis of MG based on abnormalities brought out through the neurologic history and examination. However, one or more tests are usually performed to confirm the clinical diagnosis.

Edrophonium (Tensilon) Test

The intravenous (IV) administration of up to 10 mg of edrophonium is often the first diagnostic test performed in the evaluation of a potential MG patient. However, the edrophonium test has a number of pitfalls. The most common mistake is that the physician performing the test does not have an objective parameter to measure before and after edrophonium administration. The most useful parameter is the degree of ptosis. The best indication of a positive test is a significant increase in the palpebral fissure aperture or the opening of a completely ptotic eye. If no ptosis is present, the edrophonium test may be difficult to interpret even in clear-cut cases of MG. If the patient has a severe restriction of extraocular movement

and edrophonium dramatically improves the motility, the test is considered positive. However, subjective diplopia may not resolve unless edrophonium produces orthophoria in the eyes, which is rare. Significant improvement in dysarthria or in swallowing is another indication of a positive edrophonium test. A mild improvement in limb strength or subjective well-being is not sufficient to claim a positive test. In addition, a positive edrophonium test is not specific because transient subjective improvement is reported in other neurologic disorders, such as motor neuron disease and peripheral neuropathy. Details on how to perform this test are located in the online 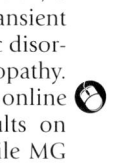 version of this chapter and elsewhere. Positive results on edrophonium testing are seen in up to 90% of juvenile MG cases (Afifi and Bell, 1993).

Electrophysiologic Testing
Repetitive Nerve Stimulation

The classic electrophysiologic demonstration of an NMJ transmission defect is the documentation of a decremental response of the compound muscle action potential (CMAP) to repetitive nerve stimulation (RNS) of a motor nerve. Decrement is attributable to failure of some muscle fibers to reach threshold and contract when successive volleys of ACh vesicles are released at the NMJ. Failure to reach the threshold EPP to achieve muscle contraction is called blocking. The percentage of decrease in amplitude and area is calculated between the first CMAP produced by a train of stimuli and each successive one. In most laboratories, five or six responses are obtained at 2 or 3 Hz, and the maximal percentage of decrement can be measured at the fourth or fifth response. A decrement of greater than 10% is considered a positive RNS study. In some patients, a decremental response can be demonstrated at baseline; in others, it is only observed after a brief period of exercise and improves after rest (Figures 145-3 and 145-4).

As with the edrophonium test, RNS does not have to be performed on every MG patient if the diagnosis is certain based on clinical findings and a positive AChR-antibody.

Single-Fiber Electromyography

Single-fiber electromyography (EMG) is a more sensitive measure of neuromuscular transmission than RNS and can be considered in select children. In MG the time required for the EPP at the NMJ to reach threshold is extremely variable. The measurement of this variability in the EPP rise time is known as jitter. The jitter value, calculated in microseconds, is the most important piece of data obtained from single-fiber EMG. Everyone, including healthy individuals, has some degree of jitter. Myasthenic patients have increased jitter values. In addition, blocking occurs in myasthenics if a muscle fiber's EPP never reaches threshold and depolarization does not occur. The frequency of blocking, expressed as a percentage, is also determined with single-fiber EMG. In healthy individuals the percentage of blocking is 0%.

Single-fiber EMG is undoubtedly the most sensitive test for MG in adults. It is abnormal in 94% of generalized and 80% of ocular MG patients. However, single-fiber EMG has several disadvantages. It is a tedious and lengthy study that requires considerable patient cooperation and is poorly tolerated by many children. Stimulated single-fiber EMG can be performed under sedation, requires less patient cooperation, and may be preferred in children, although it is still a lengthy procedure. An abnormal single-fiber electromyographic study is not specific for MG because increased jitter commonly occurs as a result of other neuromuscular diseases, including motor neuron disease, peripheral neuropathy, and many myopathies. Fortunately, it is seldom necessary to perform single-fiber

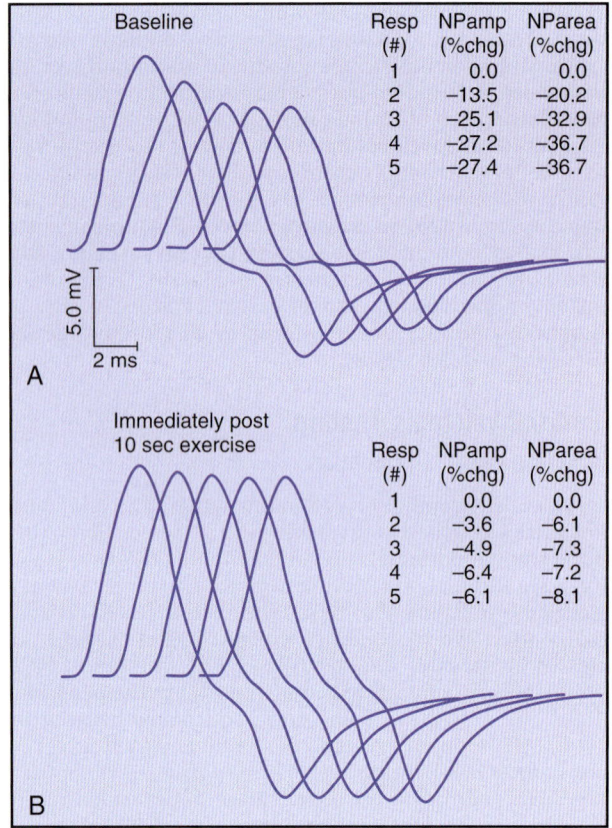

Figure 145-3. Repetitive nerve stimulation (RNS) of the ulnar nerve at 3 Hz, recorded from the adductor digiti minimi. **A,** Baseline, abnormal amplitude decrement of 27%. **B,** Immediately after 10 seconds of exercise the decrement has resolved, demonstrating *repair.* NPamp, negative peak amplitude; NParea, negative peak area; Resp, response.

EMG to diagnose MG in children. It is probably most useful in children who present difficult diagnostic dilemmas and who otherwise have normal laboratory studies for MG.

Antibody Testing
Anti-AChR Antibodies

Finding elevated AChR-antibody levels in the serum of a suspected MG patient is the most specific and reassuring diagnostic test. When the AChR-antibody assay is positive, it can be argued that no other diagnostic studies for MG are needed. Thus the clinician who is initially making the diagnosis is often in the position of performing the edrophonium and electrophysiologic tests while awaiting the serologic results.

AChR-antibody levels are not elevated in all MG patients. The assay is most helpful in adult generalized MG; it is positive in 85% of such patients. Ocular MG patients, however, have a measurable AChR-antibody in only 50% of cases. Children represent another group of MG patients who are often antibody negative. In one study, 50% of prepubertal children with autoimmune juvenile MG were seropositive. Seropositive rates of 68% and 91% were observed in peripubertal and postpubertal disease onset, respectively. Similarly, seropositivity was more common in girls with onset of juvenile MG after 11 years of age. Seronegativity was more common in pure ocular forms, mild disease, and remission (Afifi and Bell, 1993).

AChR-antibody titers correlate poorly with MG severity. Indeed, MG patients in clinical remission may still have ele-vated titers, but this is not an indication to continue immunosuppressive therapy.

Anti-MuSK Antibodies

Since 2001, IgG from 40% to 70% of seronegative generalized patients has been found to bind to the extracellular domain of muscle-specific receptor tyrosine kinase (MuSK). Marked female predominance with mean age of onset in the fourth decade has been typical, although pediatric cases have been reported. Three main patterns of anti-MuSK MG have been observed; one of them is clinically indistinguishable from anti-AChR generalized MG. The other two patterns are severe oculobulbar weakness and prominent neck, shoulder and respiratory involvement largely sparing ocular musculature. In these two phenotypic variants limb strength is relatively intact. Anti-MuSK antibodies are rarely seen in pure ocular MG. We consider testing for anti-MuSK antibodies in all suspected MG patients who are AChR-antibody negative. Anti-MuSK MG is somewhat more refractory to conventional treatment compared with anti-AChR MG.

Treatment. Most patients with juvenile MG who require maintenance therapy are treated with anticholinesterase agents with or without a variety of immunosuppressive medications. Pyridostigmine is recommended as an initial intervention. As with the adult form of the disease, corticosteroids and other immunomodulatory treatments are used, although few randomized controlled clinical trials have been performed in the pediatric MG population. Thymectomy plays an important role in treating older children at most centers. Plasmapheresis and IV gamma globulin (IVIG) are generally reserved for more refractory patients or for those in myasthenic crisis. Plasmapheresis and IVIG are also used to maximize function before thymectomy. As mentioned previously, short-term supportive care and anticholinesterase agents are usually adequate for neonatal transient MG.

Acetylcholinesterase Inhibitors

In juvenile MG the aggressiveness of management should be in accordance with disease severity. In general, management attempts should first focus on pyridostigmine. A total daily dose up to 7 mg/kg a day is delivered in 5 to 6 divided doses. Typical doses in older children and adults are 60 mg 3 to 5 times a day. If symptoms are poorly controlled on a pyridostigmine dose exceeding 300 mg/day, it is probably necessary to add immunomodulating therapy. Although weakness, a nicotinic receptor side effect, is relatively uncommon, muscarinic side effects occur frequently. The most common of these are gastrointestinal cramps and diarrhea. Oral hyoscyamine sulfate, glycopyrrolate, and over-the-counter loperamide can be prescribed on an as-needed basis or prophylactically with selected pyridostigmine doses to minimize these side effects.

Thymectomy

When a child's symptoms can no longer be controlled by anticholinesterase agents alone, a decision must be made regarding whether to pursue thymectomy or immunosuppressive therapy. There is a general consensus that generalized MG patients between puberty and 60 years of age benefit from thymectomy. However, randomized studies of thymectomy that control for medical therapy have never been performed. The use of thymectomy in very young children, in itself, is controversial because of concerns for a subsequent impairment in immune protection or an enhanced risk of cancer. A review of incidental thymectomy and thymectomy as treatment for MG in young children, however, did not find a

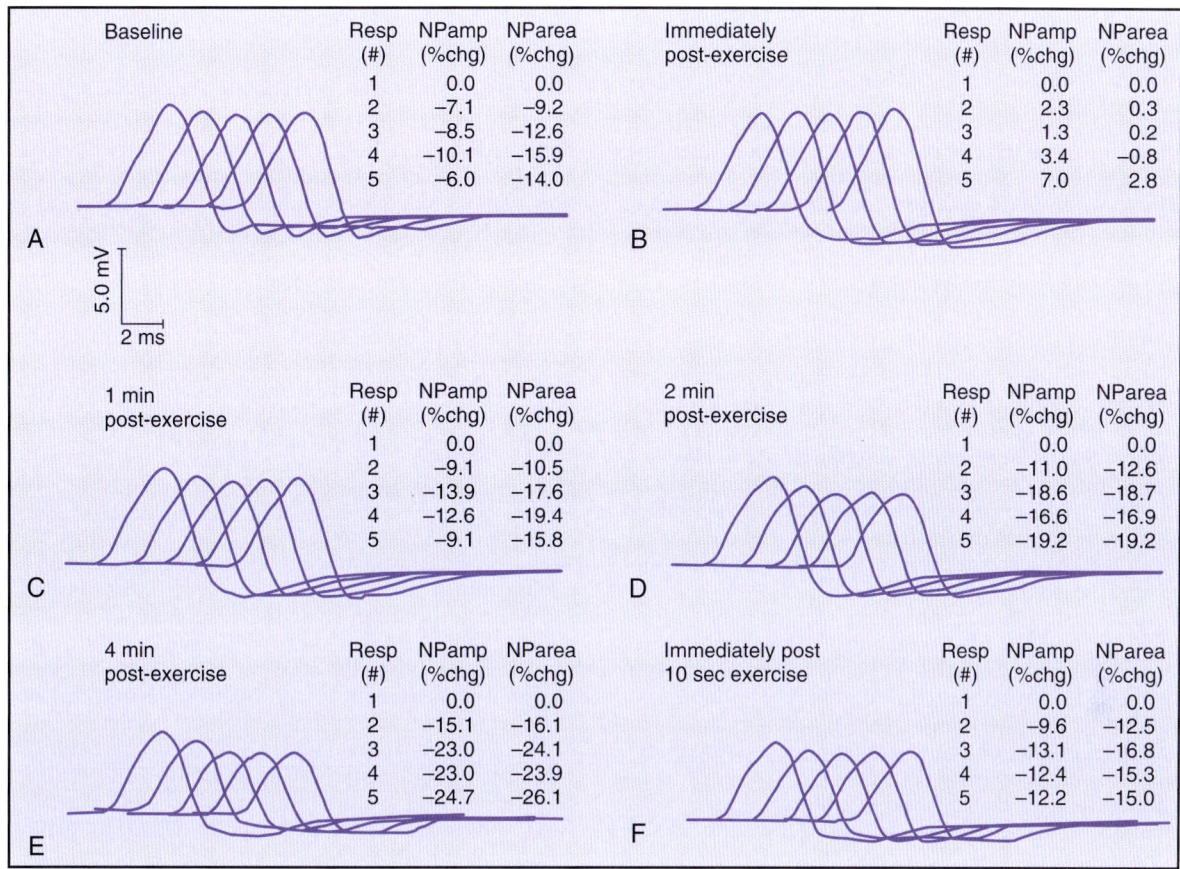

Figure 145-4. Repetitive nerve stimulation (RNS) of the ulnar nerve at 3 Hz, recorded from the adductor digiti minimi. At baseline **(A)** there is only a borderline decrement at response 4. After exercise, a 12% to 13% decrement develops immediately **(B)** at 1 minute **(C)** postexercise, and this worsens at 2 and 4 minutes **(D** and **E)**, demonstrating postexercise exhaustion. After 10 seconds of brief exercise **(F),** the decrement improves. NPamp, negative peak amplitude; NParea, negative peak area; Resp, response.

consistent association between thymectomy and these proposed risks in children older than 1 year.

Thymectomy has been widely used for the treatment of juvenile MG, showing a higher likelihood of remission when performed within 2 years of symptom onset compared with nonsurgical patients. Transsternal, transcervical, and thoracoscopic procedures are all performed and have all demonstrated benefit in clinical trials. Several studies have suggested benefit anywhere from 3 to 10 years after surgery. Favorable predictors for postoperative remission included surgery during the first year after disease onset, bulbar symptoms, onset of symptoms between ages 12 and 16 years, and the presence of other autoimmune disorders.

The presence of a thymoma is, of course, the one absolute indication for thymectomy. All newly diagnosed MG patients must undergo computed tomography or magnetic resonance imaging of the chest to search for thymoma. Routine chest radiographs may not detect up to 25% of thymic tumors. Although there is a consensus among neurologists that thymectomy should be considered in all but the youngest children with generalized MG who are not controlled on anticholinesterase agents alone, there is less enthusiasm for the procedure in pure ocular MG.

Corticosteroids

Prednisone continues to be used as an immunosuppressive agent of first choice in MG. Despite its many potential side effects, prednisone is considered by many to be the most effective oral immunosuppressive agent for the treatment of MG. Although corticosteroids can potentially suppress the immune system in a variety of ways, the exact explanation for the beneficial response in MG is unknown.

Typically, oral prednisone is initiated at 1 to 1.5 mg/kg daily. If clinical improvement occurs in the first 4 weeks, the patient can be immediately switched to an alternate-day dose of 1 to 1.5 mg/kg. Daily regimens extending beyond a month must be followed by a slower alternate-day taper. If corticosteroid therapy is initiated at moderate to high doses, an improvement is usually apparent in 2 to 3 weeks. The main concern when initiating prednisone therapy at these doses is the transient worsening that occurs in one-third to one-half of patients. The mechanism may involve a direct effect of corticosteroids to impair NMJ transmission. Thus an advised practice is to admit MG patients to the hospital for 5 to 7 days when initiating high-dose prednisone therapy. If the patient remains stable over this interval, the patient can be safely discharged on oral prednisone.

After significant improvement is observed, there should not be a rush to taper off the prednisone. Most patients remain on alternate-day dose prednisone for at least 6 to 8 months. When beginning the taper, it is best to proceed slowly by reducing the dose no faster than 5 mg every 2 weeks. When the patient's dose has been reduced to 20 mg every other day, tapering at an even slower rate is advisable. Although an attempt should be made to fully taper the patient off prednisone, it is not uncommon for patients to require low-dose therapy (5–10 mg every other day) for many years or indefinitely.

The side effects of corticosteroids are well appreciated and significant (Andrews, 2004). Children should be closely monitored for cataracts, hypertension, diabetes mellitus, weight gain, growth retardation, and cognitive or affective disturbance. Adverse effects of corticosteroids on early stages of bone mineralization and development are also of concern, emphasizing the need for "steroid-sparing" strategies in children who are refractory to tapering.

Azathioprine

Azathioprine (Imuran), an antimetabolite that blocks cell proliferation and inhibits T lymphocytes, has been used more frequently in recent years because of the side effects associated with corticosteroids. Most reports describe its use in adults. It is used most often in patients who have a relapse on prednisone or who have been on prednisone for lengthy periods in the hope that the steroid dose can be decreased or eliminated. Azathioprine is also used at times as a first-line immunosuppressive agent instead of prednisone.

Retrospective studies of azathioprine therapy have demonstrated that 70% to 90% of MG patients improve regardless of whether or not it is used as a first- or second-line immunosuppressive drug. However, the clinical response is slow, not appearing for 12 months or more. Thus if a patient already on pyridostigmine is quite weak and a rapid response is required, azathioprine is not a practical choice.

The initial dose of azathioprine in children should be no more than 25 to 50 mg daily for 1 week. If there are no side effects, the dose is increased to a target level of 2 to 3 mg/kg per day. Although azathioprine is generally well tolerated, there are three important and limiting side effects. Approximately 10% of patients have an idiosyncratic systemic reaction within the first several weeks of therapy that consists of fever, abdominal pain, nausea, vomiting, and anorexia. When the drug is stopped, the symptoms resolve quickly. If the patient is rechallenged, the symptoms invariably recur. In addition, patients can develop leukopenia and hepatotoxicity. Blood counts and hepatic enzymes need to be monitored monthly. If the white blood cell count falls below 4000 cells/mm^3, it is advisable to decrease the dose. If it falls below 3000 cells/mm^3, medication should be temporarily withheld until the cell count normalizes. Similarly, medication should be temporarily withheld if there is evidence of hepatocellular dysfunction. Although the patient can be rechallenged after the laboratory values normalize, toxicity often recurs, requiring discontinuation of the drug. Patients should be evaluated for thiopurine methyltransferase (TPMT) deficiency because this may lead to severe myelosuppression. Azathioprine dosing needs to be adjusted in hepatic and renal impairment, and potential interactions with other medications should be considered on initiation. Late development of malignancy following chronic use of azathioprine is a concern (Andrews, 2004).

Cyclosporine

Cyclosporine (Sandimmune, Neoral) is an accepted option for immunosuppressive therapy in adult MG. Data are not available on its use in juvenile MG, although it is frequently used in pediatric transplant patients. Cyclosporine inhibits helper T lymphocytes and allows the expression of suppressor T lymphocytes. It blocks the production and secretion of interleukin-2 by helper T cells. Cyclosporine has been subjected to randomized, double-blinded, placebo-controlled trials in MG. These studies demonstrated that cyclosporine was more effective than placebo in improving MG when a quantitative MG scale was used as the primary efficacy measure. Corticosteroid doses could be reduced after cyclosporine was initiated.

The onset of clinical benefit for cyclosporine is 1 to 2 months. This is somewhat faster than azathioprine and slower than prednisone. Doses for cyclosporine range between 4 and 6 mg/kg per day in two divided doses. Side effects include hirsutism, tremor, gum hyperplasia, paresthesias, and hepatotoxicity. Hypertension and nephrotoxicity are the main limitations to therapy. Over one-quarter of adult patients taking cyclosporine had serum creatinine levels increase between 30% to 70% above baseline levels, and 11% of them also developed skin cancers. Such high rates of neoplasia have not been reported in other studies. Blood pressure, renal function, and trough plasma cyclosporine levels are monitored monthly. A similar medication, tacrolimus, has also been widely used in adult patients with MG with success.

Mycophenolate Mofetil

Mycophenolate mofetil (MM; CellCept) is another immunosuppressive agent commonly used in practice at MG centers, having shown initial promise in several uncontrolled, open series demonstrating favorable responses in two-thirds of adult patients. MM had a relatively rapid onset of action, with improvement observed at a mean of 9 to 11 weeks and maximal improvement by approximately 6 months. However, in some subjects the initial response was delayed up to 40 weeks. With its more rapid onset of action and favorable side-effects profile, MM began replacing azathioprine as the first-line "steroid sparer" in many MG centers. Unfortunately, two randomized controlled studies failed to demonstrate additional efficacy for MM when added to prednisone. Study design may have been at fault in these negative trials.

MM blocks inosine monophosphate dehydrogenase, resulting in selective inhibition of B and T lymphocyte proliferation by blocking purine synthesis. It has been well tolerated in the MG population. The most common adult dosing regimen is 1 gm by mouth twice daily, although doses up to 3 gm a day have been used. It is used in the pediatric transplant population at doses of 600 mg/m^2 twice daily. Children with body surface areas greater than 1.5 gm/m^2 are dosed at 1 gm twice daily.

Main side effects are diarrhea, vomiting, increased risk for infection, and leukopenia, which is relatively uncommon. Complete blood counts are checked weekly for the first month and then less frequently. Long-term safety for MM is still in question, but there have been rare reports of primary central nervous system (CNS) lymphoma with use of MM in MG.

Cyclophosphamide

The use of cyclophosphamide (Cytoxan), a nitrogen mustard alkylating agent that blocks cell proliferation, is mainly reserved for refractory MG patients, but its reported use is limited. One study reported 42 adults who had been treated with cyclophosphamide; 23 were also on prednisone. At the time of the retrospective data analysis, 25 of the 42 patients became asymptomatic, and 12 were in complete remission off all medications. Eight of 10 children with juvenile MG improved when cyclophosphamide was added to regimens including azathioprine and corticosteroids.

The high rate and severity of toxicity are the drawbacks for cyclophosphamide. In one study, alopecia occurred in 75%, leukopenia in 35%, and nausea and vomiting in 25%. The increased risk of bladder and lymphoreticular malignancy with prolonged administration of cyclophosphamide should be of particular concern. As a result, cyclophosphamide should be considered only in the most refractory cases of juvenile MG.

Plasmapheresis

Plasma exchange is primarily employed in the short-term, acute management of severe disease, including crisis, and in readying weak patients for thymectomy. Plasmapheresis removes pathogenic antibodies from the circulation of MG patients, with improvement measured in several days rather than weeks for corticosteroids and months for immunosuppressive agents. Two other circumstances in which plasmapheresis is considered include the treatment of severely weak patients admitted for initiation of prednisone therapy and as a chronic intermittent therapy in patients with refractory disease. Plasmapheresis has been life-saving in some children.

Generally a course of plasmapheresis consists of four to six exchanges in which approximately 50 ml/kg of plasma are removed at each treatment. Decisions regarding the number of exchanges and total amount removed are largely driven by the status of the patient, including clinical response and tolerability of the hemodynamic shifts from the procedure. Improvement is often seen within 48 hours after the first or second exchange. Treatments are usually administered every other day or on no more than 2 of 3 consecutive days so that a full course is completed in 7 to 10 days (Andrews, 2004).

The main limitations of plasmapheresis are (1) IV access— a double-lumen catheter is required in younger children; (2) complications, including pneumothorax, hypotension, sepsis, and pulmonary embolism; (3) the expense of the procedure; and (4) the relatively brief clinical benefit, which persists for only a few weeks.

Intravenous Immunoglobulin

Over the last two decades, IVIG has been used by neurologists for various immune-mediated neuromuscular diseases, including MG, in which response rates of approximately 75% were observed in early retrospective series. Although no studies have focused on the pediatric population, children and adolescents have responded favorably to IVIG (Andrews, 2004).

The initial dose of IVIG is usually 2 g/kg. This can be given over 2 to 5 days. When given over the shorter interval, the infusion runs nearly continuously. A common practice is to then schedule two or three subsequent infusions of 0.4 to 1 g/kg at 2- to 4-week intervals. Patients are then reevaluated to determine whether further treatments are needed.

Advantages of IVIG over plasma exchange include relative ease of administration and favorable side-effects profile in both children and adults. Headache, transient flu-like symptoms, and hyperactivity are the adverse events most common to the pediatric population. Migraine patients are prone to develop a severe headache related to aseptic meningitis. Major complications are observed in up to 5% of adults, including cardiovascular, cerebrovascular, and deep venous thrombotic events; congestive heart failure; and acute nephrotoxicity.

Drugs to Avoid

Children, like adults with MG, are sensitive to nondepolarizing neuromuscular blocking agents. Intermediate-acting nondepolarizing blockers such as atracurium and vecuronium should be used with care. It is advisable to administer small increments of these agents, using neuromuscular monitoring as a guide. Other commonly used drugs known to exacerbate MG or interfere with neuromuscular transmission are listed in Box 145-2.

Lambert–Eaton Myasthenic Syndrome

Lambert–Eaton myasthenic syndrome (LEMS) is an acquired autoimmune disorder of neuromuscular transmission in

---

BOX 145-2 Drugs That May Worsen Myasthenia Gravis or Interfere With Neuromuscular Transmission

ANTIBIOTIC AGENTS
- Aminoglycosides
- Erythromycin
- Tetracycline
- Penicillins
- Sulfonamides
- Fluoroquinolones
- Clindamycin
- Lincomycin
- Telithromycin

ANESTHETIC AGENTS
- Neuromuscular blocking agents
- Lidocaine
- Procaine

ANTICONVULSANT AGENTS
- Phenytoin
- Mephenytoin
- Trimethadione

CARDIOVASCULAR DRUGS
- Beta blockers
- Procainamide
- Quinidine

RHEUMATOLOGIC DRUGS
- Chloroquine
- D-Penicillamine

MISCELLANEOUS
- Iodinated contrast
- Chlorpromazine
- Corticosteroids
- Lithium

---

which there is an autoimmune attack on voltage gated calcium channels (VGCC) on the presynaptic nerve terminal, ultimately resulting in a reduction in presynaptic release of ACh and defective neuromuscular transmission.

Clinical Features

LEMS begins gradually and is characterized by fatigability and weakness in a limb-girdle distribution. Unlike MG, patients may note that the weakness is worse soon after awakening, and better later in the day. While exercise can transiently improve strength, persistent exertion causes fatigue. Cranial nerve and respiratory involvement is less common than in MG. Patients also have autonomic involvement including dry mouth and eyes, impotence, blurred vision, and orthostasis (Sanders, 2003). On examination, there is a limb-girdle pattern of weakness and reduced or absent deep tendon reflexes. In only about 50% of patients can one convincingly demonstrate improvement in strength or reflexes after brief exercise. A malignancy is present in approximately 50% of adult LEMS patients. The tumor is usually a small-cell carcinoma of the lung, but other malignancies such as renal cell carcinoma and hematologic tumors occur. Malignancy is more common in men than in women, and is more likely in the setting of chronic smoking or after age 50 years. LEMS can be the presenting manifestation of a small-cell carcinoma, and can precede the detection of the tumor by months. Patients with small-cell carcinoma tend to have a more rapidly progressive course than those without malignancy, with dysarthria, difficulty chewing, weakness, dry mouth, and impotence appearing earlier in the disease course. LEMS is only rarely described in children.

Diagnostic Tests

A diagnosis of LEMS is often first suggested by findings on nerve conduction studies and repetitive nerve stimulation (RNS). The classic electrophysiologic triad of LEMS is as follows: (1) low-amplitude compound muscle action potentials (CMAPs) that increase dramatically after brief exercise, (2) decremental response at low rates of RNS (2–5 Hz), and (3) incremental response at high rates of RNS above 20 Hz. Diffusely reduced CMAPs on routine motor nerve conduction studies should raise suspicion of LEMS.

Antibody testing in LEMS for antibodies to P/Q-type VGCC is readily available and is positive in a large majority of patients with this disorder.

Treatment

As with MG, treatment of LEMS should be individualized, tailored according to clinical severity, underlying disease, and life expectancy. Upon confirmation of the diagnosis, an extensive search for an underlying malignancy is imperative. This should begin with radiologic studies and may require bronchoscopy. Initial treatment should be directed against the malignancy because this may improve neurologic manifestations. When no malignancy is found, repeat screening every 6 to 12 months is advised, especially in patients at greater risk.

Aggressive immunotherapy is easier to justify in LEMS patients without cancer because there is concern that such agents may adversely affect management of malignant disease by interfering with normal immunosurveillance. In general, a trial of pyridostigmine is the first pharmacologic intervention, although it is often of limited benefit. Ideally, drugs that enhance the presynaptic release of ACh vesicles should be used (Sanders, 2003). 3, 4-diaminopyridine (3, 4-DAP) increases the duration of the presynaptic action potential by blocking outward potassium efflux. This indirectly prolongs the activation of VGCC and increases calcium entry in nerve terminals. Most patients tolerate the drug well, and side effects such as paresthesias tend to be minor. There is a risk of seizures when daily doses exceed 100 mg. Usually doses up to 20 mg three times a day are used. Expert recommendations for laboratory monitoring include liver function tests, complete blood count (CBC), blood urea nitrogen (BUN), and creatinine every 3 months for the first year and then less frequently.

There are only a few clinical studies of immunosuppressive therapy in LEMS. Plasmapheresis, corticosteroids, and azathioprine can be effective in both neoplastic and nonneoplastic LEMS. IVIG has also been effective. In general, the regimens and doses for the immunotherapies outlined for MG can be applied to LEMS. Response to immunosuppression tends to be less dramatic for LEMS than for MG.

Botulism

Botulism is caused by a toxin produced by *Clostridium botulinum*, a gram-positive anaerobic organism found commonly in soil and agricultural products. Eight immunologically distinct toxins have been identified, with most human cases caused by types A, B, or E (Cherington, 2004). Recovery time varies between toxin types; for instance, type A toxin produces more persistent paralysis than types B and E. After binding irreversibly to receptors on presynaptic nerve terminals, the toxin is translocated across the membrane and blocks the calcium-dependent release of ACh. The action of the toxin appears independent of calcium entry. The impaired release of ACh results in failed neuromuscular transmission. The damage to nerve terminals may be permanent, resulting in a prolonged clinical recovery believed to be dependent on the formation of new neuromuscular junctions. Infantile botulism, first described in 1976, is now the most common form of the disease, representing over 70% of approximately 110 annual cases in the United States.

Infantile Botulism

Most reported cases of infantile botulism in the United States occur in California, Pennsylvania, and Utah, states with high counts of *C. botulinum* spores in the soil. After spores of *C. botulinum* are ingested, they germinate and propagate in the gastrointestinal tract, producing toxin in vivo. Consumption of honey and corn syrup has been associated with infantile botulism, but in most cases the source of infection is not evident. Infantile botulism typically presents between 6 weeks and 9 months of age, often heralded by the onset of severe constipation. A descending paralysis with cranial nerve palsy, poor suck, feeble cry, and reduced facial expressions ensues, followed by limb weakness. The child appears hypotonic, with ptosis, decreased extraocular motility, sluggish pupillary light responses, facial diplegia, weak suck, and a reduced gag response. Deep tendon reflexes and spontaneous bowel sounds are reduced. There is usually no associated fever. Both respiratory and autonomic compromise may occur. The diagnostic approach should consider other possible etiologies, including systemic infection, tick paralysis, organophosphate poisoning, Guillain-Barré syndrome, congenital myopathies, and autoimmune and congenital myasthenic conditions. Electrophysiologic studies support a presumptive diagnosis of botulism while waiting for the bacteriologic studies to return. Sensory nerve conduction studies are normal. Compound muscle action potential amplitudes are normal to reduced, with preserved motor conduction velocities. Repetitive stimulation will confirm a presynaptic defect in neuromuscular transmission. Decremental responses are variably seen on slow rates of repetitive nerve stimulation, but increments are present at rapid rates (20–50 Hz). Fibrillation potentials are seen on EMG in approximately 50% of infants, and short-duration, low-amplitude motor units in over 90%. Diagnosis is confirmed by isolation of the organism or toxin in stool samples. Toxin isolation is accomplished by the mouse neutralization test, usually performed at state health departments. Polymerase chain-reaction assays are increasingly available. In infantile botulism, the toxin is only rarely found in serum.

Treatment of infantile botulism is generally supportive, with complete recovery requiring several weeks to months. Botulism immune globulin, approved by the U.S. Food and Drug Administration (FDA) in late 2003, reduced the hospital stays for both ventilated and nonventilated children. Overall, median hospital stays fell from 40 to 23 days. Case-fatality rates of hospitalized patients in the United States are below 5%. Nasogastric or parenteral nutrition is needed if the child is unable to drink or eat. Mechanical ventilation may also be required. Aminoglycosides and other agents that impair neuromuscular transmission should be used with extreme caution. The length of hospitalization averages 4 weeks, but some infants may require supportive care for as long as 5 months.

Foodborne Botulism

The classic form of botulism almost always follows ingestion of food contaminated by preformed toxin. The classic presentation is the development of bulbar symptoms, including blurred vision, diplopia, ptosis, dysarthria, and dysphagia within 12 to 36 hours after ingestion of the contaminated food. A descending pattern of weakness follows and, in some cases, respiratory paralysis. Supportive care measures have improved survival rates, and nearly full recovery is expected for surviving patients. Treatment with antitoxin mainly plays a role in this form of botulism, but it is not likely to be effective unless administered in the first 24 to 48 hours; the antitoxin does not reverse established paralysis. Beneficial effects are more likely with type E toxin (Cherington, 2004). Use of antitoxin remains controversial because of the lack of efficacy in some cases and the 20% risk of serious allergic side effects related to the equine source. The incidence of hypersensitivity increases further with polyvalent antitoxin. Antitoxin is obtained from the Centers for Disease Control and Prevention (CDC) in Atlanta.

Wound Botulism

Wound botulism appears 4 to 14 days following infection with *C. botulinum*. Although considered rare, an increasing number of cases have been recognized in drug abusers. Wound botulism can be severe, with ventilatory support required in a majority of patients. The organism can be isolated directly when an obvious wound is present. Wound debridement, appropriate antibiotic therapy, and supportive care are the keys to management.

REFERENCES

The complete list of references for this chapter is available online at www.expertconsult.com.
See inside cover for registration details.

SELECTED REFERENCES

Afifi, A.K., Bell, W.E., 1993. Tests for juvenile myasthenia gravis: comparative diagnostic yield and prediction of outcome. J. Child Neurol. 8, 403–411.

Andrews, P.I., 2004. Autoimmune myasthenia gravis in childhood. Semin. Neurol. 24, 101–110.

Castro, D., Derisavifard, S., Anderson, M., et al., 2013. Juvenile myasthenia gravis: a twenty-year experience. J. Clin. Neuromuscul. Dis. 14, 95–102.

Cherington, M., 2004. Botulism: update and review. Semin. Neurol. 24, 155–163.

Chiang, L.M., Darras, B.T., Kang, P.B., 2009. Juvenile myasthenia gravis. Muscle Nerve 39, 423–431.

Grob, D., Brunner, N., Namba, T., et al., 2008. Lifetime course of myasthenia gravis. Muscle Nerve 37, 141–149.

Meriggioli, M.N., Sanders, D.B., 2009. Autoimmune myasthenia gravis: emerging clinical and biological heterogeneity. Lancet Neurol. 8, 475–490.

Millichap, J.G., Dodge, P.R., 1960. Diagnosis and treatment of myasthenia gravis in infancy, childhood, and adolescence: a study of 51 patients. Neurology 10, 1007–1014.

Rodriguez, M., Gomez, M.R., Howard, F.M., Jr., et al., 1983. Myasthenia gravis in children: long-term follow-up. Ann. Neurol. 13, 504–510.

Sanders, D.B., 2003. Lambert-Eaton myasthenic syndrome: diagnosis and treatment. Ann. N. Y. Acad. Sci. 998, 500–508.

E-BOOK FIGURES AND TABLES

146 Duchenne and Becker Muscular Dystrophies

Kevin Flanigan

 An expanded version of this chapter is available on www.expertconsult.com. See inside cover for registration details.

The muscular dystrophies comprise a clinically and genetically heterogeneous group of disorders, the most common of which are the allelic X-linked recessive disorders, Duchenne muscular dystrophy (DMD) and Becker muscular dystrophy (BMD). Both occur because of mutations in the *DMD* gene, encoding the dystrophin protein, and are thus known as dystrophinopathies. In general, the more severe DMD is associated with an absence of the dystrophin protein, whereas the milder BMD is associated with the presence of a partially functional dystrophin protein. Both states result in dystrophic changes in muscle, a term that refers to chronic and severe myopathic changes, including muscle fiber degeneration and regeneration but also fibrosis and fatty replacement of muscle fibers. The severity and tempo of these changes differs between DMD and BMD, but these features play a prominent role in the loss of muscle function, as noted by Guilliame Duchenne de Boulogne when he described *paralysie musculaire pseudohypertrophique ou paralysie myosclérosique*. Despite the association of his name with the syndrome, a compelling case has been made that the English physician Edward Meryon provided an earlier description of the syndrome in 1852, and claim has been made for the primacy of an even earlier description by the Italian physician Gaetano Conte in 1836. The German neurologist Peter Becker first proposed what we now know as BMD as a "benign variant" in 1952.

The more severe DMD is also the more common dystrophinopathy. A DMD incidence of 1 in 3500 live male births is frequently cited, with a citation trail leading to a 1991 estimate of population frequency in a Northern English population. However, newborn screening studies have demonstrated an incidence ranging from around 1 : 3802 to 1 : 6391, with an incidence of around 1 : 5200 found in a recent U.S. study. BMD is about one third as common, with an estimated incidence of around 1 in 18,500 male births. Rarely, *DMD* mutations may result in a third form of dystrophinopathy: X-linked dilated cardiomyopathy (XLDC), in which skeletal myopathy may be entirely absent. As the *DMD* gene is found on chromosome Xp21, the dystrophinopathies typically affect only boys, although rare cases in females occur explained by unusual genetic mechanisms such as balanced chromosomal translocations; most often, carriers are asymptomatic, although exceptions can occur.

The Dystrophin Protein

The dystrophin protein consists of multiple functional domains. In the 427-kDa muscle-specific isoform (Dp427m), the N-terminus contains an actin-binding domain (ABD1) canonically described as critical to dystrophin function, participating in binding to the filamentous F-actin of the cytoskeleton. A central rod domain consists of 24 spectrin-like repeats, and 4 hinge regions. Within this region are found a second actin-binding domain and a binding site for neuronal nitric oxide synthase (nNOS). A C-terminal cysteine-rich domain mediates binding to β-dystroglycan at the sarcolemmal membrane. Anchored by a complex of four sarcoglycan proteins (mutations in any of which cause a limb-girdle

muscular dystrophy), β-dystroglycan binds the extracellular α-dystroglycan, which in turn is engaged in glycosylation-dependent binding to extracellular matrix ligands and in particular to laminin α_2. Distal to the dystroglycan-binding region are binding sites for additional proteins, including dystrobrevin and syntrophin.

Based on this structure, a standard model of dystrophin function has been developed in which it plays a critical role as a stabilizer of the muscle membrane in the setting of significant deformational forces generated by muscle contraction. In the absence of dystrophin, the muscle membrane is damaged, as seen clinically by elevations of the muscle enzyme creatine kinase (CK) in serum. Elevated CK is typically the first biochemical sign of the disease detected by clinicians. Simultaneously, calcium influx into the muscle fiber leads to activation of calcium-dependent proteases, initiating myofiber degeneration, followed by cycles of regeneration and fibrosis and eventual loss of muscle contractile function. However, the presence of binding sites for nNOS, dystrobrevin, and syntrophin suggests that dystrophin has a significant signaling role as well. In contrast to the absence of dystrophin resulting in DMD, the protein resulting from BMD mutations retains some of these functions, resulting in the milder phenotype.

Shorter isoforms utilize promoters found in intronic regions, but generally share the same C-terminal domains. Of particular clinical relevance are the dystrophin isoforms Dp140 and Dp71, which are predominant in brain; as discussed below, mutations that result in absent expression of these isoforms are related to increased cognitive impairment in DMD patients.

The "Reading Frame Rule"

DMD is nearly always associated with an absence of dystrophin expression, whereas BMD is associated with expression of a partially functional protein (Figure 146-1). At the level of gene mutations, the difference between an absent or a partially functional dystrophin is explained by the concept of the "reading frame rule." As discussed under Molecular genetic testing, the majority of mutations responsible for dystrophinopathies consist of exonic deletions. The reading frame rule states that the number of exons deleted is not the primary determinant of disease severity. Rather, mutations that disrupt an open reading frame—commonly termed "out-of-frame" mutations—lead to termination of translation, no protein expression, and DMD. In contrast, mutations that maintain an open reading frame—or "in-frame" mutations—lead to BMD (Figure 146-2). Most often, these are single or multiple exon deletions that result in internal deletions of some portion of the central rod domain, and allow translation of the protein that still binds F-actin and β-dystroglycan. As a result, some patients with quite large deletions, particularly of the spectrin repeat–containing central rod domain, can have relatively mild disease.

This rule has proven useful in understanding phenotypic differences, with a sensitivity of 93% to 96% in predicting

DMD in large series (Flanigan et al., 2009). Importantly, it also provides a pathway for therapeutic approaches for DMD. Two examples discussed below include virally mediated microdystrophin gene therapy and antisense oligonucleotide exon-skipping therapy, both of which are directed toward expression of internally deleted dystrophin proteins from in-frame BMD-like transcripts. Exceptions to the rule occur, and are discussed in more detail in the Molecular Diagnostic section below.

Clinical Features

Duchenne Muscular Dystrophy

Boys with DMD typically present with symptoms between 2 and 5 years of age. Parents most commonly describe abnormal gait, often as toe walking immediately on gait acquisition, but gait onset may also be delayed. Recent studies show measurable differences in motor function in infants. Symptoms may only be obvious to parents in retrospect—sometimes noted only after a younger sibling is noted to show more rapid motor development—but delayed motor and developmental function can be demonstrated within the first years of life. Delayed language acquisition may be the presenting sign of DMD, and boys with language delay should have a CK level checked as part of their assessment.

By the time of presentation to the specialist, proximal weakness is typically evident to an examiner. At ages when isolated strength testing is unreliable, examination shows difficulty in climbing stairs or hopping. Attempts to arise from the floor typically elicit the Gowers' maneuver (Figure 146-3), which, although not specific (as it may be seen in the setting of any disease causing pelvic girdle weakness), is always eventually seen in DMD: a supine boy will roll over into quadruped, spread his base of support, raise his buttocks into the air before his trunk, and place one hand or both hands on his knees and walk his hands up his thighs to thrust into an upright position. Muscle enlargement is common, particularly in the calves. Originally termed "pseudohypertrophy" by Duchenne, such enlargement is often attributed to increased fibrosis and fatty replacement, but true hypertrophy of the contractile mass of muscle fibers also occurs. At presentation, heel cords are typically tight, and mild lordosis is present. Neck extension strength is often normal but the neck flexors are particularly weak, in contrast to BMD, in which neck flexor strength may be relatively preserved. Given their gait abnormalities, boys with DMD are often first referred to orthopedic physicians, or physical therapists rather than neurologists as part of their diagnostic odyssey.

The clinical course in DMD after diagnosis is stereotyped. Strength may show improvement, and motor function typically improves into the sixth or seventh year, followed by a plateau in function that may last 12 to 18 months. Thereafter, weakness progresses and leads inexorably to wheelchair dependence. This loss of ambulation historically occurred, in the precorticosteroid treatment era, by the age of 12 years (although, steroid treatment has moderately altered the natural history of disease). Wheelchair dependence is followed by progressive arm weakness, which limits independent function. It is also followed by a progressively increased risk of ventilatory insufficiency, scoliosis, and cardiomyopathy, and without supportive ventilatory therapy, death historically occurred by the age of 20 years—a figure altered by current care standards.

Arguably the best predictor of disease severity in an individual patient is the clinical course of an affected male relative carrying the same mutation. Such comparisons must take into account different treatment practices, but families with significant differences in severity between affected individuals are rare. Few clinical tests help provide prognostic information. Importantly, the level of CK elevation is not predictive of the severity of the phenotype, but rather reflects the phase of the disease process.

In addition to motor symptoms, cognitive impairment is common in DMD patients. IQ is diminished by one standard deviation in comparison to normal controls and in general does not change with age. Language development is delayed, and although the verbal IQ does improve, difficulties with expression may occur. Combined with dysarthria because of tongue hypertrophy, this may make communication challenging with age. Boys with DMD are also at an increased risk of autism, attention-deficit/hyperactivity disorder, and obsessive-compulsive disorder.

Measuring progression of skeletal muscle dysfunction is important both for clinical trials and to predict the loss of function in clinical care (see Ch. 137). In general, boys with DMD improved by most measures until the age of 7 years, after which their function begins to decline. Timed functional tests in common usage include the time to rise from the floor, the time to complete a 10-m walk/run, the time to climb a standard set of 4 stairs, and the distance covered during a 6-minute walk test (6MWT). Among these, the 10-m walk and time to rise from the floor are particularly useful in the clinic setting, as a boy taking greater than 12 seconds to walk 10 m or unable to rise from the floor is highly likely to lose the ability to ambulate independently within 1 year. The 6MWT has become the current de facto standard as both a stratification tool and an outcome measure in clinical trials. A 30-m change on the 6MWT is considered the minimal clinically significant change in the DMD population, and among DMD boys those walking less than 350 m are at a high risk for a significant functional decline within 1 year, and those walking less than <325 m are at risk for loss of ambulation. Another tool used in clinical trials is the North Star Ambulatory Assessment (NSAA), an evaluator-administered scale specifically designed for children with DMD.

Becker Muscular Dystrophy

BMD is much more clinically heterogeneous than DMD. Half of affected males demonstrate muscle weakness by age 10 years, typically in a limb-girdle pattern, but many without muscle weakness at that age recall myalgias with exertion and calf hypertrophy in childhood. Symptoms may present well into mid-adulthood or late adulthood, and may include prominent or isolated quadriceps involvement. Very mild phenotypes include cramp-myalgia syndromes, exercise-induced myoglobinuria, and asymptomatic hyperCKemia. Although isolated cognitive impairment has been reported as the predominant presenting feature of rare cases of BMD, patients with BMD have a normal IQ distribution. Two thirds of BMD children have behavioral problems, and the frequency of autism and attention-deficit disorders is increased.

Although BMD displays a significant degree of variability, patients at the more severe end of the spectrum do present in childhood, but differ from DMD patients in that they continue to ambulate beyond the age of 13 years. However, as steroid therapies have altered the natural history of DMD, prolonging the age at which loss of ambulation occurs, many clinicians choose to use the categorization of an "intermediate muscular dystrophy" (IMD) phenotype for patients who walk past the age of 12 but stop walking by age 15. In this scheme, the clinical classification of BMD applies to the patient with dystrophinopathy who loses ambulation after age 15. The use of an IMD category is helpful to describe patients who are less severe than is typical for DMD but more severe than is typical for BMD.

Laboratory Features

Serum creatine kinase (CK) is increased in both DMD and BMD, and is usually the initial diagnostic test performed when a dystrophinopathy is suspected. In DMD, it is often 50 to 100 times normal at diagnosis. Serum CK levels are generally lower in BMD, and reach a maximum around age 10 to 15 years, reflecting relatively preserved muscle mass and activity in comparison to DMD. Episodes of extremely elevated serum CK leading to myoglobinuria or a diagnosis of rhabdomyolysis have been described, most often in BMD patients at the very mild end of the phenotypic spectrum and likely reflecting the ability of these mildly affected patients to perform vigorous physical activity that leads to such episodes.

Serum CK is elevated at birth, providing a marker for newborn screening. Most such studies utilize a fluorometric CK testing assay from a dried blood spot followed by a confirmatory serum CK and subsequent genomic mutational analysis. However, a two-tiered analysis allows both CK determination and mutational analysis of DNA extracted from the same Guthrie card, improving the feasibility of newborn screening. The CK is often >1000 U/L as a neonate, then typically rises to 20,000+ (>100× normal values) in childhood, but then declines as muscle mass is lost; as a result, the serum CK level may be normal in end-stage disease.

No other clinical laboratory values besides serum CK is particularly useful in making the diagnosis. However, it is very important for clinicians to be aware that the serum aspartate aminotransferase (AST) and alanine aminotransferase (ALT) levels are always elevated in dystrophinopathies, as these enzymes are found in muscle in addition to the liver. In the setting of unexplained transaminase elevations, the serum CK should always be checked before liver biopsy. The serum level of the liver-specific gamma-glutamyl transferase has proven to be a useful marker of liver injury in the dystrophinopathy population. In assessing renal function in the DMD patient, serum creatinine or creatinine clearance may be decreased because of diminished muscle mass, and cystatin C is a more appropriate clinical marker of renal dysfunction.

Molecular Genetic Testing

***DMD* Mutation Analysis.** Mutation analysis of the *DMD* gene has largely replaced muscle biopsy as the first diagnostic test performed after serum CK testing. Testing of genomic DNA derived from lymphocytes is readily available. Detailed mutational analysis now represents the standard of care, not only because it may provide prognostic information, but also because it facilitates genetic counseling and potentially more importantly may determine suitability for specific novel therapies. Notably, DNA confirmation of an obligate carrier status is not required in the setting of a clear X-linked history consistent with that state. However, one third of DMD cases are *de novo* (consistent with the Haldane rule for an X-linked lethal disorder). Genetic counseling is essential, in part to address the risk of germline mosaicism in mothers whose lymphocyte DNA analysis is negative (up to 10%).

The *DMD* gene is, in genomic terms, the largest gene identified. Because it consists of 79 exons spread over 2.2 million bases, mutation analysis has historically been challenging. Eight different promoters have been identified, resulting in a variety of isoforms that share the same C-terminal portion of the protein. The most abundant in muscle is 427 kDa (Dp427m), but other isoforms are found in brain, retina, and in a wide variety of tissues.

Around 65% of all dystrophinopathy mutations consist of a deletion of one or more exons, and because males are hemizygous at the *DMD* locus, a polymerase chain reaction (PCR)–based test can readily detect the absence of exons. As exon lesions are clustered around "hotspots" within the gene, a limited number of exons (25 to 28) could be tested to determine whether there was a deletion. This multiplex PCR test identified 98% of patients with deletions (Beggs et al., 1990), but did not necessarily identify the full extent of the deletion, nor could be used for determining carrier status or identifying duplications. In addition, it could not identify point mutations, such as nonsense mutations, missense mutations, or small insertion/deletion mutations.

This now archaic test has been superseded by methods that interrogate all exons for copy number change, allowing complete characterization of the exon range of all duplication and deletions, as well as identification of carriers of these mutation classes. Several such methods exist, including multiplex ligation-dependent probe amplification, and comparative genomic hybridization. Clinically, the specific method used is not as important as the fact that these methods interrogate all exons, which not only confirms the extent of deletions or duplications but also has the additional benefit of allowing the identification of those rare patients with complex exon duplications or deletions (i.e., affecting noncontiguous blocks of exons). Such modern methods are typically paired with a reflex test for direct sequence analysis of all exons by either Sanger or next-generation sequencing in patients without an exon copy number change to detect point mutations. Nearly all point mutations are individually rare and random mutations, meaning that they do not occur in hotspots and sequencing must be performed across the entire coding region.

The distribution of *DMD* mutation classes varies slightly in different cohorts, but in an unselected clinic cohort of 68 index cases, exonic deletions accounted for 65% of mutations and exonic duplications for 6%; nonsense mutations for 13%; missense mutations for 4%; and small insertions/deletions for 3%. Some reported cohorts are enriched for a single mutation class because of their recruitment design, but a similar distribution of mutation classes is seen in other large aggregate collections of patients.

With these modern methods of mutation analysis, the sensitivity of mutation detection in the peripheral blood–derived genomic DNA samples is approximately 93% to 96%. Patients for whom there is a strong index of suspicion but no detectable mutation on genomic DNA analysis require muscle biopsy. This allows confirmation of the diagnosis of the dystrophinopathy (by analysis of dystrophin expression) and provides muscle tissue for mRNA extraction, necessary for detection of mutations that escape detection by current clinical blood-based assays. The standard mutational methods result in the sequencing of both exons and flanking introns, but many dystrophinopathy patients without detectable mutations within these regions have deep intronic mutations that activate cryptic splice sites and result in the inclusion of intronic sequence as a "pseudoexon" within the mRNA. Sequencing of cDNA generated by reverse transcription PCR is required for diagnosis of pseudoexon mutations and for clarification of other unusual mutations such as exon inversions, for which standard mutational analyses may prove inadequate.

It is important for clinicians to recognize that exceptions to the reading frame rule do exist, and complicate prognostication based on mutation analysis alone. One such example consists of large in-frame deletions that encompass a large part of the ABD1 domain and extend the central rod domain, and may be associated with DMD. More commonly, predicted nonsense mutations—which, by definition, should result in no dystrophin expression—may instead alter exon splice definition elements, including exon splice enhancer or exon splice suppressor sequences. Among predicted nonsense mutations, 14% are associated with BMD, nearly all of which affect pre-mRNA splicing. These mutations are found within the exons flanked by two exons that would maintain an open-reading frame, typically with the regions spanning exons 23 to 42; the resulting mature mRNA includes some proportion that excludes the nonsense-containing exon, with resultant dystrophin expression. Particularly in the absence of an informative family history regarding the implication of a given mutation, prognostication or phenotypic classification cannot rely solely on the results of mutation analysis, but must take into account the entire clinical picture, including age at presentation, consistency of the examination with the predicted phenotype, and, if available, the results of any dystrophin expression studies on muscle biopsy.

Genotype-Phenotype Correlations

All mutations that ablate expression of the Dp427m isoform result in skeletal muscle degeneration, and with the exception of some mutations in which some variability of splicing may result in low levels of reading frame restoration, the specifics of the mutation do not significantly influence skeletal muscle phenotype. However, in nonmuscle tissues, mutations may influence symptoms; for example, mutations that ablate expression of the shorter dystrophin isoforms that are expressed in brain (Dp140, Dp71) result in a higher frequency of cognitive impairment (Pane et al., 2012). When a mutation results in an open reading frame, allowing expression of a partially functional dystrophin, symptom severity may be related to the presence or absence of specific domains, such as in BMD because of in-frame rod domain mutations where cardiomyopathy onset occurs earlier in deletions affecting the amino-terminal portion of the rod domain than in those affecting the latter portion of the rod domain.

Observations from patient mutations confirm the importance of the reading frame rule while providing templates for therapeutic approaches. The identification of a mildly affected BMD patient with a very large central rod domain deletion lends credence to the potential of mini- or microdystrophin approaches for viral gene therapies. The large in-frame deletion of exons 45 to 55 may result in X-linked dilated cardiomyopathy (XLDCM) without any significant limb weakness, or may result in relatively mild BMD; either outcome suggests the utility of a therapy directed at inducing exon skipping to result in the equivalent mRNA.

Besides variation caused by underlying alternative splicing, notable exceptions to the reading frame rule can result from alternative translational initiation. Another is the only DMD founder allele mutation described in North American families.

Muscle Biopsy

The histopathologic features in DMD and BMD are not specific to the dystrophinopathies. The degree of changes depends in part on age of the patient, the muscle sampled, and where the patient lies in the disease course. In DMD patients without dystrophin, myofiber necrosis, phagocytosis, and regeneration are present from an early age, along with fibrosis and fatty replacement leading eventually to end-stage pathology. NF-kB is upregulated in DMD in infancy, before fibrosis becomes evident. In BMD, the degree of pathology is often less severe, particularly in earlier phases of the disease, where more moderate variation in myofiber size may be seen, and fibrosis may be less prominent; however, with time many BMD muscles in older patients appear indistinguishable from

DMD muscles, correlating with weakness rather than a specific clinical classification.

The importance of muscle biopsy in the diagnosis of the dystrophinopathies has declined as robust and complete mutational analysis has become available. Nevertheless, absent or altered dystrophin expression can provide an unequivocal diagnosis, and as previously noted, muscle biopsy is still required to establish the specifics of the mutational mechanism in some patients. Dystrophin protein expression can be assessed by either immunofluorescent (IF) or immunohistochemical (IHC) staining of muscle sections, or by immunoblot analysis of homogenized tissue, or by Western blot (WB) analysis (see Figure 146-1). The standard clinical practice is to perform IF or IHC staining with three antibodies, with one directed to each of the N-terminal, C-terminal, and central rod domains, as utilization of a rod domain antibody alone may give a false result in patients with in-frame deletions of exons coding for the epitope. Reproducible and specific quantification of dystrophin expression is technically challenging, and is routinely performed only in research settings. In routine clinical practice, dystrophin expression is typically expressed qualitatively. Biopsies of DMD muscle frequently demonstrate revertant fibers—found in up to 50% of biopsies—which are clusters of fibers with significant dystrophin expression that occurs because of altered mRNA splicing resulting in some mRNA with an open reading frame, resulting in the expression of dystrophin. Western blotting can provide information regarding protein size, and quantitative estimates, although absolute values as cutoffs of DMD versus BMD have not been rigorously validated.

Management of DMD and BMD

Although the dystrophinopathies commonly present because of skeletal muscle symptoms, multiple systems are affected. DMD uniformly progresses to include cardiomyopathy, impaired ventilation because of diaphragmatic and thoracic muscle weakness, diminished bone density (exacerbated by corticosteroid therapy), and gastrointestinal dysmotility. Once a boy is wheelchair dependent, cardiac and ventilatory dysfunction become more severe, scoliosis typically supervenes, and the need for adaptive therapies becomes more important. Management may be facilitated by provision of care within a multidisciplinary clinic, and published standards of care describe consensus recommendations (with an updated version in preparation) (Bushby et al., 2010a,b). At a minimum, DMD patients should be seen yearly by a neurologist or rehabilitation physician, a cardiologist, a pulmonologist, physical and occupational therapists, and a nutritionist (see also Ch. 152). Additional input may be required from endocrinologist, orthopedic surgeons, social workers, and palliative care specialists.

Pharmacologic Management

Corticosteroids. The mainstay of medical therapy for DMD is the corticosteroids prednisone and deflazacort. These are the only medications that have been shown to affect the clinical course, with a consensus that treatment with some corticosteroid regimen results in preservation of ambulation by up to 1 to 3 years. Their precise mechanism of their effect is unknown, but postulated effects include membrane stabilization, diminished fibrosis, and decreased inflammatory responses. A seminal randomized placebo-controlled trial of prednisone demonstrated that treatment with 0.75 mg/kg per day resulted in improved muscle strength by 6 months, whereas a dose twice that showed no additional benefit, with significantly more side effects. Deflazacort at an equivalent dose of 0.9 mg/kg per day has equivalent efficacy but a potentially a less pronounced side effect profile, with less weight gain. However, both drugs are associated with significant side effects, including obesity, gastrointestinal bleeding, osteoporosis (leading to increased vertebral body and long bone fracture, with the latter leading to a risk of fat embolism syndrome), short stature, delayed puberty, Cushingoid features, hypertension, cataracts, glaucoma, and emotional lability. Alternative regimens have been utilized in an effort to minimize side effects, including dosing on a schedule of 10 days on/10 days off or for the first 10 days a month. A small study of weekend dosing at 10 mg/ kg per week divided on weekend days suggested efficacy roughly equivalent to daily dosing in terms of efficacy, but showed no significant decrease in side effects. These different regimens have not been well characterized in head-to-head clinical trials, but the ongoing NIH-sponsored multicenter, multiyear FOR-DMD randomized double-blinded trial will likely answer outstanding questions regarding relative efficacy and side effects among these alternate regimens.

Despite decades of use, several issues regarding corticosteroid therapy exist. One is at what age to initiate corticosteroid therapy with treatment. Published recommendations suggest starting therapy between 2 and 5 years of age in boys whose strength has plateaued or is declining, but earlier treatment may be more beneficial. A second concern regards dose adjustments; in common practice most physicians do not adhere strictly to a 0.75-mg/kg dose of prednisone over years but instead allow the per-kilogram dose to drift down depending on tolerance and side effects. A third issue relates to the optimal use of corticosteroids after loss of ambulation, as there is increasing evidence that the use of low-dose steroids in nonambulant boys may result in diminished scoliosis and improved ventilation.

Cardiac. All patients with DMD eventually develop cardiomyopathy, the clinical importance of which is arguably increasing as ventilatory and orthopedic care continues to improve. Although a typical age of onset is often described as around 14 to 15 years, the incidence may be as high as 25% by age 6 years and 59% by 10 years. Screening echocardiograms are recommended at diagnosis or by age 6 years, then every 2 years up to age 10, and yearly thereafter. Cardiac MRI is increasingly available, and may demonstrate fibrosis and diastolic dysfunction before systolic dysfunction is noted. Cardiomyopathy is typically treated with afterload reduction, using angiotensin-converting enzyme inhibitors or angiotensin receptor blockers, with evidence that drugs should be initiated even before echocardiographic abnormalities are detected. Cardiac conduction disturbances are frequent, and the use of regular Holter monitoring may be helpful. In BMD, cardiomyopathy is also frequent, and may be severe, even necessitating cardiac transplantation, often when the skeletal muscle phenotype is more modestly affected.

Pulmonary. Pulmonary insufficiency remains the major cause of mortality, with impairment in vital capacity and airway clearance frequently leading to significant morbidity. Respiratory therapy and nocturnal ventilatory support have played key roles in extending life expectancy and improving quality of life in patients with DMD (LoMauro et al., 2015). The use of mechanical insufflator/exsufflator devices is associated with decreased pulmonary infections, and their use should be considered routine in this population. Loss of forced vital capacity becomes noticeable after loss of ambulation, and all patients in a wheelchair should be considered for yearly sleep studies and institution of bilevel positive airway pressure support.

Non-pharmacologic Management

Spine/Scoliosis. Scoliosis ultimately affects the majority of boys with DMD, accelerating after loss of ambulation.

Orthopedic consultation should be considered for boys with scoliosis notable on examination, with yearly progression assessed by x-rays. Historical retrospective data from a single clinic suggest that spine stabilization surgeries in appropriate patients, combined with nocturnal ventilation, are sufficient interventions to prolong survival into the fourth decade.

Contractures. Early institution of the use of nighttime ankle-foot orthoses (AFOs) decreases the development and progression of heel cord contractures. Dynamic splints may be preferred over fixed AFOs, as they reduce contracture progression by stretching the ankle joint and maintaining ankle position over several hours. A dynamic splint has the potential to provide a passive muscle stretch throughout the night, whereas a solid brace will maintain the ankle in a 90-degree position. Use of daytime ankle bracing is generally not recommended, as they may interfere with gait deviations that are compensatory for pelvic girdle and the extensor weakness. Other muscle groups prone to contracture and targeted for passive stretching are the iliotibial band, hip flexors, hamstrings, and elbow and finger flexors. Surgical release of Achilles tendon contractures is generally not advised when the child is still ambulatory, and may even lead to premature loss of ambulation.

Recent Advances in Dystrophinopathy Therapeutics

Multiple approaches toward correcting the pathologic features of dystrophinopathy are in development, and some are near or have reached clinical trials. These include therapies directed toward upregulation of the dystrophin surrogate utrophin, toward diminishing fibrosis, or toward modulating nNOS (which is mislocalized in muscle in the absence of dystrophin). Many of the most promising potential therapies that have already reached clinical trials are directed toward correcting the fundamental defect in DMD by inducing expression of a corrective (i.e., at least partially functional) version of the dystrophin protein (Figure 146-4).

Nonsense suppression therapies alter ribosomal recognition of premature stop codons, as first demonstrated with gentamicin treatment in the *mdx* mouse, which carries a nonsense mutation in exon 23. Gentamicin treatment of nonsense mutation associated DMD patients—accounting for around 15% of all mutations—is not practical, despite a small proof-of-principle study. The orally available nonsense suppression agent ataluren has demonstrated promising clinical efficacy into early phase clinical trials, and received conditional approval in Europe.

Exon skipping therapies are based on the reading frame rule, and seek to alter pre-mRNA splicing such that an exon flanking an out-of-frame exonic deletion excluded from the mature mRNA resulted in an in-frame transcript encoding a BMD-like protein. Targeting of a given exon may restore the reading frame for several different out-of-frame mutations; for example, exclusion of exon 51 will restore the reading frame for deletions of 13 to 50, 29 to 50, 43 to 50, 45 to 50, 47 to 50, 48 to 50, 49 to 50, 50 alone, 52 alone, and 52 to 63. Because of the clustering of exon deletions around the central rod domain deletion hotspot, targeting a limited number of exons will allow restoration of an open reading frame for a relatively large number of patients. For example, skipping of only four exons would be beneficial to around 35% of patients, including exon 51 (13.0% of patients), exon 45 (8.1%), exon 53 (7.7%), and exon 44 (6.2%), and skipping of up to two exons corrects 83% of DMD mutations.

Such skipping has been brought to human trials using antisense oligonucleotides based on two different chemistries,

2'O-methyl phosphorothioate (2'O-Me) antisense oligonucleotides or phosphorodiamidate morpholino oligomers (PMO), in each case with exon 51 as the lead target. Treatment of 12 patients with the PMO eteplirsen resulted, at 48 weeks, in a significant difference in the distance walked in the 6MWT between patients treated with the compound at the start of the study and those who initially received a placebo for 24 weeks before receiving active drug, and at 3 years in a difference between treated patients and historical controls. Similarly, treatment of 53 patients with the 2'O-Me drisapersen for 48 weeks resulted in a significant increase in 6MWT distance walked at 25 weeks in those patients treated with continuous treatment, rather than intermediate treatment or placebo. In 2016, the US Food and Drug Adminstration granted approval for Eteplirsen and denied approval for drisapersen. Studies targeting other exons are underway.

Gene transfer is directed toward the delivery of a functional version of the gene to skeletal muscle, and ultimately as well to the heart and diaphragm. Delivery of the full-length *DMD* gene in naked plasmid form proved inefficient. In contrast, various serotypes of adeno-associated viruses (AAV) show significant tropism for muscle, and can deliver transgenes that remain in the cell as episomal DNA. Because AAVs are limited in the size of transgene they can encapsidate (with a maximum capacity of around 5 kb), microdystrophin transgenes lacking large portions of the central rod domain have been developed. Although an initial trial with an early microdystrophin vector version did not show significant dystrophin expression after intramuscular injection, improved AAV vectors are in development and are reaching clinical trials.

Other approaches: In addition to these gene-directed therapies, a variety of other approaches are in or have reached clinical trials, although none have yet gained regulatory approval. Treatment with idebenone, a benzoquinone antioxidant that inhibits lipid peroxidation and stimulates mitochondrial electron flux and cellular energy production, has been shown to slow the decline in peak expiratory flow as percentage predicted, forced vital capacity, and peak cough flow in nonambulant DMD patients. Inhibition of myostatin has been shown to ameliorate disease severity in animal models of DMD. This has led to trials of myostatin inhibition by antibodies or by expression of a transgene expressing the competing protein follistatin, and studies have been published in BMD or are underway in DMD. Another approach is the use of phosphodiesterase type 5 (PDE5) inhibitors such as tadalafil or sildenafil to increase nNOS activity in skeletal muscle. Although this has been shown to be promising in animal models and can alter measures of muscle ischemia in DMD patients, it has not yet been shown to have a clinical benefit. Upregulation of the dystrophin paralog utrophin is beneficial in mouse models, and clinical development of a small-molecule upregulator is underway. Other new therapeutics are directed toward antiinflammatory pathways or membrane stabilization.

Altogether the breadth of these approaches allows the clinician to offer some optimism to the parents of a child with a new diagnosis, and can appropriately claim that the dystrophinopathies are the subject of intense clinical research with the prospect of meaningful therapies on the horizon.

SELECTED REFERENCES

Beggs, A.H., Koenig, M., Boyce, F.M., et al., 1990. Detection of 98% of DMD/BMD gene deletions by polymerase chain reaction. Hum. Genet. 86, 45–48.

Bushby, K., Finkel, R., Birnkrant, D.J., et al., 2010a. Diagnosis and management of Duchenne muscular dystrophy, part 1: diagnosis, and pharmacological and psychosocial management. Lancet Neurol. 9, 77–93.

Bushby, K., Finkel, R., Birnkrant, D.J., et al., 2010b. Diagnosis and management of Duchenne muscular dystrophy, part 2: implementation of multidisciplinary care. Lancet Neurol. 9, 177–189.

Cheuk, D.K., Wong, V., Wraige, E., et al., 2015. Surgery for scoliosis in Duchenne muscular dystrophy. Cochrane Database Syst. Rev. (10), CD005375.

Flanigan, K.M., Dunn, D.M., von Niederhausern, A., et al., 2009. Mutational spectrum of DMD mutations in dystrophinopathy patients: application of modern diagnostic techniques to a large cohort. Hum. Mutat. 30, 1657–1666.

Kamdar, F., Garry, D.J., 2016. Dystrophin-deficient cardiomyopathy. J. Am. Coll. Cardiol. 67, 2533–2546.

LoMauro, A., D'Angelo, M.G., Aliverti, A., 2015. Assessment and management of respiratory function in patients with Duchenne muscular dystrophy: current and emerging options. Ther. Clin. Risk Manag. 11, 1475–1488.

Matthews, E., Brassington, R., Kuntzer, T., et al., 2016. Corticosteroids for the treatment of Duchenne muscular dystrophy. Cochrane Database Syst. Rev. (5), CD003725.

Pane, M., Lombardo, M.E., Alfieri, P., et al., 2012. Attention deficit hyperactivity disorder and cognitive function in Duchenne muscular dystrophy: phenotype-genotype correlation. J. Pediatr. 161, 705–709 e701.

Shieh, P.B., 2015. Duchenne muscular dystrophy: clinical trials and emerging tribulations. Curr. Opin. Neurol. 28, 542–546.

147 Congenital, Limb Girdle and Other Muscular Dystrophies

Richard S. Finkel, Payam Mohassel, and Carsten G. Bönnemann

An expanded version of this chapter is available on www.expertconsult.com. See inside cover for registration details.

Muscular dystrophies (MDs) are prototypic neuromuscular disorders that often present in childhood and are characterized by progressive weakness and loss of motor function. In addition, there is often related cardiac, pulmonary, and musculoskeletal morbidity, and survival may be shortened. All MDs are caused by mutations in genes responsible for the production of proteins essential for contractile, cytoskeletal, signaling, or enzymatic function within the muscle fiber or extracellular matrix. The explosion in molecular genetics over the past three decades has brought a greater understanding of the biologic basis for these disorders and the appreciation that multiple genes, when mutated, can cause a similar phenotype. Conversely, mutations in one gene can cause very different phenotypes. Chapter 135 discusses normal muscle development and the pathophysiologic processes involved in MDs. Common themes to MDs are features of muscle fiber degeneration with inadequate cellular repair, leading to atrophy of these fibers and replacement by fat and connective tissue. As a consequence, muscles lose contractile force and become flaccid, stiff, atrophic, or hypertrophied. This results in loss of function and joint contractures in skeletal muscle, and in some instances impaired cardiac and intestinal (smooth muscle) function. Each MD has distinctive features, for reasons not well understood, where some muscles are more vulnerable and others more resistant to the intrinsic pathologic processes that cause the progressive muscle fiber deterioration. As such, patterns of muscle involvement have been identified over nearly two centuries, and this has led to the current nomenclature. Figure 147-1 presents a classification of the MDs within the overall context of muscle disorders. Chapter 137 discusses more general principles of neuromuscular disorders and Figure 137-2 illustrates the more common MDs. Duchenne and Becker MD ("dystrophinopathies") are discussed in Chapter 146. Myotonic dystrophies, a distinct category of muscle disease, are discussed in Chapter 151. This chapter discusses the other common MDs with an emphasis on pediatric presentation:

- Limb-Girdle MD (LGMD): proximal > distal weakness involving the lower > upper extremities
- Congenital MD (CMD): early onset dystrophic process, often with brain and ophthalmologic involvement, abnormal brain myelination, or extracellular matrix collagen abnormality
- Facioscapulohumeral MD (FSHD): principal involvement of the facial, scapular, humeral, peroneal, and abdominal muscles
- Emery-Dreifuss MD (EDMD): scapular, humeral, and peroneal involvement with early onset of joint contractures and often cardiac involvement
- Oculopharyngeal MD (OPMD): ocular, bulbar, and variable proximal shoulder and hip girdle involvement (onset of OPMD is typically in the adult years)

To grasp how these conditions are interrelated, it is useful to understand how the various genes and gene products (proteins) function within the muscle fiber as illustrated in

Figure 147-2. Table 147-1 categorizes these disorders based on the clinical phenotype and related genes, mode of inheritance, and name of the gene product. Each subsection below will address the relevant genes, proteins, mechanisms, and pathophysiology. The inheritance patterns—autosomal dominant, autosomal recessive, and X-linked recessive—are also discussed. Three websites listed in the selected references are particularly useful when a focused search is desired. In addition, the Online Mendelian Inheritance in Man (www.omim.org) and the Orphanet (www.orpha.net) websites provide a broad overview of all genetic conditions. The Gene Tests website (www.genetests.org) provides a comprehensive resource of genetic testing laboratories, by country, where testing for these disorders can be pursued.

DYSTROPHINOPATHIES (DUCHENNE AND BECKER MUSCULAR DYSTROPHIES AND CLINICAL VARIANTS)

The dystrophinopathies are reviewed in Chapter 146.

LIMB-GIRDLE MUSCULAR DYSTROPHIES
Definition

The limb-girdle MDs (LGMDs) consist of a diverse group of disorders within the broader field of genetic muscle diseases.

LGMD is defined as a muscular dystrophy presenting with predominantly proximal weakness, sparing facial, extraocular, and distal extremity muscles (at least early in the course of the disease). Muscle biopsy is of great importance for inclusion into this group and shows dystrophic features, including degeneration and regeneration, increased internalized nuclei, fiber size variability, increased endomysial fibrosis, and fatty replacement. However, just mild, nonspecific myopathic changes may also be seen still be consistent with the diagnostic category. Autosomal-recessive LGMDs (type 2) are more common than the autosomal-dominant (type 1) counterparts and will be discussed first in this chapter. Currently, 8 forms of type 1 and 19 forms of type 2 have been described and assigned a number and are summarized in Table 147-1.

Autosomal-Recessive Limb-Girdle Muscular Dystrophies

Classic autosomal-recessive LGMDs include the sarcoglycanopathies (LGMD 2C-F), calpainopathy (LGMD 2A), and dysferlinopathy (LGMD 2B). This order reflects their average age of onset from younger to older. Two additional more common autosomal-recessive LGMDs are attributed to mutations in the α-dystroglycanopathy gene fukutin-related protein (FKRP) (LGMD 2I), with a broad range of age of onset, and anoctamine-5 (LGMD 2L), a primarily adult-onset disease that resembles dysferlinopathy. There are a number of additional recessive LGMD forms.

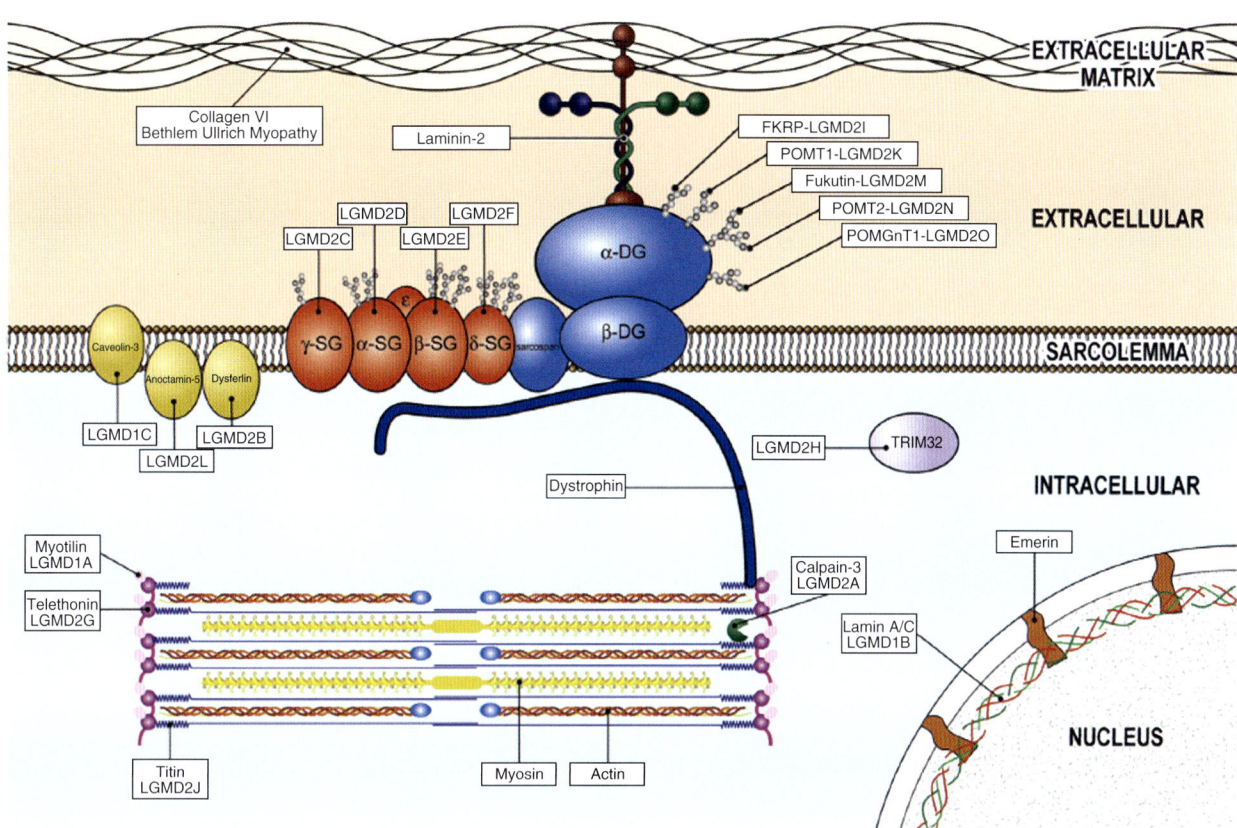

Figure 147-2. Schematic Schematic diagram illustrating a muscle fiber and the cellular localization of the gene products for the limb-girdle and congenital muscular dystrophies, with their associated disorders. DG, dystrophglycan; SG, sarcoglycan. *(Reproduced, with permission, from Wicklund MP, Kissel JT. The limb-girdle muscular dystrophies. Neurol Clin 2014;32:729–49.)*

Sarcoglycanopathies (LGMD 2C-F)

Sarcoglycanopathies were first described as autosomal-recessive disorders resembling Duchenne muscular dystrophy (DMD). In addition to the autosomal-recessive pattern of inheritance, the immunohistochemical presence of dystrophin on muscle biopsy differentiated sarcoglycanopathies from DMD. While initially referred to as SCARMD (for severe childhood autosomal-recessive muscular dystrophy), many patients with milder presentations were subsequently identified and the term SCAMRD is no longer widely used.

Sarcoglycanopathies account for 20% to 25% of all patients with muscular dystrophy but comprise roughly 50% to 60% of the more severe LGMDs as opposed to 10% to 20% of the milder forms.

Pathophysiology. See online chapter for discussion.

Genetics and Mutations. Mutations in all four major sarcoglycan genes cause four genetically separate forms of autosomal-recessive LGMD with almost indistinguishable clinical phenotypes. The majority of milder cases in sarcoglycanopathies are related to α-sarcoglycan mutation, including almost asymptomatic patients with high CK levels and lordosis. β- and γ-sarcoglycan mutations have a higher proportion of severe early childhood cases, although significant intrafamilial variability occurs. δ-Sarcoglycan mutations generally are more severe.

Clinical Features. Clinical features of the four sarcoglycanopathies overlap. They predominantly affect young children with a median age of onset around 6 to 8 years.

Time Course and Distribution of Motor Symptoms. The first symptoms generally relate to pelvic muscle weakness, evidenced by a waddling gait, which limits running, getting up from the floor, or climbing stairs. Primary toe walking may be present. Muscle cramps, pain, and exercise intolerance with or without myoglobinuria can occur. The distribution of weakness is reminiscent of dystrophinopathies. However, unlike dystrophinopathies, anterior and posterior compartments of the thigh may be equally affected. Shoulder girdle weakness ensues. Deltoid, infraspinatus, and biceps muscles are involved early in the disease. Scapular weakness tends to be more pronounced compared with dystrophinopathies (Figure 147-3). Facial and extraocular muscles are spared. Late in the disease, distal muscles may be involved. In later stages and similar to DMD, neck flexor weakness may occur. Loss of independent ambulation may occur around 12 to 16 years of age, although there is variability. CK levels are elevated 10- to 100-fold early in the course of the disease.

Cardiac Features. Cardiac involvement occurs although clinically overt dilated cardiomyopathy is only seen in a minority of patients. Cardiac failure or sudden cardiac death may occur and cardiac transplantation may become necessary. Dilated cardiomyopathy may be more common in γ- and δ-sarcoglycanopathies but cardiac involvement is reported in all sarcoglycanopathies. Subclinical cardiac involvement is more common and noticeable on electrocardiography and echocardiography.

Pulmonary Features. Symptomatic respiratory failure is not an early feature of sarcoglycanopathies. Some patients with severe early onset muscle weakness develop severe restrictive lung disease. Clinically relevant respiratory failure does not manifest while the patient is still ambulant.

Contractures and Other Signs and Symptoms. Other associated signs include calf hypertrophy and macroglossia. Achilles tendon shortening tends to be the first sign of contractures and lordosis may occur early in the course, and so toe walking can be an early manifestation. Later, more contractures involving the hip flexors, lateral tractus, and knee flexors may develop. Progressive scoliosis may worsen respiratory compromise later in the disease. Intellectual impairment is not seen.

Diagnosis. Sarcoglycanopathies can be suspected based on clinical grounds. The probability of an autosomal-recessive LGMD in boys with a Duchenne-like phenotype is 6% to 8%.

Definitive histologic diagnosis requires immunohistochemical stains with antibodies against muscle sarcoglycans and dystrophin (Figure 147-4). Histology usually shows marked degeneration and regeneration and severely dystrophic muscle. Dystrophin immunoreactivity is expected to be normal, although it can be reduced similar to BMD or female carriers of a dystrophin mutation. Western blot analysis usually shows dystrophin with a normal molecular weight and quantities within 10% of normal.

Treatment. No specific therapies are available for sarcoglycanopathies but unlike dystrophinopathies, sarcoglycanopathies are more amenable to gene therapy as discussed in the online chapter.

Disorders of α-Dystroglycan Glycosylation

Limb-Girdle Muscular Dystrophy 2I: Fukutin-Related Protein Deficiency

Fukutin-related protein (FKRP) belongs to the growing list of genes underlying the group of α-dystroglycanopathies, characterized by abnormal O-mannosyl glycosylation of α-dystroglycan, which more typically are associated with forms of CMD (Congenital Muscular Dystrophies, below). Mutations in *FKRP* cause an extremely wide spectrum of phenotypes: ranging from severe Walker-Warburg syndrome (WWS), transitional phenotypes of CMD with variable central nervous system involvement or normal brain imaging, to less severe LGMDs with Duchenne to Becker MD-like like severities that are referred to as LGMD2I. LGMD2I is one of the more common forms of LGMD, representing from 11% to 19% of all cases of LGMD in different series.

Clinical Features. The LGMD phenotype of FKRP mutations can present with severity and distribution of muscle weakness similar to DMD, with early loss of ambulation even before 10 years of age. There is a pronounced predilection for axial muscles, neck flexors, and proximal limb muscles with prominent lordosis. Predominant weakness is typically seen in shoulder adduction and internal rotation, elbow flexion, hip flexion and adduction, knee flexion, and ankle dorsiflexion. Hamstrings are generally more involved than the quadriceps. Mild facial weakness can be seen. Scapular winging is not common. There can be tongue, calf, and brachioradialis hypertrophy.

Dilated cardiomyopathy can occur even before the loss of ambulation, whereas respiratory failure necessitating nocturnal ventilatory support manifests after loss of ambulation.

Diagnosis. LGMD 2I may be clinically suspected based on features such as the peculiar hypertrophy of brachioradialis muscle and tongue and the pattern of muscle weakness. Muscle MRI may demonstrate a distinctive pattern of involvement, similar to LGMD2A (calpain-3 deficiency). Muscle biopsy shows prominently reduced α-dystroglycans and also

mild reduction of laminin α2. Although these are not specific, they can be helpful in suggesting appropriate genetic analysis of the *FKRP* gene.

Management. No specific treatments are available at this time. Similar to other MDs with a predilection for cardiomyopathy and respiratory failure, recognition, evaluation, and treatment of these complications is of utmost importance.

Other α-Dystroglycanopathies

See online chapter for discussion.

Calpainopathy (LGMD2A)

Background and Epidemiology. Calpainopathy or LGMD 2A is likely the most common juvenile onset form of LGMD and may account for 40% to 50% of all LGMD patients.

Pathophysiology, Genetics, and Mutations. *CAPN3*, the gene mutated in LGMD 2A, encodes calpain-3, a calcium-activated protease that localizes to the cytoplasm and nuclei of the cells.

Clinical Features. Calpainopathies have a characteristic clinical phenotype although variations and atypical presentations do occur. The age of onset is later than sarcoglycanopathies, between 8 and 15 years of age, with a wide range from 2 to 40 years.

Time Course and Distribution of Motor Symptoms. The first symptoms generally relate to pelvic girdle muscle weakness. Later, shoulder girdle and arm weakness becomes apparent. Minimal facial weakness is reported very late in the disease, and facial, extraocular, and pharyngeal muscles are otherwise spared. Overall, a rather thin-appearing muscle profile, with gluteus maximus and hip adductor weakness, scapular winging and high riding scapulae, wide stance, biceps atrophy, and lax abdominal muscles, is the most typical clinical appearance of patients with calpain-3 mutations (Figure 147-5). The course of the disease is progressive. Loss of independent ambulation occurs around 14 years of age or later. CK concentrations in the serum are significantly elevated. In comparison to sarcoglycanopathies or dysferlinopathies, CK levels tend to be lower on average.

Cardiac Features. No primary cardiac involvement has been attributed to *CAPN3* mutations. However, right bundle branch block has been reported.

Pulmonary Features. Respiratory failure is rare, occurring only in patients with severe and very advanced disease. Mild restrictive lung disease evidenced by reduced forced vital capacity is quite prevalent and usually asymptomatic.

Contractures and Other Signs and Symptoms. Contractures appear in the Achilles tendons and may involve the elbows and spine. In some patients, contractures may be severe earlier in the course, mimicking EDMD. Early lordosis may be seen.

Diagnosis. The clinical features can strongly suggest calpainopathy but further studies are needed for confirmation. Muscle imaging may reveal the characteristic distribution of muscle disease with selective involvement of the posterior compartment of the thigh and hip adductors, but such testing should be interpreted with caution. Muscle biopsy may show dystrophic features and type 1 fibers may appear lobulated on the oxidative stains such as NADH. Direct immunohistochemistry for calpain-3 with the current antibodies is not reliable but Western blot analysis can be informative with the calpain-3 level reduced or absent in muscle biopsy immunoblots in most patients. Mutation analysis is the most specific test.

Treatment. No specific therapies are available for calpainopathies. Findings of eosinophilic inflammation in the muscle in some LGMD2A patients have raised some interest in the use of immunosuppressive therapies. In mouse models, adenovirus-mediated gene transfer has been successful.

Dysferlinopathy (LGMD 2B)

Linkage studies have identified mutations in *DYSF*, the gene coding for dysferlin, the protein affected in LGMD 2B on chromosome 2p. *DYSF* mutations are associated with a number of distinct clinical phenotypes: a typical LGMD, a distal muscular dystrophy known as Miyoshi myopathy, and a third phenotype with early anterior tibial compartment weakness. Even in the limb-girdle phenotype, the phenotypic spectrum is broad. The majority of patients first develop weakness in late adolescence and early adulthood. However, some patients develop a congenital myopathy and some remain only mildly affected well into adulthood.

Pathophysiology. (see online)

Genetics and Mutations. (see online)

Clinical Features. Compared with sarcoglycanopathies and calpainopathies, dysferlinopathies begin later in life with weakness starting around 18 to 20 years of age but congenital disease or mild adult onset disease have been reported. Weakness is slowly progressive and ambulation is usually preserved typically into the fourth decade.

Time Course and Distribution of Motor Symptoms. In the limb-girdle dysferlinopathy (LGMD2B), the first motor symptoms occur in the pelvifemoral distribution, in particular the quadriceps, and later involve the arms. However, one can detect gastrocnemius and soleus muscle wasting and weakness early in the limb-girdle phenotype as well, causing early inability to walk on toes even in the LGMD phenotype. This unique feature, which can be demonstrated with muscle imaging, can be diagnostically helpful. The pattern of weakness in the arms is usually mild at first and involves the distal biceps. Deltoid and periscapular muscles are often spared and as a result, in contrast to sarcoglycanopathies and calpainopathy, scapular winging is not a usual feature. As in other LGMDs, facial and extraocular muscles are preserved. In the Miyoshi phenotype, the gastrocnemius and soleus muscles are affected first, manifesting as the inability to walk on toes. In the upper extremities, the muscles of the forearms are quite weak, yet the intrinsic muscles of the hand are spared. The proximal muscles are affected as the disease progresses.

CK levels tend to be very high during the early, 20 to 150 times the upper limit of normal; in the presymptomatic patients it may only be mildly elevated.

Cardiac and Pulmonary Features. Dysferlinopathies do not feature conductive or functional cardiac disease or restrictive lung.

Contractures and Other Signs and Symptoms. Contractures are not a usual feature of dysferlinopathy.

Diagnosis. The characteristic clinical presentation includes the following features: age of onset around 18 to 20 years, highly elevated CK levels, proximal lower extremity weakness in conjunction with inability to walk on toes, relative sparing of the periscapular muscles, and early gastrocnemius muscle involvement on muscle imaging. However, the significant phenotypic variation, even among family members, can be misleading.

Muscle biopsy usually shows dystrophic features but inflammation may be prominent and delay the accurate diagnosis by suggesting myositis. Immunostains for dysferlin are usually absent. However, secondary reductions and staining abnormalities for dysferlin in other dystrophic conditions are not uncommon. Likewise, calpain level may be secondarily reduced or absent in dysferlinopathy. Western blot analysis is

a more specific diagnostic test and can also be attempted and yield diagnostic information. Mutation analysis is the most specific test.

Treatment. No specific treatments are available. Judicious use of orthotics can provide help in maintenance of ambulation in many patients.

Anoctaminopathy (LGMD2L)

Recessive mutations in *ANO5* on chromosome 11, the gene encoding anoctamine-5, have recently been linked with a group of adult patients with limb-girdle muscular dystrophy. See online chapter for discussion.

Other Rare Autosomal-Recessive Limb-Girdle Muscular Dystrophies

Telethoninopathy (LGMD 2G), LGMD 2H, and titinopathy (LGMD 2J) are rare forms of LGMD that may present in childhood. Further information on these disorders can be found on the resources listed at the beginning of this chapter.

Autosomal-Recessive Conditions Presenting as LGMD

Partial Laminin α_2 Deficiency. This condition is allelic to primary laminin α_2 deficiency, the form of CMD related to severe deficiency of laminin α_2, the heavy chain of the heterotrimer laminin 211 (merosin). Primary mutations in the *LAMA2* gene on chromosome 6q are responsible. In case of complete deficiency the clinical phenotype is that of a severe CMD. MRI of the brain may show supratentorial white matter T2 hyperintensities and some children develop seizures. The clinical presentation may be that of a milder CMD or may resemble LGMD with proximal weakness only, in which case, walking may be achieved. Joint contractures can be prominent and resemble EDMD. In these cases, only a partial deficiency of laminin α_2 on muscle biopsy specimen is seen. Western blot analysis is a more sensitive measure. Patients with partial laminin α_2 deficiency almost always show subtle alterations of white matter signal on T2-weighted MRIs. Patients with the LGMD phenotype usually have a missense mutation or an in frame deletion.

X-Linked Recessive Conditions Presenting as LGMD

Some patients with emerin mutations, the protein mutated in classical X-linked EDMD, discussed below, may present with an LGMD-like presentation without cardiac involvement.

Autosomal-Dominant Limb-Girdle Muscular Dystrophies

Autosomal-dominant LGMDs are generally less common and constitute about 10% of LGMDs. They occur later in comparison to autosomal-recessive LGMDs and have a milder or moderate course. Commonly, a positive family history is evident; however, de novo mutations and germline and/or somatic mosaicism account for some patients.

In this section we will divide autosomal-dominant LGMDs into two groups: one without cardiac involvement (LGMD 1A, 1C, and 1D) and the other with cardiac involvement (LGMD 1B).

Autosomal-Dominant LGMDs Without Cardiac Involvement

Myotilinopathy-LGMD 1A. Myotilinopathy LGMD 1A mutations have been implicated in myofibrillar myopathy-3—a distal, adult-onset, autosomal-dominant myopathy.

Pathophysiology and Mutations. (see online)

Clinical Features. Onset usually is in adulthood (late 20s) with slowly progressive symptoms involving proximal leg and arm weakness. Patients have a particular nasal speech quality and dysarthria. Achilles tendon contractures may be seen. CK values may be raised 1.6- to 10-fold the upper limit of normal. Cardiac and pulmonary involvement is not a typical feature.

Diagnosis. The peculiar clinical feature of nasal speech quality in the setting of an autosomal-dominant LGMD with mildly raised CK values can suggest this diagnosis. Muscle biopsy shows dystrophic features and in some cases autophagic vacuoles; Z-line streaming and disorganization as well as rod-shaped accumulations similar to nemaline myopathies have been reported on electron microscopy. Immunohistochemistry and Western blot analysis usually show normal levels of myotilin. Mutation analysis is usually necessary.

Treatment. No specific therapies are available.

Caveolinopathy (LGMD 1C)

Pathophysiology and Genetics. Caveolin-3 mutations, the muscle-specific form of caveolin, result in LGMD 1C as well as other phenotypes. Caveolae contribute to sarcolemmal integrity, regulate ion channels, and play a role in signal transduction among other roles. Most mutations resulting in the limb-girdle phenotype are missense or microdeletions. There is significant reduction of caveolin-3 immunoreactivity in muscle biopsy specimens of heterozygous patients.

Clinical Features. Four different muscle disease phenotypes are recognized: LGMD, rippling muscle disease, asymptomatic CK elevation, and a distal myopathy. There is significant overlap. There is also significant intrafamilial variability without a typical clinical phenotype. Some patients develop weakness in early childhood, whereas others remain asymptomatic. Myalgias and cramping with exertion have been reported. Some patients have calf hypertrophy (Figure 147-6). Definite cardiac or pulmonary involvement is not typically seen.

Diagnosis. Immunohistochemistry of muscle biopsy tissue shows reduced caveolin-3 immunoreactivity. Genetic confirmation is necessary in suggestive cases.

Treatment. Supportive management can be helpful to patients.

LGMD 1D.

This particular muscular dystrophy has been genetically linked to chromosome 7q in several families with DNAJB6 mutations. See online chapter.

Autosomal-Dominant LGMDs With Cardiac Involvement

Autosomal-dominant LGMDs with cardiac involvement have a close relationship to autosomal-dominant EDMD. Desmin mutations can also present with LGMD-like phenotype (LGMD 1E) and cardiac involvement; however, they are better described as myofibrillar myopathy.

Laminopathy (LGMD 1B).

This LGMD is allelic with autosomal-dominant EDMD.

Pathophysiology and Genetics. (see online)

Clinical Features. Whereas the EDMD and CMD forms have onset in earlier childhood, the LGMD presentation of laminopathy usually occurs in the late teens and early adulthood. Most patients develop weakness in the pelvic girdle muscles. Mild facial weakness and mild anterior tibial compartment weakness may be seen. Progression is slow, and biceps and Achilles tendon contractures may develop. CK values are usually mildly elevated, 1.5- to 3-fold.

Cardiac Features. Cardiac problems may manifest in the third and fourth decades with first-degree atrioventricular (AV) block that progresses to complete AV block. Similar to the EDMD and CMD presentations of *LMNA* mutations, sudden cardiac death is a prominent risk and may be its first and only manifestation. Dilated cardiomyopathy only rarely occurs.

Diagnosis. Diagnosis is based on suggestive clinical features, the cardiac manifestations, as well as the presence of contractures and an autosomal-dominant hereditary pattern. Muscle biopsy evaluation is not particularly helpful as lamin A/C immunoreactivity appears normal even in the presence of mutations; however, it is helpful to rule out other causes of LGMD. Genetic analysis should be initiated when LGMD 1B is suspected.

Treatment. No specific treatments are available. Careful cardiac evaluation and monitoring is important to evaluate for the need for intracardiac defibrillator placement to prevent fatal cardiac arrhythmias.

Autosomal-Dominant Conditions That May Present as LGMD

Facioscapulohumeral Dystrophy (FSHD, See Below).

FSHD is the single most important entity to consider in patients with an LGMD-like presentation, especially those with an autosomal-dominant pattern of inheritance.

Myotonic Dystrophy (DM) Types 1 and 2.

Myotonic dystrophy, discussed in Chapter 152, is one of the most common MDs. Patients with myotonic dystrophy, especially DM type 2, may present with a limb-girdle pattern of muscle weakness.

Collagen VI–Related Dystrophies.

Collagen VI–related dystrophies constitute a spectrum of severities from the mild Bethlem myopathy, via intermediate severity to the more severe Ullrich CMD. For the differential diagnosis of LGMD, Bethlem myopathy is the most important to consider. Bethlem myopathy is an autosomal-dominant and rarely also a recessive disorder caused by mutations in one of three genes coding for alpha chains of collagen type VI, *COL6A1* and *A2* on chromosome 21q22.3 or *COL6A3* on chromosome 2q37.

Ullrich CMD is characterized by severe weakness concomitant with joint hyperlaxity and contractures at birth. Respiratory insufficiency, which may begin before loss of independent ambulation, also worsens over time. As a result, early detection and treatment with noninvasive bilevel positive airway pressure ventilation may be required. There are also patients presenting with phenotypes of intermediate severity (Figure 147-7). Patients in this intermediate phenotype also experience progressive respiratory insufficiency, frequently leading to the need for nighttime noninvasive ventilator support.

Diagnosis is clinically suspected based on congenital weakness and concomitant severe contractures and joint laxity. Skin findings with prominent keratosis pilaris of the extensor surfaces of the arms and legs and abnormal keloid formation may be seen (Figure 147-8). Muscle imaging may show a characteristic pattern of muscle degeneration beginning adjacent to the fascia, resulting in the typical rimming of muscles and the "central cloud" in the rectus femoris along its central fascia. Molecular testing is similar for all collagen VI–related phenotypes.

Most patients with Bethlem myopathy develop symptoms in childhood and some may have congenital weakness/ hypotonia, torticollis, or foot deformities. Weakness is usually more predominant in the proximal muscles. Early on, there may be no contractures, and joint hyperlaxity may be present. Contractures usually occur at the end of the first decade, involving the deep finger flexors and proximal joints (Figure 147-8), and when absent or minor, the phenotype can resemble LGMD. Diagnosis is usually secured by showing mutations in one of the three genes encoding one of the alpha chains of collagen type VI. Sanger sequencing as well as next-generation sequencing is available to screen for mutations in the collagen type VI genes and arrive at a specific diagnosis.

EMERY-DREIFUSS MUSCULAR DYSTROPHY

Emery-Dreifuss MD (EDMD) is characterized by a clinical triad of early contractures, muscle wasting, and weakness in a humeroperoneal distribution, and cardiomyopathy. Considerable phenotypic variability exists regarding age at onset and rate of progression. X-linked transmission and autosomal-dominant transmission are recognized. Five genes have been identified (Table 147-1). EDMD is included in this section on LGMD because of the phenotypic similarity. Mutations in *FHL1* or *STA* genes also cause EDMD (see online chapter).

Pathophysiology and Genetics

Both X-linked and autosomal-dominant EDMD result from mutations in genes coding for nuclear envelope proteins. See online chapter.

Autosomal-dominant EDMD and, very rarely, autosomal-recessive EDMD result from mutations of the *LMNA* gene, located on 1q21, which encodes two nuclear envelope proteins, lamins A and C, discussed above.

Clinical Features

Although X-linked EDMD and autosomal-dominant EDMD usually share a similar phenotype, wide clinical variation with poor genotype-phenotype correlation has been documented in both.

The onset of contractures occurs early in the disease, in the first or second decade, and often precedes weakness. Contractures are most prominent at the elbows, Achilles tendons, and posterior cervical muscles. Upper-extremity contractures often precede axial and lower extremity deformities. The arms are held in a semiflexed position. The feet are set in talipes equinus, often in association with toe walking. Posterior cervical contractures preclude full neck flexion (Figure 147-9). Contractures usually remain disproportionate to the degree of weakness and may be the major factor in functional impairment. Muscle weakness is relatively mild and slowly progressive. The distribution of motor deficits is humeroperoneal, with upper-extremity weakness (in biceps, triceps, and spinatus muscles) occurring earlier than leg weakness (in tibialis anterior and peroneal muscles). Pseudohypertrophy is not seen, and its absence helps differentiate X-linked EDMD from dystrophinopathy (BMD) clinically.

Cardiac symptoms may include palpitations, syncope, and diminished exercise tolerance. Supraventricular dysrhythmias, AV conduction block, ventricular dysrhythmias, and restrictive or dilated cardiomyopathy may evolve.

Diagnosis

The diagnosis of EDMD is suspected based upon the clinical phenotype, especially the early onset of joint contractures relative to the degree of weakness, and confirmed by genetic testing for mutations in the *LMNA*, *FHL1*, or *STA* genes.

Management

Treatment is based largely on symptoms. The high incidence of cardiac dysfunction mandates early and regular cardiology evaluations. ICD rather then pacemaker should be considered for the arrhythmogenic component of the cardiomyopathy. Mothers and sisters of males with X-linked EDMD should also receive cardiology consultation. Orthopedic interventions may be helpful in addressing limb contractures. In the late stage of EDMD, respiratory aids, including cough-assistive devices and noninvasive nocturnal respiratory support, may be helpful.

Summary and Approach to LGMD Patients

Clinical Features

Because of the significant genetic and phenotypic variability of the different LGMDs, a careful family history and examination of family members that may or may not be aware of symptoms can play an important role in narrowing the differential diagnosis. Certain diagnostically helpful clinical features need to be evaluated fully:

1. Age of onset and speed of progression may provide an important clue in patients with suspected LGMD. Earlier onset and a more severe course with elevated CK are suggestive of mutations in the sarcoglycan complex or FKRP. With later childhood-onset symptoms, calpainopathy become more likely. If symptoms first appear in adolescence or early adulthood, a dysferlinopathy should be suspected, especially if the CK levels are extremely elevated. Adult-onset symptoms that are mild with significantly elevated CK may suggest anoctaminopathy, or myotilinopathy if the CK is close to normal.
2. The distribution of muscle weakness, presence or absence of contractures, or muscle groups that are spared can be important clues. Radiologic imaging such as MRI can be helpful in discerning the distribution of myopathy. For a summary of the specific clinical features in the commonly encountered LGMDs, please refer to Table 147-2.
3. The presence or absence of cardiac features can be an important clue, especially in autosomal-dominant LGMDs.

Muscle Biopsy and Protein Studies

In LGMD patients, muscle biopsy with routine histochemical stains usually shows dystrophic features with fiber size variability, increased endomysial fibrosis, fatty replacement, as well as myofiber degeneration and regeneration. Immunohistochemistry, in addition to Western blot analysis, can be helpful in many cases. Although assessment against many antibodies can be done, these methods are at best semiquantitative and should be interpreted with caution. Major patterns of immunohistochemical reduction of expression in different LGMDs are summarized in Table 147-2.

Molecular Genetic Testing

It is preferable that all diagnoses of genetic LGMDs be confirmed by molecular genetics when available. Availability of whole-exome sequencing and simultaneous sequencing of multiple genes at relatively low cost using next-generation technology has recently provided an alternative to traditional methods and costly panels. However, some mutations with large deletions or duplications are not amenable to detection using this approach. In addition, variations of unknown significance complicate the interpretation of the results in the absence of functional data. As a result, these approaches should be used as a complement to the clinical findings and the molecular and clinical features carefully correlated. It is always important to adequately consider metabolic etiologies, for example, Pompe disease, and acquired muscle diseases as the treatment and genetic implications are so different.

Diagnostic Algorithm

The American Academy of Neurology published an evidence-based guideline in 2014 for the diagnosis and treatment of LGMD and distal MDs. The three algorithm tables for autosomal-dominant, autosomal-recessive, and X-linked LGMDs and distal MDs are reproduced as Figure 147-10.

TABLE 147-2 Characteristic Clinical and Biopsy Findings in the Limb-Girdle Muscular Dystrophies

	Helpful Clinical Features	Immunohistochemistry and Western Blot
A. Autosomal-Dominant LGMD		
LGMD 1A (myotilinopathy)	Late onset and milder disease Nasal speech quality Early contractures of the Achilles tendons	Usually normal
LGMD 1B (laminopathy)	Contractures mimicking EDMD but can be minimal Conductive cardiac disease and AV block Early childhood onset possible Common de novo mutations	Usually normal
LGMD 1C (caveolinopathy)	Highly variable May present with isolated elevated CK with none to minimal weakness	Majority of cases with reduced or absent protein
B. Autosomal-Recessive LGMD		
LGMD 2A (calpainopathy)	Juvenile onset (~10 yrs) Early periscapular weakness Muscle wasting and atrophy Hamstrings weakness Sparing of the hip abductors	IHC is not available but WB shows reduction in the majority of cases. Secondary reduction in dysferlin occurs. Eosinophilic myositis has been reported.
LGMD 2B (dysferlinopathy)	Late adolescent onset (~18 yrs) Can present with proximal and/or distal weakness Early gastrocnemius involvement, esp. on MRI Spared periscapular muscles CK levels extremely high	Possible by IHC but WB is more specific. Secondary reductions in calpainopathy occurs. Intramuscular vessels may show amyloid deposits.
LGMD 2C-F (sarcoglycanopathies)	Early childhood onset (6–8 yrs) Similar pattern to DMD/BMD except early scapular weakness Calf hypertrophy very common CK levels very high Cardiomyopathy in a subset	IHC and WB are possible. Pattern of absence of all sarcoglycan proteins may be helpful.
LGMD 2G (telethoninopathy)	Variable clinical phenotype Early anterior tibial weakness and foot drop	IHC and WB are possible.
LGMD 2H	Variable clinical phenotype LE > UE weakness Trapezius and deltoid affected	Not possible
LGMD 2I	Typically mild but early childhood onset seen Weakness in the neck flexors and axial muscles UE > LE weakness Brachioradialis, tongue, and calf hypertrophy Cardiopulmonary disease possible	IHC may show reduced α-dystroglycan and laminin α₂ but not specific.
LGMD 2L (anoctaminopathy)	Adult onset Knee flexor and extensor weakness Medial gastroc, hamstring, and quadriceps atrophy, esp. vastus medialis	Not possible Intramuscular vessels may show amyloid deposits.

AV, atrioventricular; BMD, Becker's muscular dystrophy; DMD, Duchenne's muscular dystrophy; EDMD, Emery-Dreifuss muscular dystrophy; IHC, immunohistochemistry; LE, lower extremity; LGMD, limb-girdle muscular dystrophy; UE, upper extremity; WB, Western blot.

The Jain Foundation website (www.jain-foundation.org) provides a computer-based "automated LGMD diagnostic assistant," which is a useful resource to narrow the focus of diagnostic considerations in an individual patient.

FACIOSCAPULOHUMERAL MUSCULAR DYSTROPHY

Facioscapulohumeral MD (FSHD) is inherited as an autosomal-dominant disorder with high penetrance and variable expression. Between 10% and 30% of cases represent new mutations. Prevalence is estimated at 2 to 4.5×10^{-5} (refer to Table 137-2 in Chapter 137). Clinical signs and symptoms are usually present before age 20 years and are manifested by weakness of the facial muscles, fixators of the scapula, and dorsiflexors of the ankle. Although skeletal muscle symptoms dominate the clinical picture, other systems are often involved, which implies a more widespread developmental/degenerative process.

Molecular Genetics

FSHD maps to chromosome 4q35. More than 95% of patients with FSHD have a reduced number of 3.3-kilobase tandem repeat sequences termed *D4Z4*. See online chapter for additional discussion. Testing for the number of D4Z4 tandem repeats on chromosome 4q35 is the most specific and sensitive diagnostic test for FSHD. Subtelomeric translocations between chromosomes 4q35 and 10q26 occur relatively frequently in the general population and may complicate molecular diagnosis.

Clinical Features

Clinical diagnostic criteria have been established by the Facioscapulohumeral Muscular Dystrophy Consortium. Inclusion criteria specify autosomal-dominant inheritance; bifacial weakness; and weakness of the scapular stabilizer muscles, ankle dorsiflexor muscles, or both. Supporting criteria include asymmetry of motor deficits (a finding far more common in FSHD than any other muscular dystrophy); sparing of deltoid, neck flexor, and calf muscles; and involvement of wrist extensors and abdominal muscles. Hearing loss involving high frequencies and retinal vasculopathy (Coats disease) are additional supportive findings. Exclusion criteria include eyelid ptosis, extraocular muscle weakness, skin rash, elbow contractures, cardiomyopathy, sensory loss, neurogenic changes documented in muscle biopsy, and myotonia or neurogenic motor unit potentials documented on needle electromyography.

Weakness is usually appreciated first in the facial muscles. Patients have difficulty with puckering the lips, whistling, sipping through a straw, or blowing up balloons because of weakness of the orbicularis oris muscle. Most patients have a transverse smile and limited facial expression. Weakness of the orbicularis oculi is usually asymptomatic, but the examiner can recognize facial muscle weakness by observing incomplete burying of the eyelashes with forced eyelid closure and the ease with which the closed eyelids can be pried apart. A history of sleeping with the eyes open may be offered by a parent or spouse. Facial weakness may be asymmetric (Figure 147-11).

Weakness of scapular fixation is evidenced by scapular winging, accentuated by arm extension. The scapulae ride high on the back, producing the illusion of hypertrophied trapezius muscles. Arm abduction is impaired in the presence of normal power and bulk of the deltoid muscles. Wasting of the biceps and triceps with preservation of deltoid and forearm muscles yields a "Popeye" configuration to the arms. Wasting of the clavicular head of the pectoral muscles produces a reversal of the axillary folds with a deep upward slope. Weakness of lower abdominal muscles may result in a "pot belly" when standing and a positive Beevor sign (cephalad movement of the umbilicus with neck flexion) when the patient lies supine.

Lower-extremity weakness is usually evident first in the ankle dorsiflexors, with compromised heel walking or overt footdrop. Atrophy is most prominent in the tibialis anterior muscle. Preservation or hypertrophy of the extensor digitorum brevis muscle clinically excludes a neurogenic etiology of the footdrop. Axial paraspinal muscle weakness may result in marked lumbar lordosis, especially in patients with childhood-onset FSHD.

Motor deficits are slowly progressive. Most patients remain functionally independent throughout life.

Sensorineural hearing loss is frequently documented, especially in children presenting before 10 years of age, and can often be asymptomatic. Retinal vasculopathy with telangiectasia and retinal detachment (Coats disease) may develop. Symptomatic cardiac disease is infrequently encountered. Restrictive lung disease may be seen in patients with more severe FSHD. Congenital onset of FSHD has been associated with mental retardation and epilepsy in children with the largest D4Z4 deletions. The congenital-onset, or infantile, phenotype is often severe and rapidly progressive, accompanied by sensorineural hearing loss and Coats disease. Profound weakness of facial muscles is typical (Figure 147-11).

Laboratory Findings

Creatine kinase determinations are either normal or slightly elevated; creatine kinase levels exceeding five times the laboratory norms are suggestive of an alternative diagnosis. Genetic testing has largely replaced electrodiagnostic and muscle biopsy evaluations in persons with suspected FSHD.

Diagnosis

The American Academy of Neurology published an evidence-based guideline in 2015 for the evaluation, diagnosis, and treatment of FSHD (reference below) (Figure 147-12).

Treatment

There is no definitive treatment for FSHD. Results of therapeutic trials of corticosteroids and the β-adrenergic agonist albuterol have been disappointing. Trials of the calcium blocker diltiazem and an industry-sponsored trial of monoclonal antibody directed against human myostatin failed to increase strength or function.

OCULOPHARYNGEAL MUSCULAR DYSTROPHY

Oculopharyngeal MD (OPMD) is an adult-onset, autosomal-dominant disorder, manifesting after 50 years of age, that maps to chromosome 14q11.2 and is caused by a small trinucleotide GCG repeat expansion. See online chapter.

CONGENITAL MUSCULAR DYSTROPHIES

The CMDs are a diverse group of genetically based disorders characterized by early onset of progressive hypotonia, weakness, and a variable degree of muscle contractures. There may be associated dysmorphic or dysmyelinating brain abnormalities and structural eye abnormalities. Signs and symptoms are typically evident in the neonatal period, but may present within the first year of life, before ambulation is achieved. Serum creatine kinase levels are usually elevated. Muscle biopsy abnormalities typically show features of a dystrophic process, with variation in muscle fiber size, degenerating and regenerating fibers, and an increase in endomysial and perimysial connective tissue (refer to Chapter 135). Milder myopathic changes can also be seen initially. Biopsies are also useful to exclude congenital structural or metabolic myopathies. Biopsies from suspected CMD patients should be analyzed in specialized muscle histopathology laboratories that can perform the detailed immunohistochemical staining and interpretation necessary to identify features of dystroglycanopathies, merosinopathy, and collagen type VI disorders. The CMDs are autosomal recessive, with the exceptions of de novo dominant mutations in the lamin A/C gene, and the majority of cases of Ullrich CMD.

There is no clear separation of the CMDs from the LGMDs. The latter, in a general sense, have onset after ambulation has been achieved and after 24 months of age. Different mutations within genes causing CMD can also cause LGMD (i.e., allelic heterogeneity). Additional mutations and range of related phenotypes are likely to be discovered that will blur the boundary between the CMDs and the LGMDs.

The CMDs are rare disorders, having an estimated overall prevalence of approximately 0.8 to 5.46×10^{-5} (refer to Table 137-2 in Chapter 137).

The CMD syndromes have been classified in several ways. An earlier classification of CMDs into two groups of "merosin-negative" and "merosin-positive" is no longer used as the latter group has been better characterized by the identification of several genes that comprise this clinical cluster. CMDs can be considered as those with dysmorphic brain and eye changes ("syndromic") and those with a pure muscle phenotype ("nonsyndromic"). Current classification schema combine clinical features and cellular localization of the gene product into five categories, discussed in more detail below and summarized in Table 147-1:

1. Dystroglycanopathies: 15 glycosyltransferase genes that affect glycosylation of α-dystroglycan, and *DAG1*
2. Basil lamina disorders: 4 genes—laminin α_2 (merosinopathy), integrins α_7 and α_9, and also incorporating the dystroglycanopathies
3. Extracellular matrix (collagenopathies): 3 collagen type VI genes
4. Nuclear envelope proteins: 2 genes—lamin A/C (*LMNA*) and nesprin
5. Endoplasmic reticulum: selenoprotein 1 (*SEPN1*)

Abnormalities of α-Dystroglycan

The dystroglycan complex, discussed above in the LGMD section, structurally links the intracellular dystrophin-cytoskeleton complex to the extracellular matrix (Figure 147-2). Here the discussion will focus on α-dystroglycan (ADG) and its role in CMD. CMD patients with mutations in the dystroglycan gene (*DAG1*) are extremely rare, as it believed that most of these mutations result in an embryologic lethal condition. The vast majority of ADG-related CMDs are caused by mutations in glycosyltransferase genes responsible for the glycosylation of ADG and are termed *dystroglycanopathies*. Fifteen such genes have been identified to date (Table 147-1).

Clinical Presentations of the Dystroglycanopathies

Current classification in OMIM divides the dystoglycanopathies into three syndromic categories:

1. Muscle-eye-brain phenotypes. This includes WWS, muscle-eye-brain (MEB) disease, and Fukuyama CMD. Brain abnormalities involve migrational disorders of the cortex (lissencephaly, polymicrogyria, pachygyria), gross structural defects (absence of the corpus callosum, or vermis of the cerebellum, ventriculomegaly without hydrocephalus), and posterior fossa defects (cerebellar cysts, cerebellar and brainstem hypoplasia). Eye abnormalities range from microphthalmia, retinal degeneration, cataracts, glaucoma, and anterior chamber malformation to mild myopia.
2. CMD with posterior fossa abnormalities but having normal supratentorial structures. These CMD patients may have intellectual disability.
3. LGMD and CMD phenotypes with normal brain MRI.

Unlike several of the other CMDs and LGMDs, the responsible gene cannot be inferred from the phenotype as many of these glycosyltransferase genes can present with a similar phenotype. Conversely, some of these genes can present with a broad range of phenotypes; for example, FKRP can cause CMD with a severe WWS phenotype or a milder LGMD type 2I.

Muscle Biopsy Features

See online chapter.

Fukuyama Congenital Muscular Dystrophy

Fukuyama CMD is the second most common form of muscular dystrophy in Japan, where the carrier frequency is estimated at 1 in 90. The disease is uncommon outside of Japan. Fukuyama CMD is caused by mutations in the *FKTN* gene coding

for fukutin, a protein localized to the basement membrane of muscle. Fukutin deficiency is associated with decreased immunostaining for α-dystroglycan and merosin, with preservation of the dystrophin-related complex.

Hypotonia and generalized muscle weakness are usually present before 9 months of age, and 50% of affected infants manifest a poor suck and weak cry. Facial weakness and a tented upper lip are frequent findings. Calf hypertrophy is often present. Gross motor milestones are severely delayed. Affected children often achieve independent sitting, but never gain independent ambulation. Contractures are not marked at birth, but develop by 1 year of age and involve the hips, knees, ankles, and elbows.

Mental retardation is often severe. Seizures occur in approximately 40% of affected children. Ocular abnormalities are common but not universal, and include myopia, cataracts, optic disc pallor, and retinal detachment.

Creatine kinase levels are increased. Electrodiagnostic studies reveal myopathic potentials on electromyography; nerve conduction velocities are normal. Brain imaging studies and postmortem studies reveal brain malformations, including polymicrogyria, pachygyria, and agyria of the cerebrum and cerebellum (type II cobblestone lissencephaly), with a lack of normal lamination of the cerebral cortex.

MDC1C (Fukutin-Related Protein Deficiency)

MDC1C is allelic to LGMD2I, discussed above, caused by mutations in the *FKRP* gene coding for fukutin-related protein. Symptoms usually manifest at birth or in the first few weeks of life, with hypotonia and leg muscle hypertrophy. Creatine kinase values are greatly increased (1000 to 10,000 IU/L). Children follow a regressive course that may include cardiomyopathy. Routine histochemical analysis of muscle biopsy specimens does not differentiate these patients from children with merosin-negative CMD, but immunohistochemical staining reveals partial merosin deficiency and severely reduced glycosylated α-dystroglycan.

Muscle-Eye-Brain Disease

The first description of patients with the muscle-eye-brain phenotype were from Finland but the syndrome has now been seen worldwide. Initial reports suggested that POMGNT1 was the gene causing muscle-eye-brain disease. It is now evident that this phenotype may be the result of mutations in other genes along the α-dystroglycan O-mannosyl-glycosylation pathway (Table 147-1). The clinical phenotype may be severe, dominated by neonatal hypotonia, profound developmental delay with psychomotor retardation, and ocular abnormalities. Affected children may attain independent ambulation by age 4 years. Visual failure is in the form of severe myopia, followed by retinal degeneration, glaucoma, and cataracts. Seizures are common. Central nervous system dysgenesis includes lissencephaly type II (cobblestone complex), frontal pachygyria, cerebellar hypoplasia, and occipital micropolygyria. There is severe disorganization of the cerebral and cerebellar cortices. The associated myopathy may be overshadowed by central nervous system and ocular abnormalities. Creatine kinase levels are increased, especially after the first year of life, and electromyography studies show myopathic abnormalities.

Walker-Warburg Syndrome

WWS has no ethnic predominance. The clinical stigmata are dominated by the most severe brain malformations seen in any CMD syndrome, including lissencephaly type II, hydrocephalus, occipital encephalocele, fusion of the cerebral hemispheres, absence of the corpus callosum, and hypoplasia of the cerebellum and brainstem. Ocular findings have included congenital cataracts, microphthalmia, buphthalmus, and Peter's anomaly. At birth, affected children are blind, markedly hypotonic, and poor feeders. Myopathy is manifest by mild elevations of the creatine kinase level and variable abnormalities on muscle biopsy. All affected infants manifest profound psychomotor retardation, and the median length of survival is only 4 months. Epilepsy is a common comorbidity. It is now felt that WWS and muscle-eye-brain disease represent a clinical spectrum secondary to multiple mutations in multiple genes rather than distinct diseases.

MDC1D: LARGE

CMD caused by *LARGE1* gene mutations (MDC1D) is a very rare disorder and is discussed in the online chapter.

Congenital Muscular Dystrophy With Integrin α_7 Deficiency

Integrins are transmembrane heterodimeric (α/β) receptors crucial in establishing linkages between the extracellular matrix and muscle cytoskeleton. Deficiency of integrin α_7 is a very rare disorder and is discussed in the online chapter.

Abnormalities of Extracellular Matrix Proteins

MDC1A: Laminin-α_2 (Merosin)–Negative Congenital Muscular Dystrophy ("Nonsyndromic Congenital Muscular Dystrophy")

Genetics. The *LMNA* gene encodes the extracellular matrix protein lamin α_2 (merosin). Laminin α_2–negative CMD (MDC1A) is the most commonly diagnosed of the CMD disorders and accounts for about one-quarter of cases of nonsyndromic autosomal-recessive CMDs.

Clinical Features. Patients with complete absence of merosin present as neonates with significant hypotonia and generalized trunk and limb weakness, and may have multiple joint contractures. The upper limbs are often more affected than the lower limbs, which may exhibit muscle hypertrophy. Feeding and respiratory function is usually preserved initially. Small, slow gains in motor function are expected over the first year or two, with maximal milestones usually no better than independent sitting, and occasionally standing with support, but independent ambulation would be exceptional. Flexion contractures develop initially and are followed by a progressive rigid kyphoscoliosis that often necessitates surgical correction. Feeding tubes and noninvasive ventilation support are often needed because of development of dysphagia with aspiration and respiratory insufficiency, respectively. Most patients exhibit normal brain structure, although cystic lesions have been described, and cognitive development is generally preserved. Epilepsy occurs in approximately 30% of patients.

Diagnosis. Serum creatine kinase levels are usually elevated in the neonatal period in excess of 1000 U/L but tend to decrease over years.

Characteristic changes are seen in brain MRI scans of merosin-negative CMD patients. These findings may not be evident at birth but invariably become evident by age 6 months. White-matter hyperintensity is most prominent on T2-weighted images and principally involve the centrum semiovale, while sparing other myelinated structures in the corpus callosum, internal capsule, cerebellum, and brainstem. These MRI scans are often misinterpreted as a leukodystrophy. Focal cortical dysplasia of the occipital lobes occurs in some

cases with concurrent intellectual impairment, but the extensive neuronal migration abnormalities characteristic of patients with syndromic CMD are not seen.

Electrodiagnostic studies yield nonspecific myopathic findings on electromyography. Nerve conduction studies reveal slowing of conduction velocity.

Muscle biopsy demonstrates changes consistent with a dystrophic process. Absence of immunohistochemical staining for the laminin α_2 chain on frozen muscle biopsy or skin biopsy tissue provides confirmation of the diagnosis of merosin deficiency. Genetic testing is necessary to confirm the diagnosis.

Partial merosin deficiency has been reported in patients with a less severe childhood-onset or young adult-onset LGMD phenotype. See online chapter.

Merosin-Positive, Nonsyndromic Congenital Muscular Dystrophies

This category is no longer used.

Ullrich Congenital Muscular Dystrophy and Bethlem Myopathy

They are allelic disorders caused by mutations in any of three collagen 6 genes (*COL6A1*, *COL6A2*, and *COL6A3*). Ullrich CMD and Bethlem myopathy are discussed above in the LGMD section.

Congenital Muscular Dystrophy With Early Rigid Spine Syndrome

Rigid spine syndrome (RSS) is characterized by contractures of the paraspinal muscles, which limit spine flexion, especially in the thoracolumbar segments. Onset of RSS in infancy is caused by mutations in the *SEPN1* gene. Rigid spine can be seen in other muscle disorders, including EDMD and Ullrich CMD. Infants with *SEPN1*-related CMD present initially with mild hypotonia and weakness, followed by development of rigid spine and joint contractures, especially the Achilles tendons (Figure 147-13). Despite the spine rigidity, scoliosis typically evolves and may need surgical correction. A thin body habitus with generalized decrease in muscle bulk is typical. Motor milestones are delayed but most children with *SEPN1*-related CMD eventually achieve and maintain independent ambulation. Restrictive lung disease evolves later in the course and cardiac involvement has not been described.

Diagnosis. Classic features of *SEPN1*-CMD can lead the clinician directly to request genetic testing for mutations in the *SEPN1* gene. The creatine kinase level is typically normal and the muscle biopsy can have subtle dystrophic features or have multiminicores, fiber-type disproportion, or myofibrillar changes with Mallory body–like inclusions. These findings may erroneously focus attention on other congenital myopathies.

Treatment. Management of *SEPN1-CMD* is supportive.

Lamin A/C-Associated Congenital Muscular Dystrophy

The broad spectrum of neuromuscular and nonneuromuscular disorders caused by mutations in the lamin A/C gene (*LMNA*) has been outlined earlier in the section describing Emery–Dreifuss MD. A CMD phenotype has also been identified with de novo mutations of the *LMNA* gene. See online chapter for further discussion.

Nesprin-Associated Congenital Muscular Dystrophy

This entity is discussed in the online chapter.

Approach to the Patient With an LGMD, FSHD, EDMD, and CMD

Clinical Assessment

The following clinical features should be considered when evaluating the patient with a suspected MD: age at symptom onset, distribution and extent of weakness, contractures, rigid spine, muscle atrophy or hypertrophy, microcephaly, eye abnormalities, and seizures. Feeding, respiratory, and cardiac status also should be evaluated. It is important to obtain a careful family history.

Diagnostic Studies

Diagnostic testing to consider includes creatine kinase level, electromyography, and nerve conduction studies; muscle biopsy, MR brain, and muscle imaging; and ophthalmology evaluation. The algorithms presented here and in Chapter 137 (Figure 137-1) can then be used to help focus on a small number of diagnoses and guide confirmatory genetic testing.

Treatment

Management of these patients is supportive and discussed in more detail in the online chapter. Chapters 152 and 160 provide additional information on these issues.

As the molecular genetic basis and related cellular pathophysiology of these disorders become better understood, targeted treatment strategies are likely to be developed. The age of precision medicine for the MDs as with other childhood neurologic disorders is now emerging and offers some hope to these patients.

Acknowledgments

Drs. Diana M. Escolar and Robert T. Leshner contributed the chapter on muscular dystrophies to the prior edition of this textbook. We thank them for use of portions of their chapter and some figures that have been retained here.

REFERENCES

The complete list of references for this chapter is available in the e-book at www.expertconsult.com.
See inside cover for registration details.

SELECTED REFERENCES

Bonne, G., Quijano-Roy, S., 2013. Emery-Dreifuss muscular dystrophy, laminopathies, and other nuclear envelopathies. Handb. Clin. Neurol. 113, 1367–1376.

Bonnemann, C.G., Wang, C.H., Quijano-Roy, S., et al., 2014. Diagnostic approach to the congenital muscular dystrophies. Neuromuscul. Disord. 24, 289–311.

Bushby, K.M., Collins, J., Hicks, D., 2014. Collagen type VI myopathies. Adv. Exp. Med. Biol. 802, 185–199.

Gene Reviews. Resource from the University of Washington. <www.ncbi.nlm.nih.gov/books/NBK1116/>.

Narayanaswami, P., Weiss, M., Selcen, D., et al., 2014. Evidence-based guideline summary: diagnosis and treatment of limb-girdle and distal dystrophies: report of the guideline development subcommittee of the American Academy of Neurology and the practice issues review panel of the American Association of Neuromuscular & Electrodiagnostic Medicine. Neurology 83, 1453–1463.

Tawil, R., Kissel, J.T., Heatwole, C., et al., 2015. Evidence-based guideline summary: evaluation, diagnosis, and management of facioscapulohumeral muscular dystrophy: Report of the Guideline Development, Dissemination, and Implementation Subcommittee of the American Academy of Neurology and the Practice Issues Review Panel of the American Association of Neuromuscular & Electrodiagnostic Medicine. Neurology 85, 357–364.

The Gene Table. Comprehensive compendium of genes identified to cause neuromuscular disorders. <www.musclegenetable.fr>.

The Washington University neuromuscular center searchable compendium website. <www.neuromuscular.wustl.edu>.

Wang, C.H., Bonnemann, C.G., Rutkowski, A., et al., 2010. Consensus statement on standard of care for congenital muscular dystrophies. J. Child Neurol. 25, 1559–1581.

Wicklund, M.P., Kissel, J.T., 2014. The limb-girdle muscular dystrophies. Neurol. Clin. 32, 729–749.

E-BOOK FIGURES AND TABLES

The following figures and tables are available in the e-book at www.expertconsult.com. See inside cover for registration details.

148 Congenital Myopathies

Jahannaz Dastgir, Hernan D. Gonorazky, Jonathan B. Strober, Nicolas Chrestian, and James J. Dowling

An expanded version of this chapter is available on www.expertconsult.com. See inside cover for registration details.

Congenital myopathies are a clinically and genetically heterogeneous group of neuromuscular diseases. The most common clinical presentation is in the neonatal period as the floppy infant. However, congenital myopathies can present at essentially all life stages, making them an important diagnostic consideration in all individuals with muscle weakness. The prevalence of congenital myopathies is incompletely defined. The most accurate pediatric estimate (from a North American study) is approximately 1:26,000, though this is likely a significant underestimation given the increasing recognition of the condition and the delineation of an expanded range of clinical phenotypes considered under the congenital myopathy umbrella (North et al., 2014).

Historically, congenital myopathies have been diagnosed and defined based on features observed on muscle biopsy. The first congenital myopathy described, central core disease (CCD), was by Shy and Magee in 1956. The most common histopathologic subtypes are nemaline myopathy (NM), centronuclear myopathy (CNM), core myopathy, and congenital fiber-type disproportion (CFTD). With significant improvements in the cost, availability, and diagnostic accuracy of genetic testing, a gene-based definition of congenital myopathies has recently taken shape. At present, the most accurate and parsimonious categorization for congenital myopathies incorporates clinical features, muscle biopsy findings, and genetic information.

All congenital myopathies, with very rare exceptions, are assumed to have a genetic underpinning. To date, mutations in 20+ genes have been identified as causes of congenital myopathies (Table 148-1). These genes explain disease in approximately two thirds of all cases; in other words, about one third of the genetic burden of disease remains to be solved (Colombo et al., 2015). Inheritance can be autosomal dominant, autosomal recessive, and X-linked. Although a positive family history is often elicited, many cases are sporadic, and dominant mutations in particular often present (because of the severity of symptoms) as de novo.

At present, no therapies have been defined for congenital myopathies that have been tested in controlled clinical trials (Wang et al., 2012). Therefore management has largely been symptomatic, with a strong focus on respiratory management, surgical correction of orthopedic complications, and application of physical and occupational therapy services to maximize motor function. For a select few congenital myopathies, cardiac management is also necessary. A handful of drugs, all of which seem to provide modest clinical benefit at best, have hinted at efficacy based on case-controlled studies. In addition, several candidate therapeutics have been developed in preclinical studies and are now on the cusp of assessment in the clinical arena. Efforts to evaluate these drug targets will hopefully usher in a new era of therapy for a group of previously untreatable and devastating diseases.

DIAGNOSTICS

In general, congenital myopathies are considered in the setting of low muscle tone, depressed or absent reflexes, and extremity muscle weakness, often of a long-standing nature, that exhibits limited active progression. Facial weakness is often a key additional clue (Fig. 148-1). Ultimately, the diagnosis of congenital myopathy, regardless of clinical presentation, is established through a compatible muscle biopsy result and/or through positive genetic testing. The diagnostic strategy for assessing patients with neonatal hypotonia in whom congenital myopathy is suspected follows logically from the differential diagnoses (spinal muscular atrophy (SMA) DM1, congenital myasthenic syndromes, congenital muscular dystrophies, and Prader-Willi syndrome). Studies should include serum CPK levels (typically normal to maximum two to three times elevated in congenital myopathies), chromosomal microarray, genetic testing for SMA and congenital DM1, and (where available) electromyography and nerve conduction studies (EMG/NCS) (with repetitive stimulation) to evaluate for congenital myasthenic syndrome. Muscle magnetic resonance imaging (MRI) can also provide useful data in many cases. As mentioned, the diagnosis of congenital myopathy is only truly established through a consistent muscle biopsy and/or via positive genetic testing (see below under muscle biopsy and genetics sections). Similar strategies for diagnosis should be considered in the older child, keeping in mind that there will be a shift in consideration of potential alternative diagnoses based on age. A diagnostic algorithm that highlights some discriminative clinical and biopsy features is presented in Figure 148-2.

DIAGNOSTIC TESTING FOR CONGENITAL MYOPATHIES
Muscle Biopsy

The muscle biopsy has long been the definitive diagnostic study for congenital myopathies. In fact, congenital myopathies are defined and named by the characteristic observations seen by muscle pathology analysis. Each subtype of congenital myopathy is defined as follows (Dowling et al., 2015):

Centronuclear myopathy (Jungbluth et al., 2008): The basic definition of CNM is the presence of centrally located nuclei in >25% of the muscle fibers. This number can be quite variable, and truly there is no specific threshold for establishing CNM. Central nuclei are best seen with hematoxylin/eosin (H/E) staining (Fig. 148-3, *A*), though can also be appreciated with Gomori trichrome. The diagnosis of CNM is thus usually established not only by the presence of central nuclei but also by other histopathologic features. These features include myofiber hypotrophy, type I fiber predominance, and central accumulation of staining product with oxidative stains.

Nemaline myopathy: NMs are defined on biopsy by the presence of nemaline rods or nemaline bodies. Rods are composed primarily of proliferations of Z-band lattices. By light microscopy, rods are best visualized on Gomori trichrome staining, where they appear as eosinophilic aggregates (Fig. 148-3, *B*). The signature rod-like appearance from which the disorder derives its name is best appreciated by electron microscopy. In most cases, light microscopy is sufficient for

TABLE 148-1 Classification of Congenital Myopathies by Genes

Gene	Subtype	Inheritance Pattern	Protein	Features
ACTA1	• Nemaline myopathy (NM) • Cap disease (NM variant) • Zebra body myopathy (NM variant) • Congenital fiber-type disproportion	AD, AR AD AD AD	Actin, alpha1, skeletal muscle	Onset; variable within families with variable severity. Could present severe arthrogryposis or fetal akinesia. Severe respiratory involvement out of proportion to muscle weakness rarely cardiomyopathy. One patient described with hypertonia.
TPM3	• Nemaline myopathy (NM variant) • Cap disease (NM variant) • Congenital fiber-type disproportion	AD, AR AD AD	Tropomyosin 3	Onset at birth to early adolescence. Distal leg involvement with later involvement of proximal muscle. Slow progression. Respiratory involvement out of proportion to muscle weakness. Could present mild ptosis and mild facial involvement.
TPM2	• Nemaline myopathy(NM) • Cap disease (NM variant)	AD AD	Tropomyosin 2 (beta)	Onset at birth to early childhood. Distal leg weakness, severe arthrogryposis, fetal akinesia. Cardiac involvement (bifascicular ventricular block with right bundle block and left anterior hemiblock).
TNNT1	• Nemaline myopathy (NM)	AR	Troponin T type 1 (skeletal, slow)	Older order Amish and rare Dutch and Hispanic patients. Onset at birth, 1 month of age usually starts with tremor on the jaw and lower limbs (resolves by 3 months of age). Proximal weakness with mild proximal contractures, rigid chest wall severe respiratory involvement, death usually at the age of 2 years.
NEB	• Nemaline myopathy (NM)	AR	Nebulin	Variable onset, classic form, birth onset with dysmorphic features (high-arched palate, micrognathia, lower facial weakness with marked bulbar involvement chest deformities, nasal voice, and distal leg weakness respiratory involvement out of proportion to muscle weakness).
LMOD3	• Nemaline myopathy (NM)	AR	Leiomodin 3	Onset; prenatal. Polyhydramnios, multiple joint contractures, proximal distal and lower facial weakness with marked bulbar involvement, and ophthalmoplegia. Usually neonatal death.
KBTBD13	• Nemaline myopathy (NM)	AD	Kelch repeat and BTB (POZ) domain containing protein 13	Onset; childhood. Proximal and axial involvement, slow movements, high-arched palate, and thorax deformities.
CFL2	• Nemaline myopathy (NM)	AR	Cofilin 2 (muscle)	Onset at birth to early childhood. Proximal and axial weakness, prominent neck extensors involvement. Severe scoliosis.
KLHL40	• Nemaline myopathy (NM)	AR	Kelch-like family member 40	Onset; prenatal. Polyhydramnios, severe arthrogryposis and fetal akinesia, dysmorphic faces, severe respiratory and limb involvement, ophthalmoplegia usually death at the age of 5 months.
KLHL41	• Nemaline myopathy (NM)	AR	Kelch-like family member 41	Onset; prenatal. Fetal akinesia hip and knee dislocation with severe respiratory involvement early death. Missense mutations could present with mild forms with a survival into late childhood or early adulthood.
RYR1	• Central core myopathy • Multiminicore myopathy • Core rod myopathy • Nemaline myopathy • Congenital fiber-type disproportion • Centronuclear myopathy • Congenital neuromuscular disease with uniform type 1 fiber	AD, AR AR AD, AR AR AR AR AD	Ryanodine receptor I	Variable onset and severity. Proximal weakness, ptosis, ophthalmoplegia, hyperlaxity, congenital hip dislocation, scoliosis, moderate respiratory involvement, exercise induce myalgia, MHS. Could present rigid spine syndrome, and severe arthrogryposis.

TABLE 148-1 Classification of Congenital Myopathies by Genes *(Continued)*

Gene	Subtype	Inheritance Pattern	Protein	Features
STAC3	• Native American myopathy	AR	SH3 and cysteine rich domain containing protein 3	Lumbee Indians in North Carolina. Congenital onset, dysmorphic features (telecanthus, cleft palate, downslating palpebral fissures, low ear set, ptosis), short stature, arthrogryposis proximal weakness, MHS.
SEPN1	• Multiminicore myopathy • Congenital fiber-type disproportion	AR AR	Selenoprotein N1	Onset birth to childhood. Predominant axial muscle involvement, poor head control, rigid spine, scoliosis at the age of 10 years, nocturnal hypoventilation central apnea during paradoxical sleep.
CCDC78	• Centronuclear myopathy	AD	Coiled coil domain containing protein 78	Congenital onset, distal involvement with slow progression, excessive fatigue mild to moderate cognitive impairment.
BIN 1	• Centronuclear myopathy	AR, AD	Amphiphysin	Variable onset. Severe forms present at birth or childhood. Proximal and lower facial weakness with marked bulbar involvement, ophthalmoparesis and ptosis, could present cardiomyopathy (dilated)
DNM2	• Centronuclear myopathy	AD	Dynamin 2	Variable onset. Distal muscle weakness, exercise induce myalgias, ophthalmoparesis, ptosis, lower facial weakness and marked bulbar involvement, slow progression hypertrophy of paravertebral muscles absent or reduce tendon reflexes, distal limb, contractures, scoliosis cardiomyopathy.
MTM1	• Myotubular myopathy	XR	Myotubularin 1	Onset; prenatal. Polyhydramnios, macrosomia, proximal and distal weakness with severe respiratory involvement at birth, lower facial weakness with marked bulbar involvement, usually early death, other features, bleeding diathesis, liver and gastrointestinal complications.
SPEG	• Centronuclear myopathy with dilated cardiomyopathy	AR	SPEG complex locus	Onset at birth, proximal weakness with lower face and bulbar involvement, ophthalmoplegia, hip contractures cardiomyopathy.
PTPLA (= HCDA1)	• Congenital myopathy related to PTPLA	AR	Protein tyrosine phosphatase-like (3-hydroxyacyl CoA dehydratase)	Onset birth. Lower facial and proximal weakness. Absent or reduce deep tendon reflexes. Severe presentation at onset with progressive improvement.
TTN	• Centronuclear myopathy • Congenital myopathy with fatal cardiomyopathy	AR AR	Titin	Onset, birth or infancy. Proximal and distal weakness with facial involvement. Could present asymmetric ptosis. Some with scapula-peroneal syndrome. Pseudohypertrophy of thighs and calves. Ambulation could be achieved in most of the cases. Scoliosis and absent reflexes. Cardiomyopathy (dilated)
MYH7	• Myosin storage myopathy • Myosin storage myopathy with cardiomyopathy • Congenital fiber-type disproportion	AD AR AD	Myosin, heavy chain 7, cardiac muscle	Onset at infancy or early childhood, distal weakness predominant, and week toe extensor (hanging big toe), scapular winging, mild facial involvement, cardiomyopathy (dilated or hypertrophic)
MYH2	• Myosin IIa myopathy	AD, AR	Myosin, heavy chain 2, skeletal muscle	Onset at birth, contractures, ophthalmoplegia, ptosis, mild to moderate proximal weakness
MEGF10	• Early onset myopathy, areflexia respiratory distress and dysphagia • Minicores	AR AR	Multiple EGF-like domains 10	Prenatal onset with reduced fetal movements. Proximal and distal weakness, distal contractures, scoliosis, areflexia, bulbar involvement, respiratory distress.

AD, autosomal dominant; *AR*, autosomal recessive; *XR*, X linked.
(Adapted from Kaplan JC, et al. The 2015 version of the gene table of monogenic neuromuscular disorder. *Neuromuscul Disord* 2014;24:1123–53.)

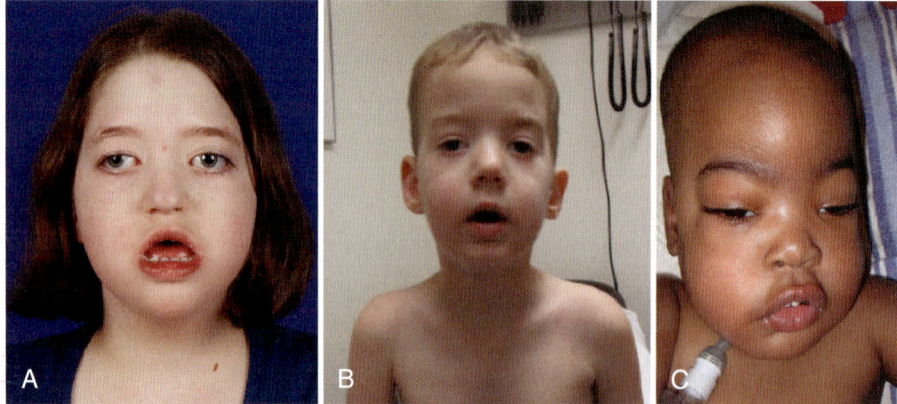

Figure 148-1. The "myopathic" facies. One of the characteristic clinical observations in many children with congenital myopathies is the so-called "myopathic" facial appearance. This can include both upper and lower facial weakness, as illustrated in these photomicrographs. *Left panel:* The patient depicted demonstrates ptosis, ocular misalignment caused by ophthalmoparesis, an inverted C-shape to her upper lip, and prominent lower facial weakness resulting in an open mouth appearance. The ultimate diagnosis in this case was nemaline myopathy caused by recessive mutation in the *LMOD3* gene. Patients with nemaline myopathy often have particularly striking lower facial weakness. *Middle panel:* This individual has ptosis, ophthalmoparesis, and moderate lower facial weakness. He has DNM2-related centronuclear myopathy. Note also the muscle atrophy present in his chest and shoulders. *Right panel:* Photograph of a young boy with myotubular myopathy caused by MTM1 mutation. He has the characteristic long face with bilateral ptosis and ophthalmoparesis.

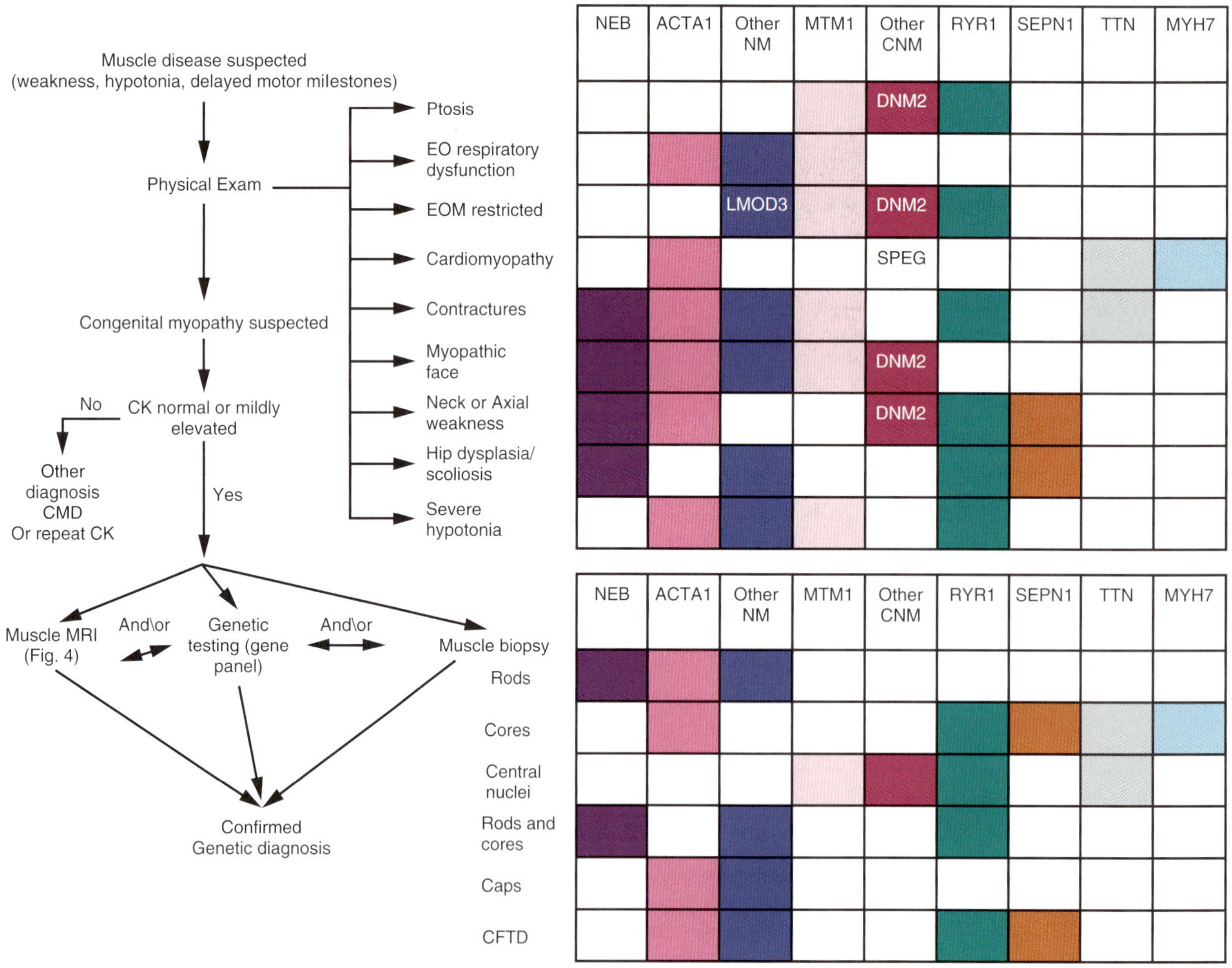

Algorithm (left):

Muscle disease suspected (weakness, hypotonia, delayed motor milestones) → Physical Exam → Congenital myopathy suspected → CK normal or mildly elevated → No → Other diagnosis CMD Or repeat CK; Yes → Muscle MRI (Fig. 4) — And\or — Genetic testing (gene panel) — And\or — Muscle biopsy → Confirmed Genetic diagnosis

Physical Exam → Ptosis, EO respiratory dysfunction, EOM restricted, Cardiomyopathy, Contractures, Myopathic face, Neck or Axial weakness, Hip dysplasia/scoliosis, Severe hypotonia

Clinical feature table:

	NEB	ACTA1	Other NM	MTM1	Other CNM	RYR1	SEPN1	TTN	MYH7
Ptosis					DNM2				
EO respiratory dysfunction									
EOM restricted			LMOD3		DNM2				
Cardiomyopathy					SPEG				
Contractures									
Myopathic face					DNM2				
Neck or Axial weakness					DNM2				
Hip dysplasia/scoliosis									
Severe hypotonia									

Muscle biopsy table:

	NEB	ACTA1	Other NM	MTM1	Other CNM	RYR1	SEPN1	TTN	MYH7
Rods									
Cores									
Central nuclei									
Rods and cores									
Caps									
CFTD									

Figure 148-2. Clinical approach to congenital myopathy, practical algorithm. *ACTA1*, ACTA1 nemaline myopathy; *CFTD*, congenital fiber-type disproportion; *CK*, creatine kinase; *CMD*, congenital muscular dystrophy; *CNM*, centronuclear myopathy; *EO*, early onset; *EOM*, extraocular movements; *MM*, mitochondrial myopathy; *MYH7*, MYH7 myopathy; *NEB*, nebulin mutation; *NM*, nemaline myopathy; *Other NM*, LMOD3, TPM2, TPM3, KBTBD13, TNNT1, KLHL40, KLHL41, and large spectrum of clinical presentation from mild to severe; *RYR1*, ryanodine receptor myopathy; *SEPN1*, SEPN1 myopathy; *TTN*, Titin myopathy.

establishing the diagnosis; however, there are instances where the rods are either poorly appreciated or else not seen at the light level and only revealed through electron microscopic analysis. In addition, there are histopathologic variants that are included within the nemaline umbrella. These include cap myopathy (where there is an accumulation of myofibrillar material sitting as a cap at the periphery of the myofiber) and zebra body myopathy (Dowling et al., 2015).

Core myopathy (Jungbluth, 2007a,b): Core myopathies are typically subdivided into CCD and multiminicore myopathy. Cores are best appreciated on light microscopy with oxidative stains such as SDH and NADH (Fig. 148-3, *C*). They are defined as areas devoid of reactivity for these enzymes and reflect areas in the myofibers that lack mitochondria. Central cores are longitudinal and often traverse the entire length of the myofiber. Minicores are typically transverse in location and usually small. Core myopathies are often also seen in the context of type I fiber predominance and type I fiber hypotrophy, both features best seen with ATPase staining. Electron microscopy is often required for evaluation of core myopathies. This is because there are other conditions that can result in absence or change of SDH/NADH staining. Most prominent among them is the targetoid staining pattern seen with neurogenic lesions. On EM, cores appear as areas of myofibril disorganization that lack mitochondria. At times there will be a ring of mitochondria around the area of disorganization (referred to as a structured core).

Congenital fiber-type disproportion: CFTD is defined by two biopsy features. The first is relative hypotrophy of type I fibers compared with type II fibers. The second is numerical predominance of type I fibers over type II fibers. The general criterion for calling CFTD is a 25% reduction in type I fiber size. Such a reduction is relatively nonspecific and can be seen in a range of disease, many of which are not primary myopathies. "True" CFTD, or CFTD caused by mutations in congenital myopathy genes, is usually characterized by much more significant reduction in type I fiber size (to <50% that of type IIs) and clear type I predominance (often >75% of fibers). CFTD can be seen by H/E staining, but is best diagnosed and evaluated using stains for fiber type (Fig. 148-3, *D*). These include enzymatic reactions (ATPase at acid pH [4.3 to 4.6] to stain type I fibers and at basic pH [9.4 to 10.2] to mark type II fibers) or immunostaining with myosin antibodies (slow myosin for type I and fast myosin for type II).

Genetics

All pediatric-onset (and most adult-onset) congenital myopathies are considered to have a genetic underpinning. It is important to establish a genetic diagnosis, even when a child has a consistent muscle biopsy, because knowledge of the specific genetic subtype greatly contributes to understanding of specific clinical features, anticipatory care requirements, and prognostication (Wang et al., 2012; North et al., 2014). Mutations in congenital myopathies span the range of inheritance patterns (X-linked, autosomal recessive, autosomal dominant) and often are caused by sporadic/de novo variants. To date, mutations in 20 genes have been identified as causal in patients with congenital myopathy (see Table 148-1). The interplay between clinical presentation, biopsy diagnosis, and genetic subtype is complex. In particular, there are several genetic causes for each histopathologic grouping (e.g., mutations in 10 genes are associated with NM), and each genetic cause can result in a variety of clinical presentations and histopathologic diagnoses (e.g., *RYR1* mutations have been described in every histopathologic subtype) (North et al., 2014). Of note, it is critically important that genetic counseling be offered to all patients with congenital myopathies and to their families,

ideally starting at the time that genetic testing is first considered (Wang et al., 2012).

Muscle Imaging (MRI or Ultrasonography)

Muscle imaging is an emerging modality for the diagnosis and care of patients with a range of neuromuscular disorders. For congenital myopathies it is used primarily as an adjunct diagnostic tool, though in the future may aid in assessment of disease status and progression. Muscle ultrasonography is the fastest and least expensive technique and offers the potential of application in the outpatient clinic and/or inpatient setting, though requires an experienced user for interpretation. Muscle MRI is widely available and does not require any particular advanced training to obtain or analyze; the downside is expense and the fact that some children (particularly those under age 5 years) may require sedation. The diagnostic value of muscle imaging lies in the fact that different genetic subtypes of myopathy present with different imaging patterns of muscle involvement. The pathognomonic patterns are best characterized with lower extremity imaging, though the value of whole-body MRI for diagnosis (particularly in the young child) is increasingly being recognized. Representative examples of muscle MRI and a diagnostic flow chart describing its application are presented in Figure 148-4.

SPECIFIC SUBTYPES OF CONGENITAL MYOPATHY
Centronuclear Myopathies

Centronuclear myopathies, even though clinically heterogeneous (particularly in terms of symptom onset and severity), often feature prominent eye muscle weakness (ptosis and ophthalmoparesis) in addition to lower facial and extremity weakness (Jungbluth et al., 2008). In infancy and childhood, these features can appear like those seen in congenital myasthenic syndromes. The extremity weakness may have significant distal involvement, including distal predominance in some individuals.

There are six established genetic causes of CNM. Mutations in myotubularin (*MTM1*) are associated with the distinctive, severe, neonatal-onset X-linked condition myotubular myopathy (XLMTM or MTM) (Das et al., 1993). Mutations in dynamin-2 (*DNM2*) are the most common cause of dominant CNM; patients typically present either in the first year or two of life (with de novo mutations) or in late childhood. Recessive causes of CNM include mutations in *RYR1*, *BIN1*, *TTN*, and *SPEG*. *RYR1* mutations are the most common and can present in infancy in a manner resembling MTM. *BIN1* mutations typically cause childhood-onset CNM, though one particular homozygous splice mutation results in a rare, rapidly progressive form. There is also a late-onset CNM in some families with dominant *BIN1* mutations. *SPEG* mutations cause a rare, severe form of CNM that also includes cardiomyopathy.

There are currently no therapies that have been proven to be efficacious for CNM. There is mounting evidence, however, including several case reports and compelling preclinical data, that acetylcholinesterase inhibitors such as pyridostigmine provide modest but definitive improvement in clinical symptomatology. Patients with mutations in *RYR1*, *DNM2*, and *MTM1* have all been reported in these case series. In terms of experimental therapies, there is considerable excitement concerning both gene therapy and enzyme replacement therapy for MTM. These strategies have shown robust disease correction in the MTM mouse model, and gene therapy additionally has been effective in a spontaneous dog model of the disease.

Nemaline Myopathies

NMs are characterized in general by the presence of significant bulbar dysfunction (because of lower face and neck flexor weakness) in the setting of additional and variable extremity weakness (North et al., 2014). The disease is noted to have significant clinical variability and has thus been classically subdivided into groups based on age of onset and clinical severity: (1) severe congenital NM (16% of NM cases), (2) intermediate congenital NM (20%), (3) typical congenital NM (46%), (4) childhood-/juvenile-onset NM (13%), and (5) adult-onset NM (4%) (North and Ryan, 1993). There is considerable overlap between the groups, though the distinctions can be helpful (e.g., individuals with severe congenital NM have a high risk of death in infancy, whereas those with typical congenital NM tend to show stabilization and even improvement).

There are 10 known genetic causes of NM. Mutations in ACTA1 are the most common dominant/de novo cause (25% of all NM), whereas those in nebulin (NEB) are the most common autosomal-recessive cause (~50% of all NM). Mutations in ACTA1 are associated with a tremendous variability in age of presentation and clinical expression, not only between different mutations in the gene but also among family members with the same mutation. They are the most common cause of severe congenital NM (severe weakness, reduced or absent fetal/neonatal movements, respiratory failure, and often death in infancy). Mutations in NEB are most frequently encountered with typical congenital NM (neonatal hypotonia, weakness, feeding difficulties, ability to eventually ambulate, static/slowly progressive course).

The specific breakdown in terms of relative prevalence of the other genetic subtypes is otherwise not well established. Some are associated primarily with specific clinical groupings. LMOD3 and KLHL40 mutations are seen almost exclusively with severe congenital NM. Dominant mutations in TPM2 and TPM3 are associated with symptoms ranging from typical congenital to mild childhood (with TPM2 mutations usually milder), whereas rare recessive mutations in TPM3 are associated with severe disease. TPM2 mutations can additionally been seen in the absence of overt weakness with distal arthrogryposis syndromes. Dominant mutations in KBTBD13 are seen with childhood-onset NM and characteristic slowness of movements. Recessive mutations in TNNT1 (Amish NM) and CFL2 (severe or typical congenital) are extremely rarely encountered. Of note, ophthalmoparesis is infrequently observed in NM (with the exception of LMOD3 mutations), and may serve as a means of distinguishing NM from other congenital myopathies.

At present, there are no specific therapies that have proven efficacious for NM. L-tyrosine has been examined in a mouse model of Acta1 and shown to increase muscle strength; a limited patient case series examining L-tyrosine found that it improves some bulbar symptoms and specifically sialorrhea. Its impact on disease course is likely limited, and true efficacy awaits more systematic clinical study. There are no other therapies currently in the clinical pipeline, though a few are at the stage of preclinical assessment.

Core Myopathies

Core myopathies can be subdivided into CCD and multiminicore disease (MmD). CCD is caused by RYR1 mutations (usually dominant/de novo) in approximately 90% of cases (Jungbluth, 2007a). The other well-described cause is dominant MYH7 mutation. Minicore disease, along with the more general categorization of myopathy with cores, has several genetic causes (Jungbluth, 2007b). Most classically, it is caused by mutations in either SEPN1 (MmD without ophthalmoparesis) or RYR1 (MmD with ophthalmoparesis). Other genetic causes include ACTA1, TTN, MEGF10, and CCDC78; biopsies in these settings typically include additional histopathologic abnormalities (such as rods or protein aggregates). In addition, there can be both cores and rods in the same biopsy (termed "core-rod" myopathy), with known causes, including TPM2, NEB, RYR1, ACTA1, and KBTBD13.

RYR1-Related Myopathies

Myopathies caused by mutations in the skeletal muscle ryanodine receptor (RYR1) are the commonest group of nondystrophic muscle conditions. These are also termed "RYR1-related myopathies," and encompass a broad clinical spectrum that spans the entire gamut of histopathologic subtypes. RYR1-related myopathies are subdivided primarily either by mode of inheritance (recessive vs. dominant/de novo) or by histopathology (CCD, MmD, CNM, etc.), though there are distinctive clinical conditions that do not classically fall into a specific grouping (e.g., axial myopathy, malignant hyperthermia, exertional rhabdomyolysis, isolated ophthalmoparesis).

CCD associated with RYR1 mutation is almost entirely caused by dominant mutations (Jungbluth, 2007a). The typical pediatric presentation for CCD is one of neonatal hypotonia, muscle hypotrophy, and extremity muscle weakness, often accompanied by significant skeletal abnormalities such as chest wall deformities, scoliosis, joint contractures, and hip dysplasia. Respiratory failure is present in some instances, though rarely requires tracheostomy and often improves. The course of disease is typically quite stable, and, although delayed, individuals often acquire all motor developmental milestones. Of note, there may be some mild facial muscle involvement, including ptosis and lower facial weakness, but ophthalmoparesis is rarely encountered. There is also a milder CCD presentation that includes minimal weakness that may only be recognized in adulthood; there are also several cases of dominant mutations causing late-onset axial myopathy. Rarely, heterozygous de novo mutations can present with extreme weakness in the perinatal period that results in death in infancy. The mutations in RYR1 that cause CCD are enriched in the C-terminal aspect of the gene. Some are additionally associated with malignant hyperthermia susceptibility (MHS), a pharmacogenetic condition of hypermetabolism and muscle breakdown in response to exposure to volatile anesthetics.

The other histopathologic subtypes (MmD, CNM, core-rod myopathy, and CFTD) are most commonly seen with recessive RYR1 mutations. The most frequently encountered recessive subtype is minicore disease, which typically presents with diffuse weakness in combination with ophthalmoparesis. Onset is usually in the neonatal period or in early childhood, and can be severe enough to result in respiratory failure with chronic ventilator support and wheelchair dependence. As with CCD, skeletal abnormalities (particularly joint contractures and scoliosis) are quite frequently encountered. These are often accompanied by severe facial weakness that can include ophthalmoparesis. Axial muscle involvement can also be quite pronounced.

At present, there are no specific treatments for RYR1-related myopathies. Salbutamol has been shown in a small case-control series to improve strength and motor function. This result has not been followed up with additional clinical trials, and the medication is not widely used in RYR1 patients. An intriguing candidate drug class is the RyCals; RyCals interact with RyR1 and augment its ability to release calcium. RyCals have yet to be tested for efficacy in patients, and have not been examined in any preclinical models of *RYR1* myopathy. One drug that has shown promising results in animal models and in patient cells is the antioxidant N-acetylcysteine (NAC). NAC is currently being evaluated in a placebo-controlled clinical trial in ambulant *RYR1* myopathy patients. Of note, dantrolene is the standard therapy for treating MH. It has yet to be tested in other dynamic *RYR1*-related phenotypes such as rhabdomyolysis. Because it reduces RyR1 calcium release, it is unlikely to be effective in the majority of instances of *RYR1* mutations that cause static muscle weakness.

SEPN1-Related Myopathies

Recessive mutations in *SEPN1* were first described in a rare muscular dystrophy subtype called rigid spine muscular dystrophy. However, *SEPN1* mutations are most typically found associated with multiminicore disease; they are also seen with other histopathologic patterns, including CFTD and Mallory Body myopathy. Regardless of histopathologic phenotype, patients with *SEPN1* mutations present a relatively uniform clinical picture. This picture includes early onset hypotonia and axial muscle weakness with relative sparing of the extremity muscles. It also includes spinal rigidity; severe, progressive scoliosis; and potentially lethal, progressive respiratory failure. These severe axial symptoms are not matched by corresponding limb weakness, with the resulting appearance often one of an ambulant patient with ventilator dependence. Patients do not have ophthalmoparesis, a distinguishing feature from *RYR1* mutations.

SEPN1 encodes selenoprotein N1 (SelN1), a selenocysteine-containing protein located in the endoplasmic reticulum. The functions of SelN1 in relation to muscle structure and function have been relatively elusive, though it seems clear that one of its major roles is to regulate oxidative stress. Based on this, the consequences of *SEPN1* mutations (which in general result in loss of SelN1 expression and/or function) are predicted to be increased basal oxidative stress, susceptibility to the consequences of oxidative species, and ultimately impaired redox related RyR1 function. As with *RYR1* myopathies, the antioxidant NAC protects *SEPN1*-patient-derived myotubes from oxidant-related death, and is now being considered for clinical trial in *SEPN1*-related myopathy patients.

Congenital Fiber-Type Disproportion

CFTD is a diagnosis applied in the context of clinical symptoms of myopathy and fiber-type disproportion on biopsy (significantly smaller type I fibers, usually type I predominance) (Clarke, 2011). The biopsy observation of CFTD often precedes or is accompanied by other pathologic features (rods, cores, etc.); in such cases, the individual is typically described as having the diagnoses corresponding to the other biopsy features (e.g., NM when rods are present). Some individuals, however, do have "pure" CFTD (usually considered when type I fibers are >40% smaller). When this occurs, the recognized genetic causes are mutations in *TPM3, TPM2, RYR1, SEPN1,* and *ACTA1*. The clinical presentations in these cases are primarily dictated by the underlying genetic cause; for example, patients with CFTD caused by *TPM3* mutations resemble those with similar mutations and NM on biopsy.

GENERAL MANAGEMENT OF CONGENITAL MYOPATHIES

General management guidelines for congenital myopathies are based on practical experience, expert opinion, and inferences from other similar neuromuscular conditions. These guidelines are summarized here, and also found in extensive detail in the recently published standards of care for congenital myopathies (Wang et al., 2012).

Respiratory

Respiratory dysfunction is the likeliest cause of morbidity and mortality in children with congenital myopathies. This relates to the fact that the diaphragm and intercostal muscles are often weakened in these conditions, leading to poor rib excursion, impaired mucus expectoration and airway clearance, and sleep apnea. The recognition of early respiratory compromise (often identified via sleep study or pulmonary function testing in both the seated and supine positions) leads to early intervention via noninvasive ventilation, typically first at night and then during daytime in more severe or progressive cases. Identifying a weak cough in patients is also an important predictor of how a child may respond to an upper respiratory infection. A weak cough can predispose to mucus plugging and bronchiectasis and hence cause risk for fatal pneumonias. This can be prevented with the use of a cough assist device (either while sick or best also when healthy) as a form of pulmonary physical therapy. A thairvest, which employs chest vibration to loosen mucus, may also be used, though it is imperative that this treatment is followed by cough assist regimen. This is so that the mucus that is loosened as a result of this procedure can actually be expectorated and not actually make things worse by being left to plug the airways.

Nutrition, Gastrointestinal, and Oromotor Management

Nutritional management guidelines for congenital myopathies are essentially nonexistent despite the fact that poor nutrition and growth are inherent to many of these conditions. Weakness in oromotor function is a contributing factor, particularly in nemaline and centronuclear myopathies. Efforts should be made to monitor patient weight and height (either erect or via ulnar length) in conjunction with calorie intake. If calorie intake is limited, or the risk of aspiration pneumonia is high, the placement of a gastrostomy tube should be discussed with families early in the disease course. Improved nutritional status has been related to improved growth and decreased respiratory problems. Yearly assessments of calcium and vitamin D levels should also be made in order to address bone health, as osteopenia is a concern in any individual with long-standing muscle weakness.

Gastrointestinal dysmotility is also a frequent problem in children with congenital myopathies. Dysmotility may present as gastroesophageal reflux, which can be managed with medication (e.g., proton pump inhibitors, H2 blockers, and antacids), nonpharmacologically (e.g., thickening of formula and adjusting feeding positions), and/or surgically (e.g., with Nissen fundoplication). Dysmotility can also present with delayed gastric emptying and constipation, symptoms that can be treated with diet modification, stool softeners/laxatives, and the use of prokinetic drugs (erythromycin or metaclopromide).

Excessive oral secretions are often a significant problem in congenital myopathies. This is related to bulbar and facial weakness and particularly seen in nemaline and CNM. Speech and occupational therapy can be used to address this, primarily through facial muscle–strengthening exercises. If this is not successful, anticholinergic drugs may be administered systemically (e.g., robinul and scopolamine), though they are not without systemic side effects (e.g., constipation). A small study has also found evidence that L-tyrosine supplementation may be helpful with sialorrhea in NM. Botulinum toxin injections and surgical management are considered in very rare circumstances when secretions are particularly debilitating, though such strategies are controversial.

Cardiac

The majority of congenital myopathy subtypes are not associated with primary cardiac involvement. Baseline and periodic follow-up cardiac evaluations, however, should be provided to all patients with congenital myopathy until the specific genetic cause has been identified. This is because certain gene mutations, such as those in *TTN, MYH7, SPEG,* and (more rarely) *ACTA1,* can cause cardiomyopathy. In addition, continued cardiac screening is indicated in settings (*SEPN1*-related myopathy, for example) where secondary right-sided heart failure is of concern because of chronic respiratory compromise.

Orthopedic

Scoliosis is a pervasive problem in these conditions and should be monitored from the initial presentation of symptoms. This can initially be done via clinical examination (with the patient assessed in forward flexion at the hip), but once any curvature is noted, routine x-rays should be obtained. Once scoliosis has been diagnosed, patients should be referred to orthopedics for the management of the progressive curvature with either a conservative (e.g., bracing/casting) or invasive/surgical approach. The management of scoliosis is essential for maintaining respiratory function.

Joint contractures are a concern for the majority of congenital myopathy patients, and may in fact be the presenting sign of patients in some individuals. Ankle contractures are typically managed with physical therapy, passive stretching, and ankle-foot orthoses, which are used in the ambulant patient to slow contracture progressive and to improve gait, and in the nonambulant patient to aid in comfort and wheelchair positioning. Surgery to release contractures is rarely indicated, as it often does not appreciably improve range of motion and can potential worsen muscle weakness. Exceptions include contractures that significantly hinder ambulation (in the setting of relatively preserved strength) and those that cause considerable discomfort (in the nonambulant patient).

Physical Therapy/Exercise

Physical therapy is mainstay of management in children with congenital myopathy. It helps with strengthening and improves range of motion. It should be utilized regularly and in a manner that matches the child's pattern of weakness. Assist devices can complement therapy services, and include gait trainers and stationary bikes.

The impact of exercise on muscle strength and motor function in congenital myopathies has yet to be formally addressed, though there is anecdotal evidence that exercise in children with myopathies is safe and potentially of benefit. Further work is necessary to establish this as a formal recommendation.

SUMMARY

Congenital myopathies represent a clinically and genetically heterogeneous group of childhood muscle disorders. With improvements in clinical recognition and genetic testing, it is now clear that these disorders represent a significant portion of childhood genetic neuromuscular disease. The availability of gene panels and whole-exome sequencing has improved diagnostics, has enabled the discovery of new myopathy genes, and has greatly broadened the genotype-phenotype spectrum of these disorders. It has also presented challenges related to disease classification and genetic variants of unknown clinical significance; in addition, the genetic cause in many individuals still remains elusive. Currently there are few, if any, therapies available for these often devastating disorders; however, work using preclinical model systems has identified several promising candidates for translation into the clinical arena. One of the key challenges in the future will be effectively translating these drugs, and factors related to disease natural history and clinical trial readiness are becoming of paramount importance as the field moves forward toward hopefully identifying meaningful therapies.

REFERENCES

The complete list of references for this chapter is available in the e-book at www.expertconsult.com.
See inside cover for registration details.

SELECTED REFERENCES

Clarke, N.F., 2011. Congenital fiber-type disproportion. Semin. Pediatr. Neurol. 18, 264–271.

Colombo, I., et al., 2015. Congenital myopathies: natural history of a large pediatric cohort. Neurology 84, 28–35.

Das, S., Dowling, J., Pierson, C.R., 1993. X-Linked centronuclear myopathy. In: Pagon, R.A., et al. (Eds.), GeneReviews® [Internet]. University of Washington–Seattle, Seattle, WA, pp. 1993–2016.

Dowling, J.J., et al., 2015. Congenital and other structural myopathies. In: Darras, B.T., et al. (Eds.), Neuromuscular Disorders of Infancy, Childhood, and Adolescence: A Clinician's Approach. Elsevier, New York, pp. 502–537.

Jungbluth, H., 2007a. Central core disease. Orphanet J. Rare Dis. 2, 25.

Jungbluth, H., 2007b. Multi-minicore disease. Orphanet J. Rare Dis. 2, 31.

Jungbluth, H., Wallgren-Pettersson, C., Laporte, J., 2008. Centronuclear (myotubular) myopathy. Orphanet J. Rare Dis. 3, 26.

North, K.N., Ryan, M.M., 1993. Nemaline myopathy. In: Pagon, R.A., et al. (Eds.), GeneReviews® [Internet]. University of Washington–Seattle, Seattle, WA, pp. 1993–2016.

North, K.N., et al., 2014. Approach to the diagnosis of congenital myopathies. Neuromuscul. Disord. 24, 97–116.

Wang, C.H., et al., 2012. Consensus statement on standard of care for congenital myopathies. J. Child Neurol. 27, 363–382.

E-BOOK FIGURES AND TABLES

The following figures and tables are available in the e-book at www.expertconsult.com. See inside cover for registration details.

Fig. 148-3. The common congenital myopathy subtypes by histopathology.

Fig. 148-4. Muscle MRI in congenital myopathies.

Fig. 148-5. *MTM-* and *DNM2*-related centronuclear myopathy.

Fig. 148-6. *ACTA1-* and *NEB*-related nemaline myopathies.

Fig. 148-7. *RYR1*-related myopathy.

149 Metabolic Myopathies

Ingrid Tein

 An expanded version of this chapter is available on www.expertconsult.com. See inside cover for registration details.

UTILIZATION OF BIOENERGETIC SUBSTRATES IN EXERCISE

Symptoms in muscle energy defects are directly related to a mismatch between the rates of adenosine triphosphate (ATP) utilization (energy demand) relative to the capacity of the muscle metabolic pathways to regenerate ATP (energy supply). This energy supply-demand mismatch impairs energy-dependent processes that power muscle contraction (weakness, exertional fatigue), mediate muscle relaxation (muscle cramping, tightness), and/or maintain membrane ion gradients necessary for normal membrane excitability (fatigue, weakness) and muscle cell integrity (muscle pain, injury, myoglobinuria). In metabolic myopathies, the specific metabolic mediators of premature fatigue, cramping, pain, and muscle injury are complex and vary among the different metabolic disorders. Disorders of glycogen, lipid, or mitochondrial metabolism may cause two main clinical syndromes in muscle: (1) acute, recurrent, reversible muscle dysfunction with exercise intolerance and acute muscle breakdown or myoglobinuria (with or without cramps), for example, mitochondrial disorders, and (2) progressive weakness, for example, fatty acid oxidation (FAO) defects and mitochondrial enzyme deficiencies (Box 149-1). Progressive weakness and recurrent myoglobinuria can also occur together in a given disorder.

Defects of energy metabolism may profoundly disrupt the function of muscle and other highly energy-dependent tissues, such as brain, nerve, heart, kidney, liver, and bowel. The limits of energy utilization in skeletal muscle are set by the adenosine triphosphatases (ATPases) that couple muscle contraction (myosin ATPase) and ion transport (calcium and sodium, potassium ATPases) to the hydrolysis of ATP to adenosine diphosphate (ADP) and inorganic phosphate (Pi). ADP and Pi in turn activate energy-producing reactions that regenerate ATP. Without this, ATP stores would be exhausted in seconds. The substrates that are used to replenish ATP are determined by the intrinsic properties of these fuels and by the intensity and duration of exercise that modulates fuel selection. The creatine kinase (CK) reaction and anaerobic glycogenolysis are the major anaerobic sources of ADP phosphorylation. Increases in ADP and AMP that occur in heavy exercise are primarily buffered by the coupled adenylate kinase (myokinase), adenylate deaminase (myoadenylate deaminase) reactions. Anaerobic glycogenolysis and phosphocreatine hydrolysis support muscle energy production with two- to fourfold higher rates than those supported by oxidative metabolism. Anaerobic energy is crucial for rapid bursts of exercise and to fuel the transition from rest to exercise. The acceleration to high rates of energy production occurs instantly for ATP, in less than a second for phosphocreatine, and within seconds for anaerobic glycogenolysis. In contrast, maximal oxidative power requires from 3 minutes (with glycogen as the oxidative substrate) to 30 minutes (for peak FAO). Anaerobic fuels are rapidly depleted and lead to the accumulation of metabolic end products such as protons and Pi that promote fatigue.

If exercise needs to be sustained for more than a few minutes, then oxidative phosphorylation is necessary and provides the most abundant source of ATP synthesis. Glycogen is the major endogenous oxidative fuel of skeletal muscle, whereas blood glucose and free fatty acids (FFA) are the major exogenous fuels. A small percentage of muscle energy needs are supplied by amino acids, predominantly branched chain amino acids, which are oxidized to a limited extent. Oxidative metabolism provides higher yields of ATP per mole of substrate, rising from 2 to 36 for glucose and from 3 to 37 per glycosyl unit of glycogen metabolized anaerobically versus oxidatively. Furthermore, the metabolic end products of oxidative metabolism, namely, CO_2 and water, are easily removed from working muscle and do not promote fatigue. The most abundant and critical fuel for the support of prolonged, moderate exercise is lipid. Carbohydrate stores in the form of muscle and hepatic glycogen and blood glucose (derived mainly from hepatic glycogenolysis) are limited and can support high-intensity exercise for only 1 to 2 hours. However, carbohydrate, particularly muscle glycogen, is critical for normal oxidative metabolism. Glycogen supports a peak rate of oxidative phosphorylation that is about twofold greater than fat. Though incompletely understood, this may be based upon a requirement for glycogen-derived pyruvate to support optimal function of the tricarboxylic acid cycle. The proportion of carbohydrate relative to lipid oxidation progressively increases as the intensity of the aerobic exercise increases until carbohydrate is the exclusive fuel of maximum oxidative metabolism. Second, glycogen is able to accelerate to maximal oxidative power output rapidly compared with other fuels. Third, the molar ratio of ATP produced to O_2 consumed is higher for glycogen (6.17) and glucose (5.98) than for fatty acids (5.61). The importance of this point lies in the fact that peak O_2 utilization in healthy humans is limited by O_2 delivery.

The combustion of fuels in oxidative metabolism involves the generation of reducing equivalents in β-oxidation, glycolysis, and the tricarboxylic acid cycle that are oxidized via the respiratory chain, where the phosphorylation of ADP is coupled to the reduction of molecular oxygen to water. Normal oxidative metabolism requires a highly integrated physiologic support system to regulate the flow of oxygen from the lungs to the respiring muscle mitochondria as well as functional mitochondria that can efficiently extract the available oxygen from blood. Muscle oxygen utilization in oxidative phosphorylation may increase 50-fold or greater from rest to peak exercise. This increase is achieved by increases in the level of oxygen extraction from oxyhemoglobin in red blood cells and in the rate of delivery of oxygenated blood to working muscle by the circulation.

The primary source of energy for resting muscle is derived from FAO. At rest, glucose utilization accounts for 10% to 15% of total oxygen consumption. Both slow and fast twitch fibers have similar levels of glycogen content at rest. The choice of the bioenergetic pathway in working muscle depends on the type, intensity, and duration of exercise (Gollnick et al., 1974), but also on diet and physical conditioning. In the first 5 to 10

BOX 149-1 Heritable Causes of Myoglobinuria

I. Biochemical abnormality known
  A. Glycolysis/glycogenolysis
    1. Phosphorylase*
    2. Phosphofructokinase
    3. Phosphoglycerate kinase*
    4. Phosphoglycerate mutase*
    5. Lactate dehydrogenase*
    6. Phosphorylase b kinase
    7. Debrancher
    8. Aldolase A deficiency*
  B. Fatty acid oxidation
    1. Carnitine palmitoyltransferase II*
    2. Long-chain acyl-CoA dehydrogenase
    3. Very long-chain acyl-CoA dehydrogenase
    4. Medium-chain acyl-CoA dehydrogenase
    5. Short-chain L-3-hydroxyacyl CoA dehydrogenase*
    6. Trifunctional protein deficiency*
    7. Medium-chain 3-ketoacyl CoA thiolase*
    8. Acyl-CoA dehydrogenase 9 (*ACAD9*)*,**
  C. Pentose phosphate pathway
    1. G6PDH*
  D. Purine nucleotide cycle
    1. Myoadenylate deaminase
  E. Respiratory chain
    1. Complex I deficiency*
    2. Coenzyme Q deficiency
    3. Complex II and aconitase*
    4. Complex III deficiency (cytochrome b)
    5. Complex IV deficiency (cytochrome oxidase deficiency)*
    6. Multiple mitochondrial DNA deletions*
II. Ryanodine receptor 1 (*RYR1*) abnormality
  1. Malignant hyperthermia
  2. Central core disease
  3. Minicore myopathy with external ophthalmoplegia
  4. King-Denborough syndrome
III. Biochemical abnormality incompletely characterized
  A. Impaired long-chain fatty acid oxidation*
  B. Impaired function of the sarcoplasmic reticulum (?) (predisposition in myotonic dystrophy, myotonia congenita, Schwartz-Jampel syndrome)
IV. Abnormal composition of sarcolemma
  A. Abnormal composition of the sarcolemma in Duchenne and Becker muscular dystrophy*
  B. Muscle-specific phosphatidic acid phosphatase deficiency (*LPIN1* mutations)*
V. Biochemical abnormality unknown
  A. Familial recurrent myoglobinuria*
  B. Repeated attacks in sporadic cases*

*Etiologies that have been documented to cause recurrent myoglobinuria beginning in childhood.
**ACAD9 deficiency also leads to mitchondrial complex I deficiency.
(Modified with permission of Tein I, DiMauro S, Rowland LP. Myoglobinuria. In: Rowland LP, DiMauro S, editors. Handbook of clinical neurology, vol. 18 (62). Myopathies. Amsterdam: Elsevier Science Publishers; 1992, pp. 553–93.)

minutes of moderate exercise, high-energy phosphates are used to first regenerate ATP. This is followed by muscle glycogen breakdown, which is indicated by a sharp rise in lactate during the first 10 minutes. Blood lactate levels then drop as muscle triglycerides and blood-borne fuels are used. After 90 minutes, the major fuels are glucose and FFAs. During 1 to 4 hours of mild to moderate prolonged exercise, muscle uptake

of FFAs increases approximately 70%, and after 4 hours, FFAs are used twice as much as carbohydrates.

The disorders discussed here have a genetic basis. The inheritance pattern, gene, gene product, and function are summarized in the following sections for each disorder. More detailed and current molecular genetic information can be obtained from the Online Mendelian Inheritance in Man (omim.org), Gene Table of Neuromuscular Disorders (musclegenetable.fr), Gene Cards human gene database (genecards.org), and MitoMap.com websites.

A fuller discussion of the history, genetic, biochemistry, and pathophysiologic aspects of these disorders can be obtained from the online version of the chapter.

MYOGLOBINURIA

Myoglobinuria is a clinical syndrome, not just a biochemical state. In the alert patient, myalgia and limb weakness are the most common presenting symptoms. Urine color is usually brownish rather than red, and the urine tests positive for both albumin and heme (a concentration of at least 4 µg/mL). There are few or no red blood cells. Myoglobin can be identified by immunochemical methods. The sarcoplasmic enzymes, including serum CK, are usually elevated to more than 100 times normal. Inconstant features include hyperphosphatemia, hyperuricemia, and hypocalcemia. If renal failure occurs, serum potassium and calcium levels may rise. If the patient is comatose or if the presenting disorder is one of acute renal failure, there may be no muscle symptoms or signs. Under these conditions, the diagnosis can be made if (1) there is renal failure and (2) the serum content of sarcoplasmic enzymes is 100 times normal. The potentially life-threatening hazards of an attack of myoglobinuria include renal or respiratory failure and cardiac arrhythmias. The etiologies of heritable myoglobinuria differ in adults compared with children. In a study of 77 adult patients aged 15 to 65 years, Tonin et al. (1990) identified the enzyme abnormality in 36 patients (47%) as follows: CPT deficiency in 17 patients; glycolytic defects in 15 patients (including PPL in 10, PPL b kinase in 4, and PGK in 1); myoadenylate deaminase in 3; and combined CPT and myoadenylate deaminase in 1. In contrast, in 100 cases of recurrent childhood-onset myoglobinuria, a lower percentage of children have been diagnosed biochemically (24%): 16 with CPT deficiency, 1 with SCHAD deficiency, and 7 with various glycolytic defects, including 2 PPL, 1 PGK, 3 PGAM, and 1 LDH deficiency. These children could be divided into two groups: a type I exertional group, in which exertion was the primary precipitating factor (56 cases), and a type II toxic group, in which infection and/or fever and leukocytosis were the primary precipitants (37 cases). The type II toxic childhood group was distinguished from the type I exertional childhood- and adult-onset groups by its etiologies, which were limited to FAO defects, as well as its slight female predominance, which contrasted with the marked male predominance in the latter two groups. The type II toxic group was further distinguished by the earlier age at onset of myoglobinuria, the presence of a more generalized disease (e.g., ictal bulbar signs, seizures, encephalopathy, developmental delay), and a higher mortality rate. Currently the most common etiology for recurrent myoglobinuria in both adults and children is CPT II deficiency (Tein et al., 1992).

GLYCOGENOSES

Only glycogenoses affecting skeletal muscle, alone or in association with other tissues, are discussed in this section (Figure 149-1). Molecular genetic analysis has led to the cloning of genes encoding the enzymes involved in the glycogenoses,

TABLE 149-2 Clinical Presentation of Muscle Glycogenoses

Type	Enzyme Defect	Affected Tissues	Clinical Presentation
II Infancy	Acid maltase	Generalized	Cardiomegaly, weakness, hypotonia, death <age 1 yr
II Childhood	Acid maltase	Generalized	Myopathy simulating Duchenne dystrophy, respiratory insufficiency
II Adult	Acid maltase	Generalized	Myopathy simulating limb girdle dystrophy or polymyositis, respiratory insufficiency
III	Debrancher	Generalized	Hepatomegaly, fasting hypoglycemia, progressive weakness
IV	Brancher	Generalized	Hepatosplenomegaly, cirrhosis of liver, hepatic failure, myopathy, cardiomyopathy, APBD
V	Muscle phosphorylase	Skeletal muscle	Intolerance to intense exercise, cramps, myoglobinuria
VII	Muscle phosphofructokinase (PFK-M)	Skeletal muscle RBC	Intolerance to intense exercise, cramps, myoglobinuria
VIII	Phosphorylase kinase	Liver	Asymptomatic hepatomegaly
VIII	Phosphorylase kinase	Liver and muscle	Hepatomegaly, growth retardation, hypotonia
VIII	Phosphorylase kinase	Skeletal muscle	Exercise intolerance, myoglobinuria
VIII	Phosphorylase kinase	Heart	Fatal infantile cardiomyopathy
IX	Phosphoglycerate kinase 1 (PGK1)	Generalized	Hemolytic anemia, seizures, mental retardation, intolerance to intense exercise, myoglobinuria
X	Muscle phosphoglycerate mutase (PGAM-M)	Skeletal muscle	Intolerance to intense exercise, myoglobinuria
XI	Muscle lactate dehydrogenase (LDH-M)	Skeletal muscle	Intolerance to intense exercise, myoglobinuria
XII	Aldolase A	Skeletal muscle RBC	Nonspherocytic hemolytic anemia, exercise intolerance, weakness
XIII	β-Enolase	Skeletal muscle	Exercise intolerance
XIV	Phosphoglucomutase 1	Skeletal muscle	Exercise intolerance, myoglobinuria

APBD, adult polyglucosan body disease; RBC, red blood cells.
(Modified with permission of DiMauro S, Lamperti C. Muscle glycogenoses. Muscle Nerve 2001;24:985, John Wiley and Sons, Inc.)

as well as their chromosomal localization (Table 149-1). Inheritance is autosomal recessive, in the majority, or X-linked recessive. In the glycogenoses, fixed weakness is the primary presentation in acid maltase, debrancher, aldolase, and brancher enzyme deficiencies, whereas exercise intolerance with cramps, myalgia, and recurrent myoglobinuria are the primary presentation in phosphorylase kinase, phosphorylase, phosphofructokinase, phosphoglycerate kinase, phosphoglyc-erate mutase, β-enolase, and lactate dehydrogenase deficien-cies (Table 149-2).

Pathophysiology (see online version for details)

The pathophysiology of glycogenoses relates more to the impairment of aerobic than anaerobic glycolysis. The energy substrates used by muscle for aerobic metabolism depend on the type, intensity, and duration of exercise, as well as on physical conditioning and diet. During low-intensity exercise the primary source of energy is derived from blood glucose and FFAs. During intense exercise, energy is derived from anaerobic glycolysis and the proportion of energy derived from carbohydrate oxidation increases, with glycogen serving as an important fuel. Fatigue occurs when glycogen stores are exhausted. Individuals with defective glycolysis/glycogenolysis are most vulnerable during the initial stages of intense exercise, and they must rest soon after beginning exercise because of muscle cramps. However, if they continue to exercise at low intensity, they are able to continue for a longer time. This is known as the *second-wind phenomenon* and has been attributed

to a metabolic switch from carbohydrate to fatty acid utiliza-tion and to increased circulation with increased availability of blood glucose from hepatic glycogenolysis.

Provocative testing with the ischemic or non-ischemic forearm exercise test has been performed traditionally to measure the change in lactate and ammonia levels in blood (see online version of this chapter for details). The sensitivity and positive predictive value of this test vary among the gly-cogenosis. Now, with the availability of gene panels for myoglobria, this testing is often omitted.

Glycolytic/Glycogenolytic Defects

The specific clinical features, laboratory tests, pathology, pathophysiology, inheritance pattern, biochemistry, molecular genetics, and treatment for each defect in this pathway with muscle involvement are presented in the online version. For a summary of the chromosomal assignment and pattern of inheritance, see Table 149-1, and for a summary of the clinical presentations, see Table 149-2.

FATTY ACID OXIDATION DISORDERS
Historical Background

FAO disorders are an important group of diseases because they are potentially rapidly fatal and a source of major mor-bidity. They present with a spectrum of clinical disorders, including recurrent myoglobinuria, progressive lipid storage myopathy, neuropathy, progressive cardiomyopathy, recurrent hypoglycemic hypoketotic encephalopathy or Reye-like syndrome, seizures, and mental retardation. All of the currently known conditions are inherited as autosomal-recessive traits. Thus there is frequently a family history of sudden infant death syndrome (SIDS) in siblings. Early recognition and prompt institution of therapy and appropriate preventive measures, and in certain cases specific therapy, may be life-saving and may significantly decrease long-term morbidity, particularly with respect to CNS sequelae. There are now at least 25 enzymes and specific transport proteins in the pathway of β-oxidation, and defects in 18 of them have been recognized to cause disease in humans. With the significant advances in biomedical technology, there has been a rapid increase in the number of subsequently diagnosed cases. The incidence for MCAD deficiency was 1 in 8930 live births in a survey from the Pennsylvania newborn screening program using tandem mass spectrometry followed by confirmation through molecular analysis for several common mutations. Identification of the individual serum acylcarnitine esters has been facilitated by electrospray ionization–tandem mass spectrometry (ESI-MS/MS) and is now being used in newborn screening for early diagnosis and treatment of FAO disorders

Fasting Adaptation

Fats constitute the most important and efficient fuel for oxidative metabolism and are the largest reserve of fuel in the body. As liver glycogen stores are depleted within a few hours of a meal and because there are no reserve stores of protein in the body, fatty acids become the predominant substrate for oxidation quite early in fasting.

Fatty acids serve three major functions. First, the partial oxidation of fatty acids by the liver produces ketones, which are an important auxiliary fuel for almost all tissues and particularly for the brain. Second, fatty acids serve as a major fuel for cardiac and skeletal muscle. Exercising muscle, during mild to moderate prolonged exercise, and resting muscle depend primarily on FAO (Gollnick et al., 1974). Third, the high rates of hepatic gluconeogenesis and ureagenesis needed for maintaining fasting homeostasis are sustained by the production of energy (ATP), reducing equivalents, and metabolic intermediates derived from FAO.

Increased Susceptibility of the Child

Children with FAO defects are most prone to decompensation, within the context of depleted glycogen and glucose reserves, during conditions that place stress on the FAO pathway for fuel generation. These conditions include prolonged exercise (particularly after 1 hour of mild to moderate aerobic exercise), fasting, infection with vomiting, and cold-induced shivering thermogenesis. After an overnight fast, children are most likely to be found comatose in the early morning hours. During infection, there may be an added problem with vomiting and decreased oral intake with shivering thermogenesis. If not recognized and therefore untreated, children may progress to a Reye-like syndrome. There are several reasons for an increased risk of problems with fasting adaptation in infants and young children. First, given the large ratio of surface area to body mass, basal energy needs in the infant are high to maintain body temperature. Shivering thermogenesis, which maintains body temperature, is highly dependent on efficient FAO. Second, infants have a larger brain compared with body size. The developing brain is highly dependent on glucose and has a high rate of metabolism; therefore, infants and children show an even earlier activation of FAO with hyperketonemia within 12 to 24 hours of fasting. Third, there is a lower activity of several key enzymes involved in energy production in the

infant compared with the older child and adult, leading to further impairment of the infant's ability to maintain glucose homeostasis.

Normal Pathway of Fatty Acid Oxidation

The pathway of mitochondrial FAO is outlined in Figure 149-2 and is described in detail in the online version.

Clinical and Biochemical Features of Identified Defects

Common Features of Fatty Acid Oxidation Disorders

Hale and Bennett (1992) suggest that there are at least four clinical and laboratory features that should lead the clinician to suspect a genetic defect in FAO: (1) acute metabolic decompensation in association with fasting, (2) chronic involvement of tissues highly dependent on efficient FAO (e.g., heart, muscle, liver), (3) recurrent episodes of hypoketotic hypoglycemia, and (4) alterations in the quantity of total carnitine or of the percentage of esterified carnitine in plasma and tissue.

Involvement of Fatty Acid Oxidation–Dependent Tissues

Hypoketotic Hypoglycemia. Tissues such as skeletal muscle, heart, and liver have high energy demands and are therefore dependent on efficient FAO. When there is a defect in hepatic ketogenesis, glucose becomes the only available fuel and thus becomes rate limiting under conditions of FAO stress when glycogen and glucose stores have been depleted. As a result, FFAs, which are liberated during fasting and cannot be metabolized because of the block, may be stored in the cytosol as triglycerides. This produces a progressive lipid storage myopathy with weakness, a hypertrophic and/or dilatative cardiomyopathy, and a fatty liver.

The pattern of hypoketotic hypoglycemia reflects the accelerated rate of glucose utilization that occurs when fatty acids cannot be used as fuels and ketone bodies are not generated to spare glucose/glycogen stores. An increase in the ratio of serum FFAs to ketones, from the normal ratio of 1:1 to greater than 2:1, therefore would suggest a block in β-oxidation.

Alterations in Plasma and Tissue Concentrations of Carnitine.

In most cases of intramitochondrial β-oxidation defects, the total carnitine concentration is decreased (<50% or normal), and the acylcarnitine fraction is increased (>50% esterified; normal is 10% to 25% in the fed state and 30% to 50% in the fasted state). In the intramitochondrial β-oxidation disorders, the excessive acyl-CoAs that accumulate proximal to the metabolic block may be converted into acylcarnitines by chain length-specific carnitine acyltransferases.

Additional Laboratory Findings

During acute catabolic crises, other biochemical derangements may be noted. A modest hyperammonemia (100 to 200 μmol/L) accompanied by threefold to fivefold elevation of liver transaminases may be documented during the Reye-like syndrome presentation. In acute myoglobinuria there are marked increases in the sarcoplasmic enzymes, including serum CK, which may rise higher than 100,000 IU/L (normal <250 IU/L). The serum concentrations of amino acids (especially taurine), creatinine, potassium, phosphate, and urate may also be increased. The hyperphosphatemia may lead to secondary hypocalcemia, which may be later followed by hypercalcemia (Tein et al., 1992). It is urgent to prevent renal failure. These changes may have deleterious renal and cardiac effects, thereby further exaggerating the damage. Lactic acidosis

TABLE 149-3 Clinical Features Associated With Specific Genetic Defects of Fatty Acid Oxidation

Deficiency	Fasting Disorder	Tissue Involved	Hypoketotic Hypoglycemia	Altered Carnitine	Dicarboxylic Acids	Reye-Like Syndrome	SIDS
LCFAUD	+	L	+	+	NR	NR	NR
OCTN2	+	H, M	+	+	NR	+	NR
CPT IA	+	K, L	+	+	NR	+	NR
TRANS	+	H, M, (Mg)	+	+	NR	+	+
CPT II (mild)	+/−	M, Mg, P	NR	+	NR	NR	NR
CPT II (severe)	+	H, M, Mg, L	+	+	NR	+	+
VLCAD/LCAD	+	H, M, Mg, L	+	+	+	+	+
ACAD9	+	B, H, L, M, Mg	+	+	+	+	NR
Trifunctional/LCHAD	+	H, M, Mg, L, N, P, R	+	+	+	+	+
Dienoyl CoA reductase	NR	M, D, B, (H)	NR	+	NR	NR	NR
MCAD	+	(Mg)	+	+	+	+	+
SCAD	+	M, B, D, H	+/−	+	+	NR	+
SCHAD	+	H, M, Mg, L	+	+	+	NR	+
ETF and ETF/Qo	+	M, H, K, B, D	+	+	+	NR	+
HMG-CoA lyase	+	B, P	+	+	+	+	+ ?

ACAD9, acyl-CoA dehydrogenase 9; B, brain; CPT, carnitine palmitoyltransferase; D, dysmorphic features; ETF, electron transfer flavoprotein; H, heart; HMG, β-hydroxy-β-methylglutaryl; K, kidney; L, liver; LCAD, long-chain acyl-CoA dehydrogenase; LCFAUD, long-chain fatty acid uptake defect; M, muscle; MCAD, medium-chain acyl-CoA dehydrogenase; Mg, myoglobinuria; N, neuropathy; NR, no case yet reported.; OCTN2, plasmalemmal high-affinity carnitine transporter; P, pancreatitis; Qo, coenzyme Q oxidoreductase; R, retinopathy; SCAD, short-chain acyl-CoA dehydrogenase; SCHAD, short-chain L-3-hydroxyacyl-CoA dehydrogenase; TRANS, carnitine acylcarnitine translocase; trifunctional, long-chain enoyl-CoA hydratase + long-chain L-3-hydroxyacyl-CoA dehydrogenase + long-chain 3-ketoacyl-CoA thiolase; VLCAD, very long-chain acyl-CoA dehydrogenase.

(Modified with permission of Tein I. Fatty acid oxidation and associated defects. American Academy of Neurology Proceedings, Seattle, 1995. Madison, WI: Omnipress.)

may also be noted during the acute catabolic presentations. Urine organic acid screening may demonstrate unusual or excessive amounts of organic acids, which may be diagnostic of a specific block in β-oxidation.

Specific Features of Individual Genetic Defects (see online version of this chapter for details)

The specific features of individual FAO disorders are outlined in the online version, and the clinical and laboratory characteristics are summarized, respectively, in Table 149-3 and Table 149-4.

Differentiating Laboratory Features

Analysis of the fatty acid intermediates in the serum or urine of affected children may suggest the site of defect, depending on the chain-length specificity and the species type of the intermediates. These intermediates often require specialized biomedical technology, which may require referral to specialized metabolic laboratories. Particularly useful are the assessment of plasma total and free carnitine, serum acylcarnitines, urine acylcarnitines and urine acylglycines, and organic acids. These intermediates may be absent at times when the child is metabolically stable and receiving adequate supplies of glucose because this would reduce the stress on the FAO pathway. They are best detected in the serum and urine of children during acute catabolic crises or during times of fasting.

Serum acylcarnitine analysis from dried blood spots by electrospray ionization–tandem mass spectrometry (ESI-MS/MS) is increasingly used in newborn screening programs and can be used to detect FAO disorders, carnitine cycle disorders, and organic acidurias. Stored dried blood spots are also a valuable source for postmortem investigations to elucidate the cause of SIDS.

Diagnostic Approaches and Screening Methods

History and Physical Examination

The key to investigation of these patients is a careful history and clinical examination. The presentation may be either acute and recurrent, or more chronic and slowly progressive. The more typical presentation is the acute one in which the child has a history of decreased oral intake during the preceding 24 to 36 hours followed by increasing lethargy and progressive obtundation or coma. The important initial investigations in a comatose child should include serum glucose and urine ketone measurements. Determination of urine ketones may be complicated because ill children are often dehydrated and will have concentrated urine that may demonstrate a relatively spurious elevation in ketones. If the blood glucose is above 3.3 mmol/L (60 mg/dL) and if it is accompanied by large amounts of urinary ketones, this tends to rule out an FAO disorder. However, if the blood glucose is less than 3.3 mmol/L and the urine ketones are trace or small in amount, this would suggest the possibility of an FAO disorder and would warrant further investigation. Most important, samples from the acute presentation, particularly before intravenous glucose therapy, should be saved for the determination of serum carnitine total and free, serum acylcarnitines, serum FFAs and ketones, urine organic acids, acylglycines, and acylcarnitines. With normal

FAO, the serum FFA/ketone ratio is 1:1. In the event of a block in FAO, this ratio increases to greater than 2:1 and is therefore useful as an initial screen. The serum and urine specimens during the acute episode can also be used to assess the integrity and hormonal regulation of the biochemical pathways involved in glucose homeostasis.

Once presumptive evidence for a defect in FAO has been established, the clinical picture, in combination with an analysis of serum acylcarnitines, urinary organic acid profiles, and urinary acylglycines, may suggest a specific site of defect and the chain-length specificity of the defect (e.g., short chain, medium chain, or long chain). Further investigations to identify the specific site of defect may include oxidation rates of [1-^{14}C]-labeled palmitate (C16), octanoate (C8), and butyrate (C4) and deuterium-labeled oleic acid in the fibroblasts to establish the chain-length specificity of the defect. Depending on the suspected site of defect, a direct enzymatic assay may then be performed for the specific enzyme (Table 149-5). These assays can be performed in cultured skin fibroblasts or in biopsied muscle specimens. However, certain of these defects may be tissue specific, such as muscle SCHAD deficiency, in which case the defect is expressed in biopsied muscle and not in fibroblasts, and therefore may be missed unless the affected tissue is examined. For the carnitine uptake defect or OCTN2 deficiency, diagnosis is confirmed by *in vitro* studies of carnitine uptake in cultured skin fibroblasts. After identification of a specific enzyme or transporter defect, molecular genetic analysis can be performed to identify the underlying mutations.

Treatment

The biochemical consequences of a defect in FAO can be divided into the following: (1) inadequate energy supply; (2) accumulation of toxic metabolites (e.g., misfolded proteins, membranotoxic long-chain acylcarnitines, increased ROS in ETFDH deficiency); (3) sequestration or loss of vital components (e.g., sequestration of Coenzyme A in the formation of excessive acyl-CoA intermediates); (4) altered production of enzyme product; (5) loss of protein-protein interaction (e.g., loss of inhibition of glutamate dehydrogenase by the SCHAD protein in SCHAD deficiency).

The mainstay of therapy is the avoidance of precipitating factors, particularly prolonged fasting. General treatment strategies are discussed next.

Avoidance of Precipitating Factors

Avoidance of precipitating factors, such as prolonged fasting, prolonged aerobic exercise (>30 minutes), and cold exposure leading to shivering thermogenesis, is key. Suggested maximal fasting periods (during stable metabolic conditions) from a European consensus panel are as follows: neonates, 3 hours, also at night; <6 months, 4 hours, also at night; >6 months, 4 hours in the daytime, 6 (to 8) hours at night in well-nourished infants; >12 months to 3 years, 4 hours in the daytime, 10 (to 12) hours at night; 4 to 7 years, 4 hours during day, 10 (to 12) hours at night (Spiekerkoetter et al., 2009). These fasting periods apply under healthy, steady-state conditions, when on a normocaloric diet, glycogen sores can be built up during the day and used for glucose production during longer fasting intervals at night. In the event of progressive lethargy or obtundation or an inability to take oral feedings because of vomiting, the child should be taken immediately to the emergency room for intravenous glucose therapy. Intravenous glucose should be provided at rates sufficient to prevent fatty acid mobilization (8 to 10 mg/kg/

min). This regimen should be continued until the catabolic cascade has been reversed and the child is able to take oral feedings again. It is prudent to institute intravenous glucose therapy as soon as there is a concern regarding the status of the child and not to wait until the occurrence of severe symptoms or a drop in blood glucose <3.3 mmol/L, as a delay may lead to serious morbidity or death. It is wise to avoid prolonged exercise (i.e., >30 minutes) because during this time there is increased fat mobilization. A high-carbohydrate load before exercise is advisable, with a rest period and repeat carbohydrate loading at 15 minutes. Avoidance of cold exposure to limit shivering thermogenesis is essential.

High-Carbohydrate, Low-Fat Diet

In general, it is advisable to institute a high-carbohydrate, low-fat diet with frequent feedings throughout the day, which would be commensurate with the nutritional needs of the child given his or her age. This goal is best achieved with the aid of a dietitian, aiming toward approximately 60% of calories from carbohydrate sources, 15% from protein, and approximately 25% to 30% from fat. Long-chain fat intake in healthy infants is 40% to 45% of total energy, and in children of school age it is 30% to 35%. Monitoring of essential fatty acid levels is important to ensure that the child is receiving adequate essential fatty acids, as these may require supplementation. See the online version for additional details.

Uncooked Cornstarch

Routine enrichment of the diet with glucose polymers or cornstarch is not recommended, but is part of oral prophylactic and therapeutic emergency management. To delay the onset of fasting overnight, the nightly institution of uncooked cornstarch, in doses similar to those used in the treatment of glycogen storage disease (1 to 2 g/kg body weight/day as a single nighttime dose), will prolong the postabsorptive state and delay fasting. Cornstarch provides a sustained release source of glucose, thereby preventing hypoglycemia and lipolysis. Cornstarch is usually initiated at 8 months of age when pancreatic enzymes are first able to function at full capacity for appropriate absorption. The initial recommended doses are generally 1.0 g/kg/day, which can be gradually increased to 1.5 to 2.0 g/kg/day by age 2 years as needed. This may lead to undesirable weight gain.

Other Treatments

Specific treatments for individual FAO disorders may include consideration of medium-chain triglyceride (MCT) oil for long-chain FAO disorders, riboflavin for the multiple acyl-CoA dehydrogenase deficiencies, carnitine for OCTN2 deficiency, and docosahexaenoic acid (DHA) for TFP/LCHAD deficiency, and prednisone, triheptanoin, PPAR agonists (bezafibrate), resveratrol, premature stop codon read-through drugs (gentamicin and ataluren), and gene therapy approaches for selected disorders, as discussed in more detail in the online version.

Clinical Monitoring

On a chronic basis, clinical monitoring of individuals with FAO disorders is very important. This should include evaluation of growth, development, neurologic examination, and diet as well as reinforcement of the prevention of risk factors and management of acute crises. Yearly ophthalmologic examinations are important for long-chain FAO disorders (e.g., pigmentary retinopathy in TFP/LCHAD deficiency) and

GA II. ECG and echocardiography are important to monitor cardiac function in long-chain disorders and OCTN2 defects. Liver ultrasonography may be important in LCHAD/TFP deficiency. Biochemical follow-up should include serum carnitine total and free and serum acylcarnitines to monitor metabolic control, and CK. Essential fatty acid and DHA status should be monitored in long-chain defects. Regular follow-up and education of the child and family is important throughout life to help prevent morbidity and mortality.

Genetics and Presymptomatic Recognition

All known FAO disorders are inherited as autosomal-recessive conditions. The inclusion of FAO disorders in newborn screening programs with comprehensive and consistent long-term follow-up is highly desirable to prevent morbidity and mortality, to implement preventative measures and treatment strategies, and to reduce the cost of care of affected patients.

MITOCHONDRIAL ENCEPHALOMYOPATHIES
(also refer to Chapter 42)

Though all of the mitochondrial encephalomyopathies that are expressed in muscle are at potential risk for the development of myopathy and exercise intolerance, the specific defects in which acute episodes of myoglobinuria have been documented to date include defects of complexes I, II, III, and IV activities as well as multiple mtDNA deletions, mtDNA depletion syndromes, and Coenzyme Q10 (CoQ10) deficiency. Mitochondrial myopathy commonly manifests with exercise intolerance and premature fatigue, which is often out of proportion to the degree of muscle weakness. The myopathy may selectively involve the extraocular muscles (progressive external ophthalmoplegia [PEO]) and/or may extend to bulbar, limb (usually proximal but may be distal), and axial muscles. Onset may occur at any age, although more severe phenotypes present earlier in life and milder phenotypes present later in life. As there is an entire chapter dedicated to the detailed discussion of the individual mitochondrial disorders (see Chapter 42), the following sections will serve to briefly summarize and highlight the key clinical, morphologic, biochemical, genetic, and physiologic features of this group of disorders.

Morphologic Considerations

Although the finding of ragged-red fibers (RRF) or ultrastructural alterations of mitochondria in muscle biopsy specimens suggests the possibility of a mitochondrial disorder, there are important limitations. These have been articulated by DiMauro (2001) as follows:

1. Nonmitochondrial disorders, such as muscular dystrophies, polymyositis, and some glycogenoses, may demonstrate RRF or ultrastructural mitochondrial abnormalities in which they likely represent secondary changes.
2. Conversely, many primary mitochondrial diseases, such as enzyme defects in metabolic pathways other than the respiratory chain (e.g., the pyruvate dehydrogenase complex [PDHC], CPT, beta-oxidation, and fumarase deficiencies), do not have RRF.

In addition, there are defects of the respiratory chain, such as Leigh syndrome secondary to cytochrome c oxidase (COX) deficiency, that tend not to have RRF. RRF are often COX negative, although not all COX-negative fibers are RRF.

A global decrease in the activity of COX is usually suggestive of a nuclear mutation in an ancillary protein required for COX assembly such as SURF1 but can also be associated with some homoplasmic mt-tRNA defects. A mosaic appearance of COX-negative fibers generally suggests an mtDNA mutation because of the variable degrees of heteroplasmy between muscle cells. There may be increased numbers of mitochondria (pleoconial myopathy), increased size (megaconial myopathy), disoriented or rarefied cristae, or osmiophilic or paracrystalline inclusions on electron microscopy. The paracrystalline inclusions are deposits of mitochondrial CK. There may also be lipid or glycogen storage on muscle biopsy, signifying a defect of terminal oxidation. It should be noted that muscle histochemistry and/or electron microscopy may be normal even in the context of genetically proven mitochondrial syndromes, particularly early in the disease course or when the biochemical abnormality does not involve complex IV (COX).

Clinical Considerations

Mitochondrial diseases are clinically heterogeneous. There may be variation in the age at onset, course, and distribution of weakness in pure myopathies. On average, the age of onset reflects the level of mutation and the severity of the biochemical defects; however, other factors, including nuclear genetic and/or environmental factors, can also affect the expression of disease. Additional features may include exercise intolerance and premature fatigue. Mitochondria and mtDNA are ubiquitous, which explains why every tissue in the body can be affected by mtDNA mutations. The most common presenting clinical features include short stature, sensorineural hearing loss, migraine headaches, opthalmoparesis, myopathy, axonal neuropathy, diabetes mellitus, hypertrophic cardiomyopathy, and renal tubular acidosis. Additional features may include stroke-like episodes, seizures, myoclonus, retinitis pigmentosa, optic atrophy, ataxia, and gastrointestinal pseuoobstruction. In the case of mtDNA mutations, there may be a diverse spectrum of associated syndromes, even in a single pedigree, because of heteroplasmy and the threshold effect whereby different tissues harboring the same mtDNA mutation may be affected to different degrees or not at all. Furthermore, the same mutation can cause different syndromes (e.g., the T8993G mutation can cause either neuropathy, ataxia, retinitis pigmentosa [NARP] or maternally inherited Leigh syndrome [MILS]) and different mutations can cause the same phenotype (e.g., A3243G mutation, single deletion, and multiple deletions of the mtDNA can all cause progressive external ophthalmoplegia [PEO]). Thus the diagnosis of mtDNA-related disorders often requires a careful synthesis of the clinical history, signs, mode of inheritance, laboratory data, neuroradiological findings, exercise physiology, muscle biopsy, muscle biochemistry with measurement of respiratory chain enzyme activities in fresh or snap-frozen muscle samples, and molecular genetics.

Biochemical Classification

Mitochondrial encephalomyopathies can be classified into five groups according to the area of mitochondrial metabolism specifically affected: (1) defects of transport, (2) defects of substrate utilization, (3) defects of the Krebs cycle, (4) defects of the respiratory chain, and (5) defects of oxidation/phosphorylation coupling (Figure 149-3) (see Chapter 42). Limitations of this classification scheme relate to the respiratory chain defects that can result from genetic defects of mtDNA, which are usually heteroplasmic, and to deletions of mtDNA or point mutations in tRNA, which affect mtDNA translation as a whole and may lead to multiple respiratory chain defects and from genetic defects of nDNA.

Physiologic Considerations (see online version of this chapter for details)

Standard exercise physiology tests, such as cycle ergometers or treadmills, can be used to detect alterations of oxidative metabolism. Maximal oxygen uptake is the most useful indicator of a patient's capacity for oxidative metabolism. Typical physiologic responses in patients with defects in oxidative metabolism are as follows (Taivassalo et al., 2003):

1. The increase of cardiac output during exercise is greater than normal relative to the rate of oxidative metabolism.
2. Oxygen extraction per unit of blood remains almost unchanged from rest to maximal exercise.
3. Ventilation is normal at rest but increases excessively relative to oxygen uptake.
4. Venous lactate, which is usually elevated at rest, increases excessively relative to workload and oxygen uptake.

Genetic Classification (see Chapter 42)

Specific defects of mtDNA and nuclear DNA with myopathy as a feature are discussed in detail in the online version (Tables 149-6 and 149-7).

Therapeutic Approaches in Mitochondrial Diseases

Overall the therapy of mitochondrial respiratory chain disorders is highly inadequate, though there are currently multiple new emerging therapeutic strategies that may hold promise for the future. The therapeutic approaches have been comprehensively reviewed.

Palliative therapy: Palliative therapy includes anticonvulsants, treatment of endocrinopathies (e.g., thyroxine, insulin), adequate nutrition (enteral feeding via gastrostomy is frequently needed), pancreatic enzyme replacement, electrolyte replacement in patients with severe renal tubulopathy, renal dialysis and/or transplantation, hearing aids, blood transfusions for sideroblastic anemia, psychological support for patients and families, and surgical procedures, for example, cochlear implants for hearing loss, pacemakers for cardiac conduction blocks, surgery for cataracts and for ptosis, and liver and cardiac transplantation for related organ failure. Valproic acid should be avoided because it inhibits cellular carnitine uptake and mitochondrial OXPHOS. Valproic acid should be absolutely avoided in Alper's disease. Other medications to be used cautiously or to be preferentially avoided include statin medications, where there should be careful monitoring of symptoms and serum CK and antiretroviral agents, which are known to cause reversible and dose-dependent mitochondrial toxicity.

General anesthesia: General anesthesia may be needed in individuals with mitochondrial disorders and requires special perioperative, intraoperative, and postoperative care. It is important to maintain normothermia, normoglycemia, and normal electrolytes. Given the impairment in lactate metabolism, lactated Ringer's solution should be avoided. It has been suggested that volatile inhalational anesthetics and depolarizing muscle relaxants should be avoided and that some individuals fail to tolerate local anesthetics. A listing of anesthetic recommendations from different investigators is provided by Rivera-Cruz (2013).

Removal of noxious metabolites: Other strategies include removal of noxious metabolites, including lowering the lactic acidosis. Though dichloroacetate (DCA) lowers serum lactic acid, a double-blind, placebo-controlled, randomized, crossover trial of DCA in a cohort of MELAS patients with the A3243G mutation had to be terminated because of significant peripheral nerve toxicity. Therefore DCA should not be used long-term in mitochondrial patients prone to peripheral neuropathy. Attempts to bypass respiratory chain blocks through the administration of electron acceptors have been disappointing.

Cofactor and metabolite supplementation: Cofactor and metabolite supplementation has been the mainstay of therapy, particularly in disorders of primary deficiencies, for example, CoQ10 deficiency and primary carnitine deficiency caused by OCTN2 deficiency. Supplementation with oral CoQ10 (10 to 30 mg/kg/day in children and 1200 to 3000 mg/day in adults) has been effective in patients with *COQ2* mutations, especially for the neurologic and renal manifestations of this disorder. In contrast, poor responses to CoQ10 supplementation have been observed in patients with *PDSS2* and *COQ9* mutations.

Other agents used include riboflavin, thiamine, folic acid, and creatine. Antioxidants and reactive oxygen species scavengers are an area of increasing interest, particularly in complex I and III deficiencies. Agents used have included vitamin E, CoQ10, idebenone, and dihydrolipoate.

Aerobic endurance and resistance exercise and physical therapy: Aerobic endurance and resistance exercise and physical therapy help to prevent deconditioning and disuse muscle atrophy and have been shown to improve exercise tolerance in patients with mtDNA mutations through mitochondrial proliferation and gene shifting, respectively, as outlined in the online version.

In a recent Cochrane review of trials with vitamin, antioxidant, and nutrient supplements (CoQ10, lipoic acid, creatine, whey-based supplement, dimethylglycine), pharmacologic agents (dichloroacetate), and exercise therapy used in mitochondrial disorders, out of 1335 abstracts, only 12 studies fulfilled criteria for randomized controlled trials (including cross-over studies) (Pfeffer et al., 2012). It was concluded that, though there were some improvements in secondary outcome measures, there was no clear evidence supporting the use of any of these interventions in mitochondrial disorders. The ideal clinical trial should be adequately powered, statistically valid, and randomized, double-blinded, placebo-controlled and include a large group of homogenous patients in terms of clinical presentation, biochemical findings, and genetic defect, ideally at a similar stage of disease progression. However, this is very difficult for mitochondrial disorders because of the marked heterogeneity of diseases with different clinical manifestations and problems, the vast number of different genetic causes that may be individually rare, and the unpredictable course of the disease.

There are a number of emerging approaches that may hold future promise.

Antioxidants: The accumulation of reactive oxygen species (ROS) is generally accepted as a major cause of mitochondrial disease pathogenesis, leading to depletion of glutathione (GSH). Therapeutic strategies have included analogs of CoQ10. Though CoQ10 in high doses is of proven value in CoQ10 biosynthesis defects, its use in other mitochondrial disorders is less certain. Other analogs of interest include idebenone, which has reportedly better blood-brain barrier penetration. Another synthetic analog is EPI-743, which has had some potentially encouraging results in open-label studies in Leigh disease and other progressive mitochondrial disorders, but the unpredictable course of the disease makes the interpretation of results challenging. A summary of ongoing or recent completed clinical trials in mitochondrial disease is provided by Rahman. N-acetylcysteine combined with metronidazole has been suggested as beneficial in ethylmalonic encephalopathy arising from mutations in the *ETHE1* gene.

Stem cells: In mitochondrial neurogastrointestinal encephalomyopathy (MNGIE) syndrome, the loss of thymidine phosphorylase (TP) activity causes toxic accumulations of the nucleosides thymidine and deoxyuridine that are incorporated by the mitochondrial pyrimidine salvage pathway and cause deoxynucleoside triphosphate pool imbalances, which in turn cause mtDNA instability. Allogenic hematopoietic stem cell transplantation to restore TP activity and to eliminate the toxic metabolites is a promising therapy for MNGIE.

Mitochondrial biogenesis: Newer pharmacologic approaches have sought to upregulate mitochondrial biogenesis. Bezafibrate, a PPAR panagonist, has been used to activate mitochondrial proliferation enhancing oxidative phosphorylation capacity per muscle mass in a murine model of mitochondrial myopathy because of cytochrome c oxidase deficiency. Other pharmacologic agents that increase mitochondrial biogenesis and are under investigation include resveratrol, which activates the sirtuin SIRT1, which in turn is responsible for NAD+-dependent deacetylation of multiple proteins, including PGC1α and the mitochondrial transcription factor TFAM. Additional agents include 5-aminoimidazole-4-carboxamide ribonucleotide (AICAR), which is a pharmacologic activator of the adenosine monophosphate kinase (AMPK)-PGC1α axis, and nicotinamide riboside, which is able to stimulate mitochondrial biogenesis by increasing NAD+ availability, leading to NAD+-dependent activation of SIRT1.

Dietary approaches: Dietary approaches include the ketogenic diet as a potential treatment, particularly for the associated epilepsy, though evidence in patients remains anecdotal.

Future pharmacologic approaches: A comprehensive review of future pharmacologic approaches to restore mitochondrial function, including mitochondrial biogenesis, mitochondrial dynamics (fission and fusion), mitophagy, and the mitochondrial unfolded protein response, is given by Andreux et al. (2013). New and powerful phenotypic assays in cell-based models as well as multicellular organisms have been developed to explore these different aspects of mitochondrial function for the development of new drugs. Translating the emerging therapies to the bedside remains challenging because of the lack of large cohorts of clinically, biochemically, and genetically homogenous individuals; natural history data; and validated meaningful outcome measures for use in clinical trials. However, the recent development of national and international mitochondrial disease consortia and several large natural history studies will lay the groundwork for these trials.

Gene therapy: Gene therapy is a highly challenging area because of heteroplasmy and polyplasmy, but approaches have been developed to decrease the ratio of mutant to wild-type mitochondrial genomes (gene shifting), converting mutated mtDNA genes into normal nuclear DNA genes, and importing cognate genes from other species. Emerging approaches in gene therapy, currently largely experimental, include the use of restriction endonucleases with mitochondrial targeting sequences, zinc finger nucleases to selectively degrade mtDNA mutations, transcription activator–like effector (TALE) nuclease and CRISPR/Cas9 mutant gene editing, rescue by overexpression of aminoacyl tRNA synthetases, and gene therapy for nuclear-encoded mitochondrial disorders.

Germline therapy: Germline therapy raises ethics issues, but may be considered in the future for prevention of maternal transmission of mtDNA mutations. Preventive therapy through genetic counseling and prenatal diagnosis is important for nuclear DNA-related disorders.

MYOADENYLATE DEAMINASE DEFICIENCY
Clinical Presentation

Myoadenylate deaminase (mAMPD) deficiency is detected in 1% to 3% of all muscle biopsies and may be characterized by exercise-related myalgia and cramps. However, the pathogenetic significance of this defect is controversial because (1) in patients with unexplained myopathy, symptoms are generally mild, ill-defined, and often subjective, and (2) more than 50% of patients had either well-defined myopathies, such as Duchenne or Becker muscular dystrophy, McArdle's disease, spinal muscular atrophy, or amyotrophic lateral sclerosis. Therefore Fishbein divided mAMPD into the following two forms: (1) a primary (hereditary) mAMPD deficiency characterized by myopathy alone with exercise intolerance, myalgia, and cramps; very low residual activity (<1% of normal); and lack of cross-reacting material (CRM) in muscle, and (2) a secondary (acquired) mAMPD deficiency associated with well-defined myopathies or neuromuscular disorders in which there is a higher residual activity and detectable CRM. Isolated mAMPD deficiency may present with recurrent myoglobinuria.

Laboratory Tests

The resting serum CK level is usually normal but may increase after exercise. The forearm ischemic exercise test demonstrates a normal rise in venous lactate but no rise in ammonia or inosine monophosphate. The EMG may be normal or may demonstrate nonspecific myopathic features.

Pathology

Muscle biopsy is usually normal; however, decreased mAMPD activity can be detected by histochemical staining.

Biochemistry and Molecular Genetics

There are three tissue-specific subunits: M (muscle), L (liver), and E (erythrocyte), which are under separate genetic control. Adult human muscle contains almost exclusively the M homotetramer. AMPD converts AMP to inosine monophosphate (IMP) and ammonia.

Acknowledgments

Part of the work described here was supported by an operating grant from the Heart and Stroke Foundation of Ontario (NA 4964) and the physicians of Ontario through the Physicians' Services Incorporated Foundation.

REFERENCES

The complete list of references for this chapter is available in the e-book at www.expertconsult.com.
   See inside cover for registration details.

SELECTED REFERENCES

Andreux, P.A., Houtkooper, R.H., Auwerx, J., 2013. Pharmacological approaches to restore mitochondrial function. Nat Rev Drug Discov 12, 465–483.

DiMauro, S., Lamperti, C., 2001. Muscle glycogenosis. Muscle Nerve 24, 984–999.

Gollnick, P.D., Piehl, K., Saltin, B., 1974. Selective glycogen depletion pattern in human muscle fibres after exercise of varying intensity and at varying pedal rates. J Physiol 241, 45–57.

Hale, D.E., Bennett, M.J., 1992. Fatty acid oxidation disorders: a new class of metabolic diseases. J Pediatr 121, 1–11.

Pfeffer, G., Majamaa, K., Turnbull, D.M., et al., 2012. Treatment for mitochondrial disorders. Cochrane Database Syst Rev (4), CD004426.

Rivera-Cruz, B., 2013. Mitochondrial diseases and aesthesia: a literature review of current options. AANA J 81, 237–243.

Spiekerkoetter U., Lindner M., Santer R., et al., 2009. Management and outcome in 75 individuals with long-chain fatty acid oxidation defects: results from a workshop. J Inherit Metab Dis 32:488–497.

Taivassalo, T., Dysgaard Jensen, T., Kennaway, N., et al., 2003. The spectrum of exercise tolerance in mitochondrial myopathies: a study of 40 patients. Brain 126, 413–423.

Tein, I., DiMauro S., Rowland L.P., 1992. Myoglobinuria. In: Rowland, L.P., DiMauro, S. (Eds). Handbook of Clinical Neurology, Vol. 18(62): Myopathies. Elsevier Science Publishers B.V., Amsterdam, pp. 553–593.

Tonin, P., Lewis, P., Servidei, S., et al., 1990. Metabolic causes of myoglobinuria. Ann Neurol 27, 181–185.

⊗ E-BOOK FIGURES AND TABLES

150 Inflammatory Myopathies

Anthony A. Amato and John T. Kissel

 An expanded version of this chapter is available on www.expertconsult.com. See inside cover for registration details.

The inflammatory myopathies are a heterogeneous group of disorders characterized pathologically by inflammation in skeletal muscle, with resulting muscle fiber damage and subsequent clinical weakness. There are two major categories of inflammatory myopathy—idiopathic and infectious (Box 150-1). Although several types of muscular dystrophy may be associated with inflammation (e.g., facioscapulohumeral dystrophy and some of the limb-girdle dystrophies), these disorders traditionally are excluded from classification of inflammatory myopathy because they result from a fundamental genetic defect. The classic idiopathic inflammatory myopathies are usually considered to be autoimmune diseases, although a genetic predisposition may exist for many of these diseases based on inherited human leukocyte antigen haplotypes.

As a group, the inflammatory myopathies are the most common acquired myopathies of childhood (Rider et al., 2013; Shah et al., 2013). The infectious myositides are the most prevalent of these conditions worldwide, with acute viral myositis clearly the most common variety in North America and Europe. In contrast, the idiopathic varieties are relatively uncommon, with a combined incidence (including adult cases) of approximately 1 in 100,000. There are four major forms of idiopathic inflammatory myopathy—dermatomyositis, polymyositis, inclusion body myositis, and immune mediated necrotizing myopathy—with dermatomyositis by far the most common form in childhood (Amato and Griggs, 2003; Amato and Greenberg, 2013; Dalakas and Holfeld, 2013). Polymyositis is relatively uncommon in children and usually is seen as an overlap syndrome with other connective tissue disorders (CTD). Immune mediated necrotizing myopathy is a recently recognized entity usually seen in the setting of other connective tissue diseases or as a paraneoplastic syndrome. More commonly it is idiopathic in nature or associated with a CTD; it may be associated with antisignal recognition antibodies. In adults, it may be seen as a rare complication of statin medications and associated with autoantibodies directed against 3-hydroxy-3-methylglutaryl coenzyme A reductase (HMGCoAR). Inclusion body myositis is exclusively a disease of adulthood and therefore is not discussed here.

IDIOPATHIC INFLAMMATORY MYOPATHIES

Although clinicians often conceptualize the idiopathic inflammatory myopathies as a single entity (e.g., polymyositis is dermatomyositis without the rash), the disorders are clinically, histologically, and pathogenetically distinct. Banker and Victor first reported the unique vascular changes of juvenile dermatomyositis and highlighted the involvement of organs other than muscle and skin. Subsequent immunologic and pathologic observations confirmed distinct pathophysiologies for each of these disorders, and recent observations have solidified this view. Although there have been occasional reports of siblings or parent/child cases of both dermatomyositis and polymyositis, most cases are sporadic.

Dermatomyositis
Clinical Features

Juvenile dermatomyositis (JDM) can present at any age, including infancy, although most cases occur between ages 5 and 14 years. Females are affected more commonly than males. Onset of weakness is typically over weeks to a few months, although fatigue, muscle aches and stiffness, decreased activity, and fever can precede the onset of weakness by months. More acute, fulminate onset (over days) or an indolent, slowly progressive course (sometimes lasting a year) also has been described. Weakness typically affects the neck flexors along with shoulder and pelvic girdle muscles first, so that the child may have difficulty getting up from the floor, riding a bicycle, running, climbing steps, or raising the arms above the head. Distal weakness is usually present, although not as severe as in proximal muscles. Complete sparing of distal strength should always lead the clinician to suspect another diagnosis, particularly one of the dystrophies. Dysphagia occurs in approximately one-third of patients; also, individuals will rarely have chewing difficulties, dysarthria, and speech delay because of oropharyngeal involvement.

The rash frequently precedes the muscle symptoms and often provides the most important clue to diagnosis. Skin changes typically involve the fingers and periorbital regions first, although any area may be involved. A purplish discoloration of the eyelids (heliotrope rash) with periorbital edema and extension on to the cheeks and forehead is typical (Fig. 150-1). On the hands, the periungual regions become erythematous and scaly, with dilated capillary loops in the nail beds (Fig. 150-2). Papular, erythematous, scaly lesions over the knuckles (Gottron sign) are characteristic, with similar lesions occurring on the elbows, knees, and malleoli. A more macular, erythematous rash may appear on the face, neck, and anterior chest (V sign) or on the shoulders and upper back (shawl sign). Subcutaneous calcifications, which do not occur in adult cases, are present in 30% to 70% of childhood cases. The calcinosis tends to develop over pressure points (e.g., buttocks, knees, elbows) but can occur anywhere and develops more commonly when the diagnosis has been delayed or the treatment inadequate. The lesions typically appear as painful, hard nodules that erupt through the skin in severe cases. Occasional patients have the characteristic rash but never develop weakness, a condition sometimes referred to as dermatomyositis sine myositis or amyopathic dermatomyositis.

Associated Manifestations. Although involvement of organs other than muscle and skin has become less common with the advent of effective immunosuppressive therapies, some children will develop clinical manifestations, in addition to weakness and rash, on the basis of the underlying vasculopathy. About 50% will have electrocardiographic abnormalities, including conduction defects and dysrhythmias pericarditis, myocarditis, and congestive heart failure can occur. Pulmonary function tests may demonstrate restrictive defects and reduced

---

BOX 150-1 The Inflammatory Myopathies

I. IDIOPATHIC
A. Juvenile dermatomyositis
B. Polymyositis
C. Immune-mediated necrotizing myopathy
D. Inclusion body myositis
E. Myositis as overlap syndrome
    1. Mixed connective tissue disease
    2. Scleroderma
    3. Systemic lupus erythematosus
    4. Rheumatoid arthritis
    5. Sjögren syndrome
F. Other inflammatory myopathies
    1. Eosinophilic myositis
    2. Focal nodular myositis
    3. Sarcoid myopathy

II. INFECTIOUS
A. Viral myositides
    1. Influenza
    2. Human immunodeficiency virus
    3. Others (coxsackievirus, parainfluenza, mumps, measles, adenovirus, herpes simplex, cytomegalovirus, hepatitis B, Epstein-Barr virus, respiratory syncytial virus, echovirus, and possibly arboviruses)
B. Parasitic myositis
    1. Trichinosis
    2. Toxoplasmosis
    3. Cysticercosis
C. Bacterial myositis
D. Fungal myositis

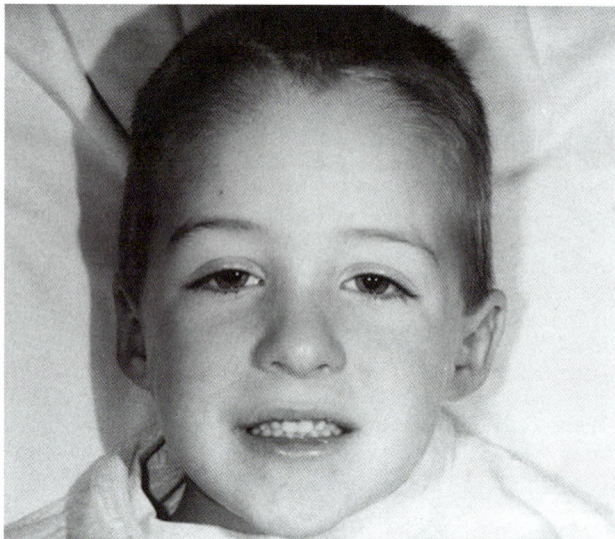

Figure 150-1. An 8-year-old male with juvenile dermatomyositis has a mild, erythematous rash over the cheeks, nasal bridge, and eyelids with mild periorbital edema. *(Courtesy of Albert Tsao, MD.)*

diffusion capacity, even in patients with no pulmonary symptoms. Approximately 10% of patients, particularly those with antibodies to histidyl transfer ribonucleic acid synthetase (Jo-1), develop frank interstitial lung disease or bronchiolitis obliterans and organizing pneumonia. Vasculopathic involvement of the gastrointestinal tract can result in malabsorption, mucosal ulceration, perforation, and hemorrhage. Dysphagia

and delayed gastric emptying, caused by inflammatory involvement of the alimentary skeletal and smooth muscles, are more common.

Arthralgias are common, but true arthritis occurs mainly in children with an "overlap" connective tissue disorder (see later in this chapter). Ophthalmic involvement on the basis of vascular changes in the retina and conjunctiva can occur. Renal compromise is rare and results from acute tubular necrosis in the setting of myoglobinuria after fulminant muscle necrosis. In contrast to adult dermatomyositis patients, children have demonstrated no definitive increased incidence of malignancy.

Laboratory Features

The laboratory evaluation of patients with inflammatory myopathy should include muscle enzyme analysis, electrodiagnostic studies, and muscle biopsy. Muscle imaging studies can indicate areas of inflammation in affected muscles but are seldom useful in making a diagnosis.

Blood Tests. Creatine kinase (CK) is the most reliable, sensitive, and specific marker for muscle destruction. The CK level is elevated in about 70% of patients sometime during the course of the disease, with levels up to 50 times normal. However, it is important to note that the CK level can be normal throughout the course of the disease and does not correlate consistently with weakness. Rarely, serum aldolase can be elevated when the serum CK is normal; serum myoglobin, lactate dehydrogenase, aspartate aminotransferase, and alanine aminotransferase can also be elevated but provide no additional information to the CK. Erythrocyte sedimentation rate is usually normal or mildly elevated and does not correlate with severity. Antinuclear antibodies occur in 25% to 50% of patients, most commonly in those with overlap syndromes.

Myositis-specific antibodies (MSA) may be present in both children and adults with myositis and are associated with specific clinical features, including providing some information about prognosis (Casciola-Rosen and Mammen, 2012; Ghiradello et al., 2013). The frequency of these antibodies differs between children and adults. For example, anti-p155/140 (TIF1-γ) and anti-NXP2 autoantibodies are more common in JDM than in adult DM, but unlike adult myositis, these antibodies are not associated with increased risk of cancer in JDM. The antisynthetase autoantibodies (i.e., anti-Jo-1), which are the most common MSA in adult myositis and associated with interstitial lung disease, are seen in less than 5% of patients with JDM.

Electromyography. Electromyography can serve to support a myopathic origin for the patient's weakness and to determine which muscle to biopsy in patients with mild weakness. However, in a child with classic rash, weakness, and an elevated CK level, electromyography is often not needed. Typical electromyographic features include increased spontaneous activity with fibrillation potentials, positive sharp waves, and, occasionally, pseudomyotonic and complex repetitive discharges, as well as small-duration, low-amplitude, polyphasic motor unit potentials, which recruit early but at normal frequencies. The amount of spontaneous activity generally reflects the ongoing disease activity.

Muscle Biopsy. Children suspected of having dermatomyositis should undergo a muscle or skin biopsy before therapy is instituted, if there is any question regarding the diagnosis. In those children with a clearly acquired disorder presenting with a classic rash, weakness, and elevated serum CK, a muscle biopsy may not be necessary.

The classic pathologic features associated with dermatomyositis include a microvasculopathy with capillary loss, perivascular and perimysial inflammation, perifascicular atrophy, and scattered areas of fibers with central areas of myofibrillar loss (Fig. 150-3). The most characteristic of these changes is perifascicular atrophy, which is present in approximately 50% of cases and is relatively specific for dermatomyositis. The inflammatory infiltrates are predominantly perimysial and perivascular, and are composed primarily of macrophages, B cells, and CD4 + cells (Fig. 150-4). One of the earliest demonstrable histologic abnormalities on light microscopy is deposition of C5b-9 complement membrane attack complex (MAC) on small blood vessels (as well as immunoglobulin M and other complement components, including C3 and C9) (Kissel et al., 1986). These immunohistochemical findings can be helpful in making a diagnosis, especially when other histologic findings are absent or equivocal. Electron microscopy typically reveals small intramuscular arterioles and capillaries with endothelial hyperplasia, microvacuoles, and cytoplasmic inclusions, but is seldom needed to make a diagnosis.

Pathogenesis (see online chapter)

Treatment. Although corticosteroids are generally regarded as the most effective therapy for dermatomyositis, there is disagreement surrounding the optimal route of administration, dosing regimen, duration of therapy, and parameters to monitor during therapy. There have been no controlled trials to examine these issues, although retrospective analyses and case series have demonstrated that prednisone reduces morbidity and improves strength and function.

Corticosteroids. Prednisone is the usual first line of treatment for dermatomyositis. Short courses of intravenous methylprednisolone (Solu-Medrol; 20 to 30 mg/kg/day or every other day for 3 to 5 days) may be the best way to initiate therapy in severely affected individuals, especially because this therapy may prevent calcinosis. After the intravenous pulses, most patients will require daily oral therapy as described later in this chapter. A more traditional starting regimen, especially for less severe cases, involves oral therapy (0.75 to 1.0 mg/kg/day), given as a single morning dose. After 3 to 6 weeks of daily prednisone, the dosage usually can sometimes be switched directly to an alternate-day regimen at the same dose, although most of the time we use daily prednisone. The high dose is maintained, and strength is carefully monitored. Although the CK level can sometimes be useful in monitoring response, it should never be the primary determinant of therapeutic decision making.

Patients should be evaluated at least monthly during this phase of treatment. When the child's strength has returned to normal or improvement has reached a plateau (usually within 4 to 6 months), the prednisone can be tapered at a rate no faster than 5 mg every 2 to 4 weeks. If an exacerbation occurs during the tapering, the prednisone dose is increased back to its original level and again given daily. When strength has recovered, the prednisone taper can be resumed. Although occasional patients will require daily dosing, or even split daily doses to maintain adequate disease control, alternate-day dosing is preferred because it is associated with fewer side effects. Most patients (approximately 80%) improve with therapy with approximately two-thirds having a complete response.

As most patients require therapy for 1 to 2 years to achieve remission, limiting the side effects of prednisone is an important part of management. Patients should be started on a low sodium, low carbohydrate, high protein, low calorie diet to limit weight gain and reduce the risk of hypertension. Calcium supplementation (1000 to 1500 mg/day) and vitamin D

reduce the risk of osteoporosis, as does physical therapy with axial exercise, as tolerated by the patient's weakness. Baseline determination of bone density through dual-energy x-ray absorptiometry scanning is indispensable in diagnosing and tracking osteoporosis in this population. Therapy with bisphosphonates should be considered in children who develop definite osteoporosis or in those expected to be on very long-term therapy. Exercise also reduces the risk of steroid myopathy. Blood pressure, serum glucose and potassium levels, and ocular status (for cataracts and glaucoma) should be assessed periodically. Hip pain in a child on prednisone must be investigated aggressively because avascular necrosis is an uncommon but devastating development in these individuals. Growth retardation and delayed puberty can occur with prolonged therapy.

Although the rash usually responds along with the muscle response, some patients occasionally require separate treatment for their skin changes. Hydroxychloroquine, chloroquine, topical steroids, topical tacrolimus, and sunscreen have been used to treat the rash when weakness is mild or not apparent. Treatment of calcinosis is more difficult. Colchicine, probenecid, warfarin, and phosphate buffers have been used with only limited success. Surgery may be indicated, but the lesions may recur or worsen despite surgery.

Other Agents. Patients who respond poorly to steroids, relapse repeatedly as prednisone is tapered, or develop intolerable side effects are candidates for alternative therapy (Table 150-1). Methotrexate is probably the drug of choice in children. In retrospective series, the majority of children refractory to prednisone improved with methotrexate therapy. In a series of 49 children with juvenile dermatomyositis initially treated aggressively with both pulsed corticosteroids and methotrexate, a prolonged, medication-free remission was attained in 28 of 49 within a median of 38 months from the time of diagnosis. Methotrexate must be used with caution because of side effects, including alopecia, stomatitis, oncogenicity, infection, interstitial lung disease, and bone marrow, renal, and liver toxicity. Pulmonary function tests, blood counts, and liver function tests must be monitored. Azathioprine, mycophenolate mofetil, cyclophosphamide, and cyclosporine have also been used in refractory patients (Table 150-1).

On the basis of a single double-blind, placebo-controlled study suggesting benefits in 15 adult dermatomyositis patients, intravenous immunoglobulin has become an important component of the treatment of dermatomyositis. Although originally used only for refractory cases, it is finding increasing use as both a steroid-sparing agent and a primary agent because of its effectiveness and low incidence of long-term side effects. Treatment is usually initiated at a dose of 2 g/kg given slowly over 2 to 5 days, with repeat infusions at 1 gm/kg at variable intervals (usually every 3 to 6 weeks) for at least 3 months. Flulike symptoms (i.e., headaches, myalgias, fever, chills, and nausea) may occur in as many as 50% of patients during the infusions but are usually mild. Rash, aseptic meningitis, transient leukopenia, renal failure, and stroke have been described rarely. A controlled trial of plasmapheresis and leukopheresis demonstrated no improvement with either modality in dermatomyositis.

Rituximab is a monoclonal antibody directed against CD20 and thus depletes B cells. A number of case reports and small series have suggested that rituximab maybe an effective therapy, but a large multicenter, double-blind, placebo-controlled trial in both adult and juvenile dermatomyositis and polymyositis failed to demonstrate efficacy (Oddis et al., 2013). However, there were flaws in the study design of this trial (e.g., crossover too early, lumping of adult and childhood polymyositis and dermatomyositis, and use of nonvalidated

TABLE 150-1 Steroid-Sparing Immunosuppressive Therapy for Inflammatory Myopathies

Agent	Route	Dose	Side Effects	Monitor
Methotrexate	PO	10–20 mg/m²/wk	Hepatotoxicity, leukopenia, alopecia, stomatitis, neoplasia	LFTs, CBC BUN, Cr
	IV	1–3 mg	Same	Same
Cyclophosphamide	PO	1–2 mg/kg/day	Leukopenia, cystitis, alopecia, infections, neoplasia	CBC, UA
	IV	50–75 mg/m²	Same, nausea and vomiting	Same
Cyclosporine	PO	0.5–7.5 mg/kg/day	Renal toxicity, hypertension, hirsutism, hepatotoxicity, infection, gum hyperplasia	BP, BUN, Cr, LFTs, drug levels
IVIG	IV	2 g/kg; may need to be repeated at dose of 1–2 g/kg/month for maintenance therapy	Fevers, chills, diaphoresis, aseptic meningitis, headache, hypotension, leukopenia	BP, BUN, Cr
Rituximab	IV	A course is typically 750 mg-meter squared (up to 1 gm) and repeated in 2 wks Courses are then repeated usually every 6-18 months	Infusion reactions (as per IVIG), infection, progressive multifocal leukoencephalopathy	Some check B-cell count before subsequent courses (but this may not be warranted)

BP, blood pressure; BUN, blood urea nitrogen; CBC, complete blood count; Cr, creatinine; IV, intravenous; IVIG, intravenous immunoglobulin; LFTs, liver function tests; PO, orally; UA, urinalysis.

outcome measures), and most experienced clinicians feel that rituximab is effective in at least some patients. Currently, this therapy probably should be reserved for only the most refractory cases. The dose is 750 mg/m² (up to 1 g), given once and then repeated in 2 weeks. The course of rituximab then is to be repeated every 6 to 18 months.

Polymyositis

Polymyositis, although common in adults, is relatively rare in children as an isolated entity. In one epidemiologic study, juvenile dermatomyositis was 10 to 20 times more common than polymyositis. When polymyositis does occur in children, it is usually in the setting of an "overlap" condition with features of another connective tissue disorder. Due to the absence of the rash, the diagnosis is often delayed compared with dermatomyositis.

Clinical Features

As with dermatomyositis, patients typically present after weeks to months of neck flexor as well as symmetric, proximal greater than distal, arm and leg weakness. Muscle pain and tenderness are common but not always present. Dysphagia occurs in approximately one-third of patients secondary to oropharyngeal and esophageal involvement. Mild facial weakness occasionally may be demonstrated. Sensation and tendon reflexes are usually preserved. As in adults, other organs, most notably the heart and lungs, can be involved, although the incidence appears to be lower in children than in adults. Congestive heart failure or conduction abnormalities and interstitial lung disease are found in rare patients, the latter more commonly in patients with serum anti-Jo-1 antibodies. Polyarthritis has been reported in as many as 45% of polymyositis patients at the time of diagnosis.

Overlap Syndromes. In children, polymyositis occurs as part of an overlap syndrome, in which the myositis is associated with another connective tissue disorder, more frequently than as an isolated entity. The common overlap syndromes that are associated with polymyositis (and often dermatomyositis) include scleroderma, mixed connective tissue disease, Sjögren syndrome, systemic lupus erythematosus, polyarteritis nodosa, and rheumatoid arthritis. Involvement of the skin, joints,

kidneys, eyes, and salivary glands is identical to that seen for each disorder in isolation (Fig. 150-5), and the serologic abnormalities are also similar. Weakness in these patients is not always due to myositis because disuse and type 2 fiber atrophy caused by chronic steroid treatment of the underlying condition can also result in muscle weakness. In these individuals, it is crucial to document the nature of the muscle involvement with serologic and electromyographic studies and often muscle biopsy. The prognosis is often related to the underlying disorder, and treatment may have to be modified based on the associated condition.

Laboratory Features

Laboratory evaluation in polymyositis is similar to that in dermatomyositis. Unlike dermatomyositis, the serum CK is essentially always elevated in polymyositis. The serum CK level can be helpful in monitoring response to therapy but only in conjunction with the physical examination. Positive antinuclear antibodies are present in approximately 30%. Muscle-specific antibodies have been reported in polymyositis as in dermatomyositis, as discussed previously. Close analysis of these reports, however, indicates that the muscle histopathology in many of the antibody-positive cases does not demonstrate invasion of nonnecrotic muscle fibers by CD8+ T lymphocytes, which some consider necessary to diagnosis polymyositis. Electromyography is similar to that in dermatomyositis, with a myopathic picture of increased spontaneous activity, small polyphasic motor units, and early recruitment.

Muscle Biopsy. The pathologic findings of polymyositis are distinct from dermatomyositis and reflect basic differences in the underlying pathophysiology. Biopsies are characterized by variability in fiber size, with scattered necrotic and regenerating fibers, and endomysial inflammation, with invasion of nonnecrotic muscle fibers by CD8+ cytotoxic/suppressor T cells and macrophages (Fig. 150-6). The invaded (and some- times noninvaded) fibers express major histocompatibility complex class 1 antigen, which is not present on normal fibers. The vascular changes of dermatomyositis are not seen. Although B lymphocytes are not common, oligoclonal plasma cells have been identified in the endomysium in polymyositis. Unlike in dermatomyositis, in which there are many plasmacytoid dendritic cells that produce interferons, polymyositis muscle biopsies have many endomysial myeloid dendritic cells that probably function as antigen-presenting cells.

✪ Pathogenesis (see online chapter)

Treatment. The treatment of children with polymyositis does not differ in any substantive way from that of dermatomyositis. Corticosteroids are the mainstay of treatment, with secondary agents used as indicated by the response. The role of intravenous immunoglobulin in polymyositis is less clear than in dermatomyositis and should probably be reserved for refractory cases. Treatment of patients with an overlap syndrome is occasionally dictated more by the degree of joint, kidney, or skin involvement than by the muscle disease. Although the majority of patients with polymyositis respond to therapy, the response is often less robust and less sustained than in dermatomyositis. Fewer patients (approximately 20%) attain a complete remission, so that more long-term therapy, along with its associated side effects from medications, is frequently required. Unfortunately, no prospective studies have examined in detail the long-term prognosis of these patients.

Congenital Inflammatory Myopathy

Over the past three decades, there have been scattered reports of infants with "congenital inflammatory myopathy" or "infantile myositis." The disorder is characterized by perinatal hypotonia and generalized weakness with elevated serum CK levels, myopathic electromyography, and striking inflammation on muscle biopsy. In one case of well-documented congenital myositis, the child was later diagnosed as having Prader-Willi syndrome. Most of the other patients did not improve with corticosteroid therapy, and it is likely that many of these cases had a form of muscular dystrophy with secondary inflammation. Inflammation on biopsy is not specific for a primary inflammatory myopathy and can be demonstrated in Duchenne, facioscapulohumeral, in some limb-girdle muscular dystrophies and Fukuyama-type muscular dystrophies, in Walker-Warburg syndrome, and in the Occidental type of congenital dystrophy with hypomyelination and laminin alpha-2 deficiency.

Other Idiopathic Inflammatory Myopathies

Several other extremely rare inflammatory myositides have been described in children. Eosinophilic myositis has been described in several children with peripheral eosinophilia and focal eosinophilic infiltration in isolated muscles. However, several reports suggest that many of these cases may actually be calpainopathy (i.e., limb-girdle muscular dystrophy type 2B. Thus diagnoses of polymyositis or eosinophilic myositis should be made with extreme caution in children and then only after the various dystrophies have been carefully considered.

Focal nodular myositis, as the name implies, is also a focal disorder associated with mononuclear infiltration in individual muscles, causing the subacute onset of focal pain, swelling, and weakness. Some patients go on to develop generalized polymyositis. Improvement has been reported after surgical excision of the mass but can also occur spontaneously. A myositis with noncaseating granulomas can occur in sarcoid myopathy, a condition that may respond partially to prednisone.

INFLAMMATORY MYOPATHY ASSOCIATED WITH INFECTIONS

Although myositis can occur after a wide variety of bacterial, parasitic, fungal, or viral infections, the viral myositides

(especially those caused by influenza), toxoplasmosis, and trichinosis are the disorders most likely to be encountered by the clinician.

Influenza Myositis

Influenza A, B, and, rarely, C are common upper respiratory tract pathogens. Acute infection usually is associated with myalgias when fever and other constitutional symptoms are present. The myalgias presumably are caused by the systemic release of cytokines, although a true myositis can develop.

Clinical Features

As respiratory symptoms subside, pain, swelling, and muscle tenderness herald the onset of myositis. The pain can be so severe as to interfere with the child's ability to walk or perform routine activities, and muscle swelling and induration may be present. Weakness can be profound and myoglobinuria has been reported. Lasting less than 1 week, the symptoms are self-limited, although rare patients have recurrent symptoms associated with different influenza types.

Laboratory Features

The CK level is usually elevated, often markedly so, whereas it is typically normal in uncomplicated influenza infection. Electromyography reveals features of an active necrotizing myopathy. Muscle biopsy is rarely indicated but indicates scattered necrotic and regenerating fibers, with occasional interstitial inflammatory cells. Influenza virus has been isolated only occasionally on culture of the muscle specimen.

Pathogenesis (see online chapter) ✪

Treatment. The disorder is usually self-limited, and treatment is supportive, with bed rest, hydration, and acetaminophen or nonsteroidal antiinflammatory drugs.

Other Viral Myositides

Acute viral myositis is not specific for influenza infection, and similar syndromes can complicate infections with coxsackievirus, parainfluenza, mumps, measles, adenovirus, herpes simplex, cytomegalovirus, hepatitis B, Epstein-Barr virus, respiratory syncytial virus, echovirus, and, possibly, arboviruses. Similar to influenza, the myositis associated with these viruses is usually self-limited and requires only supportive therapy. Acute and convalescent viral titers (3 or 4 weeks after infection), as well as blood, stool, urine, and throat cultures, can be useful in identifying the responsible virus but seldom add to the management of the muscle symptoms.

An inflammatory myopathy has also been described with infection by human immunodeficiency virus (HIV). This disorder usually develops in patients with acquired immune deficiency syndrome but also can occur in early HIV infection. It has been reported exclusively in adults, although HIV-infected children also are at risk. The presentation is similar to that of polymyositis, with subacute progressive, symmetric proximal weakness, an elevated CK level, and myopathic electromyography. The disorder must be distinguished from zidovudine (AZT) myotoxicity, HIV wasting syndrome, and other disorders that can complicate HIV infection.

Trichinosis

Trichinosis, the most common parasitic disease of skeletal muscle, is caused by the nematode Trichinella spiralis, which is ingested in inadequately cooked meat (usually pork). Most infected patients are asymptomatic.

Clinical Features

Between 2 and 12 days after ingestion, the larval form of the nematode disseminates through the bloodstream and invades the muscles. Patients develop fever, headache, abdominal pain, diarrhea, generalized myalgias, and weakness during the acute systemic reaction. Periorbital edema, ptosis, subconjunctival hemorrhage, and an erythematous urticarial or petechial rash also are often present. Myalgias and weakness peak in the third week of the infection but can last for months. Severe disease can be complicated by myocarditis, pneumonitis, and central nervous system infection.

Laboratory Features

Most patients have a marked eosinophilic leukocytosis and elevated serum creatine kinase level. Serum antibodies against T. spiralis can be demonstrated 3 to 4 weeks after infection. Electromyography demonstrates the typical features of an inflammatory myopathy. In the early stage of infection, muscle biopsy reveals infiltration of the muscle by eosinophils and polymorphonuclear leukocytes. With more chronic infection, mononuclear inflammatory cells are more common. Larvae, cysts with focal calcification, fibrosis, and granulomas may be observed months after the initial infection (Fig. 150-7).

Treatment

Thiabendazole (25 mg/kg twice daily to a maximum dose of 3 g/day) is the drug of choice for killing the larvae and adult nematode, with 7 days usually an adequate course of therapy. Thiabendazole is not effective against the encysted larvae, and mebendazole may be a better agent in this regard. As a Herxheimer-like reaction can develop after degeneration of the larvae, concurrent prednisone administration is beneficial (2 mg/kg/day for several weeks). The majority of patients respond quickly to treatment.

Toxoplasmosis

Toxoplasmosis is caused by the protozoon Toxoplasma gondii. The common mode of infection is through the ingestion of food, usually undercooked meat, contaminated with oocysts or cysts containing bradyzoites of the organism. The cysts mature and enter the bloodstream and lymphatics to invade other organs. Exposure to the organism is common worldwide, although symptomatic infection usually occurs in immunocompromised patients. Skeletal muscle involvement can occur in isolation or as part of more generalized infection.

Clinical and Laboratory Features

In most patients, symptoms are mild and nonspecific; they include fever, malaise, fatigue, and myalgias. Patients with more severe disease have lymphadenopathy, hepatosplenomegaly, uveitis, pneumonia, myocarditis, rash, or meningoencephalopathy. Weakness develops in those with significant muscle involvement. The serum creatine kinase level is elevated, and the typical myopathic picture is evident on electromyography. Muscle biopsy may reveal cysts containing the organism, along with inflammation and giant cells. The diagnosis is confirmed through serologic studies indicating immunoglobulin M reactivity to the organism.

Treatment

A combination of pyrimethamine and sulfadiazine or trisulfapyrimidines is the treatment of choice for the primary infection, although, once the organisms have become encysted in muscle, no medication is effective. Clindamycin also is an effective agent and can be used in place of sulfadiazine. The duration of therapy is variable and depends on the severity of the illness.

Cysticercosis

Cysticercosis is caused by the tapeworm Taenia solium, another organism usually transmitted through eating undercooked meat. Although central nervous system infection usually dominates the clinical picture, with focal neurologic deficits, seizures, and encephalopathy, skeletal muscles also can be involved. Weakness, myalgias, muscle tenderness, and muscle pseudohypertrophy are accompanied by an elevated creatine kinase level and eosinophilia. The biopsy is characterized by fibrosis, inflammation with eosinophils, giant cells, and encysted organisms. Praziquantel (50 mg/kg/day in three divided doses for 2 weeks) is effective against central nervous system infection, but its efficacy in muscle is less clear. Albendazole (15 mg/kg/day in divided doses for 8 days) also has been used. Niclosamide and paromomycin are useful for treating the adult worms, and corticosteroids suppress the inflammatory reaction against degenerating parasites.

Bacterial Infections

Pyomyositis refers to the multifocal abscesses associated with bacterial infection of the muscle. Although bacterial infections are more common in developing countries, they are being seen with increasing frequency in developed countries as a result of HIV infection and intravenous drug abuse.

Muscle pain, tenderness, and fever are the initial symptoms, most commonly affecting the quadriceps, glutei, and deltoids. Most patients have a neutrophilic pleocytosis, elevated erythrocyte sedimentation rate, and normal or elevated serum creatine kinase level. Blood cultures are usually negative early in the infection until the patient becomes septic. Ultrasound, computed tomography, and magnetic resonance imaging of muscle can be useful in localizing abscesses for diagnostic needle aspiration. The most common organisms are Staphylococcus aureus, streptococci, Escherichia coli, Yersinia organisms, and Legionella organisms. Pyomyositis usually arises as an extension of infection from adjacent tissues or via hematologic spread of the organisms. Early in the illness, the infection may respond to appropriate antibiotics, although more severe infections require incision and drainage.

Fungal Myositides

Fungal infection of the muscles is very uncommon and usually occurs in an immunosuppressed adult patient. Candidiasis is the most common fungal myositis and almost always is associated with disseminated disease. Diffuse muscle pain, tenderness, weakness, fever, and a papular erythematous rash are evident but may be obscured by other systemic involvement. Muscle biopsy demonstrates infiltration of the muscle by hyphal and yeast forms of the organism, inflammation, and hemorrhagic necrosis. Myositis also has been reported as complicating cryptococcal infection, sporotrichosis, actinomycosis, and histoplasmosis.

REFERENCES

The complete list of references for this chapter is available online at www.expertconsult.com.
    See inside cover for registration details.

SELECTED REFERENCES

Amato, A.A., Barohn, R.J., 2009. Evaluation and treatment of inflammatory myopathies. J. Neurol. Neurosurg. Psychiatry 80, 1060.

Amato, A.A., Greenberg, S.A., 2013. Inflammatory myopathies. Continuum (Minneap Minn) 19 (6 Muscle Disease), 1615–1633.

Amato, A.A., Griggs, R.C., 2003. Inflammatory myopathies. Curr. Opin. Neurol. 16, 569.

Casciola-Rosen, L., Mammen, A.L., 2012. Myositis autoantibodies. Curr. Opin. Rheumatol. 24, 602–608.

Dalakas, M.C., Hohlfeld, R., 2003. Polymyositis and dermatomyositis. Lancet 362, 971.

Ghirardello, A., Bassi, N., Palma, L., et al., 2013. Autoantibodies in polymyositis and dermatomyositis. Curr. Rheumatol. Rep. 15, 335.

Kissel, J.T., Mendell, J.R., Rammohan, K.W., 1986. Microvascular deposition of complement membrane attack complex in dermatomyositis. N. Engl. J. Med. 314, 331.

Oddis, C.V., Reed, A.M., Aggarwal, R., et al., 2013. Rituximab in the treatment of refractory adult and juvenile dermatomyositis and adult polymyositis: a randomized, placebo-phase trial. Arthritis Rheum. 65, 314–324.

Rider, L.G., Katz, J.D., Jones, O.Y., 2013. Developments in the classification and treatment of the juvenile idiopathic inflammatory myopathies. Rheum. Dis. Clin. North Am. 39, 877–904.

Shah, M., Targoff, I.N., Rice, M.M., et al., 2013. The clinical phenotypes of the juvenile idiopathic inflammatory myopathies. Medicine (Baltimore) 92, 25–41.

E-BOOK FIGURES AND TABLES

The following figures and tables are available in the e-book at www.expertconsult.com. See inside cover for registration details.

Fig. 150-2 Close-up view of the fingers of a 17-year-old female with juvenile dermatomyositis.

Fig. 150-3 Biceps biopsy from a patient with dermatomyositis, showing characteristic perifascicular atrophy with relative sparing of the central fascicle.

Fig. 150-4 Muscle biopsy from a patient with juvenile dermatomyositis, showing a striking focus of perivascular inflammation in a perimysial blood vessel.

Fig. 150-5 Scleroderma/dermatomyositis overlap syndrome in a 16-year-old male.

Fig. 150-6 Muscle biopsy from a patient with polymyositis, revealing endomysial inflammation surrounding and occasionally invading (top right) individual nonnecrotic muscle fibers.

Fig. 150-7 Muscle biopsy from a patient with trichinosis, documenting encysted larvae of the Trichinella organism.

151 Channelopathies: Myotonic Disorders and Periodic Paralysis

Richard T. Moxley III and Chad Heatwole

The term *channelopathies* extends to include disorders affecting all organ systems. This chapter focuses on channelopathies of skeletal muscle. It includes a number of diseases associated with mutations in the genes for specific skeletal muscle channels for chloride, sodium, calcium, and potassium ions. (Jurkat-Rott et al., 2015; Statland and Barohn, 2013; Suetterlin, Mannikko, and Hanna, 2014; Heatwole, Statland, and Logigian, 2013; Matthews et al., 2010; Cannon, 2002)

THE MYOTONIC DYSTROPHIES
Mode of Inheritance of Myotonic Dystrophy Types 1 and 2

Myotonic dystrophy types 1 and 2 (DM1 and DM2) are autosomal dominant. Anticipation (earlier onset of more severe symptoms in successive generations) occurs primarily in DM1 (see Figure 151-1) (Kamsteeg et al., 2012; Moxley, Ciafaloni, and Guntrum, 2015). Congenital myotonic dystrophy (CDM) occurs almost exclusively through maternal transmission (see Figure 151-1). DM2 occurs neither in infancy nor childhood, although teenage onset of myotonic symptoms can occur in some DM2 patients carrying concomitant mutations in the gene for the skeletal muscle chloride channel.

Myotonic Dystrophy Type 1
Clinical Features

DM1 is a multisystem, highly variable muscle disease with an incidence of 1 in 8000 individuals (see Table 151-1) (Udd and Krahe, 2012; Moxley et al., 2015). In childhood DM1 presents as a severe early congenital form or as a milder form with symptoms occurring after infancy throughout childhood years. The congenital form presents at birth with respiratory failure, poor feeding, generalized hypotonia, clubfoot deformity, and an increased risk of intracerebral hemorrhage and eventration of the diaphragm (Moxley et al., 2015). During gestation there are often reduced fetal movements and a history of polyhydramnios. There is an increased frequency of placenta previa and miscarriage, and not uncommonly a failed labor may require urgent cesarean section. During the perinatal period, infants with congenital myotonic dystrophy may require continuous ventilator support, and those remaining ventilator dependent beyond 4 weeks of age have a poor prognosis for survival, although recent advances in neonatal intensive care have allowed many affected infants to survive with subsequent slow improvement in function throughout childhood and the teen years (Moxley et al., 2015) (see Figure 151-1). During the first 2 years of life, children with congenital myotonic dystrophy are at increased risk for aspiration pneumonitis and difficulties with feeding. Mental retardation and learning disabilities are common in congenital myotonic dystrophy. Determining the degree of cognitive deficit requires careful evaluation because these patients have marked facial weakness and are unable to speak and communicate well until middle to late childhood. There is also an increased incidence of hearing loss. These problems often complicate neuropsychologic testing. The bottom panel of Figure 151-1 shows a mother with two daughters, both of whom have congenital myotonic dystrophy. Both children had delayed ability to speak and cognitive impairment. Their mother has mild ptosis, minimal grip myotonia, and minimal distal weakness. The figure legend provides follow-up information on the clinical course of all three over the subsequent 15 years (Moxley et al., 2015). The top left panel of Figure 151-1 shows another mother with classical DM1 and her infant with congenital DM1 who is not longer ventilator dependent. Figure 151-1 emphasizes the phenomenon of anticipation and the fact that almost all DM1 patients with the severe newborn onset of congenital DM1 are born to females with DM1.

The later childhood-onset form of DM1 usually is evident from nonmuscular manifestations of the disease, such as intellectual deficiency, difficulty with speech or hearing, clumsiness, or, rarely, with a cardiac dysrhythmia or postoperative apnea. DM1 patients may have an increased sensitivity to sedative medications, especially barbiturates and opiates, and occasionally experience increased muscle stiffness, myotonia during general anesthesia (Moxley et al., 2015). Cardiac arrhythmias are more common complications for the adult-onset forms of DM1. However, other nonmuscular manifestations, such as gastrointestinal hypomotility with chronic constipation, and intermittent urinary tract symptoms, such as urgency or frequent urination, are common in childhood myotonic dystrophy (Moxley et al., 2015).

Myotonic Dystrophy Type 2 (Formerly Proximal Myotonic Myopathy)
Clinical Features

DM2, proximal myotonic myopathy (PROMM) typically appears in adult life and has variable manifestations, such as early-onset cataracts (younger than 50 years), varying grip myotonia, thigh muscle stiffness, muscle pain, and weakness (hip flexors, hip extensors, abdominal muscles, or long flexors of the fingers) (Udd and Krahe, 2012). Symptoms often appear between 20 and 70 years of age, and patients and their care providers ascribe them to overuse of muscles, "pinched nerves," "sciatica," arthritis, fibromyalgia, or statin use. Younger patients may complain of stiffness or weakness when running up steps. In general, DM2 muscle pain has no consistent relationship to exercise or to the severity of myotonia found on clinical examination. The pain, which tends to come and go without obvious cause, usually fluctuates in intensity and distribution over the limbs. It can last for days to weeks. This pain seems qualitatively different from the muscle and musculoskeletal pain that occurs in patients with DM1.

TABLE 151-1 Myotonias Attributable to Unstable Nucleotide Repeat Expansion

Clinical Features	Myotonic Dystrophy of Steinert (Myotonic Dystrophy Type 1; DM1)	Myotonic Dystrophy Type 2 (Proximal Myotonic Dystrophy; DM2)
Inheritance	Dominant	Dominant
Gene defect	Chromosome 19q33, 3' untranslated region; CTG expansion affecting a protein kinase (DMPK); repeat size ranges from 50 to > 2000; normal 5–37 repeats	Chromosome 3q21.3, intron 1; CCTG expansion affecting the CNP (previously zinc finger 9 protein) gene; repeat sizes vary from 75 > 11,000; normal < 75 repeats
Age of onset	Broad range of ages (infancy to adulthood), with infant onset in most severe cases; approximately 10% begin in childhood	Broad range of ages (late childhood to late adulthood)
Myopathy	Face, eyes, forearm, hands, and legs, with generalized weakness and hypotonia in affected infants	Mild; thighs, hips, neck flexors, abdominal muscles; occasional calf muscle hypertrophy
Myotonia	Primarily affects hand and forearm muscles and tongue; often absent on clinical testing in infants and young children; occasionally affects respiratory muscles and smooth muscle, such as intestine or uterus; myotonia improves with heat and exercise; myotonia results from a decrease in chloride channel protein	Mainly in hands and thighs; varies; frequently hard paraspinal muscles detect; pain occurs sometimes with and without myotonia; myotonia improves with repeated contractions; myotonia results from a decrease in chloride protein
Provocative stimuli	Myotonia worsened by rest and cold; myotonia is relatively constant in severity and muscles affected once it develops	Myotonia worsened by rest but varies in severity, occasionally being absent on clinical examination; hand grip and thigh stiffness are usual sites
Therapy for symptoms	Bracing; cataract removal; monitoring dysrhythmias and respiratory insufficiency; pacemaker; antimyotonia therapy (mexiletine); avoid depolarizing muscle relaxants, opiates, and barbiturates with surgery	Cataract removal; occasional need for pacemaker; antimyotonia therapy often not necessary (mexiletine); monitor carefully during and after surgery for muscle rigidity and rhabdomyolysis

Early in the presentation of DM2 there is only mild weakness of hip extension, thigh flexion, and finger flexion. Myotonia of grip and thigh muscle stiffness vary from minimal to moderate severity over days to weeks. Direct percussion of forearm extensor and thenar muscles is the most sensitive clinical test for myotonia in DM2 but may be absent. Myotonia of grip is sometimes prominent and often has a jerky quality that seems to differ from that in DM1 and the nondystrophic myotonias. Myotonia is often less apparent in DM2 compared with patients with DM1. In cases of late-onset DM2, myotonia may only appear on electromyographic testing after examination of several muscles. Facial weakness is mild in DM2, as is muscle wasting in the face and limbs. Weakness of neck flexors is frequent. Trouble arising from a squat is common, especially as the disease progresses. Calf muscle hypertrophy occasionally is prominent. Other manifestations, such as excessive sweating, hypogonadism, glucose intolerance, dysphagia, cardiac conduction disturbances, and cognitive/neuropsychologic alterations may also occur and worsen over time. A higher rate of premature labor and preterm deliveries has also been reported. In contrast to DM1, respiratory insufficiency or failure and cardiac conduction disturbances are less common in DM2. Difficulty swallowing, gastrointestinal dysfunction, and cognitive disturbances do occur in DM2, but they appear to be less frequent.

At present there is no clear evidence of a congenital form of DM2 (Moxley et al., 2015). When symptoms occur in childhood, they typically are transient and relate to grip myotonia in the hands and thighs (Moxley et al., 2015). Proximal weakness, muscle pain, cataracts, and occasional cardiac dysrhythmias usually do not develop until mid or late adult life.

DM1 and DM2: Genotype–Phenotype Correlations

In general, the greater the length of the abnormal CTG expansion in circulating leukocytes, the more severe are the disease manifestations and the earlier is the onset (Moxley et al., 2015). There are important exceptions to this generalization. In DM2 there is no clear relationship between disease onset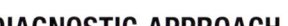

and severity and the length of the abnormal CCTG repeat in circulating leukocytes (Udd and Krahe, 2012). See the online chapter for a more detailed and helpful explanation of genotype–phenotype correlations.

DIAGNOSTIC APPROACH

The major problem in making the diagnosis of DM1 and DM2 is the tendency of clinicians to ignore these entities in their practice. DM1 can present as a floppy infant or as child with delayed motor and cognitive development (Figures 151-3 and 151-4 show the workup of an infant with congenital DM1 and the workup of a child suspected to have childhood DM1, respectively). There are long lists indicating more common causes for these presentations in infants and in childhood than DM1. If there is a low diagnostic suspicion of DM1, the clinician may not probe the family history sufficiently and may not examine the parents of the patient using a focused approach to search for characteristic features of DM1 (Tables 151-1 and 151-2). The failure to consider DM1 is the principal contributor to the diagnostic odyssey and delays DNA testing, family counseling, and appropriate management and treatment (Moxley et al., 2015).

DM1 and DM2 present primarily in adult life. The core clinical features and the multisystem manifestations can occur in isolation or combination and usually develop gradually (Moxley et al., 2015). Muscle stiffness, muscle pain, intermittent trouble with clear speech and swallowing, dropping of items, gait instability, and trouble seeing are frequent initial symptoms (Udd and Krahe, 2012). Early-onset cataracts (typically, iridescent posterior capsular cataracts) and cardiac arrhythmias are examples of multisystem manifestations that can occur early in DM1 and DM2. In contrast, patients with other hereditary myotonic disorders, such as chloride or sodium channel myotonias, do not have cardiac arrhythmias or posterior capsular cataracts. DM1 patients occasionally present with prolonged apnea or delayed-onset apnea following general anesthesia. These complications can occur in individuals with only mild clinical signs of DM1. The risk of complications after general anesthesia in DM2 patients appears to be low, but until more long-term data are available, it is prudent to monitor both DM2 and DM1 patients closely during and 24 hours or more following general anesthesia (Moxley et al., 2015).

The current gold standard to establish the diagnosis is DNA testing to identify the abnormally expanded CTG repeat in the *DMPK* gene for DM1 and the abnormally expanded CCTG repeat in the *CNBP* gene for DM2 (Kamsteeg et al., 2012; Udd and Krahe, 2012). If a patient suspected of having DM1 or DM2 has negative DNA testing, performance of a muscle biopsy may help establish the diagnosis of another myotonic disorder. However, if the muscle biopsy findings are typical for DM1 (increased central nuclei, atrophy of type-1 fibers, ringed fibers, subsarcolemmal masses) or DM2 (very small fibers, type-2 nuclear clumps, type-2 fiber atrophy), further genetic analysis, including bidirectional triplet-primed polymerase chain reaction (TP-PCR), may provide evidence of a mutation variant (Kamsteeg et al., 2012).

The diagnosis of congenital or childhood DM1 usually involves DNA testing for abnormal CTG repeat enlargement in the *DMPK* gene and usually prompts additional DNA testing of family members. Immediate counseling of the family is necessary to provide an understanding of current management of DM1 at its different stages. Parents need to know that preventive therapy and in vitro fertilization are available, along with the important supportive and symptomatic treatments (Table 151-2).

LABORATORY TESTING FOR DM1 AND DM2
DM1 Testing

Identifying the abnormally expanded CTG repeat in the *DMPK* gene isolated from circulating leukocytes establishes the diagnosis of DM1. Electromyography to detect myotonia is helpful in older children, but myotonia may be absent in infancy and early childhood. Slit-lamp examination is helpful in older children to identify the typical iridescent spokelike posterior capsular cataracts that develop early in the disease. Muscle biopsy is not necessary to diagnose DM1. Careful examination of the mothers of patients with congenital DM1 may reveal clinical signs of the disease. Creatine kinase levels are often normal or only mildly elevated in children and adults with DM1, whereas gamma glutamyltransferase levels are often high normal to significantly elevated, two- or three-fold over the upper limit of normal.

DM2 Testing

Leukocyte DNA testing is also available for DM2 (Kamsteeg et al., 2012). Slit-lamp examination to detect early cataract formation and electromyography, especially of the first dorsal interosseous, anterior tibialis, and anterior thigh muscles, are useful. Grip myotonia varies in severity and may be absent. Some patients have an elevation (twofold to eightfold) in creatine kinase and gamma glutamyltransferase levels. Muscle biopsy in DM1 and DM2 is rarely necessary for diagnosis.

TREATMENT OF DM1 AND DM2
DM1 Treatment

Table 151-2 summarizes treatment of the typical multisystem problems that occur in congenital and childhood-onset DM1. Treating patients with congenital myotonic dystrophy involves ventilatory support, use of a feeding tube, bracing for clubfoot deformities when present, and occasional corrective surgery

for foot deformities (Moxley et al., 2015). Speech problems and abdominal pain may improve with antimyotonia treatment. Mexiletine is sometimes helpful in alleviating some of the symptoms, especially in later childhood or adolescence when patients may have recurrent dislocation of the mandible and pain and muscle spasm in the masseter muscles. Electrocardiographic monitoring is necessary on a regular basis, particularly during treatment with mexiletine, to search for covert dysrhythmias. Treatment should be coordinated with the child's school to ensure that cognitive deficiencies and hearing deficits are monitored. The increased risk for cardiac dysrhythmia and apnea after administration of general anesthesia for surgery requires overnight hospitalization with monitoring. Apnea can develop several hours after a patient has been extubated. No specific limitation on physical activity is necessary during childhood provided the child has gained sufficient strength and coordination to carry out activities requested in the school environment.

DM2 Treatment

In general, the management of DM2 is similar to that of DM1, but there is less need for supportive care, such as bracing, scooters, or wheelchairs (Moxley et al., 2015). Cataracts require monitoring, and serial monitoring with an electrocardiogram (ECG) is necessary to check for covert dysrhythmia. Disturbances in cardiac rhythm are less frequent in DM2, but abnormalities do occur. Hypogonadism and insulin resistance need monitoring as in DM1. Myotonia tends to be less marked and less troublesome in DM2, but in specific circumstances antimyotonia therapy is helpful, especially if muscle stiffness is frequent and persistent or if pain is prominent. Cognitive difficulties also occur in DM2 as in DM1, but the changes are less severe than in DM1. Management of these brain symptoms is similar to that for DM1.

A frequent and difficult problem in DM2 is the peculiar muscle pain described earlier. Carbamazepine or mexiletine along with nonsteroidal antiinflammatory medications or Tylenol ameliorate this pain in some patients.

AUTOSOMAL-DOMINANT AND AUTOSOMAL-RECESSIVE MYOTONIA CONGENITA

Thomsen's disease (autosomal-dominant myotonia congenita) and Becker's disease (autosomal-recessive myotonia congenita) represent two forms of chloride channelopathies (Heatwole et al., 2013; Statland and Barohn, 2013; Suetterlin et al., 2014; Jurkat-Rott et al., 2015) (Table 151-3). The chloride channelopathies that produce myotonia as their primary symptom resemble the sodium channel disorders without periodic paralysis and may resemble mild forms of DM1 and DM2. Other causes of muscle stiffness or poor coordination, including central nervous system diseases affecting the frontal lobes, brainstem, and cerebellum, require initial consideration but are rarely confused with these channelopathies.

Clinical Features

Generalized myotonia is the major clinical symptom in dominant and recessive forms of chloride channel myotonia congenita. Recent studies indicate pain occurs in almost 30% of patients with chloride channel myotonia, and as many as 75% have mild generalized muscle weakness that is slightly greater proximally. Symptoms develop in the first or second decade of life. Myotonic stiffness occurs with sudden physical exertion after a period of rest. Repeated muscle contractions ameliorate the stiffness. This response is the "warm-up phenomenon,"

TABLE 151-3 Chloride Channel Myotonias

Clinical Features	Autosomal-Dominant Myotonia Congenita of Thomsen	Autosomal-Recessive Generalized Myotonia of Becker
Inheritance	Dominant	Recessive
Gene defect	Chromosome 7; mutation in skeletal muscle chloride channel	Chromosome 7; mutation in skeletal muscle chloride channel
Age of onset	Infancy to early childhood	Late childhood, occasionally starts earlier or begins in teens
Myopathy	Muscle hypertrophy frequent; no myopathy, although variants uncommonly develop weakness	Occasional muscle wasting and weakness can occur late; hypertrophy of muscles frequently occurs in legs
Myotonia	Generalized stiffness, especially after rest; improves with exercise; prominent myotonia of eye closure, but not paradoxical myotonia	Generalized stiffness, especially after rest; transient weakness is prominent after complete relaxation for several minutes; myotonia occurs in eyes; no paradoxical myotonia
Provocative stimuli	Prolonged rest or maintenance of the posture	Prolonged rest or maintenance of the same posture
Therapy for symptoms	Exercise; antimyotonia therapy (e.g., mexiletine); Achilles' tendon stretching helps prevent need for heel cord–lengthening surgery	Exercise; especially avoiding prolonged rest; antimyotonia therapy (e.g., mexiletine); transient weakness does not improve after mexiletine

which helps distinguish chloride channel myotonia congenita from certain forms of sodium channel myotonia that display increasing muscle stiffness with repeated contractions, a paramyotonic response. DM1 and DM2, like chloride channel myotonia, demonstrate the typical warm-up response.

In contrast to Thomsen's disease, patients with autosomal-recessive myotonia congenita (Becker's disease) have transient proximal muscle weakness. The transient weakness appears for a few seconds during the initial attempt at a specific movement after a period of inactivity. Muscle strength improves to normal after several strong contractions.

Patients have prominent muscle hypertrophy, especially in the legs, in both the autosomal-dominant and autosomal-recessive forms of myotonia congenita. Tendon reflexes, cerebellar function, sensation, and strength are normal. Myotonia can be noted with hand contraction or after eye closure. If patients lie supine for 5 to 10 minutes and suddenly arise, generalized myotonic stiffness in the proximal and paraspinous muscles becomes apparent. The estimated prevalence of autosomal-dominant myotonia congenita is 0.14/100,000, and the prevalence for autosomal-recessive myotonia congenita is 0.12/100,000.

Genetics

Point mutations in the gene for the skeletal muscle chloride channel cause both autosomal-dominant and autosomal-recessive forms of myotonia congenita (Jurkat-Rott et al., 2015). Over 100 mutations of the *CLCN1* gene have been associated with myotonia congenita.

Pathophysiology

 See the online chapter for commentary on pathophysiology.

Clinical Laboratory Tests

Evaluation of patients with suspected myotonia congenita should include consideration of other myotonic disorders, such as DM1, DM2, paramyotonia congenita, sodium channel myotonias of other types, and chondrodystrophic myotonia (Schwartz–Jampel syndrome). Distinguishing patients with chloride channel myotonia, either the autosomal-dominant or autosomal-recessive form, from those with sodium channel myotonic disorders is often difficult. Both cause myotonic

stiffness and muscle hypertrophy, especially in the legs. One distinguishing feature of sodium channel myotonia is the paradoxical myotonia of the eyelids that develops with repeated forceful eye closure. In contrast, patients with autosomal-dominant and autosomal-recessive forms of chloride channel myotonia exhibit warm-up after repeated contractions. Patients with chloride channel myotonia do not have a worsening of myotonic stiffness or paralysis after prolonged exposure of muscle to cold. To search for cold-induced paralysis, it is necessary to soak the hand or forearm muscles in cold water (15° C) for 15 to 20 minutes. If there is weakness with exercise after this cold exposure, this observation strongly favors sodium channel myotonia rather than chloride channel disease (Heatwole and Moxley, 2007). Electrodiagnostic studies should be considered in every patient suspected of having a myotonic disorder or channelopathy. Short and long exercise tests can identify differentiating patterns associated with specific channelopathies or myotonic conditions.

Treatment

Antimyotonia treatment with mexiletine is often helpful (Heatwole and Moxley, 2007). Before initiating treatment with mexiletine, a baseline ECG is necessary to identify patients with unsuspected cardiac conduction abnormalities. Side effects of mexiletine, which are usually mild and dose related, include dysgeusia, light-headedness, and diarrhea. Carbamazepine is an alternative antimyotonia medication to consider for myotonia congenita. Children with moderately severe myotonia develop heel cord shortening and contractures at their elbows. If these contractures do not respond to stretching and other physical therapy exercises, it is appropriate to initiate antimyotonia treatment even when patients do not complain of stiffness.

ACETAZOLAMIDE-RESPONSIVE SODIUM CHANNEL MYOTONIA AND MYOTONIA FLUCTUANS

Two disorders that mimic myotonia congenita and are forms of sodium channel myotonia without periodic paralysis are acetazolamide-responsive sodium channel myotonia and myotonia fluctuans (Heatwole and Moxley, 2007) (Table 151-4).

TABLE 151-4 Sodium Channel Myotonias Without Periodic Paralysis

Clinical Features	Acetazolamide-Responsive Sodium Channel Myotonia	Myotonia Fluctuans
Inheritance	Dominant	Dominant
Gene defect	Chromosome 17; mutation in skeletal muscle sodium channel	Chromosome 17; mutation in skeletal muscle sodium channel
Age of onset	First decade	First or second decade
Myopathy	Rare	Rare, muscle hypertrophy common
Myotonia	Face, paraspinal muscles, paradoxical myotonia of eyelids, grip limbs; varies in severity and often there is pain with myotonia	Face, limbs, eyelids; frequently fluctuates in severity; especially after exercise
Provocative stimuli	Fasting, cold, oral potassium, infection	Exercise–rest–exercise, oral potassium
Therapy for symptoms	Acetazolamide, mexiletine; avoid high-potassium diet; monitor during and after surgery for rigidity and rhabdomyolysis	Mexiletine; avoid high-potassium diet; monitor during and after surgery for rigidity and rhabdomyolysis

Clinical Features

Acetazolamide-responsive sodium channel myotonia often initially presents to the pediatrician rather than the neurologist with common complaints, such as clumsiness causing frequent falls, a lazy eye, growing pains, back muscle spasm, or stridor. Parents may observe that after prolonged crying, an infant or young child will have "their eyes stuck." This symptom is a manifestation of paradoxical eyelid myotonia that develops with repeated bouts of forceful closure of the eyes during crying. Myotonia is most apparent in the face, eyes, and larynx in very young patients. Stiffness in the hands, proximal limb muscles, and paraspinous muscles is more apparent in middle childhood. Muscle hypertrophy, especially in the legs, is frequent. Cerebellar function, sensory testing, tendon reflexes, and muscle strength are normal. Grip and percussion myotonia, and lid lag, are present. The severity of these complaints varies both in affected individuals within the same kindred and between kindreds. Episodes of painful muscle spasm occur in some patients, usually during or immediately after exercise. Pain is relatively infrequent in recessive and dominant chloride channel myotonias. In contrast, pain is common and can be severe in acetazolamide-responsive sodium channel myotonia and in DM2.

The clinical findings in myotonia fluctuans are similar to those described previously for acetazolamide-responsive sodium channel myotonia, with one important additional finding. The severity of the muscle stiffness fluctuates to a greater degree in this illness. On "good days" the myotonia can vanish. The fluctuating myotonia also has an interesting relationship with prolonged exercise. A phenomenon termed *exercise-induced delayed-onset myotonia* occurs. Patients report that after a period of rest following vigorous exercise, if they resume exercise "at the wrong time," severe muscle stiffness may develop. The time interval between the period of rest and the resumption of exercise is critical. If it is only a few minutes or an hour or more, stiffness does not occur. During the intermediate time interval, the fluctuation and provocation of severe myotonia happen.

The myotonic symptoms in both acetazolamide-responsive sodium channel myotonia and myotonia fluctuans tend to persist throughout a patient's lifetime. Some individuals note a lessening in severity in middle to late adulthood. This finding may represent only an adjustment to the illness and a decrease in physical activity.

Genetics

 See Table 151-4 and the Genetics section in the online chapter for more information.

Pathophysiology

See the online chapter for commentary on pathophysiology.

Clinical Laboratory Tests

Laboratories may screen for known mutations in the gene for the sodium channel in selected patients (Jurkat-Rott et al., 2015; Statland and Barohn, 2013; Suetterlin et al., 2014). The remainder of the laboratory evaluation is as described previously for chloride channel myotonia.

Treatment

Acetazolamide often controls myotonic stiffness and pain in acetazolamide-responsive sodium channel myotonia (Heatwole and Moxley, 2007). This treatment usually ameliorates the muscle pain. Annual ultrasound of the abdomen is useful to detect early formation of kidney stones, which are a common complication of acetazolamide. Dysesthesia and dysgeusia typically occur. For attacks of severe muscle spasm and pain, cyclobenzaprine can be tried. Patients undergoing surgery require monitoring during and after the procedure for signs of worsening muscle stiffness. Maintaining plasma potassium levels between 3.8 and 4.2 mEq/L helps to decrease perioperative muscle stiffness. Stress, muscle tissue damage, and bleeding all elevate plasma potassium levels and worsen myotonia. Postoperatively, intravenous diazepam or lorazepam may be necessary to decrease myotonic stiffness, especially if patients are unable to take medications by mouth. Mexiletine is an effective alternative to acetazolamide, and, if necessary, these drugs can be used in combination (Heatwole and Moxley, 2007).

The management of myotonia fluctuans is similar to that of acetazolamide-responsive sodium channel myotonia. Careful attention to the pattern and timing of exercise helps to decrease episodes of severe muscle stiffness. Intraoperative and postoperative monitoring is important, as noted previously.

THE PERIODIC PARALYSES

This section focuses on those disorders listed in Tables 151-5 and 151-6, which are associated with periodic paralyses, including channelopathies affecting the sodium, potassium, and calcium channels in skeletal muscle. See the online chapter for commentary on general classification and features of the periodic paralyses.

TABLE 151-5 Sodium Channel Myotonias With Periodic Paralysis

Clinical Features	Paramyotonia Congenita	Paramyotonia Congenita With Hyperkalemic Periodic Paralysis	Hyperkalemic Periodic Paralysis With Myotonia
Inheritance	Dominant	Dominant	Dominant
Gene defect	Chromosome 17; mutation in skeletal muscle sodium channel	Chromosome 17; mutation in skeletal muscle sodium channel	Chromosome 17; mutation in skeletal muscle sodium channel
Age of onset	First decade	First decade	First decade
Myopathy	Very rare	Rare	Infrequent
Myotonia	Especially paradoxical myotonia of the eyelids, and grip	Especially paradoxical myotonia of the eyelids, and grip	Especially paradoxical myotonia of the eyelids
Provocative stimuli	Cold exposure followed by exercise leads to focal paralysis; occasionally exercise provokes stiffness	Oral potassium load, rest after exercise mainly in morning (hyperkalemic weakness), cold exposure followed by exercise (focal paralysis)	Rest after exercise, cold, oral potassium
Therapy for symptoms	Mexiletine, mild exercise, keep patient warm	Mild exercise, thiazides, mexiletine	Thiazides, acetazolamide, sodium restriction

TABLE 151-6 Channelopathies With Hypokalemic Periodic Paralysis

Clinical Features	Andersen's Syndrome: Periodic Paralysis With Cardiac Dysrhythmia	Calcium Channel Periodic Paralysis	Sodium Channel Periodic Paralysis	Potassium Channel Periodic Paralysis	Periodic Paralysis With Thyroid Disease
Inheritance	Dominant	Dominant	Dominant	Dominant	Sporadic-occasionally dominant
Age of onset	First or second decade	First to third decade	First to third decade	Not yet determined	Third decade (males 20:1)
Myopathy	Typical; also short stature; dysmorphic features; prolonged QT interval on electrocardiogram; ventricular dysrhythmias	Moderately common late; vacuoles frequently seen on biopsy	Not yet determined	Not yet determined	Infrequent
Myotonia	No	No	No	No	No
Provocative stimuli	Rest after exercise, oral glucose	High-carbohydrate meals, rest after exercise, cold, emotional stress/excitement	High-carbohydrate meals, rest after exercise, cold, emotional stress/excitement	Usually by strenuous exercise followed by rest; less consistent provocation after high carbohydrate intake	High-carbohydrate meals, rest after exercise, acetazolamide
Therapy for symptoms	Mild exercise, glucose, high sodium intake, acetazolamide, dichlorphenamide	Acetazolamide, dichlorphenamide, potassium, spirolactone	Acetazolamide, dichlorphenamide, potassium, spirolactone	Acetazolamide	Propranolol, restoration of euthyroid state, oral potassium, spironolactone

Hyperkalemic Periodic Paralysis

Clinical Features

Table 151-5 outlines the major clinical and diagnostic features of hyperkalemic periodic paralysis and important issues in management. All three forms are autosomal dominant with high penetrance in both sexes (Cannon, 2002). Attacks begin in childhood and are usually brief, being shorter and more frequent than attacks in hypokalemic periodic paralysis. The attacks can occur with or without myotonia; in certain families, hyperkalemic paralysis occurs in combination with coexisting paramyotonia congenita (Jurkat-Rott et al., 2015; Statland and Barohn, 2013; Cannon, 2002; Heatwole and Moxley, 2007). At the onset of an attack, myalgia may develop. Patients with hyperkalemic periodic paralysis plus myotonia frequently develop muscle stiffness and prominent paradoxical myotonia of the eyelids during attacks. Similar symptoms occur in patients with hyperkalemic periodic paralysis in association with paramyotonia congenita (Jurkat-Rott et al.,

2015; Statland and Barohn, 2013). Most patients with hyperkalemic attacks manifest signs of myotonia and notice increasing muscle tension, especially in the paraspinous muscles. The estimated prevalence of hyperkalemic periodic paralysis is 0.13/100,000.

Genetics

See Table 151-5 and the Genetics section in the online chapter for more information.

Pathophysiology

See the online chapter for commentary on pathophysiology.

Clinical Laboratory Tests

The primary laboratory evaluation involves monitoring of serum electrolytes during attacks to identify hyperkalemia or hypokalemia and monitoring the ECG to search for any evidence of dysrhythmia or other conduction disturbance, such as the ECG changes that occur in Andersen–Tawil syndrome. A dominant family history helps to limit additional laboratory testing to search for secondary forms of hyperkalemia, which might lead to muscle weakness. Laboratory evaluation for secondary hyperkalemic weakness should include a search for hormonal disturbances, such as insulin deficiency or adrenal insufficiency, or toxic effects of medications, such as beta-adrenergic antagonists, alpha-adrenergic agonists, digitalis intoxication, or the use of succinylcholine. Full gene screening can be performed for mutations in the skeletal muscle sodium, chloride, calcium, and potassium channel genes to search for a mutation to account for one of the forms of nondystrophic myotonia or one of the forms of periodic paralysis (Jurkat-Rott et al., 2015; Statland and Barohn, 2013; Suetterlin et al., 2014). In patients not observed during a spontaneous attack of weakness or posing a continuing problem in definite classification of the form of periodic paralysis, it may be necessary to perform provocative testing with oral potassium loading or exercise followed by potassium challenge. Electrodiagnostic testing including short and long exercise tests may also provide diagnostic utility (Statland and Barohn, 2013).

Treatment

Attacks of weakness in hyperkalemic periodic paralysis are seldom severe enough to require emergency room evaluation. Oral glucose hastens recovery. Severe attacks usually respond to oral glucose and crystalline insulin subcutaneously. Occasionally, severe attacks may fail to respond to these treatments. Calcium gluconate is sometimes effective. Inhalation of beta-adrenergic agents, such as metaproterenol, every 15 minutes for three doses has also been utilized.

Preventive treatment includes avoidance of fasting, exposure to cold, and overexertion. A prudent consumption of frequent meals high in carbohydrate content is helpful. Diuretics that promote kaluresis, such as hydrochlorothiazide and carbonic anhydrase inhibitors, are good primary therapies (Heatwole and Moxley, 2007).

Paramyotonia Congenita
Clinical Features

Symptoms develop usually during the first decade of life and have a predilection for facial, lingual, neck, and hand muscles (see Table 151-5) (Jurkat-Rott et al., 2015; Heatwole and Moxley, 2007). Attacks of increased muscle stiffness followed by paralysis occur on exposure to cold followed by exercise. The hallmark clinical sign is paradoxical myotonia or paramyotonia, that is, stiffness that worsens with repeated muscle contraction. This sign is most prominent in the muscles of eye closure. Clinical myotonia may be restricted to the eye muscles and not be apparent in grip or after percussion. Some patients experience lid lag and diplopia. See the online chapter for commentary on rare severe variants. The estimated prevalence of this paramyotonia congenita is 0.17/100,000.

Genetics

Mutations in the gene for the skeletal muscle sodium channel in several locations cause paramyotonia congenita (Jurkat-Rott et al., 2015; Matthews et al., 2010). See the online chapter for more details.

Clinical Laboratory Tests

Standardized testing using immersion of the hand and forearm in cold water for 15 minutes followed by exercise is effective in provoking paramyotonic stiffness and paralysis in most patients. Most cooperative children can tolerate this testing. If no clear evidence of cold-induced muscle stiffness and weakness is apparent, further laboratory testing as indicated previously under hyperkalemic periodic paralysis and as noted under laboratory tests for chloride channel myotonia may be necessary. Repetitive nerve stimulation of the ulnar nerve at the wrist as a short exercise test before and after cold exposure helps to identify certain forms of sodium channel myotonia, including paramyotonia congenita, but it is uncomfortable and has been standardized only in adults. DNA analysis to search for known mutations in the gene for the sodium channel is available (Jurkat-Rott et al., 2015; Statland and Barohn, 2013; Matthews et al., 2010).

Pathophysiology

See the online chapter for commentary on pathophysiology.

Treatment

Mexiletine is usually effective in preventing attacks of cold-induced weakness (Heatwole and Moxley, 2007). Patients having the combination of paramyotonia congenita plus hyperkalemic periodic paralysis require additional treatment with either a thiazide diuretic or acetazolamide.

Hypokalemic Periodic Paralysis

Hypokalemic periodic paralysis is an autosomal-dominant disorder caused most commonly by mutations in the alpha subunit of the skeletal muscle calcium channel gene Cav1.1 (Jurkat-Rott et al., 2015; Statland and Barohn, 2013). A clinically identical form of hypokalemic periodic paralysis can also result from specific mutations of the alpha subunit of the Nav1.4 skeletal muscle sodium channel associated with hyperkalemic periodic paralysis (Jurkat-Rott et al., 2015; Statland and Barohn, 2013). Approximately 60% of cases are caused by missense mutations of the calcium channel gene, Cav1.1, and 15% to 20% of cases are caused by mutations in the sodium channel gene, Nav1.4. The estimated prevalence is 0.17/100,00.

Clinical Features

Attacks of hypokalemic periodic paralysis usually have their onset in the first or second decade, and about 60% of patients are affected before the age of 16 years (Jurkat-Rott et al., 2015; Statland and Barohn, 2013). Rarely, attacks occur in infancy. Initially, attacks tend to be infrequent but eventually may recur daily. Diurnal fluctuations in strength may develop so that patients demonstrate greatest weakness during the night or early morning hours and gradually gain strength as the day passes. During major attacks, the serum potassium level decreases but not always to below normal. There is urinary retention of sodium, potassium, chloride, and water. Oliguria or anuria develops during such attacks, and patients tend to be constipated. Sinus bradycardia and ECG signs of hypokalemia appear when the serum potassium falls below normal. Usually during the fourth and fifth decades of life, attacks become less frequent and may cease. However, repeated attacks may leave the patient with permanent residual weakness (Jurkat-Rott et al., 2015). Treatment with acetazolamide can aggravate hypokalemic periodic paralysis caused by sodium channel mutations in some but not all kindreds.

Genetics

In most kindreds familial hypokalemic periodic paralysis results from missense mutations at charged residues of the S4 voltage-sensing segments in either the L-type voltage-gated calcium channel Cav1.1 encoded by the *CACNA1S* gene or in the voltage-gated sodium channel Nav1.4.

Pathophysiology

 See the online chapter for commentary on pathophysiology.

Clinical Laboratory Tests

Evaluation of serum electrolytes and ECG during attacks of weakness is essential to diagnosis and treatment. Muscle biopsy is usually not necessary but may reveal vacuoles, especially in patients with fixed weakness. In patients not observed during attacks of weakness, it may be necessary to undertake careful provocative testing if DNA analysis does not identify the responsible mutation. This testing requires hospitalization and continuous monitoring of the ECG, as indicated in previously published protocols. Occasionally, hypokalemic paralysis develops from acquired, secondary causes. Causes for secondary hypokalemic weakness include the following: hypokalemia in association with hyperthyroidism, beta-adrenergic stimulation, excessive insulin, alkalemia, barium poisoning, poor potassium intake (e.g., alcoholics, anorexia nervosa), excessive potassium excretion (e.g., diarrhea, laxative abuse, profuse sweating during athletic training), and renal loss of potassium (e.g., renal tubular acidosis, osmotic diuresis, and medication use, such as large doses of penicillin antibiotics).

Treatment

Acute attacks may respond to oral potassium chloride. Monitoring of ECGs, serum potassium levels, and muscle strength helps determine the frequency of these doses. Milder attacks resolve spontaneously, and mild exercise of the weakened muscles speeds recovery. If a patient has a severe attack and is unable to swallow or is vomiting, very cautious intravenous infusion of potassium may be necessary. Treating physicians should keep in mind that a patient's serum potassium levels do not represent a total body deficit of potassium but rather a temporary intracellular shift. Therefore potassium replacement formulas tend to overestimate the replacement needs and result in potentially dangerous hyperkalemia. Preventive therapy for attacks of hypokalemic weakness is usually needed. A low-sodium (2–3 g/day) and low-carbohydrate (60–80 g/day) diet, avoidance of exposure to cold and overexertion, and supplemental doses of potassium chloride taken two to four times daily are preventive measures that may help. However, no convincing data are available to indicate that oral potassium chloride prevents attacks.

Acetazolamide in divided doses usually abolishes attacks of weakness in most patients when taken daily. Dichlorphenamide is another carbonic anhydrase inhibitor that is useful as preventive treatment if acetazolamide proves ineffective. Carbonic anhydrase inhibitors produce a metabolic acidosis, and despite their kaluretic action and their tendency to lower serum potassium levels, they appear to act on skeletal muscle to stabilize potassium flux, especially during insulin stimulation. There are rare familial cases of hypokalemic periodic paralysis in which acetazolamide exacerbates attacks of weakness. This weakness appears to be a consistent but not universal feature of hypokalemic periodic paralysis families carrying sodium channel mutations. In these families, triamterene or spironolactone may control the attacks.

Periodic Paralysis With Cardiac Arrhythmia: Andersen–Tawil Syndrome

Clinical Features

Andersen syndrome (Jurkat-Rott et al., 2015; Statland and Barohn, 2013) or, as recently recognized, Andersen–Tawil syndrome, is a rare inherited disorder with an estimated prevalence of 0.08/100,000 that is characterized by periodic paralysis, long QT syndrome, ventricular dysrhythmias, and skeletal developmental abnormalities. Skeletal abnormalities include low-set ears, widely spaced eyes, scoliosis, short stature, small mandibles, and fifth-digit clinodactyly (Statland and Barohn, 2013). The early reports of this disorder raised the possibility of hyperkalemia during attacks of weakness, but as more specific identification of kindreds with Andersen–Tawil syndrome has occurred, it is apparent that the disorder occurs with both hyper- and hypokalemia. One form is a variant of hypokalemic periodic paralysis. Patients with this type of hypokalemic weakness have short stature, clinodactyly, and microcephaly, and ventricular dysrhythmias (Figure 151-7). Attacks of weakness develop during the first or second decade. The attacks of limb weakness can vary from mild, resembling those in the sodium channel form of hyperkalemic periodic paralysis, to severe, resembling the typical calcium channel form of hypokalemic periodic paralysis. The major difference is that occasionally the episodes of weakness are associated with syncopal attacks and rarely sudden death. The cardiac arrhythmias and extrasystoles improve with an elevation in extracellular potassium, whereas hypokalemia tends to aggravate the cardiac dysrhythmias. Cardiac symptoms can be provoked by digitalis; are refractory to disopyramide phosphate, propranolol, and phenytoin; and may respond to imipramine. Weakness and cardiac symptoms in some patients occur following corticosteroid treatment. Patients with Andersen–Tawil syndrome have a neurocognitive phenotype, with individuals having deficits in executive function and abstract reasoning compared with their siblings. Isolated reports have also identified patients with afebrile seizures, dilated cardiomyopathies, and renal tubular defects (Statland and Barohn, 2013).

Genetics

One of the responsible mutations involves the KCNJ2 gene encoding the inward-rectifying potassium channel Kir2.1. Autosomal-dominant inheritance occurs with variable severity within families. See the online version of chapter for more information.

Pathophysiology

See the online chapter for commentary on pathophysiology.

Clinical Laboratory Tests

Periodic monitoring of the ECG (or Holter monitoring) is important to identify covert dysrhythmias. ECG can reveal premature ventricular contractions, QT interval prolongation, large U-waves, and bidirectional ventricular tachycardia. DNA testing is helpful in confirming the diagnosis. Secondary forms of periodic paralysis must be ruled out with assessments of thyroid, renal, and adrenal functions. Muscle biopsy may help to distinguish patients with Andersen–Tawil syndrome from those with other myopathic disorders, especially various congenital myopathies. Electrophysiologic cold studies are helpful in confirming the presence of skeletal muscle membrane and excitability using the exercise nerve conduction study, which can in many patients distinguish those with known sodium, chloride, and calcium channel mutations from individuals with Andersen–Tawil syndrome.

Treatment

Acetazolamide in doses used to treat sodium channel forms of hyperkalemic periodic paralysis is sometimes effective in preventing attacks of weakness. Dichlorphenamide or flecainide may provide an effective alternative if acetazolamide fails. Oral potassium repletement with ECG monitoring can be used during episodic weakness if a patient's serum potassium concentration is low (Statland and Barohn, 2013). If serum levels of potassium are high, exercise or carbohydrates may shorten an attack. Cardiac dysrhythmias are less frequent if serum potassium is permitted to range from 4 to 4.4 mEq/L. However, this elevation in potassium may be difficult to achieve because it is typically not feasible with the use of carbonic anhydrase inhibitors. In general, agents that create drug-induced hypokalemia or prolong QT intervals should be avoided. Management of the cardiac dysrhythmia is best handled by a cardiologist. Cardiac dysrhythmia in this condition is typically difficult to control and can result in sudden cardiac death.

Thyrotoxic Periodic Paralysis

Clinical Features

Attacks of thyrotoxic periodic paralysis tend to develop in the late teens and during the 20s. Thyrotoxic periodic paralysis is much more frequent in Asians and males; 95% of cases are sporadic. Precipitating factors include sleep, hot weather, and excessive physical activity. Recurrent attacks of weakness may occur in over 60% of patients who have not returned to the euthyroid state. Cardiac problems, including sinus tachycardia, atrial fibrillation, supraventricular tachycardia, and ventricular fibrillation, can occur.

Pathophysiology

See the online chapter for commentary on pathophysiology.

Genetics

The gene defect responsible for thyrotoxic hypokalemic periodic paralysis remains unclear. See the online chapter for more information.

Clinical Laboratory Tests

Measurement of thyroid function tests and the ECG are essential in establishing the diagnosis and in directing treatment. Other aspects of clinical laboratory evaluation are as described for familial hypokalemic periodic paralysis.

Treatment

Treatment consists of antithyroid therapy until the patient achieves the euthyroid state. Preventive measures should be undertaken after treatment of the acute attack as described for primary familial hypokalemic periodic paralysis. Propranolol is often effective in preventing attacks in thyrotoxic periodic paralysis. Recent studies emphasize the importance of propranolol as an initial treatment and suggest caution about the use of potassium replacement. Acetazolamide is ineffective and may worsen or precipitate symptoms in thyrotoxic hypokalemic periodic paralysis and should be avoided. In general, beta-blocking drugs are helpful to use throughout the early stages of management until the patient becomes euthyroid.

REFERENCES

The complete list of references for this chapter is available in the e-book at www.expertconsult.com.
    See inside cover for registration details.

SELECTED REFERENCES

Cannon, S.C., 2002. An expanding view for the molecular basis of familial periodic paralysis. Neuromuscl. Disord. 12 (6), 533–543.

Heatwole, C.R., Moxley, R.T. III, 2007. The nondystrophic myotonias. Neurother. 4 (2), 238–251.

Heatwole, C.R., Statland, J.M., Logigian, E.L., 2013. The diagnosis and treatment of myotonic disorders. Muscle Nerve 47 (5), 632–648.

Jurkat-Rott, K., Rudel, R., Lehmann-Horn, F., 2015. Muscle Channelopathies: Myotonias and Periodic Paralyses. In: Darras, B.T., Roydon Jones, H., Ryan, M.M., et al. (Eds.), Neuromuscular Disorders of Infancy, Childhood and Adolescence. Elsevier, London, pp. 719–734.

Kamsteeg, E.J., Kress, W., Catalli, C., et al., 2012. Best practice guidelines and recommendations on the molecular diagnosis of myotonic dystrophy types 1 and 2. Eur. J. Hum. Genet. 20 (12), 1203–1208.

Matthews, E., Fialho, D., Tan, S.V., et al., 2010. The non-dystrophic myotonias: molecular pathogenesis, diagnosis and treatment. Brain 133 (Pt 1), 9–22.

Moxley, R.T., Ciafaloni, E., Guntrum, D., 2015. Myotonic Dystrophy. In: Darras, B.T., Jones, R., Ryan, M.M., et al. (Eds.), Neuromuscular Disorders of Infancy, Childhood, and Adolescence: A Clinician's Approach. Elsevier, London, pp. 697–718.

Statland, J.M., Barohn, R.J., 2013. Muscle channelopathies: the nondystrophic myotonias and periodic paralyses. Continuum (Minneap Minn) 19 (6 Muscle Disease), 1598–1614.

Suetterlin, K., Mannikko, R., Hanna, M.G., 2014. Muscle channelopathies: recent advances in genetics, pathophysiology and therapy. Curr. Opin. Neurol. 27 (5), 583–590.

Udd, B., Krahe, R., 2012. The myotonic dystrophies: molecular, clinical, and therapeutic challenges. Lancet Neurol. 11 (10), 891–905.

E-BOOK FIGURES AND TABLES

152 Management of Children with Neuromuscular Disorders

Dennis J. Matthews, Joyce Oleszek, Julie A. Parsons, and Oren Kupfer

 An expanded version of this chapter is available on www.expertconsult.com. See inside cover for registration details.

The management of pediatric neuromuscular disorders is complex and challenging. Developing an effective management plan requires an understanding of the underlying pathophysiology, genetics, and natural history, as well as the interactions of normal maturation, treatment modalities, and the environment. Optimum management requires a multidisciplinary approach that focuses on anticipatory and preventive measures as well as active interventions to address the primary and secondary aspects of the disorder (Bushby et al., 2009). Implementing comprehensive management strategies can favorably alter the natural history of the disorder and improve function, quality of life, and longevity (Fig. 152-1). This chapter will discuss general recommendations for management of pediatric neuromuscular disorders along with specific recommendation for individual diseases.

Appropriate management of patients with neuromuscular disorders requires an accurate diagnosis, including the relevant patient and family history, and focused general, musculoskeletal, neurologic, and functional physical examinations. All diagnostic information should be interpreted, not in isolation, but within the context of relevant historical information, family history, examination findings, laboratory data, molecular diagnostic studies, electrophysiologic findings, and pathologic information, if obtained (McDonald, 2010).

Therapeutic treatment includes early intervention, age-appropriate functional training, therapy programs, play, therapeutic exercise, adjustment to disability support and transition planning. Engaging in play activities and working on developing activities of daily living are the primary mechanisms by which children with neuromuscular disorders can maintain muscle strength. The available evidence suggests that in patients with neuromuscular diseases, both strength training and aerobic exercise programs appear to be safe, without any notable deleterious effects. Gentle, low impact aerobic exercise (swimming, stationary bicycling) improves cardiovascular performance, increases muscle efficiency, and lessens fatigue (Narayanaswami et al., 2014).

Muscles can be strengthened by prescribing progressive resistance exercises, stretching and aerobic exercise. A minimum of once-a-day muscle contraction at 30% to 50% of maximal strength for 3 to 5 minutes, 3 times per week, for a single muscle group has been shown to be effective. High resistance strengthening has not demonstrated additional benefit. Patients who are participating in an exercise program need to be aware of the warning signs of overwork weakness, which includes feeling weaker rather than stronger within 30 minutes post exercise or excessive muscle soreness 24 to 48 hours after exercise, severe muscle cramping, heaviness in the extremities, and prolonged shortness of breath. Significant muscle pain or myoglobinuria in the 24-hour period after specific activity is a sign of overexertion and indicates that activity should be modified.

The management of limb contractures in patients with progressive neuromuscular disease and the role of stretching, orthotics, and surgery have been comprehensively reviewed.

Principle therapies include: 1) regularly prescribed periods of daily standing and walking if the patient is functionally capable of being upright; 2) passive stretching of muscles and joints with a daily home program; 3) positioning of the legs to promote extension and oppose joint flexion when the patient is nonweight-bearing; and 4) splinting, which can be useful measure for the prevention or delay of ankle contracture (Bushby et al., 2009).

Stretching to maintain optimal muscle resting length as well as viscoelastic properties is important for maintaining muscle function. Muscles that cross two joints, such as the gastrocnemius, hamstrings, hip flexors, biceps, and the long back extensors, are particularly prone to develop contractures. Once a contracture has developed, the treatment is active and passive range of motion exercises combined with a sustained terminal stretch on a daily basis. The intensity of stretch should be of a mild degree without discomfort. Static stretches are held 15 to 60 seconds. Sustained stretching can be obtained by splinting orthotics. Resting ankle foot orthoses (AFOs) can help to prevent or minimize progressive equinus contractures. Knee-ankle-foot orthoses (KAFOs) can be of value in late ambulatory and early nonambulatory stages to allow standing and limited ambulation for therapeutic purposes (see Fig. 152-2). A passive standing device can be used with either no or mild hip, knee, or ankle contractures.

Dynamic splinting provides tension in the desired direction with the use of springs or elastic bands. This type of splinting is often used in the hand and arm because it allows a measure of function while providing stretching. To achieve optimal joint position, it is sometimes necessary to surgically lengthen the contracted tendon.

In the upper extremity, elbow flexion contractures in dystrophic myopathies may occur soon after wheelchair transition secondary to static positioning of the arms and elbow flexion on the armrests of the wheelchair. Other associated deformities include forearm pronator tightness and wrist flexion-ulnar deviation in the later stages of the disease. Mild elbow flexion contractures of 15° or less are of no functional consequence. Severe elbow flexion contractures of greater than 60° are associated with decreased distal upper extremity function and produce difficulty when dressing. Nighttime resting splints, which promote wrist extension, metacarpophalangeal extension, and proximal interphalangeal flexion, are recommended. Daytime positioning should emphasize wrist and finger extension, but splinting should not compromise sensation or function.

Weakness is the major cause of loss of ambulation in Duchenne muscular dystrophy (DMD), not contracture formation. The primary indication for orthopedic surgical tenotomies is the provision of optimal alignment. Little evidence supports the efficacy of early prophylactic lower extremity surgery in DMD for prolonging ambulation.

The release of contractures at both the heel cord and iliotibial band may be necessary to obtain optimal alignment. Hip and knee flexion contractures generally are not severe enough

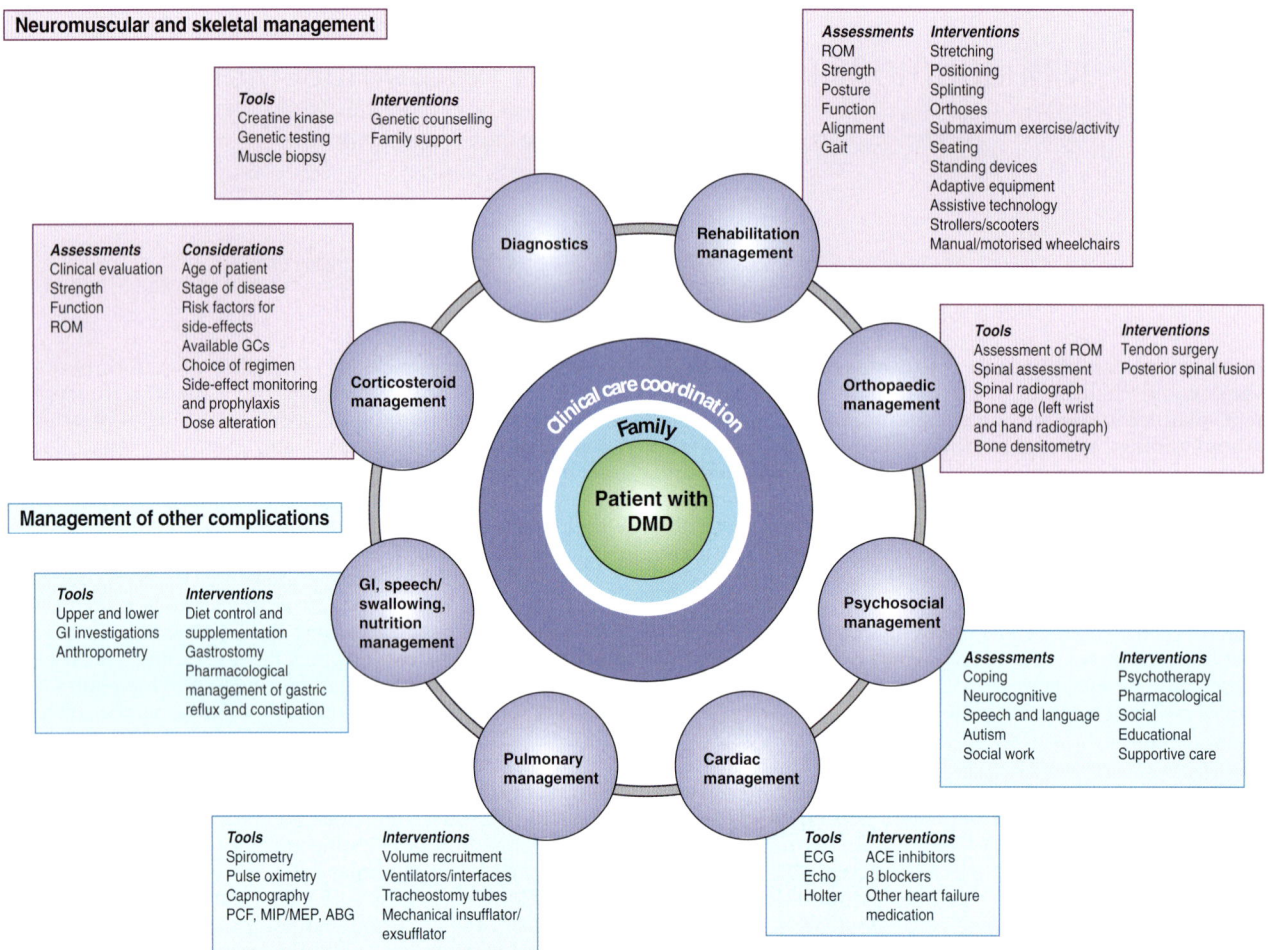

Figure 152-1. Interdisciplinary management of DMD. *(With permission from Bushby, K., Finkel, R., Birnkrant, D.J., et al., 2010. Diagnosis and management of Duchenne muscular dystrophy, part 1: diagnosis, and pharmacological and psychosocial management. Lancet Neurol 9(1), 77–79.)*

to require surgery. The ankle deformity may be corrected by either a tendo-Achilles lengthening (TAL) or a TAL combined with a surgical transfer of the posterior tibialis muscle tendon to the dorsum of the foot.

Those still ambulating independently without orthotics use their ankle equinus posturing from the gastrocnemius-soleus group to create a knee extension moment at foot contact, thus stabilizing the knee when the quadriceps muscle is weak. Several authors have cautioned against isolated heel cord tenotomies. Overcorrection of the heel cord contracture may result in immediate loss of the ability to walk without bracing unless the quadriceps are grade 4 strength or better.

Adaptive devices are frequently used to maintain function. During the early ambulatory phase, a lightweight wheelchair can be used for distances. As the weakness progresses in the late ambulatory phase, use of manual wheelchair, scooter, or power chair can be considered. As functional community ambulation declines, a power wheelchair is advocated. Generally, children can be taught to safely operate a power wheelchair at the developmental age of approximately 2 years. The initial power wheelchair prescription needs to consider the natural history of the neuromuscular disease disorder over the following 5 years, as some children will develop the need for a power recline system. In more severely disabled, the power wheelchair electronics should be sufficiently sophisticated to incorporate alternative drive control systems, environmental control adaptations, and possibly augmentative communication

systems in patients who are unable to vocalize. The power wheelchair should include: a solid custom seat and back, lateral trunk supports, hip guides, headrest, power tilt/recline, elevating or swing away leg rests, and a pressure-relieving cushion.

Upper extremity weakness can be augmented with a lap tray, extended straws, balance forearm orthoses, and environmental controls. Bathing equipment, hospital bed, and transfer devices are frequently used in nonambulatory patients.

Severe spinal deformity in progressive neuromuscular disorders leads to multiple problems, including poor sitting balance, difficulty with upright seating and positioning, pain, difficulty in parental or attendant care, and potential exacerbation of underlying restrictive respiratory compromise. Fixed pelvic obliquity (pelvic tilt) may increase the risk of developing pressure ulcers due to imbalanced seating. Increased spinal deformity may require the patient to utilize the upper extremities to support an upright position, thereby leaving the hands unable to be used for other activities.

Populations at risk for scoliosis include DMD, autosomal recessive LGMD, congenital muscular dystrophy, FSH muscular dystrophy, congenital myotonic muscular dystrophy, spinal muscular atrophy II and III, and Friedreich ataxia (Wang et al., 2007).

Close clinical monitoring is essential for children at risk for scoliosis. Baseline spinal radiography is indicated near time of wheelchair dependency and then annually for curves less than

20 degrees. Curves may progress rapidly during the adolescent growth spurt, and children will then need to be monitored every 6 months with clinical assessments and spine radiographs. Patients who are likely to require surgical arthrodesis at some point should be monitored with pulmonary function tests every 6 months.

Scoliosis progression in the thoracic spine can lead to the development of restrictive lung disease and increased need for noninvasive positive pressure ventilation, especially during sleep. Patients with DMD are expected to lose 4% of their forced vital capacity per year with an additional 4% decline for each 10 degree increase of their scoliosis. Similar reductions in pulmonary function with an increase in scoliosis have also been demonstrated in children with spinal muscular atrophy (SMA).

The management of spinal deformity with orthotics is relatively ineffective in DMD. Spinal orthoses are often reported to be uncomfortable and poorly tolerated in this population. Furthermore, vital capacity potentially can be lowered with constrictive orthoses. On the other hand, in neuromuscular diseases with spinal deformity beginning in the first decade of life such as SMA, congenital muscular dystrophy, congenital myotonic muscular dystrophy, some congenital myopathies, and congenital myasthenic syndromes, spinal orthoses are generally used to improve sitting balance.

Recent data have demonstrated markedly decreased incidence of scoliosis and progression to surgery for scoliosis in children with DMD treated with glucocorticoids. In a nonrandomized comparative cohort of 54 children, 6 of 30 (20%) of children in the glucocorticoid group developed scoliosis and had surgery, compared with 22 of 24 (92%) in the group not treated with glucocorticoids.

Surgical correction of scoliosis should be considered based upon the patient's curve progression, pulmonary function, and bone maturity. Evidence suggests that earlier surgery results in better outcomes. The beneficial effects on pulmonary function remains controversial, but the rate of decline may be slowed.

The extent of the fusion depends on the degree of spinal curvature, pelvic obliquity, and mobility. Generally, posterior spinal fusion is appropriate for curves greater than 30 degrees. If there is pelvic obliquity greater than 15 degrees, it is necessary to perform correction and stabilization from the upper thoracic region to the sacrum (Fig. 152-4).

Multidisciplinary preoperative evaluation is recommended before considering treatment for scoliosis in DMD and SMA. These evaluations are useful to prepare the patient and optimize the treatment plan to minimize surgical complications. These assessments also can prove critical for families who are trying to decide whether or not to pursue surgery. In some cases, patients are so severely compromised medically that surgery no longer is a practical option due to unacceptably high risks of postoperative complications.

At minimum, the preoperative evaluation should include pulmonary, anesthesia, cardiology, and nutritional assessments. Sleep studies are often recommended to assess for hypoxia and obstructive sleep apnea. Pulmonary evaluation helps prepare the patient and surgeon for the potential need for postoperative respiratory support that can range from supplemental oxygen to mechanical ventilation with tracheostomy.

A plan should also be in place for changes in seating equipment that will be needed after the major alteration in body contour after scoliosis surgery. Most children will no longer comfortably fit in their old custom seating systems after scoliosis correction. Resuming upright posture as soon as possible after surgery is important to help with expansion of the lungs and prevention of atelectasis and pneumonia.

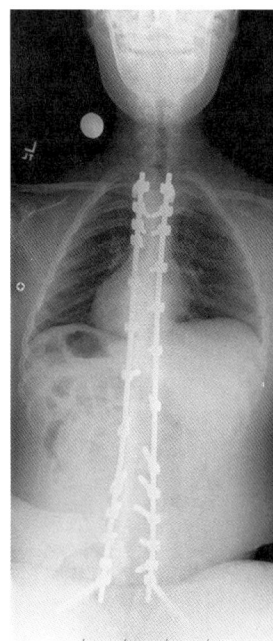

Figure 152-4. Posterior spinal fusion.

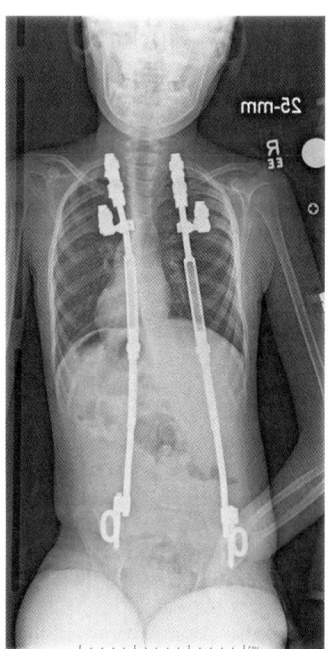

Figure 152-5. VEPTR (vertical expandable prosthetic titanium rib) implants.

For children who develop severe scoliosis at a young age (younger than 10 years), however, spinal fusion has been discouraged due to the concern that it will lead to restrictive lung disease as the child grows. Various "growth friendly" surgical options have been studied in neuromuscular patients. Growing rod treatment involves short fusions of the spine at the upper and lower ends with connecting rods that are periodically distracted (every 6 months) to maintain growth. VEPTR (vertical expandable prosthetic titanium rib) implants function in a similar manner, with fixation proximally on the ribs instead of the spine (see Fig. 152-5). Although these advances can be beneficial for some patients, they have high complication rates. A rod that can be expanded via a magnet external to the patient has recently been approved for use in the United States and may prove beneficial for young patients with neuromuscular scoliosis.

Complications occur at a high rate in neuromuscular scoliosis surgery. Surgical site infection has been reported in 5% to 15% of patients. Infection typically requires return to the operating room for debridement and prolonged antibiotic treatment. Pulmonary and gastrointestinal complications in neuromuscular scoliosis are also frequent, and seen in up to 50% of patients. Postoperative respiratory support is frequently needed as is enteral or parenteral nutritional support.

Complications are also frequent in growing rod and VEPTR surgery for neuromuscular scoliosis. These include failure of rib/spine anchors and infection. Together, these complications affect about 1 in 3 patients undergoing growing rod or VEPTR treatment. Complications appear to be less frequent in patients with SMA compared with idiopathic diagnoses, perhaps due to decreased functional demand on the nonfusion constructs.

Quality of life data after surgery for neuromuscular scoliosis is sparse. Scoliosis surgery in patients with SMA and DMD is generally thought to provide good functional results with improvements in sitting balance, caregiver burden, and patient/parent perception of self-image after surgery.

Respiratory involvement in neuromuscular disorders is variable depending on the diagnosis. It may be progressive or static. In some disorders such as Duchenne muscular dystrophy, the progression of respiratory involvement is predictable. The pathophysiology depends on the pattern of muscle weakness. Weakness of the diaphragm, accessory respiratory muscles, and pharynx can lead to impaired cough strength, recurrent pneumonia, aspiration, persistent atelectasis, restrictive lung disease, hypoventilation, obstructive sleep apnea, and chronic respiratory failure. Scoliosis can further complicate respiratory function by contributing to chest wall restriction by impairing normal chest and diaphragm mechanics.

Neonatal respiratory distress or failure is seen in many of the congenital myopathies, spinal muscular atrophy type I, and myotonic dystrophy type I. These infants often require assisted ventilation, provided either invasively or noninvasively. They may also require airway clearance with chest physiotherapy or mechanical insufflation-exsufflation (commonly referred to as cough assist). Examination findings include feeding difficulty, tachypnea, nasal flaring, accessory muscle use, thoracoabdominal asynchrony ("see-saw breathing"), weak cough, decreased air entry, crackles, and dullness to percussion.

In toddlers and children, respiratory muscle dysfunction may or may not be commensurate with other skeletal muscle function (e.g., age-appropriate developmental milestones such as sitting, crawling, and walking). Therefore a high index of suspicion for respiratory disease is needed. In toddlers or patients in whom voluntary pulmonary function testing is not possible due to cognitive or other barriers, detailed history is needed. Questions should focus on daily respiratory symptoms of cough, dyspnea, exercise tolerance (if applicable), swallowing difficulty, history of pneumonia, and difficulty with anesthesia. As diaphragm function is often more affected in the supine position and during sleep, detailed inquiries searching for sleep-disordered breathing are vital. These findings may be subtle and questions should include the presence or absence of snoring, overt apnea or gasping, abnormal respiratory patterns, restless sleep, nocturnal diaphoresis, frequent awakenings, enuresis, morning headaches, mood on awakening, and need for daytime sleep. Children whose sleep is disrupted may also experience attention deficits and hyperactivity rather than daytime somnolence. Should any concerns for impaired sleep-disordered breathing arise, referral for a formal polysomnogram (not overnight home pulse oximetry) is recommended.

In children who can complete voluntary pulmonary function tests, findings include decreased vital capacity (restrictive defect), decreased inspiratory and/or expiratory pressures, and decreased peak cough flows. Vital capacity may be further reduced in the supine position. A 20% decrease in vital capacity from prone to supine position is consistent with diaphragm dysfunction and increases the risk for sleep-disordered breathing.

Every patient with a neuromuscular disorder and known or suspected respiratory manifestations should be referred to a pulmonologist with expertise in neuromuscular disease. Frequency and nature of monitoring is determined by the underlying diagnosis, interval history, pulmonary function, and polysomnography where relevant.

Published guidelines are available for Duchenne muscular dystrophy, spinal muscular atrophy, congenital myopathies as a whole, and congenital muscular dystrophies as a whole (Finder et al., 2004; Manzur et al., 2003; Wang et al., 2012). All infants and children should receive standard immunizations. Influenza immunization should only be given using inactivated virus vaccine given by intramuscular injection and not with a live attenuated vaccine given by nasal inhalation. Infection with respiratory syncytial virus (RSV) leads to more severe RSV-related disease in infants and children with neuromuscular impairment than in those without neuromuscular impairment. Therefore passive RSV immunization with palivizumab has been recommended by some providers. Immunization with pneumococcal polysaccharide vaccine (PPSV) is recommended for those patients with respiratory disease over the age of 5 years.

Treatment of respiratory weakness is supportive and focuses on improving cough clearance, optimizing sleep-disordered breathing, and maximizing oxygenation and ventilation, all while improving quality of life. Supplemental oxygen may correct hypoxemia but may lead to worsened hypercapnia by eliminating the hypoxemic drive to breathe. Mechanical airway clearance, similar to mechanical insufflation-exsufflation, is used when peak cough flow is impaired. Daily mechanical insufflation may also play a role in maintaining chest compliance. Breath stacking, glossopharyngeal breathing, and abdominal thrusts (also called "quad cough") have been used to varying degrees of success. Other modalities of airway clearance such as inhaled bronchodilators, inhaled or oral mucolytics, and mechanical vibration (e.g., pneumatic vest or intrapulmonary percussive ventilation) have not been well-studied in neuromuscular disorders. These are often used as adjunctive therapies, especially in the setting of acute respiratory illness.

Continuous positive airway pressure (CPAP) is not recommended as it does not provide inspiratory support for normal tidal breathing. Bilevel positive airway pressure provides continuous airway pressure to maintain functional residual capacity as well as inspiratory tidal support. Settings for nocturnal use are best determined in the sleep laboratory during sleep. Progression to daytime hypercapnia and chronic respiratory failure occurs in many neuromuscular disorders. This can be managed noninvasively (with nasal or oronasal interfaces or mouthpiece ventilators) or invasively with tracheostomy. Clinical monitoring with pulse oximetry and noninvasive measurements of CO_2 can also direct mechanical ventilation strategies. Many patients are not able to tolerate noninvasive ventilation initially and may benefit from sleep psychology services for desensitization therapy.

Discussions about goals of care, end-of-life decisions, and code status should be conducted well in advance of any surgery or the development of chronic respiratory disease. This should be undertaken on a recurrent basis with providers with whom the patient and family are familiar. Enlisting the assistance of palliative care services is a vital but often neglected part of the patient's care.

Cardiac involvement is not uniform in neuromuscular diseases. Yet in some disorders such as Duchenne muscular dystrophy (DMD), Becker muscular dystrophy (BMD), some of the limb-girdle muscular dystrophies, and myotonic dystrophy, cardiac disease is a major cause of morbidity and mortality. Early diagnosis and detection of cardiac involvement provides opportunity for early therapy and intervention, which will hopefully affect positive outcomes.

In DMD, cardiac manifestations include cardiomyopathy and cardiac arrhythmia. Dystrophin is present both in the myocardium as well as in the cardiac Purkinje cells that affect conduction. Cardiomyopathy is progressive and a major source of morbidity and mortality in DMD and BMD. Myocardial disease is present before symptoms becoming apparent. By age 10, cardiomyopathy is clinically evident and virtually all boys by age 18 are affected. ECG abnormalities are present in almost all boys with DMD age 13 years and over. Most boys will have a resting tachycardia. This is possibly due to autonomic disturbance or direct involvement of the sinus node. As cardiomyopathy progresses, decreased stroke volumes can also result in tachycardia. Fibrosis localized to the posterior wall of the left ventricle has been noted in DMD but not in other muscular dystrophies.

Close cardiac monitoring is essential. Current care guidelines recommend that patients have a baseline cardiac assessment at the time of diagnosis or at least by 6 years old. Baseline assessments include electrocardiogram and a noninvasive cardiac imaging study such as echocardiogram. Subsequently, patients should have a cardiac evaluation every 2 years until the age of 10, then annually thereafter. If symptoms occur earlier than age 10, they should be evaluated more urgently. Increased frequency of evaluations should occur if ventricular dysfunction is diagnosed.

Early pharmacologic therapy is indicated. Angiotensin-converting-enzyme inhibitors such as lisinopril or enalapril to reduce afterload are typically used as first-line therapy. Alternatively, angiotensin II receptor blockers such as losartan may be used. Diuretics and beta-blockers are also appropriate as recommended by published heart failure guidelines. Patients with DMD commonly have a sinus tachycardia but should be assessed including use of event monitoring if necessary. There are a variety of opinions on routine use of cardiac MRI devices, steroid use, and appropriateness of transplant in these patients.

Although in general the BMD phenotype is milder and weakness develops more slowly, cardiac failure may progress rapidly, independent of progression of skeletal myopathy. In fact, some patients may present with cardiomyopathy and no discernable skeletal involvement. Seventy-five percent or more of BMD patients have ECG abnormalities, but resting sinus tachycardia is not typical as it is in DMD. Cardiac transplant should be considered in cases of BMD when rapid cardiac failure is diagnosed in the face of slowly progressive functional impairment.

Selected types of limb-girdle muscular dystrophy have associated cardiomyopathy and warrant referral to a cardiologist and close follow-up. Laminopathies (LMNA mutations) carry a high risk of cardiac disease including primary dilated cardiomyopathy conduction defects and both supraventricular and ventricular arrhythmias. Cardiac involvement is early, and sudden death has been reported.

Patients with dystroglycanopathies frequently have myocardial dysfunction. Patients with the fukutin-related protein (FKRP) gene develop an early dilated cardiomyopathy whereas those with the Fukuyama-type present in the second decade.

Thirty to fifty percent of patients with FKRP have cardiomyopathy. Arrhythmias have not been reported. No increased risk of cardiac involvement is seen in COL6 or SEPN1 diseases. LAMA 2 (merosin deficiency) patients develop severe heart failure, noted in about one-third of patients whether or not they are symptomatic.

Care guideline recommendations suggest that all patients undergo cardiac evaluation at the time of diagnosis. If diagnosed with dystroglycanopathy or laminopathy, annual cardiac examinations are recommended. If symptomatic, examinations every 6 months are suggested. Standard evaluations consist of ECG and echocardiogram in most patients, but because of the risk of arrhythmias and paroxysmal conductive defects in LMNA, 24-hour Holter monitoring is useful.

Tachyarrhythmia and conduction abnormalities are commonly observed in myotonic dystrophy type 1. Cardiomyopathy is not typical. Cardiac complications as a cause of death include sudden unexpected death possibly due to arrhythmias, ischemic heart disease, and progressive left ventricular dysfunction. The mean age of death is 53 years, with a third due to cardiovascular disease or sudden death. Prolonged PR and or QRS interval, second- or third-degree heart block, nonsinus rhythm noted on ECG, or an atrial tachyarrhythmia predicted sudden death in one study. Conduction defects progress and severe bradycardia or asystole may occur secondary to atrioventricular heart block.

Patients with myotonic dystrophy should be monitored with yearly ECGs and referred to cardiology if prolongation of PR or QRS complex is noted or if the patient has any cardiac symptoms. Early placement of a pacemaker or defibrillator should be considered.

Primary cardiomyopathies are rare in congenital myopathies. Some cases of nemaline myopathy have had transient cardiac failure and ECG abnormalities. Guidelines suggest that screening evaluations occur every 2 years in asymptomatic congenital myopathy patients if their genetic diagnosis is uncertain.

Kearns-Sayre syndrome is a mitochondrial myopathy featuring a triad of progressive external ophthalmoplegia, pigmentary retinopathy, and heart block. Patients may have ptosis, proximal weakness, short stature, hearing loss, and endocrine disorders. Cardiac pacemakers may be placed in patients with conduction blocks.

For any patient with neuromuscular weakness, decreased mobility, or weak abdominal muscles, constipation and reflux are chronic medical concerns. Standard treatments for constipation include dietary management, hydration, use of stool softeners, laxatives, and agents to stimulate GI motility (Ducolax, Sennakot). For acute constipation, in addition to the agents mentioned, enemas may be needed. A routine bowel management program should be introduced soon after diagnosis. Chronic constipation may require daily use of agents such as lactulose or polyethylene glycol in addition to increased fluid intake and diet modification.

H2 receptor antagonists (ranitidine, cimetidine), proton-pump inhibitors (omeprazole, lansoprazole), or antacids (magnesium or calcium carbonate) are typically used for medical management of gastroesophageal reflux. Sucralfate may be used in addition. Prokinetic agents such as metoclopramide or erythromycin may be considered if delayed gastric emptying or decreased gastric motility is diagnosed. For children on chronic corticosteroids for DMD, myasthenia gravis, or inflammatory myopathies, antacids, ranitidine or proton-pump inhibitors should be considered for GI prophylaxis.

Patients with myotonic dystrophy commonly have gastrointestinal issues. Bowel dysmotility may result in constipation and diarrhea. They have esophageal issues and are at higher risk for cholelithiasis. Liver function studies may be mildly elevated but typically not progressive Triglycerides and cholesterol may be elevated as well. DMD patients are at risk for intestinal pseudoobstruction, gastric dilatation, and dysphagia. Delayed gastric emptying in disorders such as SMA may lead to decreased oral intake.

Many neuromuscular disorders have dysphagia as another prominent feature. Palatal and pharyngeal muscles are affected in myasthenia gravis, congenital myasthenic syndromes, SMA, and congenital myopathies such as myotubular myopathy. Choking, aspiration, pocketing food, or pooling of secretions may all result from pharyngeal muscle dysfunction. Fatiguing during meals and prolonged meal times (longer than 30 min) may occur. Patients with myotonic dystrophy or facioscapulo-humeral dystrophy may have severe facial weakness leading to difficulty chewing effectively. Swallowing problems may present with coughing, aspiration pneumonia, and unintentional or unexplained weight loss.

When swallowing concerns are raised, patients should be evaluated promptly. Speech therapists, nutritionists, dentists, and gastroenterologists are all members of the multidisciplinary team who can address these issues. A swallowing study is typically indicated when there are concerns about swallow safety. As weakness progresses, recurrent pneumonias or continued weight loss may necessitate discussion regarding placement of a gastrostomy tube for feeding.

Patients with severe SMA have bulbar dysfunction. With less severe involvement, the degree of dysfunction is variable. Patients may have difficulty getting food to their mouths, limited mouth opening, fatigue with chewing, poor oral manipulation of food, and poor coordination of swallow. As patients lose head control, they are unable to use compensatory postures for swallowing. Reflux can be a life-limiting event in patients with SMA, which necessitates consideration for a Nissen procedure in addition to G-tube placement.

Careful monitoring of weight and nutritional status for neuromuscular patients is an integral part of medical management. With decreased movement and decreased calorie expenditure, patients are at risk for gaining excess weight. On the contrary, decreased oral intake due to fatigue and dysphagia can lead to weight loss. Nutrition and dietician consults are helpful in management of these issues.

Common to all neuromuscular diseases is concern for bone health. Muscle strength has a significant effect on bone density. Nonambulatory neuromuscular patients and children with chronic steroid exposure (DMD, myasthenia gravis, inflammatory myopathies) are at heightened risk for osteoporosis or osteopenia. As a result of these conditions, patients develop fractures, compression fractures, and kidney stones. According to the International Society for Clinical Densitometry guidelines (2014), if a child with risk factors for osteoporosis in the absence of trauma develops a vertebral fracture, the diagnosis of osteoporosis is confirmed. The society suggests monitoring of the spine with a lateral spine radiograph. Although there is no true consensus in terms of monitoring or prevention of osteoporosis, treatment with calcium and vitamin D is recommended. Prophylactic use of bisphosphonates has been tried without evidence that fracture rates are diminished (Quinlivan et al., 2010).

Boys with Duchenne or Becker muscular dystrophy are even at increased risk for osteopenia/osteoporosis and fractures secondary to decreased mobility and muscle weakness. The addition of steroids compounds the combined risk, resulting in significant scoliosis, osteopenia, osteoporosis, and fractures (Henricson et al, 2013).

Growth is also affected by chronic steroid use, although there are some regimens (high-dose weekend) that reportedly do not induce short stature. It is important to monitor side effects of chronic steroid use such as weight gain, Cushingoid features, hirsutism, acne, delayed growth, delayed puberty, hypertension, glucose intolerance, gastroesophageal reflux and ulcers, cataracts, disordered sleep, and behavioral changes. Vitamin D levels should also be monitored and supplemented if low.

Patients with myotonic dystrophy have multiple endocrine abnormalities, including hypothyroidism and insulin resistant diabetes. Men have hypogonadism, erectile dysfunction, decreased sperm counts, and decreased fertility. An increase in miscarriages and menstrual irregularities are common in women. Insulin-like growth factor 1 levels may be decreased as well as decreased growth hormone release. Monitoring with thyroid stimulating hormone, fasting glucose, or hemoglobin A1C should be a part of routine healthcare in these patients.

As a part of comprehensive care for neuromuscular disorders of any kind, monitoring emotional and psychosocial well-being is of upmost importance. Patients and their families face many kinds of stress—financial, social, and emotional, as well as physical. These issues should be acknowledged from very early on in the relationship so that trust and good communication are established from the outset. If the resources are available, a social worker or other qualified professional who is knowledgeable about neuromuscular disease should be introduced at the first appointment. Assessment of family and patient stressors and resources, coping skills, and emotional adjustment to the diagnosis is an ongoing, dynamic process that will continue to change over time. Continuity of care is a priority. A clinic coordinator can be very helpful to serve as a point person for a patient or family. The coordinator can provide education to the patient and family as well as the school or daycare, communicate with the medical team, offer a wide variety of resources, and ongoing support. Depending on the diagnosis and clinical presentation, palliative care may be another excellent resource to be involved early in the clinical course. Help with family and sibling support, partnering in difficult decision making, offering spiritual guidance, and dealing with loss and bereavement are a few of the palliative care services that may improve quality of life for a patient and their family.

Many neuromuscular patients will need an IEP (individual education plan) developed in conjunction with their school. An IEP is formulated to guide therapies, insure accessibility and safety, modify physical activity (if indicated), and address learning issues that may accompany such diagnoses as DMD or myotonic dystrophy.

Boys with DMD are likely to have intellectual disabilities, specifically learning disorders, and behavioral problems such as attention deficit disorder, obsessive compulsive disorder, and autism spectrum diagnoses. Depression and anxiety may be evident both in the boys as well as their families.

Congenital myotonic dystrophy patients have significant cognitive impairment, and in the noncongenital form, intelligence is generally lower (86 to 92 full-scale IQ), although IQ values vary and seem to correlate with size of the CTG repeat expansion at the DM1 gene. Other behavioral issues such as apathy, executive dysfunction, memory difficulty, and avoidant behavior are common.

Children with complex medical and genetic conditions are living longer than was predicted in the past due to better treatments and overall care. Often, the success of excellent pediatric medicine results in young adults who require ongoing, sometimes intensive, medical supervision throughout their lives. Children with DMD are living longer into adulthood due to a variety of improvements in healthcare interventions. These include multidisciplinary care, regular cardiac and respiratory monitoring, corticosteroid initiation, and assisted ventilation. Patients with neuromuscular disease present many complex transition issues and medical problems. Transitioning from a nurturing pediatric care system to a more self-directed adult care model can be very difficult for patients and their families. Adult healthcare providers may lack expertise and interest in childhood-onset disabling conditions and services can be fragmented. Preserving wellness, function, independence, activity, participation in society, and quality of life needs to be the ultimate focus, not necessarily episodic or acute care management.

A consensus policy statement, issued by the American Academy of Pediatrics, the American Academy of Family Physicians, and the American College of Physicians American Society of Internal Medicine, states that the transition of care should "maximize lifelong functioning and potential through the provision of high-quality, developmentally appropriate healthcare services that continues uninterrupted as the individual moves from adolescence to adulthood" (AAFP et al., 2002). An effective transition includes having a primary care provider with responsibility for transition planning, incorporating the necessary knowledge and skills to provide developmentally appropriate healthcare transition services, maintaining an up-to-date portable medical summary, creating a written healthcare transition plan by age 14, implementing recommended preventive service guidelines, and ensuring continuous health insurance coverage (AAFP et al., 2002). According to the 2005–2006 National Survey of Children With Special Healthcare Needs, only 41.2% of youth aged 12 to 17 years have ever talked with healthcare providers about their changing health-related needs, decreasing dependence on parents for health management, or their eventual transition to adult care.

Healthcare professionals should be aware of both positive feelings (sense of achievement) and negative feelings (anxiety about the future) about transition. It is important to provide support to address negative feelings and the progressive effects of neuromuscular disorders such as DMD. There are many barriers that challenge families, patients, and physicians alike, which greatly complicate the process. For example, the age of typical transition can be a time when cardiac and/or pulmonary status is most vulnerable in boys with DMD, thus emphasizing the importance of transition to an adult multidisciplinary clinic or providers well versed in DMD.

As young adults with disabilities transition to more independence, physicians need to educate patients and their families about potential age-related changes and medical issues. Prevention strategies require anticipation of potential secondary conditions, recognition of changes that alter function and require intervention, and an understanding of interventions that have an influence on function. This requires that adults with childhood-onset disabling chronic diseases have access to knowledgeable healthcare providers and the medical systems necessary to implement a medical home approach to management of chronic illness and disease. Environmental, communication, attitudinal, and systems barriers must be overcome.

Pain is a significant problem for most patients with neuromuscular disease, although it is not typically a direct consequence of the disease. Most commonly, the pain is caused by immobility. A significant correlation has been shown between increased pain and lower levels of general health, vitality, social function, and physical role. Pain assessment needs to be a standard aspect of care. In a study of adults with DMD, symptoms of fatigue (40.5%), pain (73.4%), anxiety (24%), and depression (19%) were reported, and individuals often had multiple conditions.

End-of-life directives are a critical part of anticipatory care. The role of palliative care to maximize quality of life in patients with progressive neuromuscular disease cannot be overlooked. Respiratory failure can occur suddenly or in association with a prolonged process. Many families are hesitant to discuss end-of-life issues during periods of medical stability, but it is important that education about ventilatory and palliative options be discussed before ventilatory failure. There is evidence that healthcare professionals underestimate the quality of life of ventilator-dependent patients with DMD. Those choosing to forgo long-term ventilation must receive palliative care and guidance.

REFERENCES

The complete list of references for this chapter is available online at www.expertconsult.com.
See inside cover for registration details.

SELECTED REFERENCES

American Academy of Pediatrics, AAFP, American College of Physicians-American Society of Internal Medicine, 2002. A consensus statement on healthcare transitions for young adults with special healthcare needs. Pediatrics 110 (6), 1304–1306.

Bushby, K., Finkel, R., et al., 2009. Diagnosis and management of Duchenne muscular dystrophy, part 2: implementation of multidisciplinary care. Lancet Neurol. 9 (2), 177–189.

Finder, J.D., Birnkrant, D., Carl, J., et al., 2004. Respiratory care of the patient with Duchenne muscular dystrophy: ATS consensus statement. Am. J. Respir. Crit. Care Med. 170 (4), 456–465.

Henricson, E.K., Abresch, T., Cnaan, A., et al., 2013. The cooperative international neuromuscular research group Duchenne natural history study: glucocorticoid treatment preserves clinically meaningful functional milestones and reduces rate of disease progression as measured by manual muscle testing and other commonly used clinical trial outcome measures. Muscle Nerve 48 (1), 55–67.

Manzur, A.Y., Muntoni, F., Simonds, A., 2003. Muscular dystrophy campaign sponsored workshop: recommendation for respiratory care of children with spinal muscular atrophy type II and III. 13th February 2002, London, UK. Neuromuscul. Disord. 13 (2), 184–189.

McDonald, C., 2010. Neuromuscular Diseases. In: Alexander, M., Matthews, D.J. (Eds.), Pediatric Rehabilitation. Demos, New York, pp. 277–333.

Narayanaswami, P., Weiss, M., et al., 2014. Evidence-based guideline summary: diagnosis and treatment of limb-girdle and distal dystrophies: report of the guideline development subcommittee of the American Academy of Neurology and the practice issues review panel of the American Association of Neuromuscular & Electrodiagnostic Medicine. Neurology 83 (16), 1453–1463.

Quinlivan, R., Shaw, N., Bushby, K., 2010. 170th ENMC International Workshop: bone protection for corticosteroid treated Duchenne muscular dystrophy. 27–29 November 2009, Naarden, The Netherlands. Neuromuscul. Disord. 20 (11), 761–769.

Wang, C.H., Dowling, J.J., North, K., et al., 2012. Consensus statement on standard of care for congenital myopathies. J. Child Neurol. 27 (3), 363–382.

Wang, C.H., Finkel, R.S., Bertini, E.S., et al., 2007. Participants of the International Conference on SMA Standard of Care. Consensus statement for standard of care in spinal muscular atrophy. J. Child Neurol. 22 (8), 1027–1049.

E-BOOK FIGURES AND TABLES

The following figures and tables are available in the e-book at www.expertconsult.com. See inside cover for registration details.

Fig. 152-2 Resting ankle foot orthoses (AFOs).
Fig. 152-3 Neuromuscular scoliosis.

153 Endocrine Disorders of the Hypothalamus and Pituitary in Childhood and Adolescence

Roger K. Long and Stephen M. Rosenthal

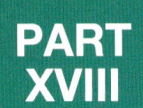 An expanded version of this chapter is available on www.expertconsult.com. See inside cover for registration details.

INTRODUCTION

Through integrated neural and hormonal signaling, the hypothalamus and pituitary regulate a broad range of physiologic processes, including statural growth, sexual maturation, lactation, metabolic actions ascribed to adrenal (glucocorticoid) and thyroid hormones, appetite, and water balance. Each of these physiologic processes involves hypothalamic/pituitary regulation of a variety of target tissues, which, in turn, regulate hypothalamic/pituitary function through feedback loops. A comprehensive endocrine approach to abnormalities of any of these physiologic loops or axes requires consideration of disorders intrinsic to the hypothalamus/pituitary or to the target tissues. This chapter will focus on those endocrine disorders specifically caused by abnormalities of the hypothalamus and pituitary.

ANATOMIC AND PHYSIOLOGIC ASPECTS

The hypothalamus is an evolutionarily conserved region of the mammalian brain. The hypothalamus is separated by the third ventricle and functions as the primary control center for a variety of physiologic processes, integrating neural and hormonal signaling. Hypothalamic nuclei are not well-demarcated regions; however, these cell groups in the walls of the third ventricle possess specific physiologic functions. The supraoptic and paraventricular nuclei produce arginine vasopressin (AVP, also known as antidiuretic hormone [ADH]) and oxytocin. Paraventricular nuclei and arcuate nuclei release thyrotropin-releasing hormone (TRH), corticotropin-releasing hormone (CRH), somatostatin (SST), growth-hormone-releasing hormone (GHRH), gonadotropin-releasing hormone (GnRH), and dopamine into the hypophysial portal circulation to regulate the synthesis and release of anterior pituitary hormones. In addition, hypothalamic neurons that regulate appetite and energy balance are also located in the paraventricular and arcuate nuclei of the hypothalamus, such as proopiomelanocortin (POMC), neuropeptide Y (NPY), and agouti-related protein (AgRP)–expressing neurons.

The pituitary (hypophysis) is housed in the sella turcica and is attached to the hypothalamus by the hypophysial stalk, which serves as an anatomic and functional link between the hypothalamus and the pituitary. The optic chiasm is situated directly anterior to the pituitary stalk (Fig. 153-1). The pituitary is small, weighing about half a gram, and is divided into the anterior lobe (adenohypophysis), which is embryonically derived from oral ectoderm (Rathke's pouch); the posterior lobe (neurohypophysis), which is a downward extension of the diencephalon; and a vestigial intermediate lobe. Six hormones,

growth hormone (GH), thyroid-stimulating hormone (TSH), adrenocorticotropic hormone (ACTH), follicle-stimulating hormone (FSH), luteinizing hormone (LH), and prolactin (PRL), are synthesized, stored, and secreted from well-differentiated distinct cell types (somatotrophs, thyrotrophs, corticotrophs, gonadotrophs, and lactotrophs) within the adenohypophysis. The neurohypophysis synthesizes, stores, and secretes AVP and oxytocin.

The blood supply in the hypothalamic–pituitary–portal system allows bidirectional hypothalamic–pituitary hormonal interaction. The superior hypophysial arteries from the internal carotid arteries form a primary plexus that travel down to the anterior pituitary as the major blood supply. The hypothalamic–pituitary–portal circulation carries the hypothalamic releasing and inhibiting hormones to the adenohypophysis. Retrograde blood flow within the internal capillary plexus (gomitoli), derived from the stalk branches of the superior hypophysial arteries, provides local hormonal feedback to the hypothalamus.

Normal development of the hypothalamus and the pituitary relies on expression of multiple homeodomain transcriptions factors, morphogenic proteins, and growth factors. Differentiation of anterior pituitary cell types requires a spatiotemporally regulated cascade of homeodomain transcription factors. Several pituitary-specific transcription factors, such as Lhx3/Lhx4 (LIM-homeobox-3 and 4), Rpx (Rathke's pouch homeobox, also known as Hesx1), Pitx (pituitary homeobox), Prop-1, Pit-1, POU1F1, Sox2, and Sox3, are important determinants of pituitary cell lineages. Mutations in these and other transcription factors can lead to either isolated or combined pituitary hormone deficiencies, with or without detectable anatomic abnormalities (Dauber et al., 2014).

HYPOTHALAMIC/PITUITARY DISORDERS OF PUBERTAL DEVELOPMENT

Normal Physiology of Puberty and Adrenarche

Puberty is the transitional period between the juvenile state and adulthood, characterized by attainment of secondary sex characteristics and reproductive capability. The control center of puberty is comprised of hypothalamic GnRH neurosecretory neurons (pulse generator). The GnRH pulse generator becomes pulsatile by midgestation, and remains active until about 6 months of age in boys and 12 to 24 months in girls. Between late infancy and the onset of puberty, the GnRH pulse generator becomes relatively quiescent as a consequence of a poorly defined central nervous system (CNS) inhibitory mechanism. After a quiescent period of approximately 10 years, the

GnRH pulse generator is disinhibited, leading to increased amplitude and frequency of LH and FSH secretion, and resulting in increased sex steroid production (estradiol and testosterone) and attainment of physical puberty. Kisspeptin and the kisspeptin receptor, also known as GPR54, have emerged as key regulators of the hypothalamic–pituitary–gonadal (HPG) axis, triggering and guiding the tempo of sexual maturation at puberty (Oakley et al., 2009). In addition, the tachykinin neurokinin B and its receptor NK3R also serve as central regulators for normal gonadatropin secretion and pubertal development, and MKRN3 appears to have an inhibitory function in pubertal regulation (Abreu et al., 2013; Bulcao et al., 2014).

The normal age of onset of secondary sexual characteristics is 8 to 13 years in girls and 9 to 14 years in boys. The appearance of secondary sexual characteristics, acceleration of growth, and the capacity of reproduction are hallmarks of puberty. In females, secondary sexual characteristics include breast development, the appearance of pubic and axillary hair, maturation of the labia, and estrogenization of the vaginal mucosa. The development of pubic and axillary hair is influenced by androgens produced in both the adrenal cortex and the ovary. Menarche usually occurs 2 to 3 years after initiation of breast development. The pubertal growth spurt, which normally occurs in the early stages of puberty for girls, can result in a gain in height of 25 cm or more. In males, puberty begins with testicular enlargement (≥2.5 cm in the longest dimension) followed by the appearance of sexual hair and phallic enlargement. The growth spurt occurs during midpuberty, which results in an average 28-cm gain in height. Abnormalities of puberty include sexual precocity and delayed or arrested puberty, each with a broad differential diagnosis.

Sexual Precocity

Sexual precocity is usually defined as the development of secondary sexual characteristics before 6 to 7 years of age in girls, and before 9 years of age in boys. Precocious puberty is defined as early puberty specifically resulting from premature reactivation of the GnRH pulse generator. Precocious puberty most commonly is idiopathic, but can result from a broad range of abnormalities, including CNS tumors, hamartoma of the tuber cinereum, congenital malformations, subarachnoid cysts, CNS infection, irradiation, and trauma. The incidence of precocious puberty is significantly higher in females. In studies of girls with precocious puberty, idiopathic precocious puberty ranges from 63% to 74%. In contrast, only 6% of boys with precocious puberty are idiopathic. Idiopathic precocious puberty is a diagnosis of exclusion and it is, thus, essential to search for underlying neurologic causes. Tumors involving the posterior hypothalamus, such as glioma, germinoma, and teratoma, can cause precocious puberty. Most of these tumors are thought to trigger early puberty by interfering with mechanisms that normally inhibit the GnRH pulse generator. Few LH/FSH-secreting adenomas have been reported. Hamartoma of the tuber cinereum, a congenital malformation, can cause central precocious puberty. Hamartomas are small lesions (4 to 25 mm), may be sessile or pedunculated, and usually do not enlarge with time (Fig. 153-2). Histologically, they appear to be composed of normal brain tissue and contain GnRH secretory neurons, which may serve as an "ectopic pulse generator."

Human chorionic gonadotropin (hCG)–secreting tumors can cause sexual precocity in boys. Such patients do not have central precocious puberty, in that they do not have premature reactivation of the hypothalamic GnRH pulse generator. Rather, the ectopic hCG interacts with the LH/hCG receptor on testicular Leydig cells, resulting in increased testosterone secretion and virilization. In girls, ovarian estrogen secretion requires both LH and FSH. Thus ectopic secretion of hCG alone causes sexual precocity only in boys.

The accurate diagnosis of precocious puberty and its cause requires a detailed history, physical examination, hormonal testing, and imaging studies of the CNS. Precocious puberty may be familial, rare gain-of-function mutations in *KISS1* and *GPR54* (*KISS1R*) have been found, and loss-of-function mutations in *MKRN3* represent the most frequent known cause of familial central precocious puberty. The occurrence of early breast and pubic hair development is often seen in girls with precocious puberty, whereas testicular enlargement and other signs of virilization are seen in boys. Hormonal analysis demonstrates increased amplitude and frequency of LH and FSH pulsatile secretion, resulting from increased pulsatile secretion of GnRH. This finding can be demonstrated either by serial sampling of LH and FSH or by single LH/FSH measurements using highly sensitive assays. Dynamic testing using GnRH or a GnRH agonist is also used routinely to diagnose precocious puberty. Magnetic resonance imaging (MRI), with particular attention to the hypothalamic–pituitary area, should be carried out in any child diagnosed with precocious puberty.

Management

If a CNS lesion that causes precocious puberty is identified, an appropriate treatment plan for that lesion should be developed. Surgical treatment of hamartomas of the tuber cinereum carries a significant risk of morbidity and mortality, whereas medical management with GnRH agonist demonstrates excellent long-term response. Rarely, the rapid progression of pubertal development is reversed or arrested after treatment of CNS disorders causing precocious puberty. More commonly, once puberty has been initiated, it will continue, despite treatment of the primary CNS disorder. Such patients require hormonal treatment with a GnRH agonist, which desensitizes pituitary GnRH receptors, leading to suppression of the HPG axis. This treatment is commonly given by regular depot intramuscular injection or implant placement. Long-term studies demonstrate resumption of normal puberty after discontinuation of a GnRH agonist.

Delayed or Arrested Puberty

Delayed puberty may be defined, in boys, by the absence of testicular enlargement by 14 years of age, and in girls, by the absence of breast development by 13 years of age. The differential diagnosis of delayed puberty can be divided into three major categories: constitutional delay in growth, hypogonadotropic hypogonadism, and hypergonadotropic hypogonadism. Constitutional delay in growth, the most common cause of delayed puberty, is a normal variant, and is thought to result from a prolonged quiescent period of the GnRH pulse generator. Such patients often have a family history of delayed puberty and have delayed skeletal maturation without evidence of endocrinopathy or other organic diseases. Hypergonadotropic hypogonadism indicates a defect at the level of the gonads. Hypogonadotropic hypogonadism indicates a defect at the level of the hypothalamus or pituitary, and can be congenital or acquired, can occur alone or in association with multiple hypothalamic and pituitary hormone deficiencies, and may be organic or functional in etiology.

Isolated Congenital Hypogonadotropic Hypogonadism

Isolated hypogonadotropic hypogonadism (IHH) caused by congenital GnRH deficiency may or may not be associated with olfactory abnormalities. IHH associated with anosmia or hyposmia is referred to as Kallmann syndrome, and is thought to be a consequence of defective embryonic migration of GnRH neurons from the olfactory placode to the hypothalamus. Kallmann syndrome is the most common form of IHH. Considerable genetic heterogeneity exists for hypogonadotropic hypogonadism with or without anosmia; it is transmitted in an X-linked, autosomal-dominant, autosomal-recessive, or oligogenic fashion with variable penetrance. Mutations in the *KAL1* gene account for half of males with X-linked hypogonadotropic hypogonadism and only 5% of sporadic IHH cases. The clinical phenotype of *KAL1* mutation includes microphallus, cryptorchidism, and anosmia. Some patients may also have unilateral renal agenesis, synkinesia (mirror movements), high-arched palate, cerebellar ataxia, and pes cavus. IHH without olfactory abnormalities (normosmic IHH) and Kallman syndrome are associated with autosomal loss-of-function mutations of the fibroblast growth factor receptor 1 (*FGFR1*) (also known as *KAL2*), and with mutations in a variety of other genes, including *FGF8* (ligand for FGFR1), prokineticin-2 (*PROK2*), and prokineticin receptor-2 (*PROKR2*). Individuals with CHARGE syndrome often manifest hypogonadotropic hypogonadism and olfactory bulb aplasia, features of Kallmann syndrome. Mutations of *CHD7* (CHARGE syndrome gene) have been identified in patients with Kallmann syndrome, suggesting that IHH caused by *CHD7* mutations is a mild variant of CHARGE syndrome. Lack of correlation between genotype and phenotype has been described in Kallmann syndrome.

Normosmic IHH is associated with mutations in a variety of genes, including the GnRH receptor, the *GNRH1* gene, *GPR54*, *TAC3*, and *TACR3*. Another form of X-linked hypogonadotropic hypogonadism is associated with adrenal hypoplasia congenita caused by defects of *DAX1*. *DAX1* encodes a transcription factor that appears to play key developmental roles in the hypothalamus, pituitary, gonad, and adrenal cortex. In addition, mutations in the beta subunits of FSH and LH have been reported in association with primary amenorrhea and hypogonadism.

Hypogonadotropic Hypogonadism Associated with Multiple Hypothalamic/Pituitary Hormone Deficiencies

Hypogonadotropic hypogonadism can also present in combination with other hypothalamic/pituitary hormone deficiencies. Mutations of pituitary transcription factors known to cause delayed puberty include *Prop-1* and *Lhx3*. Combined pituitary hormone deficiencies caused by mutations in *Prop-1* occur with an incidence of about 1 in 8000 births. Patients with mutations in *Prop-1* have combined pituitary hormone deficiencies, which may include deficiencies of GH, PRL, TSH, and gonadotropins. Such patients have hypogonadotropic hypogonadism in association with short stature and hypothyroidism. Mutations in *Lhx3* have been associated with anterior pituitary hypoplasia and complete deficits of GH, PRL, TSH, and gonadotropins. *Lhx3* mutations are also associated with decreased range of motion in the cervical spine.

Other genetic factors that lead to delayed puberty include mutations of prohormone convertase (PC1), leptin, and leptin receptor genes. A defect in PC1 has been shown to disrupt GnRH processing, and results in hypogonadotropic hypogonadism and obesity associated with impaired processing of insulin and POMC. Mutations in leptin and the leptin receptor are associated with a similar clinical picture of hypogonadotropic hypogonadism, hyperinsulinemia, and obesity. Congenital midline defects of the CNS, such as septo-optic dysplasia (SOD), empty sella syndrome, and Rathke's cyst, are often associated with hypothalamic/pituitary dysfunction, which may include hypogonadotropic hypogonadism.

Numerous CNS lesions can lead to hypogonadotropic hypogonadism, including CNS tumors, CNS infection, invasive diseases, cranial irradiation, and trauma. These CNS disorders often present with combined anterior and posterior pituitary hormone deficiencies. CNS tumors of the sella and parasellar region associated with multiple hypothalamic/pituitary hormone deficiencies include craniopharyngioma, pituitary adenomas, optic and hypothalamic gliomas, and germ-cell tumors. Delayed or arrested puberty is the second most common presenting symptom of CNS tumors after headache. Craniopharyngiomas, the most common tumor of the sella and parasellar region in children, are slow-growing, space-occupying tumors (Fig. 153-3). Most patients present before their teenage years with headache, visual loss, and multiple hypothalamic/pituitary hormone deficits. Pituitary adenomas in children with pituitary hormone hypersecretion usually present as microadenomas (<1 cm in diameter). Prolactinoma, prolactin-secreting pituitary adenoma, is the most common pituitary adenoma in the pediatric population and frequently is associated with delayed or arrested puberty. Nonsecreting microadenomas found incidentally by MRI are common in children, about 28% of children. Nonsecreting macroadenomas (>1 cm in diameter) are rare, but can also cause delayed puberty, at least in part, through elevation of prolactin as a consequence of stalk compression.

Functional Hypogonadotropic Hypogonadism

Reproductive capability is intimately linked to nutritional and metabolic homeostasis. Chronic systemic disease, malnutrition, hypothyroidism, hypercortisolism, poorly controlled diabetes mellitus, and anorexia nervosa are known to cause delayed or arrested pubertal development as a consequence of hypogonadotropic hypogonadism. Functional gonadotropin deficiency may be associated with marijuana use and may occur in some female athletes and ballet dancers. In general, weight loss to less than 80% of ideal weight may result in functional gonadotropin deficiency.

Evaluation of Delayed or Arrested Puberty

As part of an initial evaluation, basal gonadotropin levels (LH, FSH) should be measured. Elevated gonadotropins indicate primary ovarian or testicular failure, whereas low or normal gonadotropins indicate either constitutional delay or hypogonadotropic hypogonadism. A GnRH stimulation test is often useful in distinguishing patients with constitutional delay from those with hypogonadotropic hypogonadism. If hypogonadotropic hypogonadism is strongly suspected, further evaluation to identify a specific etiology should be undertaken. An important aspect of the physical examination is evaluation of the sense of smell. Any patient with proven hypogonadotropic hypogonadism should have a thorough evaluation of all hypothalamic/pituitary hormones and should undergo an MRI with particular focus on the third ventricular area.

Management

Once the etiology of delayed or arrested puberty has been established, an appropriate treatment plan can be designed. For constitutionally delayed pubertal development, short-term (3 to 6 months) low-dose sex steroid replacement may be useful to induce maturation of the GnRH pulse generator. Permanent hypogonadotropic hypogonadism requires long-term sex hormone replacement. Testosterone for boys can be administrated either by intramuscular or subcutaneous injection or topically. Long-term hormonal therapy for girls includes the use of oral, intramuscular, or transdermal estrogen and progestin cycling.

DISORDERS OF PROLACTIN SECRETION
Normal Biochemistry and Physiology of Prolactin

Regulation of prolactin secretion is distinct from that of other anterior pituitary hormones. PRL is the only pituitary hormone that is regulated predominantly by the hypothalamus through an inhibitory mechanism mediated by dopamine via the hypothalamic–pituitary–portal circulation. The principal physiologic functions of PRL are enhanced mammary gland development during pregnancy and lactation. PRL may be increased through physiologic and pathologic mechanisms. Physiologic stimuli include pregnancy, lactation, stress, sleep, and exercise. Pathologic causes of hyperprolactinemia include prolactinomas; injury to the hypothalamic–pituitary stalk; a variety of systemic disorders, including chronic renal failure and cirrhosis; and a variety of drugs.

Clinical Features and Management of Hyperprolactinemia

In postpubertal females the principal clinical feature of hyperprolactinemia, regardless of the cause, is galactorrhea, which may be unilateral or bilateral. Other clinical features may include delayed or arrested puberty and hypogonadism; menstrual irregularities, including amenorrhea in females; and gynecomastia in males secondary to hypogonadism. Prolactinoma is the most common tumor of the pituitary, comprising about 50% of anterior pituitary adenomas. Most prolactinomas are microprolactinomas, and normally do not cause significant mass effects. Macroprolactinomas are predominately found in males because of poor appreciation of hypogonadal symptoms and inability to manifest menstrual irregularities or galactorrhea, early indicators of hyperprolactinemia.

If a prolactinoma is diagnosed, therapeutic options include medical management with dopamine agonists, surgery, and adjunctive radiotherapy. Medical management is considered the principal intervention; however, microprolactinomas can be removed surgically, though with variable recurrence rates. Macroprolactinomas are less likely to be cured surgically and often require chronic dopamine agonist treatment. Dopamine agonists are effective and safe pharmacologic interventions for both micro- and macroprolactinoma. Withdrawal of medication after long-term therapy has been safe, although careful monitoring of tumor progression is necessary. Adjunctive radiotherapy has been considered beneficial in some patients with macroprolactinoma. The skill and experience of the surgeon clearly play a role in determining the optimal treatment and outcome.

HYPOTHALAMIC/PITUITARY DISORDERS OF GLUCOCORTICOID PRODUCTION

ACTH is produced in response to stimulation, principally by hypothalamic CRH, and increases adrenal production of cortisol, the principal glucocorticoid. Cortisol, in turn, regulates the production of both CRH and ACTH through negative-feedback loops. An intact hypothalamic–pituitary–adrenal (HPA) axis is essential for general homeostasis, including regulation of blood pressure and glucose, and for response to stress. Increased levels of circulating glucocorticoids lead to Cushing's syndrome, whereas hypersecretion of pituitary ACTH leads to Cushing's disease. Inadequate production of CRH/ACTH will cause adrenal glucocorticoid insufficiency.

Adrenocorticotropic Excess

Excessive production of ACTH from the pituitary arises either from CRH overproduction or from a primary ACTH-producing adenoma. The first sign of Cushing's disease in a growing child is often impaired linear growth. Other classic signs and symptoms of Cushing's disease include central obesity, buffalo hump, plethora, "moon facies," acne, striae, hypertension, hirsutism, fatigue, pubertal delay or arrest, bruising, and headache. Usually, at the time of diagnosis, ACTH-producing adenomas are significantly smaller than other pituitary adenomas (Fig. 153-4).

Determination of the cause of Cushing's syndrome can pose significant challenges. Patients with hypercortisolism will demonstrate elevated urinary cortisol excretion and loss of normal diurnal variation in plasma cortisol and ACTH. Endogenous hypercortisolism is either ACTH dependent or ACTH independent. Of the ACTH-dependent causes, Cushing's disease is most common. A rare ACTH-dependent cause is ectopic ACTH production associated with a variety of extrapituitary neoplasms. In general, patients with Cushing's disease show suppression of cortisol and ACTH only with high-dose dexamethasone administration. An MRI of the hypothalamic/pituitary area should be obtained if Cushing's disease is suspected, though small adenomas may not be visualized. Bilateral inferior petrosal sinus sampling before and after ovine CRH stimulation may be utilized to determine a pituitary source of ACTH production.

Transsphenoidal resection of pituitary adenomas has emerged as the treatment of choice for Cushing's disease (Lonser et al., 2013). Because of small size, some of these tumors are difficult to identify intraoperatively. The recurrence rate after surgery is about approximately 8%, even in the hands of skilled neurosurgeons (Lonser et al., 2013). Radiotherapy has been shown to be effective for unsuccessful transsphenoidal surgery. Other therapeutic options for recurrent Cushing's disease include repeated pituitary exploration, bilateral adrenalectomy, and the use of pharmacologic agents that directly impair cortisol synthesis and secretion.

Adrenocorticotropic Hormone Deficiency

Secondary adrenal insufficiency is defined as hypocortisolism as a consequence of ACTH deficiency. Secondary adrenal insufficiency can be isolated or occur as part of multiple hypothalamic/pituitary deficiencies. Chronic suppression of CRH and ACTH by long-term glucocorticoid therapy also can result in secondary adrenal insufficiency.

Isolated ACTH deficiency is a rare cause of secondary adrenal insufficiency, caused by either CRH deficiency or a primary decrease in ACTH production by corticotrophs. Clinical presentation is highly variable. Neonatal onset of isolated ACTH deficiency usually presents with sudden, severe episodes of hypoglycemia, sometimes with seizure and coma. Neonates may also present with prolonged cholestatic jaundice. Death may occur if treatment is not initiated promptly. Over 70% of these patients have a loss-of-function mutation in the *TPIT* gene, which encodes a transcription factor that is expressed specifically in corticotrophs and is required for expression of POMC, the precursor of ACTH. ACTH deficiency can be associated with multiple hypothalamic/pituitary hormone deficiencies as described previously.

Secondary adrenal insufficiency is characterized by an inappropriately low serum cortisol level and a nonelevated ACTH level suggestive of inadequacy of the HPA axis. Assessment of the HPA axis adequacy is challenging. A peak cortisol level after an injection of synthetic ACTH may be used to assess adrenal gland responsiveness to ACTH. However, a false normal response will occur in the setting of acute pituitary dysfunction. HPA axis integrity can be confirmed by dynamic testing protocols that measure the adrenal glucocorticoid production response to acute hypoglycemia induced by insulin injection or an overnight cortisol insufficiency caused by metyrapone treatment, an inhibitor of the last enzymatic step in cortisol production.

Cortisol (hydrocortisone) replacement is based on studies of the cortisol secretory rate in the pediatric population, which is 7 to 9 mg/m^2/day. During periods of significant stress, such as febrile illness and surgery, such patients are managed routinely with a temporary increase in glucocorticoids (given orally or parenterally) at doses up to 50 mg/m^2/day of hydrocortisone.

HYPOTHALAMIC/PITUITARY DISORDERS OF STATURAL GROWTH

Statural growth is a complex process influenced by multiple factors. Endocrine regulation of postnatal growth stems from hormones produced in the hypothalamus and the pituitary, including GHRH, SST, GH, TRH, TSH, CRH, and ACTH. Abnormal statural growth related to either GH deficiency or GH excess is discussed in this section.

Pulsatile GH secretion is regulated principally by two hypothalamic regulatory peptides, GHRH and SST. Acute glucocorticoid administration stimulates GH secretion, whereas chronically elevated glucocorticoids inhibit GH, as seen in Cushing's disease and during chronic administration of glucocorticoids. Sex steroids (estradiol and testosterone) stimulate GH secretion, contributing to a pubertal rise in GH. In addition, GH levels are decreased in hypothyroidism. The growth-promoting effects of GH are mediated principally through endocrine, autocrine, and paracrine production of insulin-like growth factors (IGFs).

Growth Hormone Deficiency

Children with congenital GH deficiency are of normal size at birth. However, after approximately 6 months of life, growth failure becomes apparent when linear growth becomes GH dependent. Usually, children with GH deficiency are short and cherubic, with a doll-like appearance. Approximately 10% to 20% of GH-deficient patients present with severe hypoglycemia in addition to short stature. In the neonatal period, hypoglycemia and microphallus strongly suggest GH deficiency.

Although abnormalities can occur at any level of the GHRH-GH-IGF-I axis, the majority of these abnormalities occur at the hypothalamic/pituitary level. In fact, most patients with GH deficiency (80% to 90%) are GHRH deficient. As with gonadotropins or ACTH, a deficiency of GH may be isolated or associated with other hypothalamic/pituitary hormone abnormalities. Isolated GH deficiency has been reported to be familial in 3% to 30% of cases. Mutations have been found in only a minority of such patients, primarily involving the *GH1* and *GHRHR* genes. Mutations in the gene *Rpx/Hesx1* are associated with septo-optic dysplasia, a common midline malformation characterized by the classical triad of optic nerve hypoplasia, midline malformations (such as agenesis of the corpus callosum and absence of the septum pellucidum), and pituitary hypoplasia with consequent panhypopituitarism. The phenotypes of mutations in the *Rpx/*

Hesx1 gene are highly variable, ranging from isolated GH deficiency without any midline defects, to the complete spectrum of the disease with panhypopituitarism.

Evaluation of a child with suspected GH deficiency includes a thorough history, physical examination, and careful review of growth charts and laboratory studies. Severe neonatal hypoglycemia is suggestive of GH deficiency. Most children with GH deficiency will have not only short stature, but also a subnormal height velocity with relative preservation of weight and head circumference. The diagnosis of GH deficiency is often difficult to make with a single blood test, in light of the pulsatile nature of GH secretion. GH-dependent IGF-I and IGF binding protein 3 (IGF-BP3) levels, and provocative tests of GH secretion have been used widely to evaluate GH status. If a diagnosis of GH deficiency is made, it is essential to evaluate all pituitary hormones, and to obtain an MRI with particular attention to the third ventricular area.

The principal treatment of children with GH deficiency is recombinant GH administered as a daily subcutaneous injection. Some children with GH deficiency on the basis of GHRH deficiency have been treated successfully with GHRH. Adequacy of treatment is determined by assessment of growth velocity and serum IGF-I and IGF-BP3 levels. Recent studies demonstrate beneficial effects of continued GH treatment (at lower doses) after final height is reached in adolescents with permanent GH deficiency. GH treatment occasionally is associated with side effects, such as increased intracranial pressure, hyperglycemia, and slipped capital femoral epiphysis.

Growth Hormone Excess

Gigantism is a rare condition caused by GH excess in children who have open epiphyses, primarily caused by increased GH production from the pituitary. GH-producing adenomas constitute up to 10% of pituitary adenomas. Ectopic GHRH overproduction is a rare cause of GH excess. In addition, McCune–Albright syndrome (MAS) can present with gigantism because of constitutively active G proteins in somatotrophs that result in increased GH secretion.

Accelerated longitudinal growth and acromegalic features (enlarged head, large hands and feet, big tongue, and broad nose) are the most prominent signs of GH excess. In girls, menstrual irregularity is common. Mass effect of the tumor can cause impaired vision and headache caused by increased intracranial pressure. Some patients also may have hyperprolactinemia as a result of cosecretion. A diagnosis of pituitary gigantism is made by demonstrating nonsuppressible GH in response to glucose loading, in association with elevated IGF-I and IGF-BP3 levels. Usually, sellar MRI will reveal a pituitary mass.

The goal of treatment in GH-secreting adenomas is normalization of GH and IGF-I levels. Transsphenoidal surgery has resulted in a greater than 80% cure rate, and thus remains the first choice of treatment. If surgery is unsuccessful, somatostatin analogs, GH receptor antagonists, and dopamine agonists can be used. Somatostatin analogs may be used as first-line treatment should the patient prefer medication over surgery (Colao et al., 2009). Radiotherapy may be beneficial to treat an adenoma that increases in size despite medical therapy.

HYPOTHALAMIC/PITUITARY DISORDERS OF THYROID FUNCTION
Normal Thyroid Physiology

Under regulation by the hypothalamus and pituitary, the thyroid gland produces thyroid hormones, which have broad effects on metabolism, growth, and CNS development. TSH is a heterodimeric glycoprotein consisting of alpha and beta subunits. The alpha subunit is common to TSH, LH, FSH, and hCG, whereas the beta subunit confers specificity. TSH acts on the thyroid gland to stimulate thyroid hormone synthesis and secretion. TSH is negatively regulated by thyroid hormones and positively regulated by TRH.

Central Hypothyroidism

Central (hypothalamic/pituitary) hypothyroidism is rare in comparison to primary hypothyroidism, and may be congenital or acquired. Signs and symptoms associated with hypothyroidism may arise insidiously and are often nonspecific. In the neonatal period, newborns may have lethargy, hypotonia, hypothermia, or prolonged jaundice. Untreated hypothyroidism during infancy and early childhood can result in developmental delay, mental retardation, and poor statural growth. Presenting symptoms in older children include weight gain, subnormal height velocity, constipation, cold intolerance, hoarse voice, dry skin, and lethargy.

Congenital TSH deficiency occurs in 1:50,000 to 150,000 newborns. Underlying etiologies include isolated TSH deficiency, developmental defects of the hypothalamus and pituitary, and familial panhypopituitarism. Isolated TSH deficiency is caused by usually autosomal-recessive mutations in the TSH beta subunit. TSH deficiency, in combination with other pituitary hormone deficiencies, is seen frequently in patients with *HESX1*, *PIT-1*, and *PROP-1* mutations or CNS insults. In addition, isolated central hypothyroidism can result from a loss-of-function mutation in the TRH receptor. Patients with congenital TSH deficiency are usually not detected by neonatal screening for hypothyroidism, as most programs are designed to screen for the hyperthyrotropinemia that accompanies primary hypothyroidism.

With respect to laboratory assessment of thyroid function, it is critical to recognize that normal ranges vary significantly with age. In particular, TSH and free T4 are relatively high in newborns in comparison to older infants, children, and adolescents. The principal goals of treating central hypothyroidism are normalization of thyroxine levels and prevention of mental retardation and growth impairment. Thus thyroxine replacement should be instituted promptly after diagnosis of hypothyroidism, regardless of etiology.

Central Hyperthyroidism

Most cases of hyperthyroidism in the pediatric population are autoimmune and TSH-independent. Central hyperthyroidism as a consequence of a pituitary TSH-secreting adenoma is exceedingly rare. Such patients may have a prominent local mass effect of the tumor. Signs and symptoms of hyperthyroidism, such as agitation, tall stature, goiter, tremor, and palpitation, are manifested in central hyperthyroidism. Biochemically, patients with central hyperthyroidism have elevated concentrations of TSH in the context of elevated T4 and T3. If a pituitary adenoma is not identifiable on imaging studies, rare selective pituitary T3 resistance attributable to inactivating mutation of thyroid hormone receptor beta should be considered. Surgical removal of the tumor is the treatment of choice for TSH-secreting pituitary adenoma. The treatment of selective pituitary T3 resistance remains a therapeutic challenge.

HYPOTHALAMIC DISORDERS OF APPETITE REGULATION AND ENERGY BALANCE

Appetite and energy balance are regulated by a complex network, in which the hypothalamus serves as the central

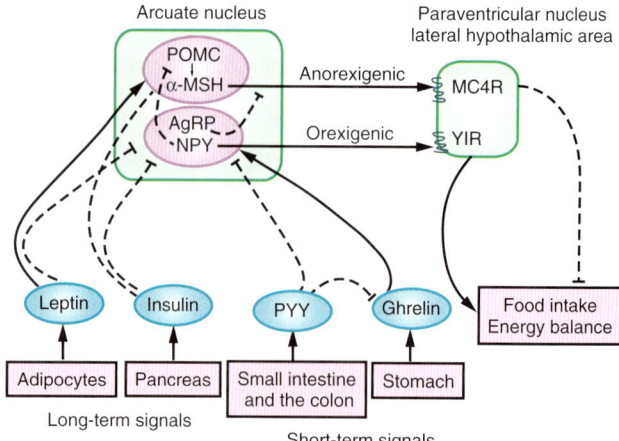

Figure 153-5. Hormonal regulation of food intake and energy balance in the hypothalamus. The dashed lines indicate inhibitory effects and the solid lines with arrows indicate stimulatory effects. Long-term signals affecting body fat mass include leptin and insulin, whereas short-term signals determining meal initiation and termination include peptide YY$_{3-36}$ and ghrelin. AgRP, agouti-related protein; α-MSH, α-melanocyte-stimulating protein; MC4R, melanocortin 4 receptor; POMC, proopiomelanocortin; PYY, peptide YY$_{3-36}$; Y1R, Y1 subtype of neuropeptide Y (NPY) receptor.

processing unit for hormonal, nutritional, and neuronal input from both peripheral tissue and higher brain centers. In humans, it is well known that hypothalamic damage can lead to excessive weight gain, hypothalamic obesity. These patients present with excessive weight gain without response to caloric restriction or exercise. Traditionally, the ventromedial hypothalamus has been viewed as the "satiety" center, because damage to the ventromedial hypothalamus can cause hyperphagic obesity. In contrast, the lateral hypothalamus has been viewed as the "feeding" center, because its disruption leads to hypophagia and weight loss.

Insights into mechanisms of hypothalamic obesity derive from advances in our understanding of hypothalamic control of appetite regulation and energy balance (Fig. 153-5). Energy storage and appetite are regulated at the hypothalamus through signaling by leptin and insulin. Both leptin and insulin affect anorexigenic and orexigenic pathways in the hypothalamus. The effects of leptin are quantitatively much greater than that of insulin, and there are complex responses of various neuron subsets within hypothalamic nuclei (Sohn et al., 2013; Morton et al., 2014). In the anorexigenic pathway, leptin maintains expression of POMC in the arcuate nuclei, and POMC-derived α-melanocyte-stimulating hormone (α-MSH) activates the melanocortin-4 receptor (MC4R) in the paraventricular nuclei and the lateral hypothalamic area. This melanocortin signal is appetite suppressing. In addition, leptin and insulin inhibit NPY and AgRP within the arcuate nuclei, both of which are appetite-stimulating peptides. NPY decreases POMC expression through the neuropeptide Y1 receptor (Y1R). AgRP is an antagonist for MC4R, competing with α-MSH for binding to the MC4R and leading to increased food intake.

Hypothalamic obesity frequently is seen in children with hypothalamic insults, such as brain tumor, surgery, irradiation, or trauma. Approximately 50% of children with craniopharyngioma develop hypothalamic obesity. Other tumors, such as germinoma, optic glioma, prolactinoma, and hypothalamic astrocytoma, also are associated with hypothalamic obesity. These patients usually have unrelenting weight gain after tumor removal or radiotherapy, without documented excessive food intake. Reduced physical activity, rather than increased energy intake, was shown to be primarily responsible for obesity in patients with craniopharyngioma. Decreased resting energy expenditure also may be present in children after brain tumor therapy, including hypothalamic irradiation (greater than 51 Gy).

Numerous examples of monogenic obesity have been described at many levels of hypothalamic control of energy balance, including leptin, leptin receptor, POMC, prohormone convertase 1/3 (PC1/3), and MC4R (Ranadive and Vaisse, 2008). Mutations in leptin and leptin receptor are extremely rare monogenic forms of morbid obesity. The children reported with leptin deficiency had normal birth weight, but became hyperphagic in infancy and developed severe obesity with undetectable levels of leptin. Exogenous administration of leptin induced sustained weight loss because of loss of fat mass. Similar results were observed in adults with congenital leptin deficiency. Mutations of the leptin receptor also are associated with severe childhood obesity associated with absent pubertal development, reduced levels of both TSH and GH, and impaired immune function. Loss-of-function mutations in *POMC* result in severe hyperphagia and obesity as a consequence of lack of MC4R activation by α-MSH, and adrenal insufficiency as a consequence of defective synthesis of ACTH. Patients may also have red hair from lack of MC1R activation by α-MSH in melanocytes. Mutations in *PC1/3*, thought to result in defective processing of POMC to α-MSH, as well as defective ACTH synthesis, lead to hyperphagia, early onset obesity, and partial ACTH deficiency. *MC4R* mutations have been found in 2.5% of obese children, representing the most common genetic defects in human obesity.

HYPOTHALAMIC/PITUITARY DISORDERS OF WATER BALANCE

Under normal circumstances, plasma osmolality is maintained within a relatively narrow range by adequate water intake, regulated by thirst, and appropriate free water excretion by the kidneys, mediated by appropriate secretion of vasopressin (AVP). AVP is produced in the magnocellular neurons, which originate in the paraventricular and supraoptic nuclei of the hypothalamus and terminate in the posterior pituitary gland. AVP exerts its antidiuretic action by binding to the X chromosome–encoded V2 vasopressin receptor (V2R) on the basolateral membrane of renal collecting duct epithelial cells. After V2R activation, the water channel aquaporin 2 (AQP-2) is shuttled to the apical membrane of collecting duct epithelial cells, resulting in increased water permeability and antidiuresis.

AVP secretion is regulated principally by changes in plasma osmolality and in effective circulating volume. AVP levels are normally low and do not increase until plasma osmolality exceeds 280 mOsm/kg, but responds to as little as 1% increases in plasma osmolality. AVP secretion also is regulated by changes in blood volume. Baroreceptors in the venous and arterial circulation become activated when stretched by increases in intravascular volume, leading to inhibition of AVP secretion. In addition, a variety of other factors affect AVP secretion. It is stimulated by pain, stress, and a variety of drugs, and is inhibited by surgery, trauma, and infiltrative processes of the hypothalamus.

Clinical disorders of water balance are common, and abnormalities in many steps involving AVP secretion and responsiveness have been described (Ranadive and Rosenthal, 2009). The focus of this section is on the principal hypothalamic/pituitary disorders of water balance, diabetes insipidus (DI), and the syndrome of inappropriate antidiuretic hormone secretion (SIADH).

Diabetes Insipidus

DI may result from a deficiency of AVP or from nephrogenic causes that manifest resistance to AVP. Central DI is rarely congenital and more frequently acquired. Congenital central DI may be associated with congenital conditions, including congenital hypopituitarism, Wolfram syndrome, and SOD, and through both autosomal-dominant and autosomal-recessive mutations in the *AVP/NPII* gene. Of the latter, the autosomal-dominant causes are more common, and are thought to be a consequence of heterozygous mutations in the *AVP/NPII* gene that lead to misfolding of the precursor AVP/NPII protein. The dominant negative effect is thought to occur as a consequence of the misfolded precursor protein, which accumulates in the endoplasmic reticulum of vasopressinergic neurons, ultimately resulting in death of these neurons. In such patients, clinical DI usually develops several months to years after birth. A rare autosomal-recessive form of central DI has been reported, resulting in a biologically inactive AVP.

Acquired forms of DI occur in association with a variety of disorders in which there is destruction or degeneration of vasopressinergic neurons. Etiologies include primary tumors (e.g., craniopharyngioma, germinoma) or metastases, infection (meningitis, encephalitis), histiocytosis, granuloma, vascular disorders, and autoimmune disorders (lymphocytic infundibuloneurohypophysitis). Acquired DI may occur in association with trauma and surgery. Idiopathic DI is a diagnosis of exclusion, and one that is made with decreasing frequency concurrent with improved sensitivity of CNS MRI and of cerebrospinal fluid and serum tumor markers.

The principal presenting sign of DI is polyuria, which, in addition to deficiency or impaired responsiveness to AVP, may result from an osmotic agent (e.g., hyperglycemia in diabetes mellitus) or from excessive water intake (primary polydipsia). Hypernatremia usually does not occur if patients have an intact thirst mechanism, adequate access to fluids, and no additional ongoing fluid losses (e.g., diarrhea). Infants with DI, in addition to polyuria and polydipsia, may be irritable and have fever of unknown origin, growth failure secondary to inadequate caloric intake, and hydronephrosis. Older children may have nocturia and enuresis. DI may not be apparent in patients with coexisting untreated anterior pituitary-mediated adrenal glucocorticoid insufficiency, as cortisol is required to generate a normal free water loss.

A diagnosis of DI can be made if screening laboratory studies reveal serum hyperosmolality concurrent with inappropriately dilute urine. However, as most patients with DI do not have hyperosmolality and hypernatremia, a standardized water deprivation test is useful to distinguish DI. If DI is indicated during the water deprivation test, then an AVP level should be obtained and AVP or a synthetic analog (desmopressin) should then be administered to distinguish AVP deficiency from AVP unresponsiveness.

Once a diagnosis of central DI is made, a brain MRI of the third ventricular area should be obtained. An absent posterior pituitary "bright spot" is seen in virtually all patients with central DI. Under normal circumstances, a posterior pituitary bright spot is seen on T1-weighted images because of stored AVP in neurosecretory granules (see Fig. 153-1). In central DI patients with an absent posterior pituitary bright spot, an otherwise-normal MRI warrants close follow up with cerebrospinal fluid tumor markers and cytology, serum tumor markers, and serial contrast-enhanced brain MRIs for early detection of an evolving occult hypothalamic-stalk lesion.

In addition to treatment of a primary disease causing central DI, the drug of choice for most patients with AVP deficiency is desmopressin. This AVP analog has markedly reduced vasopressor activity in comparison to native AVP, has a prolonged half-life, and can be administered orally, intranasally, or by subcutaneous injection.

Syndrome of Inappropriate Antidiuretic Hormone Secretion

SIADH is characterized by the inability to excrete a free water load, with inappropriately concentrated urine, and resultant hyponatremia, hypo-osmolality, and natriuresis in the absence of renal dysfunction, hypothyroidism, and adrenal insufficiency. Although most patients with SIADH have inappropriately measurable or elevated levels of plasma AVP relative to plasma osmolality, 10% to 20% of patients with SIADH do not have measurable AVP levels. This may reflect issues of assay sensitivity or may indicate a syndrome resembling SIADH, nephrogenic syndrome of inappropriate antidiuresis (NSIAD), which is associated with an activating mutation in the X-linked V2R and unmeasurable circulating levels of AVP.

Euvolemia in chronic SIADH is an important distinguishing factor in the evaluation of a patient with serum hypo-osmolality and has a bearing on treatment issues. Euvolemia in chronic SIADH is thought to represent an adaptation to water overload. Natriuresis, thought to be mediated in part through secretion of atrial natriuretic peptide, also contributes to volume regulation in chronic SIADH. Cerebral salt wasting, associated with some intracranial diseases (e.g., subarachnoid hemorrhage), is often considered in the differential diagnosis of SIADH. However, the hypo-osmolality, hyponatremia, and natriuresis in cerebral salt wasting are associated with volume contraction, which distinguishes this disorder from the euvolemic condition of SIADH.

A large number of disorders and conditions are associated with SIADH. These include disorders of the CNS (e.g., infection, trauma, cerebrovascular accident, tumors), surgery, ectopic AVP production from non-CNS tumors, medications, and pulmonary disorders. Therapy for SIADH includes treatment of the underlying disorder (or discontinuation of an offending drug) and fluid restriction. Replacement of lost body sodium also may be necessary but usually can be achieved through normal dietary salt intake. Severe hyponatremia may be associated with CNS abnormalities, including seizures, and may require treatment with hypertonic intravenous sodium chloride solution. Concurrent use of a diuretic, such as furosemide, may be indicated. Urea has been used as an osmotic diuretic in pediatric SIADH and NSIAD. A variety of nonpeptide V2R antagonists have been approved by the Food and Drug Administration for use in adults.

If SIADH and hyponatremia are acute (<48 hours), it is thought that hyponatremia can be corrected quickly. However, if SIADH and hyponatremia are chronic (>48 hours), overzealous treatment can result in CNS damage, including central pontine myelinolysis. Generally, it is recommended that plasma sodium be corrected to a "safe" level of approximately 120 to 125 mEq/L, at a rate of no greater than 0.5 mEq/L per hour, with an overall correction that does not exceed 12 mEq/L in the initial 24 hours and 18 mEq/L in the initial 48 hours of treatment.

REFERENCES

The complete list of references for this chapter is available in the e-book at www.expertconsult.com.
    See inside cover for registration details.

SELECTED REFERENCES

Abreu, A.P., Dauber, A., Macedo, D.B., et al., 2013. Central precocious puberty caused by mutations in the imprinted gene MKRN3. N. Engl. J. Med. 368, 2467–2475.

Bulcao, M.D., Nahime, B.V., Latronico, A.C., 2014. New causes of central precocious puberty: The role of genetic factors. Neuroendocrinology 100, 1–8.

Colao, A., Auriemma, R.S., Galdiero, M., et al., 2009. Effects of initial therapy for five years with somatostatin analogs for acromegaly on growth hormone and insulin-like growth factor-I levels, tumor shrinkage, and cardiovascular disease: A prospective study. J. Clin. Endocrinol. Metab. 94, 3746.

Dauber, A., Rosenfeld, R.G., Hirschhorn, J.N., 2014. Genetic evaluation of short stature. J. Clin. Endocrinol. Metab. 99, 3080–3092.

Lonser, R.R., Wind, J.J., Nieman, L.K., et al., 2013. Outcome of surgical treatment of 200 children with Cushing's disease. J. Clin. Endocrinol. Metab. 98, 892–901.

Morton, G.J., Meek, T.H., Schwartz, M.W., 2014. Neurobiology of food intake in health and disease. Nat. Rev. Neurosci. 15, 367–378.

Oakley, A.E., Clifton, D.K., Steiner, R.A., 2009. Kisspeptin signaling in the brain. Endocr. Rev. 30, 713.

Ranadive, S.A., Rosenthal, S.M., 2009. Pediatric disorders of water balance. Endocrinol. Metab. Clin. North Am. 38, 663–672.

Ranadive, S.A., Vaisse, C., 2008. Lessons from extreme human obesity: Monogenic disorders. Endocrinol. Metab. Clin. North Am. 37, 733–751.

Sohn, J.W., Elmquist, J.K., Williams, K.W., 2013. Neuronal circuits that regulate feeding behavior and metabolism. Trends Neurosci. 36, 504–512.

E-BOOK FIGURES AND TABLES

The following figures and tables are available in the e-book at www.expertconsult.com. See inside cover for registration details.

Fig. 153-1 T1-weighted magnetic resonance images of the normal hypothalamus/pituitary in an 8-year-old girl.

Fig. 153-2 Hamartoma of the tuber cinereum in a 3-year-old girl by magnetic resonance imaging.

Fig. 153-3 Craniopharyngioma in a child by magnetic resonance imaging.

Fig. 153-4 Adrenocorticotropic hormone-secreting pituitary adenoma in a 15-year-old girl by magnetic resonance imaging.

154 Disorders of the Autonomic Nervous System: Autonomic Dysfunction in Pediatric Practice

Jose-Alberto Palma, Lucy Norcliffe-Kaufmann, Cristina Fuente-Mora, Leila Percival, Christy L. Spalink, and Horacio Kaufmann

INTRODUCTION

Dysfunction of the autonomic nervous system (ANS) is an increasingly recognized health problem in the pediatric population. Patients with ANS dysfunction may present with a number of seemingly unrelated symptoms, including lightheadedness on standing, syncope, labile blood pressure, problems with sweating or thermoregulation, gastrointestinal dysmotility, bladder urgency or incontinence, and sleep abnormalities.

The vast majority of complaints in children referred to an autonomic disorders clinic correspond to physiologic responses to emotional states. Neuronal pathways connect the limbic system to the autonomic system, and as a consequence, emotions have a profound effect on autonomic outflow to the organs. In these cases, rather than a primary autonomic disorder, the symptoms result from activation of the classic "flight-or-fight" autonomic response to a perceived (but not always obvious) threat.

Autonomic dysfunction in children can be secondary to metabolic disorders, including obesity, anorexia, and diabetes. Severe, sometimes life-threatening derangements of autonomic function occur in a number of rare genetic and autoimmune disorders. Autonomic dysreflexia as a result of spinal cord lesions and afferent baroreflex failure as a result of neck tumors or as sequelae of surgery or radiotherapy can occur in children and adolescents and presents with dramatic blood pressure volatility.

ANATOMY AND PHYSIOLOGY OF THE AUTONOMIC NERVOUS SYSTEM
Anatomy of the Autonomic Nervous System

The ANS innervates most of the organs in the body and controls involuntary functions to maintain homeostasis. In 1898, physiologist John Langley divided the ANS into three branches: sympathetic, parasympathetic, and enteric. The sympathetic and the parasympathetic nervous system have opposing actions.

Efferent Autonomic Pathways

The autonomic outflow from the central nervous system (CNS) to the effector organs consists of a two-neuron pathway with one synapse in the peripheral autonomic ganglia (Fig. 154-1).

Sympathetic Efferent Pathways. The cell bodies of preganglionic *sympathetic neurons* are in the intermediolateral cell column (IML) of the thoracic and lumbar spinal cord (levels T1 through L3). Preganglionic sympathetic axons leave the spinal cord as small myelinated fibers to synapse with (post)ganglionic neurons in sympathetic ganglia close to the spinal cord. Unmyelinated axons from postganglionic neurons emerge from sympathetic ganglia to synapse with target organs. Preganglionic sympathetic neurons in the IML cell column receive direct descending excitatory inputs from hypothalamic nuclei and from the ventromedial and rostral ventrolateral medulla (RVLM). Preganglionic sympathetic axons exit the spinal cord through the ventral roots toward paravertebral or prevertebral ganglia.

Parasympathetic Efferent Pathways. The cell bodies of preganglionic *parasympathetic neurons* are located in the brainstem and at the sacral (S2-S4) level of the spinal cord. Axons of preganglionic parasympathetic neurons are myelinated and leave the brainstem or spinal cord to synapse with cell bodies of postganglionic parasympathetic neurons in autonomic ganglia close to (or within) the effector organs. Short unmyelinated postganglionic parasympathetic fibers synapse with target tissues.

Efferent Neurotransmission. Acetylcholine is the neurotransmitter of preganglionic neurons, both sympathetic and parasympathetic. Acetylcholine, via activation of nicotinic receptors, produces excitation of postganglionic neurons. The main neurotransmitter of postganglionic sympathetic neurons is norepinephrine, which activates alpha- and beta-adrenergic receptors. The sympathetic neurons innervating sweat glands release acetylcholine, which activates muscarinic receptors. The main neurotransmitter of postganglionic parasympathetic neurons is also acetylcholine, which acts on different types of muscarinic receptors (Fig. 154-1).

Afferent Autonomic Pathways

The classic descriptions of the ANS were of a purely efferent motor system. The ANS, however, has afferent pathways that run parallel to the efferent pathways and can also be divided into sympathetic and parasympathetic. *Parasympathetic* afferents are small-diameter fibers that transmit information to the CNS via the vagus (X) and glossopharyngeal (IX) nerves and have their cell bodies in the nodose and petrosal ganglia, respectively. Vagal afferents relay information from aortic, cardiac, pulmonary, and gastrointestinal receptors. Glossopharyngeal afferents carry signals from baroreceptors and chemoreceptors in the carotid sinus. Parasympathetic afferents synapse with neurons in the NTS in the brainstem.

Sympathetic afferents relay information about an array of physiologic variables, including the mechanical, thermal, chemical, metabolic, and hormonal status of the skin, muscle, joints, teeth, and viscera. They are responsible for muscular and visceral sensations, vasomotor activity, hunger, thirst, and "air hunger." These neurons synapse with neurons in lamina I of the dorsal horn of the spinal cord. Lamina I neurons in turn project densely to the IML cell column synapsing with preganglionic sympathetic neurons, forming a spino-spinal loop for autonomic reflexes.

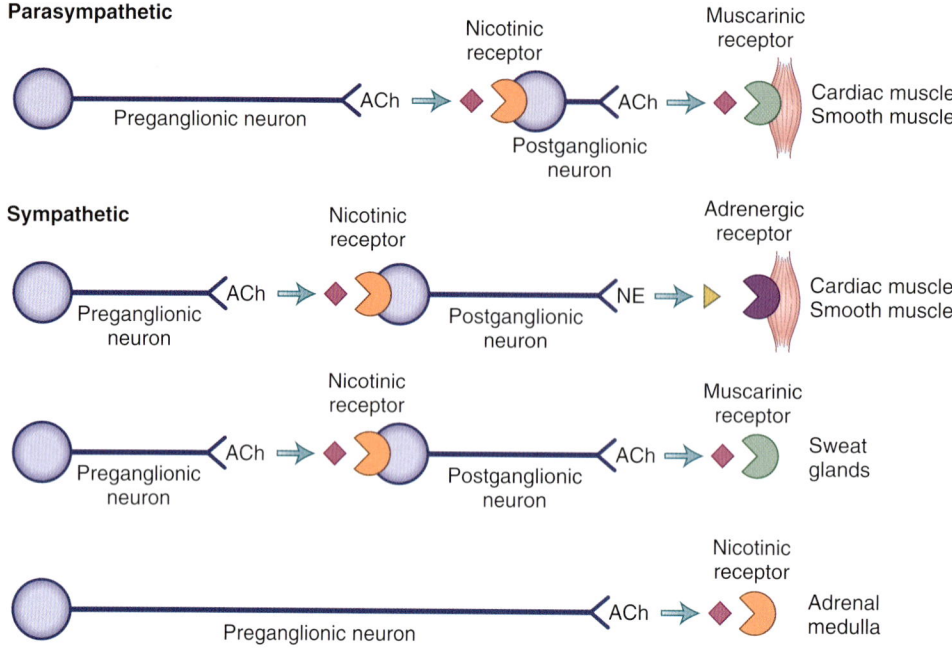

Figure 154-1. Elements of the parasympathetic and sympathetic nervous systems. Most organs receive both sympathetic and parasympathetic innervation, except for the blood vessels (only sympathetic adrenergic), the sweat glands (only sympathetic cholinergic), and the adrenal medulla (receives direct sympathetic innervation from the intermediolateral cell column in the spinal cord).

Central Nervous System Integration

Spinal, brainstem, and rostral cortical areas modulate signals from the afferent pathways, resulting in precise reflex activation or inhibition of autonomic efferent nerves. A well-studied example of an autonomic reflex pathway is the arterial baroreflex (Fig. 154-2). As with other polysynaptic autonomic reflexes, baroreflex information is integrated with other sensory information and with input from more rostral cortical areas.

CLINICAL APPROACH TO THE DIAGNOSIS OF PEDIATRIC AUTONOMIC DISORDERS
Clinical History Taking

Children with autonomic dysfunction can present with a variety of symptoms involving different organs. Detailed history taking is of paramount importance to establish a diagnosis. A structured clinical interview can provide valuable diagnostic clues. Careful review of current medications can rule out drug-induced causes. A thorough family history is key to the diagnosis of genetic disorders.

Orthostatic Intolerance

Because the sympathetic nervous system plays a crucial role maintaining blood pressure and cerebral blood flow when standing, orthostatic intolerance with symptoms of tissue hypoperfusion is the most characteristic presentation of sympathetic failure (see following discussion). The clinical interview should be framed with the goal of carefully reconstructing the events, signs, symptoms, and outcome of the syncopal/presyncopal episode.

Syncope. Most children are referred to an autonomic clinic after experiencing brief episodes of transient loss of consciousness. Although seizures are frequently suspected, syncope is much more frequent. Syncope is defined as a transient loss

of consciousness and postural tone resulting from global cerebral hypoperfusion; it is short-lived, with spontaneous recovery and no neurologic sequelae. Urinary incontinence and myoclonic jerks can occur in children with both reflex syncope and seizures, but a clear-cut aura and postictal confusion are signs of a seizure. Tongue biting is rare in syncope but common in seizures. Syncope most commonly occurs when standing, whereas seizures have no postural predilection.

Questions should aim to differentiate reflex (vasovagal) syncope—a reversible physiologic condition with a benign prognosis—from cardiac syncope or chronic impairment of sympathetic outflow. Although the latter is very infrequent in children, it does occur in genetic and immune-mediated autonomic disorders.

Orthostatic Intolerance with Orthostatic Tachycardia. The second most commonly encountered problem in an autonomic clinic is the so-called postural tachycardia syndrome (PoTS), a heterogenous syndrome common in young females. It is associated with a myriad of symptoms, including light-headedness, palpitations, tremulousness, weakness, fatigue, exercise intolerance, hyperventilation, paresthesiae, shortness of breath, anxiety, chest pain, nausea, acral coldness or pain, and difficulty concentrating. Syncope is not common in PoTS. The overlap with anxiety/panic disorders is often readily apparent.

Abnormal Gastrointestinal Motility. Constipation and diarrhea are common in children with functional autonomic disorders and are also a side effect of some medications or diets. Reduced salivation and dry mouth (xerostomia) can occur in autoimmune autonomic disorders and may result in dysphagia when eating. Autonomic diseases affecting the esophagus (e.g., achalasia) may cause dysphagia and heartburn. Abdominal distension, nausea, vomiting, and early satiety as a consequence of gastroparesis can be seen in metabolic disorders (e.g., diabetes, anorexia nervosa).

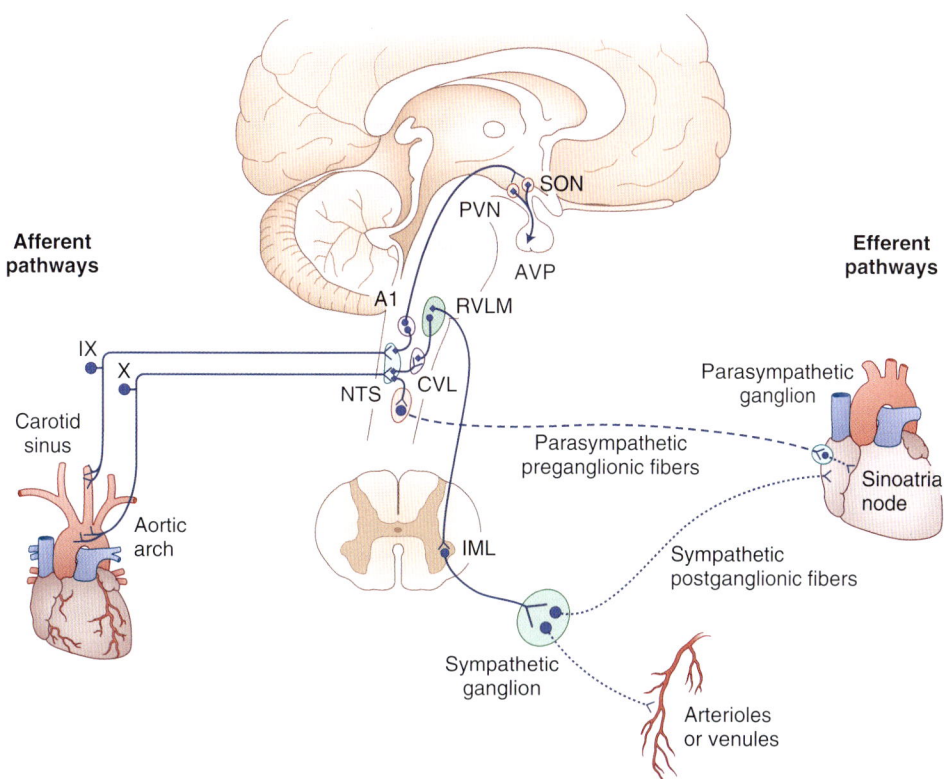

Figure 154-2. The arterial baroreflex. The arterial baroreceptors are mechanoreceptors located in the carotid sinus (innervated by the glosso-pharyngeal nerve, IX) and aortic arch (innervated by the vagus nerve, X) that respond to stretch elicited by increase in arterial pressure. Barore-ceptor afferents provide monosynaptic excitatory inputs to the nucleus of the solitary tract (NTS) in the brainstem. Barosensitive NTS neurons initiate a sympathoinhibitory pathway that involves projections from the NTS to the caudal ventrolateral medulla (CVL) that send inhibitory projec-tions to sympathoexcitatory neurons in the rostral ventrolateral medulla (RVLM). There is also direct input from the NTS to the vagal preganglionic neurons of the nucleus ambiguus (NAmb). These neurons project to the cardiac ganglion neurons that promote bradycardia. The baroreflex, via the NTS, also inhibits secretion of vasopressin by neurons of the supraoptic (SON) and paraventricular (PVN) nuclei of the hypothalamus, by inhibiting cells of the A1 noradrenergic group.

Neonatal severe constipation is a feature of Hirschsprung disease. Nausea and vomiting in response to emotional or physical stimuli occur in the rare genetic condition famil-ial dysautonomia, although such occurrences are more fre-quently a result of functional disorders (e.g., cyclic vomiting syndrome).

Genitourinary Symptoms. Urinary symptoms are frequent in children, and in most cases they are not indicative of an underlying autonomic disorder. Interpretation in young children should take into account that 10% of those younger than 8 years old suffer from daytime or nocturnal enuresis. In rare cases, daytime enuresis is attributable to detrusor overac-tivity. Urinary retention can be seen in autoimmune auto-nomic disorders and in spinal cord injury (Neveus and Sillen, 2013). In adolescents and young men, erectile dysfunction and failure to ejaculate can be a consequence of autonomic dysfunction. Milky-colored urine may represent retrograde ejaculation.

Thermoregulatory Abnormalities. Anhidrosis and hypohi-drosis are manifestations of sympathetic cholinergic failure, and lesions causing these abnormalities can occur anywhere from the level of the cerebral cortex to the eccrine sweat glands. Anhidrosis can lead to hyperthermia, heat stroke, and death. In spinal cord injury there often is a band of hyperhi-drosis above the lesion with anhidrosis below. Hypothermia may occur in hypothalamic disorders and spinal cord injury.

Hyperhidrosis (excessive sweating beyond that required for thermal homeostasis) can be generalized or focal. It should be distinguished from normal night sweats, which can occur in up to 12% of healthy children. In the vast majority of cases, hyperhidrosis is linked to anxiety. Hyperhidrosis may accom-pany episodes of paroxysmal sympathetic activation in famil-ial dysautonomia or pheochromocytoma.

Ocular Symptoms. Blurry vision and photophobia can be symptoms of abnormal autonomic innervation of the pupil. Impaired lacrimation may be a sign of autonomic impairment of the lacrimal glands.

Respiratory Symptoms. Hyperventilation is common and can be found in up to 15% of children and adolescents. Hyperventilation is frequently a feature in patients with func-tional autonomic symptoms, including PoTS and reflex syncope. Daytime symptoms of hypoventilation and central sleep apnea in children include decreased attention span, poor performance in school, and behavioral changes.

PEDIATRIC AUTONOMIC DISORDERS

Pediatric autonomic disorders can be classified in several ways. Table 154-1 depicts proposed schemes based on the patho-physiological features of autonomic dysfunction in children. In clinical practice, the main goal is to distinguish functional disorders, which are very common, from the more severe, but rare disorders.

TABLE 154-1 Classifications of Pediatric Autonomic Disorders

Etiology	Topography	Frequency	Neurotransmission
Functional Reflex (vasovagal) syncope Postural tachycardia syndrome Orthostatic intolerance without tachycardia	**Generalized** Reflex (vasovagal) syncope Postural tachycardia syndrome Orthostatic intolerance without tachycardia Hereditary sensory autonomic neuropathies Other rare genetic disorders Reflex (vasovagal) syncope Postural tachycardia syndrome Orthostatic intolerance without tachycardia Immune-mediated	**Common** Reflex (vasovagal) syncope Postural tachycardia syndrome Orthostatic intolerance without tachycardia Obesity Diabetes Anorexia nervosa Other metabolic disorders	**Pandysautonomia (adrenergic and cholinergic failure)** Autoimmune autonomic ganglionopathy Acute autonomic and sensory neuropathy Guillain-Barré syndrome Paraneoplastic neuropathies Porphyria
Inherited Hereditary sensory autonomic neuropathies Other rare genetic disorders	**Pupil** Argyll Robertson pupil Adie pupil Horner syndrome Pourfour du Petit syndrome	**Rare** Immune-mediated Traumatic Hereditary sensory autonomic neuropathies Other rare genetic disorders	**Pure adrenergic failure** Dopamine-beta hydroxylase deficiency Pure adrenergic neuropathy
Metabolic Obesity Diabetes Anorexia Other metabolic disorders	**Face** Cluster headache Harlequin syndrome Gustatory sweating		**Pure cholinergic failure** Botulism Lambert-Eaton syndrome Adie pupil Chagas disease Acute cholinergic neuropathy
Immune-mediated Autoimmune autonomic ganglionopathy Guillain-Barre syndrome Anti-NMDA receptor encephalitis Paraneoplastic autonomic neuropathy Sjögren disease	**Limbs** Raynaud phenomenon Acrocyanosis Primary idiopathic hyperhidrosis		
Infectious Chagas disease HIV Tetanus			
Neoplasia Catecholamine-secreting tumors Brainstem and posterior fossa tumors			
Trauma and malformations Spinal cord injury Traumatic brain injury Syringomyelia Arnold-Chiari			
Drugs			
Postsurgical or postradiotherapy Acquired baroreflex failure			

Functional Disorders of Unknown Origin

Reflex (Vasovagal) Syncope

Reflex syncope (i.e., the common faint, also known as vasovagal, neurally mediated, or neurocardiogenic syncope) refers to a sudden fall in blood pressure and slowing of the heart rate causing impaired cerebral perfusion that leads to a brief episode of loss of consciousness and muscle tone. Patients with reflex syncope usually describe classical prodromal signs and symptoms (pallor, diaphoresis, nausea, abdominal discomfort, yawning, sighing), and many children begin to hyperventilate in the time leading up to the faint. If blood pressure continues to fall, cerebral and retinal hypoperfusion (visual disturbances, concentration difficulties, and lightheadedness) develop just before the loss of consciousness. Scenarios likely to provoke reflex syncope are motionless standing,

elevated ambient temperatures, and dehydration. Known emotional triggers are fear, anger, blood sampling, pain, and TV programs about medical matters (Wieling et al., 2009).

The prevalence of reflex syncope in the pediatric population is high. A survey of young adults averaging 20 years of age showed that about 20% of males and 50% of females reported having experienced at least one syncopal episode in their lifetime. The median age at the first episode of reflex syncope is approximately 15 years.

In most cases, reflex syncope can be diagnosed by eyewitness accounts and careful reconstruction of the event. In cases when the diagnosis is not straightforward, prolonged tilt testing can be helpful by replicating symptoms while recording the typical acute drop in blood pressure and slowing of the heart rate (Fig. 154-4).

Key aspects of the management of young patients with reflex syncope include reassurance, advice, and patient

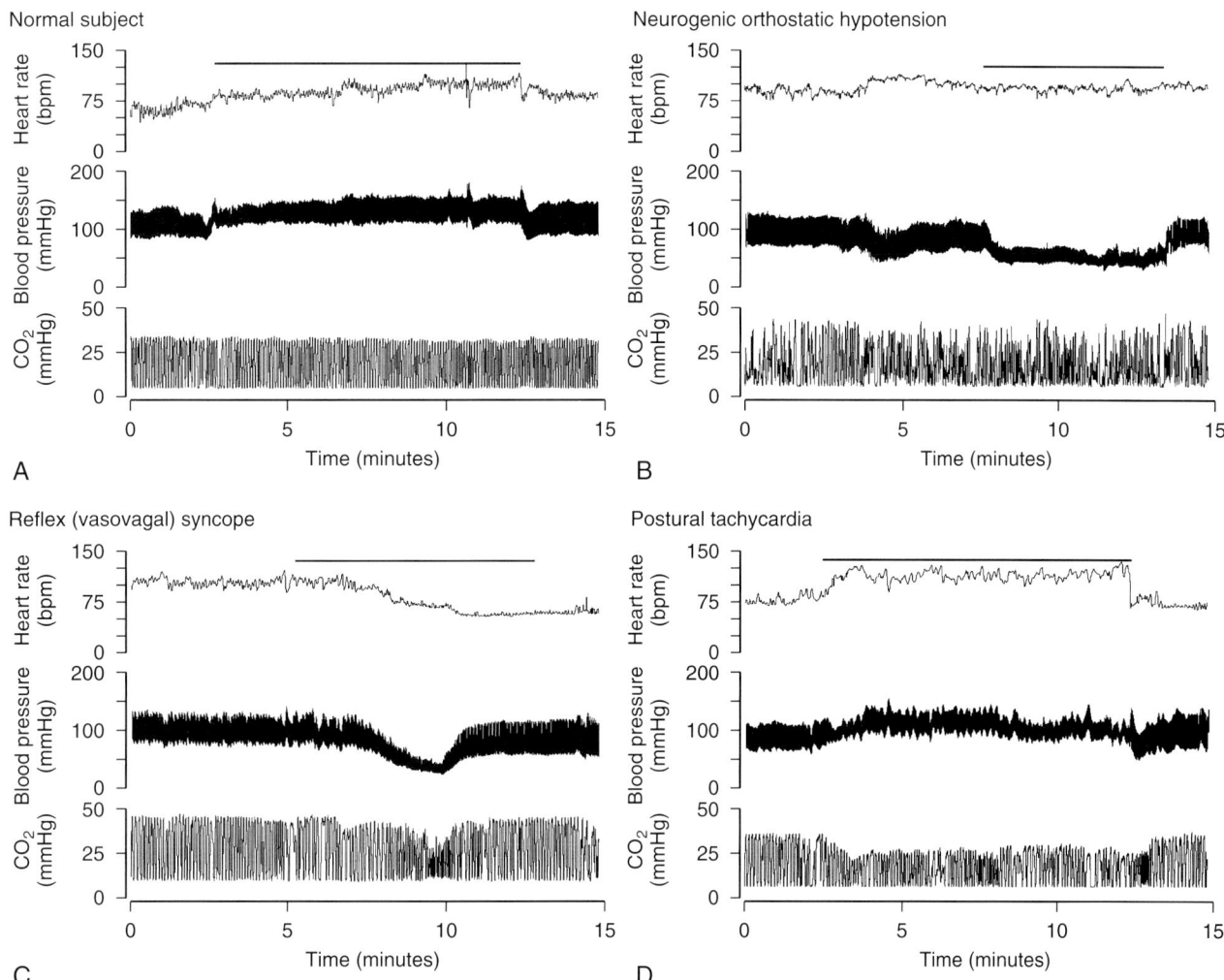

Figure 154-4. Changes in heart rate (HR), blood pressure (BP), and ventilation pattern during head-up tilt test. **A,** In a normal subject, no major changes are observed in BP, HR, or end-tidal CO_2 during the tilt test. **B,** Neurogenic orthostatic hypotension features a dramatic decrease in blood pressure and absence of compensatory increase in heart rate. Hyperventilation does not occur. **C,** Reflex (vasovagal) syncope. During the episode, a dramatic decrease in blood pressure occurred, accompanied by a decrease in HR; CO_2 levels also decreased right before and during the syncope. **D,** In postural tachycardia syndrome (PoTS), heart rate increases during tilt and CO_2 levels decrease, with no significant changes in BP. The bar above the graphs denotes the period during the 60-degree-angle head-up tilt.

education. Time should be taken to identify triggers that exaggerate venous pooling and provoke syncope. Children should be taught nonpharmacologic measures that can prevent or abort the episode, including slow breathing and muscle-tensing maneuvers to increase venous return. Increasing salt and water intake and sleeping with the head of the bed raised are helpful nonpharmacologic means to expand intravascular volume. In cases of refractory reflex syncope, the short-acting pressor agent midodrine can be used "on demand" to improve orthostatic intolerance before situations known to trigger syncope. Pacemakers are ineffective (Kaufmann and Hainsworth, 2001).

Postural Tachycardia Syndrome

Postural tachycardia syndrome (PoTS) is a complex disorder that is not well understood. It is characterized by chronic symptoms of orthostatic intolerance accompanied by a heart-rate increment within 10 minutes of standing or head-up tilt with no orthostatic hypotension. Current consensus criteria of PoTS require, at least, a heart rate increment of 40 beats/min in children aged 12 to 19 years (Fig. 154-4).

Symptoms may develop gradually or acutely, range from mild to severe, and resolve spontaneously or continue intermittently for years. Syncope is not a typical feature of PoTS. Many children with PoTS also report symptoms not attributable to orthostatic intolerance, including those of functional gastrointestinal or bladder disorders, chronic headache, fibromyalgia, and sleep disturbances.

The pathophysiology of PoTS is unclear but likely involves a combination of factors, including cardiovascular deconditioning, hyperventilation, and volume depletion. Emotional comorbidities, including somatic hypervigilance, anxiety, and depression, are common and contribute to symptom chronicity. The severity of the symptoms is often linked to the degree of hyperventilation-induced hypocapnia, which exacerbates venous pooling and tachycardia. Many patients with PoTS go on to develop additional symptoms, including constipation, bloating, bladder sensitivity disorders, and chronic headache, and despite comprehensive workup, usually no structural cause can be identified.

Management of PoTS should begin by removing any medications that produce tachycardia, including norepinephrine reuptake inhibitors and stimulants. Surreptitious use of diuretics should be ruled out in any adolescent or young adult with elevated renin levels. Exercise training and cognitive behavioral therapy are the most appropriate inventions. Correcting the standing heart rate with beta blockers or cholinesterase inhibitors may not be effective to improve symptoms (Benarroch, 2012).

Metabolic Disorders

Obesity

The prevalence of pediatric obesity (defined as a body mass index [BMI] ≥ 95th percentile for age and sex) has more than tripled during the past decades in the United States, and around 20% of children and adolescents are now overweight. Epidemiologic studies have evaluated the effect of obesity in cardiac autonomic modulation in children. Most studies show an increase in sympathetic and a decrease in parasympathetic function with abnormal cardiac circadian patterns. The pathophysiology of autonomic abnormalities in obesity is not well understood but is likely mediated by comorbidities such as sleep apnea, metabolic abnormalities, and arterial hypertension. Children with obesity as a result of genetic disorders, such as Prader-Willi syndrome, appear to have diminished parasympathetic nervous system activity.

Eating Disorders

Anorexia nervosa is a potentially life-threatening eating disorder characterized by an intense fear of gaining weight, distorted body image, and amenorrhea. It affects 0.5% to 4% of adolescent girls in the United States, and its incidence has increased over the past few decades. Children with anorexia are predisposed to arrhythmias and sudden cardiac death. Bradycardia, hypotension, and cardiac atrophy are all features of the disease. Patients have significantly lower heart rates at night and increased heart rate variability. These abnormalities are reversible after weight recovery. Bulimia nervosa affects 1% to 2% of adolescent girls in the United States and has similar cardiovascular autonomic findings.

Diabetes Mellitus

Although diabetes mellitus is one of the most common causes of autonomic dysfunction in adults, signs and symptoms of autonomic dysfunction are infrequent in pediatric patients. However, autonomic neuropathy should be considered in adolescents and young adults with long duration of type 1 diabetes mellitus, who may have early evidence of cardiovascular autonomic dysfunction.

Other Metabolic Disorders

Hypothyroidism (with symptoms of fatigue, dry skin, sleep disturbances, and constipation) and hyperthyroidism (with symptoms of fever, tachycardia, hypertension, and gastrointestinal abnormalities) can present with symptoms of autonomic dysfunction. Symptoms of Addison disease include hypotension, hyperpigmentation, and adrenal crises.

Autonomic Dysfunction Secondary to Focal Disease

Areas distributed throughout the neuraxis, including the anterior insula, anterior cingulate cortex, amygdala, hypothalamus, periaqueductal gray matter, parabrachial nucleus, and several regions of the medulla, are involved in autonomic control, particularly in cardiovascular regulation. Therefore lesions of various etiologies (e.g., trauma, hydrocephalus, demyelination, stroke, malformations, tumors) can potentially cause autonomic dysfunction.

Spinal cord injury in the pediatric population is relatively rare. More than half of pediatric spinal cord injuries occur in the cervical area. Signs and symptoms depend on the level of the lesion and whether the section is complete or incomplete. Destruction of the descending cardiovascular autonomic pathways results in (a) blunted release of norepinephrine when upright, leading to neurogenic orthostatic hypotension, and (b) loss of inhibitory and excitatory supraspinal input to the sympathetic preganglionic neurons, leading to unrestrained sympathetic activity of fibers arising below the level of the lesion (referred to as "autonomic dysreflexia"), particularly in subjects with an injury at the T6 level or above.

ACQUIRED AFFERENT BAROREFLEX FAILURE

Bilateral destruction of baroreceptor afferent neurons in the glossopharyngeal and vagus nerves that relay information to the NTS can result in afferent baroreflex failure. Patients with baroreflex failure have extremely labile blood pressure and heart rates. Many alternate between orthostatic hypotension and paroxysmal hypertension. Hyperadrenergic signs and symptoms usually dominate the clinical picture and can resemble those of a pheochromocytoma.

Causes of afferent baroreflex failure include nerve injury secondary to neck surgery or delayed effect of radiotherapy to the neck for cancer, or trauma; brainstem strokes that damage the nucleus of the solitary tract and other areas of the brainstem; and rare hereditary conditions that affect the development of afferent baroreceptor pathways, including familial dysautonomia and Moebius syndrome. Treatment involves techniques to manage stress and medications to control blood pressure. Preliminary data suggest that carbidopa, a DOPA decarboxylase inhibitor that does not cross the blood–brain barrier, may reduce norepinephrine surges and lessen blood pressure peaks.

Catecholamine-Secreting Tumors

Paragangliomas are rare neuroendocrine tumors derived from neural crest cells that arise in the peripheral ANS. Pheochromocytomas are paragangliomas that arise from chromaffin cells of the adrenal medulla. These are characterized by unpredictable paroxysmal episodes of excessive catecholamine secretion, resulting in hypertension, tachycardia, and headaches. Approximately 50% are malignant. Treatment requires surgery.

Autoimmune Autonomic Disorders

Guillain-Barré Syndrome

Guillain-Barré syndrome (GBS) is less common in children than in adults, with an incidence of 0.4 to 1.3 cases per 100,000 per year in children in the United States; it is rarely seen in children younger than 2 years old. GBS (also known as acute inflammatory demyelinating polyneuropathy) is responsible for most cases of acute and subacute flaccid paralysis in infants and children. Approximately two thirds of patients diagnosed with GBS had a respiratory or gastrointestinal infection prior the start of the symptoms. Autonomic instability with episodes of hypertension and hypotension and cardiac arrhythmia can occur. This can be life threatening, so close monitoring is required. Other autonomic symptoms such as gastrointestinal and bladder dysfunction can also be present. Treatment includes intravenous immunoglobulin (IVIG) or plasma exchange.

Autoimmune Autonomic Ganglionopathy

Autoimmune autonomic ganglionopathy is characterized by an acute-onset widespread sympathetic and parasympathetic failure. Cholinergic deficits are pronounced and include severe impairment of gastrointestinal motility, with gastroparesis and constipation, bladder retention, dry eyes, and dry mouth. Abnormal pupillary responses are common. Orthostatic hypotension can be severe. There is no motor or sensory impairment. In 30% to 50% of patients, high titers of antibodies against the neuronal ganglionic nicotinic acetylcholine receptor (AChR) are identified. In the remaining cases, other autoantibodies not yet identified are the likely cause. Patients may respond to IVIG, plasma exchange, or rituximab. Some cases in children and adolescents have been reported, although its incidence in children is unknown.

Acute Autonomic and Sensory Neuropathy

Acute autonomic and sensory neuropathy is a rare disorder in which patients develop acute-onset fine-touch and proprioceptive sensory deficits leading to severe ataxia. Autonomic involvement includes neurogenic orthostatic hypotension, lack of sweating, and urinary and fecal incontinence. Plasma norepinephrine levels are low or undetectable. In most cases a gastrointestinal or respiratory infection precedes the neuropathy, suggesting an immune-mediated process, in some cases associated with antigalactocerebrosidase or antisulfatide antibodies. IVIg and plasma exchange have been used, with varied success (Koike et al., 2010).

Anti-NMDA Receptor Encephalitis

Anti-NMDA receptor encephalitis results from antibodies against the NR1 and NR2 subunits of the NMDA receptor. Symptoms in children include behavioral and personality changes. As the diseases progresses, patients develop sleep disorders, seizures, movement disorders, and autonomic instability (tachycardia, hypertension, hypoventilation, urinary incontinence, and hypothermia or hyperthermia). It has been linked to ovarian neoplasms, although it has been described in patients without cancer (Florance et al., 2009).

Lambert-Eaton Myasthenic Syndrome

In addition to weakness and reduced or absent deep tendon reflexes, autonomic dysfunction is a recognized feature of Lambert-Eaton myasthenic syndrome (LES). Dry mouth is the most frequent autonomic symptom, followed by sweating abnormalities and impaired cardiac parasympathetic reflexes. The majority of patients have antibodies against PQ-type voltage-gated calcium channels (VGCC), and approximately 30% of patients have N-type VGCC autoantibodies. This syndrome is frequently found in association with small-cell carcinoma of the lung, but it has also been found in patients without neoplasms. Lambert-Eaton syndrome is very rare in children.

Dipeptidyl-Peptidase-Like Protein-6 (DPPX) Potassium Channel Antibody Encephalitis

Dipeptidyl-peptidase-like protein-6 (DPPX) potassium channel antibody encephalitis, a recently described autoimmune encephalitis, affects adults and young teenagers and is characterized by the presence of antibodies against DPPX, a subunit of Kv4.2 potassium channels. Main features are insidious and subacute cognitive impairment, abnormal eye movements, dysphagia, insomnia, and autonomic abnormalities, most prominently gastrointestinal symptoms (diarrhea, gastroparesis, constipation), followed by urinary symptoms, fluctuating hyperthermia/hypothermia, and asymptomatic ventricular tachycardia.

Genetic Autonomic Disorders

There are a number of rare, early-onset genetic disorders that affect the ANS. Although the extent of autonomic involvement varies, certain genetic conditions are associated with widespread autonomic dysfunction.

Hereditary Sensory and Autonomic Neuropathies

Hereditary sensory and autonomic neuropathies (HSANs) are a group of rare disorders caused by different mutations that affect different aspects of the development, function, or survival of sensory and autonomic neurons. Classification is evolving as a result of the discovery of increasing numbers of mutations and the availability of whole-exome sequencing (Table 154-2). For each HSAN type, penetrance is complete, but phenotypic expression varies markedly. Impaired pain and temperature perception are common traits.

HSAN Type 1. HSAN type 1 is the most common HSAN, but it is an adult-onset disorder. Patients have varying degrees of sensorineural hearing loss, distal anhidrosis, and episodes of lancinating pain in the limbs. There are several subtypes (Table 154-2).

HSAN Type 2. HSAN type 2 is an autosomal-recessive disorder characterized by impaired temperature, pain, and fine-touch sensation. Onset varies from birth up until the beginning of the teens. There are at least four causative gene mutations, resulting in subsequent subtype designations (A through D). Autonomic involvement varies markedly (Table 154-2).

HSAN Type 3 (Familial Dysautonomia). HSAN type 3 (familial dysautonomia, Online Mendelian Inheritance in Man database (OMIM) #223900) is an autosomal-recessive disease almost exclusively affecting children with Eastern European Jewish ancestry. Over 99% of affected patients are homozygous for the founder point mutation (6T>C change) in the gene encoding for the elongator-1 protein (ELP-1), known also as I-k B kinase-associated protein (IKAP). IKAP (ELP-1) is expressed in most cells throughout the body. The deficiency of IKAP (ELP-1) during embryogenesis affects the development of primary sensory (i.e., afferent) neurons that carry information to the CNS with cell bodies in the dorsal root and cranial nerve ganglia. Efferent (motor) neurons are mostly spared.

In contrast to other HSANs, in HSAN type 3, autonomic dysfunction dominates the clinical picture. The main autonomic defect in patients with HSAN type 3 is in the afferent (sensory) neurons that convey incoming information from the arterial baroreceptors, resulting in the unusual combination of orthostatic hypotension and paroxysmal hypertension. Although reduced in number, the efferent sympathetic nerves are functionally active. Supine plasma norepinephrine levels are normal. Stimuli that activate efferent sympathetic neurons, independently of baroreceptor afferent pathways, such as cognitive tasks and emotional arousal, dramatically increase blood pressure, heart rate, and circulating norepinephrine levels (Norcliffe-Kaufmann, Axelrod, and Kaufmann, 2010).

Episodic retching and vomiting attacks accompanied by skin blotching, diaphoresis, hypertension, and tachycardia ("dysautonomic crises") are common. These are the result of sudden increases in circulating catecholamines that are unrestrained by baroreceptor feedback. End-organ target damage (e.g., chronic kidney disease) occurs as a long-term consequence of hypertension and excessive blood pressure variability.

TABLE 154-2 Hereditary Sensory and Autonomic Neuropathies

Type	Gene	Inheritance	Onset	Autonomic Features	Sensory Features	Other Features
HSAN 1A	SPTLC1	AD	Adult	Varying degrees of distal anhidrosis	Progressive loss of pain, temperature, and fine-touch sensation; Varying degrees of sensorineural hearing loss Episodes of lancinating limb pain	One case with congenital presentation reported with severe growth and mental retardation, microcephaly, hypotonia, and respiratory insufficiency
HSAN 1B	3p24-p22 locus					Cough and gastroesophageal reflux
HSAN 1C	SPTLC2					Varying degrees of distal muscle weakness
HSAN 1D	ALT1			None		—
HSAN 1E	DMNT1			None		Early-onset dementia
HSAN 1F	ATL3			None		—
HSAN 2A	WNK1	AR	Childhood or adolescence	None	Varying degrees of progressive loss of pain, temperature, and fine-touch sensation	—
HSAN 2B	FAM134B			Varying degrees of hyperhidrosis, urinary incontinence, and pupillary abnormalities		
HSAN 2C	KIF1A			None		—
HSAN 2D	SCN9A			Urinary and fecal incontinence, reduced sweating		Lack of fungiform lingual papillae, hyposmia, hearing loss, hypogeusia, and bone dysplasia
HSAN 3	IKAP (ELP-1)	AR	Newborn	Impaired lacrimation Orthostatic hypotension Paroxysmal hypertension and vomiting episodes with skin blotching Normal or increased sweating	Impaired pain and temperature sensation with preserved fine-touch sensation	Described in Ashkenazi Jewish ancestry; Neonatal hypotonia; Respiratory and feeding difficulties; Neuropathic joints Optic neuropathy Chronic lung disease Scoliosis; Rhabdomyolysis Renal failure Varying degrees of cognitive and behavioral problems
HSAN 4	NTRK (TRKA)	AR	Newborn	Anhidrosis; Episodic hyperthermia Undetectable plasma norepinephrine	Loss of pain and temperature sensation Preserved fine-touch and vibration sensation	Frequent fractures Neuropathic joints Slow-healing wounds Varying degrees of cognitive and behavioral problems
HSAN 5	NGFβ	AR	Newborn	Variable degree of anhidrosis	Loss of pain and temperature sensation. Preserved fine touch and vibration sensation	Frequent fractures Neuropathic joints Tooth loss from gingival disease
HSAN 6	DST	AR	Newborn	Impaired lacrimation Labile blood pressure and heart rate Hyperthermia and skin-blotching episodes	Loss of pain and temperature sensation	Described in Ashkenazi Jewish ancestry; Neonatal hypotonia Respiratory and feeding difficulties, delayed psychomotor development, neuropathic joints All described patients died before age 3
HSAN 7	SCN11A	AD (only a heterozygous de novo mutation described)	Newborn	Hyperhidrosis and gastrointestinal dysfunction	Loss of pain and temperature sensation	Frequent fractures Neuropathic joints Slow-healing wounds

Superficial pain perception is severely decreased, but patients complain of abdominal discomfort and/or bone pain following fractures or surgical procedures, suggesting that some visceral pain perception is preserved. Corneal analgesia often results in abrasions and ulcerations complicated by alacrima. Patients with HSAN type 3 have been shown to have a specific type of optic neuropathy that resembles mitochondrial neuropathies.

Gait ataxia and incoordination, resulting from a lack of muscle spindle afferents, affect patients from birth and progressively worsen over time. Other features include feeding problems as a result of neurogenic dysphagia, failure to thrive, and increased frequency of rhabdomyolysis. Cognitive and behavioral issues, such as anxiety, reduced IQ, emotional overreaction, and emotional rigidity, prevent many patients from living independently. Abnormal spinal curvature, corrective spinal surgery, depressed ventilatory drive, sleep-disordered breathing, and frequent aspirations compromise respiratory function. The incidence of sudden death, particularly during sleep, is increased.

Therapeutic focus in HSAN type 3 is on reducing the catecholamine surges caused by blunted baroreceptor feedback (i.e., afferent baroreflex failure). Carbidopa is frequently used to block dopamine production outside the CNS and prevent dopamine-induced vomiting. Additional therapeutic measures include management of neurogenic dysphagia, early treatment of aspiration pneumonias, and noninvasive ventilation during sleep. Clinical trials of compounds that increase levels of IKAP (ELP-1) are under way (Palma et al., 2014).

HSAN Type 4 (Congenital Insensitivity to Pain with Anhidrosis). HSAN type 4 (OMIM #256800) is an autosomal-recessive disorder first described in children with mental retardation, insensitivity to pain, self-mutilating behavior, and unexplained fevers. A cardinal feature of the disease is complete anhidrosis in response to thermal, emotional, or direct stimulation of the skin. Self-mutilation is extremely common. Pinprick sensation is also diminished. Skin wounds and bone injuries heal poorly. Joints are susceptible to repeated trauma, resulting in neuropathic joints and osteomyelitis. Avoidance of harmful stimuli is crucial to prevent recurrent injuries but is frequently difficult to accomplish because patients usually have intellectual disability with impulsivity and reckless behaviors.

HSAN type 4 is associated with missense, nonsense, and frame-shift mutations in the gene that encodes for the neurotrophic tyrosine kinase-1 receptor (NTRK, previously known as TRK or TRKA). Skin biopsies of patients with HSAN type 4 reveal that sweat glands are preserved, but they lack sympathetic cholinergic innervation, thus the anhidrosis, which can lead to hyperthermia and death.

Patients with HSAN type 4 have very low or undetectable levels of circulating norepinephrine but normal epinephrine levels, suggesting that lack of NTRK-NGF signaling affects the development of sympathetic adrenergic neurons but spares chromaffin cells in the adrenal medulla. Interestingly, despite the very low norepinephrine levels indicating impaired or absent sympathetic activity, patients with HSAN type 4 have normal cardiovascular responses to orthostatic stress (Norcliffe-Kaufmann et al., 2015).

HSAN Type 5. Patients with HSAN type 5 (OMIM # 608654) have a selective loss of temperature and pain sensation, leading to painless fractures, bone necrosis, and neuropathic joints. The have variable degrees of sweating impairment. The disorder is caused by homozygous mutations in the nerve growth factor β (NGFB) gene. Heterozygous carriers can present in adulthood with a mild phenotype.

HSAN Type 6. Reported in a large consanguineous Ashkenazi Jewish family, HSAN type 6 is a severe autosomal-recessive disorder resulting from homozygous truncating mutations in the dystonin gene (OMIM #614653). The disorder is characterized by neonatal hypotonia, areflexia, respiratory and feeding difficulties, delayed psychomotor development, neuropathic joints, labile blood pressure and heart rate, and lack of corneal reflexes. All patients died before age 3.

HSAN Type 7. Reported in two unrelated patients (OMIM # 615548), HSAN type 7 includes the clinical features of congenital insensitivity to pain resulting in self-mutilations, slow-healing wounds, painless fractures, hyperhidrosis, and gastrointestinal dysfunction requiring parenteral nutrition. The disorder results from de novo heterozygous missense mutations in the SCN11A gene.

Other Syndromes with Sensory and Autonomic Involvement. *Navajo familial neurogenic arthropathy* was initially described in Native American (Navajo) children. It is characterized by diminished or absent sweating with variable sensory deficits, ranging from insensitivity to pain (leading to fractures, corneal injuries, and neuropathic joints) to normal sensation.

Stuve-Wiedemann syndrome (OMIM #601559), also known as neonatal Schwartz-Jampel syndrome type 2 (SJS2), is an autosomal-recessive disorder caused by mutations in the LIFR gene. It is characterized by bowing of the lower limbs, wide metaphyses with abnormal trabecular pattern, and camptodactyly (one or more fingers permanently bent as a result of fixed-flexion deformity of the proximal interphalangeal joints). Additional features include feeding and swallowing difficulties, respiratory distress, and episodes of hyperthermia, which can be fatal in the first months of life. Sensory abnormalities, including decreased sensitivity to pain and temperature, lead to corneal injury and absent deep tendon reflexes. Cognition and behavior appear to be normal. Hypertrichosis is common.

Inborn Errors of Metabolism

Dopamine Beta-Hydroxylase Deficiency. Dopamine beta-hydroxylase deficiency, a rare disorder, is caused by mutations in the gene encoding the enzyme dopamine beta-hydroxylase (DBH), which converts dopamine to norepinephrine (OMIM # 223360). Affected patients have undetectable levels of plasma norepinephrine and epinephrine, with increased dopamine levels. Newborns can show a delay in eye opening and palpebral ptosis. Hypotension, hypoglycemia, and hypothermia may occur early in life. The absence of norepinephrine leads to deficient vasoconstriction, resulting in hypotension, syncope, and reduced exercise capacity. Symptoms generally worsen in late adolescence and early adulthood. Treatment with droxidopa (Northera®), a synthetic norepinephrine precursor, replenishes norepinephrine, increases blood pressure, and improves symptoms of hypotension (Biaggioni and Robertson, 1987).

Aromatic L-Amino Acid Decarboxylase Deficiency. Aromatic L-amino acid decarboxylase deficiency, an extremely rare autosomal recessive disorder, is caused by mutations in the *DDC* gene. The enzyme aromatic L-amino acid decarboxylase (AADC) converts L-dopa and 5-hydroxytryptophan to dopamine and serotonin, respectively (OMIM #608643). Neonatal symptoms include poor feeding, lethargy, ptosis, hypothermia, hypotension, intermittent eye movement abnormalities (oculogyric crises), hypotonia, and motor symptoms such as rigidity and difficulty with movements. Diagnosis is based on measurement of AADC activity in plasma and *DDC* gene sequencing. Increased levels of urinary vanillactic acid (VLA) are diagnostic. Treatment is aimed at correcting the neurotransmitter abnormalities with different medications (e.g., dopamine agonists, monoaminoxidase inhibitors, selective serotonin reuptake inhibitors, pyridoxine, droxidopa, 5-hydroxytryptophan).

Menkes Disease. Also known as kinky-hair disease, Menkes disease is an X-linked neurodegenerative disease of impaired copper transport. It is caused by mutations in the *ATP7A* gene (OMIM #309400). Children usually present at 2 to 3 months of age with loss of developmental milestones, failure to thrive, truncal hypotonia, and epileptic and myoclonic seizures. Autonomic abnormalities are not well characterized, although orthostatic hypotension and chronic diarrhea have been reported. Decreased serum copper and serum ceruloplasmin levels can be useful in the differential diagnosis. Decreased norepinephrine levels have been found. An elevated hydroxyphenylalanine (DOPA) and dihydroxyphenylglycol (DHPG) ratio resulting from decreased activity of DBH may be observed, with higher values reflecting more severe disease. Treatment with droxidopa might be useful.

Fabry Disease. Fabry disease, an X-linked inborn error of glycosphingolipid catabolism, is caused by mutations in the *GLA* gene, resulting in deficient or absent activity of the lysosomal enzyme alpha-galactosidase A (OMIM # 301500). This leads to systemic accumulation of globotriaosylceramide (Gb3) and related glycosphingolipids in plasma and organ cells throughout the body, including autonomic and dorsal root ganglia. Clinical manifestations begin in childhood or adolescence and include severe neuropathic or limb pain, telangiectasias and angiokeratomas, and renal manifestations. Symptoms of autonomic dysfunction include sweating abnormalities (hypohidrosis or hyperhidrosis), decreased lacrimation, decreased salivation, and gastrointestinal dysmotility. The degree of cardiovascular autonomic involvement is unclear.

Porphyrias. Porphyrias are inherited defects in the biosynthesis of heme. Acute intermittent porphyria (OMIM #176000) is the most common form of porphyria and is inherited in an autosomal-dominant manner. It is characterized by acute, recurrent episodes of abdominal pain, gastrointestinal dysfunction, and neurologic impairment. Patients are asymptomatic in between episodes. Autonomic abnormalities include tachycardia, hypotension, urinary retention, and gastrointestinal symptoms (nausea, vomiting, diarrhea, or constipation). Acute attacks rarely occur before puberty and can be precipitated by medications, alcohol, infection, starvation, and hormonal changes. Increased urinary excretion of delta-aminolevulinic acid (ALA) and porphobilinogen (PBG) during the attacks supports the diagnosis.

Porphyria variegata (OMIM #176200) is also an autosomal-dominant disorder and is caused by heterozygous mutations in the gene encoding for protoporphyrinogen oxidase (PPOX). The clinical features are similar to those of acute intermittent porphyria, but with an increased frequency of skin photosensitivity and hypertrichosis.

Hirschsprung Disease

Also known as aganglionic megacolon, Hirschsprung disease is characterized by congenital absence of ganglionic cells in the myenteric and submucosal plexuses of the gastrointestinal tract. Affected patients have severe gastroparesis, leading to partial or complete bowel obstruction and dilatation of the colon. Cardiovascular autonomic dysfunction has been described. Mutations in the *RET* gene and several other identified loci increase susceptibility to the disorder.

Heterozygous mutations in the *ECE1* gene (OMIM #613870) cause Hirschsprung disease with cardiac defects and autonomic dysfunction (episodes of severe agitation in association with tachycardia, hypertension, and hyperthermia).

Congenital Central Hypoventilation Syndrome and Related Ventilatory Disorders

Congenital central hypoventilation syndrome (CCHS; OMIM #209880) is an autosomal-dominant disorder most commonly caused by mutations in the *PHOX2B, RET, GDNF, EDN3, ASCL1,* and *BDNF* genes. These patients typically present in the first hours of life with cyanosis and increased hypercapnia during sleep. They have an impairment of ventilatory and arousal responses to both hypercapnia and hypoxemia. Children with CCHS often have additional autonomic symptoms, including severe constipation, dysphagia, pupillary abnormalities, and decreased body temperature. Sympathetic activity can be exaggerated.

Pitt-Hopkins syndrome (OMIM # 610954), caused by heterozygous (sometimes de novo) mutations of the *TCF4* gene, is characterized by abnormal psychomotor development, distinctive facial features, microcephaly, clubbing, and intermittent hyperventilation followed by apnea during both wakefulness and sleep.

Allgrove Syndrome and Related Disorders

Also known as achalasia-addisonianism-alacrima syndrome, and triple-A syndrome, Allgrove syndrome is caused by mutations in the gene encoding the protein aladin (*AAAS*; OMIM #231550). It is inherited in a recessive fashion. Children present with classic symptoms of primary adrenal insufficiency, including hypoglycemic seizures and shock. Less frequently, they present with recurrent vomiting, dysphagia, and failure to thrive, or ocular symptoms associated with alacrima. At presentation, review of systems may also be positive for hyperpigmentation, developmental delay, seizures, hypernasal speech, and symptoms related to orthostatic hypotension.

Alacrima, achalasia, and mental retardation (AAMR) syndrome is an autosomal-recessive disorder caused by homozygous mutations in the *GMPPA* gene and characterized by onset of features at birth or in early infancy. Patients with AAMR do not have adrenal insufficiency.

Other Genetic Disorders with Autonomic Dysfunction

Rett Syndrome. Rett syndrome is a neurodevelopmental disorder that occurs almost exclusively in females. Autonomic dysfunction results in abnormal, irregular breathing during wakefulness and sleep, including hyperventilation, hypoventilation, and apnea; abnormal heart-rate variability; and labile blood pressure with episodic hypertension and tachycardia. Almost a third of all deaths from Rett syndrome are sudden and unexpected, which has been linked to autonomic dysregulation.

Alexander Disease. Alexander disease, an autosomal-dominant disease, is caused by mutations (usually de novo) in the gene encoding glial fibrillary acidic protein (*GFAP*; OMIM # 203450). The disorder is subclassified as infantile, juvenile, or adult onset. Patients present with seizures, megalencephaly, developmental delay, and spasticity. They have early signs of autonomic dysfunction, including constipation, episodic hypothermia, and sleep-disordered breathing. Brain MRI typically shows cerebral white-matter abnormalities affecting the frontal region; brainstem and cerebellar atrophy also can be present.

Hyperbradykininism. Hyperbradykininism is an autosomal-dominant disorder characterized by orthostatic hypotension (leading to lightheadedness upon standing and syncope), facial erythema, and purple discoloration of the legs after standing. Plasma bradykinin is elevated.

Panayiotopoulos Syndrome. Panayiotopoulos syndrome is a form of idiopathic benign childhood focal epilepsy in which the seizures are associated with signs of increased autonomic activity. Recent reports document hypertension, tachycardia, and release of vasopressin during the seizures, suggestive of activation of the central autonomic network. In rare cases, respiratory and cardiac arrest have been reported. Mutations in the *SCN1A* gene increase susceptibility for this disorder.

Congenital Alacrima. Children with congenital alacrima have markedly deficient lacrimation from infancy, leading to corneal epithelial lesions, presumably as a result of hypoplasia of the lacrimal glands. Genetic mutations have not yet been identified.

Cold-Induced Sweating Syndrome. Cold-induced sweating syndrome, an autosomal recessive disorder, presents in the neonatal period with orofacial weakness and feeding difficulties related to impaired sucking and swallowing. During the first year, most infants have episodes of unexplained fever. From childhood onward, the most disabling symptoms stem from impaired thermoregulation. Patients have hyperhidrosis, mainly of the upper body, in response to cold temperatures, and sweat very little with heat. The disorder is caused by homozygous or compound heterozygous mutations in the *CRLF1* gene or in the *CLCF1* gene (OMIM #272430 and # 610313).

REFERENCES

 The complete list of references for this chapter is available in the e-book at www.expertconsult.com.

See inside cover for registration details.

SELECTED REFERENCES

Benarroch, E.E., 2012. Postural tachycardia syndrome: a heterogeneous and multifactorial disorder. Mayo Clin. Proc. 87 (12), 1214–1225.

Biaggioni, I., Robertson, D., 1987. Endogenous restoration of noradrenaline by precursor therapy in dopamine-beta-hydroxylase deficiency. Lancet 2 (8569), 1170–1172.

Florance, N.R., Davis, R.L., Lam, C., et al., 2009. Anti–N-Methyl-D-Aspartate Receptor (NMDAR) Encephalitis in Children and Adolescents. Ann. Neurol. 66 (1), 11–18.

Kaufmann, H., Hainsworth, R., 2001. Why do we faint? Muscle Nerve 24 (8), 981–983.

Koike, H., Atsuta, N., Adachi, H., et al., 2010. Clinicopathological features of acute autonomic and sensory neuropathy. Brain 133 (10), 2881–2896.

Neveus, T., Sillen, U., 2013. Lower urinary tract function in childhood; normal development and common functional disturbances. Acta Physiol (Oxf) 207 (1), 85–92.

Norcliffe-Kaufmann, L., Axelrod, F., Kaufmann, H., 2010. Afferent baroreflex failure in familial dysautonomia. Neurology 75 (21), 1904–1911.

Norcliffe-Kaufmann, L., Katz, S.D., Axelrod, F., et al., 2015. Norepinephrine deficiency with normal blood pressure control in congenital insensitivity to pain with anhidrosis. Ann. Neurol. 77 (5), 743–752.

Palma, J.A., Norcliffe-Kaufmann, L., Fuente-Mora, C., et al., 2014. Current treatments in familial dysautonomia. Expert Opin. Pharmacother. 15 (18), 2653–2671.

Wieling, W., Thijs, R.D., van Dijk, N., et al., 2009. Symptoms and signs of syncope: a review of the link between physiology and clinical clues. Brain 132 (Pt 10), 2630–2642.

E-BOOK FIGURES AND TABLES

The following figures and tables are available in the e-book at www.expertconsult.com. See inside cover for registration details.

Fig. 154-3 Diagnostic evaluation of pediatric patients with orthostatic intolerance and transient loss of consciousness.

Fig. 154-5 Tracing of Valsalva maneuver in a healthy subject showing muscle sympathetic nerve activity (MSNA) recording from the peroneal nerve electrocardiogram (ECG) and beat-to-beat blood pressure measured with plethysmography in the finger (BP) showing the four characteristic phases of the maneuver.

Fig. 154-6 Histogram showing the incidence of reflex (vasovagal) syncope in a population of young individuals up to the age of 24.

Fig. 154-7 Catecholamine pathways. Droxidopa (L-DOPS) converts to norepinephrine as a result of the action of the enzyme dopa-decarboxylase (L-amino acid aromatic decarboxylase).

155 Disorders of Micturition and Defecation

Israel Franco and Cecile Ejerskov

An expanded version of this chapter is available on www.expertconsult.com. See inside cover for registration details.

INTRODUCTION

Our understanding of bowel and bladder control has changed dramatically in the last 20 years with the introduction of fMRI and PET scanning of the brain. In this period of time, it has become more apparent that micturition and defecation involve and interplay with numerous sites in the spinal cord, brainstem, midbrain and cortex. In this chapter, we will examine the control of storing and emptying of urine and stool from what will be a new perspective, integrating the frontal lobes into the process and moving beyond the pons on which most of the literature had focused in the past.

DISORDERS OF MICTURITION

Attainment of bowel and bladder control is an important milestone in the lives of children and their parents. When this occurs varies from geographic region to geographic region and from ethnic group to ethnic group, but the maturational order is the same regardless, with bowel control preceding bladder control, and the sequence being:

1. Nocturnal bowel control
2. Daytime bowel control
3. Daytime bladder control
4. Nocturnal bladder control

What is certain is that girls tend to achieve continence quicker than boys, irrespective of the society in which they live. Daytime control is achieved between 3 to 4 years and nighttime control between 3.5 and 4 years of age. It may be obvious that we have refrained from using the term "diurnal incontinence" and are using the term "daytime incontinence." Throughout this chapter, we will use the terminology recommended by the International Children's Continence Society to allow for the proper communication in future clinical studies and to thereby enhance reproducibility of studies and outcomes (Austin et al., 2014). We will only deal with daytime urinary incontinence in this chapter. Nocturnal enuresis is a completely different entity that is best seen as an arousal disorder in the majority of patients. In fact, some patients have an appropriate diurnal variation in antidiuretic hormone production. Many children with nocturnal enuresis have "nonmonosymptomatic nocturnal enuresis," nocturnal enuresis with daytime lower urinary tract symptoms. These entities are well discussed in consensus papers put out by the International Children's Continence Society (Neveus et al., 2010).

Voiding in the infant is a reflexive action which lacks adequate volitional control, because the frontal lobes are not yet able to properly inhibit micturition. This concept is verified in previous studies in which frontal lobe arousal was recognized even in newborns, and some even awaken before urination. The human neonate initially voids hourly, and there is evidence that there is an interrupted voiding pattern that is the result of dyssynergia between the bladder and the sphincter. By 1 to 2 years of age, children can hold their urine, but it is difficult for them to willfully relax the external

sphincter. There is a gradual expansion in bladder capacity, and by 2 to 3 years of age, the bladder capacity has reached appropriate size to withhold urination for extended periods of time.

EPIDEMIOLOGY

The prevalence of daytime incontinence varies widely from study to study. For the most part nocturnal enuresis tends to be more prevalent than daytime incontinence. A meta-analysis of 3 studies was performed giving an overall prevalence of 6.4%. The English ALSPAC longitudinal study (Heron et al., 2008) found the following trajectories for daytime incontinence over the age range 4.5 to 9.5 years:

1. Normative (86.2%); dry by 4.5 years
2. Delayed (6.9%); steadily decreasing probability of daytime incontinence from 80% at 4.5 years of age to less than 10% at 9.5 years of age
3. Persistent (3.7%); probability of daytime incontinence greater than 80% until 7.5 years of age with steady reduction to 60% at 9.5 years of age
4. Relapsing (3.2%); probability of daytime incontinence less than 10% at 5.5 years of age, increasing to 60% at 6.5 years with slow decline thereafter

There was no gender difference in the delayed group, but girls outnumbered boys in the persistent and relapsing groups. In one study that looked at children with persistent urinary incontinence who had urodynamics and imaging of their spines revealed that, if extrapolated out to 18 years of age, up to 33% of the children that were wetting at 10 years of age were likely to persist with some form of urinary symptoms. From a pediatric urologist's perspective, the child who has OAB has a very good chance of becoming an adult who continues to have problems with OAB. This correlation has been seen in two published reports in adult females.

NEUROPSYCHIATRIC COMORBIDITY

Children with elimination disorders have an increased rate of comorbid behavioral or psychological disorders. About 20% to 40% of children with daytime urinary incontinence are affected by comorbid behavioral disorder. In a large epidemiologic study of a cohort of 8213 children aged 7.5 to 9 years, children with daytime wetting had significantly increased rates of psychological problems, especially separation anxiety (11.4%), attention deficit (24.8%), oppositional behavior (10.9%), and conduct problems (11.8%). In the same cohort, 10,000 children aged 4 to 9 years were analyzed. Delayed development, difficult temperament, and maternal depression/anxiety were associated with daytime wetting and soiling. In another population-based study that included 2856 children, the incidence of incontinence was 16.9% within the previous 6 months. In a retrospective study of patients with ADHD, 20.9% wetted at night and 6.5% wetted during the day. The odds ratios were 2.7 and 4.5 times higher, respectively, which means that there is unspecific association of ADHD and both nighttime and daytime wetting. The association of urinary incontinence and lower psychological well-being in adults also has been noted in other studies. Further discussion of neuropsychiatric disorders and urinary incontinence can be found in the online version of this chapter (von Gontard and Neveus, 2006).

ANATOMY OF THE LOWER URINARY TRACT (LUT)

The three main components of the bladder are the detrusor smooth muscle, connective tissue, and urothelium. The detrusor constitutes the bulk of the bladder, and is arranged into inner longitudinal, middle circular, and outer longitudinal layers. Elastin and collagen make up the connective tissue, which determines passive bladder compliance. The detrusor maintains a baseline tension, which is modulated by hormones, local neurotransmitters, and the autonomic nervous system.

Although the urothelium was previously thought to be an inert barrier, we now know that urothelial cells participate in afferent signaling. Bladder nerves terminate close to as well as on urothelial cells. Urothelial cells have pain receptors and mechanoreceptors, which can be modulated by ATP to activate or inhibit sensory neurons. Abnormal activation of these channels by inflammation can lead to pain responses to normally nonnoxious stimuli. Urothelial cells release factors such as acetylcholine, ATP, prostaglandins, and nitric oxide that affect sensory nerves (Fig. 155-2).

The internal and external urethral sphincters (EUS) are vital for urinary continence. The internal urethral sphincter functions as a unit with the bladder base and trigone to store urine. The smooth muscle of the female EUS has less sympathetic innervation than the male, and the male EUS is larger in size. The skeletal muscle of the EUS has both slow and fast twitch fibers, of which the slow twitch fibers are more important in maintaining tonic force in the urethra.

The lower urinary tract is innervated by both the autonomic and somatic nervous systems. Sympathetic nervous system control of the lower urinary tract travels via the hypogastric nerve (T10–L2) (Fig. 155-1, sympathetic preganglionic nucleus in thoracolumbar spinal cord), whereas parasympathetic control travels via the pelvic nerve (S2–S4) (Fig. 155-1, Gert's nucleus in sacral spinal cord). The somatic motor neurons control the skeletal muscle of the EUS via the pudendal nerve (S2–S4). Its motor neurons are found in Onuf's nucleus (Fig. 155-1, sacral spinal cord) The sympathetic and somatic nervous systems promote storage of urine and stool and facilitates ejaculation (Sympathetic: Storage and Shoot), whereas the parasympathetic system promotes bladder and bowel emptying and erections (Parasympathetic: Pee, Poop, and Point).

AFFERENT MECHANISMS

The sensation of bladder fullness is carried by two types of afferent fibers via the pelvic, hypogastric, and pudendal nerves. Normal bladder sensations are carried by Aδ fibers, whereas C fibers become more important in diseased bladders. In humans, C fibers transmit pain sensations and are found in the urothelial and suburothelial layers, whereas Aδ fibers are found in the smooth muscle (Fig. 155-2).

These fibers terminate in the dorsal horn of the lumbar and sacral cord. Spinal connections in this area mediate segmental reflexes. Some of the spinal interneurons send ascending projections to two nuclei in the brainstem. The gracile

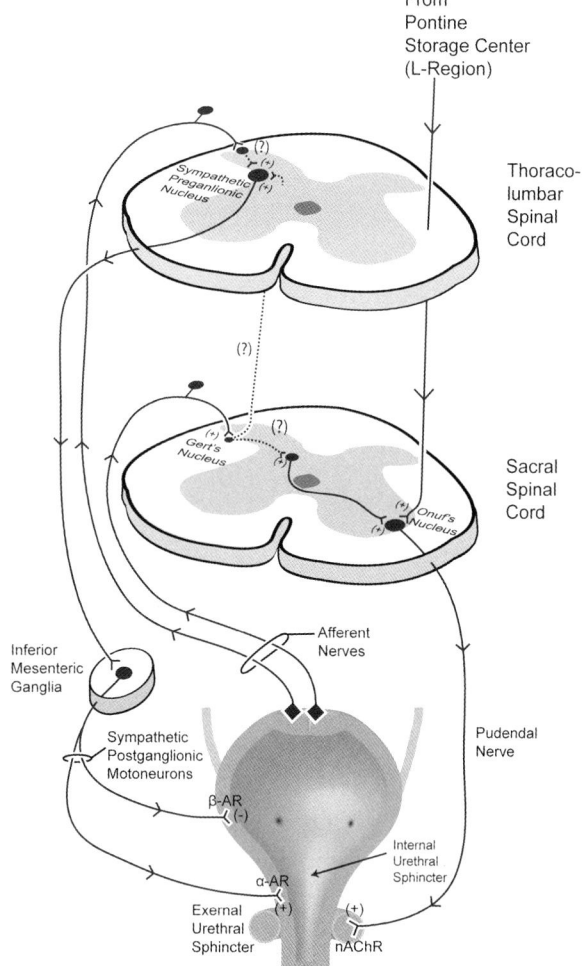

Figure 155-1. Afferent pathways for the control of micturition. *(With permission from Birder, L., de Groat, W., Mills, I., et al., 2010. Neural control of the lower urinary tract: peripheral and spinal mechanisms. Neurourol Urodyn 29, 128–139.)*

nucleus relays nociception to the thalamus and cortex. The parabrachial nucleus is a major relay center for visceral afferent information going to the amygdala and the insular cortex integrating nociceptive and autonomic inputs. A significant degree of convergence of inputs from pelvic viscera is seen at the level of the medullary reticular formation.

During bladder storage, afferent signals from the hypogastric nerve and pelvic nerve travel to the thoracolumbar and sacral spinal cord, respectively (Fig. 155-1). The hypogastric nerve sends signals via the sympathetic nervous system to block bladder contraction and contact the internal urethral sphincter. Onuf's nucleus maintains contraction of the EUS, which is coordinated with bladder storage by the pontine micturition center (PMC) in the medial pons (Fig. 155-1).

Once the bladder pressure threshold is exceeded, afferent signals travel via the pelvic nerve to synapse on interneurons in Gert's nucleus in the S1–S2 spinal cord (Fig 155-3). These interneurons send projections up to the periaqueductal gray (PAG) in the midbrain to initiate voiding, which occurs if the cerebral cortex determines that it is appropriate to void. The medial anterior frontal lobes connect to the pudendal neurons via the corticospinal tracts (pyramidal tracts). They send connections to the PAG that sends caudal projections to the PMC, which is the final efferent center of the lower urinary tract. The

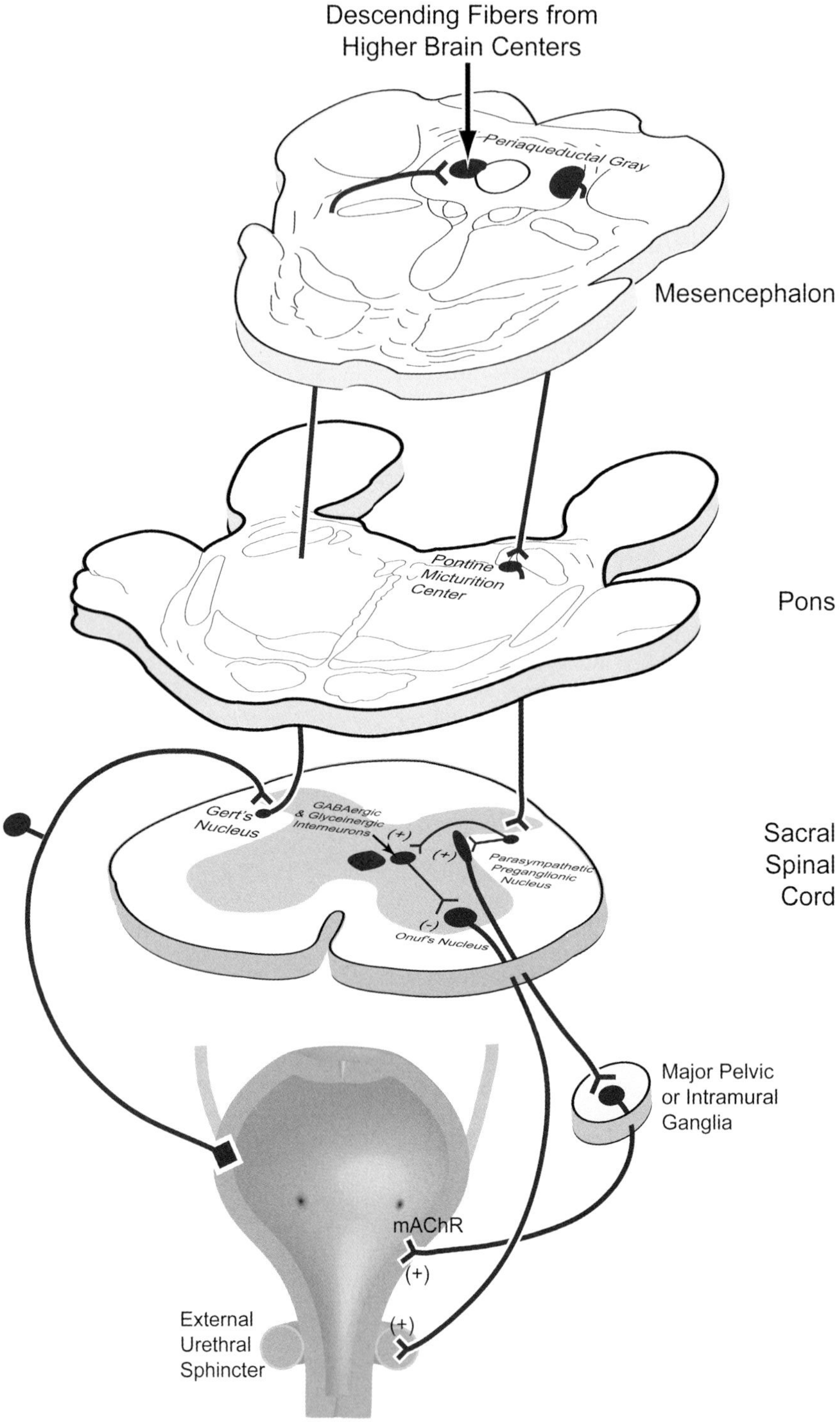

Descending Fibers from
Higher Brain Centers

Periaqueductal Gray

Mesencephalon

Pontine
Micturition
Center

Pons

Gert's
Nucleus

GABAergic
& Glycinergic
Interneurons

(+)

(+)

Parasympathetic
Preganglionic
Nucleus

Sacral
Spinal
Cord

(−)

Onuf's Nucleus

Major Pelvic
or Intramural
Ganglia

mAChR

(+)

External
Urethral
Sphincter

(+)

Figure 155-3. Efferent pathways for the control of micturition. *(With permission from Birder, L., de Groat, W., Mills, I., et al., 2010. Neural control of the lower urinary tract: peripheral and spinal mechanisms. Neurourol Urodyn 29, 128–139.)*

PMC sends projections caudally via the corticospinal tracts in the cord to the sacral parasympathetic nucleus, activating the neurons which cause bladder contraction and EUS relaxation (Fig. 155-3). Bilateral pathologic involvement of the pyramidal tract, usually in the spinal cord, results in impaired volitional control of the urethral sphincter; therefore the urethral sphincter may undergo inappropriate relaxation, or increased sphincter activity may occur during detrusor contraction. This imbalance is termed detrusor-urethral sphincter dyssynergia (Birder et al. 2010).

Disorders that affect the spinal cord and have effects on the micturition and sensation are described in the online version of this chapter.

Periaqueductal Gray (PAG) and Pontine Micturition Center (PMC)

The PAG is involved in neurobiological functions that include the control and expression of pain, analgesia, fear, anxiety, vocalization, lordosis, cardiovascular function, and reproductive behavior. Conceptually the structure may be involved in balancing or segueing information related to survival.

Forebrain projections to the PAG arise mainly from the prefrontal cortex, the insular cortex, and the amygdala. Further, the PAG receives highly organized projections from the central nucleus of the amygdala and, in turn, has reciprocal connections with the central nucleus. The PAG also projects to the thalamus, hypothalamus, brainstem, and deep layers of the spinal cord with some somatotopic organization, but projections to cortical regions have not been identified.

The central role of the PAG is evident, as it both receives sacral afferents and transmits efferent signals (via the PMC) to the sacral spinal cord. During storage, it is chronically suppressed by a net inhibition from the many other regions shown in Figure 155-4A. These include prefrontal cortex and hypothalamus, as well as insula and anterior cingulate cortex. The posterior hypothalamic region, which is involved in fight or flight (defense) responses, has direct connections to the PAG and may account for the urination reported in conscious animals during a defense response (Linnman et al., 2012).

The PMC, however. is the ultimate arbiter of lower urinary tract function, acting as a switch between the storage and voiding phases. It is believed that, for voiding to occur, the PMC requires both an excitatory signal from the PAG and a "safe" signal from the hypothalamus as suggested by Figure 155-4B.

Micturition problems with inability to empty well and urinary retention have been associated with posterior fossa tumors, discrete pontine lesions, brainstem gliomas, or vascular lesions that support the role of the dorsolateral pons (pontine reticular nucleus and the reticular formation, adjacent to the medial parabrachial nucleus, and locus coeruleus). Functional imaging shows activations near the postulated location of the PMC during voiding. PMC activity during bladder filling has also been seen, though this might be inhibitory rather than excitatory.

The area thought responsible for off-switching at the end of urination is the pontine continence center (PCC) also known as the L region described by Bradley. This area is located in the dorsolateral tegmentum. Projections form the PCC appear limited to Onuf's nucleus. Activation of this site can cause the detrusor to relax and the pelvic floor musculature and urethral sphincter to contract. A few functional imaging studies appear to localize this area ventral, lateral, or caudal to the PMC.

Insula

The cardinal feature of enteroceptive system is that the afferent input is from small diameter fibers ($A\delta$ and C). These afferents project via the spinothalamic tracts to subcortical homeostatic centers, including the hypothalamus and PAG. In humans they relay in the thalamus and converge on the nondominant anterior insula. The insula has come to be regarded as the homeostatic afferent cortex and has been shown to be activated by a range of modalities associated with visceral sensation. Insula activation has been extensively studied in the fMRI experiments carried out by other investigators and have shown a correlation between the degree of bladder filling and insula activation in healthy controls (Figure 155-5A and B). The conscious desire to void or urgency is lost in extensive frontal lobe lesions involving the insula (Griffiths and Tadic, 2008).

Anterior Cingulate Cortex (ACC)

The anterior cingulate cortex (ACC) is the cortical region associated with motivation. Motivation plays a critical role in human homeostasis. Therefore if the insula is regarded as the limbic sensory cortex, the ACC can be considered as the limbic motor cortex, the two being frequently seen to be coactivated in functional brain imaging studies. A wide range of cerebral functions has been attributed to the ACC over the years as its activation is seen with many different executive tasks but the demonstration that output was correlated with sympathetic activation led to the hypothesis that the ACC "mediates context-driven modulation of bodily arousal states."

The ACC also is the site in which pain is processed. The proximity of the nociceptive, motor, and attentional regions of ACC suggests possible local interconnections that might allow the output of the ACC pain area to command immediate behavioral reactions. Similarly, the ACC pain area might participate in the substantial interconnections between the ACC and the "fight or flight" regions of the midbrain and the periaqueductal gray matter. The anatomic connections between ACC, IC (rostral insula), SI, and SII (primary and secondary somatosensory cortices) suggest that these regions do not function independently in encoding different aspects of pain but are highly interactive.

Another key feature of the ACC is the role it plays in autonomic control. Previous fMRI studies and neuropsychological and physiologic observations have shown that a direct link exists between ACC activity and modulation of cardiac function via sympathetic output. These observations argue for control of the ACC in the production and control of behaviorally integrated patterns of autonomic activity (Critchley et al., 2003).

Prefrontal Cortex

The ventral region of prefrontal cortex (PFC) is involved in aspects of cognition, and the inferior lateral parts are involved in emotions. The orbitofrontal or prefrontal lateral cortex (PFLC) has extensive interconnections with the limbic system—the hypothalamus, amygdala, insula, and ACC. The importance of the prefrontal cortex in bladder control was established from clinical studies both by previous studies that found that acts of micturition and defecation occur in a normal manner; however, what is disturbed by this frontal lesion is the higher control of these acts. The lesion causes frequency and extreme urgency of micturition when the patient is awake and incontinence when asleep. The sensation of gradual awareness of increasing fullness of the bladder and the sensation that micturition is imminent are impaired. In the most complete form of the syndrome, the patient cannot inhibit the detrusor contraction of the micturition reflex and is forced to empty the bladder as soon as the reflex occurs. When the syndrome is less pronounced, the patient can make a conscious effort to stop the act of micturition and may or may not succeed. The lowering of the micturition reflex threshold may account for the fact that the patient does not feel the normal gradual filling of the bladder that underlies the desire to micturate; however, it cannot account for the unawareness of the sensations arising from the activity of pelvic and perineal muscles or of the sensation that urine is passing. A further discussion on the effects of strokes is in the online chapter.

Cortical areas such as the prefrontal cortex have the ability to inhibit limbic system activation and have been implicated in the therapeutic effects of distraction techniques such as hypnosis therapy and the use of placebo.

In the PFC, cortisol modulates dopaminergic projections with a remarkable degree of lateralization. Dopaminergic projections to the right hemisphere display an enhanced sensitivity to stressors that are perceived as severe and uncontrollable such as those that arise from social conflict. Thus chronic psychological stress can disinhibit reflexive circuits through a cortisol-induced right PFC dysfunction that is caused by a prolonged activation of the hypothalamic-pituitary-adrenal axis. This reduction in activity in the PFC can

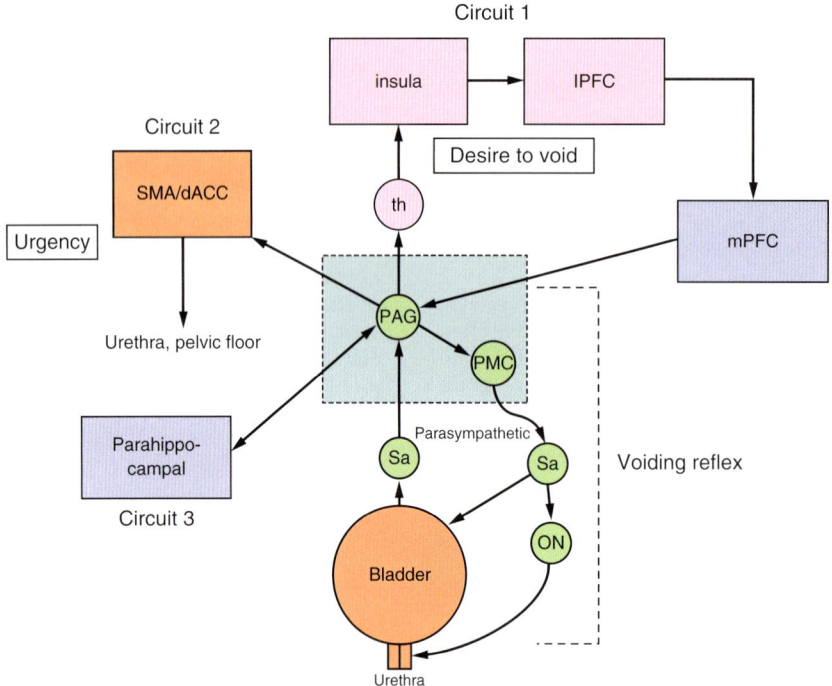

Figure 155-6. Proposed interconnections between the different areas of the cortex, midbrain, and brainstem structures that are involved in the control of micturition. Arrows show probable directions of connectivity but do not preclude movement in the opposite direction. Three circuits are described that are critical to the control of micturition. The green area is the critical transit point that includes the periaqueductal gray area (PAG) and pontine micturition center (PMC). They control contraction and relaxation of the bladder via the sacral parasympathetic regions (Sa) and Onuf's nucleus (ON). These reflexes are controlled by three cerebral neural pathways. Circuit 1 involves the thalamus (th), insula, and lateral prefrontal cortex (LPFC) that maps for desire to void, although the mPFC (medial prefrontal cortex) makes the executive decision when and where to void. Circuit 2 involves the supplemental motor area (SMA) and the dorsal anterior cingulate cortex (dACC). Here, urgency is processed as an emotion, and lesions in this area lead to urge incontinence; pain is processed here as well. Circuit 3 goes the parahippocampal area. Areas in blue are typically deactivated with filling; orange and red areas are activated with bladder filling. *(From Griffiths, D., Clarkson, B., Tadic, S.D., Resnick, N.M., 2015. Brain mechanisms underlying urge incontinence and its response to pelvic floor muscle training. J Urol 194, 708–715.)*

lead to the inability to inhibit the urge to urinate and it may lead to urge incontinence as well as fecal incontinence. The information in Figure 155-6 has been proposed as a summary illustration of the current thinking about brain control of the bladder during filling and emptying (Griffiths et al., 2015).

Efferent mechanisms—peripheral
See online chapter for discussion.
Efferent mechanisms—central
See online chapter for discussion

DIAGNOSIS
History and Physical Examination

The evaluation of the child with bowel and bladder dysfunction should start with a good history and physical examination. Generally, it is best to try to get the history from the child if he or she is cooperative, but in other cases there may be no choice but to obtain it from the parents. Crossing the legs, running to the bathroom, grabbing the penis, rubbing the clitoris, squatting, and sitting on the heels are all signs of urgency. These maneuvers trigger reflexive suppression of the voiding reflex. Urinary frequency is also another manifestation of an overactive bladder and quantifying the number of times that the patient goes to the bathroom and the amount is useful in determining whether there is true frequency. Urinary urge incontinence is another classic hallmark of overactive bladder. The physician should also ask about a history of dysuria. Dysuria without evidence of infection is usually due to

dyssynergic voiding. One should ascertain the type of stream and the strength. Whether the patient strains to void or uses the Credé maneuver is critical to know. In infants, grunting with urination may be a sign of dyssynergic voiding.

On entering the room, the physician should take close note of the interaction between the child and parent as well as the child and the physician. Excessive anxiety or inappropriate fear is something that should be noted. The parents should be questioned as to whether this type of behavior is commonly present at home or during other stressful situations. A careful history should be taken with regards to a family history of anxiety, phobias, ADD/ADHD, or depression within the first-line family members.

A thorough history of the bowel habits of the patient should be obtained from the patient directly. Documentation of the size and nature of the bowel movements should be obtained. Use of a diagram is quite beneficial, and it facilitates communication with the child. Chronic constipation can be a clue of a cord lesion, especially if it is refractory.

The presence of bladder fullness or urgency and frequency would indicate that the sensory pathways are intact. Urgency in a neurologically impaired patient is a sign of a partial suprasegmental injury whereas a complete lesion is usually associated with incontinence associated with no warning or sensation. On the other hand, the patient that does not void unless prompted may have inappropriate sensation. Those that void with Valsalva or Credé maneuver can have a myogenic failure of the detrusor or failure of the efferent pathways. Obstruction would need to be excluded as well.

Autonomic dysreflexia may occur and is discussed in the online chapter.

Peripheral motor lesions involving the conus medullaris, which anatomically is located between T12 and L1, or the cauda equina will lead the majority of patients to complain of an "obstructive" symptom and will need to strain or use the Credé maneuver to urinate. Further discussion of cauda equina, conus, and epiconus lesions are in the online chapter.

Physical Examination

Examination of the abdomen is critical in determining whether there is stool present in the colon. Examination of the back will typically reveal a normal-appearing back and anocutaneous folds. In rare instances, one will notice flattening of the buttocks or abnormal creasing at the SI joint indicative of some type of sacral anomaly. Low-lying sacral dimples are typically not of concern. Dimples that are associated with tufts of hair or if located higher up on the back are of concern and should be evaluated with an MRI of the lumbosacral spine.

Examination of the genitalia should be performed on all children with bowel and bladder dysfunction. First and foremost, one should look at the underwear when it is pulled down to help gauge the gravity of the problem. Visual inspection of the anus is a very useful tool, which allows one to assess whether the patient has skin tags, fissures, and hemorrhoids that are indicators of chronic problems with constipation or large bowel movements. Laxity of the anal sphincter is another good sign that the child is passing massive bowel movements or has a neurologic problem. Evidence of an anal wink is a sign of an intact sacral reflex arch (S2–S4) and is commonly seen as soon as the buttocks are separated to inspect the anus. Pinprick testing for sensation of the perineum and anus is critical as well. A bulbocavernosus reflex test should be performed and should be present in 98% of all males and 81% of females. Absence indicates a complete lower motor neuron lesion of the sacral cord that correlates well with perineal floor denervation. Digital rectal examination is rarely necessary in these children. If it is going to be done, then the bulbocavernosus reflex should be tested at the same time. Rectal examination neither confirms nor denies the presence of constipation.

Examination of the patients smile is another critical part of the examination in children that have evidence of a severely trabeculated bladder or evidence of severe voiding dysfunction without sacral dysraphism. Children who have Ochoa urofacial syndrome (OMIM 236730) when asked to smile will have an unusual inversion of facial expression when smiling is attempted. The face becomes contorted into a grimace that makes it appear as if the subject is sobbing and crying, thus, making it possible to recognize afflicted patients early in life (Fig. 155-8). Please see the online chapter for a more thorough discussion of this topic.

Clinical Testing

In children suspected of having a disorder of micturition or storage, the first study should be a urinalysis and urine culture to rule out infection that can lead to such symptoms. The next study should be a postvoid residual ultrasound measurement. This determines whether the patient is adequately emptying the bladder and thereby frequently helps to differentiate disorders of emptying from storage disorders, even though some children, especially those with functional voiding problems, can simultaneously have both disorders. If at all possible, uroflowmetry utilizing EMG of the perineal muscles should be done initially. Perineal EMG allows for the identification of external sphincter dyssynergia and internal sphincter

dyssynergia that can be identified utilizing the lag time, which is the delay before the initiation in urination. Internal sphincter dyssynergia has been associated with dizziness and autonomic dysfunction (hypotension on standing without concomitant increase in heart rate) with specificity rates in the high 90s for both males and females when patients are asked if they get dizzy on standing. Renal and bladder ultrasounds are next in order if there is evidence of large bladder capacities or urinary retention or an abnormal uroflowmetry. Patients that exhibit markedly abnormal uroflowmetry or ultrasonography should then have a voiding cystourethrogram if indicated or a KUB radiograph with an AP and lateral of the spine at a minimum. Blood tests evaluating renal function are indicated if the ultrasound or VCUG are abnormal. In refractory patients, it is necessary to obtain a VCUG to further delineate voiding dynamics and to make sure that anatomic problems are not missed.

Urodynamics are not necessary in patients who have functional voiding problems in the vast majority of cases. In one study, urodynamics did not offer any information that was not noted on the MRI if it was positive. If there is suspicion of a spinal problem, it is best to initially obtain a spinal MRI, and later, if a spinal abnormality is identified, then urodynamics are indicated to define the problem and to provide a baseline for future reevaluations to assess whether there is progression of the disease or before when surgery is to be done. There are noninvasive means of testing the bulbocavernosus reflex latency, but these are not done routinely in children.

Disorders of Defecation
Normal Defecation Patterns

Defecation patterns in childhood differ with age and are determined by the change from breastfeeding to solid foods. In breastfed infants, defecation occurs from six to seven times a day to once every seventh day, and, on average, three times daily. At 6 to 12 months, the average defecation rate is just lower than two times per day; at 1 to 3 years, the average defecation rate is one and a half times per day. At 3 to 12 years, the defecation rate settles at once daily. There is no difference in gender until puberty. During puberty and adulthood, the defecation rate among females is less than among males. To appreciate colorectal motility of defecation, the neurophysiology, and the various pathologic changes related hereto, it is important to understand the functional anatomy and neurophysiology of colon, rectum, and anus.

FUNCTIONAL ANATOMY OF COLON, RECTUM, AND ANUS

The main functions of the large intestine are intraluminal bacterial fermentation of nutrients resistant to digestive enzymes (e.g., short-chain fatty acids), reabsorption of water and electrolytes, and transport and storage of feces until it can be discharged from the body.

Histologically, the wall of the large intestine is made up of mucosa, submucosa, tunica muscularis, and serosa. The mucosa consists of an inner layer epithelium, underlying the lamina propria, and the muscularis mucosa. Distributed within the columnar epithelium are absorptive cells, goblet cells, and enteroendocrine cells. The lamina propria is a connective tissue rich in cells. It includes immunocompetent cells, nerve fibers, fibroblasts, lymphatic vessels, and capillaries. The muscularis mucosa is a thin layer of intestinal smooth muscle. The submucosa consists of loose connective tissue and substantial fatty tissue; here lies the submucosal plexus (Meissner's plexus), one of the plexuses of the enteric nerve system (ENS), together with larger nerves, blood, and lymph vessels. The tunica muscularis consists of the inner complete circular layer that, during contraction, divides the colon into segments—the characteristic haustra and an outer incomplete longitudinal layer, which is made up by three flat longitudinal bands, taenia coli. In the rectum, the taenia disappears, and the longitudinal muscle layer becomes complete. The feces is transported as a result of contractions in the muscle layer containing the myenteric plexus (Auerbach's plexus), the other plexus of the ENS located between the circular and the longitudinal layers. The serosa consists of a mesothelial lining resembling the visceral peritoneal surface. The rectum initially runs distally and posteriorly, then directly downward, and finally anteriorly and ends as the anus in the perineum. The rectum is closely related to the bladder. The rectum is divided into two segments: the rectal ampulla and the anal canal. As a reservoir for storage of feces, the function of the rectum is to maintain fecal continence and allow defecation at an appropriate time and place. The upper and the lower part of the anal canal are separated by a mucocutaneous zone. The lower squamous epithelium is rich in somatosensory fibers and is highly sensitive to temperature, touch, movement, and pain. The anal canal in children is estimated to be between 2.5 and 3 cm long. At the anorectal junction, the puborectalis muscle creates an angle of approximately 80 degrees, which is considered to contribute to anal continence. The continuation of the circular smooth muscle layer constitutes the internal anal sphincter (IAS), whereas the external sphincter (EAS) consists of striated muscle and hence is partly under voluntary control. With the support from the pelvic floor, the levator ani muscle and the internal and external anal sphincters maintain a higher pressure in the anal canal than in the rectal ampulla (Fig. 155-10A and B).

Colorectal Motility and Defecation

There are at least three regulatory mechanisms in the gastrointestinal tract; endocrine, paracrine, and the enteric nervous system (ENS). The scope of this paragraph is the ENS, its modulators and colorectal motility. Overall, neural control of colorectal motility is provided by the ENS, the intrinsic nervous system, modulated through the extrinsic nervous system; the lumbar sympathetic nerves; sacral parasympathetic nerves; and extrinsic sensory innervations.

THE INTRINSIC NERVOUS SYSTEM

The majority of the neural control of colorectal motility is meditated by the ENS. Auerbach's plexus mainly controls the motility, and Meissner's plexus mainly controls the secretion and blood flow. Generally, the ENS consists of sensory neurons, interneurons, and both excitatory and inhibitory motor neurons. Different neurotransmitters, neuropeptides, and other molecules either inhibit (e.g., noradrenalin, dopamine, somatostatin) or increase (e.g., acetylcholine, serotonin, histamine) motility.

THE EXTRINSIC NERVOUS SYSTEM

Indirectly, by modulating the ENS via the interneurons, the sacral parasympathetic nerves increase digestion and motility whereas the lumbar sympathetic nerves decrease digestion and motility. This is caused by an increase/decrease of vasodilation, secretion, and peristaltic activity and relaxation/constriction of the sphincters. The colorectal extrinsic sensory innervation is provided by spinal afferent neurons and a subpopulation of these, mechanosensitive afferents that are highly sensitive to intestinal distension by feces, can consequently be an important factor of conscious awareness of rectal filling, of continence, and in initiating defecation. The somatic innervation of the extrinsic anal sphincter is via a perineal branch of the S4 nerve and the pudendal nerve.

MUSCLE CONTRACTIONS AND COLORECTAL MOTILITY

Control of muscle contractions are discussed in the online version of this chapter.

Defecation, to void feces from the distal colon and rectum, is a complex process involving the previously described ENS, autonomic nervous system, and smooth and striated muscles. It is initiated when a colonic mass movement continues to rectum generating a slow distension of the rectal wall. As the distension proceeds, the filling of the rectum stimulates the rectoanal inhibitory reflex (RAIR), mediated by the ENS, and causes relaxation of the IAS. Additionally, the rectum now serves as a conduit, and the RAIR stimulates the filling of the upper anal canal. The upper anal canal's sensory innervations make it possible to detect consistency and thereby distinguish between air, solid or liquid. The filling creates the urge to defecate. Defecation will proceed with the voluntary relaxation of the puborectal muscle, straightening of the anorectal angle, and relaxation of the EAS. Defecation is normally improved by the Valsalva maneuver. As wall tension relaxes, the defecation reflex subsides and rectal compliance increases, which leads to a resting pressure of the anal canal higher than in rectum and thereby reaching continence.

CNS AND THE GUT

More than 90% of the body's serotonin (5-HT) is found in the enterochromaffin cells in the gastrointestinal canal, and plasma 5-HT has been found increased in diarrheal diseases and decreased in constipation. The 5-HT$_4$ agonist, prucalopride, is used to treat chronic constipation if laxatives prove insufficient. It has shown promising results, but research among children is lacking (Brookes et al., 2009).

Higher brain centers that influence and control defecation are the ACC, PFC, insula, the amygdala, the stria terminalis, and the hypothalamus. In humans, response to external stressors is mediated through the coordinated action of the hypothalamic-pituitary-adrenal (HPA) axis and the sympathetic branch of the autonomic nervous system. With this in mind, research in treatment with 5-HT$_3$-antagonist in irritable bowel syndrome among adults found a decrease in brain activity in the emotional motor systems with correlates to a decrease in gastrointestinal symptoms. One model for irritable bowel syndrome proposes that altered central stress circuits have been introduced. It is hypothesized that triggering of these circuits by external stressors results in the development of gut and extraintestinal symptoms in predisposed individuals. Central control of defecation and gastrointestinal function are in the same sites as that for urination (Mayer et al., 2006).

Further discussion of this topic is in the online version of the chapter.

PATIENT EVALUATION
History

Fecal incontinence, constipation and abdominal pain are the most common complaints in children seeking help. In some patients, fecal incontinence and abdominal pain may be due to constipation. But in other individuals, these symptoms may be isolated problems. Questioning should precede the same as for disorders of micturition.

As with disorders of micturition, the same questioning process should be used except that specific questions assessing alterations in bowel habits, stool mass, stool color, and stool consistency should be done. The age at onset, frequency, related circumstances (e.g., time of day, association with sleep, behavioral aspects), and alterations in bowel habits, stool mass, stool color, and stool consistency should be established. It should be determined whether the child feels stool in the rectum, has the urge to defecate, whether soiling occurs without notice, or whether the child have some sensation when he/she has an accident. It is helpful to ascertain whether the child can differentiate between passage of flatus and feces. Similarly, efferent function can be evaluated by asking questions related to volitional inhibition of defecation. Fecal incontinence is unlikely to be due to spinal cord disease in the absence of urinary symptoms or neurologic abnormalities involving the lower limbs.

Neurologic Examination

As the neural pathways are similar, neurologic evaluation of bowel incontinence parallels that described for disorders of micturition. Further insight to the examination is discussed in the online version of the chapter.

Clinical Studies

A simple flat plate of the abdomen is necessary to evaluate for constipation. An AP and lateral film should be done to look at the sacrum. In children with a history of imperforate anus, a sacral ratio less than 0.52 correlates well with spinal cord anomalies and with unfavorable prognosis in children with anorectal malformations. We also know that children with high imperforate anus have a 70% to 80% rate of neurogenic bladder dysfunction.

Current promising pediatric anorectal investigations are manometry, measuring contractility in the anus and rectum, and impedance planimetry, studies of rectal compliance. Proctoscopy and fiber optic studies of the lower bowel are efficient methods of excluding the presence of structural abnormalities. Barium enema studies sometimes are necessary, as are defecography studies, which monitor the functional events visually during defecation.

Differential Diagnosis

The most common cause of fecal incontinence is encopresis, which is not associated with neurologic dysfunction. Encopresis is fecal incontinence without organic cause for more than a month in children 4 years of age or older. Males outnumber females by 3.5 to 1. Children with fecal incontinence (or encopresis) have the highest rates of coexistent behavioral disorders: 30% to 50% of all children have clinically relevant behavioral disturbances. Many will exhibit withholding of stools that will lead to stool smearing of the underwear and, at times, outright full defecation. In some, the urge to control defecation many not be processed appropriately in executive areas, leading to inability to suppress the reflexive event. Neurogenic and other organic conditions causing bowel dysfunction must be excluded. Other causes of functional bowel problems such as irritable bowel syndrome and abdominal migraines may have their origins in the frontal lobes as well.

Lumbosacral defects may be associated with reduced or absent external sphincter function, which is demonstrated by sphincter electromyography. Denervation potentials or reduced large-amplitude potentials may be observed. In Hirschsprung disease, manometric studies demonstrate an absence of the rectoanal inhibitory reflex; that is, the internal sphincter fails to relax in response to a transient rectal distention. The relaxation wave is absent.

Management

Assessment of contributing factors, including psychosocial milieu, anorectal examination, and appropriate neurologic evaluation, is necessary for adequate management. Therapeutic approaches include dietary, behavioral, pharmacologic, and surgical methods. For fecal incontinence, the management of the concomitant constipation is paramount and a thorough bowel cleansing is in order. Education is important in achieving good outcome.

Further discussion of management techniques is included in the online version.

REFERENCES

The complete list of references for this chapter is available in the e-book at www.expertconsult.com.
See inside cover for registration details.

SELECTED REFERENCES

Austin, P.F., Bauer, S.B., Bower, W., et al., 2014. The standardization of terminology of lower urinary tract function in children and adolescents: update report from the Standardization Committee of the International Children's Continence Society. J. Urol. 191, 1863–1865 e13.

Blankstein, U., Chen, J., Diamant, N.E., et al., 2010. Altered brain structure in irritable bowel syndrome: potential contributions of pre-existing and disease-driven factors. Gastroenterology 138, 1783–1789.

Birder, L., de Groat, W., Mills, I., et al., 2010. Neural control of the lower urinary tract: peripheral and spinal mechanisms. Neurourol. Urodyn. 29, 128–139.

Brookes, S.J., Dinning, P.G., Gladman, M.A., 2009. Neuroanatomy and physiology of colorectal function and defecation: from basic science to human clinical studies. Neurogastroenterol. Motil. 21 (Suppl. 2), 9–19.

Critchley, H.D., Mathias, C.J., Josephs, O., et al., 2003. Human cingulate cortex and autonomic control: converging neuroimaging and clinical evidence. Brain 126, 2139–2152.

Critchley, H.D., Mathias, C.J., Josephs, O., et al., 2006. Human cingulate cortex and autonomic control: converging neuroimaging and clinical evidence. Brain 126, 2139–2152.

Griffiths, D., Clarkson, B., Tadic, S.D., et al., 2015. Brain mechanisms underlying urge incontinence and its response to pelvic floor muscle training. J. Urol. 194, 708–715.

Griffiths, D., Tadic, S.D., 2008. Bladder control, urgency, and urge incontinence: evidence from functional brain imaging. Neurourol. Urodyn. 27, 466–474.

Heron, J., Joinson, C., Croudace, T., et al., 2008. Trajectories of daytime wetting and soiling in a United Kingdom 4- to 9-year-old population birth cohort study. J. Urol. 179, 1970–1975.

Linnman, C., Moulton, E.A., Barmettler, G., et al., 2012. Neuroimaging of the periaqueductal gray: state of the field. Neuroimage 60, 505–522.

Mayer, E.A., Naliboff, B.D., Craig, A.D., 2006. Neuroimaging of the brain-gut axis: from basic understanding to treatment of functional GI disorders. Gastroenterology 131, 1925–1942.

Neveus, T., Eggert, P., Evans, J., et al., 2010. Evaluation of and treatment for monosymptomatic enuresis: a standardization document from the International Children's Continence Society. J. Urol. 183, 441–447.

von Gontard, A., Nevéus, T., 2006. Management of Disorders of Bladder and Bowel Control in Childhood. Mac Keith Press, London.

⊛ E-BOOK FIGURES AND TABLES

The following figures and tables are available in the e-book at www.expertconsult.com. See inside cover for registration details.

Fig. 155-2 Current concepts of sensory innervation of the bladder.

Fig. 155-4 A, Storage phase: A model of lower urinary tract control by higher brain centers. **B,** Voiding phase: A model of lower urinary tract control by higher brain centers.

Fig. 155-5 A, The response to bladder filling in normal controls at large bladder volumes. **B,** The response to bladder filling in subjects with urge incontinence at large bladder volumes.

Fig. 155-7 Current treatment options to improve bladder storage.

Fig. 155-8 Child with Ochoa urofacial syndrome.

Fig. 155-9 Anatomy of the rectum and its nervous supply.

Fig. 155-10 Functional anatomy of storage of stool and defecation.

Box 155-1 Selected Differential Diagnosis of Neurologically Induced Disorders of Micturition and Defecation

156 Poisoning and Drug-Induced Neurologic Diseases

Kristyn Tekulve, Laura M. Tormoehlen, and Laurence Walsh

INTRODUCTION

Many substances are potential nervous system toxins. Manufactured and naturally occurring agents may be ingested, inhaled, injected, or absorbed, with subsequent deleterious effects on a child's central or peripheral nervous system. Most childhood ingestions are accidental. Effects may be acute, subacute, or chronic, and may occur at any age. Neurologic dysfunction may be isolated or part of a systemic derangement. Neurotoxins are among the most commonly encountered toxins, although less common in children younger than 6 years (Mowry et al., 2014). Poisonings and drug-induced neurologic disease may mimic infection, trauma, neoplasm, psychiatric illness, or metabolic disorders.

A more detailed description of the following toxins and information about additional toxins can be found in the online version.

Emergency Evaluation

Management of the poisoned child requires immediate stabilization of the patient and appropriate corrective and supportive therapy. Physicians must review the history and examine the child carefully and have a high index of suspicion. Three-quarters of poisonings are by ingestion. Medications account for most deaths. Physical examination can establish the cause and guide therapy. Neurologic findings may result from the toxin itself or its systemic effects. Systemic effects include CNS hypoxia, cardiac dysrhythmias, gastrointestinal disturbances, and metabolic acidosis.

Management

Gastric lavage has been a mainstay of treatment; however, experts now recommend against it as it does not improve outcomes and can have severe complications, including aspiration pneumonia, laryngospasm, arrhythmias, esophageal or stomach perforation, fluid and electrolyte imbalances, and small conjunctival hemorrhages. Local poison control should be consulted if gastric lavage is considered.

Ipecac syrup works as an emetic, but there is insufficient data to recommend its use. The most common adverse effects are diarrhea, lethargy, prolonged vomiting, irritability, fever, and diaphoresis. If the vomiting is severe, Mallory–Weiss tears, pneumomediastinum, and aspiration pneumonia may result. Some experts argue that ipecac syrup may be used in rare circumstances, such as when medical care cannot be achieved within 1 hour, the toxin ingested was dangerous, there is no alteration in mental status, and the ipecac syrup would not affect further medical care. Many other experts disagree and recommend never using ipecac syrup.

Whole-bowel irrigation with large volumes of polyethylene glycol–electrolyte solutions to prevent toxin absorption has been used. There has also not been evidence to show that this improves patient outcomes. Complications of the treatment include vomiting, diarrhea, electrolyte abnormalities, aspiration, and rarely angioedema/anaphylactic reactions. It may be

considered when a sustained-release or enteric-coated preparation has been ingested, if the toxin cannot be removed by activated charcoal, or if illicit drugs are carried in the body.

Appropriate general management steps are outlined in Box 156-1; details may be found in several references (Leikin and Paloucek, 1995). Therapy for specific toxidromes is discussed with the individual agents.

Testing

The value of routine toxicologic testing in cases of possible intoxications is debated. The low sensitivity of specific tests and the inability to test for all possible agents, medicolegal concerns, cost-effectiveness, and limited use specifically for children suggest that routine testing should be limited. Ideally, history and physical examination narrow the list of possible exposures and direct specific toxicologic testing.

Other Ancillary Testing

Ancillary testing is directed by specific clinical findings. Electroencephalography (EEG) is important to exclude subtle or subclinical seizures if altered mental status is present. Neuroimaging is used if there is a suspicion of concomitant trauma or hemorrhage. It also may be helpful to detect specific radiologic patterns associated with toxins and to assess for any cerebral injury.

Neurologic Examination

Examination of a poisoned child includes initial and serial assessment of neurologic status. This assessment guides clinical management, predicts prognosis, and often identifies the offending agent. Please see the online version for specific examination findings associated with toxins (see Box 156-3).

COMMON TOXIDROMES

The neurologic examination may indicate poisonings and drug intoxications that fit clinically into one of several toxidromes (Leikin and Paloucek, 1995). The major toxidromes include the following: anticholinergic, cholinergic, sympathomimetic, serotonergic, antihistaminic, opioid, and sedative-hypnotic syndromes.

The anticholinergic syndrome has peripheral and central muscarinic signs. Peripheral muscarinic signs include tachycardia, dry skin and mucous membranes, dilated pupils, decreased gastrointestinal motility, urinary retention, and hyperthermia. Central anticholinergic signs include confusion, disorientation, agitation, hallucinations, incoordination, ataxia, and frank psychosis ("mad, hot, dry, and blind"). The anticholinergic toxidrome is caused by atropine, belladonna alkaloids, plants (jimson weed), antihistamines, low-potency phenothiazines, and antidepressants, especially tricyclic antidepressants.

Cholinergic toxidromes, which include both muscarinic and nicotinic effects, are produced by organophosphate insecticides, carbamate insecticides, nicotine, physostigmine, and their congeners. Consciousness may be severely depressed with respiratory depression; pinpoint pupils; widespread fasciculations; **s**alivation, **l**acrimation, **u**rination, **d**efecation, **g**astrointestinal distress, and **e**mesis (SLUDGE syndrome); bronchoconstriction and bronchorrhea; pulmonary edema; hypotension or hypertension; and bradycardia. Seizures may occur. Young children may not display typical peripheral cholinergic signs and symptoms.

Serotonin syndrome is traditionally described as neuromuscular abnormalities, autonomic hyperactivity, and mental status changes. The Hunter serotonin toxicity criteria are used to increase the accuracy of diagnosis. The most significant finding is clonus. Other findings associated with the syndrome include diaphoresis, agitation, hyperreflexia, and tremor (Dunkley et al., 2003). Hyperthermia is seen in severe cases (Dunkley et al., 2003). Symptoms usually occur rapidly and can be the result of a single initial medication dosage, a change in the dose, or in an overdose. Serotonin syndrome can occur after ingestion of many classes of medications. Treatment is removal of the drug source and supportive care. Benzodiazepines should be used early to control agitation. Cyproheptadine and chlorpromazine have some efficacy. Hyperthermia should be treated with sedation, intubation, and neuromuscular paralysis.

Antihistaminic agents are divided into histamine-1 and histamine-2 receptor antagonists. Both may cause significant CNS side effects at therapeutic doses, but the degree is agent-specific. Older histamine-1 blockers cause sedation, delirium, and subtle cognitive defects. Delirium is especially prominent in children. They may also have significant toxicity, including movement disorders and autonomic dysfunction. With overdose, ataxia and seizures may supervene. Toxicity may be delayed by several days. Histamine-2 blockers tend not to have significant antihistaminic side effects (except cimetidine) in children at therapeutic doses. At high doses, mental status changes predominate, especially with cimetidine.

The opioid-induced toxidrome is diagnosed and treated with naloxone. It includes CNS depression with coma, pinpoint pupils, muscle flaccidity, respiratory depression, and bradycardia. All opioid-derived agents may cause this syndrome.

Sedative-barbiturate toxidromes are manifested by lethargy/profound sedation, respiratory depression, miotic pupils, and generalized hypotonia with areflexia and ataxia. Signs and symptoms may be progressive, especially in intoxication with longer-acting agents, such as phenobarbital.

POISONS AND ENVIRONMENTAL TOXINS
Biologic Toxins

Biologic toxins include snake, arthropods (tick), insect, and fish toxins; botanic toxins; and bacterial toxins (e.g., diphtheria, tetanus, botulism) (Table 156-1, Box 156-2, and Boxes 156-4 to 156-9) (Stommel, 2008).

Snake Venom

There are two major families of poisonous snakes, Crotalids and Elapids. Crotalid venom is primarily hemotoxic, whereas Elapid venom is neurotoxic. Symptoms include fever, nausea, vomiting, diarrhea, tachycardia, altered blood coagulation, and local effects of envenomation. Neurotoxins affect the neuromuscular junction and occasionally altered states of consciousness and convulsions. Initial treatment is immobilization of the bite area and transport to the hospital. Incisions, suctions, tourniquets, and ice are not recommended. Venom extraction within 5 minutes can be beneficial. Treatment should include wound cleaning, tetanus prevention, and antivenin. Exercise hastens absorption of venom. Intravenous administration of specific antivenoms is recommended.

Tick Bites. Neurotoxins from various ticks can cause acute paralysis or ataxia through impaired acetylcholine release at the neuromuscular junction. This causes restlessness and irritability followed by progressive ataxia or symmetric ascending flaccid paralysis with loss of deep tendon reflexes. Removal of the tick early leads to reversal of the clinical manifestations within 24 hours. Insect repellents may be used as a preventive measure.

Botulism. Botulinum toxin also irreversibly blocks acetylcholine presynaptic release at the neuromuscular junction. It causes three different clinical syndromes: childhood or adult food-borne, infantile, and wound botulism (Stommel, 2008). Inhalation botulism has been rarely reported. Food-borne botulism causes gastrointestinal symptoms of diarrhea and vomiting, followed by rapidly developing progressive paralytic disease associated with visual blurring and diplopia, dysphagia, dysarthria, and subsequent weakness of extremities and intercostal muscles. Onset is within 2 days. Botulinum antitoxin has been effective in shortening the length of ventilation, feeding dysfunction, and hospitalization. It must be administered within 7 days of hospital admission. Treatment

TABLE 156-1 Selected Agents Causing Cranial Nerve Deficits

Cranial Nerve Deficit	Medications	Industrial Toxins	Biologic Toxins
General	Methotrexate, vincristine	Organic mercury, ethylene glycol	Cobra venom
Olfactory	Levodopa	–	–
Optic nerve and retina	Antibiotics, phenothiazines, antineoplastics, cyclosporine, disulfiram (retrobulbar neuritis), isoniazid, minoxidil, quinines, valproic acid, vigabatrin	Cyanide, methanol, lead, thallium, organic mercury, hexachlorophene	Lathyrus
Extraocular muscles	Botulinum A toxin, bretylium, interferon	–	*Clostridium botulinum* toxin
Mydriasis	Antihistamines, anticholinergics, nortriptyline, barium, bromides, carbamazepine, cocaine, cyclobenzaprine, glutethimide, sertraline, sympathomimetics	Ethylene glycol, benzene, cyanide	Black nightshade (*Solanum nigrum*), box thorn (*Lycium halmifolium*), lupine, morning glory, potato (leaves, stems, immature tubers), tetrodotoxin (puffer fish, others), water hemlock (*Cicuta* spp.), mescaline, peyote
Miosis	Buspirone, cholinergics, narcotics	–	–
Dysgeusia	Dipyridamole, disulfiram, selegiline, ethambutol, lithium, nedocromil, tocainide, topiramate	Dimethyl sulfoxide	Ciguatera toxin (red snapper, farm-raised salmon)
Auditory	Antibiotics, especially aminoglycosides, antifungals, antineoplastics, lithium (acute), nonsteroidal antiinflammatory drugs and salicylates, quinine antiarrhythmics, angiotensin-converting enzyme inhibitors, danazol, dantrolene, dapsone, antidepressants, digoxin, dimenhydrinate, diuretics, vitamin A	Carbon monoxide, cyanide, methanol, solvents, mercury (organic)	Tobacco (acute), lathyrus

otherwise is supportive and neuromuscular effects may linger, even after recovery.

Infantile botulism can be a severe paralytic disease affecting the limbs, trunk, bulbar musculature, and cranial nerves. It is preceded by a history of severe constipation without other gastrointestinal symptoms. It has been associated with ingestion of honey. Human-derived botulinum immune globulin (BIG) has also been effective in reducing hospitalization, ventilation, and enteral/parental feeding in infants, but it has not been shown to reduce adverse outcomes.

Tetanus. Pediatric tetanus is extremely rare in the vaccination era. Neonatal tetanus is reported, resulting from infection of the umbilical stump. Presentation is generalized rigidity and mortality is high, especially in neonates less than 10 days of age (Stommel, 2008).

Insecticides

Organophosphate and Carbamate Insecticides. Account for most childhood insecticide exposures. Poisoning is rare. Toxins can be absorbed through the skin and gastrointestinal tract, but most childhood poisonings are the result of ingestion. Toxicity produces a cholinergic syndrome within 12 to 24 hours. Salivation, lacrimation, bronchoconstriction, wheezing, and increased pulmonary secretions are all muscarinic manifestations. Peripheral nicotinic signs include muscle weakness, decreased respiratory effort, and muscle fasciculations. CNS signs are anxiety, restlessness, confusion, headache, slurred speech, ataxia, and generalized seizures. With low-dose organophosphate exposure, muscarinic signs predominate, but in more severe acute intoxication, the nicotinic and CNS signs appear. Long-term effects may include memory difficulties, attention problems, and brisk reflexes. With longer-acting agents, recovery is protracted and possibly incomplete. Rarely, a myopathy may occur.

Treatment includes decontamination, general supportive therapy, and administration of specific antidotes, including atropine and oximes. Single-dose activated charcoal is most effective if given within 1 hour after ingestion. Oximes, such as pralidoxime or obidoxime, are cholinesterase reactivators. They are beneficial if given soon after the ingestion, but can be harmful if treatment is delayed.

Insect Repellents. The most effective general insect repellent currently in use is diethyltoluamide (DEET). Preparations containing more than 20% diethyltoluamide are likely to cause neurotoxicity. Seizures (8 to 48 hours after exposure), ataxia, and tremor are the most common neurotoxic effects.

Metals

Lead. Acute lead poisoning is rare. Acute lead encephalopathy consists of listlessness, drowsiness, and irritability, followed by seizures and signs of increased intracranial pressure. Severe resultant cerebral edema often results in significant neurologic sequelae. Blood levels in acute pediatric lead encephalopathy exceed 90 mcg/dL (Kumar, 2008). Acute lead encephalopathy at any blood lead level constitutes a life-threatening emergency and should be managed accordingly (Kumar, 2008). The most important treatment is to remove the patient from the lead exposure.

Chronic lead exposure as a result of ingestion of lead paint, inhalation of automobile exhaust fumes from leaded gasoline, or inhalation of industrial pollutants may result in high levels of blood lead and is the more common form of intoxication today. Effects can include antisocial behaviors, attention-deficit/hyperactivity disorder, learning disabilities, and reduced intelligence scores. Oral succimer, intravenous ethylenediaminetetraacidic acid (EDTA), or oral meso-2,3-dimercaptosuccinic acid can be considered for children who

BOX 156-2 Selected Agents That Cause Changes in Sensorium or Seizures

MEDICATIONS

- Acetylsalicylic acid (ASA)
- Allopurinol
- Amphetamines
- Antiarrhythmics
- Antibiotics
- Anticholinergic agents
- Antidepressants
- Antiepileptic drugs
- Antifungal agents
- Antihistamines
- Antihypertensives
- Antineoplastics
- Antiparasitic agents
- Antipsychotics
- Antitubercular drugs
- Antiviral agents
- Anxiolytics
- Baclofen
- Barbiturates
- Benzodiazepines
- Beta agonists
- Beta blockers
- Bismuth subgallate
- Bromides
- Bromocriptine
- Carbinols
- Castor oil
- Chloral hydrate
- Cholinergic agents
- Cisapride
- Clomiphene
- Clonidine
- Cocaine
- Colchicine
- Cyclobenzaprine
- Cyclosporin
- Dantrolene
- Dextromethorphan
- Digitalis
- Disulfiram
- Diuretics
- Ergot alkyloids
- Erythropoietin
- Flumazenil
- Glutethimide, zolpidem
- Granisetron, nabilone
- Guaifenesin
- Hallucinogens
- Hydrogen peroxide
- Immunomodulators
- Inhalational anesthetics
- Isotretinoin
- Ketamine
- L-dopa
- Levothyroxine
- Lithium
- Lovastatin
- Mefloquin
- Methylxanthines
- Muromonab-CD3
- Nabilone
- Niacin (acute)
- Nitrous oxide
- Nonsteroidal antiinflammatory drugs, salicylates
- Omeprazole (acute)
- Opiates/opiods
- Steroids
- Sucralfate
- Sulfasalazine
- Sumatriptan
- Sympathomimetics, stimulants
- Tacrolimus
- Vitamin A

INDUSTRIAL TOXINS

- Acetone
- Acrylamide
- Alcohols (ethanol, ethylene glycol, isopropanol, methanol)
- Aluminum compounds
- Ammonium chloride (toilet bowl cleaners)
- Antifreeze components
- Benzene
- Bismuth
- Boric acid (antiseptics, insecticides)
- Camphor
- Carbon monoxide
- Cyanide
- Ethylene oxide
- Formaldehyde
- Gasoline
- Heavy metals
- Hexachlorophene
- Lindane
- Metaldehyde (snail bait, fire starters)
- Naphthalene
- Nerve agents (VX, sarin)
- Organophosphate and carbamate insecticides
- Rodenticides
- Solvents
- Zinc, manganese

BIOLOGIC TOXINS

- Baneberry (*Actaea* spp.)
- Box jellyfish (sea wasp)
- Box thorn (*Lycium halmifolium*)
- Buckeye (*Aesculus* spp.)
- Copperhead, cottonmouth, some rattlesnake venom
- Corn lily (*Helleborus* spp.)
- Daphne
- Death camus (*Zigadenus* spp.)
- Foxglove (*Digitalis purpurea*)
- Ginkgo nuts
- *Hyoscyamus niger*
- Jimson weed (*Datura stramonium*)
- Lupine
- Marijuana (*Cannabis sativa*)
- Mayapple (*Podophyllum peltatum*)
- Mescaline, peyote
- Methcathinone
- Morning glory (*Ipomoea purpurea, Rivea corymbosa*)
- Mushrooms (especially *Amanita muscaria, Pantherina, Psilocybe, Panaeolus,* and *Copelandia* spp.)
- Nutmeg
- Oleander
- Peony, *Paeonia* spp. (high doses in medicinal preparations)
- Poison hemlock (*Conium maculatum*)
- Potato (leaves, stems, immature tubers)
- Shellfish (domoic acid poisoning)
- *Shigella* toxin
- *Solanum* spp. (Jerusalem cherry or ornamental pepper, black nightshade)
- Star fruit
- Star of Bethlehem, Indian tobacco (*Lobelia inflata*)
- Strychnine ("slang nut")
- Tobacco (nicotine, acute)
- Water hemlock (*Cicuta maculata*)

BOX 156-3 Selected Agents Associated With Myopathies

- Amphetamine
- Amiodarone
- Barium
- Beta blockers
- Caffeine
- Chloroquine, hydroxychloroquine
- Cimetidine
- Clofibrate
- Cocaine
- Colchicine
- Corticosteroids: prednisone
- Cromolyn sodium
- Cyclosporine
- Diltiazem
- Doxepin
- d-Penicillamine
- Ethanol
- Etretinate
- Heroin
- Hydrogen peroxide
- Licorice
- Lovastatin
- Minoxidil
- Niacin
- Phencyclidine palmitate (PCP)
- Procainamide
- Propylthiouracil
- Pyrithioxine
- Quinolones, penicillin, nalidixic acid
- Salicylates
- Sulfasalazine
- Tiopronin
- Vincristine, paclitaxel
- Zidovudine

BOX 156-4 Selected Agents Causing Peripheral Neuropathy

MEDICATIONS
- Amiodarone
- Amitriptyline (acute polyradiculopathy)
- Antibiotics: nitrofurantoin, chloramphenicol, quinolones, aminoglycosides, polymyxin B
- Antineoplastic agents: vinca alkaloids, paclitaxel, procarbazine (mixed), cisplatin, cytosine arabinoside
- Antiparasitic agents: metronidazole, chloroquine, hydroxychloroquine
- Antitubercular agents
- Colchicine
- Dapsone (distal motor neuropathy)
- Digitoxin
- Disulfiram
- Ethanol
- Ethionamide
- Hydralazine
- Interferons (sensory)
- Nitrous oxide
- Phenytoin, fosphenytoin
- Pyridoxine (sensory)
- Streptokinase (Guillain–Barré syndrome)
- Thalidomide (sensory)

INDUSTRIAL TOXINS
- Acrylamide (sensory)
- Carbon monoxide
- Chlorophenoxy herbicides (sensory)
- Dinitrophenols
- Ethylene oxide (mixed motor, sensory)
- Heavy metals
- Organophosphate pesticides
- Solvents

BIOLOGIC TOXINS
- Cyanide (cassavism)
- Diphtheria
- Lathyrus
- Podophyllum (ingestion)
- Stonefish (Scorpaenidae)

have elevated lead levels; however, there is no improvement in later cognitive, neuropsychiatric, or behavioral measures or blood levels.

Mercury. Mercury poisoning can result from elemental, inorganic, and organic mercury exposure. Elemental mercury exposure can occur from a laboratory exposure, broken thermometer, light bulbs, or interior paint. The majority of children are asymptomatic. Headache, abdominal pain, and nausea are the most common symptoms. Rarely visual deficits and peripheral neuropathy can persist. Inorganic mercury exposure can occur acutely after accidental ingestion of an antiseptic solution containing mercury. Chronic poisoning may follow prolonged use of mercury-containing teething powders, repeated applications of ammoniated mercury ointment to the skin, or application of mercury-containing antiseptics to the oral mucosa. Acute inorganic mercury poisoning results primarily in severe gastrointestinal problems, whereas chronic or subacute mercury toxicity causes coarse tremor, irritability, and peripheral neuropathy. Symptoms and signs of acrodynia ("pink disease") include irritability and profound peripheral neuropathy.

Organic mercury poisoning has occurred as a result of ingestion of contaminated fish, grain, or pork and in occupational exposures. Symptoms include ataxia, peripheral neuropathy, choreoathetosis, visual loss, confusion, and coma.

Dimercaprol (BAL), meso-2,3-dimercaptosuccinic acid (DMSA), and 2,3-dimercapto-propanesulphonate (DMPS)

effectively chelate and remove mercury from the tissues; however, this has not been shown to reduce morbidity or mortality.

Thallium. The primary sources of thallium ingestions are rodenticides and insecticides. Thallium poisoning presents with abdominal pain, alopecia, and mixed peripheral neuropathy. Abdominal pain is usually secondary to peripheral neuropathy. Other neurologic effects of thallium include cranial neuropathies, coma, dementia, delirium, and seizures. CNS levels of thallium may continue to rise for at least a few days after the initial exposure. Cardiovascular involvement includes hypertension and myocardial damage, with shock and death occurring in massive doses. Painful distal glossitis, Mees's lines, and black thallium deposits at the base of abnormally tapered hairs may also be present. Cerebrospinal fluid protein may be elevated. Treatment is to lower thallium blood levels through hemodialysis, hemoperfusion, and/or continuous veno-venous hemofiltration. Prussian blue can help prevent absorption from the gastrointestinal tract.

Arsenic. Most arsenic toxicity occurs by contamination of the water supply. Inhalation of smoke from coal and industrial

---

BOX 156-5 Selected Agents Associated With Paralysis and Muscular Rigidity

PARALYSIS

Medications and Industrial Toxins

- Aminoglycoside antibiotics
- Beta blockers
- Chloroquine (with color vision shift)
- Cholinesterase inhibitors: neostigmine, pyridostigmine
- D-Penicillamine
- Pesticides: organophosphates, carbamates
- Pyrithioxine
- Trimethadione

BIOLOGIC TOXINS

- Cobra venom
- Poison hemlock (*Conium maculatum*)
- Scorpion fish (Scorpaenidae)
- Snake venom, ticks, botulinum toxin
- Star of Bethlehem (*Hippobroma longiflora*)
- Sweet pea (*Lathyrus odoratus*)
- Tetrodotoxin (puffer fish, blue-ringed octopus, others)

MUSCULAR RIGIDITY

- Black widow spider venom (*Latrodectus mactans*)
- Strychnine (*Strychnos nux vomica*, "slang nut")
- Tetanus toxin

BOX 156-6 Selected Agents Associated With Parkinsonism and Other Acute Extrapyramidal Reactions

MEDICATIONS

- Amiodarone
- Anticholinergic agents: benztropine
- Antidepressants (including selective serotonin reuptake inhibitors)
- Antiepileptic drugs
- Antifungal agents
- Antihistamines
- Antipsychotics and related drugs (including "novel" agents)
- Bethanechol
- Bupropion (acute)
- Buspirone
- Captopril (acute)
- Clonazepam
- Diazoxide
- Digoxin (chorea)
- Estrogen (chorea)
- Heroin
- Ketamine
- L-DOPA
- Lithium (chorea)
- l-Methyl-4-phenyl-1,2,3,6,-tetrahydropyridine (MPTP)
- Metronidazole (oculogyric crisis)
- Ofloxacin (Tourette-like syndrome)
- Opiates/opioids
- Reserpine
- Stimulants
- Sulfasalazine (chorea)
- Vinblastine

INDUSTRIAL TOXINS

- Carbon monoxide
- Metals: manganese, thallium, aluminum
- Methanol
- Trichloroethylene

BIOLOGIC TOXINS

- *Arthrinium* mycotoxin

---

wastes may also cause poisoning. Acute poisoning manifests with nausea and vomiting, abdominal pain, diarrhea, cutaneous, and neurologic findings. Severe inorganic arsenic poisoning also results in encephalopathy in older children. A Guillain–Barré-like neuropathy may follow. Other acute cutaneous findings may include facial edema, transient flushing, conjunctival hemorrhage, and maculopapular rash in intertriginous areas. Mees's lines may be found several months after exposure. Unlike thallium, arsenic typically does not cause alopecia. Treatment includes removal of the exposure. Chelation is the mainstay of acute exposure treatment. It has limited efficacy in chronic exposures.

Heavy-metal exposure, including cadmium, lead, arsenic, mercury, and thallium, may occur from intake of medicinals. Ernst and Coon provide a review of such metal toxicity in traditional Chinese medicines.

DRUGS OF ABUSE
Cocaine

Cocaine inhibits reuptake of norepinephrine, dopamine, and serotonin. Acute toxicity includes behavioral effects, hyperthermia, tremors, diaphoresis, tachycardia, cardiac dysrhythmias, myocardial infarctions, vasoconstriction, and hypertension. These effects are followed by anxiety, agitation, depression, exhaustion, and sometimes paranoid psychosis. Addiction follows continued use. Stroke, intracranial hemorrhage, vasculitis, and death have been reported. Seizures have also been reported; however, validity of the association is debated. First-line treatment for all symptoms is benzodiazepines. Alpha-antagonist treatment may follow.

Opiates

There are limited data available regarding opiate use in childhood. Symptoms of intoxication include CNS depression, miotic pupils, respiratory depression/arrest, circulatory collapse, and convulsions. Morphine sulfate can rarely cause a leukoencephalopathy. Heroin can cause a spongiform leukoencephalopathy. Treatment of opiate intoxication includes administration of naloxone and supportive care.

Cannabis

Cannabis (tetrahydrocannabinol) is usually inhaled or ingested. Tetrahydrocannabinol intoxication produces psychomotor slowing, short-term memory loss, analgesia, pupillary dilatation, conjunctival hyperemia, tachycardia, and appetite stimulation. Coma has been reported. Long-term sequelae include mild cognitive impairment, psychiatric conditions, chronic bronchitis, bone loss, cardiovascular effects, and teratogenicity. Dependency may occur.

Gamma-Hydroxybutyrate

Gamma-hydroxybutyrate is most often a "date-rape" drug. It can lead to a profound flaccid, areflexic coma. This may mimic brain death. Treatment is supportive.

Hydrocarbons

"Hydrocarbons" are a broad range of substances that are organic in nature with hydrogen and carbon as their main

BOX 156-7 Selected Agents Associated With Myoclonus

MEDICATIONS

- Antibiotics (β-lactams)
- Antidepressants
- Antineoplastics: busulfan, chlorambucil
- Carbamazepine, vigabatrin
- Clozapine
- L-DOPA
- Lidocaine
- Lithium
- Lorazepam (preterm infants)
- Methaqualone
- Morphine
- Nitroprusside
- Piperazine

INDUSTRIAL TOXINS

- Camphor
- Chlorophenoxy herbicides
- Gasoline

BIOLOGICAL TOXINS

- Buckeye (*Aesculus* spp.)
- Lupine
- Shellfish (domoic acid poisoning)

BOX 156-8 Selected Toxic Causes of Ataxia

MEDICATIONS

- Acetohexamide
- Amiodarone
- Anticholinergic agents
- Antidepressants, including selective serotonin reuptake inhibitors
- Antiepileptic drugs
- Antihistamines
- Antimicrobials, antifungals
- Antineoplastics
- Antiparasitics
- Baclofen
- Buspirone
- Dextromethorphan
- Disulfiram
- Ethanol
- Fenfluramine
- Lithium
- Lysergic acid diethylamide (LSD), phencyclidine palmitate (PCP)
- Mexiletine
- Sedatives, narcotics

INDUSTRIAL TOXINS

- Aluminum compounds
- Butyl alcohol
- Carbon monoxide
- Carbon tetrachloride
- Ethylene glycol
- Formaldehyde
- Gasoline
- Manganese
- Metaldehyde (snail bait, fire starters)
- Paradichlorobenzene (moth repellent, diaper pail deodorant)
- Rodenticides: aluminum phosphide, sodium monofluoroacetate
- Solvents

BIOLOGIC TOXINS

- Belladonna, hyoscyamine
- Buckeye (*Aesculus* spp.)
- Mayapple (*Podophyllum peltatum*)
- Mescaline, peyote
- Podophyllum (ingested)
- Poison hemlock (*Conium maculatum*)

elements. Common examples are glue, kerosene, leaded gasoline, and Freon*. Toxicity most often occurs through inhalation. The exact mechanism of hydrocarbon toxicity is unknown. Toxicity is substance- and dose-dependent. Acute effects include euphoria, disinhibition, impulsivity, headache, dizziness, and nausea. Blurred vision, tinnitus, arrhythmias, peripheral numbness, muscle weakness, and dysesthesia of the tongue have also been described. Long-term abuse may result in neuropsychiatric alterations, cerebellar dysfunction, encephalopathy, tremor, spasticity, and dementia. White matter abnormalities on MRI have been described. Treatment is symptomatic and includes removal of exposure source.

Hallucinogens

Phencyclidine (PCP) is commonly inhaled or ingested. It causes euphoria, violent behavior, extreme muscular rigidity, and exaggerated muscle strength. Vertical and horizontal nystagmus with marked pupillary dilatation is common. A syndrome of catatonic rigidity, opisthotonus, dystonic posturing, stupor or profound fluctuations in the level of consciousness, seizures, and myoclonus can occur. Extreme elevations of blood pressure are common. Intracranial hemorrhage can occur. Treatment includes sedation, hyperthermia treatment, and hypertensive management.

LSD is a hallucinogen. Intoxication results in acute personality changes, hallucinations, panic reactions, and feelings of depersonalization. Ataxia, tremors, diaphoresis, convulsions, coma, and respiratory arrest may occur. Treatment is supportive care with sedation.

Amphetamines

Amphetamines cause a sense of well-being and decreased fatigue. With toxic doses, acute paranoid psychosis may develop, with mania, hyperactivity, and severe sympathomimetic effects. The most common adverse effects in children are agitation and tachycardia. Less commonly hypertension, hyperthermia, and convulsions occur. Cerebral vasculitis, cerebral infarction, subarachnoid hemorrhage, and intracranial hemorrhage have been reported. Severe agitation or seizures may be treated with intravenous benzodiazepines; hallucinations and agitation may also be treated with haloperidol or olanzapine. Hyperthermia and hypertension should be treated aggressively.

"Ecstasy"

3,4-Methylenedioxymethamphetamine (ecstasy) both stimulates and blocks reuptake of serotonin (5-HT). It also has a lesser effect on other monoaminergic neurotransmitters. It typically causes euphoria. Acutely, it commonly causes serotonergic symptoms of confusion, hyperkinesis, and increased body temperature. Rarely, these symptoms can develop into a serotonergic syndrome. Once the acute effects wear off, depressive symptoms occur. Treatment is supportive.

BOX 156-9 Selected Agents Associated With Tremor

MEDICATIONS
- Aluminum compounds
- Aminophylline, theophylline
- Amiodarone
- Antiepileptic drugs
- Antihistamines
- Chlorambucil
- Ciprofloxacin
- Cyclosporine, tacrolimus (FK-506)
- Dextromethorphan
- Digitoxin, lidocaine
- Fenfluramine
- Levothyroxine
- Lithium
- Nortriptyline
- Piperazine
- Sympathomimetics, stimulants

INDUSTRIAL TOXINS
- Carbon tetrachloride
- Fluoride
- Metaldehyde (snail bait, fire starters)
- Organic mercury
- Pyrethrins
- Rodenticides: aluminum phosphide

BIOLOGIC TOXINS
- Hyoscyamine
- Mescaline, peyote
- Star of Bethlehem, Indian tobacco (*Lobelia inflata*)
- Tobacco (nicotine)

Emerging Drugs of Abuse

Synthetic cathinones (bath salts) can be snorted, ingested, or injected. They cause increased release and decreased reuptake of norepinephrine, serotonin, and dopamine. Sympathomimetic toxicity can result, causing symptoms of agitation, hyperthermia, tachycardia, anxiety, confusion, seizures, chest pain, nausea, palpitations, fever, diaphoresis, hypertension, dizziness, and peripheral vasoconstriction. Symptoms have a significant overlap with both serotonin and sympathomimetic syndromes. Treatment is with benzodiazepines, antipsychotic agents, and supportive care.

Synthetic cannabinoids (i.e., K2 and spice) exert their effects through the CB1 and CB2 cannabinoid receptors. Their effects include mood alteration, hallucinations, conjunctival injection, tachycardia, and dry mouth. They may also provoke anxiety and psychotic reactions. Seizures have been reported. Treatment is primary supportive.

Salvia is a hallucinogen that acts as an agonist at the kappa opioid receptor. Adverse effects include agitation, tachycardia, hypertension, seizures, leukocytosis, hyperglycemia, and elevated creatine kinase.

Barbiturates

Barbiturate intoxication produces confusion and varying degrees of sedation and coma; lesser amounts may result in ataxia. Respiratory depression, flaccid areflexia, miotic pupils, and absent brainstem reflexes occur with more severe poisoning. Activated charcoal, given repeatedly, is the most efficacious treatment along with supportive care. Hemodialysis is of unproved value but may benefit severely intoxicated patients. Renal function monitoring is recommended.

Benzodiazepines

Benzodiazepine intoxication produces ataxia and sedation at low doses, and confusion, somnolence, and coma at higher doses. Respiratory depression and hypotension may occur. The combination of benzodiazepines and other CNS depressants is potentially fatal. Treatment is supportive care and administration of flumazenil. Flumazenil-induced convulsions may occur in individuals with chronic benzodiazepine use.

Baclofen

Baclofen is a GABA B receptor agonist that is most often used to treat spasticity. Mild toxicity typically results in sedation or agitation. More severe toxicity may manifest as hypothermia, hypotonia, respiratory depression, cardiac conduction abnormalities, hyporeflexia, and/or coma. Seizures or myoclonic jerks are common. A burst suppression pattern on EEG may occur and may persist for days after ingestion (Leikin and Paloucek, 1995). The clinical picture may mimic brain death. Treatment is supportive.

Antipsychotic Agents (Neuroleptics)

Older neuroleptics include phenothiazines and butyrophenones. These can cause sedation, acute dystonic reactions, akathisia, pseudoparkinsonism, withdrawal, emergent dyskinesia, tardive dyskinesia, and neuroleptic malignant syndrome. Acute intoxication in a young child usually results in a confusional state or depressed level of consciousness. Acute dystonic reactions may manifest as an oculogyric crisis or sudden dystonic posturing of the head and neck, including opisthotonus, retrocollis, torticollis, facial grimacing, and tongue thrusting. These acute reactions are not necessarily dose related, and are usually readily reversed with the intravenous administration of diphenhydramine. Miosis, coma, hypothermia or hyperthermia, and hypotension may occur after ingestion of a large dose of either phenothiazines or butyrophenones.

Akathisia is a dose-related neurologic complication of neuroleptic treatment and is rare in children. It usually responds to treatment with benzodiazepines, beta-adrenergic blockers, or dose reduction. Tardive dyskinesia is extremely rare in children.

Neuroleptic malignant syndrome is a rare complication of neuroleptic drug therapy and is characterized by fever, muscular rigidity, autonomic dysfunction, and altered sensorium, with waxing and waning of consciousness. The patient may be in a catatonic-like stupor and may be mute. Myoglobinuria and acute renal failure may occur. Treatment consists of intensive supportive care, aggressive fluid management, and, in selected cases, dantrolene or bromocriptine administration. This syndrome can occur with both first- and second-generation antipsychotics (Belvederi et al., 2015).

The second-generation antipsychotics, such as clozapine, risperidone, olanzapine, quetiapine, ziprasidone, and sertindole, have clinically significant pharmacologic activity at multiple receptors, and fewer typical antidopaminergic side effects. They can cause acute extrapyramidal effects (clozapine and risperidone), confusion, lethargy, ataxia, seizures (clozapine), and myoclonus.

Antidepressants

Tricyclic antidepressants (i.e., amitriptyline, imipramine, and desipramine) are associated with acute toxicity and significant morbidity and mortality (Qin et al., 2014). Dry mouth, palpitations, and tachycardia are typical anticholinergic effects.

An acute encephalopathy with ataxia, hallucinations, and nystagmus can occur followed by somnolence and tremor or myoclonus. Death may occur as a result of progressive coma, seizures, and cardiac conduction defects resulting in hypotension. In acute poisoning, activated charcoal with a cathartic may be helpful. Seizures are treated with benzodiazepines. Tachyarrhythmias from prolongation of the QRS interval can be treated with sodium bicarbonate and potassium. Prolonged QTc intervals should be treated with magnesium supplementation and potassium repletion.

Selective serotonin reuptake inhibitors' neurotoxicity is generally limited to accidental ingestions or intentional overdoses. This can lead to a serotonergic syndrome, including coma and convulsions. Sedation and vomiting are the most common side effects. Paradoxical behavioral reactions and SSRI-induced hyperkinetic movement disorders are the most likely adverse neurologic effects (Qin et al., 2014). Citalopram intoxication can be associated with severe encephalopathy and seizures requiring intensive care admission. Extrapyramidal symptoms can occur from duloxetine, escitalopram, and citalopram. A neonatal withdrawal syndrome has been reported. Buproprion has the highest risk for seizures.

Lithium

Lithium carbonate is often used for the treatment of bipolar disorder. Most cases of lithium intoxication occur during the course of prolonged therapy. An acute encephalopathy can occur, but most chronic toxicity manifests as an irreversible cerebellar syndrome. This can be displayed as apathy, drowsiness, nystagmus, tinnitus, dysarthria, ataxia, coarse muscle tremors, vomiting, and diarrhea. Choreiform movements, dystonic posturing, and cogwheel rigidity may occur. Severity of symptoms does not appear to correlate well to serum concentrations, but instead to chronic exposure. Seizures and coma indicate severe toxicity. Treatment is supportive care and drug discontinuation.

Salicylates

Salicylates are present in a myriad of medicinal preparations, ranging from aspirin tablets to oil of wintergreen and long-used Chinese medicinal oils. The classic triad of acute intoxication is hyperventilation, tinnitus, and gastrointestinal irritation. Symptom onset in acute intoxications is within a few hours. Salicylates directly affect the CNS and cause central hyperventilation with respiratory alkalosis. Mortality is related to brain salicylate concentration; respiratory decompensation and subsequent worsening acidosis facilitate salicylic acid passage into the CNS.

Chronic toxicity occurs after several days of use. CNS disturbances include lethargy, coma, and convulsions; however, the predominant toxicity is pulmonary edema.

Isotonic alkaline solution, activated charcoal, management of hypoglycemia, early hemodialysis, and supportive therapy are the best treatments.

Stimulants

Stimulant medications are used to treat attention-deficit/hyperactivity disorder. They may produce increased activity and varying dyskinesias, including motor tics and chorea. Stimulants overall do not worsen tic severity or exacerbate epileptic seizures.

Atomoxetine is a nonstimulant agent approved for the treatment of attention-deficit/hyperactivity disorder. Side effects are mild and can include headache, decreased appetite, gastrointestinal disturbances, and somnolence. Atomexetine overdoses have been associated with dyskinesias and seizure activity.

Diphenhydramine

The antihistamine and anticholinergic diphenhydramine is contained commonly in over-the-counter cold/allergy remedies and in topical preparations. Neurologic side effects are sedation or paradoxical hyperactivity. Hallucinations, seizures, and death have been reported in a dose-dependent manner.

Drugs Used in Organ Transplantation
Cyclosporine

Cyclosporine is an immunosuppressant that likely has the most neurotoxicity among transplant medications (de Groen et al., 1987). It also causes nephrotoxicity and hypertension. The most common nervous system effects are headache, confusion, and seizures. Cortical blindness, hemiparesis, ataxia, and tremor are also reported. Posterior reversible encephalopathy syndrome can occur. These complications are reversible and usually dose dependent. Other factors that exacerbate cyclosporine toxicity include hypertension, fever, hypomagnesemia, hypocholesterolemia, aluminum overload, and concurrent methylprednisolone treatment (de Groen et al., 1987).

Muromonab-CD3 (OKT3)

Muromonab-CD3 (OKT3) is a murine monoclonal antibody used in acute cellular allograft rejection or graft-versus-host disease. Aseptic meningitis with fever, photophobia, cephalgia, and cerebrospinal fluid pleocytosis has been described. Other complications include cerebral edema, akinetic mutism, seizures, cerebritis, and tremor.

Tacrolimus (FK-506)

Tacrolimus (FK-506) inhibits interleukin-2 and is thought to act by inhibiting T-cell activation. Serum levels of tacrolimus are altered significantly by multiple drugs. Toxicity may be related to dosing. Symptoms include delirium, catatonia, dysphasia, seizures, peripheral neuropathy, and tremor. Posterior reversible encephalopathy syndrome can occur.

Antibiotics
Chloramphenicol

Chloramphenicol has been associated with the development of a reversible optic neuritis with long-term treatment.

Nitrofurantoin

A rare, reversible polyneuropathy can develop with prolonged nitrofurantoin treatment, particularly in the presence of impaired renal function.

Aminoglycosides

Aminoglycosides are potentially ototoxic. Symptoms may arise from oral, parenteral, or wound irrigation administration of the drug. A myasthenic-like syndrome accompanied by generalized muscle weakness may also result. This reaction usually occurs after the simultaneous administration of a neuromuscular blocking agent. It may be partially antagonized by neostigmine. These antibiotics may also cause a transient clinical deterioration in patients with myasthenia gravis.

Beta-Lactam Antibiotics

Penicillins, cephalosporins, and carbapenems may cause seizures as the result of inhibition of gamma-aminobutyric acid (GABA) receptors and are most likely to occur with renal impairment. Cefepime may provoke seizures independent of renal function, especially in those with an underlying epileptic risk. Supratherapeutic levels can lead to an acute encephalopathy and movement disorders. Effects may be magnified in a child with an altered blood–brain barrier.

Antineoplastic Drugs

Vinca Alkaloids

Neurotoxicity from vincristine and vinblastine is related to impaired nutrition, drug dosage, frequency of dosing, and duration of therapy. An axonal sensorimotor neuropathy is most common. It may worsen for weeks after treatment completion and can take months to recover (Armstrong and Gilbert, 2004). Muscle cramps, muscle weakness, cranial nerve palsies, ophthalmoparesis, ptosis, and olivocohlear bundle dysfunction can also occur (Armstrong and Gilbert, 2004). Autonomic dysfunction can present with colicky abdominal pain, paralytic ileus, constipation, and bladder atony. Generalized seizures and inappropriate secretion of antidiuretic hormone are rare complications. Temporary cortical blindness, ataxia, parkinsonism, and athetosis have been reported.

Methotrexate

Myelopathy, headache, cognitive deficits, vomiting, nuchal rigidity with aseptic meningitis, truncal ataxia, tremor, paraplegia, delirium, and somnolence have been described as complications of both intrathecal and systemic therapy with methotrexate. Methotrexate toxicity may have a genetic component. Toxicity may be improved with leucovorin rescue. A dose-dependent leukoencephalopathy is the most common CNS complication. High-dose intravenous, prolonged low-dose oral, or intrathecal therapy can provoke a typically one-time reversible acute stroke-like syndrome (Armstrong and Gilbert, 2004). MRI can show hyperintense foci on FLAIR and DWI. Meningoencephalopathy can occur as late as several months after completion of methotrexate therapy. The most devastating effect of methotrexate therapy is a subacute and usually progressive leukoencephalopathy. Clinical manifestations include mental deterioration with dementia, seizures, and focal neurologic deficits. This complication may occur between 3 and 9 months, but can occur years, after high-dose methotrexate therapy.

L-Asparaginase

L-Asparaginase therapy may produce changes in mentation, somnolence, and EEG slowing. It produces a coagulation disorder unresponsive to corrective factors. Intracranial thrombosis or hemorrhage and peripheral arterial thrombosis with headache, obtundation, hemiparesis, and seizures are also complications.

Platinum Agents

Ototoxicity is a common complication of cisplatin therapy. Dose-dependent peripheral axonal sensory neuropathy may also occur. Retinal toxicity and autonomic neuropathy are rare. Oxaliplatin typically causes an acute and chronic sensory neuropathy. Chronic oxaliplatin exposure has similar effects to cisplatinin. Carboplatin appears somewhat less toxic to the nervous system and a neuropathy is rare. Calcium and magnesium may have some protective effects.

Cytosine Arabinoside

Cytosine arabinoside is most commonly associated with cerebellar ataxia, developing within hours of treatment. This is typically self-resolving. It may also cause a change in sensorium (at high doses), and, rarely, peripheral neuropathy, myelopathy, brachial plexopathy, or transient paraplegia.

Cyclophosphamide and Ifosfamide

Cyclophosphamide and ifosfamide both may cause CNS toxicity. This toxicity is manifest as an encephalopathy with mental status changes, seizures, and ataxia. Cranial neuropathies also are possible. Improvement has been reported with methylene blue administration.

Neuroteratology

Drugs administered during pregnancy may affect the fetus. The effects of these drugs depend on the timing of administration; the dose, distribution, and metabolism in maternal tissues; placental transfer; and subsequent concentration and distribution of the drug in fetal tissues. Brain development from morphogenesis to terminal myelination represents a long period of developmental vulnerability.

Initial recognition of structural defects associated with neuroteratogens has matured into appreciation for more subtle deleterious effects of these agents. Many neuroteratogens are best thought of as neurobehavioral teratogens that cause clinically significant cognitive and behavioral alterations but minimal structural brain changes, at least on the neuroimaging level.

Despite newer clinical and imaging technologies, teratogenic risk is frequently imprecise. This discussion is limited to agents in which a neuroteratogenic effect seems likely based on human data, or in which animal data reflect a likely human scenario (e.g., some antineoplastic agents) (Table 156-2).

Fetal ethanol exposure is the most common preventable chemical cause of mental retardation in the United States. There is an estimated 6% risk that an alcoholic mother will have a child with fetal alcohol syndrome (FAS); the risk is 70% for subsequent offspring. The current CDC prevalence estimate for fetal alcohol syndrome (FASD) in infants is 0.2 to 1.9 per 1000 infants in the general population, although two recent studies report FAS prevalence in 6- to 7-year-olds of 6 to 9 per 1000 and FASD prevalence of 2% to 5% in the same group. Although most studies suggest that significant risk to the fetus occurs with maternal ethanol consumption of about two drinks per day or a few "weekend binges" during pregnancy, the neurobehavioral teratogenicity of "light" alcohol consumption (defined as 1 to 2 drinks per week or per occasion) is not clear. Regardless, a safe threshold value for alcohol consumption value has not been defined. Cardinal features of FAS are

1. prenatal and postnatal growth deficiency,
2. CNS anomalies, usually involving microcephaly and mental retardation, with irritability and restlessness in infants, and
3. craniofacial anomalies that include short palpebral fissures, frontonasal alterations, midface hypoplasia with flat midface, thin upper lip, hypoplastic maxilla, and sometimes hypoplastic mandible.

TABLE 156-2 Selected Human Neuroteratogens

Drug/Toxin	Effect on Nervous System
Aminoglycoside antibiotics	Cranial nerve VIII damage (10–15%)
Antiepileptic drugs: oxazolidinediones (trimethadione), phenytoin, valproic acid, carbamazepine)	CNS malformations, mental retardation, developmental delay, microcephaly, neural tube defect; spina bifida (1–2%)
Cisplatin	Cranial nerve III
Chloroquine, hydroxychloroquine, quinine	Hydrocephalus, optic nerve hypoplasia, cranial nerve VIII damage (10–15%)
Cocaine	CNS hemorrhage, infarction
Coumarin anticoagulants	Mental retardation, microcephaly, optic nerve hypoplasia, midline CNS malformations
Ethanol (dose-related)	Mental retardation, developmental and behavioral disabilities, dyscoordination, microcephaly, CNS midline malformations and migrational errors
Folic acid antagonists (aminopterin, methotrexate)	Cranial malformations, mental retardation
Hyperthermia	Neural tube defect, migrational errors, Möbius' syndrome
Ionizing radiation (>200 Gy)	CNS malformation, microcephaly
Lead	Learning disabilities
Maternal diabetes mellitus	Caudal regression, holoprosencephaly arhinencephalia
Organic mercury	CNS malformation, microcephaly
Solvents: gasoline, xylene, toluene (as substances of abuse)	Caudal regression malformation, CNS malformations, mental retardation
Retinoids, vitamin A	Holoprosencephaly, neural tube defect, microcephaly, posterior fossa cysts, cranial nerve palsies (II, III, VII)
Thiouracil, propylthiouracil (PTU), iodine-131	Mental retardation (congenital hypothyroidism)
Undertreated maternal phenylketonuria	Mental retardation (>90% in untreated mothers)

Partial morphologic expression of alcohol effect is referred to as partial FAS, and behavioral effects in a child without morphologic changes suggest alcohol-related neurobehavioral deficits. Fetal alcohol spectrum disorder encompasses all of these disorders. Long-term follow-up suggests that patients with FAS continue to have growth retardation, craniofacial anomalies, and cognitive and behavioral problems in school. Children with FAS had lower weight, shorter length, and smaller head circumference at 3 years of age. Decrease in intelligence quotient at 4 and 7 years of age has been reported. FAS carries worse neurodevelopmental prognosis than do the milder related phenotypes. A broad pattern of postnatal effects may occur in children with FASD, including decreased cognitive abilities, executive dysfunction, anxiety and depressive disorders, and changes in social relationships.

Several antiepileptic medications are also teratogens. Phenytoin syndrome consists of facial and digital anomalies, growth deficiency, and mental deficiency. Neurodevelopmental abnormalities may occur in up to 10% of prenatally exposed children. Carbamazepine, trimethadione, and valproic acid are also teratogenic. Neural tube defects occur in about 1% to 2% of valproate- or carbamazepine-exposed fetuses. Maternal folic acid supplementation may reduce the risk for antiepileptic drug-associated neural tube defects. The 2013 NEAD study found that children with prenatal exposure to valproic acid scored 7 to 10 points lower on IQ testing and had other cognitive deficits. To date, no reports concerning other anticonvulsants marketed in the United States provide convincing evidence for injury to the prenatal central nervous system.

Isotretinoin (Accutane) produces a characteristic pattern of malformation involving craniofacial, cardiac, thymic, and CNS structures. The CNS malformations include hydrocephalus, posterior fossa defects, and focal cortical abnormalities. The syndrome is thought to relate to isotretinoin's ability to interfere with neural crest cell development. The current recommendation is to stop oral isotretinoin at least 4 weeks before conception. There is no evidence for increased frequency of birth defects in pregnancies with topical retinoid exposures, but its use cannot be recommended. Although the evidence is strongest for the agents listed in Table 156-2, suggestive animal or human data support the teratogenicity of other substances, including antineoplastic medications (Smith et al., 2013).

Severe intrauterine methylmercury exposure may result in mental retardation, visual and hearing deficits, and a cerebral palsy–like picture. Stable low-level maternal exposure to mercury also appears to have neuropsychologic consequences at least into early school age. The U.S. National Research Council has concluded that 0.1 g/kg body weight per day probably is a safe level of methylmercury exposure for maternal–fetal pairs.

Finally, the effects of prenatal exposure to currently popular drugs of abuse, including cocaine, marijuana, and methamphetamine, are less defined. Despite this, at least regarding cocaine and marijuana, evidence supports some degree of neurobehavioral teratogenicity.

Prenatal exposure to cocaine may have both short- and long-term CNS sequelae. Infants and children may be exposed to cocaine through transplacental transfer, breast-milk ingestion, and passive inhalation. Although a consistent dysmorphic "syndrome" in cocaine-exposed neonates is not described, congenital urogenital malformations are linked more firmly to prenatal cocaine exposure. Infants exposed to cocaine prenatally have intrauterine growth retardation and reduced head circumference. Sharp waves and spikes may be seen in the neonatal EEG, and there is maturational delay in the brainstem auditory-evoked response in neonates as well. Maternal cocaine use is associated with intracranial hemorrhage and antenatal or perinatal cerebral infarction. Infants frequently are irritable and tremulous, with a high-pitched cry and sometimes hypertonia and hyperreflexia. Poor feeding, abnormal sleep patterns, inappropriate response to stimulation, and difficulties with state regulation also may be present. Long-term, there is a suggestion that prenatally exposed children are highly distractible, with poorly developed verbal, language, and motor skills, despite average test scores. Microcephaly, and increased behavioral and affective symptoms, have more recently have been demonstrated in a longitudinal study of children now at age 10 years. Unfortunately, some of these studies were poorly controlled for birth weight, which also may be a predictor of cocaine neurodevelopmental effects. The role of other confounding factors is also unclear.

Chronic marijuana use is associated with persistent cognitive dysfunction and other sequelae. To date, neurobehavioral sequelae of prenatal marijuana exposure are not agreed upon, although deleterious effects have been reported in behavior, attention, and overall IQ scores into adolescence. Neonates born to women using marijuana in the immediate prenatal period may be jittery and have an abnormal cry, symptoms that may persist for the first month of life.

Patterns of prenatal exposure are becoming better understood, and more sensitive techniques with which to test the effects of those exposures on the developing nervous system are emerging. As increasingly subtle postnatal neurobehavioral consequences are reported, the discussion will move from "if" to "how" these agents affect neurodevelopment throughout the lifespan.

CONCLUDING REMARKS AND ADDITIONAL SOURCES

The American Association of Poison Control Centers (AAPCC) compiles Toxic Exposure Surveillance System data from regional centers in the United States. This effort, combined with educational efforts by the American Academy of Pediatrics, the National Association of Medical Examiners' Pediatric Toxicology (PedTox) Registry, and local poison control center public and professional education, has significantly reduced pediatric poison-related deaths in this country. Other nations have similar programs and results.

New information concerning poisoning and drug effects on the nervous system appears rapidly. The following section lists several other sources of current toxicology information, and the phone number for AAPCC is 1-800-222-1222. Internet URLs are current as of 2015. The sites have links to other sites involving specific subtopics.

Internet Sites

- Poison Control Centers (United States)
  - Toxnet: http://toxnet.nlm.nih.gov
  - American Association of Poison Control Centers: http://www.aapcc.org/
- Poison Control Centers (International)
  - Europe: http://www.eapcct.org/
  - Asia: http://prn.usm.my/

REFERENCES

The complete list of references for this chapter is available in the e-book at www.expertconsult.com.
    See inside cover for registration details.

SELECTED REFERENCES

Armstrong, T., Gilbert, M.R., 2004. Central nervous system toxicity from cancer treatment. Curr. Oncol. Rep. 6, 11–19.

Belvederi, M., Guaglianone, A., Bugliani, M., et al., 2015. Second-generation antipsychotics and neuroleptic malignant syndrome: systematic review and case report analysis. Drugs R D. 15, 45–62.

de Groen, P.C., Aksamit, A.J., Rakela, J., et al., 1987. Central nervous system toxicity after liver transplantation. N. Engl. J. Med. 14, 861–866.

Dunkley, E.J., Isbister, G.K., Sibbritt, D., et al., 2003. The hunger serotonin toxicity criteria: simple and accurate diagnostic rules for serotonin toxicity. QJM 96, 635–642.

Kumar, N., 2008. Industrial and environmental toxins. Continuum (N Y) 14, 102–137.

Leikin, J.B., Paloucek, F.P., 1995. Poisoning and Toxicology Handbook, second ed. Lexi-Comp, Hudson, OH, pp. 1996–1997.

Mowry, J.B., Spyker, D.A., Cantilena, L.R., et al., 2014. Annual Report of the American Association of Poison Control Centers' National Poison Data System (NPDS): 31st Annual Report. Clin. Toxicol. (Phila) 52, 1032–1283.

Qin, B., Zhang, Y., Zhou, X., et al., 2014. Selective serotonin reuptake inhibitors versus tricyclic antidepressants in young patients: a meta-analysis of efficacy and acceptability. Clin. Ther. 36, 1087–1095.

Smith, E.R., Borowsky, M.E., Jain, V.D., 2013. Intraperitoneal chemotherapy in a pregnant woman with ovarian cancer. Obstet. Gynecol. 122, 481–483.

Stommel, E., 2008. Terrestrial biotoxins. Continuum (N Y) 14, 35–80.

157 Neurologic Disorders in Children with Heart Disease

Daniel J. Licht, John Brandsema, Michael von Rhein, and Beatrice Latal

 An expanded version of this chapter is available on www.expertconsult.com. See inside cover for registration details.

LIST OF ABBREVIATIONS

Heart Diagnosis	Abbreviation/Acronym
Transposition of the Great Arteries	TGA
Hypoplastic Left Heart Syndrome	HLHS
Patent Ductus Arteriosus	PDA
Tetralogy of Fallot	TOF
Ventricular Septal Defect	VSD
Atrial Septal Defect	ASD
Intact Ventricular Septum	IVS
Common AV Canal	CAVC
Double Outlet Right Ventricle	DORV
Interrupted Aortic Arch	IAA
Pulmonary Atresia	PA

INTRODUCTION

Congenital heart defects (CHDs) are among the most common birth defects with a national prevalence estimated at about 18 per 10,000 live births. The most serious heart defects (i.e., those requiring surgery in the first week of life) occur at a national prevalence of about 8 per 10,000, with transposition of the great arteries (TGA) occurring in about 4.7 and hypoplastic left heart (HLHS) in about 2.4 per 10,000 live births. Furthermore, previously healthy children can suffer from acquired cardiac disorders including endocarditis and myocarditis. Others, including those with underlying neuromuscular disorders such as Becker muscular dystrophy and Pompe disease, may have an intrinsic abnormality of myocardial function, referred to as a cardiomyopathy.

Children with cardiac disease often have neurologic complications. Acute neurologic emergencies include seizures, hypoxic-ischemic injury, arterial ischemic stroke, cerebral sinovenous thrombosis, and intracerebral hemorrhage. Evaluation and management of these neurologic conditions may be complicated due to the specific cardiac considerations and physiologic requirements.

Because the risk for the various types of brain injury are closely related to the type of heart lesion, the stage of the patient's brain development and to the perioperative management, the first part of the chapter will be organized accordingly. The second part of the chapter will cover the perioperative neurologic symptoms and will discuss the spectrum, severity, and evolution of the short-term and long-term neurodevelopmental consequences of altered fetal brain development and perioperative brain injury.

ANATOMIC CONSIDERATIONS

Severe CHDs may be categorized as either single ventricle lesions, biventricular lesions with or without aortic arch obstructions caused by atresia, stenosis, or coarctation (Table 157-1). These lesions can be complicated by intracardiac and extracardiac shunts such as septal defects (atrial and ventricular) or a patent ductus arteriosus (DA) respectively. Mixing of venous and arterial blood and altered flow patterns from malformed heart valves or obstructed outflow tracts (aortic or pulmonary arteries) lead to diminished oxygen delivery (the product of cerebral blood flow and oxygen content of the blood) to the brain and are the major contributors of altered brain growth and development. In addition, they increase the risk for acute brain injury in the form of hypoxic-ischemic injury to the cerebral white matter, stroke, and hemorrhage. Venous to arterial shunts (also known as "right to left shunts") through septal defects or shunts are sources for paradoxical embolization to the brain. Furthermore, genetic syndromes that are associated with heart defects including Trisomy 21, Alagille syndrome, Noonan syndrome, and several other conditions; carry the risk for other cerebrovascular anomalies such as Moyamoya vasculopathy (Pierpont et al. 2015) (Table 157-2).

The two most common diagnoses for high risk severe CHD are TGA and HLHS (Fig. 157-1). In TGA (Fig. 157-1C), the pathology results from the aortic trunk, which arises from the right ventricle shunting systemic venous blood (deoxygenated) to the ascending aorta and on to the neck vessels and coronary arteries (coronaries always arise from the aorta). The pulmonary artery arises from the left ventricle and shunts arterialized (oxygenated) blood to the lungs. In HLHS (Fig. 157-1B), the pathology results from obstruction of antegrade blood flow from the left atrium, either by developmental atresia of the mitral or aortic valve. The lack of antegrade flow from the left atrium results in profound growth failure of the left ventricle and ascending aorta. Thus all cardiac output, both pulmonary and systemic, is from the right ventricle via the pulmonary trunk. Blood flow to the neck vessels and coronary arteries is retrograde from the DA, which is just distal to the left subclavian artery. These flow patterns result in an ascending aorta that has an internal diameter of 1 to 2 mm and a large pulmonary trunk that is receiving twice the normal blood volume (pulmonary and systemic blood). Regulation of vascular resistance determines how much blood is directed to the systemic circulation and how much will flow to the pulmonary bed.

FETAL CIRCULATION

At birth, infants with severe CHD have evidence of fetal growth restriction. It has been noted that head circumferences are one-half to one standard deviation lower than the mean for normal populations, and their birth weight is likewise decreased. In keeping with the smaller head sizes, a study using preoperative brain magnetic resonance imaging (MRI) with diffusion tensor imaging and magnetic resonance spectroscopy on infants with and without CHD, found evidence of brain immaturity that was both structural and biochemical. Using an observational scale called the Total Maturation Scale (TMS), another study demonstrated that not only was maturation delayed, but the average maturation score for infants with CHD was equivalent to infants at 35 weeks gestation (Fig. 157-2), Work from multiple centers has demonstrated that brain immaturity, as measured by the TMS, is a leading risk factor for white matter injury (WMI) and predicts functional outcomes, as measured by the Bailey Scales of Infant Development (BSID), at 2 years of age.

To understand why full-term infants with CHD have delayed brain maturation, the cardiac anatomy and the effects of altered anatomy on fetal circulation must be considered. Oxygen delivery to the brain can be compromised by decreases in either cerebral blood flow (CBF) or a reduction in oxygen content of the blood (anemia or low oxygen saturations or both) or a combination of the two. Furthermore, placental circulation is dependent on fetal cardiac output, if cardiac output is abnormal, placental function may be compromised.

In TGA and HLHS, alterations in fetal blood flow likely lead to decreased brain oxygen delivery defined previously. In TGA, the aorta arises from the right ventricle and receives relatively desaturated blood from the vena cavae (Fig. 157-3B). The higher saturated stream from the left hepatic veins is directed normally across the foramen ovale to the left ventricle. The left ventricle, however, is connected to the pulmonary trunk and thus this higher saturated blood (approximately 65%) is delivered to the lungs and lower body by way of the DA (Fig. 157-3B). In HLHS, the fetal circulation is characterized by increased left atrial pressure (no outlet), resulting in reversal of flow across the foramen ovale (Fig. 157-3C). Left ventricular filling is impaired or nonexistent and consequently left ventricle outflow is diminished (aortic stenosis) or absent (aortic atresia). Pulmonary venous return and blood from the placenta mix at the atrial level and are ejected into the right ventricle and into the pulmonary trunk and DA (Fig. 157-3C). Although the resulting blood saturations are not as low as with TGA, a number of factors may restrict flow to the cerebral circulation. In many cases, flow to the head and neck vessels only occurs by retrograde flow into the transverse aorta and is in competition with systemic and pulmonary vascular resistance (Fig. 157-3C). Consequences of these altered flow patterns have been demonstrated on postnatal brain MRI with the TMS evaluation but more remarkably with fetal MRI (Fig. 157-4). In the fetal MRI, Limperopoulos and colleagues performed a

TABLE 157-1 CHD Grading System

Standard CHD Grading System	Diagnoses/Examples
Grade I— Two ventricle, no aortic arch obstruction	TGA/IVS, TGA/VSD, TOF, VSD, ASD, truncus arteriosis, CAVC
Grade II— Two ventricle with aortic arch obstruction	Coarctation of the aorta, VSD with coarctation, IAA
Grade III— Single ventricle with no arch obstruction	PA/IVS,
Grade IV— Single ventricle with arch obstruction	HLHS, DORV, unbalanced CAVC

TABLE 157-2 Common Genetic Syndromes With Cardiac and Nervous System Involvement (Listed According to Prevalence)

Name	Omim #	Prevalence	Percent With CHD	Involved Genes	Cardiac Diagnoses	Nervous System Involvement
Trisomy 21 (Down syndrome)	#190685	1:650–1:1000	40–50	Chromosome 21, particularly 21q22.3	AVSD, VSD, ASD	Muscular hypotonia, mental retardation, expressive language disorder, impaired hearing, Alzheimer disease
Noonan syndrome	#163950	1:1000–2500	80–90	12q24.13	PS, AVSD, hypertrophic cardiomyopathy	Mental retardation, speech and articulation difficulties
22q11.2 deletion syndrome (DiGeorge, VCF syndrome *)	#611867	1:6000	75	22q11.2	Interrupted aortic arch, truncus arteriosus, TOF, aortic arch anomalies	Feeding disorder, nonverbal learning disability, behavioral and psychiatric disorders (adulthood)
Williams-Beuren syndrome	#194050	1:8000	50–85	7q11.23	Supravalvular and valvular aortic stenosis, PS	Mental retardation/cognitive delay, sociable personality
CHARGE syndrome	#214800	1:10,000	75–80	8q12.2 (7q21.11)	TOF (33%), PDA, DORV, ASD, VSD,	CHARGE acronym: **C**oloboma, **H**eart defect, **A**tresia choanae, **R**etarded growth and development, **G**enital hypoplasia, **E**ar anomalies/deafness)
Alagille syndrome 1	#118450 (#610205)	1:70,000	85–95	20p12.2 (1p12 in Alagille syndrome 2)	Peripheral PA, TOF, PS	In some mental retardation or mild, learning disability

*Patients with a clinical diagnosis of DiGeorge, VCF syndrome (velocardiofacial), or Shprintzen syndrome most often have a 22q11 deletion (Pierpont et al., 2007).

Abbreviations: ASD–atrioventricular septal defect; AVSD–atrioventricular septal defect; DORV–double outlet right ventricle; PA–pulmonary atresia; PDA–patent ductus arteriosus; PS–pulmonary stenosis; TOF–tetralogy of Fallot; VSD–ventricular septal defect.

For a full list of genetic syndromes associated with CHD see Pierpont et al., 2007. Trisomy 13 and 18 are not listed as children usually die within the first year of life, both defects have various forms of CHD and manifest with severe mental retardation.

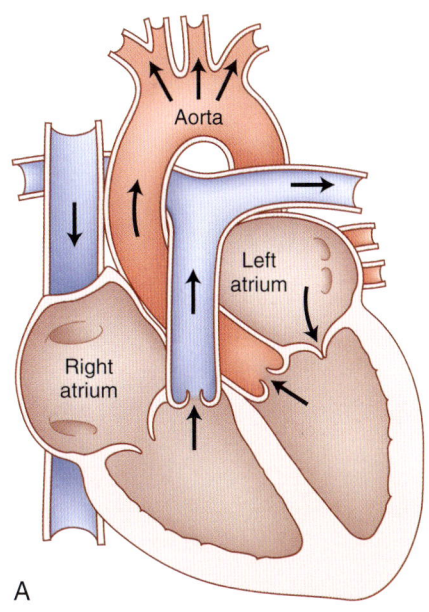
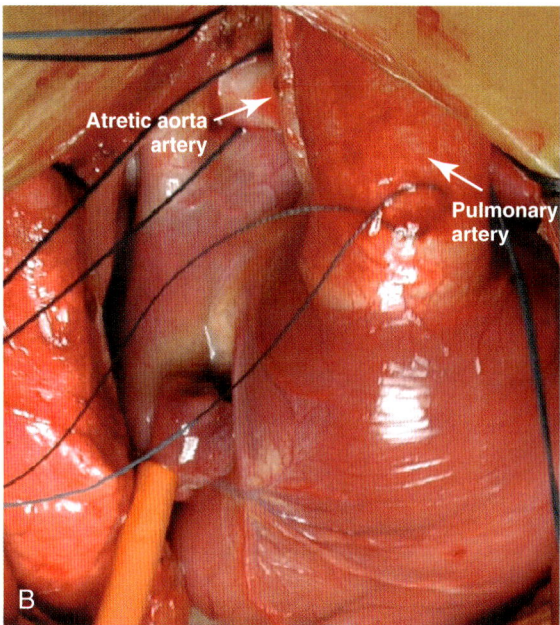
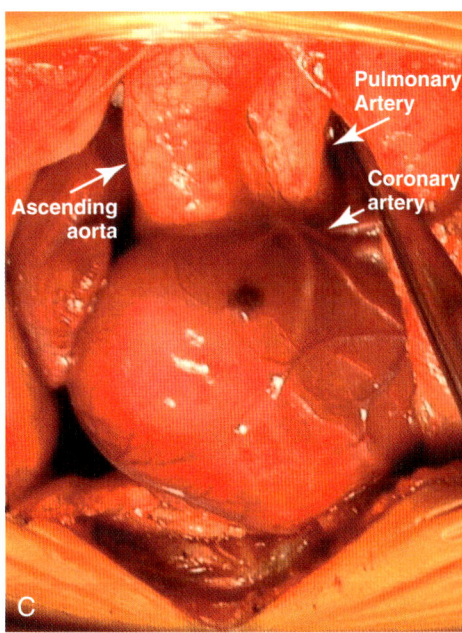

Figure 157-1. Anatomy and orientation of the great arteries. **A,** Normal orientation with the pulmonary artery crossing in front of the aorta. **B,** HLHS, a very large pulmonary artery crossing in front of an atretic aorta. **C,** TGA, aorta in front of the pulmonary artery, both normal size. *(Courtesy of Dr. Gil Wernovsky)*

cross-sectional analysis of three-dimensional brain volumes from fetal brain MRIs performed prospectively on mothers carrying fetuses with and without CHD. Starting early in the third trimester, it is clear that, in fetuses with CHD, there is a divergence from normal of total brain volume and intracranial volume growth, resulting in the postnatal phenotype of lower brain volume (Fig. 157-4).

POSTNATAL CIRCULATION
Heart Surgeries

It is convenient to think of cardiac surgery as being the sole risk for brain injury. However recent research suggests that the primary/major risks for injury are the abnormal anatomy and circulatory patterns in the fetus and newborn. Most surgical repairs and palliative procedures require cardiopulmonary bypass (CPB), whereby the chambers of the heart are isolated from the circulation by inflow (i.e., right atrium) and outflow (i.e., aortic trunk) surgical clamps, and the systemic circulation is diverted to a roller pump equipped with a membrane oxygenator via large, centrally placed cannulae.

For the more delicate surgeries involving repair of the aortic arch or the pulmonary veins, a different strategy is required. Here the suturing of the vascular structures must be accomplished in a bloodless, unencumbered field. The patient is cooled to 18°C (64.4°F) to reduce systemic and cerebral oxygen metabolism to zero (Fig. 157-5). The bypass pump is stopped and blood is drained from the body into a reservoir

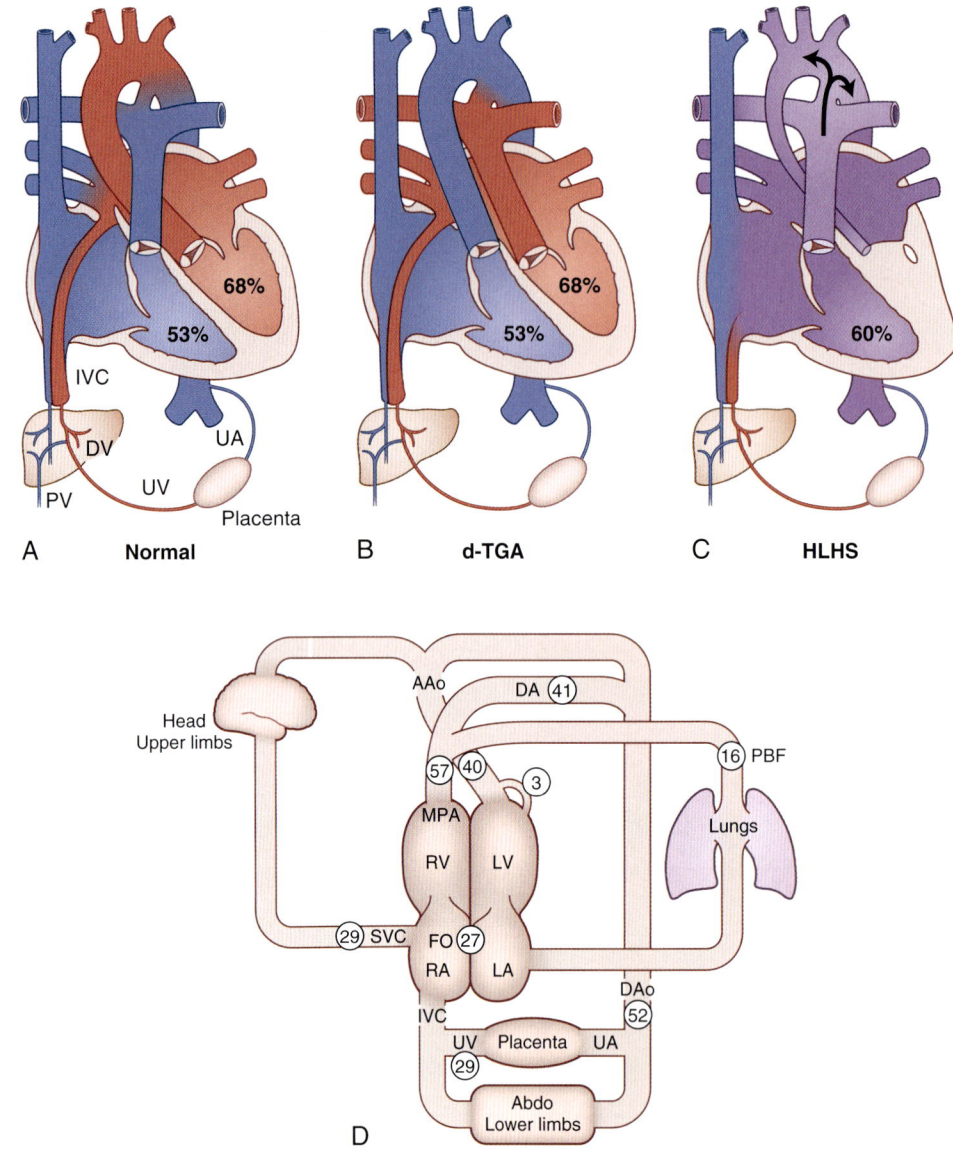

Figure 157-3. Comparative fetal circulations. **A.** Normal fetal circulation with oxygenated blood (red color) from the placenta streaming across the foramen ovale into the left-sided heart structures and out to the ascending aorta. Venous deoxygenated blood (blue) returns to the right-side of the heart. **B,** TGA anatomy with oxygenated blood circulating to the transposed pulmonary artery and on to the ductus arteriosus. Venous blood circulates to the right side of the heart and to the ascending aorta. **C,** HLCS anatomy with complete blood mixing at the level of the common atrium. All cardiac output is through the pulmonary artery to the ductus with retrograde flow to the transverse arch, neck vessels and the ascending aorta. **D,** Normal distribution of blood flow measured by phase contrast fetal MRI. *(With permission from Prsa, M., Sun, L., van Amerom, J., et al., 2014. Reference ranges of blood flow in the major vessels of the normal human fetal circulation at term by phase-contrast magnetic resonance imaging, Circ Cardiovasc Imaging 7(4), 663–670.)*

on the circuit. The cannulae are then removed from the field. Developed in the 1950s, this strategy is called Deep Hypothermic Circulatory Arrest (DHCA) was rapidly adopted in the 1970s. The use of DHCA continues today and is particularly useful for complex adult and pediatric cases involving aortic repairs.

The effect of the use of DHCA on cognitive outcomes has been hotly debated, and surgical strategies therefore altered with the stated goal of improving outcomes. There are several surgical strategies that allow for continuous cerebral blood flow throughout the case, and these have been adopted in many centers. These new surgical strategies still require cooling to 18°C, but there is continuation of antegrade cerebral circulation. The trade-off for these modifications is longer surgical and

bypass times. Both piglet and human studies have examined DHCA and continuous flow strategies and suggest that there does not seem to be a demonstrable difference between the two strategies. A randomized controlled trial of DHCA versus continuous antegrade cerebral perfusion was performed in Europe and also failed to show significant differences. A recent retrospective collaborative study examined how BSID scores changed as a result of surgical modifications over the past decades (Gaynor et al., 2015). BSID data collected from 1770 subjects from 1996 to 2009 at 22 international institutions found that, although scores have increased over time, the clinical significance of this change was dubious (0.39 points/ year or less than one-third of a standard deviation over a decade).

Perioperative Considerations

A detailed discussion of the risks associated with each surgical intervention is beyond the scope of this chapter. Typical surgical risks involving anesthetics, mechanical ventilation, bleeding, and infection are always present. Some of the perisurgical neurologic morbidity is specific to the type of heart defect or postoperative management, and not simply the conduct of the surgery itself. The following discussion is focused on specific risks related to the care of infants and children with critical CHD regardless of diagnosis. The management of other complications such as arterial ischemic stroke, intracranial hemorrhage, and venous thrombosis are discussed in other chapters (Chapters 108–113).

White Matter Injury

Neonatal heart surgery refers to surgical procedures performed on infants less than 30 days old. Survival beyond the neonatal period for these infants depends on surgical correction or palliation of their heart defect. For such patients, the mortality from these early surgeries has decreased dramatically since the late 1980s. In the more experienced centers with the highest surgical volumes, survival approaches 90% for the most complex and technically challenging surgeries. With this increase in survival, the focus of care has shifted to long-term neurologic morbidity.

Infants with severe CHD are prone to hypoxic-ischemic white matter injury (Fig. 157-6) that is not distinguishable from WMI, an injury seen primarily in premature infants. In infants with multiple forms of CHD, this injury is seen in 17% to 40% before surgery and in as high as 80% after surgery (Licht, 2015; Morton et al., 2015). Research has now demonstrated that the primary vulnerability for this injury is the brain-specific IUGR that arises as a consequence of the alterations in fetal hemodynamics created by the CHD, reviewed previously. Recent research supports the notion that not only is the surgery not the cause of WMI, but that delaying the correction/palliation of the native anatomy may increase the risk for postoperative WMI (Lynch et al., 2014).

Brain MRI is required to diagnose WMI as the lesions may be missed on CT or cranial ultrasonography. The typical white matter lesion occurs in the white matter watershed zone, is hyperintense on T1 imaging (Fig. 157-6) and may have susceptibility signal on T2* sequences, reflecting hemorrhage or mineralization. If imaging is acquired acutely, the lesions may demonstrate restricted water diffusion. MRI slice thickness is an important consideration when assessing this injury as thick slices or large interslice gaps may obscure lesions. There exist some controversy in nomenclature of these white matter lesions; some researchers view lesions with restricted water mobility on diffusion-weighted imaging as arterial ischemic stroke whereas others consider these lesions part of the spectrum of WMI. An international consortium of neurologists,

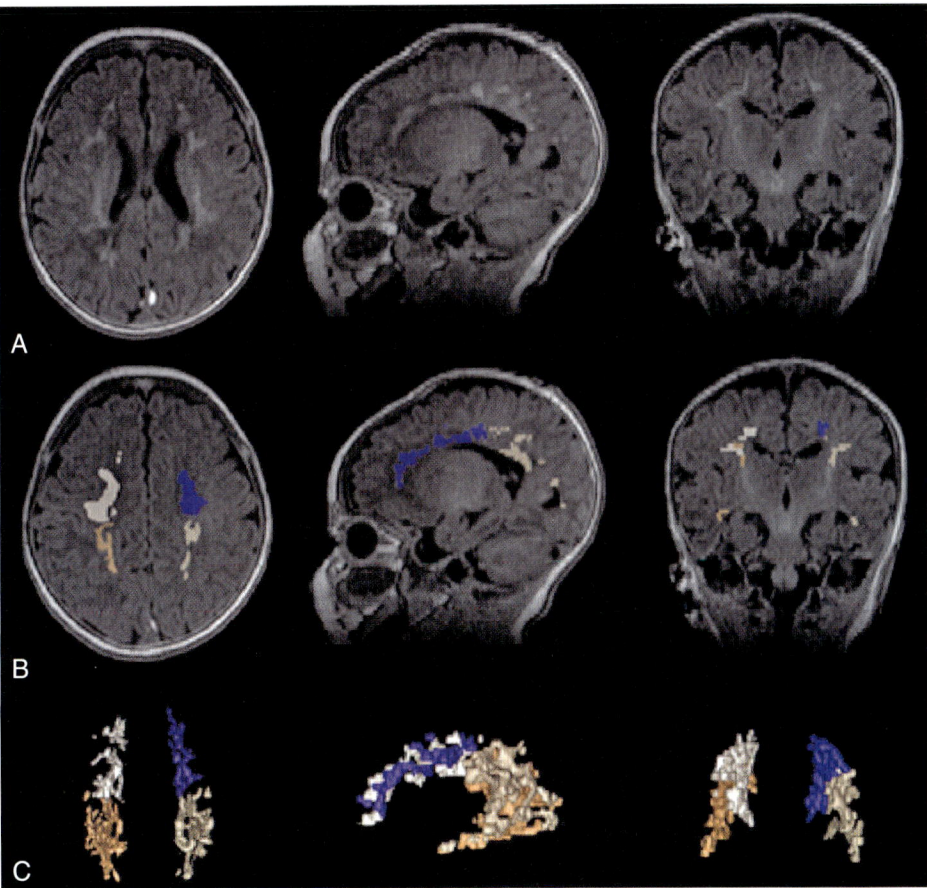

Figure 157-6. Three dimensional segmentation. **(A)** The T1-weighted image before manual PVL segmentation, **(B)** the manual segmentation, and **(C)** the volumetric reconstruction colored by quadrant, are shown in the transverse (left), sagittal (middle), and coronal (right) plane. PVL, periventricular leukomalacia. *(With permission from McCarthy, A.L., et al., 2015. Scoring system for periventricular leukomalacia in infants with congenital heart disease. Pediatr Res 78(3), 304–309.)*

cardiologists, and radiologists is in the process of establishing a universal nomenclature and standardized imaging protocol for this population.

The prevalence of preoperative and postoperative injury is different for individual cardiac diagnoses. Across centers, there appears to be a higher preoperative prevalence seen in TGA and higher rates of postoperative injury seen in HLHS. For patients with TGA, systemic oxygen saturations are lowest before surgery and rapidly normalize after corrective surgery. Proceeding to surgical correction at the earliest time possible should be protective against WMI. Conversely, for patients with HLHS or other single ventricle heart lesions, systemic oxygen saturations are typically in the mid 80% range before surgery and are not significantly higher after initial surgical palliation. In infants with ductal dependent physiology, cerebral oxygen saturations decrease on a daily basis from birth to surgery. This decrease, coupled with increasing oxygen extraction and failure of a compensatory increase in CBF, results in an increasing risk for WMI after surgery.

Arterial Ischemic Stroke

Classically, arterial ischemic stroke (AIS) is defined by a focal neurologic deficit that is related to a known arterial territory of the brain (Chapter 109). In children this definition has been expanded to include confirmatory neuroimaging (usually MRI). As infants with AIS are likely to be asymptomatic, the diagnosis is dependent on neuroimaging. The risk for AIS in CHD is not limited to the neonate requiring heart surgery. In fact, the risk for AIS in patients with single-ventricle heart defects increases with time and is reported to be greatest after the final stage of surgical palliation (the Fontan circulation, total cavopulmonary connection).

There is sparse literature on subsequent stroke occurrence in infants with severe CHD requiring newborn heart surgery. In a retrospective study, symptomatic stroke was identified in 12 of 122 infants (10%). Seizures were mostly identified after a clinical change or the occurrences of clinically observable seizures. Of these 12 infants, 6 had arterial ischemic stroke and 6 had watershed stroke. This low prevalence rate is congruent with the rate of stroke seen in another study and with the authors' experience of 2% to 4% preoperatively and 8.6% postoperatively, in mixed populations of infants with severe CHD. With such small numbers, investigation of risk factors is unlikely to be fruitful. Centrally placed catheters, such as umbilical catheters, right atrial catheters, and femoral artery catheters, are potential thrombus sources. Intracardiac and extracardiac shunts allow for paradoxical embolization and stroke. Poor heart function is another important source for intracardiac thrombus formation (discussed later).

Older children with single-ventricle heart lesions are highly predisposed to arterial ischemic stroke due to their unique anatomy. Lower extremity vascular access should be avoided if possible in patients with bidirectional Glenn physiology (superior cavopulmonary connection, Stage 2 palliation) as the inferior vena cava remains in direct communication with the systemic circulation. Fenestrations placed surgically at the time of Fontan completion act as a pressure pop-off valve but are obligate right-to-left (venous to arterial) shunts that may also allow for paradoxical emboli. Simple monitoring of systemic oxygen saturations will inform the clinician of the size of the right-to-left shunt. Long-term structural changes in the common atrium, higher central venous pressures resulting in sluggish venous blood flow, and failing ventricle function lead to increased risk for right atrial thrombi (and stroke), chylous effusions, protein losing enteropathies, congested liver, and plastic bronchitis. At the Children's Hospital of Philadelphia, it is the clinical practice to manage the single-ventricle patients

with prior unprovoked thrombotic events with life-long anticoagulation to prevent recurrence.

Intracranial Hemorrhage

Detection of intracranial hemorrhage before surgery is of obvious importance, as the cardiac surgery with cardiopulmonary bypass requires aggressive anticoagulation. At the time of birth, some amount of intracranial hemorrhage has been commonly found. These include subdural hemorrhages along the tentorial membrane and choroid plexus hemorrhages, which may have intraventricular extension. It is important to note that these hemorrhage types *do not* extend during the conduct of infant heart surgery with cardiopulmonary bypass despite the requirement for systemic anticoagulation.

Intraparenchymal hemorrhages found on preoperative head ultrasound or incidentally as part of a research protocol must be managed on a case-by-case basis because there is a paucity of information on the risk of hemorrhagic extension on cardiopulmonary bypass with this finding. At the Children's Hospital of Philadelphia, if an incidental parenchymal hemorrhage is found, surgical postponement is discussed with the surgeon and intensivist. This frequently results in the postponement of surgery. If the decision is made to postpone surgery, the patient is returned to the intensive care unit and surgery is rescheduled in 1 week with a second preoperative brain MRI.

Subdural hemorrhages are the most common clinically significant hemorrhages in the postsurgical patient, and these can occur acutely or subacutely after surgery. Anticoagulation, elevation in central venous pressures, and brain atrophy (from other injury) are all putative contributors to increased risk. Subdural hemorrhages requiring surgical intervention are uncommon in the cardiac ICU population.

Punctate microhemorrhages seen on brain MRI (Fig. 157-7) after heart surgery with cardiopulmonary bypass or after catheter-based interventional procedures are of unclear clinical significance. These microhemorrhages are unlikely to be hemorrhages at all and may be the result of micro thromboembolic material from bypass cannulation. The lesions are common, occurring in 30% to 50% of postsurgical patients. There is a single report that these lesions may contribute to the neurodevelopmental impairment that is seen in survivors of infant heart surgery.

Cerebral Sinovenous Thrombosis

Cerebral sinovenous thrombosis has been described in the CHD population, particularly in children or infants with dehydration and/or protein loss through pleural effusions or protein losing enteropathy. Management is described in Chapter 110 and includes hydration, elevation of the head of the bed when possible to promote venous drainage, and systemic anticoagulation.

Seizures

Seizures after infant heart surgery were identified as one of the significant predictors of a poor neurocognitive outcome in The Boston Circulatory Arrest Trial (BCAT). In that trial, electroencephalography (EEG) monitoring was performed on paper tracings, which were then read retrospectively. As a result, clinically silent seizures (electrographic only) were not treated. As a consequence of the findings in the BCAT, many centers have started to perform EEG monitoring (full montage or amplitude integrated EEG) after infant surgery. Seizure prevalence is quite variable after infant surgery and ranges from 5% to 26% of infants. The majority of seizures are electrographic only (as was seen in the BCAT), and status epilepticus occurs in the majority of seizures detected by EEG monitoring (85% to 100% of patients with seizures detected). Most seizures that occur after infant heart surgery are acute symptomatic seizures, and neuroimaging commonly shows WMI or AIS. Recent results from one study showed that longer duration of DHCA and/or returning to the cardiac ICU with an open chest were the most predictive risk factors for postoperative seizures after infant heart surgery.

Neurologic Sequelae of Heart Failure

Heart failure is the syndrome that results from the inability of the heart to meet the body's metabolic demands. Heart failure may be primary or secondary—that is, due to congenital or acquired cardiomyopathy or due to high flow states as seen in large hemangiomas, arterial-venous malformations (AVM), or severe anemia, among other causes. During heart failure, a child is at increased risk of neurologic injury: low cardiac output decreases cerebral perfusion, sudden arrests can lead to watershed infarction, hypoxic-ischemic brain damage, and secondary seizures or encephalopathy. Furthermore, decreased ventricular systolic function can result in stasis of blood in the heart chamber and increase the child's risk of cardioembolic events including AIS.

The degree of thrombotic risk associated with severe ventricular dysfunction is poorly defined in children. There are no guidelines to recommend the use of anticoagulation versus antiplatelet therapy. Current American College of Cardiology/American Heart Association adult heart failure guidelines (Monagle et al., 2008) suggest anticoagulating adults with heart failure and no history of atrial fibrillation or prior thromboembolic events (class IIb recommendation with level of evidence B). In children, recent guidelines suggest that anticoagulation should be considered in children with cardiomyopathy awaiting heart transplantation. Neither guideline specifies a threshold level of ventricular dysfunction where antiplatelet or anticoagulant agents would be strongly recommended. Further investigation is needed to help define the risk-to-benefit ratio of these therapies in various heart failure scenarios. At the Children's Hospital of Philadelphia, it is the clinical practice to use anticoagulation when the cardiac ejection fraction falls lower than 30%, unless there are contraindications such as a large AIS (i.e., greater than one-third of a specific vascular territory) or hemorrhage.

Mechanical Circulatory Support Devices

Children with severe heart failure may require support devices to maintain cardiopulmonary circulation. These support devices often require maintenance on anticoagulation, antiplatelet agents, or both. Complications from the underlying cardiac failure, the device itself, or the medications used to maintain the device may arise, most commonly stroke.

Extracorporeal Membrane Oxygenation (ECMO)

ECMO has been the most commonly used form of mechanical cardiopulmonary support and is a form of heart-lung bypass. There are two types of ECMO: veno-arterial ECMO supports *both* oxygenation and circulation and veno-venous ECMO supports oxygenation alone. For veno-arterial ECMO, a vascular cannula is placed into an artery (usually the right carotid artery, but it can also be the femoral artery) and a large vein. Systemic venous return is shunted into the pump and the blood is passed through an oxygenator that then returns the oxygenated blood to the arterial cannula in the patient. It is important to know that the carotid cannula is pointed down, toward the aortic arch, so that blood flows away from the brain on the right side. An intact circle of Willis allows for collateralization of blood flow. Survival of "cardiac" ECMO is improving and is listed as 66% (https://www.elso.org/Registry/Statistics.aspx) by the Extracorporeal Life Support Organization (ELSO), with 51% surviving to discharge or transfer (inferring heart transplant or other destination therapy). Neurologic complications can arise from ischemia due to carotid cannulation, hypoxic-ischemic damage, embolic arterial ischemic stroke, or intracranial hemorrhage. Sequelae including seizures and encephalopathy can arise in any of these settings.

There are many other types of ventricular assist devices (VAD) that support circulation only (without a membrane oxygenator). The FDA recently approved the Berlin Heart EXCOR Pediatric VAD under the Humanitarian Device Exemption Program. They can be used to assist the left ventricle only (systemic flow), right ventricle only (pulmonary flow), or both ventricles. Most cases involve direct cannulation of the ventricle for flow to the pump and aortic cannulation for systemic outflow. VADs are more compact than ECMO, thus providing a longer-term option for mechanical circulatory support so that the patient can be an active participant in rehabilitation. In pediatric centers, VADs are currently used almost exclusively as a bridge to cardiac transplantation, although newer impeller devices are beginning to be considered as "destination therapy" for special populations such as Duchene muscular dystrophy and other nontransplantable cardiomyopathies and in patients in whom heart transplant is not an option due to anatomic considerations.

Similar to ECMO, children supported by VADs are at significant risk of neurologic complications including AIS and intracerebral hemorrhage. The prevalence of neurologic complications varies by case series. In one study, children with short-term VAD devices were significantly more likely to suffer a stroke than those with long-term VAD devices (35% versus 13%, p = 0.02). In another series, children with left atrial cannulation were more likely to develop embolic arterial ischemic stroke than were those with left systemic apical cannulation.

There are relatively few studies of neurologic complications in children supported with ECMO versus VAD; one nonrandomized study reported a higher rate of neurologic complications with ECMO than for VAD. However, in a different study that compared an institutional experience between ECMO and the Berlin EXCOR device, the incidence of stroke was not significantly different between the two devices. A child placed on ECMO who is suspected of needing more long-term support is generally transitioned to a more mobile VAD device.

NEUROLOGIC MANAGEMENT SPECIFIC TO CARDIAC CARE

The intensivist must choose medications and management with the child's underlying cardiac status in mind when managing neurologic complications of cardiac disease. For example, a child with acute arterial ischemic stroke or cerebral sinovenous thrombosis is often placed on isotonic fluids at 1 to 1.5 times the maintenance rate for age and weight. In the child with heart failure, the fluid rate may require modification in order to avoid iatrogenic worsening of heart failure. In the management of seizures with or without status epilepticus, anticonvulsant choices should take into account the child's cardiac status. Although phenobarbital is often the medication of choice for infants and phenytoin or fosphenytoin the choice for older children, these medications can cause hypotension. Furthermore, phenytoin is a class 1B sodium channel blocker with both arrhythmogenic and antiarrhythmic properties. There are little data to guide anticonvulsant choice.

Indwelling vascular catheters are a likely source for most clots in patients cared for in the cardiac intensive care unit. For these patients, if ultrasound confirms the presence of a clot, a complete thrombophilia work up and consideration for anticoagulation is recommended in those patients with an arterial ischemic stroke (Chapter 109). An echocardiogram is helpful to evaluate for a residual intracardiac clot or fibrin stranding, as can be seen after removal of a right atrial catheter. Rarely is a transesophageal approach required for this assessment, as a transthoracic approach can usually provide adequate images in the pediatric population. For patients with significant residual right to left shunting (assessed by knowing the pulse-oxygen saturations in a patient without pulmonary disease), Doppler flow ultrasonography of the lower extremity venous system is also indicated.

SHORT AND LONG-TERM OUTCOMES
Postoperative Neurologic Findings

With improved surgical techniques and perioperative care, the prevalence of immediate postoperative complications has significantly decreased over the last decades. In the 1980s, the prevalence of perioperative neurologic abnormalities, mostly consisting of postoperative seizures, was as high as 25%. The significance of postoperative seizures as a risk factor for adverse long-term outcome has been documented already in the 1990s. Importantly, the prevalence of perioperative neurologic symptoms has dropped to around 2%, again mostly consisting of a decline in clinical seizures. However, despite this reduction, neurologic complications, often moderate to mild in severity, are still common when looking at early neurodevelopmental outcome.

The reported overall rate of neurologic complications developing in the postoperative period is quite broad, ranging from 2.3% to over 50%. This heterogeneity may be explained by different patient characteristics in the studies, including all different types of CHD or only severe ones, by the definitions of neurologic impairments, and by the variability across centers in surveillance. To address this, Bird and colleagues proposed a consensus list and definitions to help standardize terminology across centers (Bird et al., 2008). Preoperative abnormalities can persist after surgical repair or accentuate. Newly occurring neurologic abnormalities have also been described and manifest by changes of muscle tone, reflexes, or power or by movement abnormalities such as choreoathetosis.

Seizures are important neurologic symptoms that may occur preoperatively, but more frequently occur postoperatively. Postoperative seizures may have a significant influence on mortality and morbidity. The Boston Circulatory Arrest Trial demonstrated a negative effect of postoperative seizures on neurodevelopmental outcome in newborns with TGA. This has also been shown for children with a large variety of CHD diagnoses. Recently a study confirmed that postoperative seizures on amplitude integrated EEG (aEEG) predicted motor, but not cognitive, outcome at 2 years of age.

Cerebral MRI cannot always be performed during the immediate postoperative period. Thus studies have examined the use of functional bedside tools such as aEEG and NIRS to assess brain injury. Furthermore, the bedside clinical diagnosis of neurologic dysfunction may be complicated by their subtle manifestations, and further impaired by the use of sedating medications. These confounding factors can delay the accurate diagnosis of perioperative brain dysfunction. The aEEG is increasingly used as a routine monitoring, but its prognostic value for abnormal outcome remains unclear. One study

demonstrated a relationship between delayed recoveries of the background pattern on postoperative aEEGs and motor outcome.

When summarizing clinical outcome predictions for early childhood and school-age outcome, the strongest predictors are postoperative neurologic abnormalities, including seizures, as well as lower preoperative and postoperative head circumference.

Short-Term Outcome

Recent reviews summarized neurodevelopmental outcomes in children with CHD, showing a consistent pattern of global developmental impairment, characterized by motor and cognitive delay in the first 2 to 3 years with motor delay and neuromotor abnormalities being more affected than cognitive and language functions (Marino et al., 2012; Snookes et al., 2010). Of note, children with genetic disorders are at particular risk for poorer neurodevelopmental outcome (Table 157-2).

In a recent large multicenter retrospective analysis, neurodevelopmental outcome of 1700 children from 22 institutions who had undergone cardiac surgery using cardiopulmonary bypass at ages less than 9 months showed significant neurodevelopmental impairments (Gaynor et al., 2015). At a mean age of 14.5 months, the Psychomotor Development Index (PDI) and Mental Development Index (MDI) of the Bayley Scales of Infant Development II (BSID II) were lower (PDI: 77.6±18.8; MDI: 88.2±16.7) than normative means. In that study, time trends over two decades were analyzed. The rate of survivors with more complex CHD and genetic/extracardiac abnormalities increased over time. Despite this, a modest improvement of motor and cognitive function was observed after correction for a variety of cofactors. However, this improvement is not substantial and is counterbalanced by the high rate of children with complex CHD and genetic comorbidities. Another study reported on children with various types of CHD who were assessed every 6 months until the age of 36 months. Of this group, 75% had scores in the "at risk" or "delayed" range in more than one domain at more than one assessment. Nineteen percent of children who had cognitive, language, and motor scores in the average range at 1 year of age were later found to be at risk or delayed in more than 1 area. In this study, parents reported that 74% of the children had received or were actively receiving early intervention services from the state-based "Birth to 3" programs or private therapy. Importantly, although motor delay improved in children without genetic syndrome, cognitive and language delay became more evident in nonsyndromal children. In addition, in children with syndromal disorders, developmental scores decline over time, and developmental delay become more apparent. The ability to successfully achieve oral feeding was an important clinical predictor for a favorable developmental course, indicating neuronal integrity. An increase of developmental delay within early childhood has also been shown in another study in which children were followed between 8 and 24 months. The most pronounced increase in the odds to have impairments was found in the problem-solving and in the personal-social dimension.

Long-Term Outcome

School-age children with CHD may exhibit a wide range of long-term developmental impairments (Latal, 2016; Marino et al., 2012) (Table 157-7). They affect all areas of development, are most frequently mild to moderate in severity. Though they often occur in combination and can lead to significant school problems and academic difficulties. Mean IQ scores are in the low-average range, and motor difficulties

TABLE 157-7 Potential Long-Term Neurocognitive and Behavioral Problems in Children and Adolescents With CHD

Developmental Domain	Impairment
Neurology	Cerebral palsy (rare, only if significant perioperative insult has occurred) Microcephaly Mild muscular hypotonia
Motor function and visuomotor function	Fine and gross motor coordination disorder Visuoperceptual and visuomotor problems
Cognition/intellectual function	Reduced overall IQ Working memory Processing speed Poorer academic achievement
Higher order intellectual function	Higher order language functions Executive functions
Behavior	Attention-deficit disorder Emotional disorders Social interaction problems

in gross and fine motor domains occur in around 20% to 40% of the children tested. Children with motor difficulties at school age will have a higher need of therapeutic support. Language problems may manifest themselves as impaired reading abilities. The Boston Circulatory Arrest Trial, one of the largest and most comprehensive studies of long-term neurodevleopmental outcomes, showed that at age 4 and 8 years after surgery, neurodevelopmental outcomes were independent of surgical strategy (ie DHCA). In addition, hearing problems and abnormalities on neurologic examination were more frequent than in the group that did not receive DHCA. This pattern of impairment seems to persist without much "outgrowth" occurring. When these children were reexamined at adolescent age, performance scores were lower in both treatments with a significant proportion of adolescents performing lower than average, who were in need of academic or behavioral services. The pattern of mild to moderate impairments in a variety of developmental domains has been shown also in other CHD populations with varying diagnoses, persisting into adolescence. These findings consolidate the impression that regardless of type of CHD, there seems to be an increased risk for long-lasting neurodevelopmental impairments in this population.

Adolescent and Adult Outcome

The number of studies examining adolescent and adult outcome is small but growing. There is consistent evidence that with increasing academic challenges, children with CHD may be faced with more difficulties. One of the first studies examining long-term outcome demonstrated a persistence of lower IQ at 13 years of age in a small group of children with TGA. More studies followed and confirmed this finding in larger populations of children with TGA, TOF, after Fontan procedure or with mixed cardiac diagnoses. Overall IQ and other developmental domains such as executive functions and visuospatial, and motor performance remained affected (Calderon and Bellinger, 2015; Marino et al., 2012). These difficulties went along with an increased need for remedial academic or behavioral services. Of note, one study demonstrated flexibility and problem-solving executive skills to be impaired in all CHD patients in a large sample of patients aged 10 to 19 years, whereas visuospatially mediated executive

abilities were preserved in adolescents with TGA. Overall, adolescents seem to score worse on academic achievement tests, to need more supportive help, and to have a lower chance of completing mandatory schooling.

The transition into adulthood is an important phase and CHD survivors may be particularly vulnerable. There are very few studies examining this period. A recent study demonstrated that Swiss adolescents with a variety of CHD diagnosis had similar school educations and that patients were satisfied with their educational career. Only those patients with severe CHD were more likely to attend lower level education. One explanation for this favorable outcome may be the good educational support system allowing for a relatively easy transition into adulthood. Overall, the trend of poorer academic achievement described for adolescents with CHD seems to persist into adulthood, resulting in a higher rate of early unemployment and a lower rate of full-time employment. Patients with complex CHD seem to be at particular risk.

SUMMARY

As mortality rates for children and adolescents with CHD have decreased significantly, the focus has shifted toward potential acute and chronic neurologic and developmental sequelae. Infants with CHD requiring cardiac surgery may show a combination of delayed intrauterine cerebral maturation and acute preoperative and postoperative brain injuries, associated with clinical neurologic symptoms such as seizures and abnormalities on neurologic examination. The mechanisms are complex and most likely multifactorial, consisting of altered fetal hemodynamics and cerebral perfusion, leading to a delay in brain maturation that in turn seems to be a risk factors for neonatal WMI. Children may present with mild neurologic abnormalities in early childhood (typically muscular hypotonia) and may continue to show motor deficits (balance and fine motor problems). In addition children with CHD may have cognitive impairments and attention problems, as well as deficits in working memory and higher language functions, which in turn influence school performance and academic achievement. Studies in this area of the long-term outcome up to adolescence and young adulthood are needed to shed light onto the full spectrum of potential problems, as well as their effect on personal well-being, on quality of life, and on societal financial burdens. Also, parents and caregivers need to be informed about the potential short-term and long-term neurodevelopmental and behavioral problems their children may face, and interdisciplinary follow-up clinics need to be established to detect developmental problems early in order to provide timely therapeutic interventions and parental guidance.

REFERENCES

The complete list of references for this chapter is available in the e-book at www.expertconsult.com.
   See inside cover for registration details.

SELECTED REFERENCES

Bird, G.L., Jeffries, H.E., Licht, D.J., et al., 2008. Neurological complications associated with the treatment of patients with congenital cardiac disease: consensus definitions from the Multi-Societal Database Committee for Pediatric and Congenital Heart Disease. Cardiol. Young 18 (Suppl. 2), 234–239.

Calderon, J., Bellinger, D.C., 2015. Executive function deficits in congenital heart disease: why is intervention important? Cardiol. Young 25, 1238–1246.

Gaynor, J.W., Stopp, C., Wypij, D., et al., 2015. Neurodevelopmental outcomes after cardiac surgery in infancy. Pediatrics 135, 816–825.

Latal, B., 2016. Neurodevelopmental outcomes of the child with congenital heart disease. Clin. Perinatol. 43 (1), 173–185.

Licht, D.J., 2015. The path forward is to look backward in time—fetal physiology: the new frontier in managing infants with congenital heart defects. Circulation 131 (15), 1307–1309.

Lynch, J.M., et al., 2014. Time to surgery and preoperative cerebral hemodynamics predict postoperative white matter injury in neonates with hypoplastic left heart syndrome. J. Thorac. Cardiovasc. Surg. 148 (5), 2181–2188.

Marino, B.S., Lipkin, P.H., Newburger, J.W., et al., 2012. Neurodevelopmental outcomes in children with congenital heart disease: evaluation and management: a scientific statement from the American Heart Association. Circulation 126, 1143–1172.

Monagle, P., Chalmers, E., Chan, A., et al., 2008. Antithrombotic therapy in neonates and children: American College of Chest Physicians Evidence-Based Clinical Practice Guidelines (8th edition). Chest 133, 887S–968S.

Morton, P.D., Ishibashi, N., Jonas, R.A., et al., 2015. Congenital cardiac anomalies and white matter injury. Trends Neurosci. 38, 353–363.

Pierpont, M.E., Basson, C.T., Benson, D.W. Jr., et al., 2007. Genetic basis for congenital heart defects: current knowledge: a scientific statement from the American Heart Association Congenital Cardiac Defects Committee, Council on Cardiovascular Disease in the Young: endorsed by the American Academy of Pediatrics. Circulation 115, 3015–3038.

Snookes, S.H., Gunn, J.K., Eldridge, B.J., et al., 2010. A systematic review of motor and cognitive outcomes after early surgery for congenital heart disease. Pediatrics 125, e818–e827.

E-BOOK FIGURES AND TABLES

The following figures and tables are available in the e-book at www.expertconsult.com. See inside cover for registration details.

158 Neurologic Disorders Associated With Renal Diseases

Cheryl P. Sanchez, Rita D. Sheth, Robert S. Rust, Jessica L. Carpenter, and Stephen Ashwal

An expanded version of this chapter is available on www.expertconsult.com. See inside cover for registration details.

Advances in the treatment of children with kidney disease with new antihypertensive medications, dialysis, transplantation, and immunosuppressive agents have resulted in improved long-term survival and quality of life. Still, children present acutely with neurologic symptoms, and they may develop long-term neurologic disorders because of currently available treatments. This chapter reviews various aspects of the complex interrelationships between the kidneys and the brain. Four areas are discussed: (1) renal diseases that secondarily affect the nervous system, (2) diseases that affect both the kidneys and the nervous system, (3) neurologic drugs that may affect renal function in individuals with normal kidneys, and (4) drug therapy in renal disease.

RENAL DISEASES SECONDARILY AFFECTING THE NERVOUS SYSTEM

Acute Kidney Injury

Acute kidney injury (AKI) is a common problem occurring in as many as 10% to 25% of all hospital admissions in the United States, and approximately 25% to 50% of these admissions may require critical care management. Neurologic decompensation occurs as a result of the following: (1) disturbances in water homeostasis, electrolyte abnormalities, and acid–base metabolism; (2) impairment in the blood–brain barrier (BBB); (3) changes in neurotransmitter activity; and (4) derangements in drug metabolism.

Sodium and Water Disorders

Neurologic abnormalities associated with water intoxication may arise in AKI. The kidney's capacity to excrete water as dilute urine is the chief mechanism for prevention of water intoxication. In AKI, this mechanism is impaired, and neurologic dysfunction can develop within hours to days. Individuals with sodium values as low as 120 to 125 mEq/L can remain asymptomatic. Neurologic symptoms become more prevalent once the serum sodium is less than 120 mEq/L. Signs and symptoms of water intoxication are variable and include mental status changes (e.g., apathy, agitation, or confusion to obtundation), headache, nystagmus, vomiting, diaphoresis, weakness, generalized tremulousness, and seizures.

Children are at high risk for the development of brain edema from hyponatremia. Systemic aspects of water intoxication include cardiovascular compromise and pulmonary edema. These complications further jeopardize brain function. Hyponatremia may result in seizures, increasing cerebral energy demand and the rate at which toxic by-products of metabolism accumulate. Brain edema may increase intracranial pressure, further impairing cerebral circulation. Medical conditions that can lead to sodium disorders should be addressed (Table 158-1).

Hyponatremia can also be seen with acute neurologic disorders. Low serum sodium can result from excess renal sodium losses, as in cerebral salt wasting (CSW), or free-water retention, as in the syndrome of inappropriate antidiuretic hormone

(SIADH). CSW is characterized by a negative fluid balance, whereas SIADH is associated with a state of euvolemia or positive fluid balance. Distinguishing between these disorders is critical for management. Treatment of CSW is with sodium replacement and fluids and/or mineralocorticoids, whereas SIADH is treated with fluid restriction. A high index of suspicion for these disorders should exist for patients with acute brain dysfunction and down-trending or low serum sodium levels to minimize complications.

Correction of serum sodium should be done slowly to prevent complications associated with rapid osmolar shifts. Maintenance of circulation may require acute administration of fluid, in which case isotonic sodium is permissible. Volume expansion with hypotonic saline in a hyponatremic patient poses risks if the patient is actually in a sodium-depleted state. The decision to restrict fluids is appropriate if there is evidence of SIADH. Hypertonic saline should be administered in any symptomatic hyponatremic patient. Dialysis is often not necessary unless the patient is anuric or oliguric and fluid overload is the major cause of the sodium abnormality.

The rate of sodium correction is crucial. Excessively rapid correction poses the danger of central pontine myelinolysis. In children, correction at approximately 0.5 to 1 mEq/L/hour should be implemented, until the patient becomes alert and seizure-free, plasma sodium becomes 125 to 130 mEq/L, or the serum sodium level increases by 10 to 15 mEq/L, whichever occurs first. If seizures persist, or if there are signs of increased intracranial pressure (especially if these signs are worsening), the sodium concentration may be corrected at a rate of 4 to 8 mEq/L for 1 hour (if tolerated) or until seizures stop. Assuming that total body water comprises 50% of body mass, administration of 1 ml/kg of 3% NaCl solution will increase plasma sodium by approximately 1 mEq/L.

Potassium Abnormalities

During the first 48 hours of anuric AKI there is loss of as much as 70% to 80% of renal outer medullary potassium secretory channels and 35% to 40% of the activity of potassium channel inducing factor. Cardiac and pulmonary manifestations of hyperkalemia generally precede and are greater threats to survival than neurologic ones. Cardiac dysfunction is usually the earliest and most ominous sign. However, there are rare instances of hyperkalemia that present with neurologic signs such as striated muscle paralysis.

Other important causes of acute hyperkalemia include rhabdomyolysis and succinylcholine administration to susceptible individuals in the setting of acute muscle damage. Catecholamine elevation in the setting of hypothermia may produce hyperkalemia. A list of causes of potassium disorders is given in Table 158-2.

Calcium and Magnesium Abnormalities

Neurologic symptoms associated with calcium and magnesium disorders vary and depend on the rate with which these levels change. Typical symptoms of hypocalcemia include mental status changes, muscle irritability, and seizures.

TABLE 158-1 Causes of Hyponatremia and Hypernatremia

Mechanism	Source	Causative Factor/Disorder
CAUSES OF HYPONATREMIA		
Excessive NaCl loss	Gastrointestinal tract	Diarrhea
		Cystic fibrosis
	Skin	Heat stress
	Urinary tract	Salt-losing renal disease
		Adrenal insufficiency
		Diabetes mellitus
Excessive water intake	Oral	Psychogenic
	Parenteral	Acute kidney injury
	Rectal	Therapeutic error
		Coma
		Tap water enema
		Improperly mixed formula
Defective water excretion	Inappropriate antidiuretic hormone secretion	Anesthetic drugs
		Craniocerebral trauma
		Infection
		Malignancy
CAUSES OF HYPERNATREMIA		
Excess sodium intake		Improperly mixed formula or rehydration solution
		Excessive sodium bicarbonate or chloride administration during resuscitation
		Saltwater drowning
Water deficit		Diabetes insipidus
		Diabetes mellitus
		Excessive sweating
		Increased water loss
		Adipsia
		Inadequate water intake
Water deficit in excess of sodium deficit		Diarrhea
		Osmotic diuretics
		Obstructive uropathy
		Renal dysplasia

TABLE 158-2 Causes of Hypokalemia and Hyperkalemia

Mechanism	Causative Factor/Disorder
HYPOKALEMIA	
Deficient intake	Protein-calorie malnutrition
	Parenteral nutrition
Renal loss	Distal tubular acidosis
Renal disease	Proximal tubular acidosis (Fanconi's syndrome)
	Bartter's syndrome
	Interstitial nephritis
Extrarenal disease	Diabetes mellitus
	Cushing's syndrome
	Aldosteronism
	Drug administration (diuretic, aspirin, steroids)
	Hypomagnesemia
	Hypercalcemia
Shift (extracellular to intracellular)	Alkalosis
	Drugs (insulin, catecholamines)
	Parenteral nutrition
Extrarenal loss	Vomiting, diarrhea
	Fistula drainage
	Laxative abuse
	Ion-exchange resins
	Congenital alkalosis
	Increase urine output
HYPERKALEMIA	
Excessive intake	Potassium-containing salt substitutes
	Parenteral administration (excessive infusion, outdated blood)
	Gastrointestinal bleeding
DECREASED RENAL EXCRETION	
Renal disease	Oliguric kidney injury
	Chronic hydronephrosis
	Potassium-sparing diuretics
Extrarenal causes	Addison's disease
	Congenital adrenal hyperplasia
	Diabetes mellitus
	Drugs (beta blockers, heparin)
Shift (intracellular to extracellular)	Rapid cell breakdown (trauma, infection, cytotoxic agents)
	Acidosis
	Freshwater drowning

Hypercalcemia can present with lethargy, weakness, and confusion. Box 158-1 lists some of the common causes of hypocalcemia, hypomagnesemia, and hypermagnesemia.

The interactions between calcium and magnesium are complex, and each must be considered in situations where the other is present. Hypomagnesemia is a serious condition. Acute deficiency of magnesium is the cause of cramps and tetany. In critically ill patients, development of hypomagnesemia is associated with a twofold to threefold increased risk of death. Hypomagnesemia may be found in as many as 47% of patients with hypokalemia, 27% of individuals with hyponatremia, and 22% of those with hypocalcemia.

Hypermagnesemia may cause neurologic manifestations in AKI, although it is uncommon because normal renal magnesium regulation is efficient.

Chronic Kidney Disease

Current estimates of the incidence of end-stage renal disease (ESRD) in children is approximately 16 per million in the United States.

Uremic Encephalopathy

The syndrome of uremic encephalopathy is a spectrum of brain abnormalities resulting from the failure of the kidney to do the following:

1. Regulate fluids and electrolytes
2. Excrete protein catabolites and toxic substances
3. Balance endocrine secretion (Seifter and Samuels, 2011)

In developed countries, severe uremia is rare because of the availability of dialysis or renal replacement therapy. Clinical symptoms usually do not occur until the estimated glomerular filtration rate (GFR) is less than 10% of normal. High levels of uremic toxins, advanced glycation end products, inflammatory mediators, excess of parathyroid hormone, and acid–base imbalance may contribute to the development of uremic encephalopathy. Brain edema is uncommon in uremic encephalopathy.

Disturbances of endocrine function occur in uremia, with elevations of parathyroid hormone (PTH), insulin, growth hormone, glucagons, thyrotropin, prolactin, luteinizing hormone, or gastrin. Secondary hyperparathyroidism may contribute to the development of uremic encephalopathy because elevated PTH levels have been clearly linked to the reduction of mental capacity.

Clinical Features of Uremia. Clinical symptoms include seizures, encephalopathy, poor feeding, lethargy, tremulousness, and gastrointestinal autonomic dysregulation. Twitching, muscular weakness or tetany, apnea, and paresthesias also may occur. Altered mental status, tremulousness, and muscle cramping tend to occur.

Uremic encephalopathy remains a complicated condition, the pathophysiology of which is likely multifactorial.

BOX 158-1 Causes of Calcium and Magnesium Abnormalities

HYPOCALCEMIA

- Vitamin D deficiency
- Hypoparathyroidism
- Pseudohypoparathyroidism
- Hyperphosphatemia
- Magnesium deficiency
- Acute pancreatitis
- Alkalosis
- Rapid correction of acidosis

HYPERCALCEMIA

- Vitamin D excess
- Hyperparathyroidism
- Malignancy
- Medications
- Infections
- Sarcoidosis

HYPOMAGNESEMIA

- Malabsorption
- Hypoparathyroidism
- Renal tubular acidosis
- Diuretic therapy
- Primary aldosteronism
- Neonatal tetany

HYPERMAGNESEMIA

- Decreased renal function
- Magnesium-containing laxatives or enema preparations
- Maternal magnesium sulfate treatment

Encephalopathy is more common in children than in adults with uremia and may present with subtle psychiatric manifestations such as moodiness or depression. Hypocalcemic tetany and a peculiar movement disorder termed "uremic twitching" occur more commonly in children.

Neurologic manifestations to which hypermagnesemia might contribute include lethargy, depression, paresthesias, muscle weakness, and neuropathic changes in cardiac conduction, autonomic cardiovascular regulatory abnormalities, and autonomic aspects of gastrointestinal function. Conditions that might worsen uremic hypermagnesemia are hypothyroidism, Addison's disease, familial hypercalciuric hypercalcemia, and milk alkali syndrome. As with other electrolyte disturbances, clinically significant hypomagnesemia is found more commonly in infants and elderly individuals, usually in association with chronic kidney disease.

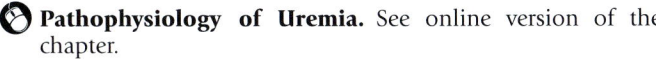 **Pathophysiology of Uremia.** See online version of the chapter.

Diagnostic Considerations in Patients With Uremia. Most cases of chronic uremia are seen in those on dialysis for ESRD. In patients with new-onset renal failure and uremia, there is a wide differential diagnosis to consider for possible causes of neurologic deterioration.

Acute uremic encephalopathy produces deterioration of higher cortical function that varies from slowly progressive to fulminant. The earliest changes include inattention, irritability, and diminished intellectual agility and are often more apparent to caregivers than to the patient. Cognitive deficits may worsen as a consequence of the duration of hemodialysis.

Tremor and asterixis are reliable early signs of uremic encephalopathy and should prompt careful mental status

evaluation. With progressive obtundation, encephalopathy becomes less intermittent, and severe disturbances of orientation, memory, cognition, judgment, and primitive reflexes (e.g., snout, root, grasp) may emerge. Transient loss of hearing or vision may develop. Seizures occurring in the later stages of acute uremia generally signify the development of other complications.

Muscle twitching or fasciculations, especially in the distal extremities, are common in acute renal failure. Such activity may be preceded by muscle aches or cramping. Restless-leg phenomenon is not uncommon in uremic encephalopathy. Tetany may develop and may not respond to calcium supplementation. Moderate to severe motor weakness may follow. Multifocal stimulus-sensitive myoclonus emerges as uremic stupor develops. In patients with chronic kidney disease, acute weakness must be distinguished from preexisting changes related to neuropathy or hyperparathyroidism. Endocrinopathies and vitamin deficiency states should be considered because most are treatable. Cardiovascular autonomic dysregulation in uremia is a cause of considerable morbidity and increases mortality risk. Some abnormalities (e.g., emotional and intellectual) may respond quickly to dialysis, whereas others (e.g., motor and sensory) respond more slowly.

Brain imaging is often normal. When present, abnormalities may be transient and of uncertain significance. Elevated lumbar cerebrospinal fluid (CSF) pressure may be found and usually resolves with dialysis. CSF protein concentration may be elevated, and pleocytosis may be found. These changes may occur without identification of any treatable process and may be a result of uremic alteration of BBB function.

Management of Uremic Encephalopathy. The primary treatment of uremic encephalopathy is dialysis. Seizures should suggest reevaluation for hypertension, electrolyte or water imbalance, infection, or intoxication (commonly, penicillin or a phenothiazine). Persistent seizures should be treated with antiseizure drugs.

Congenital Uremic Encephalopathy

Most infants with congenital uremic encephalopathy have inherited forms of nephrosis, particularly congenital nephrosis of the Finnish type. It is possible that some of the neurologic abnormalities in these infants are independently inherited developmental abnormalities or a result of the prenatal metabolic effects of nephrosis. The appearance of abnormalities may present after a latent interval. Early provision of dialysis has not been shown to prevent development of congenital uremic encephalopathy.

Infants with seizures and developmental arrest in the first year of life are at a high risk for developing epilepsy and moderate to severe motor, cognitive, language, and psychosocial delay in later childhood. Neurologic abnormalities include ataxia, choreoathetosis, facial myoclonus, hypotonicity, weakness, and hyperreflexia. If language develops, it is often compromised by dysarthria and lingual apraxia. Renal transplantation may reverse progression of uremic encephalopathy.

Stroke and Vasculopathy

Vascular accidents may cause acquired neurologic injuries in children with congenital nephrotic syndrome. Ischemic lesions appear to correlate with a history of pretransplantation hemodynamic crises and with greater duration of dialysis before renal transplantation. Attention devoted to ensuring hemodynamic stability in infants undergoing dialysis for chronic renal failure and early consideration of transplantation may improve outcome. There may be a beneficial effect of folate, pyridoxine, and cobalamin supplements for the prevention of stroke in individuals undergoing peritoneal dialysis.

Dialysis-Associated Complications

Dialysis is efficacious in the remediation or prevention of acute uremic encephalopathy and is also beneficial in the treatment of uremic peripheral neuropathy. Dialysis is associated with many potential complications. Problems related to the preparation of dialysis fluids are now seldom encountered. When they occur, they tend to manifest as seizures or decline in mental status. Dialysis side effects include headache, fatigue, allergic reactions, and hypotension. Mild to moderate headache is not uncommonly reported by older children. It is likely that dialysis headache is prompted by water and electrolyte shifts or by other aspects of dialysis disequilibrium. Risk can be reduced by adjustment of dialysis parameters. Patients with higher predialysis systolic and diastolic blood pressure may be at greater risk for headache, in addition to those who experience dialysis-related hypotension or weight loss. Metabolic abnormalities should be excluded. Headaches tend to occur after 3 to 4 hours of dialysis and often respond to acetaminophen. Hypertension or subdural hemorrhage should be considered when headache is more severe or persistent, particularly if mental status changes or new focal neurologic signs are present.

Dialysis Disequilibrium Syndrome

Dialysis disequilibrium syndrome is a rare but serious complication mostly associated with aggressive hemodialysis. Manifestations include irritability, fatigue, headache, nausea, blurred vision, muscle cramps, and tremulousness. Hypertension, elevated intraocular pressure, and asterixis are sometimes seen. The syndrome is likely to occur with recently initiated dialysis, utilization of a rapid dialysis protocol, or dialysis with ultrafiltration, especially when initial serum osmolality is high.

The term *osmotic demyelination* has been applied to some patients who experience neurologic deterioration after dialysis and are found to have pontine abnormalities on T2-weighted magnetic resonance imaging (MRI). These changes may be found with dialysis-associated seizures or mild alterations of consciousness. Repeat scans usually demonstrate the rapid and complete disappearance of these changes. Dialysis removes osmotically active molecules from blood more rapidly than they can diffuse out of the brain. This movement results in an osmotic gradient that provokes net flow of water into the brain, resulting in cerebral edema, increased intracranial pressure, and encephalopathy.

Modifications in dialysis protocols have reduced the frequency of dialysis disequilibrium. The most important element in preventing dialysis disequilibrium is early diagnosis of uremia and initiation of dialysis, so that profound azotemia (blood urea nitrogen $\geq$ 200 mg/dl) is not encountered.

Dialysis-Associated Seizures

Dialysis-associated seizures occur in 7% to 10% of children (newborn to 21 years) with ESRD. Most are generalized tonic-clonic seizures that occur during or shortly after dialysis. Risk factors include previous seizures, young age, malignant hypertension, uremic encephalopathy, dialysis disequilibrium, and congenital uremic encephalopathy. Seizures occur during the early phases of dialysis. Hemodialysis poses a greater risk for seizures than peritoneal dialysis because of more rapid clearance of electrolytes and other osmotically active solutes.

The efficacy of antiseizure drugs in treating or preventing dialysis-associated seizures is poorly defined. In individuals chronically treated with antiseizure medications, dialysis-associated seizures may be a result of dialysis-related reduction of antiseizure medication concentration.

Aluminum Toxicity and Encephalopathy (Including Dialysis Dementia)

Aluminum toxicity and dementia related to dialysis and use of aluminum phosphate binding agents in chronic kidney disease have declined over the last decade; however, aluminum can still be found in total parenteral nutrition (TPN) and some drug preservatives. Infants, children, and adults with chronic kidney disease are at risk for aluminum toxicity. See the online chapter for further discussion.

Vitamin and Cofactor Deficiencies

The B vitamins are water soluble, and most are readily dialyzable. A single dialysis session may reduce plasma thiamine concentration by as much as 40%. Patients with ESRD continue to be at risk for thiamine deficiency, which causes Wernicke's encephalopathy. Symptoms include a triad of ophthalmoplegia, encephalopathy, and ataxia. Symptomatic thiamine deficiency has been reported rarely in children probably because stores of thiamine accumulated before the development of renal disease are only gradually depleted, and considerable effort is expended by parents and caregivers to ensure good nutrition. Response to intravenous thiamine may confirm the diagnosis.

Pyridoxine deficiency is a risk factor for seizures. Hyperhomocystinuria is an important indicator of vitamin B_{12} deficiency. If found, it is associated with higher risk for pre-eclampsia, neural tube defects in offspring, atherosclerotic arterial disease, stroke, and venous thrombosis. Supplementation with B vitamins is routine to avoid these various complications. Chapters 46 and 47 review the vitamin and other micronutrient deficiency states seen in children.

Intracranial Hemorrhage

Individuals requiring chronic dialysis for renal failure have an 11-fold greater risk for cerebral hemorrhage and 4-fold greater lifetime risk for subarachnoid hemorrhage. Replacement of generalized with regional anticoagulation and use of nonheparin-based anticoagulation have reduced the risk of this serious complication. Intracranial hemorrhage must be considered in renal patients with persistent drowsiness, headache, vomiting, persistent focal neurologic signs, or meningismus.

Milder Forms of Encephalopathy

Neuropsychologic studies of children on dialysis have shown lower cognitive functioning. Abnormalities of performance IQ, short-term visual and auditory memory, attention span, memory, and speed of decision making have been documented. The risk is greatest if ESRD developed in early childhood (particularly during the first year of life) or if renal failure is of very long duration. Subtle intellectual and behavioral abnormalities, responsive to dialysis, have been detected. Sensorineural hearing abnormalities may occur in some patients with ESRD as a result of ototoxic medications given during the course of illnesses and multiple hospitalizations. Drugs used for treatment of ESRD and its complications may contribute to encephalopathy.

There is a high prevalence of depression, anxiety, and emotional stress in patients with chronic renal failure. Other confounding effects include developmental dysmaturity related to chronic hospitalization. A long-term outcome study of individuals who started dialysis before 16 years of age reported good overall quality of life despite coexistent conditions and disabilities.

Poor intellectual function should lead to identification and scrupulous correction of metabolic abnormalities. Moderate uremia may result in disturbances ranging from mild encephalopathy to mild chronic delirium or psychosis. Intellectual dysfunction, deafness, and neuropathy, unresponsive to dialysis, may improve after successful transplantation.

Uremic Peripheral Polyneuropathy

Peripheral neuropathy occurs in 65% of patients with ESRD. Somatic and autonomic nerves may be involved. As with other neurologic complications, the duration and severity of chronic kidney disease are important determinants of the occurrence and severity of neuropathy.

Electrophysiologic abnormalities consistent with neuropathy are detectable in two thirds of adults with long-standing chronic kidney disease, whether or not dialysis has been initiated. Restless-leg syndrome is among the most common presenting complaints of sensorimotor neuropathy, associated with an unpleasant sensation of crawling skin or a dull ache in the legs that is worse in the evening. Pruritus is common more likely in individuals who also complain of paresthesias.

Hearing is an important modality to be monitored in individuals with chronic kidney disease. Hearing loss may be the result of uremic axonal neuropathy, although other incompletely cleared endogenous or administered ototoxic substances may contribute to this and other neuropathic abnormalities.

Loss of deep tendon reflexes (especially the ankle jerk), diminished vibratory sense, and weakness of great toe extension are among the earliest signs of uremic neuropathy. Paradoxical heat sensation, the tendency to identify a low-temperature stimulus as being hot, is also a sensitive early sign of uremic polyneuropathy. Fully developed uremic neuropathy is a distal, symmetric polyneuropathy that involves sensory and motor modalities. Diminished sensitivity to all modalities in a glove-stocking distribution gradually develops. Pressure palsies, to which chronic renal failure/neuropathic renal disease patients are particularly subject, may alter the expected distribution of abnormalities.

In adolescents and adults on dialysis for ESRD, sudomotor changes and postural hypotension are common consequences of autonomic neuropathy. Delayed gastric emptying can occur in children with chronic kidney disease independent of age, gender, duration of disease, or blood urea nitrogen or creatinine levels. Successful renal transplantation may reverse sympathetic and parasympathetic dysfunction.

The mechanisms of nerve injury in association with end-stage kidney disease remain incompletely understood and are discussed in the online chapter.

Uremic Myopathy (Myopathy of Chronic Kidney Disease)

Muscle weakness is common in patients with ESRD. The pathogenesis is incompletely understood, and the definition and diagnostic features of the term *uremic myopathy* remain controversial. Diagnosis is often made on the basis of loss of endurance or ability for muscular exercise without muscle physiologic testing or biopsy. Muscle enzymes and electromyography tend to be normal.

Chronic and progressive muscular weakness may be the secondary consequence of "uremic" neuropathy. Uremic vasculopathy is another cause of secondary myopathy. Vascu-lar myopathy is a necrotic process that has been ascribed to severe hyperparathyroidism with calcification of blood vessels, rather than representing a consequence of autonomic neuropathy. Muscle biopsy abnormalities include atrophy, type grouping, lipidosis, glycogen depletion, and mitochondrial proliferation. Caution is needed to avoid excessive use of calcium-based phosphate binders and vitamin D analogs in the treatment of secondary hyperparathyroidism and hyperphosphatemia in patients with chronic kidney disease. Sudden cardiac death occurs in approximately 25% of adult dialysis patients as a result of multifactorial etiologies, including vascular calcification, calcium abnormalities, and high prevalence of arrhythmias. The rate in children is unknown.

Malnutrition

Protein and energy wasting are a serious problem in children with chronic kidney disease. Tube feedings and special formulas have improved growth, although motor, speech, and fine motor delays remain evident, especially in the very young. Nutritional disorders are often difficult to dissociate from the metabolic and endocrine dysfunction of chronic kidney disease.

Endocrinopathy

Secondary hyperparathyroidism with hypercalcemia or hypocalcemia may directly injure the nervous system. Parathyroid hormone excess may directly affect central neurotransmission. Studies in animals and human adults have found that encephalopathy may be prevented or ameliorated with parathyroidectomy.

Complications Associated With Renal Transplantation

The quality of life, including certain aspects of neurologic function, is generally improved after renal transplantation. Dialysis-associated complications are avoided, and neuropathy usually improves. Cognitive function, head growth, and psychomotor development also improve in many children. Survival also has been extended with kidney transplantations from deceased donors and living relatives. Transplantation entails risk for a particular set of neurologic complications that are usually associated with infection, hypertension, and medications including immunosuppressive agents.

Infection

Infections may be related to the donor organ, surgical procedure, or presence of a foreign body, including urinary stents. Infections can be severe as a result of immunosuppression during the first few weeks after transplantation. Common gram-positive bacterial infections include *Staphylococcus aureus*, coagulase-negative staphylococcus, and enterococcus; gram-negative organisms include *Escherichia coli*, *Pseudomonas*, *Klebsiella*, and *Enterobacter*.

Donor-derived or naturally acquired fungal infections can be fatal after renal transplantation. It is important to know the endemic areas where these infections can occur, travel history, and donor history. Central nervous system (CNS) infections account for 4% to 29% of CNS lesions in transplant recipients. Given the gravity of these infections, early biopsy of brain lesions and CSF collection for viral polymerase chain reaction (PCR) should be considered.

Meningoencephalitis in transplant recipients is often caused by viral infections, including Epstein–Barr virus (EBV), cytomegalovirus (CMV), West Nile virus, varicella zoster, polyoma virus JCV, and BK virus. EBV and CMV infections in the first few months after renal transplantation are less common than previously because of the use of antiviral prophylaxis.

Malignancy

Newer and more powerful immunosuppressants have decreased allograft rejection, but increased the risk of infections and malignancy. In adults, posttransplant malignancies are at least double in transplant recipients compared with the general population. The risk of developing a solid tumor is 6.7-fold higher in pediatric kidney recipients compared with the general pediatric population.

Posttransplant lymphoproliferative disorders (PTLDs) are more common in children than in adults who have received renal allografts and constitute the majority of neoplasms for which these children are at risk. Approximately 1% to 2% of pediatric kidney recipients will develop PTLD within 5 years. The use of lymphocyte-depleting antibodies has been associated with an increase in the incidence of PTLD in children, and CNS involvement carries a poor prognosis. Management includes reduction or cessation of immunosuppression and treatment with a combination of chemotherapy including rituximab (specific anti-CD20 monoclonal antibody), cranial irradiation, and intravenous (IV) ganciclovir. Approximately 72% of pediatric patients achieve CNS remission with the use of intrathecal/intraventricular rituximab in posttransplant EBV associated CNS lymphoma.

Drugs

Drug-related complications include hypertension, immunosuppression, oncogenesis, and direct neurotoxicity. The use of corticosteroids and calcineurin inhibitors, cyclosporine A and tacrolimus, can lead to posterior reversible encephalopathy syndrome (PRES). Cyclosporine A is a calcineurin inhibitor most commonly associated with neurologic side effects, including paresthesias, peripheral neuropathy, ataxia, tremor, encephalopathy, sympathetic overactivation, headaches, and seizures. Cyclosporine neurotoxicity occurs more frequently in younger children and in those who develop hypertension.

There is evidence that tacrolimus, a more potent immunosuppressant than cyclosporine A, may also have a greater tendency to engender neurotoxicities of the same variety as that associated with cyclosporine use. Tacrolimus has been associated with a posttransplantation encephalopathy that includes MRI-discernible changes in gray and white matter. This syndrome may subside without discontinuation of tacrolimus. Patients who developed neurotoxicity with calcineurin inhibitors have been safely treated with mTOR inhibitors and mycophenolate mofetil without recurrence of their neurologic symptoms. Calcineurin-treated patients also have a higher prevalence and severity of neuropathy.

Administration of the CD3 monoclonal antibody, orthoclone OKT3, to prevent renal allograft rejection may provoke headache, fever, vomiting, a flulike syndrome, hypotension, seizures, or aseptic meningitis in as many as one third of patients. These changes may be severe and can progress to coma. Severe symptoms associated with OKT3 have precluded its use in the majority of renal transplant centers, in lieu of newer and safer medications and biologic agents.

Hypertension

Hypertensive Encephalopathy

The designation *hypertensive encephalopathy* is generally reserved for hypertensive patients with alteration of consciousness with diffuse or multifocal CNS dysfunction, in whom there is no better or more complex etiologic explanation. Malignant hypertension leading to hypertensive encephalopathy can arise in association with a number of underlying illnesses, including aortic coarctation (30%) and polycystic kidneys (30%), nephritis (16%), and hemolytic-uremic syndrome (7%). The causes of malignant hypertension in children are age dependent. Increased sophistication in imaging has led to increased recognition of PRES and concomitant redesignation of cases that would previously have been designated as hypertensive encephalopathy.

More than 40% of patients with malignant hypertension develop significant neurologic complications. The risk for hypertensive encephalopathy is related to the rapidity and severity of blood pressure increases from any given baseline. Risk is higher in patients with acute renal failure. When hypertensive encephalopathy occurs in children, it carries a high risk of morbidity and mortality.

Clinical Features of Hypertensive Encephalopathy. Clinical symptoms include a combination of hypertension, headache, encephalopathy, and visual disturbances. The headache typically develops hours to days after the initiating blood pressure crisis and may be accompanied by lethargy, projectile vomiting, meningismus, or edema of the eyelids and ankles. Ophthalmoscopic findings include funduscopic evidence of arteriolar spasm or ischemic nerve fiber infarction. Papilledema is present in one third of children with hypertensive encephalopathy.

Newborns and infants with hypertensive encephalopathy can present with irritability, lethargy, and unresponsiveness. Encephalopathy in older children may consist of fluctuating confusion, irritability, and restlessness that may progress to coma. Mental status changes typically develop 12 to 36 hours after headache onset. Seizures may occur and are more commonly generalized.

Focal neurologic signs may signify more permanent injury. Unilateral infarction of some portion of the anterior optic pathways is especially characteristic. Infarction may be more common in patients who have had long-standing unrecognized hypertension. It also may occur in individuals who experience hypotensive episodes as a result of overly aggressive management of blood pressure elevation.

Pathophysiology of Hypertensive Encephalopathy. The exact nature of the pathophysiology of hypertensive encephalopathy is not fully understood, but two major theories are advocated. Both propose dysfunction of cerebral autoregulation, with one favoring excessive vasoconstriction with secondary ischemia. The other theory proposes a vasoconstrictive threshold that is exceeded, resulting in the development of transudative perivascular edema, which then compresses the regional microvasculature. Microinfarction, edema, and loss of autoregulation can occur, necessitating caution in blood pressure reduction and manipulation of cardiac output because rapid changes may result in acute cerebral infarction.

Diagnostic Considerations in Patients With Hypertensive Encephalopathy. The differential diagnosis for hypertensive encephalopathy is broad. Structural CNS lesions, encephalitis (infectious or immune mediated), and seizures should all be considered in the initial evaluation. Focal lesions, such as infarction, intracranial hemorrhage, or tumor, may be the cause of the hypertension. Alternatively, focal lesions, such as PRES or cerebral ischemia, may be the consequence of the hypertension.

Outcomes From Hypertensive Encephalopathy

Outcome in hypertensive encephalopathy is generally favorable. Encephalopathy and seizures resolve with correction of blood pressure. Visual disturbances are typically reversible but occasionally can persist. The degree and duration of the hypertensive phase are important elements in the risk for visual dysfunction, underlining the importance of early diagnosis and treatment.

Posterior Reversible Encephalopathy Syndrome

PRES is thought to represent a disorder of cerebral autoregulation occurring in the setting of acute hypertension and manifest as acute neurologic symptoms associated with stereotypical radiographic changes. The phenomenon was first described in patients with hypertension, but it is now thought to be associated with a variety of conditions and may occur in children with or without hypertension. Populations known to be at risk for PRES include children with autoimmune disease, renal or hematological disorders, and bone marrow or solid-organ transplantation. An increasing number of medications are associated with PRES. Risk is highest with immunosuppressive medications, including monoclonal antibodies, calcineurin inhibitors, steroids, and cytotoxic medications.

Clinical Features of Posterior Reversible Encephalopathy Syndrome. Clinical features of PRES include fairly sudden onset of severe headache, encephalopathy, seizures, and visual disturbance. Symptoms typically resolve spontaneously or after correction of blood pressure. Recurrent PRES is not uncommon.

Brain imaging usually illustrates fairly symmetric and extensive abnormalities within 24 hours of clinical onset that are much more apparent on MRI than on computed tomography. Changes are both cortical and subcortical and generally without diffusion restriction.

Diagnostic Considerations in Patients With Posterior Reversible Encephalopathy Syndrome. A broad differential diagnosis should be considered when making a diagnosis of PRES. Other considerations include vasculitis, hypoxic ischemic injury, infectious or immune-mediated encephalitis, acute disseminated encephalomyelitis, toxic leukoencephalopathy (e.g., methotrexate toxicity), and/or osmotic demyelination syndrome.

Management of Posterior Reversible Encephalopathy Syndrome. Management of PRES largely consists of supportive care. Severe blood pressure elevation should be treated aggressively. Blood pressure reduction is likely to be well tolerated except in the setting of chronic hypertension or cerebral vasculopathy.

Seizures should be treated aggressively, and continuous electroencephalogram (EEG) monitoring should be employed to assess for subclinical seizures. Medications should be renally dosed for children with renal insufficiency/failure. Electrolytes should be normalized, with close attention to sodium, calcium, and magnesium. Chronic anticonvulsant therapy is seldom required.

DISEASES AFFECTING BOTH KIDNEY AND NERVOUS SYSTEM

Diseases that affect both the kidney and the nervous system can be divided into four general categories:

1. Inflammatory/vascular
2. Infectious
3. Toxic or metabolic
4. Heritable disorders with brain and renal anomalies

The inflammatory/vascular illnesses, which are considered first in this section, include thrombotic thrombocytopenic purpura, hemolytic-uremic syndrome, and other thrombocytopenic microangiopathies. Additional disorders such as hepatorenal syndrome, Henoch–Schönlein syndrome, and familial amyloidosis are also reviewed. Systemic lupus erythematosus, polyarteritis nodosa, and Wegener's granulomatosis are examples of other illnesses that produce inflammatory changes in both the nervous and renal systems. The details of these illnesses are covered in Chapter 121.

Infections with a predilection for renal and neurologic involvement include bacterial infections, such as Shiga-toxin-producing *E. coli*–associated hemolytic-uremic syndrome (STEC-HUS) and *S. aureus* infections; infections with viruses such as adenovirus, enteroviruses, coxsackieviruses, and echoviruses; and infections caused by fungi such as *Candida* spp. and *Aspergillus*.

A variety of toxins ranging from metals (e.g., lead, mercury, aluminum) and illicit substances (cocaine and heroin) to household products (e.g., ethylene glycol) and insecticides such as malathion, chlorpyrifos, and dichlorvos are known to cause brain and kidney dysfunction. Rare inherited metabolic diseases are a vast category of diseases with potential for multiorgan involvement. Examples of subtypes with a predilection for kidney and brain disease include glycogen storage and lysosomal storage disorders (e.g., Gaucher disease and Fabry disease).

Many inherited disorders include brain and kidney involvement. Polycystic kidney disease is associated with an increased risk for cerebral aneurysms and arachnoid cysts.

Hereditary angiopathy with nephropathy, aneurysms, and muscle cramps syndrome (HANAC) includes kidney disease, cerebral aneurysms, and myopathy. Von Hippel–Lindau disease is a genetic disorder with a predisposition to malignancies, including CNS neoplasms, such as endolymphatic sac tumors and craniospinal hemangioblastomas, and renal masses, such as renal cysts and carcinomas. Sickle-cell disease is a chronic hematologic disorder with a high risk for cerebral vasculopathy, stroke, and kidney abnormalities ranging from proteinuria to ESRD.

Thrombotic Thrombocytopenic Purpura

The clinical diagnosis of thrombotic thrombocytopenic purpura (TTP) requires at least two major (thrombocytopenia, Coombs-negative microangiopathic anemia, or neurologic dysfunction) and two minor (fever, renal dysfunction, or circulating thrombi) manifestations, permitting the diagnosis to be made in the absence of either renal or neurologic dysfunction. Determining the boundaries between TTP and a number of other microangiopathic conditions, collectively termed thrombotic microangiopathies, was challenging until recently.

It is now understood that TTP and HUS are distinct entities. TTP-associated thrombi are rich in platelets and are found in the heart, pancreas, kidney, adrenal glands, and brain, in decreasing order of severity. HUS-associated thrombi are rich in fibrin/red cells, and they tend largely to be confined to the kidney. TTP thrombi are found in the brains and kidneys of 50% to 75% of individuals with fatal TTP. Brain thromboses of TTP occur in small arterioles, capillaries, and venules and are associated with microinfarction. Small petechial hemorrhages may be widely scattered in gray matter. Diagnostic tests are available that reliably designate most heritable and acquired TTP cases. Classification of thrombotic microangiopathies is described in the online version of the chapter (James et al., 2014).

Signs and symptoms of acute TTP usually evolve quickly and quite noticeably over 7 to 10 days. Skin purpura is the initial manifestation in more than 90% of patients. Fever usually develops early. Hemorrhage (retinal, choroidal, nasal, gingival, gastrointestinal, and genitourinary), abdominal pain, arthralgia, or pancreatitis may also develop. Neurologic findings include fatigue, confusion, headache, and varying degrees of dysfunction of vision or language. Significant laboratory findings include microangiopathic hemolytic anemia, thrombocytopenia, elevated lactate dehydrogenase, proteinuria, and microscopic hematuria. CSF chemistry, cell counts, and pressure are usually normal. Other findings associated with disseminated intravascular coagulopathy are not usually found. MRI of brain is often normal.

Plasma exchange is the therapy of choice. A survival rate of at least 80% has been found for plasma exchange, compared with 60% survival for patients randomized to plasma infusion. Plasma infusions may be used as a temporizing measure in patients with suspected TTP until plasma exchange can be instituted because of the high risk for morbidity and mortality if therapy is delayed. In addition to therapeutic plasma exchange, immunosuppressant therapy with corticosteroids is indicated in patients with acquired TTP (Blombery and Scully, 2014).

Most cases of TTP are monophasic, but 11% to 28% of patients experience one or more recurrences. Relapses can occur weeks to years after initial remission. For severe or recurrent cases, chronic plasmapheresis is useful. Rituximab can be used for initial therapy and in refractory or relapsing cases.

Hemolytic-Uremic Syndrome

HUS is a Coombs-negative thrombocytopenic microangiopathy, the onset of which is typically in early childhood. Classic HUS, also known as D + HUS or STEC-HUS, occurs with a prodrome of diarrhea and is secondary to infections with Shiga-toxin-producing *E. coli*, although other bacterial infections have been associated with D + HUS. HUS that occurs in the absence of a diarrheal illness is labeled D-HUS or atypical HUS (aHUS). aHUS is considered to be a disorder of the alternate complement pathway involving dysregulation and increased terminal complement pathway activation. Multiple genetic mutations in the complement pathway have been identified as risk factors for the development of aHUS. Other forms of D-HUS include infection-related HUS that occurs with nondiarrheal illnesses, such as HUS associated with *Streptococcus pneumoniae* infections or drug-induced HUS. Most cases occur in children younger than 5 years of age; however, HUS associated with *E. coli* outbreaks can occur in patients at any age (Trachtman, 2013). HUS that presents in infancy is often noninfectious and is secondary to familial or genetic mutations. HUS can have multisystem involvement with associated cardiac, liver, and pancreatic dysfunction (Trachtman, 2013).

Neurologic manifestations of HUS—most commonly, seizures, stroke, and varying degrees of encephalopathy—are seen in 30% to 40% of patients. Occurrence of neurologic abnormalities predicts a worse outcome, with enhanced risk for ESRD or death. It is not always clear whether such neurologic changes are the result of cerebral microangiopathy or are secondary to metabolic disturbances and hypertension. MRI of the brain may disclose focal areas of infarction with swelling and, in some patients, hemorrhage.

Treatment

Management of patients with D + HUS is supportive, with attention to fluid and electrolyte management, hypertension control, and judicious use of blood transfusions. HUS-associated renal failure usually persists for several weeks. Dialysis is required in 30% to 50% of patients and is indicative of a poorer prognosis. Patients with aHUS are more likely to develop severe AKI requiring dialysis. Most patients with D + HUS will recover renal function, as opposed to patients with aHUS, who often develop chronic kidney disease or dialysis dependency.

Patients with aHUS have a more prolonged course with a higher incidence of morbidity and mortality. Eculizumab, a complement inhibitor, has been used successfully in the treatment of patients with aHUS and is considered the first line of therapy in patients with suspected complement-mediated aHUS (Loirat et al., 2016). Renal transplantation is indicated in patients with chronic kidney disease secondary to HUS; however, patients with aHUS are at a high risk for HUS recurrence posttransplantation.

Vasculitic Diseases With Neurologic-Renal Presentations

Extended consideration of the various inflammatory disorders can be found in Chapters 109, 112, 121, 142, and 150.

Hepatorenal Syndrome

Hepatorenal syndrome (HRS) is defined as the presence of functional, potentially reversible AKI that occurs in patients with various forms of liver failure in the absence of hypovolemia or other identifiable causes for AKI. It is divided into two types. Type 1 includes patients with AKI with rapidly deteriorating renal function in association with acute severe hepatic dysfunction. It can be fulminant and carries a high risk for death. Encephalopathy is common in type 1. Type 1 hepatorenal syndrome is rare in childhood. Type 2 includes patients who manifest the combination of less severe liver and renal disease with a slow progressive course and evidence of chronic liver and concurrent kidney disease. Encephalopathy is less common in type 2 cases. Some form of hepatorenal syndrome develops in as many as 20% of patients who are in their first year of acute or subacute hepatic failure.

Clinical features include ascites, jaundice, and low arterial blood pressure, despite increased plasma volume. The hepatorenal syndrome is often precipitated by infections such as spontaneous bacterial peritonitis or with aggressive diuresis or paracentesis. Laboratory findings consistent with AKI include a rise in serum creatinine from baseline values with concurrent evidence of a prerenal state in the form of a normal urine analysis, a low urinary sodium clearance, and a high urine osmolarity.

Therapy is based on replenishing the low effective circulatory volume with fluids, albumin infusions, and correction of the vasomotor dysregulation with vasoconstrictors. Other supportive therapies include the institution of renal replacement therapies, such as hemodialysis in patients with severe hyponatremia, azotemia, or other metabolic disturbances. Combined liver–kidney transplantation may be considered when patients remain dialysis dependent or have evidence of chronic kidney disease (Sampaio, Martin, and Bunnapradist, 2014; Eason et al., 2008).

Amyloidosis

Amyloidoses are a group of rare disorders of amyloid proteins that affect the kidney and the brain. They can be divided into the heredofamilial (primary) type and those that constitute the secondary (reactive) group. Renal amyloidosis is uncommon in children and is often secondary to chronic infectious or inflammatory diseases such as familial Mediterranean fever (Bilginer, Akpolat, and Ozen, 2011). These disorders are discussed in the online chapter.

Metabolic Diseases Producing Generalized Renal and Neurologic Dysfunction

Both acute and chronic generalized nephron dysfunction may result from metabolic diseases that have primary effects on the kidney and nervous system. Diseases that are most likely to result in encephalopathy are those that produce the combination of chronic metabolic and catabolic dysfunction in association with acute renal failure. Under such conditions, the metabolic perturbation worsens more rapidly and often achieves greater severity. Systemic diseases that can provoke encephalopathy, even without renal failure (e.g., sepsis, burns, fever, ethylene glycol, lactic acidosis, or ketoacidosis), produce more fulminant, severe, and difficult-to-treat nervous system dysfunction when renal failure also occurs or was previously present. Therapeutic interventions must include attention to cerebrovascular dynamics because cardiac output is often low, and cerebral autoregulation is often compromised.

Selective Tubular Dysfunction

Many inherited diseases and intoxications produce characteristic patterns of renal tubular acidosis in association with neurologic abnormalities; glomerular function is usually preserved in these diseases. Renal tubular acidosis is generally characterized by hyperchloremia and reduced plasma bicarbonate, and is further divided into proximal (bicarbonate-wasting) or distal (defective acid-excreting) renal tubular varieties. Selective tubular dysfunction itself produces far fewer clinical manifestations than are observed in uremia. In many instances, the neurologic dysfunction is more apparent than the associated renal dysfunction, which is often overlooked.

Proximal Renal Tubular Acidosis

Proximal renal tubular acidosis (proximal RTA) refers to the condition characterized by urinary bicarbonate loss secondary to an isolated proximal tubular dysfunction, which leads to hyperchloremic non-anion-gap metabolic acidosis. Proximal RTA can occur as an adverse effect of medications, such as carbonic anhydrase inhibitors. It can occur transiently in infants and preterm babies as a result of lack of renal tubular maturation. Isolated proximal RTA can be primary in origin as a result of inherited genetic mutations, but it is more commonly seen secondary to medications or other systemic illnesses (Haque, Ariceta, and Batlle, 2011).

Clinical presentation includes a history of recurrent dehydration and failure to thrive, along with polyuria and polydipsia in older children. Laboratory evaluation will a reveal normal anion gap and metabolic acidosis. Urinary acidification will be impaired with a urine pH less than 5.5. Fractional excretion of urinary bicarbonate will be high, providing evidence of urinary bicarbonate loss. In patients with the Fanconi's syndrome, hypophosphatemia and hypokalemia may be seen. Urine studies will confirm the presence of generalized aminoaciduria along with glycosuria despite normal serum glucose.

Nephropathic Cystinosis

Nephropathic cystinosis, caused by a defective lysosomal membrane transport protein, is the most common identifiable cause of renal Fanconi's syndrome in children. Mutations in the *CTNS* gene located on 17p13.2 result in defective cystinosin. Presentation is usually that of symptoms of failure to thrive and recurrent dehydration. Laboratory evaluation is consistent with Fanconi's syndrome with progressive renal dysfunction. The diagnosis is confirmed by detection of elevated white blood cell (WBC) cystine levels, genetic analysis, and/or the presence of cystine crystals seen on slit-lamp examination (Emma et al., 2014).

Before renal transplantation was available, it was thought that neurologic abnormalities occurred only as consequences of renal dysfunction. With the prolonged survival, it has become clear that the infantile and juvenile forms may be associated with visual, intellectual, and motor abnormalities that result from cystine accumulation in the eye (cornea, conjunctiva, retina) or brain (choroid plexus, cortex). Other neurologic consequences develop at various ages from childhood to adulthood. They may include headache; autonomic abnormalities (heat intolerance, hyperthermia, abnormal sweating); poor vision and deficient visual memory; short, raspy, repetitive speech; tremor; pyramidal or extrapyramidal motor defects; and weakness. Selective impairment of visual processing is a frequent finding. Abnormal tactile recognition with astereognosis has been discerned in some patients. These subtle deficits are the likely basis of some of the school difficulties experienced by children with nephropathic cystinosis. Intellectual deficits are mild and may be static or slowly progressive.

Some patients experience severe and strikingly progressive neurologic complications. Cystinosis-related encephalopathy is an entity characterized by cerebellar and pyramidal signs, with ensuing mental deterioration, and then development of pseudobulbar or bulbar palsy with a prominent swallowing disorder. Evidence suggests that cysteamine may reverse cystinosis-related encephalopathy, improve the radiologic appearance of the brain, and prevent paroxysmal episodes.

One quarter of patients with long-standing nephropathic cystinosis develop distal lipid inclusion myopathy. This result may be the direct effect of cystine toxicity, although carnitine deficiency and other potential causes may contribute. Patients with cystinosis-related myopathy develop weakness and wasting of small hand muscles, facial weakness, and muscular dysphagia. Biopsies may indicate a vacuolar myopathy of lysosomal origin.

Additional heritable diseases that may result in a combination of neurologic and renal manifestations are listed in Table 158-6.

NEUROLOGIC DRUGS THAT MAY AFFECT RENAL FUNCTION IN INDIVIDUALS WITH NORMAL KIDNEYS

Some drugs commonly used in the management of neurologic diseases may produce disturbances of renal function that range from mild transient effects on the regulation of free-water clearance to severe parenchymal kidney injury. Important effects of selected neurologic drugs on renal function are summarized in Table 158-7.

It is well known that carbamazepine and oxcarbazepine can produce hyponatremia. Prevalence with carbamazepine treatment is approximately 5%. Mild hyponatremia is seen in 18% to 25% of oxcarbazepine-treated children, with more severe hyponatremia (i.e., <125 mM/L) seen in no more than 3%. Symptomatic hyponatremia is found in 2% or less.

The mechanism of hyponatremia with either of these drugs is unknown. Although SIADH was formerly thought to explain the effect, it has recently been shown that this is not the case (at least for carbamazepine). Clinical manifestations of hyponatremia are rare in children treated with either carbamazepine or oxcarbazepine.

Lamotrigine use in children with centrally mediated diabetes insipidus has been found to induce hyponatremia as a result of change in desmopressin requirements. Acetazolamide

TABLE 158-6 Syndromes With Kidney Malformation and Neurologic Disease

Syndrome (Inheritance)	Kidney	Neurologic	Syndrome (Inheritance)	Kidney	Neurologic
Bardet–Biedl (AR)	Congenital renal cysts Renal dysplasia	Mental retardation Visual abnormalities	Pallister–Hall (Sp)	Renal dysplasia	Tumors CNS migrational abnormalities
Beckwith/Wiedemann (Sp)	Renal dysplasia RT	Mental retardation	Partial trisomy 10S	Renal dysplasia	Mental retardation CNS migrational abnormalities
Cat's eye	Renal agenesis	Mental retardation Visual abnormalities	Rubinstein–Taybi	Renal dysplasia	Mental retardation
Cockayne's (AR)	Renal dysplasia Hypertension	Mental retardation Deafness Ataxia Peripheral neuropathy	Schinzel–Giedion	Hydronephrosis	Mental retardation Deafness Encephalopathy
Fanconi's pancytopenia (AR)	Renal hypoplasia Renal dysplasia	Mental retardation Cranial neuropathy Deafness	Short-rib polydactyly II	Renal dysplasia Renal cysts	Cervical dysplasia CNS migrational abnormalities
Fraser's (AR)	Renal agenesis	Mental retardation	Townes'	Renal hypoplasia Hydronephrosis	Deafness
Johanson–Blizzard	Renal dysplasia Hydronephrosis	Mental retardation Deafness	Trisomy 18	Hydronephrosis Renal cysts	Mental retardation CNS migrational abnormalities Neural tubule defects Hydrocephalus
Joubert's	Renal cysts	Cerebellar dysplasia			
Klippel–Feil (Sp)	Renal dysplasia	Cranial neuropathy Neural tubule defects Cervical dysplasia	Tuberous sclerosis (AD)	Renal cysts Angiomyolipomas	Tumors Mental retardation Encephalopathy
Meckel–Gruber (AR)	Renal dysplasia Renal cysts	Neural tubule defects CNS migrational abnormalities	Turner's	Renal dysplasia Horseshoe kidney Hypertension	Mental retardation Deafness
Melnick–Fraser (AD)	Renal hypoplasia Renal dysplasia	Deafness	Zellweger's (AR)	Renal cysts	Mental retardation CNS migrational abnormalities
MURCS	Renal agenesis	Cervical dysplasia Deafness			
Orofaciodigital I	Renal cysts	Mental retardation CNS migrational abnormalities Hydrocephalus Encephalopathy			

AD, autosomal dominant; AR, autosomal recessive; CNS, central nervous system; MURCS, Müllerian duct renal and cervical vertebral defects; Sp, sporadic.

may provoke a selective form of proximal renal tubular acidosis manifested by bicarbonate wasting without generalized proximal tubular dysfunction. Phenytoin, conversely, may inhibit the secretion of antidiuretic hormone, resulting in diabetes insipidus. Phenytoin-induced lupus may, in turn, produce lupus-related nephropathy.

Tricyclic drugs may interfere with the action of some antihypertensive medications and may provoke urine retention. Nifedipine may worsen the edema of renal failure.

Other drugs commonly employed for management of neurologic diseases can cause acute interstitial nephritis, including phenytoin, phenobarbital, carbamazepine, cimetidine, amphetamine, and interferon-alpha.

Valproic acid has direct effects on renal tubular ammonia metabolism. The increased renal ammoniagenesis may combine with valproate-related inhibition of hepatic ureagenesis to produce the hyperammonemia that is observed in some children with therapeutic serum valproate concentrations. Chronic valproate administration may result in proximal renal tubular dysfunction.

Acyclovir may result in acute renal failure. Coadministration of cephalosporins, which compete for tubular excretion, may increase the nephrotoxic risk of acyclovir administration.

DRUG THERAPY IN RENAL DISEASE

Renal dysfunction may have significant effects on drug disposition, including many drugs administered to treat neurologic complications of renal disease. Renal dysfunction may affect drug binding, hepatic biotransformation, or renal clearance. Drug binding (especially of acidic drugs) may be affected by poor nutrition, protein loss, or competition with the weak organic acids that accumulate in uremia. Biotransformation may be affected by changes in the free fraction of a drug or, as is the case with phenytoin, by unknown mechanisms. Renal clearance is of little importance for some drugs but of great importance for others (e.g., barbiturates, levetiracetam, gabapentin). Drug penetration into the CNS or systemic clearance may be altered in renal failure.

Drug-Induced Encephalopathy in Renal Failure

Encephalopathy is the most common consequence of pharmacologic changes with renal failure, with manifestations ranging from subtle intellectual impairment to hallucinations, agitation, confusion, delirium, or coma. Drugs most commonly implicated are antibiotics, antihistamines, antihypertensives, and neuropsychiatric medications.

TABLE 158-7 Drugs/Toxins Affecting Nervous System and Kidney

Drug	Neurologic	Renal
Analgesics	Encephalopathy Headache	Proximal renal tubular acidosis Renal Fanconi's syndrome Distal renal tubular acidosis
Arsenic	Encephalopathy Headache Peripheral neuropathy and/or myopathy	Proximal renal tubular acidosis Chronic renal failure
Burn toxin	Encephalopathy	Proximal renal tubular acidosis
Cadmium	Encephalopathy Seizures Peripheral neuropathy and/or myopathy	Proximal renal tubular acidosis Renal Fanconi's syndrome
Chromium	Encephalopathy	Acute renal failure Chronic renal failure
"Ecstasy"	Encephalopathy Seizures	Acute renal failure
Ethylene glycol	Encephalopathy	Acute renal failure Chronic renal failure
Gallium	Blindness Peripheral neuropathy and/or myopathy	Acute renal failure Chronic renal failure
Indium	Encephalopathy Seizures Peripheral neuropathy and/or myopathy	Acute renal failure Chronic renal failure
Lead	Encephalopathy Peripheral neuropathy and/or myopathy	Proximal renal tubular acidosis Renal Fanconi's syndrome
Lithium	Encephalopathy Delirium	Distal renal tubular acidosis
Mercury	Encephalopathy Myopathy	Proximal renal tubular acidosis Renal Fanconi's syndrome
Mycotoxin	Encephalopathy	Proximal renal tubular acidosis
Pentazocine	Encephalopathy Delirium Headache	Distal renal tubular acidosis
Tellurium	Encephalopathy	Acute renal failure Chronic renal failure
Tetracycline	Pseudotumor	Proximal renal tubular acidosis Renal Fanconi's syndrome
Thallium	Encephalopathy Seizures Guillain–Barré syndrome	Proximal renal tubular acidosis Renal Fanconi's syndrome Distal renal tubular acidosis
Toluene	Encephalopathy Long-tract signs Seizures Delirium Pseudotumor	Proximal renal tubular acidosis Distal renal tubular acidosis
Xylitol	Encephalopathy Seizures	Acute renal failure Chronic renal failure

Although a careful drug history is often of greater importance in ascertaining the deleterious drug than the symptom pattern or serum levels, some clinical findings are relevant. Agitation, emotional lability, and anticholinergic signs suggest antihistamines or neuroleptics. Anticholinergic effects may include life-threatening cardiorespiratory impairment. Myoclonus may result from penicillins, chelated aluminum, cyclosporine, nitroprusside, tricyclic antidepressants, phenothiazine, or meperidine. Established "toxic levels" of medications may not always represent reliable guides in renal failure because unmeasured toxic metabolites may accumulate. Therefore trial withdrawal of expendable or especially toxic medications may be necessary. Recovery from medication effects may require weeks to months.

Treatment of Seizures Associated With Renal Disease

Seizures are common problems in children with renal disease. Management generally involves treatment of precipitating causes and correction of metabolic disturbances. However, some individuals with renal disease experience prolonged seizures or develop epilepsy and require acute or chronic treatment with antiseizure medications.

Longer-term or even chronic treatment with an antiseizure medication must be undertaken when the risk for seizure recurrence is high. Usage is guided by medication level, known pharmacokinetics and pharmacodynamics of the antiseizure medication, the extent to which these are likely to be altered at a given level of reduction of renal creatinine clearance or by dialysis, and the degree of hepatic dysfunction.

Concerns About Specific Antiseizure Medication Use in the Setting of Renal Failure

Phenytoin. Renal failure mandates adjustment of dosages and/or dosing intervals of many antiseizure medications. The effects of chronic renal failure on drug disposition are greatest for phenytoin. Protein binding may decrease by as much as threefold in uremia or nephrotic syndrome as a result of hypoalbuminemia and the presence of competitive or noncompetitive inhibitors of binding (uremic or dialysis related). Conversely, the steady-state plasma concentration for a given dose of phenytoin also decreases by twofold to threefold as a result of an increase in the apparent volume of distribution and shortened half-time of elimination. It is particularly important to monitor phenytoin levels carefully in patients with renal failure because of the nonlinear kinetics of this drug and narrow therapeutic window. Levels should be followed with free-phenytoin concentrations because total phenytoin levels are unreliable. Dosing intervals should be 8 hours or less because administration of larger, less frequent doses may produce toxic symptoms. Hemodialysis has little effect on total serum phenytoin concentration but may decrease free-phenytoin levels to variable degrees. Heparinization for dialysis may displace bound phenytoin, resulting in transient toxicity.

Chronic phenytoin therapy may aggravate renal osteomalacia, especially in the setting of renal disease. Risk for osteomalacia is higher for individuals with reduced mobility.

Valproate. Although few good studies are available, valproic acid is subject to pharmacokinetic changes similar to phenytoin when administered to patients with renal failure. Valproic acid appears to be moderately dialyzable, and hence hemodialysis may be indicated with severe valproic acid poisoning. Development of valproate-associated pancreatitis with hepatic dysfunction has been suggested as a condition for which there is greater risk in children with ESRD.

Barbiturates. Phenobarbital elimination depends in part on the GFR and urine pH, but there are few data on its disposition in renal failure. Over the short term, renal failure usually has little effect on serum phenobarbital levels. Long-term phenobarbital therapy in severe renal disease may require dosage reduction. Postdialysis doses are usually necessary because phenobarbital is readily dialyzed, especially by hemodialysis. Pentobarbital, on the other hand, is poorly dialyzable.

Carbamazepine. Carbamazepine bioavailability and clearance are unlikely to be greatly affected by renal disease because it is predominantly metabolized in the liver, and less than 5% is excreted unchanged in the urine. Studies have demonstrated removal with dialysis to a moderate degree, and hence hemodialysis is recommended for severe carbamazepine poisoning.

Oxcarbazepine. The glucuronide metabolites of oxcarbazepine may accumulate in patients with severe renal dysfunction, but the concentration of the monohydroxy derivative (MDH) that provides most of the antiseizure effect accumulates because only about 25% of this metabolite is renally excreted. Creatinine clearance is a useful index for estimating dosage adjustment in the setting of renal failure. There is limited information on the efficacy of hemodialysis for oxcarbazepine.

Ethosuximide. Ethosuximide has not been well studied, perhaps because it is seldom (although sometimes) used in patients with renal disease. It is likely to be readily dialyzable.

Levetiracetam. Less than 10% of circulating levetiracetam is protein bound, and as much as 90% is excreted in the urine—more than two-thirds unchanged and the remainder as inactive metabolites. It is not metabolized in the liver; hence, in patients with renal failure, dosage must be modified in accordance with the degree of decline in creatinine clearance.

Zonisamide. Approximately two thirds of zonisamide elimination is accomplished by the kidneys, either unchanged or as a glucuronide conjugate. Renal clearance also diminishes with diminished creatinine clearance. With severe renal failure (creatinine clearance < 20 ml/minute), zonisamide accumulation may result in serum concentrations approximately one-third greater than otherwise anticipated. It must be borne in mind that the very long elimination time of this drug means that steady-state elevation will not be achieved for a considerable interval after introduction or dose modification.

Lamotrigine. Lamotrigine inactivation is the result of hepatic conjugation with ensuing elimination of the predominantly 2-*N*-glucuronate adduct. At least 94% of elimination of this metabolite is renal; hence, accumulation occurs with renal failure. The mean plasma half-life of the drug is more than 40 hours in renal failure, compared with 26 hours in patients who do not have renal or hepatic failure. It has been suggested that lamotrigine (Lamictal) may elevate risk for renal stones by twofold to fourfold, compared with the expected risk of the underlying disease.

Gabapentin. Gabapentin is not appreciably metabolized, so elimination is achieved almost entirely as unchanged drug in the urine. The usual elimination half-life of 5 to 7 hours is increased to a mean of 132 hours for creatinine clearance less than 30 ml/minute without dialysis, or to approximately 50 hours in end-stage chronic renal failure with thrice-weekly dialysis. Published dosage tables for renal failure in adults receiving hemodialysis are available.

Benzodiazepines. Benzodiazepines (especially clonazepam) are useful in controlling uremic myoclonus and may not require dosage alteration for acute administration in renal failure, although protein binding may be reduced. Diazepam and lorazepam require reduction more often than clonazepam. Diazepam is not readily dialyzable. Little information is available concerning the dialysis of other benzodiazepines.

Kidney Stones

The risk for urolithiasis is elevated with the utilization of carbonic anhydrase inhibitors, including acetazolamide, zonisamide, and topiramate. Risk may be particularly high with a positive family history of urolithiasis and elevation of the calcium : creatinine ratio, or if these medications are used in combination. The ketogenic diet is associated with risk for stones, and the diet is thought to double the risk for kidney stones associated with any particular carbonic anhydrase inhibitor.

Other Neurologic Drugs

A number of other medications commonly used in the therapy of neurologic disease should be administered with caution in patients with renal failure. Both aspirin and acetaminophen require longer interdose intervals in renal failure. Aspirin should not be administered when the GFR is less than 10 ml/minute. Both of these analgesic drugs are readily cleared by dialysis.

Acetazolamide is entirely eliminated by renal mechanisms. The dosage should be reduced for renal failure and avoided in ESRD and in patients with acidosis, hypokalemia, or urolithiasis (all of which may be worsened by its administration). Tricyclic drugs are not dialyzed well but usually do not require dosage changes in renal failure. Alpha and calcium-channel blockers are not readily cleared by dialysis. Dosage may require adjustment in severe renal failure. Haloperidol is not well dialyzed and may provoke hypotension in patients with renal failure. Lithium is a dialyzable drug that requires a longer interdose interval in renal failure. It should be avoided in patients with renal disease because of potential aggravation of renal tubular acidosis or provocation of nephrogenic diabetes insipidus or chronic interstitial fibrosis. Considerably greater detail concerning the management of drugs pertinent to neurologic and other forms of medical practice in children with renal failure is available in several previous reviews.

REFERENCES

The complete list of references for this chapter is available online at www.expertconsult.com.
    See inside cover for registration details.

SELECTED REFERENCES

Bilginer, Y., Akpolat, T., Ozen, S., 2011. Renal amyloidosis in children. Pediatr. Nephrol. 26 (8), 1215–1227.

Blombery, P., Scully, M., 2014. Management of thrombotic thrombocytopenic purpura: current perspectives. J. Blood Med. 5, 15–23.

Eason, J.D., Gonwa, T.A., Davis, C.L., et al., 2008. Proceedings of Consensus Conference on Simultaneous Liver Kidney Transplantation (SLK). Am. J. Transplant. 8 (11), 2243–2251.

Emma, F., Nesterova, G., Langman, C., et al., 2014. Nephropathic cystinosis: an international consensus document. Nephrol. Dial. Transplant. 29 (Suppl. 4), iv87–iv94.

Haque, S., Ariceta, G., Batlle, D., 2012. Proximal renal tubular acidosis: a not so rare disorder of multiple etiologies. Nephrol. Dial. Transplant. 27 (12), 4273–4287.

James, N., George, M.D., Carla, M., et al., 2014. Syndromes of Thrombotic Microangiopathy. N. Engl. J. Med. 371, 654–666.

Loirat, C., Fakhouri, F., Ariceta, G., et al., 2016. An international consensus approach to the management of atypical hemolytic uremic syndrome in children. Pediatr. Nephrol. 31 (1), 15–39.

Sampaio, M., Martin, P., Bunnapradist, S. Renal Dysfunction in End-Stage Liver Disease and Post–Liver Transplant Clinics in Liver Disease, 2014-08-01, Volume 18, Issue 3, Pages 543–560.

Seifter, J.L., Samuels, M.A., 2011. Uremic encephalopathy and other brain disorders associated with renal failure. Semin. Neurol. 31 (2), 139–143.

Trachtman, H., 2013. HUS and TTP in children. Pediatr. Clin. North Am. 60, 1513–1526.

E-BOOK FIGURES AND TABLES

The following figures and tables are available in the e-book at www.expertconsult.com. See inside cover for registration details.

159 Neurologic Disorders Associated with Gastrointestinal Diseases

Yitzchak Frank and Stephen Ashwal

 An expanded version of this chapter is available on www.expertconsult.com. See inside cover for registration details.

INTRODUCTION

The gastrointestinal (GI) tract and nervous system are interrelated. GI and liver abnormalities are associated with central nervous system (CNS) disease, and CNS abnormalities can cause GI dysfunction. The CNS depends on the GI system for the intake, absorption, and metabolism of important nutrients, including those required for normal brain function and for the removal of toxic metabolic wastes. GI impairment may interfere with these functions. Some neurologic complications of GI diseases are nutritional, such as those related to malabsorption of vitamin B_1, nicotinamide, vitamin B_{12}, vitamin D, and vitamin E. Other complications are related to the toxic effects of waste products (e.g., ammonia). Conditions affecting the GI tract may affect the CNS and the peripheral nervous system. For instance, cerebrovascular diseases can complicate hepatitis C infection and inflammatory bowel disease; encephalopathy can be caused by hepatic disease; antitumor necrosis factor alpha drugs may induce demyelination; and antigliadin antibodies, a marker of celiac disease, can be found in subjects with neurologic dysfunction of unknown cause, particularly in sporadic cerebellar ataxia, in addition to cerebral, brainstem, and peripheral nerve abnormalities. Characteristic movement disorders are key features of acquired hepatocerebral degeneration and of Whipple's disease. Multiple types of neuropathy can be found in association with hepatitis, inflammatory bowel disease, and gluten-related disorders. The severity of neurologic disease can vary—from minor cognitive changes in chronic portosystemic encephalopathy and hepatitis C to coma in acute liver failure and acute pancreatitis (Ferro and Oliveira, 2014; Datar and Wijdicks, 2014).

Conversely, central, peripheral, or enteric nervous system abnormalities may affect the GI tract. For instance, disorders of motility, such as achalasia and Hirschsprung disease, are the result of defects of innervation of the esophagus and distal large bowel or the result of primary muscle disorders or autonomic neuropathies, respectively. Dysphagia can be a symptom in many neurologic disorders, including strokes. Neurodevelopmental abnormalities are well known to be associated with gastroesophageal reflux. In addition, several drugs used to treat hepatic and GI diseases can have neurologic side effects. Likewise, drugs used in the treatment of neurologic disorders can cause hepatic dysfunction; thus, they may not be safely used or their dosage should be reduced in patients with hepatic failure.

This chapter reviews neurologic complications of the most common GI and liver diseases, including the enteric nervous system (see also Chapter 154 on the autonomic nervous system, Chapter 46 on vitamin deficiencies, and Chapter 47 on nutritional disorders).

DISORDERS ASSOCIATED WITH GASTROINTESTINAL DISEASE
The Enteric Nervous System

The enteric nervous system (ENS) is the intrinsic innervation of the GI tract. It is an elaborate network of neurons, glial cells, and connections arranged in intramuscular plexuses, and it modulates the motility, microcirculation, sphincter tone and activity, hormone secretion, and immune and inflammatory responses of the GI tract (Obermayr, Hotta, Enomoto, and Young, 2013). Please see the online chapter for discussion of the development and modulators of the ENS. Developmental disorders involving the ENS in children including dysphagia, feeding intolerance, gastroesophageal reflux, abdominal pain, and constipation.

Dysphagia. Certain groups of infants with specific developmental or medical conditions are at higher risk for developing dysphagia, including those with neurologic conditions or structural deficits (e.g., cleft lip or palate). Left untreated, these problems can lead to failure to thrive, recurrent aspiration pneumonias, gastroesophageal reflux, or the inability to establish and maintain proper nutrition and hydration.

Inhibition of gastric emptying and stimulation of colonic transit are the most frequent dysmotility responses of the GI tract to acute short-term stress. Endogenous corticotropin-releasing factor (CRF) plays a significant role in CNS mediation of stress-induced inhibition of upper GI motor function and stimulation of lower GI motor function.

Sucking, swallowing, and feeding disorders are common. Several investigations help determine the mechanism(s) causing symptoms (e.g., fiber endoscopy, videofluoroscopy, facial and swallowing electromyography, esophageal manometry). The main causes of sucking, swallowing, and feeding disorders are lesions of the brainstem (malformations of the posterior fossa, neonatal brainstem tumors, agenesis of cranial nerves, destructive lesions of the posterior brain, craniovertebral anomalies, and syndromes that involve rhombencephalic development, such as Pierre Robin sequence, CHARGE syndrome, etc.). Suprabulbar lesions, neuromuscular disorders, and anomalies or dysfunction of the esophageal, digestive, and laryngeal systems also can cause these symptoms. Management of these disorders involves treating the underlying cause, facilitating the sucking reflex, preventing the deleterious consequences of aspiration and malnutrition, and preventing posttraumatic anorexia.

Episodic Gastrointestinal Disease

Recurrent Abdominal Pain and Irritable Bowel Syndrome

Episodic GI diseases resulting from ENS dysfunction include irritable bowel syndrome, functional dyspepsia, chronic abdominal pain, and motility disorders such as gastroparesis, constipation, gastroesophageal reflux disease, and cyclic vomiting syndrome.

Patients with inflammatory bowel disease (IBD) and irritable bowel syndrome (IBS) develop long-term neuroplastic changes in the brain–gut axis that result in chronic abdominal pain. These changes are driven by peripheral mechanisms within the intestinal wall, neuronal synaptic changes, and/or increased neurotransmitter release in the spinal cord and brain. Therapeutic interventions are mainly carried out using pharmacologic agents, although interventions involving electrical stimulation have been suggested. Psychological stress factors also may play a role.

Cyclic Vomiting Syndrome and Recurrent Abdominal Pain

Cyclic vomiting syndrome (CVS; Online Mendelian Inheritance in Man [OMIM] No. 500007) is manifested by repeated episodes of vomiting lasting for hours or days, which can cause dehydration, hypochloremic alkalosis, and ketosis in an otherwise healthy-appearing child (Moses et al., 2014). Abdominal pain and fever may be present, and the patient may become pale, drowsy, and lethargic. In one study, annual incidence of CVS was 3.15 per 100,000 children per year, the median age at onset was 4 years, the median age of diagnosis was 7.42 years, and the median duration of an episode was 24 hours, with a range of up to 5 days. CVS and migraine share coexistent dysautonomias, including orthostatic intolerance and syncope.

Treatment of cyclic vomiting is by fluid and electrolyte replacement and treatment of esophagitis, which may be caused by the continued vomiting. Antimigraine, antiemetic, and antiepileptic agents have been used. Lorazepam has antiemetic and anxiolytic properties. Phenothiazines, butyrophenones, metoclopramide (Reglan), cyproheptadine, and trimethobenzamide (Tigan) may be effective as antiemetic agents but may cause extrapyramidal side effects. Ondansetron also may be considered. Beneficial effects of prophylactic therapy with propranolol and of oral or nasal sumatriptan have been described. Antiepileptic drugs (phenobarbital, valproic acid) have been suggested as ameliorating symptoms. Prophylactic therapy with valproate or amitriptyline has been described.

Irritable Bowel Syndrome

IBS is characterized by abdominal discomfort, pain, and changes in bowel habits. It is the most common cause of recurrent abdominal pain in children, affecting 10% to 15% of older children and adolescents. It is defined by the 2006 Rome III criteria for functional GI disorders, which characterize symptoms as abdominal pain associated with a change in stool form and/or frequency, that is improved by defecation, and that is not explained by structural or biochemical abnormalities. The pathophysiology of IBS is not fully understood and is discussed in the online chapter.

The diagnosis of IBS is made based on the Rome III criteria together with the exclusion of other organic causes of recurrent abdominal pain, such as IBD and celiac disease. Diagnostic testing includes routine blood studies, stool testing, celiac disease serology, abdominal ultrasonography, and breath testing to rule out carbohydrate (lactose, fructose, etc.) intolerance and small intestinal bacterial overgrowth. Colonoscopy is recommended if alarming symptoms are present or to obtain biopsies.

Management is based on a multifactorial approach and includes lifestyle modifications, stress management, behavioral and psychological treatment, dietary alterations, education, reassurance, and development of an effective patient–physician relationship (Chapter 160). Hypnotherapy and probiotics can be helpful. Antispasmodic and antidiarrheal agents may have a role in severe cases.

Infantile Colic

Infantile colic is defined as a condition in which an otherwise healthy baby cries or displays symptoms of distress frequently and for extended periods. In these instances, there is no clear cause for the discomfort. Colic usually starts within the first month of life, and, in most babies, stops before the infant is 3 to 4 months of age. In some babies it can last up to 12 months. Infantile colic is thought to be a pain syndrome. Migraine is a common cause of headache pain in childhood. An association between these two pain syndromes has been suggested.

Anatomic Gastrointestinal Disorders

Gastroesophageal Reflux

Gastroesophageal reflux (GER) is present when reflux of gastric contents causes troublesome symptoms or complications. GER occurs in about one third of all children with severe psychomotor retardation and other neurologic conditions, including myopathies and cerebral palsy, and as a sequelae of birth asphyxia. Factors related to the frequent occurrence of GER with neurologic conditions include esophageal muscle weakness, hypotonia, incoordination of the swallowing mechanism, scoliosis, and immobility.

Symptoms include pain, discomfort, irritability, and vomiting. Anemia and recurrent aspiration pneumonia also may occur. Respiratory symptoms resulting from reflux, aspiration, and laryngospasm that cause apnea, cyanosis, and stiffening (Sandifer syndrome) may be confused with seizures. In children with severe neurologic impairment, self-injurious behaviors or considerable agitation may be a marker for GER.

Esophageal pH monitoring demonstrates intermittent periods of reduced pH. Esophageal manometry may show decreased sphincter pressure and reduced peristalsis. A barium swallow may determine the presence of anatomic or functional abnormalities that mimic reflux.

Medications that enhance GI motility (e.g., metoclopramide, cisapride, ranitidine, sucralfate) usually are beneficial. Those who do not respond may benefit from gastrostomy and Nissen fundoplication, which can be done laparoscopically. Postoperative complications or recurrent gastroesophageal disease occur more frequently in neurologically impaired children.

Intestinal Pseudoobstruction

Intestinal pseudoobstruction is manifested by intestinal obstruction in the absence of mechanical blockage. Disorders causing chronic intestinal pseudoobstruction (CIPO) are listed in Box 159-1. Acute pseudoobstruction (paralytic ileus) usually occurs postoperatively or secondary to the use of medications, including anticholinergic agents, phenothiazines, tricyclic antidepressants, narcotics, and certain anticonvulsants, particularly benzodiazepines and barbiturates. Infant botulism can present as colonic ileus (Chapter 145).

BOX 159-1 Causes of Intestinal Pseudoobstruction in Children

I. ACUTE

A. Postoperative

B. Electrolyte disturbances

C. Medication effects

D. Acute infections or toxins

II. CHRONIC

A. Disorders of the Myenteric Plexus

1. Primary disorders of the myenteric plexus
   a. Developmental abnormalities—neuronal immaturity and developmental abnormalities
   b. Aganglionosis—Hirschsprung disease, segmental aganglionosis
2. Familial visceral neuropathies—multiple subtypes
3. Systemic disorders affecting the myenteric plexus
   a. Infectious—Chagas's disease, cytomegalovirus infection, infectious mononucleosis, zoster
   b. Neurologic disorders—familial dysautonomia
   c. Endocrine disorders—diabetes mellitus
   d. Gastrointestinal disorders—malabsorption syndromes

B. Disorders of Intestinal Smooth Muscle

1. Primary disorders of smooth muscle
   a. Familial visceral myopathy—various inherited forms
   b. Sporadic childhood visceral myopathies
2. Systemic disorders affecting visceral smooth muscle
   a. Muscular and myotonic dystrophies
   b. Hypothyroidism
   c. Connective tissue disorders—systemic lupus erythematosus, polymyositis/dermatomyositis

C. Small Intestinal Diverticulosis

1. With myopathic changes
2. With neuropathic changes

(Modified from Scott RB: Motility disorders. In Walker WA, et al, editors: Pediatric gastrointestinal disease, St. Louis, 1996, Mosby.)

When no recognizable etiology is found, CIPO is referred to as idiopathic (CIIPO). Clinical manifestations include recurrent episodes of bowel obstruction without a mechanical obstructive cause. Symptoms include poor feeding, vomiting, abdominal distention, megacolon, and constipation. Evaluation for pseudoobstruction requires exclusion of structural, mechanical, and pharmacologic etiologies, followed by additional studies to evaluate motor activity and motility, including breath hydrogen determination, scintigraphy, and manometric studies.

A mitochondrial neurointestinal encephalopathy may cause chronic pseudoobstruction in addition to cranial nerve abnormalities, ataxia, ophthalmoplegia, facial and limb muscle weakness, and pigmentary retinopathy. Brain MRI demonstrates diffuse leukoencephalopathy. Muscle biopsy may reveal neuropathic and myopathic changes, scattered ragged red fibers, and focal cytochrome oxidase deficiency.

Therapy and prognosis vary depending on the lesions identified by pathology; treatment includes diet modifications, parenteral nutrition, and use of cisapride.

Hirschsprung Disease

Hirschsprung disease (HSCR; OMIM 142623), or aganglionic megacolon, is a congenital disorder that is characterized by the absence of intestinal ganglion cells in the submucosal and myenteric plexuses, which causes proximal bowel distention. It is the consequence of defective migration of neural crest cells to the colonic submucosa and is one of a spectrum of neurocristopathies, a group of diverse disorders resulting from defective growth, differentiation, and migration of neural crest cells, with a wide spectrum of neurologic abnormalities. HSCR, its variants, and the key genes that regulate neural crest cell development are described in the online chapter.

Other Neurocristopathy Syndromes

Several neurocristopathy syndromes are described in the online chapter, including Down syndrome in association with HSCR, Shah-Waardenburg syndrome or Waardenburg syndrome type IVB (OMIM 613265), Mowat-Wilson syndrome (OMIM 235730), and neuroblastoma (OMIM 613013).

Other Pseudoobstruction Syndromes

Children with muscular or myotonic dystrophies may have intestinal pseudoobstruction. X-linked recessive neuropathic forms of intestinal pseudoobstruction also have been described.

Mitochondrial Neurogastrointestinal Encephalopathy (MNGIE)

Mitochondrial neurogastrointestinal encephalomyopathy (MNGIE) is a rare autosomal-recessive mitochondrial DNA depletion syndrome with heterogeneous multisystem involvement and usually presents between the first and fifth decades of life (OMIM 603041). It is characterized by peripheral neuropathy, ophthalmoplegia, ptosis, deafness, leukoencephalopathy, and GI symptoms resulting from visceral neuropathy. Clinical manifestations include progressive GI dysmotility and cachexia, accompanied by ptosis/ophthalmoplegia, hearing loss, and a demyelinating neuropathy. Although symptoms can start between the first and fifth decades, they usually begin before age 20 years (60% of individuals). Confirmatory laboratory studies include an elevated plasma lactate level and elevated plasma thymidine and deoxyuridine concentrations and reduced leukocyte thymidine phosphorylase enzyme activity. Electron microscopy of rectal biopsy tissue may suggest a mitochondrial disorder.

MNGIE is caused by mutations in the *TYMP* gene encoding thymidine phosphorylase. The diagnosis of MNGIE is made by demonstrating reduced or absent thymidine phosphorylase activity and elevated serum thymidine and deoxyuridine, along with genetic identification of the *ECGF1* gene mutation on nuclear DNA (and also mitochondrial DNA deletions).

Clinical presentation may vary, and patients can be misdiagnosed with myasthenia gravis, chronic inflammatory demyelinating polyneuropathy (CIDP), and intestinal inflammatory disease. Electromyographic testing may demonstrate demyelinating sensory and motor polyneuropathy. The most common finding on MRI is that of a diffuse leukoencephalopathy. The extent and distribution of leukoencephalopathy may not correlate with disease severity or be related to the TYMP mutations, enzyme activity, or pyrimidine levels. Magnetic resonance imaging (MRI) apparent diffusion coefficient (ADC) maps have shown moderately increased diffusivity. The leukoencephalopathy can worsen over time, regardless of the clinical course.

Acute medical events such as infections often provoke worsening of symptoms, suggesting that careful monitoring and early treatment of intercurrent illnesses may be beneficial. Anecdotal reports suggest that allogeneic hematopoietic stem cell transplantation may be beneficial.

Intussusception

Intestinal intussusception, with invagination of the gut into its distal segment, is the most common cause of bowel obstruction in children. Presenting signs and symptoms typically are abdominal, but encephalopathy with irritability, lethargy, obtundation, or coma has been described.

Malabsorption Syndromes

GI disorders associated with malabsorption can cause selected nutritional, biochemical, and vitamin deficiencies, including vitamin E and vitamin B_{12} deficiency. Neurologic involvement is present in some children. Neurologic abnormalities associated with nutritional deficiencies and specific vitamin deficiencies are reviewed in Chapters 46 and 47.

Celiac Disease

Celiac disease is an immune-mediated malabsorption syndrome characterized by permanent gluten intolerance in genetically susceptible individuals, with symptoms of chronic diarrhea, failure to thrive, weight loss, and abdominal distention (OMIM 212750). Jejunal biopsy demonstrates villous atrophy, absence of surface mucosa, and crypt hyperplasia.

Extraintestinal manifestations are becoming increasingly more common. They include numerous conditions, such as dermatitis herpetiformis, anemia, dental enamel hypoplasia, recurrent oral aphthae, short stature, osteoporosis, arthritis, neurologic problems, unexplained elevation of transaminase levels, and female infertility.

Neurologic symptoms infrequently are the presenting manifestation of celiac disease (Diaconu, Burlea, Grigore, Anton, and Trandafir, 2013). In some patients, gluten sensitivity can be present with neurologic abnormalities without meeting the strictly defined criteria for celiac disease. The most common neurologic problems are ataxia and seizures. Peripheral nervous system involvement and acute disseminated encephalomyelitis are rare complications in children and may respond to diet modification. Specific syndromes of occipital calcifications and epilepsy, and cerebellar degeneration with or without epilepsy, also have been described in children. A significant percentage of patients with Down syndrome have celiac disease.

Psychiatric abnormalities include apathy, anxiety, irritability, depressive syndromes, schizophrenia, and psychosis. There are reports of immunopathological changes in the intestinal mucosa of autistic children, but a direct association between autism and celiac disease remains uncertain. Reports of behavioral improvement in autistic children on a gluten- and casein-free diet remain controversial. Untreated patients with celiac disease can have signs of ADHD.

The pathogenesis of nervous system dysfunction in gluten enteropathy remains unclear. It may be the result of malabsorption causing folic acid, vitamin B_{12}, or vitamin E deficiencies. Hypocalcemia and hypokalemia also have been implicated. Although some patients have malabsorption, the majority of patients with neurologic symptoms do not.

Abnormalities of humoral and cell-mediated immunity suggest that celiac disease is an immunologic disorder caused by an inappropriate immune response to the gliadin component in dietary gluten. There is a genetic susceptibility, and 90% of patients have the human leukocyte antigen (HLA) DRG 3 DQ-2 haplotype. Antiendomysial, antigliadin, and antireticulin antibodies also are associated with the disease. Antitissue transglutaminase antibody assay has been used as a serologic screening test for celiac disease. Neurologic abnormalities in celiac disease may result from vasculitis involving the vascular endothelium, possibly mediated by tissue transglutaminase.

Patients with celiac disease improve after dietary withdrawal of gluten. Neurologic abnormalities can be present before the appearance of celiac disease symptoms and may progress despite a gluten-free diet. In general, there is no evidence that a gluten-free diet or vitamin supplementation reverses the neurologic abnormalities, although, in an adult series, neurologic symptoms improved or disappeared in 7 of 13 individuals within 6 months of starting a gluten-free diet.

Short Bowel Syndrome

Short bowel syndrome is a malabsorption syndrome that follows resection of a significant part of the small bowel, usually because of a congenital anomaly, necrotizing enterocolitis, inflammatory bowel disease, or ischemic injury. See the online chapter.

Inflammatory Bowel Disease

IBDs, including Crohn's disease (regional enteritis) and ulcerative colitis, occur infrequently in children. Crohn's disease is a chronic, inflammatory process that affects any region of the GI tract, mostly the small bowel, in a discontinuous fashion. Patients complain of diarrhea, rectal bleeding, abdominal pain, vomiting, and weight loss. Therapy includes antiinflammatory agents, corticosteroids, and supportive nutritional therapy. Ulcerative colitis is a chronic relapsing inflammatory disease involving the mucosa of the colon and rectum in a continuous manner. Both conditions cause extraintestinal symptoms in about 25% to 35% of patients.

Neurologic manifestations are rare and are dominated by CNS vascular complications, including arterial occlusion, vasculitis, encephalopathy, mononeuropathies, and abnormalities of the white matter. The majority of patients experience the onset of neurologic symptoms within the first 5 to 6 years after the onset of IBD symptoms. Peripheral neuropathy is the most common complication of IBD and may be immune mediated or caused by antitumor necrosis factor-alpha (TNF-α) therapy or metronidazole. Myelopathy, myopathy, myasthenia gravis, and multiple sclerosis also have been reported. Other symptoms that occur with higher frequency in children with IBS include headache, dizziness, and attention deficit hyperactivity disorder (Ben-Or, Zelnik, Shaoul, Pacht, and Lerner, 2015).

Enteric Infections

Enteric viruses and bacteria that cause primary CNS infection are reviewed in Chapters 114 to 116. A variety of systemic viral and bacterial infections may cause an encephalopathy resulting from the presence of endotoxins or electrolyte and fluid disturbances. Some of the more well-recognized entities are reviewed in this section.

Seizures and encephalopathy in infants with enteric infections and diarrhea can be caused by hyponatremia or hypernatremia (Chapter 158). Hyponatremia may cause brain swelling because sodium and chloride ions cross the brain capillaries slower than water. Treatment consists of rehydration with adequate sodium salts and avoidance of more dilute fluids. Hypokalemia can accompany diarrhea and cause neuromuscular manifestations, including hypotonia, diminished bowel sounds, weakness, lethargy, abdominal distention, and, in severe cases, rhabdomyolysis and myoglobinuria. Neuromuscular manifestations become more prominent with serum potassium levels lower than 3 mEq/L. Severe hypokalemia occurs more frequently in children younger than 24 months and in infants receiving dextrose-containing intravenous fluids without electrolyte replacement, and is related to the type of rehydration therapy.

Please see the online chapter for a discussion of the following infectious agents: *Escherichia coli*, *Campylobacter jejuni*, Nipah virus, infant botulism, shigellosis, and rotavirus infection.

The Human Microbiome and Neurologic Disorders in Children

The human body contains more than 1 trillion bacteria, and it is estimated that the number of bacteria are tenfold greater than the number of human cells. There is increasing interest in the human microbiota (the body's entire microbial population) and the human microbiome (the body's collective genomes of all microorganisms) and their relation to nervous system function in health and disease (termed the *microbiota–gut–brain, or MGB, axis*) (Mayer, Padua, and Tillisch, 2014).

Development and Role of the Human Microbiota

Over the course of the first year of life, bacterial populations colonize the gut, skin, and other regions with the predominant phyla, including actinobacteria, bacteroidetes, firmicutes, and proteobacteri. Many factors affect the development of the infant's microbiota, including the state of maternal health, gestational age, mode of delivery, prematurity, exposure to being in an intensive care unit, the nature (e.g., breast milk vs. infant formulas) and amount of nutritional intake, use of antibiotics, prolonged hospitalization, and environmental factors. For a discussion of the changes in the microbiota prenatally, postnatally, and during childhood/adolescence, please see the online chapter and the review by Borre and colleagues (2014).

Disease States and the Influences of the Microbiota and Microbiome

When there are conditions of pathologic stress or disease, intestinal dysbiosis can adversely influence gut physiology, leading to inappropriate MGB axis signaling and associated CNS dysfunction (Borre et al., 2014). The ensuing inflammatory response causes loss of intestinal integrity that promotes increased release of pathogenic bacterial constituents to the systemic circulation. These processes can activate the peripheral immune system to release proinflammatory/antiinflammatory cytokines/chemokines that alter the blood–brain barrier and impair multiple aspects of CNS function, involving the ENS and the sympathetic and parasympathetic (e.g., vagal) autonomic nervous systems. Other metabolic pathways (e.g., tryptophan-kynurenine) that participate in serotonin metabolism may mediate some of the affective behaviors attributed to alterations of the MGB axis.

The Microbiota and Immune-Mediated Nervous System Disorders. A number of immune-mediated diseases that affect the nervous system interface with the human microbiota.

Multiple Sclerosis. Translational studies have demonstrated that, in mice, commensal microbiota are essential for the development of experimental autoimmune encephalitis (EAE), a model commonly used to study CNS demyelination. Antibiotic administration modulates gut microbiota and affects EAE progression. Dietary patterns (e.g., high-fat diets) may increase EAE severity, whereas caloric restriction attenuates EAE symptoms. Such data suggest the possibility that the human microbiota may contribute to the pathogenesis of multiple sclerosis and perhaps other CNS demyelinating disorders.

Guillain–Barré Syndrome. Guillain–Barré syndrome (GBS) is frequently seen in children and is reviewed in Chapter 161. Preceding infections with bacteria or viruses, such as *Haemophilus pneumoniae*, *Mycoplasma pneumoniae*, influenza, Epstein-Barr virus, and *Campylobacter jejuni*, have been associated with this disorder. GBS results, in part, from cross-reactivity between antibodies produced by the specific infectious agent to peripheral nerve tissues. *C. jejuni* has been associated with different types of GBS. The possibility exists that modifying this enteric pathogen could alter the effects of immune-mediated GBS.

The Microbiota and Nonimmune-Mediated CNS Disorders

Autistic Spectrum Disorder. Of the neurodevelopmental disabilities, autistic spectrum disorders (ASDs) (Chapter 65) have attracted the most interest in studying the MGB axis relation (Mayer et al., 2014). Children with autism have a higher rate of GI symptoms. Numerous clinical studies in children with ASD have linked changes in the gut microbiota with behavioral disturbances, including irritability, inattentiveness, self-injurious behaviors, and mood disturbances.

Alterations in the gut microbiome composition and abnormal levels of microbial cometabolites have been described in children with ASD. An imbalance of *Bacteroidetes* and *Firmicutes* phyla was seen in autistic children. Other reports provide conflicting evidence, and it remains unclear whether these are causal or associative phenomena. Certain diets (e.g., probiotics or gluten-/casein-free) that alter the microbiota appear to improve symptoms in individual patients. Recent rodent autism model studies have provided intriguing evidence that alteration in the gut microbiome and associated changes in serum metabolites play an important role in autism-like behaviors, and that these changes were reversible by ingestion of a probiotic. Therapeutic options that have been studied for treatment of autism include diet modulation, prebiotics, probiotics, synbiotics, postbiotics, antibiotics, fecal transplantation, and activated charcoal (Mayer et al., 2014).

Attention Deficit Hyperactivity Disorder. A few studies have addressed the potential relation of the MGB axis and ADHD. Genetic predisposition and environmental exposures to certain toxins and allergic triggers are linked to an increased risk of developing or of worsening ADHD symptoms. In contrast, factors such as sugar, artificial food colorings, zinc, iron, and ω-3 fatty acids do not have established causality in ADHD, although in some children elimination diets have been shown to be effective.

Cerebral Palsy. Children with cerebral palsy have a wide range of GI symptoms, including feeding and swallowing disorders, sialorrhea, constipation, gastroesophageal reflux disease, recurrent respiratory infections secondary to aspiration, failure to thrive, and the need for gastrostomy. To date, there are no published reports of the MGB axis in affected children.

Epilepsy. GI complications frequently occur in children with epilepsy related to the genetic and metabolic diseases that cause the epilepsy or as side effects of anticonvulsants. There also are possible effects of recurrent seizures, diets such as the ketogenic diet, or vagal nerve stimulation on GI motility and function. There are no published reports of the MGB axis in children with pediatric epilepsy.

Intellectual Disability. As with cerebral palsy and epilepsy in which GI disorders are common, there is no literature on the human MGB axis.

Depression, Anxiety, Stress and Schizophrenia. The same general principles of the MGB axis as described previously have been examined in a variety of psychiatric disorders, including depression, anxiety, stress, and schizophrenia, and the reader is referred to several recently published reviews for more in-depth discussion (see the online chapter).

Therapeutic Implications

Understanding the MGB axis should allow development of new complementary treatment strategies for a wide range of pediatric neurologic disorders. There are a large number of potential therapies that could alter the gut microbiota, and the extent to which such treatments could result in improved outcomes will require extensive translational studies and carefully controlled clinical trials.

Other Gastrointestinal Diseases

Whipple's Disease

Whipple's disease is a chronic, multisystem, bacterial, inflammatory disorder caused by a soil-borne, Gram-positive bacillus, *Tropheryma whipplei*. It is a rare disease that is misdiagnosed frequently, occurs primarily in adults, and is manifested by intestinal features that include weight loss, diarrhea, malabsorption, and abdominal pain, in addition to polyarthritis, lymphadenopathy, cardiomyopathy, hyperpigmentation, hypotension, and cardiovascular, pulmonary, and neurologic dysfunction. Up to one third of patients demonstrate signs of neurologic involvement, including progressive dementia, external ophthalmoplegia, myoclonus, seizures, ataxia, hypothalamic dysfunction (sleep disorders, hyperphagia, polydipsia), and meningitis. Oculomasticatory myorhythmia, possibly caused by brainstem tegmental abnormalities, is a movement disorder nearly unique to patients with Whipple's disease. It consists of rhythmic convergence of the eyes and synchronous contractions of the eyelids, jaw, face, and neck, with characteristics resembling spinal myoclonus. The disorder responds to antibiotic therapy. This disorder is very rare in children. Please see the online chapter.

Turcot's Syndrome

Turcot's syndrome is the rare association of polyposis of the colon and malignant tumors of the CNS (glioblastomas, medulloblastomas, and anaplastic astrocytomas). See the online chapter.

Porphyria

The porphyrias are a heterogenous group of metabolic disorders characterized by abnormal heme biosynthesis and are rare in children. The abnormalities involve porphyrin metabolism in the metabolic pathway that converts glycine and succinyl-CoA to heme, which is reviewed in the online chapter.

Although all subtypes are rare, acute intermittent porphyria (AIP) is the most common form of the neuroporphyrias. It manifests with occasional neurovisceral crises resulting from overproduction of porphyrin precursors, such as aminolevulinic acid (ALA), which is released from the liver into the circulation. More than 60 mutations causing AIP have been found (OMIN 176000). Manifestation of neuropsychiatric symptoms in hepatic porphyria patients is triggered by precipitating factors, including various drugs, hormones, fasting, and other agents.

Acute porphyrias present with acute attacks consisting of severe abdominal pain, nausea, constipation, polyneuropathy mental symptoms, confusion, and seizures, and can be life-threatening. In general, presentation in childhood is uncommon. Rare recessive porphyrias usually manifest in early childhood with severe cutaneous photosensitivity and chronic hemolysis, or chronic neurologic symptoms with or without photosensitivity. Symptoms include features of autonomic neuropathy, including severe abdominal pain, vomiting, constipation, hypertension, tachycardia, and bladder dysfunction. Other symptoms are those of peripheral axonal neuropathy and neuropsychiatric symptoms. Acute porphyric neuropathy predominantly involves the motor system and can be manifested by symptoms, signs, and CSF abnormalities resembling acute Guillain-Barré syndrome.

Acute encephalopathy in patients with hepatic porphyria is manifested as a combination of neuropsychiatric symptoms with seizures, syndrome of inappropriate antidiuretic hormone secretion, and, rarely, focal CNS deficits. Neuroimaging abnormalities are uncommon, although MRI ischemic lesions have been reported, as has a posterior reversible encephalopathy syndrome.

Diagnosis is based on detection of porphyrins and their precursors in blood, urine, or feces. Measurement of urinary porphobilinogen is the best screening biochemical test for AIP, although it is nonspecific.

Treatment is mainly symptomatic and includes supportive treatment with analgesia, monitoring for and treating complications such as hypertension, prevention and treatment of water and electrolyte disorders that may result from inappropriate antidiuretic hormone production, and a high-carbohydrate diet. See the online chapter.

NEUROLOGIC DISORDERS ASSOCIATED WITH HEPATOBILIARY DISEASES

Neurologic abnormalities occur in patients with acute and chronic liver disease and include impairments of memory, attention, and executive and motor functions. These abnormalities vary in severity, being mild initially but later progressing to overt hepatic encephalopathy. Cognitive dysfunction also can be generalized or specific, including selective attention deficits and abnormalities of motor skills, language, or visuospatial skills. The etiology of the liver disease (e.g., hepatitis C virus, Wilson's disease, alcohol related) can influence the pattern of cognitive dysfunction.

Hepatitis

Encephalitis, myelitis, Guillain-Barré syndrome, mononeuritis, and polymyositis are infrequent complications of hepatitis A and B. Associated nervous system involvement from Hepatitis C virus (HCV) infection includes cerebrovascular events, encephalopathy, myelitis, encephalomyelitis, cognitive impairment, psychiatric manifestations, and peripheral neuropathy.

Treatment includes use of interferon-alpha, steroids, and plasmapheresis. Treatment of chronic hepatitis with interferon may result in the onset of neuropsychiatric symptoms in some patients.

Hepatic Encephalopathy

The most common etiology of hepatic encephalopathy (HE) in children is fulminant viral hepatitis, accounting for 50% to 75% of cases, followed by drug or toxin ingestion, including acetaminophen overdose, high-dose salicylate therapy, parenteral hyperalimentation, ingestion of isoniazid, rifampicin, halothane, alpha-methyldopa, azathioprine, erythromycin, sodium valproate, and tetracycline. Other etiologies are end-stage chronic liver disease caused by biliary atresia, α1-antitrypsin deficiency, autoimmune chronic active hepatitis, Wilson's disease, and Reye's syndrome.

HE can complicate most liver diseases, whether acute, subacute, or chronic, and can occur with or without portosystemic shunting. It is characterized by an altered state of consciousness, abnormal mental status, and neurologic abnormalities. The pathophysiology of HE is described in the online chapter.

There have been several classifications of HE. A newer classification proposes three subtypes associated with (1) acute liver failure, (2) portosystemic bypass and no intrinsic hepatocellular disease, and (3) cirrhosis and portal hypertension or portosystemic shunting. The latter is subdivided into episodic HE (subtypes: precipitated, spontaneous, recurrent), persistent HE (subtypes: mild, severe, treatment dependent), and minimal HE.

Neurologic Abnormalities

Neurologic examination may demonstrate mental status changes, motor abnormalities with pyramidal tract dysfunction, and an early parkinsonian syndrome. Other signs include ataxia, action tremor, dysarthria, and asterixis. Seizures are relatively uncommon, as are focal neurologic abnormalities and cerebral and retinal visual abnormalities. Patients with minimal HE usually have no overt neurologic abnormalities.

Fulminant Liver Failure

Fulminant liver failure is present when HE occurs within one to several weeks of the first evidence of liver disease. Cerebral edema may develop and cause increased intracranial pressure. Ammonia concentration may be elevated, resulting in psychomotor agitation, muscle twitching, mania, delirium, or seizures, especially in children. It also may contribute to the pathogenesis of cerebral edema and raised intracranial pressure.

In affected patients, 70% to 80% of cases respond to antibiotic therapy. Although the mortality rate of acute hepatic failure is high, hepatic function can be restored completely in survivors. Children with moderate or severe electroencephalogram (EEG) abnormalities on admission are more likely to require a liver transplant or die, whereas children with a normal or only mildly abnormal EEG are more likely to survive without transplantation. Management includes monitoring and treatment of hypoglycemia and of intracranial pressure, along with maintenance of adequate cerebral perfusion pressure.

Cognitive and Behavioral Abnormalities

The earliest changes of HE are subtle behavioral changes and mild impairments of intellectual function. Changes in activities of daily living; impairment of sleep–wake status, attentiveness, cognition, and consciousness; and deterioration in school performance and motor functions become increasingly apparent. Abnormalities occur in mental and motor status, including an abnormal level of consciousness; reduced attention; slow reaction speed; defects in orientation, memory, affect, perception, and judgment; and psychomotor slowing. HE is graded into four stages, with derangement of consciousness progressing from drowsiness to stupor and coma. These stages are as follows:

Grade I: altered sleep cycle, altered affect (euphoria or belligerence), mild confusion, loss of spatial orientation
Grade II: drowsy, responsive to simple commands
Grade III: stuporous, responsive only to painful stimuli
Grade IV: unresponsive to pain; decorticate or decerebrate posturing

Minimal Hepatic Encephalopathy

MHE was known formerly as subclinical hepatic encephalopathy and refers to patients with chronic liver disease who have a normal neurologic examination but have milder subcortical cognitive impairments, including deficits in attention, executive function, immediate recall, visuospatial tasks, psychomotor speed, verbal learning, and long-term memory.

Laboratory Tests

Liver function tests usually are abnormal, but derangements may not be as drastic as expected. Arterial blood ammonia may be elevated and correlates somewhat with the clinical state. Most studies have noted that the ammonia level does not correlate with the severity of encephalopathy. CSF glutamine concentration is more specific and correlates better with the stage of HE.

The EEG may assist in clinical staging. In the early stages, EEG shows reduction of the alpha rhythm with increased theta activity. With a more advanced encephalopathy and further clouding of consciousness, slower delta frequencies appear. Triphasic waves are characteristic but not specific and carry a poor prognosis. Subsequently, there is decreasing amplitude of the EEG waveforms and, finally, absent activity. CT may be normal early, and cortical atrophy may be seen later. MRI abnormalities include increased T1-weighted signal in basal ganglia regions. MRI does not correlate with laboratory indices of hepatic function, with histologic liver diagnosis, or with the neurologic status at the time of MRI acquisition. MR spectroscopy demonstrates depletion of myoinositol, preservation of N-acetylaspartate, and elevation of glutamine.

Neuropathology and Pathophysiology

Please see the online chapter.

Treatment

The treatment of HE is directed toward removal or correction of any precipitating factors, diminishing the absorption of nitrogenous substances from the intestinal tract, and minimizing portosystemic shunting. Hyperammonemia may suggest poor functional reserves, malnutrition, and impending multiorgan dysfunction. Early provision of nutritional support; correction of hypokalemia, hypovolemia, and acidosis; aggressive treatment of infection; avoidance of sedatives; and modification of portosystemic shunts may contribute to reducing the production of ammonia and thus help to prevent its damaging effects (Tapper, Jiang, and Patwardhan, 2015).

All patients should be evaluated for secondary triggers of HE. Most effective therapies are directed at reducing the ammonia concentration and treating various complications, including infections, renal and cardiovascular dysfunction, and bleeding secondary to ruptured varices, hypersplenism, or clotting factor deficiencies. Probiotics can improve minimal HE and act as prophylaxis of overt HE. Therapy is more effective for portosystemic encephalopathy and much less so for fulminant hepatic failure. Ammonia production can be reduced by decreasing dietary intake of protein, treating constipation, controlling GI tract bleeding, and reducing bacterial intestinal growth. Ammonia also can be removed from the intestines by the osmotic action of nonabsorbable disaccharides, such as lactulose. Complications of lactulose therapy include dehydration and hypernatremia. Reduction of gut ammonia also can be achieved using antibiotics such as neomycin or Rifaximin, which are active against urease-producing bacteria. Management of acute severe cerebral edema is important and is discussed in Chapter 105.

Prognosis

Prognosis of hepatic encephalopathy is guarded, in spite of improvement in intensive medical support. One-year survival is 40%, and 3-year survival is 15%. Fulminant hepatic failure has a mortality rate of 75%, and severe hepatic coma carries a substantial risk of permanent neurologic disability.

Neurologic Abnormalities Associated With Liver Transplantation

Patients undergoing liver transplantation can have serious postoperative neurologic complications, including encephalopathy, seizures, headaches, involuntary movement disorders, cortical blindness, brachial plexopathy, and peripheral neuropathy. Etiologic factors include air embolism, graft-versus-host reactions, coagulopathy-associated cerebral hemorrhage, seizures and central pontine myelinolysis resulting from severe electrolyte and metabolic changes, cerebral infarction resulting from perioperative hypotension, and meningoencephalitis or cerebral abscess resulting from opportunistic infection. Drug-induced neurologic disorders also may occur. Seizures can be the manifestations of ischemic or hemorrhagic strokes, CNS infection, or metabolic abnormalities. Neurologic complications also can be associated with cyclosporine A.

Neurologic Abnormalities in Primary Biliary Cirrhosis

Primary biliary cirrhosis (PBC) is a chronic cholestatic liver disease with an autoimmune etiology. In addition to chronic liver disease, patients have other symptoms, including fatigue and cognitive dysfunction, in particular, memory and concentration difficulties. Please see the online chapter for additional discussion.

Reye's Syndrome

Reye's syndrome is a now-uncommon syndrome characterized by an acute encephalopathy with fatty infiltration of various organs, including the liver, kidney, and heart. The syndrome is associated with viral illnesses, such as influenza B and varicella, and salicylate therapy.

Several metabolic conditions, including fatty-acid oxidation defects (e.g., carnitine deficiency, organic acidurias, medium-chain acyl coenzyme A dehydrogenase deficiency), can cause recurrent Reye's syndrome–like episodes. In Reye's-like syndromes that are a result of inborn errors of metabolism, hypoglycemia, hypoketonemia, elevated ammonia, and organic aciduria often are evident. The most commonly diagnosed metabolic disorder has been medium-chain acyl coenzyme A dehydrogenase deficiency. Because Reye's syndrome is now very rare, any child suspected of manifesting this disorder should undergo investigations for inborn errors of metabolism.

Clinical presentation involves an antecedent viral infection, followed by vomiting and marked changes in sensorium that may start with a hyperexcitable stage and progress to lethargy and coma with decorticate posturing. The latter symptoms are secondary to increased intracranial pressure and central herniation as a result of brain edema. Clinical staging systems, consisting of four or five stages, are based on the cephalocaudal progression of brainstem dysfunction secondary to increased intracranial pressure, or EEG criteria. Laboratory abnormalities include marked elevations of hepatic transaminases, prolongation of the prothrombin time,

hyperammonemia, hypoglycemia, increases in plasma fatty acid levels, elevation of plasma lactate, and reduced phosphorus concentrations. Imaging findings and pathology are reviewed in the online chapter. The most important therapeutic measure is reduction of intracranial pressure, as reviewed in Chapter 105.

Hepatolenticular Degeneration: Wilson's Disease

Wilson's disease (OMIM 27790) is a rare autosomal-recessive disease presenting in late childhood or adolescence and results from a defect in copper metabolism, secondary to ATP7B gene mutations on chromosome 13q14.3–q21.1, which codes for a copper-transporting adenosine triphosphatase. The basic defect in Wilson's disease is the impaired biliary excretion of copper, resulting in the accumulation of copper in the liver, cornea, and brain. Manifestations include liver dysfunction (acute or chronic hepatitis, cirrhosis, acute hepatic failure), neuropsychiatric disease, and Kayser–Fleischer rings.

Diagnosis is clear if two of the following symptoms are present: Kayser–Fleischer rings, typical neurologic symptoms, and low serum ceruloplasmin levels. Serum ceruloplasmin levels are low (<20 mg/dL), serum copper levels are decreased (<20 μg/dL), and 24-hour urinary excretion is increased (>100 μg/24 hours). Liver biopsy using radioactive 64Cu or 67Cu can be performed to determine hepatic copper levels.

Neurologic manifestations are gradual in onset. Dystonia is the most common feature. Dysarthria, tremors, and psychiatric manifestations start more commonly during the second decade of life. Three subsets of patients have been recognized: (1) pseudoparkinsonian patients with dilation of the third ventricle who have bradykinesia, rigidity, cognitive impairment, and an organic mood syndrome; (2) pseudosclerosis patients with focal thalamic lesions, ataxia, tremor, and reduced functional capacity; and (3) dyskinesia patients with focal abnormalities of the putamen and globus pallidus, dyskinesias, dysarthria, and an organic personality syndrome.

Psychiatric disorders are common and include mania, psychosis, depression, and schizophrenia. Almost all patients with neurologic and psychiatric manifestations develop corneal Kayser–Fleischer rings, a granular brown pigmentation of the cornea caused by copper deposition in Descemet's membrane, which can be visualized by slit-lamp examination.

Seizures are uncommon and can occur at any stage. In children, deterioration in school achievement and the development of behavioral and conduct disorders begin insidiously and progress slowly. Neurologic manifestations have been reported in children as young as 6 years of age, although, traditionally, children younger than age 10 years have the hepatic form of the disease, whereas children older than 10 years have neurologic involvement.

See the online chapter for a review of imaging abnormalities.

Treatment is directed at reducing systemic copper levels with a low-copper diet and with anticopper medications. The drugs used include zinc, which blocks intestinal copper absorption; penicillamine and trientine, both of which are chelators that increase urinary excretion of copper; and tetrathiomolybdate, which forms a tripartite complex with copper and protein and blocks copper absorption from the intestine or renders blood copper nontoxic. Because of its efficacy and lack of toxicity, zinc is considered by some to be the treatment of choice for maintenance therapy, for treatment of the presymptomatic patient, and for treatment of the pregnant patient.

For patients with mild liver failure, combined treatment with trientine and zinc is effective.

For patients with neurologic disease, tetrathiomolybdate is preferred to penicillamine by some groups because it provides rapid, safe control of copper. Patients treated with penicillamine are at great risk of serious permanent neurologic worsening or side effects. Pyridoxine should be given concurrently in those patients receiving penicillamine. A reduction of clinical symptoms usually is achieved with therapy, but the degree of recovery is variable.

Progressive Hepatocerebral Disease

Alpers's syndrome is a heterogeneous group of disorders affecting young children, manifested by progressive neurologic degeneration with seizures, brain atrophy with neuronal necrosis, and sometimes liver disease; it is reviewed in Chapter 48.

Bilirubin Encephalopathy: Kernicterus

Hyperbilirubinemia affects term and late-preterm infants in the first week of life, but is generally mild (Bhutani and Johnson-Hamerman, 2015). Chronic neurologic sequelae are seen in a subset of infants.

Many infants who now develop kernicterus are not those with Rhesus disease, and they often have no documented evidence of hemolytic disease. Rather, they are term and late-preterm infants who have been discharged from the nursery as "healthy newborns," yet returned with extreme hyperbilirubinemia and have then developed the classic findings associated with kernicterus. The term *kernicterus* describes the neuropathology of bilirubin-induced brain injury (including the yellow staining of the deep nuclei of the brain) and the clinical finding associated with this condition. Another term that can be used to describe the clinical condition is *bilirubin encephalopathy*.

Bilirubin is the end product of the catabolism of heme and is transported in plasma bound to albumin and converted in the liver to an excretable conjugated form, which is then excreted into the bile, transported to the small intestine, further degraded by intestinal bacteria, and excreted in the stool. A number of neonatal disorders may lead to much higher concentrations of unconjugated bilirubin. These include hemolytic diseases of the newborn caused by blood group incompatibility (but also some hemoglobinopathies), hemorrhage, polycythemia, inherited or acquired defects of conjugation, and hypothyroidism. Premature infants are more susceptible to hyperbilirubinemia. The risk for bilirubin encephalopathy also depends on the etiology of hyperbilirubinemia. The level of total serum bilirubin that may lead to acute bilirubin encephalopathy (ABE) and to kernicterus depends on a number of variables, including the gestational age and the serum albumin. In a full-term baby this level is equal to or more than 20 mg/dl, although in infants without risk factors neurotoxicity may be observed at higher bilirubin levels.

Pathophysiology of Hyperbilirubinemia. This is discussed in the online chapter.

Neuropathology. This is discussed in the online chapter.

Clinical Manifestations. The sequence of acute bilirubin encephalopathy (ABE) consists of three phases. Acute symptoms are characterized by lethargy, hypotonia, and poor sucking and swallowing responses. If untreated, the later stage of ABE is more severe and includes hypertonia, possible fever (secondary to muscular contraction), and a high-pitched cry. The hypertonia is evident in the extensor muscle groups and is manifested by backward arching of the neck (retrocollis) and trunk (opisthotonos). The condition can progress to apnea, coma, seizures, and death. Central apneic events may be a sign of bilirubin-induced neurotoxicity. Clinical manifestations of ABE in preterm infants are similar but more subtle than those of term infants.

Chronic bilirubin encephalopathy (CBE, kernicterus) defines the permanent neurologic sequelae of bilirubin toxicity and is manifested by extrapyramidal motor abnormalities (e.g., chorea, dystonia, or ballismus) that may fluctuate—athetoid cerebral palsy, auditory impairment, and oculomotor impairment, especially paralysis of upward gaze.

Auditory impairment, usually high-frequency bilateral hearing loss, is common because the auditory pathway is the part of the nervous system most sensitive to bilirubin toxicity. Dental dysplasia is another complication of kernicterus and affects only the deciduous teeth. The permanent teeth may not be affected.

Intellectual deficits can vary from severe intellectual disability to isolated symptoms and also to subtle bilirubin-induced neurologic dysfunction (BIND). Characteristic features may not become apparent until after 1 year of age. Some patients may have a delayed onset of several years before developing a movement disorder. BIND is a constellation of more subtle neurodevelopmental abnormalities caused by bilirubin neurotoxicity, without classical kernicterus. These include abnormal central auditory processing, cognitive dysfunction, and alterations in muscle, sensorimotor and visual function.

Laboratory Testing. Determination of blood bilirubin, albumin, and pH levels may give an indication of the risk of kernicterus. Auditory brainstem response (ABR) testing provides early detection of bilirubin neurotoxicity. Neuroimaging hallmarks of kernicterus include high-intensity lesions in the globus pallidus and in the subthalamic nucleus on MRI T2-weighted imaging. These abnormalities are different from those seen with neonatal hypoxia-ischemia, which affects the cortex, thalamus, periventricular white matter, caudate nucleus, and putamen.

Management. The essential aspect of bilirubin encephalopathy management is the early detection of at-risk neonates. Phototherapy and exchange transfusion are the treatment of choice for hyperbilirubinemia (see the online chapter).

REFERENCES

The complete list of references for this chapter is available in the e-book at www.expertconsult.com.
    See inside cover for registration details.

SELECTED REFERENCES

Ben-Or, O., Zelnik, N., Shaoul, R., et al., 2015. The neurologic profile of children and adolescents with inflammatory bowel disease. J. Child Neurol. 30 (5), 551–557.

Bhutani, V.K., Johnson-Hamerman, L., 2015. The clinical syndrome of bilirubin induced neurologic dysfunction. Semin. Fetal Neonatal Med. 20, 5–13.

Borre, Y.E., O'Keeffe, G.W., Clarke, G., et al., 2014. Microbiota and neurodevelopmental windows: implications for brain disorders. Trends Mol. Med. 20 (9), 509–518.

Datar, S., Wijdicks, E.F., 2014. Neurologic manifestations of acute liver failure. Handb Clin Neurol. 120, 645–659.

Diaconu, G., Burlea, M., Grigore, I., et al., 2013. Celiac disease with neurologic manifestations in children. Rev. Med. Chir. Soc. Med. Nat. Iasi 117 (1), 88–94.

Ferro, J.M., Oliveira, S., 2014. Neurologic manifestations of gastro-intestinal and liver diseases. Curr. Neurol. Neurosci. Rep. 14 (487), 1–12.

Mayer, E.A., Padua, D., Tillisch, K., 2014. Altered brain-gut axis in autism: comorbidity or causative mechanisms? Bioessays 36 (10), 933–939.

Moses, J., Keilman, A., Worley, S., et al., 2014. Approach to the diagnosis and treatment of cyclic vomiting syndrome: a large single-center experience with 106 patients. Pediatr. Neurol. 50 (6), 569–573.

Obermayr, F., Hotta, R., Enomoto, H., et al., 2013. Development and developmental disorders of the enteric nervous system. Nat. Rev. Gastroenterol. Hepatol. 10 (1), 43–57.

Tapper, E.B., Jiang, Z.G., Patwardhan, V.R., 2015. Refining the ammonia hypothesis: a physiology-driven approach to the treatment of hepatic encephalopathy. Mayo Clin. Proc. 90 (5), 646–658.

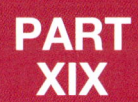
160 Counseling Children with Neurologic Disorders and Their Families

David J. Michelson and Robin D. Clark

 An expanded version of this chapter is available on www.expertconsult.com. See inside cover for registration details.

INTRODUCTION

Clinicians treating a child with neurologic symptoms have the same fundamental goals as do the child's family: an accurate diagnosis and a plan for treating the disease; improving the child's symptoms, quality of life, and functioning; and minimizing the child's suffering. Good communication between clinicians and family members is vital to defining, clarifying, and meeting these goals, but in some circumstances, communication is difficult or breaks down, leading instead to confusion, misunderstanding, frustration, and dissatisfaction. Whether dealing with questions about a minor complaint in the clinic setting or with questions of critical importance in the intensive care unit, clinicians have a tendency to put themselves in the limited role of information providers—obtaining and conveying information about symptoms and treatment options. However, as the complexity and emotional intensity of discussions about illness increase, so too does the difficulty of maintaining clear communication.

Patients often express dissatisfaction with clinicians, saying that they did not feel listened to or understood during their interactions. Clinicians tend to interrupt, focus on the few symptoms initially elicited, and launch into biomedical explanations without exploring how the information fits with the patient's culture and perspective (Searight and Gafford, 2005). Patients and their families are often more capable of understanding medical issues and wish to play a more prominent role in decision making than clinicians estimate. Even discussions of informed consent are too often judged by patients to be hurried, limited, and unsatisfying (Elwyn et al., 2014). In situations where emotions run particularly high, such as giving bad news or negotiating differences of opinion, clinicians fare even worse.

Skills important to communication with patients can be taught through mentoring and focused practice, with self-awareness and self-reflection being the keys to success (Kern et al., 2005). Such efforts have shown positive and enduring results, particularly when integrated into training programs. A commitment to improved communication skills takes an investment of time and a willingness to engage with intense, often unpleasant emotional reactions, but ultimately leads to improved outcomes and a greater sense of satisfaction for both clinicians and patients.

THE CLINICIAN–PATIENT RELATIONSHIP

Society invests physicians (and many allied health professionals) with the responsibility to use their knowledge and experience for their patients' benefit, putting their patients' interests ahead of almost all other concerns. Trust is required if patients are going to provide clinicians access to their most private information and emotional states. Nevertheless, there has been a steady trend toward placing more emphasis on patient autonomy and self-determination. Paternalistic, doctor-centered approaches to directing patient care are increasingly giving way to more balanced and collaborative models.

Although trust is the foundation of good communication, patients may initially place only a small amount of trust in a clinician based solely on the clinician's professional title. Lower degrees of implicit trust may derive from a patient's own negative experiences or from a negative cultural perspective. A clinician can build on and solidify trust over time through use of communication skills that demonstrate interest, respect, and empathy.

COMMUNICATION SKILLS

Even when a clinician focuses on information delivery, such as reviewing the results of a diagnostic test, the delivery is more likely to succeed if tailored to the needs of the family. Each family member may have differing levels of education, levels of trust in the medical profession, and perceptions of illness and death. The implications of a medical diagnosis, including the benefits and risks involved in testing and treatment decisions, depend greatly on the individual. Collaborative decision making depends on developing the interviewing and listening skills needed for understanding the perspective of each person involved.

Communication is easier and more efficient when relationships have developed and matured over time, but clinicians can engender trust in even brief encounters by paying attention to showing respect, interest, empathy, support, and a willingness to forge a partnership (Box 160-1). Compassionate care requires the clinician to be sensitive to the patient's immediate needs, rather than the clinician's agenda for the discussion (Epstein, Siegel, and Silberman, 2008).

NONVERBAL COMMUNICATION

Clinicians show attentiveness, respect, and empathy, or lack thereof, through nonverbal behaviors as much as through words. Frequent eye contact, relaxed and open facial expressions and body postures, a warm and inviting tone of voice, and supportive head nods and encouraging semiverbal comments are important for conveying interest in what families have to say. Attentive silence also has a positive influence.

BOX 160-1 Communication Skills

RESPECT

- Introduce the medical team and have the family members introduce themselves, discuss the purpose of the meeting, and give the name of the child for whom the meeting is being held.
- Be "in the moment" and genuine, show interest, and take your time.
- Shake hands if culturally appropriate, sit down, and make eye contact.
- Use positive, engaged body postures, with your shoulders and head leaning forward, your hands relaxed on your lap, and with nothing in between you and the family.
- Consider leaving your pager and phone outside of the meeting space or turning them off so that calls and messages do not interrupt anyone.
- Acknowledge things the family is doing well and the family's strengths.

EMPATHY

- Respond to emotions, identify and reflect them, and give them time to develop.
- Reframe emotional responses as communicating ideas.

SUPPORT

- Talk about the clinician–patient relationship as an ongoing partnership.

BOX 160-2 PEARLS for Difficult Conversations

PARTNERSHIP

- We will work together to deal with this.

EMPATHY

- I wish that things had turned out differently.

APOLOGY/APPRECIATION

- I'm sorry that I don't have better news.
- You are handling this news quite well.

REFLECTION

- You seem upset by what I just told you.

LEGITIMATION (VALIDATION)

- It is understandable that you feel angry right now.

SUPPORT

- I will do what I can to help.

Postures that suggest emotional distance, disinterest, or disapproval (e.g., crossing one's arms on the chest, standing by the door, frequently looking away) can undermine sincere efforts to establish rapport. The setting can also facilitate or detract from a sense of intimacy with the clinician. Clinicians should sit at a similar level to others, at a distance that is neither too close nor too far, and there should be as few distracting objects between the family and the clinician as possible. Some situations call for exceptions. Family members who are agitated or paranoid may perceive efforts to sustain eye contact or sit close to them as threatening or provocative.

CONVEYING EMPATHY

Demonstrating empathy is particularly important. Clinicians can communicate empathy through nonverbal expressions of attention and through the use of active listening techniques, encouraging comments, and repetition of things the patient says. Asking patients about nonmedical aspects of their lives, including their hopes and worries, gives the clinician important insights and communicates that the clinician values their feelings.

Identifying and affirming emotional responses also demonstrates empathy. Clinicians may be reluctant to address strong emotional responses directly, worrying that doing so will take too much time or be seen as an invasion of privacy. However, expressions of empathy can encourage patients to get to the heart of their concerns.

Responding to a strong emotion, such as fear, anger, or sadness, can be difficult, but a structured approach can be helpful (Box 160-2). Clinicians can use reflective statements to encourage patients and family members to express themselves and are particularly important when patients and family members are feeling guilt or shame about the subject matter. Clinicians can validate emotional responses as understandable and common. Such expressions convey understanding

without suggesting that the person's response is one that the clinician agrees with.

Angry responses, especially those directed at clinicians, are difficult to handle. Validating such anger usually has the effect of diminishing it, rather than fueling it, and can be done in a supportive and respectful way. Clinicians should bear in mind that anger is a natural response to pain, loss, and fear, and that it can feel as if it is directed personally at the clinician even when the real cause is the situation. A defensive response from a clinician is likely to be counterproductive, escalating the person's anger. It is important for clinicians to remain empathetic while also maintaining enough detachment from the interaction to monitor their own reactions.

Clinicians can demonstrate empathy and concern toward patients through promises to continue to be involved. Families appreciate hearing that clinicians are primarily interested in their child's well-being and will provide them with support in whatever way they can.

PROVIDING INFORMATION

As with any interaction, advanced preparation is useful. Clinicians should consider their own emotional response to the situation, the patient, and the family and how best to make the discussion productive. For example, a clinician who had trouble with a particular family member in a prior interaction may choose to take a different approach in talking with the family, to speak to the difficult person individually, or even to ask another clinician to lead the discussion. Having time to prepare written information regarding the disease, treatment options, or support groups will help the family members recall the information they receive in the discussion.

It is helpful to provide preemptive counseling about diagnostic tests or procedures with highly consequential results. Families benefit from having at least a basic understanding of the possible results, including the ongoing uncertainty of an ambiguous or nondiagnostic result. The pretest discussion can build a solid foundation for the discussion of the test results. Clinicians should discuss important or ambiguous test results in person, in a dedicated counseling session whenever possible, rather than relay them over the phone. Optimally, posttest discussions should occur as soon as possible after results are available and be structured to allow other members of the medical team and family who wish to be involved in decision making to participate. Unanticipated medical problems can arise with such acuity that families and clinicians must discuss test results and treatments with little time to prepare and plan.

Clinicians should still do what they can to help families feel that they have time to consider their options. When families are uncertain of how to proceed with treatment, it may be possible in some cases to use temporizing measures to extend the time window for making a more definitive decision.

The location chosen for discussions should be as quiet, comfortable, and private as possible. In both the outpatient and inpatient settings, having a dedicated consultation room for such discussions is ideal. However, even when only the examination or patient room is available, sitting down before beginning discussions can increase relaxation and indicate that the clinician considers the conversation important enough not to rush. Facial tissues, paper and pens for taking notes, and water should be available.

Whether it is appropriate for minor children to be present during discussions of their diagnosis, prognosis, and treatment will depend largely on their age and maturity. Clinicians should strive to follow the parents' wishes. A child-life specialist may be an available resource for explaining medical procedures to children in an age-appropriate manner. Clinicians should also ask parents about whether they wish for members of their extended families to be included in discussions. Clinicians may wish to invite the participation of other staff members who have been involved in caring for the patient, including physicians, bedside nurses, therapists, social workers, and chaplains. All participants should introduce themselves by name and title and/or relationship to the patient.

Because family members may have heard or understood previously conveyed medical information differently from clinicians, from one another, or from other sources (such as the Internet), it is useful to begin discussions by asking family members to summarize the child's condition. This not only gives the clinician a sense of how much family members already know, what their concerns and beliefs are, and where further discussion needs to start, but also informs clinicians of the type of language the family members feel comfortable using to discuss medical issues. Clinicians should also ask, early on, what families are hoping to learn from the discussion. Clinicians may use this to propose an overview of their goals for the discussion, keeping expectations to a manageable size and offering to address other topics at another time.

Being mindful of an overall plan for the session can improve the consistency with which basic principles of good communication are followed. A six-step method, known by the acronym SPIKES, has proven to be an effective tool for delivering bad news (Kaplan, 2010) (Box 160-3).

Clinicians may find it quite natural to launch into long, complex discussions of medical issues, but it is unlikely that families will understand or retain what they hear. Families appreciate receiving information in small, digestible amounts expressed in words with which they are familiar. Clinicians can employ a number of methods to improve understanding and retention: telling a personal anecdote, drawing illustrations, or providing the family with written (or online) resources for later review. Clinicians should also ensure that families understand when and why important information, such as the patient's diagnosis or prognosis, is uncertain. Clinicians who use an "ask-tell-ask" paradigm with each new topic that they introduce find that it allows them to tailor the information provided to the needs of the family and to check for any misunderstandings or gaps that need correction. It is also generally helpful for clinicians to adhere to a consistent template for keeping conversations organized.

When clinicians anticipate that they are going to say something that will be emotionally difficult for the family to process, they should introduce the topic gradually, with frequent pauses to allow for questions. Before revealing information that may be distressing, an effort can be made to lessen

---

BOX 160-3 The Six Steps of SPIKES

S—SET UP THE SESSION
- Arrange for privacy.
- Involve significant others.
- Sit down.
- Make a connection with the patient.
- Manage time constraints and interruptions.

P—ASSESS THE FAMILY'S PERCEPTION
- "Before you tell, ask"—ask the family members to summarize their current understanding of the situation.

I—OBTAIN THE PATIENT'S INVITATION
- Some patients do not want full information.

K—GIVE KNOWLEDGE TO THE FAMILY
- Warn the patient that bad news is coming.
- Speak at the level of comprehension of the patient.
- Use nontechnical words when possible.
- Avoid excessive bluntness.
- Give information in small chunks and check for understanding.

E—ADDRESS EMOTIONS WITH EMPATHY
- Observe for emotional responses.
- Identify the emotion and the reason for it; ask if unsure.
- Acknowledge emotions with empathic and validating statements.

S—STRATEGIZE AND SUMMARIZE
- Ask if the family is ready to discuss plans.
- Check for misunderstandings and unrealistic expectations.
- Frame treatment options in terms of specific patient goals.

---

their surprise through the use of a "warning shot" that allows them to better prepare to hear what you have to say. The expression "I'm sorry to tell you this" should be used cautiously because families may misinterpret the word "sorry" as an apology or as an expression of pity, causing them to react with anger or mistrust.

Pauses after statements with great impact give listeners time to process the information and their emotional response to it, whether disbelief, sadness, or anger. Clinicians should view a patient's silence after hearing bad news as an opportunity for them to show the patient empathy. Nonverbal signs of support can help to convey empathy better than words alone. In the context of difficult treatment decisions, clinicians should try to help families express their feelings about their goals for treatment, particularly whether they place more value on quality of life and avoidance of treatment side effects or on the child having the greatest possible chance of response to treatment. Clinicians can then frame their discussion of treatment options in terms of how each may or may not help the family achieve their goals. Medical decisions should be made based on scientific knowledge and standards of care, but they should reflect the personal, cultural, and spiritual values of the family. It is particularly important to check that families understand the purpose, risk, and potential for benefit of any treatments before they are considered mutually agreed upon (Jeoung, Yang, Bak, Lim, and Sim, 2014).

When the prognosis is uncertain, it can be difficult to make the risks understandable with the use of statistical descriptions alone, even when simplified. Using a diagram such as a single darkened circle out of 10 to convey the significance of a 10% risk can help avoid misunderstandings. It is also important to make it clear when the outcome is unclear. Families may come away from discussions believing that a clinician described the prognosis as absolutely positive or negative, despite efforts to convey uncertainty.

Understandably, families experience grief when they perceive that a child's diagnosis implies any chance that the child will not be healthy, not recover, or not survive. It is important to try to point out positive and negative aspects of the situation, even when the prognosis is dire, and to avoid statements that convey abandonment. Even when a child's condition is beyond hope of cure, the family will still be focused on hope that treatments can achieve other important goals, such as pain control and symptom relief.

SPECIFIC CHALLENGES
Low Health Literacy

Communication with one or more family members may be difficult because of a language barrier, low literacy, or impairments in receptive or expressive language skills. Nearly one fifth of adults living in the United States speak a language other than English at home, and many who speak English as a second language may only reluctantly admit to doing so less than fluently. Information given to patients and families, whether verbally or in written materials, is above their level of comprehension about half of the time. Asking family members for the highest grade they completed in school will often overestimate their reading comprehension level. Men are more likely than women to have lower health literacy but are less likely to identify as such when asked.

Several measures of health literacy have been designed for research purposes, but one tool that is particularly easy to administer quickly is the Rapid Evaluation of Adult Literacy in Medicine–Revised (REALM-R). This screening test asks subjects to read aloud the following list of eight words: *osteoporosis, allergic, jaundice, anemia, fatigue, directed, colitis, constipation.* Subjects unable to pronounce more than six of these words correctly are likely to have reading abilities at the sixth-grade level or lower. Other measures, which may take more time to administer, assess subjects for other aspects of health literacy, including numeracy and familiarity with medical concepts (Duell, Wright, Renzaho, and Bhattacharya, 2015). Clinicians can use information about health literacy to tailor how they convey spoken and written medical information.

Family Discord

Family members may have differing opinions and values and struggle to agree on treatment decisions. When such conflicts arise, the clinician should try to express empathy for all points of view while looking for common ground. If the discussion threatens to become disruptive, the clinician may choose to restrict further discussion of that topic (Cannarella Lorenzetti, Jacques, Donovan, Cottrell, and Buck, 2013).

Alternate Belief Systems

Families may ask that a child be shielded from some medical information or decisions, contrary to more prevalent views of patient autonomy, or may ask that medical decisions be made on the basis of an alternate belief system, such as faith healing or traditional medicine/folk remedies. The reasoning behind any treatment decision should be made clear through discussion—what initially appears to be lack of cooperation with recommendations may be a result of lack of understanding or fear of the unknown.

Spirituality

Religious and spiritual faith play a major role in shaping the goals and values of many families, and it is usually helpful to broach the subject when exploring a family's worldview and sources of support. Views on illness, medicine, death, and dying can vary greatly between religions and even within sects of a religion. Patients and families often derive comfort from the opportunity to seek counsel from spiritual leaders when facing difficult decisions. In many cultures, there is crossover between the roles of healthcare providers and spiritual leaders, and some families may look to a clinician as a source of spiritual support. It can be appropriate to accept offers to pray with families if clinicians are able to do so based on genuinely held faith, but it may be a violation of interpersonal boundaries for clinicians to spontaneously offer to do so (D'Souza, 2007). It is perfectly acceptable and appropriate for clinicians to decline such requests respectfully, instead referring families to spiritual support services.

Difficult Patients

Clinicians may encounter family members with whom they find it especially difficult to build rapport and partnership. A family member's particular emotional response to grief, such as anger, may cause difficulties. It may be family members with disorders, such as alcoholism or hypochondriasis, with whom clinicians struggle to feel empathy. Clinicians should cultivate self-awareness of how they respond to patients and reflect on what they are responding to, whether it is reasonable, and whether they can overcome those reactions.

If a person becomes inappropriately angry during an interaction, a clinician may choose to attempt to continue to engage with the person, giving warnings and choices that indicate a willingness to continue listening if boundaries are respected. However, when there are reasonable safety concerns, it may be wiser for clinicians to avoid further confrontation and either walk away from the conversation or call for help from security officers. Demonstrations of extreme anger are unusual but can occur as a defensive reaction to other intense emotions, such as fear, or may reflect an underlying pathology in the person, such as substance abuse or a personality disorder.

Occasionally, frustration and anger boil over to the point of family members becoming verbally abusive or physically threatening toward one another, toward clinicians, or toward other staff. A family member with a psychiatric disorder or substance abuse problem is particularly likely to behave inappropriately. If clinicians are unable to defuse a potentially dangerous situation, they should put their own safety first, carefully withdraw from the room, and seek help.

Uncertain Test Results

Communicating test results is difficult enough in general, and especially so when the interpretation is uncertain. Genetic tests are particularly likely to be of uncertain significance. There are common phenotypes with variable genetic bases (e.g., nonsyndromic global developmental delay), genotypes with highly variable phenotypic expression (e.g., Marfan syndrome), and genetic mutations with incomplete penetrance (e.g., *BRCA1* mutations). As genetic screening tests become more sensitive for previously unreported copy-number changes and mutations, these tests are reporting an ever-increasing number of genetic variants of unknown significance (VUSs). As with any test, it is important that the ordering physician understand and consider the sensitivity and specificity of a genetic test before it is ordered (see Chapter 161). For example, a patient with Angelman syndrome resulting from a *UBE3A* mutation in a splice site, detectable through traditional Sanger sequencing of the whole gene, might initially escape diagnosis when tested by whole-exome sequencing or with a multigene panel using a next-generation sequencing platform.

When a screening test reveals a VUS, the initial step toward reducing the uncertainty of its significance is parental testing to determine whether the variant was inherited or arose *de novo*. If the VUS was inherited and the carrier parent is unaffected, it is more likely that the VUS is benign. However, it can still be the cause of the disorder if there is a second mutation elsewhere in the same gene or if the variation has reduced penetrance or expressivity in the parent.

The nature of genetic disorders also lends itself to parents experiencing shame and guilt. This may lead to denial—for example, a father refusing to be tested for carrier status, not wanting to know if he bears direct responsibility for his child's illness. Test results may also reveal unexpected information. When a patient with an autosomal-recessive condition is hemizygous for an uncommon mutation or has extensive homozygosity, it suggests consanguinity or even incest. Parental testing may reveal nonpaternity of the father. Ideally, clinicians should address these and other issues in pretest counseling.

Terminal Illnesses

Discussing an illness that is likely to be terminal is uniquely challenging for families and for clinicians. Studies have shown that clinicians are more than twice as likely to overestimate a patient's survival as to underestimate it, and that their overestimates are greater when they are familiar with the patient. When discussing prognosis, it is best for clinicians to avoid giving a specific time frame, such as the average life expectancy, without also discussing the range of outcomes and the possibility of exceptions, including both shorter and longer survival.

Clinicians are also likely to offer treatments that they themselves believe to be futile and not discuss prognosis at all, not wanting to broach such anxiety-provoking topics or to deprive families of their hope for a cure. Understandably, clinicians tend to assume that families will want to pursue treatment options that will lead to recovery from illness, even when reaching that goal requires significant pain and suffering. It is always better to explore this upfront, so that the necessary trade-offs are clear. When no treatment options are likely to result in recovery, or survival, it is even more important to discuss this with families and help them focus on other goals for the patient. Families may or may not choose a second round of chemotherapy after relapse of a cancer; they may or may not want resuscitation performed if an attempt at extubation fails. There is not necessarily a path that suits all families, and by listening carefully, clinicians can guide families toward the path that best fits their values. Palliative care specialists are particularly experienced and comfortable with discussing these issues.

Avoiding difficult discussions about advanced care and resuscitation increases the likelihood that clinicians will maintain their default position, ready to make all efforts to prolong life, regardless of the potential for the child to return to an acceptable quality of life. If doctors find it difficult to discuss the limited benefits of a test or treatment, patients and their families may have unrealistic expectations and make decisions that are not in the patient's best interest.

Clinicians may avoid having a full discussion about the short- and long-term consequences of an illness, even avoiding the topic completely, when they themselves are unused to dealing with grief. With training, clinicians can learn to remain supportive in the face of even the strongest emotional responses that patients and family members experience in response to bad news. Helping to guide people through their denial, depression, anger, and bargaining, leading them toward ultimate acceptance and peace of mind, can become a very rewarding aspect of medical practice (Back, Arnold, and Tulsky, 2009).

REFERENCES

The complete list of references for this chapter is available in the e-book at www.expertconsult.com.

See inside cover for registration details.

SELECTED REFERENCES

Back, A., Arnold, R., Tulsky, J., 2009. Mastering communication with seriously ill patients: Balancing Honesty with Empathy and Hope. Cambridge University Press., New York.

Cannarella Lorenzetti, R., Jacques, C.H., Donovan, C., et al., 2013. Managing difficult encounters: understanding physician, patient, and situational factors. Am. Fam. Physician 87 (6), 419–425.

D'Souza, R., 2007. The importance of spirituality in medicine and its application to clinical practice. Med. J. Aust. 186 (10 Suppl), S57–S59.

Duell, P., Wright, D., Renzaho, A.M., et al., 2015. Optimal health literacy measurement for the clinical setting: A systematic review. Patient Educ. Couns. 98 (11), 1295–1307.

Elwyn, G., Lloyd, A., May, C., et al., 2014. Collaborative deliberation: a model for patient care. Patient Educ. Couns. 97 (2), 158–164.

Epstein, R., Siegel, D., Silberman, J., 2008. Self-monitoring in clinical practice: A challenge for educators. J. Contin. Educ. Health Prof. 28, 5–13.

Jeoung, Y.O., Yang, T.K., Bak, Y.I., et al., 2014. An ideal model of informed consent communication. Korean J. Med. Educ. 26 (1), 9–17.

Kaplan, M., 2010. SPIKES: a framework for breaking bad news to patients with cancer. Clin. J. Oncol. Nurs. 14 (4), 514–516.

Kern, D.E., Branch, W.T., Jr., Jackson, J.L., et al., the General Internal Medicine Generalist Educational Leadership Group, 2005. Teaching the psychosocial aspects of care in the clinical setting: practical recommendations. Acad. Med. 80, 8–20.

Searight, H.R., Gafford, J., 2005. Cultural diversity at the end of life: issues and guidelines for family clinicians. Am. Fam. Physician 71, 515–522.

E-BOOK FIGURES AND TABLES

The following figures and tables are available in the e-book at www.expertconsult.com. See inside cover for registration details.

Box 160-4 Template for Discussions.
Box 160-5 Discussing Complex Outcomes.

161 Approaches to Personalized Medicine in Pediatric Neurology

Bruce R. Korf

 An expanded version of this chapter is available on www.expertconsult.com. See inside cover for registration details.

INTRODUCTION

The idea of personalized medicine offers the prospect of customization of medical management with unprecedented precision (Collins and Varmus, 2015; Hamburg and Collins, 2010). This includes use of testing to precisely define a diagnosis, choose the most appropriate treatment, and tailor drug dosage to individual metabolism. In addition it entails development of new treatments based on knowledge of pathophysiology. It can also entail predictive testing and formulation of an individualized management plan to reduce risk.

Genomic testing permits diagnoses to be made that had previously been elusive in spite of intensive medical evaluation. In some cases this opens the door to treatments targeted at the disease mechanism and may reveal subgroups of patients who will respond particularly well or poorly to the treatment. It can also be used to guide administration of a drug at a dosage that will minimize side effects and maximize efficacy. In some cases, genomic testing may reveal individuals who are at risk of disease well in advance of signs or symptoms, allowing anticipatory guidance or even efforts to prevent or delay disease. This chapter reviews some of the applications of genomics to pediatric neurology and briefly considers the application of nongenomic approaches as well.

GENOMIC DIAGNOSIS

The mainstay of the genomic approach is the ability to provide testing, either to diagnose a rare Mendelian disorder, to assess risk of a common multifactorial disorder, or to determine individual patterns of drug metabolism. Until recently, genetic diagnosis was limited to analysis at the two extremes of genetic variation: single-nucleotide changes and large-scale chromosomal abnormalities. Changes within a gene may alter the amino acid sequence of a protein, completely eliminate protein production, or alter patterns of splicing of the messenger RNA. Copy-number changes may occur on a larger scale, deleting or duplicating whole exons or groups of exons, or even entire genes or groups of genes, up to complete chromosomes. The major approaches to detection of genetic variants are summarized in Table 161-1.

The plummeting cost of genome sequencing has offered a new approach to genome-scale diagnosis (Bamshad et al., 2011). The protein-encoding portion of the genome, referred to as the *exome*, amounts to less than 1.5% of the 3.15 billion base pairs of the haploid genome yet harbors most of the known variants that account for disease. Exome sequencing can usually be performed for under $1000, although the analysis of the tens of thousands of variants that are found in any individual may cost many times that amount. Further advances in sequencing are bringing the cost of whole-genome sequencing to a comparable level and may further increase the sensitivity of analysis. Exome or genome sequencing can reveal pathogenic mutations without prior knowledge of the target

gene (Yang et al., 2014). Interpretation can be complicated by the finding of variants of unknown significance. In addition, incidental findings of pathogenic mutations that predict disorders other than those that explain the phenotype also may result. These possibilities necessitate careful pretest and posttest counseling.

Although genetic counseling should be available when any genetic test is done, it is especially important when doing genome sequencing, given the complexity of the analysis and potential findings. Pretest counseling includes informing the patient about what the testing can and cannot accomplish, including the overall likelihood of achieving a diagnosis. The possibility of finding a variant of unknown significance must be discussed because patients are often unprepared for ambiguous results such as these. Testing also includes the possibility of incidental findings, such as discovery of unexpected genetic variants that predict medical problems different from those that prompted testing (Green et al., 2013). Some patients may decline to be informed of incidental findings, but such information offers potential for learning about potentially life-changing findings. There is also a need to inform patients about revealing potentially unexpected family relationships, for example, unexpected consanguinity. After the test results are available, counseling again should be provided to inform the patient of results and to put the results in perspective. There is the potential to identify multiple genetic variants of possible medical significance, so the session may be a long one, and most laypersons are not well versed in the concepts of genome sequencing. Findings may also have implications for other family members, which needs to be discussed and may require follow up.

THERAPEUTICS

Genetic and genomic information can be used to guide drug therapy in three ways. First, precise definition of a medical condition at the genetic level can result in treatment that targets the underlying pathogenesis, with improved efficacy and reduced likelihood of side effects. Second, the manner in which drugs are absorbed, metabolized, and excreted is, to a large extent, under genetic control. Recognition of an individual's pattern of interacting with a drug can result in optimization of dosage, again improving efficacy and avoiding side effects. Also, some rare "idiosyncratic" side effects occur only in individuals with specific at-risk genotypes; recognition of such individuals allows the physician to avoid administration of the offending drugs, preventing potentially devastating adverse reactions.

Targeted Treatment

Since the advent of molecular genetic approaches, the genes that underlie neurogenetic disorders have gradually come to light. This in turn reveals molecular mechanisms of disease

TABLE 161-1 Major Approaches to Genetic Diagnosis

Mode of Analysis	Introduced	Applications	Limitations	Current Status
Unbanded chromosomal analysis	Late 1950s–1960s	Detection of aneuploidy	Unable to visualize small structural changes	Obsolete
Banded chromosomal analysis	Late 1960s–1970s	Detection of aneuploidy, large deletions, duplications, structural rearrangements	Limited resolution	Still in use
Fluorescence in situ hybridization	1990s	Detection of small deletions or duplications, characterization of unknown chromosomal rearrangements	Requires prior knowledge of region of concern	Still in use
Cytogenomic microarray	2000s	Detection of copy-number variants	Does not detect balanced structural rearrangements	First-line test for congenital anomalies, intellectual disability
Genetic linkage analysis	1980s	Determination of segregation of mutation in a family; does not require identification of specific mutation	Genetic recombination can lead to errors; requires family study	Rarely used clinically
Single-gene-mutation analysis	1980s–1990s	Identification of mutation in specific gene	Identification of variants of unknown significance; need to know target gene in advance; some mutations not readily detectable	Still in use
Exome/genome sequencing	2010s	Identification of pathogenic variants across genome	Variants of unknown significance; incidental findings; does not detect structural rearrangements	Emerging technology

that can guide the development of specific treatments. Medical treatment for some complications of tuberous sclerosis complex is now available, and clinical trials are under way for many other neurogenetic disorders, such as neurofibromatosis, Duchenne muscular dystrophy, and various forms of epilepsy. Some of these treatments target biochemical pathways involved in disease; some target the abnormal gene.

Disease Stratification

Genetic studies also have the potential to inform drug therapy for common multifactorial disorders. Cancer is one area where this concept of disease stratification based on genotype has made significant progress. There are now increasing numbers of drugs that target specific tumor proteins that only are effective if those proteins are altered as a result of gene mutation. Genomic sequencing of tumors is now being done on a wide scale in an effort to identify other such targets; in some cases it is becoming routine clinical practice, and the information is being used to inform both prognosis and treatment.

Pharmacogenetics

The study of genes that control drug metabolism is referred to a pharmacogenetics (de Wildt, Tibboel, and Leeder, 2014). Exogenous chemicals, including drugs, undergo metabolic changes in three phases. Phase I reactions are chemical changes in the drug, principally oxidation, reduction, or hydrolysis. These are carried out by multiple groups of enzymes, such as the family of cytochrome c oxidases, monoamine oxidase, and NADPH cytochrome P450 reductase. Phase II reactions involve conjugation of chemical groups onto the drug, such as glucuronidation, acetylation, methylation, and conjugation with glutathione. Phase III reactions involve active transport of the conjugated drug out of the cell, usually through action of ABC-type transporters, a family of ATP-dependent cell mem-

brane proteins responsible for pumping conjugated chemicals out of the cell.

Many of the enzyme systems involved in these reactions are encoded by genes that exist in various forms in the population (i.e., exhibit genetic polymorphism). These genetic variants may lead to either increased or decreased activity of the corresponding enzymes. The effect of such a variant on drug metabolism depends on the nature of the reaction and its role in metabolism of the drug. For example, some phase I reactions are required to convert a biologically inert drug to one that effectively interacts with its target, whereas others function to inactivate a drug. If the reaction activates a drug, a variant that increases activity will result in higher levels of the active drug in the system, and potentially toxicity; a variant that decreases activity will result in lack of sufficient active drug, and hence inadequate treatment. If the reaction inactivates a drug, the opposite will occur; reduced enzyme activity will lead to higher levels and potential toxicity, increased activity in rapid metabolism, and lower levels of the active drug. Some pharmacogenetic polymorphisms that are relevant to neurologic practice are listed in Table 161-2.

PREVENTION

Genomics offers the possibility of identification of risk factors for disease in advance of development of signs and symptoms, with the hope of maintaining good health as long as possible.

Newborn Screening

The paradigm of newborn screening is that of detection of a treatable disorder before onset of symptoms to avoid irreversible damage. A successful program is predicated on the availability of an inexpensive but accurate screening test, an effective treatment, and knowledge of the natural history of the disorder. The advent of tandem mass spectrometry has

TABLE 161-2 Major Pharmacogenetic Polymorphisms of Interest in Pediatric Neurology

Drug	Enzyme/Gene	Comments
Amitriptyline, desipramine, nortriptyline	CYP2D6/CPY2C19	Ultrarapid or slow metabolizers require dosage adjustment or alternative drug
Azathioprine	Thiopurine methyltransferase	Slow metabolizers at risk of fatal bone marrow suppression; rapid metabolizers may have inadequate treatment
Carbamazepine	HLA-B*15:02	Increased risk of Stevens-Johnson syndrome
Phenytoin	HLA-B*15:02 CYP2C19	Increased risk of Stevens-Johnson syndrome Dosage adjustment
Clopidogrel	CYP2C19	Intermediate or poor metabolizers: choose alternative drug
Warfarin	CYP2C9, VKORC1	Dosage adjustment based on genotype

allowed a significant increase in the number of disorders for which screening is possible without increasing the cost of testing. In the United States, state departments of public health run most screening programs, and the specific disorders to be screened are determined on a state-by-state basis. During the past decade, however, a systematic evidence-based effort has been under way to standardize at least the core panel. Recently the possibility of screening based on genomic sequencing has been in consideration. This offers the opportunity to vastly increase the numbers of conditions that could be detected but also raises significant challenges, such as the identification of variants of unknown significance or incidental findings. There is also the potential of discovery of variants that indicate a risk for a late-onset disorder. Typically, one does not do genetic testing of children for conditions that do not manifest until later in life. It is not known how such findings will affect the child and the parent–child relationship, or the way a child with such a risk should be followed by care providers. These issues are currently under study, and newborn DNA sequencing is not yet ready for routine clinical implementation.

Risk Assessment

Genetic factors contribute to common disorders via a complex interaction of multiple genes and the environment. Approaches such as genome-wide association studies have revealed hundreds of gene loci that are associated with common disorders. There are several important caveats to keep in mind when genetic variants are used for risk assessment. First, in most cases the odds of disease in an individual who carries a specific variant usually are only modestly different from the odds for one who does not carry the variant. Second, the proportion of the genetic contribution to a disease accounted for by a specific variant may be small. Genome-wide association is based on the assumption that common variants (found in 1%-5% of the population) account for most of the genetic contribution to common disease. It is possible that at least some of the contribution is comprised of a constellation of rare variants

that may be almost unique to an individual—the "dark side" of personalized medicine (i.e., that risk is so personal it will never be possible to know for any individual). A third caveat is that case-control studies are done in specific populations, and results may not generalize to people of different ethnic backgrounds, a point that may not be appreciated by a layperson looking at information from a direct-to-consumer site. Fourth, genetic factors do not operate on their own to contribute to disease risk; thus there is concern that an individual could interpret risk to be low on the basis of genomic testing and ignore commonsense advice. Finally, the specific combinations of genetic and nongenetic factors that determine risk are not entirely known, and risk calculations may be based on proprietary algorithms, leading to different conclusions from the same data set. These caveats notwithstanding, individualized risk assessment has been marketed both through health professionals and to the public. Currently, the U.S. Food and Drug Administration is exploring the role it might play in regulating genetic testing, which has put a hold on direct-to-consumer genomic testing for disease risk assessment. It is likely that this landscape will continue to evolve in the coming years as the costs of genotyping decline, knowledge of disease associations increases, and the regulatory landscape is clarified.

FUTURE PROSPECTS

The modern era of genomic medicine is in its infancy, and predictions are especially hazardous given the rapid pace of technological change along with changes in the context in which healthcare is provided. Indeed, some of the technologies that are fueling the personalized medicine approach are also catalyzing overall change in healthcare delivery.

Genome Sequencing

As the price of genome sequencing decreases, it is likely that there will be increasing pressure to provide access on a routine basis. It should be noted that the cost of sequencing is only part of the overall cost of providing sequence-based genomic analysis. The informatics analysis currently exceeds the cost of sequencing itself, but that may change as approaches to analysis of genomic data advance. At least three issues will need to be addressed before routine genomic sequencing is offered: clinical utility, timing, and data storage.

Patient Engagement

Although the focus in this chapter is on application of genomics to personalized medicine, there are many other areas of technology that may also be applied to the personalization of healthcare. These include imaging devices that provide highly precise data on both anatomy and physiology and may be placed in the hands of physicians or even patients at low cost. Advances also include portable and even wearable devices that track data in real time, such as physical activity, heart rate, and oxygenation (Topol, Steinhubl, and Torkamani, 2015). There is even a possibility of development of devices that will diagnose common conditions by themselves, without the need for intervention by a health professional.

These devices may be coupled with increasingly powerful and popular social networking and health-coaching systems. People already wear activity trackers and share their level of physical activity through social networking. Health coaches will be able to access real-time data and offer individualized advice on issues such as diet and exercise, and even optimal use of medical care. Social networking is also being used for patients to share their experiences with the healthcare system and to assist one another in diagnosis and treatment of chronic illness. Although the quality of data that can be acquired by portable devices or self-reporting may be less than that obtained through more systematic professionally guided approaches, the sheer volume of data may lead to insights and even discoveries that would not have been made in conventional epidemiologic studies.

These approaches may supplant direct professional involvement in some areas of healthcare as less expensive and more accessible alternatives become available. This is exemplified by the availability of direct-to-consumer genomic data. It may be argued that the quality of care currently provided by such approaches is far inferior to that available with professional guidance. If the quality gradually improves, however, such models may eventually supplant existing approaches, along the lines of a "disruptive technology" that replaces traditional approaches because of lower cost, easier access, and comparable or better outcomes. Such a model raises complex questions regarding the ability to provide pretest and posttest genetic counseling, although new approaches to counseling may be developed as part of the model.

FINAL COMMENTS

The revolution in healthcare represented by personalized medicine has been the subject of much hype and reactionary cynicism. The genome sequence was completed more than 10 years ago, and although there are tangible medical applications, such as cytogenomic microarray analysis and cancer sequencing, these advances are a long way from having transformed healthcare. It is clear that the path from sequencing the genome to clinical application is arduous; some promised advances will prove to be unrealistic and some eventual applications will be ones we cannot dream of today. A statement that has become known as Amara's law is apt here: We tend to overestimate the effects of a technology in the short run and underestimate its effects in the long run.

REFERENCES

The complete list of references for this chapter is available in the e-book at www.expertconsult.com.
    See inside cover for registration details.

SELECTED REFERENCES

Bamshad, M.J., Ng, S.B., Bigham, A.W., et al., 2011. Exome sequencing as a tool for Mendelian disease gene discovery. Nat. Rev. Genet. England. 12 (11), 745–755.

Collins, F.S., Varmus, H., 2015. A new initiative on precision medicine. N. Engl. J. Med. 372 (9), 793–795.

de Wildt, S.N., Tibboel, D., Leeder, J.S., 2014. Drug metabolism for the paediatrician. Arch. Dis. Child. BMJ Publishing Group Ltd and Royal College of Paediatrics and Child Health. 99 (12), 1137–1142.

Green, R.C., Berg, J.S., Grody, W.W., et al., 2013. ACMG recommendations for reporting of incidental findings in clinical exome and genome sequencing. Genet Med. 15 (7), 565–574.

Hamburg, M.A., Collins, F.S., 2010. The path to personalized medicine. N. Engl. J. Med. 363 (4), 301–304.

Topol, E.J., Steinhubl, S.R., Torkamani, A., 2015. Digital medical tools and sensors. JAMA 313 (4), 353–354.

Yang, Y., Muzny, D.M., Xia, F., et al., 2014. Molecular findings among patients referred for clinical whole-exome sequencing. JAMA 312 (18), 1870–1879.

162 Pediatric Neurorehabilitation Medicine

Michael J. Noetzel and Nico U. F. Dosenbach

An expanded version of this chapter is available on www.expertconsult.com. See inside cover for registration details.

INTRODUCTION

Rehabilitation is the process of restoration after injury or disease, with the goal of maximizing an individual's ability to function in a typical manner. The application of rehabilitation extends far beyond the traditional bounds of medicine because one of its chief aims is to restore personal and social identity (Noetzel, 2003). The principles and challenges of pediatric neurorehabilitation are best understood in the context of the International Classification of Functioning, Disability, and Health. Impairment is the loss or abnormality of physiologic, psychological, or anatomic structure or function, whereas disability, the lack or restricted ability to perform a task, is dependent on the individual's environment. Thus one of the ways in which neurorehabilitation can be carried out is to modify or adapt the environment. Disability does not flow solely or directly from the type and degree of impairment. Instead, disability is a three-dimensional construct, consisting of functional impairment, activity limitations, and participation restrictions. Each dimension is the result of interaction between the biologic features intrinsic to the individual's medical condition and the physical and social environment (Noetzel, 2012). The concept of dependency also plays a fundamental role in rehabilitation. Degree of dependency is a critical element in the cost of rehabilitation care, as well as in quality of life.

The disablement/dependency paradigm in pediatric neurorehabilitation emphasizes progress toward appropriate functional outcomes (Noetzel, 2003). Thus therapeutic interventions should be based primarily on the disablement and resultant activity limitations, as opposed to the underlying pathologic process, and rehabilitation techniques should be transferrable from one child to another despite differences in diagnosis. Similarly, the process of neurorehabilitation logically involves a multidisciplinary team working in collaboration with the patient and the patient's family. Finally, the paradigm provides a framework that can be expanded to encompass all aspects of neurorehabilitation inherent in the practice of child neurology. For example, the paradigm works just as well in describing an adolescent with seizures (impairment) who is prohibited from driving an automobile (disablement) and relies on his parents for rides (dependency) as it does for a child with a spinal cord injury causing paraplegia and impaired ambulation.

MECHANISMS UNDERLYING FUNCTIONAL RECOVERY IN THE NERVOUS SYSTEM

The degree of recovery after injury to the nervous system is variable but often incomplete. A better understanding of the cellular and molecular bases of neuronal dysfunction and the mechanisms by which recovery of function occurs is the framework upon which development of any pediatric neurorehabilitation program must rest (Noetzel, 2003). Based upon increasing scientific evidence (Johnston, 2009), we now recognize that significant biologic modification in response to injury and developmental aberrations exist within the nervous

system that are more dynamic than suggested by prior studies (Dosenbach and Noetzel, 2014). Additionally, meaningful recovery of function continues for an extended period of time, longer than previously recognized (Noetzel, 2012). These findings stand in contrast to former beliefs that recovery essentially was a biphasic process in that early improvement was due to reversibility of factors affecting dysfunctional, as opposed to dead, tissue. Later improvements in functional capabilities were attributed to behavior modification. Presently, however, there is strong evidence that changes in neuronal circuitry within the central nervous system (CNS) also mediate later recovery of function (Johnston, 2009), although there remains ongoing debate concerning the relative contributions of brain reorganization and functional adaptation.

Resolution of Temporary Dysfunction

Rapid recovery of function within hours to days after CNS injury likely relates to resolution of temporary dysfunction caused by mild tissue hypoxia, elevated intracranial pressure, edema, small contusions, and reversible depression of metabolic activity in areas remote from the primary injury (Dosenbach and Noetzel, 2014). Focal brain injury results in depressed metabolic activity in noncontiguous brain areas, secondary to a decrease in transmitter synthesizing enzymes in regions of damage. The concept of diaschisis similarly has evolved to explain uninvolved brain areas that are rendered temporarily nonfunctional when deprived of appropriate input from a remote injured CNS region. Recovery of function presumably transpires as a result of increased neurotransmitter synthesis or elevated production of receptors. In addition, cellular and molecular mechanisms at the systems level are initiated within 1 to 5 days after injury to help mediate recovery.

Plasticity of the Nervous System

Although, individual brain regions contribute specialized computations, all human behaviors are the emergent property of networks distributed through cerebral cortex, subcortical structures, and even the cerebellum (Dosenbach and Noetzel, 2014). Abilities such as executive control, attention, and movement are supported by widespread networks and not localized to specific brain areas (Carter, et al., 2012). The brain's organization into functional networks allows a certain degree of malleability both during development and in reaction to damage. Plasticity is a term that encompasses multiple capabilities of the nervous system to encode information in response to learning, as well as adapting to environmental changes (Johnston, 2009). In the context of rehabilitation, plasticity may relate both to redundancy within the brain's functional network architecture, as well as injury-driven reorganization of brain networks. These redundancies in connectivity and computational specialization allow functional networks to reorganize into new network states that enable the best possible performance (Dosenbach and Noetzel, 2014). For example, during the initial subacute recovery phase in adult stroke patients, widespread activations throughout the motor system are observed. Patients with good functional recovery gradually develop activation patterns focused in perilesional areas—that is, patterns of more typical activation, even though task performance relies on different functional neuroanatomy (Dosenbach and Noetzel, 2014).

Reorganization of Neuronal Connections

The proposed events of neural reorganization that emerge in response to injury are well-recognized, normal developmental processes, which are reactivated or potentiated in response to CNS damage (Noetzel, 2012). After the immediate postinjury period, functional recovery starts to occur through modification of active neural connections, three of which have been suggested as the most promising examples of reorganization mechanisms. Axonal regeneration, whereby damaged axons regrow to their normal target, serves as a dominant process of recovery in the peripheral nervous system, but its role in restoration of brain function is debatable. Axon retraction and synaptic pruning are the second mechanisms by which neuronal reorganization transpires. During early development, certain axons project branches that ultimately will be retracted. Similarly, maturation of the cerebral cortex in early postnatal life is characterized by an initial proliferation of synapse formation, followed by activity-dependent pruning of excessive synapses. Research now indicates that these normal retraction and pruning processes may not occur if nervous system injury is sustained early on, thus providing a mechanism for retention of function.

Collateral sprouting involves axonal outgrowth from undamaged neurons and the establishment of synaptic contact at sites vacated by degenerating neurons. This process typically is confined to brain regions normally innervated by nerve cells sharing common features with the injured neurons, and axonal growth cones rarely migrate into novel nervous system domains. Collateral sprouting is influenced by growth and apoptotic factors, in particular activation of genes responsible for molecular growth-promoting programs. As such the magnitude and rate of sprouting after acute CNS injury appears much greater in the immature brain.

A potential final mechanism involved in modifying neural connections consists of neural progenitor cells, which retain the capacity to proliferate, divide, and differentiate after injury. Damage in the CNS initiates a cascade of molecular signals that recruit migrating neuroblasts into the injured areas. Whether these cells actually promote restoration of function in humans has not been established.

Functional Recovery Through Adaptation

Recovery long past the onset of injury primarily is dependent on functional substitution in which an altered strategy is adapted to achieve a goal. It is a recovery of the "ends" and not a restoration of the "means to that end," in that the action performed is modified in order to fit the capabilities of undamaged nerve cells. The tissue subserving this recovery does not alter its intrinsic properties but utilizes novel strategies to complete the task. Because functional substitution is highly dependent on new learning and repetitive problem-solving, neurorehabilitation can influence greatly on this type of recovery.

PRINCIPLES OF PEDIATRIC NEUROREHABILITATION

Pediatric rehabilitation has several guiding principles based upon the nature of recovery and reorganization mechanisms, as well as the age and developmental level of the patients requiring treatment (Box 162-1) (Noetzel, 2003). The

rehabilitation process requires a coordinated transdisciplinary team working to provide integrated evaluations and therapeutic interventions. Because injury to or malformation of the brain and spinal cord accounts for the majority of children referred for rehabilitation, child neurologists are uniquely positioned to contribute in a meaningful way to the discipline of rehabilitation (Noetzel, 2003). Issues such as home accessibility, psychosocial adaptation, and school reintegration mandate that the team include individuals who can address these all-important considerations. In addition, the rehabilitation process should concentrate on strategies designed to effect functional improvement. The team must have a clear understanding of the physical, emotional, cognitive, and social consequences of a child's injury (Noetzel, 2012). The degree, extent, and rate of recovery, which varies significantly among children, as well as differences in functioning from setting to setting and task to task, mandate continual assessment. Neurorehabilitation is a spiral management process in which a treatment program is initiated and then constantly revised and updated, based on therapy-mediated improvements.

Another essential principle is that reassessments must be guided by a detailed understanding of normative maturation. Typical developmental milestones can be identified as sequential goals (Noetzel, 2003). In addition, as a result of injury or illness, the pediatric patient typically loses age-appropriate developmental capabilities. Thus the manner in which therapy can be provided and the individual's ability to respond to it will be limited. This is most notable early on in patients who lack skills necessary to learn complex strategies upon which functional substitution is predicated (Noetzel, 2012). Finally, an understanding of cognitive development allows more accurate prediction of the long-term effects of cerebral injury sustained by young children, especially in cortical areas subserving functions that mature later such as executive functioning and emotional and attentional control.

Equally important in pediatric rehabilitation is the core principle of family-centered care, recognizing that the child's family is a constant presence in the rehabilitation process, available to provide comfort and reassurance during times of stress (Dosenbach and Noetzel, 2014). Practical management decisions must be endorsed by the family, whose members should be expected to participate in therapy programs.

A final guiding principle is that intervention should begin as soon as possible. Coma is not a contraindication to the initiation of rehabilitation strategies, and once the patient is medically stable, therapy should be instituted (Noetzel, 2012). This early phase of intervention is designed to limit maladaptive movement patterns and to prevent, or at least minimize, complications that can take months to resolve if not promptly addressed.

MEDICAL ASPECTS OF ACUTE PEDIATRIC REHABILITATION MANAGEMENT

In any child with an acquired nervous system injury, the risk for compromised nutrition is high. Causes include: a hypermetabolic state resulting from trauma and/or infection; delayed gastric emptying and intestinal dysmotility; oral pharyngeal dysfunction; and underestimation of caloric requirements necessary for repair and growth (Noetzel, 2003). Oropharyngeal dysfunction and swallowing difficulties mandate a detailed evaluation by a feeding team.

Fever and associated infection often affect acute management (Noetzel, 2012). In those with intracranial trauma, the possibility of CNS infection must be considered (Noetzel, 2003). Sinusitis is a relatively common infection secondary to the frequent need for long-term nasogastric tube utilization.

Dysautonomia characterized by simultaneous and paroxysmal sympathetic and muscle overactivity typically follows severe traumatic brain injury, with an incidence of 5% to 12%. Autonomic changes include marked tachycardia, hyperventilation, hypertension, fever, and increased sweating; motor disturbances include posturing, dystonia, rigidity and spasticity. Evidence-based treatment paradigms for dysautonomia in pediatric patients do not exist. Bromocriptine, propranolol, clonidine, and midazolam may be beneficial, although intrathecal baclofen is clearly effective in children who are resistant to oral medications (Noetzel, 2012).

Damage to the pituitary and hypothalamic glands can produce the syndrome of inappropriate antidiuretic hormone secretion (SIADH), or conversely, central diabetes insipidus (Noetzel, 2012). Gastrointestinal disorders in acquired nervous system injury range from delayed gastric emptying and intestinal stasis to hemorrhage secondary to esophagitis and ulcers (Noetzel, 2003). In severe CNS trauma, long bone and other skeletal fractures are common. Such fractures may not be apparent early on in the comatose patient or in spinal cord injury (SCI) but reveal themselves during the course of treatment.

COMPREHENSIVE PEDIATRIC REHABILITATION PROGRAMS

Once medical issues have stabilized, the direction in which the rehabilitation process should proceed must be addressed. In some children, recovery has been sufficiently rapid for discharge to outpatient or day treatment programs. For others whose progress has been very slow, a subacute nursing center with less intense therapy is reasonable. A dedicated pediatric rehabilitation program is indicated for most children and adolescents with moderate to severe acute neurologic injury whose management issues typically include:

- Inability to walk, climb stairs, or perform wheelchair transfers
- Dependence in self-care activities
- Receptive/expressive aphasia
- Cognitive or perceptual motor dysfunction
- Incontinence of bowel or bladder
- Limited functional performance due to pain
- Severe neuromuscular deconditioning secondary to prolonged ventilatory support

Eligibility criteria for admission to comprehensive neurorehabilitation services include: a primary condition that is medically stable, but mandates intensive rehabilitation; the premorbid physical and cognitive level of the child indicates potential for meaningful recovery; the patient is responsive to verbal or visual stimuli and has sufficient alertness to participate in rehabilitation; and the diagnosis allows an expectation for improvement with the potential to achieve clearly identifiable treatment goals within a reasonable time period (Box 162-2) (Noetzel, 2003).

A comprehensive pediatric rehabilitation program is a highly intensive service with an initial minimum of 3 hours of therapy each day. As recovery proceeds and endurance improves, treatment is expanded to a full day. The program is supervised by a physician with specialized training and experience in rehabilitation medicine. Rehabilitation nursing care/supervision must be provided 24 hours a day. In addition to physical and occupational therapists and speech-language pathologists, most teams also include social workers, childlife specialists, music therapists, chaplains, orthotists, and

dieticians. In any program with a large number of children with acquired brain injury, psychologists and neuropsychologists are essential, as psychological support and neurocognitive assessment and intervention will be required at frequent intervals. Written evaluations should: measure progress; determine impediments to recovery and potential solutions; readjust established goals; develop and implement discharge plans; and facilitate transition into the community (Dosenbach and Noetzel, 2014).

REHABILITATION TREATMENT OF MOTOR IMPAIRMENT
Overview

Almost every patient requiring acute neurorehabilitation will manifest motor impairments or alterations in tone (Noetzel, 2003). In pediatrics, spasticity is most commonly found in children with cerebral palsy, but spasticity can result from any brain or spinal cord disorder causing damage to or abnormal development of nerves or pathways controlling motor movement. In adults motor rehabilitation is predicated on long-standing therapies designed to improve performance (Dosenbach and Noetzel, 2014). Similar interventions are endorsed in pediatric patients despite lack of strong empirical evidence to substantiate or quantify the actual benefit (Noetzel, 2012). Pediatric rehabilitation includes physical, occupational, and speech therapy and utilization of assistive devices and/or medications to reduce elevated tone and facilitate postural alignment. Aerobic conditioning, muscle strengthening, and task-specific training strategies assume greater importance as recovery proceeds. Innovative techniques for improving motor outcome, such as constraint-induced movement therapy (CIMT) and direct stimulation of the CNS, recently have been introduced (Dosenbach and Noetzel, 2014).

Treatment of Spasticity

In the early phase after CNS injury, reduced tone typically is encountered; over time, the pattern often evolves into spasticity as part of the upper motor neuron syndrome. Spasticity is characterized by excessive and inappropriately timed activation of skeletal muscles, which interferes with normal voluntarily movement. In most children, spasticity impairs passive movement and static postural alignment and is accompanied by deficient activation of voluntary movement, resulting in weakness, clumsiness, and reduced exercise tolerance. Invariably, these deficits cause excessive energy expenditure compared with able-bodied children (Noetzel, 2012). Spasticity eventually reduces protein synthesis in muscles and impairs longitudinal growth, causing contractures and bony deformities.

Treatment of spasticity should be predicated upon establishing goals that improve a child's functional capabilities, most commonly either upper-extremity use in activities of daily living or movement to achieve ambulation. Improvement of head, neck, and trunk posture by reducing spasticity may improve oral feeding and provide better breath support for speech. However, spasticity may impart advantages, including maintenance of muscle bulk and tone, support of circulatory function, and assistance in transfers and ambulation.

Rehabilitation Therapy

Early on the focus of relieving spasticity is to minimize joint and muscle contractures with a secondary goal of eliminating painful spasms (Noetzel, 2003). Management in comatose or obtunded patients combines proper positioning, range of motion exercises (ROM), and splinting (Fig. 162-1). As recovery ensues, specific affected muscles are targeted. Heat, cold, water, and electrical stimulation are effective adjuncts with few side effects or contraindications (Noetzel, 2012).

Positioning is designed to facilitate proper postural alignment and symmetry and to correct weight-bearing distribution throughout the body. Tone-inhibiting techniques can use gravity to stretch muscles and promote relaxation. In the latter stages of recovery, proper position facilitates active contraction of functionally weak muscles (Noetzel, 2003). Other mainstays are casting and splinting, designed to prevent formation or worsening of contractures in spastic extremities (Noetzel, 2012). Inhibitive casting also may lower tone via several mechanisms. Splints or orthotics may be utilized to produce functional benefits (Fig. 162-2). For example, an appropriately designed wrist/finger extension splint may improve hand activities such as keyboarding.

Equipment is an important adjuvant, especially in patients with chronic motor deficits. Standing frames allow a child with reduced weight-bearing ability to be placed in an appropriate position to minimize the development of contractures, improve bone maturation and increase pulmonary function. Deficits in static and dynamic balance may prevent independent ambulation, mandating the use of walkers and crutches (Fig. 162-3). For recreational activities, more creative assistive devices have further enhanced the independence of patients with motor disability (Fig. 162-4).

Oral Medications

Despite the fact that a large number of antispasticity medications have been available for many years, data currently available (Table 162-1) are too limited to conclude that any of these agents is truly effective in reducing spasticity in acutely brain-injured pediatric patients. In children with spastic cerebral palsy, data on tone reduction efficacy exist, but whether oral antispasticity medication can improve functional

capabilities has not been determined (Delgado, et al., 2010). Moreover, the side effects of antispasticity medication in children are concerning (Table 162-1). Thus antispasticity medication should be utilized only when severe spasticity cannot be managed by other modalities and continued use must be justified by ongoing demonstrable benefit. Finally, antispasticity medication should be prescribed in those situations

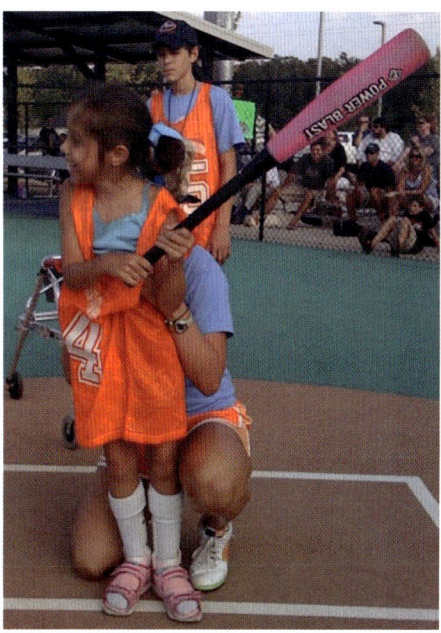

Figure 162-2. Ankle-foot orthotics. Ankle-foot orthotics often are appropriate for children starting to make gains in functional ambulation. *(Courtesy of Dr. Janice E. Brustrom-Hernandez and Anna Marie Champion.)*

TABLE 162-1 Oral Antispasticity Medications

Drug	Mechanism	Dosage	Side Effects	Studies
Baclofen (oral)	GABA-B agonist inhibits at spinal cord level	2–7 yr; max 40 mg 8–11 yr; max 60 mg >12 yr; max 80 mg; divided three to four times a day; increase every 3 days	2 + sedation, confusion 2 + weakness, ± seizure control	DBPC (adult)
Clorazepate	Facilitates GABA	>9–12 yr; max 60 mg/day >12 yr; max 90 mg/day; divided twice a day to three times a day; increase weekly	1–2 + sedation 1–2 + weakness	DBPC (adult)
Clonazepam	Facilitates GABA	<10 yr or 30 kg; max 0.1–0.2 mg/kg/day >10 yr or 30 kg; max 20 mg/kg/day; divided twice a day to three times a day; increase every 3 days	3 + sedation 2 + weakness	Open trial only
Diazepam	Facilitates GABA	<12 yr; 0.1–0.8 mg/kg/day >12 yr; 6–30 mg/day; divided three times a day to four times a day; increase weekly	3 + sedation 2 + weakness, dizziness	DBPC (child/adult)
Dantrolene	Interferes with skeletal muscle contraction by interruption of calcium release from sarcoplasmic reticulum	>5 yr; 12 mg/kg/day divided twice a day to four times a day Adult; max 400 mg/day; increase every 4–7 days	1 + sedation 3 + weakness, hepatotoxicity, GI complaints	DBPC (child/adult)
Tizanidine	Alpha-2 adrenergic agonist with presynaptic inhibition	0.2–0.3 mg/kg/day divided three to four time a day; night dosing helpful for sleep Adult max 36 mg; increase weekly	2 + sedation 1 + weakness, hypotension	DBPC (adult)

DBPC: double-blind, placebo-controlled; GABA: gamma-aminobutyric acid; GI: gastrointestinal.

in which meaningful functional goals can be achieved, as opposed to mere clinical ones—i.e., decreased resistance to stretch. Exceptions to the above "rule" include medications to facilitate hygiene, improve positioning, reduce caregiver demands and ease proper fitting of orthotics.

Commonly employed medications treating spasticity in pediatrics include diazepam, baclofen, tizanidine, and dantrolene (Table 162-1). Baclofen usually is well tolerated and has been moderately effective in reducing spasticity in spinal cord injury, with lesser benefit in brain injury from trauma or stroke. In cerebral palsy, baclofen studies have demonstrated significant reduction in spasticity and improved use of extremities. Sudden withdrawal of the medication has been associated with seizures and hallucinations. Although there have been numerous controlled trials of tizanidine in adults with spasticity, studies in children are few (Table 162-1). The usefulness of clonidine is limited mainly to patients with acute brain injury resulting in hypertension, tachycardia, and autonomic dysfunction, given its propensity to cause hypotension and bradycardia. Dantrolene sodium is the least sedating of the antispasticity medications, but requires careful titration to minimize the potential for severe generalized weakness and a limited duration of treatment due to the risk of hepatic injury (Noetzel, 2012). Newer agents such as gabapentin and pregabalin, both GABA analogs, as well as modafinil lack convincing data to establish that any of them reduce spasticity or improve quality of life in children (Noetzel, 2012).

Neuromuscular Blockade: Alcohol, Phenol, and Botulinum Toxin Injections

Neuromuscular blockade with phenol and alcohol causes axonal degeneration, with tone reduction lasting up to 1 to 3 years, but they are utilized relatively infrequently due to the need for sedation or anesthesia, as electrical stimulation is necessary to identify the target nerve (Noetzel, 2012). Intramuscular injection of botulinum toxin inhibits the release of the neurotransmitter acetylcholine responsible for transforming nerve impulses into muscle contraction. Studies on children with cerebral palsy have documented reduction in spasticity and modest functional improvement after injections in the arms and legs (Noetzel, 2012).

The limitation in movement must be the result of spasticity and not from a fixed contracture (Box 162-3). In addition, there should be sufficient underlying strength so that weakening of the problem muscle does not produce paresis. A clinically apparent effect is most notable 2 to 4 weeks after injection, and ongoing benefit typically lasts 3 to 4 months or longer. The total maximum dose of botulinum that can be administered at a single time is limited, and there must be appropriate spacing between injections in order to minimize antibodies developing to the toxin. Botulinum injections can be employed with other therapies and typically are coupled with an intensification of therapy and/or serial casting in order to secure maximum benefit (Fig. 162-1) (Noetzel, 2012). Pain on injection and transient flu-like syndromes have been noted; with increasing use, systemic botulism, resulting in deterioration in respiratory and oral-motor function, has occurred.

Intrathecal Baclofen Therapy

In patients with more extensive spasticity, intrathecal baclofen pump (ITB) therapy can be employed. Components include: a pump implanted under the skin on the abdomen, which infuses the drug at a predetermined rate; a catheter, which delivers drug to the intrathecal space of the spinal cord (with

the tip placed between T2 and C6 for maximum efficacy); and a programmer for adjustable and precise dosing (Noetzel, 2003). ITB therapy should be considered in children whose spasticity interferes with function or care, those who have painful spasticity-related spasms, and individuals unable to tolerate side effects from oral medications (Box 162-4). Because intrathecal baclofen diffuses directly into the spinal cord, the doses are much smaller than those taken orally, and the potential for systemic side effects is reduced. ITB therapy is not the optimal treatment if: spasticity predominantly affects the arms or is focal; trunk control is poor; and families cannot fully commit to the requirements of therapy maintenance (Box 162-4) (Noetzel, 2012). The pump reservoir is refilled percutaneously every 2 to 6 months, and the battery life of 5 to 7 years mandates pump replacement at the end of that time. Contraindications in patient selection include hypersensitivity to baclofen, unrealistic expectations of benefit, and small size/low weight.

ITB therapy complications due to surgical implantation and refilling procedures include CNS infection and peritonitis; device-related complications also may occur (Box 162-5). Side effects, such as somnolence, dizziness, and hypotonia, have been reported. Signs of overdose range from itching, excessive weakness, and ascending low tone to respiratory depression, seizures, and coma. Withdrawal is a medical emergency, presenting as altered mental status, spasticity and rigidity that may advance to rhabdomyolysis, organ failure, and death. Management of withdrawal is predicated on prompt recognition, institution of oral baclofen or tizanidine, and, in severe cases, intravenous benzodiazepines or propofol. Cyproheptadine can be a useful adjunct in the management of serotonergic syndrome symptoms.

Selective Dorsal Rhizotomy

Selective dorsal rhizotomy (SDR) is designed to reduce moderate to severe lower-extremity spasticity by minimizing aberrant muscle spindle input believed to trigger muscle overactivity. Bone covering the first two lumbar segments is removed. Afferent fibers in the dorsal roots from L1 to S2 are dissected, and those rootlets that demonstrate excessive activity are severed. Studies have demonstrated that the combination of SDR and intensive post operative PT is beneficial in reducing spasticity in children with diplegic cerebral palsy and produces gains in strength, gait speed, and overall gross motor function (Noetzel, 2012).

Patients most suitable for SDR are those between the ages of 4 and 10 with spastic diplegia or mild quadriplegia who have some degree of ambulatory capability (Box 162-6) (Noetzel, 2003). Most have a history of prematurity or evidence of periventricular leukomalacia on imaging studies. Those unsuitable for SDR include patients with spasticity from congenital or neonatal CNS infection and head trauma or hypoxic brain injury outside the newborn period (Box 162-6). In addition, children with very weak abdominal muscles and those with predominant dystonia or ataxia are less likely to benefit from SDR.

Orthopedic Surgery

Even with optimal treatment, spasticity may progress to cause contractures and bony deformities necessitating orthopedic intervention such as tendon releases for fixed contractures at the ankle, surgery to correct hip subluxation or dislocation, and instrumentation for scoliosis. The benefit of orthopedic surgery is most pronounced in patients who have achieved some degree of skeletal maturation.

Treatment of Dystonia and Other Hyperkinetic Movement Disorders

A number of movement disorders have been recognized in children after traumatic brain injury and stroke (Dosenbach and Noetzel, 2014). Management is predicated upon the type of movement disorder, but unfortunately most medications have proven to be ineffective or of minimal benefit. For children with acquired dystonia, trihexyphenidyl, tetrabenazine, and botulinum toxin injections often are utilized.

ACQUIRED BRAIN INJURY

Traumatic brain injury, together with stroke, hypoxic/ischemic injury, brain tumor, and CNS infection, account for about 75% of all pediatric admissions to an acute neurorehabilitation service (Noetzel, 2012). Even though the primary injury may be focal, brain damage is typically widely distributed in most patients. Secondary injury from cerebral edema, hypoxia, or ischemia, often in the setting of elevated intracranial pressure, may inflict additional diffuse damage, especially in infants with nonaccidental trauma. Although the pathology of acquired brain injury is variable, certain neurorehabilitation issues require attention in almost every child recovering from this type of injury.

Behavioral Disturbances

Behavioral aberrations are a nearly universal consideration and can be observed in all stages of recovery (Noetzel, 2012). Agitation, characterized as nonpurposeful, random, motor and verbal activity, is common early in recovery. Emotional regression and impaired information processing likewise often are observed and may persist for weeks or months. Sedative medications usually are without benefit and, in fact, symptoms may be aggravated by further clouding the sensorium. In the middle stages of recovery, patients often have limited understanding of their own deficits and intolerance to sensory stimulation (Noetzel, 2003). Hyperactivity and impulsivity are typical manifestations seen in a child 3 to 8 years old; in older children and adolescents, the behavioral theme is one of decreased motivation and poor initiation of action, combined with lethargy. Therapeutic intervention and management strategies require ongoing careful assessment of the patient's attention and arousal patterns. Medications with adverse cognitive or behavioral side effects should be withdrawn when possible. Careful modulation of a child's surroundings may be beneficial, avoiding either overstimulation or prolonged sensory deprivation. Alerting, orienting, and preparing a child for any therapy activity is important. In addition, it is essential to monitor the child's response so as to determine which environmental adaptations are beneficial (Noetzel, 2003).

In some children with acquired brain injury, aberrant behavior persists and medication may need to be prescribed, recognizing that the use of pharmacologic agents to manage behavior in this clinical setting has not been investigated in a scientifically rigorous manner. The most pressing behavioral issues of aggression and severe agitation have been treated with beta blockers, carbamazepine, and tricyclic antidepressants, as well as clonidine, amantadine, and buspirone (Noetzel, 2012). Stimulants may have a role in children with underarousal and slow cognitive processing.

Communication and Cognitive Deficits

Deficits in communication and cognition are exceedingly common and represent the largest cause of long-term disability, most often affecting memory and learning of new information. Agents acting upon the various neurotransmitter systems have been employed to establish an appropriate level of arousal and sustained attention. Although not overwhelming, the results do demonstrate a likely overall beneficial effect. Efficacy of pharmacologic intervention with respect to memory and learning has not been demonstrated (Noetzel, 2012).

Therapeutic interventions for communication and cognitive impairment should be initiated in the acute care setting, with the main focus on providing sensory modulation. Cognitive retraining should pervade all aspects of the therapy process. Finally, rehabilitation should be predicated not only on enhancing preserved function, but also on remediating residual deficits, utilizing standardized tests to establish a structured intervention program (Noetzel, 2003).

Postinjury Seizures

Seizures resulting from brain trauma commonly occur within the first 7 to 10 days after injury. The risk is highest in children under the age of 3 years and those with a severe injury or any nonaccidental brain injury. The incidence of posttraumatic epilepsy (PTE) is less than 1%; severity of brain injury and the presence of early seizures are the most important predictive factors for PTE (Noetzel, 2012). Early seizures do not mandate treatment, but recurrent seizures can be treated with levetiracetam, especially in patients with raised intracranial pressure and those with risk factors for late seizures, such as intraparenchymal hemorrhage and penetrating cerebral injury. There is, however, no convincing evidence in children that prophylactic therapy prevents PTE. In contrast, epilepsy as a long-term complication occurs in 15% to 20% of childhood acute ischemic stroke patients, with large cortical infarcts imposing the highest risk. In patients with seizures at stroke onset, anticonvulsants are warranted, with the choice of medication dictated by seizure semiology and EEG findings.

PEDIATRIC STROKE

There is increasing recognition of the incidence, severity, and functional impact of pediatric stroke and of the consequent rehabilitation needs of survivors. Disability caused by pediatric stroke and its influence on a child's quality of life endures over decades (Dosenbach and Noetzel, 2014). Although brain damage from a stroke is not progressive, the resultant functional deficits typically evolve over time, commensurate with nervous system maturation. Permanent motor and cognitive dysfunction is seen in the majority of pediatric stroke survivors, with deficits ranging from 50% to 90%.

Novel Rehabilitation Strategies-Overview

Fueled by a growing understanding of brain reorganization stategies, various novel rehabilitation treatments are currently in different stages of development and efficacy testing, mostly in adults (Carmichael, 2010). Because stroke recovery utilizes some of the same systems-level, neuronal and molecular mechanisms as learning, theraputic interventions demonstrated to improve learning are being applied to stroke patients.

Novel stroke rehabilitation treatments can be grouped into three basic categories. First, many are practice programs that build on existing therapy paradigms but incorporate novel technologies or vary some of the specifics of training. A second group has as its foundation electrical stimulation of the nervous system. Finally, medications are being tested in the hope that they might boost recovery from stroke. Although most novel rehabilitation treatments have focused on improving motor outcome, efforts are under way to extend these therapies into other domains such as the restoration of sensory, language, attentional, and executive deficits (Dosenbach and Noetzel, 2014). However, these interventions have not demonstrated any lasting benefit over convential therpies in the small number of pediatric patients enrolled. There is increasing interest in the potential use of stem cell therapy (Chapter 15).

Practice Based Therapies—Constraint Induced Movement Therapy and Robot Assisted Therapy

In pediatrics, intervention with CIMT has focused on children with hemiparesis from presumed perinatal stroke, utilizing a bivalvedcast to restrain the more functional arm (Fig. 162-5). CIMT can result in lasting improvements in motor function compared with standard, less intense treatment. A recent study found slightly better outcomes for CIMT compared with dose-matched bimanual intensive therapy immediately after the treatment period, but these differences were not sustained at 12-month follow up (Sakzewski, et al., 2011). Robot-assisted therapy may eventually allow convenient delivery of the high volume of repetitions needed to effect use-dependent neural plasticity (Noetzel, 2012) and currently is being investigated in children with cerebral palsy and stroke.

Stimulation of the Nervous System to Improve Stroke Recovery

Numerous studies have demonstrated that functional neuro-anatomy of the brain's distributed systems can be reshaped by task practice (Lewis, et al., 2009), but repetitive training is time consuming. Thus there is significant interest in directly stimulating the nervous system to bypass or at least enhance task practice. Transcranial magnetic stimulation (TMS), which uses rapidly shifting magnetic fields to induce small currents, has been well studied in pediatric patients. Repetitive TMS (rTMS) can increase or decrease the excitability of underlying cortex and appears to induce a local state of heightened use-dependent neuroplasticity via several molecular and cellular mechanisms, including both GABA and glutamate levels. Evidence for clinical efficacy of rTMS is limited to small-scale studies in children with chronic paresis after stroke (Kirton,

et al., 2008). More research is needed before it can become a mainstream treatment, but rTMS appears to have great potential.

Medications to Improve Stroke Recovery

Efforts to find neurorehabilitative medications have focused on compounds shown to improve use-dependent neuroplasticity and learning, including selective serotonin reuptake inhibitors, stimulants, and agents that increase dopamine. In the best trial to date, adults with moderate to severe motor deficits who were randomized to 90 days of standard rehabilitative care plus 20 mg of fluoxetine daily had significantly better outcomes compared with standard care plus placebo. Thus it may be reasonable to consider fluoxetine treatment in teenagers who have suffered a motor stroke (Dosenbach and Noetzel, 2014). Stimulant medications and dopamine also induce neuroplasticity and improve stroke recovery in animal models, but no data exists to determine whether pediatric patients might benefit from their use during stroke recover.

SPINAL CORD INJURY

About 20% of acute SCI patients are under 20 years of age. Although trauma accounts for the vast majority of SCI in children, demyelination, infarction, and tumors contribute to cases of myelopathy. The neurologic examination with suspected SCI entails a sensory evaluation of dermatomes and strength assessment in key muscles in the arms and legs. An understanding of motor movement and reflexes, as they relate to spinal level, aids in the examination (Table 162-2). The assigned level of injury is the lowest segment at which sensory and motor responses are intact bilaterally. The American Spinal Injury Association provides criteria defining the extent of injury that not only informs rehabilitation decisions (Box 162-7), but also has predictive value because mobility and independence in activities of daily living outcomes correlate with the level of functional motor activity.

Medical Issues

Pulmonary complications such as ventilator failure, pulmonary edema, pneumonia, and aspiration are a major source of morbidity and mortality in the acute stage of SCI. Patients with high cervical injuries (C1–C4) typically require lifelong

TABLE 162-2 Neurologic Examination to Determine the Spinal Level of Injury

Spinal Level	Cutaneous Sensation	Motor Function	Working Muscles	Reflex
C5	Lateral upper arm	Elbow flexion	Biceps, deltoid	Biceps
C6	Anteromedial arm/thumb	Wrist extension	Extensor carpi ulnaris/radialis	Brachioradialis
C7	Posterior forearm/middle finger	Elbow extension	Triceps	Triceps
C8	Fourth/fifth fingers	Finger flexion	Flexor digitorum sublimis	
T12	Lower abdomen	None	None	
L1	Groin	Weak hip flexion	Iliopsoas	
L2	Anterior upper thigh	Full hip flexion	Iliopsoas and sartorius	
L3	Anterior distal thigh/knee	Knee extension	Quadriceps	Knee jerk
L4	Medial leg	Knee flexion/hip adduction	Medial hamstrings	Knee jerk
L5	Lateral leg/medial knee	Foot dorsiflexion/eversion	Anterior tibial/peroneals	Ankle jerk
S1	Sole of foot	Foot plantar flexion	Gastrocnemius/soleus	Ankle jerk
S2	Posterior leg/thigh	Toe flexion	Flexor hallucis	Anal wink
S3	Middle of buttock	None	None	Anal wink

ventilator support because respiratory muscles are innervated by cranial nerve XI and C2–C4. Individuals with injuries from C3–C5 have varying degrees of ventilator compromise depending on diaphragmatic function, whereas damage at the C6–C7 level usually allows for eventual discontinuation of ventilator support.

Once spinal shock resolves, bladder spasticity with detrusor hyperreflexia produces elevated voiding pressures and impaired emptying, with the potential for renal damage. Treatment consists of intermittent catheterization and anticholinergic medications. Bowel dysfunction in SCI almost always takes the form of constipation and incomplete evacuation of stool, thus a bowel management program, with stool softeners and suppositories, as well as digital stimulation, is important.

Other concerns in children with SCI include heterotopic ossification, hypercalcemia, and deep vein thrombosis (DVT), the latter of which occurs in 10% of adolescents. In adults with SCI, thromboprophylaxis with low molecular weight heparin is recommended for the first 3 months; data are less compelling in children.

Rehabilitation Strategies

Childhood SCI produces greater disability than a similar injury in an adult. In addition to the profound multisystem trauma that often occurs in an SCI, in a child there is secondary impairment created by the disruption of normal development, physical growth, and psychosocial maturation. Although rehabilitation goals are dictated by specific deficits in bodily function, the overriding aim is to treat the needs of the whole child and maximize the potential for future independence. Patients with C1–C4 injuries require significant adaptive equipment, typically with activating switches. In most cervical cord injuries, a power wheelchair is indicated, with the method of control determined by the level of injury. Appropriate splinting and orthotics may facilitate greater independence in feeding and upper-extremity dressing. With slightly lower injury levels, patients have adequate arm extension and improved hand function, which are critical for wheelchair propulsion (Fig. 162-6), the ability to self-transfer, and participation in bowel and bladder training programs. Programs and equipment designed to assist ambulation are predicated on residual muscle function in the trunk and legs. Finally, regardless of injury level, pressure relief is necessary, and patients, as well as their caretakers, need to be instructed in this maneuver to minimize development of decubitus ulcers.

FUTURE DIRECTIONS

Pediatric neurorehabilitation has improved dramatically over the last quarter century. Our understanding of the mechanisms of recovery has accelerated, leading to the hope that this knowledge can be translated into specific neurologic therapies that can serve as the basis for restorative rehabilitation. The more immediate need is to upgrade the neurorehabilitation treatments we provide for our patients. Few of the currently employed interventions, medications, and physical modalities implemented in the rehabilitation of children have been subjected to rigorous scientific research with appropriate control subjects. Most investigations involve limited populations, with little regard for the influence of normal development on recovery; many fail to recognize that achievement of functional goals is the only meaningful outcome. Double-blinded protocols, utilizing quantifiable clinically relevant outcomes, are essential for the growth of rehabilitation and improving the care we provide to neurologically injured children.

REFERENCES

The complete list of references for this chapter is available in the e-book at www.expertconsult.com.
See inside cover for registration details.

SELECTED REFERENCES

Carmichael, S.T., 2010. Translating the frontiers of brain repair to treatments: starting not to break the rules. Neurobiol. Dis. 37 (2), 237–242.

Carter, A.R., Shulman, G.L., Corbetta, M., 2012. Why use a connectivity-based approach to study stroke and recovery of function? Neuroimage 62 (4), 2271–2280.

Delgado, M.R., Hirtz, D., Aisen, M., et al., 2010. Practice parameter: pharmacological treatment of spasticity in children and adolescents with cerebral palsy (an evidence-based review); report of the Quality Standards Subcommittee of the American Academy of Neurology and the Practice Committee of the Child Neurology Society. Neurology 74, 336–343.

Dosenbach, N.U.F., Noetzel, M.J., 2014. Rehabilitation of children after stroke. In: Stein, J., Harvey, R.L., Winstein, C.J., et al. (Eds.), Stroke Recovery and Rehabilitation, 2nd ed. Demos Medical, New York, pp. 699–734.

Johnston, M.V., 2009. Plasticity in the developing brain: implications for rehabilitation. Dev. Disabil. Res. Rev. 15 (2), 94–101.

Kirton, A., Chen, R., Friefeld, S., et al., 2008. Contralesional repetitive transcranial magnetic stimulation for chronic hemiparesis in subcortical paediatric stroke: a randomized trial. Lancet Neurol. 7 (6), 507–513.

Lewis, C.M., Baldassarre, A., Committeri, G., et al., 2009. Learning sculpts the spontaneous activity of the resting human brain. Proc. Natl. Acad. Sci. U.S.A. 106 (41), 17558–17563.

Noetzel, M.J., 2003. Acute pediatric neurorehabilitation. In: Winn, H.R. (Ed.), Youman's Neurological Surgery, 5th ed. Elsevier Science, Philadelphia, pp. 3783–3791.

Noetzel, M.J., 2012. Pediatric neurorehabilitation medicine. In: Swaiman, K.F., Ashwal, S., Ferriero, D.M., et al. (Eds.), Swaiman's Pediatric Neurology: Principles and Practice, 5th ed. Elsevier Science, Philadelphia, pp. e234–e249.

Sakzewski, L., Ziviani, J., Boyd, R.N., 2011. Best responders after intensive upper-limb training for children with unilateral cerebral palsy. Arch. Phys. Med. Rehabil. 92 (4), 578–584.

E-BOOK FIGURES AND TABLES

The following figures and tables are available in the e-book at www.expertconsult.com. See inside cover for registration details.

163 Pain Management and Palliative Care

John Colin Partridge and Elizabeth E. Rogers

 An expanded version of this chapter is available on www.expertconsult.com. See inside cover for registration details.

PAIN MANAGEMENT

Introduction

Pain has been defined as "an unpleasant sensory and emotional experience associated with actual or potential tissue damage, or described in terms of such damage" from thermal, chemical, or mechanical stimuli. Nociception, or pain perception, is the series of electrochemical events after the tissue damage or injury, excluding any emotional correlates of the noxious sensation. Acute pain is common in pediatric medical encounters, and chronic pain affects an estimated 15% to 30% of children. Only 20% of patients achieve effective relief of chronic pain.

Historical Background

Studies from the 1970s into the 1990s documented undertreatment of pediatric patients compared with adults undergoing uncomfortable diagnostic procedures (e.g., lumbar puncture) and even for major surgical procedures. Newborn infants have both the neurophysiologic basis necessary to experience and remember pain and an intact and functional opiate receptor system. Appropriately, routine pain assessment is now standard of care, and there is consensus on the need to prevent and treat pain in pediatric patients (Hall and Anand, 2014).

Physiology

Nociceptors transduce a noxious stimulus into electrical sensory nerve activity, and the sensory information is projected to the central nervous system via several types of fibers to the dorsal root and on to the medial and lateral divisions of the dorsolateral fasciculus, then forming synapses within the laminae of spinal cord gray matter (Simons and Tibboel, 2006). Neurons within the spinal cord relay information via the long ascending tracts to various portions of the brain, including the locus ceruleus, thalamus, hypothalamus, anterior and posterior cingulate gyrus, amygdala, insular cortex, and somatosensory cortex, forming what has been termed the "pain matrix."

Developmental Differences

Fetal stress responses to pain have been documented as early as 18 weeks' gestation, with peripheral, spinal, and supraspinal capacity for afferent pain transmission by 26 weeks' gestation (Lee et al., 2005). Neonates demonstrate characteristic facial expressions, aversive body movements, alterations in cardiac activity, and changes in cry in response to painful stimuli. Nociceptive receptors are fewer in number in children; so tissue damage must be more significant before a pain response is elicited. Young infants may perceive pain more intensely than older children or adults because inhibitory pathways develop later than afferent excitatory pathways. Inadequately treated pain in premature infants is associated with adverse short-term effects (e.g., more postoperative com-

plications); the accompanying physiologic changes (increases in heart rate, blood pressure, cardiac variability, autonomic tone, venous pressure, cerebral blood flow, and intrathoracic and intracranial pressure) may augment the risks for intraventricular hemorrhage or white-matter injury in the immature brain. Repetitive pain may lead to accentuated neuronal apoptosis, wind-up, pain syndromes, long-term behavioral changes, and diminished visual-perceptual abilities at school age (Grunau et al., 2009).

Clinical Assessment

Infants and children demonstrate nonspecific but consistent behavioral, physiologic, and autonomic responses to pain (Box 163-1). There is no single, uniform, standard technique for assessing pain in neonates or children. Biochemical responses to pain, (cortisol, catecholamines, beta-endorphins, insulin, glucagon, renin-aldosterone, growth hormone, and prolactin) are not specific to pain.

Self-report, usually by linear analog scale, is regarded as most reliable among children having sufficient cognitive capacity. For preverbal patients, pain assessment is best achieved using multidimensional scales, including behavioral, physiologic, and autonomic responses. Behavioral observational scales are used for pain assessment with children under the age of 4 or with cognitive impairment. Toddlers and preschool children can often use standardized, semiquantitative pain assessment tools (poker chips, cartoons of faces, a pain thermometer, and colors or words) to rate pain intensity. Children of 8 years or older can effectively use questionnaires or visual analog scales designed for adults. Newer studies are investigating the use of near-infrared spectroscopy and EEG to monitor neonatal cortical pain responses.

Management

Pain, acute or chronic, should be assessed regularly and treated aggressively with nonpharmacologic methods and appropriate analgesics with around-the-clock dosing tailored to individual patient needs. In neonates, nonnutritive sucking (with or without sucrose), distraction, breastfeeding, swaddling, kangaroo care, contralateral tactile stimulation, massage, acupuncture, music therapy, and multisensorial stimulation can decrease the pain severity and needs for pharmacologic treatment. Nonpharmacologic interventions should be developmentally appropriate for older patients.

When pharmacologic management is required, regular doses should be ordered at appropriate intervals with added "as necessary" medication for breakthrough pain (Howard et al., 2008). Doses should be titrated according to response. Mild pain that is unresponsive to cognitive techniques or sucrose in neonates can be treated with nonsteroidal antiinflammatory (NSAIDs) drugs or acetaminophen. For moderate pain, oral "weaker" opioids or combinations of opioids and NSAIDs or acetaminophen can be used. Severe pain requires more aggressive parenteral opioids such as morphine or

BOX 163-1 Responses to Painful Stimuli

BEHAVIORAL RESPONSES TO PAIN

1. Crying, whimpering
2. Facial expressions: brow bulge, eye squeeze, and deepening of the nasolabial folds
3. Active movement and attempts to withdraw from the painful stimulus
   a. Thrashing
   b. Tremulousness
   c. Limb withdrawal, flexion
   d. Bicycling
   e. Arching
4. Disorganized behavior; limpness and flaccidity
5. Flexor reflexes; leg withdrawal
6. Exaggerated reactivity
7. State changes
   a. Decreased sleep periods
   b. Rapid changes in state cycles
   c. Decreased rapid eye movement (REM) sleep

PHYSIOLOGIC/AUTONOMIC RESPONSES

1. Changes in heart rate and variability
2. Respiratory rate and quality
3. Fluctuations in blood pressure
4. Decreased transcutaneous oxygen and carbon dioxide levels
5. Oxygen desaturation
6. Increased intracranial pressure
7. Palmar sweating
8. Pallor
9. Flushing
10. Pupillary dilatation
11. Increased catabolic state

TABLE 163-2 Dosage Guidelines for Analgesics

Drug	Dose	Interval (Hr)	Route
NONOPIOID ANALGESICS			
Sucrose	0.2 mL of 30% solution*		PO
Acetaminophen	10–15 mg/kg	4	PO, PR
	Maximal daily dose		
	Infants: <75 mg/kg		
	Neonates >32 wks: 60 mg/kg		
	Neonates 28–32 wks: 40 mg/kg		
Ibuprofen	6–10 mg/kg	6	
Naproxen	5–6 mg/kg	8–12	PO, PR
Aspirin[†]	10–15 mg/kg	4–6	
Ketorolac	0.5 mg/kg	8	IV
OPIOID ANALGESICS (INITIAL DOSES AND INTERVALS)			
Morphine[‡]	Bolus: 0.1 mg/kg	2–4	IV
	Infusion		
	Children: 0.03 mg/kg/hr		IV
	Infants: 0.01–0.03 mg/kg/hr		IV
	Term neonates: 0.005–0.02 mg/kg/hr		IV
	Preterm neonates: 0.002–0.01 mg/kg/hr		IV
	Oral immediate release: 0.3 mg/kg	3–4	PO
	Oral sustained release		
	20–35 kg: 10–15 mg/kg	8–12	PO
	35–50 kg: 15–30 mg/kg	8–12	PO
Oxycodone	0.1–0.2 mg/kg	3–4	PO
Methadone	0.1 mg/kg	4–8	IV, PO
Fentanyl	Bolus: 0.5–1.0 µg/kg	1–2	IV
	Infusion		
	Children: 0.05–2.0 µg/kg/hr		IV
	Infants: 1–2 µg/kg/hr		IV
	Term neonates: 0.05–2 µg/kg/hr		IV
	Preterm neonates: 0.05–1 µg/kg/hr		IV
	Transdermal: Children: 12.5 µg/hr		TD
Hydromorphone	Bolus: 0.02 mg/kg	2–4	IV
	Infusion: 0.006 mg/kg/hr		IV
	Oral 0.04–0.08 mg/kg	3–4	PO

*Optimal dose not established.
[†]Restricted use for antiplatelet or anti-inflammatory effect.
[‡]No ceiling effect for severe pain.
IV, intravenous; PO, by mouth; PR, rectal; TD, transdermal.
(Adapted from: Berde, C.B., Sethna, N.F., 2002. Analgesics for the treatment of pain in children. N Engl J Med 347, 1094–1103; Stevens, B. et al., 2000. Treatment of pain in the neonatal intensive care unit. Pediatr Clin North Am 47, 633–650; Holder, K.A., Patt, R.B., 1995. Taming the pain monster: pediatric postoperative pain management. Pediatr Ann 24, 164–168; Tobias, J.D., 2000. Weak analgesics and nonsteroidal anti-inflammatory agents in the management of children with acute pain. Pediatr Clin North Am 47:527–543.)

fentanyl. Intractable pain or unacceptable toxicities of pain medications may require nerve blocks or intraspinal anesthetic infusions. For prolonged pain, neuropathic pain, addictive behavior, history of addiction, or complicated family or psychosocial issues, referral to a multidisciplinary pain service consultation may be helpful.

Types of Pain Medications

Aspirin, Acetaminophen, and NSAIDs

Aspirin is used less commonly as an analgesic in pediatrics because of its association with Reye's syndrome. NSAIDs are most effective as preemptive agents or for treatment of mild to moderate pain of somatic origin. Acetaminophen is used widely for minor pain and discomfort. Ibuprofen and naproxen have gained wide acceptance in pediatric use and are equally effective. For children who cannot tolerate oral dosing, ketorolac is available. Concurrent use of NSAIDs can reduce opioid dosing needed for effective analgesia. The use of more than one NSAID concurrently offers little therapeutic advantage and increases side effects. Dosage guidelines and maximal doses are summarized in Table 163-2.

Opioids

Opioids are the mainstay of treatment of severe pain, operative procedures, postoperative pain relief, and chronic painful medical conditions in neonates and children. Agonist-antagonist drugs are not recommended as they may precipitate withdrawal if given concomitantly with full agonists, and they have have limited routes of administration. Suggested guidelines for opiate-naive patients are shown in Table 163-2.

As opiate agonists have no therapeutic ceiling, dosages should be adjusted to meet the patient's individual needs. Clinicians should not hesitate to treat pain aggressively out of fear for later addiction. Increased risks for respiratory depression in young infants younger than 6 months of age require close cardiorespiratory, and oxygen saturation monitoring. Methadone, a long-acting opioid agonist, has been utilized in combination therapy for children with cancer pain. Fentanyl is the drug most often used for short procedures because of its rapid onset, peak effect, and short duration of action.

Opioids may be administered subcutaneously, orally, rectally, transdermally, or intranasally, or by patient-controlled analgesia in children over age 7 years. For some procedures, oral transmucosal or transdermal fentanyl provides an alternative for conscious sedation, although emesis is a frequent side effect. Rectal administration can be utilized when oral dosing is contraindicated; intramuscular injection should be a last resort. Tolerance may develop more rapidly with continuous infusions and with use of synthetic opioids. Opiate withdrawal can occur when opioids are discontinued abruptly after several days of exposure. Although considered safe, bolus opioids are associated with an increased incidence of severe intraventricular hemorrhage, white matter injury, and short-term neurodevelopmental abnormalities.

Procedural Sedation and Analgesia

Methods such as perioperative preparation, relaxation training, distraction, guided imagery, cognitive interventions, and hypnosis may reduce the need for pharmacologic treatment for minor procedures. More uncomfortable procedures require deeper sedation, more appropriately performed by anesthesiologists, intensivists, or emergency physicians experienced in deep sedation techniques and monitoring. The American Academy of Pediatrics has defined two levels of sedation for procedures that are less deep than general anesthesia: 1) conscious sedation, a medically controlled state of depressed consciousness that preserves protective reflexes, airway, and responses to physical stimuli or verbal commands; and 2) deep sedation, involving depressed consciousness or unconsciousness when the patient is not easily aroused, cannot protect the airway, or respond to physical stimuli or verbal commands (Committee on Drugs, 2002).

Analgesia

Topical analgesia such as EMLA (eutectic mixture of topical anesthetics, prilocaine, and lidocaine) can reduce the discomfort of minor procedures. For very brief procedures, ethyl chloride or fluoromethane can provide limited analgesia. Local anesthetics or peripheral nerve blocks should be used for lumbar punctures, difficult intravenous cannulation, suturing, or procedures involving prolonged pain. For surgical procedures, fentanyl is preferable because of its faster onset, shorter duration, and lack of a histamine-inducing effect. For longer duration procedures, morphine remains the preferable agent. Ketamine induces profound analgesia while maintaining spontaneous respiratory activity, airway tone, and protective reflexes; it may be the drug of choice for emergency procedures when the patient has not fasted. When used in conjunction with propofol for short-term procedural sedation, doses and side effects are reduced.

Sedation

Benzodiazepines are the most commonly used drugs for sedating children, particularly in pediatric intensive care. Midazolam is the preferred drug for procedural sedation given its rapid onset of action, short half-life, and potent sedative and anxiolytic effects. For painful procedures, benzodiazepine sedation should be accompanied by opioid analgesia, and patients should be monitored for hypoxia or respiratory depression. Barbiturates are regarded as the sedatives of choice for diagnostic imaging in children younger than 3 years of age but provide no analgesia. Chloral hydrate, an acceptably safe sedative without analgesic efficacy, can be used for nonpainful procedures such as electroencephalograms and diagnostic imaging in children younger 3 years of age, although it has a long half-life and concerns about potential carcinogenicity.

Given at subanesthetic doses, intravenous ultrashort-acting agents (etomidate, methohexital, propofol, remifentanil, and thiopental) can be used for procedural analgesias but should be used only by certified practitioners due to risks for oversedation or rapid swings in consciousness.

Types of Pain
Neuropathic Pain

Neuropathic pain is seldom responsive to opioids, often requiring multiple modalities for effective pain relief. Analgesic agents recommended for first-line medications for neuropathic pain in pediatric patients are gabapentinoids, tricyclic antidepressants, and serotonin noradrenaline reuptake inhibitors. For moderate to severe pain, tramadol and controlled-release opioid analgesics are recommended as second-line medications, with cannabinoids now recommended as third-line treatments. Other drugs for management of neuropathic pain include methadone, less efficacious anticonvulsants (e.g., lamotrigine), tapentadol, or botulinum toxin. Phantom pain after amputation may respond to preemptive regional anesthesia, antiepileptics, tricyclic antidepressants, calcitonin, topical agents, or intrathecal medication. Nerve trauma may be treated with injected local anesthetics, steroids, neurolysis, antiepileptics, tricyclic antidepressants, or mexiletine. Neuropathies after chemotherapy can be treated with antiepileptics, tricyclic antidepressants, or mexiletine.

Pain in Children With Significant Neurological Impairment

Children with cerebral palsy or developmental delays do experience pain despite some reports of blunted pain responses or insensitivity to pain. Pain from spasticity and muscle spasms can be treated with diazepam, dantrolene, oral baclofen, or botulinum toxin. Oral analgesia is the preferred route as intramuscular injections may be more painful in children with decreased muscle mass. Subcutaneous and transdermal administration can be used for chronic administration. Patients with neurologic impairment are more likely to have pain discounted or denied and thus may have pain treated ineffectively. In patients too impaired to communicate pain levels, behavioral responses should be regarded as effective surrogate indications for analgesic treatment. Analgesic needs must be balanced by the recognition that systemic opioids may have undesirable side effects such as respiratory depression or constipation.

Migraine and Headache

NSAIDs or weak analgesics can be given for mild to moderate pain from tension headaches and to many children with migraine attacks. Once a chronic pattern is established, cognitive-behavioral techniques such as biofeedback and relaxation therapy may help alleviate headaches. Practitioners should be aware of the possible development of medication overuse headache when NSAIDS or opiates are used chronically (Lewis et al., 2002, Lewis et al., 2004). Sumatriptan is an effective and safe abortive treatment; dihydroergotamine and ibuprofen may help interrupt episodes. Other drugs studied for prevention of migraine include beta-blockers, calcium-channel blockers, and antidepressants. For migraine, the hallmark of effective control is treatment early in an attack.

Summary

Pain in pediatric patients is often underrecognized and undertreated. Relief of pain is one of the most important aspects of ethical pediatric care. Judicious use of nonpharmacologic modalities, analgesics, and anxiolytics to treat pain is recommended until further research indicates the medications and dosing schedules that relieve pain and pose the least side effects or neurodevelopmental risks.

PALLIATIVE CARE
Introduction

At least 500,000 children suffer life-threatening medical conditions such as extreme prematurity, heritable disorders, or acquired diseases warranting palliative care services; of these, 15,000 die each year (Feudtner et al., 2011; Himelstein et al., 2004). Nearly half of pediatric deaths and over 70% of deaths from chronic complex conditions occur in hospital; of these, nearly half occur in an intensive care setting. It is estimated that only 5000 to 7000 children receive hospice care or formal palliative care services and that another 10,000 to 15,000 children could benefit from them. Recent population-based studies have documented that 15% of pediatric hospital deaths are from neurologic or neuromuscular diseases. Neuromuscular disorders cause 3% to 4% of childhood deaths in all age groups but account for 18% of deaths of children with complex chronic conditions (Feudtner, 2007). A third of the children referred for palliative care have neuromuscular conditions, and another 41% have genetic or congenital conditions that may have neurologic consequences (Ho and Straatman, 2013).

Children with neuromuscular disorders tend to be referred for palliative care earlier than those with other chronic diseases (cancer, human immunodeficiency virus, cystic fibrosis, sickle cell disease, or chronic lung disease); however, 30% to 35% of children with metabolic diseases, muscular dystrophy, severe cerebral palsy, and posttraumatic brain injury receive only end-of-life care. Some neurologists may feel they lack the training or experience in addressing the complex needs of dying children or communicating bad news to young patients and their families.

Historical Background

Palliative care as an adjunct to modern medical care began with the founding of St. Christopher's Hospice by Cecily Saunders in 1967. Although the first pediatric hospices started in 1982, it is only recently that widespread institution of pediatric palliative care has been recommended, including in intensive care settings. Pediatric palliative care is a cost-effective way to care for dying children, decreasing procedures and intensive care days, increasing support, and facilitating withholding or withdrawing aggressive measures.

Definitions of Palliative Care

Best provided by a multidisciplinary team (Box 163-3), the focus of palliative care is to provide comprehensive, compassionate, and developmentally appropriate care that optimizes the quality of life by meeting the physical, psychological, emotional, social, and spiritual needs of the child as the disease progresses. The intent is a decent or good death, free from avoidable distress and suffering for patients, families, or caregivers.

Components of Palliative Care
Identifying the Need

Children with neuromuscular diseases and their family members have palliative care needs that differ from those of

---

BOX 163-3 Interdisciplinary Team for Palliative Care

- Primary care provider, community pediatricians, subspecialists
- Pediatric registered nurses/case managers
- Pediatric social worker
- Child life therapist
- Spiritual care counselor
- Home health aides
- Pediatric medical consultants
- Physical/occupational therapists
- Clinical pharmacist
- Clinical dietitian
- Volunteers
- Insurers/payers
- Other providers
- Regional centers
- Durable medical equipment companies
- Community pharmacies

---

dying adults. A series of questions can help inform the counseling process and considerations about the appropriateness of further interventions of changing the goals of care when necessary. First, what has been the child's health status and quality of life previously? Second, how likely is the child to survive the current life-threatening condition? Third, what degree of suffering is entailed if the child survives in the short term? Fourth, what is the anticipated quality of life in the future and how long is it expected to endure? Fifth, how likely are future crises or deteriorations? Discussions about treatment options should assist the child and parents in selecting which measures should or should not be done (Feudtner 2007).

Critically ill or dying children benefit from being with and comforted by their parents. Providers should allow time for the family to nurture their child and recognize the emotional stress of anticipating neurologic compromise or death. Providers should attempt to give parents and, when appropriate, children some sense of control in their care.

Transition in Goals of Care

Palliative care should not be restricted to children expected to die soon when therapeutic interventions fail or are withdrawn. Providers should learn to recognize when needs for palliative care become more salient with neurodegenerative diseases or progressive neuropathies or as complications from a static encephalopathy impinge on quality of life. In conditions associated with a predictably shortened life span (e.g., trisomy 13 and 18, neurodegenerative diseases, anencephaly, and many inborn errors of metabolism), the primary focus of care is limited to optimizing quality of life. For diseases with less certain prognoses (for example, traumatic or hypoxic brain injury, some central nervous system or spinal tumors, congenital myopathies and neuropathies), it is appropriate to introduce palliative care at an early stage that can soften the effect of nonintervention discussions *later* in the disease trajectory. With older children, it is important to address future choices for care before the neurologic status deteriorates and bars them from participating in healthcare decisions. Parents must be given the information necessary to decision making and be made aware of the limits of our prognostic ability. An essential step is to clarify, and reassess periodically, the goals of continuing, rather than limiting, ongoing interventions as the chances for cure lessen.

Levels of Care

A shift from curative to palliative treatment goals does not imply that all ongoing medical interventions must be abandoned. It is important to clarify specific measures that will continue to be utilized, as well as what level of nonintervention appears most appropriate. An order proscribing all or selected resuscitative measures in the event of a cardiac or respiratory arrest (a "Do not resuscitate" or "Do not attempt resuscitation" order) is often an appropriate first step; it is not a half-hearted resuscitation ("slow code") order. It should be discussed with parents and the healthcare team before being written. Withholding of life-sustaining measures involves an agreement not to institute medically indicated measures given that more aggressive interventions would not improve a grim prognosis or quality of life. Interventions deemed futile are not required and should be discontinued. Withdrawal of life-sustaining measures involves the discontinuation of current medical interventions deemed either futile or no longer appropriate to the child's best interests.

Communication

Patterns of communication sensitive to the child's developmental status and to the parents' emotional state are critical to good palliative care. The degree to which the child can participate in decision making increases as children develop sufficient cognitive capacity (over the age of 7). Pictures, stories, toys, music, or other family rituals can help younger children communicate their preferences. Whenever the child has the cognitive capacity to participate, it is important for providers to allow the child the time to express hopes, dreams, and fears. Infections of the nervous system, hypoxia-ischemia, neurodegenerative diseases, or traumatic brain injury may limit older children's decision-making capacity.

Conversations about changing the goals of care when the disease progresses are best held by continuity providers over a period of time, allowing patients or parents time for questions, second opinions, reflection, and informed decision making. To minimize the sense of giving up or abandoning their child, it is critical that parents understand that the goal of care will be to do everything that *should* be done rather than everything that *can* be done.

The primary focus is what is important to the child and the family: longer life, pain-free, time with family members, specific desires, environment and setting, time to say goodbye in ways that respect family values. A structured approach can help physicians deliver difficult news and negotiate goals of care (Box 163-4).

Communications should be simple, direct, clear, and honest explanations that relate the expected outcomes of each treatment option. It is critical to avoid promising outcomes

---

BOX 163-4 Protocol for Palliative Care Communications

SPIKES: A PROTOCOL FOR DELIVERING BAD NEWS AND NEGOTIATING GOALS OF CARE
- **S**etting: create environment conducive to communication
- **P**erception: determine what the family knows
- **I**nvitation: determine how the family would like information delivered
- **K**nowledge: provide information
- **E**motions: empathetically support patient
- **S**ummarize: set realistic goals, make a treatment plan, and follow through
- **R**epeat: review and revise frequently

---

that are not reasonably feasible, overwhelming the parents, or leaving them in despair.

Healthcare Decision Making

Children usually have no previously documented preferences for healthcare decisions; the first issue is to identify who will be making healthcare decisions. In general, advanced directives are not relevant in pediatrics; parents are assumed to be the primary proxy decision makers for young children, although their discretion is not limitless. Older children themselves have the right to determine what quality of life means to them, with support from their parents and physicians.

Parents (or competent adolescents) determine the quantity of information necessary for to informed decision making. If decisions seem not to reflect a full understanding of the disease, the goals of care and expected outcomes should be readdressed. Decisions that do not concur with the provider's choices should be respected when taken in the child's best interests. Ethics committee consultation can help clarify impediments to decision making, the limits to parental decision making, or the need to advocate for the child or refer to child welfare. The resulting care plan should be disseminated to the healthcare team and any limitations to care clearly documented.

Persistent Vegetative State

Although there is no consensus as to whether children in a persistent vegetative state experience pain and suffering, it seems prudent to treat suggestive signs and symptoms. Decisions to withdraw or withhold life-sustaining measures should be made only when neurodiagnostic testing and a sufficient period of observation suggest there is no chance for a meaningful recovery. Decisions involving the withholding of fluids or hydration remain controversial, even when deemed appropriate responses to the child's medical situation.

Environment for Death and Dying

When parents prefer continued inpatient care, a private space for families to gather before and after the child's death is recommended (e.g., a separate comfort care room) but should not impede nursing medical attention to pain and symptoms. Elective transfer to a lower level of care or to a hospice may be preferred and feasible despite concerns about changing care providers late in their child's disease. Death at home from neuromuscular disorders is preferred by an increasing proportion (25%) of children and parents. Plans for a death at home require a continuity provider skilled in managing pain and suffering and able to provide 24-hour coverage from discharge through the child's death and the parents' bereavement.

Support During Dying

When death is near, providers can commit to aggressive treatment of pain or suffering and help parents envision the child's imminent death and the likely timing. Overall support when a child is dying involves a balance between respect for privacy and close, but noninvasive, attention to the child's and the family's needs in collaboration with primary care pediatricians, social workers, clergy, and psychologists or psychiatrists.

Assessment and Treatment of Symptoms

Providers should reevaluate the efficacy of pain and symptom management as the disease progresses. Many neurologists will feel comfortable treating seizures, insomnia, and depression in dying patients but may prefer to have primary care

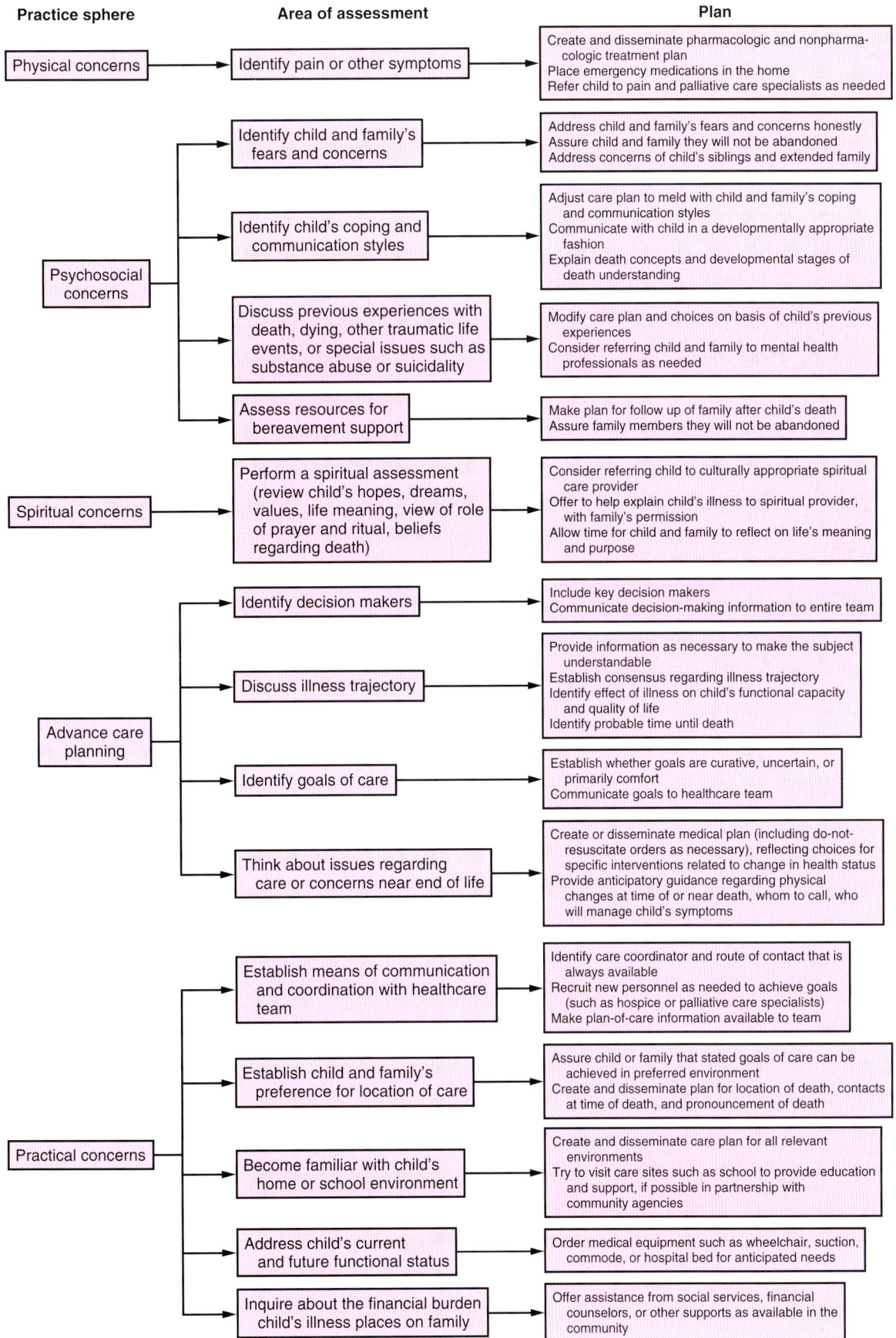

Figure 163-3. Essential elements in the approach to pediatric palliative care.

pediatricians or palliative care specialists manage other frequently encountered end-of-life symptoms (dyspnea, anxiety, fatigue, fever, bleeding, nausea, skin breakdown, anorexia, dehydration, and constipation).

Pain should be treated aggressively with analgesics. Terminal sedation with opioids is effective and justifiable in alleviating severe or unremitting pain at the end of life despite risks of suppressing respiratory drive and thereby hastening death. Fears of addiction to opioids are unwarranted. Paralytics are not appropriate when life support is being withdrawn. Anxiolytics may help terminal agitation and perhaps air hunger experienced in the terminal phases.

Developmental, Emotional and Spiritual Concerns

Care for a dying child requires candor, openness, and an emotional availability to the child's experience of illness and imminent death in a developmentally appropriate manner. Children come to understand death as a change of being by age 3 and as a universal fact of living by age 5 to 6; by age 8 to 9, they have gained a concept of their personal mortality. Developmentally appropriate interactions that respect the children's spiritual nature will allow providers to explore issues of love, hope, security, loneliness, and concepts of the legacy that the child will leave to family and friends. Family routines and rituals add structure and a sense of normality and should be encouraged as the medical condition worsens.

Bereavement

Children are aware of dying and disease; they understand much more about death and dying than adults often realize and do not need to be protected from death and dying as much as they need help making it understandable. Parents often regret not having talked with the child about death. Dying children may grieve about their impending death, the loss of functional status, or the inability to participate in current or future events. They may fear how their family members will cope after their death. When heritable neuromuscular disorders pose a future risk to affected siblings, particular care is necessary to deal with concerns about subsequent pregnancies or fears of future illness.

Providers should allow family members the opportunity to spend time grieving with their deceased child alone, with time to talk and time to be silent. It may be helpful to celebrate their child's life, recap the family's experience, value their loss and emotions, and help them contact family members and friends. Parents should be offered religious observances, social services support, family support groups, or other supportive measures to help them cope. Funerals can help siblings remember and value the dead child. Psychological counseling may help parents and siblings work through the emotional trauma.

Follow-Up Conference

Many physicians arrange a postdeath conference to see how the parents are coping. Clarification of the diagnosis, etiology, end-of-life events, and (when relevant) autopsy results can provide solace, an opportunity to address parents' questions about their decisions, a method of reducing guilt, time to detail the implications of heritable neurologic disorders and to offer referrals for counseling or support.

Barriers to Palliative Care

Providers may encourage treatments with little hope of a favorable outcome, abandoning them only when death seems inevitable. A late transition from curative care to palliative care is a frequent problem. For many pediatric neurologic diagnoses, it is difficult to predict which children will die of their disease or the quality of life as the disease progresses. Parents' recognition that death is inevitable often lags behind their understanding of the diagnosis.

Summary

Neurologists can offer children and their families the comprehensive palliative care that can improve children's and families' experience of end-of-life care (Fig. 163-3). Primary-care neurologists should develop expertise in the palliative care of children with life-threatening neuromuscular conditions. Consultant neurologists should coordinate their palliative care efforts with primary pediatric providers, palliative care specialists, and the interdisciplinary team.

REFERENCES

The complete list of references for this chapter is available in the e-book at www.expertconsult.com.
See inside cover for registration details.

SELECTED REFERENCES

Committee on Drugs, American Academy of Pediatrics, 2002. Guidelines for monitoring and management of pediatric patients during and after sedation for diagnostic and therapeutic procedures. Pediatrics 110, 836–838.

Feudtner, C., Kang, T.I., Hexem, K.R., et al., 2011. Pediatric palliative care patients: a prospective multicenter cohort study. Pediatrics 127, 1094–1101.

Feudtner, C., 2007. Collaborative communication in pediatric palliative care: a foundation for problem-solving and decision making. Pediatr. Clin. North Am. 54, 583–607.

Grunau, R.E., Whitfield, M.F., Petrie-Thomas, J., et al., 2009. Neonatal pain, parenting stress and interaction, in relation to cognitive and motor development at 8 and 18 months in preterm infants. Pain 143, 138–146.

Hall, R.W., Anand, K.J., 2014. Pain management in newborns. Clin. Perinatol. 41 (4), 895–924. [Epub 2014 Oct 7].

Himelstein, B.F., Hilden, J.M., Boldt, A.M., et al., 2004. Pediatric palliative care. N. Engl. J. Med. 350, 1752–1762.

Ho, C., Straatman, L., 2013. A review of pediatric palliative care service utilization in children with a progressive neuromuscular disease who died on a palliative care program. J. Child Neurol. 28, 40–44.

Howard, R., Carter, B., Curry, J., et al., 2008. Analgesia review. Paediatr. Anaesth. 18 (Suppl. 1), 64–78.

Lee, S.J., Ralston, H.J., Drey, E.A., et al., 2005. Fetal pain: a systematic multidisciplinary review of the evidence. JAMA 294, 947–954.

Lewis, D.W., Ashwal, S., Dahl, G., et al., 2002. Practice parameter: evaluation of children and adolescents with recurrent headaches: report of the Quality Standards Subcommittee of the American Academy of Neurology and the Practice Committee of the Child Neurology Society. Neurology 59, 490–498.

Lewis, D.W., Ashwal, S., Hershey, A., et al., 2004. Practice parameter: pharmacologic treatment of migraine headache in children and adolescents: report of the American Academy of Neurology Quality Standards Subcommittee and the Practice Committee of the Child Neurology Society. Neurology 63:2215–2224.

Simons, S.H., Tibboel, D., 2006. Pain perception development and maturation. Semin. Fetal Neonatal Med. 11 (4), 227–231. [Epub 2006 Apr 18].

E-BOOK FIGURES AND TABLES

The following figures and tables are available in the e-book at www.expertconsult.com. See inside cover for registration details.

Fig. 163-1 Questions to address prognostic uncertainty in palliative care decisions for children.

Fig. 163-2 Model for concurrent components of palliative care.

Box 163-2 Examples of Neuromuscular Conditions that may be Appropriate for Pediatric Palliative Care.

Table 163-1 Examples of Pain Assessment Scales for Differing Developmental Ages.

164 Ethical Issues in Child Neurology

David L. Coulter

 An expanded version of this chapter is available on www.expertconsult.com. See inside cover for registration details.

INTRODUCTION

The task of ethics in general is to understand how human beings should behave in regard to other persons and to society: to understand what is right and what is wrong. The philosophic study of ethics parallels the growth and development of human society. Morality is understood as the set of generally accepted rules and guidelines for acceptable conduct in society. These social conventions about what is right and wrong constitute the common morality (Beauchamp and Childress, 2012). Philosophic ethics can be thought of as the attempt to develop a rational basis for morality. Although ethics (as a form of philosophy) strives for universal truth, it is inextricably linked to the realities of the human societies whose morality it seeks to understand. Distinguishing between "moral" and "ethical" behavior is often difficult (Bernat, 2008). Perhaps moral behavior may be thought of as a personal attempt to conduct one's life in conformity with the common morality, whereas ethical behavior may be thought of as a more theoretical or rational attempt to apply philosophic thinking to what is right and wrong. In other words, ethics is a systematic attempt to understand how to live and act morally in a social context.

Ethics addresses all aspects of human behavior. Bioethics considers the interaction between biology and ethics. It is defined as the systematic study of the moral dimensions of the life sciences and health care, and it includes consideration of the health- and science-related moral issues in the areas of public health, environmental health, population ethics, and animal care. Clinical ethics is a subcategory of bioethics that refers to the day-to-day moral decision making of those caring for patients. More specifically, clinical ethics refers to the identification, analysis, and resolution of moral problems that arise in the care of a particular patient (Jonsen, Siegler, and Winslade, 2015). Medical ethics is a subcategory of clinical ethics that refers to the moral behavior of physicians (and is thus distinguishable from nursing ethics, social work ethics, and pastoral ethics).

Neuroethics is a concept that cuts across most of these distinctions. As an area of bioethics, it considers the interaction between the neurosciences and clinical neurology and ethics in all of the same areas of study as for bioethics, noted previously. As a clinical discipline, it addresses the care of patients with neurologic disorders. As an area of medical ethics, it refers most directly to the moral behavior of neurologists and neurosurgeons. Thus child neurologists interested in ethics need to be knowledgeable about the general approaches to ethics, the emerging scope of bioethics, and the more specific approaches to ethics in medicine, nursing, and other health-related disciplines.

The goal of this chapter is to provide child neurologists interested in ethics with the tools they need to identify, analyze, and resolve moral problems they may encounter in the care of children and adolescents with neurologic disorders. The first part covers the most significant theoretical approaches to ethics as they apply to child neurology. The second part considers the varied duties of the child neurologist working with patients with morally problematic issues. These tools should help child neurologists to frame the ethical problems that arise in their work. Developing a framework for the analysis and identifying the key ethical question or questions are the first step in approaching these cases. The next step is to consider the most relevant and appropriate ethical approach, which may vary considerably from case to case. The final step is to synthesize all of the available information (usually through discussion with colleagues, patients, and family) and attempt to answer the question as it was framed.

THEORETICAL APPROACHES TO ETHICS

Philosophy may be a search for truth, but the fact is that there is no one, true, universal approach to ethics. Physicians who want to act ethically should be aware of the several major ethical theories that compete for attention in contemporary medical practice. Two ethical theories in particular dominate thinking in Western philosophy. Utilitarianism is derived from the writings of Jeremy Bentham and John Stuart Mill. Deontology is derived mainly from the writings of Immanuel Kant. Elements of both theories persist in modern ethical approaches to clinical problems, usually in somewhat modified form. Most physicians will find themselves using utilitarian thinking on some occasions and deontological thinking on other occasions, or using some combination of both when it is necessary to resolve an ethical dilemma in clinical practice.

A number of other ethical approaches have been developed more recently and also deserve consideration. As a general statement, probably no one theory or approach is optimal in every case in medical practice. A skillful physician will recognize which approach is best suited to the challenges of a specific ethical situation. Knowledge about these several ethical theories thus provides the physician with a kind of "ethical toolkit," from which to select the approach that is most likely to be helpful in analyzing the specific issues present in a particular case.

UTILITARIANISM

The essence of utilitarian theory is the idea that the morality of an action is determined mainly by its consequences: the morally right action is the one that produces the best result. Of course, the result of an action may be quite complex and challenging to identify. An action that helps one person may harm another person. Withdrawing support from a child in a vegetative state undoubtedly harms the child because it results in the child's death, but the action may help the family grieve and may allow society to use limited medical resources to help other patients. The utility principle states that one should act to produce the best overall balance of positive and negative consequences of the act. This idea is embedded in the concept of balancing risks and benefits to achieve the best overall result.

Utilitarian theory is often cited to justify actions that are most likely to increase happiness, but other desirable results are also possible. Individuals may wish to act in such a way as to increase personal quality of life, enjoyment of and satisfaction with life, success in a preferred career, and general knowledge and understanding, or to strengthen personal relationships. Lawyers and policymakers use the utility principle to produce the best overall balance of justice and fairness for society.

Utilitarian thinking is almost intuitive in many aspects of ordinary life. Understanding this form of thinking is important because it may help avoid the potential pitfalls that can result from uncritical application of the theory. Perhaps the most familiar situation is the use of utilitarian theory to justify the killing of defective newborns. Although theoretically logical, such arguments are morally repugnant to persons who apply a different moral standard based on some other approach to ethics. Another problem with utilitarian theory is its failure to protect minorities, which results from its emphasis on producing the greatest good for the majority. The needs of children with rare neurologic disorders can be overlooked if utilitarian thinking allocates scarce medical resources primarily to children with more common and less debilitating disorders.

DEONTOLOGY

The term *deontology* is derived from the root *deon*, meaning "duty," and deontological theory is based on the importance of duty. Duty is based more on the intentions that lead a person to act than on the outcomes or consequences of the action. Utilitarian thinking is mostly situational and depends on the specific aspects of a given situation; deontological thinking strives to be more universal and to emphasize decisions that would apply in all relevant situations. Thus Kant's categorical imperative states that we should act only in a way that is consistent with a universal law or obligation. Using people as means to an end implies that different actions (or reactions) are needed, depending on the end or outcome that is desired; therefore, the actions are not universally applicable. For this reason, deontological thinking stipulates that we should treat all people as "ends" and not as means to an end. This could cause problems in thinking about the morality of organ transplantation if the organ donor is thought of only as a means to the end of survival for the recipient. Clearly, deontological thinking imposes a duty to respect the rights and value of the donor as much as those of the recipient because anyone could be either a donor or a recipient.

Deontological thinking emphasizes duties and obligations, but these may conflict. For example, physicians may have different and competing obligations toward patients, families, hospitals, insurance companies, and society. The attempt to describe duties leads to formulation of general or universal rules for moral action, but these rules may also conflict. Rules may be too abstract and impractical to apply to real-life situations. Deontologically based rules do not take into account the messiness of human relationships, a point that it is essential to keep in mind when considering the ethics of care discussed later in this chapter.

Common Morality and Natural Law

What are the universal rules that spring from deontological thinking? Most Western philosophers would argue that these rules can be derived from the application of reason—from rational, logical thinking about the nature of human existence. The general argument is that all rational persons would agree that these rules are essential to govern and guide the moral actions of individuals in a cohesive society. The common morality represents the socially approved norms of human conduct that form the basis of ethical theory. This common-sense understanding of what is needed for individuals to behave in society is not derived from theory, but rather forms the basis for potentially competing theories.

Natural law theory is an ancient approach to deriving universal rules through the application of reason. For Thomas Aquinas, natural law sprang from man's participation in God's eternal law and was brought into being by the application to action of human intelligence and reasoning. This application leads first to the principle that all things desire that which is good; therefore, good is to be pursued and evil is to be avoided. Good things are those to which man has a natural inclination, such as life (existence), social interaction, family life, and civil government. To pursue these good things, one should act fairly, love God, and love other persons. Secondary precepts or rules (such as the Ten Commandments) follow from these basic principles.

Secular interpretations of natural law are as old as Aristotle and are still used in some forms of legal theory. Beauchamp and Childress do not define any specific rules as part of their concept of the common morality, but they do define four principles that are not absolute and that need to be specified based on actual circumstances (Beauchamp and Childress, 2012). These four principles may be seen to correlate with the precepts of natural law:

1. Do good (beneficence).
2. Avoid evil (nonmaleficence).
3. Act fairly (justice).
4. Love one another (autonomy).

Whatever the source of the common morality, it is the basis for principlism, the ethical theory based on the application of principles to specific situations.

Principlism

Principlism is an approach to ethical problems that is based on the application of the four principles of beneficence, nonmaleficence, justice, and autonomy. It is more of a practical guide than an abstract theory, and it has found widespread acceptance in a variety of settings. It was adopted explicitly in the Belmont Report, which forms the foundation for research ethics in the United States. Although principlism is perhaps the best-known approach to clinical ethical problems, it is by no means the only approach. Understanding principlism is necessary to consider these alternative systems.

The principle of autonomy has become preeminent in Western society, although it may be less prominent in Eastern or religiously oriented societies that place a greater value on social harmony. Physicians need to keep this in mind when caring for patients from other cultures. An autonomous choice is one that is based on sufficient knowledge of the facts involved, the ability to understand the situation, and the independence to choose without undue influence of other people. Autonomous individuals can determine for themselves what they think is best, and this principle states that other people should respect these choices, even when they do not agree with or approve of them. Autonomy is the basis for the concept of informed consent, which requires that a patient has the capacity or competence to understand the issues, full disclosure of all of the information needed to make a decision, and freedom from any coercion that might influence the decision.

In general, persons younger than 18 years of age are not considered to have the capacity to make fully autonomous choices, although their preferences should be considered and respected, if possible. American law recognizes that persons 18 years of age and older are fully competent, unless a judge has determined otherwise. This recognition is critically important for young adults with neurologic disorders (such as intellectual disability) that may affect their capacity to make fully autonomous decisions. If capacity is in doubt, the family will need to initiate legal proceedings to obtain guardianship when the person becomes 18 years old. A young adult (over 18 years) with a neurologic disorder that results in limited competence is unable to give informed consent, but that individual's parents cannot give consent for him or her unless they have obtained guardianship. Failure to obtain guardianship when it is necessary can interfere seriously with timely medical treatment. It should be noted that this age threshold is arbitrary and may differ in other countries.

The principle of beneficence encourages physicians to do good or to act in the best interest of the patient whenever possible. This principle can also be interpreted to suggest that physicians should seek to promote an optimal quality of life or satisfaction with life. Considerable debate exists about how to define and measure quality of life. Objective measures are based on the judgments of others, whereas subjective measures are based on the opinions of the patient about what constitutes a satisfying life. In general, preference is given to subjective judgments when they can be known with reasonable certainty.

The principle of nonmaleficence encourages physicians to avoid doing harm to patients and dates back to Hippocrates ("*primum non nocere*"). It is related logically to the principle of beneficence. Both principles are considered when physicians attempt to strike a balance between providing a benefit for the patient (doing good) and not imposing a burden (avoiding harm). This balance may become especially problematic when the same action could produce a good, or desired, effect, along with a bad, or undesired, effect. The classic example is prescription of sufficient medicine to reduce pain while knowing that it may also cause the patient to stop breathing. This problem is known as the situation of double effect. In Catholic moral theory (which contains the most explicit analysis of such situations), an action that causes double effects is morally justifiable only if it meets all of the following criteria:

1. The action itself is not morally wrong (such as killing would be).
2. The intent is to produce the good effect, even though the bad effect may be expected.
3. The good effect is not based on achieving the bad effect.
4. The benefit to be obtained is greater than the harm that might occur.

This concept is admittedly difficult to apply in practice. Evaluation of each criterion may be arguable in a specific situation. Perhaps the best that can be expected is that physicians will make a good-faith effort to adhere to the principles involved and seek to obtain the optimal balance between benefit and harm for the patient and family.

The principle of justice requires that equals be treated equally, but the basis for an equal distribution of resources may be arguable. Should resources be distributed according to need, effort, merit, contribution to society, or some other factor? Utilitarian, libertarian, communitarian, and egalitarian approaches have been proposed to answer this question. Rawls suggests that resources should be distributed to ameliorate the effects of life's inherently unfair natural and social lotteries. It may be simply bad luck ("losing the lottery") that a child is born with a disabling condition or is born into poverty. If the child is not responsible for this condition, then society should act to remedy the situation. According to this rule, unfair situations would presumably have priority over merely unfortunate situations. How many resources should be provided to those who have been unfairly deprived? The limits of this redistribution policy may be the extent to which it disables or impoverishes the rest of society.

Jonsen et al. (2015) suggest that ethical issues can be analyzed by asking the following four questions (which are, in fact, practical applications of the four principles discussed previously):

1. What are the medical indications for treatment? (principle of beneficence)
2. What are the patient's preferences? (principle of autonomy)
3. What effect on the patient's quality of life can be reasonably anticipated? (principle of beneficence)
4. What are the burdens and benefits that may affect the family and society? (principles of justice and nonmaleficence)

The questions may be somewhat hierarchic, in the sense that medical indications and patient preferences are usually more important than potential social burdens, but physicians should not be too rigid about this. In fact, asking (and answering) these four questions in a particular case is an excellent way to make sure that the relevant issues are identified and evaluated. These issues can then be considered by the caregiving team, patient, and family. Resolution of the issues may vary from case to case, but at least everyone involved will be able to see how the decision was determined.

Virtue or Character Ethics

Virtue can be described as a trait that has positive moral or social value. According to Aristotle, virtuous behavior requires both the right motive and the right action. In other words, wanting (or intending) to do the right thing is not enough by itself. This idea is somewhat at variance with pure deontological thinking, as described previously. In virtue theory, following a presumably universal rule is not necessarily a moral or virtuous act if it produces a bad result. Similarly, doing right for the wrong reason is not necessarily a moral or virtuous act if the motive itself was not virtuous.

The catalog of virtues not surprisingly varies from one writer to another. Pellegrino and Thomasma (1993) suggest eight virtues that are necessary for sound medical practice:

1. Fidelity to trust (trustworthiness)
2. Compassion (understanding the patient's feelings)
3. Prudence (clinical judgment)
4. Justice (in the sense of love and altruism)
5. Fortitude (sustained courage in the face of difficulty or despair)
6. Temperance (balance in one's life, perhaps also Osler's sense of equanimity)
7. Integrity (personal honesty and wholeness)
8. Effacement of self-interest (putting the patient's interests first)

They argue that these eight virtues are necessary but not sufficient for physicians to practice ethically. Possessing these virtues provides evidence of good intent but they must be linked to ethical action. They suggest that principlism, although not specifically part of virtue theory, can provide a guide for virtue-based ethical action.

Ethics of Care

Care-based ethical thinking is prominent in nursing practice but may be unfamiliar to physicians. It arose as somewhat of an alternative to deontological, rule-based thinking that depends on adherence to more or less rigid principles. It also arose from feminist research studies comparing male and female approaches to ethical dilemma. Gilligan (1982) found that males were more likely to look for rules to follow and to insist on adherence to these rules. Females were more likely to look for some situation-based way to resolve a dilemma, taking into consideration the person's feelings and significant relationships. This "feminine" way is not exclusively reserved for women (or for nurses), of course. Rather, it provides an alternative and perhaps more subjective way to evaluate an ethical problem that is especially relevant when a rule-based approach seems to be inappropriate or unhelpful.

Somewhat obviously, care-based ethics does not have any fixed rules. In fact, this perspective challenges the idea that impartial or universal rules should guide ethical action. Instead, it looks at the particularity of the patient and the specific clinical situation and seeks to find answers that fit this unique case. Care-based ethics accepts the fact that emotions have important moral value and must be considered carefully. It also emphasizes the patient's human relationships and the mutual interdependence of the patient, family, and all members of the caregiving team. A care-based approach to an ethical dilemma would say something like, "That can't be the only possible ethical solution. There must be another way to resolve this problem that is acceptable to everyone here. We all want to do what's best for the patient, so let's think about what that means. Maybe we could start by understanding what the patient is feeling and by talking to the family. We should also talk about how we feel about all of this. Let's brainstorm some ideas and think about what they would involve. Maybe we need to talk to some more people and get more information. If we keep working at it, we'll find a way."

This approach will sound familiar to anyone who has been involved in difficult cases in the intensive care unit, which emphasizes the ubiquity and usefulness of this way of thinking in clinical practice. Perhaps an awareness of the sound ethical foundation of care-based ethics will also help clinicians give this way of thinking attention and consideration.

Casuistry

Casuistry, or case-based ethics, is another alternative to utilitarian or rule-based ethical approaches. It rejects the very idea of a "moral calculus" that can be analyzed impartially, based on abstract concepts. Instead of a "top-down" approach, based on pure theory, it takes a "bottom-up" approach, based on the particularity of specific cases. Casuistry looks at specific cases and emphasizes points of agreement about those cases. It recognizes that moral intuition may be more important than adherence to principles. It is common knowledge that members of hospital ethics committees often agree on what needs to be done but cannot always say with clarity why they feel that way (or what ethical theory they relied on to make a particular judgment) or whether they share some degree of social commonality. This moral intuition may also reflect the influence of the "common morality" described previously. By looking at the particularities of a specific case, casuistry is also sensitive to contextual influences and individual differences.

The method of casuistry is somewhat analogous to the method of case law used in the United States. One first identifies several key cases about which there is a consensus regarding the proper ethical approach. These are cases that have had careful scrutiny in the past and are still believed to be instructive. New cases are then compared with these key cases, selecting those past cases that have the greatest similarity to the current case. One then seeks to develop a consensus about how to resolve the current case, based on how these past cases were resolved. Each new case that is resolved in this way goes into the body of case experience, so that the consensus is revised and modified incrementally in the light of evolving and accruing clinical experience.

One can see that casuistry is very similar to what an experienced clinician does naturally, drawing on his or her experience in past cases to sort out the issues in a new case. One has to be careful about which past cases to consider and to what extent the decisions made in those cases apply to the current case. Experience in past cases may also be conflicting, and it may be difficult to sort out the similarities and differences compared with the current case. One also has to be careful about how much weight should be given to one past case compared with another past case. In a very real sense, every new case is different (as every clinician knows), but there is still much to be learned from past experience. Casuistry provides a sound ethical foundation for using this clinical experience in resolving ethical dilemmas.

Spirituality

Spirituality is variously defined, but it can be understood as a belief system that focuses on intangible elements that impart vitality and meaning to one's life. Because it is based on beliefs, or faith statements, it is not provable through logical argument. Spirituality in medicine is often based on religious beliefs but it need not be. As an expression of ultimate concern, it reflects the elements of our lives that are the most important and make life worth living. Most people have some spiritual beliefs that become prominent when their health is threatened; yet these beliefs are often not considered by physicians and other health-care providers. Physicians may anticipate that patients would have certain beliefs based on knowledge of their religious background, but individual differences exist, even within a religious tradition. A more direct understanding of the patient's spirituality would be preferable.

One approach to understanding the patient's spirituality is the "three ways of looking." The first look is to see the person subjectively as an individual human being. Compassion requires distance and objectivity, but this first look requires closeness and subjectivity. It is an attempt to understand the patient's spiritual beliefs. The second look is to recognize in the other person that which we know to be central to our own existence. With the second look, we can value in the patient that which we most value in ourselves. These values include living, freedom, tolerance, respect, happiness, and satisfaction with life. Physicians would then seek to protect for their patients the values that they would protect for themselves. The third look is more elusive and is an attempt to grasp, through our relationship with another person, the transcendence or divinity that is the basis of our spiritual existence. This third look comes when it is least expected, often in the vulnerability of a frustrating or challenging ethical situation. When we are open to it, it can provide insight, enrichment, and ethical guidance.

The three ways of looking can be the basis for a spiritual approach to medical ethics. Three precepts can be identified:

1. Respect in others what I value in myself. This precept is similar to the principle of autonomy but is based on the mutuality of spiritual sharing between physician and patient.
2. Do the most loving thing possible. When we love in the patient what we love in ourselves, we will strive to do that which is best for all. Love—not just duty, convention, rules, or cost containment—is the basis for action.
3. Seek guidance from the source of my own and the other person's being, through deep reflection, prayer, advice, or sharing. Thoughtful physicians often do this in difficult ethical situations but may not recognize the spiritual nature of these reflections.

These precepts do not appear to depend on any specific religious tradition and should be applicable in all cultures and religions. One need not be religious to apply them to one's practice. They avoid the relativity of accepting cultural practices at face value by providing a general structure for applying differing cultural beliefs to specific clinical situations. Spirituality cannot and must not be coerced or imposed on others, but physicians who are open to the role of spirituality in the lives of their patients may find these precepts useful in considering difficult ethical challenges.

ETHICAL RESPONSIBILITIES

Child neurologists have duties as physicians, as pediatricians, and as neurologists. These categories overlap to some extent. Physicians in general have duties that are reflected in the Hippocratic Oath and the Code of Ethics of the American Medical Association (AMA). Pediatricians have duties as primary care physicians and as caregivers for minor children in a family context. Neurologists have duties as specialists to provide consultation and to maintain expertise in the field.

Duties as a Physician

The AMA Code of Ethics is but one example of ethical codes that professional societies and organizations in many countries espouse. It is a document that has been revised over the years and includes opinions and statements on a variety of current issues. It is a good starting point for considering a physician's duties. Additional guidance may be found in descriptions of the virtues needed for medical practice. These include the need for trustworthiness, compassion, empathy, prudent clinical judgment, altruism, fortitude, temperance, integrity, and primacy of the patient's interest. Indeed, many of these virtues are implicit in the principles delineated by the AMA.

Many professional societies have developed ethical codes or guidelines that are specific for their field. The websites of the American Academy of Pediatrics (www.aap.org), the American Academy of Neurology (www.aan.com), and the Child Neurology Society (www.childneurologysociety.org) may be consulted for the most up-to-date statements about the ethical responsibilities of members of these societies.

Conflicts may arise in applying these principles during ordinary practice. For example, physicians should generally tell the truth, but what if truth-telling would appear to be harmful to the patient? There are no easy answers. The application of a care-based ethical approach may be useful in such situations. A carefully considered amount of information may be provided in such a way and in a particular context, taking into account the physician–patient relationship, so that all involved will understand the information being conveyed and be able to use it to benefit the patient.

Consider this example. A 5-week-old infant had severe neonatal hypoxic-ischemic encephalopathy and remains on a ventilator. The magnetic resonance image shows extensive brain damage. To maintain optimal care and plan for the future, the clinical team has recommended a tracheostomy and gastrostomy. The neurologist is asked to provide an estimate of the child's developmental potential, knowing that the family is also looking into withdrawal of life support and organ donation after cardiac death. The neurologist realizes the great difficulty in predicting outcomes in this context but also is aware of the literature that predicts severe neurologic disability in this case. How should the neurologist present this information? Emphasizing the small but real possibility of an outcome that might be better than expected could help the family choose to maintain support and plan for rehabilitation. Emphasizing the greater possibility of a poor outcome will likely result in the child's death. Ultimately, it is the family's decision to make, but the neurologist's role in telling the truth, and how it is told, about the prognosis will have a significant influence on the family's decision and on the child's life.

Physicians are often called upon to write letters for patients. These letters may be used to secure benefits for the patient in school, work, or other settings. Letters may also be requested to assist the patient or family in obtaining insurance coverage for tests or treatments, or in obtaining help with housing and utilities (heat, electricity, or telephone services). In general, physicians would seem to be required to do what is best for the patient, but what if this seems to conflict with a duty to respect the law and to do what is best for the community?

Consider this example. A 10-year-old boy had Lyme meningoencephalitis 5 years ago and now is experiencing problems in school. The neurologist has recommended neuropsychological testing to help define the child's school-related needs, but the family's insurance company has stated that it will not cover testing for educational purposes. The neurologist is asked to write a letter to support the request for insurance authorization for the testing. Should the neurologist request the testing to define the cognitive implications of possible chronic Lyme encephalopathy (because the insurance company will cover neuropsychological testing for medical indications), even though the neurologist does not believe that the child has this condition?

In a more general sense, is it ever ethical to lie to an insurance company for the benefit of the patient? The question puts so many ethical principles in conflict that no single answer can be given that would apply in every case. One way to approach the question is through virtue ethics. Compassion and effacement of self-interest might support lying for the benefit of the patient, but following the virtues of integrity and fidelity to trust might indicate otherwise. In this context, each physician would have to develop a balancing of these virtues that he or she can live with in good conscience.

Physicians are often requested by insurance companies to prescribe older, cheaper drugs or to use generic products instead of new brand-name products. Indeed, in some insurance arrangements (such as full capitation), physicians may receive a financial benefit by limiting the cost of the patient's care. Should a physician order expensive tests or prescribe expensive treatments anyway, if they are believed to be in the patient's best interest? How much is a physician responsible for the overall cost of health care in society, and how should this responsibility be balanced against the responsibility to do what is best for the patient?

Consider this example. A 14-year-old girl with epilepsy had a breakthrough seizure after having been well controlled for several years. She had been taking brand-name oxcarbazepine but was recently switched to the generic equivalent. The neurologist checks the blood level and finds that it has dropped from 20 to 10 mg/dl. Should the neurologist rewrite the prescription to specify brand name only (which increases the cost of health care in general), or just increase the dose of the generic product?

Physicians are members of their community, and ethical questions can arise in the course of fairly ordinary activities. For example, suppose a physician is in church and observes a young child who is being presented for baptism. The physician suspects the child may be showing signs of autism, which the child's parents do not seem to recognize. Knowing the importance of early diagnosis and treatment of autism, should the physician say something to the family or to the minister? This may be a situation where spiritual ethics might help guide the physician toward an answer.

Clearly, application of general principles of medical ethics to complicated clinical situations is anything but straightforward. Nonetheless, physicians should make a genuine effort to do the best they can. The requirement to make the patient's interests paramount would appear to be the defining standard in most cases. In doubtful or difficult situations, consultation or discussion with one's colleagues (either formally or informally) is probably a good idea.

Duties as a Pediatrician

Many (but not all) child neurologists have trained as pediatricians and have some experience with the roles and responsibilities of a pediatrician. Most also have frequent contact with referring pediatricians who provide primary care for the patients seen in neurologic practice. The role of a pediatrician often involves primary care in the United States, but in other countries and other settings the pediatrician is a specialist who manages diseases involving other parts of the body. Child neurologists interact regularly with pediatric specialists involved in the care of children with complex disorders. Thus there is an overlap between the duties of the child neurologist and the pediatrician that warrants some exploration.

Primary care involves the longitudinal management of all of the health issues of the child and family and requires a commitment to being accessible, available, and capable. Effective primary care is compassionate, culturally competent and sensitive, and comprehensive, and includes coordination and oversight of all of the child's health problems. Most child neurologists do not provide this type of primary care. Many do, however, provide many of the same elements of care for children whose neurologic problems constitute the main health issues. These include older children and adolescents who are otherwise healthy but have ongoing neurologic problems and patients with complex neurologic problems whose general health problems are fairly straightforward. Child neurologists have no obligation to take on this role and may confine their role to that of a consultant. Those who do take on this role would seem to have the same duties as those of a primary care physician, as listed earlier, except that their duties are limited to management of the child's neurologic problems.

All physicians who care for children (including pediatricians and child neurologists) have a duty to understand and respect the child's status as a minor. This duty has two elements: one involves promoting the child's emerging development into an adult, and the other involves protecting the child from harm. Promoting the child's development involves an understanding of normal child development and helping the child succeed as much as possible. Child neurologists ordinarily monitor the child's progress in school and provide whatever assistance is possible to secure special education and therapeutic resources needed to promote the child's development. Although the primary responsibility rests with the parents and the school, the child neurologist should be available and capable of providing help when needed.

Because children are not capable of making sound judgments about their own best interests, others must judge for them what is in their best interests. Social convention and the law generally recognize that parents are the best judge of what is in the child's best interest, but this recognition is not absolute. A substantial body of law and regulation governs when and in what circumstances a parent's rights may be superseded. Consideration of these laws and regulations is beyond the scope of this chapter. Child neurologists may be called upon to give an opinion about what medical care is in the child's best interest. They may also be asked about whether they believe the child is capable of independent judgment. Persons who are 18 years old are usually assumed to be fully autonomous adults who are capable of giving informed consent for medical treatment. Many neurologic patients with significant intellectual disabilities are not capable, however; therefore, others must be designated as guardians for them. The child neurologist should be aware of what is involved in determining the need for guardianship and assist the patient and family in whatever way is appropriate.

The United Nations has formulated a declaration on the rights of children, the Convention on the Rights of the Child, which contains 54 articles that stipulate the rights of the child to life, safety, health, education, and a decent standard of living. Article 23 states that a mentally or physically disabled child should enjoy a full and decent life in conditions that ensure dignity, promote self-reliance, and facilitate the child's active participation in the community. It further recognizes the rights of the disabled child to special care. Article 24 states that the child should have access to quality health services, including primary care, preventive health care, and treatment of health conditions. Although the Convention's declaration is not legally binding, it provides a strong moral statement about the internationally accepted obligations of states to protect the best interests of all children. Awareness of this international consensus may be helpful to physicians who are advocating for children under their care.

Duties as a Neurologist

Child neurologists are specialists or subspecialists and have duties that correspond to this role. They provide longitudinal care for children and adolescents with chronic neurologic disorders, and this includes corresponding duties that resemble those of primary care, as described previously. They also provide consultative opinions about diagnosis and treatment, both in outpatient and inpatient settings. As a consultant, the child neurologist has a duty to provide a fair, impartial, accurate, and (as much as possible) evidence-based statement about the facts of the case. The child neurologist's principal role in evaluating ethical dilemmas is to clarify the facts. This is a critical role because accurate data are essential for making sound ethical decisions. Indeed, poor or questionable ethical decisions often are attributable to inadequate specialized medical information regarding the diagnosis, treatment, and/or prognosis of a case. This problem is illustrated well in cases when the patient is in a vegetative state. Some may consider such a state permanent and hopeless after only a few weeks and seek to withdraw life-sustaining treatment. The child neurologist, acting as a consultant in such a case, would inform the family and caregivers about the published data indicating that the vegetative state is not considered permanent until 3 months after an anoxic injury and 12 months after a traumatic brain injury. The family may be given some slim hope for possible recovery of consciousness before these time periods, which may call for continued treatment and rehabilitation.

The role of an expert consultant has certain limitations. For the most part, child neurologists are experts in child neurology and not in ethics. The child neurologist should distinguish between opinions regarding the neurologic data and opinions regarding the ethical issues involved in cases that present ethical dilemmas. The child neurologist's opinion about the ethical issues is one voice among many and is not necessarily the most important or determining opinion. Normally, the family's opinion about the ethical issues is the most important. The views of the extended family and the family's religious or faith or cultural community are often important. In many cases, the views of individuals who have had long-term, close, and personal relationships with the patient (e.g., friends, personal attendants, or group home staff) also deserve consideration. Child neurologists, in addition to other physicians and nurses involved in such cases, should be careful not to impose their own ethical opinions or attempt to override the expressed opinions of the patient's family and friends.

The child neurologist also has a duty to maintain expertise in the field. This is a duty that is shared with all medical specialists. Expertise is maintained through continuing education, which may involve reading journals, attending conferences, and discussing issues or cases with colleagues who may have more knowledge or experience regarding the issues in question.

Research

Many child neurologists are involved in research, which carries additional ethical duties. One of the challenges for child neurologists involved in clinical research is to separate their ethical obligations as investigators from their ethical obligations as physicians responsible for treating patients who may be enrolled as subjects in the neurologist's research study. This challenge is harder than it may seem. In the United States research ethics is based on the Belmont Report, which adopted the principles of autonomy, nonmaleficence, beneficence, and justice (see earlier discussion) as the basis of research ethics. In general, the researcher's principal ethical obligation is to protect the rights and welfare of the research subject. Poorly designed research studies are inherently unethical because they are not likely to produce sound scientific results, and thus they place the patient subject at risk for harm without the prospect of benefit. The researcher's ethical obligation as an investigator to pursue well-designed scientific studies is secondary to his or her obligation to protect the subject involved in the research. When the research subject is also a patient, this means that the child neurologist investigator's clinical duties to the patient are ordinarily stronger than his or her duties to enroll subjects in the research study.

In the United States federally sponsored research is governed by the Code of Federal Regulations, which stipulates the roles and responsibilities of researchers and institutions involved in clinical research. Researchers are required to obtain review and approval of the research study by a properly constituted Institutional Review Board for the Protection of Human Subjects in Research (IRB). Child neurologists involved in clinical research have legal and ethical obligations to follow these rules and regulations. In general, ethical issues in research should be considered when the study is being designed, not just at the end of the process when IRB review and approval are formally requested. The researcher should be knowledgeable about ethical issues in research. If the researcher has questions about ethical aspects of study design or protocol development, most IRBs will provide assistance. Building ethics into the study from the beginning will usually prevent problems later during the process of IRB approval and during continuing review and oversight of the study.

SYNTHESIS

The child neurologist striving to do the right thing and to avoid doing the wrong thing will listen to many voices conveying a variety of messages. Some of these voices are internal and reflect the several theoretical approaches that provide a "best fit" for the patient's problem. The neurologist's mind will hear different ways of conceptualizing the problem, perhaps from an ethics of care or a utilitarian perspective, or some other approach. Experience teaches that clinical ethics is not procrustean, that no theory or approach will fit every clinical situation. Every case is unique and provides lessons that can be stored away in memory and called upon another day. Drawing upon his or her knowledge about ethics derived from careful study and the knowledge that can only come from having been at the bedside of many sick children over the years, the neurologist will struggle to derive a sense of harmony that will be helpful when a decision must be made.

The child neurologist also listens to the external voices of others who are involved in the clinical situation. Foremost among them is the voice of the family. When love is present, families usually find a way to deal with whatever life hands them. It may not be the "right" way (the way others want them to take), but it is a way that works for them and deserves respect. At any given point in time, most people are doing the best they can, given their skills and abilities and the pressures and limitations they face. When physicians seek to understand the situation from the family's point of view, they may be able to help them do the best they can for themselves and for their child. The neurologist will also hear the voices of other patients and families he or she has treated and followed over the years, who were in a similar situation in the past and whose subsequent history speaks to the wisdom of decisions that were made. The child neurologist also will hear the voices of other caregivers involved in a particular case, especially those of the nurses who have a more intimate relationship with the patient and family. In some cases, the voices of long-time friends, pastoral ministers, and staff who have cared for the patient before the present situation arose will need to be heard and considered carefully. The soft but insistent voices of insurance administrators and utilization reviewers may also be softly or stridently audible.

Synthesizing all of these arguments and perspectives is never easy and perhaps benefits most from a deep sense of humility.

REFERENCES

The complete list of references for this chapter is available in the e-book at www.expertconsult.com.
    See inside cover for registration details.

SELECTED REFERENCES

Beauchamp, T.L., Childress, J.F., 2012. Principles of Biomedical Ethics, 7th ed. Oxford University Press, New York.

Bernat, J.L., 2008. Ethical Issues in Neurology, third ed. Lippincott, Williams & Wilkins, Philadelphia.

Gilligan, C., 1982. In a Different Voice. Harvard University Press, Cambridge, MA.

Jonsen, A.R., Siegler, M., Winslade, W.J., 2015. Clinical Ethics: a Practical Approach to Ethical Decisions in Clinical Medicine, 8th ed. McGraw-Hill (LANGE), New York.

Pellegrino, E., Thomasma, D., 1993. The Virtues in Medical Practice. Oxford University Press, New York.

165 Transitional Care for Children with Neurologic Disorders

Carol S. Camfield, Peter R. Camfield, and Lawrence W. Brown

 An expanded version of this chapter is available on www.expertconsult.com. See inside cover for registration details.

INTRODUCTION

Neurologic disorders of childhood often persist into adulthood. Although many have a good medical and social outcome, 20% to 30% are complex with physical, psychiatric, or developmental problems complicated by societal stigma. The problem is compounded as more children with chronic neurologic diseases now survive into adulthood with advances in diagnosis, treatment, technology and management that continue to create a new "natural history." Child neurologists need to facilitate the transition of all youth with neurologic disorders as they enter to adult healthcare (Brown and Roach, 2013).

The distinction between transfer and transition is important (Camfield and Camfield, 2011). Transfer is the formal handing over of care from a pediatric to an adult healthcare system. The relationship with the child neurologist ends with a detailed referral letter to an adult care provider and responsibility for care is transferred. Transition is a long-term, purposeful, planned process beginning in childhood to prepare youth and their families for the adult healthcare system. Over a period of years the adolescent becomes knowledgeable about his or her medical condition and as independent as possible. Ideally, they become able to evaluate the adequacy of their care. The child neurologist actively participates in the transition process and develops and maintains a relationship with the adult healthcare team to prepare for the eventual transfer.

Pediatric care includes intensive involvement with the family. Adult medical care is focused firmly on the individual, not their caregiver(s). Adolescents and young adults move from family-centered pediatric care dominated by their parents, a change that they may find difficult after years of a well-established relationship. Many of these young people have never developed full knowledge about their neurologic disorder, may not even know their diagnosis or treatment plan, and are unprepared to cope with the adult healthcare system.

In 2014 the Child Neurology Society convened a panel to identify common principles underlying the process of transition to adult care that could help to clarify the process for neurologists and caregivers. The panel outlined eight critical points that are shown in Box 165-1.

This chapter attempts to outline: 1) barriers to transfer; 2) the natural history of several disorders that evolve during or after adolescence; and 3) models that have been used for "transition."

BARRIERS TO CARE

The family, patient, pediatric neurologist, and adult neurologist have an underlying inertia to initiate the process of transition. Legal issues of confidentiality and age of consent are encountered. Electronic interchange of patient information currently is often awkward with differences in computing technology. Changes in insurance coverage in some countries (especially the United States) are of grave concern.

Many worries cause barriers to transition (Box 165-2). Families may fear the unknown and the passing of their own responsibility to their child and new adult healthcare team. They are attached and comfortable with the pediatric service (often described as holistic, attentive, understanding, and knowledgeable). Parents of an adolescent with significant physical or intellectual disability understand that normal independence is precluded (he or she remains a "child"). They may fear that this reality will not be respected by the adult healthcare team. Interestingly, parents are typically more anxious about transition than the adolescent.

For the child neurologist, transition/transfer means a loss of the long-term attachment associated with years of working with these families. There is often a nagging feeling of not having done everything possible to "cure" the child during the pediatric years. Adult service may be viewed as less holistic, particularly for management of comorbidities. Discussion of transition takes time and reimbursement may be inadequate for "nonmedical" counseling. There may be difficulty finding appropriate expert adult primary or subspecialty care.

The adult neurologist faces other challenges. No professional wants to convince reluctant youths and families of their "credentials" or justify their model of care. It may be difficult for them because many child neurologists have not dealt with issues from sexuality and relationships to vocational challenges, from potential of death from the neurologic illness to end-of-life issues. Some patients have disorders that are rarely seen in adulthood; a whole new set of information is needed. The expectations for psychosocial care may be very difficult to meet, especially in a setting with little help from other professionals such as social workers. These issues cannot be easily addressed in a short visit.

An American study documented barriers to transition by a Delphi survey (Peter et al., 2009). Internal medicine providers (n = 241) rated highest concerns about lack of training in congenital and childhood-onset conditions, lack of family involvement, difficulty meeting patients' psychosocial needs, needing access to a super specialist, lack of training in the care of adolescents, facing disability and end-of-life issues during youth, financial pressures limiting visit time, and families' high expectations.

Other issues in adult care relate to the setting. The office is rarely set up for youth who are intellectually disabled or disruptive, and consultation rooms are often inadequate for parents or a power wheel chair. Young people with intellectual disability present a special problem for the adult healthcare system, even if the adult provider is comfortable with their limitations in providing a clear history or cooperating with the examination. Unless there is guardianship, does the patient or parent decide what is best? Office visits may need to be longer than usual for good cooperation.

The pediatric model of care emphasizes a "medical home" that is optimal especially for those with rare, complex, difficult to treat medical problems involving multiple specialties. This is less common for adults who may suffer if there is no designated individual with overall responsibility for care. In

---

BOX 165-1 Principles for Transition for Child Neurologists (from the Child Neurology Society ref 16)

1. The pediatric neurology team should start to discuss the expectation of future transition to the adult care system beginning at an early age, no later than early adolescence.
2. This discussion should be continued annually and documented in the medical record and communicated to other healthcare providers. Reassessment of self-management skills can help to gradually allow the adolescent to assume more responsibility for his or her own care.
3. This phased transition planning should occur at scheduled visits rather than acute care visits and allow for sufficient time to deal with emerging issues such as sexuality, driving, and graduation from secondary education.
4. For those with intellectual disability, the child neurology team should begin the discussion of the youth's expected legal competency by age 14, support interventions to maximize this decision-making ability, and support caregivers who must address the legal implications of the assessment. This might include guardianship and power of attorney.
5. The child neurology team should collaborate with the youth and family, primary healthcare provider, and others on an annual basis to address comprehensive needs. Although the child neurologist is not responsible for healthcare finances and legal concerns, education, employment, and community-based adult services, he/she is obligated to make sure that a comprehensive transition plan is developed and updated.
6. The child neurology team is responsible for the neurologic component of the transition plan and should update it yearly.
7. Appropriate adult providers, whether neurologists or others, should be identified in collaboration with the youth and family before the anticipated time of transfer. The child neurology team coordinates the transfer, preferably utilizing a transition packet that documents the diagnosis, supportive testing, previous drug trials and past procedures, current management, and any protocols for emergency care.
8. The child neurology team should directly communicate with the identified adult providers to ensure successful transfer and document the youth's transfer (i.e., completion of transition) into the medical record.

BOX 165-2 Barriers to Care

1. Family
   - Fear of the unknown
   - Comfort and attachment to pediatric service
   - Personal negative past personal experiences with adult care
   - Behavioral/psychiatric difficulties within family
   - Cultural and racial barriers attached to the family's financial and socioeducational background
   - Child with intellectual handicap or severe disabilities perceived always as a "child"
2. Child neurologist
   - Loss of long-term professional "friendship" and sharing relationship with family members
   - Adolescent and family resistance to transfer
   - Nagging feeling that care was not as complete as possible
   - Difficulty identifying appropriate adult healthcare providers perceived as excellent and compassionate
   - Long wait lists for entrance into the adult system
   - Financial reimbursement, institutional support for transition/transfer services
   - Reminder of personal mortality
3. Adult Neurologist
   - Reluctance of family and adolescent to change
   - Insufficient time and reimbursement for complex care
   - The challenge of dealing with "taboo" subjects such as sexuality, potential of death, and longevity
   - Possible insufficient of knowledge of the natural history and management of rare, chronic neurologic diseases of childhood
   - Unease with youth with intellectual disability and the complexity of deciding who is the decision maker
   - Lack of multidisciplinary clinics

---

addition, multidisciplinary clinics are common in pediatrics but rare in adult medicine, which may lead to fragmented, incomplete care.

In the next section, we provide examples of transition/transfer issues for a variety of childhood neurologic disorders.

Disorders that May be Dangerous to Society if Untreated

Attention deficit with or without hyperactivity (ADHD or ADD) is important because it is so common and persists into adulthood in approximately 30% of individuals. It may exist as a single diagnosis or as a comorbidity of other disorders. For example, 20% of children with epilepsy also have ADHD, as do more than 50% with Tourette Disorder, possibly 20% with cerebral palsy, and 40% of survivors of some brain tumors. The symptoms have a profound effect on adult functioning, including accidents, substance abuse, and suicide. In 2012 Montano noted, "The current literature reveals a number of barriers to continuity of care of ADHD, including disparities and inadequacies in ADHD education in primary care and internal medicine residencies, prohibitive prescribing practices with respect to stimulants, inadequate clinic staffing, lack

of support by college health services, inadequate health insurance coverage, and failure to conduct transitional planning. Without improved continuity of care and adherence to medication, adolescents and young adults with ADHD are at greater risk of academic, social, and vocational difficulties, as well as behavioral problems, including substance abuse, unsafe driving, and criminal activity." (Montano et al., 2012.)

Barkley compared 149 children with ADHD who were followed into young adulthood to a matched cohort of "community" controls. Only two thirds with ADHD completed high school compared with all of the controls. ADHD subjects were more likely to have been involved with a pregnancy (38% versus 4%) and have a driver's license suspension (41% versus 26%). Automobile accident rates in those with ADHD are alarming, and the effect of ADHD is similar to moderate alcohol intoxication according to studies using driving simulators. The combination of mild alcohol intoxication and ADHD is even more striking. Adults with ADHD are more competent drivers if they take stimulant medication. Effective management of ADHD in young adults can dramatically reduce the rate of substance abuse. Therefore sophisticated adult care is needed to continue to optimize treatment for ADHD.

Disorders that are Potentially Lethal in Childhood and Young Adulthood and Have Emerging Treatments Leading to Increased Survival Well into Adulthood

Treatment advances have allowed improved function and prolonged survival in some conditions such as boys with

Duchenne muscular dystrophy. Affected boys can now walk well into their teenage years and 85% survive to age 35 years or longer since the addition of positive pressure ventilation. However, the burden of disease increases with longevity and is further complicated if there is significant learning and/or intellectual disability. Sleep-related breathing disorders, cardiomyopathy, and progressive restrictive lung disease from scoliosis are among the challenging issues. Adult neurology, rehabilitation, pulmonary medicine, and cardiology all need to be involved along with many allied health professionals and social workers. These services are typically well coordinated in a pediatric hospital, but it is rare to find comparable adult comprehensive programs. As more youths are surviving with formally fatal disorders, "taboo" issues such as sexuality management, life-threatening cardiopulmonary complications, and end-of-life care need to be discussed more fully (Barkley et al., 2006). Goals for young adult life require innovative solutions as do satisfying daily activities, acceptance by peers, coping with difficulties, and establishing optimism.

Disorders that Are Problematic and "Static" in Childhood but Progress in Adulthood

The brain lesions causing cerebral palsy (CP) are not progressive. They are permanent and associated with evolving movement disorders that limit activities (Backman and Conaway, 2014). Comorbidities are frequent: 50% of patients have intellectual disability and/or epilepsy. Over 90% live beyond 18 years of age, and many are able to successfully adapt to adult life; however, others face monumental challenges. Learning or behavioral problems often become troublesome as the child reaches school age and may persist into adulthood, resulting in low educational attainment, decreased employment, limited finances, living with family, reduced social opportunities, and overall poor quality of life. Limitations in coordination, strength, and mobility gradually lead to curbing activities with peers. Associated epilepsy may be intractable. Unfortunately, there is increasing evidence that mobility for children with cerebral palsy worsens in adulthood. An initial survey of 226 adults with cerebral palsy was repeated after an interval of 7 years. Depending on the type of CP, one-third to three-fourths of patients reported increased walking difficulties that included pain, fatigue, and decreased balance. Others have noted a variety of progressive orthopedic problems in adults with cerebral palsy frequently complicated by musculoskeletal pain. Young adults with cerebral palsy between ages 20 to 22 years were twice as likely to rate their health as poor (21%) compared with those who were 15 to 16 years old (9%).

Some studies have been more optimistic. A cohort of patients who underwent dorsal rhizotomy in early childhood seemed to have stable gaits 20 years later. Nonetheless, a comprehensive program that includes adult neurology would appear to be necessary to optimize management of a myriad of needed services, including orthopedic surgery, gastroenterology, pulmonary medicine, pain management, physical, occupational and speech therapy, and social services.

Disorders Diagnosed in Childhood with Their Most Serious Manifestations in Adulthood

Neurofibromatosis 1 (NF1) is a complex disorder for transition/transfer. Most patients are diagnosed in childhood and followed by child neurologists without progressive problems unless they have an optic pathway glioma; however, the effect of NF1 in adulthood may be profound. A recent meta-analysis

of eight studies relating NF1 with adult health-related quality of life found that NF1 decreases all aspects of quality of life compared with the general population. Medical complications and visible cosmetic effects were strong predictors of quality of life.

During the school years, learning/behavior problems, sometimes autistic spectrum disorder, headache, and epilepsy are the focus of clinicians. Schwannomas become increasingly prominent with age, but many of the really serious complications begin in adulthood with sarcomas, renal failure and cerebrovascular disease. In our experience, referral is infrequent between the pediatric and adult neurology services. Primary care physicians are left to provide overall medical care but may not have the detailed knowledge to coordinate comprehensive care. Most guidelines for NF1 management have focused on children and have not been recently updated nor have they recognized that life expectancy now approaches the seventh decade.

Different issues exist for children with tuberous sclerosis complex (TSC) (De Waele et al., 2015). Recent improved understanding of the pathophysiology has lead to new therapies. One of the most promising is mTOR inhibitors which have potential for treatment of subependymal giant cell astrocytoma as well as renal angiomyolipoma, lymphangioleiomyomatosis, and facial angiofibromas, all problems that span the ages between childhood and adulthood.

Renal disease is the most common cause of mortality after the age of 30 with renal cysts, angiomyolipomas, fat-poor lesions, and malignant tumors causing chronic renal disease. These problems become nearly universal in adulthood.

Epilepsy is typically a persistent problem. In infancy, TSC may present with infantile spasms. During childhood and adulthood seizures are focal or secondarily generalized. Autism, learning disorders, intellectual disabilities, ADHD, or other psychiatric disorders ordinarily present in childhood but persist.

There are few "birth-to-death" programs for neurocutaneous disorders that ensure optimal long-term care, and such multidisciplinary clinics are unusual. The need for TSC patient advocacy along with an awareness and knowledge of the upcoming treatment advances underlies the requirement for continued lifelong surveillance. There are presently no clinical guidelines for patient management of TSC; however, a recent consensus statement by international experts describes a standardized, routine "surveillance" program for life.

Disorders that Are Cured in Childhood but Have Neurologic Sequelae that Persist into Adulthood

An increasing number of children survive brain cancers due to improvements in early diagnosis, surgery, radiotherapy and chemotherapy. Oncologists may continue to follow these patients for problems related to the late effects of chemotherapy and second malignancies, but many continue to have significant neurologic problems. It is critical to have neurologic involvement in their care. Ongoing surveillance by adult neurologists is increasingly important now that so many children with brain tumors survive into adulthood. Unfortunately, long-term survival does not necessarily equate to optimal outcome; a large cohort of childhood brain tumor survivors was compared with their siblings. Over 1800 cases were followed for a median of 19 years; survivors were much less likely to graduate from college, more likely to be unemployed, and much less likely to be married than their siblings. Of those with medulloblastoma, more than 40% of survivors had neuropsychiatric problems. One other study from a single center suggested that about 50% of survivors of childhood brain tumors were "disabled." The long-term neurologic issues may be complex and include intractable epilepsy or remote vasculitis from radiation. Clearly, adult neurologic expertise is required.

Disorders that May/May Not Remit in Childhood but Have Persistent Effects on Adult Social Function

As a group, children with epilepsy have very high rates of poor social outcome in adulthood, rates that are higher than other pediatric chronic disease comparisons and population controls (Borlot et al., 2014; Geerlings et al., 2015). Adult consequences of pediatric epilepsy are reviewed in Chapter 62. A critical observation is that social outcome appears to be independent of seizure remission, although those with persistent seizures may have even greater problems. Although the main focus is always seizure control, optimizing quality of life is critical if children with epilepsy are expected to live fulfilling lives. Identifying and treating comorbidities must begin in childhood but is a lifelong concern.

Disorders that May Be Uncomfortable for Adult Care

Youth with intellectual disability are at particular risk for care discontinuity as they approach adulthood. Lack of communication skills, disruptive behavior, and inadequate medical insurance are particularly challenging for adult neurologists. As these young people become adults, their parents age, and siblings move away. When placed in an institution or a group home with high rates of staff turnover, many intellectually handicapped adults soon become "well known by no one." The link with their medical records may be broken, and the original diagnosis and management become unfamiliar or unknown to their caretakers and physicians.

Caretakers may not be aware of new approaches to diagnosis or treatment. For example, profoundly handicapped adults with untreated phenylketonuria may still benefit from a low phenylalanine diet with improved quality of life. Organizing transition and transfer for this type of patient is a major challenge. A strong case can be made for a birth-to-death clinic, although institutional barriers are to be expected.

Disorders in Childhood Treated in a Way that is Difficult to Replicate in Adult Medicine

Adult care rarely uses the "medical home" model that brings together specialists working together with families and community resources. Such care is ideally suited to the many children now surviving with neurologic disorders who would have died 20 to 30 years ago. Without major efforts at coordination, their complex care easily becomes fragmented and suboptimal. For example, gastrostomy tubes are well accepted in pediatrics and have been a major contributor to longevity. Dietary/nutrition support for tube feeding may not be available in adult care settings nor is there often familiarity with the ketogenic diet or other special diets for metabolic disorders. There are many young people with disorders in this category; examples include progeria, craniosynostosis syndromes, Ondine's curse, Down syndrome, serious head injury, and neural tube defects.

POOR OR LITTLE DEVELOPMENT OF THE TRANSITION PROCESS YIELDS POOR OUTCOME

There is very little literature about the unsatisfactory transition for youth with neurologic disorders. Examples from other chronic diseases suggest that the effect may be devastating. For example, youths with type 1 diabetes dropped attendance rates within 2 years of transfer to adult clinics from 94% to 57%; 21% were lost to follow up. Only 40% of those with asymptomatic ulcerative colitis adhered to their medication regime after transfer to the adult setting. Renal transplant patients are another example. One study tracked 20 young adult kidney transplant recipients and found that medical outcomes sharply deteriorated in the 36 months after transfer. One third lost their transplant; nonadherence to immunosuppressant medications was suspected as the primary cause.

Models of Care for Transition

An optimal model of transitional care has not been identified in general or specifically for neurologic patients. The Kaiser Permanente Patient Risk Stratification Pyramid is a method to stratify patients with long-term health conditions and defines the appropriate level of required care. This approach divides the population of patients with chronic conditions into three groups based on their level of risk and degree of need.

For those with relatively low healthcare needs (Level 1), adult care might be provided by a family physician with sufficient knowledge, skills, and confidence; this may encompass 70% to 80% of youths with chronic neurologic conditions. A multidisciplinary team, including a nurse practitioner, might be optimal. Level 2 indicates a need for more structured assisted care or care management for a single or multiple conditions. These youths have increased risk because their condition is unstable or is likely to deteriorate unless they receive specialist disease management. Transfer from the pediatric neurologist to adult specialist care is appropriate.

For the most complex conditions (Level 3), management of multiple, high intensity conditions through case managers, nurse practitioners, and super specialists should be provided along with care from an array of professionals to plan and coordinate services. As suggested in the Child Neurology Foundation report, this does not have to be an adult neurologist, but it is essential to have a designated "captain." Beyond medical needs, additional issues to be addressed over time include the individual's cognitive function and level of competence, personal and family psychosocial issues, the degree of support from family and friends, community resources, capacity to navigate and engage with the medical system, ethnicity and language that may create barriers/challenges, and end-of-life care, power of attorney, and creation of wills and trusts.

A variety of transition/transfer models has been described in Box 165-3 (Carrizosa et al., 2014).

1. Abandonment of Specialized Care or "Fend for Yourself"

This approach places the burden for ongoing care entirely on the youth's pediatrician or family physician. Unfortunately, this physician may have had limited involvement in the child's chronic disorder and is unlikely to have full, current knowledge of the disease. The youth and family may not be particularly attached to the provider or may doubt his or her competence.

An alternative is a group of family physicians who might develop a special interest in chronic neurologic disorders (preferably with an able nurse practitioner as a case manager)

BOX 165-3 Models for Transitional Care

1. Abandonment of specialized care or "fend for yourself"
2. Referral to adult rehabilitation program
3. Referral to adult neurologist or internist
4. Referral to an internal medicine/pediatric subspecialist
5. Referral to a nurse-run transition clinic
6. A formal transition clinic with pediatric and adult neurologists and other professionals
7. Referral to a professionally moderated Internet support group

(From: Carrizosa, J., An, I., Appleton, R., Camfield, P., Von Moers, A., 2014. Models for transition clinics. Epilepsia 55(Suppl 3), 46–51.)

and, as a group, follow transferred youth with neurologic problems. To be successful, multidisciplinary consultation would need to be available with financial compensation adequate for the additional time needed.

2. Referral to an Adult Rehabilitation Program

These programs are typically oriented toward a single consultation or short-term intervention. Examples would be management for gait difficulties, repetitive strain injury, or wheel chair assessment. Care in this setting is generally multidisciplinary, but long-term follow up is unusual. "Botox" treatment for spasticity may be an exception. Rehabilitation programs are found in large tertiary centers and cities more often than in smaller hospitals or communities.

3. Referral to an Adult Neurologist or Internist

This is generally a consultation model with follow-up visits. It begins with a request for consultation to an adult specialist. Although follow-up visits may be scheduled with the specialist, they may require a new referral from the primary care physician.

There are limitations to this approach. Few adult internists or neurologists are trained or interested in the long-term care of developmental brain disorders. Financial pressures limiting visit time and high expectations of the family are particularly problematic. Many adult neurologists and internists are uncomfortable treating patients with intellectual disability and worry about not having easy access to appropriate subspecialists.

4. Referral to an Internal Medicine/Pediatric Subspecialist

We are unaware of published literature about the effectiveness of a neurology transition program that uses the United States model of a fully accredited Internal Medicine/Pediatrics residency program. The concept is that during a "med/peds" residency, training is offered in comprehensive care for children, adolescents, and adults with chronic health disorders. This model allows for 2 to 4 years before transfer to an adult specialist or return to the family physician. During this period, the youth has time to mature, gain skills to manage medical care, and recognize when and where to seek additional help for health issues. Families have time to establish estate planning and learn to relinquish their responsibility for their child, allowing the young adult to "grow up."

5. Referral to a Nurse-Run Transition Clinic

This model was described in Edmonton, Alberta. A pediatric epileptologist completes a referral to the adult care team. The patient and family meet jointly with the pediatric and adult epilepsy nurses for several visits to prepare for their initial and long-term visits with the adult epilepsy team.

6. A Joint Pediatric/Adult Transition Clinic

We favor this approach (Camfield et al., 2012). Careful initial review in such a transition clinic may revise the original diagnosis, reconsider medications, investigate surgical options, and address comorbidities. Adherence can be addressed along with potential side effects to medications and potential lifestyle alterations. Counseling may include sexuality, life expectancy, newer treatments, and ways to improve quality of life with the opportunity for increased maturity and self-esteem in addition to realistic long-term goals. In 1997 Appleton first described such a program for youth with epilepsy in the United Kingdom. There were 120 "transitioned" patients—37% with intellectual disability. Patients were seen several times by the clinic staff of a pediatric and adult neurologist, as well as a nurse practitioner. During these visits a new diagnosis emerged for 10%, and medication was changed 22% of patients. After an average of two visits, the pediatric neurologist bowed out leaving the youth to be followed in the adult care system. The pediatric neurologist continued to be available for consultation to the adult staff.

7. Internet-Based Support Groups

Encouragement for youth and families to align with a professionally moderated, disease-specific online support group or organization will hopefully permit very long-term access to new developments in treatment. Such a connection is not a replacement for a transition process.

CONCLUSIONS

More information is needed about the long-term outcome of neurologic diseases in children and the best way to manage transition and transfer. The optimal age to begin the transition process is not known, but starting in early adolescence seems appropriate. The best time for transfer may vary from high school graduation to completion of college or when the young adult is fully emancipated. The success of any transition program will surely be strongly related to the enthusiasm and commitment of the physicians and other healthcare professionals who are involved. Personal contact between providers in the pediatric and adult settings is likely the most important ingredient to success. Given the intensity of treatment for children with chronic neurologic disorders, it is essential to transition satisfactorily to adult medicine.

REFERENCES

The complete list of references for this chapter is available online at www.expertconsult.com.
    See inside cover for registration details.

SELECTED REFERENCES

Backman, J.A., Conaway, M., 2014. Adolescents with cerebral palsy: transitions to adult healthcare services. Clin. Pediatr. (Phila) 53 (4), 356–363.

Barkley, R.A., Fischer, M., Smallish, L., et al., 2006. Young adult outcome of hyperactive children: adaptive functioning in major life activities. J. Am. Acad. Child Adolesc. Psychiatry 45, 192–202.

Borlot, F., Tellez-Zenteno, J.F., Allen, A., et al., 2014. Epilepsy transition: challenges of caring for adults with childhood-onset seizures. Epilepsia 55 (10), 1659–1666.

Brown, L.W., Roach, E.S., 2013. Outgrowing the child neurologist: facing the challenges of transition. JAMA Neurol. 70, 496–497.

Camfield, P., Camfield, C., Pohlmann-Eden, B., 2012. Transition from pediatric to adult epilepsy care: a difficult process marked by medical and social crisis. Epilepsy Curr. 12 (Suppl. 3), 13–21.

Camfield, P.R., Camfield, C.S., 2011. Transition to adult care for children with chronic neurologic problems. Ann. Neurol. 69 (3), 437–444.

Carrizosa, J., An, I., Appleton, R., et al., 2014. Models for transition clinics. Epilepsia 55 (Suppl. 3), 46–51. doi:10.1111/epi.12716.

De Waele, L., Lagae, L., Mekahli, D., 2015. Tuberous sclerosis complex: the past and the future. Pediatr. Nephrol. 30 (10), 1771–1780. doi:10.1007/s00467-014-3027-9.

Geerlings, R.P.I., Aldenkamp, A.P., de With, P.H.N., et al., 2015. Transition in adolescents with epilepsy. Epilepsy Behav. 51, 182–190.

Montano, C.B., Young, J., 2012. Discontinuity in the transition from pediatric to adult healthcare for patients with attention deficit hyperactivity disorder. Postgrad. Med. 124, 23–32.

Peter, N.G., Forke, C.M., Ginsburg, K.R., et al., 2009. Transition from pediatric to adult care: internists' perspectives. Pediatrics 123 (2), 417–423.

166 Practice Guidelines in Pediatric Neurology

David J. Michelson, Gary Gronseth, and Stephen Ashwal

 An expanded version of this chapter is available on www.expertconsult.com. See inside cover for registration details.

INTRODUCTION

Clinical practice guidelines (CPGs), practice parameters, and practice advisories are documents developed to address the need of practitioners for guidance in making medical decisions. High-quality CPGs are written by panels of authors, including topic experts, using a formalized process to reach consensus recommendations based on a systematic review (SR) of available clinical evidence regarding the benefits and harms of different treatment options. The last half century has seen CPGs evolve along with the field of evidence-based medicine and come to play an increasingly important and highly scrutinized role in medical practice and health care policy.

HISTORY

The first SRs were efforts to analyze the combined data from multiple small clinical trials. Concurrently, authors began to use SRs of evidence as the basis for practice recommendations. Evidence-based medicine (EBM) emerged from work done in the 1970s that uncovered wide geographic variations in care received by seemingly similar groups of patients. An EBM Working Group report in 1992 advocated for a greater emphasis on rigorous and systematic evaluation of high-quality scientific medical evidence for understanding causation, prognosis, diagnostic accuracy, and treatment effects (Eddy, 2005).

Within a few years, dozens of medical specialty societies and disease-specific societies began publishing practice guidelines. However, these guidelines continued to rely more heavily on the beliefs of the authors, or on expert consensus, than on empirical evidence. Governmental agencies and insurance providers, acting on their interest in improving patient outcomes and slowing the rising cost of healthcare, began to take an active role in the guideline development process. In 1989 the U.S. Congress established the Agency for Health Care Policy and Research (AHCPR), later renamed the Agency for Healthcare Research and Quality (AHRQ), which currently provides support for a network of centers that produce systematic reviews for public and private groups and maintains the National Guideline Clearinghouse (http://www.guideline.gov), a searchable online CPG database.

Private and international organizations have also been significant contributors to the field in EBM development. The Cochrane Collaboration produces systematic reviews following protocols that emphasize transparency and scientific rigor. The Scotland-based Guidelines International Network (GIN) library has collected more than 6000 guidelines from around the world (http://www.G-I-N.net).

Several dozen guidelines with particular relevance to child neurologists have been developed in the last 20 years, mostly through the work of what is now called the Guideline Development, Dissemination, and Implementation (GDDI) subcommittee of the American Academy of Neurology (AAN), often with involvement and endorsement by the Child Neurology Society (CNS) (Table 166-1) (Hurwitz et al., 2015).

DEVELOPMENT PROCESS

Over the years, guidelines have come to play a more prominent role in healthcare practice, administration, and law. Private and government insurers are supporting guidelines for their potential to reduce practice variations, improve the quality of care, and reduce healthcare costs by discouraging ineffective or harmful practices. Hospitals are using guidelines as the basis for quality assessments and computer-based decision support tools. Lawyers working both sides of malpractice suits are attempting to introduce guidelines into evidence as the accepted standards of appropriate care.

Many previously published guidelines fall short because of limitations in the scientific evidence upon which they are based. Even when developers can overcome the difficulty and expense involved in reviewing all available studies, there may still be a lack of sufficiently rigorous, unbiased, consistent, and generalizable evidence to support more than vague recommendations. CPG development groups may only be able to produce specific recommendations by relying on expert opinion.

The process of guideline development may also suffer from a lack of transparency, inclusiveness, or consistency, diminishing the actual or apparent reliability of the result. Perception that one or more authors of a guideline are biased by self-interest can diminish the acceptance of a guideline by both practitioners and the public.

Conflicts of interest (COIs) can be academic, intellectual, and financial. The American Thoracic Society defined COI as "a divergence between an individual's private interests and his or her professional obligations such that an independent observer might reasonably question whether the individual's professional actions or decisions are motivated by personal gain, such as financial, academic advancement, clinical revenue streams, or community standing" (Schünemann et al., 2009).

The evidence available to guideline developers may also suffer from COIs. Many published clinical trials are industry sponsored and conducted to obtain U.S. Food and Drug Administration (FDA) approval for a new medication or clinical indication. Although these studies tend to be of high quality, they are more likely to show favorable results than independently done studies and to use socioeconomically homogenous populations, exclude patients with important medical comorbidities, utilize relatively brief follow-up periods that may underestimate risks, and rely on surrogate endpoints that may overestimate benefits (Avorn, 2005). These shortcomings have reduced the generalizability of even very recent guidelines. With evidence lacking, imperfect, or disputed, and guideline developers making recommendations based on some estimation of expert consensus, multiple guidelines on a subject have been published with conflicting recommendations.

Concerns about CPG quality prompted the U.S. Congress to direct the Secretary of Health and Human Services to contract with AHRQ and the Institute of Medicine (IOM) of the

TABLE 166-1 Selected Practice Guidelines Related to Child Neurology

Year	Type	Topic	Developer	References
1995	E	Persistent vegetative state	AAN	[62]
1996	E	Simple febrile seizures	AAP	[63]
1996	T	Seizure-free patients	AAN	[64]
1999	T	Simple febrile seizures	AAP	[65]
1999	T	Closed head injury	AAP, AAFP	[66]
1999	E	Tuberous sclerosis	NTSA	[67]
2000	E	Autism	AAN, CNS	[68]
2000	E	Attention deficit disorder	AAP	[69]
2000	E	First nonfebrile seizure	AAN, CNS, AES	[70]
2000	T	Status epilepticus	SEWP	[71]
2001	T	Attention deficit disorder	AAP	[72]
2002	E	Neuroimaging neonates	AAN, CNS	[73]
2002	E	Recurrent headaches	AAN, CNS	[74]
2003	E	Hypertonia	TFCMD	[75]
2003	T	Severe TBI	AAN	[76]
2003	E	Global developmental delay	AAN, CNS	[41]
2003	T	Severe TBI	CNS, others	[77]
2003	T	Guillain-Barré syndrome	AAN	[78]
2003	T	First unprovoked seizure	AAN, CNS	[79]
2004	E	Cerebral palsy	AAN, CNS	[42]
2004	T	Epilepsy	AAN, AES	[80, 81]
2004	E/T	Migraine headaches	SFEMC	[82]
2004	T	Migraine headaches	AAN, CNS	[83]
2004	T	Infantile spasms	AAN, CNS	[84]
2005	T	Duchenne muscular dystrophy	AAN, CNS	[85]
2006	T	Epilepsy	ILAE	[86]
2006	E	Status epilepticus	AAN, CNS	[87]
2007	E/T	Spinal muscular atrophy	ICSMASC	[88]
2008	T	Stroke	AHA	[45]
2008	E	Antiepileptic drug levels	ILAE	[89]
2009	E	Microcephaly	AAN, CNS	[90]
2010	T	Cerebral palsy	AAN, CNS	[91]
2010	T	Cerebral palsy	CPI	[92, 93]
2010	T	Congenital muscular dystrophy	ISCCCMD	[94]
2011	E	Simple febrile seizure	AAP	[95]
2011	E	Brain death	AAP, CNS, SCCM	[47]
2012	E/T	Traumatic brain injury	CNS, AAP, others	[48]
2012	T	CVST	FSPN, EPNS	[96]
2012	E/T	Epilepsy	NICE	[97]
2012	T	Infantile spasms	AAN, CNS	[98]
2012	E/T	Insomnia in autism	ATN	[99]
2013	T	VNS for epilepsy	AAN	[100]
2013	T	Prolonged seizures	NLAE, BSEDM	[101]
2014	T	Status epilepticus	MGMSECI	[102]
2013	E/T	Sports concussion	AAN	[40]
2015	E/T	Congenital muscular dystrophy	AAN, AANEM	[103]
2015	T	Infantile spasms	ILAE	[104]

AAFP, American Academy of Family Physicians; AAN, American Academy of Neurology; AAP, American Academy of Pediatrics; AES, American Epilepsy Society; ATN, Autism Treatment Network; BSEDM, Belgian Society for Emergency and Disaster Medicine; CNS, Child Neurology Society; CPI, Cerebral Palsy Institute; CVST, cerebral venous sinus thrombosis; E, evaluation; EPNS, European Pediatric Neurology Society; FSPN, French Society of Pediatric Neurology; ICSMASC, International Conference on Spinal Muscular Atrophy Standard of Care; ISCCCMD, International Standard of Care Committee for Congenital Muscular Dystrophy; ILAE, International League Against Epilepsy; MGMSECI, Multidisciplinary Group on Management of Status Epilepticus in Children in India; NICE, National Institute for Health and Clinical Excellence; NTSA, National Tuberous Sclerosis Association; SCCM, Society of Critical Care Medicine; SFEMC, French Society for the Study of Migraine Headache; SMA, spinal muscular atrophy; T, treatment; TFCMD, Task Force on Childhood Motor Disorders; VNS, vagus nerve stimulator.

BOX 166-2 Institute of Medicine (IOM) Standards for Developing "Trustworthy" Guidelines

1. Transparency
   a. Details regarding clinical practice guideline (CPG) development and funding should be explicit and public.
2. Conflict of Interest (COI)
   a. Potential guideline development group (GDG) members should declare all potential COIs.
   b. COIs should be reported and discussed by the GDG before any member joins the group.
   c. Each member should explain how COIs could influence their work.
   d. Members should take steps to minimize their current and future COIs.
   e. Ideally, members should not have COIs, but when necessary, those who do should be a minority of the group and should not serve as the chair or cochairs of the group.
   f. Funders should have no role in CPG development.
3. GDG Composition
   a. GDGs should be multidisciplinary and balanced.
   b. Patient and public involvement should be facilitated.
   c. GDGs should adopt strategies for increasing effective participation of patient and consumer representatives.
4. CPG–Systematic Review (SR) Intersection
   a. CPG developers should use SRs that meet standards set by the IOM.
   b. When SRs are conducted specifically for a CPG, the GDG and SR team should interact regarding the scope, approach, and output of both processes.
5. Establishing Evidence Foundations for and Rating Strength of Recommendations
   a. Each recommendation should be accompanied by:
      i. the reasoning underlying the recommendation, including
         1. a clear description of potential benefits and harms;
         2. a summary of relevant available evidence (and evidentiary gaps), a description of the quality (including applicability), quantity (including completeness), and consistency of the aggregate available evidence; and
         3. an explanation of the part played by values, opinion, theory, and clinical experience in deriving the recommendation.

      ii. a rating of the level of confidence in (certainty regarding) the evidence underpinning the recommendation;
      iii. a rating of the strength of the recommendation in light of the preceding bullets; and
      iv. a description and explanation of any differences of opinion regarding the recommendation.
6. Articulation of Recommendations
   a. Recommendations should be articulated in a standardized form that makes clear what actions are recommended and under what circumstances.
   b. Strong recommendations should be worded to facilitate evaluation of compliance.
7. External Review
   a. External reviewers should include scientific and clinical experts, interested organizations (e.g., healthcare, specialty societies) and agencies (e.g., federal government), patients, and representatives of the public.
   b. The confidentiality of authorship of external reviews by individuals and/or organizations should be maintained unless waived.
   c. The GDG should record its responses to all reviewers' comments.
   d. A draft of the CPG should be made available to the general public for comment and reasonable notice of impending publication should be provided to interested public stakeholders.
8. Updating
   a. The CPG publication date, date of pertinent SR, and proposed date for future CPG review should be documented in the CPG.
   b. Literature should be monitored regularly to evaluate the continued validity of the CPG.
   c. CPGs should be updated when new evidence suggests the need for modification of clinically important recommendations.

(Adapted from Institute of Medicine (IOM). Clinical Practice Guidelines We Can Trust. Washington, DC: The National Academies Press; 2011.)

National Academy of Sciences to research the most objective, scientifically valid, and consistent methods for producing SRs and CPGs. The IOM's report "Clinical Practice Guidelines We Can Trust," published in 2011, outlined eight recommendations for improving the transparency and validity of the guideline development process (Box 166-2) (IOM, 2011).

THE AMERICAN ACADEMY OF NEUROLOGY PROCESS

The AAN GDDI subcommittee produces guidelines according to a process manual that has incorporated each of the IOM report's recommendations (AAN, 2011).

Choosing Topics and Panelists

AAN guidelines may be written to address any number of the decision points facing practitioners in the management of patients with neurologic disorders, including how diagnostic tests should be used, how to choose the most appropriate medical and surgical treatments, and how to apply test results to counseling about prognosis.

Topics for AAN guidelines can be suggested by anyone, but typically come from physicians interested in serving as guideline authors, physician or patient interest groups and organizations, and members of the AAN GDDI and Practice committees. These nominations are rated by a topic expert designated by the GDDI based on relevance, prevalence, degree of practice variation or controversy, financial implications, feasibility of the project, and the potential for changes in treatment to improve patient care and outcomes.

Once a topic is selected, the GDDI then uses the same factors to decide whether the topic and its time-sensitivity warrant the production of a full SR, a more focused SR, a full CPG that uses a full SR, or a practice advisory focused on one or two clinical questions, based on a focused SR.

Next, a writing panel made up of volunteer subject experts and GDDI members serving as process experts is assembled, with careful attention to minimizing and balancing COIs. For full systematic reviews and guidelines, the panel includes at least one patient or patient representative. The writing panel formulates a protocol with an introduction to the topic, the clinical questions the panel will try to answer, and the search strategy the researchers will use for collecting scientific evidence. Clinical questions are written in PICO format, specifying the population (P) or type of patient involved, the intervention (I) experienced by the patient (e.g., treatment, risk factor, or positive test result), the co-intervention (C) that serves as a comparator to the intervention (e.g., no-treatment or different treatment, lack of the risk factor, or negative test result), and the outcome (O) by which the effect of the intervention is being assessed.

For fully IOM-compliant products, the panel protocol is posted for public review and the framework and PICO questions are revised based on the comments received.

Collecting and Grading Evidence

The search strategy for fully IOM-compliant products must query more than one database, including the so-called "gray literature," which refers to results of clinical studies and literature reviews that are never published as articles in medical journals, but are nonetheless available (www.graylit.org/about). Including data from unpublished studies may help to counter some of the bias that leads to studies showing less benefit and more harm from treatments or tests being more likely either to be rejected for publication or to never be submitted in the first place. Most clinical trials performed in academic centers are now registered with the National Institutes of Health (NIH), and their protocols are published and maintained on an online site (www.clinicaltrials.gov) so that the investigators can be asked for study data even when the study is never completed or never published.

The AAN process calls for an explicit search strategy to be laid out, for the abstracts of all papers identified by that search to be reviewed by at least two people for relevance, and then for the full text of all remaining papers to be reviewed by at least two people for relevance and stratification of the evidence into one of four classes based on characteristics of the study design that are relevant to bias. Different criteria are applied to studies addressing different clinical questions. For randomized, controlled clinical trials (RCTs) pertaining to the effectiveness of a treatment, studies can receive the highest rating (lowest risk of bias), class I, only when they are done in a sample of patients representative of the population, use masked or objective outcome assessments, exclude or adjust for substantial differences between treatment groups in relevant baseline characteristics, use appropriate concealment allocation, prospectively define no more than two primary outcome measures, have clearly defined exclusion and inclusion criteria, and follow at least 80% of enrolled subjects to completion of the study, adequately accounting for dropouts. Studies that fail to meet one or more of these criteria will be downgraded to class II (moderate risk of bias) or class III (high risk of bias). Uncontrolled case series are given the lowest rating (very high risk of bias), class IV (Table 166-4).

The rationale for classifying evidence relates to the likelihood that given methods will affect the internal and external validity of the study's results and conclusions. When there are multiple studies pertaining to a question, particularly when they reach conflicting conclusions, greater weight should be given to studies providing stronger evidence (i.e., ones that because of their methodology are more likely to accurately reflect reality). For treatment trials, biases affecting internal validity lead to an underestimation or overestimation of the effectiveness of interventions. These biases frequently involve improper use of control groups, blinding, and randomization. External validity is lower when a study's results cannot easily be generalized to real-world patients and clinical settings, as a result of such factors as the exclusion of representative patients, high costs, and onerous burdens on patients and caregivers.

Drawing Conclusions

Each study is then abstracted for a measure of the strength of the association between the intervention and outcome pair. For treatment trials, such association measures might be relative or absolute risk or odds differences between the treatment and control groups, with the precision in measurement shown by 95% confidence intervals (CIs) or by p-values (from which the 95% CI can usually be estimated). For relative risks or odds, a 95% CI that does not cross the value 1 is statistically equivalent to a p-value of less than 0.05. A study may or may not show a statistically significant association between interventions and outcomes, but the width of the CI should also be considered. A study may have great precision (narrow CI) and show significance ($p < 0.5$) but still lack clinical relevance

TABLE 166-4 American Academy of Neurology Process

CONFIDENCE IN EVIDENCE

Confidence	Evidence
High	At least 2 consistent class I studies
Moderate	1 class I or at least 2 class II studies
Low	1 class II or at least 2 class III studies
Very Low or Unknown	Insufficient for a higher rating

LEVELS OF RECOMMENDATIONS

Recommendation Level	Level U	Level C	Level B	Level A
Wording	None	May	Should	Must
Adherence expected to affect	Few	Some	Most	Nearly all
Variation in patient preferences	Large			Minimal
Cost	Prohibitive			Minimal
Availability	Limited			Universal
Value of benefit relative to risk	Too close to call	Small	Moderate	Large
Confidence in evidence	Very low	Low	Moderate	High
Strength of principle-based inferences	Not plausible	Plausible	Convincing	Compelling

The recommendation level is anchored by the lowest of the confidence in evidence and the strength of principle-based inferences. The recommendation level can be decreased for any factor. The recommendation level can be increased only for a value of the benefit relative to risk that is moderate or large and can only increase by one level. With the exception of the unusual circumstance of recommendations derived solely from first principles, the level of recommendation can never attain level A without high confidence in evidence.

(Adapted from AAN. Clinical Practice Guideline Process Manual. 2011 Ed. St. Paul: The American Academy of Neurology; 2011.)

because of actually small or clinically irrelevant differences in outcome. A study lacking both precision (wide CI) and statistical significance ($p > 0.5$) may be inconclusive, rather than negative, suggesting that an intervention could be clinically important if measured more precisely. If a great deal of the identified evidence suffers from lack of precision, a meta-analysis to combine the results of comparably performed studies may be appropriate.

The AAN uses the Grading of Recommendations Assessment, Development and Evaluation (GRADE) process for determining the confidence in the evidence, modified by using the class of the supporting evidence as an anchor point. First, interventions are assigned an initial level of confidence based on the class of evidence supporting their association with an outcome. This serves as an anchor limiting how much a recommendation can be upgraded or downgraded based on other factors that are then considered. The confidence can be downgraded by one level if the panel feels that there are additional factors limiting confidence in the evidence, including biological implausibility, the number and consistency of studies, their statistical precision, their generalizability, and their potential for being skewed by reporting bias. Similarly, the panel members may decide to raise their confidence in the evidence by one level if supporting factors are present, such as a large effect size, a dose–response relationship, and a bias that tends to minimize effect size.

To complete an evidence report or systematic review, the writing panel must summarize the collected evidence for each PICO question into conclusions that account for the class of evidence found, the strength and precision of the measures of association, the populations to which the findings apply, and the consistency, or lack thereof, between studies. The AAN uses language in writing its conclusions that is directly tied to the confidence in the evidence. For example, if there are multiple, consistent class I studies showing a clinically meaningful association between a treatment and improved clinical outcomes supporting high confidence, the panel is prompted to conclude that it is "highly likely" that the treatment is effective. If there is a single class I study or there are multiple class II studies showing a similar association supporting moderate confidence, the panel will conclude that it is "likely" that the treatment is effective, and so on. The panel may exclude negative studies lacking the precision to exclude a meaningful association (high risk of random error) when drawing conclusions, even if those studies were rated highly for class of evidence (low risk of systematic error).

Writing Recommendations

If the writing panel had intended to draft a clinical practice guideline or advisory, and the evidence review was able to identify evidence of good quality and consistency, the writing panel then begins the process of formulating recommendations. Each recommendation is rated according to the level of the panel's confidence in making it. The levels imply the obligation of practitioners to follow the recommendations. High-level (level A) recommendations direct practitioners toward things that they "must" or "must not" do. Moderate-level (level B) recommendations suggest to practitioners things that they "should" or "should not" do. Low-level (level C) recommendations imply that practitioners "may" or "may choose not to" decide to follow them. The lowest-level recommendation (level U) is assigned when there is insufficient evidence and rationale for choosing between available options (Table 166-4).

The author panel then drafts a set of recommendations, starting with the clinical questions and considering the available evidence in a realistic context. Each recommendation is

rated for the strength of deductive inference behind it, based on how well it can be related to accepted principles of medicine, related clinical evidence, and deductive reasoning. Recommendations considered at this stage can be based on this deductive process alone, rather than on conclusions from the evidence review. Each recommendation is assigned an overall rating based on the lower of the two ratings, the level of confidence (high, medium, low, very low) and the level of plausibility (compelling, convincing, plausible, or not plausible). The panel then systematically considers additional factors affecting the relative value of an intervention (the benefits [effect size], risks [tolerability and safety], availability, cost, and presence [or lack] of alternatives) and the variation expected in patient preferences. Only a large relative value can raise the level of confidence in a recommendation, and even then it can do so by only one level and cannot raise a recommendation up to level A. Interventions that might otherwise be worthy of a level U recommendation may also be designated level R (research-only) if concerns about costs or risks are such that the panel feels that patients should only receive the intervention in the context of ongoing research.

Often, the AAN uses a modified Delphi technique to reach consensus between the guideline development group (GDG) members regarding the wording and rating of the level of recommendations. The Delphi process involves GDG members anonymously answering a series of questions intended to determine the soundness of the recommendation and the relative importance of the factors that might influence the strength of the recommendation. The GDG responses are summarized and then presented to each member again, along with any commentary, and another round of rating is carried out. This rating and summarization process is repeated until consensus is obtained ($\geq 80\%$ agreement), up to a maximum of three voting rounds. Because the process maintains participant anonymity, it reduces some negative group dynamics, including the tendency for opinion to be strongly influenced by participants with greater authority, reputation, or personality, and the tendency for participants to avoid changing their opinions out of fear of appearing inconsistent.

Some important clinical questions cannot be answered with current data, and some studies, even if conceivable, are unlikely to ever be financially or ethically feasible. Clinical context sections in some recent AAN guidelines have provided discussions by the authors of what is common in clinical practice without making specific recommendations. In the absence of sufficient evidence to support strong recommendations, the AAN has typically opted to lay out the limitations of the evidence and leave decisions regarding the best course of action to individual neurologists, who are those with the best understanding of their patients' values and circumstances.

Once the author panel has finalized the wording and grading for its recommendations, the guideline is vetted by the AAN staff working with the GDDI subcommittee, including the staff EBM methodologist; reviewed by other members of GDDI committee; posted online with invitations for public comments; reviewed by the AAN Practice committee; and finally submitted for publication to the AAN's official academic journal, *Neurology*. At each step, the feedback received and the reasoning behind any modifications made or not made in response are documented. Finally, the manuscript is submitted to the AAN Board of Directors and to any cooperating professional and patient-centered organizations for endorsement.

Dissemination efforts beyond publication in *Neurology* include press releases and official AAN written and electronic announcements directed at AAN members and the public. An archive of prior guidelines and educational materials for patients and practitioners, including summary pages and slide sets, are freely available for download on the AAN website (http://www.aan.com/Guidelines).

The GDDI considers whether or not to update previously published AAN guidelines every 2 years, based on whether sufficient and compelling new evidence is identified by an interim literature search that would significantly change prior recommendations. If a guideline appears to still be valid, the panel may vote to reaffirm it. If a guideline no longer appears to be valid, the panel may decide to either retire it or nominate it for revision.

LAW AND ETHICS

Many clinicians have a reflexive objection to the idea of being obligated by a clinical practice guideline to take specific actions in the care of their patients, feeling that rote application of "cookbook" standards of care cannot adequately substitute for their use of their own clinical judgment, incorporating their experience, their knowledge of disease pathophysiology, and their understanding of the nuances in their patients' characteristics and individual values and preferences.

There has been little demonstrable effect of guidelines on the frequency with which defensive medicine is practiced. It has been suggested that CPGs would be more widely accepted, and that greater improvements in the cost-effectiveness of care could be realized, if it was clear that CPG recommendations could serve as an effective defense against malpractice claims. However, most malpractice trials take place in state courts, which tend to look to customary local practices, rather than to recommendations from a CPG, for the standards of care to which they will compare the actions of physician defendants (Avraham and Schanzenbach, 2010). Courts in most states will not hold practitioners liable for care that is judged customary, even if it is not optimal or evidence-based.

However, the U.S. federal legal system has allowed the submission of CPGs as expert testimony even if not as evidence. CPGs have been introduced into court proceedings both to defend a practitioner's actions and to suggest negligence. In one case, a court ruled a physician's care negligent for following a guideline without consideration of his patient's specific circumstances (Recupero, 2008).

Because of ongoing concerns about their legal implications, all guidelines produced by the AAN carry a general disclaimer that their recommendations, even when worded as strongly as possible, should be considered suggestions rather than explicit directives. Nevertheless, some specific AAN guidelines anticipated to be controversial or upsetting to particular interest groups have been submitted to the AAN's legal team before their publication to be vetted for wording that might be unnecessarily provocative.

GUIDELINE UTILIZATION

There have been several studies done regarding awareness and acceptance of guidelines; these studies suggest that practitioners value them, but do not follow their advice (Davis and Taylor-Vaisez, 1997). A general obstacle to guideline utilization is the consideration of how decisions for real patients must usually account for far greater complexity, nuance, and specificity than clinical trials, meta-analyses, or guidelines can cover. Financial incentives to order unnecessary tests and treatments probably play a smaller role in the overutilization of services than do inclinations to perform defensive medicine out of concern for potential lawsuits. Guidelines may adversely affect their own adoption by lacking clearly actionable language or simply because they rely on a weak base of evidence.

It is clear that the most successful strategies for changing practitioner behavior use financial incentives, such as those that can be directed by hospitals and insurers (Rosenthal and Dudley, 2007). The pay-for-performance incentives and penalties incorporated into the 2008 Affordable Care Health Care law are driving sweeping systematic changes in physician participation in electronic health record (EHR) systems, registries, and quality improvement (QI) measurement efforts. Guidelines can suggest improvements in standards for practice when based on evidence of benefit verus harm that is clear, strong, and generalizable. For example, studies have shown that patients treated in accordance with CPG recommendations for asthma (Licska, Sands, and Ong, 2012) tend to have better health, shorter hospital stays, lower short-term costs, and lower rates of early rehospitalization.

Ongoing research in measuring the impact of guidelines will involve the use of electronic medical records (EMRs) to assess implementation and outcomes. Additional research will address the most effective ways for hospitals and practice groups to integrate guideline recommendations into the care of patients, such as through prompts generated in EMRs and assignment (especially of noncontroversial and strongly supported recommendations) to physician extenders such as nurse practitioners.

CONCLUSION

When developed using methodologically sound processes, clinical practice guidelines can provide clinicians, researchers, and administrators with a clear picture of the state of the art in the evaluation, diagnosis, and management of a disease. In addition, systematic reviews and guidelines, by providing a clear accounting of the quality of the existing evidence, can suggest where the need for additional information is greatest. Because recommendations can only be as strong as the evidence will support, the growing interest in evidence-based guidelines is naturally stoking interest in creating a stronger evidence base. In 2010 the U.S. Congress established the nonprofit Patient-Centered Outcomes Research Institute (PCORI), which has already provided more than $1 billion to fund comparative effectiveness research projects to "provide information about which approaches to care might work best, given [patients'] particular concerns, circumstances, and preferences" (http://www.pcori.org).

The methods used for disseminating and implementing CPGs are undergoing rapid changes, with some trends having unintended consequences. Healthcare providers share the interest of consumers and payers in identifying and minimizing practices that are questionable or outright harmful. However, institutions must take care to ensure that practitioners do not end up feeling overburdened with levels of regulation of unproven value. The coming years, with additional insights from studies assessing the impact of CPGs on outcomes, will see these competing interests brought into better balance.

REFERENCES

The complete list of references for this chapter is available in the e-book at www.expertconsult.com.
> See inside cover for registration details.

REFERENCES

American Academy of Neurology (AAN), 2011. Clinical Practice Guideline Process Manual, 2011 Ed. The American Academy of Neurology, St. Paul, MN.

Avorn, J., 2005. FDA standards – good enough for government work? NEJM 353 (10), 969–972.

Avraham R., Schanzenbach M., 2010. The Impact of Tort Reform on Private Health Insurance Coverage. Am Law Econ Rev. 12 (2), 263–4.

Davis, D.A., Taylor-Vaisez, A., 1997. Translating guidelines into practice: A systematic review of theoretic concepts, practical experience and research evidence in the adoption of clinical practice guidelines. CMAJ 157, 408–416.

Eddy, D.M., 2005. Evidence-based medicine: A unified approach. Health Aff. 24 (1), 9–17.

Hurwitz B.A., Hurwitz K.B., Ashwal S., 2015. Child neurology practice guidelines: past, present, and future. Pediatr. Neurol. 52 (3), 290–301.

Institute of Medicine (IOM), 2011. Clinical Practice Guidelines We Can Trust. The National Academies Press, Washington, DC.

Licska, C., Sands, T., Ong, M., 2012. Using a knowledge translation framework to implement asthma clinical practice guidelines in primary care. Int. J. Qual. Health Care 24, 538–546.

Recupero, P.R., 2008. Clinical practice guidelines as learned treatises: understanding their use as evidence in the courtroom. J. Am. Acad. Psychiatry Law 36 (3), 290–301.

Rosenthal, M.B., Dudley, R.A., 2007. Pay-for-performance: will the latest payment trend improve care? JAMA 297 (7), 740–744.

Schünemann, H.J., Osborne, M., Moss, J., et al., 2009. An official American Thoracic Society Policy statement: managing conflict of interest in professional societies. Am. J. Respir. Crit. Care Med. 180 (6), 564–580.

E-BOOK FIGURES AND TABLES

The following figures and tables are available in the e-book at www.expertconsult.com. See inside cover for registration details.

167 Special Education Law as it Relates to Children with Neurologic Disorders

Kathleen A. Hurwitz

 An expanded version of this chapter is available on www.expertconsult.com. See inside cover for registration details.

HISTORY

Special education case law carried out by individual states and the federal legislation for the education of children with disabilities has its roots in the Fourteenth Amendment of the U.S. Constitution. This post-Civil War proposal insured that no state could deprive a person to life, liberty, or property without due process of law. Defining educational laws for children with special needs took its next big leap during the civil rights movement in the 1950s and 1960s. The equal rights amendments and the desegregation laws opened the door for children with disabilities to fall under the umbrella of antidiscrimination legislation. Educators, families, physicians, and disabled children have lobbied for education provisions that provide the best possible learning environment for special needs children.

Physicians and allied healthcare providers who deliver diagnostic and prognostic information to patients and families are compelled to understand current special education laws. In 1992 the American Academy of Pediatrics put forward a policy statement that called upon all pediatricians and pediatric subspecialists to provide a "medical home" for their patients. The medical home concept is particularly relevant for children with special needs. The statement advocates that physicians develop a "coordinated, comprehensive plan" for each child and involve community resources, including schools and educators in that plan. The physician needs to "claim responsibility" and oversee the implementation of the child's care plan. Expansion and inclusion of healthcare services during school hours is increasingly falling under the jurisdiction of public education. Children with complex medical needs who frequently are sustained on technological devices require physician input for their care during school hours. In anticipation of the clinician's changing role, a working knowledge of the evolution of the legislative process as it pertains to special needs education is presented in this chapter.

SPECIAL EDUCATION CASE LAW

Special education law developed in state courts. A chronologic review is presented to give a historical perspective. These changing state rulings are precursors to federal legislation (Table 167-1).

Brown v the Board of Education (1954) was a class action suit that was a plea for racial desegregation. African American parents who had attempted to enroll their children in neighborhood schools with Anglo American students had been refused. They were required to attend segregated schools. Previously, "separate but equal" facilities were acceptable as long as they were equivalent. The Supreme Court ruled that in "the field of education separate but equal has no place. Separate educational facilities are inherently unequal."

In *Hobson v Hanson (1969)*, the first objection to the use of standardized testing as part of tracking students was challenged. Ninety percent of students in Washington, DC, were African American. However, they were given Intelligent Quotient (IQ) testing benchmarked to Anglo American standards. Children were placed based on socioeconomics and race as opposed to their learning aptitude. The legal decision abolished Washington, DC's tracking system. IQ testing in a child's native language was first tested in *Diana v State Board of Education (1970)* (Reynolds, 2007). Civil rights groups brought suit on behalf of a bilingual student who was placed in a classroom for the mentally retarded. The child, Diana, had been tested in English and not in her native language, Spanish. The case never was heard because a decree was issued that IQ testing must be performed in the child's primary language.

Lau v Nichols (1974) was a case involving Chinese-speaking students who claimed that they could not take advantage of certain educational opportunities because instruction was only in English. The court ruled that supplemental English be provided or instruction be carried out in the native language.

In 1979, *Larry P. v Riles* clarified testing of African American children. Larry P., one of six African American children, brought suit against the California Superintendent of Schools, claiming overrepresentation of African American children in classes for the mentally retarded. The children were placed in these classes solely on IQ testing. The court's ruling favored the plaintiffs and restricted IQ testing for African American children. It was ruled that testing could only be performed if: 1) the court had received a request; 2) the test was validated for identifying cognitive delays; 3) the test was not racially or culturally biased; 4) the test was administered in a nonbiased environment; and 5) an open public hearing was held regarding the test.

Stanford Binet and WISC-R testing procedures were evaluated in the Illinois case, *PASE v. Hannon (1980)*. Cultural bias was on trial for each test question. Very few biased questions were found. The case never became historically significant because the state of Illinois banned the IQ testing of African American children as part of a settlement in a desegregation case.

High school competency testing as a requirement for graduation has been challenged in Florida. *Debra P. v Turlington (1984)* challenged the fact that a disproportionate number of African American children were failing their exit examinations. Because students taking the test started school when Florida was still segregating students, the court found for the plaintiffs. The courts also placed an injunction and the test was not required for graduation.

Mills v Board of Education of the District of Columbia (1972) is a landmark case for special needs children. Seven children brought suit against the schools because they were excluded

TABLE 167-1 Summary of Case Laws

Case	Complaint	Ruling
Brown v Board of Education (1954)	Unable to enroll African American students in neighborhood school	Separate schools are inherently unequal
Hobson v Hanson (1969)	Objection to using Intelligent Quotient (IQ) testing for tracking students	Abolished tracking system
Diana v Board of Education (1970)	IQ testing in nonnative language	IQ testing must be in native language
Lau v Nicholas (1974)	Instruction not in native language	Supplemental English or instruction in native languages required
Larry P. v Riles (1979)	Overrepresentation of African Americans in EMR classes	Courts severely restructured IQ testing
PASE v. Hannon (1980)	Cultural bias in IQ tests	Very few culturally biased questions
Debra P. v Turlington (1984)	High school competency testing for graduation	Requires adequate notification to student before enforced
Mills v Board of Education (1972)	Excluded from school based on behavior, hyperactivity, and mental retardation	Free and appropriate education to all children regardless of disability type
Pennsylvania Association for Retarded Children v Pennsylvania (1972)	Excluded from classroom	Must include all children in education process and attempt to educate alongside nonhandicapped children if possible
Pennsylvania v Battle (1980)	Related service terminated at end of school year	Must be continued year round if a negative or regressive effect would result from termination
Board of Education of the Hendrick Hudson Central School District, Westchester County, et al. v Rowley (1982)	Deaf student requested an interpreter even though meeting IEP goals	No; the program in place was adequate
Timothy v Rochester (1989)	Severely handicapped and thought to be uneducable	Free and appropriate education upheld
N.B. v Warwick School (2004)	Parents wanted a different education program for autistic child and not the school-offered program	School providing program with a reasonable prediction of success was adequate

from public education based on their disabilities. These were issues of behavior, hyperactivity, and mental retardation. Many of the students excluded had not received a fair hearing. The court found in favor of the children; thus began "a free and appropriate education" for all children regardless of the disability. The case predated but greatly influenced the federal 1965 legislation called the "Education for all Handicapped Children Act" of 1975.

Defining a free and public education in the least restrictive environment became clearer from the case, *Pennsylvania Association for Retarded Children v Pennsylvania*. Thirteen mentally retarded children on behalf of all such children sued for a free and appropriate education under the equal protection clause. The court developed the concept of a least restrictive environment. A regular public classroom was a better choice for educational training than a special education classroom, which in turn, was preferable to a separate educational facility.

Battle v Pennsylvania (1980) extended benefits and services to disabled children beyond the traditional 180-day school year. The court supported the claim that discontinuing special education and programs, particularly self-help skills during recesses, could have a negative, regressive effect on children. This legal precedent protects interruption of much needed services.

The *Board of Education of the Hendrick Hudson Central School District, Westchester County, et al. v Rowley (1982)* was ultimately heard by the Supreme Court and interpreted the legal language of a "free and appropriate education" more clearly. Amy Rowley, a deaf student with two deaf parents, was enrolled in a regular classroom with an Individual Education Plan

(IEP) in place. She thrived in her environment, yet her parents requested an interpreter. The lower courts supported her parents because of a discrepancy between her performance and potential. However, the Supreme Court felt the program in place was "benefitting" her and fell under the definition of a free and appropriate education.

Accessibility of education for children with disabilities was tested in the courts in 1989. In *Timothy W. v Rochester*, it was ruled that the severity of a disability was not at the interpretation of the state. Timothy was severely mentally retarded, a spastic quadriplegic, cortically blind, and thought to be uneducable. Timothy's right to a free and appropriate education was upheld (Murdick et al., 2007).

N.B. v Warwick School Committee (2004) has important ramifications for child advocates. The parents of an autistic child brought suit against a school district. The child in question had an IEP that supported a program called Treatment and Education of Autistic and Related Communicatively Handicapped Children (TEACH). The parents preferred a program that promoted "discrete trials" and enrolled their child at their own expense into such a program and were requesting reimbursement. The court found in favor of the school. The school was not required to provide the requested program but rather any program as long as it had a "reasonable prediction" of success.

Federal Legislation

Federal legislation for children with disabilities emerged from a combination of social, political, and legal pressures. In the late 1960s and early 1970s, over 8 million disabled children attended U.S. public schools (Wright et al., 2007). However, the special education needs of each child were not being provided in any consistent manner. Some states had exclusionary practices whereas others were struggling to meet the demands without appropriate classification procedures in place. Parental advocacy groups, education leaders, and lawmakers realized the need for federal legislation.

The first program of federal assistance to local school districts was defined in the Elementary and Secondary Education Act of 1965 (P.L. 89-10). Title 1 of this statute provided federal funding for schools based upon the number of students living at or below the poverty level. The No Child Left Behind Act of 2002 replaced this legislation.

The Handicapped Children's Early Education Assistance Act of 1968 (P.L. 95-538) provided for educational programs for disabled young children. Demonstration projects or educational models were to be funded, established, and measured for their success in providing educational services. This act also funded research institutes to study behavioral, cognitive, and emotional functioning of children. In 1982 funding was also provided for the evaluation of children with autism.

The Vocational Rehabilitation Act of 1973 (P.L. 93-112) provided services for the educationally handicapped (physical or mental) to promote independent functioning or employability. Section 504 of this act protected against discrimination of services. It ensured that children who may not meet "special education" definitions can have appropriate classroom modifications. This is important for children with medical conditions who cannot meet the full demands of a classroom. Children with attention deficit disorder or attention deficit hyperactivity disorder are an example of those needing a "504" in place. This "504" can provide extra time for testing, frequent breaks, etc. (Osborne and Russo, 2006).

Access to a minor's academic records is defined in the Family Education Rights and Privacy Act (1974). Parents of minors or 18-year-old students must provide a written request to review their records. If they believe the record to be incorrect they can request that the record be amended. A hearing can be called if the school disputes the amendment. Law enforcement records must be maintained separately and are not included in a student's file (Family Education Rights and Privacy Act, 1974, Pub. L No. 93-380).

In the early 1970s, Congress recognized that over 1.5 million children were excluded from school based on their disabilities. Therefore P.L. 142, known as The Education of All Handicapped Children Act (1975), was passed. This act included the all-important inclusion of an Individual Education Plan (IEP) for every child in special education. It was mandated that the child's education be carried out in the least restrictive environment and that parents be given informed consent regarding testing and evaluation results. Testing and reports were to be conducted and discussed in the child's native language. Due process must be provided for conflict and disagreement, and placement in special education must be nondiscriminatory. The concept of "zero reject" was established in P.L. 142. No child regardless of the disability could be excluded (Murdick et al. 2007).

This act was expanded as P.L. 101 to 476, as the Individuals with Disabilities Education Act of 1990 (IDEA). Just before this, the Americans with Disability Act of 1990 (P.L. 101-336) was passed. The Americans with Disability Act mandated the elimination of discriminations for individuals with disabilities. It prevented the disabled from being discriminated against in employment and required that public school services (e.g., field trips, after school activities, and school facilities) be physically accessible to all disabled students. Passage of this act also required private entities to provide public services to all disabled individuals. Effective telecommunications and

BOX 167-1 Summary of Individuals with Disabilities Education Act

1. Age 3 to 21 that are disabled
2. Free and appropriate education
3. Least restrictive environment
4. Related services
5. Public school must search and find children who qualify
6. Nondiscriminatory testing
7. Individual Education Plan (IEP) for every qualified child
8. IEP's are transferable
9. Transition program from infant to preschool
10. Personnel development
11. Transition programs for after high school graduation
12. Confidentiality

closed-captioning services were also mandated for the speech and hearing impaired.

Individuals with Disabilities Education Act (IDEA)

The seminal legislation in protecting disabled children's educational rights is embodied in federal statutes 101 to 426, 102 to 119, 105 to 17 and 108 to 445, the Individuals with Disabilities Acts of 1990, 1991, 1997, and 2004. This act is divided into four sections. The first, Part A, is composed of definitions. Part B houses the important laws and bulk of the legislation. Part C refers to infants and toddlers, and Part D refers to the national activities that exist to improve special education.

The essence of this act, Part B, contains the legislative components important to physicians. Any state that receives federal funding must include these essential components (Box 167-1). The act states who qualifies for special education in Section B. Any child between the ages of 3 to 21 who has been evaluated under this act's standards who is mentally retarded, speech or hearing impaired, deaf, a victim of traumatic brain injury, visually impaired, orthopedically impaired, autistic, possesses another health impairment, or is learning disabled qualifies for special education if the preexisting impairment influences the learning potential of the child.

Children with disabilities are entitled to a free and appropriate education. Free literally means "no charge." The child and his parents cannot be refused a service or billed for a service if it is covered under this act or if it is part of the child's IEP. The school can provide the least expensive form of the service. Medicaid or MediCal or private insurance can be billed for services covered under this act as long as it does not financially injure the family. Schools cannot charge for transportation to public or private facilities if the service is part of an agreed IEP. Appropriate education has been tested at the court level. In *Board of Education of the Hendrick Hudson Central School District, Westchester County, et al. v Rowley (1982)*, an appropriate education must have "a reasonably calculated benefit to the child's education." A child's "educability" and prognosis does not exclude him from the process as seen in *Timothy v N.H. (1987)*. Section 504 of the Rehabilitation Act of 1973 included modification and support for children with "other health impairments." Children with allergies, asthma, diabetes, attention deficient and hyperactivity disorder, etc., who do not qualify for an IEP are entitled to accommodations to protect their right to a free and appropriate education.

The term "least restrictive environment" is the general education classroom. A classroom with an aide for the child is less restrictive than a special education classroom, followed by a special school. The most restrictive setting would be a home environment.

The Individuals with Disabilities Education Act includes "related services" and covers a child's need for services as long as the child qualifies for special education and the services are necessary to meet the education goals set forth in the IEP. The services covered are transportation, counseling, physical, occupational and speech therapy, recreation and enrichment programs, and school nurse services. Transportation includes "door to bus" assistance but not transportation from school to after-care programs unless it is a part of the IEP. Counseling services do not include psychiatric services because these services fall under medical need unless they are required for the achievement of educational goals. Equal opportunity to participate in extracurricular activities must be provided, if appropriate. Health or nursing services such as intermittent catheterization, suctioning, etc., are included. Medical services that must be performed by a licensed physician are not provided. Drug abuse programs are not considered related services. Various classroom modifications, for example an air conditioner, are covered if maintaining body temperature in a brain-injured child is required for that individual to meet their IEP goals.

Public schools and educational agencies must search, find, and identify children with special educational needs as per the Individuals with Disabilities Education Act. Children in private schools and homeless children are included. Nondiscriminatory testing and assessment is guaranteed by this act. The testing process must be free of cultural or language barriers and be administered by a person who is trained and speaks the student's native language. Importantly, no single testing modality can be used solely to qualify a child for special education. Multiple evaluations and inputs must be performed before a child qualifies for special education.

An IEP must exist for every child that qualifies for special education. The IEP is a legal document that must be followed or the local public agency (school) can be cited for noncompliance. The IEP is reviewed every year and evaluated every 3 years. All confidential material must be made available to parents. The IEP team includes the child's parents, the child if appropriate, one regular education teacher (only if the child will be participating at some level in a regular classroom), a special education teacher, an individual from the school who is responsible for overseeing the performance of the others, an individual (usually a school psychologist) who can interpret the testing tools and their instructional implications, and, lastly, persons who also may contribute to the IEP process. Current (2004) amendments to the IEP do not require, for example, the presence of a physical therapist, an occupational therapist, etc., unless that particular service is being provided. The IEP, as an education plan for the disabled child, needs to include the following: a general statement regarding the child's current capabilities, annual goals, a statement regarding "related services," the approximate time spent out of a "regular" classroom, modifications needed for mandated assessments, the projected date of commencement of the plan, how progress will be measured, and a method to keep parents regularly informed.

An IEP is transferable. It travels with the child between schools and between states. This continues until a new plan is adopted or the current one is accepted. Provided services can be continued through summer recesses. The summer IEP is separate from the school year and may be completely different. The student must be at risk for "substantial regression" if recess services are to be provided.

Children with disabilities, at the age of 14, need an IEP that includes transition planning. By age 16, the transition process must be in action. Transition IEPs include vocational planning, assessment of activities of daily living, employment plans, and access to community services. Credentials and diplomas should be offered to special education students. An IEP diploma, the minimum requirement for armed services vocational training, can be earned. The diploma also can be used for seeking employment.

Part C of this act addresses infants and toddlers (up to 2 years) with disabilities. The Individualized Family Service Plan (IFSP) must be adopted, planned, and implemented by the local public agency and carefully mirrors an IEP. Federal grants are available for developing interagency systems in individual states for these services. The IFSP is a legal document specifying: the current status of the child's abilities; a statement of a family's resources and concerns; a plan for measurable treatment outcomes; a specific early intervention service plan based on research evidence; the location of the services; dates of commencement; and the name of the "service coordinator" who will oversee the IEP.

Part D of this act includes national activities to improve education of disabled children. Parent training, personnel improvement, and preparation and grants for research fall under this portion of the act.

HEALTH INSURANCE PORTABILITY AND ACCOUNTABILITY ACT OF 1996 (HIPAA)

The Health Insurance Portability and Accountability Act (HIPAA) was enacted to protect health-insured individuals from preexisting penalties and privacy violations when changing jobs and hence health insurance carriers. Schools that provide health services that are federally funded (catheterization, tracheostomy care, suctioning, and medication administration) are under HIPAA law guidelines.

No Child Left Behind Act (NCLB)

The No Child Left Behind Act was signed into law in 2002 (No Child Left Behind Act 2002, Pub. L No. 107 to 110). The Individuals with Disabilities Education Act of 2004 aligns itself with this act. The No Child Left Behind Act replaced the Elementary and Secondary Education Act of 1965 and is a huge paradigm shift from previous legislation. Federal funding to schools, based on the Education Act of 1965, was preferentially given to schools with the greatest number of children whose family incomes were near or lower than the poverty level. The No Child Left Behind Act distributes federal funding to schools that are in need of improvement based on student performance. Children with disabilities were expected to be included in this annual progress assessment of academic proficiency. Adequate progress must be made, and if a school fails for two consecutive years, the students and their parents may transfer to a nonfailing school. The sending school district must provide transportation until it is no longer a failing school for two consecutive years. This applies to all children in the school, regardless of disabilities.

INTERNATIONAL SPECIAL EDUCATION

Educational programs for children with disabilities vary widely internationally and approaches in several different countries are described in this section.

Canada

The Constitution Act is the legal document that gives the provinces of Canada the control of educational policies and their funding. Within the act, the Canadian Charter of Rights and Freedoms is the highest law of the country. So, the laws of any province regarding special education cannot be in violation of these fundamental rights outlined in the Charter of Rights and Freedoms. Passage by a province of their Education Act outlines the powers, responsibilities, and specific education laws for that province, and the minister of education enforces these laws. In the Education Act, special education, suspension, and expulsion resolutions are defined. Special needs schools are available for children with physical, mental, behavior, and communication disorders, as well as for gifted children.

China

The United States special education laws have been adopted by China in many ways (Kritzer, 2012). The 1975 Education for All Handicapped Children Act and IDEA Act have served as models for China. Interestingly, despite the large number of children with disabilities in China, the percentage of children receiving services in China is much lower than in the United States (Worrell et al., 2009). China excludes children who have learning disabilities, emotional behavioral disorders, language impairments, and other health impairments from receiving special education services. A lack of experienced professionals, of diagnostic technology, and of delivery systems decreases the number of children who are properly identified and who ultimately receive services.

China's law, The Compulsory Education Law (CEL) issued in 1986, demands that all children attend school at the age of 6. However, in remote areas of China, the CEL-2006 requires only children from the age of 7 to attend. The length of mandated education in China is 9 years. Children with disabilities are entitled to the same number of years of education (Worrell, 2009). Unfortunately, China's legislation does not guarantee financial support for schools or for the agencies that provide services for disabled children. Class size can reach 70 to 90 students per class, preventing special education children from having their needs met (Worrell, 2009).

Infants and toddlers are excluded from special education services unlike in the United States. Some large cities in China, however, do have programs to teach parents with challenged infants and toddlers on how to provide services. China's beliefs and ideology are contradictory to an IEP so that the unique needs of a child are not readily defined and addressed.

India

Special education has moved from segregation to integration through government laws and policies. India's Integration and Education of Disabled Children (IEDC) law was written in 1974. In 1991 there were 1200 special schools for disabled children that included children with visual impairments, intellectual disabilities, and orthopedic problems. In 1992 a new IEDC program was approved, and financing was provided to integrate disabled students into regular classrooms. Teacher training began and intensive teacher education was undertaken. Selected teachers at a given school were given a 1-year training program. They were then designated as resource teachers. In 1996 the government of India enacted the Persons with Disabilities Act, ensuring opportunities for, protecting the rights of, and allowing for full participation for all citizens. Education, employment, and rehabilitative services were covered for the blind, those with cured leprosy, and those with hearing impairment, motor disability, intellectually disability, and mental illness. Free and appropriate education until the age of 18 was included (National Policy for Persons with Disabilities, 2006).

Challenges occurred with attempts to integrate students and implement education. Because of poverty, access, and religious beliefs, many children did not receive services. The prevailing belief among many Hindus in India is that the disabilities a child or individual possessed were the result of past deeds in a former life and assisting the disabled could interfere with "karma." Therefore many disabled students did not receive education and inclusion.

Israel

Israel has very comprehensive special education programs for its citizens. The Special Education Law (SEL) of 1988 provided landmark legislation. A child with special needs is defined as "a person aged 3 to 21 whose capacity for adapted behavior is limited due to faulty physical, mental, psychological, or behavioral development and is in need of special education." A special education placement committee decides a child's educational needs. The committee includes a social worker, pediatrician, psychologist, minister of education services, and a representative of the National Special Education Parents Organization. A parent has no legal right to attend the meeting, but if the parent does not agree with the placement committee's decision, he or she has 21 days to request an appeal. Individual Educational Programs are developed for each child (Gumpel, 1996).

Italy

Since 1977, children with special education needs in Italy have an opportunity for inclusion with an Individual Educational Program. Special needs schools, separate from the parent school, have essentially been discontinued. All students, since 1987, are entitled to secondary education. In 1992 the Italian Parliament approved the Disabled Persons Bill (L.104/92), which allows inclusion education from preschool to university. A functional dynamic profile is developed utilizing public health doctors. Infants and children with disabilities are involved in education from birth to 19 years of age. Classrooms are composed of 20 students, and no more than 25 students are allowed in a classroom that contains a disabled student.

Japan

Japanese laws for special education began after World War II. The School Education Law of 1947 stated that special needs children should receive education with similar expected goals of ordinary children. Ultimately, the School Education Law made school attendance for all disabled children mandatory. In 1994 the law extended compulsory education to all students between the ages of 6 to 15 years.

Multiple school arrangements are available in Japan. The severely disabled attend special education schools, and students are given individual education plans. The National Institution for Special Education (NISE) was founded in 1991 and oversees the education of special needs children. Furthermore, special classes exist as well as resource learning classes for students with milder disabilities. Schools exist for children with vision, hearing, or orthopedic impairment as well as for those who are intellectually disabled and children who fall under the category of being "sickly" (Ministry of Education, Culture, Sports, Science and Technology, 2015).

REFERENCES

The complete list of references for this chapter is available in the e-book at www.expertconsult.com.
See inside cover for registration details.

SELECTED REFERENCES

Family Education Rights and Privacy Act of 1974, Pub. L No. 93-380. 1974.

Gumpel, T., 1996. Special Education education law in Israel. J. Spec. Educ. 29, 457–468.

Kritzer, J.B., 2012. Comparing Special Education in the United States and China. Int. J. Spec. Educ. 27 (2), 52–56.

Ministry of Education, Culture, Sports, Science and Technology. Special support education in Japan: education for children with special needs. <http://www.mext.go.jp/a_menu/shotou/tokbetu/material/001.pdf>; Retrieved 1 March 1 2015.

Murdick, N.L., Gartin, B.C., Crabtree, T., 2007. A free appropriate education. In: Special Education Education Lawlaw, second ed. MerrilMerrill Prentice Hall, New Jersey, pp. 56–57.

National Policy for Persons with Disabilities. Ministry of Social Justice and Empowerment. Government of India, 2006.

No Child Left Behind Act of 2002, Pub. L No. 107-110.

Osborne, A.G., Russo, C.T., 2006. Section 501 of the Rehabilitation Act of 1973. In: Special Education Education and the lLaw. Corwin Press, CAThousand Oaks, CA, pp. 10–16.

Reynolds, C.R., 2007. Diana v State Board of Education. In: Reynolds, C.R., Fletcher-Janzen, E. (Eds.), Encyclopedia of Special Special Educationeducation, third ed. Wiley, New York, pp. 724–725.

The Education for All Handicapped Children Act of 1975, Pub. L No. 94-142.

Vocational Rehabilitation Act of 1973. Section 504, Pub. L No. 93-112.

Worrell, J., Taber, M., 2009. Special Education practice in China and the United States: what is to come next? Int. J. Spec. Educ. 24 (3), 132–142.

Wright, P., 2007. History of special education law. In: Special Education Law, second ed. Virginia: Harbor House Law Press, Virginia, pp. 11–16.

168 Measurement of Health Outcomes in Pediatric Neurologic Disorders

Annette Majnemer and F. Virginia Wright

This chapter focuses on outcome measurement from the perspective of rehabilitation specialists such as occupational therapists, physical therapists, speech language pathologists, and psychologists. The general principles described apply to all outcome measures; however, specific examples and considerations for specialized areas such as educational or psychiatric assessment are not provided. Most standardized measures require either formal training according to the tool's guidelines and certification protocols or expertise in child development, in addition to clinical experience in the components that are being assessed.

OUTCOME MEASURES: PURPOSE, PROPERTIES, PRIORITIZING

An outcome is something that follows as a consequence or result of a process, which may be a disease, treatment, or service. An outcome measure is a tool that evaluates or determines the result of a disease, activity, or program. Outcome assessment using the appropriate tool(s) enables objective determination of changes in a neurologic condition over time or changes related to an intervention or program.

Identifying the purpose of outcome measurement in a given situation is essential because this will guide the selection of the most appropriate outcome measure(s). Whether in clinical practice or research, the evaluator must first consider what areas (domains) are most important to measure. These considerations always need to be accompanied by the question "why" to ensure that the outcome results will have direct relevance. Once what needs to be measured has been determined, the assessment tools that best align with the concepts (constructs) of interest within the targeted domains can be chosen.

It also is essential when selecting an outcome measure to know the intended purpose of the tool itself. With the recognition of the strong importance of being able to measure outcomes, tools have been created to measure particular outcomes and are typically identified as such in the corresponding validation literature that pertain to them. Examples include the Gross Motor Function Measure (observational measure) and Pediatric Evaluation of Disability Inventory (parent-report questionnaire). For an outcome measure to be used for change detection, the tool must contain items that have potential for change in the clinical group being measured and also have a response-option format that will permit change detection. Dichotomous (yes/no) response scales are not sufficiently sensitive to change, whereas response sets with five to seven options, although more difficult to score, enhance detection of small but potentially meaningful changes (Streiner, Norman, and Cairney, 2014).

There are two other categories of measures that users need to be aware of. *Discriminative measures* differentiate children as having or not having a particular characteristic or skill level (e.g., delayed or not delayed). Most of these measures have normative values for comparison. Although these can be useful at the initial assessment (e.g., Bruininks-Oseretsky Test of Motor Proficiency, Battelle Developmental Inventory), their application to outcome measurement needs to be approached with caution because they may lack item and response characteristics needed to detect change. Predictive tools are meant to classify children into categories with respect to their future status (Streiner et al., 2014). For example, the Alberta Infant Motor Scales and the General Movement Assessment are used to predict future motor ability in young infants. These measures are typically not well suited to evaluate change.

As part of this selection process, the properties of candidate measures need to be considered. They need to be age appropriate and applicable to the child's condition, appropriately scaled, and psychometrically sound and feasible. Measures must produce consistent and reproducible results (reliable), whether tested by independent evaluators (interrater reliability) or repeatedly by the same evaluator (test-retest reliability). The tester's experience or training or the child's level of attention or lack of engagement can contribute to measurement error. Subscales items should aggregate well together to represent particular attributes of interest (internal consistency). It is imperative that assessment tools are actually measuring what they are intending to measure (valid). Content may be verified by experts to ensure it has the attributes of interest (face validity), and results may be compared with other gold-standard measures of a similar construct (concurrent validity) or a gold standard in the future (predictive validity). Gold-standard measures often do not exist for children, and therefore the potential correlations will be less than perfect.

Validity also can be estimated by determining that the measurement tool behaves as expected. It may differentiate between children with low and high performance levels (discriminant validity). Finally, if an outcome measure is to be used to evaluate change over time, it must have evidence of being sensitive to change (responsiveness). This is important to verify when clinicians want to use the tool to evaluate treatment effectiveness; it is also important for researchers who are conducting an intervention trial (Streiner et al., 2014).

The clinical or research priorities for outcome measurement should also influence the selection of measures. In clinical practice, the functions of the clinician will guide the choice of the best-fitting outcome tools. In acute hospital-based care, providers focus on diagnosis and need to consider the health-related attributes they must identify. In a rehabilitation center, specialists provide intensive interventions and need to focus on the child- and family-related attributes they expect to change. In the home or community setting, the focus is on integration and child/family adaptation to the real-life context, and therefore assessment will focus on the activities/areas in which the clinician can make a difference.

Assessment results should inform clinical decisions and promote greater accountability and a reflective practice approach. The outcome measures selected by providers should inform their goals for intervention plans that are unique and specific to the child and family and their needs and priorities. After treatment or following a period of evolution of the neurologic condition, reassessment is helpful in determining whether there are clinically meaningful changes and whether treatment goals should continue in the same direction or need to be realigned. For the family, the findings on their child's assessment offer objective quantitative information regarding abilities (strengths), areas of challenge, and changes documented over time.

In research endeavors, investigators need to select valid outcome measures to address their hypotheses. In pediatric neurology, these questions could relate to the underlying biologic mechanisms of disability, determinants of brain recovery or brain organization, validation of new diagnostic tools, treatment efficacy, quality and benefit of services, or knowledge-translation efforts (Majnemer and Limperopoulos, 2002). Researchers need to be specific in formulating their questions, and may use a *patient intervention comparison outcome* (PICO) format for question formulation (Thebane, Thomas, and Paul, 2009). For example, if the researcher wanted to evaluate the efficacy of botulinum toxin, the PICO question might be: Will there be a significant improvement (the *comparison*) in range of motion, gross motor function, participation, and quality of life (the *outcomes*) in preschoolers with spastic diplegia (the *patients*) 3 months after treatment with botulinum toxin (the *intervention*)? The researcher may want to determine which children benefit most, and may evaluate how specific attributes of the child (e.g., age, baseline motor/cognitive function) or environment (e.g., family support, access to interventions) affect the outcomes. These attributes would also need to be specifically measured.

One other priority is that the outcome measurement process and the actual measures selected need to reflect and support a child- and family-centered philosophy of practice. This means using tools that elicit information directly from participants themselves about what they experience and do (performance) in their daily lives in addition to using observational measures that show what the child can do (capability) in the clinical setting. With respect to parent or child report questionnaires, it is important to ensure the measures will be acceptable as far as content, format, and wording. For example, a validated measure of family stress created 30 years ago, developed for a context that is very different from today's extended-family and multicultural environment, may no longer be optimal from the standpoint of response comfort or relevance.

Being family centered requires that the clinician think carefully about the relative burden of assessment to ensure that the measurement that is done is worth the time and effort expended and also fits with the information needs of the child and/or parent. It is important to explain to families the rationale for measurement and to discuss the measurement approach(es). This information sharing helps to optimize family engagement in the outcomes process at the outset of a new intervention block. Sufficient time needs to be provided to allow for discussion of results as they occur. This ongoing dialogue helps families develop realistic expectations regarding their child's progress, outcome, and goals. The well-targeted intervention planning that results from this collaborative and systematic process is expected to result in a more efficient intervention-delivery process and potentially better outcomes.

It is important to recognize that standard items within measures "typically focus on selected aspects of health and frequently do not include items that directly reflect a client's unique needs and goals" (McDougall and Wright, 2009, p. 1363), even though they may be valuable in providing an overall picture of the child's abilities and be sensitive to change. Integration of standard item measurement tools and individualized measures such as the Canadian Occupational Performance Measure (COPM) and/or Goal Attainment Scaling (GAS) (Cusick et al., 2006) is a powerful way of bringing child and family outcome priorities into a comprehensive and collaborative measurement approach. For these two goal measures, the child or caregiver (for younger children) selects the specific activities that he or she feels are problematic and important to improve. The child's present abilities are rated preintervention using the measure's specific scoring approach, and re-evaluated using the same goal-specific rating scale is done at targeted follow-up periods.

ICF AS A FRAMEWORK FOR OUTCOME MEASUREMENT

Given the breadth of areas and domains that can be measured, the number of measures available, and the growth in the number of new measures being developed, it can be daunting to determine which areas to measure and to examine how the measures interrelate in terms of a child's health and functioning. These relationships are critical in understanding how a child and family are doing and will influence goal setting and planning of interventions. The International Classification of Functioning, Disability and Health (ICF) framework developed by the World Health Organization (2007) serves well as a template for conceptualizing the priority outcome areas to measure for a given child and family. The ICF language offers a way of moving beyond the notion of disability (formerly thought of as the absence of health) and reframing it as functioning (in terms of body functions/structure, activity and participation) and the relationship to health (Table 168-1). The ICF framework looks at the child's abilities and the effects of the social and physical environment on a child's functioning and health. Use of an ICF diagram (as illustrated in the following scenario describing a 3-year-old with cerebral palsy) to plan the measures used by a clinician/team for a child provides awareness of the current emphasis (and relative balance) of a measurement/goal/intervention focus and added clarity on how one might adjust the focus and balance at times of re-evaluation.

As an illustration of the use of an ICF-based outcome measurement approach, consider the scenario of a child who is age 3 and has monoplegic cerebral palsy (right leg) with spasticity in her right calf muscles resulting in mildly impaired walking and running (consistent with a definition of mobility in Gross Motor Function Classification Level I [GMFC I]). The parents describe an increasing tightness in her ankle when they put her socks and shoes on, a tendency to toe walk that has become more pronounced, tripping and occasionally falling, and a reluctance to try new physical activities. It is this last observation that worries the parents most because they fear she is starting to be excluded from activities in her preschool class and neighborhood. Physical examination by her pediatric neurologist revealed that she is an ideal candidate for botulinum toxin injections. Although the area of outcome measurement pertaining to this intervention relates directly to changes (gains) in body function/structure (spasticity, range of motion) (Fig. 168-1), the parents' observations make it clear that evaluating changes in gross motor skills (activities such as running, going down hills, ascending/descending stairs) and doing new activities/keeping up with peers (participation

TABLE 168-1 Components of the ICF–Children and Youth Version (ICF-CY)

Components of the ICF	Description	Abnormalities	Examples
1. FUNCTIONING AND HEALTH			
Body structure	Anatomic parts of the body	Impairments	Periventricular leukomalacia, spinal muscular atrophy
Body function	Physiologic functions of the body or psychological functions	Impairments	Spasticity, decreased attention span, poor short-term memory
Activities and participation	Activity (A)—execution of a task/action Participation (P)—involvement in life situation or role	Activity limitations and participation restrictions	Walking (A), mobility in all environments (P); reading (A), education (P); brushing teeth (A), self-care (P)
2. CONTEXTUAL FACTORS			
Personal factors	Internal influences on functioning and health	Can be facilitator or obstacle	Lifestyle preferences, age, gender
Environmental factors	External influences on functioning and health	Can be facilitator or obstacle	Family functioning, peer support, health-care services, policies, resources,

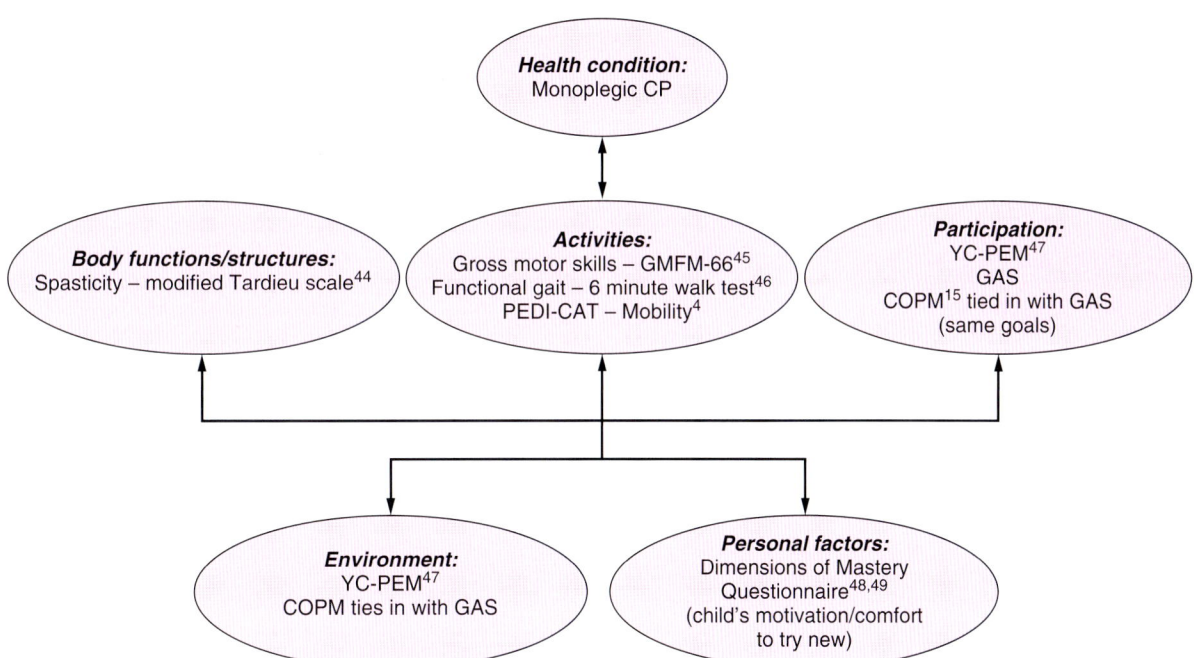

Figure 168-1. An example of the application of the ICF framework to a child with cerebral palsy. *(Based on the WHO International classification of functioning, disability and health. Geneva, Switzerland: World Health Organization; 2001.)*

or mobility in the playground and in gym activities) is also critical as evidence that the intervention is working. Two well-validated measures that physical or occupational therapists can administer are the Gross Motor Function Measure-66 (GMFM-66) and the Pediatric Evaluation of Disability Inventory's (PEDI-CAT's) Mobility Domain, parent-report questionnaire that directly address gross motor skills and functional abilities in young children with cerebral palsy. Collectively these provide measurement of what the child can do (GMFM-66: ICF Activity) and how the child is able to integrate those skills into daily life (PEDI-CAT: ICF Activities and Participation). There is also a recently published parent report measure that delves more deeply into a young child's participation in the environment, the Young Children's Participation and Environment Measure (YC-PEM), which was adapted from the Participation and Environment Measure for Children and Youth (PEM-CY). This measure was incorporated into the assessment because

it considers the role of the environment as a facilitator or barrier to participation. Finally, GAS could be used with these measures to highlight two or three well-operationalized individualized goals focused on important everyday activities, with outcome specifications tailored directly to the parent's hopes and expectations.

A word of caution in using the ICF framework for the linking of outcome measures is that there is a lack of incorporation of the overarching concept of quality of life (QOL) in the model (McDougall et al., 2010). Although enhancement of a child's QOL is at the core of the care clinicians provide, there will be times when changes in QOL will be seen as a direct goal of an intervention, whereas in other scenarios, higher QOL/life satisfaction may be an outcome of a series of interventions over a longer time frame.

Tables 168-2–168-6 provide examples of measures that can be used to assess children with physical disabilities (Table 168-2), intellectual disabilities (Table 168-3), and global developmental delays (Table 168-4), and generic measures of activities and participation (Table 168-5) and health and quality of life (Table 168-6). These tables are available in the online version of this chapter.

CHILD'S AGE AND STAGE AS A DETERMINANT OF MEASUREMENT FOCUS

Child development is a dynamic process marked by ongoing change. When evaluating a child, it is essential that relevant activities and life roles are evaluated based on the stage of the child's development (i.e., chronologic age), not the level of functioning or mental age. A second important principle is that evaluation of the outcomes of children with neurologic disorders requires periodic assessment at key transition points because their development, functioning, and health are continuously changing and evolving, even if their health condition is static. Difficulties at each stage of development may be identified, with the expectation of periodic utilization of additional services to enhance outcomes (Majnemer and Mazer, 2004). Finally, evaluators should seek to identify strengths within the child at a particular developmental stage because capitalizing on these strengths can enhance motivation, takes advantage of the child's abilities and competencies, and is more solutions-focused. This would include strengths within the family as well. In rehabilitation interventions, there is increasing interest in applying a strengths-based approach to promote positive youth development, meaningful participation, and resilience. The following websites offer additional information on these concepts:

http://www.acywr.org/2011/09/the-strength-based -approaches-backgrounder/

http://humanservices.ucdavis.edu/academy/pdf/strength_ based.pdf

In practice, a uniform template of specific measures is not applied to all children of all ages. Rather, the child's stage of development will influence the scope and focus of assessment, and the neurologic disorder and its associated impairments that manifest at each stage of development will guide selection of the most important measures. For example, in a 3-year-old with Down syndrome, it would be appropriate to ask the child to build a block tower to examine fine motor control (e.g., grasp, release, eye–hand coordination, proximal control, motor planning); however, at 13 years of age this activity would not be age appropriate. Rather, observations carried out during assessment of everyday tasks such as dressing, writing, and eating would be helpful in evaluating fine motor control, and use of standardized measures such as the Purdue Pegboard Test can provide objective and age-appropriate measurement of unilateral and bilateral manual dexterity.

For *newborns,* the primary focus is sensorimotor, such as the neonate's response to auditory and visual stimuli; the quality and symmetry of the infant's movements in prone, supine, and supported sitting; muscle tone; primitive reflex patterns; and behavioral state (e.g., lethargy, irritability). Many standardized neonatal neurobehavioral assessments (see review in Majnemer and Snider, 2005) are available and can be used in the neonatal intensive care unit. Feeding efficiency, an emerging life skill with important consequences for growth and development, may also be assessed.

In *infancy,* standardized evaluation tools such as the Bayley Scales of Infant and Toddler Development (Bayley-III, 3rd edition) are meant to assess the developmental abilities of infants and toddlers (up to 42 months), focusing predominantly on gross motor and fine motor skill development and cognitive abilities but also expressive and receptive language skills, social-emotional development, and adaptive behavior. At this stage, all domains of development begin to unfold, and delays in particular areas may gradually manifest themselves.

Preschool age is marked by rapid changes in developmental abilities across all domains, and children also become independent in basic self-care activities such as eating, toileting, and dressing. Children are able to communicate their needs and participate in conversations. At this developmental stage, important preacademic skills are also achieved, such as listening to instructions and attending to task demands, basic writing and copying, interacting socially with other children, and separating from caregivers. Measurement must be holistic and cover the spectrum of developmental and functional expectations.

At *school age,* there is increasing emphasis on functioning and health. Outcome measurement focuses on educational achievement, oral and written communication, independence in daily living skills to include domestic chores, mobility in all environments, socialization, and community engagement. By *adolescence,* personal identity formation, preferences and motivation, and life choices shape these areas, influencing functional potential. Environmental resources and supports, such as availability of aids and adaptations and accessibility of and participation in adaptive programs and activities, exert important influences on functioning and health. Therefore measurement at school age and adolescence is increasingly focused on activities and participation and personal and environmental factors, as framed by the ICF, and less on developmental impairments.

Reflecting back on the scenario of the 3-year-old child receiving botulinum toxin injections, and thinking instead about a school-aged child (e.g., an 11-year-old) with the same diagnosis and similar body function/structures issues in her right leg, although the areas of priority for measurement are likely similar, the actual measures that are used will need to differ to ensure that the measurement focus and perspective are optimal. First, it would be of value to use activity and participation measures that allow self-report by the child herself (instead of or in addition to the parent). In this regard, although the PEDI-CAT would apply as far as content for evaluating the aspect of gross-motor-related functional abilities, at the time of writing this chapter, the child report version had not been validated, and therefore it would still be necessary to have the caregiver as the proxy reporter of the child's abilities on the PEDI-CAT. An alternative might be use of the well-validated Activities Scale for Kids questionnaire. This outcome tool is a good content fit from the viewpoint of advanced motor skills and has a validated version that allows school-aged children to self-report on abilities. Second, although the GMFM-66 will serve well to capture the child's stand and walk/run/jump abilities in the 3-year old child, the ceiling effect that is present with children in the category of GMFC I who are ages 7 and up is a key issue. Hence, to be able to measure this area, an outcome measure for advanced gross motor skills is necessary. At present, one of the few possibilities in this outcome-measure category is a new observational tool known as the Challenge. Third, a shift from the YC-PEM to the PEM-CY (which the YC-PEM was modeled after) would allow age-suitable measurement of the participation and environment outcome areas. Finally, it will be important to capture priority goals directly from the child using the COPM or GAS and then work with the child and parent together to allow these goals to guide the intervention offered.

Irrespective of age or stage of development, a holistic view of the child's functioning and health in the context of the personal (e.g., lifestyle, intrinsic motivation, sociodemographic factors) and environmental (e.g., family functioning and well-being, peer support, resources in the community, societal attitudes) factors that can positively or negatively influence functioning is needed. This enables the clinician to capture a complete picture of the child's abilities and disabilities, which will then inform the next steps in intervention and health promotion.

NEW DIRECTIONS IN OUTCOME MEASUREMENT

One of the important considerations in using outcome measures that relates to the psychometric properties of the measures is the actual clinical meaning or interpretation of the changes that are observed. Change-score magnitude needs to be considered in light of the measure's reliability and the estimated measurement error. As the awareness of the importance of this concept has grown, recent outcome-measure validation studies have tended to place greater emphasis on reporting the minimum detectable change (MDC) or minimum detectable difference (MDD) estimates. For example, the MDC_{95} estimate for the GMFM-66 is 2.5 points, meaning that the user can have 95% confidence that a change of more than this will reflect true change and not measurement error. These estimates are still emerging for many of the commonly used pediatric outcome measures.

A related concept pertains to the minimum clinically important difference (MCID) (Streiner et al., 2014). Although it is often confused with MDC (Stratford and Riddle, 2013), this concept relates to what children, parents, and clinicians deem to be a meaningful change. Thus although it is fully reliant on the strength of the measure as far as reliability and related MDC, it goes a step beyond and takes child/parent priorities into account. There have been attempts to establish the MCID within different diagnostic groups for measures such as the PEDI and GMFM, and when these values are available, they at least give users some benchmarks to consider. However, at this point, caution is advised when using these values to signify intervention success because these estimates are at best only an average value across a group of parents/children and have been based upon statistical or consensus methods that are still in early conceptual stages (Copay et al., 2007).

An important new direction in outcome measurement is the concept of patient-reported outcomes (PROs). PROs include any report of the status of a patient's health condition that comes directly from the patient, without interpretation of the patient's response by the clinician or anyone else. These are self-report measures that are completed by the youth or by a proxy, typically a parent. PROs allow patients (or their proxies, if they cannot report for themselves) to describe and assess a number of attributes, such as symptoms, functional status, participation in life roles, health perceptions and quality of life, environmental facilitators and barriers, and satisfaction with services.

Numerous global initiatives promote the use of PROs as an emerging priority for clinical and research measurement. At the National Institutes of Health (NIH) in the United States, person-centered medicine and outcome research (PCOR) emphasizes the conduct of research that compares the benefits and harms of interventions to prevent, diagnose, and treat health conditions, and researchers are expected to apply PROs in the real-life context. NIH has funded research programs such as PROMIS, which is focused on PROs in health care and rehabilitation. In Canada, the strategy for patient-oriented research (SPOR) has been launched by the Canadian Institutes of Health Research; PROs are integral to SPOR programs. The United Kingdom has policies in place to promote the use of PROs and a focus on patient experience frameworks. In reality, PROs are not often used in clinical practice but can be instrumental to allow patient voices to be heard and to identify outcome status or factors influencing outcomes, and they can be influential in setting goals and making treatment decisions based on patient priorities and values.

Finally, a challenge for selection of outcome measures is that this is a growing area in which new measures will continue to be developed to address identified measurement gaps or issues related to existing measures. The concept of a toolbox of measures (Koene et al., 2013) that can apply to a clinical group or intervention has been advocated across rehabilitation settings, providing a cohesive approach and common language to outcome measurement across the international community. The reader is referred to an earlier paper for an example of how this concept pertains to cerebral palsy (Wright and Majnemer, 2014). Within any outcomes toolbox, there will also need to be space for a few new emerging measures (e.g., the Focus on the Outcomes of Communication under Six and the YC-PEM) that may fill important measurement gaps and have foundational evidence of psychometric strength; current work on responsiveness and MCID may also be worth considering for the toolbox, either as a replacement for or addition to the measures for given clinical situations (e.g., the use of the Challenge mentioned earlier to replace the GMFM-66 for children with cerebral palsy at GMFC I).

In summary, outcome measurement is essential to characterizing a child's functioning and health. The ICF provides a universal framework to ensure that outcomes are viewed holistically, across the spectrum of the child's functioning and in the context of personal and environmental factors that can influence outcomes. Outcome measurement provides essential individualized information to children and families regarding the child's current status and how it evolves over time; it also provides clinicians objective feedback about the changes that can be documented in response to interventions. Managers also benefit from outcome measurement as part of quality improvement, and researchers use standardized measures to answer their research questions. Selecting the most appropriate measures can be a daunting task and is best achieved in collaboration with patients and families and team members across health disciplines.

REFERENCES

The complete list of references for this chapter is available in the e-book at www.expertconsult.com.
  See inside cover for registration details.

SELECTED REFERENCES

Copay, A.G., Subach, B.R., Glassman, S.D., et al., 2007. Understanding the minimum clinically important difference: a review of concepts and methods. Spine J. 7, 541–546.

Cusick, A., McIntyre, S., Novak, I., et al., 2006. A comparison of goal attainment scaling and the Canadian Occupational Performance Measure for paediatric rehabilitation research. Pediatr. Rehabil. 9 (2), 149–157.

Koene, S., Jansen, M., Verhaak, C.M., et al., 2013. Towards the harmonization of outcome measures in children with mitochondrial disorders. Dev. Med. Child Neurol. 55, 698–706.

Majnemer, A., Limperopoulos, C., 2002. Importance of outcome determination in pediatric rehabilitation. Dev. Med. Child Neurol. 44, 773–777.

Majnemer, A., Mazer, B., 2004. New directions in the outcome evaluation of children with cerebral palsy. Semin. Pediatr. Neurol. 11 (1), 11–17.

Majnemer, A., Snider, L., 2005. A comparison of developmental assessments of the newborn and young infant. Ment. Retard. Dev. Disabil. Res. Rev. 11, 68–73.

McDougall, J., Wright, V., 2009. The ICF-CY and goal attainment scaling: benefits of their combined use for pediatric rehabilitation practice. Disabil. Rehabil. 31, 1362–1372.

McDougall, J., Wright, V., Rosenbaum, P., 2010. The ICF Model of Functioning and Disability: Incorporating Quality of Life and Human Development. Dev. Neurorehabil. 13 (3), 204–211.

Streiner, D.L., Norman, G.R., Cairney, J., 2014. Health measurement scales: a practical guide to their development and use. fifth ed. Oxford University Press, London.

Thebane, L., Thomas, T., Paul, J., 2009. Posing the research questions: not so simple. Can. J. Anaesth. 56, 71–79.

World Health Organization, 2007. International classification of functioning, disability and health-child and youth version. World Health Organization, Geneva, Switzerland.

Wright, F.V., Majnemer, A., 2014. The concept of a toolbox of outcome measures for children with cerebral palsy: why, what, and how to use? J. Child Neurol. 29, 1055–1065.

E-BOOK FIGURES AND TABLES

The following figures and tables are available in the e-book at www.expertconsult.com. See inside cover for registration details.

Table 168-2 Measures Commonly Used for Children with Physical Disabilities

Table 168-3 Measures Commonly Used for Children and Youth with Intellectual Disabilities

Table 168-4 Measures Commonly Used for Young Children with Global Developmental Delays

Table 168-5 Generic Measures of Activities and Participation That May Be Relevant for Children with Neurologic Disorders

Table 168-6 Generic Measures of Health and Quality of Life That May Be Relevant for Children with Neurologic Disorders

169 The Influence of Computer Resources on Child Neurology

Michael M. Segal and Steven M. Leber

An expanded version of this chapter is available on www.expertconsult.com. See inside cover for registration details.

As computer technology becomes more integrated into our lives, much of the information that we use now, including summarization of knowledge in textbooks, will be accessed primarily electronically. This chapter examines how such changes are unfolding in the ways we communicate and discuss information, in the ways we marshal information to diagnose and treat patients, and in the ways we educate newcomers to the field and keep experienced clinicians up to date. Table 169-1 in the online version of the chapter lists websites of interest to child neurologists.

CLINICAL DISCUSSIONS AND GROUPS

Throughout medical history, doctors have talked to one another, patients have talked to one another, and doctors and patients have talked to each other. With the advances in information technology, such communications have become faster, cheaper, and, in some situations, more anonymous. For over a century, doctors have used conferences, journals, and textbooks to exchange information. Recent innovations in technology have moved such discussions to the Internet and made them more instantaneous. These have used listservs (discussions sent by e-mail to groups of subscribers) and web-based forums that are organized by topic, in which people post questions, answers, and news.

Speeding up communication is no small thing. It can take one or two decades for therapeutic advances to become part of routine clinical practice (http://archive.ahrq.gov/research/findings/factsheets/translating/tripfac/trip2fac.html). The ability to learn of such advances and hear considered responses from leaders in the field within days, results not only in an increased speed of learning of new advances but also in attention directed to potential problems in published interpretations of research. Web forums and listservs are also popular, in part, because they have created an environment that encourages spontaneity and sharing of hypotheses.

The specifics of the technology of listservs versus forums seem not to matter much. What matters most is the community. The Child-Neuro listserv (http://www-personal.umich.edu/~leber/c-n/e-mailUM.html) was established in 1993, using what is now antiquated technology—using text-format messages distributed individually or in daily digests. Nevertheless, the Child-Neuro listserv continues to be the core Internet discussion group in the field, whereas more technologically sophisticated web-based discussion services, such as Sermo (http://www.sermo.com/), have less influence because they do not have the same presence of experts. It is too early to be able to assess the utility of the Child Neurology Society's new "Open Forum" web-based service.

The technology for discussions among patients is often newer, since the communities are newer, the numbers are greater, and the needs for privacy are lower. In the past, patients had much less contact with one another due to difficulty finding each other and the reluctance to disclose illness to people they knew personally. As a result of the anonymity of the Internet and the ability to find others with similar problems through search engines, patient-to–patient discussions have proliferated. Since these discussions are new, they have tended

to use newer Web-based forum technologies. Communities such as PatientsLikeMe (http://www.patientslikeme.com/) and Brain Talk (http://braintalkcommunities.org/) have become meta-sites for people with neurologic diseases. Some forums offer advanced community capabilities. For example, PatientsLikeMe allows users to search for others with similar symptoms, an ability that can be used for identifying hypotheses to test in controlled studies. In addition to these meta-sites, there are communities for individual disorders, such as attention deficit disorder (http://www.addforums.com/forums/index.php) and periodic paralysis (http://www.periodicparalysis.org/).

Another innovation enabled by the Internet is medical blogging. Blogs, the shorthand term for "weblogs," are websites on which articles, commentary, and other forms of textual, graphic, or multimedia content are posted. Blogs are often run by a single individual, providing a personal perspective and a top-down structure. As the costs associated with blogging have fallen essentially to the cost of the time involved, blogs have proliferated. In medicine, blogs have tended to cover medical practice and common diseases; blogs covering rare diseases would have very small audiences, and online communities make more sense as forums for such communication. However, there is quite a continuum. Blogs are sometimes a group effort and typically include some discussion in each thread, and discussion groups often have several regulars who sustain the discussion. So, in actuality, there are hybrids between pure blogs and pure discussions that have evolved to meet the needs of individual communities.

One of the important innovations in online discussions is the breaking down of the separateness of doctor-to-doctor and patient-to-patient discussions to create doctor-to-patient discussions. Doctor-to-patient discussions are of course the core of medical practice, but sharing such discussions among wider communities has value. An advantage of the Internet is the ability to have doctor-to-patient discussions with anonymity that one cannot achieve by group visits to doctors. The main barriers to doctor-to-patient discussions on the Internet are the absence of physical examination and medical records from other doctors, making the doctor less confident about giving advice, as well as the lack of incentives for physicians to provide such assistance with commitment and consistency. However, this may be merely an issue of creating the proper incentives and structures. One of the authors of this chapter has spent a significant amount of time in recent years interacting with patients on a variety of sites as part of an effort to uncover the molecular mechanism of attention deficit disorder (Segal, 2014). The patients would make little progress by themselves because they lack the deep expertise of the doctors in understanding the biology of disease. The doctors would stagnate without the patients' descriptions of their clinical symptoms. The combination is much more effective. In the past, progress could be made by studying the patients in a large clinical practice and hearing their observations personally, but such a process is difficult to arrange for less common diseases. Now, the ability to have such interactions is much accelerated. A doctor can post a query and get responses from many patients within days and, furthermore, can get a sense of how many of the regular participants respond in a particular way. Such interactions allow patients to partner with doctors, not only in decisions on treatment, but also in advances in understanding pathophysiology.

A patient-centered movement that calls itself "Health 2.0" has touted patient-to-patient discussions as a replacement for many types of doctor-to-patient interactions and replacing top-down "information therapy." Health 2.0 is the exchange of information in Internet forums "that get richer as more people use them" by "harnessing collective intelligence" (http://patients.aan.com/news/?event = read&article_id = 5277), whereas information therapy involves more traditional instructional materials provided by doctors. However, drawing a distinction between Health 2.0 and information therapy may be more theoretical than real. For example, the patients in the listserv of a prototypical Health 2.0 group, the Periodic Paralysis Association, asked the doctors associated with the listserv to write an "owner's manual" for hypokalemic periodic paralysis (http://simulconsult.com/resources/hypopp.html), a prototypical information therapy type of resource. The patients used the listserv to collect questions for which they wanted answers, both for their own education and to educate physicians caring for them. Yet the patients made very clear that they wanted the responses—that is, the content—to be written by people whom they and their physicians trust as experts. Far from guarding their realm as a patient-to-patient self-empowerment organization, the patients encouraged two doctors to participate in the listserv, one motivated by a research interest in the area and the other motivated by having one of the diseases himself. This ability to add doctor-to-patient interactions and mix Health 2.0 and information therapy shows how some of the rigid conceptions of the types of medical information on the Internet are evolving into more flexible approaches that are better at meeting the needs of patients. There is an important need to institutionalize resources valued by patients such as "owner's manuals" into a meta-site covering many diseases and thus known widely and trusted in the field.

The discussion groups described previously involve groups of patients, groups of doctors, and sometimes a few doctors and many patients. Yet in medical practice, a different type of exchange predominates: discussions about one patient in a clinical chart. With only a bit of exaggeration, one could characterize an electronic health record (EHR) as a privacy-protected blog about one patient. Despite the simplicity of blogs, they have the ability to incorporate a wide variety of types of external content. Currently, however, EHRs have a lot of standardized, nonpertinent material that distracts the reader from the main points. However, one should expect improvements in the EHRs of the future; as discussed later in "Diagnostic Decision Support," it is possible to use computerized tools to reintroduce pertinence to EHRs and do so in ways that leverage large amounts of information.

There is much discussion about automating some types of doctor-to-patient interactions using e-mail and telemedicine. This is most extensively implemented so far in radiology, in which the subtleties of patient interaction are largely absent and reimbursement issues are most clearly defined. It is widely expected that such techniques will expand. Using telemedicine in radiology and psychiatry, however, is more practical than in in some areas of neurology in which physical examination plays a much large role. In other areas, however, such as epilepsy and movement disorders, the history and observation of the patient is more important than hands-on examination, and telemedicine may be boon for patient-centered health care (Joshi, 2014). Over the years, it is expected that telemedicine will increase, driven by provisions for reimbursement, technology and services for physical examination and patient monitoring, and secure options for such online interactions.

On a more basic level, many patients already are using e-mail to communicate with their physicians. Electronic communication between patients and healthcare providers is advantageous, in that the communications can be thought out carefully in advance, posted and read at convenient times, and saved for future reference and for the medical record. Supplemental information (e.g., medication instructions and handouts going from doctors to patients, or videos of patients' events going from patients to doctors) can be attached or linked. "Asynchronous communication" also avoids "phone tag," long telephone queues and holds, and long distance phone charges, a difficulty for many patients. However, the use of e-mail to convey sensitive information raises numerous security and privacy concerns, particularly given the legal right of employers to access their employees' e-mail. A potential solution to many of the problems posed by e-mail lies in the development of comprehensive, password-protected patient portals for doctor-to-patient interaction. Most commercial EHRs have built-in portals with secure messaging; having at least 5% of a provider's patients use the portal is now a requirement of the Centers for Medicare and Medicaid Services (CMS) Meaningful Use Stage 2 requirements (http://www.cms.gov/Regulations-and-Guidance/Legislation/EHRIncentivePrograms/downloads/Stage2_EPCore_17_UseSecureElectronicMessaging.pdf).

WIKIS

Wikis are a type of web content with no real analog in the precomputer age. A wiki is a document that can be edited independently by many people using a simple set of web page formatting tags. The prototypical and dominant wiki is the collection called Wikipedia.

The advantage of Wikipedia is that the wide participation has resulted in millions of pages of content, with many popular articles having material contributed by many different authors, none of whom is paid. The disadvantage of Wikipedia is that battles can erupt over controversial issues and editing of pages can be banned by editors with a particular perspective despite the existing information being false or misleading.

In medicine, a key concern about Wikipedia is that articles are often written by people who are not medical professionals, sometimes resulting in content that is dubious or very incomplete. Although Wikipedia has articles on thousands of diseases, many physicians will prefer wikis with authorship restricted to doctors, but there is not much content of this sort for child neurology.

As with traditional narrative content, a promising future direction for wikis is finding some way of getting doctors and patients "on the same page." One such example is having a doctor who has a particular disease write material that combines both the doctor's and patient's perspectives, resulting in a full understanding that comes from living with the disease from both perspectives.

As with Internet forums, the chief difficulty in achieving the desired doctor-to-patient collaboration is creating financial and professional models for inducing the doctor to write patient-directed material. Due to the value of such material, it seems likely that this will be achieved, but it remains to be seen what incentives will get doctors involved in such patient-directed materials. Such helpful but hard-to-monetize resources are an example of the benefit of large, integrated health organizations (Christensen et al., 2008).

DIAGNOSTIC DECISION SUPPORT

The basic difficulty with diagnosis is that medical information is typically organized by disease, yet the process of diagnosis begins with a collection of findings and considers which diseases best fit with these findings. Some of the resources for diagnostic decision support, such as flow charts and diagnosis confirmation protocols, existed long before computers. These approaches are very useful in situations in which a particularly salient finding is present or a particular diagnosis is being considered. However, for the more general case, we now have access to novel approaches to decision support that did not exist in the precomputer age and can improve both diagnostic accuracy and cost-effectiveness of workups. These new approaches include automated search and diagnostic software. Although in the past people argued about whether such resources were useful, with the proliferation of newly recognized genetic disorders and the advent of inexpensive genome sequencing, little doubt remains that such computerized approaches are needed.

The advantage of automated search is the ability to process huge amounts of information collected in an inexpensive, automated process of searching accessible web pages (e.g., Google; http://www.google.com/) or adding some natural language processing (e.g., Isabel; http://www.isabelhealthcare .com/). The disadvantage of search is that many of the subtleties of the information are lost or jumbled, including information about timing and onset, absent findings, frequency of findings, and treatability. Such subtleties can be used in a diagnostic software approach, but a "curation" process of collecting information manually in a standardized format is needed to characterize diseases, and tradeoffs must be made as to level of granularity to characterize findings (e.g., Simul-Consult: http://www.simulconsult.com/; and Phenomizer: http://compbio.charite.de/phenomizer/). Furthermore, there are many subtleties to how we think of patient findings such as how we group them (e.g., including orthostatic changes in blood pressure as part of the disease or considering it incidental) and with what level of granularity the clinician should describe findings (should weakness be described as proximal vs. distal, rapid vs. slow onset, and so forth).

Another advantage of diagnostic software is the ability to offer advice prospectively on which findings or laboratory tests would be most useful and cost-effective to distinguish among likely diagnoses. This is important in getting doctors and insurers to focus on evidence relevant to decisions about whether a test should be covered by insurance. Software also offers the ability to link such recommendations about useful tests to resources such as the Genetic Testing Registry (http://www.ncbi.nlm.nih.gov/gtr/) and the NextGxDx gene test shopping service (https://www.nextgxdx.com/). The ability to suggest useful findings is also important in promoting communication among medical specialties. For example, a radiologist can begin from a diagnostic software session begun by a neurologist, using a display of useful radiologic findings to ensure that the findings most useful to the neurologist are commented on explicitly.

One area in which doctors need help is in interpreting genetic tests. Increasingly, we face situations in which a mutation is found in a gene or an abnormality is found on a chromosomal test, but it is not clear whether the result is pathogenic or incidental. Such information is a key proprietary resource of companies that have interpreted many genetic tests, but such information is being increasingly centralized in the ClinVar database (http://www.ncbi.nlm.nih.gov/clinvar/), which allows genome interpretation software to tap into such listings via automated queries.

A basic philosophic issue is developing about interpretation of whole exome and whole genome testing. Is this similar to a single gene test, in which the laboratory returns an answer, or is it more similar to an MRI, in which the neurologist provides detailed information to the radiologist, and the ultimate diagnosis is made by the neurologist, not the radiologist? Clinical diagnostic decision support software that can also do genome analysis in a clinical context can be a crucial way of empowering the neurologist to interpret genome results with appropriate clinical correlation (Segal, 2015). Clinicians who know the patient can often check findings (such as crying without tears or a molar tooth sign on MRI) that were not recognized as useful to check until results became available from genomic analysis of the patient.

TREATMENT DECISION SUPPORT

Treatment is a more straightforward software task than diagnosis because one already knows the diagnosis. If the disease is unfamiliar, software simplifies access to narrative text, calculators, and flow charts to help with treatment. Even when the disease is familiar, integration of computer programs into the workflow can enhance fine-tuned management and increase safety and improve outcomes.

Examples of freestanding or integrated applications include calculators (such as automated anticoagulation calculators), drug information and interactions, flowcharts, look-up tables, nomograms, and automated guidelines and protocols (e.g., an online ordering system that might recommend deep vein thrombosis prophylaxis in an adult in bed for longer than 2 days, or a patient-controlled anesthesia pump that puts an upper limit on the amount of morphine infused).

The difficulties in deciding about treatment typically arise from lack of data and from conflicts between data sources. Perhaps the most useful recent advance in treatment decision making has been the ability of groups of healthcare professionals to address specific treatment questions, review the medical literature, and make these systematic reviews widely and easily available via the Internet (http://en.wikipedia.org/wiki/Systematic_review). The best known collection is the Cochrane Database of Systematic Reviews section of the Cochrane Library (http://www.cochranelibrary.com/). Yet even when clear recommendations have been formulated, they often are not used (McGlynn et al., 2003). Why is this the case?

First, even when guidelines exist, it takes extra effort for the practitioner to look for them and remember to use them. However, "guideline execution engines" are being developed to address this issue; these are programs integrated into EHRs that translate clinical guidelines into recommendations (http://en.wikipedia.org/wiki/Guideline_execution_engine). Examples might include alerts about drug interactions and dosage errors, disease management pathways (e.g., reminders to obtain surveillance laboratory tests in patients on certain medications or renal ultrasounds in patients with tuberous sclerosis) and automatic retrieval of relevant systematic reviews. A meta-analysis of clinical decision support systems for treatment or screening revealed that 68% of these support systems improved clinical practice and that the only ones that did so were those in which decision support was automatically supplied to the clinicians as part of their normal workflow; none of the support systems in which clinicians were required to seek out the help of the support system improved clinical practice (Kawamoto et al., 2005). Other features associated with improvement in clinical practice for treatment and screening were:

1. Computerized systems compared with manual systems
2. Systems integrated into the charting or order system, rather than acting as standalone applications
3. Systems that prompted clinicians for reasons when they chose to override automated recommendations, rather than allowing bypass of recommendations without recording a reason
4. Systems that provided recommendations rather than those that simply assessed risk (e.g., "Patient is at high risk of coronary artery disease; recommend initiation of beta-blocker therapy" rather than simply "Patient is at high risk of coronary artery disease")

5. Systems that provided decision support at the location and time of decision making compared with those providing support away from the point of care

Some 94% of clinical support systems that incorporated these key features were associated with improvement in clinical practice. Paper-based clinical guidelines do not have the influence of guidelines that are integrated into a clinical management system.

The second reason why these clinical protocols are not used is that there are so few of them, and even the ones we have are based on limited information and often do not give definitive guidance. For example, the American Academy of Neurology and Child Neurology Society have a total of only 12 treatment guidelines for child neurology on their websites (https://www.aan.com/Guidelines/home/ByTopic?topicId=14 and http://www.childneurologysociety.org/resources/practice-parameters; accessed 11 April 2016). Moreover, guidelines frequently do not exist or apply to the individual patient in front of us and the specific clinical question being asked (Gronseth and French, 2008). The patient in front of us is not the "average patient" addressed in the study and may have secondary diagnoses that affect treatment. Establishing recommendations can be very difficult (e.g., Smeets et al., 1999; regarding initiation of anti-epileptic medications), particularly for rare diseases. We are hopeful that, as medical records are digitized, medical information will become more easily abstracted, coded, and shared, aiding generation of better information about diseases, treatments, and outcomes. However, the complexities of coding information at appropriate levels of granularity are far from trivial, particularly because medical knowledge is in a constant state of flux.

EDUCATION

Education is an area likely to be transformed in major ways by computer technology. Many of the information resources discussed previously, from narrative resources to wikis to decision support, are already being used in education. The ability of the web to disseminate video is of huge importance to teaching areas of neurology that are very visual, such as movement disorders and epilepsy; even the ability to provide still images at low cost is very helpful for neurocutaneous diseases and neuroimaging. The ability of diagnostic decision support software to highlight useful findings and link to resources about them is crucial to enabling such just-in-time education.

Several online educational resources relevant to child neurology are listed in the table accompanying the online version of this chapter.

The web has also facilitated case-based education by allowing many training programs to share interesting clinical cases. The Child Neurology Society and the Professors of Child Neurology have been running such a program since 2008 (http://www.childneurologysociety.org/resources/continuing-education/cns-case-studies), making use of the web to include images and to hyperlink the cases directly to articles in the literature and to diagnostic software.

Decision support software is also useful in teaching in a very concrete context how we approach differential diagnosis. Typically, medical students are taught to make diagnoses by collecting all relevant information, thinking about it, and constructing a differential diagnosis. In reality, the process is far more iterative (Bowen, 2006). One collects a bit of information, forms hypotheses, and then collects more information based on the hypotheses and continues in this manner, refining the differential diagnosis iteratively. Using diagnostic software, one can show this process in a very concrete way and illustrate other factors that are important in diagnostic thinking such as frequency of findings, treatability, and time information. Diagnosis turns out to be far more complex than the way it is presented in medical schools, and the ability to demonstrate this in a very concrete fashion with diagnostic software makes it easier to convey these complexities to students.

PERSPECTIVES

One of the big questions about computerization in medicine is whether the new medium will change the type of medical information used. For new tools, such as diagnostic software, the use of the tool at all is a real change. But the wider question is how traditional narrative material will be changed by the Internet. Will we move away from authoritative sources and toward a social networking approach in which information is amplified by the community of users? The examples discussed in this chapter suggest that both doctors and patients want some mix of certification and social networking approaches and that the successful resources will be those that merge these to combine the solidity of expertise with the nimbleness of a vigorous community.

It seems clear that most of our information will be on the Internet, and new approaches to information will become common. We expect a rapid move toward interoperability among information resources, jumping not only from software to narrative resources but also from narrative resources to software to obtain advice tailored to an individual patient.

CONFLICT OF INTEREST

Dr. Segal is the founder of SimulConsult. He acknowledges that his interest in promoting use of the software poses a potential conflict of interest. Dr. Leber has no conflicts of interest.

REFERENCES

The complete list of references for this chapter is available online at www.expertconsult.com.
See inside cover for registration details.

SELECTED REFERENCES

Bowen, J.L., 2006. Educational strategies to promote clinical diagnostic reasoning. N. Engl. J. Med. 355, 2217–2225.

Christensen, C.M., Grossman, J.H., Hwang, J., 2008. The Innovator's Prescription: A Disruptive Solution for Health Care. McGraw-Hill, New York.

Gronseth, G., French, J., 2008. Practice parameters and technology assessments: what they are, what they are not, and why you should care. Neurology 71 (20), 1639–1643.

Joshi, C., 2014. Telemedicine in pediatric neurology. Pediatr. Neurol. 51, 189–191.

Kawamoto, K., Houlihan, C.A., Balas, E.A., et al., 2005. Improving clinical practice using clinical decision support systems: a systematic review of trials to identify features critical to success. BMJ 330 (7494), 765.

McGlynn, E.A., Asch, S.M., Adams, J., et al., 2003. The quality of healthcare delivered to adults in the United States. N. Engl. J. Med. 348, 2635–2645.

Segal, M.M., 2014. We cannot say whether attention deficit hyperactivity disorder exists, but we can find its molecular mechanisms. Pediatr. Neurol. 51, 15–16.

Segal M.M., 2015. Genome interpretation: Clinical correlation is recommended. Appl. Transl. Genom. 6, 26–27.

Smeets, R., Talmon, J., Meinardi, H., et al., 1999. Validating a decision support system for anti-epileptic drug treatment. Part I: initiating anti-epileptic drug treatment. Int. J. Med. Inform. 55 (3), 189–198.

E-BOOK TABLE

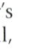

The following figures and tables are available in the e-book at www.expertconsult.com. See inside cover for registration details.

Table 169-1 Selected Websites of Interest to Pediatric Neurologists

170 Education and Training of Child Neurologists and Workforce Issues

David K. Urion

 An expanded version of this chapter is available on www.expertconsult.com. See inside cover for registration details.

INTRODUCTION

This chapter considers two interrelated issues: how should child neurologists ideally be educated and trained in terms of their early development and introduction to the field, and how do these issues of education and training have an influence upon the workforce for the first half of the current century? Consideration of the issues of education and training, as well as the workforce in child neurology, directly affects the very nature and identity of child neurology. How we educate and train those who will follow us, to whom we are accountable for the content and outcome of that education, and how we deploy the workforce we thus prepare define our very essence as child neurologists.

The term most frequently used these days is "training," but we must consider this in a broader sense. We are not limiting the notion of "training" to the acquisition of a set of skills and knowledge, a craft. Skills and knowledge are necessary but not sufficient. The training of child neurologists must also include the development of habits of mind, ethical and moral considerations, and the cultivation of certain virtues. Russell Gruen and his colleagues have argued quite persuasively that the evolution of the profession of medicine has been one of the constant extensions of domains of professional obligation into what had previously been domains of professional aspiration. Individual patient care was the sole domain of professional obligation for a long period of time. As time passed, he argues that access to care becomes a domain of professional obligation—whether or not all children have access to child neurology care becomes our professional obligation. Direct socioeconomic influences then became our professional obligation—do our patients have access to insurance coverage, and does their family's socioeconomic status have an influence upon their health? Gruen then argues that broader socioeconomic influences and global health issues are still in the domain of professional aspiration, not currently normative for us, but that this will likely change as time goes on.

This concept of "training" is more akin to the notion of "formation" that was prevalent in the 19th century among the so-called liberal professions—medicine, law, the clergy, and the military. In those days, "formation" meant taking individuals and engaging them in a process in which they obtained not only the knowledge and skills necessary for a profession, but also a world view, a set of attitudes and beliefs, a common set of reference values and virtues, which were all recognized as essential to the profession. Another central feature to this calculus was the independence of the profession: it determined its own standards for becoming a member of the profession, as well as that which was needed to remain a member of the profession. The profession argued that it was the guarantor of skills and proficiency, ethical behavior and practice, and the public could, and should, be reassured by that. Although the use of the term "formation" has fallen out of currency, the broadness of the concept it embraces is one we should still

continue—it allows us to consider historical approaches before formal programs in child neurology evolved and to contemplate a generation of our forebears that became child neurologists through pathways other than our current mode of education and training, the residency program. It also allows us to think more broadly about the nature of child neurologists and what skills, attributes, and virtues they need to be successful, competent, and compassionate practitioners of the art and science of child neurology for the 21st century.

This chapter will use the framework of the development of child neurology training from the vantage point of how training evolved in the United States. It is but one example of the development of the field as a paradigm for consideration. Child neurology training has evolved differently across the globe based on how regional socioeconomic, cultural, and religious factors have influenced the development of different medical specialties.

HISTORICAL ASPECTS

Unlike most other pediatric subspecialties, child neurology in the United States emerged from the evolution of certain adult neurology practitioners, who became particularly interested in the problems and disorders that were particular to children in the context of their discipline. This contrasts with most other pediatric subspecialties, whose history is one of pediatricians becoming increasingly interested in a specific set of disorders and a subspecialty organizing itself in that emergent fashion. This maintains itself today by the organization of the certifying bodies of pediatric subspecialties. Most derive their authority from the American Board of Pediatrics. Child neurologists are certified instead by the American Board of Psychiatry and Neurology. Even the preferred name for our discipline subtly demonstrates this. One is a pediatric cardiologist and is board certified as such. Our discipline is populated by people who usually refer to themselves as child neurologists and whose certification is in neurology with special competence in child neurology. The distinction is not merely semantic but is foundational in terms of identity.

It is beyond the scope of this chapter to consider in detail the founders of child neurology; the reader is referred to the excellent text by that name for a biographic compendium (Ashwal, 1990). We can, however, note several pathways that emerged in the evolution of the discipline. The vast majority of the early practitioners of what became our discipline began as adult neurologists who developed abiding interests in the neurologic disorders of children. They, in turn, began to gather like-minded younger physicians around them and what we can consider the first era of child neurology formation ensued. Informal and centered around one or two charismatic teachers, these schools of child neurology emerged at some of the larger university teaching hospitals of the early 20th century. The disciples of these schools then moved out across the country, taking their traditions, interests, and approaches with them. The late Dr. David Clark likened this era of child neurology to tracing bloodlines in racehorses. One could trace many of these early leaders back to their original progenitor. Thus one could say that Charles Barlow, for example, personified the education he received from Douglas Buchanan, and the Boston Children's Hospital child neurology program could have been considered in the mid-20th century as a branch of the University of Chicago tree. The American schools of child neurology emanated from individuals such as Philip Dodge in Boston and then St. Louis and Sidney Carter in New York.

The argument could be made that during this period, individuals chose places in which to be formed in child neurology based upon the leadership and the school of child neurology that was represented there. Although this was undoubtedly fruitful for the development of career interests, it did not assure the public that formation in child neurology would be broad, inclusive, and comprehensive in all places in which it was being undertaken.

As child neurology emerged as a distinctive discipline within neurology, it was argued that it represented a competence sufficiently separable to be distinguished from adult neurology. Thus whereas adult neurologists were being certified by the American Board of Psychiatry and Neurology (ABPN) by 1935, it was not until the late 1950s that a set of examinations were promulgated by the ABPN to determine the competence an applicant had in that field.

In response to this, we can see that places in which child neurologists were being prepared began to respond to these early standards. The ABPN has argued since its inception that one of its chief fiduciary responsibilities is to the public; the standards for board certification create a body of persons in whom the public can trust in terms of competence, ethics, and professional behavior. The emergence of a separable competence in child neurology extended that approach. The ABPN was thus a public guarantor of the general competence of an individual to practice child neurology.

Supported by efforts from the United States government, child neurology programs took on a sort of mixed self-organization—some in response to the mandates of the certification examination of the ABPN, some in response to the mandates inherent in various parts of federal funding, particularly training grants which incentivized research into large domains such as intellectual disability. The meeting of those standards, however, was left to the individual programs with great leeway.

The disadvantages of this relatively unstructured approach became obvious, not just in child neurology but across almost all domains of medicine. Thus the last quarter of the 20th century saw increasing requirements of programs on the part of bodies such as the ABPN and the Accreditation Council for Graduate Medical Education (ACGME). Most of these requirements, however, were time-based; that is, the chief metric was so many months of a given type of rotation. One needed to do 1 year of adult neurology, for example, and rotations in psychiatry, to be eligible for the ABPN examination. Theorists of professional education refer to this as an industrial model of education. So much time on the assembly line assures the product.

CURRENT APPROACHES

Among child neurology educators, this led to a general dissatisfaction with the variability in training that could still occur with this time-based, examination-referenced approach. In addition, there was a feeling that the public needed to be assured that there was sufficient consistency across child neurology programs that they could be confident that any child neurologist their child saw was well prepared and

broadly informed. Robert Rust edited an issue of *Seminars in Neurology* (Rust, 2011), which attempted to describe the corpus of knowledge that a child neurologist should have in a broad spectrum of domains of clinical practice. Each section was authored by a recognized expert in that domain. One could thus argue that the community of scholars was making a statement about what was essential to the practice of child neurology at the beginning of the new century.

The Professors of Child Neurology subsequently formed a working group that undertook to convert this set of essays and outlines into a framework of the knowledge that was viewed as essential to the practice of child neurology, a so-called "Universal Curriculum." The name cited the normative nature of the material—that is, an organization representing the academic training programs and departments, divisions and sections of child neurology across the country had endorsed this as the corpus of knowledge and skills required to practice child neurology in the new century.

A similar process is also happening in Canada. The Royal College of Physicians and Surgeons has embraced this concept under the rubric "competency by design." Competency is to be demonstrated in each of the CanMEDS roles: medical expert, communicator, collaborator, manager/leader, scholar, advocate, and professional. From a pedagogic viewpoint, this effort shifts the emphasis from time-based, rotation-based metrics of training to the achievement of mastery in a given domain, independent of the time spent on a rotation devoted to that area of expertise.

This happened in parallel to the movement by the ACGME to create "Milestones," a developmentally oriented approach to specific domains of performance for persons in training, which would chart their progress from absolute beginner to mastery of a given domain. Each recognized specialty represented in the ACGME was asked to convene a group that would work with the staff to draft a set of milestones relevant to that specialty. The child neurology milestones which were developed (Child Neurology Milestones, 2015) were very pragmatic and focused by and large on observable, verifiable behaviors. Other specialties, such as pediatrics, created Milestones frameworks that were oriented toward pedagogic theory such as Bloom's taxonomy of adult learning (Pediatrics Milestones, 2015).

The authors of the Universal Curriculum subsequently demonstrated how it could project onto the child neurology milestones. This allows the more granular Universal Curriculum to be used for the mandated reporting of resident progress through the milestones, which all programs must report to the ACGME on an annual basis (Urion et al., submitted). Child neurology therefore has two interrelated metrics to assess the progress of individuals through the course of their formation toward the established goal of being capable of the independent practice of child neurology. For those programs that find using the milestones themselves convenient, this can be done directly. For those who find that they think along the lines of the Universal Curriculum, this can be used and then translated into milestones.

Table 170-1 demonstrates some examples of the child neurology milestones; it should be noted that the levels do not correspond to years in training, but rather steps along a road toward basic competence to practice independently (level 4 in any given milestone) or the further step of contributing to the scholarly literature in a given domain (level 5). It is anticipated that graduates of child neurology training programs will achieve level 5 competences in perhaps one or two domains, likely to be the focus of their careers. One of the further implications of the milestones system would be a gradual move toward more individualized models of formation. In the past, residency has been viewed as a time-based

TABLE 170-1 Two Examples of Child Neurology Milestones

Example 1: Patient Care—Obtaining History in a Neonate With a Neurologic Disorder				
Level 1	*Level 2*	*Level 3*	*Level 4*	*Level 5*
• Obtains a perinatal and developmentally appropriate neurologic and behavioral history	• Obtains a complete and relevant perinatal and developmentally appropriate neurologic and behavioral history • Elicits patient contribution in addition to family as appropriate based on cognitive level and cultural norms	• Obtains a complete, relevant, and organized perinatal and developmentally appropriate neurologic and behavioral history • Integrates patient and parent/caregiver contribution into history • Incorporates information from readily available sources external to the encounter (e.g., medical records	• Efficiently obtains a complete, relevant, and organized perinatal and developmentally appropriate neurologic and behavioral history • Synthesizes patient, parent/caregiver, and external source contribution into history	• Incorporates information from sources difficult to access external to the encounter (e.g., teachers, social workers)

Example 2: Patient Care—Evaluation of a Pediatric Patient With a Neuroimmunologic and White Matter Disorder				
Level 1	*Level 2*	*Level 3*	*Level 4*	*Level 5*
• Recognizes when a patient may have a neuroimmunologic or white matter disorder	• Diagnoses and manages patients with common neuroimmunologic and white matter disorders	• Recognizes patients with uncommon neuroimmunologic and white matter disorders • Manages acute presentations of neuroimmunologic and white matter disorders	• Diagnoses patients with uncommon neuroimmunologic and white matter disorders	• Manages patients with uncommon neuroimmunologic and white matter disorders • Engages in scholarly activity in neuroimmunologic or white matter disorders (e.g., teaching, research)

(With permission from the Child Neurology Milestone Project, a joint initiative of the Accreditation Council for Graduate Medical Education and the American Board of Psychiatry and Neurology, 2015.)

progression: so many months of ward or consult services, so many months of elective rotations in allied disciplines, and the like, with everyone spending equal amounts of time on all rotations. The milestones would allow individuals to progress at rates commensurate with their own achievement of expertise and would ideally spend time in various areas of clinical work commensurate with their need for the development of expertise in that area. The implications of this for organizing clinical services with a workforce within a hospital thus not automatically placed on a given service for a set length of time are profound and potentially disruptive to long established modes of health service delivery in teaching hospitals.

Table 170-2 demonstrates examples of goals established within the Universal Curriculum. These are perhaps more familiar in appearance to most child neurologists and represent identifiable goals of instruction and mastery of various parts of clinical child neurology practice. They are, in a sense, agnostic to means of instruction and learning, as well as the organization of that learning. Thus although they can be associated with the milestones, they might also readily map onto another structure being discussed by medical educators and certifying bodies, the Entrustable Professional Activities (EPA) (ten Cate, 2005).

In the EPA model, one considers an activity such as performing a lumbar puncture. The activity, from its start to finish, includes many elements. The resident must know that the lumbar puncture results are essential to the diagnosis of the patient at hand (medical knowledge and a sound differential diagnosis). The resident must be able to explain the rationale for this test to the family (communication skills and professionalism in conduct). The resident must assemble the needed personnel (working in multidisciplinary team), and then be able to execute the procedure skillfully (technical skills). It has been argued that an EPA model of education

TABLE 170-2 Two Examples of the Universal Curriculum

Example 1: Demyelinating Disorders
1. Recognition of patterns of lesion localization identified on brain, optic nerve or spinal cord MRI characteristic of multiple sclerosis (MS), neuromyelitis optica (NMO), CNS vasculitis, other inflammatory CNS disorders (e.g., infection, sarcoidosis), and disorders of cerebral white matter that are metabolic or malignant in origin
2. Identification of clinical "red flags," including persistent headache and raised intracranial pressure that should prompt consideration of central nervous system (CNS) vasculitis
3. Appropriate use of diagnostic tests including brain, optic nerve, and/or spinal MRI, CSF examination, and multimodal evoked potentials
4. Familiarity with intravenous corticosteroid use and appreciation of second-line therapies including IVIG, plasma exchange, and other immunosuppressant or immunomodulatory therapies
5. Referral for rehabilitation services as appropriate

Example 2: Relapsing CNS Inflammatory Diseases
1. Knowledge of current diagnostic criteria for multiple sclerosis (MS), neuromyelitis optica (NMO), and CNS vasculitis
2. Familiarity with established MS treatments including interferon beta 1a, interferon beta 1b, and glatiramer acetate
3. Recognition of new and emerging MS therapies including natalizumab, fingolimod, teriflunamide, and dimethyl fumarate
4. Knowledge of treatment algorithms for MS, NMO, and CNS vasculitis
6. Appreciation of key genetic and environmental risk factors for pediatric MS (e.g., HLA-DRB1 haplotype, vitamin D deficiency, and viral exposures)
7. Recognition of emerging biomarkers (e.g., anti-MOG antibodies) and neuroimaging advances (e.g., DTI and OCT) in CNS inflammatory diseases
5. Appropriate involvement of a multidisciplinary care team

more closely captures what goes on for a child neurologist in actual practice, given the synthetic nature of multiple separate skills and attributes which must come into play,and thus is a more proximate and direct measure of an individual's readiness for clinical practice. Recent investigations have supported this assertion (Johnston, 2003).

Regardless of the measures used to determine a resident's progress through formation, the previously-noted Universal Curriculum and Milestones represent the current state of the conversation in the profession about what constitutes the body of knowledge, skills, and professional attributes that are considered necessary for the effective, compassionate, and ethical practice of child neurology.

EDUCATION AND TRAINING PRECEDING CHILD NEUROLOGY

It is worth considering, for a moment, the current dialogue regarding the necessary formation that precedes child neurology formation. At present, the ABPN requires 2 years of formation before child neurology formation itself can begin. The most common pathway is 2 years of general pediatrics, organized in such a fashion that the person will be eligible for board certification in general pediatrics (that is, certain critical rotations must be accomplished in those 24 months). A less frequently used path is 1 year of general pediatrics and 1 year of internal medicine, the latter in a program that leads to board eligibility in internal medicine (that is, rotations must be supervised by board certified internists and not by family medicine specialists, for example). A so-called third path, with 1 year of general pediatrics and 1 year of neuroscience research, approved at the discretion of the local child neurology residency program director, requires approval at the ABPN as well. This latter pathway was designed to both assist individuals with significant research interests and also to help address a perceived lack of child neurologists with basic, clinical, or translational science expertise.

CURRENT WORKFORCE ISSUES

This leads us into the consideration of workforce issues. After a period of substantial growth in the last quarter of the last century, child neurology approached and then reached what we might consider "zero population growth"—as many people were leaving the field annually through retirement or death as were entering.

This steady state, however, is a bit deceptive. Numbers of persons in practice or board certified is a less important measure from the standpoint of the families served by a child neurologist; access to child neurology care is more closely determined by the amount of time a given person spends seeing patients. This is the "full-time equivalent" measure of which organizations are so fond. Despite its provenance as a term, we might consider what the implications of this are for child neurology.

Recent surveys have shown that the mean clinical FTE (that is, the average amount of time spent seeing patients) of a retiring child neurologist was just lower than 0.7; that is, most people leaving the practice were spending more than two-thirds of their time seeing patients. The average clinical FTE of persons joining child neurology is slightly over 0.4. (Child Neurology Society/American Academy of Pediatrics survey on Child Neurology, 2015) This means that in order to keep the same amount of clinical time available across the country, we would need to add nearly two child neurologists to the roster for every one that dies or retires. Thus our "zero population growth" actually represents a likely progressive decline in the

number of available clinical child neurologists expressed as clinical FTE across the country. Given the nature of the disorders that child neurologists see, the increasing acuity reported on most hospital services, and the increasing number of treatment options available for previously untreatable diseases, our current staffing and training models would seem to be on a collision course with access to care.

A separate issue is that of the distribution of child neurologists. Child neurologists are generally unequally distributed across the country, tending to center in urban/exurban/suburban areas, often close to the children's hospitals in which they trained. This geographic distribution creates huge challenges for access to child neurology care, with families from rural areas of the country having to travel great distances in order to see a child neurologist. In addition, urban populations often have very poor access to specialty pediatric care, including child neurology, despite geographic proximity. Given the observation that urban and rural populations bear a greater burden of conditions that predispose to neurologic disorders (higher rates of premature births and lower birth weights of full term infants), this makes this lack of access all the more problematic.

United States programs that provide incentives to primary care physicians to practice in medically underserved areas (primarily through loan forgiveness) do not apply directly to child neurologists. The federal calculation of medically underserved is based upon all physicians in a region, weighted toward primary care providers. The calculation is not made in a specialty-specific fashion. Thus one could be in an area that is adequately staffed by primary care providers but be the only child neurologist serving that jurisdiction, and still not be considered in a medically underserved area. Yet anyone who practices as the only child neurologist, or part of a very small group, covering all of a state on the high plains or in northern New England, might disagree. Recent surveys show that practicing in such settings is viewed as stressful by those who do and undesirable by those who are starting. Incentivizing work in such areas through loan forgiveness might not be an entirely sufficient means of helping with this issue of maldistribution, but it is a necessary one. Experience in primary care settings suggests it can be very helpful in establishing a sustainable medical community.

Regardless of issues of distribution, is the workforce we are creating likely to meet the needs of the country? If we assume for a moment that child neurologists are likely to work as parts of larger treatment teams as changes occur in the practice of medicine in this century, we need to consider what patients need to be under the direct care of a child neurologist, what patients are likely to need a single or intermittent consultation by a child neurologist with care being shared with a primary care provider, and what patients might be effectively managed within a primary care provider's office if there were sufficient transfer of information and knowledge from a child neurologist to that primary care provider.

No matter how much primary care can be optimized, it is unlikely that patients with certain disorders will ever have anyone except a child neurologist responsible for that portion of their care. Children with complex neurogenetic disorders, multiple sclerosis, intractable epilepsy, brain tumors, or neuromuscular disorders, for example, will continue to require their care come from child neurologists.

There are children with other disorders that are likely to prompt a consultation with a child neurologist because they are not seen frequently enough by a primary care provider to produce clinical comfort and expertise. We could consider entities such as tic disorders, more readily controlled epilepsies, language disorders, cerebral palsy, or neurodevelopmental disabilities in this realm. Once a diagnosis has been established, it is conceivable that a child neurologist could transfer the care of this patient back to a pediatrician, with some suggestions for the next steps, along with a willingness to either consult remotely with the provider or see the patient again if something does not go as predicted.

Then there are disorders that are sufficiently prevalent that we would expect them to be the domain of a primary care provider, yet in many parts of the country are now routinely sent to child neurologists with minimal attempts by the primary care provider at management. Disorders such as attention deficit-hyperactivity disorder (present in 5% to 7.5% of the childhood population), headache (25% of the childhood population will seek medical consultation at least once for a headache), or febrile seizures, now prompt child neurology referral in many parts of the country. Given the prevalence of these disorders, no rational system of child neurology formation or workforce could possibly meet such a demand; it inevitably leads to issues of access, justice, and quality.

These three domains interact in terms of access issues. If a child neurology practice or clinic is receiving large numbers of referrals for the third category, then access to appointments for the first category and sufficient time to manage the second category will inevitably suffer.

There are certain experiences that suggest this might be changed. Intentional instruction, targeted continuing medical education, and mutually developed treatment paradigms with built-in specialists support for primary care providers have been demonstrated to decrease the rate of specialist referral, produce noninferior or better clinical outcomes, and enhance family satisfaction and engagement. In one study, overall costs were also driven down, thus meeting the so-called "triple aim" of the Institute for Healthcare Improvement (Berwick et al., 2000).

The challenge with such models is one of scale (could these be extended over larger segments of the population) and compensation. (These studies were done under experimental conditions, and child neurologists were compensated for their time by the study; if these initiatives were to be extended, a way for third party payers to compensate child neurologists for information transfer without actually seeing a patient would need to be developed.) The evolution of Accountable Care Organizations, beyond the scope of this chapter, is likely to create incentives for such approaches.

Shifting dynamics in demographics of child neurologists are also likely to change issues of access. The child neurology workforce is an increasingly female one, and this raises issues of work-life balance and the challenges of raising a family while practicing a demanding specialty. Recent studies have suggested that despite assertions of sharing domestic responsibilities in dual professional couples, greater than 50% of those tasks are usually performed by the woman in a different-gender couple. This, in turn, often leads to less than full-time employment, which for our considerations here would have influence upon total FTE in child neurology, and access to care.

FUTURE WORKFORCE ISSUES

If we do some basic calculations, we can estimate the number of child neurologists that might be needed for the most optimistic model of distributed or shared care (which makes the lowest use of direct patient visits and maximizes the sharing of child neurology knowledge across various treatment paradigms as noted previously). If we assume that the average child neurologist in this second decade of the century is 0.6 FTE clinical (which would be the average based upon recent survey data), given a current membership of 1800, we have 1080 FTE child neurologists in terms of clinical practice. If we imagine that workforce seeing patients 5 days a week for 48 weeks each year, we have 240 patient-seeing days per FTE. The current childhood population of the United States is roughly 74 million. If we estimate that roughly 10% of that population will seek neurologic consultation at least once per year (given numbers of persons with intellectual disability, epilepsy, cognitive disorders, headache, and neurogenetics disorders), we find that the average child neurologist would need to see just over 28 patients per day in order to accommodate those needs (7.4 million ÷ (1080 x 240) = 28.5). If we are more conservative in that number and say that only 5% of the population will need to be seen by a child neurologist, this still leads to over 14 patients being seen each day. Both of these models presume a single annual visit, not currently viewed as sufficient for most neurologic disorders under the care of child neurologists.

Thus our current workforce is not sufficient to cover the needs of the country. If the workforce continues to evolve in the direction of less than full-time clinical practice for most child neurologists, this gap will continue to grow.

It is beyond the scope of this chapter to address means of addressing this situation. Although we have made enormous progress as a profession in terms of training that meets individual learning needs and through assessment can assure the public of the high quality of child neurologists, we face enormous challenges in access.

REFERENCES

The complete list of references for this chapter is available online at www.expertconsult.com.

See inside cover for registration details.

SELECTED REFERENCES

Ashwal, S. (Ed.), 1990. The founders of child neurology. Norman Neurosciences in conjunction with the Child Neurology Society, Novato, CA.

Berwick, D.M., Nolan, T.W., Whittington, J., 2000. The triple aim: care, health, and cost. Health Aff. 27 (3), 759–769.

Child Neurology Milestones. <https://www.acgme.org/acgmeweb/portals/0/pdfs/milestones/childneurologymilestones.pdf>.

Child Neurology Society/American Academy of Pediatrics survey on Child Neurology. 2015. Unpublished data from surveyors.

Johnston, K.C., 2003. Responding to the ACGME's competency requirements: an innovative instrument from the University of Virginia's neurology residency. Acad. Med. 78 (12), 1217–1220.

Pediatrics Milestones. <https://www.acgme.org/acgmeweb/Portals/0/PDFs/Milestones/PediatricsMilestones.pdf>.

Rust, R.S., 2011. Child neurology training in the 21st century. Semin. Pediatr. Neurol. 18 (2), 57–58.

ten Cate, O., 2005. Entrustability of professional activities and competency-based training. Med. Educ. 39 (12), 1176–1177.

Urion, D.K., et al., Submitted. Correlations between the child neurology Milestones and the Child Neurology Universal Curriculum. Manuscript in preparation for *Neurology*.

DENVER II

DIRECTIONS

DATE
NAME
BIRTHDATE
HOSP.NO.

1. Try to get child to smile by smiling, talking or waving to him. Do not touch him.
2. When child is playing with toy, pull it away from him. Pass if he resists.
3. Child does not have to be able to tie shoes or button in the back.
4. Move yarn slowly in an arc from one side to the other, about, 6'' above child's face.
   Pass if eyes follow 90° to midline. (Past midline; 180°)
5. Pass if child grasps rattle when it is touched to the backs or tips of fingers.
6. Pass if child continues to look where yarn disappeared or tries to see where it went. Yarn should be dropped quickly from sight from tester's hands without arm movement.
7. Pass if child picks up raisin with any part of thumb and a finger.
8. Pass if child picks up raisin with the ends of thumb and index finger using an overhand approach.

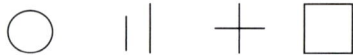

9. Pass any enclosed form. Fail continuous round motions
10. Which line is longer? (Not bigger.) Turn paper upside down and repeat. (3/3 or 5/6)
11. Pass any crossing lines.
12. Have child copy first. If failed, demonstrate.

When giving items 9, 11 and 12, do not name the forms. Do not demonstrate 9 and 11.

13. When scoring, each pair (2 arms, 2 legs, etc.) counts as one part.
14. Point to picture and have child name it. (No credit is given for sounds only.)

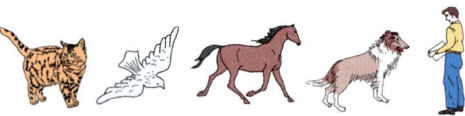

15. Tell child to: Give block to Mommy; put block on table; put block on floor. Pass 2 of 3.
    (Do not help child by pointing, moving head or eyes.)
16. Ask child: What do you do when you are cold? ..hungry? ..tired? Pass 2 of 3.
17. Tell child to: Put block on table; under table; in front of chair; behind chair.
    Pass 3 of 4. (Do not help child by pointing, moving head or eyes.)
18. Ask child: If fire is hot, ice is ?; Mother is a woman, Dad is a ?; a horse is big, a mouse is?. Pass 2 of 3.
19. Ask child: What is a ball? ..lake? ..desk? ..house? ..banana? ..curtain? ..ceiling? ..hedge? ..pavement?
    Pass if defined in terms of use, shape, what it is made of or general category (such as banana is fruit, not just yellow). Pass 6 of 9.
20. Ask child: What is a spoon made of? ..a shoe made of? ..a door made of? (No other objects may be substituted.) Pass 3 of 3.
21. When placed on stomach, child lifts chest off table with support of forearms and/or hands.
22. When child is on back, grasp his hands and pull him to sitting. Pass if head does not hang back.
23. Child may use wall or rail only, not person. May not crawl.
24. Child must throw ball overhand 3 feet to within arm's reach of tester.
25. Child must perform standing broad jump over width of test sheet. (8-1/2 inches)
26. Tell child to walk forward, ⚬⚬⚬⚬➤heel within 1 inch of toe.
    Tester may demonstrate. Child must walk 4 consecutive steps, 2 out of 3 trials.
27. Bounce ball to child who should stand 3 feet away from tester. Child must catch ball with hands, not arms, 2 out of 3 trials.
28. Tell child to walk backward, ◄⚬⚬⚬⚬ toe within 1 inch of heel.
    Tester may demonstrate. Child must walk 4 consecutive steps, 2 out of 3 trials.

DATE AND BEHAVIORAL OBSERVATIONS (how child feels at time of test, relation to tester, attention span, verbal behavior, self-confidence, etc.):

A

Figure A-1ab. **Denver II.** *(From Frankenburg WK, Dodds JB, Archer P, et al. The Denver II: A major revision and restandardization of the Denver Developmental screening test. Pediatrics 1992;89:91.)*

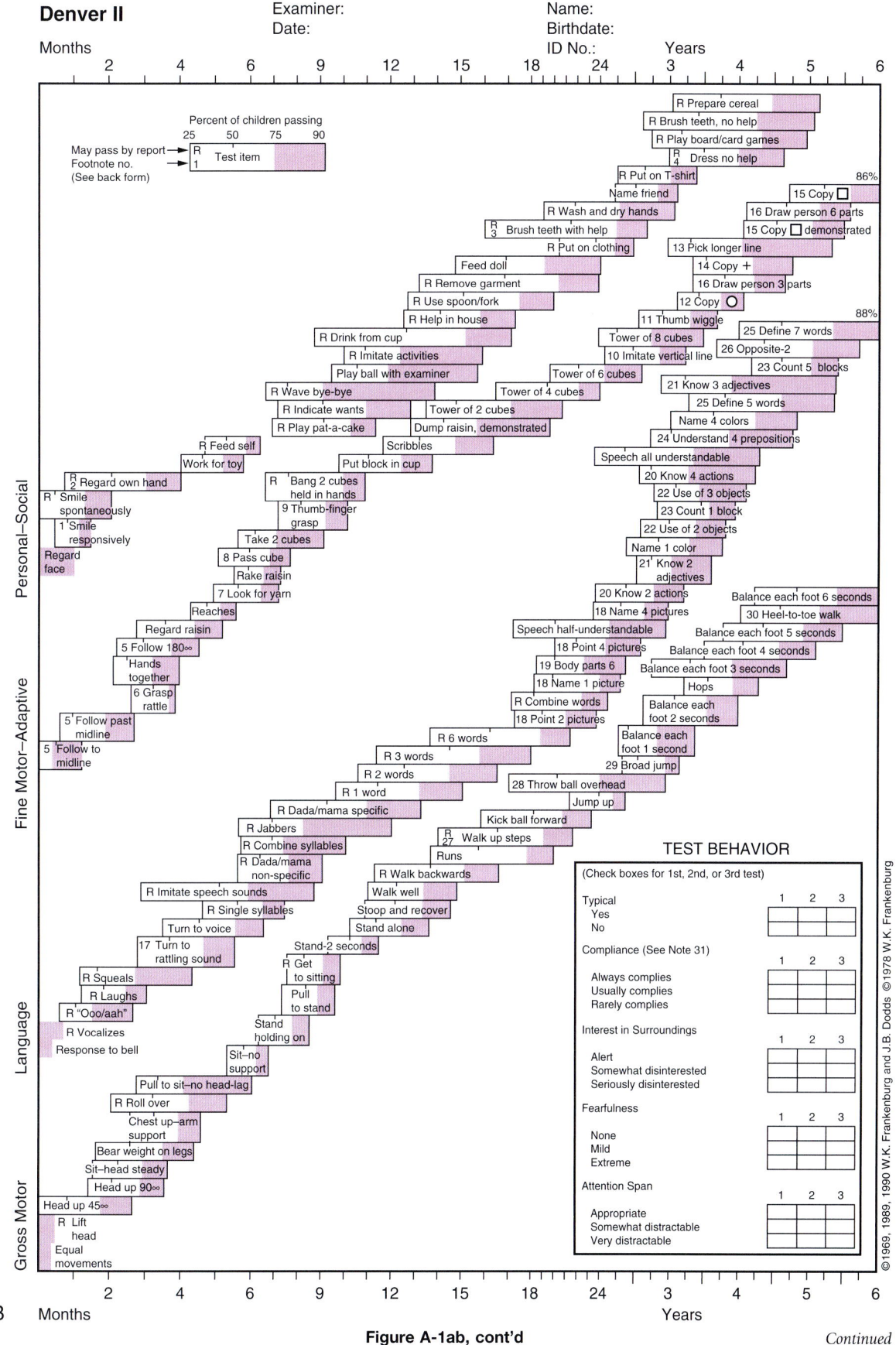

Figure A-1ab, cont'd

Continued

CHECKLIST FOR DOCUMENTATION OF BRAIN DEATH EXAMINATION IN INFANTS AND CHILDREN

Age of Patient	Timing of first exam	Inter-exam. interval
Term newborn 37 weeks gestational age and up to 30 days old	First exam may be performed 24 hours after birth OR following cardiopulmonary resuscitation or other severe brain injury	At least 24 hours Interval shortened because ancillary study (section 4) is consistent with brain death
31 days to 18 years old	First exam may be performed 24 hours following cardiopulmonary resuscitation or other severe brain injury	At least 12 hours OR Interval shortened because ancillary study (section 4) is consistent with brain death

Section 1. PREREQUISITES for brain death examination and apnea test

A. IRREVERSIBLE AND IDENTIFIABLE Cause of Coma (Please check)

Traumatic brain injury   Anoxic brain injury   Known metabolic disorder   Other (Specify) _____

B. Correction of contributing factors that can interfere with the neurologic examination	Examination One		Examination Two	
a. Core Body Temp is over 95° F (35° C)	Yes	No	Yes	No
b. Systolic blood pressure or MAP in acceptable range (Systolic BP not less than 2 standard deviations below age appropriate norm) based on age	Yes	No	Yes	No
c. Sedative/analgesic drug effect excluded as a contributing factor	Yes	No	Yes	No
d. Metabolic intoxication excluded as a contributing factor	Yes	No	Yes	No
e. Neuromuscular blockade excluded as a contributing factor	Yes	No	Yes	No

If ALL prerequisites are marked YES, then proceed to section 2, OR

_____ confounding variable was present. Ancillary study was therefore performed to document brain death. (Section 4).

Figure A-2. Checklist for documentation of brain death examination in Infants and Children.

Section 2. Physical Examination (Please check)	Examination One		Examination Two	
NOTE: SPINAL CORD REFLEXES ARE ACCEPTABLE	Date/ time:		Date/ Time:	
a. Flaccid tone, patient unresponsive to deep painful stimuli	Yes	No	Yes	No
b. Pupils are midposition or fully dilated and light reflexes are absent	Yes	No	Yes	No
c. Corneal, cough, gag reflexes are absent	Yes	No	Yes	No
Sucking and rooting reflexes are absent (in neonates and infants)	Yes	No	Yes	No
d. Oculovestibular reflexes are absent	Yes	No	Yes	No
e. Spontaneous respiratory effort while on mechanical ventilation is absent	Yes	No	Yes	No

The _____ (specify) element of the exam could not be performed because_____.

Ancillary study (EEG or radionuclide CBF) was therefore performed to document brain death. (Section 4).

Section 3. APNEA Test	Examination One	Examination Two
	Date/ Time_____	Date/ Time_____
No spontaneous respiratory efforts were observed despite final $PaCO_2 \geq 60$ mm Hg and a ≥ 20 mm Hg increase above baseline. (Examination One) No spontaneous respiratory efforts were observed despite final $PaCO_2 \geq 60$ mm Hg and a ≥ 20 mm Hg increase above baseline. (Examination Two)	Pretest $PaCO_2$: _____ Apnea duration: _____min Posttest $PaCO_2$: _____	Pretest $PaCO_2$: _____ Apnea duration: _____min Posttest $PaCO_2$: _____

Apnea test is contraindicated or could not be performed to completion because_____.

Ancillary study (EEG or radionuclide CBF) was therefore performed to document brain death. (Section 4).

Section 4. ANCILLARY testing is required when (1) any components of the examination or apnea testing cannot be completed; (2) if there is uncertainty about the results of the neurologic examination; or (3) if a medication effect may be present. **Ancillary testing can be performed to reduce the inter-examination period however a second neurologic examination is required. Components of the neurologic examination that can be performed safely should be completed in close proximity to the ancillary test**	Date/Time: _____
Electroencephalogram (EEG) report documents electrocerebral silence OR	Yes No
Cerebral Blood Flow(CBF) study report documents no cerebral perfusion	Yes No
Section 5. Signatures	
Examiner One	
I certify that my examination is consistent with cessation of function of the brain and brainstem. Confirmatory exam to follow.	

_____   _____

(Printed Name)   (Signature)

Figure A-2, cont'd

Continued

_____   _____   _____   _____

(Specialty)   (Pager #/License #)   (Date mm/dd/yyyy)   (Time)

Examiner Two

I certify that my examination and/or ancillary test report confirms unchanged and irreversible cessation of function of the brain and brainstem. The patient is declared brain dead at this time.

Date/Time of death: _____

_____   _____

(Printed Name)   (Signature)

_____   _____   _____   _____

(Specialty)   (Pager #/License #)   (Date mm/dd/yyyy)   (Time)

Figure A-2, cont'd

Index

Page numbers followed by "*f*" indicate figures, "*t*" indicate tables, "*b*" indicate boxes, and "*e*" indicate online content.